Fetal and Neonatal
PHYSIOLOGY

Fetal and Neonatal PHYSIOLOGY

VOLUME 2 / THIRD EDITION

Richard A. Polin, M.D.

Professor of Pediatrics
Columbia University College of Physicians and Surgeons
Director, Division of Neonatology
Children's Hospital of New York-Presbyterian
New York, New York

William W. Fox, M.D.

Professor of Pediatrics
University of Pennsylvania School of Medicine
Division of Neonatology
Children's Hospital of Philadelphia
Philadelphia, Pennsylvania

Steven H. Abman, M.D.

Professor of Pediatrics
University of Colorado School of Medicine
Director, Pediatric
Heart Lung Center
The Children's Hospital
Denver, Colorado

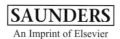

SAUNDERS
An Imprint of Elsevier

SAUNDERS
An Imprint of Elsevier

The Curtis Center
Independence Square West
Philadelphia, Pennsylvania 19106-3399

Volume 1   ISBN   9997628268
Volume 2   ISBN   9997628314
Two-volume set   ISBN   0-7216-9654-6

FETAL AND NEONATAL PHYSIOLOGY

Notice

Medicine is an ever-changing field. Standard safety precautions must be followed, but as new research and clinical experience broaden our knowledge, changes in treatment and drug therapy may become necessary or appropriate. Readers are advised to check the most current product information provided by the manufacturer of each drug to be administered to verify the recommended dose, the method and duration of administration, and contraindications. It is the responsibility of the treating physician, relying on experience and knowledge of the patient, to determine dosages and the best treatment for each individual patient. Neither the Publisher nor the editor assumes any liability for any injury and/or damage to persons or property arising from this publication.

The Publisher

First Edition 1992. Second Edition 1998. Third Edition 2004.

Library of Congress Cataloging-in-Publication Data

Fetal and neonatal physiology/ [edited by] Richard A. Polin, William W. Fox, Steven H. Abman. — 3rd ed.
      p. ; cm.
      Includes bibliographical references and index.
      ISBN 0-7216-9654-6 (set)   ISBN 9997628268 (v. 1)   ISBN 9997628314 (v. 2)
        1. Fetus—Physiology. 2. Infants (Newborn)—Physiology. I. Polin, Richard A. (Richard Alan).
        II. Fox, William W.   III. Abman, Steven H.
      [DNLM: 1. Fetus—physiology.   2. Infant, Newborn—physiology.   3. Maternal-Fetal
      Exchange—physiology.   WQ 210.5 F4173 2004]
   RG610.F46 2004
   612.6'47-dc21

                                                                    2003042443

Acquisitions Editor: Judith Fletcher
Developmental Editor: Jennifer Shreiner
Project Manager: Jeffrey Gunning

Cover illustration courtesy of Jay S. Greenspan, M.D.

Printed in the United States of America

Last digit is the print number: 9   8   7   6   5   4   3   2   1

This book is dedicated to our wives and children:

Helene, Allison, Mitchell, Jessica, and Gregory Polin
Laurie, Will, Jon, James, and Lauren Fox
Carolyn, Ryan, Lauren, Mark, and Megan Abman

CONTRIBUTORS

Soraya Abbasi, M.D.
Clinical Professor of Pediatrics, University of Pennsylvania
School of Medicine; Neonatologist, Pennsylvania Hospital,
Philadelphia, Pennsylvania
Evaluation of Pulmonary Function in the Neonate

Steven H. Abman, M.D.
Professor of Pediatrics, University of Colorado School of
Medicine; Director, Pediatric Heart Lung Center,
The Children's Hospital, Denver, Colorado

S. Lee Adamson, Ph.D.
Professor of Obstetrics and Gynecology, University of Toronto
Faculty of Medicine; Senior Scientist, Samuel Lunenfeld
Research Institute of Mount Sinai Hospital, Toronto,
Ontario, Canada
Regulation of Umbilical Blood Flow

N. Scott Adzick, M.D.
C. Everett Koop Professor of Pediatric Surgery, University of
Pennsylvania School of Medicine; Surgeon-in-Chief, Children's
Hospital of Philadelphia, Philadelphia, Pennsylvania
Fetal Wound Healing; Pathophysiology of Neural Tube Defects

Kurt H. Albertine, Ph.D.
Professor of Pediatrics, Medicine, and Neurobiology and
Anatomy, and Director, Pediatrics Fellowship Training
Curriculum, University of Utah School of Medicine; Training
Director, Children's Health Research Center, Salt Lake City, Utah
Impaired Lung Growth After Injury in Premature Lung

Benjamin A. Alman, M.D., F.R.C.S.C.
Associate Professor and Canadian Research Chair, University of
Toronto Faculty of Medicine; Surgeon, Hospital for Sick
Children, Toronto, Ontario, Canada
Defective Limb Embryology

Steven M. Altschuler, M.D.
President and Chief Executive Officer, The Children's Hospital
of Philadelphia, Philadelphia, Pennsylvania
Development of the Enteric Nervous System

Page A. W. Anderson, M.D.
Professor of Pediatrics, Department of Pediatrics, Division
of Cardiology, Duke University School of Medicine and
Duke University Medical Center, Durham, North Carolina
**Cardiovascular Function During Development and the Response to
Hypoxia**

Russell V. Anthony, Ph.D.
Hill Professor, Animal Reproduction and Biotechnology
Laboratory, Department of Biomedical Sciences, Colorado State
University, Fort Collins; Perinatal Research Facility, Department
of Pediatrics, University of Colorado Health Sciences Center,
Aurora, Colorado
Angiogenesis

Elisabeth A. Aron, M.D.
Visiting Scientist, Colorado State University, Fort Collins; Senior
Instructor and Women's Reproductive Health Research Scholar,
University of Colorado Health Sciences Center, Denver, Colorado
Angiogenesis

Ahmet R. Aslan, M.D.
Research Scholar in Pediatric Urology, Albany Medical College,
Albany, New York; Attending in Urology, Haydarpasa Numune
Hospital, Istanbul, Turkey
Testicular Development; Testicular Descent

Jeanette M. Asselin, R.R.T., M.S.
Manager, Neonatal Pediatric Research, Children's Hospital and
Research Center at Oakland, Oakland, California
High-Frequency Ventilation

Richard L. Auten, Jr., M.D.
Associate Professor of Pediatrics, Department of Pediatrics,
Duke University School of Medicine, Durham, North Carolina
Mechanisms of Neonatal Lung Injury

Mary Ellen Avery, M.D., Sc.D.(Hon.)
Professor Emeritus, Harvard Medical School; Thomas Morgan
Rotch Distinguished Professor of Pediatrics, Children's Hospital,
Boston, Massachusetts
Historical Perspective [Surfactant]

Ellis D. Avner, M.D.
Gertrude Lee Chandler Tucker Professor and Chairman,
Department of Pediatrics, Case Western Reserve University
School of Medicine; Chief Medical Officer, Rainbow Babies and
Children's Hospital, and Chair for Excellence in Pediatrics,
Rainbow Babies and Children's Corporation, Cleveland, Ohio
Embryogenesis and Anatomic Development of the Kidney

H. Scott Baldwin, M.D.
Katrina Overall McDonald Chair in Pediatrics, Professor of
Pediatrics (Cardiology) and Cell and Development Biology,
Vice Chair of Laboratory Sciences in Pediatrics, Vanderbilt
University Medical Center, Nashville, Tennessee
Molecular Determinants of Embryonic Vascular Development

Philip L. Ballard, M.D., Ph.D.
Professor of Pediatrics, University of Pennsylvania School of
Medicine; Director of Neonatal Research, Children's Hospital of
Philadelphia, Philadelphia, Pennsylvania
Hormonal Therapy for Prevention of Respiratory Distress Syndrome

Eduardo Bancalari, M.D., M.D.
Professor, Departments of Pediatrics and Obstetrics-Gynecology,
University of Miami School of Medicine; Director, Division of
Neonatology, Jackson Memorial Hospital, and Chief, Newborn
Services/Perinatal Intensive Care Unit, Jackson Memorial
Medical Center, Miami, Florida
Pathophysiology of Chronic Lung Disease

David J. P. Barker, M.D., Ph.D., F.R.S
Professor of Clinical Epidemiology, University of Southampton Faculty of Medicine; Director, Medical Research Council Environmental Epidemiology Unit, Southampton General Hospital, Southampton, England
Fetal Origins of Adult Disease

Pierre M. Barker, M.B., Ch.B., M.D., M.R.C.P.
Associate Professor, Department of Pediatrics, University of North Carolina at Chapel Hill School of Medicine; Medical Director, Children's Clinics, UNC Children's Hospital, Chapel Hill, North Carolina
Regulation of Liquid Secretion and Absorption by the Fetal and Neonatal Lung

Frederick C. Battaglia, M.D.
Professor of Pediatrics and Obstetrics-Gynecology, University of Colorado School of Medicine, Aurora, Colorado
Mechanisms Affecting Fetal Growth

Gary K. Beauchamp, Ph.D.
Adjunct Professor, School of Veterinary Medicine, and School of Arts and Sciences, University of Pennsylvania; Director and Member, Monell Chemical Senses Center, Philadelphia, Pennsylvania
Development of Taste and Smell in the Neonate

Jacqueline Beesley, Ph.D.
Weston Laboratory, Institute of Reproductive and Developmental Biology, Division of Paediatrics, Obstetrics and Gynaecology, Imperial College Faculty of Medicine, London, United Kingdom
Apoptosis and Necrosis

Corinne Benchimol, D.O.
Clinical Assistant Professor, Department of Pediatrics, Division of Pediatric Nephrology, Mount Sinai School of Medicine of The City University of New York; Mount Sinai Hospital, New York, New York
Potassium Homeostasis in the Fetus and Neonate

Laura Bennet, M.D., Ph.D.
Senior Research Fellow, Liggins Institute, University of Auckland, Auckland, New Zealand
Responses of the Fetus and Neonate to Hypothermia

Robert A. Berg, M.D.
Associate Professor, University of Arizona College of Medicine; Director, Pediatric Intensive Care Unit, University Medical Center, Tucson, Arizona
Developmental Pharmacology of Adrenergic Agents

Gerard T. Berry, M.D.
Professor and Vice Dean for Research, Jefferson Medical College, Thomas Jefferson University, Philadelphia, Pennsylvania
Pathophysiology of Metabolic Disease of the Liver

Carol Lynn Berseth, M.D.
Director, Medical Affairs North America, Mead Johnson Nutritionals, Evansville, Indiana
Digestion-Absorption Functions in Fetuses, Infants, and Children

Vinod K. Bhutani, M.D.
Professor of Pediatrics, Section of Newborn Pediatrics, Pennsylvania Hospital; Pediatrician, Pennsylvania Hospital, and Senior Physician, Children's Hospital of Philadelphia, Philadelphia, Pennsylvania
Evaluation of Pulmonary Function in the Neonate

Stan R. Blecher, M.D., F.C.C.M.G.
Professor Emeritus, University of Guelph Faculty of Medicine, Guelph, Ontario, Canada
Genetics of Sex Determination and Differentiation

Arlin B. Blood, B.S.
Research Assistant, Center for Perinatal Biology, Loma Linda University Medical School, Loma Linda, California
Perinatal Thermal Physiology

David L. Bolender, Ph.D.
Associate Professor, Department of Cell Biology, Neurobiology and Anatomy, Medical College of Wisconsin, Milwaukee, Wisconsin
Basic Embryology

Robert D. H. Boyd, M.B., B.Ch., F.R.C.P., F.F.P.H., F.R.C.P.C.H., F.Med.Sci.
Professor of Pediatrics, University of London Faculty of Medicine, and Principal, St. George's Hospital Medical School; Honorary Consultant, St. George's Hospital, London, England
Mechanisms of Transfer Across the Human Placenta

Robert A. Brace, Ph.D.
Professor Emeritus of Reproductive Medicine, University of California, San Diego, School of Medicine, La Jolla, California
Fluid Distribution in the Fetus and Neonate

Eileen D. Brewer, M.D.
Professor of Pediatrics and Head, Pediatric Renal Section, Baylor College of Medicine; Chief Renal Service, Texas Children's Hospital, Houston, Texas
Urinary Acidification

Patrick D. Brophy, M.D., F.R.C.P.C., F.A.A.P.
Assistant Professor of Pediatrics, University of Michigan Medical School, Ann Arbor, Michigan
Functional Development of the Kidney *In Utero*

Delma L. Broussard, M.D.
Director, Regulatory Affairs International, Merck Research Laboratories, Merck & Co., Inc., West Point, Pennsylvania
Development of the Enteric Nervous System

John C. Bucuvalas, M.D.
Professor of Pediatrics, University of Cincinnati College of Medicine; Medical Director, Liver Transplantation, and Attending Physician, Cincinnati Children's Hospital Medical Center, Cincinnati, Ohio
Bile Acid Metabolism During Development

Douglas G. Burrin, Ph.D.
USDA Children's Nutrition Research Center, Baylor College of Medicine, Houston, Texas
Trophic Factors and Regulation of Gastrointestinal Tract and Liver Development

Bridgette M. P. Byrne, M.D., M.R.C.P.I., M.R.C.O.G.
Senior Lecturer, Royal College of Surgeons in Ireland; Consultant Obstetrician and Gynaecologist, Coombe Women's Hospital, Dublin, Ireland
Regulation of Umbilical Blood Flow

Anne Grete Byskov, M.Sc., Ph.D., D.Sc.
Professor of Reproductive Physiology, August Krogh Institute, University of Copenhagen; Head, Laboratory of Reproductive Biology, Juliane Marie Centre, Rigshospitalet, Copenhagen, Denmark
Differentiation of the Ovary

Mitchell S. Cairo, M.D.
Professor of Pediatrics, Medicine, and Pathology, Columbia
University College of Physicians and Surgeons; Director,
Pediatric Blood and Marrow Transplantation, and Director,
Pediatric Cancer Research, Children's Hospital of
New York–Presbyterian, New York, New York
Neonatal Neutrophil Normal and Abnormal Physiology

Barbara Cannon, Ph.D.
Professor, The Wenner-Gren Institute, Stockholm University,
Stockholm, Sweden
Brown Adipose Tissue: Development and Function

Michael S. Caplan, M.D.
Associate Professor of Pediatrics, Northwestern University
Feinberg School of Medicine, Chicago; Chairman, Department
of Pediatrics, Evanston Northwestern Healthcare, Evanston,
Illinois
**Pathophysiology and Prevention of Neonatal Necrotizing
Enterocolitis**

Neil Caplin, M.B., B.S.
Endocrinology and Diabetes, Princess Margaret Hospital
for Children, Perth, Australia
Pathophysiology of Hypoglycemia

Susan E. Carlson, Ph.D.
Professor of Dietetics and Nutrition and Professor of
Pediatrics, University of Kansas School of Medicine,
Kansas City, Kansas
Long Chain Fatty Acids in the Developing Retina and Brain

David P. Carlton, M.D.
Associate Professor, Department of Pediatrics, University of
Wisconsin School of Medicine; Chief, Division of Neonatology,
University Hospital, Madison, Wisconsin
Pathophysiology of Edema

William J. Cashore, M.D.
Professor of Pediatrics, Brown University Medical School;
Associate Chief of Pediatrics, Women and Infants' Hospital of
Rhode Island, Providence, Rhode Island
Bilirubin Metabolism and Toxicity in the Newborn

Tinnakorn Chaiworapongsa, M.D.
Research Fellow, Perinatology Research Branch, National
Institute of Child Health and Human Development, National
Institutes of Health, Bethesda, Maryland
Fetal and Maternal Responses to Intrauterine Infection

Sylvain Chemtob, M.D., Ph.D., F.R.C.P.C.
Professor of Pediatrics, Pharmacology, and Ophthalmology,
University of Montreal, Faculty of Medicine; Neonatologist,
Hôpital Ste. Justine, Montreal, Quebec, Canada
Basic Pharmacologic Principles

Robert L. Chevalier, M.D.
Benjamin Armistead Professor and Chair, Department of
Pediatrics, University of Virginia School of Medicine,
Charlottesville, Virginia
Response to Nephron Loss in Early Development

Sadhana Chheda, M.D., D.T.M.H., M.B.B.S.
Staff Neonatologist, Providence Memorial Hospital, Sierra
Medical Center, Las Palmas Medical Center, and Del Sol Medical
Center, El Paso, Texas
Immunology of Human Milk and Host Immunity

Robert D. Christensen, M.D.
Professor and Chairman, Department of Pediatrics, University of
South Florida College of Medicine; Physician-in-Chief, All
Children's Hospital, St. Petersburg, Florida
Developmental Granulocytopoiesis

David H. Chu, M.D., Ph.D.
Teaching Assistant, The Ronald O. Perelman Department of
Dermatology, New York University School of Medicine, New
York, New York
Structure and Development of the Skin and Cutaneous Appendages

Robert Ryan Clancy, M.D.
Professor of Neurology and Pediatrics, University of
Pennsylvania School of Medicine; Director, Pediatric Regional
Epilepsy Program, Children's Hospital of Philadelphia,
Philadelphia, Pennsylvania
Electroencephalography in the Premature and Full-Term Infant

M. Thomas Clandinin, Ph.D.
Professor of Nutrition, Department of Agricultural Food and
Nutritional Science, University of Alberta, Edmonton, Alberta,
Canada
Aceretion of Lipid in the Fetus and Newborn

David A. Clark, M.D.
Professor and Chairman, Department of Pediatrics, Albany
Medical College; Director, Children's Hospital at Albany Medical
Center, Albany, New York
**Development of the Gastrointestinal Circulation in the Fetus and
Newborn**

Jane Cleary-Goldman, M.D.
Maternal-Fetal Medicine Fellow, Columbia Presbyterian Medical
Center, Sloane Hospital for Women, New York, New York
Physiologic Effects of Multiple Pregnancy on Mother and Fetus

Ronald I. Clyman, M.D.
Professor of Pediatrics, University of California, San Francisco,
School of Medicine; Senior Staff, Cardiovascular Research
Institute, San Francisco, California
Mechanisms Regulating Closure of the Ductus Arteriosus

Pinchas Cohen, M.D.
Professor, Department of Pediatrics, David Geffen School of
Medicine at UCLA, Los Angeles, California
Growth Factor Regulation of Fetal Growth

Howard E. Corey, M.D.
Director, Children's Kidney Center of New Jersey, Morristown
Memorial Hospital, Morristown, New Jersey
Renal Transport of Sodium During Early Development

Robert B. Cotton, M.D.
Professor of Pediatrics, Vanderbilt University School of
Medicine, Nashville, Tennessee
**Pathophysiology of Hyaline Membrane Disease (Excluding
Surfactant)**

Beverly J. Cowart, Ph.D.
Adjunct Assistant Professor of Otolaryngology (Research),
Jefferson Medical College, Thomas Jefferson University;
Member and Director, Monell-Jefferson Taste and Smell Clinic,
Monell Chemical Senses Center, Philadelphia, Pennsylvania
Development of Taste and Smell in the Neonate

Richard M. Cowett, M.D.
Professor of Pediatrics, Northeastern Ohio Universities College
of Medicine, Rootstown, Ohio
**Role of Glucoregulatory Hormones in Hepatic Glucose Metabolism
During the Perinatal Period**

Timothy M. Crombleholme, M.D.
Associate Professor of Pediatric Surgery, University of
Pennsylvania School of Medicine; Attending Pediatric Surgeon,
Children's Hospital of Philadelphia, and Fetal Surgeon, Center
for Fetal Diagnosis and Therapy at Children's Hospital of
Philadelphia, Philadelphia, Pennsylvania
Pathophysiology of Neural Tube Defects

James E. Crowe, Jr., M.D.
Associate Professor of Pediatrics, Vanderbilt University School
of Medicine, Nashville, Tennessee
B-Cell Development

Leona Cuttler, M.D.
Professor of Pediatrics, Case Western Reserve University School
of Medicine; Division Chief, Pediatric Endocrinology, Rainbow
Babies and Children's Hospital, Cleveland, Ohio
**Luteinizing Hormone and Follicle-Stimulating Hormone Secretion in
the Fetus and Newborn**

Mary E. D'Alton, M.D.
Willard C. Rappeleye Professor of Obstetrics and Gynecology
and Chair, Department of Obstetrics and Gynecology, Columbia
University College of Physicians and Surgeons; Director of
Services, Sloane Hospital for Women, New York Presbyterian
Hospital, New York, New York
Physiologic Effects of Multiple Gestation on Mother and Fetus

Enrico Danzer, M.D.
Fetal Surgery Research Fellow, Center for Fetal Diagnosis and
Treatment/University of Pennsylvania School of
Medicine/Children's Hospital of Philadelphia, Philadelphia,
Pennsylvania
Pathophysiology of Neural Tube Defects

Diva D. De León, M.D.
Assistant Professor of Pediatrics, University of Pennsylvania
School of Medicine; Attending Physician, Children's Hospital of
Philadelphia, Philadelphia, Pennsylvania
Growth Factor Regulation of Fetal Growth

Maria Delivoria-Papadopoulos, M.D.
Professor of Pediatrics, Physiology, and Obstetrics and
Gynecology, Drexel University College of Medicine; Chief,
Division of Neonatal-Perinatal Medicine, St. Christopher's
Hospital for Children, Philadelphia, Pennsylvania
Oxygen Transport and Delivery

George A. Diaz, M.D. Ph.D.
Assistant Professor, Department of Human Genetics and
Pediatrics, Mount Sinai School of Medicine of The City
University of New York, New York, New York
Molecular Genetics: Developmental and Clinical Implications

Chris J. Dickinson, M.D.
Professor of Pediatrics, University of Michigan Medical School,
Ann Arbor, Michigan
Development of Gastric Secretory Function

John P. Dormans, M.D.
Professor of Orthopaedic Surgery, University of Pennsylvania
School of Medicine; Chief, Orthopaedic Surgery, Children's
Hospital of Philadelphia, Philadelphia, Pennsylvania
**The Growth Plate: Embryologic Origin, Structure, and Function;
Common Musculoskeletal Conditions Related to Intrauterine
Compression: Effects of Mechanics on Endochondral
Classification**

David J. Durand, M.D.
Neonatologist, Children's Hospital and Research Center,
Oakland, California
High-Frequency Ventilation

**A. David Edwards, M.A., M.B.B.S., F.R.C.P., F.R.C.P.C.H.,
F.Med.Sci.**
Chairman of Division of Paediatrics, Obstetrics and
Gynaecology, and Professor of Neonatal Medicine, Imperial
College London; Group Head, Medical Research Council
Clinical Sciences Centre, Hammersmith Hospital, London,
United Kingdom
Apoptosis and Necrosis

John F. Ennever, M.D., Ph.D.
Associate Clinical Professor of Pediatrics, Columbia University
College of Physicians and Surgeons; Associate Attending,
Children's Hospital of New York–Presbyterian, New York, New York
Mechanisms of Action of Phototherapy

Robert P. Erickson, M.D.
Professor of Cellular and Molecular Biology and Holsclaw
Family Professor of Human Genetics and Inherited Disease,
Department of Pediatrics, University of Arizona College of
Medicine, Tucson, Arizona
Genetics of Sex Determination and Differentiation

Bulent Erol, M.D.
Attending Surgeon and Fellow, Children's Hospital of
Philadelphia, Philadelphia, Pennsylvania
**The Growth Plate: Embryologic Origin, Structure, and Function;
Common Musculoskeletal Conditions Related to Intrauterine
Compression: Effects of Mechanics on Endochondral
Classification**

Mohamed A. Fahim, Ph.D.
Professor of Physiology, Department of Physiology, Faculty of
Medicine and Health Sciences, Al Ain, United Arab Emirates
Functional Development of Respiratory Muscles

Leonard G. Feld, M.D., Ph.D., M.M.M.
Professor of Pediatrics, UMDNJ–New Jersey Medical School;
Chairman of Pediatrics, Atlantic Health System, Morristown,
New Jersey
Renal Transport of Sodium During Early Development

Miguel Feldman, M.D.
Director, Neonatal Intensive Care Unit, Hillel-Jaffe Medical
Center, Hadera, Israel
Accretion of Lipid in the Fetus and Newborn

Lucas G. Fernandez, M.D.
Postdoctoral Research Assistant, University of Virginia Health
System, Charlottesville, Virginia; Associate Professor, University
of Zulia, Maracaibo, Venezuela
Development of the Renin-Angiotensin System

Douglas G. Field, M.D.
Assistant Professor of Pediatrics, Pennsylvania State University
College of Medicine; Attending, Department of Pediatrics,
Division of Pediatric Gastroenterology and Nutrition, Penn State
Children's Hospital, Milton S. Hershey Medical Center, Hershey,
Pennsylvania
Fetal and Neonatal Intestinal Motility

Delbert A. Fisher, M.D.
Professor Emeritus, Pediatrics and Medicine, David Geffen
School of Medicine at UCLA, Los Angeles, California;
Vice President, Science and Innovation, Quest Diagnostics,
Nichols Institute, San Juan Capistrano, California
Fetal and Neonatal Thyroid Physiology

William W. Fox, M.D.
Professor of Pediatrics, University of Pennsylvania School of
Medicine; Attending, Division of Neonatology, Children's
Hospital of Philadelphia, Philadelphia, Pennsylvania
Assisted Ventilation: Physiologic Implications and Complications

Hans-Georg Frank, Dr. Med.
Associate Professor, Department of Anatomy II, University of Technology Aachen Medical Faculty, Aachen; CSO, AplaGen GmbH, Baesweiler, Germany
Placental Development

Philippe S. Friedlich, M.D.
Assistant Professor of Clinical Pediatrics, University of Southern California Keck School of Medicine; Medical Director, Neonatal Intensive Care Unit, Children's Hospital Los Angeles, Los Angeles, California
Pathophysiology of Shock in the Fetus and Neonate; Regulation of Acid-Base Balance in the Fetus and Neonate

Aaron L. Friedman, M.D.
Professor and Chairman, Department of Pediatrics, University of Wisconsin School of Medicine; Medical Director, University of Wisconsin Children's Hospital, Madison, Wisconsin
Transport of Amino Acids During Early Development

Joshua R. Friedman, M.D., Ph.D.
Instructor, Department of Pediatrics, University of Pennsylvania School of Medicine; Fellow, Division of Gastroenterology and Nutrition, Children's Hospital of Philadelphia, Philadelphia, Pennsylvania
Pathophysiology of Gastroesophageal Reflux

Marianne Garland, M.B., Ch.B.
Assistant Professor of Pediatrics, Columbia University College of Physicians and Surgeons; Assistant Attending in Pediatrics, Children's Hospital of New York–Presbyterian, New York, New York
Drug Distribution in Fetal Life

Maria-Teresa Gervasi, M.D.
Chief, Operative Unit of Obstetrics, Department of Obstetrics and Gynecology, Ospedale Regionale Ca' Foncello-Treviso, Treviso, Italy
Fetal and Maternal Responses to Intrauterine Infection

James B. Gibson, M.D., Ph.D.
Associate Professor, Department of Pediatrics, University of Arkansas for Medical Sciences; Attending Geneticist, Arkansas Children's Hospital, Little Rock, Arkansas
Pathophysiology of Metabolic Disease of the Liver

P. D. Gluckman, M.B., Ch.B., M.Med.Sc., D.Sc., F.R.S., F.R.S.N.Z., F.R.A.C.P., F.R.C.P.C.H.
Director, Liggins Institute for Medical Research, University of Auckland Faculty of Medicine, Auckland, New Zealand
Growth Hormone and Prolactin

Michael J. Goldberg, M.D.
Professor and Chairman, Department of Orthopaedics, Tufts University School of Medicine; Orthopaedist in Chief, Tufts–New England Medical Center, Boston, Massachusetts
Defective Limb Embryology

Armond S. Goldman, M.D.
Emeritus Professor, Department of Pediatrics, Division of Immunology/Allergy/Rheumatology, University of Texas Medical Branch, Galveston, Texas
Immunology of Human Milk and Host Immunity

Gary W. Goldstein, M.D.
Professor of Neurology, Pediatrics, and Environmental Health Sciences, Johns Hopkins University School of Medicine; President and CEO, Kennedy Krieger Institute, Baltimore, Maryland
Development of the Blood-Brain Barrier

R. Ariel Gomez, M.D.
Professor of Pediatrics and Biology; Vice President for Research and Graduate Studies, University of Virginia, Charlottesville, Virginia
Development of the Renin-Angiotensin System

Bernard Gondos, M.D.
Clinical Professor of Pathology, David Geffen School of Medicine at UCLA, Los Angeles; Senior Scientist, Sansum Medical Research Institute, Santa Barbara, California
Testicular Development

Denis M. Grant, Ph.D.
Professor and Chair, Department of Pharmacology, Faculty of Medicine, and Associate Dean for Research, Faculty of Pharmacy, University of Toronto; Director, Institute for Drug Research, Toronto, Ontario, Canada
Pharmacogenetics

Lucy R. Green, Ph.D.
Lecturer, Centre for Fetal Origins of Adult Disease, University of Southampton; Princess Anne Hospital, Southampton, England
Programming of the Fetal Circulation

Jay S. Greenspan, M.D.
Professor and Vice Chairman, Department of Pediatrics, Jefferson Medical College; Thomas Jefferson University; Director of Neonatology, A.I. duPont Hospital for Children, Thomas Jefferson University Hospital, Philadelphia, Pennsylvania
Assisted Ventilation: Physiologic Implications and Complications

Adda Grimberg, M.D.
Assistant Professor, Department of Pediatrics, University of Pennsylvania School of Medicine; Attending Physician, Division of Pediatric Endocrinology, Children's Hospital of Philadelphia, Philadelphia, Pennsylvania
Hypothalamus: Neuroendometabolic Center

Justin C. Grindley, Ph.D.
Research Instructor, Division of Pediatric Cardiology, Vanderbilt University School of Medicine, Nashville, Tennessee
Molecular Determinants of Embryonic Vascular Development

Ian Gross, M.D.
Professor of Pediatrics, Yale University School of Medicine; Director of Perinatal Medicine, Newborn Special Care Unit, Yale–New Haven Children's Hospital New Haven, Connecticut
Hormonal Therapy for Prevention of Respiratory Distress Syndrome

Jean-Pierre Guignard, M.D.
Professor of Pediatric Nephrology, Lausanne University Faculty of Medicine; Director, Division of Pediatric Nephrology, Center Hospitalier Universitaire Vaudois, Lausanne, Switzerland
Postnatal Development of Glomerular Filtration Rate

Alistair J. Gunn, M.B., Ch.B., Ph.D., F.R.A.C.P.
Associate Professor, Liggins Institute, Department of Paediatrics, University of Auckland, Auckland, New Zealand
Responses of the Fetus and Neonate to Hypothermia

Gabriel G. Haddad, M.D.
Professor of Pediatrics and Neuroscience and University Chairman, Department of Pediatrics, Albert Einstein College of Medicine of Yeshiva University; Pediatrician-in-Chief, Children's Hospital of Montefiore, Bronx, New York
Basic Mechanisms of Oxygen-Sensing and Response to Hypoxia

J. Nathan Hagstrom, M.D.
Assistant Professor of Pediatrics, University of Connecticut School of Medicine, Farmington; Attending Physician, Connecticut Children's Medical Center, Hartford, Connecticut
Developmental Hemostasis; Pathophysiology of Bleeding Disorders in the Newborn

xii Contributors

Kathrin V. Halpern, B.A.
Research Coordinator, Division of Orthopaedic Surgery,
Children's Hospital of Philadelphia, Philadelphia, Pennsylvania
**Embryologic Origin, Structure, and Function; Common
    Musculoskeletal Conditions Related to Intrauterine Compression:
    Effects of Mechanics on Endochondral Ossification**

K. Michael Hambidge, M.D., Sc.D.
Professor Emeritus, Department of Pediatrics, Section of
Nutrition, University of Colorado School of Medicine;
The Children's Hospital, Denver, Colorado
Zinc in the Fetus and Neonate

Margit Hamosh, Ph.D.
Professor of Pediatrics (Emeritus), Georgetown University
School of Medicine; formerly Chief, Division of Developmental
Biology and Nutrition, Georgetown University Medical Center,
Washington, District of Columbia
Human Milk Composition and Function in the Infant

Mark A. Hanson, M.D., D.Phil., Cert.ED., F.R.C.O.G
British Heart Foundation Professor of Cardiovascular Science,
University of Southampton Faculty of Medicine; Director,
Center for Fetal Origins of Adult Disease, and Director, Fetal
Origins of Adult Disease Research Division, Princess Anne
Hospital, Southampton, England
Programming of the Fetal Circulation

Aviad Haramati, Ph.D.
Professor and Director of Education, Department of Physiology
and Biophysics, Georgetown University School of Medicine,
Washington, District of Columbia
Role of the Kidney in Calcium and Phosphorus Homeostasis

Richard Harding, M.D., D.Sc.
Professor, Department of Physiology, Monash University Faculty
of Medicine, Melbourne, Victoria, Australia
Physiologic Mechanisms of Normal and Altered Lung Growth

Mary Catherine Harris, M.D.
Associate Professor of Pediatrics, University of Pennsylvania
School of Medicine; Attending, Children's Hospital of
Philadelphia, Philadelphia Pennsylvania
Cytokines and Inflammatory Response in the Fetus and Neonate

Musa A. Haxhiu, M.D., Ph.D.
Professor of Pediatrics, Medicine, and Anatomy, Case Western
Reserve University School of Medicine, Cleveland, Ohio;
Professor, Department of Physiology and Biophysics, Howard
University School of Medicine, Washington, District of Columbia
Regulation of Lower Airway Function

William W. Hay, Jr., M.D.
Professor, Department of Pediatrics, University of Colorado
School of Medicine; Director, Neonatal Clinical Research Center,
and Scientific Director, Perinatal Research Center, University of
Colorado Health Sciences Center, Aurora, Colorado
Fetal Requirements and Placental Transfer of Nitrogenous Compounds

Anthony R. Hayward, M.D., Ph.D.
Director, Division of Clinical Research, National Center for
Research Resources, National Institutes of Health, Bethesda,
Maryland
T-Cell Development

William C. Heird, M.D.
Professor of Pediatrics, Children's Nutrition Research Center,
Baylor College of Medicine, Houston, Texas
Protein and Amino Acid Metabolism and Requirements

Emilio Herrera, Ph.D.
Professor of Biochemistry and Molecular Biology, School of
Experimental Sciences and Health, University of San
Pablo–CEU, Madrid, Spain
Maternal-Fetal Transfer of Lipid Metabolites

Harry R. Hill, M.D.
Professor of Pathology, Pediatrics and Internal Medicine,
University of Utah, Salt Lake City, Utah
Host Defense Mechanisms Against Bacteria

A. Craig Hillemeier, M.D.
Professor and Chair, Department of Pediatrics, Pennsylvania
State University College of Medicine; Medical Director, Penn
State Children's Hospital, Milton S. Hershey Medical Center,
Hershey, Pennsylvania
Fetal and Neonatal Intestinal Motility

Kurt Hirschhorn, M.D.
Professor of Pediatrics, Human Genetics, and Medicine, Mount
Sinai School of Medicine of The City University of New York;
Attending Pediatrician, Mount Sinai Hospital, New York,
New York
Molecular Genetics: Developmental and Clinical Implications

Steven B. Hoath, M.D.
Professor of Pediatrics, University of Cincinnati College of
Medicine; Medical Director, Skin Sciences Institute, Children's
Hospital Medical Center, Cincinnati, Ohio
Physiologic Development of the Skin

David A. Horst, M.D.
Assistant Professor, Baylor College of Medicine, Houston,
Texas
Bile Formation and Cholestasis

Tracy E. Hunley, M.D.
Assistant Professor of Pediatrics, Vanderbilt University School of
Medicine; Attending Pediatric Nephrologist, Vanderbilt
Children's Hospital, Nashville, Tennessee
Pathophysiology of Acute Renal Failure in the Neonatal Period

Christian J. Hunter, B.S.
Medical Student/Graduate Student, Loma Linda University
School of Medicine, Loma Linda, California
Perinatal Thermal Physiology

Shahid M. Husain, M.D., F.R.C.P.C.H.
Senior Lecturer, Barts and the London School of Medicine and
Dentistry, Queen Mary College, University of London;
Consultant Neonatologist, Homerton University Hospital,
London, England
**Calcium, Phosphorus, and Magnesium Transport Across
    the Placenta**

Susan M. Hutson, M.D., Ph.D.
Professor of Biochemistry, Wake Forest University School of
Medicine, Winston-Salem, North Carolina
Vitamin K Metabolism in the Fetus and Neonate

Machiko Ikegami, M.D., Ph.D.
Professor of Pediatrics, University of Cincinnati College of
Medicine; Attending, Division of Pulmonary Biology, Cincinnati
Children's Hospital Medical Center, Cincinnati, Ohio
**Pathophysiology of Respiratory Distress Syndrome and Surfactant
    Metabolism**

Terrie E. Inder, M.B., Ch.B., M.D., F.R.A.C.P.
Associate Professor in Pediatrics, University of Melbourne;
Neonatal Neurologist, Royal Women's and Children's Hospitals,
Murdoch Childrens Research Institute, Melbourne, Australia
Pathophysiology of Intraventricular Hemorrhage in the Neonate

Alan H. Jobe, M.D., Ph.D.
Professor of Pediatrics, University of Cincinnati College of
Medicine; Attending, Division of Neonatology Pulmonary
Biology, Cincinnati Children's Hospital, Cincinnati, Ohio
**Antenatal Factors That Influence Postnatal Lung Development and
Injury; Pathophysiology of Respiratory Distress Syndrome and
Surfactant Metabolism; Surfactant Treatment**

Lois H. Johnson, M.D.
Clinical Professor of Pediatrics in the Associated Faculty,
University of Pennsylvania School of Medicine; Associate
Physician, Section of Newborn Pediatrics, Pennsylvania
Hospital, Philadelphia, Pennsylvania
Vitamin E Nutrition in the Fetus and Neonate

Michael V. Johnston, M.D.
Professor of Neurology and Pediatrics, Johns Hopkins
University School of Medicine; Chief Medical Officer, Kennedy
Krieger Institute, Baltimore, Maryland
Development of Neurotransmitters

Richard B. Johnston, Jr., M.D.
Professor of Pediatrics and Associate Dean for Research
Development, University of Colorado School of Medicine,
Denver, Colorado
Host Defense Mechanisms Against Fungi

Deborah P. Jones, M.D.
Associate Professor, Department of Pediatrics, University of
Tennessee Health Sciences Center; Director of Dialysis Services,
Department of Pediatrics, LeBonheur Children's Medical
Center; Attending Physician, St. Jude Children's Research
Hospital, Memphis, Tennessee
Developmental Aspects of Organic Acid Transport

Peter Lloyd Jones, Ph.D.
Assistant Professor of Pediatrics, University of Colorado School
of Medicine, Denver, Colorado
The Extracellular Matrix in Development

Pedro A. Jose, M.D., Ph.D.
Professor of Pediatrics and Physiology and Biophysics,
Georgetown University School of Medicine, Washington,
District of Columbia
Postnatal Maturation of Renal Blood Flow

Satish C. Kalhan, M.B.B.S., F.R.C.P., D.C.H.
Professor, Department of Pediatrics, Case Western Reserve
University School of Medicine; Attending Neonatologist and
Director, Robert Schwartz M. D. Center for Metabolism and
Nutrition, MetroHealth Medical Center, Cleveland, Ohio
**Metabolism of Glucose and Methods of Investigation in the Fetus
and Newborn**

Subas Kallapur, M.B.B.S., M.D.
Assistant Professor of Pediatrics, University of Cincinnati
College of Medicine; Attending, Cincinnati Children's Hospital,
Cincinnati, Ohio
**Antenatal Factors That Influence Postnatal Lung Development
and Injury**

Stanley Kaplan, Ph.D.
Professor Emeritus, Departments of Cellular Biology,
Neurobiology, and Anatomy, Medical College of Wisconsin,
Milwaukee, Wisconsin
Basic Embryology

Saul J. Karpen, M.D., Ph.D.
Associate Professor of Pediatrics and Molecular and Cellular
Biology, Baylor College of Medicine; Director, Texas Children's
Liver Center, Baylor College of Medicine/Texas Children's
Hospital, Houston, Texas
Bile Formation and Cholestasis

Sudha Kashyap, M.B.B.S., D.C.H.
Professor of Clinical Pediatrics, College of Physicians and
Surgeons, Columbia University; Attending Physician,
Department of Pediatrics, Children's Hospital of New York,
Columbia-Presbyterian Medical Center, New York, New York
Protein and Amino Acid Metabolism and Requirements

Frederick J. Kaskel, M.D., Ph.D.
Professor of Pediatrics and Vice Chairman for Affiliate and
Network Affairs, Albert Einstein College of Medicine of Yeshiva
University; Director of Pediatric Nephrology, Children's Hospital
at Montefiore, Bronx, New York
Role of the Kidney in Calcium and Phosphorus Homeostasis

Lorraine E. Levitt Katz, M.D.
Assistant Professor of Pediatrics, University of Pennsylvania
School of Medicine; Attending, Endocrinology/ Diabetes
Division, Children's Hospital of Philadelphia, Philadelphia,
Pennsylvania
Growth Factor Regulation of Fetal Growth

Peter Kaufmann, M.D.
Professor of Anatomy, University of Technology Aachen
Medical Faculty, Department of Anatomy II, Aachen,
Germany
Placental Development

Susan E. Keeney, M.D.
Associate Professor, Department of Pediatrics, University of
Texas Medical Branch, Galveston, Texas
Immunology of Human Milk and Host Immunity

Laurie Kilpatrick, Ph.D.
Associate Member, Joseph Stokes Jr. Research Institute, Division
of Allergy and Immunology, Children's Hospital of Philadelphia,
Philadelphia, Pennsylvania
Cytokines and Inflammatory Response in the Fetus and Neonate

John P. Kinsella, M.D.
Professor, Department of Pediatrics, University of Colorado
School of Medicine; Attending, Section of Neonatology,
The Children's Hospital; and Director, ECMO Services, and
Director, Pediatric Advisory Group, Flight for Life Emergency
Medical Transport, Denver, Colorado
Physiology of Nitric Oxide in the Developing Lung

Margaret L. Kirby, Ph.D.
Professor of Pediatrics—Neonatology, Duke University School
of Medicine, Durham, North Carolina
Development of the Fetal Heart

Charles S. Kleinman, M.D.
Professor of Pediatrics, Diagnostic Imaging, and Obstetrics and
Gynecology, Yale University School of Medicine; Attending
Pediatrician and Section Chief, Pediatric Cardiology,
Yale-New Haven Hospital, New Haven, Connecticut
**Cardiovascular Function During Development and the Response
to Hypoxia**

Barry A. Kogan, M.D.
Professor of Surgery and Pediatrics, Albany Medical College; Chief,
Division of Urology, Albany Medical Center, Albany, New York
Testicular Development; Testicular Descent

Otakar Koldovský, M.D., Ph.D. (deceased)
Formerly Professor of Pediatrics and Physiology, University of
Arizona College of Medicine, Tucson, Arizona
Digestion-Absorption Functions in Fetuses, Infants, and Children

Valentina Kon, M.D.
Associate Professor of Pediatrics, Vanderbilt University School
of Medicine, Nashville, Tennessee
Pathophysiology of Acute Renal Failure in the Neonatal Period

Ernest A. Kopecky, Ph.D.
Senior Clinical Scientist, Department of Medical Research,
Purdue Pharma L.P., Stamford, Connecticut
Maternal Drug Abuse: Effects on Fetus and Neonate

Helen M. Korchak, Ph.D.
Research Professor of Pediatrics and Biochemistry/Biophysics,
University of Pennsylvania School of Medicine; Children's
Hospital of Philadelphia, Philadelphia, Pennsylvania
Stimulus-Response Coupling in Phagocytic Cells

Gideon Koren, M.D., F.R.C.P.C.
Professor of Pediatrics, Pharmacology, Pharmacy, Medicine, and
Medical Genetics, University of Toronto Faculty of Medicine;
Director, Motherisk Program, and Senior Scientist, Hospital for
Sick Children, Toronto, Ontario, Canada
Maternal Drug Abuse: Effects on Fetus and Neonate

Nancy F. Krebs, M.D.
Associate Professor and Head, Section of Nutrition, Department
of Pediatrics, University of Colorado School of Medicine;
Medical Director, Department of Nutrition, The Children's
Hospital, Denver, Colorado
Zinc in the Fetus and Neonate

Thomas J. Kulik, M.D.
Professor, Department of Pediatrics, University of Michigan
Medical School; Medical Director, Pediatric Cardiothoracic
Intensive Care Unit, C.S. Mott Children's Hospital, Ann Arbor,
Michigan
Physiology of Congenital Heart Disease in the Neonate

Jessica Katz Kutikov, M.D.
Medical student, University of Pennsylvania School of Medicine,
Philadelphia, Pennsylvania
Hypothalamus: Neuroendometabolic Center

Timothy R. La Pine, M.D.
Adjunct Assistant Professor of Pathology and Pediatrics,
University of Utah School of Medicine, Salt Lake City, Utah
Host Defense Mechanisms Against Bacteria

Miguel Angel Lasunción, Ph.D.
Associate Professor of Biochemistry and Molecular Biology,
University of Alcalá Faculty of Medicine, Alcalá de Henares;
Head, Biochemical Investigation Service, Hospital Ramón y
Cajal, Madrid Spain
Maternal-Fetal Transfer of Lipid Metabolites

John Laterra, M.D., Ph.D.
Professor, Departments of Neurology, Oncology, and
Neuroscience, John Hopkins University School of Medicine;
Department of Neurology, John Hopkins Hospital; Director of
Neuro-Oncology, Kennedy Kriegen Institute, Baltimore, Maryland
Development of the Blood-Brain Barrier

P. C. Lee, Ph.D.
Professor of Pediatrics, Pharmacology and Toxicology, Medical
College of Wisconsin; Director, Pediatric Gastrointestinal and
Nutrition Laboratory, Medical College of Wisconsin, Milwaukee,
Wisconsin
Development of the Exocrine Pancreas

Fred Levine, M.D., Ph.D.
Associate Professor, Department of Pediatrics, University of
California, San Diego, School of Medicine; Rebecca and John
Moores UCSD Cancer Center, La Jolla, California
Basic Genetic Principles

David B. Lewis, M.D.
Associate Professor of Pediatrics, Stanford University School of
Medicine; Attending Physician, Lucile Salter Packard Children's
Hospital at Stanford, Palo Alto, California
Host Defense Mechanisms Against Viruses

Chris A. Liacouras, M.D.
Associate Professor, University of Pennsylvania School of
Medicine; Attending Physician, Division of Pediatric
Gastroenterology, Children's Hospital of Philadelphia,
Philadelphia, Pennsylvania
Pathophysiology of Gastroesophageal Reflux

Michael A. Linshaw, M.D.
Associate Professor of Pediatrics, Harvard Medical School;
Pediatrician, Massachusetts General Hospital for Children,
Boston Massachusetts
Concentration and Dilution of the Urine

George Lister, M.D.
Professor of Pediatrics and Anesthesiology, Department of
Pediatrics, Section of Critical Care, Yale University School of
Medicine; Director, Pediatric Intensive Care Unit, and
Attending Pediatrician and Section Chief, Pediatric
Critical Care Medicine, Yale-New Haven Children's Hospital,
New Haven, Connecticut
**Cardiovascular Function During Development and the Response
to Hypoxia**

Cynthia A. Loomis, M.D., Ph.D.
Assistant Professor, Department of Dermatology and Cell
Biology; Tisch Hospital, Department of Dermatology,
NYU School of Medicine, New York, New York
**Structure and Development of the Skin and Cutaneous
Appendages**

John M. Lorenz, M.D.
Professor of Clinical Pediatrics, Columbia University
College of Physicians and Surgeons; Attending,
Children's Hospital of New York-Presbyterian, New York,
New York
**Fetal and Neonatal Body Water Compartment Volumes with
Reference to Growth and Development**

Steven Lobritto, M.D.
Hepatologist, Pediatrics and Adults, New York-Presbyterian
Hospital, New York, New York
Organogenesis and Histologic Development of the Liver

Ralph A. Lugo, Pharm.D.
Associate Professor of Pharmacy and Adjunct Associate
Professor of Pediatrics, University of Utah College of Pharmacy
and School of Medicine, Salt Lake City, Utah
Basic Pharmacokinetic Principles

Akhil Maheshwari, M.D.
Fellow in Neonatal-Perinatal Medicine, University of South
Florida College of Medicine, St. Petersburg, Florida
Developmental Granulocytopoiesis

Marilyn J. Manco-Johnson, M.D.
Professor of Pediatrics, University of Colorado School of
Medicine; Attending, The Children's Hospital, Denver,
Colorado
**Pathophysiology of Neonatal Disseminated Intravascular Coagulation
and Thrombosis**

Carlos B. Mantilla, M.D., Ph.D.
Assistant Professor of Anesthesiology, Mayo Medical School;
Senior Associate Consultant, Department of Anesthesiology,
Mayo Clinic, Rochester, Minnesota
Functional Development of Respiratory Muscles

M. Michele Mariscalco, M.D.
Assistant Professor of Pediatrics, Baylor College of Medicine,
Houston, Texas
Integrins and Cell Adhesion Molecules

László Maródi, M.D., Ph.D., D.Sc.
Professor and Chairman, Department of Pediatrics,
Division of Infectious Disease and Pediatric Immunology,
University of Debrecen Faculty of Medicine, Debrecen,
Hungary
Host Defense Mechanisms Against Fungi

Karel Maršál, M.D., Ph.D.
Professor of Obstetrics and Gynecology, University of Lund
Faculty of Medicine; Attending, Department of Obstetrics and
Gynecology, University Hospital, Lund, Sweden
Fetal and Placental Circulation During Labor

Richard J. Martin, M.B., F.R.A.C.P.
Professor of Pediatrics, Reproductive Biology, Physiology, and
Biophysics, Case Western Reserve University School of
Medicine; Director of Neonatology, Rainbow Babies and
Children's Hospital, Cleveland, Ohio
**Regulation of Lower Airway Function; Pathophysiology of Apnea of
Prematurity**

Dwight E. Matthews, Ph.D.
Professor and Chairman, Department of Chemistry, and
Professor of Medicine, School of Medicine, University of
Vermont, Burlington, Vermont
General Concepts of Protein Metabolism

Marcia McDuffie, M.D.
Associate Professor of Microbiology, University of Virginia
School of Medicine, Charlottesville, Virginia
T-Cell Development

Jane E. McGowan, M.D.
Associate Professor of Pediatrics, Johns Hopkins University
School of Medicine, Baltimore, Maryland
Oxygen Transport and Delivery

James McManaman, Ph.D.
Assistant Professor, Obstetrics and Gynecology, University of
Colorado Health Sciences Center, Denver, Colorado
Physiology of Lactation

Huseyin Mehmet, Ph.D.
Head, Weston Laboratory, Senior Lecturer in Neurobiology,
Imperial College London, London, United Kingdom
Apoptosis and Necrosis

Julie A. Mennella, Ph.D.
Member and Director of Education Outreach, Monell Chemical
Senses Center, Philadelphia, Pennsylvania
Development of Taste and Smell in the Neonate

Andrew Metinko, M.D.
Director, Pediatric Critical Care Services, Swedish Medical
Center, Seattle, Washington
Neonatal Pulmonary Host Defense Mechanisms

Martha J. Miller, M.D., Ph.D.
Associate Professor of Pediatrics, Case Western Reserve
University School of Medicine; Attending, Rainbow Babies and
Children's Hospital, Cleveland, Ohio
Pathophysiology of Apnea of Prematurity

Paul Monagle, M.B.B.S., M.Sc., F.R.A.C.P, F.R.C.P.A., F.C.C.P.
Associate Professor, Department of Paediatrics, University of
Melbourne; Director, Division of Laboratory Services, Head of
Haematology, Royal Children's Hospital, Melbourne, Victoria,
Australia
Developmental Hemostasis

Jacopo P. Mortola, M.D.
Professor of Physiology, McGill University Faculty of Medicine,
Montreal, Quebec, Canada
Mechanics of Breathing

Glen E. Mott, Ph.D.
Professor, Department of Pathology, University of Texas Health
Science Center, San Antonio, Texas
**Lipoprotein Metabolism and Nutritional Programming in the Fetus
and Neonate**

M. Zulficar Mughal, M.B., Ch.B., F.R.C.P., F.R.C.P.C.H., D.C.H.
Department of Child Health, University of Manchester;
Consultant Paediatrician and Honorary Senior Lecturer in Child
Health, Department of Paediatrics, Saint Mary's Hospital for
Women and Children, Manchester, United Kingdom
Calcium, Phosphorus, and Magnesium Transport Across the Placenta

Susan E. Mulroney, Ph.D.
Associate Professor, Department of Physiology, Georgetown
University School of Medicine, Washington, District of Columbia
Role of the Kidney in Calcium and Phosphorus Homeostasis

Upender K. Munshi, M.B.B.S., M.D.
Assistant Professor, Department of Pediatrics, Albany Medical
College, Albany, New York
**Development of the Gastrointestinal Circulation in the Fetus
and Newborn**

Leslie Myatt, Ph.D.
Professor, Department of Obstetrics-Gynecology, Division of
Maternal-Fetal Medicine, University of Cincinnati College of
Medicine, Cincinnati, Ohio
Regulation of Umbilical Blood Flow

Margaret A. Myers, M.D.
Clinical Assistant Professor of Pediatrics, University of
Pennsylvania School of Medicine; Associate Clinical Director,
Newborn Infant Center, Children's Hospital of Philadelphia,
Philadelphia, Pennsylvania
Development of Pain Sensation

Ran Namgung, M.D., Ph.D.
Professor, Department of Pediatrics, Yonsei University College of
Medicine, Seoul, Korea
Neonatal Calcium, Phosphorus, and Magnesium Homeostasis

Michael R. Narkewicz, M.D.
Associate Professor of Pediatrics and Hewit-Andrews Chair in
Pediatric Liver Disease, University of Colorado School of
Medicine; Medical Director, The Pediatric Liver Center,
The Children's Hospital, Denver, Colorado
Neonatal Cholestasis: Pathophysiology, Etiology, and Treatment

Heinz Nau, Ph.D.
Professor, School of Veterinary Medicine, University of
Hannover, Hannover, Germany
**Physicochemical and Structural Properties Regulating Placental Drug
Transfer**

Jan Nedergaard, Ph.D.
Professor, The Wenner-Gren Institute, Stockholm University,
Stockholm, Sweden
Brown Adipose Tissue: Development and Function

Margaret C. Neville, Ph.D.
Professor of Physiology and Biophysics, Professor of Cell and
Developmental Biology, and Professor of Obstetrics and
Gynecology, University of Colorado School of Medicine, Denver,
Colorado
Physiology of Lactation

Heber C. Nielsen, M.D.
Professor of Pediatrics, Tufts University School of Medicine;
Attending, Tufts–New England Medical Center, Boston,
Massachusetts
Homeobox Genes

Lawrence M. Nogee, M.D.
Associate Professor of Pediatrics, Johns Hopkins University
School of Medicine, Baltimore, Maryland
Genetics and Physiology of Surfactant Protein Deficiencies

Shahab Noori, M.D.
Assistant Professor of Pediatrics, University of Southern
California Keck School of Medicine; Neonatologist, USC
Division of Neonatal Medicine, Department of Pediatrics,
Children's Hospital Los Angeles, Women's and Children's
Hospital, and LAC+USC Medical Center, Los Angeles,
California
Pathophysiology of Shock in the Fetus and Neonate

Errol R. Norwitz, M.D., Ph.D., F.A.C.O.G.
Assistant Professor, Harvard Medical School; Attending,
Brigham and Women's Hospital, Boston, Massachusetts
Pathophysiology of Preterm Birth

Victoria F. Norwood, M.D.
Associate Professor of Pediatrics, University of Virginia School
of Medicine; Chief, Pediatric Nephrology, University of Virginia
Health System, Charlottesville, Virginia
Development of the Renin-Angiotensin System

Edward S. Ogata, M.D., M.M.
Professor of Pediatrics and Obstetrics and Gynecology,
Northwestern University Feinberg School of Medicine;
Chief Medical Officer, Children's Memorial Hospital, Chicago,
Illinois
Carbohydrate Metabolism During Pregnancy

Robin K. Ohls, M.D.
Associate Professor of Pediatrics, University of New Mexico
School of Medicine; Director, Neonatal-Perinatal Fellowship
Program, Division of Neonatology, University of New Mexico
Children's Hospital, Albuquerque, New Mexico
Developmental Erythropoiesis

Thomas A. Olson, M.D.
Associate Professor of Pediatric Hematology/Oncology, Emory
University School of Medicine, Atlanta, Georgia
**Developmental Megakaryocytopoiesis in Fetal and Neonatal
Physiology**

Taher I. Omari, Ph.D.
Affiliate Senior Lecturer, Department of Paediatrics, University
of Adelaide, Adelaide, Australia; Senior Research Officer, Centre
for Paediatric and Adolescent Gastroenterology, Women's and
Children's Hospital, North Adelaide, Australia
Gastrointestinal Motility

James F. Padbury, M.D.
Professor and Vice Chair, Department of Pediatrics, Brown
University Medical School; Chief of Pediatrics, Women and
Infant's Hospital of Rhode Island, Providence, Rhode Island
Developmental Pharmacology of Adrenergic Agents

Mark R. Palmert, M.D., Ph.D.
Assistant Professor of Pediatrics, Case Western Reserve
University School of Medicine; Attending, Division of Pediatric
Endocrinology and Metabolism, Rainbow Babies and Children's
Hospital, University Hospitals of Cleveland, Cleveland, Ohio
**Luteinizing Hormone and Follicle-Stimulating Hormone Secretion in
the Fetus and Newborn Infant**

Elvira Parravicini, M.D.
Assistant Professor of Pediatrics in Neonatology, Columbia
University College of Physicians and Surgeons;
Attending–Neonatology, Children's Hospital of
New York–Presbyterian, New York, New York
Neonatal Neutrophil Normal and Abnormal Physiology

Gilberto R. Pereira, M.D.
Professor of Pediatrics, University of Pennsylvania School of
Medicine; Neonatologist, Children's Hospital of Philadelphia,
Philadelphia, Pennsylvania
Nutritional Assessment [Intrauterine and Postnatal Growth]

Jeff M. Perlman, M.B., Ch.B.
Professor of Pediatrics, University of Texas Southwestern
Medical Center; Medical Director, Neonatal Intensive Care Unit,
Parkland Hospital, Dallas, Texas
**Cerebral Blood Flow in Premature Infants: Regulation, Measurement,
and Pathophysiology of Intraventricular Hemorrhage**

Anthony F. Philipps, M.D.
Professor and Chair, Department of Pediatrics, University of
California, Davis, School of Medicine; Attending, UCD Children's
Hospital, Sacramento, California
**Oxygen Consumption and General Carbohydrate Metabolism
in the Fetus**

Arthur S. Pickoff, M.D.
Professor and Chair, Department of Pediatrics, Wright State
University School of Medicine; Pediatric Cardiologist, Children's
Medical Center, Dayton, Ohio
Developmental Electrophysiology in the Fetus and Neonate

C. S. Pinal, Ph.D.
Biology Santa Cruz Research Fellow, The Liggins Institute,
University of Auckland, Auckland, New Zealand
Growth Factor Regulation of Fetal Growth

David Pleasure, M.D.
Professor of Neurology and Pediatrics, University of
Pennsylvania School of Medicine; Director, Joseph Stokes, Jr.
Research Institute, and Senior VP for Research, Children's
Hospital of Philadelphia, Philadelphia, Pennsylvania
**Trophic Factor and Nutritional and Hormonal Regulation of Brain
Development**

Jeanette Pleasure, M.D.
Associate Professor of Pediatrics, Drexel University College of
Medicine; Attending Neonatologist, Hahnemann Hospital and
St. Christopher's Hospital for Children, Philadelphia,
Pennsylvania
**Trophic Factor and Nutritional and Hormonal Regulation of Brain
Development**

Sabine Luise Plonait, M.D., M.R.C.P.(UK), D.C.M.
Private Practice; Instructor, DRU Nursing School; Freelance
Researcher, RUI, Berlin, Germany
**Physicochemical and Structural Properties Regulating Placental Drug
Transfer**

Richard A. Polin, M.D.
Professor of Pediatrics, Columbia University College of
Physicians and Surgeons; Director, Division of Neonatology,
Children's Hospital of New York–Presbyterian, New York,
New York

Daniel H. Polk, M.D.
Professor of Pediatrics, Northwestern University Feinberg
School of Medicine; Associate Chief, Neonatology, Children's
Memorial Hospital, Chicago, Illinois
Fetal and Neonatal Thyroid Physiology

Scott L. Pomeroy, M.D., Ph.D.
Associate Professor of Neurology, Harvard Medical School;
Senior Associate in Neurology, Children's Hospital, Boston,
Massachusetts
Development of the Nervous System

Fred Possmayer, Ph.D.
Professor, Departments of Obstetrics/Gynaecology and
Biochemistry, University of Western Ontario Faculty of
Medicine; CIHR Group in Fetal and Neonatal Health and
Development, London, Ontario, Canada
Physicochemical Aspects of Pulmonary Surfactant

Martin Post, Ph.D.
Professor of Pediatrics, Physiology, Laboratory Medicine, and
Pathobiology, University of Toronto Faculty of Medicine; Head,
Lung Biology and Integrative Biology Programs, Hospital for
Sick Children, Toronto, Ontario, Canada
**Molecular Mechanisms of Lung Development and Lung Branching
Morphogenesis**

Gordon G. Power, M.D.
Professor of Physiology and Research Professor of Internal
Medicine, Loma Linda University School of Medicine, Loma
Linda, California
Perinatal Thermal Physiology

Jorge A. Prada, M.D.
Assistant Professor, Department of Obstetrics and Gynecology,
Division of Maternal-Fetal Medicine, University of Cincinnati
College of Medicine, Cincinnati, Ohio
Calcium-Regulating Hormones

Guy Putet, M.D.
Professor of Pediatrics, Claude Bernard University Faculty of
Medicine; Head, Department of Neonatology, Hospices Civils de
Lyon, Lyon, France
Lipids as an Energy Source for the Premature and Full-Term Neonate

Theodore J. Pysher, M.D.
Professor (Clinical) of Pathology, University of Utah School of
Medicine; Medical Director of Laboratories, Primary Children's
Medical Center, Salt Lake City, Utah
Impaired Lung Growth After Injury in Premature Lung

Graham E. Quinn, M.D., M.S.C.E.
Professor of Ophthalmology, University of Pennsylvania School
of Medicine; Attending Ophthalmologist, Children's Hospital of
Philadelphia, Philadelphia, Pennsylvania
**Retinal Development and the Pathophysiology of Retinopathy
of Prematurity**

Marlene Rabinovitch, M.D.
Dwight and Vera Dunlevie Professor of Pediatrics and Professor
(by courtesy) of Developmental Biology, Stanford University
School of Medicine; Research Faculty, Cancer Biology Program;
Research Director, Wall Center for Pulmonary Vascular Disease;
Pediatric Cardiologist, Lucile Packard Children's Hospital,
Stanford, California
Developmental Biology of the Pulmonary Vasculature

Scott H. Randell, Ph.D.
Assistant Professor of Medicine and Cell and Molecular
Physiology, University of North Carolina at Chapel Hill School
of Medicine; UNC Cystic Fibrosis/Pulmonary Research and
Treatment Center, Chapel Hill, North Carolina
**Structure of Alveolar Epithelial Cells and the Surface Layer During
Development**

Timothy R. H. Regnault, Ph.D.
Assistant Professor, Department of Pediatrics, Division of
Perinatal Medicine, University of Colorado School of Medicine,
Aurora, Colorado
**Fetal Requirements and Placental Transfer of Nitrogenous
Compounds**

**Michael J. Rieder, M.D., Ph.D., F.R.C.P.C., F.A.A.P., F.R.C.P.
(Glasgow)**
Professor and Chair, Division of Clinical Pharmacology,
Departments of Paediatrics, Physiology, Pharmocology and
Medicine, University of Western Ontario; Section Head,
Paediatric Clinical Pharmacology, Department of Paediatrics,
Children's Hospital of Western Ontario, London, Ontario,
Canada
Drug Excretion During Lactation

Henrique Rigatto, M.D.
Professor of Pediatrics, Physiology, and Reproductive Medicine,
University of Manitoba Faculty of Medicine; Director of
Neonatal Research, Health Sciences Centre, Winnipeg,
Manitoba, Canada
**Control of Breathing in Fetal Life and Onset and Control of Breathing
in the Neonate**

Natalie E. Rintoul, M.D.
Clinical Associate, University of Pennsylvania School of
Medicine; Attending Physician, Division of Neonatology,
Children's Hospital of Philadelphia, Philadelphia,
Pennsylvania
Pathophysiology of Neural Tube Defects

Jean E. Robillard, M.D.
Professor and Dean, University of Iowa Roy J. and Lucille A.
Carver College of Medicine, Iowa City, Iowa
Functional Development of the Kidney *In Utero*

Julian Robinson, M.D.
Assistant Professor of Pediatrics, Columbia University College of
Physicians and Surgeons; Attending, New York–Presbyterian
Hospital, New York, New York
Pathophysiology of Preterm Birth

Roberto Romero, M.D.
Chief, Perinatology Research Branch, National Institute of Child
Health and Human Development, National Institutes of Health,
Bethesda, Maryland
Fetal and Maternal Responses to Intrauterine Infection

Seamus A. Rooney, Ph.D., Sc.D.
Professor of Pediatrics, Yale University School of Medicine,
New Haven, Connecticut
**Regulation of Surfactant-Associated Phospholipid Synthesis
and Secretion**

James C. Rose, Ph.D.
Professor, Department of Obstetrics and Gynecology, Wake
Forest University School of Medicine, Winston-Salem,
North Carolina
**Development of the Corticotropin-Releasing Hormone–Corticotropin/
β-Endorphin System in the Mammalian Fetus**

Charles R. Rosenfeld, M.D.
Professor of Pediatrics and Obstetrics/Gynecology, University of
Texas Southwestern Medical Center; Director of Neonatal
Medicine, Parkland Memorial Hospital; Children's Medical
Center, Dallas, Texas
Regulation of Placental Circulation

xviii Contributors

Arthur J. Ross III, M.D., M.B.A.
Professor of Surgery and Pediatrics and Associate Dean, Western Clinical Campus, University of Wisconsin Medical School; Director of Medical Education, Gundersen Lutheran Medical Foundation, La Crosse, Wisconsin
Organogenesis of the Gastrointestinal Tract

Colin D. Rudolph, M.D., Ph.D.
Professor, Department of Pediatrics, Medical College of Wisconsin; Chief, Department of Pediatric Gastroenterology, Hepatology and Nutrition, Milwaukee, Wisconsin
Gastrointestinal Motility

Rakesh Sahni, M.B., B.S., M.D.
Associate Professor of Clinical Pediatrics, Columbia University College of Physicians and Surgeons; Associate Attending Pediatrician, Children's Hospital of New York–Presbyterian, New York, New York
Temperature Control in Newborn Infants

Harvey B. Sarnat, M.D., F.R.C.P.C.
Professor of Pediatrics (Neurology) and Pathology (Neuropathology), David Geffen School of Medicine at UCLA; Director, Pediatric Neurology, Cedars-Sinai Medical Center, Los Angeles, California
Ontogenesis of Striated Muscle

Lisa M. Satlin, M.D.
Professor of Pediatrics, Mt. Sinai School of Medicine of The City University of New York; Chief, Division of Pediatric Nephrology, Mount Sinai Medical Center, New York, New York
Potassium Homeostasis in the Fetus and Neonate

Ola Didrik Saugstad, M.D., Ph.D.
Professor of Pediatrics, University of Oslo Faculty of Medicine; Director, Department of Pediatric Research, University of Oslo Hospital, Oslo, Norway
Physiology of Resuscitation

Kurt R. Schibler, M.D.
Associate Professor of Pediatrics, University of Cincinnati College of Medicine; Attending, Children's Hospital Medical Center, Cincinnati, Ohio
Developmental Biology of the Hematopoietic Growth Factors; Mononuclear Phagocyte System

Karl Schulze, M.D.
Associate Professor of Clinical Pediatrics/Special Lecturer in Pediatrics, Columbia University College of Physicians and Surgeons, New York, New York
Temperature Control in Newborn Infants

Jeffrey Schwartz, Ph.D.
Senior Lecturer, School of Molecular and Biomedical Science, University of Adelaide, Adelaide, Australia; Adjunct Assistant Professor, Department of Obstetrics and Gynecology, Wake Forest University School of Medicine, Winston-Salem, North Carolina
Development of the Corticotropin-Releasing Hormone–Corticotropin/ β-Endorphin System in the Mammalian Fetus

Gunnar Sedin, M.D., Ph.D.
Professor of Perinatal Medicine, Department of Women's and Children's Health, Perinatal Research Laboratory and Neonatal Intensive Care, Uppsala University; Attending Neonatologist, Uppsala University Children's Hospital, Uppsala, Sweden
Physics and Physiology of Human Neonatal Incubation

Jeffrey L. Segar, M.D.
Associate Professor, Department of Pediatrics, University of Iowa Roy J. and Lucille A. Carver College of Medicine, Iowa City, Iowa
Neural Regulation of Blood Pressure During Fetal and Newborn Life

Istvan Seri, M.D., Ph.D.
Professor of Pediatrics, University of Southern California Keck School of Medicine; Head, USC Division of Neonatal Medicine, Women's and Children's Hospital, USC–LAC Medical Center, and Children's Hospital Los Angeles, Los Angeles, California
Pathophysiology of Shock in the Fetus and Neonate; Regulation of Acid-Base Balance in the Fetus and Neonate

Kenneth Setchell, Ph.D.
Professor of Pediatrics, University of Cincinnati College of Medicine; Professor of Pediatrics, Director, Clinical Mass Spectrometry, Cincinnati Children's Hospital Medical Center, Cincinnati, Ohio
Bile Acid Metabolism During Development

Thomas H. Shaffer, Ph.D.
Professor of Physiology and Pediatrics, Temple University School of Medicine and Professor of Pediatrics, Thomas Jefferson University, Jefferson Medical College, Philadelphia, Pennsylvania; Director, Nemours Research Lung Center, Alfred I. du Pont Hospital for Children, Wilmington, Delaware
Upper Airway Structure: Function, Regulation, and Development; Assisted Ventilation: Physiologic Implications and Complications; Liquid Ventilation

Philip W. Shaul, M.D.
Professor of Pediatrics and Lowe Foundation Professor of Pediatric Critical Care Research, University of Texas Southwestern Medical Center at Dallas, Dallas, Texas
Physiology of Nitric Oxide in the Developing Lung

Jayant P. Shenai, M.D.
Professor of Pediatrics, Vanderbilt University School of Medicine, Nashville, Tennessee
Vitamin A Metabolism in the Fetus and Neonate

Colin P. Sibley, Ph.D.
Professor of Child Health and Physiology, Academic Unit of Child Health, University of Manchester; St. Mary's Hospital, Manchester, England
Mechanisms of Transfer Across the Human Placenta

Gary C. Sieck, Ph.D.
Professor of Physiology and Anesthesiology, Mayo Medical School; Chair, Department of Physiology and Biophysics, Mayo Clinic, Rochester, Minnesota
Functional Development of Respiratory Muscles

Theresa M. Siler-Khodr, Ph.D.
Professor of Obstetrics-Gynecology, University of Texas Health Science Center at San Antonio, San Antonio, Texas
Endocrine and Paracrine Function of the Human Placenta

Faye S. Silverstein, M.D.
Professor of Pediatrics and Neurology, University of Michigan Medical School, Ann Arbor, Michigan
Development of Neurotransmitters

Rebecca A. Simmons, M.D.
Assistant Professor of Pediatrics, University of Pennsylvania School of Medicine; Attending Neonatologist, Children's Hospital of Philadelphia, Philadelphia, Pennsylvania
Cell Glucose Transport and Glucose Handling During Fetal and Neonatal Development

Emidio M. Sivieri, M.S.
Biomedical Engineer, Neonatal Pulmonary Function Laboratory, Newborn Pediatrics, Pennsylvania Hospital/University of Pennsylvania School of Medicine, Philadelphia, Pennsylvania
Evaluation of Pulmonary Function in the Neonate

Harold C. Slavkin, D.D.S.
Dean, University of Southern California School of Dentistry, Los Angeles, California
Regulation of Embryogenesis

Evan Y. Snyder, M.D., Ph.D.
Professor and Director, Program in Stem Cell and Regeneration
Biology, The Burnham Institute, La Jolla, California; Attending
Neonatologist, Department of Neonatology, University of
California, San Diego, La Jolla, California; Attending
Neonatologist, Division of Newborn Medicine, Department of
Pediatrics, Children's Hospital, Boston, Boston, Massachusetts
Stem Cell Biology

Jeanne M. Snyder, Ph.D.
Professor, Department of Anatomy and Cell Biology, University
of Iowa Roy J. and Lucille A. Carver College of Medicine,
Iowa City, Iowa
Regulation of Alveolarization

Michael J. Solhaug, M.D.
Professor of Pediatrics and Associate Professor of Physiology,
Eastern Virginia Medical School, Norfolk, Virginia
Postnatal Maturation of Renal Blood Flow

Kevin W. Southern, Ph.D., M.B.Ch.B., M.R.C.P.
Senior Lecturer in Pediatric Respiratory Medicine, University of
Liverpool Faculty of Medicine; Honorary Consultant in
Paediatric Respiratory Medicine, Royal Liverpool Children's
Hospital, Liverpool, England
**Regulation of Liquid Secretion and Absorption by the Fetal
and Neonatal Lung**

Adrian Spitzer, M.D.
Professor of Pediatrics, Albert Einstein College of Medicine of
Yeshiva University; Attending, Children's Hospital at Montefiore,
Montefiore Medical Center, Bronx, New York
Role of the Kidney in Calcium and Phosphorus Homeostasis

Alan R. Spitzer, M.D.
Professor of Pediatrics and Chief, Division of Neonatology, State
University of New York at Stony Brook School of Medicine;
Director of Neonatology, Stony Brook University Hospital,
Stony Brook, New York
Assisted Ventilation: Physiologic Implications and Complications

Charles A. Stanley, M.D.
Professor of Pediatrics, University of Pennsylvania School of
Medicine; Chief, Division of Endocrinology/Diabetes, Children's
Hospital of Philadelphia, Philadelphia, Pennsylvania
Pathophysiology of Hypoglycemia

F. Bruder Stapleton, M.D.
Ford/Morgan Professor and Chair, University of Washington
School of Medicine; Pediatrician-in-Chief, Children's Hospital
and Regional Medical Center, Seattle, Washington
Developmental Aspects of Organic Acid Transport

Dennis Styne, M.D.
Professor, Department of Pediatrics, University of California,
Davis, School of Medicine; Chief, Pediatric Endocrinology, UCD
Medical Center, Sacramento, California
Endocrine Factors Affecting Neonatal Growth

William E. Sweeney, Jr., M.D.
Assistant Professor, Department of Pediatrics, Case Western
Reserve University School of Medicine; Director, Renal
Development and Center for Childhood PKD Laboratory,
Department of Pediatric Nephrology, Rainbow Babies and
Children's Hospital, Cleveland, Ohio
Embryogenesis and Anatomic Development of the Kidney

Norman S. Talner, M.D.
Professor of Pediatrics, Department of Pediatrics, Division of
Cardiology, Duke University Medical Center, Durham,
North Carolina
**Cardiovascular Function During Development and the Response to
Hypoxia**

Paul S. Thornton, M.B., B.Ch., M.R.C.P.I.
Medical Director, Department of Endocrinology and Diabetes,
Cook Children's Medical Center, Fort Worth, Texas
Ketone Body Production and Metabolism in the Fetus and Neonate

William Edward Truog, M.D.
Professor of Pediatrics, University of Missouri–Kansas City
School of Medicine; Sosland Family Endowed Chair in Neonatal
Research and Attending Neonatologist, Children's Mercy
Hospital, Kansas City, Missouri
Pulmonary Gas Exchange in the Developing Lung

Reginald C. Tsang, M.B.B.S.
Professor Emeritus of Pediatrics, University of Cincinnati
College of Medicine; Children's Hospital Medical Center,
Cincinnati, Ohio
**Calcium, Phosphorus, and Magnesium Transport Across the Placenta;
Neonatal Calcium, Phosphorus, and Magnesium Homeostasis**

Alda Tufro, M.D., Ph.D.
Associate Professor of Pediatrics, Department of Pediatrics,
Division of Nephrology, Albert Einstein College of Medicine of
Yeshiva University, Bronx, New York
Development of the Renin-Angiotensin System

Nicole J. Ullrich, M.D., Ph.D.
Clinical Fellow in Neuro-Oncology, Children's Hospital, Boston,
Massachusetts
Development of the Nervous System

Socheata Un, M.A., J.D.
Medical Student, University of Kansas School of Medicine,
Kansas City, Kansas
Long Chain Fatty Acids in the Developing Retina and Brain

John E. Van Aerde, M.D., Ph.D.
Clinical Professor of Pediatrics and Director, Division of
Neonatology, University of Alberta Faculty of Medicine;
Regional Director for Newborn Services, Capital Health,
Edmonton, Alberta, Canada
Accretion of Lipid in the Fetus and Newborn

Carmella van de Ven, M.A.
Senior Staff Research Associate, Columbia University, New York,
New York
Neonatal Neutrophil Normal and Abnormal Physiology

Johannes B. van Goudoever, M.D., Ph.D.
Attending, Department of Neonatology, Erasmus Medical
Center, Sophia Children's Hospital, Rotterdam, The Netherlands
General Concepts of Protein Metabolism

Robert C. Vannucci, M.D.
Professor of Pediatrics (Pediatric Neurology), Pennsylvania State
University School of Medicine, Hershey, Pennsylvania
Perinatal Brain Metabolism

Susan J. Vannucci, Ph.D.
Research Director, Pediatric Critical Care Medicine, Morgan
Stanley Children's Hospital of New York, New York, New York
Perinatal Brain Metabolism

Minke van Tuyl, M.D.
Research Fellow, Hospital for Sick Children, Toronto, Ontario,
Canada
**Molecular Mechanisms of Lung Development and Lung Branching
Morphogenesis**

Joseph J. Volpe, M.D.
Bronson Crothers Professor of Neurology, Harvard Medical
School; Neurologist-in-Chief, Children's Hospital, Boston,
Massachusetts
Pathophysiology of Intraventricular Hemorrhage in the Neonate

Reidar Wallin, Ph.D.
Professor, Department of Internal Medicine, Wake Forest
University School of Medicine, Winston-Salem, North Carolina
Vitamin K Metabolism in the Fetus and Neonate

David Warburton, D.Sc., M.D., F.R.C.P.
Professor of Pediatrics and Surgery, University of Southern
California Keck School of Medicine; Professor of Craniofacial
Biology, University of Southern California School of Dentistry;
Leader, Developmental Biology Program, Children's Hospital Los
Angeles Research Institute, Los Angeles, California
Regulation of Embryogenesis

Robert M. Ward, M.D.
Professor of Pediatrics, University of Utah School of Medicine;
Director, Pediatric Pharmacology Program, University of Utah
Hospital, Salt Lake City, Utah
Basic Pharmacokinetic Principles

Joern-Hendrik Weitkamp, M.D.
Fellow, Pediatric Infectious Diseases, Vanderbilt University
Medical Center, Nashville, Tennessee
B-Cell Development

Steven L. Werlin, M.D.
Professor of Pediatrics, Medical College of Wisconsin,
Milwaukee, Wisconsin
Development of the Exocrine Pancreas

Lynne A. Werner, Ph.D.
Professor, Department of Speech and Hearing Sciences,
University of Washington School of Medicine, Seattle, Washington
Early Development of the Human Auditory System

Susan E. Wert, Ph.D.
Associate Professor of Pediatrics, University of Cincinnati
College of Medicine; Director, Molecular Morphology Core,
Division of Pulmonary Biology, Cincinnati Children's Hospital
Medical Center, Cincinnati, Ohio
Normal and Abnormal Structural Development of the Lung

Lars Grabow Westergaard, M.D., D.M.Sc.
Associate Professor, Obstetrics and Gynecology, University of
Southern Denmark; Associate Professor, Department of
Obstetrics and Gynecology, Odense University Hospital,
Odense, Denmark
Differentiation of the Ovary

Jeffrey A. Whitsett, M.D.
Professor of Pediatrics, University of Cincinnati College of
Medicine; Director, Neonatology and Pulmonary Biology,
Cincinnati Children's Hospital Medical Center, Cincinnati, Ohio
Composition of Pulmonary Surfactant Lipids and Proteins

Michaelann Wilke, B.Sc.
Doctoral Candidate, Nutrition and Metabolism, University of
Alberta, Edmonton, Alberta, Canada
Accretion of Lipid in the Fetus and Newborn

John V. Williams, M.D.
Assistant Professor, Division of Pediatric Infectious Diseases,
Department of Pediatrics, Vanderbilt University; Assistant
Professor, Division of Pediatric Infectious Diseases, Department
of Pediatrics, Vanderbilt University Medical Center, Nashville,
Tennessee
B-Cell Development

Dermot H. Williamson, D.Phil. (deceased)
Formerly Medical Research Council (UK), External Scientific
Staff, and University Research Lecturer, Metabolic Research
Laboratory, University of Oxford, Radcliffe Infirmary, Oxford,
England
Ketone Body Production and Metabolism in the Fetus and Neonate

Jerry A. Winkelstein, M.D.
Eudowood Professor of Pediatrics and Professor of Medicine
and Pathology, Johns Hopkins University School of Medicine;
Director, Division of Immunology, Department of Pediatrics,
Johns Hopkins Hospital, Baltimore, Maryland
The Complement System of the Fetus and Neonate

Jeremy S. D. Winter, M.D., F.R.C.P.C.
Professor and Head, Section of Endocrinology and Metabolism,
Department of Pediatrics, University of Alberta Faculty of
Medicine, Edmonton, Alberta, Canada
Fetal and Neonatal Adrenocortical Physiology

Douglas A. Woelkers, M.D.
Assistant Professor, Department of Reproductive Medicine,
University of California, San Diego, San Diego, California
**Maternal Cardiovascular Disease and Fetal Growth and
Development**

Marla R. Wolfson, Ph.D.(Physiol.)
Associate Professor of Physiology and Pediatrics and Chair,
Physiology Graduate Studies, Temple University School of
Medicine; Attending, Temple University Children's Hospital,
Philadelphia, Pennsylvania
**Upper Airway Structure: Function, Regulation, and Development;
Liquid Ventilation**

Robert P. Woroniecki, M.D.
Assistant Professor of Pediatrics, Pediatric Nephrology, Albert
Einstein College of Medicine of Yeshiva University; Research
Fellow, Pediatric Nephrology, Children's Hospital at
Monte Fiore, Bronx, New York
Role of the Kidney in Calcium and Phosphorus Homeostasis

Walid K. Yassir, M.D.
Assistant Professor of Orthopaedics, Tufts University School of
Medicine; Pediatric Orthopaedic Surgeon, Tufts–New England
Medical Center, Boston Floating Hospital for Children, Boston,
Massachusetts
Defective Limb Embryology

Stephen Yip, M.D., Ph.D.
Resident, Neurosurgery, Vancouver General Hospital, Vancouver,
British Columbia, Canada
Stem Cell Biology

Mervin C. Yoder, M.D.
Professor of Pediatrics and of Biochemistry and Molecular
Biology, Indiana University School of Medicine; Attending
Hematologist, James Whitcomb Riley Hospital for Children,
Indianapolis, Indiana
**Biology of Stem Cells and Stem Cell Transplantation; Developmental
Biology of the Hematopoietic Growth Factors**

Sharla Young, Ph.D.
Postdoctoral Fellow, National Institute of Child Health and
Human Development, National Institutes of Health, Bethesda,
Maryland
**Development of the Corticotropin-Releasing Hormone–Corticotropin/
β-Endorphin System in the Mammalian Fetus**

Stephen L. Young, M.D.
Professor of Medicine, Duke University School of Medicine,
Durham, North Carolina
**Structure of Alveolar Epithelial Cells and the Surface Layer During
Development**

Dan Zhou, Ph.D.
Instructor, Department of Pediatrics, Albert Einstein College of
Medicine of Yeshiva University, Bronx, New York
Basic Mechanisms of Oxygen-Sensing and Response to Hypoxia

PREFACE TO THE THIRD EDITION

With the publication of the third edition of *Fetal and Neonatal Physiology*, we welcome a new (third) editor, Dr. Steven Abman. Dr. Abman is Professor of Pediatrics at the University of Colorado School of Medicine and Director of the Pediatric Heart Lung Center in the Department of Pediatrics. In addition to his expertise as an editor, he brings considerable experience in basic science investigations in fetal and neonatal pulmonary and cardiovascular physiology.

The challenges posed by preparation of the new edition were immense. Within each major section, the increase in the amount of information—especially at the molecular level—has been staggering. In addition, new topics that were not covered in the second edition needed to be included. Therefore, we faced difficult decisions in determining both the content and the length of the book. As a general rule, we eliminated clinical material that is thoroughly covered in one of the many excellent textbooks of neonatology. However, there are 30 completely new chapters ranging in scope from apoptosis and angiogenesis to stem cells in development. In addition, almost all of the other chapters have been updated and extensively rewritten. As before, advancements in developmental physiology are discussed in the context of changing concepts in normal human physiology.

There are many people to whom we owe special thanks. First of all, we wish to express our gratitude to all the individuals who agreed to write chapters for the third edition. The quality of the chapters is outstanding, and we recognize the time and effort each of them required. We are also indebted to Heidi Kleinbart at the Children's Hospital of New York and to Ellen Ramsay at the Children's Hospital of Philadelphia for their organizational skills and editorial assistance. In addition, we offer our thanks to Jennifer Shreiner at Saunders for her tremendous help with the development and organization of the book. Finally, we want to thank our friend and senior editor Judy Fletcher, who was instrumental in the development of the third edition and served as the "irresistible force" that kept our textbook—the "immovable object"—on target for size and completion date.

Richard A. Polin
William W. Fox
Steven H. Abman

PREFACE TO THE FIRST EDITION

When I was young my teachers were the old.
I gave up fire for form till I was cold.
I suffered like a metal being cast.
I went to school to age to learn the past.

Now I am old my teachers are the young.
What can't be molded must be cracked and sprung.
I strain at lessons fit to start a suture.
I go to school to youth to learn the future.

ROBERT FROST

The first definitive treatise dealing with the care of the newborn infant dates back to the second century A.D. Considering its antiquity, it is startling that Soranus of Ephesus' work persisted as an acceptable way to treat newborn infants until relatively recent times. It is only during the last 100 years that physiologists have directed their attention to the fetus and newborn infant.

The reader of this work will soon appreciate that we have not attempted to reproduce another clinical textbook of neonatal/perinatal medicine. In contrast, we have tried to make our book appropriate for individuals interested in a "readable," in-depth presentation of fetal and neonatal developmental physiology. Clinical topics are presented only when discussion of disease pathophysiology seems appropriate. As can be appreciated from its size (28 sections, 190 chapters), we have tried to make the book both comprehensive and current. Most authors have focused their discussions on the developmental physiology of a single organ system. In addition, we have included several sections (e.g., Genetics and Embryology) that contain information relevant to the development of all body systems. Almost every chapter contains a detailed discussion of the "normal" adult physiology as well as a description of the physiologic differences that exist in the fetus and neonate. Where appropriate, the discussion is directed at biochemical, cellular, or molecular levels. The minor degree of chapter overlap that remains was done purposely so that the reader could obtain viewpoints on the same issue from individuals with different perspectives.

The progress made in fetal and neonatal medicine since the publication of Smith and Nelson's classic textbook, *the Physiology of the Newborn Infant*, has been astounding. At the time of the last edition (1976), infants weighing less than 750 gm rarely survived and most of the survivors demonstrated neurological deficits. Many centers did not even attempt to ventilate infants of that birth weight. Although the lipid composition of surfactant was relatively known at that time, effective artificial surfactant preparations were not available. In 1976, little was understood about the pathophysiology of diseases such as bronchopulmonary dysplasia, intraventricular hemorrhage, and necrotizing enterocolitis. Furthermore, drugs were not routinely available to treat apnea of prematurity or patency of the ductus arteriosus. The last edition of Smith and Nelson's book includes a quote from Dr. Clement Smith that appeared in the third edition: "The very passage of the normal infant through the valley of the shadow (of birth) is a striking example of the physiological resiliency of the newborn infant." Today, clinicians do not have to rely solely upon the inherent resiliency of the newborn infant. We have at our disposal new and better drugs to support the circulation, treat infection, and improve pulmonary function. Even the smallest neonates can be fed intravenously with dextrose and amino acid solutions that are tailored to their physiology and that produce little in the way of metabolic derangements. Technologic advancements in life support (extracorporeal membrane oxygenation and high-frequency ventilation) now allow us to keep infants alive who would previously not have survived. Despite these seeming "breakthroughs," fetal and neonatal medicine ought to be perceived as being in its infancy as a specialty. In the next 10 years, molecular biology techniques should have an enormous impact on the day-to-day practice of our subspecialties. Genetically engineered products are already being used to correct physiologic deficiencies associated with preterm birth, and gene transplantation has recently been used to correct an inborn error of metabolism. We hope this textbook will provide a clear understanding of the physiologic basis for these and future clinical and technologic advancements.

In keeping with the spirit of the poem quoted at the beginning of the preface, we expect this book will be used by both new and established investigators. Young investigators will find the text a comprehensive foundation upon which to formulate new questions. Established investigators will be able to learn not only about future directions of research in their field, but also about alternative approaches taken by other investigators interested in similar problems.

As with the preparation of any large textbook, there are many people who deserve special recognition. First of all, we would like to recognize the help of the section editors, who greatly assisted us in identifying authors considered to be at the "cutting edge" of their respective fields. We would also like to thank each of the chapter authors who expended an enormous amount of time and effort in the preparation of material for their sections. Next we would like to thank Carol Miller for her editorial assistance and help with the typing and re-typing of the manuscripts. We greatly appreciate the many individuals at the W.B. Saunders Company, without whom the project would not have come to fruition. We are especially indebted to Lisette Bralow, who oversaw production of the book from its inception, and Lawrence McGrew, for his advice, assistance, and considerable help in organizing each of the chapters. Lastly, we gratefully acknowledge the contributions of earlier authors (Barcroft, Smith, Dawes, Nelson, and others), for it was their efforts that served as a foundation for the subspecialty of neonatology and that first attracted us (and countless others) to enter the field.

Richard A. Polin
William W. Fox

CONTENTS

VOLUME 1

I

Genetics and Embryology   1

1 Basic Genetic Principles   1
Fred Levine

2 Molecular Genetics: Developmental and Clinical Implications   16
George A. Diaz and Kurt Hirschhorn

3 Basic Embryology   25
David L. Bolender and Stanley Kaplan

4 Regulation of Embryogenesis   41
Harold C. Slavkin and David Warburton

5 The Extracellular Matrix in Development   52
Peter Lloyd Jones

6 Stem Cell Biology   57
Evan Y. Snyder and Stephen Yip

7 Homeobox Genes   65
Heber C. Nielsen

8 Apoptosis and Necrosis   72
Huseyin Mehmet, Jacqueline Beesley, and A. David Edwards

9 Angiogenesis   79
Elisabeth A. Aron and Russell V. Anthony

II

Placenta and Intrauterine Environment   85

10 Placental Development   85
Peter Kaufmann and Hans-Georg Frank

11 Regulation of Placental Circulation   97
Charles R. Rosenfeld

12 Pathophysiology of Preterm Birth   103
Julian N. Robinson and Errol R. Norwitz

13 Mechanisms of Transfer Across the Human Placenta   111
Colin P. Sibley and Robert D. H. Boyd

14 Endocrine and Paracrine Function of the Human Placenta   122
Theresa M. Siler-Khodr

15 Fetal and Maternal Responses to Intrauterine Infection   131
Roberto Romero, Tinnakorn Chaiworapongsa, and Maria-Teresa Gervasi

16 Maternal Cardiovascular Disease and Fetal Growth and Development   142
Douglas A. Woelkers

17 Fetal Origins of Adult Disease   160
David J. P. Barker

18 Physiologic Effects of Multiple Pregnancy on Mother and Fetus   165
Jane Cleary-Goldman and Mary E. D'Alton

III

Developmental Pharmacology and Pharmacokinetics   179

19 Basic Pharmacologic Principles   179
Sylvain Chemtob

20 Basic Pharmacokinetic Principles   190
Ralph A. Lugo and Robert M. Ward

21 Physicochemical and Structural Properties Regulating
Placental Drug Transfer 197
Sabine Luise Plonait and Heinz Nau

22 Pharmacogenetics 211
Denis M. Grant

23 Drug Distribution in Fetal Life 218
Marianne Garland

24 Developmental Pharmacology of Adrenergic
Agents 227
James F. Padbury and Robert A. Berg

25 Maternal Drug Abuse: Effects on Fetus
and Neonate 234
Ernest A. Kopecky and Gideon Koren

26 Drug Excretion During Lactation 249
Michael J. Rieder

IV

Intrauterine and Postnatal Growth 259

27 Circulatory and Metabolic Changes Accompanying
Fetal Growth Restriction 259
Frederick C. Battaglia

28 Endocrine Factors Affecting Neonatal Growth 266
Dennis M. Styne

29 Human Milk Composition and Function
in the Infant 275
Margit Hamosh

30 Physiology of Lactation 284
Margaret C. Neville and James McManaman

31 Nutritional Assessment 291
Gilberto R. Pereira

V

Perinatal Iron, Mineral, and Vitamin Metabolism 303

32 Calcium-Regulating Hormones 303
Jorge A. Prada

33 Calcium, Phosphorus, and Magnesium Transport
Across the Placenta 314
Shahid M. Husain, M. Zulficar Mughal, and Reginald C. Tsang

34 Neonatal Calcium, Phosphorus, and Magnesium
Homeostasis 323
Ran Namgung and Reginald C. Tsang

35 Zinc in the Fetus and Neonate 342
K. Michael Hambidge and Nancy F. Krebs

36 Vitamin A Metabolism in the Fetus and Neonate 347
Jayant P. Shenai

37 Vitamin E Nutrition in the Fetus and Newborn 353
Lois H. Johnson

38 Vitamin K Metabolism in the Fetus and Neonate 369
Reidar Wallin and Susan M. Hutson

VI

Lipid Metabolism 375

39 Maternal-Fetal Transfer of Lipid Metabolites 375
Emilio Herrera and Miguel Angel Lasunción

40 Accretion of Lipid in the Fetus and Newborn 388
*John E. Van Aerde, Michaelann S. Wilke, Miguel Feldman,
and M. Thomas Clandinin*

41 Brown Adipose Tissue: Development
and Function 404
Jan Nedergaard and Barbara Cannon

42 Lipids as an Energy Source for the Premature
and Full-Term Neonate 415
Guy Putet

43 Ketone Body Production and Metabolism in the Fetus
and Neonate 419
Dermot H. Williamson and Paul S. Thornton

44 Long Chain Fatty Acids in the Developing Retina
and Brain 429
Socheata Un and Susan E. Carlson

45 Lipoprotein Metabolism and Nutritional Programming
in the Fetus and Neonate 440
Glen E. Mott

VII

Carbohydrate Metabolism 449

46 Metabolism of Glucose and Methods of Investigation
in the Fetus and Newborn 449
Satish C. Kalhan

47 Carbohydrate Metabolism During Pregnancy 464
Edward S. Ogata

48 Oxygen Consumption and General Carbohydrate Metabolism in the Fetus 465
Anthony F. Philipps

49 Role of Glucoregulatory Hormones in Hepatic Glucose Metabolism During the Perinatal Period 478
Richard M. Cowett

50 Cell Glucose Transport and Glucose Handling During Fetal and Neonatal Development 487
Rebecca A. Simmons

51 Pathophysiology of Hypoglycemia 494
Charles A. Stanley and Neil Caplin

VIII

Protein Metabolism 501

52 General Concepts of Protein Metabolism 501
Dwight E. Matthews and Johannes B. van Goudoever

53 Fetal Requirements and Placental Transfer of Nitrogenous Compounds 509
William W. Hay, Jr., and Timothy R. H. Regnault

54 Protein and Amino Acid Metabolism and Requirements 527
William C. Heird and Sudha Kashyap

IX

Thermoregulation 541

55 Perinatal Thermal Physiology 541
Gordon G. Power, Arlin B. Blood, and Christian J. Hunter

56 Temperature Control in Newborn Infants 548
Rakesh Sahni and Karl Schulze

57 Physics and Physiology of Human Neonatal Incubation 570
Gunnar Sedin

58 Responses of the Fetus and Neonate to Hypothermia 582
Alistair J. Gunn and Laura Bennet

X

Skin 589

59 Structure and Development of the Skin and Cutaneous Appendages 589
David H. Chu and Cynthia A. Loomis

60 Physiologic Development of the Skin 597
Steven B. Hoath

XI

Fetal and Neonatal Cardiovascular Physiology 613

61 Development of the Fetal Heart 613
Margaret L. Kirby

62 Molecular Determinants of Embryonic Vascular Development 621
H. Scott Baldwin and Justin C. Grindley

63 Cardiovascular Function During Development and the Response to Hypoxia 635
Page A. W. Anderson, Charles S. Kleinman, George Lister, and Norman S. Talner

64 Developmental Electrophysiology in the Fetus and Neonate 669
Arthur S. Pickoff

65 Developmental Biology of the Pulmonary Vasculature 690
Marlene Rabinovitch

66 Development of the Gastrointestinal Circulation in the Fetus and Newborn 701
David A. Clark and Upender K. Munshi

67 Physiology of Congenital Heart Disease in the Neonate 705
Thomas J. Kulik

68 Neural Regulation of Blood Pressure During Fetal and Newborn Life 717
Jeffrey L. Segar

69 Programming of the Fetal Circulation 727
Lucy R. Green and Mark A. Hanson

70 Physiology of Nitric Oxide in the Developing
Lung 733
John P. Kinsella and Philip W. Shaul

71 Mechanisms Regulating Closure of the Ductus
Arteriosus 743
Ronald I. Clyman

72 Regulation of Umbilical Blood Flow 748
S. Lee Adamson, Leslie Myatt, and Bridgette M. P. Byrne

73 Fetal and Placental Circulation During Labor 758
Karel Maršál

74 Physiology of Resuscitation 765
Ola Didrik Saugstad

75 Pathophysiology of Shock in the Fetus
and Neonate 772
Shahab Noori, Philippe S. Friedlich, and Istvan Seri

XII

The Lung 783

76 Normal and Abnormal Structural Development
of the Lung 783
Susan E. Wert

77 Regulation of Alveolarization 794
Jeanne M. Snyder

78 Physiologic Mechanisms of Normal and Altered
Lung Growth 802
Richard Harding and Stuart B. Hooper

79 Molecular Mechanisms of Lung Development
and Lung Branching Morphogenesis 812
Minke van Tuyl and Martin Post

80 Regulation of Liquid Secretion and Absorption
by the Fetal and Neonatal Lung 822
Pierre M. Barker and Kevin W. Southern

81 Upper Airway Structure: Function, Regulation,
and Development 834
Thomas H. Shaffer and Marla R. Wolfson

82 Regulation of Lower Airway Function 842
Richard J. Martin and Musa A. Haxhiu

83 Functional Development of Respiratory Muscles 848
Gary C. Sieck, Carlos B. Mantilla, and Mohamed A. Fahim

84 Mechanics of Breathing 864
Jacopo P. Mortola

85 Pulmonary Gas Exchange in the Developing Lung 870
William Edward Truog

86 Oxygen Transport and Delivery 880
Maria Delivoria-Papadopoulos and Jane E. McGowan

87 Control of Breathing in Fetal Life and Onset
and Control of Breathing in the Neonate 890
Henrique Rigatto

88 Basic Mechanisms of Oxygen-Sensing and Response
to Hypoxia 900
Dan Zhou and Gabriel G. Haddad

89 Pathophysiology of Apnea of Prematurity 905
Martha J. Miller and Richard J. Martin

90 Evaluation of Pulmonary Function in the
Neonate 919
Soraya Abbasi, Emidio M. Sivieri, and Vinod K. Bhutani

91 Pathophysiology of Hyaline Membrane Disease
(Excluding Surfactant) 926
Robert B. Cotton

92 Mechanisms of Neonatal Lung Injury 934
Richard L. Auten, Jr.

93 Impaired Lung Growth After Injury in Premature
Lung 942
Kurt H. Albertine and Theodore J. Pysher

94 Antenatal Factors That Influence Postnatal Lung
Development and Injury 949
Alan H. Jobe and Suhas Kallapur

95 Pathophysiology of Chronic Lung Disease 954
Eduardo Bancalari

96 Assisted Ventilation: Physiologic Implications
and Complications 961
*Jay S. Greenspan, Thomas H. Shaffer, William W. Fox,
and Alan R. Spitzer*

97 High-Frequency Ventilation 979
David J. Durand and Jeanette M. Asselin

98 Liquid Ventilation 985
Thomas H. Shaffer and Marla R. Wolfson

Index   i

VOLUME 2

XIII

Surfactant 1003

99 Historical Perspective 1003
Mary Ellen Avery

100 Composition of Pulmonary Surfactant Lipids and Proteins 1005
Jeffrey A. Whitsett

101 Physicochemical Aspects of Pulmonary Surfactant 1014
Fred Possmayer

102 Structure of Alveolar Epithelial Cells and the Surface Layer During Development 1034
Scott H. Randell and Steven L. Young

103 Regulation of Surfactant-Associated Phospholipid Synthesis and Secretion 1041
Seamus A. Rooney

104 Pathophysiology of Respiratory Distress Syndrome and Surfactant Metabolism 1055
Alan H. Jobe and Machiko Ikegami

105 Hormonal Therapy for Prevention of Respiratory Distress Syndrome 1069
Ian Gross and Philip L. Ballard

106 Surfactant Treatment 1074
Alan H. Jobe

107 Genetics and Physiology of Surfactant Protein Deficiencies 1085
Lawrence M. Nogee

XIV

Physiology of the Gastrointestinal Tract in the Fetus and Neonate 1095

108 Trophic Factors and Regulation of Gastrointestinal Tract and Liver Development 1095
Douglas G. Burrin

109 Organogenesis of the Gastrointestinal Tract 1101
Arthur J. Ross III

110 Development of the Enteric Nervous System 1110
Delma L. Broussard and Steven M. Altschuler

111 Development of Gastric Secretory Function 1117
Chris J. Dickinson

112 Gastrointestinal Motility 1125
Taher I. Omari and Colin D. Rudolph

113 Fetal and Neonatal Intestinal Motility 1139
Douglas G. Field and A. Craig Hillemeier

114 Development of the Exocrine Pancreas 1142
Steven L. Werlin and P. C. Lee

115 Digestion-Absorption Functions in Fetuses, Infants, and Children 1151
Otakar Koldovský and Carol Lynn Berseth

116 Pathophysiology of Gastroesophageal Reflux 1163
Joshua R. Friedman and Chris A. Liacouras

117 Pathophysiology and Prevention of Neonatal Necrotizing Enterocolitis 1169
Michael S. Caplan

XV

Liver and Bilirubin Metabolism 1175

118 Organogenesis and Histologic Development of the Liver 1175
Steven Lobritto

119 Bile Acid Metabolism During Development 1179
John C. Bucuvalas and Kenneth Setchell

120 Bile Formation and Cholestasis 1186
David A. Horst and Saul J. Karpen

121 Bilirubin Metabolism and Toxicity in the Newborn 1199
William J. Cashore

122 Mechanisms of Action of Phototherapy 1205
John F. Ennever

123 Pathophysiology of Metabolic Disease of the Liver 1211
James B. Gibson and Gerard T. Berry

124 Neonatal Cholestasis: Pathophysiology, Etiology, and Treatment 1218
Michael R. Narkewicz

XVI

The Kidney 1223

125 Embryogenesis and Anatomic Development of the Kidney 1223
William E. Sweeney, Jr., and Ellis D. Avner

126 Functional Development of the Kidney *In Utero* 1229
Patrick D. Brophy and Jean E. Robillard

127 Postnatal Maturation of Renal Blood Flow 1242
Michael J. Solhaug and Pedro A. Jose

128 Development of the Renin-Angiotensin System 1249
Victoria F. Norwood, Lucas G. Fernandez, Alda Tufro, and R. Ariel Gomez

129 Postnatal Development of Glomerular Filtration Rate 1256
Jean-Pierre Guignard

130 Renal Transport of Sodium During Early Development 1267
Leonard G. Feld and Howard E. Corey

131 Potassium Homeostasis in the Fetus and Neonate 1279
Corinne Benchimol and Lisa M. Satlin

132 Role of the Kidney in Calcium and Phosphorus Homeostasis 1286
Robert P. Woroniecki, Susan E. Mulroney, Aviad Haramati, Adrian Spitzer, and Frederick J. Kaskel

133 Transport of Amino Acids During Early Development 1294
Aaron L. Friedman

134 Developmental Aspects of Organic Acid Transport 1299
Deborah P. Jones and F. Bruder Stapleton

135 Concentration and Dilution of the Urine 1303
Michael A. Linshaw

136 Urinary Acidification 1327
Eileen D. Brewer

137 Response to Nephron Loss in Early Development 1330
Robert L. Chevalier

138 Pathophysiology of Acute Renal Failure in the Neonatal Period 1335
Tracy E. Hunley and Valentina Kon

XVII

Fluid and Electrolyte Metabolism 1341

139 Fluid Distribution in the Fetus and Neonate 1341
Robert A. Brace

140 Fetal and Neonatal Body Water Compartment Volumes with Reference to Growth and Development 1351
John M. Lorenz

141 Pathophysiology of Edema 1357
David P. Carlton

142 Regulation of Acid-Base Balance in the Fetus and Neonate 1361
Philippe S. Friedlich and Istvan Seri

XVIII

Developmental Hematopoiesis 1365

143 Biology of Stem Cells and Stem Cell Transplantation 1365
Mervin C. Yoder

144 Developmental Biology of the Hematopoietic Growth Factors 1374
Mervin C. Yoder and Kurt R. Schibler

145 Developmental Granulocytopoiesis 1388
Akhil Maheshwari and Robert D. Christensen

146 Developmental Erythropoiesis 1397
Robin K. Ohls

147 Developmental Megakaryocytopoiesis in Fetal and Neonatal Physiology 1421
Thomas A. Olson

XIX

Hemostasis 1435

148 Developmental Hemostasis 1435
Paul Monagle and J. Nathan Hagstrom

149 Pathophysiology of Bleeding Disorders in the
Newborn 1447
J. Nathan Hagstrom

150 Pathophysiology of Neonatal Disseminated
Intravascular Coagulation and Thrombosis 1460
Marilyn J. Manco-Johnson

XX

Developmental Immunobiology 1475

151 Host Defense Mechanisms Against Bacteria 1475
Timothy R. La Pine and Harry R. Hill

152 Host Defense Mechanisms Against Fungi 1487
László Maródi and Richard B. Johnston, Jr.

153 Host Defense Mechanisms Against Viruses 1490
David B. Lewis

154 T-Cell Development 1512
Marcia McDuffie and Anthony R. Hayward

155 B-Cell Development 1518
*James E. Crowe, Jr., Joern-Hendrik Weitkamp,
and John V. Williams*

156 Mononuclear Phagocyte System 1523
Kurt R. Schibler

157 Neonatal Neutrophil Normal and Abnormal
Physiology 1538
*Elvira Parravicini, Carmella van de Ven,
and Mitchell S. Cairo*

158 The Complement System of the Fetus and
Neonate 1549
Jerry A. Winkelstein

159 Cytokines and Inflammatory Response in the Fetus
and Neonate 1555
Laurie Kilpatrick and Mary Catherine Harris

160 Integrins and Cell Adhesion Molecules 1572
M. Michele Mariscalco

161 Stimulus-Response Coupling in Phagocytic
Cells 1591
Helen M. Korchak

162 Fetal Wound Healing 1604
N. Scott Adzick

163 Immunology of Human Milk and Host
Immunity 1610
Sadhana Chheda, Susan E. Keeney, and Armond S. Goldman

164 Neonatal Pulmonary Host Defense Mechanisms 1620
Andrew Metinko

XXI

Neurology 1675

165 Development of the Nervous System 1675
Scott L. Pomeroy and Nicole J. Ullrich

166 Development of the Blood-Brain Barrier 1699
John Laterra and Gary W. Goldstein

167 Development of Neurotransmitters 1706
Michael V. Johnston and Faye S. Silverstein

168 Perinatal Brain Metabolism 1713
Robert C. Vannucci and Susan J. Vannucci

169 Electroencephalography in the Premature and
Full-Term Infant 1726
Robert Ryan Clancy

170 Cerebral Blood Flow in Premature Infants:
Regulation, Measurement, and Pathophysiology
of Intraventricular Hemorrhage 1745
Jeffrey M. Perlman

171 Pathophysiology of Intraventricular Hemorrhage
in the Neonate 1757
Terrie E. Inder and Joseph J. Volpe

172 Pathophysiology of Neural Tube Defects 1772
*Enrico Danzer, Natalie E. Rintoul,
Timothy M. Crombleholme, and N. Scott Adzick*

173 Trophic Factor and Nutritional and Hormonal
Regulation of Brain Development 1785
Jeanette Pleasure and David Pleasure

174 Development of Pain Sensation 1792
Margaret A. Myers

XXII

Special Sensory Systems in the Fetus and Neonate 1797

175 Retinal Development and the Pathophysiology of Retinopathy of Prematurity 1797
Graham E. Quinn

176 Early Development of the Human Auditory System 1803
Lynne A. Werner

177 Development of Taste and Smell in the Neonate 1819
Beverly J. Cowart, Gary K. Beauchamp, and Julie A. Mennella

XXIII

Orthopedics 1829

178 The Growth Plate: Embryologic Origin, Structure, and Function 1829
Bulent Erol, Kathrin V. Halpern, and John P. Dormans

179 Common Musculoskeletal Conditions Related to Intrauterine Compression: Effects of Mechanics on Endochondral Ossification 1838
Kathrin V. Halpern, Bulent Erol, and John P. Dormans

180 Defective Limb Embryology 1844
Walid K. Yassir, Benjamin A. Alman, and Michael J. Goldberg

181 Ontogenesis of Striated Muscle 1849
Harvey B. Sarnat

XXIV

Endocrine Function 1871

PITUITARY

182 Hypothalamus: Neuroendometabolic Center 1871
Adda Grimberg and Jessica Katz Kutikov

183 Growth Factor Regulation of Fetal Growth 1880
Diva D. De León, Pinchas Cohen, and Lorraine E. Levitt Katz

184 Growth Hormone and Prolactin 1891
P. D. Gluckman and C. S. Pinal

185 Luteinizing Hormone and Follicle-Stimulating Hormone Secretion in the Fetus and Newborn Infant 1896
Leona Cuttler and Mark R. Palmert

186 Development of the Corticotropin-Releasing Hormone–Corticotropin/β-Endorphin System in the Mammalian Fetus 1907
James C. Rose, Jeffrey Schwartz, and Sharla Young

ADRENAL

187 Fetal and Neonatal Adrenocortical Physiology 1915
Jeremy S. D. Winter

THYROID

188 Fetal and Neonatal Thyroid Physiology 1926
Daniel H. Polk and Delbert A. Fisher

XXV

Ovary and Testis 1935

189 Genetics of Sex Determination and Differentiation 1935
Robert P. Erickson and Stan R. Blecher

190 Differentiation of the Ovary 1941
Anne Grete Byskov and Lars Grabow Westergaard

191 Testicular Development 1950
Ahmet R. Aslan, Barry A. Kogan, and Bernard Gondos

192 Testicular Descent 1956
Ahmet R. Aslan and Barry A. Kogan

Index   i

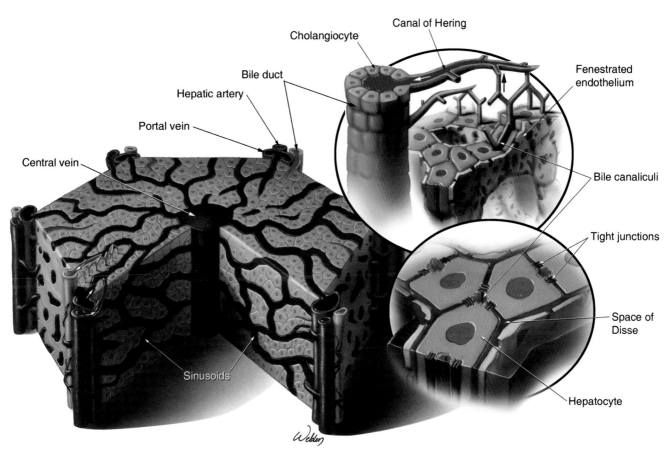

Canal of Hering

Cholangiocyte

Bile duct

Hepatic artery

Portal vein

Central vein

Fenestrated
endothelium

Bile canaliculi

Tight junctions

Space of
Disse

Sinusoids

Hepatocyte

Weldon

Figure 120–1

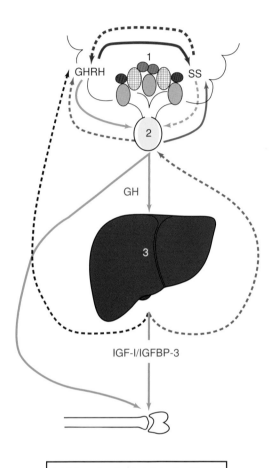

GHRH   1   SS

2

GH

3

IGF-I/IGFBP-3

Inhibitory feedback (all dashed lines)

Stimulatory feedback (all solid lines)

Ultrashort feedback

Short feedback

Long feedback

Primary hormonal action

Figure 182–2

Surfactant

Mary Ellen Avery

Historical Perspective

In 1929, a Swiss physician, Kurt von Neergaard,[1] wrote, "New notions on a fundamental principle of respiratory mechanics: the retractile force of the lung, dependent on the surface tension in the alveoli." He speculated that atelectasis of the newborn could result from "considerable retractive force of surface tension in the lungs." He carried out experiments demonstrating that an excised lung inflated with air had considerably greater transpulmonary pressure than the same lung extended to the same volume with liquid.[1] That simple, straightforward experiment was reproduced independently in the 1950s by Mead and associates[2] at the Harvard School of Public Health. The stage was set for understanding which physical and chemical forces were involved in incurring the unique properties of the alveolar lining layer, namely, the ability to augment elastic recoil of the lung at large lung volumes and the ability to reduce surface tension and stabilize air-filled spaces arranged in parallel at low lung volumes (and thus to act as an antiatelectasis factor).[2]

In the late 1940s, George Anderson and Peter Gruenwald,[3, 4] both pathologists at Johns Hopkins University, studied lungs at autopsy and commented on the airless state that was seen. They described the lungs as "liver-like" and, in the case of Gruenwald, noted that the lungs could be expanded with liquid without significant change, but when they were expanded with air, they achieved a "Swiss cheese pattern" of overdistended air spaces and atelectasis.[3, 4] I had the privilege as a medical student and, later, as a resident of hearing from both these pathologists, and I realized how very important was the contribution of pathologists in stimulating clinicians to relate the baby's clinical course to the findings at autopsy. It was not until the early 1950s that Herbert Miller[5] at Yale University, and Blystad and associates[6] in Boston, described the clinical correlations of elevated respiratory rates and retractions that small premature infants showed before their demise from atelectasis with hyaline membranes. It was Herbert Miller[5] who first said that membranes could not result from the aspiration of amniotic fluid, as had been previously surmised, because they were not seen in babies who died in the first hours of life but took time after birth to develop. Gitlin and Craig,[7] working in Boston, demonstrated the fibrin content of the membranes and deduced that the proteinaceous material had to have come from the circulation.

Totally independently of these clinical and pathologic observations, the respiratory physiologists at the Harvard School of Public Health were repeating von Neergaard's experiments and were making estimates of lung surface areas on the basis of an assumed surface tension of 50 dyne/cm (the equivalent of serum). The results of those calculations revealed the estimated areas to be one-tenth of that estimated by histologists, and it was clear that there had to be a better explanation for the differences.[8]

The better explanation came from an unlikely source, the Chemical Defense Establishment in Porton, England, where Pattle[9] was assigned. Pattle[9] had been stationed there to study the role of antifoam agents in the prevention of pulmonary edema induced by certain war gases. He needed a measure of bubble stability and expressed bubbles from the lung into a drop of saline to measure their life span. He noted that bubbles expressed from the lung seemed to have a much longer life span than bubbles from serum, from other tissues, or even from ordinary detergents. He wrote a description of his findings in a now famous article entitled "Properties, Function, and Origin of the Alveolar Lining Layer," published in the *Proceedings of the Royal Society of London* in 1958.[10] He had noted that bubbles expressed from the lungs of fetal guinea pigs did not have the stability of those found in term mammalian lungs and then suggested that one of the difficulties with which a premature baby has to contend is the increased surface forces in the immature lung.

The turning point in all this was the work of John Clements,[11] who was working at the Army Chemical Center in Edgewood, Maryland. Clements proceeded to measure surface tension in a somewhat more sophisticated way with a Wilhelmy balance that allowed him to ascertain the changes of surface tension with surface area. It was Christmas 1957, when I drove to Edgewood and visited Clements. I saw the surface balance, returned to Boston, and decided to explore the reason that lungs of infants who died of hyaline membrane disease never had foam in their airways. It is obvious that the reason they lacked foam was that they did not have surfactants with the capacity to reduce surface tension when surface area was reduced. It was straightforward to demonstrate the deficiency in surfactants on a surface film balance modeled after that of Clements. The following is a quotation from the publication I co-wrote with Mead[12]:

"Low surface tension in the lining of the lung permits stability of the alveoli at end-expiration. Lacking such a material, the lung is predisposed to atelectasis. Measurements of the surface tension of lung extracts confirm the presence of a very surface-active substance in lungs of infants over 1,000–2,000 gm and in children and adults. In lung extracts of immature infants and infants dying with hyaline membrane disease, surface tension is higher than expected. This deficiency of surface-active material may be significant in the pathogenesis of hyaline membrane disease."

Meanwhile, Sue Buckingham joined me,[13] with the idea that the alveolar Type II cells could be the source of production of surface-active lipids, because these cells contained osmiophilic lamellar inclusions. She showed a temporal correspondence in mice between the appearance of the osmiophilic bodies and the capacity of lung extracts to lower surface tension. Many studies since then support the concept that the osmiophilic or lamellar bodies are sites of storage for the phospholipids, which are attached to apoproteins that facilitate secretion and spreading on the alveolar surface.

The subsequent years were characterized by work from many laboratories, analyzing the lipid composition of materials expressed from the lung. The finding that lung lipid could be identified in amniotic fluid suggested to Gluck and Kulovich[14] that sampling amniotic fluid in the last trimester of pregnancy may allow ascertainment of the maturity of the lung. The use of the lecithin/sphingomyelin ratio led to the important and clinically useful test to guide obstetricians in the likelihood of an infant's being born with or without adequate quantities of pulmonary surfactants. That same year, 1973, Richard King and colleagues[15] identified a surfactant-specific protein, which subsequently led to extensive exploration of the three or more proteins that are associated with lipids and can be recovered from lung lavage liquid.

As of early 1995, four surfactant-associated proteins had been discovered and fully defined by identification of their respective genes. Surfactant protein A (SP-A) is hydrophilic and extensively modified after translation. SP-B is hydrophobic and has been found deficient in congenital alveolar proteinosis. SP-C, the smallest of the peptides, has a covalent linkage with the phospholipids and enhances their uptake by the alveolar Type II cells. SP-D resembles SP-A and serves as an opsonin to enhance uptake of bacteria and viruses by macrophages. The sites of synthesis, methods of degradation, and aspects of hormonal regulation have been explored and reviewed extensively.[16-18]

SURFACTANT REPLACEMENT

Glucocorticoids play an essential role in both lung maturation and the synthesis of lipid and protein components of pulmonary surfactants.[19, 20] Knowledge of hormonal influences in the timing of organ maturation began with the observations of Moog,[21] who in 1953 described the influence of the pituitary-adrenal system on the differentiation of phosphatase in the duodenum of the suckling mouse. Extensive experience with the use of antenatal glucocorticoids to accelerate lung maturation followed the pioneering observations of Liggins,[22] who in 1969 noted the survival at a younger age of premature lambs of ewes that had received glucocorticoids before delivery. Many controlled clinical trials, which were reviewed in 1990 by Crowley and co-workers,[23] established both the safety and the efficacy of antenatal corticosteroids. It appears that the effects of the combined use of prenatal corticosteroids and postnatal surfactant replacement are additive. It is as if the steroids "condition" the lung by increasing the surface area over which the surfactants, which are instilled as a liquid into the trachea, can spread and exert their effects.

A new chapter in the history of surfactant discovery was heralded when Fujiwara[24] presented his initial experience in an article in *Lancet* in 1980. He and others, notably Forrest Adams in Los Angeles and Goran Enhorning in Toronto,[25, 26] had spent the previous decade analyzing various mixtures of phospholipids in animal models and then testing them *in vitro*. They finally decided that mixtures composed only of phospholipids would not have the requisite surface properties to stabilize airways effectively. Fujiwara decided to use artificial surfactant (material derived from minced cow lungs), which consisted of lipids and lipid-associated proteins. He enriched the material with added dipalmitoylphosphatidylcholine (DPPC) and called it TA surfactant, after Tokyo, where the pharmaceutical house was located, and Akita, where he was working at the time.

Fujiwara's experience was distinguished from that of many investigators who attempted to treat surfactant-deficiency states with aerosolized DPPC; he used natural surfactants from cow lungs, and he instilled them as a liquid into the trachea and

enhanced distribution by changing the position of the infant from one side to the other. After the instillation of 3 to 5 mL of material, he could demonstrate distribution in all the lobes of the lung and, impressively, a prompt increase in oxygenation. Thus, it was evident that the material was distributed to the gas-exchanging surfaces of the lungs because it resulted in a prompt and sustained improvement in oxygenation. Fujiwara demonstrated that, in some infants, a single instillation in the first hour of life or after the establishment of hyaline membrane disease could produce improved oxygenation that persisted for 2 to 3 days, which was long enough for the baby to acquire the capacity to synthesize endogenous surfactant.

These observations were not immediately acclaimed because the experience was not a prospective, randomized, controlled one. Nevertheless, many investigators in various parts of the world in the mid-1980s were encouraged to conduct prospective, randomized, controlled trials, not only with TA surfactant but also with other mixtures of materials, mostly those derived from calf lung lavage. Other sources of surfactant have included human amniotic fluid, as evaluated by Merritt and colleagues,[27] and porcine lung extracts, which were studied by Robertson and others[28] in Europe. Meanwhile, TA surfactant was licensed in Japan in 1988 and is widely used. Other preparations, including a totally synthetic mixture known as Exosurf, are licensed in the United States. Exosurf was invented by John Clements, who proposed that an alcohol (hexadecanol) be added to the principal phospholipid in pulmonary surfactant, DPPC. He also added tyloxapol to facilitate dispersion.

The natural surfactants from bovine or porcine sources have been used extensively. Short-term benefits are evident with early administration, and continuing evaluation is under way to assess long-term benefits and safety.

Thus, in the years from identification of a deficiency of surfactants in the lungs of infants who died of hyaline membrane disease, to clinical trials, and now to the wide availability of natural and synthetic surfactants for treatment, the odyssey from bench to bedside to pharmacy has been accomplished.

REFERENCES

1. von Neergaard K: Neue Auffassungen uber einen Grundbergriff der Atemmechanik: die Retraktion-skraft der Lunge, abhangig von der Oberflachenspannung in den Alveolen. Z Gesamte Exp Med 66:373, 1929.
2. Mead J, et al: Surface tension as a factor in pulmonary volume-pressure hysteresis. J Appl Physiol 10:191, 1957.
3. Gruenwald P: Surface tension as a factor in the resistance of neonatal lungs to aeration. Am J Obstet Gynecol 53:996, 1947.
4. Tra-Dinh-De, Anderson G: Hyaline-like membranes associated with diseases of the newborn lungs: a review of the literature. Obstet Gynecol Surv 8:1, 1953.
5. Miller HC, Hamilton TR: The pathogenesis of the "vernix membrane": relation to aspiration pneumonia in stillborn and newborn infants. Pediatrics 3:735, 1949.
6. Blystad W, et al: Pulmonary hyaline membranes in newborn infants. Pediatrics 8:5, 1951.
7. Gitlin D, Craig JM: The nature of the hyaline membrane in asphyxia of the newborn. Pediatrics 17:64, 1956.
8. Radford EP: Recent studies of mechanical properties of mammalian lungs. *In* Remington JW (ed): Tissue Elasticity. Washington, DC, American Physiological Society, 1957.
9. Pattle RE: Properties, function and origin of the alveolar lining layer. Nature 175:1125, 1955.
10. Pattle RE: Properties, function and origin of the alveolar lining layer. Proc R Soc Lond 148:217, 1958.
11. Clements JA, et al: Pulmonary surface tension and the mucous lining of the lungs: some theoretical considerations. J Appl Physiol 12:262, 1958.
12. Avery ME, Mead J: Surface properties in relation to atelectasis and hyaline membrane disease. Am J Dis Child 97:517, 1959.
13. Buckingham S, Avery ME: The time of appearance of lung surfactant in the fetal mouse. Nature 193:688, 1962.
14. Gluck L, Kulovich MV: Lecithin/sphingomyelin ratios in amniotic fluid in normal and abnormal pregnancy. Am J Obstet Gynecol 115:539, 1973.
15. King RJ, et al: Isolation of apoproteins from canine surface active material. Am J Physiol 224:788, 1973.
16. Wright JR, Clements JA: Metabolism and turnover of lung surfactant: state of the art. Am Rev Respir Dis 136:426, 1987.

17. VanGolde LMG, et al: The pulmonary surfactant system: biochemical aspects and functional significance. Physiol Rev *68*:374, 1988.
18. Jobe A, Ikegami M: Surfactant for the treatment of respiratory distress syndrome: state of the art. Am Rev Respir Dis *136*:1256, 1987.
19. Jobe AH, et al: Beneficial effects of the combined use of prenatal corticosteroids and postnatal surfactant on preterm infants. Am J Obstet Gynecol *168*:508, 1993.
20. Avery ME: Historical overview of antenatal steroid use. Pediatrics *85*:133, 1995.
21. Moog F: The influence of the pituitary-adrenal system on the differentiation of phosphatase in the duodenum of the suckling mouse. J Exp Zool *124*:329, 1953.
22. Liggins GC: Premature delivery of foetal lambs infused with glucocorticoids. J Endocrinol *45*:515, 1969.
23. Crowley P, et al: The effects of corticosteroid administration before preterm delivery: an overview of the evidence from controlled trials. Br J Obstet Gynaecol *97*:11, 1990.
24. Fujiwara T, et al: Artificial surfactant therapy in hyaline membrane disease. Lancet *1*:55, 1980.
25. Adams FH, Enhorning G: Surface properties of lung extracts. I. A dynamic alveolar model. Acta Physiol Scand *68*:23, 1966.
26. Enhorning G: Pulsating bubble technique for evaluating pulmonary surfactant. J Appl Physiol *43*:198, 1977.
27. Merritt TA, et al: Randomized, placebo-controlled trial of human surfactant given at birth versus rescue administration in very low birth weight infants with lung immaturity. J Pediatr *118*:581, 1991.
28. Collaborative European Multicenter Study Group: A two year follow-up of the babies enrolled in a European multicenter trial of porcine surfactant replacement for severe neonatal respiratory distress syndrome. Eur J Pediatr *151*:372, 1992.

Jeffrey A. Whitsett

Composition of Pulmonary Surfactant Lipids and Proteins

In vertebrates, adaptation to a nonaqueous respiratory environment was achieved by the development of lungs, which provide an extensive surface area for gas exchange. The unique physicochemical boundary between respiratory gases and the respiratory epithelium creates a region of high surface tension generated by the unequal distribution of molecular forces on water molecules at the air-liquid interface. Unopposed, this surface tension creates collapsing forces that cause atelectasis and respiratory failure. Pulmonary surfactant creates a lipid layer separating alveolar gas from the aqueous phase, decreasing these surface forces. It is not surprising that pulmonary surfactant is found in all air-breathing vertebrates studied, including animals as phylogenetically divergent as the lung fish and humans. Synthesis and secretion of an abundance of phospholipid-rich material accompany the maturation of lung before birth in the human. The lack of pulmonary surfactant in premature infants results in respiratory distress syndrome (RDS) after birth. Likewise, loss of surfactant function related to lung injury causes acute respiratory failure postnatally. The structure and function of the surfactant complex have important implications for treatment of RDS and other pulmonary diseases. This chapter considers the phospholipid and protein components that play critical roles in surfactant function and pulmonary homeostasis.

FORMS OF PULMONARY SURFACTANT

Pulmonary surfactant is composed primarily of phospholipids, but it also contains proteins and carbohydrates. These components are present in distinct macromolecular aggregates whose structural forms are likely conferred by the relative abundance of proteins and phospholipids, as well as by the impact of mechanical forces on the surfactant material accompanying the respiratory cycle. Tubular myelin is a highly surface-active material sedimenting at relatively low gravitational forces and consists primarily of phospholipids and proteins (Fig. 100-1). Various lamellar and vesicular forms of surfactant that lack the highly organized structures of tubular myelin can also be isolated from the lung. Although the forms of surfactant may be influenced by procedures designed to isolate or identify them (and thus represent artifactual structures), it is likely that these diverse structures are generated *in vivo* and play distinct roles in surfactant function and homeostasis.

LIFE CYCLE OF PULMONARY SURFACTANT

Surfactant lipids and proteins are synthesized, stored, and secreted by Type II alveolar epithelial cells (Fig. 100-2). Surfactant lipids and proteins are routed through the endoplasmic reticulum, Golgi apparatus, and multivesicular bodies before storage in lamellar bodies. Lamellar bodies are secreted into the air space in response to stretch, as well as various secretagogues, including purinoreceptor and adrenergic agonists. As lamellar bodies unravel in the air space, tubular myelin is formed under the influence of extracellular calcium ions, surfactant proteins A and B (SP-A and SP-B). Tubular myelin is an abundant, large aggregate form of surfactant, likely serving as a reservoir from which surfactant monolayers or multilayers are generated at the alveolar surface. Rapid spreading and stability of these lipid films are determined by the influence of SP-B and SP-C, which serve to maintain phospholipids at the air-liquid interface, thereby reducing surface tension. Small vesicular forms, likely produced by the molecular forces produced during compression and decompression of surfactant during the respiratory cycle, are taken up by Type II cells and are either reused or catabolized. A fraction of surfactant is taken up by alveolar macrophages and is degraded in a process requiring signaling via granulocyte-macrophage colony-stimulating factor (GM-CSF). Evidence demonstrates the important role of both GM-CSF and SP-D in the regulation of surfactant phospholipid concentrations in the alveolus.[1]

ISOLATION OF PULMONARY SURFACTANT

Surface-active material is usually isolated by differential sedimentation of material collected by washing the lung with isotonic saline solutions.[2-4] Centrifugation at low forces is used to remove mononuclear cells, which, in the normal lung, are primarily alveolar macrophages. Some surface-active material, specifically large tubular myelin forms, generally sediment at low gravitational forces. Higher-speed centrifugation or buoyant density separation is then used to isolate subfractions of surfactant containing various physical forms. The organization and separation of pulmonary surfactant are highly dependent on the concentration of calcium used during preparation. Calcium enhances the aggregation of surfactant and creates material with higher buoyant density.[5, 6] The dense tubular myelin-rich material (large aggregate

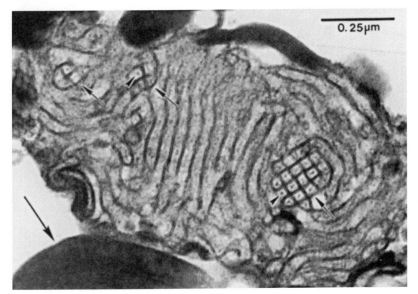

Figure 100–1. Aggregate forms of alveolar surfactant. Lamellar bodies, the intracellular form of surfactant, are secreted into the alveolar lumen as concentrically arranged layers of tightly packed, phospholipid-rich membranes (*large arrow*). Here they are converted into tubular myelin, a lattice-like arrangement of intersecting tubules (*small arrows*) and associated matrix material (*arrowheads*). Transmission electron micrograph of glutaraldehyde–tannic acid–osmium tetroxide–fixed material from the neonatal mouse lung. (×124,200.)

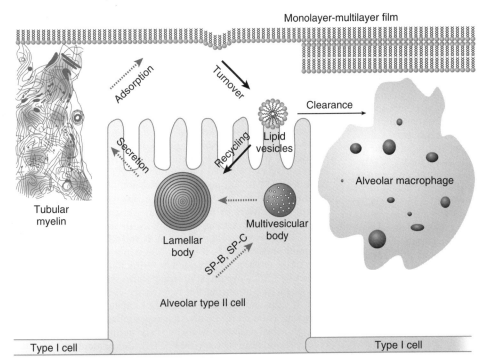

Figure 100–2. Life cycle of pulmonary surfactant. Pulmonary surfactant lipids and proteins are synthesized by Type II epithelial cells. Surfactant proteins and lipids are transported from endoplasmic reticulum, Golgi, multivesicular bodies to lamellar bodies. Surfactant protein B (SP-B) and SP-C are proteolytically processed during transit to lamellar bodies, in which the active peptides are stored with phospholipids before secretion. After secretion, lamellar bodies unwind, and, in the presence of extracellular calcium and SP-A, form tubular myelin (large aggregate surfactant) from which monolayers and multilayers of phospholipids are produced to lower surface tension at the air-liquid interface. Small vesicles are produced during the respiratory cycle that are taken up and are recycled by Type II cells or catabolized by alveolar macrophages.

surfactant) is enriched in SP-A, SP-B, and SP-C and is highly active as a pulmonary surfactant.[7, 8] Less surface-active fractions containing primarily smaller or less dense vesicular forms (small aggregate forms) are relatively depleted of protein and are less surface active than tubular myelin. These vesicular forms may represent catabolic products generated from tubular myelin or from the lipids of the surface multilayers and monolayers that are formed during the respiratory cycle and are destined for uptake and catabolism by alveolar macrophages or reutilization by Type II epithelial cells.

COMPOSITION

The general composition of lung surfactant has been determined in numerous species, including reptiles, fish, birds, amphibians, and mammals. The composition of pulmonary surfactant is, in general, quite similar among diverse species and is rich in phosphatidylcholine and other lipids; proteins generally contribute less than 10% of its mass. The general composition of mammalian surfactant[9-11] is represented in Figure 100–3.

Lipid Components

Surfactant is composed primarily of *phospholipid*, which represents approximately 80 to 90% of its mass. Lesser amounts of glycolipids and neutral lipids are detected in approximately equal amounts. Phospholipid is the primary surface tension-lowering component of pulmonary surfactant. The phospholipids are thought to form a surface monolayer derived from tubular myelin or other aggregate forms present in the alveolus. Phosphatidylcholine is the most abundant phospholipid in surfactant and is uniquely enriched in disaturated forms of

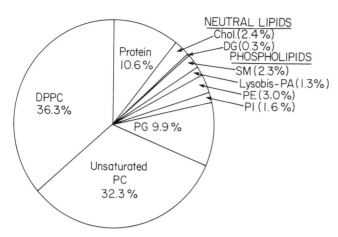

Figure 100–3. Composition of bovine pulmonary surfactant obtained from lung lavage. Components are expressed percentage of weight. Chol = cholesterol; DG = diacylglycerol; DPPC = dipalmitoylphosphatidylcholine, PA = phosphatidic acid; PC = phosphatidylcholine, PE = phosphatidylethanolamine; PG = phosphatidylglycerol; PI = phosphatidylinositol; SM = sphingomyelin. (Adapted from Possmayer F. et al: Can J Biochem Cell Biol *62*:1121, 1984.)

TABLE 100–1

Phospholipid Composition of Human Surfactant and Lamellar Bodies (% wt/wt)

	Surfactant	Lamellar Bodies
Phosphatidylcholine	73	71
Phosphatidylethanolamine	3	8
Phosphatidylglycerol	12	10
Phosphatidylinositol and phosphatidylserine	6	6
Sphingomyelin	4	2
Others	2	3

Adapted from Harwood JL: Prog Lipid Res *26*:211, 1987.

palmitoylphosphatidylcholine (Table 100–1). In human surfactant isolated from lung minces, phosphatidylcholine represents 80% of the total phospholipid, of which 70% is present as the palmitoylphosphatidylcholine; 55% of this lipid species is in the form of disaturated palmitic acid acyl groups or disaturated phosphatidylcholine.[11] Phosphatidylglycerol generally represents 5 to 10% of surfactant phospholipids. Phosphatidylglycerol is also capable of reducing surface tension at an air-liquid interface; however, its precise role in surfactant function remains unclear. Phosphatidylglycerol is not a prerequisite for surface-tension lowering, because surfactant from newborn rabbits lacking phosphatidylglycerol is highly functional at birth. It is possible that phosphatidylinositol provides the acidic phospholipid components required for optimal surface properties in the phosphatidylglycerol-deficient lung. Other phospholipids, including phosphatidylinositol, phosphatidylserine, phosphatidylethanolamine, lysophosphatidylcholine, and sphingomyelin, are present in relatively low amounts in pulmonary surfactant. Glycolipids are also present in pulmonary surfactant and have been partially characterized in rabbit surfactant. Neutral lipids are present primarily as cholesterol esters and acylglycerol fatty acids. The biologic functions of these components, present in relatively low amounts, have not been determined with certainty.[9-12]

The molecular structures of phosphatidylcholine and phosphatidylglycerol are represented in Figure 100–4. Several aspects of their structures are critical for surface tension reduction at the alveolar-air interface. Each molecule consists of a three-carbon glycerol backbone. The C_1 carbon is modified by the addition of polar head groups (relatively more hydrophilic residues). In the case of pulmonary surfactant, the most abundant head groups are choline and glycerol. The C_2 and C_3 carbons of the glycerol backbone contain acyl groups of long chain fatty acid chains that

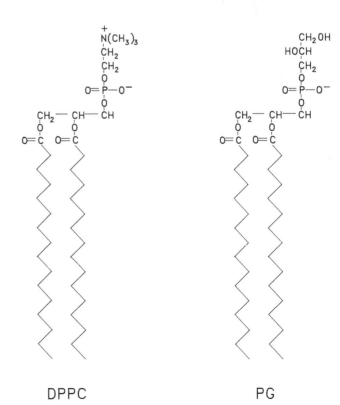

Figure 100–4. Molecular structures of dipalmitoylphosphatidylcholine (DPPC) and phosphatidylglycerol (PG). Phospholipid molecules pack densely, forming membrane monolayers, bilayers, and vesicles and other aggregate forms. Strong molecular interactions occur between polar head groups. Distinct interactions occur among atoms composing the more hydrophobic acyl chains.

TABLE 100-2

Fatty Acid Composition of Phospholipids in Human Surfactant

Acyl Chains	Percentage of Weight/Weight (%)
14:0	3
16:0 (dipalmitoylphosphatidylcholine [DPPC])	81
16:1	6
18:0	3
18:1	5
18:2	2
Others	Trace

Adapted from Harwood JL: Prog Lipid Res *26*:211, 1987.

are highly hydrophobic and lacking in significant charge. The polar head groups (choline, glycerol, and inositol) of the phospholipids produce charge-dependent interactions among neighboring phospholipid molecules and with water. In contrast, the acyl groups are energetically more stable in a nonaqueous environment and are tightly associated with neighboring phospholipid molecules by interactions between carbon and hydrogen atoms of the acyl chains. Hence, these molecules are inherently insoluble in aqueous environments and form various complex structures including membrane monolayers, bilayers, multilayers, micelles, inverted micelles, and vesicles.

The surface properties of surfactant phospholipids (spreading, stability, and surface tension reduction) are influenced by certain factors, including the degree of saturation of the acyl chains, which alter the tightness of packing of phospholipid molecules in membranes. The fatty acid composition of the phospholipids in pulmonary surfactants has been determined for various species (Table 100–2).[10] The structure of the acyl chains and the composition of the major phospholipids are important determinants of the organization of the membranes. The acyl chains present in phosphatidylcholine isolated from pulmonary surfactant are uniquely enriched in palmitic acid (C16) with disaturated acyl chains. Enrichment of these phospholipid species at the surface would result in a densely packed monolayer, creating an interface with extremely low surface tension. Saturated acyl chains contain no methylene (C=C) bonds, and the carbon atoms are fully hydrogenated. Membranes containing such lipids pack densely through the hydrophobic interactions of the acyl chains. The ordering of phospholipid molecules in the surfactant membrane is also highly dependent on temperature. Surfactant lipids are present in a gel or crystalline state at the physiologic temperatures of homeothermic organisms because the transition temperature (temperature of melt) of dipalmitoylphosphatidylcholine is approximately 41°C. Therefore, dipalmitoylphosphatidylcholine would be present in a relatively rigid state at 37°C. However, the presence of minor lipids, proteins, and unique phospholipid acyl chains alters the packing characteristics of the phospholipids. The relative abundance of the major lipid classes, their acyl chain length, and compositions, including the proportion of molecular species with unsaturated acyl chains, therefore comprise a unique mixture in pulmonary surfactant that may alter the surface properties of the surfactant monolayer and its aggregate forms. The characteristics of rapid adsorption and stability during compression of pulmonary surfactant are not properties inherent in the phospholipids alone, and they require the presence of surfactant proteins for these characteristics. The hydrophobic surfactant proteins, SP-B and SP-C, play critical roles in the organization of phospholipids and are required for full surface-active properties of the lipids in surfactant.

Composition of Lamellar Bodies

Surface-active material can also be isolated from its primary intracellular storage site in lamellar bodies of alveolar Type II

cells. Lamellar bodies are highly enriched in phospholipids and generally contain approximately 10 to 12 mg phospholipid/mg protein. Lipid composition of lamellar bodies is similar to surfactant isolated from lung lavage.[10] SP-B and SP-C are highly enriched in lamellar bodies and are co-secreted with phospholipids into the air space.

Developmental Changes in Phospholipid Composition

The phospholipid composition of alveolar lavage material changes during perinatal development. Increased phospholipid synthesis and secretion occur with advancing gestation and are influenced by various hormonal and cellular factors.[12] Because pulmonary secretions contribute a significant volume to amniotic fluid, increased phospholipid in amniotic fluid accompanying advancing gestation has been used for determining the relative maturity of the fetal lung and therefore for predicting the risk of RDS in premature infants. The phosphatidylcholine content of amniotic fluid increases during the latter one-third of human gestation. The ratio of lecithin (phosphatidylcholine) to sphingomyelin, otherwise known as the *L/S ratio*, has been useful in the clinical assessment of risk of RDS.[13] Surfactant content in amniotic fluid can be determined by certain procedures that predict pulmonary maturity.[14,15] Various amniotic fluid assays are useful in predicting surfactant function or lack of respiratory distress in preterm infants, including the L/S ratio, lamellar body counts, quantitation of phosphatidylglycerol, disaturated phosphatidylcholine, or phosphatidylcholine and fluorescence anisotropy. Changes in total phospholipid content and in the relative abundance of phospholipid species also accompany respiratory failure in infants and adults.[16]

Proteins

The characteristics and nomenclature of surfactant proteins have been reviewed previously.[17-19] Surface-active fractions isolated from lung lavage by differential sedimentation contain numerous polypeptides, which include both serum and nonserum proteins. At present, four distinct surfactant-associated proteins have been purified from surfactant, and their primary structures have been discerned. These proteins have been designated SP-A, SP-B, SP-C, and SP-D (Table 100–3). Complementary DNAs and genes encoding these surfactant proteins have been isolated and characterized. The role of each of the proteins in surfactant function and pulmonary homeostasis has been clarified in gene-targeted mice and in clinical observations in children and adults. The precise abundance of each of the proteins in pulmonary surfactant or surfactant subfraction has not been determined with certainty. Nevertheless, SP-A, SP-B, SP-C, and SP-D account for most of the nonserum proteins present in the lipid-associated fraction isolated from lung lavage.

Surfactant-Associated Proteins: Collectins
Surfactant Protein A and Surfactant Protein D

SP-A is the most abundant nonserum lipid-associated protein in pulmonary surfactant.[4] SP-A is a member of a related family of polypeptides termed the *collectins* that includes SP-D, mannose-binding lectin, conglutinin, and CL-43. These proteins share collagenous and lectin-containing domains that bind complex carbohydrates. SP-A is a 26,000- to 35,000-dalton glycoprotein that undergoes sulfhydryl-dependent oligomerization and other posttranslational modifications, accounting for the significant molecular heterogeneity of its isoforms in pulmonary surfactant. Two human SP-A genes have been identified, each consisting of five exons contained within approximately 4.5 kB of DNA.[20] The SP-A locus consists of two coding sequences and a noncoding sequence on human chromosome 10.[21,22] The entire polypeptide sequence of SP-A has been deduced from the gene and cDNAs encoding the human proteins (Fig. 100–5).[20] SP-A is first synthesized as a 248-amino terminal precursor peptide from which a

TABLE 100-3

Human Surfactant Proteins

Protein	Monomeric Size	Oligomers	mRNA (kB)	Chromosome	Amino Acids in Precursor (Approximate)
SP-A	30,000–36,000	Octadecamers	2.2	10	248
SP-B	8,000	Dimers	2.0	2	381
SP-C	3,800	Dimers	0.9	8	191
SP-D	43,000	Tetramers/dodecamers	1.3	10	374

SP = surfactant protein.

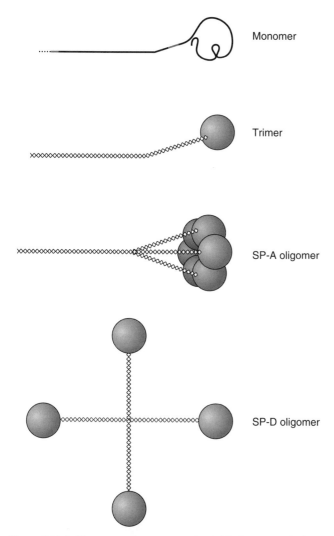

Figure 100–5. Human surfactant protein A (SP-A) is encoded by genomic DNA on chromosome 10. Translation of the mRNA produces a monomer that forms trimers. Further, oligomerization via the amino terminal collagen-like domain (*hatched area*) results in hexamers and larger assembled forms such as octadecamers found in association with tubular myelin in the alveolus. SP-D is formed by a similar process from the SP-D gene locus, also located on chromosome 10; SP-D monomers form trimers that are organized into tetramers and dodecamers.

small signal sequence is cleaved. The remaining amino-terminal domain of the mature SP-A peptide contains an extensive collagen-like region composed of approximately 10,000 daltons. A discrete carboxy-terminal globular domain is homologous to other mammalian lectins (carbohydrate-binding proteins) and is structurally related to those in SP-D, mannose-binding lectin, and

other members of the collectin family of polypeptides.[23] SP-A binds carbohydrates, phospholipids, and glycolipids that are surface components of numerous pathogens including bacteria, viruses, and fungi.[24, 25]

Functions of Surfactant Protein A. Although the functions of SP-A have not been clarified precisely, *in vitro* and *in vivo* studies demonstrated many different biologic activities intrinsic to the molecule. SP-A binds carbohydrates and aggregates phospholipids in a calcium-dependent manner.[26-28] Mixtures of phospholipids, SP-A, and SP-B form tubular myelin-like structures *in vitro*.[29] SP-A enhances the biophysical activity of surfactant phospholipid-rich extracts.[26] *In vitro*, SP-A binds Type II epithelial cells and macrophages and is internalized by receptor-mediated endocytosis.[30, 31] After uptake, SP-A is detected in multivesicular bodies and vesicles closely associated with lamellar bodies.[30] Receptor binding and internalization support the concept that SP-A is reused or is involved in cell signaling. Although *in vitro* findings supported a role for SP-A in surfactant homeostasis,[32-34] gene-targeting experiments in transgenic mice do not support its importance in surfactant metabolism *in vivo*.[35] In contrast, studies in SP-A null mice support a critical role for SP-A in innate host defense of the lung.[24] SP-A is a member of the calcium-dependent lectins (collectins) that serve as opsonins, enhancing binding, phagocytosis, and killing of various bacterial, fungal, and viral pathogens. SP-A enhances binding or uptake of group B streptococci and subtypes of *Haemophilus influenzae*, *Staphylococcus aureus,* and *Pseudomonas aeruginosa* by alveolar macrophages and is therefore an important defense molecule in the neonatal and mature lung.[24] In the presence of pathogens, SP-A activates alveolar macrophages *in vitro* and *in vivo,* enhancing opsonization, oxidant production, and killing of pathogens.[36]

Transgenic SP-A–deficient mice, in which the SP-A gene was targeted by homologous recombination, survive postnatally.[35] Although SP-A–deficient mice do not form tubular myelin, intracellular and extracellular surfactant phospholipid content, uptake of phospholipid by lung tissue, phospholipid secretion, and surfactant function are not altered by the absence of SP-A. Thus, SP-A plays a critical role in innate host defense of the lung, but it does not play an important role in surfactant function or homeostasis *in vivo*.

Control of Surfactant Protein A Content. Like other surfactant proteins, SP-A is synthesized by respiratory epithelial cells in the developing fetal lung, and its expression increases in late gestation.[37] SP-A is detected in nonciliated cells in tracheal bronchial glands, as well as in bronchiolar and alveolar epithelial cells of the lung. In humans, expression of SP-A increases with advancing gestational age in association with the maturation of Type II epithelial cells occurring in the latter part of gestation. SP-A appears in increasing concentrations in amniotic fluid during advancing gestation. Like the L/S ratio, SP-A is a useful marker of fetal lung maturity in humans.[38, 39] SP-A synthesis in human fetal lung cultures is enhanced by numerous hormonal factors, including epidermal growth factor, interferon-γ, interleukin-1, and cyclic adenosine monophosphate (cAMP).[37,40] Glucocorticoids both stimulate and inhibit human SP-A synthesis by distinct mechanisms, which include transcriptional enhancement and decreased mRNA stability *in vitro*.[41] Transcription of the SP-A gene, as well as the genes encoding SP-B and SP-C, are regulated by elements located in the 5' region of the gene that bind to nuclear transcription factor thyroid transcription factor-1 (TTF-1), a homeodomain-containing member of the Nkx2.1 family of proteins. Binding of TTF-1 to regulatory elements in target genes confers lung epithelial specificity to their transcription. TTF-1 also regulates the transcription of other genes expressed exclusively in the respiratory epithelium, including SP-B, SP-C, and the Clara cell secretory protein.[42] Inhibitory effects of transforming growth factor-β and insulin on SP-A expression have been observed in human fetal lung explant culture.[43,44] SP-A content in alveolar lavage is induced by oxygen exposure, interleukin-4, and silicosis, and SP-A accumulates in the lavage fluid from patients with alveolar proteinosis.[45-47] Although GM-CSF–deficient mice develop pulmonary alveolar proteinosis, the relative abundance of surfactant protein mRNAs is not altered, a finding supporting the concept that GM-CSF plays an important role in surfactant clearance.[1, 48] Studies in humans demonstrated that pulmonary alveolar proteinosis is associated with neutralizing antibodies against GM-CSF or mutations in the GM-CSF receptor.[49]

In summary, SP-A is an abundant pulmonary host defense protein that is strongly associated with surfactant phospholipids and is required for formation of tubular myelin. SP-A plays important roles in innate defense against bacterial, fungal, and viral pathogens, enhancing opsonization and killing of respiratory pathogens by alveolar macrophages.[24]

Surfactant Protein D. SP-D, a member of the collectin family of polypeptides, shares structural motifs with SP-A and related family members.[24, 25] A single human SP-D gene is located in close proximity to the SP-A genes on chromosome 10. SP-D is slightly larger than SP-A, and it is composed of 43-kDa monomers containing an approximately 15,000-kDa collagenous region that forms trimers and higher-ordered complexes that are found in the alveoli (see Fig. 100–5). Unlike SP-A, SP-B, and SP-C, SP-D expression is not restricted to cells within the lung. SP-D mRNA and protein have been detected in various organs, including the gastrointestinal tract, pancreas, bile duct, cervical glands, and other sites.[50] In the lung, SP-D is expressed by Type II epithelial cells in the alveoli, nonciliated bronchiolar, and tracheal-bronchial epithelial cells, including cells lining tracheal-bronchial glands. SP-D is less abundant and less strongly associated with surfactant phospholipids than SP-A, SP-B, or SP-C. SP-D can be isolated from both lipid-containing and non–lipid-containing fractions of alveolar surfactant, and it is not required for the formation of tubular myelin or lamellar bodies.

Role of Surfactant Protein D in Innate Host Defense of the Lung and Regulation of Surfactant Homeostasis. The C-terminus of SP-D consists of a globular carbohydrate recognition domain that binds molecules on the surface of bacterial, viral, and fungal pathogens. SP-D has high affinity for various bacterial lipopolysaccharides, complex carbohydrates, and lipids.[25] SP-D binds and agglutinates various bacterial (including *Escherichia coli*, *Salmonella*, and *Pseudomonas*), fungal, and viral (influenza A, adenovirus, and respiratory syncytial virus) pathogens, and it enhances their uptake and killing by alveolar macrophages.[24,25] Thus, SP-D serves as an important role in pathogen recognition critical to innate defense of the lung against infection. *In vivo*, SP-D–deficient mice are susceptible to various pulmonary pathogens. SP-D enhances the clearance of pathogens and suppresses inflammatory responses after infection of the lung.[24] SP-D also plays important roles in the regulation of surfactant phospholipid pool size and in the suppression of oxidant production by alveolar macrophages in the lung.[51] Deletion of SP-D in transgenic mice caused emphysema, macrophage activation, accumulation of oxygen reactive

species, and pulmonary lipidosis. Alveolar and tissue surfactant lipid pool sizes were markedly increased in the absence of SP-D. Thus, SP-D plays a critical role in the regulation of surfactant lipid homeostasis, inflammatory responses, and innate host defense. Because SP-D influences inflammation and cytokine responses after exposure to various pulmonary pathogens, it is also highly likely that SP-D influences subsequent acquired immune responses after infection.

Regulation of Surfactant Protein D. Unlike the other surfactant proteins, SP-D expression is not directly regulated by TTF-1 and is expressed in many organs in various cell types.[50] SP-D content in fetal lung and amniotic fluid increases with advancing gestational age, and its content is enhanced by glucocorticoids in experimental models. SP-D expression is enhanced by allergens and interleukin-4. SP-D concentrations in alveolar fluid are decreased in various clinical conditions associated with severe pneumonitis, including cystic fibrosis.[24, 52] Like other surfactant components, SP-D accumulates in the pulmonary alveolar proteinosis associated with GM-CSF deficiency and silicosis.[1,24]

Surfactant Protein B. SP-B is a small hydrophobic polypeptide comprising 79 amino acids (Fig. 100–6).[53] A single human SP-B gene is composed of 10 exons, spanning approximately 10 kB of DNA located on chromosome 2.[54] Analysis of cDNAs encoding SP-B demonstrates that the SP-B polypeptide is produced by proteolytic processing of an approximately 40,000- to 46,000-dalton glycosylated precursor comprising 381 amino acids.[55-57] The active peptide found in the airway forms sulfhydryl-dependent oligomers that include dimers and tetramers. Proteolytic processing of proSP-B occurs in Type II epithelial cells (during routing of the proSP-B from endoplasmic reticulum to multivesicular bodies) and during transport from multivesicular bodies and lamellar bodies before secretion. Immunostaining with antibodies generated against SP-B co-localizes with apical intracellular inclusions in Type II cells and stains material in the lumen of alveolar and airway structures.[58, 59] Although the functions of SP-B have not been elucidated with certainty, SP-B is tightly associated with surfactant phospholipids and is required for formation of tubular myelin in the presence of SP-A, phospholipids, and calcium.[29] SP-B is highly fusogenic,[60] generating phospholipid membranes from vesicular lipid forms; SP-B enhances spreading and stability of surfactant. SP-B converts vesicular lipids in the lumen of multivesicular bodies to the tightly packed membrane sheets observed in the lamellar bodies.[61] Although SP-B enhances the uptake of phospholipid vesicles by Type II epithelial cells *in vitro*, when present with SP-A, it also enhances formation of tubular myelin.[62] Increasing evidence supports the concept that SP-B is critical for the enhancement of surface properties of surfactant phospholipids. SP-B is an important component of surfactant replacement mixtures made by organic solvent extraction of pulmonary surfactant or lung minces.

Surfactant Protein B is Required for Lung Function at Birth: Hereditary SP-B Deficiency. Studies in SP-B gene-targeted mice, and in full-term infants bearing mutations in the SP-B gene, demonstrated that SP-B is required for pulmonary function at birth.[61,63] Although pulmonary structure is normal, mice lacking SP-B die of respiratory distress immediately after birth. Decreased lung volumes, lack of hysteresis, and atelectasis were associated with the lack of lamellar bodies and accumulation of aberrant multivesicular bodies within Type II cells. Decreased surfactant activity, lack of tubular myelin, and the synthesis of an abnormal proSP-C precursor demonstrated that SP-B is required for both intercellular and extracellular routing of surfactant lipids and proteins. Full-term human infants with mutations in the SP-B gene generally develop respiratory distress within hours after birth, with clinical and radiologic findings typical of that seen in preterm infants with RDS. Respiratory failure is generally pro-

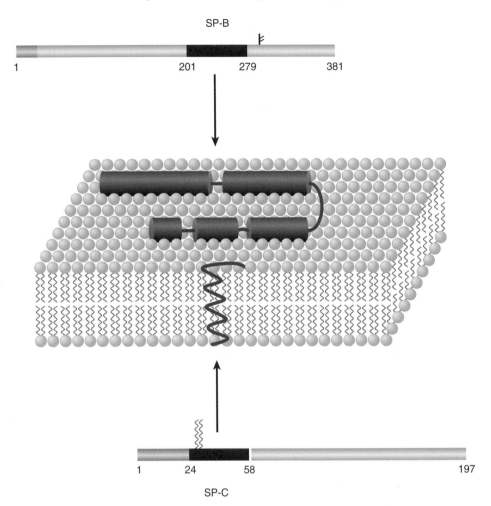

Figure 100–6. Human surfactant protein B (SP-B) is encoded by a single gene located on chromosome 2 and comprises approximately 9.5 kB of genomic DNA. The active peptide comprises 79 amino acids. The mRNA is approximately 2.0 kB in length and is translated to a preproprotein of approximately 39,000 daltons that is proteolytically processed and glycosylated. The active peptide is generated from proSP-B during proteolytic processing to form the M_r = 8000 (79-amino acid) peptide, and its oligomers are tightly associated with phospholipids in the airway. Human SP-C is encoded by a gene locus located on chromosome 8 that comprises approximately 3.5 kB of genomic DNA. The active peptide comprising 35 to 36 amino acids is encoded by a single exon and is palmitoylated. The mRNA is approximately 0.9 kB and is translated to proSP-C (M_r ~22,000), which is proteolytically processed to an M_r = 3800 monomer and its oligomers found in the airway. SP-B and SP-C are tightly associated with phospholipid membranes in the alveolus.

gressive and is not responsive to exogenous surfactant replacement therapy; these infants die of respiratory failure in spite of intensive ventilatory support. In SP-B–deficient infants, alveolar spaces are filled with proteinaceous material[63] that consists primarily of surfactant proteins and abnormally processed proSP-C. The disorder is generally inherited in an autosomal recessive manner. The most common mutation, SP-B[121ins], creates an unstable mRNA, resulting in lack of SP-B protein production. More than 15 distinct mutations in the SP-B gene have been associated with respiratory failure in infants.[64] The disorder is generally lethal in the first months of life, but it has been treated by lung transplantation. In summary, SP-B is required for packaging and processing of surfactant lipids and proteins intracellularly and for organization, function, and homeostasis of surfactant lipids and proteins in the alveolar space.

Regulation of Expression of Surfactant Protein B. SP-B mRNA increases with advancing gestation in the human fetal lung, Type II alveolar cells, and nonciliated respiratory epithelial cells in the distal respiratory tract.[65] In fetal lung, SP-B synthesis is stimulated by cAMP, interleukin-1, and glucocorticoids.[37, 40, 66, 67] The concentration of SP-B in human amniotic fluid increases with advancing gestation in association with an increased L/S ratio and phosphatidylglycerol.[68] Like SP-A, SP-B expression is also regulated by the homeodomain-containing nuclear protein, TTF-1, that controls transcription of the SP-B gene.[42]

Surfactant Protein C. SP-C is the most hydrophobic protein isolated from pulmonary surfactant (see Fig. 100–6).[18, 19] Like SP-A and SP-B, SP-C is relatively abundant in the dense surfactant fractions obtained by lung lavage. SP-C consists of 35 to 36 amino

acids, most of which are hydrophobic residues valine, leucine, and isoleucine.[69] cDNAs and genomic DNA encoding SP-C have been isolated and characterized.[70, 71] In the human, the SP-C gene comprises approximately 3 kB of contiguous DNA and consists of 6 exons located on chromosome 8. Allelic variations and differential RNA splicing are likely to account for the molecular heterogeneity at these loci.[72] The precursor contains neither an amino terminal signal sequence nor amino acid sequences predicting the addition of asparagine-linked carbohydrate. SP-C is palmitoylated and is transported through the endoplasmic reticulum to multivesicular bodies with proSP-B. Both proSP-C and proSP-B are processed during transport to lamellar bodies; SP-B is required for proteolytic processing of proSP-C. The active 35- to 36-amino acid SP-C peptide is stored in lamellar bodies and is associated with surfactant lipid in the alveolus. Synthesis of SP-C is restricted to Type II alveolar cells in the lung.

SP-C and mixtures of SP-B and SP-C enhance the rate of absorption of surfactant phospholipids and confer important surfactant-like properties to the lipids,[18, 19, 53, 73] but they are not required for formation of lamellar bodies or tubular myelin. SP-C is taken up by alveolar epithelial cells; addition of SP-C peptides enhances uptake of phospholipid vesicles by Type II epithelial cells *in vitro*.[62, 74] SP-C is highly enriched in organic solvent extracts of surfactant and, like SP-B, is present in the surfactant extracts used for replacement therapy of RDS in infants.

Role of Surfactant Protein C in Surfactant Function and Homeostasis. Studies in SP-C gene targeted mice and in humans bearing mutations in the SP-C gene demonstrate the important role of SP-C in surfactant function and pulmonary homeostasis.[73]

Although SP-C gene targeted mice survive perinatally, abnormalities in the stability of surfactant film formed from SP-C–deficient mice, demonstrate the role of SP-C in recruiting phospholipids to monolayers/multilayers, SP-C is required for the stability of phospholipid films during dynamic compression.[75] Formation of lamellar bodies and of tubular myelin is not perturbed in SP-C–deficient mice. However, SP-C–deficient mice develop interstitial lung disease associated with emphysema, epithelial cell dysplasia, and inflammation.[73, 76] Likewise, humans bearing mutations in the SP-C gene develop various forms of acute and chronic pulmonary disease including acute RDS and idiopathic pulmonary fibrosis.[77,78] SP-C mutations are generally inherited as an autosomal dominant disorder and have been associated with the pathologic diagnoses of usual interstitial pneumonitis, nonspecific interstitial pneumonitis, and desquamating interstitial pneumonitis.

Regulation of Surfactant Protein C Synthesis. SP-C synthesis and mRNA content increase in association with Type II cell maturation in fetal lung, and SP-C expression is restricted to Type II cells in the postnatal lung.[37, 66, 67] SP-C mRNA is detected early in embryonic lung development (postconception day 10) in the mouse and at 10 to 12 weeks' gestation in the human.[79] SP-C mRNA is enhanced by glucocorticoids and cAMP.[66, 67] As with the SP-A and SP-B genes, the transcription of the SP-C gene is lung epithelial cell specific and requires TTF-1.[42]

Role of Surfactant Proteins in Surfactant Replacement Preparations. The structures of each of the major surfactant proteins are quite distinct and support the concept that each plays a unique role in the structure and function of surfactant. Although the surfactant phospholipids themselves provide the molecules critical for the reduction of surface tension in the alveolus, they do not have the properties inherent in pulmonary surfactant. At physiologic temperatures, the surfactant lipids themselves are in a highly organized gel-crystalline state that is not capable of rapidly forming a surface film. Phospholipid molecules alone fail to spread and respread rapidly during compression and decompression. Their adsorption rates to surfaces are slow and do not generate the surface tension–lowering film necessary to maintain surface forces during the respiratory cycle. It is increasingly apparent that SP-B and SP-C interact with surfactant phospholipids to produce surfactant with unique physicochemical properties, thus allowing formation and stability of the surfactant film during the respiratory cycle.

Both SP-B and SP-C confer important surfactant-like activity to phospholipids and are present in preparations used for treatment of surfactant-deficient states.[80-82] Preparations containing SP-A have not been used widely for clinical studies. Human surfactant isolated from amniotic fluid, containing SP-A, SP-B, or SP-C, as well as various other human proteins, was previously used for exogenous surfactant replacement.[83] Surfactant extracts based on organic solvent extracts of lung or surfactant preparations contain SP-B and SP-C (but not SP-A). Survanta, Curosurf, Alveofact, and Infasurf are examples of such preparations. SP-B and SP-C, when mixed with phospholipids, appear to be sufficient to generate the surface-active properties of pulmonary surfactant and therefore may be useful in future development of surfactant replacement preparations for treatment of surfactant-deficient states. A protein-free phospholipid-rich preparation, Exosurf, was also an effective therapy for RDS.[84]

Other Alveolar Proteins

Detailed analysis of material obtained by lung lavage, such as by two-dimensional gel electrophoresis and sensitive silver staining techniques, reveals hundreds of serum and nonserum proteins. Precise abundance, cellular source, and role of each of these proteins in lung function have not been determined. The alveolar fluid contains certain molecules that may play a role in host defense: SP-D, fibronectin, lysozyme, antiproteases, immunoglobulins (particularly IgA), defensins, mucins, and Clara cell proteins. Products of Type I and Type II epithelial cells, alveolar macrophages, and lymphocytes are likely to contribute to the heterogeneity of proteins found in the alveolar lavage from the normal lung; however, the identity and functions of these proteins have not been clarified. It is also increasingly apparent that surfactant homeostasis may be disrupted by the presence of blood or serum proteins, including albumin and fibrin.[84-87] Thus, homeostatic mechanisms that exclude nonsurfactant proteins from the alveolus are likely to be highly critical for the function of surfactant and therefore for gas exchange after birth.

REFERENCES

1. Trapnell BC, Whitsett JA: GM-CSF regulates pulmonary surfactant homeostasis and alveolar macrophage-mediated innate host defense. Annu Rev Physiol 64:775, 2002.
2. King RJ, Clements JA: Surface active materials from dog lung. I. Methods of isolation. Am J Physiol 223:707, 1972.
3. King RJ, Clements JA: Surface active materials from dog lung. II. Composition and physiological correlations. Am J Physiol 223:715, 1972.
4. King RJ, et al: Isolation of apoproteins from canine surface active material. Am J Physiol 224:788, 1973.
5. Sanders RL, et al: Isolation of lung lamellar bodies and their conversion of tubular myelin figures in vitro. Anat Rec 198:485, 1980.
6. Benson BJ, et al: Role of calcium ions in the structure and function of pulmonary surfactant. Biochim Biophys Acta 793:1827, 1984.
7. Magoon MW, et al: Subfractionation of lung surfactant. Implications for metabolism and surface activity. Biochim Biophys Acta 750:18, 1983.
8. Wright JR, et al: Protein composition of rabbit alveolar surfactant subfractions. Biochim Biophys Acta 791:320, 1984.
9. Possmayer F, et al: Pulmonary surfactant. Can J Biochem Cell Biol 62:1121, 1984.
10. Harwood JL. Lung surfactant. Prog Lipid Res 26:211, 1987.
11. Shelly SA, et al: Biochemical composition of adult human lung surfactant. Lung 160:195, 1982.
12. Rooney SA: Lung surfactant. Environ Health Perspect 55:205, 1984.
13. Gluck L, et al: Diagnosis of respiratory distress syndrome by amniocentesis. Am J Obstet Gynecol 109:440, 1971.
14. Hallman M, et al: Phosphatidylinositol and phosphatidylglycerol in amniotic fluid: Indices of pulmonary maturity. Am J Obstet Gynecol 125:613, 1976.
15. Hallman M: Antenatal diagnosis of lung maturity. In Robertson B, et al (eds): Pulmonary Surfactant. Amsterdam, Elsevier, 1984, pp 419–448.
16. Hallman M, et al: Evidence of lung surfactant abnormality in respiratory failure. Study of bronchoalveolar lavage: surface activity, phospholipase activity and plasma myoinositol. J Clin Invest 70:673, 1982.
17. Possmayer F: A proposed nomenclature for pulmonary surfactant-associated proteins. Am Rev Respir Dis 138:990, 1988.
18. Weaver TE: Pulmonary surfactant-associated proteins. Gen Pharmacol 19:361, 1988.
19. Hawgood S: Pulmonary surfactant apoproteins: a review of protein and genomic structure. Am J Physiol 257:L13, 1989.
20. White RT, et al: Isolation and characterization of the human surfactant apoprotein gene. Nature 317:361, 1985.
21. Bruns G, et al: The 35 kd pulmonary surfactant-associated protein is encoded on chromosome 10. Hum Genet 76:58, 1987.
22. Katyal SL, et al: Characterization of a second human pulmonary surfactant-associated protein SP-A gene. Am J Respir Cell Mol Biol 6:446, 1992.
23. Drickamer K, et al: Mannose-binding proteins isolated from rat liver contain carbohydrate recognition domains linked to collagenous tails. J Biol Chem 267:6878, 1986.
24. Crouch E, Wright JR: Surfactant proteins A and D and pulmonary host defense. Annu Rev Physiol 63:521, 2001.
25. Reid KB: Interactions of surfactant protein D with pathogens, allergens and phagocytes. Biochim Biophys Acta 1408:290, 1998.
26. Hawgood S, et al: Effects of a surfactant-associated protein and calcium ions on the structure and surface activity of lung surfactant lipids. Biochemistry 24:184, 1985.
27. Haagsman HP, et al: The major lung surfactant protein, SP 28–36, is a calcium-dependent, carbohydrate-binding protein. J Biol Chem 262:13877, 1987.
28. Voss T, et al: Macromolecular organization of natural and recombinant lung surfactant protein SP 28–36. J Mol Biol 201:219, 1988.
29. Suzuki Y, et al: Reconstitution of tubular myelin from synthetic lipids and proteins associated with pig pulmonary surfactant. Am Rev Respir Dis 140:75, 1989.
30. Ryan RM, et al: Binding and uptake of pulmonary surfactant protein (SP-A) by pulmonary type II epithelial cells. J Histochem Cytochem 37:429, 1989.
31. Kuroki Y, et al: Alveolar type II cells expressing a high affinity receptor for pulmonary surfactant protein A. Proc Natl Acad Sci USA 85:5566, 1988.

32. Wright IR, et al: Surfactant apoprotein M_r = 26,000–36,000 enhances uptake of liposomes by type II cells. J Biol Chem 262:2888, 1987.

33. Dobbs LG, et al: Pulmonary surfactant and its components inhibit secretion of phosphatidylcholine from cultured rat alveolar type II cells. Proc Natl Acad Sci USA 84:1010, 1987.

34. Rice WR, et al: Surfactant-associated protein inhibits phospholipid secretion from type II cells. J Appl Physiol 63:692, 1987.

35. Korfhagen TR, et al: Altered surfactant function and structure in SP-A gene targeted mice. Proc Natl Acad Sci USA 93:9594, 1996.

36. Tenner AJ, et al: Human pulmonary surfactant protein (SP-A), a protein structurally homologous to C1Q, can enhance Fcr-mediated and Cr1-mediated phagocytosis. J Biol Chem 264:13923, 1989.

37. Ballard PL: Hormonal regulation of pulmonary surfactant. Endocr Rev 10:165, 1989.

38. King RJ, et al: Appearance of apoproteins of pulmonary surfactant in human amniotic fluid. J Appl Physiol 39:735, 1975.

39. Hallman M, et al: Surfactant proteins in the diagnosis of fetal lung maturity. I. Predictive accuracy of the 35 kDa protein, the lecithin/sphingomyelin ratio and phosphatidylglycerol. Am J Obstet Gynecol 158:531, 1988.

40. Dhar V, et al: Interleukin-1 alpha upregulates the expression of surfactant protein-A in rabbit lung explants. Biol Neonate 71:46, 1997.

41. Boggaram V, et al: Regulation of expression of the gene encoding the major surfactant protein (SP-A) in human fetal lung in in vitro–disparate effects of glucocorticoids on transcription and on messenger RNA stability. J Biol Chem 264:11421, 1989.

42. Bohinski RJ, et al: Lung-specific surfactant protein B gene promoter is a target for thyroid transcription factor 1 and hepatocyte nuclear factor 3 indicating common mechanisms for organ-specific gene expression along the foregut axis. Mol Cell Biol 14:5671, 1994.

43. Whitsett JA, et al: Differential effects of epidermal growth factor and transforming growth factor on synthesis of M_r = 35,000 surfactant-associated protein in fetal lung. J Biol Chem 262:7908, 1987.

44. Snyder JM, Mendelson CR: Insulin inhibits the accumulation of the major lung surfactant apoprotein in human fetal lung explants maintained in vitro. Endocrinology 120:1250, 1987.

45. Nogee LM, et al: Increased synthesis and mRNA of surfactant protein A in oxygen-exposed rats. Am J Respir Cell Mol Biol 1:119, 1989.

46. Kawada H, et al: Alveolar type II cells, surfactant protein A (SP-A) and the phospholipid components of surfactant in acute silicosis in the rat. Am Rev Respir Dis 140:460, 1989.

47. Ross GF, et al: Structural relationships of the major glycoproteins from human alveolar proteinosis surfactant. Biochim Biophys Acta 911:294, 1987.

48. Dranoff G, et al: Involvement of granulocyte-macrophage colony-stimulating factor in pulmonary homeostasis. Science 264:713, 1994.

49. Kitamura T, et al: Idiopathic pulmonary alveolar proteinosis as an autoimmune disease with neutralizing antibody against granulocyte/macrophage colony-stimulating factor. J Exp Med 190:875, 1999.

50. Madsen J, et al: Localization of lung surfactant protein D on mucosal surfaces in human tissues. J Immunol 164:5866, 2000.

51. Wert SE, et al: Increased metalloproteinase activity, oxidant production, and emphysema in surfactant protein D gene-inactivated mice. Proc Natl Acad Sci USA 97:5972, 2000.

52. Postle AD, et al: Deficient hydrophilic lung surfactant proteins A and D with normal surfactant phospholipid molecular species in cystic fibrosis. Am J Respir Cell Mol Biol 20:90, 1999.

53. Weaver TE, Conkright JJ: Function of surfactant proteins B and C. Annu Rev Physiol 63:555, 2001.

54. Pilot-Matias TJ, et al: Structure and organization of the gene encoding human pulmonary surfactant proteolipid SP-B. DNA 8:75, 1989.

55. Hawgood S, et al: Nucleotide and amino acid sequences of pulmonary surfactant protein SP 18 and evidence for cooperation between SP 18 and SP 28–36 in surfactant lipid adsorption. Proc Natl Acad Sci USA 84:66, 1987.

56. Glasser SW, et al: cDNA and deduced amino acid sequence of human pulmonary surfactant-associated proteolipid SPL(Phe). Proc Natl Acad Sci USA 84:4007, 1987.

57. Jacobs KA, et al: Isolation of a cDNA clone encoding a high molecular weight precursor to a 6-kDa pulmonary surfactant-associated protein. J Biol Chem 262:9808, 1987.

58. Suzuki Y, et al: A monoclonal antibody to the 15,000 dalton protein associated with porcine pulmonary surfactant. Exp Lung Res 11:61, 1986.

59. Weaver TE, et al: Identification of surfactant proteolipid SP-B in human surfactant and fetal lung. J Appl Physiol 65:982, 1988.

60. Rice WR, et al: Surfactant peptides stimulate uptake of phosphatidylcholine by isolated cells. Biochim Biophys Acta 1006:237, 1989.

61. Clark JC, et al: Targeted disruption of the surfactant protein B gene disrupts surfactant homeostasis, causing respiratory failure in newborn mice. Proc Natl Acad Sci USA 92:7794, 1995.

62. Horowitz AD, et al: Roles of SP-A, SP-B and SP-C in modulation of lipid uptake by pulmonary epithelial cells in vitro. Am J Physiol 270:L69, 1996.

63. Nogee LM, et al: A mutation in the surfactant protein B gene responsible for fatal neonatal respiratory disease in multiple kindreds. J Clin Invest 93:1860, 1994.

64. Nogee LM, et al: Allelic heterogeneity in hereditary surfactant protein B (SP-B) deficiency. Am J Respir Crit Care Med 161:973, 2000.

65. Phelps DS, Floros J: Localization of surfactant protein synthesis in human lung by in situ hybridization. Am Rev Respir Dis 137:939, 1988.

66. Whitsett JA, et al: Glucocorticoid enhances surfactant proteolipid Phe and pVal synthesis and RNA in fetal lung. J Biol Chem 262:15618, 1987.

67. Liley HG, et al: Regulation of messenger RNAs for the hydrophobic surfactant proteins in human lung. J Clin Invest 83:1191, 1989.

68. Pryhuber GS, et al: Ontogeny of surfactant proteins A and B in human amniotic fluid as indices of fetal lung maturity. Pediatr Res 30:597, 1991.

69. Johansson J, et al: Hydrophobic 3.7 kDa surfactant polypeptide: structural characterization of the human and bovine forms. FEBS Lett 232:61, 1988.

70. Warr RG, et al: Low molecular weight human pulmonary surfactant protein (SP5): isolations characterization and cDNA and amino acid sequences. Proc Natl Acad Sci USA 84:7915, 1987.

71. Glasser SW, et al: cDNA, deduced polypeptide structure and chromosomal assignment of human pulmonary surfactant proteolipid: SPL(pVal). J Biol Chem 263:9, 1988.

72. Glasser SW, et al: Two genes encoding human pulmonary surfactant proteolipid SP-C. J Biol Chem 268:10326, 1988.

73. Whitsett JA, Weaver TE: Hydrophobic surfactant proteins in lung function and disease. N Engl J Med 347:2141, 2002.

74. Horowitz AD, et al: Distinct effects of SP-A and SP-B on endocytosis of SP-C by pulmonary epithelial cells. Am J Physiol 273:L159, 1997.

75. Glasser SW, et al: Pneumonitis and emphysema in SP-C gene targeted mice. J Biol Chem 2003.

76. Glasser SW, et al: Altered stability of pulmonary surfactant in SP-C-deficient mice. Proc Natl Acad Sci USA 98:6366, 2001.

77. Nogee LM, et al: A mutation in the surfactant protein C gene associated with familial interstitial lung disease. N Engl J Med 344:573, 2001.

78. Thomas AQ, et al: Heterozygosity for a surfactant protein C gene mutation associated with usual interstitial pneumonitis and cellular nonspecific interstitial pneumonitis in one kindred. Am J Respir Crit Care Med 165:1322, 2002.

79. Wert SE, et al: Transcriptional elements from the human SP-C gene direct expression in the primordial respiratory epithelium of transgenic mice. Dev Biol 156:426, 1993.

80. Whitsett JA, et al: Hydrophobic surfactant-associated protein in whole lung surfactant and its importance for biophysical activity in lung surfactant extracts used for replacement therapy. Pediatr Res 20:460, 1986.

81. Taeusch HW, et al: Characterization of bovine surfactant for infants with respiratory distress syndrome. Pediatrics 77:572, 1986.

82. Robertson B, Lachmann B: Experimental evaluation of surfactants for replacement therapy. Exp Lung Res 14:279, 1988.

83. Hallman M, et al: Isolation of human surfactant from amniotic fluid and a pilot study of its efficacy in respiratory distress syndrome. Pediatrics 71:473, 1983.

84. Tooley WH, et al: Lung function in prematurely delivered rabbits treated with a synthetic surfactant. Am Rev Respir Dis 136:651, 1987.

85. Ikegami M, et al: A protein from airways of premature lambs that inhibits surfactant function. J Appl Physiol 57:1134, 1984.

86. Holm BA, et al: Surface property changes from interactions of albumin with natural lung surfactant and extracted lung lipids. Chem Phys Lipids 38:287, 1985.

87. Seeger W, et al: Alteration of surfactant function due to protein leakage: special interaction with fibrin monomer. J Appl Physiol 58:326, 1985.

101 Physicochemical Aspects of Pulmonary Surfactant

When an infant is born, he or she must clear the lungs of fetal pulmonary fluid, inflate the alveoli with air, and establish air breathing. These functions are facilitated by the presence of pulmonary surfactant. By lowering the surface tension in the lung to low values, surfactant reduces the work of breathing and stabilizes the terminal air spaces, particularly at low lung volumes. The net effect is to increase air space and thereby to enhance gaseous exchange. The obvious success of surfactant replacement therapy for prematurely delivered infants with the respiratory distress syndrome (RDS), who lack sufficient surfactant of their own, emphasizes the critical role of surfactant during the neonatal period.[1-3] Surfactant is also being used to treat meconium aspiration and to help wean infants during treatment with extracorporeal membrane oxygenation[4-8] (see Chap. 106). Considerable evidence indicates that surfactant dysfunction contributes to pulmonary instability in acute lung injury and acute RDS (ARDS) and that surfactant therapy could prove beneficial.[6,9-15]

It is generally appreciated that the physicochemical properties of pulmonary surfactant are critical for normal lung function. However, the mechanisms by which this lipid-protein complex adsorbs to form a surface active film that stabilizes the lung are still not completely understood. Improved insights into the mechanisms by which surfactant lowers surface tension in the lung could lead both to superior "designer" surfactants and to improved applications of clinical management. Since the 1960s, it has generally been concluded that surfactant stabilizes the lung by generating a surface monolayer highly enriched in the disaturated lecithin, dipalmitoyl-*sn*-phosphatidylcholine (DPPC). More recently, new techniques and new approaches have combined to indicate that this paradigm is not only oversimplified, but may be flawed. As elaborated later, certain surfactant properties can best be explained in terms of multilayers rather than monolayers. In addition, it has become apparent that, under appropriate circumstances, the low surface tensions required to stabilize our terminal air spaces can be attained with unsaturated phosphatidylcholine (PC) in the absence of gel-phase disaturated phospholipids such as DPPC. This chapter attempts to clarify our current understanding of pulmonary surfactant compositional function *in vitro* and *in vivo*.

SURFACTANT COMPOSITION

Natural Pulmonary Surfactants

Surfactant can be isolated through bronchoalveolar lavage followed by centrifugation. Although some variation exists among species and with different disease states,[16-20] the composition given in Figure 101-1 for bovine surfactant is representative. Mammalian surfactants normally contain approximately 80 to 85% phospholipid, 5 to 10% neutral lipids, and 5 to 10% weight/weight–specific surfactant apoproteins. Phospholipid classes include PC approximately 80%, phosphatidylglycerol (PG) plus phosphatidylinositol 10 to 15%, and phosphatidylethanolamine 1 to 3%, with lesser amounts of sphingomyelin, lyso-*bis*-phosphatidic acid, and lyso-PC. The neutral lipid fraction includes cholesterol, cholesterol esters, diacylglycerol, triacylglycerol, and some free fatty acids.[18,20] The surfactant-associated proteins (SPs) consist of SP-A and SP-D, which are hydrophilic glycoproteins, and SP-B and SP-C, which are low

molecular weight hydrophobic proteins that dissolve with the lipids in organic solvents such as chloroform:methanol.[21-24]

Electrospray ionization mass spectroscopy and high-pressure liquid chromatography analyses have been used to estimate molecular species distribution of individual phospholipids in pulmonary surfactant for numerous animal species.[20,25,26] PC and PG molecular species for bovine surfactant are listed in Table 101-1. Such analyses show the PC fraction for different animal surfactants is high in DPPC (35 to 55%), with significant amounts (5 to 20%) of palmitoyl-myristoyl PC (PMPC), palmitoyl-palmitoleoyl PC (PPPC), palmitoyl-oleoyl PC (POPC), and palmitoyl-linoleoyl PC (PLPC). PG molecular species are high in palmitoyl-oleoyl-PG (POPG) (25 to 35%), with substantial amounts of dipalmitoyl-PG (DPPG) and palmitoyl-linoleoyl-PG (PLPG).

Surfactant Proteins

The SPs are described in detail in Chapter 100. In the human, SP-A is a 228-amino acid hydrophilic protein. As a result of glycosylation and other secondary modifications, apparent molecular weights of 28 to 36 kDa are observed with polyacrylamide gel electrophoresis under reducing conditions. SP-A contains four functional domains: a short N-terminal region involved in sulfhydryl-dependent oligomerization, a collagen-like region, a neck region that forms coiled-coil oligomers, and an approximately 130-amino acid C-terminal globular carbohydrate recognition domain.[27] SP-A forms trimers resulting from triple helical formation within the collagen-like domain, coiled-coil interactions within the neck region, and sulfhydryl-dependent and perhaps other interactions in the short N-terminal region. Furthermore, six of these triple-helix subunits combine to form a bouquet-like structure containing 18 monomers. Collagen consists of Gly-X-Y repeats where Y is often hydroxyproline. The collagen-like region of SP-A contains an extra amino acid that produces a kink in this structure. As a result of this kink, the collagenous region forms the stalks and stems of the bouquet. The C-terminal carbohydrate recognition domain forms structures resembling three-petaled flowers. The resulting oligomeric form is approximately 20 nm long and at its widest point is approximately 20 nm across.[28] Polyacrylamide gel electrophoresis of SP-A under nonreducing conditions shows that SP-A recovered from the alveolus is predominantly present as large oligomers of up to 640 kDa. SP-A is a member of the C-type lectin (carbohydrate-binding) superfamily, which contains mannose-binding protein and the collectins (*col*lagen-*lectins*).[27,29] SP-A binds lipids and is isolated with natural surfactant. Its role in the biophysical functions of surfactant is discussed in a later section.

SP-D also contains collagenous and calcium-dependent lectin domains, and like SP-A, is a member of the C-lectin superfamily.[21,30,31] As in the case of SP-A, the collagen-like and neck-like regions of SP-D promote trimerization. SP-D contains four of these trimers, which are bound at their N-terminus through disulfide bonds. The resulting structure of SP-D forms a cruciform oligomer consisting of 4 trimers in a total of 12 subunits. Some SP-D is present in larger oligomeric forms (6 to 8 trimers). Each monomer has a molecular weight of approximately 43 kDa, yielding an overall molecular weight of 500 kDa or more. SP-D does not bind to surfactant lipids as well as SP-A and is predominantly found in the supernatant arising after

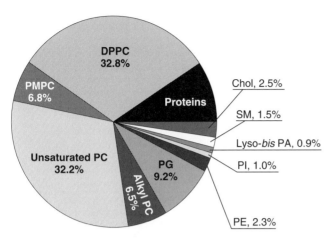

Figure 101–1. The composition of bovine pulmonary surfactant. Alkyl-PC = alkylphosphatidylcholine; Chol = cholesterol; DPPC = dipalmitoylphosphatidylcholine; PA = phosphatidic acid; PC = phosphatidylcholine; PE = phosphatidylethanolamine; PG = phosphatidylglycerol; PI = phosphatidylinositol; PMPC = palmitoylmyristoylphosphatidylcholine; SM = sphingomyelin. (Modified from Possmayer, F. et al. [1984] *Can J Biochem Cell Biol* 62 [11], 1121–1133; unpublished data courtesy of Dr. K. Rodriguez Capote.)

TABLE 101-1

Major Molecular Species for Phosphatidylcholine and Phosphatidylglycerol in Bovine Lipid Extract Surfactant Determined by Electrospray Ionization Spectrometry

Phosphatidylcholine (PC) molecular species	% Total
Palmitoyl, myristoyl-PC (16:0, 14:0)*	9.2±0.3
O-palmityl, palmitoyl-PC (16:0a,14:0)†	5.4±0.7
Palmitoyl, palmitoleoyl-PC (16:0, 16:1)	13.0±1.0
Palmitoyl, palmitoyl-PC (16:0, 16:0)	40.0±1.7
Palmitoyl, linoleoyl-PC (16:0, 18:2)	4.6±0.7
Palmitoyl, oleoyl-PC (16:0, 18:1)	22.8±1.0
Stearoyl, linoleoyl-PC (18:0, 18:2), plus oleoyl, oleoyl-PC (18:1, 18:1)	2.7±0.7
Stearoyl, oleoyl-PC (18:0, 18:1)	1.8±0.4

Phosphatidylglycerol (PG) molecular species	% Total
Palmitoyl, palmitoleoyl-PG (16:0, 16:1)	6.4±0.6
Palmitoyl, palmitoyl-PG (16:0, 16:0)	23.1±0.6
Palmitoyl, linoleoyl-PG (16:0, 18:2)	7.6±0.5
Palmitoyl, oleoyl-PG (18:0, 18:1)	48.2±3.4
Stearoyl, linoleoyl-PG (18:0, 18:2) plus oleoyl, oleoyl-PG (18:1, 18:1)	7.0±0.7
Stearoyl, oleoyl-PG (18:0, 18:1)	7.7±0.7

* Numerical representations for the fatty acyl groups are given in brackets.
† Alkyl, acyl-PC.
Unpublished data from Rodrigues Capote K, and Possmayer, F.

centrifugation of lung lavages. SP-D exhibits different lectin properties from SP-A and selectively binds phosphatidylinositol rather than DPPC. SP-D has a relatively weak biophysical role compared to SP-A. SP-A and SP-D have important roles in the innate host defense system.[21,32]

SP-B is a low molecular weight hydrophobic protein, 79 amino acids long, present in surfactant as a disulfide-dependent dimer of approximately 18 kDa. Mature SP-B is produced by N-terminal and C-terminal proteolytic processing of a larger proprotein of approximately 42 kDa.[33–38] SP-B is cysteine rich and is very basic (positively charged). The 18-kDa SP-B dimer appears to be a membrane-associated protein that binds to the surface of lipid bilayers.[24,35,39] SP-B deficiency arising from natural human mutations or deliberate gene disruption in mice results in neonatal respiratory distress leading to death.[10,24,40,41]

Pro–SP-C (approximately 21 kDa) is also proteolytically processed. Mature SP-C is present in surfactant as a monomer of 35 amino acids with a molecular weight of 4.2 kDa. SP-C is not only the most hydrophobic protein known, but it also contains two palmitic acid moieties that are acylated to two adjacent cysteine groups near the amino terminus. In some species, such as mink and canine, SP-C contains only one cysteine and therefore a single palmitate. SP-C has a short, 12-amino acid moderately hydrophilic N-terminal region, terminating in positively charged arginine and lysine groups. The remaining 23 amino acids form a hydrophobic α-helix composed primarily of aliphatic amino acids (leucine, isoleucine, and valine). This α-helix is of appropriate length to act as a membrane spanning domain.[24,42,43] SP-C appears to be unique in that no similar protein has yet been identified.

Therapeutic Surfactants

As indicated earlier, SP-B and SP-C can dissolve in organic solvents and are isolated with the lipids in lipid extracts of pulmonary surfactant. Organic solvent lipid extracts, containing SP-B and SP-C but not SP-A, are the basis of the so-called *second generation* clinical preparations. These surfactants should not be called "natural" or "animal" surfactants. Rather, they should be referred to as "modified natural" or "animal-based" surfactants,[44]

and, because of processing differences, such preparations are not equivalent.[1,13,45] Survanta, also known as Beractant (Abbott Laboratories, United States), Curosurf (Chiesi Pharmaceuticals, Italy), and HL-10 (Leo Pharmaceuticals, Denmark) are obtained from minced bovine or porcine (Curosurf) lung. Alveofact (Boehringer-Ingelheim, Germany), BLES (bovine lipid extract surfactant, BLES Biochemicals, Canada), and Infasurf, also referred to as CLSE (calf lung surfactant extract, Forest Laboratories, United States) are obtained by lavage or foaming (BLES) techniques. Infasurf is obtained from neonatal calves, whereas the other bovine preparations are from mature calves or adult cows. Because neutral lipids (mainly cholesterol) reduced the ability to attain low surface tensions during compression with the available techniques, they were removed from BLES, Curosurf, and Survanta. Survanta has very little SP-B compared with the other animal-based surfactants, but palmitic acid and tripalmitin are added to enhance surface film formation.[46–49] The available animal experimental literature would suggest that Infasurf promotes a faster and more effective response than Survanta, although one head-to-head clinical trial comparing these surfactants showed no difference in death or incidence of pneumothorax (air leak).[50]

In addition to these modified animal surfactants, two protein/peptide-based surfactants have been developed.[51] Surfaxin (Discovery Laboratories, United States) contains KL4 (a 21-amino acid peptide containing a series of 5 amino acid repeats, each with a lysine followed by 4 leucines), DPPC, dioleoyl-PC, and palmitic acid. Although designed to mimic SP-B, a surface membrane protein, KL4 acts as a transmembrane peptide.[52] Venticute (Byk Gulden Pharmaceuticals, Germany) contains recombinant human SP-C (rSP-C) produced in *Escherichia coli*, plus DPPC, dioleoyl-PC, and palmitic acid. Palmitic acid enhances phospholipid adsorption and can enhance the ability of these preparations to attain low surface tensions *in vitro*. However, the effectiveness of adding palmitate has been questioned because this fatty acid is taken up almost instantaneously by lung tissue.[53]

At least two artificial, wholly synthetic, protein-free surfactants, Pneumactant, also known as ALEC (artificial lung expanding compound, Britannia Pharmaceuticals, United Kingdom) and Exosurf (Burroughs-Wellcome, United States) are available. ALEC, which contains DPPC:POPG (7:3), was named for Dr. Alec Bangham of Cambridge, who developed this artificial preparation. Exosurf, developed by Dr. John A. Clements, a pioneer in the surfactant field, consists of DPPC, hexadecanol (a long chain alcohol that acts as a spreading agent), and tyloxapol, a detergent introduced to ensure consistent formulations. Clinical trials show that these surfactants have biologic activity with premature neonates, but the effects are slow compared with those of the lipid extract surfactants, a finding consistent with a secondary effect arising from phospholipid uptake and recycling by Type II cells.[51] Exosurf recovered from premature lungs possesses enhanced surface activity consistent with the equilibration with endogenous surfactant apoproteins.[54] Comparisons indicate that natural surfactant–based extracts are more effective than the wholly synthetic preparations in reducing death and morbidity.[2,55]

LUNG BIOLOGY OF PULMONARY SURFACTANT

The present view of the life cycle of pulmonary surfactant is depicted in Figure 101-2. Surfactant is produced in the Type II cells of the alveoli, assembled and stored in lamellar bodies.[56-61] These organelles are composed of a limiting membrane and concentric or parallel phospholipid lamellae apparently composed primarily of phospholipid bilayers. Lamellar bodies contain surfactant lipids, SP-B, and SP-C, but relatively low amounts of SP-A.[62-64] SP-A is also secreted from Type II cells via the normal constitutive secretory pathway, which bypasses lamellar bodies.[65] Once secreted into the alveolar hypophase, lamellar bodies interact with calcium and SP-A to form the unique structure known as *tubular myelin*.[56,59,66-68] Tubular myelin consists of long, rectangular, stacked tubes composed mainly of phospholipid bilayers. The corners of these tubes appear fused, giving cross-sections of tubular myelin a lattice-like appearance (Fig. 101-3). Tubular myelin–enriched surfactant fractions adsorb readily to form a film at the air-liquid interface, a finding suggesting that this structure acts as an important monolayer-generating source.[61,69] The surfactant monolayer is ultimately responsible for lowering surface tension at the air-liquid interface.

As described elsewhere, surfactant obtained through lung lavage (washing) can be separated into numerous fractions by density gradient or differential centrifugation. Two major fractions, known as large surfactant aggregates (LAs) and small surfactant aggregates (SAs), also known as heavy and light surfactant subtypes, are readily isolated.[61,70,71] The heavy LA subtype contains lamellar bodies, tubular myelin, and multilamellar vesicles of various sizes. The light subtype is composed mainly of small unilamellar vesicles. Time course studies conducted shortly after birth and pulse-labeling experiments have established that the small vesicles are metabolic products of the larger, heavier forms. These observations support the view that SAs, presumably generated from the surface film during repeated compression and expansion, represent spent surfactant in transit to the Type II cells. Surfactant lipids are taken up by Type II cells and are partially degraded, presumably by lysosomes, but they are also recycled into lamellar bodies. Considerable recycling of surfactant constituents occurs with newborn animals, and this feature likely explains in part the success of surfactant therapy for RDS. Certainly, without recycling, more frequent retreatment would be required. Compositional studies have shown the LA and SA surfactant subtypes exhibit similar phospholipid profiles, but only the heavier subtype possesses significant amounts of the surfactant apoproteins.[72,73] Not surprisingly, the heavier LA forms show superior surface activity.[74,75]

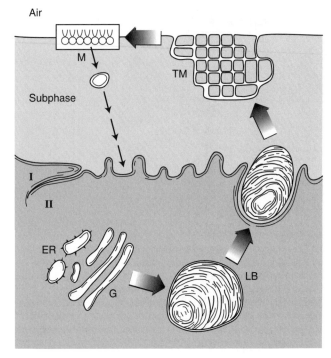

Figure 101–2. Diagrammatic representation of the biologic life cycle of pulmonary surfactant. Pulmonary surfactant is synthesized in Type II alveolar cells and assembled into lamellar bodies (LB). After exocytosis, lamellar bodies form tubular myelin (TM), which is thought to be a major source of the surface film. Tubular myelin consists of long rectangular hollow tubes composed of phospholipid bilayers that are fused together at the corners. A cross-sectional view with a lattice-like appearance is shown. Tubular myelin is thought to be the major source for phospholipid adsorption to create a film at the air-water interface. Although shown as a single monolayer (M), there is evidence of surfactant multilayers. The surface monolayer reduces surface tension. Vesicles formed from the surface during repeated compression and expansion are taken up by the Type II cells for degradation and recycling into lamellar bodies. I = Type I cell; II = Type II cell; ER = endoplasmic reticulum; G = Golgi apparatus. (From Possmayer, F. et al. [1984] *Can J Biochem Cell Biol* 62 [11], 1121-1133; modified from Goerke, J. [1974] *Biochim Biophys Acta* 344 [3-4], 241-261.)

SURFACE TENSION AND LUNG MECHANICS

Initial evidence of the importance of surface tension in pulmonary function was reported in 1929 by von Neergaard, who observed that a greater pressure difference was required to keep lungs inflated with air than with fluid.[76] Figure 101-4 presents data from a more recent pressure-volume relationship study on excised lungs.[77,78] When air is introduced stepwise into a lung, there is an initial modest increase in lung volume, followed by a more rapid elevation to total lung capacity. As the pressure difference is lowered, considerably more air remains in the lungs at any given pressure than during inflation. This is known as *hysteresis* (literally, "lagging behind"). Furthermore, at zero pressure, a new initial volume is obtained that is larger than the volume observed during the initial inflation. Filling the lung with saline eliminates surface tension forces. Under these circumstances, the lung expands readily and uniformly, and little hysteresis is observed.

This simple experiment permits us to draw three important conclusions. First, the work done against surface tension forces

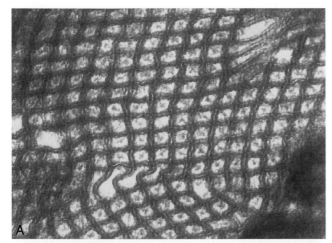

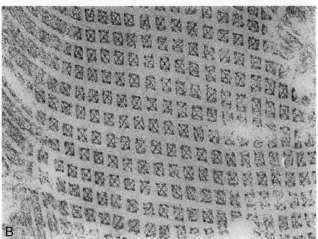

Figure 101–3. Tubular myelin. **A,** Electron micrograph showing cross-section of tubular myelin from bovine surfactant. Tubular myelin consists of fused tubes that, in this case, extend perpendicular to the plane of the image. The squares are approximately 50 nm across. **B,** Structures remaining after acetone washing to remove phospholipids. The X-shaped structures are thought to be surfactant-associated protein As that interact with the phospholipids via their carbohydrate recognition domains. (From Nag, K. et al. [1999] *J Struct Biol* 126 [1], 1-15.)

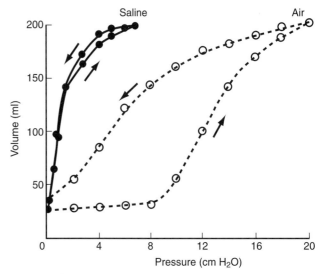

Figure 101–4. Pressure-volume relationships in cat lungs. Air filling (*open circles*): a considerable pressure is required before the lungs begin to expand to maximum volume. On deflation, the lung remains more open than during inflation. This effect is known as hysteresis. Some air is left in the lung at zero pressure. Saline filling (*closed circles*): the lung inflates from zero pressure to a similar maximum volume as with air. Little hysteresis is present during deflation. (From Clements, J.A. [1962] *Physiologist* 5 (1), 11-28, in Radford, E.P., Jr. [1957] In *Tissue Elasticity* (Remington, J.W., ed.), pp. 177-190, American Physiology Society.)

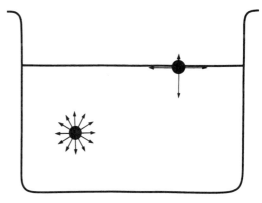

Figure 101–5. Diagrammatic representation of surface tension. A molecule of water within the bulk phase is attracted by all molecules surrounding it, but molecules of water at the surface experience a net attraction into the bulk phase (From Possmayer, F. et al. [1984] *Can J Biochem Cell Biol* 62 [11], 1121-1133.)

constitutes a major part of the effort required to inflate the lung.[76] Assuming that the pressure required to inflate the lung to half-maximal volume with air represents both surface forces and tissue elasticity, whereas the pressure needed to achieve this volume with saline functions primarily against tissue elasticity, it can be seen that more than two-thirds of the work can be accounted for by lung surface tension resistance. Second, the difference in the pressure-volume relationships during inflation and deflation indicates surface tension changes during this cycle. Finally, the observation that the air-filled lung retains some air on deflation suggests that surface tension must be low at low lung volumes.[77,79,80]

SURFACE TENSION

Surface tension arises from the attractive forces between molecules.[81-85] A molecule in the bulk phase is subject to attractive forces from the molecules around it, resulting in a net force of zero (Fig. 101-5). Molecules at the surface are attracted by the molecules below (and to either side) but in the upward direction

only by the weak attractive forces of water vapor and air. As a result, all the molecules at the surface experience a net attraction (downward) into the bulk phase. Work is required to move a molecule from its lower energy state in the bulk phase to the more energetic state at the surface. With water, the work or the energy required to move sufficient molecules to the surface to expand it by 1 cm² at 37°C is 70 mJ/cm² or 70 erg/cm². Because of the difference in energy of surface molecules, the most stable situation arises with a minimum surface area. This is why materials with high surface tension, such as water or mercury, form spherical droplets. One can also think of surface tension in terms of a thin elastic film of liquid at the surface that resists expansion (or works toward contraction) of the surface area. This may be more readily understood by considering a bubble blown in water. The pressure difference across the surface of such a bubble is described by the well-known Law of Young and Laplace:

$$\Delta P = 2\gamma / r \qquad [1]$$

where P = pressure in milliNewtons per meter squared (mN/m^2), r = the radius in meters, and γ = the surface tension in milliNewtons per meter (mN/m). Because of the attractive forces on molecules at the surface, there is a force or a tension in the surface film that resists expansion of the bubble and consequently acts to contract the surface area. This contractive force is known as the *surface tension* and has a value of 70 mN/m or 70 dyne/cm for water at 37°C (72 mN/m at 25°C).

Surface tension can be altered by the presence of a second substance in the liquid. Because of hydrogen bonding, water has a high γ. The γ of ethanol is less than that of water. With a water:ethanol solution, the water molecules interact less strongly with ethanol than with one another, and hydrogen bonding is reduced. Consequently, a molecule of ethanol at the surface of a water:ethanol solution will experience less attraction into the bulk phase than a water molecule. This replacement of some surface water with ethanol molecules results in a reduction in γ. The difference in attractive forces between surface molecules of water and ethanol results in a second effect. Because ethanol molecules at the surface experience less attraction into the bulk phase, there will be a small but definite net accumulation of ethanol molecules at the surface. The resulting increase in the surface concentration of ethanol generates slightly lower γs than would be predicted from the bulk concentrations. Conversely, the presence of substances such as sodium chloride in water produces a slight increase in γ, likely because water molecules have a stronger association to the sodium and chloride ions in the bulk phase. Therefore, water molecules require even more potential energy to attain the surface than with pure water.

The surface tension–reducing capacity of surfactant is the result of its phospholipid constituents. Phospholipids contain *hydrophilic* (water-attracting) polar head groups and *hydrophobic* (water-repelling) fatty acyl groups. Such molecules are known as *amphipathic* (literally, "feeling both ways"). Phospholipids are essentially insoluble, existing in aqueous dispersions as aggregates such as liposomes. Figure 101–6 shows a monomolecular film of PCs or "lecithins" spread at the air-liquid interface. Numerous different PC molecular species, with palmitate (16:0) at the sn-1 position but differing in the fatty acids at the sn-2 position of the glycerol moiety, are depicted (sn = stereospecific numbering). The polar phosphorylcholine groups interact with water, whereas the hydrophobic fatty acyl moieties

extend toward the air. Interactions between these molecules are weaker than the attractive interactions between water molecules. As in the case of ethanol, these lipids reduce γ by displacing water from the surface.

PC monolayers can be formed by spreading the lipids at the air-water interface using an organic solvent such as chloroform. As more phospholipid is spread, γ falls until a surface tension of approximately 23 mN/m is attained. Application of additional phospholipids will not decrease γ further. Although PC dispersions adsorb to form a monolayer relatively slowly, under appropriate conditions and with long time periods, γs of approximately 23 mN/m can be obtained. Because of the presence of the SPs, surfactant adsorbs quite rapidly, again to a final γ of approximately 23 mN/m. This value of approximately 23 mN/m is known as the *equilibrium surface tension* for phospholipid monolayers. At equilibrium surface tension the air-liquid interface can no longer spontaneously accept more phospholipid molecules (i.e., the surface is "saturated" with phospholipid). The precise equilibrium surface tension depends on the composition of the film and the temperature, but 23 mN/m is used for discussion purposes.

Dry or partially hydrated DPPC crystals placed on a water surface or mixed as a dispersion will spread to form a monolayer, again to a final equilibrium surface tension of 23 mN/m. It appears that as the DPPC head groups become fully hydrated, they can either remain at the surface, where they spread to form a monolayer, or they can form vesicles with other hydrated DPPC molecules. The rate of monolayer formation from DPPC increases manyfold at 41°C.[86-89] This temperature dependence of monolayer formation can be understood by considering bilayer structure, which is the molecular basis of biologic membranes (Fig. 101–7). As hydrated DPPC bilayers are heated, the palmitic acids change from a relatively ordered state in which all carbon-carbon bonds are extended in the all-*trans* configuration to a disordered fluid state in which some of the carbon bonds are in the *gauche* configuration. Below the critical transition temperature (T_c) of 41°C, the acyl groups are packed together in a regular pattern, and the phospholipid molecules are relatively motionless, although they may rotate in an axis roughly perpendicular to the bilayer. At T_c, the fatty acyl groups gain sufficient thermal energy, so the ordered acyl chains start to move and become disordered and fluid (i.e., the chains "melt"). The individual phospholipid molecules become more mobile, allowing them to diffuse rapidly relative to one another in their plane of the bilayer.

It is clear from cell biology studies that membrane fluidity is essential for life. Membrane lipids possess high proportions of phospholipids with unsaturated phospholipids at their sn-2 position. As can be seen from Figure 101–6, double bonds introduce a kink in the fatty acid. This reduces the ability of

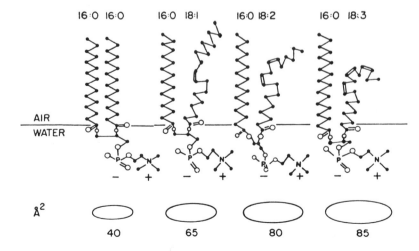

16:0 16:0   16:0 18:1   16:0 18:2   16:0 18:3

AIR
WATER

$Å^2$

40   65   80   85

Figure 101–6. Orientation of various molecular species of phosphatidylcholine (PC) at the air-water interface. The hydrophobic fatty acyl groups extend into the air, whereas the hydrophilic polar phosphorylcholine groups interact with water via their positive and negative charges. Because of kinks at the double bonds, PCs with unsaturated fatty acids occupy a larger average molecular size, as indicated by *ovals* below the molecules. Unsaturated PCs cannot pack as well as dipalmitoylphosphatidylcholine, the molecule on the extreme *left*. (From Possmayer, F. et al. [1984] *Can J Biochem Cell Biol* 62 [11], 1121–1133.)

the phospholipid to pack closely in monolayers or bilayers. Consequently, T_c for phospholipids containing unsaturated fatty acids is much lower than for saturated phospholipids with fatty acids of similar length. Reducing the chain length of saturated fatty acids also lowers T_c. The concept of ordered and fluid fatty acyl chains is important for understanding the principles involved in alveolar stabilization as explained in the next section.

In summary, surface tension arises from the difference in attractive forces on molecules at an interface. The term *surface tension* is applied to air-liquid interfaces; *interfacial tension* is used for other interfaces. Molecules at a surface possess excess potential energy relative to molecules in the bulk phase. All the molecules at the surface experience an attraction into the bulk phase. This force is perpendicular to the surface. Clearly, the most stable situation arises with a minimum surface area. This is why water and mercury form droplets. One can think of γ in terms of the work required to expand the surface area. One can also consider γ in terms of an elastic film of surface molecules, in which the attraction of molecules into the bulk phase resists expansion and works toward minimizing surface area. This contractile force produces a pressure difference across bubbles or alveoli, which is equal to twice the surface tension divided by the radius (law of Young and Laplace; Equation 1). The surface tension of water at 37°C is 70 mN/m.

A monolayer of phospholipids at the air-liquid interface (see Fig. 101-6) lowers γ by replacing water at the surface. Phospholipids are amphipathic molecules possessing hydrophilic polar head groups and hydrophobic fatty acyl chains. Phospholipids such as PC are essentially insoluble in water and readily form lipid bilayers, which are the structural basis of biologic membranes. The gel-to-liquid crystalline T_c marks the temperature at which the fatty acyl groups in a bilayer change from an ordered state to a disordered fluid state (see Fig. 101-7). Membrane fluidity is essential for membrane processes compatible with life. Below T_c, PC forms monolayers either from crystals placed at the surface or from dispersions in the bulk phase at an extremely slow rate. T_c is lowered by reducing the acyl chain length or introducing double bonds. Mixing DPPC, which has a T_c of 41°C, with unsaturated phospholipids reduces T_c and allows increased adsorption at 37°C.[90-93] However, such adsorption is still insufficient to stabilize the alveoli.

The equilibrium surface tension of 23 mN/m is attained when all available sites at the air-water interface are "fully" occupied by PCs. Equilibrium surface tension is the lowest γ that can be achieved by spreading sufficient phospholipid on the surface with an organic solvent. A similar γ is achieved when natural surfactant, which adsorbs rapidly, is injected below the subphase. Under equilibrium conditions, phospholipids cannot spontaneously enter the monolayer unless a similar amount of phospholipid leaves the surface.

REDUCTION OF SURFACE TENSION BY PULMONARY SURFACTANT

An important physicochemical difference exists between soluble and insoluble surface films. The γ of a bubble blown in a 50% ethanol solution is 30 mN/m. (The surface concentration of ethanol is slightly higher than the bulk concentration.) Increasing the bubble size does not affect γ because ethanol molecules are soluble and move into the surface film almost instantaneously. Likewise, reducing the bubble surface area does not affect the surface concentration of ethanol or γ. However, phospholipid films are insoluble, and reducing the size of the bubble leads to lateral compression of the monolayer. Slow *dynamic* (in the sense of continuous) *lateral compression* of the PC film depicted in Figure 101-6 results in closer packing of the surface phospholipids and a fall in γ because the phospholipid molecules are forced closer to one another and more water is excluded from the surface. However, phospholipid films such as that in Figure 101-6, which contain a high proportion of unsaturated fatty acids, are not very stable at 37°C. Because of the fluid nature of the fatty acids, such films can withstand limited dynamic compression only to a γ of approximately 20 mN/m.[85, 94-96] Further reduction in surface area does not produce a concomitant reduction in γ, but it results in the expulsion of PCs from the two-dimensional monolayer (into a collapse phase of uncertain structure). With dynamic compression, γ can be driven slightly below equilibrium, but when dynamic compression ceases (i.e., surface area is held constant), γ returns to its equilibrium state. This increase in γ is thought to arise from loss of unsaturated PC molecules from the surface, thereby relieving the strain resulting from film overcompression. Such molecules can form bilayer structures such as vesicles, which are lost from the surface. However, as discussed later, it is clear that, especially with surfactant, some of the lipid material can remain associated with the surface monolayer.

In contrast to unsaturated PCs, films of DPPC are quite stable at 37°C and can be compressed until γ approaches 0 mN/m. This film stability is attributed to the ability of the saturated palmitic acids to pack closely, thus allowing the DPPC molecules to organize into a highly ordered, two-dimensional surface gel at this temperature. Experimental evidence of the differences in the physicochemical properties of gel and fluid phospholipid monolayers is outlined in Figure 101-8, which depicts the effects of compressing DPPC (see Fig. 101-8*A*) or 1-stearoyl, 2-oleoyl-PC (SOPC) (see Fig. 101-8*B*) monolayers on a Langmuir-Wilhelmy surface balance (see Fig. 101-8*C*). The Langmuir-Wilhelmy surface balance introduced by John Clements[79] provided some of the first direct experimental evidence of pulmonary surfactant. Figure 101-8*A* shows a so-called *compression isotherm* (i.e., compression at constant temperature) for DPPC monolayers spread at low surface concentration with organic solvent, which is then allowed to evaporate. Compressing the film from "lift off," the point on the right side of the graph at which a significant decrease in γ is first noted, results in a slow progressive decrease in γ. At a certain point (γ ~60 mN/m [70% surface area] for the curve at 25°C), there is a sharp decrease in slope. This leads to a slowly increasing plateau, which then curves upward as surface area is reduced further. As the monolayer is compressed still further, surface tension falls to approximately 0 mN/m, at which the DPPC monolayer collapses. At 37°C, because of increased mobility of the acyl groups, greater compression is required to reach the initial plateau, but the curves become identical as γ declines.

This DPPC isotherm contrasts with that for SOPC, which has a T_c of 6°C. With this unsaturated PC at 37°, the gradual plateau at

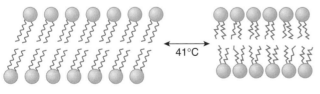

41°C

Gel-crystalline   Liquid-crystalline

Figure 101-7. Diagrammatic representation of the phase transition from the gel-crystalline to the liquid-crystalline state of a bilayer of dipalmitoylphosphatidylcholine (DPPC). The hydrophobic palmitates interact together, and the polar phosphorylcholine groups interact with the water. At 41°C, the acyl groups gain sufficient thermal energy to twist, rotate, and move laterally. This "fluidity" permits the individual DPPC molecules to diffuse relative to one another while remaining in the same leaflet.

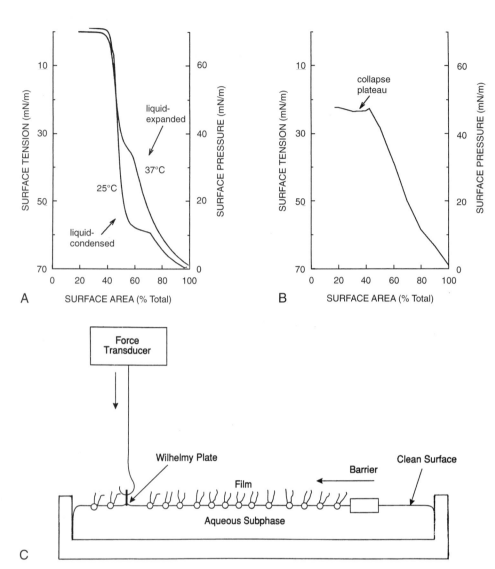

Figure 101–8. Effect of compression on surface tension of a dipalmitoylphosphatidylcholine (DPPC) monolayer or a monolayer of 1-stearoyl, 2-oleoylphosphatidylcholine (SOPC) on a Langmuir-Wilhelmy surface balance. **A,** Surface tension/surface pressure relationship for DPPC monolayers at 25° and 37°C. The liquid-expanded (LE) and liquid-condensed (LC) phase regions are indicated. Because of thermal agitation at 37°C, the liquid-expanded region extends to a lower γ (higher surface pressure). Surface tensions of approximately 0 mN/m are attained with both monolayers at approximately 50% original area. **B,** Surface tension/surface pressure versus area curve for SOPC at 37°C. Only the liquid-expanded state is observed, before the collapse point is attained at approximately 45% surface area reduction. Further surface area reduction results in a collapse plateau at which surface tension is not lowered further. **C,** Diagrammatic representation of a Langmuir-Wilhelmy surface balance. The barrier is used to compress the film. The Wilhelmy plate is used to monitor surface tension. (A and C, Modified from Goerke, J. and Clements, J.A. [1986] In *Handbook of Physiology, Section 3: The Respiratory System* [Vol. III, Part 1] [Fishman, A.P., ed.], pp. 247–261, American Physiological Society. B, Modified from Hawco, M.W. et al. [1981] *J Appl Physiol* 51 [2], 509–515.)

low γ is not observed (see Fig. 101–8*B*). Furthermore, it is apparent that SOPC monolayers cannot withstand sufficient lateral pressure to lower the surface tension to very low levels. At approximately 20 mN/m, further compression squeezes SOPC molecules out of the monolayer into a collapse phase. The lowest surface tension attained (~20 mN/m) is only slightly below the equilibrium surface tension of 23 mN/m. Electron microscopic studies indicate that compressed DPPC monolayers near 0 mN/m are relatively solid and collapse as structures resembling small ice floe sheets as the barrier progresses near 0 mN/m. SOPC monolayers collapsing at γ approximately 20 mN/m appear more like fluid pools.[97]

The behavior of DPPC and SOPC monolayers can be readily understood in terms of the generalized phase diagram for phospholipids below T_c depicted in Figure 101-9. The interpretation of such curves is based on extensive work with fatty alcohols and fatty acids, as well as phospholipids.[89, 98-102] At low surface concentrations, DPPC molecules act as a two-dimensional gas and have no discernible effect on γ. As surface area decreases to approximately 120 Å²/molecule, the DPPC molecules interact with each other such that they become more erect. This marks the *liquid-expanded* (LE) state, which continues to approximately 80 Å², at which some of the molecules become compressed into

the *liquid-condensed* (LC) state, giving rise to an LE/LC coexistence plateau. As more of the LE molecules become tightly packed and assume the LC state, γ decreases more rapidly with surface area reduction. This continues until γ approaches 0 mN/m at approximately 40 Å², at which the monolayer acts like a solid LC gel. Because SOPC at 37°C is far above T_c, only the LE phase is observed during monolayer compression, and the monolayer collapses near equilibrium surface tension. Below its T_c of 6°C, SOPC can be compressed to low γs.[95] It has been suggested that, at high compression, DPPC monolayers can be transformed to a more tightly packed LC solid state by altering head group orientation to create less tilt in the molecules, but this is controversial.[99, 100, 103]

Our appreciation of the molecular interactions occurring during monolayer compression has been greatly improved by the development of fluorescence imaging microscopy, Brewster angle microscopy, and atomic force microscopy. DPPC films in the LE/LC coexistence plateau can be examined directly on the monolayer to reveal kidney bean–shaped LC condensed structures as dark probe-excluding regions with fluorescence imaging microscopy and thickened monolayer regions with Brewster angle microscopy. Such structures can also be observed on *Langmuir-Blodgett films* deposited from the monolayer as elevated regions using atomic force microscopy (Fig. 101-10).

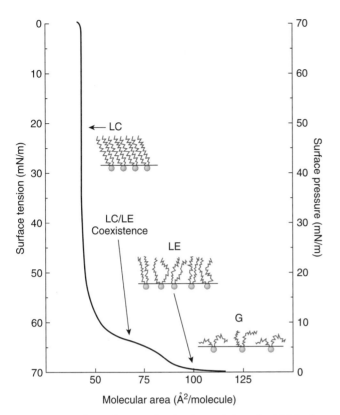

Figure 101–9. Phase diagram for dipalmitoylphosphatidylcholine showing a diagrammatic representation of the gaseous phase (G), the liquid-expanded (LE) phase, the LE:LC coexistence plateau, and the liquid-condensed (LC) phase. (Modified from Kaganer, V.M. et al. [1999] *Rev Modern Phys* 71, 779–819.).

Although the kidney bean structure in Figure 101–10A is obviously an LC gel-phase structure, some explanation is needed for the BLES floral-shaped structure in Figure 101–10B. This is also an LC gel-phase structure that arises through segregation (i.e., phase separation) of the gel-phase phospholipids DPPC and DPPG. Fluid constituents remain in the LE phase.[104-106] The kidney bean shape of the DPPC LC structures (see Fig. 101–10A) and the floral shape of the BLES LC structures (see Fig. 101–10B) observed using atomic force microscopy arise through line tension, which is the two-dimensional equivalent of surface tension. Water and mercury form spherical droplets because of high surface tension (large interfacial tension between air and water). A high line tension would cause the shape of the domain to be spherical.[102] In fact, this occurs with CLSE, which has cholesterol. DPPC and BLES domains have low line tensions between LE and LC, and as a result, their domains take up a longer perimeter.

The manner in which surfactant films benefit the lung can be considered in terms of both high lateral surface pressure and low surface tension. High surface pressure resists decreases in alveolar surface area by acting as a monomolecular surface "splint." Low surface tensions stabilize the lung by reducing the pressure gradient across the alveolar lining layer. This may also function to reduce transudation of interstitial fluid into alveolar spaces.[107,108] Surface pressure is related to surface tension by Equation 2, which states that the surface pressure, π, is equal to the surface tension of a clean surface (γ_o) minus the surface tension of the surface containing the film (γ):

$$\pi = \gamma_o - \gamma \qquad [2]$$

It should be evident from this equation that applying a lateral pressure on a monolayer produces a corresponding decrease in surface tension. For historical reasons, surfactant specialists normally express this kind of information as surface tension (left axis in Fig. 101–8A, B), whereas physical chemists normally use surface pressure (right axis). As indicated earlier, films compressed to surface tensions below equilibrium[82,84,109,110] (23 mN/m for phospholipids) are no longer in thermodynamic equilibrium and are theoretically capable of returning to their equilibrium surface tension by shedding molecules from the compressed monolayer. However, although inherently metastable, films containing a high proportion of DPPC can remain at surface tensions near 0 mN/m for long periods (i.e., many minutes). This is more than sufficient to stabilize the alveoli during breathing.

As discussed further later, it is clear that the surface tension of the alveolar lining layer *in vivo* falls to values very near 0 mN/m during expiration. This low surface tension is important for stabilizing the alveoli and preventing their collapse. Such low surface tensions could not be achieved experimentally through compression of fluid phospholipid films such as those with compositions similar to that of pulmonary surfactant on Langmuir-Wilhelmy balances (see Fig. 101–8C). This led to the concept that the alveolar surface lining must be covered by a film highly enriched in DPPC, which is the major tenet of the classical model mentioned at the beginning of this chapter.[48,49,107,109-113] Because removing surfactant from the lung disrupts the surface film, this enrichment could not be directly measured by chemical analysis but was inferred from physical measurements. It is generally held that the fluid lipid components could contribute to the surfactant adsorption, which is very slow at 37°C for DPPC. However, DPPC:unsaturated phospholipid mixtures adsorb relatively slowly in the absence of surfactant apoproteins. The fluid lipid constituents could also be important for the transport of surfactant components within the Type II cells and for secretion of lamellar bodies.

In summary, phospholipids are amphipathic molecules that contain hydrophilic polar head groups and hydrophobic acyl chains. Amphipathic molecules form insoluble monolayers in which surface concentration can be increased by dynamic lateral compression. Dynamic compression can be exerted by a barrier, as with the Langmuir-Wilhelmy surface balance (see Fig. 101–8C). Lateral compression also increases when the surface area of a bubble (or an alveolus) is reduced by decreasing the volume. In either case, the resulting increase in the surface concentration of the amphipathic molecules produces a decrease in γ.

Dynamic compression of DPPC monolayers results in highly ordered, closely packed, gel-like LC films. Compressed DPPC monolayers can reduce γs to near 0 mN/m. Furthermore, such monolayers can remain at low γs for long periods (i.e., these films are very stable). In contrast, monolayers composed of phospholipids with bilayer gel to liquid-crystalline T_cs significantly lower than 37°C cannot be compressed to low surface tensions with conventional balances at biologic temperatures. Such fluid films collapse at surface tensions only slightly below their equilibrium tension of approximately 23 mN/m and tend to return to equilibrium once dynamic compression ceases.[114-117]

It can be shown that the surface pressure of a monolayer is equal to the surface tension of the clean surface minus the surface tension of the surface containing the film (see Equation 2). For water, which has a surface tension of 70 mN/m at 37°C, surface pressure can vary from 0 mN/m (clean surface) to near 70 mN/m (corresponds to a surface tension of 0 mN/m).

ROLE OF SURFACTANT IN ALVEOLAR STABILITY

Theoretical calculations based on measurements of transpulmonary pressure and morphologic considerations with normal and saline-filled lungs indicate that surface tension varies during lung inflation and deflation and falls to very low values during expiration.[77,79,118-120] Studies in detergent-rinsed and fluorocarbon-filled lungs, in which surface tension is altered by the

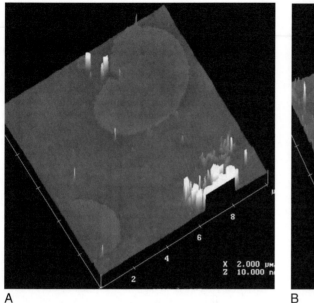 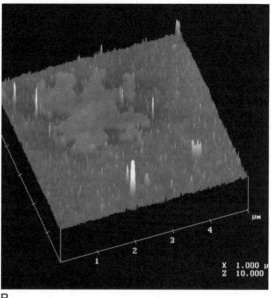

A   B

Figure 101–10. Atomic Force Microscopy images of dipalmitoylphosphatidylcholine (DPPC) (**A**) and bovine lipid extract surfactant (BLES) (**B**) monolayers in the liquid-expanded (LE):liquid-condensed (LC) coexistence region. The kidney bean–shaped LC structure in **A** is aproximately 6 μm long and extends approximately 1.2 nm above the plane of the LE phase. The BLES LC structure in **B** is approximately 7 nm long and is floral shaped. It extends approximately 1.7 nm above the LE phase. The nature of the small spikes in the *insert* is not known. SP-A = surfactant-associated protein A. (Unpublished data from Nag, K., Peterson, N., and Possmayer, F.)

remaining detergent or fluorocarbon, support the view of low alveolar surface tension.

More direct evidence was obtained by Samuel Schürch and his co-workers[119, 122-125] by monitoring the spreading properties of fluorocarbon or silicone oil test droplets deposited on the lung's alveolar surfaces *in situ*.[119,122-125] Such droplets spread to form a thin lens when surface tension of the droplet is similar to that of the underlying phase. When surface tension of the underlying substrate is lower than the test droplet, the droplet adopts a more nearly spherical shape (this is the reason water forms droplets on Teflon-coated materials). Calibration of the test droplets with DPPC monolayers on the Langmuir-Wilhelmy surface balance allowed precise estimation of the surface tension of the alveolar lining layer *in situ*. These microdroplet studies revealed that lung volume alterations corresponding to quiet breathing (e.g., between 40 and 50% total lung capacity) were associated with only modest increases in γ from 1 to 5 mN/m. Large inflations to total lung capacity resulted in alveolar surface tensions of approximately 30 mN/m, slightly higher than the equilibrium value of 23 mN/m. When lung volume was reduced to functional residual capacity, which is 40% of total lung capacity, γ fell to less than 1 mN/m. Furthermore, when the lung was held at this volume, surface tension remained at this low value for several minutes before increasing gradually. Even after 1 hour, γ at functional residual capacity remained at less than 10 mN/m. These measurements showed that the surface film covering the alveolar lining layer is very stable in the sense that it returns to equilibrium surface tension only very slowly. This property would minimize pressure differences between small and large alveoli and would prevent collapse of the smaller units. These observations reinforced the view that the endogenous surface monolayer must be highly enriched with DPPC and were considered consistent with the classical model of surfactant function.

The functional significance of the presence of a lipid-protein complex capable of generating low surface tensions within the lungs can be readily demonstrated through surfactant supplementation of surfactant-deficient lungs. Treatment of prematurely delivered rabbit fetuses of 27 days' gestation (term, 31 days) with natural or lipid extract surfactant increases survival. Surfactant administra-

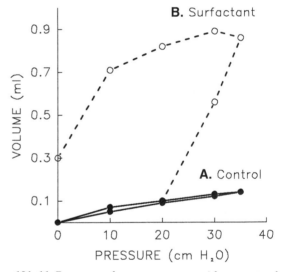

Figure 101–11. Pressure-volume maneuvers with prematurely delivered rabbit fetuses of 27 days' gestation (term, 31 days). Control inflation (*A, closed circles*) shows little increase in lung volume or hysteresis. Lipid extract surfactant administration (*B, open circles*) results in a marked increase in lung volume and prominent hysteresis. (Data from Metcalfe, I.L. et al. [1982] *J Appl Physiol* 53 [4], 838–843.)

tion results in a four- to fivefold increase in inflation during pressure-volume loops (Fig. 101–11)[126-128] (see Chap. 106). Similar observations have been made with prematurely delivered fetuses of other species and with adult lungs made surfactant deficient through lavage. Administration of lipid mixtures similar to those present in surfactant has little immediate effect. This finding emphasizes the role of the SPs in surfactant function.[1,49,51,129]

Studies in which surfactant-deficient animals or prematurely delivered infants are treated with natural or lipid extract surfactants *in vivo* prove more difficult to interpret but clearly indicate increased compliance resulting in an increase in lung volume.[1,126,130] Clinically, this can readily be monitored by a rapid increase in arterial oxygen tension, a finding indicating enhanced gaseous exchange.[131] Studies by Bachofen and Schürch[121] would indicate that, in addition to promoting lung expansion, surface tension reduction of the alveolar lining layer influences lung alveolar morphology. At low lung volumes, alveolar septa are elongated, thereby maximizing alveolar surface area. At high surface tensions of 20 to 30 mN/m, these septa are contracted through extensive folding, resulting in 30 to 50% decreases in alveolar surface area. The combined abilities of surfactant to increase compliance and optimize alveolar surface area would appear to explain the rapid (<30-minute) increases in gaseous exchange often noted on treatment of surfactant-deficient infants and would have important implications for ARDS.

TECHNIQUES FOR INVESTIGATING SURFACTANT FUNCTION

Discussion of the mechanisms involved in surfactant function requires a brief introduction into the technical approaches used and their limitations.

Langmuir-Wilhelmy Balance

The Langmuir-Wilhelmy surface balance illustrated earlier (see Fig. 101–8C) is an excellent tool for examining spread films because film composition and the amount of material deposited can be controlled accurately.[49,132] This approach is readily combined with other techniques such as fluorescence imaging, Brewster angle microscopy, and grazing angle x-ray diffraction. By drawing mica sheets, glass slides, or cover slips perpendicular to the plane of the film, one can deposit *Langmuir-Blodgett films,* which are useful for atomic force microscopy, time-of-flight secondary ion mass spectroscopy, or autoradiography. Because of the large subphase, the Langmuir-Wilhelmy approach is not convenient for studying adsorbed films. Temperature control at 37°C is difficult. Compression rates can be altered, but experimentally productive compression and expansion rates are limited. In addition, Langmuir-Wilhelmy studies require considerable expertise and scrupulous cleanliness, and they take a long time to conduct. However, the major limitation of the Langmuir-Wilhelmy balance studies is that it has become apparent that, at the high surface pressures required to generate γs approaching 0 mN/m (values critical for surfactant function *in vivo*), film material "creeps" onto the Teflon barriers and walls.[115,133] This difficulty is particularly problematic with spread monolayers containing cholesterol and becomes more significant at physiologic temperatures. This situation is often referred to as "leakage" because frank film leakage did occur with early balance studies before Teflon tapes were introduced.

Pulsating Bubble Surfactometer

The pulsating bubble surfactometer (PBS), introduced by G. Enhorning,[134,135] is an artificial alveolus model. The key component is a small cuvette in which a bubble communicating with the atmosphere is drawn into the surfactant suspension to be tested.[49,85,132,136] This device can be thought of as a bubble on a tube model. With the commercial version of this apparatus, the pulled bubble diameter is maintained for 10 seconds to measure adsorption and then is pulsated at 20 cycles/minute with 50% surface area change. Bubble radius and the pressure difference across the bubble are recorded. Using the law of Young and Laplace (see Equation 1), a microchip controls bubble radius and generates γ at a minimum and maximum radius.

An important feature of the PBS is that it monitors surface activity at compression rates and ratios comparable to those in the alveolus *in vivo*. In practice, the Enhorning PBS is an easily

learned, rapid method for testing small (~25 µL) surfactant samples at 37°C for physiologically important parameters. It is therefore superb as a screening device, especially for animal or clinical samples. An apparent disadvantage is that, at γs approximating zero, the bubble tends to flatten, thus losing its spherical shape. This can affect calculation of γ, although the error appears to be small. In any case, γ is clearly quite low.[136] The major difficulty is that it has become apparent that some fluid can remain in the capillary when the bubble is created. This produces a variable increase in effective surface area.[137] This effect would be particularly serious for samples containing hydrophilic nonsurfactant proteins, for example in inhibitory studies. As with the Langmuir-Wilhelmy balance, leakage can occur in which material creeps up the polyacrylamide capillary. This leakage limits the usefulness of the PBS for mechanistic studies, although it is very useful for monitoring surfactant effectiveness.

Captive Bubble Tensiometer

The captive bubble tensiometer (CBT) or surfactometer combines many of the advantages of the Langmuir-Wilhelmy balance with those of the PBS. With this device, introduced by S. Schürch,[119,133,138] an air bubble is introduced into the surfactant sample in an air-tight chamber where it floats up to a hydrophilic agar ceiling. The agar gel is highly hydrated and so cannot accept phospholipid material from the adsorbed film. Film leakage appears to be negligible. The CBT can be used to study adsorption, after which quasistatic or dynamic compression and expansion curves can be generated by increasing and decreasing pressure in the chamber. Surface area and surface tension are obtained from bubble shape, which is recorded with a video camera.[139]

The original CBT designed by Schürch used an air-tight syringe. More recent versions using gas-type plastic cuvettes have been introduced that are convenient for film spreading experiments. With such studies, it is important to change the subphase numerous times to remove the organic spreading solvent. Although both experiments and analysis with the CBT are slow, the availability of an apparently leak-proof system for studying surfactant at any temperature is an important advantage. This device has proved pivotal in studies challenging the classical model for surfactant function.

ROLE OF SURFACTANT-ASSOCIATED PROTEINS IN THE PHYSICOCHEMICAL FUNCTIONS OF PULMONARY SURFACTANT

As indicated by the law of Young and Laplace (see Equation 1) the pressure difference across an alveolus is inversely related to the radius. If the surface tension in the alveolus were 70 mN/m, the surface tension of water at 37°C, the pressure difference across the alveolus would be considerable, promoting alveolar instability. The mechanical properties of the lung suggest that the alveoli are covered with a phospholipid monolayer highly enriched in DPPC. However, at less than the bilayer T_c of 41°C, DPPC adsorbs and spreads only slowly at the air-liquid interface.[87-91, 109, 140, 141] Thus, considered in terms of the classical model, the situation faced by the lung is that surfactant must contain fluid lipids and other substances (i.e., apoproteins) that facilitate rapid adsorption and spreading of DPPC without interfering with the ability of this disaturated phospholipid to reduce the surface tension to near 0 mN/m when the surface film is under dynamic compression during expiration.

In vitro studies indicate that surfactant apoproteins augment the surface activity of surfactant lipids in three distinct ways. First, they promote adsorption and spreading of surfactant lipids at the air-water interface. This forms a surface-active film that lowers γ toward equilibrium. Second, SPs modify the properties of the surface film and facilitate its ability to attain low surface tensions near 0 mN/m during film compression. Third, SPs enhance respreading or reinsertion of phospholipids from collapse phase.

Adsorption

The processes by which phospholipids adsorb (i.e., form surface-active films) at the air-water interface is poorly understood. Long chain molecules such as phospholipids have very low critical micellar concentrations. The critical micellar concentration for DPPC of approximately 10^{-10} mol/L[109] means that DPPC in excess of this low concentration forms aggregates. The tendency of phospholipids to form aggregates arises from the so-called *hydrophobic effect*, which states that the high energetic cost of water:hydrocarbon interactions drives lipids to adopt specific aggregate forms in which water:fatty acid contact is minimized. Phospholipids such as saturated PC and unsaturated PC are shaped like cylinders with similar diameters for the polar head group and the hydrophobic diacylglycerol moieties.[142] Hydration of phospholipid films dried on the walls of a test tube with water or saline above T_c results in the formation of planar bilayer sheets that minimize water:hydrocarbon contact. If these sheets had ends (i.e., if the structures remained *open*), water:hydrocarbon interactions would still occur. However, such sheets curve to produce vesicles (also known as liposomes), which are *closed* structures. Depending on the preparative conditions, multilamellar vesicles of various sizes are generated, but in each case the structures are closed, engulfing some of the aqueous phase. Below T_c, hydration proceeds very slowly. This is why it is often stated that DPPC alone cannot be an effective pulmonary surfactant. Introducing short chain phospholipids, unsaturated phospholipids (which have low T_cs), or cholesterol will decrease T_c of the mixture. In each case, the resulting vesicles are closed structures. Applying energy in the form of ultrasound using bath or probe sonicators will convert multilamellar vesicles into smaller unilamellar vesicles. This results in an increase in the surface area of the vesicle available for adsorptive processes, as reviewed by Hope and colleagues.[142]

In view of the foregoing considerations, it should not be surprising that surfactant film formation is thought to proceed not through individual phospholipid molecules, but through mechanisms whereby vesicles interacting with the surface rapidly donate many of their phospholipids to the interface. Observations by Schürch and co-workers[143] indicate that the porcine lipid extract surfactant Curosurf adsorbs in discrete, sudden bursts, corresponding to approximately 10^{14} phospholipid molecules.[143] This finding suggests a cooperative mechanism whereby film formation involves the collective transport of subphase material into the surface film. The collective transport of large amounts of lipid into the surface monolayer does not imply that all the lipids in a particular surface vesicle will become incorporated into the monolayer. As elaborated later, it has become evident that considerable amounts of lipid can remain associated with the monolayer as functional multilayers.

Phospholipid Adsorption

Studies of surfactant phospholipid adsorption are considered both in the absence and in the presence of surfactant apoproteins. Phospholipid adsorption characteristics change dramatically at the bilayer transition temperature T_c. Below T_c, dried phospholipid films hydrate extremely slowly, and, as a result, DPPC alone fails to generate surface-active films at physiologic temperatures lower than the T_c of 41°C. In addition, vesicles of saturated PCs prepared from above their T_c adsorb very slowly below their T_c. This rate increases slowly as a function of temperature and increases markedly once T_c is attained. For example, DPPC vesicles (prepared above 41°C) at 1.0 mmol/L do not attain equilibrium in 15 minutes below 41°C, but they

achieve equilibrium in approximately 1.5 minutes at all temperatures above T_c.[140] Likewise, dimyristoyl PC vesicles prepared above the T_c of 23.5°C attain equilibrium at significant rates only at this temperature or higher. DPPC adsorption at 37°C can be enhanced by addition of fluid-phase phospholipids such as unsaturated PC, unsaturated phosphatidylethanolamine, unsaturated phosphatidylinositol, or unsaturated PG, which lowers T_c of the mixture below 41°C.[84, 144, 145] PG is particularly effective in increasing DPPC adsorption.[146] Dialkyl phosphono analogues of DPPC, which are diethers rather than diacyl phospholipids, adsorb more readily than DPPC.[147]

It has long been thought that cholesterol present in mammalian surfactant at 2 to 10% weight/weight (which corresponds to 8 to 20 mole%) could play a critical role in surfactant phospholipid adsorption. In this context, it has been known for some time that cholesterol interacts with saturated PC, sphingomyelin, and sphingoid-based glycolipids to form a liquid-ordered L_o phase, which possesses properties between LE and LC.[148,149] This distinct liquid-ordered phase is the physicochemical basis of membrane rafts and caveolae, plasma membrane (and likely other cellular membrane) structures with numerous important roles, including cell signaling.[150, 151] As mentioned earlier, cholesterol is removed from Curosurf and BLES and is not included in any of the current artificial synthetic surfactants. At present, no distinct physiologic functions or advantages can be attributed to this sterol in replacement surfactants. Adding (returning) cholesterol to BLES enhances adsorption and surface activity on the PBS at 25°C, but this difference is negated at 37°C.[93] The cholesterol content of rat and human surfactant is changed during vigorous exercise, although the physiologic significance is unknown.[20, 152, 153] Cholesterol levels are also altered in animals in torpor (temporary programmed decreases in body temperature), but again, the significance is not clear.[20, 154]

Addition of certain other lipids such as palmitic acid, hexadecanol, or dipalmitoylglycerol to DPPC markedly enhances adsorption *in vitro*.[155, 156] As indicated earlier, palmitic acid is added to Surfactant-TA and Survanta, whereas hexadecanol is used as a spreading agent in Exosurf. However, as explained later, because of nonsurfactant protein inhibition, the *in vivo* efficacy of monolayer formation is dubious.

In addition to bilayers, certain phospholipids and phospholipid mixtures can form nonbilayer phases.[142] It has been suggested that a hexagonal II phase could be involved in surfactant adsorption. DPPC:phosphatidylethanolamine mixtures that can form a hexagonal II phase do adsorb rapidly.[157, 158] However, evidence of a role for a hexagonal II phase in surfactant adsorption is lacking.[159]

Phospholipid Adsorption with Surfactant Proteins

The increased fluidity arising from introduction of non–gel-phase phospholipids and cholesterol can explain, in part, the rapid adsorption of pulmonary surfactant. However, the overall effects are relatively small. This has led to the conclusion that the ability of natural and modified pulmonary surfactant to adsorb sufficiently rapidly to stabilize the terminal air spaces can be attributed to the low molecular weight hydrophobic proteins SP-B and SP-C. Early studies demonstrating organic solvent extracts adsorbed rapidly were instrumental in the development of the modified natural surfactant used clinically.[129, 145, 156, 159-163] Such preparations contain SP-B and SP-C, but not SP-A. SP-B and SP-C, alone or together, greatly enhance adsorption of DPPC-containing mixtures to the equilibrium γ of 23 mN/m.[156, 164-170] Whether SP-B or SP-C is more effective depends on the experimental conditions, but SP-B appears to have a greater effect with phospholipid mixtures closely mimicking natural surfactant.[168, 169, 171, 172] SP-A has only a minor effect on adsorption of DPPC or DPPC-containing lipid mixtures but greatly enhances film formation of mixtures containing SP-B in a calcium-dependent manner.[166,173-175] The carbohydrate recognition domain of SP-A is important for this function.[27] SP-A does not influence phospholipid adsorption rate in the presence of SP-C.

The manner by which either SP-B or SP-C promotes adsorption of surfactant phospholipids is not known. These low molecular weight hydrophobic proteins can be thought of as bilayer breakers, which disrupt the bilayer structure in such a way that they permit cooperative flow of bilayer phospholipids to the surface monolayer. It is likely separate mechanisms are involved. The 79-amino acid SP-B has three intrapeptide and one interpeptide disulfide bonds. Each monomer has four or five amphipathic helices with hydrophobic amino acids on one face of the protein and hydrophilic amino acids on the other side. SP-B thus acts as a membrane surface protein, with the hydrophobic face buried in the membrane, whereas the hydrophilic residues can interact with phospholipid head groups or with the surrounding water. In addition to the intermolecular disulfide bridge at Cys 48 of the homodimer, SP-B (a dimer) is stabilized by salt bridges (Glu 51 of one SP-B monomer and Arg 52 of the other chain, and vice versa).[176,177] The dimeric nature of SP-B is important for its surface activity.

Several properties of SP-B could contribute to its bilayer-disrupting propensity. SP-B surfactant lipid mixtures can form discoidal disks approximately 50 nm in diameter,[179] similar to those observed in serum high density lipoprotein fractions.[180] These disks are thought to represent bilayer sheets with SP-B dimers associating with the fatty acyl perimeters to minimize aqueous contact. Discoidal fractions have been reported in natural surfactant and in reconstituted systems. Whether these discoidal particles are directly involved in phospholipid adsorption is not known.

SP-B possesses *fusogenic properties* that could contribute to its ability to enhance phospholipid adsorption. Phospholipid vesicles containing SP-B aggregate through membrane:membrane interactions and allow the phospholipids in the outer bilayer leaflets to flow onto the corresponding leaflet of the adjacent vesicle.[35,181] Lipid mixing should be distinguished from true fusion, in which the surface bilayers of the two vesicles combine to become a single membrane and the intravesicular aqueous compartments form a common pool.[142,182] Thus, SP-B–mediated lipid mixing is correctly referred to as *hemifusion*. Because air is considerably less polar than water, vesicular hemifusion with the air-water interface could generate a monolayer. However, the molecular details are still vague. SP-B enhancement of DPPC adsorption is greater in the presence of acidic phospholipids such as PG. SP-B contains eight conserved positive residues, but only one conserved negative residue and so could interact with PG. Calcium also promotes adsorption of systems containing SP-B.[92,169,181]

SP-A, SP-B, DPPC, and calcium can combine to reconstitute tubular myelin, a natural surfactant form consisting of stacked square tubules hemi-fused at the corners[179,183] (see Fig. 101–3). Tubular myelin may represent the most active form for surfactant adsorption, because the rate at which natural surfactant preparations adsorb varies with tubular myelin content.[69] However, because it is not possible to purify this surfactant form, this conclusion cannot be validated.

PL adsorption is also enhanced in the presence of SP-C. SP-C is a 4.2-kDa monomeric protein with a short, 12-amino acid N terminus, ending in Lys-Arg, which marks initiation of a 23-amino acid α-helical segment, terminating in Met 35.[42] It has been reported that removal of the two palmitates esterified to Cys 4 and Cys 5 hampers the ability of SP-C to promote phospholipid adsorption to variable extents.[184-186] Depalmitoylated SP-C can dimerize readily and forms large β-sheet aggregates that could account, in part, for the difference in activity.[187-189] Neutralizing the membrane surface lysine initiating the α-helix greatly diminishes SP-C surface activity.[190,191]

To this point, the adsorption of surfactant phospholipids to a clean surface has been considered. Phospholipid adsorption to a

partially occupied surface can occur by a different mechanism. In these experiments, DPPC:PG mixtures containing SP-B or SP-C were spread to a surface tension of 50 mN/m.[192,193] This surface film accelerated subsequent incorporation of lipids from DPPC:PG unilamellar vesicles and resulted in rapid lowering of surface tension to equilibrium. Lipid insertion was triggered by injecting calcium ions into the subphase. This triggering effect arose because calcium ions neutralize the negative charge on PG and thus minimize charge repulsion between surface and subphase phospholipids. SP-B is considerably more effective than SP-C in promoting the "pulling up" of lipids into the surface film. This mechanism could involve interaction of surface lipids with the nonlamellar structures discussed earlier. Such a mechanism could be important in lipid insertion during inspiration when surface tension rises to more than the equilibrium value. The dimeric nature of SP-B enhances surface properties.[178] Removal of the palmitates from SP-C has little effect on SP-C–mediated incorporation of lipids from DPPC:PG into the monolayer. Surprisingly, lipid insertion from neutral DPPC:PC unilamellar vesicles into DPPC:PG:SP-C–containing monolayers was slower with palmitoylated SP-C.[194]

Surface Tension during Film Compression

Surfactant apoproteins modify the properties of model surfactant films and facilitate their ability to attain low γ during film compression. In this context, the term *surface activity* is defined as the ability to reduce surface tension, and the same term is used for γ reduction through adsorption (i.e., 70 mN/m to equilibrium 23 mN/m) and for γ reduction during film compression (i.e., to values lower than equilibrium). The term *compressibility* can be used to describe the degree to which surfactant films lower γ during surface area reduction. Unsaturated phospholipids at equilibrium surface tension are highly compressible: little reduction in γ occurs with large decreases in surface area. Thus, compressibility is inversely related to the slope of the γ versus surface area reduction curve. Good surfactants have low compressibility: γ falls markedly during surface area reduction. The low compressibility of good surfactant films resembles DPPC. This is why the classical model concluded that surfactant monolayers were enriched in DPPC. Addition of the low molecular weight apoprotein SP-B or SP-C leads to decreased compressibility, so smaller surface area reductions are required to lower γ from equilibrium to near zero.[171,175,195-197] As in the case of adsorption, SP-A decreases compressibility of surfactant films containing SP-B but not films with SP-C. The manner in which SPs contribute to decreased surfactant compressibility is not understood.

The classical model of surfactant function argues that, for a film to achieve the low γs near 0 mN/m required to stabilize the terminal airspaces, the surface monolayer must be highly enriched with DPPC. Two mechanisms have been proposed for producing this purported DPPC enrichment: (1) the squeezeout of non-DPPC fluid phospholipids during film compression and (2) selective DPPC adsorption.

Squeezeout

This model proposes that, during surface area reduction, gel-phase phospholipids are retained, whereas fluid-phase lipids are selectively expelled from surface monolayers. This hypothesis arose primarily from Langmuir-Wilhelmy balance studies showing that DPPC is the only major lipid component in surfactant that could sustain sufficient surface pressure to generate γ near zero with surface balances. DPPC monolayers at equilibrium require approximately 12% surface area reduction to lower γ to near zero.[133] Both spread and adsorbed surfactant model systems lacking SP-B and SP-C exhibit high compressibility and require high compression ratios (surface area reduction) to attain low γ. As indicated earlier, compressibility is markedly reduced by the presence of the hydrophobic apoproteins.

Selective DPPC Adsorption

Selective DPPC adsorption means that the initial adsorbed surfactant monolayer contains a higher proportion of DPPC than the bulk phase surfactant. The basis of this proposed phenomenon can be best understood by comparing theoretical and experimental surface area reductions required to compress surfactant monolayers from equilibrium surface tension to γs less than 2.0 mN/m during the initial compression. DPPC monolayers require approximately 12% surface area reduction to lower γ from 23 mN/m to less than 2 mN/m.[129, 133] Theoretically, DPPC:PG (70:30) mixtures with 1% SP-B or SP-C at equilibrium would require 30% surface area reduction for squeezeout of the fluid PG (assumes perfect squeezeout), resulting in a pure DPPC film (Fig. 101–12). A further 12% surface area reduction of the

remaining DPPC (70%) in the monolayer would require an 8.4% (0.12 × 70) area reduction to approach zero, resulting in a total area reduction of 38.4% (30 + 8.4). Applying the same reasoning to BLES, which contains approximately 35% DPPC, it would require at least 65% (100% total phospholipid 35% DPPC) surface area reduction to expel the non-DPPC components from the monolayer. To achieve γ of zero, the remaining DPPC would have to be compressed 4.2% (35 × 0.12) of the surface area. Thus, a minimum total surface area reduction of 69.2% (65 + 4.2) would be required to achieve low γ. Table 101–2 shows that the surface area reductions observed during the first quasistatic compression of films adsorbed on a CBT are considerably lower than theoretical.[129] Interpreted in terms of the classical theory, these studies suggest that SP-B and SP-C promote selective DPPC adsorption. This corresponds to a change in surface monolayer composition. However, these inferences are indirect, and the results could indicate a change in surface film organization.

Surface Tension during Film Expansion

Compression of spread DPPC monolayers at equilibrium results in a reduction in γ to near zero. However, with repeated compression and expansion cycles, greater compression ratios are required, particularly if compression is allowed to continue once low γ is attained. This results from low reinsertion of DPPC molecules into the monolayer after collapse. Addition of non-DPPC phospholipids improves respreading, although larger compression ratios are required for the squeezeout of the non-DPPC components. However, in the absence of the low molecular weight hydrophobic proteins, respreading remains poor.[132, 171, 196-199] These observations demonstrate that SP-B and SP-C promote reinsertion of surfactant lipids. In addition, in the presence of these apoproteins, compressibility decreases during cycling. For example, CBT studies show that Curosurf or BLES films adsorb at low concentrations, requiring 50 to 60% surface area reduction to attain γ near zero during the first quasistatic compression, but approximately 20% during the fifth compression.[129, 175, 200] The ability of SP-B and SP-C to augment surface activity during cycling can be observed with spread monolayers, but it is more pronounced with surfactant material in excess of a single monolayer. These observations are best explained by the presence of surfactant multilayers, as discussed in the next section.

Evidence Counter to the Classical Model for Surfactant Function

The classical model argues that surfactant adsorption results in monolayers containing DPPC and non-DPPC lipids. This model suggests that repeated compression and expansion of the mono-

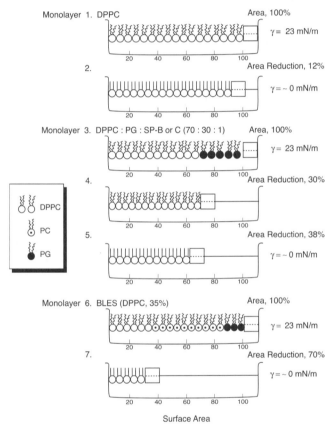

Figure 101–12. Representation of the theoretical surface area reductions required for various monolayers to reduce surface tension from approximately 23 mN/m (equilibrium) to near 0 mN/m. See text for explanation of calculations. *Monolayer 1,* Dipalmitoylphosphatidylcholine (DPPC) alone at equilibrium, 23 mN/m. Surface area reduction of approximately 12% leads to *monolayer 2,* which shows DPPC alone after compression to near 0 mN/m. *Monolayer 3,* DPPC: phosphatidylglycerol (PG) (70:30) with 1% surfactant-associated protein B (SP-B) or SP-C at 23 mN/m. Surface area reduction of 30% leads to *monolayer 4,* after squeezeout of PG. Only DPPC remains. Compressing monolayer 4, an additional 12% leads to *monolayer 5,* which contains DPPC alone after squeezeout of PG and compression to near 0 mN/m. *Monolayer 6,* Bovine lipid extract surfactant (BLES) at 23 mN/m. Compression of 70% leads to *monolayer 7,* showing BLES after squeezeout of unsaturated phosphatidylcholine (PC) and PG and compression to near 0 mN/m. (Modified from Possmayer, F. et al. [2001] *Comp Biochem Physiol A Mol Integr Physiol* 129 [1], 209–220.)

TABLE 101-2

Theoretical and Observed Surface Area Reductions Required to Reduce Surface Tension from Equilibrium (23 mN/m) to <2 mN/m

Film Composition	Surface Area Reduction Required	
	Theoretical (%)	*Observed (%)*
DPPC	—	12
DPPC/PG/SP-B (70:30:1)	38	20
DPPC/PG/SP-C	38	30
BLES	69	30
BLES plus SP-A	69	25

BLES = bovine lipid extract surfactant; DPPC = dipalmitoylphosphatidylcholine; PG = phosphatidylglycerol; SP = surfactant-associated protein.

layer result in refining because of squeezeout of fluid non-DPPC lipids, resulting in enrichment in DPPC.[107, 113, 201] This process would require incorporation of fresh surfactant during cycling to replace material lost by squeezeout. The classical model readily explained observations with the Langmuir-Wilhelmy surface balance and the PBS in which repeated compression and expansion cycles led to lowering of γ to low values. The squeezeout hypothesis was proposed to explain the original classical model when it was introduced.[107, 113, 201] The selective adsorption model, conversely, arose only because more recent observations with the CBT indicated that the surface activity of adsorbed films during the first compression could not be explained by the DPPC content of natural surfactant or its extracts (see Table 101–2).[112, 116, 119, 129]

Although the classical model considers surfactant from the perspective of a single monolayer, considerable more recent experimental evidence is most readily explained in terms of functional multilayers, which can provide surfactant phospholipids to the surface monolayer.[132, 159, 200, 202] Multilayers can be characterized as *adsorption reservoirs*, generated during film formation, and *compression reservoirs*, generated during film surface area reduction.

Adsorption Reservoirs

Figure 101–13 presents a CBT washout experiment that presents evidence for the formation of functional multilayers during surfactant adsorption.[200] A bubble was introduced into a BLES-1% SP-A (1.0 mg/mL) dispersion in saline-1.5 mmol/L calcium chloride. After adsorption to equilibrium, the CBT chamber was sealed, and the subphase was washed repeatedly to remove surfactant material not associated with the surface film. An initial quasistatic compression (see Fig. 101–13, point 1) was then performed to γ approximately 1.0 mN/m. Quasistatic expansion of the bubble led to increases in γ to just above equilibrium. This γ was maintained even though the surface area was expanded well

beyond the original value. Because the subphase had been depleted of surfactant, the excess material required to maintain γ near equilibrium must originate from a *surface-associated surfactant reservoir*. After relaxation, a second quasistatic compression (see Fig. 101–13, point 2) was performed, followed by a second expansion. Again, γ remained near equilibrium. This also occurred with a third compression, but after the fourth maneuver, γ increased above equilibrium, a finding indicating that the surface-associated reservoir was being depleted. Surface area reduction to attain γ near zero for each compression was 20 to 25%, although BLES contains approximately 35% DPPC. The final compressed monolayer was approximately fivefold larger than that obtained with the initial compression, a finding indicating the reservoir formed during adsorption contained functional surfactant corresponding to at least four monolayers.

Further evidence of the existence of the surface-associated multilayers that can act as surfactant reservoirs has been obtained through electron microscopy of surfactant systems in rabbit and guinea pig lung *in situ*[138, 200] and *in vitro*.[203] The presence of a surface-associated reservoir has also been deduced from autoradiographic examination of Langmuir-Blodgett films from model and lipid extract surfactants and from radioactive studies on monolayers spread from adsorbed BLES films using filter paper-supported wet bridges.[204, 205] These studies indicate the presence of surface-associated lipid aggregate complexes that are generated during adsorption.[206, 207] Existence of a surfactant reservoir created during adsorption would serve to explain the remarkable bulk concentration dependence of surfactant observed in numerous studies.[173, 175, 200] For example, whereas 50 to 60% surface area reduction is required to reduce γ from equilibrium to near zero during the first compression with BLES at 50 μg/mL, only 22.5 to 25% surface area reduction is required to reduce γ to near zero at bulk concentrations of 250 to 300 μg/mL. Addition of SP-A to BLES at low concentration greatly improves surface activity.[175, 200, 208]

Compression Reservoirs

The existence of surface-associated reservoirs, formed during film compression, that could supply phospholipid to the surface monolayer during film expansion would provide an efficient means for surfactant respreading. Evidence of such reservoirs is available from fluorescence imaging and atomic force microscopy. For example, fluorescence imaging studies reveal that compression of model systems such as DPPC:DPPG, DPPG:POPG, and DPPC:POPC:POPG results in loss of material from the surface into the bulk phase during collapse. Inclusion of either SP-B or SP-C (or synthetic analogues thereof) results in film buckling and formation of large folds or buds that extend into the subphase.[197, 209-217] As the surface is expanded again, the folds are incorporated into the surface monolayer with minimal loss of material over many compression and expansion cycles. Examination of Langmuir-Blodgett films deposited under compression reveals large irregular plates divided by thin spaces with phospholipid multilayers containing protein.[189, 197, 212, 215-218] In addition to the folds noted earlier, buds that grew into stacked bilayers have been noted, particularly with lipid extract surfactants and similar systems.[104-106, 219]

Compression reservoirs that function in phospholipid reinsertion into the monolayer during film expansion not only provide a plausible function for SP-B and SP-C, but also explain why adsorbed films and films spread in excess of a single monolayer remain more surface active during cycling. SP-B and SP-C also promote uptake of phospholipid vesicles from the bulk phase.[192, 193] Such uptake can occur only when γ rises above equilibrium.

Phase Transitions and the Classical Model

Further evidence incompatible with the classical model arises from fluorescence imaging studies. Dark probe-excluding

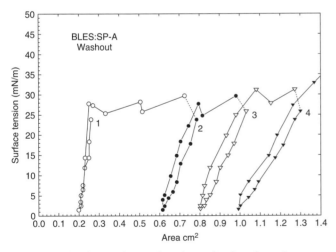

Figure 101–13. Physicochemical evidence for the adsorption surface-associated reservoir. After washing the subphase (*1*), the film (*open circles*) compressed to low tension. The bubble surface tension increases as surface area is increased but remains close to equilibrium. After a brief relaxation period (*2*), the film (*closed circles*) is compressed to low tension a second time. The bubble is again expanded, allowed to relax, and expanded a third time (*3, open triangles*). After the fourth compression, surface area expansion (*4, closed triangles*) leads to high surface tension, indicating that the surface-associated reservoir has been depleted (see text for further details). BLES:SP-A = bovine lipid extract surfactant:surfactant-associated protein A. (From Schürch, S. et al. [1995] The surface-associated surfactant reservoir in the alveolar lining. *Biol Neonate* 67, 61–76.)

regions, apparently LC domains, are observed during compression of DPPC:1% fluorescent probe on Langmuir-Wilhelmy balances (see earlier). Probe-excluding LC domains can also be observed with natural surfactant, lipid extract surfactants, and the phospholipid fraction from the calf surfactant CLSE. The classical model would imply that compression to high surface pressures (low γ) would result in nearly complete elimination of fluid probe-containing LE phase, leaving only dark LC phase in the monolayer. Fluorescence imaging studies with CLSE and porcine surfactant lipid extracts reveal probe-excluding domains that appear at γ near 60 mN/m and attain 33 to 40% total surface area around γ near 40 mN/m. However, these LC domains diminish and disappear around γ near 30 to 40 mN/m;[104, 106, 159, 219] This behavior suggests that lateral phase separation occurs at high γs (low surface pressures), but it is followed by a loss of LE and LC phases resulting from phospholipid remixing at lower γs (higher surface pressures). This phase remixing (co-dissolving) can be attributed to the cholesterol present in these extracts. Cholesterol appears to serve to maintain the monolayer in a more fluid phase capable of reaching relatively (but not very) low γ. These studies provided no evidence for generalized exclusion of non-DPPC lipids leading to monolayer enrichment in DPPC as required by the classical model.

Further evidence contrary to the classical model was obtained with fluorescence studies employing BLES or the phospholipid fraction from CLSE (no cholesterol). Such films readily attain γ near zero during compression while containing less than 40% surface area probe-excluding regions.[159, 220] This level of LC phase is comparable to the DPPC mole fraction. The ability of LE:LC-containing phospholipid monolayers to achieve γ of approximately zero in the presence of more than 60% LE phase is incompatible with the classical model, which would predict that only LC phase would be present at low γs.

The classical model evolved from the observations that DPPC was the only major surfactant component that could achieve and maintain surface tensions below equilibrium during monolayer compression. Such studies were normally conducted using the Langmuir-Wilhelmy balance introduced by Clements.[79] Studies by Hall's group have demonstrated that the ability to achieve γ near zero depends not only on monolayer composition but also on the rate at which the film is compressed. As stated earlier, phospholipid monolayers can be compressed dynamically to surface tensions below their equilibrium surface tensions, but above T_c, surface tension will rapidly return to equilibrium. However, compressing POPC ($T_c = -6°C$) or dimyristoyl PC (DMPC) ($T_c = 24.5°C$) at rates of 32% of initial area/second permits such films to reduce to approximately 2 mN/m.[221, 222] Furthermore, such rapidly compressed films can maintain γ below equilibrium for many minutes. Once compressed rapidly across the equilibrium γ of approximately 23 mN/m threshold, monolayers can be compressed or expanded more slowly without losing this remarkable property. Such rates are inaccessible on the Langmuir trough, which is normally compressed at approximately 3% total surface area/minute, but are readily attainable with the pulsating and captive bubble surfactometers and correspond to those in the lung. As emphasized later, films below γ equilibrium are metastable (also true for DPPC) but remain at low tensions for periods much longer than required to stabilize the terminal air spaces during breathing or with high-frequency (fixed-volume) ventilation.

The mechanism by which spread monolayers of fluid-phase phospholipid attains this remarkable metastable state is not understood. Hall and co-workers suggested that as fluid LE monolayers are compressed beyond equilibrium, they can either collapse to three-dimensional multilayers or form a disordered phase that, although thermodynamically metastable, is kinetically trapped for long periods.[159] A possible analogy for this kinetically trapped metastable phase may be glass, which is an amorphous

(nonordered) solid. The observation that single-component fluid phospholipid monolayers can be compressed into viscous metastable phases raises the question of whether either the gel-phase lipid DPPC or surfactant apoproteins may be required in the lung. A possible explanation is that these surfactant components facilitate transformation of LE phase to the viscous state. Such an interpretation would be consistent with evidence from compression and expansion cycles as described earlier. Regardless of the interpretation, it should be clear that the rapid compression studies provide further strong evidence against the absolute requirement for a monolayer highly enriched in gel-phase phospholipids such as DPPC, as argued by the classical model. (After tornadoes, straws are sometimes reported to be found stuck through barn boards. It thus appears that rapid motion can alter physical stiffness.)

In summary, it is evident that surfactant apoproteins play essential roles in the biophysical functions of pulmonary surfactant. These low molecular weight hydrophobic proteins enhance surfactant lipid adsorption so surfactant can form phospholipid films at the rates required by the lung. Observations have suggested that surfactant films can act as functional multilayers. Evidence has been obtained for both adsorption reservoirs and compression reservoirs that can provide surfactant phospholipids to the surface monolayer during film expansion. SP-B, SP-C, and SP-A plus SP-B contribute to the formation of these reservoirs, but the mechanisms involved are not clear. The classical model for surfactant function implies that, during film compression, LC regions consisting primarily of DPPC increase and coalesce as a single gel-phase monolayer at γ near zero. Fluorescence studies on porcine and calf surfactant extracts do not observe a large increase in LC phase. Rather, at a critical surface pressure, LC phase lipids appear to dissolve again (remix) with the fluid components. This behavior is not predicted by the classical model.

Other studies have demonstrated that monolayers consisting of the phospholipid fraction from calf surfactant can be compressed to low surface tensions without the anticipated large increase in LC gel phase. The observation that low surface tensions (high surface pressures) can be achieved in the presence of LE and LC phases is counter to the classical theory.

Finally, studies using CBT have shown that monolayers of fluid lipids such as DMPC and POPC can achieve γs near zero at 37°C when compressed at rapid rates that are similar to those occurring in the lung. It is suggested that when fluid monolayers are compressed slowly, they collapse. However, when compressed rapidly enough, fluid monolayers can be kinetically trapped as an amorphous solid that collapses very slowly. Such monolayers, although metastable by definition (they are below equilibrium γ), could stabilize the alveoli. The existence of such metastable monolayers is opposite to the requirement for the DPPC-enriched monolayer proposed by the classical model.

SURFACTANT INACTIVATION

In addition to surfactant deficiency, such as occurs in neonatal RDS, alveolar stability can also be compromised through surfactant inactivation. Numerous natural and synthetic materials including meconium (fetal feces), lysophospholipids (produced by phospholipase A_2), pulmonary edema fluid, and nonsurfactant proteins can inhibit surfactant function *in vitro*.[11, 49, 155, 223-230] Although the importance of surfactant inhibition in ARDS is recognized, the mechanisms are not well understood. Considerable effort has been devoted toward examining the effects of serum proteins on surfactant function. Acute lung injury arising from certain insults results in disruption of the capillary-endothelial integrity leading to increased protein influx into alveolar spaces.[11, 71, 230] The enhanced permeability and increased protein oncotic pressure antagonize the efforts of the alveolar epithelium to remove fluid from the alveoli. In addition, by inhibiting surfactant function, serum proteins increase the hydrostatic pressure gradient across the alveolar surface, possibly further promoting pulmonary edema. Perhaps not surprisingly, wholly artificial surfactants lacking surfactant apoproteins are very susceptible to protein inhibition.[155,231,232] The ability of several clinical preparations to resist protein inhibition correlates with their SP-B content.[233-235] SP-C–based surfactant preparations show resistance to meconium.[224]

SP-A is not present in the lipid extract surfactants used clinically. However, addition of SP-A to lipid extract surfactant effectively reverses *in vitro* inhibition resulting from serum proteins.[174,236] SP-A does not block surfactant inhibition resulting from nonprotein inhibitors such as lysophospholipids. Lysophospholipids can sensitize lipid extract surfactant to inhibition by proteins.[228] SP-A deletion knock-out studies demonstrate that SP-A is not essential for normal lung function. There is evidence indicating that this collectin can play a role in reversing surfactant inhibition by proteins *in vivo*[237-240] as well as *in vitro*, but this remains controversial.

Surfactant inactivation varies with both the particular serum protein examined and the surfactant preparation employed. This finding indicates that protein inactivation could involve several mechanisms. Some proteins, for example, albumin, appear to inhibit surfactant by adsorbing rapidly, thereby monopolizing the air-water interface. Surfactant inhibition is readily reversed by increasing the concentration of lipid extract surfactant. This reversal of protein inhibition is nonstoichiometric and cannot be readily explained by competition.[230,241] Albumin binds free fatty acids, but whether this property is involved in surfactant inhibition is not known. Studies indicate albumin interferes with surfactant respreading from compression reservoirs.[213] However, this interference and the ability of albumin to compete with surfactant for the air-water interface only occur at surface tensions higher than those observed in the lung.[121,124,133] A possible explanation is that several inhibiting mechanisms occur during acute lung injury and ARDS. For example, lyso-PC at low concentration does not inhibit surfactant but can sensitize it to protein inhibition.[228,242] The C-reactive peptide, an acute phase protein, can bind the phosphorylcholine-head groups of PC and DPPC.[243] Inhibition by C-reactive protein can be reversed by phosphorylcholine, which is water soluble. The reason that C-reactive protein can inhibit surfactant, whereas SP-A, which also binds DPPC, blocks protein inhibition, is not understood.

Fibrinogen and fibrin monomers are particularly effective in inactivating surfactant.[11,229] These proteins appear to inactivate surfactant by sequestering surfactant constituents, such as surfactant apoproteins, in the hyaline membranes characteristic of respiratory distress.[244-246] Procoagulant activity increases in RDS and ARDS. The ability of the lung to remove fibrin-based clots is also compromised in ARDS. These observations further emphasize the complexity of the relationship between lung injury and surfactant inactivation. Studies *in vitro* have reported surfactant inhibition by proteins and meconium can be reversed by high molecular weight dextran[247] or polyethylene glycol.[248] Attempts to overcome surfactant inactivation *in vivo* have been variable.[249,250] Surfactant is also inactivated by oxidative stress. Superoxide and hydroxyl radicals likely react with surfactant lipids and SPs.[251-253] SPs can also be affected by nitration.[254,255] SP-A (and SP-D) has been reported to block lipid oxidation by free radicals.[252] In addition, SP-A can reverse the inhibitory effects of surfactant oxidation.[256]

Artificial surfactant preparations lacking surfactant apoproteins are susceptible to inactivation by serum proteins. Addition of the low molecular weight hydrophobic proteins, particularly SP-B, results in resistance to inhibition by serum proteins. SP-A is capable of resisting surfactant inactivation by serum proteins *in vitro*, and this may be important *in vivo*. SP-A may also be important in preventing and reversing surfactant inactivation during oxidative stress.

CONCLUSION

This chapter discusses the physicochemical principles governing surfactant function. These principles provide insight into the design of exogenous surfactants for clinical use. It is apparent that different optimizing strategies will be required to develop exogenous surfactants for treating neonatal and adult respiratory distress. However, the precise requirements for acute lung injury and ARDS must still be defined.

It is clear an effective exogenous surfactant must adsorb rapidly at 37°C and spread quickly to form a surface film with an equilibrium surface tension of approximately 23 mN/m. Excellent spreading within the terminal air spaces is important for exogenous surfactant to ensure adequate distribution.[257] In addition to rapid adsorption and good spreading, exogenous surfactants should achieve low surface tensions with the dynamic compressions produced during normal breathing or mechanical ventilation. The highest γs that can be attained during inspiration and expiration while still compatible with adequate lung function are not known.[121] Effective exogenous surfactants must resist inactivation by serum proteins, other inhibitors, and oxidative stress. This is particularly true for acute lung injury and ARDS. Therapeutic surfactants should also be resistant to film overcompression at low surface tensions. In addition, considerable benefit would accrue if the exogenous preparations could resist conversion from the highly active LA subtype to the poorly active SA form. Exogenous surfactants could also contribute by modulating conversion of endogenous surfactant, thereby maintaining a high proportion in the active LA form.

The artificial synthetic surfactants used clinically can become "activated" in the lung through interaction with endogenous surfactant apoproteins.[1,54] This interaction should be optimized in the design of exogenous preparations. The ability of exogenous surfactant to act as "substrate" for recycling into lamellar bodies and secretion as "new" surfactant must also be considered. It is thought that recycling of artificial surfactant components and mixing with endogenous surfactant apoproteins explain their effectiveness in RDS. Their inability to act directly may explain why artificial surfactants have not proven effective with ARDS. The use of synthetic lipid molecules that resist degradation by secreted phospholipids or cellular catabolic systems could prove useful.[147] However, such lipid analogues must be recycled appropriately and should not accumulate within cells.

It has become evident that peptides or peptoids that can mimic the activities of specific surfactant apoproteins are required for exogenous treatment, especially for the treatment of ARDS.[39,258-261] Therefore, this chapter closes with a recapitulation of the nature of the surfactant apoproteins and emphasizes their proposed roles in surfactant function. SP-A by itself has little effect on phospholipid adsorption. However, SP-A markedly enhances the phospholipid adsorption observed in the presence of SP-B and calcium.[92,166,208,236] In the presence of SP-B, SP-A counteracts serum protein inhibition of surfactant function. SP-A preferentially binds gel-phase lipids demonstrating a very high preference for DPPC.[27,28] Although only small amounts are present in lamellar bodies, SP-A is an important constituent of tubular myelin. Tubular myelin structures can be formed *in vitro* with DPPC, PG, SP-A, SP-B, and calcium.[179,183] Its ability to interact with DPPC would explain SP-A's role in maintaining the integrity of LAs. SP-A could also contribute to formation of a surface-associated surfactant reservoir.[200]

SP-A and SP-D are members of the collectin superfamily and have important roles in the innate host defense system.[21,22,29,31,32] *In vitro* studies indicate that SP-A can play an important role in regulating alveolar levels of surfactant lipids, but this is controversial because SP-A–deficient knock-out mice have normal surfactant levels and turnover.

SP-B is a low molecular weight hydrophobic protein that is an important constituent of the lipid extract surfactant used clinically.[24,35,132] SP-B deficiencies resulting from gene disruption in mice or human SP-B mutations are associated with neonatal pulmonary complications and death.[10, 40] SP-B enhances the adsorption of surfactant lipids. In addition to promoting adsorption to clean surfaces, SP-B present in partially filled monolayers can assist in the "incorporation" of phospholipid from vesicles in the subphase. SP-B can stabilize surface monolayers at low surface tensions hindering the return to the equilibrium surface tension of 23 mN/m. With DPPC-PG, SP-A, and calcium, SP-B is involved in the formation of tubular myelin *in vitro*. The ability of SP-B to promote hemifusion of phospholipid vesicles indicates that SP-B may be responsible for forming the lattice corners of tubular myelin. SP-B contributes to the formation of adsorption and compression reservoirs.

Like SP-B, SP-C is present in the lipid extract surfactants used clinically.[42] Recombinant SP-C is the only apoprotein present in the synthetic SP-C–containing surfactant Ventacute. SP-C enhances phospholipid adsorption. Surface SP-C can also promote the uptake of phospholipid vesicles into the surface film until equilibrium is attained. SP-C contributes to the mechanical stability of surface films compressed to low surface tensions. SP-C also promotes the uptake of phospholipids from a surface-associated surfactant reservoir during monolayer expansion. This property appears to resist the decrease in surface activity of surfactant films subjected to repeated overcompression at low surface tensions. The palmitoyl groups esterified to N-terminal cysteines of SP-C appear important for these latter functions.

This chapter reviews the physicochemical functions of pulmonary surfactant with emphasis on the SPs. Although a great deal has been learned about the nature and properties of these apoproteins, further experimentation will be required to confirm some of the suggested mechanisms proposed in this review. A more complete understanding of these mechanisms is clearly essential for producing optimal surfactants for clinical application.

ACKNOWLEDGMENTS

I would like to thank Mr. Brent Moyer, Ms Angela Brackenbury, and Drs. Kaushik Nag, Amiya Panda, Karina Rodriguez Capote, and Ruud Veldhuizen for helpful comments and discussions. Comments from the Graduate Biochemistry Membrane Protein class of the University of Western Ontario are also appreciated. I would like to express special thanks to Dr. Kaushik Nag and Dr. Karina Rodriguez Capote for assistance with some of the figures. This review was supported by a Group Grant from the Canadian Institutes of Health Research.

REFERENCES

1. Jobe, A.H. (1993) Pulmonary surfactant therapy. *N Engl J Med* 328 (12), 861–868.
2. Soll, R.F. and Blanco, F. (2002b) Natural surfactant extract versus synthetic surfactant for neonatal respiratory distress syndrome (Cochrane Review). (Vol. 2002), The Cochrane Library.
3. Soll, R.F. (2002a) Prophylactic natural surfactant extract for preventing morbidity and mortality in preterm infants (Cochrane Review). (Vol. 2002), The Cochrane Library.
4. Curley, A.E. and Halliday, H.L. (2001) The present status of exogenous surfactant for the newborn. *Early Hum Dev* 61 (2), 67–83.
5. Jobe, A.H. and Ikegami, M. (2000) Lung development and function in preterm infants in the surfactant treatment era. *Annu Rev Physiol* 62, 825–846.
6. McCabe, A.J. et al. (2000) Surfactant: a review for pediatric surgeons. *J Pediatr Surg* 35 (12), 1687–1700.
7. Robertson, B. and Halliday, H.L. (1998) Principles of surfactant replacement. *Biochim Biophys Acta* 1408 (2–3), 346–361.
8. Wiswell, T.E. (2001) Expanded uses of surfactant therapy. *Clin Perinatol* 28 (3), 695–711.
9. Frerking, I. et al. (2001) Pulmonary surfactant: functions, abnormalities and therapeutic options. *Intensive Care Med* 27 (11), 1699–1717.
10. Griese, M. (1999) Pulmonary surfactant in health and human lung diseases: state of the art. *Eur Respir J* 13 (6), 1455–1476.
11. Gunther, A. et al. (2001) Surfactant alteration and replacement in acute respiratory distress syndrome. *Respir Res* 2 (6), 353–364.
12. Lesur, O. et al. (1999) Acute respiratory distress syndrome: 30 years later. *Can Respir J* 6 (1), 71–86.
13. Lewis, J.F. and Veldhuizen, R.A. (2003) The role of exogenous surfactant in the treatment of acute lung injury. *Annu Rev Physiol* 65, 613–642.
14. Lewis, J.F. and Jobe, A.H. (1993) Surfactant and the adult respiratory distress syndrome. *Am Rev Respir Dis* 147, 218–233.
15. Spragg, R.G. (2000) Surfactant replacement therapy. *Clin Chest Med* 21 (3), 531–541, ix.
16. Akino, T. (1992) Lipid components of the surfactant system. In *Pulmonary Surfactant: from Molecular Biology to Clinical Practice* (Robertson, B. et al., eds.), pp. 19–31, Amsterdam, Elsevier.
17. Batenburg, J.J. and Haagsman, H.P. (1998) The lipids of pulmonary surfactant: dynamics and interactions with proteins. *Prog Lipid Res* 37 (4), 235–276.
18. Cockshutt, A.M. and Possmayer, F. (1992) Metabolism of surfactant lipids and proteins in the developing lung. In *Pulmonary Surfactant: From Molecular Biology to Clinical Practice* (Robertson, B. et al., eds.), pp. 339–377, Amsterdam, Elsevier.
19. Van Golde, L.M. et al. (1988) The pulmonary surfactant system: biochemical aspects and functional significance. *Physiol Rev* 68 (2), 374–455.
20. Veldhuizen, R. et al. (1998) The role of lipids in pulmonary surfactant. *Biochim Biophys Acta* 1408, 90–108.
21. Crouch, E. and Wright, J.R. (2001) Surfactant proteins A and D and pulmonary host defense. *Annu Rev Physiol* 63, 521–554.
22. Haagsman, H.P. and Diemel, R.V. (2001) Surfactant-associated proteins: functions and structural variation. *Comp Biochem Physiol A Mol Integr Physiol* 129 (1), 91–108.
23. Hawgood, S. and Poulain, F.R. (2001) The pulmonary collectins and surfactant metabolism. *Annu Rev Physiol* 63, 495–519.
24. Weaver, T.E. and Conkright, J.J. (2001) Function of surfactant proteins B and C. *Annu Rev Physiol* 63, 555–578.
25. Kahn, M.C. et al. (1995) Phosphatidylcholine molecular species of calf lung surfactant. *Am J Physiol* 269 (5 Pt 1), L567–573.
26. Postle, A.D. et al. (2001) A comparison of the molecular species compositions of mammalian lung surfactant phospholipids. *Comp Biochem Physiol A Mol Integr Physiol* 129 (1), 65–73.
27. McCormack, F.X. (1998) Structure, processing and properties of surfactant protein A. *Biochim Biophys Acta* 1408 (2–3), 109–131.
28. Palaniyar, N. et al. (2001) Domains of surfactant protein A that affect protein oligomerization, lipid layer structure and surface tension. *Comp Biochem Physiol A Mol Integr Physiol* 129 (1), 109–127,
29. LeVine, A.M. and Whitsett, J.A. (2001) Pulmonary collectins and innate host defense of the lung. *Microbes Infect* 3 (2), 161–166.
30. Hakansson, K. and Reid, K.B. (2000) Collectin structure: a review. *Protein Sci* 9 (9), 1607–1617.
31. Vaandrager, A.B. and van Golde, L.M. (2000) Lung surfactant proteins A and D in innate immune defense. *Biol Neonate* 77 (Suppl 1), 9–13.
32. McCormack, F.X. and Whitsett, J.A. (2002) The pulmonary collectins, SP-A and SP-D, orchestrate innate immunity in the lung. *J Clin Invest* 109 (6), 707–712.
33. Clark, H.W. et al. (2000) Collectins and innate immunity in the lung. *Microbes Infect* 2 (3), 273–278.
34. Crouch, E. et al. (2000) Collectins and pulmonary innate immunity. *Immunol Rev* 173, 52–65.
35. Hawgood, S. et al. (1998) Structure and properties of surfactant protein B. *Biochim Biophys Acta* 1408 (2–3), 150–160.
36. Lawson, P.R. and Reid, K.B. (2000) The roles of surfactant proteins A and D in innate immunity. *Immunol Rev* 173, 66–78.
37. Reid, K.B. (1998) Interactions of surfactant protein D with pathogens, allergens and phagocytes. *Biochim Biophys Acta* 1408 (2–3), 290–295.
38. Tino, M.J. and Wright, J.R. (1998) Interactions of surfactant protein A with epithelial cells and phagocytes. *Biochim Biophys Acta* 1408 (2–3), 241–263.
39. Walther, F.J. et al. (2000) Surfactant protein B and C analogues. *Mol Genet Metab* 71 (1–2), 342–351.
40. Cole, F.S. et al. (2001) Genetic disorders of neonatal respiratory function. *Pediatr Res* 50 (2), 157–162.
41. Weaver, T.E. and Beck, D.C. (1999) Use of knockout mice to study surfactant protein structure and function. *Biol Neonate* 76 Suppl 1, 15–18.
42. Johansson, J. (1998) Structure and properties of surfactant protein C. *Biochim Biophys Acta* 1408 (2–3), 161–172.
43. Whitsett, J.A. and Baatz, J.E. (1992) Hydrophobic surfactant proteins SP-B and SP-C: molecular biology, structure, and function. In *Pulmonary Surfactant: From Molecular Biology to Clinical Practice* (Robertson, B. et al., eds.), pp. 685–703, Amsterdam, Elsevier.
44. Jobe, A. and Ikegami, M. (1987) Surfactant for the treatment of respiratory distress syndrome. *Am Rev Respir Dis* 136 (5), 1256–1275.
45. Jobe, A.H. (1997) Surfactant treatment. In *Fetal and Neonatal Physiology* (Vol. 2) (Polin, R.A. and Fox, W.W., eds.), pp. 1321–1335, Philadelphia, W.B. Saunders Company.
46. Bernhard, W. et al. (2000) Commercial versus native surfactants. Surface activity, molecular components, and the effect of calcium. *Am J Respir Crit Care Med* 162 (4 Pt 1), 1524–1533.
47. Fujiwara, T. and Robertson, B. (1992) Pharmacology of exogenous surfactant. In *Pulmonary Surfactant: From Molecular Biology to Clinical Practice* (Robertson, B. et al., eds.), pp. 561–592, Amsterdam, Elsevier.
48. Notter, R.H. et al. (2002) Component-specific surface and physiological activity in bovine-derived lung surfactants. *Chem Phys Lipids* 114 (1), 21–34.
49. Notter, R.H. and Wang, Z. (1997) Pulmonary surfactant: physical chemistry, physiology, and replacement. *Rev Chem Engineering* 13 (4), 1–118.

50. Clark, R.H. et al. (2001) A comparison of the outcomes of neonates treated with two different natural surfactants. *J Pediatr* 139 (6), 828-831.
51. Robertson, B. et al. (2000) Synthetic surfactants to treat neonatal lung disease. *Mol Med Today* 6 (3), 119-124.
52. Nilsson, G. et al. (1998) Synthetic peptide-containing surfactants—evaluation of transmembrane versus amphipathic helices and surfactant protein C polyvalyl to poly- leucyl substitution [In Process Citation]. *Eur J Biochem* 255 (1), 116-124.
53. Tabor, B. et al. (1990) Rapid clearance of surfactant-associated palmitic acid from the lungs of developing and adult animals. *Pediatr Res* 27 (3), 268-273.
54. Jobe, A.H. and Ikegami, M. (1993) Surfactant metabolism. *Clin Perinatol* 20 (4), 683-696.
55. Jobe, A.H. (2000) Which surfactant for treatment of respiratory-distress syndrome. *Lancet* 355 (9213), 1380-1381.
56. Fehrenbach, H. (2001) Alveolar epithelial type II cell: defender of the alveolus revisited. *Respir Res* 2 (1), 33-46.
57. Mulugeta, S. et al. (2002) Identification of LBM180, a lamellar body limiting membrane protein of alveolar type II cells, as the ABC transporter protein ABCA3. *J Biol Chem* 277 (25), 22147-22155.
58. van Golde, L.M.G. et al. (1994) The pulmonary surfactant system. *NIPS* 9, 13-20.
59. Williams, M.C. (1992) Morphologic aspects of the surfactant system. In *Pulmonary Surfactant: From Molecular Biology to Clinical Practice* (Robertson, B. et al., eds.), pp. 87-107, Amsterdam, Elsevier.
60. Wright, J.R. and Dobbs, L.G. (1991) Regulation of pulmonary surfactant secretion and clearance. *Annu Rev Physiol* 53, 395-414.
61. Wright, J.R. (1990) Clearance and recycling of pulmonary surfactant. *Am J Physiol* 259 (2 Pt 1), L1-12.
62. Farrell, P.M. et al. (1990) Relationships among surfactant fraction lipids, proteins and biophysical properties in the developing rat lung. *Biochim Biophys Acta* 1044 (1), 84-90.
63. Froh, D. et al. (1990) Lamellar bodies of cultured human fetal lung: content of surfactant protein A (SP-A), surface film formation and structural transformation *in vitro*. *Biochim Biophys Acta* 1052 (1), 78-89.
64. Oosterlaken-Dijksterhuis, M.A. et al. (1991) Surfactant protein composition of lamellar bodies isolated from rat lung. *Biochem J* 274 (Pt 1), 115-119.
65. Ikegami, M. and Jobe, A.H. (1993) Surfactant metabolism. *Semin Perinatol* 17 (4), 233-240.
66. Beckmann, H.-J. and Dierichs, R. (1984) Extramembranous particles and structural variations of tubular myelin figures in rat lung surfactant. *J Ultrastr Res.* 86, 57-66.
67. Nag, K. et al. (1999) Correlated atomic force and transmission electron microscopy of nanotubular structures in pulmonary surfactant. *J Struct Biol* 126 (1), 1-15.
68. Voorhout, W.F. et al. (1991) Surfactant protein A is localized at the corners of the pulmonary tubular myelin lattice. *J Histochem Cytochem* 39, 1331-1336.
69. Benson, B.J. et al. (1984) Role of apoprotein and calcium ions in surfactant function. *Exp Lung Res* 6 (3-4), 223-236.
70. Gross, N.J. (1995) Extracellular metabolism of pulmonary surfactant: the role of a new serine protease. *Annu Rev Physiol* 57, 135-150.
71. Lewis, J.F. and Veldhuizen, R.A. (1995) Factors influencing efficacy of exogenous surfactant in acute lung injury. *Biol Neonate* 67 (Suppl 1), 48-60.
72. Baritussio, A. et al. (1994) SP-A, SP-B, and SP-C in surfactant subtypes around birth: reexamination of alveolar life cycle of surfactant. *Am J Physiol* 266 (4 Pt 1), L436-447.
73. Putman, E. et al. (1995) Pulmonary surfactant subtype metabolism is altered after short-term ozone exposure. *Toxicol Appl Pharmacol* 134 (1), 132-138.
74. Putz, G. et al. (1994) Surface activity of rabbit pulmonary surfactant subfractions at different concentrations in a captive bubble. *J Appl Physiol* 77 (2), 597-605.
75. Veldhuizen, R.A. et al. (1996) Surfactant-associated protein A is important for maintaining surfactant large-aggregate forms during surface-area cycling. *Biochem J* 313 (Pt 3), 835-840.
76. von Neergaard, K. (1929) Neue Auffassungen über einen Grundbegriff der Atemmechanik. Die Retraktionskraft der Lunge, abhangig von der Oberflachenspannung in den Alveolen. *Z Gesammte Exp Med* 66, 373-394.
77. Clements, J.A. (1962) Surface phenomena in relation to pulmonary function. *Physiologist* 5 (1), 11-28.
78. Radford, E.P., Jr. (1957) Recent studies of mechanical properties of mammalian lungs. In *Tissue Elasticity* (Remington, J.W., ed.), pp. 177-190, Bethesda, MD, American Physiological Society.
79. Clements, J. (1957) Surface tension of lung extracts. *Proc Soc Exp Biol Med* 95, 170-172.
80. Pattle, R. (1955) Properties, function and origin of the alveolar lining layer. *Nature* 175, 1125-1126.
81. Adam, N.K. (1941) *The Physics and Chemistry of Surfaces*, Oxford, U.K., Oxford University Press.
82. Adamson, A.W. (1982) *Physical Chemistry of Surfaces*, New York, John Wiley & Sons.
83. Defay, R. and Prigogine, I. (1966) *Surface Tension and Adsorption*, New York, John Wiley & Sons.
84. Gaines, G.L. (1966) *Insoluble Monolayers at Liquid-Gas Interfaces*, New York, Interscience Publishers, John Wiley & Sons.
85. Notter, R.H. (2000) *Lung Surfactants. Basic Science and Clinical Applications*, Marcel Dekker, Inc.
86. Bois, A.G. and Albon, N. (1985) Equilibrium spreading of L-alpha-dipalmitoyl lecithin below the main bilayer transition temperature: can it be measured? *J Colloid Interface Sci* 104, 579-582.
87. Lawrie, G.A. et al. (1996) Spreading properties of dimyristoyl phosphatidylcholine at the air/water interface. *Chem Phys Lipids* 79 (1), 1-8.
88. Philips, M.C. and Hauser, H. (1974) Spreading of solid glycerides and phospholipids at the air/water interface. *J Colloid Interface Sci* 49, 31-39.
89. Vilallonga, F. (1968) Surface of L-alpha-dipalmitoyl lecithin at the air-water interface. *Biochim Biophys Acta* 163 (3), 290-300.
90. Meban, C. (1981) Effect of lipids and other substances on the adsorption of dipalmitoyl phosphatidyl choline. *Pediatr Res* 15, 1029-1031.
91. Notter, R.H. et al. (1982) Path dependence of adsorption behavior of mixtures containing dipalmitoyl phosphatidylcholine. *Pediatr Res* 16 (7), 515-519.
92. Yu, S.-H. and Possmayer, F. (1992) Effect of pulmonary surfactant protein B (SP-B) and calcium on phospholipid adsorption and squeeze-out of phosphatidylglycerol from binary phospholipid monolayers containing dipalmitoylphosphatidylcholine. *Biochim Biophys Acta* 1126, 26-34.
93. Yu, S.H. and Possmayer, F. (1993) Adsorption, compression and stability of surface films from natural, lipid extract and reconstituted pulmonary surfactants. *Biochim Biophys Acta* 1167 (3), 264-271.
94. Hawco, M.W. et al. (1981) Exclusion of fluid lipid during compression of monolayers of mixtures of dipalmitoylphosphatidylcholine with some other phosphatidylcholines. *Biochim Biophys Acta* 646 (1), 185-187.
95. Hawco, M.W. et al. (1981) Lipid fluidity in lung surfactant: monolayers of saturated and unsaturated lecithins. *J Appl Physiol* 51 (2), 509-515.
96. Keough, K.M.W. (1984) Physical chemical properties of some mixtures of lipids and their potential for use in exogenous surfactant. *Prog Respir Res* 18, 257-262.
97. Tchoreloff, P. et al. (1991) A structural study of interfacial phospholipid and lung surfactant layers by transmission electron microscopy after Blodgett sampling: influence of surface pressure and temperature. *Chem Phys Lipids* 59 (2), 151-165.
98. Denicourt, N. et al. (1989) The liquid condensed diffusional transition of dipalmitoylphosphoglycerocholine in monolayers. *Biophys Chem* 33 (1), 63-70.
99. Denicourt, N. et al. (1994) The main transition of dipalmitoylphosphatidylcholine monolayers: A liquid expanded to solid condensed high order transformation. *Biophys Chem* 49, 153-162.
100. Albrecht, O. et al. (1978) Polymorphism of phospholipid monolayers. *Le Journal de Physique* 39, 301-313.
101. Trauble, H. et al. (1974) Respiration—a critical phenomenon? Lipid phase transitions in the lung alveolar surfactant. *Naturwissenschaften* 61 (8), 344-354.
102. Kaganer, V.M. et al. (1999) Structure and phase transitions in Langmuir monolayers. *Rev Modern Phys* 71, 779-819.
103. Brumm, T. et al. (1994) Conformational changes of the lecithin headgroup in monolayers at the air/water interface. *Eur Biophys J* 23, 289-295.
104. Discher, B.M. et al. (1996) Lateral phase separation in interfacial films of pulmonary surfactant. *Biophys J* 71 (5), 2583-2590.
105. Discher, B.M. et al. (1999b) Phase separation in monolayers of pulmonary surfactant phospholipids at the air-water interface: composition and structure. *Biophys J* 77 (4), 2051-2061.
106. Nag, K. et al. (1998) Phase transitions in films of lung surfactant at the air-water interface. *Biophys J* 74 (6), 2983-2995.
107. Clements, J.A. (1977) Functions of the alveolar lining. *Am Rev Respir Dis* 115 (6 Pt 2), 67-71.
108. Engstrom, P.C. et al. (1989) Surfactant replacement attenuates the increase in alveolar permeability in hyperoxia. *J Appl Physiol* 67 (2), 688-693.
109. Bangham, A.D. (1987) Lung surfactant: how it does and does not work. *Lung* 165 (1), 17-25.
110. Keough, K.M.W. (1992) Physical chemistry of pulmonary surfactant in the terminal air spaces. In *Pulmonary Surfactant: From Molecular Biology to Clinical Practice* (Robertson, B. et al., eds.), pp. 109-164, Amsterdam, Elsevier.
111. Goerke, J. and Clements, J.A. (1986) Alveolar surface tension and lung surfactant. In *Handbook of Physiology, Section 3: The Respiratory System* (Vol. III, Part 1) (Fishman, A.P., ed.), pp. 247-261, Bethesda, MD, American Physiological Society.
112. Perez-Gil, J. and Keough, K.M.W. (1998) Interfacial properties of surfactant proteins. *Biochim Biophys Acta* 1408 (2-3), 203-217.
113. Watkins, J.C. (1968) The surface properties of pure phospholipid to those of lung extracts. *Biochim Biophys Acta* 152, 293-306.
114. Egberts, J. et al. (1989) Minimal surface tension, squeeze-out and transition temperatures of binary mixtures of dipalmitoylphosphatidylcholine and unsaturated phospholipids. *Biochim Biophys Acta* 1002 (1), 109-113.
115. Goerke, J. and Gonzales, J. (1981) Temperature dependence of dipalmitoyl phosphatidylcholine monolayer stability. *J Appl Physiol* 51 (5), 1108-1114.
116. Goerke, J. (1998) Pulmonary surfactant: Functions and molecular composition. *Biochim Biophys Acta* 1408 (2-3), 79-89.
117. Hildebran, J.N. et al. (1979) Pulmonary surface film stability and composition. *J Appl Physiol* 47 (3), 604-611.
118. Bachofen, H. et al. (1994) Disturbance of alveolar lining layer: effects on alveolar microstructure. *J Appl Physiol* 76 (5), 1983-1992.
119. Schürch, S. et al. (2001) Surface activity in situ, in vivo, and in the captive bubble surfactometer. *Comp Biochem Physiol A Mol Integr Physiol* 129 (1), 195-207.
120. Wilson, T.A. and Bachofen, H. (1982) A model for mechanical structure of the alveolar duct. *J Appl Physiol* 52 (4), 1064-1070.

121. Bachofen, H. and Schürch, S. (2001) Alveolar surface forces and lung architecture. *Comp Biochem Physiol A Mol Integr Physiol* 129 (1), 183-193.

122. Bachofen, H. et al. (1987) Relations among alveolar surface tension, surface area, volume, and recoil pressure. *J Appl Physiol* 62 (5), 1878-1887.

123. Schürch, S. et al. (1976) Direct determination of surface tension in the lung. *Proc Natl Acad Sci USA* 73 (12), 4698-4702.

124. Schürch, S. et al. (1978) Direct determination of volume- and time-dependence of alveolar surface tension in excised lungs. *Proc Natl Acad Sci USA* 75 (7), 3417-3421.

125. Schürch, S. (1982) Surface tension at low lung volumes: dependence on time and alveolar size. *Respir Physiol* 48, 339-355.

126. Jobe, A.H. and Ikegami, M. (2001) Biology of surfactant. *Clin Perinatol* 28 (3), 655-669, vii-viii.

127. Metcalfe, I.L. et al. (1982) Lung expansion and survival in rabbit neonates treated with surfactant treatment. *J Appl Physiol* 53 (4), 838-843.

128. Yamada, T. et al. (1990) Effects of surfactant protein—A on surfactant function in preterm ventilated rabbits. *Am Rev Respir Dis* 142 (4), 754-757.

129. Possmayer, F. et al. (2001) Surface activity in vitro: role of surfactant proteins. *Comp Biochem Physiol A Mol Integr Physiol* 129 (1), 209-220.

130. Kelly, E. et al. (1993) Compliance of the respiratory system in newborn infants pre- and postsurfactant replacement therapy. *Pediatr Pulmonol* 15 (4), 225-230.

131. Milner, A.D. (1993) How does exogenous surfactant work? *Arch Dis Child* 68 (3 Spec No), 253-254.

132. Veldhuizen, E.J. and Haagsman, H.P. (2000) Role of pulmonary surfactant components in surface film formation and dynamics. *Biochim Biophys Acta* 1467 (2), 255-270.

133. Schürch, S. et al. (1989) A captive bubble method reproduces the in situ behavior of lung surfactant monolayers. *J Appl Physiol* 67 (6), 2389-2396.

134. Enhorning, G. (1977) Pulsating bubble technique for evaluating pulmonary surfactant. *J Appl Physiol* 43 (2), 198-203.

135. Enhorning, G. (2001) Pulmonary surfactant function studied with the pulsating bubble surfactometer (PBS) and the capillary surfactometer (CS). *Comp Biochem Physiol A Mol Integr Physiol* 129 (1), 221-226.

136. Hall, S.B. et al. (1993) Approximations in the measurement of surface tension on the oscillating bubble surfactometer. *J Appl Physiol* 75 (1), 468-477.

137. Putz, G. et al. (1994) Comparison of captive and pulsating bubble surfactometers with use of lung surfactants. *J Appl Physiol* 76 (4), 1425-1431.

138. Schürch, S. et al. (1998) Formation and structure of surface films: captive bubble surfactometry. *Biochim Biophys Acta* 1408 (2-3), 180-202.

139. Schoel, W.M. et al. (1994) The captive bubble method for the evaluation of pulmonary surfactant: surface tension, area, and volume calculations. *Biochim Biophys Acta* 1200 (3), 281-290.

140. Lee, S. et al. (2001) Equilibrium and dynamic interfacial tension measurements at microscopic interfaces using a micropipet technique. 2. Dynamics of phospholipid monolayer formation and equilibrium tensions at the water-air interface. *Langmuir* 17, 5544-5550.

141. Schwarz, G. and Zhang, J. (2001) Chain length dependence of lipid partitioning between the air/water interface and its subphase: thermodynamic and structural implications. *Chem Phys Lipids* 110 (1), 35-45.

142. Hope, M.J. et al. (1998) Cationic lipids, phosphatidylethanolamine and the intracellular delivery of polymeric, nucleic acid-based drugs (review). *Mol Membr Biol* 15 (1), 1-14.

143. Schürch, S. et al. (1994) Surface activity of lipid extract surfactant in relation to film area compression and collapse. *J Appl Physiol* 77 (2), 974-986.

144. Notter, R.H. et al. (1983) Comparative adsorption of natural lung surfactant, extracted phospholipids, and artificial phospholipid mixtures to the air-water interface. *Chem Phys Lipids* 33 (1), 67-80.

145. Notter, R.H. (1984) Surface chemistry of pulmonary surfactant: The role of individual components. In *Pulmonary Surfactant* (Robertson, B. et al., eds.), pp. 17-65, Amsterdam, Elsevier Science Publishers.

146. Obladen, M. et al. (1979) Surfactant substitution. *Eur J Pediatr* 131 (4), 219-228.

147. Skita, V. et al. (1995) Bilayer characteristics of a diether phosphonolipid analog of the major lung surfactant glycerophospholipid dipalmitoyl phosphatidylcholine. *J Lipid Res* 36 (5), 1116-1127.

148. Brown, D.A. and London, E. (1997) Structure of detergent-resistant membrane domains: does phase separation occur in biological membranes? *Biochem Biophys Res Commun* 240 (1), 1-7.

149. London, E. and Brown, D.A. (2000) Insolubility of lipids in triton X-100: physical origin and relationship to sphingolipid/cholesterol membrane domains (rafts). *Biochim Biophys Acta* 1508 (1-2), 182-195.

150. Anderson, R.G. and Jacobson, K. (2002) A role for lipid shells in targeting proteins to caveolae, rafts, and other lipid domains. *Science* 296 (5574), 1821-1825.

151. Nanjundan, M. and Possmayer, F. (2003) Pulmonary phosphatidic acid phosphatase and lipid phosphate phosphohydrolase (PAP/LPP). *Am J Physiol Lung Cell Mol Physiol* 284, L1-L23.

152. Doyle, I.R. et al. (2000) Composition of alveolar surfactant changes with training in humans. *Respirology* 5 (3), 211-220.

153. Orgeig, S. et al. (1995) Effect of hyperpnea on the cholesterol to disaturated phospholipid ratio in alveolar surfactant of rats. *Exp Lung Res* 21 (1), 157-174.

154. Orgeig, S. and Daniels, C.B. (2001) The roles of cholesterol in pulmonary surfactant: insights from comparative and evolutionary studies. *Comp Biochem Physiol A Mol Integr Physiol* 129 (1), 75-89.

155. Holm, B.A. et al. (1988) A biophysical mechanism by which plasma proteins inhibit lung surfactant activity. *Chem Phys Lipids* 49 (1-2), 49-55.

156. Tanaka, Y. et al. (1986) Development of synthetic lung surfactants. *J Lipid Res* 27, 475-485.

157. Perkins, W.R. et al. (1996) Role of lipid polymorphism in pulmonary surfactant. *Science* 273 (5273), 330-332.

158. Yu, S.-H. et al. (1984) Artificial pulmonary surfactant: Potential role for hexagonal H-II phase in the formation of a surface active monolayer. *Biochim Biophys Acta* 776, 37-47.

159. Piknova, B. et al. (2002) Pulmonary surfactant: phase behavior and function. *Curr Opin Struct Biol* 12 (4), 487-494.

160. Fujiwara, T. et al. (1980) Artificial surfactant therapy in hyaline-membrane disease. *Lancet* 1 (8159), 55-59.

161. Metcalfe, I.L. et al. (1980) Pulmonary surfactant-associated proteins: their role in the expression of surface activity. *J Appl Physiol* 49 (1), 34-41.

162. Suzuki, Y. (1982) Experimental studies on the pulmonary surfactant: reconstitution of surface-active material. *J Lipid Res* 23, 53-61.

163. Notter, R.H. and Shapiro, D.L. (1987) Lung surfactants for replacement therapy: biochemical, biophysical, and clinical aspects. *Clin Perinatol* 14 (3), 433-479.

164. Suzuki, Y. (1982) Effect of protein, cholesterol, and phosphatidylglycerol on the surface activity of the lipid-protein complex reconstituted from pig pulmonary surfactant. *J Lipid Res* 23 (1), 62-69.

165. Takahashi, A. and Fujiwara, T. (1986) Proteolipid in bovine lung surfactant: its role in surfactant function. *Biochem Biophys Res Commun* 135 (2), 527-532.

166. Hawgood, S. et al. (1987) Nucleotide and amino acid sequences of pulmonary surfactant protein SP 18 and evidence for cooperation between SP 18 and SP 28-36 in surfactant lipid adsorption. *Proc Natl Acad Sci USA* 84 (1), 66-70.

167. Yu, S.H. and Possmayer, F. (1986) Reconstitution of surfactant activity by using the 6 kDa apoprotein associated with pulmonary surfactant. *Biochem J* 236 (1), 85-89.

168. Yu, S.H. and Possmayer, F. (1988) Comparative studies on the biophysical activities of the low-molecular-weight hydrophobic proteins purified from bovine pulmonary surfactant. *Biochim Biophys Acta* 961 (3), 337-350.

169. Yu, S.H. and Possmayer, F. (1990) Role of bovine pulmonary surfactant-associated proteins in the surface-active property of phospholipid mixtures. *Biochim Biophys Acta* 1046 (2), 233-241.

170. Wang, Z. et al. (1996) Roles of different hydrophobic constituents in the adsorption of pulmonary surfactant. *J Lipid Res* 37 (4), 790-798.

171. Wang, Z. et al. (1996) Differential activity and lack of synergy of lung surfactant proteins SP-B and SP-C in interactions with phospholipids. *J Lipid Res* 37 (8), 1749-1760.

172. Possmayer, F. and Yu, S.-H. (1990) Role of the low molecular weight proteins in pulmonary surfactant. *Prog Respir Res* 25, 54-63.

173. Chung, J. et al. (1989) Effect of surfactant-associated protein-A (SP-A) on the activity of lipid extract surfactant. *Biochim Biophys Acta* 1002 (3), 348-358.

174. Cockshutt, A.M. et al. (1990) Pulmonary surfactant-associated protein A enhances the surface activity of lipid extract surfactant and reverses inhibition by blood proteins in vitro. *Biochemistry* 29 (36), 8424-8429.

175. Rodriguez Capote, K. et al. (2001) Surfactant protein interactions with neutral and acidic phospholipid films. *Am J Physiol Lung Cell Mol Physiol* 281 (1), L231-242.

176. Zaltash, S. et al. (2000) Pulmonary surfactant protein B: a structural model and a functional analogue. *Biochim Biophys Acta* 1466 (1-2), 179-186.

177. Zaltash, S. et al. (2001) Membrane activity of (Cys48Ser) lung surfactant protein B increases with dimerisation. *Biol Chem* 382 (6), 933-939.

178. Veldhuizen, E.J. et al. (2000) Dimeric N-terminal segment of human surfactant protein B (dSP-B(1-25)) has enhanced surface properties compared to monomeric SP-B(1-25). *Biophys J* 79 (1), 377-384.

179. Williams, M.C. et al. (1991) Changes in lipid structure produced by surfactant proteins SP-A, SP-B, and SP-C. *Am J Respir Cell Mol Biol* 5 (1), 41-50.

180. Brouillette, C.G. et al. (2001) Structural models of human apolipoprotein A-I: a critical analysis and review. *Biochim Biophys Acta* 1531 (1-2), 4-46.

181. Poulain, F.R. et al. (1996) Kinetics of phospholipid membrane fusion induced by surfactant apoproteins A and B. *Biochim Biophys Acta* 1278 (2), 169-175.

182. Duzgunes, N. and Bentz, J. (1988) Fluorescence assays for membrane fusion. In *Spectroscopic Membrane Probes* (Vol. 1) (Loew, L., ed.), pp. 117-159, Boca Raton, FL, CRC Press.

183. Suzuki, Y. et al. (1989) Reconstitution of tubular myelin from synthetic lipids and proteins associated with pig pulmonary surfactant. *Am Rev Respir Dis* 140, 75-81.

184. Qanbar, R. and Possmayer, F. (1995) On the surface activity of surfactant-associated protein C (SP-C): effects of palmitoylation and pH. *Biochim Biophys Acta* 1255 (3), 251-259.

185. Qanbar, R. et al. (1996) Role of the palmitoylation of surfactant-associated protein C in surfactant film formation and stability. *Am J Physiol* 271 (4 Pt 1), L572-580.

186. Wang, Z. et al. (1996) Acylation of pulmonary surfactant protein-C is required for its optimal surface active interactions with phospholipids. *J Biol Chem* 271 (32), 19104-19109.

187. Gustafsson, M. et al. (2001) The palmitoyl groups of lung surfactant protein C reduce unfolding into a fibrillogenic intermediate. *J Mol Biol* 310 (4), 937-950.

188. Szyperski, T. et al. (1998) Pulmonary surfactant-associated polypeptide C in a mixed organic solvent transforms from a monomeric alpha-helical state into insoluble beta-sheet aggregates. *Protein Sci* 7 (12), 2533-2540.

189. Ross, M. et al. (2002) Kinetics of phospholipid insertion into monolayers containing the lung surfactant proteins SP-B or SP-C. *Eur Biophys J* 31 (1), 52-61.
190. Creuwels, L.A. et al. (1995) Neutralization of the positive charges of surfactant protein C. Effects on structure and function. *J Biol Chem* 270 (27), 16225-16229.
191. Creuwels, L.A. et al. (1997) The pulmonary surfactant system: biochemical and clinical aspects. *Lung* 175 (1), 1-39.
192. Oosterlaken-Dijksterhuis, M.A. et al. (1991) Characterization of lipid insertion into monomolecular layers mediated by lung surfactant proteins SP-B and SP-C. *Biochemistry* 30 (45), 10965-10971.
193. Oosterlaken-Dijksterhuis, M.A. et al. (1991) Interaction of lipid vesicles with monomolecular layers containing lung surfactant proteins SP-B or SP-C. *Biochemistry* 30, 8276-8281.
194. Creuwels, L.A. et al. (1993) Effect of acylation on structure and function of surfactant protein C at the air-liquid interface. *J Biol Chem* 268 (35), 26752-26758.
195. Nag, K. et al. (1999) SP-B refining of pulmonary surfactant phospholipid films. *Am J Physiol* 277 (6 Pt 1), L1179-1189.
196. Wang, Z. et al. (1995) Dynamic surface activity of films of lung surfactant phospholipids, hydrophobic proteins, and neutral lipids. *J Lipid Res* 36 (6), 1283-1293.
197. Takamoto, D.Y. et al. (2001) Interaction of lung surfactant proteins with anionic phospholipids. *Biophys J* 81 (1), 153-169.
198. Veldhuizen, E.J. et al. (2001) Effect of the hydrophobic surfactant proteins on the surface activity of spread films in the captive bubble surfactometer. *Chem Phys Lipids* 110 (1), 47-55.
199. Veldhuizen, E.J. et al. (2000) The role of surfactant proteins in DPPC enrichment of surface films. *Biophys J* 79 (6), 3164-3171.
200. Schürch, S. et al. (1995) The surface-associated surfactant reservoir in the alveolar lining. *Biol Neonate* 67, 61-76.
201. Bangham, A.D. et al. (1979) The physical properties of an effective lung surfactant. *Biochim Biophys Acta* 573 (3), 552-556.
202. Zasadzinski, J.A. et al. (2001) The physics and physiology of lung surfactants. *Curr Opin Colloid Interface Sci* 6, 506-513.
203. Sen, A. et al. (1988) Localization of lipid exchange sites between bulk lung surfactants and surface monolayer: freeze fracture study. *J Colloid Interface Sci* 126, 355-360.
204. Yu, S.-H. and Possmayer, F. (2001) Effect of pulmonary surfactant protein SP-A on adsorption of cholesterol and dipalmitoylphosphatidylcholine into the monolayer. *Biophys J* 80, 545A.
205. Yu, S.-H. and Possmayer, F. (2003) Lipid compositional analysis of pulmonary surfactant monolayers and monolayer-associated reservoirs. *J Lipid Res* 44, 621-629.
206. Yu, S.H. and Possmayer, F. (1998) Interaction of pulmonary surfactant protein A with dipalmitoylphosphatidylcholine and cholesterol at the air/water interface. *J Lipid Res* 39 (3), 555-568.
207. Yu, S.H. et al. (1999) Interactions of pulmonary surfactant protein SP-A with monolayers of dipalmitoylphosphatidylcholine and cholesterol: roles of SP-A domains. *J Lipid Res* 40 (5), 920-929.
208. Schürch, S. et al. (1992) Pulmonary SP-A enhances adsorption and appears to induce surface sorting of lipid extract surfactant. *Am J Physiol* 263 (2 Pt 1), L210-218.
209. Amrein, M. et al. (1997) A scanning force- and fluorescence light microscopy study of the structure and function of a model pulmonary surfactant. *Eur Biophys J* 26 (5), 349-357.
210. Lipp, M.M. et al. (1998) Coexistence of buckled and flat monolayers. *Phys Rev Lett* 81, 1650-1653.
211. Bourdos, N. et al. (2000) Analysis of lung surfactant model systems with time-of-flight secondary ion mass spectrometry. *Biophys J* 79 (1), 357-369.
212. Ding, J. et al. (2001) Effects of lung surfactant proteins, SP-B and SP-C, and palmitic acid on monolayer stability. *Biophys J* 80 (5), 2262-2272.
213. Warriner, H.E. et al. (2002) A concentration-dependent mechanism by which serum albumin inactivates replacement lung surfactants. *Biophys J* 82 (2), 835-842.
214. Kramer, A. et al. (2000) Distribution of the surfactant-associated protein C within a lung surfactant model film investigated by near-field optical microscopy. *Biophys J* 78 (1), 458-465.
215. Diemel, R.V. et al. (2002) Multilayer formation upon compression of surfactant monolayers depends on protein concentration as well as lipid composition: an atomic force microscopy study. *J Biol Chem* 277 (24), 21179-21188.
216. von Nahmen, A. et al. (1997) The phase behavior of lipid monolayers containing pulmonary surfactant protein C studied by fluorescence light microscopy. *Eur Biophys J* 26, 359-369.
217. Post, A. et al. (1995) Pulmonary surfactant protein C containing lipid films at the air-water interface as a model for the surface of lung alveoli. *Mol Membr Biol* 12, 93-99.
218. Krol, S. et al. (2000) Formation of three-dimensional protein-lipid aggregates in monolayer films induced by surfactant protein B. *Biophys J* 79 (2), 904-918.
219. Discher, B.M. et al. (1999a) Neutral lipids induce critical behavior in interfacial monolayers of pulmonary surfactant. *Biochemistry* 38 (1), 374-383.
220. Piknova, B. et al. (2001) Discrepancy between phase behavior of lung surfactant phospholipids and the classical model of surfactant function. *Biophys J* 81 (4), 2172-2180.
221. Crane, J.M. and Hall, S.B. (2001) Rapid compression transforms interfacial monolayers of pulmonary surfactant. *Biophys J* 80 (4), 1863-1872.
222. Laderas, T.G. et al. (2002) Persistent metastability of rapidly compressed monolayers at the air-water interface. *Biophys J* 82, 152A.
223. Moses, D. et al. (1991) Inhibition of pulmonary surfactant function by meconium. *Am J Obstet Gynecol* 164 (2), 477-481.
224. Herting, E. et al. (2001) Resistance of different surfactant preparations to inactivation by meconium. *Pediatr Res* 50 (1), 44-49.
225. Enhorning, G. et al. (1992) Phospholipases introduced into the hypophase affect the surfactant film outlining a bubble. *J Appl Physiol* 73 (3), 941-945.
226. Kobayashi, T. et al. (1991) Inactivation of exogenous surfactant by pulmonary edema fluid. *Pediatr Res* 29 (4 Pt 1), 353-356.
227. Holm, B.A. et al. (1991) Inhibition of pulmonary surfactant function by phospholipases. *J Appl Physiol* 71 (1), 317-321.
228. Cockshutt, A.M. and Possmayer, F. (1991) Lysophosphatidylcholine sensitizes lipid extracts of pulmonary surfactant to inhibition by serum proteins. *Biochim Biophys Acta* 1086 (1), 63-71.
229. Seeger, W. et al. (1985) Alteration of surfactant function due to protein leakage: special interaction with fibrin monomer. *J Appl Physiol* 58 (2), 326-338.
230. Holm, B.A. (1992) Surfactant inactivation in adult respiratory distress syndrome. In *Pulmonary Surfactant: From Molecular Biology to Clinical Practice* (Robertson, B. et al., eds.), pp. 665-684, Amsterdam, Elsevier.
231. Hall, S.B. et al. (1992) Importance of hydrophobic apoproteins as constituents of clinical exogenous surfactants. *Am Rev Respir Dis* 145 (1), 24-30.
232. Venkitaraman, A.R. et al. (1991) Biophysical inhibition of synthetic phospholipid-lung surfactant apoprotein admixtures by plasma proteins. *Chem Phys Lipids* 57 (1), 49-57.
233. Seeger, W. et al. (1993) Surfactant inhibition by plasma proteins: differential sensitivity of various surfactant preparations. *Eur Respir J* 6 (7), 971-977.
234. Friedrich, W. et al. (2000) Surfactant protein SP-B counteracts inhibition of pulmonary surfactant by serum proteins. *Eur J Med Res* 5 (7), 277-282.
235. Mbagwu, N. et al. (1999) Sensitivity of synthetic surfactants to albumin inhibition in preterm rabbits. *Mol Genet Metab* 66 (1), 40-48.
236. Venkitaraman, A.R. et al. (1990) Enhancement of biophysical activity of lung surfactant extracts and phospholipid-apoprotein mixtures by surfactant protein A. *Chem Phys Lipids* 56 (2-3), 185-194.
237. Yukitake, K. et al. (1995) Surfactant apoprotein A modifies the inhibitory effect of plasma proteins on surfactant activity in vivo. *Pediatr Res* 37 (1), 21-25.
238. Strayer, D.S. et al. (1996) Antibody to surfactant protein A increases sensitivity of pulmonary surfactant to inactivation by fibrinogen in vivo. *Am J Respir Crit Care Med* 153 (3), 1116-1122.
239. Elhalwagi, B.M. et al. (1999) Normal surfactant pool sizes and inhibition-resistant surfactant from mice that overexpress surfactant protein A. *Am J Respir Cell Mol Biol* 21 (3), 380-387.
240. Ikegami, M. et al. (2001) The collagen-like region of surfactant protein A (SP-A) is required for correction of surfactant structural and functional defects in the SP-A null mouse. *J Biol Chem* 276 (42), 38542-38548.
241. Holm, B.A. et al. (1999) Multiple mechanisms of lung surfactant inhibition. *Pediatr Res* 46 (1), 85-93.
242. Cockshutt, A.M. et al. (1991) The role of palmitic acid in pulmonary surfactant: enhancement of surface activity and prevention of inhibition by blood proteins. *Biochim Biophys Acta* 1085 (2), 248-256.
243. McEachren, T.M. and Keough, K.M. (1995) Phosphocholine reverses inhibition of pulmonary surfactant adsorption caused by C-reactive protein. *Am J Physiol* 269 (4 Pt 1), L492-497.
244. Seeger, W. et al. (1993) Lung surfactant phospholipids associate with polymerizing fibrin: loss of surface activity [published erratum appears in Am J Respir Cell Mol Biol 1993 Oct;9(4):following 462]. *Am J Respir Cell Mol Biol* 9 (2), 213-220.
245. Gunther, A. et al. (1994) Clot-embedded natural surfactant: kinetics of fibrinolysis and surface activity. *Am J Physiol* 267 (5 Pt 1), L618-624.
246. Gunther, A. et al. (1999) Cleavage of surfactant-incorporating fibrin by different fibrinolytic agents. Kinetics of lysis and rescue of surface activity. *Am J Respir Cell Mol Biol* 21 (6), 738-745.
247. Tashiro, K. et al. (2000) Dextran reduces surfactant inhibition by meconium. *Acta Paediatr* 89 (12), 1439-1445.
248. Taeusch, H.W. et al. (1999) Nonionic polymers reverse inactivation of surfactant by meconium and other substances. *Am J Respir Crit Care Med* 159 (5 Pt 1), 1391-1395.
249. Campbell, H. et al. (2002) Polyethylene glycol (PEG) attenuates exogenous surfactant in lung-injured adult rabbits. *Am J Respir Crit Care Med* 165 (4), 475-480.
250. Lu, K.W. et al. (2001) Polyethylene glycol/surfactant mixtures improve lung function after HCl and endotoxin lung injuries. *Am J Respir Crit Care Med* 164 (8 Pt 1), 1531-1536.
251. Gilliard, N. et al. (1994) Exposure of the hydrophobic components of porcine lung surfactant to oxidant stress alters surface tension properties. *J Clin Invest* 93 (6), 2608-2615.
252. Bridges, J.P. et al. (2000) Pulmonary surfactant proteins A and D are potent endogenous inhibitors of lipid peroxidation and oxidative cellular injury. *J Biol Chem* 275 (49), 38848-38855.
253. Cifuentes, J. et al. (1995) Interaction of surfactant mixtures with reactive oxygen and nitrogen species. *J Appl Physiol* 78 (5), 1800-1805.
254. Zhu, S. et al. (2000) Carbon dioxide enhances nitration of surfactant protein A by activated alveolar macrophages. *Am J Physiol Lung Cell Mol Physiol* 278 (5), L1025-1031.

255. Zhu, S. et al. (2001) Increased levels of nitrate and surfactant protein a nitration in the pulmonary edema fluid of patients with acute lung injury. *Am J Respir Crit Care Med* 163 (1), 166–172.
256. Rodriguez Capote, K. and Possmayer, F. (2002) SP-A restores the surface activity of oxidized pulmonary surfactant. *Biophys J* 82, 2554-Pos.
257. Jobe, A.H. (1995) Techniques for administering surfactant. In *Surfactant Therapy for Lung Disease* (Robertson, B. and Taeusch, H.W., eds.), pp. 309–324, New York, Marcel Dekker.
258. Johansson, J. et al. (2001) Artificial surfactants based on analogues of SP-B and SP-C. *Pediatr Pathol Mol Med* 20 (6), 501–518.
259. Robertson, B. et al. (2000) Prospects for a new synthetic surfactant. *Acta Biomed Ateneo Parmense* 71 (Suppl 1), 409–412.
260. Possmayer, F. et al. (1984) Pulmonary surfactant. *Can J Biochem Cell Biol* 62 (11), 1121–1133.
261. Goerke, J. (1974) Lung surfactant. *Biochim Biophys Acta* 344 (3–4), 241–261.

Scott H. Randell and Stephen L. Young

Structure of Alveolar Epithelial Cells and the Surface Layer During Development

This chapter offers a morphologic description of the developmental anatomy of the alveolar epithelium and the alveolar interfacial (surfactant) layer. When possible, it includes data from human studies, but the fundamental process of alveolar epithelial maturation appears to be common to most mammals, and we have also drawn freely from animal data. There are several illnesses and developmental anomalies that affect *in utero* development of the pulmonary epithelium, but they are beyond the scope of this chapter and are described in the literature.[1]

HISTORICAL PERSPECTIVE

In 1953, Low and Daniels[2] resolved a riddle of the lung: Are alveolar capillaries exposed directly to alveolar air? With the new technology of electron microscopy, they demonstrated conclusively the presence of a thin alveolar membrane consisting of capillary endothelium, lung interstitium, and a continuous covering of (Type I) epithelium (Fig. 102-1).[2] Even before the anatomic work of these investigators, physiologic considerations predicted the presence of a surface-active alveolar lining layer. Terry[3] had proposed, in 1926, that a thin film overlay the alveolar epithelium. By 1929, von Neergaard's experiments[4] had proven that surface forces had a profound influence on the mechanical properties of lungs, and evidence mounted during the next 30 years that surface tension at the alveolar air-liquid interface must be extraordinarily low,[5] especially at low lung volumes. Macklin[6] hypothesized that the alveolar lining film functioned to remove particulates, maintain a favorable surface tension, protect the alveolar septa from desiccation, and suppress invading microorganisms. Early histologists had recognized the granular pneumonocyte (now known as the Type II cell) as a lung secretory cell, and Macklin correctly proposed that it was the source of an alveolar lining layer. He speculated that "... [the film's] mechanism of production insured a constancy of volume, thickness, weight and solid content...."[6] Despite the soundness of the physiologic experiments, the morphology of the surfactant lining layer remained controversial because a lining layer could not be demonstrated microscopically. Light microscopy was unable to resolve whether the observed carbohydrate-rich lining of alveoli was the result of a mucoid surface layer or of cell membranes. Electron microscopy initially failed because aqueous solutions and organic solvents used for tissue processing washed away the lipid-rich lining layer. By using perfusion fixation methods, Weibel and Gil[7] were finally able to demonstrate remnants of the interfacial film in situ. Later refinements[8] showed details of an unbroken superficial alveolar lining, probably a pure phospholipid monolayer, on top of an aqueous

hypophase containing reserves of newly secreted material and pools of exhausted surfactant (Fig. 102-2).

IN UTERO DEVELOPMENT OF THE ALVEOLAR EPITHELIUM

The mammalian lung begins as a tiny foregut pouch formed at the level of the pharynx. During early organogenesis, the lung anlage consists of clumps of endodermally derived, pluripotent, columnar to cuboidal epithelial cells, which are surrounded by mesenchyme. Important developmental signals are exchanged between the mesenchyme and the epithelium. Clever tissue recombination experiments showed that the development of an organ-specific epithelium is controlled by its mesenchyme and that, in the lung, branching morphogenesis of the bronchial tree is dependent on the presence of surrounding bronchial mesenchyme.[9] Epithelial cytodifferentiation also depends on intimate contact with mesenchymal cells, and it is clear that mesenchymal-epithelial cell interactions are important in the regulation of development (and possibly of repair in the adult).

The several stages of human lung development[10] (see Chap. 76) serve as a useful framework for describing important steps in epithelial cell development (Fig. 102-3). The *glandular* (or pseudoglandular) stage of human lung development ends at 16 weeks of gestation. At this time, conducting airways to the level of the terminal bronchioles are surrounded by a loosely packed investment of mesenchyme, which includes a few blood vessels. The airways are lined with pluripotent, glycogen-rich, and morphologically undifferentiated epithelial cells that have a columnar to cuboidal shape. Sixteen weeks of gestation marks the onset of the *canalicular* period, during which the respiratory bronchioles and alveolar ducts of the gas exchange region of the lung are formed. The mesenchyme becomes more condensed, blood vessels proliferate, and the epithelium overlying capillaries thins, the hallmark of Type I epithelial cell differentiation.

After 24 to 28 weeks, the *saccular* period begins. Large and primitive forms of the future alveoli are present (hence the term *saccular*), which are lined by squamous Type I cells and cuboidal Type II cells. At about 25 weeks of gestation, the human lung has the potential for the support of gas exchange, although successful unassisted ventilation is unlikely because the lung and its surfactant system are still underdeveloped.

There are significant species differences in the timing of alveolar epithelial cell differentiation. In laboratory rodents and in lambs, the first appearance of Type II cell lamellar bodies occurs at approximately 80% of gestation, whereas in humans their appearance at 24 weeks marks 60% of gestation. The most

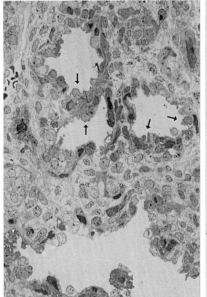
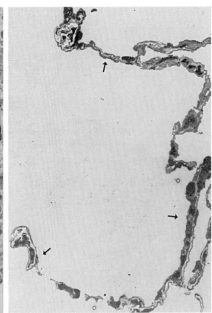

Figure 102–1. Electron micrographs of fetal (week 25, *left panel*) and adult *(right panel)* human lungs taken at the same magnification. The dramatic expansion of the air spaces, the thinning of the interstitium, and the extreme thinning of the epithelial cells *(arrows)* are some of the critical developmental changes that enable the lung efficiently to bring blood into contact with air.

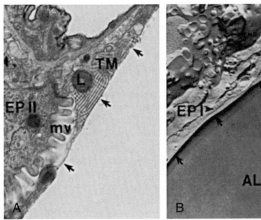
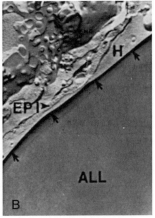

Figure 102–2. A, Electron micrograph of a perfusion-fixed adult rat lung. A Type II cell (EP II) can be seen with microvilli (mv), and the alveolar lining layer is apparently visible *(arrows)*. In the hypophase fluid are lamellar forms (L) and tubular myelin (TM), which is in contact with the surface. **B,** A freeze fracture micrograph, en face view, of the lining layer (ALL), hypophase fluid (H), and a Type I cell (EP I). (**A,** Courtesy of Robert Mercer, PhD; **B,** from Manabe T: J Ultra Res *69*:86, 1979.)

remarkable maturational timing belongs to the marsupials, in which Type II cell lamellar bodies occur in time for the marsupial's precocious transition to air breathing. Lamellar bodies appear in female offspring slightly earlier than they appear in males, partly because androgens exert an inhibitory influence on alveolar epithelial maturation.[11] The details of the several mechanisms that govern phenotypic expression in the epithelium are incompletely understood, and we can expect more insight from research in the next several years (see Chap. 79). Human Type II cells at 24 weeks of gestation or rat Type II cells at 19 days of gestation can be recognized by their cuboidal appearance, apical intercellular junctions, microvilli, and a few lamellar bodies. They have a large and dispersed cytoplasmic pool of glycogen that displaces organelles toward the cell periphery. The cells are rich in the organelles of synthesis, such as granular endoplasmic reticulum, polyribosomes, and the Golgi apparatus, with its associated

vesicles. Impressive changes in Type II cell morphology occur during late gestation, with a rapid loss of glycogen and proliferation of the cellular structures used for surfactant production and secretion (Fig. 102–4).

Biochemical markers supplement morphology in the study of lung development, and they have been used to study cellular parental lineage and the timing of cellular differentiation of the lung's distal epithelium. Wuenschell and co-workers[12] demonstrated coexpression of markers characteristic of neuroendocrine cells, Clara cells, and type II cells during the glandular stages of human lung development when only conducting airways were present. Later, these markers were restricted to their respective cell lineages. Funkhouser and colleagues[13] produced a monoclonal antibody against a (nonsurfactant) cell surface antigen, which localized to Type II cells in adult lung. These investigators found that this antigen was present on airway lining cells even during the earliest stage of lung development in rats, when only the bronchial buds were present.[13] The significance of the early appearance of undifferentiated airway cells that share phenotypic traits with structurally mature Type II cells is unknown. The cells may be acquiring an antigen relatively specific to the Type II cell (as in the case of surfactant-related proteins), or they may contain an epitope that is present on pluripotent cells and persists into adulthood on Type II cells only.

Williams and co-workers[14] described a monoclonal antibody directed against a surface antigen of Type I cells, and this reagent was useful to clarify the timing of Type I cell differentiation. Their studies demonstrated expression of Type I cell antigens on distal bronchial epithelial cells early during development, when no squamous cells and only cuboidal cells were present. This finding of Williams and co-workers suggested a direct lineage of the early saccular epithelium to Type I cells, instead of a transformation from Type II to Type I epithelium.

Type II cells are usually considered the precursors of Type I cells both during development and during repair of the injured epithelium in adults.[15, 16] The principal method for classifying Type I cells is by their attenuated plates of cytoplasm. The Type I cell covers more than 90% of the alveolar surface area,[17] and the cytoplasm is so attenuated that most organelles appear to be grouped within the perinuclear region. The Type I cell volume is also about five times as large as the Type II cell, with its large volume consisting mainly of cytoplasm. Although the volume of organelles such as mitochondria or rough endoplasmic reticulum

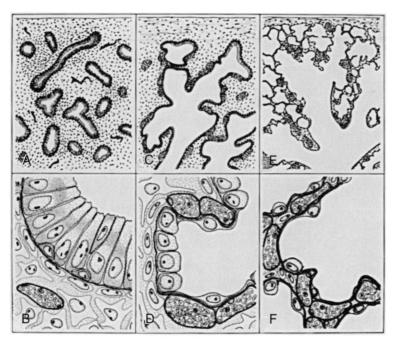

Figure 102–3. Drawing that illustrates the light microscopic appearance of human lung during the glandular (**A, B**), canalicular (**C, D**), and saccular (**E, F**) stages of *in utero* development. Undifferentiated columnar cells of the early bronchi (**B**) rest on a basal lamina, which has been emphasized by the *heavy line*. Mesenchymal cells and capillaries are present below the basal lamina. **D,** The epithelium overlying proliferating blood vessels thins to a squamous Type I morphology, and the most distal cells retain a cuboidal shape. At the saccular stage (**E, F**), the septa are thinned, and the air spaces are lined by differentiated Type I and Type II cells. The low- and high-magnification drawings are shown at approximately the same magnification in each panel.

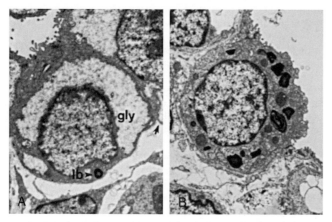

Figure 102–4. Electron micrographs of rat lung illustrating Type II cells during development. The earliest morphologically recognizable Type II cell (**A**) has large pools of glycogen (gly) and small lamellar bodies (lb). A foot process *(arrow)* can be seen perforating the basement membrane. At the time of birth (**B**), the Type II cell undergoes a rapid depletion of glycogen and acquires many lamellar bodies.

is reduced per unit volume of cytoplasm, the absolute volume of such organelles per cell is about the same as for Type II cells.[18]

INTRACELLULAR METABOLISM OF SURFACTANT

Details of the biochemistry of surfactant lipids and the four surfactant-related proteins are given in Chapter 100. *De novo* lipid biosynthesis occurring in the endoplasmic reticulum of Type II cells has been demonstrated by *in vivo* injection of tritiated choline. After they are synthesized in the endoplasmic reticulum, surfactant lipids must be transported to the lamellar bodies, but the structural pathway for this process is incompletely understood. Autoradiographic studies have demonstrated that [3H]choline radiolabel appears in multivesicular bodies after its appearance in the endoplasmic reticulum and before it is found in lamellar bodies.[19] Thus, there is morphologic and biochemical evidence placing the multivesicular body in the pathways leading to lamellar body production, yet knowledge of its role

remains incomplete.[20] Two morphologic types of multivesicular bodies are visible in Type II cells: one has vesicles plus an electron-lucent background, and the other is composed of vesicles within an electron-dense matrix (Fig. 102–5). Lamellar bodies have no vesicles, but they do have a limiting membrane, a thin rim of granular material, many phospholipid-rich lamellae, and often a central core of granular material (see Figs. 102–4 and 102–8). An intermediate, possibly immature, form of lamellar bodies is recognized that contains both lamellae and vesicles (Table 102–1).

Pathways of protein biosynthesis and cellular packaging by Type II cells have also been described. Investigators have demonstrated that Type II cells use intracellular pathways of cellular protein metabolism noted in other cell types, with the exception of the possible synthetic role played by the Type II cell multivesicular body.[19] Proteins for export, namely, surfactant apoproteins, are synthesized in the endoplasmic reticulum, and several studies indicate that extensive posttranslational protein modifications occur in the *trans*-Golgi region.[19,21,22]

Biochemical studies indicate an extensive recycling of surfactant lipid and protein.[23,24] Morphologic descriptions of the recycling pathways remain incomplete, but there is evidence that endocytosed components can be directed into lamellar bodies, presumably for re-secretion. Multivesicular bodies appear to be part of the endocytic pathway and may function as a nexus among synthetic, recycling, and degradation systems.[25] Electron-lucent multivesicular bodies are the structures that first receive freshly endocytosed membrane markers such as cationic ferritin or lectins.[20] About 30 minutes later, these markers are found within lamellar bodies, the mature secretory and storage granules of the Type II cells. Autoradiographic studies[26] of radiolabeled lipid and surfactant protein instilled into rat lungs revealed recycling of both components, although lipid and protein were differently localized to electron dense (protein) and electron lucent (lipid) multivesicular bodies. Lamellar bodies were a later recipient of both labels.

ORGANIZATION OF THE TYPE II CELL DURING DEVELOPMENT

Three-dimensional views of Type II cells obtained from rats from gestational day 20 to adulthood have demonstrated the pattern

Figure 102–5. Electron micrographs of multivesicular bodies (**A, B**) and composite forms (**C, D**) from rat lung Type II cells. The mature lamellar body (**E**) contains no vesicles. The magnifications vary, multivesicular bodies are about 0.2 μm, composite forms are about 0.5 μm, and lamellar bodies average about 1 μm. (From Young SL, et al: Am J Anat *174*:1, 1985.)

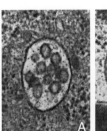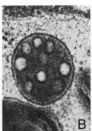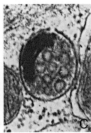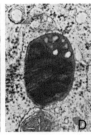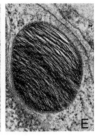

TABLE 102-1

Morphologic Forms of Surfactant

Intracellular	Extracellular

Lamellar body
   Composite forms
   Mature forms
	Tubular myelin
	
	Interfacial monolayer
	Vesicles

of spatial organization of the cells' organelles during differentiation. At the earliest time points studied, the composite bodies and the few mature lamellar bodies are both localized to the basal side of the cell. Later in life, there is an increased number of lamellar bodies, which are distributed throughout Type II cells.[27] The composite forms, which may represent immature lamellar bodies, are always polarized toward the basal part of Type II cells, away from the alveolar air border. Their numbers peak at the time of the rapid appearance of lamellar bodies, around the time of birth, in rats. Multivesicular bodies with an electron-lucent background are usually polarized toward the apical side of rat Type II cells.

GESTATIONAL CHANGES IN ALVEOLAR BASAL LAMINA

The basal lamina may exert important influences on overlying epithelial cells. On gestational day 19 in rats, the basal lamina is continuous, but as cellular maturation proceeds, Type II cells extend cytoplasmic foot processes through interruptions of the basal lamina. Some of those foot processes become closely apposed to interstitial lipofibroblasts (see Fig. 102–4).[28-30] The appearance of foot processes parallels increasing cellular lipid synthesis (and cytodifferentiation). Transient, gender-related differences observed in Type II cell lipid synthesis have also been observed in foot process number.[28] Steroids accelerate the appearance of foot processes and enhance Type II cell differentiation and surfactant lipid and apoprotein synthesis. Foot processes rapidly decrease in number after birth, but they reappear during repair of the injured alveolar epithelium in human adults.[31] These observations imply that foot processes are one of the structures through which mesenchymal (or fibroblastic) factors influence epithelial cell function and vice versa.

The basal lamina underlying the alveolar epithelium in adults is polyanionic.[29] The anionicity of the basal lamina decreases with increasing gestational age in rats, and there is a shift of anionic sites from the interstitial side of the basement membrane to the epithelial side of the basement membrane.[29] The basal lamina is more anionic beneath Type I than Type II cells. The causes and functional consequences of these features of the alveolar basal lamina are largely unknown, but they may be important in view of the substantial effects of different substrates on the Type II cell's appearance *in vitro*.[32] Reported details of the biochemical composition of the alveolar basal lamina indicate substantial species variations as well as developmental programming.[33]

BIRTH AND THE TRANSITION TO AIR BREATHING

Secretion of surfactant begins *in utero*, and serial analysis of amniotic fluid reflects an accumulation of the lipid and apoprotein parts of surfactant, which are released into the fetal alveolus (saccule) and are carried out of the lung by the evolving lung liquid.

Immediately after birth, the lung must function as the organ of gas exchange, and dramatic events occur that, in a matter of moments, convert the fluid-filled newborn lung to one that is gas filled. Fluid adsorption and surfactant production are two major tasks for the alveolar, and possibly the bronchiolar, epithelium. Both events must occur to achieve normal gas exchange after birth. Fluid adsorption from the fetal alveolar space begins in early labor and is augmented by adrenergic hormones.[34] There are few morphologic correlates of fluid transport across the alveolar epithelium, although ultrastructural studies suggest the possibility of a paracellular route through cell junctions, a transcellular route through the endocytic vesicles of Type I cells, or a basolateral exit in which lung fluid is transported by alveolar epithelial cells or by Clara cells.[35]

By the end of gestation, the lung of the newborn rat pup has twice as many Type II cells per gram of dry tissue when compared with the adult lung, and each Type II cell has about half the adult volume of lamellar bodies. At birth, there is no evidence of an overload on Type II cell lamellar body production, because the intracellular lamellar body pools are not depleted at any time during the postnatal period.[36, 37] However, large changes are found in the alveolar surfactant lipid pools, which represent substantial alveolar accumulation of newly synthesized surfactant.[37, 38]

Surfactant exists in several recognizable morphologic forms (see Table 102-1), although technical challenges in the preservation of these lipid-rich structures leave questions about artifacts and make quantitation of the different forms difficult. Perhaps the best-recognized form of surfactant is the intracellular lamellar body (see Figs. 102-4, 102-8, and 102-9). Modern methods of tissue fixation for electron microscopy now preserve about 75% of the tissue lipids, but even so, the open spaces of lamellar body profiles seen in most preparations are likely to be artifacts. The characteristic lamellae may represent a large sheet of a phospholipid bilayer, draped and folded to appear almost circular in some profiles. Freeze fracture techniques, which do not fix or extract lipids, have been used to demonstrate that the lipid layers of the lamellar body completely fill the lamellar body. When cells are prepared in that fashion, no structures are present that suggest insertion of protein into the lipid membranes (Fig. 102-6). Lamellar bodies are bounded by a limiting bilayer membrane, and although there are some variations, many human lamellar bodies contain a thin rim of granular material beneath the bounding membrane plus pools of granular material within the central core of the lamellar body. The biochemical composition of each lamellar body subcompartment is unknown, although the lamellae probably represent lipid and the core material stains for protein and enzyme activities, such as acid phosphatase. Although surfactant protein A (SP-A) has been immunolocalized to lamellar bodies, the precise amount or location of the surfactant apoprotein molecules within the lamellar bodies is not known.

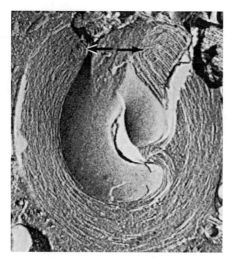

Figure 102–6. Freeze fracture of rat lung Type II cell lamellar body. The folding of the lamellae is seen at the *arrows.* (From Williams MC: Exp Lung Res 4:37, 1982.)

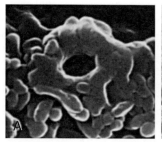 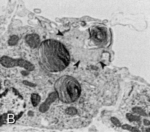

Figure 102–7. A, Scanning electron micrograph showing the plasma membrane pit, which probably corresponds to the secretory pore formed during lamellar body extrusion. **B,** Transmission electron micrograph showing a secretory event and the broad base of F-actin *(arrowheads)* beneath the secretory granule. (From Kliewer M, et al: Exp Lung Res 9:351, 1985.)

THE SECRETORY EVENT

During exocytosis, the limiting membrane of the lamellar body fuses with the apical plasma membrane of the Type II cell, and a dense band of F-actin forms at the cytoplasmic face of the lamellar body being secreted (Fig. 102-7).[39] Between 15 and 50 lamellar bodies are secreted per rat Type II cell per hour, although the cell is capable of much faster secretion after β-adrenergic stimulation.[40] The freshly secreted lamellar body, stripped of its surrounding membrane, enters the acidic alveolar hypophase liquid, which has a high calcium content.[41] The next series of morphologic transformations probably occurs within a few hundred milliseconds by unknown, but presumably spontaneous, mechanisms. Several lamellar bodies (from a few to at least 24) together contribute closed tubular sheets of membranous material to a lung-specific structure called *tubular myelin* (Fig. 102-8). This unique and highly ordered array has an absolute requirement for calcium ions and can be reversibly disassembled by ethylene glycol tetra-acetic acid.[42] High-magnification electron micrographs of tubular myelin membranes reveal regular spacing of small globular profiles on short stalks (Fig. 102-9), which decorate the lipid bilayers. These images are consistent with high-resolution micrographs using rotary shadowing of pure SP-A oligomers,[43] and immunoelectron microscopy suggests that SP-A is localized at the "corners" of tubular myelin.[44]

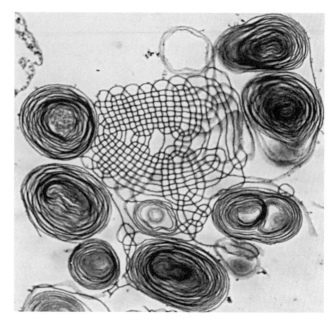

Figure 102–8. Transmission electron micrograph of lamellar bodies forming tubular myelin in the (fluid-filled) air space of a fetal rat.

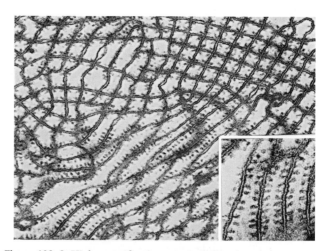

Figure 102–9. High-magnification transmission electron micrograph of tubular myelin. Regularly spaced globular profiles on short stalks that decorate the lipid bilayers are probably surfactant protein A (*inset* shows a section parallel to the tubular structure at higher magnification). (Courtesy of C. Kuhn III, MD.)

Recombination experiments have also revealed the "lollipop" appearance of the decorations of phospholipid membranes when SP-A is added to phospholipid mixtures. Fully developed tubes with 90-μm intersecting membranes can be generated by addition of SP-A plus SP-B to phospholipid mixtures.[45]

ESTABLISHMENT OF THE AIR-LIQUID INTERFACE

Both freeze fracture and transmission electron micrographic images are in agreement about the structure of tubular myelin, which supports use of current methods of preparation of surfactant for transmission electron microscopy. Serial section reconstructions provided an indication of the size of some tubular myelin collections and revealed uninterrupted tubes of more than 12 μm in length.[46] Such large sizes for tubular myelin aggregates explain why these structures are easily sedimented at low centrifugal force. Tubular myelin is an unstable form of surfactant that may be specialized to enhance lipid insertion into the alveolar interfacial film. Adsorption rates of lipids from tubular myelin are very rapid, permitting insertion of saturated phospholipids into an interfacial film within the time taken by a single breath. Lipid insertion into the surfactant film uses some mechanism that involves a direct contact of the tubules with the surface layer, and at least one of the apoproteins, SP-A, is dissociated from the lipid during that adsorption step.[47,48]

DESORPTION AND RECYCLING OF SURFACTANT

The interfacial film of surfactant is subject to high pressures (low surface tension) at low lung volumes, and desorption of surfactant lipid occurs. The morphologic forms that may represent desorbed surfactant are poorly understood, in part because the physical techniques for their isolation likely cause artifacts. There is some evidence that surfactant material that is ready to be recycled is shaped like collapsed disks or liposomal vesicles.[23,49] From the point of desorption of surfactant to reuptake and recycling within the Type II cell, morphologic information is sparse. Studies in adult rats demonstrated an increase in the vesicular surfactant forms after a period of large tidal volume ventilation.[50] These observations are consistent with the proposal of Magoon and co-workers[23] that the extracellular cycling of surfactant includes the formation of tubular myelin and other aggregated forms that are the precursors to the interfacial monomolecular film. Desorption of material from the interfacial film may then contribute to the intra-alveolar pool of small vesicular forms.

CHANGES IN ALVEOLAR SURFACTANT AT THE START OF AIR BREATHING

While *in utero*, the lung is fluid filled, and no air-liquid interface is present. The initiation of air breathing at birth must be accompanied by formation of an adequate interfacial surfactant layer and the initiation of mechanisms for its maintenance. Experiments with newborn rats and rabbits demonstrated dramatic (10-fold) increases in the amount of phospholipid recoverable from bronchial lavage during the first postnatal day (Fig. 102–10).[37, 38] The separation of lavageable phospholipids into aggregated and nonaggregated classes by differential centrifugation showed that the aggregated forms (including tubular myelin) represented a relatively stable amount of lipid, but the class of lavageable lipid that had liposomal forms increased greatly until a stable adult ratio between aggregated and nonaggregated lipid was achieved by the end of the first postnatal day (see Fig. 102–10). These observations are consistent with the hypothesis that newly secreted surfactant is highly aggregated, and spent surfactant produced by respiratory cycling differs in having the physical appearance of small vesicles.

POSTNATAL MATURATION

From gestational day 19 to day 22 (in rats), the glycogen content of maturing Type II cells decreases rapidly, and lamellar body and mitochondrial volumes increase. The Type II cell at birth provides the lung with a higher surfactant content (per gram of dry lung weight) than at any other time of life, but the Type II cell is still immature.[51] In rats, the Type II cell volume density of lamellar bodies nearly doubles from birth to adulthood (Fig. 102–11). Clara cells undergo a late gestational differentiation similar to that of the Type II cell pattern.[52] Nuclear size, glycogen content, and granular endoplasmic reticulum content decrease, whereas agranular endoplasmic reticulum, mitochondria, and secretory granule content increase. Most of these changes occur postnatally for this cell type, thus placing Clara cell differentiation somewhat later than Type II cell differentiation.

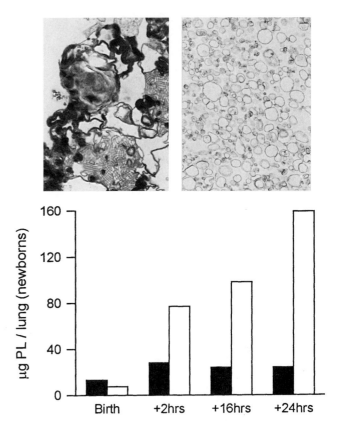

Figure 102–10. The onset of air breathing at birth produces large changes in the alveolar pool of phospholipids. The electron micrographs show the highly aggregated forms of newly secreted surfactant (*upper left panel*) and the vesicular forms that are probably spent surfactant (*upper right panel*). The amount of phospholipid in each fraction is shown in the bar graph with an equal amount of aggregated (*dark bars*) and vesicular (*open bars*) forms at birth to a marked increase in the vesicular forms after a few hours of air breathing. (From Spain CL, et al: Pediatr Res *21*:5, 1987.)

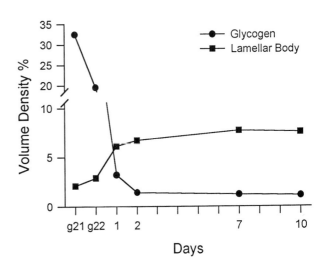

Figure 102–11. Changes in the percentage of composition of Type II components, glycogen, and lamellar bodies. (Adapted from Massaro GD, et al: Am J Physiol *251*:R470, 1986.)

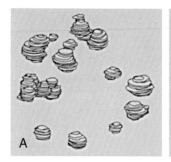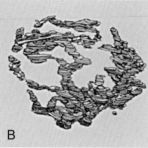

Figure 102–12. Three-dimensional reconstructions of the mitochondria of single Type II cells from a rat on the day of birth (**A**) and an adult rat (**B**). Both are approximately the same magnification.

An interesting postnatal change also occurs in Type II cell mitochondria. As noted in quantitative stereologic studies, the volume density of mitochondria increases postnatally (see Fig. 102–11), but the changing shapes and configuration of mitochondria have not been readily appreciated. Three-dimensional studies reveal that Type II cell mitochondria are isolated spheric organelles at gestational day 22 in rats and that, by adulthood, they assume a branched, interconnected morphology (Fig. 102–12).[27] These changes are similar to those found in mitochondria from widely divergent cell types in which transitions between metabolically quiescent and active states occur, such as exponentially growing yeast or housefly flight muscle during metamorphosis.

ACKNOWLEDGMENT

This work is supported by National Institutes of Health grant HL-32188 and by Veterans Affairs Research Funds.

REFERENCES

1. Stocker JT: The respiratory tract. *In* Stocker JT, Dehner LP (eds): Pediatric Pathology. Philadelphia, Lippincott Williams & Wilkins, 2001, pp 445–518.
2. Low FN, Daniels CW: Electron microscopy of the rat lung. Anat Rec *113*:437, 1952.
3. Terry RJ: Evidence of free fluid in the pulmonary alveoli. Anat Rec *32*:223, 1926.
4. von Neergaard K: Neue Retraktionskraft uber einen Grundbegriff der Attemechanik. Z Ges Exp Med *66*:373, 1929.
5. Clements JA: Surface phenomena in relation to pulmonary function. Physiologist *5*:11, 1962.
6. Macklin CC: The pulmonary alveolar mucoid film and the pneumocytes. Lancet *1*: 1099, 1954.
7. Weibel ER, Gil J: Electron microscopic demonstration of an extracellular duplex lining layer of alveoli. Respir Physiol *4*:42, 1968.
8. Nakamura H, et al: Monomolecular surface film and tubular myelin figures of the pulmonary surfactant in hamster lung. Cell Tissue Res *241*:523, 1985.
9. Spooner BS, Wessells NK: Mammalian lung development: interactions in primordium formation and bronchial morphogenesis. J Exp Zool *175*:445, 1970.
10. Burri P: Development and growth of the human lung. In Fishman AP, Fisher AB (eds): Handbook of Physiology, Vol 1. Bethesda, MD, American Physiological Society, 1985, pp 1–46.
11. Nielsen H, Torday JS: Sex differences in fetal rabbit pulmonary surfactant production. Pediatr Res *15*:1245, 1981.
12. Wuenschell, CW, et al: Embryonic mouse lung epithelial progenitor cells co-express immunohistochemical markers of diverse mature cell lineages. J Histochem Cytochem *44*:113, 1996.
13. Funkhouser JD, et al: Monoclonal antibody identification of a type ii alveolar epithelial cell antigen and expression of the antigen during lung development. Dev Biol *119*:190, 1987.
14. Williams MC, et al: Expression of cell-specific markers for alveolar epithelium in fetal rat lung. Am J Respir Cell Mol Biol *2*:533, 1990.
15. Adamson IYA, Bowden DH: Derivation of type I epithelium from type II cells in the developing rat lung. Lab Invest *32*:736, 1975.
16. Evans MJ, et al: Transformation of alveolar type ii cells to type i cells following exposure to NO$_2$. Exp Mol Pathol *22*:142, 1975.
17. Crapo JD, et al: Cell number and cell characteristics of the normal human lung. Am Rev Respir Dis *125*:332, 1982.
18. Harris JB, et al: Rat lung alveolar type I epithelial cell injury and response to hyperoxia. Am J Respir Cell Mol Biol *4*:115, 1991.
19. Chevalier G, Collet AJ: In vivo incorporation of choline-H, leucine-H, and galactose-H in alveolar type II pneumocytes in relation to surfactant synthesis: a quantitative radioautographic study in mouse by electron microscopy. Anat Rec *174*:289, 1972.
20. Williams MC: Vesicles within vesicles: what role do multivesicular bodies play in alveolar type II cells? Am Rev Respir Dis *135*:744, 1987.
21. Voorhout WF, et al: Intracellular processing of pulmonary surfactant protein B in an endosomal/lysosomal compartment. Am J Physiol *263*:L479, 1992.
22. Whitsett JA, et al: Glycosylation and secretion of surfactant-associated glycoprotein A. J Biol Chem *260*:15273, 1985.
23. Magoon MW, et al: Subfractionation of lung surfactant. Biochim Biophys Acta *750*:18, 1983.
24. Wright JR: Clearance and recycling of pulmonary surfactant. Am J Physiol *259*:L1, 1990.
25. Young SL, et al: Cellular uptake and processing of surfactant lipids and apoprotein SP-A by rat lung. J Appl Physiol *66*:1336, 1989.
26. Young SL, et al: Recycling of surfactant lipid and apoprotein-A studied by electron microscopic autoradiography. Am J Physiol *265*:L19, 1993.
27. Young SL, et al: Three dimensional reconstruction and quantitative analysis of rat lung type II cells: a computer based study. Am J Anat *174*:1, 1985.
28. Adamson IYA, King GM: Epithelial-mesenchymal interactions in postnatal rat lung growth. Exp Lung Res *8*:261, 1985.
29. Brody JS, et al: Alterations in alveolar basement membranes during postnatal lung growth. J Cell Biol *95*:394, 1982.
30. Grant MM, et al: Alterations in lung basement membrane during fetal growth and type II cell development. Dev Biol *97*:173, 1983.
31. Kawanami O, et al: Structure of alveolar epithelial cells in patients with fibrotic lung disorders. Lab Invest *46*:39, 1982.
32. Shannon JM, et al: Functional differentiation of alveolar type II epithelial cells in vitro: effects of cell shape, cell-matrix interactions and cell-cell interactions. Biochim Biophys Acta *931*:143, 1987.
33. Wang Y, et al: Detection of chondroitin sulfates and decorin in developing fetal and neonatal rat lung. Am J Physiol *282*:L484, 2002.
34. Olver RE: Fetal lung liquids. Fed Proc *36*:2669, 1977.
35. Widdicombe JH, et al: Structural changes associated with fluid absorption by dog tracheal epithelium. Exp Lung Res *10*:57, 1986.
36. Faridy EE, et al: Relationship between lung intra and extracellular DSPC in fetal and neonatal rats. Respir Physiol *45*:55, 1981.
37. Spain CL, et al: Alterations of surfactant pools in fetal and newborn rat lungs. Pediatr Res *21*:5, 1987.
38. Stevens PA, et al: Changes in quantity, composition, and surface activity of alveolar surfactant at birth. J Appl Physiol *63*:1049, 1987.
39. Tsilibary EC, Williams MC: Actin and secretion of surfactant. J Histochem Cytochem *31*:1298, 1983.
40. Kliewer M, et al: Secretion of surfactant by rat alveolar type II cells: morphometric analysis and three-dimensional reconstruction. Exp Lung Res *9*:351, 1985.
41. Eckenhoff RG, Somlyo AP: Rat lung type II cell and lamellar body: elemental composition in situ. Am J Physiol *254*:C614, 1988.
42. Benson BJ, et al: Role of apoprotein and calcium ions in surfactant function. Exp Lung Res *6*:223, 1984.
43. Voss T, et al: Macromolecular organization of natural and recombinant lung surfactant protein SP-36. J Mol Biol *201*:219, 1988.
44. Voorhout WF, et al: Surfactant protein A is localized at the corners of the pulmonary tubular myelin lattice. J Histochem Cytochem *39*:1331, 1991.
45. Suzuki Y, et al: Reconstruction of tubular myelin from synthetic lipids and proteins associated with pig pulmonary surfactant. Am Rev Respir Dis *140*:75, 1989.
46. Young SL, et al: Three-dimensional reconstruction of tubular myelin. Exp Lung Res *18*:497, 1992.
47. Wright JR, et al: Uptake of lung surfactant subfractions into lamellar bodies of adult rabbit lungs. J Appl Physiol *60*:817, 1986.
48. Wright JR, et al: Surfactant apoprotein M_r = 26,000–36,000 enhances uptake of liposomes by type II cells. J Biol Chem *262*:2888, 1987.
49. Wright JR, et al: Protein composition of rabbit alveolar surfactant subfractions. Biochim Biophys Acta *791*:320, 1984.
50. Savov J, et al: Mechanical ventilation of rat lung: effect on surfactant forms. Am J Physiol *277*:L320, 1999.
51. Massaro GD, et al: Perinatal anatomic development of alveolar type II cells in rats. Am J Physiol *251*:R470, 1986.
52. Plopper CG, et al: Cytodifferentiation of the nonciliated bronchiolar epithelial (Clara) cell during rabbit lung maturation: an ultrastructural study. Am J Anat *167*:329, 1983.

Seamus A. Rooney

Regulation of Surfactant-Associated Phospholipid Synthesis and Secretion

Lung surfactant is composed largely of lipids, of which phospholipids account for at least 80% of the total. Phosphatidylcholine (PC) is by far the most abundant phospholipid in surfactant and accounts for approximately 80% of its total phospholipid. At least 50% and often as much as 85% of the PC in surfactant preparations consist of the disaturated, surface-active species.[1] Phosphatidylglycerol is the second most abundant phospholipid in surfactant. It represents approximately 13% of the total phospholipid. In some situations, phosphatidylglycerol is replaced by phosphatidylinositol, and there appears to be a reciprocal relationship between the amounts of these two acidic phospholipids in surfactant. The focus in this chapter is on the biosynthesis of the major surfactant phospholipids—PC and disaturated PC. Biosynthesis of the acidic phospholipids—phosphatidylglycerol and phosphatidylinositol—is also discussed. The biosynthesis of other typical membrane phospholipids found in very low amounts in surfactant—phosphatidylethanolamine, sphingomyelin, phosphatidylserine, and cardiolipin—is beyond the scope of this chapter but is discussed elsewhere.[2]

Even though surfactant has a characteristic phospholipid composition, it contains no unique phospholipid component. Although present in relatively large amounts in surfactant, disaturated PC and phosphatidylglycerol are also found in nonsurfactant fractions of the lung[1] and, indeed, in other organs of the body.[3] Thus, it is difficult to study the synthesis of surfactant-associated phospholipids specifically. Of course, rates of substrate incorporation into phospholipids in surfactant-enriched fractions (e.g., lamellar bodies) can be measured, but this is of little help when enzyme activities are to be determined. Studies can be carried out in isolated Type II pneumocytes, which are the cellular sites of surfactant phospholipid biosynthesis, but even the Type II cell synthesizes phospholipid for membranes, as well as for surfactant. Therefore, in most studies it has not been possible to distinguish between synthesis of membrane phospholipids and synthesis of those associated with surfactant, and the data must be interpreted accordingly. In contrast, secretion of specific surfactant-associated phospholipids can be studied relatively easily. This is because membrane phospholipids are not secreted to any appreciable extent. Thus, the lipids secreted by cultured Type II cells have the typical profile of surfactant-associated phospholipids.[1] This is also true of lipids recovered in lung lavage.[1]

PATHWAYS IN THE BIOSYNTHESIS OF PHOSPHOLIPIDS AND FATTY ACIDS

The pathways in the biosynthesis of PC, phosphatidylglycerol, and phosphatidylinositol are illustrated in Figure 103–1. Phospholipid biosynthesis begins with the biosynthesis of phosphatidic acid (PA). This phospholipid occupies a central position in glycerolipid biosynthesis; it is the common lipid precursor of all other glycerophosphatides as well as acylglycerols. The glycerophosphate backbone of PA originates from the triose phosphate, dihydroxyacetone phosphate, an intermediate in glycolysis. Dihydroxyacetone phosphate is metabolized to 1-acylglycerol 3-phosphate by two pathways: acylation followed by reduction or reduction followed by acylation. There is

evidence that both pathways exist in the lung and are involved in the synthesis of PC and phosphatidylglycerol in Type II cells.[4] PA is subsequently synthesized by further acylation of 1-acylglycerol 3-phosphate.

Numerous nonlipid precursors can be incorporated into phospholipids during the biosynthesis of PA.[1] Glucose, derived from dietary sources through the blood or from glycogen degradation in the lung, can be incorporated into phospholipids through the glycolytic pathway and dihydroxyacetone phosphate. Glycerol can be incorporated after phosphorylation to glycerol 3-phosphate by the action of glycerol kinase. Fatty acids are incorporated into phospholipids during the previously described acylation steps, as well as in subsequent reacylation reactions.

PC and the acidic phospholipids, phosphatidylglycerol and phosphatidylinositol, are synthesized from PA by different mechanisms. In the case of PC biosynthesis, PA is first dephosphorylated, and the resulting diacylglycerol (DAG) is combined with cytidine diphosphocholine (CDPcholine) to form PC. CDPcholine arises from choline after initial phosphorylation and subsequent transfer to cytidine triphosphate (CTP) in reactions catalyzed by choline kinase and choline-phosphate cytidylyltransferase (CCT), respectively. Choline is essentially a vitamin in that it is not synthesized in the body but is obtained from dietary sources, often in the form of PC.[5,6]

Although disaturated PC can be synthesized by the foregoing de novo mechanism, there is also evidence that it can be synthesized by remodeling of the 1-saturated-2-unsaturated molecular species. At least half of lung and Type II cell disaturated PC is synthesized by remodeling.[4,7] As shown in Figure 103–1, at least two remodeling mechanisms have been described. Both involve initial deacylation of de novo synthesized 1-saturated-2-unsaturated PC. The resulting 1-acyl-2-lysophosphatidylcholine (lysolecithin) is then either reacylated by reaction with a saturated acyl-coenzyme A (acyl-CoA) or transacylated in a reaction in which two molecules of lysophosphatidylcholine react to form one molecule each of PC and glycerophosphocholine. Of the two remodeling mechanisms, only the reacylation pathway is of any quantitative importance.[4,7,8]

In the synthesis of phosphatidylglycerol and phosphatidylinositol, PA reacts with CTP to form CDPdiacylglycerol. This intermediate then reacts with either inositol or glycerol 3-phosphate to form phosphatidylinositol or phosphatidylglycerophosphate, respectively. The last substance does not accumulate but is immediately dephosphorylated to phosphatidylglycerol.

Fatty acids are clearly integral components of phospholipids and consequently of surfactant. Fatty acids may be synthesized de novo in the lung or supplied from extrapulmonary sources by the blood.[9,10] Although fetal and adult lungs can synthesize fatty acids de novo, the relative contributions of de novo synthesis and exogenous sources to the supply of fatty acids for surfactant synthesis are not known.[7,9] In view of the poor blood supply to the lungs during fetal life, it is likely that de novo synthesis is of quantitative importance at that stage of development. The fatty acid biosynthesis pathway is illustrated in Figure 103–2. Starting from citrate, an intermediate in the Krebs cycle, long chain fatty acid biosynthesis is accomplished by just three enzymes: adenosine triphosphate (ATP)-citrate lyase, acetyl-CoA carboxylase, and

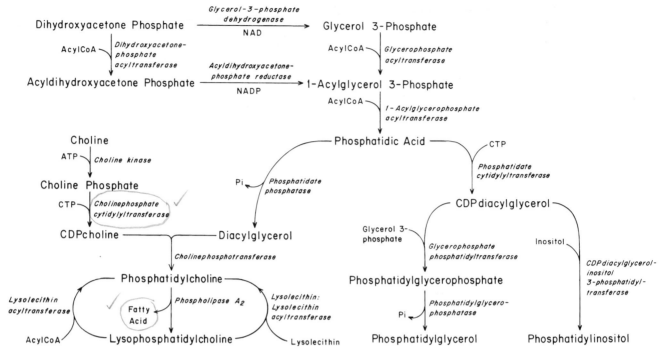

Figure 103–1. Pathways in the biosynthesis of phosphatidylcholine, phosphatidylglycerol, and phosphatidylinositol. (From Rooney SA: Am Rev Respir Dis *131*:439, 1985.)

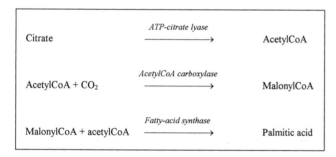

Figure 103–2. Enzymes involved in fatty acid biosynthesis.

fatty-acid synthase (FAS). FAS catalyzes seven distinct biochemical reactions, four of which are repeated for the addition of each 2-carbon unit. In bacteria and plants, the seven reactions are carried out by separate proteins, but in animals and yeasts, they are carried out by single multifunctional proteins.[11, 12] The 16-carbon fatty acid, palmitic acid, is the usual product of *de novo* fatty acid biosynthesis in mammals. All the reactions illustrated in Figures 103-1 and 103-2 have been shown to occur in the lung. Most of the enzymes listed have been assayed in isolated Type II cells.[1]

DEVELOPMENTAL AND HORMONE-INDUCED CHANGES IN LUNG PHOSPHOLIPID CONTENT AND BIOSYNTHESIS

Normal Development

There is an increase in surfactant production toward the end of gestation as the fetus prepares for extrauterine life.[1] The amount of total and disaturated PC in lung lavage from fetal rabbits increases 10-fold between days 27 and 31 (full term) of gestation, and there is a further increase of similar magnitude immediately after birth (Table 103-1). At the same time, the composition of the phospholipids recovered in lung lavage changes substantially. As shown in Figure 103-3, PC increases from less than 30%

of the total phospholipid at 27 days' gestation to almost 70% at term and to 80% or more after birth. During this period, sphingomyelin decreases from almost 40% of the total at 27 days' gestation to less than 10% at term and to 1 to 2% after birth. As shown in Table 103-1, this results in a dramatic increase in the ratio of PC (lecithin) to sphingomyelin (*L/S ratio*). Because fetal lung fluid contributes to amniotic fluid, measurement of the L/S ratio in human amniotic fluid, obtained by amniocentesis, is widely used to predict the degree of fetal lung maturity and hence the optimal time for elective delivery.[13, 14] There is also a developmental increase in the amount of phosphatidylglycerol in late-gestation fetal lung lavage,[15] and measurement of this phospholipid in human amniotic fluid can provide an additional assessment of the extent of fetal lung maturity.[13]

The prenatal increase in surfactant PC appears to be largely the result of increased synthesis, whereas the massive increase immediately after birth is caused by increased secretion in response to labor and ventilation (see later). The rate of incorporation of radiolabeled choline into total or disaturated PC in fetal lung has been used extensively to assess the rate of synthesis of these phospholipids. A major problem in the interpretation of such data is that unless the intracellular pool sizes of choline, choline phosphate, and CDPcholine are known, rates of radiolabeled choline incorporation are not necessarily synonymous with rates of synthesis. Despite this caveat, rates of choline incorporation into PC in fetal lung have correlated quite well with other parameters of synthesis such as increased mass of PC and increased enzyme activities.[8] As shown in Figure 103-4, there is a developmental increase in the rate of choline incorporation into PC in fetal rat lung, and this continues into newborn life. Similar developmental increases have been reported in other species.[1, 8] CCT is a major rate-regulatory enzyme in the biosynthesis of PC,[2, 16] and there is a developmental increase in its activity in the lung either at the end of gestation or immediately after birth.[8] A developmental increase in CCT activity has also been reported in isolated Type II cells,[17] and the increase in activity is accompanied by increased enzyme mass, mRNA content, and mRNA stability,[18, 19] a finding indicating increased expression of the CCT gene.

TABLE 103-1

Developmental Changes in Phospholipid Content and Composition of Rabbit Lung Lavage

	Phospholipid Content (μg Phosphorus/g Lung Dry Wt)		
Gestational Age (d)	*Total Phosphatidylcholine*	*Disaturated Phosphatidylcholine*	L/S Ratio*
27	2.6	1.3	0.8
28	5.4	3.0	1.9
29	7.4	3.4	5.1
30	8.4	4.2	4.3
31	25.4	13.4	9.9
+ 1†	274.0	147.0	31.1
+ 2†	389.0	208.0	39.2
Adult	264.0	143.0	<50.0

Data from refs. 274–276.

* L = phosphatidylcholine (lecithin) as % of total phospholipid: S = sphingomyelin as % of total phospholipid.

† Newborn animals at 1 and 2 days of age.

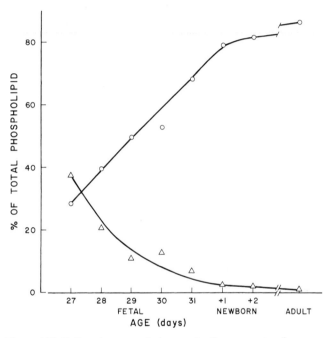

Figure 103-3. Developmental changes in the amounts of phosphatidylcholine (*circles*) and sphingomyelin (*triangles*) in rabbit lung lavage. (From Rooney SA: *In* The Surfactant System and the Neonatal Lung. Mead Johnson Symposium on Perinatal and Developmental Medicine No. 14. Evansville, IN, Mead Johnson, 1979, pp 19-24.)

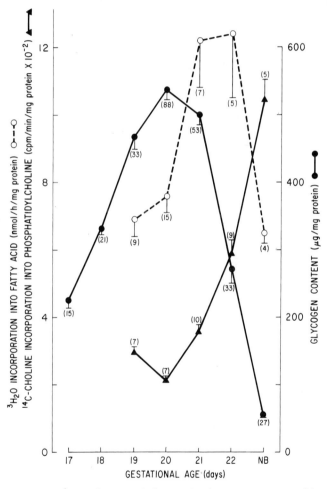

Figure 103-4. Developmental changes in glycogen content and in rates of ^3H_2O incorporation into fatty acids and of [^{14}C]choline incorporation into phosphatidylcholine in developing fetal rat lung. (From Rooney SA, et al: Pediatr Res *20*:545, 1986.)

There is a developmental increase in lung fatty acid biosynthesis during late fetal life. The rate of *de novo* fatty acid biosynthesis can be assessed by measuring the rate of ^3H_2O incorporation into fatty acids. The problem of pool size does not arise in this situation because intracellular and extracellular water become equally labeled. A developmental increase in the rate of fatty acid synthesis in fetal rat lung has been reported using this method.[20, 21] As shown in Figure 103-4, the increase occurs between days 19 and 21 of gestation and is followed by a decrease after birth. The increase in fatty acid biosynthesis coincides with the increase in PC biosynthesis (see Fig. 103-4). The increase in *de novo* fatty acid synthesis in fetal rat lung is accompanied by a similar developmental increase in FAS activity.[22, 23] The increase in FAS activity results from increased gene expression because there is a corresponding developmental increase in the level of FAS mRNA.[24, 25] There is a similar developmental

increase in FAS expression in late-gestation fetal rabbit lung.[26] In contrast to FAS, no changes or minor and inconsistent developmental increases in the activities and mRNA levels of ATP-citrate lyase and acetyl-CoA carboxylase have been reported.[20, 22-25] Therefore, the developmental increase in *de novo* fatty acid biosynthesis is mediated by the increase in FAS expression.

As is also shown in Figure 103-4, there is a developmental increase followed by a decrease in lung glycogen content of fetal rat lung. Similar developmental changes in lung glycogen have been reported in other species.[1] Parallel developmental changes in the enzymes controlling glycogen synthesis and degradation have also been reported.[22, 27, 28] The temporal relationship between glycogen depletion and increased PC synthesis, which has also been reported in isolated fetal Type II cells,[29] prompted speculation that glycogen provides substrate or energy for surfactant phospholipid biosynthesis in the fetal lung.[27, 29, 30] However, a direct relationship between glycogen depletion and increased phospholipid synthesis has not been proven. The reciprocal relationship that exists between fetal lung glycogen content and PC biosynthesis also exists between glycogen and fatty acid biosynthesis (see Fig. 103-4). Glycogen is therefore just as likely to provide substrate or energy for the biosynthesis of fatty acids as for that of phospholipids.

Influence of Hormones

Lung maturation and surfactant production in the fetus can be accelerated by certain hormones and growth factors.

Glucocorticoids

In 1969, Liggins[31] reported that administration of dexamethasone to fetal lambs resulted in delivery of live animals as early as 117 to 123 days of gestation, although term is approximately 147 days. Because such premature fetuses were born alive and had partly expanded lungs, he suggested that the hormone "accelerated appearance of pulmonary surfactant, possibly as a result of premature activity of enzymes involved in a biosynthetic pathway." That the glucocorticoid did increase the amount of surfactant was soon demonstrated by deLemos and colleagues,[32] who measured lung pressure-volume relationships and the surface activity of lung extracts in the same species. Shortly thereafter, similar findings were reported in the rabbit,[33] a species in which accelerated morphologic maturation of the fetal lung was also observed.[34] Within 3 years of the initial observation, Liggins and Howie[35] reported the first successful use of glucocorticoids in the prevention of respiratory distress syndrome (RDS) in human infants. Since that time, there has been intense investigation in many laboratories into the mechanism by which glucocorticoids accelerate fetal lung maturation and stimulate surfactant production.

The influence of glucocorticoids on surfactant phospholipid synthesis and the related biochemical parameters of fetal lung maturation were studied in several species. Experimental models included intact animals and explants of fetal lung in organ culture. Direct injection of fetal rabbits with cortisol or administration of betamethasone to pregnant rabbits results in an increase in the amount of surfactant phospholipid in fetal lung lavage. There is an increase in the amount of total phospholipid and PC, an increase in PC as a percentage of the total phospholipid, and an increase in the L/S ratio.[36, 37] Similarly, glucocorticoid administration *in vivo* increases the rate of PC biosynthesis in fetal rabbit,[37] rat,[21] mouse,[38] baboon,[39] and human[40] lung; and culture of fetal rat,[41] rabbit,[42] baboon,[43] and human[44] lung explants in the presence of the hormone results in the same effect and also increases the amounts of total PC,[44,45] disaturated PC,[45, 46] and phosphatidylglycerol.[45] Glucocorticoids also stimulate fatty acid biosynthesis in fetal lung. They increase the rate of *de novo* fatty acid biosynthesis in fetal rat,[21] rabbit,[47] and human[48] lung. In addition, the hormone has been reported to accelerate the glycogen developmental profile (see Fig. 103-4) in fetal lung. Thus, glucocorticoids increase lung glycogen content at the time of the normal developmental increase in this parameter[21] and decrease it later in gestation at the time of the normal developmental decrease.[21,37,38]

Despite the early prediction by Liggins[31] that glucocorticoids accelerate enzyme activity, there was initially considerable controversy and confusion with respect to the effects of glucocorticoids on enzymes of lipid biosynthesis in the fetal lung. Eventually, it was established that the hormones increase the activity of two lipogenic enzymes in fetal lung in late gestation-CCT and FAS. CCT activity increases in fetal rabbit,[36, 37, 49] rat,[46, 50, 51] and mouse[38] lung tissue and in fetal rat Type II cells[52] after injection of the mother with glucocorticoids. It also increases in fetal rabbit,[53] rat,[54] and human[55] lung explants treated with glucocorticoids in culture. Similarly, FAS activity increases in fetal rat lung tissue[22] and in isolated Type II cells[56] after maternal injection with dexamethasone and in response to the same hormone in cultured explants of fetal rat[25] and human[57] lung. However, unlike in rats and humans, it has been reported that betamethasone does not increase FAS activity in fetal lamb lung.[58] Whether that is the result of a species difference or a function of gestational age needs to be investigated. Glucocorticoids do not increase the activities of ATP-citrate lyase[25] or acetyl-CoA carboxylase.[22] Thus, as in the case of normal development, the glucocorticoid-induced increase in fetal lung fatty acid biosynthesis is entirely the result of increased FAS activity.

The situation with respect to other enzymes of phospholipid synthesis is less clear. Fetal lung phosphatidate phosphatase activity has been reported to increase with glucocorticoid administration in the rabbit and mouse but not in the rat.[8, 59] Glucocorticoids were also shown to increase cholinephosphotransferase activity in a few studies, but it was not a consistent finding.[8, 59] Similarly, lysolecithin acyltransferase, lysolecithin:lysolecithin acyltransferase, and glycerophosphate phosphatidyltransferase activities have been reported to increase in some studies, but not in others.[59]

The finding that glucocorticoid effects occur in cultured explants indicates that the hormone acts directly on the lung. Glucocorticoid receptors have been demonstrated in fetal and adult lung,[60] and data indicate that the effects of glucocorticoids on PC synthesis and CCT and FAS activities are directly mediated by the receptor. Stimulation of PC synthesis in the rat,[61] rabbit,[42] and human[44] and of CCT[54, 55] and FAS[48,62] activities in the rat and human depends on glucocorticoid concentration. The EC_{50} values (concentration at which 50% of the maximal stimulation is achieved) are of the same order of magnitude,[42,44,54,63] or even lower,[62] than the dissociation constant (K_d) values for specific binding of the glucocorticoid to the nuclear receptor. Furthermore, the order of potency of various steroids in producing the previously described effects is the same as that of their binding to the receptor.[42, 54, 62] Glucocorticoid stimulation of PC synthesis[42] and of CCT[64] and FAS[62, 64] activities in fetal lung explants is not apparent until after exposure to the hormone for about 12 hours. Maximal stimulation is achieved in 20 to 36 hours. This time course is consistent with induction of new protein synthesis. The stimulatory effects of the hormone are antagonized by actinomycin D[42,54,62] and cycloheximide,[42,65] and this finding again shows that the action of the hormone involves increased transcription and induction of new protein synthesis.

Glucocorticoid stimulation of CCT activity (a direct effect on the lung) is clearly receptor mediated and dependent on mRNA and protein synthesis. However, quantification by immunotitration[66] and Western blotting[51] revealed that the amount of the CCT protein is not increased by the hormone. Similarly, glucocorticoids have no effect on CCT mRNA content,[19] although small increases have been reported in some studies.[43,67] As discussed in detail later, the preponderance of the evidence suggests that the effect of the hormone results from the activation of existing enzyme, rather than increased expression of the CCT gene. Conversely, the glucocorticoid-induced increase in FAS activity in fetal lung is clearly the result of increased gene expression. The increase in activity is accompanied by an increase in the amounts of FAS protein[56, 57, 62, 68] and mRNA[25, 56, 57, 69] in the rat and human, whereas lung FAS mRNA content is decreased in glucocorticoid-insufficient fetal mice.[70] The glucocorticoid-induced increase in FAS mRNA results from both increased transcription[56, 57, 68] and mRNA stability.[57, 71] Increased transcription is the predominant mechanism in the rat, whereas increased mRNA stabilization predominates in the human.[57, 68, 71] Glucocorticoid-induced transcription of the FAS gene has been reported to be mediated by an 89–base pair fragment in the promoter region.[72] It is therefore clear that the increase in FAS activity in fetal lung is the result of increased expression of the FAS gene. FAS is the only enzyme involved in lipid synthesis that is induced by glucocorticoids in fetal lung. Consistent with a role for FAS in surfactant production, the glucocorticoid-induced increase in its expression is more pronounced in Type II cells than in other lung cells.[56, 57] As discussed later, there is evidence that increased FAS activity accounts for the stimulatory effects of glucocorticoids on PC synthesis and CCT activity.

Although maternal injection with glucocorticoid results in increased CCT[52] and FAS[56] activities in fetal Type II cells (the site of surfactant synthesis within the lung), this action of the hormone is not the result of a direct effect on the Type II cell. Adult Type II cells contain glucocorticoid receptors,[73] and glucocorticoids have stimulatory effects on some parameters in Type II cells,[74-76] including stimulation of surfactant secretion (see later). However, glucocorticoids have little effect on parameters of PC synthesis when either adult[77] or fetal[67, 78] Type II cells are cultured with the hormone. Data indicate that the effects of glucocorticoids on surfactant lipid synthesis are mediated by mesenchymal factors. The maximum effect of cortisol on FAS expression in fetal rat Type II cells requires a fibroblast-conditioned medium.[67] In early studies,[79] a factor released from fibroblasts, fibroblast-pneumonocyte factor (FPF), was proposed to mediate the effect of glucocorticoids, but FPF has never been isolated or characterized. However, other factors are known to be released from fibroblasts, and one or more of those may be the active ingredient in a fibroblast-conditioned medium. Indeed, keratinocyte growth factor (KGF), also called fibroblast growth factor 7, stimulates surfactant phospholipid synthesis, CCT activity, and FAS expression in fetal rat Type II cells.[80] Administration of KGF *in vivo* also increases the amount of disaturated PC in the lungs of preterm rabbits.[81] Dexamethasone increases KGF expression in fetal lung fibroblasts, and an anti-KGF antibody blocks the glucocorticoid-induced increase in PC synthesis in fetal rat Type II cells cultured with fibroblast-conditioned medium.[82] Although involvement of other factors is also possible,[82] such data suggest that KGF may have a major role in mediating the effects of glucocorticoids on stimulation of surfactant synthesis.

Thyroid Hormone

Thyroid hormone has been reported to accelerate surfactant phospholipid production in several species. Direct injection of fetal rabbits with thyroxine (T_4) results in accelerated morphologic lung maturation, as well as increased amounts of surfactant in lung lavage.[8, 83] T_4 also increases the L/S ratio in fetal lamb tracheal fluid.[84] Administration of triiodothyronine (T_3) to pregnant rats results in increased biosynthesis of total and disaturated PC as well as increased CCT activity in the fetal lung.[46] The effect of thyroid hormone is a direct effect on the lung because both PC synthesis and CCT activity are increased in fetal rat lung explants exposed to T_3 or T_4 in culture.[41, 46, 61] T_3 also increases PC synthesis in explants of fetal rabbit[85] and human[44] lung. Fetal lungs of genetically hypothyroid mice are less mature and contain less surfactant than normal.[86, 87]

Thyroid hormone receptors are present in adult and fetal lung and in Type II cells.[88] Half-maximal stimulation of PC synthesis in fetal rabbit and human lung explants is achieved at a concentra-

tion of T_3 that is almost identical to the Kd for binding of the hormone to the nuclear receptor.[44, 85] The relative potencies of various thyroid hormone analogues in stimulating PC biosynthesis and in binding to the receptor are also the same,[44, 85] and the stimulatory effect of T_3 is abolished by actinomycin D and cycloheximide.[85] These data indicate that the stimulatory effect of thyroid hormone in fetal lung is receptor mediated and involves increased gene expression. The gene or genes induced by thyroid hormone remain to be identified.

Several of the stimulatory effects of thyroid hormone in fetal lung are similar to those of glucocorticoids. However, the effects of the two hormones on certain parameters of surfactant phospholipid synthesis have been reported to be additive,[44, 61, 85, 89] a finding suggesting that glucocorticoids and thyroid hormone act through different mechanisms. Furthermore, these two hormone types have opposite effects on other developmental parameters in fetal lung. Thyroid hormone and glucocorticoids both accelerate the normal developmental decrease in fetal lung glycogen content; however, the normal developmental increase in glycogen (which occurs earlier in gestation [see Fig. 103–4]) is accelerated by glucocorticoids but is prevented by thyroid hormone in the fetal rat.[21] Furthermore, the glucocorticoid-accelerated increase is antagonized by thyroid hormone.[21] Similarly, although dexamethasone accelerates the normal developmental increase in *de novo* fatty acid biosynthesis in fetal rat lung, both the normal increase and the stimulatory effect of the glucocorticoid on this parameter are antagonized by thyroid hormone.[21] T_3 does not stimulate *de novo* fatty acid biosynthesis or FAS activity in fetal rat or human lung explants.[22, 48, 62] Furthermore, it diminishes the stimulatory effect of glucocorticoid on FAS activity in fetal rat[22, 62] but not human[48] lung.

A major difficulty in studying the effects of thyroid hormone on the fetal lung *in vivo* is that, in most species, T_4 does not easily cross the placenta. In early studies, therefore, T_4 was administered directly to the fetus.[83] However, directly injecting the fetus, even with saline, causes stress, which itself stimulates surfactant production,[36] so in that model some effects of thyroid hormone may have been masked. Administration of a relatively high dose of T_3 to pregnant rats results in elevated levels of the hormone in the fetal serum, and this model has been employed to examine effects of thyroid hormone on surfactant synthesis *in vivo*.[46] In the same *in vivo* model, antagonism between the effects of glucocorticoids and thyroid hormone on fatty acid biosynthesis, FAS activity, and glycogen accumulation has been observed.[21, 22] In contrast, although the stimulatory effect of T^3 on PC synthesis in cultured fetal lung[44, 61, 85] occurs at a concentration consistent with receptor mediation, the inhibitory effect of thyroid hormone on FAS in the same model requires a much higher hormone concentration.[62] The physiologic relevance of the inhibitory effects of thyroid hormone is therefore not clear.

Thyrotropin-Releasing Hormone

In an effort to overcome the problem of poor placental transfer of thyroid hormone, thyrotropin-releasing hormone (TRH), a tripeptide that readily crosses the placenta, was administered to pregnant rabbits and was found to increase the amount of surfactant phospholipid in lung lavage from the fetuses.[90] TRH has been reported to have a similar effect in the fetal lamb,[91] and it has also been noted to accelerate functional and morphologic lung maturation in the fetal rabbit.[92] A combination of TRH and cortisol is more effective than either hormone alone in the fetal rabbit[93] and lamb.[91, 94] However, a combination of TRH and betamethasone is no more effective than betamethasone alone in prevention of RDS in premature human newborns (see Chap. 108)[95-97] Although there are contradictory data on its effect on PC biosynthesis,[43, 90] TRH was reported to increase CCT mRNA content markedly in fetal baboon lung explants.[43]

Estrogen

Clinical data suggest that low estrogen levels are associated with an increase in the incidence of RDS,[8,98,99] and in one early study, administration of estrogen to pregnant women resulted in an increase in the amniotic fluid L/S ratio.[100] In that study, estrogen was just as effective as dexamethasone.[100] In animal studies, estrogen has been reported to stimulate surfactant production in the late-gestation fetal rabbit[101-104] and rat[105,106] but not in the lamb.[107] The most dramatic changes are found in the fetal rabbit when the hormone is administered to the pregnant doe. In this model, the hormone increases the amount of surfactant phospholipid in lung lavage[101] and the rate of PC synthesis[102,104] and CCT activity in the lung.[102,104,108] In addition, it decreases lung glycogen content.[53,103] *In vivo* administration of estrogen also accelerates morphologic maturation of the fetal rabbit[103] and rat[106] lung.

Estrogen increases PC synthesis[53,105,109] and CCT activity[53] and decreases glycogen[105] in organ cultures of fetal rat and rabbit lung. However, the effects in organ culture are less pronounced than those occurring *in vivo*, they are apparent only at relatively high hormone concentrations,[53,105] and they do not appear to be mediated by an estrogen receptor.[53] It is therefore not clear that the stimulatory effects of estrogen occur directly on the lung. Thus, although estrogen clearly stimulates fetal lung surfactant synthesis, particularly in the rabbit, the mechanism by which this occurs and its physiologic significance are not known.

Prolactin

There is a developmental increase in blood prolactin levels, and infants with RDS have lower levels of this hormone than controls at the same gestational age.[8,110] Although a temporal relationship does not prove cause and effect, such clinical observations led to the hypothesis that prolactin has a role in fetal lung maturation and surfactant production. Support for this notion comes from the observation that administration of prolactin to fetal rabbits led to an increase in the amounts of total phospholipid, total PC, and disaturated PC in fetal lung tissue.[111] Lung lavage was not examined, so surfactant-associated phospholipids were not specifically measured.[111] In other studies, prolactin had no effect on lung PC content or synthesis in the fetal rabbit[112] or on surfactant content in the fetal rabbit[113] or lamb.[112] The lung has prolactin receptors,[114,115] and prolactin was reported to stimulate PC synthesis in cultured explants of fetal rat[116] but not fetal rabbit[117] or human[118] lung. In the rat and human systems, it enhanced the stimulatory effect of glucocorticoids.[116,118] In view of these conflicting data in both *in vivo* and cultured lung systems, a role for prolactin in regulation of surfactant production has not been established.

Other Hormones and Growth Factors

In addition to KGF,[80-82] other hormones and growth factors that have been reported to stimulate surfactant phospholipid production in fetal lung include corticotropin,[8] corticotropin-releasing hormone,[43] epidermal growth factor (EGF),[119,120] parathyroid hormone,[121] leptin,[122] insulin-like growth factor,[123] and gastrin-releasing peptide.[123] Platelet-activating factor (PAF) has been reported to decrease lung glycogen in the fetal rabbit *in vivo*,[124] and there is a temporal relationship between the decrease in glycogen content and increased PAF concentration in cultured human fetal lung explants.[125] However, a role for PAF in regulation of surfactant phospholipid synthesis has not been established. Cyclic adenosine monophosphate (cAMP), which is clearly involved in regulation of surfactant secretion (see later), may also have a regulatory role in its synthesis.[8] cAMP increases FAS expression in human,[126] but not in rat,[68] fetal lung explants. Vitamin D was reported to stimulate surfactant synthesis in fetal rat Type II cells[127] but it did not increase FAS expression.[68]

Numerous agents have been reported to inhibit surfactant phospholipid synthesis in the late-gestation fetal lung. Infants of diabetic mothers are particularly prone to RDS.[128] In animal models, fetuses of rats and rabbits made diabetic by administration of streptozotocin and alloxan exhibit delayed lung maturation and decreased surfactant, as determined by several criteria.[129-132] However, although the infants of diabetic mothers are hyperinsulinemic and hyperglycemic, in the animal models the fetuses generally have high glucose levels, but insulin levels are often normal. It is therefore not clear whether the delayed lung maturation is the result of the increased insulin or the high glucose concentration. Infusion of insulin into fetal rhesus monkeys leads to hyperinsulinemia without elevated glucose levels, but there is no evidence of delayed lung maturation in such animals.[133] Conversely, hyperinsulinemia with hypoglycemia in the fetal rat[134] and lamb[135] does reduce surfactant production. In cultured fetal lung systems, insulin does not decrease PC synthesis,[136,137] but it diminishes the stimulatory effect of glucocorticoids on both PC synthesis[137] and CCT activity.[138] A high glucose concentration has also been reported to decrease surfactant production and morphologic maturation in cultured fetal rat lung explants.[139,140]

It is known that premature male infants are more prone to RDS than female infants.[141] The lungs of female fetuses tend to be about 1 week more mature than those of males, as determined by the amniotic fluid L/S ratio and disaturated PC content.[142] There is also evidence of this female advantage in fetal lung maturation and surfactant synthesis in rats[143-145] and, to a lesser extent, in rabbits,[146,147] but not in monkeys.[148,149] There are reports that this maturational difference may result from inhibition of surfactant production in male fetuses by androgens.[150,151] More recent studies suggest that the androgen effect is caused by enhancement of lung morphogenesis and branching earlier in gestation,[152] and it may be mediated by changes in the relative amounts of EGF and transforming growth factor-β (TGF-β) receptors in fibroblasts.[153]

TGF-β$_1$ was reported to antagonize the dexamethasone-induced increase in FAS expression in human fetal lung explants,[154] an effect that appears to be mediated at the transcription level.[72] Retinoic acid was reported to antagonize the stimulatory effect of glucocorticoids on FAS expression in fetal rat lung explants, but retinoic acid on its own had no effect.[68] In contrast, retinoic acid was reported to increase the amount of fetal lung surfactant phospholipid and rate of PC synthesis.[155] Vitamin A–deficient fetal rats were reported to have a reduced amount of surfactant phospholipid, an effect accompanied by decreased FAS expression but normal CCT activity.[156]

MECHANISM OF REGULATION OF FETAL LUNG PHOSPHATIDYLCHOLINE BIOSYNTHESIS

Numerous studies in the developing fetal lung, in isolated Type II cells, and in other organs established that CCT is a major rate-regulatory enzyme in *de novo* PC biosynthesis.[2,4,16] As shown in Figure 103-1, CCT catalyzes the conversion of choline phosphate to CDPcholine. The size of the choline phosphate pool is larger than that of choline or CDPcholine in both whole lung and Type II cells.[4] As discussed earlier, there is a developmental increase in CCT activity in association with increased PC biosynthesis in the developing lung. Glucocorticoids, thyroid hormone, and estrogen, which stimulate PC synthesis and increase PC content in fetal lung, also increase CCT activity.

The developmental increase in fetal lung CCT activity is largely the result of increased expression of the CCT gene,[18,19] although activation of existing enzyme may also be involved.[157,158] In contrast, although the stimulatory effect of glucocorticoids on fetal lung CCT activity is dependent on new protein and mRNA synthesis, CCT is not the protein that is induced by the hormone: CCT enzyme mass[51, 66] and mRNA content[19] are not increased by glucocorticoids in the fetal lung. The effect of glucocorticoids on CCT activity is caused by activation of existing enzyme, rather than by synthesis of new CCT. How is CCT activated?

CCT belongs to a group of proteins called amphitropic[159] or ambiquitous,[160] the activities of which are regulated by interconversion between a soluble and a membrane-bound form. There is considerable evidence that CCT activity is regulated by reversible membrane association: the membrane-bound form is active, whereas the soluble form is inactive and requires lipid for activation.[2, 161] The curvature and other physical properties of the membrane are critical in the interaction with CCT.[162, 163] Physiologic activation of CCT in many systems is believed to involve translocation of the enzyme from the cytosol to membranes.[164] Translocation from cytosol to microsomes has been reported in association with increased PC synthesis in choline-depleted Type II cells.[165] However, translocation is not always involved in CCT activation, because activation without translocation has been reported.[2, 166] There is little evidence that translocation has a role in hormonal stimulation of CCT activity in the fetal lung. The stimulatory effects of dexamethasone on CCT in the fetal rat[54] and of estrogen in the fetal rabbit[108] are clearly not the result of translocation. The bulk of the enzyme is in the cytosolic fraction, and the subcellular distribution is not altered by the hormones. Estrogen increases only the CCT activity in the cytosol and has no effect on activities in the microsomal or mitochondrial fractions.[108] Similarly, dexamethasone does not alter the subcellular distribution of CCT in fetal lung Type II cells, although in that study, most of the activity was in the microsomal fraction.[52]

It is clear, however, that hormonal activation of CCT is mediated by endogenous lipids. Fetal lung CCT activity can be increased severalfold by inclusion of fatty acids,[167] as well as phospholipids,[108, 168, 169] in the assay mixture, and when the enzyme is assayed in the presence of sufficient lipid to achieve maximal activation in vitro, the stimulatory effects of glucocorticoids,[46, 51, 54, 64, 66] T_3,[46] and estrogen[102, 104, 108] are considerably reduced or completely abolished. Because the lipids would be expected to activate any newly synthesized CCT just as much as existing enzyme, these data are consistent with the concept that it is the catalytic activity, rather than the amount of CCT, that is increased by the hormones. CCT activity in fetal lung cytosol is markedly decreased by extraction of lipids with solvents that do not cause protein denaturation.[51, 108, 157] Lipid extraction under the same conditions completely abolishes the stimulatory effects of betamethasone in the rat[51] and of estrogen in the rabbit.[108] CCT activity and the stimulatory effects of the hormones are fully restored on re-addition of the appropriate lipid extract.[51, 108] Furthermore, the stimulatory effects of the hormones can be switched from the treated to the control groups by interchanging the added lipids.[51, 108] Such data establish that the stimulatory effects of those hormones are mediated by a lipid factor. Indeed, betamethasone elevates the levels of some phospholipids and fatty acids in fetal rat lung.[51] Estrogen also increases phospholipid levels in fetal rabbit lung, but its effect on fatty acids has not been examined.[108]

As discussed earlier, glucocorticoids enhance fatty acid biosynthesis and increase expression of the FAS gene in late-gestation fetal lung. Indeed, FAS is the only gene for a lipogenic enzyme that is known to be induced by glucocorticoid in fetal lung. Inhibition of fatty biosynthesis in fetal rat lung explants completely abolishes the stimulatory effect of dexamethasone on CCT activity.[64] This finding suggests that the stimulatory effect of glucocorticoids on CCT activity in fetal lung is mediated by induction of the FAS gene. Whether FAS induction also accounts for the estrogen- and thyroid hormone–induced increases in CCT activity is a question that remains to be investigated.

It is not clear at present whether the glucocorticoid effect on CCT activity is mediated by free fatty acids, by the lipids into which they become incorporated, or possibly by other fatty acid metabolites. The observations that linoleic acid was the fatty acid that was increased to the greatest extent by betamethasone in fetal rat lung and the same fatty acid was the most effective in activating CCT in vitro led to the suggestion that glucocorticoid stimulation of fetal lung CCT activity is mediated by linoleic acid.[170] However, linoleic acid is an essential fatty acid that is not synthesized by mammals. It is consequently difficult to reconcile the notion that glucocorticoid activation of CCT is mediated by induction of FAS with the concept that it is also mediated by linoleic acid. In summary, although there is compelling evidence that the stimulatory effect of glucocorticoids on CCT activity results from increased FAS expression and is mediated by endogenous lipids, the precise identity of the activator(s) remains to be established.

There are three CCT isoforms: α, β_1, and β_2. The β isoforms are splice variants of the same gene, but CCTα is encoded by a different gene.[166, 171] There are some sequence differences among the three isoforms, but the catalytic and membrane-binding domains are highly conserved.[166] All three isoforms are enzymatically active and are regulated by reversible membrane association.[166] The membrane-bound form of CCTα has been reported to be largely associated with the nucleus in some systems,[2, 16, 166] but it is also found in association with endoplasmic reticulum,[171] especially in the lung, where it is entirely extranuclear.[172, 173] In contrast, CCTβ_1 and CCTβ_2 are associated with the endoplasmic reticulum.[16, 171] CCTα is widely expressed,[171] and it is the most extensively investigated of the three isoforms. The three CCT isomers are expressed in fetal lung, but only CCTα is expressed in adults.[171] Therefore, an interesting question that has not yet been addressed is whether one or both of the CCTβ isoforms may have a role in regulation of PC synthesis during fetal lung development.

Although the glucocorticoid-induced increase in CCT activity appears to be primarily the result of enzyme activation, the possibility of increased synthesis cannot be discounted entirely. In contrast to the effect of estrogen in fetal rabbit lung, in which stimulation of CCT is completely abolished by inclusion of phosphatidylglycerol in the in vitro assay mixture,[102, 104, 108] glucocorticoid stimulation of CCT activity in rat and mouse lung is not completely abolished by inclusion of activating lipids.[38, 46, 51, 54, 64, 66] Indeed, although markedly reduced, the stimulatory effect of dexamethasone remained statistically significant even in the presence of phosphatidylglycerol.[38, 54] In human lung explants, increased CCT activity in response to dexamethasone was even more pronounced and became statistically significant only when phosphatidylglycerol was included in the assay mixture.[55] That the stimulatory effect of the hormone was apparent when the enzyme was maximally activated in vitro suggests an increase in enzyme mass. As discussed earlier, CCT mRNA was reported to be increased in some studies,[43, 67] although that was not a consistent finding.[19]

Apart from CCT, it is possible that other enzymes have regulatory roles in phospholipid biosynthesis, at least under some circumstances. In one study,[174] mice overexpressing CCT in the lungs had only modest increases in PC synthesis and content, a finding suggesting that other steps in the PC biosynthetic pathway may also be important in its regulation. As discussed earlier, activities of fetal lung phosphatidate phosphatase, cholinephosphotransferase, lysolecithin acyltransferase, lysolecithin:lysolecithin acyltransferase, and glycerophosphate phosphatidyltransferase have been reported to be increased in some studies either during normal development or after hormone treatment. Data suggest that glycerophosphate acyltransferase, an enzyme catalyzing an early step in glycerophospholipid synthesis (see Fig. 103–1), has a regulatory role in

Type II cells isolated from adult rats[175] and rabbits.[176] There is also evidence that choline kinase and phosphatidate phosphatase are regulatory enzymes in other organs.[2] However, rate-regulatory roles for these and other enzymes have not been established in the fetal lung.

SECRETION OF SURFACTANT-ASSOCIATED PHOSPHOLIPIDS

Lamellar inclusion bodies are the secretory organelles of the Type II pneumocyte. The phospholipid composition of isolated lamellar bodies is virtually identical to that of surfactant.[1] After their biosynthesis, surfactant phospholipids are stored in lamellar bodies and are finally secreted into the alveolar lumen by the process of regulated exocytosis.[177-181] A lamellar body in the process of exocytosis is shown in Figure 103–5. It is possible that there is also some constitutive secretion of surfactant lipids; the basal secretion of phospholipids that is observed in isolated Type II cells cultured without secretagogues may well be a constitutive process. However, secretion of surfactant appears to be a slow process, with little difference between regulated and constitutive mechanisms.[182]

Surfactant secretion has been measured in several systems ranging from intact animals *in vivo* to isolated Type II cells in culture.[177-180] Isolated Type II cells have been the model of choice for most studies on the regulation of surfactant secretion. Most such studies have been carried out on Type II cells isolated from adult animals, but surfactant secretion in fetal and newborn Type II cells[76,183-185] has also been investigated. In most studies, secretion of surfactant phospholipid has been assessed biochemically by labeling the intracellular PC pool with [³H]choline during overnight culture of the cells and then measuring the amount of [³H]PC or disaturated PC released into the medium. However, cell physiologic and fluorescent techniques have been used to study surfactant secretion and membrane fusion kinetics in single Type II cells.[182,186-189]

Various physiologic and pharmacologic agents stimulate surfactant secretion in isolated Type II cells, and there are also

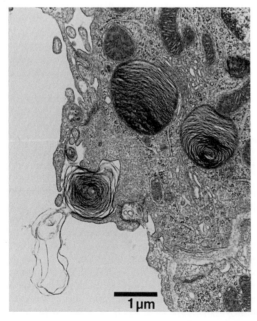

Figure 103–5. Exocytosis of a lamellar body by an adult rat Type II cell. This electron micrograph was generated by Dr. Stephen L. Young at Duke University. (From Rooney SA, et al: FASEB J 8:957, 1994.)

agents that inhibit it.[177-180] Well-established surfactant secretagogues in cultured Type II cells include the following: β-adrenergic, adenosine A_{2B}, and $P2Y_2$ receptor agonists; agents such as tetradecanoylphorbol acetate (TPA); cell-permeable DAGs; forskolin and cholera toxin, which bypass receptors and activate downstream signaling steps; and the ionophores ionomycin and A23187, which promote calcium (Ca^{2+}) influx into the cell (Fig. 103–6).

A working model of the signal-transduction mechanisms that mediate surfactant secretion is shown in Figure 103–6. The signaling mechanisms consist of three distinct pathways, although there is overlap and interactions among them.[177,190] The first mechanism involves activation of adenylate cyclase (AC), generation of cAMP and subsequent activation of cAMP-dependent protein kinase (protein kinase A [PKA]). This pathway is activated by agonists such as terbutaline and the adenosine analogue N-ethylcarboxyamidoadenosine (NECA) that bind to β-adrenergic and adenosine A_{2B} receptors, respectively, both of which are coupled to AC through the G-protein G_s. The AC pathway is also activated by cholera toxin, which permanently activates G_s, and by forskolin, which directly activates AC.

The second mechanism involves direct or indirect activation of protein kinase C (PKC). TPA and cell-permeable DAGs directly activate PKC. ATP and uridine triphosphate (UTP) activate PKC by binding to $P2Y_2$ receptors that are coupled to phospholipase C-$β_3$ (PLC-$β_3$) through G_q. Activation of PLC-$β_3$ results in hydrolysis of phosphatidylinositol bisphosphate and formation of DAG, which then activates PKC. PKC, in turn, activates phospholipase D (PLD),[191] which hydrolyzes PC to form choline and PA. Phosphatidate phosphatase converts PA to DAG (see Fig. 103–1), which further activates PKC. The PLD loop may provide a mechanism whereby surfactant secretion is sustained for a prolonged period. PA itself may also have a signaling role,[192] although that possibility has not been investigated in the Type II cell. In addition to acting through $P2Y_2$ receptors, ATP also stimulates surfactant secretion by the cAMP pathway; ATP, but not UTP, promotes cAMP formation in the Type II cell.[193] This effect of ATP is not the result of direct action at the adenosine A2B receptor.[177] Whether it is caused by catabolism to adenosine with consequent activation of A_{2B} receptors[194] or by activation of an unidentified AC-coupled receptor[177,195] has not been established.

The third mechanism involves elevation of intracellular Ca^{2+} levels. This can be accomplished by increasing the level of inositol triphosphate (IP_3), the other product of the action of PLC-$β_3$; IP_3 promotes mobilization of Ca^{2+} from intracellular stores.[196] It can also be accomplished by ionophores that promote Ca^{2+} influx into the cell from the medium. Ca^{2+} activates a Ca^{2+}/calmodulin-dependent protein kinase (CaCM-PK) and may also act synergistically with DAG to activate some PKC isoforms. Protein phosphorylation by PKA, PKC, or CaCM-PK ultimately leads to surfactant secretion.

Secretion is an indispensable step in the overall homeostasis of surfactant.[179,197] Failure of secretion would likely lead to a drastic deficiency in surfactant. Because severe surfactant deficiency is probably incompatible with life, it is likely that there is sufficient redundancy so a fatal defect in surfactant secretion does not occur. This would account for the number of potential physiologic agonists that can stimulate surfactant secretion and would also explain the multiple signaling mechanisms.

There is a developmental increase in agonist-induced surfactant secretion in fetal and neonatal rat Type II cells.[183,185] The response to the $P2Y_2$ agonist UTP is negligible in early newborn cells, but it increases with age,[185] and the response to ATP, terbutaline, NECA, and TPA also increases with age.[183] Dexamethasone significantly increases the response to terbutaline, NECA, ATP, and UTP in early newborn rat Type II cells while causing a small decrease in the basal rate of surfactant secretion.[76] This effect is mediated by the glucocorticoid receptor and is probably the result of induction of a signaling step downstream of the receptors that is common to the different signaling pathways.[76] Thus, in addition to stimulation of surfactant synthesis, regulation of its secretion may be an additional function of glucocorticoids in the developing lung.

There are many subtypes and isomers of the receptors and other signaling proteins shown in Figure 103–6, and there is increasing information on the identity of those involved in surfactant secretion. Of the three β-receptors, β_3 is not expressed in the lung,[198] but the β_1 and β_2 genes are both expressed in the Type II cell.[199,200] However, pharmacologic data suggest that surfactant secretion is regulated by the β_2 receptor.[201,202] There are four subtypes of adenosine receptors, A_1, A_{2A}, A_{2B}, and A_3,[203] and all four are expressed in the Type II cell.[199] Agonist and antagonist potency data and the observation that adenosine agonists that stimulate surfactant secretion also enhance cAMP formation make it clear that it is the adenosine A_{2B} receptor that regulates surfactant secretion.[195] P2 receptors are divided into two major groups: P2X receptors are ion channels, whereas P2Y receptors are metabotropic and are coupled to G-proteins.[204] To date, seven mammalian P2X and seven P2Y receptors have been cloned.[205,206] There is good evidence that the P2 purinoceptor responsible for stimulation of surfactant secretion is P2Y$_2$,[177,195] which was termed P$_{2u}$ in an older nomenclature system.[204] The P2Y$_2$ receptor is expressed in the Type II cell,[193,199,207] ATP and UTP are equally potent at P2Y$_2$ receptors,[204] and both nucleotides stimulate surfactant secretion in Type II cells with similar EC$_{50}$ values.[193] Additional agonist potency order data are also consistent with involvement of the P2Y$_2$ receptor in surfactant secretion.[193,208,209]

There are four subfamilies of mammalian PLC: β,γ, δ, and ε.[210] P2Y$_2$ receptors are coupled to PLC-β,[211] of which there are four isoforms: β_1, β_2, β_3, and β_4.[212] PLC-β_3 is the only PLC-β isomer expressed in the Type II cell[199] and therefore the one involved in regulation of surfactant secretion. The P2Y$_2$ receptor is also coupled to PLC-β_3 in other systems.[211] Twelve PKC isoforms are currently known to exist: α, βI, βII, δ, ε, γ, η θ, ζ, λ/ι, μ, and ν.[213] PKCμ and PKCν are structurally different from the other PKCs[214,215] and have been designated as a new class of protein kinases, protein kinase D (PKD), of which there are currently three members.[216] In this system, PKCμ becomes PKD1. The α, βI, βII, δ, η, θ, and ζ isoforms of PKC as well as PKD1 are expressed in the Type II cell.[199,217] PKD1 is activated by the P2Y$_2$ agonists ATP and UTP as well as by TPA and a cell-permeable DAG, dioctanoylglycerol, in the Type II cell.[218] This finding suggests a physiologic role for PKD1 in regulation of surfactant secretion. TPA and dioctanoylglycerol also activate PKCs α, βI, βII, δ, and η;[217,218] however, because both agonists are nonphysiologic, the significance of this in terms of regulation of surfactant secretion is not clear. PKD is involved in several signaling pathways and has been reported to be downstream of PKC.[216] However, in Type II cells, there is no evidence that any PKC isomers other than PKD1 are activated by P2Y$_2$ agonists.[218]

The specific isomers of other signaling proteins (see Fig. 103–6) involved in regulation of surfactant secretion have not been identified. There are two mammalian PLDs, PLD1 and PLD2,[219] and both are expressed in the Type II cell.[181] However, the PLD isomers involved in surfactant secretion are not known. Eight of the nine membrane-associated mammalian AC isoforms are expressed in the lung,[220,221] and AC-II and AC-IV, but not AC-I, are expressed in the Type II cell.[222] Whether other ACs are also expressed in the Type II cell is not known, and the AC isoforms involved in surfactant secretion have not been identified. There is currently no information of the subunits or isomers of PKA[223]

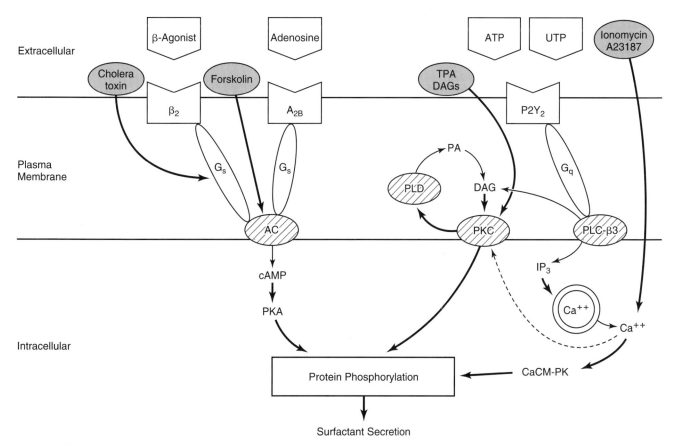

Figure 103–6. Schematic representation of signal transduction mechanisms mediating surfactant phospholipid secretion in Type II cells. See text for explanation and abbreviations. (Modified from Rooney SA, et al: FASEB J 8:957, 1994.)

and CaCM-PK[224, 225] that are expressed in the Type II cells or are involved in surfactant secretion.

Other signaling mechanisms may also be involved in surfactant secretion.[181] For instance, data suggest involvement of phospholipase A_2 as well as a PC-specific PLC in ATP- and TPA-mediated secretion.[177] High- and low-density serum lipoproteins stimulate PC secretion by activation of receptors coupled to PKC through G_i.[226, 227] Mastoparan, an agent that activates several signaling mechanisms, is a powerful surfactant secretagogue, and there are indications that its effect is also mediated in part by G_i.[228] Mitogen-activated protein (MAP) kinase activation is not involved in surfactant secretion, although this enzyme is often downstream of PKC activation,[229] and it is activated by $P2Y_2$ agonists in numerous systems.[181, 230, 231] Although ATP and TPA activate the MAP kinase cascade in Type II cells,[232] MAP kinase inhibitors do not antagonize agonist-stimulated PC secretion.[181,232,233] Involvement of the MAP kinase cascade in SP-A inhibition of surfactant secretion has also been discounted.[180,233] Experiments with inhibitors similarly suggest that tyrosine kinase signaling does not have a role in regulation of surfactant secretion,[181] although it is involved in P2 receptor signaling in other systems.[231]

Distal steps in the surfactant secretory pathway have been incompletely studied. As shown in Figure 103-6, all the signal-transduction pathways are believed to result in phosphorylation of proteins after activation of specific protein kinases. There is virtually no information on the identity of the proteins phosphorylated in response to surfactant secretagogues, although TPA[234] and terbutaline[235] were reported to promote phosphorylation of certain proteins in Type II cells. Relatively little is known of the steps beyond protein phosphorylation that ultimately result in exocytosis of lamellar bodies;[177] there is essentially no information on whether the SNARE (soluble NSF [N-ethylmaleimide–sensitive fusion protein] attachment protein receptor) paradigm of vesicle (lamellar body) docking and membrane fusion[236, 237] applies to surfactant secretion.[177] However, some of the proteins involved in the SNARE exocytosis mechanism are phosphorylated,[236, 237] and it is possible that such proteins are the site of action of the protein kinases involved in surfactant secretion. There is also evidence of a role for synexin in fusion of lamellar bodies with the cell membrane in Type II cells,[238, 239] and it has been suggested that both synexin and the SNARE mechanism may be independently involved in mediating surfactant secretion.[239]

Little is known about the physiologic regulation of surfactant secretion.[177, 181] Two physiologic factors are known to stimulate surfactant secretion *in vivo*: ventilation/exercise, which stimulates secretion in both adults[240-243] and newborns,[244, 245] and labor, which stimulates secretion in newborns.[246] Ventilation-induced surfactant secretion is thought to result from a direct mechanical effect on the lung,[247] and *in vitro* experiments have shown that stretch increases surfactant secretion in Type II cells.[248] There is also evidence that ventilation causes stretch of Type I cells, and the Type I cell then acts as a mechanotransducer to stimulate surfactant secretion by the Type II cell.[189] There is an extensive literature on the mechanisms by which the effects of physical forces are transduced.[247] There is evidence of the involvement of at least three signaling pathways: activation of AC, PLC and MAP kinase. Although, as discussed earlier, MAP kinase is not involved in regulation of surfactant secretion,[181,232,233] both AC and PLC are involved (Fig. 103-6).

There is direct evidence of a physiologic role for the AC signaling mechanism in regulation of surfactant secretion. A physiologic role for β-receptor activation is suggested by the finding that the stimulatory effects of ventilation[241] and labor[249] are antagonized by β-antagonists. A similar role for the adenosine A_{2B} receptor is suggested by the finding that the ventilation-induced increase in surfactant secretion in newborn rabbits is attenuated by an adenosine receptor antagonist.[244] Finally, although atropine blocks the effect of ventilation *in vivo*,[240, 244, 245] a finding suggesting cholinergic regulation, there is substantial evidence that cholinergic regulation of surfactant secretion is mediated by activation of β-receptors on the Type II cell in response to catecholamines released from the adrenal medulla.[177] β-agonists,[241,250] cholinergic agonists,[240, 244, 250] and adenosine[251] all stimulate surfactant secretion *in vivo*.

There is currently no direct evidence that PLC activation has a physiologic role. As shown in Figure 103-6, PLC-β_3 is central to both the PKC and CaCM-PK signaling pathways. Apart from ATP, UTP, and possibly lipoproteins,[227] the only well-established surfactant secretagogues that activate the PKC signaling pathway are the nonphysiologic agonists TPA and cell-permeable DAGs, whereas those that activate the CaCM-PK pathway are the equally unphysiologic ionophores ionomycin and A23187. It is highly likely that some physiologic agonist activates those signaling mechanisms, and it is tempting to speculate that ATP or UTP may be such an agonist. Currently, there is no information on whether the $P2Y_2$ receptor on the Type II cell has a physiologic role in regulation of surfactant secretion, but there is good evidence that the $P2Y_2$ receptor has such a role in many other systems.[204, 205, 252, 253] Activation of P2Y receptors is one of the mechanisms by which the effect of mechanical force is transduced;[254] a mechanical stimulus promotes release of ATP and UTP in airway epithelial and other cells.[254-256] The nucleotides then activate P2Y receptors on either the same or adjacent cells in an autocrine or paracrine manner.[253, 254, 256] Mechanical stimulation activates PLC in airway epithelial and other cells,[257, 258] and the stretch-induced increase in surfactant secretion in Type II cells is accompanied by elevated intracellular Ca^{2+} levels.[248] Thus, there is a reasonable possibility that the stimulatory effect of ventilation on surfactant secretion is mediated by the Type II cell $P2Y_2$ receptor and therefore by the PKC or CaCM-PK signaling pathways. Based on tissue culture data, ATP levels in bronchoalveolar lavage fluid[259] are sufficient to stimulate surfactant secretion.

SECRETION OF SURFACTANT PROTEINS

Secretion of the protein components of surfactant has been less extensively investigated than that of the phospholipids. Lamellar bodies are enriched in the hydrophobic proteins, SP-B and SP-C,[260] and these organelles have a central role in the overall processing of both proteins.[261] Secretion of SP-B and SP-C in rat Type II cells is stimulated by the same agonists that stimulate PC secretion: terbutaline, NECA, ATP, TPA, and ionomycin.[262] A combination of agonists and a PKC inhibitor have the same effects on secretion of SP-B and SP-C as on that of PC.[262] In addition, there is evidence that *in vivo* secretion of SP-B and PC have similar kinetics.[263] Therefore, secretion of surfactant phospholipids and of hydrophobic proteins is similarly regulated, and secretion of both involves exocytosis of lamellar bodies.

In contrast, secretion of SP-A and SP-D occurs by a different mechanism. Although there are conflicting data with respect to the distribution of SP-A between lamellar bodies and other compartments of the Type II cell,[180,264-266] there is general agreement that secretion of SP-A occurs independently of lamellar bodies. SP-A secretion in isolated Type II cells is usually not stimulated by agonists that stimulate PC secretion,[184, 262, 265, 267] although in two studies it was stimulated by TPA.[268, 269] Furthermore, both *in vivo*[270, 271] and tissue culture[266] experiments suggest that newly synthesized SP-A is secreted independently of lamellar bodies. Lamellar bodies are devoid of SP-D,[272, 273] and secretion of SP-D is not stimulated by surfactant phospholipid secretagogues in isolated Type II cells.[262,267,268]

In summary, secretion of surfactant phospholipids, SP-B, and SP-C occurs largely by regulated exocytosis of lamellar bodies, whereas secretion of SP-A and SP-D occurs independently of lamellar bodies and is either not regulated or is regulated by a different mechanism from that of the phospholipids and hydrophobic proteins.

REFERENCES

1. Rooney SA: Phospholipid composition, biosynthesis, and secretion. *In* Parent RA (ed): Comparative Biology of the Normal Lung. Boca Raton, FL, CRC Press, 1992, p 511.
2. Kent C: Eukaryotic phospholipid biosynthesis. Annu Rev Biochem 1995;64:315.
3. Mason RJ: Disaturated lecithin concentration of rabbit tissues. Am Rev Respir Dis 1973;107:678.
4. Rooney SA: Regulation of surfactant phospholipid biosynthesis. *In* Rooney SA (ed): Lung Surfactant: Cellular and Molecular Processing. Austin, TX, Landes, 1998, p 29.
5. Zeisel SH, Blusztajn JK: Choline and human nutrition. Annu Rev Nutr 1994;14:269.
6. Blusztajn JK: Choline, a vital amine. Science 1998;281:794.
7. Batenburg JJ: Surfactant phospholipids: synthesis and storage. Am J Physiol 1992;262:L367.
8. Rooney SA: The surfactant system and lung phospholipid biochemistry. Am Rev Respir Dis 1985;131:439.
9. Rooney SA: Fatty acid biosynthesis in developing fetal lung. Am J Physiol 1989;257:L195.
10. Coleman RA: Placental metabolism and transport of lipid. Fed Proc 1986;45:2519.
11. Wakil SJ, et al: Fatty acid synthesis and its regulation. Annu Rev Biochem 1983;52:537.
12. Smith S: The animal fatty acid synthase: one gene, one polypeptide, seven enzymes. FASEB J 1994;8:1248.
13. Dubin SB: The laboratory assessment of fetal lung maturity. Am J Clin Pathol 1992;97:836.
14. Burkhart AE, et al: Neonatal outcome when delivery follows a borderline immature lecithin to sphingomyelin ratio. J Perinatol 2000;20:157.
15. Hallman M, Gluck L: Formation of acidic phospholipids in rabbit lung during perinatal development. Pediatr Res 1980;14:1250.
16. Kent C: CTP:phosphocholine cytidylyltransferase. Biochim Biophys Acta 1997;1348:79.
17. Zimmermann LJ, et al: Regulation of phosphatidylcholine synthesis in fetal type II cells by CTP:phosphocholine cytidylyltransferase. Am J Physiol 1993;264:L575.
18. Hogan M, et al: Increased expression of CTP:phosphocholine cytidylyltransferase in maturing type II cells. Am J Physiol 1994;267:L25.
19. Hogan M, et al: Regulation of phosphatidylcholine synthesis in maturing type II cells: increased mRNA stability of CTP:phosphocholine cytidylyltransferase. Biochem J 1996;314:799.
20. Maniscalco WM, et al: De novo fatty acid synthesis in developing rat lung. Biochim Biophys Acta 1982;711:49.
21. Rooney SA, et al: Thyroid hormone opposes some glucocorticoid effects on glycogen content and lipid synthesis in developing fetal rat lung. Pediatr Res 1986;20:545.
22. Pope TS, Rooney SA: Effects of glucocorticoid and thyroid hormones on regulatory enzymes of fatty acid synthesis and glycogen metabolism in developing fetal rat lung. Biochim Biophys Acta 1987;918:141.
23. Batenburg JJ, et al: Phosphatidylcholine synthesis in type II cells and regulation of the fatty acid supply. Prog Respir Res 1990;25:96.
24. Batenburg JJ, Whitsett JA: Levels of mRNAs coding for lipogenic enzymes in rat lung upon fasting and refeeding and during perinatal development. Biochim Biophys Acta 1990;1006:329.
25. Xu ZX, et al: Glucocorticoid regulation of fatty acid synthase gene expression in fetal rat lung. Am J Physiol 1993;265:L140.
26. Das DK: Fatty acid synthesis in fetal lung. Biochem Biophys Res Commun 1980;92:867.
27. Maniscalco WM, et al: Development of glycogen and phospholipid metabolism in fetal and newborn rat lung. Biochim Biophys Acta 1978;530:333.
28. Bhavnani BR: Ontogeny of some enzymes of glycogen metabolism in rabbit fetal heart, lungs, and liver. Can J Biochem Cell Biol 1983;61:191.
29. Carlson KS, et al: Temporal linkage of glycogen and saturated phosphatidylcholine in fetal lung type II cells. Pediatr Res 1987;22:79.
30. Farrell PM, Bourbon JR: Fetal lung surfactant lipid synthesis from glycogen during organ culture. Biochim Biophys Acta 1986;878:159.
31. Liggins GC: Premature delivery of foetal lambs infused with glucocorticoids. Endocrinology 1969;45:515.
32. deLemos RA, et al: Acceleration of appearance of pulmonary surfactant in the fetal lamb by administration of corticosteroids. Am Rev Respir Dis 1970;102:459.
33. Kotas RV, Avery ME: Accelerated appearance of pulmonary surfactant in the fetal rabbit. J Appl Physiol 1971;30:358.
34. Kikkawa Y, et al: Morphologic development of fetal rabbit lung and its acceleration with cortisol. Am J Pathol 1971;64:423.
35. Liggins GC, Howie RN: A controlled trial of antepartum glucocorticoid treatment for prevention of the respiratory distress syndrome in premature infants. Pediatrics 1972;50:515.
36. Rooney SA, et al: Studies on pulmonary surfactant: effects of cortisol administration to fetal rabbits on lung phospholipid content, composition and biosynthesis. Biochim Biophys Acta 1976;450:121.
37. Rooney SA, et al: Effects of betamethasone on phospholipid content, composition and biosynthesis in fetal rabbit lung. Biochim Biophys Acta 1979;572:64.
38. Brehier A, Rooney SA: Phosphatidylcholine synthesis and glycogen depletion in fetal mouse lung. Exp Lung Res 1981;2:883.
39. Bunt JE, et al: Metabolism of endogenous surfactant in premature baboons and effect of prenatal corticosteroids. Am J Respir Crit Care Med 1999;160:1481.
40. Bunt JE, et al: The effect in premature infants of prenatal corticosteroids on endogenous surfactant synthesis as measured with stable isotopes. Am J Respir Crit Care Med 2000;162:844.
41. Gross I, et al: Fetal lung in organ culture. III. Comparison of dexamethasone, thyroxine, and methylxanthines. J Appl Physiol 1980;48:872.
42. Gross I, et al: Corticosteroid stimulation of phosphatidylcholine synthesis in cultured fetal rabbit lung: evidence for de novo protein synthesis mediated by glucocorticoid receptors. Endocrinology 1983;112:829.
43. Emanuel RL, et al: Direct effects of corticotropin-releasing hormone and thyrotropin-releasing hormone on fetal lung explants. Peptides 2000;21:1819.
44. Gonzales LW, et al: Glucocorticoids and thyroid hormone stimulate biochemical and morphological differentiation of human fetal lung in organ culture. J Clin Endocrinol Metab 1986;62:678.
45. Xu ZX, Rooney SA: Influence of dexamethasone on the lipid distribution of newly synthesized fatty acids in fetal rat lung. Biochim Biophys Acta 1989;1005:209.
46. Gross I, et al: Glucocorticoid-thyroid hormone interactions in fetal rat lung. Pediatr Res 1984;18:191.
47. Maniscalco WM, et al: Dexamethasone increases de novo fatty acid synthesis in fetal rabbit lung explants. Pediatr Res 1985;19:1272.
48. Gonzales LW, et al: Glucocorticoid stimulation of fatty acid synthesis in explants of human fetal lung. Biochim Biophys Acta 1990;1042:1.
49. Freese WB, Hallman M: The effect of betamethasone and fetal sex on the synthesis and maturation of lung surfactant phospholipids in rabbits. Biochim Biophys Acta 1983;750:47.
50. Post M, et al: The cellular mechanism of glucocorticoid acceleration of fetal lung maturation: fibroblast-pneumocyte factor stimulates choline-phosphate cytidylyltransferase activity. J Biol Chem 1986;261:2179.
51. Mallampalli RK, et al: Betamethasone activation of CTP:cholinephosphate cytidylyltransferase in vivo is lipid dependent. Am J Respir Cell Mol Biol 1994;10:48.
52. Post M: Maternal administration of dexamethasone stimulates cholinephosphate cytidylyltransferase in fetal type II cells. Biochem J 1987;241:291.
53. Khosla SS, et al: Influence of sex hormones on lung maturation in the fetal rabbit. Biochim Biophys Acta 1983;750:112.
54. Rooney SA, et al: Glucocorticoid stimulation of choline-phosphate cytidylyltransferase activity in fetal rat lung: receptor-response relationships. Biochim Biophys Acta 1986;888:208.
55. Sharma AK, et al: Hormonal regulation of cholinephosphate cytidylyltransferase in human fetal lung. Biochim Biophys Acta 1993;1170:237.
56. Beneke S, Rooney SA: Glucocorticoids regulate expression of the fatty acid synthase gene in fetal rat type II cells. Biochim Biophys Acta 2001;1534:56.
57. Wagle S, et al: Hormonal regulation and cellular localization of fatty acid synthase in human fetal lung. Am J Physiol 1999;277:L381.
58. Jobe AH, et al: Combined effects of fetal beta agonist stimulation and glucocorticoids on lung function of preterm lambs. Biol Neonate 1997;72:305.
59. Rooney SA: Biochemical development of the lung. *In* Warshaw JB (ed): The Biological Basis of Reproductive and Developmental Medicine. New York, Elsevier, 1983, p 239.
60. Ballard PL: Hormones and Lung Maturation. Berlin, Springer-Verlag, 1986.
61. Gross I, Wilson CM: Fetal lung in organ culture. IV. Supra-additive hormone interactions. J Appl Physiol 1982;52:1420.
62. Pope TS, et al: Hormonal effects on fatty-acid synthase in cultured fetal rat lung: induction by dexamethasone and inhibition of activity by triiodothyronine. Biochim Biophys Acta 1988;959:169.
63. Ballard PL, et al: Corticosteroid binding by fetal rat and rabbit lung in organ culture. J Steroid Biochem 1984;21:117.
64. Xu ZX, et al: Glucocorticoid induction of fatty-acid synthase mediates the stimulatory effect of the hormone on choline-phosphate cytidylyltransferase activity in fetal rat lung. Biochim Biophys Acta 1990;1044:70.
65. Viscardi RM, et al: Cholinephosphate cytidylyltransferase in fetal rat lung cells: activity and subcellular distribution in response to dexamethasone, triiodothyronine, and fibroblast-conditioned medium. Exp Lung Res 1989;15:223.
66. Rooney SA, et al: Dexamethasone increases the activity but not the amount of choline-phosphate cytidylyltransferase in fetal rat lung. Biochim Biophys Acta 1990;1044:385.
67. Batenburg JJ, Elfring RH: Pre-translational regulation by glucocorticoid of fatty acid and phosphatidylcholine synthesis in type II cells from fetal rat lung. FEBS Lett 1992;307:164.
68. Xu ZX, et al: Glucocorticoid stimulation of fatty-acid synthase gene transcription in fetal rat lung: antagonism by retinoic acid. Am J Physiol 1995;268:L683.

69. Fraslon C, Batenburg JJ: Pre-translational regulation of lipid synthesizing enzymes and surfactant proteins in fetal rat lung in explant culture. FEBS Lett 1993;325:285.

70. Muglia LJ, et al: Proliferation and differentiation defects during lung development in corticotropin-releasing hormone–deficient mice. Am J Respir Cell Mol Biol 1999;20:181.

71. Xu ZX, Rooney SA: Glucocorticoids increase fatty-acid synthase mRNA stability in fetal rat lung. Am J Physiol 1997;272:L860.

72. Lu Z, et al: Transcriptional regulation of the lung fatty acid synthase gene by glucocorticoid, thyroid hormone and transforming growth factor-β1. Biochim Biophys Acta 2001;1532:213.

73. Ballard PL, et al: Glucocorticoid binding by isolated lung cells. Endocrinology 1978;102:1570.

74. Ambrose MP, Hunninghake GW: Corticosteroids increase lipocortin I in alveolar epithelial cells. Am J Respir Cell Mol Biol 1990;3:349.

75. Isohama Y, et al: Dexamethasone increases β₂-adrenoceptor-regulated phosphatidylcholine secretion in rat alveolar type II cells. Jpn J Pharmacol 1997;73:163.

76. Isohama Y, Rooney S: Glucocorticoid enhances the response of type II cells from newborn rats to surfactant secretagogues. Biochim Biophys Acta 2001;1531:241.

77. Post M, et al: Effects of cortisol and thyroxine on phosphatidylcholine and phosphatidylglycerol synthesis by adult rat lung alveolar type II cells in primary culture. Biochim Biophys Acta 1980;618:308.

78. Post M, et al: Alveolar type II cells isolated from fetal rat lung organotypic cultures synthesize and secrete surfactant-associated phospholipids and respond to fibroblast-pneumonocyte factor. Exp Lung Res 1984;7:53.

79. Smith BT, Post M: Fibroblast-pneumonocyte factor. Am J Physiol 1989;257:L174.

80. Chelly N, et al: Keratinocyte growth factor enhances maturation of fetal rat lung type II cells. Am J Respir Cell Mol Biol 1999;20:423.

81. Ikegami M, et al: Keratinocyte growth factor increases surfactant pool sizes in premature rabbits. Am J Respir Crit Care Med 1997;155:155.

82. Chelly N, et al: Role of keratinocyte growth factor in the control of surfactant synthesis by fetal lung mesenchyme. Endocrinology 2001;142:1814.

83. Wu B, et al: The effect of thyroxine on the maturation of fetal rabbit lungs. Biol Neonate 1973;22:161.

84. Nwosu UC, et al: Effect of in utero intravenous administration of thyroxine and other hormones on the lung fluid lecithin/sphingomyelin ratio in the fetal lamb. Am J Obstet Gynecol 1980;138:459.

85. Ballard PL, et al: Thyroid hormone stimulation of phosphatidylcholine synthesis in cultured fetal rabbit lung. J Clin Invest 1984;74:898.

86. deMello DE, et al: Delayed ultrastructural lung maturation in the fetal and newborn hypothyroid (Hyt/Hyt) mouse. Pediatr Res 1994;36:380.

87. Ansari MA, et al: Effect of prenatal glucocorticoid on fetal lung ultrastructural maturation in hyt/hyt mice with primary hypothyroidism. Biol Neonate 2000;77:29.

88. Lindenberg JA, et al: Triiodothyronine nuclear binding in fetal and adult rabbit lung and cultured lung cells. Endocrinology 1978;103:1725.

89. Smith BT, Sabry K: Glucocorticoid-thyroid synergism in lung maturation: a mechanism involving epithelial-mesenchymal interaction. Proc Natl Acad Sci USA 1983;80:1951.

90. Rooney SA, et al: Thyrotropin-releasing hormone increases the amount of surfactant in lung lavage from fetal rabbits. Pediatr Res 1979;13:623.

91. Liggins GC, et al: Synergism of cortisol and thyrotropin-releasing hormone in lung maturation in fetal sheep. J Appl Physiol 1988;65:1880.

92. Devaskar U, et al: Transplacental stimulation of functional and morphologic fetal rabbit lung maturation: effect of thyrotropin-releasing hormone. Am J Obstet Gynecol 1987;157:460.

93. Oulton M, et al: Gestation-dependent effects of the combined treatment of glucocorticoids and thyrotropin-releasing hormone on surfactant production by fetal rabbit lung. Am J Obstet Gynecol 1989;160:961.

94. Moraga FA, et al: Maternal administration of glucocorticoid and thyrotropin-releasing hormone enhances fetal lung maturation in undisturbed preterm lambs. Am J Obstet Gynecol 1994;171:729.

95. Ballard RA, et al: Antenatal thyrotropin-releasing hormone to prevent lung disease in preterm infants: North American Thyrotropin-Releasing Hormone Study Group. N Engl J Med 1998;338:493.

96. Collaborative Santiago Surfactant Group: Collaborative trial of prenatal thyrotropin-releasing hormone and corticosteroids for prevention of respiratory distress syndrome. Am J Obstet Gynecol 1998;178:33.

97. Crowther CA, et al: Australian collaborative trial of antenatal thyrotropin-releasing hormone: adverse effects at 12-month follow up. Pediatrics 1997;99:311.

98. Parker CR, et al: Ontogeny of unconjugated estriol in fetal blood and the relation of estriol levels at birth to the development of respiratory distress syndrome. Pediatr Res 1987;21:386.

99. Stovall WS, et al: Serum unconjugated estriol level as a predictor of pulmonary maturity. Am J Obstet Gynecol 1985;153:568.

100. Spellacy WN, et al: Human amniotic fluid lecithin/sphingomyelin ratio changes with estrogen or glucocorticoid treatment. Am J Obstet Gynecol 1973;115:216.

101. Khosla SS, Rooney SA: Stimulation of fetal lung surfactant production by administration of 17β-estradiol to the maternal rabbit. Am J Obstet Gynecol 1979;133:213.

102. Khosla SS, et al: Stimulation of phosphatidylcholine synthesis by 17β-estradiol in fetal rabbit lung. Biochim Biophys Acta 1980;617:282.

103. Khosla SS, et al: Effects of estrogen on fetal rabbit lung maturation: morphological and biochemical studies. Pediatr Res 1981;15:1274.

104. Possmayer F, et al: Hormonal induction of pulmonary maturation in the rabbit fetus: effects of maternal treatment with estradiol-17β on the endogenous levels of cholinephosphate, CDP-choline and phosphatidylcholine. Biochim Biophys Acta 1981;664:10.

105. Gross I, et al: The influence of hormones on the biochemical development of fetal rat lung in organ culture. I. Estrogen. Biochim Biophys Acta 1979;575:375.

106. Thuresson-Klein ASA, et al: Estrogen stimulates formation of lamellar bodies and release of surfactant in the rat fetal lung. Am J Obstet Gynecol 1985;151:506.

107. Andujo O, et al: Failure to detect a stimulatory effect of estradiol-17β on ovine fetal lung maturation. Pediatr Res 1987;22:145.

108. Chu AJ, Rooney SA: Stimulation of cholinephosphate cytidylyltransferase activity by estrogen in fetal rabbit lung is mediated by phospholipids. Biochim Biophys Acta 1985;834:346.

109. Adamson IYR, et al: Accelerated fetal lung maturation by estrogen is associated with an epithelial-fibroblast interaction. In Vitro 1990;26:784.

110. Parker CR Jr, et al: Prolactin levels in umbilical cord blood of human infants: relation to gestational age, maternal complications, and neonatal lung function. Am J Obstet Gynecol 1989;161:795.

111. Hamosh M, Hamosh P: The effect of prolactin on the lecithin content of fetal rabbit lung. J Clin Invest 1977;59:1002.

112. Ballard PL, et al: Failure to detect an effect of prolactin on pulmonary surfactant and adrenosteroids in fetal sheep and rabbits. J Clin Invest 1978;62:879.

113. van Petten GR, Bridges R: The effects of prolactin on pulmonary maturation in the fetal lamb and rabbit. Am J Obstet Gynecol 1979;134:711.

114. Amit T, et al: Specific binding sites for prolactin and growth hormone in the adult rabbit lung. Mol Cell Endocrinol 1987;49:17.

115. Josimovich JB, et al: Binding of prolactin by fetal rhesus cell membrane fractions. Endocrinology 1977;100:557.

116. Mullon DK, et al: Effect of prolactin on phospholipid synthesis in organ cultures of fetal rat lung. Biochim Biophys Acta 1983;751:166.

117. Cox MA, Torday JS: Pituitary oligopeptide regulation of phosphatidylcholine synthesis by fetal rabbit lung cells. Lack of effect with prolactin. Am Rev Respir Dis 1981;123:181.

118. Mendelson CR, et al: Multihormonal regulation of surfactant synthesis by human fetal lung in vitro. J Clin Endocrinol Metab 1981;53:307.

119. Fisher DA, Lakshmanan J: Metabolism and effects of epidermal growth factor and related growth factors in mammals. Endocr Rev 1990;11:418.

120. Goetzman BW, et al: Prenatal exposure to epidermal growth factor attenuates respiratory distress syndrome in rhesus infants. Pediatr Res 1994;35:30.

121. Rubin LP, et al: Parathyroid hormone (PTH) and PTH-related protein stimulate surfactant phospholipid synthesis in rat fetal lung, apparently by a mesenchymal-epithelial mechanism. Biochim Biophys Acta 1994;1223:91.

122. Torday JS, et al: Leptin mediates the parathyroid hormone-related protein paracrine stimulation of fetal lung maturation. Am J Physiol 2002;282:L405.

123. Fraslon C, Bourbon JR: Comparison of effects of epidermal and insulin-like growth factors, gastrin releasing peptide and retinoic acid on fetal lung cell growth and maturation in vitro. Biochim Biophys Acta 1992;1123:65.

124. Hoffman DR, et al: Platelet-activating factor induces glycogen degradation in fetal rabbit lung in utero. J Biol Chem 1988;263:9316.

125. Hoffman DR, et al: The role of platelet-activating factor in human fetal lung maturation. Am J Obstet Gynecol 1986;155:70.

126. Gonzales LW, et al: Glucocorticoid and cAMP increase fatty acid synthetase mRNA content in human fetal lung explants. Biochim Biophys Acta 1994;1215:49.

127. Nguyen TM, et al: Evidence for a vitamin D paracrine system regulating maturation of developing rat lung epithelium. Am J Physiol 1996;271:L392.

128. Bourbon JR, Farrell PM: Fetal lung development in the diabetic pregnancy. Pediatr Res 1985;19:253.

129. Bose CL, et al: Delayed fetal pulmonary maturation in a rabbit model of the diabetic pregnancy. J Clin Invest 1980;66:220.

130. Mulay S, McNaughton L: Fetal lung development in streptozotocin-induced experimental diabetes: cytidylyl transferase activity, disaturated phosphatidyl choline and glycogen levels. Life Sci 1983;33:637.

131. Singh M, Feigelson M: Effects of maternal diabetes on the levels, synthetic rates and activities of synthetic enzymes of surface-active phospholipids in perinatal rat lung. Biochim Biophys Acta 1983;753:53.

132. Sosenko IRS, et al: Functional delay in lung maturation in fetuses of diabetic rabbits. J Appl Physiol 1980;48:643.

133. Rooney SA, et al: Lung surfactant in the hyperinsulinemic fetal monkey. Lung 1981;161:313.

134. Pignol B, et al: Lung maturation in the hyperinsulinemic rat fetus. Pediatr Res 1987;21:436.

135. Warburton D, et al: Primary hyperinsulinemia reduces surface active material flux in tracheal fluid of fetal lambs. Pediatr Res 1981;15:1422.

136. Gross I, et al: The influence of hormones on the biochemical development of fetal rat lung in organ culture. II. Insulin. Pediatr Res 1980;14:834.

137. Smith BT, et al: Insulin antagonism of cortisol action on lecithin synthesis by cultured fetal lung cells. J Pediatr 1975;87:953.

138. Rooney SA, et al: Insulin antagonism of dexamethasone-induced stimulation of cholinephosphate cytidylyltransferase in fetal rat lung in organ culture. Lung 1980;158:151.

139. Gewolb IH, Torday JS: High glucose inhibits maturation of the fetal lung in vitro: morphometric analysis of lamellar bodies and fibroblast lipid inclusions. Lab Invest 1995;73:59.

140. Gewolb IH, et al: High glucose causes delayed fetal lung maturation as measured by fluorescence anisotropy. Biochem Biophys Res Commun 1993;193:794.

141. Perelman RH, et al: Discordance between male and female deaths due to the respiratory distress syndrome. Pediatrics 1986;78:238.

142. Torday JS, et al: Sex differences in fetal lung maturation. Am Rev Respir Dis 1981;123:205.

143. Adamson IYR, King GM: Sex related differences in cellular composition and surfactant synthesis of developing fetal rat lungs. Am Rev Respir Dis 1984;129:130.

144. Adamson IYR, King GM: Sex differences in development of fetal rat lung. I. Autoradiographic and biochemical studies. Lab Invest 1984;50:456.

145. McCoy DM, et al: Identification of sex-specific differences in surfactant synthesis in rat lung. Pediatr Res 1999;46:722.

146. Kotas RV, Avery ME: The influence of sex on fetal lung maturation and on the response to glucocorticoid. Am Rev Respir Dis 1980;121:377.

147. Nielsen HC, Torday JS: Sex differences in fetal rabbit pulmonary surfactant production. Pediatr Res 1981;15:1245.

148. Perelman RH, et al: Fetal lung development in male and female nonhuman primates. Pediatr Res 1986;20:987.

149. Truog WE, et al: Differential effect of sex in experimental hyaline membrane disease in newborn monkeys. Am Rev Respir Dis 1981;124:435.

150. Nielsen HC, et al: Dihydrotestosterone inhibits fetal rabbit pulmonary surfactant production. J Clin Invest 1982;69:611.

151. Torday JS: Androgens delay human fetal lung maturation in vitro. Endocrinology 1990;126:3240.

152. Levesque BM, et al: Dihydrotestosterone stimulates branching morphogenesis, cell proliferation, and programmed cell death in mouse embryonic lung explants. Pediatr Res 2000;47:481.

153. Dammann CE, et al: Androgen regulation of signaling pathways in late fetal mouse lung development. Endocrinology 2000;141:2923.

154. Beers MF, et al: TGF-β1 inhibits surfactant component expression and epithelial cell maturation in cultured human fetal lung. Am J Physiol 1998;275:L950.

155. Fraslon C, Bourbon JR: Retinoids control surfactant phospholipid biosynthesis in fetal rat lung. Am J Physiol 1994;266:L705.

156. Chailley-Heu B, et al: Mild vitamin A deficiency delays fetal lung maturation in the rat. Am J Respir Cell Mol Biol 1999;21:89.

157. Chu AJ, Rooney SA: Developmental differences in activation of cholinephosphate cytidylyltransferase by lipids in rabbit lung cytosol. Biochim Biophys Acta 1985;835:132.

158. Zimmermann LJ, et al: Regulation of CTP:phosphocholine cytidylyltransferase by cytosolic lipids in rat type II pneumocytes during development. Pediatr Res 1995;38:864.

159. Johnson JE, Cornell RB: Amphitropic proteins: regulation by reversible membrane interactions. Mol Membr Biol 1999;16:217.

160. Nemat-Gorgani M, Wilson JE: Ambiquitous behavior: a biological phenomenon of general significance? Curr Top Cell Regul 1980;16:45.

161. Lykidis A, et al: Lipid activation of CTP: phosphocholine cytidylyltransferase alpha: characterization and identification of a second activation domain. Biochemistry 2001;40:494.

162. Attard GS, et al: Modulation of CTP:phosphocholine cytidylyltransferase by membrane curvature elastic stress. Proc Natl Acad Sci USA 2000;97:9032.

163. Davies SM, et al: Regulation of CTP: phosphocholine cytidylyltransferase activity by the physical properties of lipid membranes: an important role for stored curvature strain energy. Biochemistry 2001;40:10522.

164. Clement JM, Kent C: CTP:phosphocholine cytidylyltransferase: insights into regulatory mechanisms and novel functions. Biochem Biophys Res Commun 1999;257:643.

165. Tesan M, et al: Regulation of CTP:phosphocholine cytidylyltransferase activity in type II pneumocytes. Biochem J 1985;232:705.

166. Cornell RB, Northwood IC: Regulation of CTP:phosphocholine cytidylyltransferase by amphitropism and relocalization. Trends Biochem Sci 2000;25:441.

167. Feldman DA, et al: Activation of CTP:phosphocholine cytidylyltransferase in rat lung by fatty acids. Biochim Biophys Acta 1981;665:53.

168. Feldman DA, et al: The stimulation and binding of CTP:phosphorylcholine cytidylyltransferase by phosphatidylcholine-oleic acid vesicles. Biochim Biophys Acta 1985;429:429.

169. Feldman DA: The role of phosphatidylglycerol in the activation of CTP:phosphocholine cytidylyltransferase from rat lung. J Biol Chem 1978;253:4980.

170. Mallampalli RK, et al: Betamethasone activation of CTP:cholinephosphate cytidylyltransferase is mediated by fatty acids. J Cell Physiol 1995;162:410.

171. Lykidis A, et al: Distribution of CTP:phosphocholine cytidylyltransferase (CCT) isoforms: identification of a new CCTβ splice variant. J Biol Chem 1999;274:26992.

172. Ridsdale R, et al: CTP:phosphocholine cytidylyltransferase alpha is a cytosolic protein in pulmonary epithelial cells and tissues. J Biol Chem 2001;276:49148.

173. Tseu I, et al: Cell cycle regulation of pulmonary phosphatidylcholine synthesis. Am J Respir Cell Mol Biol 2002;26:506.

174. Li J, et al: Effect of CTP:phosphocholine cytidylyltransferase overexpression on the mouse lung surfactant system. Am J Respir Cell Mol Biol 2002;26:709.

175. Haagsman HP, et al: Synthesis of phosphatidylcholines in ozone-exposed alveolar type II cells isolated from adult rat lung: is glycerolphosphate acyltransferase a rate-limiting enzyme? Exp Lung Res 1988;14:1.

176. Holm BA, et al: Type pneumocyte changes during hyperoxic lung injury and recovery. J Appl Physiol 1988;65:2672.

177. Rooney SA: Regulation of surfactant secretion. In Rooney SA (ed): Lung Surfactant: Cellular and Molecular Processing. Austin, TX, Landes, 1998, p 139.

178. Chander A, Fisher AB: Regulation of lung surfactant secretion. Am J Physiol 1990;258:L241.

179. Wright JR, Dobbs LG: Regulation of pulmonary surfactant secretion and clearance. Annu Rev Physiol 1991;53:395.

180. Mason RJ, Voelker DR: Regulatory mechanisms of surfactant secretion. Biochim Biophys Acta 1998;1408:226.

181. Rooney SA: Regulation of surfactant secretion. Comp Biochem Physiol A Mol Integr Physiol 2001;129:233.

182. Frick M, et al: Secretion in alveolar type II cells at the interface of constitutive and regulated exocytosis. Am J Respir Cell Mol Biol 2001;25:306.

183. Griese M, et al: Ontogeny of surfactant secretion in type II pneumocytes from fetal, newborn, and adult rats. Am J Physiol 1992;262:L337.

184. Froh D, et al: Secretion of surfactant protein A and phosphatidylcholine from type II cells of human fetal lung. Am J Respir Cell Mol Biol 1993;8:556.

185. Gobran LI, Rooney SA: Adenylate cyclase–coupled ATP receptor and surfactant secretion in type II pneumocytes from newborn rats. Am J Physiol 1997;272:L187.

186. Haller T, et al: Dynamics of surfactant release in alveolar type II cells. Proc Natl Acad Sci USA 1998;95:1579.

187. Haller T, et al: Fusion pore expansion is a slow, discontinuous, and Ca²⁺-dependent process regulating secretion from alveolar type II cells. J Cell Biol 2001;155:279.

188. Mair N, et al: Exocytosis in alveolar type II cells revealed by cell capacitance and fluorescence measurements. Am J Physiol 1999;276:L376.

189. Ashino Y, et al: [Ca²⁺]ᵢ oscillations regulate type II cell exocytosis in the pulmonary alveolus. Am J Physiol 2000;279:L5.

190. Griese M, et al: Signal-transduction mechanisms of ATP-stimulated phosphatidylcholine secretion in rat type II pneumocytes: interactions between ATP and other surfactant secretagogues. Biochim Biophys Acta 1993;1167:85.

191. Rooney SA, Gobran LI: Activation of phospholipase D in rat type II pneumocytes by ATP and other surfactant secretagogues. Am J Physiol 1993;264:L133.

192. Waggoner DW, et al: Structural organization of mammalian lipid phosphate phosphatases: implications for signal transduction. Biochim Biophys Acta 1999;1439:299.

193. Gobran LI, et al: P₂ᵤ purinoceptor stimulation of surfactant secretion coupled to phosphatidylcholine hydrolysis in type II cells. Am J Physiol 1994;267:L625.

194. Matsuoka I, et al: Adenine nucleotide-induced activation of adenosine A₂B receptors expressed in Xenopus laevis oocytes: involvement of a rapid and localized adenosine formation by ectonucleotidases. Mol Pharmacol 2002;61:606.

195. Rooney SA: Role of purinoceptors in the regulation of lung surfactant secretion. In Turner JT, et al (eds): The P₂ Nucleotide Receptors. Totowa, NJ, Humana Press, 1998, p 291.

196. Berridge MJ, et al: The versatility and universality of calcium signalling. Nat Rev Mol Cell Biol 2000;1:11.

197. Rooney SA, et al: Molecular and cellular processing of lung surfactant. FASEB J 1994;8:957.

198. Barnes PJ: Beta-adrenergic receptors and their regulation. Am J Respir Crit Care Med 1995;152:838.

199. Gobran LI, et al: PKC isoforms and other signaling proteins involved in surfactant secretion in developing rat type II cells. Am J Physiol 1998;274:L901.

200. Isohama Y, et al: Changes in β₁- and β₂-adrenoceptor mRNA levels in alveolar type II cells during cultivation. Biochem Mol Biol Int 1995;36:561.

201. Fabisiak JP, et al: Interactions of beta adrenergic antagonists with isolated rat alveolar type II pneumocytes. I. Analysis, characterization and regulation of specific beta adrenergic receptors. J Pharmacol Exp Ther 1987;241:722.

202. Ewing CK, et al: Characterization of the β-adrenergic receptor in isolated human fetal lung type II cells. Pediatr Res 1992;32:350.

203. Fredholm BB, et al: Nomenclature and classification of adenosine receptors. Pharmacol Rev 2001;53:527.

204. Ralevic V, Burnstock G: Receptors for purines and pyrimidines. Pharmacol Rev 1998;50:413.

205. Burnstock G, Williams M: P2 purinergic receptors: modulation of cell function and therapeutic potential. J Pharmacol Exp Ther 2000;295:862.

206. Zhang FL, et al: P2Y₁₃: identification and characterization of a novel Gαi-coupled ADP receptor from human and mouse. J Pharmacol Exp Ther 2002;301:705.

207. Rice WR, et al: Cloning and expression of the alveolar type II cell P₂ᵤ-purinergic receptor. Am J Respir Cell Mol Biol 1995;12:27.

208. Gilfillan AM, Rooney SA: Functional evidence for involvement of P_2 purinoceptors in the ATP stimulation of phosphatidylcholine secretion in type II alveolar epithelial cells. Biochim Biophys Acta 1988;959:31.

209. Griese M, et al: A_2 and P_2 purine receptor interactions and surfactant secretion in primary cultures of type II cells. Am J Physiol 1991;261:L140.

210. Rhee SG: Regulation of phosphoinositide-specific phospholipase C. Annu Rev Biochem 2001;70:281.

211. Strassheim D, Williams CL: $P2Y_2$ purinergic and M_3 muscarinic acetylcholine receptors activate different phospholipase C-β isoforms that are uniquely susceptible to protein kinase C–dependent phosphorylation and inactivation. J Biol Chem 2000;275:39767.

212. Rhee SG, Bae YS: Regulation of phosphoinositide-specific phospholipase C isozymes. J Biol Chem 1997;272:15045.

213. Dempsey EC, et al: Protein kinase C isozymes and the regulation of diverse cell responses. Am J Physiol 2000;279:L429.

214. Van Lint J, et al: Expression and characterization of PKD, a phorbol ester and diacylglycerol-stimulated serine protein kinase. J Biol Chem 1995;270:1455.

215. Hayashi A, et al: PKCν, a new member of the protein kinase C family, composes a fourth subfamily with PKCμ. Biochim Biophys Acta 1999;1450:99.

216. Van Lint J, et al: Protein kinase D: an intracellular traffic regulator on the move. Trends Cell Biol 2002;12:193.

217. Linke MJ, et al: Surfactant phospholipid secretion from rat alveolar type II cells: possible role of PKC isozymes. Am J Physiol 1997;272:L171.

218. Gobran LI, Rooney SA: Surfactant secretagogue activation of protein kinase C isoforms in cultured rat type II cells. Am J Physiol 1999;277:L251.

219. Gomez-Cambronero J, Keire P: Phospholipase D: a novel major player in signal transduction. Cell Signal 1998;10:387.

220. Sunahara RK, et al: Complexity and diversity of mammalian adenylyl cyclases. Annu Rev Pharmacol Toxicol 1996;36:461.

221. Jourdan KB, et al: Characterization of adenylyl cyclase isoforms in rat peripheral pulmonary arteries. Am J Physiol 2001;280:L1359.

222. Pian MS, Dobbs LG: Evidence for G$\beta\gamma$-mediated cross-talk in primary cultures of lung alveolar cells: pertussis toxin–sensitive production of cAMP. J Biol Chem 1995;270:7427.

223. Rubin CS: A kinase anchor proteins and the intracellular targeting of signals carried by cyclic AMP. Biochim Biophys Acta 1994;1224:467.

224. Hanks SK, Hunter T: Protein kinases 6: the eukaryotic protein kinase superfamily: kinase (catalytic) domain structure and classification. FASEB J 1995;9:576.

225. Means AR: Regulatory cascades involving calmodulin-dependent protein kinases. Mol Endocrinol 2000;14:4.

226. Voyno-Yasenetskaya TA, et al: Low density lipoprotein- and high density lipoprotein–mediated signal transduction and exocytosis in alveolar type II cells. Proc Natl Acad Sci USA 1993;90:4256.

227. Pian MS, Dobbs LG: Lipoprotein-stimulated surfactant secretion in alveolar type II cells: mediation by heterotrimeric G proteins. Am J Physiol 1997;273:L634.

228. Joyce-Brady M, et al: Mechanisms of mastoparan-stimulated surfactant secretion from isolated pulmonary alveolar type 2. cells. J Biol Chem 1991;266:6859.

229. Malarkey K, et al: The regulation of tyrosine kinase signalling pathways by growth factor and G-protein-coupled receptors. Biochem J 1995;309:361.

230. Weisman G, et al: $P2Y_2$ receptors regulate multiple signal transduction pathways in monocytic cells. Drug Develop Res 2001;53:186.

231. Boarder MR, Hourani SM: The regulation of vascular function by P2 receptors: multiple sites and multiple receptors. Trends Pharmacol Sci 1998;19:99.

232. Edwards YS, et al: Osmotic stress induces both secretion and apoptosis in rat alveolar type II cells. Am J Physiol 1998;275:L670.

233. White MK, Strayer DS: Surfactant protein A regulates pulmonary surfactant secretion via activation of phosphatidylinositol 3-kinase in type II alveolar cells. Exp Cell Res 2000;255:67.

234. Warburton D, et al: Protein phosphorylation and dephosphorylation in type II pneumocytes. Am J Physiol 1991;260:L548.

235. Zimmerman UJP, et al: Secretagogue-induced proteolysis of cAMP-dependent protein kinase in intact rat alveolar epithelial type II cells. Biochim Biophys Acta 1996;1311:117.

236. Turner KM, et al: Protein phosphorylation and the regulation of synaptic membrane traffic. Trends Neurosci 1999;22:459.

237. Lin RC, Scheller RH: Mechanisms of synaptic vesicle exocytosis. Annu Rev Cell Dev Biol 2000;16:19.

238. Chander A, Wu RD: In vitro fusion of lung lamellar bodies and plasma membrane is augmented by lung synexin. Biochim Biophys Acta 1991;1086:157.

239. Chander A, et al: Synexin and GTP increase surfactant secretion in permeabilized alveolar type II cells. Am J Physiol 2001;280:L991.

240. Oyarzun MJ, Clements JA: Ventilatory and cholinergic control of pulmonary surfactant in the rabbit. J Appl Physiol 1977;43:39.

241. Oyarzun MJ, Clements JA: Control of lung surfactant by ventilation, adrenergic mediators and prostaglandins in the rabbit. Am Rev Respir Dis 1978;117:879.

242. Dietl P, et al: Mechanisms of surfactant exocytosis in alveolar type II cells in vitro and in vivo. News Physiol Sci 2001;16:239.

243. Nicholas TE, et al: Surfactant homeostasis in the rat lung during swimming exercise. J Appl Physiol 1982;53:1521.

244. Rooney SA, Gobran LI: Adenosine and leukotrienes have a regulatory role in lung surfactant secretion in the newborn rabbit. Biochim Biophys Acta 1988;960:98.

245. Lawson EE, et al: Augmentation of pulmonary surfactant by lung expansion at birth. Pediatr Res 1979;13:611.

246. Rooney SA, et al: Stimulation of surfactant production by oxytocin-induced labor in the rabbit. J Clin Invest 1977;60:754.

247. Wirtz HR, Dobbs LG: The effects of mechanical forces on lung functions. Respir Physiol 2000;119:1.

248. Wirtz HRW, Dobbs LG: Calcium mobilization and exocytosis after one mechanical stretch of lung epithelial cells. Science 1990;250:1266.

249. Marino PA, Rooney SA: The effect of labor on surfactant secretion in newborn rabbit lung slices. Biochim Biophys Acta 1981;664:389.

250. Abdellatif MM, Hollingsworth M: Effect of oxotremorine and epinephrine on lung surfactant secretion in neonatal rabbits. Pediatr Res 1980;14:916.

251. Ekelund L, et al: Release of fetal lung surfactant: effects of xanthines and adenosine. *In* Andersson KE, Persson CGA (eds): Anti-asthma Xanthines and Adenosine. Amsterdam, Excerpta Medica, 1985, p 202.

252. Pintor J, et al: Research on purines and their receptors comes of age. Trends Pharmacol Sci 2000;21:453.

253. Lazarowski ER, Boucher RC: UTP as an extracellular signaling molecule. News Physiol Sci 2001;16:1.

254. Sauer H, et al: Mechanical strain-induced Ca^{2+} waves are propagated via ATP release and purinergic receptor activation. Am J Physiol 2000;279:C295.

255. Grygorczyk R, Hanrahan JW: CFTR-independent ATP release from epithelial cells triggered by mechanical stimuli. Am J Physiol 1997;272:C1058.

256. Lazarowski ER, et al: Direct demonstration of mechanically induced release of cellular UTP and its implication for uridine nucleotide receptor activation. J Biol Chem 1997;272:24348.

257. Felix JA, et al: Stretch increases inositol 1,4,5-trisphosphate concentration in airway epithelial cells. Am J Respir Cell Mol Biol 1996;14:296.

258. Kulik TJ, et al: Stretch increases inositol trisphosphate and inositol tetrakisphosphate in cultured pulmonary vascular smooth muscle cells. Biochem Biophys Res Commun 1991;180:982.

259. Rice WR, et al: Effect of oxygen exposure on ATP content of rat bronchoalveolar lavage. Pediatr Res 1989;25:396.

260. Oosterlaken-Dijksterhuis MA, et al: Surfactant protein composition of lamellar bodies isolated from rat lung. Biochem J 1991;274:115.

261. Weaver TE: Synthesis, processing and secretion of surfactant proteins B and C. Biochim Biophys Acta 1998;1408:173.

262. Gobran LI, Rooney SA: Regulation of SP-B and SP-C secretion in rat type II cells in primary culture. Am J Physiol 2001;L1413.

263. Henry M, et al: Surfactant protein B metabolism in newborn rabbits. Biochim Biophys Acta 1996;1300:97.

264. Ochs M, et al: Intracellular and intraalveolar localization of surfactant protein A (SP-A) in the parenchymal region of the human lung. Am J Respir Cell Mol Biol 2002;26:91.

265. Rooney SA, et al: Secretion of surfactant protein A from rat type II pneumocytes. Am J Physiol 1993;265:L586.

266. Osanai K, et al: Trafficking of newly synthesized surfactant protein A in isolated rat alveolar type II cells. Am J Respir Cell Mol Biol 1999;21:929.

267. Mason RJ, et al: Maintenance of surfactant protein A and D secretion by rat alveolar type II cells in vitro. Am J Physiol 2002;282:L249.

268. Xu X, et al: KGF increases SP-A and SP-D mRNA levels and secretion in cultured rat alveolar type II cells. Am J Respir Cell Mol Biol 1998;18:168.

269. Dobbs LG, et al: Secretion of surfactant by primary cultures of alveolar type II cells isolated from rats. Biochim Biophys Acta 1982;713:118.

270. Ikegami M, et al: Surfactant protein A metabolism in preterm ventilated lambs. Am J Physiol 1992;262:L765.

271. Ikegami M, et al: Surfactant protein A labeling kinetics in newborn and adult rabbits. Am J Respir Cell Mol Biol 1994;10:413.

272. Crouch E, et al: Surfactant protein D. Increased accumulation in silica-induced pulmonary lipoproteinosis. Am J Pathol 1991;139:765.

273. Voorhout WF, et al: Immunocytochemical localization of surfactant protein D (SP-D) in type II cells, Clara cells, and alveolar macrophages of rat lung. J Histochem Cytochem 1992;40:1589.

104 Pathophysiology of Respiratory Distress Syndrome and Surfactant Metabolism

OVERVIEW

The pathophysiology of respiratory distress syndrome (RDS) and the surfactant system have been closely linked from the initial description of abnormal surfactant function in RDS by Avery and Mead in 1959[1] to the development of surfactant treatment for RDS.[2] This chapter focuses on the pathophysiology of RDS from the perspective of surfactant metabolism and function. The effects of surfactant treatment on the initial pathophysiologic events and on surfactant metabolism are also reviewed. Clinical aspects of surfactant treatment for RDS and its resolution are covered in other chapters.

LUNG STRUCTURE OF THE PRETERM WITH RESPIRATORY DISTRESS SYNDROME

Lung structure is the substrate on which surfactant functions. The preterm lung changes structure as it matures, and the structural maturation of the lung affects the responses of the lung to surfactant and the lung complications that may occur after preterm birth. The lung of the term infant contains about 30% of the 300 million alveoli that are present in the adult lung (Fig. 104-1).[3, 4] The fetal lung at the margin of viability at 24 weeks' gestation has just matured beyond the canalicular stage to be in the early saccular stage of lung development.[5] The saccular lung has undifferentiated distal air saccules with a poorly developed capillary microvasculature. The surface area of the developing human lung does not increase very much before 30 weeks' gestation, and alveolar septation of the distal saccules does not begin until about 32 weeks. However, the rate of alveolar formation then is very high until term. After birth, the rate of alveolar septation decreases until alveolar development ceases at 18 to 24 months of age. The early lung maturation that commonly occurs in preterm infants with maternal glucocorticoid treatment accelerates mesenchymal involution and increases surfactant, but it may delay alveolar septation.[6, 7] A major factor in determining how the preterm lung will respond to treatment and injury is the structural maturation of the lung at delivery.

OVERVIEW OF SURFACTANT METABOLISM

The general scheme of surfactant metabolism as it is understood in the adult lung is the basis for the discussion of surfactant metabolism in the preterm lung with RDS (Fig. 104-2).[8] More extensive descriptions of the surfactant lipids and proteins, the biophysics of surfactant function, and regulation of synthesis and secretion are found in other chapters in this section. Surfactant lipids are synthesized from precursors, such as palmitic acid, that are transported from the circulation into Type II cells. The lipids are processed through the Golgi apparatus to multivesicular bodies that associate with the mature forms of the surfactant proteins SP-B and SP-C and are stored in the form of membrane-enclosed lipid/protein structures called *lamellar bodies*. Lamellar bodies localize to the apical (air) surface of the Type II cell and are secreted by exocytosis either constitutively or when they are stimulated by secretagogues such as β-agonists and purines or by mechanical stretch. The other surfactant proteins,

SP-A and SP-D, are secreted primarily independently of the lamellar bodies.

Surfactant also has an extracellular life cycle once it is secreted to the thin fluid hypophase in the healthy lung. The SP-A associates with the lipids and SP-B and SP-C secreted as lamellar bodies to form tubular myelin and other loose lipid arrays that are macroaggregated lipoprotein forms.[9] These large lipoprotein aggregates are the forms that facilitate adsorption of surfactant to the air-water interface. The surfactant film is multilayered and is continuously replenished from the surfactant in the hypophase.[10] Lipids are cleared from the air spaces as small liposomal vesicles that contain the phospholipids but essentially no surfactant proteins. The surfactant proteins also are cleared by macrophages and Type II cells, but their forms for clearance have not been characterized. About half of the lipids and proteins are catabolized by alveolar macrophages in the adult mouse lung, and the other half of them are catabolized by Type II cells.[11] However, the Type II cells also take up phospholipids, SP-B, SP-C, and SP-A and recycle them through multivesicular bodies back to lamellar bodies for re-secretion.

The important concept is that the surfactant lipids and proteins are dynamically cycling from the Type II cell to the surfactant layer and back to the Type II cell. In the adult rabbit lung, in which measurements have been made, the rate of synthesis of surfactant phosphatidylcholine is 1.5 μmol/kg/hour, 0.5 μmol/kg/hour is recycled back from the air space, and about 2 μmol/kg/hour is secreted into an alveolar pool of about 10 μmol/kg.[12] About 25% of the phospholipids are recycled in the adult. At steady state, the alveolar surfactant pool is replaced every 5 hours, a finding demonstrating that the surfactant is a very metabolically active pool. The airway clearance rates and efficiencies of recycling for SP-A, SP-B, and SP-C are similar to those for the lipids in the adult lung.[13-15] As will be apparent, the recycling pathways are important for surfactant treatment strategies.

Characteristics of Surfactant in the Preterm

Composition

The composition of surfactant and the characteristics and function of the surfactant proteins are discussed extensively in Chapters 103 and 104. We focus on the composition of surfactant in the preterm. The surfactant recovered from the air spaces of preterm animals with RDS has less saturated phosphatidylcholine relative to total phospholipids.[16] The lower amount of saturated phosphatidylcholines results in a surfactant with decreased surface activity. The surfactant of a mature animal or human contains about 8% phosphatidylglycerol and very little phosphatidylinositol. In contrast, surfactant from the preterm contains much more phosphatidylinositol than phosphatidylglycerol.[17] These two acidic phospholipids are interchangeable in terms of surfactant function, but the lack of phosphatidylglycerol in surfactant indicates lung immaturity or injury to the Type II cells. Based on the phospholipids in amniotic fluid from normal pregnancies, the lecithin/sphingomyelin (L/S) ratio increases beginning at about 34 weeks' gestation.[18] The L/S ratio measures primarily saturated phosphatidylcholine relative to

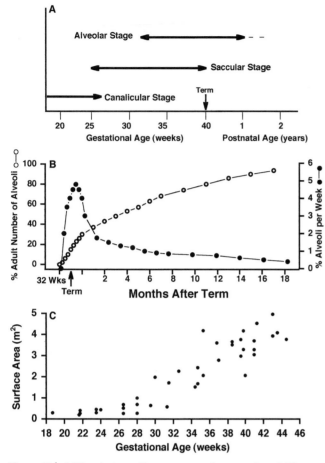

Figure 104–1. The timing of lung structural maturation. **A,** The stages of lung development from 20 weeks' gestation to 2 years, as adapted from Burri. **B,** Alveolar number and weekly rate of accumulation of alveoli are expressed as a percentage of the adult number of alveoli. The curves assume that the term infant has 30% of the adult number of alveoli. The curves are based on measurements of Langston et al. **C,** The large increase in lung surface area does not occur until after the saccular lung begins to alveolarize. (*A,* Redrawn from Burri PH: Structural aspects of prenatal and postnatal development and growth of the lung. *In* McDonald JA [ed]: Lung Growth and Development. New York, Marcel Dekker, 1997, pp 1–35; *B,* redrawn from Hislop AA, et al: Early Hum Dev *13*:1, 1997; *C,* redrawn from Langston C, et al: Am Rev Respir Dis *129*:607, 1984.)

sphingomyelin, a lipid not specific to the fetal lung surfactant. The phosphatidylinositol content of amniotic fluid increases after 28 weeks' gestation to peak at 35 weeks' gestation, and phosphatidylglycerol does not begin to increase until after 34 weeks' gestation.[17] Infants with early lung maturation presumably resulting from fetal stress can rapidly increase the amounts of saturated phosphatidylcholine, decrease phosphatidylinositol, and increase phosphatidylglycerol to have a surfactant composition comparable to that of mature lung. Infants recovering from RDS have increasing amounts of phosphatidylglycerol in the surfactant. In contrast, RDS that progresses to bronchopulmonary dysplasia (BPD) results in surfactant with a delayed appearance of phosphatidylglycerol, presumably because of injury to Type II cells.[19]

The protein content of surfactant from the preterm lung is low relative to the amount of surfactant lipid. In general, Type II cells with lamellar bodies appear in the human lung after about 22 weeks, but there is very little surfactant protein mRNA expres-

sion until later in gestation. The timing of gene expression and protein secretion in the normal human preterm fetus can be inferred from the increases in the proteins in amniotic fluid.[20] SP-A increases after 32 weeks' gestation, and SP-B increases after 34 weeks' gestation. In animal models, SP-A and SP-B mRNA expression is low until late in gestation, and then it increases rapidly to term. SP-B protein must be extensively processed before it enters lamellar bodies. With induced lung maturation in fetal sheep, both the mRNA and the protein processing of SP-B increase in parallel.[21] SP-D mRNA in the lung also is low until late gestation, and amniotic fluid levels of SP-D do not change very much with advancing gestation.[22] SP-A and SP-D in amniotic fluid may also come from nonpulmonary sources because these innate host defense proteins are made in locations other than the lung.

In contrast to other surfactant proteins, SP-C mRNA is highly expressed at the tips of branching airways during early lung development.[23] SP-C mRNA also is expressed in the developing Type II cells before SP-C is found in the fetal airways. Incompletely processed SP-C is in tissue before mature SP-C is measurable in the secreted surfactant in the fetal rabbit, and the ratio of mature SP-C to saturated phosphatidylcholine increases about 10-fold over 2 days' gestation in the rabbit.[24] SP-C has not been measured in human amniotic fluid.

Surfactant Pool Size

During normal gestation, the lungs store progressively larger amounts of surfactant in the maturing Type II cells. The appearance of surfactant in the fetal air spaces lags behind the accumulation of surfactant in the fetal lung tissue. After about 34 weeks, the surfactant is secreted by the fetus, and large amounts of surfactant can be isolated from amniotic fluid at term. The term infant has a large excess of surfactant that facilitates rapid pulmonary adaptation to air breathing. The amount of surfactant in the lung saccules in infants of less than 32 weeks' gestation and in the developing alveoli and small airways after 32 weeks depends on the physiologic events experienced by the fetus or newborn. With labor and the stress of delivery, some of the lamellar bodies are secreted into the fetal lung fluid, and surfactant concentration increases as fetal lung fluid volume decreases.[25] More surfactant is secreted after the initiation of ventilation in response to stretch, increased catecholamines, and purinoceptor agonists. In the preterm sheep, the fetal surfactant stores in the Type II cells are secreted within about 30 minutes of ventilation after birth.[26]

The only direct measurements of surfactant pool sizes of infants were made by alveolar lavage of lungs of infants who died of RDS soon after birth and before mechanical ventilation was available.[27] The lavages contained about 5 mg/kg surfactant. Measurements by bronchoalveolar lavage in preterm rabbits and lambs with severe RDS yield values less than about 3 mg/kg. The differences in phospholipid composition between exogenous surfactant given as treatment and the endogenous surfactant have been used to estimate the pool size. By measuring the change in phosphatidylglycerol, Hallman and associates[28] estimated a surfactant pool size of about 9 mg/kg for infants with RDS. Similar measurements by Griese and colleagues[29] yielded a surfactant pool size estimate of 20 mg/kg. A more recent measurement using dipalmitoylphosphatidylcholine labeled with the stable isotope ^{13}C yielded a value of 5.6 mg/kg.[30] These techniques assume good mixing of the treatment surfactant with the endogenous pool, no loss of the treatment surfactant from the alveolar pool, and the accuracy of samples taken by airway aspirates. None of these assumptions are strictly valid, and Jacobs and colleagues[26] found in a preterm lamb model that the techniques used clinically overestimated the endogenous pool size by at least twofold.

The endogenous pool size of surfactant is the major determinant of lung compliance in preterm animals (Fig. 104–3).[31, 32]

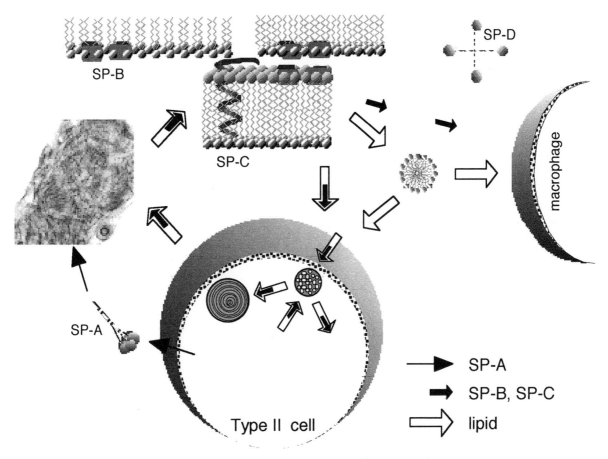

Figure 104–2. Diagram of the major metabolic pathways of surfactant. SP = surfactant protein.

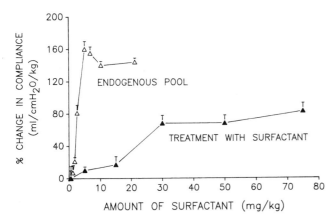

Figure 104–3. Compliance changes in relation to surfactant pool sizes. The curve for the endogenous pool was measured for alveolar washes of ventilated preterm rabbits that were 27 to 29 days' gestational age at delivery. The increase in compliance includes a surfactant effect, as well as any spontaneous lung structural maturation that occurred over the 2-day interval. The curve for treatment with surfactant gives the responses of 27-day gestation rabbits to treatment with natural rabbit surfactant. (Data from refs. 31 and 32.)

Very preterm infants with severe RDS probably have surfactant pools of less than 5 mg/kg. Although not measured in humans, term newborn animals have surfactant pools on the order of 100 mg/kg. In contrast, the surfactant pool size in the adult human was measured to be only about 4 mg/kg.[33] Therefore, preterm infants have perhaps 5% of the amount of surfactant in the term newborn lung, but they have amounts comparable to the healthy adult human. This issue is addressed relative to surfactant function subsequently in this chapter.

Changes in Surfactant Pool Size After Birth

The pool sizes of surfactant that can be recovered by alveolar lavage increase slowly after birth in preterm ventilated monkeys and sheep. In monkeys recovering from RDS, the surfactant increases from about 5 mg/kg toward term values by 3 to 4 days of age (Fig. 104–4).[34, 35] There are no direct measurements of surfactant pool size in infants recovering from RDS. An indirect estimate of the changes in surfactant concentration in airway samples was reported by Hallman and co-workers.[36] The concentration of surfactant was similar for infants without RDS and for infants with RDS who were treated with surfactant. Infants with RDS have a progressive increase in surfactant concentration over about 4 days.

Surfactant treatments with the commonly used dose of 100 mg/kg do not result in large or sustained increases in alveolar surfactant pool size. Soon after administration, most of the lipids can no longer be recovered by lavage. For example, in sheep, only about 25% of the treatment dose is recovered 5 hours after treatment.[37] In preterm ventilated baboons, about 20% of the treatment amount of surfactant was recovered 24 hours later.[38] Infants with RDS had a mean surfactant pool size of 17 mg/kg at 33 hours after an initial 100 mg/kg surfactant treatment, based on measurements with stable isotopes.[30] The increase in alveolar surfactant that accompanies the resolution of RDS does not occur in preterm ventilated baboons that are developing BPD.[39] In these animals, the alveolar pool size after surfactant treatment at birth and 6 days of ventilation was about

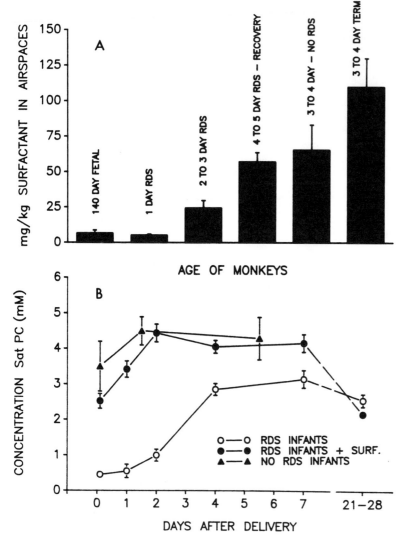

Figure 104–4. Changes in surfactant pool sizes with resolution of respiratory distress syndrome (RDS). **A,** The amount of surfactant recovered by alveolar lavage from mechanically ventilated preterm monkeys with RDS is shown relative to age and stage of the disease. **B,** The concentrations of saturated phosphatidylcholine (Sat PC) in airway samples from infants with RDS, infants with RDS treated with surfactant, and infants without RDS are graphed relative to age from birth. The concentrations of Sat PC approached values for healthy preterm infants by 4 to 7 days. (*A,* Data from refs. 34 and 35; *B,* data from ref. 36.)

30 mg/kg, and this had not increased after two surfactant treatments and 14 days of ventilation. The alveolar content of the surfactant proteins SP-A and SP-D also were very low in these preterm baboons.[40] Nevertheless, the lung tissue content of saturated phosphatidylcholine increased about fourfold, and the tissue content of SP-A and SP-D were increased, findings indicating a defect in surfactant processing and secretion.

Surfactant Metabolism

To understand how the alveolar surfactant pool is maintained in the lung, it is helpful to divide metabolism into the anabolic components of synthesis and secretion and the catabolic activities of uptake, degradation, and recycling. There is no information about surfactant metabolic activity in adult humans. Stable isotopes were used to evaluate surfactant metabolism in infants. Although these measurements have certain limitations, they provide information that corroborates the more complete measurements that have been made in term and preterm animals. Most metabolic studies have focused on saturated phosphatidylcholine because it is the major component of surfactant and is primarily responsible for the biophysical properties of surfactant.

Measurements of synthesis of surfactant phospholipids generally involve the intravascular injection of labeled precursors. The labeled precursors are taken up by Type II cells and are incorporated into phosphatidylcholine, which is transacylated to increase the amount of *de novo* synthesized saturated phos-

phatidylcholine. The surfactant lipids together with SP-B and SP-C are processed and packaged by multivesicular bodies to the storage-secretion granule, the lamellar body (see Fig. 104-2).[41] Secretion can be measured by recovering the labeled surfactant components from the air spaces; this approach evaluates the overall kinetics of synthesis and secretion. The absolute amount of a surfactant component that is synthesized cannot be easily determined because the radiolabeled precursor is diluted into the plasma pool and is further diluted by the precursor pool in the Type II cell. However, the net kinetics of synthesis and secretion provides critical information for understanding why surfactant deficiency requires a certain number of days to resolve in infants with RDS.

After term delivery and ventilation of lambs, an intravascular injection of radiolabeled palmitic acid is incorporated into lung phosphatidylcholine within minutes.[42] However, radiolabeled surfactant is not detected in the air spaces for about 5 hours, and the amount of radiolabeled surfactant continues to accumulate in the air spaces for 30 to 40 hours (Fig. 104-5).[43] A similar curve for accumulation of *de novo* synthesized surfactant was measured for ventilated preterm lambs with mild RDS. Subsequent surfactant treatment of these preterm lambs demonstrated a large dilution of the endogenous surfactant. Surfactant lipids labeled with [13C]glucose could not be detected in airway samples of surfactant-treated very preterm baboons until 24 hours of age, after a [13C]glucose infusion for the first 24 hours after

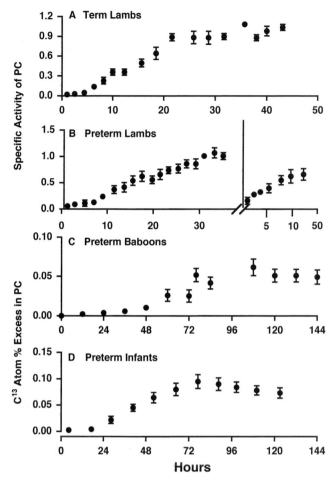

Figure 104–5. Time course of appearance of *de novo* synthesized surfactant phosphatidylcholine (PC) in airway samples of term lambs, preterm lambs, preterm baboons, and preterm infants. **A,** Labeling of saturated PC in airway samples of ventilated term lambs given [³H]palmitic acid as a bolus intravascular injection at birth. Data are means ± SE of specific activities (CPM/μmol PC) normalized to the maximal values for each animal. **B,** Labeling of saturated PC in airway samples of ventilated preterm lambs given a single intravascular injection of [³H]palmitic acid at birth and not treated with surfactant until about 38 hours of age. The discontinuity in the curve demonstrates the fall in the specific activity after treatment with surfactant. **C,** Labeling of PC in airway samples of preterm surfactant-treated baboons that were ventilated for 6 days. The animals received [¹³C]glucose by intravascular infusion for the first 24 hours of age, and the ¹³C in the palmitate of PC is expressed as [¹³C]atom % excess. **D,** Labeling of PC in airway samples of preterm surfactant-treated and mechanically ventilated infants with RDS after an intravascular infusion of [¹³C]glucose for the first 24 hours of life. The label in the PC is expressed as atom % excess. (*A* and *B,* Data from ref. 43; *C,* data from ref. 44; *D,* data from ref. 45.)

birth.[44] The peak accumulation of [¹³C]glucose in phosphatidylcholine was at about 100 hours. The curve for the preterm baboon has a longer delay in detection than the curve for the preterm sheep because the radiolabel was not given as a pulse label, and time was required for enough label to reach the system to be detected. Preterm surfactant-treated infants given infusions of [¹³C]palmitic acid and [¹³C]glucose had curves similar to the baboons for the detection of surfactant lipids in airway samples (see Fig. 104–5).[45] The consistent conclusion is that secretion is

delayed for hours after synthesis, and surfactant made shortly after birth is secreted gradually over a prolonged period. The curves are not altered very much by surfactant treatment or by age after birth when the labeled precursor is given.[44] Antenatal glucocorticoids may increase lipid synthesis, but this conclusion is not secure because precursor pools may be altered by the glucocorticoids.[45] Surfactant treatment does not inhibit *de novo* synthesis of lipids or the surfactant proteins in preterm lungs. Surfactant treatment also does not alter the ultrastructure of Type II cells or the volume fraction of lamellar bodies in Type II cells.[46] The labeling and timing of phosphatidylcholine secretion measured with stable isotopes were similar for infants with RDS ventilated with conventional or high-frequency oscillatory ventilation.[47]

The other half of the metabolic equation is the loss of surfactant from the lung. This measurement has three components that include uptake and catabolism of surfactant components from the air space by Type II cells and macrophages and recycling by Type II cells. Very little surfactant is lost from adult lungs to the lymph or vascular space unless there is lung injury, and minimal amounts of surfactant are lost by suctioning the airways unless there is edema fluid. In the term lamb, a trace dose of surfactant given at birth had a half-life of about 6 days, longer than values of about 10 hours for adult animals.[48] Almost all of a trace dose of surfactant given to preterm lambs with mild RDS was recovered in the lungs after 24 hours of ventilation, a finding demonstrating minimal catabolism (Fig. 104–6).[49] However, only 20% of the labeled surfactant was still in the air spaces, and 80% was associated with the lung tissue. Similar measurements in preterm lambs with more severe RDS that were treated with surfactant demonstrated a 30% loss of the surfactant used for treatment by 24 hours and only 14% of the surfactant recovered by alveolar lavage.[50] This rate of loss of surfactant from the lungs yields a biologic half-life of about 48 hours. The percentage of a treatment dose of surfactant that remains in the air spaces is decreased with a high tidal volume ventilation or with high-frequency oscillatory ventilation in preterm lambs.[51, 52] The amount of surfactant lost from the lungs is increased by ventilator-induced lung injury. Surfactant-treated and ventilated preterm baboons that were developing BPD retained only 4% of the treatment in the air spaces, and about 80% of the surfactant was lost from the lungs by 6 days, yielding a half-life of about 60 hours.[38] These results indicate that the term and preterm lung degrades surfactant lipids slowly, and injury can increase the loss of surfactant from the lungs.

There is no information in the preterm regarding where degradation of surfactant occurs. The normal preterm lung at birth contains very few macrophages and essentially no granulocytes. However, inflammation and injury rapidly recruit inflammatory cells to the lung, which may then increase the loss of surfactant. A significant amount of a treatment dose of surfactant that becomes associated with the lung tissue probably is in Type II cells. In the term newborn rabbit, more than 90% of the surfactant phospholipids are recycled back into the Type II cells for re-secretion.[53] In the only estimate available, ventilated preterm lambs with mild RDS had a turnover time for surfactant phosphatidylcholine of about 13 hours.[49] These animals had no measurable surfactant catabolism, a finding indicating very efficient recycling.

Measurements of surfactant clearance and biologic half-life in animals were estimated from the amount of labeled surfactant that remained in the lung tissue and in the air space after an interval of time. The only practical measurement in the human is to give a trace or treatment dose of surfactant containing a stable isotope and to follow the change in concentration of the label in the surfactant sampled by aspiration of the air spaces. This measurement gives an integrated assessment of the mixing of the exogenous label with the endogenous air space and a delayed

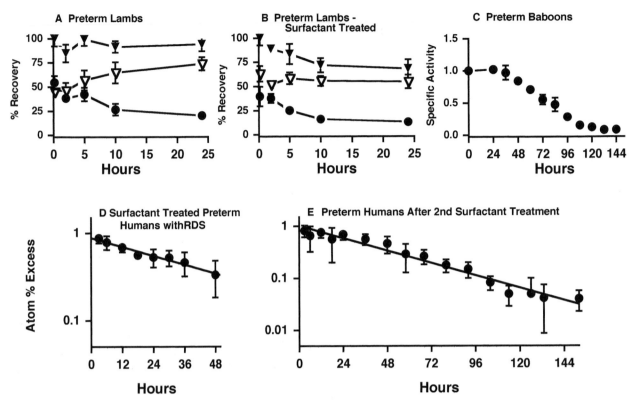

Figure 104–6. Loss of labeled phosphatidylcholine (PC) given into the airways of preterm lambs not treated with surfactant (**A**), preterm lambs treated with surfactant (**B**), preterm surfactant-treated baboons (**C**), and surfactant-treated preterm infants (**D** and **E**). All animals and infants were mechanically ventilated and had respiratory distress syndrome (RDS). **A**, The preterm lambs received a trace dose of natural sheep surfactant labeled with [3H]dipalmitoylphosphatidylcholine. Recoveries in alveolar washes, lung tissue, and the total lungs (alveolar and tissue) were measured 2, 5, 10, and 24 hours after birth. **B**, Preterm lambs were treated at birth with 100 mg/kg of natural sheep surfactant, containing radiolabeled phosphatidylcholine, and the lambs were ventilated for periods to 24 hours for measurements of the percentage of recovery of the phosphatidylcholine from the surfactant used for treatment. **C**, Curve for specific activity of phosphatidylcholine in airway samples of preterm baboons treated at birth with [14C]dipalmitoylphosphatidylcholine-labeled surfactant. The specific activities were normalized to the values for the surfactant used to treat the baboons. **D**, Curve for atom % excess in airway samples for [13C]dipalmitoylphosphatidylcholine labeled surfactant used to treat preterm ventilated infants with RDS. The atom % excess in the initial surfactant dose given after delivery fell exponentially for 48 hours. **E**, A second dose given at about 2 days of age resulted in a similar curve. (*A*, Data from ref. 49; *B*, data from ref. 50; *C*, data from ref. 38; *E*, data from ref. 30.)

mixing with tissue pools of surfactant. A decrease in the concentration of the label in the airway sample represents dilution of the label with surfactant from the lung, but it does not necessarily measure catabolism. Such measurements have been made in surfactant-treated preterm ventilated baboons and in infants with RDS (see Fig. 104–6).[30,38] In baboons, the concentration of labeled lipid (specific activity) did not change for about 24 hours, a finding indicating that very little endogenous surfactant was present. However, independent information from preterm lambs and baboons indicates that only about 20% of the surfactant would have been in the air spaces at 24 hours and 25% of the surfactant would have been lost from the lung compartment.[49,50] Subsequently, the specific activity decreased exponentially, yielding a biologic half-life of about 30 hours. The biologic half-life values for infants with RDS measured with [13C]dipalmitoylphosphatidylcholine were 34±9 hours after surfactant treatment at a mean of 4.6 hours of age and were similar after a second dose of surfactant was given at a mean age of 37 hours. The consistency of the indirect measurements in humans and the animals indicates that surfactant catabolism is slow in the preterm with RDS. The treatment dose of surfactant does not remain in the air space but becomes part of the overall metabolic pool of surfactant.

The surfactant proteins SP-A, SP-B, and SP-C are cleared from the air spaces and the lung compartment of adult animals in parallel with the surfactant lipids.[14] The proteins are recycled with an efficiency somewhat lower than that of the lipids, and degradation of SP-A occurs about equally in macrophages and Type II cells.[11] The preterm ventilated lamb lung clears SP-A from the air spaces more rapidly than the lipids.[54] The lipophilic proteins SP-B and SP-C are cleared from the air spaces and from the lung compartment similarly to saturated phosphatidylcholine in ventilated preterm lamb lungs (Fig. 104–7).[37,52] SP-B clearance is similar in lambs ventilated with a conventional style of ventilation or with high-frequency oscillatory ventilation.

Lung Injury with Mechanical Ventilation in Respiratory Distress Syndrome

The lungs of infants who have died of RDS have alveolar atelectasis, alveolar and interstitial edema, and hyaline membranes, primarily in distorted small airways. *Hyaline membranes* are a coagulum of cell debris, surfactant, and serum proteins, and they indicate epithelial injury and large amounts of soluble and insoluble proteins in the air spaces. The earliest anatomic lesion identified in the lungs of infants who died of RDS shortly after birth was epithelial disruption in the small airways.[55] In preterm surfactant-deficient rabbits, bronchiolar epithelial injury develops within minutes of delivery and ventilation, and this injury is prevented with surfactant treatment (Fig. 104–8).[56] The epithelial damage occurs because the small airways of the immature

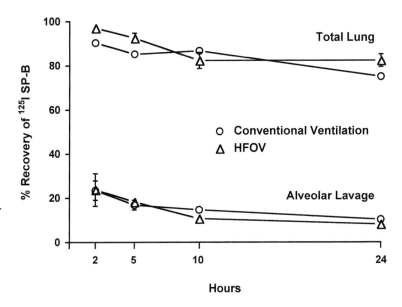

Figure 104–7. Recoveries of [^{125}I]surfactant protein B (SP-B) from the alveolar lavages and total lungs (alveolar and tissue) of preterm surfactant-treated and ventilated lambs. The lambs were conventionally ventilated or were ventilated with high-frequency oscillatory ventilation (HFOV). Although there was minimal loss of SP-B from the lungs, the amount of SP-B recovered by alveolar lavage was low. (Data from ref. 52.)

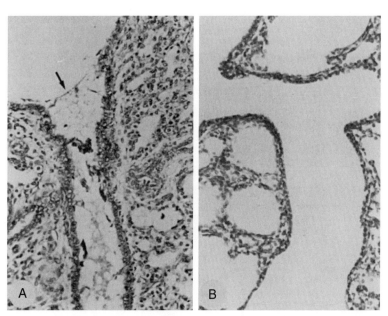

Figure 104–8. Bronchiolar-epithelial injury. **A,** Lungs from preterm ventilated rabbits had fluid-filled airways with epithelial tears in the absence of surfactant treatment. **B,** With surfactant treatments, the bronchiolar epithelium remained intact, and fluid was cleared from the airways and alveoli. (From Lachmann B, et al: Pediatr Res *16*:921, 1982.)

lung are compliant and distort during the ventilation of preterm lungs. Lung fluid clearance is not complete, and small airways are fluid filled at end expiration. Ventilation requires high peak pressures for the noncompliant lung to achieve relatively normal tidal volumes and carbon dioxide removal.

The ventilated preterm lung has both endothelial and epithelial abnormalities that lead to proteinaceous pulmonary edema after delivery and ventilation.[57] In preterm lambs ventilated for the first 3 hours of life, 11.5%/hour of the labeled albumin mixed with the fetal lung fluid at birth left the lung, and 1.7%/hour of the labeled albumin given intravascularly at birth was recovered from the air spaces, a finding demonstrating the bidirectional movement of albumin across an injured alveolar epithelium.[58] Because net protein in the alveolar washes increased more than fourfold, the dominant direction of protein movement was from the intravascular compartment to the air spaces. The rate of protein accumulation in the air spaces was striking in preterm ventilated rabbits. About 2 to 3% of the intravascularly injected and labeled albumin was recovered from the air spaces within 20 minutes of birth. The leakage was not homogeneous.[59] Leakage involved an increasing number of saccules with time and appeared to occur directly into the alveoli, rather than at the bronchiolar level.

Lung gas volumes of infants with RDS can be low because the lung has not yet developed sufficiently to hold much gas or because distal air spaces are uninflated. Another cause of the volume loss in the lungs of infants with RDS is alveolar edema. After 3 hours of ventilation, the total lung capacity was 48 mL/kg in preterm monkeys without RDS and 19 mL/kg for monkeys with RDS.[60] The lungs were flash frozen and were evaluated by light and scanning electron microscopy. The lungs of the animals with RDS showed overexpansion of the distal airways and under-expanded and fluid-filled alveolar spaces (Fig. 104–9). By scanning electron microscopy, the alveoli of the animals with RDS were filled with proteinaceous liquid, and the interstitium was swollen by edema fluid (Fig. 104–10). The monkeys with RDS had alveolar and interstitial edema because of the combination of slow clearance of fetal lung fluid after birth and the entrance of proteinaceous edema into the air spaces.

Four variables are important determinants of the amount of edema formation: gestational age, positive end-expiratory pressure, tidal volume, and surfactant treatment. In preterm animal models, the protein leaks from the vascular space to the alveolar space and from the alveolar space to the vascular space increased as gestation decreased (Fig. 104–11).[61] A variable in

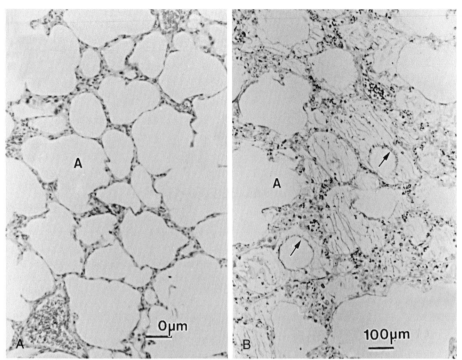

Figure 104–9. A, Light micrograph of lung tissue from a preterm monkey lung without respiratory distress syndrome (RDS). The alveoli and alveolar ducts (indicated by A) are air filled. **B,** In contrast, lung tissue from a monkey with RDS has some air-filled alveoli, and other alveoli are completely or partially filled with proteinaceous material. The *arrows* indicate partially filled alveoli. (From Jackson JC, et al: Am Rev Respir Dis *143*:865, 1991.)

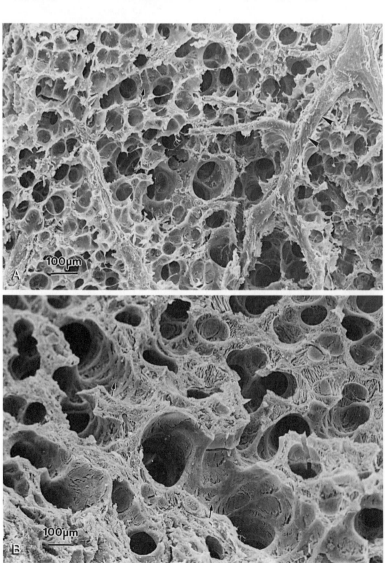

Figure 104–10. Scanning electron micrographs of frozen, dehydrated lung tissue from a preterm monkey without respiratory distress syndrome (RDS) (**A**) and from a preterm monkey at the same gestational age with RDS (**B**). The lung from the animal with RDS has dilated alveolar ducts and interstitial and alveolar edema. (From Jackson JC, et al: Am Rev Respir Dis *143*:865, 1991.)

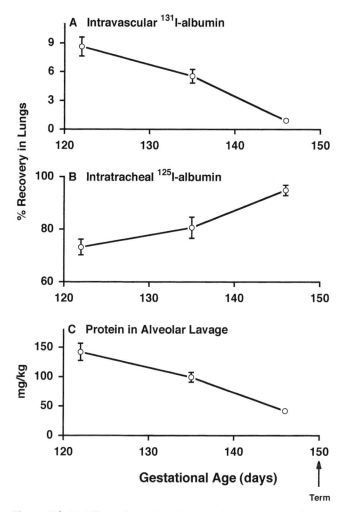

Figure 104–11. Effect of gestational age on the movement of labeled albumin and protein in and out of the air spaces of preterm lambs. Peak ventilatory pressures were held constant at the three gestational ages for 3 hours of ventilation. The more preterm lambs were treated with surfactant to achieve similar ventilatory pressures. **A,** [^{131}I]Albumin was given into the vascular space, and the net recovery in alveolar washes and in the total lung (sum of parenchyma plus alveolar wash) decreased as gestational age increased toward term. **B,** [^{125}I]Albumin was given into the airways at birth, and the amount that was lost from the lungs decreased as gestation increased. **C,** The total amount of protein in alveolar washes decreased as gestation increased. (Data from ref. 61.)

ventilated animals is the pressure needed to achieve an adequate tidal volume and gas exchange, pressure that decreases as gestational age increases. Therefore, an explanation of the increased leak is the barotrauma caused by the ventilatory requirements needed to support the more immature animals (Fig. 104–12).[62] In the mature lung, pulmonary edema occurs after lung overdistention using high-pressures (*volutrauma*). High pressures are not required to injure the immature surfactant-deficient lung, because nonuniform inflation results in focal overdistention. Without surfactant treatment, pulmonary edema can occur with relatively low tidal volume ventilation.[51] The end-expiratory volume of the preterm lung also is an important variable in injury. Ventilation of preterm lambs with the same tidal volume results in different amounts of protein recovery from the airways, depending on the positive end-expiratory pressure used to support end expiratory lung volume.[63]

The severity of the surfactant deficiency also influences the development of pulmonary edema. Egan and colleagues[64] reported that surfactant-sufficient preterm lambs and goats did not lose large molecular weight substances from the air spaces, whereas surfactant-deficient animals did. Treatment of premature lambs with surfactant decreased the protein leakage from the vascular space to the air spaces. Surfactant treatment also decreased the endothelial leak of plasma proteins. Surfactant can protect the lung from injury caused by high tidal volumes that would otherwise injure the surfactant-deficient lung.[51] The major effect of surfactant is probably by increasing the uniformity of lung expansion.[65]

SURFACTANT FUNCTION IN THE ALVEOLUS

Surfactant Forms in the Alveolus

Surfactant in the alveolus is present in different structural forms that have different characteristics and functions.[8] After secretion, the lamellar bodies unravel to form the elegant structure called *tubular myelin*. This lipoprotein array has SP-A at the corners of the lattice and requires at least SP-A, SP-B, and the phospholipids for its unique structure. Tubular myelin and other loose surfactant lipoprotein arrays in the hypophase generate the surface film within the alveolus and small airways. New surfactant enters the surface film, and "used" surfactant leaves as small vesicles, which then are cleared from the air spaces. The major differences in composition between the surface-active tubular myelin and the biophysically inactive small vesicles are that the small forms contain very little SP-A, SP-B, or SP-C.

Preceding and after birth, surfactant is secreted to yield an alveolar pool that primarily consists of lamellar bodies and tubular myelin. During neonatal transition to air breathing, the percentage of surface-active forms falls as the small vesicular forms increase (Fig. 104–13).[66] At steady state, approximately 50% of the surfactant in the air spaces is in a surface-active form, and 50% is in the inactive vesicular form. The total surfactant pool size is not equivalent to the amount of active surfactant. The maintenance of surfactant function depends on the preservation of the active forms of surfactant in the air space.

Surfactant Inactivation

Surfactant inactivation or surfactant inhibition is a complex concept because it is the integrated result of multiple factors that can alter the alveolar forms and biophysical properties of the surfactant in the air spaces (Table 104–1).[67] The net effects can be a decrease in the effective pool size, a degradation of the surface tension–lowering properties of the surfactant, or both. Injury to the alveolar epithelium and edema change the environment where surfactant acts. The mechanisms that contribute to surfactant inactivation vary with the type of lung injury. The biophysically active surfactant pool can be depleted by an increased rate of conversion to the inactive vesicular forms. This conversion is accelerated by proteinaceous edema and inflammatory products, probably because proteases degrade surfactant proteins.[68] Ventilation styles that use large tidal volumes and no positive end-expiratory pressure can deplete the active surfactant pool, and high-frequency oscillatory ventilation can preserve the surfactant in adult animal models.[69] However, in surfactant-treated preterm lambs, ventilation with high-frequency oscillation did not have an advantage over conventional ventilation.[52] Meconium and bilirubin can accelerate the conversion to inactive surfactant forms, and surfactant with less surfactant protein is inactivated more quickly.

Another mechanism of inactivation is the removal of the surfactant by sequestration into clots or hyaline membranes. Surfactant is a thromboplastin and activates clotting, and *in vitro* the clot will capture most of the pulmonary surfactant that is in

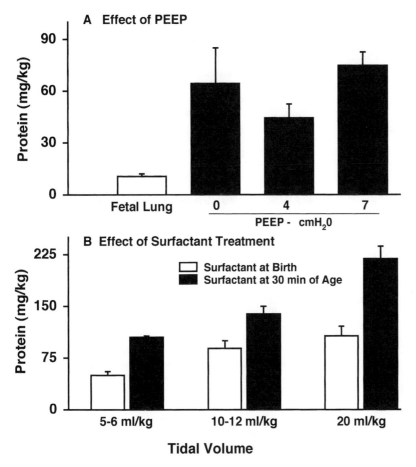

Figure 104–12. Effect of positive end-expiratory pressure (PEEP), tidal volumes, and surfactant on the amount of protein recovered in alveolar lavages of ventilated preterm lambs. **A,** Lambs were ventilated for 7 hours to similar Pco$_2$ values after surfactant treatment with PEEP values of 0, 4, or 7 cm H$_2$O. In comparison with the protein in the alveolar lavages of unventilated fetal animals, all ventilated animals had increased protein in alveolar lavages. However, the protein was higher with the use of 0 or 7 cm H$_2$O PEEP than with 4 cm H$_2$O PEEP. **B,** Preterm lambs were ventilated for 30 minutes after birth with different tidal volumes and were then ventilated with a tidal volume of 10 mL/kg until the lambs were 6 hours old. Some lambs were treated with surfactant at birth, and others were treated at 30 minutes of age. The high tidal volume of 20 mL/kg increased the protein recovered by alveolar lavage, and surfactant treatment decreased protein recovery at all tidal volumes. (**A,** Data from ref. 62; **B,** data from ref. 51.)

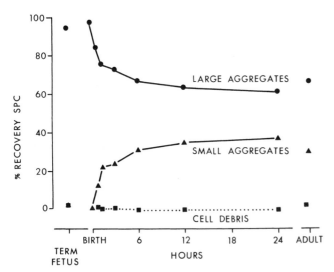

Figure 104–13. Changes in surfactant aggregate size distribution with time after birth. Surfactant suspensions recovered by alveolar wash from term rabbit fetuses and at various ages after birth were fractionated by centrifugation. The large aggregates were recovered by centrifugation at 80,000 times gravity for 90 minutes, and the small aggregates were the fraction that did not pellet. The distribution of saturated phosphatidylcholine (SPC) in fractions is also indicated for alveolar washes from adult rabbits. (Redrawn from Bruni R, et al: Biochim Biophys Acta *958*:255, 1988.)

TABLE 104–1

Mechanisms of Surfactant Inactivation and Substances That Contribute to Inactivation

Form conversions in air spaces
   Normal process of alveolar metabolism
   Increased conversion with proteinaceous edema (proteases?)
   Ventilation, meconium, decreased surfactant protein content
Removal of surfactant from alveolar pool
   Clots and hyaline membranes
Inhibitors of adsorption and film stabilization
   Proteins
      Edema fluid
      Plasma
      Fibrinogen, monomers
      Albumin
      Laminin
      Hemoglobin
   Lipids
      Lysophosphatidylcholine
      Cholesterol
      Red cell membranes
   Other inactivators
      Meconium
      Bilirubin
      Oxidizing agents
      Amino acids

the plasma.[67] Although most soluble proteins can interfere with surface adsorption and film formation, the products of clot lysis are particularly inhibitory.[70] Albumin is not as inhibitory as fibrinogen, although it is the protein that is in the highest concentration in edema and inflammatory fluid. Hemoglobin and other protein products of lung injury also are inhibitors. The phenomenon of interference with film formation by soluble proteins is dependent on both the relative and absolute concentrations of the surfactant and the inhibiting proteins.[71] If surfactant concentrations are high, potent inhibitors at high concentration will have little adverse effect when tested *in vitro*. However, when surfactant concentrations are low, low concentrations of inhibitors can severely degrade surfactant function. Surfactants that contain low amounts of surfactant proteins also are more sensitive to inactivation by soluble proteins.

Lung function deteriorates when inactivation interferes with sufficient surfactant to alter the function of the surfactant at the air-fluid interface. Therefore, inactivation can be a severe problem when the surfactant pool size is small, as in RDS. Airway samples from infants taken at the time of intubation for the treatment of RDS had very high minimal surface tensions (Fig. 104–14).[72] Inhibition of surfactant function was contributing to the problem because the airway samples contained surfactant with good function that could be isolated by centrifugation. The soluble proteins from these airway samples inhibited natural surfactant more than did proteins from airway samples from infants without RDS. The importance of surfactant inactivation can be demonstrated using a preterm ventilated lamb model of RDS (Fig. 104–15).[73] Lambs at less than 125 days' gestation (term is 150 days) have a surfactant pool of less than 1 mg/kg and thus are severely surfactant deficient. Ventilation for 30 minutes causes severe lung injury, and surfactant treatment then results in improved oxygenation and a fall in minimal surface tensions of the surfactant in airway samples. However, decreased oxygenation occurs because these animals have progressive lung injury. Most of these adverse effects can be avoided by giving the surfactant before ventilating the animal and using a low tidal volume and gentle style of ventilation.[51]

These inhibitory effects can be interpreted in the clinical context of the progressive deterioration in lung function after birth in infants with severe RDS. The infants with RDS have low surfactant pool sizes, and with ventilation they develop edema, inflammation, and lung injury. The combination of clot formation (hyaline membranes) and increased soluble inhibitory proteins depletes the functional surfactant pool and results in progressive respiratory failure.

Inactivation phenomena depend on the type of surfactant being tested. The animal source surfactants in clinical use have in common organic solvent extraction steps that remove nonspecific contaminating proteins (primarily plasma-derived proteins), SP-A, and SP-D. SP-B and SP-C are retained in the surfactant in variable amounts, along with the phospholipids and neutral lipids. The only functional abnormality in surfactant from mice that lack SP-A is increased sensitivity to inhibition.[74] The addition of SP A to an organic solvent-extracted surfactant made that surfactant less sensitive to inactivation by albumin and fibrinogen.[75] The potent inactivation of surfactant by fibrinogen was reversed by 0.5% SP-A. Addition of SP-A to surfactant containing SP-B and SP-C preserved the *in vivo* function of the surfactant in the presence of plasma when the mixture was used to treat preterm rabbits.[76, 77] These observations may have direct clinical relevance because Hallman and colleagues[36] reported that soluble proteins in airway samples from infants with RDS were much more inhibitory to surfactant samples with low SP-A/saturated phosphatidylcholine ratios than were surfactant samples with higher ratios. These investigators also found that for infants with birth weights less than 1 kg, death or

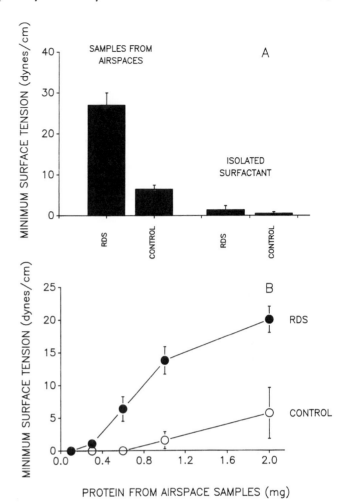

Figure 104–14. Minimum surface tensions of airway samples from infants with respiratory distress syndrome (RDS) and control infants (**A**) and inhibition of surfactant by air space protein (**B**). Samples from infants with RDS had high minimum surface tensions, whereas control samples had low minimum surface tensions. After isolation of surfactant by centrifugation, the surfactant had low minimum surface tensions from both RDS and control infants. Increasing amounts of the supernatant protein fractions from airway samples were added to a constant amount of natural sheep surfactant (**B**). Protein fractions from infants with RDS had higher inhibitory activity than proteins from the control infants. (From Ikegami M, et al: J Pediatr *102*:443, 1983.)

BPD correlated with airway samples with low SP-A/saturated phosphatidylcholine ratios.

SP-B and SP-C also influence the sensitivity of lipid mixtures to inactivation.[78] Synthetic surfactants that lack these surfactant proteins are sensitive to inactivation by albumin or fibrinogen. Addition of native SP-B and SP-C improved resistance to inactivation.[79] Recombinant SP-C and lipids and mixtures of SP-B and SP-C and lipids are less sensitive to protein inactivation than are lipid mixtures alone, although these combinations are not as resistant as natural surfactant.

Quality of Surfactant from the Preterm

The preterm infant with RDS has surfactant with properties that are inferior to surfactant from the mature lung, and this further compounds the problem of a small pool size of surfactant.[16]

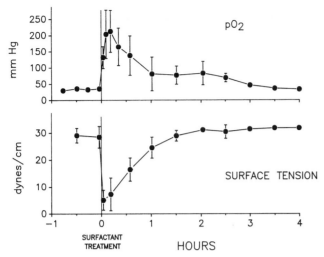

Figure 104–15. Surface tension versus clinical response to surfactant treatment of lambs. Sequential values for partial pressure of oxygen (Po₂) and minimum surface tensions from birth to treatment at about 45 minutes with surfactant and then for the subsequent 4 hours are given. The immature lambs had severe respiratory failure despite ventilatory support and 100% O₂. After surfactant treatment, Po₂ values increased, and surface tensions of airway samples were low. Subsequently, the respiratory function of the lambs deteriorated in parallel with increasing minimum surface tension values in the airway samples. (From Ikegami M, et al: J Appl Physiol 57:1134, 1984.)

Surfactant from the preterm with RDS has a different composition from surfactant from the mature or adult lung. The phosphatidylglycerol content is lower, the phosphatidylinositol content is higher, and the percentage of saturated phosphatidylcholine is lower. Surfactant from the preterm that has been separated from the inhibitory effects of edema fluid is intrinsically different in function from surfactant from the mature lung. Surfactant from the preterm is less dense than surfactant from term or adult lungs because it contains less SP-A relative to saturated phosphatidylcholine. The alveolar pool from preterm lambs with RDS has a higher percentage of the surfactant in inactive forms than more mature lambs, and *in vitro* conversion rates from active to inactive forms are more rapid. The surfactant from the preterm also is more sensitive to inactivation *in vitro* by

soluble proteins, most likely because of a lower surfactant protein content. Furthermore, when surfactants from the preterm lambs or baboons are tested in preterm surfactant-deficient rabbit lungs, they are less effective at improving compliance than is surfactant from term animals.[16, 38] Therefore, surfactant from the preterm is intrinsically less effective and more susceptible to inactivation than is surfactant from the mature lung.

Surfactant Function with Surfactant Treatment

The surfactants used clinically are organic solvent extracts of alveolar washes or lung tissue. These surfactants contain no SP-A, the amount of SP-B and SP-C is variable, and processing and sterilization disrupt the lipoprotein structural arrays. The clinical surfactants are more sensitive to inactivation by plasma proteins than is natural surfactant. There are counterbalancing phenomena of improved function after exposure of the surfactants to the preterm lung. When surfactant is recovered by alveolar wash after surfactant treatment of preterm lambs with RDS, the surfactant has enhanced function.[80] This improved function can be demonstrated by comparing the surfactant used to treat the lambs with the surfactant recovered from the lambs for effects on surfactant-deficient rabbit lungs (Fig. 104–16). The very preterm lung cannot improve the function of surfactant used for treatment, whereas the more mature lung can. The mechanism for the enhanced function probably is the mixing of the surfactant used for treatment with small amounts of endogenous surfactant lipids and proteins. Many hours after treatment, the enhanced function of surfactant can occur by recycling of components from the surfactant used for treatment through the Type II cells. The sensitivity of the surfactants used clinically to inactivation also can be modulated after exposure to the preterm lung.[81] The surfactants become less susceptible to inactivation if they are mixed with 5 or 10% by weight natural surfactant. Therefore, small endogenous surfactant pools can interact with the large doses of surfactant used clinically to result in an improved surfactant. This activation phenomenon will not occur if the lung is injured.

Surfactant and Innate Host Defenses

The lung of the infant with RDS is not inflamed at birth unless there was chorioamnionitis and infection before birth. However, the initiation of ventilation in the preterm lung initiates inflammation.[62] The initiation of ventilation results in nonuni-

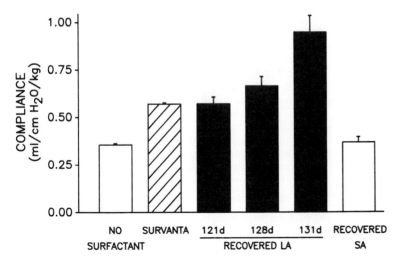

Figure 104–16. Surfactant function after surfactant treatment. Preterm lambs were treated with 100 mg/kg Survanta and were ventilated for several hours. Surfactant was recovered by alveolar wash and was divided by differential centrifugation into the large aggregate (LA) surface-active fraction and the small aggregate (SA) inactive forms. These surfactant fractions were then used to treat preterm surfactant-deficient rabbits in comparison with an untreated control group and a Survanta-treated group. The large aggregates from the more mature lambs at 128 and 131 days' gestation had enhanced function relative to Survanta. The small aggregates from all gestational ages were ineffective. (From Ikegami M, et al: Am Rev Respir Dis 148:837, 1993.)

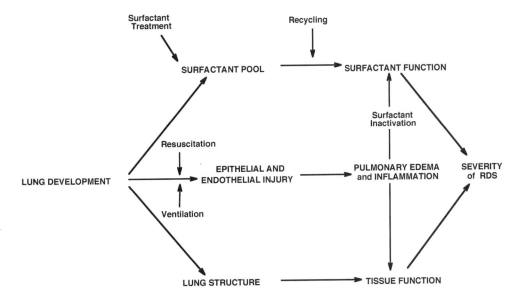

Figure 104–17. Flow diagram of the major variables influencing the clinical course of respiratory distress syndrome (RDS).

form inflation of the surfactant-deficient lung and stretch-mediated injury. If the tidal volume is high or the functional residual capacity is too high or too low, then lung injury will occur. The use of oxygen also may initiate an inflammatory response. Surfactant treatment decreases the severity of this initial inflammation, in part by its mechanical effects on the lungs to make lung inflation more uniform. However, surfactant also can have effects on the inflammatory response because of its multiple innate host defense functions.[82] The preterm lung is severely deficient in SP-A and SP-D. These proteins opsonize a variety of organisms and promote phagocytosis while suppressing inflammation in the adult lung. The hydrophobic proteins SP-B and SP-C can mitigate oxidant-induced injury. The potential for surfactant components to modulate the inflammation that accompanies RDS has not been well characterized.

Model for the Initial Events in Respiratory Distress Syndrome

The preterm infant born at less than 30 weeks' gestation and destined to develop RDS has a saccular lung and a small surfactant pool (Fig. 104–17). Antenatal glucocorticoid treatment can increase the surfactant pool and can increase the structural potential for gas exchange.[83] The techniques used for resuscitation and initiating ventilation influence the initial epithelial and endothelial injury, and subsequent ventilation may further aggravate the injury.[84] The small surfactant pool can be inhibited by the products of the injury and initial inflammation that enter the air spaces. Surfactant treatment can decrease the initial lung injury and can increase the surfactant pool size. The surfactant used for treatment becomes substrate for the recycling metabolic pathways. The initial severity of RDS then is a reflection of the reciprocal interactions of surfactant function altered by surfactant inhibition acting on the lung tissue. Surfactant function can be improved with surfactant treatment or by decreasing lung injury. Lung tissue function is determined by the stage of development and the amount of lung injury. These effects are occurring to different degrees in different lung regions because the injury that occurs with RDS is not uniformly distributed throughout the lung.

REFERENCES

1. Avery ME, Mead J: Surface properties in relation to atelectasis and hyaline membrane disease. Am J Dis Child 97:517, 1959.
2. Jobe AH: Pulmonary surfactant therapy. N Engl J Med 328:861, 1993.
3. Langston C, et al: Human lung growth in late gestation and in the neonate. Am Rev Respir Dis 129:607, 1984.
4. Hislop AA, et al: Alveolar development in the human fetus and infant. Early Hum Dev 13:1, 1986.
5. Burri PH: Structural aspects of prenatal and postnatal development and growth of the lung. In McDonald JA (ed): Lung Growth and Development. New York, Marcel Dekker, 1997, p 1.
6. Bunton TE, Plopper CG: Triamcinolone-induced structural alterations in the development of the lung of the fetal rhesus macaque. Am J Obstet Gynecol 148:203, 1984.
7. Massaro DJ, Massaro GD: The regulation of the formation of pulmonary alveoli. In Bland RD, Coalson JJ (eds): Chronic Lung Disease in Early Infancy, Vol 137. New York, Marcel Dekker, 2000, p 479.
8. Wright JR, Dobbs LG: Regulation of pulmonary surfactant secretion and clearance. Annu Rev Physiol 53:395, 1991.
9. McCormack FX: Structure, processing and properties of surfactant protein A. Biochim Biophys Acta 1408:109, 1998.
10. Schurch S, et al: Formation and structure of surface films: captive bubble surfactometry. Biochim Biophys Acta 1408:180, 1998.
11. Gurel O, et al: Macrophage and type II cell catabolism of SP-A and saturated phosphatidylcholine in mouse lung. Am J Physiol 280:L1266, 2001.
12. Jacobs HC, et al: Reutilization of surfactant phosphatidylcholine in adult rabbits. Biochim Biophys Acta 837:77, 1985.
13. Ueda T, et al: Clearance of surfactant protein A from rabbit lungs. Am J Respir Cell Mol Biol 12:89, 1995.
14. Ueda T, et al: Clearance of surfactant protein B from rabbit lungs. Am J Physiol 268:L636, 1995.
15. Ikegami M, et al: Clearance of SP-C and recombinant SP-C in vivo and in vitro. Am J Physiol 274:L933, 1998.
16. Ueda T, et al: Developmental changes of sheep surfactant: in vivo function and in vitro subtype conversion. J Appl Physiol 76:2701, 1994.
17. Hallman M, et al: Phosphatidylinositol and phosphatidylglycerol in amniotic fluid: indices of lung maturity. Am J Obstet Gynecol 125:613, 1976.
18. Kulovich MV, et al: The lung profile: normal pregnancy. Am J Obstet Gynecol 135:57, 1979.
19. Obladen M: Alterations in surfactant composition. In Merritt TA, et al (eds): Bronchopulmonary Dysplasia, Vol 4. Boston, Blackwell Scientific 1988, p 131.
20. Pryhuber GS, et al: Ontogeny of surfactant protein-A and protein-B in human amniotic fluid as indices of fetal lung maturity. Pediatr Res 30:597, 1991.
21. Bachurski CJ, et al: Intra-amniotic endotoxin increases pulmonary surfactant components and induces SP-B processing in fetal sheep. Am J Physiol 280:L279, 2001.
22. Miyamura K, et al: Surfactant proteins A (SP-A) and D (SP-D)—levels in human amniotic fluid and localization in the fetal membranes. BBA-Lipid Lipid Metab 1210:303, 1994.
23. Wert SE, et al: Transcriptional elements from the human SP-C gene direct expression in the primordial respiratory epithelium of transgenic mice. Dev Biol 156:426, 1993.
24. Ross GF, et al: Surfactant protein C (SP-C) levels in fetal and ventilated preterm rabbit lungs. Am J Physiol 277:L1104, 1999.
25. Faridy EE, Thliveris JA: Rate of secretion of lung surfactant before and after birth. Respir Physiol 68:269, 1987.

26. Jacobs H, et al: Accumulation of alveolar surfactant following delivery and ventilation of premature lambs. Exp Lung Res 8:125, 1985.

27. Adams FH, et al: Lung phospholipid of the human fetus and infants with and without hyaline membrane disease. J Pediatr 77:833, 1970.

28. Hallman M, et al: Effect of surfactant substitution on lung effluent phospholipids in respiratory distress syndrome: evaluation of surfactant phospholipid turnover, pool size, and the relationship to severity of respiratory failure. Pediatr Res 20:1228, 1986.

29. Griese M, et al: Pharmacokinetics of bovine surfactant in neonatal respiratory distress syndrome. Am J Respir Care Med 152:1050, 1995.

30. Torresin M, et al: Exogenous surfactant kinetics in infant respiratory distress syndrome: a novel method with stable isotopes. Am J Respir Crit Care Med 161:1584, 2000.

31. Ikegami M, et al: Relationship between alveolar saturated phosphatidylcholine pool sizes and compliance of preterm rabbit lungs: the effect of maternal corticosteroid treatment. Am Rev Respir Dis 139:367, 1989.

32. Seidner S, et al: Corticosteroid potentiation of surfactant dose response in preterm rabbits. J Appl Physiol 64:2366, 1988.

33. Rebello CM, et al: Alveolar and tissue surfactant pool sizes in humans. Am J Respir Crit Care Med 154:625, 1996.

34. Jackson JC, et al: Surfactant quantity and composition during recovery from hyaline membrane disease. Pediatr Res 20:1243:1247, 1986.

35. Jackson JC, et al: Developmental changes of surface active material in newborn non-human primates. Am Rev Respir Dis 129:A204, 1984.

36. Hallman M, et al: Surfactant protein-A, phosphatidylcholine, and surfactant inhibitors in epithelial lining fluid: correlation with surface activity, severity of respiratory distress syndrome, and outcome in small premature infants. Am Rev Respir Dis 144:1376, 1991.

37. Ikegami M, Jobe AH: Surfactant protein-C in ventilated premature lamb lung. Pediatr Res 44:860, 1998.

38. Seidner SR, et al: Abnormal surfactant metabolism and function in preterm ventilated baboons. Am J Respir Crit Care Med 158:1982, 1998.

39. Janssen DJ, et al: Surfactant phosphatidylcholine half-life and pool size measurements in premature baboons developing BPD. Pediatr Res 52:724, 2002.

40. Awasthi S, et al: Surfactant proteins A and D in premature baboons with chronic lung injury: evidence for an inhibition of secretion. Am J Respir Crit Care Med 160:942, 1999.

41. Weaver TE, Conkright JJ: Function of surfactant proteins B and C. Annu Rev Physiol 63:555, 2001.

42. Jobe A, et al: Surfactant metabolism of newborn lamb lungs studied in vivo. J Appl Physiol 49:1091, 1980.

43. Jobe AH, et al: Saturated phosphatidylcholine secretion and the effect of natural surfactant on premature and term lambs ventilated for 2 days. Exp Lung Res 4:259, 1983.

44. Bunt JE, et al: Metabolism of endogenous surfactant in premature baboons and effect of prenatal corticosteroids. Am J Respir Crit Care Med 160:1481, 1999.

45. Bunt JE, et al: The effect in premature infants of prenatal corticosteroids on endogenous surfactant synthesis as measured with stable isotopes. Am J Respir Crit Care Med 162:844, 2000.

46. Pinkerton KE, et al: Surfactant treatment effects on lung structure and type II cells of preterm ventilated lambs. Biol Neonate 77:243, 2000.

47. Merchak A, et al: Endogenous pulmonary surfactant metabolism is not affected by mode of ventilation in premature infants with respiratory distress syndrome. J Pediatr 140:693, 2002.

48. Glatz T, et al: Metabolism of exogenously administered natural surfactant in the newborn lamb. Pediatr Res 16:711, 1982.

49. Jobe AH, et al: Surfactant phosphatidylcholine metabolism and surfactant function in preterm, ventilated lambs. Am Rev Respir Dis 139:352, 1989.

50. Ikegami M, et al: Surfactant metabolism in surfactant-treated preterm ventilated lambs. J Appl Physiol 67:429, 1989.

51. Wada K, et al: Tidal volume effects on surfactant treatment responses with the initiation of ventilation in preterm lambs. J Appl Physiol 83:1054, 1997.

52. Ikegami M, et al: Effects of ventilation style on surfactant metabolism and treatment response in preterm lambs. Am J Respir Crit Care Med 157:638, 1998.

53. Jacobs H, et al: The significance of reutilization of surfactant phosphatidylcholine. J Biol Chem 258:4156, 1983.

54. Ikegami M, et al: Surfactant protein-A metabolism in preterm ventilated lambs. Am J Physiol 262:L765, 1992.

55. Robertson D: Pathology and pathophysiology of neonatal surfactant deficiency. In Robertson B, et al (eds): Pulmonary Surfactant. Amsterdam, Elsevier Science, 1984, p 383.

56. Lachmann B, et al: Combined effects of surfactant substitution and prolongation of inspiration phase in artificially ventilated premature newborn rabbits. Pediatr Res 16:921, 1982.

57. Normand IC, et al: Passage of macromolecules between alveolar and interstitial spaces in foetal and newly ventilated lungs of the lamb. J Physiol 210:151, 1970.

58. Jobe A, et al: Permeability of premature lamb lungs to protein and the effect of surfactant on that permeability. J Appl Physiol 55:169, 1983.

59. Robertson B, et al: Leakage of protein in the immature rabbit lung; effect of surfactant replacement. Respir Physiol 61:265, 1985.

60. Jackson JC, et al: Mechanisms for reduced total lung capacity at birth and during hyaline membrane disease in premature newborn monkeys. Am Rev Respir Dis 142:413, 1990.

61. Jobe A, et al: Lung protein leaks in ventilated lambs: effects of gestational age. J Appl Physiol 58:1246, 1985.

62. Naik AS, et al: Effects of ventilation with different positive end-expiratory pressures on cytokine expression in the preterm lamb lung. Am J Respir Crit Care Med 164:494, 2001.

63. Michna J, et al: Positive end-expiratory pressure preserves surfactant function in preterm lambs. Am J Respir Crit Care Med 160:634, 1999.

64. Egan EA, et al: Fetal lung liquid absorption and alveolar epithelial solute permeability in surfactant deficient, breathing fetal lambs. Pediatr Res 18:566, 1984.

65. Pinkerton KE, et al: Lung parenchyma and type II cell morphometrics: effect of surfactant treatment on preterm ventilated lamb lungs. J Appl Physiol 77:1953, 1994.

66. Bruni R, et al: Postnatal transformations of alveolar surfactant in the rabbit: changes in pool size, pool morphology and isoforms of the 32–38 kDa apolipoprotein. Biochim Biophys Acta 958:255, 1988.

67. Jobe AH: Surfactant-edema interactions. In Weir EK, Reeves JT (eds): The Pathogenesis and Treatment of Pulmonary Edema. Armonk, NY, Futura Publishing, 1998, p 113.

68. Ueda T, et al: Surfactant subtypes: in vitro conversion, in vivo function, and effects of serum proteins. Am J Respir Crit Care Med 149:1254, 1994.

69. Kerr CL, et al: Effects of high-frequency oscillation on endogenous surfactant in an acute lung injury model. Am J Respir Crit Care Med 164:237, 2001.

70. Gunther A, Seeger W: Resistance to surfactant inactivation. In Robertson B, Taeusch HW (eds): Surfactant Therapy for Lung Disease. New York, Marcel Dekker, 1995, p 269.

71. Holm BA, Enhorning G, Notter RH: A biophysical mechanism by which plasma proteins inhibit lung surfactant activity. Chem Phys Lipids 49:49, 1988.

72. Ikegami M, et al: Surfactant function in the respiratory distress syndrome. J Pediatr 102:443, 1983.

73. Ikegami M, et al: A protein from airways of premature lambs that inhibits surfactant function. J Appl Physiol 57:1134, 1984.

74. Korfhagen TR, et al: Altered surfactant function and structure in SP-A gene targeted mice. Proc Natl Acad Sci USA 93:9594, 1996.

75. Cockshutt AM, et al: Pulmonary surfactant-associated protein-A enhances the surface activity of lipid extract surfactant and reverses inhibition by blood proteins in vitro. Biochemistry 29:8424, 1990.

76. Yukitake K, et al: Surfactant apoprotein A modifies the inhibitory effect of plasma proteins on surfactant activity in vivo. Pediatr Res 37:21, 1995.

77. Rider ED, et al: Treatment responses to surfactants containing natural surfactant proteins in preterm rabbits. Am Rev Respir Dis 147:669, 1993.

78. Seeger W, et al: Differential sensitivity to fibrinogen inhibition of SP-C-based vs SP-B-based surfactants. Am J Physiol 262:L286, 1992.

79. Hall SB, et al: Importance of hydrophobic apoproteins as constituents of clinical exogenous surfactants. Am Rev Respir Dis 145:24, 1992.

80. Ikegami M, et al: Changes in exogenous surfactant in ventilated preterm lamb lungs. Am Rev Respir Dis 148:837, 1993.

81. Chen C, et al: Exogenous surfactant function in very preterm lambs with and without fetal corticosteroid treatment. J Appl Physiol 78:955, 1995.

82. Crouch EC: Collectins and pulmonary host defense. Am J Respir Cell Mol Biol 19:177, 1998.

83. Jobe AH, Ikegami M: Fetal responses to glucocorticoids. In Mendelson CR (ed): Endocrinology of the Lung. Totowa, NJ, Humana Press, 2000, pp 45–57.

84. van Marter LJ, et al: Rate of bronchopulmonary dysplasia as a function of neonatal intensive care practices. J Pediatr 120:938, 1992.

Ian Gross and Philip L. Ballard

105

Hormonal Therapy for Prevention
of Respiratory Distress Syndrome

Over the past 20 years, a multifaceted approach to the prevention of respiratory distress syndrome (RDS) of the newborn has evolved. This involves prenatal prediction of fetal lung maturation by examination of the amniotic fluid, use of prenatal hormone therapy to accelerate fetal lung maturation, and provision of postnatal surfactant replacement therapy. This chapter reviews the clinical evidence that glucocorticoids accelerate fetal lung maturation and act synergistically with postnatal surfactant therapy to decrease the incidence of RDS and other neonatal disorders. Guidelines for the use of prenatal glucocorticoid therapy are provided.

BIOLOGIC CONSIDERATIONS

Several hormones have been shown to influence aspects of fetal lung maturation both *in vivo* and *in vitro* (Table 105-1).[1, 2] Glucocorticoids are the most important of the stimulatory agents; they increase synthesis of all components of surfactant and accelerate morphologic development. Endogenous fetal corticosteroids have a physiologic role in modulating the rate of lung development and likely cause precocious maturation under conditions of *in utero* stress. Corticoid levels increase in newborn infants who have respiratory disease or other illnesses, and this response may contribute to the resolution of RDS that normally occurs after a few days. Prenatal corticosteroid therapy for prevention of RDS achieves levels of circulating glucocorticoid activity comparable with those during the postnatal surge and thus is considered to mimic a physiologic stress response.[3] In the absence of endogenous fetal and maternal corticosteroids (as occurs in homozygous mice genetically engineered with a knockout of either the corticotropin-releasing hormone or glucocorticoid receptor), the lung is structurally and biochemically immature at birth, and affected animals die of respiratory failure.[4, 5] Effects in the developing lung represent one of many examples of the role of glucocorticoids in modulating tissue differentiation and helping to prepare the fetus for birth.

Glucocorticoids act by binding to specific receptors in lung cells. The receptor-glucocorticoid complex binds to regulatory elements in the promoter of target genes and increases (or in some cases decreases) synthesis of mRNA and protein.[6] Because effects are receptor mediated, responses occur at physiologic levels of glucocorticoid (e.g., 10–100 nM cortisol), and higher doses of steroid evoke little additional response. The peak fetal plasma concentration of glucocorticoid after maternal betamethasone treatment (12 mg) is estimated to result in 75% or greater occupancy of receptors.[3] From *in vitro* studies using high-resolution gel electrophoresis, it is estimated that at least 2% of the proteins in human fetal lung are regulated by glucocorticoids.[7] Glucocorticoids are known to induce the four surfactant-associated proteins, at least two lipogenic enzymes, ion and water transport proteins (Na^+,K^+-adenosine triphosphatase [ATPase], Na^+ channel, aquaporins), elastin, and a limited number of other proteins; however, most glucocorticoid-responsive proteins of fetal lung have not been identified.[8]

Although an increase in transcription of responsive genes in cultured lung occurs within 1 to 2 hours of corticosteroid exposure, accumulation of new proteins usually requires 12 to 24 hours. The earliest effect on pulmonary function in the fetal lamb occurred between 8 and 15 hours after treatment; optimal responses were observed at 48 hours and persisted for at least 7 days.[9] Thus, there may not be an observable benefit of glucocorticoid administration in those situations in which the infant is delivered shortly after therapy is initiated.[10, 11] It is known that receptor-bound glucocorticoid is necessary for continuing hormone action[1, 2] and that glucocorticoid action *in vitro* is often reversible on removal of hormone (e.g., induction of surfactant proteins in cultured lung and in fetal sheep).[12, 13] Therefore, some glucocorticoid responses may be of limited duration *in utero*. Clinically, reduction of RDS appears to diminish 7 to 10 days after hormone administration is completed.[11] If the infant is delivered after this time, there may be no therapeutic benefit. For this reason, retreatment has been used for women with recurring premature labor, and, as is discussed later in this chapter, the efficacy and safety of this practice are currently being investigated.[14]

Glucocorticoids also regulate gene expression by an indirect process termed *transrepression* in which the corticosteroid-receptor complex interacts with transcription factors such as activator protein-1 (jun/fos) and NFκB, regulators of cytokine production. This interaction blocks up-regulation of the cytokine-chemokine cascade in response to various stimuli and is the mechanism for the antiinflammatory effects of glucocorticoids.[15] Possible involvement of the transrepression mechanism in glucocorticoid effects on fetal lung development are not known but are possible given that several cytokines are known to inhibit surfactant production.

The physiologic role and mechanism of other hormones that stimulate lung development (see Table 105-1) have been less extensively studied. An increased level of the second messenger cyclic AMP (cAMP) stimulates Type II cell differentiation and induces surfactant lipids and surfactant-associated proteins A and B in cultured lung.[12] Some evidence suggests that treatment of fetal animals with terbutaline or other β-agonists, particularly in combination with glucocorticoid, enhances lung maturation. It is possible that cAMP-mediated effects occur clinically after treatment with β-agonists, prostaglandins or their inhibitors, or agents that inhibit phosphodiesterases (e.g., xanthine derivatives), but no possible clinical benefit or harm has been documented. Thyroid hormones stimulate surfactant lipid synthesis in cultured tissue and in fetal lambs, acting in a synergistic manner with glucocorticoids (and prolactin *in vivo*).[16-18] Nuclear receptors for triiodothyronine (T_3) are present in fetal lung cells, and the properties of thyroid hormone's stimulatory effects (e.g., response with physiologic concentrations of hormone) are consistent with a receptor-mediated process.[19] Target proteins for thyroid hormones in fetal lung, except for one lipogenic enzyme (choline-phosphate cytidylyltransferase), are unknown. Clinically, injection of thyroid hormone into amniotic fluid has been reported to cause a slow increase in the lecithin:sphingomyelin ratio, but clinical benefit and safety have not been investigated.[20] Combined glucocorticoid and thyrotropin-releasing hormone (TRH) treatment, however, may be a potentially useful clinical approach for prevention of newborn lung disease in some circumstances (see later discussion).

TABLE 105-1

Hormones That Influence Fetal Lung Maturation in Animal and Culture Models

Stimulation

Glucocorticoids
Cyclic adenosine monophosphate
Thyroid hormones/thyrotropin-releasing hormone
Epidermal growth factor
Retinoic acid
Bombesin-related peptides
Parathyroid hormone-related peptide
Lipopolysaccharide
? Estrogen

Inhibition

Insulin/hyperglycemia/?butyrate
Tumor-necrosis factor alpha
Transforming growth factor β
Interleukin-1
Phorbol esters
Androgen

Several agents have an inhibitory effect on levels of surfactant components *in vitro* (see Table 105-1). Tumor necrosis factor-α (TNF-α), transforming growth factor β, and activators of protein kinase C (e.g., phorbol esters and lipopolysaccharide [endotoxin]) are of particular interest because they are involved in the etiology of lung inflammation and infection. A negative effect of these agents on levels of surfactant proteins A and B has been observed in cultured lung, even with combined treatment with glucocorticoids. It is possible that down-regulation of surfactant components contributes to the pathobiology of newborn lung diseases (e.g., meconium aspiration, bronchopulmonary dysplasia, and pneumonia).

CLINICAL EVIDENCE FOR THE EFFECTIVENESS OF PRENATAL GLUCOCORTICOID THERAPY

The effects of glucocorticoids on lung maturation and perinatal outcome have been extensively studied. Liggins and Howie[21] reported in 1972 that there was a significant reduction in the incidence of RDS and mortality in premature infants after maternal treatment with glucocorticoids. However, despite the positive effects noted in that study and many others, some obstetricians continued to question the effectiveness and safety of the use of prenatal glucocorticoids for the prevention of RDS. In 1993 it was estimated that only about 15% of preterm infants between 500 and 1500 g birth weight were receiving prenatal glucocorticoid therapy in the United States.[22] In 1994, the National Institutes of Health (NIH) convened a Consensus Conference[22] to examine the data and make recommendations relating to glucocorticoid therapy, fetal maturation, and perinatal outcome. The clinical information used was primarily the comprehensive meta-analysis of published randomized trials of Crowley[23, 24] and several observational databases. The latter consisted of treatment and outcome information that was prospectively collected from five registries, including multicenter surfactant trials, and involved more than 30,000 low birth weight infants. The major findings of these two sources of information are reviewed in this chapter, as well as the recommendations of this NIH Consensus Conference.

Impact of Prenatal Glucocorticoids on the Incidence of Respiratory Distress Syndrome

Meta-analysis[24] (Fig. 105-1) revealed that glucocorticoid therapy significantly reduced the overall incidence of RDS by about 50%.

The effect was greatest in those infants who delivered from 1 to 7 days after the initiation of maternal treatment. There was a trend toward decreased RDS in babies born less than 24 hours, or more than 7 days, after initiation of therapy, but the differences were not statistically significant.

Steroids were effective over a wide gestational age range. There was a significant reduction in the incidence of RDS in babies born before 31-weeks' gestation. Babies born after 34 weeks are a heterogeneous group; some have lungs that are quite mature. There was a trend toward decreased RDS in this age group. The effectiveness of glucocorticoids in infants born before 28-weeks' gestation has been a source of controversy. Although it has been questioned whether the incidence of RDS is decreased,[25] there is benefit in terms of diminished severity of RDS, decreased mortality, and a lower incidence of intraventricular hemorrhage.

The U.S. Collaborative Antenatal Steroid Therapy trial[10] found that male fetuses were not responsive to glucocorticoid therapy. However, this finding has not been borne out in other studies, and meta-analysis reveals that there is a significant decrease in RDS in both male and female infants.

Effect of Prenatal Glucocorticoids on Complications Associated With Premature Birth

According to the results of meta-analysis, as set out in Figure 105-2, prenatal glucocorticoid therapy results in decreased early neonatal mortality as well as a reduction in two major complications of prematurity, intraventricular hemorrhage (IVH), and necrotizing enterocolitis (NEC). The observational database did not support the decrease in NEC, but it did find a decreased incidence of IVH, even in infants born less than 24 hours after the first dose of steroid. The diminution in these two complications of prematurity may relate to the fact that steroid-treated babies have a more benign clinical course, but there may also be specific maturational effects of glucocorticoids on the gut and brain. The intestine, like the lung, arises from the embryonic endodermal tube, and in animals glucocorticoids induce specific enzymes in the developing gut and cause precocious maturation of closure (restricted passage of intact proteins).[3]

When glucocorticoid therapy for the prevention of RDS was first proposed, there were major concerns regarding potential toxicity, particularly to the developing brain. Studies in newborn rats, with brains that are at approximately the same stage of development as a third trimester human, had shown that administration of large doses of glucocorticoid results in a reduction in brain cell number, particularly in the cerebellum, where cells are undergoing rapid mitosis. The doses and relative exposure time in these animal studies, however, far exceeded those used in the clinical trials. Long-term follow-up studies of infants exposed to prenatal glucocorticoids have revealed no adverse effects on developmental outcome. At 12 years of age, there are no deficits in motor skills, language, cognition, memory, or scholastic achievement despite greater survival of smaller infants in the steroid-treated group.[26, 27] In fact, meta-analysis of three published studies reveals a trend toward decreased neurologic abnormalities at follow-up. There also appear to be no adverse effects on physical growth or health. These studies did not involve repeated weekly courses of glucocorticoids. As discussed later in this chapter, major concerns exist about fetal toxicity when repeated courses of steroids are administered to pregnant women.

Effects of Prenatal Glucocorticoids on Neonatal and Maternal Infection

One area of concern in glucocorticoid therapy is its impact on infection. Meta-analysis indicates that there is a small increase in maternal infection (odds ratio [OR], 1.15) and a slight reduction in neonatal infection (OR, 0.80), but neither of these effects is statistically significant. When steroids are administered in the

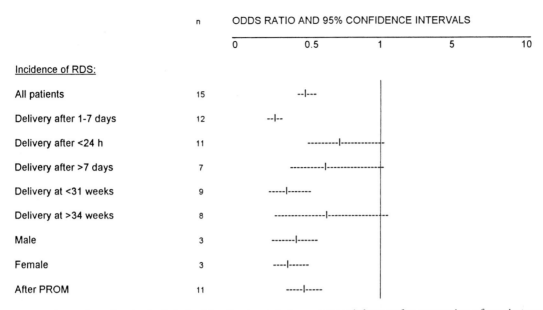

Figure 105–1. Meta-analysis of randomized clinical trials of antenatal glucocorticoid therapy for prevention of respiratory distress syndrome. A significant reduction in the incidence of respiratory distress syndrome is indicated if the mean and 95% confidence interval are below 1.0. (*n* = number of trials evaluated.) (Data from ref. 24.)

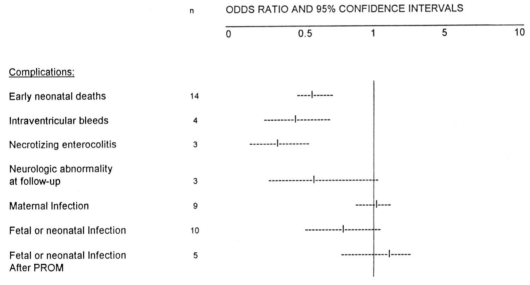

Figure 105–2. Meta-analysis of clinical trials of prenatal glucocorticoids—effects on perinatal complications. Therapy is associated with a significant reduction in deaths, intraventricular hemorrhage, and necrotizing enterocollitis. (n = number of trials evaluated.) (Data from ref. 24.)

presence of premature rupture of the membranes (PROM), there is a trend toward an increase in fetal and neonatal infection (OR, 1.46), but this effect is also not statistically significant.

Effects of Prenatal Glucocorticoids in the Presence of Premature Rupture of the Membranes

Although the risk of fetal or neonatal infection may be somewhat increased, analysis of the randomized trials reveals that glucocorticoids decrease the incidence of RDS in the presence of PROM. Evidence from the observational database indicates that glucocorticoid therapy in patients with PROM results in a decrease in intraventricular hemorrhage and overall mortality. Thus, the overall maternal-infant benefit:risk ratio for steroid therapy is also favorable with PROM .

Use of Glucocorticoids in Complicated Pregnancies

Liggins and Howie[21] reported that fetal mortality increased when steroids were administered to women with hypertension and proteinuria. However, this observation was not confirmed in two subsequent trials, and apparently Liggins and Howie's results arose from mismatched groups in terms of severity of preeclampsia.[10, 28]

Glucocorticoid administration may complicate the management of diabetes in pregnancy and the decision to use steroids in this situation is a matter of clinical judgment.

There is little information on the effectiveness of glucocorticoid therapy in pregnancies complicated by multiple gestation, intrauterine growth retardation, or hydrops fetalis. In these circumstances, fetuses should probably receive routine steroid therapy.

Recommendations of the 1994 NIH Consensus Conference

Prenatal glucocorticoid therapy clearly has several significant benefits for the premature infant. These are summarized in Table 105-2. The recommendations of the 1994 NIH Consensus Conference are listed in Table 105-3. These recommendations were drafted after review and discussion of the relevant data and provide authoritative guidelines. With the publication and dissemination of these guidelines, there appears to be no reason to withhold steroid therapy in patients who meet the recommended criteria.

Since the 1994 NIH Consensus Conference, attention has focused on the question of dexamethasone-specific toxicity, the impact of repeated courses of prenatal glucocorticoids and the effects of combinations of hormones. A review of these topics follows.

REPEATED COURSES OF PRENATAL GLUCOCORTICOIDS

Results of both experimental[12] and clinical studies (see Fig. 105-1) suggest that some of the effects of prenatal glucocorticoids on fetal lung development diminish after about a week. A question has arisen about what to do if a pregnant mother is given a course of steroids because she is at risk for premature delivery, but the pregnancy then continues without such deliv-

---

TABLE 105-2

Benefits of Antenatal Glucocorticoid Therapy

From meta-analysis of published studies:

Decreased respiratory distress syndrome
Decreased incidence of intraventricular hemorrhage
Decreased incidence of necrotizing enterocolitis
Decreased mortality
A trend toward better neurologic and intellectual function at
  follow-up

From observational database:

Decreased respiratory distress syndrome
Decreased incidence of intraventricular hemorrhage, even if delivery
  occurs less than 24 hours after initiation of therapy
Decreased mortality

From individual studies:

Decreased incidence of clinically significant patent ductus arterious
Decreased duration (and cost) of hospitalization

TABLE 105-3

Summary of Recommendations of the National Institutes of Health NIH Consensus Development Conference: The Effect of Corticosteroids for Fetal Maturation on Perinatal Outcomes

All fetuses between 24 and 34 weeks' gestation that are at risk for
  preterm delivery are candidates for treatment.
The decision should not be altered by fetal race, gender, or availability
  of surfactant therapy.
Prenatal corticosteroids should be given unless immediate delivery is
  anticipated.
Tocolytic therapy is not a contraindication.
In the absence of clinical chorioamnionitis, antenatal corticosteroids
  are recommended in patients with premature rupture of membranes
  at less than 32 weeks' gestation
Treatment is recommended in complicated pregnancies, unless
  evidence suggests that it will have an adverse effect on the mother.

(*Note:* Although the Consensus Conference recommended either dexamethasone or betamethasone, the currently recommended regimen is betamethasone, 12 mg q 24 h × 2 doses intramuscularly)

---

ery having occurred. It was the practice of some obstetricians to give repeated, even weekly, courses of steroid in this situation until the pregnancy progressed beyond the stage where the infant would have been born prematurely.

Animal studies in various species have shown that multiple courses of prenatal glucocorticoids do result in greater enhancement of lung maturation than a single course, but that there is also associated toxicity, particularly growth retardation.[29] A retrospective analysis of the data derived from a multicenter randomized clinical trial of prenatal TRH plus glucocorticoid compared with glucocorticoid alone (both dexamethasone and betamethasone were used) has provided relevant clinical information.[30, 31] This analysis revealed that compared with infants who received one course of glucocorticoid, those who were exposed to two courses had lower birth weights, and administration of three courses was associated with increased risk of death and evidence of adrenal suppression. The increased infant mortality was not explained by maternal factors or the occurrence of other preterm morbidities, but was associated with early severe lung disease that may reflect, in part, glucocorticoid-induced lung hypoplasia. Furthermore, administration of two or three courses did not result in improved outcome in terms of RDS, IVH, or chronic lung disease. These findings are consistent with preliminary reports of decreased head circumference and delayed psychomotor development associated with exposure to multiple courses of prenatal glucocorticoids. Furthermore, a recent clinical trial in which pregnant women were randomized to receive either a single course or weekly courses of prenatal glucocorticoid treatment found that there was no significant difference in outcome (defined as occurrence of death, RDS, chronic lung disease, severe IVH, periventricular leukomalacia [PVL], NEC, or proven sepsis.)[14] Investigators in other trials are currently examining different regimens of repeated prenatal hormone treatment.

An NIH Consensus Conference in 2000[32] revisited the issue of prenatal steroids and recommended that repeat courses should not be used routinely. Given the current state of knowledge in this area, we recommend that an initial course of prenatal betamethasone should be administered if there is concern that premature delivery will occur. If the pregnancy continues, one additional course of betamethasone may be considered if threatened premature delivery recurs 10 or more days later.

DEXAMETHASONE-SPECIFIC TOXICITY

Prenatal dexamethasone therapy was found, in one study, to result in a higher incidence of PVL than prenatal betamethasone. In a retrospective analysis, Baud and colleagues[33] examined the effects of dexamethasone, betamethasone, or no prenatal steroid therapy on the incidence of RDS, IVH, PVL, and NEC. Administration of either of the two glucocorticoids resulted in a decrease in all these complications of prematurity, except PVL. Although betamethasone-treated infants produced fewer cases of PVL than infants who were treated with nonsteroidal agents, those who had been exposed to prenatal dexamethasone produced more. It was suggested that the sulfites in dexamethasone were responsible for this effect and *in vitro* studies support this possibility.[34] However, sulfites are present in many medications that are routinely given to neonates. An alternative explanation relates to the method of administration of these two glucocorticoids. Dexamethasone is usually given intravenously, whereas betamethasone is administered intramuscularly as a slowly released mixture of phosphate and acetate forms. The higher peak blood levels of dexamethasone may be responsible for the toxicity, perhaps mediated by a mechanism that does not involve receptor binding to DNA.[35]

The apparent increased CNS-related risk associated with prenatal dexamethasone therapy is also supported by recent follow-up observations related to postnatal use of this cortico-steroid. Treatment of infants using dexamethasone to prevent bronchopulmonary disease, particularly in the first few days after birth, is associated with increased cerebral palsy and other abnormal neuromotor outcomes. This adverse effect of postnatal dexamethasone likely reflects the relatively high dosage used, intravenous administration, delayed clearance due to liver imma-turity, and prolonged treatment regimens.

SYNERGISM BETWEEN PRENATAL GLUCOCORTICOID AND POSTNATAL SURFACTANT THERAPIES

Several animal studies have demonstrated the benefit of prenatal glucocorticoid combined with postnatal surfactant therapy. Work by Fiascone and colleagues[36] and Ikegami and co-workers,[37] in which prematurely delivered fetal rabbits were ventilated and lung compliance was measured, found that both prenatal glucocorticoid treatment and postnatal natural surfac-tant treatment resulted in a significant improvement in lung compliance. However, the combination of steroid and surfactant produced a greater effect than did either therapy alone. These results are consistent with the observations that glucocorticoids increase nonsurfactant components of lung compliance, such as tissue elasticity, in addition to enhancing surfactant production. Glucocorticoids also accelerate the development of lung parenchymal structure, decreasing mesenchymal volume and septal thickness, and these changes themselves can increase tissue compliance.[37, 38] It is also possible that the enhanced alve-olarization resulting from glucocorticoid treatment provides a better substrate for surfactant therapy.

Clinical data also support the positive interaction between prenatal glucocorticoid and postnatal surfactant therapy. Kari and associates[39] randomized patients with threatened preterm delivery, at less than 32-weeks' gestation, to prenatal glucocorti-coid therapy or placebo. All babies born before 33 weeks who required ventilation with greater than 40% oxygen also received postnatal surfactant. As shown in Table 105–4, the infants who were exposed to prenatal steroids had significantly less respira-tory disease, as well as a lower incidence of IVH and PVL.

COMBINED HORMONAL TREATMENT FOR THE PREVENTION OF RESPIRATORY DISTRESS SYNDROME

Even with optimal glucocorticoid treatment, some infants develop RDS. In an effort to enhance lung maturation, the effects of combinations of hormones have been studied in experimen-tal models.[16-18] There is evidence that thyroid hormones stimu-late lung development and may act synergistically with

TABLE 105-4

Prenatal Glucocorticoid Effects in the Era of Postnatal Surfactant Therapy

	Dexamethasone (n = 41)	Placebo (n = 38)
Gestational age (wk)	29.9 + 2.0	29.8 + 2.3
Respiratory distress syndrome —incidence	44%	79%*
Received surfactant	22%	53%*
Days ventilated	2.0	5.3*
Days in oxygen	2.0	7.0*
Intraventricular hemorrhage or periventricular leukomalacia	10%	46%*

* $p < 0.05$.
Infants born 1 to 14 days after glucocorticoid treatment were analyzed.
(Data from ref. 39.)

glucocorticoid. Triiodothyronine is the most active thyroid hormone in terms of surfactant phospholipid production, but it does not cross the placenta well, whereas TRH administered to the mother is transferred to the fetus and increases TSH, tri-iodothyronine, and thyroxine levels in cord blood.[40-42] The com-bination of glucocorticoid and TRH has been evaluated in a number of randomized clinical trials.

A series of trials was completed before widespread availability of surfactant. These studies generally found that there was a decreased incidence of RDS, chronic lung disease, and mortality in babies who delivered from 1 to 10 days after the initiation of maternal therapy with TRH and glucocorticoid compared with glucocorticoid alone.[43] However, three large trials that also incor-porated postnatal surfactant therapy were subsequently pub-lished.[44-46] These trials, which included an "intention to treat" analysis, all indicated that there was no additional benefit when TRH was added to glucocorticoid therapy. Collectively, these findings suggest that a combination of prenatal glucocorticoid and postnatal surfactant is an effective therapy, which is not enhanced by the addition of TRH.[47]

Surfactant therapy is, unfortunately, not routinely available to infants in some parts of the world due to its cost. In situations in which surfactant is not available, there may still be a role for pre-natal TRH plus glucocorticoid therapy.[47]

CONCLUSIONS

Development of the fetal lung is influenced by a number of hor-mones and agents that either accelerate or inhibit differentiation. Endogenous and administered corticosteroids modulate the developmental process, acting through glucocorticoid receptors to induce a network of gene products involved in cellular differ-entiation and production of surfactant. Animal and clinical data demonstrate that the advent of surfactant therapy has further enhanced the benefits of prenatal glucocorticoid administration for lung maturation. Optimal management of premature infants currently consists of prenatal hormone administration followed by postnatal surfactant therapy, if indicated. Betamethasone is the glucocorticoid of choice. The 2000 NIH Consensus Conference[32] recommended that repeat courses should not be used routinely. One or possibly two courses of betamethasone should be given if a pregnancy is complicated by threatened pre-mature labor. This approach has had a significant impact on the prevention or amelioration of RDS and other major complica-tions in prematurely born infants.

REFERENCES

1. Kresch MJ, Gross I: The biochemistry of fetal lung surfactant. Clin Perinatol *14*:481, 1987.
2. Ballard PL: Hormonal regulation of pulmonary surfactant. Endocr Rev *10*:165, 1989.
3. Ballard PL, Ballard RA: Scientific basis and therapeutic regimens for use of ante-natal glucocorticoids. Am J Obstet Gynecol *173*:254, 1995.
4. Muglia L, et al: Corticotropin-releasing hormone deficiency reveals major fetal but not adult glucocorticoid need. Nature *373*:427, 1995.
5. Cole TJ, et al: GRKO mice express an aberrant dexamethasone-binding gluco-corticoid receptor, but are profoundly glucocorticoid resistant Mol Cell Endocrinol *173*:193, 2001.
6. Venkatesh VC, Ballard PL: Glucocorticoids and gene expression. Am J Respir Cell Mol Biol *4*:301, 1991.
7. Odom MW, et al: Hormonally regulated proteins in cultured human fetal lung: analysis by two-dimensional polyacrylamide gel electrophoresis. Am J Physiol *259*:L283, 1990.
8. Ballard PL: The glucocorticoid domain in the lung and mechanisms of action. *In* Mendelson CR (ed): Endocrinology of the Lung: Development and Surfactant Synthesis. Totowa NJ, Humana Press, 2000, p 1.
9. Ikegami M: Minimum interval from fetal betamethasone treatment to postnatal lung responses in preterm lambs. Am J Obstet Gynecol *174*:1408, 1996.
10. Collaborative Group on Antenatal Steroid Therapy: Effects of antenatal dexa-methasone administration on the prevention of respiratory distress syndrome. Am J Obstet Gynecol *141*:276, 1981.

11. Liggins GC: The prevention of RDS by maternal betamethasone administration. *In* 70th Ross Conference Report. Lung Maturation and the Prevention of Hyaline Membrane Disease. Columbus, OH, Ross Laboratories, 1976, p. 1989.
12. Liley HG, et al: Regulation of messenger RNAs for the hydrophobic surfactant proteins in human lung. J Clin Invest *83*:1191, 1989.
13. Tan RC, et al: Developmental and glucocorticoid regulation of surfactant protein mRNAs in preterm lambs. Am J Physiol. *277*:L1142, 1999.
14. Guinn DA, et al: Single vs. weekly courses of antenatal corticosteroids for women at risk of preterm delivery: a randomized controlled trial. JAMA *286*:1581, 2001.
15. Adcock IM, Caramori G: Cross-talk between pro-inflammatory transcription factors and glucocorticoids. Immunol Cell Biol *79*:376, 2001.
16. Gross I, et al: Glucocorticoid-thyroid hormone interactions in fetal rat lung. Pediatr Res *18*:191, 1984.
17. Gonzales LW, et al: Glucocorticoids and thyroid hormones stimulate biochemical and morphological differentiation of human fetal lung in organ culture. J Clin Endocrinol Metab *62*:678, 1986.
18. Liggins GC, et al: Synergism of cortisol and thyrotropin-releasing hormone in lung maturation in fetal sheep. J Appl Physiol *65*:1880, 1988.
19. Gonzales LK, Ballard PL: Identification and characterization of nuclear T3-binding sites in fetal human lung. J Clin Endocrinol Metab *53*:21, 1981.
20. Romaguera J, et al: Responsiveness of L-S ratio of the amniotic fluid to intra-amniotic administration of thyroxine. Am Obstet Gynecol Scand *69*:519, 1990.
21. Liggins GC, Howie RN: A controlled trial of antepartum glucocorticoid treatment for prevention of the respiratory distress syndrome. Pediatrics *50*:515, 1972.
22. Consensus Development Conference on the Effect of Corticosteroids for Fetal Maturation on Perinatal Outcomes. National Institutes of Health. JAMA *273*:413, 1995.
23. Crowley P: Promoting pulmonary maturity. *In* Chalmers IM, Keirse MJNC (eds): Effective Care in Pregnancy. Vol 1. Oxford, UK, Oxford University Press, 1989, p. 746.
24. Crowley P: Antenatal corticosteroid therapy: a meta-analysis of the randomized trials, 1972 to 1994. Am J Obstet Gynecol *173*:322, 1995.
25. Garite TJ, et al: A randomized, placebo controlled trial of betamethasone for the prevention of respiratory distress syndrome at 24 to 28 weeks' gestation. Am J Obstet Gynecol *166*:646, 1992.
26. Smolders-de Haas H, et al: Physical development and medical history of children who were treated antenatally with corticosteroids to prevent respiratory distress syndrome: a 10 to 12 year follow-up. Pediatrics *86*:65, 1990.
27. Schmand B, et al: Psychological development of children who were treated antenatally with corticosteroids to prevent respiratory distress syndrome. Pediatrics *86*:58, 1990.
28. Gamsu HR, et al: Antenatal administration of betamethasone to prevent respiratory distress syndrome in preterm infants: report of a UK multicentre trial. Br J Obstet Gynaecol *96*:401, 1989.
29. Ikegami M, et al: Repetitive prenatal glucocorticoids improve lung function and decrease growth in preterm lambs. Am J Respir Crit Care Med *156*:178, 1997.
30. Banks BA, Cnaan A, Morgan M, et al: Multiple courses of antenatal corticoids and outcome of premature neonates. Am J Ob Gynecol *181*:709, 1999.
31. Banks BA, et al: Multiple courses of antenatal corticosteroids are associated with early severe lung disease in preterm neonates. J Perinatol *22*:101, 2002.
32. Antenatal Corticosteroids revisited: Repeat courses. NIH Consensus Statement Online *17*:2, 2000. Accessed August 17-18, 2000.
33. Baud O, et al: Antenatal glucocorticoid treatment and cystic periventricular leucomalacia in very premature infants. N Engl J Med *341*:1190, 1999.
34. Baud O, et al: Neurotoxic effects of fluorinated glucocorticoid preparations on the developing mouse brain: role of preservatives. Pediatr Res *50*:706, 2001.
35. Thebaud B, et al: Postnatal glucocorticoids in very preterm infants: "The good, the bad and the ugly"? Pediatrics. *107*:413, 2001.
36. Fiascone JM, et al: Betamethasone increases pulmonary compliance in part by surfactant independent mechanisms in preterm rabbits. Pediatr Res *22*:730, 1987.
37. Ikegami M, et al: Corticosteroids and surfactant change lung function and protein leaks in the lungs of ventilated premature rabbits. J Clin Invest *79*:1371, 1987.
38. Schellenberg JC, Liggins GC: Growth, elastin concentration and collagen concentration of perinatal rat lung: effects of dexamethasone. Pediatr Res *21*:603, 1987.
39. Kari MA, et al: Prenatal dexamethasone treatment in conjunction with human surfactant therapy—a randomized placebo-controlled multicenter study. Pediatrics *93*:730, 1994.
40. Roti E, et al: Human cord blood concentrations of thyrotropin, thyroglobulin, and iodothyronines after maternal administration of thyrotropin-releasing hormone. J Clin Endocrinol Metab *53*:813, 1981.
41. Moya F, et al: Effect of maternal administration of thyrotropin releasing hormone on the preterm fetal pituitary-thyroid axis. J Pediatr *119*:966, 1991.
42. Ballard PL, Ballard RA, Creasy RK, et al: Plasma thyroid hormones and prolactin in premature infants and their mothers after prenatal treatment with thyrotropin-releasing hormone. Pediatr Res. *32*:673, 1992.
43. Moya FR, Gross I: Combined hormonal therapy for the prevention of respiratory distress syndrome and its consequences. Sem Perinatol. *17*:267, 1993.
44. Ballard RA, et al: Antenatal thyrotropin-releasing hormone to prevent lung disease in preterm infants. N Engl J Med *338*:493, 1998.
45. Collaborative Santiago Surfactant Group: Collaborative trial of prenatal thyrotropin-releasing hormone and corticosteroids for prevention of respiratory distress syndrome. Am J Obstet Gynecol *178*:33, 1998.
46. Alfirevic Z, et al: Two concurrent randomised trials of antenatal thyrotropin-releasing hormone for fetal maturation: stopping before the due date. Br J Obstet Gynecol 106:898, 1999.
47. Gross I. and Moya FR: Is there a role for antenatal TRH in the prevention of neonatal respiratory disorders. Semin Perinatol 25:406, 2001.

106

Alan H. Jobe

Surfactant Treatment

A brief history of the development of surfactant for the treatment of respiratory distress syndrome (RDS) provides perspective on how this major therapeutic advance occurred. In 1959, not long after surfactant had been identified as critical to maintaining lung inflation at low transpulmonary pressures,[1,2] Avery and Mead[3] reported that saline extracts from the lungs of preterm infants with RDS lacked the low surface tensions characteristic of pulmonary surfactant. After unsuccessful attempts to treat infants with RDS with aerosolized phospholipids,[4] intratracheal administration of surfactant recovered from the air spaces of mature animal lungs was found to improve lung expansion and ventilation in preterm animals.[5,6] The clinical potential of surfactant treatment for RDS was demonstrated by Fujiwara and colleagues[7] in a nonrandomized study in 1980, using a surfactant prepared from an organic solvent extract of bovine lung (surfactant TA). Small, investigator-initiated, randomized, controlled trials testing surfactants prepared from bovine alveolar lavage or human amniotic fluid demonstrated significant decreases in pneumothorax and death by 1985.[8-10] Subsequent

multicenter trials demonstrated decreased death rates and complications of RDS,[11] and wide, although still investigational, use of surfactant for RDS began in 1989. A synthetic surfactant was approved for the treatment of the syndrome in the United States in 1990, and surfactant from bovine lung was approved in 1991. These surfactants represented a new class of drug developed specifically for preterm infants. Subsequently, synthetic surfactants that contain no protein were found to be less effective than surfactants isolated from animals lungs.[12,13] Current research is focused on the optimal timing of surfactant treatments using surfactants from animal lungs and on the development of synthetic surfactants that contain recombinant surfactant proteins.

SURFACTANTS FOR CLINICAL USE

Surfactants for clinical use were developed empirically by testing surface properties of mixtures of lipids and proteins with the goal to emulate the properties of natural surfactant.[14] Although dipalmitoyl phosphatidylcholine is the principal surface active component of surfactant, it is not an effective surfactant because it is a solid at 37°C and does not spread or adsorb to a surface.[15] If spread from an organic solvent, dipalmitoyl phosphatidylcholine forms a stable film with an equilibrium surface tension similar to that of natural surfactant. On surface compression, values approaching 0 dynes/cm can be achieved. However, surface tensions increase to high values with surface expansion because of the insolubility of dipalmitoyl phosphatidylcholine. Surface adsorption can be enhanced by adding other components, such as dioleoyl phosphatidylcholine, phosphatidylglycerol, or cholesterol. Simple mixtures of dipalmitoyl phosphatidylcholine with other lipids can have surface properties similar to those of a natural surfactant.[16]

Two synthetic surfactants were extensively evaluated in clinical trials and were in clinical use until about the year 2000. A 7:3 weight ratio of dipalmitoyl phosphatidylcholine and unsaturated phosphatidylglycerol (ALEC) was used in England.[17] This surfactant is similar to the prototype mixtures found *in vitro* to have reasonable adsorption properties because of the fluidization of the dipalmitoyl phosphatidylcholine provided by the unsaturated phosphatidylglycerol.[15] The other synthetic surfactant to be used clinically was Exosurf, a mixture of dipalmitoyl phosphatidylcholine, hexadecanol, and tyloxapol. Synthetic surfactants were not as effective as surfactants and are no longer widely used clinically.[13]

Highly surface active surfactants could be recovered from animal lungs, and these surfactants were effective replacement agents in preterm surfactant-deficient lungs, demonstrating that formulations for clinical use could come from animal sources.[18] The surfactants from natural sources are of two general types: surfactants recovered from alveolar lavages and surfactants recovered from minced lungs. The surfactant first used clinically by Fujiwara and colleagues[7] was prepared by saline extraction of minced lungs. The saline extract was then further extracted with organic solvents to yield phospholipids, neutral lipids, and small amounts of the hydrophobic surfactant proteins SP-B and SP-C. This lipid extract contains all the components of natural surfactant except SP-A, but it has increased amounts of unsaturated phospholipids and neutral lipids that interfere with its surface properties. Synthetic lipids were added to improve surface properties and the effects on surfactant-deficient lungs.[14] This surfactant, initially named surfactant TA and subsequently called Surfacten (Japan) or Survanta (elsewhere) was developed using the strategy to "fortify" a lung extract to approximate natural surfactant. Another surfactant made from lung minces (Curosurf)

was developed using the opposite strategy of removal of the components that interfere with function from the lipid extract by liquid-gel chromatography.[19] Curosurf contains 99% polar lipids, mainly phospholipids, and 1% SP-B plus SP-C, with the neutral lipids removed by the chromatography step.

Another approach to making an animal source surfactant is to recover surfactant from alveolar lavages and prepare organic solvent extracts of that material. Surfactant from lavages can be recovered by relatively simple techniques, and highly effective surfactants can be prepared from the organic solvent extract. A surfactant called Infasurf that is made from lavage from calf lungs has been extensively tested in the United States.[20] Another lavage-derived surfactant called Alveofact is in use in Europe. The organic solvent extraction step is essential to confer sterility and to remove nonessential proteins that might be sensitizing. Other surfactants are being made in other regions of the world.

PHYSIOLOGIC EFFECTS OF SURFACTANT TREATMENT ON PRESSURE-VOLUME CURVES

The pressure-volume curve is used to assess the static effects of surfactant on the lung because it encapsulates the essence of the physiologic effects of surfactant on the preterm lung (Fig. 106–1).[21] When comparing control animals with natural surfactant-treated animals, surfactant decreases the *opening pressure*, defined as the pressure at which the lung begins to fill above dead space volume. The opening pressure of preterm surfactant-deficient rabbit lungs decreased from about 20 to 15 cm H_2O with sheep surfactant in this example. The explanation for this effect is that the surfactant-deficient immature lung resists inflation because of the high surface tensions at the interfaces of gas and fluid in small airways. If surfactant is added, the resistance to fluid movement in small airways drops and expansion of lung units is facilitated. The major effect of natural surfactant treatment is the 2.5-fold increase in lung volume at 30 cm H_2O. Because dead space volume should not change with surfactant treatment, this increase in volume represents the recruitment of 2.5-fold more surface area for gas exchange. The definition of maximal lung volumes (V_{max}) in preterm lungs is dictated by the characteristics of the preterm lamb. In the mature lung, V_{max} can be defined by the limits of expansion of the lung matrix. In contrast, in the preterm the lung continues to expand linearly with increasing pressure until rupture occurs.[22] The result is that the potential gas volume of the preterm lung cannot be achieved because inflation pressures needed to recruit the volume exceed

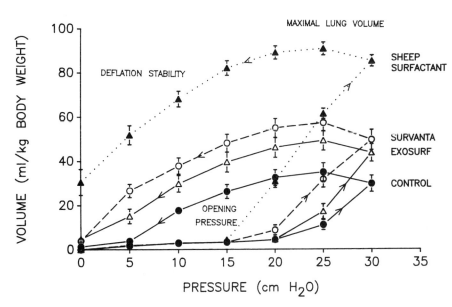

Figure 106–1. Pressure-volume curves for 27-day preterm rabbit lungs treated with three surfactants in comparison to control lungs. The curves were measured after a 30-minute period of ventilation. Sheep surfactant has more pronounced effects on opening pressure, maximal lung volumes, and deflation stability than do the surfactants used clinically. (Data from Rider ED, et al: J Appl Physiol *73*:2089, 1992. Figure republished from Jobe AH: N Engl J Med *328*:851, 1993. Copyright 1993, Massachusetts Medical Society. All rights reserved.)

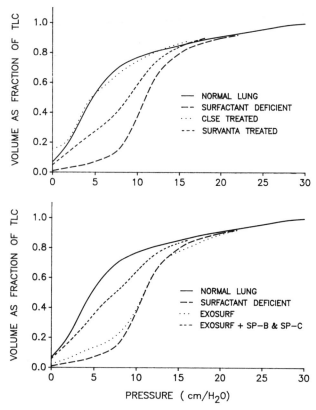

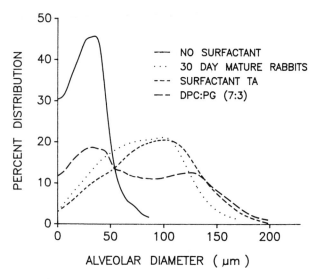

Figure 106–3. Alveolar size distributions for 30-day gestation mature rabbits, 27-day preterm rabbits receiving no surfactant, and preterm rabbits treated with surfactant TA and a dipalmitoyl phosphatidylcholine:phosphatidylglycerol synthetic surfactant (DPG:PG). The lungs were immersed in formalin at a deflation pressure of 10 cm H_2O for fixation before the measurements were made. (From Fujiwara T: Surfactant replacement in neonatal respiratory distress syndrome. *In* Robertson B, et al [eds]: Pulmonary Surfactant. Amsterdam, Elsevier Science Publishers, 1984, pp 480–503.)

Figure 106–2. Deflation limbs of pressure-volume curves for rat lungs normalized as a fraction of total lung capacity (TLC) measured at 30 cm H_2O. The curves in the upper frame are for normal rat lungs, rat lungs made surfactant deficient by saline lavage, and the subsequent improvement in deflation stability for the lavaged lungs treated with Survanta and an extract of calf lung lavage (CLSE). The lower frame shows the improvement of the deflation curve of surfactant-depleted lungs when SP-B and SP-C were added to Exosurf. (From Hall SB, et al: Am Rev Respir Dis *145*:24, 1992.)

rupture pressures. Surfactant also stabilizes the lung during deflation and maintains a lung volume at 5 cm H_2O pressure in excess of the V_{max} achieved in control animals at 30 cm H_2O. Surfactants used clinically improved the static pressure-volume curves relative to control lungs; however, the effects on opening pressures, maximal volumes, and volumes on deflation were less striking than with the natural surfactant.[21]

Normal mature surfactant-sufficient lungs can be made surfactant deficient by repetitive lavage and then used to test surfactant.[23] Surfactant effects are measured as the restoration of the maximal lung volume and the improvement in deflation stability of the lungs. An organic solvent extracted calf lavage surfactant (CLSE) completely restored deflation stability to lavaged rat lungs, whereas partial effects were noted with Survanta (Fig. 106–2). Addition of the surfactant proteins SP-B and SP-C to Exosurf improved deflation lung volumes, illustrating the importance of the surfactant proteins for surfactant function.

Evaluation of degree and uniformity of inflation is another way to assess surfactant effects on the lung. Based on the simplest model of alveoli as two interconnecting spheres, surfactant deficiency will cause alveolar (or small airway) instability characterized by collapse of units with small radii and dilation of units with large radii. This instability results from Laplace's law: pressure at the surface of an alveolus = 2 × surface tension/radius. Because the alveolus is open to atmospheric pressure, the pres-

sure outside must be balanced by the pressure on the inner surface or the alveolus will collapse. The forces acting on the alveolus are chest wall elasticity, lung tissue elasticity, and surface tensions at the alveolar surface. All alveoli are not the same size. Therefore, Laplace's law predicts that the retractive force of surface tension will be greater on the small alveoli than on the large alveoli, with the result being collapse of the small alveoli with further filling of the large alveoli. Surfactant, however, has the unique property of variable surface tension depending on the rate and amount of surface area compression. As alveolar radius decreases, surface tension falls, preventing collapse of the small alveolus. This stabilizing influence is lost in the absence of surfactant.

The scaling up of the alveolar model results in the concept of interdependence, in which each alveolus depends on the normal position and elasticity of the neighboring alveolar walls to maintain normal shape and volume. If adjacent alveoli collapse, the alveolus either tends to overexpand and distort or to collapse. In surfactant-deficient states, the more normal alveoli tend to overexpand as other regional alveoli collapse, generating a nonhomogeneously inflated lung. The interdependence relationships are disrupted by surfactant deficiency. Surfactant treatment improves uniformity of inflation, minimizing the small airway dilation and promoting alveolar inflation. Fujiwara[14] demonstrated that surfactant treatment of 27-day preterm rabbits resulted in a distribution of alveolar sizes comparable to those of term rabbits (Fig. 106–3). Surfactant treatment resulted in more normal lung as evaluated morphometrically 24 hours after delivery in preterm lambs receiving continuous mechanical ventilation.[24] The alveoli of the lambs not treated with surfactant were shallow, and alveolar ducts were dilated. Most of these abnormalities were prevented with surfactant treatment (Fig. 106–4). This effect on uniformity of lung expansion may be essential for decreasing lung injury with surfactant treatment.

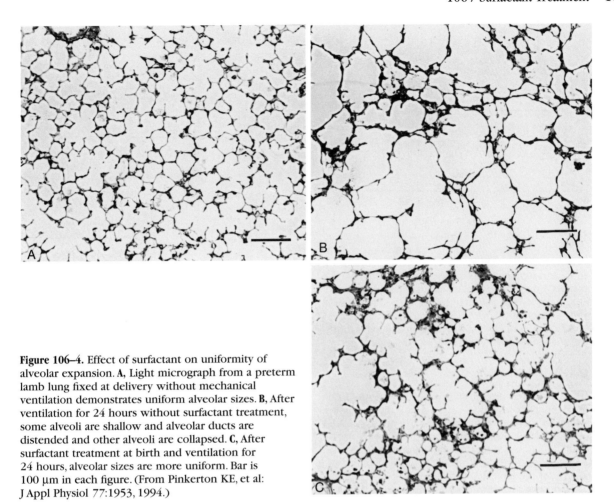

Figure 106–4. Effect of surfactant on uniformity of alveolar expansion. **A,** Light micrograph from a preterm lamb lung fixed at delivery without mechanical ventilation demonstrates uniform alveolar sizes. **B,** After ventilation for 24 hours without surfactant treatment, some alveoli are shallow and alveolar ducts are distended and other alveoli are collapsed. **C,** After surfactant treatment at birth and ventilation for 24 hours, alveolar sizes are more uniform. Bar is 100 μm in each figure. (From Pinkerton KE, et al: J Appl Physiol 77:1953, 1994.)

EFFECTS OF SURFACTANT TREATMENT ON DYNAMIC LUNG FUNCTION

If surfactant treatment were to completely normalize lung function, then functional residual capacity (FRC) should increase, the time constant for inflation should decrease, and the time constant for expiration should increase. These effects all occur to variable degrees, probably depending on factors related to the disease process in each infant, the style of ventilatory management, and the surfactant used to treat the infant. FRC in infants with RDS increased by about 150% to approach a normal value after surfactant treatment in one report.[25] In another report, FRC increased from 7.6 ml/kg to 15.4 ml/kg 1 hour after surfactant treatment.[26] The effect of surfactant treatment on FRC depends on the positive end-expiratory pressure (PEEP) used to ventilate the infant, and FRC can be too high after surfactant treatment, resulting in CO_2 retention.[27]

Compliance uniformly increased in animal models of surfactant treatment.[28] Compliance did not increase in infants soon after surfactant treatment in most clinical reports. For example, Davis and associates[29] reported no change in compliance for mechanical breaths with surfactant treatments, although spontaneous breaths after surfactant treatment demonstrated improved compliance. There are several explanations for this inconsistency. The animal models of RDS are ventilated in a standard fashion often with control of tidal volume. In clinical practice, tidal volumes were seldom measured until recently when the trend has been to decrease the tidal volumes used for mechanical ventilation. Large tidal volumes or high FRC may mask a compliance effect of surfactant treatment. Kelly and associates[30] found no improvement in dynamic compliance after treatment of infants with surfactant, and static compliance decreased as a result of lung volume recruitment. When the ventilator pressures were lowered, consistent improvements in both static and dynamic compliance occurred. Figure 106–5 illustrates what probably is occurring in many infants. Surfactant treatment increases lung volumes at both low and high transpulmonary pressures. Over a range of pressures, the curves are relatively parallel and the calculated compliance does not change with surfactant treatment. By lowering pressures, mechanical ventilation becomes more efficient and compliance improves. If peak inspiratory pressures and/or positive end-expiratory pressures are too high, compliance will decrease after surfactant treatment because the lung is overinflated.

Another variable in the compliance response is the type of surfactant used for treatment. A synthetic surfactant without surfactant proteins may not demonstrate improved compliance in the first few hours after treatment. In contrast, treatment with animal source surfactants can result in rapid improvements in compliance. These different responses between synthetic surfactants and surfactant from animal lungs have been noted in preterm animal models[31] and in clinical practice.[32] Differences in acute physiologic responses between the surfactants from animal lungs that are now used clinically are not as large, and differences in longer term outcomes have not been convincingly demonstrated.

Surfactant treatments also can have effects on the time constants for lung inflation and deflation. The stiff, atelectatic lung of the infant with RDS does not inflate easily, and deflation to low

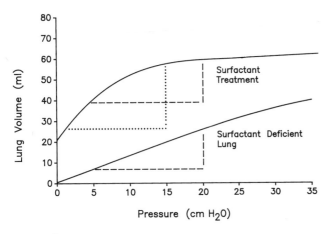

Figure 106–5. Idealized deflation limbs of static pressure-volume curves for a surfactant-deficient lung and surfactant-treated lung. The surfactant treatment has increased lung volume and deflation stability. Compliances calculated over the pressure range of 5 to 20 cm H_2O as indicated by the dashed lines are similar despite surfactant treatment. By lowering ventilatory pressures to 15 over 2 cm H_2O, however, as indicated by the dotted lines, compliance has improved with surfactant treatment.

lung volumes is rapid because the elastic recoil properties of the lungs are not counterbalanced by surfactant. With mechanical ventilation, inspiratory times and peak pressures are used empirically to adjust tidal volumes. The time constant for expiration (defined as the time required for the lung to empty two thirds of its volume calculated from the peak tidal volume to FRC) is a passive property of the lung that is not controlled by the clinician. Although measurements of expiratory time constants have not been reported for surfactant-treated infants, Curosurf treatment of preterm rabbits increased the mean expiratory time constant from 25 ± 6 milliseconds for controls to 50 ± 9 milliseconds for treated animals.[33] In other experiments using preterm rabbits, the expiratory time constant increased as the SP-B content of Survanta increased.[34] Increases in expiratory time constants in surfactant-treated infants ventilated at rapid rates could significantly increase expiratory lung volumes to the point of lung overdistention, resulting in decreased compliance and carbon dioxide retention. The combination of surfactant treatment and a ventilatory style that promotes air trapping may mask surfactant treatment effects.

OXYGENATION RESPONSE TO SURFACTANT

Although compliance may or may not improve soon after surfactant treatment, the consistent response to surfactant treatment is an improvement in oxygenation.[11] That effect occurs in preterm animals within seconds to minutes after surfactant treatment (Fig. 106–6).[28] Surfactant treatments decrease pulmonary vascular resistance in infants with RDS.[35] Although the fall in pulmonary vascular resistance may reverse the ductal shunt (from right-to-left to left-to-right) and decrease hypoxic shunt,[36] this effect is probably delayed in most clinical situations until after the initial oxygenation response has occurred.[37] The rapid improvement in oxygenation results from the acute increase in lung volume with surfactant instillation.

CLINICAL TRIALS OF SURFACTANT FOR RESPIRATORY DISTRESS SYNDROME

The use of surfactant in preterm infants is the most thoroughly studied therapy in neonatal care. The clinical trials have been

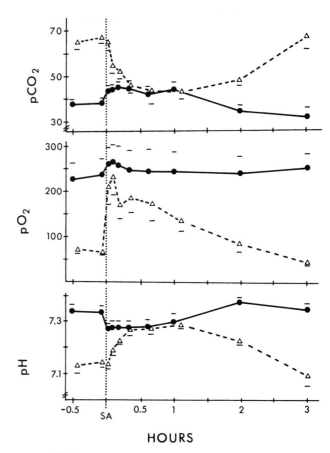

Figure 106–6. Blood gas and pH responses of very preterm lambs to treatment with 100 mg/kg natural sheep surfactant (●). Preterm lambs were delivered at about 121 days' gestation (term is 150 days) and treated either at birth (●) or after ventilation for about 30 minutes (Δ) with surfactant by tracheal instillation. Untreated lambs had P_{CO_2} values greater than 100 mm Hg and P_{O_2} values less than 50 mm Hg by 1 hour of age. Oxygenation improved very rapidly after surfactant treatment at 30 minutes of age. (Reproduced from Jobe AH, et al: J Clin Invest 67:370, 1981, by copyright permission of The American Society for Clinical Investigation.)

compiled by Soll using the technique of meta-analysis.[38] Two strategies for the use of surfactant have been evaluated: One involves treating infants at high risk of RDS in the delivery room concurrently with the initiation of breathing and resuscitation. The other involves treating infants at 2 to 24 hours of age after a diagnosis of RDS has been made. Treatment in the delivery room is referred to as *prevention* or *prophylactic treatment* because the goal is to prevent both RDS and any injury to the preterm surfactant-deficient lung that might result from mechanical ventilation. The odds ratio for death by 28 days of age was about 0.6 for either treatment strategy.[11] With surfactant treatment, the absolute decrease in death from any cause was 30 to 40%.

The major pulmonary complications of RDS are air leaks (pneumothorax and pulmonary interstitial emphysema) and the chronic lung disease of infants called *bronchopulmonary dysplasia*. Surfactant treatment results in a striking decrease in pneumothorax and other air leaks. The incidence of bronchopulmonary dysplasia was not consistently lower, although it was reduced in individual studies. A problem with the reported incidence of bronchopulmonary dysplasia is that the severity of the lung disease was not quantified. Many tiny preterm infants have a supplemental oxygenation requirement and some radiographic abnormalities at 28 days of age, but they need no oxygen

Prophylactic Surfactant Treatment Versus Control

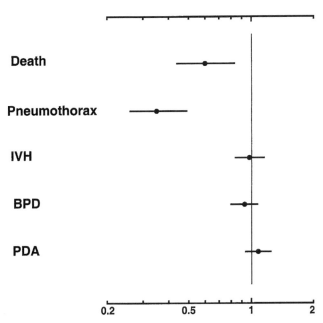

Figure 106–7. Odds ratios and 95% confidence intervals from meta-analysis of clinical trials of natural surfactant treatments given at birth for respiratory distress syndrome (RDS). (Data from Soll RF: Cochrane Library, 2003:1)

or other treatment for lung disease at discharge.[39] Another problem is that more infants treated with surfactant survive, and these survivors may have the highest risk of bronchopulmonary dysplasia. Egberts and de Winter[40] point out that the incidence of bronchopulmonary dysplasia is decreased if the calculation is based on survivors rather than on infants randomized.

An initial hope was that the improved cardiopulmonary stability and oxygenation resulting from surfactant treatment would protect preterm infants from the nonpulmonary complications of prematurity, such as patent ductus arteriosus, severe intraventricular hemorrhage, and necrotizing enterocolitis. Unfortunately, treatment has not consistently decreased the frequency of patent ductus arteriosus or severe intraventricular hemorrhage. Large decreases in intraventricular hemorrhage after surfactant treatment have been reported in individual trials (Fig. 106–7),[41] suggesting that other aspects of neonatal care may be interacting with surfactant therapy to influence the incidence of this complication. A thorough analysis of the available data on the possible association of intraventricular hemorrhage with surfactant treatment did not lead to any direct links.[42] Necrotizing enterocolitis and retinopathy of prematurity were not tabulated for the meta-analyses, but no trends were reported in the individual trials. One study found a decrease in retinopathy of prematurity in the infants treated with surfactant.[43] Infants treated with surfactant generally perform as well as or better than control infants when assessed at long-term follow-up.[44-46] After treatments with a lung source surfactant, infants needed less supplemental oxygen at 6 months and had less wheezing at 12 and 24 months of age relative to control infants.[47] In this study, less cerebral palsy also was diagnosed in surfactant-treated infants.

TIMING OF SURFACTANT TREATMENT

In the initial trials, surfactant was administered 6 to 24 hours after birth when a diagnosis of severe RDS could be made accurately. In contrast, delivery room treatment was considered to be optimal only if given before the infant breathed or received positive-pressure ventilation.[48] This delivery room strategy was based on information from surfactant treatment of preterm animals demonstrating airway epithelial damage with very short-term ventilation of the surfactant-deficient lung.[49] The two treatment strategies have been compared in eight trials using different surfactants.[50] There were no differences in the incidences of intraventricular hemorrhage, bronchopulmonary dysplasia, or patent ductus arteriosus. Delivery room treatment decreased pneumothorax, and this outcome would be expected because early treatment protected the infant from pneumothorax for the period before treatment. The important difference is a decrease in death with prophylactic surfactant relative to treatment of RDS. In the more recent trials, delivery room treatment has been delayed until after the infant has stabilized for a few minutes and the treatment of RDS has been done sooner after birth. Therefore, the two treatment strategies are approaching each other in time. Treating infants at birth has two disadvantages: (1) a number of the infants are treated unnecessarily because they would not have developed RDS, and (2) instillation of a large volume of surfactant can interfere with normal resuscitative efforts. Kendig and co-workers[48] demonstrated that surfactant treatment within the first 15 minutes after birth was equivalent and perhaps preferable to treatments before the infant is allowed to breathe. A reasonable approach is to treat most infants as soon as clinical signs of RDS appear. Waiting for the disease to progress to establish the diagnosis more firmly before beginning treatment will minimize the efficacy of the therapy and increase complications. Delivery room treatment is most appropriate for the smallest infants who are at the highest risk of RDS and should be given only by a person experienced in both neonatal resuscitation and the administration of surfactant.

REPETITION OF TREATMENT

Multiple doses of surfactant have been given in most trials because the response to an individual dose can be transient. In preterm animals, exogenously administered surfactant is not lost from the lungs,[51] but its function can be inhibited by soluble proteins and other factors in the small airways and alveoli. Multiple doses are thought to be useful because they can overcome this functional inactivation of surfactant. Multiple doses of surfactant have been compared with single-dose treatments. In one trial, second and third doses given 12 and 24 hours after an initial treatment at about 6 hours of age reduced the frequency of pneumothorax from 18% with a single dose to 9% with three doses ($p < .01$), and the death rate at 28 days decreased from 21 to 13% ($p < .05$).[52] In the other study of 75 large infants with RDS (mean birth weight, 1900 g), those who received multiple doses had better oxygenation during the first several days of life.[53] An unresolved question is whether all infants treated with surfactant would benefit from subsequent treatments. All recent trials have used re-treatments. Although most infants respond favorably to treatment, about 20% of infants thought to have RDS will have little or no response. These infants may have other diseases, such as pneumonia, pulmonary hypoplasia, or congenital heart disease. Structural immaturity of the lungs and birth asphyxia with decreased cardiovascular performance can also blunt the response to surfactant. A re-treatment because the initial response to treatment was poor is reasonable if other causes of respiratory failure have been excluded. Other infants will have such a good response that they have minimal residual lung disease. In clinical practice, re-treatment should be individualized and considered for infants with enough residual lung disease to put them at risk for complications such as pneumothorax. The major reason for re-treatment is probably to overcome inhibition of surfactant resulting from lung injury. If treatment is given early in the clinical course and a gentle approach to ventilation is used, then significant lung injury can be avoided. The dose of 100 mg/kg surfactant that is normally used is large relative to the endogenous pool in a normal lung and it is metabolized slowly.[51] Therefore, re-treatment with surfactant will not be for inadequate amounts of surfactant but for inadequate surfactant function. On average, infants with RDS receive less than two doses of surfactant.

COMPLICATIONS OF SURFACTANT TREATMENT

The complications associated with the administration of surfactant are listed in Table 106-1. This documentation of treatment complications resulted from the extensive data collection required for the Survanta Treatment Investigational New Drug program in 1990 and 1991.[54] Similar problems associated with surfactant treatments were reported by Horbar and colleagues[55] for the comparison trial of Survanta and Exosurf. The treatment procedures combine positioning of the infant, manipulation of the endotracheal tube, and instillation of suspensions of surfactant in a 3- to 5-ml/kg vehicle. The explanations for these acute physiologic effects are related to the handling of the infant and the acute effects of the surfactant on the lungs. Manipulation of the head, neck, and endotracheal tube can cause vagal responses resulting in bradycardia and cyanosis. The bolus of fluid can acutely obstruct airways leading to cyanosis, bradycardia, and carbon dioxide retention. If surfactant is rapidly distributed to the distal lung, lung compliance can improve; and if the amount of mechanical ventilation is not decreased, then increased Po_2 and decreased Pco_2 can result. Reflux of some of the material up the endotracheal tube is frequent. These acute effects of surfactant are easily dealt with by adjustments in the ventilator and probably have no long-term effect on outcome. Of more concern are the reports of transient changes in blood pressure, cerebral blood flow velocities, and electrocortical depression after surfactant treatments.[56-58] The mechanisms and importance of these effects are not known.

The only severe complication consistently associated with surfactant treatment is pulmonary hemorrhage. The overall relative risk for pulmonary hemorrhage after surfactant therapy was 1.47 (95% confidence interval 1.05 to 2.07) in the clinical trials.[59] Incidences ranged from 1 to 5% of treated infants. The presence of a patent ductus arteriosus with a left-to-right shunt resulting in elevated pulmonary vascular pressures has been linked to pulmonary hemorrhage in several trials. Although this association has not been identified in other trials, increased pulmonary vascular pressures leading to stress failure of alveolar capillaries is the likely explanation for the pulmonary hemorrhage.[60] The pulmonary hemorrhage after surfactant treatment does not often occur at the time of treatment. In general, hemorrhage occurs in the smallest infants a number of hours after a surfactant treatment

improved lung function. Pulmonary hemorrhage is frequent in autopsies of infants who have died of RDS. The association of pulmonary hemorrhage with surfactant treatment may result from the decreased death rate in tiny preterm infants receiving surfactant, which allows pulmonary hemorrhage to become apparent clinically. Surfactant treatment after pulmonary hemorrhage can improve subsequent lung function.[61] This result is consistent with the concept that pulmonary hemorrhage inactivates surfactant. Although not well documented, pulmonary hemorrhage seems to be less frequent in recent years. Perhaps changes in ventilation style toward the use of better lung inflation, lower tidal volumes, and acceptance of higher carbon dioxide levels have contributed to the decrease in pulmonary hemorrhage.

ROUTINE CLINICAL USE OF SURFACTANT

The randomized, controlled trials demonstrate that surfactant decreases death when used to treat infants with RDS. There was no assurance, however, that general clinical use would result in similar effects. Several reports of the probable effect of surfactant introduction on outcomes for preterm infants have been published. Incidences of death and other major neonatal complications were analyzed for the period before surfactant introduction (before 1989) and after general clinical availability. Horbar and colleagues[62] reported outcomes for 2870 infants weighing 601 to 1300 g before surfactant and 1413 infants after surfactant was available. Mortality decreased from 28% before surfactant to 20% after surfactant was introduced. This decreased mortality was associated with an increase in the duration of ventilation and length of hospitalization. Of perhaps more importance is the information on secondary outcomes (Fig. 106-8). Surfactant treatments were not associated with increased incidences of intraventricular hemorrhage, bronchopulmonary dysplasia, sepsis, or patent ductus arteriosus. Beneficial secondary effects were decreased necrotizing enterocolitis, air leak, and severe retinopathy of prematurity. The increase in apnea probably resulted from the survival of more small infants. This favorable clinical experience was not replicated in a compilation of data for 5629 infants weighing 500 to 1500 g from 14 centers.[63]

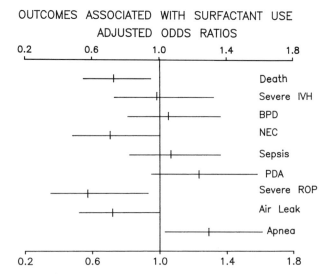

OUTCOMES ASSOCIATED WITH SURFACTANT USE
ADJUSTED ODDS RATIOS

Figure 106–8. Adjusted odds ratios for infants before and after the introduction of surfactant for the treatment of RDS. The odds ratios and 95% confidence limits are from Horbar and colleagues.[62] IVH = intraventricular hemorrhage; BPD = bronchopulmonary dysplasia; NEC = necrotizing enterocolitis; PDA = patent ductus arteriosus; ROP = retinopathy of prematurity.

TABLE 106-1

Problems Associated with Administering Surfactant: Percent of 17,641 Infants Treated*

Problem	%
Cyanosis	3.7
Bradycardia	4.2
Tachycardia	0
Increased O_2	3.3
Decreased O_2	16.6
Increased Pco_2	0.5
Decreased Pco_2	0.1
Reflux	14.6
Others	2.7
At least 1 event	30.4

* Data from reference 54.

Although death decreased by 30% after the introduction of sur-factant, intraventricular hemorrhage increased from 17 to 23% (adjusted risk ratio 1.4, with 95% confidence interval of 1.2 to 1.6). Nevertheless, the effect on death was extrapolated to result in a 5% decline in mortality nationwide and can explain 80% of the decline in infant mortality between 1989 and 1990. The use of surfactant also decreased overall costs for both survivors and the infants who died. Palta and co-workers[64] also noted a decrease in death with the introduction of surfactant and that intraventricular hemorrhage decreased, but this outcome was associated primarily with increased use of antenatal cortico-steroids. The incidence of bronchopulmonary dysplasia in-creased, perhaps because more small infants were surviving. The epidemiology is important for understanding how the introduc-tion of a new therapy affects overall outcomes.

ADMINISTRATION OF SURFACTANT

The instillation procedures used in the trials to treat RDS were selected empirically based on the techniques of treatment for preterm animal models of RDS. Surfactant can be given in the delivery room soon after delivery and intubation as a single bolus into the endotracheal tube followed by mechanical ventilation to infants at risk of developing RDS.[48] For infants with RDS, surfac-tant has been given by a variety of bolus injection schemes that include positioning the chest of the infant in an effort to opti-mize distribution. These treatment procedures were standard-ized for each clinical trial such that each surfactant in current use is given by a somewhat different technique. The essence of the treatment techniques is the instillation of surfactant into the proximal or distal trachea with positioning of the chest. The only clinical trial comparing treatment techniques found that there were no differences in short-term efficacy if the surfactant dose was divided into 2 or 4 aliquots for administration or if two or four chest positioning maneuvers were used.[65]

The goals of the treatment technique are to get the surfactant into an infant's lungs with as little physiologic disturbance as possible. This clinical treatment goal may conflict with the ulti-mate goal of an optimal pulmonary outcome. At the level of the alveolus the primary goal is to achieve as uniform a distribution of surfactant as possible. If distribution were perfectly uniform, expansion of the lung should be uniform and result in normal alveolar expansion. The physiologic result should be decreased oxygen and pressure needs and less lung injury. In contrast, if the distribution of surfactant were primarily to one lobe or one lung, that lung volume would expand if pressures were not decreased. The inflated lung would tend to overexpand and potentially be injured.[14] If the pressures were decreased, the untreated lung would lose whatever gas volume it was receiving and become more atelectatic. At the alveolar level, alveoli are interdependent in that if a group of alveoli collapse, the adjacent alveoli may overinflate and distort[24] (see Figs. 106–3 and 106–4). The fre-quent occurrence of bronchopulmonary dysplasia following sur-factant treatment may result in part from the nonhomogeneous distribution of surfactant, contributing to focal lung injury.

Most experimental studies of surfactant distribution have used radiolabeled surfactant components (primarily dipalmitoyl phos-phatidylcholine) or other easily measured substances mixed with surfactant.[66] The distribution of the material has been meas-ured by external scanning of radioactivity,[67] autoradiograms of lung slices,[68] or the content of the marked material in lung pieces of various sizes.[69] Each technique has different strengths and weaknesses, giving only partial information about surfactant distribution. In the only attempt to measure distribution in infants, Charon and colleagues[67] mixed technetium-sulfur colloid with surfactant and treated eight infants using a four-bolus, four-position treatment technique. They found relatively homoge-neous distributions in all infants that did not correlate with

clinical response. Subsequently, van der Bleek and colleagues[70] reported that microaggregated technetium-albumin mixed with surfactant appeared to be uniformly distributed by external scan-ning of the lungs of saline-lavaged rabbits. When the lungs were divided into 200 pieces and distribution per piece was meas-ured, however, the distribution was not homogeneous. Analysis of lung pieces does not provide information about alveolar dis-tribution. For example, if the preterm human lung at 32 weeks' gestational age were cut into 200 pieces for a distribution meas-urement, each piece would contain about 200,000 saccules. Therefore, even if distribution to lung pieces were homoge-neous, significant inhomogeneities may exist at the alveolar level.

VARIABLES THAT INFLUENCE SURFACTANT DISTRIBUTION

Surfactant has the biophysical properties of adsorption to an air-fluid interface and rapid spreading over a surface. Therefore, it is logical to anticipate that surfactant will facilitate its own distri-bution by this spreading behavior. Davis and associates[71] used external scanning to measure the kinetics of surfactant or saline distribution to the lungs of saline-lavaged piglets after instillation of a single 3.3-ml/kg dose. They found that surfactant began to distribute within 5 seconds of dosing, with substantial distribu-tion to the lung fields within 20 seconds. In contrast, saline did not distribute as rapidly, and multiple filling defects were noted on the scans. These results demonstrate rapid spreading of sur-factant with a more uniform ultimate distribution than for saline alone. Kharasch and colleagues[68] compared surfactant and saline as carriers to spread pentamidine in the lungs of hamsters after airway instillation of 0.25-ml/kg volumes. After 4 hours of spon-taneous ventilation, the lungs were removed and sliced and autoradiograms were used to demonstrate distribution patterns. Surfactant resulted in 40% of the lung areas being labeled versus 21% for the saline-treated animals. Therefore, surfactant facilitated its own distribution within the lungs. Oetomo and colleagues[72] treated single lobes of rabbit lungs with surfactant and found virtually no migration to other lobes after 10 hours of spontaneous ventilation. This result demonstrated that surfac-tant did not spread between bronchi. Therefore, theoretically the most uniform distribution would be achieved if each bronchus at each branching level received surfactant in proportion to the surface area that the bronchus served.

The surfactants used clinically are given as suspensions in volumes that range from 2.5 to 5 ml/kg. Intuitively, the larger the volume administered, the more likely multiple bronchi will be filled, and the better the distribution is likely to be. Large volumes, however, are much more likely to cause airway obstruc-tion, respiratory distress, cyanosis, and other undesirable side effects. Gilliard and co-workers[73] found that instillation of 1.5 ml/kg surfactant into ventilated rabbits with normal lungs resulted in a nonuniform distribution. Increasing surfactant con-centration did not improve the distribution. The same amount of surfactant suspended in 15 ml/kg resulted in a homogeneous dis-tribution. However, with lung injury, the distribution was volume independent and reasonably uniform. This result was interpreted to mean that with severe lung injury, the alveoli were flooded and provided a fluid volume to facilitate surfactant distribution. Similar observations were made in the saline-lavaged rabbit model of lung injury by van der Bleek and colleagues.[70] They found poor distributions in unlavaged and lavaged rabbits when surfactant was instilled in a volume of 2.4 ml/kg. The distribution was only marginally improved when a suspension volume of 8 ml/kg was used, and distribution improved significantly when 16 ml/kg was instilled. These results demonstrate that in an unin-jured lung a large volume is needed to achieve a good distribu-tion. The alveolar edema associated with RDS may help better distribute the surfactant. Large volumes are not realistic for clinical practice, and some nonhomogeneity of surfactant distribution is an inevitable consequence of the present treatment techniques.

If surfactant distribution can be improved by increasing the treatment volume, and the administration of large volumes over short treatment intervals results in respiratory complications, a logical approach on first impression would be to deliver surfactant to the lungs more slowly. This approach has been evaluated in two animal models of RDS. Segerer and associates[74] reported that 4 ml/kg of a surfactant suspension given as a bolus through the endotracheal tube in 10 seconds to saline-lavaged rabbits resulted in a reasonably uniform distribution. In contrast, infusion of the same volume of surfactant over 45 minutes by means of the pressure monitoring channel in an endotracheal tube resulted in an extremely nonhomogeneous distribution. Ueda and associates[75] compared the four-aliquot, four-position techniques used clinically and a two-position technique with half the dose given in the left lateral position and the other half in the right lateral position with a slow infusion in preterm lambs with RDS. The infusion-treated group received 2 ml/kg surfactant in the right lateral position over 15 minutes followed by 2 ml/kg in the left lateral position over 15 minutes. All three groups of lambs had improvements in Po_2 and lung mechanics, although the responses were not as large with surfactant infusion. The bolus treatments delivered surfactant quite uniformly to the different lobes of the sheep lung, whereas infusion resulted primarily in upper lobe localization (Fig. 106–9). The animals received a second treatment 2 hours after the initial treatment, and the second treatment localized to the same lung pieces that received the majority of the surfactant with the initial treatments. This result indicated that the first treatment determines primarily which lung volumes will open, and the second treatment tends to treat the same lung volumes that were initially treated. Pulmonary blood flow was relatively uniform across the lung pieces of the bolus-treated animals. In contrast, blood flow decreased to the lung pieces that received the most surfactant by infusion probably because of overinflation of those lung regions. In the injured lung, instilled surfactant goes preferentially to lung regions that are partially inflated and not to atelectatic or overinflated areas.[76]

Surfactant distributes to the lungs by bulk movement of the suspension down the airways and by spreading. The style of ventilation immediately after treatment could affect the distribution. In clinical practice, conventional volume ventilation is routinely used after surfactant treatments. Walther and colleagues[77] reported that surfactant instilled into the airways of preterm lambs distributed similarly with conventional or high-frequency ventilation. In contrast, Heldt and coworkers[78] found that high-frequency ventilation seemed to delay surfactant delivery to distal air spaces in preterm rabbits. Different ventilation strategies may affect surfactant treatment techniques and distribution. Surfactant can be delivered to the lungs by aerosol, but in practice the surfactant goes primarily to the ventilated lung regions resulting in a nonuniform distribution.[79] The surfactant dose that can be delivered by aerosol also is low.

VENTILATION EFFECTS ON SURFACTANT TREATMENT RESPONSES

Although mechanical ventilation and the use of PEEP is routine in infants with RDS, the selection of ventilatory style remains controversial. The interaction between ventilatory management and surfactant treatment has not been studied extensively, although in experimental animals the style of ventilation is an important variable in the response of the preterm lung to surfactant treatment.[21] In clinical practice, surfactant does not have equivalent effects in different neonatal units, and the differences probably can in part be explained by ventilatory management.[80] Lung

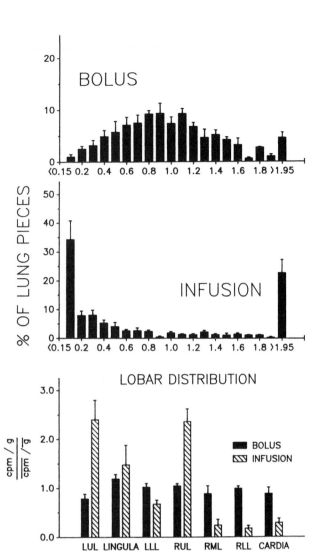

Figure 106–9. Distribution of surfactant by a bolus technique in comparison with a 30-minute infusion to preterm ventilated lamb lungs. The 100-mg/kg dose of lung extract surfactant was radiolabeled, and the amount of surfactant recovered in lung pieces or by lobe was measured. Bolus treatment resulted in about 40% of the lung pieces containing within ± 25% of the mean amount of surfactant. In contrast, infusion resulted in 7% of the pieces of lung receiving within ± 25% of the mean. The majority of the infused surfactant was found in the upper lobes. (Redrawn from Ueda T, et al: J Appl Physiol 76:45, 1994.)

injury is induced by ventilation of the normal lung at volumes close to maximal lung volume.[81] With surfactant deficiency, ventilation at low lung volumes (below the normal FRC) also causes progressive injury and pulmonary edema.[82] If alveolar expansion is optimized in the saline lavaged rabbit model of surfactant deficiency, the effectiveness of surfactant treatments is enhanced. These effects also depend on the type of surfactant used for treatment. Surfactants that contain lipids only are not effective at improving compliances or pressure volume curves of preterm rabbits.[83] Addition of the surfactant proteins SP-B and SP-C improves function, but the enhanced function is evident only if PEEP is used to ventilate the animals. The use of PEEP in the preterm rabbit model also resulted in striking decreases in the leak of albumin from the vasculature to the lungs.

The equipment used for the mechanical ventilation of preterm infants and the ventilatory techniques have changed since surfactant was tested clinically in the 1980s. Most trials of

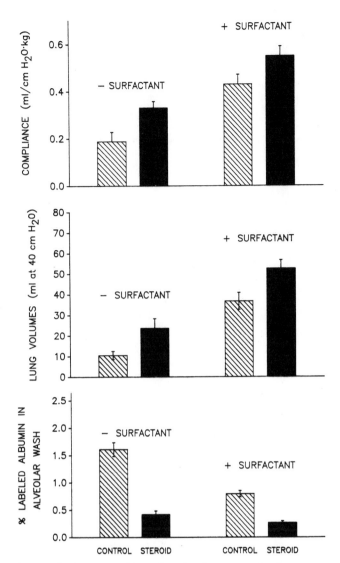

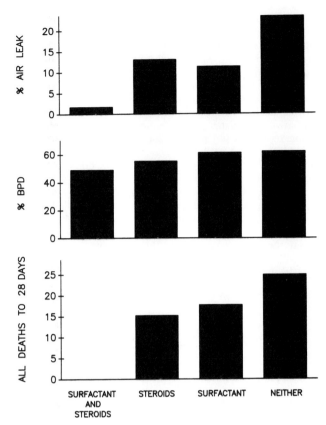

Figure 106–11. Combined effects of prenatal corticosteroids and postnatal surfactant on death, air leaks, and bronchopulmonary dysplasia (BPD) for infants randomized to Survanta or placebo treatment. (Data from Jobe AJ, et al: Am J Obstet Gynecol *168*:508, 1993.)

Figure 106–10. Postnatal lung function in preterm lambs randomized to prenatal cortisol and postnatal surfactant treatments. Each treatment increased postnatal compliances, increased lung volumes, and decreased pulmonary edema as measured by the amount of intravascular ^{125}I albumin that was recovered by alveolar wash. The lambs that received both treatments had responses that were approximately the sum of the surfactant and cortisol responses. (Data from Ikegami M, et al: J Appl Physiol *70*:2268, 1991.)

ventilation now focus on very low birth weight infants at highest risk of bronchopulmonary dysplasia. These infants usually have RDS and have been treated with surfactant before trial enrollment. Examples are the trials comparing high-frequency oscillation with conventional ventilation.[84, 85] The newer management approaches of trying to keep the FRC relatively high (the open lung strategy) while ventilating with low tidal volumes (4–6 ml/kg) to achieve carbon dioxide values higher than the normal range (greater than 50 mm Hg) depend on good surfactant function. If surfactant is deficient, FRC cannot be maintained without excessive PEEP. Surfactant treatment before the initiation of high-frequency oscillation improves respiratory stabilization.[86] The use of continuous positive airway pressure (CPAP) is also becoming more common as a way to decrease the need for mechanical ventilation and perhaps to decrease the severity of bronchopulmonary dysplasia.[87] An advantage of CPAP

is the avoidance of intubation, but surfactant cannot be given without intubation. Verder and colleagues[88] have found that elective intubation followed surfactant treatment and extubation to CPAP can decrease the need for mechanical ventilation in infants with RDS. The best timing for the combination of surfactant treatment with CPAP or mechanical ventilation in very low birth weight infants remains to be defined.

SURFACTANT–MATERNAL CORTICOSTEROID INTERACTIONS

Prenatal corticosteroid therapy decreases the incidence of death and the incidence and severity of RDS as well as other complications of prematurity.[89] Prenatal corticosteroids and postnatal surfactant both decrease RDS or death by similar amounts. The question of clinical relevance is how these two effective therapies interact. The two therapies have additive effects on postnatal lung function in animal models (Fig. 106–10). After fetal cortisol exposure, preterm lambs treated with surfactant have improved lung compliance, increased lung volumes, and decreased alveolar edema relative to lambs receiving either treatment.[90] Prenatal corticosteroid treatment of preterm rabbits also resulted in an enhanced postnatal response to surfactant. Corticosteroid-exposed rabbits required less surfactant for larger compliance responses than did control animals.[91] If the only effects of prenatal corticosteroids on the developing lung were to increase surfactant, prenatal corticosteroids and postnatal surfactant treatments would be acting by the same mechanism. Experiments in developing animals indicate that the primary effects of prenatal corticosteroid treatments are on lung structure, causing increased lung gas volumes that resulted in improved ventilation and better responses to surfactant treatment.

Randomized, controlled trials of the interactions between postnatal surfactant and prenatal corticosteroids are not available because these therapies were developed in different eras. It is no longer ethical to randomize infants to either surfactant or prenatal corticosteroids. Retrospective evaluations of the surfactant trial databases demonstrate that there is a beneficial interaction between prenatal corticosteroids and postnatal surfactant. In one report, treatment with surfactant or prenatal corticosteroids decreased air leak and death similarly (Fig. 106–11). Those infants who received both treatments, however, had the best outcome.[92] Kari and associates[93] also found that infants with RDS randomized to receive maternal corticosteroids had a better response to postnatal surfactant than did infants with RDS not receiving prenatal corticosteroids. The combined use of antenatal corticosteroids and postnatal surfactant are major contributions to the improved outcomes of preterm infants.

REFERENCES

1. Clements JA: Surfactant tension of lung extracts. Proc Soc Exp Biol Med 95:170, 1957.
2. Pattle RE: Properties, function and origin of the alveolar lining layer. Nature 175:1125, 1955.
3. Avery ME, Mead J: Surface properties in relation to atelectasis and hyaline membrane disease. Am J Dis Child 97:517, 1959.
4. Chu J, et al: Neonatal pulmonary ischemia: I. Clinical and physiological studies. Pediatrics 40(Suppl):709–782, 1967.
5. Enhorning G, Robertson B: Lung expansion in the premature rabbit fetus after tracheal deposition of surfactant. Pediatrics 50:58, 1972.
6. Robertson B, Enhorning G: The alveolar lining of the premature newborn rabbit after pharyngeal deposition of surfactant. Lab Invest 31:54, 1974.
7. Fujiwara T, et al: Artificial surfactant therapy in hyaline-membrane disease. Lancet 1:55, 1980.
8. Hallman M, et al: Exogenous human surfactant for treatment of severe respiratory distress syndrome: a randomized prospective clinical trial. J Pediatr 106:963, 1985.
9. Enhorning G, et al: Prevention of neonatal respiratory distress syndrome by tracheal instillation of surfactant: a randomized clinical trial. Pediatrics 76:145, 1985.
10. Shapiro DL, et al: Double-blind, randomized trial of a calf lung surfactant extract administered at birth to very premature infants for prevention of respiratory distress syndrome. Pediatrics 76:593, 1985.
11. Jobe AH: Pulmonary surfactant therapy. N Engl J Med 328:861, 1993.
12. Ainsworth SB, et al: Randomized controlled trial of early treatment of respiratory distress syndrome with pumactant (ALEC) or poractant alfa (Curosurf) in infants of 25 to 29 weeks' gestation. Lancet 355:1387, 2000.
13. Soll RF, Blanco F: Natural surfactant extract versus synthetic surfactant for neonatal respiratory distress syndrome. Cochrane Database of Systemic Reviews, The Cochrane Library 1, 2003.
14. Fujiwara T: Surfactant replacement in neonatal respiratory distress syndrome. In Robertson B, et al (eds): Pulmonary Surfactant. Amsterdam, Elsevier Science Publishers, 1984, pp 480–503.
15. Notter RH: Surface chemistry of pulmonary surfactant: the role of individual components. In Robertson B, et al (eds): Pulmonary Surfactant. Amsterdam, Elsevier Science Publishers, 1984, pp 17–65.
16. Notter RH, et al: Lung surfactant replacement in premature lambs with extracted lipids from bovine lung lavage: effects of dose, dispersion technique, and gestational age. Pediatr Res 19:569, 1985.
17. Morley CJ: Surfactant treatment for premature babies—a review of clinical trials. Arch Dis Child 66:445, 1991.
18. Egan EA, et al: Natural and artificial lung surfactant replacement therapy in premature lambs. J Appl Physiol 55:875, 1983.
19. Robertson B, et al: Structural and functional characterization of porcine surfactant isolated by liquid-gel chromatography. In von Muller WP (ed): Progress in Respiration Research, vol 25. Basel, Karger, 1990, pp 237–246.
20. Bloom BT, et al: Comparison of Infasurf (calf lung surfactant extract) to Survanta (beractant) in the treatment and prevention of respiratory distress syndrome. Pediatrics 100:31 1997.
21. Rider ED, et al: Different ventilation strategies alter surfactant responses in preterm rabbit. J Appl Physiol 73:2089, 1992.
22. ElKady T, Jobe AH: Corticosteroids and surfactant increase lung volumes and decrease rupture pressures of preterm rabbit lungs. J Appl Physiol 63:1616, 1987.
23. Bermel MS, et al: Lavaged excised rat lungs as a model of surfactant deficiency. Lung 162:99, 1984.
24. Pinkerton KE, et al: Lung parenchyma and type II cell morphometrics: effect of surfactant treatment on preterm ventilated lamb lungs. J Appl Physiol 77:1953, 1994.
25. Goldsmith LS, et al: Immediate improvement in lung volume after exogenous surfactant: alveolar recruitment versus increased distention. J Pediatr 119:424, 1991.
26. Dinger J, et al: Functional residual capacity and compliance of the respiratory system after surfactant treatment in premature infants with severe respiratory distress syndrome. Eur J Pediatr 161:485, 2002.
27. Dinger J, et al: Effect of positive end-expiratory pressure on functional residual capacity and compliance in surfactant-treated preterm infants. J Perinat Med 29:137, 2001.
28. Jobe AH, et al: Duration and characteristics of treatment of premature lambs with natural surfactant. J Clin Invest 67:370, 1981.
29. Davis JM, et al: Changes in pulmonary mechanics after the administration of surfactant to infants with respiratory distress syndrome. N Engl J Med 319:476, 1988.
30. Kelly E, et al: Compliance of the respiratory system in newborn infants pre- and post-surfactant replacement therapy. Pediatr Pulmonol 15:225, 1993.
31. Cummings JJ, et al: A controlled clinical comparison of four different surfactant preparations in surfactant-deficient preterm lambs. Am Rev Respir Dis 145:999, 1992.
32. Choukroun ML, et al: Pulmonary mechanics in ventilated preterm infants with respiratory distress syndrome after exogenous surfactant administration: a comparison between two surfactant preparations. Pediatr Pulmonol 18:273, 1994.
33. Noack G, et al: Passive expiratory flow-volume recordings in immature newborn rabbits. Respiration 57:1, 1990.
34. Mizuno K, et al: Surfactant protein-B supplementation improves in vivo function of a modified natural surfactant. Pediatr Res 37:271, 1995.
35. Kaapa P, et al: Pulmonary hemodynamics after synthetic surfactant replacement in neonatal respiratory distress syndrome. J Pediatr 123:115, 1993.
36. Clyman RI, et al: Increased shunt through the patent ductus arteriosus after surfactant replacement therapy. J Pediatr 100:101, 1982.
37. Heldt GP, et al: Closure of ductus arteriosus and mechanics of breathing in preterm infants after surfactant replacement therapy. Pediatr Res 25:305, 1989.
38. Soll RF: Prophylactic natural surfactant extract for preventing morbidity and mortality in preterm infants. Cochrane Database of Systematic Reviews 1, 2003.
39. Jobe A, Bancalari E: NICHD/NHLBI/ORD Workshop Summary—Bronchopulmonary Dysplasia. Am J Respir Crit Care Med 163:1723 2001.
40. Egberts J, de Winter JP: Meta-analyses of surfactant and bronchopulmonary dysplasia revisited. Lancet 344:882, 1994.
41. Fujiwara T, et al: Surfactant replacement therapy with a single post-ventilatory dose of a reconstituted bovine surfactant in preterm neonates with respiratory distress syndrome: final analysis of a multicenter, double-blind, randomized trial and comparison with similar trials. Pediatrics 86:753, 1990.
42. Gunkel JH, Banks PLC: Surfactant therapy and intracranial hemorrhage: review of the literature and results of new analyses. Pediatrics 92:775, 1993.
43. Repka MX, et al: Calf lung surfactant extract prophylaxis and retinopathy of prematurity. Ophthalmology 99:531, 1992.
44. Vaucher YE, et al: Neurodevelopmental and respiratory outcome in early childhood after human surfactant treatment. Am J Dis Child 142:927, 1988.
45. Dunn MS, et al: Two-year follow-up of infants enrolled in a randomized trial of surfactant replacement therapy for prevention of neonatal respiratory distress syndrome. Pediatrics 82:543, 1988.
46. Ware J, et al: Health and developmental outcomes of a surfactant controlled trial: follow-up at 2 years. Pediatrics 85:1103, 1990.
47. Survanta Multidose Study Group: Two-year follow-up of infants treated for neonatal respiratory distress syndrome with bovine surfactant. J Pediatr 124:962, 1994.
48. Kendig JW, et al: Comparison of two strategies for surfactant prophylaxis in very premature infants: a multicenter randomized trial. Pediatrics 101:1006, 1998.
49. Robertson B: Pathology and pathophysiology of neonatal surfactant deficiency. In Robertson B, et al (eds): Pulmonary Surfactant. Amsterdam, Elsevier Science Publishers, 1984, pp 384–418.
50. Suresh GK, Soll RF: Current surfactant use in premature infants. Clin Perinatol 28:671 2001.
51. Jobe AH, Ikegami M: Surfactant therapy. Clin Perinatol 20:683, 1993.
52. Speer CP, et al: Randomized European multicenter trial of surfactant replacement therapy for severe neonatal respiratory distress syndrome: single versus multiple doses of Curosurf. Pediatrics 89:13, 1992.
53. Dunn MS, et al: Single versus multiple-dose surfactant replacement therapy in neonates of 30 to 36 weeks' gestation with respiratory distress syndrome. Pediatrics 86:564, 1990.
54. Zola EM, et al: Treatment Investigational New Drug experience with Survanta (beractant). Pediatrics 91:546, 1993.
55. Horbar JD, et al: A multicenter randomized trial comparing two surfactants for the treatment of neonatal respiratory distress syndrome. J Pediatr 123:757, 1993.
56. van de Bor M, et al: Cerebral blood flow velocity after surfactant instillation in preterm infants. J Pediatr 118:285, 1991.
57. Hellstrom-Westas L, et al: Cerebroelectrical depression following surfactant treatment in preterm neonates. Pediatrics 89:643, 1992.
58. Rey M, et al: Surfactant bolus instillation: effects of different doses on blood pressure and cerebral blood flow velocities. Biol Neonate 66:16, 1994.
59. Raju TNK, Langenberg P: Pulmonary hemorrhage and exogenous surfactant therapy: a metaanalysis. J Pediatr 123:603, 1993.

60. Costello ML, et al: Stress failure of alveolar epithelial cells studied by scanning electron microscopy. Am Rev Respir Dis *145*:1446, 1992.
61. Pandit PB, et al: Surfactant therapy in neonates with respiratory deterioration due to pulmonary hemorrhage. Pediatrics *95*:32, 1995.
62. Horbar JD, et al: Decreasing mortality associated with the introduction of surfactant therapy: an observational study of neonates weighing 601 to 1300 grams at birth. Pediatrics *92*:191, 1993.
63. Schwartz RM, et al: Effect of surfactant on morbidity, mortality, and resource use in newborn infants weighing 500 to 1500 g. N Engl J Med *330*:1476, 1994.
64. Palta M, et al: Mortality and morbidity after availability of surfactant therapy. Arch Pediatr Adolesc Med *148*:1295, 1994.
65. Zola EM, et al: Comparison of three dosing procedures for administration of bovine surfactant to neonates with respiratory distress syndrome. J Pediatr *122*:453, 1993.
66. Jobe A. Techniques for administering surfactant. *In* Robertson B (ed): Surfactant Therapy for Lung Disease. New York, Marcel Dekker, 1995 (vol 84).
67. Charon A, et al: Factors associated with surfactant treatment response in infants with severe respiratory distress syndrome. Pediatrics *83*:348, 1989.
68. Kharasch VS, et al: Pulmonary surfactant as a vehicle for intratracheal delivery of technetium sulfur colloid and pentamidine in hamster lungs. Am Rev Respir Dis *144*:909, 1991.
69. Jobe AH, et al: Surfactant and pulmonary blood flow distributions following treatment of premature lambs with natural surfactant. J Clin Invest *73*:848, 1984.
70. van der Bleek J, et al: Distribution of exogenous surfactant in rabbits with severe respiratory failure: the effect of volume. Pediatr Res *34*:154, 1993.
71. Davis JM, et al: Short-term distribution kinetics of intratracheally administered exogenous lung surfactant. Pediatr Res *31*:445, 1992.
72. Oetomo SB, et al: Surfactant treatments alter endogenous surfactant metabolism in rabbit lungs. J Appl Physiol *68*:1590, 1990.
73. Gilliard N, et al: Effect of volume and dose on the pulmonary distribution of exogenous surfactant administered to normal rabbits or to rabbits with oleic acid lung injury. Am Rev Respir Dis *141*:743, 1990.
74. Segerer H, et al: Pulmonary distribution and efficacy of exogenous surfactant in lung-lavaged rabbits are influenced by the instillation technique. Pediatr Res *34*:490, 1993.
75. Ueda T, et al: Distribution of surfactant and ventilation in surfactant treated preterm lambs. J Appl Physiol *76*:45, 1994.
76. Diemel RV, et al. *In vitro* and *in vivo* intrapulmonary distribution of fluorescently labeled surfactant. Crit Care Med *30*:1083, 2002.
77. Walther FJ, et al: A comparison of high-frequency oscillation superimposed onto backup mechanical ventilation and conventional mechanical ventilation on the distribution of exogenous surfactant in premature lambs. Pediatr Res *22*:725, 1987.
78. Heldt GP, et al: Distribution of surfactant, lung compliance, and aeration of preterm rabbit lungs after surfactant therapy and conventional and high-frequency oscillatory ventilation. Pediatr Res *31*:270, 1992.
79. Henry MD, et al: Ultrasonic nebulized in comparison with instilled surfactant treatment of preterm lambs. Am J Respir Crit Care Med *154*:366, 1996.
80. Hallman M, et al: Association between neonatal care practices and efficacy of exogenous human surfactant: results of a bicenter randomized trial. Pediatrics *91*:552, 1993.
81. Dreyfuss D, Saumon G: Ventilator-induced injury. *In* Tobin MJ (ed): Principles and Practice of Mechanical Ventilation. New York, McGraw-Hill, 1994, pp 793–812.
82. Froese AB, et al: Optimizing alveolar expansion prolongs the effectiveness of exogenous surfactant therapy in the adult rabbit. Am Rev Respir Dis *148*:569, 1993.
83. Rider ED, et al: Treatment responses to surfactants containing natural surfactant proteins in preterm rabbits. Am Rev Respir Dis *147*:669, 1993.
84. Johnson AH, et al: High-frequency oscillatory ventilation for the prevention of chronic lung disease of prematurity. N Engl J Med *347*(9):633, 2002.
85. Courtney SE, et al: High-frequency oscillatory ventilation versus conventional mechanical ventilation for very-low-birth-weight infants. N Engl J Med *347*:643, 2002.
86. Plavka R, et al: Early versus delayed surfactant administration in extremely premature neonates with respiratory distress syndrome ventilated by high-frequency oscillatory ventilation. Intensive Care Med *28*:1483, 2002.
87. Polin RA, et al: Newer experience with CPAP. Semin Neonatol *7*:379, 2002.
88. Verder H, et al: Nasal continuous positive airway pressure and early surfactant therapy for respiratory distress syndrome in newborns of less than 30 weeks' gestation. Pediatrics *103*:E24, 1999.
89. Crowley P: Prophylactic corticosteroids for preterm birth (Cochrane Review). The Cochrane Library, Issue 3, 2001. Oxford: Update Software.
90. Ikegami M, et al: Corticosteroid and thyrotropin-releasing hormone effects on preterm sheep lung function. J Appl Physiol *70*:2268, 1991.
91. Seidner S, et al: Corticosteroid potentiation of surfactant dose response in preterm rabbits. J Appl Physiol *64*:2366, 1988.
92. Jobe AH, et al: Beneficial effects of the combined use of prenatal corticosteroids and postnatal surfactant on preterm infants. Am J Obstet Gynecol *168*:508, 1993.
93. Kari MA, et al: Prenatal dexamethasone treatment in conjunction with rescue therapy of human surfactant: a randomized placebo-controlled multicenter study. Pediatrics *93*:730, 1994.

107

Lawrence M. Nogee

Genetics and Physiology of Surfactant Protein Deficiencies

The principal cause of the respiratory distress syndrome (RDS) in prematurely born infants is an inability to produce sufficient amounts of pulmonary surfactant due to immaturity.[1] Surfactant phospholipids, in combination with specific proteins, help to reduce alveolar surface tension at the air-liquid interface and prevent end-expiratory collapse. The risk of RDS is related to gestational age; more immature infants are at highest risk, although full-term infants may also develop RDS.[2, 3] Investigators have recognized that RDS in some full-term infants may result from inherited abnormalities in the genes encoding some of the specific surfactant proteins. Hereditary surfactant protein B (SP-B) deficiency is an autosomal recessive cause of neonatal respiratory failure resulting from loss of function mutations in the gene encoding SP-B. More recently, mutations in the SP-C gene have been associated with lung disease of more variable onset and severity. Although these conditions are rare, they are associated with significant morbidity and mortality, and it is important that they be recognized in a timely fashion, to counsel families of affected infants appropriately. Surfactant protein deficiencies provide insights into the roles of these proteins in normal lung function and surfactant homeostasis, and they demonstrate how genetic mechanisms may contribute to the development of more common forms of lung disease.

PULMONARY SURFACTANT PROTEINS

The hydrophobic SP-B and SP-C have important roles in enhancing the surface tension–lowering properties of surfactant phospholipids.[4, 5] Both SP-B and SP-C are found in varying amounts in the mammalian-derived surfactant preparations used to treat premature infants with RDS.[4] SP-B and SP-C are both derived from proteolytic processing of precursor proteins that are encoded by single genes on chromosomes 2 and 8, respectively, with the genetic loci referred to as *SFTPB* and *SFTPC*.[6, 7] The mature forms of SP-B and SP-C are routed to lamellar bodies, the storage organelles for surfactant in the alveolar Type II cell, and they are secreted along with surfactant phospholipids.[8]

Pulmonary surfactant also contains two larger glycoproteins, SP-A and SP-D, which are members of the collectin family, with both collagenous and carbohydrate binding lectin-like domains.[9] The principal roles of SP-A and SP-D in the lung are likely related to local host cell defense.[10,11] Both SP-A and SP-D bind to a wide array of microorganisms and facilitate their uptake or killing by alveolar macrophages.[11] Genetically engineered SP-A– and SP-D–deficient mice do not develop neonatal respiratory disease, but they do appear to have an increased susceptibility to infection with various organisms that are relevant to human neonates, including group B streptococci and respiratory syncytial virus.[12-14] SP-D–deficient mice also develop lung disease as they age; both emphysema and fibrosis suggest a role in regulating chronic inflammation, and lipoproteinosis suggests a possible role in surfactant homeostasis.[15-17] Two genes and a pseudogene for SP-A and a single gene for SP-D are located on chromosome 10.[18] Mutations in the SP-A and SP-D genes associated with human lung disease have not yet been reported.

HEREDITARY SURFACTANT PROTEIN B DEFICIENCY

Clinical Aspects

Hereditary SP-B deficiency was recognized as a cause of neonatal lung disease in 1993, with a report of three siblings who each developed severe parenchymal neonatal lung disease that proved fatal despite maximal medical therapy.[19] As in the initial report, the most common presentation for hereditary SP-B deficiency is a full-term infant who develops symptoms and signs of respiratory distress consistent with surfactant deficiency within the first several hours of life, without other risk factors for lung disease. Air leak and pulmonary hypertension are common. The radiographic findings are usually those associated with surfactant deficiency, although this has not been examined systematically.[20,21] Suspected diagnoses have included RDS, transient tachypnea of the newborn, pneumonia, persistent pulmonary hypertension, and meconium aspiration.[22] Although SP-B–deficient infants usually have very severe lung disease, often requiring support with extracorporeal membrane oxygenation when available, the initial severity of respiratory disease can be quite variable. Some affected infants have not required mechanical ventilation for several weeks, and the factors responsible for the variability in the severity of the initial lung disease in affected infants are unclear. Affected infants may have an initial positive response to surfactant replacement therapy, but their lung disease subsequently worsens with diminished response to subsequent doses. Glucocorticoids may improve the lung disease in some affected infants, perhaps because these patients have mutations that allow for some SP-B production.[23] The lung disease in SP-B deficiency is progressive, with an escalating need for respiratory support and persistent and worsening alveolar and interstitial infiltrates radiographically. The disease is rapidly fatal; more than 80% of affected infants die within 3 months despite aggressive supportive measures.[24,25]

Molecular Genetics and Epidemiology

The SP-B gene contains 11 exons, of which the first 10 contribute to the coding sequence. The gene is transcribed into a 2-kB mRNA that directs the synthesis of a 381-amino acid pre-proprotein. The first 23 amino acids constitute a signal peptide that is removed co-translationally. Mature SP-B corresponds to codons 201 (encoding phenylalanine) to 279 (encoding methionine) of the mRNA, and it is encoded in exons 6 and 7 of the gene[26] (Fig. 107-1). The first and most common mutation identified involves a substitution of three bases (GAA) for one (C) in codon 121 of the SP-B mRNA, located in exon 4 of the SP-B gene, leading to a net insertion of two bases and is termed 121ins2. The 121ins2 mutation causes a frameshift and introduces a premature codon for the termination of translation in exon 6, thus completely precluding production of mature SP-B (Fig. 107-2). The resulting transcript is also unstable, and this feature accounts for the lack of SP-B mRNA.[27]

Many other mutations resulting in SP-B deficiency have since been identified in the SP-B gene (see Fig. 107-1).[23,25,28-31] Identified SP-B gene mutations are loss of function mutations that result in markedly reduced or absent amounts of mature SP-B, although some allow for production of proSP-B. However, the normal processing of the proSP-B–containing mutations to mature SP-B is hindered, resulting in the lack of mature SP-B in lung tissue and tracheal secretions of affected infants.[25] Affected infants have mutations on both SP-B alleles consistent with the autosomal recessive inheritance pattern.

ProSP-B contains three tandem domains with structural homology to the saposins, lysosomal proteins that bind lipids and activate lysosomal hydrolases.[32] Mature SP-B corresponds to the middle domain of the proprotein,[33] and mutations in this region could theoretically result in the production of a SP-B protein with abnormal surface properties. However, a synthetic peptide containing one such mutation (R236C) was able to augment surface tension lowering normally in an *in vitro* system,[34] a finding suggesting that the disease in infants with this mutation also resulted from impaired processing of proSP-B containing the mutation. Mature SP-B forms higher-order oligomers dependent on sulfhydryl bond formation as well as ionic interactions.[35,36] Mutations that prevent oligomerization of SP-B could also in theory result in an SP-B with decreased activity, and they could possibly even act in a dominant negative fashion to interfere with SP-B from a normal allele. Such a mechanism for SP-B deficiency has not been recognized to date.

The exact incidence of SP-B deficiency is unknown. The number of reported cases is relatively small (~75),[19,23,25,28-31,37-42] and population-based studies to determine the incidence of disease have not been performed. A carrier frequency of approximately 1 in 1000 individuals has been reported for the 121ins2 mutation.[43,44] Because this mutation has accounted for approximately two-thirds of the mutant alleles identified, this finding implies that the frequency of any SP-B gene mutation in the population is approximately 1 in 600. Given that SP-B deficiency is an autosomal recessive disorder, if both parents have a mutation, they have a 25% chance of having an affected child. The predicted incidence of disease would thus be approximately 1 in 1.4 million (600 × 600 × 4), an incidence indicating that SP-B deficiency is a very rare disease, although this is probably an underestimate. Most studies to date have focused on children with either the 121ins2 mutation or very severe lung disease, and children with mutations resulting in milder disease may have been underrecognized.

The 121ins2 mutation has been found mainly in persons of Northern European descent; therefore, a common ancestral origin may account for the finding of a common mutation (*founder effect*).[24] A similar genetic background for chromosomes containing the 121ins2 mutation was found by analyzing genetic markers within and near the SP-B gene consistent with this hypothesis.[45] However, two other SP-B gene mutations (122delC and 122delT) have been identified within five nucleotides of the site of the common mutation, and a single nucleotide polymorphism is located within 30 base pairs of the site of the 121ins2 mutation, a finding suggesting that this region of the SP-B gene could also be a "hot spot" for mutation.[30,40] Clusters of mutations have also been identified in exons 2 and 9. Other mutations that have been observed in more than one unrelated individual include the 122delT mutation in persons of Middle Eastern descent, the 1043ins3 mutation in Asians, and a splicing mutation (c.479G>T) in French-Canadians. The frequencies of these mutations and the incidence of the disease in these populations have not been determined.

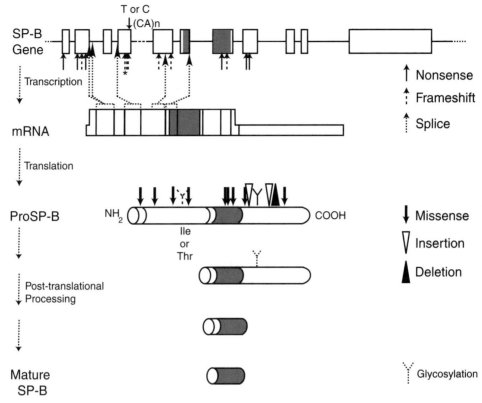

Figure 107–1. Surfactant protein B (SP-B) gene, protein synthesis, and posttranslational processing of SP-B and mutations in the SP-B gene. The normal transcription, translation, and processing of SP-B are outlined with the SP-B gene at the *top*, with the 11 exons represented by *boxes* and the introns represented by *lines*. The locations of a coding polymorphism resulting in either isoleucine (Ile) or threonine (Thr) in exon 4 and variable nucleotide repeat sequences ([CA]n) in intron IV are indicated. Untranslated regions of the mRNA are indicated by the *narrower rectangles*. Regions corresponding to mature SP-B are *shaded*. *Arrows* indicate the locations of known nonsense and frameshift mutations in the SP-B gene that result in absent SP-B mRNA and protein. The location of the 121ins2 mutation is indicated with an *asterisk*. Mutations that interfere with normal SP-B mRNA splicing are indicated by *arrows* pointing to the location in the gene and indicating the affected exon on the mRNA. Missense mutations or in-frame deletions or insertions that interfere with the processing of proSPB to mature SP-B are indicated by their location in the SP-B proprotein.

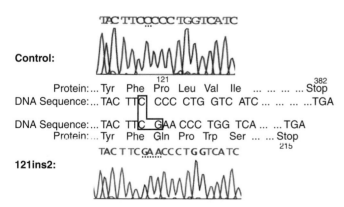

Figure 107–2. DNA sequence analysis of the surfactant protein B (SP-B) gene and the 121ins2 mutation. The SP-B gene DNA sequence in the region of exon 4 with the corresponding protein sequences and sequencing chromatograms are shown with the normal SP-B gene sequence on *top* and the 121ins2 mutation on the *bottom*. The substituted bases are indicated by a *box*, and the results of the substitution on the SP-B coding sequence are shown.

Laboratory Findings

Given the importance of SP-B in surfactant function *in vitro* and in animal models, it was not entirely surprising that a complete lack of SP-B was associated with lung disease consistent with surfactant deficiency. Unexpectedly, certain secondary changes have been observed in the composition or metabolism of other surfactant components in the lung fluid and tissue of infants with hereditary SP-B deficiency, a finding indicating a role for SP-B (or proSP-B) in surfactant metabolism that had been unanticipated. These secondary changes include ultrastructual changes, a relative paucity of surfactant phospholipids, in particular phosphatidylglycerol, and abnormal processing of the SP-C precursor protein (proSP-C) to mature SP-C.[27, 46] ProSP-C is proteolytically processed at both its amino and carboxy-termini to yield the 35-amino acid mature SP-C. The lung tissues of SP-B–deficient infants contain abundant amounts of proSP-C–derived proteins of intermediate size. Although the exact nature of these peptides has not been determined, their reactivity with antisera directed against amino-terminal proSP-C epitopes suggests that they represent incompletely or aberrantly processed proSP-C.[47] (Fig. 107-3). The finding of these peptides in bronchoalveolar lavage fluid from affected infants and the intense extracellular staining

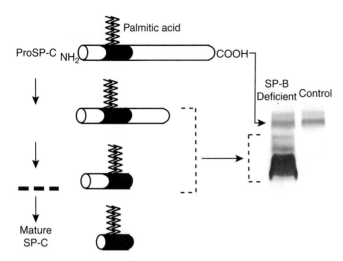

Figure 107–3. Aberrant processing of prosurfactant protein C (ProSP-C) in surfactant protein B (SP-B) deficiency. The normal processing of proSP-C to mature SP-C is shown on the *left*, with the portion corresponding to mature SP-C *shaded*. A *dashed line* indicates the site of the presumed block in proSP-C processing that occurs in the absence of SP-B, with the accumulation of immunoreactive peptides in the lung tissue from an SP-B–deficient infant in the Western blot *inset on the right*; such peptides are not present in lung tissue from a control infant.

observed with anti–proSP-C antisera indicate that these abnormal proSP-C peptides are secreted. This incomplete processing of proSP-C may also result in a relative deficiency of mature SP-C in affected infants, such that infants with hereditary SP-B deficiency have more global surfactant deficiency, although the block in SP-C processing does not appear to be complete.[48] The mechanisms underlying these secondary changes in phospholipids and SP-C metabolism are unknown. However, ultrastructural examination of the lungs of affected infants reveals a lack of normally formed lamellar bodies, the intracellular storage organelles of surfactant, with abundant abnormal-appearing lipid vesicles. Tubular myelin, the lattice-like extracellular form of surfactant whose formation requires SP-B as well as SP-A and calcium, is also not found in lung tissue of affected infants.[49, 50] A possible mechanism to account for these observations is that intracellular expression of SP-B (or proSP-B) is needed for lamellar body biogenesis. Because the final steps in processing of proSP-C to mature SP-C take place in a late cellular compartment, the inability to form these organelles resulting from the lack of SP-B results in incompletely processed proSP-C and inadequate packaging of surfactant components for secretion.

The histopathologic findings in the lungs of SP-B–deficient infants are largely nonspecific and include alveolar Type II cell hyperplasia, interstitial fibrosis, and diffuse alveolar damage. A finding that may be quite prominent is an accumulation of granular eosinophilic material with entrapped foamy macrophages filling distal air spaces. This histopathologic picture is similar to that seen in adults with alveolar proteinosis, a disease in which there is accumulation of surfactant phospholipids and proteins (including SP-B) in the air spaces. The term *congenital alveolar proteinosis* was thus used to distinguish infants with neonatal-onset, fatal disease from the adult disorder in which the onset and progression of disease are more gradual.[51-54] In SP-B–deficient infants, the proteinosis material does not contain SP-B, but it does stain intensely with antisera to SP-A and proSP-C, and it likely contains a relative paucity of surfactant phospholipids as well as abundant incompletely processed proSP-C. These aberrantly processed SP-C peptides would contain both

hydrophobic and hydrophilic epitopes and would likely not be very surface active, and they are present in large enough amounts that they could interfere with normal surfactant function and contribute to the pathophysiology of the lung disease. The exact mechanisms leading to the extracellular accumulations of SP-A, incompletely processed proSP-C, and other proteins leading to the appearance of alveolar proteinosis are not well understood. However, findings of alveolar proteinosis may be patchy within the lungs of SP-B–deficient infants or even not observed, although immunostaining for SP-A or proSP-C may make the proteinosis material more evident (Fig. 107–4).[25] Moreover, not all neonates with findings of alveolar proteinosis have hereditary SP-B deficiency as the basis for their lung disease.[55, 56] Similar histopathologic findings may result from other mechanisms, including deficiencies of granulocyte-macrophage colony stimulating factor or its receptor.[57] Thus, the term congenital alveolar proteinosis should *not* be used synonymously with hereditary SP-B deficiency.

Partial and Transient Surfactant Protein B Deficiency

Although SP-B deficiency results in severe disease, rare children with a relatively milder phenotype have been identified. These children have had mutations in their SP-B genes that allow for the production of some SP-B and thus have had a partial deficiency.[23, 31] These observations suggest that a critical level of SP-B is needed for normal lung function, although the precise level of SP-B needed for normal lung function is unknown. Whether the small amount of mature SP-B (~8 to 10% of control levels) or some retained function of proSP-B accounted for the milder phenotype is unclear. Additionally, severe neonatal lung disease was observed in a child who had undetectable amounts of SP-B in bronchoalveolar lavage fluid during his acute illness and an SP-B mutation on only one allele with an apparently normal second SP-B allele. The child's lung disease gradually improved in association with increased amounts of SP-B detected in subsequent bronchoalveolar lavage samples, a finding suggesting that the mutation on one allele contributed to transient SP-B deficiency.[28] Thus, loss of function mutations on even one allele (haploinsufficiency) for SP-B could predispose to neonatal lung disease should other factors (e.g., prematurity or inflammation) delay or reduce SP-B expression.

This hypothesis is supported by experiments with genetically engineered mice unable to produce SP-B. Similar to human infants with nonsense or frameshift SP-B mutations, SP-B–deficient mice do not have detectable SP-B mRNA or protein in their lungs, and they die of respiratory insufficiency within minutes of birth.[58] SP-B–deficient mice also have secondary abnormalities in their lungs similar to those observed in human infants with hereditary SP-B deficiency, including aberrant processing of proSP-C and abnormal lamellar body formation.[58, 59] Mice heterozygous for a null SP-B allele have half normal levels of SP-B mRNA and protein and do not have neonatal respiratory disease.[60] However, these SP-B–haploinsufficient mice were more susceptible to pulmonary oxygen toxicity than their wild-type littermates.[61, 62] In contrast to these observations, pulmonary function tests in seven human adult carriers for the 121ins2 mutations did not differ from controls, nor have the parents of affected infants generally had a history of neonatal lung disease.[63] Larger, population-based studies will be necessary to determine whether carrying one abnormal SP-B allele is a risk factor for lung disease.

Other Surfactant Protein B Gene Variants and Lung Disease

Although it is rare, SP-B deficiency demonstrates the essential role of SP-B in normal surfactant metabolism. Given its critical

SP-B   ProSP-C

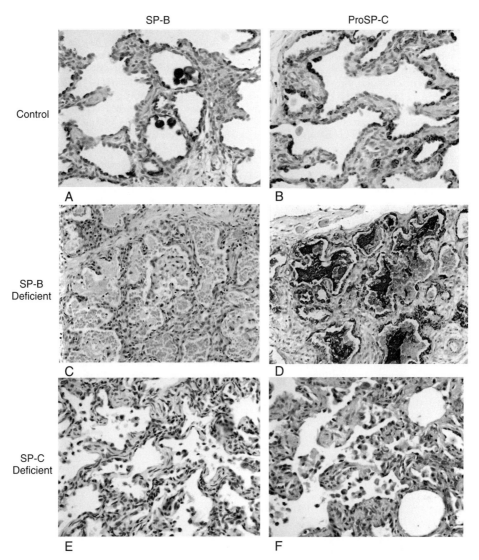

Control

A   B

SP-B
Deficient

C   D

SP-C
Deficient

E   F

Figure 107–4. Immunohistochemical staining of lung tissue. Lung tissue was immunostained for mature surfactant protein B (SP-B; *left*) and proSP-C (*right*). Lung tissue from a control infant who died of chronic lung disease demonstrates positive staining for both mature SP-B (**A**) and proSP-C (**B**) observed in alveolar epithelial cells (*top row*). In contrast, absent staining for mature SP-B (**C**), but intense staining for proSP-C in the alveolar epithelium and extracellular proteinaceous material (**D**) is observed lung tissue from an SP-B–deficient infant who was homozygous for the 121ins2 mutation (*middle row*). Staining for mature SP-B is also markedly reduced (**E**), as is staining for proSP-C (**F**) in tissue from a patient with an SP-C mutation on the allele that resulted in the skipping of an exon and production of an abnormal proSP-C protein (*bottom row*). (Courtesy of Dr. Susan Wert, Children's Hospital Medical Center, Cincinnati, OH.)

role, SP-B is a reasonable candidate gene to account for possible genetic variation observed in more common lung diseases such as RDS. Certain variants in the SP-B gene have been identified that could potentially affect SP-B expression. A single nucleotide polymorphism has been identified in codon 131, which encodes either threonine (Thr) or isoleucine (Ile).[25, 26, 40, 64, 65] The 131Thr allele, but not 131Ile, has a potential additional recognition site for N-linked glycosylation. Whether glycosylation at this site significantly affects proSP-B structure or its routing through the cell is unknown. However, the 131Thr allele was associated with an increased risk of acute RDS in adults and an increased risk of neonatal RDS in premature infants.[66-68] Alterations in the SP-B gene resulting in small differences in SP-B function or metabolism could thus be important in the pathogenesis of other lung diseases. Exon 8 contains an alternative splice site whose utilization would result in a SP-B proprotein with four amino acids deleted from the carboxy-terminal domain.[37, 69] This splice

variant has been detected in normal human lung tissue and in increased in amounts in lung tissue from patients with various lung diseases.[69] It is not known whether this alternative transcript is translated or whether the resulting proprotein would be processed normally. Further studies are needed to address these questions, as well as whether the increase in the use of the alternative splice site is a consequence of or contributes to lung disease.

The fourth intron of the SP-B gene also contains a variable nucleotide tandem repeat sequence, and allelic variants containing different numbers of repeats have been characterized.[70] An increased risk of RDS in infants with alleles that differ from the predominant allele alone or in association with polymorphic variants in the SP-A gene loci has been observed in some studies.[67, 70-74] These variants are not currently known to affect SP-B expression directly, and the mechanism by which these intron IV allelic variants would affect RDS risk is unclear. One possibility is that they are linked to other variations in the SP-B gene with direct functional importance. Other single nucleotide polymorphisms have also been identified in both coding and noncoding regions of the SP-B gene whose functional significance likewise remains unknown.[40, 56, 66, 75]

Currently hereditary SP-B deficiency has only been shown to result from a primary inability to produce SP-B caused by mutations in the SP-B gene. However, other mechanisms that impair SP-B production such as mutations in genes for the enzymes needed for the proper processing of proSP-B to mature SP-B, or to accelerate SP-B catabolism, could result in deficiency of SP-B and similar lung disease. Fatal neonatal lung disease inherited in an autosomal recessive fashion, associated with reduced or undetectable amounts of SP-B in the bronchoalveolar lavage fluid or lung tissue of affected children, but without mutations identified to account for the lack of SP-B, has been reported.[56, 76] Absent lamellar bodies were also observed in association with fatal lung disease in children in whom no SP-B gene defects were identified.[77] These observations support the notion of genetic or locus heterogeneity resulting in SP-B deficiency. Apparent SP-B deficiency may be also observed in diseases resulting from other mechanisms. Reduced immunostaining for SP-B was observed in lung tissue from two patients who had a mutation in their SP-C gene, although SP-B was readily detected by Western blotting (see Fig. 107–4).[48] Thus, mutations in other genes may affect SP-B metabolism, and there may be important intracellular interactions between SP-B and SP-C. A comprehensive approach to the evaluation of children with severe neonatal lung disease of unclear origin, including ultrastructural examination and collection of frozen as well as fixed tissue from biopsy and autopsy studies, will be essential to elucidating novel mechanisms of lung disease.

Evaluation of Infants with Suspected Hereditary Surfactant Protein B Deficiency

Clinical features that distinguish SP-B deficiency from reversible causes of neonatal respiratory failure have not been identified. Full-term infants with respiratory distress that is not explained by history and does not improve after the first week of life or infants who have died of lung disease of unclear origin should be suspected of having the disorder. Although a family history of neonatal lung disease may prompt suspicion of a genetic disorder, a positive family history is often absent, given the autosomal recessive inheritance pattern. The differential diagnosis includes RDS, infection, persistent pulmonary hypertension, unrecognized cardiac malformations, and developmental anomalies of the lung such as alveolar capillary dysplasia.

Routine laboratory findings in SP-B–deficient infants are nonspecific. Tracheal aspirate samples for lecithin/sphingomyelin ratios have been reported as being low and within the normal range, but they have not been systematically evaluated because such testing is not routinely done on full-term infants.[54, 78] Unfortunately, specific tests that may be helpful in establishing a diagnosis are not widely available, or they are available only on a research basis. The presence or absence of SP-B in tracheal aspirate or bronchoalveolar lavage fluid can be analyzed by either enzyme-linked immunosorbent assay or Western blot assays, although the sensitivity and specificity of such testing are unknown, and the potential for both false-positive and false-negative results exists. Pulmonary immaturity or injury to alveolar Type II cells may be associated with decreased production of all surfactant components. Conversely, exogenous surfactant preparations used to treat infants with RDS contain SP-B in varying amounts, and because most polyclonal antisera do not distinguish among human, bovine, and porcine SP-B, recent treatment with a surfactant preparation containing exogenous SP-B could lead to a falsely positive result. Finally, some mutations could

allow for some SP-B production, and the SP-B levels that distinguish such infants from unaffected infants are unknown.

A definitive diagnosis may be made through genetic testing. Such testing is noninvasive and can be performed rapidly, and a finding of mutations on both alleles is diagnostic for the disorder. However, the sensitivity of genetic testing is limited by the number of mutations that may result in disease. A relatively rapid assay for the 121ins2 mutation may be performed by amplification of the region containing the mutation by polymerase chain reaction and restriction analysis for a novel site introduced by the mutation. Assays for this mutation are available in clinical diagnostic laboratories as well as on a research basis. However, the disease may result from as yet unknown mutations, and tests for other previously identified mutations may be unavailable outside research laboratories because such mutations have generally been found in only one kindred.

A diagnosis of SP-B deficiency may be established by immunohistochemical staining of lung tissue for the surfactant proteins. Intense staining of extracellular material using antisera directed against proSP-C has been consistently observed in affected children (see Fig. 107–4).[25] In contrast, the absence of staining for mature SP-B is consistent with the diagnosis, but not definitive. Absent staining for mature SP-B has been observed in children in whom mutations in the SP-B gene were not identified or in whom other mechanisms for their lung disease were subsequently identified.[48, 56] Moreover, positive staining for proSP-B or mature SP-B does not exclude the diagnosis, because variable intensity of staining for both proSP-B and mature SP-B may be observed in association with mutations that allow for some SP-B production.[25] The exact sensitivity and specificity of staining for SP-B have not been determined. A limitation of method is that it requires a lung biopsy in a critically ill, unstable child, or it is limited to a postmortem approach. Such studies can, however, be performed on archived lung specimens, thus allowing for retrospective diagnosis of children who died years earlier. Unfortunately, antisera directed against proSP-C are not widely available, and such testing is currently confined to research laboratories.

It is likely that other inherited disorders may result in abnormal surfactant production and may present with the nonspecific phenotype of RDS. This could result from mutations in the genes for other important enzymes and factors needed for the proper production, intracellular routing, and packaging, secretion, and metabolism of other surfactant components. For example, haploinsufficiency for thyroid transcription factor-1 (TTF-1, also known as NKx2.1) resulting from loss of function mutations on one allele or a gene deletion has been associated with neonatal respiratory disease in full-term infants.[79-81] Similar to the nonspecific appearance of a sepsis-like illness and metabolic disturbances in children with inborn errors of intermediary metabolism, children with inborn errors of lung cell metabolism may present with a nonspecific picture of neonatal respiratory distress and radiographically diffuse lung disease. Elucidation of these inborn errors should enhance our understanding of normal surfactant metabolism and may provide clues to the pathogenesis of lung diseases outside the neonatal period.

Treatment

Unfortunately, hereditary SP-B deficiency is a fatal disease with limited treatment options. Purified preparations of SP-B are not available for replacement therapy. Replacement therapy with exogenous surfactants containing SP-B has been attempted, but it did not alter the course in an antenatally diagnosed infant treated from birth with more than 80 doses of surfactant.[78] Because exogenous replacement surfactants contain variable amounts of SP-B as well as other surfactant components, the amount of SP-B administered may have been insufficient or repeated treatment with surfactant lipids, and SP-C may have been toxic. Even if a preparation of purified SP-B were available, exogenous replacement therapy could be ineffective because it seems likely from the secondary disturbances in SP-C processing and lamellar body biogenesis that SP-B has a critical intracellular role in the packaging and processing of surfactant. Exogenously administered SP-B may not reach the intracellular compartments needed to correct these intracellular deficits, or endogenous proSP-B synthesis may be necessary. Gene therapy may thus eventually be a potential treatment option for the disorder. Viral vectors capable of directing SP-B expression have been generated and tested in *in vitro* and animal systems.[82-84] Among the obstacles that need to be overcome before gene therapy may be considered for human infants include the need for sustained expression within individual cells and throughout the lung and limitation of the potential toxicity of the viral vectors.

Lung transplantation is the only therapy that has proven effective to date. Lung transplantation requires long-term immunosuppressive therapy with continued risks of infection and rejection. The procedure is costly and is available only at a limited number of medical centers. Thus, it usually requires long-distance transport of a critically ill, unstable child. The availability of donor lungs is also limited, and given the severity of the lung disease, death may occur before donor lungs become available. Despite these obstacles, SP-B–deficient infants have received lung transplants with correction of the underlying biochemical abnormalities and survival for up to 8 years after receipt of the transplant, although the ultimate prognosis for these children remains unknown.[46] Because SP-B deficiency is a fatal disorder, compassionate care is an appropriate option once a diagnosis is established. The parents of affected children should also be referred for formal genetic counseling, because there is a 25% recurrence risk for subsequent pregnancies, and prenatal diagnosis may be an option if the mutations responsible for disease in a family are identified.[85]

SURFACTANT PROTEIN C MUTATIONS AND LUNG DISEASE

SP-C is a 35-amino acid, extremely hydrophobic protein that also enhances the surface tension–lowering properties of surfactant phospholipids. SP-C is encoded by a small (<3.5 kB) gene on human chromosome 8 that contains 6 exons, of which the last is untranslated. The gene directs the synthesis of a 900-base pair mRNA that is translated into a proprotein (proSP-C) of either 191 or 197 amino acids, depending on alternative splicing at the beginning of the fifth exon. SP-C is extensively posttranslationally modified, including the palmitoylation of cysteine residues at positions 5 and 6 of mature SP-C, such that it is a proteolipid.[6,86] ProSP-C is proteolytically processed at both the amino- and carboxy-termini to yield the 35-amino acid mature SP-C that is secreted into the air spaces. ProSP-C does not contain a signal peptide, and the domain corresponding to mature SP-C is thought to anchor it in the membrane such that proSP-C is an integral membrane protein. Because of its importance in surfactant function, that SP-C deficiency owing to loss of function mutations could also result in neonatal lung disease resembling RDS is a reasonable hypothesis. To date, no patients with such mutations and RDS have been identified. Moreover, mice genetically engineered to be unable to produce SP-C do not develop neonatal lung disease, although the surfactant from such animals is unstable at low lung volumes.[87] Thus, SP-C does not appear to be essential for normal neonatal lung function.

Mutations in the SP-C gene have been identified in association with human lung disease. In contrast to SP-B deficiency, the phenotype of these patients has generally involved their presentation with signs of lung disease after the neonatal period.[48,88] The lung disease has generally involved predominant interstitial

pneumonitis progressing to pulmonary fibrosis. The course of patients with SP-C mutations has, however, been quite variable; some patients present in early infancy, yet others remain asymptomatic well into adulthood. In familial cases, the disease has been transmitted as an autosomal dominant condition with a high degree of (but not complete) penetrance.[88] Mutations have been identified on only one allele in affected individuals, and the identified mutations are ones that would be predicted to result in an abnormal form of proSP-C, as opposed to null mutations (i.e., missense or in-frame insertions or deletions, as opposed to nonsense mutations.) A proposed pathogenesis for the lung disease associated with SP-C gene mutations involves the mutation causing abnormal folding of proSP-C leading to exposure of hydrophobic epitopes, potential aggregation, and accumulation of misfolded protein early in the secretory pathway, with secondary toxicity to the alveolar Type II cells.[89,90] Because proSP-C self-associates in the secretory pathway, production of abnormal proSP-C from one allele could have a dominant negative effect of SP-C metabolism.[90,91] The potential for misexpression of abnormal SP-C to result in lung disease is demonstrated by the observations that transgenic animals that overexpressed mature SP-C without the flanking domains of the protein died of a marked disruption of lung development.[92] This finding suggests that some SP-C mutations could result in neonatal lung disease. In support of this concept, 4 of 10 patients with SP-C mutations in preliminary report had symptoms as neonates.[93] The incidence and prevalence of lung disease associated with SP-C gene mutations are unknown. Because mutations need be on only one allele to cause disease, *de novo* mutations may result in sporadic disease.

SUMMARY

Hereditary SP-B deficiency is a rare disorder that causes fatal lung disease in full-term infants and demonstrates an essential role for SP-B in normal lung metabolism. Mutations in the SP-C gene are associated with sporadic and familial lung disease of variable severity and age of onset. The pathophysiology of the lung diseases resulting from the lack of SP-B and SP-C, or from abnormally folded proSP-C, is incompletely understood. Environmental factors and other genes that may have roles in modifying the course of these diseases need to be identified, and more effective treatments are necessary. The essential role of SP-B implicates it as a candidate gene by which genetic variability can either directly cause or contribute to lung disease in neonates as well as in older children and adults.

ACKNOWLEDGMENTS

I wish to thank Drs. Timothy Weaver, Jeffrey A. Whitsett, Aaron Hamvas, and F. Sessions Cole for their collaboration, along with Susan Wert, who also provided photographs of immunostained lung tissue. This work is supported by grants from the National Institutes of Health (HL-54703, HL-65174, HL-56387) and the Eudowood Foundation.

REFERENCES

1. Farrell PM, Avery ME: Hyaline membrane disease. Am Rev Respir Dis *111*:657, 1975.
2. Miller HC, Futrakul P: Birth weight, gestational age, and sex as determining factors in the incidence of respiratory distress syndrome of prematurely born infants. J Pediatr *72*:628, 1968.
3. Usher RH, et al: Risk of respiratory distress syndrome related to gestational age, route of delivery, and maternal diabetes. Am J Obstet Gynecol *111*:826, 1971.
4. Whitsett JA, et al: Hydrophobic surfactant-associated protein in whole lung surfactant and its importance for biophysical activity in lung surfactant extracts used for replacement therapy. Pediatr Res *20*:460, 1986.
5. Johansson J, et al: The proteins of the surfactant system. Eur Respir J 7:372, 1994.
6. Weaver TE: Synthesis, processing and secretion of surfactant proteins B and C. Biochim Biophys Acta *1408*:173, 1998.
7. Nogee LM: Genetics of the hydrophobic surfactant proteins. Biochim Biophys Acta *1408*:323, 1998.

8. Voorhout WF, et al: Biosynthetic routing of pulmonary surfactant proteins in alveolar type II cells. Microsc Res Tech 26:366, 1993.
9. Crouch EC: Collectins and pulmonary host defense. Am J Respir Cell Mol Biol 19:177, 1998.
10. Crouch E, et al: Collectins and pulmonary innate immunity. Immunol Rev 173:52, 2000.
11. Crouch E, Wright J: Surfactant proteins A and D and pulmonary host defense. Annu Rev Physiol 63:521, 2001.
12. LeVine AM, et al: Surfactant protein A–deficient mice are susceptible to group B streptococcal infection. J Immunol 158:4336, 1997.
13. LeVine AM, et al: Surfactant protein-A enhances respiratory syncytial virus clearance in vivo. J Clin Invest 103:1015, 1999.
14. LeVine AM, et al: Surfactant protein-A binds group B streptococcus enhancing phagocytosis and clearance from lungs of surfactant protein-A-deficient mice. Am J Respir Cell Mol Biol 20:279, 1999.
15. Korfhagen TR, et al: Surfactant protein-D regulates surfactant phospholipid homeostasis in vivo. J Biol Chem 273:28438, 1998.
16. Botas C, et al: Altered surfactant homeostasis and alveolar type II cell morphology in mice lacking surfactant protein D. Proc Natl Acad Sci USA 95:11869, 1998.
17. Wert SE, et al: Increased metalloproteinase activity, oxidant production, and emphysema in surfactant protein D gene-inactivated mice. Proc Natl Acad Sci USA 97:5972, 2000.
18. Floros J, Hoover RR: Genetics of the hydrophilic surfactant proteins A and D. Biochim Biophys Acta 1408:312, 1998.
19. Nogee LM, et al: Brief report: deficiency of pulmonary surfactant protein B in congenital alveolar proteinosis. N Engl J Med 328:406, 1993.
20. Herman TE, et al: Surfactant protein B deficiency: radiographic manifestations. Pediatr Radiol 23:373, 1993.
21. Newman B, et al: Congenital surfactant protein B deficiency—emphasis on imaging. Pediatr Radiol 31:327, 2001.
22. Nogee LM, et al: Phenotypic variability in hereditary surfactant protein B (SP-B) deficiency. Am J Respir Crit Care Med 161:A523, 2000.
23. Ballard PL, et al: Partial deficiency of surfactant protein B in an infant with chronic lung disease. Pediatrics 96:1046, 1995.
24. Hamvas A, et al: Pathophysiology and treatment of surfactant protein-B deficiency. Biol Neonate 67:18, 1995.
25. Nogee LM, et al: Allelic heterogeneity in hereditary surfactant protein b (SP-B) deficiency. Am J Respir Crit Care Med 161:973, 2000.
26. Pilot-Matias TJ, et al: Structure and organization of the gene encoding human pulmonary surfactant proteolipid SP-B. Dna 8:75, 1989.
27. Beers MF, et al: Pulmonary surfactant metabolism in infants lacking surfactant protein B. Am J Respir Cell Mol Biol 22:380, 2000.
28. Klein JM, et al: Transient surfactant protein B deficiency in a term infant with severe respiratory failure. J Pediatr 132:244, 1998.
29. Tredano M, et al: Compound SFTPB 1549C–>GAA (121ins2) and 457delC heterozygosity in severe congenital lung disease and surfactant protein B (SP-B) deficiency. Hum Mutat 14:502, 1999.
30. Somaschini M, et al: Hereditary surfactant protein B deficiency resulting from a novel mutation. Intensive Care Med 26:97, 2000.
31. Dunbar AE 3rd, et al: Prolonged survival in hereditary surfactant protein B (SP-B) deficiency associated with a novel splicing mutation. Pediatr Res 48:275, 2000.
32. Hawgood S, et al: Structure and properties of surfactant protein B. Biochim Biophys Acta 1408:150, 1998.
33. Guttentag SH, et al: Surfactant protein B processing in human fetal lung. Am J Physiol 275:L559, 1998.
34. Mbagwu N, et al: Sensitivity of synthetic surfactants to albumin inhibition in preterm rabbits. Mol Genet Metab 66:40, 1999.
35. Beck DC, et al: Ablation of a critical surfactant protein B intramolecular disulfide bond in transgenic mice. J Biol Chem 275:3371, 2000.
36. Beck DC, et al: The role of homodimers in surfactant protein B function in vivo. J Biol Chem 275:3365, 2000.
37. Nogee LM, et al: A mutation in the surfactant protein B gene responsible for fatal neonatal respiratory disease in multiple kindreds. J Clin Invest 93:1860, 1994.
38. Ball R, et al: Fatal familial surfactant protein B deficiency (letter). Arch Dis Child 73:F53, 1995.
39. de la Fuente AA, et al: Congenital alveolar proteinosis in the Netherlands: a report of five cases with immunohistochemical and genetic studies on surfactant apoproteins. Pediatr Pathol Lab Med 17:221, 1997.
40. Lin Z, et al: An SP-B gene mutation responsible for SP-B deficiency in fatal congenital alveolar proteinosis: evidence for a mutation hotspot in exon 4. Mol Genet Metab 64:25, 1998.
41. Williams GD, et al: Surfactant protein B deficiency: clinical, histological and molecular evaluation. J Paediatr Child Health 35:214, 1999.
42. Andersen C, et al: Recurrent familial neonatal deaths: hereditary surfactant protein B deficiency. Am J Perinatol 17:219, 2000.
43. Cole FS, et al: Population-based estimates of surfactant protein B deficiency. Pediatrics 105:538, 2000.
44. Hamvas A, et al: Population-based screening for rare mutations: high-throughput DNA extraction and molecular amplification from Guthrie cards. Pediatr Res 50:666, 2001.
45. Nogee LM, et al: Evidence for a common ancestral origin for the most frequent mutation responsible for surfactant protein B (SP-B) deficiency. Pediatr Res 47:370A, 2000.

46. Hamvas A, et al: Lung transplantation for treatment of infants with surfactant protein B deficiency. J Pediatr 130:231, 1997.
47. Vorbroker DK, et al: Aberrant processing of surfactant protein C in hereditary SP-B deficiency. Am J Physiol 268:L647, 1995.
48. Nogee LM, et al: A mutation in the surfactant protein C gene associated with familial interstitial lung disease. N Engl J Med 344:573, 2001.
49. Williams MC, et al: Changes in lipid structure produced by surfactant proteins SP-A, SP-B, and SP-C. Am J Respir Cell Mol Biol 5:41, 1991.
50. deMello DE, et al: Ultrastructure of lung in surfactant protein B deficiency. Am J Respir Cell Mol Biol 11:230, 1994.
51. Coleman M, et al: Pulmonary alveolar proteinosis: an uncommon cause of chronic neonatal respiratory distress. Am Rev Respir Dis 121:583, 1980.
52. Knight DP, Knight JA: Pulmonary alveolar proteinosis in the newborn. Arch Pathol Lab Med 109:529, 1985.
53. Schumacher RE, et al: Pulmonary alveolar proteinosis in a newborn. Pediatr Pulmonol 7:178, 1989.
54. Moulton SL, et al: Congenital pulmonary alveolar proteinosis: failure of treatment with extracorporeal life support. J Pediatr 120:297, 1992.
55. deMello DE, et al: Molecular and phenotypic variability in the congenital alveolar proteinosis syndrome associated with inherited surfactant protein B deficiency. J Pediatr 125:43, 1994.
56. Lin Z, et al: Aberrant SP-B mRNA in lung tissue of patients with congenital alveolar proteinosis (CAP). Clin Genet 57:359, 2000.
57. Dirksen U, et al: Human pulmonary alveolar proteinosis associated with a defect in GM-CSF/IL-3/IL-5 receptor common beta chain expression. J Clin Invest 100:2211, 1997.
58. Clark JC, et al: Targeted disruption of the surfactant protein B gene disrupts surfactant homeostasis, causing respiratory failure in newborn mice. Proc Natl Acad Sci USA 92:7794, 1995.
59. Stahlman MT, et al: Lamellar body formation in normal and surfactant protein B-deficient fetal mice. Lab Invest 80:395, 2000.
60. Clark JC: Decreased lung compliance and air trapping in heterozygous SP-B-deficient mice. Am J Respir Cell Mol Biol 16:46, 1997.
61. Tokieda K, et al: Surfactant protein-B-deficient mice are susceptible to hyperoxic lung injury. Am J Respir Cell Mol Biol 21:463, 1999.
62. Tokieda K, et al: Surfactant protein B corrects oxygen-induced pulmonary dysfunction in heterozygous surfactant protein B-deficient mice. Pediatr Res 46:708, 1999.
63. Yusen RD, et al: Normal lung function in subjects heterozygous for surfactant protein-B deficiency. Am J Respir Crit Care Med 159:411, 1999.
64. Glasser SW, et al: cDNA and deduced amino acid sequence of human pulmonary surfactant-associated proteolipid SPL(Phe). Proc Natl Acad Sci USA 84:4007, 1987.
65. Jacobs KA, et al: Isolation of a cDNA clone encoding a high molecular weight precursor to a 6-kDa pulmonary surfactant-associated protein. J Biol Chem 262:9808, 1987.
66. Lin Z, et al: Polymorphisms of human SP-A, SP-B, and SP-D genes: association of SP-B Thr131Ile with ARDS. Clin Genet 58:181, 2000.
67. Makri V, et al: Polymorphisms of surfactant protein B encoding gene: modifiers of the course of neonatal respiratory distress syndrome? Eur J Pediatr 161:604, 2002.
68. Marttila R, et al: Surfactant protein B polymorphism and respiratory distress syndrome in premature twins. Hum Genet 112:18, 2003.
69. Lin Z, et al: An alternatively spliced surfactant protein B mRNA in normal human lung: disease implication. Biochem J 343:145, 1999.
70. Floros J, et al: Dinucleotide repeats in the human surfactant protein-B gene and respiratory-distress syndrome. Biochem J 305:583, 1995.
71. Haataja R, et al: Surfactant proteins A and B as interactive genetic determinants of neonatal respiratory distress syndrome. Hum Mol Genet 9:2751, 2000.
72. Haataja R, et al: Respiratory distress syndrome: evaluation of genetic susceptibility and protection by transmission disequilibrium test. Hum Genet 109:351, 2001.
73. Kala P, et al: Association of pulmonary surfactant protein A (SP-A) gene and respiratory distress syndrome: interaction with SP-B. Pediatr Res 43:169, 1998.
74. Veletza SV, et al:. Racial differences in allelic distribution at the human pulmonary surfactant protein B gene locus (SP-B). Exp Lung Res 22:489, 1996.
75. Cole FS, et al: Genetic disorders of neonatal respiratory function. Pediatr Res 50:157, 2001.
76. Tryka AF, et al: Absence of lamellar bodies with accumulation of dense bodies characterizes a novel form of congenital surfactant defect. Pediatr Dev Pathol 3:335, 2000.
77. Cutz E, et al: Deficiency of lamellar bodies in alveolar type II cells associated with fatal respiratory disease in a full-term infant. Am J Respir Crit Care Med 161:608, 2000.
78. Hamvas A, et al: Surfactant protein B deficiency: antenatal diagnosis and prospective treatment with surfactant replacement. J Pediatr 125:356, 1994.
79. Iwatani N, et al: Deletion of NKX2.1 gene encoding thyroid transcription factor-1 in two siblings with hypothyroidism and respiratory failure. J Pediatr 137:272, 2000.
80. Krude H, et al: Choreoathetosis, hypothyroidism, and pulmonary alterations due to human NKX2-1 haploinsufficiency. J Clin Invest 109:475, 2002.
81. Pohlenz J, et al: Partial deficiency of thyroid transcription factor 1 produces predominantly neurological defects in humans and mice. J Clin Invest 109:469, 2002.
82. Yei S, et al: Adenoviral-mediated gene transfer of human surfactant protein B to respiratory epithelial cells. Am J Respir Cell Mol Biol 11:329, 1994.

83. Korst RJ, et al: In vitro and in vivo transfer and expression of human surfactant SP-A– and SP-B–associated protein cDNAs mediated by replication-deficient, recombinant adenoviral vectors. Hum Gene Ther 6:277, 1995.

84. Strayer MS, et al: Targeting type II and Clara cells for adenovirus-mediated gene transfer using the surfactant protein B promoter. Am J Respir Cell Mol Biol 18:1, 1998.

85. Stuhrmann M, et al: Prenatal diagnosis of congenital alveolar proteinosis (surfactant protein B deficiency). Prenat Diagn 18:953, 1998.

86. Johansson J: Structure and properties of surfactant protein C. Biochim Biophys Acta 1408:161, 1998.

87. Glasser SW, et al: Altered stability of pulmonary surfactant in SP-C-deficient mice. Proc Natl Acad Sci USA 98:6366, 2001.

88. Thomas AQ, et al: Heterozygosity for a surfactant protein C gene mutation associated with usual interstitial pneumonitis and cellular nonspecific interstitial pneumonitis in one kindred. Am J Respir Crit Care Med 165:1322, 2002.

89. Nogee LM: Abnormal expression of surfactant protein C and lung disease. Am J Respir Cell Mol Biol 26:641, 2002.

90. Wang WJ, et al: Biosynthesis of surfactant protein C (SP-C): sorting of SP-C proprotein involves homomeric association via a signal anchor domain. J Biol Chem 277:19929, 2002.

91. Conkright JJ, et al: Secretion of surfactant protein C, an integral membrane protein, requires the N-terminal propeptide. J Biol Chem 276:14658, 2001.

92. Conkright JJ, et al: Overexpression of surfactant protein-C mature peptide causes neonatal lethality in transgenic mice. Am J Respir Cell Mol Biol 26:85, 2002.

93. Nogee LM, et al: Mutations in the surfactant protein C gene associated with interstitial lung disease. Chest 121:20S, 2002.

SECTION XIV

Physiology of the Gastrointestinal Tract in the Fetus and Neonate

108

Douglas G. Burrin

Trophic Factors and Regulation of Gastrointestinal Tract and Liver Development

FETAL AND NEONATAL GASTROINTESTINAL AND LIVER GROWTH

Nature of Growth

To understand the role of trophic factors in fetal and neonatal gastrointestinal (GI) and hepatic growth, it is important first to consider the nature of growth. The fetal and neonatal period is the most dynamic period of postconceptual growth and includes critical developmental milestones, such as gastrulation, organogenesis, morphogenesis, cellular differentiation, and functional maturation, all of which are described in detail in other chapters in this section. In the case of the intestine, this includes formation of the gut tube, the appearance of villi and digestive enzymes, and the development of swallowing and mature motility patterns.[1] Growth at the tissue and cellular level is characterized by increased cell numbers (i.e., hyperplasia) and increased cellular size (i.e., hypertrophy). Intestinal growth also involves expansion of the number and size of crypt and villus units (Fig. 108-1).[2] Moreover, the timing and characteristics of fetal and neonatal GI and liver growth are coordinated with the events of birth and weaning to ensure survival of the organism. The regulation of the timing and nature of GI and liver growth is complex and involves multiple and often redundant factors. Among these factors are intrinsic cell programs or signals arising from gene expression, as well as extracellular signals (e.g., peptide growth factors, hormones, nutrients, and microbes) that originate from surrounding cells, the circulation, and the gut lumen.

The application of molecular biologic techniques in model organisms such as the mouse, zebrafish, fruit fly, and nematode have revealed that genetic regulatory factors have a critical influence on early organogenesis and morphologic development of the gut, pancreas, and liver.[3-5] These types of studies have identified a group of key homeodomain transcription factor genes, including *hox*, *pdx1*, and *cdx2*, along with the *GATA* family and winged-helix family genes.[6,7] Another important aspect of growth in the gut is the continual proliferation, migration, and loss of epithelial cells along the mucosal surface. In the intestine, this process involves four cell lineages (absorptive enterocyte, goblet, Paneth, and endocrine) that differentiate from one pluripotent stem cell located in the crypt.[8] Recent studies have identified a transcription factor, named math1, that is important for lineage cell commitment in the intestine.[9] The homeodomain transcription factors are also involved in the anteroposterior pattern formation of demarcations in muscular sphincters and regional epithelial morphology along the length of the gut.[1,10] Genetic regulation through homeodomain factors also influences functional maturation of the intestine that occurs during the late gestation and neonatal periods. For example, the expression of lactase-phlorizin hydrolase, a key enzyme involved in digestion of lactose, is up-regulated by a synergistic interaction between Cdx2 and HNF1 transcription factors.[11]

Environmental Influences

Normal GI growth and development during fetal life is critical to facilitate the successful adaptation from nutritional support through umbilical circulation to that of oral ingestion of breast-milk. An increase in circulating fetal glucocorticoid concentration just before and during vaginal birth is an important trigger of gut functional development.[12] In the neonatal period, growth of the GI tract is influenced by multiple physiologic factors that serve to prepare the developing neonate for separation from maternal nutritional support (i.e., weaning). In addition, several important environmental cues signal adaptive changes in GI function to facilitate postweaning survival. For example, the microbial colonization of the gut may serve to prime intestinal lymphoid cell development for normal innate immune function.[13,14] During these processes, extracellular signals, such as peptide growth factors, are often considered to be the major trophic factors that influence growth. However, the term *trophic* actually means "of or pertaining to nutrition," and in the case of the gut, nutrients present in both amniotic fluid and breast milk are a major trophic influence. There are numerous extracellular trophic signals including foods, nutrients, peptide growth factors, gut peptide hormones, steroid and thyroid hormones, microbes, and neural inputs. The cells within the fetal and neonatal GI tract and liver are influenced by extracellular signals from multiple sources including blood-borne factors in the circulation (e.g., hormones that act through endocrine mechanisms); luminal factors derived from amniotic fluid, mammary secretions, or microbes; and local factors secreted through autocrine or paracrine mechanisms from surrounding cells (Fig. 108-2).

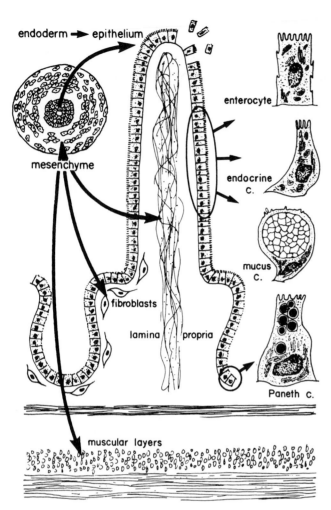

Figure 108–1. Ration of some of the key substrates and nutrients supplied to the gut through the diet and the blood that have been shown to play a role in oxidative metabolism, polyamine synthesis, cell proliferation, inflammation, and mucin production in the intestinal mucosa. (PUFA = polyunsaturated fatty acid; SCFA = short-chain fatty acid.) (From Haffen K, Kedinger M, Simon-Assmann P: Cell contact dependent regulation of enterocytic differentiation. *In* Lebenthal E (ed): Human Gastrointestinal Development. New York, Raven Press, 1989, p. 20)

Some earlier studies have revealed novel insights into the role of mesenchymal cells and luminal microbes on intestinal epithelial growth and differentiation. Mesenchymal cell interactions are mediated through local secretion of tissue growth factors (e.g., fibroblast growth factor [FGF], hepatocyte growth factor [HGF], keratinocyte growth factor [KGF], insulinlike growth factor [IGF]) and basement membrane proteins (laminins, collagens, proteoglycans).[15-17] The extracellular matrix protein, laminin, may be particularly critical for expression of Cdx-2 and induction of epithelial differentiation genes, such as lactase. Interaction between the integrin receptors on the basal surface of epithelial cells with basement membrane proteins can also affect differentiation and cell death. Studies have shown that disruption of the integrin-receptor binding through protease degradation leads to detachment of epithelial cells from the basement membrane and activation of anoikis-mediated apoptotic signaling pathways.[18] Symbiotic relationships between commensal microorganisms and their mammalian host, such as ruminants, are well known. Yet interest is rapidly growing in how these environmental influences also affect the health and disease of the human gut. Studies in conventional and germ-free animals demonstrated that the presence of intestinal microbes exerts a trophic effect on the gut, as evidenced by increased epithelial cell proliferation, mucosal thickness, and lymphoid cell density. Studies with germ-free mice monoassociated with specific bacterial species (e.g. *Bacteroides thetaiotamicron*) have shown how microbes can alter particular pathways of intestinal differentiation.[19] The neonatal gut is sterile, but colonization occurs rapidly during early postnatal life and plays a critical role in development of mucosal immune function. Microbes also produce bioactive molecules and substrates, including toxins and short-chain fatty acids, which influence the proliferation and function of mucosal epithelial and immune cells. The aim of this chapter is to provide a brief overview of some of the major trophic factors in these categories and discuss their relevance to the growth and development of the fetal and neonatal gut and liver. Most of the references cited in this chapter are review articles and the number of original articles listed is limited due to space constraints.

MAJOR TROPHIC FACTORS

Nutrients

Enteral Versus Parenteral

Nutrition is perhaps the most potent trophic stimulus of GI tract growth. The diet acts directly by supplying nutrients for growth and oxidative metabolism of the mucosal epithelial cells, but it also acts indirectly by triggering the release of local growth factors, gut hormones, and activating neural pathways. Maternal malnutrition and neonatal starvation causes reduced gut tissue mass, shortened villi, generalized increased catabolism, and decreased protein synthesis.[20-22] However, the route of nutrient input, either enteral or parenteral, has a critical impact on the trophic response. In the late-gestation fetus, the onset of amniotic fluid swallowing coincides with increased intestinal growth and development. Studies in fetal sheep and pigs have shown that preventing this process by esophageal ligation suppresses intestinal growth.[12, 23] In the neonate, total parenteral nutrition (TPN) leads to significantly reduced growth and atrophy of the intestinal mucosa.[24] The TPN-induced intestinal atrophy is associated with reduced gut DNA and protein mass, cell proliferation, villous height and protein synthesis, and increased apoptosis and proteolysis. Studies with neonatal animals and human infants show that lack of enteral nutrition is also associated with reduced secretion of many gut peptide hormones and growth factors.[24, 25] Animal studies have shown that several growth factors and gut peptides can prevent intestinal atrophy when coinfused with TPN, but few of these studies have been done with neonatal animals. The practice of feeding small volumes of enteral nutrition, known as *minimal enteral feeding* or *trophic feeding*, has been shown to enhance GI motility and other functions.[26] However, the precise relationship between enteral feeding level and gut function has not been established. Studies in neonatal piglets suggest that an enteral intake of between 20 and 40% of the total nutrient intake is necessary to maintain normal growth.[24] An additional consideration is whether to provide enteral nutrition orally, intragastrically, intraduodenally, as a bolus, or continuously. Studies in piglets suggest that, in comparison with continuous feeding, bolus feeding resulted in increased gut growth; however, this does not appear to be linked to secretion of trophic gut peptides.[24]

Breast Milk Versus Formula

The relative significance of milk-borne trophic factors has been one of the most intensely studied areas of pediatric nutrition and gastroenterology.[24,27-31] Many trophic peptide growth factors discussed in this chapter are present in breast milk but not in infant formulas and have been implicated in the beneficial outcomes of

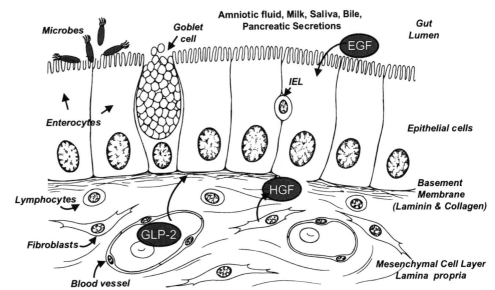

Figure 108–2. Organization of various cell types and structural architecture of intestinal mucosa. Sites of input and expression of selected extracellular factors within the intestinal mucosa are shown. (EGF = epidermal growth factor; GLP-2 = glucagonlike peptide 2; HGF = hepatocyte growth factor).

breast-fed infants. Studies have assessed the relative trophic effect of colostrum and mature milk compared with formula in neonatal animal studies in which macronutrient intake was controlled. These studies have largely confirmed that idea that breast milk has a greater trophic effect on the GI tract than formula, as measured by typical indices of structural and cellular growth. However, the most significant advantage of breast milk on the neonatal intestine may not be related to growth but to mucosal barrier and immune function. There is considerable evidence suggesting that immunoprotective factors in breast milk (e.g., secretory immunoglobulin A, lactoferrin, oligosaccharides) act to modulate mucosal immune function and bacterial colonization, thereby limiting the incidence of infection, sepsis, and necrotizing enterocolitis (NEC).[32-38] Many trophic factors in milk are polypeptides that survive digestion, retain their biologic activity, and interact with specific receptors present on the mucosal epithelium of neonates. Several studies have shown that these milk-borne growth factors stimulate neonatal intestinal growth when given in purified and recombinant forms either orally or systemically. Moreover, in preterm neonates, the presence of increased intestinal permeability could facilitate the intestinal absorption of milk-borne peptide growth factors; however, there are limited instances in which this process has been found to be physiologically significant.

Macronutrients

The chemical form and nutrient composition can also influence the impact of enteral nutrition on GI growth and function.[21,22,24] Some studies indicate that enteral nutrition in a complex, polymeric form is more trophic to the small intestine than in a simpler, more elemental form. The dietary restriction of protein and energy generally suppresses gut growth and mucosal immune function. The enteral infusion of individual nutrients, by themselves, can have a trophic stimulus on the gut if administered in a sufficiently large amount. However, several specific nutrients have trophic actions when used as supplements to a complete diet, among which are glutamine, arginine, threonine, leucine, nucleotides (NTs), short chain fatty acids (SCFAs), long chain polyunsaturated fatty acids (LC-PUFAs) and retinoic acid.

Glutamine is a key intestinal oxidative fuel that is extensively metabolized and oxidized to CO_2 by intestinal tissues when fed either enterally or parenterally.[24,39] However, several studies have shown that enteral and parenteral glutamine also stimulates intestinal growth and enhances function in health and disease.[40,41] Studies in cultured intestinal epithelial cells indicate that glutamine, but not other nonessential amino acids, specifically stim-

ulates cell proliferation, activates mitogenic intracellular signaling pathways,[42] and may be a critical precursor for glucosamine and arginine synthesis.[43] Arginine is an essential amino acid for neonates and may be an important substrate for maintenance of intestinal nitric oxide synthesis, blood flow, and immune function. Some studies have shown that enteral arginine supplementation can reduce the incidence of NEC in neonates.[40] Other nonessential amino acids, including glutamate, proline, and ornithine, have been shown to have stimulatory actions on the gut, perhaps because they are precursors for glutamine and arginine synthesis.[44] Threonine is also a key nutrient for the intestine, because it is used for the synthesis of threonine-rich mucins by goblet cells. The intestinal threonine use by goblet cells appears to be dependent on enteral rather than parenteral route. Studies in liver cells have shown that glutamine and leucine specifically activate anabolic intracellular signaling pathways, involving cell hydration, protein synthesis, and cell death.[45-47]

Nucleotides, which are ubiquitous, low-molecular-weight, intracellular compounds that are integral to numerous biochemical processes, are especially important as precursors for nucleic acid synthesis in rapidly dividing cells, such as epithelial and lymphoid cells in the mucosa.[48] Nucleotides consist of a purine or pyrimidine base, which can be synthesized within cells *de novo* from glutamine, aspartic acid, glycine, formate, and carbon dioxide as precursors, or they can be salvaged from the degradation of nucleic acids and nucleotides. Human milk is an excellent source of dietary nucleotides for infants during the first months of life, and its nucleotide content is markedly higher than that of cow's milk and most infant formulas. Numerous reports show that dietary supplementation with nucleosides, nucleotides, or nucleic acids supports small intestinal mucosal function, growth, and morphology.

SCFAs, largely in the form of acetate, propionate, and butyrate, are produced by microbial fermentation of carbohydrates in the large bowel.[49] Colonic epithelial cells derive most (60-70%) of their energy from SCFAs, and butyrate is the preferred oxidative fuel compared with glucose, glutamine, or ketone bodies. The diet of the human neonate is largely devoid of fiber, yet the production of SCFAs from large bowel microbial fermentation increases with the degree of microbial colonization and postnatal age.[14] Normal substrates for colonic SCFA production in neonates include endogenous secretions and malabsorbed dietary carbohydrates, such as lactose and oligosaccharides.[50] Oligosaccharides are the second most abundant carbohydrate in human milk but are substantially lacking in cow's milk and infant formulas.[33] There is considerable evidence for the specific intestinal trophic effects of SCFAs. Intraluminal and systemic infusions of SCFAs have a stimulatory effect on intestinal mucosal proliferation, gene expression, blood flow, and gut hormone secretion, yet studies with cultured colonic tumor cell lines indicate that butyrate induces differentiation and apoptosis, thereby suppressing neoplasia.[24, 51, 52]

There is considerable interest in dietary LCFAs, because breast milk generally contains higher concentrations of n-3 LC-PUFAs than are found in formulas. As a result, many infant formulas are now being formulated with these fatty acids. Interest in the n-3 LC-PUFAs or ω-3 fatty acids, particularly docosahexanoic acid (DHA), eicosapentaenoic acid (EPA), and arachidonic acid (AA), has been heightened by recent studies showing that supplementing these fatty acids can lower the incidence and inflammatory effects of NEC in neonatal infants and rats.[53] There is limited information regarding the intestinal trophic effects of either n-3 LC-PUFAs or other LCFAs in developing animals. However, a series of studies have demonstrated that n-3 LC-PUFAs enhance intestinal adaptation after small-bowel resection, and their effects were greater than those of less saturated oils; they also found that medium-chain triglycerides are less trophic than long-chain triglycerides.[24] In contrast, studies with neonatal piglets indicated that one LCFA, oleic acid, can cause significant mucosal injury and increased permeability, and that this effect is more severe in newborn than in 1-month-old piglets.[54]

Gastrointestinal Hormones

The gut is one of the largest endocrine organs in the body and secretes numerous peptide hormones primarily in response to nutrient ingestion, but also in response to stage of development and disease. Many gut hormones discussed in this section have been implicated in the stimulation of gut and liver growth in response to enteral nutrition. Gastrin is secreted from the G-cells within the antrum of the stomach and acts primarily to stimulate proliferation of parietal and enterochromaffin-like cells within the gastric mucosa.[55] Cholecystokinin (CCK) is expressed in endocrine cells of the gut and in neurons within the gut and brain; its primary target tissues are the pancreas and gallbladder.[55] There is structural homology between gastrin and CCK with respect to both the peptide sequence and receptor function. Studies have shown that hypogastrinemia, produced by antrectomy and targeted disruption of the gastrin gene, leads to atrophy of the gastric mucosal cells. CCK stimulates pancreatic growth and cell proliferation, and these trophic effects have been attributed exclusively to interaction through the CCK-A receptor. The neonate exhibits hypergastrinemia and comparatively high gastric pH, yet gastrin secretion is induced by feeding.[25] The development of pentagastrin-responsive gastric acid secretion occurs within 1 week in neonatal piglets and can be prematurely induced with glucocorticoids, consistent with up-regulation of gastrin receptor expression with age.[23] The trophic effects of gastrin are most evident in the stomach and are mediated by increased ornithine decarboxylase (ODC) activity and cell proliferation.[56] Gastrin-releasing peptide (GRP) is a 27-amino acid peptide with a C-terminus region that is structurally related to bombesin, a 14-amino acid neuropeptide found in amphibian skin.[57] Gastrin-releasing peptide is secreted from neurons located throughout the GI tract in response to vagal stimulation. Bombesin is also found in milk, and both oral and systemic administration to suckling animals stimulates intestinal growth.[24, 29]

Glucagonlike peptide 2 (GLP-2) is a product of the intestinal proglucagon gene expressed in the enteroendocrine "L" cells located predominantly in the distal intestine.[58] GLP-2 is secreted in response to feeding, especially carbohydrate, and studies in fetal and neonatal piglets suggest an ontogenic increase in GLP-2 secretion.[59] GLP-2 has significant trophic effects on the neonatal gut that are mediated by increased cell proliferation, protein synthesis, blood flow, and glucose transport. Peptide YY (PYY) is secreted from the same enteroendocrine cell as the glucagonlike peptides GLP-1 and 2, and together these hormones have been implicated as factors responsible for the so-called ileal-brake phenomenon. Studies indicate that PYY stimulates gut growth in some, but not all, cases and does not stimulate proliferation of cultured epithelial cells. Neurotensin is a 13-amino-acid peptide secreted from the enteroendocrine "N" cells located exclusively in the gut within the distal small intestine.[60] Neurotensin expression is markedly increased during the neonatal period, and secretion is stimulated specifically by ingestion of fat. Administration of neurotensin stimulates gut growth in animals following small bowel resection even in the absence of enteral nutrients.

Tissue Growth Factors

Tissue growth factors can be generally categorized as polypeptides that are secreted locally and act through paracrine or autocrine mechanisms to affect cellular growth and function. However, several tissue growth factors are also present in the blood and GI secretions and thus may act through an endocrine mechanism, for example, IGF-I. Moreover, many of these growth factors are present in breast milk and thought to influence neonatal gut growth.[24, 27-31, 61] Among the best known of these is EGF, a member of a family of peptides that includes transforming growth factor-alpha (TGF-α), amphiregulin, heparin-binding EGF, epiregulin (EPR), betacellulin (BTC), neuregulin (NRG), and neuregulin 2 (NRG2).[62] These factors act as ligands for membrane-bound EGF receptor and other EGF-related (ErbB family) receptors that become activated through phosphorylation on binding. EGF is widely distributed in most body fluids (notably mammary, salivary, biliary, and pancreatic secretions), but is not produced in epithelial cells, in contrast to its homologue, TGF-α. Most of the EGF family peptides are trophic to the gut, stimulating cell proliferation and suppressing apoptosis; however, they also modulate several other physiologic functions including accelerated tooth eruption, decreased gastric acid secretion, increased mucus secretion and gastric blood flow, reduced gastric emptying, and increased sodium and glucose transport.[63-65,80] EGF also has been found to increase mucosal growth and functional adaptation following intestinal resection, diarrhea, and TPN and to prevent the incidence of NEC. Enteral nutrition stimulates GI secretion, resulting in the release of EGF into the gut lumen where it is postulated to play a protective role, whereas TGF-α functions in the maintenance of epithelial cell proliferation and migration in the healthy gut.[65] EGF appears to be more trophic to the gut when it is given intravenously than when given enterally, perhaps because the EGF receptor is localized to the basolateral membrane. However, many neonatal animal studies have shown that oral EGF administration augments gut growth and functional development.[24] These findings, combined with recent evidence from transgenic mice, support the idea that both local expression and milk-borne ingestion of EGF and TGF-α play a physiologic role in neonatal gut growth and development.

The IGF family of peptides includes insulin, IGF-I, and IGF-II.[24, 28, 66-68] The biologic actions of insulin are mediated through the insulin receptor, whereas the actions of both IGF-I and IGF-II are largely mediated through the Type I IGF receptor. The insulin and Type I IGF receptors are present in epithelial cells; they are more abundant on the basolateral than apical membrane, and they are more abundant in proliferating crypt cells than in differentiated enterocytes. Although insulin secretion is confined to the pancreas, both IGF-I and IGF-II are expressed throughout the body, including the gut. However, within the intestinal mucosa, expression of both IGF-I and II appears to be localized to mesenchymal cells in the lamina propria, although epithelial cells may also produce IGF-II. The expression of IGF-I and II in the gut is highest in the fetal and neonatal period and declines with age. In addition, insulin, IGF-I, and IGF-II are present in milk, and IGF-I is also found in salivary, biliary, and pancreatic secretions and in amniotic fluid. Numerous studies have shown that either administering IGF systemically or increasing its expression locally (as in transgenic mice) stimulates intestinal growth and function in normal animals and under conditions of TPN administration, gut resection, dexamethasone treatment, sepsis, and radiation therapy. The expression of IGF-binding proteins has been shown to inhibit IGF action in gut tissues. Some studies in fetal and neonatal animals given pharmacologic oral doses of insulin and IGF-I have demonstrated a stimulation of gut growth, disaccharidase activity, and glucose transport.[24,69] Others however have shown only limited effects of oral IGF on the neonatal gut, thus suggesting that the IGFs may not play a physiologic role in the neonate. GH has a major influence on IGF-I expression during postnatal growth, and studies in postweanling rodents indicate that hypophysectomy results in gut atrophy, whereas transgenic overexpression of GH in mice increases gut growth.[24,67,70] However, the significance of GH in neonatal gut and liver growth may be limited by the abundance and responsiveness of the GH-receptor. Studies with hypophysectomized neonatal rats suggest some degree of pituitary-dependent intestinal growth and development. Other studies in rats demonstrate that GH treatment does not prevent TPN-induced intestinal atrophy but may augment intestinal growth after massive small bowel resection.[63]

TGF-β is structurally unrelated to TGF-α and is found in three major forms (TGFβ 1-3) in mammalian tissues.[71] TGF-β expression has been found throughout the small intestine in both lamina propria and epithelial cells; the levels are low in neonates and increase with age. In contrast, the levels of TGF-β-2 are high in early milk and decline as lactation progresses. At least five receptors (Types I-V) have been found to bind one or more of the various TGF-β ligands, although the Type I and II receptors appear to mediate the effects on cell proliferation. TGF-β is a potent inhibitor of epithelial cell proliferation and may also induce differentiation. TGF-β has been implicated as an intermediate signal whereby butyrate suppresses proliferation and induces differentiation of colonic epithelial cells. TGF-β also stimulates epithelial cell migration and production of extracellular matrix proteins such as collagen through induction of connective tissue growth factor, thus making it a critical factor in the process of restitution of the epithelium following mucosal damage.[72] This latter function of TGF-β may play an important role in the intestinal inflammatory response, as evidenced by the fact that its expression is up-regulated in inflammatory bowel disease and that TGF-β–deficient transgenic mice develop inflammatory disease.

HGF, vascular endothelial growth factor, FGF, and KGF are expressed in the gut tissues, where they may play a role in mucosal growth and repair.[24] HGF is expressed by mesenchymal but not epithelial cells, whereas the HGF receptor (c-met) is found in epithelial cells; the c-met receptor is localized on the basolateral membrane. Studies with cultured intestinal epithelial cells demonstrate that HGF stimulates cell proliferation and wound closure proliferation but decreases transepithelial resistance.[73,74] HGF is found in human milk mononuclear cells and partially accounts for the stimulatory effect of human milk on intestinal cell proliferation. Studies in rats have shown that HGF, given either systemically or orally, increased gut growth and nutrient transport after massive small bowel resection.

VEGF is expressed in the small intestine, predominantly in the lamina propria mast cells.[24] A recent report indicates that the receptor (flt-1) for the VEGF 165 amino acid isoform is present in intestinal epithelial cells; however, VEGF did not stimulate cell proliferation of these cells. Another recent report, in mice, demonstrated that VEGF and FGF-2 reduce the rate of crypt cell apoptosis following total body irradiation treatment. FGF and the FGF receptors have been found in intestinal tissues, yet their function remains poorly understood. Both VEGF and FGF-2 have been implicated in angiogenesis during intestinal repair.[75] Increased local expression of KGF has been found in patients with inflammatory bowel disease, and administration of KGF enhanced mucosal healing in rats following induction of colitis.[76] The trefoil factors are a family of peptides (TFF1–TFF3) that play an important protective role in gut.[77] TFF3 is expressed and secreted from goblet cells of the small and large intestine; these peptides interact with mucins on the apical cell surface. Trefoil peptides have been shown to promote cell migration and suppress apoptosis through activation of intracellular signaling pathways linked to mitogen-activated kinase and the EGF receptor; however, TFF receptors have not been identified.

Glucocorticoids and Thyroid Hormones

The role of glucocorticoids and thyroid hormones on neonatal intestinal development has been studied extensively, especially in rodents.[78] The impact of glucocorticoids, particularly dexamethasone, on human intestinal growth and development has received considerable attention in the past decade because of their influence on pulmonary function in premature infants.[79] Studies in fetal animals suggest that increased endogenous glucocorticoid levels are critical signals that stimulate GI development and growth.[23] The prenatal cortisol surge is an important signal for development of the neonate, and premature birth precludes the exposure to this key intestinal maturation signal. This idea is supported by studies in infants and piglets showing that premature birth results in insufficient intestinal maturation of intestinal lactase and lactose digestive capacity.[12,50] Numerous studies demonstrate how glucocorticoids stimulate neonatal intestinal development and maturation, especially with regard to disaccharidase expression.[78] However, their effects on neonatal mucosal growth, *per se*, as indicated by cell proliferation, cell cycle, protein turnover, and apoptosis are not completely understood. Studies *in vivo* and *in vitro* suggest that glucocorticoids inhibit intestinal mucosal growth by suppressing cell proliferation and increasing protein catabolism.[24] Likewise, triiodothyronine (T_3) induces apoptosis in primary intestinal cell cultures. Studies have also shown a link between local intestinal thyroid-stimulating hormone expression and intraepithelial lymphocyte development. The epithelial expression of both thyroid-releasing hormone receptors, coupled with the fact that thyroid-releasing hormone is present in milk, may also provide a connection between breast milk and mucosal immune function in the neonate.[30]

REFERENCES

1. Montgomery RK, et al: Development of the human gastrointestinal tract: twenty years of progress. Gastroenterology *116*:702, 1999.
2. Cheng H, Bjerknes M: Whole population cell kinetics and postnatal development of the mouse intestinal epithelium. Anat Rec *211*:420, 1985.
3. Roberts DJ: Molecular mechanisms of development of the gastrointestinal tract. Dev Dyn *219*:109, 2000.
4. Simon TC, Gordon JI: Intestinal epithelial cell differentiation: new insights from mice, flies and nematodes. Curr Opin Genet Dev *5*:577, 1995.
5. Bates MD, et al: Novel genes and functional relationships in the adult mouse gastrointestinal tract identified by microarray analysis. Gastroenterology *122*:1467, 2002.
6. Beck F, et al: Homeobox genes and gut development. Bioessays *22*:431, 2000.
7. Scharfmann R: Control of early development of the pancreas in rodents and humans: implications of signals from the mesenchyme. Diabetologia *43*:1083, 2000.
8. Bjerknes M, Cheng H: Clonal analysis of mouse intestinal epithelial progenitors. Gastroenterology *116*:7, 1999.
9. Yang Q, et al: Requirement of Math1 for secretory cell lineage commitment in the mouse intestine. Science *294*:2155, 2001.

10. Beck F: Homeobox genes in gut development. Gut *51*:450, 2002.
11. Mitchelmore C, et al: Interaction between the homeodomain proteins Cdx2 and HNF1alpha mediates expression of the lactase-phlorizin hydrolase gene. Biochem J; *346*:529, 2000.
12. Sangild, PT, et al: How does the foetal gastrointestinal tract develop in preparation for enteral nutrition after birth? Livestock Production Science *66*:141, 2000.
13. Brandtzaeg PE: Current understanding of gastrointestinal immunoregulation and its relation to food allergy. Ann NY Acad Sci *964*:13, 2002.
14. Mackie RI, et al: Developmental microbial ecology of the neonatal gastrointestinal tract. Am J Clin Nutr *69*:1035S, 1999.
15. Ilieva A, et al: Pancreatic islet cell survival following islet isolation: the role of cellular interactions in the pancreas. J Endocrinol *161*:357, 1999.
16. Kedinger M, et al: Intestinal epithelial-mesenchymal cell interactions. Ann N Y Acad Sci *859*:1, 1998.
17. Beaulieu JF: Integrins and human intestinal cell functions. Front Biosci *4*:D310, 1999.
18. Frisch SM, Screaton RA: Anoikis mechanisms. Curr Opin Cell Biol *13*:555, 2001.
19. Hooper LV, et al: How host-microbial interactions shape the nutrient environment of the mammalian intestine. Annu Rev Nutr *22*:283, 2002.
20. Raul F, et al: Longitudinal distribution of brush border hydrolases and morphological maturation in the intestine of the preterm infant. Early Hum Dev *13*:225, 1986.
21. Raul F, Schleiffer R: Intestinal adaptation to nutritional stress. Proc Nutr Soc *55*:279, 1996.
22. Jenkins AP, Thompson RP: Mechanisms of small intestinal adaptation. Dig Dis *12*:15, 1994.
23. Trahair JF, Sangild PT: Systemic and luminal influences on the perinatal development of the gut. Equine Vet J Suppl:40, 1997.
24. Burrin DG, Stoll B: Key nutrients and growth factors for the neonatal gastrointestinal tract. Clin Perinatol *29*:65, 2002.
25. Berseth CL: Minimal enteral feedings. Clin Perinatol *22*:195, 1995.
26. McClure RJ: Trophic feeding of the preterm infant. Acta Paediatr Suppl *90*:19, 2001.
27. Hamosh M: Bioactive factors in human milk. Pediatr Clin North Am *48*:69, 2001.
28. Donovan SM, Odle J: Growth factors in milk as mediators of infant development. Annu Rev Nutr *14*:147, 1994.
29. Koldovsky O: Hormonally active peptides in human milk. Acta Paediatr Suppl *402*:89, 1994.
30. Grosvenor CE, et al: Hormones and growth factors in milk. Endocr. Rev. *14*:710, 1993.
31. Buts JP: Bioactive factors in milk. Arch Pediatr *5*:298, 1998.
32. Claud EC, Walker WA: Hypothesis: inappropriate colonization of the premature intestine can cause neonatal necrotizing enterocolitis. FASEB J *15*:1398, 2001.
33. Kunz C, et al: Oligosaccharides in human milk: structural, functional, and metabolic aspects. Annu Rev Nutr *20*:699, 2000.
34. Dai D, et al: Role of oligosaccharides and glycoconjugates in intestinal host defense. J Pediatr Gastroenterol Nutr *30*(Suppl 2):S23, 2000.
35. Rodriguez-Palmero M, et al: Nutritional and biochemical properties of human milk: II. Lipids, micronutrients, and bioactive factors. Clin Perinatol *26*:335, 1999.
36. Garofalo RP, Goldman AS: Expression of functional immunomodulatory and anti-inflammatory factors in human milk. Clin Perinatol *26*:361, 1999.
37. Bernt KM, Walker WA: Human milk as a carrier of biochemical messages. Acta Paediatr Suppl *88*:27, 1999.
38. Dai D, Walker WA: Protective nutrients and bacterial colonization in the immature human gut. Adv Pediatr *46*:353, 1999.
39. Burrin DG, Stoll B: Modulators of gut growth and intestinal well-being. *In* Lifschitz CH (ed): Pediatric Gastroenterology and Nutrition in Clinical Practice. New York, Marcel Dekker, 2001, pp 75–112.
40. Neu J, et al: Glutamine: clinical applications and mechanisms of action. Curr Opin Clin Nutr Metab Care *5*:69, 2002.
41. Neu J: Glutamine in the fetus and critically ill low birth weight neonate: metabolism and mechanism of action. J Nutr *131*:2585S, 2001.
42. Rhoads, M. Glutamine signaling in intestinal cells. JPEN J Parenter Enteral Nutr *23*:S38, 1999.
43. Wu G, et al: Arginine nutrition in development, health and disease. Curr Opin Clin Nutr Metab Care *3*:59, 2000.
44. Gardiner KR, et al.: Novel substrates to maintain gut integrity. Nutr Res Rev *8*:43, 1995.
45. Kimball SR, Jefferson LS: Control of protein synthesis by amino acid availability. Curr Opin Clin Nutr Metab Care *5*:63, 2002.
46. Haussinger D, et al: Glutamine and cell signaling in liver. J Nutr *131*:2509S, 2001.
47. van Sluijters DA, et al: Amino-acid-dependent signal transduction. Biochem J *351*:545, 2000.
48. Carver JD: Dietary nucleotides: effects on the immune and gastrointestinal systems. Acta Paediatr Suppl *88*:83, 1999.
49. Cummings JH, Macfarlane GT: Role of intestinal bacteria in nutrient metabolism. JPEN J Parenter Enteral Nutr *21*:357, 1997.
50. Kien CL: Digestion, absorption, and fermentation of carbohydrates in the newborn. Clin Perinatol *23*:211, 1996.
51. Hague A, et al: Butyrate acts as a survival factor for colonic epithelial cells: further fuel for the in vivo versus in vitro debate. Gastroenterology *112*:1036, 1997
52. Velazquez OC, et al: Butyrate and the colonocyte. Production, absorption, metabolism, and therapeutic implications. Adv Exp Med Biol *427*:123, 1997.
53. Caplan MS, Jilling T: The role of polyunsaturated fatty acid supplementation in intestinal inflammation and neonatal necrotizing enterocolitis. Lipids *36*:1053, 2001.
54. Crissinger KD, et al: An animal model of necrotizing enterocolitis induced by infant formula and ischemia in developing piglets. Gastroenterology *106*:1215, 1994.
55. Walsh JH: Gastrointestinal hormones. *In* Johnson LR, et al (eds): Physiology of the Gastrointestinal Tract. New York, Raven Press, 1994, pp 1–128.
56. Johnson LR, McCormick SA: Regulation of gastrointestinal mucosal growth. *In* Johnson LR, et al (eds): Physiology of the Gastrointestinal Tract. New York, Raven Press, 1994, pp 611–641.
57. Dockray GJ: Physiology of enteric neuropeptides. *In* Johnson LR, et al (eds): Physiology of the Gastrointestinal Tract. New York, Raven Press, 1994, pp 169–209.
58. Drucker DJ: Gut adaptation and the glucagon-like peptides. Gut 50:428, 2002.
59. Burrin DG, et al: Glucagon-like peptide 2: A nutrient-responsive gut growth factor. J Nutr *131*:709, 2001.
60. Evers BM: Expression of the neurotensin/neuromedin N gene in the gut. *In* Greeley GH Jr (ed): Gastrointestinal Endocrinology. Totowa, NJ, Humana, 1999, 425–438.
61. Polk DB, Barnard JA: Hormones and growth factors in intestinal development. *In* Sanderson I, Walker WA (eds): Development of the Gastrointestinal Tract. Hamilton, Ontario, Decker, 2000, pp 37–56.
62. Barnard JA, et al: Epidermal growth factor–related peptides and their relevance to gastrointestinal pathophysiology. Gastroenterology *108*:564, 1995.
63. Thompson JS: Epidermal growth factor and the short bowel syndrome. JPEN J Parenter Enteral Nutr *23*:S113, 1999.
64. Wong WM, Wright NA: Epidermal growth factor, epidermal growth factor receptors, intestinal growth, and adaptation. JPEN J Parenter Enteral Nutr *23*:S83, 1999.
65. Seare NJ, Playford RJ: Growth factors and gut function. Proc Nutr Soc *57*:403, 1998.
66. MacDonald RS: The role of insulin-like growth factors in small intestinal cell growth and development. Horm Metab Res *31*:103, 1999.
67. Lund PK: Molecular basis of intestinal adaptation: the role of the insulin-like growth factor system. Ann NY Acad Sci *859*:18, 1998.
68. Hill DJ, et al: Growth factors and the regulation of fetal growth. Diabetes Care *21*(Suppl 2):B60, 1998.
69. Kimble RM, et al: Enteral IGF-I enhances fetal growth and gastrointestinal development in oesophageal ligated fetal sheep. J Endocrinol *162*:227, 1999.
70. Ney DM: Effects of insulin-like growth factor-I and growth hormone in models of parenteral nutrition. JPEN J Parenter Enteral Nutr *23*:S184, 1999.
71. Podolsky DK: Peptide growth factors in the gastrointestinal tract. *In* Johnson LR, et al (eds): Physiology of the Gastrointestinal Tract. New York, Raven Press, 1994, pp 129–167.
72. Podolsky DK: Mucosal immunity and inflammation. V. Innate mechanisms of mucosal defense and repair: the best offense is a good defense. Am J Physiol 277:G495, 1999.
73. Nusrat A, et al: Hepatocyte growth factor/scatter factor effects on epithelia. Regulation of intercellular junctions in transformed and nontransformed cell lines, basolateral polarization of c-met receptor in transformed and natural intestinal epithelia, and induction of rapid wound repair in a transformed model epithelium. J Clin Invest 93:2056, 1994.
74. Goke M, et al: Intestinal fibroblasts regulate intestinal epithelial cell proliferation via hepatocyte growth factor. Am J Physiol *274*:G809, 1998.
75. Jones MK, et al: Gastrointestinal mucosal regeneration: role of growth factors. Front Biosci *4*:D303, 1999.
76. Farrell CL, et al: The effects of keratinocyte growth factor in preclinical models of mucositis. Cell Prolif *35*(Suppl 1):78, 2002.
77. Podolsky DK: Mechanisms of regulatory peptide action in the gastrointestinal tract: trefoil peptides. J Gastroenterol *35*(Suppl 12):69, 2000.
78. Henning SJ, et al: Ontogeny of the intestinal mucosa. *In* Johnson LR, et al (eds): Physiology of the Gastrointestinal Tract. New York, Raven Press, 1994, pp 571–610.
79. Yeung MY, Smyth JP: Hormonal factors in the morbidities associated with extreme prematurity and the potential benefits of hormonal supplement. Biol Neonate *81*:1, 2002.
80. Uribe JM, Barrett KE: Non-mitogenic actions of growth factors: an integrated view of their role in intestinal physiology and pathophysiology. Gastroenterology *112*:255, 1997.

109 Organogenesis of the Gastrointestinal Tract

Prenatal morphogenesis comprises a series of events that begins with fertilization and ends with parturition—the act of expulsion of the fetus from the uterus. The prenatal period is generally divided into an embryonic period (gestational weeks 1-10), a fetal period (gestational weeks 11-28), and a perinatal period (gestational weeks 29-40). Blastogenesis (formation of the primary germ cell layers) occurs during the embryonic period. The majority of organogenesis occurs during the fetal period, although some occurs earlier than the tenth gestational week. This chapter details the events of organogenesis of the gastrointestinal tract.

The gastrointestinal tract develops from the primitive digestive tube, which is derived from the dorsal or intraembryonic portion of the yolk sac. The digestive tube develops after the initial development of the embryo and contains all three distinct germ cell layers (ectodermal, mesodermal, and endodermal); however, it consists primarily of endodermal components. At 3.5 weeks' gestation, the gut becomes distinct from the yolk sac. Before that time, the yolk sac is broadly attached to the midgut of the digestive tube. The connection of the yolk sac to the digestive tube is through the vitelline (omphalomesenteric) duct, and the digestive tube is suspended from the dorsal wall of the embryo by the dorsal mesentery. Additionally, the anterior portion of the gut is suspended from the ventral body wall by a ventral mesentery. The digestive tube is closed anteriorly by the buccopharyngeal membrane and posteriorly by the cloacal membrane.

A good understanding of the boundaries and distribution of the foregut, midgut, and hindgut can be obtained by understanding that there are three major arteries supplying the digestive tube. The celiac axis is responsible for the foregut, the superior mesenteric artery supplies the midgut, and the inferior mesenteric artery supplies the hindgut. The anatomic boundaries of the digestive tube are the anterior aspects of the foregut, including the pharynx and oral cavity; the posterior aspects of the foregut, including the esophagus, stomach, and upper duodenum; the midgut, which develops into the distal duodenum, the jejunum and ileum, the cecum, appendix, and transverse colon; and the hindgut, which differentiates into the descending colon, the sigmoid colon, and the upper two-thirds of the rectum.

ESOPHAGUS

Organogenesis

At 22 to 23 days' gestation, a median ventral diverticulum is first noted within the region of the posterior confines of the developing foregut. This diverticulum, which is destined to become the cranial end of the fetus' esophagus and trachea, is termed the *tracheal diverticulum.* The diverticulum becomes groovelike as it elongates concurrently with the proliferation of endodermal cells at its lateral aspect. This phenomenon forms lateral ridges, which themselves ultimately create a division between the trachea and the esophagus occurring at 34 to 36 days' gestation. Muscular and submucosal layers are present at this time point, and it is at this stage in development that tracheoesophageal anomalies such as the relatively common tracheoesophageal fistula occur. As these tracheoesophageal folds continue to develop, a spindle-shaped dilation occurs along the caudal aspect of the foregut—this structure ultimately becomes the

stomach. The foregut between this dilation and the tracheal diverticulum is the *developing esophagus.* Elongation of the developing esophagus occurs first craniad and then caudad so that it is ascent of the pharynx rather than descent of the stomach that accounts for most esophageal growth. By 7 weeks' gestation, the final, relative length of esophagus is achieved. Additionally, any tracheoesophageal anomalies are present and, theoretically, identifiable at this stage of development.[1]

Anomalies of Embryogenesis

Esophageal atresia and *tracheoesophageal fistula* are commonly found in association. In the most common form of this anomaly, there is a blind proximal esophageal pouch associated with a distal tracheoesophageal fistula. As shown in Figure 109-1, other, less common configurations can be observed. Interruption of the events responsible for elongation and separation of the esophageal and tracheal tubes during the fourth fetal week is thought to lead to the development of this anomaly. The most full-blown manifestation of this disease of embryogenesis is a complete communication between the esophagus and trachea, or *laryngotracheoesophageal cleft.*

Most presentations of *esophageal stenosis* in children and adults result from an acquired anomaly rather than a congenital defect. However, a narrowing of the esophagus is occasionally found in the middle to distal third of the esophagus and presents as either a web or a long segment of narrowed esophagus. This anomaly likely results from incomplete recanalization of the esophagus. Another form of esophageal stenosis is one created by the presence of abnormal tissue rests within the esophageal wall. Often called an *esophageal ring,* this is commonly respiratory tissue and often contains cartilage as well as ciliated epithelium.[2] This lesion is generally found within the lower third of the esophagus.

Esophageal duplications may be in direct communication with the esophagus or they may lie within the mediastinum completely separate from the esophagus. It is generally believed that intramural duplications or those that communicate directly with the esophagus are examples of faulty recanalization of the esophageal lumen (as suggested by the Bremer theory of duplications), whereas the etiology of those duplications lying free within the mediastinum-thorax is not so easily understood.[3] Results of separate studies by Bentley and Smith[4] and by McLetchie and partners have suggested that the developmental error underlying the formation of these cysts occurs during the formation of the notochord (at 18 to 19 days' gestation) before development of the foregut itself has begun.[4,5] Attachment of endodermal cells to the developing notochord permits formation of such enterogenous cysts.

As already noted, during the development of the esophagus the lining is initially columnar epithelium, which later becomes ciliated as the transition is made to the final stratified squamous epithelium. As this differentiation proceeds, if glandular columnar epithelium develops instead of the stratified squamous epithelium, gastric-type epithelium can occur within the esophagus. Termed *heterotopic mucosa,* this is a particularly common finding, and as many as 70% of clinically normal people are known to have such ectopic mucosa at some point within their esophagus.[6] Intraesophageal thyroid tissue has also been described;[7] the embryogenesis of this phenomenon is obscure.

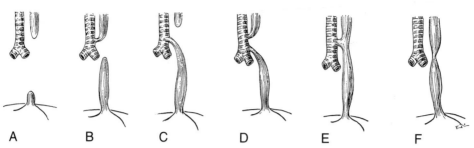

Figure 109–1. A–F, Types of esophageal atresia and tracheoesophageal fistula. Type *C,* with a blind proximal esophageal pouch and distal tracheoesophageal fistula, is the most common presentation (85%) of this anomaly. Type *A,* isolated esophageal atresia and type *E,* isolated (H-type) tracheoesophageal fistula constitute about 10% of this entity. (From Gross RE: The Surgery of Infancy and Childhood. Philadelphia, WB Saunders Co, 1953, p 76.)

Because it is known that the elongation of the esophagus is a phenomenon that creates the "descent" of the stomach, one can conceptualize that cessation of the elongation before the time that the stomach has reached the appropriate level would result in a situation in which a portion of the stomach remains in the thorax. This is a true *congenital short esophagus,* and the fact that a portion of the stomach remains supradiaphragmatic needs to be distinguished from a similar condition in which the supradiaphragmatic stomach is the result of a hiatal hernia.

STOMACH

Organogenesis

At 4- to 5-weeks' gestation, a fusiform dilation at the caudal region of the foregut is first noted. There remains disagreement within the literature about whether the initial fusiform dilation destined to become the stomach occurs before or after the initial appearance of the tracheal diverticulum; however, it is known that the initial enlargement of the stomach is in a ventrodorsal direction.[1] The stomach begins its development at the C3 to C5 level. Because of the marked cephalic growth of the foregut, "descent" of the stomach occurs so that its eventual final location is in the region between T10 and L3. Although still unproved, it is generally believed that as the stomach develops, its dorsal border grows more rapidly than the ventral border does so that a 90° clockwise rotation occurs on its longitudinal axis. As a result of this leftward rotation, the dorsal border of the stomach becomes the greater curvature of the organ, whereas the ventral border rotates toward the right and becomes the lesser curvature. The end result is that the original left side of the stomach becomes its ventral surface and the original right side of the stomach becomes its dorsal surface; the pylorus rotates upward and to the right and the cardia rotates downward and to the left. There have been studies challenging this classic hypothesis, and the suggestion has been made that the left side of the stomach becomes the greater curvature (this anatomic orientation could result from accelerated growth only, with no actual rotation).[1] Although both hypotheses have solid foundations, it seems that the rotational hypothesis better explains why the left vagus supplies the anterior portion of the stomach and the right vagus innervates the posterior wall. Regardless, it is known that the final position of the longitudinal axis of the stomach is transverse to the longitudinal axis of the body itself and that this process is completed by approximately 8 weeks' gestation.

Anomalies of Embryogenesis

Total agenesis of the stomach is an anomaly not encountered in otherwise viable infants. *Microgastria* is not uncommonly encountered and is believed to be the result of a failure or arrest of appropriate development of the caudal portion of the embryologic foregut. It is almost always associated with an enlarged esophagus and incomplete gastric rotation.[8] Although the mucosa of the gastric wall is normal, there may be other associated gastrointestinal anomalies—most frequently, incomplete rotation. Asplenia is a common concurrent finding, which is not unexpected because embryologically the spleen is derived from the dorsal mesogastrium, which has an intimate relationship with the developing stomach. *Gastric atresias,* almost always partial and in the form of membranous diaphragms, have been encountered, as have been complete, solid atresias of a portion of the stomach. Discontinuity of the stomach may occur in cases of such solid atresias. These atresias tend to be located within the antral and pyloric regions, and infants present as newborns with complete gastric outlet obstruction. Incomplete prepyloric membranes also occur. The embryologic characteristics of gastric atresias are considered to be different from those encountered within the duodenum, because there is no solid phase of epithelial occlusion of the stomach during development. It has been suggested that areas of endodermal redundancy may be the origin of small, weblike membranous diaphragms, whereas the larger zones of atresia are thought to be due to local attenuation of the developing endodermal tube during the formation of the pylorus. In this instance, endodermal proliferation fails to keep up with the elongating foregut.[1] Others have suggested that an *in utero* vascular accident (as occurs with other small and large intestinal atresias) is the cause of the solid atresias found within the gastric region; however, most clinicians favor the former theory.[9]

Pyloric stenosis results from hypertrophy of the muscularis of the pyloric channel, especially the circular muscle. It was for a long period considered to be a developmental defect of the pyloric musculature and thus congenital. Because this anomaly generally occurs at about 3 weeks of life and has not been known to occur earlier than the fourth or fifth day of life, it is no longer considered to be a true congenital defect. Its pathogenesis remains, essentially, unexplained.

Most *gastric duplications* occur along the greater curvature or on the anteroposterior walls of the stomach. Communications to the stomach are not always present, and the mucosal lining is generally gastric. Several embryologic theories have been suggested, which include the persistence of vacuoles within the primitive foregut epithelium[3] and the persistence of embryonic diverticula.[10] However, as with the esophagus, larger duplications as well as those that lie completely outside the normal gastric wall are likely the result of faulty separation of the notochord and endoderm.[5]

Acute gastric *volvulus* in children is a rare condition. Chronic gastric volvulus is encountered more frequently. Gastric volvulus is the result of errors in gastric rotation that lead to laxity or lack of the normal attachments of the stomach to the body. These attachments include the gastrophrenic ligaments, the gastrocolic ligament, the short gastric vessels, and the retroperitoneal fixation of the duodenum. The volvulus itself is classified according to the plane of rotation. If the stomach rotates on its long axis, it is called an *organoaxial volvulus*. In this situation, the greater curvature generally passes anteriorly but can be displaced posteriorly. A less common volvulus is mesenteroaxial volvulus, and rotation here is on an axis from the greater to the lesser curvature. In this instance, the pylorus and cardia commonly rotate anteriorly, although rotation in the opposite direction is also possible.

The most common *heterotopic mucosal tissue* found within the stomach is pancreatic; it is most frequently found within the antral region. Heterotopic tissue often presents as a 1- to 2-cm diameter mass within the submucosal layers. Both translocation of the embryonic pancreatic cells and metaplasia *in situ* have been postulated as the cause of this anomaly. On rare occasions, heterotopic intestinal epithelium has been observed. Some have suggested that the presence of such epithelium (generally columnar epithelial cells with a striated border and interspersed goblet cells) is due to metaplasia induced by gastritis.[11] Conversely, there is clearly some embryologic basis for this phenomenon, as such cells are found in abundance within the pylorus and cardia of fetuses and newborns.[12] It is thought that this heterotopic tissue results from the persistence of a primitive form of gut epithelium.

DUODENUM

Organogenesis

Although the histogenesis of the duodenum is not significantly different from that of the rest of the small bowel, the organogenesis is quite different in many regards. The duodenum's development begins early in the fourth week of gestation, at which time it is the most caudal portion of the foregut and the most cranial portion of the midgut. This junction of the foregut and midgut is at a region just distal to the entry of the bile duct. The duodenal loop, which is convex throughout organogenesis and later life, is originally oriented in an anterior fashion. However, when gastric rotation takes place, the duodenal loop also rotates to the right so that the duodenum ends up lying with its loop convex to the right. The duodenum's rotation results in movement of the duodenum and pancreas to the right upper quadrant, at which point they are pressed against the posterior abdominal wall so that fusion of peritoneal structures with the posterior abdominal wall results in the duodenum becoming retroperitoneal. As it represents a watershed between the foregut and the midgut, its blood supply is derived from both the celiac and superior mesenteric arterial trees. Unlike the rest of the midgut, the duodenum is not herniated into the extracoelomic cavity because of mesenteric-retroperitoneal attachments that anchor it in the right upper quadrant.

Duodenal mucosal proliferation begins around the fourth week of gestation, and an exuberant amount of duodenal epithelial proliferation occurs through the tenth week of gestation. The cellular proliferation is so abundant that at 5 to 6 weeks of gestation complete duodenal occlusion routinely occurs. This occlusion is an epithelial proliferative formation rather than a stage of anatomic "narrowing" during the gut's development. Epithelial proliferation is the basis for most current theories of duodenal atresia-stenosis as well as the basis for the Bremer theory of duplications.[3] Furthermore, at this time, the proliferating epithelia bulge into the antimesenteric mesenchyme so that budlike diverticula appear in the embryo. These diverticula also appear in other regions of the small bowel, but to a lesser extent. Such diverticula resorb into the gut wall at a later time during development, but they may play a role in the pathogenesis of duplications (the Lewis and Thyng theory of gastrointestinal duplications).[10]

Anomalies of Embryogenesis

The duodenum may be involved in many different manifestations of disordered embryogenesis. *Duodenal atresia* results from a failure of recanalization during the solid stage of duodenal development. If the lumen does not re-form as a result of revacuolization of the epithelial plug, an atresia will result. Atresias commonly occur in the second or third portion of the duodenum, with the site of atresia located just distal to the opening of the bile duct. The duodenum may or may not be in continuity (Fig. 109-2). Similarly, if the vacuolization process has been incomplete, a *duodenal stenosis* may exist. Although duodenal atresia may often be a solid phenomenon, webs, either partial or complete, may also create obstruction within the duodenal region. Duodenal webs are also thought to result from a failure of recanalization. Duodenal obstruction of a partial or complete nature may occur secondary to an *annular pancreas* or *incomplete intestinal rotation*. In this anomaly, the cecum overlies the second portion of the duodenum and obstruction results from peritoneal attachments (Ladd bands), which run from the cecum to the lateral body wall. Obstruction of the duodenum can also be created by a *preduodenal portal vein* that arises from abnormal development of vitelline vein anastomoses. This anomaly is commonly associated with other serious malformations that are often of a rotational variety.

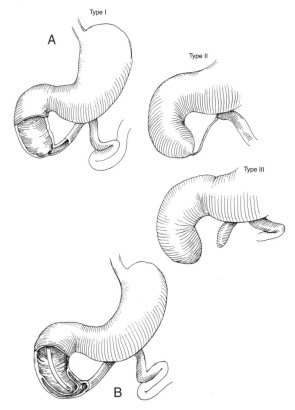

Figure 109-2. A, B, Duodenal atresia-stenosis, an anomaly of failure of duodenal recanalization, may be seen in several ways. Type I may be either a complete or incomplete membrane, and the membrane may be more proximally based (so-called windsock anomaly) as seen in **B.** (From Ross AJ III: Intestinal atresia. *In* Nora PF [ed]: Operative Surgery, 3rd ed. Philadelphia, WB Saunders Co, 1990, p 1042.)

PANCREAS

Organogenesis

Organogenesis of the pancreas is very closely related to that of the duodenum. During the fifth week of gestation, two buds appear as diverticula of endodermal cells emanating from the more caudal region of the foregut. The two endodermal buds are termed the *dorsal and ventral pancreatic anlagen*, and their eventual fusion creates the pancreas. The ventral anlage normally develops at the site of entry of the bile duct into the duodenum, and during the duodenum's rotation to the right this ventral anlage is carried dorsally along with the bile duct. Although initially this ventral anlage lies on the same side and below the dorsal primordium, this rotation permits the ventral anlage to fuse with the proximal portion of the dorsal anlage by the seventh week of gestation. The course of the ventral pancreatic anlage may be widely variable; errors in this rotation commonly lead to pancreatic anomalies.

Most of the pancreas is derived from the dorsal bud; the ventral bud is responsible for forming only the uncinate process in the inferior portion of the head of the pancreas. The pancreatic ducts normally anastomose as the two anlagen fuse. The main pancreatic duct (duct of Wirsung) is derived from the former duct of the ventral bud and the distal portion of the dorsal bud. The portion of the duct more proximal to the dorsal bud eventually becomes the accessory pancreatic duct (duct of Santorini), lying approximately 2 cm cranial to the main duct (Fig. 109–3).

Anomalies of Embryogenesis

Annular pancreas is a well-known cause of duodenal obstruction and a commonly encountered error in development (Fig. 109-4). One finds a thin, flat band of tissue surrounding the second portion of the duodenum. The tissue of this band is histologically

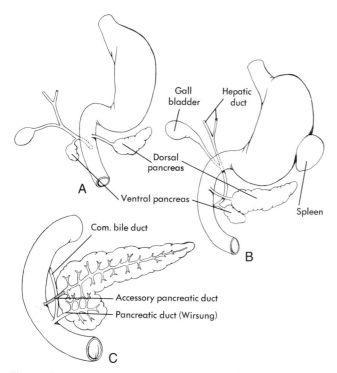

Figure 109–3. A–C, The migration of the ventral pancreatic anlage and subsequent relationship of the dorsal and ventral anlagen and pancreatic ducts are depicted. (From Allan FD: Essentials of Human Embryology. New York, Oxford University Press, 1969.)

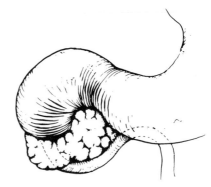

Figure 109–4. Failure of appropriate migration of the ventral pancreatic anlage leads to anomalies such as annular pancreas with resultant duodenal obstruction. (From Schnaufer L: Duodenal atresia, stenosis, and annular pancreas. *In* Welch KJ, et al [eds]: Pediatric Surgery, 4th ed. Copyright © 1986 by Year Book Medical Publishers, Chicago.)

normal, and it is noted to be continuous with the head of the pancreas. The annular pancreas need not be complete and, as such, may manifest as a duodenal stenosis rather than a complete duodenal obstruction. Furthermore, intrinsic duodenal stenosis or atresia, or both, have been noted to occur in addition to the annular pancreas itself. A number of theories regarding the embryogenesis of this anomaly have been proposed. Although none completely explains all the intricacies involved in the embryogenesis of annular pancreas, there is no question that an aberration in the rotation of the ventral anlage has a key role.

Another common pancreatic anomaly is that of *variations of the pancreatic ducts.* Normally, the main duct (duct of Wirsung) and accessory duct (duct of Santorini) open into the duodenum and are interconnected. Obliteration of one or the other duct or the complete separation of one from the other is not at all uncommon so that the main drainage occurs through the accessory duct. *Complete agenesis* of the pancreas has not been reported in otherwise viable newborns, and *partial agenesis* of the pancreas is an exceedingly rare anomaly.

MIDGUT

Organogenesis

The midgut consists of small bowel beginning with the duodenum distal to the point of entry of the ampulla of Vater. It also includes the cecum and appendix as well as the ascending colon and right one-half to two-thirds of the transverse colon. The midgut is supplied by the superior mesenteric artery and is thus also defined as that portion of bowel supplied by the superior mesenteric artery. The midgut is also defined from an embryologic standpoint as that portion of gut that opens ventrally into the yolk sac. The organogenesis of the midgut is one of the most fascinating aspects of development and was first described in 1923 by Dott, whose sketches remain the standard index for understanding the development of the appropriate intraabdominal rotational anatomy.[13]

By the beginning of the sixth week of development, elongation of the midgut occurs at a rate faster than that of the elongation of the embryonic body itself. This is seen especially at the cranial end of the midgut. The result is a U-shaped ventral loop of gut (the midgut loop), which projects anteriorly and enters the extraembryonic coelom of the developing body stalk. Conceptually, one could consider this a huge physiologic umbilical hernia. The apex of this loop entering the extraembryonic coelom (marked by the yolk stalk) is directly in line with the superior mesenteric arterial axis and is termed the *omphalomesenteric duct.* The midgut proximal to this point is termed the *prearterial segment* (signifying that it is proximal to the superior mesenteric artery), whereas bowel distal to this point is the *postarterial segment.* Developmentally, the prearterial segment of bowel is small bowel, whereas the postarterial segment is mostly colon. Following the appearance of the U-shaped ventral loop of the midgut, a counterclockwise (approximately 90°) rotation begins. While bowel is herniated into the extraembryonic coelom, most growth occurs within the prearterial segment so that jejunum and ileum develop at a rate proportionately greater than that of the colon. Within the postarterial segment, a cecal bud forms at 6- to 7-weeks' gestation. Beginning at about 10-weeks' development, the bowel begins to return to the embryonic abdominal cavity. The return of the bowel to the abdomen occurs rather suddenly and rapidly; the forces that dictate this phenomenon remain unknown. It has been postulated that external pressure forces the mass of bowel back through the umbilical ring, but this has not been substantiated. Both the prearterial and postarterial bowel segments rotate a total of 270° counterclockwise before their rotation is completed. Although much of the rotation of the postarterial segment occurs during the time of its return into the body cavity, it is believed that the prearterial segment rotates 180° while it remains herniated. It is the prearterial segment that enters first, passing posteriorly to the superior mesenteric artery during its return. This segment is followed by the cecum and colon (postarterial), which come to lie in front of the superior mesenteric artery. The terminal prearterial segment enters last (Fig. 109-5).

Formal fixation begins after the midgut has returned to the abdominal cavity (approximately the twelfth gestational week). The cecum and developing appendix lie in the subhepatic region at this time point, but further growth of the ascending colon forces the cecum down into the right lower quadrant. The force of the mesenteries of the ascending and descending colons against the posterior abdominal wall fuses these surfaces. As a result, the ascending and descending colons come to lie in the retroperitoneal space. The attachments of the fascial fusion planes of the right and left colon are termed the *fascial fusion planes of Toldt.*

The apex of the cecum does not grow as rapidly as the rest of the cecal pouch, which ultimately results in the development of the appendix. The appendix generally lies on the medial aspect of the cecum. During rotation and fixation of the cecum, however, the appendix can become retrocecal or retrocolic. A similar form of fusion occurs in the midgut portion of the duodenum, which attaches to the retroperitoneum in the left upper quadrant, termed the *ligament of Treitz.* As a result of the attachments of the right and left colon and the midgut duodenum, the small bowel mesentery becomes fan-shaped with a very broad oblique line of attachment from the left upper quadrant to the right lower quadrant (Fig. 109-6). This broad-based attachment limits the mobility of the mesentery and prevents midgut volvulus from occurring around the superior mesenteric artery. When the intestinal rotation is incomplete (i.e., malrotated), mesenteric attachment may not be sufficient to prevent the development of midgut volvulus. Errors in rotational development need operative correction to avoid this potentially lethal problem (Fig. 109-7).

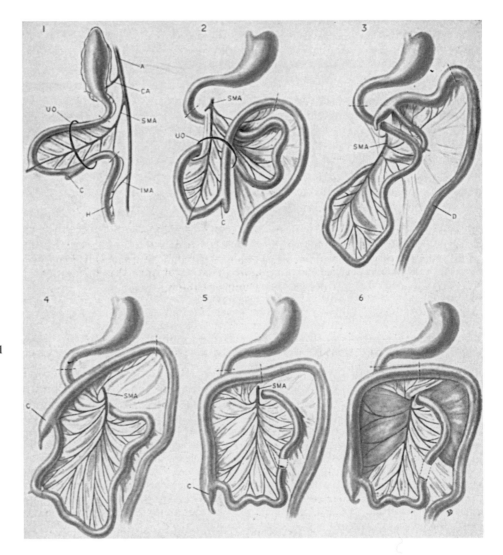

Figure 109–5. Shown are the normal rotation and fixation of the developing midgut. **1,** Herniation into the extraembryonic coelom at week 5. **2,** At week 10, initial rotation has taken place, and the midgut begins its return into the abdominal cavity. **3–5,** Completion of the 270° counterclockwise rotation of the prearterial and postarterial segments. **6,** Final fixation. (From Gross RE: The Surgery of Infancy and Childhood. Philadelphia, WB Saunders Co, 1953, p 131.)

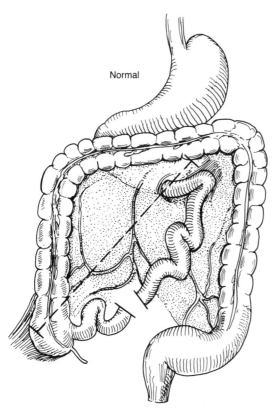

Figure 109–6. Normal rotation and fixation of the midgut are shown. Note the broad-based fixation between the left upper and right lower quadrants, which fixes the superior mesenteric artery such that it cannot be the "root" of a volvulus. (From Ross AJ III: Malrotation of the intestine. *In* Nora PF [ed]: Operative Surgery, 3rd ed. Philadelphia, WB Saunders Co, 1990, p 1048.)

Anomalies of Embryogenesis

Failure of the midgut to return to the abdominal cavity is a frequently encountered congenital anomaly known as *omphalocele.* This developmental arrest is associated with a small abdominal cavity. It is unclear whether the small abdominal cavity is due to failure of the development of the body wall by appropriate migration of the lateral body folds medially or to failure of the return of the intestinal contents, or both. The amount of intestine herniated varies from a small amount that is barely distinguishable from an umbilical hernia to a massive anomaly containing the entire midgut and liver. Unless ruptured, the omphalocele is covered by a sac consisting of both peritoneum and amnion, and the umbilical cord is seen to enter the large exomphalos. In this anomaly, midgut rotation does not occur, so all children with omphalocele have an incompletely rotated intestine. Omphalocele needs to be distinguished from *gastroschisis,* in which there is an abdominal wall defect lateral (usually to the right) to the intact umbilical cord. Gastroschisis is thought to be due to a rupture of the lateral umbilical ring at the site of regression of the right umbilical vein during development (Fig. 109–8). In this situation, in addition to the intact umbilical cord, there is no membrane covering the herniated bowel, which is generally thick, matted, and leathery. Rotation in this anomaly is similarly incomplete (Fig. 109–9). Meckel diverticulum is another commonly noted embryologic anomaly that arises from the remains of the vitelline (*omphalomesenteric*) duct or embryonic yolk stalk. This anomaly is a fingerlike pouch approximately 5 cm long arising from the antimesenteric border of the ileum some

40 to 50 cm proximal to the ileocecal junction. It is found in approximately 2 to 3% of the normal population. As many as 24 variations of persistent vitelline duct anomalies have been described. In addition to the uncomplicated variety of Meckel diverticulum, the tip of the vitelline duct remnant can be attached to the body wall or another intra-abdominal structure. Volvulus or obstruction, or both, can occur at this site. Additionally, this diverticulum may be patent, creating an *omphaloileal fistula* (connecting the ileum with the umbilicus). A mucosal remnant may persist, creating either an *umbilical sinus* or *polyp.* Furthermore, cystic remnants may persist along the length of the vitelline duct lying within the body wall or within the abdominal cavity itself (Fig. 109–10).

Anomalies of midgut rotation are generally referred to as *malrotations.* If the extent of midgut rotation is less than the full 270°, the mesentery may be incompletely based, allowing the bowel to rotate on the superior mesenteric artery axis, creating a volvulus-type picture. The number of possible anomalies of rotation is bewildering; however, all intestinal malrotations have the risk of volvulus.

Congenital intestinal atresia and *stenosis* are common anomalies. The observations of Louw and Barnard[14] have clearly demonstrated that such atresias are due to late intrauterine mesenteric vascular accidents. On rare occasions, jejunoileal atresia may be due to a failure of recanalization of the intestinal lumen occluded by epithelial cells. Atresia of the colon is far less common than atresia of the ileum or jejunum. Its cause is generally accepted as being similar to that of jejunoileal stenosis-atresia.

Duplications of the intestinal tract have been broadly categorized as cystic duplications and tubular duplications.[15] Cystic duplications are far more common and generally do not communicate with the intestinal tract, whereas tubular duplications communicate with the intestinal lumen. Duplications are almost invariably located on the mesenteric side of the bowel. When duplications enlarge, they can compress (and possibly obstruct) adjacent bowel or create a mass effect, or both. Most duplications are located within the small intestine, most commonly

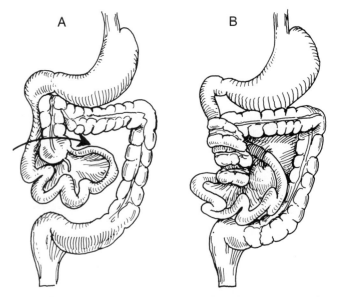

Figure 109–7. A, Malrotated bowel with the cecum overlying the duodenum. Bands from the cecum to the right upper quadrant could obstruct the duodenum. **B,** The lack of fixation in *A* permits the bowel to volvulize—note how the entire axis of the superior mesenteric artery is compromised. (From Ross AJ III: Malrotation of the intestine. *In* Nora PF [ed]: Operative Surgery, 3rd ed. Philadelphia, WB Saunders Co, 1990, p 1048.)

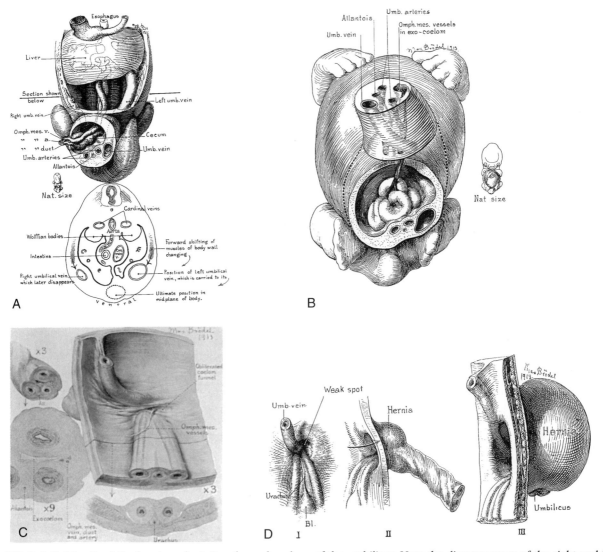

Figure 109–8. A–D, Max Brodel's drawings depicting the embryology of the umbilicus. Note the disappearance of the right umbilical vein and the resultant weak spot to the right side of the umbilicus. It is proposed that rupture at this weak spot is the cause of gastroschisis, thus explaining the usual finding of the defect occurring to the right of an infant's umbilical cord. (From Cullen TS: The Umbilicus and Its Diseases. Philadelphia, WB Saunders Co, 1916, p 745.)

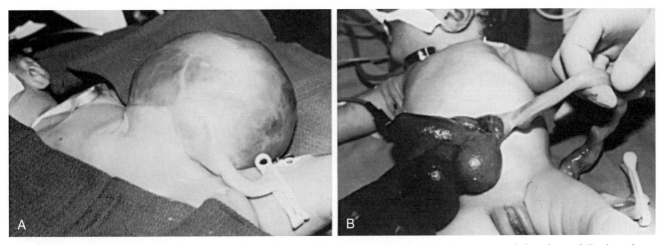

Figure 109–9. A, A baby with a large hepato-omphalocele. Note that the defect includes an intact sac and that the umbilical cord enters the sac. **B,** A baby with gastroschisis. Note the defect is to the right of an intact umbilical cord normally situated on the abdominal wall. Also note the absence of a sac and the thick, matted bowel.

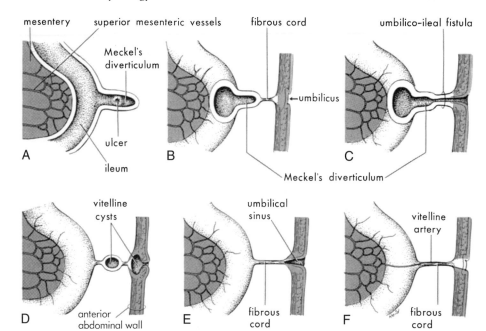

Figure 109–10. A–F, Meckel diverticulum and other anomalies of a persistent omphalomesenteric duct are shown. It is easily appreciated how **B** through **F** can be the focus of either volvulus or obstruction from an adhesive band. (From Moore KL: The Developing Human, 4th ed. Philadelphia, WB Saunders Co, 1988, p 236.)

within the ileum. Most have mucosa resembling that of the adjoining gut. Duplications are generally thought to arise from (1) a failure of normal regression of the known embryonic diverticula with persistence of the transitory diverticula noted during embryogenesis (Lewis and Thyng theory); (2) traction between endoderm and overlying structures during early embryogenesis (Bentley and McLetchie theory; Fig. 109–11); (3) errors of recanalization of epithelial plugs within the small intestine (Bremer theory); or (4) adherence of the endodermal walls lining the developing gut to create a double lumen.[3-5,10]

HINDGUT

Organogenesis

The hindgut comprises that region of the digestive tube that is supplied by the inferior mesenteric artery. The watershed region between the superior and inferior mesenteric arteries is located in the mid- to distal transverse colon. This region, as well as the descending colon, sigmoid colon, rectum, and superior portion of the anal canal, is a derivative of the hindgut. The epithelium of the urinary bladder and most of the urethra are derivatives of the hindgut as well.

It is well known that the growth of the postarterial limb lags behind that of the prearterial limb so that at week 10 of gestation, when the intestines return to the abdominal cavity, the caliber of the large intestine is much smaller than that of the small intestine! Transient occlusion of the colon by a solid epithelial plug probably occurs between the fifth and eighth weeks of gestation.[1]

Developmentally, the most complex region of the hindgut is its most terminal portion, the cloaca. At approximately day 13 of development, a ventral diverticulum, the *allantois*, forms. The future cloacal region is located at the junction of the allantoic stalk and the hindgut. The gut posterior to the allantois (tailgut) remains small and disappears by about the sixth week of devel-

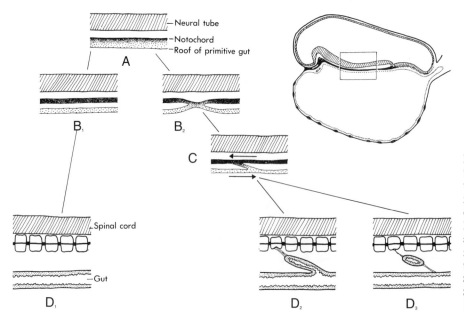

Figure 109–11. Abnormal separations of the notochord from the endoderm at week 4 (A, B₂, C) can result in the formation of an enteric duplication, either cystic (D₃) or diverticular (D₂). Normal is depicted in A, B₁, D₁. It can be appreciated why a vertebral malformation is often seen concurrent to the enteric duplication. (From Gray SW, Skandalakis JE: Embryology for Surgeons. Philadelphia, WB Saunders Co, 1972, p 173.)

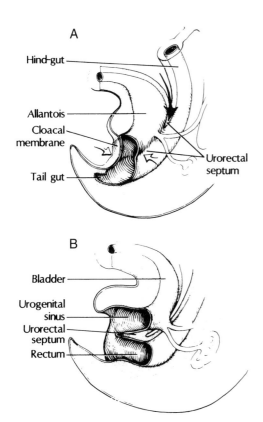

A

Hind-gut

Allantois

Cloacal
membrane

Tail gut

Urorectal
septum

B

Bladder

Urogenital
sinus

Urorectal
septum

Rectum

Figure 109–12. A, B, Descent of the urorectal septum is demonstrated. This results in the partitioning of the distal hindgut, or cloaca, into a urogenital sinus and rectum. It can be appreciated how deviations in the descent of this septum can lead to anorectal malformations, which often include urogenital anomalies as well. (From Ziegler MM, et al: Cloacal exstrophy. *In* Welch KJ, et al [eds]: Pediatric Surgery, 4th ed. Copyright © 1986 by Year Book Medical Publishers, Chicago.)

opment. Although the cloaca is lined with endoderm, it is in direct contact with an ectodermally lined structure termed the *proctodeum* (anal pit). The area of contact between the ectodermal and endodermal surfaces is termed the *cloacal membrane*. Thus, the cloaca proper has the allantois ventrally and the cloacal membrane, an ectodermal-endodermal interface, posteriorly.

As organogenesis proceeds, the cloaca becomes partitioned by a mesenchymal-mesodermal wedge termed the *urorectal septum*. This structure begins development in the angle between the allantois and the hindgut and proceeds in a cephalic to caudal direction moving toward the cloacal membrane (Fig. 109–12). The septum stimulates lateral cloacal ridge development and fusion, and by week 7 of development it reaches and fuses with the cloacal membrane. This results in the formation of a perineal body, which divides the cloacal membrane into a caudal anal membrane and a larger ventral urogenital membrane. Anatomically, this creates a rectum and upper anal canal dorsally and a urogenital sinus ventrally. At approximately 8 weeks of development, the anal membrane (proctodeum) ruptures. The caudal portion of the digestive tract (the anal canal) is now in communication with the amniotic cavity. The superior two-thirds of the

anal canal is derived from the hindgut and the inferior third from the proctodeum. The junction is noted by the pectinate line. This pectinate line represents not only the junction of the proctodeum's ectoderm and the hindgut's endoderm but also the region of vascular watershed between these two structures. The superior rectal artery supplies the upper portion of the anal canal (from the inferior mesenteric artery), and the inferior rectal artery supplies the lower third (from the internal pudendal artery). The urorectal septum descent also defines a cloacal sphincter, the posterior aspect of which develops into the external anal sphincter, and the anterior aspect becomes part of the transversus perinei superficialis, the bulbospongiosus, the ischiocavernosus, and the urogenital diaphragm. In females, the fusion of the müllerian ducts (to form the uterus and vagina) moves down the urorectal septum and reaches the urogenital sinus at week 16 of development. In the male, the urogenital diaphragm is eventually obliterated by the fusion of the genital folds, and the sinus itself becomes incorporated into the urethra.

The obvious complex development of the cloacal region makes it easy to understand why anorectal malformations are common. Most arise from abnormal partitioning of the cloaca by the urorectal septum and its descent to create anorectal and urogenital structures. More often than not, it would seem that many of the anomalies can be explained by a dorsal (posterior) deviation of this septum, which leads to anomalies such as imperforate anus with rectourethral fistula. These anomalies would develop at approximately 6 to 8 weeks' gestation (Fig. 109–13).

Anomalies of Embryogenesis

The most common disorder of embryogenesis involving the hindgut is generally referred to as *imperforate anus.* Found more commonly in males, anorectal malformations result from the abnormal development of the urorectal septum so that there is incomplete separation of the cloaca into its urogenital and anorectal components. As a result, the anal canal may end blindly or there may be an ectopic opening on the perineum, almost always directed anteriorly toward or into the vulva in females or into the scrotum or urethra in males (see Fig. 109–13). The anorectal malformations are commonly categorized as either low or high, determined by whether the blind end of the rectum is above or below, respectively, the level of the levator musculature. The high type of lesion is more common than the low and, generally, more complex. In its most complete form (usually encountered in females) one is left with a *persistent cloaca.* In this anomaly, only a single perineal hole is present, which functions as a common outlet for the intestinal, urinary, and reproductive tracts.

The congenital lack of ganglion cells within the myenteric plexus of the bowel is termed *congenital aganglionic megacolon,* or *Hirschsprung disease.* Congenital megacolon results from the failure of neuromyenteric cells to migrate normally into the wall of the colon and, in most cases, the rectosigmoid is the only bowel involved. This anomaly probably arises between the sixth and eighth weeks of gestation. The "normal" bowel is the proximal dilated bowel that results from the aganglionic bowel's inability to undergo parasympathetic-mediated relaxation. Total colonic and total intestinal aganglionosis have been reported. The aberrant developmental stimulus leading to the lack of the parasympathetic ganglion cells is unclear.

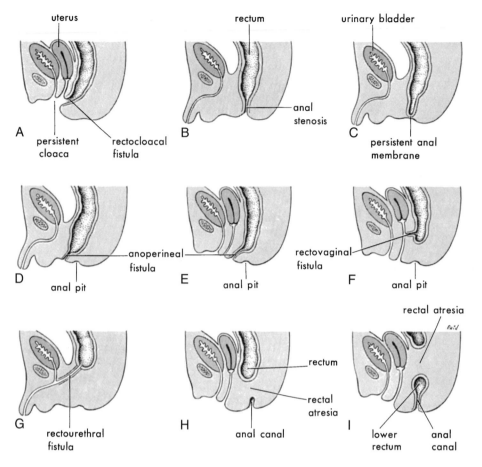

Figure 109–13. Various anorectal anomalies are shown. **A,** Persistent cloaca, a common confluence of the intestinal, urinary, and reproductive tracts, results from failure of descent of the urorectal septum. **B–E,** Manifestations of low-type imperforate anus. **F–H,** Manifestations of high-type imperforate anus. **I,** Rectal atresia (rare). (From Moore KL: The Developing Human, 4th ed. Philadelphia, WB Saunders Co, 1988, p 241.)

REFERENCES

1. Gray SW, Skandalakis JE: Embryology for Surgeons. Philadelphia, WB Saunders Co, 1972.
2. Paulino F: Congenital esophageal stricture due to tracheobronchial remnants. Surgery 53:547, 1963.
3. Bremer JL: Congenital Anomalies of the Viscera. Cambridge, MA, Harvard University Press, 1957.
4. Bentley JFR, Smith JR: Developmental posterior enteric remnants and spinal malformations. Arch Dis Child 35:76, 1960.
5. McLetchie NGB, et al: Genesis of gastric and certain intestinal diverticula and enterogenous cysts. Surg Gynecol Obstet 99:135, 1954.
6. Schridde H: Über Magenschleimhaut-Insein vom Bau der Cardialdrusenzone und Fundus-Drusen-Region und der unteren, osophagealen Cardialdrusen gleichende, Drusen im obersten Oesophagusabschnitt. Virchow Arch Pathol Anat 175:1, 1904.
7. Porto G: Esophageal nodule of thyroid tissue. Laryngoscope 70:1336, 1960.
8. Velasco AL, et al: Management of congenital microgastria. J Pediatr Surg 25:192, 1990.
9. Campbell JR: Other conditions of the stomach. In Welch KJ, et al: Pediatric Surgery. 4th ed. Chicago, Year Book Medical Publishers, 1986: p 821.
10. Lewis FT, Thyng FW: Regular occurrence of intestinal diverticula in embryos of the pig, rabbit, and man. Am J Anat 7:505, 1907.
11. Magnus NA: Observations on the presence of intestinal epithelium in the gastric mucosa. J Pathol Bacteriol 44:389, 1937.
12. Salenius P: On the ontogenesis of the human gastric epithelial cells. A histologic and histochemical study. Acta Anat (Basel) 50(Suppl 46):1, 1962.
13. Dott NM: Anomalies of intestinal rotation: their embryology and surgical aspects with the reports of 5 cases. Br J Surg 11:251, 1923.
14. Louw JN, Barnard CN: Congenital intestinal atresia: observation on its origin. Lancet 2:1065, 1955.
15. Holcomb GW III, et al: Surgical management of alimentary tract duplications. Ann Surg 209:167, 1989.

Delma L. Broussard and Steven M. Altschuler

110 Development of the Enteric Nervous System

Multiple maturational milestones, including coordination of sucking and swallowing, effective gastric emptying, propagation of small intestinal contents, and colonic elimination, are necessary for successful enteral feeding of the infant. Symptoms consistent with poor gastrointestinal motility, such as vomiting, abdominal distention, and constipation, are common in the preterm infant. Developmental patterns of gastrointestinal motility have been described in both animals and humans. This chapter reviews the physiology of gastrointestinal movements, the extrinsic innervation of the gut, and the development of the intrinsic neural tissue of the gut, the enteric nervous system (ENS).

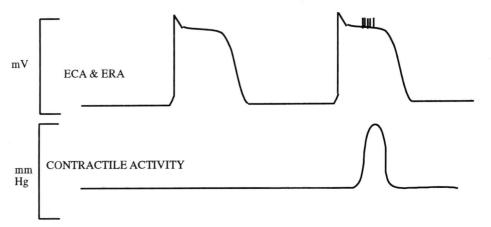

Figure 110–1. Schematic of pacemaker electrical control activity (ECA) with electrical response activity (ERA) in the second cycle. The ERA results from depolarization of the ECA beyond a threshold potential and produces a smooth muscle contraction. (Modified from Sarna SK, Otterson ME: Gastroenterol Clin North Am *18*:383, 1989.)

PHYSIOLOGY OF GASTROINTESTINAL CONTRACTIONS

Myogenic Control

Neurochemical, humoral, and mechanical stimuli control smooth muscle contractile activity. Smooth muscle cells generate spontaneous electrical activity through a fluctuation in resting membrane potential. These periodic depolarizations are below the membrane potential necessary to initiate a contraction and are known as *slow waves, electrical control activity, basic electrical rhythm*, or *pacesetter potentials*. Contractions occur only when a slow wave, following neural or chemical stimulation, exceeds the excitation threshold necessary for an action potential. Following depolarization of a smooth muscle cell, there is an increase in intracellular calcium. Calcium binds to calmodulin, a regulatory protein, and permits binding of the contractile proteins actin and myosin, resulting in a contraction. Therefore, the action potential, referred to as *electrical response activity* or *spike potential*, occurs against the background of the slow wave (Fig. 110-1).[1] Slow waves control the timing, speed, and direction of intestinal contractions.[2]

Neural Control

Central Nervous System

The central nervous system (CNS) and neural tissue within the intestinal wall, known as the ENS, control gastrointestinal motor, secretory, and vascular activities. The CNS and ENS consist of afferent (sensory) neurons, efferent (motor) neurons that synapse directly with effector cells (muscle secretory cells, blood vessels), and interneurons, which integrate messages from the afferent neurons and program the efferent neurons. The sensory fibers travel closely with parasympathetic preganglionic fibers in the vagus nerve and sympathetic postganglionic fibers in the splanchnic nerves. Their neuronal cell bodies are located in the nodose and dorsal root ganglia, respectively. Vagal afferents terminate in the mucosal and muscular layers of the gastrointestinal tract from the soft palate to the descending colon, as well as the liver, gallbladder, and pancreas.[3-5] Splanchnic afferents innervate the serosal surface and the bowel mesentery, as well as its mucosal and muscular layers.[6]

Gastrointestinal motor innervation is provided by the sympathetic and parasympathetic divisions of the autonomic nervous system (Fig. 110-2). Postganglionic neurons of the sympathetic division are located in the prevertebral position on either side of the spinal cord, and the ganglia of the parasympathetic division are within the gastrointestinal tract. Preganglionic sympathetic and parasympathetic neurons are located in spinal cord segments T2 through L2 (sympathetic) and in the medulla and sacral spinal cord (parasympathetic).

Most parasympathetic innervation of the gut is supplied by the vagus; the sacral nerves innervate only from the middle of the transverse colon to the rectum. Vagal efferents terminate primarily within the enteric ganglia.[7,8] Because the vagus nerve innervates most of the gut, organization of its projections within the brain stem has been studied extensively. Neural tracer studies have demonstrated a viscerotopic organization of afferent projections within the vagal sensory nucleus and the nucleus tractus solitarii (NTS), as well as efferent fibers within the motor nuclei, the dorsal motor nucleus (DMN) of the vagus nerve, and the nucleus ambiguus (NA) of the rat.[3,4,9-13]

The NTS is the first synaptic site for vagal afferent fibers of the alimentary tract through cranial nerves IX and X. Within the NTS are interneurons involved in the coordination of afferent and efferent information to control esophageal and gastrointestinal motor activity. Afferent fibers, depending on their site of origin with the rat gastrointestinal tract, project to the distinct subnuclei within the NTS. For example, the central subnucleus (NTS_{cen}) has been implicated in the coordination of esophageal peristalsis using organ-specific injections of neural tracers.[3,14-16] In the rat, esophageal vagal afferents terminate in the NTS_{cen} and its neurons (esophageal premotor neurons) project directly to esophageal motoneurons located in the compact formation of the nucleus ambiguus (NA_c)[17,18] The efferent neurons for the striated muscle of the esophagus are located in the nucleus ambiguus, and the smooth muscle efferents originate in the dorsal motor nucleus of the vagus nerve in the rat.

Identification of anatomic circuits that project to specific bowel segments has enabled investigation of neurotransmitters, which may be involved in the control of esophageal and other gastrointestinal motor activities in animal models. Pseudorabies virus (PRV), a swine neurotropic herpesvirus that undergoes retrograde axonal transport, has been instrumental in the colocalization of neurotransmitters within the brain-stem neurons involved in esophageal peristalsis.[16] Following injection of the virus into an end organ, active infection develops within a neuronal cell body following retrograde transport. The virus replicates and subsequently undergoes retrograde transport to the synapsing afferent terminals. (Specific transsynaptic retrograde transport to first-, second-, and third-order neurons is a function of postinjection time.) The virus can be localized immunohistochemically using specific PRV antisera.

Several neurotransmitters have been implicated as mediators of synaptic transmission in the brain-stem–esophageal swallowing circuit, including the excitory amino acid (EAA) glutamate (GLU).[19-21] GLU binds to a family of receptors that includes the *N*-methyl-D-aspartate (NMDA) receptor class. Pharmacologic studies demonstrate that the application of GLU-agonist NMDA to the rat NTS_{cen}[20-22] and NA_c[23] stimulates esophageal motor activity. NMDA is a heteromeric protein composed of several

Structural Relations of the Autonomic Nervous System

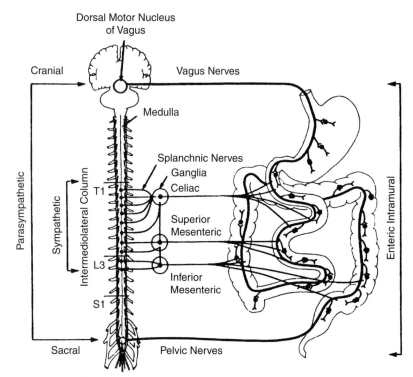

Figure 110–2. Organization of the projections of the autonomic nervous system to the gut. The enteric nervous system is within the bowel wall. (Adapted from Wood JD, Wingate DL: Gastrointestinal neurobiology: The little brain in the gut. *In* American Gastroenterological Association Undergraduate Teaching Project in Gastroenterology and Liver Disease. Timonium, MD, Milner-Fenwich, 1988, p 1.)

subunits, of which NMDA R1 is a subunit necessary for a functional receptor. The demonstration of the colocalization of NMDA R1 mRNA and PRV immunoreactive (PRV-IR) neurons in the esophageal premotor neurons (NTS_{cen}) and esophageal motoneurons (NA_c),[24] adds further support to this hypothesis.

Enteric Nervous System

Although the CNS plays a significant role in the control of gastrointestinal movements, central innervation of the gastrointestinal tract is relatively sparse when compared with the large number of ENS neuronal fibers. The ENS is unique, compared with other peripheral nervous system ganglia, because of its ability to mediate reflex activity independent of the CNS. The ENS is a complex system of neurons, which integrates extrinsic neuronal and humoral stimuli to produce stereotypic patterns that regulate motility, secretion, and vascular flow. For example, contraction of an orad segment of bowel to a food bolus is coordinated with relaxation of a caudad segment to attain peristalsis. Consequently, the ENS has been referred to as the "little brain" in the gut (Fig. 110–3).[25]

The ENS consists of two major plexuses—the myenteric (Auerbach), located between the external circular and longitudinal muscle layers, and the submucosal (Meissner); it also includes six relatively minor plexuses, occupying different layers of the bowel wall (Fig. 110-4).[26] The density of each plexus varies according to location in the gastrointestinal tract and by animal species.[27-29] The importance of the ENS is supported by abnormal myoelectrical recordings from the small intestine following chemical ablation of the myenteric neurons.[30] Additionally, extrinsically denervated bowel can still mix and propel foodstuffs, and an autotransplanted small-bowel segment does not cause obstruction.[31]

The ENS and CNS ganglia share ultrastructural and neurochemical similarities. Neither the enteric ganglia nor the CNS ganglia contain connective tissue or blood vessels.[32, 33] The enteric glia, support cells of enteric neurons, have processes that abut the basal lamina surrounding the myenteric plexus, analogous to the pia-astroglial border of the brain.[34] The internal structure of the enteric glia consists of high concentrations of cytoskeletal protein glial fibrillary acidic protein (GFAP), which is also a marker for astroglia.[35] The functions of enteric glia are not clear; however, selective destruction of enteric glia in niacin-deficient mice results in diarrhea.[36] The anatomic, structural, and chemical similarities of enteric glia and astroglia support the hypothesis that their roles are analogous.[34]

Neurotransmitters

Many CNS neurotransmitters are also found in the ENS. Acetylcholine (ACh) is the most abundant excitatory neurotransmitter mediating smooth muscle contractions in the ENS. Although many other enteric neurotransmitters have been suggested by immunocytochemical, pharmacologic, and electrophysiologic studies, not all have met the criteria for a neurotransmitter. These criteria include (1) a pharmacologic response to exogenous application of the potential neurotransmitter, (2) a mechanism for transmitter uptake and synthesis, (3) storage in presynaptic vesicles, and (4) a physiologic action following the neurotransmitter release by nerve stimulation.

Nitric oxide (NO), which is a gas, has been shown to mediate nonadrenergic noncholinergic (NANC) relaxation in gastrointestinal smooth muscle. There are several proposed mechanisms for the effects of NO. NO mediates relaxation through an increase in 5′-cyclic guanosine monophosphate (cGMP).[38, 39] Other studies suggest that NO does not act alone but may interact with other inhibitory neurotransmitters such as vasoactive intestinal peptide (VIP) to mediate its effects.[40] NO synthase (NOS), the enzyme responsible for NO synthesis, has been demonstrated in the ENS of several animal species.[41-45] There is also electrophysiologic evidence for NO in the human gastrointestinal tract,[37, 46, 47] as well as immunocytochemical labeling of NO-containing enteric neurons in the developing human intestine.[48]

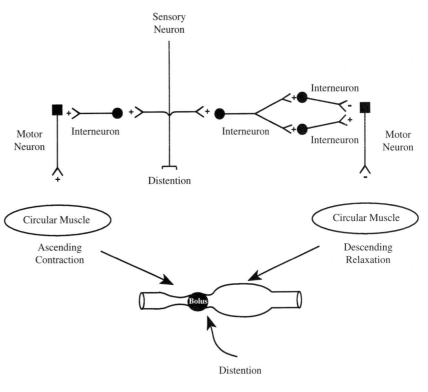

Figure 110–3. Schematic of intestinal peristalsis of a food bolus, illustrating the local coordination of sensory and motor information within the enteric nervous system. (Modified from Makhlouf GM: Regulation of muscle function by neuro-peptides. In Fisher R, et al [directors]: American Gastroenterological Association Postgraduate Course 1992: Gastrointestinal Motility Disorders—What's New and What to Do! Philadelphia, WB Saunders Co, 1992.)

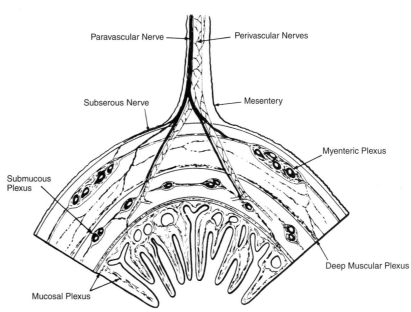

Figure 110–4. Arrangement of enteric plexuses in whole mounts of intestine. In addition to the large myenteric and submucosal plexuses, several smaller plexuses are shown. (From Furness JB, Costa M: Arrangement of enteric plexuses. In Furness JB, Costa M [eds]: The Enteric Nervous System. New York, Churchill Livingstone, 1987.)

Pyloric stenosis is the most common cause of gastroduodenal obstruction in infancy. The pathophysiology of antropyloric muscle hypertrophy and decreased neuronal fibers is not known. Animal and human studies have suggested that NO may play a role in pyloric stenosis. NO,[49] VIP,[50] and substance P[51] fibers have been found to be decreased in the circular muscle layer of infants with hypertrophic pyloric stenosis. Although several neurotransmitters are decreased in the circular muscle layer of infants with pyloric stenosis, a transgenic neuronal NOS gene–deficient mouse phenotypically expresses hypertrophy of the circular muscle of the pylorus and marked enlargement of the stomach as its only phenotypic abnormalities.[52] Unlike the ubiquitous distribution of NO in wild-type mice, homozygous mutant mice do not have NO-positive fibers in the myenteric

plexus or circular muscle of the stomach or pylorus. NO deficiency has also been described in aganglionic segments of patients with Hirschsprung disease.[53]

Intestinal guinea pig muscle tension studies have implicated glutamate as a potential excitatory neurotransmitter in the gut. Longitudinal muscle strips associated with the myenteric plexus (LMMP) contract in the presence of exogenous glutamate, an abundant excitatory amino acid neurotransmitter in the CNS.[54-57] This contraction can be inhibited by agents that antagonize the CNS glutamate receptor NMDA and by drugs that block cholinergic receptors. Glutamate can be synthesized from exogenous L-glutamine in myenteric neurons and released from myenteric neurons following neuronal depolarization in vitro.[58] These data support an excitatory glutamate neural pathway in the myenteric plexus through NMDA-type receptors and suggest that glutamatergic neurons are interneurons initiating contraction through cholinergic motoneurons. *In situ* hybridization studies have localized the NMDA receptor gene to the neurons of the guinea pig taenia coli myenteric plexus[59] and rat intestine.[60] The NMDA receptor has also been implicated in colonic peristalsis.[61] These studies support the concept that glutamate is a neurotransmitter in the ENS that mediates its effects through NMDA receptors, but further studies are necessary to confirm a functional NMDA receptor. CNS astroglia take up neuronally released glutamate and convert it to glutamine, through the enzyme glutamine synthetase.[62] Our laboratory[63] and that of Jessen and Mirsky[35] have demonstrated the presence of glutamine synthetase in enteric glia, the support cells of enteric neurons. However, further studies are needed to confirm the uptake of glutamate by enteric glia.

Development of the Enteric Nervous System

Enteric neurons and glial elements are derived from the migration of neural crest cells.[64-66] Early investigations of the origin of the ENS, using quail-chick chimeras, demonstrated that vagally derived neural crest cells migrated throughout the entire bowel, but sacral emigres were found only in the postumbilical hindgut.[71] Because the neural crest émigrés are not recognized as neurons or glia as they first enter the bowel, novel labeling methods have been developed to more specifically trace the migration of neural crest cells. Fluorescent dye DiI (1,1-dioctadecyl-3,3,3′,3′-tetramethylindocarbocyanine perchlorate) or retrovirus LZ10, constructed with *lac Z* reporter gene and detected with ß-galactosidase immunoreactivity, was injected by Pomeranz and colleagues[67] into the neural tube of chick embryos before neural crest migration. Injections into the vagal crest level resulted in labeled cells in the avian stomach and duodenum. Injections into the sacral crest resulted in labeled cells in the postumbilical bowel; however, injections into the truncal crest localized to the sympathetic ganglia and not to the bowel wall. DiI tracer experiments have also demonstrated that the murine gut is colonized by the vagal and sarcal regions of the neural crest.[68-69]

The premigratory neural crest cells are multipotent; therefore, factors that determine their differentiation have been of interest.[70] Premigratory chick crest cells replaced with those of quails (or the reverse) in younger embryos demonstrate that the phenotypic expression of the grafted crest cells is independent of the site of origin and determined by the migration pathway of the host embryo.[66, 71, 72] Phenotypic expression of the neural crest cells is dictated by the enteric microenvironment at the site of terminal differentiation. This is illustrated by the transient expression of the catecholaminergic neuronal phenotype by crest-derived cells that colonize the rodent bowel.[73] Transiently catecholaminergic (TC) cells are found in the murine and rat foregut at embryo days 9.5 and 11, respectively. During their migration through the vagal nerve pathway, TC cells express tyrosine hydroxylase (TH), aromatic L-amino acid decarboxylase, dopamine β-hydroxylase, catecholamine storage, and norepinephrine transport as is seen in other sympathetic neurons. When these cells reach the bowel, they no longer express the catecholaminergic phenotype. Differentiated neurons express serotonergic and peptidergic neurotransmitters (e.g., serotonin, substance P, and neuropeptide Y) .

Hirschsprung Disease

Hirschsprung disease is a gastrointestinal disorder manifested by intestinal obstruction, as a result of the absence of neural crest–derived enteric ganglia in the terminal hindgut. It is a common disease occurring in 1 in 5000 live births. Patients with Hirschsprung disease commonly present with partial or complete obstruction during the first year of life. The cellular mechanisms for this disease are not known, but animal models such as the lethal spotted (*ls/ls*) mouse, in which congenital aganglionosis is an autosomal recessive trait, have suggested possible mechanisms.[74] As is seen in association with Hirschsprung disease, the colon of the *ls/ls* mouse is dilated proximal to the aganglionic segment, which acts as a functional obstruction. The aganglionosis develops as a result of failure of precursors of enteric neurons[75] and enteric glia[76] to colonize the bowel wall. Neurotropins[77] and laminin,[78] in addition to other molecules, may play a role in the control of enteric neuron migration and differentiation. After reaching the gut, neural crest cells express a 110-kD cell-surface laminin-binding protein, which is not detected in ENS precursor cells.[78] It has been hypothesized that laminin interacts with the laminin-binding protein to cause neural crest cells to terminate migration. Neural crest cells from the *ls/ls* mouse can colonize the colonic walls of normal mice, but not the distal colon of *ls/ls* mice.[79] Examination of the aganglionic segment of *ls/ls* bowel reveals that there is an overabundance of laminin and other components of the extracellular matrix in the gut wall.[80] It has been hypothesized that the accumulation of laminin could result in premature cessation of migration of crest-derived cells and, therefore, the absence of ganglionic cell bodies in the distal colonic segments of *ls/ls* mice. The 110-kD laminin-binding protein may promote neurite extension.[78] The inhibition of cranial-to-caudal migration of vagal enteric neuroblasts to the large intestine of *ls/ls* mice suggests that a defect in the mesenchyme of the large intestine prevents colonization.[81] In vitro studies of the effects of neuronal development on smooth muscle cells from normal and aganglionic human bowel have suggested that the aganglionic colon is a less favorable environment for neuronal growth because of a membrane-linked factor.[82]

Genetic and molecular studies in both animals and humans have proposed that specific genes may be responsible for regulating the migration of enteric neurons. In the mouse, the homeobox-containing gene, *Hoxa-4*, is expressed in various developing tissues, including the mesodermal layer of the gut. Exploration of the function of *Hoxa-4* has used a transgenic mouse expressing multiple copies of the *Hoxa-4* gene, which demonstrates congenital megacolon as its phenotype.[83] However, the pathogenesis of the bowel lesions of transgenic and lethal spotted mice is different. In this transgenic mouse model, crest-derived cells can enter the terminal colon, but their development is abnormal, resulting in hypoganglionosis. The *ls/ls* mouse has an abnormality of the extracellular matrix that prevents normal migration into the terminal bowel.

Pedigree studies have demonstrated that Hirschsprung disease is a heterogenous genetic disorder with autosomal dominant, autosomal recessive, and polygenic forms, as well as a few cases that result from environmental factors.[84] One autosomal dominant form has been mapped to human chromosome 10q11.1.[85] This region contains the *RET* proto-oncogene, a protein tyrosine kinase gene expressed in the cells derived from the neural crest. Mutations in the *RET* gene of Hirschsprung disease in both sporadic and familial cases have now been identified.[86,87] These data suggest that *RET* plays a critical role in the development of the mammalian ENS. However, the existence of Hirschsprung disease families without linkage to the *RET* gene suggests that there are additional genes affected in patients with Hirschsprung disease.[88]

Another susceptible chromosome in an inbred Mennonite kindred with Hirschsprung disease is chromosome 13q22.[89] Extensive molecular and genetic studies have implicated the endothelin-B (ET$_B$) receptor gene (*EDNRB*) as a gene candidate for Hirschsprung disease susceptibility within a subset of this family. Endothelins are a group of peptides that bind to two receptors, including ET$_B$. The ET$_B$ receptor is expressed in the human colon, particularly in the myenteric plexus, mucosa, ganglia, and blood vessels of the submucosa,[90] areas that may be abnormal in Hirschsprung disease. Targeted disruption of the *EDNRB* gene in the mouse results in aganglionic megacolon.[91]

Following the transfection of a mutant *EDNRB* haplotype (identified in this pedigree) into a cell line, the resulting mutant did not demonstrate a normal ET_B-induced intracellular Ca^{2+} response, further supporting the susceptibility of this gene in Hirschsprung disease. These data suggest that *EDNRB* is important in the normal development of enteric ganglion in some patients with Hirschsprung disease.

Intestinal Motor Activity

The stomach and small intestine exhibit periodic motor activity during fasting. A migrating band of contractions of maximum spiking frequency and pressures is observed throughout the fasting small intestine. This is known as the migrating motor complex (MMC) or interdigestive motor complex (Fig. 110-5).[92] The MMC is a recognizable pattern of cyclic groups of caudally migrating contractions or myoelectric activity of the antrum and small intestine that occurs in mammals in the fasted state.[92,93] The MMC consists of four phases—phase I, a period of quiescence, characterized by an absence of action potentials; phase II, a period of irregular contractile and myoelectric activity; phase III, maximal-amplitude regular contractions occurring at the frequency of the slow wave; and phase IV, a brief period of contractile activity before the start of phase I.[93-95] The MMC is thought to sweep residual products of digestion toward the colon, serving as a housekeeper.[96]

The MMC is primarily controlled by local enteric mechanisms.[2] Denervation of the extrinsic nerves to the gut does not stop initiation of the MMC cycle,[97-101] but the MMC cycle's duration becomes more variable, suggesting that the extrinsic nerves modulate periodicity. It is hypothesized that the MMC is under local control by the ENS, which has a neuronal circuit that periodically activates smooth muscle cells to contract at their maximal frequency.[99,102] Intraluminal calories disrupt MMC activity at all levels of the bowel and initiate generalized irregular contractions—the fed pattern—in the stomach and small intestine (Fig. 123-6).[93] Introduction of nutrients into the bowel lumen results in a fed pattern in all areas of the bowel, including a noncontiguous bowel loop. The fed pattern does not occur, however, if the noncontiguous bowel is extrinsically denervated.[103] This suggests that initiation of the fed motor pattern requires regulation by extrinsic nerves or humoral factors. The caloric content of the ingested nutrient influences gastrointestinal motility. Fats reduce spiking amplitude and intestinal transit[104] to a greater extent than carbohydrates and protein.[105]

Development of Intestinal Motility

Animal studies of the fetal development of small intestinal motility, using chronically implanted electrodes, have demonstrated a progressive increase in the duration of spiking activity in dogs and sheep to a well-defined propulsive motor pattern.[106] Three stages of development of intestinal myoelectrical activity in the fetuses of several species have been identified. Stage 1 is characterized by unorganized spiking activity. In Stage 1, there is a high percentage of retrograde propagation of low-amplitude spike bursts, suggesting that its main motor function is to mix intestinal contents. Stage 2, the fetal pattern, exhibits occasional cyclic spike bursts superimposed on slow waves that propagate aborally or orally. When Stage 2 is associated with distally propagated phases of spiking activity recurring at short intervals, intraluminal contents may be propelled slowly for storage in the ileum and colon. Stage 3 resembles the adult MMC pattern.

Comparison of small bowel motility patterns of ungulates (the gastrointestinal motility patterns of which mature prenatally) with species with small intestinal motility patterns that develop postnatally demonstrate parallel development of the ENS and CNS. Ungulates have full CNS maturity at the time of birth, which allows them to run with the herd soon after birth. In dog and rat pups that are born blind, deaf, and poikilothermic, maturation of the CNS and ENS is mainly postnatal.[107] Intestinal motor activity develops according to a species-specific, gestation-dependent pattern and is independent of birth.

The first studies in human fetuses to investigate intestinal transit used amniography. McLain[108] showed there was no transit of contrast down the intestine until 30-weeks' gestation. Thereafter, an increasing aboral transit and propagation rate were seen as the pregnancy progressed. Subsequent manometric studies in infants illustrated a gestationally dependent pattern of development of small intestinal motility, with developmental

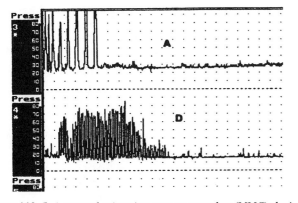

Figure 110–5. A normal migrating motor complex (MMC) during fasting in a human subject. The recording was obtained with intraluminal miniature pressure transducers spaced 8 cm apart in the antrum *(A)* and duodenum *(D)*. High-amplitude contractions are distally propagated. (Scale bar = 2 min.) (From Broussard DL: Clin Perinatol *22*:39, 1995.)

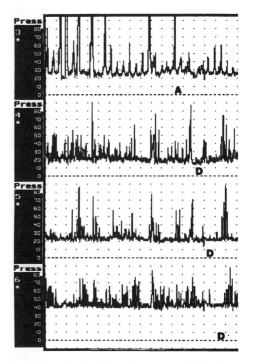

Figure 110–6. Antroduodenal motility pattern following a meal. Generalized spiking activity in the antrum *(A)* and duodenum *(D)* observed with miniature pressure transducer catheter. (Scale bar = 2 min.) (From Broussard DL: Clin Perinatol *22*:39, 1995.)

stages similar to those of dogs and sheep.[109, 110] Increasing gestational age resulted in an increase in both duration and propagation of phase II contractions before the development of the MMC pattern.[110, 111] The amplitude of contractions is also increased with gestational age.[110-112] The cycle time of the MMC is shorter in the term infant than in the adult,[111, 113] suggesting that there is further maturation of the MMC in infancy.

REFERENCES

1. Sarna SK: Gastrointestinal electrical activity: Terminology. Gastroenterology 68:1631, 1975.
2. Sarna SK: Cyclic motor activity; migrating motor complex. Gastroenterology 89:894, 1985.
3. Altschuler SM, et al: Viscerotopic representation of the upper alimentary tract in the rat: sensory ganglia and nuclei of the solitary and spinal trigeminal tracts. J Comp Neurol 283:248, 1989.
4. Altschuler SM, et al: Representation of the cecum in the lateral dorsal motor nucleus of the vagus nerve and commissural subnucleus of the nucleus tractus solitarii in rat. J Comp Neurol 304:261, 1991.
5. Appia F, et al: Convergence of sensory information from abdominal viscera in the rat brain stem. Am J Physiol 251:G169, 1986.
6. Leek BF: Abdominal and pelvic visceral receptors. Br Med Bull 2:163, 1977.
7. Kirshgessner AL, Gershon MD: Identification of vagal efferent fibers and putative target neurons in the enteric nervous system of the rat. J Comp Neurol 285:38, 1989.
8. Berthoud H-R, et al: Simultaneous labeling of vagal innervation of the gut and afferent projection form the visceral forebrain with DiI injected into the dorsal vagal complex in the rat. J Comp Neurol 1:301, 1990.
9. Dennison SJ, et al: Viscerotopic localization of preganglionic parasympathetic cell bodies of origin of the anterior and posterior subdiaphragmatic vagus nerves. J Comp Neurol 197:259, 1981.
10. Dennison SJ, et al: Redefinition of the location of the dorsal (motor) nucleus of the vagus in the rat. Brain Res Bull 6:77, 1981.
11. Kalia M, Mesulam MM: Brain stem projections of sensory and motor components of the vagus complex in the cat: I. The cervical vagus and nodose ganglion. J Comp Neurol 193:435, 1980.
12. Kalia M: Brain stem localization of vagal preganglionic neurons. J Auton Nerv Syst 3:451, 1981.
13. Kalia M, Sullivan JM: Brainstem projections of sensory and motor components of the vagus nerve in the rat. J Comp Neurol 211:248, 1982.
14. Cunningham ET, Sawchenko PE: Central neural control of esophageal motility: a review. Dysphagia 5:35, 1990.
15. Barrett R, et al: Brain stem localization of esophageal premotor neurons in the rat as determined by the transneuronal passage of pseudorabies virus. Gastroenterology 107:728, 1994.
16. Card JP, et al: Neurotropic properties of pseudorabies virus: Uptake and transneuronal passage in the rat central nervous system. J Neurosci 10:1974, 1990.
17. Rinaman L, et al: Ultrastructural demonstration of a gastric monosynaptic vagal circuit in the nucleus of the solitary tract in rat. J Neurosci 9:1985, 1989.
18. Ross CA, et al: Projections from the nucleus tractus solitarii to the rostral ventrolateral medulla. J Comp Neurol 242:511, 1985.
19. Hashim MA, Bieger D: Excitatory amino acid receptor–mediated activation of solitarial deglutitive loci. Neuropharmacology 28:913, 1989.
20. Kessler JP, et al: Swallowing responses induced by micro-injection of glutamate and glutamate agonists into the nucleus tractus solitarius of ketamine-anesthetized rats. Exp Brain Res 83:151, 1990.
21. Kessler JP, Jean A: Evidence that activation of N-methyl-D-aspartate (NMDA) and non-NMDA receptors within the nucleus tractus solitarii triggers swallowing. Eur J Pharmacol 201:59, 1991.
22. Tell F, Jean A: Bursting discharges evoked in vitro, by solitary tract stimulation or application of N-methyl-D-aspartate, in neurons of the rat nucleus tractus solitarii. Neurosci Lett 124:221, 1991.
23. Kessler JP, Involvement of excitatory amino acids in the activity of swallowing-related neurons of the ventro-lateral medulla. Brain Res 603:353, 1993.
24. Broussard DL, et al: Expression of N-methyl-D-aspartate (NMDA) receptor mRNA in the brainstem circuit controlling esophageal peristalsis. Mol Brain Res 27:329, 1994.
25. Wood JD: Intrinsic neural control of intestinal motility. Ann Rev Physiol 43:33, 1981.
26. Furness JB, Costa M: Arrangement of enteric plexuses. In Furness JB, Costa M (eds): The Enteric Nervous System. New York, Churchill Livingstone, 1987, pp 6–25.
27. Christensen J, et al: Arrangement of the myenteric plexus throughout the gastrointestinal tract of the opossum. Gastroenterology 86:890, 1983.
28. Christensen J, Rick GA: Nerve cell density in submucous plexus throughout the gut of cat and opossum. Gastroenterology 89:1064, 1985.
29. Christensen J, et al: Comparative anatomy of the myenteric plexus of the distal colon in eight mammals. Gastroenterology 86:706, 1984.
30. Holle GE, Forth W: Myoelectric activity of small intestine after chemical ablation of myenteric neurons. Am J Physiol 258:G519, 1990.
31. Sarna SK, Otterson MF: Small intestinal physiology and pathophysiology. In Ouyang A (ed): Clinics in Gastroenterology. Philadelphia, WB Saunders Co, 1989, pp 375–404.
32. Gabella G: Ultrastructure of the nerve plexuses of the mammalian intestine: The enteric glial cells. Neuroscience 6:425, 1981.
33. Komuro T, et al: An ultrastructural study of neurons and nonneuronal cells in the myenteric plexus of the rabbit colon. Neuroscience 7:1797, 1982.
34. Gershon MD, Rothman TP: Enteric glia. Glia 4:195, 1991.
35. Jessen KJ, Mirsky R: Astrocyte-like glia in the peripheral nervous system: An immunohistochemical study of enteric glia. J Neurosci 3:2206, 1983.
36. Aikawa H, Suzuki K: Enteric gliopathy in niacin-deficiency induced by CNS gliotoxin. Brain Res 334:354, 1985.
37. Stark ME, Szurszewski JH: Role of nitric oxide in gastrointestinal and hepatic function and disease. Gastroenterology 103:1928, 1992.
38. Wolin MS, et al: A kinetic analysis of the regulation of the purified soluble enzyme by protoporphyrin IX, heme, and nitrosyl-heme. J Biol Chem 257:13312, 1982.
39. Gruetter CA, et al: Relationship between cyclic guanosine 3':5'-monophosphate formation and relaxation of coronary arterial smooth muscle by glyceryl trinitrate, nitroprusside, nitrite and nitric oxide: effects of methylene blue and methemoglobin. J Pharmacol Exp Ther 219:145, 1981.
40. Grider JR, et al: Stimulation of nitric oxide from muscle cells by VIP: prejunctional enhancement of VIP release. Am J Physiol 25:G774, 1992.
41. Bredt DS, et al: Localization of nitric oxide synthase indicating a neuronal role for nitric oxide. Nature 347:768, 1990.
42. Llewellyn-Smith IJ, et al: Ultrastructural localization of nitric oxide synthase immunoreactivity in guinea pig enteric neurons. Brain Res 577:337, 1992.
43. Dawson JM, et al: Nitric oxide synthase and neuronal NADPH diaphorase are identical in brain and peripheral tissues. Proc Natl Acad Sci U S A 88:7797, 1991.
44. Conklin JL, et al: Characterization and mediation of inhibitory junction potentials from opossum lower esophageal sphincter. Gastroenterology 104:1439, 1993.
45. Murray J, et al: Nitric oxide: Mediator of nonadrenergic noncholinergic responses of opossum esophageal muscle. Am J Physiol 261:G401, 1991.
46. Stark ME: Nitric oxide mediates inhibitory nerve input in human and canine jejunum. Gastroenterology 104:398, 1993.
47. Burleigh DE: ng-nitro-L-arginine reduces nonadrenergic, noncholinergic relaxations of human gut. Gastroenterology 102:679, 1992.
48. Timmermans J-P, et al: Nitric oxide synthase immunoreactivity in the enteric nervous system of the developing human digestive tract. Cell Tissue Res 275:235, 1994.
49. Vanderwinden JM, et al: Nitric oxide synthase activity in infantile hypertrophic pyloric stenosis. N Engl J Med 327:511, 1992.
50. Malmfors G, Sundler F: Peptidergic innervation in infantile hypertrophic pyloric stenosis. J Pediatr Surg 21:303, 1986.
51. Tam PKH: An immunochemical study with neuron-specific enolase and substance P of human enteric innervation—the normal developmental pattern and abnormal deviations in Hirschsprung's disease and pyloric stenosis. J Pediatr Surg 21:227, 1986.
52. Huang PL, et al: Targeted disruption of the neuronal nitric oxide synthase gene. Cell 75:1273, 1993.
53. Bealer JF, et al: Nitric oxide is deficient in the aganglionic colon of patients with Hirschsprung's disease. Pediatrics 93:647, 1994.
54. Luzzi S, et al: Agonists, antagonists and modulators of excitatory amino acid receptors in the guinea pig myenteric plexus. Br J Pharmacol 95:1271, 1988.
55. Frye GD: Interaction of ethanol and L-glutamate in the guinea pig ileum myenteric plexus. Eur J Pharmacol 192:1, 1991
56. Campbell BG, et al: N-methyl-D-aspartate receptor-mediated contractions of the guinea pig ileum longitudinal muscle/myenteric plexus preparation: modulation by phencyclidine and glycine receptors. J Pharmacol Exp Ther 257:754, 1991.
57. Shannon HE, Sawyer BD: Glutamate receptors of the N-methyl-D-aspartate subtype in the myenteric plexus of the guinea pig ileum. J Pharmacol Exp Ther 251:518, 1989.
58. Wiley JW, et al: Evidence for a glutamatergic neural pathway in the myenteric plexus. Am J Physiol 261:G693, 1991.
59. Broussard DL, et al: Expression of a NMDA gene in guinea pig myenteric plexus. Neuroreport 5:973, 1994.
60. Burns GA, et al: Expression of mRNA for the N-methyl-D-aspartate (NMDAR1) receptor by enteric neurons of the rat. Neurosci Lett 170:87, 1994.
61. Cosentino M, et al: N-Methyl-D-aspartate receptors modulate neurotransmitter release and peristalsis in the guinea pig isolated colon. Neurosci Lett 183:139, 1995.
62. Schousboe A: Transport and metabolism of glutamate and GANA in neurons and glial cells. Int Rev Neurobiol 22:1, 1981.
63. Broussard DL, et al: Electrophysiologic and molecular characterization of guinea pig enteric glia. J Neurosci Res 34:24, 1993.
64. Yntema CL, Hammond WS: The origin of intrinsic ganglia of trunk viscera from vagal neuronal crest in the chick embryo. J Comp Neurol 101:515, 1954.
65. LeDouarin NM, Teillet MA: The migration of neural crest cells to the wall of the digestive tract in avian embryo. J Embrol Exp Morphol 30:31, 1973.
66. LeDouarin NM, Teillet MA: Experimental analysis of the migration and differentiation of neuroblasts of the autonomic nervous system and of neuroecto-

dermal mesenchymal derivatives, using a biological cell marking technique. Dev Biol 41:162, 1974.

67. Pomeranz HD, et al: Colonization of the post-umbilical bowel by cells derived from the sacral neural crest: Direct tracing of cell migration using an intercalating probe and a replication-deficient retrovirus. Development 111:647, 1991.

68. Serbedzija GN, et al: Vital dye labeling demonstrates a sacral neural crest contribution to the enteric nervous system of chick and mouse embryos. Development 111:857, 1991.

69. Gershon MD, et al: From neural crest to bowel: development of the enteric nervous system. J Neurobiol 24:199, 1993.

70. Baroffio A, et al: Clone-forming ability and differentiation potential of migratory neural crest cells. Proc Natl Acad Sci U S A 85:5325, 1988.

71. LeDouarin NM: The Neural Crest. Cambridge, Cambridge University Press, 1982.

72. Rothman TP, et al: Developing potential of neural crest–derived cells migrating form segments of developing quail bowel back-grafted into younger chick host embryos. Development 109:411, 1990.

73. Baetge G, et al: Development and persistence of catecholaminergic neurons in cultured explants of fetal murine vagus nerves and bowel. Development 110:689, 1990.

74. Lane PW: Association of megacolon with two recessive spotting genes in the mouse. J Hered 57:29, 1966.

75. Rothman TP, Gershon MD: Regionally defective colonization of the terminal bowel by; the precursors of enteric neurons in lethal spotted mutant mice. Neuroscience 12:1293, 1984.

76. Rothman TP, et al: Colonization of the bowel by the precursors of enteric glia: studies of normal and congenitally aganglionic mutant mice. J Comp Neurol 252:493, 1986.

77. Baetge G, et al: Transiently catecholaminergic (TC) cells in the bowel of fetal rats and mice: precursors of non-catecholaminergic enteric neurons. Dev Biol 132:353, 1990.

78. Pomeranz HD, et al: Expression of a neurally related laminin binding protein by neural crest-derived cells that colonize the gut: relationship to the formation of enteric ganglia. J Comp Neurol 313:625, 1991.

79. Jacobs-Cohen RJ, et al: Inability of neural crest cells to colonize the presumptive aganglionic bowel of ls/ls mutant mice: requirement for a permissive microenvironment. J Comp Neurol 255:425, 1987.

80. Payette RF, et al: Accumulation of components of basal laminae: association with the failure of neural crest cells to colonize the presumptive aganglionic bowel of ls/ls mutant mice. Dev Biol 125:341, 1988.

81. Kapur RP, et al: A transgenic model for studying development of the enteric nervous system in normal and aganglionic mice. Development 116:167, 1992.

82. Langer JC, et al: Smooth muscle from aganglionic bowel in Hirschsprung's disease impairs neuronal development in vitro. Cell Tissue Res 276:181, 1994.

83. Tennyson VM, et al: Structural abnormalities associated with congenital megacolon in transgenic mice that overexpress the Hoxa-4 gene. Dev Dyn 198:28, 1993.

84. Badner JA, et al: A genetic study of Hirschsprung disease. Am J Hum Genet 46:568, 1990.

85. Angrist M, et al: A gene for Hirschsprung disease (megacolon) in the pericentromeric region of human chromosome-10. Nat Genet 4:351, 1993.

86. Edery P, et al: Mutations of the RET proto-oncogene in Hirschsprung's disease. Nature 367:378, 1994.

87. Romeo G, et al: Point mutations affecting the tyrosine kinase domain of the RET proto-oncogene in Hirschsprung's disease. Nature 367:377, 1994.

88. Puffenberger EG, et al: A missense mutation of the endothelin-b receptor gene in multigenic Hirschsprung's disease. Cell 79:1257, 1994.

89. Puffenberger EG, et al: Identity-by-descent and association mapping of a recessive gene for Hirschsprung disease on human chromosome 13q22. Hum Mol Genet 3:1217, 1994.

90. Inagaki H, et al: Localization of endothelinlike immunoreactivity and endothelin binding sites in human colon. Gastroenterology 101:47, 1991.

91. Hosoda K, et al: Targeted and natural (piebald-lethal) mutations of endothelin-b receptor gene produce megacolon associated with spotted coat color in mice. Cell 79:1267, 1994.

92. Szurszewski JH: A migrating electric complex of the canine small intestine. Am J Physiol 217:1757, 1969.

93. Code CF, Marlett JA: The interdigestive myoelectric complexes of the stomach and small bowel of dogs. J Physiol (Lond) 246:289, 1975.

94. Carlson GM, et al: Mechanism of propagation of intestinal interdigestive myoelectric complex. Am J Physiol 222:1027, 1972.

95. Wingate DL: Backwards and forwards with the migrating complex. Dig Dis Sci 26:641, 1981.

96. Code CF, Schlegel J: The gastrointestinal interdigestive housekeeper: Motor correlates of the interdigestive myoelectric complex of the dog. In Daniel EE, ed: Proceedings of the IV International Symposium on GI Motility. Vancouver, Mitchell Press Ltd., 1973.

97. Marik F, Code CF: Control of the interdigestive myoelectric activity in dogs by the vagus nerves and pentagastrin. Gastroenterology 679:387, 1975.

98. Marlett JA, Code CF: Effects of celiac and superior mesenteric ganglionectomy on interdigestive myoelectric complex in dogs. Am J Physiol 237:E432, 1979.

99. Ormsbee HIS, et al: Mechanism of propagation of canine migrating motor complex—a re-appraisal. Am J Physiol 240:G141, 1981.

100. Sarna S, et al: The enteric mechanisms of initiation of migrating myoelectric complexes (MMCs) in dogs. Gastroenterology 84:814, 1983.

101. Bueno L, et al: Propagation of electrical spiking activity along the small intestine: Intrinsic versus extrinsic neural influences. J Physiol (Lond) 292:15, 1979.

102. Itoh Z, et al: Neurohormonal control of gastrointestinal motor activity in conscious dogs. Peptides 2:223, 1981.

103. Sar MG, Kelly KA: Myoelectric activity of the autotransplanted canine jejunoileum. Gastroenterology 81:303, 1981.

104. Gregory PC, et al: The influence of intestinal infusion of fats on small intestinal motility and digesta transit in pigs. J Physiol 379:27, 1986.

105. Dooley CP, et al: Variations in gastric and duodenal motility during gastric emptying of liquid meals in humans. Gastroenterology 87:1114, 1984.

106. Bueno L, Ruckebusch Y: Perinatal development of intestinal myoelectrical activity in dogs and sheep. Am J Physiol 237:E61, 1979.

107. Ruckebusch Y: Development of digestive motor patterns during perinatal life. Mechanism and significance. J Pediatr Gastroenterol Nutr 5:523, 1986.

108. McLain CR: Amniography studies of the gastrointestinal motility of the human fetus. Am J Obstet Gynecol 86:1079, 1963.

109. Wozniak ER, et al: The development of fasting small intestinal motility in the human neonate. In Roman C (ed): Gastrointestinal Motility. Lancaster, UK, MTP Press, 1984, pp 265–270.

110. Bisset WM, et al: Ontogeny of fasting small intestinal motor activity in the human infant. Gut 29:483, 1988.

111. Berseth CL: Gestational evolution of small intestine motility in preterm and term infants. J Pediatr 115:646, 1989.

112. Morriss FHJ, et al: Ontogenic development of gastrointestinal motility: IV. Duodenal contractions in preterm infants. Pediatrics 78:1106, 1986.

113. Tomomasa T, et al: Nonmigrating rhythmic activity in the stomach and duodenum of neonates. Biol Neonate 48:1, 1985.

Chris J. Dickinson

111

Development of Gastric Secretory Function

The development of the human stomach is complex because of the many roles it plays in the digestive process. The stomach serves as a reservoir for food and regulates the flow of nutrients into the small bowel. Additionally, the stomach is a secretory organ that continues digestive processes that were initiated in the mouth. Although hydrochloric acid is the major gastric secretory product, the stomach also secretes mucus, pepsinogen, bicarbonate, intrinsic factor, prostaglandins, and regulatory peptides. This chapter outlines gastric organogenesis and gives an overview of the regulation of gastric secretion, with emphasis on developmental studies in humans and animal models.

In interpreting the data currently available regarding the development of gastric secretory capability, several points should be kept in mind. First, although the mechanisms regulating gastric acid secretion are consistent across species, the relative contribution of individual components is quite variable. Second, considerable gaps remain in our understanding of the development of gastric secretory processes in humans. Third, although there have been numerous advances in understanding the molecular mechanisms that regulate the development of the small intestine and the digestive enzymes (e.g., sucrase-isomaltase and lactase), much less is known regarding the development of gastric secretory function.

ORGANOGENESIS AND CELL DIFFERENTIATION

The human stomach derives from the endoderm of the foregut at about 4 weeks' gestation. As the gastric pouch continues to grow, the dorsal portion of the stomach enlarges at a more rapid rate than does the ventral border, producing the greater curvature. As this disproportionate growth continues, the stomach eventually undergoes a 90° rotation clockwise to assume the adult position by 8 weeks. The final J shape of the human stomach is not seen until 22 weeks.[1] Fetal ultrasound studies have greatly refined this process and can be used to detect abnormalities in gut function very early in gestation.[2] Histologically, the stomach is initially lined with stratified or pseudo-stratified epithelium.[3,4] At 6 to 9 weeks, the first gastric pits appear,[5,6] followed by the development of glands at about 12 weeks' gestation, when the first primitive parietal cells can be recognized. The antral glands develop slightly later than those of the fundus but are present by 13 weeks' gestation. At 12 to 13 weeks, the glands contain virtually no parietal cells but an abundance of mucous and endocrine cells. The gastric glands then expand toward the fully developed mature structures. In the hamster, the glands appear to multiply by dichotomous branching.[7,8] In humans, the gastric glands appear to mature in a similar fashion and are very convoluted during this process, which is complete by 5 to 6 months of gestation.[6]

For many years it was unclear whether the various secretory cells of the stomach (mucous, acid-secreting parietal, pepsin-secreting chief, and endocrine cells) arose from a common progenitor cell or whether there were multiple stem cells. It is now known that a multipotent stem cell (known as the isthmus), is located in the middle region of the gastric pit.[9-14] is located in the middle region of the gastric pit.[9-14] Investigators also know that neck cells of neonatal mice can be grafted into the subcutaneous tissue of nude mice and it will differentiate into all four cell types.[15] This is consistent with a multipotent stem cell model analogous to that of the small intestinal crypt. (Fig. 111–1). It is interesting that grafts from embryonic day 14 mice maintain the axial patterning of gastric glands despite the fact that they are in a different endocrine environment. Although these grafts do develop parietal and chief cells, there is a delay in the appearance of differentiated endocrine cells, suggesting that extragastric factors may be required for their development.

These data have led investigators to search for genes that might regulate gastric differentiation. Unfortunately, no such gene has yet been identified, but several things are known. First, the *N-myc* gene is necessary for development of the stomach, since *n-myc* knock-out mice have a poorly developed gut.[16] Second, GATA-4 is known to be expressed first in primitive endoderm and then in definitive gastric endoderm. GATA-4null blastocysts develop an abnormal gastric epithelium that has a squamous morphology.[17] Third, Sonic-Hedgehog, an endoderm-derived signaling molecule, is overexpressed in the GATA-4–deficient cells.[17] Fourth, the nuclear transcription factor SP-1 is expressed in large quantities in the developing gut and is responsible for basal and gastrin-mediated transcription of some important genes, such as the proton pump H+/K+-ATPase.[18,19] It is likely that over the coming years other important transcription factors necessary for gastric development will be identified in mouse models.

The regulation of gastric development took a leap forward when the human fetal stomach was studied in organ culture.[20] Overall cell division decreased after 12 to 17 weeks' gestation and became concentrated in the neck region. Unlike the mature human stomach, the fetal stomach can grow in serum-free media, suggesting that the fetal stomach contains all the growth factors necessary for growth.

Other studies have confirmed that all the epithelial cells of the gastric gland (mucous, parietal, chief/zymogen, and soon) arise from stem cells in the neck region. A stem cell in the neck gives rise to pre-pit/premucous, preparietal, and prezymogen cells.[11-13] These premucous cells then migrate up the gland to the surface, where they eventually are shed into the lumen. The prezymogen cells migrate down into the base of the gland, where they differentiate into pepsin-secreting chief cells and eventually undergo apoptosis. These cells also secrete intrinsic factor in rodents but not humans. Preparietal cells differentiate in the neck and migrate only a very short distance into the large, acid-secreting mature parietal cell. Transgenic experiments confirm that all three cell types are monoclonal and thus arise from a common precursor.[21] Parietal cell ablation experiments demonstrate a block in the differentiation of the other two cell types, suggesting that a balance between the cell types is maintained by interactions among the cells.[22]

REGULATION OF ACID SECRETION IN ADULTS

Since the discovery of the acidic nature of gastric secretions by Beaumont in 1826, investigators have sought to determine the regulation of their release in humans.[23] It is now known that the parietal cell utilizes H+/K+-ATPase to secrete hydrochloric acid into the lumen of the stomach. Furthermore, several stimuli regulate acid secretion in mammals. These include neurogenic input (primarily via the vagus) and endocrine or paracrine effects from somatostatin-producing D cells, gastrin-producing G cells, histamine-containing enterochromaffin-like (ECL) cells, and other peptide hormones. An overview of the regulation of gastric acid secretion is necessary to understand the developmental changes seen in humans and animal models (Fig. 111–2). It should be noted that although these regulatory mechanisms are seen in a wide variety of mammalian species, the relative contribution of individual components has intraspecies variation. Thus, animal models may not entirely reflect human physiology. Moreover, it has also been shown that the contribution of these inputs can vary during development.

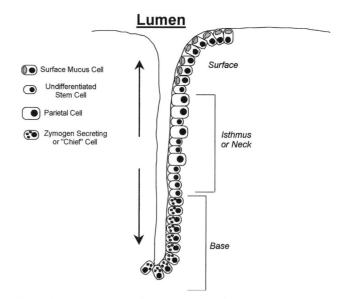

Figure 111–1. Representation of a gastric gland. The gastric gland is divided into three contiguous and overlapping areas: surface, isthmus or neck, and base. Unlike in the small intestine, gastric stem cells are located in the middle of the gland. As differentiation progresses, the three main cell types migrate to different areas.

As shown in Figure 111–2, the regulation of gastric acid secretion is quite complex. Excellent reviews of this topic have been published elsewhere but an overview is provided here.[24] As noted by Beaumont and Pavlov,[23, 25] the central nervous system during the cephalic phase of gastric acid secretion can stimulate acid secretion via specific sites in the medulla and the vagus nerve.[26, 27] The predominant vagal effect is mediated by acetylcholine released from postganglionic fibers and muscarinic receptors. Acetylcholine has multiple effects, including a direct stimulatory effect on the parietal cell. Acetylcholine also stimulates the release of somatostatin from D cells, which provides a brake on acid secretion via multiple pathways. In addition to acetylcholine, gastrin-releasing peptide (GRP) is secreted from postganglionic vagal nerve fibers and directly stimulates gastrin release[28] via GRP receptors on G cells.[29, 30] Vasoactive intestinal polypeptide (VIP) is also released from vagal postganglionic fibers, but, unlike GRP, VIP does not have a direct effect on the G cell. VIP stimulates somatostatin release[31] from D cells, which, in turn, inhibits gastrin secretion. Other candidate peptides regulating the cephalic phase of acid secretion include calcitonin gene–related peptide and corticotropin-releasing hormone.

During the gastric phase of a meal, antral distention evokes low levels of gastrin release that is inhibited by low doses of the muscarinic antagonist atropine but enhanced by atropine at higher doses.[32] Other studies show that low-dose atropine depresses gastrin release in response to feeding in both intact and vagotomized dogs, suggesting that this effect is mediated by local neural reflexes.[33] Gastrin is also released by the presence of food in the stomach. Neurotoxins, such as tetrodotoxin, GRP antagonists, and atropine, abolish both stimulation of gastrin release and inhibition of somatostatin release, indicating that peptone-induced gastrin release is mediated, in part, by both cholinergic and GRP neurons. However, other groups have shown that amino acids and amines also stimulate gastrin release from isolated canine G cells.[34] Circulating gastrin is the principal mediator of postprandial gastric acid secretion in adult humans.[35] Gastrin stimulates acid secretion by a direct effect on the parietal cell or by stimulating the release of histamine from ECL cells, which, in turn, enhances acid secretion.

The entry of chyme into the small intestine initiates the intestinal phase of the acid secretory process. The primary stimulatory factors in the small bowel are distention and the products of protein digestion, and these contribute relatively little to overall gastric acid secretion. The presence of food, especially fat, does initiate several inhibitory mechanisms. Duodenal fat releases intestinal cholecystokinin (CCK), which stimulates the release of somatostatin from gastric D cells.[36] Somatostatin has several inhibitory effects on gastric acid secretion, including suppression of release of gastrin from G cells, histamine release from ECL cells, and acid secretion from parietal cells. Although many other peptides released during the intestinal phase of digestion can inhibit gastric acid secretion, it appears that many of their effects are mediated by gastric D cells.[37] As the stomach empties, the continued secretion of acid is no longer buffered by the presence of food, and luminal pH drops. This lower pH has no direct effects on the G cell, parietal cell, or ECL cell but does cause a release of somatostatin from D cells to provide an inhibitory feedback loop for acid secretion.

NEONATAL PARIETAL CELL SECRETION

At birth, the gastric pH is greater than 2, probably secondary to the alkaline nature of swallowed amniotic fluid.[38, 39] However, by several hours of age the stomach begins to secrete acid and the pH falls. Unfortunately, the amount of acid produced in the human neonatal stomach has been difficult to determine since

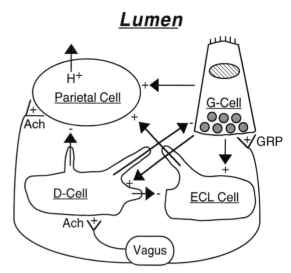

Lumen

Figure 111–2. Regulation of gastric acid secretion. See also text. The acid-secreting parietal cell is regulated by inputs from the vagus nerve and three main cell types found in gastric mucosa: gastrin-secreting G cells, somatostatin-secreting D cells, and enterochromaffin-like (ECL) cells that secrete histamine. Vagal postganglionic fibers release acetylcholine (ACh) that directly stimulates acid secretion from parietal cells and somatostatin release from D cells. Other vagal gastrin-releasing peptide (GRP)-containing fibers stimulate gastrin secretion from G cells. Gastrin is post-translationally processed to its biologically active forms within secretory granules that release their contents into the circulation. Increases in plasma gastrin enhance acid secretion from parietal cells, histamine release from ECL cells, and somatostatin release from D cells. Unlike gastrin, which acts in an endocrine fashion, somatostatin and histamine are released from D and ECL cells in a paracrine manner. Histamine stimulates acid secretion from parietal cells, whereas somatostatin inhibits secretion of acid from parietal cells and inhibits the release of gastrin from G cells and histamine from ECL cells.

many studies have not included important parameters to quantify acid secretion accurately, such as body weight.[38, 39] Most studies agree that acid secretion increases from birth to day 10 and then declines again over the next 20 days.[40, 41] Acid production then slowly increases toward adult levels by about 3 months of age.[42] To examine gastric acid secretion more thoroughly, investigators have examined acid secretion in the absence (basal acid output, BAO) or presence of secretagogues such as gastrin (maximal acid output, MAO). As with previous studies, Euler and associates[43, 44] demonstrated that the BAO of full-term infants was very low during the first 5 hours of life when compared with basal values of infants 4 to 14 hours of age. Basal acid secretion then increased in the infants from 6 to 8 hours of life. It is interesting that administration of pentagastrin did not increase acid production over basal levels. The investigators concluded that either acid secretion was already at maximal levels or that the acid secretory apparatus was insensitive to gastrin at this stage of development. Euler found that infants had elevated levels of serum gastrin that did not fall despite the increase in acid secretion. This suggested that the normal inhibitory effect of acid on gastrin release mediated by somatostatin was also not fully functional. Recent studies in neonates demonstrate that the proton pump H^+,K^+-ATPase is expressed at low levels as early as 25 weeks' gestation. H^+,K^+-ATPase gene expression increases in concert with gastric acid secretion, gestational age, and postnatal age.[45]

Hyman and others investigated acid secretion in 34 healthy 7-day-old preterm infants of less than 37 weeks' gestation and found that BAO was proportional to body weight but less than that of term infants.[46,47] BAO then gradually increased from 1 to 4 weeks of age and varied with postgestational but not postconceptual age, suggesting that extrauterine factors were involved. Hyman has suggested that feeding may play a primary role in this effect, but this has not been experimentally confirmed. Although there is no acid secretory response to pentagastrin in term infants at birth, preterm infants demonstrate this effect at 1 week of age. Unlike the effect of age on BAO, MAO in preterm infants increases with postgestational age and postconceptual age but remains far below that seen in older children and adults.[48-50]

To investigate the acid secretory capacity of the neonatal stomach in response to other stimuli, investigators examined MAO in response to the histamine analogue betazole.[51] They noted that BAO was low within the first 24 hours of life but that there was a two to threefold increase in acid output in response to betazole, which is consistent with other studies. Betazole-stimulated MAO, however, was much lower than that seen in older infants, suggesting that the acid secretory apparatus was not functionally mature at this early stage in development.

MECHANISMS FOR DIMINISHED PARIETAL CELL FUNCTION IN THE NEONATE: ANIMAL MODELS

To explore the mechanisms that regulate the development of gastric acid secretory capacity, investigators have turned to animal models to examine each of the individual components in the acid secretory apparatus. In human neonates, BAO is quite low at birth but rises shortly thereafter. Moreover, the acid secretory response is sensitive to meals but not to exogenous gastrin stimulation despite high plasma gastrin levels. Johnson has extensively studied the development of acid secretion in the rat and noted a similar pattern in the ontogeny of gastric acid secretion.[52] One theme common to all animal models is that the development of gastric acid secretion depends on the maturation of the parietal cell and those cells important for the regulation of acid secretion (outlined earlier).

Parietal Cell

In the mouse, gastric glands are first seen on fetal day 18, at which time there is no ultrastructural evidence of distinct parietal cells nor alpha or beta H^+,K^+-ATPase subunit expression.[53,54] On fetal day 19 in the mouse, parietal cells can be identified, and both subunits of H^+,K^+-ATPase are now associated with apical membranes. Marino and colleagues examined H^+,K^+-ATPase expression as well as expression of a second enzyme, carbonic anhydrase II, that generates a H^+ within the parietal cell in the rat.[18] They noted that H^+,K^+-ATPase expression was present in 1-week-old pups, slowly increased over the next 7 weeks of development, and was limited to parietal cells. Conversely, carbonic anhydrase II was expressed in many cell types within the gastric mucosa at high levels shortly after birth. Carbonic anhydrase expression then declined slowly over the next several weeks but maintained high levels of expression in parietal cells. Hervatin and colleagues[55] examined H^+,K^+-ATPase activity in the developing rat and detected enzymatic activity on fetal day 19 although most of the enzyme was in the inactive state. H^+,K^+-ATPase activity rose from fetal day 19 to birth and then to almost zero by day 12 of life. Activity then rose over the next several weeks to adult levels, and the enzyme was found primarily in the active state. Other studies in the mouse[53,54] and rabbit[56] also detect the presence of functional H^+,K^+-ATPase early in gestation. Unlike in the rat, basal acid secretion in pigs is present at birth, but there is little response to secretagogues until 1 week of age.[57] In summary, it appears that the parietal cells are present at birth and contain the machinery necessary to secrete acid, albeit at diminished levels when compared with mature parietal cells.

Other investigators have examined the ability of the parietal cell to respond to gastrin, histamine, and acetylcholine. The receptors and postreceptor mechanisms for these secretagogues appear to develop with age; however, their patterns of development are both cell- and species-specific.[58-62] Despite the presence of parietal cells and functional H^+,K^+-ATPase at birth, basal acid secretion is very low at birth.[58,59] In the adult, basal acid secretion is controlled largely by vagal cholinergic inputs. Thus the low level of basal acid secretion suggests that these animals lack muscarinic receptors shortly after birth. However, muscarinic receptors are found at 70% to 80% of adult levels from birth onward and are functional, in that they can stimulate the release of pepsin from chief cells.[58] Investigators have hypothesized that this may reflect a low level of receptors on parietal cells or a failure of the parietal cell to develop postreceptor mechanisms that mediate the response. It is interesting that histamine and gastrin do not stimulate acid or pepsin secretion until day 20 of life.[59] Nevertheless, in neonates, protein hydrolysate formulas can stimulate gastric acid secretion twofold via unknown mechanisms.[63] Injection of corticosterone into 8-day-old pups prior to the natural steroid burst seen at weaning around day 21 prematurely induces basal acid secretion and the acid secretory response to all three secretagogues.

In other studies in the developing rat, investigators measured the binding of gastrin to its receptor and found no specific binding until day 20 of life; the receptor number was increased by treatment with corticosteroids.[64-66] The parietal cell response to histamine is more variable in its time of presentation but is documented to occur between 14 and 20 days of life in rats.[51,59] Although investigators can describe the presence of receptors in developing gastric mucosa and note the effects of secretagogues on acid secretion, it has been very difficult to examine postreceptor mechanisms in the developing animal. To determine that the changes in second messengers reflect changes in a particular cell type requires the use of isolated cell systems and large quantities of tissue. Thus this important area remains relatively unexplored.

INTRINSIC FACTOR SECRETION FROM PARIETAL CELLS

In humans, the parietal cell secretes intrinsic factor,[67] and investigators have examined its ontogeny to gain insight into the development of the parietal cell. Marino and associates[47] found that basal intrinsic factor production was similar in term and preterm infants. Conversely, term infants had much higher gastric acid secretion than preterm infants, suggesting that the development of these processes in human parietal cells was not linked. Other investigators have examined histamine-stimulated intrinsic factor secretion and noted low levels at birth that increase to normal adult values by 2 weeks of age.[51] Again, there was a dissociation between the maturation of intrinsic factor secretion and gastric acid secretion—histamine-stimulated acid secretion did not reach adult levels even at 2 to 3 months of age. In the rat, intrinsic factor is a product of the chief cell, and thus it is difficult to use the rat as a suitable model for human development.[67,68]

G-CELL FUNCTION

Gastrin-producing G cells can be detected in the human fetus as early as 12 weeks of gestation.[69] It is interesting that most of these early G cells also express thyroid-releasing hormone (TRH), and the number of TRH-positive G cells increases to reach a maximum between 26 and 36 weeks' gestation.[69] Thereafter, the number of TRH-positive G cells decreases, and none are found in the mature human stomach. Moreover, there is no known physiologic role for TRH in the developing stomach, and

TRH is not found in G cells of other developing animals. In the rat, gastrin immunoreactivity is detected in the pancreatic islets before it is seen in the gastric antrum.[70] As fetal development proceeds, gastrin expression increases in the antrum and decreases in the islets. It appears that fetal pancreatic gastrin, in combination with transforming growth factor α, plays an important role in islet neogenesis.[71]

Human plasma gastrin levels in the neonate are approximately three times higher than those found in adults and pregnant women.[42] Unfortunately, the physiologic significance of neonatal hypergastrinemia is not known. It has been suggested that these elevated levels may play a role in the growth and development of the gastrointestinal tract.[72] To explore the role of gastrin in gut development, two groups have developed gastrin-deficient mice.[73-75] These mice are viable and develop normally with normal weight gain. This suggests that gastrin is not a vital hormone. However, both basal and stimulated gastric acid secretions are severely impaired in homozygous animals. Furthermore, there is a reduction in gastric mucosal thickness, with reductions in all three cell types. Although CCK can bind to the gastrin receptor, CCK does not substitute for gastrin since both gastrin-deficient and gastrin receptor–deficient mice have a similar gastric phenotype.[76]

Antral gastrin content increases in the developing rat until weaning. Early weaning or administration of corticosteroids or thyroid hormone increases antral gastrin content and promotes the maturation of the gastric mucosal gastrin receptors.[52,55,65] It is unknown whether a similar phenomenon also occurs in the human stomach with a change in diet, but human plasma gastrin levels do remain elevated for several months after birth while infants are primarily milk fed.[77] The cause of neonatal hypergastrinemia is multifactorial, and the rat seems to provide a suitable model for study (Fig. 111–3). A milk-based diet that is high in known gastrin secretagogues such as amino acids and calcium[78] may account for some of the hypergastrinemia. In both rats and humans there is diminished gastric acid secretion due to a diminished number of functional parietal cells. In mature humans this inhibits somatostatin secretion, which increases gastrin secretion. Consistent with this is the finding that the somatostatin content of the rat gastric antrum is low at birth and increases gradually until weaning at around day 21.[79] Moreover, infusion of somatostatin does not inhibit gastrin release in newborn rat pups until day 18 of life, suggesting that somatostatin receptor or postreceptor mechanisms are functionally mature until weaning.[80] The combined effect of low somatostatin content and diminished response to exogenous somatostatin prior to weaning suggests that somatostatin plays a major role in neonatal hypergastrinemia.

The exact nature of the role that gastrin plays in neonatal gastric acid secretion also is not fully elucidated. For example, gastrin is the primary mediator of gastric acid secretion during a meal in mature humans.[35] However, it has been unclear whether this is a direct effect on the parietal cell, because H_2 receptor antagonists block much of this response. This suggests that gastrin's effects on acid secretion are mediated via histamine release from ECL cells. In other species, it appears that gastrin has a more direct effect on the parietal cell. In the developing rat, gastrin-stimulated acid secretion is not blocked by H_2 receptor antagonists but is partially attenuated in mature animals.[81] It is currently unknown whether gastrin exerts its effects directly on the parietal cell of human infants or whether its effects are mediated by histamine release.

Gastrin, as is the case with other regulatory neuropeptides, is initially synthesized as a large, biologically inactive precursor termed *progastrin* (Fig. 111–4). Endoproteolytic processing of progastrin within G cells results in the formation of a glycine-extended form of gastrin (G-Gly) that is found in high concentrations in the developing rat gastric antrum.[82] G-Gly serves as a

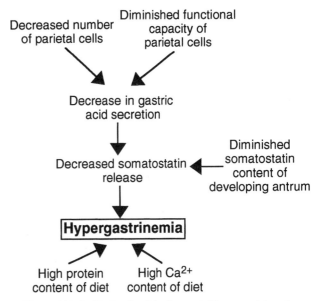

Figure 111–3. Mechanism(s) of neonatal hypergastrinemia.

substrate for the amidation enzyme, peptidyl-glycine α-amidating monooxygenase (PAM), that catalyzes the formation of fully processed, mature, amidated gastrin.[83] Gastrin (G-NH_2) requires its carboxyl-terminal amide moiety for full biologic activity mediated by gastrin/CCK_B receptors. Indeed, removal of the carboxyl-terminal amide in gastrin completely abolishes its acid stimulatory effects mediated by standard gastrin/CCK_B receptors, and the immediate precursor of amidated gastrins, G-Gly, is at least four orders of magnitude less potent than G-NH_2 in stimulating acid secretion from gastric parietal cells.[84] Nevertheless, interest in the physiologic effects of G-Gly has been fueled by the observations that G-Gly is stored in brain and gut tissues,[85] secreted with G-NH_2 from antral G cells into the circulation, and achieves concentrations in plasma roughly equivalent to those of G-NH_2.[86] Moreover, G-Gly is seen in greater concentrations than G-NH_2 during development and in some malignant tissues that express gastrin, such as Zollinger-Ellison tumors and colon cancers.[87, 88] Finally, biosynthetic studies suggested that G-Gly may be a distinct end-product of progastrin processing.[89] Thus, the evidence pointed to G-Gly's role as a growth factor but not as a direct acid secretagogue.

To further characterize the potential trophic effects of G-Gly, we examined whether G-Gly might function as a growth factor in a fashion that could be distinguished from its relatively weak effects on the standard gastrin/CCK_B receptor.[84] We compared the abilities of G-NH_2 and G-Gly to stimulate DNA synthesis.[90] Both G-NH_2 and G-Gly stimulated [^{3}H]thymidine incorporation in a dose-dependent fashion. As expected, the stimulation induced by G-NH_2 was completely reversed by selective gastrin/CCK_B receptor antagonists. In further studies, we characterized a distinct receptor and signaling cascade for G-Gly.[91] However, the inability of investigators to isolate a cDNA encoding the putative G-Gly receptor has hampered further study in this area. Other data help confirm the role that G-Gly may play in gastrointestinal physiology. G-Gly can stimulate growth in an autocrine fashion.[92] Although acute administration of G-Gly has no effect on gastric acid secretion,[84, 93] chronic administration of G-Gly markedly enhances stimulated but not basal acid secretion from isolated parietal cells and *in vivo*. This action of G-Gly is mediated via an increase in the expression of H^+,K^+-ATPase within gastric parietal cells.[94] G-Gly may play a role in the growth of the colon.[95,96] Indeed, gastrin-deficient mice have a diminished colonic proliferative index, and transgenic mice overexpressing G-Gly have

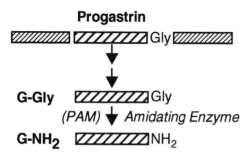

Figure 111–4. Progastrin post-translational processing. Progastrin (*top*) is sequentially processed to a glycine-extended form of gastrin (G-Gly). G-Gly then serves as a substrate for the amidation enzyme (peptidyl-glycine α-amidating monooxygenase [PAM]), which catalyzes the formation of amidated gastrin (G-NH$_2$). The c-terminal amide moiety is necessary for G-NH$_2$ binding to the gastrin/CCK$_B$ receptor. Developing tissues often contain more G-Gly than G-NH$_2$ before maturation of PAM.

enhanced colonic proliferation.[97] These observations suggest that growth-related receptors for G-Gly work in concert with G-NH$_2$ to enhance the functional development of the gut (Fig. 111–5).

D-CELL FUNCTION

In the fetal human, somatostatin has been found as early as 8 weeks' gestation.[98, 99] However, unlike gastrin, somatostatin exerts its effects in a paracrine manner and therefore the release of gastric somatostatin may not result in an increase in plasma levels. Thus it has been difficult to describe carefully the development of gastric D-cell function in humans.

Gastric D-cell development, however, has been studied in animal models. In the rat, antral G cells can be detected at day 19 of gestation, but D cells are not clearly identified until day 4 of life.[79, 100, 101] Gastric somatostatin concentrations increase slowly from birth to weaning at day 21.[79] At day 21, there is a marked increase in gastric acid secretion, which is followed by an abrupt increase in gastric somatostatin content on day 24 that is more marked in the antrum than in the fundus.[79] Others have noted similar changes in somatostatin gene expression,[102] suggesting that peptide content is closely linked to gene expression. As is the case with the development of G-cell function, diet and glucocorticoids play a similar role in the development of D-cell content.[100, 103] Rabbits and sheep are similar to humans in that immunoreactive somatostatin can be detected during fetal development although at levels much lower than that seen in mature animals.[104, 105] The rabbit stomach also demonstrates a marked reduction in somatostatin and an increase in gastrin content in the third trimester that coincides with the development of acid secretion.[104]

To explore the effect of somatostatin on gastric development, investigators created a mouse deficient in the somatostatin receptor subtype found in the stomach (SSTR-2).[106] SSTR-2 mice developed and gained weight normally but have a marked increase in gastric acid secretion that was abolished by an anti-gastrin antibody. This is similar to the effect seen in humans overexpressing gastrin and confirms the inhibitory role of somatostatin on gastrin release and gastric acid secretion.

ENTEROCHROMAFFIN-LIKE CELLS

There are few data concerning histamine-secreting ECL cells during development. Histamine is synthesized from histidine via the action of histidine decarboxylase (HDC). HDC activity is first seen in the developing rat at day 10 of life.[59] Gastrin stimulation

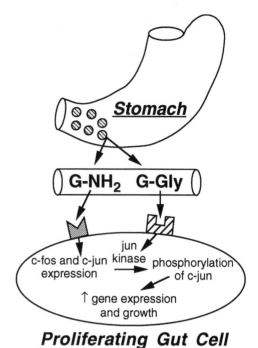

Proliferating Gut Cell

Figure 111–5. Mechanisms of G-NH$_2$ and G-Gly trophic effects. Amidated gastrin (G-NH$_2$) and its glycine-extended precursor (G-Gly) are released from G cells in the gastric antrum into the circulation. G-NH$_2$ acts through gastrin/CCK$_B$ receptors to enhance the expression of c-fos and c-jun. G-Gly, via another distinct receptor and jun kinase, phosphorylates and thus bioactivates c-jun. c-fos and phosphorylated c-jun then induce the expression of other genes necessary for the proliferation of gut cells.

of HDC activity is first noted on day 16 of life.[59] However, other investigators can detect the presence of immunoreactive histamine on embryonic day 16 in the rat gastric muscular layer and on embryonic day 18 within the mucosa.[107] From embryonic day 18 the number of histamine-positive cells increases, and at birth many of these have the paracrine-like processes that are characteristic of mature ECL cells. The number of mature ECL cells increases from birth to weaning, when their numbers and distribution are similar to that seen in a mature animal.[107] Since mature ECL cells express gastrin/CCK$_B$ receptors, it is likely that the diminished number of gastrin receptors found in the developing rat reflect not only a loss of receptors on the parietal cell but also on ECL cells.[52, 55, 65] This has not been tested experimentally, but because gastrin is an important regulator of histamine release from ECL cells, it suggests that histamine secretion might also be diminished.

Histamine's effects on gastric acid secretion are mediated via histamine2 receptors (H$_2$R). As was the case for gastrin- and SSTR-2–deficient mice, H$_2$R-deficient mice are viable and grow normally.[106] However, unlike the gastrin-deficient mice, these mice have unexplained normal gastric acid secretion. They do have an elevated serum gastrin and an increase in gastric mucosal thickness that contains increased numbers of small parietal cells.

SUMMARY OF REGULATION OF GASTRIC ACID SECRETION IN DEVELOPMENT

From the various human and animal studies, it appears that at birth there is diminished gastric acid secretion from parietal cells (see Fig. 111–3). The reasons for this include a decrease in the number of cell surface receptors and a diminished number of fully functional parietal cells.[52] This lack of acid production results in a decrease in somatostatin release that further increases gastrin secretion. One clinical implication of these observations is that since gastric acid secretion is requisite to the formation of duodenal ulcers, one would expect to see a low incidence of this condition in neonates. Moreover, the lack of acid production also contributes to the relatively low incidence of erosive esophagitis in infants with gastroesophageal reflux.

CHIEF CELL FUNCTION

In humans, the primary function of the chief cell is to secrete the proteolytic enzyme pepsin. Pepsin is packaged and stored in the chief cell within secretory granules in an inactive or zymogen (pepsinogen) form. Immunoreactive pepsinogen can be detected in the human fetus by 8 weeks of gestation,[108] and chief cells can be identified by the end of the 13th week.[3] Peptic activity can be seen in the fetal stomach by 16 weeks of gestation.[4] Peptic activity increases thereafter, and thus premature infants weighing 1 kg have approximately one half the gastric peptic activity of term infants.[109] There are several different forms of pepsinogen in humans, but the primary type is pepsinogen IV.[108] Pepsin is the primary enzyme responsible for gastric proteolytic activity in humans; however, other species secrete proteolytic enzymes, such as chymosin, that are not found in humans.[110] Thus, it is difficult to use animal models to examine the total gastric proteolytic activity for insight into human development.

Like gastric acid secretion, the secretion of pepsinogen appears to be diminished in the rat pup prior to weaning.[111] The rat chief cell response to carbachol is present at birth, but the amount of pepsinogen secreted is very low.[111] As is the case with the development of gastric acid secretion, the development of pepsinogen secretion is sensitive to corticosteroids.[112] Although thyroxine has a similar effect, this effect is mediated by an increase in endogenous glucocorticoid levels.[111]

GASTRIC LIPASE

Although not generally thought of as an organ responsible for fat absorption, the neonatal stomach secretes a lipase distinct from that found in the pancreas. It is not surprising that gastric lipase has a lower pH optimum than does pancreatic lipase.[113-115] Moreover, gastric lipase is somewhat more important in the neonate than in the adult because of the relative pancreatic insufficiency seen in newborns infants.[116] Although lingual lipase is the major source of gastric lipolytic activity in the rat,[117] it appears that there is little lingual lipase in humans.[118] Human gastric lipase is synthesized in gastric fundic chief cells and co-secreted with pepsinogen.[119,120] In humans, gastric lipase appears as early as 10 to 13 weeks after conception, consistent with the development of early gastric glands.[121] In preterm infants, gastric lipolytic activity is low at 24 to 26 weeks' gestation but increases to reach a peak around 32 weeks' gestation.[122] Thereafter, gastric lipase activity slowly declines until term and remains level throughout infancy.[122,123] In adults, lipase secretion is stimulated by agents such as gastrin that promote pepsin secretion from chief cells, but this has not been studied in human neonates.

REFERENCES

1. Hawass NE, et al: Morphology and growth of fetal stomach. Invest Radiol 26:998, 1991.
2. Sase M, et al: Fetal gastric size in normal and abnormal pregnancies. Ultrasound Obstet Gynecol 19:467, 2002.
3. Montgomery RK, et al: Development of the human gastrointestinal tract: twenty years of progress. Gastroenterology 116:702, 1999.
4. Deren JS: Development of structure and function in the fetal and newborn stomach. Am J Clin Nutr 24:144, 1971.
5. Salenius P: On the ontogenesis of the human gastric epithelial cells. Acta Anat (Basel) 50:1, 1962.
6. Delemos C: The ultrastructure of endocrine cells in the corpus of the stomach of human fetuses. Am J Anat 148:359, 1977.
7. Wright N, Alison M (eds): Morphological Aspects of Cell Renewal Systems. Oxford, Clarendon Press, 1984.
8. Hattori T, Fujita S: Fractographic study on the growth and multiplication of the gastric gland of the hamster. Cell Tissue Res 153:145, 1974.
9. Rubin W, et al: The normal human gastric epithelia. A fine structural study. Lab Invest 19:598, 1968.
10. Matsuyama M, Susuki H: Differentiation of immature mucus cells into parietal, argyrophil, and chief cells in stomach grafts. Science 169: 1970.
11. Karam SM: Lineage commitment and maturation of epithelial cells in the gut. Frontiers in Biosci 4:D286, 1999.
12. Karam SM: Cell lineage relationship in the stomach of normal and genetically manipulated mice. Braz Med Biol Res 31:271, 1998.
13. Karam SM: Dynamics of epithelial cells in the corpus of the mouse stomach. IV. Bidirectional migration of parietal cells ending in their gradual degeneration and loss. Anat Rec 236:314, 1993.
14. Karam SM, et al: Gastric epithelial morphogenesis in normal and transgenic mice. Am J Physiol 272:G1209, 1997.
15. Rubin DC, et al: Use of isografts to study proliferation and differentiation programs of mouse stomach epithelia. Am J Physiol 267:G27, 1994.
16. Stanton BR, et al: Loss of N-myc function results in embryonic lethality and failure of the epithelial component of the embryo to develop. Genes Dev 6:2235, 1992.
17. Jacobsen CM, et al: Genetic mosaic analysis reveals that GATA-4 is required for proper differentiation of mouse gastric epithelium. Dev Biol 241:34, 2002.
18. Marino LR, et al: H(+)-K(+)-ATPase and carbonic anhydrase II gene expression in the developing rat fundus. Am J Physiol 259:G108, 1990.
19. Saffer JD, et al: Developmental expression of Spl in the mouse. Mol Cell Biol 11: 2189, 1991.
20. Menard D, et al: Maturation of human fetal stomach in organ culture. Gastroenterology 104:492, 1993.
21. Lorenz RG, Gordon JI: Use of transgenic mice to study regulation of gene expression in the parietal cell lineage of gastric units. J Biol Chem 268:26559, 1993.
22. Li Q, et al: Diphtheria toxin–mediated ablation of parietal cells in the stomach of transgenic mice. J Biol Chem 271:3671, 1996.
23. Beaumont W: Experiments and Observations on the Gastric Juice and the Physiology of Digestion. Birmingham, AL, Gryphon Editions, 1883.
24. Hersey SJ, Sachs G: Gastric acid secretion. Physiol Rev 75:155, 1995.
25. Pavlov IP: The Work of the Digestive Glands. London, Charles Griffen, 1902.
26. Gillespie IE: Effect of antrectomy and vagotomy with gastrojejunostomy and antrectomy with vagotomy on the spontaneous and maximal gastric acid output in man. Gastroenterology 38:361, 1960.
27. Feldman M, Richardson CT: Total 24-hour gastric acid secretion in patients with duodenal ulcer. Comparison with normal subjects and effects of cimetidine and parietal cell vagotomy. Gastroenterology 90:540, 1986.
28. Dockray GJ, et al: The neuronal origin of bombesin-like immunoreactivity in the rat gastrointestinal tract. Neuroscience 4:1561, 1979.
29. Sugano K, et al: Stimulation of gastrin release by bombesin and canine gastrin-releasing peptides. Studies with isolated canine G cells in primary culture. J Clin Invest 79:935, 1987.
30. Schepp W, et al: Bombesin-like peptides stimulate gastrin release from isolated rat G-cells. Reg Peptides 28:241, 1990.
31. Schubert ML: The effect of vasoactive intestinal polypeptide on gastric acid secretion is predominantly mediated by somatostatin. Gastroenterology 100:1195, 1991.
32. Schiller LR, et al: Distention-induced gastrin release: effects of luminal acidification and intravenous atropine. Gastroenterology 78:912, 1980.
33. Hirschowitz BI, Gibson RG: Stimulation of gastrin release and gastric secretion: effect of bombesin and a nonapeptide in fistula dogs with and without fundic vagotomy. Digestion 18:227, 1978.
34. DelValle J, Yamada T: Amino acids and amines stimulate gastrin release from canine antral G-cells via different pathways. J Clin Inves 85:139, 1990.
35. Feldman M, et al: Role of gastrin heptadecapeptide in the acid secretory response to amino acids in man. J Clin Invest 61:308, 1978.
36. Seal A, et al: Immunoneutralization of somatostatin and neurotensin: effect on gastric acid secretion. Am J Physiol 255:G40, 1988.
37. Wershil BK: Gastric function. In Walker WA, et al (eds): Pediatric Gastrointestinal Disease: Pathophysiology, Diagnosis, Management. Philadelphia, BC Decker, 1991, pp 256–265.
38. Avery GB, et al: Gastric acidity in the first day of life. Pediatrics 37:1005, 1966.
39. Baron JH: The clinical use of gastric function tests. Scand J Gastroenterol 6:9, 1970.
40. Ames MD: Gastric acidity in the first ten days of life in the prematurely born baby. Am J Dis Child 100:123, 1960.
41. Ahn CI, Kim YJ: Acidity and volume of gastric contents in the first week of life. J Korean Med Assoc 6:948, 1963.
42. Christie DL: Gastric secretion. In Labenthal E (ed): Textbook of Gastroenterology and Nutrition in Infancy New York, Raven Press, p 109, 1981.
43. Euler AR, et al: Increased serum gastrin concentrations and gastric acid hyposecretion in the immediate newborn period. Gastroenterology 72:1271, 1977.

44. Euler AR, et al: Basal and pentagastrin-stimulated acid secretion in newborn human infants. Pediatr Res 13:36, 1979.

45. Grahnquist L, et al: Early development of human gastric H,K-adenosine triphosphatase. J Pediatr Gastroenterol Nutr 30:533, 2000.

46. Hyman PE et al: Gastric acid secretory function in preterm infants. J Pediatr 106:467, 1985.

47. Marino L, et al: Parietal cell function of full-term and premature infants: unstimulated gastric acid and intrinsic factor secretion. J Pediatr Gastroenterol Nutr 3:23, 1984.

48. Hyman PE, et al: Effect of enteral feeding on the maintenance of gastric acid secretory function. Gastroenterology 84:341, 1983.

49. Euler AR, et al: Basal and pentagastrin-stimulated gastric acid secretory rates in normal children and in those with peptic ulcer disease. J Pediatr 103:766, 1983.

50. Lari J, et al: Response to gastrin pentapeptide in children. J Pediatr Surg 3:682, 1968.

51. Agunod M, et al: Correlative study of hydrochloric acid, pepsin, and intrinsic factor secretion in newborns and infants. Am J Dig Dis 14:400, 1969.

52. Johnson LR: Functional development of the stomach. Annu Rev Physiol 47:199, 1985.

53. Pettitt JM, et al: Gastric parietal cell development: expression of the H+/K+ATPase subunits coincides with the biogenesis of the secretory membranes. Immunol Cell Biol 71:191, 1993.

54. Morley GP, et al: The mouse gastric H,K-ATPase beta subunit. Gene structure and coordinate expression with the alpha subunit during ontogeny. J Biol Chem 167:1165, 1992.

55. Hervatin F, et al: Ontogeny of rat gastric H+-K+-ATPase activity. Am J Physiol 252:G28, 1987.

56. Yee LF, et al: Mechanisms of gastric acid secretion in the fetal rabbit. Surgery 118:199, 1995.

57. Xu RJ, Cranwell PD: Development of gastric acid secretion in pigs from birth to thirty-six days of age: the response to pentagastrin. J Dev Physiol 13:315, 1990.

58. Seidel ER, Johnson LR: Ontogeny of gastric mucosal muscarinic receptor and sensitivity to carbachol. Am J Physiol 246:G550, 1984.

59. Ikezaki M, Johnson LR: Development of sensitivity to different secretagogues in the rat stomach. Am J Physiol 244:G165, 1983.

60. Garzon B, et al: Biphasic development of pentagastrin sensitivity in rat stomach. Am J Physiol 242:G111, 1982.

61. Ackerman SH, Shindledecker RD: Maturational increases and decreases in acid secretion in the rat. Am J Physiol 247:G638, 1984.

62. Gespach C, et al: Development of sensitivity to cAMP-inducing hormones in the rat stomach. Am J Physiol 247:G231, 1984.

63. Harada T, et al: Meal-stimulated gastric acid secretion in infants. J Pediatr 104:534, 1984.

64. Takeuchi K, et al: Mucosal gastrin receptor. V. Development in newborn rats. Am J Physiol 240:G163, 1981.

65. Peitsch W, et al: Mucosal gastrin receptor. VI. Induction by corticosterone in newborn rats. Am J Physiol 240:G442, 1982.

66. Speir GR, et al: Mucosal gastrin receptor. VII. Up-and-down regulation. Am J Physiol 242:G243, 1982.

67. Schepp W, et al: Intrinsic factor secretion from isolated gastric mucosal cells of rat and man—two different patterns of secretagogue control. Agents Actions 14:522, 1984.

68. Dieckgraefe BK, et al: Developmental regulation of rat intrinsic factor mRNA. Am J Physiol 254:G913, 1988.

69. Grasso S, et al: Gastrin (G) cells are the cellular site of the gastric thyrotropin-releasing hormone in human fetuses and newborns. A chromatographic, radioimmunological, and immunocytochemical study. J Clin Endocrinol Metab 74:1421, 1992.

70. Brand SJ, et al: Complete tyrosine-O-sulphation of gastrin in neonatal rat pancreas. Nature 309:456, 1984.

71. Wang TC, et al: Pancreatic gastrin stimulates islet differentiation of transforming growth factor alpha–induced ductular precursor cells. J Clin Invest 92:1349, 1993.

72. Majumdar AP, Johnson LR: Gastric mucosal cell proliferation during development in rats and effects of pentagastrin. Am J Physiol 242:G135, 1982.

73. Hinkle KL, Samuelson LC: Lessons from genetically engineered animal models. III. Lessons learned from gastrin gene deletion in mice. Am J Physiol 277:G500, 1999.

74. Friis-Hansen L, et al: Impaired gastric acid secretion in gastrin-deficient mice. Am J Physiol 274:G561, 1998.

75. Koh TJ, et al: Gastrin deficiency results in altered gastric differentiation and decreased colonic proliferation in mice. Gastroenterology 113:1015, 1997.

76. Langhans N, et al: Abnormal gastric histology and decreased acid production in cholecystokinin-B/gastrin receptor–deficient mice. Gastroenterology 112:280, 1997.

77. Euler AR, et al: Human newborn hypergastrinemia: an investigation of prenatal and perinatal factors and their effects on gastrin. Pediatr Res 12:652, 1978.

78. Lichtenberger L: A search for the origin of neonatal hypergastrinemia. J Pediatr Gastroenterol Nutr 3:161, 1984.

79. Koshimizu T: The development of pancreatic and gastrointestinal stomato-statin-like immunoreactivity and its relationship to feeding in neonatal rats. Endocrinology 112:911, 1983.

80. Johnson LR, Guthrie PD: Proglumide inhibition of trophic action of pentagastrin. Am J Physiol 246:G62, 1984.

81. Ackerman SH: Ontogeny of gastric acid secretion in the rat: evidence for multiple response systems. Science 217:75, 1982.

82. Marino LR, et al: Development of gastrin synthesis and posttranslational processing mechanisms in rats. Am J Physiol 254:G87, 1988.

83. Dickinson C, Yamada T: Gastrin-amidating enzyme in the porcine pituitary and antrum: characterization of molecular forms and substrate specificity. J Biol Chem 266:334, 1991.

84. Matsumoto M, et al: Biological activity of progastrin posttranslational processing intermediates. Am J Physiol 252:G315, 1987.

85. Del Valle J, et al: Progastrin and its glycine-extended posttranslational processing intermediates in human gastrointestinal tissues. Gastroenterology 92:1908, 1987.

86. DelValle J, et al: Glycine-extended processing intermediates of gastrin and cholecystokinin in human plasma. Gastroenterology 97:1159, 1989.

87. Ciccotosto GD, et al: Expression, processing, and secretion of gastrin in patients with colorectal carcinoma. Gastroenterology 109:1142, 1995.

88. Kochman M, et al: Post-translational processing of gastrin in neoplastic human colonic tissues. Biochem Biophys Res Commun 189:1165, 1992.

89. Varro A, et al: Pathways of processing of the gastrin precursor in rat antral mucosa. J Clin Invest 95:1642, 1995.

90. Seva C, et al: Growth-promoting effects of glycine-extended progastrin. Science 265:410, 1994.

91. Todisco A, et al: Gastrin and glycine-extended processing intermediates induce different programs of early gene activation. J Biol Chem 270:28337, 1995.

92. Negre F, et al: Autocrine stimulation of AR4-2J rat pancreatic tumor cell growth by glycine-extended gastrin. Int J Cancer 66:653, 1996.

93. Higashide S, et al: Glycine-extended gastrin potentiates gastrin-stimulated gastric acid secretion in rats. Am J Physiol 270:G220, 1996.

94. Kaise M, et al: Glycine-extended progastrin intermediates induce H+,K+-ATPase α-subunit gene expression through a novel receptor. J Biol Chem 270:11155, 1995.

95. Dickinson CJ: Relationship of gastrin processing to colon cancer. Gastroenterology 109:1384, 1995.

96. Stepan V, et al: Glycine-extended gastrin exerts growth-promoting effects on human colon cancer cells. Mol Med 5:147, 1999.

97. Koh T, et al: Overexpression of glycine-extended gastrin in transgenic mice results in increased colonic proliferation. J Clin Invest 103:1119, 1999.

98. Stein BA, et al: The ontogeny of regulatory peptide-containing cells in the human fetal stomach. J Histochem Cytochem 31:1117, 1983.

99. Bryant MG, et al: Development of intestinal regulatory peptides in the human fetus. Gastroenterology 83:47, 1982.

100. Okahata H, et al: Development of gastric somatostatin-like immunoreactivity in response to corticosterone acetate and dietary changes in young rats. Acta Endocrinol 112:383, 1986.

101. Onolfo JP, Lehy T: Comparative development of gastrin and somatostatin cell populations in the pancreas, stomach, and duodenum of the rat during the perinatal period. Anat Rec 218:416, 1987.

102. Zingg HH, et al: Developmental expression of the rat somatostatin gene. Endocrinology 115:90, 1984.

103. Okahata H, et al: Influence of diet on the development of antral gastrin-like immunoreactivity in the stomach of rats. Acta Endocrinol (Copenh) 120:374, 1989.

104. Yee LF, et al: Roles of gastrin and somatostatin in the regulation of gastric acid secretion in the fetal rabbit. J Surg Res 63:364, 1996.

105. Grabau BJ, et al: Developmental regulation of gastric somatostatin secretion in the sheep. Endocrinology 140:603, 1999.

106. Martinez V, et al: High basal gastric acid secretion in somatostatin receptor subtype 2 knockout mice. Gastroenterology 114:1125, 1998.

107. Nissinen MJ, et al: Ontogeny of histamine-immunoreactive cells in rat stomach. Cell Tissue Res 267:241, 1992.

108. Hirsch-Marie H, et al: Immunochemical study and cellular localization of human pepsinogens during ontogenesis and in gastric cancers. Lab Invest 34:623, 1976.

109. Keene MFL, Hewer EE: Digestive enzymes of the human fetus. Lancet 1:767, 1929.

110. Foltmann B: Chymosin: a short review on foetal and neonatal gastric proteases. Scand J Clin Lab Invest Suppl 210:65, 1992.

111. Tseng CC, et al: Hormonal effects on development of the secretory apparatus of parietal cells. Am J Physiol 253:G284, 1987.

112. Yahav PC, et al: Ontogeny of pepsin secretory response to secretagogues in isolated rat gastric glands. Am J Physiol 250:G200, 1986.

113. Bodmer MW, et al: Molecular cloning of a human gastric lipase and expression of the enzyme in yeast. Biochim Biophys Acta 909:237, 1987.

114. DeNigris SJ, et al: Secretion of human gastric lipase from dispersed gastric glands. Biochim Biophys Acta 836:67, 1985.

115. Tiruppathi C, Balasubramanian KA: Purification and properties of an acid lipase from human gastric juice. Biochim Biophys Acta 712:692, 1982.

116. Hamosh M, et al: Fat digestion in the newborn. Characterization of lipase in gastric aspirates of premature and term infants. J Clin Invest 67:838, 1981.

117. Liao TH, et al: Gastric lipolysis in the developing rat. Ontogeny of the lipases active in the stomach. Biochim Biophys Acta 754:1, 1983.

118. Sarles J, et al: Human gastric lipase: ontogeny and variations in children. Acta Paediatr *81*:511, 1992.
119. Abrams CK, et al: Gastric lipase: localization in the human stomach. Gastroenterology *95*:1460, 1988.
120. Moreau H, et al: Immunocytolocalization of human gastric lipase in chief cells of the fundic mucosa. Histochemistry *91*:419, 1989.
121. Menard D, et al: Ontogeny of human gastric lipase and pepsin activities. Gastroenterology *108*:1650, 1995.
122. Lee PC, et al: Development of lipolytic activity in gastric aspirates from premature infants. J Pediatr Gastroenterol Nutr *17*:291, 1993.
123. DiPalma J, et al: Lipase and pepsin activity in the gastric mucosa of infants, children, and adults. Gastroenterology *101*:116, 1991.

112

Taher I. Omari and Colin D. Rudolph

Gastrointestinal Motility

The process of digestion and absorption of nutrients begins with the ingestion of complex foods. Food is moved through the digestive tract lumen, where it undergoes sequential mechanical disruption and chemical digestion. During passage through the intestine, products of digestion including simple sugars, amino acids, peptides, and fatty acids are absorbed across the mucosal surface into the bloodstream. In each portion of the gastrointestinal tract, the coordinated contractions of the muscles surrounding the digestive tract lumen are responsible for the process of breaking large particles of food into smaller digestible fragments, mixing and stirring lumen contents, and propelling luminal contents down the digestive tract. Chewing or mastication begins the process of breaking down food so it can safely progress through the esophagus into the stomach. In the stomach, food is divided into small particles and is mixed into a suspension with gastric secretions, thus increasing the surface area for enzymatic digestion in the stomach and intestine. In the intestine, mixing and churning within the intestinal lumen ensure that the digested simple nutrients contact the mucosal border and allow absorption.

This chapter focuses on the development of *gastrointestinal motility*, which describes the coordinated contractions of gastrointestinal muscle that facilitate the mechanical digestion, mixing, and propulsion of food as it moves through the gastrointestinal lumen. The embryologic and functional development of the gastrointestinal smooth muscle and neural plexus is discussed elsewhere in this book.

SUCKING AND SWALLOWING

Ingestion of milk by the newborn infant depends on the ability to (1) suck and express milk from the breast or bottle into the oral cavity, (2) swallow and propel milk from the oral cavity into the pharynx and then from the pharynx into the esophagus, and (3) coordinate sucking and swallowing with breathing. As shown in Figure 112-1, the oral and pharyngeal chambers of the neonate and adult are anatomically different. In the neonate, the tongue is enlarged relative to the size of the oral cavity, and there are also additional sucking pads (dense fatty tissue) located laterally to the tongue. The larynx lies higher in the neonate, thereby reducing the size of the pharyngeal chamber and allowing the top of the epiglottis to overlap the soft palate. This positioning of the epiglottis provides added airway protection by diverting liquid laterally around the laryngeal opening.[1,2] Sucking and swallowing depend on both the anatomic integrity of the feeding apparatus and the maturation of highly complex oropharyngeal neuromuscular control mechanisms. Very premature newborn infants are usually unable to take oral feedings, thus necessitating the use of enteral feeding tubes. As described later in this chapter, this deficiency probably relates to impaired coordination of suck and swallow rather than functional immaturity of the esophageal phase of swallowing.

Oral Phase of Swallowing

The sequence of normal adult deglutition is as follows: (1) food is firstly chewed, mixed with saliva, and positioned on the anterior surface of the tongue (preparatory phase); (2) the tongue rolls posteriorly, making sequential contact with the palate and propelling the bolus into the pharynx (oral phase); (3) pharyngeal constrictors contract sequentially and propel the bolus through the relaxed upper esophageal sphincter (UES) and into the esophagus (pharyngeal phase); and (4) esophageal peristalsis propels the bolus down the length of the esophagus through the relaxed lower esophageal sphincter (LES) into the stomach (esophageal phase). The sequence of normal infant deglutition is essentially the same, with the exception of the preparatory phase, which involves the expression of a liquid meal into the oral cavity by sucking.

The small size and shape of the infant oral cavity facilitate sucking. The buccal fat pads and palate stabilize the lateral and superior walls of the cavity. To suck, the lips seal over the nipple, and the tongue presses against the soft palate to form a closed chamber in the oral cavity around the nipple (Fig. 112-2). The large tongue is pulled inferiorly like a piston, creating a negative suction in the oral cavity while the gums synchronously appose to produce a positive expression pressure.[3] This sucking action is essentially the same during bottle and breast-feeding, with the exception of the tongue, which is projected further forward during breast sucking.[3] Milk expressed into the oral cavity collects either over the base of the tongue (and vallecula) or between the midtongue and the hard palate.[4]

These coordinated sucking movements are not present until about 28 weeks' gestation in the human. Mouthing and patterns of lingual extension and retraction are present *in utero* at 15 weeks' gestation[5] and are sometimes still seen at 6 months of age.[1] Single sucks can be recorded manometrically at 28 weeks' gestation, and these develop into sucking bursts by 31 weeks (Fig. 112-3).[6] A mature sucking pattern that adequately expresses milk from a breast or nipple is not present until 32 to 34 weeks' gestation.

Intraoral pressures generated during sucking and patterns of sucking change with maturity. Intraoral pressures range from -50 to -225 mm Hg[7] and are up to 40% lower in preterm infants.[8] The use of pacifiers to stimulate nonnutritive sucking during enteral feeding in preterm infants can augment suck pressures by 15 to 25%[8,9] but it does not speed the maturation of the infant's acquisition of mature suck and swallow skills, a process that appears to depend on neuromaturation related to postconceptual age.[10] Premature infants suck in short 6- to 9-second

INFANT

ADULT

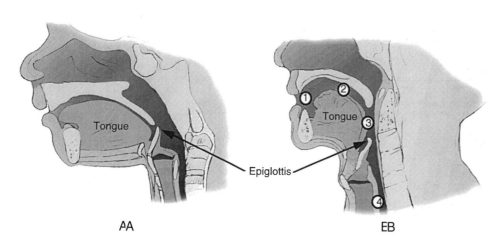

AA

EB

Figure 112–1. Comparative diagrams of the anatomy of the mouth and pharynx of neonates (**A**) and adults (**B**). Note the reduction in the relative size of the pharyngeal chamber and overlap between the soft palate and the epiglottis. The numbers on the figure refer to the phases of swallowing in the adult: (*1*) preparatory, (*2*) oral, (*3*) pharyngeal, and (*4*) esophageal. (From Rudolph CD: *In* Hyman PE, Di Lorenzo C (eds): Pediatric Gastrointestinal Motility Disorders. New York, Academy Professional Information Services, 1994, p 37.)

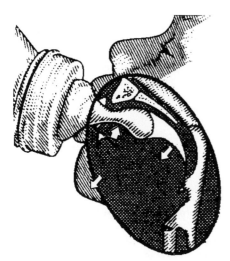

Figure 112–2. Mechanism of sucking from a nipple. The lips seal the anterior oral cavity, and the tongue seals against the palate to close the posterior opening of the oral cavity. The tongue and jaw descend with sucking, to create negative intraoral pressure. (From Bu'Lock F, et al: Dev Med Clin Neurol *32*:669, 1990.)

bursts of 8 to 10 sucks per burst,[8, 10] newborn term infants demonstrate a similar burst pattern of 14 sucks per burst,[8,10] and older term infants exhibit a more constant sucking pattern with frequencies of 8 to 11 sucks per minute.[7, 11]

As the infant matures, the oral cavity enlarges, thus allowing manipulation of pureed spoon feedings. At 3 to 4 months of age, tongue movements develop that move a food bolus from the front of the tongue back toward the pharynx. At 6 months, infants occlude their lips to remove pureed foods from a spoon and move the food toward the midline with their tongue for chewing. As alveolar ridges and teeth develop over the next year, the infant develops increased tongue mobility that allows lateralization of solid foods for mature mastication.[12,13]

Pharyngeal Swallowing

The exquisite pattern of muscular contractions that produce the swallowing action is centrally integrated by two regionally distinct groups of medullary interneurons—the nucleus tractus solitarius (ventrally located) and the nucleus ambiguus (dorsally located)—that form the *swallowing center*. The nucleus tractus solitarius receives inputs from cortical fibers and peripheral sensory fibers originating in the pharynx, larynx, and esophagus. The nucleus tractus solitarius acts as a pattern generator and precisely regulates the sequence of motor nuclei excitation that leads to pharyngeal and esophageal contraction. The nucleus ambiguus receives some sensory input but predominantly acts as a relay station for the sequential activation of motor neurons responsible for pharyngeal and esophageal contraction and UES and LES relaxation.[14, 15]

Swallowing reflexes are triggered when the contents of the oral cavity are propelled posteriorly toward the pharynx. This is achieved by highly complex contractions of the longitudinal and transverse intrinsic lingual musculature of the tongue.[1] Swallowing is initiated by distal elevation of the tongue, followed by a posteriorly propagated peristaltic-like wave along the medial portion of the tongue.[3, 16] Abnormal tongue movements such as incomplete peristaltic contractions and tremulous contractions are frequent in premature infants and diminish as infants approach term.[3] If these poorly coordinated lingual movements fail to clear the oral cavity of its contents, the residue may overflow into the oropharynx, and if the airway is not protected, aspiration may occur.

As the oral contents enter the pharynx, a pharyngeal swallow is triggered. In term infants, the time delay between initial suck and pharyngeal contraction is 500 milliseconds,[17] and suck–oral transit time is 900 milliseconds, whereas pharyngeal transit time is 600 milliseconds.[4] The phasic relationship between sucking and swallowing is not constant; preterm and newborn infants demonstrate one to four sucks per swallow,[3,5,17] whereas older term infants demonstrate one to two sucks per swallow.[3, 4] During pharyngeal swallowing, the vellum and laryngeal musculature elevate, thus closing the nasopharynx and epiglottis and forming a conduit for passage of the milk bolus through the pharyngoesophageal junction. In adults, contraction of pharyngeal musculature does not actively propel the food bolus. Instead, the pressure wave associated with pharyngeal contraction occurs after the bolus has passed and functions predominantly to clear the pharynx of food residues.[18] Uncoordinated pharyngeal contraction may lead to the retention of food bolus residues in the pharynx.

Coordination of Swallowing with Breathing

In utero, the pharynx is a conduit for fluid. The human fetus ingests up to 750 mL of amniotic fluid per day.[19] Swallowing of

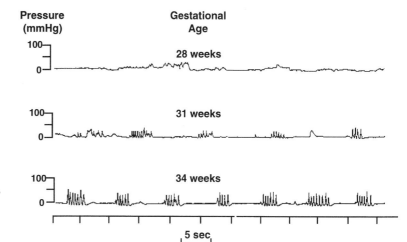

Figure 112–3. Intraoral pressure recordings of sucking patterns in premature infants during active sleep. Between 28 and 34 weeks' postmenstrual age, sucking develops from poorly coordinated low-amplitude sucks to higher-amplitude burst sucking. (From Hack MM, Esterbrook MM: Early Hum Dev *11*:133-140, 1985).

amniotic fluid contributes to amniotic fluid homeostasis,[20,21] and the swallowed fluid appears to be trophic for mucosal development of the gastrointestinal tract.[22] Postnatally, however, the pharynx performs a dual function regulating the passage of food (into the esophagus) and air (into the larynx). As discussed earlier, anatomic differences between the newborn and adult larynx provide some protection of the airway in the neonate.[23] The laryngeal inlet is located high in the pharynx in the newborn, at the level of cervical vertebrae C1 to C3. The tip of the epiglottis often extends into the nasopharynx, thus separating the respiratory passages and digestive conduit. During the third year of life, the larynx descends to the adult C3 to C5 location, creating a longer common passageway for the airway and digestive tracts in the oropharynx. This anatomic arrangement facilitates phonation but increases the risk of aspiration during swallowing. Although swallowing and respiration must be precisely controlled in the newborn, the prevention of aspiration becomes more difficult with growth.

Neonates possess an airway inhibitory mechanism that is triggered 200 milliseconds before pharyngeal swallowing and lasts approximately 600 milliseconds.[17] In mature term infants, the ratio of swallowing to breathing is usually 1:1.[3] In contrast, newborn and preterm infants rarely synchronize breathing and swallowing. In the newborn, unstable breathing, prolonged inhibition, and depressed respiratory rate and minute volume occur frequently during periods of rapid swallowing.[5,11,17] Premature infants exhibit bursts of rapid swallowing interpolated with periods of rapid breathing.[3,24] Episodes of apnea, bradycardia, and oxygen desaturation are common during burst swallowing.[24] The poor coordination of breathing and swallowing seen in premature and newborn infants indicates that the interneuronal pathways between the medullary swallow and respiratory centers that synchronize respiratory inhibition are not fully functional.

ESOPHAGEAL MOTILITY

The motility of the esophagus, comprising the UES and LES and the esophageal body, has been well characterized in premature infants from 26 weeks' gestation to term. The major features of esophageal motility are summarized in Figure 112-4.

Upper Esophageal Sphincter

UES pressure is generated predominantly by tonic contraction of the cricopharyngeus muscle. During swallowing, the cricopharyngeus muscle is inhibited and produces relaxation. Approximately 100 milliseconds after relaxation, the UES is opened by the intrabolus pressure and the superior excursion of the hyoid

and larynx.[25,26] Studies of term infants and children (2 months to 7 years) have demonstrated UES pressures comparable to those of adults (40 to 50 mm Hg) and UES relaxation in response to swallowing.[27,28,29] UES function has been investigated in premature infants at gestational ages as young as 33 weeks. In these infants, UES resting tone ranged from 2 to 28 mm Hg, and the UES was found to relax appropriately in response to dry swallow.[30] In addition, the magnitude of UES resting pressure is dependent on the behavioral state, with periods of apparent comfort associated with significantly lower UES pressures than periods of activity and apparent discomfort or abdominal straining.[30] These findings are consistent with effect of behavior and arousal reported in older children and adults.[27,31,32]

Esophageal Body

Swallowing initiates primary peristaltic esophageal contractions, which can be measured as pressure wave sequences propagated in an aboral direction along the length of the esophageal body. Normal primary esophageal peristalsis has been recorded in the premature infant down to 26 weeks' gestation[33-35] and in term infants.[36] The premature infant also exhibits esophageal body contractions that occur spontaneously and are not triggered by the usual mechanisms (i.e., swallowing or esophageal distention). These spontaneous contractions are usually propagated in a nonperistaltic fashion (i.e., retrograde, synchronous, or incomplete propagation).[33-35] Similar spontaneous esophageal motor activity has been observed in adults, but these events are far less common and are usually associated with the occurrence of the migrating motor complex (MMC) of the small intestine.[37] These motor patterns occur as a background to what appears to be normal, mature, primary and secondary peristalsis and therefore do not appear to impair esophageal function, at least in the healthy infant. An example tracing illustrating swallow-related peristaltic and spontaneous nonperistaltic contractions is shown in Figure 112-4.

Lower Esophageal Sphincter

The LES functions as a physical esophagogastric antireflux barrier and comprises two sphincter mechanisms: the intrinsic smooth muscle sphincter and the crural diaphragm, which provides extrinsic support and squeeze. Both sphincter components work together and contribute to LES pressure. Early reports concluded that premature infants have poor LES tone because of immaturity of sphincter control mechanisms.[38-41] However, it has since been shown that, in premature infants, the LES generates tonic pressures that are sufficiently higher than intragastric pressure to maintain

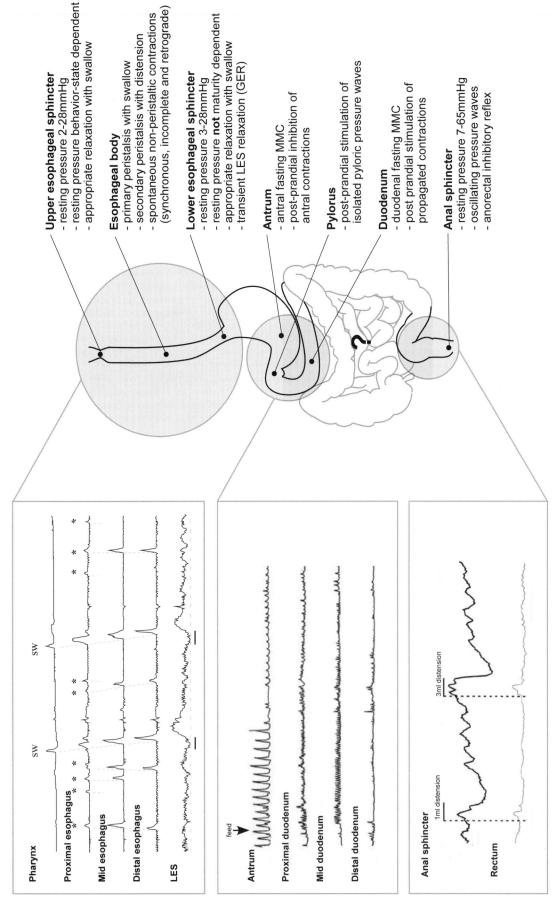

Upper esophageal sphincter
- resting pressure 2-28mmHg
- resting pressure behavior-state dependent
- appropriate relaxation with swallow

Esophageal body
- primary peristalsis with swallow
- secondary peristalsis with distension
- spontaneous non-peristaltic contractions (synchronous, incomplete and retrograde)

Lower esophageal sphincter
- resting pressure 3-28mmHg
- resting pressure **not** maturity dependent
- appropriate relaxation with swallow
- transient LES relaxation (GER)

Antrum
- antral fasting MMC
- post-prandial inhibition of antral contractions

Pylorus
- post-prandial stimulation of isolated pyloric pressure waves

Duodenum
- duodenal fasting MMC
- post prandial stimulation of propagated contractions

Anal sphincter
- resting pressure 7-65mmHg
- oscillating pressure waves
- anorectal inhibitory reflex

Pharynx

SW SW

Proximal esophagus

Mid esophagus

Distal esophagus

LES

feed
Antrum

Proximal duodenum

Mid duodenum

Distal duodenum

Anal sphincter

1ml distension

3ml distension

Rectum

Figure 112–4. Patterns of gastrointestinal motility described in the premature neonate and example tracings (*left*) of esophageal, antroduodenal, and anorectal motility recorded with perfusion manometry. *Top tracing,* esophageal motility; two pharyngeal swallows (sw) trigger primary peristalsis, which is propagated down the length of the esophagus. The swallows also trigger lower esophageal sphincter (LES) relaxation (*black bars*). Spontaneous nonperistaltic contractions (incomplete and synchronous) are also shown (*asterisks*). *Middle tracing,* antroduodenal response to feeding; feeding inhibits antral contraction and stimulates duodenal contraction. *Bottom tracing,* anorectal motility; rectal balloon distention initiates reflex relaxation of the anal sphincter. GER = gastroesophageal reflux; MMC = migrating motor complex.

effective esophagogastric competence (5 to 10 mm Hg).[33-35, 42, 43] Contrary to early reports indicating that LES pressure increases with maturation,[42] more recent evaluations showed no such pattern of maturation.[44] The LES relaxes with swallow to allow passage of a food bolus (see Fig. 112-4). This swallow-related relaxation lasts for 3 to 6 seconds, during which the LES pressure drops to within 2 to 4 mm Hg of intragastric pressure. Swallow-related relaxation is well developed in the premature infant.[33-35] In addition to swallow-related relaxation, the LES exhibits transient LES relaxation (TLESR) (see later).

Sphincteric Mechanisms of Gastroesophageal Reflux

Gastroesophageal reflux (GER) results when stomach contents (liquid, gas, or liquid and gas in combination) are expelled into the esophageal lumen. This is a normal physiologic phenomenon that often occurs during or after feeding. Abnormally frequent GER, poor clearance of GER from the esophageal lumen, or exposure of GER to airway structures may lead to the manifestation of GER disease, which has numerous clinical presentations including feeding problems with or without weight loss, irritability, and obstructive apnea. GER is common in premature infants, and it was originally thought that this related to poor LES competence resulting from immaturity of neural control mechanisms. As described previously, more recent studies in these infants showed that mechanisms of sphincter competence are well developed, and GER usually occurs in association with complete sphincter relaxation. Certain motor mechanisms of GER triggering have been identified; these include predominantly swallow-related LES relaxation in association with failed peristalsis, prolonged inhibition of LES tone, and esophageal contraction by multiple swallowing and TLESRs, which are triggered in the absence of swallowing (Fig. 112-5).[34] TLESR is by far the most common mechanism of GER triggering (see Fig. 112-5), and it has been described in all age groups from 26-week premature infants[33] through to adults.[45] Compared with normal swallow-related LES relaxations, TLESRs occur independently of pharyngeal swallowing, are prolonged in duration (>10 seconds), relax more completely (lower nadir), and are associated with inhibition of the esophageal body and crural diaphragm. Physiologically, TLESRs serve to vent gases from the stomach during belching to prevent gastrointestinal bloating.[45, 46] TLESRs are also stimulated in response to gastric distention after a meal, most commonly in the early postprandial period and reducing in frequency after the first postprandial hour;[47] this is also the case in infants (see Fig. 112-5).[48]

Neurophysiologically, TLESRs occur by a vagovagal reflex initiated by stretch-sensitive receptors located in the smooth muscle of the stomach wall, particularly the cardia of the stomach, which is the region most sensitive to TLESR triggering.[49] The stretch-sensitive sensory nerve fibers of the afferent arm of the reflex pathway terminate in the brain stem (nucleus tractus solitarius) and ultimately synapse with vagal motor neurons (dorsal motor nucleus of the vagus nerve and nucleus ambiguus) projecting to the LES, esophagus, pharynx, and crural diaphragm.[46] In premature infants, TLESRs have the same characteristics (duration, nadir pressure) as those described in adults,[35] a finding indicating that the basic integrative mechanisms underlying TLESR are well developed in these infants.

GASTRIC MOTILITY

The motility of the stomach is less completely characterized in infants. Gastric emptying, gastric pacemaker activity (by electrogastrography), and antropyloric motility have been evaluated in infants down to 27 to 30 weeks. The predominating patterns of gastric motility are summarized in Figure 112-4.

The stomach is divided into two myoelectrically distinct regions: (1) the proximal stomach, consisting of the fundus and orad third of the corpus; and (2) the distal stomach, comprising the remaining corpus, antrum, and pylorus. Each of these regions exhibits a distinct pattern of contractile activity that contributes to the storage and mechanical breakdown of ingested foods and facilitates the selective emptying of solids and liquids into the duodenum.

Control of Gastric Emptying

Ingestion of a meal inhibits the tone of the fundus and contraction of the antrum. This mechanism enables the stomach to function as a food reservoir and to undergo substantial changes in volume without significantly altering intragastric pressure. Gastric tone is best measured by a barostat, a device that records the volume of air contained within a bag placed in the proximal stomach and maintained at a constant pressure. In adults, gastric volume can increase by more than 400% in response to a meal.[50] In the newborn term neonate, the mechanisms responsible for proximal gastric relaxation function poorly, but compliance quickly doubles in the first 3 postnatal days.[51] Gastric inhibition is normally triggered by swallowing; this is known as *receptive relaxation* and aids the passage of the food bolus into the stomach.[52, 53] Esophageal or gastric distention also triggers gastric inhibition; this is known as *adaptive relaxation* and is mediated by a vagovagal reflex initiated by excitation of highly sensitive gastric mechanoreceptors. In the cat, esophageal or gastric distention produces long-lasting inhibition of gastric tone that is absent in the presence of vagal cooling.[54] Mechanoreceptor excitation occurring with distention of the proximal stomach also triggers local or vagal reflexes that stimulate motility of the antrum.[55, 56]

Intraduodenal infusion of nutrients decreases fundic tone, suppresses antral contraction, and stimulates the pylorus to contract phasically and tonically (isolated pyloric pressure waves).[57, 58] These changes in the pattern of motility act to slow gastric emptying and are regulated by neural feedback. Changes in the physical or chemical nature of intraluminal contents are detected by mucosal receptors located in or immediately below the gastric, duodenal, and small intestinal epithelium. Although mucosal receptors with specificity for carbohydrates, pH, amino acids, short and long chain fatty acids, temperature, and touch have been described (mostly in the cat), most mucosal receptors in most species are multimodal and are excited by both mechanical and chemical stimuli. Afferent signals originating at these receptors are transmitted to the brain stem (nucleus tractus solitarius), principally by unmyelinated vagal afferent fibers. The liver also contains receptors to detect osmotic, ionic, nutrient (glucose, amino acids and sugars), pressure-volume, and temperature changes in the portal circulation and possesses a rich vagal afferent innervation that may alter gastric contraction by vagovagal pathways.[59-62] Various hormones also alter gastric emptying. For example, the products of protein or fat digestion stimulate the release of cholecystokinin from the small intestinal mucosa. Cholecystokinin increases satiety, inhibits gastric motility (possibly by excitation of gastroduodenal vagal mucosal mechanoreceptors), and stimulates duodenal contraction.

Liquid Emptying

Liquids empty from the stomach faster than solids; fluids pass around solids, whereas solids must be reduced into smaller particles.[63] During initial filling, the greater curvature of the gastric sinus bulges downward, a posture that facilitates the separation of liquids and solids and favors selective liquid emptying across the pylorus.[63] Liquid emptying is regulated by the pressure gradient

Mechanisms of GER Triggering

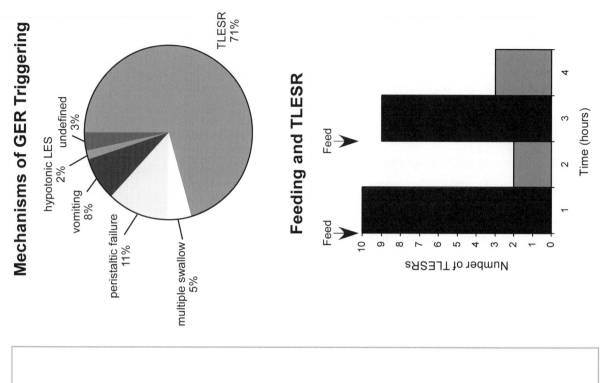

Feeding and TLESR

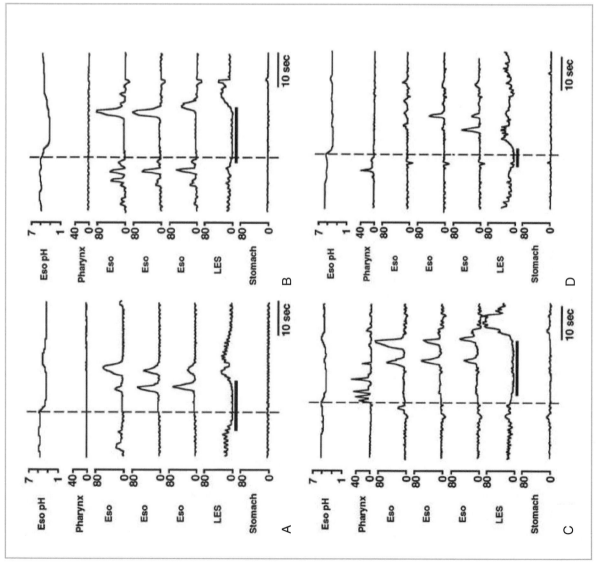

◀ **Figure 112–5.** Mechanisms of acid gastroesophageal reflux (GER) in premature infants. *Manometric tracings*, transient lower esophageal sphincter relaxation (TLESR) (**A** and **B**), prolonged LES relaxation during multiple swallowing (**C**), and failed peristalsis during normal swallow-related LES relaxation (**D**). In all cases, LES relaxation initiates acid GER, which is indicated by the drop in esophageal pH (onset marked by *dotted line*). *Pie chart*, the proportion of acid GER triggered by different mechanisms; TLESR is the predominant reflux mechanism, and LES hypotonicity is the least common mechanism. *Graph*, the relationship between feeding and TLESRs; gastric distention by feeding resulted in an increased rate of TLESR by vagovagal mechanisms. Data are from two hourly-fed premature infants. Eso = esophagus.

between the stomach and the duodenum generated by tonic contraction of the proximal stomach;[64] the pylorus also has a profound effect on gastric emptying through the action of isolated pyloric pressure waves, leading to pulsatile transpyloric flow.[65-67]

Solid Emptying

Solid food is processed by the distal stomach. After initial liquid emptying, the bulge of the greater curvature of the gastric sinus is reduced, and the antrum assumes a tubular posture, bringing solids into line with the pylorus.[63] Movement of gastric contents from the corpus into the antrum is regulated by vagal mechanoreceptors in the antrum that inhibit corpus tone in a reflex manner.[54] Distally propagating antral contractions occur at a frequency of two to three per minute, and these serve to break up digestible solids and sweep particles toward the gastric opening. The passage of solid particles across the pylorus is exquisitely controlled. Particles larger than 1 mm in diameter are usually blocked by pyloric contractions, some of which can be followed by retrograde flow from the duodenum, which returns particles to the antrum to be broken down further.[63,64]

Gastric Emptying in Neonates

Gastric emptying in neonates is generally considered a function of fluid (milk) flow across the pylorus. On acidification, however, milk separates into a semisolid curd and liquid whey fraction. This may account for differences in gastric emptying of formulas containing different ratios of casein and whey. The presence of milk in the fundus stimulates gastric contraction that empties the milk into the duodenum. Gastric emptying rates of term and preterm infants have been extensively evaluated using ultrasonographic, scintigraphic, marker dilution, and breath test techniques. Gastric emptying is biphasic, that is, it has a rapid linear phase followed by a slower exponential phase. Measurements of 50% emptying times in premature infants fed on breast milk range from 25 to 72 minutes.[68-71]

Feedback regulation of gastric emptying rate in response to the duodenal nutrient infusion is exhibited by infants as young as 32 weeks' gestation.[72] As in adults,[73] increased caloric density of feedings slows gastric emptying,[74,75] and long chain triglycerides produce greater inhibition than medium chain triglycerides.[74] In term infants, starch solutions do not inhibit gastric emptying as effectively as isocaloric glucose solutions because of the lack of pancreatic amylase responsible for hydrolyzing starch into glucose.[76] There is a profound but unexplained difference between gastric emptying of expressed breast milk and of infant formula. Despite being isocaloric, breast milk can empty at double the rate of infant formula.[68-70] Breast milk contains various regulator peptides such as gastrin, growth factors, and cytokines. In addition, feedings of breast milk alter the postprandial expression of gut peptides in the plasma compared with formula feedings.[77] The effects of these factors on gastric motility have not been evaluated. Nonnutritive influences such as feed temperature, nonnutritive sucking, phototherapy, and position do not affect the gastric emptying rate.[78-80] The effect of gestational age on gastric emptying rate is not clear. Newell and associates[68] reported that infants ranging from 25 to 36 weeks' gestation exhibit similar rates of emptying, whereas

Gupta and Brans[81] found that gastric emptying in term infants is faster than in preterm infants in the first 12 hours of life. Studies in premature infants have shown that nasogastric feeding or intraduodenal feed infusion inhibits antral motility (see Fig. 112–4) and stimulates isolated pyloric pressure waves.[82] As previously mentioned, isolated pyloric pressure waves serve to regulate fluid flow across the gastric outlet.

SMALL INTESTINAL MOTILITY

Direct measurement of small intestinal motility in infants has been limited to studies of the duodenum. The major motility patterns characterized in premature infants are shown in Figure 112–4.

The *small intestine* is a long, tubular structure lined with absorptive epithelium, surrounded by layers of smooth muscle. The innermost layer is a thin layer underlying the mucosa, the muscularis muscosa. The middle and thickest layer, the circular muscle layer, is arrayed circumferentially so contraction narrows the lumen, whereas contraction of the thinner, outermost longitudinal layer foreshortens the intestine. Between the mucosa and each layer of muscle lies a meshwork of nerve fibers and ganglia that integrate varied contractile responses, depending on the input of sensory signals from the lumen and mechanoreceptors in the muscles, as well as extrinsic input from vagal and sympathetic nerves. During the fifth to eighth week of gestation, circular muscle layers develop in the small intestine; the longitudinal muscle is not present until 10 weeks' gestation. The neurons migrate to the bowel as neural crest cells and differentiate through gestation. Mature phenotypes are achieved in the third trimester. During fetal morphogenesis, the small intestine elongates, reaching a length of approximately four times the heel-to-crown length at birth (200 to 250 cm) and subsequently elongates to about 6 m in the adult.[83,84] The small intestine is segmented into the following: a relatively short proximal segment, the retroperitoneal duodenum; a middle region, the jejunum; and a distal portion, the ileum. Mucosal functions vary in each region of the small intestine; however, regional differences in the organization of the muscle and nerve in each region are not well characterized. Most studies of small intestinal patterns of contraction have focused on the duodenum and jejunum, but limited studies of the ileum demonstrate different organization and control of patterns of contraction.[85,86]

Small Intestinal Contraction

The smooth muscle cells of the small intestine are connected by gap junctions to form a syncytium. Between the muscle layers, specialized cells known as the *interstitial cells of Cajal* generate slow-wave oscillations of membrane potential that are transmitted through the syncytium (Fig. 112–6). The slow wave is propagated rapidly around the circumference of a ring of bowel but not longitudinally, thereby creating the conditions for the simultaneous contraction of a localized ring of bowel around the lumen. However, the slow-wave depolarizations do not cause muscle contraction. Further depolarization to a *threshold potential* is stimulated by the release of acetylcholine from nerves, thus triggering a rapid influx of calcium into the cells and generating a *spike potential* associated with contraction of the muscle cells. Thus, the slow wave determines the maximal rate of contraction for each segment of the intestine, but the linkage of slow-wave depolarization with the actual occurrence of contractions depends on neural activity. In humans, the slow-wave frequency decreases from about 12 per minute in the duodenum to 8 per minute in the ileum. Slow waves propagate longitudinally down the bowel at a rate of 60 to 100 cm per minute.

As a ring of muscle contracts around the lumen, it generates force that is measured as a change in pressure in the lumen. The intrinsic neural plexus integrates excitatory and inhibitory input from mucosal sensory receptors, mechanoreceptors, and extrinsic vagal and sympathetic nerves to determine whether a segment of the intestine contracts. Sequential, coordinated contraction of rings of bowel along the longitudinal axis of the small intestine result in regions of high lumen pressure and low lumen pressure that mix and move the contents of the small intestine. In humans, most contractions involve only 1 to 4 cm of bowel at a time and last about 5 seconds.[87]

Coordination of Small Intestinal Contraction

During fasting, small intestinal contractions are grouped into characteristic patterns (Fig. 112-7). The MMC consists of patterns of contractions that migrate aborally from the antrum to the cecum.[88, 89] In each region of the bowel, a period of no contractile activity (Phase 1) is followed by irregular activity (Phase 2) and by then strong, regular contractions at the slow-wave frequency (Phase 3). The bowel then again becomes quiescent. In the adult human, this pattern recurs every 45 to 180 minutes. Phase 3 activity lasts from 6 to 10 minutes and occupies 5 to 10% of the total MMC cycle, whereas Phase 2 activity occupies 20 to 30% of the MMC cycle. The migration velocity of the MMC along the small intestine is 4 to 6 cm per minute in the proximal intestine and decreases to 1 to 2 cm per minute in the ileum. The absence of this MMC pattern is associated with the development of bacterial overgrowth of the small intestine,[90] probably because the entire luminal contents, including bacteria, are swept out of the bowel during the migration of the strong Phase 3 contractions down the bowel.

Feeding, bowel distention, and various other stimuli disrupt the fasting MMC pattern with a more irregular pattern of contractions (see Fig. 112-7). During this irregular pattern of contractile activity, intestinal chyme is mixed and churned, but the net effect is to propel the nonabsorbed contents aborally from the stomach to the cecum within 2 to 12 hours after feeding.[91, 92] The period of disruption by a meal varies with the size and content of the meal. Meals containing fat disrupt the MMC for a longer period

than meals that contain equivalent amounts of energy in the form of protein or carbohydrate.[92] Vagotomy inhibits the conversion from a fasting to fed pattern, a finding suggesting that sensory input from the vagus initiates a reflex alteration of intestinal contractile patterns or suppresses the interdigestive patterns. Local factors are also important because the infusion of glucose into an isolated denervated loop of the small intestine can disrupt the fasting motor pattern.[93] The MMC pattern returns after the meal is conveyed down the small intestine. In most mammals, the MMC pattern is present only during fasting, but in ruminants, after weaning, the MMC persists postprandially.[94] In the pig, the MMC persists after fasting when food is taken ad libitum, but if pigs are fed only once per day, large meals disrupt the MMC cycle.[89]

Several other patterns of small intestinal contractile activity have been described. Migrating clusters of contractions that last less than 2 minutes and migrate about 20 to 30 cm are observed after the ingestion of indigestible substrates such as cellulose, laxatives, and enterotoxins or in partial obstruction. In the ileum, high-amplitude contractions lasting up to 15 seconds occur on exposure of mucosa to short chain fatty acids, bile acids, and laxatives.[85, 86] These contractions appear to clear the ileum of refluxed fecal contents and therefore may also be important for the prevention of bacterial overgrowth of the small intestine. Vomiting is often preceded by vagal nerve–mediated, retrograde giant migrating contractions that are two to three times larger in amplitude and four to six times longer in duration than the usual short-duration phasic contraction. These contractions usually begin in mid–small intestine and rapidly propagate to the antrum at a velocity of 10 to 12 cm per second, thereby clearing intestinal contents into the stomach.[95]

Ontogeny of Coordinated Small Bowel Contraction

The ontogeny of organized patterns of contraction of the small intestine was first studied in fetal and newborn lambs and dogs

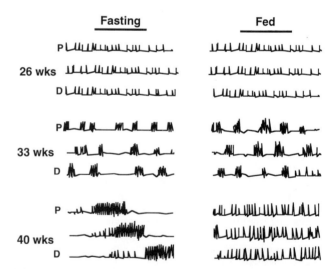

Figure 112–7. Examples of fasted and fed intraluminal pressure recordings from the upper small intestine at increasing gestational age in human infants. At 26 weeks, a random disorganized pattern is present with low-amplitude contractile waves. There is no change in pattern with feeding. At 33 weeks, there are prolonged clusters of contractions with intervening quiescence. Cluster activity persists after feeding, with a decrease in the periods of quiescence. At 40 weeks' gestation, there is an organized migrating motor complex. Feeding results in an irregular, disorganized contractile pattern. In normal newborn infants, cluster patterns can persist after feeding. P = proximal; D = distal.

Contractile force

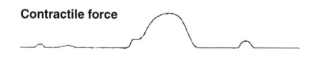

Membrane potential

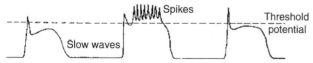

Figure 112–6. Diagram of the electrical and mechanical activity of smooth muscle showing the relationship between fluctuations in membrane potential and contractile force. (Adapted from Read N: *In* McCallum R, Champion M (eds): Gastrointestinal Motility Disorders: Diagnosis and Treatment. Baltimore, Williams & Wilkins, 1990, pp 23-36.)

(see Fig. 112-7; Fig. 112-8).[96] Electrodes implanted on the intestine revealed slow-wave electrical rhythms at the earliest time recorded, the beginning of the third trimester. Episodic spike contractions occurred episodically throughout the bowel, but no organized contractions were observed. As gestation progressed, this pattern of unorganized activity was replaced by a pattern described as the *fetal burst* pattern. Clusters of spike activity progressed for distances along the intestine in a pattern similar to the migrating cluster pattern observed in adult intestine. In the older fetus, the clusters became more organized and tended to migrate aborally for longer distances. In the lamb, an MMC pattern emerges before birth, whereas in the dog, this pattern is not observed until 10 days after birth.

Since these early fetal studies, the ontogeny of small bowel contractile activity in the human premature infant has been well studied using intraluminal perfused catheter techniques.[97-100] A similar sequence of development of increasingly coordinated activity begins with disorganized, low-amplitude, irregular contractile activity at 25 to 30 weeks' gestation. Between 30 and 33 weeks, rhythmic clusters of activity are observed that rarely migrate over large distances. From 33 to 36 weeks, migrating clusters with higher amplitudes of contraction are present. There are increasing periods of time with no contractile activity. By

36 weeks' gestation, the mature MMC pattern is detected, with quiescent periods (Phase 1) and irregular (Phase 2) and regular (Phase 3) contractions sequentially occurring in an aborally migrating pattern along the intestine. The length of time between episodes of Phase 3 activity increases from 25 to 45 minutes in newborns[98,102] to 60 minutes at about age 2 years[101] and to about 100 to 150 minutes in adolescents and adults.[103] The duration of Phase 3 does not change significantly after birth. Migration velocities of 2 to 4 cm per minute and mean amplitudes of contraction of 20 mm Hg in newborns increase to nearly double these values in adulthood.[90] Cluster activity persists after birth but becomes less common through childhood.

As patterns of coordinated contraction mature, the bowel also appears to undergo maturation in the responses to various factors that alter motility. In the term infant, feeding abruptly interrupts the MMC with the onset of irregular contractions,[104,105] although some cluster activity may persist. In older premature infants, an irregular pattern of activity replaces the fetal burst pattern, but in infants less than 30 weeks' gestation, feeding has little effect on intestinal motor patterns. As is observed in adults, in preterm infants of about 33 weeks' gestation, the length and degree of interruption of the fasting patterns vary with the amount of calories delivered to the bowel.[106] Alterations in response to pharmacologic agents also mature with age. Erythromycin initiates an almost immediate MMC pattern in adults and newborn infants[107] but not in premature infants before 31 weeks' gestation (Fig. 112-9).[108,109]

The factors controlling the ontogeny of small intestinal motility remain unclear. The maturation of the enteric nervous system is likely an important factor. Hormonal changes may also play a role. Morriss and associates[108] noted an increase in duodenal contraction in those infants exposed to prenatal maternal corticosteroids. There is some evidence that early feeding of preterm infants promotes postnatal maturation of intestinal motor activity.[110] The nutrient exposure in the feedings may replace exposure to the nutrients and growth factors in swallowed amniotic fluid. The effects of a lack of swallowed amniotic fluid on fetal development of small bowel motility has not been studied. Assessment of the maturity of small bowel motility may be useful to predict feeding readiness of preterm infants. Those infants with less mature patterns of small intestinal motility and without conversion of motility patterns after feeding appear to be less tolerant of feeding challenges.[111] Monitoring of intestinal motility may provide a rational approach for determining the stage of

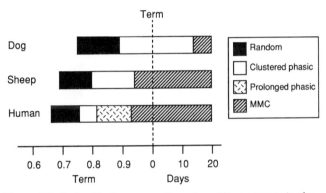

Figure 112–8. Qualitative maturation of motility patterns in the dog, sheep, and human. MMC = migrating motor complex. (From Bisset W, et al: Gut *29*:483–488.)

Figure 112–9. Schematic representations of motor activity recorded in a very preterm infant (**A**), a preterm infant (**B**), and a term infant (**C**). In all three figures, motor activity recorded from the most proximal port is shown in the *top line;* motor patterns in each *lower line* were recorded from sites 2.5 cm distal to the one above it. Where the line is flat, motor quiescence was present. The *dark bars* show the duration and amplitude of contractions. In the very preterm infant (**A**), motor activity occurs independently in each lead before and after the administration of erythromycin (*arrow*). In the preterm infant (**B**), the administration of erythromycin (*arrow*) results in an increase in the amplitude of contractions in the antrum and the duodenum and in an increase in motor activity that migrates distally, as indicated by the *asterisks*. In the term infant (**C**), erythromycin (*arrow*) also causes the appearance of migrating activity identified by the *asterisks;* however, the overall duration of each episode is longer than that seen in the preterm infant. (From Jadcherla SR, Berseth CL: J Pediatr Gastroenterol Nutr *34*:16-22, 2002.)

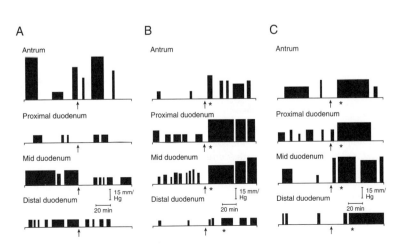

gut neuromaturation and the relative risk of feeding for each preterm infant. Technical improvements in the methods of monitoring small intestinal motor activity will be required before this approach can be adapted for routine clinical use.

COLONIC AND ANORECTAL MOTILITY

Colonic motility has not been directly measured in infants because of the technical difficulty of performing such measurements. Our understanding of the development of colonic motility is therefore limited and is based on measurements performed in older children and animal models. Anorectal motility has been well characterized, however, and the major features are described in Figure 112-4.

Colon

The *colon* is a region of the digestive tract that is largely inaccessible and is difficult to investigate. The placement of probes by anal intubation and endoscopic techniques is widely used; however, this requires bowel preparation, which cleanses the colon of its normal fecal and bacterial environment and has unpredictable effects on motility. Nevertheless, investigations of colonic transit and contractile activity in children and adults have provided some insight into colonic function in health and disease.[112] Colonic transit is usually very slow, constituting two-thirds of total mouth to anus transit time (34 to 55 hours in normal adults).[112] This allows the colon sufficient time to carry out its primary function, the facilitation of transmural exchange of water and electrolytes.

Unless extreme circumstances prevail, the colon is in a continuous digestive state and does not exhibit interdigestive motility patterns such as the MMC. Instead, the colon exhibits specific patterns of motility that result in either mass movement or mixing of ileal effluent. Mass movement is achieved by high-amplitude propagated contractions (HAPCs). HAPCs are seen in the entire colon, exhibit contraction amplitudes of greater than 80 mm Hg, last longer than 10 seconds, and are propagated in an aboral direction over at least 30 cm at approximately 1 cm per second (Fig. 112-10). Although highly effective in moving colonic intraluminal contents, HAPCs occur infrequently in adults, usually six times a day in the cleansed colon[113] and twice a day in the normal unprepared colon.[114] In children, HAPCs occur more often and are more likely to be associated with defecation.[115]

Other types of motility that are more frequently seen include independent contractions of individual or multiple colonic segments (Fig. 112-11). These contractions move the colonic contents over short distances, both aborally and orally, to facilitate mixing. These segmental or nonpropagating contractions are not normally seen in infants but are expressed in older children.[116] The expression of colonic motility follows a circadian rhythm occurring after awakening and then cyclically during the day. Both adults and children demonstrate an immediate postprandial colonic response that manifests as an increase in colonic motility in direct response to nutrient (predominantly fats and carbohydrates) contact with the duodenojejunal mucosa and perhaps gastric distention. The mechanism for this response is unclear but may involve both vagal and endocrine systems. The duration of this response increases with age; it lasts 30 minutes in infants[115,116] and 2 hours in adults.[117] In children less than 4 years of age, the postprandial response consists solely of HAPCs, whereas children older than 4 years exhibit 60% HAPCs and 40% segmental contractions.[115,116]

Little information is available regarding the prenatal development of colonic motility. In rhesus primates, the postprandial increase in colonic motility observed in the full-term infant is similar to the human and adult response. In the preterm rhesus primate, there is a lesser response to meals, a finding suggesting that the colonic response to meals matures late in gestation.[118,119] This finding may explain why the first meconium bowel movement is delayed by up to 3 days in premature infants (see the following section, on the anorectum). Fetal hypoxemia frequently provokes passage of meconium by the full-term infant *in utero*, with resultant risks of meconium aspiration.[120,121] In contrast, even severe hypoxia rarely causes *in*

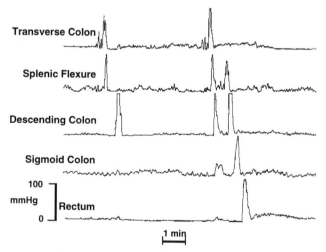

Figure 112-10. Postprandial high-amplitude propagated contractions observed in a child. Pressures are recorded in the transverse colon, splenic flexure, descending colon, sigmoid colon, and rectum. (From Di Lorenzo C, et al: Gut *34*:803-807, 1993.)

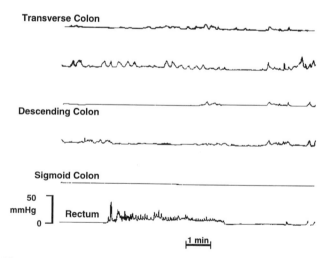

Figure 112-11. Colonic nonpropagating contractions in a child. There are nonpropagating contractions in the transverse colon and a rectal motor complex in the rectum lasting 6 minutes. (From Di Lorenzo C, et al: Gut *34*:803-807, 1993.)

utero meconium passage in the premature infant,[122] a finding that further supports the contention that colonic motility is deficient in the preterm infant.

Anorectum

The *anorectum* is an anatomically complex region. Fecal continence depends on the ability to perceive rectal filling and then to retain rectal contents until the appropriate moment for defecation arises. Neonates usually defecate immediately on entry of stool into the rectum. The ability to delay defecation until a socially appropriate time requires coordination of the muscles of the sigmoid colon, rectum, levator ani, puborectalis (U-shaped striated muscle passing around the distal rectum), and anal canal. This is usually learned with toilet training. Normal full-term neonates pass their first meconium stool within 48 hours of birth, whereas premature infants may experience a delay of more than a week before their initial defecation.[119,120,123]

The rectum acts as receptacle for fecal matter that arrives as a consequence of colonic HAPCs. In adults, the rectum has a resting pressure of 6 mm Hg and demonstrates three different patterns of phasic contraction: (1) isolated prolonged contractions (10 to 20 seconds' duration); (2) cluster contractions lasting 1 to 2 minutes and occurring every 20 to 30 minutes (10 to 12 seconds' duration); and (3) the rectal motor complex, a series of phasic contractions at the rectosigmoid junction lasting 10 minutes and occurring cyclically every 50 to 300 minutes, depending on the time of day (see Fig. 112-10).[124] During defecation, rectal contraction serves to position fecal material to the proximal anal canal. Extrusion of the feces is achieved by relaxation of the anal canal in combination with straining (contraction of diaphragmatic and abdominal muscles) and propagated colorectal contractions. In addition, the puborectalis muscle relaxes and the levator ani muscles contract, causing the pelvic floor to descend, opening the anorectal angle, and assisting fecal passage.[122,125-128]

The anal canal measures 3 to 4 cm in adults and 1.25 to 2 cm in neonates. It consists of two sphincteric muscle groups: the external striated sphincter and the thicker internal smooth muscle sphincter. The external sphincter is under voluntary control of the pudendal nerve, whereas the internal sphincter is under both parasympathetic and sympathetic autonomic control. Resting anal sphincter tone is predominantly (85%) generated by the internal smooth muscle sphincter. The external striated muscle sphincter plays only a partial role in generating resting tone but can generate squeeze pressures that double the pressure in the anal canal. The ability to develop adequate squeeze pressure is essential in the maintenance of fecal continence because it overrides the effect of involuntary internal sphincter relaxation. It is thought that contraction of the external sphincter during internal sphincter relaxation allows the rectal contents to be sampled by receptors at the border of the anal canal that allow discrimination among solid, liquid, and gas.[127,129,130]

Anorectal Motility in Neonates

Basal pressure of the anal sphincter is 0 to 74 mm Hg in newborn infants and 15 to 98 mm Hg in older children and adults.[131—133] The internal sphincter contracts rhythmically 8 to 14 times per minute (oscillating pressure waves) and relaxes through a local reflex in response to balloon distention of the rectal wall, the *rectoanal reflex* (see Fig. 112-4).[134] The threshold volume of air required to produce rectoanal reflex relaxation is 2 to 3.5 mL in infants,[135,136] 11 mL in older children,[132] and 20 mL in adults.[128] The anorectal relaxation reflex is present[134,135,136] and can be elicited in infants as young as 28 to 30 weeks' gestation.[136,137] The anorectal reflex is absent in infants and children with Hirschsprung disease as a result of the lack of intrinsic innervation of the rectum.[138]

OVERVIEW OF THE DEVELOPMENT MOTILITY IN THE INFANT

Numerous investigations performed since the 1980s have characterized patterns of gastrointestinal motility in older preterm and term infants (>31 weeks' gestation) and, in some instances, in infants as young as 26 weeks' gestation. As shown in Figure 112-12, we now have an almost complete picture of the relative maturation of the motor patterns and reflexes of greatest importance to appropriate functioning of the gastrointestinal tract, with the exception of the colon. The gastrointestinal tract itself exhibits "mature" motility patterns in most regions, with some notable exceptions, including impairment of lingual function, ability to generate sucking pressures, and patterns and coordination of suck and swallow. This immaturity is the most likely cause of delays and difficulties in establishing full oral feeding; however, this deficiency is easily overcome in most infants with nasogastric tube feeding. Once nutrients enter the stomach, it appears that an appropriate fed antroduodenal motility response ensures regulated delivery of nutrients to the duodenum and mixing of luminal contents with gastrointestinal secretions. Despite these normal fed patterns, there is a delay in development of the fasting MMC that may lead to bacterial overgrowth or may contribute to feeding intolerance associated with slow intestinal transit. Well-developed esophageal motility allows for effective esophageal volume clearance in response to GER; however, if materials (feedings, oral secretions, or refluxate) come into contact with airway structures (made more likely by poor coordination of swallowing and breathing), then this may lead to significant complications including apnea and aspiration.

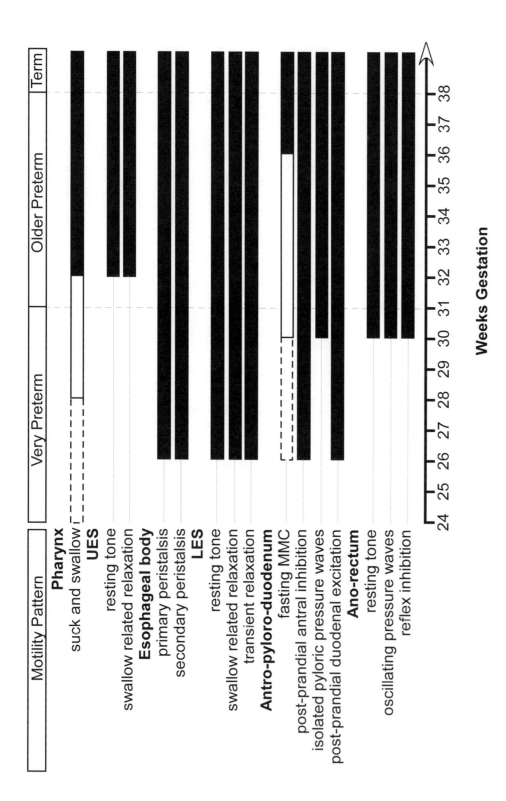

| Motility Pattern | Very Preterm | Older Preterm | Term |

Pharynx
suck and swallow

UES
resting tone
swallow related relaxation

Esophageal body
primary peristalsis
secondary peristalsis

LES
resting tone
swallow related relaxation
transient relaxation

Antro-pyloro-duodenum
fasting MMC
post-prandial antral inhibition
isolated pyloric pressure waves
post-prandial duodenal excitation

Ano-rectum
resting tone
oscillating pressure waves
reflex inhibition

24 25 26 27 28 29 30 31 32 33 34 35 36 37 38

Weeks Gestation

not characterised

absent or very immature

immature

mature

◀ **Figure 112–12.** Pictorial summary of the understanding of the relative maturity of predominant gastrointestinal motility patterns in very premature, older premature, and term infants. LES = lower esophageal sphincter; MMC = migrating motor complex; UES = upper esophageal sphincter.

REFERENCES

1. Stevenson RD, Allaire JH: The development of normal feeding and swallowing. Pediatr Clin North Am *39*:1439-1453, 1991.
2. Morris SE: The Normal Acquisition of Oral Feeding Skills: Implications for Assessment and Treatment. New York, Therapeutic Media, 1982.
3. Bu'Lock F, et al: Development of coordination of sucking, swallowing and breathing. Dev Med Clin Neurol *32*:669-678, 1990.
4. Newman LA, et al: Videofluoroscopic analysis of the infant swallow. Investigative Radiology. *26*:870-873, 1991.
5. Bamford O, et al: The relationship between rhythmic swallowing and breathing during suckle feeding in term neonates. Pediatr Res. *31*:619-624, 1992.
6. Hack ME, Robertson SS: Development of sucking rhythm in preterm infants. Early Hum Dev *11*:133-140, 1985.
7. McGowan JS, et al: Developmental patterns of normal nutritive sucking in infants. Dev Med Clin Neurol *33*:891-897, 1991.
8. Bernbaum JC, et al: Nonnutritive sucking during gavage feeding enhances growth and maturation in premature infants. Pediatrics *71*:41-45, 1983.
9. Field T, et al.: Nonnutritive sucking during tube feedings: effect on preterm neonates in an intensive care unit. Pediatrics 70:381-384, 1982.
10. Hanlon MB, et al: Deglutition apnoea as indicator of maturation of suckle feeding in bottle-fed preterm infants. Dev Med Child Neurol *39*:534-542, 1997.
11. Mathew OP, Bhatia J: Sucking and breathing patterns during breast- and bottle-feeding in term neonates. Am J Dis Child *143*:588-592, 1989.
12. Stolovitz P, Gisel E: Circumoral movements in response to three different food textures in children 6 months to 2 years of age. Dysphagia 6:17-25, 1991.
13. Sheppard J, Mysak E: Ontogeny of infantile oral reflexes and emerging chewing. Child Dev *55*:831-843, 1984.
14. Dodds WJ: The physiology of swallowing. Dysphagia *3*:171-178, 1989.
15. Miller AJ: The search for the central swallowing pathway: the quest for clarity. Dysphagia 8:185-194, 1993.
16. Bosma JF, et al: Ultrasound demonstration of tongue motions during suckle feeding. Dev Med Clin Neurol *32*:223-229, 1990.
17. Koenig JS, et al: Coordination of breathing, sucking, and swallowing during bottle feedings in human infants. J Appl Physiol 69:1623-1629, 1990.
18. Kahrilas PJ, et al: Pharyngeal clearance during swallowing: a combined manometric and videofluoroscopic study. Gastroenterology *103*:128-136, 1992.
19. Pritchard JA: Fetal swallowing and amniotic fluid volume. Obstet Gynecol 28:606-610, 1966.
20. Sherman DJ, et al: Fetal swallowing: correlation of electromyography and esophageal fluid flow. Am J Physiol *258*:R1386-R1394, 1990.
21. Brace RA: Amniotic fluid volume and its relationship to fetal fluid balance: review of experimental data. Semin Perinatol *10*:103-112, 1986.
22. Trahair J, Harding R: Ultrastructural anomalies in the fetal small intestine indicate that fetal swallowing is important for normal development: an experimental study. Virchows Arch A Pathol Anat *420*:305-312, 1992.
23. Laitman J, Reidenberg J: Specialization of the human upper respiratory and upper digestive systems as seen through comparative and developmental anatomy. Dysphagia 8:318-325, 1993.
24. Mathew OP: Respiratory control during nipple feeding in preterm infants. Pediatr Pulmonol 5:220-224, 1988.
25. Cook I, et al.: Opening mechanisms of the human upper eesophageal sphincter. Am J Physiol *257*:G748-G759, 1989.
26. Jacob P, et al: Upper esophageal sphincter opening and modulation during swallowing. Gastroenterology 97:1469-1478, 1989.
27. Davidson GP, et al: Monitoring of upper oesophageal sphincter pressure in children. Gut 32:607-611, 1991.
28. Willing J, et al: Effect of gastro-oesophageal reflux on upper oesophageal sphincter motility in children. Gut *34*:904-910, 1993.
29. Willing J, et al: Stain Induced augmentation of upper oesophageal sphincter pressure in children. Gut 35:159-164, 1994.
30. Omari T, et al: Measurement of upper esophageal sphincter tone and relaxation during swallowing in premature infants. Am. J. Physiol *277*:G862-G866, 1999.
31. Cook I, et al: Measurement of upper esophageal sphincter pressure: effect of acute emotional stress. Gastroenterology 93:526-532, 1987.
32. Kahrilas P, et al: Effect of sleep, spontaneous gastroesophageal reflux and a meal on upper esophageal sphincter pressure in normal human volunteers. Gastroenterology 92:466-471, 1987.
33. Omari T, et al: Characterisation of esophageal body and lower esophageal sphincter motor function in the very premature neonate. J Pediatr *135*:517-521, 1999.
34. Omari TI, et al: Mechanisms of gastroesophageal reflux in healthy premature infants. J Pediatr *133*:650-654, 1998.
35. Omari TI, et al: Characterisation of relaxation of the lower oesophageal sphincter in healthy premature infants Gut *40*:370-375, 1997.
36. Gryboski J: Esophageal motility in infants and children. Pediatrics *31*:382-395, 1963.
37. Janssens J, et al: Bursts of non-deglutitive simultaneous contractions may be a normal oesophageal motility pattern. Gut *34*:1021-1024, 1993.
38. Boix-Ochoa J, Canals J: Maturation of the lower oesophagus. J Ped Surg *11*:749-756, 1976.
39. Gryboski J: Suck and swallow in the premature infant. Pediatrics *43*:96-102, 1969.
40. Gryboski J, et al: Esophageal motility in infants and children. Pediatrics *31*:382-395, 1963.
41. Gryboski J, et al: Esophageal motility in infants and children. Pediatrics *31*:382-395, 1983.
42. Newell S, et al: Maturation of the lower oesophageal sphincter in the preterm baby. Gut 29:167-172, 1988.
43. Omari TI, et al: Esophageal body and lower esophageal sphincter function in healthy premature infants. Gastroenterology *109*:1757-1764, 1995.
44. Davidson GP, Omari TI: Reflux in children. Baillieres Clin Gastroenterol *14*:839-855, 2000.
45. Mittal R, et al: Transient lower esophageal relaxation. Gastroenterology *109*:601-610, 1995.
46. Holloway RH: The anti-reflux barrier and mechanisms of gastro-oesophageal reflux. Baillieres Clin Gastroenterol *14*:681-699, 2000.
47. Holloway RH, et al: Gastric distension: a mechanism for post-prandial gastroesophageal reflux. Gastroenterology 89:779-784, 1985.
48. Omari TI, et al: Mechanisms of gastro-oesophageal reflux in preterm and term infants with reflux disease. Gut *51*:475-479, 2002.
49. Franzi SJ, et al: Response of canine lower esophageal sphincter to gastric distension. Am J Physiol *259*:G380-385, 1990.
50. Ropert A, et al: Simultaneous assessment of liquid emptying and proximal gastric tone in humans. Gastroenterology *105*:667-674, 1993.
51. Di Lorenzo C, et al: Postnatal maturation of gastric response to distension in newborn infants. Gastroenterology *107*:A1222, 1994.
52. Lind JF, et al: Motility of the gastric fundus. Am J Physiol *201*:197-202, 1961.
53. Cannon WB, Lieb CW: The receptive relaxation of the stomach. Am J Physiol 29:267-273, 1911.
54. Abrahamsson H, Jansson G: Vago-vagal gastro-gastric relaxation in the cat. Acta Physiol Scand 88:289-295, 1973.
55. Grundy D, et al: A permissive role for the vagus nerves in the genesis of antro-antral reflexes in the ferret. J Physiol (Lond) *381*:377-384, 1986.
56. Andrews PLR, et al: Reflex excitation of antral motility induced by gastric distention in the ferret. J Physiol (Lond) 298:79-84, 1980.
57. Heddle R, et al: The motor mechanisms associated with slowing of the gastric emptying of a solid meal by a intraduodenal lipid infusion. J Gastroenterol Hepatol 4:437-447, 1989.
58. Azpiroz F, Malagelada JR: Intestinal control of gastric tone. Am J Physiol *249*:G501-G509, 1985.
59. Ewart WR: Hepatic afferents affecting ingestive behaviour. *In* Booth DA (ed): Neurophysiology of Ingestion. Oxford, Pergamon Press, 1993, pp 33-46.
60. Grundy D, Scratcherd T: Sensory afferents from the gastrointestinal tract. *In* Wood JD (ed): Handbook of Physiology. Bethesda, MD, American Physiological Society, 1989, pp 593-620.
61. Grundy D: Vagal afferent mechanisms of mechano- and chemoreception. *In* Ritter S, et al (eds): Neuroanatomy and Physiology of Abdominal Vagal Afferents. Pullman, WA, CRC Press, 1992, pp 179-192.
62. Blackshaw LA, Grundy D: Gastrointestinal mechanoreception in the control of ingestion. *In* Booth DA (ed): Neurophysiology of Ingestion. Oxford, Pergamon Press, 1993, pp 57-78.
63. Brown BP, et al: The configuration of the human gastroduodenal junction in the separate emptying of liquids and solids. Gastroenterology *105*:433-440, 1993.
64. Kelly K: Gastric Emptying of liquids and solids: roles of proximal and distal stomach. Am J Physiol *238*:G71-G76, 1980.
65. Malbert CH, Mathis C: Antropyloric modulation of transpyloric flow of liquids in pigs. Gastroenterology *107*:37-46, 1994.
66. Edelbroek M, Ph.D. dissertation, University of Utrecht, Netherlands, 1993.
67. Horowitz M, Dent J: The study of gastric mechanics and flow: a mad hatter's tea party starting to make sense. Gastroenterology *107*:302-305, 1994.
68. Newell SJ, et al: Ultrasonic assessment of gastric emptying in the preterm infant. Arch Dis Child 69:32-36, 1993.
69. Ewer AK, et al: Gastric emptying in preterm infants. Arch Dis Child *71*:F24-F27, 1994.
70. Cavell B: Gastric emptying in preterm infants. Acta Paediatr Scand 68:725-730, 1979.
71. Barnett CB, et al: Reproducibility of the ^{13}C-octanoic acid breath test for the assessment of gastric emptying in premature infants. J Pediatr Gastroenterol Nutr 29:26-30, 1999.

72. Berseth CL, Ittmann PI: Antral and duodenal motor responses to duodenal feeding in preterm and term infants. J Pediatr Gastroenterol Nutr 14:182-186, 1992.

73. Hunt J, Stubbs D: The volume and energy content of meals as determinants of gastric emptying. J Physiol (Lond) 245:209-225, 1975.

74. Seigel M, et al: Effect of fat and carbohydrate composition on the gastric emptying of isocaloric feedings in premature infants. Gastroenterology 89:785-790, 1985.

75. Siegel M, et al: Effect of caloric density on gastric emptying in premature infants. J Pediatr 104:118-122, 1984.

76. Husband J, et al: Gastric emptying of starch meals in the newborn. Lancet 53:290-292, 1970.

77. Lucus A, et al.: Breast vs bottle: endocrine responses are different with formula feeding. Lancet 56:1267-1269, 1980.

78. Blumenthal I, et al: Effect of feed temperature and phototherepy on gastric emptying in the neonate. Arch Dis Child 55:562-574, 1980.

79. Costalos C, et al: Is it necessary to warm infants' feeds? Arch Dis Child 54:899-901, 1979.

80. Szabo JS, et al: Effect of non-nutritive and nutritive suck on gastric emptying in premature infants. J Pediatr Gastroenterol Nutr 4:348-351, 1985.

81. Gupta M, Brans YW: Gastric retention in neonates. Pediatrics 62:26-29, 1978.

82. Hassan BB, et al: Patterns of antropyloric motility in fed healthy preterm infants. Arch Dis Child 87:F95-9, 2002.

83. Reiquim C, et al: Normal and abnormal small bowel length. Am J Dis Child 109:447-451, 1965.

84. Siebert J: Small-intestine length in infants and children. Am J Dis Child 134:593-595, 1980.

85. Quigley E, et al: Motility of the terminal ileum and ileocecal sphincter in healthy humans. Gastroenterology 87:857-866, 1984.

86. Kamath P, et al: Short chain fatty acids stimulate motility in the canine ileum. Am J Physiol 253:G427-433, 1987.

87. Weisbrodt N: Motility of the small intestine. In Johnson L (ed): Gastrointestinal Physiology. St. Louis, CV Mosby, 1991, pp 50-56.

88. Code C, Marlett J: The interdigestive myo-electric complex of the stomach and small bowel of dogs. J Physiol (Lond) 246:289-309, 1975.

89. Sarna S: Cyclic motor activity: migrating motor complex. Gastroenterology 89:894-913, 1985.

90. Vantrappen G, et al: The interdigestive motor complex of normal subjects and patients with bacterial overgrowth of the small intestine. J Clin Invest 59:1158-1166, 1977.

91. Read N, et al: Relationship between postprandial motor activity in the human small intestine and the gastrointestinal transit of food. Gastroenterology 86:721-727, 1984.

92. Eeckhout C, et al: Local disorganisation of the interdigestive migrating motor complex (MMC) by perfusion of a Thiry-Vella loop. Gastroenterology 76:1127-1131, 1979.

93. Ruckebusch Y, Bueno L: The effect of weaning on the motility of the small intestine in the calf. Br J Nutr 30:491-499, 1973.

94. Stewart J, et al: Intestinal myoelectric activity after activation of central emetic mechanisms. Am J Physiol 233:E131-E137, 1977.

95. Bueno L, Ruckebusch Y: Perinatal development of intestinal myoelectrical activity of the small intestine in dogs and sheep. Am J Physiol 237:E61-E67, 1979.

96. Milla P, Fenton T: Small intestinal motility patterns in the perinatal period. J Pediatr Gastroenterol Nutr 2(Suppl 1):S141-S144, 1983.

97. Bisset W, et al: Ontongeny of fasting small intestinal motor activity in the human infant. Gut 29:483-488, 1988.

98. Berseth C: Gestation evolution of small intestine motility in preterm and term infants. J Pediatr 115:646-651, 1989.

99. Amarnath R, et al: Postnatal maturation of small intestinal motility in preterm and term infants. J Gastrointest Motil 1:138-143, 1989.

100. Tomomasa T, et al: Nonmigrating rhythmic activity in the stomach and duodenum of neonates. Biol Neonate 48:1-9, 1985.

101. Cucchiara S, et al: Abnormalities of gastrointestinal motility in children with nonulcer dyspepsia and in children with gastroesophageal reflux disease. Dig Dis Sci 36:1066-1073, 1991.

102. Pineiro-Carrero V, et al: Abnormal gastroduodenal motility in children and adolescents with recurrent functional abdominal pain. J Pediatr 113:820-825, 1988.

103. Tomomasa T, et al: Gastroduodenal motility in neonates: response to human milk compared with cow's milk formula. Pediatrics 80:434-438, 1987.

104. Berseth C: Neonatal small intestinal motility: motor responses to feeding in term and preterm infants. J Pediatr 117:777-782, 1990.

105. Koenig W, et al: Manometrics for preterm and term infants: a new tool for old questions. Pediatrics 95:203-206, 1995.

106. Tomomasa T, et al: Erythromycin increases gastric antral motility in human premature infants. Biol Neonate 48:1-9, 1993.

107. Sudarshan R, Berseth C: Prokinetic effects of erythromycin in preterm and term infants are related to gestational age. Pediatr Res 37:124A, 1995.

108. Morriss F, et al: Ontogenic development of gastrointestinal motility. IV. Duodenal contraction in preterm infants. Pediatrics 78:1106-1113, 1986.

109. Jadcherla SR, Berseth CL: Effect of erythromycin on gastroduodenal contractile activity in developing neonates. J Pediatr Gastroenterol Nutr 34:16-22, 2002.

110. Berseth C, Nordyke C: Enteral nutrients promote postnatal maturation of intestinal motor activity in preterm infants. Am J Physiol 264:G1046-G1051, 1993.

111. Berseth C, Nordyke C: Manometry can predict feeding readiness in preterm infants. Gastroenterology 103:1523-1528, 1992.

112. Sarna S: Physiology and pathophysiology of colonic motor activity. I. Dig Dis Sci 36:827-862, 1991.

113. Proano M, et al: Transit of solids through the human colon: regional quantification in the unprepared colon. Am J Physiol 258:G856-G862, 1990.

114. Narducci F, et al: Twenty-four hour manometric recording of colonic motor activity in humans. Gut 28:17-25, 1987.

115. Soffer E, et al: Prolonged ambulant monitoring of human colonic motility. Am J Physiol 257:G601-G606, 1989.

116. Di Lorenzo C, et al: Inhibition of high-amplitude propagated contractions (HAPCs) characterized maturation of colonic motility. Gastroenterology 104:A617, 1993.

117. Di Lorenzo C, et al: Colonic manometry differentiates causes of intractable constipation in children. J Pediatr 120:690-695, 1992.

118. Sarna S: Physiology and pathophysiology of colonic motor activity. II. Dig Dis Sci 35:998-1018, 1991.

119. Cannon R, Cheung A: Development of methodology for recording colonic myoelectrical activity in the primate. Biomater Artif Cells Artif Organs 17:81-92, 1989.

120. Sherry S, Kramer I: The time of passage of the first stool and first urine by the newborn infant. J Pediatr 46:158-159, 1955.

121. Verma A, Dhanireddy R: Time of first stool in extremely low birth weight (<1000g) infants. J Pediatr 122:626-629, 1993.

122. G. Gregory, et al: Meconium aspiration in infants: a prospective study. J Pediatr 85:848-852, 1974.

123. Matthew O, Warshaw J: Relevance of the gestational age distribution of meconium passage in utero. Pediatrics 64:30-31, 1979.

124. Clark D: Times of first void and first stool in 500 newborns. Pediatrics 60:457-459, 1977.

125. Smout AJPM, Akkermans LMA: Normal and Disturbed Motility of the Gastrointestinal Tract. Petersfield, Hampshire, UK: Wrightson Biomedical Publishing, 1992.

126. Goei R: Defecography: A Radiological Study on Anorectal Function and Related Disorders. Limburg, Netherlands, Rijksunversiteit, 1990.

127. Mahieu P, et al: Defaecography. I. Description of a new procedure and results in normal patients. Gastrointest Radiol 9:247-251, 1984.

128. Read NW, Sun WM: Disordered anorectal motor function. In Dent J (ed): Practical Issues in Gastrointestinal Motor Disorders. London, Bailliere Tindall, 1991, pp 479-503.

120. Read NW, Bannister JJ: Anorectal manometry: techniques in health and anorectal disease. In Henry MM, Swash M (eds): Coloproctology and the Pelvic Floor. London, Butterworth, 1985, pp 65-87.

130. Duthie HL, Bennett RC: The relations of sensation in the anal canal to the function of the anal sphincter: a possible factor in anal continence. Gut 4:179-182, 1963.

131. Sun WM, Read NW: Anorectal function in normal subjects: the effect of gender. Int J Colorectal Dis 4:188-196, 1989.

132. Loening-Baucke V: Anorectal manometry and biofeedback training. In Hyman PE (ed): Pediatric Gastrointestinal Motility Disorders. New York, Academy Professional Information Services, 1994, pp 231-252.

133. Mishalany H, et al: Report on the first international symposium of anorectal manometry. J Pediatr Surg 24:356-359, 1989.

134. Benninga MA, et al: Characterisation of anorectal pressure and the anorectal inhibitory reflex in healthy preterm and term infants. J Pediatr 139:233-237, 2001.

135. Lopez-Alonso M, Ribas J: Technical improvement for anorectal manometry in newborns. J Pediatr Surg 26:1215-1218, 1991.

136. Bowes KL, Kling S: Anorectal manometry in premature infants. J Pediatr Surg 14:533-535, 1979.

137. Holschneider AM, et al: The development of anorectal continence and its significance in the diagnosis of Hirschsprung's disease. J Pedriatr Surg 11:151-156, 1976.

138. Loening-Baucke V, et al: Anorectal manometry for the exclusion of Hirschsprung's disease in neonates. J Pediatr Gastroenterol Nutr 4:596-603, 1985.

Fetal and Neonatal Intestinal Motility

During fetal development, nutrients are provided by placental circulation; at birth, the intestinal tract is called on to ingest, transport, and assimilate nutrients necessary for survival. In preterm infants these functions are often compromised to varying degrees. This has led to an interest in determining the developmental sequence of events within the gastrointestinal tract involved in the digestive sequence.

Ingestion of food and its presentation into the intestinal tract are the functions of suck and swallow reflexes. Many difficulties that arise in this area are due to the complex integration required of the skeletal muscle of the oropharynx or its integration with the smooth muscle of the esophagus. The stomach is responsible for receiving and storing ingested nutrients and initiating mechanical trituration. There is increasing evidence that the changing dietary requirements during the first year of life are accompanied by basic changes in gastric physiology during that same period of time. The primary responsibility of the small intestine is to deliver nutrients close to the intestinal mucosa, which has the regional specialization necessary to absorb various intestinal contents. The colon, particularly in early life, has a limited role in delivering nutrients to the body. It primarily stores the nutrients that are not absorbed in the small intestine and packages them into a form that is suitable for defecation.

ESOPHAGUS

Sucking consists of organized movements of skeletal muscular origin. The primary purpose of sucking is to create a fluid bolus that can be transported into the esophagus where a monophasic peristaltic smooth muscle contraction transports the bolus into the stomach. A coordinated suck-and-swallow mechanism does not usually begin until the 30th week of gestation or later. There are certainly many indications from *in utero* studies that the fetus is able to swallow amniotic fluid as early as 15 to 20 weeks' gestation.[1, 2] The mouthing and poorly coordinated sucking performed by the midgestational fetus and the early preterm infant reflect the inability of this age group to coordinate the oral, pharyngeal, and esophageal phases of swallowing. As the newborn reaches 34 to 36 weeks' gestational age, it is able to undertake bursts of at least 30 sucks. At this stage, the infant generates sufficient intraoral pressure to form a bolus and is better able to coordinate the suck-and-swallow mechanism with breathing. Initiating oral feedings in premature infants before effective sucking and coordinated swallowing are developed places the neonate at risk for aspiration. The degree of sophistication of the neural processes responsible for the skeletal muscle involved in sucking and swallowing often develops later than the integration required for satisfactory performance of the more distal smooth muscle aspects of the intestinal tract. This often results in infants' requiring nasogastric tube feedings to receive adequate nutrition.

After a bolus has passed to the hypopharynx, relaxation of the upper esophageal sphincter is required. Inability to relax the upper esophageal sphincter at the appropriate time can result in reflux of food into the oral or nasal pharynx. As a bolus passes the upper esophageal sphincter, it enters the smooth muscle portion of the esophagus, which in the human infant is the distal one-half to two-thirds of the esophagus. Here a peristaltic wave transports (or pushes) the ingested nutrient into the stomach.

In the distal esophagus is found a tonic region of muscle called the *lower esophageal sphincter*. This sphincter inhibits the reflux of gastric contents into the esophagus. The lower esophageal sphincter must relax at the appropriate time to allow ingested foodstuffs entrance to enter into the stomach. There has been great interest in the lower esophageal sphincter's ability to inhibit gastroesophageal reflux in the neonate. It appears from animal studies that the muscle in this area is able to generate stress similar to muscle from this region in the adult; however, it may be at a mechanical disadvantage in generating lower esophageal sphincter pressures.[3] It is also possible that much of the gastroesophageal reflux seen in the infant may be due to inappropriate relaxation.[4-6]

GASTRIC MOTOR FUNCTION

The stomach acts as a reservoir for ingested food, begins mechanical trituration of ingested food, and empties the nutrients into the small intestine. Various regions of the stomach are responsible for these different physiologic functions. The proximal region of the stomach, known as the *fundus*, through a process of receptive relaxation or gastric accommodation, is able to receive relatively large volumes of ingested nutrients with only small increases in pressure. This allows the fundus of the stomach to serve as a reservoir for the ingested nutrients. This function is mediated to a large extent by the central nervous system through the action of the vagus nerve, which mediates inhibitory neurotransmitters during gastric distention. Receptive relaxation during the newborn period has received little study, although it is likely that this area may be important in the pathophysiology of certain events such as gastroesophageal reflux during infancy. It has also been proposed that the fundus can facilitate emptying of liquids from the stomach by developing low-grade tonic contractions that enhance gastric emptying effects, which are primarily due to coordinated antral-pyloric peristalsis. One study has shown that the neuroregulatory mechanisms that result in the coordination of antral-pyloric motility and gastric emptying are developed by 30 weeks' postgestational age.[7]

The most distal portion of the stomach is known as the *antrum* and is responsible for the mechanical trituration or mixing and grinding of ingested foodstuffs, which occur before gastric emptying. Although newborns rarely ingest solids, the formation of curds from ingested milk products may require some trituration before they are emptied from the stomach. The antrum participates in a peristaltic sequence with the pylorus and duodenum to promote emptying of food. This implies that the antrum and pylorus do more than simply act as a filter to prohibit large food particles from leaving the stomach. Data from newborn animal models suggest that newborn antral smooth muscle does not have the ability to use the same calcium stores for contraction as in the adult.[8] It is possible that this contributes to the newborn antral smooth muscle's relative inability to contract with short, transient contractions and makes it more likely that contractions will occur in a prolonged tonic fashion.[8]

To attempt to compare the rates of gastric emptying in the preterm infant to those of the term infant and the adult is in many respects similar to comparing apples and oranges because the composition of diet and method of feeding are so different. In adults, the most important factor in determining the rate of gastric emptying of a liquid is the liquid caloric density. Additionally, the rate of gastric emptying is controlled by feedback from the small intestine. Stimulation of duodenal receptors by acid, fat, carbohydrate, tryptophan, or increasing osmolarity decreases rates of gastric emptying. Similarly, the stimulation of ileal receptors by acid, fat, and carbohydrate may decrease gastric emptying, apparently by humoral mechanisms.[9,10]

Similar to these adult studies, there is evidence in studies of term infants that suggest that increasing caloric density is associated with slower rates of gastric emptying.[11,12] In that regard, Siegel and colleagues performed a series of careful studies evaluating the effects of caloric density[13] and the nutrient content of formula[14] on gastric emptying in infants ranging in gestational age from 32 to 39 weeks. Incremental increases of caloric density from 0.2 to 0.66 cal/mL decreased the rate of gastric emptying, indicating that feedback control mechanisms were comparable with those in the adult.[15] In term neonates, starch-containing solutions empty at a rate similar to that of water.[11,12] This finding is most likely explained by the slower rates of starch hydrolysis caused by the low amylase concentrations in the proximal intestine of the infant,[16] resulting in glucose's not being released in the duodenum; therefore, gastric emptying is not reduced accordingly. A similar lack of effect of complex carbohydrates on gastric emptying is seen in adults with pancreatic insufficiency.[17]

Clinical experience suggests that gastric emptying is delayed in preterm infants. It is oftentimes not clear whether this is due to a primary problem with gastric motor function or whether it reflects the inability of the duodenum to receive the gastric contents. Studies comparing gastric emptying rates in preterm and term infants are difficult to evaluate, but this suggests that gastric emptying is slower in preterm infants than in term infants.[18,19] One study evaluated gastric electrical activity and gastric emptying in preterm and term infants and showed that gastric electrical activity and gastric emptying show an intrinsic maturation depending on gestational age.[20]

It is unclear whether formulas of different composition and roughly the same caloric content are emptied at different rates by the newborn. In adults, it has been suggested that triglycerides of various chain lengths exert variable effects on gastric emptying, with medium chain triglycerides being less inhibitory than long chain triglycerides. Similar findings have been demonstrated in infants of 30 weeks' gestation[13] or longer; however, other studies have not confirmed these differences. One study showed no gastric electrical activity or gastric emptying in preterm infants fed either a standard preterm formula or protein hydrolysate formula.[21]

Nonnutritive sucking does not appear to have much influence on gastric emptying times in the infant.[22] Various other nonnutritive factors, such as formula temperature,[23,24] phototherapy,[23] and position,[18] have been shown to have no effect on gastric emptying times in infants who are examined within reasonable limits of physiologic variation. However, it has been shown that elevated bilirubin levels can decrease rates of gastric emptying.[25] Systemic illness can also decrease rates in newborn infants, as is demonstrated by dilution markers in infants with respiratory distress syndrome.[26]

The use of pharmacologic agents to accelerate gastric emptying in infants should be reserved for those instances when one is certain that no other underlying abnormality exists. Although metoclopramide has been shown to increase the gastric emptying rate in preterm and term infants,[27,28] it has also been shown to cross the blood-brain barrier. Its very high incidence of central nervous system side effects in older children and its relatively low therapeutic efficacy have largely led to its abandonment as a front-line therapeutic agent. Similarly, cisapride[29] and low-dose erythromycin[30] may increase emptying rates in preterm infants, although clinical success attributable to these agents has not been consistently observed.[31] One study showed that low dose erythromycin accelerated gastric emptying and improved feeding intolerance in preterm infants.[32] Nasojejunal feedings bypass the stomach, allowing enteral feeding even if gastric emptying is delayed; however, because intestinal motility also is immature, the nasojejunal feeding may provide only limited improvement in feeding tolerance.[33,34]

SMALL INTESTINE

In contradistinction to the esophagus and stomach, both of which tend to have more regionalized motor function, the small intestine can be viewed as a hollow tube consisting of supporting tissue, three muscle layers, and mucosa that absorbs nutrients. The three layers of muscle are identified as the muscularis mucosae, the internal circular muscle layer, and the external longitudinal muscle layer. Most evaluations of small intestinal motility center on the role of the internal circular muscle layer in the generation of intraluminal pressure, which results from contraction of this muscle layer.

These muscle layers are closely regulated and have their motor activity coordinated by the enteric nervous system, which is modulated by the central nervous system and a variety of neurohumoral agents. In the normal adult it has become clear that there are at least two different types of small intestinal motor activity. One occurs during the fasting state. This type of motor activity consists of clusters of phasic activity that migrate down the intestinal tract at periodic intervals. These migrating clusters of phasic motor activity normally occur every 1 to 2 hours and are known as migratory motor complexes (MMCs). One of the primary functions of these MMCs is to act as an "intestinal housekeeper" to move forward intestinal contents that have been left behind and to stop bacterial counts from increasing to high levels in the proximal small intestine. In the postprandial period after food is ingested, this periodicity of MMCs changes into what appears to be a continuous series of seemingly sporadic contractions that occur throughout the intestine. It is thought that this activity is responsible for the mixing and churning of ingested nutrients as they leave the stomach. It is also likely that the somewhat random-appearing nature of these contractions is actually a rather sophisticated series of peristaltic cascades that results in propulsion of nutrients through the small intestine.

When one examines movement of foodstuffs through the small intestine, it is important to understand what is being described. There are techniques to measure actual transit time of foodstuffs from the proximal to the distal small intestine, but the measurements of contractile activity in the small intestine do not necessarily equate with transit times. The actual motor activity that is responsible for the movement of foodstuffs in the postprandial period through the small intestine has not been well characterized and is poorly quantitated in most clinical settings. This is because the peristaltic sequences that are responsible for the movement of foodstuffs through the small intestines are not monophasic but consist of a multitude of contractions that coordinate peristalsis, retroperistalsis, and mixing in a manner that ultimately results in movement of food in an aboral direction. Most quantitative analysis of small intestinal motor activity consists of analysis of MMCs, most of which occur in the fasting period.[35]

It has been noted by Amaranth and colleagues[36] and by Berseth[37] that few infants display a pattern consistent with a true MMC. They tend to have episodes of motor inactivity interspersed with nonmigrating phasic motor activity. This nonmigrating motor activity has been demonstrated in up to 60% of the recording time in both term and preterm infants. It has been shown that these episodes of nonmigrating activity change with gestational age in that episodes lengthen in duration and increase in overall frequency.[37]

The sporadic contractions seen in the adult intestine in the postprandial state are not as predictable as in the preterm infant[38] in whom one can see no change, an increase, or a decrease in the intestine in response to feeding. Berseth and Nordyke[39] have noted that as the infant increases in gestational age, the likelihood of a mature feeding pattern increases. They have suggested that the presence of such a pattern may predict which infants are more likely to tolerate enteral feedings.[38] It has also been suggested that infants who have difficulty tolerating feedings are more likely to show an immature feeding pattern after enteral feedings.[40] A more recent study showed that term infants have increased duodenal motor activity postprandially like adults, while most preterm infants have decreased duodenal motor activity.[41]

In adults, initiation of an MMC is coincident with a rise in serum motilin levels. Intravenous motilin in an adult can cause the premature appearance of an MMC,[42, 43] as can erythromycin, which competitively binds to the motilin receptor.[44] Because MMCs are rarely seen in extremely preterm infants, Jadcherla and Berseth studied the correlation of small intestinal motor activity with serum motilin levels. They found that even when MMCs did occur in infants, there was no rise in serum motilin levels.[45] However, it was demonstrated that the administration of erythromycin did initiate MMCs in infants of 32-weeks' gestation, suggesting that motilin receptors are available at that age. More recently, Jadcherla and Berseth showed that erythromycin, a motilin-receptor agonist, increased antral and duodenal contractions in term and preterm infants whose gestational ages were 32 weeks and older.[46]

Initiation of enteral feedings tends to bring about a more rapid maturation of motor patterns in the preterm infant.[47, 48] It is possible that in preterm infants lacking MMCs during the fasting phase, there is a defect in the "housekeeping" function of small intestinal motor activity, which may predispose to bacterial overgrowth. Some clinicians have speculated that this may be a predisposing factor to necrotizing enterocolitis.

COLONIC MOTILITY

Colonic motility has not received as much study as the functions of upper areas of the gastrointestinal tract, although it is known that its embryologic development occurs in concert with that of the small intestine. Peristaltic waves in the colon can be seen early in gestation. Meissner and Auerbach plexuses are present by the 10th to 12th weeks. The distribution of ganglion cells has been studied quite fully in infants because of the pathophysiology associated with colonic aganglionosis. It is now believed that aside from the well-described area of hypoganglionosis present within the first 10 mm of the anal valve, a normal distribution of ganglion cells exists in the premature infant as young as 24 weeks' gestation.[49] More than 98% of normal newborns pass meconium within the first 36 to 48 hours. However, preterm infants weighing less than 1 kg oftentimes do not pass stool in the first 3 days.[50] It has been noted that high-amplitude propagating contractions in the colon are a good indicator of normal bowel function and passage of fecal material. These high-amplitude propagating contractions (HAPCs) have been noted to decrease in frequency from several an hour after a meal in toddlers to just a few per day in adults.[51,52] Very little is known about HAPCs during the newborn period. Work done on colonic motility of newborn rhesus primates suggested that the term newborn colon exhibits responses to feeding similar to those seen in the adult colon, whereas the response in the preterm primate is less well defined. This suggests that the colonic response matures late in gestation.[53]

REFERENCES

1. Pritchard J: Fetal swallowing and amniotic fluid volume. Obstet Gynecol 28:606, 1996.
2. Gryboski JD: The swallowing mechanisms of the neonate: 1. Esophageal and gastric motility. Pediatrics 31:382, 1965.
3. Hillemeier AC, et al: Developmental characteristics of the lower esophageal sphincter in the kitten. Gastroenterology 89:760, 1985.
4. Werlin SL, et al: Mechanisms of gastroesophageal reflux in children. J Pediatr 97:244, 1980.
5. Kawahanah H, et al: Mechanisms responsible for gastroesophageal reflux in children. Gastroenterology 113:399, 1997.
6. Omari TI, et al: Mechanisms of gastroesophageal reflux in preterm and term infants with influx disease. Gut 51:475, 2002.
7. Hassan BB, et al: Patterns of antropyloric motility in fed healthy preterm infants. Arch Dis Child Fetal Neonatal Ed 87:F95, 2002.
8. Hillemeier AC, et al: Developmental characteristics of the kitten antrum. Gastroenterology 101:339, 1991.
9. Lin H, et al: Gastric emptying of solid food is mostly potently inhibited by carbohydrate in the canine distal ileum. Gastroenterology 102:793, 1992.
10. Read N, et al: Effect of infusion of nutrient solutions into the ileum on gastrointestinal transit and plasma levels of neurotensin and enteroglucagon. Gastroenterology 86:274, 1984.
11. Costalos C, et al: Gastric emptying of Caloreen meals in the newborn. Arch Dis Child 55:883, 1980.
12. Husband J, et al: Gastric emptying of starch meals in the newborn. Lancet 2:290, 1970.
13. Siegel M, et al: Effect of caloric density on gastric emptying in premature infants. J Pediatr 104:118, 1984.
14. Siegel M, et al: Effect of fat and carbohydrate composition on the gastric emptying of isocaloric feedings in premature infants. Gastroenterology 89:785, 1985.
15. Sidebottom R, et al: Effects of long-chain vs. medium-chain triglycerides on gastric emptying time in premature infants. J Pediatr 102:448, 1983.
16. Zoppi G, et al: Exocrine pancrease function in premature and full term neonates. Pediatr Res 6:880, 1972.
17. Long W, Weiss J: Rapid gastric emptying of fatty meals in pancreatic insufficiency. Gastroenterology 67:920, 1974.
18. Cavell B: Gastric emptying in preterm infants. Acta Paediatr Scand 68:725, 1979.
19. Siegel MM: Gastric emptying time in premature and compromised infants. J Pediatr Gastroenterol Nutr 2(Suppl):S136, 1983.
20. Riezzo G, et al: Gastric electrical activity and gastric emptying in term and preterm infants. Neurogastroenterol Motil 12:223, 2000.
21. Riezzo G, et al: Gastric electrical activity and gastric emptying in preterm infants fed standard and hydrolyzed formulas. J Pediatr Gastroenterol Nutr 33:290, 2001.
22. Szabo J, et al: Effect of non-nutritive and nutritive suck on gastric emptying in premature infants. J Pediatr Gastroenterol Nutr 4:348, 1985.
23. Blumenthal I, et al: Effect of feed temperature and phototherapy on gastric emptying in the neonate. Arch Dis Child 55:562, 1980.
24. Costalos C, et al: Is it necessary to warm infants' feeds? Arch Dis Child 54:899, 1979.
25. Costalos C, et al: Effects of jaundice and phototherapy on gastric emptying in the newborn. Biol Neonate 46:57, 1984.
26. Yu VYH: Effect of body position on gastric emptying in the neonate. Arch Dis Child 50:500, 1975.
27. Hyman P, et al: Gastric emptying in infants: response to metoclopramide depends on the underlying condition. J Pediatr Gastroenterol 7:181, 1988.
28. Sankaran K, et al: Use of metoclopramide in preterm infants. Dev Pharmacol Ther 5:114, 1982.
29. Janssens G, et al: Long-term use of cisapride (Propulsid) in premature infants of less than 34 weeks gestational age. J Pediatr Gastroenterol Nutr 11:420, 1990.
30. Tomomasa T, et al: Erythromycin increases gastric antral motility in human premature infants. Biol Neonate 63:349, 1993.
31. Costalos C, et al: Erythromycin as a prokinetic agent in preterm infants. J Pediatr Gastroenterol Nutr 34:23, 2002.
32. Oei J, Lui K: A placebo controlled trial of low-dose erythromycin to promote fetal tolerance in preterm infants. Acta Paediatr 90:904, 2001.
33. Liang I, et al: Nasogastric compared with nasoduodenal feeding in low birth-weight infants. Arch Dis Child 61:138, 1986.
34. Van Caillie M, Powell G: Nasoduodenal versus nasogastric feedings in the very low birthweight infant. Pediatrics 56:1065, 1975.
35. Szurszewski JH: A migrating electronic complex of the canine small intestine. Am J Physiol 217:1757, 1969.
36. Amaranth RP, et al: Postnatal maturation of small intestinal motility in preterm infants. J Gastroint Motil 1:138, 1989.
37. Berseth CL: Gestational evolution of small intestinal motility in preterm and term infants. J Pediatr 115:646, 1989.
38. Al Tawil YS, et al: Motor activity responses to bolus feeding differ in preterm and term infants. J Pediatr Gastroenterol Nutr 19:126, 1995.
39. Berseth CL, Nordyke C: Manometry can predict feeding readiness in preterm infants. Gastroenterology 103:1523, 1992.
40. Berseth CL, McCoy HH: Birth asphyxia alters neonatal small intestinal motility in term infants. Pediatrics 90:669, 1992.
41. al Tawil Y, Berseth CL: Gestational and postnatal maturation of duodenal motor responses to intragastric feeding. J Pediatr 129:374, 1006.
42. Janssen J, et al: Pancreatic polypeptide is not involved in the regulation of the migrating motor complex in man. Regul Pept 3:41, 1982.
43. Houghton LA, et al: Motor activity of the gastric antrum, pylorus and duodenum under fasted conditions and after a liquid meal. Gastroenterology 94:1276, 1988.
44. Tomomasa T, et al: Developmental changes in agonist-mediated gastric smooth muscle contraction in the rabbit. Pediatr Res 26:458, 1989.
45. Jadcherla SR, Berseth CL: Cycling of plasma motilin and pancreatic polypeptide concentrations with migrating activity is blunted in term infants. Pediatr Res 35:128A, 1994.
46. Jadcherla SR, Berseth CL: Effect of erythromycin on gastroduodenal contractile activity in developing neonates. J Pediatr Gastroenterol Nutr 34:13, 2002.
47. Berseth CL: Effect of early feeding on maturation of the preterm infant's small intestine. J Pediatr 120:947, 1992.
48. Berseth CL, Nordyke CK: Enteral nutrients promote postnatal maturation of intestinal motor activity in preterm infants. Am J Physiol 264:G1046, 1993.
49. Weinberg AG: The anorectal myenteric plexus, its relation to hypoganglionosis of the colon. Am J Clin Pathol 54:637, 1970.

50. Verma A, Ramasubbareddy D: Time of first stool in extremely low birth weight (≤1000 grams). J Pediatr *122*:626, 1993.
51. Di Lorenzo C, et al: Age-related changes in colon motility. J Pediatr *127*:593, 1995.
52. Staiano A, et al: Esophageal motility in children with Hirschsprung's disease. Am J Dis Child 145:310, 1991.
53. Mulvihill S, et al: Trophic effect of amniotic fluid on fetal gastrointestinal development. J Surg Res *40*:291, 1986.

114

Steven L. Werlin and P. C. Lee

Development of the Exocrine Pancreas

EMBRYOLOGY AND HISTOGENESIS OF THE HUMAN PANCREAS

The dorsal and ventral anlagen of the human pancreas develop as evaginations of the primitive foregut during the fifth week of gestation (Fig. 114-1).[1] The larger dorsal anlage, which develops into the tail, body, and part of the head of the pancreas, grows directly from the duodenum. The ventral anlage develops from one or two buds from the primitive liver and eventually forms the major part of the head of the pancreas. At about 17 weeks' gestation, the dorsal and ventral anlagen fuse as the buds develop and the gut rotates. The ventral duct forms the proximal portion of the major pancreatic duct of Wirsung. The dorsal duct forms the distal portion of the duct of Wirsung and the accessory duct of Santorini. Variations in fusion account for the variety of developmental abnormalities of the pancreas.

Histologic examination of the early pancreas reveals predominantly undifferentiated epithelial cells, which by 9 to 12 weeks' development form a lobular-tubular pattern; zymogen granules are absent but the Golgi apparatus is present.[2, 3] Primitive acini containing rough endoplasmic reticulum and recognizable zymogen granules are present by 14 to 16 weeks. Golgi vesicles become prominent at this time. Activity of secretory enzymes is first detectable at this age. By 16 to 20 weeks' development, large numbers of zymogen granules are present. As the pancreas matures, the luminal volume decreases and acinar cell volume increases. Connective tissue continues to decrease both throughout gestation and in the postnatal period. By 20 weeks' gestation, acinar cells contain mature-appearing zymogen granules, well-developed endoplasmic reticulum, and highly developed basolateral membranes. The pancreas from the 6-day-old rat shows a similar increase in acinar volume and small lumina. Stroma con-

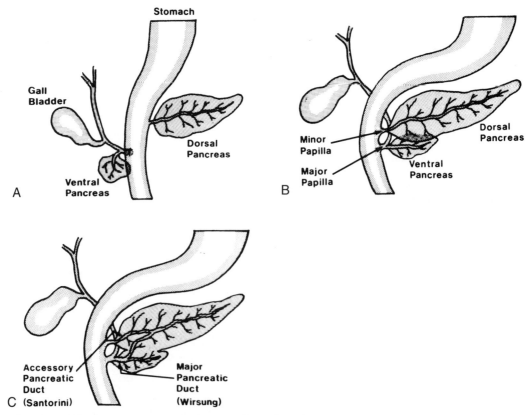

Fig. 114–1. Development of the human pancreas. **A,** Gestational age, 6 weeks; **B,** gestational age, 7–8 weeks. The ventral pancreas has rotated but has not yet fused with the dorsal pancreas. **C,** The ventral and dorsal pancreatic ductal systems have fused. (In Kelley VC [ed]: Practice of Pediatrics. Vol V, Philadelphia, Harper & Row, 1987.)

tinues to decrease, and acinar cells have a mature appearance. Postnatally, the volume of the exocrine pancreas continues to grow, nearly tripling in size during the first year of life from 5.5 g to 14.5 g.[4] The adult pancreas weighs 85 g. During the first 4 months, the ratio of acinar cells to connective tissue increases fourfold.

Centroacinar and duct cells (which are responsible for water, electrolyte, and bicarbonate secretion) are also found by 20 weeks. The ductal system contains less than 5% of the volume of the exocrine pancreas. The actual volume of the ductal system is only 0.5% of total pancreatic volume. In the postnatal period, luminal volume increases, along with the increase in acinar cell volume.

Islets are first identifiable at 12 to 16 weeks, at which time immunoreactive insulin is present in β cells. Mixed cells, those with characteristics of both acinar and islet cells that are only rarely seen in the adult, may be found.[5] Endocrine cells of the fetus, but not the adult, may contain more than one hormone, and more than one hormone may also be found within a single granule. The histologic appearance of the pancreas in an infant born at term is similar to that of the adult.

The signals controlling both cytodifferentiation, the process by which pancreatic cells differentiate into the various structural elements, and morphogenesis have not been well described in the human, but abundant information on these processes now being derived from studies on rodents is discussed later in this chapter.

Although duodenal and stool protease activity has been clearly demonstrated by many investigators, the time of first appearance of digestive enzymes in the fetal pancreas has been variably described. Unfortunately, until recently much of the available data not only were derived from methods no longer considered scientifically acceptable but also were contradictory. Only studies using modern techniques are reviewed here.

Lieberman found proteolytic activity, both in the pancreas of the 500-g fetus after activation of pancreatic homogenate with enterokinase and in the meconium from fetuses of similar age.[6] Track and colleagues found that trypsin, chymotrypsin, phospholipase A, and lipase were all present in the 14-cm (14-week) fetus in low concentrations, and these steadily increased with gestational age but amylase was not found.[3] Jodl and colleagues found increasing chymotrypsin activity in the stools collected from 42 low birth weight infants ranging in size from 750 to 2570 g with gestational age.[7] Chymotrypsin activity was low at birth, peaked at age 3 days, then declined slightly. Similarly, Mullinger and Palasi[8] detected trypsin and chymotrypsin in the stool of neonates. A wide day-to-day variation of enzyme concentration is found.

Using immunohistochemical techniques, Carrere and colleagues[9] demonstrated that trypsinogen and chymotrypsinogen are present in all acinar cells at week 16 of gestation and progressively increase in concentration until birth. In contrast, lipase-containing cells were scattered until week 21. Fukayama and co-workers[10] found pancreatic secretory trypsin inhibitor in the fetal pancreas at 10 weeks of gestation.

Using electrophoresis and immunohistochemistry with monoclonal antibodies, Davis and colleagues[11] demonstrated that pancreatic amylase is present in amniotic fluid at 14 weeks of gestation. Immunologic activity is present in the pancreas at 16 weeks of gestation. In contrast, Mally and colleagues[12] were unable to detect amylase mRNA in the human fetal pancreas. Thus, amylase, lipase, trypsinogen, and chymotrypsinogen are present in the fetal pancreas by 16 weeks' gestation, the time of rapid development of zymogen granules.

Human mucin gene expression *(Muc 1)* was evaluated in the fetal pancreas by Batra and colleagues[13], who found that *Muc 1* mRNA, a marker for differentiation of pancreatic cells, was not detectable until 18- to 19-weeks' gestation. In adults, *Muc 1* expression correlates with the differentiation state of pancreatic tumors.

ONTOGENY OF NONHUMAN PANCREAS

Many of our concepts concerning human pancreatic development are based on studies performed in rodents. Although the time span is different, the developmental stages of rat and human pancreas are believed to be similar. Pictet and Rutter[14] and others[15,16] have documented and correlated the morphologic, histologic, ultrastructural, and biochemical development of the rat pancreas and have defined several distinct prenatal developmental periods.[14-16]

Using the combination of embryo microdissection and reverse transcriptase polymerase chain reaction to measure low-level gene expression, Gittes and Rutter[17] related the onset of cell-specific gene expression to morphogenesis within 2 to 3 hours. They found expression of pancreas-specific transcripts in the foregut before formation of the pancreas. Insulin and glucagon were detected 10 to 12 hours before evagination of the pancreatic bud, but only in the area destined to become pancreas. Carboxypeptidase was first detected at 10.5 days and amylase at 12 days, both after the formation of the pancreas. Early expression of endocrine protein suggests a possible role in ontogenesis.

Hisaoka and colleagues[18] have related pancreatic morphogenesis and organization of the extracellular matrix. Throughout fetal development, epithelial compartments are separated by the basement membrane components (laminin and Type IV collagen) present at the epithelial mesenchyme interface. Spatial distribution of Types I and III collagen changes with time. Laminin-1 expression is important in the induction of exocrine cell differentiation.[19] These extracellular matrix components are presumed to play a role in the regulation of differentiation. Organ culture studies have shown that local mesenchymal factors, but not nerves or hormones, are required for morphogenesis and cytodifferentiation, which themselves are separable events.

The proliferating cell nuclear antigen (PCNA), a protein associated with DNA polymerase Δ, is expressed during the S phase of the cell cycle. Activity of PCNA is related to ³H-thymidine uptake.[20] Using monoclonal antibody immunostaining, Elsasser and colleagues[20] demonstrated that the percentage of PCNA-positive cells was high at 16 days' gestation (60%), declined (to below 10%) at birth, increased to 30% at age 5 days, and then fell slowly until the pup weaned, at which time a precipitous fall to the adult level (below 5%) occurred (60 days). This was highly correlated with ³H-thymidine uptake.

Oates and Morgan[21] examined the proliferation of various cell compartments during rat development both *in vivo* and *in vitro*. They found that the acinar cell population was predominantly mononuclear at birth but after weaning became progressively binuclear. Before weaning, acinus formation was due to mononuclear acinar cell and duct cell proliferation. Pour[22] found that in Syrian hamsters primordial pancreatic cells most resembled centroacinar cells and that transitional cells could be found in the fetal pancreas.

The shape of the mature acinar cell is pyramidal with a basal nucleus. The most prominent organelles in the fasted state are large numbers of zymogen granules, located apically. Abundant rough endoplasmic reticulum (RER, the location of protein synthesis) and Golgi apparatus (the nidus of packaging proteins for export) are present. Junctional complexes join adjacent acinar cells. The apical membrane contains abundant microvilli projecting into the lumen. The final three-dimensional structure of the exocrine pancreas consists of a complex series of branching ducts surrounded by grapelike clusters of acinar cells. The ontogeny of cell surface glycoproteins is critical for normal cell-cell interactions and morphogenesis.[23,24] Studies of the ontogeny of lectin-binding patterns have clearly demonstrated that the primitive pancreatic cells most resemble the centroacinar cells. Stage-specific polylactosamine (carbohydrate) antigens have been described in many organs, including the pancreas. These antigens are thought to be important for cell-to-cell communication and recognition.[25]

The expression of the mature phenotype can first be detected at a gestational age of 15 days, the onset of the differentiated stage. Inhibition of glycoprotein synthesis (with tunicamycin therapy) in pancreatic rudiments between days 15 and 17 delays histogenesis, as well as the normal increase in amylase found at this age.[26] At 17 days, acinar lumina are first seen coincident with differentiation of the apical and basolateral domains of the acinar cell membrane. The adult pattern is fully developed at age 19 days.

The temporal profiles of secretory proteins in the prenatal pancreas have been defined in the rodent.[27-29] Until day 14 of gestation, little or no secretory product, specific mRNA for secretory proteins, or zymogen granules are found. From days 14 to 18, synthesis of embryonic proteins (found in a wide variety of other fetal tissues, but not in zymogen granules) continues. A constant low level of a few pancreas-specific secretory proteins is found. From days 18 to 21, a rapid increase in specific mRNA transcripts occurs, followed by a nonparallel increase in pancreas-specific proteins and zymogen granules.[30,31] RNA synthesis peaks at day 18 followed by a peak in protein synthesis 1 day later. During this period, although total pancreatic protein synthesis increases only 25%, synthesis of some pancreas-specific proteins (e.g., amylase and chymotrypsinogen) increases by more than 100%. During the final days of gestation and during early neonatal life, synthesis of secretory proteins accounts for more than 90% of all pancreatic protein synthesis.

The appearance of the various secretory proteins is not parallel, suggesting independent regulation of gene expression.[28,29] Amylase and chymotrypsinogen appear synchronously at day 15. Other proteins that also appear in pairs are trypsinogen and procarboxypeptidase B, and specific lipase and procarboxypeptidase A. Nonspecific lipase and ribonuclease accumulate independently. Amylase-specific mRNA increases 600-fold at a gestational age between 14 and 20 days, coincident with the already described 1000-fold increase in amylase-specific activity. Synthesis of secretory proteins is regulated at the level of transcription.

Le Huerou and colleagues[32] studied the postnatal developmental profile of mRNA transcripts coding for chymotrypsinogen, trypsinogen, lipase, and amylase and the expression of these proteins in the calf. Specific mRNA levels of amylase, lipase, and trypsin increased with age; chymotrypsin mRNA decreased from birth until day 28 and then increased at day 119 back to the level found in the newborn. Specific activities of the proteins did not necessarily parallel mRNA levels. At day 119, levels of trypsinogen, lipase, and amylase mRNAs were markedly increased; the level of chymotrypsinogen mRNA remained decreased when compared with the level found in the animal born at term. All four mRNAs were increased in weaned animals but to differing degrees. Thus, in the cow, these genes are differently expressed during development.

Payne and colleagues[33] demonstrated the presence of at least three different lipases, one of which may be identical to the zymogen granule membrane protein GP3. Each lipase appears to be under different regulatory control, both prenatally and postnatally. Yang[34] and co-workers have also shown discoordinate expression of pancreatic lipase and two related proteins in the human fetal pancreas.

Thus, the timing of initiation of synthesis of individual proteins is different, and the final levels are also different. Although the curves for the appearance of each protein are quite similar, they are time shifted. The final adult level of each enzyme is unrelated to the onset of synthesis or to the peak fetal level. Concentrations of enzyme change considerably after birth.[27] The level of secretory protein in the mature pancreas represents the balance between synthesis and secretion. In addition, the presence of mRNA does not necessarily indicate an abundance of its translational product.

SECRETION FROM THE EXOCRINE PANCREAS

Although there is a continuous slow basal secretion of pancreatic enzymes, physiologically significant secretion occurs only after stimulation by a secretagogue. A large number of agents have been described that are effective secretagogues in the experimental animal, but probably only acetylcholine and cholecystokinin (CCK) are of significance in humans. Acetylcholine is released locally in the pancreas after vagal stimulation. CCK is synthesized and stored in the intestinal amine precursor uptake and decarboxylation (APUD) cells and released after ingestion of a protein or fatty meal.

The secretagogue then interacts with its specific receptor on the acinar cell membrane. Intracellular second and third messengers include Ca^{2+}, protein kinase C, diacylglycerol, and inositol phosphates.[35,36] This complex and as yet inadequately understood process eventually leads to fusion of zymogen granules and cell membranes and to exocytosis of pancreatic protein into the ductal system. GP2 is the most abundant glycoprotein in zymogen granule membranes. Scheele and partners[37] have proposed that luminal factors, including the process of assembly and disassembly of a matrix (containing GP2 and proteoglycans), perform critical functions during storage and secretion of pancreatic secretory proteins. Regulation by CCK and secretin is critical. A portion of GP2 is cleaved by protein kinase C and released into the pancreatic duct during stimulated secretion.[38]

Although nonparallel secretion of pancreatic proteins has also been described, at the present time, most authors consider that nonparallel secretion is probably the exception and not the norm.[39]

Fluid and electrolyte secretion from the centroacinar and ductal cells are controlled by secretin, the first gastrointestinal hormone to be identified. Intracellular messengers in this system are cyclic adenosine monophosphate (cAMP) and protein kinase A. The concentrations of bicarbonate and chloride in pancreatic secretion depend on the flow rate. At lower flow rates, the concentration of bicarbonate is low and that of chloride is high.[39] As the rate increases, bicarbonate secretion increases and chloride secretion decreases, whereas sodium and potassium secretions remain constant.

The pancreas synthesizes more than 20 proteins specifically designed for export. After synthesis, it must segregate those proteins designated for export from those synthesized for internal use. Classic studies have demonstrated the synthetic pathway using the pulse-chase technique. Newly synthesized proteins travel from the endoplasmic reticulum to the Golgi apparatus, where they are "packaged" to the condensing vacuoles and then converted into mature zymogen granules in the apical portion of the cell. There is little or no processing of individual proteins from the time they leave the rough endoplasmic reticulum until the time they leave the cell. In rodents this entire process takes less than 1 hour. Molecular chaperones or chaperonins are involved in the transit process as they are in other cell types.[40]

ONTOGENY OF SECRETORY FUNCTION IN THE HUMAN

Because of both the technical difficulties and the ethical concerns about performing invasive procedures on healthy infants, few studies of pancreatic secretory function in the human infant have been published. Because direct collection of pancreatic juice is not possible in the infant and young child, pancreatic secretions must be collected in the duodenum in the fasted or basal state, after indirect stimulation with a meal, or after direct stimulation with secretagogues such as secretin or cholecystokinin, or both. Pancreatic function may be determined indi-

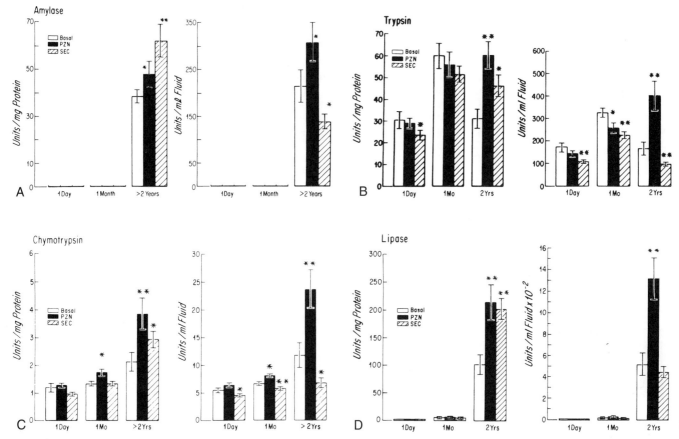

Fig. 114–2. Effect of cholecystokinin and secretin on specific activities of pancreatic enzymes in duodenal fluid in infants and children. **A,** Amylase; **B,** trypsin; **C,** chymotrypsin; **D,** lipase.

rectly by the measurement of pancreatic enzymes in stool and by fat balance studies.

In a series of studies, Zoppi and colleagues[41-44] measured stimulated pancreatic secretion in normal infants and children. In premature infants who have not been fed (gestational age 32 weeks), duodenal trypsin, lipase, and amylase were present in levels considerably lower than those found in term infants. Enzyme levels were even lower at 24 hours. The levels found at age 1 week depended on the carbohydrate of the ingested formula. Infants fed a high-starch formula had higher amylase levels; those fed a high-glucose formula had lower amylase but higher trypsin and lipase levels. Although infants fed a low-fat formula had the highest trypsin levels and no change in lipase, secretion of trypsin was lower than that found in older children and adults. The major problems with these early studies are the qualitative nature of the collections and the lack of separation between the pancreatic and salivary amylase and lipase isoenzymes. Thus, the presence and changes of concentration of either or both of these enzymes may have been due to contamination with the salivary isoenzyme.

In a small group of older children, Zoppi and associates[42] demonstrated that amylase secretion continues to increase with age (the oldest child studied was 13 years old), whereas output of lipase, proteinases, fluid, and bicarbonate was independent of age. A good correlation was found between protein secretion and enzyme activity. Norman and co-workers measured pancreatic secretion in eight healthy full-term infants aged 3 to 15 days after a test meal of breast milk.[45] Although the trypsin:chymotrypsin ratio was relatively constant, the levels of the individual enzymes varied considerably between infants. Salivary but not pancreatic amylase was present in low levels.

Lebenthal and Lee[46] studied basal and stimulated pancreatic secretion in groups of well premature and full-term neonates, infants 1 month of age, and toddlers 2 years of age (Fig. 114–2). Results obtained from full-term and premature infants were similar, and data were pooled in the report. Although total protein content was similar in the pancreatic secretions collected from the duodenum of all three groups, each of the five individual secretory proteins studied had its own developmental profile. Trypsin was low at 1 day, but at 1 month it was similar to the level seen at 2 years. Chymotrypsin remained low at 1 month. Carboxypeptidase was low both at 1 day and at 1 month when compared with the level found at 2 years. Amylase was not detected until age 2 years. Similarly, lipase was undetectable at 1 day and at 1 month. Thus, the ontogeny of the various enzymes is not parallel, a finding that has also been documented in rodents. Responses to secretin and CCK were poor in the newborn and infant. Responses at 1 month were similar, whether the infants were fed a cow's milk–based formula or a soy formula.

These data confirm previous reports concerning proteinases but are contradictory with respect to amylase and lipase. It has clearly been shown that pancreatic amylase is present early in gestation. Similarly, salivary amylase is secreted in high concentration in the newborn. Serum pancreatic isoamylase and isolipase are both low at birth and increase with age. These findings suggest that the newborn pancreas can synthesize but not secrete amylase. The failure to find any amylase may reflect the fasted state of the infants. A similar argument can be constructed to explain the extremely low levels of lipase.

Enzyme secretion is decreased in the infant and young child, and secretion of water and bicarbonate is blunted as well. An increase in ductal cell function also occurs with increasing age. Secretion of water increases 10 times by age 9 months.[44]

Despite this pancreatic insufficiency just described, the human newborn infant and the premature infant absorb both fat and carbohydrate with seemingly little difficulty. In elegant studies, Fomon and colleagues[47] evaluated fat absorption in a group of infants ingesting various formulas. Although an adult-type coefficient of fat absorption was not seen until age 4 to 6 months of life, "clinically" important malabsorption was not seen unless an additional pancreatic insult, such as cystic fibrosis, was present. The lack of significant malabsorption is almost certainly due to the presence of the nonpancreatic (lingual and gastric) lipases.

Although the ontogeny of complex carbohydrate digestion and absorption has not yet been as carefully examined as that of fat absorption, there is some information regarding the ability of the newborn to digest starches. There is only a minimal rise in blood sugar after the ingestion of cooked starch. Intestinal hydrolysis of starch is rapid in the 1-year-old; at age 6 months, hydrolysis of amylopectin is incomplete and duodenal amylase activity is low. Despite the poor duodenal hydrolysis of starch, only minimal carbohydrate is found in the stool of infants fed formulas containing complex carbohydrates. This seeming paradox has been explained as being secondary to salvage of colonic carbohydrate by bacterial fermentation and absorption of short chain organic acid products.[48] It is also clear that the digestibility of starches, modified starches, and complex carbohydrates varies considerably. Levitt and colleagues[49] have shown in adults that the increase in breath hydrogen after ingestion of meals containing complex carbohydrates varied considerably, suggesting that a large amount of fermentable material escapes small bowel absorption even in the adult. Neonates also have the enzyme glucoamylase in the brush border of the intestine, which aids in the digestion of starch and increases intraluminal glucose by removing glucose units from the nonreducing ends of molecules of starch.

It is clear that most infants, even those who are premature, thrive on formulas that contain glucose polymers or corn syrup solids as their carbohydrate source. It has been our experience, which is supported by a small number of published case reports, that some infants develop watery diarrhea when fed such formulas.[50-52] This diarrhea resolves when the formula is changed to one containing an alternative carbohydrate.

Diet modulates pancreatic enzyme secretion in the human as it does in the animal models discussed later in this chapter. Although these changes may occur at the level of synthesis, some changes reported to occur in animals clearly occur faster than can be explained by changes in synthesis. Feeding a soy-based formula to premature infants increases stimulated pancreatic secretion of lipase and trypsin compared with infants fed a cow's milk–based formula.[53] Total parenteral nutrition induces reversible pancreatic atrophy in animals and pancreatic hyposecretion in humans. Despite this potential problem, clinical experience has demonstrated that extended parenteral nutrition seems to have no long-term deleterious effects on pancreatic function in the human infant. Thus, as in the animal models described later in this chapter, some changes in pancreatic enzyme secretion are programmed, and others are inducible by diet.

ONTOGENY OF RODENT EXOCRINE PANCREATIC SECRETION

The pancreas of the newborn rat is both histologically and ultrastructurally fully developed; it is packed with secretory proteins. Although it appears poised to secrete, it is functionally immature. Immaturity has been documented at a number of steps along the stimulus-secretion chain. Responsiveness to cholinergic and peptidergic (e.g., CCK) secretagogues in a manner similar to, but not identical with, the adult gland does not occur until age 24 to

48 hours.[54-56] The newborn pancreas, although unresponsive to cholinergic agents and to CCK, does respond with increased secretion of amylase to the calcium ionophore A23187, suggesting that the secretory mechanism distal to calcium mobilization is intact.[56-57] In contrast, Chang and Jamieson[58] failed to find responsiveness to A23187 in fetal pancreas.

Dumont and colleagues[59] have defined the ontogeny of the muscarinic receptor. Receptor density, low in the fetal and newborn periods, steadily increases with age, reaching maximal levels at age 1 month; it then decreases steadily until age 1 year. They found a parallel increase in secretory response and receptor density.

The ontogeny of the CCK receptor has been similarly evaluated by Leung and associates[60] and Werlin and co-workers.[61] Binding of radiolabeled CCK also rises rapidly (from low levels at birth), reaching levels of the mature pancreas at age 3 weeks. In contrast, Chang and Jamieson[58] found that the postnatal increase in secretory responsiveness was not associated with increased CCK binding. They found that in both the fetal and neonatal pancreas, CCK mobilized calcium. These receptors were shown by Hadjiivanova and colleagues[62] to be of the A or intestinal type that just after birth are already coupled to G proteins. These authors also demonstrated that CCK-A glycoforms were different prenatally. LeMeuth and colleagues[26] showed that in the cow the CCK-A receptor predominated at birth, but later the CCK-B receptor predominated. Results of these studies suggest that decreased receptor density cannot explain the lack of secretory responsiveness in the immature pancreas and that the immaturity is distal to calcium mobilization. The absence of the zymogen granule membrane protein GP2 in the fetus may contribute to secretory unresponsiveness.[13]

The ontogeny of the vasoactive intestinal polypeptide (VIP) receptor has been described in rats and calves. In the rat, VIP receptors are present at day 19 of gestation.[32, 63] In the cow, a single class of receptors is present at birth; however, at 28 and 119 days after birth, two classes (high-affinity and low-affinity) receptors are found.

Because protein phosphorylation appears to play an important role in the pancreatic response to secretagogues, the roles of protein kinases have been examined. Calcium-calmodulin-dependent protein kinase increases in parallel with responsiveness to secretagogues from the late fetal to the newborn period.[64] Similarly, protein kinase C was found to be low in the term fetus. Levels increased in the newborn period, reaching adult values by age 2 days.[65] Newborn rat pancreas was unresponsive to 12-0-tetradecanoylphorbol acetate (TPA), an activator of protein kinase C, but the 2-day-old pancreas responded to TPA with increased amylase secretion. These studies of protein kinases suggest immaturity of the secretory response to regulatory peptides at a number of levels.

Thus, immaturity both of receptors to secretagogues and of protein kinases is found in the neonatal rat. At this time, the lack of responsiveness to secretagogues in the neonatal rat cannot be attributed to any one pharmacologic deficiency and may in fact be multifactorial.

EFFECTS OF DIET AND WEANING IN RODENTS

Dakka and colleagues[66] found that a protein-free, carbohydrate-rich diet had no effect on mRNA coding for elastase isoenzymes; however, trypsinogen isoenzyme mRNA levels increased slightly. Because this same dietary manipulation decreases cationic trypsinogen synthesis, the trypsinogen genes must be under different translational and transcriptional control.

Wicker and Puigserver[67] showed that in the rat fed a high-fat diet in which lipase synthesis increased within 24 hours, amylase synthesis did not increase and peptidase synthesis increased by day 5. Lipase-specific mRNA increased fourfold on day 1 followed by a second 6.5-fold increase on day 4. Amylase mRNA levels remained unchanged. Because of the biphasic increase in lipase and lipase-specific mRNA, those authors postulated that the first phase was due to an increase in mRNA synthesis and the second phase to increased translation, possibly secondary to hormonal influences.

The pancreatic content of exportable proteins and zymogen granules falls dramatically after birth.[16, 68] This fall is not preprogrammed but rather relates to feeding and stimulation of secretion.[69-70] Alterations in diet, time of weaning, and time of first feeding all affect the levels of secretory proteins in predictable ways.

Studies in which the diets of immature animals are altered have shown that the changes in concentrations of various pancreatic enzymes are not all preprogrammed. The molecular basis for many of these effects has been reviewed.[71] Changing the diet from high fat–low carbohydrate to high carbohydrate–low fat by early weaning increases chymotrypsin and lipase and decreases amylase. Delaying weaning, by prolonged nursing, postpones these changes in enzyme concentration. Animals weaned on a high-fat diet similar to mother's milk demonstrated changes in enzyme patterns similar to those found in animals prematurely weaned. Interestingly, the changes found with early weaning are similar to those induced with glucocorticoids, and premature weaning induces an increase in corticosteroid levels in the infant rat. Changes in diet after 21 days of age induce characteristic changes in pancreatic enzyme composition; thus, increasing the dietary intake of starch increases amylase, increasing intake of fat increases lipase, and increasing protein intake increases trypsin. Thus, glucocorticoids may modulate some effects of feeding; however, others seem to be preprogrammed.

REGULATORY FACTORS

Plasma CCK (CCK-8 + CCK-33 + CCK-39) levels were measured before and following breast-feeding in 4-day-old infants.[72] A significant increase was seen immediately after a meal, followed by a decrease to basal levels at 10 minutes and a secondary increase at 30 and 60 minutes following feeding. This biphasic rise is not seen in older children or adults. Plasma gastrin-34 levels increased by 50% 5 and 10 minutes after the onset of suckling and immediately after breast-feeding in 3-day-old infants. Previous studies that failed to find a gastrin response to feeding examined only the period after feeding. Postprandial levels of 11 regulatory hormones were measured by Salmenpera and colleagues[73] in 9-month-old infants who had been fed exclusively by either breast or bottle. The basal level and postprandial rise in CCK were lower in breast-fed than in bottle-fed infants.

In the rat colon, CCK mRNA is found in the fetus, is absent at birth, and then increases steadily until adulthood.[74] CCK is present in low amounts in the rat fetal colon. Immediately after birth, the rat small intestine contains CCK-like bioactivity. In the pig, CCK immunoreactivity is found in the small intestine at 6 to 8 weeks' gestation.[75] In the guinea pig, plasma CCK levels are low at birth but rise to near adult levels at day 15.[76] Thus, CCK is present in the gut and is presumably available to participate in the regulation of pancreatic growth in the fetus.

Progastrin and gastrin are present in many species, including humans, in both fetal and adult states.[77] In the human fetal pancreas, the levels of gastrin and progastrin are low when compared with findings in other species. In the mouse, the gastrin gene is first expressed at 9.5 to 10 days' gestation, whereas immunoreactivity does not develop until day 20. The gastrin gene is unique among those expressed by the pancreas in that it is active in the fetus but inactive in the adult, except when the Zollinger-Ellison syndrome develops. Thus, CCK and gastrin, both trophic agents for the pancreas, are present at birth when the rate of pancreatic growth is the greatest.

Iovanna and associates[78] demonstrated that CCK controls gene expression at the translational level. Using cloned cDNA probes to quantify concentrations of specific mRNA transcripts, Renaud and co-workers[79] found that long-term stimulation with CCK and cerulean (a CCK analogue) resulted in stimulation of mRNA synthesis for genes coding for trypsinogen and chymotrypsinogen but not amylase.

Pancreatic growth in the mature animal can be altered by a variety of agents, diets, and experimental procedures.[80] The trophic effects of CCK, gastrin, and CCK-like peptides have been well documented. In the adult rat, the postprandial CCK level regulates ornithine decarboxylase and secretory protein gene expression at the translational level. Treatment of rats with the CCK antagonist L364718 not only prevents the trophic effects of exogenous CCK but also causes pancreatic atrophy, suggesting that CCK is necessary for growth and maintenance of the gland.[81] When given to the immature rat, this agent did not alter normal growth but did block the trophic effects of exogenous CCK.[82] CCK-induced growth is mediated by a single-type variety of type A receptors with both high- and low-affinity states.[83-86]

Glucocorticoids induce pancreatic hypertrophy in the mature rat, with particular increases in concentrations of amylase and chymotrypsin. Hydrocortisone also potentiates the trophic effect of cerulean, a CCK analogue. Although secretin has only a mildly trophic effect, it potentiates the trophic effect of CCK. Secretin infusion increases synthesis of lipase. Although high doses of cholinergic agents induce hypertrophy in rat pancreas, the physiologic importance of this effect is uncertain. Epidermal growth factor (EGF), which is found in high levels in the pancreas, can be either trophic or not trophic.[87] Pancreatic biliary diversion, small bowel resection, and ingestion of raw soy flour all induce pancreatic growth in the mature animal.

Although there are published studies concerning the roles of many of the previously discussed agents and treatments on the immature pancreas, interpretation and comparison of these studies present numerous difficulties in data analysis, including that (1) the various agents tested were given in different doses, at different ages, and for different lengths of time and (2) the animals were evaluated for effects on growth in different ways. A major fact often overlooked is that the growth rate and the rates of synthesis of both DNA and protein vary considerably with developmental ages.[88]

Werlin and colleagues have shown that the concentrations of DNA and protein in immature rat pancreas do not parallel the rates of their synthesis.[88] DNA concentration increases rapidly from a low level in the first day of life, peaks between ages 3 and 14 days, then slowly falls to a lower adult level. In contrast, DNA synthesis decreases in the first 24 hours, peaks at age 3 days at a rate 30 times that observed in the adult, then falls slowly to the adult value. Similarly, protein concentration that is nearly as high at birth as in the adult, plummets at day three before it slowly begins to rise to adult levels. Protein synthesis, in contrast, is as low at birth (as it is in the adult) but is three to five times higher at all intermediate ages tested.

Despite these controversies and the gaps in our knowledge, a great deal has been learned concerning the effects of many agents on the growth of the exocrine pancreas in the developing animal. CCK and CCK-like peptides have a variety of effects that seem to be age dependent. DNA synthesis is not increased by CCK before age 28 days, and variable effects on growth have been described depending on age, dosage, and CCK analogue studied.[89-91] The potent specific CCK antagonist L364718 blocks the effects of exogenous cerulean on the growth of the neonatal rat pancreas, but when given alone it has no effect. This suggests that endogenous CCK is not a controlling factor in the growth of the neonatal rat pancreas.[92]

CCK action is mediated by CCK receptors. Of the two types of CCK receptors (A and B), the adult rat pancreas has only Type A, which mediates pancreatic growth in adult rats. Miyasaka and partners[93] found that the Otsuka Long-Evans Tokushima fatty (OLETF) rats lack the CCK-A receptor gene. Despite this defect, pancreatic growth in the immediate postnatal life is normal although the pancreas is slightly smaller at 5 to 6 weeks of age. However, in later growth at 24 to 25 weeks, OLETF rats showed a significantly lower protein-DNA content than the wild-type strain, which suggests that the CCK-A receptor plays a small role in the early postnatal growth of the pancreas but is required for later cell growth. Thus, CCK might not be important in regulating pancreatic growth in early postnatal life.

The role of gastrin is likewise questioned. In a study by Ballinger and colleagues,[94] administration of a specific gastrin antagonist, CI-988, to neonates for 5 days reduced stomach growth but not pancreatic growth. Thus although pharmacologic doses of gastrin and CCK are trophic for the neonatal exocrine pancreas, it is unclear whether they play a role in the early development of the exocrine pancreas.

Hydrocortisone decreases protein synthesis in the first week of life but has no effect on DNA synthesis in the immature animal.[88] Other studies have described hypertrophy and hyperplasia or hypertrophy alone,[89,94] depending on age. Cerulean and hydrocortisone potentiate each other's trophic effects. The lack of increase in DNA synthesis in the suckling animal after treatment with either CCK or hydrocortisone may be due to the finding that synthesis is already proceeding at the maximum rate possible.

A temporal relationship exists between corticosterone levels, cytoplasmic corticosteroid receptors, and increases in pancreatic secretory products in the developing rat pancreas.[94, 95] Corticosterone levels and dexamethasone binding increase from birth, reach a peak at about age 25 days, then decrease to adult levels. Increases in circulating levels of steroids precede increases in receptor density, which increases sharply after age 15 days. These increases parallel those of both amylase and hydrolase activities, which can be induced by exogenous steroids. The pancreatic glucocorticoid receptor is under autologous control by glucocorticoid. Early weaning, which augments corticosterone levels, causes similar changes in the content of exportable proteins in the pancreas. The highest density of steroid receptors occurs at age 21 to 28 days, the period of peak responsiveness of the pancreas to hydrocortisone. Thus, glucocorticoids clearly modulate postnatal pancreatic development.[96]

Thyroxine (T_4) induces precocious increases of amylase, lipase, chymotrypsin, and trypsin in neonatal rats; however, chemical thyroidectomy retards pancreatic development.[97] Endogenous T_4 peaks between days 10 and 16, the time point when amylase levels are also increasing. T_4 induces maturation of secretory function by modulating the maximum binding capacity of high-affinity CCK receptors. In the immature animal, thyroid hormone acts both directly on the pancreatic acinar cell and indirectly through the adrenal system.[98]

Pancreatic duct cells have high levels of epidermal growth factor (EGF).[99] Parenteral but not oral EGF increases pancreatic amylase in suckling rabbits.[100] Inhibition of ornithine decarboxylase (and thus polyamine metabolism) inhibits stimulated pancreatic growth.[101] The role of polyamines in normal pancreatic growth and development is not established. Secretin increases DNA, amylase, and chymotrypsin in 6-day-old rats.[102] The effects of PYY and somatostatin, which are antitrophic to the pancreas in mature animals, have not been studied in developing animals.

Bombesin induces hypertrophy and hyperplasia in newborn rats.[103] In adult animals, the effects of bombesin were thought to be mediated by CCK. Studies by Rosewicz and colleagues[104] have demonstrated that bombesin regulates pancreatic gene expression at the level of mRNA and that this effect is not mediated by CCK. Borysewicz and associates[105] have shown that in the immature animal bombesin acts directly on the pancreas.

The developmental profiles of a number of other proteins and peptides have been studied in a variety of experimental animals using immunohistochemistry, radioimmunoassay, and molecular biology techniques. Recently, we demonstrated that short term hypoxia in newborn rats delayed the maturation of pancreatic exocrine enzymes.[106] Exactly how this can be translated to human infants is not known at present, however.

Other regulatory factors have also been implicated in rodent pancreatic exocrine development. Transforming growth factor alpha (TGFα) appears after birth and increases progressively with age in the exocrine pancreas.[107] TGF-α thus may have a functional role in pancreatic development. Artificially mutated TGF-β receptor in mice leads to a pancreas with acinar hyperplasia and atypia.[108] In addition, overexpression of TGF-β interferes with acinar differentiation.[109] TGF-β added to rat embryonic pancreatic rudiments resulted in differential gene activation.[110] Fibroblast growth factors (FGFs) and FGF receptors (FGFRs) are important mediators of epithelial-mesenchyme interactions. FGFs are expressed throughout rat pancreatic development. In mesenchyme-free culture of embryonic pancreatic epithelium, addition of FGFs promotes growth, morphogenesis, and cytodifferentiation of exocrine pancreatic cells.[111] In the presence of mesenchyme, growth and development of pancreatic epithelium progresses without the addition of FGFs. Abrogation of FGFR-2IIIb in the system attenuates both growth and development.

FETAL ANTIGENS

Fetoacinar protein (FAP) is a specific acinar cell antigen found only in the exocrine pancreas, associated with ontogenesis in the Syrian golden hamster and in humans. In the human fetus, FAP is present at 9- to 10-weeks' gestation.[112] The highest concentrations are found at ages 15 to 25 weeks when acinar cell proliferation is most intense. FAP synthesis then progressively decreases. The levels found in adults are lower than those in the fetus. FAP is found in high concentration in amniotic fluid. FAP can also be considered an oncodevelopmental antigen, because in pancreatic cancer and in some cases of chronic pancreatitis, FAP is elevated. Although the developmental role of this protein is still not known, FAP has been shown to be a variant of bile salt-dependent lipase, differing only by a decrease in O-glycosylation.[113] It is not known whether this decrease in O-glycosylation changes enzyme activity or function.

A second fetal antigen, fetal antigen 1 (FA1), is found in both the exocrine and endocrine fetal pancreas and hepatocytes.[114] FA1 is found in high concentration in the fetal venous blood and amniotic fluid during the second and third trimesters. At 7 weeks' gestation, FA1 is found in 94% of the ductal epithelial cells. By week 17, only 64% of the duct cells test positive for FA1 by immunoperoxidase staining, decreasing to only 11% in the 4-month-old infant. The role or roles and controls of FA1 in pancreatic development are not known.

PROTO-ONCOGENES

Viral oncogenes have been shown to be responsible for the development of many cancers. Cellular oncogenes, which are homologues of viral oncogenes, are critical for the regulation of normal cell growth and differentiation. The extreme conservation found in these genes suggests that they play important roles in the normal cell. Oncogenes are present during fetal development and generate growth-promoting signals in the normal cell and after organ injury. During prenatal and postnatal development in the mouse, these various oncogenes have different patterns of expression.

There have been only a few studies of oncogenes in the pancreas, and most have related to pancreatic cancer.[115] *C-H-ras* has

PANCREATIC CELL DIFFERENTIATION

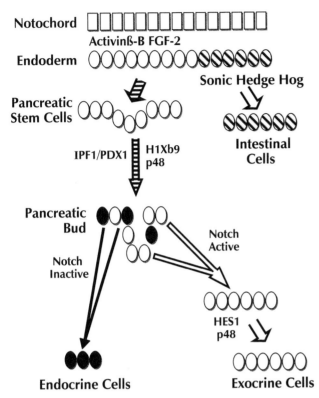

Fig. 114–3. Origin of the exocrine and endocrine cell lineages in the developing pancreas. This model is based on descriptions from various reports (e.g., see Kim and Hebrok,[121] Crisera[123]). *Arrows* in the diagram indicate the sequential activities based on the appearance of specific cell markers in the developing mouse pancreas. (Adapted from Edlund[122]).

been observed in the human embryo between 12 and 18 weeks' gestation. Calve and colleagues[116] demonstrated that at 12 to 48 hours following subtotal pancreatectomy, the oncogenes *c-myc* and *c-ras* in adult rat pancreas were overexpressed, at the same time that secretory protein expression was decreased. Thus, repression and derepression of genes occur during the recovery from subtotal pancreatectomy. Silverman and co-workers[117] found increased levels of mRNAs for *c-myc, c-raf*-1, and *c-Ki-ras* following both pancreatectomy and pancreatitis induced by camostat mesylate. Increased expression of these cellular oncogenes was also found in azaserine-induced adenomas and carcinomas. Lu and Lodsdon[118] have shown that the secretagogues CCK, bombesin, and carbachol stimulate the expression of the cellular oncogenes, *c-myc, c-fos,* and *c-jun,* which are members of the "immediate early gene" nuclear oncogene family, because their expression is rapid and transient. The oncogene *c-Ki-ras* is elevated in human and experimental pancreatic cancers. Point mutations in Ki-*ras* oncogenes are frequent in pancreatic cancer.[119] The c-*erb*B-2 proto-oncogene is overexpressed in the head of the pancreas in a subgroup of patients with chronic pancreatitis.[120]

HOMEOBOX GENES

Studies at the molecular levels have identified specific transcription factors and homeobox genes responsible for the precise transcriptional programs in guiding the proper differentiation of the pancreas. Using the gene knock-out and other techniques in mice, various genes that are essential for normal pancreatic development have been delineated. Although a detailed description of these processes would be outside the scope of the present discussion, a brief outline is important in understanding the intricate steps involved and their implications in congenital defects of the exocrine pancreas. For more precise and comprehensive accounts, readers are referred to the reviews by Kim and Hebrok,[121] Edlund,[122] and Crisera and colleagues.[123]

In early embryonic development, the notochord is in contact with the dorsal endoderm of the primitive foregut (Fig. 114–3). At the appropriate stage (about 8 days postconception in mice), part of the notochord neighboring the future pancreatic cells in the primitive foregut produces activin β-B (a member of TGF β) and FGF-2. At the same time, the dorsal and ventral endoderm exhibits a programmed activation of the hedgehog (HH) genes (sonic hedgehog [*shh*] and indian hedgehog [*ihh*]). The presence of activin β-B and FGF-2 suppresses HH gene expression at the dorsal endodermal site designated the protopancreas and allows pancreatic development to proceed. The ventral endoderm also undergoes similar changes although it is never in contact with the notochord, suggesting an as yet unknown mechanism independent of the notochord. Transient expression of *H1Xb9* and *P48* in the dorsal and ventral endoderm and of *P48* perhaps also in the notochord together with attenuation of *HH* gene expression sets the stage for pancreatic evagination to form pancreatic stem cell pouches in both the dorsal and ventral endoderm. Simultaneously, in these pancreatic stem cells, insulin promoter factor 1/pancreas duodenum homeobox 1 (*IPF1/PDX1*) expression is activated and fully expressed. The expression of *IPF1/PDX1* is required if further morphogenesis and difference are to occur. Thus the *IPF1(/PDX1)* mutation in humans does not result in pancreas formation.[124] Further differentiation of pancreatic cells hinges on Notch pathway signaling. In cells where Notch signaling is lacking, differentiation into endocrine cells occurs. In cells where Notch signaling is present, these cells become the progenitors for pancreatic exocrine cells. Mutations within the gene *JAG1* that encodes a ligand for Notch receptor(s) has been shown to cause Alagille syndrome.[125] In this regard, pancreatic insufficiency is found in 41% of patients with Alagille syndrome. *JAG1* is expressed in the pancreas. Notch receptors and their ligands play important roles in development. It is therefore highly suggestive that *JAG1* mutation in subjects with Alagille syndrome might also cause pancreatic abnormality in such individuals. Active notch signaling subsequently leads to expression of *Hes1* and *P48* genes in these cells. P48 [the DNA binding part of the pancreatic transcription factor (PTF1)] is critically required for the final maturation of exocrine cells. In relation to this, we have shown that in T4 stimulated precocious development of exocrine pancreatic enzymes in rats, T4 apparently acts through PTF1.[126]

Dysfunction of signaling events has been used successfully in deciphering the molecular steps in pancreatic differentiation, but the associated variety of congenital malformations has provided even more valuable knowledge for human diseases. In addition to the documented absence of pancreas in an *IPF1*-deletion human infant,[127] other forms such as annular pancreas, ectopic pancreas, pancreatic hypoplasia, and absence of exocrine cells might be expected and explainable by defects of one or more signaling pathways involved.[125,128]

REFERENCES

1. Moore KL: The Developing Human. Philadelphia, WB Saunders Co, 1982.
2. Lucia M, et al: The developing human fetal pancreas: an ultrastructural and histochemical study with special reference to exocrine cells. J Anat *117*:619, 1974.
3. Track NS, et al: Enzymatic, functional and ultrastructural development of the exocrine pancreas II. The human pancreas. Comp Biochem Physiol *51A*:95, 1975.

4. Schulz DM, et al: Weight of organs of fetuses and infants. Arch Pathol *74*:244, 1962.
5. Lukinius A, et al: Ultrastructural studies of the ontogeny of fetal human and porcine endocrine pancreas, with special reference to colocalization of the four major islet hormones. Dev Biol *153*:376, 1992.
6. Lieberman J: Proteolytic enzyme activity in fetal pancreas and meconium, demonstration of plasminogen and trypsinogen activators in pancreatic tissue. Gastroenterology *50*:183, 1966.
7. Jodl J, et al: Chymotryptic activity in stool of low birth weight infants in the first week of life. Acta Pediatr Scand *64*:619, 1975.
8. Mullinger M, Palasi M: Tryptic and chymotryptic activity of stools of newborn infants. Pediatrics *38*:657, 1966.
9. Carrere J, et al: Immunohistochemical study of secretory proteins in the developing human pancreas. Differentiation *51*:55, 1992.
10. Fukayama M, et al: Immunohistochemical localization of pancreatic secretory trypsin inhibitor in fetal and adult pancreatic and extra pancreatic tissues. J Histochem Cytochem *34*:227, 1986.
11. Davis MM, et al: Pancreatic amylase expression in human pancreatic development. Hybridoma *5*:137, 1986.
12. Mally MI, et al: Developmental gene expression in the human fetal pancreas. Pediatr Res *36*:537, 1994.
13. Batra BK, et al: Human *Muc 1* mucin gene expression in the fetal pancreas. Pancreas *7*:391, 1992.
14. Pictet R, Rutter WJ: Development of the embryonic endocrine pancreas. *In* Steiner DF, Freinkel N (eds): Handbook of Physiology, Section 7, Endocrinology. Vol 1. Washington, DC, American Physiological Society, 1972, pp 25–66.
15. Park I, Bendayan M: Development of the endocrine cells in the rat pancreatic and bile duct system. Histochem J *25*:807, 1993.
16. Ermak TH, Rothman SS: Large decrease in zymogen granule size in the postnatal rat pancreas. J Ultrastruct Res *70*:242, 1980.
17. Gittes GK, Rutter WJ: Onset of cell-specific gene expression in the developing mouse pancreas. Dev Biol *89*:1128, 1992.
18. Hisaoka M, et al: Pancreatic morphogenesis and extracellular matrix organization during rat development. Differentiation *53*:163, 1993.
19. Crisera C, et al: Expression and role of laminin-1 in mouse pancreatic organogenesis. Diabetes *49*:936, 2000.
20. Elsasser HP, et al: Growth of rat pancreatic acinar cells quantitated with a monoclonal antibody against the proliferating cell nuclear antigen. Cell Tissue Res *276*:603, 1994.
21. Oates PS, Morgan RGH: Cell proliferation in the exocrine pancreas during development. J Anat *167*:235, 1989.
22. Pour PM: Pancreatic centroacinar cells. Int J Pancreatol *15*:51, 1994.
23. Jamieson JD: Plasmalemmal glycoproteins and basal lamina: involvement in pancreatic morphogenesis. *In* Hoffman J, Giebisch G (eds): Membranes in Growth and Development. New York, Alan R Liss, 1982.
24. Barresi G, et al: Peanut lectin binding sites in human foetal and neonatal pancreas. Eur J Histochem *37*:329, 1993.
25. Tuo XH, et al: Stage-specific expression of cancer-associated type 1 and type 2 chain. Polylactosamine antigens in the developing pancreas of human embryos. Cancer Res *52*:5744, 1992.
26. LeMeuth V, et al: Differential expression of A- and B- subtypes of cholecystokinin/gastrin receptors in the developing calf pancreas. Endocrinology *133*:1182, 1993.
27. Sanders TG, Rutter WJ: The developmental regulation of amylolytic and proteolytic enzymes in the embryonic rat pancreas. J Biol Chem *249*:3500, 1974.
28. Kemp JD, et al: Protein synthesis during the secondary developmental transition of the embryonic rat pancreas. J Biol Chem *247*:3941, 1972.
29. Van Nest GA, et al: Proteins synthesized and secreted during rat pancreatic development. J Cell Biol *86*:784, 1980.
30. Harding JD, Rutter WJ: Rat pancreatic amylase mRNA. J Biol Chem *253*:8736, 1978.
31. Przybyla AE, et al: Accumulation of the predominant pancreatic mRNAs during embryonic development. J Biol Chem *254*:2154, 1979.
32. Le Huerou-Luron I, et al: Gastric and pancreatic enzyme activities and their relationship with some gut regulatory peptides during postnatal development and weaning in calves. J Nutr *122*:1434, 1992.
33. Payne RM, et al: Rat pancreatic lipase and two related proteins: enzymatic properties and mRNA expression during development. Am J Physiol *266*:G914, 1994.
34. Yang Y, et al: Discoordinate expression of pancreatic lipase and two related proteins in the human fetal pancreas. Pediatr Res *47*:184, 2000.
35. Grossman A: An overview of pancreatic exocrine secretion. Comp Biochem Physiol *78B*:1, 1984.
36. Nishizuka Y: Studies and perspectives of protein kinase C. Science *233*:305, 1986.
37. Scheele GA, et al: Role of the GP2/THP family of GPI anchored proteins in membrane trafficking during regulated exocrine secretion. Pancreas *9*:139, 1994.
38. Wagner AC, Williams JA: Pancreatic zymogen granule membrane proteins: molecular details begin to emerge. Digestion *55*:191, 1994.
39. Scheele G, Kern H: Cellular compartmentation, protein processing and secretion in the exocrine pancreas. *In* Go VLW, et al (eds): The Pancreas. 2nd ed. New York, Raven Press, 1993:121–150.
40. Velez-Granell CS, et al: Molecular chaperones in pancreatic tissue: the presence of cpn 10, cpn 60 and hsp 70 in distinct compartments along the secretory pathway of the acinar cells. J Cell Sci *107*:539, 1994.
41. Hadorn B, et al: Quantitative assessment of exocrine pancreatic function in infants and children. J Pediatr *73*:39, 1968.
42. Zoppi G, et al: Protein content and pancreatic enzyme activities of duodenal juice in normal children and in children with exocrine pancreatic insufficiency. Helv Paediatr Acta *23*:577, 1968.
43. Zoppi G, et al: The electrolyte and protein contents and outputs in duodenal juice after pancreozymin and secretin stimulation in normal children and in patients with cystic fibrosis. Acta Paediatr Scand *59*:692, 1970.
44. Zoppi G, et al: Exocrine pancreas function in premature and full term infants. Pediatr Res *6*:880, 1972.
45. Norman A, et al: Bile acids and pancreatic enzymes during absorption in the newborn. Acta Paediatr Scand *61*:571, 1972.
46. Lebenthal E, Lee PC: Development of functional response in human exocrine pancreas. Pediatrics *66*:556, 1990.
47. Fomon SJ, et al: Excretion of fat by normal full-term infants fed various milks and formulas. Am J Clin Nutr *23*:1299, 1970.
48. Shulman RJ, et al: Utilization of dietary cereal by young infants. J Pediatr *103*:23, 1983.
49. Levitt MD, et al: H$_2$ excretion after ingestion of complex carbohydrates. Gastroenterology *92*:383, 1987.
50. Lilibridge CB, Townes PL: Physiologic deficiency of pancreatic amylase in infancy: a factor in iatrogenic diarrhea. J Pediatr *82*:279, 1973.
51. Fisher SE, et al: Chronic protracted diarrhea: intolerance to dietary glucose polymers. Pediatrics *67*:271, 1981.
52. Fagundes-Neto U, et al: Tolerance to glucose polymers in malnourished infants with diarrhea and disaccharide intolerance. Am J Clin Nutr *41*:228, 1985.
53. Lebenthal E, et al: The development of pancreatic function in premature infants after milk-based and soy-based formulas. Pediatr Res *15*:1240, 1981.
54. Larose L, Morisset J: Acinar cell responsiveness to urecholine in the rat pancreas during fetal and early postnatal growth. Gastroenterology *73*:530, 1977.
55. Doyle CM, Jamieson JD: Development of secretagogue response in rat pancreatic acinar cells. Dev Biol *65*:11, 1978.
56. Werlin SL, Grand RJ: Development of secretory mechanisms in rat pancreas. Am J Physiol *236*:E446, 1979.
57. Werlin SL, Stefaniak J: Maturation of secretory function in rat pancreas. Pediatr Res *16*:123, 1982.
58. Chang A, Jamieson JD: Stimulus-secretion coupling in the developing exocrine pancreas: secretory responsiveness to cholecystokinin. J Cell Biol *103*:2353, 1986.
59. Dumont Y, et al: Parallel maturation of the pancreatic secretory response to cholinergic stimulation and the muscarinic receptor population. Br J Pharmacol *73*:347, 1981.
60. Leung YK, et al: Maturation of cholecystokinin receptors in pancreatic acini rats. Am J Physiol *250*:G594, 1986.
61. Werlin SL, et al: Ontogeny of secretory function and cholecystokinin binding capacity in immature rat pancreas. Life Sci *40*:2237, 1987.
62. Hadjiivanova C, et al: Pharmacological and biochemical characterization of cholecystokinin/gastrin receptors in developing rat pancreas. Eur J Biochem *204*:273, 1992.
63. Le Meuth V, et al: Characterization of binding sites for VIP-related peptides and activation of adenylate cyclase in developing pancreas. Am J Physiol *260*:G265, 1991.
64. Gorelick FS, et al: Calcium-calmodulin-stimulated protein kinase in developing pancreas. Am J Physiol *253*:G469, 1987.
65. Shimizu K, et al: Immature stimulus-secretion coupling in the developing exocrine pancreas and ontogenic changes of protein kinase C. Biochim Biophys Acta *968*:186, 1988.
66. Dakka N, et al: Regulation by a protein-free carbohydrate-rich diet of rat pancreatic mRNAs encoding trypsin and elastase isoenzymes. Biochem J *268*:471, 1990.
67. Wicker C, Puigserver A: Changes in mRNA levels of rat pancreatic lipase in the early days of consumption of a high-lipid diet. Eur J Biochem *180*:563, 1989.
68. Harb JM, et al: Effects of cholecystokinin octapeptide and hydrocortisone on the exocrine pancreas of fed and fasted 24-hour-old rats: an electron microscopic study. Exp Mol Pathol *37*:92, 1982.
69. Lee PC, et al: Effect of early weaning and prolonged nursing on development of rat pancreas. Pediatr Res *16*:470, 1982.
70. Merchant Z, et al: Pancreatic exocrine enzymes during the neonatal period in post mature rats. Int J Pancreat *2*:325, 1987.
71. Le Huerou-Luron I, et al: Molecular aspects of enzyme synthesis in the exocrine pancreas with emphasis on development and nutritional regulation. Proc Nutr Soc *52*:301, 1993.
72. Uvnas-Moberg K, et al: Plasma cholecystokinin concentrations after breast feeding in healthy 4 day old infants. Arch Dis Child *68*:46, 1993.
73. Salmenpera L, et al: Effects of feeding regimen on blood glucose levels and plasma concentrations of pancreatic hormones and gut regulatory peptides at 9 months of age: comparison between infants fed with milk formula and infants exclusively breast-fed from birth. J Pediatr Gastroenterol Nutr *7*:651, 1988.
74. Luttichau HR, et al: Developmental expression of the gastrin and cholecystokinin genes in rat colon. Gastroenterology *104*:1092, 1993.

75. Alumets J, et al: Ontogeny of endocrine cells in porcine gut and pancreas. Gastroenterology 85:1359, 1983.

76. Joekel CS, et al: Postnatal development of circulating cholecystokinin and secretin, pancreatic growth, and exocrine function in guinea pigs. Int J Pancreatol 13:1, 1993.

77. Bardram L, et al: Progastrin expression in mammalian pancreas. Proc Natl Acad Sci U S A 87:298, 1990.

78. Iovanna JL, et al: Transcriptional regulation by cholecystokinin-pancreozymin in rat pancreas. Regul Pept 33:165, 1991.

79. Renaud W, et al: Regulation of concentrations of mRNA for amylase, trypsinogen I and chymotrypsinogen B in rat pancreas by secretagogues. Biochem J 235:305, 1986.

80. Hakanson R, et al: Trophic effects of gastrin and cholecystokinin. Z Gastroenterol 26:265, 1991.

81. Nylander AG, et al: Pancreatic atrophy in rats produced by the cholecystokinin-A receptor antagonist devazepide. Scand J Gastroenterol 27:743, 1992.

82. Zucker KA, et al: Effects of the CCK receptor antagonist L364, 718 on pancreatic growth in adult and developing animals. Am J Physiol 257:G511, 1989.

83. Hoshi H, Logsdon CD: Both low and high affinity CCK receptor states mediate trophic effects on rat pancreatic acinar cells. Am J Physiol 265:G1177, 1993.

84. Povoski SP, et al: Stimulation of in vivo pancreatic growth in the rat is mediated specifically by way of cholecystokinin A receptors. Gastroenterology 107:1135, 1994.

85. Rivard N, et al: Pancreas growth, tyrosine kinase, PtdIns 3-kinase, and PLD involve high-affinity CCK-receptor occupation. Am J Physiol 266:G62, 1994.

86. Wank SA, et al: Cholecystokinin receptor family. Ann N Y Acad Sci 713:49, 1994.

87. Loser CHR, Folsch UR: Epidermal growth factor (EGF) fails to stimulate pancreatic growth and pancreatic polyamine metabolism in rats. Z Gastroenterol 32:216, 1994.

88. Werlin SL, et al: DNA and protein synthesis in developing rat pancreas. Pediatr Res 22:34, 1987.

89. Werlin SL, et al: Effects of cholecystokinin and hydrocortisone on DNA and protein synthesis in immature rat pancreas. Pancreas 3:274, 1988.

90. Werlin SL, Stefaniak J: Effects of hydrocortisone and cholecystokinin octapeptide on neonatal rat pancreas. J Pediatr Gastroenterol Nutr 1:591, 1982.

91. Morisset J: Symposium: Physiology of the gastrointestinal tract: regulation of function and metabolism. J Dairy Sci 76:2080, 1993.

92. Wisner JR, et al: Chronic administration of a potent cholecystokinin receptor antagonist, L-364,718, fails to inhibit pancreas growth in preweanling rats. Pancreas 5:434, 1990.

93. Miyasaka K, et al: Role of cholecystokinin (CCK)-A receptor for pancreatic growth after weaning: a study in a new rat model without gene expression of the CCK-A receptor. Pancreas 12:351, 1996.

94. Ballinger A, et al: Gastrin effects on growth and exocrine secretion in the neonatal rat pancreas. Pancreas 14:295, 1997.

95. Grossman A, et al: Role of steroids in secretion modulating effect of triamcinolone and estradiol on protein synthesis and secretion from the rat exocrine pancreas. J Steroid Biochem 19:1069, 1983.

96. Lu RB, et al: Developmental changes of glucocorticoid receptors in the rat pancreas. J Steroid Biochem 26:213, 1987.

97. Lu RB, et al: Thyroxine effect on exocrine pancreatic development in rats. Am J Physiol 254:G315, 1988.

98. Yoon H, Lee PC: Autologous regulation of pancreatic glucocorticoid receptors in suckling rats. Pancreas 7:226, 1992.

99. Vaughan TJ, et al: Expression of epidermal growth factor and its mRNA in pig kidney, pancreas and other tissues. Biochem J 279:315, 1991.

100. O'Loughlin EV, et al: Effect of epidermal growth factor on ontogeny of the gastrointestinal tract. Am J Physiol 249:G674, 1985.

101. Folsch UR, et al: Polyamines in pancreatic growth. Digestion 46:345, 1990.

102. Polk PF, et al: Effect of secretin on growth of stomach, small intestine, and pancreas of developing rats. Dig Dis Sci 35:749, 1990.

103. Lehy T, et al: Stimulating effect of bombesin on the growth of gastrointestinal tract and pancreas in suckling rats. Gastroenterology 90:1942, 1986.

104. Rosewicz S, et al: Effects of bombesin on pancreatic digestive enzyme gene expression. Endocrinology 130:1451, 1992.

105. Borysewicz R, et al: Direct effect of bombesin on pancreatic and gastric growth in suckling rats. Reg Pept 41:157, 1992.

106. Lee PC, et al: Neonatal hypoxia in the rat: Effects on exocrine pancreatic development. J Pediatr Gastroenterol Nutr 34:542, 2002.

107. Hormi K, et al: Developmental expression of transforming growth factor-α in the upper digestive tract and pancreas of the rat. Regul Peptides 55:67, 1995.

108. Bottinger E, et al: Expression of a dominant-negative mutatnt TGF-beta type II receptor in transgenic mice reveals essential roles for TGF-beta in regulation of growth and differentiation in the exocrine pancreas. EMBO J 16:2621, 1997.

109. Sanvito F, et al: TGF-beta 1 influences the relative development of exocrine and endocrine pancreas in vitro. Development 120:3451, 1994.

110. Battelino T, et al: TGF-beta activataes genes identified by differential mRNA display in pancreatic rudiments. Pflugers Archiv- Euro J Physiol. 439(Suppl 3):R26, 2000.

111. Miralles F, et al: Signaling through fibroblast growth factor receptor 2b plays a key role in the development of the exocrine pancreas. Proc Natl Acad Sci U S A 96:6267, 1999.

112. Albers GHR, et al: Fetoacinar pancreatic protein in the developing human pancreas. Differentiation 34:210, 1987.

113. Mas E, et al: Human fetoacinar pancreatic protein: an oncofetal glycoform of the normally secreted pancreatic bile-salt-dependent lipase. Biochem J 289:609, 1993.

114. Tornehave D, et al: Fetal antigen 1 (FA1) in the human pancreas: cell type expression, topological and quantitative variations during development. Anat Embryol 187:335, 1993.

115. Mellersh H, et al: Expression of the proto-oncogenes C-H-ras and N-ras in early second trimester human fetal tissues. Biochem Biophys Res Commun 141:510, 1986.

116. Calve EL, et al: Changes in gene expression during pancreatic regeneration: Activation of c-myc and H-ras oncogenes in the rat pancreas. Pancreas 6:150, 1991.

117. Silverman JA, et al: Expression of c-myc, c-raf-1, and c-Ki-ras in azaserine-induced pancreatic carcinomas and growing pancreas in rats. Mol Carcinog 3:379, 1990.

118. Lu L, Lodsdon CD: CCK, bombesin, and carbachol stimulate c-fos, c-jun, and c-myc oncogene expression in rat pancreatic acini. Am J Physiol 263:G327, 1992.

119. Lemoine NR, et al: Ki-ras oncogene activation in preinvasive pancreatic cancer. Gastroenterology 102:230, 1992.

120. Friess H, et al: A subgroup of patients with chronic pancreatitis over express the c-erb B-2 protooncogene. Ann Surg 220:183, 1994.

121. Kim SK, Hebrok M. Intercellular signals regulating pancreas development and function. Genes and Development 15:111, 2001.

122. Edlund H: Pancreas: how to get there from the gut? Curr Opin Cell Biol 11:663, 1999.

123. Crisera CA, et al: Molecular approaches to understanding organogenesis. Semin Pediatr Surg 8:109, 1999.

124. Stoffers DA, et al: Pancreatic agenesis attributable to a single nucleotide deletion in the human IPF1 gene sequence. Nat Genet 15:106, 1997.

125. Jones EA, et al: JAGGED1 expression in human embryos: correlation with the Alagille syndrome phenotype. J Med Genet 37:658, 2000.

126. Lee PC, Mao XC: Thyroxine control of pancreatic amylase gene expression: modulation of PTF1 binding activity. Mol Cell Endocrinol 101:287, 1994.

127. Stoffers DA, et al: Pancreatic agenesis attributable to a single nucleotide deletion in the human IPF1 gene sequence. Nature Genet 15:106, 1997.

128. St-Onge L, et al: Pancreas development and diabetes. Current Opinion in Genetics and Development. 9:295, 1999.

Otakar Koldovský* and Carol Lynn Berseth

115

Digestion-Absorption Functions in Fetuses, Infants, and Children

Various functions of the human gastrointestinal tract undergo substantial changes during perinatal development. Changes in the digestive and absorptive processes of the three main nutrients—carbohydrates, proteins, and lipids—are reviewed in detail here. Reviews of other functions appear in the literature.[1-6]

* Deceased.

DIGESTION AND ABSORPTION OF CARBOHYDRATES

Digestion of Polysaccharides

Prenatal Period

Salivary[7] and pancreatic amylase activity has been demonstrated in 22-week-old fetuses.[8] Pancreatic amylase is increased in 27-week-old fetuses but still constitutes only 30% of the activity found in neonates.[8] The presence of both salivary and pancreatic amylase has been observed in amniotic fluid in the 16th to 18th weeks of pregnancy.[9]

Postnatal Period

In addition to the classic enzymes capable of digesting starches and glucose polymers (i.e., salivary and pancreatic α-amylase, intestinal glucoamylase), an enzyme present in breast milk, α-amylase,[10-12] also may participate in digestion.[13-15] This can survive the relatively mild acidity and the lower activity of pepsin in the stomach of the newborn infant (see Fig. 115–5). Amylase in saliva is present in lower concentrations in children than in adults.[16-18] Electrophoretic analysis of sera[19-21] and urine[22] from infants and children demonstrates the presence of salivary α-amylase only. During the postnatal period, the activity of salivary amylase increases earlier than that of the pancreas (see farther on).

Large numbers of reports (Fig. 115–1) show that the *amylase content of the pancreatic tissue*,[23-25] or duodenal juice,[26-32] and its rate of secretion after standardized stimulation with secretin[30] or pancreozymin-secretin[28, 33-36] or after a meal[27, 32] is lower in young infants and increases considerably during postnatal life. The *digestion of starch* in the newborn infant has been examined by both carbohydrate tolerance type and balance studies. Gastric administration of a starch solution results in a slow, small increase in blood glucose levels in neonates; an equicaloric amount of glucose solution administered to the same children evokes a greater, earlier increase, with an earlier return to starting values within 120 minutes.[37, 38]

Feedings of maltose and dextrin-maltose are followed by increases in blood glucose concentrations that are intermediate to those observed in infants fed either starch or glucose.[38] In infants younger than 6 months, amylopectin hydrolysis is incomplete, but in 1-year-old children, amylopectin is rapidly hydrolyzed into glucose, maltose, maltotriose, and branched dextrins. Although the digestion of starch in infants is considerable, the tolerance of young infants to large quantities is limited. This limitation may vary in individual infants.[39]

Glucoamylase, an intestinal brush-border enzyme,[40] removes glucose units from the nonreducing ends of molecules of starch and dextran. This enzyme, which is present in the developing small intestine,[41] exhibits activity in a baby at the age of 1 month[42] that is comparable to the activity in young adults.[43, 44]

Recent investigations have shown that oligosaccharides in human milk and formula survive transit through the gastrointestinal tract and are recovered in both feces and urine.[45] The latter observation is consistent with the uptake that has been described for lactose.[46] Many of these oligosaccharides have been found to function as prebiotics, and their malabsorption may contribute to host defense.

Digestion of Disaccharides

Prenatal Period

Data from numerous laboratories,[47-55] which are summarized schematically in Figure 115–2, show that activity of sucrase and lactase is lower in young fetuses than in specimens from the small intestinal mucosa of adults. Activity of sucrase increases earlier than does that of lactase. This interesting observation, for which there is still no explanation, was made as early as 1910.[56, 57] In all other mammals, sucrase appears later than lactase.[58] The jejunoileal gradient of sucrase is expressed in 3- to 4-month-old fetuses (Fig. 115–3),[48, 49, 59-61] and that of lactase[59, 62] has been demonstrated in 5-month-old fetuses. These gradients increase during later prenatal and postnatal development.[49, 52, 54, 55, 61, 62] Sucrase activity is present in the fetal colon and disappears before birth[49] (see Fig. 115–3). The presence of lactase in the fetal colon (13 to 20 weeks of age) has been described previously.[63]

Sucrase-isomaltase in the human fetal intestine is present in a different form from that in adults, and it differs in degree of glycosylation (different electrophoretic mobility)[64] and in the size of the polypeptide.[65] In fetuses younger than 30 weeks' gestation, it is present as one large (enzymatically active) polypeptide,[54, 65, 66] In adults,[40] this molecule is split, most probably by the action of pancreatic proteases, into two smaller polypeptides—sucrase and isomaltase. Triadou and Zweibaum[54] demonstrated the presence of two subunits in fetuses older than 30 weeks' gestation. The fetal enzyme as its proform and its two subunits have faster electrophoretic motility than does the enzyme in adult subjects (removal of sialic acid residues from fetal enzymes emphasizes this difference). The difference in polypeptide length in fetuses and adults can be related to low activity of pancreatic proteases in the fetal intestinal lumen. Appearance of sucrase and isomaltase activities correlates with the appearance of mRNA.[67-69]

Villa and coworkers[70] confirmed that intestinal lactase phlorizin hydrolase (LPH) is low between 14 and 20 weeks of gestation and exhibits a relatively high level of activity at 37 weeks; amounts of LPH mRNA correlated with the enzymatic activity. Culture of fetal jejunal explants for 5 days induces by itself a twofold increase in LPH mRNA without any significant change in lactase enzymatic activity. This increase may reflect the loss of a negative transcriptional regulation operative in vivo and suggests an additional post-transcriptional regulatory compo-

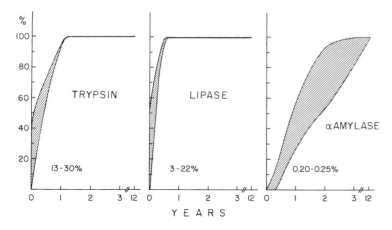

Figure 115–1. Composite figure depicting rate of secretion (per unit body weight per unit time) of pancreatic enzymes into duodenum as reported from various laboratories (see text). Data are given as a percentage of the values found in adults. The shaded areas denote the range of postnatal increase. The numbers in the left corner of each panel denote the rate of secretion found in neonates compared with that found in adults.

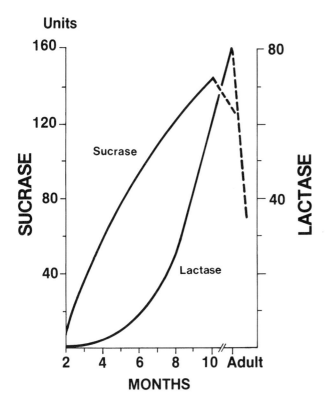

Figure 115–2. Composite graph depicting sucrase and lactase activity in the small intestine of human fetuses as reported from different laboratories.[8, 41, 47, 53, 55, 59-62, 66] Activity is expressed as μmol/min/g protein.

nent. The addition of hydrocortisone (50 ng/mL) during culture induces a doubling of lactase activity without variation in LPH mRNA, indicating a post-transcriptional modulation by hydrocortisone. Results suggest a complex developmental regulation of human intestinal lactase and that the perinatal increase in lactase activity could be modulated at a post-transcriptional level by hydrocortisone. Wang and colleagues[68] confirmed the expression of lactase mRNA in the small intestine of 9- to 18-week-old fetuses at a low level. It is interesting that lactase mRNA was not dectectable in the colon of adult subjects, whereas it was detectable at low levels in fetal colon.

Postnatal Period

Lactose Digestion. Several studies have characterized the changes of lactose digestion capacity in the first weeks of life. Newborn (premature and term) infants have a limited capacity to absorb lactose, as judged by the presence of reducing substances in the feces[71-73] and urine[46] and by the results of lactose tolerance tests.[48, 74, 75] Studies using breath hydrogen tests indi-

cate low absorption in preterm[76] but not in term infants.[77] Lactose malabsorption has been reported to be more common in breast-fed infants than in bottle-fed infants (even though lactose concentration in the milk is similar).[71, 73, 78, 79] Douwes and colleagues,[80] however, using the breath hydrogen test, did not confirm that observation. In term infants, the absorption capacity increases within the first few days of life,[75] but (using the breath hydrogen test) about 25% of 1-week-old term infants still exhibit lactose malabsorption.[80] Growth-retarded term infants all demonstrate a decreased ability to absorb lactose.[81] In premature infants, the lactose absorption capability increases more slowly.[48, 74, 81, 82] Some of the lactose malabsorbed in the small intestine of term and preterm infants is salvaged in the colon by bacterial fermentation.[76, 77, 83, 84] Moreover, studies suggest that colonic fermentation activity is adequate for colonic salvage of lactose even during the second week of life.

Using a stable isotope method for serial assessment of lactose carbon assimilation, Kien and associates[85, 86] demonstrated efficient absorption of lactose in premature infants (30 to 32 weeks' gestation and 11 to 36 days of age). In spite of that finding, when Erasmus and associates fed 130 preterm infants standard preterm formula with and without lactase, they showed that lactase-treated infants grew faster the first ten days of life but similarly thereafter, suggesting that limitations in lactose absorption are short-lived in the preterm infant.[87] In fact, infants absorb 98% of lactose from lactose-containing formulas[88] and have similar feeding tolerance to those fed a lactose-free formula.[89] However, term infants fed lactose-free formula have higher calcium intake and retention than those fed lactose-containing formula.[90]

Another approach to evaluating postnatal changes in lactase activity in infants involves the determination of its activity together with that of sucrase activity in jejunal fluid. This method is based on an earlier study demonstrating a positive correlation between the activity of disaccharidases in the fluid and a corresponding intestinal biopsy specimen in children 1 to 12 years of age.[91] Jejunal fluid lactase activity and its properties in children closely reflect the activity of the microvillus membrane enzyme.[92] More recent studies have investigated disaccharidase activity in jejunal fluid of preterm infants.[93, 94] In those studies, lactase activity was within the normal range for older infants and children within the first week of life. Sucrase/lactase ratios fell during the second and third week of life, suggesting a further increase in lactase activity. The results of this study by Mayne and colleagues,[94] as well as those quoted previously,[77, 80] raise questions about the reasons for the reduced lactose absorption in preterm infants. Transient lactose intolerance in infants may also be associated with various pathologic states, such as gastroenteritis, neonatal surgery, cycstic fibrosis, and protracted diarrhea,[95-99] as well as fluorescent light–treated jaundiced infants.[100]

Digestion of α-Disaccharides. The enteral absorption of sucrose and maltose from a peroral load (as judged from blood glucose curves) was similar in 2-week-old premature infants fed diets in

Figure 115–3. *Left*, Development of active glucose transport in human fetuses as studies *in vitro* using the everted sacs technique.[61,69] Abscissa equals age in postconceptional weeks. Ordinate equals (S/M) ratio of concentration of glucose in serosal fluid to glucose in mucosal fluid at the end of a 60-minute incubation period. Vertical brackets represent 2 SEM. *Right*, Sucrase activity of the jejunum (○), ileum (●), and colon (X) of human fetuses. Activity given as milligrams of glucose liberated/60 minutes/g w.w.[49,61]

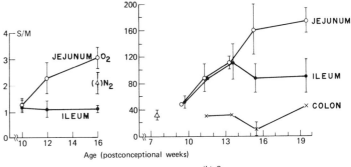

(a) Glucose transport   (b) Sucrase

Age (postconceptional weeks)

which the carbohydrate was either lactose or predominantly sucrose.[48] The activity of various α-disaccharidases does not change until late in life in healthy subjects, as reported earlier.[4]

Absorption of Monosaccharides

Prenatal Period

The active transport of hexoses has been demonstrated using the everted sac *in vitro* technique in freshly obtained human fetuses. Transport increased between the 10th and 18th weeks of gestation (see Fig. 115–3).[49,66,69,101] Malo and Berteloot[102] demonstrated a fully functional sodium-dependent D-glucose co-transport system with a proximodistal gradient of activity in brush-border membrane vesicles isolated from the jejunum and ileum of 17- to 20-week-old normal human fetuses. Later, Malo[103,104] demonstrated the existence of two distinct sodium-dependent D-glucose carriers in the human jejunum during the early gestation period, which were differentiated not only by their kinetic properties, but also by differences in their substrate and inhibitor specificities. In the proximal small intestine, high-affinity, low-capacity and low-affinity, high-capacity systems were present; in the distal small intestine, only a single carrier was detected. Developmental and regional expression of mRNAs encoding sodium-dependent and facilitative glucose transporter proteins in human fetal and adult small intestine was studied by Davidson and colleagues.[105] The abundance of mRNAs encoding the sodium glucose co-transporter isoform SGLT1 and the facilitative glucose transporter isoforms GLUT2 and GLUT5 exhibited highest levels in adult small intestine, but the levels of GLUT1 mRNA were found to be higher in fetal than in adult small intestine. Immunohistochemical analysis of the fetal small intestine showed that GLUT5 was localized along the intercellular junctions of the developing villus. Wang and coworkers[68] also demonstrated expression of sodium-dependent glucose transporter mRNA in the small intestine of fetuses between 9 and 18 weeks of gestational age. The sodium-dependent glucose transporter mRNA is also expressed in the fetal colon but in lower levels than in the adult colon.

Postnatal Period

Several types of data are available to evaluate the absorption rate of monosaccharides during postnatal development. Figure 115–4 summarizes the data from multiple studies in which the rate of glucose absorption under steady-state conditions was determined in infants[97,106,107] and adults.[108–115] These data indicate that glucose absorption in infants is less efficient than in adults. K_m and V_{max} of glucose absorption are related to gestational age and appear to be affected by diet and exposure to glucocorticoids.[116,117] Rouwet and colleagues have shown that carrier-mediated monosaccharide absorption increases the first 2 postnatal weeks in infants born at 28 to 30 weeks' gestation.[118] The galactose absorption rate reaches adult values between 4 and 8 years of age.[119]

DIGESTION AND ABSORPTION OF PROTEIN

Digestion

Proteolysis in the Stomach

Gastric Acidity

Prenatal Period. The first traces of gastric acidity appear in 4-month-old fetuses.[120] Studies by Kelly and Brownlee[121] and Kelly and associates[122] indicate that the human fetus has the potential to produce gastric acid and gastrin from the middle of the second trimester. Parietal cell activity was noted in the body, antrum, and pyloric regions in all the fetal specimens (ranging from 13 to 28 weeks) examined; this activity was much more limited in the infant specimens (2 to 21 weeks).[123]

Postnatal Period. The pH of gastric fluid in newborn infants is usually neutral or slightly acid, and the acidity increases within

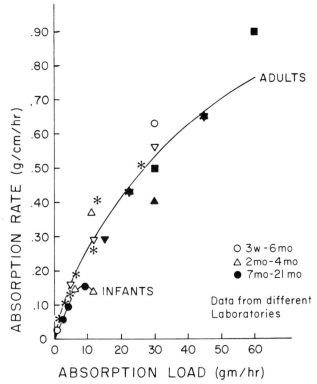

Figure 115–4. Rate of glucose absorption from the perfused jejunum in infants and adults. Symbols and references: Infants (△) 2 to 4 months old,[107] (●) 7 to 21 months old,[97] (○) 3 weeks to 6 months old.[106] Adults: (■),[108] (□),[110] (●),[111,112] (▼),[112] (*),[113] (△),[114] (▲).[115] The concentration of the glucose solution administered to infants varied between 0.15% and 16%; to adults, between 0.12% and 10%. Data for infants compiled by Younoszai,[310] for adults compiled by Fordtran and Ingelfinger.[311] (From Koldovský O: Digestion and absorption. *In* Stave U [ed]: Perinatal Physiology. New York, Plenum, 1978, p 317.)

several hours of birth.[124, 125] Kelly and associates[122] recorded intragastric pH continuously in preterm infants (24 to 29 weeks of gestation) receiving parenteral nutrition during the first 5 days and in the third week of life. As the infants became more mature (in terms of both gestation and postnatal age), intragastric pH decreased. All the infants were able to maintain a gastric pH, less than 4 from the first day of life. The actual pH of the stomach contents in infants is substantially influenced by food intake. The entry of milk into the infant's stomach causes a sharp increase in the pH of the gastric contents and a slower return to lower pH values than in older children and adults (Fig. 115–5).[126-128] These findings not only stress the importance of defining the time after feeding when pH is determined, but also show that the gastric acidity of the newborn infant is unsuitable for optimal pepsin action but might be favorable for the action of other enzymes and peptide substances.

Mouterde and coworkers[129] reported that gastric acid outflow doubled between 0 and 2 months and 2 and 12 months of age. Hydrochloric acid secretion was found to be much lower in premature infants than in full-term infants.[130] No change was seen in basal and pentagastrin-stimulated output of acid in term neonates between days 1 and 2 of life; furthermore, the basal acid secretion was no different from the stimulated one.[131, 132] These results suggest that gastric acid secretion in the newborn infant is maximal under basal conditions, or that newborn parietal cells are unresponsive to pentagastrin. The concentration and output of titratable acid following histamine stimulation are

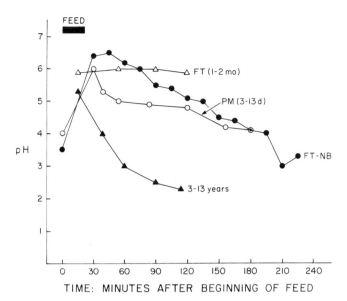

Figure 115–5. Effect of feeding on pH values of the stomach contents of infants of different ages. (○) 10 premature infants, 3 to 13 days old;[16] (●) 25 full-term newborn infants;[128] (△) infants 1 to 2 months old;[125] (▲) children 3 to 13 years old.[125] (From Koldovský O: Digestion and absorption. *In* Stave U [ed]: Perinatal Physiology. New York, Plenum, 1978, p 317.)

low in the neonate; values increase through the third week of life.[133] Output values show a brief decline in the third to fourth week of life, with a second sustained rise continuing into the second and third months of life. Although the concentration data for 2- to 3-month-old infants and adults do not overlap, output values show some overlap. The increase of stimulated acid output occurs between the first and second year of life; a similar increase is observed for basal output.[134]

Proteolytic Activity

Prenatal Period. Proteolytic activity has been described as present in fetuses older than 16 weeks' gestation.[24,135] The peptic activity of newborn infants is low and is in proportion to the degree of maturity.[136] It increases in the fundus about fourfold after food intake on the second day of postnatal life.[135] Immunoelectrophoretic analysis of fetal gastric mucosal extracts indicates the presence of progastricsin in the third month of gestation and pepsinogen by the fourth month.[137] Slow-moving protease is believed to be the main acid proteinase in the human stomach at birth.[138] Reid and colleagues,[139] using immunohistochemical methods, studied the presence of several aspartic proteinases in the fetal stomach. The slow-moving protease appeared to be the dominant enzyme from 12 weeks of gestation onward. Although progastricsin was also present at this time, pepsinogen and cathepsin did not appear until 17 to 18 weeks' gestation.

Postnatal Period. The output of pepsin is diminished in the newborn infant and increases until the third month of life. The range of values found in the second and third months of life is less than the range of adult values.[133,134,140] A five times lower outflow of pepsin was reported in infants 0 to 2 months old than in infants 2 to 12 months old.[129] In contrast, pepsin activity in the biopsy specimen from the stomachs of infants and children did not change between the ages of 6 months and 15 years.[141] Yahav and associates[142] demonstrated that formula feeding evoked an increase of pepsin activity in the stomach content of 3- to 4-week-old orogastrically fed premature infants.

No substantial digestion of protein was found in specimens of gastric content taken from 5- to 8-day-old infants.[128] The probable explanation for this finding is that the pepsin (which is present

in low levels at that time) is almost completely inactivated at the high pH levels that were found in the newborn stomach at various intervals after feeding (see Fig. 115–5). In older infants (13 to 44 days of age), traces of hydrolyzed protein were found in stomach contents; cow's milk protein was hydrolyzed to a greater degree than were the proteins of human milk.[143]

Pancreatic Proteolytic Enzymes

Prenatal Period. Pancreatic enzymes begin to form at about the third fetal month,[24] and pancreatic secretion starts at the beginning of the fifth month of gestation.[144] Biochemical studies on the activity of trypsinogen and chymotrypsinogen at various gestational ages have been reported in detail.[137,145] Immunoreactive trypsin 1 and immunoreactive chymotrypsin A were detected in amniotic fluids taken at 17 to 18 weeks of pregnancy.[146]

Postnatal Period. Various reports show relatively modest differences in the concentration of trypsin (compared with amylase and lipase) when collected after simple fasting, during food digestion,[26,29,147-151] or after pancreozymin-secretin stimulation during postnatal development[28,33,34] (see Fig. 115–1). Similarly, no substantial difference was observed in premature infants between the ages of 2 days and 7 weeks.[29,152] Levels of trypsin concentration encountered during the first 2 years of life are reached by the age of 3 months.[153] Using the N-benzoyl-L-tyrosyl paraaminobenzoic acid (NBT-PABA) test, Bujanover and associates[154] demonstrated that chymotryptic activity was low in the newborn infant (3 days of age) and increased gradually, approaching the levels of older children at about 6 months.

The effect of feedings on pancreatic proteolytic enzyme activity has been variable. In one group of children, the concentration of trypsin did not increase[147]; however, in two other studies,[155,156] a decrease in enzyme activity occurred that was not seen in adults. From birth onward, the concentration of chymotrypsin (after pancreozymin-secretin stimulation) increases approximately threefold and reaches adult levels in 3-year-old children.

Serial measurement of fecal chymotrypsin concentrations in preterm infants (23 to 32 weeks' gestation) during the first 4 weeks of life demonstrated values generally similar to those found in term infants. A chymotrypsin concentration peak, seen in term infants at age 4 days, did not occur in this study until day 8, suggesting a slower initiation of pancreatic exocrine function in the preterm infant. Median fecal chymotrypsin concentrations calculated for each infant (using data from stools passed between day 2 and day 12 of life) were significantly lower in infants who were small for gestational age (SGA) when compared with those who were appropriate for gestational age (AGA).[157] It is interesting that fecal excretion of chymotrypsin in healthy infants (1 week to 5 months of age) was lower in breast-fed than in bottle-fed infants.[158]

Feeding a high-protein diet to premature infants evoked a substantial increase of trypsin at the ages of both 1 week and 1 month, compared with values found in infants on a diet with a lower protein content.[159] Premature infants fed soy-based formula for 1 month exhibited higher trypsin activity after cholecystokinin-pancreozymin stimulation than did those fed a milk-based formula.[160] The presence of protease inhibitors in the colostrum and milk[161-164] might play a role in the processing of protein in the gastrointestinal tract of breast-fed infants. However, a recent study has shown that this is not the case.[165]

Proteolytic and Peptidase Activity in the Small Intestinal Mucosa

During fetal development, protease and aminopeptidase activity in the jejunum does not change markedly between the 8th and 17th weeks of gestation, but in the ileum there is a pronounced increase.[166] Enzyme activity capable of breaking down peptone is present in the small intestine of 7- to 10-week-old fetuses and rises slightly after the 14th week of gestation.[8]

Dipeptidase (glycyl-glycine) is present in the small intestine of 2-month-old fetuses; it increases in the third month of gestation.[167, 168] This and other dipeptidases (substrates alanyl-glutamic acid, alanyl-proline, glycyl-leucine, and glycylvaline) are present in the small intestine of fetuses aged 11 to 23 weeks without any pronounced developmental changes. Lichnovsky and Lojda[51] published an extensive study on fetal development of brush-border enzymes using material obtained from 45 fetuses aged 4 to 22 weeks of intrauterine life. In the embryonal developmental period (to week 8), the activity of proteases was mainly detected on the luminal surface of the primitive pseudostratified columnar epithelium of the intestine anlage. The highest activity was displayed by dipeptyl peptidase IV (DPP IV). Beginning with the eighth week, villi are formed from the duodenum up to the ileum, and after week 9, differentiation of Lieberkühn crypts is observed. The activity of proteases was high (especially DPP IV) in the differentiating microvillus zone of primitive enterocytes. Gradient of apex-base activity of the villus was maximal on the apex of the villi.

Absorption of Proteins and their Degradation Products

Questions related to immune functions are reviewed in another chapter; for a review, see Walker.[169] Proteins are present in the amniotic fluid. About 50% of its volume is swallowed by the fetus daily;[170] thus, the protein amount obtainable at or near term from the amniotic fluid is about one fifth of the daily protein gain by the fetus. A fairly wide spectrum of protein is transferred to the fetus by this process—human serum albumin, immunoglobulin G (IgG), IgA, chorionic gonadotropin, and growth hormone.[170]

Various studies have indicated increased small intestinal permeability for intact food proteins during the neonatal period,[171-175] but passage of proteins has also been demonstrated in older children and even in adults.[176] The serum of infants contains a higher percentage of antibodies to food antigens than does the serum of adults,[177] which suggests that food proteins are absorbed intact in sufficient quantities for an immunologic response. Based on determination of serum concentration, the absorption of β-lactoglobulin was considered to be higher in preterm infants than in full-term infants.[173]

Various immunoglobulins are present in the lumen of the upper segment of the small intestine in infants and children.[178,179] Information about digestion and absorption of protein in infants has been obtained using three different methodologic approaches: (1) balance studies, (2) analysis of intestinal contents during absorption of a test meal, and (3) observation of changes in various nitrogen metabolites in blood during absorption. The last-mentioned approach is not reviewed.

Balance Studies

Various reports[180-188] show that about 85% of the food nitrogen in infants is absorbed from the gut independent of age (0 to 150 days), type of diet, or maturity. There have been theoretical concerns that preterm infants would absorb protein better if they were given partially hydrolyzed protein. However, a recent study has shown that nitrogen retention is similar in preterm infants fed partially hydrolyzed formula and standard preterm formula.[189] This similarity of nitrogen retention is reflected by similar growth rates.[190]

Analysis of Intestinal Contents During Absorption of Test Meal

Borgstrom and colleagues[147, 148] found that the absorption of protein at the duodenal level was about the same in 1- to 2-week-old full-term and 1- to 4-week-old premature infants, although the 1-week-old premature infants had lower trypsin values.

Hirata and associates[191,192] introduced a tube into the ileocecal region and analyzed the protein level (quantitatively and qualitatively) during digestion in infants fed breast milk or whole cow's

milk. The protein nitrogen concentration in the ileocecal contents of 1- to 5-month-old infants fed whole cow's milk formula was more than three times higher than that found in breast-fed infants. When the protein concentration in cow's milk formula was reduced, there ceased to be a difference between formula-fed and breast-fed infants. Furthermore, these investigators found unsplit casein in the ileal contents of infants fed 3.3% protein cow's milk. Using this technique, they determined the maximum digestibility of cow's milk casein in infants of different ages. Digestion and absorption of cow's milk casein increased with age (Fig. 115–6). Their data agree with the calculation[155] that adults can digest about 1.6 g of casein/kg body weight/hr; the corresponding value in children was lower (1 g). A single study[193] has suggested that the colon of infants can assimilate proteins.

Juvonen and associates[194] evaluated macromolecular absorption in children fed cow's milk–based formula by measuring serum concentrations of human milk α-albumin after a human milk feeding. Undetectable or low values were found; no significant differences were found between the ages of 2 and 24 months. Kuitunen and associates[195] confirmed that in preterm (32 to 36 weeks of gestational age) infants, absorption of α-lactalbumin was small (0.1% of the amount given) but significant for a few months after birth; later, it decreased rapidly. This group also demonstrated absorption of bovine β-lactoglobulin in these infants following introduction of cow's milk. Using human α-lactalbumin as a marker protein, other investigators[14] demonstrated that its concentration in serum after a human milk feed was correlated negatively with maturity and postnatal age (between days 7 and 42 after delivery). They also concluded that intrauterine growth retardation causes a delayed postnatal decrease in macromolecular absorption.

Absorption of amino acids was studied *in vitro* using the everted sac technique in human 12- to 18-week-old fetuses. L-Alanine was actively transported. This transport was found to be specific; D-alanine was not transported.[131] Malo[196] has demonstrated that the characteristics of the uptake pathways in 17- to

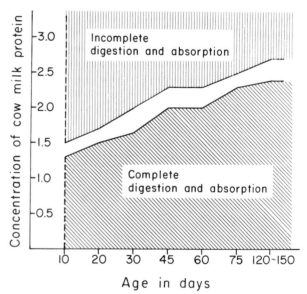

Figure 115–6. Change of digestion and absorption of cow's milk protein in infants during the first 4 postnatal months of life. Digestion and absorption were considered complete when analysis of ileal contents showed absence of undigested casein and both the nitrogen protein concentration and the nitrogen protein/total nitrogen ratio were the same as in infants of corresponding age fed breast milk.[228] (From Koldovský O: Digestion and absorption. *In* Stave U [ed]: Perinatal Physiology. New York, Plenum, 1978, p 317.)

20-week-old human fetuses (sodium requirement and the proximodistal gradient of activity for amino acids in jejunal and ileal brush-border membrane vesicles) are already established at this developmental stage.

DIGESTION AND ABSORPTION OF LIPIDS

Lipolytic Activities of the Gastrointestinal Tract

Prenatal Period

Tachibana[197] was the first investigator to demonstrate the presence of lipase in the stomachs of fetuses in the fourth month of gestation; its activity increased with subsequent development. Menard and colleagues[198] reported the appearance of lipase at 10 weeks' gestation. They confirmed its increase with subsequent fetal development. Lipase is localized in the fundus of the stomach;[198, 199] only low activity can be detected in the antrum.[200] Lipase immunoreactivity appears in the pancreas at the 21st week of pregnancy; 5 weeks later, immunoreactivity for trypsinogens and chymotrypsinogen can be demonstrated. Lipase labeling is first observed in a few of the acini dispersed in the pancreas and then spreads out progressively to be present in all the acini at 2 weeks of fetal life. Intensities of lipase increase greatly at birth. The ontogenesis of carboxyl ester hydrolase does not follow that of lipase.[146] The presence of pancreatic lipase activity in the small intestine has been reported.[182, 201] Esterase activity (substrate α-naphthylacetate) was detected in the fetal small intestine.[200]

Postnatal Period

Milk Lipolytic Activities

Bile Salt–Stimulated Lipase. At the beginning of the 20th century, it was already reported that human milk contains esterolytic activity that is not detectable in bovine milk.[202] Freudenberg[203] showed that the digestion of long-chain triglycerides proceeded only in the presence of bile salts by an enzyme, later classified as bile salt–stimulated lipase (BSSL), which is present in human colostrum[203] and in preterm[204] and term milk.[120, 126, 204-212] Based on an *in vitro* assay,[208] it was estimated that it can hydrolyze all triglycerides in the small intestine in 30 minutes. Estimates based on a different assay in which milk was used as substrate and at the same time as a source of enzyme[206] give values that are substantially lower but still of considerable magnitude. These investigators have determined that in milk produced during the first 2 weeks of lactation, 40% of triglycerides are hydrolyzed within 2 hours, and during later lactation, only 20% of triglycerides are hydrolyzed. This apparent decrease is caused by an increase in milk fat content during lactation, rather than a real change in absolute BSSL activity.

Properties of BSSL make it suitable to survive in the stomach with little or no loss of activity and to act in the duodenum when activated by bile acids (cholate, chenodeoxycholate) in concentrations close to those found in the infant duodenum.[120,206,208,209,213] Thus, at a low bile salt concentration, the action of milk BSSL may facilitate fat absorption.[214] BSSL hydrolyzes long-chain triglycerides with no positional specificity and thus hydrolyzes 2-monoacylglycerol.[208, 209] This property, to hydrolyze 2-monoacylglycerol, makes this enzyme complementary to the pancreatic lipase that delivers as its main products fatty acids and 2-monoacylglycerol. The significance of the presence of BSSL for the digestion of milk lipids is supported further by studies on low birth weight preterm infants (3 to 6 weeks old) fed raw or heat-treated (pasteurized or boiled) human milk. Fat from the former was absorbed more (74%) than the latter two (54% and 46%).[215] The effect of heat processing of human milk on absorption of fat was considered for a long time, with rare exception,[216] as not clinically significant, probably based on an older report that found no difference in fat absorption in preterm infants fed human milk subjected to various heat treatments.[217]

Lipoprotein Lipase. Milk also contains a serum-activated lipoprotein lipase (LPL).[203, 204, 210, 218-221] The presence of LPL in milk is considered to reflect a leakage of enzymes from the mammary tissue.[222] Its activity is inhibited by bile salts. Milk lipids are hydrolyzed by LPL to a limited extent, causing hydrolytic rancidity on storage of milk.[125, 218] Although the concentration of BSSL activity in milk does not change during the duration of lactation, LPL activity increases during lactation,[211] exhibiting a peak around the third week of life.[204] LPL has been implicated in the prolonged neonatal jaundice of breast-fed infants. Fresh milk samples from mothers of jaundiced infants exhibit an increased level of LPL.[218, 220, 223] Feeding preheated milk is followed by the rapid disappearance of hyperbilirubinemia.[234] The relationship between the high activity of LPL in milk and jaundice is not simple, because high levels of LPL in mother's milk are not always associated with jaundice.[224, 225]

Other Lipases. There are several reports describing the presence of other less-defined esterolytic activities in human milk.[162, 218, 226-230]

Preduodenal Lipases. The presence of lipase activity in the gastric content of fetuses,[201] preterm and full-term neonates, and adults has been well documented.[231-238] Part, but not all, of its activity can be attributed to lingual origin. At the end of the last century, von Ebner[239] described the presence of serous glands located on the proximal dorsal site of the tongue. According to the studies of Hamosh and colleagues,[240-242] these glands are the source of lingual lipase. The existence of gastric lipase in humans has been proved,[243-246] and gastric lipase has been purified from the stomach contents of newborn[237] and adult human subjects.[233, 247] It exhibits a considerable resistance to acid inactivation.[243] Substantial catalytic activity is found in the pH range of 3.5 to 6.5.[232,237] This is in the range found in the infant's stomach after food intake (see Fig. 115-5). The release of these lipases is stimulated by feeding.[234, 248] Milk triglycerides are hydrolyzed mainly to diglycerides and fatty acids.[233,235,245,246,249]

Hydrolysis of medium chain triglycerides (trioctanoin) occurs five times faster than that of long chain triglycerides (triolein).[250] The outer positions, 1 and 3, are split, as is the inside one, position 2. Preduodenal lipases are slightly activated by low concentrations of bile salts, but higher concentrations of bile salts lead to an almost complete inhibition. Furthermore, they exhibit partial stereospecificity for sn-3 esters over sn-1 esters.[251] Lipase activity is present in gastric aspirates as early as 6 months of gestation and increases substantially around 8 to 9 fetal months.[237] Medium chain and long chain triglycerides are hydrolyzed in the stomachs of preterm infants, and released medium chain acids are absorbed directly from the stomach.[236,252,253] It is interesting that gastric lipase activity expressed per volume of gastric aspirate does not change when long chain triglycerides are fed, but this activity decreases considerably (by 85%) when medium chain triglycerides are fed.[236]

Lipase activity (substrate ³H triolein) in biopsy specimens of the gastric body was found to be similar in subjects between the ages of 5 and 19 months and 2 and 4, 6 and 10, 11 and 13, and 15 and 26 years. Lipase activity was low or undetectable in the gastric antrum and in duodenal tissue or duodenal bulb tissue.[141] Using another substrate (tributyrin), it was shown that lipase activity in gastric aspirates collected from premature infants was lower at birth in infants at 26 weeks and less, peaked at 30 to 32 weeks, and declined to lower levels at term. Continuous feeding, as opposed to intermittent parenteral alimentation, appeared to promote the development of this lipase activity.[254]

Pancreatic Lipases. In adults, pancreatic juice contains two enzymes that are active against neutral lipids. The so-called pancreatic lipase is more active against insoluble, emulsified substrates than against soluble ones. The second lipase, also called pancreatic carboxylase esterase, is more active against micellar or soluble substrates than against insoluble, emulsified substrates. In contrast to the first lipase, it is strongly stimulated by bile salts. Colipase removes the inhibiting effect of bile salts on lipase. Studies usually do not differentiate between these lipases.[26, 28, 29, 32-34, 36, 151, 160, 255-257] Generally, lipases show the lowest values after birth (see Fig. 115-1). The increase toward adult values occurs within the first 6 months of life, which is earlier than in the case of amylase. Premature and very low birth weight infants have lower values than do full-term neonates.[36, 258] During the first week of life, lipase activity increases about fourfold in premature infants.[36]

In healthy preterm infants between days 3 and 40 postnatally, this activity increased linearly (both in infants at gestational age 29 to 32 and 33 to 36 weeks).[259] At 1 month of age, values reached 35% of values found in 2- to 6-week-old babies. Premature infants fed soy-based formula at the age of 1 month exhibited higher lipase activity in the duodenal fluid after cholecystokinin-pancreozymin-secretin stimulation than did premature infants fed milk-based formula.[160]

Bile Acids

Bile acids play an essential role in the processes of digestion and absorption of dietary lipids. Information about bile acids is not included here, as it is the subject of another chapter.

Studies on Fat Absorption (Retention)

Various laboratories have studied absorption of fat in infants.[48, 72, 115, 183-187, 216, 217, 255, 260-299] Absorption of fat from breast milk increases slightly during the first month in full-term infants, achieving values close to 90%. In premature infants, absorption values are close to those found in full-term infants.[186,188,219,261,300]

Fat absorption from cow's milk in full-term infants also increases postnatally, but values are somewhat lower than those given for breast milk in corresponding age groups; the difference disappears around 6 months of age.[294] In premature infants, absorption during the first weeks of life is substantially lower and reaches the 80% value around 10 weeks of postnatal life.[261]

In studies on absorption of butterfat or olive oil, or both, lower absorption in premature infants was found in both 2-month-old infants[278] and 5-week-old infants.[273] In other studies using various cow's milk–based formulas, the lower absorption rate in premature infants was observed up to 2.5 months of age.[268, 269] Data obtained in various laboratories demonstrate the dependency of fatty acid absorption on chain length and the degree of saturation in premature and term infants.* This dependency reported in older studies was confirmed in premature infants,[251] but another report[302] concluded that the absorption of long chain and medium chain triglycerides from two infant formulas, as well as weight gain, was the same in preterm infants.[302] In full-term infants, fat absorption values from formulas in which some cow's milk fat was replaced by vegetable fat are closer to those reported from breast milk fat. Although absorption of long chain fatty acid triglycerides is lower during the first 6 weeks of life, medium chain fatty acid triglycerides and short chain fatty acid triglycerides are already absorbed quite efficiently in premature infants soon after birth.[184-187,260,290,303]

The importance of milk lipase in the digestion of fat was first suggested by the study of Freudenberg,[203] demonstrating decreased fat absorption in those infants fed heat-processed milk (thus, presumably with inactivated milk lipase), compared with those fed raw milk. Another study[303] brings additional support for the role of milk lipase. Preterm infants (26 to 33 weeks) retained more fat when fed a mixture of standard preterm formula and fresh human milk (3:2) than did those fed the stan-

dard preterm formula only. Other studies, in which the fat retention was found to be lower in low birth weight infants fed a long chain triglyceride containing formula nasojejunally than in those fed nasogastrically,[286] support the concept that lipid processing in the stomach by lingual lipase is important.

Preterm neonates fed a lard-modified formula achieved the same low fat absorption coefficient as those fed a standard formula.[304] In both groups, fecal lipids consisted almost completely of free fatty acids, whose composition was highly correlated with the corresponding formula's fatty acid composition. Both groups had similar relative amounts and compositions of fecal cholesterol esters and triglycerides. Plasma long chain fatty acid compositions correlated with those of the corresponding formulas. Therefore, Verkade and colleagues[305] suggested that extensive intestinal hydrolysis and limited absorption of dietary lipids was at least partly due to lipolysis in the colon. Furthermore, the appearance of triglycerides in the colon may have been caused by a rapid small intestinal passage relative to small intestinal lipolysis. By comparing the plasma triacylglycerol total and sn-2 position fatty acid levels in breast-fed and formula-fed term infants, Innis and associates[306] provided evidence that palmitic acid from human milk is absorbed as sn-2 monoacylglycerol in infants receiving breast milk. Breast-fed infants have a significantly higher proportion of acetic acid in the fecal short chain fatty acid spectra than the bottle-fed infants.[307-309] According to Siigur and colleagues,[309] this may be related to a different composition of the intestinal microflora and may be associated with protection against diarrhea and respiratory infection in the infant.

REFERENCES

1. Berseth CL: Gastrointestinal motility in the neonate. Clin Perinatol 23:179, 1996.
2. Grand RJ, et al: Progress in gastroenterology: development of the human gastrointestinal tract; a review. Gastroenterology 70:790, 1976.
3. Goldman AS: Modulation of the gastrointestinal tract of infants by human milk. Interfaces and interactions. An evolutionary perspective. J Nutr 130:426S, 2000.
4. Koldovskoy O: Developmental, dietary and hormonal control of intestinal disaccharidases in mammals (including man). In Randle PJ (ed): Carbohydrate Metabolism and Its Disorders. London, Academic Press, 1981, pp 481–522.
5. Lebenthal E, Leung YK: Feeding the premature and compromised infant: gastrointestinal considerations (review). Pediatr Clin North Am 35:215, 1988.
6. Milla PJ: Gastrointestinal motility disorders in children (review). Pediatr Clin North Am 35:311, 1988.
7. Smith CA: The Physiology of the Newborn Infant. Springfield, IL, Charles C Thomas, 1959.
8. Fomina LS: Soderzhanije nekotorikh fermentov v kishechnikje i drugikh organakh ploda chelovjeka. Vopr Med Khim 6:176, 1960.
9. Wolf RO, Taussig L: Human amniotic fluid isoamylases: functional development of fetal pancreas and salivary glands. Obstet Gynecol 41:337, 1973.
10. Aw SE, et al: Chromatographic purification of isoenzymes of human α-amylases. Biochem Biophys Acta 168:362, 1968.
11. Fridhandler L, et al: Column-chromatographic studies of isoamylases in human serum, urine and milk. Clin Chem 20:547, 1974.
12. Got R, et al: Les isoamylases du colostrum humain. Clin Chim Acta 22:545, 1968.
13. Heitlinger LA, et al: Mammary amylase: a possible alternate pathway of carbohydrate digestion in infancy. Pediatr Res 17:15, 1983.
14. Jones JB, et al: α-Amylase in preterm human milk. J Pediatr Gastroenterol Nutr 1:43, 1982.
15. Lindberg T, Skude G: Amylase in human milk. Pediatrics 70:235, 1982.
16. Mayer WB: Comparison of amylase concentration in saliva of infants and adults. Bull Johns Hopkins Hosp 44:246, 1929.
17. Nicory C: Salivary secretion in infants. Biochem J 6:387, 1922.
18. Rossiter MA, et al: Amylase content of mixed saliva in children. Acta Paediatr Scand 63:389, 1974.
19. Skude G: Sources of the serum isoamylases and their normal range of variation with age. Scand J Gastroenterol 10:577, 1975.
20. Kamaryt VJ, Fintajslova O: Die Entwicklung der Speichel- und Pankreas-Amylase bei Kindern im Laufe des ersten Lebensjahres. Z Klin Chem Klin Biochem 8:564, 1970.
21. Laxova R: Antenatal development of amylase isoenzymes. J Med Genet 9:321, 1972.
22. Tye JG, et al: Differential expression of salivary (AMY₁) and pancreatic (AMY₂) human amylase loci in prenatal and postnatal development. J Med Genet 13:96, 1976.

* References 127, 185, 216, 264, 270, 271, 278, 287, 292, 293, 297, 299, 301.

23. Hess AF: The pancreatic ferments in infants. Am J Dis Child 4:205, 1912.
24. Keene MFL, Hewer EE: Digestive enzymes of the human foetus. Lancet 1:767, 1924.
25. Matas AJ, et al: Insulin and amylase content of human neonatal pancreas (abstract). Fed Proc 34:864, 1975.
26. Andersen DH: Pancreatic enzymes in the duodenal juice in the celiac syndrome. Am J Dis Child 63:643, 1942.
27. Auricchio S, et al: Studies on intestinal digestion of starch in man. II. Intestinal hydrolysis of amylopectin in infants and children. Pediatrics 39:853, 1967.
28. Delachaume-Salem E, Sarles H: Normal human pancreatic secretion in relation to age. Biol Gastro-Enterol 2(Suppl 2):135; Arch Fr Mal Appar Digest 59:135, 1970.
29. Farber S, et al: Pancreatic function and disease in early life. I. Pancreatic enzyme activity and the celiac syndrome. J Clin Invest 22:827, 1943.
30. Gibbs GE: Secretion test with bilumen gastroduodenal drainage in infants and children. Pediatrics 5:941, 1950.
31. Ingomar CJ, Tersley E: Chronic diarrhoeas in infancy and childhood. II. Enzyme content of duodenal juice. Arch Dis Child 42:289, 1969.
32. Klumpp TG, Neale AV: The gastric and duodenal contents of normal infants and children. Am J Dis Child 40:1215, 1930.
33. Hadorn B, et al: Quantitative assessment of exocrine pancreatic function in infants and children. J Pediatr 73:39, 1968.
34. Lebenthal E, Lee PC: Development of functional response in human exocrine pancreas. Pediatrics 66:556, 1980.
35. Menard D, et al: Differential effect of epidermal growth factor and hydrocortisone in human fetal colon. J Pediatr Gastroenterol Nutr 10:13, 1990.
36. Zoppi G, et al: Exocrine pancreas function in premature and full-term neonates. Pediatr Res 6:880, 1972.
37. Anderson TA, et al: Carbohydrate tolerance studies with 3-day-old infants. J Lab Clin Med 79:31, 1972.
38. Husband J, et al: Gastric emptying of starch meals in the newborn. Lancet 2:290, 1970.
39. de Vizia B, et al: Digestibility of starches in infants and children. J Pediatr 85:50, 1975.
40. Semenza G: Intestinal oligo- and disaccharidases. In Randle PJ, et al (eds): Carbohydrate Metabolism and Its Disorders. London, Academic Press, 1981, pp 425–479.
41. Eggermont E: Enzymic activities in meconium from human foetuses and newborns. Biol Neonate 10:266, 1966.
42. Eggermont E: The hydrolysis of the naturally occurring α-glucosides by the human intestinal mucosa. Eur J Biochem 9:483, 1969.
43. Kerzner B, Sloan HR: Mucosal glucoamylase activity (letter to editor). J Pediatr 99:388, 1981.
44. Lebenthal E, Lee PC: Glucoamylase and disaccharidase activities in normal subjects and in patients with mucosal injury of the small intestine. J Pediatr 97:389, 1980.
45. Haworth JC, McCredie D: Chromatographic separation of reducing sugars in the urines of newborn babies. Arch Dis Child 31:189, 1956.
46. Chaturvedi P, et al: Survival of human milk oligosaccharides in the intestine of infants. Adv Exp Med Biol 501:315, 2001.
47. Heilskov NSC: Studies on animal lactase. II. Distribution in some of the glands of the digestive tract. Acta Physiol Scand 24:84, 1951.
48. Jarrett EC, Holman GH: Lactose absorption in the premature infant. Arch Dis Child 41:525, 1966.
49. Jirsova V, et al: Development of invertase activity in the intestines of human fetuses: appearance of jejunoileal differences. Biol Neonate 13:143, 1986.
50. Lacroix B, et al: Early organogenesis of human small intestine: scanning electron microscopy and brush border enzymology. Gut 25:925, 1984.
51. Lichnovsky V, Lojda Z: Early prenatal development of the brush border enzymes in the embryonal intestine. Acta Univ Palacki Olomuc Fac Med 134:27, 1992.
52. Raul F, et al: Longitudinal distribution of brush border hydrolases and morphological maturation in the intestine of the preterm infant. Early Hum Dev 13:225, 1986.
53. Sheehy TW, Anderson PR: Fetal disaccharidases. Am J Dis Child 121:464, 1971.
54. Triadou N, Zweibaum A: Maturation of sucrase-isomaltase complex in human fetal small and large intestine during gestation. Pediatr Res 19:136, 1985.
55. Zweibaum A, et al: Sucrase-isomaltase: a marker of foetal and malignant epithelial cells of the human colon. Int J Cancer 32:407, 1983.
56. Ibrahim J: Die Doppelzuckerfermente (Lactase, Maltase, Invertin) beim menschlichen Neugeborenen und Embryo. I. Mitteilung. Hoppe-Seylers Z Physiol Chem 66:19, 1910.
57. Ibrahim J, Kaumheimer L: Die Doppelzuckerfermente (Lactase, Maltase, Invertin) beim menschlichen Neugeborenen und Embryo. II. Mitteilung. Hoppe-Seylers Z Physiol Chem 66:37, 1910.
58. Koldovsky O: Nutrition and the development of digestion and absorption. In Rechcigl M (ed): Handbook of Nutritional Requirements in a Functional Context, Vol II. Boca Raton, CRC Press, 1981, pp 129–161.
59. Antonowicz I, et al: Development and distribution of lysosomal enzymes and disaccharidases in human fetal intestine. Gastroenterology 67:51, 1974.
60. Dahlqvist A, Lindberg T: Development of the intestinal disaccharidase and alkaline phosphatase activities in the human foetus. Clin Sci 30:517, 1966.
61. Jirsova V, et al: The development of the functions of the small intestine of the human fetus. Biol Neonate 9:44, 1966.
62. Antonowicz I, Lebenthal E: Developmental pattern of small intestinal enterokinase and disaccharidase activities in the human fetus. Gastroenterology 72:1299, 1977.
63. Menard D, Pothier P: Differential distribution of digestive enzymes in isolated epithelial cells from developing human fetal small intestine and colon. J Pediatr Gastroenterol Nutr 6:509, 1987.
64. Auricchio S, et al: Human fetal intestinal brush border (BB) sucrase oligoaminopeptidase and dipeptidylaminopeptidase (abstract). Pediatr Res 15:1193, 1981.
65. Skovbjerg H: High molecular weight pro-sucrase-isomaltase in human fetal intestine. Pediatr Res 16:948, 1982.
66. Sebastio G, et al: The biosynthesis of intestinal sucrase-isomaltase in human embryo is most likely controlled at the level of transcription. Biochem Biophys Res Commun 149:830, 1987.
67. Auricchio S, et al: Intestinal glycosidase activities in the human embryo, fetus, and newborn. Pediatrics 35:944, 1965.
68. Wang Y, et al: Expression of human intestinal mRNA transcripts during development: analysis by a semi-quantitative RNA polymerase chain reaction method. Pediatr Res 36:514, 1994.
69. Koldovskoy O, et al: Transport of glucose against a concentration gradient in everted sacs of jejunum and ileum of human fetuses. Gastroenterology 48:185, 1965.
70. Villa M, et al: The expression of lactase enzymatic activity and mRNA in human fetal jejunum: effect of organ culture and of treatment with hydrocortisone. FEBS Lett 301:202, 1992.
71. Counahan R, Walker-Smith J: Stool and urinary sugars in normal neonates. Arch Dis Child 51:517, 1976.
72. Davidson M, Bauer CH: Patterns of fat excretion in feces of premature infants fed various preparations of milk. Pediatrics 25:375, 1960.
73. Whyte RK, et al: Faecal excretion of oligosaccharides and other carbohydrates in normal neonates. Arch Dis Child 53:913, 1978.
74. Boellner SW, et al: Impairment of intestinal hydrolysis of lactose in newborn infants. Pediatrics 36:542, 1965.
75. Cook GC: Lactase activity in newborn and infant Baganda. Br Med J 1:527, 1967.
76. MacLean WC, Fink BB: Lactose malabsorption by premature infants: magnitude and clinical significance. J Pediatr 97:383, 1980.
77. MacLean WC, et al: Lactose assimilation by full-term infants: relation of (^{13}C) and H$_2$ breath tests with fecal (^{13}C) excretion. Pediatr Res 17:629, 1983.
78. Davidson AGF, Mullinger M: Reducing substances in neonatal stools detected by Clinitest. Pediatrics 46:632, 1970.
79. Heine W, et al: Lactose and protein absorption from breast milk and cow's milk preparations and its influence on the intestinal flora. Acta Paediatr Scand 66:699, 1977.
80. Douwes AC, et al: Sugar malabsorption in healthy neonates estimated by breath hydrogen. Arch Dis Child 55:512, 1980.
81. Fekete M, et al: Lactose absorption in growth retarded newborn infants. Acta Paediatr Acad Sci Hung 10:303, 1969.
82. Weaver LT, et al: Neonatal intestinal lactase activity. Arch Dis Child 61:896, 1986.
83. Kien CL, Liechty EA: Colonic bacterial (BAC) salvage of carbohydrate energy (CE) in premature infants: a mutually beneficial symbiosis (abstract). Pediatr Res 23:307, 1988.
84. Kien CL, et al: Dietary carbohydrate assimilation in the premature infant: evidence for a nutritionally significant bacterial ecosystem in the colon. Am J Clin Nutr 46:456, 1987.
85. Kien CL, et al: Efficient assimilation of lactose carbon in premature infants. J Pediatr Gastroenterol Nutr 15:253, 1992.
86. Kien CL, et al: Comparison of methods for estimating fecal carbohydrate excretion in premature infants. J Pediatr Gastroenterol Nutr 17:276, 1993.
87. Erasmus HD, et al: Enhanced weight gain in preterm infants receiving lactase-treated feeds: a randomized, double-blind, controlled trial. J Pediatr 141:532, 2002.
88. Kien CL, et al: Effects of lactose intake on digestion and colonic fermentation in preterm infants. J Pediatr 133:401, 1998.
89. Kwinta P, et al: Influence of the lactose free and lactose containing diet on prevalence of gram-negative sepsis and feeding intolerance in very low birth weight infants: double blind randomized trial. Przegl Lek 59;Suppl 1:63, 2002.
90. Moya M, et al: A metabolic balance study in term infants fed lactose-containing or lactose-free formula. Acta Paediatr 88:1211, 1999.
91. Aramayo LA, et al: Disaccharidase activities in jejunal fluid. Arch Dis Child 58:686, 1983.
92. Quak SH, et al: The nature of small bowel luminal fluid lactase. Clin Chim Acta 204:145, 1991.
93. Mayne A, et al: Postnatal development of disaccharidase activities in jejunal fluid of preterm neonates. Lancet 2:622, 1983.
94. Mayne AJ, et al: Postnatal development of disaccharidase activities in jejunal fluid of preterm neonates. Gut 27:1357, 1986.
95. Bartrop RW, Hull D: Transient lactose intolerance in infancy. Arch Dis Child 48:963, 1973.
96. Greene HL, et al: Protracted diarrhea and malnutrition in infancy: changes in intestinal morphology and disaccharidase activities during treatment with total intravenous nutrition or oral elemental diets. J Pediatr 87:695, 1975.
97. James WP: Sugar absorption and intestinal motility in children when malnourished and after treatment. Clin Sci 39:305, 1970.

98. Prinsloo JG, et al: Lactose absorption and mucosal disaccharidases in conva-lescent pellagra and kwashiorkor children. Arch Dis Child 46:474, 1971.
99. Rossi TM, et al: Extent and duration of small intestinal mucosal injury in intractable diarrhea of infancy. Pediatrics 66:730, 1980.
100. Bakken AF: Temporary intestinal lactase deficiency in light-treated jaundiced infants. Acta Paediatr Scand 66:91, 1977.
101. Levin R, et al: Electrical activity across human foetal small intestine associated with absorption processes. Gut 9:206, 1968.
102. Malo C, Berteloot A: Proximodistal gradient of Na+-dependent D-glucose trans-port activity in the brush border membrane vesicles from the human fetal small intestine. FEBS Lett 220:201, 1987.
103. Malo C: Kinetic evidence for heterogeneity in Na+ D-glucose cotransport systems in the normal human fetal small intestine. Biochim Biophys Acta 938:181, 1988.
104. Malo C: Separation of two distinct Na+ D-glucose cotransport systems in the human fetal jejunum by means of their differential specificity for 3-O-methylglucose. Biochim Biophys Acta 1022:8, 1990.
105. Davidson NO, et al: Human intestinal glucose transporter expression and localization of GLUT 5. Am J Physiol 262:C795, 1992.
106. Lugo-de-Rivera C, et al: Studies on the mechanism of sugar malabsorption in infantile infectious diarrhea. Am J Clin Nutr 25:1248, 1972.
107. Torres-Pinedo R, et al: Studies on infant diarrhea. II. Absorption of glucose and net fluxes of water and sodium chloride in a segment of the jejunum. J Clin Invest 45:1916, 1966.
108. Cummins AJ, Jussila R: Comparison of glucose absorption rates in the upper and lower human small intestine. Gastroenterology 29:982, 1955.
109. Fordtran JS, et al: The kinetics of water absorption in the human intestine. Trans Assoc Am Phys 74:195, 1961.
110. Fordtran JS, et al: Sugar absorption tests, with special reference to 3-O methyl-D-glucose and D-xylose. Ann Intern Med 57:883, 1962.
111. Gray GM, Ingelfinger FJ: Intestinal absorption of sucrose in man: interrelation of hydrolysis and monosaccharide product absorption. J Clin Invest 45:388, 1966.
112. Holdsworth CD, Dawson AM: The absorption of monosaccharides in man. Clin Sci 27:371, 1964.
113. Schedl HP, Clifton JA: Kinetics of intestinal absorption in man: normals and patients with sprue. In Proceedings of the Second World Congress of Gastroenterology, Vol II. Basel, S Karger, 1963, pp 728–748.
114. Talley RB, et al: Small intestinal glucose, electrolyte, and water absorption in cirrhosis. Gastroenterology 47:382, 1964.
115. Vinnik IE, et al: The effect of diabetes mellitus and insulin on glucose absorp-tion by the small intestine in man. J Lab Clin Med 66:131, 1965.
116. Shulman RJ: In vivo measurements of glucose absorption in preterm infants. Biol Neonate 76:10, 1999.
117. Murray RD, et al: Comparative absorption of [13C] glucose and [13C] lactose by premature infants. Am J Clin Nutr 51:59, 1990.
118. Rouwet EV, et al: Intestinal permeability and carrier-mediated monosaccha-ride absorption in preterm neonates during the early postnatal period. Pediatr Res 51:64, 2002.
119. Beyreiss K, et al: Besonderheiten der Resorption und des Stoffwechsels von Kohlenhydraten bei Früh und Neugeborenen. Wiss Z Friedrich-Schiller Univ Jena Math-Naturwiss Reihe 21:683, 1972.
120. Blackberg L, et al: Bile salt–stimulated lipase in human milk and carboxyl ester hydrolase in pancreatic juice: are they identified enzymes? FEBS Lett 136:284, 1981.
121. Kelly EJ, Brownlee KG: When is the fetus first capable of gastric acid, intrinsic factor and gastrin secretion? Biol Neonate 63:153, 1993.
122. Kelly EJ, et al: Gastric secretory function in the developing human stomach. Early Hum Dev 31:163, 1992.
123. Kelly EJ, et al: Immunocytochemical localisation of parietal cells and G cells in the developing human stomach. Gut 34:1057, 1993.
124. Wolman IJ: Gastric digestive secretions in infancy and childhood: a review. Am J Med Sci 206:770, 1943.
125. Wolman IJ: Gastric phase of milk digestion in childhood. Am J Dis Child 71:394, 1946.
126. Castberg HB, Hernell O: Role of bile salt–stimulated lipase in lipolysis in human milk. Milchwissenschaft 30:71, 1975.
127. Harries JT, Fraser AJ: The acidity of the gastric contents of premature babies during the first fourteen days of life. Biol Neonate 12:186, 1968.
128. Mason S: Some aspects of gastric function in the newborn. Arch Dis Child 37:387, 1962.
129. Mouterde O, et al: Gastric secretion in infants: application to the study of sudden infant death syndrome and apparently life-threatening events. Biol Neonate 62:15, 1992.
130. Mignone F, Castello D: Ricerche sulla secrezione gastrica di acido cloridrico nell'immaturo. Minerva Pediatr 13:1098, 1961.
131. Euler AR, et al: Basal and pentagastrin-stimulated acid secretion in newborn human infants. Pediatr Res 13:36, 1979.
132. Ghai OP, et al: An assessment of gastric acid secretory response with maximal augmented histamine stimulation in children with peptic ulcer. Arch Dis Child 40:77, 1965.
133. Agunod M, et al: Correlative study of hydrochloric acid, pepsin, and intrinsic factor secretion in newborns and infants. Am J Digest Dis 14:400, 1969.
134. Rodbro P, et al: Parietal cell secretory function in early childhood. Scand J Gastroenterol 2:209, 1967.

135. Wagner H: The development to full functional maturity of the gastric mucosa and the kidneys in the fetus and newborn. Biol Neonate 3:257, 1961.
136. Werner B: Peptic and tryptic capacity of the digestive glands in newborns: a comparison between premature and full-term infants. Acta Paediatr 35(Suppl 6):1, 1948.
137. Hirsch-Marie H, et al: Immunochemical study and cellular localization of human pepsinogens during ontogenesis and in gastric cancers. Lab Invest 34:623, 1976.
138. Foltmann B, Axelsen NH: Gastric proteinases and their zymogens: phylo-genetic and developmental aspects. In Mildner P, Ries B (eds): Enzyme Regulation and Mechanism of Action. Oxford, Pergamon Press, 1980, pp 271–280.
139. Reid WA, et al: Immunolocalisation of aspartic proteinases in the developing human stomach. J Dev Physiol 11:299, 1989.
140. Rodbro P, et al: Gastric secretion of pepsin in early childhood. Scand J Gastroenterol 2:257, 1967.
141. Di Palma J, et al: Lipase and pepsin activity in the gastric mucosa of infants, children, and adults. Gastroenterology 101:116, 1991.
142. Yahav J, et al: Meal-stimulated pepsinogen secretion in premature infants. J Pediatr 110:949, 1987.
143. Berfenstam R, et al: Protein hydrolysis in the stomachs of premature and full-term infants. Acta Paediatr 44:348, 1955.
144. Koshtoyants CS: Beitrag zur Physiologie des Embryos (Embryosecretin). Pfluegers Arch Gesamte Physiol 227:359, 1931.
145. Lieberman J: Proteolytic enzyme activity in fetal pancreas and meconium. Gastroenterology 50:183, 1966.
146. Carrere J, et al: Immunohistochemical study of secretory proteins in the devel-oping human exocrine pancreas. Differentiation 51:55, 1992.
147. Borgstrom B, et al: Enzyme concentration and absorption of protein and glucose in duodenum of premature infants. Am J Dis Child 99:338, 1960.
148. Borgstrom B, et al: Digestive studies in children. Am J Dis Child 101:454, 1961.
149. Davidson WC: The duodenal contents of infants in health, and during and fol-lowing diarrhea. Am J Dis Child 29:743, 1925.
150. Heikura S, et al: Cholic acid and chenodeoxycholic acid concentrations in serum during infancy and childhood. Acta Paediatr Scand 69:659, 1980.
151. Veghelyi PV: Pancreatic enzymes: normal output and comparison of different methods of assay. Pediatrics 3:749, 1949.
152. Madey S, Dancis J: Proteolytic enzymes of the premature infant. Pediatrics 4:177, 1949.
153. Guilbert PW, Barbero GJ: The importance of trypsin in infancy and childhood. II. Clinical considerations. Am J Med Sci 227:672, 1954.
154. Bujanover Y, et al: The development of the chymotryptic activity during post-natal life using the bentiromide test. Int J Pancreatol 3:53, 1988.
155. Lindberg T: Proteolytic activity in duodenal juice in infants, children, and adults. Acta Paediatr Scand 63:805, 1974.
156. Norman A, et al: Bile acids and pancreatic enzymes during absorption in the newborn. Acta Paediatr Scand 61:571, 1972.
157. Kolacek S, et al: Ontogeny of pancreatic exocrine function. Arch Dis Child 65:178, 1990.
158. Ben RA, et al: Fecal chymotrypsin in infants fed different diets (letter to the editor). J Pediatr Gastroenterol Nutr 16:104, 1993.
159. Zoppi G, et al: The electrolyte and protein contents and outputs in duodenal juice after pancreozymin and secretin stimulation in normal children and in patients with cystic fibrosis. Acta Paediatr Scand 59:692, 1970.
160. Lebenthal E, et al: The development of pancreatic function in premature infants after milk-based and soy-based formulas. Pediatr Res 15:1240, 1981.
161. Barkholt-Pedersen V, et al: On the properties of trypsin inhibitors from human and bovine colostrum. FEBS Lett 17:23, 1971.
162. Heyndrickx GV: Further investigations on the enzymes in human milk. Pediatrics 31:1019, 1963.
163. Laskowski M Jr, Laskowski M: Crystalline trypsin inhibitor from colostrum. J Biol Chem 190:563, 1951.
164. Lindberg T: Protease inhibitors in human milk. Pediatrics 13:969, 1979.
165. Henderson TR, et al: Gastric proteolysis in preterm infants fed mother's milk or formula. Adv Exp Med Biol 501:403, 2001.
166. Heringova A, et al: Proteolytic and peptidase activities of the small intestine of human fetuses. Gastroenterology 51:1023, 1966.
167. Blum E, et al: Die proteolytischen Fermente menschlicher Embryonen in den verschiedenen Stadien der Entwicklung. Bull Biol Med Exp USSR 1:113, 1936.
168. Lindberg T: Intestinal dipeptidases: characterization, development and distri-bution of intestinal dipeptidases of the human foetus. Clin Sci 30:505, 1966.
169. Walker W: Development of the intestinal mucosal barrier. J Pediatr Gastroenterol Nutr 34:S33, 2002.
170. Gitlin D, et al: The turnover of amniotic fluid protein in the human concep-tus. Am J Obstet Gynecol 113:632, 1972.
171. Anderson A, et al: Intestinal absorption of antigenic proteins by normal infant. Proc Soc Exp Biol Med 23:180, 1925.
172. Lippard VW, et al: Immune reactions induced in infants by intestinal absorp-tion of incompletely digested cow's milk protein. Am J Dis Child 51:562, 1936.
173. Roberton DM, et al: Milk antigen absorption in the preterm and term neonate. Arch Dis Child 57:369, 1982.
174. Tainio V-M, et al: Plasma antibodies to cow's milk are increased by early weaning and consumption of unmodified milk, but production of plasma IgA

and IgM cow's milk antibodies is stimulated even during exclusive breast feeding. Acta Paediatr Scand 77:807, 1988.

175. Walzer M: Studies in absorption of undigested proteins in human beings. I. A simple direct method of studying the absorption of undigested protein. J Immunol 14:143, 1927.

176. Gruskay FL, Cooke RE: The gastrointestinal absorption of unaltered protein in normal infants and in infants recovering from diarrhea. Pediatrics 16:763, 1955.

177. Rothberg RM: Immunoglobulin and specific antibody synthesis during the first weeks of life of premature infants. J Pediatr 75:391, 1969.

178. Hjelt K, et al: Concentrations of IgA, IgM, secretory IgM, IgD and IgG in the upper jejunum of children without gastrointestinal disorders. J Pediatr Gastroenterol Nutr 7:867, 1988.

179. Lebenthal E, et al: Immunoglobulin concentrations in duodenal fluid of infants and children. Am J Dis Child 134:834, 1980.

180. Brown GA, et al: Nonlipid formula components and fat absorption in the low-birth-weight newborn. Am J Clin Nutr 49:55, 1989.

181. Feinstein MS, Smith CA: Digestion of protein by premature infants. Pediatrics 7:19, 1951.

182. Fomon SJ: Nitrogen balance studies with normal full-term infants receiving high intakes of protein. Pediatrics 28:347, 1961.

183. Gordon HH, et al: Respiratory metabolism in infancy and in childhood. Am J Dis Child 54:1030, 1937.

184. MacLaurin JC, et al: Fat calcium and nitrogen balance in full-term infants. Postgrad Med J 51:45, 1975.

185. Roy CC, et al: Correction of the malabsorption of the preterm infant with a medium-chain triglyceride formula. J Pediatr 86:446, 1975.

186. Soderhjelm L: Fat absorption studies in children. I. Influence of heat treatment of milk on fat retention by premature infants. Acta Paediatr Scand 41:207, 1952.

187. Widdowson EM: Absorption and excretion of fat, nitrogen, and minerals from "filled" milks by babies one week old. Lancet 2:1099, 1965.

188. Zoula J, et al: Nitrogen and fat retention in premature infants fed breast milk, "humanized" cow's milk, or half-skimmed cow's milk. Acta Paediatr Scand 55:26, 1966.

189. Picaud JC, et al: Nutritional efficacy of preterm formula with a partially hydrolyzed protein source: a randomized study. J Pediatr Gastroenterol Nutr 32:555, 2001.

190. Szajewska H, et al: Extensive and partial protein hydrolysate preterm formulas: the effect on growth rate, protein metabolism indices, and plasma amino acid concentrations. J Pediatr Gastroenterol Nutr 32:303, 2001.

191. Hirata Y: Studies in infant nutrition. Pediatr Jpn 1:67, 1958.

192. Hirata Y, et al: Digestion and absorption of milk protein in infant's intestine. Kobe J Med Sci 11:103, 1965.

193. Heine W, et al: Evidence for colonic absorption of protein nitrogen in infants. Acta Paediatr Scand 76:741, 1987.

194. Juvonen P, et al: Macromolecular absorption and cows' milk allergy. Arch Dis Child 65:300, 1990.

195. Kuitunen OOM, et al: Human α-lactalbumin and bovine β-lactoglobulin absorption in premature infants. Pediatr Res 35:344, 1994.

196. Malo C: Multiple pathways for amino acid transport in brush-border membrane vesicles isolated from the human fetal small intestine. Gastroenterology 100:1644, 1991.

197. Tachibana T: Fetus: I. Enzymes in the digestive tract. Trypsinogen in the pancreas. II. A peptone-splitting enzyme in the intestinal canal. III. Lipase in the stomach (abstract). Chem Zentr 23:52, 1929.

198. Menard D, et al: Ontogeny of human gastric lipase and pepsin activities. Gastroenterology 108:1650, 1995.

199. Sarles J, et al: Human gastric lipase: ontogeny and variations in children. Acta Paediatr 81:511, 1992.

200. Pelichova H, et al: Fetal development of non-specific esterases and alkaline phosphatases activities in the small intestine of man. Biol Neonate 10:281, 1966.

201. Tachibana T: Lung lipase in the human fetus and the newborn child. Supplement: other intestine lipases (abstract). Chem Zentr 25:5454, 1930.

202. Marfan AB: Allaitment naturel et allaitment artificiel. Presse Med 9:13, 1901.

203. Freudenberg E: Die Frauenmilch-Lipase. Basel, Karger, 1953.

204. Mehta NR, et al: Lipases in preterm human milk: ontogeny and physiologic significance. J Pediatr Gastroenterol Nutr 1:317, 1982.

205. Fredrikzon B, et al: Bile salt-stimulated lipase in human milk: evidence of activity in vivo and of a role in the digestion of milk retinol esters. Pediatr Res 12:1048, 1978.

206. Hall B, Muller DPR: Studies on the bile salt stimulated lipolytic activity of human milk using whole milk as source of both substrate and enzyme. I. Nutritional implications. Pediatr Res 16:251, 1982.

207. Hall B, et al: Studies of lipase activity in human milk. Proc Nutr Soc 38:114A, 1979.

208. Hernell O: Human milk lipase. III. Physiological implications of the bile salt-stimulated lipase. Eur J Clin Invest 5:267, 1975.

209. Hernell O, Blackberg L: Digestion of human milk lipids: physiologic significance of sn-2 monoacylglycerol hydrolysis by bile salt-stimulated lipase. Pediatr Res 16:882, 1982.

210. Hernell O, Olivecrona T: Human milk lipases. I. Serum-stimulated lipase. J Lipid Res 15:367, 1974.

211. Hernell O, et al: Breast milk composition in Ethiopian and Swedish motherso. IV. Milk lipases. Am J Clin Nutr 30:508, 1977.

212. Jubelin J, Boyer J: The lipolytic activity of human milk. Eur J Clin Invest 2:417, 1972.

213. Wang C-S: Human milk bile salt-activated lipase: further characterization and kinetic studies. J Biol Chem 256:10198, 1981.

214. Olivecrona T, Hernell O: Are the lipases in human milk important for fat digestion in the newborn? In Rommel K (ed): Lipid Absorption: Biochemical and Clinical Aspects. Proceedings of an International Conference held at Titisee, The Black Forest, Germany, May 1975. London, MTP Press, 1976, pp 315–320.

215. Williamson S, et al: Effect of heat treatment of human milk on absorption of nitrogen, fat, sodium, calcium, and phosphorus by preterm infants. Arch Dis Child 53:555, 1978.

216. Williams ML, et al: Calcium and fat absorption in neonatal period. Am J Clin Nutr 23:1322, 1970.

217. Southgate DAT, Barrett IM: The intake and excretion of calorific constituents of milk by babies. Br J Nutr 20:363, 1966.

218. Luzeau R, et al: Nonesterified fatty acids and the titratable acidity of breast milk: consequences for collection conditions in milk banks. Arch Fr Pediatr 40:449, 1983.

219. Luzeau R, et al: Demonstration of a lipolytic activity in human milk that inhibits the glucuroconjugation of bilirubin. Biomedicine 21:258, 1974.

220. Luzeau R, et al: Activite á de la lipoproteine lipase dans les laits de femme inhibiteurs in vitro de la conjugaison de la bilirubine. Clin Chim Acta 59:133, 1975.

221. Wang C-S, et al: Studies on the substrate specificity of purified human milk lipoprotein lipase. Lipids 17:278, 1982.

222. Hamosh M, Scow RO: Lipoprotein lipase activity in guinea pig and rat milk. Biochim Biophys Acta 231:283, 1971.

223. Poland RL, et al: High milk lipase activity associated with breast milk jaundice. Pediatr Res 14:1328, 1980.

224. Constantopoulos A, et al: Breast milk jaundice: the role of lipoprotein lipase and the free fatty acids. Eur J Pediatr 134:35, 1980.

225. Odievre M, Luzeau R: Lipolytic activity in milk from mothers of unjaundiced infants. Acta Paediatr Scand 67:49, 1978.

226. Chandran RC, et al: Lysozyme, lipase and ribonuclease in milk of various species. J Dairy Sci 51:606, 1968.

227. Heyndrickx GV: Investigations on the enzymes in human milk. Ann Pediatr (Basel) 198:356, 1962.

228. Sumtsov BM: Esterase activity and protein composition of the milk. Pediatrica 37:31, 1959.

229. Tarassuk NP, et al: Lipase action in human milk. Nature (Lond) 201:298, 1964.

230. Wuthrich SR, et al: Untersuchungen über Milchenzyme. I. Enzyme in Kuhmilch und Frauenmilch. Z Unters Lebens Forsch 124:336, 1964.

231. Bank S, et al: Hydrolysis of fat by human gastric juice. Gut 5:480, 1964.

232. Blackberg L, et al: On the source of lipase activity in gastric contents. Acta Paediatr Scand 66:473, 1977.

233. Cohen M, et al: Lipolytic activity of human gastric and duodenal juice against medium and long-chain triglycerides. Gastroenterology 60:1, 1971.

234. Fredrikzon B, Hernell O: Role of feeding on lipase activity in gastric contents. Acta Paediatr Scand 66:479, 1977.

235. Gargouri Y, et al: Importance of human gastric lipase for intestinal lipolysis: an in vitro study. Biochim Biophys Acta 879:419, 1986.

236. Hamosh M: A review: fat digestion in the newborn; role of lingual lipase and preduodenal digestion. Pediatr Res 13:615, 1979.

237. Hamosh M, et al: Fat digestion in the newborns: characterization of lipase in gastric aspirates of premature and term infants. J Clin Invest 66:838, 1981.

238. Schoenheyder F, Volqvartz K: The gastric lipase in man. Acta Physiol Scand 11:349, 1946.

239. von Ebner K: Die acinosen Drusen der Zunge und ihre Beziehungen zu den Geschmacksorganen. In Hoelliker V (ed): Handbuch D Geweblehre d Menschen, Vol 3. Graz, Austria, Leuschner & Lubensky, 1899, pp 18–38.

240. Fink CS, et al: Fat digestion in the stomach: stability of lingual lipase in the gastric environment. Pediatr Res 18:248, 1984.

241. Hamosh M, Burns WA: Lipolytic activity of human lingual glands (Ebner). Lab Invest 37:603, 1977.

242. Hamosh M, et al: Pharyngeal lipase and digestion of dietary triglyceride in man. J Clin Invest 55:908, 1975.

243. de Nigris SJ, et al: Secretion of human gastric lipase from dispersed gastric glands. Biochim Biophys Acta 836:67, 1985.

244. Moreau H, et al: Human preduodenal lipase is entirely of gastric fundic origin. Gastroenterology 95:1221, 1988.

245. Salzman-Mann C, et al: Lipolytic activity in esophageal and gastric aspirates from infants with esophageal atresia (abstract). Fed Proc 37:854, 1978.

246. Salzman-Mann C, et al: Congenital oesophageal atresia: lipase activity is present in the oesophageal pouch and in the stomach. Dig Dis Sci 27:124, 1982.

247. Fredrikzon B, Blackberg L: Lingual lipase: an important lipase in the digestion of dietary lipids in cystic fibrosis. Pediatr Res 14:1387, 1980.

248. Fredrikzon B, et al: Lingual lipase: its role in lipid digestion in infants with low birthweight and/or pancreatic insufficiency. Acta Paediatr Scand 296(Suppl):75, 1982.

249. Olivecrona T, et al: Gastric lipolysis of human milk lipids in infants with pyloric stenosis. Acta Paediatr Scand 62:520, 1973.

250. Liao TH, et al: Preduodenal fat digestion in the newborn infant: effect of fatty acid chain length on triglyceride hydrolysis (abstract). Clin Res 28:820, 1980.

251. Jensen RG, et al: Stereospecificity of premature human infant lingual lipase. Lipids 17:570, 1982.

252. Faber J, et al: Absorption of medium chain triglycerides in the stomach of the human infant. J Pediatr Gastroenterol Nutr 7:189, 1988.

253. Hamosh M, et al: Medium chain fatty acids (MCFA) are absorbed directly from the stomach of premature infants (abstract). Pediatr Res 21:429, 1987.

254. Lee P-C, et al: Development of lipolytic activity in gastric aspirates from premature infants. J Pediatr Gastroenterol Nutr 17:291, 1993.

255. Droese W: Untersuchungen über den Gallensauren- und Lipasengehalt im Duodenalsaft von Säuglingen. Monatsschr Kinderheilkd 100:233, 1952.

256. Tachibana T: Physiological investigation of fetus: supplementary research of ferments in digestive organ; lipase in pancreas. Jpn J Obstet Gynecol 11:92, 1928.

257. Vazquez C: La funcion pancreatica del recien nacido. Rev Espan Pediatr 7:75, 1951.

258. Katz L, Hamilton JR: Fat absorption in infants of birth weight less than 1,300 gm. J Pediatr 85:608, 1974.

259. Boehm G, et al: Activities of trypsin and lipase in duodenal aspirates of healthy preterm infants: effects of gestational and postnatal age. Biol Neonate 67:248, 1995.

260. Droese W: Über die Fetttoleranz der Säuglinge. Klinisch-experimentelle Untersuchung des Gallensauren- und Lipasengehaltes im Duodenalsaft. Ann Paediatr 178:121, 1952.

261. Lavy U, et al: Role of bile acids in fat absorption in low birth-weight infants (abstract). Pediatr Res 5:387, 1971.

262. Signer E, et al: Role of bile salts in fat malabsorption of premature infants. Arch Dis Child 49:174, 1974.

263. Barltrop D, Oppe TE: Absorption of fat and calcium by low birth weight infants from milks containing butterfat and olive oil. Arch Dis Child 48:496, 1973.

264. Barnes LA, et al: Calcium and fat absorption from infant formulas with different fat blends. Pediatrics 51:217, 1974.

265. Blomstrand R, Lindquist B: Intestinal absorption of carbon-labeled oleic acid in normal infants and in congenital bile duct atresia. Acta Paediatr Helv 10:627, 1955.

266. Blomstrand R, et al: Intestinal absorption of carbon-labeled oleic acid and palmitic acid in normal infants and in cystic fibrosis of pancreas. Acta Paediatr Helv 10:640, 1955.

267. de Curtis M, et al: Effect of non-nutritive suckling (NNS) on energy, nitrogen and fat balance in preterm infants (abstract). Pediatr Res 20:1038, 1986.

268. Droese W, Stolley H: Probleme des Fettstoffwechsels in der Sauglingsernahrung. Fette Seifen Anstrichm 62:281, 1960.

269. Droese W, Stolley H: Kuhmilchfett und pflanzliches Fett in der Ernahrung des jungen, gesunden Säuglings. Dtsch Med Wochenschr 17:855, 1961.

270. Filer LJ, et al: Triglyceride configuration and fat absorption by the human infant. J Nutr 99:293, 1969.

271. Fomon SJ, et al: Excretion of fat by normal full-term infants fed various milks and formulas. Am J Clin Nutr 23:1299, 1970.

272. Gompertz SM, Sammons HG: The origin of faecal lipids: the composition of faecal fats in human subjects. Clin Chim Acta 8:591, 1963.

273. Gordon HH, McNamara H: Fat excretion of premature infants: I. effect on fecal fat of decreasing fat intake. Am J Dis Child 62:328, 1941.

274. Hanmer OJ, et al: Fat as an energy supplement for preterm infants. Arch Dis Child 57:503, 1982.

275. Hanna FM, et al: Calcium-fatty acid absorption in term infants fed human milk and prepared formulas simulating human milk. Pediatrics 45:216, 1970.

276. Holt LE Jr: Celiac disease—what is it? J Pediatr 46:369, 1955.

277. Holt LE, et al: A study of the fat metabolism of infants and young children. I. Fat in the stools of breast-fed infants. Am J Dis Child 17:241, 1919.

278. Holt LE, et al: Studies in fat metabolism. I. Fat absorption in normal infants. J Pediatr 6:427, 1935.

279. Johnson AL, et al: "Tween 20" and fecal fat in premature infants. Am J Dis Child 80:545, 1950.

280. Lavy U: Personal communication. Cited in Watkins JB: Bile acid metabolism and fat absorption in newborn infants. Pediatr Clin North Am 21:501, 1974.

281. Luther G, Schreier K: Untersuchungen zur Resorption einzelner Fettsauren an Säuglingen. Klin Wochenschr 41:189, 1963.

282. Milner RDG, et al: Fat absorption by small babies fed two filled milk formulae. Arch Dis Child 50:654, 1975.

283. Morales S, et al: Absorption of fat and vitamin A in premature infants. I. Effect of different levels of fat intake on the retention of fat and vitamin A. II. Effect of particle size on the absorption of these substances. Pediatrics 6:86, 1950.

284. Ocklitz HW, Reinmuth B: Fettbilanzstudien bei Frühgeborenen. Z Kinderheilkd 82:321, 1959.

285. Ricour C, Rey J: Study of the oil and micellar phases during fat digestion in the normal child. Rev Eur Etudes Clin Biol 15:287, 1970.

286. Roy RN, et al: Impaired assimilation of nasojejunal feeds in healthy low-birth-weight newborn infants. J Pediatr 90:431, 1977.

287. Scheppe KJ, et al: Fettadaptierte Milchfertignährung im Kinderkrankenhaus. Med und Ernährung 6:80, 1965.

288. Senterre J, Lambrechts A: Nitrogen, fat and mineral balances in premature infants fed acidified or nonacidified half-skimmed cow milk. Biol Neonate 20:107, 1972.

289. Snyderman SE, et al: The absorption of short-chain fats by premature infants. Arch Dis Child 30:83, 1955.

290. Snyderman SE, et al: Absorption of fat and vitamin A in premature infants. III. Effect of surface active agents on the absorption of these substances. Pediatrics 12:158, 1953.

291. Southgate DAT, et al: Absorption and excretion of calcium and fat by young infants. Lancet 1:487, 1969.

292. Tantibhedhyangkui P, Hashim SA: Medium-chain triglyceride feeding in premature infants: effects on fat and nitrogen absorption. Pediatrics 55:359, 1975.

293. Tidwell HC, et al: Studies in fat metabolism. J Pediatr 6:481, 1935.

294. van de Kamer JH, Weijers HA: Malabsorption syndrome. Fed Proc 7(suppl):333, 1961.

295. Watkins JB, et al: Bile salt metabolism in newborn infants (abstract). Pediatr Res 6:432, 1972.

296. Watson WC: Intestinal hydrogenation of dietary fatty acids. Clin Chim Acta 12:340, 1965.

297. Welsch H, et al: Fettersorption aus Frauenmilch beim Neugeborenen. Klin Wochenschr 43:902, 1965.

298. Wollaeger EE, et al: Total solids, fat and nitrogen in the feces. III. A study of normal persons taking a test diet containing a moderate amount of fat: comparison with results obtained with normal persons taking a test containing a large amount of fat. Gastroenterology 9:272, 1947.

299. Yamashita F, et al: Absorption of medium chain triglyceride in the low birth weight infant: an evaluation of MCT milk formula for low birth weight infant nutrition using the Latin square technique. Kurume Med J 16:191, 1969.

300. Jarvenpaa A-L: Feeding the low-birth-weight infant. IV. Fat absorption as a function of diet and duodenal bile acids. Pediatrics 72:684, 1983.

301. Watkins JB, et al: Characterization of newborn fecal lipid. Pediatrics 53:511, 1974.

302. Hamosh M, et al: Gastric lipolysis and fat absorption in preterm infants: effect of medium-chain triglyceride or long-chain triglyceride–containing formulas. Pediatrics 83:86, 1989.

303. Alemi B, et al: Fat digestion in very low-birth-weight infants: effect of addition of human milk to low-birth-weight formulas. Pediatrics 68:484, 1981.

304. Verkade HJ, et al: Fat absorption in premature infants: the effect of lard and antibiotics. Eur J Pediatr 149:126, 1989.

305. Verkade HJ, et al: Fat absorption in neonates: comparison of long-chain-fatty-acid and triglyceride compositions of formula, feces, and blood. Am J Clin Nutr 53:643, 1991.

306. Innis SM, et al: Evidence that palmitic acid is absorbed as sn-2 monoacylglycerol from human milk by breast-fed infants. Lipids 29:541, 1994.

307. Bullen CC, et al: Bifidobacteria in the intestinal tract of infants: an *in vivo* study. J Med Microbiol 9:325, 1976.

308. Midtvedt A-C, et al: Development of five metabolic activities associated with the intestinal microflora of healthy infants. J Pediatr Gastroenterol Nutr 8:559, 1988.

309. Siigur U, et al: Faecal short-chain fatty acids in breast-fed and bottle-fed infants. Acta Paediatr 82:536, 1993.

310. Younoszai MK: Jejunal absorption of hexose in infants and adults (editorial). J Pediatr 85:446, 1974.

311. Fordtran JS, Ingelfinger FJ: Absorption of water, electrolytes, and sugars from the human gut. *In* Code CF (ed): Handbook of Physiology: 6. Alimentary Canal. Vol III. Washington, DC, American Physiological Society, 1968, pp 1457–1490.

116 Pathophysiology of Gastroesophageal Reflux

COMPONENTS OF THE ANTIREFLUX MECHANISM

There is normally a pressure gradient between the stomach and the esophagus that, in the absence of other factors, would propel gastric contents into the esophagus. To counteract this gradient, there is a *high-pressure zone* at the gastroesophageal junction.[1] This high-pressure zone reflects the combined activities of two sphincters: the lower esophageal sphincter and the crural diaphragm. The activities of these two sphincters are constantly changing to prevent reflux despite changes in gastric, abdominal, and thoracic pressures. The high-pressure zone must also relax to allow passage of material across the gastroesophageal junction during swallowing, vomiting, eructation, and esophageal distention.

High-Pressure Zone

Manometrically, the high-pressure zone is characterized by the following two components: a tonically elevated basal pressure and a respiratory-induced pressure oscillation, both of which are of greater magnitude than the pressure simultaneously found in the adjacent stomach and esophagus (Fig. 116–1).[2-4] The basal pressure within the high-pressure zone can be accounted for by an intrinsic smooth muscle sphincter located at the distal esophagus known as the *lower esophageal sphincter.* Pressure changes in the high-pressure zone associated with respiratory oscillations are primarily the result of active diaphragmatic contractions that occur during inspiration.[4, 5] The combined activities of both an internal sphincter (the lower esophageal sphincter) and an external sphincter (the crural diaphragm) allow the high-pressure zone to modify the gastroesophageal pressure gradient during a variety of physiologic processes, such as deglutition, esophageal distention, and abdominal straining.[5-9]

Lower Esophageal Sphincter

The lower esophageal sphincter is a muscular structure with distinctive mechanical and electrical characteristics, unique responses to drugs and hormones, and specialized neural innervation.[10-24] The muscles of the lower esophageal sphincter appear thicker than those of the more proximal esophagus when they are examined by ultrasound.[25] The innervation of the lower esophageal sphincter is unique in that the myenteric

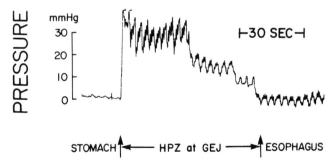

Figure 116–1. High-pressure zone (HPZ) at the gastroesophageal junction (GEJ) as measured by the station pull-through technique.[2, 3] This zone is characterized by an elevated basal pressure and an oscillating pressure wave corresponding to respiratory rate.

plexus occupies multiple muscle planes, in contrast to the adjacent esophagus, in which the plexus lies only between the circular and longitudinal muscle layers.[26]

The activity of the lower esophageal sphincter has been studied in a feline model in which esophageal distention results in changes in sphincter tone. During esophageal distention, the baseline high-pressure zone decreases to gastric baseline pressure; simultaneously, the magnitude of the respiratory-induced oscillations in the high-pressure zone is markedly reduced (Fig. 116–2). This observation suggests that the response of the sphincter mechanism to esophageal distention involves a relaxation of the intrinsic lower esophageal sphincter. These events provide an ideal situation for the transit of a swallowed bolus through the gastroesophageal junction.

The neural pathways controlling such rapid changes in lower esophageal sphincter tone have been characterized. During swallowing, afferent signals from the pharynx travel to the nucleus solitarius in the medulla. Efferent signals then travel from the adjacent dorsal vagal nucleus and the nucleus ambiguus through the vagus nerve to the esophagus, thereby mediating both esophageal peristalsis and lower esophageal sphincter relaxation to propel swallowed material into the stomach.[27]

Measurements of lower esophageal pressure have also revealed high-amplitude ($\leq$80 mm Hg) fluctuations in sphincter tone. These fluctuations occur at a frequency of approximately three per minute, and they correspond to the activity of the migrating motor complex of the stomach. Thus, the lower esophageal sphincter allows the high-pressure zone to compensate for wide variations in gastric pressure caused by the motor activity of the stomach.[28]

The region of the stomach just below the lower esophageal sphincter also contributes to the intrinsic antireflux barrier. The smooth muscle fibers of this region form a sling around the greater curvature of the stomach.[29] Although they are not strictly part of the lower esophageal sphincter, the sling fibers help to prevent reflux by acting as a flap valve in which fundic distention presses the closed end of the sling against the distal esophagus.[30]

Crural Diaphragm

The crural diaphragm is distinguished from the costal diaphragm by its attachment to the vertebral column rather than the rib cage. Because the esophagus passes through the crural diaphragm, diaphragmatic contractions create an external sphincter mechanism at the gastroesophageal junction. The activity of the crural diaphragm varies with the respiratory cycle, thereby compensating for variations in thoracic and abdominal pressure that would otherwise favor gastroesophageal reflux during inspiration (see Fig. 116–1). The activity of the crural diaphragm is increased or decreased in various other physiologic settings to allow forward passage of swallowed material but to prevent gastroesophageal reflux despite changes in abdominal pressure (see later). Indeed, in the absence of the lower esophageal sphincter (after resection), the crural diaphragm alone is able to maintain the high-pressure zone.[31]

In mammals, swallowing, distention of the esophagus, eructation, vomiting, regurgitation, and rumination are associated with an inhibition of diaphragmatic electrical activity, thereby facilitating passage of material through the gastroesophageal junction.[5, 32-38] A consistent finding associated with transit through the gastroesophageal junction is that inhibition of the

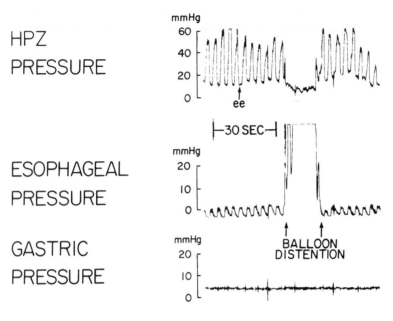

Figure 116–2. Effect of esophageal balloon distention on high-pressure zone (HPZ) pressure in a cat. During the period of balloon distention, baseline end-expiratory (ee) HPZ pressure decreases to the level of gastric pressure, and there is a marked reduction in the magnitude of the respiratory-induced oscillations in HPZ pressure.

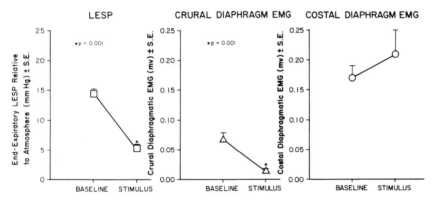

Figure 116–3. Summary of the effect of distention of the lower esophagus on intrinsic lower esophageal sphincter (LES) tone and diaphragmatic electromyographic (EMG) activity. It can be seen that distention (stimulus) caused a decrease in the activity of the crural diaphragm, together with a decrease in LES pressure (LESP). In contrast, the activity of the costal diaphragm does not change significantly.

crural diaphragm occurs to a much greater degree than that of the costal diaphragm (Fig. 116–3). In a feline model, swallowing and esophageal balloon distention resulted in concurrent relaxation of the lower esophageal sphincter and inhibition of crural inspiratory activity. The respiratory-induced oscillations in high-pressure zone pressure were abolished secondary to inhibition of crural inspiratory activity, whereas relaxation of the lower esophageal sphincter resulted in a decrease in baseline end-expiratory pressure. Costal diaphragmatic activity remained unchanged and allowed continued ventilation with little change in the respiratory rate or intrapleural pressure (Fig. 116–4). During periods of increased intra-abdominal pressure, such as the Valsalva maneuver, coughing, straight-leg raising, or abdominal compression, there is an increase in crural diaphragmatic tone, thereby compensating for the increased pressure gradient favoring gastroesophageal reflux.[39]

In summary, the manometrically defined high-pressure zone at the gastroesophageal junction depends on the tone generated by the intrinsic lower esophageal sphincter and on the magnitude of crural diaphragmatic contraction. Transit of material through the gastroesophageal junction is most likely to occur during simultaneous relaxation of the lower esophageal sphincter and inhibition of the crural diaphragm.

MECHANISMS OF GASTROESOPHAGEAL REFLUX

In theory, gastroesophageal reflux occurs in either of the following two situations: relaxation of the high-pressure zone (either transiently or for longer periods) or elevation of the gastroesophageal pressure gradient above that of the high-pressure zone (Fig. 116–5A). Using techniques that allow for simultaneous and continuous recording of lower esophageal sphincter pressure (manometry) and esophageal pH, investigators have been able to distinguish these two possibilities.[6–9,38–45] It has become clear that gastroesophageal reflux is almost always associated with a transient relaxation of the high-pressure zone involving decreased activity in both the lower esophageal sphincter and the crural diaphragm. However, the converse is not true; most transient relaxations are not associated with reflux events. Transient relaxations of the high-pressure zone occur in normal subjects, but it appears that those with gastroesophageal reflux disease have both a higher frequency of relaxations and an increased rate of reflux per episode of relaxation. Other factors must therefore also play a role in the pathogenesis of reflux disease, such as transient increases in intra-abdominal pressure, impaired clearance of refluxed material, or the presence of hiatal hernia.

Transient Relaxation of the High-Pressure Zone

As illustrated in Figure 116–5, most episodes of gastroesophageal reflux occur during transient relaxation of the high-pressure zone (see Fig. 116–5A).[8,9,46,47] Transient relaxation is caused by an abrupt collapse of pressure in the high-pressure zone in the absence of a swallow or primary esophageal peristalsis. Pressure in the high-pressure zone before and immediately after these episodes is always greater than gastric pressure. The pressure

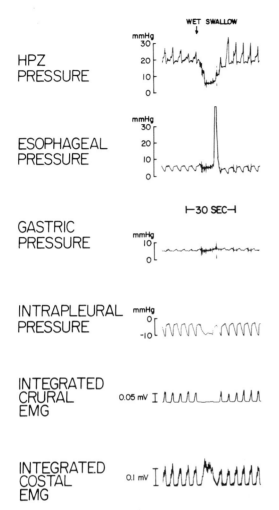

WET SWALLOW

HPZ
PRESSURE

ESOPHAGEAL
PRESSURE

├─30 SEC─┤

GASTRIC
PRESSURE

INTRAPLEURAL
PRESSURE

INTEGRATED
CRURAL
EMG

INTEGRATED
COSTAL
EMG

Figure 116–4. Effect of a wet swallow on high-pressure zone (HPZ) pressure and diaphragmatic activity. The wet swallow was induced by a bolus injection of water into the posterior pharynx. The swallow results in an esophageal contraction, with a simultaneous relaxation of the intrinsic lower esophageal sphincter and inhibition of integrated crural electromyographic (EMG) activity. The combination of these events results in end-expiratory HPZ pressure decreasing to gastric baseline and an absence of respiratory-induced oscillations in HPZ pressure. The costal diaphragm remains active during the swallow, thus allowing ventilation to continue. (From Altschuler SM, et al: Am J Physiol *249:*G586, 1985.)

profile of the high-pressure zone during transient relaxation is similar to that observed during a swallow and is characterized by decreases in both lower esophageal sphincter activity and crural diaphragm activity (Fig. 116-6). The physiologic role of transient relaxations is to allow eructation (belching) to occur, consistent with the finding that gastric distention can trigger transient relaxations.[48-52]

Other triggers for transient relaxation remain unclear. Swallow-induced and transient relaxations of the high-pressure zone are identical manometrically, and, in humans, transient relaxations frequently occur within a few seconds of a previous swallow-induced relaxation or in association with an incomplete peristaltic sequence (Fig. 116-7).[1, 8, 52-54] In an experimental model using the opossum, transient relaxations were produced by stimuli that tended to be less vigorous than the threshold required for inducing a full deglutition sequence or for the induction of secondary esophageal peristalsis.[55] Aggressive pharyngeal

stroking tended to cause a full deglutition reflex, whereas a single pharyngeal stroke was most commonly associated with isolated lower esophageal sphincter relaxation. Electrical stimulation of the central end of the superior laryngeal nerve (vagal afferent stimulation) or the peripheral end of the cervical vagus (vagal efferent stimulation) at high frequencies resulted in a normal deglutition sequence, whereas low-frequency stimulation resulted in isolated lower esophageal sphincter relaxation. Studies in humans have shown that transient relaxation is frequently associated with mylohyoid and pharyngeal activity of a much lower magnitude than that observed during a swallow or with a nonperistaltic esophageal contraction.[53] As a result of these studies, it has been suggested that transient relaxations occur by the same neural pathways as swallowing-associated relaxation (see earlier) and may be induced by a long train of sub-threshold stimuli originating in the pharynx.[55]

Studies in both normal subjects and in patients with gastro-esophageal reflux disease have shown that most reflux episodes occur during transient relaxations.[49-51] Although transient relaxations of the high-pressure zone may last from 10 to 45 seconds, the actual episodes of reflux occur only during the period when the baseline high-pressure zone pressure is zero and there is a lack of respiratory-related pressure oscillations (see Fig. 116-6). Why are transient relaxations associated with gastroesophageal reflux disease in some subjects and not in others? Studies of transient relaxations in patients with and without reflux symptoms have found only a slight increase in the frequency of relaxations in those with symptoms.[51] Some of these patients, and children in particular, may have delayed gastric emptying resulting in gastric distention, which, in turn, may produce transient relaxations of the lower esophageal sphincter.[56-59] A more important difference appears to be an increase in the percentage of transient relaxations that result in reflux from 40 to 50% in physiologically normal persons to 60 to 70% in patients with gastroesophageal reflux disease.[51] Possible causes of this difference are discussed later.

Intra-abdominal Pressure Transients

Although transient relaxation of the high-pressure zone is the major criterion for episodes of gastroesophageal reflux in both physiologically normal persons and symptomatic patients, other mechanisms must contribute to reflux in symptomatic patients.[1, 9, 46, 47] Some of these mechanisms are illustrated in Figure 116-5. Active increases in abdominal pressure occur during coughing, straining, and changes in position. In physiologically normal persons, an increase in crural diaphragm activity during active increases in abdominal pressure is thought to prevent episodes of gastroesophageal reflux.[39] In contrast, during passive abdominal compression (which may occur frequently in neonates and infants), crural diaphragmatic activity is inhibited and the activity of the lower esophageal sphincter is increased, thus leaving the lower esophageal sphincter as the sole barrier to gastroesophageal reflux (Fig. 116-8). This adaptive response involves a vagally mediated increase in lower esophageal sphincter pressure in excess of the transmitted pressure increase in the stomach.[60] The degree to which failure of these responses to active or passive increases in intra-abdominal pressure is responsible for symptomatic gastroesophageal reflux remains to be determined.

Spontaneous Free Gastroesophageal Reflux

Before the development of the sleeve sensor device to measure high-pressure zone transient relaxations and the simultaneous recording of esophageal pH, a depressed basal high-pressure zone pressure was considered the major factor leading to episodes of gastroesophageal reflux. A low resting high-pressure

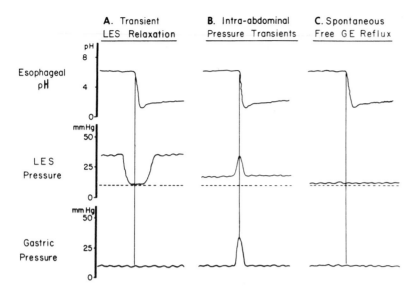

Figure 116–5. A–C, Schematic representation of different mechanisms of gastroesophageal (GE) reflux using the sleeve sensor to monitor high-pressure zone (HPZ) lower esophageal sphincter (LES) pressure. Episodes of GE reflux occur during transient relaxation of the HPZ (**A**), during increases in intra-abdominal pressure that overcomes HPZ pressure (**B**), or as spontaneous reflux across an atonic HPZ (**C**). (From Dodds WJ, et al: N Engl J Med *307*:1547, 1982.)

zone pressure was primarily attributed to a hypotonic intrinsic lower esophageal sphincter,[17] which allows free reflux of gastric contents into the esophagus. Strawczynski and colleagues[61] demonstrated that lower esophageal sphincter pressure is normally decreased in infants compared with that in adults. In addition, studies in the opossum have illustrated that lower esophageal pressure is depressed at birth and gradually achieves normal levels later in life.[62]

The presence of a hypotonic lower esophageal sphincter has also been observed in patients with neurologic impairment, connective tissue disorders such as scleroderma, previous surgery of the gastroesophageal junction, and esophagitis.[1,47] An alteration in central neural input to the lower esophageal sphincter or an impairment of the contractile function of the lower esophageal sphincter muscle is likely present in these patients.[1,56] In many cases, it is difficult to establish the sequence of cause and effect, because reflux esophagitis itself causes esophageal dysmotility. Likewise, although hiatal hernia can exacerbate gastroesophageal reflux, it may be a secondary result of esophageal shortening caused by chronic esophagitis.[1] Although episodes of gastroesophageal reflux are now known to occur infrequently by the mechanism of a hypotonic lower esophageal sphincter, this mechanism may be important with regard to chalasia of infancy and in other patients with the previously mentioned disorders.

GASTROESOPHAGEAL REFLUX IN THE NEONATAL PERIOD

The mechanisms of gastroesophageal reflux in the neonate, and in particular in premature infants, have been less well described than in adults. Regurgitation is very common in this age group; up to 40 to 60% of normal 0- to 4-month-old infants regurgitate some amount of most of their feeds.[63] Basic mechanical considerations provide some explanation for the high frequency of regurgitation in infants. Newborns spend most of their time in the supine position, which has been shown to promote gastroesophageal reflux. The newborn full-term infant's esophageal length is only 8 to 10 cm, and the intra-abdominal esophagus is less than a centimeter, thereby facilitating passage of refluxed material to a relatively higher anatomic level than in adults.

Esophageal pH monitoring, the current standard for the diagnosis of gastroesophageal reflux in adults, is of limited value in

infants because gastric acid is buffered by frequent feedings. Nonetheless, it is possible to measure esophageal pressures in neonates and even premature infants and to identify ways in which their antireflux mechanisms differ from those of adults.[64-66] As suggested by prenatal ultrasound images of fetuses swallowing amniotic fluid, the primary esophageal mechanisms are present at an early stage. Manometric studies of both premature and full-term neonates have confirmed normal primary esophageal peristalsis. Moreover, even premature infants as young as 33 weeks' postmenstrual age have been found to have a normal lower esophageal high-pressure zone.[64-66] However, premature infants have an elevated frequency of synchronous (i.e., nonperistaltic) esophageal contractions in the absence of a swallow, and this lack of coordination may lead to inadequate clearance of refluxed material.[64,65] As in adults, it appears that transient relaxations of the high-pressure zone are the primary mechanism of gastroesophageal reflux in neonates.[64-67] Thus, it appears that the high frequency of gastroesophageal reflux in neonates reflects both anatomic factors and immaturity of the esophageal clearance mechanisms.

Manifestations of Gastroesophageal Reflux in the Neonate

Neonatal gastroesophageal reflux is considered pathologic if it is associated with growth failure resulting from poor feeding, excessive regurgitation, pulmonary complications, or neurobehavioral manifestations, such as severe irritability or Sandifer syndrome. In these cases, there is generally a clear temporal association of the symptoms with feeding times or episodes of regurgitation. Somewhat more controversial is the potential relationship between gastroesophageal reflux and apnea of prematurity. Several studies using pH monitoring and polysomnography have not demonstrated a correlation between gastroesophageal reflux and apneic spells.[68-74] As mentioned earlier, these studies are limited by the inability of pH monitoring to detect nonacid gastroesophageal reflux. However, a study in which an intraluminal impedance technique was used to detect both acid and nonacid gastroesophageal reflux also failed to demonstrate a correlation between gastroesophageal reflux and apnea.[75] Thus, it is not clear that measures directed toward reducing gastroesophageal reflux will be effective in reducing the frequency or severity of apnea of prematurity.

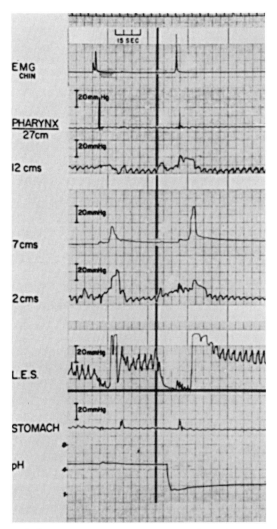

Figure 116–6. Comparison of swallow-induced high-pressure zone (HPZ) lower esophageal sphincter (L.E.S.) relaxation with transient relaxation of the HPZ. The swallow-related HPZ relaxation *(left of the dark vertical line)* is associated with a submental electromyographic (EMG) spike, a pharyngeal contraction, and an esophageal peristaltic contraction. The presence of the esophageal peristaltic contraction prevents the occurrence of gastroesophageal reflux. The *dark vertical line* indicates the start of a transient HPZ relaxation. The relaxation is of longer duration than the swallow-induced HPZ relaxation. An episode of gastroesophageal reflux occurs (esophageal pH falls from 5 to 1) when baseline HPZ pressure approaches 0 and there is no respiratory-related oscillation in HPZ pressure. (From Mittal RK, McCallum RW: Gastroenterology 95:593, 1988. Copyright 1988 by the American Gastroenterological Association.)

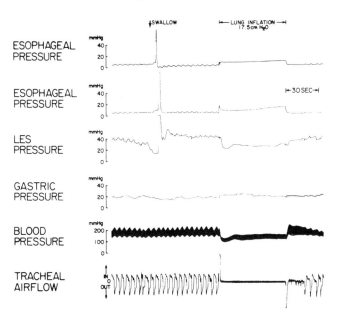

Figure 116–7. Effect of static lung inflation on high-pressure zone (HPZ) lower esophageal sphincter (LES) pressure. Lung inflation induces a reflex relaxation of HPZ pressure that persists for the duration of the stimulus. During the lung inflation, there is no spontaneous respiration and thus an absence of respiratory oscillation in HPZ pressure. The HPZ relaxation induced by lung inflation is not associated with any esophageal motor events. The swallow-induced HPZ relaxation is terminated by a contraction of the LES. (Courtesy of J.T. Boyle, MD.)

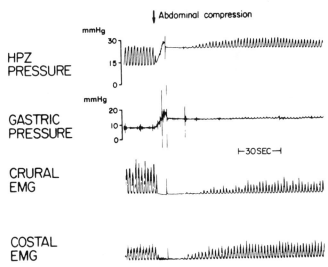

Figure 116–8. Effect of abdominal compression on the high-pressure zone (HPZ) pressure profile. With the onset of abdominal compression, end-expiratory HPZ pressure increases and crural and costal diaphragmatic electromyographic (EMG) activity decreases. The crural diaphragmatic EMG activity remains inhibited for the duration of the stimulus, whereas costal activity returns to baseline levels. As a result of the inhibition of crural EMG activity, there is a decrease in the magnitude of the respiratory-induced oscillations in HPZ pressure. The increase in end-expiratory HPZ pressure is greater than the increase in gastric pressure induced by the abdominal compression, a finding indicating the lower esophageal sphincter has undergone an adaptive response during the period of abdominal compression. (From Boyle JT, et al: Am J Physiol 253:G315, 1987.)

REFERENCES

1. Mittal RK, Balaban DH: The esophagogastric junction. N Engl J Med *336*:924, 1997.
2. Pope CE: A dynamic test of sphincter strength: its application to lower esophageal sphincter. Gastroenterology *52*:799, 1967.
3. Welch RW, Gray JE: Influence of respiration on recordings of lower esophageal sphincter pressure in humans. Gastroenterology *83*:590, 1982.
4. Boyle JT, et al: Role of the diaphragm in genesis of lower esophageal sphincter pressure in the cat. Gastroenterology *88*:723, 1985.
5. Altschuler SM, et al: Simultaneous reflex inhibition of lower esophageal sphincter and crural diaphragm in cats. Am J Physiol *249*:G586, 1985.
6. Winans CS: Alterations of lower esophageal sphincter characteristics with respiration and proximal esophageal balloon distention. Gastroenterology *62*:380, 1972.
7. Dodd WJ, et al: Effect of esophageal movement on intraluminal esophageal pressure recording. Gastroenterology *67*:592, 1974.
8. Dent J, et al: Mechanism of gastroesophageal reflux in recumbent asymptomatic human subjects. J Clin Invest *65*:256, 1980.
9. Dodds WJ, et al: Mechanism of gastroesophageal reflux in patients with reflux esophagitis. N Engl J Med *307*:1547, 1982.
10. Rattan S, Goyal RK: Neural control of the lower esophageal sphincter: influence of the vagus nerves. J Clin Invest *54*:899, 1974.
11. Goyal RJ, Rattan S: Genesis of basal sphincter pressure: effect of tetrodotoxin on lower esophageal sphincter pressure in opossum in vivo. Gastroenterology *71*:62, 1976.
12. Fournet J, et al: Sympathetic control of lower esophageal sphincter function in the cat. J Clin Invest *63*:562, 1979.
13. Biancani P, et al: Lower esophageal sphincter mechanics: anatomic and physiologic relationships of the esophagogastric junction of cat. Gastroenterology *82*:468, 1982.
14. Behar J, et al: Neural control of the lower esophageal sphincter in the cat: studies on the excitatory pathways to the lower esophageal sphincter. Gastroenterology *82*:680, 1982.
15. Reynolds JC, et al: Electrically coupled intrinsic responses of feline lower esophageal sphincter. Am J Physiol *243*:G415, 1982.
16. Robinson BA, et al: Differences in cytochrome c oxidase capacity in smooth muscle of opossum esophagus and lower esophageal sphincter. Gastroenterology *87*:1009, 1984.
17. Biancani P, et al: Vasoactive intestinal polypeptide: a neuro-transmitter of lower esophageal sphincter relaxation. J Clin Invest *73*:963, 1984.
18. Reynold RPE, et al: Lower esophageal sphincter function in the cat: role of central innervation assessed by transient vagal blockage. Am J Physiol *246*:G346, 1984.
19. Reynolds JC, et al: A lower esophageal sphincter reflux involving substance P. Am J Physiol *246*:G346, 1984.
20. Zeleer E, Weisbrat NW: Electrical and mechanical activity in the lower esophageal sphincter of the cat. Am J Physiol *246*:G243, 1984.
21. Holloway RH, et al: Motilin: a mechanism incorporating the opossum lower esophageal sphincter into the migrating motor complex. Gastroenterology *89*:507, 1985.
22. Corazziari E, et al: Effect of bombesin on lower esophageal sphincter pressure in humans. Gastroenterology *83*:10, 1982.
23. Holloway RH, et al: Electrical control activity of the lower esophageal sphincter in unanesthetized opossums. Am J Physiol *252*:G511, 1987.
24. Hillemeir C, et al: Developmental characteristics of the lower esophageal sphincter in the kitten. Gastroenterology *89*:760, 1985.
25. Liu J-B, et al: Transnasal US of the esophagus: preliminary morphologic and function studies. Radiology *184*:721, 1992.
26. Sengupta A, et al: Atypical localization of myenteric neurons in the opossum lower esophageal sphincter. Am J Anat *180*:342, 1987.
27. Thor KD, et al: Reappraisal of the flap valve mechanism in the gastroesophageal junction: a study of a new valvuloplasty procedure in cadavers. Acta Chir Scand *153*:25, 1987.
28. Dent J, et al: Interdigestive phasic contractions of the human lower esophageal sphincter. Gastroenterology *84*:453, 1983.
29. Liebermann-Meffert M, et al: Muscular equivalent of the lower esophageal sphincter. Gastroenterology *76*:31, 1979.
30. Goyal RK, Ratten S: Nature of vagal inhibitory innervation to the lower esophageal sphincter. J Clin Invest *55*:1119, 1975.
31. Klein WA, et al: Sphincterlike thoracoabdominal high pressure zone after esophagogastrectomy. Gastroenterology *105*:1362, 1993.
32. Duron B: Inhibitory reflex from the oesophagus to the crura of the diaphragm. Bull Physiol Pathol Respir *11*:105, 1975.
33. Harding R, Titchen DA: Oesophageal and diaphragmatic activity during sucking in lambs. J Physiol (Lond) *321*:317, 1981.
34. Detroyer A, Rosso J: Reflex inhibition of the diaphragm by esophageal afferent. Neurosci Lett *30*:43, 1982.
35. Monges H, et al: Dissociation between the electrical activity of the diaphragmatic dome and crural muscular fibers during esophageal distention, vomiting and eructation. An electromyographic study in the dog. J Physiol Paris *64*:541, 1978.
36. Mittal RK, et al: Electrical and mechanical inhibition of the crural diaphragm during transient relaxation of the lower esophageal sphincter. Gastroenterology *96*:A347, 1989.
37. Tan LK, Miller AD: Innervation of periesophageal region of the cat's diaphragm: implication for studies of control of vomiting. Neurosci Lett *68*:339, 1986.
38. Titchen DA: Diaphragmatic and oesophageal activity in regurgitation in sheep: an electromyographic study. J Physiol (Lond) *292*:381, 1979.
39. Mittal RK, et al: Human lower esophageal sphincter pressure response to increased intra-abdominal pressure. Am J Physiol *258*:G624, 1990.
40. Dodds WJ: Instrumentation and methodology for intraluminal esophageal manometry. Arch Intern Med *136*:513, 1976.
41. Dodds WJ: Movement of the feline esophagus associated with respiration and peristalsis: an evaluation using tantalum markers. J Clin Invest *52*:1, 1973.
42. Dent J: A new technique for continuous sphincter pressure measurement. Gastroenterology *72*:263, 1976.
43. Dent J, et al: Factors that influence induction of gastroesophageal reflux in normal human subjects. Dig Dis Sci 33:270, 1988.
44. Dent J, et al: Interdigestive phasic contraction of the human lower esophageal sphincter. Gastroenterology *84*:453, 1983.
45. Linchan JH, et al: Sleeve device functions as a Starling resistor to record sphincter pressure. Am J Physiol *248*:G251, 1985.
46. Werlin SL, et al: Mechanisms of gastroesophageal reflux in children. J Pediatr *97*:244, 1980.
47. Williams TA, et al: Mechanisms of gastroesophageal reflux in recumbent neurologically impaired children. Gastroenterology *96*:547, 1989.
48. Holloway RH, et al: Gastric distention: a mechanism for post-prandial gastroesophageal reflux. Gastroenterology *89*:779, 1985.
49. Kahrilas PJ, et al: Upper esophageal sphincter function during belching. Gastroenterology *91*:133, 1986.
50. Wyman JB, et al: Control of belching by the lower esophageal sphincter. Gut *31*:639, 1990.
51. Mittal RK, et al: Transient lower esophageal sphincter relaxation. Gastroenterology *109*:601, 1995.
52. Mittal RK, McCallum RW: Characteristics and frequency of transient relaxations of the lower esophageal sphincter in patients with reflux esophagitis. Gastroenterology *95*:543, 1988.
53. Mittal RK, McCallum RW: Characteristics and frequency of lower esophageal sphincter relaxations in humans. Am J Physiol *252*:G636, 1987.
54. Longhi EH, Jordan PH Jr: Pressure relationships responsible for reflux in patients with hiatal hernia. Surg Gynecol Obstet *129*:734, 1969.
55. Paterson WG, et al: Experimental induction of isolated lower esophageal sphincter relaxation in anesthetized opossums. J Clin Invest *77*:1187, 1986.
56. Holloway RH, et al: Gastric distention: a mechanism for postprandial gastroesophageal reflux. Gastroenterology *89*:779, 1985.
57. Werlin SL, et al: Mechanisms of gastroesophageal reflux in children. J Pediatr *97*:244, 1980.
58. Sutphen JL, Dillard VL: Dietary caloric density and osmolality influence gastroesophageal reflux in infants. Gastroenterology *97*:601, 1989.
59. DiLorenzo C, et al: Gastric emptying with gastro-esophageal reflux. Arch Dis Child *62*:449, 1987.
60. Boyle JT, et al: Responses of feline gastroesophageal junction to changes in abdominal pressure. Am J Physiol *253*:G315, 1987.
61. Strawczynski H, et al: The behavior of the lower esophageal sphincter in infants and its relationship to gastroesophageal regurgitation. J Pediatr *64*:17, 1964.
62. Cohen S: Developmental characteristics of lower esophageal sphincter function: a possible mechanism for infantile chalasia. Gastroenterology *67*:252, 1974.
63. Martin AJ, et al: Natural history and familial relationships of infant spilling to 9 years of age. Pediatrics *109*:1061, 2002.
64. Omari TI, et al: Esophageal body and lower esophageal sphincter function in healthy premature infants. Gastroenterology *109*:1757, 1995.
65. Omari TI, et al: Characterisation of relaxation of the lower oesophageal sphincter in healthy premature infants. Gut *40*:370, 1997.
66. Kawahara H, et al: Mechanisms responsible for gastroesophageal reflux in children. Gastroenterology *113*:399, 1997.
67. Omari T, et al: Mechanism of gastroesophageal reflux in premature infants with chronic lung disease. J Pediatr Surg *34*:1795, 1999.
68. Walsh KJ, et al: Gastroesophageal reflux in infants: relation to apnea. J Pediatrics *99*:197, 1981.
69. Newell SJ, et al: Gastroesophageal reflux in preterm infants. Arch Dis Child *64*:780, 1989.
70. Kahn A, et al: Sleep apneas in acid esophageal reflux in control infants and in infants with apparent life-threatening events. Biol Neonate *57*:144, 1990.
71. Paton JY, et al: Observations on gastro-oesophageal reflux, central apnoea and heart rate in infants. Eur J Pediatr *149*:608, 1990.
72. de Ajuriaguerra M, et al: Gastroesophageal reflux and apnea in prematurely born infants during wakefulness and sleep. Am J Dis Child *145*:1132, 1991.
73. Arad-Cohen N, et al: The relationship between gastroesophageal reflux and apnea in infants. J Pediatr *137*:321, 2000.
74. Peter CS, et al: Gastroesophageal reflux and apnea of prematurity: no temporal relationship. Pediatrics *109*:8, 2002.
75. Barrington KJ, et al: Apnea at discharge and gastro-esophageal reflux in the preterm infant. J Perinatol *22*:8, 2002.

Michael S. Caplan

Pathophysiology and Prevention of Neonatal Necrotizing Enterocolitis

Neonatal necrotizing enterocolitis (NEC) is an ischemic and inflammatory necrosis of bowel that primarily afflicts premature neonates after the initiation of enteral feeding.[1] Despite the significant morbidity and mortality associated with NEC, the pathophysiology has remained poorly understood. The disease presents clinically in premature neonates with variable symptoms of intestinal bleeding, emesis, abdominal distention, lethargy, apnea, and bradycardia and with signs of abdominal tenderness, thrombocytopenia, metabolic acidosis, tachycardia, respiratory failure, and, if severe, shock.[2] Clues to the origin are suggested by the pathologic changes observed in surgical specimens and autopsy material, including coagulation necrosis (suggesting some component of ischemic injury), inflammation (acute or chronic), and, less commonly, ulceration, hemorrhage, reparative change, bacterial overgrowth, edema, and pneumatosis intestinalis.[3]

Whereas most cases of NEC are diagnosed in premature neonates, full-term infants with specific underlying risk factors are at risk of developing this disease.[4-7] Previous studies have identified birth asphyxia, polycythemia, exchange transfusion, intrauterine growth restriction, cyanotic congenital heart disease, myelomeningocele, gastroschisis, and intrauterine cocaine exposure as potential events leading to the development of intestinal injury.[8] Nonetheless, the presentation of NEC in these cases is typically different from that in premature infants, with the onset in the first days after delivery and the course often less dramatic. For these reasons, the pathophysiology in full-term infants may be quite different from that in the premature neonate and will therefore not be considered further in this chapter.

PREMATURITY: THE MAJOR RISK FACTOR FOR NECROTIZING ENTEROCOLITIS

The multifactorial theory has been suggested to explain the pathophysiology of neonatal NEC and purports that several risk factors (prematurity, formula feeding, ischemia or asphyxia, and bacterial colonization) result in the final common pathway of bowel necrosis. More than 90% of cases of NEC occur in premature infants, whereas stratification studies have shown that gestational age and birth weight inversely correlate with a higher incidence of disease.[9-11] Although epidemiologic observations suggest an association of intestinal ischemia, infection, and feeding practice in the development of NEC, the presence of these factors is less consistent than the observation of prematurity. Although there are many differences between preterm and full-term neonates, the specific underlying mechanisms responsible for the predilection of NEC in the premature condition remain incompletely elucidated. Studies in humans and animals have identified alterations in multiple components of intestinal host defense,[12-14] motility,[15-18] bacterial colonization,[19-23] blood flow regulation,[24-26] and inflammatory response,[27-29] and these may contribute to the development of intestinal injury in this unique population (Table 117-1).

Host Defense

Intestinal *host defense* involves a complex combination of factors that function to prevent intraluminal pathogens and toxins from

---

TABLE 117-1

Premature Infant: Factors that May Increase Susceptibility to Necrotizing Enterocolitis

Compromised Intestinal Host Defense
Physical barriers
  Skin
  Mucus membranes
  Epithelia or microvilli
  Tight junctions
  Mucin
Immune factors
  Neutrophils
  Macrophages
  Eosinophils
  Lymphocytes (including intraepithelial lymphocytes)
  Secretory immunglobulin A
Biochemical factors
  Antimicrobial proteins (trefoil factor, defensins/crytidins)
  Oligosaccharides
  Glutamine
  Lactoferrin
  Polyunsaturated fatty acids
  Nucleotides
  Growth factors (epidermal growth factor, transforming growth factor, insulin-like growth, factor, erythropoeitin)
  Gastric acid
  Cytokines

Intestinal Dysmotility
Migratory motor complexes

Bacteria
Patterns of colonization or overgrowth
Pathogenicity of organisms

Altered Autoregulation of Intestinal Circulation
Basal vascular resistance
Response to stress

Disordered Inflammatory Response
Increased proinflammatory response to stimuli
Suppressed antiinflammatory components

---

resulting in disease while allowing for normal absorption of nutrients. This intricate system includes the following: (1) physical barriers such as skin, mucus membranes, intestinal epithelia and microvilli, epithelial cell tight junctions, and mucin; (2) immune cells such as polymorphonuclear leukocytes, macrophages, eosinophils, and lymphocytes, and secretory immunoglobulin A (IgA); and (3) various biochemical factors.[14, 30-38] Although not exhaustively studied, many of these important functions appear to be abnormal in the premature infant and may therefore put this population at risk for NEC. Intestinal permeability to macromolecules including immunoglobulins, proteins, and carbohydrates is known to be greater in neonates compared with older children and adults, and in premature infants this permeability may be more pronounced.[36, 39] Although mucosal permeability is beneficial for developing animals to augment passive immunity and nutrient absorption, the precise mechanisms accounting for these differences are poorly understood. The microvilli and tight junctional barrier may be deficient in the premature infant, but the data are inconclusive.[40] It is known that intestinal mucus, a complex gel consisting of water, electrolytes, mucins, glycoprotein, immunoglobulins, and glycolipids, protects against bacterial and toxin invasion, and it is abnormal in developing animals and perhaps premature infants.[32,41] Additionally, key bacteriostatic proteins are secreted from epithelium that bind to or inactivate the function of invading organisms. Intestinal trefoil factor is one such molecule that appears to be developmentally regulated and therefore deficient in the premature neonate.[42-44] Human defensins (or cryptidins) are bacteriostatic proteins synthesized and secreted from Paneth cells that protect against bacterial translocation and are altered in premature infants and those with NEC.[45,46]

Immunologic host defense is abnormal in developing animals.[47-49] It is known that intestinal lymphocytes are decreased in neonates (B and T cells) and do not approach adult levels until 3 to 4 weeks of life. Newborns have markedly reduced secretory IgA in salivary samples, reflecting the decreased activity presumed in intestine.[50,51] Breast milk feeding provides significant supplementation; formula-fed neonates have impaired intestinal humoral immunity, and this deficiency may predispose to the increased incidence of infectious diseases noted in this population.[52,53] A complete review on the importance of breast milk on immunologic host defense can be found in Chapter 163, and additional detail on developmental immunobiology is included in Chapters 151 to 161 of this textbook.

Several biochemical factors that are present in the intestinal milieu play an important role in the maintenance of gut health and integrity. Substances such as lactoferrin,[54] glutamine,[55,56] growth factors such as epidermal growth factor,[27] transforming growth factor-β,[57] insulin-like growth factor,[58] and erythropoietin,[59,60] gastric acid, oligosaccharides,[61] polyunsaturated fatty acids,[62,63] nucleotides,[64] and many others affect mucosal barrier function, intestinal inflammation, and the viability of intraluminal bacteria. Many of these factors are deficient or absent in the preterm neonate, especially in those patients not receiving breast milk feedings. Intensive research is ongoing to define the specific role of each on gut integrity and the development of intestinal inflammation and necrosis.

Motility

The premature infant has altered gastrointestinal motility; full-term newborn motility patterns or *migratory motor complexes* do not appear until 34 to 35 weeks' gestation.[15,65] Abnormal peristaltic activity may allow for bacterial overgrowth that could increase endotoxin exposure and predispose the infant to NEC. Furthermore, dysmotility causes intestinal dilatation and compromised intestinal blood flow, with further ischemic stress to compromised intestinal circulation.

Bacterial Colonization

Premature infants hospitalized in the neonatal intensive care unit have different patterns of gut bacterial colonization than healthy breast-fed term infants.[66] Although there have been epidemics of NEC described associated with specific bacteria (e.g., *Clostridium* sp., *Escherichia coli*, *Klebsiella* sp., *Staphylococcus epidermidis*), most cases occur endemically and demonstrate a variety of bacterial isolates from stool cultures.[23,67] Blood cultures are positive in only 20 to 30% of affected cases, and this likely represents the degree of mucosal damage at presentation. At birth, the intestine is a sterile environment, and no cases of NEC have been described *in utero,* a finding supporting the importance of bacterial colonization in the pathophysiology. Breast-fed infants develop colonization by several species by 1 week of age that includes anaerobic species of bifidobacteria and lactobacilli,

whereas the hospitalized, extremely premature infant intestine has less species diversity and fewer anaerobes.[53,68-70] This imbalance may allow for pathologic proliferation, binding, and invasiveness of otherwise nonpathogenic intestinal bacteria. It remains unclear whether bacterial translocation into submucosa is a prerequisite for disease or, rather, the activation of the Toll-like receptors from endotoxin and other bacterial cell wall products is adequate to initiate the final common pathway of intestinal injury.[21,71-73] Nonetheless, certain bacteria such as adherent *E. coli* produce disease in a rabbit model of NEC, whereas nonpathogenic strains of gram-positive organisms prevent disease.[74] Furthermore, preliminary work has suggested that early colonization by probiotics (facultative anaerobes, such as bifidobacteria and lactobacilli) reduces the risk of NEC in animal and human studies.[19,75] In summary, bacterial colonization is an important factor in the initiation of intestinal injury, but the specific events in the pathophysiology are not well delineated.

Intestinal Blood Flow Regulation

Early observations on the pathophysiology of NEC suggested that profound intestinal ischemia was a critical predisposing factor.[76,77] Similar to the diving reflex observed in aquatic mammals, it was hypothesized that in periods of stress, blood flow was diverted away from the splanchnic circulation, with resulting intestinal necrosis. Although early epidemiologic observations identified asphyxia as an important risk factor, subsequent studies have shown that most cases of NEC are not associated with profound impairment in intestinal perfusion.[2] In animal models, studies have shown that the reperfusion after intestinal ischemia is required in the initiation of bowel necrosis,[78,79] and, therefore, experimentation on the role of intestinal ischemia on the pathophysiology of NEC is focused on this construct.

Neonatal animals have been shown to have differences in the intestinal circulation that may predispose them to NEC. The basal intestinal vascular resistance is elevated in the fetus and decreases significantly soon after birth, thus allowing for rapid increase in intestinal blood flow.[24] Intestinal and somatic growth is dramatic in developing animals, and therefore sufficient flow is mandatory. Investigators have shown that this change in the resting vascular resistance is dependent on the balance between the dilator (nitric oxide) and constrictor (endothelin) molecules and the myogenic response.[80,81] Perhaps more relevant than basal vascular tone, studies have shown that the newborn has alterations in response to circulatory stress, resulting in compromised intestinal flow or vascular resistance. In response to hypotension, newborn animals (3-day-old but not 30-day-old swine) appear to have defective pressure-flow autoregulation, resulting in compromised intestinal oxygen delivery and tissue oxygenation.[25,26,82] In addition, in the presence of arterial hypoxemia, the newborn intestinal circulatory response differs from that in older animals. Although intestinal vasodilation and increased intestinal perfusion occur after modest hypoxemia, severe hypoxemia causes vasoconstriction, intestinal ischemia, and hypoxia, mediated in part by loss of nitric oxide production. There are multiple chemical mediators (nitric oxide, endothelin, substance P, norepinephrine, and angiotensin) that affect intestinal vasomotor tone, and in the stressed newborn, abnormal production of these mediators may result in compromised circulatory autoregulation, leading to perpetuation of intestinal ischemia and tissue necrosis.[83-85]

Enteral Alimentation

Enteral alimentation has long been considered an important risk factor on the initiation of NEC; more than 90% of cases presented in premature infants after feedings were introduced. Although the onset of disease used to occur several days after the first feeding, in reports of extremely low birth weight infants from the 1990s, NEC was often diagnosed several weeks later.[9, 86] Whereas the precise relationship between enteral feedings and NEC remains poorly understood, studies have identified the importance of breast milk (versus formula), the volume and rate of feeding advancement, osmolality, and substrate fermentation as important factors.[87-90]

Breast milk feeding appears to reduce the incidence of NEC in human studies and in carefully controlled animal models.[11, 20] Breast milk contains multiple bioactive factors that influence host immunity, inflammation, and mucosal protection including secretory IgA, leukocytes, lactoferrin, lysozyme, mucin, cytokines, growth factors, enzymes, oligosaccharides, and polyunsaturated fatty acids, which are absent in neonatal formula preparations and are discussed in detail in Chapter 163. Specific intestinal host defense factors acquired from breast milk such as epidermal growth factor, polyunsaturated fatty acids, platelet-activating factor (PAF) acetylhydrolase, IgA, and macrophages are effective in reducing the incidence of disease in animals,[27,62,91,92] and some of these factors have been effective in human trials.[51, 63] Nonetheless, breast milk is not completely protective against NEC in premature infants; the largest prospective trial identified a reduction by 50% in most birth weight–specific groups.[11, 93] Because most premature infants receive breast milk by the nasogastric route after artificial collection by mothers and subsequent freezing, it has been suggested that the lack of the normal maternal-infant physical interaction during feeding interferes with specific milk immunity and thereby reduces the protection against the neonate's microbial flora.

Specific components of milk feedings have been implicated to cause mucosal injury in the high-risk neonate. Studies have shown that hyperosmolar formula resulted in NEC, and the addition of medication to feedings can markedly increase osmolality.[94, 95] Animal studies have shown that short chain fatty acids such as propionic or butyric acid can damage developing intestine, and colonic fermentation leading to production of these acids by the host microflora may occur in situations of carbohydrate malabsorption.[96-98] This pathway may be especially problematic in the premature infant, deficient in lactase activity and other brush-border enzymes.

Different approaches to feeding have been associated with the initiation of NEC. Early studies suggested that rapid volume increases with full-strength formula made the incidence of disease more prevalent, and protocols were designed to limit feeding advancement. Several studies have shown that early, hypocaloric, or trophic feedings are safe and improve gastrointestinal function in very low birth weight infants.[99-102] Feeding advancement has been evaluated, and the results suggest that judicious volume increase may be safer. It has been postulated that overdistention of the stomach with aggressive volumes may compromise splanchnic circulation and may lead to intestinal ischemia.

In summary, the premature neonate has several unique features that may increase susceptibility to NEC, but the precise interrelationship of these factors in the final common pathway of intestinal necrosis remains unclear.

FINAL COMMON PATHWAY: THE INFLAMMATORY CASCADE

Based on a growing body of evidence obtained from humans and from animal and tissue experimentation, the final common pathway of intestinal injury appears to result from the activation of the inflammatory cascade.[38, 103, 104] This cascade involves a complex balance of proinflammatory and antiinflammatory endogenous mediators, receptors, signaling pathways, second messengers, and a variety of downstream effects that ultimately results in end-organ damage in certain circumstances (Fig. 117-1).

Inflammation can be initiated by a variety of factors, most notably the exposure to the bacterial cell wall product, endotoxin. After endotoxin stimulation of the Toll receptor family in animals, tissue, or cells, several mediators are rapidly produced, including PAF, tumor necrosis factor, and interleukin-1 (IL-1).[105-109] In intestine, subsequent events lead to chemotaxis, transmigration, and activation of leukocytes and to synthesis and release of many products from epithelial and inflammatory cells such as IL-6, IL-8, IL-10, IL-18, arachidonic acid metabolites, thromboxanes, leukotrienes, prostaglandins, nitric oxide, endothelin-1, and oxygen free radicals.[110-117] If counterregulatory responses are insufficient, pathologic changes to gut mucosa occur and may include accentuated apoptosis of epithelial cells, perturbation of tight junctional proteins and complexes, increased mucosal permeability, bacterial translocation, alterations of vascular tone and microcirculation, and additional neutrophil infiltration and accumulation. The process may then be perpetuated by the activation of the secondary inflammatory response, and the final common pathway will result in intestinal necrosis. Whereas these events remain localized in some cases, in others this activation results in the systemic inflammatory response syndrome, in which patients develop capillary leak, hypotension, metabolic acidosis, thrombocytopenia, renal failure, respiratory failure, and, often, death.[118]

Although endotoxin is a well-characterized activator of inflammation, additional factors may play a role in stimulating the NEC cascade in premature infants. Asphyxia or ischemia-reperfusion activates the early mediators of inflammation in many tissues including intestine. Neonatal animal studies have shown that the stress of formula feeding with hypoxia stimulates phospholipase A_2 gene expression, intestinal PAF production, and stimulation of apoptosis and the inflammatory response with resulting NEC.[104, 119] Therefore, many of the purported risk factors for NEC may activate the inflammatory response that results in the final common pathway described earlier.

The evidence suggests that the premature neonate may have an abnormal balance between proinflammatory and antiinflammatory mediator production, thereby increasing the predisposition for diseases such as NEC. PAF is a potent phospholipid inflammatory mediator that is associated with NEC in several experimental models and human analyses.[120-124] PAF infusion causes intestinal necrosis in animals, and PAF receptor antagonists prevent injury after hypoxia, endotoxin challenge, tumor necrosis factor infusion, and ischemia-reperfusion.[125-127] It has been shown that neonates are markedly deficient in their ability to degrade PAF because of decreased activity of the PAF-specific enzyme PAF acetylhydrolase.[28] PAF acetylhydrolase is present in breast milk but absent in commercial formula, and this may in part explain the beneficial effects of breast milk feeding. IL-10 is an antiinflammatory cytokine thought to be important in reducing intestinal inflammation and possibly NEC in animals and humans.[128, 129] In neonatal rats, maternal milk feedings increased IL-10 and reduced the incidence of NEC, whereas in human milk specimens, significant percentages of NEC patient-pairs were deficient in this important cytokine. Studies have compared proinflammatory response to endotoxin and IL-1 in different cell lines and have found that IL-8 response is significantly higher in fetal intestinal epithelium compared with mature, adult intestine.[29] These results suggest that the neonatal balance of the inflammatory response may be weighted toward the proinflammatory side and is more likely to result in the pathologic outcome of NEC.

In conclusion, NEC is a multifactorial disease without one clear and precise cause. The well-described epidemiologic risk factors including bacterial colonization, intestinal ischemia or hypoxia, and formula feeding stimulate a final common pathway that results in intestinal injury in a subset of premature infants. Premature infants differ from term infants and older patients in multiple ways, including the complex system of intestinal host

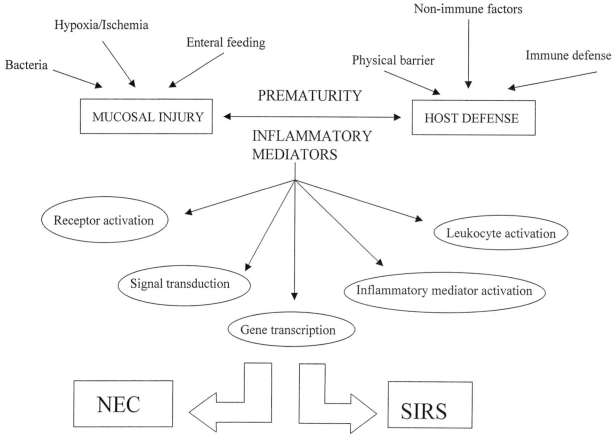

Figure 117–1. Hypothetical events leading to the final common pathway of inflammatory mediator activation and necrotizing enterocolitis (NEC) in premature infants. Note the important balance between host defense and mucosal injury in the pathway. SIRS = systemic inflammatory response syndrome.

TABLE 117-2

Published Reports of Successful Strategies to Prevent Intestinal Injury or Necrotizing Enterocolitis

Animals	Humans
Breast milk	Breast milk
Immunoglobulin A	Immunoglobulins A and G
Steroids	Steroids
Probiotics	Probiotics
Polyunsaturated fatty acids	Polyunsaturated fatty acids
Antibiotics	Antibiotics
Platelet-activating factor acetylhydrolase	
Trefoil factor	
Epidermal growth factor	
Platelet-activating factor receptor antagonists	
Leukocyte depletion	
Oxygen radical scavengers	

defense, intestinal motility, bacterial colonization patterns, autoregulation of splanchnic blood flow, and the regulation of the inflammatory cascade. Because each case of NEC is different, and the importance of each of the complex factors may vary between cases, no single approach has been completely successful in preventing this dreaded disease. Although preventing prematurity would be the most successful approach to preventing NEC, several strategies have been tested in humans and animals, with intriguing results (Table 117-2). Future trials in high-risk premature infants will be needed to reduce

significantly this morbidity and mortality that currently plague neonatal intensive care units worldwide.

REFERENCES

1. Caplan MS, MacKendrick W. Necrotizing enterocolitis: a review of patho-genetic mechanisms and implications for prevention. Pediatr Pathol *13*:357-69, 1993.
2. Walsh MC, Kliegman RM. Necrotizing enterocolitis: treatment based on staging criteria. Pediatr Clin North Am *33*:179-201, 1986.
3. Ballance WA, et al. Pathology of neonatal necrotizing enterocolitis: a ten-year experience. J Pediatr *117*:S6-13, 1990.
4. Rodin AE, et al. Necrotizing enterocolitis occurring in full-term neonates at birth. Arch Pathol *96*:335-8, 1973.
5. Wiswell TE, et al. Necrotizing enterocolitis in full-term infants: a case-control study. Am J Dis Child *142*:532-5, 1988.
6. Martinez-Tallo E, et al. Necrotizing enterocolitis in full-term or near-term infants: risk factors. Biol Neonate *71*:292-8, 1997.
7. Bolisetty S, Lui K. Necrotizing enterocolitis in full-term neonates. J Paediatr Child Health *37*:413-4, 2001.
8. Lopez SL, et al. Time of onset of necrotizing enterocolitis in newborn infants with known prenatal cocaine exposure. Clin Pediatr *34*:424-9, 1995.
9. Uauy RD, et al. Necrotizing enterocolitis in very low birth weight infants: biodemographic and clinical correlates. National Institute of Child Health and Human Development Neonatal Research Network. J Pediatr *119*:630-8, 1991.
10. Ryder RW, et al. Necrotizing enterocolitis: a prospective multicenter investi-gation. Am J Epidemiol *112*:113-23, 1980.
11. Lucas A, Cole TJ. Breast milk and neonatal necrotising enterocolitis Lancet *336*:1519-23, 1990.
12. Furlano RI, Walker WA. Immaturity of gastrointestinal host defense in new-borns and gastrointestinal disease states. Adv Pediatr *45*:201-22, 1998.
13. Bines JE, Walker WA. Growth factors and the development of neonatal host defense. Adv Exp Med Biol *310*:31-9, 1991.
14. Walker WA. Role of nutrients and bacterial colonization in the development of intestinal host defense. J Pediatr Gastroenterol Nutr *30*:S2-7, 2000.

15. Berseth CL. Gestational evolution of small intestine motility in preterm and term infants. J Pediatr *115*:646-51, 1989.
16. Berseth CL. Neonatal small intestinal motility: motor responses to feeding in term and preterm infants. J Pediatr *117*:777-82, 1990.
17. Berseth CL. Gut motility and the pathogenesis of necrotizing enterocolitis. Clin Perinatol *21*:263-70, 1994.
18. Bueno L, Ruckebusch Y. Perinatal development of intestinal myoelectrical activity in dogs and sheep. Am J Physiol *237*:E61-7, 1979.
19. Caplan MS, et al. Bifidobacterial supplementation reduces the incidence of necrotizing enterocolitis in a neonatal rat model. Gastroenterology *117*:577-83, 1999.
20. Caplan MS, et al. Role of asphyxia and feeding in a neonatal rat model of necrotizing enterocolitis. Pediatr Pathol *14*:1017-28, 1994.
21. Deitch EA. Role of bacterial translocation in necrotizing enterocolitis. Acta Paediatr Suppl *396*:33-6, 1994.
22. Duffy LC, et al. Concordance of bacterial cultures with endotoxin and interleukin-6 in necrotizing enterocolitis. Dig Dis Sci *42*:359-65, 1997.
23. Duffy LC, et al. Bacterial toxins and enteral feeding of premature infants at risk for necrotizing enterocolitis. Adv Exp Med Biol *501*:519-27, 2001.
24. Nowicki PT, Miller CE. Autoregulation in the developing postnatal intestinal circulation. Am J Physiol *254*:G189-93, 1988.
25. Nowicki PT, et al. Effects of ischemia and reperfusion on intrinsic vascular regulation in the postnatal intestinal circulation. Pediatr. Res. 1993;33:400-4.
26. Nowicki PT. Effects of sustained flow reduction on postnatal intestinal circulation. Am J Physiol *275*:G758-68, 1998.
27. Dvorak B, et al. Epidermal growth factor reduces the development of necrotizing enterocolitis in a neonatal rat model. Am J Physiol *282*:G156-64, 2002.
28. Caplan M, et al. Serum PAF acetylhydrolase increases during neonatal maturation. Prostaglandins *39*:705-14, 1990.
29. Nanthakumar NN, et al. Inflammation in the developing human intestine: a possible pathophysiologic contribution to necrotizing enterocolitis. Proc Natl Acad Sci U S A *97*:6043-8, 2000.
30. Haller D, et al. Non-pathogenic bacteria elicit a differential cytokine response by intestinal epithelial cell/leucocyte co-cultures. Gut *47*:79-87, 2000.
31. Kagnoff MF. Immunology of the intestinal tract. Gastroenterology *105*:1275-80, 1993.
32. Laboisse CL. Structure of gastrointestinal mucins: searching for the Rosetta stone. Biochimie *68*:611-7, 1986.
33. Pang KY, et al. Development of the gastrointestinal mucosal barrier. V. Comparative effect of calcium binding on microvillus membrane structure in newborn and adult rats. Pediatr Res *17*:856-61, 1983.
34. Pang KY, et al. Development of the gastrointestinal mucosal barrier: evidence for structural differences in microvillus membranes from newborn and adult rabbits. Biochim Biophys Acta *727*:201-8, 1983.
35. Pang KY, et al. Development of gastrointestinal mucosal barrier. VII. In utero maturation of microvillus surface by cortisone. Am J Physiol *249*:G85-91, 1985.
36. Udall JN, et al. Development of gastrointestinal mucosal barrier. I. The effect of age on intestinal permeability to macromolecules. Pediatr Res *15*:241-4, 1981.
37. Udall JN, Jr. Gastrointestinal host defense and necrotizing enterocolitis. J Pediatr *117*:S33-43, 1990.
38. Hsueh W, et al. Platelet-activating factor, tumor necrosis factor, hypoxia and necrotizing enterocolitis. Acta Paediatr Suppl *396*:11-7, 1994.
39. Weaver LT, Laker MF, Nelson R. Intestinal permeability in the newborn. Arch Dis Child *59*:236-41, 1984.
40. Smith SD, et al. Unique characteristics of the neonatal intestinal mucosal barrier. J Pediatr Surg *27*:333-6, 1992.
41. Snyder JD, Walker WA. Structure and function of intestinal mucin: developmental aspects. Int Arch Allergy Appl Immunol *82*:351-6, 1987.
42. Lin J, et al. Expression of intestinal trefoil factor in developing rat intestine. Biol Neonate *76*:92-7, 1999.
43. Sands BE, Podolsky DK. The trefoil peptide family. Annu Rev Physiol *58*:253-73, 1996.
44. Tan XD, et al. Characterization of a putative receptor for intestinal trefoil factor in rat small intestine: identification by in situ binding and ligand blotting. Biochem Biophys Res Commun *237*:673-7, 1997.
45. Salzman NH, et al. Enteric defensin expression in necrotizing enterocolitis. Pediatr Res *44*:20-6, 1998.
46. Ouellette AJ. Paneth cells and innate immunity in the crypt microenvironment. Gastroenterology *113*:1779-84, 1997.
47. Guy-Grand D, et al. The mouse gut T lymphocyte, a novel type of T cell: nature, origin, and traffic in mice in normal and graft-versus-host conditions. J Exp Med *148*:1661-77, 1978.
48. Rieger CH, Rothberg RM. Development of the capacity to produce specific antibody to an ingested food antigen in the premature infant. J Pediatr *87*:515-8, 1975.
49. Perkkio M, Savilahti E. Time of appearance of immunoglobulin-containing cells in the mucosa of the neonatal intestine. Pediatr Res *14*:953-5, 1980.
50. Roberts SA, Freed DL. Neonatal IgA secretion enhanced by breast feeding. Lancet *2*:1131, 1977.
51. Eibl MM, et al. Prevention of necrotizing enterocolitis in low-birth-weight infants by IgA-IgG feeding. N Engl J Med *319*:1-7, 1988.
52. Villalpando S, Hamosh M. Early and late effects of breast-feeding: does breast-feeding really matter? Biol Neonate *74*:177-91, 1998.
53. Wold AE, Adlerberth I. Breast feeding and the intestinal microflora of the infant: implications for protection against infectious diseases. Adv Exp Med Biol *478*:77-93, 2000.
54. Lee WJ, et al. The protective effects of lactoferrin feeding against endotoxin lethal shock in germfree piglets. Infect Immun *66*:1421-6, 1998.
55. Neu J, et al. Enteral glutamine supplementation for very low birth weight infants decreases morbidity. J Pediatr *131*:691-9, 1997.
56. Neu J, et al. Glutamine: clinical applications and mechanisms of action. Curr Opin Clin Nutr Metab Care *5*:69-75, 2002.
57. Neurath MF, et al. Experimental granulomatous colitis in mice is abrogated by induction of TGF-beta-mediated oral tolerance. J Exp Med *183*:2605-16, 1996.
58. Riegler M, et al. Effect of growth factors on epithelial restitution of human colonic mucosa in vitro. Scand J Gastroenterol *32*:925-32, 1997.
59. Juul SE, et al. Why is erythropoietin present in human milk? Studies of erythropoietin receptors on enterocytes of human and rat neonates. Pediatr Res *46*:263-8, 1999.
60. Ledbetter DJ, Juul SE. Erythropoietin and the incidence of necrotizing enterocolitis in infants with very low birth weight. J Pediatr Surg *35*:178-81, 2000.
61. Dai D, et al. Role of oligosaccharides and glycoconjugates in intestinal host defense. J Pediatr Gastroenterol Nutr *30*:S23-33, 2000.
62. Caplan MS, et al. Effect of polyunsaturated fatty acid (PUFA) supplementation on intestinal inflammation and necrotizing enterocolitis (NEC) in a neonatal rat model. Pediatr Res *49*:647-52, 2001.
63. Carlson SE, et al. Lower incidence of necrotizing enterocolitis in infants fed a preterm formula with egg phospholipids. Pediatr Res *44*:491-8, 1998.
64. Tanaka M, et al. Exogenous nucleotides alter the proliferation, differentiation and apoptosis of human small intestinal epithelium. J Nutr *126*:424-33, 1996.
65. Bisset WM, et al. Ontogeny of fasting small intestinal motor activity in the human infant. Gut *29*:483-8, 1988.
66. Lawrence G, et al. Pathogenesis of neonatal necrotising enterocolitis. Lancet. *1*:137-9, 1982.
67. Peter CS, et al. Necrotising enterocolitis: is there a relationship to specific pathogens? Eur J Pediatr *158*:67-70, 1999.
68. Tomkins AM, et al. Diet and the faecal microflora of infants, children and adults in rural Nigeria and urban U.K. J Hyg (Lond) *86*:285-93, 1981.
69. Rubaltelli FF, et al. Intestinal flora in breast- and bottle-fed infants. J Perinat Med *26*:186-91, 1998.
70. Gewolb IH, et al. Stool microflora in extremely low birthweight infants. Arch Dis Child Fetal Neonatal Ed *80*:F167-73, 1999.
71. Yoshimura A, et al. Cutting edge: recognition of gram-positive bacterial cell wall components by the innate immune system occurs via Toll-like receptor 2. J Immunol *163*:1-5, 1999.
72. Deitch EA, et al. Endotoxin-induced bacterial translocation and mucosal permeability: role of xanthine oxidase, complement activation, and macrophage products. Crit Care Med *19*:785-91, 1991.
73. Birchler T, et al. Human Toll-like receptor 2 mediates induction of the antimicrobial peptide human beta-defensin 2 in response to bacterial lipoprotein. Eur J Immunol *31*:3131-7, 2001.
74. Panigrahi P, et al. Occurrence of necrotizing enterocolitis may be dependent on patterns of bacterial adherence and intestinal colonization: studies in Caco-2 tissue culture and weanling rabbit models. Pediatr Res *36*:115-21, 1994.
75. Hoyos AB. Reduced incidence of necrotizing enterocolitis associated with enteral administration of Lactobacillus acidophilus and Bifidobacterium infantis to neonates in an intensive care unit. Int J Infect Dis *3*:197-202, 1999.
76. Alward CT, et al. Effects of asphyxia on cardiac output and organ blood flow in the newborn piglet. Pediatr Res *12*:824-7, 1978.
77. Touloukian RJ, et al. The pathogenesis of ischemic gastroenterocolitis of the neonate: selective gut mucosal ischemia in asphyxiated neonatal piglets J Pediatr Surg *7*:194-205, 1972.
78. Schoenberg MH, Beger HG. Reperfusion injury after intestinal ischemia. Crit Care Med *21*:1376-86, 1993.
79. Crissinger KD. Animal models of necrotizing enterocolitis. J Pediatr Gastroenterol Nutr *20*:17-22, 1995.
80. Nankervis CA, Nowicki PT. Role of endothelin-1 in regulation of the postnatal intestinal circulation. Am J Physiol *278*:G367-75, 2000.
81. Nankervis CA, Nowicki PT. Role of nitric oxide in regulation of vascular resistance in postnatal intestine. Am J Physiol *268*:G949-58, 1995.
82. Nowicki PT, et al. Intestinal blood flow and O2 uptake during hypoxemia in the newborn piglet. Am J Physiol *251*:G19-24, 1986.
83. Nowicki PT, Minnich LA. Effects of systemic hypotension on postnatal intestinal circulation: role of angiotensin. Am J Physiol *276*:G341-52, 1999.
84. Reber KM, et al. Newborn intestinal circulation: physiology and pathophysiology. Clin Perinatol *29*:23-39, 2002.
85. Nankervis CA, et al. Age-dependent changes in the postnatal intestinal microcirculation. Microcirculation *8*:377-87, 2001.
86. Brown EG, Sweet AY. Preventing necrotizing enterocolitis in neonates. JAMA *240*:2452-4, 1978.
87. Stoll BJ, et al. Epidemiology of necrotizing enterocolitis: a case control study. J Pediatr *96*:447-51, 1980.
88. Kamitsuka MD, et al. The incidence of necrotizing enterocolitis after introducing standardized feeding schedules for infants between 1250 and 2500 grams and less than 35 weeks of gestation. Pediatrics *105*:379-84, 2000.

89. Tyson JE, Kennedy KA. Minimal enteral nutrition for promoting feeding tolerance and preventing morbidity in parenterally fed infants. Cochrane Database Syst Rev 2, 2000.

90. Di Lorenzo M, et al. An intraluminal model of necrotizing enterocolitis in the developing neonatal piglet. J Pediatr Surg 30:1138-42, 1995.

91. Caplan MS, et al. The role of recombinant platelet-activating factor acetylhydrolase in a neonatal rat model of necrotizing enterocolitis. Pediatr Res 42:779-83, 1997.

92. Pitt J, et al. Protection against experimental necrotizing enterocolitis by maternal milk. I. Role of milk leukocytes. Pediatr Res 11:906-9, 1977.

93. Kliegman RM, et al. Necrotizing enterocolitis in neonates fed human milk. J Pediatr 95:450-3, 1979.

94. Willis DM, et al. Unsuspected hyperosmolality of oral solutions contributing to necrotizing enterocolitis in very-low-birth-weight infants. Pediatrics 60:535-8, 1977.

95. White KC, Harkavy KL. Hypertonic formula resulting from added oral medications. Am J Dis Child 136:931-3, 1982.

96. Butel MJ, et al. Clostridial pathogenicity in experimental necrotising enterocolitis in gnotobiotic quails and protective role of bifidobacteria. J Med Microbiol 47:391-9, 1998.

97. Clark DA, et al. Necrotizing enterocolitis: intraluminal biochemistry in human neonates and a rabbit model. Pediatr Res 19:919-21, 1985.

98. Clark DA, Miller MJ. Intraluminal pathogenesis of necrotizing enterocolitis. J Pediatr 117:S64-7, 1990.

99. Dunn L, et al. Beneficial effects of early hypocaloric enteral feeding on neonatal gastrointestinal function: preliminary report of a randomized trial. J Pediatr 112:622-9, 1988.

100. Slagle TA, Gross SJ. Effect of early low-volume enteral substrate on subsequent feeding tolerance in very low birth weight infants. J Pediatr 113:526-31, 1988.

101. Schanler RJ, et al. Feeding strategies for premature infants: randomized trial of gastrointestinal priming and tube-feeding method. Pediatrics 103:434-9, 1999.

102. Troche B, et al. Early minimal feedings promote growth in critically ill premature infants. Biol Neonate 67:172-81, 1995.

103. Caplan MS, MacKendrick W. Inflammatory mediators and intestinal injury. Clin Perinatol 21:235-46, 1994.

104. Caplan MS, Jilling T. New concepts in necrotizing enterocolitis. Curr Opin Pediatr 13:111-5, 2001.

105. O'Neill LA. The interleukin-1 receptor/Toll-like receptor superfamily: signal transduction during inflammation and host defense. Sci STKE 2000:RE1-9, 2000.

106. Medzhitov R. Toll-like receptors and innate immunity. Nat Rev Immunol 1:135-45, 2001.

107. Read RC, Wyllie DH. Toll receptors and sepsis. Curr Opin Crit Care 7:371-5, 2001.

108. Tracey KJ, et al. Shock and tissue injury induced by recombinant human cachectin. Science 234:470-4, 1986.

109. Benveniste J. PAF-acether, an ether phospho-lipid with biological activity. Prog Clin Biol Res 282:73-85, 1988.

110. Hsueh W, et al. Sequential release of leukotrienes and norepinephrine in rat bowel after platelet-activating factor: a mechanistic study of platelet-activating factor-induced bowel necrosis. Gastroenterology 94:1412-8, 1988.

111. Hsueh W, et al. Release of leukotriene C4 by isolated, perfused rat small intestine in response to platelet-activating factor. J Clin Invest 78:108-14, 1986.

112. Cueva JP, Hsueh W. Role of oxygen derived free radicals in platelet activating factor induced bowel necrosis. Gut 29:1207-12, 1988.

113. Ford H, et al. The role of inflammatory cytokines and nitric oxide in the pathogenesis of necrotizing enterocolitis. J Pediatr Surg 32:275-82, 1997.

114. Hammerman C, et al. Amelioration of ischemia-reperfusion injury in rat intestine by pentoxifylline-mediated inhibition of xanthine oxidase. J Pediatr Gastroenterol Nutr 29:69-74, 1999.

115. Wallace JL, et al. Reduction of gastrointestinal injury in acute endotoxic shock by flurbiprofen nitroxybutylester. Eur J Pharmacol 280:63-8, 1995.

116. Tan X, et al. PAF and TNF increase the precursor of NF-kappa B p50 mRNA in mouse intestine: quantitative analysis by competitive PCR. Biochim Biophys Acta 1215:157-62, 1994.

117. Sun X, et al. P-selectin–deficient mice are protected from PAF-induced shock, intestinal injury, and lethality. Am J Physiol 273, 1997.

118. Takakuwa T, et al. Assessment of inflammatory cytokines, nitrate/nitrite, type II phospholipase A2, and soluble adhesion molecules in systemic inflammatory response syndrome. Res Commun Mol Pathol Pharmacol 98:43-52, 1997.

119. Caplan MS, et al. The platelet-activating factor receptor antagonist WEB 2170 prevents neonatal necrotizing enterocolitis in rats. J Pediatr Gastroenterol Nutr 24:296-301, 1997.

120. Caplan MS, et al. Role of platelet activating factor and tumor necrosis factor-alpha in neonatal necrotizing enterocolitis. J Pediatr 116:960-4, 1990.

121. Caplan MS, et al. Hypoxia, PAF, and necrotizing enterocolitis. Lipids. 26:1340-3, 1991.

122. Hsueh W, et al. Platelet-activating factor-induced ischemic bowel necrosis: an investigation of secondary mediators in its pathogenesis. Am J Pathol 122:231-9, 1986.

123. Gonzalez-Crussi F, Hsueh W. Experimental model of ischemic bowel necrosis: the role of platelet-activating factor and endotoxin. Am J Pathol 112:127-35, 1983.

124. Rabinowitz SS, et al. Platelet-activating factor in infants at risk for necrotizing enterocolitis. J Pediatr 138:81-6, 2001.

125. Mozes T, et al. Platelet-activating factor: an endogenous mediator of mesenteric ischemia-reperfusion-induced shock. Am J Physiol 257:872-7, 1989.

126. Sun XM, Hsueh W. Bowel necrosis induced by tumor necrosis factor in rats is mediated by platelet-activating factor. J Clin Invest 81:1328-31, 1988.

127. Caplan MS, et al. Hypoxia causes ischemic bowel necrosis in rats: the role of platelet-activating factor (PAF-acether). Gastroenterology 99:979-86, 1990.

128. Edelson MB, et al. Circulating pro- and counterinflammatory cytokine levels and severity in necrotizing enterocolitis. Pediatrics 103:766-71, 1999.

129. Lindsay JO, et al. The prevention and treatment of murine colitis using gene therapy with adenoviral vectors encoding IL-10. J Immunol 166:7625-33, 2001.

Liver and Bilirubin Metabolism

118

*Steven Lobritto**

Organogenesis and Histologic Development of the Liver

The liver is the largest internal organ of the body, comprising approximately 6% to 7% of the total weight of an adult. The organ is unique in that it receives both a venous blood supply, predominantly from the intestines, pancreas, and spleen, and an arterial blood supply from the aorta. Together, this blood supply delivers nutrients, hormones, toxins, and oxygen to the liver tissues.[1] The hepatocytes, organized into linear plates, are exposed to these blood elements on their basal surface, which abuts a plexus of sinusoidal capillaries.[2-4] The hepatocytes are the predominant cellular element of the liver but are supported by interactions with other cellular components, including cholangiocytes, stellate cells, Kupffer cells, Ito cells, endothelial cells, and hematopoietic elements. An intercellular matrix that provides both structural integrity as well as pathways for intracellular communications supports these cellular elements.[5-7]

The hepatocytes perform various secretory and metabolic functions, including but not limited to detoxification of drugs and toxins, synthesis of key serum proteins (albumin, clotting factors, complement, apolipoproteins, etc.), synthesis and metabolism of dietary lipids, glucose homeostasis, and bile production.[8-12] Distortion of the normal architecture of the liver either by chronic disease states or congenital malformations can have a significant impact on the ability of the liver to perform these complex functions. As expected, the developmental steps necessary to ensure proper hepatic organization and function involve multiple and complex communications between the cellular and matrix components of the organ during organogenesis of the liver.[13-16] Investigators continue to discover new intracellular signals (specific growth factors and transcription factors) that appear to combine to initiate and propagate the transformation of fetal endodermal tissue into differentiated hepatic cellular elements and a functioning organ. This chapter summarizes some of the experiments by means of molecular genetics, molecular biology techniques, and tissue explant culture techniques that have shed light on our understanding of early steps in hepatic development.

EARLY EMBRYOGENSIS: AN OVERVIEW

Recent important discoveries have helped clarify some of the steps involved in the early development of the liver and the specific messengers and tissue signals that orchestrate this process, as well as the maturation of the hepatocytes.[13,17] Specific signaling molecules, hormones, growth factors, transcriptional factors, and intracellular matrix interactions have been shown to contribute to the

induction of pluripotential primitive tissues into cells committed to a hepatic fate. In addition, these molecules are critical to the maturation of the cells into specialized epithelium, and they contribute to the proper organization of these cells into the correct configuration comprising the fully functioning organ. Much of this work has been derived from observations in genetically altered mice and tissue culture systems. During the third to fourth week of gestation, a bud of proliferating endodermal tissue is observed originating from the ventral foregut constituting the hepatic diverticulum. The primitive cells of this bud, referred to as hepatoblasts, appear to be bipotential, with the ability to differentiate into either mature hepatocytes or cholangiocytes.[18] These cells are in contact with embryonic cardiac mesoderm, and they abut the septum transversum mesenchyme.[13,17] The hepatoblasts migrate as cords into the septum transversum, closely associated with primitive sinusoidal endothelial cells. As the process progresses, the sinusoidal structure is established, initially lacking the fenestrations observed at later stages of maturity. The undifferentiated hepatoblasts have few organelles at this stage, with a high nuclear-to-cytoplasmic ratio; scant, rough endoplasmic reticulum; and few lysosomes.[11] Intercellular communication appears to be mediated via cell surface adhesions with other hepatoblasts and surrounding mesenchymal cells. The anterior vitelline vessels of the yolk sac are the initial source of sinusoidal blood.[19] Early synthesis and secretion of alpha-fetoprotein, transferrin, and alpha$_1$-antitrypsin can be observed from these immature prehepatic cells.[20]

LATE EMBRYOGENESIS: AN OVERVIEW

Early in the second month of gestation, the hepatoblasts gradually begin to differentiate into mature hepatocytes, with the necessary intercellular components (rough endoplasmic reticulum and Golgi apparatus) to conduct their multiple synthetic and metabolic functions.[11] These cells also acquire polarity with the increased production of specific membrane-associated proteins and transmembrane transporters.[21] This process creates both a basolateral hepatocyte domain with clusters of these membrane-associated receptors and transporters for protein secretion, in association with sinusoidal vessels, and an apical hepatocyte domain constituting the bile canaliculi, with transporters related to bile secretion.[22] Both these surfaces develop a microvillous architecture, presumably to optimize surface area for extracellular contact. Other hepatoblasts are thought to develop into cholangiocytes that organize into the hepatic biliary system.[23,24] The intrahepatic bile ducts are formed from periportal hepatoblasts constituting the ductal plate. Differentiation and maturation of the intrahepatic ducts occur via interactions with periportal

---

*This chapter is based on the work of Dr. Stuart S. Kaufman, which appeared in the previous edition of this book.

connective tissue, glucocorticoid hormones, and basal laminar components.[18] Intrahepatic hematopoiesis increases at this stage and appears to progress with interactions between maturing hepatocytes and undifferentiated mesenchymal elements.[25-27]

SPECIFIC INTERACTIONS PROMOTING HEPATOGENESIS

The initial induction of the ventral foregut to commit to a hepatic fate has been shown in embryo tissue transplant studies in the chick to be a function of interactions of this endodermal region with cardiac mesoderm[28] (Table 118-1). The growth factors found to mediate this process produced by cardiac mesoderm are fibroblast growth factors (FGF)-1 and -2. Further studies with purified FGFs and FGF inhibitors confirmed this interaction.[29] The specificity of FGF for this region appears to be related to the fact that FGF migration is limited by high-affinity interactions with extracellular matrix.[30,31] In fact, without this induction stimulus, the fate of the ventral foregut that normally gives rise to the hepatic diverticulum will default to a pancreatic fate.[32] Specifically, FGF stimulation of the ventral foregut endoderm inhibits pancreatic genes and induces liver genes in this bipotential precursor cell population.

The induction stimulus provided by FGF is not sufficient to stimulate hepatocyte differentiation. Hepatocyte differentiation appears to be a function of a second induction stimulus from another mesoderm-derived tissue, the septum transversum mesenchyme. The signal proteins for this interaction appear to be bone morphogenetic proteins (BMP).[33] Specifically, BMP-2, BMP-4, and BMP-7 are produced by the septum transversum mesenchyme cells. Further studies with a BMP signal inhibitor, Noggin, demonstrated that BMP as well as FGF was needed to achieve hepatoblast induction from ventral gut endoderm.[33] The stimulatory effects of FGFs are focused on the prehepatic endodermal tissue by a network of transcription factors expressed in embryonic gut tissue. One such molecule is hepatocyte nuclear factor (HNF) 3B.[34] These transcription factors appear to be important mediators of hepatocyte differentiation; they bind to specific hepatic gene enhancer regions, promoting gene expression and cellular differentiation.[35]

The importance of the interaction between the septum transversum mesenchyme and the developing prehepatic endoderm cannot be overemphasized. The septum transversum mesenchyme is the source of BMP signaling, leading to induction of hepatoblast differentiation and propagation of the hepatocyte maturation process.[36] Extracellular matrix components of the septum transversum mesenchyme aid in the regulation of differentiation by binding and concentrating signaling molecules.[37,38] In addition, extracellular matrix components can mediate intracellular communication directly through interactions with integrins, focal adhesion kinase, and other signaling molecules.[7,39] Hepatocyte growth factor (HGF) is a potent hepatocyte proliferation stimulant that affects cell migration as well as differentiation.[40,41] These are but a few of the recognized components of the septum transversum mesenchyme and its extracellular matrix that are part of an integrated and diverse signaling process ensuring integrity to the hepatocyte maturation process and the overall hepatic structural organization.[42]

HEPATIC VASCULAR ANATOMY

During fetal development, highly oxygenated blood is delivered to the liver through the falciform ligament from the placenta via the umbilical vein.[1,43,44] The blood supply to the right lobe is derived from the right branch of the portal vein. The left branch of the portal vein connects via the portal sinus to the umbilical vein. The blood supply to the left lobe of the liver is derived from direct branches off the umbilical vein. This difference in blood oxygen saturation gives preferential dominance to the left lobe *in utero*. The umbilical vein continues past these branch points as the ductus venosus, delivering well-oxygenated blood to the inferior vena cava, which is directed across the patent foramen ovale to the left side of the heart.[19,43,45] At birth, the ductus venosus and umbilical veins obliterate, and the normal adult hepatic vascular supply is established.

INTRAHEPATIC VASCULAR DEVELOPMENT

In the adult, the portal vein enters the liver and branches into smaller and smaller vessels that travel within the portal tracts, along with branches of the hepatic artery and the interlobular bile ducts. The portal veins terminate in the sinusoids of the liver that are characterized by fenestrated endothelial epithelium. Sinusoids are separated by single cell–thick sheets of hepatocytes, referred to as the hepatic plates. Therefore, the hepatocytes are directly exposed to portal blood, permitting transfer of macromolecules. The sinusoidal blood empties into the central branches of the hepatic veins, which terminate into the left, right, and middle hepatic veins and return blood to the inferior vena cava and back to the heart. This important anatomic arrangement is critical for proper gland function and is under the control of a number of factors during hepatic development.[1,46]

Angioblasts, or primitive precursors to functional endothelial cells, have been found in an intermediate position between the prehepatic endoderm and the surrounding septum transversum mesenchyme[13] (see Table 118-1). These endothelial cell precursors intermingle with hepatoblasts as the endoderm organizes into the hepatic bud. The development of this cell population is under the influence of vascular endothelial growth factor 2.[47,48] Observations in transgenic mice and explant systems of liver bud tissue suggest that angioblasts stimulate development of the hepatic bud in endodermal tissues before the local blood vessels are formed.[49] The origin of the angioblast cells remains unknown. The current thinking is that vessel anatomy does not follow a rigid predetermined pattern, but rather vasculogenesis appears to be guided by local needs and flow dynamics. The vascular endothelium may well be equally important in providing signaling to the surrounding tissue, affecting the differentiation of organ cell precursors and the ultimate structural integrity of the organ.[50,51]

BILIARY DUCT DEVELOPMENT

In the adult liver, mature hepatocytes secrete bile into the canaliculi, which are small channels along the apical surface created by clusters of adjacent hepatocytes. These channels coalesce into a network of intrahepatic bile ducts and eventually into the main hepatic ducts lined by biliary epithelial cells or cholangiocytes. Bile is exported from the liver and stored and concentrated in the gallbladder for excretion during a meal.

The origin of biliary cells appears to be bipotential hepatoblasts originating at the hepatic bud[18] (see Table 118-1). Under the influence of the transcription factor HNF-6 (and its effect on HNF-1B) these cells undergo differentiation and proliferation.[52]

TABLE 118-1

Liver Cell Derivations

Cell Type	Tissue of Origin
Hepatocytes	Foregut endoderm, bipotential hepatoblast
Endothelial cells	Septum transversum mesenchyme, angioblast
Biliary epithelial cells	Foregut endoderm, bipotential hepatoblast
Hematopoietic cells	Septum transversum mesenchyme
Kupffer cells	Yolk sac and bone marrow
Ito cells	Septum transversum mesenchyme

These subsets of hepatoblasts strongly express biliary-specific cytokeratins.[24] The biliary precursor cells form the ductal plate that is characterized as a continuous, single-layered ring around the portal mesenchyme, which proliferates into a bilayer. Focal dilatations of the ductal plate along the bilayer give rise to the bile ducts. The newly formed ducts are incorporated into the hepatic mesenchyme. The whole process is moderated by biliary precursor cell interactions with neighboring cells and with matrix proteins, including laminin, fibronectin, and collagen types I and IV.[37,38,53,54] The process of bile duct formation also appears to be influenced by interactions with the nearby developing blood vessels, as evidenced by abnormalities in bile duct morphology observed with genetic deficiencies in the vascular Notch pathways.[55]

HEPATIC HEMATOPOIESIS

The yolk sac contributes significantly to early fetal hematopoiesis.[25] The yolk sac delivers blood from the anterior vitelline vessels to the developing sinusoids of the liver. Around the sixth week of gestation, the earliest hematopoietic elements appear to differentiate from the undifferentiated mesenchymal cells derived from the septum transversum[56] (see Table 118-1). These cells appear to interact with the developing hepatocytes and may derive trophic signals stimulating growth and development.[26] This stimulatory effect appears to change with time, diminishing as the hepatocyte matures.[57] Hematopoietic elements produced in the liver migrate through regulated temporary migration pores (not between the intact endothelial cell lining of the sinusoids), a process termed diapedesis.[2,3] Interesting new evidence suggests that hepatocytes themselves may be derived from multipotential bone marrow cells as well as from prehepatic endoderm.[58,59] As the hepatocyte matures and differentiates into the cells responsible for serum protein production, there appears to be a diminished role for intrahepatic hematopoiesis, which is then assumed by the marrow.

SINUSOIDAL CELLS—KUPFFER AND ITO CELLS

Kupffer cells are manifested during the second month of gestation. These specialized cells residing on sinusoidal surfaces of the endothelium have macrophage-like activity.[3] These cells appear to originate from both the embryonic yolk sac and from the bone marrow at later stages of development[60] (see Table 118-1). The position of these cells permits regulation of migration across the endothelium of the sinusoid.

Ito cells are specialized cells that reside in the perisinusoidal space of Disse between the endothelial cells and the developing hepatocytes of the hepatic plate.[61] These cells appear to originate from the undifferentiated mesenchyme of the septum transversum[4] (see Table 118-1). These cells store fat and vitamin A. Along with endothelial cells, these cells are involved with the production and secretion of basement membrane collagen and may therefore contribute to fibrosis in chronic liver injury.[61,62]

ACINAR ORGANIZATION

The functional unit of the liver is known as the acinus. This functional unit is defined by the hepatic blood flow from the portal vein branches within adjacent portal tracts, through the hepatic sinusoids separated by hepatocyte plates, terminating in the central branches of the hepatic veins. These basic units of function are recognized in the second and third months of gestation as the cell elements of the liver differentiate and as the matrix elements proliferate. In the mature liver, the hepatocytes within this functional unit perform different operations depending on their position within the acinus. The hepatocytes within the

acinus have been divided into three zones. Zone one cells are closest to the portal tracts and therefore receive blood with the highest nutrient and oxygen content. These cells appear to be best suited to extract bile acids, perform gluconeogenesis, produce glycogen, synthesize and secrete protein, and metabolize lipids.[63-67] Zone three cells are located adjacent to the branches of the hepatic vein. Zone three hepatocytes appear to have a higher capacity to perform glycolysis, have higher cytochrome P450 expression, and perform various metabolic reactions, including drug detoxification, glycosylation events, and ureagenesis.[10,68-70] Zone two cells are intermediate in position, and the hepatocytes in this zone appear to express activities similar to the cells of the other two zones depending on their relative proximity.

Investigations of the differences in the functions of the cells within these defined zones have led to two likely overlapping theories.[71] The first assumption is that differences in the oxygen and macromolecule content of the blood supply to these zones may influence the development and differentiation of hepatocytes. The second theory is that regional differences in cell signaling and matrix element interactions influence hepatocyte differentiation in local populations. Modulators of gene function and expression within the hepatocytes of a particular zone ultimately will define and refine their respective functions.[72] In addition, intercellular communications between adjacent hepatocyte populations will further affect hepatocyte differentiation and regional coordination of function. The likely conclusion is that both of these influences are responsible for the observed differences and similarities in hepatocyte function within the acinus.

REGULATION OF FETAL LIVER GROWTH AND MATURATION

As cell differentiation proceeds, the fetal liver also undergoes growth and structural organization. The molecules stimulating these processes are poorly understood. The process seems to be under the influence of circulating hormones and various growth factors (Table 118-2). Specifically, growth hormone and its gestational homologue placental lactogen are believed to be important stimuli for hepatocellular hyperplasia.[73,74] Furthermore, insulin, cortisol, and thyroid hormone have been shown to alter protein production and growth factor receptor expression in the developing liver and may be important mediators of growth and maturation of the organ both *in utero* and postpartum.[75-77] In part, the effect of these hormones is a function of their effect on the production and binding of secondary messenger molecules, the insulin-like growth factors.[73,75-80] Differential production and binding of these messengers may contribute to cell growth and replication, cell migration, and tissue organization and maturation.

Other molecules contributing to cell hyperplasia, migration, and tissue organization are hepatocyte growth factor and epidermal growth factor (Table 118-2). Hepatocyte growth factor has emerged as an important tissue-specific signaling molecule between epithelial and mesenchyme tissues. This molecule is a

TABLE 118-2

Stimuli of Hepatocellular Development

Hormonal	Growth hormone, placental lactogen
	Thyroid hormone
	Cortisol
	Insulin
Growth Factors	Insulin-like growth factor I
	Insulin-like growth factor II
	Hepatocyte growth factor
	Epidermal growth factor

ligand for the c-met proto-oncogene product of receptor tyrosine kinase and originates from mesenchymal tissues.[81] As such, this paracrine molecule supports organogenesis, mature organ regeneration, and neoplastic processes.[81,82] Hepatocyte growth factor and the expression of its receptor in liver and other tissues have been demonstrated in association with tissue injury, suggesting a focused tissue-specific regeneration response.[82] The diverse biologic functions of this multipotent polypeptide now lead investigators to consider it a key molecule for tissue organization, organogenesis, and organ repair.

Epidermal growth factor has been identified as a key molecule involved with liver regeneration and may play a role in embryogenesis and fetal growth, since receptors have been found in fetal tissues.[83,84] The liver appears to modulate serum levels of this molecule, providing efficient clearance and degradation of the internalized protein.[85] Also, extensive data indicate interactions between epidermal growth factor and other circulating hormones.[84] Growth hormone increases epidermal growth factor binding in the liver.[86] Thyroid and steroid hormones modulate both epidermal growth factor and its receptors in multiple tissues.[87] Epidermal growth factor stimulates hormone release from the pituitary, the placenta, and the adrenal gland but inhibits hormone production by the gonads and thyroid. The effect on fetal growth and development may be mediated by gene activation, or it may be a function of other protein interactions.[88] The significance of this molecule on hepatic growth and maturation has yet to be proved.

CONCLUSIONS

In summary, the development of the liver from primitive endoderm and mesoderm is a complicated yet orchestrated process that mandates continued intercellular and matrix signaling. Our current knowledge of the multitude of contributing messengers to this process is likely just the tip of the "organogenesis iceberg." The expanding knowledge base of the steps ensuring proper hepatocyte differentiation, growth, and organization will permit the application of learned techniques to promote regeneration and restoration of the damaged mature organ. In addition, by increasing the knowledge of the signaling pathways governing normal growth and development of the liver, we may expand our understanding and ability to manage the uncontrolled growth of hepatic malignancies. The key to the evolution of this process in the short term is our expanding technical expertise with tissue culture systems and transgenic animal models.

REFERENCES

1. Valette PJ, De Baere T: Biliary and vascular anatomy of the liver. J Radiol 83:221, 2002.
2. Zamboni L: Electron microscopic studies of blood embryogenesis in humans. I. The ultrastructure of the fetal liver. J Ultrastruct Res 12:509, 1965.
3. Bankston PW, Pino RM: The development of the sinusoids of fetal rat liver: morphology of endothelial cells, Kupffer cells, and the transmural migration of blood cells into the sinusoids. Am J Anat 159:1, 1980.
4. Enzan H, et al: Fine structure of hepatic sinusoids and their development in human embryos and fetuses. Acta Pathol Jpn 33:447, 1983.
5. Quondamatteo F, et al: Fibrillin-1 and fibrillin-2 in human embryonic and early fetal development. Matrix Biol 21:637, 2002.
6. Chagraoui J, et al: Fetal liver stroma consists of cells in epithelial-to-mesenchymal transition. Blood 101:2973, 2002.
7. Schwartz MA: Integrin signaling revisited. Trends Cell Biol 11:466, 2001.
8. Diehl-Jones WL, Askin DF: The neonatal liver. Part 1: embryology, anatomy, and physiology. Neonatal Netw 21:5, 2002.
9. Prip-Buus C, et al: Hormonal and nutritional control of liver fatty acid oxidation and ketogenesis during development. Biochem Soc Trans 23:500, 1995.
10. Buhler R, et al: Zonation of cytochrome P450 isozyme expression and induction in rat liver. Eur J Biochem 204:407, 1992.
11. Kanamura S, et al: Fine structure and function of hepatocytes during development. J Electron Microsc Tech 14:92, 1990.
12. Hepatocyte heterogeneity and liver function. Revis Biol Celular 19:1, 1989.
13. Zaret KS: Regulatory phases of early liver development: paradigms of organogenesis. Nat Rev Genet 3:499, 2002.
14. Shiojiri N: [Molecular mechanisms of liver development]. Seikagaku 74:285, 2002.
15. Schrem H, et al: Liver-enriched transcription factors in liver function and development. Part I: the hepatocyte nuclear factor network and liver-specific gene expression. Pharmacol Rev 54:129, 2002.
16. Zaret KS: Hepatocyte differentiation: from the endoderm and beyond. Curr Opin Genet Dev 11:568, 2001.
17. Duncan SA: Mechanisms controlling early development of the liver. Mech Dev 120:19, 2003.
18. Shiojiri N: Development and differentiation of bile ducts in the mammalian liver. Microsc Res Tech 39:328, 1997.
19. Silver M, et al: Placental blood flow: some fetal and maternal cardiovascular adjustments during gestation. J Reprod Fertil Suppl 31:139, 1982.
20. Jones CT, Rolph TP: Metabolism during fetal life: a functional assessment of metabolic development. Physiol Rev 65:357, 1985.
21. Feracci H, et al: The establishment of hepatocyte cell surface polarity during fetal liver development. Dev Biol 123:73, 1987.
22. Gallin WJ: Development and maintenance of bile canaliculi in vitro and in vivo. Microsc Res Tech 39:406, 1997.
23. Alison MR, et al: Pluripotential liver stem cells: facultative stem cells located in the biliary tree. Cell Prolif 29:373, 1996.
24. Lemaigre FP: Development of the biliary tract. Mech Dev 120:81, 2003.
25. Fukuda T: Fetal hemopoiesis. II. Electron microscopic studies on human hepatic hemopoiesis. Virchows Arch B Cell Pathol 16:249, 1974.
26. Medlock ES, Haar JL: The liver hemopoietic environment: I. Developing hepatocytes and their role in fetal hemopoiesis. Anat Rec 207:31, 1983.
27. Timens W, Kamps WA: Hemopoiesis in human fetal and embryonic liver. Microsc Res Tech 39:387, 1997.
28. Le Douarin NM, Teillet MA: Experimental analysis of the migration and differentiation of neuroblasts of the autonomic nervous system and of neurectodermal mesenchymal derivatives, using a biological cell marking technique. Dev Biol 41:162, 1974.
29. Jung J, et al: Initiation of mammalian liver development from endoderm by fibroblast growth factors. Science 284:1998, 1999.
30. Crossley PH, Martin GR: The mouse Fgf8 gene encodes a family of polypeptides and is expressed in regions that direct outgrowth and patterning in the developing embryo. Development 121:439, 1995.
31. Szebenyi G, Fallon JF: Fibroblast growth factors as multifunctional signaling factors. Int Rev Cytol 185:45, 1999.
32. Deutsch G, et al: A bipotential precursor population for pancreas and liver within the embryonic endoderm. Development 128:871, 2001.
33. Rossi JM, et al: Distinct mesodermal signals, including BMPs from the septum transversum mesenchyme, are required in combination for hepatogenesis from the endoderm. Genes Dev 15:1998, 2001.
34. Bossard P, Zaret KS: GATA transcription factors as potentiators of gut endoderm differentiation. Development 125:4909, 1998.
35. Duncan SA: Transcriptional regulation of liver development. Dev Dyn 219:131, 2000.
36. Houssaint E: Differentiation of the mouse hepatic primordium. I. An analysis of tissue interactions in hepatocyte differentiation. Cell Differ 9:269, 1980.
37. Baloch Z, et al: Ontogenesis of the murine hepatic extracellular matrix: an immunohistochemical study. Differentiation 51:209, 1992.
38. Amenta PS, Harrison D: Expression and potential role of the extracellular matrix in hepatic ontogenesis: a review. Microsc Res Tech 39:372, 1997.
39. Renshaw MW, et al: Focal adhesion kinase mediates the integrin signaling requirement for growth factor activation of MAP kinase. J Cell Biol 147:611, 1999.
40. Sonnenberg E, et al: Expression of the met-receptor and its ligand, HGF-SF, during mouse embryogenesis. EXS 65:381, 1993.
41. Birchmeier C, et al: Tyrosine kinase receptors in the control of epithelial growth and morphogenesis during development. Bioessays 15:185, 1993.
42. Maher JJ, Bissell DM: Cell-matrix interactions in liver. Semin Cell Biol 4:189, 1993.
43. Rudolph AM: Hepatic and ductus venosus blood flows during fetal life. Hepatology 3:254, 1983.
44. Nagano K, et al: Patent ductus venosus. J Gastroenterol Hepatol 14:285, 1999.
45. Edelstone DI: Regulation of blood flow through the ductus venosus. J Dev Physiol 2:219, 1980.
46. Gouysse G, et al: Relationship between vascular development and vascular differentiation during liver organogenesis in humans. J Hepatol 37:730, 2002.
47. Millauer B, et al: High affinity VEGF binding and developmental expression suggest Flk-1 as a major regulator of vasculogenesis and angiogenesis. Cell 72:835, 1993.
48. Quinn TP, et al: Fetal liver kinase 1 is a receptor for vascular endothelial growth factor and is selectively expressed in vascular endothelium. Proc Natl Acad Sci U S A 90:7533, 1993.
49. Matsumoto K, et al: Liver organogenesis promoted by endothelial cells prior to vascular function. Science 294:559, 2001.
50. Lammert E, et al: Role of endothelial cells in early pancreas and liver development. Mech Dev 120:59, 2003.
51. Weinstein B: Building the house around the plumbing. Bioessays 24:397, 2002.
52. Clotman F, et al: The onecut transcription factor HNF6 is required for normal development of the biliary tract. Development 129:1819, 2002.

53. Shah KD, Gerber MA: Development of intrahepatic bile ducts in humans. Possible role of laminin. Arch Pathol Lab Med *114*:597, 1990.
54. Terada T, Nakanuma Y: Expression of tenascin, type IV collagen and laminin during human intrahepatic bile duct development and in intrahepatic cholangiocarcinoma. Histopathology *25*:143, 1994.
55. Li L, et al: Alagille syndrome is caused by mutations in human *Jagged1*, which encodes a ligand for *Notch1*. Nat Genet *16*:243, 1997.
56. Emura I, et al: Four types of presumptive hemopoietic stem cells in the human fetal liver. Arch Histol Jpn *46*:645, 1983.
57. Nessi AC, et al: Foetal haemopoiesis during the hepatic period. I. Relation between in vitro liver organogenesis and erythropoietic function. Anat Rec *200*:221, 1981.
58. Austin TW, Lagasse E: Hepatic regeneration from hematopoietic stem cells. Mech Dev *120*:131, 2003.
59. Petersen BE, et al: Bone marrow as a potential source of hepatic oval cells. Science *284*:1168, 1999.
60. Janossy G, et al: Separate ontogeny of two macrophage-like accessory cell populations in the human fetus. J Immunol *136*:4354, 1986.
61. Enzan H, et al: Immunohistochemical identification of Ito cells and their myofibroblastic transformation in adult human liver. Virchows Arch *424*:249, 1994.
62. Fujita M, et al: Extracellular matrix regulation of cell-cell communication and tissue-specific gene expression in primary liver cultures. Prog Clin Biol Res *226*:333, 1986.
63. Tanaka T, et al: Quantitative analysis of endoplasmic reticulum and cytochrome P-450 in hepatocytes from rats injected with methylcholanthrene. Eur J Cell Biol *74*:20, 1997.
64. Aggarwal SR, et al: Glucagon stimulates phosphorylation of different peptides in isolated periportal and perivenous hepatocytes. FEBS Lett *377*:439, 1995.
65. McCashland TM, et al: Zonal differences in ethanol-induced impairments in hepatic receptor binding. Alcohol *10*:549, 1993.
66. Lawrence GM, et al: Histochemical and immunohistochemical localization of hexokinase isoenzymes in normal rat liver. Histochem J *16*:1099, 1984.
67. Hildebrand R: Quantitative and qualitative histochemical investigation on NADP+-dependent dehydrogenases in the limiting plate and the residual parenchyma surrounding terminal hepatic venules. Histochemistry *80*:91, 1984.
68. de Groot H, Littauer A: Hypoxia, reactive oxygen, and cell injury. Free Radic Biol Med *6*:541, 1989.
69. Takahashi T, et al: Induction of cytochrome P-4502E1 in the human liver by ethanol is caused by a corresponding increase in encoding messenger RNA. Hepatology *17*:236, 1993.
70. Lupp A, et al: Developmental expression of cytochrome P450 isoforms after transplantation of fetal liver tissue suspension into the spleens of adult syngeneic rats. Exp Toxicol Pathol *50*:41, 1998.
71. Groothuis GM, Meijer DK: Hepatocyte heterogeneity in bile formation and hepatobiliary transport of drugs. Enzyme *46*:94, 1992.
72. Gumucio JJ, et al: The isolation of functionally heterogeneous hepatocytes of the proximal and distal half of the liver acinus in the rat. Hepatology *6*:932, 1986.
73. Strain AJ, et al: Regulation of DNA synthesis in human fetal hepatocytes by placental lactogen, growth hormone, and insulin-like growth factor I/somatomedin-C. J Cell Physiol *132*:33, 1987.
74. Hill DJ, et al: Placental lactogen and growth hormone receptors in human fetal tissues: relationship to fetal plasma human placental lactogen concentrations and fetal growth. J Clin Endocrinol Metab *66*:1283, 1988.
75. Rajaratnam VS, et al: Maternal diabetes induces upregulation of hepatic insulin-like growth factor binding protein-1 MRNA expression, growth retardation and developmental delay at the same stage of rat fetal development. J Endocrinol *152*:R1, 1997.
76. Forhead AJ, et al: Control of hepatic insulin-like growth factor II gene expression by thyroid hormones in fetal sheep near term. Am J Physiol *275*:E149, 1998.
77. Unterman T, et al: Circulating levels of insulin-like growth factor binding protein-1 (IGFBP-1) and hepatic mRNA are increased in the small for gestational age (SGA) fetal rat. Endocrinology *127*:2035, 1990.
78. Serna J, et al: Differential and tissue-specific regulation of (pro)insulin and insulin-like growth factor-I mRNAs and levels of thyroid hormones in growth-retarded embryos. Growth Regul *6*:73, 1996.
79. Coulter CL, et al: Role of pituitary POMC-peptides and insulin-like growth factor II in the developmental biology of the adrenal gland. Arch Physiol Biochem *110*:99, 2002.
80. Briese V, Hopp H: [Somatomedins—insulin-like growth factors.] J Zentralbl Gynakol *111*:1017, 1989.
81. Matsumoto K, Nakamura T: Emerging multipotent aspects of hepatocyte growth factor. J Biochem (Tokyo) *119*:591, 1996.
82. Nakamura T: Hepatocyte growth factor as mitogen, motogen and morphogen, and its roles in organ regeneration. Princess Takamatsu Symp *24*:195, 1994.
83. Marti U, et al: Biological effects of epidermal growth factor, with emphasis on the gastrointestinal tract and liver: an update. Hepatology *9*:126, 1989.
84. Fisher DA, Lakshmanan J: Metabolism and effects of epidermal growth factor and related growth factors in mammals. Endocrinol Rev *11*:418, 1990.
85. Hoath SB, et al: Characterization of hepatic epidermal growth factor receptors in the developing rat. Biochim Biophys Acta *930*:107, 1987.
86. Jansson JO, et al: Growth hormone enhances hepatic epidermal growth factor receptor concentration in mice. J Clin Invest *82*:1871, 1988.
87. Perheentupa J, et al: Hormonal modulation of mouse plasma concentration of epidermal growth factor. Acta Endocrinol (Copenh) *107*:571, 1984.
88. Murray MA, et al: Epidermal growth factor stimulates insulin-like growth factor-binding protein-1 expression in the neonatal rat. Endocrinology *133*:159, 1993.

John C. Bucuvalas and Kenneth Setchel

119

Bile Acid Metabolism During Development

Bile acids serve critical roles in fat digestion, generation of bile flow, lipid metabolism, and excretion of xenobiotics. This chapter reviews bile acid metabolism and physiology with special attention to bile acid metabolism during early life.

PHYSIOLOGIC FUNCTION OF BILE ACIDS

Bile acids are amphipathic sterols formed in the liver by stereospecific additions and modifications to cholesterol (Fig. 119-1). Bile acids self-associate to form micelles with a lipid-soluble interior and a water-soluble exterior. In bile and in the intestinal lumen, bile acids form mixed micelles by interacting with lipids and cholesterol.[1-3] Formation of mixed micelles permits removal of amphipathic and lipid-soluble xenobiotics from the liver and facilitates intestinal fat digestion. Furthermore, bile acids play a critical role in cholesterol metabolism because cholesterol excretion into bile depends on formation of mixed micelles, and bile acid synthesis accounts for one half of net cholesterol removal.[4-6] Bile acids are a major driving force in the cellular formation of bile because secretion of osmotically active bile acids into bile stimulates water flow and canalicular bile formation (Table 119-1).[7,8]

CHEMICAL STRUCTURE AND PROPERTIES OF BILE ACIDS

Bile acids have a chemical structure similar to that of cholesterol and are made up of a steroid nucleus connected to an aliphatic side chain.[9] The nuclear structure is composed of three 6-carbon rings, identified as A, B, and C, fused to a 5-carbon ring identified as D. For both cholesterol and bile acids, two methyl groups project from the steroid nucleus. Although the chemical structure of the steroid nucleus for bile acids is similar to cholesterol, their physical structure and properties differ. Cholesterol is a flat, water-insoluble molecule, whereas the predominant human bile acids are kinked and water soluble. The kinked structure reflects a β-configuration of the hydrogen atom at C5. The number and orientation of hydroxyl groups determine the capability of bile acids to form micelles and solubilize lipids. As a result of the stereospecific addition of hydroxyl groups to carbons of the steroid nucleus, the α side of the predominant human bile acids is hydrophobic, whereas the β side is hydrophilic. When the predominant human bile acids self-associate in bile to form micelles, the β side forms a water-soluble exterior, and the α side forms a lipid-soluble interior.

In humans, the aliphatic side chain of bile acids is composed of five carbons. Bile acids with a side chain containing five

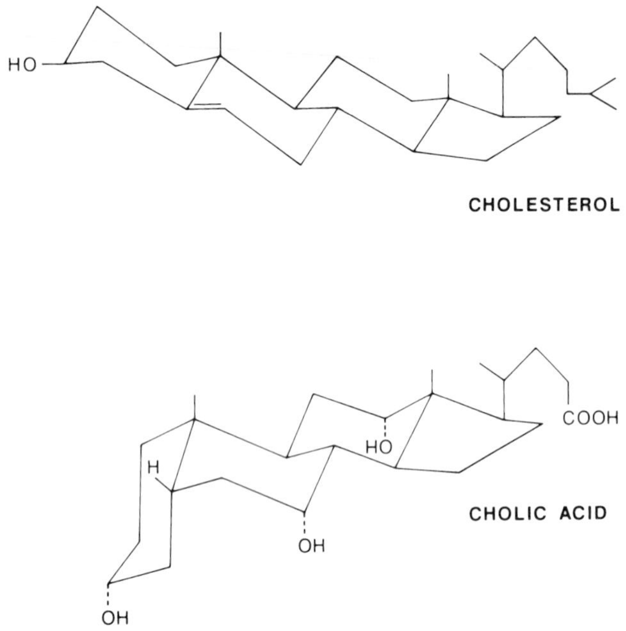

Figure 119–1. Steric diagram of cholesterol and cholic acid.

TABLE 119-1

Physiologic Roles of Bile Acids

Excretion of biliary lipids and toxins
Cholesterol metabolism
Excretion of biliary lipids and toxins
Bile formation
Fat digestion

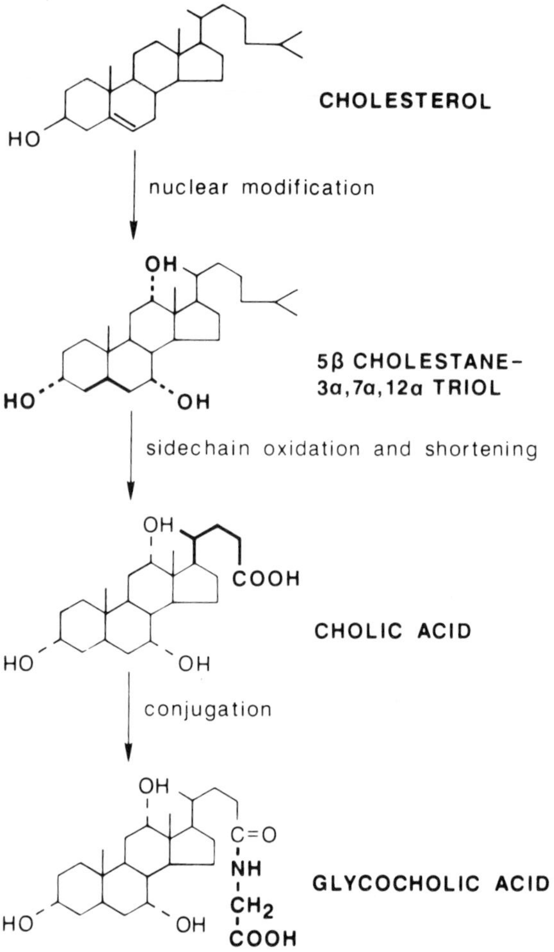

Figure 119–2. Summary of critical chemical modifications involved in the conversion of cholesterol to a conjugated trihydroxy bile acid (glycocholic acid).

carbons are called cholanoic acids and comprise the primary human bile acids, cholic acid and chenodeoxycholic acid. Precursors for the primary bile acids have 8-carbon side chains and are called cholestanoic acids.

Cholic and chenodeoxycholic acid form conjugates by the formation of amides between the carboxyl group of the bile acid side chain and the amino group of taurine or glycine. Formation of conjugates with taurine or glycine lowers the negative log of dissociation constant (pKa) of the carboxyl group and increases the solubility of bile acids in water at the pH present in the intestinal lumen. By remaining soluble at physiologic pH, conjugated bile acids are not passively absorbed by the small intestine. As a result, the intraluminal concentration of bile acids exceeds the critical micellar concentration, and fat digestion is facilitated. To a lesser degree, bile acids form conjugates by esterification with glucuronate, sulfate, glucose, and N-acetylglucosamine.

BILE ACID SYNTHESIS

The primary bile acids—cholic acid and chenodeoxycholic acid—are synthesized from cholesterol in the liver. Conversion of cholesterol to bile acid involves nuclear modification, side chain alteration, and conjugation (Fig. 119–2).[9] Nuclear ring changes include stereospecific hydroxylation and oxidoreduction of the 3β-hydroxyl group. The side chain is hydroxylated and shortened to form the unconjugated C24 bile acid. Finally, conjugation with glycine and taurine and, to a lesser extent, glucuronic and sulfuric acids completes the process. Biotransformation of the side chain or nucleus may occur first, although current models are based on the assumption that nuclear modification precedes side chain changes.

Sequential deconjugation and 7α-dehydroxylation, oxidoreduction, and epimerization of the primary bile acids by endogenous bacteria take place primarily in the jejunum and ileum. The products are referred to as the secondary bile acids: deoxycholic acid, ursodeoxycholic acid, and lithocholic acid. The secondary bile acids are reabsorbed passively in the small intestine and colon. Lithocholate, the product of 7α-dehydroxylation of chenodeoxycholic acid, can be hepatotoxic and has been proposed to contribute to the development of liver disease associated with inflammatory bowel disease or total parenteral nutrition.[10, 11]

Cholesterol biosynthesis is closely coupled to bile acid metabolism. The conversion of hydroxymethylglutaryl-coenzyme A (HMG-CoA) to mevalonic acid by HMG-CoA reductase is the rate-limiting step in cholesterol biosynthesis (Fig. 119–3).[12] Once formed in the liver, cholesterol can be inserted into cell membranes, incorporated into lipoproteins, converted into bile acids, or excreted as biliary cholesterol. Because bile acids are critical to dissolve biliary cholesterol, both routes for cholesterol removal (secretion in bile and biotransformation to bile acids) are closely linked to bile acid metabolism.[2, 5, 12]

Cholesterol 7α-hydroxylase is a mixed-function oxidase associated with the endoplasmic reticulum that catalyzes the conversion of cholesterol to 7α-hydroxycholesterol.[13–15] Generation of 7α-hydroxycholesterol occurs preferentially from newly synthesized cholesterol, and the reaction product is totally committed to bile acid synthesis.[13, 16] Nuclear modification proceeds with the isomerization of the Δ⁵ double bond and oxidation

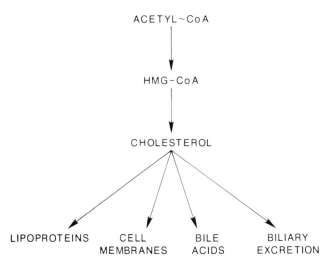

Figure 119–3. Simplified scheme of cholesterol biosynthesis from acetyl coenzyme A (CoA) and the ultimate fate of newly synthesized cholesterol. HMG = hydroxymethylglutaryl. (From Brown MS, Goldstein JL: Science *232*:34, 1986. The Nobel Foundation, 1986.)

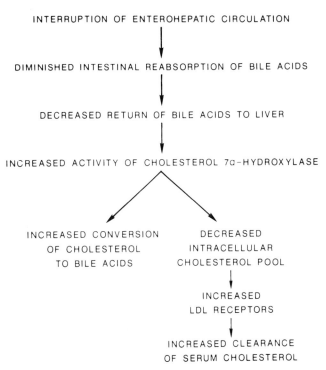

Figure 119–4. Effect of interruption of the enterohepatic circulation on cholesterol and bile acid metabolism. LDL = low density lipoprotein.

of the 3β-hydroxyl to form 7α-hydroxy-4-cholesten-3-one.[17] 12α-Hydroxylation of 7α-hydroxy-4-cholesten-3-one then occurs in compounds destined to form cholic acid. The microsomal mixed-function oxidase that catalyzes 12α-hydroxylation is the major branch point for cholic or chenodeoxycholic acid synthesis.[13, 15, 18] Despite its apparent importance, the 12α-hydroxylase does not appear to control the ratio of cholic to chenodeoxycholic acid. This ratio may be more strongly influenced by differential rates of cycling of specific bile acids through the enterohepatic circulation. Nuclear modification is completed by two cytosolic enzymes: Δ^4-3-oxosteroid 5β-reductase, which performs stereospecific reduction of Δ^4 double bond, and 3α-hydroxysteroid dehydrogenase, which reduces the 3-oxo group.[19] The 27-carbon product that is formed is saturated, and all hydroxyl groups project below (α) the steroid nucleus.

The initial step in side chain modification is 27-hydroxylation by a mitochondrial enzyme.[5, 20] (The presence of a 26-cholesterol hydroxylase and conversion of 26-hydroxycholesterol to 3β-hydroxy-5-cholenoic acid by peroxisomes have been demonstrated *in vitro.*) Oxidation of the C27 hydroxyl to a carboxylic acid group results in formation of dihydroxy or trihydroxy 5β-cholestanoic acid. By a series of reactions similar to those involved in β-oxidation of fatty acids, the side chain is shortened by peroxisomal enzymes to the final products, cholic or chenodeoxycholic acid.[21]

The first step in conjugation of cholic and chenodeoxycholic acid with glycine or taurine is the formation of the bile acid–CoA thioester by the microsomal enzyme cholyl-CoA ligase. Glycine or taurine is then conjugated to the intermediate product by bile acid–CoA-amino acid *N*-acyltransferase.[22] The transferase has an increased affinity for taurine, but the final ratio of glycine to taurine conjugates depends on the relative abundance of the free amino acids in the liver.[22, 23] Because many mature mammals show decreased biosynthetic capacity for taurine, glycine conjugates predominate, particularly when dietary taurine is limited.[24] Conjugation of free bile acids to glycine or taurine markedly decreases their pKa from 6 to 4.0 or 2.0. The lower pKa reduces the proportion of bile acids, with protonated carboxylic acid groups present at the pH found in the intestinal lumen, and it significantly increases the solubility of bile acid monomers. As a result of the decreased pKa, passive absorption of conjugated bile acids is diminished, and conjugated bile acids remain at concentrations higher than their critical micellar concentrations at which they can facilitate fat digestion and absorption.

Regulation of Bile Acid Synthesis

Bile acid synthesis is regulated to maintain bile acid pool size and to compensate for intestinal loss. Cholesterol 7α-hydroxylase is the rate-limiting enzyme in the conversion of cholesterol to bile acids and is critical to regulation of bile acid pool size. Interruption of the enterohepatic circulation by establishment of biliary fistula or ileal resection decreases bile acid return to the liver (Fig. 119–4).[9, 25, 26] When the enterohepatic circulation is interrupted, mRNA levels and enzyme activity of cholesterol 7α-hydroxylase increase.[9, 25] With increased conversion of cholesterol to bile acids, intracellular cholesterol is depleted. Depletion of the cholesterol pool induces synthesis of low density lipoprotein (LDL) receptors.[4, 9, 25, 26] The increased number of LDL receptors permits more effective clearance by LDLs from the blood and is the basis for the use of bile acid resin (e.g., cholestyramine) to treat hypercholesterolemia.[4, 25]

Intraduodenal infusion of taurocholate to rats with bile duct fistula inhibits the conversion of cholesterol to bile acids by 90%.[27] Incubation of microsomes from cultured or isolated hepatocytes with bile acids does not directly inhibit cholesterol 7α-hydroxylase. Information indicates, however, that hydrophobic bile acids may suppress cholesterol 7α-hydroxylase activity by altering binding of liver nuclear proteins to a bile acid–responsive element of the cholesterol 7α-hydroxylase gene.[18]

ENTEROHEPATIC CIRCULATION OF BILE ACIDS

An efficient enterohepatic circulation conserves bile acids and maintains the bile acid pool. The enterohepatic circulation, which consists of two mechanical pumps (gallbladder and small intestine) and two chemical pumps (hepatocyte and ileal brush border), effectively conserves the bile acid pool (Fig. 119–5). In the fasted state, most of the bile acid pool is concentrated in the gallbladder. In response to a meal or hormonal stimuli, the gallbladder contracts, and bile acids are secreted into the intestine. In the small intestine, bile acids are present at concentrations greater than their critical micellar concentration; this permits mixed micelle formation with dietary fat and allows efficient digestion and mucosal absorption of fat. Approximately 90% of the intraluminal bile acids are reabsorbed in the small intestine and return to the liver via the portal vein. In the intestine, unconjugated bile acids are conserved by passive uptake, whereas conjugated bile acids are conserved by carrier-mediated active uptake. Passive absorption of unconjugated bile acids occurs in the small intestine and colon. For passive absorption to occur, bile acids must be protonated and remain in solution. At the pH of the small intestine, approximately 50% of unconjugated bile acids (but only negligible amounts of conjugated bile acids) are protonated. Conservation of taurine and glycine conjugates of bile acids depends on a sodium/bile acid co-transport system present on the ileal brush border. To compensate for fecal losses, 0.2 to 0.5 g of bile acids is synthesized from cholesterol in the liver.

The cellular mechanisms for bile acid transport have been an area of intense investigation. In the hepatocyte, a sodium/bile acid transport protein present on the sinusoidal membrane of the hepatocyte actively transports bile acids from sinusoidal blood into the hepatocyte. Bile acid uptake is influenced by the chemical structure of the steroid nucleus and by side chain charge and length.[19, 28-30] Intracellular transport of bile acids, which occurs via a vesicular-dependent or vesicular-independent pathway, is poorly understood but likely involves bile acid-binding proteins. Bile acids are actively secreted across the canalicular membrane into the bile canaliculus. Bile acids secreted into the canalicular space stimulate movement of water into the canaliculus and are the principal driving force for bile secretion. The electrochemical gradient across the canalicular domain of the plasma membrane was previously thought to drive bile acid

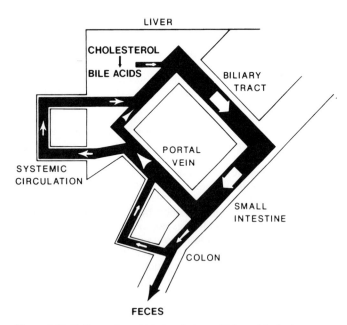

Figure 119–5. Enterohepatic circulation of bile acids during development. *Arrows* indicate the direction of bile acid movement. The width of the *shaded lines* is proportional to the amount of bile acid delivered to organs, circulation, and biliary tract.

secretion. Studies have shown that canalicular secretion of bile acids occurs via an adenosine triphosphate (ATP)-dependent transporter.[31-33]

BILE ACID METABOLISM DURING DEVELOPMENT

Immaturity of the systems involved in bile acid synthesis and the enterohepatic circulation has been demonstrated in fetal and developing animals.[34, 35] In this section, bile acid synthesis, the placenta as an excretory organ, and the enterohepatic circulation of bile acids during development are discussed.

Bile Acid Synthesis During Development

Bile acids are detected in human fetuses by 14 weeks' gestation, and similar to adults, bile acids are synthesized from cholesterol in the liver during prenatal and perinatal life. In premature and full-term infants, bile acid pool size is decreased, resulting in duodenal bile acid concentrations less than the critical micellar concentration. Intraluminal concentrations are increased two- to threefold in term compared with premature infants, a finding reflecting expansion of pool size and increased secretion of bile acids.[36, 37] Increased pool size is associated with a 30- to 40-fold increase in cholesterol 7α-hydroxylase activity and increased capacity to convert cholesterol to bile acids.[38, 39] Bile acid pool size continues to increase, and by 7 weeks, it is similar to that for adults when corrected for body surface area.[40]

In meconium and in bile collected from newborn infants and from aborted fetuses, there is an increased ratio of chenodeoxycholic acid to cholic acid, a predominance of taurine conjugates, and the presence of bile acids with hydroxylations at C1, C2, C6, or C4 (Table 119–2).[41-43] Although meconium is readily available for analysis, careful interpretation of the results is necessary. Because no bacteria are present in meconium, the extracted bile acids are either products of fetal synthetic pathways or, to a lesser degree, maternal bile acid transferred transplacentally. The presence of bile acids in meconium reflects their biosynthetic rate and their rate of reabsorption. A bile acid that is poorly absorbed by the intestine may be sequestered in meconium over time and may accumulate to a concentration out of proportion to its rate of synthesis. Nevertheless, examination of meconium is a useful tool to examine bile metabolism during development. These observations imply that pathways for bile acid synthesis differ in fetal compared with normal adult liver.

The predominance of chenodeoxycholic acid in the newborn infant contrasts with the adult, in whom cholic acid is the most abundant bile acid. Differential cycling through the enterohepatic circulation may explain this phenomenon, but the enterohepatic cycle is poorly developed at this stage of development.[34] 12α-Hydroxylase activity is not decreased compared with other hydroxylases, a finding implying that decreased 12α-hydroxylation is not responsible for the altered ratio.[44] An alternative pathway favoring chenodeoxycholic acid production may explain its predominance in fetal life. 3β-Hydroxy-5-cholenoic acid, which has a side chain resembling that of cholic acid and a nuclear structure identical to that of cholesterol, is present in fetal bile, and this indicates that side chain modification can precede nuclear hydroxylation and isomerization (Fig. 119–6). Preferential shunting of 3β-hydroxy-5-cholenoic acid into pathways favoring chenodeoxy-

TABLE 119-2
Unusual Characteristics of Fetal Bile Acids

Increased chenodeoxycholic acid/cholic acid ratio
Increased taurine conjugates
Hydroxylation at C1, C4, C6, C2

cholic acid may provide an explanation for the altered ratio detected in fetal bile and meconium.[41-43,45]

The increased proportion of taurine to glycine conjugates in fetal bile contrasts with the adult, in whom glycoconjugates predominate.[4] These findings may reflect differential handling of conjugates by the enterohepatic circulation or increased bioavailability of taurine during development. Increased hepatic uptake of taurine in developing rats compared with mature rats supports the latter possibility.[46] The physiologic significance of the increase in taurine conjugates during development remains uncertain. Because of the lower pKa, tauroconjugates are more likely to remain in micellar solution and increase fat absorption. Nevertheless, clinical studies have failed to demonstrate improved fat absorption in infants despite increased tauroconjugates.[47,48] Taurine may serve a cytoprotective role because conjugation of potentially hepatotoxic bile acids with taurine decreases the cytotoxic effects of these compounds.[49]

Bile acids with hydroxyl groups on carbons 1 and 6 in the sterol nucleus are detected in adults with cholestasis and in fetal bile and meconium.[41,42,45] The physiologic significance of these unusual bile acids remains uncertain, but they may be the final products of alternative pathways, converting potentially toxic compounds (e.g., lithocholate) to less damaging dihydroxy and trihydroxy bile acids. For example, there is evidence that the fetal liver is capable of synthesizing hepatotoxic compounds such as lithocholate by conversion of cholesterol to 3β-hydroxy-5-cholenoic acid and then to lithocholic acid.[42] In the fetal liver, protection against the hepatotoxic effects of lithocholate may result from removal by the placenta, from conjugation with taurine, or from activation of C1, C4, or C6 hydroxylases, which convert lithocholate to less toxic forms.

Studies have detected a mixture of short chain bile acids in meconium.[41] Their physiologic significance and their origin remain uncertain, but their presence emphasizes the complexity of bile acid metabolism by the fetus.

Role of the Placenta in Bile Acid Metabolism

The prenatal liver has limited capacity to detoxify xenobiotics, and because the fetus exists in a closed system, the placenta assumes a critical role in excretory function *in utero*. Bile acid concentrations are greater in human fetal arterial compared with cord venous serum, a finding suggesting placental clearance of bile acids and transfer of bile acids from fetal to maternal circulation.[50] Because the fetal intestine is sterile and the formation of secondary bile acids requires bacterial enzymes, the presence of secondary bile acids in human and sheep fetal circulation implies maternal-to-fetal transfer of bile acids.[51] A carrier-mediated bile acid transport system similar to that found on liver canalicular membranes has been demonstrated using human placental membrane vesicles.[52] These findings imply that the placenta may protect the fetus from accumulation of potentially

toxic bile acids and may indirectly play a role in regulation of cholesterol and bile acid metabolism.

Enterohepatic Circulation During Development

In infants and immature animals, the cellular mechanisms for generating bile flow and for bile acid uptake are immature and may explain, in part, the predisposition of the neonate to cholestatic liver disease as well as diminished fat absorption (see Fig. 119-5). Serum bile acids are elevated in human infants younger than 6 months old and in developing rats, a finding implying ineffective hepatic clearance.[53,54] Studies using perfused liver, isolated hepatocytes, and plasma membrane vesicles demonstrated diminished sodium/bile acid co-transport in immature compared with mature rats.[55,56] In rat liver, mRNA for the sodium/bile acid transporter protein is undetectable until 18 days' gestation. Message levels increase during late gestation and early postnatal life. Increased message levels coincide with functional expression of sodium-dependent bile acid transport activity, a finding implying transcriptional regulation.[57] Decreased bile flow and bile acid secretion have been demonstrated in developing liver from several experimental animals.[58-60] During development, functional expression of ATP and potential sensitive bile acid transport across canalicular membranes are decreased. The appearance of ATP and potential sensitive bile acid secretion are associated with the emergence of a canalicular membrane protein (M_r = 100 kDa) believed to be the bile acid carrier protein.[57,61,62] Coincident with the appearance of the carrier protein is a shift in distribution of bile from the liver to the intestinal lumen, a finding implying increased canalicular secretion of bile acids.[38] Ileal reabsorption of bile acids is diminished in immature compared with mature animals, with detectable carrier-mediated transport activity appearing just before weaning.[63-66]

Bile acid transport and metabolism have a coordinated appearance and maturation of the systems (Fig. 119-7). Increased activity of the enzymes involved in bile acid synthesis increases pool size in late gestation. In rats, hepatic transport of bile acids across the basolateral and canalicular membrane is detected around birth, with rapid maturation of the function in the canalicular domain. Just before weaning, carrier-mediated ileal transport is observed, and finally there is maturation of the sodium/bile acid co-transporter on the basolateral liver plasma membrane. The role of external factors (thyroid hormone, corticosteroids, weaning) in the coordination of this maturation process in rats has not been examined extensively. Data from other systems (e.g., intestinal sucrase, lactase), however, show that the appearance of enzyme activity can be modulated by hormonal stimuli, but the target cell is not dependent on external factors for expression of its specialized function.[44]

ALTERED BILE ACID METABOLISM

Acquired or congenital defects in the enterohepatic circulation of bile acids alter cholesterol and bile acid metabolism and affect intraluminal fat digestion, hepatic function, and bile flow (Table 119-3). These disorders are best understood by examining the individual steps in the enterohepatic circulation of bile acids. In contrast, inherited defects in bile acid biosynthesis are considered rare, but advances in techniques for characterization and identification of bile acids and their metabolites have permitted their identification.[13]

Alteration in Enterohepatic Circulation of Bile Acids

Cholestasis, defined as diminished or absent bile flow, is associated with decreased bile acid secretion and accumulation of bile acids within hepatocytes. Bile acid retention promotes liver

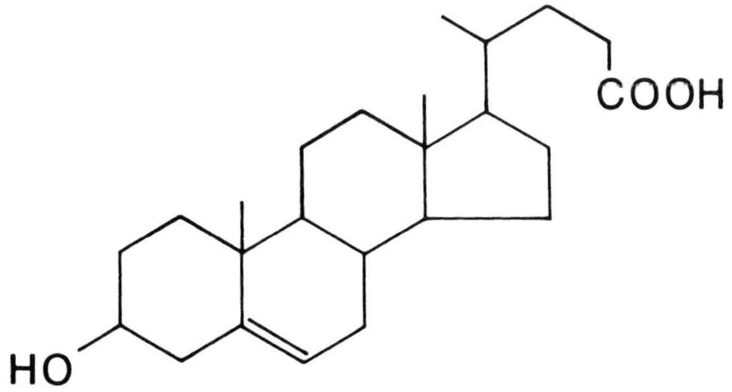

Figure 119–6. Chemical structure of 3β-hydroxy-5-cholenoic acid.

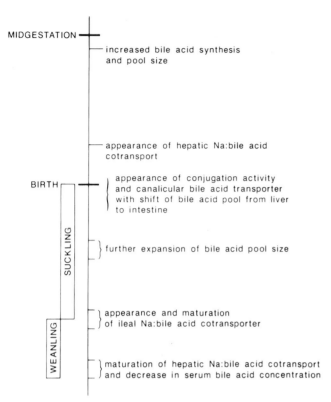

Figure 119–7. Timetable indicating the appearance of the enzyme and membrane transport systems involved in bile acid metabolism during fetal and neonatal development.

TABLE 119-3

Defects in Bile Acid Metabolism

Alteration of enterohepatic circulation of bile acids
Cholestasis
Intestinal bacterial overgrowth
Increased fecal loss of bile acids
Bile acid synthetic defects
Nuclear modification
Side chain oxidation and shortening

injury in patients with cholestasis by interfering with mitochondrial function.[67] Hepatotoxicity is increased with hydrophobic compared with hydrophilic bile acids. Treatment with ursodeoxycholic acid, a hydrophilic bile acid, benefits patients with cholestasis. Ursodeoxycholic acid may exert its beneficial effects by replacing cytotoxic bile acids and changing the composition of the bile acid pool by a direct hepatoprotective effect, by influencing the enterohepatic circulation of endogenous bile salts, or by enhancing bile flow.[68, 69] Sulfated bile acids and bile acids with altered patterns of hydroxylation (e.g., C1, C6) are detected in patients with cholestasis and in fetal bile, a finding implying activation of metabolic pathways not expressed or of minor importance in the normal liver.[42, 70, 71] Their physiologic significance remains uncertain, but the additional hydroxyl groups may increase hydrophilicity and may permit increased urinary excretion of potentially toxic bile acids.

In patients with altered intestinal flora (e.g., bacterial overgrowth, inflammatory bowel disease), increased amounts of lithocholate have been detected in duodenal fluid and biliary bile.[10, 11, 72, 73] These observations imply that increased production and absorption of the potential hepatotoxin lithocholate are seen with conditions that alter bacterial metabolism of bile acids.

Increased fecal losses of bile acids occur when intestinal reabsorption is decreased. Intestinal malabsorption of bile acids may result from mucosal abnormalities, changes in the intestinal milieu (decreased pH), or the presence of bile acid resins (cholestyramine). Surgical resection or inflammatory disease of the terminal ileum decreases the surface area available for carrier-mediated bile acid uptake.[11] Deconjugation of bile acids in association with bacterial overgrowth raises their pKa and favors formation of insoluble bile acids that precipitate within the lumen.[4] Similarly, the decreased intraluminal pH seen with cystic fibrosis leads to formation of insoluble bile acid precipitates.[74] These precipitates are less efficiently absorbed by the terminal ileum. Cholestyramine is an anion exchange resin that binds bile acids within the intestinal lumen, thereby decreasing access to the ileal transporter. In each clinical setting, the decreased amount of bile acids returning to the liver via a portal vein stimulates cholesterol 7α-hydroxylase activity and leads to increased synthesis of bile acids. The liver has a tremendous capacity to synthesize bile acids and may increase its basal synthetic rate 5- to 10-fold. When fecal losses exceed the compensatory capacity of the liver, however, bile acid pool size decreases, resulting in lithogenic bile and steatorrhea secondary to diminished intraluminal bile acid concentrations.

Inherited Defects in Bile Acid Biosynthesis

Defects in bile acid biosynthesis have profound effects on gastrointestinal and hepatobiliary physiology because bile acids play a critical role in establishing bile flow and fat digestion. For all disorders involving the transformation of cholesterol to bile acids, the loss of feedback inhibition of primary bile acids on cholesterol 7α-hydroxylase activity results in accumulation of bile acid precursors and their potentially toxic metabolites.

Disorders in bile acid synthesis have been identified in infants with neonatal cholestasis.[71, 75-77] In all, six defects leading to impaired primary bile acid synthesis have been identified thus far.[78-80] Three of these involve modifications to the sterol ring.[78-80] Deficiencies in the function of the 3β-hydroxy-C27-steroid dehydrogenase/isomerase[78] (caused by at least 16 different mutations in the gene encoding this enzyme,[81] the second step in nuclear modification of cholesterol), and in the function of the Δ^4-3-oxosteroid 5β-reductase[79] (the enzyme responsible for catalyzing the stereospecific reduction of Δ^4 double bond), have been detected.[71] More recently, a mutation in the gene encoding the oxysterol 7α-hydroxylase enzyme was found to cause severe and lethal liver disease of infancy.[80] In all defects, normal primary bile acids were absent, and abnormal bile acid metabolites were detected in urine by fast atom bombardment mass spectrometry. Defects involving reactions associated with the sterol side chain oxidation include the sterol 27-hydroxylase enzyme causing cerebrotendinous xanthomatosis (an amidation defect in which glycine and taurine conjugated bile acids are not formed),[79] and a 2-methylacyl-CoA racemase deficiency,[82,83] the obligate enzyme for isomerization of 25R-trihydrocoprostanoic acid to 25S-trihydrocoprostanoic acid before its import to the peroxisome for subsequent β-oxidation. These side chain defects generally present with less severe cholestasis and are manifest more as fat-soluble vitamin malabsorption or neurologic syndromes. Administration of primary bile acids results in clinical, biochemical, and histologic improvement.[84] The rationale for treatment with primary bile acids is based on supposition that increased bile acid pool size provides the driving force for bile secretion, decreases cholesterol 7α-hydroxylase activity, and diminishes the accumulation of hepatotoxic bile acid metabolites.[75]

REFERENCES

1. Havel RJ: Lowering cholesterol, 1988. J Clin Invest *81*:1653, 1988.
2. Salen G, Shefer S: Bile acid synthesis. Annu Rev Physiol *45*:679, 1983.
3. Einarsson K, et al: Influence of age on secretion of cholesterol and synthesis of bile acids by the liver. N Engl J Med *313*:277, 1985.
4. Hofmann AF: Chemistry and enterohepatic circulation of bile acids. Hepatology 5:4S, 1984.
5. Bilhartz LE, Dietschy JM: Bile salt hydrophobicity influences cholesterol recruitment from rat liver in vivo when cholesterol synthesis and lipoprotein uptake are constant. Gastroenterology *95*:771, 1988.
6. Tint GS, et al: Effect of ursodeoxycholic acid and chenodeoxycholic acid in cholesterol and bile acid metabolism. Gastroenterology *91*:1007, 1986.
7. Reuben A: Bile formation: sites and mechanisms. Hepatology 5:15S, 1984.
8. Strange RC: Hepatic bile flow. Physiol Rev *64*:1055, 1984.
9. Hoffman AF: Bile acids. *In* Arias IM, et al (eds): The Liver: Biology and Pathobiology, 3rd ed. New York, Raven Press, 1994.
10. Fouin-Fortunet H, et al: Hepatic alterations during total parenteral nutrition in patients with inflammatory bowel disease: a possible consequence of lithocholate toxicity. Gastroenterology *82*:932, 1982.
11. Capron JP, et al: Metronidazole in prevention of cholestasis associated with total parenteral nutrition. Lancet *1*:446, 1983.
12. Brown MS, Goldstein JL: A receptor-mediated pathway for cholesterol homeostasis. Science *232*:34, 1986.
13. Setchell KDR, Street J: Inborn errors of bile acid synthesis. Semin Liver Dis 7:85, 1987.
14. Myant NB, Mitropoulos KA: Cholesterol 7α-hydroxylase. J Lipid Res *18*:135, 1977.
15. Hansson R, Wikvall K: Hydroxylations in biosynthesis and metabolism of bile acids. J Biol Chem *255*:1643, 1980.
16. Schwartz CC, et al: Multicompartmental analysis of cholesterol metabolism in man. J Clin Invest *61*:408, 1978.
17. Wikvall K: Purification and properties of a 3β-hydroxy-Δ-C_{27}-steroid oxidoreductase from rabbit liver microsomes. J Biol Chem *256*:3376, 1981.
18. Chiang JY, Stroup D: Identification and characterization of a putative bile acid-responsive element in cholesterol 7 alpha-hydroxylase gene promoter. J Biol Chem *269*:17502, 1994.
19. Van Dyke RW, et al: Bile acid transport in cultured rat hepatocytes. Am J Physiol *243*:G482, 1982.
20. Bjorkheim I: Mechanism of bile acid biosynthesis in mammalian liver. *In* Daniellson H, Sjovall J (eds): Sterols and Bile Acids. Amsterdam, Elsevier Science Publishers, 1985, pp 231–278.
21. Bjorkheim I, et al: Role of peroxisomes in the biosynthesis of bile acids. Scand J Clin Lab Invest *177*:23, 1985.
22. Vessey DA: The biochemical basis for the conjugation of bile acids with glycine or taurine. Biochem J *174*:621, 1978.
23. Killenberg PG, Jordan JT: Purification and characterization of bile acid-CoA: amino acid N-acyltransferase from rat liver. J Biol Chem *253*:1005, 1978.
24. Wright CE, et al: Taurine biological update. Annu Rev Biochem *55*:427, 1986.
25. Everson GT: Bile acid metabolism and its role in human cholesterol balance. Semin Liver Dis *12*:420, 1992.
26. Stange EF, et al: Feedback regulation of bile acid synthesis in the rat by dietary vs. intravenous cholate or taurocholate. Hepatology 8:879, 1988.
27. Heuman DM, et al: Regulation of bile acid synthesis. II. Effects of bile acid feeding on enzymes regulating hepatic cholesterol and bile acid synthesis in the rat. Hepatology 8:892, 1988.
28. Scharschmidt BF, Stephens FE: Transport of sodium, chloride and taurocholate by cultured rat hepatocytes. Proc Natl Acad Sci USA *78*:986, 1981.
29. Duffy MC, et al: Direct determination of driving forces for taurocholate uptake into rat liver plasma membrane vesicles. J Clin Invest *72*:1470, 1983.
30. Blitzer BL, Boyer JL: Cellular mechanisms of bile formation. Gastroenterology *82*:346, 1982.
31. Graf J, et al: Isolated rat hepatocyte couplets: a primary secretory unit for electrophysiologic studies of bile secretory function. Proc Natl Acad Sci USA *81*:6516, 1984.
32. Meier PJ, et al: Mechanisms of taurocholate transport in canalicular and basolateral rat liver plasma membrane vesicles. J Biol Chem *259*:10614, 1984.
33. Meier PJ, Stieger B: Canalicular membrane adenosine triphosphate-dependent transport systems. Prog Liver Dis *11*:27, 1993.
34. Balistreri WF, Heubi JE: Bile acid metabolism: relationship of bile acid malabsorption and diarrhea. J Pediatr Gastroenterol Nutr 2:105, 1983.
35. Balistreri WF, et al: Immaturity of the enterohepatic circulation in early life: factors predisposing to "physiologic" maldigestion and cholestasis. J Pediatr Gastroenterol Nutr 2:346, 1983.
36. Watkins JB, et al: Bile acid metabolism in the newborn: measurement of pool size and synthesis by stable isotope technique. N Engl J Med *288*:431, 1973.
37. Watkins JB, et al: Bile salt metabolism in the human premature infant. Gastroenterology *69*:706, 1975.
38. Little JM, et al: Taurocholate pool size and distribution in the fetal rat. J Clin Invest *63*:1042, 1979.
39. Subbiah MTR, Hassan AS: Development of bile acid biogenesis and its significance in cholesterol homeostasis. Adv Lipid Res *19*:137, 1982.
40. Heubi JE, et al: Bile salt metabolism in the first year of life. J Lab Clin Med *100*:127, 1982.
41. Lester R, et al: Diversity of bile acids in the fetus and newborn infant. J Pediatr Gastroenterol Nutr 2:355, 1983.
42. Setchell KDR, et al: Hepatic bile acid metabolism during early development revealed from the analysis of human fetal gallbladder bile. J Biol Chem *263*:16637, 1988.
43. Gustafsson J: Bile acid biosynthesis during development: hydroxylation of C-27 sterols in human fetal liver. J Lipid Res *27*:801, 1986.
44. Henning SJ: Postnatal development: coordination of feeding, digestion and metabolism. Am J Physiol *241*:G199, 1981.
45. Colombo C, et al: Biliary bile acid composition of the human fetus in early gestation. Pediatr Res *21*:197, 1987.
46. Bucuvalas JC, et al: Enhanced uptake of taurine by basolateral plasma membrane vesicles isolated from developing liver. Pediatr Res *23*:172, 1988.
47. Watkins JB: Feeding the low-birth weight infant: effects of taurine, cholesterol and human milk on bile acid kinetics. Gastroenterology *85*:793, 1983.
48. Okamato E, et al: Role of taurine in feeding the low-birth-weight infant. J Pediatr *104*:936, 1984.
49. Dorvil NP, et al: Taurine prevents cholestasis induced by lithocholic acid sulfate in guinea pigs. Am J Clin Nutr *37*:221, 1983.
50. Watkins JB: Placental transport: bile acid conjugation and sulfation in the fetus. J Pediatr Gastroenterol Nutr 2:365, 1983.
51. Hardy KJ, et al: Bile acid metabolism in fetal sheep: perinatal changes in the bile acid pool. J Physiol (Lond) *309*:1, 1980.
52. Dumaswala R, et al: Characterization of a specific transport mechanism for bile acids on the brush border membrane of human placenta. Am J Physiol *264*:G1016, 1993.
53. Belknap WL, et al: Physiologic cholestasis. II. Serum bile acid levels reflect the development of the enterohepatic circulation in rats. Hepatology *1*:613, 1981.
54. Suchy FJ, et al: Physiologic cholestasis: elevation of the primary serum bile acid concentrations in normal infants. Gastroenterology *80*:1037, 1981.
55. Suchy FJ, Balistreri WF: Uptake of taurocholate by hepatocytes isolated from developing rats. Pediatr Res *16*:282, 1982.
56. Suchy FJ, et al: Taurocholate transport and Na+-K+-ATPase activity in fetal and neonatal rat liver plasma membrane vesicles. Am J Physiol *251*:G665, 1986.
57. Suchy FJ: Hepatocellular transport of bile acids. Semin Liver Dis *13*:235, 1993.
58. Tavaloni N, et al: Postnatal development of bile secretory physiology in the dog. J Pediatr Gastroenterol Nutr *4*:256, 1985.
59. Shaffer EA, et al: Postnatal development of hepatic bile formation in the rabbit. Dig Dis Sci *30*:558, 1985.
60. Piccoli DA, et al: Bile salt secretion in the developing rat: implications for cholestasis. Gastroenterology *90*:1801, 1986.
61. Sippel CJ, et al: Isolation and characterization of the canalicular bile acid transport protein of rat liver. Am J Physiol *258*:G728, 1990.
62. Suchy FJ: Bile formation: mechanisms and development. *In* Suchy FJ (ed): Liver Disease in Children. St Louis, CV Mosby, 1994.
63. Little JM, Lester R: Ontogenesis of intestinal bile salt absorption in the neonatal rat. Am J Physiol *239*:G319, 1980.
64. Heubi JE, Fondacaro JD: Postnatal development of intestinal bile salt transport in the guinea pig. Am J Physiol *243*:G189, 1982.
65. Barnard JA, et al: Ontogenesis of taurocholate transport by rat ileal brush border membrane vesicles. J Clin Invest *75*:869, 1985.
66. Moyer MS, et al: Ontogeny of bile acid transport in brush border membrane vesicles from rat ileum. Gastroenterology *90*:1185, 1986.
67. Radominska A, et al: Bile acid metabolism and the pathophysiology of cholestasis. Semin Liver Dis *13*:219, 1993.
68. van Berge-Henegouwen GP: Therapy with ursodeoxycholic acid in cholestatic liver disease. Scand J Gastroenterol *200*:15S, 1993.
69. Rudolph G, et al: Effect of ursodeoxycholic acid on the kinetics of cholic acid and chenodeoxycholic acid in patients with primary sclerosing cholangitis. Hepatology *17*:1028, 1993.
70. Summerfield JA, et al: Identification of bile acids in the serum and urine in cholestasis. Biochem J *154*:507, 1976.
71. Setchell KDR, O'Connell NC: Disorders of bile acid synthesis and metabolism: a metabolic basis for liver disease. *In* Suchy FJ, et al (eds): Liver Disease in Children. Philadelphia, Lippincott Williams & Wilkins, 2001, pp 701–734.
72. Oelberg DG, et al: Lithocholate glucuronide is a cholestatic agent. J Clin Invest *73*:1507, 1984.
73. Roberto E, et al: Luminal events of lipid absorption in protein calorie malnourished children: relationship with nutritional recovery and diarrhea; alteration in bile acid content of duodenal aspirates. Am J Clin Nutr *27*:778, 1974.
74. Boyle BT, et al: Effect of cimetidine and pancreatic enzymes on serum and fecal bile acids and fat absorption in cystic fibrosis. Gastroenterology *78*:950, 1980.
75. Suchy FJ: Bile acids for babies? Diagnosis and treatment of a new category of metabolic liver disease. Hepatology *18*:1274, 1993.
76. Setchell KDR, O'Connell NC: Disorders of bile acid synthesis and metabolism. *In* Walker WA, et al (eds): Pediatric Gastrointestinal Disease. Hamilton, Canada, BC Decker, 2000, pp 1138–1170.
77. Bove K, et al: Bile acid synthetic defects and liver disease. Pediatr Dev Pathol 3:1, 2000.
78. Clayton PT, et al: Familial giant cell hepatitis associated with synthesis of 3β, 7α-dihydroxy- and 3β,7α,12α-trihydroxy-5-cholenoic acids. J Clin Invest *79*:1031, 1987.

79. Setchell KDR, et al: Δ⁴-3-Oxosteroid 5β-reductase deficiency described in identical twins with neonatal hepatitis: a new inborn error in bile acid synthesis. J Clin Invest 82:2148, 1988.
80. Setchell KDR, et al: Identification of a new inborn error in bile acid synthesis: mutation of the oxysterol 7α-hydroxylase gene causing severe neonatal liver disease. J Clin Invest 102:1690, 1998.
81. Cheng JB, et al: Molecular genetics of 3β-hydroxy-Δ⁵-C₂₇-steroid oxidoreductase deficiency in 16 patients with loss of bile acid synthesis. J Clin Endocrinol Metab 4:1833, 2003.
82. Setchell KDR, et al: Neonatal liver disease in two siblings caused by failure to racemize trihydroxycholestanoic acid: identity of gene mutation and effect of cholic acid therapy. Gastroenterology 124:217, 2003.

83. Setchell KDR, et al: Neonatal liver disease in two siblings caused by a failure to racemize (25R)trihydroxycholestanoic acid due to a gene mutation in 2-methylacyl-CoA racemase: effectiveness of cholic acid therapy in preventing liver and neurological disease. In Bile Acids from Genomics to Disease Therapy: Falk Symposium No. 129. Lancaster, UK, Kluwer Academic Publishers, 2003.
84. Jacquemin E, et al: Long-term effects of bile acid therapy in children with defects of primary bile acid synthesis: 3β-hydroxy-C27-steroid dehydrogenase/isomerase and Δ⁴-3-oxosteroid 5β-reductase deficiencies. In van Berge Henegouwen GP, et al (eds): Biology of Bile Acids in Health and Disease. Dordrecht, Kluwer Academic Publishers, 2001, pp 278–282.

120

David A. Horst and Saul J. Karpen

Bile Formation and Cholestasis

The liver, the largest organ in the body, performs three main functions: (1) metabolism and detoxification, (2) serum protein synthesis, and (3) bile secretion. Infants, especially premature infants, are particularly susceptible to damage elicited by impairments in bile flow (cholestasis), yet the underlying mechanisms are poorly understood. To comprehend fully the molecular mechanisms that form bile and how cholestasis develops when these mechanisms are perturbed, it is necessary to understand hepatic macroanatomy and microanatomy, cell organization, membrane transport functions, and hepatic development. A detailed understanding of the determinants of bile formation will help medical practitioners to understand its relevance to the care and treatment of cholestatic infants.

ANATOMY OF THE LIVER

Hepatic Blood Flow

The adult liver receives 20 to 25% of the cardiac output via two inputs: 70% of the blood entering the liver comes from the intestines via the portal circulation, and the remainder is provided by the hepatic artery.[1] The portal circulation brings nutrients, toxic substances, endobiotics, and xenobiotics from the digestive tract into the sinusoidal space bathing the hepatocytes. Blood from the portal vein and blood from the hepatic artery mix in the periportal sinusoids and flow toward the central vein, bathing each hepatocyte and allowing for uptake of nutrients, drugs, and toxins from blood (Fig. 120-1). After modification by the hepatocytes, sinusoidal blood exits via the central vein into the hepatic vein and eventually empties into the systemic circulation via three hepatic veins. The well-oxygenated blood from the hepatic artery mixes with portal blood that has relatively low oxygen content immediately in the periportal sinusoidal region. Thus, a gradient exists within the microanatomic zonal architecture of the liver lobule, whereby the periportal area is exposed to the highest oxygen tension and levels of nutrients. The biliary tree is supplied exclusively by the hepatic artery via an extensive peribiliary vascular plexus that provides nutrients to the cholangiocytes.[2]

As displayed in Figure 120-1, the functional unit of the liver is the hepatic lobule. Portal triads consisting of a portal vein, hepatic artery, and bile duct form the corners of each roughly hexagonal lobule. Bile forms within canaliculi and flows in a countercurrent fashion toward bile ducts within the portal triads. The flow of bile toward the portal triad is facilitated by the active secretion of biliary solutes into the canalicular space and is propelled by contraction of the microvilli on the apical membrane.[3,4]

Cellular Composition of the Liver

More than 80% of the cells in the liver are hepatocytes. The remaining nonparenchymal cells include cholangiocytes, Kupffer cells, hepatic stellate cells, and Pit cells, as well as sinusoidal endothelial cells. Hepatocytes contain a relatively large number of organelles, which participate in manifold synthetic, metabolic, nutritional, and detoxifying functions.[5] Fifteen per cent of the cell volume is endoplasmic reticulum, and each hepatocyte contains more than 1000 mitochondria, 300 lysosomes and peroxisomes, 50 Golgi complexes, and an organized cytoskeleton.[5-7] Kupffer cells, the resident macrophages in the liver, are present within sinusoids and can migrate within the lumen.[8] Hepatic stellate cells are perisinusoidal, with cytoplasmic extensions around the sinusoidal endothelial lining. They express neuroendocrine markers and therefore may have a neural crest origin.[9] In addition to representing the largest pool of retinol (vitamin A) in the body, stellate cells produce and maintain the extracellular matrix, control the microvascular tone, and have a role in fibrosis, cirrhosis, and regeneration.[5] Pit cells are located on the endothelial lining and have natural killer activity. Sinusoidal endothelial cells function in many types of metabolic processes in the liver, but they have functional differences (e.g., fenestrae) from typical vascular endothelial cells.[10]

Hepatocyte Polarity and Membrane Domains

Hepatocytes have a distinct polarity, and their plasma membrane can be divided into three domains: the sinusoidal (basolateral), the intercellular, and the canalicular (apical) membranes. The basolateral and intercellular membrane domains are contiguous and in direct contact with sinusoidal blood via the subendothelial space, the space of Disse (see Fig. 120-1). Thirty-five per cent of the total hepatocyte surface consists of basolateral membrane. Unlike most other endothelia, the sinusoidal endothelial layer has no basement membrane, and it contains fenestrae that are approximately 1000 Å in diameter, allowing for direct contact between sinusoidal blood and the hepatocyte membranes. This facilitates the uptake of relatively large proteins and particles (e.g., lipoprotein complexes) from the blood by the hepatocyte.

Approximately 15% of the hepatocyte plasma membrane is the canalicular membrane that is in contact with bile. The canalicular membrane contains vastly different lipid composition and resident transporter proteins from the sinusoidal membrane. In general, the prime determinants of the secretion of bile occur at the canalicular membrane as a result of recently identified res-

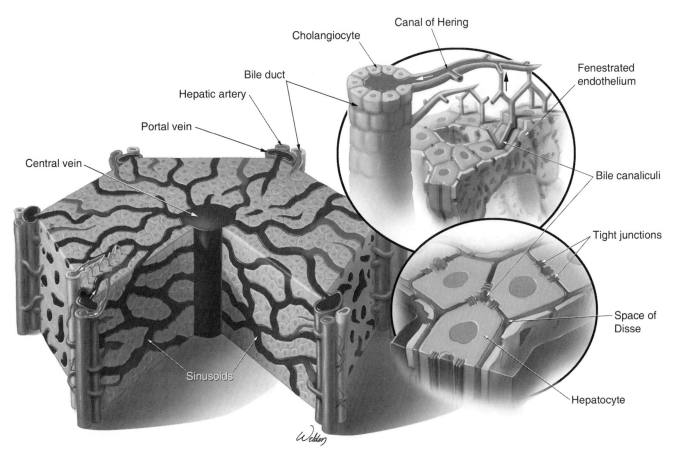

Figure 120–1. Schematic view of the liver lobule. (See also color plate section). The central vein is shown in the center of the lobule, separated by cords of hepatocytes forming sinusoids from six portal areas at the periphery. The portal areas contain a portal vein, hepatic artery, and bile duct. Blood flow is toward the center of the lobule, whereas bile flows toward the portal triads at the margins. Note the hepatic artery providing oxygenated blood to the hepatic sinusoids as well as the peribiliary plexus. *The top inset* provides a more detailed view of the fenestrated endothelium and the connections between intercellular canaliculi and the canals of Hering. The *lower inset* emphasizes the separate basolateral and canalicular membranes, as well as the junctional complexes. (Illustration by Scott Weldon: © 2003, Saul J. Karpen, Baylor College of Medicine.)

ident biliary solute transporter proteins that transport various substances from the hepatocyte interior into bile.

Fifty per cent of the plasma membrane of the hepatocyte is adjacent to other hepatocytes but still in continuity with the basolateral surface, and thus it is exposed to sinusoidal blood. This is termed the *intercellular domain*, and it is separated from the canalicular membrane by specialized junctional complexes stabilized by actin-containing microfilaments.[4, 11] These cell:cell tight junctions (zonula occludens) form the only anatomic barrier between the blood bathing the sinusoidal membrane and the canalicular membrane. In addition to defining the polarity of the hepatocyte, these tight junctions can determine the permeability of the barrier between blood and bile, and they allow for intercellular communication.[12] These multipartite junctional complexes contribute to the low permeability of the tight junctions and form a negatively charged barrier that usually allows for passage of small charged ions but not proteins. In models of cholestasis, the junctional complex may be altered to allow bile contents to cross the anatomic barrier and to reflux back into sinusoidal blood.[13]

Bile Formation

Bile is secreted across the apical membrane into bile canaliculi, which are small (0.75-μm) channels formed by half-tubules from the apical surface of two adjacent hepatocytes (see Fig. 120–1).

Bile ductules are channels that collect bile directly from transition zones adjacent to the liver parenchyma, the canals of Hering, and drain into the terminal branches of the biliary tree. The system of bile ducts resembles an inverted root system. The terminal branches are called interlobular bile ducts or, more recently, the terminal bile ducts.[14] Area ducts are the first grossly visible ducts, coalescing into segmental ducts, then into the right and left hepatic ducts that ultimately drain into the common hepatic duct.[15] Bile is stored in the gallbladder and is subsequently secreted into the common bile duct via the cystic duct. The gallbladder, unlike the relatively rigid ducts of the biliary tree, is readily distensible and is large enough to hold 30 to 50 mL of bile in adult humans.[16] In the interlobular region, the ducts become lined with a polarized, cuboidal epithelium of cholangiocytes, which transitions to columnar cells in larger septal duct units.

Approximately 5% of the cells in the liver are cholangiocytes. These bile duct epithelial cells line the intrahepatic biliary tree and modify bile after its secretion from hepatocytes. Cholangiocytes are polar cells capable of active transport at their basolateral and apical membranes. Cholangiocytes deliver fluids and electrolytes in response to hormonal secretion (primarily secretin) released by the duodenum into the portal bloodstream after stimulation by acidic pH, fatty acids, and bile acids.[17] They express several transporters, including cystic fibrosis transmembrane conductance regulator (CFTR) and a chloride/bicarbonate exchanger on their apical membrane. CFTR transports chloride and is defective in cystic fibrosis, which, when mutated, can result in neonatal cholestasis.[18, 19] The chloride/bicarbonate exchanger works with chloride secretion to alkalinize the ductular bile and to increase fluid secretion.[20, 21] The morphology, secretion, and response to injury of cholangiocytes are heterogeneous.[22, 23] As cholangiocytes progress from cuboidal to columnar epithelium along the biliary tree, these cells express various enzymes and hormone receptors.[22, 24, 25] Moreover, the cytoplasmic/nuclear ratios of the epithelial cells increase as the ducts progress to the common bile duct and empty into the intestine.[25]

DEVELOPMENT OF THE LIVER AND BILIARY TREE

The human liver is derived from the foregut endoderm, specifically the liver diverticulum, and the septum transversum.[26, 27] The liver diverticulum penetrates the septum transversum in a cranioventral direction. The septum transversum is made of loosely joined mesenchyme cells in a collagen-rich environment and a capillary plexus from the branches of the vitelline veins, and it defines the area of the embryonic cavity for ingrowth of the hepatic bud.[26-28] Secreted proteins and cellular interactions with the mesenchyme are necessary for differentiation of the endoderm into hepatoblasts and then hepatocytes.[28-32] The main liver cells, hepatocytes and cholangiocytes, appear to share a common progenitor cell, the hepatoblast. The differential expression of several transcription factors plays an essential role in induction, early growth, and differentiation of the liver and biliary tree (Table 120-1).[28] Between the third and fourth weeks of gestation, the diverticulum divides into a hollow caudal section and a solid cranial hepatic section. The larger hepatic section differentiates into proliferating cords of hepatocytes and the intrahepatic bile ducts. The early hepatocytes grow in thick epithelial sheets between the vitelline veins to form a system of plates. Initially, the plates are three to five cells thick, and they do not complete progression to one-cell-thick plates until 5 years of age.[33] The vitelline veins develop into the sinusoids. The smaller cystic section of the diverticulum develops into the extrahepatic bile ducts including the gallbladder, the common duct, and the cystic duct through elongation and recanalization.[34-37] The epithelial lining of the extrahepatic bile ducts begins as solid cords of epithelial cells that are continuous between the duodenal epithelium and the primitive hepatic cords. Sequential vacuolization produces a patent gallbladder and ductal system by the third month of gestation.[38]

The development of the intrahepatic bile ducts is distinct from the formation of the extrahepatic ducts, and it is a poorly understood process. The intrahepatic bile ducts develop from the primitive hepatocytes around the branches of the portal vein.[39-41] Starting at approximately 6 weeks of gestation, a single layer of hepatocytes surrounding the portal vein appears to transform into bile duct–type cells.[42, 43] This transformation begins at the hilum and spreads to the periphery. By the seventh week of gestation, a second layer of primitive hepatocytes transforms into similar cells and produces a double-walled cylinder with a slitlike lumen lined with cuboidal epithelial cells in the vicinity of the portal vein.[43-48] This structure, the ductal plate, remodels and differentiates into tubules radially from the porta hepatis. Remodeling of the porta hepatis into tubular bile ducts is complete by 12 weeks of gestation, by forming a patent and continuous passage to the lumen of the digestive tract.[43, 49]

Little is known about the molecular signals that direct biliary tract development. Analysis of several gene deletion models suggests roles for transcription factors, cell signaling molecules, and laterality genes (see Table 120-1). The portal tract mesenchyme plays a critical role in differentiation of hepatoblasts into biliary epithelial cells.[28] For example, hepatocyte cell cultures from adult liver will not form biliary epithelial layers in the absence of mesenchyme cells.[50]

TABLE 120-1

Transcription Factor	Function	References
Foxa 1–3(Hnf3α–γ)	Early foregut morphogenesis	254–259
Hex	Early liver bud morphogenesis, earliest known effector of developing liver	260, 261
Prox1	Early liver bud morphogenesis	262
Hgf	Liver bud growth, protective for apoptosis	263
Hlx	Hepatoblast, liver bud growth	264
Smad2, 3	Liver bud growth, mediate Tgf-β signaling	265
Hnf6	Morphogenesis of biliary ducts, restricts biliary commitment from hepatoblasts	266
Hnf1β	Morphogenesis of biliary ducts	267
Hnf4	Essential for hepatocyte differentiation	268

Blood flow through the liver changes around the time of birth. Before birth, the ductus venosus shunts blood from the left umbilical vein to the inferior vena cava. After birth, it collapses and begins to atrophy, eventually forming the ligamentum venosum, which is continuous with the ligamentum teres, the remnant of the left umbilical vein (Fig. 120–2).

COMPOSITION OF BILE

The normal adult liver secretes approximately 600 to 800 mL of bile a day; accurate measurements of bile flow in infants have yet to be reported.[51] Dissolved solids are 3% of bile by weight, and bile acids are the predominant organic solute at biliary concentrations of 20 to 30 mmol/L. Four bile acids make up greater than 95% of the bile acid pool, and they are categorized as either primary or secondary. Primary bile acids are synthesized in hepatocytes from cholesterol, and secondary bile acids are formed by metabolism of primary bile acids by colonic bacteria via enzymatic 7α-dehydroxylation. The primary bile acids are cholic acid (CA; 3α,7α–,12α-trihydroxy-5β-cholanic acid) and chenodeoxycholic acid (CDCA; 3α,7α-dihydroxy-5β-cholanic acid). The more hydrophobic secondary bile acids are deoxycholic acid (DCA; 3α,12α-dihydroxy-5β-cholanic acid) and lithocholic acid (LCA; 3α–hydroxy-5β-cholanic acid). More than 95% of bile acids are conjugated via their side chain to either glycine or taurine, in a 3:1 ratio that may be influenced by the availability of dietary taurine.[52, 53] At high concentrations, bile acids can solubilize phospholipid membranes, and the affinity of each bile acid for membranes is a function of its hydrophobicity. The more hydrophobic monohydroxy bile acids (LCA is the prototype) are poorly soluble, even in their conjugated form, and they are strong detergents and are therefore more detrimental to hepatocytes and their membranes.[54, 55] Hydrophobic, but not hydrophilic, bile acids have also been shown to decrease activity of cholesterol 7α-hydroxylase, the rate-limiting step in bile acid synthesis.[56, 57]

In addition to bile acids, several other solutes are present in bile (Fig. 120–3). Phospholipid and cholesterol are the next two most prevalent components, at 7 mmol/L and 2 to 3 mmol/L, respectively. Phospholipids make up 17% of the solute in bile, and virtually all phospholipids in bile are phosphatidylcholine (~95%). Three per cent of biliary solutes are cholesterol (2 to 3 mmol/L), almost entirely in the free or unesterified form. Dietary plant-derived sterols (phytosterols) are present at small concentrations.[58] Vitamins, steroids, drugs, xenobiotics, and other lipophilic products of lipid metabolism are also present as a small fraction of bile.[59] Organic anions of endogenous origin

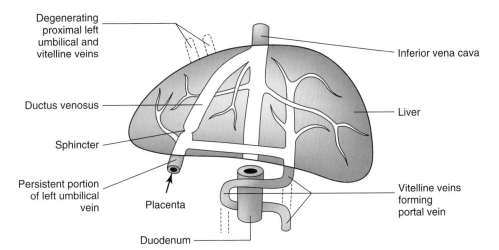

Figure 120–2. Dorsal view of the liver demonstrating the venous circulation at 7 weeks' gestation. Note the path from the umbilical vein through the ductus venosus to the inferior vena cava and the vitelline veins forming the portal vein. (Adapted from Moore, K.L., in *The Developing Human.* 1982, WB Saunders Co: Philadelphia. p. 301.)

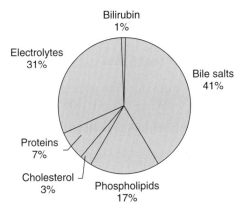

Figure 120–3. Solute composition of human bile. Bile acids are the most prevalent solute, followed by phospholipids and cholesterol. Conjugated bilirubin makes up a small fraction of biliary solute loads. (Adapted from Vlahcevic, Z.R., et al., in *Hepatology: A Textbook of Liver Disease*, D. Zakim, Boyer, T., Editors. 1996, WB Saunders: Philadelphia. p. 381.)

are secreted into bile. Bilirubin, present at a concentration of 0.2 mmol/L, gives bile its yellow color and is mostly excreted in its diglucuronide form. Glutathione is present at relatively high concentrations of 5 to 10 mmol/L in the cytosol of hepatocytes and is used in many reducing reactions, and glutathione and glutathione conjugates are actively secreted into bile. The tripeptide reduced glutathione is important as a primary driving force of the bile acid–independent proportion of bile flow.[60] Inorganic salts are present in concentrations similar to those in plasma. Drugs and toxins that are normally secreted into bile are retained within hepatocytes during any form of cholestasis, thus accentuating liver disease.

The main lipid components of bile (bile acids, phospholipid, and cholesterol) form multicomponent vesicles or mixed micelles in the canalicular lumen. Unconjugated, lipophilic bilirubin may also be part of these micelles. Mixed micelles of phosphatidylcholine and bile acid are formed in a phospholipid/bile acid ratio of 2:1. Their shape depends on the relative bile acid concentration. At higher concentrations, the micelles are globular aggregates. As the bile acid concentration decreases, they form rods and long cylinders.[61] When bile is supersaturated with cholesterol, it may exist in several phases. These include mixed micelles, lamellar phases, and solid crystals. More concentrated bile favors micelle formation, and dilution favors the bilayer or lamellar phase. The formation of sludge and gallstones is generally the result of imbalances in bile acid/cholesterol:phospho-

lipid ratios,[61] and the normal ratios of cholesterol, phospholipids, and bile acids in neonatal bile are not known. Finally, bile is the main route of excretion of divalent heavy metals, including copper, manganese, iron, and zinc.[62]

BILE FORMATION AND THE ENTEROHEPATIC CIRCULATION OF BILE ACIDS

The main determinant of bile flow is the enterohepatic circulation of bile acids, and the rate-limiting step is the secretion of bile acids from the hepatocyte across the canalicular membrane and into the canalicular lumen. Bile acids are concentrated up to 1000-fold in bile after active transport by hepatocytes. The hepatocyte depends on the recirculation of bile acids to maintain the bile acid pool, which is 3 to 4 g in adult humans. Each bile acid circulates 6 to 10 times a day, and only a small fraction, approximately 0.5 g, is lost daily in the feces.[63] Overall, this is a tremendously efficient process; greater than 95% of bile acids excreted by the hepatocyte are ultimately returned to the liver and are resecreted into bile.[64] Bile acids are absorbed in the terminal ileum via a specific transporter in the apical membrane of the ileal enterocyte, are returned to the liver via the portal blood, and are imported back in to the hepatocyte via high-affinity transport mechanisms resident in the sinusoidal membrane.

The amount of bile acids made *de novo* by the liver is generally limited to the daily amount lost in feces.[65] The primary bile acids, CA and CDCA, are synthesized from cholesterol by two interacting biosynthetic pathways in humans.[66, 67] The enzyme cholesterol 7α–hydroxylase initiates and is the rate-limiting step in the *neutral pathway*, which primarily results in the synthesis of CA.[68,69] Sterol 27-hydroxylase initiates the *acidic pathway*, which leads primarily to the formation of CDCA. Bile acids regulate their own synthesis. In rats, creation of a fistula to divert the normal secretion of bile acids away from the duodenum or luminal sequestration of bile acids with cholestyramine leads to a several-fold increase in cholesterol 7α-hydroxylase activity and bile acid synthesis that can then be abolished by intraduodenal infusion of bile acids.[70-74] Cloning of cholesterol 7α-hydroxylase has facilitated studies that demonstrate negative feedback regulation of the enzyme by bile acids at the transcriptional level.[56,57,75]

In addition to bile acid–dependent bile flow, two other main factors in bile flow, depending on the species, contribute approximately equally to the overall flow of bile.[76] These are bile acid–independent bile flow and ductular (cholangiocyte) secretion.[51] The mechanisms underlying bile flow have largely been ascribed to membrane transporters (see later). There is a linear relationship between the secretion of bile acids and bile flow (Fig. 120–4).[77-80] The normal liver has a large functional reserve for the excretion of bile acids, with the ability to increase its basal excretion rate

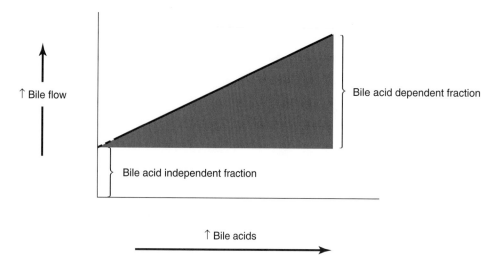

Figure 120–4. Bile acid-dependent bile flow (BADF) and bile acid-independent flow (BAIF) Note the linear relationship between bile acid secretion and BADF. The majority of bile flow is BADF that is reduced with smaller bile acid pool sizes, such as those of infants. The contribution made by BAIF to total bile flow is approximately 25% and is estimated by the extrapolation of the relation between biliary flow and bile acid excretion to the y-axis, the imaginary point at which there is no bile acid secretion.

by approximately eightfold.[81] Bile acids increase bile flow by several mechanisms, but mostly by creating an osmotic driving force for water, electrolytes, and other solutes brought into bile, and different bile acids have varying choleretic potency. Notably, pharmacologic increases in the bile acid pool size (e.g., by treatment with ursodeoxycholic acid [UDCA]) increase bile flow.

In contrast to the bile acid–dependent bile flow that is regulated by the bile acid pool size and the efficiency of the enterohepatic circulation, the bile acid–independent bile flow is mainly related to the liver cell mass, although it can be increased by the secretion of organic anions into bile.[82, 83] The transport of glutathione, of glutathiuone conjugates, and of organic anions is the primary determinant of bile acid-independent bile flow.[84,85] Bile acid-independent bile flow is stimulated by hormones, UDCA, and certain drugs, and it mainly reflects ion and non-bile acid solute transport into the canalicular space.[86-89] The non–bile acid canalicular membrane transporters likely play important roles in driving bile acid-independent bile flow. Ductular secretion is stimulated mainly by secretin-induced ion secretion, which further alkalinizes and dilutes the bile.[19, 90-93] Active absorption and excretion of various solutes provide additional alteration of the composition of bile.[94] The ductular contribution to overall bile flow varies according to species. For example, secretin is a potent choleretic agent in humans and in dogs, but it has little effect in rodents.[52,66,67,95]

Water can flow from the sinusoids to the lumen of the bile canaliculi via transcellular, paracellular, or transcytotic pathways. The paracellular route from the sinusoidal space to the canalicular lumen via the tight junctions between cells is responsible for most of the water movement. The transcellular and transcytotic or vesicular mechanisms make up a relatively limited contribution to fluid transport.[96, 97] Moreover, studies show that human and rat cholangiocytes express aquaporins. These channels contribute to active biliary water transport via their secretin-dependent exocytic insertion into the apical membrane.[98,99]

MOLECULAR DETERMINANTS OF BILE FLOW

Transporters and Their Regulation

Since the early 1990s, the gene products responsible for driving hepatobiliary transport, and hence bile formation, have been identified.[100] Both sinusoidal and canalicular membrane transporters are responsible for the coordinated transport of many different organic anions, drugs, toxins, endobiotics, and bile acids that ultimately are metabolized by hepatocytes and are secreted into bile (Fig. 120-5). This new information has led to greater comprehension of the mechanisms underlying basic hepatic

functions, including a molecular understanding of intermediary metabolism, cholesterol homeostasis, drug and toxin disposal, bile acid recirculation, and bile formation, as well as the identification of mutations in canalicular transporter genes in select rare forms of pediatric cholestasis.[101-103] The transporters responsible for delivering the main biliary solutes have been identified (compare Figs. 120-3 and 120-5). Taken together, alterations in the expression and activities of hepatobiliary transporter genes will have substantial effects on bile flow and biliary constituents that, if prolonged, will likely lead to adverse nutritional and hepatic consequences.

Regulation of Basolateral Transporters

NTCP

First-pass hepatic extraction of conjugated bile acids from sinusoidal blood is 75 to 90% efficient.[104] Approximately 75% of the uptake of bile acids across the basolateral membrane is a sodium (Na+)-dependent process in rodents, and it is likely similar in humans.[105, 106] The NTCP gene product (Na+-taurocholate-co-transporting polypeptide, SLC10A1) is expressed exclusively in hepatocytes and is responsible for the Na+-mediated high-affinity import of conjugated bile acids into the hepatocyte.[107] The NTCP gene product is considered to be the major means for the hepatic uptake of bile acids from portal blood.[63, 108, 109] The NTCP gene has significant regulation primarily at the transcriptional level, evident mainly during cholestasis and inflammation.

The rat and mouse NTCP genes appear to be regulated in similar fashion in experimental models of inflammation and cholestasis.[110, 111] In virtually all models of inflammation, (cecal ligation and puncture, injection of endotoxin, or the endotoxin-related cytokines tumor necrosis factor-α, interleukin-1β) or cholestasis (bile duct ligation, bile acid feeding), NTCP RNA levels are rapidly and profoundly repressed, leading to markedly reduced bile acid import during these states.[112-120] Thus, during periods of significant hepatocyte "vulnerability" to the continued importation of bile acids, the hepatocyte responds by transcriptionally suppressing NTCP expression. NTCP RNA levels are markedly suppressed in conditions in which intracellular bile acid concentrations rise, thereby initiating a negative feedback loop to protect the hepatocyte from bile acid–induced hepatocyte damage and apoptosis.[110,111,117,120,121]

The identification of a nuclear receptor for bile acids, the farnesoid X receptor (FXR; NR1H4) proved vital in understanding how the hepatocyte responds to bile acid excess. FXR is essential for protection of hepatocytes from excess bile acid loads. Feeding of FXR+/+ or FXR+/- mice 1% CA led to a coordinated response

Figure 120–5. Composite schematic of select hepatobiliary transporters involved in bile formation. The hepatocyte is oriented with sinusoidal (BLOOD) transporters on the *left* and canalicular (BILE) on the *right*. *Arrows* connote general directions that the listed solutes may be transported. The resident canalicular transporters are responsible for active secretion of nearly all components of bile. BA = bile acids; BSEP = bile salt export pump; MDR = multidrug resistance protein; MRP = multidrug resistance–related protein; NTCP = Na+/taurocholate co-transporting polypeptide; OA = organic anion; OATP = organic anion transporting polypeptide; OC = organic cation; PL = phospholipid; XOL = cholesterol.

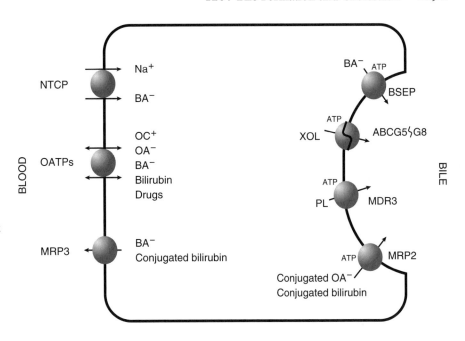

designed to help unload the hepatocyte of excess bile acids, including a marked reduction of NTCP RNA levels.[120] Conversely, FXR$^{-/-}$ mice fed the same diet did not initiate these hepatoprotective pathways and maintained high levels of NTCP RNA expression, which led to continued importation of bile acids, accumulation of intracellular bile acids, and rapid bile acid–induced hepatocellular damage and apoptosis.[120] Taken together, the combined rapid suppression of NTCP expression in inflammation and cholestasis leads to hepatocyte protection from bile acid excess, but it obligately reduces bile acid–dependent bile flow and thus contributes to the nutritional consequences of cholestasis. Given the normally low expression of NTCP RNA in developing rodents and the high serum bile acid levels in infancy, it is likely that the regulation of NTCP RNA expression plays an important role in the sick, premature infant.[122,123]

OATP Family

Approximately 25% of bile acid uptake by the hepatocyte is by Na+-independent mechanisms.[63] The family of organic anion transporting polypeptide (OATP) proteins is composed of at least a dozen members, and these proteins are the principal means of transport of many different substances across the basolateral membrane. Among the more notable substances are bile acids, organic anions, organic cations, drugs, toxins, and unconjugated bilirubin. In addition to the hepatocyte basolateral membrane, OATP family members participate in solute transport in other epithelia including kidney, intestine, choroid plexus, and retina.[63,124] These 12-membrane spanning proteins are multispecific transporters, typically function bidirectionally, and therefore likely regulate both the import and the export of solutes from blood to hepatocyte and vice versa. Their hepatic expression is therefore critically linked to the ability of the hepatocyte to metabolize many amphipathic organic molecules adequately, including xenobiotics, drugs, hormones, bilirubin, and bile acids. Some NTCP gene regulators are OATP gene regulators, especially regarding bile acid transport and metabolism, a finding suggesting common nuclear regulation to coordinate physiologic processes.[125] The expression and regulation of most OATP family members during development, inflammation, and cholestasis are generally unknown.

An important human Na+-independent bile acid transporter is OATP-C (SLC21A6), which transports taurocholate at a slightly lower affinity than human NTCP, and it may also transport

unconjugated bilirubin into the hepatocyte.[126,127] RNA levels of the rat homologue of the human OATP-C gene are rapidly and profoundly suppressed in models of sepsis and cholestasis, a finding suggesting similar means of regulation to the rat NTCP gene.[128,129] The actual molecular mediators of OATP-C regulation in cholestasis and sepsis remain to be determined. These findings suggest that repression of both NTCP and OATP-C expression likely occurs in the sick, septic, premature infant and leads to reduced bile flow and hyperbilirubinemia.

MRP3

Basolateral efflux of bile acids from the hepatocyte across the basolateral membrane into the sinusoidal blood is minimal under physiologic conditions. Several investigators identified multidrug resistance protein 3 (MRP3/ABCC3) as an important component of the hepatic response to cholestasis by exporting retained bile acids and conjugated organic anions across the basolateral membrane.[130] Both rat and human MRP3 gene products can transport bile acids as well as various conjugated organic anions, including conjugated bilirubin.[131,132] Normally, MRP3 expression is low and is restricted to the basolateral membrane of cholangiocytes and perivenous hepatocytes.[133-135] However, in cholestatic rat liver, MRP3 expression is markedly up-regulated.[133,135-140] MRP3 expression is up-regulated in human and rodent models in which the canalicular transporter MRP2 (ABCC2; see later) is mutated.[137,141] The significant overlap in substrate specificities between MRP2 and MRP3 transporters thereby permits compensatory basolateral export of typical MRP2 substrates when canalicular MRP2 expression is impaired. However, the actual role of MRP3 induction in human liver is not clear, because analysis of human liver biopsy samples from cholestatic patients did not show significant activation of MRP3 RNA levels.[142]

Regulation of Canalicular Transporters

BSEP

Canalicular bile acid transport is the rate-limiting step in the transport of bile acids from the sinusoidal blood through the hepatocyte and into the bile. The 1000-fold concentration gradient for bile acids across the canalicular membrane is maintained by adenosine triphosphate (ATP)–dependent transport.[143,144] The canalicular bile acid transporter has been cloned from rat, mouse, and human and is designated the canalicular bile salt export pump, or BSEP (ABCB11).[145-148] The human BSEP gene has been identified in persons with progressive familial intrahepatic cholestasis type 2 (PFIC2; see later), a disease that presents in infancy with cholestasis, high serum bile acid concentrations, and low γ-glutamyltranspeptidase (GGT) serum levels.[149] Mutations in the BSEP gene can eliminate canalicular BSEP expression and can decrease biliary bile acid levels to less than 1% of normal in BSEP−/− knock-out mice and humans.[150,151] In contrast to basolateral transporters, expression of BSEP is maintained during cholestasis in rats, possibly as a protective mechanism.[152]

MRP2

The multidrug resistance related protein 2, MRP2 (ABCC2), is expressed on the canalicular membrane of hepatocytes, as well as on the apical membrane of enterocytes and kidney.[153,154] The MRP2 gene product exports glutathione, sulfated and glucuronidated conjugates of drugs, toxins, and bilirubin, and it is likely responsible for the majority of bile acid–independent bile flow across the canaliculus.[155] Mutation of MRP2 leads to reduced bile acid–independent bile flow in rodent models and to elevated serum levels of conjugated bilirubin seen in the Dubin-Johnson syndrome.[155-157]

MRP2 RNA levels are profoundly suppressed in rodent models of sepsis and cholestasis.[119,158-161] MRP2 RNA levels are essentially normal in human liver biopsies from cholestatic patients, but they are reduced in liver biopsies from patients infected with hepatitis C virus.[142,162] Mice fed diets enriched with CA or UDCA showed increased hepatic MRP2 RNA expression.[163] Human and rat MRP2 RNA expression is increased in response to redox reagents, toxins, and drugs, and it is decreased in response to inflammatory cytokines.[112,164-170]

MDR3

Phosphatidylcholine is transferred from the outer leaflet of the canalicular membrane into bile by the phospholipid translocator ("flippase") MDR3 (ABCB4; Mdr2 in rodents).[171] Phospholipids are critical to the formation of micelles that protect the biliary tree from hydrophobic bile acids. Mdr2−/− knock-out mice lack phospholipids in their bile, leading to ductular damage and cholestasis.[172] Mutations in the human MDR3 gene cause PFIC type 3 (PFIC3), a cholestatic disease of infancy with high serum bile acid levels and increased GGT levels indicative of biliary damage.[173]

ABCG5 and ABCG8

Two other transporters worthy of note that have been identified are ABCG5 and ABCG8. These two half-ABC transporters are unique in that they are targeted to the canalicular membrane together as a heterodimer that transports cholesterol into bile.[174-177] A mutation in either ABCG5 or ABCG8 results in defective biliary sterol transport and leads to the human disease sitosterolemia.[178,179]

Developmental Expression of Transporter Genes

Ntcp mRNA is first detectable during the latter stages of rodent gestation; there is a significant increase in mRNA postnatally, reaching adult levels by 1 to 4 weeks.[180,181] In contrast, the expression of rodent Oatp2 and Oatp4 could be detected only at the mRNA level or the protein level during the first 4 weeks after birth.[182-184] The ontogenic expression of the canalicular transporters has also been studied in rats, and the MRP2 gene is expressed earlier in liver development that BSEP.[185] BSEP mRNA and protein are not expressed until after birth, but MRP2 mRNA is weakly expressed, and protein is strongly expressed in the 16-day-old fetus. Reduced neonatal expression of bile acid transporters is a likely contributor to perinatal hypercholanemia (cholestasis).

BILE FORMATION IN THE NEONATE

The placenta plays a major role in detoxification and excretion of lipophilic organic anions and bile acid metabolism before its abrupt removal at birth, when the functional immaturity of the fetal liver becomes evident.[186] The liver is both a hematopoetic and a hepatic organ until birth, when it begins its major transition to its adult role as the primary site for metabolism and detoxification in the body. The immaturity of neonatal bile acid metabolism is clinically significant because adequate bile acid synthesis and secretion are essential for hepatic bile formation and for intestinal fat and fat-soluble vitamin absorption.

Bile acids have been isolated from human gallbladder and liver as early as 14 to 16 weeks' gestation.[187] After 22 to 26 weeks' gestation, the main bile acids in human fetal gallbladder are the taurine-conjugated dihydroxy bile acids, principally TCDCA. The trihydroxy bile acid TCA and small amounts of glycocholate appear at 28 weeks' gestation, and TCA is the principal bile acid at birth.[188] Taurine conjugates predominate in the fetus and neonate until the adult pattern of predominant glycine conjugation is achieved at 2 to 7 months.[189] Animal studies show that conjugation of bile acids in the third trimester is markedly less than in newborns or adults.[190,191]

Studies in fetal sheep and dogs using tracer doses of [14C]cholesterol demonstrated that only TCA and TCDCA were synthesized by the fetus in both species.[192,193] There was no synthesis of the secondary bile acids LCA and DCA, likely reflecting the requirement of postnatal colonic bacteria for their formation. Recovery of labeled secondary bile acids occurred only when the maternal bile acid pool was labeled. External biliary drainage resulted in increased conversion of cholesterol to bile acids, showing some degree of autonomous regulation of primary bile acid synthesis. These studies indicate some degree of functionality and regulation of the fetal enterohepatic circulation. The fetus' ability to absorb bile acids from the intestinal lumen was studied using [14C]taurocholate in utero and showed significant passive reabsorption of conjugated bile acids occurring in the proximal jejunum and poorly developed active reabsorption of taurocholate in the fetal ileum.[194] Fetal serum bile acids are low compared with adults, likely owing to clearance by the placenta and immature absorption from the intestinal lumen.[195,196] Bidirectional transfer of bile acids between the maternal and fetal circulations is mediated by specific transport mechanisms of brush-border and basal membranes of the human placental syncytiotrophoblast.[197]

When compared with the adult, the near-term human fetus is substantially deficient in bile acid pool size, gallbladder concentrating function, and intestinal absorption.[192,198] Stable isotope techniques determined that the term infant's CA pool size and synthesis rates were roughly half of adult levels.[199] CA pool and synthesis rates studies in premature infants from 32 to 36 weeks' gestation are approximately one third of the already reduced levels in term neonates.[200] It is likely that premature infants less than 32 weeks' gestation have even lower bile acid pool sizes, although this has not been tested. Significantly, premature infants who were retrospectively grouped by antenatal maternal treatment with dexamethasone or phenobarbital had bile acid pool sizes approximating those of the term neonate. In another study, cortisone administration to suckling rats on day 13 of life resulted in adult levels of CA conjugation on day 14, 7 days earlier than the usual increase at the time of weaning.[201] These data suggest a role for adrenal hormones in the maturation of the enterohepatic circulation of bile acids.

Serum levels of bile acids after birth follow a characteristic developmental pattern. During the first week of life, serum concentrations of the primary bile acids, CA and CDCA, progressively increase to reach concentrations that are significantly higher than in physiologically normal older children and adults.[123,202] In contrast to the transient physiologic hyperbilirubinemia of the newborn, serum bile acid levels do not decline to levels comparable to those of adults until 6 months of age.[123] High serum bile acids are not indicative of increased synthesis or recirculation, but they reflect impaired hepatic uptake. Taken together with the aforementioned smaller pool size and decreased intestinal absorption, this situation leads to *physiologic cholestasis* (or *physiologic hypercholanemia*) of infancy.[194, 203, 204] The mechanisms underlying physiologic cholestasis have been well studied in developing rodents. Basolateral uptake of bile acids is markedly diminished in the fetal and neonatal hepatocyte. The rate-limiting step in enterohepatic circulation of bile acids is also affected, because there is an almost complete lack of acinar gradient in suckling rats.[205,206] Reduced bile acid uptake is correlated with impaired expression of Ntcp RNA levels, protein concentration, and bile acid transport.[181] Na+-dependent taurocholate uptake begins at fetal day 20 and increases to adult levels by 3 to 4 weeks postnatally in membrane vesicles isolated from fetal and newborn rat livers.[207] In human infants, bile acid pool sizes, intraluminal concentrations, and secretion rates increase in infancy, and they reach maturation at the end of the first year of life.[204,208]

The biliary tree's response to hormones important to the postcanalicular modification of bile also undergoes maturation. The biliary epithelium does not respond to secretin or glucagon stimulation in the newborn dog at 3 days, and the response is only 30 to 45% of adult levels at 4 to 6 weeks.[209,210] High serum levels of secretin, glucagon, and vasoactive intestinal peptide suggest decreased numbers of receptors or decreased activity and postreceptor response.[211] Currently, very little is known about cholangiocyte function in human neonates.

In addition to maturation of the intrahepatic determinants of bile duct secretion, bile flow into the duodenum depends on active contraction of the main biliary storage organ, the gallbladder. Fasting gallbladder volume is larger, and contraction occurs more readily, in term infants than in premature infants.[212, 213] Significant contraction was observed in infants who weighed more than 1300 g or who were 31 weeks' postconceptual age, whereas infants 27 to 32 weeks' postconceptual age showed no postprandial gallbladder contraction.[214] Studies in newborn piglets found decreased intraluminal pressure at similar gallbladder volumes and less increase in pressure with cholecystokinin stimulation in newborn than in adult gallbladders.[215] Moreover, *in situ*, the neonatal gallbladders were 3 to 12 times less compliant. These models suggest that intraluminal pressure may not be enough to overcome the resistances offered by the common bile duct and sphincter of Oddi. In addition, the ability of the fetal and neonatal gallbladder to concentrate bile acids is less when compared with adults. Duodenal bile acid concentration measured after stimulation with either milk feeding or magnesium sulfate is reduced when compared with an older child.[216] In several studies of term human neonates, intraluminal bile acid concentrations of 1 to 2 mmol/L were measured after meal stimulation without significant variation during the course of the day.[204] Bile secretion appears to be unresponsive to postprandial stimulation in the neonate.

CONGENITAL CHOLESTATIC DISORDERS

Before the identification and cloning of specific genes responsible for defects in canalicular transport, a general descriptive classification for patients identified as having a defect in hepatic secretory function was that of PFIC. Bile flow is critically dependent on canalicular transport of bile acids, and failure will lead to the clinical picture of PFIC: hepatocyte retention of bile acids and cell damage with progressive liver failure and fat malabsorption. Biochemical markers in this situation are high serum bile acids and low biliary bile acids. Although biliary bile acids are seldom measured in patients, there exists a correlation between low biliary bile acids and normal serum levels of

GGT,[151, 217] which, when elevated, is generally considered to be an indicator of a damaged biliary tract. Historically, inclusion of GGT levels has been part of the descriptive classification of the three types of PFIC.

FIC1 Deficiency (PFIC1)

The phenotype of FIC1 deficiency is similar to BSEP deficiency (PFIC2) in its low-normal GGT levels despite impairment of bile flow. However, it differs in that there are extrahepatic manifestations, including pancreatitis and intestinal malabsorption. Patients do not have neonatal hepatitis, and their cholestasis is initially relatively mild. The genotype maps to chromosome 18, and the gene, FIC1, has been cloned.[218] FIC1 is a canalicular P-type ATPase that participates in maintaining the distribution of aminophospholipids between the inner and outer leaflets of the plasma membrane.[219] Unlike BSEP that is mainly expressed in the liver, the FIC1 gene is also expressed in pancreas and intestine with relatively low levels in the liver at the canalicular membrane. The connection between loss of this function and the clinical manifestations of FIC1 deficiency are being studied. As would be expected, the extrahepatic manifestations in patients with FIC1 may not be cured by liver transplantation.

BSEP Deficiency (PFIC2)

A mutation in the resident canalicular bile acid transporter, BSEP, has been identified as the cause of PFIC2.[149] Patients with a deficiency of BSEP usually present in the first few months of life with neonatal hepatitis and worsening pruritus, high serum bile acid levels, and progressive intrahepatic cholestasis with normal GGT levels. The disease progresses to end-stage liver disease by 2 to 10 years of age, a finding emphasizing the importance of BSEP in canalicular bile acid transport, the rate-determining step in bile flow. Transplantation is curative and is the only available therapy.

MDR3 Deficiency (PFIC3)

Patients with this deficiency have impairment of bile flow with high GGT, also known as high-GGT PFIC. The bile acid/phospholipid ratio in bile is elevated, and the patient has portal inflammation and bile duct proliferation. MDR3 is the canalicular transporter responsible for secretion of phospholipids (mainly phosphatidylcholine) that are components of mixed micelles. Impairment of phospholipid transport would be expected to create highly detergent, hydrophobic bile, as an explanation for the increased GGT levels. It has been shown to be mutated in patients with this phenotype.[173]

Dubin-Johnson Syndrome

The phenotype of Dubin-Johnson syndrome is a relatively benign increase in serum and intracellular conjugated bilirubin levels. Other organic anions, conjugated and glutathione-reduced products of drug metabolism, also accumulate. Mrp 2 (ABCC2) is the mutated canalicular transporter that is normally responsible for secretion of these substances.[220]

Disorders of Bile Acid Synthesis

Congenital defects in bile acid synthesis lead to an accumulation of potentially hepatotoxic atypical bile acids and cholestasis secondary to decreased primary bile acids that are essential for driving bile flow. The consequences may be rapid development of liver dysfunction, even liver failure, in infancy. Disorders of bile acid synthesis are responsible for approximately 2 to 3% of cases of liver disease in infants and children.[221] At least six specific enzymatic defects related to modification of the cholesterol nucleus or side chain have been characterized. Their phenotypic expression is twofold, either cholestasis or symptoms of fat-soluble vitamin malabsorption and nutritional deficiencies. Significantly, a defect in cholesterol 7α-hydroxylase, the initial and rate-limiting enzyme in the classic pathway of bile acid synthesis, has been linked to high serum levels of low density lipoprotein cholesterol, increased hepatic cholesterol content, and decreased fecal excretion of bile acids in human adults.[222] These defects are readily detectable by analyzing urine for abnormal bile acid species. Treatment with CA therapy is curative, as long as it is instituted promptly.

ACQUIRED CHOLESTATIC DISORDERS

Cholestasis is defined as impairment in bile flow, yet we have no direct means of clinically measuring bile flow. Thus, no standard diagnostic blood test exists for cholestasis, although elevated serum levels of both conjugated bilirubin and serum bile acids serve as practical clinical markers of cholestasis.[122] Clinically, cholestatic infants are typically jaundiced, with dark urine and pale stools. In cases of severe liver disease and hepatocyte destruction, patients may have evidence of significant hepatocellular synthetic dysfunction, including hypoalbuminemia, coagulopathy, hypoglycemia, and elevated levels of conjugated bilirubin and serum bile acids. Elevations of alanine aminotransferase or aspartate aminotransferase suggest hepatocellular damage, and elevated GGT or alkaline phosphatase is indicative of damage to the biliary tract. As expected, cholestatic patients have profoundly altered bile acid metabolism and recirculation, with a common feature of retained biliary constituents within hepatocytes. Conversion to secondary bile acids via sulfation and glucuronidation becomes more prominent.[223] Separating cholestatic disorders anatomically into extrahepatic (e.g., biliary atresia) and intrahepatic (e.g., Alagille syndrome) disorders is clinically useful for determining their causes. Published reviews refer to the differential diagnosis of neonatal cholestasis.[122,224]

Intracellular accumulation of bile acids, especially hydrophobic bile acids, can be toxic to the liver and other tissues, even at submicellar concentrations.[54, 55] Infusing LCA in rats or oral feeding of LCA in rabbits causes cholestasis.[225-227] Concentrations in the micromolar range in rats, perfused rat liver, primary human hepatocytes, and artificial membrane preparations can disturb membrane lipids and can cause proteins to dissociate from the lipid bilayer by a detergent-like mechanism.[55, 228-232] Accumulation of bile acids can increase calcium fluxes across intracellular and plasma membranes and can alter the metabolic activity of mitochondria,[233-239] and intracellular accumulation of submicellar concentrations of bile acids can lead to hepatocellular apoptosis by nondetergent mechanisms, findings suggesting a need for adequate regulation of bile acid levels.[240]

Total Parenteral Nutrition–Associated Cholestasis

Since the 1970s, the care and ultimate survival of premature infants have been greatly enhanced by the use of total parenteral nutrition (TPN). Although it is generally well tolerated, infants who require TPN in substantial amounts or for prolonged periods can develop a particularly aggressive form of liver disease within the first few weeks of life, TPN-associated cholestasis (TPNAC). The infants most at risk for TPNAC are usually extremely low birth weight (<1000 g) infants with inadequate bowel function typically resulting from extensive surgical resections. TPNAC presents clinically with hepatomegaly, conjugated hyperbilirubinemia, and intrahepatic cholestasis reminiscent of the histologic findings associated with bile acid–mediated hepatotoxicity.[241-243] The origin of TPNAC is unknown, but clinical studies suggest a combination of many factors, including prematurity, repeated bouts of sepsis, damaged and inadequate bowel function, hydrophobic

bile acids, and various TPN components.[242-245] TPNAC may be reversible if infants are capable of enteral nutrition, but the rapid development of hepatomegaly, cirrhosis, fibrosis, and progression to end-stage liver disease in as many as 65% of the most severely affected infants receiving long-term TPN may occur as early as 4 to 6 months of age.[122, 241, 246] The only available treatment for severe, medically intractable TPNAC in those patients who cannot be adequately fed is liver or small bowel transplantation.

Sepsis-Associated Cholestasis

Bacterial infections in the neonate are important because of their prevalence. In some situations, cholestasis and jaundice may be the only clinical signs of infection. In 1933, Dunham reported the concept of jaundice as a presenting sign of infection in neonates.[247] Sepsis-associated cholestasis does not require direct infection of the liver. Bile flow is reduced, leading to cholestasis and conjugated hyperbilirubinemia, generally without significant elevation of transaminases in the early stages.[248-250] The molecular mechanisms underlying sepsis-associated reduction in bile flow and cholestasis have become clearer, with evidence supporting cytokine-mediated suppression of the expression of key hepatobiliary transporter genes.[251-253] The activation of these sepsis-induced pathways, combined with physiologic cholestasis of infancy, likely makes neonates more susceptible to cholestasis during infection.

SUMMARY

The anatomy of the liver and the microanatomy of the hepatic lobule direct the liver's abilities to act as a bioactive filter and modifier as well as a bile secretory organ. The formation of bile is determined mainly by active transport of bile acids and other biliary solutes across the canalicular membrane of the hepatocyte. Alterations in the expression of both sinusoidal and canalicular transporters directly affects bile flow and composition, with clinical consequences evident as cholestasis and hyperbilirubinemia in the infant. Neonates are particularly prone to develop cholestasis, likely because of an inherent developmental immaturity of the multiple components necessary to form bile (mainly the enterohepatic circulation of bile acids, hepatobiliary transport, and intermediary metabolism), combined with relatively poor hepatoprotective responses. Recognition that infants with seemingly "innocent" cholestasis may rapidly develop cirrhosis and even end-stage liver disease can only help clinicians in determining the timing of potentially lifesaving therapies.

REFERENCES

1. Lautt, W.W. and C.V. Greenway, Conceptual review of the hepatic vascular bed. Hepatology, 1987. 7(5):952-963.
2. Ohtani, O., The peribiliary portal system in the rabbit liver. Arch Histol Jpn, 1979. 42(2):153-167.
3. Watanabe, S. and M.J. Phillips, Ca²⁺ causes active contraction of bile canaliculi: direct evidence from microinjection studies. Proc Natl Acad Sci USA, 1984. 81(19):6164-6168.
4. Oshio, C. and M.J. Phillips, Contractility of bile canaliculi: implications for liver function. Science, 1981. 212(4498):1041-1042.
5. Desmet, V.J., Organizational Principles, In The Liver: Biology and Pathobiology, I.M. Arias, Boyer, J.L., Chisari, F.V., Fausto, N., Schachter, D., Shafritz, D.A., Editors. 2001, Lippincott Williams & Wilkins: Philadelphia. p. 3–15.
6. Reddy, V.J., Rao M.S., Hepatic ultrastructure and adaptation, In Pathogenesis of liver diseases, E. Farber, Phillips, M. J., Kaufman, N., Editors. 1987, Williams & Wilkins: Baltimore. p. 11–42.
7. Feldmann, G., The cytoskeleton of the hepatocyte. Structure and functions. J Hepatol, 1989. 8(3):380–386.
8. MacPhee, P.J., E.E. Schmidt, and A.C. Groom, Evidence for Kupffer cell migration along liver sinusoids, from high-resolution in vivo microscopy. Am J Physiol, 1992. 263(1 Pt 1):G17–23.
9. Niki, T., et al., Class VI intermediate filament protein nestin is induced during activation of rat hepatic stellate cells. Hepatology, 1999. 29(2):520-527.
10. Yokota, S., Functional differences between sinusoidal endothelial cells and interlobular or central vein endothelium in rat liver. Anat Rec, 1985. 212(1):74-80.

11. Marceau, N., et al., Role of different epithelial cell types in liver ontogenesis, regeneration and neoplasia. In Vitro Cell Dev Biol, 1989. 25(4):336–341.

12. Anderson, J.M. and C.M. Van Itallie, Tight junctions and the molecular basis for regulation of paracellular permeability. Am J Physiol, 1995. 269(4 Pt 1):G467-75.

13. Fallon, M.B., et al., Altered hepatic localization and expression of occludin after common bile duct ligation. Am J Physiol, 1995. 269(4 Pt 1):C1057-462.

14. Saxena, R., N.D. Theise, and J.M. Crawford, Microanatomy of the human liver—exploring the hidden interfaces. Hepatology, 1999. 30(6):1339–1346.

15. Boyer, J.L., Nathanson, M.H., Bile Formation, In Schiff's Diseases of the Liver, E.R. Schiff, Sorrell, M.F., Maddrey, W.C, Editors. 1999, Lippincott-Raven: Philadelphia. p. 119–146.

16. Jones, A.L., Anatomy of the normal liver, In Hepatology: A Textbook of Liver Disease, D. Zakim, Boyer, T., Editors. 1996, WB Saunders: Philadelphia. p. 1–32.

17. Kim, M.S., K.Y. Lee, and W.Y. Chey, Plasma secretin concentrations in fasting and postprandial states in dog. Am J Physiol, 1979. 236(5):E539–E544.

18. Tizzano, E.F. and M. Buchwald, CFTR expression and organ damage in cystic fibrosis. Ann Intern Med, 1995. 123(4):305–308.

19. Cohn, J.A., et al., Localization of the cystic fibrosis transmembrane conductance regulator in human bile duct epithelial cells. Gastroenterology, 1993. 105(6):1857–1864.

20. Strazzabosco, M., A. Mennone, and J.L. Boyer, Intracellular pH regulation in isolated rat bile duct epithelial cells. J Clin Invest, 1991. 87(5):1503–1512.

21. Martinez-Anso, E., et al., Immunohistochemical detection of chloride/bicarbonate anion exchangers in human liver. Hepatology, 1994. 19(6):1400–1406.

22. Marzioni, M., et al., Functional heterogeneity of cholangiocytes. Semin Liver Dis, 2002. 22(3):227–240.

23. Alpini, G., et al., Morphological, molecular, and functional heterogeneity of cholangiocytes from normal rat liver. Gastroenterology, 1996. 110(5):1636–1643.

24. Lakehal, F., et al., Phase I and phase II drug-metabolizing enzymes are expressed and heterogeneously distributed in the biliary epithelium. Hepatology, 1999. 30(6):1498–1506.

25. Benedetti, A., et al., A morphometric study of the epithelium lining the rat intrahepatic biliary tree. J Hepatol, 1996. 24(3):335–342.

26. Severn, C.B., A morphological study of the development of the human liver. I. Development of the hepatic diverticulum. Am J Anat, 1971. 131(2):133–158.

27. Moore, K.L., In The Developing Human. 1982, WB Saunders Co: Philadelphia. p. 231–233.

28. Zaret, K.S., Regulatory phases of early liver development: paradigms of organogenesis. Nat Rev Genet, 2002. 3(7):499–512.

29. Cascio, S. and K.S. Zaret, Hepatocyte differentiation initiates during endodermal-mesenchymal interactions prior to liver formation. Development, 1991. 113(1):217–225.

30. Houssaint, E., Differentiation of the mouse hepatic primordium. I. An analysis of tissue interactions in hepatocyte differentiation. Cell Differ, 1980. 9(5):269–279.

31. Reif, S. and E. Lebenthal, Extracellular matrix modulation of liver ontogeny. J Pediatr Gastroenterol Nutr, 1991. 12(1):1–4.

32. Guguen-Guillouzo, C., et al., Modulation of human fetal hepatocyte survival and differentiation by interactions with a rat liver epithelial cell line. Dev Biol, 1984. 105(1):211–220.

33. Morgan, J.P., Hartroft W.S., Juvenile liver age at which one cell thick plates predomonate in the human liver. Arch Pathol, 1961. 71:86–88.

34. Elias, H., Origin and early development of the liver of various vertebrates. Acta Hepatologica, 1955. 3:1–56.

35. Elias, H., The early embryology of the liver of vertebrates. Anat Anz, 1955. (101):153–167.

36. Wilson J.W., G.C.S., Leduc E.H., Histogenesis of the liver. Ann NY Acad Sci, 1963. 111:8–24.

37. Severn, C.B., A morphological study of the development of the human liver. II. Establishment of liver parenchyma, extrahepatic ducts and associated venous channels. Am J Anat, 1972. 133(1):85–107.

38. Karpen, S.J., Suchy, F.J., Structural and Functional Development of the Liver, In Liver Disease in Children, F.J. Suchy, Editor. 2001, Lippincott Williams & Wilkins: Philadelphia.

39. Jorgensen, M.J., The ductal plate malformation. Acta Pathol Microbiol Scand Suppl, 1977. 257:1–87.

40. Bloom, W., The embryogenesis of human bile capillaries and ducts. Am J Anat, 1926. 36:451–465.

41. Elias, H., Sherrick, J.C., In The Development of the Human Liver: Morphology of the Liver. 1969, Academic Press: New York. p. 233–261.

42. Desmet, V.J., Intrahepatic bile ducts under the lens. J Hepatol, 1985. 1(5):545–559.

43. Crawford, J.M., Development of the intrahepatic biliary tree. Semin Liver Dis, 2002. 22(3):213–226.

44. Gall, J.A. and P.S. Bhathal, Development of intrahepatic bile ducts in rat foetal liver explants in vitro. J Exp Pathol (Oxford), 1990. 71(1):41–50.

45. Shiojiri, N., The origin of intrahepatic bile duct cells in the mouse. J Embryol Exp Morphol, 1984. 79:25–39.

46. Shiojiri, N. and Y. Nagai, Preferential differentiation of the bile ducts along the portal vein in the development of mouse liver. Anat Embryol (Berl), 1992. 185(1):17–24.

47. Aterman, K., The stem cells of the liver: a selective review. J Cancer Res Clin Oncol, 1992. 118(2):87–115.

48. Van Eyken, P., et al., The development of the intrahepatic bile ducts in man: a keratin-immunohistochemical study. Hepatology, 1988. 8(6):1586–1595.

49. Vijayan, V. and C.E. Tan, Developing human biliary system in three dimensions. Anat Rec, 1997. 249(3):389–398.

50. Michalopoulos, G.K., et al., Histological organization in hepatocyte organoid cultures. Am J Pathol, 2001. 159(5):1877–1887.

51. Fitz, J.G., Cellular mechanisms of bile secretion, In Hepatology: A Textbook of Liver Disease, D. Zakim, Boyer, T., Editors. 1996, WB Saunders Co: Philadelphia. p. 362–376.

52. Hardison, W.G., Relation of hepatic taurine pool size to bile-acid conjugation in man and animals. Prog Clin Biol Res, 1983. 125:407–417.

53. Batta, A.K., et al., The effect of tauroursodeoxycholic acid and taurine supplementation on biliary bile acid composition. Hepatology, 1982. 2(6):811–816.

54. Drew, R. and B.G. Priestly, Choleretic and cholestatic effects of infused bile salts in the rat. Experientia, 1979. 35(6):809–811.

55. Scholmerich, J., et al., Influence of hydroxylation and conjugation of bile salts on their membrane-damaging properties: studies on isolated hepatocytes and lipid membrane vesicles. Hepatology, 1984. 4(4):661–666.

56. Stravitz, R.T., et al., Transcriptional regulation of cholesterol 7 alpha-hydroxylase mRNA by conjugated bile acids in primary cultures of rat hepatocytes. J Biol Chem, 1993. 268(19):13987–13993.

57. Twisk, J., E.M. Lehmann, and H.M. Princen, Differential feedback regulation of cholesterol 7 alpha-hydroxylase mRNA and transcriptional activity by rat bile acids in primary monolayer cultures of rat hepatocytes. Biochem J, 1993. 290(Pt 3):685–691.

58. Hay, D.W. and M.C. Carey, Chemical species of lipids in bile. Hepatology, 1990. 12(3 Pt 2):6S-14S; discussion 14S-16S.

59. Cornelius, C., Comparative bile pigment metabolism in vertebrates, In Bile Pigments and Jaundice, J. Ostrow, Editor. 1986, Marcel Dekker: New York. p. 601.

60. Ballatori, N. and A.T. Truong, Glutathione as a primary osmotic driving force in hepatic bile formation. Am J Physiol, 1992. 263(5 Pt 1):G617-624.

61. Carey, M.C. and J.T. Lamont, Cholesterol gallstone formation. I. Physical-chemistry of bile and biliary lipid secretion. Prog Liver Dis, 1992. 10:139–163.

62. Dijkstra, M., et al., Bile secretion of cadmium, silver, zinc and copper in the rat: involvement of various transport systems. Life Sci, 1996. 59(15):1237–1246.

63. Meier, P.J. and B. Stieger, Bile salt transporters. Annu Rev Physiol, 2002. 64:635–661.

64. Carey, M.C., Duane, WC, Enterohepatic circulation, In The Liver: Biology and Pathobiology, I.M. Arias, Editor. 1994, Raven Press: New York. p. 719–768.

65. Hofmann, A.F., Bile acids: the good, the bad, and the ugly. News Physiol Sci, 1999. 14:24–29.

66. Axelson, M. and J. Sjovall, Potential bile acid precursors in plasma: possible indicators of biosynthetic pathways to cholic and chenodeoxycholic acids in man. J Steroid Biochem, 1990. 36(6):631–640.

67. Vlahcevic, Z.R., D.M. Heuman, and P.B. Hylemon, Regulation of bile acid synthesis. Hepatology, 1991. 13(3):590–600.

68. Shefer, S., et al., Feedback regulation of bile acid biosynthesis in the rat. J Lipid Res, 1969. 10(6):646–655.

69. Mosbach, E.H., et al., Bile acid synthesis in the isolated, perfused rabbit liver. J Clin Invest, 1971. 50(8):1720–1729.

70. Shefer, S., et al., Regulatory effects of sterols and bile acids on hepatic 3-hydroxy-3-methylglutaryl CoA reductase and cholesterol 7alpha-hydroxylase in the rat. J Lipid Res, 1973. 14(5):573–580.

71. Danielsson, H., K. Einarsson, and G. Johansson, Effect of biliary drainage on individual reactions in the conversion of cholesterol to taurochlic acid. Bile acids and steroids 180. Eur J Biochem, 1967. 2(1):44–49.

72. Ericson, S., Biliary excretion of the bile acids and cholesterol in bile fistula rats. Proc Soc Exp Biol Med, 1957. 94:578.

73. Bergstrom S., et al., On the regulation of bile acid formation in the rat liver. Acta Physiol Scand, 1958. 43:1.

74. Thompson, J.C., Vars, H. M., Biliary excretion of cholic acid and cholesterol in hyper-, hypo- and euthyroid rats. Proc Soc Exp Biol Med, 1953. 83:246.

75. Hoekman, M.F., et al., Transcriptional regulation of the gene encoding cholesterol 7 alpha-hydroxylase in the rat. Gene, 1993. 130(2):217–223.

76. Boyer, J.L. and J.R. Bloomer, Canalicular bile secretion in man. Studies utilizing the biliary clearance of (14C)mannitol. J Clin Invest, 1974. 54(4):773–781.

77. Egger, G., et al., Bile formation in the intact pig. Am J Vet Res, 1974. 35(9):1203–1208.

78. Erlinger, S., et al., Effect of inhibitors of sodium transport on bile formation in the rabbit. Am J Physiol, 1970. 219(2):416–422.

79. Shaw, H.M. and T. Heath, The significance of hormones, bile salts, and feeding in the regulation of bile and other digestive secretions in the rat. Aust J Biol Sci, 1972. 25(1):147–154.

80. Paumgartner, G., et al., Taurocholate excertion and bile formation in the isolated perfused rat liver: an in vitro-in vivo comparison. Naunyn Schmiedebergs Arch Pharmacol, 1974. 285(2):165–174.

81. Paumgartner, G., et al., Elaboration of hepatocytic bile. Bull NY Acad Med, 1975. 51(4):455–471.

82. Herz, R., G. Paumgartner, and R. Preisig, Bile salt metabolism and bile formation in the rat with a portacaval shunt. Eur J Clin Invest, 1974. 4(3):223–228.

83. Prandi, D., M. Dumont, and S. Erlinger, Influence of portacaval shunt on bile formation in the rat. Eur J Clin Invest, 1974. 4(3):197–200.

84. Ballatori, N. and A.T. Truong, Multiple canalicular transport mechanisms for glutathione S-conjugates. Transport on both ATP- and voltage-dependent carriers. J Biol Chem, 1995. 270(8):3594–3601.

85. Meier, P.J., et al., Evidence for carrier-mediated chloride/bicarbonate exchange in canalicular rat liver plasma membrane vesicles. J Clin Invest, 1985. 75(4):1256–1263.

86. Graf, J., Canalicular bile salt-independent bile formation: concepts and clues from electrolyte transport in rat liver. Am J Physiol, 1983. 244(3):G233–246.

87. Thomsen, O.O., J.A. Larsen, and H. Orskov, Insulin-induced choleresis in relation to insulin concentrations in plasma and bile in the cat. Scand J Gastroenterol, 1982. 17(2):297–303.

88. Thomsen, O.O. and J.A. Larsen, The effect of glucagon, dibutyrylic cyclic AMP and insulin on bile production in the intact rat and the perfused rat liver. Acta Physiol Scand, 1981. 111(1):23–30.

89. Thomsen, O.O. and J.A. Larsen, Interaction of insulin, glucagon, and DBcAMP on bile acid-independent bile production in the rat. Scand J Gastroenterol, 1982. 17(5):687–693.

90. Ishii, M., B. Vroman, and N.F. LaRusso, Isolation and morphologic characterization of bile duct epithelial cells from normal rat liver. Gastroenterology, 1989. 97(5):1236–1247.

91. Alpini, G., et al., Biliary physiology in rats with bile ductular cell hyperplasia: evidence for a secretory function of proliferated bile ductules. J Clin Invest, 1988. 81(2):569–578.

92. Fitz, J.G., et al., Regulation of membrane chloride currents in rat bile duct epithelial cells. J Clin Invest, 1993. 91(1):319–328.

93. Lenzen, R., G. Alpini, and N. Tavoloni, Secretin stimulates bile ductular secretory activity through the cAMP system. Am J Physiol, 1992. 263(4 Pt 1):G527–532.

94. Chenderovitch, J., Secretory function of the rabbit common bile duct. Am J Physiol, 1972. 223(3):695–706.

95. Fini, A. and A. Roda, Chemical properties of bile acids. IV. Acidity constants of glycine-conjugated bile acids. J Lipid Res, 1987. 28(7):755–759.

96. Lake, J.R., et al., Biliary excretion of fluid-phase markers by the isolated perfused rat liver: role of transcellular vesicular transport. J Clin Invest, 1985. 76(2):676–684.

97. Scharschmidt, B.F., et al., Fluid phase endocytosis by cultured rat hepatocytes and perfused rat liver: implications for plasma membrane turnover and vesicular trafficking of fluid phase markers. Proc Natl Acad Sci USA, 1986. 83(24):9488–9492.

98. Marinelli, R.A., et al., Secretin promotes osmotic water transport in rat cholangiocytes by increasing aquaporin-1 water channels in plasma membrane: evidence for a secretin-induced vesicular translocation of aquaporin-1. J Biol Chem, 1997. 272(20):12984–12988.

99. Marinelli, R.A., et al., Secretin induces the apical insertion of aquaporin-1 water channels in rat cholangiocytes. Am J Physiol, 1999. 276(1 Pt 1):G280–286.

100. Jansen, P.L., Foreword: from classic bile physiology to cloned transporters. Semin Liver Dis, 2000. 20(3):245–250.

101. Borst, P. and R.O. Elferink, Mammalian ABC transporters in health and disease. Annu Rev Biochem, 2002. 71:537–592.

102. Jansen, P.L., M. Muller, and E. Sturm, Genes and cholestasis. Hepatology, 2001. 34(6):1067–1074.

103. Thompson, R. and P.L. Jansen, Genetic defects in hepatocanalicular transport. Semin Liver Dis, 2000. 20(3):365–372.

104. Meier, P.J., Molecular mechanisms of hepatic bile salt transport from sinusoidal blood into bile. Am J Physiol, 1995. 269(6 Pt 1):G801–812.

105. Schwarz, L., et al., Proceedings: kinetics of the uptake of taurocholic acid by isolated rat liver cells. Naunyn Schmiedebergs Arch Pharmacol, 1975. 287 Suppl:R82.

106. Reichen, J. and G. Paumgartner, Uptake of bile acids by perfused rat liver. Am J Physiol, 1976. 231(3):734–742.

107. Hagenbuch, B., et al., Functional expression cloning and characterization of the hepatocyte Na+/bile acid cotransport system. Proc Natl Acad Sci USA, 1991. 88(23):10629–10633.

108. Hagenbuch, B., B.F. Scharschmidt, and P.J. Meier, Effect of antisense oligonucleotides on the expression of hepatocellular bile acid and organic anion uptake systems in Xenopus laevis oocytes. Biochem J, 1996. 316(Pt 3):901–904.

109. Wolkoff, A.W. and D.E. Cohen, Bile Acid Regulation of Hepatic Physiology. I. Hepatocyte transport of bile acids. Am J Physiol, 2003. 284(2):G175–179.

110. Karpen, S.J., Transcriptional regulation of sinusoidal transporters, In Hepatobiliary Transport: From Bench to Bedside, S. Matern et al., Editors. 2001, Kluwer Academic: London. p. 22–31.

111. Karpen, S.J., Bile acid-mediated feedback inhibition of the rat ntcp promoter, In Falk Symposium: Biology of Bile Acids in Health and Disease, v.B. Henegouwen, Editor. 2001, Kluwer Academic: London. p. 95–104.

112. Denson, L.A., et al., Interleukin-1 beta suppresses retinoid transactivation of two hepatic transporter genes involved in bile formation. J Biol Chem, 2000. 275(12):8835–8843.

113. Denson, L.A., et al., The orphan nuclear receptor, shp, mediates bile acid-induced inhibition of the rat bile acid transporter, ntcp. Gastroenterology, 2001. 121(1):140–147.

114. Li, D., et al., Interleukin-1 beta-mediated suppression of RXR:RAR transactivation of the Ntcp promoter is JNK-dependent. J Biol Chem, 2002. 277(35):31416–31422.

115. Trauner, M., et al., Endotoxin downregulates rat hepatic ntcp gene expression via decreased activity of critical transcription factors. J Clin Invest, 1998. 101(10):2092–2100.

116. Gartung, C., et al., Down-regulation of expression and function of the rat liver Na+/bile acid cotransporter in extrahepatic cholestasis. Gastroenterology, 1996. 110(1):199–209.

117. Gartung, C., et al., Expression of the rat liver Na+/taurocholate cotransporter is regulated in vivo by retention of biliary constituents but not their depletion. Hepatology, 1997. 25(2):284–290.

118. Green, R.M., D. Beier, and J.L. Gollan, Regulation of hepatocyte bile salt transporters by endotoxin and inflammatory cytokines in rodents. Gastroenterology, 1996. 111(1):193–198.

119. Kim, P.K., et al., Intraabdominal sepsis down-regulates transcription of sodium taurocholate cotransporter and multidrug resistance-associated protein in rats. Shock, 2000. 14(2):176–181.

120. Sinal, C.J., et al., Targeted disruption of the nuclear receptor FXR/BAR impairs bile acid and lipid homeostasis. Cell, 2000. 102(6):731–744.

121. Zollner, G., et al., Induction of short heterodimer partner 1 precedes down-regulation of Ntcp in bile duct-ligated mice. Am J Physiol, 2002. 282(1):G184–191.

122. Karpen, S.J., Update on the etiologies and management of neonatal cholestasis. Clin Perinatol, 2002. 29(1):159–180.

123. Suchy, F.J., et al., Physiologic cholestasis: elevation of the primary serum bile acid concentrations in normal infants. Gastroenterology, 1981. 80(5 Pt 1):1037–1041.

124. Hagenbuch, B. and P.J. Meier, The superfamily of organic anion transporting polypeptides. Biochim Biophys Acta, 2003. 1609(1):1–18.

125. Karpen, S.J., Nuclear receptor regulation of hepatic function. J Hepatol, 2002. 36(6):832–850.

126. Kullak-Ublick, G.A., et al., Hepatic transport of bile salts. Semin Liver Dis, 2000. 20(3):273–292.

127. Cui, Y., et al., Hepatic uptake of bilirubin and its conjugates by the human organic anion transporter SLC21A6. J Biol Chem, 2001. 276(13):9626–9632.

128. Kakyo, M., et al., Molecular characterization and functional regulation of a novel rat liver-specific organic anion transporter rlst-1. Gastroenterology, 1999. 117(4):770–775.

129. Abe, T., et al., Identification of a novel gene family encoding human liver-specific organic anion transporter LST-1. J Biol Chem, 1999. 274(24):17159–17163.

130. Borst, P., et al., A family of drug transporters: the multidrug resistance-associated proteins. J Natl Cancer Inst, 2000. 92(16):1295–1302.

131. Hirohashi, T., et al., ATP-dependent transport of bile salts by rat multidrug resistance-associated protein 3 (Mrp3). J Biol Chem, 2000. 275(4):2905–2910.

132. Hirohashi, T., H. Suzuki, and Y. Sugiyama, Characterization of the transport properties of cloned rat multidrug resistance-associated protein 3 (MRP3). J Biol Chem, 1999. 274(21):15181–15185.

133. Donner, M.G. and D. Keppler, Up-regulation of basolateral multidrug resistance protein 3 (Mrp3) in cholestatic rat liver. Hepatology, 2001. 34(2):351–359.

134. Nies, A.T., et al., Expression of the multidrug resistance proteins MRP2 and MRP3 in human hepatocellular carcinoma. Int J Cancer, 2001. 94(4):492–9.

135. Scheffer, G.L., et al., Tissue distribution and induction of human multidrug resistant protein 3. Lab Invest, 2002. 82(2):193–201.

136. Kool, M., et al., MRP3, an organic anion transporter able to transport anti-cancer drugs. Proc Natl Acad Sci USA, 1999. 96(12):6914–6919.

137. Konig, J., et al., Characterization of the human multidrug resistance protein isoform MRP3 localized to the basolateral hepatocyte membrane. Hepatology, 1999. 29(4):1156–1163.

138. Hirohashi, T., et al., ATP-dependent transport of bile salts by rat multidrug resistance-associated protein 3 (Mrp3). J Biol Chem, 2000. 275(4):2905–2910.

139. Ogawa, K., et al., Characterization of inducible nature of MRP3 in rat liver. Am J Physiol, 2000. 278(3):G438–446.

140. Soroka, C.J., et al., Cellular localization and up-regulation of multidrug resistance-associated protein 3 in hepatocytes and cholangiocytes during obstructive cholestasis in rat liver. Hepatology, 2001. 33(4):783–791.

141. Akita, H., H. Suzuki, and Y. Sugiyama, Sinusoidal efflux of taurocholate correlates with the hepatic expression level of Mrp3. Biochem Biophys Res Commun, 2002. 299(5):681–687.

142. Zollner, G., et al., Hepatobiliary transporter expression in percutaneous liver biopsies of patients with cholestatic liver diseases. Hepatology, 2001. 33(3):633–646.

143. Nishida, T., et al., Rat liver canalicular membrane vesicles contain an ATP-dependent bile acid transport system. Proc Natl Acad Sci USA, 1991. 88(15):6590–6594.

144. Muller, M., et al., ATP-dependent transport of taurocholate across the hepatocyte canalicular membrane mediated by a 110-kDa glycoprotein binding ATP and bile salt. J Biol Chem, 1991. 266(28):18920–18926.

145. Gerloff, T., et al., The sister of P-glycoprotein represents the canalicular bile salt export pump of mammalian liver. J Biol Chem, 1998. 273(16):10046–10050.

146. Green, R.M., F. Hoda, and K.L. Ward, Molecular cloning and characterization of the murine bile salt export pump. Gene, 2000. 241(1):117–123.

147. Lecureur, V., et al., Cloning and expression of murine sister of P-glycoprotein reveals a more discriminating transporter than MDR1/P-glycoprotein. Mol Pharmacol, 2000. 57(1):24–35.

148. Noe, J., et al., Characterization of the mouse bile salt export pump overexpressed in the baculovirus system. Hepatology, 2001. 33(5):1223-1231.

149. Strautnieks, S.S., et al., A gene encoding a liver-specific ABC transporter is mutated in progressive familial intrahepatic cholestasis. Nat Genet, 1998. 20(3):233-238.

150. Wang, R., et al., Targeted inactivation of sister of P-glycoprotein gene (spgp) in mice results in nonprogressive but persistent intrahepatic cholestasis. Proc Natl Acad Sci USA, 2001. 98(4):2011-2016.

151. Jansen, P.L., et al., Hepatocanalicular bile salt export pump deficiency in patients with progressive familial intrahepatic cholestasis. Gastroenterology, 1999. 117(6):1370-1379.

152. Lee, J.M., et al., Expression of the bile salt export pump is maintained after chronic cholestasis in the rat. Gastroenterology, 2000. 118(1):163-172.

153. Keppler, D. and J. Konig, Hepatic canalicular membrane 5: Expression and localization of the conjugate export pump encoded by the MRP2 (cMRP/cMOAT) gene in liver. FASEB J, 1997. 11(7):509-516.

154. Kullak-Ublick, G.A., U. Beuers, and G. Paumgartner, Hepatobiliary transport. J Hepatol, 2000. 32(1 Suppl):3-18.

155. Keppler, D., J. Konig, and M. Buchler, The canalicular multidrug resistance protein, cMRP/MRP2, a novel conjugate export pump expressed in the apical membrane of hepatocytes. Adv Enzyme Regul, 1997. 37:321-333.

156. Tsujii, H., et al., Exon-intron organization of the human multidrug-resistance protein 2 (MRP2) gene mutated in Dubin-Johnson syndrome. Gastroenterology, 1999. 117(3):653-660.

157. Paulusma, C.C., et al., A mutation in the human canalicular multispecific organic anion transporter gene causes the Dubin-Johnson syndrome. Hepatology, 1997. 25(6):1539-1542.

158. Trauner, M., et al., The rat canalicular conjugate export pump (Mrp2) is down-regulated in intrahepatic and obstructive cholestasis. Gastroenterology, 1997. 113(1):255-264.

159. Vos, T.A., et al., Up-regulation of the multidrug resistance genes, Mrp1 and Mdr1b, and down-regulation of the organic anion transporter, Mrp2, and the bile salt transporter, Spgp, in endotoxemic rat liver. Hepatology, 1998. 28(6):1637-1644.

160. Kubitz, R., et al., Regulation of the multidrug resistance protein 2 in the rat liver by lipopolysaccharide and dexamethasone. Gastroenterology, 1999. 116(2):401-410.

161. Wielandt, A.M., et al., Induction of the multispecific organic anion transporter (cMoat/mrp2) gene and biliary glutathione secretion by the herbicide 2,4,5-trichlorophenoxyacetic acid in the mouse liver. Biochem J, 1999. 341 (Pt 1):105-111.

162. Hinoshita, E., et al., Decreased expression of an ATP-binding cassette transporter, MRP2, in human livers with hepatitis C virus infection. J Hepatol, 2001. 35(6):765-773.

163. Fickert, P., et al., Effects of ursodeoxycholic and cholic acid feeding on hepatocellular transporter expression in mouse liver. Gastroenterology, 2001. 121(1):170-183.

164. Fromm, M.F., et al., The effect of rifampin treatment on intestinal expression of human MRP transporters. Am J Pathol, 2000. 157(5):1575-1580.

165. Stockel, B., et al., Characterization of the 5'-flanking region of the human multidrug resistance protein 2 (MRP2) gene and its regulation in comparison with the multidrug resistance protein 3 (MRP3) gene. Eur J Biochem, 2000. 267(5):1347-1358.

166. Hagenbuch, N., et al., Effect of phenobarbital on the expression of bile salt and organic anion transporters of rat liver. J Hepatol, 2001. 34(6):881-887.

167. Denson, L.A., et al., Organ-specific alterations in RAR alpha:RXR alpha abundance regulate rat Mrp2 (Abcc2) expression in obstructive cholestasis. Gastroenterology, 2002. 123(2):599-607.

168. Johnson, D.R. and C.D. Klaassen, Regulation of rat multidrug resistance protein 2 by classes of prototypical microsomal enzyme inducers that activate distinct transcription pathways. Toxicol Sci, 2002. 67(2):182-189.

169. Kast, H.R., et al., Regulation of multidrug resistance-associated protein 2 (ABCC2) by the nuclear receptors pregnane X receptor, farnesoid X-activated receptor, and constitutive androstane receptor. J Biol Chem, 2002. 277(4):2908-2915.

170. Dussault, I., et al., Peptide mimetic HIV protease inhibitors are ligands for the orphan receptor SXR. J Biol Chem, 2001. 276(36):33309-33312.

171. Oude Elferink, R.P. and A.K. Groen, Mechanisms of biliary lipid secretion and their role in lipid homeostasis. Semin Liver Dis, 2000. 20(3):293-305.

172. Smit, J.J., et al., Homozygous disruption of the murine mdr2 P-glycoprotein gene leads to a complete absence of phospholipid from bile and to liver disease. Cell, 1993. 75(3):451-462.

173. de Vree, J.M., et al., Mutations in the MDR3 gene cause progressive familial intrahepatic cholestasis. Proc Natl Acad Sci USA, 1998. 95(1):282-287.

174. Yu, L., et al., Disruption of Abcg5 and Abcg8 in mice reveals their crucial role in biliary cholesterol secretion. Proc Natl Acad Sci USA, 2002. 99(25):16237-16242.

175. Yu, L., et al., Overexpression of ABCG5 and ABCG8 promotes biliary cholesterol secretion and reduces fractional absorption of dietary cholesterol. J Clin Invest, 2002. 110(5):671-680.

176. Graf, G.A., et al., Coexpression of ATP-binding cassette proteins ABCG5 and ABCG8 permits their transport to the apical surface. J Clin Invest, 2002. 110(5):659-669.

177. Wittenburg, H. and M.C. Carey, Biliary cholesterol secretion by the twinned sterol half-transporters ABCG5 and ABCG8. J Clin Invest, 2002. 110(5):605-609.

178. Berge, K.E., et al., Accumulation of dietary cholesterol in sitosterolemia caused by mutations in adjacent ABC transporters. Science, 2000. 290(5497):1771-1775.

179. Lee, M.H., et al., Identification of a gene, ABCG5, important in the regulation of dietary cholesterol absorption. Nat Genet, 2001. 27(1):79-83.

180. Arrese, M., et al., Maternal cholestasis does not affect the ontogenic pattern of expression of the Na+/taurocholate cotransporting polypeptide (ntcp) in the fetal and neonatal rat liver. Hepatology, 1998. 28(3):789-795.

181. Hardikar, W., M. Ananthanarayanan, and F.J. Suchy, Differential ontogenic regulation of basolateral and canalicular bile acid transport proteins in rat liver. J Biol Chem, 1995. 270(35):20841-20846.

182. Li, N., et al., Tissue expression, ontogeny, and inducibility of rat organic anion transporting polypeptide 4. J Pharmacol Exp Ther, 2002. 301(2):551-560.

183. Guo, G.L., D.R. Johnson, and C.D. Klaassen, Postnatal expression and induction by pregnenolone-16alpha-carbonitrile of the organic anion-transporting polypeptide 2 in rat liver. Drug Metab Dispos, 2002. 30(3):283-288.

184. Gao, B. and P.J. Meier, Organic anion transport across the choroid plexus. Microsc Res Tech, 2001. 52(1):60-64.

185. Zinchuk, V.S., et al., Asynchronous expression and colocalization of Bsep and Mrp2 during development of rat liver. Am J Physiol, 2002. 282(3):G540-548.

186. Little, J.M., et al., Bile-salt metabolism in the primate fetus. Gastroenterology, 1975. 69(6):1315-1320.

187. Bongiovanni, A.M., Bile acid content of gallbladder of infants, children and adults. J Endocrinol Metab, 1965. 25:678-685.

188. Sharp, H.L. and B.L. Mirkin, Effect of phenobarbital on hyperbilirubinemia, bile acid metabolism, and microsomal enzyme activity in chronic intrahepatic cholestasis of childhood. J Pediatr, 1972. 81(1):116-126.

189. Challacombe, D.N., S. Edkins, and G.A. Brown, Duodenal bile acids in infancy. Arch Dis Child, 1975. 50(11):837-843.

190. deBelle, R.C., et al., Bile acid conjugation in fetal hepatic organ cultures. Am J Physiol, 1976. 231(4):1124-1128.

191. Jordan, J.T. and P.G. Killenberg, Development of enzymatic conjugation and sulfation of bile acids in hamster liver. Am J Physiol, 1980. 238(5):G429-433.

192. Jackson, B.T., et al., Fetal bile salt metabolism. I. The metabolism of sodium cholate-14C in the fetal dog. J Clin Invest, 1971. 50(6):1286-12294.

193. Smallwood, R.A., P. Jablonski, and J.M. Watts, Bile acid synthesis in the developing sheep liver. Clin Sci Mol Med, 1973. 45(3):403-406.

194. Grand, R.J., J.B. Watkins, and F.M. Torti, Development of the human gastrointestinal tract: a review. Gastroenterology, 1976. 70(5 Pt 1):790-810.

195. Itoh, S., et al., Foetomaternal relationships of serum bile acid pattern estimated by high-pressure liquid chromatography. Biochem J, 1982. 204(1):141-145.

196. Moyer, M.S., et al., Ontogeny of bile acid transport in brush border membrane vesicles from rat ileum. Gastroenterology, 1986. 90(5 Pt 1):1188-1196.

197. Dumaswala, R., et al., An anion exchanger mediates bile acid transport across the placental microvillous membrane. Am J Physiol, 1993. 264(6 Pt 1):G1016-1023.

198. Smallwood, R.A., et al., Fetal bile salt metabolism. II. Hepatic excretion of endogenous bile salt and of a taurocholate load. J Clin Invest, 1972. 51(6):1388-1397.

199. Watkins, J.B., et al., Bile-salt metabolism in the newborn. Measurement of pool size and synthesis by stable isotope technic. N Engl J Med, 1973. 288(9):431-434.

200. Watkins, J.B., et al., Bile salt metabolism in the human premature infant: preliminary observations of pool size and synthesis rate following prenatal administration of dexamethasone and phenobarbital. Gastroenterology, 1975. 69(3):706-713.

201. Suchy, F.J., S.M. Courchene, and W.F. Balistreri, Ontogeny of hepatic bile acid conjugation in the rat. Pediatr Res, 1985. 19(1):97-101.

202. Boehm, G., et al., Bile acid concentrations in serum and duodenal aspirates of healthy preterm infants: effects of gestational and postnatal age. Biol Neonate, 1997. 71(4):207-214.

203. Lester, R., Physiologic cholestasis. Gastroenterology, 1980. 78(4):864-865.

204. Balistreri, W.F., J.E. Heubi, and F.J. Suchy, Immaturity of the enterohepatic circulation in early life: factors predisposing to "physiologic" maldigestion and cholestasis. J Pediatr Gastroenterol Nutr, 1983. 2(2):346-354.

205. Suchy, F.J., et al., Absence of an acinar gradient for bile acid uptake in developing rat liver. Pediatr Res, 1987. 21(4):417-421.

206. Suchy, F.J. and W.F. Balistreri, Uptake of taurocholate by hepatocytes isolated from developing rats. Pediatr Res, 1982. 16(4 Pt 1):282-285.

207. Suchy, F.J., et al., Taurocholate transport and Na+-K+-ATPase activity in fetal and neonatal rat liver plasma membrane vesicles. Am J Physiol, 1986. 251 (5 Pt 1):G665-673.

208. Heubi, J.E., W.F. Balistreri, and F.J. Suchy, Bile salt metabolism in the first year of life. J Lab Clin Med, 1982. 100(1):127-136.

209. Tavoloni, N., Bile secretion and its control in the newborn puppy. Pediatr Res, 1986. 20(3):203-208.

210. Tavoloni, N., M.J. Jones, and P.D. Berk, Postnatal development of bile secretory physiology in the dog. J Pediatr Gastroenterol Nutr, 1985. 4(2):256-267.

211. Suchy, F.J., Structure and function of the developing liver, in Liver Disease in Children, F.J. Suchy, Editor. 1994, Mosby: St Louis. p. 129-144.

212. Ho, M.L., et al., Gallbladder volume and contractility in term and preterm neonates: normal values and clinical applications in ultrasonography. Acta Paediatr, 1998. 87(7):799-804.

213. Halpern, Z., et al., Characteristics of gallbladder bile of infants and children. J Pediatr Gastroenterol Nutr, 1996. 23(2):147–150.

214. Lehtonen, L., et al., Gall bladder contractility in preterm infants. Arch Dis Child, 1993. 68(1 Spec No):43–45.

215. Kaplan, G.S., et al., Gallbladder mechanics in newborn piglets. Pediatr Res, 1984. 18(11):1181–1184.

216. Ricour, C. and J. Rey, Study of the hydrolysis and micellar solubilization of fats during intestinal perfusion. I. Results in the normal child. Rev Eur Etud Clin Biol, 1972. 17(2):172–178.

217. Bull, L.N., et al., Genetic and morphological findings in progressive familial intrahepatic cholestasis (Byler disease [PFIC-1] and Byler syndrome): evidence for heterogeneity. Hepatology, 1997. 26(1):155–164.

218. Carlton, V.E., A.S. Knisely, and N.B. Freimer, Mapping of a locus for progressive familial intrahepatic cholestasis (Byler disease) to 18q21-q22, the benign recurrent intrahepatic cholestasis region. Hum Mol Genet, 1995. 4(6):1049–1053.

219. Ujhazy, P., et al., Familial intrahepatic cholestasis 1: studies of localization and function. Hepatology, 2001. 34(4 Pt 1):768–775.

220. Paulusma, C.C., et al., Congenital jaundice in rats with a mutation in a multidrug resistance-associated protein gene. Science, 1996. 271(5252):1126–1128.

221. Setchell, K.D., O'Connell, N. C., Disorders of bile acid synthesis and metabolism, In Liver Disease in Children, F.J. Suchy, Sokol, R. J., Balistreri, W. F., Editors. 2001, Lippincott Williams & Wilkins: Philadelphia. p. 701–733.

222. Pullinger, C.R., et al., Human cholesterol 7alpha-hydroxylase (CYP7A1) deficiency has a hypercholesterolemic phenotype. J Clin Invest, 2002. 110(1):109–117.

223. Javitt, N.B., Cholestasis in infancy: status report and conceptual approach. Gastroenterology, 1976. 70(6):1172–1181.

224. Balistreri, W.F., Neonatal cholestasis. J Pediatr, 1985. 106(2):171–184.

225. Javitt, N.B. and S. Emerman, Effect of sodium taurolithocholate on bile flow and bile acid excretion. J Clin Invest, 1968. 47(5):1002–1014.

226. Holsti, P., Cirrhosis of the liver induced in rabbits by gastric instillation of 3-monohydroxycholanic acid. Nature, 1960. 186:250.

227. Oelberg, D.G., et al., Lithocholate glucuronide is a cholestatic agent. J Clin Invest, 1984. 73(6):1507–1514.

228. Miyai, K., et al., Subcellular pathology of rat liver in cholestasis and choleresis induced by bile salts. I. Effects of lithocholic, 3beta-hydroxy-5-cholenoic, cholic, and dehydrocholic acids. Lab Invest, 1977. 36(3):249–258.

229. Schmucker, D.L., et al., Hepatic injury induced by bile salts: correlation between biochemical and morphological events. Hepatology, 1990. 12(5):1216–1221.

230. Miyazaki, K., F. Nakayama, and A. Koga, Effect of chenodeoxycholic and ursodeoxycholic acids on isolated adult human hepatocytes. Dig Dis Sci, 1984. 29(12):1123–1130.

231. Ohta, M., S. Kanai, and K. Kitani, The order of hepatic cytotoxicity of bile salts in vitro does not agree with that examined in vivo in rats. Life Sci, 1990. 46(21):1503–1508.

232. Yousef, I.M. and M.M. Fisher, In vitro effect of free bile acids on the bile canalicular membrane phospholipids in the rat. Can J Biochem, 1976. 54(12):1040–1046.

233. Zimniak, P., et al., Taurine-conjugated bile acids act as Ca2+ ionophores. Biochemistry, 1991. 30(35):8598–8604.

234. Anwer, M.S., et al., Hepatotoxic bile acids increase cytosolic Ca++ activity of isolated rat hepatocytes. Hepatology, 1988. 8(4):887–891.

235. Beuers, U., M.H. Nathanson, and J.L. Boyer, Effects of tauroursodeoxycholic acid on cytosolic Ca2+ signals in isolated rat hepatocytes. Gastroenterology, 1993. 104(2):604–612.

236. Sokol, R.J., et al., Role of oxidant stress in the permeability transition induced in rat hepatic mitochondria by hydrophobic bile acids. Pediatr Res, 2001. 49(4):519–531.

237. Rodrigues, C.M., et al., A novel role for ursodeoxycholic acid in inhibiting apoptosis by modulating mitochondrial membrane perturbation. J Clin Invest, 1998. 101(12):2790–2799.

238. Rodrigues, C.M., et al., Ursodeoxycholic acid may inhibit deoxycholic acid-induced apoptosis by modulating mitochondrial transmembrane potential and reactive oxygen species production. Mol Med, 1998. 4(3):165–178.

239. Rodrigues, C.M., et al., Ursodeoxycholic acid prevents cytochrome c release in apoptosis by inhibiting mitochondrial membrane depolarization and channel formation. Cell Death Differ, 1999. 6(9):842–854.

240. Guicciardi, M.E. and G.J. Gores, Bile acid-mediated hepatocyte apoptosis and cholestatic liver disease. Dig Liver Dis, 2002. 34(6):387–392.

241. Teitelbaum, D.H. and T. Tracy, Parenteral nutrition-associated cholestasis. Semin Pediatr Surg, 2001. 10(2):72–80.

242. Btaiche, I.F. and N. Khalidi, Parenteral nutrition-associated liver complications in children. Pharmacotherapy, 2002. 22(2):188–211.

243. Kelly, D.A., Liver complications of pediatric parenteral nutrition–epidemiology. Nutrition, 1998. 14(1):153–157.

244. Touloukian, R.J. and J.H. Seashore, Hepatic secretory obstruction with total parenteral nutrition in the infant. J Pediatr Surg, 1975. 10(3):353–360.

245. Rager, R. and M.J. Finegold, Cholestasis in immature newborn infants: is parenteral alimentation responsible? J Pediatr, 1975. 86(2):264–269.

246. Suita, S., et al., Complications in neonates with short bowel syndrome and long-term parenteral nutrition. JPEN J Parenter Enteral Nutr, 1999. 23 (5 Suppl):S106–S109.

247. Dunham, E.C., Septicemia in the newborn. Am J Dis Child, 1933. 45:229–253.

248. Moseley, R.H., Sepsis-associated cholestasis. Gastroenterology, 1997. 112(1): 302–306.

249. Koopen, N.R., et al., Molecular mechanisms of cholestasis: causes and consequences of impaired bile formation. Biochim Biophys Acta, 1998. 1408(1):1–17.

250. Trauner, M., P. Fickert, and G. Zollner, Genetic disorders and molecular mechanisms in cholestatic liver disease: a clinical approach. Semin Gastrointest Dis, 2001. 12(2):66–88.

251. Denson, L.A., et al., Interleukin-1beta suppresses retinoid transactivation of two hepatic transporter genes involved in bile formation. J Biol Chem, 2000. 275(12):8835–8843.

252. Trauner, M., P.J. Meier, and J.L. Boyer, Molecular pathogenesis of cholestasis. N Engl J Med, 1998. 339(17):1217–1227.

253. Trauner, M., P. Fickert, and R.E. Stauber, Inflammation-induced cholestasis. J Gastroenterol Hepatol, 1999. 14(10):946–959.

254. Weinstein, D.C., et al., The winged-helix transcription factor HNF-3 beta is required for notochord development in the mouse embryo. Cell, 1994. 78(4):575–588.

255. Ang, S.L. and J. Rossant, HNF-3 beta is essential for node and notochord formation in mouse development. Cell, 1994. 78(4):561–574.

256. Ruiz i Altaba, A., et al., Sequential expression of HNF-3 beta and HNF-3 alpha by embryonic organizing centers: the dorsal lip/node, notochord and floor plate. Mech Dev, 1993. 44(2-3):91–108.

257. Monaghan, A.P., et al., Postimplantation expression patterns indicate a role for the mouse forkhead/HNF-3 alpha, beta and gamma genes in determination of the definitive endoderm, chordamesoderm and neuroectoderm. Development, 1993. 119(3):567–578.

258. Ang, S.L., et al., The formation and maintenance of the definitive endoderm lineage in the mouse: involvement of HNF3/forkhead proteins. Development, 1993. 119(4):1301–1315.

259. Sasaki, H. and B.L. Hogan, Differential expression of multiple fork head related genes during gastrulation and axial pattern formation in the mouse embryo. Development, 1993. 118(1):47–59.

260. Martinez Barbera, J.P., et al., The homeobox gene Hex is required in definitive endodermal tissues for normal forebrain, liver and thyroid formation. Development, 2000. 127(11):2433–2445.

261. Keng, V.W., et al., Homeobox gene Hex is essential for onset of mouse embryonic liver development and differentiation of the monocyte lineage. Biochem Biophys Res Commun, 2000. 276(3):1155–1161.

262. Sosa-Pineda, B., J.T. Wigle, and G. Oliver, Hepatocyte migration during liver development requires Prox1. Nat Genet, 2000. 25(3):254–255.

263. Schmidt, C., et al., Scatter factor/hepatocyte growth factor is essential for liver development. Nature, 1995. 373(6516):699–702.

264. Hentsch, B., et al., Hlx homeo box gene is essential for an inductive tissue interaction that drives expansion of embryonic liver and gut. Genes Dev, 1996. 10(1):70–79.

265. Weinstein, M., et al., Smad proteins and hepatocyte growth factor control parallel regulatory pathways that converge on beta1-integrin to promote normal liver development. Mol Cell Biol, 2001. 21(15):5122–5131.

266. Clotman, F., et al., The onecut transcription factor HNF6 is required for normal development of the biliary tract. Development, 2002. 129(8):1819–1828.

267. Coffinier, C., et al., Bile system morphogenesis defects and liver dysfunction upon targeted deletion of HNF1beta. Development, 2002. 129(8): 1829–1838.

268. Li, J., G. Ning, and S.A. Duncan, Mammalian hepatocyte differentiation requires the transcription factor HNF-4alpha. Genes Dev, 2000. 14(4):464–474.

William J. Cashore

Bilirubin Metabolism and Toxicity in the Newborn

Hyperbilirubinemia is probably the most common clinical diagnosis encountered in well newborns. Although the origin of neonatal jaundice is usually "idiopathic," and the outcome is nearly always benign, a rational approach to the diagnosis and treatment of neonatal hyperbilirubinemia (including the decision not to treat) requires some understanding of factors governing production, disposal, and toxicity of bilirubin in the newborn.

BILIRUBIN PRODUCTION

Bilirubin is a catabolic byproduct of hemoglobin from senescent or hemolyzed red cells. Only a small proportion of bilirubin produced in the newborn results from ineffective erythropoiesis; most is produced from the breakdown of circulating red blood cells, and a small fraction derives from catabolism of heme-containing molecules in other cells. As red blood cells are sequestered and destroyed in the reticuloendothelial system, the globin chains are removed. The α double bond of the heme molecule is broken, the iron atom at the center of the heme skeleton is reused, and a molecule of carbon monoxide is removed from the heme ring and is excreted, converting the remaining portion of the heme ring to biliverdin. Conversion of heme to biliverdin is catalyzed by heme oxygenase, which occurs as two isozymes widely distributed in various body tissues.[1] Heme oxygenase-1 (HMOX-1) is inducible in the reticuloendothelial system by hemin[2] and in the lung by inflammatory or oxidative stress, such as toxins in cigarette smoke.[3] The constitutive isozyme HMOX-2 appears to serve "resident" antioxidant- and carbon monoxide–mediated cell messenger functions in lung, vascular endothelium, and the central and autonomic nervous system.[4-5] Although both isozymes produce carbon monoxide and biliverdin as a precursor to bilirubin, HMOX-1 is more likely to play an active role by induction in response to hemolysis.

The catabolism of 1 mol of heme to 1 mol of bilirubin releases 1 mol of carbon monoxide, so the rate of bilirubin formation can be estimated from the rate of carboxy hemoglobin production or by trace gas analysis of carbon monoxide in expired breath.[5-8]

Biliverdin reductase catalyzes the conversion of biliverdin to bilirubin in the presence of reduced nicotinamide adenine dinucleotide or nicotinamide adenine dinucleotide phosphate, by transfer of two hydrogen ions to the centrally located C_{10} carbon atom of biliverdin. Two forms of biliverdin reductase, A and B, have been identified. Biliverdin reductase A is ubiquitous in human tissues,[9] and therefore it is readily available when the constitutive isozyme of HMOX-2 produces biliverdin from heme pigments at multiple sites. Biliverdin reductase B is found predominantly in fetal liver,[10] where it would potentially have an important role in modulating the metabolic effects of antenatal and perinatal hemolysis. Compared with healthy adults or older children, newborn infants exhibit an increased rate of bilirubin production. Preterm infants have higher rates of bilirubin production than term newborns.

TRANSPORT, CONJUGATION, AND EXCRETION OF BILIRUBIN

Bilirubin Transport and Uptake

The serum concentration of bilirubin depends on its rate of elimination, as well as its rate of production. In the adult, the hepatic uptake, conjugation, and excretion of bilirubin are highly efficient, so newly formed bilirubin entering the circulation from the tissues is usually cleared from the plasma within minutes. In the newborn, conjugation and excretion of bilirubin are less efficient for several reasons. During fetal life, normal bowel function is not yet established. The hepatic conjugating system is somewhat dormant until after birth, both because the bowel is a no-exit pathway for bilirubin in the fetus and because unconjugated bilirubin, more fat soluble and less water soluble than conjugated bilirubin, can more easily recross the placenta to the maternal circulation for disposal by the maternal liver.[11, 12] Impaired maternal liver function late in pregnancy will sometimes lead to jaundice at birth, even if the infant does not have the same liver disease as the mother.[13]

For a few days after birth, the infant is not yet fully fed, frequent normal stools are not yet produced, and the system for the uptake, enzymatic conjugation, and biliary excretion of bilirubin is not yet fully functioning. Nearly all newborns have some elevation of serum unconjugated bilirubin after birth, and many have levels that would be abnormal at any other time in life.[14]

The transport and conjugating system of unconjugated bilirubin is complex, is shared by several other substances, and is not understood in full detail. New bilirubin leaving the reticuloendothelial system is tightly bound to albumin in the extracellular fluid and the plasma.[15] The albumin-bilirubin complex is in equilibrium with a very low concentration of unbound or free bilirubin, generally found in nanomolar concentrations at or below the limits of water solubility for unconjugated bilirubin.[15-16] Reversible dissociation of bilirubin from albumin appears necessary to explain some of the physiologic behavior of unconjugated bilirubin in the circulation, the liver, and the brain.

Albumin delivers bilirubin to fenestrated sites in the hepatic sinusoids within the space of Disse,[16] probably by passage of the bilirubin-albumin complex through the fenestrae and dissociation of bilirubin from albumin at the hepatic cell surface. Intracellular transport of unconjugated bilirubin is facilitated by a cytosolic form of glutathione S-transferase (GST), probably GSTA-2,[17-18] which was generically called *ligandin* when it was first identified.[19] The ligandin-mediated function of intracellular transport appears to be shared between bilirubin and other hepatically metabolized molecules of low water solubility or similar molecular weight.[18-20] It is not clear whether the initial passage of bilirubin across the basolateral portion of the hepatocyte membrane is carrier mediated, contact mediated, or caused by diffusion of free bilirubin.[16]

Conjugation of Bilirubin

Bilirubin is transported within the hepatocyte to the smooth endoplasmic reticulum, where its carboxyl groups are conjugated with glucuronic acid. Conjugation of bilirubin is catalyzed by bilirubin uridine diphosphate glucuronyl transferase (UDPGT-1),[21] one of a family of enzymes that catalyzes the hepatic glucuronidation of certain endogenously produced or exogenously introduced small molecules, such as bilirubin, barbiturates, and phenols.[22] Conjugation of bilirubin and similar small molecules increases their aqueous solubility in preparation for their canalicular transport to the bile.

The first step in the conjugation of bilirubin is the formation of bilirubin monoglucuronide, which is sufficiently water soluble for canalicular transport, and in some infants it may be the predominant form of conjugated bilirubin in fetal and early neonatal life. Addition of another molecule of glucuronic acid to its second carboxyl group forms bilirubin diglucuronide, the fully conjugated form of bilirubin and the main component of "direct-reacting" bilirubin.

Genetic Variations in Bilirubin Conjugation

More than 50 mutations and polymorphisms in the gene for UDPGT-1 have been identified in association with clinical findings of severe, prolonged, or recurrent unconjugated hyperbilirubinemia.[23] In general, the identified mutations have an autosomal recessive pattern of inheritance, but the combined effects of heterozygosity for different mutations may produce clinical disease in some persons. Several genetic lesions of UDPGT-1 have distinctive clinical phenotypes, whereas others show variable patterns of unconjugated hyperbilirubinemia. The age of onset and severity of clinical jaundice may be related to (1) the rate of bilirubin production, (2) nutritional status, (3) developmental regulation of liver functions, and (4) intercurrent illness, as well as specific mutations in the conjugating enzyme. All mutations and polymorphisms of clinical importance can cause severe or prolonged neonatal jaundice, especially if the rate of bilirubin production is increased by hemolysis. Clinical syndromes (or phenotypes) associated with specific types of UDPGT-1 mutations include those discussed in the following subsections.

Crigler-Najjar Syndrome Type I

Crigler-Najjar syndrome Type I is an autosomal recessive disorder in which no functioning UDPGT-1 is produced. Several nonsense mutations that stop synthesis or delete key amino acid sequences of the enzyme have been described.[23] The most common variant (also found in the congenitally jaundiced Gunn rat) appears to be a single guanosine deletion at nucleotide 1206, resulting in a frame shift and deletion of 115 to 150 amino acids from the COOH-terminal of the protein. This defect prevents the binding of glucuronide for conjugation with bilirubin and related compounds. Severe, prolonged unconjugated hyperbilirubinemia begins in infancy and persists throughout life, usually at levels of 20 to 45 mg/dL or higher, and with eventual signs of central nervous system injury in nearly all cases. The nonsense or "stop" codons causing Type I Crigler-Najjar syndrome preclude pharmacologic induction of the enzyme, so gene replacement and liver transplantation are the only effective long-term therapies.

Crigler-Najjar Syndrome Type II

Crigler-Najjar syndrome Type II is a conjugating defect resulting from numerous single-site missense or insertion mutations that may retard the synthesis of the enzyme or may impair the glucuronide binding of its COOH-terminal.[23-25] Although small amounts of bilirubin conjugates may be found in hepatocytes and bile, unconjugated hyperbilirubinemia may be severe in the newborn period and may persist or recur in adulthood. Peak or intermittent bilirubin levels are usually 6 to 20 mg/dL, but they are occasionally higher in newborns. Insertion or substitution mutations in exons 1, 2, 4, and 5 have been associated with the clinical diagnosis of Type II Crigler-Najjar syndrome. Enzyme synthesis or activity may be induced or enhanced by phenobarbital, with an increase in bilirubin conjugates and a decrease in plasma total and unconjugated bilirubin.

Gilbert Syndrome

Gilbert syndrome is a milder form of unconjugated hyperbilirubinemia with occasional severe neonatal hyperbilirubinemia, followed by peak levels that are usually approximately 1 to 6 mg/dL, persisting or recurring in older children and adults with the syndrome.[23] The most common genotype associated with Gilbert syndrome is an insertion of two extra bases (TA) in the 5′ promoter region of the gene for UDPGT-1, resulting in a sequence of A (TA) 7 TAA instead of the normal A (TA) 6 TAA.[26, 27] This polymorphism has a high carrier rate in some families and ethnic groups, and polymorphisms incorporating other "abnormal" numbers of 5 to 8 TA repeat sequences in the TATAA portion of the promoter have been described in patients and their family members with Gilbert syndrome.[26]

A variant form of the syndrome is caused by a substitution of adenine for guanine at nucleotide 211 in exon 1, with a glycine 71-to-argine substitution in the N-terminal (bilirubin-binding region) of the enzyme. This and several less common substitution mutations are associated with prolonged breast-feeding jaundice and a clinical diagnosis of Gilbert syndrome in several Japanese kindreds, most of whom show no mutations in the TATAA sequence.[28]

Newborns with Gilbert syndrome mutations may have severe hyperbilirubinemia and even kernicterus, especially if they have a concurrent hemolytic disorder such as ABO incompatibility or glucose-6-phosphate dehydrogenase deficiency.[27] Adults with this syndrome have mild recurrent jaundice, often exacerbated by intercurrent illness such as viral infections. Enzyme synthesis and activity can be increased and bilirubin levels decreased by administration of phenobarbital.

Persons heterozygous for two or more of the mutations associated with Crigler-Najjar or Gilbert syndrome may have neonatal or subsequent jaundice of intermediate severity, usually responsive to enzyme induction with phenobarbital. Exact classification of these mixed, heterozygous cases of unconjugated hyperbilirubinemia as manifestations of Gilbert or Crigler-Najjar syndrome may be difficult by clinical evaluation or even by determination of genotype in some patients.

Hepatic and Enteric Excretion of Bilirubin

Conjugated bilirubin is excreted into canalicular bile via the multispecific organic anion transport system (C-MOAT) located in the canalicular membrane within the apical region of the hepatocyte.[29] The C-MOAT system shares genetic and structural homologies with the multidrug resistant (MDR) family of proteins,[30] and with GST,[31] but it incorporates a different GST isozyme than that involved in basolateral intracellular ligandin transport of unconjugated bilirubin.

In the small bowel, bilirubin may be transiently deconjugated by bacterial and brush-border enzymes before further metabolism to other heme-derived compounds. Further metabolism occurs mainly in the large bowel and requires bulk transport of bile products by peristalsis and additional chemical changes in the molecule by bacterial enzymes. Because bilirubin β-glucuronidase is indigenous to the small bowel brush border, some bilirubin in the small bowel is deconjugated by β-glucuronidase, reabsorbed at the brush border, and recirculated to the blood in a loop of excretion and reabsorption known as the enterohepatic recirculation of bilirubin.[32, 33] Some cases of protracted unconjugated hyperbilirubinemia, especially as seen in premature infants, surgical patients, or infants not responding to phototherapy, may in part result from a large enterohepatic recirculation of bilirubin before the infant is fully fed or fully colonized by normal intestinal flora.

Maturation of the hepatic conjugating system, elimination of bile products in the stool, and an eventual close matching of the rates of bilirubin production and excretion allow plasma unconjugated bilirubin to decrease to normal adult levels in most newborns within 2 to 4 weeks. Persistent hyperbilirubinemia results if the rate of excretion fails to match the rate of bilirubin formation.

Clinical Considerations: Neonatal Hyperbilirubinemia

Neonatal hyperbilirubinemia may be defined as an elevation of plasma bilirubin two standard deviations or greater than the expected mean value for an infant's age. (For convenience and as a guide to management, some clinicians use 90th percentile values.) In most cases of neonatal jaundice, elevation of the indirect or unconjugated form of bilirubin predominates. Hyperbilirubinemia may result from various combinations of increased bilirubin production, delayed or deficient glucuronidation, or increased reabsorption of unconjugated bilirubin (see earlier). Most surveys of the range of "normal" bilirubin levels in North American newborns identify "upper limits" of normal as approximately 14 to 15 mg/dL (240 to 255 μmol/L) at 3 to 5 days of age. Age-specific assessment of plasma bilirubin levels showing rates of increase greater than 0.2 to 0.25 mg/dL/hour (3.5 to 4.3 μmol/L/hour) or 5 to 6 mg/dL (85 to 100 μmol/L) per day may help to predict subsequent peak levels above the normal range.

Early visible jaundice (>7 to 10 mg/dL in 12 to 24 hours) may result from an antenatal or perinatal hemolytic disorder, of which the two most common are maternofetal ABO or Rh incompatibility. Infants with visible jaundice on their first postnatal day should be evaluated for evidence of hemolysis and followed for an increased risk that their subsequent peak bilirubin values will rise above the normal range. Persistent hyperbilirubinemia without signs of hemolysis may be an exaggeration of the physiologic pattern, but it may also result from a hereditary disorder of bilirubin conjugation or from reabsorption of bilirubin from the small bowel. Hereditary conjugating defects may first present with apparently mild early jaundice, which then becomes prolonged and more severe until it is diagnosed and treated. Increased enterohepatic circulation of bilirubin may present with persistent unconjugated hyperbilirubinemia, usually mild to moderate but occasionally severe, and sometimes lasting several weeks, especially in breast-fed infants.

Newborns with jaundice on their first day should be evaluated for hemolysis and for their rate of increase in plasma bilirubin. All newborns should be screened for jaundice before hospital discharge, at least by careful examination and documentation of the appearance and extent of cutaneous jaundice, or by a more quantitative approach such as skin colorimetry or a rapid test for total serum bilirubin. Early discharged infants (<48 hours) should be reassessed for jaundice, feeding, hydration, and weight at a visit with a medical care provider 48 to 72 hours after discharge.

TOXICITY OF UNCONJUGATED BILIRUBIN

Uptake of bilirubin by tissues, based on a hypothetical equilibrium among bilirubin dianion (B^{2-}), monovalent anion (BH^-), and bilirubin acid (BH_2), is as follows:

$$B^{2-} \xrightarrow{H+} BH^- \xrightarrow{H+} BH_2 \rightarrow (BH_2)_n \text{ (precipitate)}$$

Stepwise addition of two protons to the propionic acid groups of B^{2-} would proceed through intermediate formation to BH^- to form bilirubin acid, a less soluble compound potentially able to aggregate at membrane surfaces and bind to membrane lipids. Wennberg postulated reversible binding of BH^- with cell membranes at physiologic pH.[64]

Brodersen[15,45,57,63] proposed the formation and aggregation of bilirubin acid by net acquisition of two protons,

$$B^{2-} + 2H^+ \rightarrow BH_2$$

when bilirubin is in a supersaturated condition at high plasma concentrations. The latter mechanism would be consistent with the deposition of bilirubin particles in the tissues, especially with severe acidosis.

It is well established both experimentally and epidemiologically that unconjugated bilirubin is toxic to the central nervous system, even though the exact mechanism of bilirubin toxicity is still not known.[34] The most likely situation involves the entry or deposition of unconjugated unbound bilirubin in the central nervous system, followed by bilirubin-induced disruption of several neuronal cell functions. The unconjugated, unbound fraction of bilirubin appears to be the toxin. Studies *in vitro* and in animal models show that albumin binding reduces or abolishes toxicity, and water-soluble conjugated or isomeric forms of bilirubin appear nontoxic or less toxic than bilirubin IX-α, the predominant unconjugated form.[35,36]

Strictly speaking, the term *kernicterus* refers to bilirubin staining of the basal ganglia and cranial nerve nuclei found at autopsy. The term is often applied as well to the long-term neurologic sequelae of children with evidence of bilirubin encephalopathy in the newborn period. The term *bilirubin encephalopathy* is more appropriately applied to the acute clinical findings, which appear mild and reversible at times but are not always clinically evident, even in some newborns with severe hyperbilirubinemia who later show neurologic signs of bilirubin intoxication.

Entry of Bilirubin into the Brain

The blood-brain barrier, a combination of capillary endothelial tight junctions, a dense pericapillary sheath composed of glial foot processes, and a series of selective transport systems,[36-39] is normally impermeable to albumin and therefore to most albumin-bound small molecules, including unconjugated bilirubin.[36,37,40] This means that the newborn can tolerate a substantial elevation of plasma unconjugated bilirubin without immediate significant risk of neurologic injury. It is also probable that the blood-brain barrier is relatively impermeable to the various forms of conjugated bilirubin and the more commonly found isomers of unconjugated bilirubin, all of which appear more water soluble than bilirubin IX-α. The decreased permeability of bilirubin conjugates and isomers is not experimentally proved, but it is highly probable in view of the normal physiology of the blood-brain barrier, which tends to admit small fat-soluble molecules with varying degrees of capillary permeability and to exclude many water-soluble nonelectrolytes unless they are actively transported.[38-39] The increased solubility conferred on bilirubin by albumin binding, conjugation, and isomerization may afford the term newborn with idiopathic or physiologic jaundice a high degree of protection against significant brain injury.

Several clinical circumstances may increase the risk of bilirubin entry and toxicity in the brain. These include the following: (1) injury to the blood-brain barrier;[37,41,42] (2) a very high unconjugated bilirubin concentration, exceeding the bilirubin-binding capacity of plasma proteins;[36,43] and (3) displacement of unbound bilirubin from albumin by competing small molecules.[44,45]

Injury to the blood-brain barrier appears more common in premature than in term infants and is more likely to occur in sick infants than in asymptomatic ones. Several known mechanisms for permeating the blood-brain barrier are clinically relevant. The best studied of these is hyperosmolarity. Several investigators have shown that local hyperosmolarity increases capillary permeability to albumin and thereby allows the albumin-bilirubin complex to cross the blood-brain barrier.[41,42,46-49] Other postulated mechanisms for blood-brain barrier injury include the following: seizures, meningitis, or sepsis with endotoxemia; hypertension that exceeds the autoregulatory capacity of the blood-brain barrier; severe respiratory acidosis;[50] and perhaps intracranial hemorrhage in the premature infant. All of these mechanisms may allow leakage of plasma contents from brain capillaries into the brain substance, and it is possible that under these circumstances bilirubin binding to albumin may be ineffective or only partially protective.

Bilirubin is bound tightly to albumin up to a molar ratio of 1 and somewhat tightly up to a molar ratio of 2. (A molar ratio of 1.0 indicates that approximately 8.3 mg of bilirubin is bound to each gram of albumin; thus, in a newborn with a plasma albumin concentration of 3 gm/dL, 24.9 mg/dL can be bound.) Impaired

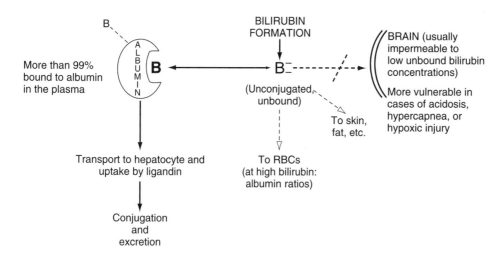

Figure 121–1. Diagram of the albumin binding and tissue distribution of unconjugated bilirubin. Most of the circulating bilirubin is bound to albumin; a low concentration of unbound bilirubin is in equilibrium between albumin and the tissues. (From Cashore WJ, Stern L: Obstet Gynecol Annu 8:313, 1979.)

binding with an increased free bilirubin concentration may occur if the bilirubin/albumin ratio in the circulation exceeds 1 or if the primary binding sites on albumin are occupied by competing small molecules. If the serum albumin concentration is low, or if the newborn is critically ill, plasma binding of bilirubin to albumin is impaired.[51] Most cases of "low bilirubin" kernicterus have occurred in infants who were very premature or critically ill.[52] Red blood cells and tissue provide some alternate binding sites, but the circulating ratio of bilirubin to albumin appears to be the most critical factor for the binding of bilirubin to albumin in the plasma and its equilibrium with extravascular tissues. The distribution of bilirubin between albumin and the tissues is shown in Figure 121–1.

Certain drugs compete for albumin binding sites with bilirubin, and in high concentrations they may displace free bilirubin. Several *in vitro* and animal models exist for this phenomenon; however, the best-documented example in human infants involved the use of sulfisoxazole, a tightly bound drug, as a prophylactic antibiotic in premature nurseries.[53] Even without exposure to sulfisoxazole, kernicterus at low circulating bilirubin concentrations was observed in some premature nurseries in the late 1960s and early 1970s.[54, 55] The precise epidemiology of this finding is not known, but it appeared to result from a combination of critical illness and certain nursery practices. For example, a survey of one large nursery[56] revealed a high incidence of low bilirubin kernicterus during a period in the 1970s when benzoyl alcohol was routinely used in many intravenous solutions and medications as an antibacterial preservative. There was a marked decline in kernicterus in the same nursery once the use of that additive was discontinued. The decreasing frequency of low bilirubin kernicterus in the 1980s was therefore most likely associated with better support of ventilation and blood pressure and less frequent use of hypertonic or displacing medications in extremely low birthweight infants.[56]

Affinity of Bilirubin for Nerve Cells

Bilirubin has a high affinity for several of the phospholipids that abound in cell membranes, and it forms complexes with these phospholipids in pure preparations,[57] as well as in liposomes and membrane vesicles.[58,59] The inclusion of protein in membrane vesicles increases the binding of bilirubin to the membranes.[59] Bilirubin also binds to synaptosomes.[60] In ultrastructural studies of neurons in experimental kernicterus, bilirubin particles are first taken up by distal axons and later into nerve cell bodies by an apparent process of retrograde uptake.[61] This ultrastructural finding in experimental kernicterus gives added significance to the affinity of bilirubin for synaptosomes[60] and to the electrophysiologic finding of nerve conduction impairment (see later).

Where and how does bilirubin bind to the cell membrane? Is it reversibly bound, or it is precipitated? Is it intracellular or extracellular? The finding of intracellular bilirubin in some cases of bilirubin toxicity, including those occurring after asphyxia, may not be typical of the "average" case. Some symptomatic infants improve with treatment, and some patients have died with postmortem disappearance of bilirubin from their basal ganglia, a finding implying that the initial aggregation and binding of bilirubin to neurons may be extracellular. In the experimental studies mentioned earlier, bilirubin embeds in bilayered membranes and may partition its nonpolar and polar groups between the inside and the outside of the membrane. The surfactant behavior of bilirubin at membrane surfaces also implies that the nonpolar portion of the bilirubin molecule may embed within the membrane, thus leaving the polar groups exposed. It is not clear what conditions are needed to transfer bilirubin from the outside to the inside of the cell, but Mayor and associates[60] and Vasquez and colleagues[62] found that bilirubin partitions between the outer membranes of synaptosomes and mitochondrial membranes within synaptosomes.

The chemical form of bilirubin in the tissues should influence its binding there and its toxicity. Brodersen[15, 57, 63] proposed a model of bilirubin toxicity in which bilirubin acid, which is nearly insoluble in water, precipitates in an "unfriendly" extracellular environment, such as tissues subjected to acidosis. In this model, the solubility of bilirubin is extremely pH dependent. Therefore, with sufficient exposure time, bilirubin begins to aggregate in the tissues in an essentially irreversible manner at the lower range of physiologic pH and in the absence of adequate intravascular albumin binding.[15, 51, 63] Bilirubin toxicity then results from irreversible aggregation of bilirubin acid in the central nervous system. This hypothesis is consistent with the pH dependence of bilirubin solubility, with the low solubility of bilirubin acid, and with the appearance of bilirubin aggregates and crystals in the brain in some cases of fatal bilirubin encephalopathy.

Another hypothesis is that reversible binding of bilirubin to membranes may be mediated by the monovalent anion of bilirubin acid. This form of unconjugated bilirubin, existing in low concentrations at physiologic pH, could potentially bind reversibly with cell membranes.[64] It could then revert to bilirubin dianion (B^{2-}) and become more water soluble at normal plasma pH, or it could acquire a second proton to form bilirubin acid if plasma pH were decreased (e.g., under conditions of severe asphyxia). The nonpolar portion of this form of bilirubin could insert into the bilayered lipid membrane, with the anionic polar portion exposed at the membrane-aqueous interface. In this model, multiple bilirubin molecules distributed at the membrane surface could have surfactant properties,[65] which not only lower the surface tension but also decrease membrane polarity[60] and alter ion transport channels. This hypothesis is consistent with the observation that bilirubin binding to liposomes and red blood cell membranes is reversible and is proportional to the hydrogen ion concentration in a direct linear fashion,[64] rather than to the square of the hydrogen ion concentration, as would be expected if bilirubin acid were the only form bound to membranes. Surfactant-mediated cation transport would also be consistent with several other observations of bilirubin effects on cells and cell membranes, including a decrease in vasopressin stimulated water and sodium (Na^+) transport,[66] intracellular accumulation of excess water and sodium,[67] and lowering of membrane potential.[60] Reversible binding (rather than irreversible membrane aggregation of bilirubin) would also be more consistent with the reversibility of jaundice and early bilirubin toxicity, with the slow disappearance of bilirubin from the skin (and even the brains) of severely jaundiced newborns, and with the observation noted earlier that bilirubin external to the cell equilibrates between the outer membranes and the inner mitochondria of synaptosomes.[60,62] If the binding of bilirubin to cells and aggregation of bilirubin in tissues proceed by a stepwise addition of protons to bilirubin dianion, perhaps the monovalent anion would be the chemical form of bilirubin initially and reversibly bound to cell membranes that is responsible for the reversible binding of bilirubin to skin and red blood cells, among others. The monovalent anion may also be involved in some of the subtle, nonspecific findings of bilirubin toxicity *in vitro* and *in vivo*. With longer exposure, higher "free" bilirubin concentrations, or more extreme physiologic conditions such as metabolic acidosis, the addition of a second proton would form bilirubin acid. This form of bilirubin can irreversibly aggregate in tissues and is associated with more drastic signs of bilirubin cellular toxicity. Therefore, the two hypotheses for bilirubin toxicity at the molecular level are potentially compatible, depending on the conditions employed for *in vitro* studies or the clinical situations encountered.

Toxicity of Bilirubin to Cells

Bilirubin reduces cellular viability and affects many different cellular processes *in vitro*. An extensive review of bilirubin toxicity by Karp[34] documented the effects of bilirubin on many different enzymatic reactions in multiple cell lines and over a wide range of extracellular bilirubin concentrations, with no single pattern of enzyme dysfunction emerging as a final common pathway for bilirubin toxicity. In the studies reviewed by Karp and in many subsequent *in vitro* studies, the experimental concentrations of unconjugated bilirubin often exceeded the assumed normal concentrations of tissue bilirubin *in vivo* and often exceeded the estimated solubility of unconjugated bilirubin IX-α at physiologic pH. Many cell lines other than neurons have been studied, and the extrapolation of bilirubin toxicity in other kinds of cells to the neurotoxicity of bilirubin remains controversial.

Based on these earlier *in vitro* studies and some more recent clinical observations of bilirubin effects in the central nervous system, several studies of bilirubin toxicity have focused more selectively on certain aspects of cell function. Some of these studies have also made more successful use of whole brain, brain slices, nerve cell cultures, or subfractions of neurons to investigate specific aspects of bilirubin toxicity with potentially greater clinical relevance. Among others, these more recent studies include investigations of water and ion transport, enzyme activation and function, and nerve conductivity and neurotransmitter metabolism.

Several *in vitro* studies have noted impairment of water and ion exchange. Brem and colleagues[66] found that bilirubin inhibits vasopressin-stimulated water and Na^+ transport across the toad bladder membrane, and the effect of bilirubin on ion and water transport in this model is distal to the action of membrane cyclic

adenosine monophosphate. Corchs and associates[67] noted inhibition of potassium (K^+) transport and increased Na^+ and water retention in cultured Ehrlich ascites cells exposed to bilirubin, and Elias and coworkers[68] found that unconjugated bilirubin inhibits *para*-aminohippurate transport in renal cortical slices. Although these experiments were not performed on nerve cells, the findings of decreased ion and water transport are consistent with the neuronal swelling and pyknosis sometimes seen in kernicteric brains,[61,69] as well as with the lowering of membrane potential and decreased action potential found in synaptosomes[60] and in brain slices (see later).[70]

Studies of bilirubin effects on selected neuronal transport functions and enzymatic reactions have possible clinical relevance. *In vitro*, bilirubin has widespread effects on protein phosphorylation, possibly by noncompetitive binding to lysine residues on the catalytic subunits of protein kinases.[71] Bilirubin impairs the phosphorylation of proteins and the activation of several protein kinases both *in vitro* and *in vivo*.[71-74] In synaptic vesicles, bilirubin decreases the phosphorylation of synapsin I, an intermediary activated by protein kinase that enables protein for the synthesis and release of neurotransmitters.[73] In whole brain studies in newborn rabbits, bilirubin also inhibits the phosphorylation of protein kinase.[74] Although older studies demonstrating uncoupling of mitochondrial oxidative phosphorylation *in vitro*[75] were not fully supported by *in vivo* investigations of brain metabolism,[35,76] studies of cultured neuroblastoma cells have shown impairment of mitochondrial action as well as decreased activity of Na^+,K^+-adenosine triphosphatase (ATPase), decreased thymidine uptake, and decreased methionine incorporation.[77,78] In summary, studies of whole brain, isolated neurons and other cells, and synaptic vesicles have demonstrated decreased activity of protein kinase and Na^+,K^+-ATPase, decreased phosphorylation of intermediary proteins and enzymes, and decreased mitochondrial function, substrate transport, and cell viability.

Bilirubin may impair the conductive properties of nerve cell membranes at both the cellular and the functional level. *In vitro* and *in vivo* studies have demonstrated lowered membrane potentials and impaired nerve conduction and transmission in at least the early phases of bilirubin toxicity. As noted earlier, unconjugated bilirubin lowers membrane potential in synaptosomes,[60] and it decreases action potentials in hippocampal brain slices.[70] In adult rats *in vivo*, unbound bilirubin crosses the blood-brain barrier,[49] lowers cortical electroencephalographic (EEG) amplitudes, and even abolishes the cortical EEG tracing.[49,79] In some whole animal studies, entry of bilirubin into the brain was associated with biochemical evidence of impaired brain metabolism (e.g., decreased glucose and glycogen, increased lactate),[79,80] whereas in other studies of bilirubin transfer into whole brain, neurobehavioral and brain stem conduction abnormalities were noted before biochemical evidence of profound neuronal damage could be documented.[76,81] The apparently discrepant results observed in whole animal studies may be related to differences in species, maturation, and methodology. Some experimental observations of changes in tone, behavior, and brain stem conduction in animal studies without evidence of severe irreversible damage to neurons are consistent with the observation of reversible neurobehavioral changes in some newborn infants as hyperbilirubinemia resolves.

In striatal synaptosomes, bilirubin decreases the uptake of tyrosine and the synthesis of dopamine from tyrosine in response to potassium chloride–stimulated depolarization.[82-84] This effect of bilirubin appears to be dose related, so at high extracellular bilirubin concentrations, the transport of tyrosine and synthesis of new dopamine are effectively abolished. Bilirubin also decreases dopamine reuptake in striatal synaptosomes and acetylcholine release from hippocampal synaptosomes.[85] The decrements in resting membrane potential, in neurotransmitter response to depolarization, in brain slice action potential, and in cortical EEG amplitude are all consistent with the surfactant properties of bilirubin and with disturbances in cation exchange noted previously. Further experimental studies of bilirubin-membrane interactions should be carried out to verify whether leakage or transport of cations across lipid membranes in the presence of membrane- or enzyme-bound bilirubin could be a final common pathway for the altered polarity and nerve conduction observed in experimental bilirubin toxicity.

Clinical Considerations: Kernicterus and Bilirubin Encephalopathy

The clinical aspects of bilirubin encephalopathy have been discussed elsewhere by several authors.[86,87] Clinically proven cases of kernicterus are too infrequent for accurate determination of its true incidence in the general population or even in subgroups considered at increased risk.[88] Currently, it is not clear whether recent concern over a possible increase in the incidence of kernicterus related to altered treatment guidelines, early discharge, or an increase in glucose-6-phosphate dehydrogenase–deficient newborns corresponds to an actual increase in the disorder.[87,88] Diagnostic imaging of the midbrain and basal ganglia is now possible in the newborn period and may help to localize or characterize suspected kernicteric lesions.[89] Because dystonic or choreoathetoid cerebral palsy may result from conditions other than hyperbilirubinemia,[87] brain imaging techniques should currently be considered adjunctive rather than specifically diagnostic of kernicterus.

REFERENCES

1. Kutty RK, et al: Chromosomal localization of the human oxygenase genes: heme-oxygenase-1 (HMOX-1) maps to chromosome 22q 12 and heme-oxygenase-2 (HMOX-2) maps to chromosome 16 p 13.3. Genomics 20:513, 1994.
2. Yoshida T, et al: Human heme oxygenase cDNA and induction of its mRNA by hemin. Eur J Biochem 171:457, 1988.
3. Yamada M, et al: Microsatellite polymorphism in the heme oxygenase-1 promoter is associated with susceptibility to emphysema. Am J Hum Genet 66:187, 2000.
4. Dennery PA, et al: Oxygen toxicity and iron accumulation in the lungs of mice lacking heme oxygenase-2. J Clin Invest 101:1001, 1998.
5. Zakhary R, et al: Heme oxygenase 2: endothelial and neuronal localization and role in endothelium-dependent relaxation. Proc Natl Acad Sci USA 93:795, 1996.
6. Maisels MJ, et al: Endogenous production of carbon monoxide in normal and erythroblastotic newborn infants. J Clin Invest 50:1, 1971.
7. Bartoletti AL, et al: Pulmonary excretion of carbon monoxide in the human infant as an index of bilirubin production I. Effects of gestational age and postnatal age and some common neonatal abnormalities. J Pediatr 94:952, 1979.
8. Dennery PA, et al: Drug therapy: neonatal hyperbilirubinemia. N Engl J Med 344:581, 2001.
9. Meera Khan P, et al: Electrophoretic characterization and genetics of human biliverdin reductase (BLVR:EC 1.3.1.24); assignment of BLVR to the p-14 cen region of human chromosome 7 in mouse-human somatic cell hybrids. Biochem Genet 21:123, 1983.
10. Saito F, et al: Mapping of the newly identified biliverdin-IX beta-reductase gene (BLVRB) to human chromosome 19q 13.13-q 13.2 by fluorescence in situ hybridization. Cytogenet Cell Genet 71:179, 1995.
11. Lester R, et al: Transfer of bilirubin 14C across monkey placenta. Pediatrics 32:416, 1963.
12. Schenker S, et al: Bilirubin metabolism in the fetus. J Clin Invest 43:32, 1964.
13. Lipsitz PJ, et al: Maternal hyperbilirubinemia and the newborn. Am J Dis Child 126:525, 1973.
14. Maisels MJ, Gifford KL: Normal serum bilirubin levels in the newborn and the effect of breastfeeding. Pediatrics 78:837, 1987.
15. Brodersen R: Aqueous solubility, albumin binding, and tissue distribution of bilirubin. In Ostrow JD (ed): Bile Pigments and Jaundice. New York, Marcel Dekker, 1986, pp 157–181.
16. Sorrentino D, Berk PD: Mechanistic aspects of hepatic bilirubin uptake. Semin Liver Dis 8:119, 1988.
17. Board PG, Webb GC: Isolation of a cDNA clone and localization of human glutathione S-transferase 2 genes to chromosome band 6 p 12. Proc Natl Acad Sci USA 84:2377, 1987.
18. Chow NWI: Human glutathione S-transferases: the H(a) multigene family encodes products of different but overlapping substrate specificities. J Biol Chem 263:12797, 1988.
19. Levi AG, et al: Two hepatic cytoplasmic protein fractions, Y and Z, and their possible role in the hepatic uptake of bilirubin, sulfobromophthalein, and other anions. J Clin Invest 48:2156, 1969.
20. Crawford JM, et al: Formation, hepatic metabolism, and transport of bile pigments: a status report. Semin Liver Dis 8:105, 1988.
21. Ritter JK, et al: A novel complex locus UGT1 encodes human bilirubin, phenol, and other UDP-glucuronyl transferase isozymes with identical carboxyl termini. J Biol Chem 267:3257, 1992.
22. Burchell B, et al: The UDP glucuronosyl transferase gene superfamily: suggested nomenclature based on evolutionary divergence. DNA Cell Biol 10:487, 1991.
23. Kadakol A, et al: Genetic lesions of bilirubin uridine-diphosphoglucuronate glucuronosyltransferase (UGT1A1) causing Crigler-Najjar and Gilbert syndrome: correlation of genotype to phenotype. Hum Mutat 16:297, 2000.
24. Moghrabi N, et al: Identification of an A-to-G missense mutation in exon 2 of the UGT1 gene complex that causes Crigler-Najjar syndrome type 2. Genomics 18:171, 1993.
25. Yamamoto K, et al: Analysis of bilirubin uridine 5-prime-diphosphate (UDP)–glucuronosyltransferase gene mutation in seven patients with Crigler-Najjar syndrome type II. J Hum Genet 43:111, 1998.
26. Beutler E, et al: Racial variability in the UDP-glucuronosyltransferase 1 (UGT1A1) promoter: a balanced polymorphism for regulation of bilirubin metabolism. Proc Natl Acad Sci USA 95:8170, 1998.
27. Kaplan M, et al: Gilbert syndrome and glucose-6-phosphate dehydrogenase deficiency: a dose-dependent genetic interaction crucial to neonatal hyperbilirubinemia. Proc Natl Acad Sci USA 94:12128, 1997.
28. Maruo Y, et al: Prolonged unconjugated hyperbilirubinemia associated with breast milk and mutations of the bilirubin uridine diphosphate-glucuronosyltransferase gene. Pediatrics 106:59, 2000.
29. van Kuijck MA, et al: Assignment of the canalicular multispecific anion transporter gene (CMOAT) to human chromosome 10q 24 and mouse chromosome 19P2 by fluorescent in situ hybridization. Cytogenet Cell Genet 77:285, 1997.
30. Buschman E, et al: Mdr2 encodes P-glycoprotein expressed in the bile canalicular membrane as determined by isoform-specific antibodies. J Biol Chem 267:180, 1992.
31. Kobayaski K, et al: Mechanism of glutathione S-conjugated transport in canalicular and basolateral rat liver plasma membranes. J Biol Chem 265:7737, 1990.
32. Gregus Z, Klaasen CD: Enterohepatic circulation of toxicants. In Preisig R, et al (eds): The Liver, Quantitative Aspects of Structure and Function. Aulendorf, Germany, Editio Cantor, 1976, pp. 363–369.
33. Billing BH: Intestinal and renal metabolism of bilirubin including enterohepatic circulation. In Ostrow JD (ed): Bile Pigments and Jaundice. New York, Marcel Dekker, 1986, pp. 255–269.
34. Karp WB: Biochemical alterations in neonatal hyperbilirubinemia and bilirubin encephalopathy: a review. Pediatrics 64:361, 1979.
35. Diamond I, Schmid R: Oxidative phosphorylation in experimental bilirubin encephalopathy. Science 155:1288, 1967.
36. Diamond I, Schmid R: Experimental bilirubin encephalopathy. The mode of entry of bilirubin into the central nervous system. J Clin Invest 45:678, 1966.
37. Chiueh EE, et al: Entry of 3H norepinephrine, 125I albumin, and Evans blue from blood into brain following unilateral osmotic opening of the blood-brain barrier. Brain Res 145:291, 1978.
38. Ohno KK, et al: Lower limits of cerebral vascular permeability to nonelectrolytes in the conscious rat. Am J Physiol 235:H299, 1978.
39. Pardridge WM, Mietus LJ: Kinetics of neutral amino acid transfer through the blood-brain barrier of the newborn rabbit. J Neurochem 38:955, 1982.
40. Lee C, et al: Permeability of the blood-brain barrier for 125I-albumin bound bilirubin in newborn piglets. Pediatr Res 25:452, 1989.
41. Levine RL, et al: Entry of bilirubin into the brain due to opening of the blood-brain barrier. Pediatrics 69:255, 1982.
42. Bratlid D, et al: Effect of serum hyperosmolarity on opening of blood-brain barrier for bilirubin in rat brain. Pediatrics 71:909, 1983.
43. Lee C, et al: Postnatal maturation of the blood-brain barrier for unbound bilirubin in newborn piglets. Brain Res 689:233, 1995.
44. Øie S, Levy G: Effect of sulfisoxazole on pharmacokinetics of free and plasma protein bound bilirubin in experimental unconjugated hyperbilirubinemia. J Pharm Sci 68:6, 1979.
45. Brodersen R: Competitive binding of bilirubin and drugs to human serum albumin, studied by enzymatic oxidation. J Clin Invest 54:1353, 1974.
46. Rapaport SI, et al: Testing of a hypothesis for osmotic opening of the blood-brain barrier. Am J Physiol 223:323, 1972.
47. Rapaport SI, et al: Regional cerebrovascular permeability to [14C]sucrose after osmotic opening of the blood-brain barrier. Brain Res 150:653, 1978.
48. Burgess GH, et al: Brain bilirubin deposition and brain blood flow during acute urea-induced hyperosmolarity in newborn piglets. Pediatr Res 19:537, 1985.
49. Wennberg RP, Hance AJ: Experimental bilirubin encephalopathy: Importance of total protein, protein binding, and blood brain barrier. Pediatr Res 20:789, 1986.
50. Bratlid D, et al: Effect of acidosis on bilirubin deposition in rat brain. Pediatrics 73:431, 1984.
51. Cashore WJ, et al: Reserve albumin and bilirubin toxicity index in infant serum. Acta Paediatr Scand 72:415, 1983.
52. Cashore WJ, Oh W: Unbound bilirubin and kernicterus in low birth weight infants. Pediatrics 69:481, 1982.
53. Harris RC, et al: Kernicterus in premature infants associated with low concentrations of bilirubin in the plasma. Pediatrics 21:875, 1958.

54. Keenan WJ, et al: Kernicterus in small sick premature infants receiving phototherapy. Pediatrics 49:652, 1972.
55. Gartner LM, et al: Kernicterus: high incidence in premature infants with low serum bilirubin concentrations. Pediatrics 45:906, 1970.
56. Jardine DS, Rogers I: Benzyl alcohol, kernicterus, intraventricular hemorrhage, and mortality in preterm infants. Pediatrics 83:153, 1989.
57. Brodersen R: Bilirubin: solubility and interaction with albumin and phospholipid. J Biol Chem 254:2364, 1979.
58. Eriksen EF, et al: Bilirubin-liposome interaction. J Biol Chem 256:4269, 1981.
59. Leonard M, et al: The interactions of bilirubin with model and biological membranes. J Biol Chem 264:5648, 1989.
60. Mayor F Jr, et al: Effect of bilirubin on the membrane potential of rat brain synaptosomes. J Neurochem 47:363, 1986.
61. Chen HC, et al: An electron microscopic and radioautographic study of experimental kernicterus. II. Bilirubin movement within neurons and release of waste products via astroglia. Am J Pathol 64:45, 1971.
62. Vasquez J, et al: Interaction of bilirubin with the synaptosomal plasma membrane. J Biol Chem 263:1255, 1988.
63. Brodersen R: Bilirubin transport in the newborn infant, reviewed with relation to kernicterus. J Pediatr 96:349, 1980.
64. Wennberg RP: The importance of free bilirubin acid salt in bilirubin uptake by erythrocytes and mitochondria. Pediatr Res 23:443, 1988.
65. Cowger ML: Mechanism of bilirubin toxicity on tissue culture cells: factors that affect toxicity, reversibility by albumin, and comparisons with other respiratory poisons and surfactants. Biochem Med 5:1, 1971.
66. Brem AS, et al: Effects of bilirubin on transepithelial transport of sodium, water, and urea. Kidney Int 27:51, 1985.
67. Corchs JS, et al: Inhibition of K^+ influx in Ehrlich ascites cells by bilirubin and ouabain. Experientia 38:1069, 1982.
68. Elias MM, et al: Inhibitory effect of unconjugated bilirubin on PAH transport in kidney cortex slices. Biochim Biophys Acta 693:265, 1982.
69. Ahdab-Barmada M, Moosy J: The neuropathology of kernicterus in the premature neonate. Diagnostic problems. J Neuropathol Exp Neurol 43:45, 1984.
70. Hansen TWR, et al: Short-term exposure to bilirubin reduces synaptic activation in rat transverse hippocampal slices. Pediatr Res 23:453, 1988.
71. Hansen TWR, et al: Bilirubin has widespread inhibitory effects on protein phosphorylation. Pediatr Res 39:1072, 1996.
72. Amit Y, Bonek A: Bilirubin inhibits protein kinase C and protein kinase C-mediated phosphorylation of endogenous substrates in human skin fibroblasts. Clin Chim Acta 223:103, 1993.
73. Hansen TWR, et al: Bilirubin decreases phosphorylation of Synapsin I: a synaptic-vesicle associated neuronal phosphoprotein, in intact synaptosomes from rat cerebral cortex. Pediatr Res 23:219, 1988.
74. Morphis L, et al: Bilirubin-induced modulation of cerebral protein phosphorylation in neonate rabbits in vivo. Science 218:156, 1982.
75. Zetterstrom R, Ernster L: Bilirubin, an uncoupler of oxidative phosphorylation in isolated mitochondria. Nature 178:1335, 1956.
76. Brann BS IV, et al: The in vivo effect of bilirubin and sulfisoxazole on cerebral oxygen, glucose, and lactate metabolism in newborn piglets. Pediatr Res 22:135, 1987.
77. Amit Y, et al: Bilirubin toxicity in a neuroblastoma cell line N-115. I. Effects on Na^+-K^+ ATPase, [^{3}H] thymidine uptake, L-[^{35}S] methionine incorporation, and mitochondrial function. Pediatr Res 25:364, 1989.
78. Amit Y, et al: Bilirubin toxicity in a neuroblastoma cell line N-115. II. Delayed effects and recovery. Pediatr Res 25:369, 1989.
79. Wennberg RP, et al: Bilirubin-induced changes in brain energy metabolism after osmotic opening of the blood-brain barrier. Pediatr Res 30:473, 1991.
80. Roger C, et al: Effects of bilirubin infusion on local cerebral glucose utilization in the immature rat. Brain Res Dev Brain Res 76:115, 1993.
81. Hansen TWR, et al: Changes in piglet auditory brainstem response amplitudes without increases in serum or cerebrospinal fluid neuron-specific enolase. Pediatr Res 32:524, 1992.
82. Cashore WJ, Kilguss NV: Inhibition of synaptosomal tyrosine uptake by bilirubin (abstract). Pediatr Res 25:209A, 1989.
83. Cashore WJ, et al: Effects of bilirubin and albumin on dopamine synthesis in striatal synaptosomes (abstract). Pediatr Res 25:210A, 1989.
84. Amato MM, et al: Dose-effect relationship of bilirubin on striatal synaptosomes in rats. Biol Neonate 66:288, 1994.
85. Ochoa ELM, et al: Interactions of bilirubin with isolated presynaptic nerve terminals: functional effects on the uptake and release of neurotransmitters. Cell Mol Neurobiol 13:69, 1993.
86. Cashore WJ: The neurotoxicity of bilirubin. Clin Perinatol 17:437, 1990.
87. Maisels MJ, Newman TB: Kernicterus in otherwise healthy, breast-fed term newborns. Pediatrics 96:730, 1995.
88. Watchko JF, Claasen D: Kernicterus in premature infants: current prevalence and relationship to NICHD phototherapy study exchange criteria. Pediatrics 93:996, 1994.
89. Penn AA, et al: Kernicterus in a full-term infant. Pediatrics 93:1003, 1994.

John F. Ennever

122 Mechanisms of Action of Phototherapy

The use of light as a treatment for neonatal jaundice was first described nearly 50 years ago. In their initial report in 1958, Cremer and colleagues[1] demonstrated that exposure of jaundiced infants to sunlight reduced serum bilirubin levels. They found that the greater the time the jaundiced infants spent in the sun, the greater the decline in serum bilirubin levels. Realizing the seasonal limitation of sunlight phototherapy, Cremer and colleagues designed an artificial source for this new treatment. Guided by the results of their *in vitro* studies, which showed that the photodestruction of bilirubin was maximal with blue light, they constructed the first phototherapy unit.

Remarkably, despite the passage of a half century and the publication of nearly one thousand papers, phototherapy is still delivered in essentially the same way as the first phototherapy unit.[2] Over the years, many investigators have tried a variety of light sources, including fluorescent, tungsten, and halogen lamps and light-emitting diodes, as well as fiberoptic delivery systems.[3-12] The contradictory results no doubt have been a source of confusion for the physician who must not only make the decision of when to begin phototherapy, but also with what device. The primary reason for the contradictory results of *apparently* well-done clinical studies is that neonatal hyperbilirubinemia has multiple causes, and jaundiced infants have

varying natural clinical courses. Therefore, small studies may produce statistically significant but physiologically irrelevant results. In addition, lamps with seemingly similar names (e.g., blue, Super Blue, Special Blue) have significantly different spectral outputs. Finally, many past studies did not report light intensities, and those that did used detectors with markedly different response characteristics.

In contrast to the lack of any significant improvement in the clinical application of phototherapy since 1958, a great deal more is now known about what occurs to bilirubin when it absorbs a therapeutic photon or two.[13-17] In addition, investigators have a reasonably good idea of the fate of the various photoproducts of bilirubin in infants.[18-22] In general, a physician can use phototherapy without understanding the photochemistry and physiology of bilirubin but cannot critically evaluate the often confusing literature. The purpose of this chapter is to provide a framework for this evaluation.

STRUCTURE OF BILIRUBIN

Bilirubin is the end product of the breakdown of heme. The formation of bilirubin from heme occurs in two steps. The first and rate-limiting step is oxidation at the α carbon bridge in heme by

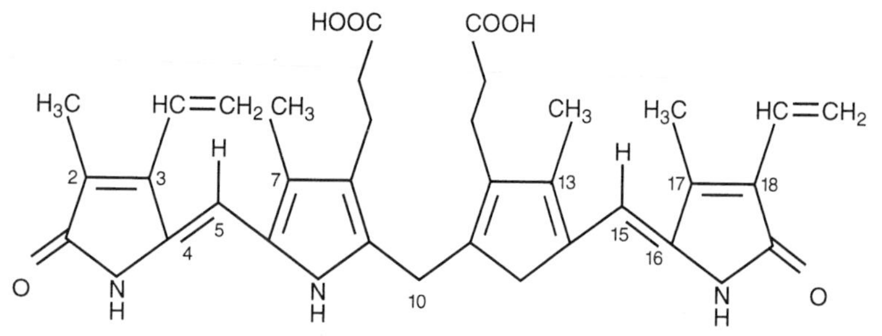

Figure 122–1. Molecular formula of bilirubin IXα. The carbon atoms are numbered according to standard nomenclature. Both exocyclic double bonds at carbons 4 and 15 are in the Z configuration.

the enzyme heme oxygenase, a microsomal enzyme present in a variety of organs, including spleen, liver, and bone marrow. This reaction yields three products: biliverdin, carbon monoxide, and Fe^{3+}. In the second step, biliverdin is converted to bilirubin by the enzyme biliverdin reductase. The formal name given to bilirubin is bilirubin IXα; the IX designation indicates that it is a derivative of protoporphyrin IX (the name of heme without iron), and the α indicates that the ring was opened at the α carbon bridge.

Bilirubin is a chain of four pyrrole rings joined by three carbon bridges (Fig. 122–1). The middle carbon bridge is singly bonded to the middle two pyrrole rings. The outer two carbon bridges are doubly bonded to the outer two pyrrole rings. Each of these two outer double bonds can have one of two arrangements, or *configurations*, called Z, from the German word zusammen (together), or E, from the German word entgegen (opposite). The configuration of these two double bonds in bilirubin IXα is Z because that is their configuration in the parent molecule heme. Thus, the complete name for bilirubin is 4Z,15Z-bilirubin IXα. Bilirubin is nearly insoluble in water despite having several polar groups (Fig. 122–1), due to its three-dimensional structure, as represented in Figure 122–2. With both bonds in the Z configuration, all the polar groups on the molecule are involved in internal hydrogen bonds, and so 4Z,15Z-bilirubin IXα is hydrophobic and lipophilic and is thus able to pass freely through biologic membranes. If the particular membrane is the placenta, this property allows for maternal clearance of fetal bilirubin, but if the membrane is the endothelial lining composing the blood-brain barrier, this property is detrimental.

These same physicochemical properties also limit the excretability of bilirubin. Nature has developed two mechanisms to deal with this lipophilic, potentially toxic molecule. One is a temporizing measure: Albumin binds bilirubin and safely transports it to the liver, where the final detoxification occurs. In the liver, bilirubin is chemically modified by the addition of one or two molecules of glucuronic acid, making it water-soluble enough to be excreted in urine and bile. Glucuronide conjugates of bilirubin are not as free as unconjugated bilirubin to pass through biologic membranes, such as the placenta. In fetal life, little bilirubin conjugation occurs in the liver, and the enzyme β-glucuronidase is present in the fetal gastrointestinal tract to hydrolyze any bilirubin conjugates that are made. The shift from fetal to neonatal life requires activation of the hepatic bilirubin conjugation machinery and a reduction in the activity of the intestinal β-glucuronidase. During this transitional phase, some infants require an additional means of detoxifying bilirubin until the capacity of the normal biochemical pathway can meet the demand. This alternative mechanism is photochemical detoxification.

ABSORPTION OF LIGHT BY BILIRUBIN

The primary event in phototherapy is the absorption of a photon by a bilirubin molecule. The probability that a photon will be absorbed by bilirubin is defined by the bilirubin absorption spectrum (Fig. 122–3). For example, a photon with a wavelength

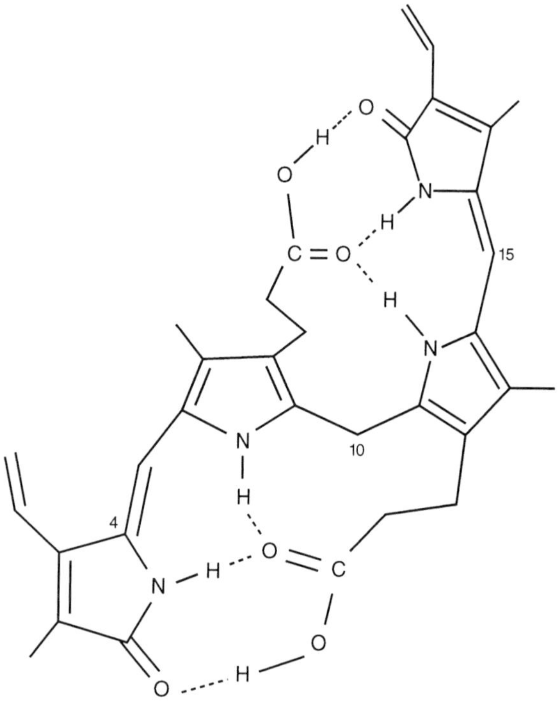

Figure 122–2. A representation of the three-dimensional structure of 4Z, 15Z-bilirubin IXα. Carbon atoms are numbered as in Figure 122–1. The hydrogen bonds are represented as dotted lines.

of 450 nm (blue) has a high probability of being absorbed by bilirubin, a photon at 510 nm (green) has a much lower probability, and a photon at 650 nm (red) has no chance of being absorbed. If infants were as optically simple as a test tube containing bilirubin bound to human albumin, it would be easy to choose the optimal light source to use in the treatment of neonatal jaundice. One would merely pick the lamp that has a spectral output closely matching the absorption spectrum of bilirubin.[23]

Figure 122–4 shows the spectral output of many of the lamps commonly used in the treatment of neonatal jaundice. From a comparison of the emission spectra of these lamps with the absorption spectrum of bilirubin, one would predict that the Special Blue lamps would be the best, whereas the green lamps would have little efficacy. However, studies show that Special Blue lights are not as clinically effective as predicted, and green lamps are more clinically effective than predicted.[8-11] The major reason is that the absorption maximum of bilirubin in infants is not the same as *in vitro* but is shifted toward longer wavelengths (to the right) (see Fig. 122–3). Several factors contribute to this shift. One is that the albumin to which bilirubin is bound *in vivo* also has long-chain fatty acids bound to it, shifting the bilirubin absorption maximum from 450 nm to about 475 nm.[24] Another

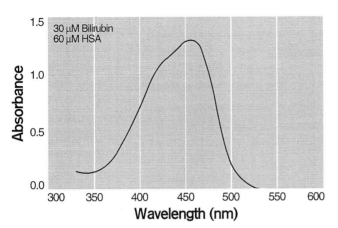

Figure 122–3. Absorption spectrum for bilirubin bound to defatted human serum albumin at pH 7.4.

factor is that longer (green) wavelengths penetrate deeper into the skin than shorter (blue) wavelengths, shifting the *effective* absorption spectrum of bilirubin to higher wavelengths. The effective absorption maximum of bilirubin is probably around 480 nm in jaundiced infants. In a small clinical trial, Donzelli and coworkers[4] found a new narrow-spectrum fluorescent lamp with a peak emission at 480 nm to be more effective than Special Blue lamps. Although these two phenomena (the shift in the absorption maximum of bilirubin by the binding of long-chain fatty acids to albumin and the deeper skin penetration of long wavelength light) are the major factors that shift the optimal

wavelength of light from the *in vitro* maximum at 450 nm to longer wavelengths, the photochemical reactions that occur subsequent to the absorption of the photons are also important variables in determining which wavelengths of light are most effective. An appreciation of these factors requires an understanding of the photochemistry of bilirubin.

PHOTOCHEMISTRY OF BILIRUBIN

When bilirubin absorbs a photon of light, the photon's energy produces an excited state of bilirubin, a state in which the molecule cannot remain for long. Once in an excited state, bilirubin can lose this excess energy and return to a normal (or ground) state by re-emission of a photon (about 0.1% of the time), production of heat (about 80% of the time), or photochemical reaction, which changes the bilirubin molecule (about 20% of the time).[16] Bilirubin can undergo three types of photochemical reactions: configurational isomerization, structural isomerization, and photo-oxidation.

Configurational Isomerization

The most likely photochemical reaction to occur when native 4Z,15Z-bilirubin absorbs a photon is a change in the configuration of one of the double bonds from a Z configuration to an E configuration. In this photochemical reaction, the number and types of atoms in the bilirubin molecule do not change (just the configuration of chemical groups about one of the double bonds); thus, the product is a *configurational isomer* of bilirubin. Bilirubin has four possible configurational isomers: 4Z,15Z (the native form); 4Z,15E; 4E,15Z; and 4E,15E. An isomer in the E

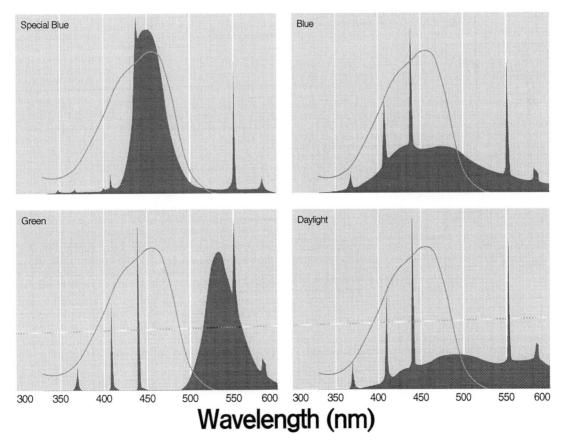

Figure 122–4. Emission spectra for commonly used fluorescent lamps. All were 20-watt, 24-inch lamps. The ordinate axis is an arbitrary linear scale but is the same for all spectra. The sharp peaks in the emission spectra are the mercury emission lines. The absorption spectrum for bilirubin bound to defatted human serum albumin is shown as a dotted curve.

configuration can absorb a photon and return to the *Z* configuration; thus, the *Z* to *E* isomerization is photochemically reversible. In addition, the *E* configurations are less stable than the *Z* and can spontaneously revert to the more stable *Z* configuration. The complete reaction scheme can be drawn as follows:

4Z,15Z–BR

hv, Δ   hv   hv   hv, Δ

4E,15Z–BR   4Z,15E–BR

hv   hv, Δ

hv, Δ   hv

4E,15E–BR

where hv represents absorption of a photon of frequency v, and Δ represents a thermal (i.e., nonphotochemical) reaction.

The isomers of bilirubin that contain double bonds in the *E* configuration are more water soluble than the native (all *Z*) bilirubin. This is because the half of the molecule with the *E* configuration is no longer able fully to hydrogen bond (Fig. 122–5). The isomer with both double bonds in the *E* configuration is even more water soluble because all the intramolecular hydrogen bonds are disrupted. Although the *E* isomers of bilirubin can spontaneously reisomerize to the *Z* configuration, when bound to albumin they are stable for hours at 37°C. In infants treated with phototherapy, the overwhelming majority of the configurational isomers in the serum is the 4Z,15E isomer, because binding to human albumin favors the formation of 4Z,15E over 4E,15Z.[25] The *E* isomers of bilirubin appear as normal unconjugated bilirubin in all standard assays of serum bilirubin.

Because the configurational isomerizations are photochemically reversible when bilirubin is irradiated in a closed system (e.g., a test tube in which nothing is removed), an equilibrium is established in which the amount of the isomers remains constant. The position of this equilibrium depends on the wavelength (i.e., color) of light used in the irradiation, ranging from 40% of the 4Z,15E isomer at 390 nm (near ultraviolet) to 7% at 510 nm (green). This effect of the color of light on the amount of the configurational isomer at equilibrium is also observed in infants treated with phototherapy: The serum concentration of the 4Z,15E isomer is highest in infants treated with Special Blue lamps, least in infants treated with green lamps, and intermediate in infants treated with daylight lamps.[20, 26, 27] In addition, it has been shown that a doubling of the light intensity while keeping the color of light the same has no effect on the percentage of serum bilirubin present as the configurational isomer.[28] These observations have led to the conclusion that in terms of the 4Z,15E isomer, jaundiced infants act like a closed system. In other words, once the 4Z,15E isomer is formed, it has nowhere to go.

Structural Isomerization

The other photochemical isomerization reaction of bilirubin involves a rearrangement of the molecule in which the double-bonded side group (—CH=CH₂) on the pyrrole ring on the left reacts with the adjacent pyrrole ring, forming a new structure with a seven-membered ring, generally called lumirubin (Fig. 122–6).[21, 29]

The formation of lumirubin requires that the side group involved in the cyclization process be located on the inside. Therefore, this reaction can occur only on the left half of the bilirubin IXα molecule, because the group on the right half of the molecule is located on the outside (see Fig. 122–1). An important feature of lumirubin is that its formation from native bilirubin is

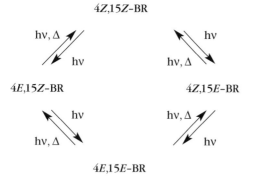

A

B

Figure 122–5. Structure of 4Z,15E-bilirubin IXα. *A*, Linear representation. *B*, Three-dimensional representation. The hydrogen bonds are represented as dotted lines. Carbon atoms are numbered as in Figure 122–1.

essentially irreversible. Lumirubin does not spontaneously reisomerize back to native bilirubin, and although the photochemical formation of bilirubin from lumirubin is possible, the rate of this process is too slow to have any biologic importance.

Lumirubin is more water-soluble than native bilirubin because of the disruption of the hydrogen bonding on the left half of the molecule (see Figure 122–6). Lumirubin is more polar than the 4Z,15E or the 4E,15Z isomer. On reversed-phase chromatography, the polarity of lumirubin is intermediate to that of bilirubin monoglucuronide and bilirubin diglucuronide. The extinction coefficient of lumirubin is about 30% lower than that of native bilirubin, so that clinical assays that measure absorbance to estimate serum bilirubin concentration give slight underestimates of the total pigment present. Lumirubin does not react in the van den Bergh diazo reaction, so this clinical assay completely misses the presence of lumirubin. Except in the presence of cholestasis (in which phototherapy should not be used in any case), however, the serum concentration of lumirubin is generally low compared with that of native bilirubin, so this error is of little clinical importance.

Photo-oxidation

From the time of the discovery of phototherapy in the mid-1950s until the late 1970s (when the photoisomerization of bilirubin was first described), it had generally been assumed that the principal mechanism by which phototherapy worked to lower serum bilirubin in jaundiced infants was through the photo-oxidation of bilirubin, a process well-characterized *in vitro*. The reasoning at the time was that the photo-oxidation products of bilirubin would be of sufficient polarity that they would be rapidly excreted in the urine and bile. Not until 1984 were

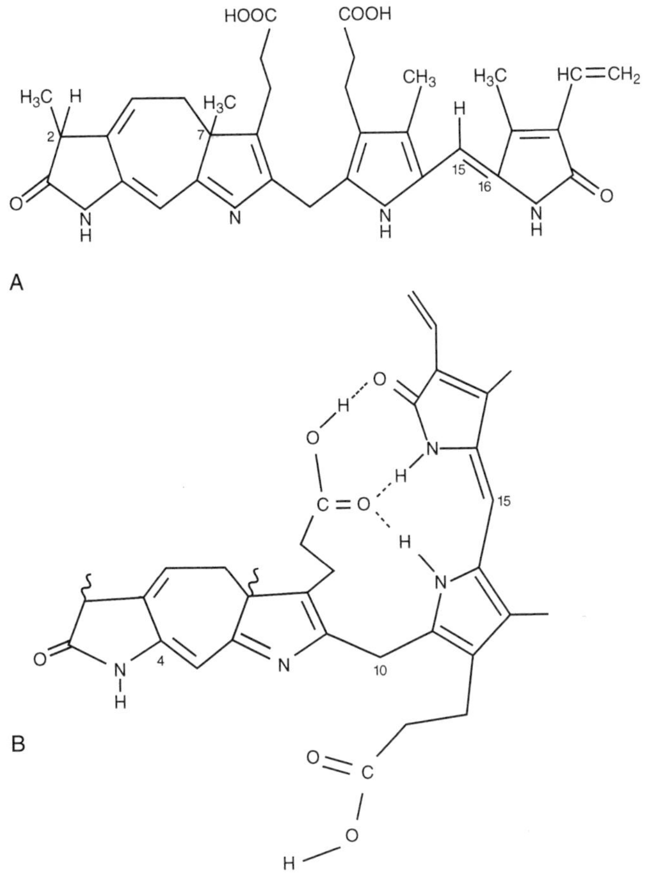

A

B

Figure 122–6. Structure of lumirubin. *A,* Linear representation. *B,* Three-dimensional representation. The hydrogen bonds are represented as dotted lines. Carbon atoms are numbered to correspond to the numbering in the parent bilirubin molecule.

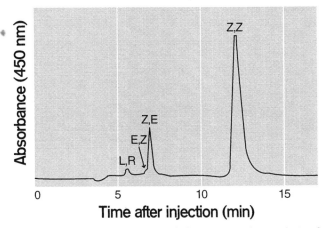

Figure 122–7. High-pressure liquid chromatographic analysis of serum from an infant treated with phototherapy.

bilirubin photo-oxidation products first identified in the urine of jaundiced infants undergoing phototherapy.[30] Current evidence suggests that although photo-oxidation clearly occurs during phototherapy, it is probably not quantitatively as important as the other isomerization reactions.

FORMATION OF BILIRUBIN PHOTOPRODUCTS *IN VIVO*

In the absence of light, the only isomer of bilirubin found in the serum of jaundiced infants is the native $4Z,15Z$ species. Infants treated with phototherapy accumulate other isomers in their serum. Within approximately 4 hours of starting phototherapy, the relative concentration of the various photoisomers reaches a steady state.[28] Figure 122–7 shows a high-pressure liquid chromatogram of serum from an infant treated with phototherapy. In general, three photoisomers are detected: $4Z,15E$; $4E,15Z$; and lumirubin. Neither *E*-lumirubin nor the $4E,15E$ configurational isomer is usually detectable in serum samples. The $4Z,15E$ isomer is typically 15% to 20% of the total pigment in the serum, the $4E,15Z$ isomer 1% to 2%, and lumirubin 2% to 4%. It should be noted that this type of chromatographic analysis does not detect any of the photo-oxidation products that may be present in the serum; however, the total concentration of these colorless products is probably much less than that of lumirubin.

HOW PHOTOTHERAPY WORKS

The goal of phototherapy is to reduce the amount of bilirubin present in a jaundiced infant. Three steps occur between turning on the lights and achievement of this goal: absorption of light by

the bilirubin molecule, photoconversion of bilirubin by any of three possible photochemical reactions, and excretion of the photoproducts. Although a great deal is understood about the first two steps, information about the third is incomplete. The two routes of photoproduct elimination are urinary excretion and biliary excretion. The relative contribution of these two routes is not known with certainty. The only quantitative data available are from the study of two patients with Crigler-Najjar type I syndrome, which clearly demonstrated that the major route of pigment elimination during phototherapy is into the bile.[31]

Precise quantitation of the relative excretion of the various bilirubin photoproducts has not been possible. The current belief is that the major photoproduct excreted in newborn infants is the structural isomer lumirubin, and that the more rapidly formed configurational isomer $4Z,15E$-bilirubin is excreted slowly, if at all. Among the data supporting this belief are the fact that the half-life of the $4Z,15E$ isomer is much longer (at least 15 hours[18]) than the half-life of lumirubin (less than 2 hours[19]). The other isomers at low or undetectable levels in the serum during phototherapy have unknown excretion rates, but their contribution to bilirubin elimination is thought to be negligible. The theory that the excretion of lumirubin is the principal route of pigment elimination during phototherapy is supported by the finding that lumirubin is the major bilirubin species in both urine[20,21] and aspirates of duodenal bile.[19]

The observation that the higher the dose of phototherapy, the more rapidly bilirubin levels decline,[7,9,32-34] although of obvious clinical importance, also supports the hypothesis that excretion of lumirubin is more important to bilirubin elimination than excretion of the configurational isomers. In that regard, Tan[33,34] demonstrated that the rate of bilirubin decline is proportional to the dose of phototherapy, and that the maximum rate occurs at a high dose of phototherapy (more than 40 μwatts/cm²/nm in the 425- to 475-nm range). Others have shown that far lower doses (approximately 6 μwatts/cm²/nm) are sufficient to reach the maximum level of $4Z,15E$ isomer in the serum.[28] A doubling of this low dose does not change the serum concentration of the configurational isomer. In contrast, higher-dose phototherapy does result in higher serum concentrations of lumirubin. These results are consistent with the *in vitro* observations noted previously. The formation of the $4Z,15E$ isomer from native bilirubin is a photochemically reversible reaction, so that the concentration of this photoproduct quickly reaches a maximum, regardless of how much light is given. In human infants, no more than 6 μwatt/cm²/nm is necessary to reach this maximum. In contrast, the formation of lumirubin from bilirubin is an essentially irreversible reaction, so the more intense the light, the more lumirubin is formed.

The fact that a relationship exists between the dose of phototherapy and the rate of decline in serum bilirubin, and that the

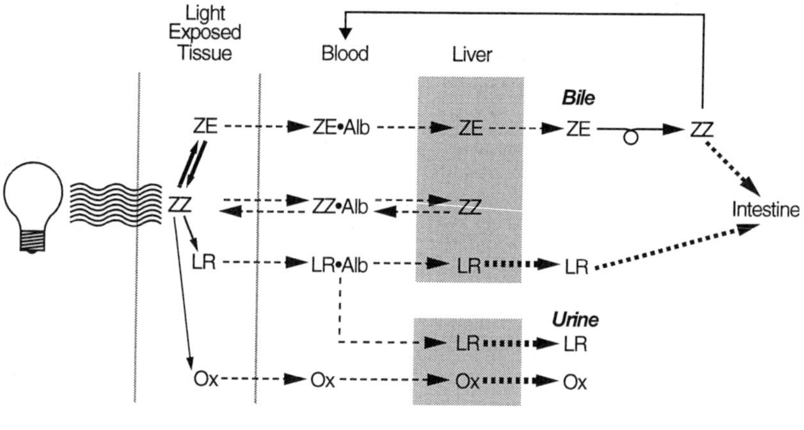

Figure 122–8. Schematic representation of how phototherapy works. ZZ = 4Z, 15Z-bilirubin; ZE = 4Z, 15E-isomer; LR = lumirubin; Ox = photo-oxidation products; Alb = albumin. The relative thickness of *arrows* represents relative rates of reactions or processes.[15]

maximum decline occurs at high doses, is good evidence that the configurational isomer is not the principal route of bilirubin elimination. The dose-response relationship is consistent with the formation and excretion of lumirubin as the principal excretory pathway. It is also consistent, however, with photo-oxidation of bilirubin being an important pathway. It is possible, although unlikely, that future work will show that the photo-oxidation is even more important than photoisomerization.

Figure 122–8 schematically summarizes how phototherapy may work to eliminate bilirubin in jaundiced infants.[15] In light-exposed tissues, native 4Z,15Z-bilirubin absorbs light and undergoes one of three types of photochemical reactions: configurational isomerization to form principally the 4Z,15E isomer, structural isomerization by a two-step process to form lumirubin, or photo-oxidation to form one or more products. Configurational isomerization is the most likely photochemical reaction to occur, and photo-oxidation is the least. The bilirubin isomers are then transported from their site of formation in the peripheral tissues bound to albumin. Both lumirubin and the photo-oxidation products can be excreted via the kidney into the urine. All of the bilirubin isomers, including native bilirubin, are taken up by the liver. Lumirubin is excreted rapidly into bile, the 4Z,15E isomer is excreted much more slowly (or not at all), and native 4Z,15Z-bilirubin is completely blocked. Any of the 4Z,15E isomer that is excreted into the bile rapidly reisomerizes back to native bilirubin, some of which can be reabsorbed from the small bowel back into the circulation.

Available data suggest that the rate-limiting step in the elimination of bilirubin by phototherapy is the formation of lumirubin, rather than its excretion.[19,22] Two factors influence the rate of lumirubin formation: the spectrum and total dose of light delivered to the jaundiced infant. The dose of light delivered is the product of the light intensity and surface area exposed. Although use of the optimal spectrum may offer some therapeutic improvement,[4] it is clear that phototherapy can be significantly improved when the dose is increased by delivering light to a larger surface area.[9,32] Because phototherapy is now used less frequently, but on more severely jaundiced infants, it is critically important that optimal doses of light be used.[35]

REFERENCES

1. Cremer RJ, et al: Influence of light on the hyperbilirubinaemia of infants. Lancet 1:1094, 1958.
2. Dobbs RH, Cremer RJ: Phototherapy (looking back). Arch Dis Child 50:833, 1975.
3. Ayyash H, et al: Green or blue light phototherapy for neonates with hyperbilirubinaemia. Arch Dis Child 62:843, 1987.
4. Donzelli GP, et al: One-day phototherapy of neonatal jaundice with blue-green lamp. Lancet 346:184, 1995.
5. Eggert P, et al: On the efficacy of various irradiation regimens in phototherapy of neonatal hyperbilirubinemia. Eur J Pediatr 147:525, 1988.
6. Sbrana G, et al: Phototherapy in the management of neonatal hyperbilirubinemia: efficacy with light sources emitting more than 500 nanometers. Pediatrics 80:395, 1987.
7. Tan KL: Efficacy of bi-directional fiber-optic phototherapy for neonatal hyperbilirubinemia. Pediatrics 99:E13, 1997.
8. Tan KL: Efficacy of "high-intensity" blue-light and "standard" daylight phototherapy for non-haemolytic hyperbilirubinemia. Acta Paediatr 81:870, 1992.
9. Tan KL: Comparison of the efficacy of fiberoptic and conventional phototherapy for neonatal hyperbilirubinemia. J Pediatr 125:607, 1994.
10. Sedman DS, et al: A new blue light-emitting phototherapy device: a prospective randomized controlled study. J Pediatr 136:771, 2000.
11. Vecchi C, et al: Phototherapy for neonatal jaundice: clinical equivalence of fluorescent green and 'special' blue lamps. J Pediatr 108:452, 1986.
12. Warshaw JB, et al: A comparison of fluorescent and nonfluorescent light sources for phototherapy. Pediatrics 65:795, 1980.
13. Ennever JF: Blue light, green light, white light, more light: treatment of neonatal jaundice. Clin Perinatol 17:467, 1990.
14. Lightner DA, McDonagh AF: Molecular mechanisms of phototherapy for neonatal jaundice. Acc Chem Res 17:417, 1984.
15. McDonagh AF, Lightner DA: 'Like a shriveled blood orange'—bilirubin, jaundice, and phototherapy. Pediatrics 75:443, 1985.
16. McDonagh AF, Lightner DA: Phototherapy and the photobiology of bilirubin. Semin Liver Dis 8:272, 1988.
17. Onishi S, et al: The separation of configurational isomers of bilirubin by high pressure liquid chromatography and the mechanism of jaundice phototherapy. Biochem Biophys Res Commun 90:890, 1979.
18. Ennever JF, et al: Phototherapy for neonatal jaundice: in vivo clearance of bilirubin photoproducts. Pediatr Res 19:205, 1985.
19. Ennever JF, et al: Rapid clearance of a structural isomer of bilirubin during phototherapy. J Clin Invest 79:1674, 1987.
20. Agati G, et al: Bilirubin photoisomerization products in serum and urine from a Crigler-Najjar type I patient treated by phototherapy. J Photochem Photobiol B 47:181, 1998.
21. Onishi S, et al: Demonstration of a geometric isomer of bilirubin-IXα in the serum of a hyperbilirubinaemic newborn infant and the mechanism of jaundice phototherapy. Biochem J 190:533, 1980.
22. Onishi S, et al: Metabolism of bilirubin and its photoisomers in newborn infants during phototherapy. J Biochem (Tokyo) 100:789, 1986.
23. Ennever JF, et al: Phototherapy for neonatal jaundice: in vitro comparison of light sources. Pediatr Res 18:667, 1984.
24. Malhotra V, et al: Fatty acid enhancement of the quantum yield for the formation of lumirubin from bilirubin bound to human albumin. Pediatr Res 21:530, 1987.
25. McDonagh AF, et al: Phototherapy for neonatal jaundice: stereospecific and regioselective photoisomerization of bilirubin bound to human serum albumin and NMR characterization of intramolecular cyclized photoproducts. J Am Chem Soc 104:6867, 1982.
26. Costarino AT, et al: The effect of spectral distribution on the isomerization of bilirubin in vivo. Pediatrics 107:125, 1987.
27. Ennever JF, et al: Differences in bilirubin isomer composition in infants treated with green and white light phototherapy. J Pediatr 109:119, 1986.
28. Costarino AT, et al: Bilirubin photoisomerization in premature neonates under low- and high-dose phototherapy. Pediatrics 75:519, 1985.
29. McDonagh AF, et al: Phototherapy for neonatal jaundice: configurational isomers of bilirubin. J Am Chem Soc 104:6865, 1982.
30. Lightner DA, et al: Bilirubin photooxidation products in the urine of jaundiced infants receiving phototherapy. Pediatr Res 18:696, 1984.
31. Callahan EW, et al: Phototherapy of severe unconjugated hypebilirubinemia: formation and removal of labeled bilirubin derivatives. Pediatrics 46:841, 1970.
32. Garg AK, et al: A controlled trial of high-intensity double-surface phototherapy on a fluid bed versus conventional phototherapy in neonatal jaundice. Pediatrics 95:914, 1995.
33. Tan KL: The nature of the dose-response relationship of phototherapy for neonatal hyperbilirubinemia. J Pediatr 90:448, 1977.
34. Tan KL: The pattern of bilirubin response to phototherapy for neonatal hyperbilirubinemia. Pediatr Res 16:670, 1982.
35. Maisels MJ: Phototherapy—traditional and nontraditional. J Perinatol 21(Suppl):S93, 2001.

James B. Gibson and Gerard T. Berry

123 Pathophysiology of Metabolic Disease of the Liver

The liver plays a central role in body metabolism. Hepatocytes, functionally heterogeneous in their spatial distribution along the tracts from the periportal to the centrilobular zones, are the principal "players" in a complex process that involves (1) transport of water and solutes across membrane bilayers; (2) biosynthesis of small and complex molecules, the latter of which are largely destined for export; (3) interconversion of metabolites assimilated from ingested food, such as amino acids; (4) catabolism of decaying macromolecules; (5) oxidation of fuels such as fatty acids, the most important energy source for hepatocytes; and (6) export synthesis of glucose, as well as its storage form, glycogen. In short, most of the cellular or subcellular processes that biochemists have classically considered the chemical reactions of intermediary metabolism take place in the liver.

Each hepatocyte possesses many different organelles (each with its own limiting membrane bilayers), which allow for the orderly, compartmentalized, and regulated execution of these many processes of anabolism and catabolism. When a metabolic function is perturbed because of a gene defect, the defective or absent protein may exert its detrimental effect on the hepatocyte by allowing the accumulated toxin initially to poison the entire cell. More often, however, the pathologic process has its origin in the organelle in which the enzyme or protein is defective. A cascade of secondary perturbations leads to the clinically recognized impairment or disease phenotype.

INBORN ERRORS OF METABOLISM

Many inborn errors of metabolism affect the liver.[1,2] In some of these biochemical genetic disorders, such as phenylketonuria (PKU), the enzyme function in the hepatocyte is defective, but the complications related to accumulation of phenylalanine metabolites are extrahepatic. Other disease types globally affect the hepatocyte or damage one or more organelles. In addition to hepatocytes, the liver contains other cell populations, such as the Kupffer cells, which also can be affected as a result of biochemical genetic disease; this may lead to alterations in hepatic function or size. In this chapter, we review the metabolic diseases that primarily affect liver function and result in clinical disease during the extended neonatal period. The biochemical genetic diseases are divided into those with and those without hepatic complications. Mechanisms of hepatic injury, including discrete involvement of organelles (as evidenced by biochemical or pathologic findings) are discussed for diverse disorders of amino acid, ammonia, organic acid, carbohydrate, glycogen, fatty acid, complex lipid, cholesterol, bile salt, glycosaminoglycan, glycoprotein, and metal metabolism.

Timing of the Presentation of Inborn Errors of Metabolism

Inborn errors of metabolism are most commonly classified as either so-called small molecule diseases, in which the pathophysiology is usually a result of either the presence of a toxic intermediate or the absence of a necessary substrate, or large molecule or complex macromolecule disorders, often termed storage diseases. This division is artificial in that all of the biochemical genetic diseases arise as a result of abnormalities in protein structure or enzymatic function. In turn, these abnor-malities are due to alterations in nuclear or mitochondrial genes and their expression. The division into toxic and storage diseases is useful for several reasons, including predicting the existence of symptomatic prenatal disease and the broad category of hepatocellular function.

Most disorders of intermediary metabolism do not show signs in the fetus. The placenta and maternal circulation provide a constant supply of calories, which reduces the metabolic stress on the affected pathway of the fetus. Maternal hepatic function is also a means of elimination of many of the toxic metabolites that would otherwise cause symptoms. The free exchange of metabolites from the affected fetus to the maternal circulation has been demonstrated in a number of disorders. For example, maternal prenatal sampling of maternal urine showed increased concentrations of pathognomonic compounds in a case of 3-hydroxy-3-methylglutaryl coenzyme A lyase deficiency.[3] Recently, a subset of fatty oxidation disorders has been recognized to cause maternal liver disease during the pregnancy of a homozygous affected fetus.[4]

The most notable exceptions to the general rule of detoxification are those disorders that may be associated with dysmorphic features, such as deficiencies in pyruvate carboxylase, pyruvate dehydrogenase, or the electron transport chain. Renal cystic changes are seen in multiple acyl coenzyme A dehydrogenase defects[5] and in the carbohydrate-deficient glycoprotein syndrome.[6] Peroxisomal disorders may have a combination of dysmorphic features and hepatocellular involvement by birth.[7]

A few storage disorders may appear with prenatal or peripartum clues caused by the accumulation of normal cellular materials as the result of a block at one or more steps of their degradation. I-cell disease[8] and mucopolysaccharidosis, type VII[9] are examples in which the disease may be evident at birth. The glycogen storage disorders that result from defects in the degradation of the carbohydrate polymer may present in a manner similar to a toxic or energy deficit disorder in the very young infant.[1,10] The recognition of accumulated material in the liver and in other tissues or the secondary alteration of the somatic structure as a result of the perturbations in metabolism may take months to occur.

Each inborn error of metabolism can arise as the result of more than one DNA mutation within the gene. Each mutation can have different effects on the phenotype as a result of varying levels of residual function of the affected protein. In the case of multimeric proteins, the net activity of the complex may be different based on the structure of the altered subunits. The residual activity, the net metabolic stress on the body (in the case of catabolic errors in intermediary metabolism), and the amount of substrate combine to determine the timing of the recognition of the altered phenotype. In rare cases, the clinical phenotype of the disorder in the infant can be very different from that in the more mature individual.[11]

Categories of Inborn Errors of Metabolism Involving the Liver in the Fetal or Neonatal Period

Table 123–1 outlines many of the disorders that have a known disturbance in the structure or function of the liver as a result of inborn errors of metabolism, which may be seen in early infancy. Not all the cases of each of these disorders demonstrate hepatic manifestations by 6 months of age. Selected examples of these

TABLE 123-1

Inborn Errors of Metabolism with Hepatic Disease Presenting in the Neonatal Period

Disease Category	Disorder	Enzyme	References
Carbohydrate metabolism	Galactosemia	galactose-1-phosphate uridyltransferase	1, 2, 20
	Hereditary fructose intolerance	fructose 1-phosphate aldolase	1, 2, 25
	Fructose 1,6-bisphosphatase deficiency	fructose 1,6-bisphosphatase	1, 2
	Glycogen synthase defect	glycogen synthase	1, 2, 10
	Glycogen storage disease (GSD), type I	glucose-6-phosphatase	1, 2, 10
	GSD, type III	amylo-1,6-glucosidase (debrancher enzyme)	1, 2, 10
	GSD, type IV	amylo 1, 4 ->1, 6 transglucosidase (brancher enzyme)	1, 2, 10
	Transaldolase deficiency	transaldolase	93
Aminoacidopathy and urea cycle enzyme disorders	Tyrosinemia, type I	fumarylacetoacetate hydrolase	1, 2, 37–39
	Ornithine transcarbamylase deficiency	ornithine transcarbamylase	1, 2, 31, 32
	Argininosuccinic acidemia	argininosuccinate lyase	1, 2, 31, 32, 75
	Citrullinemia	argininosuccinate synthase	1, 2, 31, 32
	Carbamyl phosphate synthase deficiency	carbamyl phosphate synthetase	1, 2, 31, 32
	N-acetyl glutamate synthase deficiency	N-acetyl glutamate synthetase	1, 2, 32, 74
	Hyperornithinemia-hyperammonemia-homocitrullinuria (HHH) syndrome	possibly mitochondrial ornithine transporter	1, 2, 76, 77
	Lysinuric protein intolerance	dibasic amino acid transporter	1, 2, 78
Organic acidurias and fatty acid oxidation defects	Propionic acidemia	propionyl-coenzyme A carboxylase	1, 2, 43, 44
	Methylmalonic acidemia	L-methylmalonyl coenzyme A mutase; D-methylmalonyl coenzyme A racemase; adenosylcobalamin synthase; cobalamin oxidoreductases	1, 2
	Maple syrup urine disease	branch chain oxoacid dehydrogenase	1, 2
	Carnitine palmitoyltransferase-1 (CPT-1) deficiency	carnitine palmitoyltransferase-1	1, 2, 45
	Carnitine palmitoyltransferase-2 (CPT-2) deficiency	carnitine palmitoyltransferase-2	1, 2, 48, 49
	Carnitine-acylcarnitine translocase deficiency	carnitine-acylcarnitine translocase	1, 2, 46, 47
	Long-chain acyl-Co A dehydrogenase deficiency	long-chain acyl coenzyme A dehydrogenase	1, 2, 50
	Long-chain 3-hydroxy acyl-Co A dehydrogenase deficiency	long-chain 3-hydroxy acyl coenzyme A dehydrogenase	1, 2, 50, 51
	Medium chain acyl-CoA dehydrogenase deficiency	medium chain acyl coenzyme A dehydrogenase	1, 2, 50, 52–54
	HMG CoA lyase deficiency	β-hydroxy-β-methyl glutaryl coenzyme A lyase	1, 2, 50
	Mevalonic acidemia	mevalonate kinase	94
Mitochondrial energy production/lactic acidosis	Electron transport chain (ETC) deficiencies	complexes I, II, III, IV (cytochrome c oxidase), V (ATPase) of the ETC	1, 2, 63–65, 79–81, 95
	GRACILE syndrome	BCS1L gene defect	29
	Pyruvate carboxylase deficiency	pyruvate carboxylase	1, 2
	PEPCK deficiency	phosphoenolpyruvate carboxykinase	1, 2
	Lipoamide dehydrogenase deficiency	lipoamide dehydrogenase	96
Storage disorders	Gaucher, type II	β-glucosidase	1, 2, 73
	Niemann Pick, type A	acid sphingomyelinase	1, 2, 69
	Niemann Pick, type C	cholesterol metabolism	1, 2, 71, 72
	Sialidosis, type II	neuraminidase	1, 2, 82
	Galactosialidosis	protective protein deficiency	1, 2, 83
	Sialic acid transport disorder (infantile free sialic acid storage disease)	lysosomal membrane transporter	1, 2, 84, 85
	I-cell disease	N-acetylglucosaminyl-1-phosphotransferase	1, 2, 86, 87
	GM1 gangliosidosis	β-galactosidase	1, 2
	Multiple sulfatase deficiency	arylsulfatases A, B, C	1, 2
	Wolman disease	acid lipase	1, 2
	Farber disease type I	ceramidase	1, 2
	Mucopolysaccharidosis, type VII	β-glucuronidase	1, 2, 9
	GSD, type II (Pompe disease)	acid maltase	1, 2, 10

TABLE 123-1

Inborn Errors of Metabolism with Hepatic Disease Presenting in the Neonatal Period—Cont'd

Disease Category	Disorder	Enzyme	References
Other synthetic failure	Congenital disorders of glycosylation	includes phosphomannomutase (type 1), N-acetylglucosaminyl-transferase II (type II)	1, 88–90
	Glycine-N-methyltransferase	glycine-N-methyltransferase	97
	Smith-Lemli-Opitz syndrome	7-dehydrocholesterol reductase	61
Peroxisomal biosynthesis and function	Zellweger disease	peroxisomal biogenesis defects	1, 2, 56–58
	Infantile Refsum disease	peroxisomal biogenesis defects	1, 2, 56–58
	Bile salts synthetic defects	Δ^4-3-oxosteroid 5β reductase defect; 3β-hydroxy-Δ5 steroid dehydrogenase-isomerase; bile acid amidation; oxysterol 7α-hydroxylase	1, 21, 92 1, 61, 91
Metal metabolism	Neonatal iron storage disease/perinatal hemochromatosis	see text; possible Δ^4-3-oxosteroid 5β reductase defect	1, 27

HMG = 3-hydroxy-3-methylglutaryl; GRACILE- = gracile syndrome of growth retardation, aminoaciduria, cholestasis, iron overload, lactic acidosis and early death; PEPCK = phosphoenolpyruvate carboxykinase; GM1 = generalized gangliosidosis.

disorders are discussed briefly in the subsection on mechanisms of pathogenesis.

A few examples of metabolic diseases in which the liver serves the primary role in maintaining normal extrahepatic concentrations of metabolites and in which the signs are exclusively extrahepatic have been delineated (Table 123–2). Phenylketonuria is the most widely recognized portion of the spectrum of hyperphenylalaninemias due to defects in phenylalanine hydroxylase. The enzymatic blockage prevents the conversion of phenylalanine to tyrosine. Consequences of the increased phenylalanine and lowered tyrosine concentrations include alterations in the transport of neutral aromatic amino acids into the brain and the production of neurotransmitters. As a result, mental retardation and seizures can occur. By lowering the blood phenylalanine concentration, many of the effects on cognition can be prevented or reversed. Hepatic size, synthetic functions, and laboratory tests (except that for hydroxylase) are normal.[12]

Nonketotic hyperglycinemia (NKH) is due to defects in the glycine cleavage system. Although the system is found in brain and kidney, the great majority of the activity is expressed in liver. The failure of the cleavage system results in the accumulation of glycine in all tissues; however, the pathology is due to the role of glycine as a neurotransmitter and its effects on the modulation of other neurotransmitter pathway activities. Unlike PKU, in which no symptoms are seen in the early neonatal period, infants with NKH may present with intractable seizures within hours of birth. Glycine levels are already high, implying intrauterine effects. The liver in these patients is unremarkable.[13]

MECHANISMS OF HEPATIC INJURY OR ENLARGEMENT

The metabolic processes within the hepatocyte, as in any cell, are closely regulated and interactive; they are responsive to

external as well as internal stimuli. Central to the well-being of any cell are adequate stores of energy or the means to produce energy from readily available substrates as needed. With this energy, the cell maintains its homeostasis, grows, synthesizes material for export, exports, transports, and recycles unneeded or decaying materials. All these processes are affected by one or more biochemical genetic disorders.

Compartmentalization of cellular functions is a necessary part of the synthetic and degradative pathways, and is an essential for the production and maintenance of electrochemical gradients in energy production. Hepatic metabolism is quantitatively and even qualitatively different in the periportal inflow zone compared with the perivenous outflow area. Periportal cells are responsible for the majority of gluconeogenesis, glycogen synthesis by the indirect pathway, urea synthesis, and fatty acid oxidation. Glycolysis, the synthesis of glycogen from glucose or glutamine, and possibly from odd-chain fatty acids, occurs predominantly in perivenous hepatocytes.[14] This regionalization may allow for discontinuous histopathologic findings during an acute and less than massive metabolic insult. As the degree of hepatic injury becomes more severe, or as the duration of repeat injury increases and fibrosis occurs, the distinctions become less obvious.[15]

Hepatic Pathophysiology

For many of the biochemical genetic disorders, a common histologic appearance and laboratory perturbations exist, precluding exact diagnosis without the use of extraordinary testing. The common pathophysiologic pathways of hepatic injury include inflammation, necrosis, and cholestasis as the result of alterations in homeostasis; steatosis as the result of the accumulation of intermediates and the response to metabolic stress; and the accumulation of relatively nontoxic macromolecules, which usually

TABLE 123-2

Examples of Inborn Errors of Metabolism with Primarily Hepatic Functional Defects and Major Extrahepatic Complications

Disease	Defective Enzyme	Organ Systems	Complications
Phenylketonuria	Phenylalanine hydroxylase	Brain	retardation, seizures
Nonketotic hyperglycinemia	Glycine cleavage enzyme complex	Brain	seizures

alter cellular function on the basis of mass effects rather than chemical composition. It is also clear that the pathophysiology in some instances is different with many metabolic diseases if the patient is a newborn infant rather than a child or an adult.

Cholestasis and Hepatobiliary Disease

Cholestasis can result from multiple groups of metabolic disorders. Defects in bile acid metabolism, absence of peroxisomes, and disorders of amino acid, lipid, carbohydrate, or complex molecule degradation, metal metabolism, and transport can lead to the recognition of cholestasis in a neonate.

Cystic Fibrosis. Cystic fibrosis, an extremely common autosomal recessive disease, is due to defects in the cystic fibrosis transmembrane conductance regulator (CFTR), whose gene is located on chromosome 7q31.2[16] Although respiratory disease, pancreatic exocrine insufficiency, and failure to thrive are easily recognized as components of the clinical spectrum, hepatobiliary disease may be seen in very early infancy with impaired intrahepatic and extrahepatic biliary drainage. CFTR is localized to the intrahepatic biliary epithelium[17] and is a regulator of cholangiocellular bile production.[18] Cholestasis is felt to be secondary to defective chloride transport across this epithelium. Focal biliary cirrhosis can occur early, with later evidence of steatosis and fibrosis. In a minority of patients, prolonged neonatal jaundice with cirrhotic change is seen.[19]

Other transport system defects also can cause a cholestatic change in the liver. Mutations in the FIC1 gene altering the function(s) of the FIC1 member of the aminophospholipid transporters result in Byler disease. While the exact function of the transporter is unknown, it must play a role in canalicular bile salt excretion.[18]

Hepatocellular Necrosis

Hepatocellular necrosis manifesting with jaundice, edema, ascites, hepatic synthetic failure, or hepatic encephalopathy is a common pathology due to catabolic errors. Laboratory studies show variable degrees of elevation of serum transaminases, hypoglycemia, hyperammonemia, hypofibrinogenemia, and hypoprothrombinemia. The clinical picture is similar to that of sepsis, and the laboratory findings can be indistinguishable from those of a severe viral hepatitis.

Galactosemia. Galactosemia is a typical example of a disorder in this group. Classic galactosemia is due to a severe deficiency of hepatic galactose-1-phosphate uridyl transferase (GALT) activity. As a result of significant impairment of the function of the enzyme, a syndrome of neonatal-onset toxicity occurs when the at-risk infant is exposed to significant amounts of dietary lactose or galactose. The toxic metabolites are galactose-1-phosphate (a substrate of the enzyme) and galactitol (the result of aldose reductase activity on the sugar).[20] Because there is trapping of cellular phosphate as galactose-1-phosphate, hepatic intracellular ATP/ADP ratios may be altered. Interference with other enzymatic systems has been postulated. Both mechanisms can lead to severe acute hepatocellular damage, which is reversible if treated immediately. The acute manifestations of the disease in the neonatal period often are noted within a few days of the onset of milk feedings. Vomiting and diarrhea are common. Most patients present with jaundice due to an unconjugated hyperbilirubinemia. Severe hemolysis occurs in some patients so that the clinical presentation resembles erythroblastosis fetalis. Ascites has been a prominent early finding. With the progression of hepatic disease, bile stasis, pseudoacinar formation, and portal fibrosis are seen. An end-stage cirrhotic liver can result whose histology is indistinguishable from that of other metabolic etiologies. Laboratory findings include derangements of hepatic function, albuminuria, hyperaminoaciduria, hyperchloremic metabolic acidosis, hypergalactosuria, and elevated blood galactose concentrations. There is increased production and elimination of galactitol and the presence of increased concentrations of tissue galactose-1-phosphate. In the untreated state, alterations in carbohydrate composition of glycoproteins can be seen paralleling the congenital disorders of glycosylation.[21]

The other affected organ systems in the neonate include the lens of the eye, the central nervous system (CNS), the immune system, and the renal tubules. Increased synthesis of galactitol in the lens is associated with cataract formation. CNS findings in the infant include alterations in the level of consciousness and hypotonia. Cerebral edema and increased intracranial pressure can occur. A high frequency of *Escherichia coli* sepsis has been noted with fulminant courses.[22] An inhibition of leukocyte bactericidal activity is a possible mechanism.[23] With prompt supportive therapy and the elimination of lactose and galactose from the diet, the acute toxicity syndrome resolves. Chronic, or long-term, effects of GALT deficiency occur in the central nervous system (CNS) and ovary.[20]

Hereditary Fructose Intolerance. HFI usually presents with vomiting and often is accompanied by postprandial hypoglycemia. Symptoms are related to the ingestion of fructose or sucrose. The pathophysiology includes phosphate trapping[24] as in galactosemia, with resultant similar intrahepatic pathologic progression in the face of additional carbohydrate. Beneficial effects from the withdrawal of the offending carbohydrates are seen in 2 to 3 days.[25]

Neonatal Iron Storage Disease. Also called perinatal hemochromatosis, this disorder results from severe prenatal hepatic disease. There is no single etiology for the disease, nor is there a clear genetic link to any single enzymatic defect.[26] A defect in Δ^4-3-oxosteroid 5β-reductase has been postulated in several cases.[27] At present, the evidence seems to favor the alternative that fetal liver disease leads to abnormal fetoplacental iron handling. The liver shows diffuse fibrosis with hepatocellular nodular regeneration and ductal transformation.[26] Siderosis in the apical cytoplasm of the tubular hepatocytes is typical.[28] Laboratory findings include hypoglycemia, hypoalbuminemia, nonconsumptive bleeding diathesis, anemia, and acanthocytosis. Generally, serum transaminase levels are low. Hyperbilirubinemia occurs during the first few days of life. The hypoglycemia and low transaminases point to loss of hepatocyte mass. Synthetic insufficiency causes low levels of clotting factors and hypoalbuminemia. Hyperbilirubinemia is due to increased extravasated blood, impaired hepatic synthesis, and decreased excretory capacity. Other organ systems can be affected by renal cystic changes, myofibromatosis, splenomegaly, nephromegaly, and pancreatic islet hyperplasia. Some patients have had Down syndrome (reviewed in reference 26). A newer syndrome, GRACILE, reported in Finnish infants, presents with growth retardation, lactic acidemia, anemia, and hemochromatosis. The defect is in the BCS1L gene, involved in the assembly of complex III of the respiratory chain, and has been mapped to a locus on 2q33.37.[29,30]

Urea Cycle Enzyme Disorders. Urea cycle enzyme disorders may appear as early as 1 to 3 days of age.[31] Infants show combinations of vomiting, lethargy, increased respiratory drive, and CNS dysfunction that may progress to seizure activity. Their glucose concentrations are normal, with normal or slightly alkalotic blood pHs. Markedly elevated plasma or blood ammonia concentrations are a common feature. Blood urea nitrogen concentrations are low. The common pathogenesis is an inability to detoxify ammonia, which is produced as the result of the catabolism of amino acids. Thus either protein ingestion or catabolic stress can trigger hyperammonemia. The presentation of the individual disorders is nonspecific, and specialized laboratory testing such as quantitative plasma amino acid analysis and measurement of urinary orotic acid concentration is used to separate the diseases. The cycle of ureagenesis involves intestinal, renal, and hepatic compartments. In the liver, the enzymes are localized within the mitochondrial matrix. In biopsied material examined by electron microscopy, pleomorphic mitochondria with swollen cristae and electron-dense matrices are seen. Other hepatocellular changes include alterations in the appearance of the endoplasmic reticulum.[32] Chronic injury, as the result of either prolonged hyperammonemia or repeated episodes of metabolic crisis, causes portal fibrosis.[33] Synthetic function of the liver is normal, although elevations in serum transaminases can occur. Such elevations may be present between episodes of hyperammonemia and despite the use of ammonia-trapping agents and enhancers of alternative nitrogen metabolic pathways. In the acute hyperammonemic crisis, detoxification by hemodialysis or hemofiltration may be essential.

α_1-Antitrypsin Deficiency. In α_1-antitrypsin deficiency due to the *PI ZZ* phenotype, the protein has a lysine residue instead of a glutamic acid at position 342.[34] The altered protein is not secreted, because the reactive loop center of one molecule is inserted into the β-pleated sheet structure of a second molecule. This protein is retained within the endoplasmic reticulum,[35] as is reflected by the accumulation of periodic acid–Schiff (PAS)–positive diastase-resistant material. In some susceptible individuals, the accumulation of the abnormal protein damages the endoplasmic reticulum or Golgi membranes, leading to hepatocellular damage and cirrhosis.[36]

Tyrosinemia. Tyrosinemia type I can present in early infancy with varying degrees of hepatomegaly, mild elevation of serum transaminases, and a normal serum bilirubin concentration. Common features also include abnormalities of coagulation; clotting factors are often markedly reduced. Vitamin K does not correct the disorder. Renal dysfunction with a range from mild tubular disease to overt renal failure is seen.[37] Specialized testing shows the hypertyrosinemia, increased excretion of succinylacetone, and elevated serum α-fetoprotein concentration. The hepatic disease is progressive and advances from microscopic cirrhosis, which can be seen in the first weeks of life,[38] to macronodular cirrhosis with regenerating nodules.[39] Hepatocellular carcinomas are extremely frequent. In this disorder, biochemical abnormalities may be seen prenatally.[40] The biochemical defect is a defect in fumarylacetoacetate hydrolase. The molecular mechanism of the hepatic and renal damage is not known, although the intracellular compartmentalization of toxic metabolites has been proposed to induce local damage.[41] The inhibition of 4-hydroxyphenylpyruvate dioxygenase by fumarylacetoacetate is a major factor in the recognized biochemical abnormalities. Treatment with 2-(nitro-4-trifluoromethylbenzoyl)-1,3-cyclohexanedione (NTBC) limits fumarylacetoacetate accumulation[42] but may not prevent the progression to hepatocellular carcinoma. The elevations of succinylacetone are responsible for the acute peripheral neuropathic crises that are seen in the disease.[41]

Steatosis

Steatosis can be associated at some point in the natural history of a number of the organic acidopathies that result from enzymatic defects in the metabolism of branch chain amino acids or odd chain fatty acids. Propionic acidemia, due to defects in either subunit of the heterodimeric propionyl coenzyme A carboxylase, is a prototype for these diseases. Affected infants present with severe metabolic acidosis, refusal to feed, vomiting, and alterations in CNS function.[43,44] Hepatomegaly is found in a fraction of the patients. At autopsy, the livers have shown fatty infiltration and necrosis, and the reticuloendothelial cells may have increased iron deposits.[43] The exact mechanism of the fat deposition is unknown but may relate to an imbalance between the rate of fat synthesis and the rate of export of lipoproteins. Laboratory findings of a metabolic ketoacidosis with hyperammonemia and hyperglycinemia are characteristic during the initial presentation and subsequent metabolic crises.

Almost all the disorders of β-oxidation of fatty acids (from defects in carnitine palmitoyltransferase 1,[45] carnitine/acylcarni-

tine translocase,[46,47] and carnitine palmitoyltransferase II[48-50] to the utilization of hydroxy-,[51] medium chain or short chain fatty acids[52-55]) have been associated with some degree of hepatic dysfunction and fat accumulation. In the majority of cases, when histologic studies have been performed the accumulation occurs as macrovesicular lipid storage. Hypothetical mechanisms of fat accumulation in these disorders include effects of a constant supply of fatty acids with a block in their utilization, increased concentration of glycerol, and net intracellular accumulation.

Hepatic Pathology Resulting from Peroxisomal Disease

The absence of hepatocyte organelles and their functions can result in recognized hepatic disease in late fetal or early infant life. The best-characterized group of these disorders includes those due to the peroxisomal diseases, which comprise a group of disorders with effects on multiple viscera, skeletal development, and the central nervous system.[56-58] *Zellweger disease*, the paradigm for peroxisomal disorders, is caused by biosynthetic defects in the formation of the peroxisome. As a result, more than 50 enzymes involved in multiple pathways can be perturbed. The peroxisomes are responsible for the oxidation of amino acids, alcohols, dicarboxylic acids, pipecolic acid, and phytanic acid, as well as very long chain fatty acids. They are also essential for the synthesis of bile acids, phospholipids such as the plasmalogens, and cholesterol, and they are a major reservoir of superoxide- and hydrogen peroxide–degrading enzymes.[58] Zellweger disease was also called cerebrohepatorenal disease because of the organ systems involved in the neonate. The infants have distinct dysmorphic features, as well as hypotonia, hepatomegaly, and neurodegeneration. Neuronal migratory defects are often seen. The liver has micronodular cirrhosis and fibrosis on examination. The laboratory abnormalities are explained by the missing multiple enzyme functions. Diagnosis can be strongly suspected by the constellation of physical findings and is confirmed by the abnormalities in very long chain fatty acid metabolism. The dysmorphia varies with the severity of the defect. For example, infantile Refsum disease, considered to be a milder phenotype of the peroxisomal biogenesis disorders,[7] generally presents with failure to thrive and milder degrees of hepatocellular dysfunction in older infants or toddlers with dysmorphic facial features.

Hepatic Disease Due to Glycosylation Defects

Disorders of glycosylation result from various defects in the formation or processing of the carbohydrate residues attached by N- or O-linkages of peptides. These disorders can be considered "prelysosomal" storage disorders, as improperly glycosylated proteins initially accumulate in the endoplasmic reticulum. This may in turn lead to cellular dysfunction via the unfolded peptide response.[59,60] The most common hepatic pathology is steatosis, but hydrops and severe hepatocellular dysfunction have been reported.[61] Common clinical manifestations include failure to thrive, gastrointestinal dysfunction or dysmotility, hypotonia, cognitive delays, and alterations in fat distribution.[62]

Hepatic Disease Due to Mitochondrial Depletion

Multiple reports[63-65] have described infants with severe or fatal hepatic disease of early onset due to *mitochondrial depletion*. In some cases, increased fat has been seen histologically[63]; however, ultrastructural examination of other patients' tissues has shown increased numbers of mitochondria with morphologic abnormalities, and even glycogen storage within the mitochondria.[65,66] Focal biliary necrosis has been reported, but fibrosis is a later finding.[66] Lactic acidosis, hypoglycemia, and synthetic defects also have been reported. In all cases, activities of the electron transport chain complexes with subunits encoded by mitochondrial DNA have been reduced. The amount of mitochondrial DNA has been reduced to less than 10% of normal.

TABLE 123-3

Mechanisms of Hepatic Injury and Enlargement

Category	Examples	Findings and Hypothetical Mechanisms	Comments
Hepatocellular inflammation and necrosis/cholestasis	α1-Antitrypsin deficiency	ER and Golgi damage; storage of PAS-positive material	
	Bile acid synthesis diseases	secondary membrane injury	
	Galactosemia	phosphate trapping	
	Hereditary fructose intolerance	phosphate trapping	
	Tyrosinemia	micronodular cirrhosis; see text	
	Neonatal iron storage disease	hepatocellular mass and function	
	Smith-Lemli-Opitz	low cholesterol	
	Congenital disorders of glycosylation	abnormal vacuoles; episodic elevated transaminases; ER trafficking defect	
	Long chain acyl coenzyme A dehydrogenase defect	?loss of mitochondrial function	
	UCEDs	mitochondrial dysfunction; see text	Hyperammonemia
	Oxidative phosphorylation	mitochondrial failure and energy depletion	
Steatosis	Fructose 1,6-biphosphatase deficiency	mechanism uncertain; ? due to conversion of amino acids and excess glycerol; diffuse steatosis	Failure of gluconeogenesis
	Fructose-1 phosphate aldolase		
	Methylmalonic acidemia; propionic acidemia; glutaric acidemia, type II		
	Long chain acyl coenzyme A dehydrogenase defect	macrovesicular panlobar steatosis, abnormal mitochondria	
	Long chain 3-hydroxy acyl coenzyme A dehydrogenase defect	macrovesicular panlobar steatosis, abnormal mitochondria	
	Medium chain acyl coenzyme A dehydrogenase defect	macrovesicular steatosis	
	Glycogen storage disease, type I	glycogen and fat; no fibrosis or with progression to fibrosis	
	Congenital disorders of glycosylation		
Storage of complex macromolecules	Niemann-Pick disease type A	lipid-filled Kupffer and parenchymal cells	
	Gaucher, type II	Kupffer cells	
	Sialidosis	Kupffer cells more vacuolated than hepatocytes	
	Galactosialidosis	Kupffer cells and hepatocytes	
	I-cell disease	periportal fibroblasts; Kupffer cells and hepatocytes may be normal	
	Niemann-Pick disease type C	abnormal histiocytes; giant cell transformation; cholestasis	Also cholestatic jaundice
	GM$_1$ gangliosidosis	not adequately documented	
	Multiple sulfatase	perilobular cells and bile ducts more involved than Kupffer or periportal cells	
	Farber disease	granulomatous infiltrates with vacuolar storage material	Primary defect unknown
	Glycogen storage disease, type I	see above	
	Congenital disorders of glycosylation	lysosomal vacuoles with electron-dense material	Possibly nonprogressive

ER = endoplasmic reticulum; PAS = periodic acid–Schiff; UCEDS = urea cycle enzyme defects.

Mutations in the deoxyguanosine kinase gene have been identified in some patients.[67,68]

Hepatic Disease Due to Storage Disorders

Material either synthesized within the cell or accumulated through endocytic processes as part of the body's recycling of macromolecules is the sine qua non of the heterogeneous *storage disorders*. In the glycogen storage diseases (GSDs) types I, III, or IV presenting in early infancy, there is accumulation of glycogen as well as fat. GSD type I should also be thought of as a steatosis disorder.[10] In Niemann-Pick type A, sphingomyelin accu-mulates in hepatocytes, as well as in the reticuloendothelial elements,[69,70] but in Niemann-Pick type C, the accumulated material includes both sphingomyelin and cholesterol.[71,72] In the latter disorder, hepatocellular necrosis and a progression to fibrosis can also occur,[72] blurring the distinctions made here about disorders primarily associated with hepatocytic dysfunction or storage with minimally altered hepatocytes. The accumulation and storage of glucocerebroside in Kupffer cells in Gaucher disease[73] and of glycolipids and complex lipids in other disorders lead to liver enlargement but relatively little hepatocellular functional abnormality. Patterns of storage within the liver and a description of the appearance of the stored material for some of the disorders are included in Table 123-3. In many cases, the histopathology and histochemical staining patterns can identify the disorder.

SUMMARY

A wide variety of catabolic and anabolic inborn errors of metabolism potentially affecting the liver are recognized in the prenatal or extended neonatal period. In some cases, the intrahepatic pathophysiology has been delineated, but in the majority only the broader features are currently comprehended. Our understanding of these disorders on molecular, subcellular, and organ system bases is already being aided by molecular biologic techniques *in vitro* and in transgenic animal models. Additional inborn errors of metabolism are being described at an ever-increasing rate, and our sophistication at recognizing their presentations in the very young patient is growing. Increased awareness of inborn errors of metabolism, their earlier diagnosis, our greater understanding of their pathophysiology, and new therapeutic approaches will help alter the practice of perinatal medicine in affected patients.

REFERENCES

1. Saudabray JM, Chapentier C: Clinical phenotypes: diagnosis/algorithms. *In* Scriver CR, et al (eds): The Metabolic and Molecular Bases of Inherited Disease, 8th ed. New York, McGraw-Hill, 2001, pp 1327–1403.
2. Burton BK: Inborn errors of metabolism: the clinical diagnosis in early infancy. Pediatrics 79:359, 1987.
3. Duran M, et al: 3-Hydroxy-3-methylglutaryl coenzyme A lyase deficiency: postnatal management following prenatal diagnosis by analysis of maternal urine. J Pediatr 95:1004, 1979.
4. Treem WR: Mitochondrial fatty acid oxidation and acute fatty liver of pregnancy. Semin Gastrointest Disease 13:55, 2002.
5. Frerman FE, Goodman SI: Defects of electron transfer flavoprotein and electron transfer flavoprotein-ubiquinone oxidoreductase: glutaric aciduria type II. *In* Scriver CR, et al (eds): The Metabolic and Molecular Bases of Inherited Disease, 8th ed. New York, McGraw-Hill, 2001, pp 2357–2365.
6. Strømme P, et al: Postmortem findings in two patients with the carbohydrate-deficient glycoprotein syndrome. Acta Paediatr Scand Suppl 375:55, 1991.
7. Gould SJ, et al: The peroxisome biogenesis disorders. *In* Scriver CR, et al (eds): The Metabolic and Molecular Bases of Inherited Disease, 8th ed. New York, McGraw-Hill, 2001, pp 3181–3217.
8. Spritz RA, et al: Neonatal presentation of I-cell disease. J Pediatr 93:954, 1978.
9. Machin GA: Hydrops revisited: literature review of 1414 cases published in the 1980s. Am J Med Genet 34:366, 1989.
10. Chen Y-T: Glycogen storage diseases. *In* Scriver CR, et al (eds): The Metabolic and Molecular Bases of Inherited Disease, 8th ed. New York, McGraw-Hill, 2001, pp 1521–1551.
11. Tazawa Y, et al: Infantile cholestatic jaundice associated with adult-onset type II citrullinemia. J Pediatr 138:735, 2001.
12. Scriver CR, Kaufman S: Hyperphenylalaninemia: phenylalanine hydroxylase deficiency. *In* Scriver CR, et al (eds): The Metabolic and Molecular Bases of Inherited Disease, 8th ed. New York, McGraw-Hill, 2001, pp 1667–1724.
13. Hamosh A, Johnston MV: Nonketotic hyperglycinemia. *In* Scriver CR, et al (eds): The Metabolic and Molecular Bases of Inherited Disease, 8th ed. New York, McGraw-Hill, 2001, pp 2065–2078.
14. Van den Berghe G: The role of the liver in metabolic homeostasis: implications for inborn errors of metabolism. J Inherit Metab Dis 14:407, 1991.
15. Badizadegan K, Perez-Atayde AR: Focal glycogenosis of the liver in disorders of ureagenesis: its occurrence and diagnostic significance. Hepatology 26:365, 1997.
16. Tanner MS, Taylor CJ: Liver disease in cystic fibrosis. Arch Dis Child 72:281, 1995.
17. Cohn JA, et al: Localization of the cystic fibrosis transmembrane conductance regulator in human bile duct epithelial cells. Gastroenterology 105:1857, 1993.
18. Ferenci P, et al: Hepatic transport systems. J Gastroenterol Hepatol 17:S105, 2002.
19. Valman HB, et al: Prolonged neonatal jaundice in cystic fibrosis. Arch Dis Child 46:805, 1971.
20. Holton JB, et al: Galactosemia. *In* Scriver CR, et al (eds): The Metabolic and Molecular Bases of Inherited Disease, 8th ed. New York, McGraw-Hill, 2001, pp 1553–1587.
21. Stibler H, et al: Carbohydrate-deficient transferring in galactosaemia. Acta Pediatr 86:1377, 1997.
22. Levy HL, et al: Sepsis due to *Escherichia coli* in neonates with galactosemia. N Engl J Med 297:823, 197
23. Litchfield WJ, Wells WW: Effects of galactose on free radical reactions of polymorphonuclear leukocytes. Arch Biochem Biophys 188:26, 1978.
24. Van Den Berghe G, et al: The mechanism of adenosine triphosphate depletion in the liver after a load of fructose. A kinetic study of liver adenylate deaminase. Biochem J 162:601, 1977.
25. Steinmann B, et al: Disorders of fructose metabolism. *In* Scriver CR, et al (eds): The Metabolic and Molecular Bases of Inherited Disease, 8th ed. New York, McGraw-Hill, 2001, pp 1489–1520.
26. Knisely AS: Neonatal hemochromatosis. Adv Pediatr 39:383, 1992.
27. Shneider BL, et al: Delta 4-3-oxosteroid 5-beta-reductase deficiency causing neonatal liver failure and hemochromatosis. J Pediatr 125:845, 1994.
28. Silver MM, et al: Hepatic morphology and iron quantitation in perinatal hemochromatosis. Am J Pathol 143:1312, 1993.
29. Visapaa I, et al.: Assignment of the locus for a new lethal neonatal metabolic syndrome to 2q33-37. Am J Hum Genet 63:1396, 1998.
30. de Lonlay P, et al: A mutant mitochondrial respiratory chain assembly protein causes complex III deficiency in patients with tubulopathy, encephalopathy and liver failure. Nature Genet 29:57, 2001.
31. Batshaw ML: Inborn errors of urea synthesis. Ann Neurol 35:133, 1994.
32. Brusilow SW, Horwich AL: Urea cycle enzymes. *In* Scriver CR, et al (eds): The Metabolic and Molecular Bases of Inherited Disease, 8th ed. New York, McGraw-Hill, 2001, pp 1909–1963.
33. Rowe PC, et al: Natural history of symptomatic partial ornithine transcarbamylase deficiency. N Engl J Med 314:541, 1986.
34. Jeppsson J-O: Amino acid substitution Glu-Lys in α_1-antitrypsin Pi Z. FEBS Lett 65:195, 1976.
35. Lomas DA: Loop-sheet polymerization: the structural basis of Z α_1-antitrypsin accumulation in the liver. Clin Sci 86:489, 1994.
36. Lomas DA, et al: The mechanism of Z α_1-antitrypsin accumulation in the liver. Nature 357:605, 1992.
37. Kvittingen EA: Hereditary tyrosinemia type I—an overview. Scand J Clin Lab Invest 46(Suppl 184):27, 1986.
38. Perry TL, et al: Hypermethioninemia: a metabolic disorder associated with cirrhosis, islet cell hyperplasia, and renal tubular degeneration. Pediatrics 36:236, 1965.
39. Dehner LP, et al: Hereditary tyrosinemia type I (chronic form): pathological findings in the liver. Hum Pathol 20:149, 1989.
40. Hostetter MK, et al: Evidence for liver disease preceding amino acid abnormalities in hereditary tyrosinemia. N Engl J Med 308:1265, 1983.
41. Mitchell GA, et al: Hypertyrosinemia. *In* Scriver CR, et al (eds): The Metabolic and Molecular Bases of Inherited Disease, 8th ed. New York, McGraw-Hill, 2001, pp 1777–1805.
42. Lindstedt S, et al: Treatment of hereditary tyrosinemia type 1 by inhibition of 4-hydroxyphenylpyruvate dioxygenase. Lancet 340:813, 1992.
43. Wolf B, et al: Propionic acidemia: a clinical update. J Pediatr 99:835, 1981.
44. Lehnert W, et al: Propionic acidemia: clinical, biochemical and therapeutic aspects. Experience in 30 patients. Eur J Pediatr 153:S68, 1994.
45. Treem WR, et al: Primary carnitine deficiency due to a failure of carnitine transport in kidney, muscle and fibroblasts. N Engl J Med 319:1331, 1988.
46. Ogler de Baulny H, et al: Neonatal hyperammonemia caused by a defect of carnitine-acylcarnitine translocase. J Pediatr 127:723, 1995.
47. Stanley CA, et al: Brief report: a deficiency of carnitine-acylcarnitine translocase in the inner mitochondrial membrane. N Engl J Med 327:19, 1992.
48. Demaugre F, et al: Infantile form of carnitine palmitoyltransferase II with hepatomuscular symptoms and sudden death: physiopathological approach to carnitine palmitoyltransferase II deficiencies. J Clin Invest 87:859, 1991.
49. Hug G, et al: Lethal neonatal multiorgan deficiency of carnitine palmitoyltransferase II. N Engl J Med 325:1882, 1991.
50. Roe CR, Ding J: Mitochondrial fatty acid oxidation disorders. *In* Scriver CR, et al (eds): The Metabolic and Molecular Bases of Inherited Disease, 8th ed. New York, McGraw-Hill, 2001, pp. 2297–2326.
51. Martins E, et al: Lethal dilated cardiomyopathy due to long-chain 3-hydroxyacyl-CoA dehydrogenase deficiency. J Inherit Metab Dis 19:373, 1995.
52. Wilcken B, et al: Neonatal symptoms in medium chain acyl coenzyme A dehydrogenase deficiency. Arch Dis Child 69:292, 1993.
53. Iafolla AK, et al: Medium chain acyl-coenzyme A dehydrogenase deficiency: clinical course in 120 affected children. J Pediatr 124:409, 1994.
54. Kirk JM, et al: Neonatal presentation of medium-chain acyl-CoA dehydrogenase deficiency in two families. J Inherit Metab Dis 19:370, 1996.
55. Bennett MJ, et al: Fatal hepatic short-chain L-3-hydroxyacyl-coenzyme A dehydrogenase deficiency: clinical, biochemical, and pathological studies on three subjects with this recently identified disorder of mitochondrial β-oxidation. Pediatr Dev Pathol 2:337, 1999.
56. Moser HW: Peroxisomal diseases. Adv Pediatr 36:1, 1989.
57. Fournier B, et al: Peroxisomal disorders: a review. J Inherit Metab Dis 17:470, 1994.
58. Moser AB, et al: Phenotype of patients with peroxisomal disorders subdivided into sixteen complementation groups. J Pediatr 127:13, 1995.
59. Shang J, et al: Extension of lipid-linked oligosaccharides is a high-priority aspect of the unfolded protein response: endoplasmic reticulum stress in Type 1 congenital disorder of glycosylation fibroblasts. Glycobiology 12:307, 2002.
60. Kaufman RJ: Orchestrating the unfolded protein response in health and disease. J Clin Invest 110:1389, 2002.
61. Clayton PT: Inborn errors presenting with liver dysfunction. Semin Neonatol 7:49, 2002.
62. Jaeken J, et al: Defects of N-glycan synthesis. *In* Scriver CR, et al (eds): The Metabolic and Molecular Bases of Inherited Disease, 8th ed. New York, McGraw-Hill, 2001, pp 1601–1622.

63. Mazziotta MRM, et al: Fatal infantile liver failure associated with mitochondrial DNA depletion. J Pediatr *121*:896, 1992.
64. Maaswinkel-Moolj PD, et al: Depletion of mitochondrial DNA in the liver of a patient with lactic acidemia and hypoketotic hypoglycemia. J Pediatr *128*:679, 1996.
65. Bakker HD, et al: Depletion of mitochondrial deoxyribonucleic acid in a family with fatal neonatal liver disease. J Pediatr *128*:683, 1996.
66. Mandel H, et al: The hepatic mitochondrial DNA depletion syndrome: ultrastructural changes in liver biopsies. Hepatology *34*:776, 2001.
67. Mandel H, et al: The deoxyguanosine kinase gene is mutated in individuals with depleted hepatocerebral mitochondrial DNA. Nature Genet *29*:337, 2001.
68. Salviati L, et al: Mitochondrial DNA depletion and dGK gene mutations. Ann Neurol *52*:311, 2002
69. Schuchman EH, Desnick RJ: Niemann-Pick disease types A and B: acid sphingomyelinase deficiencies. *In* Scriver CR, et al (eds): The Metabolic and Molecular Bases of Inherited Disease, 8th ed. New York, McGraw-Hill, 2001, pp 3589–3610.
70. Weisz B, et al: Niemann-Pick disease: newer classification based on genetic mutations of the disease. Adv Pediatr *41*:415, 1994.
71. Patterson MC, et al: Niemann-Pick disease type C: a lipid trafficking disorder. *In* Scriver CR, et al (eds): The Metabolic and Molecular Bases of Inherited Disease, 8th ed. New York, McGraw-Hill, 2001, pp 3611–3633.
72. Kelly DA, et al: Niemann-Pick disease type C: diagnosis and outcome in children with particular reference to liver disease. J Pediatr *123*:242, 1993.
73. Beutler E: Gaucher's disease. N Engl J Med *325*:1354, 1991.
74. Pandya AL, et al: N-Acetylglutamate synthetase deficiency: clinical and laboratory observations. J Inherit Metab Dis *14*:685, 1991.
75. Zimmerman A, et al: Severe liver fibrosis in argininosuccinic aciduria. Arch Pathol Lab Med *110*:136, 1986.
76. Smith L, et al: Hyperornithinemia, hyperammonemia, homocitrullinuria (HHH) syndrome: presentation as acute liver disease with coagulopathy. J Pediatr Gastroenterol Nutr *15*:431, 1992.
77. Winters M, et al: Unique hepatic ultrastructural changes in a patient with hyperornithinemia, hyperammonemia, homocitrullinuria. Pediatr Res *14*:583, 1980.
78. Simell O, et al: Lysinuric protein intolerance. Am J Med *59*:229, 1975.
79. Lombes A, et al: Clinical and molecular heterogeneity of cytochrome c oxidase deficiency in the newborn. J Inherit Metab Dis *19*:286, 1996.
80. Vilaseca MA, et al: Fatal hepatic failure with lactic acidemia, Fanconi syndrome and defective activity of succinate: cytochrome c reductase. J Inherit Metab Dis *14*:285, 1991.

81. Edery P, et al: Liver cytochrome c oxidase deficiency in a case of neonatal-onset liver failure. Eur J Pediatr *153*:190, 1994.
82. Wilcken B, et al: Sialuria: a second case. J Inherit Metab Dis *10*:97, 1987.
83. Sewell AC, et al: Clinical heterogeneity in infantile galactosialidosis. Eur J Pediatr *146*:528, 1987.
84. Mancini GMS, et al: Sialic acid storage disorders: observations on clinical and biochemical variation. Dev Neurosci *13*:327, 1991.
85. Sewell AC, et al: The spectrum of free neuraminic acid storage disease in childhood: clinical, morphological and biochemical observations in three non-Finnish patients. Am J Med Genet *63*:203, 1996.
86. Patriquin HB, et al: Neonatal mucolipidosis II (I-cell disease): clinical and radiologic features in three cases. Am J Roentgenol *129*:37, 1977.
87. Aula P, et al: Prenatal diagnosis and fetal pathology of I-cell disease (mucolipidosis type II). J Pediatr *87*:22,1, 1975.
88. Jaeken J, et al: Carbohydrate-deficient glycoprotein syndrome II: a deficiency in Golgi localized N-acetyl-glucosaminyltransferase II. Arch Dis Child *71*:123, 1994.
89. Tan J, et al: Mutations in the MGTAT2 gene controlling complex N-glycan synthesis cause carbohydrate-deficient glycoprotein syndrome II, an autosomal recessive disease with defective brain development. Am J Hum Genet *59*:810, 1996.
90. Conradi N, et al: Liver pathology in the carbohydrate-deficient glycoprotein syndrome. Acta Paediatr Scand Suppl *375*:50, 1991.
91. Setchell KDR: Δ⁴-3-Oxosteroid 5β reductase deficiency described in identical twins with neonatal hepatitis: a new inborn error in bile acid synthesis. J Clin Invest *82*:2148, 1993.
92. Daugherty CC, et al: Resolution of liver biopsy alterations in three siblings with bile acid treatment of an inborn error of bile acid metabolism. Hepatology *18*:1096, 1993.
93. Verhoeven NM, et al: Transaldolase deficiency: liver cirrhosis associated with a new inborn error in the pentose phosphate pathway. Am J Human Genet *68*:1086, 2001.
94. Hinson DD, et al: Hematologic abnormalities and cholestatic liver disease in two patients with mevalonate kinase deficiency. Am J Med Genet *78*:408, 1998.
95. Valnot I, et al: Mutations of the SCO1 gene in mitochondrial cytochrome c oxidase deficiency with neonatal-onset hepatic failure and encephalopathy. Am J Human Genet *67*:1104, 2000.
96. Shaag A, et al: Molecular basis of lipoamide dehydrogenase deficiency in Ashkenazi Jews. Am J Med Genet *82*:177, 1999.
97. Mudd SH, et al: Glycine N-methyltransferase deficiency: a novel inborn error causing persistent isolated hypermethioninaemia. J Inherit Metab Dis *24*:448, 2001.

124

Michael R. Narkewicz

Neonatal Cholestasis: Pathophysiology, Etiology, and Treatment

Neonatal cholestasis (prolonged conjugated hyperbilirubinemia) is the end result of a variety of insults in the newborn infant. The large list of possible causes and the heterogeneous nature of the disorders associated with the development of neonatal cholestasis present a unique diagnostic challenge to clinicians caring for newborn infants. The list of potential causes of neonatal cholestasis mandates a rapid exclusion of the treatable infectious, metabolic, and surgical disorders for which early treatment or intervention may result in rapid improvement. However, despite the long list of possible causes and recent advances in diagnosis, in up to 75% of cases the ultimate etiology of neonatal cholestasis is frequently classified as either idiopathic neonatal hepatitis or biliary atresia.

This chapter reviews the underlying physiology that results in the propensity for the development of cholestasis in the infant, the pathophysiology that leads to hepatic injury, and the consequences thereof.

Neonatal cholestasis can be defined as a reduction in the normal flow of bile. Although this definition is helpful from a pathophysiologic standpoint, a more useful and practical defini-

tion of neonatal cholestasis is any direct hyperbilirubinemia accounting for more than 20% of the total bilirubin. In general, this definition is useful except in certain rare conditions in which total bile acids are significantly elevated in the face of a normal direct bilirubin.

ONTOGENY OF BILE FLOW AND THE PHYSIOLOGIC CHOLESTASIS OF THE NEONATE

The newborn infant has an inherent propensity to develop cholestasis independent of the cause. This is caused in part by the *physiologic cholestasis* (relative physiologic reduction of bile flow compared with older children and adults) of the neonate. An age-related lag in bile acid secretion has been demonstrated in many species[1-3] and confirmed by the findings of decreased hepatic taurocholate clearance in dogs, monkeys, and sheep.[2,3] These findings have been confirmed in human infants by the demonstration that fasting serum bile acids are elevated after birth and gradually decline to adult levels only by the first 6 to 12 months of life.[4] The many physiologic and developmental factors that may contribute to physiologic cholestasis in the neonate are discussed later.

Bile is a fluid mixture of electrolytes, organic anions (primarily bile acids and bilirubin), cholesterol, lecithin, and protein. *In utero*, the placenta accomplishes detoxification and excretion of lipophilic protein-bound substances such as bilirubin or bile acids by allowing exchange with the maternal liver. Thus, *in utero*, there is no obligate physiologic requirement for the development of a significant *fetal* hepatic excretory function or bile formation. However, analysis of human fetal bile and *in vitro* studies of bile acid formation by liver homogenates have shown that primary bile acid synthesis is present by the 10th week of gestation. The developmental pattern of the enzymes for many of the steps of bile acid synthesis have been studied in the developing rat. These studies show that bile acid synthetic enzymes are present by day 13 in the fetal rat and increase synchronously 30- to 40-fold by the time of weaning.[5] Biliary bile acid concentration is quite low early in the human fetus and rises throughout most of gestation.[6,7] However, the large proportion of chenodeoxycholic acid in fetal bile is different from the predominance of cholic acid in infant and adult bile.[8,9]

Bile formation is an energy-dependent active solute transport process at the canalicular level with passive following of water.[10] One of the major stimulants of bile flow is the *bile acid pool size*. Thus, the low concentrations of fetal biliary bile acids are consistent with a small fetal bile acid pool. The fetus has a small bile acid pool (101 ± 13 μmol/kg) compared with the neonate (214 ± 26 μmol/kg).[11] The neonate's pool is also quite reduced, at only 30% of the adult bile acid pool size. One factor contributing to the small size in the fetus is the functional isolation of the fetal intestinal bile acid pool resulting from poor intestinal motility and the lack of active bile acid transport. The specific ileal bile acid transport system is absent or reduced in the fetus and develops very slowly, gradually appearing over the first several months of life.[12] Therefore, in the fetus and neonate, bile acids excreted into the intestine can be conserved only by limited passive absorption, resulting in the prolongation of the reduced bile acid pool of the neonate.[13] These findings have also been confirmed in human infants by the demonstration of a small pool of cholic acid in the neonate that increases with age.[14]

There are two components to bile flow: bile acid-dependent (flow that increases with increasing bile acid supply) and bile acid-independent (basal flow that is not altered by bile acid supply). During early life, bile flow is virtually all the result of bile acid-dependent bile flow.[15] This differs from the adult, in whom bile acid-independent bile flow accounts for a significant proportion of bile flow. Thus, in the fetus and neonate, the small bile acid pool size and the dependence on bile acid-dependent bile flow result in diminished bile flow and contribute to the physiologic cholestasis of the neonate and the propensity to develop cholestasis. Decreased intraluminal concentration of bile acids in low birth weight infants provides additional evidence for impaired bile acid secretion in human infants.[16,17]

Confounding the regulation of bile flow by bile acids is the restricted ability of hepatocytes to take up bile acids actively, as shown by a reduced uptake of taurocholate in hepatocytes from suckling rats.[18] In the rat, hepatocyte taurocholate uptake increases fourfold by 8 weeks of age.[18] In addition, serum bile acids are three- to fourfold higher in suckling rats compared with adult rats.[19] Somewhat surprisingly, all of the hepatocytes across the lobule take up a radiolabeled bile acid analogue in suckling rats, whereas it is taken up only by periportal hepatocytes in the adult rat.[19] Further work has shown that the appearance of taurocholate transport is related to the ontologic appearance of a sodium-dependent bile acid transporter localized to the basolateral membrane.[20] This transporter is absent in fetal and newborn rat liver, and its appearance parallels the ability of hepatocytes to take up taurocholate actively in a sodium-dependent manner.

Likewise, there is a reduction in canalicular membrane transport of taurocholate in 7-day-old versus 14-day-old suckling rats. This transporter is also reduced in canalicular membranes from the 7-day-old rat.[21] Because the rate-limiting step for bile flow appears to be secretion at the canalicular membrane, this latter process may be most important in the physiology of cholestasis in the infant.[22]

Another factor that contributes to the low rates of neonatal bile flow may be low fetal glutathione levels. Glutathione is the major organic anion, other than bile acids, that is excreted into bile. There is a gradual increase in hepatic glutathione after birth that precedes the appearance of glutathione in bile and the appearance of bile acid-independent bile flow.[23] In the neonate, the primary bile acids cholic and chenodeoxycholic acid are synthesized and conjugated for the most part with taurine. During the first month of life, the increase in bile acid pool size is mainly the result of increased synthesis of these primary bile acids.

Hormonal factors are also important in the developmental changes in bile formation and flow. Bile formation is increased by cyclic adenosine monophosphate and glucagon and, to a lesser extent, by secretin, cholecystokinin, and histamine.[24] In addition, prenatal maternal administration of dexamethasone has been shown to increase the bile acid pool size in the premature infant.[25] The ability of these hormones to up-regulate bile secretion is limited in the infant. Both secretin and glucagon have minimal effect on bile flow in 3-day-old dogs; however, the response to these hormones increases until adulthood.[26] Some of this effect may result from the decreased motility of the biliary tract in the neonate.[27] The other contribution to bile flow comes from contraction of the gallbladder. In pigs, the newborn gallbladder has a lower intraluminal pressure and a lower responsiveness to cholecystokinin, and it is less compliant when compared which that of adults.[28] The reason is a lack of adequate smooth muscle, which results in a reduced ability to overcome the resistance in the bile duct and the sphincter of Oddi,[28] contributing to reduced bile flow in the neonate.

Multiple canalicular transport proteins for bile acids have been identified and characterized, including several adenosine triphosphate (ATP)-dependent transporters involved in bile acid excretion (sister gene of P-glycoprotein, multidrug resistance gene *MDR3*, ecto-ATPase, and the multispecific organic anion transporter-canalicular multidrug resistance protein cMOAT). In the rat, ecto-ATPase protein is low at birth,[29] and it increases rapidly, providing an additional explanation for the physiologic cholestasis of the neonate. Defects in all the canalicular proteins have been described in genetic syndromes of cholestasis that can present in the neonate.[30]

Thus, combinations of the foregoing factors result in the neonate's predisposition to cholestasis and probably contribute to the large list of diverse conditions that can result in the development of neonatal cholestasis.

MECHANISMS OF HEPATIC INJURY IN CHOLESTASIS

Although infants with cholestasis can recover without any long-term hepatic consequences, many infants develop significant liver disease. Work by several investigators has demonstrated that the accumulation of bile acids can alone lead to hepatic injury.[31] Accumulation of bile acids in hepatocytes leads to apoptosis through both the Fas death receptor pathway[32] and via mitochondrial injury.[33] Low hepatocyte glutathione leads to more bile acid-mediated hepatocyte injury,[34] suggesting that infants may be more prone to hepatic injury from cholestasis given their low liver glutathione concentrations.[35] Hydrophobic "toxic" bile acids lead to increased oxidant injury and can stimulate subsequent fibrosis.[36] These animal data are consistent with the severe hepatic injury seen in children with inherited defects in bile acid metabolism[37] and bile salt transport,[38] which result in the accumulation of toxic bile acid metabolites and liver failure and which can be averted with treatment.

Consequences of Inadequate Bile Flow

Steatorrhea and Malnutrition

Bile acids aid in the solubilization of dietary fat and are important in the activation of pancreatic colipase to lipase for the absorption of dietary lipids. The subsequent monoglycerides and free fatty acids are then incorporated into mixed micelles, which are formed in the presence of bile acids for absorption. The reduction in bile flow that accompanies cholestasis may result in inadequate concentrations of intraluminal bile acids for effective fat absorption, with consequent malabsorption of dietary fats, lipids, and fat-soluble vitamins.[39-41] Thus, *steatorrhea* is invariably present in infants with significant cholestasis and contributes to the malnutrition that is often observed. Other factors that contribute to malnutrition in these children include abnormalities in carbohydrate and amino acid metabolism, anorexia, recurrent infections, early satiety, and increased resting energy expenditure.[42] Infant formulas with significant quantities of medium-chain triglycerides (MCT) provide better energy balance, because MCT absorption is not dependent on intraluminal bile acid concentration. MCT oil–predominant formulas (50% to 60% of fat calories as MCT) *providing 120% of recommended caloric intake* have been used successfully to promote growth in children with chronic cholestasis.[43] In selected cases, continuous enteral infusion feeding of up to 140% of recommended caloric intake and 4 g/kg/day of protein lead to improved nutritional status in children with severe chronic liver disease awaiting liver transplantation, without adverse clinical or biochemical effects.[44]

Fat-Soluble Vitamin Deficiency

The intestinal absorption of vitamins A, D, E, and K requires adequate intraluminal concentrations of bile acids, and thus malabsorption of fat-soluble vitamins is a common consequence of cholestasis. The goals of evaluation and supplementation of fat-soluble vitamins are to prevent deficiency states and to replete stores to prevent long-term consequences if a deficiency state exists.

Nutritional Consequences of the Retention of Bile and its Constitutents

Hyperlipidemia

Hyperlipidemia and the later development of xanthomas are a frequent complication of severe intrahepatic cholestasis. Hypercholesterolemia is frequently noted at presentation in infants with intrahepatic cholestasis. This is caused by regurgitation of biliary lipids into the plasma, combined with a secondary increase in hepatic cholesterol synthesis.[45] Because the primary defect is poor bile flow, treatment is directed at attempts to increase bile flow and the conversion of cholesterol to bile acids, with agents such as cholestyramine, phenobarbital, or ursodeoxycholic acid. The cholesterol synthesis–blocking agents (lovastatin, simvastatin) act by inhibiting 3-hydroxy-3-methylglutaryl (HMG)-CoA reductase, the rate-limiting enzyme. However, they do not alter the basic pathophysiology of the hyperlipidemia in cholestasis and are potentially hepatotoxic, thus are not recommended for use in neonatal cholestasis.

Accumulation of Copper, Manganese, or Aluminum

Because copper, manganese, and aluminum are excreted primarily in the bile, these trace metals can accumulate and result in high serum levels during cholestasis. Very high serum and hepatic copper levels have been observed.[46] Although copper reduction has not been clearly demonstrated to improve the outcome of cholestasis, low-copper diets and the elimination or reduction of copper from parenteral nutrition solutions are recommended.[47,48]

Manganese has been shown to accumulate in the livers and globus pallidus of infants with biliary atresia and has been associated with the development of cholestasis in rats given high doses parenterally.[49-51] As with copper, reduction or elimination of manganese from parenteral alimentation solutions and monitoring of plasma manganese levels is recommended for infants with cholestasis who are receiving parenteral nutrition.[52]

Aluminum is excreted to a significant extent in bile and has been shown to be hepatotoxic in large doses.[53,54] Therefore, the use of aluminum-containing medications such as aluminum hydroxide antacids or sucralfate should be avoided. Furthermore, aluminum contaminants in parenteral nutrition comstituents[55] must be viewed with caution until further data about potential toxicity are available.

Minerals

Deficiencies of calcium, phosphorus, magnesium, zinc, selenium, and iron deficiency states have been described in association with cholestasis or cirrhosis.[42] Whether screening for deficiency on a routine basis or preventive supplementation with foods rich in these minerals is the appropriate management has not been studied in a prospective manner.

General Care

Infants with cholestasis of early onset (less than 1 year of age) have been shown to score lower on a variety of objective tests of mental development.[56] The origin of these differences is probably multifactorial in nature. Routine pediatric care should continue to include monitoring the physical and mental development of infants with cholestasis. Immunizations on a standard schedule are appropriate for most infants with cholestatic liver disease. Because of the chronic nature of most of the disorders that cause neonatal cholestasis, attention to the unique stresses involved in being a cholestaele patient and caring for a child with a chronic medical problem is an important part of the long-term care of these children and their families.

REFERENCES

1. Little J, et al: Taurocholate pool size and distribution in the fetal rat. J Clin Invest *63*:1042, 1979.
2. Hardy K, et al: Bile acid metabolism in fetal sheep: perinatal changes in the bile acid pool. J Physiol *309*:1, 1980.
3. Smallwood R, et al: Fetal bile salt metabolism: II. Hepatic excretion of endogenous bile salt and a taurocholate load. J Clin Invest *51*:1388, 1982.
4. Suchy F, et al: Physiologic cholestasis: elevation of the primary serum bile acid concentration in normal infants. Gastroenterology *80*:1037, 1981.
5. Whitehouse MW, et al: Catabolism in vitro of cholesterol: some comparative aspects. Arch Biochem Biophys *98*:305, 1962.
6. Haber LR, et al: Bile acid conjugation in organ culture of human fetal liver. Gastroenterology *74*:1214, 1978.
7. Colombo C, et al: Biliary bile acid composition of the human fetus in early gestation. Pediatr Res *21*:197, 1987.
8. Setchell KDR, Russell DW: Ontogenesis of bile acid synthesis and metabolism. *In* Suchy FJ (ed): Liver Disease in Children. St Louis, Mosby–Year Book, 1994, pp 81–104.
9. Karpen SJ, Suchy FJ: Structural and functional development of the liver. *In* Suchy FJ, et al (eds): Liver Disease in Children. Philadelphia, Lippincott Williams & Wilkins, 2001, pp 1–22.
10. Blitzer BL, Boyer JL: Cellular mechanisms of bile formation. Gastroenterology *82*:346, 1982.
11. Watkins J: Placental transport: bile acid conjugation and sulfation in the fetus. J Pediatr Gastroenterol Nutr *2*:365, 1983.
12. DeBelle R, et al: Intestinal absorption of bile salts: immature development in the neonate. J Pediatr *94*:472, 1979.
13. Stahl G, et al: Passive jejunal bile salt absorption alters the enterohepatic circulation in immature rats. Gastroenterology *104*:163, 1993.
14. Vlahcevic Z, et al: Kinetics and pool size of primary bile acids in man. Gastroenterology *61*:85, 1971.
15. Tavoloni N, et al: Postnatal development of bile secretory physiology in the dog. J Pediatr Gastroenterol Nutr *4*:256, 1985.

16. Heubi J, et al: Bile salt metabolism in the first year of life. J Lab Clin Med *100*:127, 1982.

17. Watkins J, Perman J: Bile acid metabolism in infants and children. Clin Gastroenterol *6*:201, 1977.

18. Suchy F, Balistreri W: Uptake of taurocholate by hepatocytes isolated from developing rats. Pediatr Res *16*:282, 1982.

19. Suchy F, et al: Absence of a hepatic lobular gradient for bile acid uptake in the suckling rat. Hepatology *3*:847, 1983.

20. Ananthanarayanan M, et al: An ontogenically regulated 48-kDa protein is a component of the Na$^+$-bile acid cotransporter of rat liver. Am J Physiol *261*:G810, 1991.

21. Novak DA, et al: Postnatal expression of the canalicular bile acid transport system of rat liver. Am J Physiol *260*:G743, 1991.

22. Meier PJ: The bile secretory pole of hepatocytes. J Hepatol *9*:124, 1989.

23. Ballatori N, Truong A: Relation between biliary glutathione excretion and bile acid–independent bile flow. Am J Physiol *256*:G22, 1989.

24. Nathanson MH, Boyer JL: Mechanisms and regulation of bile formation. Hepatology *14*:551, 1991.

25. Watkins JB: Bile salt metabolism in the human premature infant. Preliminary observations of pool size and synthesis rate following prenatal administration of dexamethasone and phenobarbital. Gastroenterology *69*:706, 1975.

26. Tavoloni N: Bile secretion and its control in the newborn puppy. Pediatr Res *20*:203, 1986.

27. Cox KL, et al: Biliary motility: postnatal changes in guinea pigs. Pediatr Res *21*:170, 1987.

28. Kaplan GS, et al: Gallbladder mechanics in newborn piglets. Pediatr Res *18*:1181, 1984.

29. Hardikar W, et al: Differential ontogenic regulation of basolateral and canalicular bile acid transport proteins in rat liver. J Biol Chem *270*:20841, 1995.

30. Shneider BL: Genetic cholestasis syndromes. J Pediatr Gastroenterol Nutr *28*:124, 1999.

31. Jaeschke H, et al: Mechanisms of hepatotoxicity. Toxicol Sci *65*:166, 2002.

32. Faubion WA, et al: Toxic bile salts induce rodent hepatocyte apoptosis via direct activation of Fas. J Clin Invest *103*:137, 1999.

33. Yerushalmi B, et al: Bile acid–induced rat hepatocyte apoptosis is inhibited by antioxidants and blockers of the mitochondrial permeability transition. Hepatology *33*:616, 2001.

34. Gumpricht E, et al: Glutathione status of isolated rat hepatocytes affects bile acid–induced cellular necrosis but not apoptosis. Toxicol Appl Pharmacol *164*:102, 2000.

35. Mohan P, et al: Ontogeny of hepatobiliary secretion: role of glutathione. Hepatology *19*:1504, 1994.

36. Sokol RJ, et al: Role of oxidant stress in the permeability transition induced in rat hepatic mitochondria by hydrophobic bile acids. Pediatr Res *49*:519, 2001.

37. Setchell K, et al: 4-3-Oxosteroid 5β-reductase deficiency described in identical twins with neonatal hepatitis—a new inborn error in bile acid synthesis. J Clin Invest 82, 1988.

38. Strautnieks SS, et al: A gene encoding a liver-specific ABC transporter is mutated in progressive familial intrahepatic cholestasis. Nat Genet *20*:233, 1998.

39. Sokol R, et al: Mechanisms causing vitamin E deficiency during chronic childhood cholestasis. Gastroenterology *85*:1172, 1983.

40. Weber A, Roy C: The malabsorption associated with chronic liver disease in children. Pediatrics *70*:73, 1972.

41. Badley B, et al: Diminished micellar-phase lipid in patients with chronic nonalcoholic liver disease and steatorrhea. Gastroenterology *58*:781, 1970.

42. Feranchak AP, et al: Medical and nutritional management of cholestasis. *In* Suchy FJ, et al (eds): Liver disease in Children. Philadelphia, Lippincott Williams & Wilkins, 2001, pp 195–237.

43. Kaufmann S, et al: Nutritional support for the infant with EHBA. J Pediatr *110*:679, 1987.

44. Charlton C, et al: Intensive enteral feeding in advanced cirrhosis: reversal of malnutrition without precipitation of hepatic encephalopathy. Arch Dis Child *67*:603, 1992.

45. Sabesin S: Cholestatic lipoproteins: their pathogenesis and significance. Gastroenterology *83*:704, 1982.

46. Evans J, et al: Liver copper levels in intrahepatic cholestasis of childhood. Gastroenterology *75*:875, 1978.

47. Farrell M, et al: Serum sulfated lithocholate as an indicator of cholestasis during parenteral nutrition in infants and children. JPEN *6*:30, 1982.

48. Sinatra R: Does total parenteral nutrition produce cholestasis? Neonatal Cholestasis. Proceedings of the 87th Ross Laboratories Conference on Pediatric Research, Columbus, OH, 1984.

49. Ayotte P, Plaa G: Biliary excretion in Sprague-Dawley and Gunn rats during manganese bilirubin–induced cholestasis. Hepatology *8*:1069, 1988.

50. Bayliss E, et al: Hepatic concentrations of zinc, copper and manganese in infants with EHBA. Clin Res *36*:225A, 1988.

51. Ikeda S, et al: Manganese deposition in the globus pallidus in patients with biliary atresia. Transplantation *69*:2339, 2000.

52. Hambidge M, et al: Plasma manganese concentrations in infants and children receiving parenteral nutrition. JPEN *13*:168, 1989.

53. Williams J, et al: Biliary excretion of aluminum with aluminum osteodystrophy with liver disease. Ann Intern Med *104*:782, 1986.

54. Klein G, et al: Aluminum loading during TPN. Am J Clin Nutr *35*:1425, 1982.

55. Klein G, et al: Intravenous aluminum loading induces cholestasis (abstract). Hepatology *6*:1127, 1986.

56. Stewart SM, et al: Mental development and growth in children with chronic liver disease of early and late onset. Pediatrics *82*:167, 1988.

SECTION XVI

The Kidney

125

William E. Sweeney, Jr., and Ellis D. Avner

Embryogenesis and Anatomic Development of the Kidney

EMBRYOLOGIC FEATURES OF THE MAMMALIAN RENAL EXCRETORY SYSTEM

The embryogenesis of most viscera such as the liver proceeds as a direct process from a clearly defined anlage. However, the differentiation of the definitive mammalian kidney, or metanephros, is unable to take place unless it has been preceded by the successive formation and involution of two embryonic kidneys, the pronephros and the mesonephros.

Formation of the Metanephros

The *pronephros* is the functional kidney in early vertebrates, including *Amphioxus, Cyclostoma,* and larval forms of certain primitive fishes.[1-4] In the human, the pronephros is a rudimentary, nonfunctional kidney that appears during the third week of development (eight- to nine-somite stage) and regresses by the fifth week. The pronephric duct, which arises from fusion of pronephric tubular buds, persists as a remnant after pronephric tubular regression. It becomes the mesonephric duct, which, in turn, evolves into the ureteric bud (UB), which is required for the formation of the metanephros. The *mesonephros* appears in the third to fourth week of gestation immediately caudal to the last of the pronephric tubules. The mesonephros is the second transient kidney of higher vertebrates but is the definitive functioning kidney of fish and amphibians. Mesonephric nephrons develop a glomerulus-like filtering apparatus and tubular system and constitute the first definitive renal functional unit in the human embryo. As with the pronephros, the mesonephros degenerates in a cephalocaudal direction from the 5th to the 12th week of gestation and ceases to exist as an excretory organ. In addition to the distal end of the mesonephric duct, which gives rise to the UB, other mesonephric structures participate in genitourinary development. In the male, mesonephric tubules in the area of the gonad form the efferent ductules, whereas the mesonephric duct gives rise to the epididymis and the ductus deferens. In the female, the mesonephric duct completely disappears during the third month, whereas some mesonephric tubules persist as the epiopheron and paraoopheron, which have no known function but may become cystic, neoplastic, or both.

The formation of the metanephros gives rise to the permanent kidney in humans as well as in other mammals, reptiles, and birds. The metanephros develops from the reciprocal inductive interaction of the epithelial UB with the mesenchymal nephrogenic blastema or metanephric mesenchyme (MM). The UB in the human embryo arises from the dorsal aspect of the caudal end of the mesonephric duct in the fourth to fifth week of gestation. It extends dorsally into the caudalmost portion of the nephrogenic cord and then draws the MM in a cranial direction. The upward movement of the MM from a pelvic position to its final lumbar position is complete by the eighth embryonic week. On emerging from the pelvis, the metanephros undergoes a 90° rotation so the original ventral hilum takes its final medial position.

Normal development and embryogenesis of the UB are fundamental to renal organogenesis. The patterned migration and division of the UB determine the elaborate three-dimensional branching pattern of the mammalian kidney and are responsible for formation of the urinary collecting system. Further, the specific induction of MM by the ampullary portion of the UB is responsible for individual nephron formation (*nephrogenesis*). The two basic organogenetic processes of pattern formation (architectonics) and nephrogenesis occur simultaneously during the period of UB ampullary activity, which, in the human embryo, extends from week 6 through week 36 of gestation.

RENAL ARCHITECTONICS

The morphogenesis of the collecting system and the distinct zonal arborization of the developing kidney are controlled by the patterned divisions of the nephron-inducing UB.[4,5] The renal pelvis, calyces, and intrarenal collecting ducts arise from phases of rapid dichotomic branching of the UB, which alternate with phases of enlargement and structural reorganization (Fig. 125-1). Dilation of the early generations of UB branches and final structural modification of the pelvis, calyces, and papillae occur concomitant with the formation of functional nephron units and probably result from accumulation of urine.

During renal embryogenesis, the pattern of UB branching determines the topographic distribution of nephrons and the elaborate patterns of arborization by which they attach to successive branches of the cortical collecting ducts. Differences in embryonic behavior of the ampullae of UB branches make it possible to divide the structural development of the human kidney artificially into the following four periods[4]: period 1 (embryonic weeks 5 through 14), in which ampullae actively divide and induce formation of nephrons only when they are not carrying an attached nephron (Fig. 125-2); period 2 (embryonic weeks 14 to 15 through 20 to 22), when ampullae rarely divide but induce new nephrons while they are carrying an attached nephron, resulting in arcade formation (Fig. 125-3); period 3 (embryonic weeks 20 to 22 through 32 to 36), in which ampullae do not divide but induce new nephron formation when they are not carrying an attached nephron (Fig. 125-4); and period 4 (embryonic weeks 32 to 36 through adult life), when ampullae are inactive and do not divide or induce formation of new nephrons. All renal growth from period 4 through adulthood is secondary to enlargement of existing structures and expansion of interstitial tissue. The actual differentiation of individual nephrons occurs continuously and without variation in pattern during the different periods of ampullary activity.

The programmed stages of UB division and induction result in a predictable pattern of nephron arborization in the newborn kidney (Fig. 125-5). The connecting tubules of all nephrons in the mature kidney are connected to the last two to three generations of collecting ducts produced by UB divisions (13th to 15th generation of UB branches). The segregation of all nephron attachments to the terminal collecting duct appears to arise as a result of a unique growth process.[6] Because nephrons are successively attached to the UB within a zone of accelerated interstitial growth, they advance with the ampullae. As the ampullae divide, nephrons of different ages and at different stages of development are carried along one ramification of an extending UB branch. The nephron attachments are thus carried along in a centrifugal fashion from generation to generation of UB branches.

The development of the renal vascular system parallels the branching pattern of UB division and nephron induction.[4, 5, 7, 8] Branches of the aorta and vena cava invade the MM soon after initial UB division. Such branches proliferate, arborize, and extend to the periphery of the developing kidney, at which point they merge into a subcapsular network. At approximately 14 embryonic weeks, arterial branches at the future corticomedullary junction elongate at right angles to the basic centrifugal branching to form the arcuate arteries. Branches of the interlobar arteries directly supply the medulla as the vasa recta and return to the corticomedullary area as venules, which drain into the interlobar veins. The vascular supply of the human fetal kidney is similar to that of the newborn kidney by 15 embryonic weeks.

NEPHROGENESIS

Nephrogenesis is a complex process involving the coordinated growth and differentiation of endothelial, mesangial, neuronal, and epithelial cells that occurs throughout the previously noted periods of renal architectonic development. Cytodifferentiation and spatial assembly of different cells during nephron formation are governed by complex interactive events and changing gene expression patterns among transcription factors and proto-oncogenes, polypeptide growth factors and their receptors, cell adhesion molecules, and extracellular matrix (ECM) glycoproteins, ECM receptor molecules, and ECM degrading proteases. These reciprocal signals coordinate developmental processes such as cell proliferation, apoptosis, migration, adhesion, differentiation, vascularization, and neurogenesis that occur simultaneously

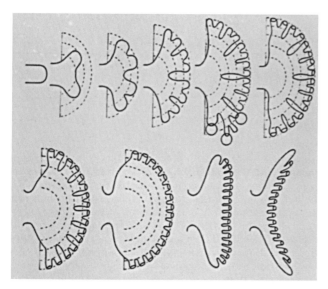

Figure 125–1. Development of a minor calyx and papilla. After the dilation of the first three to five generations of the ureteric bud that forms the renal pelvis and major calyces, a second series of three to five generations of ureteric bud divisions occurs in rapid succession. This second series of rapidly formed short tubules expands to produce the cavity of the minor calyx, whereas the tubules of the next generations expand to become the cribriform plate that covers the papillary surface. It is believed that the definitive cup shape of the calyx and the conical form of the papilla are formed by the combination of intratubular pressure generated by urine formation and the extratubular pressure generated by enlargement and differentiation of nephrons distally. (From Potter EL: Normal and Abnormal Development of the Kidney. Chicago, Year Book Medical Publishers, 1972.)

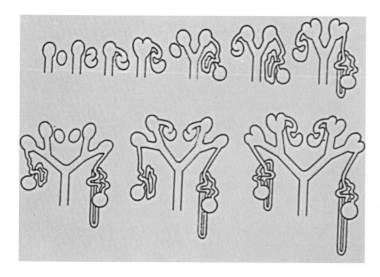

Figure 125–2. Period 1 of nephron formation (embryonic weeks 5 to 14). Ampullae actively divide and induce formation of nephrons only when not carrying an attached nephron. (From Potter EL: Normal and Abnormal Development of the Kidney. Chicago, Year Book Medical Publishers, 1972.)

during nephrogenesis. Experimental studies have provided some insight into the molecular basis of mammalian nephron formation and thereby provide a basis for exploration of the pathoembryologic characteristics of renal developmental abnormalities.

Stages of Nephron Formation

Normal nephron development encompasses four progressive stages that follow embryonic inductive interaction of the metanephric blastema and the UB (Fig. 125-6). Ultrastructural glomerular, proximal tubular, and distal nephron development can be seen in the larger context of this framework of overall nephrogenesis. Concomitant with branching of the UB, the tips of the UB branches induce epithelialization of the MM and subsequent development of the nephron from the glomerulus through the distal tubule. Nephron development proceeds through a series of intermediate forms, known as the comma-shaped and S-shaped bodies, before elongation and eventual fusion with the duct. The S-shaped body is generally regarded as the precursor of two distinct processes, that is, glomerulogenesis and tubulogenesis, which are related to the spatial segmentation of the S-shaped body. Glomerular development proceeds from the differentiation of two distinct visceral and parietal epithelial layers during the S-shaped vesicle stage when mesenchymal invagination and development of capillary loops through vasculogenesis and angiogenesis occur.[9] This is followed by the progressive development of specialized epithelial intercellular connections and basal lamina formation with consequent endothelial fenestration and basilar modification of visceral epithelium into foot processes and slit pores.[10-12]

Nephronegenesis begins as condensations of induced MM cells surrounding the ampullary tip of the UB are phenotypically and structurally converted to an epithelial vesicle. The proximal tubule and loop of Henle arise from the lower and middle limb of the S-shaped body, and the distal tubule arises from the upper limb, which ultimately fuses with the collecting duct. Continued branching of the UB and inductions of new nephrons proceed in a radial fashion, such that the first nephrons that develop lie near the corticomedullary junction and the final nephrons form in the outer cortex.

Control and Modulation of Renal Organogenesis

Basic questions about the critical molecular and cellular events that control normal and abnormal nephrogenesis have largely been addressed with *in vitro* model systems and manipulation of targeted "developmental" genes *in vivo*.[13] Model systems that have proved valuable in this regard include both transfilter and whole organ murine metanephric organ culture, isolated mature renal cell lines, isolated embryonic UB and MM cell lines, and *in vivo* models including zebrafish, *Xenopus,* and the generation of transgenic and genetically engineered mice.[14-22] These approaches have provided important insight into the regulation and modulation of renal organogenesis by characterizing the following: (1) the normal differentiation of the intermediate mesoderm, which gives rise to the wolffian duct, UB, MM, and gonadal tissue; (2) induction of the UB outgrowth from the wolffian duct; (3) regulation of growth and branching of the UB by the MM; (4) early nephron morphogenesis and epithelialization; (5) ECM remodeling and cell adhesion changes that pattern early nephron morphogenesis and epithelialization; and (6) the process of nephron vascularization. To date, studies have identified more than 300 genes (e.g., secreted growth factors, tyrosine kinase receptors, transcription factors, extracellular components, proteases) involved in renal developmental pathways. A detail compilation of the regulatory pathways of renal development is beyond the scope of this chapter, and the following discussion highlights only those studies that are

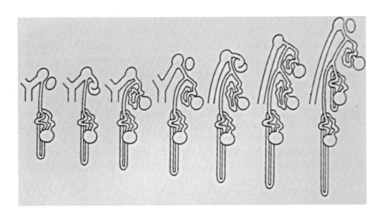

Figure 125-3. Period 2 of nephron formation (embryonic weeks 14 to 15 through 20 to 22). Ampullae no longer actively divide and become capable of inducing new nephrons, even though they already carry an attached nephron. Although two nephrons may be attached to each terminal ampulla temporarily, the connecting piece of the more mature nephron shifts to communicate only with the connecting piece of the younger nephron. In this fashion, arcades of four to six nephrons become attached to each tubule. (From Potter EL: Normal and Abnormal Development of the Kidney. Chicago, Year Book Medical Publishers, 1972.)

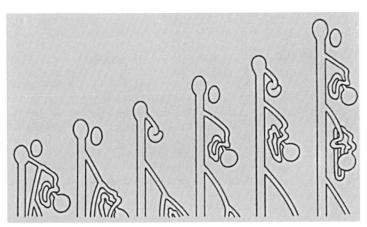

Figure 125-4. Period 3 of nephron formation (embryonic weeks 20 to 22 through 32 to 36). During this period, ampullae branch rarely, induce formation of new nephrons when not already carrying nephrons, and permit attachment of new nephrons only behind the active growth zone at the junction of ampulla and collecting tubule. This results in direct attachment of nephrons to the terminal portion of each collecting tubule. (From Potter EL: Normal and Abnormal Development of the Kidney. Chicago, Year Book Medical Publishers, 1972.)

supported by multiple models (especially knockout mice), provide novel insights, or raise interesting new questions regarding renal organogenesis. An exhaustive, regularly updated review of the molecular basis of kidney development can be found in the Kidney Developmental Database.[23]

Normal Differentiation of the Intermediate Mesoderm

Disruption in any of the sequential steps of pronephros development and involution, mesonephros development, and metanephric induction leads to altered or complete absence of kidney development. Normal differentiation of the intermediate mesoderm has been shown in targeted gene deletion experiments to depend on several transcription factors. Loss of function in *Lim1*[24] or *Pax2*[25] results in the absence or abnormal formation of the wolffian duct, thus preventing normal UB formation leading to renal agenesis.

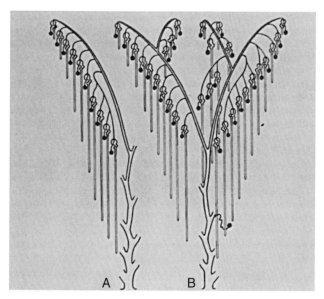

Figure 125–5. Nephron arborization in the newborn kidney. The programmed periods of ureteric bud division and induction result in a predictable pattern of nephron arborization in the newborn kidney. **A,** The most common arrangement, whereas **B,** possible variations. (From Potter EL: Normal and Abnormal Development of the Kidney. Chicago, Year Book Medical Publishers, 1972.)

Predetermination of the MM is genetically programmed before contact with the UB. The MM has developmental options restricted to either remaining a mesenchymal stroma or being converted into epithelial tubules. Loss of *WT-1*, a tumor suppressor gene normally expressed in uninduced mesenchyme, results in the loss of the MM cell population caused by apoptosis.[26] The MM of *WT-1* –/– embryos demonstrates the presence of both *Pax2* and glial cell line–derived neurotrophic factor (GDNF) mRNA but is unable to undergo tubulogenesis when recombined with wild-type UB. However, the UB from *WT-1* –/– animals is able to induce nephron formation in wild-type MM.[27]

Induction of the Ureteric Bud Outgrowth from the Wolffian Duct

One of the first-recognized regulators of UB outgrowth was limb deformity (*ld*). Through alternate splicing events, *ld* encodes a group of phosphoproteins, the formins, that are all expressed in the UB and MM. The primary defect in the *ld* –/– mutant is arrested or incomplete formation of the UB, although the urogenital deformities are expressed with differing degrees.[28] The exact role of these proteins in UB branching is unknown.

The UB develops as an outgrowth of the wolffian duct in response to GDNF secreted by the MM.[29, 30] GDNF binds a glycosylphosphatidyl-inositol–linked protein GRFa-1, which subsequently binds Ret tyrosine kinase receptors expressed on the surface of the wolffian duct.[31, 32] GDNF functions as a chemoattractant for RET-expressing cells providing guidance cues that ensure proper alignment of the UB with the MM.[33] GDNF-soaked beads can attract multiple UBs. Failure to control positioning of the UB growth and subsequent branching may lead to a variety of urogenital syndromes.[34]

Regulation of Growth and Branching of the Ureteric Bud by the Metanephric Mesenchyme

As noted previously, the programmed dichotomous branching of actively inducing UB ampullae leads to the formation of the collecting system and the three-dimensional architectonics of the mature kidney. Once the UB enters the MM, it undergoes elongation and multiple dichotomous branching events until it reaches the limiting edges of the MM. Various *in vitro* model systems have been use to identify a long list of putative regulators of the elongation and branching of the UB. However, the relative importance of specific growth factors and ECM components is still unclear due to the limitations of the model systems used and the apparent redundancy of growth processes in renal development. What

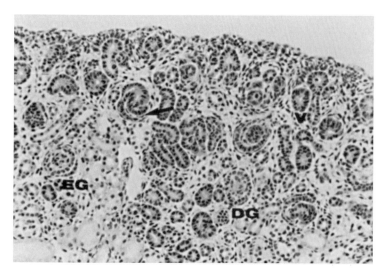

Figure 125–6. The stages of normal nephron formation. Stage 1 is characterized by the formation of the primitive renal vesicle (V), which is composed of simple columnar epithelial cells after aggregation of metanephrogenic mesenchyme. Stage 2 is defined as the development of the S-shaped tubule, which arises from dual indentations of the renal vesicle and is characterized by early mesenchymal invasion of the developing glomerular tuft *(arrow)*. Stage 3 is defined by the development of the early glomerulus (EG), which forms from cell proliferation and evagination of the lower cleft of the S-shaped tubule. Stage 4 is defined by the definitive glomerulus (DG), which develops from the early glomerulus and is characterized by highly differentiated visceral and parietal epithelial cells, as well as mesangial and endothelial cells.

is becoming increasingly clear is that the process of elongation is separate from the process of branching. Bone morphogenic protein 2 (BMP2),[35] BMP4,[36] and activin[37] all inhibit UB branching but do not affect elongation. The GDNF/c-Ret system that induces UB formation from the wolffian duct remains essential for continued branching once the UB has entered the MM. The addition of GDNF-blocking antibodies prevents bud formation in culture,[38] whereas the addition of exogenous GDNF increases the number of buds and increases proliferation and expression of c-Ret and Wnt-11 in the bud tips.[39]

Early studies suggested the necessity for direct contact of the UB with the MM for nephrogenesis to occur. More recent studies have demonstrated that a soluble factor in the conditioned medium of a MM cell line is a potent promoter of UB branching morphogenesis.[21, 40] The soluble factor has been identified as pleiotrophin,[41] a 18-kDa heparin-binding protein, initially discovered as a fibroblast proliferative factor.[42] In a three-dimensional culture system, pleiotrophin alone is capable of inducing isolated UB cell lines or, in the presence of GDNF or isolated rat UBs, of undergoing branching morphogenesis.

In addition to growth factors, UB elongation and branching require specific matrix components. *In vitro* and *in vivo* studies demonstrate a requirement for heparin-binding sulfate glycosaminoglycans.[43, 44] UB arborization also depends on laminin expression and the expression of matrix receptors such as integrins,[45] matrix metalloproteinases (MMPs), and tissue inhibitors of metalloproteinases (TIMPs).[46] Branching and elongation require tightly regulated remodeling of the ECM. Evidence suggests that gradients of matrix-bound positive and negative elongation and branching factors exist in the MM and along the UB.[36, 46, 47] Regulation of proliferation, apoptosis, and morphogenic molecules at UB branch tips, branch points, and along the stalk is crucial for establishing a controlled branching pattern.

Early Nephron Morphogenesis and Epithelialization

Nephron formation begins with the invasion of the MM by the UB, a burst of proliferation of the MM cells, and "induction" or condensation of the MM at the tips of the branching UB. To date, the use of mice with targeted mutations has conclusively identified a few important molecules involved in the early events of nephron formation and epithelialization, but these data provide little information regarding the orchestration of nephrogenesis beyond the S stage. These results demonstrate that nephrogenesis becomes "frozen" at the condensation stage in mice with homozygous mutations in *Wnt 4*[48] or *Foxd1* (originally BF-2)[49] and *Emx2*.[50] The epithelialization of MM is delayed or reduced in mice lacking expression of cadherin 6, and many tubules that form do not fuse to the UB.[51]

This induction process of MM must be initiated by secreted signals at the tip or ampullae of the UB because contact is not required. *In vivo* and *in vitro* UB cells have been shown to secrete fibroblast growth factor 2 and 9, transforming growth factor-α, TIMP1, TIMP2, and MMP2.[52] Conditioned medium from an isolated UB cell line was found to trigger mesenchyme to epithelial conversion of isolated MM grown in three-dimensional gel cultures.[53] The MM generated several differentiated epithelial cell types, cysts, tubules, and segmented nephrons. Isolation and purification of the UB-conditioned medium demonstrated that it contained fibroblast growth factor 2, which was required for MM survival, and leukemia inhibitory factor, a member of the interleukin-6 cytokine family, which initiated an epithelialization program through activation of signal transducer and activator of transcription 3 (STAT3).[54] *In vitro*, at least three interleukin-6 family members can substitute for leukemia inhibitory factor, and all can bind to their own receptor or heterodimerize with gp130 receptors and activate STAT3, again demonstrating a remarkable degree of redundancy.[54]

The development of chemically defined serum-free medium to promote nephrogenesis in organ culture models provided the opportunity to explore the role of soluble growth factors in nephron growth and differentiation.[14, 55-59] During experimental nephrogenesis, transferrin and prostaglandin E$_1$ have major roles in organotypic metanephric growth and differentiation.[57, 59] Additional organ culture studies have suggested important roles for certain polypeptide growth factors in segmental nephron differentiation.[60-63] Thus, epidermal growth factor and transforming growth factor-α increase overall renal growth and specific differentiation of distal nephron elements (thick ascending limb to early distal tubule, collecting tubule) but retard epithelial differentiation of glomeruli and proximal tubules. These effects are mediated by the tyrosine kinase activity of the epidermal growth factor receptor.[63] Insulin-like growth factors I and II stimulate overall renal growth and promote segmental differentiation of tubular, but not glomerular epithelia. Transforming growth factor-β globally retards growth and differentiation of all nephron segments.[60, 61] Postinductive nephrogenesis thus appears to be regulated by the overall balance of certain local autocrine or paracrine growth factor systems. Alterations in the critical balance of positive or negative regulatory factors may produce a variety of hypoplastic or dysplastic nephropathies.[13]

Extracellular Matrix Remodeling and Cell Adhesion

The ECM has been implicated as a mediator of epithelial-mesenchymal interactions in many embryogenic processes. Although the signal transmitted during induction of nephron formation is unknown, it is clear that changes in the composition of the ECM of the metanephrogenic mesenchyme are central to early nephron morphogenesis. At the earliest stages of nephron induction, fibronectin and collagens type I and type III are lost from condensed mesenchymal aggregates.[64] Tubulogenesis is accompanied by the synthesis of type IV and type V collagen, laminin, heparan sulfate proteoglycan, and entactin, which localize to developing tubular basement membranes.[65-69] Laminin A-chain expression appears to be a critical factor in establishing epithelial cell polarity in the developing metanephros.[70] In addition, tenascin, a matrix protein implicated in epithelial growth after embryonic epithelial-mesenchymal interaction in mammary, tooth, and vibrissa development,[71] has been identified in mesenchymal stroma surrounding differentiating renal epithelial cells.[72]

The MMPs are a growing family of ECM-degrading enzymes that are required for the remodeling process. Their genes and those encoding for their natural inhibitors, the TIMPs, are tightly regulated during embryonic development and morphogenesis.[73] The type IV collagenases, MMP2 and MMP9, MT1-MMP (activates MMP2) and TIMP1, TIMP2, and TIMP3 are spatially and temporally regulated during nephrogenesis and tubular differentiation. The expression pattern of these collagenases changes from basolateral to apical during tubule segmentation, and this apical expression persists in mature kidneys. This evidence suggests that these substances play a critical role in renal tubule differentiation and other, as yet undefined, tubular functions in mature kidneys.[74]

Nephron Vascularization

The mechanisms guiding the complex organization of the renal vasculature are unknown, and the origin of renal endothelial cells remains uncertain. The renal vasculature may differentiate from angioblasts by vasculogenesis, or it may develop from extrarenal mesenchyme vessels by angiogenesis. As previously noted, the first sign of nephron vascularization is the appearance of endothelium-like cells within the lower crevice of the S-shaped body. Grafting of mesenchymal explants onto avian chorioallantoic membranes after *in vitro* induction has indicated that invading vascular elements are nonmesenchymal endothelial cells.[75]

After grafting, uninduced mesenchymes as well as undifferentiated areas of induced explants remain avascular.[76] This finding implies that differentiation imparts angiogenesis-stimulating activity to the MM. In this regard, a specific heparin-binding angiogenesis factor has been isolated and characterized from the embryonic murine metanephros.

Studies have provided evidence that vasculogenesis may also contribute to the formation of the renal vasculature. Angioblasts have been identified in avascular MM,[77,78] and avascular embryonic kidneys develop capillaries when they are exposed to increasing levels of endogenous or exogenous vascular endothelial growth factor.[79]

Progress in identifying crucial regulatory molecules involved in renal organogenesis has been remarkable. The use of genetically engineered animals and the development of new models have provided insights into the complexities of renal development. Future progress will require the development of cell lines and transgenic models with inducible gene expression, so the temporal expression, relative prioritization, and interaction of specific signaling pathways can be elucidated. These ongoing studies of the molecular and cellular biology of renal development will form the basis for future investigations into the molecular mechanisms of gene activation and signal transduction in renal embryogenesis and will provide insight into the complex processes that underlie normal and abnormal renal organogenesis.

ACKNOWLEDGMENT

Our studies as described in this chapter were supported by grants R01-DK34891 and R01-DK44875 from the National Institutes of Health.

REFERENCES

1. Dubois AM: The embryonic kidney. *In* Rouiller C, Muller AF (eds): The Kidney. New York, Academic Press, 1969, pp 1-59.
2. McCory WW: Developmental Nephrology. Cambridge, MA, Harvard University Press 1972, pp 1-51.
3. McCory WW (ed): Renal structure and development. *In* Holiday MA, et al (eds): Pediatric Nephrology, 2nd ed. Baltimore, Williams & Wilkins, 1987, pp 31-44.
4. Potter EL: Normal and Abnormal Development of the Kidney. Chicago, Year Book Medical Publishers, 1972, pp 3-82.
5. Oliver J: Nephrons and Kidneys: A Quantitative Study of Development and Evolutionary Mammalian Renal Architectonics. New York, Harper & Row, 1968, p 148.
6. Peter K: Untersuchungen über Bau und Entwicklung der Niere. Jena, Germany, Fischer, 1909.
7. Lewis OJ: The development of the blood vessels of the metanephros. J Anat 92:84, 1958.
8. Ljungqvist A: Fetal and postnatal development of the intrarenal arterial pattern in man. Acta Paediatr Scand Suppl 52:443, 1963.
9. Kanwar YS, et al: Relevance of renal-specific oxidoreductase in tubulogenesis during mammalian nephron development. Am J Physiol 282:F752, 2002.
10. Kazimierczal J: Development of the renal corpuscle and the juxtaglomerular apparatus. Acta Pathol Microbiol Scand Suppl 218:1, 1971.
11. Reeves W, et al: Differentiation of epithelial foot processes and filtration slits: sequential appearance of occluding junctions, epithelial polyanion, and slit membranes in developing glomeruli. Lab Invest 39:90, 1978.
12. Suzuki Y: An electron microscopy of the renal differentiation. II. Glomerulus. Keio J Med 8:129, 1959.
13. Fouser L, Avner ED: Normal and abnormal nephrogenesis. Am J Kidney Dis 21:64, 1993.
14. Avner ED, et al: Renal epithelial development in organotypic culture. Pediatr Nephrol 2:92, 1988.
15. Merlino GT: Transgenic animals in biomedical research. FASEB J 5:2996, 1991.
16. Saxen L, Sariola H: Early organogenesis of the kidney. Pediatr Nephrol 1:385, 1987.
17. Saxen L: Organogenesis of the Kidney. Cambridge, England, Cambridge University Press, 1987.
18. Woychik RP, et al: An inherited limb deformity created by insertional mutagenesis in a transgenic mouse. Nature 318:36, 1985.
19. Barros EJ, et al: Differential tubulogenic and branching morphogenetic activities of growth factors: implications for epithelial tissue development. Proc Natl Acad Sci U S A 92:4412, 1995.
20. Rauchman MI, et al: An osmotically tolerant inner medullary collecting duct cell line from an SV40 transgenic mouse. Am J Physiol 265:F416, 1993.
21. Sakurai H, et al: An in vitro tubulogenesis system using cell lines derived from the embryonic kidney shows dependence on multiple soluble growth factors. Proc Natl Acad Sci U S A 94:6279, 1997.
22. Dressler GR: Kidney development branches out. Dev Genet 24:189, 1999.
23. Davies JA: The Kidney Development Database. Dev Genet 24:194, 1999.
24. Shawlot W, Behringer RR: Requirement for Lim1 in head-organizer function. Nature 374:425, 1995.
25. Torres M, et al: Pax-2 controls multiple steps of urogenital development. Development 121:4057, 1995.
26. Kreidberg JA, et al: WT-1 is required for early kidney development. Cell 74:679, 1993.
27. Donovan MJ, et al: Initial differentiation of the metanephric mesenchyme is independent of WT1 and the ureteric bud. Dev Genet 1999, 24:252.
28. Maas R, et al: Deficient outgrowth of the ureteric bud underlies the renal agenesis phenotype in mice manifesting the limb deformity (ld) mutation. Dev Dyn 199:214, 1994.
29. Vega QC, et al: Glial cell line-derived neurotrophic factor activates the receptor tyrosine kinase RET and promotes kidney morphogenesis. Proc Natl Acad Sci U S A 93:10657, 1996.
30. Sainio K, et al: Glial-cell-line-derived neurotrophic factor is required for bud initiation from ureteric epithelium. Development 124:4077, 1997.
31. Treanor JJ, et al: Characterization of a multicomponent receptor for GDNF. Nature 382:80, 1996.
32. Ehrenfels CW, et al: Perturbation of RET signaling in the embryonic kidney. Dev Genet 24:263, 1999.
33. Tang MJ, et al: The RET-glial cell-derived neurotrophic factor (GDNF) pathway stimulates migration and chemoattraction of epithelial cells. J Cell Biol 142:1337, 1998.
34. Pope JCT, et al: How they begin and how they end: classic and new theories for the development and deterioration of congenital anomalies of the kidney and urinary tract, CAKUT. J Am Soc Nephrol 10:2018, 1999.
35. Lyons KM, et al: Colocalization of BMP 7 and BMP 2 RNAs suggests that these factors cooperatively mediate tissue interactions during murine development. Mech Dev 50:71, 1995.
36. Miyazaki Y, et al: Bone morphogenetic protein 4 regulates the budding site and elongation of the mouse ureter. J Clin Invest 105:863, 2000.
37. Ball EM, Risbridger GP: Activins as regulators of branching morphogenesis. Dev Biol 238:1, 2001.
38. Davies JA, et al: Neurturin: an autocrine regulator of renal collecting duct development. Dev Genet 24:284, 1999.
39. Pepicelli CV, et al: GDNF induces branching and increased cell proliferation in the ureter of the mouse. Dev Biol 192:193, 1997.
40. Qiao J, et al: Branching morphogenesis independent of mesenchymal-epithelial contact in the developing kidney. Proc Natl Acad Sci USA 96:7330, 1999.
41. Sakurai H, et al: Identification of pleiotrophin as a mesenchymal factor involved in ureteric bud branching morphogenesis. Development 128:3283, 2001.
42. Milner PG, et al: A novel 17 kD heparin-binding growth factor (HBGF-8) in bovine uterus: purification and N-terminal amino acid sequence. Biochem Biophys Res Commun 165:1096, 1989.
43. Davies J, et al: Sulphated proteoglycan is required for collecting duct growth and branching but not nephron formation during kidney development. Development 121:1507, 1995.
44. Bullock SL, et al: Renal agenesis in mice homozygous for a gene trap mutation in the gene encoding heparan sulfate 2-sulfotransferase. Genes Dev 12:1894, 1998.
45. Zent R, et al: Involvement of laminin binding integrins and laminin-5 in branching morphogenesis of the ureteric bud during kidney development. Dev Biol 238:289, 2001.
46. Pohl M, et al: Matrix metalloproteinases and their inhibitors regulate in vitro ureteric bud branching morphogenesis. Am J Physiol 279:F891, 2000.
47. Nigam SK: Determinants of branching tubulogenesis. Curr Opin Nephrol Hypertens 4:209, 1995.
48. Stark K, et al: Epithelial transformation of metanephric mesenchyme in the developing kidney regulated by Wnt-4. Nature 372:679, 1994.
49. Hatini V, et al: Essential role of stromal mesenchyme in kidney morphogenesis revealed by targeted disruption of winged helix transcription factor BF-2. Genes Dev 10:1467, 1996.
50. Miyamoto N, et al: Defects of urogenital development in mice lacking Emx2. Development 124:1653, 1997.
51. Mah SP, et al: Kidney development in cadherin-6 mutants: delayed mesenchyme-to-epithelial conversion and loss of nephrons. Dev Biol 223:38, 2000.
52. Barasch J, et al: Tissue inhibitor of metalloproteinase-2 stimulates mesenchymal growth and regulates epithelial branching during morphogenesis of the rat metanephros. J Clin Invest 103:1299, 1999.
53. Barasch J, et al: Ureteric bud cells secrete multiple factors, including bFGF, which rescue renal progenitors from apoptosis. Am J Physiol 273:F757, 1997.
54. Barasch J, et al: Mesenchymal to epithelial conversion in rat metanephros is induced by LIF. Cell 99:377, 1999.
55. Avner ED, Sweeney WE Jr: Polypeptide growth factors in metanephric growth and segmental nephron differentiation. Pediatr Nephrol 4:372, 1990.
56. Avner ED, et al: Metanephric development in serum-free organ culture. In Vitro Cell Dev Biol 18:675, 1982.
57. Avner ED, et al: Growth factor requirements of organogenesis in serum-free metanephric organ culture. In Vitro Cell Dev Biol 21:297, 1985.
58. Ekblom P, et al: Organogenesis in a defined medium supplemented with transferrin. Cell Differ 10:281, 1981.
59. Ekblom P, et al: Transferrin as a fetal growth factor: acquisition of responsiveness related to embryonic induction. Proc Natl Acad Sci USA 80:2651, 1983.

60. Avner ED: Polypeptide growth factors and the kidney: a developmental perspective. Pediatr Nephrol *4*:345, 1990.
61. Hammerman MR, et al: Growth factors and kidney development. Pediatr Nephrol 7:616, 1993.
62. Risau W, Ekblom P: Growth factors and the embryonic kidney. *In* Serrerro G, Hayashi J (eds): Cellular Endocrinology: Hormonal Control of Embryonic and Cellular Differentiation. New York, AR Liss, 1986, pp 147–156.
63. Pugh JL, et al: Tyrosine kinase activity of the EGF receptor in murine metanephric organ culture. Kidney Int *47*:774, 1995.
64. Ekblom P, et al: Shift in collagen type as an early response to induction of the metanephric mesenchyme. J Cell Biol *89*:276, 1981.
65. Avner ED, et al: Development of renal basement membrane glycoproteins in metanephric organ culture. Lab Invest *48*:263, 1983.
66. Bonadio JF, et al: Localization of collagen types IV and V, laminin, and heparan sulfate proteoglycan to the basal lamina of kidney epithelial cells in transfilter metanephric culture. Am J Pathol *116*:289, 1984.
67. Ekblom P, et al: Role of mesenchymal nidogen for epithelial morphogenesis in vitro. Development *120*:2003, 1994.
68. Lash JW, et al: Biosynthesis of proteoglycans in organ cultures of developing kidney mesenchyme. Exp Cell Res *147*:85, 1983.
69. Ekblom P, et al: Induction of a basement membrane glycoprotein in embryonic kidney: possible role of laminin in morphogenesis. Proc Natl Acad Sci USA 77:485, 1980.

70. Ekblom M, et al: Transient and locally restricted expression of laminin A chain mRNA by developing epithelial cells during kidney organogenesis. Cell *60*:337, 1990.
71. Chiquet-Ehrismann R, et al: Tenascin: an extracellular matrix protein involved in tissue interactions during fetal development and oncogenesis. Cell *47*:131, 1986.
72. Aufderheide E, et al: Epithelial-mesenchymal interactions in the developing kidney lead to expression of tenascin in the mesenchyme. J Cell Biol *105*:599, 1987.
73. Lenz O, et al: Matrix metalloproteinases in renal development and disease. J Am Soc Nephrol *11*:574, 2000.
74. Legallicier B, et al: Expression of the type IV collagenase system during mouse kidney development and tubule segmentation. J Am Soc Nephrol *12*:2358, 2001.
75. Sariola H: Interspecies chimeras: an experimental approach for studies on embryonic angiogenesis. Med Biol *63*:43, 1985.
76. Sariola H, et al: Differentiation and vascularization of the metanephric kidney grafted on the chorioallantoic membrane. Dev Biol *96*:427, 1983.
77. Tufro-McReddie A, et al: Oxygen regulates vascular endothelial growth factor-mediated vasculogenesis and tubulogenesis. Dev Biol *183*:139, 1997.
78. Abrahamson DR, et al: Origins and formation of microvasculature in the developing kidney. Kidney Int Suppl *67*:S7, 1998.
79. Tufro A: VEGF spatially directs angiogenesis during metanephric development in vitro. Dev Biol *227*:558, 2000.

Patrick D. Brophy and Jean E. Robillard

126

Functional Development of the Kidney *In Utero*

The improvement in the management of high-risk deliveries and the enhanced survival rates of preterm infants have created a daunting task for today's neonatologist. With the rapidly increasing knowledge of the molecular and biochemical mechanisms influencing nephrogenesis, it has become apparent that a keen understanding of the physiology of the fetal kidney is fundamental to designing effective therapies for these youngsters.

RENAL MATURATION: NEPHRON FORMATION

Mammalian renal development proceeds through a preordained group of developmental steps that mimic its evolutionary origin.[1,2] This results in the formation of a series of transitional structures before ultimately generating the final adult kidney.[3] In human-like mammals, the excretory system initially forms as a single epithelial duct that arises from the mesoderm. As the nephric duct extends caudally in the developing mammal, renal tubular development begins in the most anterior portion otherwise known as the pronephric tubules.[3] These are nonfunctional organs that appear around the third week of gestation. The pronephros undergoes complete involution within 2 weeks of its development. Stage 2 occurs in the posterior developing renal system with subsequent development of the mesonephros or mesonephric tubules. The mesonephros in humans consists of 20 pairs of glomeruli and does have tubules that are relatively thick walled. By week 5 of gestation, the mesonephric kidney is a functional unit and can form urine. The final stage of development of the adult or metanephric kidney results when an outgrowth called the *ureteric bud* or metanephric diverticulum buds from the caudal end of the nephric duct itself. This occurs in conjunction with the degeneration of the mesonephros around 11 to 12 weeks of gestation. The development of the metanephros or final stage of renal maturation in the human is dependent on reciprocal interaction between the nephric ureteric bud and the undifferentiated mesenchymal cell mass known as the *anlagen.* This has also been referred to as the nephrogenic blastema. The ureteric bud grows toward the metanephric mesenchyme based on signals emanating from the mesenchyme itself. In reciprocation, the inductive signals from the ureteric bud begin the process of converting the mesenchyme into the components of the adult kidney. The subsequent mesenchymal cells aggregate around the advancing ureteric bud and form polarized epithelial vesicles.[1-3] This launches the development of a dichotomous branching structure and the development and epithelialization of the kidney that result in collecting system and tubular development, as well as glomerular development (Fig. 126–1).

MOLECULAR AND CELLULAR REGULATION OF KIDNEY ORGANIC GENESIS

Although early regionalization in the nephric duct begins the patterning of the entire urogenital system, it is beyond the scope of the present chapter; the reader is referred to an excellent review by Dressler.[3] A series of complex, and as yet poorly understood, molecular interactions form the basis of events that allow formation of the metanephros or kidney proper (Fig. 126–2).[4] The conversion of the kidney anlagen into the metanephros itself requires spatial and temporarily regulated patterning of genes (both up-regulation and repression) and proteins that encode adhesion molecules, transcription factors, structural proteins, growth factors and receptors, and extracellular matrix components.[5] To meet these complex requirements, the metanephric mesenchyme must become committed to develop into nephron cells and all the specialized cells that compose the adult kidney. Some of the primary genes involved in the initiation of these processes include transcription factors such as the homeobox (*Hox*) and paired box (*PAX*) genes along with the Wilms' tumor (*WT1*) suppressor gene (Fig. 126–3).[6]

The *PAX-2* gene is critical for early urogenital development. The PAX-2 protein specifies the noninduced metanephric mesenchyme.[7] Immunocytochemical studies have also demonstrated PAX-2 proteins in the ureteric bud, in the nuclei of condensed mesenchyme cells, in comma-shaped bodies, and in the early

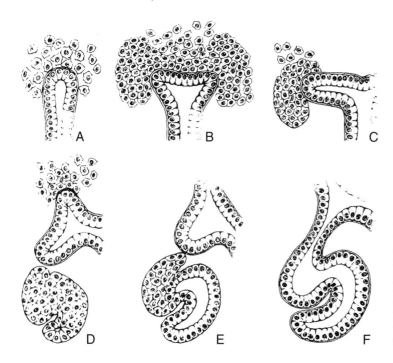

Figure 126–1. Schematic representation of the development of kidney tubules in the metanephros. **A,** Epithelial ureteric bud surrounded by loose mesenchyme. **B** and **C,** Condensed mesenchyme cells starting the process of epithelial differentiation. **D** and **E,** Mesenchymal cells differentiate into epithelial cells and form first comma-shaped (**D**) and then S-shaped (**E**) bodies. **F,** S-shaped body fuses with the terminal end of the ureteric bud. (From Ekblom P, et al: Proc Natl Acad Sci USA 77:485, 1980.)

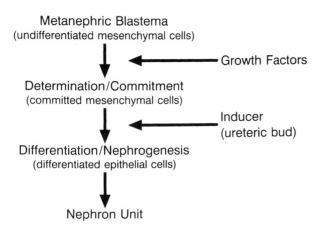

Figure 126–2. Development of the metanephros. (Adapted from Bacallao R, Fine FG: J Physiol 257:F913, 1989.)

collecting duct epithelium.[8] Once the initial structures and mature tubules form, the levels of PAX-2 decrease.[9] Studies with transgenic mice that overexpress PAX-2 have demonstrated abnormalities, which include microcystic tubular dilation and atrophic glomeruli.[10] Other PAX proteins (PAX-8) also have a similar pattern of expression in the human embryonic kidney, and their expression appears to be somewhat more extended than that of PAX-2 before they are down-regulated in the mature glomerulus.[11]

The *WT1* gene is an early marker of metanephric mesenchyme. Additionally, *WT1* is essential for the survival of the metanephric mesenchyme. Its expression appears to be regulated temporally and spatially in various tissues, and the presence of at least four different isoforms, generated by alternate splicing, adds a measure of complexity to its expression.[3] *WT1* is found in uninduced mesenchyme and in subsequent condensed mesenchyme, S-shaped bodies, and glomerular epithelial cells (podocytes). WT1 knockout mice have no renal or genital development. Mutations of the

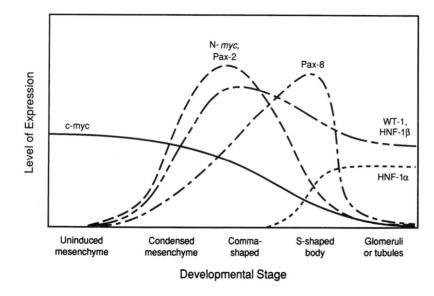

Figure 126–3. Temporal expression of selected transcription factors during early nephrogenesis. HNF = hepatocyte nuclear factor; WT-1 = Wilms' tumor suppressor gene. (From Igarashi P: Curr Opin Nephrol Hypertens 3:308, 1994.)

WT1 gene have been associated with developmental abnormalities in the developing human.[12,13] In addition to these important transcription factors, several other lines of evidence suggest that the winged helix factors, foxC1 and foxC2, are requisites for proper ureteric bud outgrowth.[14] In addition, bone morphogenic protein 4 appears to have an inhibitory action on ureteric bud outgrowth, although the mechanisms by which it is mediated remain unclear.[7] Although *PAX-2* and *WT1* genes are known to play important roles in regulation in early nephrogenesis, other oncogenes such as proto-oncogene *c*-myc are widely expressed during renal embryogenesis and are also detected in the uninduced mesenchyme and in early epithelial structures.[15] No expression of *n*-myc is noted in uninduced mesenchyme; however, it is rapidly up-regulated in early epithelial differentiation, and it is subsequently decreased after formation of the S-shaped body.[16] The continuous overexpression of *c*-myc in transgenic mice is associated with cyst formation as well as tubular hyperplasia.[17] Understandably, we mention only a few of the more importantly described transcription factors in the initiation and development of the ureteric bud metanephric mesenchyme interaction. It appears that genes such as *PAX-2*, *WT1*, *c*-myc, and *n*-myc, among others, are involved in the development of specialized renal epithelial cells and may, in fact, affect the development of other renal cell lineages. Other transcription factors have been associated with the subsequent development of stromal cells (BF2), endothelial cells, and subsequent mesangial cells.[3,18] The maintenance of epithelial phenotypes, although initiated by transcription factors such as Pax-2, seems to be maintained by other transcription factors such as Pax-8, NHF, and Kid 1.

Although transcription factors play an important role in renal development, growth factors also act synergistically in kidney cell differentiation.[4,19] In addition, growth factors play a critical role in modulating renal development as well as in setting up morphogenic gradients that polarized epithelial cells appear to traverse in response to these ligands.[2,19] One of the most important growth factors demonstrated in the developing kidney is glial-derived neurotrophic factor, which is required for a proper ureteric bud outgrowth. It provides the ligand and signal to the Ret oncogene receptor in the ureteric bud.[7] Other growth factors, such as transforming growth factor-α (TGF-α) and TGF-β, platelet-derived growth factor, insulin-like growth factors (IGFs), basic fibroblast growth factor, and epidermal growth factors, have also been shown to influence renal organogenesis.[20-24] Experimental modification and treatment of metanephric organ cultures with TGF-α antibody have been demonstrated to block cell growth and differentiation, whereas TGF-β has been shown to stimulate extracellular matrix deposition.[21,25] Platelet-derived growth factor has been implicated in the development of the glomerular vascular stock.[26] In addition, midkines such as pleotrophin have been demonstrated to be involved in early renal development.[27] A role for IGF in renal organogenesis has been demonstrated.[28,29] Both IGF-I and IGF-II receptors are present in developing mammalian kidneys.[19,22] Other molecules such as angiotensin II (AII) have also been implicated in cell replication and growth, and they influence the expression of other growth factors such as platelet-derived growth factor, TGF-β, and oncogenes.[30-35]

With the development of the first metanephric nephron, the first sign of human renal tubular function begins to appear at approximately 9 to 12 weeks of gestation, whereas the human loop of Henle becomes functional and tubular reabsorption is initiated by 14 weeks' gestation. In the human fetus, new nephrons are formed up to the 36th week of gestation, resulting in the full renal mass.[1,2] Although nephrogenesis is complete at birth in full-term infants, nephron formation continues after birth in the preterm infant.[36] This has significant implications when medications are administered that may affect renal function and when renal physiology within this patient group is considered.

RENAL BLOOD FLOW

The primary experimental work in understanding renal blood flow and dynamics has been carried out in large mammalian animals such as sheep. Kidneys of newborns receive approximately 15% of cardiac output, whereas the fetal kidneys receive a minimum amount (~3%).[37,38] Renal blood flow in fetal sheep is about 1 to 2 ml/minute/g kidney weight.[39,40] A high state of renal vascular resistance and low filtration fraction exist with this relatively low rate of renal blood flow when compared with newborn animals.[40,41]

At the moment of birth in lambs, there appears to be an immediate increase in renal blood flow; however, there is also redistribution from the inner cortex to outer superficial cortex in newborns compared with the fetal animals.[38,39] In the weeks after birth, there appears to be an associated rise in arterial blood pressure that contributes to an increase in renal blood flow with a corresponding decrease in renal vascular resistance (Fig. 126–4).[40-42] These factors do not appear to account for the primary driving force for the postnatal changes in renal hemodynamics because the rise in arterial blood pressure is often of a lesser magnitude than the rise in renal blood flow. Thus, it would appear that various other factors including the renin-angiotensin system, renal neurovascular changes, and intrinsic molecules such as prostaglandins, atrial natriuretic peptide (ANP), and adenosine may play additional roles. This appears to be supported by the ability of the adult kidney to maintain a relatively consistent renal blood flow despite alterations in perfusion pressure greater than 80 to 150 mm Hg.[43] The phenomenon has been termed *autoregulation.*[43] In addition, the fetal kidney also appears to exhibit some moderate degree of autoregulation despite a low perfusion pressure in the fetus of 40 to 60 mm Hg.[44,45] Previous studies using arginine vasopressin (AVP) infusions in examining fetal renal blood flow demonstrated an ability to maintain homeostatic blood flow in spite of an increase in the fetal arterial blood pressure by approximately 15%.[46] This phenomenon cannot be reproduced in perfused renal sheep kidneys that have been isolated.[45] Perhaps this finding could be indicative of the role the neurovascular bundle plays in moderating some of these issues.

FACTORS CONTROLLING RENAL HEMODYNAMICS

The renin-angiotensin system has been the focus of a significant amount of scrutiny. It has been demonstrated that AII is an important growth factor and is a requisite of normal nephrogenesis. Although previous reports demonstrated that renin does not cross the placenta and fetal renin-angiotensin appears to be autonomous, more recent works have shown that, in protein-restricted mothers, intrarenal AII is suppressed in the perinatal period. In fact, it has been suggested that maternal dietary protein restriction leads to impairment of the perinatal renal angiotensin system. This not only impairs nephrogenesis but also leads to adult hypertension, with the presence of a reduced nephron mass.[47-51] The fetus is able to release renin into the fetal circulation, and, in general, the fetal plasma renin levels are higher than maternal levels.[48-52] In addition, fetuses are able to generate AII when renin release is stimulated.[48,50] Various studies have demonstrated that the renin-angiotensin system has the ability to regulate fetal blood pressure and renal blood flow.[53-58] Investigators have shown that AII administered intravenously to the fetus can increase arterial blood pressure and can subsequently decrease umbilical flow. The degree to which AII can induce vasoconstrictor and vasopressor responses is less in fetus than in the adult sheep. This is thought to result from higher receptor occupancy by indigenous AII in the fetal animal.[u] The glomerular filtration rate (GFR) remains constant, although there is a decrease in the renal blood flow in fetal sheep administered

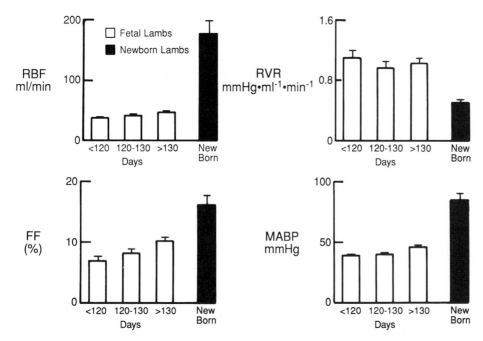

Figure 126–4. Changes in renal hemodynamics and arterial blood pressure during fetal and postnatal periods. FF = filtration fraction; MABP = mean arterial blood pressure; RBF = renal blood flow; RVR = renal vascular resistance. Values are means ± SEM. (From Robillard JE, et al: Pediatr Res *15:*1248, 1981.)

AII.[57] These studies taken together suggest that AII acts primarily through an increased tone in the efferent arteriole.[60] These data are also supported in adults. Furthermore, administration of the AII subtype ATI receptor blocker, losartan, in third trimester fetal sheep causes a decrease in fetal blood pressure, with a subsequent fall in renal vascular resistance and a corresponding rise in renal blood flow.[45] This also results in a significant decrease in glomerular filtration, a finding that certainly supports the hypothesis that maintenance of arterial blood pressure and regulation of fetal glomerular flow require a normal angiotensin system.[45] Similar results have also been noted in the fetus after administration of the angiotensin-converting enzyme inhibitor captopril.[61]

The renin-angiotensin system also appears to play a significant homeostatic and modulatory role in fetal cardiovascular and renal responses to blood loss.[62-67] There is a substantial rise in renin and angiotensin levels in fetal animals that have a rapid reduction in their fetal blood volume.[65-67] These responses appear to be tempered during prolonged hemorrhage.[66]

The importance of an intact renin-angiotensin system during human fetal development is a topic of renewed interest. The concept of perinatal programming has become a favored hypothesis of many investigators. With the postulate that low-protein diets can lead to a decreased renal mass and subsequent hypertension in adult life, these theories have been gathering credence. In support of the key role of the renin-angiotensin system is the observation that the administration of captopril to hypertensive pregnant women can have a significantly deleterious effect on fetal development, with serious complications.[68-72] Similar effects have been demonstrated with ATI receptor blockers such as losartan.[47] Some of the harmful fetal effects demonstrated with angiotensin-converting enzyme inhibitors include fetal hypotension, renal tubular dysplasia, pulmonary hypoplasia (likely secondary to anuria-oligohydramnios), growth retardation, hypocalvaria, increased fetal and neonatal mortality, and patent ductus arteriosus.[68, 69, 71] Animal studies have supported this evidence, with increased rates of fetal loss (especially later in gestation) and induction of gross morphologic changes in developing kidneys.[73-75] Similar abnormalities have been shown in rats administered an ATI receptor antagonist.[76] With the clinical data demonstrating an increased risk of hypertension in persons of lower socioeconomic status, it appears that the attention to intrauterine growth environments and the impact on the renin-

angiotensin system will become a priority in trying to deduce the role that environment plays in the development of hypertension later in life.[47]

Renal Sympathetic Nervous System

Studies have suggested that circulating catecholamines and the sympathetic nervous system play a role in the hemodynamics of the developing renal system.[77-81] The general consensus suggests that the overall sympathetic state appears to be increased renal vascular tone.[77-81] Studies in fetal lambs have corroborated this with the demonstration that fetal renal vasculature seems to be more sensitive to α_1-adrenoceptor stimulation than in either newborn or adult sheep.[81, 82] These data are supported by the observation that low-level renal nerve stimulation can produce a greater fall in renal blood flow and a subsequent larger rise in renal vascular resistance in fetal versus newborn lambs.[79] Stimulation of the renal sympathetic system at higher levels is associated with greater renal vasoconstriction in newborn lambs than fetuses. Furthermore, the renal vasculature appears to be less responsive to renal nerve stimulation in newborn piglets than it is in adult counterparts.[79, 83]

With maturation of the renal system, there may be an associated down-regulation of β_2-adrenoceptors in the renal vessels. This would be consistent with other vascular beds in the developing body. In accordance with these findings, there is an associated renal vasodilation[84] with α_1-adrenoceptor blockade and subsequent nerve stimulation in fetal sheep. This is independent of cholinergic or dopaminergic receptors, but it is inhibited by β_2-adrenoceptor antagonists (specific and nonspecific).[79, 85, 86] It would appear that norepinephrine activates β_2-adrenoceptors to produce renal vasodilation of the fetal renal vasculature. These results have been replicated using intrarenal infusions of norepinephrine in the presence of α_1-adrenoceptor blocking agents.[85]

Previous work demonstrated an impairment of the cardiopulmonary reflex control of renal sympathetic nerve activity during the newborn period. Rather than the central integration of vasoefferent input, these investigators suggested that there is a delayed maturation of the cardiopulmonary reflex needed to change the renal sympathetic nerve activity observed in early development. Furthermore, it appears to be dependent on the intrinsic alterations in baroreceptor function, rather than incomplete central integration. Thus, there may be a totally different arm of control over renal sympathetic nerve stimulation based on baroreceptor function.[87]

Prostaglandins

With the advent of selected cyclooxygenase-2 inhibitors and a better understanding of the prostaglandin synthetic pathway, it has become apparent that prostaglandins are inherently important in the regulation of renal function.[88-91] Past investigators demonstrated and suggested that prostaglandins produced within the fetal kidney were involved in renal hemodynamic regulation and function.[90,91] Clinical support for these hypotheses is present, with the relatively consistently recognized decrease in renal output after indomethacin administration in preterm and term infants with patent ductus arteriosus. Studies in fetal sheep have demonstrated that inhibition of prostaglandin synthesis during fetal life can produce a significant decrease in blood flow with a subsequent rise in renal vascular resistance and arterial blood pressure.[91, 92] The use of prostaglandin synthetase inhibitors to stop preterm labor has been associated with oligohydramnios.[93] This effect is likely secondary to a decrease in fetal urinary output resulting from decreased fetal renal blood flow.[91] These observations have also been correlated in pregnant women whose fetuses have low urinary output immediately after exposure to maternal indomethacin administration.[93] There are also detractors of this hypothesis suggesting that indomethacin interactions are mediated by an increase in plasma AVP concentrations and do not necessarily depend on changes in renal blood flow.[94-96] Contrary to this belief, Seyberth and colleagues demonstrated that prolonged indomethacin therapy can transiently reduce renal blood flow in very low birth weight infants with symptomatic patent ductus arteriosis.[97] Therefore, in the newborn period, a reduction in renal blood flow does appear to be a direct effect of indomethacin. In general, it appears that the high circulating plasma levels of the vasodilatory prostaglandins counteract the highly activated vasoconstricted state of neonatal microcirculation.[97] Thus, the renal vasoconstrictor effect by prostaglandins synthesis inhibitors can certainly be detrimental, especially in the immature kidney.

Kallikrein-Kinin System

The neonatal kidney possesses a higher expression of the β_2-bradykinin receptors compared with the adult counterpart. Bradykinin is a vasodilator and diuretic peptide produced by the kallikrein enzymes in the collecting tubules of the kidney. Its primary effect is exerted via these β_2-receptors. Renal expression of kallikrein is initially low at birth, but it rapidly rises in the postnatal period. The excretion of bradykinin in the urine also correlates with a rise in the renal blood flow. Blockade of the β_2-receptor in the rabbit has been shown to inhibit the vasodilator effect and to allow renal vasoconstriction.[98, 99] In the adult, the intrarenal kinins apparently act in a paracrine fashion and influence renal hemodynamics, along with sodium and water excretion in the kidney.[100] In the developing rat kidney, kallikrein immunoreactivity is localized to the intracortical nephrons within the distal tubules.[101] The kallikrein expression follows a central fugal pattern of nephron maturation. This finding suggests that the kinins may contribute to a preferential distribution of blood flow toward the inner cortex during early development. Findings in fetal sheep as well as in rats and humans all support the apparent increase in activity of the kallikrein system after birth.[102-104]

Nitric Oxide

The overall relevance of nitric oxide and its role in different kidney functions have not been fully elucidated.[105-108] Certainly, it appears that nitric oxide is involved in the regulation of prox-

imal reabsorption of fluid and salt and phosphorus; however, its underlying specific functions and its role under basal conditions are still unclear.[109] Nitric oxide definitely plays a role in regulating the renal vascular endothelium during development, and this role has been elucidated in fetal sheep and newborn piglets.[105,106] Nitric oxide was initially designated endothelium-derived relaxing factor by Frischcott and Zwodski.[107] It had previously been thought to exist, based on pioneering studies looking at the effect of sodium nitroprusside in isolated kidneys.[108] It is clear that nitric oxide plays an extensive role in normal renal function. For example, when nitric oxide is inhibited in third trimester fetal sheep, there is an increase in renal vascular resistance, a decrease in GFR, and a decline in urinary excretion of sodium.[105] Similar outcomes have also been demonstrated in newborn piglets after inhibition of nitric oxide formation.[106]

Atrial Natriuretic Factor

Atrial natriuretic factor, otherwise known as ANP, has potent diuretic, natriuretic, and vasodilatory effects.[110] ANP is secreted by cardiac myocytes and can increase GFR, inhibit renin and aldosterone release, and relax and increase vascular permeability.[111-115] Although the precise role of ANP in the regulation of fluid and sodium homeostasis remains elusive, evidence suggests that ANP plays a role in physiologic adaptation of the fetus and neonates to a changing environment.[111] ANP appears to be involved in the regulation of blood pressure and fluid volume. ANP levels decrease in the perinatal period, with a subsequent increase during the first couple of weeks of postnatal life in the rat.[116-119] This is the opposite of the plasma ANP concentration, which is elevated in the first days of life and decreases as maturation progresses.[111] With these data, it appears that ANP likely plays a primary role in the natriuresis and diuresis that occur postnatally. After the initial diuresis, the neonate enters a stage of positive sodium balance that is required for proper somatic growth.[111]

Various stimuli have been observed to increase ANP levels in the fetus. Circulating ANP levels are detectable by midgestation in fetal sheep and are normally greater in the fetus than in maternal circulation.[113, 120-124] In addition, premature infants have higher ANP levels than full-term neonates.[114] Certain stimuli are known to increase fetal plasma ANP levels, including acute volume expansion and blood transfusions in the human fetus.[111] Furthermore, induction of atrial tachycardia in the fetal lamb resulted in hydrops and increased plasma ANP concentrations. The renal effects of infused ANP are blunted in the fetus compared with the adult.[111]

Overall, the effects of ANP in the fetus are similar to those in the adult in that ANP decreases arterial pressure and blood volume in both.[125] There is also an increase in fetal urinary flow and electrolyte excretion, and there is a notable vasodilation in the renal splanchnic bed.[112, 121, 126-128] The effects of ANP in the renal vasculature in the fetus appeared to be mediated by high-affinity binding sites for a membrane-bound guanylate cyclase with subsequent increased production of cyclic guanosine 3',5'-monophosphate.[129] ANP not only binds guanylate cyclase receptor, but it also binds to an even greater number of receptors that are not coupled to the guanylate cyclase system. These have been classified as clearance receptors and are believed to contribute to the regulation of plasma ANP by removal of this hormone from the plasma.[111]

Endothelin

There are three known indigenous isoforms of endothelin in humans. These are designated ETI to ETIII.[130] The actions of these isoforms are mediated by two known receptor subtypes ETA and ETB. Both are subtypes belong to a G-protein–coupled receptor superfamily.[130] In humans, ETA receptors are present

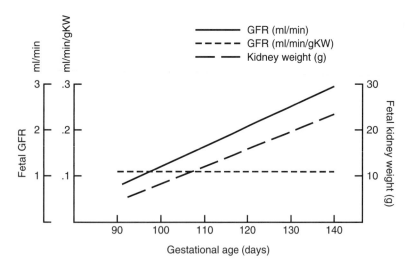

Figure 126–5. Developmental changes in glomerular filtration rate (GFR) during the last trimester of gestation in fetal sheep (term 145 days). GFR is expressed in ml/minute (*solid line*) and ml/minute/g kidney weight (*short dashed lines*). Kidney weight is expressed in grams (*long dashed lines*). (From Robillard JE, et al: Am J Obstet Gynecol *122*:601, 1975.)

mainly on vascular smooth muscle cells and are chiefly responsible for contraction. The responsiveness of ET recombinant receptors can vary depending on the species and the vascular bed.[130] Endothelin itself is a 21-amino acid peptide.[131] Infusions of endothelin in adults increase blood pressure and decrease cardiac output. Endothelin may have complex interactions and may be regulated by other vasoactive hormones including angiotensin, AVP, epinephrine, and potentially thrombin.[132,133] In addition to these phenomena, endothelin stimulation may enhance the release of endothelin-derived relaxing factors (nitric oxide or prostaglandins).[130]

In the fetus, endothelin acts a potent vasoconstrictor of the fetal circulation.[134] In addition, it is known to increase fetal blood pressure and may induce hypoxemia and acidemia consistent with its effect on the umbilical blood vessels.[134] Endothelin has been found in maternal blood, amniotic fluid, and fetal circulation.[135-138] In contrast to adults, endothelin increases urinary flow rates and urinary electrolyte excretion in the fetus.[134, 139] This finding suggests that fetal endothelin has minimal vasoconstrictive effects on renal afferent arterioles, in contrast to its known hemodynamic effects on the adult.[139] Once again, there may be a blunted effected in the fetus overall.[130]

GLOMERULAR FILTRATION

The adaptation of the fetus to the postnatal environment requires a preprogrammed change in the GFR of the kidneys. The GFR is known to be low during fetal life and increases with gestational age.[140-144] However, over the latter part of gestation, when kidneys are corrected for weight in fetal body weight, the GFR remains relatively consistent (Fig. 126–5). With the onset of birth, during day 1 of life the GFR of preterm infants reflects the intrauterine stage of development obtained by the fetus. There is a direct correlation between the GFR and the gestational age of newborn infants delivered between 27 and 43 weeks of gestation.[145, 146] In the first 24 hours after birth, the GFR/kg body weight in near-term fetal sheep is 1.14 ± 0.08 ml/minute/kg, and, in preterm sheep, the GFR/kg body weight is 1.07 ± 0.12 ml/minute/kg. These measurements are similar to those in fetal sheep.[143,145]

The maturation of GFR during fetal life is a result of the combination of all the events that occur during the change from fetal to extrauterine life. Many of the potential stressors that the neonate faces during adaptation to extrauterine life can have a detrimental effect on renal output.[99] Certainly, neonatal adversity such as hypoxemia may change the overall renal status and may alter the transition to extrauterine life. In general, multiple factors oppose and promote filtration including change in the

renal vascular resistance, increasing nephron mass, and modification of the forces involved in the process of ultrafiltration and subsequent development of concentration gradients through proper sodium and urea deposition. In puppies, lambs, and guinea pigs, the GFR rises consistently in the weeks after birth.[141, 143, 147-149] In the lamb, the rise in GFR occurs within the first few hours postnatally.[150, 151] There is a gradual increase in GFR in the first week of life (Fig. 126–6).[150-152] The rapidity of the GFR rise is indicative of a functional rather than a morphologic change occurring within the kidney.[151, 153] Current opinion is that there is enhanced glomerular perfusion, which results in the recruitment of the more superficial cortical nephrons that make up the nephron masses.[39, 40] To complicate matters even further, the fetus is exposed to various medications in the clinical environment that can inhibit or alter the vasoactive forces at work in the subsequent development of GFR.

TUBULAR FUNCTION

Although the sequence of development of renal tubules is becoming better understood, the sentinel events that allow differentiation and specification of the proximal versus the other portions of the tubules remain elusive. As the underlying mechanisms of polarization and perhaps the contribution of mechanoreception, flow kinetics, and cell-cell interactions become better understood, we will continue to develop an appreciation of tubular function and, with it, the transporters that make up the homeostatic mechanisms that allow maintenance of fluid and electrolytes in the fetus and throughout life.[154]

Sodium

The fetal excretion of sodium is greater than later on in life. This pattern has also been observed in premature infants and in the ovine fetus as well. In this model, sodium reabsorption ranges between 85 and 95% and increases with gestational age. In the adult, more than 99% of the filtered sodium load is reabsorbed in the renal tubules, and thus the fractional excretion of sodium is relatively low compared with the fetal and neonatal periods.[140-143] Various factors have been thought to contribute to the high rate of sodium excretion by the immature kidney. These include, but are not limited to, the presence of circulating natriuretic factors, the relative insensitivity to tubular reabsorption of sodium, the large extracellular fluid volume, and the relative renal tubular maturity in the fetus and neonate.[36,155-159] In addition, mechanisms that are not clearly understood may play a role in a differential sodium reabsorption between a proximal and a distal portion of

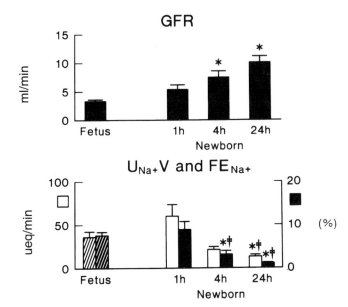

GFR

U~Na+~V and FE~Na+~

Figure 126–6. Changes in glomerular filtration rate (GFR) (*upper panel*) and urinary excretion of sodium ($U_{Na+}V$) and fractional excretion of sodium (FE_{Na+}) (*lower panel*) during the transition from fetal to newborn life. *$p < .05$ when compared with fetal values. ‡$p < .05$ when compared with newborn values at 1 hour. Values are expressed as means ± SEM. (From Nakamura KT, et al: Pediatr Res *21*:229, 1987.)

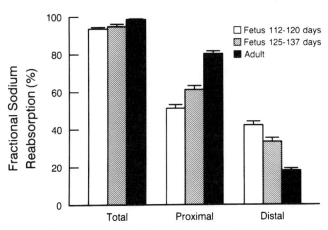

Figure 126–7. Fractional sodium reabsorption in different renal tubular segments in two groups of fetal sheep and in nonpregnant ewes. Values are means ± SEM. (From Lumbers ER, et al: Can J Physiol Pharmacol *66*:697, 1988.)

the nephron.[160] In the fetal sheep, a significantly greater fraction of filtered sodium load is reabsorbed in the distal portion of the nephron than the proximal portion; this is the opposite of that which occurs in the adult kidney (Fig. 126–7).

As the renal tubular cells differentiate into their respective portions of the nephron, an associated maturation and an obligatory change occur in the function and abundance of many membrane proteins responsible for ion transport and nutrient transport in the nephron. These obligatory changes are based on the requirements of that particular portion of the tubule. The epithelium of the tubules needs and acquires a polarized state resulting in a distribution of exchangers, pumps, and channels with the ability to perform vectorial ion and nutrient transport (Fig. 126–8). Preliminary observations from our laboratory suggest that there may be a fetal time course whereby sodium exchangers change from apical to basolateral positioning within the developing tubules. The mechanism underlying these changes is unclear at this time. Although it may have less of an impact in the fetus, the proximal tubule still retains the ability to absorb the greatest amount of sodium in the fetus and neonate.

The sodium/hydrogen exchanger (NHE) likely plays the most important regulatory role in this process.[161] This exchanger mediates the electroneutral exchange of 1 sodium for 1 hydrogen and thereby also plays a role in the acidification of urine. At least four different isoforms, referred to as NHE1, NHE2, NHE3, and NHE4, have been isolated.[162-164] NHE3 is thought to be the isoform that is present at the apical or luminal membrane in the kidney and is therefore likely responsible for the bulk of transepithelial sodium reabsorption. NHE1 has been localized along the lateral plasma membrane of multiple nephron segments and does not appear to contribute to the transepithelial sodium transport.[165] The function of this particular transporter seems to be more consistent with cell volume regulation, growth, and pH defense.[166] NHE4 is found mainly in the collecting tubules of the kidney, a feature suggesting that it may play a specialized role in rectifying cell volume in response to extreme osmotic fluctuations that occur in this area of the kidney.[167]

Both fetal sheep and rabbits demonstrate a maximal uptake rate or an increased maximal velocity that is low in the fetus when compared with older animals.[168, 169] The K_m value or the Michaelis constant for sodium is not significantly different when compared with that in older animals. Perhaps the most interesting feature of this maturation is that a significant proportion of the increasing NHE3 activity or maximal velocity is noted in the first 24 hours after birth, a time when the greatest amount of sodium reabsorption occurs.[156, 169] Previous studies demonstrated that long-term infusion of cortisol during the last trimester of gestation of fetal sheep could increase the NHE3 maximal velocity by 60%, with a subsequent fourfold rise in renal

Figure 126–8. Distribution of membrane ion transporters in proximal tubular cells. The Na⁺/H⁺ exchanger and other Na⁺-dependent carriers are localized in the brush-border membrane (luminal side), and the Na⁺,K⁺-ATPase pump (α- and β-subunits) is located in the basolateral membrane. (Adapted from Aperia A, Celsi G: *In* Seldin DW, Giebisch G [eds]: The Kidney: Physiology and Pathophysiology, Vol 1. New York, Raven Press, 1992, pp 803–828.)

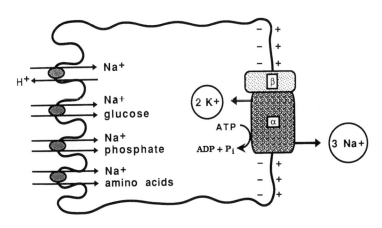

cortex mRNA levels of NHE3.[170-173] This finding is corroborated by other studies, and it indicates that glucocorticoids likely play an important role in the increase of NHE activity during the transition to the newborn life (Jean Robillard, personal observation).

The interdependence of various sodium channels has become partially clarified with the understanding of how the NHE transporters may affect the sodium, potassium–adenosine triphosphatase (Na^+,K^+-ATPase) channels. These enzymes are responsible for active sodium transport in eukaryotic cells. In the mature kidney, they are located in the basolateral membrane of renal tubular cells. The Na^+,K^+-ATPase pump consists of both catalytic and regulatory subunits. Three isoforms are catalytic (α_1, α_2, α_3), and two isoforms comprise the regulatory subunit (β_1 and β_2).[174] *In situ* hybridization techniques have demonstrated that all catalytic and regulatory subunits are present throughout all the nephron segments in the mature kidney.[175] This finding has been confirmed by Western blot analysis as well.[176] During fetal life, there is a relative gradient increase of mRNA in both α_1- and β-subunits, with minimal changes noted in α_2-subunits in the fetal rat cortex.[177] These changes have been noted to parallel the rise of Na^+,K^+-ATPase activity in the whole kidney and in various single-nephron segments during postnatal maturation.[178-181] The interdependence of Na^+,K^+-ATPase and NHE channels may be related to the increase in sodium filtrate associated with renal maturation. The increase in sodium filtrate may be an important factor in influencing the postnatal rise in Na^+,K^+-ATPase. Thus, NHE activity, which is the major sodium entry channel in the proximal tubule, may precede the rise in Na^+,K^+-ATPase activity.[182] Additional studies in rats have demonstrated that an increase or decrease in NHE activity can stimulate or inhibit Na^+,K^+-ATPase activity, respectively.[180, 183] It appears that a localization of the Na^+,K^+-ATPase channel within the developing proximal tubule may move from the apical face to the basolateral face with increasing maturity of the tubule; however, data are limited (Jean Robillard, personal observation).

Glucose

Interest in the effect of maternal hypoglycemia on multiple organ systems has grown substantially since the early 1990s. In general, the reabsorption capacity for glucose is quite high in the fetus. This work has been done in guinea pigs, fetal sheep, and newborn puppies.[184-186] In fetal sheep compared with adult sheep, investigators noted that the corrected T_m/GFR (the maximal tubule excretory capacity of the kidneys for glucose) is greater in the fetus than in adult sheep.[185] This is also true of the renal plasma threshold for glucose, which is greater during fetal life and increases with gestational age.[185] Glucose transport has been investigated using α-methyl-D-glucopyranoside, which shares a D-glucose carrier present in the proximal tubule of the brush-border membrane but does not interact with the D-glucose transport system at the basolateral border.[187] It has been demonstrated that transport of α-methyl-D-glucopyranoside by the kidneys in near-term rat fetuses has adult characteristics.[187] The uptake is sodium dependent and can be inhibited by phlorhizin. The sodium-dependent glucose transport system in fetal rabbit proximal tubules, late in gestation, is stereospecific, electrogenic, cation specific, and pH sensitive.[188]

Organic Acids and Bases

The ability for the fetal and neonatal kidney to handle organic acids and bases is limited. Secretion of the organic acid *p*-aminohippurate is quite low in both fetal and neonatal periods.[189, 190] There is some evidence to suggest that the fetal kidney can secret organic bases but to a significantly lesser degree than adults.[191] It is thought that these findings reflect immature tubular secretory pathways present during development. These phenomena may also be explained by the finding that the juxtamedullary circula-

tion shunts blood through the vasa recta, thereby decreasing the peritubular circulation perfusing the secretory cells.[191] As the kidney matures, the blood flow changes and allows for improved secretory capability of the kidney itself.

Potassium

Potassium secretion by the kidney is low early in gestation and increases toward term.[160] The fractional potassium reabsorption measured in near-term fetal sheep ($67.08 \pm 9.72\%$; $n = 13$) is similar to levels in newborn lambs ($58.3 \pm 4.76\%$ $n = 12$) and also in adult ewes ($52 \pm 7.6\%$; $n = 5$).[152] These data suggest that the secretory pathways for potassium appear to be mature during late fetal life.[155,156,192] In general, it appears that potassium excretion depends on tubular reabsorption and secretion after filtration across the glomerular membrane. It has been thought that the increase in potassium secretion as the fetus approaches term results from a larger tubular surface area available for potassium secretion. In addition, there may also be a contribution from an increase in Na^+,K^+-ATPase activity or an increase in the sensitivity of fetal nephron to aldosterone that enhances potassium excretion.[155,156,192] Furthermore, as the urinary flow increases through the fetal kidneys, an increased gradient may allow for removal of more potassium in the urine. Certainly, from a clinical standpoint, it is not uncommon to have high potassium levels in the immediate neonatal period, especially in preterm infants.

Acid-Base Homeostasis

Without the presence of an appropriate functioning kidney in the adult, acid-base balance is unattainable. The kidney itself is responsible for reabsorption of the entire filtered bicarbonate load in proximal portions of the nephron and is also responsible for secretion of hydrogen ions and the generation of new bicarbonate through the urinary buffering systems of titratable acid and ammonium. Without the presence of these homeostatic mechanisms, the other metabolic processes of life, including growth and development, are severely restricted.

Within the fetus, the kidney is also involved in regulation of acid-base balance. The urinary pH is always less than the plasma pH.[144,193] There is an age-dependent increase in excretion rates of titratable acid and ammonium associated with the rise in acid excretion.[144] It has been demonstrated that 80 to 100% of filtered bicarbonate load is reabsorbed by the fetal sheep.[144,194,195] This bicarbonate absorption provides the driving force for chloride reabsorption in the mature proximal tubule and also requires the presence of adequate carbonic anhydrase activity in these same segments. Both bicarbonate and chloride reabsorption have been noted to increase with age in the ovine fetus.[144,193] This finding may reflect increasing carbonic anhydrase activity, because inhibition with acetazolamide produces significant increase in bicarbonate excretion and also an increase in urinary pH.[195] Corroborating this hypothesis is the observation that carbonic anhydrase is present in human fetal kidney in the late gestational phase.[196] Although there is a blunted renal response in the fetus to metabolic acidosis compared with the adult, the qualitative response of increased hydrogen ion excretion is similar to that found in the adult animal.[197, 198] In the presence of fetal hyperglycemia, the resulting metabolic acidosis has not been noted to cause a change in the excretion rate of urinary buffers or urinary pH in the fetus, a finding suggesting that the placental regulation of fetal acid-base balance is sufficient and contributes a portion of the buffering capabilities and capacity required by the fetus.[199]

Phosphate

Fetal plasma is noted to contain a greater concentration of inorganic phosphate when compared with maternal plasma. This is inversely related to gestational age. The importance of phosphorus to the fetus is validated by the observation that it is transported across the placenta from the mother to the fetus against a concentration gradient.[200] There appears to be a unique sodium-phosphorus co-transporter in kidneys of growing animals that differs from the sodium–inorganic phosphorus-2 transporter, which is known to be modulated by dietary phosphorus intake. This co-transporter is thought to contribute to the high rate of renal phosphorus reabsorption during renal development.[201] In the fetal sheep, between 60 and 100% of phosphorus is reabsorbed; the concentration of inorganic phosphorus in fetal urine is quite low.[194] The fetal kidney responds to parathyroid hormone with an increase of urinary excretion of calcium and cyclic adenosine monophosphate.[202] There is a blunted and limited effect of parathyroid hormone on the urinary excretion rate of phosphorus during fetal life.[203] Thus, hyperphosphatemia may result in the presence of relative parathyroid insufficiency during fetal life that may compound the already low fetal renal clearance of phosphorus.

CONCENTRATION CAPACITY OF THE FETAL KIDNEY

During the last trimester of gestation, the fetal sheep has a urinary flow rate of approximately 600 to 1200 ml/day of urine, which works out to be 0.5 to 1.0 ml/minute.[41, 77, 141, 204] The urinary flow rate in human fetuses increases 10-fold from 0.1 ml/minute at 20 weeks to 1 ml/minute at 40 weeks, with a subsequent reduction to 0.1 ml/minute in the neonate.[205]

Because the fetus has not been exposed to a high protein load and has had little requirement to set up a concentration gradient, fetal urine is usually hypotonic with respect to fetal plasma. The range of osmolality is 100 to 250 mOsm/kg H_2O. However, the fetal kidney can adapt to its environment. The fetal kidney is able to produce diluted or concentrated urine, depending on the state of hydration of the mother as well as the fetus. One sees a fall in urinary flow rate and a decrease in free water clearance when mannitol is administered to pregnant ewes or when the mother has been deprived of water.[206, 207-209] Direct infusion of AVP into the fetus also appears to cause a decrease in fetal free water clearance.[210, 211] Free water clearance has been directly correlated with the transfer of fluid across the placenta. Therefore, a decrease in net fluid transfer across the placenta from the mother to the fetus results in decreased fetal urine production and may account for increased osmolality and decreased urine flow *in utero* in response to fetal stress.[212, 213] Although this may partially explain the decrease in urine flow rates in conditions of stress, other neuroendocrine pathways may also play a role. The kidney is not able to concentrate urine to adult levels until well after birth. Various factors are thought to contribute to the inability of the fetal kidney to concentrate urine.[214] A decrease in sensitivity of the collecting ducts to the circulating AVP clearly is one such factor. Thus, the actions of vasopressin are hindered, and the fetus has an obligatory water loss. There are also limitations in the movement of urea and the reabsorption of sodium and chloride along the ascending limb of Henle owing to structural immaturity and a preferential distribution of blood flow to the inner cortex. These factors result in a high flow through the vasa recta and prevent generation of a medullary concentration gradient. In addition, the fetus (as a general rule) has not had a sufficiently high protein intake to generate significant amounts of urea for the initial production of a concentration gradient in the medulla.

Although the fetal kidney has a decreased ability to concentrate the urine because of what appears to be decreased responsiveness to AVP, the fetus can synthesize or secrete AVP.[215,216] Both synthesis and secretion of AVP occur during the last trimester of gestation.[216] In fetal sheep, during the last trimester of gestation, both the volume and osmolality receptor controls of AVP secretion are fully functional.[217] In fact, AVP levels are known to be increased in fetal circulation after hemorrhage, hypoxemia,

diuretic administration, or osmotic stimulus.[218-221] An AVP challenge administered to fetal animals demonstrates the increased sensitivity to AVP when compared with the adult nephron.[46] Under these conditions, the urinary osmolality is approximately one-third of what the adult animals would obtain for the same plasma AVP concentration.[46] Additionally, there may be a decreased coupling between AVP receptor binding and cyclic adenosine monophosphate generation or an overall reduced number of AVP receptors that contribute to the hyporesponsiveness of the immature kidney to this hormone.[222, 223] Although ovine fetuses in early gestation do exhibit antidiuretic responses to AVP, this response is markedly varied.[65, 211, 224] Previous studies demonstrated that when the V_2 receptor for AVP is activated, fetal renal water reabsorption can increase early in gestation.[225] The V_1 receptors do not seem to participate in this response.[226] The expression and activation of collecting duct–specific water channels influence the ability of the activated V_2 receptor to increase water reabsorption. Various aquaporins (AQPs, membrane water channels) have been isolated and cloned.[227] Within the kidney, AQP-2, the collecting duct AQP, has been demonstrated to be the AVP-regulated water channel.[228, 229] It has been localized to the apical membrane of collecting duct cells, and its expression is regulated directly by the V_2 receptor.[230] AQP-2 is expressed in the medulla of the rat embryo as early as day 18, and by the time of birth, the overall distribution of AQP-2 in the newborn kidney is similar to that observed in the adult kidney.[231] These data provide support for studies that have demonstrated a role for AVP in the regulation of water balance in the fetus.

FACTORS INFLUENCING TUBULAR FUNCTION

Although fetal kidney hemodynamic status and vasculature are affected by endocrine factors such as AVP, aldosterone, renin, AII, prostaglandins, and ANP, these hormones also have a graded effect on tubular function in the developing fetus.

Aldosterone

Aldosterone is a salt-retaining steroid hormone that is produced in the adrenal cortex. It has been demonstrated to cross the placenta easily from the maternal circulation into the fetus.[232, 233] Accordingly, the fetal component of aldosterone accounts for approximately 60% of the total that has been noted in fetal circulation of guinea pigs and approximately 80% in sheep.[234, 235] As may be expected, there is a correlation between fetal plasma aldosterone levels and both plasma renin activities and potassium levels. Renal aldosterone levels also correlate with the ratio of urinary sodium to urinary potassium; the ratio decreases during fetal maturation as the plasma aldosterone level rises.[156] The responsiveness of the fetus to aldosterone occurs in the same order of magnitude as it does in the adult and is also known to decrease plasma renin activity.[236-238] However, some evidence suggests that aldosterone-mediated tubular sodium reabsorption and potassium secretion are not coupled during development. Contrary to the antinatriuretic effect of aldosterone on the fetal kidney, there is no noted increase in potassium excretion.[236] These findings have also been extended to the newborn animal.[239] Further evidence that the fetal kidney is less responsive to aldosterone infusion is the observation that the fractional excretion of sodium is greater than 1% during either long-term or short-term aldosterone infusion in the fetus when compared with the adult.[240] At this point, it is unclear whether this is a receptor-mediated effect of aldosterone in the renal tubules or whether other factors may interfere with aldosterone action on the fetal renal tubule.

Renin-Angiotensin System

With respect to its tubular function, the renin-angiotensin system appears to have a similar effect on fetal and adult kidneys. As expected, there is an inverse correlation between plasma renin activity and urinary sodium excretion.[52, 192] Furosemide administration in fetal sheep causes both water and salt loss and stimulates renin release and a subsequent decrease in sodium reabsorption.[54] The factors that could be responsible for this result include a direct effect of the renin-angiotensin system on the renal tubular sodium absorption and the establishment of tubular feedback mechanisms from the macula densa on reabsorption of sodium in the kidney.

Kallikrein-Kinin System

Although kallikrein excretion and sodium excretion have an inverse relationship during development, this may represent an epiphenomenon based on plasma aldosterone levels.[103, 241] The effect on sodium excretion may be apparent because infusion of exogenous aldosterone has also been noted to increase urinary kallikrein excretion in near-term fetal sheep.[103] Thus, a direct role of the kallikrein on these phenomena is unclear.

Prostaglandins

There may be a role for prostaglandins in modulating fetal and neonatal sodium homeostasis. It is known that urinary excretion of prostaglandins is increased during fetal life and subsequently decreases in the neonatal period.[91, 242] Prostaglandins E_2 and I_2 are known to be natriuretic in adult animals. Indomethacin, a cyclooxygenase inhibitor, decreases sodium excretion in the adult, but it causes increased sodium and chloride loss when administered to fetal sheep, despite a noted decrease in renal blood flow.[91] Because of the complex nature of other vasoactive peptides and hormones activated at the time of fetal development, it is difficult to delineate the specific role of prostaglandins in this process, and further investigation is required.

Atrial Natriuretic Peptide

It has been demonstrated that the renal responsiveness to ANP changes with advancing fetal age. Administration of ANP to fetal sheep increases excretion of potassium, calcium, chloride, and water and is also known to enhance sodium excretion by decreasing proximal sodium reabsorption.[120, 121] Toward the end of the third trimester of gestation, the fetal kidney exhibits a minimal or modest natriuretic response to ANP infusion without changes in urine volume or GFR.[127, 243] However, other data suggest that ANP may be involved in regulation of urinary sodium excretion and urinary flow rates.[112] These data also indicate that ANP is involved in the maintenance of arterial pressure in near-term fetal sheep.[112] Younger fetuses (those in the mid-third trimester) exhibit greater diuresis and natriuresis in response to ANP infusions, associated with a significant increase in GFR.[128, 244] The seemingly contradictory results may indicate that these responses are not necessarily caused by a reduced ANP receptor number, but they may depend on an increased proportion of ANP clearance receptors in older fetuses, thus providing a feedback control mechanism for this response.[113]

Cortisol

As previously discussed, steroid hormones such as cortisol are known to have an effect on the developing fetus. The administration of cortisol to fetal sheep between days 126 and 135 is associated with an elevation in GFR and a corresponding decrease in phosphate reabsorption by almost 50% of the filtered load.[245] It is thought that this increased phosphate excretion occurs because the filtered load exceeds the maximum threshold for phosphate reabsorption. Cortisol decreases proximal sodium reabsorption, but it enhances distal absorption; the overall effect is no change in total fractional sodium reabsorption. Similar results were not demonstrated after the administration of cortisol to younger fetal sheep from days 111 to 120.[246] Thus, the glucocorticoid hormones may promote maturation of the sodium pump closer to term.[173, 247] In keeping with this line of thought, the administration of dexamethasone (in rat) and glucocorticoid (in sheep) accelerate postnatal development of the tubular reabsorptive capacity for sodium, potassium, and water and increase NHE3 expression.[73, 248] The degree to which the stress responses induced by preterm birth affect these processes is difficult to assess in isolation. An appreciation of all the factors together and the potential complex interaction of these factors is necessary to understand the renal transition from the fetal to the neonatal environment.

REFERENCES

1. McCrory WW: Embryologic development of the kidney. *In* McCrory WW (ed): Developmental Nephrology. Cambridge, MA, Harvard University Press, 1972, pp 1-50.
2. Potter EL: Development of the kidney. *In* Potter EL (ed): Normal and Abnormal Development of the Kidney. Chicago, Year Book Medical Publishers, 1972, pp 3-79.
3. Dressler GR: Development of the excretory system. *In* Rossant J, Tam P (eds.): Mouse Development, Patterning, Morphogenesis and Organogenesis. New York, Academic Press, 2002, pp 395-420.
4. Bacallao R, Fine FG: Molecular events in the organization of renal tubular epithelium: from nephrogenesis to regeneration. Am J Physiol *257*:F913, 1989.
5. Igarashi P: Transcription factors and apoptosis in kidney development. Curr Opin Nephrol Hypertens *3*:308, 1994.
6. Clapp WL, Abrahamson DR: Regulation of kidney organogenesis: homeobox genes, growth factors, and Wilms' tumor. Curr Opin Nephrol Hypertens *2*:419, 1993.
7. Brophy PD, et al: Regulation of ureteric bud outgrowth by Pax2-dependent activation of the glial derived neurotrophic factor gene. Development *128*:4747, 2001.
8. Dressler GR, Douglass EC: Pax-2 is a DNA-binding protein expressed in embryonic kidney and Wilms' tumor. Proc Natl Acad Sci U S A *89*:1179, 1992.
9. Eccles MR, et al: Expression of the PAX2 gene in human fetal kidney and Wilms' tumor. Cell Growth Differ *3*:279, 1992.
10. Dressler GR, et al: Deregulation of Pax-2 expression intransgenic mice generates severe kidney abnormalities. Nature *362*:65, 1993.
11. Poleev A, et al: PAX 8, a human paired box gene: isolation and expression in developing thyroid, kidney and Wilms' tumors. Development *116*:611, 1992.
12. Rauscher FJ III: The WT1 Wilms' tumor gene product: a developmentally regulated transcription factor in the kidney that functions as a tumor suppressor. FASEB J *7*:896, 1993.
13. Kreidberg JA, et al: WT-1 is required for early kidney development. Cell *74*:679, 1993.
14. Kume T, et al: The murine winged helix transcription factors, Foxc1 and Foxc2, are both required for cardiovascular development and somitogenesis. Genes Dev *15*:2470, 2001.
15. Mugrauer G, Ekblom P: Contrasting expression patterns of three members of the myc family of protooncogenes in the developing and adult mouse kidney. J Cell Biol *112*:13, 1991.
16. Mugrauer G, et al: N-myc proto-oncogene expression during organogenesis in the developing mouse as revealed by in situ hybridization. J Cell Biochem *107*:1325, 1988.
17. Trudel M, et al: C-myc as an inducer of polycystic kidney disease in transgenic mice. Kidney Int *39*:665, 1991.
18. Hatini V, et al: Essential role of stromal mesenchyme in kidney morphogenesis revealed by targeted disruption of Winged Helix transcription factor BF-2. Genes Dev *10*:1467, 1996.
19. Hammerman MR, et al: Growth factors and metanephrogenesis. Am J Physiol *262*:F523, 1992.
20. Toback FG, et al: Kidney epithelial cells release growth factors in response to extracellular signals. Pediatr Nephrol *4*:363, 1990.
21. Avner ED, Sweeney WE Jr: Polypeptide growth factors in metanephric growth and segmental nephron differentiation. Pediatr Nephrol *4*:372, 1990.
22. Hirvonen H, et al: The n-myc proto-oncogene and IGF-II growth factor mRNAs are expressed by distinct cells in human fetal kidney and brain. J Cell Biol *108*:1093, 1989.
23. Sariola H, et al: Dependence of kidney morphogenesis on the expression of nerve growth factor receptor. Science *254*:571, 1991.
24. Sariola H, et al: Differentiation and vascularization of the metanephric kidney grafted on the chorioallantoic membrane. Dev Biol *96*:426, 1983.
25. Rogers SA, et al: Metanephric transforming growth factor-alpha is required for renal organogenesis in vitro. Am J Physiol *262*:F533, 1992.
26. Alpers CE, et al: Developmental patterns of PDGF B-chain, PDGF-receptor, and alpha-actin expression in human glomerulogenesis. Kidney Int *42*:390, 1992.

27. Sakurai H, et al: Identification of pleiotrophin as a mesenchymal factor involved in ureteric bud branching morphogenesis. Development *128*:3283, 2001.

28. Hammerman MR: The growth hormone-insulin-like growth factor axis in the kidney. Am J Physiol *257*:F503, 1989.

29. Rogers SA, et al: Insulin-like growth factors I and II are produced in the metanephros and are required for growth and development in vitro. J Cell Biochem *113*:1447, 1991.

30. Khairallah PA, et al: Effects of angiotensin II on DNA, RNA and protein synthesis. *In* Genest J, Koiw E (eds): Hypertension. Berlin, Springer-Verlag, 1972, pp 212–220.

31. Millan MA, et al: Novel sites of expression of functional angiotensin II receptors in the late gestation fetus. Science *244*:1340, 1989.

32. Naftilan AJ, et al: Induction of platelet-derived growth factor A-chain and c-myc gene expressions by angiotensin II in cultured rat vascular smooth muscle cells. J Clin Invest *83*:1419, 1989.

33. Naftilan AJ, et al: Angiotensin II induces c-fos expression in smooth muscle via transcriptional control. Hypertension *13*:706, 1989.

34. Bobik A, et al: Angiotensin II and noradrenaline increase PDGF-BB receptors and potentiate PDGF-BB stimulated DNA synthesis in vascular smooth muscle. Biochem Biophys Res Commun *166*:580, 1990.

35. Taubman MB, et al: Angiotensin II induces c-fos mRNA in aortic smooth muscle: role of Ca++ mobilization and protein kinase C activation. J Biol Chem *264*:526, 1989.

36. Kleinman LI: Developmental renal physiology. Physiologist *25*:104, 1982.

37. Rudolph AM, Heymann MA: Control of the fetal circulation. *In* Hafez ES (ed): The Mammalian Fetus: Comparative Biology and Methodology. Springfield, IL, Charles C Thomas, 1973, pp 5–19.

38. Paton JB, et al: Cardiac output and organ blood flows in the baboon fetus. Biol Neonate *22*:50, 1973.

39. Aperia A, et al: Renal hemodynamics in the perinatal period: a study in lambs. Acta Physiol Scand *99*:261, 1977.

40. Robillard JE, et al: Ontogeny of single glomerular perfusion rate in fetal and newborn lambs. Pediatr Res *15*:1248, 1981.

41. Gruskin AB, et al: Maturational changes in renal blood flow in piglets. Pediatr Res *4*:7, 1970.

42. Jose PA, et al: Intrarenal blood flow distribution in canine puppies. Pediatr Res *5*:335, 1971.

43. Jose PA, et al: Autoregulation of renal blood flow in the puppy. Am J Physiol *229*:983, 1975.

44. Smith FG: The Growth and Functional Development of the Fetal Kidney. B.Sc.(hon) thesis, University of New South Wales, Sydney, Australia, 1982.

45. Stevenson KM: Endocrine and Other Influences on the Regulation of Fetal and Neonatal Na+ Balance. Ph.D. thesis, University of New South Wales, Sydney, Australia, 1995.

46. Robillard JE, Weitzman RE: Developmental aspects of the fetal renal response to exogenous arginine vasopressin. Am J Physiol *238*:F407, 1980.

47. Ingelfinger JR, Woods LL: Perinatal programming, renal development, and adult renal function. Am J Hypertens *15*:46S, 2002.

48. Broughton-Pipkin F, et al: Renin and angiotensin-like levels in foetal, newborn and adult sheep. J Physiol (Lond) *241*:575, 1974.

49. Broughton-Pipkin F, et al: Factors influencing plasma renin and angiotensin II in the conscious pregnant ewe and its foetus. J Physiol (Lond) *243*:619, 1974.

50. Smith FG Jr, et al: The renin angiotensin system in the fetal lamb. Pediatr Res *8*:611, 1974.

51. Stevens AD, Lumbers ER: Effect on maternal and fetal renal function and plasma renin activity of a high salt intake by the ewe. J Dev Physiol *8*:267, 1986.

52. Stevens AD: Factors Affecting Renal Function and the Renin Angiotensin System in the Sheep Fetus. Thesis, University of New South Wales, Sydney, Australia, 1987.

53. Iwamoto HS, Rudolph AM: Effects of endogenous AII on the fetal circulation. J Dev Physiol *1*:283, 1979.

54. Lumbers ER, Stevens AD: The effects of furosemide, saralasin and hypotension on fetal plasma renin activity and on fetal renal function. J Physiol (Lond) *393*:479, 1987.

55. Lumbers ER, Reid GC: The action of vasoactive compounds in the foetus and the effect of perfusion through the placenta on their biological activity. Aust J Exp Biol Med Sci *56*:11, 1978.

56. Ismay MJA, et al: The action of angiotensin II on the baroreflex response of the conscious ewe and the conscious fetus. J Physiol (Lond) *288*:467, 1979.

57. Robillard JE, et al: Comparison of the adrenal and renal responses to angiotensin II in fetal lambs and adult sheep. Circ Res *50*:140, 1982.

58. Berman W Jr, et al: Effects of pharmacologic agents on umbilical blood flow in fetal lambs in utero. Biol Neonate *33*:225, 1978.

59. Robillard JE: Changes in renal vascular reactivity to angiotensin II during development in fetal, newborn and adult sheep: role of AII vascular receptors occupancy (abstract). Pediatr Res *17*:355A, 1983.

60. Levens NR, et al: Role of the intrarenal renin-angiotensin system in the control of renal function. Circ Res *48*:157, 1981.

61. Lumbers ER, et al: The effects of a converting enzyme inhibitor (captopril) and angiotensin II on fetal renal function. Br J Pharmacol *110*:821, 1993.

62. Iwamoto HS, Rudolph AM: Role of renin-angiotensin system in response to hemorrhage in fetal sheep. Am J Physiol *240*:H848, 1981.

63. Gomez RA, Robillard JE: Developmental aspects of the renal response to hemorrhage during converting-enzyme inhibition in fetal lambs. Circ Res *54*:301, 1984.

64. Gomez RA, et al: Developmental aspects of the renal response to hemorrhage during fetal life. Pediatr Res *18*:40, 1984.

65. Robillard JE, et al: The dynamics of vasopressin release and blood volume regulation during fetal hemorrhage in the lamb fetus. Pediatr Res *13*:606, 1979.

66. Brace RA, Cheung CY: Fetal cardiovascular and endocrine response to prolonged fetal hemorrhage. Am J Physiol *251*:R417, 1986.

67. Broughton-Pipkin F, et al: Changing basal and stimulated activity of the renin-angiotensin system during the second half of gestation in the anaesthetised piglet. Q J Exp Physiol *71*:277, 1986.

68. Pryde PG, et al: Angiotensin-converting enzyme inhibitor fetopathy. J Am Soc Nephrol *3*:1575, 1993.

69. Rosa FW, et al: Neonatal anuria with maternal angiotensin-converting enzyme inhibition. Obstet Gynecol *74*:371, 1989.

70. Hanssens M, et al: Fetal and neonatal effects of treatment with angiotensin-converting enzyme inhibitors in pregnancy. Obstet Gynecol *78*:128, 1991.

71. Boutroy M-J: Fetal effects of maternally administered clonidine and angiotensin-converting enzyme inhibitors. Dev Pharmacol Ther *13*:199, 1989.

72. Martin RA, et al: Effect of ACE inhibition on the fetal kidney: decreased renal blood flow. Teratology *46*:317, 1992.

73. Broughton-Pipkin F, et al: The effect of captopril (SQ14,225) upon mother and fetus in the chronically cannulated ewe and in the pregnant rabbit. J Physiol (Lond) *323*:415, 1982.

74. Ferris TF, Weir EK: Effect of captopril on uterine blood flow and prostaglandin E synthesis in the pregnant rabbit. J Clin Invest *71*:809, 1983.

75. Minsker DH, et al: Maternotoxicity and fetotoxicity of an angiotensin-converting enzyme inhibitor, enalapril, in rabbits. Fundam Appl Toxicol *14*:461, 1990.

76. Friberg P, et al: Renin-angiotensin system in neonatal rats: induction of a renal abnormality in response to ACE inhibition or angiotensin II antagonism. Kidney Int *45*:485, 1994.

77. Robillard JE, Nakamura KT: Neurohormonal regulation of renal function during development. Am J Physiol *254*:F771, 1988.

78. Robillard JE, et al: Effects of renal denervation on renal responses to hypoxemia in fetal lambs. Am J Physiol *250*:F294, 1986.

79. Robillard JE, et al: Ontogeny of renal hemodynamic response to renal nerve stimulation in sheep. Am J Physiol *252*:F605, 1987.

80. Robillard JE, et al: Functional role of renal sympathetic innervation during fetal and postnatal development. News Physiol Sci *7*:130, 1992.

81. Guillery EN, et al: Ontogenic changes in renal response to alpha 1-adrenoceptor stimulation in sheep. Am J Physiol *267*:R990, 1994.

82. Matherne GP, et al: Ontogeny of alpha-adrenoceptor responses in the renal vascular bed of sheep. Am J Physiol *254*:R277, 1988.

83. Buckley NM, et al: Renal circulatory effects of adrenergic stimuli in anesthetized piglets and mature swine. Am J Physiol *237*:H690, 1979.

84. DiBona GF: The functions of the renal nerves. Rev Physiol Biochem Pharmacol *94*:76, 1982.

85. Nakamura KT, et al: Ontogeny of renal beta-adrenoceptor mediated vasodilation in sheep: comparison between endogenous catecholamines. Pediatr Res *22*:465, 1987.

86. Whitsett JA, et al: Developmental aspects of α- and β-adrenergic receptors. Semin Perinatol *6*:125, 1982.

87. Merrill DC, et al: Sympathetic responses to cardiopulmonary vagal afferent stimulation during development. Am J Physiol *277*:H1311, 1999.

88. Pace-Asciak CR: Prostaglandin biosynthesis and catabolism in the developing fetal sheep kidney. Prostaglandins *13*:661, 1977.

89. Pace-Asciak CR: Biosynthesis and catabolism of prostaglandins during animal development. Adv Prostaglandin Thromboxane Leukot Res *1*:35, 1976.

90. Terragno NA, et al: Prostacyclin (PGI2) production by renal blood vessels: relationship to an endogenous prostaglandin synthesis inhibitor (EPSI)(abstract). Clin Res *26*:545A, 1978.

91. Matson JR, et al: The effects of inhibition of prostaglandin synthesis on fetal renal function. Kidney Int *20*:621, 1981.

92. Kirshon B, et al: Indomethacin therapy in the treatment of symptomatic polyhydramnios. Obstet Gynecol *75*:202, 1990.

93. Hendricks SK, et al: Oligohydramnios associated with prostaglandin synthetase inhibitors in preterm labour. Br J Obstet Gynaecol *97*:312, 1990.

94. Walker MPR, et al: Indomethacin-induced urinary flow rate reduction in the ovine fetus is associated with reduced free water clearance and elevated plasma arginine vasopressin levels. Am J Obstet Gynecol *167*:1723, 1992.

95. Arnold-Aldea SA, et al: The effect of the inhibition of prostaglandin synthesis on renal blood flow in fetal sheep. Am J Obstet Gynecol *165*:185, 1991.

96. Stevenson KM, Lumbers ER: Effects of indomethacin on fetal renal function, renal and umbilicoplacental blood flow and lung liquid production. J Dev Physiol *17*:257, 1992.

97. Seyberth HW, et al: Effects of prolonged indomethacin therapy on renal function and selected vasoactive hormones in very low birth weight infants with symptomatic patent ductus arteriosis. J Pediatr *103*:979, 1983.

98. Toth-Heyn P, Guignard J-P: Endogenous bradykinin regulates renal function in the newborn rabbit. Biol Neonate *73*:330, 1998.

99. Toth-Heyn P, et al: The stressed neonatal kidney: from pathophysiology to clinical management of neonatal vasomotor nephropathy. Pediatr Nephrol *14*:227, 2000.

100. Bhoola KD, et al: Bioregulation of kinins: kallikreins, kininogens, and kininases. Pharmacol Rev *44*:1, 1992.

101. El-Dahr SS, Yosipiv IV: Developmentally regulated kallikrein enzymatic activity and gene transcription rate in maturing rat kidneys. Am J Physiol 265:F146, 1993.

102. El-Dahr SS, Chao J: Spatial and temporal expression of kallikrein and its mRNA during nephron maturation. Am J Physiol 262:F704, 1992.

103. Robillard JE, et al: Developmental aspects of the renal kallikrein-kinin activity in fetal and newborn lambs. Kidney Int 22:594, 1982.

104. Vio CP, et al: Kallikrein excretion: relationship with maturation and renal function in human neonates at different gestational ages. Biol Neonate 52:121, 1987.

105. Bogaert GA, et al: Effects of endothelium-derived nitric oxide on renal hemodynamics and function in the sheep fetus. Pediatr Res 34:755, 1993.

106. Solhaug MJ, et al: Endothelium-derived nitric oxide modulates renal hemodynamics in the developing piglet. Pediatr Res 34:750, 1993.

107. Furchgott RF, Zawadzki JV: The obligatory role of endothelial cells in the relaxation of arterial smooth muscle by acetylcholine. Nature 288:373, 1980.

108. Bastron RD, Kaloyanides GJ: Effect of sodium nitroprusside on function in the isolated and intact dog kidney. J Pharmacol Exp Ther 181:244, 1972.

109. Persson PB: Nitric oxide in the kidney. Am J Physiol Regul Integr Comp Physiol 283:R1005, 2002.

110. DeBold AJ: Atrial natriuretic factor: an overview. Fed Proc 45:2081, 1986.

111. Walsh: Hormonal control of renal function during development. In Walsh (ed): Campbell's Textbook of Urology. Philadelphia, Elsevier Science, 2002, pp 1772–1774.

112. Cheung CY: Role of endogenous atrial natriuretic factor in the regulation of fetal cardiovascular and renal function. Am J Obstet Gynecol 165:1558, 1991.

113. Dodd A, et al: Ontogeny of ovine fetal renal atrial natriuretic factor receptors. Life Sci 54:1101, 1994.

114. Cheung CY, Roberts VJ: Developmental changes in atrial natriuretic factor content and localization of its messenger ribonucleic acid in ovine fetal heart. Am J Obstet Gynecol 169:1345, 1993.

115. Kikuchi K, et al: Ontogeny of atrial natriuretic polypeptide in the human heart. Acta Endocrinol 115:211, 1987.

116. Wei Y, et al: Developmental changes in the rat atriopeptin hormonal system. J Clin Invest 79:1325, 1987.

117. Wu J, et al: Perinatal expression of the atrial natriuretic factor gene in rat cardiac tissue. Am J Physiol 255:E388, 1988.

118. Scott JN, Jennes L: Distribution of atrial natriuretic factor in fetal rat atria and ventricles. Cell Tissue Res 248:479, 1987.

119. Toshimori H, et al: Immunohistochemical study of atrial natriuretic polypeptides in the embryonic, fetal and neonatal rat heart. Cell Tissue Res 248:627, 1987.

120. Smith FG, et al: Atrial natriuretic factor during fetal and postnatal life: a review. J Dev Physiol 12:55, 1989.

121. Robillard JE, et al: Ontogeny of the renal response to natriuretic peptide in sheep. Am J Physiol 254:F634, 1988.

122. Cheung CY, et al: Atrial natriuretic factor in maternal and fetal sheep. Am J Physiol 252:E279, 1987.

123. Ervin MG, et al: Ovine fetal and adult atrial natriuretic factor metabolism. Am J Physiol 254:R40, 1988.

124. Tulassay T, et al: Role of atrial natriuretic peptide in Na+ homeostasis in premature infants. J Physiol (Lond) 109:1023, 1986.

125. Brace RA, Cheung CY: Cardiovascular and fluid responses to atrial natriuretic factor in the sheep fetus. Am J Physiol 253:R561, 1987.

126. Varille VA, et al: Renal hemodynamic response to atrial natriuretic factor in fetal and newborn sheep. Pediatr Res 25:291, 1989.

127. Brace RA, et al: Fetal cardiovascular, endocrine, and fluid responses to atrial natriuretic factor infusion. Am J Physiol 257:R580, 1989.

128. Shine PF, et al: Action of atrial natriuretic peptide in the immature ovine kidney. Pediatr Res 22:11, 1987.

129. Fujino Y, et al: Ovine maternal and fetal glomerular atrial natriuretic factor receptors: response to dehydration. Biol Neonate 62:120, 1992.

130. Davenport AP, Battistini B: Classification of endothelin receptors and antagonists in clinical development. Clin Sci 103:1S, 2002.

131. Yanagisawa M, et al: Primary structure, synthesis, and biological activity of rat endothelin, an endothelium-derived vasoconstrictor peptide. Proc Natl Acad Sci USA 85:6964, 1988.

132. Goetz KL, et al: Cardiovascular, renal, and endocrine responses to intravenous endothelin in conscious dogs. Am J Physiol 255:R1064, 1988.

133. Emori T, et al: Secretory mechanism of immunoreactive endothelin in cultured bovine endothelial cells. Biochem Biophys Res Commun 160:93, 1989.

134. Cheung CY: Regulation of atrial natriuretic factor release by endothelin in ovine fetuses. Am J Physiol 267:R380, 1994.

135. Usuki S, et al: Increased maternal plasma concentration of endothelin-1 during labor pain or on delivery and the existence of a large amount of endothelin-1 in amniotic fluid. Gynecol Endocrinol 4:85, 1990.

136. Nisell H, et al: Maternal and fetal levels of a novel polypeptide, endothelin: evidence for release during pregnancy and delivery. Gynecol Obstet Invest 30:129, 1990.

137. Nakamura T, et al: Immunoreactive endothelin concentrations in maternal and fetal blood. Life Sci 46:1045, 1990.

138. Haegerstrand A, et al: Endothelin: presence in human umbilical vessels, high levels in fetal blood and potent constrictor effect. Acta Physiol Scand 137:541, 1989.

139. Han SP, et al: Effects of endothelin on regional haemodynamics in conscious rats. Eur J Pharmacol 159:303, 1989.

140. Rankin JHG, et al: Measurement of fetal renal inulin clearance in a chronic sheep preparation. J Appl Physiol 32:129, 1972.

141. Robillard JE, et al: Interrelationship between glomerular filtration rate and renal transport of Na+ and chloride during fetal life. Am J Obstet Gynecol 128:727, 1977.

142. Lumbers ER, Stevens AD: Factors influencing glomerular filtration rate in the fetal lamb. J Physiol (Lond) 298:28, 1979.

143. Robillard JE, et al: Maturational changes in the fetal glomerular filtration rate. Am J Obstet Gynecol 122:601, 1975.

144. Kesby GJ, Lumbers ER: Factors affecting renal handling of Na+, hydrogen ions, and bicarbonate by the fetus. Am J Physiol 251:F226, 1986.

145. Leake RD, et al: Inulin clearance in the newborn infant: relationship to gestational and postnatal age. Pediatr Res 10:759, 1976.

146. Guignard J-P, et al: Glomerular filtration rate in the first three weeks of life. J Pediatr 87:268, 1975.

147. Spitzer A, Brandis M: Functional and morphologic maturation of the superficial nephrons: relationship to total kidney function. J Clin Invest 53:279, 1974.

148. Merlet-Benichou C, deRouffignac C: Renal clearance studies in fetal and young guinea pigs: effect of salt loading. Am J Physiol 232:F178, 1977.

149. Kleinman LI, Lubbe RJ: Factors affecting the maturation of glomerular filtration rate and renal plasma flow in the newborn dog. J Physiol (Lond) 223:395, 1972.

150. Nakamura KT, et al: Renal hemodynamics and functional changes during the transition from fetal to newborn life in sheep. Pediatr Res 21:229, 1987.

151. Smith FG, Lumbers ER: Changes in renal function following delivery of the lamb by caesarian section. J Dev Physiol 10:145, 1988.

152. Smith FG, Lumbers ER: Comparison of renal function in term fetal sheep and newborn lambs. Biol Neonate 55:309, 1989.

153. Smith FG: Factors Influencing Fetal and Neonatal Fluid Balance. Ph.D. thesis, University of New South Wales, Sydney, Australia, 1987.

154. Dressler GR: Tubulogenesis in the developing mammalian kidney. Trends Cell Biol 12:390, 2002.

155. Lumbers ER: A brief review of fetal renal function. J Dev Physiol 6:1, 1983.

156. Robillard JE, et al: Role of aldosterone on renal Na+ and potassium excretion during fetal life and newborn period. Dev Pharmacol Ther 1:201, 1980.

157. Siegel SR, Oh W: Renal function as a marker of human fetal maturation. Acta Paediatr Scand 65:481, 1976.

158. Aperia A, et al: Sodium excretion in relation to Na+ intake and aldosterone excretion in newborn pre-term and full-term infants. Acta Paediatr Scand 68:813, 1979.

159. Spitzer A: The role of the kidney in Na+ homeostasis during maturation. Kidney Int 217:539, 1982.

160. Lumbers ER, et al: Proximal and distal tubular activity in chronically catheterized fetal sheep compared with the adult. Can J Physiol Pharmacol 66:697, 1988.

161. Bianchini L, Pouyssegur J: Na+/H+ exchangers: structure, function and regulation. In Schlondorff D, Bonventre J (eds): Molecular Biology of the Kidney in Health and Disease. New York, Marcel Dekker, 1995.

162. Orlowski J, et al: Molecular cloning of putative members of the Na/H exchanger gene family. J Biol Chem 267:9331, 1992.

163. Tse C-M, et al: Cloning and sequencing of a rabbit cDNA encoding an intestinal and kidney-specific Na+/H+ exchanger isoform (NHE-3). J Biol Chem 267:9340, 1992.

164. Tse C-M, et al: Cloning and expression of a rabbit cDNA encoding a serum-activated ethylisopropylamiloride-resistant epithelial Na+/H+ exchanger isoform (NHE-2). J Biol Chem 268:11917, 1993.

165. Biemesderfer D, et al: Immunocytochemical characterization of Na+-H+ exchanger isoform NHE-1 in rabbit kidney. Am J Physiol 263:F833, 1992.

166. Sardet C, et al: Molecular cloning, primary structure, and expression of the human growth factor-activatable Na+/H+ antiporter. Cell 56:271, 1989.

167. Bookstein C, et al: A unique Na+-hydrogen exchange isoform (NHE-4) of the inner medulla of the rat kidney is induced by hyperosmolarity. J Biol Chem 269:29704, 1994.

168. Beck JC, et al: Ontogeny of Na/H antiporter activity in rabbit renal brush border membrane vesicles. J Clin Invest 87:2067, 1991.

169. Guillery EN, et al: Maturation of proximal tubule Na+/H+ antiporter activity in sheep during the transition from fetus to newborn. Am J Physiol 267:F537, 1994.

170. Baum M, Quigley R: Glucocorticoids stimulate rabbit proximal convoluted tubule acidification. J Clin Invest 91:110, 1993.

171. Kinsella JL, et al: Glucocorticoid activation of Na+/H+ exchange in renal brush border vesicles: kinetic effects. Am J Physiol 248:F233, 1985.

172. Nathanielsz PW: Adrenocorticotropin. In Nathanielsz PW (ed): Fetal Endocrinology: An Experimental Approach. Amsterdam, North-Holland Publishing Company, 1976, pp 125–150.

173. Guillery EN, et al: Role of glucocorticoids in the maturation of renal cortical Na+/H+ exchanger activity during fetal life in sheep. Am J Physiol 268:F710, 1995.

174. Sweadner KJ: Isoenzymes of the Na+/K+-ATPase. Biochim Biophys Acta 988:185, 1989.

175. Ahn KY, et al: Differential expression and cellular distribution of mRNAs encoding alpha- and beta-isoforms of Na+-K+-ATPase in rat kidney. Am J Physiol 265:F792, 1993.

176. Tumlin JA, et al: Expression of Na-K-ATPase alpha- and beta-subunit mRNA and protein isoforms in the rat nephron. Am J Physiol 266:F240, 1994.
177. Orlowski J, Lingrel JB: Tissue-specific and developmental regulation of rat Na,K-ATPase catalytic alpha isoform and beta subunit mRNAs. J Biol Chem 263:10436, 1988.
178. Davis PW, Dixon RL: Selective postnatal development of Na, K-activated-adenosine triphosphatase in rabbit kidneys (35202). Proc Soc Exp Biol Med 136:95, 1979.
179. Fukuda Y, et al: Ontogeny of the regulation of Na+,K+-ATPase activity on the renal proximal tubule cell. Pediatr Res 30:131, 1991.
180. Schwartz GJ, Evan AP: Development of solute transport in rabbit proximal tubule: III. Na-K-ATPase activity. Am J Physiol 246:F845, 1984.
181. Schmidt U, Horster M: Na-K-activated ATPase: activity maturation in rabbit nephron segments dissected in vitro. Am J Physiol 233:F55, 1977.
182. Larsson SH, Aperia A: Renal growth in infancy and childhood—experimental studies of regulatory mechanisms. Pediatr Nephrol 5:439, 1991.
183. Fukuda Y, Aperia A: Differentiation of Na+-K+ pump in rat proximal tubule is modulated by Na+-H+ exchanger. Am J Physiol 255:F552, 1988.
184. Merlet-Benichou C, et al: Functional and morphologic patterns of renal maturation in the developing guinea pig. Am J Physiol 241:F618, 1981.
185. Robillard JE, et al: Maturation of the glucose transport process by the fetal kidney. Pediatr Res 12:680, 1978.
186. Arant BS Jr, et al: The renal reabsorption of glucose in the developing canine kidney: a study of glomerulotubular balance. Pediatr Res 8:638, 1974.
187. Lelievre-Pegorier M, Geloso JP: Ontogeny of sugar transport in fetal rat kidney. Biol Neonate 38:16, 1980.
188. Beck JC, et al: Characterisation of the fetal glucose transporter in rabbit kidney: comparison with the adult brush border electrogenic Na+-glucose symporter. J Clin Invest 82:379, 1988.
189. Alexander DP, Nixon DA: Plasma clearance of p-aminohippuric acid by the kidneys of foetal, neonatal and adult sheep. Nature 194:483, 1962.
190. Buddingh F, et al: Long-term studies of the functional development of the fetal kidney in sheep. Am J Vet Res 32:1993, 1971.
191. Elbourne I, Lumbers ER: Organic acid and base excretion by the fetal kidney (abstract). Proc Aust Phys Pharm Soc 18:15P, 1987.
192. Stevens AD, Lumbers ER: The relationship between plasma renin activity and renal electrolyte excretion in the fetal sheep. J Dev Physiol 3:101, 1981.
193. Robillard JE, et al: Influence of fetal extracellular volume contraction on renal reabsorption of bicarbonate in fetal lambs. Pediatr Res 11:649, 1977.
194. Hill KJ, Lumbers ER: Renal function in adult and fetal sheep. J Dev Physiol 10:149, 1988.
195. Robillard JE, et al: In vivo demonstration of renal carbonic anhydrase activity in the fetal lamb. Biol Neonate 34:253, 1978.
196. Lonnerholm G, Wistrand PJ: Carbonic anhydrase in the human fetal kidney. Pediatr Res 17:390, 1983.
197. Smith FG Jr, Schwartz A: Response to the intact lamb fetus to acidosis. Am J Obstet Gynecol 106:52, 1970.
198. Kesby GJ, Lumbers ER: The effects of metabolic acidosis on renal function of fetal sheep. J Physiol (Lond) 396:65, 1988.
199. Smith FG, Lumbers ER: Effects of maternal hyperglycemia on fetal renal function in sheep. Am J Physiol 255:F11, 1988.
200. Economou-Mavrou C, McCance RA: Calcium, magnesium and phosphorus in foetal tissues. Biochem J 68:573, 1958.
201. Smith FG Jr, et al: Parathyroid hormone in foetal and adult sheep: the effect of hypocalcemia. J Endocrinol 53:339, 1972.
202. Davicco MJ, et al: Parathyroid hormone-related peptide increases urinary phosphate excretion in fetal lambs. Exp Physiol 77:377, 1992.
203. Silverstein DM, et al: A growth-regulated renal mRNA induces phosphate transport in oocytes (abstract). Pediatr Res 37:370A, 1995.
204. Brace RA, Moore TR: Diurnal rhythms in fetal urine flow, vascular pressures, and heart rate in sheep. Am J Physiol 261:R1015, 1991.
205. Rabinowitz R, et al: Measurement of fetal urine production in normal pregnancy by real-time ultrasonography. Am J Obstet Gynecol 161:1264, 1989.
206. Lumbers ER, Stevens AD: Changes in fetal renal function in response to infusions of a hyperosmotic solution of mannitol to the ewe. J Physiol (Lond) 343:439, 1983.
207. Bell RJ, et al: Gestation-dependent aspects of the response of the ovine fetus to the osmotic stress induced by maternal water deprivation. Q J Exp Physiol 69:187, 1984.
208. Ross MG, et al: Maternal dehydration-rehydration: fetal plasma and urinary responses. Am J Physiol 255:E674, 1988.
209. Stevens AD, Lumbers ER: The effect of maternal fluid intake on the volume and composition of fetal urine. J Dev Physiol 7:161, 1985.
210. Woods LL, et al: Role of arginine vasopressin in fetal renal response to hypertonicity. Am J Physiol 251:F156, 1986.
211. Lingwood B, et al: The effects of antidiuretic hormone on urine flow and composition in the chronically cannulated ovine fetus. Q J Exp Physiol 63:315, 1978.
212. Lumbers ER, et al: Measurement of net transplacental transfer of fluid to the fetal sheep. J Physiol (Lond) 364:289, 1985.
213. Wintour EM, et al: The value of urine osmolality as an index of stress in the ovine fetus. J Dev Physiol 7:347, 1985.
214. Rees L, et al: Continuous urine collection in the study of vasopressin in the newborn. Horm Res 17:134, 1983.
215. Froger JL, et al: Antidiuretic activity in the fetal and newborn rabbit hypophysis. Biol Neonate 30:224, 1976.
216. Levina SE: Endocrine features in development of human hypothalamus, hypophysis and placenta. Gen Comp Endocrinol 11:151, 1968.
217. Leake RD, et al: Maternal fetal osmolar homeostasis: fetal posterior pituitary autonomy. Pediatr Res 13:841, 1979.
218. Weitzman RE, et al: Arginine vasopressin response to an osmotic stimulus in the fetal sheep. Pediatr Res 12:35, 1978.
219. Rurak DW: Plasma vasopressin levels during haemorrhage in mature and immature fetal sheep. J Dev Physiol 1:91, 1979.
220. Rurak DW: Plasma vasopressin levels during hypoxemia and the cardiovascular effects of exogenous vasopressin in foetal and adult sheep. J Physiol (Lond) 277:341, 1978.
221. Siegel SR, et al: Effects of furosemide and acute salt loading on vasopressin and renin secretion in the fetal lamb. Pediatr Res 14:869, 1980.
222. Joppich R, et al: Effect of antidiuretic hormone and dibutyryl cAMP upon the urinary concentrating capacity in neonatal piglets. Pediatr Res 14:1234, 1980.
223. Schlondorff D, et al: Vasopressin responsiveness of renal adenylate cyclase in newborn rats and rabbits. Am J Physiol 234:F16, 1978.
224. Wintour EM, et al: Regulation of urine osmolality in fetal sheep. Q J Exp Physiol 67:427, 1982.
225. Ervin MG, et al: Vascular effects alter early-gestation fetal renal responses to vasopressin. Am J Physiol 266:R722, 1994.
226. Ervin MG, et al: V1 and V2 receptor contributions to ovine fetal renal and cardiovascular responses to vasopressin. Am J Physiol 262:R636, 1992.
227. Agre P, et al: Aquaporin CHIP: the archetypal molecular water channel. Am J Physiol 265:F463, 1993.
228. Fushimi K, et al: Cloning and expression of apical membrane water channel of rat kidney collecting tubule. Nature 361:549, 1993.
229. Sasaki S, et al: Cloning, characterization and chromosomal mapping of human aquaporin of collecting duct. J Clin Invest 93:1250, 1994.
230. Hayashi M, et al: Expression and distribution of aquaporin of collecting duct are regulated by vasopressin V2 receptor in rat kidney. J Clin Invest 94:1778, 1994.
231. Baum MA, et al: The perinatal expression of aquaporin-2 (AQP-2) in developing rat kidney (abstract). Pediatr Res 37:359A, 1995.
232. Bayard F, et al: Transplacental passage and fetal secretion of aldosterone. J Clin Invest 49:1389, 1970.
233. Siegel SR, et al: Transplacental transfer of aldosterone and its effects on renal function in the fetal lamb. Pediatr Res 15:163, 1981.
234. Giry J, Delost P: Placental transfer of aldosterone in the guinea-pig during late pregnancy. J Steroid Biochem 10:541, 1979.
235. Wintour EM, et al: Placental transfer of aldosterone in the sheep. J Endocrinol 86:305, 1980.
236. Robillard JE, et al: Effects of aldosterone on urinary kallikrein and Na+ excretion during fetal life. Pediatr Res 190:1048, 1985.
237. Lingwood B, et al: Effect of aldosterone on urine composition in the chronically cannulated ovine foetus. J Endocrinol 76:553, 1978.
238. Ganong WF, Mulrow PJ: Rate of change in Na+ and potassium excretion after injection of aldosterone into the aorta and renal artery of the dog. Am J Physiol 195:337, 1958.
239. Ito Y, et al: The role of aldosterone in renal electrolyte transport during development (abstract). Pediatr Res 18:370A, 1984.
240. Horisberger J-D, Diezi J: Effects of mineralocorticoids on Na+ and K+ excretion in the adrenalectomized rat. Am J Physiol 245:F89, 1983.
241. Robillard JE, et al: Renal and adrenal responses to converting-enzyme inhibition in fetal and newborn life. Am J Physiol 244:R249, 1983.
242. Walker DW, Mitchell MD: Prostaglandins in urine of foetal lambs. Nature 271:161, 1978.
243. Hargrave BY, et al: Renal and cardiovascular effects of atrial natriuretic peptide in fetal sheep. Pediatr Res 26:1, 1989.
244. Castro R, et al: Fetal renal response to atrial natriuretic factor decreases with maturation. Am J Physiol 260:R346, 1991.
245. Hill KJ, et al: The actions of cortisol on fetal renal function. J Dev Physiol 10:85, 1988.
246. Wintour EM, et al: Cortisol is natriuretic in the immature ovine fetus. J Endocrinol 106:R13, 1985.
247. Dobrovic-Jenik D, Milkovic S: Regulation of fetal Na+/K+-ATPase in rat kidney by corticosteroids. Biochim Biophys Acta 942:227, 1988.
248. Slotkin TA, et al: Fetal dexamethasone exposure accelerates development of renal function: relationship to dose, cell differentiation and growth inhibition. J Dev Physiol 17:55, 1992.

Michael J. Solhaug and Pedro A. Jose

127

Postnatal Maturation of Renal Blood Flow

Newborn mammals, including humans, exhibit lower renal blood flow when compared with their adult counterparts.[1,2] The low neonatal renal blood flow is maintained by a high renal vascular resistance and establishes the newborn's unique renal functional state characterized by a low glomerular filtration rate. The unique renal hemodynamic state at birth affects the clinical management of the newborn. The low renal blood flow and resultant low glomerular filtration rate contribute to the newborn's altered pharmacokinetics of renally excreted medications,[3] as well as avid tubular sodium reabsorption in the distal nephron, which blunts the ability to excrete an acute saline load in the term infant.[4] The newborn's renal hemodynamic state modifies the development and severity of pathophysiologic conditions, such as acute renal failure resulting from adverse perinatal events and the complications of respiratory distress syndrome.[5] Gaining an understanding of the regulation of renal blood flow in the newborn may provide insights into creating therapies directed at the prevention and treatment of pathologic conditions in the neonate.

The postnatal maturation of renal hemodynamics involves a progressive increase in renal blood flow to reach adult capability.[1,6-8] The major factor influencing the maturational increase in renal blood flow is the synchronous drop in renal vascular resistance, which occurs most notably in the immediate postnatal period.[7,9] Renal blood flow in the postnatal developing kidney is influenced by structural factors, such as the number of existing vascular channels, as well as functional factors, offered by the glomerular resistance vessels.[10] Several studies confirmed that, in the developing kidney, the functional maintenance of vascular tone (principally through a balance of vasoactive factors) is the paramount mechanism of the modulation of renal hemodynamics.[11-13] The maturational changes in renal blood flow and renal vascular resistance must proceed normally to achieve adult capability for fully integrated renal-cardiovascular homeostasis. Disruption of the maturation of renal hemodynamics may lead to inadequate renal-cardiovascular function in the adult and may produce pathologic conditions such as hypertension.

CHARACTERISTICS OF RENAL BLOOD FLOW IN THE IMMATURE KIDNEY

Total Renal Blood Flow

In most mammalian species, renal blood flow in the neonate is lower than in the adult when compared on the basis of body weight, kidney weight, or surface area.[1] In human newborns and infants, total renal blood flow has been determined by the clearance of *p*-aminohippurate (PAH), which measures effective renal plasma flow (ERPF)[6] and by Doppler ultrasonography.[14,15] Renal blood flow measured by Doppler and ERPF by clearance of PAH is lowest in newborns, and it correlates with gestational age. The increase in renal blood flow after birth in preterm infants is influenced by postconceptional rather than postnatal age. ERPF increases from 20 ml/minute/1.73 m^2 at 30 weeks' gestation to 45 ml/minute/1.73 m^2 by 35 weeks' gestation and 83 ml/minute/1.73 m^2 at term gestation.[16] During the first 3 months of postnatal life, ERPF increases rapidly to 300 ml/minute/1.73 m.^{2} Thereafter, ERPF increases gradually, reaching values of 650 ml/minute/1.73 m^2 by 12 to 24 months of age (Fig. 127-1).[6,17] However, the clearance of PAH underestimates ERPF in the neonatal period because the renal extraction of PAH is only 60% during the first 3 months of age compared with 95% by 5 months of age.[18] The low renal extraction of PAH in the neonate[9,19,20] has been attributed to shunting of blood to non–PAH-extracting tissues (e.g., relatively greater medullary blood flow, intracortical efferent arteriovenous shunting).

Intrarenal Blood Flow

The renal vasculature is characterized by two capillary networks—the glomerular and peritubular capillary systems—linked in series with each other. The major sites of renal vascular resistance are the glomerular arterioles. Blood enters the glomerulus via the afferent arteriole that arises from the interlobular artery, and it exits via the efferent arteriole. Vasoconstriction or vasodilation at these sites regulates blood flow to the glomerulus (hence, glomerular filtration rate) as well as the intrarenal distribution between the cortex, which contains all the glomeruli, and the medulla, which contains vasa recta and tubules but not glomeruli. In the mature kidney, the afferent arteriole of inner cortical nephrons accounts for the entire preglomerular resistance to blood flow, whereas in superficial cortical nephrons, the interlobular arteries offer the largest resistance to blood flow.[21,22] Blood flow to each region of the kidney (cortical, medullary, and papillary) increases with maturation.[9,20,23-27] The distribution of intrarenal blood flow in the young, however, is different from that reported in adults. The neonatal kidney has a greater percentage of blood flow to the inner cortical and medullary areas than does the adult kidney. The low extraction ratio of PAH in infants younger than 3 months of age may be related to a relatively greater perfusion of juxtamedullary nephrons. As total renal blood flow reaches adult levels with maturation, a greater fraction of renal blood flow is received by the outer cortical nephrons. The duration of this maturational period varies from species to species.

Autoregulation of Renal Blood Flow in the Young

The mature kidney exhibits autoregulation; that is, renal blood flow remains constant even though renal perfusion pressure (determined by mean arterial pressure) varies throughout a range from low to high. Autoregulation depends on intrarenal mechanisms and is modulated by intrarenal factors. In the newborn, the range of autoregulation is set at lower perfusion pressures than seen in the adult, and the renal pressure-flow relationship changes with renal growth.[28-31] Autoregulation of renal blood flow is less efficient in the young than in the adult. Furthermore, uninephrectomy impairs the autoregulatory response in young rats but does not affect this response in adult rats. This reduced autoregulatory efficiency in the neonate is apparently the result of prostaglandin-dependent renin release, which causes vasoconstriction at lower levels of perfusion pressure.[29]

Maturational relationships between tubular flow and glomerular filtration rate (tubuloglomerular feedback) also occur with growth. The tubuloglomerular feedback mechanism is maximally sensitive at a tubular flow range that corresponds to the normal operating range. As the glomerular filtration rate increases with maturation, the maximal response and flow range

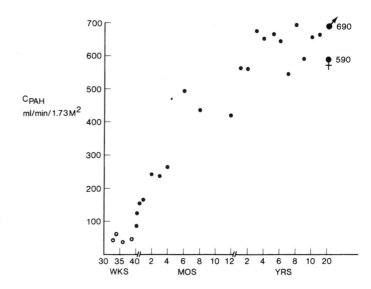

Figure 127–1. The clearance of *p*-aminohippurate (C_{PAH}) with age. (From Rubin MI, et al: Reproduced from the Journal of Clinical Investigation *28*:1144-1162, 1949, by copyright permission of the American Society for Clinical Investigation.)

also increase so the relative sensitivity of the tubuloglomerular feedback mechanism is unaltered during growth.[32] The relative roles of endothelial cell, smooth muscle, and tubuloglomerular feedback have not been defined in the developing animal.

REGULATION OF POSTNATAL RENAL HEMODYNAMICS

The low renal blood flow of the neonate and the increase that occurs with maturation are the result of a combination of effects, including alterations in cardiac output, perfusion pressure, and renal vascular resistance. Lower cardiac output and perfusion pressure may partially account for the decreased renal blood flow noted in the newborn infant. In the dog, however, cardiac output corrected for body weight is highest in the youngest puppies, which also have the lowest renal blood flow per body weight.[20, 33] The proportion of cardiac output distributed to the kidneys is about 4 to 6% in the first 12 hours of life and increases to 8 to 10% in the first week of life. In comparison, 25% of cardiac output is distributed to the kidneys in the normal adult. Systemic vascular resistance decreases markedly after birth. This may cause a redistribution of blood flow to organs other than the kidney and may immediately contribute to the low neonatal renal blood flow. Systemic vascular resistance gradually increases with maturation and therefore is not a factor in the increase in renal blood flow with age. Renal vascular resistance, however, is the most important regulating component contributing to postnatal renal hemodynamics. Gruskin and colleagues[7] demonstrated that, in the developing piglet, the major factor influencing the maturational increase in renal blood flow was an 86% decrease in renal vascular resistance. Renal vascular resistance in the developing kidney is influenced by *structural* factors, the number and size of vascular channels, as well as by *functional* vasoactive factors, the modulators of the resistance offered by the glomerular arterioles (Fig. 127–2).[10, 34, 35]

Role of Anatomic Development

The contribution of structural changes to the maturational changes of renal vascular resistance in the developing kidney is an important consideration. Renal vascular resistance in the developing kidney is a function of the number of existing vascular channels, as well as the arteriolar resistance offered by each channel.[10, 34, 35] The main structural development that could influence renal hemodynamics postnatally is the addition of vascular channels by nephrogenesis, resulting in a decrease in renal vascular resistance. The increase in renal blood flow after birth is

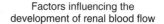

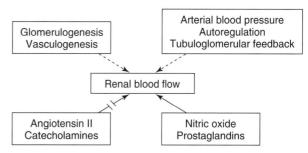

Figure 127–2. Factors that influence the development of renal blood flow include anatomic factors (glomerulogenesis and vasculogenesis), physical factors (arterial blood pressure, myogenic autoregulatory response), and vasoactive factors (autoregulation, tubuloglomerular feedback, angiotensin II, catecholamines, renal nerves, nitric oxide, and prostaglandins). Other vasoactive agents can regulate renal blood flow; however, renal vascular resistance in the newborn regulated by vasoactive agents is probably the result of a balance between the vasoconstrictor influences of angiotensin II and catecholamines or renal nerves and the vasodilatory influences of nitric oxide and prostaglandins.

caused by development and formation of new glomeruli and vascular remodeling. This increase may play a role in the postnatal renal hemodynamic development of several of the mammalian species in which nephrogenesis continues after birth, such as canines, swine, and rodents. Renal blood flow, however, continues to increase in these species long after glomerulogenesis has completed.[6, 19, 20, 36] In addition, the increase in the diameter of resistance vessels during maturation is greater in the kidneys than in other organs.[37] Evan and colleagues,[34] in studies in canine puppies, revealed substantial differences, both quantitative and qualitative, between neonatal and adult renal vasculature.[10] However, morphologic changes in renal resistance vessels cannot account for the rapid decreases in renal vascular resistance that occur in the period of renal hemodynamic maturation. Specifically, in humans, nephrogenesis is completed at 34 weeks' gestation, yet renal blood flow continues to rise and renal vascular resistance continues to decrease with postnatal age, a finding indicating that the functional vasoactive characteristics of the immature renal vessels determine this alteration. Several studies confirmed the major contribution of the functional vasoactive attributes of the developing renal vasculature in altering renal blood flow.[9, 12, 13, 38, 39] Thus, although structural development may contribute to the changes in developing kidney by decreasing renal vascular resistance during nephrogenesis, the functional vasoactive changes of the resistance vessels are the main factors producing the maturational changes in renal hemodynamics.

Role of Vasoactive Factors

High renal vascular resistance accounts for the low renal blood flow at birth, and the increase in renal blood flow with maturation mainly results from the progressive reduction in renal vascular resistance.[7, 9, 11, 13, 19, 20] Vasoactive factors modulate renal blood flow through the alteration of renal vascular resistance by (1) the extent of participation of resistance vessels (interlobular artery and afferent and efferent arterioles, (2) the intrinsic properties of immature resistance renal vasculature, and (3) neurohormonal factors unique to the immature kidney. The site of high renal vascular resistance in the newborn animal has been localized mainly to the preglomerular resistance vasculature, the interlobular artery, and the afferent arteriole.[40] In older animals, increases in renal blood flow are associated with a decrease in resistance in all the glomerular vessels: the interlobular, afferent, and efferent arterioles.[8] The decrease in renal vascular resistance with age may be modulated by developmental changes in the intrinsic properties of the renal resistance vasculature. However, little is known about the myogenic internal vasoactive capabilities of these vessels or about any developmental differences in resistance vessel responsiveness to vasoactive factors. Ultimately, the characteristics of postnatal renal hemodynamics are considered to be a balance of neurohormonal vasoactive factors. Both the vasoconstrictors and the vasodilators producing this immature renal condition have differing effects, intrarenal levels, and sites of action compared with the mature adult. Several vasoactive agents participate in the regulation of renal blood flow in the postnatal maturing kidney, including adenosine, arginine vasopressin (AVP), angiotensin II, atrial and other natriuretic peptides, bradykinin, endothelin, nitric oxide (NO), prostaglandins, renal nerves, and the adrenergic nervous system.

Adenosine

The intrarenal vasodilator action of adenosine has been implicated as an important mediator of tubuloglomerular feedback in the adult, and it may play a role in protection of the outer medulla from hypoxia. Tubuloglomerular feedback is important in the renal autoregulation of glomerular filtration rate and blood flow. Adenosine, formed by the breakdown of adenosine triphosphate, can be a renal vasodilator. Several adenosine receptor subtypes have been cloned: A_1, A_{2A}, A_{2B}, and A_3.[41] In the adult, adenosine decreases the glomerular filtration rate and increases renal blood flow apparently by reducing efferent vascular resistance.[42-44] In one study, intrarenal adenosine reduced cortical blood flow via adenosine A_1 receptors and increased medullary blood flow via adenosine A_2 receptors.[45] The stimulation of renal adenosine A_1 receptors is associated with inhibition of renin release and constriction of afferent arterioles, whereas adenosine A_2 receptors promote renin release and dilate afferent and efferent arterioles. Xanthines block all the adenosine receptor subtypes. In the adult, methylxanthines produce no consistent change in renal blood flow. Theophylline, however, via its adenosine receptor blocking property (independent of phosphodiesterase inhibition), increases renal vascular resistance in newborn rabbits.[46] The role of adenosine receptors in the control of renal blood flow during development remains to be determined. It is possible that adenosine A_2 receptors may act to modulate the high neonatal renal vascular resistance.[47]

Arginine Vasopressin

AVP functions as an intrarenal vasoconstrictor. There are three major AVP receptor subtypes: V_{1a}, V_{1b}, and V_2.[41] The V_2 receptors found in collecting ducts of the kidney increase hydraulic conductivity. V_{1a} receptors in arterioles mediate vasoconstriction, whereas V_{1b} receptors in pituitary corticotrophs and the limbic system may mediate corticotroph responsiveness and control of emotional processes. In conscious dogs, AVP has been shown to vasodilate the kidney via V_2 receptors.[48] AVP has the potential to contribute to the increased renal vascular resistance present in the neonate through its action on vascular and glomerular V_1 receptors. The role it plays in regulating basal renal hemodynamics remains to be defined. Infusion of synthetic AVP does not alter renal blood flow and renal vascular resistance in fetal sheep. AVP may still play a role, however, in certain stress-induced reductions in renal hemodynamics. For example, the marked decrease in renal blood flow and renal vascular resistance has been closely correlated with the rise in plasma AVP during hemorrhage but not with hypoxemia.[49]

Angiotensin II

The highly activated renin-angiotensin system, through the vasoconstriction of angiotensin II, contributes to the high renal vascular resistance in the very immature kidney.[26, 50-54] Circulating renin and angiotensin II levels are high in most neonatal mammals, including humans, and they decrease with age.[51, 53, 54] Although angiotensin II has been thought to be an important vasoconstrictor in the developing renal vasculature,[55] it has been difficult to demonstrate a role for angiotensin II in the increased renal vascular resistance in the immature kidney. Systemic infusion of an angiotensin-converting enzyme inhibitor in conscious fetal and newborn sheep produced similar decreases in mean arterial pressure in both age groups. However, inhibition of the converting enzyme in newborn sheep—although decreasing renal vascular resistance—did not change renal blood flow.[56] Osborn and colleagues in piglets,[57] and Jose and colleagues in puppies,[30] were unable to demonstrate significant alterations in either renal vascular resistance or renal blood flow with administration of the nonselective angiotensin receptor antagonist saralasin. The role of the renin-angiotensin system in the regulation of developing renal hemodynamics has been clarified with the use of nonpeptide antagonists of angiotensin II receptors. There are four angiotensin II receptors: AT1, AT2, AT3, and AT4.[41] In rodents, there are two AT1 receptors: AT1a and AT1b. AT1a and AT2 receptors are differentially expressed during development. AT2 but not AT1 receptors are expressed in the very immature fetal structures, a finding implicating a role in nephrogenesis.[54, 58-60] Angiotensin II, perhaps via AT1 but more probably via the AT2 receptor, may be involved in fetal renal development including angiogenesis. The AT2 receptor gene is expressed to the greatest extent in fetal kidneys; its expression decreases rapidly after birth in the rat.[58, 60-63] In young rats treated with the angiotensin-converting enzyme inhibitor enalapril, the normal increase in glomerular surface area associated with maturation is inhibited.[64] Abnormalities in renal development are noted in human infants and neonatal rats treated with angiotensin-converting enzyme inhibitors. In neonatal rats, AT1, but not AT2, receptor antagonists produce renal defects similar to those noted with angiotensin-converting enzyme inhibitors, a finding further attesting to the importance of this receptor subtype in kidney development.[55, 60, 61, 65, 66] However, disruption of both AT1 and AT2 receptors can lead to malformations of the kidney and urinary tract.[60] AT1 receptors, which mediate vasoconstriction, are expressed at later stages in the glomerulus, resistance arterioles, and medulla,[58, 67] including the period of hemodynamic development. The intrarenal infusion of a non–peptide-specific AT1 receptor antagonist produces greater increases in renal blood flow in newborn piglets, a finding suggesting that angiotensin II is a more important renal vasoconstrictor in the 3-week-old developing piglet than the adult pig.[55] AT2 receptors, in contrast, may be vasodilatory.[68] This may explain the inability of angiotensin-converting enzyme inhibition to affect renal blood flow in newborn piglets.[69] Thus, angiotensin II, via the AT1 receptor, plays an important role in the regulation of renal blood flow in the immediate postnatal period, whereas other factors such as the adrenergic receptors may become more important later during development (see later). In contrast to the apparently increased vasoconstrictor effect of angiotensin II, via AT1 receptors in the immediate neonatal period, angiotensin II may actually be needed to maintain glomerular filtration rate in the neonatal rabbit. Interruption of the renin-angiotensin system in neonatal rabbits decreases glomerular filtration rate without affecting renal blood flow.[70]

Atrial and Other Natriuretic Peptides

There are several natriuretic peptides: atrial natriuretic peptide (ANP), brain natriuretic peptide (BNP), and C-type natriuretic peptide (CNP).[71] ANP and BNP (originally described in brain) are produced in the atria and ventricles, whereas CNP is found mainly in the brain, pituitary gland, vascular endothelium, kidney, and female genitourinary tract. ANP is present in both atria and ventricles of the fetus in several species, and circulating levels of this peptide in plasma are significantly elevated compared with those of the adult.[72-74] Within the first few weeks of life, however, the plasma concentrations of ANP fall to adult levels. During the early developmental period, the release of ANP appears to respond to various stimuli that are associated with volume overload. The most important vascular and renal effects of ANP in mature animals are as follows: (1) vasodilation and decrease in mean blood pressure; (2) increase in renal blood flow, glomerular filtration rate, and filtration fraction; (3) inhibition of sodium and water reabsorption in both proximal and distal tubules; and (4) decreased concentrating ability. Although ANP may play a role in sodium and volume homeostasis during the perinatal period, its role in the regulation of renal hemodynamics is uncertain. In rabbits, clear age differences in the renal response to intravenous infusions of α-human ANP have been noted. In response to ANP, newborn rabbits demonstrate a decrease in diuresis and kaliuresis and no change in natriuresis, whereas an immediate increase in diuresis, natriuresis, and kaliuresis occurs in adult rabbits.[75] The infusion of recombinant ANP into fetal sheep results in minimal declines in mean arterial blood pressure. In contrast, significant decreases in blood pressure and increments in heart rate have been observed in newborn and adult sheep during continuous infusion of pharmacologic doses of ANP. ANP reduces renal blood flow in fetal and newborn sheep. This effect, however, decreases with maturation,[76] and its significance is not clear. Several natriuretic peptide receptors have been cloned: NPR-A, NPR-B, NPR-C, and NPR-D.[77] ANP and BNP bind to NPR-A, whereas CNP binds to NPR-B receptors. Both receptors generate cyclic guanosine monophosphate; NPR-C, which has an equal affinity to all the natriuretic peptides, is not linked to cyclic guanosine monophosphate. NPR-C acts as a clearance receptor to regulate circulating levels of natriuretic peptides but may also generate NO. NPR-D has been identified only in eels. Systemic clearance of ANP is increased in the newborn and decreases with development.[78] The decreased effects of ANP in the newborn period cannot be explained by increased clearance of ANP or by decreased production of cyclic guanosine monophosphate.[79]

Bradykinin

Bradykinin is the major functional vasodilator produced by the kallikrein-kinin system. Bradykinin exerts its effects via B₁ and B₂ receptors.[41] Under physiologic conditions, most of the effects of bradykinin are mediated by the B_2 receptor. NO may, in part, mediate the vasodilation of bradykinin.[80, 81] Kallikreins are proteinases that liberate vasoactive kinins from the protein precursor kininogen. The bradykinin-synthesizing enzyme, kininase II, is identical to angiotensin-converting enzyme, which produces angiotensin II. Although bradykinin may play a role in renal morphogenesis,[82-84] the role of this vasodilator in the renal hemodynamics is less certain. Several studies indirectly suggest that bradykinin may participate in the maturational increase in renal blood flow. Urinary kallikrein excretion corrected for either renal mass or glomerular filtration rate increases with maturation.[85, 86] Kininase II mRNA and enzymatic activity are low in newborn rat kidney and peak at 2 to 3 weeks of age.[87] However, studies have failed to demonstrate a significant role for bradykinin in immature renal hemodynamics. Newborn and 6-week-old lambs failed to show any renal hemodynamic response to acute intrarenal injection of a selective kinin B_2 antagonist.[88] Long-term administration of the same B_2 antagonist to neonatal rats from birth to 3 weeks did not alter the maturational increase in renal blood flow.[89] The possibility remains, however, that bradykinin opposes the basal vasoconstriction of angiotensin II in the immature rat kidney.[89]

Endothelin

Endothelin, one of the vasoconstricting factors produced by the endothelium, is one of the most potent endogenous vasoconstrictor, second only to urotensin II. There are three different endothelin peptides encoded by three distinct genes: endothelin-1 (ET-1), endothelin-2 (ET-2), and endothelin-3 (ET-3). ET-1 produces renal vasoconstriction in both the afferent and efferent arterioles. Two ET receptors, ETA and ETB, mediate endothelin action in the kidney. However, it is most likely that ETA receptors facilitate the ET-1 vasoconstrictor action; endothelins can also mediate vasodilation.[90, 91] On the basis of pharmacologic evidence, two types of ETB receptors have been postulated: ETB1, which is a relaxant; and ETB2, which is a constrictor. In ETB knock out mice, both vasodilatory and vasoconstrictor effects of ETB receptors were eliminated, a finding suggesting that the ETB1 and ETB2 receptors are the same receptor.[90] The differences in ETB1 and ETB2 actions are related to the sites where these receptors are expressed. Thus, ETB (ETB1) receptors expressed in endothelial cells (tunica intima) cause vasodilation because of their linkage to NO and prostaglandins, whereas ETB receptors expressed in vascular smooth muscle cells (tunica media) cause vasoconstriction.[92,93] In full-term infants, the urinary excretion of ET-1 remains constant in the first month of life; in premature infants, ET-1 excretion increases with maturation such that, after the first week, postnatal values exceed those found in older children.[94] In newborn rabbits, ET-1 failed to change renal hemodynamics at doses that decreased renal blood flow in adults; however, at higher doses, exogenous endothelin induced a marked reduction in renal blood flow and glomerular filtration rate in the newborn as well.[95] Blockade of endogenous ET-1 activity in newborn rabbits by ET-1 antiserum increased renal vascular resistance and decreased renal blood flow.[96] These studies suggest that ET-1 may not be responsible for the increased renal vascular resistance in the newborn period. Rather, ET-1, via endothelial ETB, may function as a renal vasodilator to counteract the vasoconstrictor effects of other systems (e.g., angiotensin II and catecholamines). The finding that ETA and ETB blockade in the newborn increases renal blood flow but does not affect glomerular filtration indicates that endothelin is probably not an important factor in the increase of renal blood flow with age.[97]

Nitric Oxide

NO is an important endogenous regulator of renal hemodynamics in the immature kidney, and it functions as a critical vasodilator to counterbalance highly activated vasoconstrictors, such as

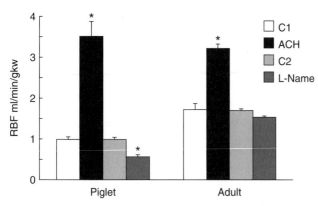

Figure 127–3. Comparison of the renal blood flow (RBF) responses in immature and adult renal vasculature to vasoactive agents that act on the nitric oxide (NO) synthesizing enzyme, nitric oxide synthase (NOS). RBF responses were directly measured by electromagnetic flow probe in anesthetized 3-week-old piglets and adults ($n = 4$) during the sequential intrarenal infusions of NOS stimulation with acetylcholine, 0.05 μg/kg/minute (ACH), and NOS inhibition with L-NAME, 3 μg/kg/minute (L-NAME) with interval control periods (C1 and C2). The immature kidney demonstrates lower baseline RBF in both control periods. RBF responses were greater in the immature kidney to NOS stimulation, ACH, and inhibition, L-NAME. gkw = gram kidney weight. *$p < .05$ versus others within each group. (Modified from Solhaug MJ, et al: Pediatr Nephrol *10*:529, 1996.)

angiotensin II.[55] The immature renal vasculature is highly responsive to alterations of the NO synthesizing enzyme, NO synthase (NOS). Figure 127–3 demonstrates the renal blood flow responses of the 3-week-old piglet to sequential intrarenal infusions of acetylcholine, an NOS stimulator, and L-NAME, an arginine analogue that competitively inhibits NOS.[12] Several reports identify NO as a vital participant in postnatal developing renal hemodynamics under physiologic and pathophysiologic conditions.[12,98,99] The intrarenal infusion of the NOS inhibitor, L-NAME, in both whole animals (3-week-old piglets and newborn lambs)[36,100] and isolated perfused kidneys (newborn rabbits),[101] produces greater renal hemodynamic responses than the adult. These data suggest that renal NO production by NOS is greater in young animals than in adults. This increased NO production is supported by the distinct developmental patterns in the postnatal maturing porcine kidney of two NOS isoforms: neuronal NOS in the macula densa and endothelial NOS in the glomerular resistance arterioles. The ability of NO to counteract the effects of vasoconstrictor agents under physiologic conditions suggests that NO may be even more important in pathologic conditions (e.g., perinatal hypoxemia).[99] In newborn rabbits, the renal blood flow responses to L-NAME are significantly greater during hypoxemia. These conditions induce an intense renal vasoconstriction, mediated by angiotensin II, often resulting in vasomotor acute renal failure.[5] Thus, NO may serve to protect the immature kidney from the deleterious effects of adverse perinatal events that lead to vasomotor acute renal failure.

Prostaglandins

Arachidonic acid is an essential fatty acid that is metabolized through different pathways: 5-lipoxygenase leads to formation of leukotrienes, 15-lipoxygenase leads to formation of lipoxins, cytochrome P450 leads to formation of epoxy-20:3, and cyclooxygenase (COX) leads to formation of prostaglandins and thromboxanes. In rats, arachidonic acid metabolism in the kidney shifts from a lipoxygenase-dependent to a cytochrome

P450–dependent pathway during development.[102] Two COX isoforms are present in the kidney: COX-1 and COX-2. COX-1 is found in the renal vasculature, glomeruli, and collecting ducts across species lines.[103] However, COX-2 intrarenal localization is species dependent. In rats and dogs, COX-2 localizes to tubules, macula densa, and thick ascending limb of the loop of Henle, whereas in humans, COX-2 co-localizes with COX-1.[104,105] Several therapeutic agents such as nonsteroidal antiinflammatory drugs, including aspirin and indomethacin, nonselectively inhibit both COX-1 and COX-2. The selective COX-2 inhibitors celecoxib and rofecoxib have been developed. Although COX-1 may not undergo postnatal regulation, COX-2 is highest after birth (between 1 and 2 weeks in rats) and declines with age.[103,106-108] COX-2 involvement in nephrogenesis may contribute to renal dysgenesis syndromes associated with COX inhibition. In fetal kidneys, COX-2 strongly localizes to tubular structures, which differ from the adult.[98,99] Selective COX-2 inhibition leads to disruption of nephrogenesis in both mice and rats.[109] Genetic ablation of COX-2 results in severe morphologic abnormalities, including impaired glomerulogenesis, cortical dysplasia, and diffuse tubular cyst formation.[110] These studies confirm the teratogenic potential of prenatal use of nonsteroidal antiinflammatory drugs and selective COX-2 inhibitors leading to acute renal failure and renal dysgenesis.[111-113]

In spite of the increasing information about the role of COX isoforms in nephrogenesis, the functional vasoactive role of the COX products (prostaglandins) in the immature kidney is uncertain. In fact, the relation of specific COX isoforms to renal function is not well understood. In general, thromboxanes and leukotrienes vasoconstrict the kidney, whereas prostaglandins and lipoxins vasodilate it. Cytochrome P450 metabolites of arachidonic acid can act as vasoconstrictors or vasodilators. Renal prostaglandin production is increased during the perinatal period. In preterm infants, the urinary excretion of prostaglandin E and a prostacyclin metabolite is five times that noted at term and is 20 times greater than that observed in physiologically normal children.[113] Glomerular prostaglandin synthesis and adenylate cyclase response to prostaglandin E_2 also decrease with maturation.[114,115] Moreover, when prostaglandin synthesis is inhibited by indomethacin in the unstressed adult or neonate, blood flow is either unchanged or redistributed to the outer cortex. Therefore, if prostaglandin synthesis was deficient in the newborn infant, one could expect a pattern of blood flow converse to that normally found in the neonatal kidney.[57] Likewise, the increased renal blood flow found in the uninephrectomized young rat is not maintained by increased prostaglandin or decreased thromboxane effects.[29] Although neonatal rabbits may be more sensitive to the vasoconstrictor effects of acetylsalicylic acid,[116] prostaglandin inhibition does not alter basal renal blood flow in the immature piglet kidney.[12] Moreover, the COX inhibitor ibuprofen does not affect renal blood flow in preterm neonates.[117] Thus, in the newborn, as in adults, prostaglandins play little or no role in the control of renal blood flow in the normal animal at rest. Prostaglandins may, however, attenuate renal vasoconstriction in pathologic conditions. In contrast, prostaglandins may be important in the fetus in the regulation of renal blood flow under both basal and stress conditions.[118] In young and adult rats, the major pathway of arachidonic acid metabolism in glomeruli occurs via the lipoxygenase pathway[114]; however, the effects of this pathway on basal renal blood flow during development remain to be determined. Moreover, the renal development of the eight prostanoid receptors has not been determined.[41,119]

Renal Nerves and the Adrenergic System

The influence of renal innervation and the adrenergic nervous system is both maturation and species dependent. The renal circulation of the pig is under tonic neural vasoconstrictor influence, whereas that of the sheep is not. As such, renal denervation does not alter basal renal blood flow in fetal lambs but does result in an increase in renal blood flow in piglets. Overall, the renal vascular bed of the newborn seems to be more sensitive, but less reactive, than that of the adult in response to renal nerve stimulation.[120, 121] Low-level stimulation of the renal nerve of fetal sheep and 1- to 2-week-old piglets results in a greater increase in renal vascular resistance than in their adult counterparts. During higher levels of renal nerve stimulation, however, renal vascular resistance increases to a greater extent in older animals than in younger animals. In the presence of α-adrenergic blockade, renal nerve stimulation induces an increase in renal blood flow in fetal and newborn lambs but not in adults. This effect is apparently the result of a greater density of α- (versus β-) adrenergic receptors in neonatal sheep. After the immediate newborn period, the neonatal renal circulation is more sensitive to α-adrenergic stimulation in several species (dogs, pigs, guinea pigs, sheep) compared with adults.[14, 122, 123] An age-dependent increase in renal blood flow and a concomitant decrease in renal vascular resistance with α-adrenergic blockade have been shown in piglets[122] and in canine puppies.[13, 123] Isolated renal vessels of fetal lambs, studied *in vitro*, are also more sensitive and reactive to α-adrenergic agonists than are their newborn or adult counterparts. The rabbit seems to be an exception in that the renal vasculature in the adult is more sensitive to catecholamines compared with newborns. β-Adrenergic agonists increase renal blood flow to a greater extent in neonatal than in adult sheep. An opposite effect has been noted in piglets. The renal vasodilator effect of dopamine increases with maturation in several species (pigs, dogs, sheep).[123-125] The earlier reports of apparent absence of ontogenic differences in the renal catecholamine response in sheep can now be attributed to bolus versus constant intrarenal infusions. Fetal and newborn sheep are more responsive to the vasoconstrictor effects of α-adrenergic ligands and less responsive to the vasodilator effects of dopaminergic ligands.[26, 122, 126, 127]

CONCLUSION

The low renal blood flow in the young is the result of several factors, including smaller size, decreased number of glomeruli, lower systemic pressure, and higher renal vascular resistance. The increased renal vascular resistance in the newborn is probably caused by increased activity of the renin-angiotensin system as well as increased sensitivity to vasoconstrictor catecholamines. The latter is the result of receptor and postadrenergic receptor mechanisms. Critical vasodilators, such as NO, may act to counterbalance these vasoconstrictor forces. The increase in renal blood flow with age presumably occurs as the vasoconstrictor influences decline. New ligands and receptors continue to be discovered, but their roles, if any, in the development of renal blood flow remain to be determined.

REFERENCES

1. McCrory WW: Developmental Nephrology. Cambridge, MA, Harvard University Press, 1972.
2. Yared A, Ichikawa I: Renal blood flow and glomerular filtration rate. *In* Barratt TM, et al (eds): Pediatric Nephrology. Baltimore, Williams & Wilkins, 1999, pp 62-78.
3. Loebstein R, Koren G: Clinical pharmacology and therapeutic drug monitoring in neonates and children. Pediatr Rev 19:423-428, 1998.
4. Solhaug MJ, et al: Role of renal interstitial hydrostatic pressure in the blunted natriuretic response to saline loading in the piglet. Pediatr Res 28:460-463, 1990.
5. Toth-Heyn P, et al: The stressed neonatal kidney: from pathophysiology to clinical management of neonatal vasomotor nephropathy. Pediatr Nephrol 14:227-239, 2000.
6. Rubin ML, et al: Maturation of renal function in childhood: clearance studies. Clin Invest 28:1144, 1949.
7. Gruskin AB, et al: Maturational changes in renal blood flow in piglets. Pediatr Res 4:7-13, 1970.
8. Ichikawa I, et al: Maturational development of glomerular ultrafiltration in the rat. Am J Physiol 236:F465-F471, 1979.
9. Kleinman LI, Lubbe RJ: Factors affecting the maturation of glomerular filtration rate and renal plasma flow in the newborn dog. J Physiol 223:397, 1972.
10. Evan AP: Maturation of the vascular system of the puppy kidney. *In* Spitzer A (ed): The Kidney During Development: Morphology and Function. New York, Masson, 1982.
11. Aschinberg LC, et al: Neonatal changes in renal blood flow distribution in puppies. Am J Physiol 228:1453-1461, 1975.
12. Solhaug MJ, et al: Nitric oxide in the developing kidney. Pediatr Nephrol 10:529-539, 1996.
13. Jose P, et al: Sensitivity of the neonatal renal vasculature to epinephrine. Am J Physiol 226:796-799, 1974.
14. Pezzati M, et al: Renal blood flow velocity in preterm and term neonates during the fourth day of life: changes in relation to gestational age and birth weight. Biol Neonate 73:19-23, 1998.
15. Pokharel RP, et al: Neonatal renal artery blood flow velocities using color Doppler ultrasonography. Kobe J Med Sci 43:1-12, 1997.
16. Fawer CL, et al: Maturation of renal function in full-term and premature neonates. Helv Paediatr Acta 34:11-21, 1979.
17. Hayton WL: Maturation and growth of renal function: dosing renally cleared drugs in children. AAPS Pharm Sci 2:E3, 2000.
18. Calcagno PL, Rubin ML: Renal extraction of para-aminohippurate in infants and children. J Clin Invest 42:1632, 1963.
19. Horster M, Valtin H: Postnatal development of renal function: micropuncture and clearance studies in the dog. J Clin Invest 50:779-795, 1971.
20. Jose PA, et al: Intrarenal blood flow distribution in canine puppies. Pediatr Res 5:335-344, 1971.
21. Tonder Heyeraas KJAK: Interlobular arterial pressure in the rat kidney. Ren Physiol Biochem 2:214, 1979.
22. Ulfendahl HR, Woolliest M: Renal circulation and lymphatics. *In* Seldin DW, Giebisch G (eds): The Kidney: Physiology and Pathophysiology. New York, Lippincott, William & Wilkins, 1992, pp 1017-1047.
23. Aperia A, et al: Maturational changes in glomerular perfusion rate and glomerular filtration rate in lambs. Pediatr Res 8:758-765, 1974.
24. Calcagno PL, Jose PA: Maturation of renal blood flow. *In* Contributions to the 5th Congress of Nephrology. Basel, Karger, 1974, pp 21-27.
25. Olbing H, et al: Postnatal changes in renal glomerular blood flow distribution in puppies. J Clin Invest 52:2885-2895, 1973.
26. Robillard JE, Nakamura KT: Neurohormonal regulation of renal function during development. Am J Physiol 254:F771-F779, 1988.
27. Roman RJ, Smits C: Laser-Doppler determination of papillary blood flow in young and adult rats. Am J Physiol 251:F115-F124, 1986.
28. Buckley NM, et al: Renal blood flow autoregulation in developing swine. Am J Physiol 245:H1-H6, 1983.
29. Chevalier RL, et al: Endogenous prostaglandins modulate autoregulation of renal blood flow in young rats. Am J Physiol 253:F66-F75, 1987.
30. Jose PA, et al: Autoregulation of renal blood flow in the puppy. Am J Physiol 229:983-988, 1975.
31. Roman RJ, Kaldunski ML: Renal cortical and papillary blood flow in spontaneously hypertensive rats. Hypertension 11:657-663, 1988.
32. Briggs JP, et al: Quantitative characterization of the tubuloglomerular feedback response: effect of growth. Am J Physiol 247:F808-F815, 1984.
33. Driscoll DJ, et al: The comparative hemodynamic effects of propranolol in chronically instrumented puppies and adult dogs. Biol Neonate 41:8-15, 1982.
34. Evan AP Jr, et al: Development of the intrarenal vascular system of the puppy kidney. Anat Rec 194:187-199, 1979.
35. John E, et al: Quantitative changes in the canine glomerular vasculature during development: physiologic implications. Kidney Int 20:223-229, 1981.
36. Solhaug MJ, et al: Endothelium-derived nitric oxide regulates renal hemodynamics in the developing piglet. Pediatr Res 34:750-754, 1993.
37. Jayka S: The problem of dormant fetal organs: the kidneys, lungs, and gut. Biol Neonate 3:343, 1961.
38. Oh W, et al: Renal and cardiovascular effects of body tilting in the newborn infant: a comparative study of infants born with early and late cord clamping. Biol Neonate 10:76-92, 1966.
39. Elinder G, et al: Effect of isotonic volume expansion on glomerular filtration rate and renal hemodynamics in the developing rat kidney. Acta Physiol Scand 108:411-417, 1980.
40. Spitzer A, Edelmann CM Jr: Maturational changes in pressure gradients for glomerular filtration. Am J Physiol 221:1431-1435, 1971.
41. Alexander SPH, et al: 2001 nomenclature supplement. Trends Pharmacol Sci 23(Suppl);1-146, 2001.
42. Edlund A, et al: Renal effects of local infusion of adenosine in man. Clin Sci (Lond) 87:143-149, 1994.
43. Hall JE, Granger JP: Renal hemodynamics and arterial pressure during chronic intrarenal adenosine infusion in conscious dogs. Am J Physiol 250:F32-F39, 1986.
44. Navar LG, et al: Direct assessment of renal microcirculatory dynamics. Fed Proc 45:2851-2861, 1986.
45. Agmon Y, et al: Disparate effects of adenosine A1- and A2-receptor agonists on intrarenal blood flow. Am J Physiol 265:F802-F806, 1993.

46. Gouyon JB, et al: Renal effects of low-dose aminophylline and enprofylline in newborn rabbits. Life Sci 42:1271-1278, 1988.

47. Elnazir B, et al: Postnatal development of the pattern of respiratory and cardiovascular response to systemic hypoxia in the piglet: the roles of adenosine. J Physiol 492:573-585, 1996.

48. Naitoh M, et al: Arginine vasopressin produces renal vasodilation via V2 receptors in conscious dogs. Am J Physiol 265:R934-R942, 1993.

49. Weismann DN, Robillard JE: Renal hemodynamic responses to hypoxemia during development: relationships to circulating vasoactive substances. Pediatr Res 23:155-162, 1988.

50. Osborn JL, et al: Regulation of plasma renin in developing piglets. Dev Pharmacol Ther 1:217-228, 1980.

51. Pelayo JC, et al: The ontogeny of the renin-angiotensin system. Clin Perinatol 8:347-359, 1981.

52. Sulyok E, et al: Postnatal development of renin-angiotensin-aldosterone system, RAAS, in relation to electrolyte balance in premature infants. Pediatr Res 13:817-820, 1979.

53. Wallace KB, et al: Postnatal development of the renin-angiotensin system in rats. Am J Physiol 238:R432-R437, 1980.

54. Gomez RA: Role of angiotensin in renal vascular development. Kidney Int Suppl 67:S12-16, 1998.

55. Solhaug MJ, et al: Nitric oxide and angiotensin II regulation of renal hemodynamics in the developing piglet. Pediatr Res 39:527-533, 1996.

56. Robillard JE: Renal and adrenal responses to converting-enzyme inhibition in fetal and newborn life. Am J Physiol 244:R249-R256, 1983.

57. Osborn JL, et al: Effect of saralasin and indomethacin on renal function in developing piglets. Am J Physiol 238:R438-R442, 1980.

58. Ciuffo GM, et al: Glomerular angiotensin II receptor subtypes during development. Am J Physiol 265:F264-F271, 1993.

59. Norwood VF, et al: Differential expression of angiotensin II receptors during early renal morphogenesis. Am J Physiol 272:R662-R668, 1997.

60. Matsusaka T, et al: The renin angiotensin system and kidney development. Annu Rev Physiol 64:551-561, 2002.

61. Shanmugam S, et al: Ontogeny of angiotensin II type 2 (AT2) receptor mRNA in the rat. Kidney Int 47:1095-1100, 1995.

62. Tufro-McReddie A, et al: Ontogeny of type 1 angiotensin II receptor gene expression in the rat. J Clin Invest 91:530-537, 1993.

63. Yoo KH, et al: Regulation of angiotensin II AT1 and AT2 receptors in neonatal ureteral obstruction. Am J Physiol 273:R503-R509, 1997.

64. Fogo A, et al: Importance of angiogenic action of angiotensin II in the glomerular growth of maturing kidneys. Kidney Int 38:1068-1074, 1990.

65. Friberg P, et al: Renin-angiotensin system in neonatal rats: induction of a renal abnormality in response to ACE inhibition or angiotensin II antagonism. Kidney Int 45:485-492, 1994.

66. Shotan A, et al: Risks of angiotensin-converting enzyme inhibition during pregnancy: experimental and clinical evidence, potential mechanisms, and recommendations for use. Am J Med 96:451-456, 1994.

67. Gimonet V, et al: Nephrogenesis and angiotensin II receptor subtypes gene expression in the fetal lamb. Am J Physiol 274:F1062-F1069, 1998.

68. Carey RM, et al: Role of the angiotensin AT2 receptor in blood pressure regulation and therapeutic implications. Am J Hypertens 14:98S-102S, 2001.

69. Nilsson AB, et al: Acute renal responses to angiotensin-converting enzyme inhibition in the neonatal pig. Pediatr Nephrol 14:1071-1076, 2000.

70. Prevot A, et al: The effects of losartan on renal function in the newborn rabbit. Pediatr Res 51:728-732, 2002.

71. Walther T, et al: Natriuretic peptide system in fetal heart and circulation. J Hypertens 20:785-791, 2002.

72. Tulassay T, et al: Role of atrial natriuretic peptide in sodium homeostasis in premature infants. J Pediatr 109:1023-1027, 1986.

73. Wei YF, et al: Developmental changes in the rat atriopeptin hormonal system. J Clin Invest 79:1325-1329, 1987.

74. Chevalier RL: The moth and the aspen tree: sodium in early postnatal development. Kidney Int 59:1617-1625, 2001.

75. Semmekrot BA, et al: Age differences in renal response to atrial natriuretic peptide in rabbits. Life Sci 46:849-856, 1990.

76. Robillard JE, et al: Ontogeny of the renal response to natriuretic peptide in sheep. Am J Physiol 254:F634-F641, 1988.

77. Takei Y, Hirose S: The natriuretic peptide system in eels: a key endocrine system for euryhalinity? Am J Physiol 282:R940-951, 2002.

78. Chevalier RL, et al: Inhibition of ANP clearance receptors and endopeptidase 24.11 in maturing rats. Am J Physiol 260:R1218-R1228, 1991.

79. Norling LL, et al: Maturation of cGMP response to ANP by isolated glomeruli. Am J Physiol 262:F138-F143, 1992.

80. Matsumura Y, et al: Renal haemodynamic and excretory responses to bradykinin in anaesthetized dogs. Clin Exp Pharmacol Physiol 26:645-650, 1999.

81. Siragy HM, et al: Bradykinin B2 receptor modulates renal prostaglandin E2 and nitric oxide. Hypertension 29:757-762, 1997.

82. Toth-Heyn P, et al: Role of bradykinin in the neonatal renal effects of angiotensin converting enzyme inhibition. Life Sci 62:309-318, 1998.

83. el Dahr SS, et al: Fetal ontogeny and role of metanephric bradykinin B2 receptors. Pediatr Nephrol 14:288-296, 2000.

84. el Dahr SS: Ontogeny of the intrarenal kallikrein-kinin system: proposed role in renal development. Microsc Res Tech 39:222-232, 1997.

85. Godard C, et al: Urinary prostaglandins, vasopressin, and kallikrein excretion in healthy children from birth to adolescence. J Pediatr 100:898-902, 1982.

86. Vio CP, et al: Kallikrein excretion: relationship with maturation and renal function in human neonates at different gestational ages. Biol Neonate 52:121-126, 1987.

87. Yosipiv IV, et al: Ontogeny of somatic angiotensin-converting enzyme. Hypertension 23:369-374, 1994.

88. Patel A, Smith FG: Renal haemodynamic effects of B2 receptor agonist bradykinin and B2 receptor antagonist HOE 140 in conscious lambs. Exp Physiol 85:811-817, 2000.

89. el Dahr SS, et al: Role of bradykinin B2 receptors in the developmental changes of renal hemodynamics in the neonatal rat. Am J Physiol 269:F786-F792, 1995.

90. Kedzierski RM, Yanagisawa M: Endothelin system: the double-edged sword in health and disease. Annu Rev Pharmacol Toxicol 41:851-876, 2001.

91. Hunley TE, Kon V: Update on endothelins—biology and clinical implications. Pediatr Nephrol 16:752-762, 2001.

92. Sharifi AM, Schiffrin EL: Endothelin receptors mediating vasoconstriction in rat pressurized small arteries. Can J Physiol Pharmacol 74:934-939, 1996.

93. Li XX, et al: Adrenergic and endothelin B receptor-dependent hypertension in dopamine receptor type-2 knockout mice. Hypertension 38:303-308, 2001.

94. Sulyok E, et al: Urinary endothelin excretion in the neonate: influence of maturity and perinatal pathology. Pediatr Nephrol 7:881-885, 1993.

95. Semama DS, et al: Effects of endothelin on renal function in newborn rabbits. Pediatr Res 34:120-123, 1993.

96. Semama DS, et al: Role of endogenous endothelin in renal haemodynamics of newborn rabbits. Pediatr Nephrol 7:886-890, 1993.

97. Chin A, et al: Effects of tezosentan, a dual endothelin receptor antagonist, on the cardiovascular and renal systems of neonatal piglets. J Pediatr Surg 36:1824-1228, 2001.

98. Simeoni U, Helig JJ: Nitric oxide (NO) and normal and pathologic renal development. Pediatr Med Chir 19:313-315, 1997.

99. Ballevre L, et al: Role of nitric oxide in the hypoxemia-induced renal dysfunction of the newborn rabbit. Pediatr Res 39:725-730, 1996.

100. Sener A, Smith FG: Renal hemodynamic effects of L-NAME during postnatal maturation in conscious lambs. Pediatr Nephrol 16:868-873, 2001.

101. Simeoni U, et al: Postnatal development of vascular resistance of the rabbit isolated perfused kidney: modulation by nitric oxide and angiotensin II. Pediatr Res 42:550-555, 1997.

102. Li D, et al: Arachidonic acid metabolic pathways regulating activity of renal Na+K+ATPase are dependent. Am J Physiol Renal Physiol 278:F823-F829, 2000.

103. Khan KN, et al: Cyclooxygenase-2 expression in the developing human kidney. Pediatr Dev Pathol 4:461-466, 2001.

104. Khan KN, et al: Pharmacology of cyclooxygenase-2 inhibition in the kidney. Kidney Int 61:1210-1212, 2002.

105. Komhoff M, et al: Localization of cyclooxygenase-1 and -2 in adult and fetal human kidney: implication for renal function. Am J Physiol 272:F460-F468, 1997.

106. Ogawa T, et al: Developmental changes in cyclooxygenase mRNA expression in the kidney of rats. Pediatr Nephrol 16:618-622, 2001.

107. Zhang MZ, et al: Cyclooxygenase-2 in rat nephron development. Am J Physiol 273:F994-1002, 1997.

108. Vio CP, et al: Postnatal development of cyclooxygenase-2 in the rat kidney. Immunopharmacology 44:205-210, 1999.

109. Komhoff M, et al: Cyclooxygenase-2-selective inhibitors impair glomerulogenesis and renal cortical development. Kidney Int 57:414-422, 2000.

110. Norwood VF, et al: Postnatal development and progression of renal dysplasia in cyclooxygenase-2 null mice. Kidney Int 58:2291-2300, 2000.

111. Peruzzi L, et al: Neonatal end-stage renal failure associated with maternal ingestion of cyclo-oxygenase-type-1 selective inhibitor nimesulide as tocolytic. Lancet 354:1615, 1999.

112. Cuzzolin L, et al: NSAID-induced nephrotoxicity from the fetus to the child. Drug Saf 24:9-18, 2001.

113. Arant BS: Renal disorders of the newborn infant. Contemp Issues Nephrol 12:111, 1984.

114. Bensman A, et al: Synthesis of prostaglandins and lipoxygenase products by rat glomeruli during development. Biol Neonate 52:149-156, 1987.

115. Judes C, et al: Effect of prostaglandin E2 on adenylate cyclase activity in isolated glomeruli and tubules during postnatal maturation of rat renal cortex. Biol Neonate 53:113-120, 1988.

116. Drukker A, et al: The renal hemodynamic effects of aspirin in newborn and young adult rabbits. Pediatr Nephrol 16:713-718, 2001.

117. Romagnoli C, et al: Effects of prophylactic ibuprofen on cerebral and renal hemodynamics in very preterm neonates. Clin Pharmacol Ther 67:676-683, 2000.

118. Matson JR, et al: Effects of inhibition of prostaglandin synthesis on fetal renal function. Kidney Int 20:621-627, 1981.

119. Breyer MD, Breyer RM: G protein-coupled prostanoid receptors and the kidney. Annu Rev Physiol 63:579-605, 2001.

120. Buckley NM, et al: Renal circulatory effects of adrenergic stimuli in anesthetized piglets and mature swine. Am J Physiol 237:H690-H695, 1979.

121. Robillard JE, et al: Ontogeny of renal hemodynamic response to renal nerve stimulation in sheep. Am J Physiol 252:F605-F612, 1987.

122. Solhaug MJ, et al: Interaction between nitric oxide and renal sympathetic nerves in the regulation of renal hemodynamics in the developing piglet. FASEB J 9:A72, 1995.

123. Felder RA, Jose PA: Development of adrenergic and dopamine receptors in the kidney. *In* Strauss J (ed): Homeostasis, Nephrotoxicity, and Renal Anomalies in the Newborn. The Hague, The Netherlands, Martinus-Nijhoff, 1986, pp 3–10.
124. Nguyen LB, et al: Renal effects of low to moderate doses of dopamine in newborn piglets. J Pediatr Surg 34:996–9999, 1999.
125. Cheung PY, Barrington KJ: Renal dopamine receptors: mechanisms of action and developmental aspects. Cardiovasc Res 31:2–6, 1996.
126. Guillery EN, et al: Ontogenic changes in renal response to alpha 1-adreno-ceptor stimulation in sheep. Am J Physiol 267:R990–R998, 1994.
127. Segar JL, et al: Ontogeny of renal response to specific dopamine DA1-receptor stimulation in sheep. Am J Physiol 263:R868–R873, 1992.

Victoria F. Norwood, Lucas G. Fernandez, Alda Tufro, and R. Ariel Gomez

128 Development of the Renin-Angiotensin System

In adult animals, the *renin-angiotensin system* (RAS) regulates arterial blood pressure, renal hemodynamics, and fluid and electrolyte balance.[1,2] The angiotensin peptides are generated by a series of enzymatic reactions depicted in Figure 128–1. Renin, produced by the juxtaglomerular cells of the kidney, is released into the circulation, where it acts on angiotensinogen to generate angiotensin I. Angiotensin I is subsequently cleaved by angiotensin-converting enzyme (ACE) to form the octapeptide angiotensin II. Most of the known actions of the RAS are exerted through the binding of angiotensin II to cell membrane–bound receptors, AT1 and AT2. Alternative pathways for the generation of angiotensin peptides also exist (see Fig. 128–1). These pathways and the actions of smaller angiotensin peptides, previously thought to be degradation products, are areas of investigative interest.[3]

In addition to the endocrine effects of the circulating RAS, a locally acting intrarenal RAS regulates renal function by paracrine or autocrine effects.[4] The existence of an extrarenal tissue RAS remains controversial, although components of the system have been localized in numerous different tissues.[5,6] Although the hemodynamic effects of the RAS garnered the greatest interest in the past, it is now apparent that angiotensin II is also involved in normal and abnormal growth processes.[7,8] These actions are preserved across the phylogenetic scale and appear to be of major importance in the attainment of normal nephrovascular architecture.[9] These developmental properties, in addition to the classic physiologic actions of the RAS, are essential functions of the RAS in the fetus and newborn.

MOLECULAR BIOLOGY OF THE RENIN-ANGIOTENSIN SYSTEM COMPONENTS

Angiotensinogen

Angiotensinogen is a 55- to 60-kDa glycoprotein precursor of the angiotensin peptides and is the only known substrate for renin.[10] Angiotensinogen is encoded by a single gene on human chromosome 1, and its mRNA product encodes a prohormone. Removal of the leader peptide results in a mature protein of which the angiotensin I decapeptide is the amino terminus.[10]

Renin

Renin is an aspartyl protease with a unique substrate, angiotensinogen. Renin substrate specificity is so stringent that only homologous angiotensinogen is cleaved efficiently.[11] Human renin is encoded by a single gene and is synthesized as an inactive single polypeptide precursor molecule, preprorenin. Removal of the signal peptide results in prorenin, which is subsequently glycosylated and is stored in immature granules before further processing into mature active renin. Renin is thought to

be secreted by two pathways: a constitutive pathway for prorenin and a regulated pathway for mature renin.[12] Therefore, prorenin may be a reservoir for local generation of active renin and angiotensin II. Renin is mainly synthesized in the kidney vasculature. However, extrarenal production of renin has been demonstrated in adrenal, liver, gonads, and brain, although in much lower abundance.[13] The characterization, regulation, and roles of extrarenal renin are areas of active investigation.

Angiotensin-Converting Enzyme

ACE is a zinc-containing protease that cleaves carboxy-terminal dipeptides from small peptides, most notably angiotensin I and bradykinin. Human ACE is the product of a single gene that ultimately produces two extensively glycosylated polypeptides: a larger form found in endothelial cells and most somatic tissues and a smaller form found in testis.[14] ACE has hydrophobic amino acids at the N-terminus that provide an anchor to the cell membrane. The soluble form of ACE present in plasma and seminal fluid is derived from membrane-bound ACE by posttranslational cleavage of the C-terminal region.[15]

Angiotensin II

Angiotensin II is an octapeptide resulting from ACE-mediated cleavage of angiotensin I. Angiotensin II is a short-lived molecule (half-life = 15 seconds),[16] the actions of which are mediated through membrane receptors. Angiotensin II regulates blood pressure and fluid and electrolyte homeostasis through various actions. Most notably, angiotensin II is an extremely potent vasoconstrictor; intravenous infusion results in a pressor response within 15 seconds that lasts for 3 to 5 minutes.[16] Several peptidases rapidly degrade angiotensin II into several active and inactive metabolites (see Fig. 128–1). Although the fates and actions of these metabolites largely remain unknown, it has been shown that angiotensin (1–7) exerts regulatory effects on both vasculature and the kidney. In contrast to the vasoconstrictor and growth promoting actions of angiotensin II, angiotensin (1–7) inhibits cell growth and causes diuresis and natriuresis.[17,18]

Angiotensin II Receptors

Angiotensin II receptors have been located by radioligand binding in every angiotensin II–responsive tissue or cell type. Two major receptor subtypes have been identified: AT1 and AT2.[19] Both receptors have substrate affinity in the nanomolar range and a maximal binding capacity that varies widely among tissues.[19]

AT1 receptors contain seven transmembrane domains that provide coupling to G-proteins.[19] Stimulation of AT1 by angiotensin II induces hydrolysis of inositol phosphates, increases

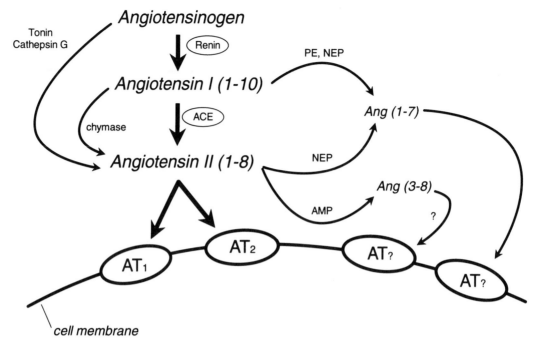

Figure 128–1. The renin-angiotensin cascade. The *thick arrows* depict the traditional enzymatic cascade. The *thin arrows* depict alternative processing pathways for angiotensin (Ang) generation. ACE = angiotensin-converting enzyme; AMP = aminopeptidase; AT = angiotensin receptor; NEP = neutral endopeptidase; PE = prolyl endopeptidase. Angiotensin III (2–8) is omitted for clarity. (From Gomez RA, Norwood VF: Am J Kidney Dis *26*:409, 1995.)

intracellular calcium (Ca^{2+}) and diacylglycerol, inhibits adenylate cyclase, and releases arachidonic acid metabolites.[20] Most of the known actions of angiotensin II are mediated by AT1 and are reviewed later.[19]

AT2 receptors are not coupled to G-proteins.[21, 22] Studies suggest that AT2 binding activates a phosphotyrosine phosphatase, thereby inactivating mitogen-activated protein (MAP) kinase and decreasing cyclic guanosine monophosphate levels.[21, 23] In addition, a growth-inhibitory function has been described for AT2.[21,24] The role for AT2 and other putative receptor subtypes during development remains elusive. AT2 has seven transmembrane domains, but the glycosylated protein is only 32% homologous to the AT1 receptor.[25] AT2 mRNA is abundant in fetal tissues but decreases rapidly after birth.[25]

MATURATIONAL CHANGES IN COMPONENT ACTIVITY

The major components of the renin-angiotensin cascade are present during fetal and newborn life, but their anatomic distributions and activities are in most cases quite different from those seen in the adult mammal. These differences are likely to represent distinct and highly specialized functions of the RAS within many different tissues in the growing, differentiating, and maturing fetus. Although little information exists regarding the components of the RAS in human fetal or infant tissues, several animal models have been successfully studied.

Angiotensinogen

In mature animals, the primary source of angiotensinogen is the liver. However, in the fetal rat liver, angiotensinogen mRNA levels are almost undetectable.[26] In contrast, angiotensinogen is expressed at relatively high levels in the yolk sac and fetal placenta, as well as fetal brain, fat, and kidney,[26] and circulating levels of angiotensinogen are similar to or higher than those seen in adult animals.[27]

In the human fetus, cord angiotensinogen levels are low.[28] Levels rise in the neonatal period and are higher in the infant

than the adult.[28] In newborn rats, there is a 20-fold increase in the expression of angiotensinogen in the liver within 24 hours of birth, and this expression remains elevated until the pups are weaned.[26] Concomitantly, circulating angiotensinogen levels rise quickly after birth.[29]

The production of angiotensinogen by the adult liver is regulated by various physiologic stimuli. Salt depletion, sex steroids, thyroxine, and angiotensin II stimulate angiotensinogen expression, whereas it is suppressed by insulin.[30-33] The fetal liver is also clearly responsive to hormonal stimuli. In the rat, dexamethasone or thyroxine administration stimulates fetal liver angiotensinogen expression.[34]

The functional importance of angiotensinogen in the fetus remains unclear, and the secretion of the protein from its various sources has not been determined. However, its presence in the yolk sac and placenta implies potential actions in the control of fetal perfusion and fluid and electrolyte transport. Its presence in numerous developing organs may also suggest a role in tissue morphogenesis and blood flow regulation.[35]

Overall, these studies indicate that, as the animal matures, angiotensinogen synthesis and regulation mature in preparation for the transition from fetal to extrauterine life. These changes in angiotensinogen availability are accompanied by adjustments in the control of blood flow patterns, blood pressure, and salt and water homeostasis.

Renin

As with angiotensinogen, renin expression and activity are markedly different during fetal and neonatal life compared with the mature animal. Renin is observed early in human development, first localized to the mesonephros at 5 to 6 weeks of gestation.[36] By 8 weeks of gestation, renin is found within the metanephros, several weeks before the onset of fetal urine production.[36] Although renin production is strictly localized to the juxtaglomerular apparatus in the normal adult, its localization is more widely distributed within the developing renal microvasculature. At 14 to 15 days of gestation in the mouse, renin-containing cells can be found distributed in the metanephric mesenchyme as single isolated cells, but by embryonic day 18, they are associated with the vasculature.[37] At 15 to 17 days of gestation in the rat, renin is found in the aorta and main renal arteries.[38, 39] By 19 to 20 days, renin is found in the arcuate and interlobular arteries and afferent arterioles.[40] After birth, renin expression decreases in the larger vessels until it remains only in the classic juxtaglomerular location.[39, 40] This developmental pattern of renin expression has been found in every species examined, including humans.[36]

The major source of circulating renin during fetal life is the kidney,[41] and fetal plasma renin concentration and activity are elevated compared with newborns that likewise have higher levels than adults.[42-44] In preterm infants, plasma renin activity is high and inversely correlates with gestational age.[45] At birth, plasma renin activity increases further for several weeks and then begins a slow decline through infancy and childhood until adult levels are reached by 6 to 9 years of age.[42]

Renin release is modulated by many different positive and negative stimuli, and control of this process is well established in the late-gestation fetus and the newborn.[46, 47] The principal mechanisms controlling renin release are the macula densa mechanism, the baroreceptor, the sympathetic nervous system, and various hormonal mechanisms. The macula densa mechanism is active in fetal and newborn lambs,[48, 49] and it stimulates renin release on detection of decreased sodium and chloride delivery to the distal tubule. The fetal and newborn renal baroreceptor respond to decreases in renal perfusion pressure with appropriate increases in renin secretion.[50] The sympathetic nervous system, acting through the renal nerves and cell-surface β-adrenergic receptors, also stimulates renin production and release in the fetus and neonate.[51, 52] Both humoral and intracellular signals including angiotensin II, cyclic adenosine monophosphate, Ca^{2+}, and prostaglandins also mediate the release of renin from its lysosomal storage pools and are active during development.[53,54] These stimuli result in changes in renin release that are qualitatively similar to those seen in adults. The physiologic, pharmacologic, and pathophysiologic factors that affect the RAS during development are shown in Table 128-1.[46] The end result of these integrated regulatory mechanisms is a precise and physiologically responsive control system that accurately governs renin secretion in the immature animal.

Angiotensin-Converting Enzyme

In contrast to renin expression, ACE activity is relatively low during fetal life and increases slowly as term approaches.[55] After delivery, renal ACE activity in the rat increases to a maximum within the first 2 weeks, followed by a decline to adult values by 1 to 2 months.[56, 57] In human infants, plasma ACE levels are similar to those seen in adults.[28] At every age studied, ACE has the same substrate affinity.[55] However, the maximum velocity (V_{max}) of the enzyme is fourfold lower in fetal than in adult tissues, a finding suggesting that increasing ACE activity during development is the result of the production of more enzyme rather than further activation of preexisting enzyme.[55] During renal organogenesis, ACE is first detected in proximal tubules, endothelial cells invading the S-shaped glomerulus, and the afferent and efferent arteriolar endothelium of more mature glomeruli.[58] With maturation, ACE is predominantly expressed by proximal tubules and peritubular capillaries.[58] The presence of vascular and intraglomerular ACE during nephrogenesis suggests that local angiotensin production may be necessary for normal development of the glomerulus and renal microvasculature.

Angiotensin II

Under most circumstances, renin secretion is the rate-limiting step in the production of angiotensin II. Accordingly, the high

TABLE 128-1

Factors that Increase and Decrease the Activity of the Renin-Angiotensin System in the Fetus and Newborn Mammal

Increase	Decrease
Prematurity	Volume expansion
Vaginal delivery	Indomethacin
Furosemide	Phenylephrine
Hemorrhage	Cortisol
Hypotension	Arginine vasopressin
Hypoxemia	Recumbent position
Aortic constriction	Exchange transfusion (replacement)
Exchange transfusion (withdrawal)	
Upright position	

Adapted from Gomez RA, et al: Pediatr Nephrol 5:80, 1991.

levels of active renin during development result in angiotensin II concentrations in the fetus that are twice those of maternal plasma.[28] Circulating angiotensin II levels remain high during the newborn period and decrease with age, paralleling the changes in active renin. In addition, the enzymes responsible for degradation of angiotensin II, the angiotensinases, are relatively inactive in the developing animal, and, therefore, high circulating levels of angiotensin II are maintained during early life.[59]

Angiotensin Receptors

The physiologic effects of angiotensin II require interaction of the peptide with its receptors. Two major receptor subtypes have been identified—AT1 and AT2—that have widely divergent patterns of tissue distribution and second-messenger signaling mechanisms. Both subtypes are developmentally regulated and are found in fetal membranes as early as 10 days of gestation in the rat.[60] During embryonic life, the AT2 subtype predominates and is expressed in most mesenchymal tissues.[61] AT1 receptors are also present, although in significantly fewer numbers.[61] In the fetal rat kidney at 14 days of gestation (the beginning of metanephric development), 80% of angiotensin receptors are the AT2 subtype and are localized to the undifferentiated renal mesenchymal cells.[62] By 17 days of gestation, AT1 expression has increased and is found primarily in deep, more mature glomeruli, but also diffusely throughout the nephrogenic cortex.[62, 63] At birth, AT1 and AT2 are equally prevalent. AT2 continues to be expressed in undifferentiated cells or differentiating structures, whereas AT1 predominates in glomeruli, arteries, and vasa recta.[62-64] After birth, AT2 is rapidly down-regulated, but it remains detectable at low levels in the adult adrenal gland, renal glomeruli, and nephrons.[65] AT1 persists in the renal microvasculature, mesangial cells, and proximal tubules, where it is maintained throughout adulthood.[62-64] The differential regulation of AT1 and AT2 is schematically represented in Figure 128-2.

The functions of the angiotensin II receptors during fetal and neonatal renal development and maturation remain incompletely studied, but they are likely to include various differentiation and growth effects as well as the well-accepted roles of vasoconstriction, renal hemodynamic control, and fluid and electrolyte balance. The AT1 receptor is linked to certain G-protein-associated second-messenger systems (phospholipase C in vascular smooth muscle, phospholipase A_2 in proximal tubules, and adenylcyclase in adrenal cortex) through which smooth muscle contraction, Na^+ reabsorption, and aldosterone secretion, respectively, are mediated.[19] Few of these effects have been studied in the developing human. The effects of AT1 on cell growth and organ development are discussed later. The effects of AT2 during renal development are very poorly understood. To date, there has been no identified second-messenger signaling system for AT2 in the developing kidney, and its function there is entirely unknown.

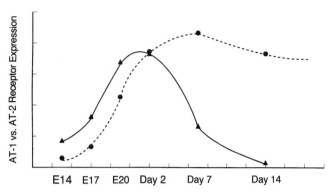

Figure 128–2. Relative expression of renal angiotensin receptor AT1 and AT2 mRNAs and receptor proteins during rat metanephric development. AT2 expression (*triangles*) is higher than AT1 expression (*circles*) at the onset of renal development. Both subtypes increase during prenatal development, although AT1 expression increases more dramatically and surpasses AT2 expression around birth. After birth, AT2 expression is down-regulated, whereas AT1 persists for the remainder of life.

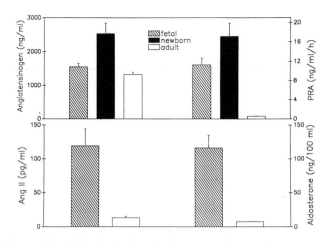

Figure 128–3. Circulating levels of angiotensinogen, plasma renin activity (PRA), angiotensin II (Ang II), and plasma aldosterone in fetal cord blood, newborn infants, and physiologically normal adults. (From Tufro-McReddie A, Gomez RA: Semin Nephrol *13*:519, 1993; data from Godard C, et al: Nephron *17*:353, 1976.)

It has been hypothesized that AT2 may modulate programmed cell death in the developing kidney because of its localization to poorly differentiated structures.

The classic representation of the RAS is that of circulating renin acting on constitutively secreted angiotensinogen to produce circulating angiotensin II. This endocrine system is highly functional and is up-regulated during development. As shown in Figure 128–3, circulating levels of angiotensinogen, renin, angiotensin II, and aldosterone are all higher in developing animals than in adults.[66] Evidence supports the additional existence of local, or tissue, RASs that may generate angiotensin II for paracrine or autocrine functions.[4, 67] Because all components of the RAS are present early in the developing embryo and are found in the kidney before the onset of fetal urine production, it is possible that the local system may regulate growth and differentiation of developing nephrons. Once kidney structures are formed, the RAS then begins to regulate renal hemodynamics and Na+ transport.

FUNCTIONAL EFFECTS OF ANGIOTENSIN II DURING DEVELOPMENT

The production of angiotensin II by the active renin-angiotensin cascade in the fetus and newborn results in systemic and local effects that control systemic blood pressure, renal hemodynamics, and fluid and electrolyte homeostasis by interaction of angiotensin II with its receptors. In addition, evidence supports the role of angiotensin II in various growth and developmental processes that are important to the care of the maturing infant. Although the role of angiotensin II in the maintenance of physiologic processes has been more thoroughly studied in adults,[19] appropriate functional responses to stimuli of the RAS have been well established during development. Hypotension, aortic constriction, hemorrhage, furosemide, ACE inhibition, sympathetic nervous system activity, prostaglandins, vasopressin, and atrial natriuretic peptide can all influence renin secretion and thereby the production of angiotensin II in the fetus (see Table 128–1).

Blood Pressure Control

The role of angiotensin II in the control of systemic blood pressure is exerted through effects on several systems (Fig. 128–4). Blood pressure is increased by elevations in both peripheral vascular resistance and cardiac output, which, in turn, are increased

by both heart rate and stroke volume. The direct vasoconstrictor effects of angiotensin II, mediated by AT1 receptor–initiated increases in vascular intracellular Ca2+, provide an exceedingly powerful mechanism for raising systemic pressure rapidly by increasing small vessel resistance. Additional mechanisms by which angiotensin II can increase blood pressure include alterations in cardiac output through AT1-mediated increases in myocardial contractility and centrally mediated increases in sympathetic nervous system activity to increase heart rate. Angiotensin II directly stimulates proximal tubular Na+ reabsorption and also leads to intrarenal vasoconstriction that ultimately results in further Na+ and water reabsorption and extracellular volume expansion. An additional long feedback loop allows angiotensin II to stimulate aldosterone secretion and thereby increase distal renal Na+ reabsorption. Meanwhile, angiotensin II in the central nervous system stimulates thirst and salt appetite and thus further increases extracellular volume. These aggregate effects of angiotensin II provide a closely balanced and integrated endocrine and paracrine system capable of very tight regulation of arterial blood pressure and body fluid homeostasis. Studies in genetically engineered animals have confirmed the primary role of the RAS in blood pressure regulation. Disruptions of the genes for angiotensinogen,[68] renin,[69] ACE,[70, 71] or the AT1A receptor[72] in mice result in marked decreases in blood pressure. These findings confirm the importance of the RAS in the normal regulation of blood pressure and illustrate that no other mechanism completely compensates for the lack of angiotensin II activity.

The potency of angiotensin II changes with development. The pressor response to exogenous angiotensin II is lower in fetal and newborn lambs than in adults,[73] and it may be caused by occupancy of the receptors by high concentrations of endogenous angiotensin II as well as maturational differences in receptor density or function. The hypotensive response to fetal hemorrhage is mediated in part by angiotensin II, but it also increases as maturation proceeds. A 20% reduction in fetal placental blood volume results in hypotension in young fetuses but has no effect near term, a finding suggesting that the control of fetal blood pressure by the RAS increases with maturation.[74]

As in the adult, alterations in the activity of the RAS during early life may lead to pathologic situations. In the human infant,

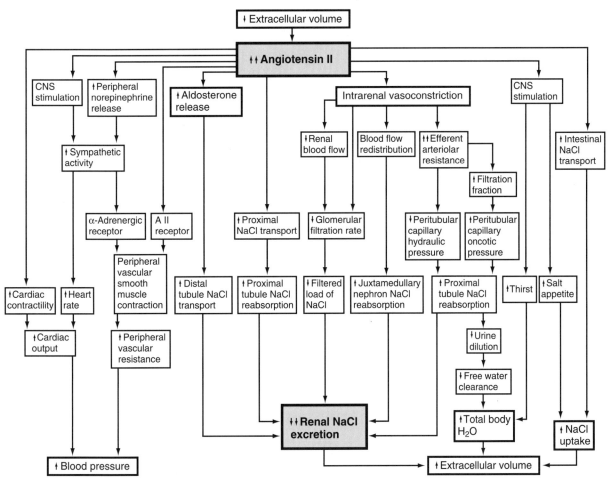

Figure 128–4. The integration of angiotensin II (A II) effects to maintain arterial pressure and extracellular fluid volume. (From Ballerman BJ, et al: *In* Brenner BM, Rector FC (eds): The Kidney, 4th ed. Philadelphia, WB Saunders, 1991, pp 510–583.)

hypertension usually results from activation of the RAS. Renal artery thromboembolism secondary to umbilical artery catheter use, coarctation of the aorta, renal artery stenosis, obstructive uropathy (especially ureteropelvic junction obstruction), glucocorticoid administration, and bronchopulmonary dysplasia all stimulate angiotensin II production. For these infants, ACE inhibitors such as captopril or enalapril are the pharmacologic treatments of choice. However, the potency of these drugs is enhanced in the first 6 months of life, and care must be taken to avoid hypotension and oliguria.[75] Effective reductions in blood pressure have been obtained with doses much lower than those required by older infants. Current recommendations suggest a starting captopril dose of 0.05 mg/kg with rapid increases until the appropriate effect is obtained. Adverse effects of these drugs include neutropenia, rash, hyperkalemia, and decreased glomerular filtration rate (GFR) necessitating careful follow-up for infants requiring these medications. Although also of likely benefit in the treatment of hypertension, the angiotensin-receptor blockers have not yet been systematically evaluated in infants or young children.

Renal Hemodynamics

The intrarenal actions of angiotensin II include control of renal blood flow, GFR, and tubular Na+ excretion. The effects on renal blood flow and GFR are primarily mediated through AT1 receptors in the afferent and efferent arterioles, with the dominant vasoconstriction occurring in the efferent arteriole.[4] As in adult animals, administration of angiotensin II to fetal lambs decreases renal blood flow and maintains GFR by increasing efferent arteriolar tone.[73] Within the adult glomerulus, angiotensin II binding to mesangial cell AT1 receptors results in contraction and decreased filtration by decreasing the surface area available for filtration.[76] This response may serve as a counterbalance to the increase in GFR caused by efferent arteriolar constriction. AT1 receptors are also present in fetal mesangial cells,[77] but their role in intraglomerular hemodynamic control is unknown. Treatment of the fetus with ACE enzyme inhibitors decreases renal vascular resistance and GFR by decreasing efferent arteriolar tone.[78] When given on a long-term basis to fetuses, ACE inhibitors can dramatically decrease fetal GFR and urine flow,[78] and may explain the neonatal anuria and renal compromise seen in human infants exposed to these drugs *in utero*. The use of these drugs during the second and third trimesters of pregnancy is associated with renal dysplasia, oligohydramnios, pulmonary hypoplasia, and renal failure in the fetus, features that make these drugs contraindicated during pregnancy.[79] These effects are most likely the result of loss of angiotensin II–dependent blood flow to the fetal kidney, as well as inhibition of the angiotensin II–dependent renal growth effects in the developing kidney, as described later.

An important function of the RAS in mature animals is the intrarenal mechanism of *tubuloglomerular feedback*. In this system, distal nephron flow is coupled to GFR at the single-nephron level, with the goal of maintaining appropriate extracellular volume. Changes in distal nephron flow rate or chloride concentration are sensed by the macula densa; increased distal

TABLE 128–2

Proposed Mediators of Angiotensin II Growth Effects

Proto-oncogenes (c-fos, c-myc, c-jun)
Growth factors (insulin-like growth factor I, transforming growth factor-β, platelet-derived growth factor, basic fibroblast growth factor, epidermal growth factor)
Kinases (mitogen-activated protein MAP kinases, S6 kinase)
Phosphatases (phosphotyrosine phosphatase)
Intracellular calcium
Mechanical deformation

From Gomez RA: Exp Nephrol 2:259, 1994.

tubular salt or flow triggers renin secretion by the juxtaglomerular cells and subsequent afferent and efferent arteriolar constriction and decreased GFR, thereby preventing excessive loss of water or solute. Microperfusion studies have shown that angiotensin II enhances tubuloglomerular feedback by activation of AT1 receptors on the luminal membrane of macula densa cells, a finding suggesting multiple mechanisms for the RAS in this process.[80] The tubuloglomerular feedback mechanism has been shown to be functioning in adolescent rats (30 days of age),[81] but it has not been studied in younger animals. Tubuloglomerular feedback is counterbalanced by another intrarenal system, known as *glomerulotubular balance,* in which changes in single-nephron Na+ delivery induce proportional changes in Na+ and water reabsorption. This mechanism may be mediated by direct modulation of Na+ reabsorption by proximal tubular cells or by changes in postglomerular blood flow, both of which are in part controlled by AT1 receptors. The juxtaposition of these control systems results in the tightly regulated Na+ and fluid balance necessary for survival in an environment in which intake may vary widely.

Fluid and Electrolyte Balance

Angiotensin II mediates the control of systemic fluid and electrolyte balance through various mechanisms, some directly affecting renal hemodynamics or tubular transport and others indirectly altering intake or output of water and solutes. In the brain, angiotensin II, through AT1 receptors, stimulates thirst, salt appetite, and vasopressin release, all of which increase extracellular fluid volume.[82] AT1 receptors in the adrenal cortex respond to angiotensin II stimulation by production and secretion of aldosterone that subsequently enhances basolateral Na+, potassium–adenosine triphosphatase (Na+,K+-ATPase), and Na+ channel activity in the distal nephron resulting in increased Na+ reabsorption. Although the fetal adrenal gland responds to angiotensin II stimulation by secretion of aldosterone, the rise in plasma aldosterone is less than that seen in adult animals, a finding suggesting relative insensitivity of the fetal adrenal gland to angiotensin II stimulation.[73] In the proximal tubule, AT1 receptors activate both luminal and basolateral Na+ transport mechanisms including the Na+/H+ antiporter,[83] the Na+/bicarbonate co-transporter,[84] and Na+K+-ATPase,[85] all of which result in net Na+ reabsorption. In the cortical collecting duct, angiotensin II, acting through AT1 receptors, stimulates H+-ATPase activity, a finding suggesting additional roles for angiotensin II in the control of acid-base balance.[86] An additional mechanism by which angiotensin II controls fluid and electrolyte balance is via control of peritubular blood flow. The capillaries that compose the peritubular network are downstream from the glomerulus, having branched from the efferent arteriole. As a result, factors that affect afferent and efferent blood flow and GFR directly affect peritubular flow. Efferent vasoconstriction decreases postglomerular flow and hydrostatic pressure and increases peritubular oncotic pressure, resulting in enhanced Na+ and water reabsorption. Therefore, the net effect of angiotensin II

stimulation in the renal tubule is to encourage Na+ and water reabsorption.

Although direct evidence of the function of the various components of the tubular RAS in the fetus and newborn is not available, it is likely that the relative immaturity of all or some of these control mechanisms may account for the negative Na+ and water balance seen in premature infants. The relatively poor capacity for Na+ reabsorption seen in the immature newborn explains the tendency for these infants to develop hyponatremia when they are given diets with Na+ contents appropriate for older infants. As maturation proceeds, renal reabsorptive capacity for Na+ increases, and the term infant maintains a positive Na+ balance on various diets. In fact, acquisition of adequate Na+ stores is required for cellular growth and bone mineralization.[87] It has been hypothesized that the ongoing deposition of Na+ into growing bone may be the mechanism driving the higher set point for the RAS in the developing animal.[87]

Angiotensin II as a Growth Factor

The role of angiotensin II as a modulator of growth is now well established in various cardiovascular and renal cell types and tissues. These effects have important implications for organogenesis, tissue maturation, glomerulosclerosis, and aging. In vascular smooth muscle cells, angiotensin II stimulation of AT1 receptors elicits hypertrophic,[88, 89] hyperplastic,[90] or dual effects.[91] In contrast, the AT2 receptor inhibits proliferation in coronary endothelial cells.[92] Angiotensin II has also been shown to induce angiogenesis in the chick embryo chorioallantoic membrane.[93] Taken together, these experimental models suggest a vital role for angiotensin II in the architectural development and growth of the renal vasculature. Supporting this suggestion is a study documenting marked thickening, truncation, and rarefaction of the renal microvasculature after postnatal treatment with AT1, but not AT2, inhibitors.[94] Likewise, deletion of the AT1A receptor subtype in the inbred mouse,[95] deletion of angiotensinogen[68] or ACE,[96] and double deletion of AT1A and AT1B receptors[97, 98] result in abnormal renal microvasculature, whereas deletion of AT2 has no effect.[99]

Within the various cell types of the nephron, angiotensin II has both hypertrophic and proliferative effects. The type of growth response to angiotensin II appears to be both species specific and cell specific, as well as developmentally regulated. Human and murine fetal mesangial cells respond to angiotensin II with proliferation,[77] whereas adult mesangial cells respond primarily with hypertrophy.[100, 101] Proximal tubular cells from rabbits, mice, and pigs all respond to angiotensin II by increasing cell size and protein content,[88, 102] whereas medullary thick ascending limb cells proliferate in response to the peptide.[103] The mechanisms by which angiotensin II exerts these effects remain incompletely understood, but to date all have been ascribed to the AT1 receptor.[100, 101] These responses may be mediated directly by angiotensin II, or they may involve various growth factors, proto-oncogenes, kinases, and phosphatases, as described in Table 128–2.[8]

The growth effects of angiotensin II have also been explored in whole animal models. Blockade of the neonatal rat AT1 receptor with losartan results in decreased ratios of kidney to body weight and suppressed renal cell proliferation.[54] Similar results have been shown using ACE inhibitors.[104] The kidneys from treated animals exhibited fewer, smaller glomeruli and tubular dilation as well as vascular malformations.[94, 105] Kidneys from animals receiving an AT2-specific inhibitor showed no abnormalities,[94] a finding indicating that the nephrogenic effects of angiotensin II are mediated through AT1. The lack of AT2 effect in this model is most likely the result of the rapid downregulation of this receptor after birth.

Transgenic animals carrying targeted disruptions of components of the RAS raise new questions regarding the importance of angiotensin II in renal developmental processes. Animals lacking angiotensinogen,[68] ACE,[71] or both AT1A and AT1B receptors[97,98] have increased neonatal death and progressive development of renal arterial and cortical disease. Abnormalities include juxtaglomerular hypertrophy, delayed glomerular maturation, tubular atrophy, arterial and arteriolar wall thickening, and interstitial fibrosis. AT2[99,106] homozygous null mice have no renal abnormalities on some genetic backgrounds, but various genitourinary abnormalities on other backgrounds, suggesting that AT2 control of renal development may be modified by other factors.[107] These results imply a central role for angiotensin II and its receptors in the appropriate development of the kidney and in the maintenance of structural integrity of the adult kidney.

Unfortunately, the growth effects of angiotensin II have also been demonstrated in human infants, in whom ACE inhibition during pregnancy has been associated with intrauterine growth retardation, renal dysplasia and anuria, pulmonary hypoplasia, bony malformations, and neonatal death.[79] These drugs are consequently contraindicated during pregnancy. Although nephrogenesis is complete in the human fetus by 32 to 36 weeks of gestation, further growth and maturation of glomeruli and tubules occur until approximately 2 years of age. This brings into question the safety of ACE or other angiotensin II inhibitors during infancy. Premature and full-term newborns are very responsive to ACE inhibition, and they require lower doses and have more significant problems with decreased GFR, hyponatremia, and hyperkalemia than do older children.[75] These effects are reasonable given the highly activated state of the RAS during development and the known effects of RAS blockade. The potential effects of ACE inhibitors on renal growth and differentiation in premature and newborn infants have not been defined. Therefore, the risks of these agents must be carefully weighed against the benefits of managing renin-mediated hypertension.

SUMMARY

The RAS is present and active at the earliest phases of development and appears to acquire different functions as maturation proceeds. Initially, the complex interplay between the mitogenic and trophic effects of angiotensin II and other growth mediators suggests an important role for angiotensin II in the tightly regulated processes of organogenesis and remodeling in the fetus. Along with other organ systems, these coordinated effects direct the kidney to become a properly differentiated and architecturally organized organ. At a slightly later time during development, coincident with differentiation and maturation of the kidney, the RAS gains the capability to control water and solute balance and then renal hemodynamics. After birth, these mechanisms become more tightly regulated and efficient and allow the maintenance of homeostasis in the extrauterine environment.

REFERENCES

1. Keeton TK, Campbell WB: The pharmacologic alteration of renin release. Pharmacol Rev 31:81, 1981.
2. Peach MJ: Renin-angiotensin system: biochemistry and mechanisms of action. Physiol Rev 57:313, 1977.
3. Ferrario CM, et al: Angiotensin-(1-7): a new hormone of the angiotensin system. Hypertension 18(Suppl 3):126, 1991.
4. Navar LG, et al: Effects of locally formed angiotensin II on renal hemodynamics. Fed Proc 45:1448, 1986.
5. Campbell DJ: Circulating and tissue angiotensin systems. J Clin Invest 79:1, 1987.
6. Von Lutterotti N, et al: Renin is not synthesized by cardiac and extrarenal vascular tissues: a review of experimental evidence. Circulation 89:458, 1994.
7. Norman JT: The role of angiotensin II in renal growth. Renal Physiol Biochem 14:175, 1991.
8. Gomez RA: Angiotensin receptors: relevance in development and disease states. Exp Nephrol 2:259, 1994.
9. Gomez RA, Norwood VF: Developmental consequences of the renin-angiotensin system. Am J Kidney Dis 26:409, 1995.
10. Lynch KR, Peach MJ: Molecular biology of angiotensinogen. Hypertension 17:263, 1991.
11. Dzau VJ, et al: Molecular biology of the renin-angiotensin system. Am J Physiol 255:F563, 1988.
12. Hsueh WA, Baxter JD: Human prorenin. Hypertension 17:469, 1991.
13. Deschepper CF, et al: Analysis by immunocytochemistry and in situ hybridization of renin and its mRNA in kidney, testis, adrenal, and pituitary of the rat. Proc Natl Acad Sci U S A 83:7552, 1986.
14. Soubrier F, et al: Two putative active centers in human angiotensin I–converting enzyme revealed by molecular cloning. Proc Natl Acad Sci U S A 85:9386, 1988.
15. Soubrier F, et al: Molecular biology of the angiotensin I converting enzyme. II. Structure-function: gene polymorphism and clinical implications. J Hypertens 11:599, 1993.
16. Peach MJ: Pharmacology of angiotensin II. In Kidney Hormones. London, Academic Press, 1986, pp 273-308.
17. Freeman EJ, et al: Angiotensin-(1-7) inhibits vascular smooth muscle cell growth. Hypertension 28:104, 1996.
18. Handa RK, et al: Renal actions of angiotensin-(1-7): in vivo and in vitro studies. Am J Physiol 270:F141, 1996.
19. Timmermans PBMWM, et al: Angiotensin II receptors and angiotensin II receptor antagonists. Pharmacol Rev 45:205, 1993.
20. Timmermans PBMWM, et al: Angiotensin II receptors and functional correlates. Am J Hypertens 5:221S, 1992.
21. Yamada T, et al: Angiotensin II type 2 receptor mediates programmed cell death. Proc Natl Acad Sci U S A 93:156, 1996.
22. Mukoyama M, et al: Characterization of a rat type 2 angiotensin II receptor stably expressed in 293 cells. Mol Cell Endocrinol 112:61, 1995.
23. Bottari SP, et al: The angiotensin AT2 receptor stimulates protein tyrosine phosphatase activity and mediates inhibition of particulate guanylate cyclase. Biochem Biophys Res Commun 183:206, 1992.
24. Nakajima M, et al: The angiotensin II type 2 (AT2) receptor antagonizes the growth effects of the AT1 receptor: gain-of-function study using gene transfer. Proc Natl Acad Sci U S A 92:10663, 1995.
25. Kambayashi Y, et al: Molecular cloning of a novel angiotensin II receptor isoform involved in phosphotyrosine phosphatase inhibition. J Biol Chem 268:24543, 1993.
26. Gomez RA, et al: Fetal expression of the angiotensinogen gene. Endocrinology 123:2298, 1988.
27. Jelinek J, et al: The renin-angiotensin system in the perinatal period in rats. J Dev Physiol 8:33, 1986.
28. Godard C, et al: The renin-angiotensin-aldosterone system in mother and fetus at term. Nephron 17:353, 1976.
29. Robillard JE, et al: Renal hemodynamics and functional adjustments to postnatal life. Semin Perinatol 12:143, 1988.
30. Kalinyak JE, Perlman AJ: Tissue-specific regulation of angiotensinogen mRNA accumulation by dexamethasone. J Biol Chem 262:460, 1987.
31. Chang E, Perlman AJ: Angiotensinogen mRNA: regulation by cell cycle and growth factors. J Biol Chem 263:5480, 1988.
32. Ellison KE, et al: Androgen regulation of rat renal angiotensinogen mRNA expression. J Clin Invest 83:1941, 1989.
33. Klett C, Hackenthal E: Induction of angiotensinogen synthesis and secretion by angiotensin II. Clin Exp Hypertens 12:2027, 1987.
34. Everett AD, et al: Hepatic angiotensinogen gene regulation in the fetal and pregnant rat. Pediatr Res 30:252, 1991.
35. Wilkes B, et al: Evidence for a functional renin-angiotensin system in full-term fetoplacental unit. Am J Physiol 249:E366, 1985.
36. Celio M, et al: Ontogeny of renin immunoreactive cells in the human kidney. Anat Embryol 173:149, 1985.
37. Lopez MLSS, et al: Embryonic origin and lineage of juxtaglomerular cells. Am J Physiol 281:F345, 2001.
38. Richoux AS, et al: Earliest renin-containing cell differentiation during ontogenesis in the rat: an immunocytochemical study. Histochemistry 88:41, 1987.
39. Pupilli C, et al: Spatial association of renin-containing cells and nerve fibers in developing rat kidney. Pediatr Nephrol 5:690, 1991.
40. Gomez RA, et al: Maturation of the intrarenal renin distribution in Wistar-Kyoto rats. J Hypertens 4(Suppl 5):S31, 1986.
41. Symonds EM, Farler I: Plasma renin levels in the normal and anephric fetus. Biol Neonate 23:133, 1973.
42. Stalker HP, et al: Plasma renin activity in healthy children. J Pediatr 89:256, 1976.
43. Hiner LB, et al: Plasma renin activity in normal children. J Pediatr 89:258, 1976.
44. Sassard J, et al: Plasma renin activity in normal subjects from infancy to puberty. J Clin Endocrinol Metab 40:524, 1975.
45. Richer C, et al: Plasma renin activity and its postnatal development in preterm infants. Biol Neonate 31:305, 1977.
46. Gomez RA, et al: Molecular and cellular aspects of renin during kidney ontogeny. Pediatr Nephrol 5:80, 1991.
47. Pelayo JC, et al: The ontogeny of the renin-angiotensin system. Clin Perinatol 8:2:347, 1981.
48. Stevens AD, Lumbers ER: The relationship between plasma renin activity and renal electrolyte excretion in the fetal sheep. J Dev Physiol 3:101, 1981.
49. Siegel SR: The effects of salt loading on the renin-angiotensin control of blood pressure in the newborn lamb. Pediatr Res 17:210, 1983.
50. Guillery EN, Robillard JE: The renin-angiotensin system and blood pressure regulation during infancy and childhood. Pediatr Clin North Am 40:61, 1993.
51. Page WA, et al: Renal nerves modulate kidney renin gene expression during the transition from fetal to newborn life. Am J Physiol 262:R459, 1992.
52. Smith FG, et al: Role of renal sympathetic nerves in lambs during the transition from fetal to newborn life. J Clin Invest 88:1988, 1991.

53. Everett AD, et al: Renin release and gene expression in intact rat kidney microvessels and single cells. J Clin Invest 86:169, 1990.
54. Tufro-McReddie A, et al: Angiotensin II type 1 receptor: role in renal growth and gene expression during normal development. Am J Physiol 266:F911, 1994.
55. Wallace KB, et al: Development of angiotensin-converting enzyme in fetal rat lungs. Am J Physiol 236:R57, 1979.
56. Costerousse O, et al: Regulation of ACE gene expression and plasma levels during rat postnatal development. Am J Physiol 267:E745, 1994.
57. Wallace KB, et al: Angiotensin-converting enzyme in developing lung and kidney. Am J Physiol 234:R141, 1978.
58. Mounier F, et al: Ontogenesis of angiotensin-I converting enzyme in human kidney. Kidney Int 32:684, 1987.
59. Wallace KB, et al: Angiotensin II metabolism by tissues from developing rats. Pediatr Res 15:1088, 1981.
60. Jones C, et al: Characterization of angiotensin II receptors in the rat fetus. Peptides 10:459, 1989.
61. Grady EF, et al: Expression of AT₂ receptors in the developing rat fetus. J Clin Invest 88:921, 1991.
62. Norwood VF, et al: Differential expression of angiotensin II receptors during early renal morphogenesis. Am J Physiol 272:R662, 1997.
63. Tufro-McReddie A, et al: Ontogeny of type 1 angiotensin receptor gene expression in the rat. J Clin Invest 91:530, 1993.
64. Ciuffo GM, et al: Glomerular angiotensin II receptor subtypes during development of rat kidney. Am J Physiol 265:F264, 1993.
65. Ozono R, et al: Expression of the subtype 2 angiotensin (AT₂) receptor protein in rat kidney. Hypertension 30:1238, 1997.
66. Tufro-McReddie A, Gomez RA: Ontogeny of the renin-angiotensin system. Semin Nephrol 13:519, 1993.
67. Levens NR, et al: Role of the intrarenal renin-angiotensin system in the control of renal function. Circ Res 48:157, 1981.
68. Kim H-K, et al: Genetic control of blood pressure and the angiotensinogen locus. Proc Natl Acad Sci U S A 92:2735, 1995.
69. Yanai K, et al: Renin-dependent cardiovascular functions and renin-independent blood brain barrier functions revealed by renin-deficient mice. J Biol Chem 275:5, 2000.
70. Esther CR Jr, et al: Mice lacking angiotensin-converting enzyme have low blood pressure, renal pathology, and reduced male fertility. Lab Invest 74:953, 1996.
71. Krege JH, et al: Male-female differences in fertility and blood pressure in ACE-deficient mice. Nature 375:146, 1995.
72. Ito M, et al: Regulation of blood pressure by the type 1A angiotensin II receptor gene. Proc Natl Acad Sci USA 92:3521, 1995.
73. Robillard JE, et al: Comparison of the adrenal and renal responses to angiotensin II in fetal lambs and adult sheep. Circ Res 50:140, 1982.
74. Gomez RA, Robillard JE: Developmental aspects of the renal responses to hemorrhage during converting-enzyme inhibition in fetal lambs. Circ Res 54:301, 1984.
75. O'Dea RF, et al: Treatment of neonatal hypertension with captopril. J Pediatr 113:403, 1988.
76. Ausiello DA, et al: Contraction of cultured rat glomerular cells of apparent mesangial origin after stimulation with angiotensin II and arginine vasopressin. J Clin Invest 65:754, 1980.
77. Ray PE, et al: Angiotensin II stimulates human fetal mesangial cell proliferation and fibronectin biosynthesis by binding to AT₁ receptors. Kidney Int 45:177, 1994.
78. Lumbers ER, et al: The effects of a converting enzyme inhibitor (captopril) and angiotensin II on fetal renal function. Br J Pharmacol 110:821, 1993.
79. Sedman AB, et al: Recognition and management of angiotensin converting enzyme inhibitor fetopathy. Pediatr Nephrol 9:382, 1995.
80. Wang H, et al: Angiotensin II enhances tubuloglomerular feedback via luminal AT1 receptors on the macula densa. Kidney Int 60:1851, 2001.
81. Briggs JP, et al: Quantitative characterization of the tubuloglomerular feedback response: effect of growth. Am J Physiol 247:F808, 1984.
82. Hogarty DC, et al: The role of angiotensin, AT₁ receptor and AT₂ receptors in the pressor, drinking and vasopressin responses to central angiotensin. Brain Res 586:289, 1992.
83. Bloch RD, et al: Activation of proximal tubular Na⁺-H⁺ exchange by angiotensin II. Am J Physiol 263:F135, 1992.
84. Geibel J, et al: Angiotensin II stimulates both Na⁺-H⁺ exchange and Na⁺/HCO₃ cotransport in the rabbit proximal tubule. Proc Natl Acad Sci U S A 87:7917, 1990.
85. Garvin JL: Angiotensin stimulates bicarbonate transport and Na⁺/K⁺ ATPase in rat proximal straight tubules. J Am Soc Nephrol 1:1146, 1991.
86. Tojo A, et al: Angiotensin II regulates H⁺-ATPase activity in rat cortical collecting duct. Am J Physiol 267:F1045, 1994.
87. Spitzer A: The role of the kidney in sodium homeostasis during development. Kidney Int 21:539, 1982.
88. Wolf G, Neilson EG: Angiotensin II induces cellular hypertrophy in cultured murine proximal tubular cells. Am J Physiol 259:F768, 1990.
89. Holycross BJ, et al: Angiotensin II stimulates increased protein synthesis, not increased DNA synthesis, in intact rat aortic segments, in vitro. J Vasc Res 30:80, 1993.
90. Dubey RK, et al: Culture of renal arteriolar smooth muscle cells: mitogenic responses to angiotensin II. Circ Res 71:1143, 1992.
91. Itoh H, et al: Multiple autocrine growth factors modulate vascular smooth muscle cell growth response to angiotensin II. J Clin Invest 91:2268, 1993.
92. Stoll M, et al: The angiotensin AT2 receptor mediates inhibition of cell proliferation in coronary endothelial cells. J Clin Invest 95:651, 1995.
93. Le Noble FAC, et al: Evidence for a novel angiotensin II receptor involved in angiogenesis in chick embryo chorioallantoic membrane. Am J Physiol 264:R460, 1993.
94. Tufro-McReddie A, et al: Angiotensin II regulates nephrogenesis and renal vascular development. Am J Physiol 269:F110, 1995.
95. Inokuchi S, et al: Hyperplastic vascular smooth muscle cells of the intrarenal arteries in angiotensin II type 1a receptor null mutant mice. Kidney Int 60:722, 2001.
96. Hilgers KF, et al: Aberrant renal vascular morphology and renin expression in mutant mice lacking angiotensin-converting enzyme. Hypertension 29:216, 1997.
97. Oliverio MI, et al: Reduced growth, abnormal kidney structure, and type 2 (AT₂) angiotensin receptor-mediated blood pressure regulation in mice lacking both AT₁ₐ and AT₁ᵦ receptors for angiotensin II. Proc Natl Acad Sci U S A 95:15496, 1998.
98. Tsuchida S, et al: Murine double nullizygotes of the angiotensin type 1A and 1B receptor genes duplicate severe abnormal phenotypes of angiotensinogen nullizygotes. J Clin Invest 101:755, 1998.
99. Hein L, et al: Behavioural and cardiovascular effects of disrupting the angiotensin II type-2 receptor gene in mice. Nature 377:744, 1995.
100. Anderson PW, et al: Angiotensin II causes mesangial cell hypertrophy. Hypertension 21:29, 1993.
101. Orth SR, et al: Angiotensin II induces hypertrophy and hyperplasia in adult human mesangial cells. Exp Nephrol 3:23, 1995.
102. Wolf G, et al: Angiotensin stimulates cellular hypertrophy of LLC-PK₁ cells through the AT₁ receptor. Nephrol Dial Transplant 8:128, 1993.
103. Wolf G, et al: Angiotensin II is a mitogen for a murine cell line isolated from medullary thick ascending limb of Henle's loop. Am J Physiol 268:F940, 1995.
104. Friberg P, et al: Renin-angiotensin system in neonatal rats: induction of a renal abnormality in response to ACE inhibition or angiotensin II antagonism. Kidney Int 45:485, 1994.
105. Spence SG, et al: Defining the susceptible period of developmental toxicity for the AT₁-selective angiotensin II receptor antagonist losartan in rats. Teratology 51:367, 1995.
106. Ichiki T, et al: Effects on blood pressure and exploratory behaviour of mice lacking angiotensin II type-2 receptor. Nature 377:748, 1995.
107. Nishimura H, et al: Role of the angiotensin type 2 receptor gene in congenital anomalies of the kidney and urinary tract, CAKUT, of mice and men. Mol Cell 3:1, 1999.

129

Jean-Pierre Guignard

Postnatal Development of Glomerular Filtration Rate in Neonates

The production of urine begins with the formation of an ultrafiltrate of plasma by the glomerulus. The function of the tubule is to modify this ultrafiltrate to allow an efficient excretion of waste products and a retention of those substances required to maintain body fluid volume and homeostasis. Glomerular filtration is also essential for the elimination of drugs. Alterations in glomerular filtration rate (GFR) have severe consequences on the body fluid homeostasis. The assessment of GFR can thus be of great value in various neonatal conditions because an estimate of GFR may be required to prescribe fluids, electrolytes, or drugs excreted by the kidney. This chapter reviews the factors that regulate GFR and the methods available to assess GFR in the newborn infant.

PHYSIOLOGY OF GLOMERULAR FILTRATION

Urine formation starts by the production of an ultrafiltrate of plasma across the permselective glomerular capillary wall. The glomerular capillary behaves as if it were a filtering membrane containing aqueous pores with a diameter of 7.5 to 10 nm. The wall of the glomerular capillary consists of three layers: (1) the endothelial cell lining of the glomerular capillaries; (2) the glomerular basement membrane, composed of connective, noncellular tissues; and (3) the visceral epithelial cells of the Bowman capsule. The endothelial cells have many circular formations (holes) with a diameter of 50 to 100 nm. The capillary endothelium acts as a screen to prevent blood cells and platelets from entering into contact with the basement membrane. Under the endothelium, the basement membrane forms a continuous layer that probably behaves as the filtration barrier of large molecules. It is formed of negatively charged glycoproteins, mainly Type IV collagen, laminin, and fibronectin. The basement membrane is the main filtration barrier. The epithelium is formed by highly specialized cells called podocytes, which are attached to the basement membrane by foot processes known as *pedicels*. Adjacent pedicels are separated by filtration slits measuring about 25 by 60 nm in width, and each gap is bridged by a thin diaphragm. The diaphragms, in turn, contain rectangular "pores" with a dimension of 4 by 14 nm. Thus, the filtration slits with their diaphragms could also constitute a filtration barrier. The podocytes may help in the phagocytosis of macromolecules. The size of the apertures in the glomerular filtration "barrier" is not the only factor that limits the passage of compounds through the glomerular capillary wall. The shape of the molecule, its flexibility and deformability, and its electrical charge also play important roles. The molecular weight (MW) cut-off for the glomerular filter is about 70,000. Thus, 69,000-MW albumin passes through the filter in minute quantities. Smaller molecules pass the filter more easily. Molecules with MW less than 7000 pass freely. The glomerular ultrafiltration thus initially contains small solutes and ions in the same concentration as present in the plasma.

The central part of the glomerular tuft is composed of irregularly shaped cells, the mesangial cells, that hold the delicate glomerular structures. By contracting, the mesangial cells can modify the filtering surface area of the glomerular capillaries. The mesangial cells also act as phagocytes to prevent the accumulation in the basement membrane of macromolecules that have escaped from the capillaries.

The rate of ultrafiltration is governed by several factors: the balance of Starling forces across the capillary wall, the rate at which plasma flows into the glomerular capillaries, the permeability of the glomerular capillary wall to water and small solutes, and the total surface area of the capillaries. The ultrafiltration coefficient (K_f) is defined as the product of the glomerular capillary permeability and the area of the capillary available for filtration. The permeability of the glomerular capillaries is about 100 times greater than the permeability of other capillaries elsewhere in the body. The mean hydrostatic pressure within the glomerulus favors filtration. It is opposed by the oncotic pressure in the glomerular capillary. ΔP and $\Delta \pi$ represent the glomerular transcapillary hydrostatic and oncotic pressure, respectively. The net ultrafiltration pressure (P_{UF}) is defined as $\Delta P - \Delta \pi$. GFR is proportional to the sum of the Starling forces across the glomerular capillaries ($\Delta P - \Delta \pi$) times the K_f:

$$GFR = K_f(\Delta P - \Delta \pi)$$

In normal conditions, P_{UF} and GFR are highly dependent on the arterial pressure within the glomerular capillaries, on renal blood flow (RBF), and on the glomerular plasma flow rate. The

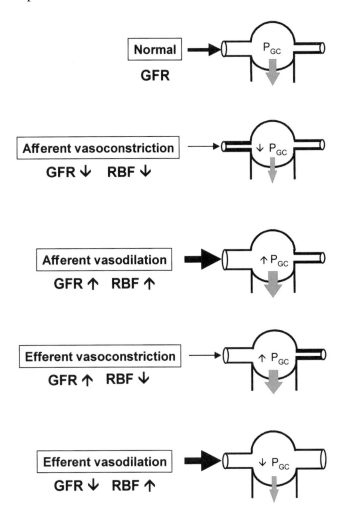

Figure 129–1. Effects of changes in the afferent or efferent arteriolar tone on renal blood flow (RBF) and glomerular filtration rate (GFR). P_{GC} = glomerular capillary hydraulic pressure.

transcapillary hydrostatic pressure is also regulated by the balance between the afferent and efferent arteriolar resistance (Fig. 129–1). Pathologic conditions and drugs can affect GFR by modifying the pressure within the glomerular capillary (severe hypotension), the K_f (drugs, diseases), or the oncotic pressure within the glomerular capillary (changes in plasma proteins).

Vasoactive Agents

Several vasoactive agents modulate GFR and RBF during fetal and postnatal life.[1] Such agents include angiotensin II, the prostaglandins, atrial natriuretic peptide, endothelin, nitric oxide, bradykinin, and adenosine. Sympathetic nerves can also affect vascular tone. All these factors modulate GFR by affecting afferent or efferent vascular tone (see Fig. 129–1), as well as mesangial contractility. The main actions of the vasoactive agents are as follows:

Angiotensin II: This peptide is a potent constrictor of the efferent arterioles and, to a lesser extent, of the afferent arterioles. It therefore increases the glomerular hydrostatic pressure and GFR, while decreasing RBF. Facilitation of angiotensin II release occurs during hypotension or hypovolemia. In these instances, increased angiotensin II levels maintain an effective transglomerular pressure gradient and prevent a decrease in GFR by constricting the efferent arterioles.[1]

Prostaglandins: The prostaglandins, in particular prostaglandins E_2 and I_2, are of major importance for maintaining the GFR of the newborn kidney perfused at low arterial pressures. They vasodilate the afferent arterioles and dampen the renal vasoconstrictor effects of both angiotensin II and sympathetic nervous stimulation on the afferent arteriole.[1]

Atrial natriuretic peptide: This peptide causes vasodilation of the afferent arteriole and vasoconstriction of the efferent arteriole, thus increasing GFR without significantly affecting RBF.[2]

Nitric oxide: The endothelium-derived nitric oxide decreases the renal vascular resistance, thus increasing both GFR and RBF. This autacoid is released from the vascular endothelial cells throughout the body. In the kidney, it prevents excessive vasoconstriction when vasoconstrictive forces are overstimulated.[3]

Bradykinin: This vasodilator and diuretic peptide is produced in the kidney by the effect of the enzyme kallikrein on kininogen. Bradykinin exerts its renal effects via β_2-receptors, the expression of which is higher in neonatal than in adult kidneys, a finding suggesting a role for this peptide during renal development. Bradykinin vasodilates the newborn kidney, as evidenced by the renal vasoconstriction that results from bradykinin by β_2-receptor blockade.[4]

Endothelin: This peptide released from endothelial cells constricts the afferent and the efferent arterioles, thereby decreasing both GFR and RBF. Surprisingly, circumstantial evidence suggests that, at low endogenous concentrations, endothelin may actually vasodilate the glomerular vessels in fetuses and neonates.[5]

Norepinephrine and epinephrine: Released from the adrenal medulla, these substances constrict the afferent and efferent arterioles and thus decrease GFR and RBF.

Sympathetic nervous stimulation: Overactivation of this system increases the tone of the afferent arterioles and decreases RBF and GFR. Overstimulation probably occurs in severe disturbances as induced by acute hemorrhage, fetal distress, and asphyxia.

Autoregulation of Glomerular Filtration Rate and Renal Blood Flow

Autoregulation is necessary to prevent abrupt changes in GFR and RBF when blood pressure varies acutely. Two systems are responsible for renal autoregulation: (1) a myogenic mechanism and (2) a tubuloglomerular feedback mechanism.

The myogenic mechanism refers to the intrinsic ability of arteries to constrict when blood pressure rises and to vasodilate when it decreases. This phenomenon prevents excessive changes in RBF and GFR when blood pressure varies.

The tubuloglomerular feedback mechanism involves the macula densa and the juxtaglomerular cells. The macula densa cells sense the changes in sodium chloride delivery to the distal tubule that follow changes in blood pressure. A drop in blood pressure and its consequent decrease in sodium chloride delivery stimulate angiotensin II formation by the juxtaglomerular cells. By constricting the efferent arteriole, angiotensin II increases the intraglomerular hydrostatic pressure and thus returns GFR toward normal levels.

CONCEPT OF CLEARANCE

The most common measurement of GFR is based on the concept of *clearance,* which relates the quantitative urinary excretion of a substance per unit time to the volume of plasma that, if "cleared" completely of the same contained substance, would yield a quantity equivalent to that excreted in the urine. The clearance (C) of a substance (x) is expressed by the following formula:

$$C = U_x \cdot V/P_x$$

where U_x represents the urinary concentration of the substance, V the urine flow rate, and P_x the plasma concentration. For its clearance to be equal to the rate of glomerular filtration, a substance must have the following properties: (1) it must be freely filterable through the glomerular capillary membranes, that is, not be bound to plasma proteins or sieved in the process of ultrafiltration; (2) it must be biologically inert and neither reabsorbed nor secreted by the renal tubules; and (3) it must be nontoxic and not alter renal function when infused in quantities that permit adequate quantification in plasma and urine.

Several substances, endogenous or exogenous, have been claimed to have the foregoing properties: inulin, creatinine, iohexol, ethylenediaminetetraacetic acid, diethylenetriaminepentaacetic acid (DTPA), and sodium iothalamate. The experimental evidence that this is true has been produced only for inulin. The most commonly used markers in neonates are creatinine and inulin.

GLOMERULAR MARKERS

Inulin

Inulin, a fructose polysaccharide derived from dahlia roots and Jerusalem artichokes, has an Einstein-Stokes radius of 1.5 nm and a MW of approximately 5200. It diffuses as would a spheric body of such radius. Inulin is inert, is not metabolized, and can be recovered quantitatively in the urine after parenteral administration.

The rate of excretion of inulin is directly proportional to, and a linear function of, the plasma concentration of inulin over a wide range. The clearance of inulin (U • [V/P]) is consequently independent of its plasma concentration. Evidence that inulin is neither reabsorbed nor secreted by the renal tubules has been obtained in experimental micropuncture studies showing that (1) the concentration of inulin was identical in the Bowman space fluid and plasma, (2) 99.3% of inulin injected in the proximal tubule could be collected in the distal tubule, and (3) the rate of recovery was the same when the peritubular plasma was loaded with inulin.[6]

The renal excretion of inulin thus occurs exclusively by glomerular filtration, so its clearance is the most accurate index of GFR. Estimates of inulin clearance provide the basis for a standard reference against which the route or mechanisms of excretion of other substances can be ascertained.

Inulin as a Marker of Glomerular Filtration Rate in Neonates

Studies comparing the clearance of inulin with that of other glomerular markers have led to the hypothesis that glomerular pore size is related to body size, and inulin may not be freely filtered by the immature glomerulus.[7] This hypothesis has not been confirmed by studies of inulin handling in rats[8] or fetal lambs,[9] both of which failed to demonstrate any restriction to the filtration of inulin. The same conclusion was reached from studies in preterm infants that showed that higher MW inulin did not accumulate in the plasma of very immature babies infused with inulin for several days and thus excluded any retention of the larger molecules.[10,11]

In clinical practice, sinistrin, a readily soluble preparation of polyfructosan with side branching (extracted from bulbs of *Urginea maritima*), is more widely used. The clearance of sinistrin is identical to that of inulin. Because complicated analytical methods are required for its measurement, inulin and sinistrin cannot be used for routine clinical purposes. Numerous other potential glomerular markers have consequently been investigated. In neonates, only creatinine has been used broadly to assess GFR.

Creatinine

Creatinine is the anhydride of creatine, a compound that exists in skeletal muscle as creatine phosphate. It has a MW of 113. Conversion of creatine to creatinine is nonenzymatic and irreversible. The serum creatinine level reflects total body supplies of creatine and correlates with muscle mass.[12] Creatinine is excreted through the kidneys in quantities proportional to the serum content. The renal excretion of endogenous creatinine is very similar to that of inulin in humans and several animal species. However, in addition to being filtered through the glomerulus, creatinine is secreted in part by the renal tubular cells. In spite of this, creatinine clearance correlates well with inulin clearance when the GFR is normal. This agreement results from the balance of two factors: (1) excretion rate of creatinine is higher than the filtered rate because of the occurrence of tubular secretion of creatinine, and (2) the measured plasma creatinine is higher than the true creatinine because of the presence of noncreatinine chromogens that interfere with the colorimetric analysis of creatinine (*Jaffe reaction*).

Overestimation of GFR by creatinine clearance is usually more evident at low GFR. As GFR falls progressively during the course of renal disease, the renal tubular secretion of creatinine contributes an increasing fraction to urinary excretion, so that creatinine clearance may substantially exceed the actual GFR.

The use of creatinine clearance to estimate GFR may be unreliable when one studies uremic patients. Creatinine is uniformly distributed in the body water,[13] and it diffuses into the gut. At a normal plasma concentration, the amount of creatinine entering the gut is negligible; it may become significant during renal failure when the plasma creatinine increases.[14] This phenomenon may also explain why creatinine clearance overestimates true GFR in patients with renal failure.

Creatinine as a Marker of Glomerular Filtration Rate in Neonates

The plasma creatinine concentration varies during the first postnatal weeks.[15-17] It is elevated at birth and decreases rapidly during the first week of life (Fig. 129–2); values stabilize around 0.40 mg/dl (35 µmol/l; range, 0.14 to 0.70 mg/dl [12 to 61 µmol/l]) on the fifth postnatal day in term infants and somewhat later in very low birth weight infants.[17, 18] The elevated plasma creatinine concentration at the time of birth reflects maternal creatinine levels. Indeed, a perfect equilibrium between fetal and maternal plasma creatinine concentrations has been observed throughout gestation.[19, 20] In very premature neonates, the elevated plasma creatinine at birth increases transiently; the highest levels are reached by the third day of life (Fig. 129–3 and Table 129–1).[21, 22] The plasma urea also rises significantly over time, but it does so in a more variable manner (see Fig. 129–3). This postnatal transient increase in plasma creatinine values is probably the consequence of creatinine reabsorption (back diffu-

sion) across leaky tubules,[23] as suggested by studies in piglets and newborn rabbits.[23,24] Plasma creatinine levels may take a month to reach *neonatal* levels in very low birth weight infants.[17,18]

Iohexol

Iohexol is a nonionic contrast agent with a MW of 821 Da that appears to be eliminated exclusively by glomerular filtration. In spite of reports showing a significant correlation between the plasma disappearance curve of iohexol and the standard clearance of inulin, its usefulness in clinical pediatric practice remains to be demonstrated. It should not be used in the neonatal period.

Iothalamate Sodium

Iothalamate sodium has a MW of 637 Da. It is only minimally bound to plasma proteins,[25] and its clearance is independent of variations in plasma activity. It is not excreted in the urine of the aglomerular fish.[26] The clearance of iothalamate was initially shown to correlate well with that of inulin. However, later studies unequivocally demonstrated that iothalamate is actively secreted by the renal tubules and perhaps also undergoes tubular reabsorption in humans and animal species.[27] The agreement of iothalamate clearance with inulin clearance appears to be a fortuitous cancellation of errors between tubular excretion and protein binding.[28] Iothalamate sodium has rarely been used in human neonates and in neonatal animal studies. Its use during the first month of life should be avoided.

Technetium 99m Diethylenetriaminepenta-acetic Acid

Technetium 99m-DTPA (Tc 99m DTPA) is excreted mainly by glomerular filtration.[28] Its clearance approximates that of other glomerular markers.[29] Although certain commercial preparations have been shown to contain impurities that bind to plasma proteins (thus causing errors when measuring GFR),[30] this agent is useful for imaging and for split renal function measurements. It cannot, however, be considered a marker of absolute GFR in clinical or experimental studies. The uptake and excretion of Tc 99m DTPA appear to vary considerably in neonates; delayed and normal uptake and excretion of the tracer have been described in healthy infants. Reliable information can, however, be obtained after 1 month of life.

Chromium 51 Ethylenediaminetetraacetic Acid

Chromium 51 Ethylenediaminetetraacetic acid has a MW of 292 Da. It is a glomerular marker with a clearance identical to that of DTPA. Useful information cannot be obtained with this agent before the end of the neonatal period.[31]

CLINICAL ASSESSMENT OF GLOMERULAR FILTRATION RATE IN NEONATES

Standard Clearances

Inulin Clearance

Classic inulin clearance studies have been performed in premature and term neonates to provide data on (1) the reliability of inulin as a marker of GFR in human neonates, (2) the development of GFR in early postnatal life, and (3) the effect of disease states on GFR.

In the classic method, inulin is administered as a priming dose to achieve plasma concentrations close to 300 to 400 mg/l and is constantly infused to maintain such levels. Accurate urine collection is performed using bladder catheterization, spontaneous voiding into plastic bags, or a collection tray.[32-34] The clearance study is performed over 3 to 4 hours.

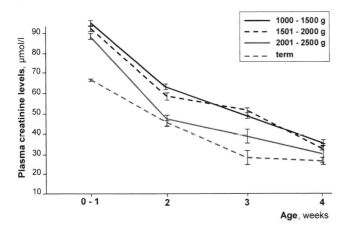

Figure 129–2. Plasma creatinine concentrations (µmol/l) during the first weeks of life. (From Bueva A, Guignard JP: Pediatr Res *36*:572, 1994.)

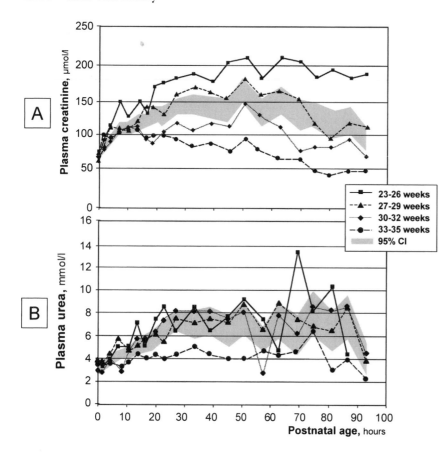

Figure 129–3. Changes in plasma creatinine (**A**) and urea (**B**) concentrations during the first 100 hours of life of premature neonates of variable gestational age. The *shaded area* represents 95% confidence intervals (CIs) for the mean plasma creatinine or urea of all infants. (Adapted from Miall LS, et al: Pediatrics 6:104, 1999.)

TABLE 129-1

Changes in Plasma Creatinine over Time for Different Gestation Groups

Group *Gestation age (wk)*	Birth *Plasma Creatinine (μmol/l)**	Peak *Plasma Creatinine (μmol/l)**	Time to Peak *Plasma Creatinine (h)**
23–26	67–92	195–247	40–78
27–29	65–89	158–200	28–51
30–32	60–69	120–158	25–40
33–45	67–79	99–140	8–23

*95% confidence intervals.
Adapted from Miall LS, et al: Pediatrics *104*: e76, 1999.

Several studies[10, 11] clearly demonstrated that inulin is freely filtered in even the most immature of human patients. The standard inulin clearance must thus be considered the reference test in human neonates to which all other methods of estimating GFR should be compared.

Creatinine Clearance

Creatinine is the most commonly used marker of GFR. Its clearance has been claimed to approximate true GFR in both term and preterm neonates. The validity of creatinine clearance has been assessed in low birth weight infants (mean birth weight, 1600 g; range, 1040 to 2275 g; postnatal age, 10 hours to 10 days). A significant correlation was found (r = 0.738) between inulin and creatinine clearance, but the scatter of values was substantial.[35] In infants with the lowest GFR (C_{in} < 12.5 ml/minute/1.73 m²), creatinine clearance overestimated true GFR, whereas it underestimated it in infants with higher filtration rates. A substantial underestimation of GFR by creatinine clearance has usually been reported in preterm and mature neonates.[36, 37] Measurement of creatinine by a manual resin adsorption method, rather than by the

automated method, improved the correlation.[37] Several factors can account for the variability of creatinine clearance determinations in very premature infants. These factors fall into two major categories: (1) those related to the transport of creatinine by the premature kidney and (2) those affecting the accuracy of plasma creatinine assays. Because of the low-normal levels of creatinine in the blood of neonates, small variations in laboratory measurement may spuriously alter the estimated concentration. Most clinical laboratories determine creatinine with the Jaffe reaction, which may be affected by many interfering substances, such as bilirubin. Values obtained by this method greatly overestimate the true creatinine concentration at values lower than 1.0 mg/dl.[38] Modifications of the classic Jaffe technique have improved its specificity. Enzymatic techniques have been shown to be specific; their major drawback for routine use in neonates is interference by bilirubin. High-pressure liquid chromatography[38,39] and dilution mass spectrometry[40] both provide reliable results. They cannot yet be used routinely.

Inaccuracies in determining the true creatinine concentration in neonates, as well as uncertainties in renal tubular handling, point to a possible drawback in the use of creatinine as a glomerular marker, at least in very low birth weight infants. With these limitations in mind, the true creatinine clearance probably remains the best index of GFR for routine use.[16,41,42]

Estimation of Glomerular Filtration Rate Without Urine Collection

Constant Infusion of Inulin Without Urine Collection

The constant infusion technique[43] assumes that the rate of intravenous infusion needed to maintain the plasma concentration of inulin at a constant level is equal to the rate of its excretion. At constant plasma levels, after inulin has equilibrated in its diffusion space, the U • V/P clearance must be equal to the rate of infusion (I) divided by the plasma concentration: C = U • [V/P] = I/P. To accelerate the achievement of a steady plasma concentration of inulin, a loading dose of inulin precedes the constant intravenous infusion. An estimate of the extracellular fluid volume (where inulin distributes) and of GFR is required to select the correct loading dose and infusion rate.

Conflicting results have been produced in studies in which inulin was constantly infused for only a few hours. Although Cole and Leake and their colleagues[44,45] found an excellent correlation between the constant infusion method and the standard clearance of inulin (r = 0.999), Alinei and Guignard[46,47] found that the infusion method without urine collection greatly overestimated the true GFR. The overestimation, close to 30%, declined with time, but it remained substantial after 3 hours of infusion.

In later studies in which inulin was constantly infused for only 80 minutes after a bolus injection, Coulthard[48] also failed to demonstrate a good correlation between the infusion technique without urine collection and the standard clearance of inulin. This occurred in infants with a stable plasma inulin concentration. A closer inspection of the data, however, showed that the plasma concentration of inulin still reflected the size of the bolus, thus demonstrating that equilibrium had not been reached. In the same study, Coulthard[48] demonstrated that reliable estimates of GFR could be obtained, provided inulin was constantly infused for 24 hours, with or without bolus injection at the start of the test. This method has the obvious advantage of eliminating the need for urine collection. Its main disadvantage is that it requires a constant infusion of long duration, as well as careful supervision of the test. Should the infusion stop for a moment, a long extra period of infusion would be necessary because the plasma inulin falls exponentially but only rises again asymptomatically.[44] The constant infusion method also has the disadvantage of not reflecting acute changes in GFR. A short 1- to 3-hour constant infusion technique was used by Leake and Trygstad[49] to define the relationship between inulin clearance and gestational age. A significant correlation was found, as previously demonstrated by Fawer and co-workers[32] in neonates studied by the standard inulin clearance technique.

Single-Injection (Plasma Disappearance Curve) Technique

The mathematical model for this technique is an open two-compartment system.[50] The glomerular marker is injected in the first compartment, equilibrates with the second compartment, and is excreted from the first compartment by glomerular filtration. The plasma disappearance curve of the marker follows two consecutive patterns. In the first, the plasma concentration falls rapidly, but at a progressively diminishing rate. This reflects distribution of the tracer in both compartments, as well as its renal excretion. In the second, the slope of the decline of the plasma concentration reflects the rate of its renal excretion only. During this phase, the marker concentration decreases at the same exponential rate in all the compartments where it is distributed. To obtain a well-defined plasma disappearance curve, and therefore an accurate calculation of the plasma clearance, numerous blood

samples are required. Extension of the sampling period to 4 to 5 hours improves the precision of the results.

The single-injection method has been used in neonates, most often by using inulin as a glomerular marker. Inulin is injected intravenously at a dose of 100 mg/kg, and the plasma concentration is measured at regular intervals over a few hours. The measured concentrations are plotted on semilogarithmic paper and are analyzed by hand or by computer. Simplified techniques have been proposed that are based on a single-compartment model. They obviate the need for frequent blood sampling, but they are less accurate.

Results comparing data obtained by the single-injection technique with those obtained by the standard inulin clearance method are conflicting. Early studies using the plasma disappearance curve of inulin or polyfructosan claimed it to be a reliable index of GFR.[51] Later studies, however, questioned the validity of the single-injection technique in neonates. A 30% overestimation of true GFR was described by Fawer and colleagues[52] in neonates 1 to 3 days old, but not in older infants 4 to 20 days of age. The overestimation in the younger neonates was ascribed to incomplete equilibration of inulin in its diffusion space during the 130 minutes of the test.

From his studies in preterm babies, Coulthard[48] also concluded that the single-injection technique overestimated GFR and had a large coefficient of variation. In addition, he warned that because of the prolonged half-life of inulin in preterm babies, the technique would produce an erroneous fall in inulin clearance if the test were repeated within 1 day.

Simple Creatinine Clearance Method in Neonates Without Urine Collection

A formula often used to estimate GFR in children is

$$\text{GFR (ml/min)} \times 1.73 \text{ m}^2 = k \cdot L/P_{Cr}$$

where k is a constant, L (cm) represents body length, and P_{Cr} (mg/dl) is the plasma creatinine concentration. This formula is based on the assumption that creatinine excretion is proportional to body height and is inversely proportional to plasma creatinine.[53] The value of factor k can be obtained from the formula $k = \text{GFR} \cdot L/P_{Cr}$. Under steady-state conditions, k should be directly proportional to the muscle component of body weight, which correlates reasonably well with the daily urinary creatinine excretion rate. The value of k has been determined in term and low birth weight neonates, using the 8- to 12-hour creatinine clearance as an estimate of GFR in the formula $k = C_{Cr} \cdot L/P_{Cr}$.[54] The mean value of k, calculated in 118 low birth weight infants with a corrected age of 25 to 105 weeks, was 0.33 ± 0.01. It rose to 0.45 in full-term infants up to 18 months.[53] When the plasma creatinine was expressed in micromoles per liter, the corresponding values were 29 and 40, respectively. In both groups, a large scatter of values for k was observed, which the authors ascribed to the variability in body composition, differences in diet and creatinine excretion, errors in collection of urine, and inaccuracies in the measurement of creatinine. In spite of these limitations, the formula was claimed to be useful, because it correlated well with the inulin single-injection technique.[54] The same conclusion was reached by Zacchello and co-workers,[55] who compared results obtained from the formula (using a k value of 0.55) and the standard 24-hour creatinine clearance. It is unfortunate that the $k \cdot L/P_{Cr}$ formula has not been validated in neonates by comparing its results with those given by the standard U • V/P inulin clearance.

The accuracy of the $k = L/P_{Cr}$ formula as an estimate of GFR has been questioned.[46,56] In a study in infants younger than 1 year of age, the value of k varied from 0.17 to 0.82 (15 to 72 when P_{Cr} was given in µmol/L), even though it was derived from the standard inulin clearance. Factor k was found to vary markedly with the state of hydration. Moreover, the regression line relating the clearance estimated from the formula with the

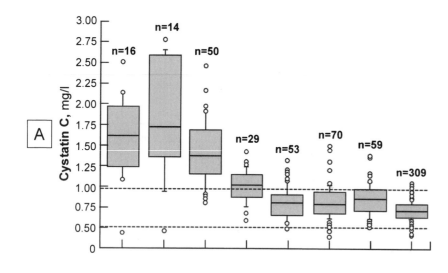

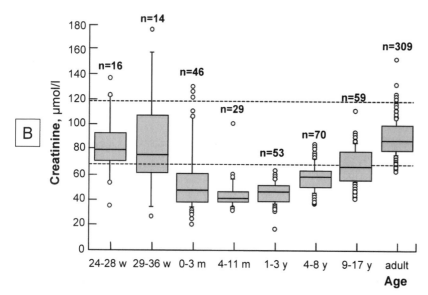

Figure 129–4. Box plot distributions showing (**A**) cystatin C and (**B**) creatinine values (10th, 25th, 50th, and 90th centiles) across the age groups. The categories of 24 to 28 weeks and 29 to 36 weeks refer to gestational ages of preterm babies. *Dotted lines* indicate the 95% confidence interval of the adult range. Preterm babies born between 24 and 36 weeks' gestation were 1 day old. (Adapted from Finney H, et al: Arch Dis Child *82*:71, 2000.)

results obtained from the standard inulin clearance differed significantly from the identity line.[46]

It is true that the k • L/P_{Cr} formula may be more informative clinically than the plasma creatinine alone because the creatinine value, in addition to renal function, is critically dependent on the percentage of muscle mass. Caution should be exercised, however, when using the formula as an estimate of GFR in studies aimed at defining pathophysiologic mechanisms in neonates.

Detection of an Abnormal Glomerular Filtration Rate by Cystatin C

Cystatin C, a nonglycosated 13-kDa basic protein, is a proteinase inhibitor involved in the intracellular catabolism of proteins.[57] It is produced by all nucleated cells, freely filtered across the glomerular capillaries, almost completely reabsorbed, and catabolized in the renal proximal tubular cells. Its production rate is apparently constant and independent of inflammatory conditions, muscle mass, and gender. When the particle-enhanced immunonephelometry assay is used for its determination in blood, no interference from bilirubin, hemoglobin, triglycerides, and rheumatoid factor could be observed.[58] Cystatin C does not appear to cross the placental barrier, and there is no correlation between maternal and neonatal serum cystatin C levels.[59] Cystatin C concentrations are highest at birth and then decrease, to stabilize after 12 months of age (Fig. 129-4). It is uncertain whether cystatin C is significantly higher in premature infants as

compared with term infants.[60, 61] In the study of Randers and associates,[62] mean values of 1.63 ± 0.26 mg/l (× ± SD) were recorded during the first month of life, 0.95 ± 0.22 mg/l during months 1 to 12, and 0.72 ± 0.12 mg/l after the first year of life. The concentration of cystatin C has been claimed to offer a greater sensitivity than creatinine in detecting an abnormal GFR in newborn infants, as well as in children or adults. Whether this advantage is clinically significant is doubtful, however. The use of cystatin C to predict GFR has important drawbacks. Because cystatin C is not excreted in the urine, the GFR predicted from its plasma concentration cannot be verified by its clearance. In children, cystatin C has also been shown to be less reliable than the Schwartz formula in distinguishing impaired from normal GFR.[63] In addition, the assessment of GFR by the Schwartz formula has the obvious advantage of providing rational semiquantitative values of GFR related to the body surface area.

DEVELOPMENT OF GLOMERULAR FILTRATION RATE

Glomerular Filtration Rate at Birth

GFR is low at birth. Standard inulin clearance studies performed by Guignard and co-workers[32,34,64] on the first 2 days of life indicated that GFR related to the body surface area increases rapidly from the 28th to the 35th week of gestation (Fig. 129-5). At the 35th week of gestation, GFR reaches a plateau that is maintained

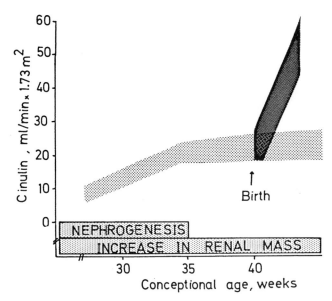

Figure 129–5. Maturation of glomerular filtration rate in relation to conceptional age. C_{inulin} = inulin clearance. (From Guignard JP: *In* Gruskin AB, Norman ME [eds]: Pediatric Nephrology. The Hague, The Netherlands, Martinus Nijhoff, 1981.)

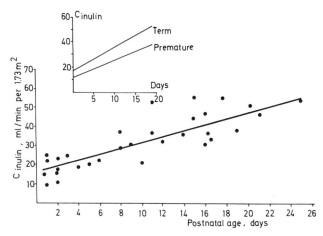

Figure 129–6. Postnatal maturation of glomerular filtration rate in term and preterm neonates. C_{inulin} = inulin clearance. (From Guignard JP: *In* Gruskin AB, Norman ME [eds]: Pediatric Nephrology. The Hague, The Netherlands, Martinus Nijhoff, 1981.)

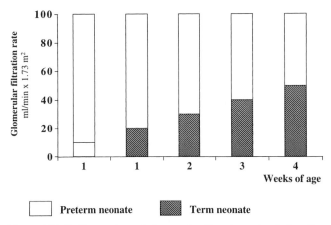

Figure 129–7. Maturation of glomerular filtration rate during the first month of life of newborn infants. The *open columns* represent normal adult values. (From Guignard JP, Drukker A: Clinical Nephrology. *In* Barratt TM, et al [eds]: Pediatric Nephrology. Baltimore, Lippincott Williams & Wilkins, 1999.)

up to the time of birth, a finding reflecting the parallel increase in kidney size and function. In these studies, GFR approximated 20 ml/minute × 1.73 m² at birth in term infants and 12 to 13 ml/minute × 1.73 m² in preterm infants of 28 to 30 weeks of gestation. Low values of GFR of 0.85 ml/kg/minute, as assessed by the inulin constant infusion technique, were also recorded by Van der Heijden and colleagues[65] on the second day of life of neonates. Using standard creatinine clearance techniques to assess GFR, Siegel and Oh[42] and Gallini and associates[22] reported somewhat lower values of GFR in 2-day-old premature infants with gestational age of less than 30 weeks. This underestimation of GFR by the clearance of creatinine was also observed by Coulthard and co-workers.[36] Such an underestimation can be accounted for by the reabsorption of creatinine across leaky immature tubules.[19, 23] In all these studies performed on the first days of life, GFR correlated with gestational age.

Maturation of Glomerular Filtration Rate in the First Month of Life

A rapid increase in GFR takes place in the first month of life. As shown in Figure 129-6, inulin clearance doubles in the first 15 days of life.[32, 34, 64, 65] The rate of increase in GFR is somewhat lower in the most premature infants. In spite of this impressive increase in GFR, as expressed in milliliters per minute per 1.73 m², the values achieved at 1 month of life are still only 50% of the adult values (Fig. 129-7). This can be considered a state of "physiologic" renal insufficiency. Using the 24-hour constant infusion method in preterm infants, van der Heijden and colleagues[66] confirmed that GFR increases rapidly after birth; the postnatal increase is independent of body weight.

A similar pattern of maturation was observed in 66 physiologically stable term and premature infants undergoing creatinine clearance studies. The lowest values of creatinine clearance were observed in the infants with the lowest birth weight (mean birth weight, 1332 ± 40 g; mean gestational age, 31.3 ± 0.5 weeks). This was true both for absolute values of creatinine clearance and for values expressed in relation to the body surface area. The progressive increase in creatinine clearance observed in the first 15 days of life also correlated significantly with postnatal age.[18, 67, 68] The study by Gallini and associates[22] confirmed the

occurrence of a steady increase in creatinine clearance over the first 52 days of life, at which time values close to 42 ml/minute × 1.73 m² and 27 ml/minute × 1.73 m² were recorded in term neonates and neonates born at less than 27 weeks of gestational age, respectively (Fig. 129-8).

Determinants of the Postnatal Increase in Glomerular Filtration Rate

Several factors account for the striking postnatal maturation of GFR: (1) a decrease in renal vascular resistance and consequent increase in RBF, (2) an increase in systemic blood pressure and in glomerular plasma flow rate, (3) an increase in the effective filtration pressure, and (4) an increase in the K_f.

1. Renal vascular resistance is elevated at birth.[69] It decreases rapidly in the first postnatal weeks. In rats, both afferent and efferent arteriolar resistances decrease by a factor of 3 during maturation.[70] The elevated renal vascular resistance is mainly the result of the high activity of vasoactive agents and hormones and the relative responsiveness of the newborn infant to these vasoconstrictor and vasodilator substances. The decrease is associated with a rise in RBF

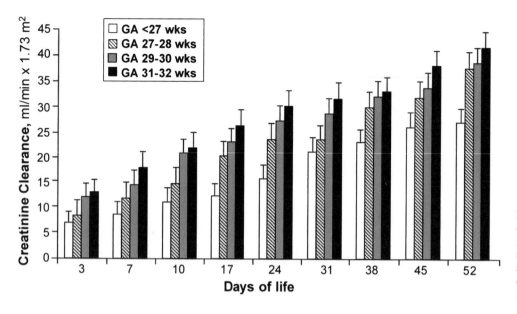

Figure 129–8. Creatinine clearance during the first 52 days of life. Values are given as times ± SE. GA = gestational age. (Adapted from Gallini F, et al: Pediatr Nephrol *15*:119, 2000.)

TABLE 129-2

Normal Mean Arterial Blood Pressure in the Newborn Infant*

Age	<1.0 kg	1.0–1.5 kg	>2.5 kg
Birth	33 ± 15	39 ± 18	49 ± 19
1 weeks	41 ± 15	47 ± 18	60 ± 19
2 weeks	45 ± 15	50 ± 18	64 ± 19
4 weeks	48 ± 15	53 ± 18	68 ± 19

*Mean ± 95% confidence limits for single measurements; measurement via umbilical artery catheterization or by Dynamap.
From Ong WH, et al: Semin Neonatol *3*:149, 1998.

and an improvement in glomerular plasma flow rate. In human neonates, the maturational increase in GFR parallels the increase in RBF.[132] Improved RBF and glomerular plasma flow rate also probably explain the 30% immediate increase in inulin clearance associated with delayed clamping of the umbilical cord.[71]

2. The striking increase in systemic blood pressure occurring during the first weeks of life (Table 129–2) is associated with an increase in the glomerular capillary hydrostatic pressure. This favors filtration. Creatinine clearances measured on the first 2 days of life in neonates of 28 to 43 gestational weeks have been shown to correlate significantly with blood pressure.[18,132]

3. The low oncotic pressure present in newborn infants resulting from low plasma protein concentrations favors the ultrafiltration pressure. Furthermore, because the glomerular hydrostatic pressure increases more rapidly than the oncotic pressure during development, the effective filtration pressure rises. Because of the low systemic blood pressure, the glomerular capillary hydraulic pressure is extremely low in early life and increases in parallel with blood pressure. The glomerular transcapillary hydraulic pressure difference increases by 10 mm Hg from the third week of life to adulthood in rats.[72] In guinea pigs, the effective filtration pressure increases 2.5 times in the first 50 days of life.[73] Increases in glomerular capillary hydraulic pressure and glomerular transcapillary hydraulic pressure difference could contribute to changes in GFR during early maturation.

4. The K_f reflects both the surface and the permeability of the filtration barrier. Maturational changes in K_f also account for the postnatal rise in GFR. The K_f is low in the newborn. It is significantly lower in 40- to 64-day-old rats than in adult

animals.[74,75] The glomerular basement membrane surface area has been shown to increase 3.5-fold from birth to adulthood in rats,[76] whereas the glomerular capillary cross-sectional area increased 10-fold from 3 weeks to adulthood in dogs.[77] A 40% increase in glomerular corpuscular diameter has been observed in humans from birth to adulthood.[78] If they correspond to increases in the glomerular filtering area, these changes should improve GFR. The increases in the area of the endothelial fenestrae observed in growing rats can also explain the postnatal rise in GFR. From studies in 1- and 6-week-old dogs, Goldsmith and colleagues[79] concluded that both an increase in the glomerular filtering area and pore density accounted for the postnatal increase in GFR.

The increase in the number of negatively charged sites in the glomerular basement membrane[80] and the 2.5-fold increase in GBM thickness[75] observed in growing rats could account for the decreased permeability to large molecules (proteins) in the first postnatal weeks of human neonates. Clearance studies in human infants infused with inulin or polyfructosides with variable MWs have clearly shown that the high-MW inulin did not accumulate in preterm infants (birth weight of 850 to 1250 g) infused with inulin for 2 to 10 days.[10] The filterability of inulin (MW 5200) appears similar in neonates and older children. This does not, however, exclude subtle changes in glomerular capillary permeability during growth. Experimental studies on isolated rat glomeruli also failed to demonstrate an increase in glomerular hydraulic permeability during growth.[81]

FACTORS THAT CAN IMPAIR GLOMERULAR FILTRATION RATE IN THE PERINATAL PERIOD

The low GFR of the very low birth weight infant is maintained by a delicate balance of intrarenal vasoconstrictor and vasodilator forces. Vasoactive disturbances can easily reduce the already low GFR in preterm neonates, so these infants are prone to develop vasomotor nephropathy and acute renal failure. The main causes of renal failure in the neonate are prerenal and include hypotension, hypovolemia, hypoxemia, and perinatal asphyxia. Other causes include the administration of angiotensin-converting enzyme inhibitors, nonsteroidal antiinflammatory drugs, and tolazoline. Artificial ventilation also impairs GFR. In all these situations, the interaction between the vasoconstrictive and vasodilation forces that are stimulated are rather complex. Several of the vasoconstrictor or vasodilatory forces indeed differ in their effects on the systemic and the intrarenal circulations.

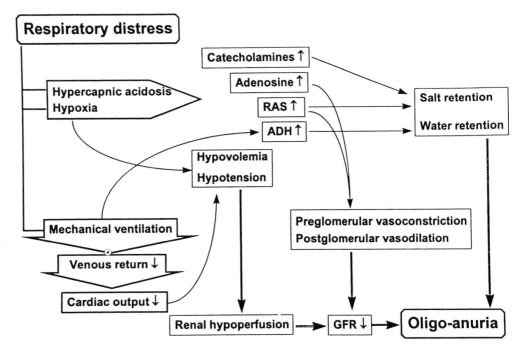

Figure 129–9. The main pathways of renal impairment in respiratory distress. ADH = antidiuretic hormone; GFR = glomerular filtration rate; RAS = renin-angiotensin system. (From Toth-Heyn P, et al: Pediatr Nephrol *14*:227, 2000.)

With regard to *hypovolemia and hypotension,* contraction of blood volume and hypotension, with or without failure of the cardiac pump, promote the release of vasoconstricting agents such as angiotensin II, vasopressin, and catecholamines. These substances can decrease GFR.

Perinatal hypoxemia and asphyxia are common causes of impaired GFR in neonates. The renal vasoconstriction is the consequence of the overactivation of the renin-angiotensin system, intrarenal adenosine, vasopressin, and the catecholamines.[82] Other conditions that impair GFR by stimulating vasoconstrictive forces are hypothermia, hyperthermia, and severe respiratory or metabolic acidosis.[82]

Ventilation of human neonates and newborn animals with continuous positive airway pressure has deleterious effects on renal function resulting from decreased venous return and low cardiac output, increased renal sympathetic nervous activity, and high serum vasopressin levels.[83] The main pathways of renal dysfunction in respiratory disorders are illustrated in Figure 129–9.

ACE inhibitors can lead to a dramatic fall in mean arterial pressure accompanied by persistent oliguria.[82] The oliguric renal insufficiency is similar to that observed in fetuses and neonates of women who are administered angiotensin-converting enzyme inhibitors shortly before birth. It is explained by the interference with the renin-angiotensin system, which is physiologically overactive during fetal and neonatal life.[82]

High prostaglandin activity is physiologically necessary to maintain sufficient perfusion of the newborn kidney. Serum prostaglandin levels are also high in infants with chronic cardiac failure, patent ductus arteriosus, and all instances of hypotension and hypovolemia. Prostaglandin synthesis inhibitors, used prenatally to prevent the premature onset of labor or after birth to promote the closure of a hemodynamically active patent ductus arteriosus, reduce GFR and RBF.[65] This effect is usually transient. In experimental immature animals, cyclooxygenase-nonselective and cyclooxygenase-2–selective inhibitors appear to impair GFR and RBF similarly.[84]

CONCLUSION

Glomerular filtration is the first essential step in urine formation. Its maintenance within narrow limits is mandatory and requires subtle autoregulatory mechanisms that involve the action of autacoids, vasoactive substances, and intrinsic myogenic mechanisms. Because not only pathologic changes but also physiologic changes in GFR during maturation may affect body fluid homeostasis and the excretion of drugs by the neonate, an estimation of GFR will help the neonatologist to rationally prescribe fluids, electrolytes, and drugs.

REFERENCES

1. Guignard JP, et al: Vasoactive factors in the immature kidney. Pediatr Nephrol *5*:443, 1991.
2. Semmerkrot BA, et al: Age differences in renal response to atrial natriuretic peptide in rabbits. Life Sci *46*:849, 1990.
3. Ballèvre L, et al: Role of nitric oxide in the hypoxemia-induced renal dysfunction of the newborn rabbit. Pediatr Res *39*:725, 1996.
4. Toth-Heyn P, Guignard JP: Bradykinin in the newborn kidney. Nephron *9*:571, 2002.
5. Semama DS, et al: Role of endogenous endothelin in renal hemodynamics of newborn rabbits. Pediatr Nephrol *7*:886, 1993.
6. Marsh D, Frasier C: Reliability of inulin for determining volume flow in rat renal cortical tubules. Am J Physiol *209*:283, 1965.
7. Arturson G, et al: Human glomerular membrane porosity and filtration pressure: dextran clearance data analysed by theoretical models. Clin Sci *40*:137, 1971.
8. Harris CA, et al: Composition of mammalian glomerular filtrate. Am J Physiol *227*:972, 1974.
9. Rankin JHG, et al: Measurement of fetal renal inulin clearance in a chronic sheep preparation. J Appl Physiol *32*:129, 1972.
10. Coulthard MG, Ruddock V: Validation of inulin as a marker for glomerular filtration in preterm babies. Kidney Int *23*:407, 1983.
11. Wilkins BH: The glomerular filterability of polyfructosan-S in immature infants. Pediatr Nephrol *6*:319, 1992.
12. Sutphen JL: Anthropometric determinants of creatinine excretion in preterm infants. Pediatrics *69*:719, 1982.
13. Schloerb PR: Total body water distribution of creatinine and urea in nephrectomized dogs. Am J Physiol *199*:661, 1960.
14. Jones JD, Burnett PD: Implication of creatinine and gut flora in the uremic syndrome: induction of "creatininase" in colon contents of the rat by dietary creatinine. Clin Chem *18*:280, 1972.
15. Feldman H, Guignard JP: Plasma creatinine in the first month of life. Arch Dis Child *57*:123, 1982.
16. Sertel H, Scopes J: Rates of creatinine clearance in babies less than one week of age. Arch Dis Child *48*:717, 1973.
17. Stonestreet BS, Oh W: Plasma creatinine levels in low-birth-weight infants during the first three months of life. Pediatrics *61*:788, 1978.
18. Bueva A, Guignard JP: Renal function in preterm neonates. Pediatr Res *36*:572, 1994.
19. Guignard JP, Drukker A: Why do newborn infants have a high plasma creatinine? Pediatrics *103*:1, 1999.
20. Forestier F, et al: Blood chemistry of normal human fetuses at mid-trimester of pregnancy. Pediatr Res *21*:579, 1987.

21. Miall LS, et al: Plasma creatinine rises dramatically in the first 48 hours of life in preterm infants. Pediatrics 104:e76, 1999.

22. Gallini F, et al: Progression of renal function in preterm neonates with gestational age ≤32 weeks. Pediatr Nephrol 15:119, 2000.

23. Matos P, et al: Creatinine reabsorption by the newborn rabbit kidney. Pediatr Res 44:639, 1998

24. Alt JM, et al: Perinatal development of tubular function in the pig. Q J Exp Physiol 69:693, 1984.

25. Anderson CF, et al: Iothalamate sodium 125I vs cyanocobalamin Co 57 as a measure of glomerular filtration rate in man. JAMA 204:653, 1968.

26. Griep RJ, Nelp WB: Mechanism of excretion of radioiodinated sodium iothalamate. Radiology 93:807, 1969.

27. Odlind B, et al: Is 125I iothalamate an ideal marker of glomerular filtration? Kidney Int 27:9, 1985.

28. Russell CD: Radiopharmaceuticals used to assess kidney function and structure. In Tauxe WN, Dubowski EV (eds): Nuclear Medicine in Clinical Urology and Nephrology. Norwalk, CT, Appleton-Century-Crofts, 1985, pp 5–31.

29. Chervu LR, Blaufox MD: Renal radiopharmaceuticals: an update. Semin Nucl Med 12:224, 1982.

30. Russell CD, Dubowski EV: Measurement of renal function with radionuclides. J Nucl Med 30:2053, 1989.

31. Piepsz A, et al: Estimation of normal chromium-51 ethylene diamine tetraacetic acid clearance in children. Eur J Nucl Med 21:12, 1994.

32. Fawer CL, et al: Maturation of renal function in full-term and premature neonates. Helv Paediatr Acta 34:11, 1979.

33. Coulthard MG: Device for continuous urine collections in the newborn. Arch Dis Child 57:322, 1982.

34. Guignard JP, et al: Glomerular filtration rate in the first three weeks of life. J Pediatr 87:268, 1975.

35. Stonestreet BS, et al: Validity of endogenous creatinine clearance in low birthweight infants. Pediatr Res 13:1012, 1979.

36. Coulthard MG, et al: Creatinine and urea clearances compared to inulin clearance in preterm and mature babies. Early Hum Dev 11:11, 1985.

37. Wilkins BH: A reappraisal of the measurement of glomerular filtration rate in pre-term infants. Pediatr Nephrol 6:323, 1992.

38. Huang YC, Chiou WL: Creatinine XII: comparison of assays of low serum creatinine levels using high-performance liquid chromatography and two picrate methods. J Pharmacol Sci 72:836, 1983.

39. Del-Razo LM, Jauge P: Quantification of creatinine in urine and plasma by reversed phase HPLC. J Liquid Chromatogr 8:1983, 1985.

40. Welsh J, et al: Determination of serum creatinine by isotope dilution mass spectrometry as a candidate definitive method. Anal Chem 58:1681, 1986.

41. Ross B, et al: Renal function of low birth weight infants during the first two months of life. Pediatr Res 11:1162, 1977.

42. Siegel SR, Oh W: Renal function as a marker of human fetal maturation. Acta Paediatr Scand 65:481, 1976.

43. Earle DP Jr, Berliner RW: A simplified clinical procedure for measurement of glomerular filtration rate and renal plasma flow. Proc Soc Exp Biol Med 62:262, 1946.

44. Cole BR, et al: Measurement of renal function without urine collection. N Engl J Med 287:1109, 1972.

45. Leake RD, et al: Inulin clearance in the newborn infant: relationship to gestational and postnatal age. Pediatr Res 10:759, 1976.

46. Alinei P, Guignard JP: Assessment of glomerular filtration rate in infants. Helv Pediatr Acta 42:253, 1987.

47. Guignard JP: Assessment of renal function without urine collection. Arch Dis Child 52:424, 1977.

48. Coulthard MG: Comparison of methods of measuring renal function in preterm babies using inulin. J Pediatr 102:923, 1983.

49. Leake RD, Trygstad CW: Glomerular filtration rate during the period of adaptation to extrauterine life. Pediatr Res 11:959, 1977.

50. Sapirstein LA, et al: Volumes of distribution and clearances of intravenously injected creatinine in the dog. Am J Physiol 181:330, 1955.

51. Svenningsen NW: Single injection polyfructosan clearance in normal and asphyxiated neonates. Acta Paediatr Scand 64:87, 1975.

52. Fawer CL, et al: Single injection clearance in the neonate. Biol Neonate 35:321, 1979.

53. Schwartz GJ, et al: The use of plasma creatinine concentration for estimating glomerular filtration rate in infants, children, and adolescents. Pediatr Clin North Am 34:571, 1987.

54. Brion LP, et al: A simple estimate of glomerular filtration rate in low birth weight infants during the first year of life: noninvasive assessment of body composition and growth. J Pediatr 109:698, 1986.

55. Zacchello G, et al: Simple estimate of creatinine clearance from plasma creatinine in neonates. Arch Dis Child 57:297, 1982.

56. Arant BS Jr: Estimating glomerular filtration rate in infants. J Pediatr 104:890, 1984.

57. Olafsson I: The human cystatin C gene promotor: functional analysis and identification of heterogeneous mRNA. Scand J Clin Lab Invest 55:597, 1995.

58. Erlandsen EJ, et al: Evaluation of the Dade Behring N Latex Cystatin C assay on the Dade Behring Nephelometer II system. Scand J Clin Lab Invest 59:1, 1999.

59. Cataldi L, et al: Cystatin C in healthy women at term pregnancy and in their infant newborns: relationship between maternal and neonatal serum levels and reference values. Am J Perinatol 16:287, 1999.

60. Harmoinen A, et al: Reference intervals for cystatin C in pre- and full-term infants and children. Pediatr Nephrol 15:105, 2000.

61. Finney H, et al: Reference ranges for plasma cystatin C and creatinine measurements in premature infants, neonates, and older children. Arch Dis Child 82:71, 2000.

62. Randers E, et al: Reference interval for serum cystatin C in children. Clin Chem 45:1856, 1999.

63. Martini SS, et al: Glomerular filtration rate: measure creatinine and height rather than cystatin C. Acta Paediatr (in press).

64. Guignard JP, John E: Renal function in the tiny premature infant. Clin Perinatol 13:377, 1986.

65. Van der Heijden AJ, et al: Renal function impairment in preterm neonates related to intrauterine indomethacin exposure. Pediatr Res 24:644, 1988.

66. Van der Heijden AJ, et al: Glomerular filtration rate in the preterm infant: the relation to gestational and postnatal age. Eur J Pediatr 148:24, 1988.

67. Sonntag J, et al: Serum creatinine concentration, urinary creatinine excretion and creatinine clearance during the first 9 weeks in preterm infants with a birth weight below 1500 g. Eur J Pediatr 155:815, 1996.

68. Gordjani N, et al: Serum creatinine and creatinine clearance in healthy neonates and prematures during the first 10 days of life. Eur J Pediatr 148:143, 1988.

69. Gruskin AB: Maturational changes in renal blood flow in piglets. Pediatr Res 4:7, 1970.

70. Ichikawa I, et al: Maturational development of glomerular ultrafiltration in the rat. Am J Physiol 26:F465, 1979.

71. Oh W, et al: Renal function and blood volume in newborn infants related to plasma transfusion. Acta Paediatr Scand 55:197, 1966.

72. Allison ME, et al: Hydrostatic pressure in the rat kidney. Am J Physiol 223:975, 1972.

73. Spitzer A, Edelmann CM Jr: Maturational changes in pressure gradients for glomerular filtration. Am J Physiol 221:1431, 1971.

74. Tucker BJ, Blantz RC: Factors determining superficial nephron filtration in the mature-growing rat. Am J Physiol 232:F97, 1977.

75. Larsson L, Maunsbach AB: The ultrastructural development of the glomerular filtration barrier in the rat kidney: a morphometric analysis. J Ultrastruct Res 72:392, 1980.

76. Knutson DW, et al: Estimation of relative glomerular capillary surface area in normal and hypertrophic rat kidneys. Kidney Int 14:437, 1978.

77. John E, et al: Quantitative changes in the canine glomerular vasculature during development: physiologic implications. Kidney Int 20:223, 1981.

78. Fetterman GH, et al: The growth and maturation of human glomeruli from term to adulthood: studies by microdissection. Pediatrics 35:601, 1965.

79. Goldsmith DI, et al: Glomerular capillary permeability in developing canines. Am J Physiol 251:F528, 1986.

80. Reeves WH, et al: Assembly of the glomerular filtation surface: differentiation of anionic sites in glomerular capillaries of newborn rat kidney. J Cell Biol 85:735, 1980.

81. Savin VJ, et al: Ultrafiltration coefficient of isolated glomeruli of rats aged 4 days to maturation. Kidney Int 28:926, 1985.

82. Toth-Heyn P, et al: The stressed neonatal kidney: from pathophysiology to clinical management of neonatal vasomotor nephropathy. Pediatr Nephrol 14:227, 2000.

83. Tulassay T, et al: Effects of continuous airway pressure on renal function in prematures. Biol Neonate 43:152, 1983.

84. Guignard JP: The adverse renal effects of prostaglandin-synthesis inhibitors in the newborn rabbit. Semin Perinatol 26:398, 2002.

Renal Transport of Sodium During Early Development

The regulation of intra- and extracellular sodium is a prerequisite to life in a nonaqueous environment. While mature animals maintain sodium homeostasis, immature animals must maintain a positive balance of sodium. This positive sodium balance is achieved by at least two complementary mechanisms.

First, newborn animals universally prefer to ingest a salt solution rather than sodium-free water.[1] In the term rat, this "sodium preference" can be demonstrated by day 5 of life.[2] Second, developing nephrons tend to retain sodium. In the term infant, approximately 65% of ingested sodium is retained rather than excreted by the kidneys.[3,4] Together, "salt preference" and "renal immaturity" promote a positive sodium balance.

Several investigations have associated sodium transport with somatic growth.[5-9] Bickel and associates[10] evaluated the relative abundances of renal sodium transporters in young lean and obese Zucker rats by semiquantitative immunoblotting. The abundances of the α_1-subunit of Na^+,K^+-ATPase, the thiazide-sensitive Na-Cl co-transporter (NCC or TSC), and the β-subunit of the epithelial sodium channel (ENaC) were all significantly higher in the kidneys of obese rats. There were no differences for the sodium-hydrogen exchanger (NHE3), the bumetanide-sensitive Na-K-2Cl co-transporter (NKCC2 or BSC1), the type II sodium-phosphate co-transporter (NaPi-2), or the α-subunit of ENaC.

Leptin, an adipose-induced hormone, up-regulates the expression of the erythrocyte sodium-hydrogen exchanger (NHE1).[11] In normal individuals, insulin also induces the expression of erythrocyte NHE1. In contrast, insulin has no effect on NHE1 activity of erythrocytes from obese individuals.[12] These findings suggest a link between obesity, insulin resistance, and hypertension on the one hand and the active renal transport of sodium on the other.

To better understand sodium handling by the kidney during development, investigators have traditionally used clearance methods to measure the fractional excretion of sodium (FE_{Na}) and the free water clearance (C_{H_2O}). These studies point to the distal tubule as the site of the most avid sodium conservation. Using modern techniques of molecular biology and targeted proteomics, more recent investigations have now established the cellular basis of these earlier observations.

Fractional Excretion of Na (FE_{Na}) During Development

Sodium handling by the kidney may be expressed as the clearance of sodium divided by the clearance of creatinine (FE_{Na}).

$$[\text{Urinary concentration of sodium } (U_{Na}, \text{mg/dl})$$
$$\times \text{ urine volume (ml)/unit time] / [creatinine or inulin clearance}$$
$$\times \text{ plasma sodium concentration } (P_{Na}, \text{mg/dl})] \text{ becomes}$$
$$[U_{Na} \times P_{cr}]/ [U_{cr} \times P_{Na}] \times 100\%$$

FE_{Na} measures renal tubular sodium transport "normalized" for the glomerular filtration rate (GFR). As GFR rises dramatically after birth, FE_{Na} is a useful measurement, particularly in the newborn infant.

Several studies have indicated that FE_{Na} varies inversely with the gestational and postconceptional age.[13,14] The entire spectrum of FE_{Na} related to gestational age is shown in Figure 130-1 and summarized in Table 130-1.

In the human, the fetus produces large amounts of sodium-rich urine with a mean FE_{Na} of 12.8%.[3-8] Healthy premature infants, particularly those less than 30 weeks' gestational age, continue to excrete large amounts of sodium (average FE_{Na} 5%) (Fig. 130-2)[15] and are at risk for negative sodium balance.[16] All preterm infants of less than 30 weeks have a negative sodium balance (Fig. 130-3).[15] The incidence decreases to 45 to 70% by 32 weeks' gestation and to 0 to 29% after 36 weeks.[16,17]

Vanpeé and colleagues compared the FE_{Na} in infants with a gestational age of 25 to 30 weeks to values found in a cohort of older infants with a gestational age of 31 to 34 weeks.[18] During the first 2 weeks, FE_{Na} fell rapidly in both groups, eventually reaching the low levels found in full-term infants 4 to 6 weeks after birth (Fig. 130-4).[18] In very sick preterm infants of less than 30 weeks' gestation, negative sodium balance persisted through the first week of life. In infants greater than 33 weeks' gestation, a positive sodium balance was achieved by days 2 to 4 of life.

In the full-term infant, the FE_{Na} decreases from 3.4 to 1.5% in the first few hours of life and to even lower values in the subsequent 24 to 48 hours. In most cases, urine sodium excretion over the first few days of life still exceeds the dietary sodium intake (breast milk or low-salt formula) by the infant.[19]

These observations suggest that maturation of the renal tubules is crucial for the newborn infant to conserve sodium. Additional studies (see later) indicate that the major site for sodium conservation by the kidney is the distal portion of the nephron.

Sodium supplementation may prevent a negative sodium balance in the neonate (Fig. 130-5).[20] In very low birth weight infants (<1.3 kg at birth) between 2 and 6 weeks of age on a low-sodium intake (≤2 mEq/kg/day), the incidence of hyponatremia (≤130 mEq/l) is nearly 40%.[21] A sodium supplementation of approximately 3 mEq/kg/day (provided until a postnatal age of 6 to 7 weeks) will reduce the occurrence of hyponatremia to less than 2%.

However, it is unclear that sodium supplementation is beneficial for the neonate. First, sodium supplementation may interfere with the capacity of the kidney to conserve sodium. In the neonatal rat, GFR does not increase following 1% volume expansion. In nonsupplemented animals, urine sodium excretion increases minimally. In rats that chronically receive sodium supplementation, urine sodium excretion increases markedly, similar to that of the adult.[22] The investigators suggested that the limited sodium in maternal milk may condition the tubules toward antinatriuresis.

Second, excessive administration of sodium to full-term newborn infants can result in extracellular volume expansion, edema, and in some cases life-threatening hypernatremia.[23] Fortunately, hypernatremia in preterm infants is rare and usually is related to excessive insensible water loss, not to sodium administration.[14] Hypernatremia typically occurs in the first postnatal week when transcutaneous water losses are high.

Clearance Studies in Animals

Newborn animals have a blunted response to saline loading.[24] Banks[25] compared the effects of saline volume expansion on renal tubular reabsorption between newborn and adult animals. Proximal and distal tubule function was estimated by the distal

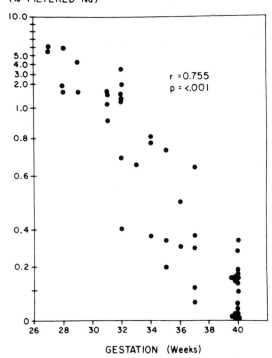

Figure 130–1. Scattergram showing the indirect correlation between the fractional excretion of sodium and gestational age. (From Siegel SR, Oh W: Acta Paediatr Scand *65*:481, 1976.)

nephron blockade technique using ethacrynic acid and amiloride. During saline infusion, which increased extracellular volume by approximately 30% for both age groups, total nephron fractional Na reabsorption was 0.91 for the adult and 0.98 for the puppy ($p < .01$). However, proximal tubule fractional Na reabsorption was greater in the adult (0.64) than in the puppy (0.48, $p < .01$), whereas distal nephron fractional Na reabsorption was much greater in the newborn (0.51) than in the adult (0.26, $p < .01$).

Using renal micropuncture re-collection techniques in proximal tubules of guinea pigs, Schoeneman and Spitzer[26] found a low proximal fractional reabsorption at all ages; however, there was a higher whole kidney fractional reabsorption in newborn when compared with adult animals. Based on these studies, the tendency to retain an intravenous sodium load was primarily due to enhanced sodium reabsorption in segments beyond the proximal convoluted tubule.

These observations suggest that factors affecting the function of the distal tubule are mainly responsible for developmental changes in sodium conservation by the nephron. These factors may include the distal delivery of sodium, the activity of natriuretic factors, the secretion of or renal response to aldosterone, and the expression of sodium transport proteins.

TABLE 130–1

Fractional Excretion of Sodium (F_{Na}) at Different Postconceptual Ages for Infants of Different Birth Weights[13]

Weight (g)	1–2 d (%)	8–9 d (%)	15–16 d (%)
1000–1500	2	1.4	0.7
1501–2000	2.2	0.8	0.4
2001–2500	0.4	0.6	0.2
>2500	1.0	0.6	0.3

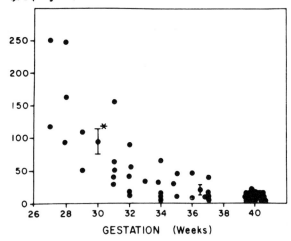

Figure 130–2. Urinary sodium excretion in newborns from 27 to 40 weeks' gestational age. Circles with bars at 30 and 37 weeks are mean values for 27- to 32-, and 33- to 40- week-gestation infants. The * indicates a significant difference between the groups. (From Siegel SR, Oh W: Acta Paediatr Scand *65*:481, 1976.)

Clearance Studies in the Neonate

Aperia and collaborators[27] studied preterm (<35 weeks' gestation) and full-term infants under maximal water diuresis following an oral load of sodium chloride. Both groups were unable to excrete the sodium load as efficiently as older children (8 to 14 years).[28] In term infants, the renal response to an oral sodium load of 2.2 mEq/kg body weight is poor in the immediate postnatal period. The urinary sodium excretion rate per hour corrected for body surface area (0.1 to 3 mEq/h/1.73 m²) is only about 10% of that found in older children (16 mEq/h/1.73 m²). However, the renal response to an oral sodium load reaches the latter value by 10 to 13 months of age and remains constant thereafter (Fig. 130–6).[29]

Sulyok and coworkers[30] also studied preterm and full-term neonates, although the conditions of maximal water diuresis

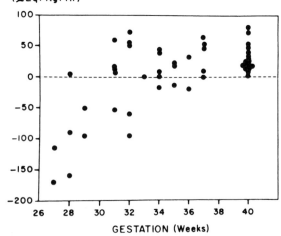

Figure 130–3. Sodium balance is represented by the difference in sodium intake and excretion of infants at 27 to 40 weeks' gestational age. (From Siegel SR, Oh W: Acta Paediatr Scand *65*:481, 1976.)

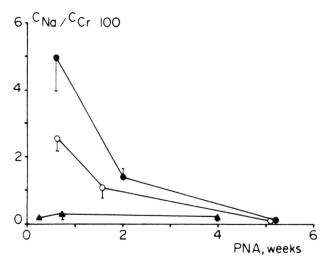

Figure 130–4. Fractional sodium excretion ($FE_{Na} = C_{Na}/_{cr} \times$ 100%) in infants with a gestational age of 28 weeks (*closed circles*) and 32-week (*open circles*) and full-term (*triangles*) infants. There was a significant difference between the 28- and 32-week groups at 1 week of age. (From Vanpeé M, et al: Acta Paediatr Scand 77:191, 1988.)

were not met. Sodium delivery to the distal tubule was significantly greater and distal sodium reabsorption was significantly less in premature than in full-term infants, suggesting the inability of the distal tubule to handle the increased sodium load secondary to defective proximal tubule sodium reabsorption. However, the fractional distal tubule reabsorption in preterm infants rose to full-term values of approximately 85% by 2 weeks after birth.[31]

Rodriquez-Soriano and associates[32] studied premature (<34 weeks' gestation) and full-term infants during maximal water diuresis. Distal tubule sodium reabsorption was significantly higher, and sodium delivery was significantly greater, in the more immature infants (Fig. 130-7).[32] Fractional distal sodium reabsorption, however, was significantly lower (82%) than in full-term infants (92%) (Fig. 130–8).[32] Therefore, a

PRETERM INFANTS

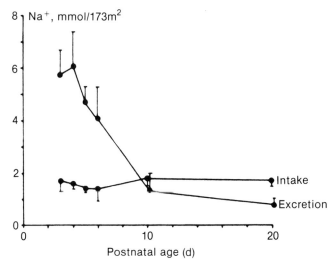

Figure 130–5. Average hourly sodium intake and excretion in preterm infants 3 to 21 days' postnatal age. Each circle represents the average of four to nine observations. (From Aperia AS et al: Acta Paediatr Scand 68:813, 1979.)

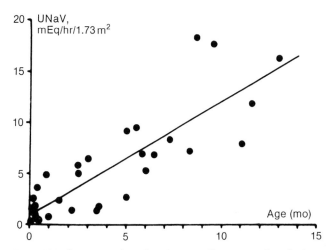

Figure 130–6. Average hourly urinary sodium excretion during the first 13 months of life. Correlation coefficient = 0.764. (From Aperia A, et al: Acta Paediatr Scand 64:393, 1975.)

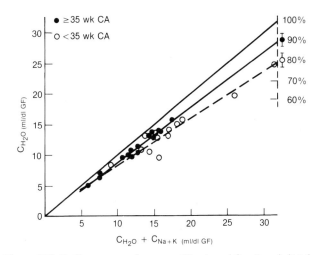

Figure 130–7. Free water clearance (C_{H_2O}) and fractional distal sodium delivery ($C_{H_2O} + C_{Na+K}$). (From Rodriquez-Soriano J, et al: Pediatr Res 17:1013, 1983.)

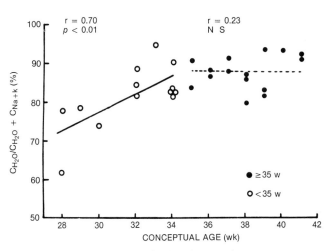

Figure 130–8. Percentage of distal sodium reabsorption versus conceptual age (gestation + postnatal age). (From Rodriquez-Soriano J, et al: Pediatr Res 17:1013, 1983.)

lower percentage of the sodium load presented to the distal tubule was reabsorbed in preterm than in term infants.

These findings suggest that both proximal and distal tubule reabsorption of sodium are inversely related to gestational age, and that the major site of adaptation to extrauterine life is the distal tubule. In the premature newborn infant, sodium reabsorptive capacity lags behind the increase of GFR ("glomerular-tubular imbalance"). The high excretion of β_2-microglobulin (a small peptide reabsorbed entirely in the proximal tubule) found in the preterm infant supports this proposition. In infants with gestational ages greater than 33 weeks, sodium reabsorption is more efficient, suggesting glomerular-tubular balance. In healthy full-term neonates, there is an enhanced ability of the distal tubule to reabsorb sodium, which explains the blunted sodium excretory response to a sodium load.[33]

Transport Studies

Plasma sodium is freely filtered by the glomerulus ("filtered load") and is then reabsorbed along the renal tubule, by means of transport systems that are unique to the individual nephron segments (proximal tubule, loop of Henle, distal tubule). The bulk of the filtered load is reabsorbed by the proximal tubule. The proximal tubule is a relatively permeable epithelium with both low-resistance paracellular and transcellular pathways. In the rat proximal tubule, approximately one third of sodium is reabsorbed by active transport, one third is reabsorbed by electrical transference and one third is reabsorbed by solvent drag.[34] Both active as well as passive transport forces change with maturation.

Passive Transport During Development. Studies in newborn puppies, guinea pigs, rabbits, and rats have revealed developmental changes in proximal sodium reabsorption.[35-38] In the guinea pig, the single-nephron glomerular filtration rate (SNGFR) and the rate of proximal fluid reabsorption increase 20-fold between 1 and 40 days of age.[40] During the same period of time, the length of the proximal tubule increases sixfold. Therefore, the rate of sodium and fluid reabsorption per millimeter of tubule length increases about fourfold during development. However, the fractional sodium reabsorption along the proximal convoluted tubule remains constant at about 60%.[39,40] Without a change in fractional sodium reabsorption in this segment, fractional reabsorption in segments distal to this site must also remain unchanged.[40]

A significant portion of the reabsorption of sodium in young animals is due to passive transport. The leakage of the proximal tubule epithelium to various molecular species is referred to as the reflection coefficient (lower values equal increased permeability). During development, the proximal tubule has a lower reflection coefficient for microperoxidase and mannitol[41] than that in adult animals. This finding may be due in part to changes in membrane permeability with development.

In renal proximal tubule brush-border membrane vesicles (BBMVs), early uptake of ^{22}Na is more rapid in BBMV from kidneys of 7-day-old than of adult rats. Furthermore, fluorescence polarization studies reveal that lipids from BBMV of 7-day-old rats

are more fluid than lipids from BBMV of adult rats.[42] These differences are likely due to age-related changes in the lipid composition of the membranes. These differences in turn could influence the transport and permeability characteristics of the developing tubular membrane. These findings would explain, in part, the alterations of renal BBMV solute transport with growth.

Spitzer and colleagues[38,40] have estimated Starling's hydraulic fluxes ("passive forces") across the proximal convoluted tubule of young and adult rabbits (Table 130–2). By subtracting the passive flux from the total reabsorptive volume flux, one may estimate the relative contribution of active and passive forces to the reabsorption of solute during development.

The reabsorptive flow rate per unit of hydrostatic pressure ($J_{\Delta P}$) is greater in young than in mature animals, possibly due to a higher tubular membrane permeability in the young animal.[40-42] Spitzer and associates estimated that the hydrostatic pressure–driven flow in the young animal accounts for 7% of the total proximal convoluted tubule reabsorptive flow (J_V) (0.33 nl/min · mm), compared with only 0.6% in the mature animal ($J_V = 1.2$ nl/min · mm) (Fig. 130–9 and Table 130–2).[38,40]

The peritubular capillary oncotic pressure is low in the immature animal due to a low plasma oncotic pressure. This results in a two- to threefold lower reabsorptive flow per unit of applied oncotic pressure ($J_{\Delta\Pi}$) in immature animals compared with adults (0.14 versus 0.38 nl/min · mm) (see Fig. 130–9 and Table 130–2).[40] Therefore, in newborn animals, oncotic pressure–driven flow accounts for 42% of total absorptive flow compared with 32% in adult animals.[40,43] The total reabsorptive flow (J_V) of the young animal is nearly four times lower, and the sum of the hydrostatic ($J_{\Delta P}$)- and oncotic ($J_{\Delta\Pi}$)-driven flow is about 2.5 times lower than that in the adult.

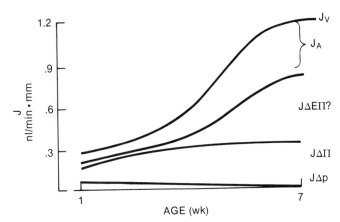

Figure 130–9. Developmental time course of net reabsorptive flow (J_V), oncotic ($J_{\Delta\pi}$) and hydrostatic ($J_{\Delta P}$) pressure-driven flows, and possible course of development of active transcellular flux (J_A) and of fluxes driven by cell-generated effective osmotic and ionic gradients ($J_{\Delta\pi E}$). (From Barac-Nieto M, Spitzer A: Pediatr Nephrol 2:356, 1988.)

TABLE 130–2

Estimates of Hydraulic Fluxes Across the Proximal Convoluted Tubules of Young and Adult Rabbits

	$J_{\Delta P}$	$J_{\Delta\Pi}$	$J_{\Delta P} + J_{\Delta\Pi}$	J_V	Non-Starling
Young	0.023 (7%)	0.14 (42%)	0.163 (49%)	0.33	0.167 (51%)
Adult	0.007 (0.6%)	0.38 (32%)	0.387 (32%)	1.2	0.813 (68%)

$J_{\Delta P}$ = hydrostatic pressure-driven flow, nl/min · mm; $J_{\Delta\Pi}$ = oncotic pressure-driven flow, nl/min · mm; $J_{\Delta P} + J_{\Delta\Pi}$ = total pressure-driven flow, nl/min · mm; J_V = reabsorptive volume flux, ml/min · mm; Non-Starling = active transport + passive transport due to transepithelial effective osmotic and ionic gradient. Since the latter term is negligible,[25] "non-Starling" forces are mainly due to active transport.

In summary, active and passive forces may contribute equally to the reabsorption of solute across the immature proximal tubule. With development, protein transport carriers mature and play an increasingly important role in solute reabsorption (see Fig. 130–9).[40,43] For example, if total flow is 50 pEq/min · mm in the young animal, 25 pEq/min · mm would occur by active transport. Conversely, if total flow is 180 pEq/min · mm in the mature animal, 60 pEq/min · mm would be accounted for by active processes.[40]

Active Transport During Development. Different sets of transport proteins are distributed to the apical and basolateral surfaces of the plasma membranes of renal epithelium.[43] The asymmetric distribution of membrane proteins is generated by an intracellular machinery that addresses the moieties to the appropriate domain. The extracellular environment regulates the protein sorting by conveying the positional information that creates the plasma membrane domains. These interactions are mediated by macromolecular assemblies of cell adhesion molecules, cytoskeleton, and signaling molecules.

To determine the ontogeny of sodium transport proteins in embryonic rat tissue, Schmitt and associates[44] used *in situ* hybridization and immunohistochemistry to localize the Na-Pi co-transporter type 2 (NaPi-2), the bumetanide-sensitive Na-K-2Cl co-transporter (NKCC2), the thiazide-sensitive Na-Cl co-transporter (NCC), the Na-Ca exchanger (NaCa), the epithelial sodium channel (rENaC), and 11β-hydroxysteroid dehydrogenase. These proteins were first observed in the post–S-shape stages. NKCC2 was initially expressed at the macula densa region and was observed later extending along the nascent ascending limb of the loop of Henle (TAL). In comparison, NaPi-2 expression along the proximal tubular part of the loop of Henle was observed later in development. The NCC was initially found at the distal end of the nascent distal convoluted tubule (DCT) and later extended toward the junction with the TAL. Strong co-expression of rENaC and 11β-hydroxysteroid dehydrogenase was observed in early nascent connecting tubule (CT) and collecting ducts and later also in the distal portion of the DCT.

The sodium transporters do not contribute equally to the maintenance of sodium balance. In knockout mice, severe salt wasting results from loss of function of the NKCC2 in the thick ascending limb, or of the ENaC in the collecting duct. However, knockout mice with loss of function of the proximal absorptive Na+-H+ exchanger (NHE) do not exhibit severe salt wasting.[45] Apparently, the severity of Na dysregulation is unrelated to the basal rate of absorption of NaCl in a given nephron segment. At least for some nephron segments, a tubuloglomerular feedback mechanism may lower the rate of sodium delivery to compensate for a lower rate of sodium reabsorption.[45]

Na+,K+-ATPase

Bistritzer and coworkers[46] measured Na+,K+-ATPase activity in cord red blood cells of newborn infants at different gestational ages. Red blood cell Na+,K+-ATPase activity was significantly lower ($p < .01$) in preterm babies with a gestational age below 35 weeks, compared with those aged 35 weeks and above: 2.3 ± 0.8 and 6.7 ± 1.3 nmol NADH/min/mg protein, respectively. Two weeks after birth, regardless of gestational age, the enzyme activity of the preterm babies increased to values similar to those observed in the term neonates at birth. These findings suggest that the Na+,K+-ATPase enzyme system undergoes important developmental changes.

Basolateral Na+,K+-ATPase provides the electrochemical driving force for solute reabsorption along the proximal tubule and the remainder of the nephron. In animals, the increase in active transport with maturation of the kidney parallels the threefold increase in Na+,K+-ATPase activity/millimeter tubule length during maturation.[47-50] The activity of Na+,K+-ATPase has been shown to increase in rats during development and to increase fol-

lowing aldosterone treatment.[51] Glucocorticoids can increase the rate of Na+,K+-ATPase production and may account for some of the increase in postnatal sodium handling in premature infants when compared with unborn fetuses at the same developmental age.[52] However, the activity of this enzyme system is not rate-limiting for sodium transport, as the increase in the tubular membrane area precedes the increase in Na+,K+-ATPase activity.[53,54]

In addition to enzyme activity, the distribution of the Na+,K+-ATPase to the basolateral tubular membrane also appears to be developmentally regulated. In the distal nephron, mRNA expression for the β2-subunit is expressed apically and is down-regulated postnatally, whereas mRNA expression for the β1-subunit is expressed basolaterally and is up-regulated after birth.[55,56]

Symporters

In primordial prokaryotic cells, families of transport proteins arose to serve a variety of cellular functions, including the regulation of cell pH and the provision of carbohydrate for cellular energy. The protein sequences have been conserved and through evolution modified proteins that now perform additional tasks, including the bulk transport of solutes.

In the proximal tubule, the filtered solutes glucose, phosphate, and amino acids are transported from the lumen into the tubular cells by proteins (symporters or antiporters) located in the brush-border luminal membrane.[57-60] Sodium travels down an electrochemical gradient, and the solutes are coupled to the movement of sodium. Bicarbonate is reabsorbed via the apical NHE3 and the basolateral Na-bicarbonate co-transporter (NBC).

PROXIMAL TUBULE

Sodium-Hydrogen Exchanger (NHE)

Neonates have a lower serum bicarbonate level than do adults owing to a lower renal threshold for bicarbonate. Eighty percent of bicarbonate reabsorption occurs in the proximal tubule, in which proton secretion is predominantly mediated by an electroneutral luminal NHE.

The NHEs are plasma membrane proteins that are either sensitive (NHE1, NHE2, and NHE4) or insensitive (NHE3) to inhibition by amiloride. Their pattern of expression differs. NHE1 is transcribed in all tissues tested and functions in the regulation of intracellular pH and cell volume. NHE2 is highly expressed in the kidney and gastrointestinal tract and may play a role in sodium reabsorption. NHE3 is expressed in the kidney and contributes to sodium and bicarbonate reabsorption, and NHE4 is expressed mainly in the stomach. The renal NHE are sorted either to the apical (NHE3) or to the basolateral (NHE1, NHE 4) membranes.[61,62]

Housekeeping Role

NHE3 plays a "housekeeping role" in maintaining the cell actin cystoskeleton. Members of the ezrin (VIL2)-radixin (RDX)-moesin (MSN) (ERM) protein family are highly concentrated in the apical aspect of polarized epithelial cells. These cells are studded with microvilli containing bundles of actin filaments, which must attach to the membrane to assemble and maintain the microvilli. The ERM proteins, together with merlin, the NF2 gene product, join integral membrane and cytoskeletal proteins and bind directly to actin. Actin cytoskeleton reorganization requires the activation of NHE3 (SLC9A3).[63]

Na Reabsorption

Schultheis and coworkers.[64] created knockout mice lacking NHE3 function. Homozygous mutant mice survived but had slight diarrhea and mild acidosis. As expected, bicarbonate and fluid absorption were low in proximal convoluted tubules, the blood pressure was low, and there was a severe absorptive defect in the intestine. These findings indicate that NHE3 is the major absorptive NHE in kidney and intestine, and that lack of the exchanger impairs acid-base balance and Na$^+$–fluid volume homeostasis.

It is important to note that the mutant mice were not severely hyponatremic. Two mechanisms may account for their ability to maintain sodium balance. First, sodium transporters other than NHE were induced. Plasma aldosterone was increased in NHE3-deficient mice, and expression of both renin and the AE1 (Slc4a1) chloride-bicarbonate exchanger mRNAs were induced in kidney. In the colon, epithelial Na$^+$ channel activity was increased and colonic H$^+$,K$^+$-ATPase mRNA was induced. Presumably, the high activity of these induced transporters compensated for the loss of function of NHE.

Second, the reduction in proximal fluid absorption was accompanied by a proportional decrease in the GFR. Compensation of the transport defect by a reduction in filtered load was so efficient that clinically symptomatic Na losses were not observed.[45,64]

Developmental Changes

The V_{max} of embryonic apical membrane NHE3 is threefold lower than that in the adult, suggesting a lower abundance or turnover rate.[65] Na-H activity increases during the transition from fetus to newborn sheep.[66] The administration of glucocorticoid to the mother increases V_{max} to the adult level.

To examine the maturation of apical NHE3 antiporter activity in rat proximal convoluted tubules, Shah and associates[67] perfused rat proximal convoluted tubules *in vitro*. Na$^+$-H$^+$ antiporter activity was assayed as the proton secretory rate on luminal sodium removal. Na$^+$-H$^+$ antiporter activity was 121.2 ± 18.4 pmol/mm × min in neonatal and 451.8 ± 40.6 pmol/mm × min in adult proximal convoluted tubules ($p < .001$). Adult renal cortical NHE3 mRNA abundance was 10-fold greater than that in 1-day-old neonates ($p < .001$). There was a comparable developmental increase in renal brush-border membrane vesicle NHE3 protein abundance ($p < .001$). These observations indicate an age-related increase in rat apical membrane Na$^+$-H$^+$ antiporter activity, renal cortical NHE3 mRNA, and brush-border membrane vesicle NHE3 protein abundance.

The abundance of mRNA for the basolateral NHE1 and NHE4 and the pH-dependent renal sodium uptake is higher in 2- to 4-week-old rats than in the adult.[68] The functional significance of this observation is unclear, as the major mechanism for the transport of HCO$_3^-$ across the basolateral membrane is via the electrogenic Na$^+$-HCO$_3^-$ co-transporter (NBC).

Sodium Bicarbonate Co-Transporter (NBC)

Molecular cloning experiments have so far identified three NBC isoforms (NBC-1, NBC-2, and NBC-3) in the kidney.[69] Under normal conditions, all appear to mediate the co-transport of Na$^+$ and HCO$_3^-$. In addition, they may be functionally altered in certain pathophysiologic states. For example, NBC-1 may be up-regulated in metabolic acidosis and potassium depletion, and also in response to glucocorticoid excess, and may be down-regulated in response to HCO$_3^-$ loading, or alkalosis.[70] Mutations in the *SLC4A4* gene for NBC cause proximal renal tubular acidosis, with bilateral glaucoma, cataracts, and band keratopathy. Such mutations may increase the bicarbonate concentration in the corneal stroma, which would facilitate calcium deposition, leading to band keratopathy.[71]

Na-Pi Type IIa (NaPi-2)

In the intestine and the kidney, the apical sodium Na-Pi co-transport is the rate-limiting step for the reabsorption of phosphate.[72] Three different Na-Pi-co-transporters have been identified:

1. Type I co-transporters, such as NPT1 (SLC17A1), are found mainly in proximal tubule and do not appear to be regulated by dietary phosphate levels. These proteins also show anion channel function and may play a role in secretion of organic anions;

2. Type II co-transporters, such as NaPi-3 (SLC34A1), determine Na$^+$-dependent transcellular Pi movements in the renal proximal tubule (type IIa) and in the small intestine (type IIb); and

3. Type III co-transporters are expressed in many different tissues, where they serve housekeeping functions. Type III transporters also can function as membrane receptors for primate retroviruses.

The Na-Pi symporters derive from ancient lineage. A NaPi-II homologue cloned from *Vibrio cholerae* is a functional Pi transporter when expressed in *Xenopus* oocytes.[73]

In the small intestine, expression of IIb protein varies in response to altered Pi intake and levels of 1,25(OH$_2$) vitamin D$_3$. In the proximal tubule, Pi intake, vitamin D levels, and parathyroid hormone all regulate the expression of the IIa co-transporter.

Contribution of NaPi-II to Sodium Reabsorption

The NHE is the major apical sodium transporter in the proximal convoluted tubule. The relative contribution of other transport systems to the reabsorption of sodium can be estimated using "targeted proteomics." In this method, the kidneys of genetically deficient mice with loss of NHE3 function are probed for renal sodium transporters. Brooks and associates[74] used semiquantitative immunoblotting to estimate the percentage change in abundance of each transporter in knockout compared with wild-type mice. In NHE3 knockout mice, three changes were identified that could compensate for the loss of NHE3-mediated sodium absorption: (1) in the proximal tubule, the sodium-phosphate co-transporter NaPi-2 was markedly up-regulated; (2) in the collecting duct, the 70-kDa form (aldosterone-stimulated) of the γ-subunit of the epithelial sodium channel ENaC was up-regulated; and (3) glomerular filtration was significantly reduced. These findings suggest that the NaPi-2 transport system plays an important role in sodium as well as phosphate handling by the kidney.

Na-Pi During Development

The renal tubules of the neonate have a high rate of phosphate reabsorption. To determine the mechanism, Woda and colleagues[75] performed renal micropuncture experiments in acutely thyroparathyroidectomized adult (>14-wk-old) and juvenile (4-wk-old) male Wistar rats in the presence and absence of parathyroid hormone (PTH). Pi reabsorption was greater in proximal convoluted (PCT) and straight tubules (PST) of the juvenile compared with adult rats, whether or not PTH was present. These findings were consistent with a greater Pi uptake in brush-border membrane (BBM) vesicles from both superficial and outer juxtamedullary cortices of juvenile animals. This high rate of Pi uptake is due to a high V_{max} of the NaPi-2 symporter.

In kidneys of newborn rats, the appearance of NaPi-2 protein and mRNA coincides with the development of the brush border (assessed by actin staining) on proximal tubular cells. Traebert and colleagues[76] found that NaPi-2 was not detectable in the nephrogenic zone or in the outgrowing straight sections of proximal tubules, which lack a brush border. In 13-day-old suckling rats, strong NaPi-2 staining was seen in the BBM of convoluted proximal tubules of all nephron generations. In contrast, in 22-day-old weaned rats, NaPi-2 staining in the BBM of superficial nephrons was weaker than that in the BBM of juxtamedullary nephrons. Western blotting demonstrated that the overall abundance of NaPi-2 protein in the BBM of 22-day-old rats was decreased to approximately 70% of that in 13-day-old rats. These observations suggest a greater abundance of NaPi-2 in newborn compared with mature animals.

Woda and colleagues[75] found that dietary phosphate restriction in juvenile rats resulted in a significant increase in phosphate reabsorption in the PCT and PST segments. NaPi-2 expression in the proximal tubule BBM was also increased, as was the expression of intracellular NaPi-2 protein. In addition, dietary phosphate restriction in the juvenile rat was associated with up-regulation of BBM NaPi-2 expression, which was associated with a further increase in proximal tubular phosphate reabsorption.

The ancient molecular lineage and the high plasticity of NaPi-2 suggest an important role in maintaining sodium as well as phosphate homestasis.

DISTAL TUBULE

The thick ascending limb of the loop of Henle in neonates has only 20% of the capacity to transport sodium compared with adults.[77, 78] Like the proximal tubule, Na+,K+-ATPase activity is significantly lower in the differentiating basolateral membrane of the thick ascending limb. This accounts for an isotonic fluid delivered to the early distal tubule in the immature kidney, in contrast to a hypo-osmotic fluid delivered in the adult kidney.

Aperia and Elinder studied distal tubular sodium reabsorptive capacity in immature (24-day-old) and mature (40-day-old) rats during hydropenia and following volume expansion.[79] Under hydropenic conditions, the fraction of filtered sodium entering the early distal tubule was higher, although it was similar in the late distal tubule in the young compared with mature rats (Fig. 130–10).[79] This indicates that immature nephrons deliver a greater fraction of sodium from the ascending loop of Henle but also have a higher fractional reabsorption of sodium along the distal tubule.

Epithelial Sodium Channel

Canessa and colleagues[80, 81] cloned and characterized subunits of a rat ENaC that had the functional properties of the distal renal sodium channel—high sodium selectivity, low conductance, and amiloride sensitivity. The functional channel is composed of at least three subunits, alpha (SCNN1A), beta (SCNN1B), and gamma (SCNN1G). The three subunits show sequence similarities to one another, indicating descent from a common ancestral gene. Each encodes a protein containing two transmembrane domains, with intracellular amino and carboxyl termini.

In the distal nephron, ENaC mediates electrogenic Na transport and is the rate-limiting step of sodium reabsorption. In the

adult, ENaC is expressed all along the connecting tubule (70% of the distal convolution) and the cortical collecting duct.[82]

Regulation of ENaC by Aldosterone and Angiotensin II

The level of sodium reabsorption is primarily determined by the action of aldosterone on ENaC in the distal nephron. To conserve sodium, aldosterone must first bind to the mineralocorticoid receptor (MR). MR-deficient knock out mice develop symptoms of pseudohypoaldosteronism, such as weight loss, dehydration, and renal sodium wasting. By day 8, MR-deficient knockout mice develop hyperkalemia, hyponatremia, and high circulating levels of renin, angiotensin II, and aldosterone. GFR is similar to controls but the FE_{Na} is more than eightfold higher.[83]

In an aldosterone-sensitive renal cell line (A6), aldosterone regulates sodium reabsorption by short- and long-term processes. In the short term, aldosterone regulates sodium transport by inducing expression of the small G-protein K-Ras2A, by stimulating the activity of methyltransferase and S-adenosylhomocysteine hydrolase to activate Ras by methylation, and, possibly, by subsequent activation by K-Ras2A of phosphatidylinositol phosphate-5-kinase (PIP-5-K) and phosphatidylinositol-3-kinase (PI-3-K), which ultimately activate ENaC. In the long term, aldosterone regulates sodium transport by altering trafficking, assembly, and degradation of EnaC.[84, 85]

Brooks and co-workers[86] examined renal homogenates from mice in which the gene for the angiotensin II type 1a [AT(1a)] receptor had been deleted to determine which sodium transporters and channels are regulated by the AT(1a) receptor. In mutant compared with wild-type mice maintained on a low-NaCl diet, the abundance of the thiazide-sensitive co-transporter and the three subunits of the amiloride-sensitive ENaC was markedly increased. There were no significant changes in the abundances of the proximal tubule NHE or the Na+-K+-2Cl- co-transporter of the thick ascending limb. These observations suggest that angiotensisn II directly alters renal sodium transport independently of aldosterone secretion.

Ontogeny of ENaC

The total expression of ENaC subunits is very low in the embryonic rat kidney but rises rapidly to adult levels by the first postnatal day.[87] ENaC is expressed in a variety of tissues, including lung and kidney. In knock out mice that do not express ENaC subunits, severe hyponatremia and/or failure to clear pulmonary fluid may occur (Table 130–3).[87-92] These findings indicate that EnaC is critically important to sodium balance.

Cation-Cl Cotransporters (CCC)

The CCC mediate the coupled movement of Na and/or K to that of Cl across membranes of epithelial cells. Eight CCC have been identified to date: two Na-K-Cl co-transporters (NKCC), four K-Cl co-transporters (KCC), one Na-Cl co-transporter (NCC), and one CCC interacting protein (CIP). All the NKCC and KCC are inhibited by loop diuretics.[93]

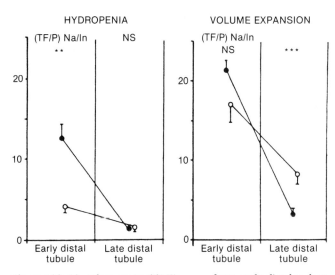

Figure 130–10. Changes in $(TF/P)_{Na/inulin}$ from early distal to late distal tubule in hydropenic and volume-expanded 24-day-old (*closed circles*) and 40-day-old (*open circles*) rats. NS = no significant difference; ** = $p < .01$; *** = $p < .001$. (From Aperia A, Elinder G: Am J Physiol *240*:F487, 1981.)

TABLE 130-3		
Epithelial Sodium Channel (ENaC) Subunit Loss of Function Mutations		
Type	Lung	Kidney
a-ENaC	Failure of pulmonary fluid clearance	Salt-wasting, metabolic acidosis, and high aldosterone
b-ENaC	Cleared fluid	Compensated on normal sodium intake but PHA-1 on low sodium
g-ENaC	Fluid problems	Severe hyperkalemia

Na-K-Cl

The Na-K-Cl co-transporters are a family of integral membrane proteins that mediate the coupled transport of Na$^+$,K$^+$, and Cl$^-$ across the plasma membrane. Quaggin and colleagues[94] observed that the kidney-specific Na-K-Cl co-transporter, (previously called NKCC2) mediates active reabsorption of sodium chloride in the thick ascending limb of the loop of Henle and is the site of action of the clinically important diuretics furosemide and bumetanide. The protein of the transporter gene, symbolized as SLC12A1 in human and mouse, is structurally related (64% amino acid identity in the mouse) to another Na-K-Cl co-transporter (SLC12A2, previously called NKCC1), which is expressed in many tissues, including the basolateral membrane of secretory epithelia, where it mediates active chloride secretion.

Na-Cl Co-transporter (NCC)

The thiazide-sensitive NCC of the distal convoluted tubule is the principal mediator of sodium and chloride reabsorption in this nephron segment, accounting for a significant fraction of net renal sodium reabsorption. Simon and colleagues[95] and others[96] have associated Gitelman's syndrome of inherited hypokalemic alkalosis with mutations in the electroneutral sodium-chloride transporter. Gamba and associates[97] have cloned this transporter from rat kidney. Simon and co-workers[95] have cloned the human homologue, which they designated TSC for thiazide-sensitive Na-Cl co-transporter, and showed that the protein is encoded by 26 exons. The human protein showed 89% identity with the rat homologue and 63% identity with the flounder homologue.

Mastroianni and co-workers[98] also cloned the *SLC12A3* gene. The predicted protein sequence of 1021 amino acids (112 kDa) showed a structure common to other members of the Na-K-Cl co-transporter family: a central region harboring 12 transmembrane domains and the two intracellular hydrophilic amino and carboxyl termini. The expression pattern of the gene confirmed the kidney specificity. By fluorescence *in situ* hybridization, these investigators mapped the gene to 16q13.

In the NCC knockout mice, the abundance of the 70-kDa form of the γ-subunit of ENaC was higher than in controls. However, the abundance of other sodium transport proteins was similar to that of wild-type mice. Compared with the renal Na transporters of the NCC knockout mouse, the renal Na transporters of NH3 knockout mice undergo extensive adaptation. This observation suggests that NHE3 is more important for bulk sodium transport than is NCC.[74]

REGULATORY SYSTEMS

Development changes in a variety of endocrine and paracrine systems (e.g., the renin-angiotensin-aldosterone system, prostaglandins, catecholamines, atrial natriuretic peptide, glucocorticoids, the kallikrein-kinin system, nitric oxide, and endothelin) may influence the renal handling of sodium. Detailed reviews have been published.[99, 100]

Renin-Angiotensin-Aldosterone System

Studies in the Fetus

In the fetus, the expression of renin in the kidney is different from that in the adult. Reddi and associates[101] observed a shift in renin distribution from interlobar and arcuate arteries in the fetus to the afferent arterioles in the adult. In addition, these investigators identified seven types of renin distribution along the afferent arterioles. In type I, renin was distributed continuously along the whole length of the afferent vessel. This pattern was most frequently observed in the fetus. In type II, renin extended upstream from the glomerulus but did not occupy the whole length of the arteriole. This type was relatively constant throughout postnatal life. In type III, renin was present as bands along the afferent vessel; it was most frequently observed in the fetal and early perinatal periods. In type IV, renin was restricted to the "classic" juxtaglomerular localization. It was the most frequent type observed in the adult rat. In type V, no renin was found in the arteriole. It was the second most frequent type observed in the adult rat. The distribution of renin-expressing cells was spatially and temporally associated with the development of blood vessels. During this process, renin-expressing cells were distributed along the whole of the newly formed vessel. As the vessel matured, renin-expressing cells became restricted to the juxtaglomerular portion of the afferent arteriole.

In chronically catheterized fetal sheep, the renin-angiotensin system (RAS) is active during intrauterine life.[102] Levels of angiotensin II (AII) in fetal sheep are similar to those in maternal sheep. The fetal kidney, like other vascular beds, has high levels of the AT2 angiotensin receptor subtype. With maturation, the proportion of the AT1 receptor subtype increases.

Blockade of the fetal RAS with angiotensin-converting enzyme (ACE) inhibitors or with the nonpeptide AII antagonist losartan causes a fall in fetal GFR and a rise in renal blood flow (RBF). AII reverses the fall in GFR even though RBF decreases. Lumbers[102] observed that the fraction of the filtered sodium load reabsorbed by the proximal tubule was not affected when the fetal RAS was blocked by captopril or losartan. High doses of infused AII had no effect on renal reabsorption of sodium in the short term, but in the long term depressed fractional proximal reabsorption. These studies suggest that the renin-angiotensin system is active in the fetus but that the proximal renal tubule is resistant to the sodium-retaining effects of AII.

Studies in the Neonate

After birth, the kidneys of newborn animals become sensitive to the salt-retaining effects of AII. FE$_{Na}$ in rat pups given daily injections of the ATI receptor inhibitor losartan is higher than in control animals administered vehicle.[103]

Plasma renin activity (PRA)[104, 105] and plasma aldosterone (PA) concentrations[106, 107] are higher in newborn animals and humans. Sulyok and co-workers studied the relationship of PRA, PA, and urinary aldosterone excretion (UAE) in sodium-supplemented and nonsupplemented infants with a mean gestational age of 31 weeks.[108] Among nonsupplemented infants, PRA, PA, and UAE increased dramatically from week 1 to week 3 postnatally and then gradually decreased over the subsequent 2 weeks of the study (Fig. 130–11).[108] In contrast, there was no consistent change in the supplemented group, with values similar to those of full-term neonates. In fact, PRA, PA, and UAE were significantly higher in nonsupplemented versus supplemented infants at a postnatal age of 2 to 4 weeks. Godard and co-workers also found PRA to be inversely correlated with urinary sodium excretion in full-term infants.[109] Highest values were noted in the first 2 days of life and decreased over the subsequent week.[109]

Aperia and associates have shown that the pattern of urinary aldosterone excretion was similar in preterm (less than or equal to 34 weeks' gestation) and full-term infants. During the first 3 postnatal weeks, UAE was higher in both groups compared with normal adult values (Fig. 130–12).[110] Since aldosterone affects tubular sodium and potassium transport in opposite directions, the urinary sodium/urinary potassium ratio (U$_{Na}$/U$_K$ or U$_K$/U$_{Na}$) has been used to assess the effect of this hormone on distal tubular transport. It is interesting that the urinary potassium/sodium ratio showed a linear relationship to UAE with time only in term infants, whereas the ratio in the preterm group showed a correlation to UAE only after 10 days of age. The hyponatremia found at 2 weeks of age in the premature infants corresponded to the highest UAE and a low urinary potassium/sodium ratio.

There seemed to be an impaired end-organ response to aldosterone, with improvement with increasing postnatal age. Since the absolute urinary sodium excretion was similar in both

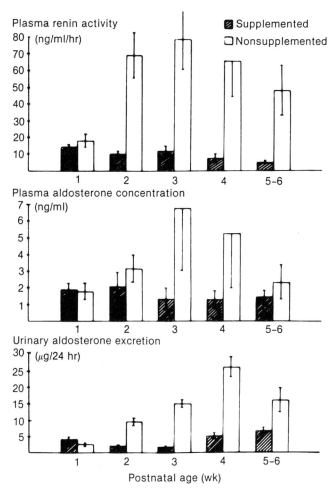

Figure 130–11. Plasma renin activity, plasma aldosterone concentration, and urinary aldosterone excretion in preterm infants with and without sodium supplementation in the first 5 to 6 weeks of life. (From Sulyok E, et al: *In* Spitzer A [ed]: The Kidney During Development. New York, Masson, 1982, pp 273–281.)

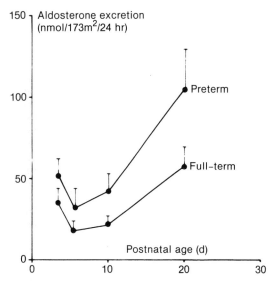

Figure 130–12. Changes in urinary aldosterone excretion in the first 30 days postnatally in preterm and full-term infants. (From Aperia A, et al: Acta Paediatr Scand *68*:813, 1979.)

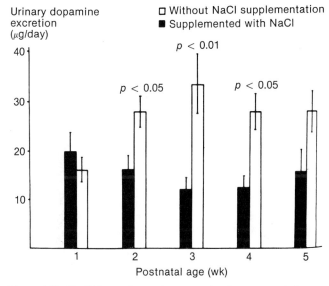

Figure 130–13. Urinary dopamine excretion in preterm infants with and without sodium supplementation in the first 5 weeks of life. (From Sulyok E, et al: Pediatr Res *19*:5, 1985.)

groups, factors other than sodium balance contributed to the hyponatremia found in very premature infants. The lack of renal tubular sensitivity to aldosterone may be related to lack of receptors or lack of Na^+,K^+-ATPase activity in the premature infant. However, Stephenson and co-workers found that immature rats (in contrast to older animals) were essentially insensitive to subcutaneously injected aldosterone.[111] In addition, there were equivalent high-affinity aldosterone-binding sites in both groups of rats. They concluded that the resistance of immature rat kidneys to aldosterone was not a defect in signal presentation or receptors but was rather a postreceptor phenomenon.

Prostaglandins

Renal prostaglandin (PGE) production, as measured by urinary PGE_2 and PGI_2, is highest in preterm neonates and decreases with increasing gestational and postnatal age.[112] PGE concentrations decrease progressively with postnatal age in sodium-supplemented premature infants but show no significant change with advancing age in a nonsupplemented group.[113] The steady decline in PGE concentrations in the sodium-supplemented group corresponds to decreased activity in the renin-angiotensin-aldosterone system under similar conditions. From the studies, Ertl suggested that increased PGE synthesis would be needed to offset the vasoconstrictor effect resulting from activa-

tion of the renin-angiotensin system in order to maintain normal blood pressure and reduce renal vascular resistance.[113] In premature neonates, inhibition of prostaglandin synthesis with indomethacin can significantly reduce glomerular blood flow and glomerular filtration, but the role of prostaglandin synthesis inhibition in renal tubular sodium handling is minimal.[114]

Catecholamines

Both neuronally derived and locally produced (renal tubular cells) catecholamines exert control over renal sodium handling. Tubule cells possess receptors for dopamine, norepinephrine, and epinephrine. There is an association between increased sodium excretion and increased dopamine excretion in nonsupplemented preterm infants (Fig. 130–13).[115, 116] Conversely, supplemented infants show no increase in dopamine excretion. These studies demonstrate that the renal sympathetic nervous system enhances sodium reabsorption. However, its relationship to the renin-angiotensin-aldosterone system still requires additional investigations.

The intravenous administration of dopamine to sick premature infants increases sodium excretion and PRA without a significant change in PA.[117] This could be interpreted as an unresponsiveness of the adrenal gland to additional stimulation. Even though there are age-related differences in the effect of dopamine administration, the results are similar to those reported in adults.

To sort out the differences in the renal response to endogenous versus exogenous dopamine, metoclopramide was given to premature infants to block dopamine production.[118] Urinary sodium excretion was increased in the low-salt intake group, whereas there was no change in the high dietary sodium group. There was also no effect on PRA in either group. Conversely, PA concentration and UAE decreased. These data suggested that increased urinary sodium excretion was due to metoclopramide suppression of aldosterone secretion in these young infants. Therefore, endogenous dopamine stimulated renal tubular sodium reabsorption, increased aldosterone production, and possibly played a role in restoration of positive sodium balance in premature infants with late hyponatremia.

Studies in fetal sheep have examined the role of renal innervation in the development of sodium homeostasis. The relative distribution of α_1-adrenoceptors (which modulate tubular sodium and water reabsorption) and α_2-adrenoceptors (which modulate sodium, water, and potassium excretion) changes during development.[119] Stimulation of α_1-adrenoceptors in fetal, newborn, and adult sheep showed a maximal ability to decrease urine flow and sodium excretion in newborn sheep, with significantly less conservation of sodium in fetal sheep.[120] The ability to reabsorb sodium and water in the immediate postnatal period is, in part, mediated by development of the renal response to catecholamines. Incomplete development of this system in premature neonates may play a role in the hyponatremia of prematurity.

Atrial Natriuretic Peptides

Atrial natriuretic peptide (ANP) is detectable early in fetal development.[121] The distribution of ANP is relatively widespread in both atria and ventricles during early development and localizes to the right atrium near the time of birth.[122] Circulating levels of ANP increase throughout gestation, continue to increase after birth for 7 to 10 days, and are higher in premature infants than in term neonates.[123] The highest ANP levels are seen in the most premature neonates, particularly those with respiratory disease.[124] Atrial natriuretic peptide concentrations are elevated in the plasma of sodium-supplemented infants (Fig. 130–14).[125] Although the exact mechanism modulating this increase is unknown, it may be secondary to an expanded extracellular fluid volume because of the augmented sodium diet. The lower value in infants on a low-sodium diet may be a response of the premature kidney to conserve sodium for tissue growth.

Although circulating levels of ANP are high during development and in the newborn period, the renal natriuretic and diuretic response to ANP is blunted. Possible reasons for this blunted response include the following: (1) lower renal perfusion pressure seen in fetal and newborn kidneys[126]; (2) incompletely developed system of ANP receptors in the kidney[127]; and/or (3) inhibition of ANP effect by high circulating levels of angiotensin II and aldosterone.

The importance of ANP in sodium handling in the young animal is unclear. Deloof and colleagues[128] placed pregnant rats on either a high-sodium or a normal sodium diet. The high-sodium diet was not associated with a change in the plasma ANP concentrations but significantly decreased the plasma aldosterone concentrations in both the maternal and fetal rats. In response to the high-salt diet, the density and affinity of total

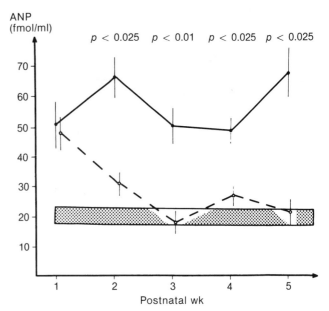

Figure 130–14. Plasma atrial natriuretic peptide (ANP) concentrations in preterm infants on a low (*dashed line*) and a high (*solid line*) sodium intake. The *stippled area* is ANP values for 7- to 10-day-old full-term infants. (From Tulassay T, et al: J Pediatr *109*:1023, 1986.)

ANP, ANPb, and ANPc receptors were not altered in the maternal isolated renal glomeruli or the adrenal zona glomerulosa membranes, or the fetal adrenal gland and kidney membrane preparations. These results suggest that ANP is not involved in the regulation of water and electrolyte balance in maternal and fetal rats during salt-loaded intake.

Digoxin-like immunoreactive substances in both the urine and plasma have been suggested to be natriuretic by virtue of their known inhibition of Na$^+$,K$^+$-ATPase activity *in vitro*.[129] Ebara and colleagues found a correlation between these substances and FE$_{Na}$ in preterm infants.[129] The urine and plasma concentrations of digoxin-like immunoreactive substances remained elevated for 4 weeks in infants of 24 to 29 weeks' gestation and decreased in those infants with a gestational age greater that 30 weeks. Additional studies will be required to assess the significance of this study.[130]

SUMMARY

Primordial cells have developed specialized proteins to aid in the maintenance of cellular integrity, pH, and metabolism. More evolved cell types have co-opted and modified these ancient proteins to serve a variety of functions useful to the organism as a whole, including the bulk transport of solutes across epithelial cell membranes. In immature animals, the transport proteins not only maintain homeostasis but also promote growth.

Newborn animals maintain a positive balance for sodium. Clearance studies have indicated that the distal tubule is mostly responsible for the adaptation to extrauterine life. Due to advances in molecular biology, a variety of specialized sodium transporters are now recognized. Studies performed using targeted proteomics have revealed the special importance of ENaC and the NCC proteins in maintaining sodium balance.

Some investigators have postulated the existence of growth-specific transporters that are not expressed in the adult. Future studies will determine exactly how these proteins are sorted, distributed, and regulated. The contribution of regulatory paracrine systems such as the renin-angiotensin system can then be rigorously investigated.

REFERENCES

1. Chevalier RL: The moth and the aspen tree: sodium in early postnatal development. Kidney Int 59:1617, 2001.
2. Bernstein IL, Courtney L: Salt preference in the preweaning rat. Dev Psychobiol 20:443, 1998.
3. Aperia A, et al: Renal response to an oral sodium load in newborn full-term infants. Acta Paediatr Scand 61:670, 1972.
4. Aperia A, et al: Renal control of sodium and fluid balance in newborn infants during intravenous maintenance therapy. Acta Paediatr Scand 64:725, 1975.
5. Forbes GB: Human Body Composition—Growth, Aging, Nutrition, and Activity. New York, Springer-Verlag, 1987, p 132.
6. McCance RA, Widdowson EM: The response of the newborn puppy to water, salt and food. J Physiol 141:81, 1958.
7. Forbes GB: Human Body Composition—Growth, Aging, Nutrition, and Activity. New York, Springer-Verlag, 1987, pp 23–27.
8. Haycock GB, Aperia A: Salt and the newborn kidney. Pediatr Nephrol 5:65, 1991.
9. Robillard JE, et al: Regulation of sodium metabolism and extracellular fluid volume during development. Clin Perinatol 19:15, 1992.
10. Bickel CA, et al: Increased renal Na-K-ATPase, NCC, and beta-ENaC abundance in obese Zucker rat. Am J Physiol Renal Physiol 281:F639, 2001.
11. Konstantinou-Tegou A, et al: The effect of leptin on Na(+)-H(+) antiport (NHE 1) activity of obese and normal subjects' erythrocytes. Mol Cell Endocrinol 183:11, 2001.
12. Kaloyianni M, et al: The effect of insulin on Na$^+$-H$^+$ antiport activity of obese and normal subjects' erythrocytes. Cell Physiol Biochem 11:253, 2001.
13. Bueva A, Guignard JP: Renal function in preterm neonates. Pediatr Res 36:572, 1994.
14. Wilkins BH: Renal function in sick, very low birth weight infants. 3. Sodium, potassium, and water excretion. Arch Dis Child 67:1154, 1992.
15. Siegel SR, Oh W: Renal function as a marker of human fetal maturation. Acta Paediatr Scand 65:481, 1976.
16. Al-Dahhan J, et al: Sodium homeostasis in term and preterm neonates. I. Renal aspects. Arch Dis Child 58:335, 1983.
17. Engelke SC, et al: Sodium balance in very low-birth-weight infants. J Pediatr 93:837, 1978.
18. Vanpeé M, et al: Postnatal development of renal function in very low birth-weight infants. Acta Paediatr Scand 77:191, 1988.
19. Wilkinson AW, et al: Metabolic changes in the newborn. Lancet 1:983, 1962.
20. Solyok E, et al: Relationship between the postnatal development of the renin-angiotensin-aldosterone system and electrolyte and acid-base status of the NaCl-supplemented premature infants. In Spitzer A (ed): The Kidney During Development. New York, Masson, 1982, pp 273–281.
21. Roy RN, et al: Late hyponatremia in very low birthweight infants (<1.3 kilograms). Pediatr Res 10:526, 1976.
22. Muchant DG, et al: Chronic sodium loading augments the natriuretic response to acute expansion in the preweaned rat. Am J Physiol 269:R15, 1995.
23. Taitz LS, Byers HD: High calorie/osmolar feeding and hypertonic dehydration. Arch Dis Child 47:257, 1972.
24. Goldsmith DI, et al: Hemodynamic and excretory response of the neonatal canine kidney to acute volume expansion. Am J Physiol 237:F392, 1979.
25. Banks RO: Segmental nephron sodium and potassium reabsorption in newborn and adult dogs during saline expansion. Proc Soc Exp Biol Med 173:231, 1983.
26. Schoeneman MJ, Spitzer A: The effect of intravascular volume expansion on proximal tubular reabsorption during development. Proc Soc Exp Biol Med 165:319, 1980.
27. Aperia A, et al: Developmental study of the renal response to an oral salt load in preterm infants. Acta Paediatr Scand 63:517, 1974.
28. Berg U: Urine elimination of an oral salt and fluid load in healthy children. Acta Paediatr Scand 62:505, 1973.
29. Aperia A, et al: Development of renal control of salt and fluid homeostasis during the first year of life. Acta Paediatr Scand 64:393, 1975.
30. Sulyok E, et al: On the mechanism of renal sodium handling in newborn infants. Biol Neonate 37:75, 1980.
31. Sulyok E, et al: Postnatal development of renal sodium handling in premature infants. J Pediatr 95:787, 1979.
32. Rodriquez-Soriano J, et al: Renal handling of sodium in premature and full-term neonates: a study using clearance methods during water diuresis. Pediatr Res 17:1013, 1983.
33. Rodriquez-Soriano J, et al: Renal handling of water and sodium in infancy and childhood: a study using clearance methods during hypotonic saline diuresis. Kidney Int 20:700, 1981.
34. Horster M, Larsson L: Mechanisms of fluid absorption during proximal tubule development. Kidney Int 10:348, 1976.
35. Horster M, Valtin H: Postnatal development of renal function: micropuncture and clearance studies in the dog. J Clin Invest 50:779, 1971.
36. Aperia A, Larsson L: Correlation between fluid reabsorption and proximal tubule ultrastructure during development of the rat kidney. Acta Physiol Scand 105:11, 1979.
37. Celsi G, et al: Proximal tubular reabsorption and Na-K-ATPase activity in remnant kidney of young rats. Am J Physiol 251:F588, 1986.
38. Spitzer A, Brandis M: Functional and morphologic maturation of the superficial nephrons. Relationship to total kidney function. J Clin Invest 53:297, 1974.
39. Schwartz GJ, Evan AP: Development of solute transport in rabbit proximal tubule. I. HCO$_3^-$ and glucose absorption. Am J Physiol 245:F382, 1983.
40. Barac-Nieto M, Spitzer A: The relationship between renal metabolism and proximal transport during ontogeny. Pediatr Nephrol 2:356, 1988.
41. Kaskel FJ, et al: Factors affecting proximal tubular reabsorption during development. Am J Physiol 252:F188, 1987.
42. Meadow MS, Lipkowitz MS: Developmental changes of renal brush border membrane ionic permeability. Biochim Biophys Acta 1191:219, 1994.
43. Van Adelsberg J: Protein targeting: the molecular basis of vectorial transport in the kidney. Semin Nephrol 18:152, 1998.
44. Schmitt R, et al: Developmental expression of sodium entry pathways in rat nephron. Am J Physiol 276:F367, 1999.
45. Schnermann J: Sodium transport deficiency and sodium balance in gene-targeted mice. Acta Physiol Scand 173:59, 2001.
46. Bistritzer T, et al: Sodium potassium adenosine triphosphatase activity in preterm and term infants and its possible role in sodium homeostasis during maturation. Am J Physiol Renal Physiol 281:F639, 2001.
47. Schwartz GJ, Evan AP: Development of solute transport in rabbit proximal tubule. III. Na-K-ATPase activity. Am J Physiol 246:F845, 1984.
48. Schmidt U, Horster M: Na-K-activated ATPase: activity maturation in rabbit nephron segments dissected in vitro. Am J Physiol 233:F55, 1977.
49. Igarashi Y, et al: Effect of betamethasone on Na-K-ATPase activity and basal and lateral cell membranes in proximal tubular cells during early development. Am J Physiol 245:F232, 1983.
50. Aperia A, Larsson L: Induced development of proximal tubular NaKATPase, basolateral cell membranes and fluid reabsorption. Acta Physiol Scand 121:133, 1984.
51. Aperia A, et al: Hormonal induction of Na-K-ATPase in developing proximal tubular cells. Am J Physiol 241:F356, 1981.
52. Fukuda Y, et al: Ontogeny of the regulation of Na$^+$,K$^+$-ATPase activity on the renal proximal tubule cell. Pediatr Res 30:131, 1991.
53. Evan AP, et al: Development of solute transport in rabbit proximal tubule. II. Morphologic segmentation. Am J Physiol 245:F391, 1983.
54. Wijkhuisen A, et al: Birth-related change in energy metabolism enzymes and Na$^+$,K$^+$-ATPase activity in proximal convoluted tubular cells. Am J Physiol Cell Physiol 272:C787, 1997.
55. Burrow CR, et al: Expression of the β$_2$-subunit and the apical localization of the Na$^+$,K$^+$-ATPase in metanephric kidney. Am J Physiol Renal Physiol 277: F391, 1999.
56. Guillery EN, et al: Posttranscriptional upregulation of Na(+)-K(+) ATPase activity in newborn guinea pig renal cortex. Am J Physiol 273:F254, 1997.
57. Kinne R, et al: Sugar transport by renal plasma membrane vesicles: characteristics of the systems in brush-border microvilli and basolateral plasma membranes. J Membr Biol 21:275, 1975.
58. Evers J, et al: Phenylalanine uptake by isolated renal brush border vesicles. Biochim Biophys Acta 426:598, 1976.
59. Hoffman H, et al: Phosphate transport by isolated renal brush border vesicles. Pflügers Arch 362:147, 1976.
60. Roth KS, et al: The ontogeny of sugar transport in kidney. Pediatr Res 12:1127, 1978.
61. Brant SR, et al: Physical and genetic mapping of a human apical epithelial Na$^+$/H$^+$ exchanger (NHE3) isoform to chromosome 5p15.3.69. Genomics 15:668, 1993.
62. Biemesderfer D, et al: Monoclonal antibodies for high-resolution localization of NHE3 in adult and neonatal rat kidney. Am J Physiol 273:F289, 1997.
63. Murthy A, et al: NHE-RF, a regulatory cofactor for Na(+)-H(+) exchange, is a common interactor for merlin and ERM (MERM) proteins. J Biol Chem 273:1273, 1998.
64. Schultheis PJ, et al: Renal and intestinal absorptive defects in mice lacking the NHE3 Na(+)/H(+) exchanger. Nature Genet 19:282, 1998.
65. Beck JC, et al: Ontogeny of Na/H antiporter activity in rabbit renal brush border membrane vesicles. J Clin Invest 87:2067, 1991.
66. Guillery EN, et al: Maturation of the proximal tubule Na/H antiporter activity in sheep during the transition from fetus to newborn. Am J Physiol 267:F537, 1994.
67. Shah M, et al: Ontogeny of Na$^+$/H$^+$ antiporter activity in rat proximal convoluted tubules. Pediatr Res 48:206, 2000.
68. Collins JF, et al: Ontogeny of basolateral membrane Na-hydrogen exchange (NHE) activity and mRNA expression of NHE-1 and NHE-4 in rat kidney and jejunum. Biochim Biophys Acta 1368:147, 1998.
69. Soleimani M, Burnham CE: Physiologic and molecular aspects of the Na$^+$:HCO$_3^-$ cotransporter in health and disease processes. Kidney Int 57:371, 2000.
70. Burnham CE, et al: Cloning and functional expression of a human kidney Na$^+$:HCO$_3^-$ cotransporter. J Biol Chem 272:19111, 1997.
71. Igarashi T, et al: Mutations in SLC4A4 cause permanent isolated proximal renal tubular acidosis with ocular abnormalities (letter). Nature Genet 23:264, 1999.
72. Murer H, et al: Molecular mechanisms in proximal tubular and small intestinal phosphate reabsorption (Plenary Lecture). Mol Membr Biol 18:3, 2001.
73. Werner A, Kinne RK: Evolution of the Na-P(i) cotransport systems. Am J Physiol Regul Integr Comp Physiol 280:R301, 2001.
74. Brooks HL, et al: Profiling of renal tubule Na$^+$ transporter abundances in NHE3 and NCC null mice using targeted proteomics. J Physiol 530:359, 2001.
75. Woda C, et al: Renal tubular sites of increased phosphate transport and NaPi-2 expression in the juvenile rat. Am J Physiol Regul Integr Comp Physiol 280:R1524, 2001.

76. Traebert M, et al: Distribution of the sodium/phosphate transporter during postnatal ontogeny of the rat kidney. J Am Soc Nephrol 10:1407, 1999.
77. Horster M: Loop of Henle functional differentiation in vitro perfusion of the isolated thick ascending segment. Pflügers Arch 378:15, 1978.
78. Horster M: Expression of ontogeny in individual nephron segments. Kidney Int 22:550, 1982.
79. Aperia A, Elinder G: Distal tubular sodium reabsorption in the developing rat kidney. Am J Physiol 240:F487, 1981.
80. Canessa CM, et al: Epithelial sodium channel related to proteins involved in neurodegeneration. Nature 361:467, 1993.
81. Canessa CM, et al: Amiloride-sensitive epithelial Na(+)-channel is made of three homologous subunits. Nature 367:463, 1994.
82. Biner HL, et al: Human cortical distal nephron: distribution of electrolyte and water transport pathways. J Am Soc Nephrol 13:836, 2002.
83. Berger S, et al: Mineralocorticoid receptor knockout mice: pathophysiology of Na⁺ metabolism. Proc Natl Acad Sci U S A 95:9424, 1998.
84. Eaton DC, et al: Mechanisms of aldosterone's action on epithelial Na⁺ transport. J Membr Biol 184:313, 2001.
85. Stockland JD: New ideas about aldosterone signaling in epithelia. Am J Physiol Renal Physiol 282:F559, 2002.
86. Brooks HL, et al: Targeted proteomic profiling of renal Na(+) transporter and channel abundances in angiotensin II type 1a receptor knockout mice. Hypertension 39:470, 2002.
87. Vahashkari VM, et al: Developmental regulation of ENaC subunit mRNA levels in rat kidney. Am J Physiol Cell Physiol 274:C1661, 1998.
88. Barker PM, et al: Role of gamma ENaC subunit in lung liquid clearance and electrolyte balance in newborn mice. Insights into perinatal adoption and pseudohypoaldosteronism. J Clin Invest 102:1634, 1998.
89. Pradervand S, et al: Salt restriction induces pseudohypoaldosteronism type 1 in mice expressing low levels of the beta-subunit of the amiloride-sensitive epithelial sodium channel. Proc Natl Acad Sci U S A 96:1732, 1999.
90. Hummler E, et al: Early death due to defective neonatal lung liquid clearance in alpha ENaC-deficient mice. Nature Genet 12:325, 1996.
91. Hummler E, et al: A mouse model for the renal salt-wasting syndrome pseudohypoaldosteronism. Proc Natl Acad Sci U S A 94:111710, 1997.
92. McDonald FJ, et al: Disruption of the beta subunit of the epithelial Na⁺ channel in mice: hyperkalemia and neonatal death associated with a pseudohypoaldosteronism phenotype. Proc Natl Acad Sci U S A 96:1727, 1999.
93. Isenring P, Forbush B: Ion transport and ligand binding by the Na-K-Cl cotransporter; structure-function studies. Comp Biochem Physiol A Mol Integr Physiol 130:487, 2001.
94. Quaggin SE, et al: Localization of the renal Na-K-Cl cotransporter gene (Slc12a1) on mouse chromosome 2. Mammal Genome 6:557, 1995.
95. Simon DB, et al: Gitelman's variant of Bartter's syndrome, inherited hypokalaemic alkalosis, is caused by mutations in the thiazide-sensitive Na-Cl cotransporter. Nat Genet 12:24, 1996.
96. Takeuchi K, et al: Association of a mutation in thiazide-sensitive Na-Cl cotransporter with familial Gitelman's syndrome. J Clin Endocrino Metab 81:4496, 1996.
97. Gamba G, et al: Molecular cloning, primary structure, and characterization of two members of the mammalian electroneutral sodium-(potassium)-chloride cotransporter family expressed in the kidney. J Biol Chem 269:17713, 1994.
98. Mastroianni N, et al: Molecular cloning, expression pattern, and chromosomal localization of the human Na-Cl thiazide-sensitive cotransporter (SLC12A3). Genomics 35:486, 1996.
99. Gomez A, et al: Endocrine paracrine control: vasoactive substances. In Holliday MA, et al (eds): Pediatric Nephrology, 3rd ed. Baltimore, Williams and Wilkins, 1994, pp 79-99.
100. Celsi G, Aperia A: Endocrine paracrine control: sodium, chloride, and water excretion. In Holliday MA, et al (eds): Pediatric Nephrology, 3rd ed. Baltimore, Williams & Wilkins, 1994, pp 99-116.
101. Reddi V, et al: Renin-expressing cells are associated with branching of the developing kidney vasculature J Am Soc Nephrol 9:63, 1998.
102. Lumbers ER: Functions of the renin-angiotensin system during development. Clin Exp Pharmacol Physiol 22:499, 1995.
103. Chevalier RL, et al: Endogenous angiotensin II inhibits natriuresis following acute expansion in the neonatal rat. Am J Physiol 270:393, 1996.
104. Kotchen TA, et al: A study of the renin-angiotensin system in newborn infants. J Pediatr 80:938, 1972.
105. Drukker A, et al: The renin angiotensin system in newborn dogs: developmental patterns and response to acute saline loading. Pediatr Res 14:304, 1980.
106. Beitins IZ, et al: Plasma aldosterone concentration at delivery and during the newborn period. J Clin Invest 51:386, 1972.
107. Kowarski A, et al: Plasma aldosterone concentration in normal subjects from infancy to adulthood. J Clin Endocrinol Metab 38:489, 1974.
108. Sulyok E, et al: Relationship between the postnatal development of the renin-angiotensin-aldosterone system and electrolyte and acid-base status of the NaCl-supplemented premature infants. In Spitzer A (ed): The Kidney During Development. New York, Masson, 1982, pp 273-281.
109. Godard C, et al: Plasma renin activity related to sodium balance, renal function and urinary vasopressin in the newborn infant. Pediatr Res 13:742, 1979.
110. Aperia A, et al: Sodium excretion in relation to sodium intake and aldosterone excretion in newborn pre-term and full-term infants. Acta Paediatr Scand 68:813, 1979.
111. Stephenson G, et al: Ontogeny of renal mineralocorticoid receptors and urinary electrolyte responses in the rat. Am J Physiol 247:F665, 1984.
112. Arant BS: Functional immaturity of the newborn kidney: paradox or prostaglandin? In Strauss J (ed): Homeostasis, Nephrotoxicity, and Renal Anomalies in the Newborn. Boston, Nijhoff, 1984, pp 271-278.
113. Ertl T, et al: The effect of sodium chloride supplementation on the postnatal development of plasma prostaglandin E and F2 values in premature infants. J Pediatr 101:761, 1982.
114. Robillard JE, et al: Mechanisms regulating renal sodium excretion during development. Pediatr Nephrol 6:205, 1992.
115. Sulyok E, et al: The influence of NaCl supplementation on the postnatal development of urinary excretion of noradrenaline, dopamine, and serotonin in premature infants. Pediatr Res 19:5, 1985.
116. Sulyok E: Dopaminergic control of neonatal salt and water metabolism. Pediatr Nephrol 2:163, 1988.
117. Sulyok E, et al: The effect of dopamine administration on the activity of the renin-angiotensin-aldosterone system in sick preterm infants. Eur J Pediatr 143:191, 1985.
118. Sulyok E, et al: The effect of metoclopramide administration on electrolyte status and activity of renin-angiotensin-aldosterone system in premature infants. Pediatr Res 19:912, 1985.
119. Gitler MS, et al: Characterization of renal α-adrenoceptor subtypes in the sheep during development. Am J Physiol 260:R407, 1991.
120. Guillery EN, et al: Ontogenic changes in renal response to α₁-adrenoceptor stimulation in sheep. Am J Physiol 267:R990, 1994.
121. Smith FG, et al: Atrial natriuretic factor during fetal and postnatal life: a review. J Dev Physiol 12:55, 1989.
122. Mercadier JJ, et al: Atrial natriuretic factor messenger ribonucleic acid and peptide in the human heart during ontogenic development. Biochem Biophys Res Commun 159:777, 1989.
123. Tulassay T, et al: Atrial natriuretic peptide and extracellular fluid volume contraction after birth. Acta Physiol Scand 76:444, 1987.
124. Stephenson TJ, Broughton-Pipkin F: Atrial natriuretic peptide in the premature newborn. Biol Neonate 66:22, 1994.
125. Tulassay T, et al: Role of atrial natriuretic peptide in sodium homeostasis in premature infants. J Pediatr 109:1023, 1986.
126. Robillard JE, et al: Ontogeny of the renal response to natriuretic peptide in sheep. Am J Physiol 254:F634, 1988.
127. Chevalier R, et al: Renal effects of atrial natriuretic peptide infusion in young and adult rats. Pediatr Res 24:333, 1988.
128. Deloof S, et al: Eur J Endocrinol 142:524, 2000.
129. Ebara H, et al: Digoxin-like immunoreactive substances in urine and serum from preterm and term infants: relationships to renal excretion of sodium. J Pediatr 108:760, 1986.
130. Crambert G, et al: Inhibition of rat Na⁺/K⁺-ATPase isoforms by endogenous digitalis extracts from neonatal human plasma. Clin Exp Hypertens 20:669, 1998.

Corinne Benchimol and Lisa M. Satlin

131 Potassium Homeostasis in the Fetus and Neonate

Potassium (K^+) is the most abundant intracellular cation. Maintenance of a high intracellular K^+ concentration (100 to 140 mEq/l) is essential for many basic cellular processes, including cell growth and division, DNA and protein synthesis, conservation of cell volume and pH, and optimal enzyme function. The steep gradient between potassium concentration in the cell and that in the extracellular fluid is the major determinant of the resting membrane potential across the cell membrane, and thus it affects neuromuscular excitability and contractility. Approximately 98% of the total body potassium content in the adult resides within cells, primarily muscle (Fig. 131-1), whereas the remaining 2% is located in the extracellular fluid. The potassium concentration in the extracellular fluid is tightly regulated by mechanisms that govern the *internal* distribution between the intracellular and extracellular compartments and the *external* balance between intake and output.

POTASSIUM HOMEOSTASIS

The homeostatic goal of the adult is to remain in zero potassium balance. Thus, of the typical daily potassium intake of 1 mEq/kg body weight, approximately 90 to 95% is ultimately eliminated from the body in the urine; the residual 5 to 10% of the daily potassium load is lost through the stool (see Fig. 131-1). Normally, the amount of potassium lost through sweat is negligible.

In contrast to the situation in the adult, the fetus and newborn must conserve potassium for growth. In fetal life, this need is met by the active transport of potassium across the placenta from mother to fetus.[1] Indeed, the fetal potassium concentration is maintained at levels exceeding 5 mEq/l even in the presence of maternal potassium deficiency.[1,2]

Postnatal growth is associated with an increase in total body potassium from approximately 8 mEq/cm body height at birth to more than 14 mEq/cm body height by 18 years of age.[3,4] The rate of accretion of body potassium per kilogram body weight in the neonate is faster than in later childhood (Fig. 131-2), a finding reflecting an increase in both cell number and potassium concentration (at least in skeletal muscle) with advancing age.[4-6] Given the requirement of the growing organism for potassium conservation, it is not unexpected that infants maintain a state of positive potassium balance.[7] This tendency to retain potassium early in postnatal life is reflected in the higher plasma potassium values in infants (particularly preterm neonates).[7,8]

Urinary potassium excretion varies considerably, depending in large part on dietary intake. Children and adults ingesting a usual diet containing sodium in excess of potassium excrete urine with a sodium/potassium ratio greater than 1.[7,9] Although breast milk and commercially available infant formulas generally provide a sodium/potassium ratio of approximately 0.5 to 0.6, the urinary sodium/potassium ratio in the newborn up to 4 months of age generally exceeds 1. This high ratio may reflect the greater requirement of potassium over sodium for growth. In fact, some premature and full-term newborns may excrete urine with a sodium/potassium ratio greater than 2, a finding suggesting significant salt wasting and a relative hyporesponsiveness of the neonatal kidney to mineralocorticoid activity.[7] Because of the many vital processes dependent on potassium homeostasis, multiple complex and efficient mechanisms have developed to regulate total potassium balance and distribution.

REGULATION OF INTERNAL POTASSIUM BALANCE

The task of maintaining potassium homeostasis is complex, in large part because the daily dietary intake of potassium in the adult (~100 mEq) typically approaches or exceeds the total potassium normally present within the extracellular fluid space (~70 mEq in 17 l of extracellular fluid with a potassium concentration ~4 mEq/l) (see Fig. 131-1). To maintain zero balance in the adult, all the dietary intake of potassium must be ultimately eliminated, a task performed primarily by the kidney. However, renal excretion of potassium is rather sluggish, requiring several hours to be accomplished. Although only approximately 50% of an oral load of potassium is excreted during the first 4 to 6 hours after it is ingested, life-threatening hyperkalemia is not generally observed during this period because of the rapid (within minutes) hormonally mediated translocation of extracellular potassium into cells, particularly muscle and liver. The buffering capacity of the combined cellular storage reservoirs, capable of sequestering up to approximately 3500 mEq of potassium, is vast compared with the extracellular pool (see Fig. 131-1).

Cells must expend a significant amount of energy to maintain the steep potassium and sodium concentration gradients across their cell membranes. Sodium-potassium-adenosine triphosphatase (Na^+,K^+-ATPase), an enzyme present on the surface of essentially all eukaryotic cells, catalyzes the hydrolysis of cytosolic ATP, thereby providing energy for the active extrusion of sodium from cells in exchange for the uptake of potassium in a ratio of 3:2, respectively. A cell interior negative potential is created by the unequal cation exchange ratio and the subsequent backdiffusion of potassium out of the cells through potassium channels in the plasma membrane.

The activity of the sodium-potassium pump varies widely among different tissues; it is highest in transporting cells such as kidney tubules and nervous tissue. Differences in pump activity among distinct tissues may be related to the unique catalytic α- and glycosylated β-subunits they express. Maturational studies of Na^+,K^+-ATPase in erythrocytes, intestine, and kidney show lower activities in the newborn compared with the adult, consistent with the low intracellular potassium concentration measured in muscle and other nonsecretory tissues during early life.[5, 10-12] Indeed, low birth weight infants frequently exhibit nonoliguric hyperkalemia during the first 48 hours after birth, despite the intake of negligible amounts of potassium.[13-16] This phenomenon has been attributed mainly to a shift of potassium from the intracellular to the extracellular space, presumably resulting, at least in part, from low Na^+,K^+-ATPase activity.[12,15]

Na^+,K^+-ATPase is regulated by numerous circulating hormones that exert short-term and long-term control over its activity.[17] Whereas long-term stimulation of pump activity is generally mediated by changes in gene and protein expression, short-term regulation generally results from alterations in the phosphorylation status of the pump or changes in the subcellular or cell surface distribution of pumps.[17] Thus, regulation of internal potassium balance in the neonate may be influenced by developmental stage-specific expression of potassium transporters and channels, receptors, and signal transduction mechanisms.

The chemical, physical, and hormonal factors that acutely influence the *internal* balance of potassium are listed in Table 131-1. Potassium uptake into cells is acutely stimulated by

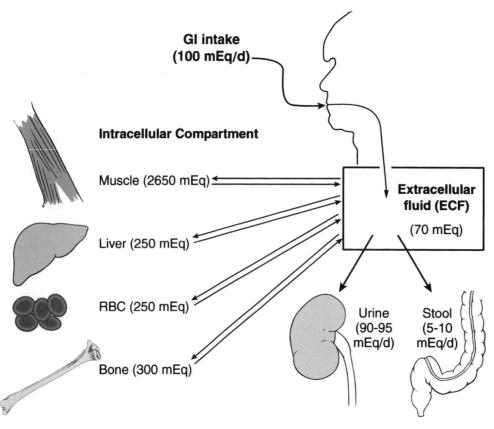

Figure 131–1. Potassium homeostasis in the adult: *internal* and *external* balance. *External* potassium balance is maintained by the urinary (90 to 95%) and fecal (5 to 10%) excretion of the daily potassium intake of approximately 1 mEq/kg/day in the typical adult. *Internal* potassium balance depends on the distribution of potassium between the extracellular fluid compartment (ECF) and the vast intracellular storage reservoirs provided by muscle, liver, erythrocytes (RBC), and bone. GI = gastrointestinal.

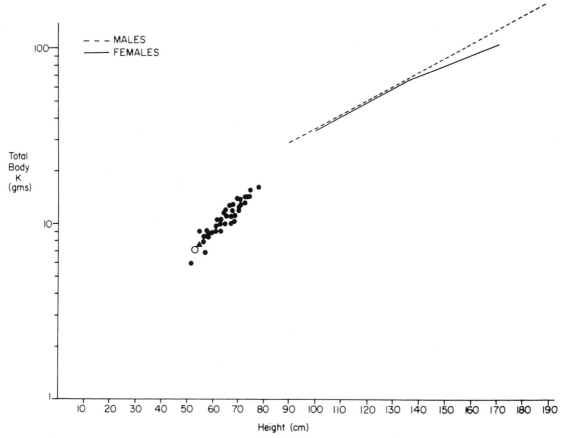

Figure 131–2. Relationship between total body potassium (gms) and height (cm) for infants and children. The rate of accretion of body potassium in the neonate is faster than in later childhood, likely reflecting both an increase in cell number and potassium concentration, at least in skeletal muscle, with advancing age. (From Flynn MA, et al: Pediatr Res *6*:239, 1972.)

TABLE 131-1

TABLE 131-1

Factors, Relevant to the Infant, Which Acutely Regulate the *Internal* Balance of Potassium

	Effect on Cell Uptake of Potassium
Physiologic Factors	
Plasma K concentration	
Increase	Increase
Decrease	Decrease
Insulin	Increase
Catecholamines	
α-Agonists	Decrease
β-Agonists	Increase
Pathologic Factors	
Acid-base balance	
Acidosis	Decrease
Alkalosis	Increase
Hyperosmolality	Enhances cell efflux
Cell breakdown	Enhances cell efflux

insulin, β₂-adrenergic agonists, and alkalosis and is impaired by α-adrenergic agonists, acidosis, and hyperosmolality. Generally, deviations in extracellular potassium concentration arising from fluctuations in internal distribution are self-limited as long as the endocrine regulation of *internal* balance and mechanisms responsible for regulation of *external* balance are intact.

Plasma Potassium Concentration

The active cellular potassium uptake in large part determines the intracellular pool of potassium. An increase in plasma potassium, either secondary to a dietary or parenteral potassium load or resulting from a chronic progressive loss of functional renal mass, decreases the concentration gradient (dependent on the ratio of intracellular to extracellular potassium concentration) against which the Na^+,K^+-ATPase pump must function and thus favors an increase in cellular potassium uptake. In those cells of the kidney and colon specifically responsible for potassium secretion, the resulting increase in intracellular potassium enhances secretion, and hence excretion, by promoting potassium diffusion into the tubular lumen down its concentration gradient.

Hormones

Insulin, the most important hormonal regulator of *internal* potassium balance, lowers plasma potassium by promoting the cellular uptake of the cation, specifically in skeletal muscle and liver.[18] This insulin-induced response is independent of the hormonal effects on glucose metabolism.[19] The mechanism of insulin action may involve stimulation of translocation of the α_2-subunit of Na^+,K^+-ATPase from the intracellular space to the plasma membrane, thereby inducing an increase in pump activity.[20, 21] Basal insulin secretion is necessary to maintain fasting plasma potassium concentration within the normal range. An increase in plasma potassium in excess of 1.0 mEq/l in the adult induces a significant increase in peripheral insulin levels to aid in the rapid disposal of the potassium load, yet a more modest elevation of approximately 0.5 mEq/l is without effect.[22]

The effect of epinephrine on potassium balance is biphasic and is characterized by an initial increase, followed by a prolonged fall in plasma potassium to a final value lower than baseline. The initial transient rise in plasma potassium results from α-adrenergic receptor stimulation causing release of potassium from hepatocytes.[23,24] β₂-Receptor stimulation, via stimulation of adenylate cyclase leading to generation of the second messenger cyclic adenosine monophosphate, activates Na^+,K^+-ATPase and thus promotes enhanced uptake of potassium by skeletal and

cardiac muscle, effects that are inhibited by the β₂-blocker propranolol.[23, 25, 26] The observation that the potassium-lowering effects of insulin and epinephrine are additive suggests that their responses are mediated by different signaling pathways.

Aldosterone is best known for its effect on transporting tissue, increasing potassium secretion in distal segments of the nephron and colon (see later). Thyroid hormone may also promote the cellular uptake of potassium secondary to its long-term stimulation of sodium-potassium pump activity.[17]

Acid-Base Balance

It is well known that the transcellular distribution of potassium and acid-base balance are interrelated.[27] Whereas acidemia (increase in extracellular hydrogen ion concentration) is associated with an increase in plasma potassium secondary to potassium release from the intracellular compartment, alkalemia (decrease in extracellular hydrogen ion concentration) results in a shift of potassium into cells and a consequent decrease in plasma potassium. However, the reciprocal changes in plasma potassium that accompany acute changes in blood pH differ widely among the four major acid-base disorders; metabolic disorders cause greater disturbances in plasma potassium than do those of respiratory origin, and acute changes in pH result in larger changes in plasma potassium than do chronic conditions.[27]

Acute metabolic acidosis after administration of a mineral acid that includes an anion that does not readily penetrate the cell membrane, such as the chloride of hydrochloric acid or ammonium chloride, and consistently results in an increase in plasma potassium. As excess extracellular protons, unaccompanied by their nonpermeant anions, enter the cell where neutralization by intracellular buffers occurs, potassium (or sodium) is displaced from the cells, thus maintaining electroneutrality. However, comparable acidemia induced by acute organic anion acidosis (lactic acid in lactic acidosis, acetoacetic and β-hydroxybutyric acids in uncontrolled diabetes mellitus) may not elicit a detectable change in plasma potassium.[27-29] In organic acidemia, the associated anion diffuses more freely into the cell and thus does not require a shift of potassium from the intracellular to the extracellular fluid.

In respiratory acid-base disturbances, in which carbon dioxide and carbonic acid readily permeate cell membranes, little transcellular shift of potassium occurs because protons are not transported in or out in association with potassium moving in the opposite direction.[27]

Changes in plasma bicarbonate concentration, independent of the effect on extracellular pH, can reciprocally affect plasma potassium concentration. Movement of bicarbonate (outward at a low extracellular bicarbonate concentration and inward at a high extracellular bicarbonate concentration) between the intracellular and extracellular compartments may be causally related to a concomitant transfer of potassium. This may account for the less marked increase in plasma potassium observed during acute respiratory acidosis, a condition characterized by an acid plasma pH with an elevated serum bicarbonate (hence inward net bicarbonate and potassium movement), as compared with acute metabolic acidosis with a low serum bicarbonate concentration (hence outward net bicarbonate and potassium movement).

Other Factors

Many other pathologic perturbations alter the *internal* potassium balance. An increase in plasma osmolality secondary to severe dehydration causes water to shift out of cells. The consequent increase in intracellular potassium concentration exaggerates the transcellular concentration gradient and favors movement of this cation out of cells. The effect of hyperosmolality on potassium balance becomes especially troublesome in

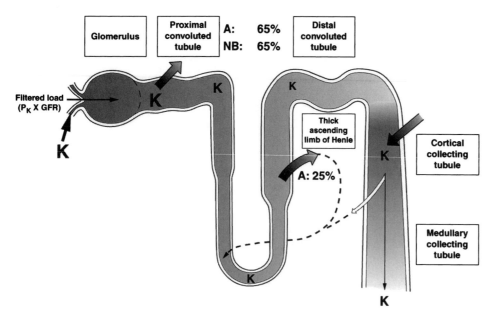

Figure 131–3. Tubular sites of potassium (K) transport along the nephron. The percentages of filtered potassium reabsorbed along the proximal tubule and thick ascending limb of the loop of Henle are indicated for the adult (A) and, when known, the newborn (NB). *Arrows* identify the direction of net potassium transport as either out of (reabsorption) or into (secretion) the urinary fluid. GFR = glomerular filtration rate.

patients with hyperglycemic diabetics, in whom the absence of insulin exacerbates the hyperkalemia.

REGULATION OF EXTERNAL POTASSIUM BALANCE

Renal Contribution

The kidney is the major excretory organ for potassium. In adults, urinary potassium excretion parallels dietary intake (see Fig. 131-1), and the speed of renal adaptation depends on the baseline potassium intake and the magnitude of the change in dietary potassium intake. Extreme adjustments in the rate of renal potassium conservation cannot be achieved as rapidly as for sodium, nor are the adjustments as complete; whereas urinary sodium can be virtually eliminated within 3 to 4 days of sodium restriction, there is a minimum urinary potassium loss of about 5 mEq/day in the adult, even after several weeks of severe potassium restriction. An increase in dietary potassium intake is matched by a parallel increase in renal potassium excretion within hours, yet maximal rates of potassium excretion are not attained for several days after increasing potassium intake. In adults, renal potassium excretion follows a circadian rhythm, presumably determined by hypothalamic oscillators, and it is characterized by maximum output during times of peak activity.[30] It is unknown whether a circadian cycle of urinary potassium excretion prevails in infancy.

The processes involved in renal potassium handling in the fully differentiated kidney include filtration, reabsorption, and secretion (Fig. 131-3).[31] Filtered potassium is reabsorbed almost entirely in proximal segments of the nephron, and urinary potassium is derived predominantly from distal potassium secretion. Therefore, potassium balance, at least in the adult, is maintained by renal secretion rather than reabsorption.

The renal potassium clearance is low in newborns, even when it is corrected for their low glomerular filtration rate.[7, 8] Infants, like adults, can excrete potassium at a rate that exceeds its glomerular filtration when given a potassium load, a finding indicating the capacity for net tubular secretion.[32] However, the rate of potassium excretion per unit body weight in response to exogenous potassium loading is less in newborn than older animals.[33, 34] Clearance studies in saline-expanded dogs also provide indirect evidence of a diminished secretory and enhanced reabsorptive capacity of the immature distal nephron to potassium.[35] In general, the limited potassium secretory capacity of the immature kidney becomes clinically relevant only under conditions of potassium excess. As stated earlier, under normal circumstances, potassium retention by the newborn kidney is appropriate and is required for somatic growth.

Sites of Potassium Transport Along the Nephron

Potassium is freely filtered at the glomerulus. Approximately 65% of the filtered load of potassium is reabsorbed along the proximal tubule of the suckling rat, a fraction similar to that measured in the adult (see Fig. 131-3).[36-39] Reabsorption is passive in this segment, closely following water reabsorption, and is driven, in part, by the positive transepithelial voltage that prevails along part of the proximal tubule.

Only approximately 10% of the filtered load of potassium reaches the early distal tubule of the adult, a finding reflecting significant further net reabsorption of this cation in the thick ascending limb of the loop of Henle (TALH; see Fig. 131-3).[37] In contrast, up to 35% of the filtered load of potassium reaches the superficial distal tubule of the 2-week-old rat.[36] The observations in the maturing rodent that the fractional reabsorption of potassium along the loop of Henle, expressed as a percentage of delivered load, increases by 20% between the second and sixth weeks of postnatal life, and that both the diluting capacity and TALH Na+,K+-ATPase activity increase after birth are consistent with a developmental maturation of potassium absorptive pathways in this segment.[36, 40, 41] However, direct functional analysis of the potassium transport capacity of the TALH in the developing nephron has not been performed.

The avid potassium reabsorption characteristic of the fully differentiated TALH is mediated by an Na+,K+-2Cl co-transporter that translocates a single potassium ion into the cell accompanied by a sodium and two chloride ions (Fig. 131-4A). This secondary active transport is ultimately driven by the basolateral Na+,K+-ATPase that generates an electrochemical gradient favoring sodium entry at the apical membrane. Activity of the Na+,K+-2Cl transporter requires the presence of a parallel potassium conductance in the urinary membrane. Diuretics such as furosemide and bumetanide that inhibit the Na+,K+-2Cl co-transporter block potassium reabsorption at this site and uncover potassium secretion, leading to profound urinary potassium losses.

The luminal secretory potassium channel present in the TALH (and cortical collecting duct) that mediates baseline potassium secretion is encoded by the *ROMK* (rat outer medullary K+ channel) gene.[31, 42] Mutations in *ROMK* have been identified in

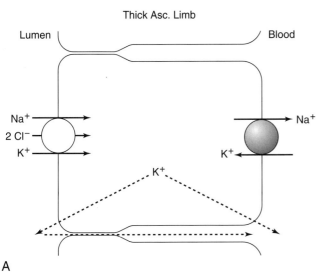

A

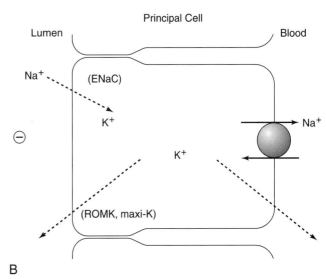

B

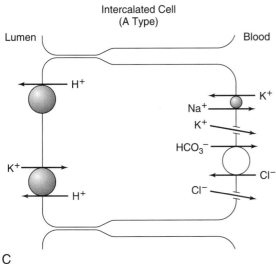

C

Figure 131–4. Potassium (K) transport pathways in specific renal tubular cells. **A,** In the thick ascending limb of the loop of Henle, potassium is avidly absorbed by specialized luminal sodium-potassium-chloride (Na^+-K^+-$2Cl^-$) co-transport. A luminal secretory potassium channel, encoded by the *ROMK* gene, in this cell, allows potassium to recycle back into the tubular fluid, thereby ensuring a continuous and abundant supply of potassium for the co-transporter. **B,** In the principal cell of the collecting duct, potassium is pumped into the cell in exchange for sodium by the basolateral sodium-potassium-adenosine triphosphatase (Na^+,K^+-ATPase). After entry into and accumulation in the cell, potassium is secreted preferentially across the apical membrane through the potassium secretory channel *ROMK* under baseline conditions, a process driven by a favorable electrochemical gradient. The electrochemical gradient is composed of two components: the cell-to-lumen concentration, or chemical gradient, and the cell-to-lumen electrical gradient. The latter is generated by apical sodium entry through epithelial amiloride-sensitive sodium channels (ENaCs) and its electrogenic basolateral extrusion. **C,** Intercalated cells in the collecting duct mediate potassium absorption via apical H^+,K^+-ATPase, a pump that catalyzes the exchange of a single proton for potassium. HCO_3^- = bicarbonate.

TABLE 131–2

Factors Regulating the *External* Balance of Potassium

Renal Factors

Potassium intake/plasma potassium concentration
Tubular flow rate
Distal sodium delivery and transepithelial voltage
Hormones (mineralocorticoids, vasopressin)
Acid-base balance

Gastrointestinal Tract Factors

Stool volume
Hormones (mineralocorticoids)

patients with Barrter syndrome, an inherited familial disease characterized by hypokalemic metabolic alkalosis, hyperreninism, and hyperaldosteronism but normal blood pressure.[43] The tubular defects present in Barrter syndrome are similar to those induced by the administration of loop diuretics.

Under baseline conditions in the adult, regulated potassium secretion by the distal tubule and the collecting duct contributes prominently to urinary potassium excretion, which can approach 20% of the filtered load (see Fig. 131–3).[31] Potassium secretion by the collecting duct requires potassium to be actively transported into principal cells in exchange for sodium at the basolateral membrane by the action of Na^+,K^+-ATPase (see Fig. 131–4B). Potassium accumulates within the cell and then passively diffuses across the apical membrane through secretory potassium channels. The magnitude of potassium secretion in the cortical collecting duct is determined by its electrochemical gradient and the apical permeability to this cation. The electrochemical gradient is established by the potassium concentration gradient between the cell and lumen, and lumen negative voltage, generated by apical sodium entry through epithelial sodium channels (ENaCs) and its basolateral electrogenic extrusion. Two apical potassium-selective channels have been functionally identified in the fully differentiated principal cell. The potassium channel encoded by *ROMK* is considered to mediate baseline potassium secretion, whereas the high-conductance, stretch- and calcium-activated maxi-K channel has been proposed to regulate flow-stimulated potassium secretion.[44] Any factor that enhances the electrochemical driving force or increases the apical membrane permeability to potassium will favor potassium secretion.

The direction and magnitude of net potassium transport in the distal nephron vary according to physiologic need. Thus, in response to potassium depletion, as may follow long-term ingestion of a potassium-restricted diet, the distal nephron may reabsorb potassium. Potassium reabsorption is mediated by apical H^+, K^+-ATPase, an enzyme that exchanges a single potassium ion for a proton (see Fig. 131-4C), present at the apical membrane of acid-base–transporting intercalated cells.

Potassium secretion in the cortical collecting duct is low early in life and cannot be stimulated by high urinary flow rates.[45] Although Na^+, K^+-ATPase activity in neonatal collecting duct segments is only approximately 50% of that measured in the mature nephron, cell potassium content of this segment is similar at both ages, consistent with a low membrane permeability of the neonatal collecting duct to potassium.[11, 40, 46] Electrophysiologic analysis has confirmed the absence of functional potassium secretory channels in the luminal membrane of the neonatal cortical collecting duct.[47] ROMK mRNA and protein are first detectable in the second week of postnatal life in the rodent, immediately preceding the appearance of functional channels and potassium secretion in this segment.[45,47-49]

Indirect evidence suggests that the neonatal distal nephron absorbs potassium. Saline-expanded newborn dogs were found to absorb 25% more of the distal potassium load than adult animals.[33] Functional analysis of the rabbit collecting duct has shown that the activity of apical H^+, K^+-ATPase in neonatal intercalated cells is equivalent to that in mature cells.[50] The latter data alone do not predict transepithelial potassium absorption under physiologic conditions. However, high distal tubular fluid potassium concentrations, as measured *in vivo* in the young rat, may facilitate lumen-to-cell potassium absorption mediated by H^+, K^+-ATPase.[36]

The major factors that influence the *external* balance of potassium are listed in Table 131-2 and are discussed in the following sections.

Potassium Intake and Cellular Potassium Content

Ingestion of a potassium-rich meal is rapidly followed by enhanced urinary excretion of potassium. The increase in potassium entry into principal cells from the basolateral (blood) side maximizes the concentration gradient favoring apical potassium secretion. Simultaneously, the increase in circulating levels of plasma aldosterone that accompanies potassium loading enhances the electrochemical driving force favoring potassium secretion in the distal tubule and cortical collecting duct, as described later. It has also been suggested that a reflex increase in potassium excretion via vagal afferents follows activation of potassium-specific sensors in the gut or hepatic portal circulation, a control system that may be regulated in the absence of change in the plasma potassium concentration.[30]

Chronic potassium loading leads to *potassium adaptation,* an acquired tolerance to an otherwise lethal acute potassium load.[31] This adaptation occurs in the renal distal tubule and collecting duct, as well as the colon; the rate of potassium secretion in these segments varies directly with body stores of potassium. A similar adaptive response is seen in renal insufficiency such that potassium balance is maintained during the course of many forms of progressive renal disease. The mechanisms underlying this adaptation in the principal cell include not only an increase in the density of apical membrane potassium channels, but also an increase in the number of conducting sodium channels and activity of the basolateral sodium-potassium pump. The latter two processes result in increases in transepithelial voltage and the intracellular potassium concentration, events that enhance the driving force favoring potassium diffusion from the cell into the urinary fluid.

When potassium intake is chronically reduced, potassium secretion by principal cells falls as reabsorption by intercalated cells increases. Stimulation of H^+, K^+-ATPase activity in intercalated cells results not only in potassium retention, but also in urinary acidification and metabolic alkalosis.

Tubular Flow Rate

High rates of urinary flow in the mature, but not the neonatal or weanling, distal nephron stimulate potassium secretion.[45] Thus, volume expansion and diuretics, both of which increase tubular fluid flow rate, enhance potassium secretion in the fully differentiated kidney. The higher the urinary flow rate in the distal nephron the slower the rate of rise of tubular fluid potassium concentration because secreted potassium is rapidly diluted in urine of low potassium concentration. Maintenance of a low tubular fluid potassium concentration maximizes the potassium concentration gradient (and thus the chemical driving force) favoring net potassium secretion. Evidence suggests that high tubular fluid flow rates recruit the maxi-K channel in the collecting duct to secrete potassium, thereby enhancing urinary potassium excretion.[44] The absence of flow-stimulated potassium secretion early in life has been proposed to result, at least in part, from the absence of calcium- and stretch-activated maxi-K channels in the collecting duct.[44]

Distal Sodium Delivery and Transepithelial Voltage

As predicted from the principal cell model (see Fig. 131-4B), an increase in sodium absorption enhances the electrochemical driving force for potassium diffusion into the lumen. The magnitude of passive apical sodium entry and its electrogenic basolateral extrusion determine the apical membrane electrical potential and rate of basolateral sodium-potassium exchange. The dependence of potassium secretion on distal sodium delivery becomes evident at tubular fluid sodium concentrations less than 30 mEq/l, a value lower than that at which potassium secretion falls sharply.[51,52] *In vivo* measurements of the sodium concentration in distal tubular fluid generally exceed 35 mM/l both in adult and suckling rats and thus should not restrict distal potassium secretion.[36,41,51,53]

Extracellular volume expansion or administration of many diuretics (osmotic diuretics, carbonic anhydrase inhibitors, loop and thiazide diuretics) is accompanied by an increase in excretion of both sodium and potassium. The kaliuresis is mediated not only by the increased delivery of sodium to the distal nephron, but also by the increased tubular fluid flow rate, which maximizes the chemical driving forces, as described earlier, favoring potassium secretion. Other potassium-sparing diuretics, such as amiloride and triamterene, block distal sodium reabsorption, which reduces the electrical potential gradient favoring potassium secretion.

Sodium delivered to the distal nephron is generally accompanied by chloride. Chloride reabsorption, which occurs predominantly via the paracellular pathway, tends to reduce the lumen-negative potential that would otherwise drive potassium secretion. When sodium is accompanied by an anion less reabsorbable than chloride, such as bicarbonate (in proximal renal tubular acidosis), β-hydroxybutyrate (in diabetic ketoacidosis), or carbenicillin (during antibiotic therapy), luminal electronegativity is maintained, thereby eliciting more potassium secretion than occurs with comparable sodium delivered with chloride.

Hormones

Mineralocorticoids stimulate sodium reabsorption and potassium secretion in principal cells of the distal tubule and cortical collecting duct.[54] Aldosterone action requires its initial binding to the mineralocorticoid receptor, followed by translocation of the hormone-receptor complex to the nucleus in which specific genes are stimulated to code for physiologically active proteins (e.g., Na^+, K^+-ATPase). Early effects of an elevation in circulating levels of mineralocorticoids include increases in the permeability of the luminal membrane to sodium, basolateral Na^+, K^+-ATPase activity, intracellular potassium concentration, and transepithelial voltage (increased lumen negativity), the latter resulting from enhanced sodium reabsorption.[31] Late steroid-induced effects include increases in number of basolateral sodium-potassium pumps and conducting apical potassium channels. Thus, mineralocorticoids affect both the luminal permeability and the electrochemical gradient across the distal nephron and favor potassium secretion. A reduction in plasma concentration of aldosterone results in a fall in urinary potassium secretion by mechanisms opposite to those just described.

Plasma aldosterone concentrations in the newborn are high compared with those in the adult.[55] Yet, clearance studies in fetal and newborn animals demonstrate a relative insensitivity of the immature kidney to the hormone.[7, 56-58] The density of aldosterone binding sites, receptor affinity, and degree of nuclear binding of hormone-receptor are believed to be similar in mature and immature rats.[58] Thus, the early hyposensitivity to aldosterone is considered to represent a postreceptor phenomenon.

Acid-Base Balance

Disorders of acid-base homeostasis can induce changes in tubular potassium secretion. Acute metabolic acidosis causes the urine pH and potassium excretion to decrease, whereas both acute respiratory alkalosis and metabolic alkalosis result in increases in urine pH and potassium excretion. Chronic metabolic acidosis has variable effects on urinary potassium excretion.

The alkalosis-induced stimulation of potassium secretion reflects two direct effects on principal cells: (1) the stimulation of Na^+,K^+-ATPase activity and basolateral potassium uptake and (2) an increase in the permeability of the apical membrane to potassium resulting from an increase in duration of time the potassium-selective channels remain open.[31] Alkalosis also decreases acid secretion in intercalated cells, thereby reducing hydrogen-potassium countertransport.

Acute metabolic acidosis results in a reduction in cell potassium concentration and inhibition of apical potassium channel activity.[31] The effect of chronic metabolic acidosis on potassium secretion is more complex and may be influenced by modifications of the glomerular filtrate (e.g., chloride and bicarbonate concentrations), tubular fluid flow rate, and circulating aldosterone levels.[31] The latter two factors may lead to an increase rather than a decrease in potassium secretion and excretion.

Contribution of the Gastrointestinal Tract

Under normal conditions in the adult, 5 to 10% of daily potassium intake is excreted in the stool (see Fig. 131-1). The primary site of regulation of intestinal potassium transport is the colon.[59] Because of water absorption in the upper gastrointestinal tract, the colon is generally presented with a low volume of fluid containing a high potassium concentration (90 mEq/l). The direction of net potassium transport in the colon, as in the distal nephron, is determined by the balance of potassium secretion and absorption. Potassium secretion requires the basolateral uptake of this cation by the Na^+,K^+-ATPase and Na-K-2Cl co-transporter (functionally similar to that present in the urinary membrane of the TALH), and its secretion across the apical membrane through potassium channels. Potassium absorption is mediated by a colonic apical K^+-ATPase.

Factors that increase stool potassium content by activating transport pathways in the colon include hormones (aldosterone, glucocorticoids), epinephrine, and prostaglandins.[60, 61] Indomethacin and dietary potassium restriction reduce potassium secretion. Diarrheal illnesses are typically associated with hypokalemia, despite an associated reduction in renal potassium excretion. Both mucosal inflammation and stimulation of potassium secretion, as prevails in the case of rotavirus enteritis, may contribute to inappropriate colonic potassium excretion.

Potassium adaptation in the colon is demonstrated by increased fecal potassium secretion after potassium loading and renal insufficiency. Whereas stool potassium averages approximately 5 to 10% of dietary intake in normal adults, fecal potassium excretion may triple in patients with severe renal insufficiency.[60]

Net colonic potassium absorption is higher early in life than in the adult because of a high activity of the apical potassium absorptive pumps.[59, 62] This has been proposed to reflect a selective β-adrenergic stimulation of apical H^+,K^+-ATPase.[63] Thus, the gastrointestinal tract of the infant, like the kidney, is poised for potassium absorption, not secretion, as is characteristic of the adult.

REFERENCES

1. Serrano CV, et al: Potassium deficiency in the pregnant dog. J Clin Invest 43:27, 1964.
2. Dancis J, Springer D: Fetal homeostasis in maternal malnutrition: potassium and sodium deficiency in rats. Pediatr Res 4:345, 1970.
3. Butte NF, et al: Body composition during the first 2 years of life: an updated reference. Pediatr Res 47:578, 2000.
4. Flynn MA, et al: Total body potassium in normal children. Pediatr Res 6:239, 1972.
5. Dickerson JWT, Widdowson EM: Chemical changes in skeletal muscle during development. Biochem J 74:247, 1960.
6. Rutledge MM, et al: A longitudinal study of total body potassium in normal breastfed and bottle-fed infants. Pediatr Res 10:114, 1976.
7. Sulyok E, et al: Relationship between maturity, electrolyte balance and the function of the renin-angiotensin-aldosterone system in newborn infants. Biol Neonate 35:60, 1979.
8. Satlin LM: Regulation of potassium transport in the maturing kidney. Semin Nephrol 19:155, 1999.
9. Rodriguez-Soriano J, et al: Renal handling of water and sodium in infancy and childhood: a study using clearance methods during hypotonic saline diuresis. Kidney Int 20:700, 1981.
10. Bistritzer T, et al: Sodium potassium adenosine triphosphatase activity in preterm and term infants and its possible role in sodium homeostasis during maturation. Arch Dis Child Fetal Neonatal Ed 81:F184, 1999.
11. Constantinescu AR, et al: Na^+,K^+-ATPase-mediated basolateral rubidium uptake in the maturing rabbit cortical collecting duct. Am J Physiol 279:F1161, 2000.
12. Stefano JL, et al: Decreased erythrocyte Na^+,K^+-ATPase activity associated with cellular potassium loss in extremely low birth weight infants with nonoliguric hyperkalemia. J Pediatr 122:276, 1993.
13. Gruskay J, et al: Nonoliguric hyperkalemia in the premature infant weighing less than 1000 grams. J Pediatr 113:381, 1988.
14. Lorenz JM, et al: Potassium metabolism in extremely low birth weight infants in the first week of life. J Pediatr 131:81, 1997.
15. Sato K, et al: Internal potassium shift in premature infants: cause of nonoliguric hyperkalemia. J Pediatr 126:109, 1995.
16. Shaffer SG, et al: Hyperkalemia in very low birth weight infants. J Pediatr 121:275, 1992.
17. Therien AG, Blostein R: Mechanisms of sodium pump regulation. Am J Physiol 279:C541, 2000.
18. McDonough AA, et al: Skeletal muscle regulates extracellular potassium. Am J Physiol 282:F967, 2002.
19. Zierler KL, Rabinowitz D: Effect of very small concentrations of insulin on forearm metabolism. Persistence of its actions on potassium and free fatty acids without its effects on glucose. J Clin Invest 43:950, 1964.
20. Ewart HS, Klip A: Hormonal regulation of the Na^+,K^+-ATPase: mechanisms underlying rapid and sustained changes in pump activity. Am J Physiol 269:C295, 1995.
21. Hundal HS, et al: Insulin induces translocation of the alpha 2 and beta 1 subunits of the Na^+/K^+-ATPase from intracellular compartments to the plasma membrane in mammalian skeletal muscle. J Biol Chem 267:5040, 1992.
22. Dluhy RG, et al: Serum immunoreactive insulin and growth hormone response to potassium infusion in normal man. J Appl Physiol 33:22, 1972.
23. DeFronzo RA, et al: Epinephrine and potassium homeostasis. Kidney Int 20:83, 1981.
24. Williams ME, et al: Impairment of extrarenal potassium disposal by alpha-adrenergic stimulation. N Engl J Med 311:145, 1984.
25. Rosa RM, et al: Adrenergic modulation of extrarenal potassium disposal. N Engl J Med 302:431, 1980.
26. Williams ME, et al: Catecholamine modulation of rapid potassium shifts during exercise. N Engl J Med 312:823, 1985.
27. Adrogue HJ, Madias NE: Changes in plasma potassium concentration during acute acid-base disturbances. Am J Med 71:456, 1981.
28. Fulop M: Serum potassium in lactic acidosis and ketoacidosis. N Engl J Med 300:1087, 1979.
29. Graber M: A model of the hyperkalemia produced by metabolic acidosis. Am J Kidney Dis 22:436, 1993.
30. Rabinowitz L: Aldosterone and potassium homeostasis. Kidney Int 49:1738, 1996.
31. Giebisch G: Renal potassium transport: mechanisms and regulation. Am J Physiol 274:F817, 1998.
32. Tuvdad F, McNamara H, Barnett H: Renal response of premature infants to administration of bicarbonate and potassium. Pediatrics 13:4, 1954.
33. Lorenz JM, et al: Renal response of newborn dog to potassium loading. Am J Physiol 251:F513, 1986.

34. McCance RA, Widdowson EM: The response of the newborn piglet to an excess of potassium. J. Physiol. *141*:88, 1958.
35. Kleinman LI, Banks RO: Segmental nephron sodium and potassium reabsorption in newborn and adult dogs during saline expansion. Proc Soc Exp Biol Med *173*:231, 1983.
36. Lelievre-Pegorier M, et al: Developmental pattern of water and electrolyte transport in rat superficial nephrons. Am J Physiol *245*:F15, 1983.
37. Malnic G, et al: Micropuncture study of distal tubular potassium and sodium transport in rat nephron. Am J Physiol *211*:529, 1966.
38. Malnic G, et al: Microperfusion study of distal tubular potassium and sodium transfer in rat kidney. Am J Physiol *211*:548, 1966.
39. Solomon S: Absolute rates of sodium and potassium reabsorption by proximal tubule of immature rats. Biol Neonate *25*:340, 1974.
40. Schmidt U, Horster M: Na+,K+-activated ATPase: activity maturation in rabbit nephron segments dissected in vitro. Am J Physiol *233*:F55, 1977.
41. Zink H, Horster M: Maturation of diluting capacity in loop of Henle of rat superficial nephrons. Am J Physiol *233*:F519, 1977.
42. Giebisch G: Physiological roles of renal potassium channels. Semin Nephrol *19*:458, 1999.
43. Simon DB, Lifton RP: The molecular basis of inherited hypokalemic alkalosis: Bartter's and Gitelman's syndromes. Am J Physiol *271*:F961, 1996.
44. Woda CB, et al: Flow-dependent K+ secretion in the cortical collecting duct is mediated by a maxi-K channel. Am J Physiol *280*:F786, 2001.
45. Satlin LM: Postnatal maturation of potassium transport in rabbit cortical collecting duct. Am J Physiol *266*:F57, 1994.
46. Satlin LM, et al: Postnatal maturation of the rabbit cortical collecting duct. Pediatr Nephrol *2*:135, 1988.
47. Satlin LM, Palmer LG: Apical K+ conductance in maturing rabbit principal cell. Am J Physiol *272*:F397, 1997.
48. Benchimol C, et al: Developmental expression of ROMK mRNA in rabbit cortical collecting duct. Pediatr Res *47*:46, 2000.
49. Zolotnitskaya A, Satlin LM: Developmental expression of ROMK in rat kidney. Am J Physiol *276*:F825, 1999.
50. Constantinescu A, et al: H-K-ATPase activity in PNA-binding intercalated cells of newborn rabbit cortical collecting duct. Am J Physiol *272*:F167, 1997.
51. Good DW, Wright FS: Luminal influences on potassium secretion: sodium concentration and fluid flow rate. Am J Physiol *236*:F192, 1979.
52. Stokes JB: Potassium secretion by cortical collecting tubule: relation to sodium absorption, luminal sodium concentration, and transepithelial voltage. Am J Physiol *241*:F395, 1981.
53. Aperia A, Elinder G: Distal tubular sodium reabsorption in the developing rat kidney. Am J Physiol *240*:F487, 1981.
54. Schwartz GJ, Burg MB: Mineralocorticoid effects on cation transport by cortical collecting tubules in vitro. Am J Physiol *235*:F576, 1978.
55. Van Acker KJ, et al: Renin-angiotensin-aldosterone system in the healthy infant and child. Kidney Int *16*:196, 1979.
56. Aperia A, et al: Sodium excretion in relation to sodium intake and aldosterone excretion in newborn pre-term and full-term infants. Acta Paediatr Scand *68*:813, 1979.
57. Robillard JE, et al: Effects of aldosterone on urinary kallikrein and sodium excretion during fetal life. Pediatr Res *19*:1048, 1985.
58. Stephenson G, et al: Ontogeny of renal mineralocorticoid receptors and urinary electrolyte responses in the rat. Am J Physiol *247*:F665, 1984.
59. Aizman RI, et al: Ontogeny of K+ transport in rat distal colon. Am J Physiol *271*:G268, 1996.
60. Bia MJ, DeFronzo RA: Extrarenal potassium homeostasis. Am J Physiol *240*:F257, 1981.
61. Rechkemmer G, et al: Active potassium transport across guinea-pig distal colon: action of secretagogues. J Physiol *493*:485, 1996.
62. Aizman R, et al: Potassium homeostasis: ontogenic aspects. Acta Paediatr *87*:609, 1998.
63. Aizman R, et al: Beta-adrenergic stimulation of cellular K+ uptake in rat distal colon. Acta Physiol Scand *164*:309, 1998.

132

Robert P. Woroniecki, Susan E. Mulroney, Aviad Haramati, Adrian Spitzer, and Frederick J. Kaskel

Role of the Kidney in Calcium and Phosphorus Homeostasis

CALCIUM

Calcium (Ca^{2+}), the most abundant mineral in the body, accounts for about 2% of total body weight.[1] Ca^{2+} plays both a structural role as a constituent of the bone and tooth matrices and a functional role in processes as diverse as blood coagulation and signal transduction. For these to take place, the concentration of Ca^{2+} must be maintained at the millimolar level in the blood and at the micromolar level in the cells. Extracellular Ca^{2+} homeostasis is dependent on complex interactions among several hormones (parathyroid hormone [PTH], vitamin D, and calcitonin) and multiple organs (the gastrointestinal tract, bone, and kidney). Intracellular Ca^{2+} concentration is the product of entry through as yet poorly characterized Ca^{2+} channels, exit via energized Ca^{2+} extruding transporters, and intracellular buffering.

More than 98% of human Ca^{2+} is in bone. The remaining 2% is in the intracellular (~0.75%) and extracellular (~0.25%) fluid compartments. In plasma, approximately 50% of total Ca^{2+} is in a free or ionized form and is available for transport and cellular metabolism; the rest is bound to proteins (~40%) and anions, such as citrate, phosphate, and bicarbonate (~10%).[2] Less than 2% of the filtered load of Ca^{2+} is excreted in the urine.[3] The largest part of the cellular Ca^{2+} (1 to 5 mmol) is restricted to the external surface of the cell membrane; only approximately 0.5 mmol is in the intracellular compartment. Most of the intracellular Ca^{2+} is sequestered in the endoplasmic reticulum and mitochondria, and the rest is bound to cytoplasmic proteins and ionic ligands. The fraction of ionized Ca^{2+} is four times lower in the intracellular than the extracellular compartment.[4,5] Further-more, the fraction of free intracellular Ca^{2+} available for signaling and various cellular processes is approximately 10^{-4}–fold lower than that present in the extracellular milieu.[6]

Renal Handling of Calcium

The kidney contributes to the maintenance of Ca^{2+} homeostasis by regulating Ca^{2+} reabsorption. Clearance studies in humans and animals have shown that if the filtered load of Ca^{2+} is increased (by infusing Ca^{2+}), absolute calcium reabsorption increases, as does urinary Ca^{2+} excretion. Sodium (Na^+) and Ca^{2+} excretion often increases or decreases in parallel.[7] The relationship between Na^+ and Ca^{2+} reabsorption is maintained during various conditions that ultimately alter Ca^{2+} excretion, including the use of furosemide and thiazide diuretics, metabolic acidosis and metabolic alkalosis, phosphate depletion, PTH administration, and volume depletion or repletion.

Most Ca^{2+} (70 to 80%) is reabsorbed passively, through the intercellular spaces of the proximal tubule and the thick ascending limb of the loop of Henle (TAL). The remaining 20 to 30% is reabsorbed via an active transcellular Ca^{2+} transport route in the distal segments of the nephron.[8]

Paracellular Calcium Transport

In the proximal tubules and the TAL, Ca^{2+} moves by diffusion between the renal epithelial cells, across the tight junctions. The rate of transport depends on the magnitude of the electrochemical gradient, the Ca^{2+} permeability coefficient, the delivery of Ca^{2+} to the transport site, and the rate of Ca^{2+} extrusion from the interstitium.[9]

Transcellular Calcium Transport

Transport Across the Luminal Membrane

The epithelial Ca^{2+} channel (ECaC), exclusively expressed in 1,25-dihydroxyvitamin D_3 $(1,25(OH)_2D_3)$–responsive tissues (i.e., kidney, intestine, and placenta), is the initial, rate-limiting step in the process of transcellular Ca^{2+} transport (Fig. 132–1).[10] ECaC belongs to a superfamily of Ca^{2+} channels that includes the vanilloid receptor and transient receptor potential channels. ECaC consists of six transmembrane-spanning domains, including a pore-forming hydrophobic stretch between domains 5 and 6. The amino (N)-terminal and carboxy (C)-terminal tails of ECaC have putative motifs for protein kinase C phosphorylation, binding to PDZ domain–containing proteins (a molecular scaffold that contains multiprotein signaling complexes), and binding to proteins that interact with ankyrin repeats, which play a role in protein-protein interaction.[11-13] The distinctive functional properties of ECaC include constitutively activated Ca^{2+} permeability, with high selectivity for Ca^{2+} hyperpolarization-stimulated and Ca^{2+}-dependent feedback regulation of channel activity, and $1,25(OH)_2D_3$–induced gene activation. ECaC is approximately 100 times more permeable to Ca^{2+} than to Na^+.[14] ECaC activity is down-regulated by Ca^{2+} influx through the channel and is blocked by micromolar concentrations of magnesium (Mg^{2+}). Ca^{2+} transporter 1 (CaT1) from rat intestine shares an 80% homology with ECaC.[15] ECaC and CaT1 originate from two distinct genes juxtaposed on chromosome 7q35, suggesting evolutionary gene duplication. Human ECaC is encoded by gene *ECAC1*, whereas CaT1 is encoded by *ECAC2*.[16,17] Finally, Ca^{2+} may enter the cell through pinocytosis[18] and through a less well-characterized Ca^{2+}–chloride (Cl^-) co-transporter.[19]

Calcium Buffering Within the Cell

In the cytosol, nearly all Ca^{2+} is bound to calbindins, a vitamin D_3–dependent calmodulin superfamily of proteins.[20] Calbindin-D28K is mainly expressed in the kidney, and calbindin-D9K is primarily expressed in the gut.[21] Calbindin-D28K helps to maintain appropriately low, nontoxic cytosolic Ca^{2+} levels during changes in transcellular Ca^{2+} transport without interfering with Ca^{2+} signaling.[22,23] Studies indicate that it may also act as a Ca^{2+} sensor.[24]

Inside the cell, calmodulin directly interacts with a calmodulin-binding isoleucine-glutamine (IQ) motif present in the C-tail of ECaC and CaT1 channels. Deletion of the first eight amino acids of the IQ motif in the C-terminal tail of the Ca^{2+}-channel subunit a1C eliminates Ca^{2+}-dependent inactivation of voltage-gated, L-type Ca^{2+} channels.[25] There is also Ca^{2+}-dependent interaction between calmodulin and a novel site in the C-terminal domain of the 1A subunit of P/Q-type Ca^{2+} channels (calmodulin-binding domain). In the presence of low concentrations of intracellular Ca^{2+} chelators, Ca^{2+} influx through P/Q-type channels enhances channel inactivation, increases recovery from inactivation, and produces a long-lasting facilitation of the Ca^{2+} current.[26] Ca^{2+} "shuttling" across the intracellular organelles such as mitochondria or endoplasmic reticulum depends on a Ca^{2+} electrochemical gradient, driven by internally negative membrane potential across the inner mitochondrial or endoplasmic reticular membrane.

Calcium Transport Across the Basolateral Membrane

The extrusion of Ca^{2+} across the basolateral membrane into the interstitium occurs against an electrochemical gradient and, as such, is an energy-dependent process. The transport is primarily mediated by the Na^+/Ca^{2+} exchanger (NCX)[27] and, to a lesser extent, by the Ca^{2+}-adenosine triphosphatase (ATPase) (PMCA).[28]

Three genes encode NCX mRNA in mammalian tissues: *NCX1, NCX2,* and *NCX3*.[29] Only NCX1 isoforms (alternatively spliced NACA2 (exons B, C, D), NACA3 (exons B and D), and NACA6 (exons A, C, D) have been identified in the kidney. Expression is restricted to the distal nephron, where it is localized along the basolateral membrane.[30] Undisturbed function of this exchanger is a prerequisite for transcellular Ca^{2+} transport.[31]

PMCA belongs to a class of P-type, ion-motive ATPase proteins with molecular weights ranging from 120,000 to 140,000 Da. Four different PMCA isoforms, encoded by separate genes, have been cloned.[32] PMCA1 and PMCA4 are ubiquitously expressed, whereas PMCA2 and PMCA3 are more tissue specific. The plasma membrane Ca^{2+}-ATPase is found in humans along the distal convolution and, in contrast to other species, along the cortical collecting duct.[33] PMCA1 and PMCA4 are housekeeping isoforms involved in the maintenance of cellular Ca^{2+} homeostasis. They have 10 transmembrane domains, very short extracellular loops, and internal COOH and NH_2 termini. PMCA plays a role in cytosolic acidification, which, in turn, is a signal for activation of the sarcoplasmic reticulum Ca^{2+}-ATPase and other cellular functions in muscle.

Another mechanism of Ca^{2+} extrusion from the cell is an Na^+-Ca^{2+} countertransporter driven by the Na^+ concentration gradient across the basolateral membrane maintained by Na^+, potassium (K^+)-ATPase $(Na^+,K^+$-ATPase). Ca^{2+} removal by this exchanger is slowed when extracellular Na^+ concentration is diminished or when Na^+,K^+-ATPase is inhibited with ouabain.[34]

Regulation of Calcium Transport

Parathyroid Hormone

PTH stimulates tubular reabsorption of Ca^{2+} in the distal segments of the nephron by increasing the apical Ca^{2+} channels' open probability. PTH binds to two types of receptors: PTH1, which also binds the PTH-related peptide (PTHrP),[35] and PTH2, which binds only PTH.[36] The PTH1 receptor is the predominant receptor found in the kidney, and it is expressed in glomeruli and all tubule segments, except the TAL. The PTH2 receptor is distributed primarily in brain, lung, pancreas, and vasculature (including the vascular pole of the glomerulus). Signal transduction for both PTH and PTHrP is via adenylate cyclase and phospholipase C.[37,38]

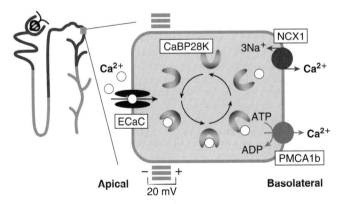

Figure 132–1. Model of transcellular calcium (Ca^{2+}) transport by cells lining the distal part of the nephron. Entry of Ca^{2+} is facilitated by the apical Ca^{2+} channel (ECaC). In the cell, Ca^{2+} binds to calbindin-D_{28K} (CaBP28K) and diffuses through the cytosol to the basolateral membrane. There, Ca^{2+} is extruded via a Na^+/Ca^{2+} exchanger (NCX1) and a Ca^{2+}-adenosine triphosphatase (PMCA1b). (Adapted from Hoenderop JG: Am J Physiol *267*:F352–F360, 2000.)

Parathyroid Hormone–Related Peptide

The PTHrP was first isolated from tumors and was found to mediate the hypercalcemia of malignancy. Subsequently, it has been identified in many different normal tissues and now is thought to play an autocrine/paracrine role in cell Ca^{2+} regulation. In the kidney, PTHrP is expressed in the proximal and distal convoluted tubules and CCD.

Calcium-Sensing Receptor

Ca^{2+}-sensing receptor (CaSR) plays a critical role in Ca^{2+} homeostasis by inducing changes in PTH secretion and renal Ca^{2+} reabsorption in response to variations in the extracellular concentration of Ca^{2+} ($[Ca^{2+}]_0$). The human CaSR is encoded by six exons of the CaSR gene located on chromosome 3q13.3-21.[39] The receptor is expressed abundantly in the parathyroid glands and, to a lesser extent, along the length of the kidney tubule.[40] Activation of the CaSR can couple the $[Ca^{2+}]_0$ signal to several different intracellular effectors. The best-described pathway involves $G_{q/11}$, which activates phospholipase C. This results in inosotol triphosphate generation, which causes the release of Ca^{2+} from intracellular stores, and diacylglycerol formation, which leads to protein kinase C activation. Mutations in CaSR are associated with familial hypocalciuric hypercalcemia, neonatal severe hyperparathyroidism, and autosomal dominant hypocalcemia.[41-45]

Vitamin D

The classic action of vitamin D is to stimulate transcription by binding to nuclear receptors. The physiologic actions of vitamin D are mediated by its metabolite 1,25-dihydroxyvitamin D_3 ($1,25[OH]_2D_3$), which is formed by 1-hydroxylation of $25(OH)_2D_3$ in proximal tubules. Vitamin D stimulates the synthesis of the rate-limiting gatekeeper ECaC by transcriptional and possibly posttranscriptional activation.[46] Expression of the vitamin D–dependent Ca^{2+} binding proteins calbindin-D28K (localized in the distal convoluted tubule, connecting tubule, CCD) and calbindin-D9K (localized primarily in the gut, but also in basolateral membranes of the TAL, the distal convoluted tubule, the connecting tubule, and the intercalated cells of the collecting duct) is up-regulated by $1,25(OH)_2D_3$, independently of PTH.[47-49] Vitamin D–dependent Ca^{2+}-binding protein, PMCA, and NCX are abundant in the distal nephron.[50-52] Vitamin D also accelerates the effect of PTH by stimulating the synthesis of Cl^- channels[53,54] and thus promoting Cl^- entry into the cells. The ensuing cell hyperpolarization results in an increase in the open probability of the Ca^{2+} channels.

Calcitonin

Calcitonin is a 32–amino acid peptide that may exert either hypercalcemic or hypocalcemic effects. In pharmacologic doses, it induces hypercalciuria and lowers serum Ca^{2+} concentration.[55,56] At physiologic concentrations, however, it decreases Ca^{2+} excretion by stimulating Ca^{2+} reabsorption in the medullary ascending limb and the distal convoluted tubule.[57,58] Calcitonin acts via receptor adenylate cyclase and inosotol triphosphate, and it is a major regulator of renal 1,25-hydroxylase gene expression.[59] The calcitonin receptor is partially homologous with Type 1 PTH/PTHrP and PTH2 receptors.

Plasma Calcium Concentration

Hypercalcemia. Hypercalcemia results in an increase in Ca^{2+} excretion caused by a net increase in the filtered load and a decrease in tubular reabsorption. Hypocalcemia has opposite effects on glomerular filtration rate (GFR) and urinary Ca^{2+} excretion. Hypercalcemia, in the presence of intact parathyroid glands, decreases the glomerular ultrafiltration coefficient (K_f) and thus causes a decline in GFR. Yet, the filtered load of Ca^{2+} may increase as a result of the elevation in serum Ca^{2+} concentration.[60,61] Hypercalcemia also causes a decline in the tubule reabsorption of Ca^{2+} by PTH-independent mechanisms.[62] This effect is mediated by stimulation of the CaSR, which inhibits the

apical K^+ channel and K^+ recycling, necessary for the activity of the $Na^+,K^+,2Cl^-$ transporter.[63] Decreased activity of the transporter decreases the lumen-positive potential difference and thus Na^+, Ca^{2+}, and Mg^{2+} reabsorption. In addition, there is a decrease in intestinal Ca^{2+} absorption brought about by diminished synthesis of $1,25(OH)_2D_3$.

Hypocalcemia. In hypocalcemic conditions, there is an increase in PTH secretion that results in the mobilization of Ca^{2+} from the bone and soft tissues. This produces a fall in PTH that, in turn, promotes a decrease in fractional excretion of Ca^{2+} and a decline in net Ca^{2+} excretion. The CaSR is thought to play a significant role in the enhancement of Ca^{2+} reabsorption in the TAL.[63] Decreased Ca^{2+} concentration in the vasa recta contributes to enhanced extrusion of Ca^{2+} at the basolateral membrane. Hypocalcemia also stimulates the production of $1,25(OH)_2D_3$, which increases the intestinal absorption of Ca^{2+}.

Phosphate and Magnesium. Hypophosphatemia produces a decrease in PTH resulting from an increase in plasma Ca^{2+} concentration. The ensuing hypercalciuria is, however, only partially corrected by the administration of PTH, a finding suggesting a direct effect of phosphate (PO_4^{3-}) deprivation on renal Ca^{2+} transport.[64] Phosphate infusion enhances Ca^{2+} reabsorption in the distal nephron and reduces Ca^{2+} excretion, even in the setting of volume expansion. Mg^{2+} infusion produces an increase in Ca^{2+} excretion that is not corrected by PTH infusion.[65]

Volume Status. Expansion of intravascular space produces natriuresis and increases Ca^{2+} excretion by inhibiting Na^+ (and, therefore, Ca^{2+}) reabsorption in the proximal tubule and Ca^{2+} reabsorption in the distal tubule. This effect, which is independent of circulating PTH levels,[66] is used in treating patients with hypercalcemia. Contraction of the extracellular volume increases proximal tubular reabsorption of Na^+ (and Ca^{2+}) and results in decreased Ca^{2+} excretion.

Acid-Base Status. Both acute and chronic metabolic acidosis have been shown to induce the release of Ca^{2+} from bone and to inhibit distal reabsorption of Ca^{2+}, resulting in hypercalciuria.[67] The effect of acidosis on tubular transport is mediated by a reduction in ECaC activity.[68,69] Metabolic alkalosis increases Ca^{2+} reabsorption in proximal tubule and decreases Ca^{2+} excretion.[70]

Insulin, Glucagon, and Glucose. Ca^{2+} excretion is enhanced by glucose infusion. Insulin infusion and hyperinsulinemia are associated with reduced proximal reabsorption of Na^+, water, and Ca^{2+}, but only Ca^{2+} excretion is increased. Insulin induces a rise in near-membrane Ca^{2+} but not of free intracellular Ca^{2+} in muscle cells. The rise in near-membrane Ca^{2+} is the result of an increase in influx through L-type Ca^{2+} channels.[71,72] Glucagon has a natriuretic and calciuretic effect secondary to increases in renal blood flow and GFR.[73]

Mineralocorticoids. Acute mineralocorticoid excess is associated with the retention of Na^+, but not Ca^{2+}.[104] Chronic mineralocorticoid excess, conversely, results in an escape from Na^+ retention (after 3 to 5 days) and a concomitant rise in Ca^{2+} excretion.[74] This is the case in the Bartter syndrome, which is characterized by high aldosterone levels, salt wasting, hypokalemic alkalosis, hypercalciuria, and normal plasma Mg^{2+} levels. These manifestations are consequent to genetic defects in the $Na^+-K^+-2Cl^-$ transporter or the ATP-sensitive K^+ channel (ROMK) in the TAL[75] and are similar to those consequent to the administration of loop diuretics. The Gitelman syndrome is also associated with salt wasting and hypokalemia but, unlike in the Bartter syndrome, the excretion of Ca^{2+} is reduced and the plasma level of Mg^{2+} is high. The genetic defect resides in the thiazide-sensitive Na^+-Cl^- co-transporter of the distal convoluted tubule encoded by the human thiazide-sensitive Na^+-Cl^- co-transporter (SLC12A3) gene. Reduced function of this co-transporter results in an increase in Ca^{2+} reabsorption because of stimulation of the basolateral extrusion of Ca^{2+} through the NCX transporter and a decrease in Mg^{2+} reabsorption because of inhibition of an apical Na^+/Mg^{2+} exchanger.[76]

Diuretics. Loop diuretics (furosemide, ethacrynic acid, and bumetanide) cause an increase in the fractional excretion of Ca^{2+} by inhibiting both active NaCl reabsorption and the development of a lumen-positive potential difference in the TAL.[77] The decrease in transepithelial voltage reduces passive, paracellular Ca^{2+} absorption. The effect of membrane hyperpolarization on transcellular Ca^{2+} transport is less certain. When combined with extracellular volume expansion, the hypercalciuric effect of the loop diuretics can be used to lower plasma Ca^{2+} levels.[78] Thiazide diuretics cause a fall in urinary Ca^{2+} excretion. Part of this effect may result from enhanced proximal tubular reabsorption secondary to volume depletion; however, a direct enhancement of distal tubular Ca^{2+} reabsorption by thiazide diuretics has also been demonstrated.[79,80] This latter effect is likely the result of the hyperpolarization of the membrane and an increase in the open probability of the Ca^{2+} channels, both favoring entry of Ca^{2+} into the cells. Thiazide diuretics can reduce Ca^{2+} excretion in the absence of PTH or volume contraction. They increase Ca^{2+} reabsorption and inhibit Na^+ reabsorption, thus revealing the dissociation in the transport of these ions in distal nephron.[81]

Autocrine and Paracrine Calcitropic Hormones

Arginine Vasopressin. This is the key regulator of water reabsorption in the distal nephron. In addition, it has a Ca^{2+}-sparing effect, mediated by an increase in the paracellular transport.[82]

Prostaglandin E_2. This predominant autacoid in the cortical collecting duct has a dual effect on Ca^{2+} transport. By interacting with apical and basolateral prostaglandin receptors EP2 or EP4 receptors, prostaglandin E_2 stimulates Ca^{2+} transport, whereas via interaction with basolateral EP3 receptors, it inhibits the stimulatory action of other calcitropic hormones.[83] The G-protein–coupled EP3 receptor modulates cyclic adenosine monophosphate (cAMP): via G_1 activation, it inhibits adenylyl cyclase, and via G_s activation, it stimulates adenylyl cyclase activity.[84] The molecular mechanism by which EP2/-4 stimulate and EP3 inhibits the action of calcitropic hormones is unknown.

Adenosine. Acting via apical A1 receptors,[46] adenosine increases transcellular Ca^{2+} transport to the same extent as PTH, arginine vasopressin, and prostaglandin E_2.

Adenosine Triphosphate. ATP inhibits the action of stimulatory calciotropic hormones. The effect is mediated via both apical and basolateral P2y receptors.[85]

Nitric Oxide. Nitric oxide activates Ca^{2+} reabsorption via cyclic guanosine monophosphate.[86]

Thyroid Hormone. Ca^{2+} uptake is increased in renal brush-border membrane vesicles from hyperthyroid rats and is decreased in those from hypothyroid rats.[87]

Fetal and Neonatal Aspects of Renal Transport of Calcium

Ca^{2+} is vital for the adequate mineralization, growth, and development of the fetal skeleton. Approximately 30 g of Ca^{2+} is transferred via the human placenta from the mother to the fetus, mainly during the third trimester. Toward the end of gestation, the Ca^{2+} levels in fetal plasma (total and ionized) are higher than they are in the mother.[88] Hormones such as calcitonin, PTH, and PTHrP have been found in maternal and fetal circulations, and they originate from mother, fetus, and placenta.[89] PTHrP has been found in the parathyroid glands of fetal sheep, in a 7-week-old human fetus, and in human placenta.[90] This protein is reported to stimulate placental Ca^{2+} transfer from mother to fetus in animals and in humans.[91] However, fetal PTH is not required for transplacental Ca^{2+} transfer.[92] The placenta has most of the G-protein–coupled receptors that bind the calcitropic hormones. CaSR is expressed in both villous and extravillous regions of the human placenta and contributes to the local control of transplacental Ca^{2+} transport and to the regulation of placental development.[93] Polycystin-2, a ubiquitous transmembrane glyco-

protein, mutated in autosomal dominant polycystic kidney disease, is present in term human syncytiotrophoblast, in which it behaves as a nonselective cation channel. Fetal renal cortex adenylate cyclase activity increases in response to PTH, as evidenced by an increase in urinary cAMP excretion after PTH administration in fetal sheep preparations[94] and by adenylate cyclase responsiveness in fetal rabbit[95] and fetal rat kidney preparations.[96] PTH infusion into fetal lambs results in a rise in plasma Ca^{2+}, a decline in plasma phosphate, and increases in urinary flow rate and urinary Ca^{2+} excretion.[97] Several studies in young animals, as well as in premature and term human neonates, revealed an increase in PTH levels during hypocalcemia and a calcemic response to PTH.[90,98] Yet, premature infants given exogenous PTH had minimal increases in urinary cAMP until day 6 of life, a finding suggesting a maturational delay in response to PTH by the nephron. Perfusion of isolated newborn guinea pig kidneys with a PTH-containing solution increased Ca^{2+} reabsorption and cAMP excretion, but it did not affect the reabsorption of phosphate.[99] Similar effects have been observed in full-term human newborns.[100]

Vitamin D–dependent Ca^{2+}-binding proteins, thought to be involved in transepithelial Ca^{2+} transfer, have been found in human kidneys as early as 14 weeks of gestation.[101] Yet, the major function of the kidneys in fetal Ca^{2+} homeostasis appears to be the production of $1,25(OH)_2D_3$, rather than renal regulation of Ca^{2+} excretion.[102] The urinary Ca^{2+}/creatinine ratio (mmol/mmol) was reported to increase from 0.05 to 1.2 in term neonates and from 0.3 to 2.3 in preterm neonates during the first week of life. Children older than 1 year of age have a mean urinary Ca^{2+}/creatinine ratio (mmol/mmol) of 0.40, and school-age children have a ratio of less than 0.21.[103] These findings suggest that the fractional excretion of Ca^{2+} is high in newborns, especially in those born prematurely.[104] However, the high excretion rates observed in these infants may have been caused, at least in part, by a low phosphate intake because these children were largely breast-fed.[105] Urinary Ca^{2+} excretion in preterm neonates has been also found to vary directly with urinary flow rate and with urinary Na^+ excretion. Yet, young animals given a saline load had an attenuated natriuretic response but a similar calciuretic response when compared with adult animals.[106] This finding suggests linked proximal tubular Ca^{2+} and Na^+ reabsorptive mechanism and an unlinked distal mechanism in newborn animals.[107]

PHOSPHORUS

Phosphate homeostasis, like that of Ca^{2+}, involves the integrated action of several hormonal systems and certain key factors. Because phosphorus is an important constituent of bone and other tissues, an adequate supply of phosphate is required for proper growth and development. During the perinatal period, this metabolic demand is met by the maintenance of positive phosphate balance as a consequence of a relatively high intake of phosphate, efficient intestinal phosphate absorption, and reduced urinary losses of phosphate.[108] The kidney plays a critical role in this process by limiting the urinary excretion of phosphate through enhanced tubular phosphate reabsorption.[109] Indeed, the rate of tubular phosphate reabsorption largely determines the levels of phosphate in the extracellular fluid and, ultimately, regulates phosphate homeostasis.

Approximately 80% of the total body phosphorus is present in the skeleton, with the remainder being in muscle, soft tissues, and extracellular fluids. Two-thirds of the circulating phosphorus pool is in the form of organic phosphates (e.g., esters and phospholipids), and one-third exists as inorganic phosphate, essentially all in the form of orthophosphate.[110] Most orthophosphates circulate as free phosphate in a 4:1 ratio of dibasic (HPO_4^{2-}) to monobasic ($H_2PO_4^-$) forms; these, together with the small amounts of phosphate complexes (with Ca^{2+} and Mg^{2+}) and phosphate bound to protein, are reported as the plasma phosphate concentration. The plasma phosphate concentration is highest in infants (4.5 to 9.3 mg/dl) and is higher in children (4.5 to 6.5 mg/dl) than in adults (3.0 to 4.5 mg/dl).[110] The elevated level of plasma phosphate in neonates is essential for proper skeletal mineralization, and it is a consequence, primarily, of a relatively high rate of tubular phosphate reabsorption. This section focuses on the adaptations in the renal handling of phosphate and response to regulators of phosphate transport that facilitate the renal retention of phosphate during growth and development.

Renal Handling of Phosphate

General Characteristics

Approximately 90% of plasma phosphate is freely filterable across the glomerular capillary, and 10% is bound to proteins. However, because of the Donnan effect and correction for plasma water, the ultrafiltrate phosphate concentrations are similar to those found in normocalcemic plasma.[111] Thus, the filtered load of phosphate can be appropriately estimated as the product of the plasma phosphate concentration and the GFR.

Under normal conditions, the kidneys reabsorb 75 to 85% of the filtered phosphate load and excrete the remainder. The tubular reabsorption of phosphate is a saturable process characterized by a transport maximum (TmPi). Accordingly, at filtered loads less than the TmPi, phosphate excretion is minimal. However, the TmPi is not a fixed value, but rather is influenced by the actions of hormones, dietary phosphate, and other factors. To facilitate comparison of TmPi values from individuals or animals of different sizes, values are normalized by kidney or body mass or, more commonly, by the GFR. On this basis, the TmPi/GFR in infants,[112,113] and in neonatal animals,[106,114,115] is greater than in corresponding adults. Furthermore, in contrast to the adult, the developing animal has a renal threshold that is far greater than the normal plasma phosphate concentration. Therefore, the newborn can maintain avid phosphate reabsorption in the presence of high plasma phosphate levels.

Nephron Sites of Phosphate Transport

The bulk of filtered phosphate is reabsorbed in the proximal convoluted tubule (Fig. 132-2). In adult animals under normal conditions, 60 to 70% of the filtered phosphate load is reabsorbed in that segment,[108,116] and the rate of reabsorption could increase to 85 to 90% of the filtered load in states of phosphate retention such as hypoparathyroidism[116] and dietary phosphate deprivation.[117-119] Significant phosphate reabsorption also occurs in segments beyond the proximal convoluted tubule, such as the proximal straight tubule (pars recta),[120-122] the distal convoluted tubule,[118,123] and the cortical collecting tubule,[124] particularly in states of phosphate conservation.[117,119,125,126]

The postnatal period of rapid growth and development may represent a state of phosphate conservation that involves avid phosphate reabsorption in several nephron segments. Results of micropuncture experiments indicate that a proportionally greater fraction of the filtered phosphate load is reabsorbed in the early part of the proximal convoluted tubule of newborn guinea pigs compared with adults.[127] In the neonatal rat, fractional phosphate reabsorption along the proximal convoluted tubule is reduced until 3 weeks of age, and then it equals or even exceeds the rate seen in older rats.[128] More recently, an intrinsic, PTH-independent adaptation to enhance phosphate reabsorption was observed in juvenile rats in both the proximal convoluted tubule and the proximal straight tubule segments.[129]

Because direct measurements of phosphate transport in the various segments of the distal nephron of developing animals have not been reported, it is not possible to localize further the sites of enhanced phosphate transport during development. However, the descending and ascending limbs of the loop of Henle probably do not contribute to the reabsorption of phosphate because the permeability of these segments to phosphate is very low.[116]

Heterogeneity of phosphate reabsorption between superficial and juxtamedullary nephrons is another important element to consider in the tubular handling of phosphate by the newborn. The intrinsic capacity to transport phosphate in single-nephron proximal tubules, *in vivo,* is greater in deep than in superficial nephrons.[130] This observation could have significant implications for the developmental period, in view of the centrifugal pattern of nephron maturation. Because nephrogenesis begins in the juxtamedullary region and continues with the development of outer cortical nephrons,[131] the relative preponderance of deep nephrons (with a higher capacity for phosphate transport) in the immature kidney may contribute to the high capacity for phosphate reabsorption during development.[109]

Tubular Sites of Phosphate Reabsorption

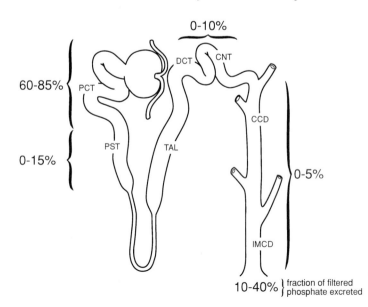

Figure 132–2. Tubular sites of phosphate reabsorption along the nephron. The percentages refer to the ranges of tubular phosphate reabsorption in adult animals. The low end occurs under high dietary phosphate conditions, and the high end reflects dietary phosphate restriction. The higher reabsorptive rates also occur during the perinatal period, when avid phosphate retention is integral to proper growth. CCD = cortical collecting duct; DCT = distal convoluted tubule; IMCD = inner medullary collecting duct; PCT = proximal convoluted tubule; PST = proximal straight tubule; TAL = thick ascending limb of the loop of Henle.

Transcellular Phosphate Transport

The rate-limiting step in the transcellular transport of phosphate is the movement of phosphate across the luminal membrane into the renal tubular cell (Fig. 132–3).[132] Phosphate enters the renal tubule cell via a Na^+-coupled, electroneutral, secondary active transport process, which is dependent on an electrochemical gradient for Na^+ generated by an Na^+,K^+-ATPase pump on the basolateral membrane of the proximal tubular cell.[133] Carrier proteins, specific for Na^+ phosphate co-transport, span the lipid bilayer and transport phosphate across the brush-border membrane into the cell. Once inside the cell, inorganic phosphate can be incorporated into many organic compounds through one of several biosynthetic pathways, or it can simply pass through the cell. The amount of phosphate leaving the cell can vary, depending on the metabolic demands of the cell. Once the intracellular phosphate pool increases, phosphate exits the cell passively down the concentration gradient across the basolateral membrane.[133] This process involves an anion countertransport, and it may also use an Na^+-independent phosphate transporter. These actions are facilitated by the electrical potential across the basolateral membrane.[111]

Na^+-dependent phosphate uptake increases in proximal tubule brush-border membrane vesicles of neonatal rats 14 to 21 days of age, as a consequence of a rise in the affinity of the Na^+-phosphate co-transporter.[134] This maturational increase in proximal tubular phosphate reabsorption in the rat appears to be intimately related to the weaning process, and it can be prevented by either early weaning or prolonged weaning.[135] Studies of the kinetics of phosphate transport in juvenile rats[136] and in the developing guinea pig[137] report that the maximum velocity of phosphate uptake is higher in newborns than in adults, possibly as a consequence of an increased number of Na^+-phosphate co-transporters in the neonatal kidney.

Studies using magnetic resonance techniques on isolated kidney cells have reported lower intracellular phosphate concentrations in kidneys of neonates compared with adults,[138] despite the known higher rate of phosphate entry into the tubular cells. This finding suggests that the rate of basolateral phosphate efflux must also be higher in the newborns and may

contribute to their high reabsorptive capacity for phosphate. The concentration of intracellular phosphate has been directly correlated with postnatal age and dietary phosphate supply and inversely correlated with the TmPi. However, it is not significantly altered when TmPi is increased or decreased because of changes in the demand for phosphate that result from reductions in the rate of body growth or bone mineralization. This finding suggests that variations in intracellular phosphate concentration do not contribute to those renal adaptations.

The isolation and cloning of specific Type II renal Na^+-phosphate (NaPi-2) co-transporters, in various species,[139, 140] have led to further elucidation of the mechanisms regulating these phosphate transporters. A study of the distribution of NaPi-2 transporters during postnatal ontogeny in the rat kidney demonstrated that NaPi-2 transporters are present when the brush border develops, and NaPi-2 transporters are not detectable in the nephrogenic zone or in the outgrowing straight sections of proximal tubules, which lack a brush border. Expression of NaPi-2 was greater in 13-day-old rats than in 22-day-old rats, and by 6 weeks of age, the pattern of NaPi-2 abundance corresponded to that in the adult rat kidney.[141]

Studies on the NaPi-2 protein in adult rats have reported that both NaPi-2 transporter mRNA and protein are up-regulated in response to a low-phosphate diet in rat proximal tubule brush-border membranes.[142] Furthermore, up-regulation of NaPi-2 mRNA and protein has also been shown to occur in parathyroidectomized rats on normal or low-phosphate diets,[143] a finding suggesting that regulation of cellular phosphate transport by PTH involves both transcriptional and translational events. Findings in juvenile rats demonstrated that renal NaPi-2 transporter expression is significantly greater in juveniles than adult rats, and there is a developmental decrease in the transporter protein into young adulthood.[129] These changes coincide directly with changes in the tubular reabsorption of phosphate.[129] Thus, although it is possible that other unique transporters may play a role during development, these findings indicate that up-regulation of NaPi-2 transporters is a key adaptation facilitating avid phosphate uptake in the developing animal.

Factors Influencing Renal Phosphate Transport

For many years, the limited ability of the newborn to excrete phosphate was thought to be a consequence of the reduced GFR. Although this may be a limiting factor in the very early postnatal period, studies performed in weaned rats,[114] newborn guinea pigs,[106] and older infants indicated that the reduced urinary excretion of phosphate occurs because of a high rate of tubular phosphate reabsorption, independent of GFR.

The principal hormonal regulator of renal phosphate transport is PTH. PTH is released in response to decreased plasma Ca^{2+} levels and acts on the kidney to increase Ca^{2+} and to decrease phosphate reabsorption. In the adult animal, the latter effect occurs through a direct action of PTH on both proximal[125, 144] and distal nephron segments.[123, 125, 126] In adult rats, nephron heterogeneity also plays a role in the tubular response to PTH, in that the deep nephrons elicit a greater phosphaturic response than do superficial nephrons.[118]

The response of the newborn infant and immature animal to the phosphaturic, but not hypocalciuric, effect of PTH is attenuated compared with the adult.[108, 129, 145] This reduced sensitivity to PTH occurs despite normal circulating levels of PTH postnatally.[146] Researchers have demonstrated that the blunted phosphaturic effect of PTH in the juvenile animal is restored to adult levels when growth hormone (GH) is suppressed,[147] an effect that is mediated through NaPi-2 transporters.[148] This finding indicates that the PTH mechanism is intact, and there is avid reabsorption of phosphate in proximal and distal segments of the nephron in the juvenile animal[129] that is regulated by GH in the young animal.[148]

Transepithelial Transport of Phosphate

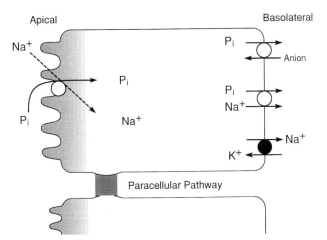

Figure 132–3. Model of transepithelial phosphate transport in renal proximal tubular cells. Phosphate enters the cells via a sodium-phosphate co-transporter located on the apical brush-border membrane. Phosphate may be used in cellular metabolic processes, or it may exit the cells via sodium-dependent and sodium-independent carriers.

One of the most important regulators of renal phosphate transport is dietary phosphate. In response to an increase in dietary phosphate, the urinary excretion of phosphate increases in the adult to maintain near-zero balance. This is associated with a rapid decrease in NaPi-2 transporters,[142] a decreasing phosphate uptake in brush-border membrane vesicles in adult rats,[149] and a reduced tubular capacity to reabsorb phosphate.[116] The juvenile rat responds to a dietary phosphate load, but relatively less phosphate is excreted compared with the adult, and the TmPi remains significantly greater than in adults.[147]

Dietary phosphate restriction elevates phosphate reabsorption in the adult animal,[116, 147] through increases in phosphate transport in the proximal tubule[118, 121, 125, 129] and distal segments.[118, 119, 129] This adaptation to enhance tubular phosphate reabsorption during dietary phosphate deprivation is also present in immature dogs[115] and rats.[129,147] Indeed, studies in the immature rat have shown that the adaptive increase in phosphate reabsorption is far greater than that observed in the phosphate-deprived adult, and it is PTH independent.[129,147] Moreover, this increase occurs despite the already high rate of phosphate transport in the immature animal. The elevated TmPi in the phosphate-deprived newborn serves to maintain avid reabsorption of phosphate and to facilitate the accelerated rate of growth, which occurs on the restoration of phosphate to the diet.[129,147]

Thyroid hormone may also be integral to proper phosphate homeostasis in the young animal. The kidney is a target organ for thyroid hormone and contains the iodothyronine diodinase enzyme that converts the main circulating hormone thyroxine to the more potent triiodothyronine. Increases in thyroid hormone have been shown to stimulate Na^+-dependent phosphate transport in the adult rat. This effect is probably related to the hormone's ability to up-regulate the maximal velocity of the transporter. Thyroid hormone may also be involved in the maturational increase in the affinity of the proximal tubule brush-border phosphate uptake that occurs with weaning.[150,151]

GH is a key factor regulating renal phosphate reabsorption, particularly in the postnatal period. GH hypersecretion is associated with hyperphosphatemia and a reduction in the urinary excretion of phosphate.[152-154] Conversely, GH deficiency (dwarfism) is associated with an attenuated growth rate and an increased excretion of phosphate.[153] When GH-deficient individuals are given GH injections, growth rate acutely increases, and phosphate excretion is diminished.[153] Studies in adult dogs[154] and rats[157] have reported that administration of GH increases the tubular reabsorption of phosphate independent of parathyroid hormone. Conversely, when adult animals are hypophysectomized, phosphate excretion increases, and the TmPi decreases.[155] It is not known whether the increase in phosphate retention results directly from the GH binding to renal GH receptors or indirectly from GH activation of renal insulin-like growth factor I (IGF-I). Indeed, IGF-I is also capable of directly increasing phosphate reabsorption *in vitro*[156] and *in vivo*.[157]

Results from animal studies have established an important link between the growth-promoting effects of GH and renal phosphate reabsorption. Blocking the pulsatile secretion of GH using a specific synthetic antagonist to GH-releasing hormone significantly attenuates the growth rate and reduces the positive phosphate balance in juvenile rats.[158, 159] These effects are associated with a reduced proximal and distal tubule phosphate reabsorption[148] and decreased TmPi, down to levels observed in adult animals.[159] GH or IGF-I replacement prevents the reduction in TmPi in GH-suppressed juvenile rats. Suppression of GH has no effect on phosphate handling in adult rats. In addition, suppression of GH release in weaning and juvenile rats produces a phosphaturic response to PTH comparable to that observed in adult rats and drives the increase in tubular phosphate reabsorption in response to dietary phosphate deprivation.[129] These findings indicate that many of the adaptations to conserve phosphate in the developing animal are facilitated, directly or indirectly, by GH.

REFERENCES

1. Nordin BEC: Nutritional considerations. *In* Nordin BEC (ed): Calcium, Phosphate, and Magnesium Metabolism. Edinburgh, Churchill Livingstone, 1976, pp 1-112.
2. Toffaletti J, et al: Separation and quantitation of serum constituents associated with calcium by gel filtration. Clin Chem 22:1968-1972, 1976.
3. Kelepouris E: Renal handling of calcium. Am J Nephrol 8:226-234, 1988.
4. Lee CO, et al: Cytosolic calcium ion activity in epithelial cells of Necturus kidney. Nature 287:859-861, 1980.
5. Murphy E, Mandel LJ: Cytosolic free calcium levels in rabbit proximal kidney tubules. Am J Physiol 242:C124-C128, 1982.
6. Birnbaumer L, et al: On the molecular basis and regulation of cellular capacitative calcium entry: roles for Trp proteins. Proc Natl Acad Sci U S A 93:15195-15202, 1996.
7. Friedman PA: Calcium transport in the kidney. Curr Opin Nephrol Hypertens 8:589-595, 1999.
8. Bindels RJ: Calcium handling by the mammalian kidney. J Exp Biol 184:89-104, 1993.
9. Friedman PA: Mechanisms of renal calcium transport. Exp Nephrol 8:343-350, 2000.
10. Hoenderop JG, et al: Epithelial calcium channel: gate-keeper of active calcium reabsorption. Curr Opin Nephrol Hypertens 9:335-340, 2000.
11. Hoenderop JG, et al: Molecular mechanism of active Ca^{2+} reabsorption in the distal nephron. Annu Rev Physiol 64:529-549, 2002.
12. Hoenderop JG, et al: Molecular identification of the apical Ca^{2+} channel in 1, 25-dihydroxyvitamin D3-responsive epithelia. J Biol Chem 274:8375-8378, 1999.
13. Hoenderop JG, et al: Localization of the epithelial $Ca^{(2+)}$ channel in rabbit kidney and intestine. J Am Soc Nephrol 11:1171-1178, 2000.
14. Vennekens R, et al: Permeation and gating properties of the novel epithelial $Ca^{(2+)}$ channel. J Biol Chem 275:3963-3969, 2000.
15. Peng JB, et al: Molecular cloning and characterization of a channel-like transporter mediating intestinal calcium absorption. J Biol Chem 274:22739-22746, 1999.
16. Muller D, et al: Gene structure and chromosomal mapping of human epithelial calcium channel. Biochem Biophys Res Commun 275:47-52, 2000.
17. Barley NF, et al: Epithelial calcium transporter expression in human duodenum. Am J Physiol 280:G285-G290, 2001.
18. Fernando KC, Barritt GJ: Pinocytosis in 2,5-di-tert-butylhydroquinone-stimulated hepatocytes and evaluation of its role in Ca^{2+} inflow. Mol Cell Biochem 162:23-29, 1996.
19. Ziyadeh FN, et al: Relationships between calcium and chloride transport in frog skin glands. Am J Physiol 251:F647-F654, 1986.
20. Varghese S, et al: Transcriptional regulation and chromosomal assignment of the mammalian calbindin-D28k gene. Mol Endocrinol 3:495-502, 1989.
21. Christakos S, et al: Vitamin D-dependent calcium binding proteins: chemistry, distribution, functional considerations, and molecular biology. Endocr Rev 10:3-26, 1989.
22. Feher JJ, et al: Role of facilitated diffusion of calcium by calbindin in intestinal calcium absorption. Am J Physiol 262:C517-C526, 1992.
23. Koster HP, et al: Calbindin-D28K facilitates cytosolic calcium diffusion without interfering with calcium signaling. Cell Calcium 18:187-196, 1995.
24. Berggard T, et al: Calbindin D28k exhibits properties characteristic of a Ca^{2+} sensor. J Biol Chem 277:16662-16672, 2002.
25. Zuhlke RD, et al: Calmodulin supports both inactivation and facilitation of L-type calcium channels. Nature 399:159-162, 1999.
26. Lee A, et al: Ca^{2+}/calmodulin binds to and modulates P/Q-type calcium channels. Nature 399:155-159, 1999.
27. Bindels RJ, et al: Role of Na^+/Ca^{2+} exchange in transcellular Ca^{2+} transport across primary cultures of rabbit kidney collecting system. Pflugers Arch 420:566-572, 1992.
28. van Baal J, et al: Localization and regulation by vitamin D of calcium transport proteins in rabbit cortical collecting system. Am J Physiol 271:F985-F993, 1996.
29. Nicoll DA, et al: Cloning of a third mammalian Na^+-Ca^{2+} exchanger, NCX3. J Biol Chem 271:24914-24921, 1996.
30. van Baal J, et al: Localization and regulation by vitamin D of calcium transport proteins in rabbit cortical collecting system. Am J Physiol 271:F985-F993, 1996.
31. Philipson KD, et al: Molecular regulation of the $Na^{(+)}$-Ca^{2+} exchanger. Ann NY Acad Sci 779:20-28, 1996.
32. Brown EM, et al: Cloning and characterization of an extracellular $Ca^{(2+)}$-sensing receptor from bovine parathyroid. Nature 366:575-580, 1993.
33. Biner HL, et al: Human cortical distal nephron: distribution of electrolyte and water transport pathways. J Am Soc Nephrol 13:836-847, 2002.
34. Friedman PA, et al: Sodium-calcium interactions in the renal proximal convoluted tubule of the rabbit. Am J Physiol 240:F558-F568, 1981.
35. Juppner H: Molecular cloning and characterization of a parathyroid hormone/parathyroid hormone-related peptide receptor: a member of an ancient family of G protein-coupled receptors. Curr Opin Nephrol Hypertens 3:371-378, 1994.

36. Usdin TB, et al: Identification and functional expression of a receptor selectively recognizing parathyroid hormone, the PTH2 receptor. J Biol Chem 270:15455-15458, 1995.

37. Hoare SR, Usdin TB: Molecular mechanisms of ligand recognition by parathyroid hormone 1 (PTH1) and PTH2 receptors. Curr Pharm Des 7:689-713, 2001.

38. Hoare SR, et al: Evaluating the signal transduction mechanism of the parathyroid hormone 1 receptor: effect of receptor-G-protein interaction on the ligand binding mechanism and receptor conformation. J Biol Chem 276:7741-7753, 2001.

39. Aida K, et al: Molecular cloning of a putative Ca(2+)-sensing receptor cDNA from human kidney. Biochem Biophys Res Commun 214:524-529,1995.

40. Loffing J, et al: Distribution of transcellular calcium and sodium transport pathways along mouse distal nephron. Am J Physiol 281:F1021-F1027, 2001.

41. Pearce SH, et al: Calcium-sensing receptor mutations in familial hypocalciuric hypercalcaemia with recurrent pancreatitis. Clin Endocrinol (Oxf) 45:675-680, 1996.

42. Pearce SH, et al: A familial syndrome of hypocalcemia with hypercalciuria due to mutations in the calcium-sensing receptor. N Engl J Med 335:1115-1122, 1996.

43. Pearce SH, Brown EM: Disorders of calcium ion sensing. J Clin Endocrinol Metab 81:2030-2035, 1996.

44. Pollak MR, et al: Familial hypocalciuric hypercalcemia and neonatal severe hyperparathyroidism: effects of mutant gene dosage on phenotype. J Clin Invest 93:1108-1112, 1994.

45. Pollak MR, et al: Autosomal dominant hypocalcaemia caused by a Ca(2+)-sensing receptor gene mutation. Nat Genet 8:303-307, 1994.

46. Hoenderop JG, et al: Calcitriol controls the epithelial calcium channel in kidney. J Am Soc Nephrol 12:1342-1349, 2001.

47. Borke JL, et al: Co-localization of erythrocyte Ca++-Mg++ ATPase and vitamin D-dependent 28-kDa-calcium binding protein. Kidney Int 34:262-267, 1988.

48. Bindels RJ, et al: Calbindin-D9k and parvalbumin are exclusively located along basolateral membranes in rat distal nephron. J Am Soc Nephrol 2:1122-1129, 1991.

49. Bindels RJ, et al: Immunocytochemical localization of calbindin-D28k, calbindin-D9k and parvalbumin in rat kidney. Contrib Nephrol 91:7-13, 1991.

50. Taylor AN, et al: Immunocytochemical localization of vitamin D-dependent calcium-binding protein in renal tubules of rabbit, rat, and chick. Kidney Int 21:765-773, 1982.

51. Magosci M, et al: Localization of mRNAs coding for isozymes of plasma membrane Ca(2+)-ATPase pump in rat kidney. Am J Physiol 263:F7-14, 1992.

52. Yu AS, et al: Identification and localization of renal Na(+)-Ca2+ exchanger by polymerase chain reaction. Am J Physiol 263:F680-F685, 1992.

53. Bindels RJ, et al: Active Ca2+ transport in primary cultures of rabbit kidney CCD: stimulation by 1,25-dihydroxyvitamin D3 and PTH. Am J Physiol 261:F799-F807, 1991.

54. van Baal J, et al: Localization and regulation by vitamin D of calcium transport proteins in rabbit cortical collecting system. Am J Physiol 271:F985-F993, 1996.

55. Pak CY, et al: Renal effects of porcine thyrocalcitonin in the dog. Endocrinology 87:262-270, 1970.

56. Pondel M: Calcitonin and calcitonin receptors: bone and beyond. Int J Exp Pathol 81:405-422, 2000.

57. Shimizu T, et al: Effects of PTH, calcitonin, and cAMP on calcium transport in rabbit distal nephron segments. Am J Physiol 259:F408-F414, 1990.

58. Carney S, Thompson L: Acute effects of calcitonin on rat renal electrolyte transport. Am J Physiol 240:F12-F16, 1981.

59. Shinki T, et al: Calcitonin is a major regulator for the expression of renal 25-hydroxyvitamin D3-1alpha-hydroxylase gene in normocalcemic rats. Proc Natl Acad Sci USA 96:8253-8258, 1999.

60. Edwards BR, et al: Effect of calcium infusion on renal tubular reabsorption in the dog. Am J Physiol 227:13-18, 1974.

61. Humes HD, et al: Evidence for a parathyroid hormone-dependent influence of calcium on the glomerular ultrafiltration coefficient. J Clin Invest 61:32-40, 1978.

62. Massry SG, et al: Role of serum Ca, parathyroid hormone, and NaCl infusion on renal Ca and Na clearances. Am J Physiol 214:1403—1409, 1968.

63. Brown EM, Hebert SC: A cloned Ca(2+)-sensing receptor: a mediator of direct effects of extracellular Ca2+ on renal function? J Am Soc Nephrol 6:1530-1540, 1995.

64. Wong NL, et al: Renal tubular transport in phosphate depletion: a micropuncture study. Can J Physiol Pharmacol 58:1063-1071, 1980.

65. Massry SG, et al: Effect of MgCl2 infusion on urinary Ca and Na during reduction in their filtered loads. Am J Physiol 219:881-885, 1970.

66. Agus ZS, et al: Regulation of urinary calcium excretion in the rat. Am J Physiol 232:F545-F549, 1977.

67. Bushinsky DA, et al: Effects of in vivo metabolic acidosis on midcortical bone ion composition. Am J Physiol 277:F813-F819, 1999.

68. Bindels RJ, et al: Effects of pH on apical calcium entry and active calcium transport in rabbit cortical collecting system. Am J Physiol 266:F620-F627, 1994.

69. Vennekens R, et al: Modulation of the epithelial Ca2+ channel ECaC by extracellular pH. Pflugers Arch 442:237-242, 2001.

70. Marone CC, et al: Effects of metabolic alkalosis on calcium excretion in the conscious dog. J Lab Clin Med 101:264-273, 1983.

71. DeFronzo RA, et al: The effect of insulin on renal handling of sodium, potassium, calcium, and phosphate in man. J Clin Invest 55:845-855, 1975.

72. Bruton JD: Insulin increases near-membrane but not global Ca2+ in isolated skeletal muscle. Proc Natl Acad Sci U S A 96:3281-3286, 1999.

73. Levy M, Starr NL: The mechanism of glucagon-induced natriuresis in dogs. Kidney Int 2:76-84, 1972.

74. Lemann J Jr, et al: Studies of the acute effects of aldosterone and cortisol on the interrelationship between renal sodium, calcium and magnesium excretion in normal man. Nephron 7:117-130, 1970.

75. Simon DB, Lifton RP: Mutations in Na(K)Cl transporters in Gitelman's and Bartter's syndromes. Curr Opin Cell Biol 10:450-454, 1998.

76. Lemmink HH: Novel mutations in the thiazide-sensitive NaCl cotransporter gene in patients with Gitelman syndrome with predominant localization to the C-terminal domain. Kidney Int 54:720-730, 1998.

77. Bourdeau JE, et al: Inhibition of calcium absorption in the cortical thick ascending limb of Henle's loop by furosemide. J Pharmacol Exp Ther 221:815-819, 1982.

78. Suki WN, et al: Acute treatment of hypercalcemia with furosemide. N Engl J Med 283:836-840, 1970.

79. Costanzo LS: Mechanism of action of thiazide diuretics. Semin Nephrol 8:234-241, 1988.

80. Stanton BA: Cellular actions of thiazide diuretics in the distal tubule. J Am Soc Nephrol 1:832-836, 1990.

81. Friedman PA: Codependence of renal calcium and sodium transport. Annu Rev Physiol 60:179-197, 1998.

82. van Baal J, et al: Vasopressin-stimulated Ca2+ reabsorption in rabbit cortical collecting system: effects on cAMP and cytosolic Ca2+. Pflugers Arch 433:109-115, 1996.

83. van Baal J, et al: Endogenously produced prostanoids stimulate calcium reabsorption in the rabbit cortical collecting system. J Physiol (Lond) 497:229-239, 1996.

84. Hatae N: Prostaglandin receptors: advances in the study of EP3 receptor signaling. J Biochem (Tokyo) 131:781-784, 2002.

85. Nilius B, et al: Modulation of the epithelial calcium channel, ECaC, by intracellular Ca2+. Cell Calcium 29:417-428, 2001.

86. Hoenderop JG, et al: The epithelial calcium channel, ECaC, is activated by hyperpolarization and regulated by cytosolic calcium. Biochem Biophys Res Commun 261:488-492, 1999.

87. Kumar V, Prasad R: Molecular basis of renal handling of calcium in response to thyroid hormone status of rat. Biochim Biophys Acta 1586:331-343, 2002.

88. Lafond J, et al: Hormonal regulation and implication of cell signaling in calcium transfer by placenta. Endocrinology 14:285-294, 2001.

89. Kovacs CS, et al: Calcitropic gene expression suggests a role for the intraplacental yolk sac in maternal-fetal calcium exchange. Am J Physiol 282:E721-E732, 2002.

90. Garel JM, Barlet JP: The effects of calcitonin and parathormone on plasma magnesium levels before and after birth in the rat. J Endocrinol 61:1-13, 1974.

91. Seki K, et al: Parathyroid hormone-related protein during pregnancy and the perinatal period. Gynecol Obstet Invest 37:83-86, 1994.

92. Kovacs CS, et al: Fetal parathyroids are not required to maintain placental calcium transport. J Clin Invest 107:1007-1015, 2001.

93. Bradbury RA, et al: Localization of the extracellular Ca(2+)-sensing receptor in the human placenta. Placenta 23:192-200, 2002.

94. Kooh SW: Parathyroid hormone responsiveness in the sheep fetus and newborn lamb. Can J Physiol Pharmacol 58:934-939, 1980.

95. Linarelli LG, et al: The effect of parathyroid hormone on rabbit renal cortex adenyl cyclase during development. Pediatr Res 7:878-882, 1973.

96. Weatherley AJ, et al: The transfer of calcium during perfusion of the placenta in intact and thyroparathyroidectomized sheep. Placenta 4:271-277, 1983.

97. Durand D, et al: The effect of 1 alpha-hydroxycholecalciferol on the placental transfer of calcium and phosphate in sheep. Br J Nutr 49:475-480, 1983.

98. Cruikshank DP, et al: Alterations in vitamin D and calcium metabolism with magnesium sulfate treatment of preeclampsia. Am J Obstet Gynecol 168:1170-1176, 1993.

99. Johnson V, Spitzer A: Renal reabsorption of phosphate during development: whole kidney events. Am J Physiol 251:F251-F256, 1986.

100. Connelly JP, et al: Studies of neonatal hypophosphatemia. Pediatrics 30:425, 1962.

101. Brun P, et al: Vitamin D-dependent calcium-binding proteins (CaBPs) in human fetuses: comparative distribution of 9K CaBP mRNA and 28K CaBP during development. Pediatr Res 21:362-367, 1987.

102. Moore ES, et al: Role of fetal 1,25-dihydroxyvitamin D production in intrauterine phosphorus and calcium homeostasis. Pediatr Res 19:566-569, 1985.

103. Ghazali S, Barratt TM: Urinary excretion of calcium and magnesium in children. Arch Dis Child 49:97-101, 1974.

104. Karlen J, et al: Renal excretion of calcium and phosphate in preterm and term infants. J Pediatr 106:814-819, 1985.

105. Senterre J, Salle B: Renal aspects of calcium and phosphorus metabolism in preterm infants. Biol Neonate 53:220-229, 1988.

106. Brown DR, Steranka BH: Renal cation excretion in the hypocalcemic premature human neonate. Pediatr Res 15:1100-1104, 1981.

107. Noguchi A: Physiologic response to calcium infusion in newborn and adult dogs. Miner Electrolyte Metab 9:87-92, 1983.

108. Spitzer A, Barac-Nieto M: Ontogeny of renal phosphate transport and the process of growth. Pediatr Nephrol 16:763-771, 2001.

109. Haramati A: Phosphate handling by the kidney during development: functional immaturity or unique adaptations for growth? News Physiol Sci 4:234-238, 1989.

110. Key LL, Carpenter TO: Metabolism of calcium, phosphorus, and other divalent ions. *In* Ichikawa I (ed): Pediatric Textbook of Fluids and Electrolytes. Baltimore, Williams & Wilkins, 1990, pp 98–106.
111. Jones DP, Chesney RW: Tubular function. *In* Holliday MA, et al (eds): Pediatric Nephrology, 3rd ed. Baltimore, Williams & Wilkins, 1994, pp 117–149.
112. Brodehl J, et al: Postnatal development of tubular phosphate reabsorption. Clin Nephrol 17:163–171, 1982.
113. Senterre J, Salle B: Renal aspects of calcium and phosphorus metabolism in preterm infants. Biol Neonate 53:220–229, 1988.
114. Haramati A, et al: Developmental changes in the tubular capacity for phosphate reabsorption in the rat. Am J Physiol 255:F287–F291, 1988.
115. Russo JC, Nash MA: Renal response to alterations in dietary phosphate in the young beagle. Biol Neonate 38:1–10, 1980.
116. Suki WN, et al: Renal transport of calcium, magnesium, and phosphate. *In* Brenner BM (ed): The Kidney, 6th ed. Philadelphia, WB Saunders, 2000, pp 520–575.
117. Awazu M, et al: Effect of phosphate infusion on proximal tubule phosphate reabsorption in phosphate-deprived and respiratory alkalotic rats. Miner Electrolyte Metab 13:393–396, 1987.
118. Haramati A, et al: Adaptation of deep and superficial nephrons to changes in dietary phosphate intake. Am J Physiol 244:F265–F269, 1983.
119. Pastoriza-Munoz E, et al: Effect of phosphate deprivation on phosphate reabsorption in rat nephron: Role of PTH. Am J Physiol 244:F140–F149, 1983.
120. Berndt TJ, Knox FG: Nephron site of resistance to the phosphaturic effect of PTH during respiratory alkalosis. Am J Physiol 249:F919–F922, 1985.
121. Brazy PC, et al: Comparative effects of dietary phosphate, unilateral nephrectomy, and parathyroid hormone on phosphate transport by the rabbit proximal tubule. Kidney Int 17:788–800, 1980.
122. Webster SK, et al: Effect of dexamethasone on segmental phosphate reabsorption in phosphate-deprived rats. Am J Physiol 251:F576–F580, 1986.
123. Pastoriza-Munoz E, et al: Effect of parathyroid hormone on phosphate reabsorption in rat distal convolution. Am J Physiol 235:F321–F330, 1978.
124. Sharegi GR, Agus ZS: Phosphate transport in the light segment of rabbit cortical collecting tubule. Am J Physiol 242:F379–F384, 1982.
125. Haas JA, et al: Nephron sites of action of nicotinamide on phosphate reabsorption. Am J Physiol 246:F27–F31, 1984.
126. Webster SK, et al: Effect of dexamethasone on segmental phosphate reabsorption in phosphate-deprived rats. Am J Physiol 251:F576–F580, 1986.
127. Kaskel FJ, et al: Renal reabsorption of phosphate during development: tubular events. Pediatr Nephrol 2:129–134, 1988.
128. Lelievre-Pegorier M, et al: Developmental pattern of water and electrolyte transport in rat superficial nephrons. Am J Physiol 245:F15–F21, 1983.
129. Woda C, et al: Renal tubular sites of increased phosphate transport and NaPi-2 expression in the juvenile rat. Am J Physiol 280:R1524–R1533, 2001.
130. Haramati A: Tubular capacity of phosphate reabsorption in superficial and deep nephrons. Am J Physiol 248:F729–F733, 1985.
131. Speller AM, Moffat DB: Tubulo-vascular relationships in the developing kidney. J Anat 123:487–500, 1977.
132. Hammerman MR: Phosphate transport across renal proximal tubular cell membranes. Am J Physiol 251:F385–F398, 1986.
133. Murer H: Cellular mechanisms of proximal tubular Pi reabsorption: some answers and more questions. J Am Soc Nephrol 2:1649–1665, 1992.
134. Lelievre-Pegorier M, et al: Transport of phosphate, D-glucose, and L-valine in newborn rat kidney brush border. Am J Physiol 245:F367–F373, 1983.
135. Lelievre-Pegorier M, Merlet-Benichou C: Effect of weaning on phosphate transport maturation in the rat kidney: clearance and brush border membrane studies. Pediatr Nephrol 7:807–814, 1993.
136. Ladas JG, et al: Regulation of renal proximal tubule phosphate transport during development. Proc Soc Exp Biol Med 208:210, 1995.
137. Neiberger R, et al: Renal reabsorption of phosphate during development: transport kinetics in BBMV. Am J Physiol 257:F268–F274, 1989.
138. Barac-Nieto M, et al: Role of intracellular phosphate in the regulation of renal Pi transport during development. Pediatr Nephrol 7:819–822, 1993.
139. Werner A, et al: Cloning and expression of cDNA for a Na-Pi co-transport system of kidney cortex. Proc Natl Acad Sci U S A 88:9608–9612, 1991.
140. Magagnin SA, et al: Expression cloning of human and rat renal cortex Na/Pi cotransporter. Proc Natl Acad Sci U S A 90:5979–5983, 1993.
141. Traebert M, et al: Distribution of the sodium/phosphate transporter during postnatal ontogeny of the rat kidney. J Am Soc Nephrol. 10:1407–1415, 1999.
142. Levi M, et al: Cellular mechanisms of acute and chronic adaptation of rat renal Pi transporter to alterations in dietary Pi. Am J Physiol 267:F900–F908, 1994.
143. Kempson SA, et al: Parathyroid hormone action on phosphate transporter mRNA and protein in rat renal proximal tubules. Am J Physiol 268:F784–F791, 1995.
144. Brazy PC, et al: Comparative effects of dietary phosphate, unilateral nephrectomy, and parathyroid hormone on phosphate transport by the rabbit proximal tubule. Kidney Int 17:788–800, 1980.
145. Webster SK, Haramati A: Developmental changes in the phosphaturic response to parathyroid hormone in the rat. Am J Physiol 249:F251–F255, 1985.
146. Toverud SU, et al: Circulating parathyroid hormone concentrations in normal and vitamin D-deprived rat pups determined with an N-terminal–specific radioimmunoassay. Bone Miner 1:145–155, 1986.
147. Mulroney SE, Haramati A: Renal adaptations to changes in dietary phosphate during development. Am J Physiol 258:F1650–F1656, 1990.
148. Woda C, et al: Renal tubular sites of increased phosphate transport and NaPi-2 expression in the juvenile rat. Am J Physiol 280:R1524–R1533, 2001.
149. Cheng LC, et al: Renal adaptation to phosphate load in the acutely thyroparathyroidectomized rat: rapid alteration in brush border membrane phosphate transport. Am J Physiol 246:F488–F494, 1984.
150. Euzet S, et al: Maturation of rat renal phosphate transport: effect of triiodothyronine. J Physiol (Lond) 488:449–457, 1995.
151. Euzet S, et al: Effect of 3,5,3'-triiodothyronine on maturation of rat renal phosphate transport: kinetic characteristics and phosphate transporter messenger ribonucleic acid and protein abundance. Endocrinology 137:3522–3530, 1996.
152. Cammani F: Increased renal tubular reabsorption of phosphorus in acromegaly. Clin Endocrinol Metab 28:999–1003, 1968.
153. Corvilain J, Abramow M: Some effects of human growth hormone on renal hemodynamics and on tubular phosphate transport in man. J Clin Invest 41:1230–1234, 1962.
154. Corvilain J, Abramow M: Effect of growth hormone on tubular transport of phosphate in normal and parathyroidectomized dogs. J Clin Invest 43:1608–1612, 1964.
155. Caverzasio J, et al: Tubular adaptation to Pi restriction in hypophysectomized rats. Pflugers Arch 392:17–21, 1981.
156. Caverzasio J, Bonjour JP: Insulin-like growth factor I stimulates Na-dependent Pi transport in cultured kidney cells. Am J Physiol 257:F712–F717, 1989.
157. Caverzasio J, et al: Stimulatory effect of insulin-like growth factor-1 on renal Pi transport and plasma 1,25-dihydroxyvitamin D_3. Endocrinology 127:453–459, 1990.
158. Mulroney SE, et al: Antagonist to growth hormone-releasing factor inhibits growth and renal phosphate reabsorption in immature rats. Am J Physiol 257:F29–F34, 1989.
159. Haramati A, et al: Regulation of renal phosphate reabsorption during development: implications from new model of growth hormone deficiency. Pediatr Nephrol 4:387–391, 1990.

Aaron L. Friedman

133 Transport of Amino Acids During Early Development

GENERAL FEATURES

The reclamation of filtered amino acids by the proximal tubule of the kidney undergoes a process of maturation coincident with other changes in renal function.[1] To understand the ontogeny of renal amino acid transport, it is useful to review general features of renal amino acid transport.

Glomerular filtrate contains amino acids in concentrations essentially identical to those in plasma. It is from this filtered load

that amino acids are reabsorbed exclusively by the proximal tubule. Glycine and taurine are reabsorbed in later segments of the proximal tubule, but for most amino acids, more than 80% of reabsorption occurs in the early proximal tubule.[2, 3] This reclamation of amino acids back into the extracellular space is not merely movement across a single plasma membrane but is passage through a cell layer–transepithelial transport.

Figure 133-1 depicts a proximal tubule cell with its major reabsorptive surface, the brush-border membrane, oriented into the

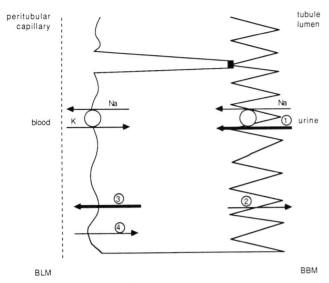

Figure 133–1. Representation of process involved in transepithelial transport of amino acids by the renal proximal tubule: (1) sodium amino acid co-transport; (2) efflux back into tubule lumen (backleak); (3) efflux from tubule to peritubular space (extracellular space) and return to plasma; (4) transport from peritubular space into tubule cell. *Circle with opposite-pointing arrows* = Na+,K+-ATPase; BBM = brush border; BLM = basolateral membrane.

lumen of the tubule and the other membrane that any reabsorbed solute must transverse, the basolateral membrane. The net flux for amino acids is from the tubule lumen to the peritubular capillary. Hence the heavier arrows in the figure are pointed in that direction. The net flux is composed of movement into the cell from the lumen and the interstitial space surrounding the basolateral membrane, as well as movement back into the tubule lumen and out of the cell into the surrounding interstitium. This view is somewhat simplistic in that it does not take into account any contribution made by intracellular metabolic processes or the possibility of amino acid movement by paracellular processes across the tight junction. However, Figure 133–1 does define the general components of transepithelial amino acid transport.

The net movement across the renal proximal tubule cell is primarily an active transport process requiring energy.[4] Passive diffusion plays a small role. For every amino acid studied thus far, the movement across the brush-border membrane is inextricably tied to sodium (Na^+) transport. The present model suggests that energy is expended by the cell to pump Na^+ from the cell into the extracellular space. This is performed at the basolateral membrane by sodium–potassium–adenosine triphosphatase (Na^+,K^+-ATPase). The extrusion of Na^+ creates an inward driving force for Na^+ (down a concentration gradient) at the brush-border membrane. Thus, amino acids and Na^+ are co-transported. In studies with brush-border membrane vesicles, in which transport across the brush-border membrane can be studied, amino acid accumulation in the vesicles is nearly completely blunted when Na^+ is excluded from the external medium.[4-6]

Transport characteristics of the brush-border carrier (transporter) for amino acids and Na^+ suggest that the transporter is saturable. In other words, increasing the concentration of amino acids to greater than a certain level does not lead to significant further accumulation. All amino transporters follow Michaelis-Menten kinetics, meaning that under proper experimental conditions, it should be possible to determine the maximal velocity (V_{max}) of transport and the concentration at which half-maximal velocity occurs (K_m). The V_{max} can be viewed as a measure of

transport capacity, with the higher the V_{max}, the greater the capacity. The K_m is a measure of affinity. The lower the K_m, the more avidly the substrate is "attracted" to the transporter. As Scriver and others have pointed out, the transporters have a higher affinity for the L-isomers of amino acids, and they demonstrate specificity.[7] In many instances, groups of amino acids are transported by the same carrier. Group-specific carriers are, with respect to any single amino acid, high-capacity but low-affinity systems. In a disease such as cystinuria, a group carrier is often involved, and most patients excrete excessive quantities of cystine, ornithine, lysine, and arginine. There are also more selective transporters for single amino acids that have lower capacities but higher affinities.

Transport properties at the basolateral membrane resemble those of the brush-border membrane, although Na^+-*independent* transport may play a greater role in transport at the basolateral membrane. Efflux properties are less well understood, although diffusion down a concentration gradient (intracellular → extracellular) may be important in the transepithelial movement of amino acids from the tubule lumen to the extracellular space. With respect to the reclamation of amino acids by the proximal tubule, and thereby the final amino acid concentration in the urine, the important features are the filtered load of amino acids and the transport capability, especially the proximal tubule brush-border membrane transporter properties.

DEVELOPMENTAL ASPECTS

It is generally recognized that very young developing mammals (including humans) have "physiologic" aminoaciduria. As the term suggests, there is more amino acid in the urine as compared with that in adults, and this aminoaciduria is not pathologic. Perhaps the term *developmental aminoaciduria* would be more appropriate, because the failure of the young mammal to reabsorb amino acids to the degree seen in the adult appears to be a developmental process.

The excretion of amino acids by humans is measured by numerous methods. Using any method, the hyperexcretion of amino acids by the human infant can be documented. Table 133–1 shows the normal range of urinary amino acid excretion in infants, children, and adults as measured after a timed collection (μmol amino acid/g creatinine/24 hours). Two other techniques for quantitating the excretion of amino acids have been employed. Scriver and Rosenberg[7] proposed the following renal clearance method:

$$(C_{AA}) \text{ clearance of amino acids} = \frac{\text{(U) urine concentration (μmol/mL)} \times \text{volume (ml/minute)}}{\text{(P) plasma concentration (μmol/ml)}}$$

and Silbernagel[3] quantified excretion by determining the fractional excretion (FE) of amino acids:

$$FE = \frac{C_{AA}}{C_{cr}} = \frac{U_{AA} \times P_{cr}}{P_{AA} \times U_{cr}}$$

where C_{AA} = amino acid clearance, C_{cr} = creatinine clearance, U_{AA} = urine amino acid concentration, P_{cr} = plasma creatinine concentration, P_{AA} = plasma amino acid concentration, and U_{cr} = urine creatinine concentration.

Fractional excretion and clearance data clearly indicate that higher concentrations of amino acids are present in the urine of newborn infants. Importantly, however, these data also suggest that the excess amino acids are not secondary to higher filtered loads. What then could be the cause of this maturational delay in the reabsorptive capacity of the proximal tubule of the infant?

Scriver and colleagues,[8] in their discussion of the expression of mutations that could lead to hereditary disorders of tubular transport, postulated at least three mechanisms to explain the

TABLE 133-1

Plasma and Urine Amino Acids*

	Plasma (μmol/l) Normal Ranges by Age			
	<1 mo	*1–24 mo*	*2–18 y*	*>18 y*
Taurine	46–492	15–143	10–170	54–210
Aspartic acid	20–129	0–23	1–24	1–25
Threonine	90–329	24–174	35–226	60–225
Serine	99–395	71–186	69–187	58–181
Glutamic acid	62–620	10–133	5–150	10–131
Glutamine	376–709	246–1182	254–823	205–756
Sarcosine	0	0	0	0
Proline	110–417	52–298	59–369	97–329
Glycine	232–740	81–436	127–341	151–490
Alanine	131–710	143–439	152–547	177–583
Citrulline	10–45	3–35	1–46	12–55
Valine	86–190	64–294	74–321	119–336
Cystine	17–98	16–84	5–45	5–82
Methionine	10–60	9–42	7–47	10–42
Cystathionine	0–3	0–5	0–3	0–3
Isoleucine	26–91	31–86	22–107	30–108
Leucine	48–160	47–155	49–216	72–201
Tyrosine	55–147	22–108	24–115	34–112
Phenylalanine	38–137	31–75	26–91	35–85
β-Alanine	0–10	0–7	0–7	0–12
Homocysteine	0	0	0	0
Tryptophan	0–60	23–71	0–79	10–140
Ethanolamine	0–115	0–4	0–7	0–7
Ornithine	48–211	22–103	10–163	48–195
Lysine	92–325	52–196	48–284	48–284
1-Methylhistidine	0–43	0–44	0–42	72–124
Histidine	30–138	41–101	41–125	41–125
3-Methylhistidine	0–5	0–5	0–5	0
Anserine	0	0	0	0
Carnosine	0	0	0	0
Arginine	6–140	12–133	10–140	15–128
	0–91	0–63	3–45	0–53

	Urine (mmol/g Creatinine) Normal Values	
	<1 y	*>1 y*
Taurine	0.64 ± 1.16	0.83 ± 0.69
Aspartic acid		
Threonine	0.47 ± 0.38	0.17 ± 0.12
Serine	1.43 ± 0.80	0.48 ± 0.28
Glutamic acid	0.10 ± 0.21	0.05 ± 0.07
Glutamine	1.30 ± 0.70	0.61 ± 0.37
Sarcosine		
Proline	0.57 ± 0.78	0.07 ± 0.04
Glycine	5.07 ± 3.10	1.48 ± 0.98
Alanine	0.92 ± 0.49	0.46 ± 0.37
Citrulline	0.04 ± 0.03	0.02 ± 0.01
Valine	0.10 ± 0.08	0.06 ± 0.05
Cystine	0.16 ± 0.15	0.05 ± 0.03
Methionine	0.28 ± 0.23	0.07 ± 0.06
Cystathionine		
Isoleucine	0.14 ± 0.10	0.05 ± 0.04
Leucine	0.16 ± 0.11	0.08 ± 0.06
Tyrosine	0.33 ± 0.23	0.18 ± 0.12
Phenylalanine	0.16 ± 0.10	0.09 ± 0.06
β-Alanine		
Homocysteine		
Tryptophan	0.10 ± 0.12	0.07 ± 0.07
Ethanolamine		
Ornithine	0.08 ± 0.07	0.05 ± 0.06
Lysine	0.52 ± 0.69	0.21 ± 0.19
1-Methylhistidine	0.13 ± 0.22	0.25 ± 0.20
Histidine	1.34 ± 0.01	0.96 ± 0.54
3-Methylhistidine	0.23 ± 0.08	0.32 ± 0.13
Anserine		
Carnosine		
Arginine	0.07 ± 0.06	0.04 ± 0.06

*Urine values are given as mmol/g creatinine in a 24-hour urine collection. Plasma values are given as concentration in μmol/l.
From University of Wisconsin Metabolic Program, with permission of Dr. Jon Wolff. See also references. 3 and 7.

developmental tubular differences seen in the infant. The first of the possible developmental differences could be at the brush-border membrane transporter site (see *site 1* in Fig. 133–1). Diminished transporter function could lead to a decrease in amino acid influx and an increase in amino acid excretion. An increase in amino acid exit at site 2 in Figure 133–1, that is, increased backflux into the lumen, could represent a second developmental difference that could explain developmental aminoaciduria. A third possibility (see Fig. 133–1, *site 3*) is a decrease in efflux. This would lead to increased intracellular concentrations of amino acids that would then result in increased backflux into the tubule lumen or a direct inhibitory effect on transporters to reduce the amount of amino acid carried into the proximal tubule cell, or both. A further possibility discussed by Scriver and colleagues deals with the metabolic fate of amino acids. In disease states, it is possible that intracellular accumulation may occur because the metabolic end-point of an amino acid may be blocked, leading to diminished metabolic "runout" and abnormal intracellular accumulation. This last possibility is not likely to explain developmental aminoaciduria because amino acids that do not undergo metabolic change or incorporation into protein are excreted in high quantities in the young of many mammalian species (see Table 133–1). Certain amino acids seem to contribute more to the high urinary amino acid excretion than do others.[9] This finding suggests that a single defect such as altered energy use cannot explain the developmental changes seen. Rather, it is more likely that any developmental effect is related to the maturation of influx or efflux capabilities and that the influx-efflux transport systems "mature" at separate rates.

Numerous laboratories have studied the ontogeny of amino acid transport. Early studies by Baerlocher and associates[10, 11] examined glycine and proline transport in rat kidney cortex slices (Long-Evans rat) from neonatal animals. Their work were consistent with the presence of a low-affinity, high-capacity transporter at birth and the emergence of a high-affinity, low-capacity system at 1 week of age for proline and 2 weeks of age for glycine. Studies by Segal and co-workers[12] in Sprague-Dawley rats found similar glycine uptake systems in the newborn and the adult Sprague-Dawley rat. Roth and associates[13] reexamined glycine transport in isolated rat tubule segments, and Reynolds and co-workers[14] reexamined glycine transport in the cortex slice. Both groups of investigators found high- and low-affinity uptake systems in newborn and adult renal tissues. However, the efflux of glycine from rat cortex slides[12] or from isolated rat tubule segments[13] was slower in the newborn than in the adult. These data, along with work reported by Meadow and colleagues,[15] suggest that slowed efflux is an important determinant of intracellular amino acid pools and therefore of transepithelial transport in the newborn.

Cystine is another amino acid whose fractional excretion is higher in the immature animal and in the human neonate. Studies with cystine have shed light on additional aspects relevant to amino acid transport. Hwang and co-workers[16] and Foreman and colleagues[17] documented the presence of two transport systems for cystine (high-affinity, low-capacity, and low-affinity, high-capacity). In the report by Foreman and co-workers,[17] the affinity for cystine was actually *higher* in the newborn infant than in the adult, but the V_{max} (capacity) was much lower. This could clearly lead to a decrease in renal cystine reabsorption. These authors further commented on the metabolic potential of the neonatal proximal tubule. Cystine is reduced intracellularly to cysteine. In their studies, tubules from the immature kidney metabolized cystine just as readily as did those from adult kidneys. Therefore, at least for cystine (and perhaps other intracellularly metabolized amino acids), the explanation for developmental aminoaciduria does not rest with an altered intracellular metabolic process. In the same study,

Foreman investigated the effect of lysine on cystine transport. Lysine inhibited the high-affinity system in the immature kidney tissue just as it did in tissue from adult animals. These data suggest that the properties of shared transport for cystine and dibasic amino acids (lysine, ornithine, citrulline) are intact even in the newborn. This group of studies points to the luminal brush-border membrane as another important site responsible for developmental aminoaciduria (see Fig. 133–1).

A structure-function analysis of amino acid transporters has resulted in classification of transporters into four genetic families:

1. GAT family: Na+- and chloride-dependent transporters
2. CAT family: cationic amino acid transporters
3. Glutamate transporters
4. rBAT family: cationic-neutral amino acid transporters

Further follow-up of these gene families has demonstrated two different membrane protein structures. GAT, CAT, and glutamate families have multiple transmembrane domains and are considered carriers, whereas rBAT family members are considered activators or part of oligomeric carriers. These findings raise an interesting question regarding maturation of amino acid transporters. No information is yet available on the maturation of these transport systems.[18, 19]

Chesney and colleagues studied the ontogeny of the transport system for the β–amino acid taurine in the rat. Using dietary alterations to help uncover the adaptive response of the kidney to taurine, most of these investigations focused on the brush-border membrane vesicle. The results of these studies can be summarized as follows:

1. Thin renal cortex slices from young rats demonstrated greater accumulation of taurine than did cortical slices from adult rats. This observation is especially striking considering that urinary excretion and fractional excretion of taurine during the first 28 days of life in the rat are much greater than those of the mature rat.[20]
2. Studies with cortical slices and proximal tubule segments revealed two transport systems—a high-affinity, low-capacity system and a low-affinity, high-capacity system.[21-23] Thus, maturation of a specific transport system could not explain the developmental taurinuria present in the young mammal.
3. Experiments using brush-border membrane vesicles (isolating the apical portion of the proximal renal tubule) revealed no difference in transport kinetics between the adult and the still-maturing 28-day-old rat.[24, 25]
4. In dietary alteration studies in which the mother was fed a low-, normal-, or high-taurine diet, taurine excretion in the 14- and 21-day-old pup mirrored dietary intake in the mother. With a low-taurine diet in the mother, urinary excretion of taurine was reduced in the 14- or 21-day-old pup. A similar positive correlation was seen with a high-taurine diet.[26]
5. This adaptation to dietary intake was reflected in the brush-border membrane, with an increase in V_{max} seen at the brush-border membrane during low dietary taurine intake. This adaptation was observed in rats ranging in age from 14 days to maturity.[25-28]
6. A plausible explanation for the finding of developmental taurinuria (but similar transport kinetics between young [≥14 days] and mature animals) is that efflux from the proximal tubule cell is diminished in the maturing animal (see *site 3* in Fig. 133–1), thereby resulting in an increased back-leak of amino acid into the tubule lumen and into the urine.
7. Total taurine accumulation was lower in brush-border vesicles prepared from 7-day-old rats compared with any other age studied (14-, 21-, 28-day-old or mature 60-day-old rats). Further, no dietary influence on taurine uptake could

be demonstrated in 7-day-old pups. These findings suggest that, in the most immature animal, the developmental aminoaciduria observed may in part result from diminished uptake across the brush-border membrane and not just diminished efflux across the basolateral membrane.[27]

Amino acids are transported across the renal epithelium primarily by NaCl co-transport systems.[29] Studies examining proline transport in experimental animals revealed a reduced uptake of proline in the immature animal and a less pronounced characteristic uptake pattern in the immature animal, attributed to differences in Na^+ permeability and Na^+-K^+ exchange activity in the immature versus the mature animal.[30,31] A faster or higher accumulation of Na^+ would more quickly dissipate the extracellular-to-intracellular Na^+ gradient, thereby reducing the driving force for Na^+-dependent transport, such as amino acid transport. In this way, amino acid accumulation by the renal epithelium of the very young rat could be diminished. Such a hypothesis could explain the aminoaciduria, diminished brush-border vesicle accumulation of amino acids, and failure of the brush border to demonstrate an adaptive response to a dietary deficiency.

Protein phosphorylation has been proposed as a controlling factor for amino acid transport. Intracellular protein kinases, including protein kinase A, protein kinase C, and calcium calmodulin–dependent protein kinase, have been shown to modulate amino acid transport. Studies by Zelikovic and associates showed that (1) exogenous and endogenous calcium-dependent protein kinases inhibit proline uptake in brush-border membrane vesicles and (2) differential regulation of calcium-dependent and calcium-independent protein kinase C isoenzymes exists during development.[32-34] Taken together, these data point to a role for age-related changes in calcium-dependent protein kinases and their differential regulation during development in the maturation of renal amino acid transport.

On the whole, studies in the developing animal point to maturational events at both the brush border and basolateral membrane that are necessary for the efficient reabsorption of amino acid seen in the adult mature animal. At present, the two most likely explanations are (1) diminished efflux at the basolateral membrane leading to backleak into the tubule urine (see *site 3* in Fig. 133-1) and (2) diminished apical transport in the most immature animals (see *site 1* in Fig. 133-1). Of course, questions remain. (1) Is there a qualitative, generalized membrane difference that could explain developmental aminoaciduria? (2) What is the maturational signal?

The interest in developmental amino acid transport is not merely the study of a fascinating biologic question. Geggel and associates[35] reported abnormal retinograms and low plasma taurine levels in infants receiving long-term taurine-free parenteral nutrition. More recently, Zelikovic and colleagues[36] reported that low birth weight infants receiving total parenteral nutrition can become taurine depleted, in part because of immaturity of the reabsorptive function of the proximal tubule. For some amino acids, such as taurine, the kidney may be the major regulator of that amino acid's body pools. With immaturity (developmental aminoaciduria), the kidney may not be able to adapt sufficiently during periods of deficient intake, and body stores of certain amino acids will be depleted. This could lead to important growth and maturational effects.

Much remains to be learned, but the studies to date of developmental renal amino acid transport suggest that at least two aspects of transport across the proximal tubule undergo change in the postnatal period: diminished efflux from the tubular epithelial cell and diminished transport into the tubular epithelial cell in the infant compared with those in the adult. Future study likely will focus on the exact membrane changes that underlie this developmental change.

REFERENCES

1. Guillery EN, et al: Functional development of the kidney in utero. In Polin RA, Fox WW (eds): Fetal and Neonatal Physiology. Philadelphia, WB Saunders, 1998, pp 1560-1573.
2. Zelikovic I: Aminoaciduria and Glycosuria. In Barratt TM, et al (eds): Pediatric Nephrology. Baltimore, Williams & Wilkins, 1994, pp 507-527.
3. Silbernagel S: Amino acids and oligopeptides. In Seldin DW, Giebisch G (eds): The Kidney: Physiology and Pathophysiology. New York, Raven Press, 1992, pp 2889-2920.
4. Silbernagel S: Renal transport of amino acids. Klin Wochenschr 57:1009, 1979.
5. Ullrich KJ, et al: Sodium dependence of amino acid transport in the proximal convolution of the rat kidney. Pflugers Arch 351:49, 1974.
6. Ullrich KJ: Sugar, amino acid and Na cotransport in the proximal tubule. Annu Rev 41:181, 1979.
7. Scriver CR, Rosenberg LE: Distributions of amino acids in body fluids. In Amino Acid Metabolism and Its Disorders. Philadelphia, WB Saunders, 1973, pp 39-60.
8. Scriver CR, et al: Genetic aspects of renal tubular transport: diversity and topology of carriers. Kidney Int 9:149, 1976.
9. Brodehl J, Gellissen K: Endogenous renal transport of free amino acids in infancy and childhood. Pediatrics 421:395, 1968.
10. Baerlocher KE, et al: Ontogeny of iminoglycine transport in mammalian kidney. Proc Natl Acad Sci U S A 65:1009, 1970.
11. Baerlocher KE, et al: The ontogeny of amino acid transport in rat kidney. I. Effect on distribution ratios and intracellular metabolism of proline and glycine. Biochim Biophys Acta 249:353, 1971.
12. Segal S, et al: Separate transport systems for sugars and amino acids in developing rat kidney cortex. Proc Natl Acad Sci U S A 68:372, 1971.
13. Roth KS, et al: Ontogeny of glycine transport in isolated rat renal tubules. Am J Physiol 233:F241, 1977.
14. Reynolds R, et al: On the development of glycine transport systems by rat renal cortex. Biochim Biophys Acta 511:274, 1978.
15. Meadow ME, et al: Renal brush border membrane vesicles from newborn rat by free flow electrophoresis and their prolive uptake. Biochem J 214:209, 1983.
16. Hwang SM, et al: Developmental pattern of cystine transport in isolated rat renal tubules. Biochim Biophys Acta 690:145, 1978.
17. Foreman JW, et al: Developmental aspects of cystine transport in the dog. Pediatr Res 20:593, 1986.
18. McGivan JD, Pastor-Anglader M: Regulatory and molecular aspects of mammalian amino acid transport. Biochem J 299:321, 1994.
19. Molandro MS, Kilberg MS: Molecular biology of mammalian amino acid transporters. Annu Rev Biochem 65:305, 1996.
20. Chesney RW, Jax DK: Developmental aspects of renal β-amino acid transport. I. Ontogeny of taurine reabsorption and accumulation in rat renal cortex. Pediatr Res 13:854, 1979.
21. Chesney RW, Jax DK: Developmental aspects of renal β-amino acid transport. II. Ontogeny of uptake and efflux processes and effect of anoxia. Pediatr Res 13:861, 1979.
22. Friedman AL, et al: Developmental aspects of renal β-amino acid transport. III. Characteristics of transport in isolated renal tubules. Pediatr Res 15:10, 1981.
23. Friedman AL, et al: Renal adaptation to alteration in dietary amino acid intake. Am J Physiol 245:F159, 1983.
24. Chesney RW, et al: Renal adaptation to altered dietary sulfur amino acid intake occurs at the luminal brush border membrane. Kidney Int 24:588, 1983.
25. Chesney RW, et al: Developmental aspects of renal β-amino acid transport. IV. Brush border membrane response to altered intake of sulfur amino acids. Pediatr Res 18:611, 1984.
26. Chesney RW, et al: Divergent membrane maturation in rat kidney: exposure to dietary taurine manipulation. Int J Pediatr Nephrol 6:93, 1985.
27. Chesney RW, et al: Developmental aspects of renal β-amino acid transport. V. Brush border membrane transport in nursing animals-effects of age and diet. Pediatr Res 20:980, 1986.
28. Chesney RW, et al: Renal adaptation to dietary amino acid alteration is expressed in immature renal brush border membranes. Pediatr Nephrol 2:146, 1988.
29. Chesney RW, et al: Factors affecting the transport of β-amino acids in rat renal brush border membrane vesicles: the role of external chloride. Biochim Biophys Acta 812:702, 1985.
30. Goldman DR, et al: L-Proline transport by newborn rat kidney brush border vesicles. Biochem J 178:253, 1979.
31. Zelikovic I, Chesney RW: Development of renal amino acid transport. Semin Nephrol 9:49, 1989.
32. Chesney RW, et al: Renal amino acid transport: cellular and molecular events from clearance studies to frog eggs. Pediatr Nephrol 7:574, 1993.
33. Zelikovic I, Przekwas J: The role of protein phosphoregulation in renal amino acid transport. Pediatr Nephrol 7:621, 1993.
34. Zelikovic I, et al: Ca++ dependent protein kinases inhibit proline transport across the rat renal brush border membrane. Am J Physiol 268:F155, 1995.
35. Geggel HS, et al: Nutritional requirement for taurine in patients receiving long term parenteral nutrition. N Engl J Med 312:142, 1985.
36. Zelikovic I, et al: Taurine depletion in very low birth weight infants receiving prolonged total parenteral nutrition: the role of immaturity. J Pediatr 116:301, 1990.

134 Developmental Aspects of Organic Acid Transport

Renal tubular capacity for organic acid secretion undergoes prenatal and postnatal maturation, as do glomerular filtration and other tubular functions. Organic acids include endogenous compounds, such as uric acid, hippurate, and prostaglandins, as well as many exogenous acids, such as diuretics and antibiotics (Table 134-1). Because many drugs are secreted by the organic acid transporter, the development of this system is important. Studies of the developmental aspects of renal organic anion transport primarily have concentrated on renal tubular transport of p-aminohippurate (PAH), the standard substrate for clearance studies. The original developmental studies of organic anion transport often use the tissue slice technique. In this method, the uptake of radiolabeled compounds into tissue slices can be quantified and expressed as a slice/media (S/M) ratio. Because the patterns of postnatal development of renal organic acid secretion may differ among species, care must be exercised in generalizing findings to humans.

Organic acids (or anions), such as PAH, are secreted by the proximal tubule. The net direction of movement is from the basolateral (blood side) membrane of the proximal tubular cell and then out into the proximal tubular fluid. The relative magnitude of organic acid transport along the proximal tubule segments (S1, S2, and S3) is species dependent.[1] PAH secretion is accomplished by two basic steps. At the basolateral membrane, exchange of extracellular organic anions with α-ketoglutarate allows the transport of substrate against a concentration gradient. Basolateral transport of PAH is indirectly dependent on basolateral sodium as a result of the coupling of PAH transport to a dicarboxylic acid (α-ketoglutarate).[2] This so-called *tertiary active transport* is linked to sodium because the dicarboxylic acid is co-transported along with three sodium ions. Sodium dicarboxylate transport is maintained by a sodium, potassium, adenosine triphosphatase (Na^+, K^+-ATPase)–generated sodium gradient (Fig. 134-1). Once inside the proximal tubular cell, in the second step of PAH secretion, PAH exits the cell in exchange for an anion at the luminal membrane by the organic anion/OH^- antiporter, a transport system shared with urate in some species.[3] An additional luminal voltage-driven efflux mechanism for PAH secretion has been proposed as an alternative pathway for luminal organic acid exit along its concentration gradient.[3]

The gene for the organic anion transporter has been isolated in humans, with four isoforms identified thus far: OAT1, OAT2, OAT3, and OAT4.[4] The protein has 551 amino acids and 12 transmembrane domains, and it shares nearly 50% structural homology with the flounder OAT (fOAT). There is also structural homology of the OAT family of transporters with the organic cation transporters (OCT). There are shared substrates between the two systems as well: verapamil, clonidine, cimetidine, cortisol, and aldosterone. OAT1 is exclusively localized to the basolateral membrane of the proximal renal tubule and is the PAH/dicarboxylate exchanger also elucidated by physiologic studies.[5] OAT3 is a lower affinity organic anion transporter also found along the basolateral membrane of the proximal renal tubule. Whereas the two systems share substrates, they are distinct. The Michaelis-Menten constant (K_m) values for PAH are 9.3 μM for OAT1 and 87.2 μM for OAT3.

Developmental expression of mRNA for each OAT isoform was studied in the rat. Levels of mRNA were low at birth. OAT1 expression, which was primarily localized to the kidney, reached adult levels by day 30 of life.[6] Alternatively, OAT2 mRNA did not increase until after day 30. OAT3 mRNA levels increased rapidly during the first 10 days of life. The impact of developmental differences among the three transporters has not been elucidated.[6]

The ability of the kidney to produce a concentration gradient of organic anions is present in early gestation. Both mesonephros and metanephros of the developing chick are able to accumulate PAH.[7] Organic acid transport of the chick mesonephros peaks as early as 9 days after fertilization and then begins to decline by 17 days, when the metanephros displays significant PAH accumulation. Uptake of ^{3}H-PAH in tissue slices from fetal mice increases from 24% of adult values in 16-day-old fetuses to 79% in 19-day-old fetuses.[8] Organic cation concentration has a different pattern of maturation. Maximal PAH-concentrating ability peaks before that of organic bases or tetraethylammonium (the standard substrate) in both the mesonephros and the metanephros of the chick embryo. Similarly, the uptake of radiolabeled tetraethylammonium into tissue slices is only 24% of adult values in 19-day-old fetal mice, whereas PAH is 79% of adult values.[8]

Studies performed in newborn humans,[9] dogs,[10] and rats[11] demonstrate a gradual increase in renal extraction of PAH with age. When PAH transport is examined using renal tissue slices from rabbits, S/M ratios peak at approximately 150% of adult values by 1 month of age and then decline to values similar to those in adults by 3 months of age. Both clearance and renal extraction of PAH are reduced in human infants and neonates. Calcagno and Rubin[9] found PAH extraction and clearances in infants 3 months of age and younger to be approximately 30% lower than values in older children. Postnatal maturation of PAH clearance and extraction has been found in most animal species studied. In the neonatal puppy, clearance studies indicate that the maximal tubular transport of PAH gradually increases by 10-fold over the first 8 weeks of life, although values are still reduced compared with those in adult animals.[12] Parallel studies, using the tissue slice technique, demonstrated a rather dramatic peak in the S/M ratio of PAH at 4 weeks of age, after which the S/M ratio declined to adult values over the next several weeks. Kim and colleagues[13] found S/M ratios for PAH to be 3.23 ± 0.27 in tissue slices from 2-day-old rats compared with 6.93 ± 0.337 in 10-day-old rats and 4.94 ± 0.28 in 14-day-old rats. By 20 days of age, S/M ratios were still less than adult levels.

This apparent discrepancy between *in vivo* and *in vitro* findings may be explained by the somewhat artificial nature of the slice method as well as the possible contributions made by maturational differences in PAH efflux and protein binding. Cole and co-workers[14] found different maturational patterns in PAH uptake, efflux, and ligandin binding. Consistent with previous reports, there was a gradual increase in intracellular/media PAH ratios in rabbit cortical slices up to 4 weeks of age, at which time the ratio exceeded levels in adults and then declined to adult values by 10 weeks of age. The rate of ^{14}C-labeled PAH uptake reached adult values by 4 weeks of age and was maintained at adult levels from 6 to 10 weeks to adulthood. Efflux of PAH in fetal, 2-week-old, and 4-week-old rabbits was lower than in adult animals and attained adult levels by 6 weeks of age. In addition, ligandin levels were lower in immature animals and gradually increased with age. Thus, developmental patterns of PAH transport, observed *in vitro*, may be the result of the sum of changes in efflux and transport as well as the fraction of protein-bound PAH at a given age.

TABLE 134-1

Example of Common Organic Acids Secreted by Proximal Tubule

Exogenous acids

Furosemide
Thiazides
Acetazolamide
Antimicrobials
    Penicillins
    Cephalosporins
Azidothymidine
Salicylates
Indomethacin
Probenecid
Iodinated contrast media
Morphine

Endogenous acids

Uric acid
Hippurates
Oxalate
Prostaglandins
Bile salts
Benzoates
Cyclic adenosine monophosphate

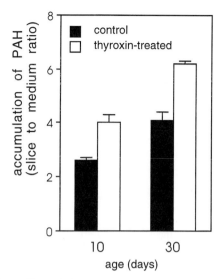

Figure 134–2. Effect of thyroid hormone treatment on *p*-aminohippurate (PAH) accumulation by renal cortical slices from 10- and 30-day-old rats. (Modified from Braunlich H: Pediatr Nephrol *2*:151, 1988.)

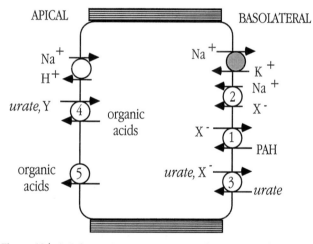

Figure 134–1. Schematic representation of organic acid transport by the renal proximal tubular cell: (1) basolateral anion exchanger specific for p-aminohippurate (PAH) with α-ketoglutarate as the primary anion exchanged for PAH; (2) coupled co-transport of organic acids such as ketoglutarate with sodium; (3) facilitated transport of uric acid or anion exchange for anions of different specificity; (4) bidirectional luminal urate-anion exchanger; (5) probenecid-sensitive pathway driven by the inside negative potential favors PAH exit. X = α-ketoglutarate; Y = chloride, bromide, losartan, lactate, furosemide, probenecid.

Enhancement of PAH transport occurs when organic acids (substrates for the transport system) are administered to animals before the study. In rabbits, the S/M ratios of PAH increase from birth to 4 weeks of age and then gradually decline to adult levels.[15] When procaine penicillin was given to 2- and 4-week-old rabbits for 3 consecutive days, there was an increase in PAH transport in the 2-week-old animals but not in the 4-week-old animals, a finding suggesting that administration of organic acids to immature animals may induce maturation of the tubular transport process.[15] In addition, when pregnant animals received daily procaine penicillin during the last half of their pregnancy, S/M ratios of PAH in the offspring were markedly increased when compared with those in age-matched controls during the first 2 postnatal weeks, after which time values were equal to those in controls.[15] Subsequent studies have corroborated these findings.[16,17] There may be species-related or compound-related differences in the response to organic acid exposure. Stopp and Braunlich[17] failed to induce increases in PAH transport after treatment of neonatal (5-day-old) rats with sulfamethoxypyridazine, cyclopenthiazide, and phenobarbital, although 2-week-old rabbits did exhibit increases in PAH transport after administration of these compounds.

In vivo administration of triiodothyronine (T₃) enhances PAH uptake into cortical tissue slices from weanling rats without affecting PAH uptake of adult slices.[18] Other investigators have found conflicting responses of PAH secretion to T₃. Braunlich[19] demonstrated that T₃ stimulates PAH transport in both 10- and 30-day-old rats (Fig. 134-2). The stimulatory action of T₃ on PAH transport can be prevented by the simultaneous administration of inhibitors of protein synthesis, neomycin and azauracil. Pretreatment of rats with thyroid-stimulating hormone does not have an effect on PAH accumulation.[19] One may conclude that the effect of T₃ on PAH uptake is dependent on protein synthesis (possibly reflecting synthesis of new transporters) and that pharmacologic rather than physiologic doses are required to stimulate PAH transport.

Kinetic analysis of age-related changes in PAH transport in tissue slices has revealed that transporter affinity (K_m) for PAH remains constant at 0.50 mM, whereas the maximal PAH uptake increases as a function of age.[20] The stimulatory effect of organic anions on renal tubular secretion of PAH during early development is related to their ability to increase the maximal transport capacity for PAH rather than to an effect on K_m.[17] There appears to be no detectable effect on efflux. It is speculated that *de novo* synthesis of new transporters occurs both with maturation and after exposure to organic acids.

Na⁺,K⁺-ATPase activity increases with renal maturation. Developmental increases in the activity of this pump provide an additional influence on the renal tubular capacity for organic acid transport. Ouabain (inhibitor of Na⁺,K⁺-ATPase) exposure reduces PAH uptake into renal tissue slices. Stopp and Braunlich[21] demonstrated that addition of ouabain reduced PAH accumulation in renal cortical slices from 5-, 15-, 33-, and 53-day-old rats. In comparison with adult animals, immature animals exhibited a greater fraction of ouabain-sensitive transport. The ratio of ouabain-insensitive to ouabain-sensitive PAH transport increased from 1:4 in 5-day-old animals to 3:2 in adult animals.[18] In addition, after administration of organic acids, a greater proportion of PAH accumulation was found to be ouabain insensitive.

Rapid renal growth as well as the possibility of postnatal nephrogenesis in some species could explain some of the maturational changes observed in PAH secretion. Schwartz and colleagues[22] measured PAH uptake in isolated cortical tubules from 8- and 16-day-old rabbits. Transport capacity was then standardized for tubule length. An almost fivefold increase in transport capacity was observed in the older animals. Although tubular elongation could explain a fraction of the increasing transport of PAH observed with maturation, acquisition of transport sites was the major factor. Additional studies revealed that penicillin pretreatment increases intrinsic transport capacity by 89%.

Age-related changes in organic anion excretion result from increases in intrinsic renal tubular transport capacity and, to a lesser extent, increases in glomerular filtration and renal blood flow. Exposure to similar organic compounds stimulates the immature renal tubule to enhance transport, probably by increasing the density of transporters. Many drugs, such as antibiotics and diuretics, are secreted by the organic anion transport system. The newborn is less able to eliminate drugs when their elimination is dependent on renal tubular secretion.[23] Continued administration of some drugs, however, such as the penicillins, to the developing kidney may result in alterations of drug clearance by the mechanism of substrate stimulation. Such changes may require modification of drug dosage or dosing interval.[24] In addition, PAH clearance is not a reliable estimation of renal plasma flow in the newborn animal because of the reduced tubular secretion observed with immaturity.

URIC ACID TRANSPORT

Uric acid is freely filtered at the glomerulus; however, a wide variation in urate handling has been observed in different species.[1] For example, in the monkey, human, rat, and mongrel dog, the fractional excretion of urate is less than 100%, a finding indicating net reabsorption. In other species, such as the rabbit and pig, urate excretion is greater than the filtered rate, a finding indicative of net secretion. Species-dependent differences in net urate excretion and the parallel presence of both secretory and reabsorptive processes along the proximal tubule make characterization of the precise mechanisms of urate transport elusive.

The net reabsorption of urate across the proximal tubular epithelium involves a luminal anion exchange transporter, which is inhibited by SITS (4-acetamido-4′-isothio-cyanostilbene-2,2′-disulfonic acid), DIDS (4,4′-diisothiocyanostilbene-2,2′-disulfonic acid), probenecid, and furosemide.[1] Anions such as OH^-, bicarbonate, chloride, lactate, and some dicarboxylic acids are exchanged for urate by movement down their electrochemical gradient. Two basolateral mechanisms for urate transport are considered: an anion exchange system separate from the basolateral system for PAH and a facilitated carrier, which enables movement of urate down its electrochemical gradient. This process is driven by the inside-negative membrane potential. Although the basolateral anion exchanger is not shared with PAH, it is probably coupled to ketoglutarate in a manner similar to the PAH exchanger. Studies performed in brush-border membrane vesicles failed to demonstrate direct sodium dependence of urate transport; however, sodium is required for the intracellular movement of the anion that is exchanged for urate. Urate secretion occurs through a basolateral anion exchanger. This transporter is not affected by the presence of PAH. Once inside the cell, urate may

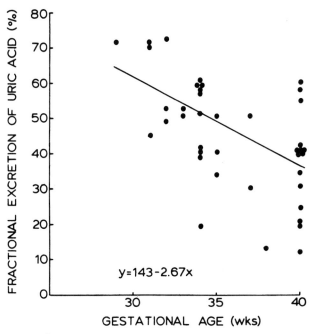

Figure 134–3. Fractional excretion of uric acid during the first day of life in infants according to gestational age. (From Stapleton FB: J Pediatr *103*:290, 1983.)

exit by a passive luminal mechanism or may use the luminal anion exchange transporter.[25] Those species in which urate secretion is the primary directive force appear to lack the luminal anion exchange system, although this remains under debate because a PAH- and probenecid-inhibitable system for urate transport is suggested by some studies.[3] In addition, some species appear to possess a common basolateral system for PAH and urate. Thus, discrimination among these organic acid transport mechanisms remains difficult and somewhat confusing.

The human renal urate anion exchanger gene (*URAT1*) has been identified.[26] As predicted, the urate-anion exchanger exhibits 42% homology with the OAT4 organic anion exchanger and has a similar predicted structure with 12 transmembrane domains. Immunohistochemical analyses localized the protein to the luminal membrane of the proximal tubule, consistent with its role to mediate luminal reabsorption of urate. Using the *Xenopus* oocyte functional expression system, intracellular to extracellular chloride stimulated urate transport, as did organic anions. PAH did not have an effect on urate accumulation. Probenecid, phenylbutazone, nonsteroidal antiinflammatory drugs, diuretics, and losartan inhibited urate uptake.[26]

Details regarding the maturational pattern of uric acid transport are limited. Clearance studies have been performed in humans and mongrel puppies. Newborns have higher serum uric acid levels as well as elevated urinary urate excretion. As a rule, uric acid clearance increases and fractional excretion decreases during childhood.[27] Values for the fractional excretion of urate in 3- to 4-day-old term newborns were 20 to 59% compared with 13 to 26% in older infants up to 1 year of age and 11 to 17% in children aged 1 to 7 years. When fractional excretion of uric acid was examined during the first 24 hours of life in newborns of differing gestational ages, mean fractional excretion was $61.24 \pm 12.21\%$ in infants at 29 to 33 weeks' gestation, $44.52 \pm 15.23\%$ in neonates at 34 to 37 weeks' gestation, and $38.19 \pm 13.61\%$ in term infants (Fig. 134–3).[28] Serum uric acid levels and uric acid clearances were not significantly different among infants of differing gestational age.

In the mongrel dog, plasma uric acid decreases with age in a manner similar to that in humans. Stapleton and Arant[29]

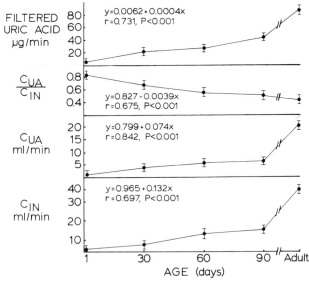

Figure 134–4. Patterns of renal clearance of uric acid (C_{UA}) and inulin (C_{IN}) in mongrel puppies during early development compared with values in adult dogs.

demonstrated that the clearance of uric acid increased and fractional excretion of uric acid decreased as a function of postnatal age (Fig. 134-4). Uric acid clearance increased from 0.39 ml/minute at 1 day of age to 3.72, 5.54, and 6.3 ml/minute at 30, 60, and 90 days of age, still lower than the adult value of 20.16 ml/minute. At 1, 30, 60, and 90 days of age, the fractional excretion of urate was 83%, 69%, 57%, and 51%, compared with the adult value of 44%. Decreased fractional excretion of urate in the presence of an increased filtered load can be explained by either increased reabsorption or decreased secretion with increasing age. Studies done to date have not answered this question; however, the net reabsorption of urate in the mongrel dog increased from 0.2 µg/minute at 1 day of age to 8.8, 11.9, and 22.2 µg/minute at 30, 60, and 90 days, respectively. Adult animals exhibited a net reabsorption of urate of 39 µg/minute.[24]

Urate uptake has been measured using tissue slices obtained from fetal and newborn mice.[5] Accumulation of ^{14}C-labeled uric acid by slices from 16-day fetuses was 49% of adult levels and increased to 79% of adult values at 19 days' gestation. At day 1 postnatal age, a transient decline in urate accumulation to 58% of adult values was observed; however, urate accumulation increased to 70% of adult values by 7 to 8 postnatal days.[8] This developmental pattern was similar to that observed for PAH. In contrast to PAH, however, uric acid uptake into renal cortical slices is not enhanced by pretreatment of neonatal animals with acetate or procaine penicillin.[23]

The mechanisms responsible for the increase in net tubular urate reabsorption associated with maturation are not fully understood. One may anticipate that nonspecific cellular events, as well as increased transport capacity of either or both luminal and basolateral transport systems for urate, could account for the decrease in fractional excretion with increasing age; however, these events have yet to be characterized by kinetic or molecular studies.

REFERENCES

1. Burckhardt G, Pritchard JB: Organic anion and cation antiporters. *In* Seldin DW, Giebisch G (eds): The Kidney: Physiology and Pathophysiology. Philadelphia, Lippincott Williams & Wilkins, 2000, pp 193–222.
2. Shimada H, et al: Indirect coupling to Na⁺ of *p*-aminohippuric acid uptake into rat renal basolateral vesicles. Am J Physiol *253*:F795, 1987.
3. Pritchard JB, Miller DS: Mechanisms mediating renal secretion of organic anions and cations. Physiol Rev *73*:765, 1993.
4. Motohashi H, et al: Gene expression levels and immunolocalization of organic ion transporters in the human kidney. J Am Soc Nephrol *13*:866, 2002.
5. Kojima R, et al: Immunolocalization of multispecific organic anion transporters, OAT1, OAT2, and OAT 3 in rat kidney. J Am Soc Nephrol *13*:848, 2002.
6. Buist SC, et al: Gender-specific and developmental influences on the expression of rat organic anion transporters. J Pharmacol Exp Ther *301*:145, 2002.
7. Rennick BR: Development of renal accumulation of organic ions by chick embryo. Am J Physiol *217*:247, 1969.
8. Diezi J, Michoud-Hausel P: Fetal development of renal tubular transports and ATPase activity. Proceedings of the 7th International Congress of Nephrology, 1978, pp 263–266.
9. Calcagno PL, Rubin MI: Renal extraction of *para*-aminohippurate in infants and children. J Clin Invest *42*:1632, 1963.
10. Kleinman LI, Lubbe RJ: Factors affecting the maturation of renal PAH extraction in the newborn dog. J Physiol *23*:411, 1972.
11. Horster M, Lewy JE: Filtration fraction and extraction of PAH during neonatal period in the rat. Am J Physiol *219*:1061, 1970.
12. Hook JB, et al: Functional maturation of renal PAH transport in the dog. Can J Physiol Pharmacol *48*:169, 1970.
13. Kim JK, et al: In vivo analysis of organic ion transport in renal cortex of the newborn rat. Pediatr Res *6*:600, 1972.
14. Cole BR, et al: Maturation of *p*-aminohippuric acid transport in the developing rabbit kidney: interrelationships of the individual components. Pediatr Res *12*:992, 1978.
15. Hirsch GH, Hook JB: Maturation of renal organic acid transport: substrate stimulation by penicillin. Science *165*:909, 1969.
16. Pegg DG, et al: Substrate stimulation of aminohippuric acid transport: effect on uptake and runout. Proc Soc Exp Biol Med *149*:546, 1975.
17. Stopp M, Braunlich H: In vitro analysis of drug-induced stimulation of renal tubular *p*-aminohippurate (PAH) transport in rats. Biochem Pharmacol *29*:983, 1980.
18. Hirsch GH, Hook JB: Stimulation of *p*-aminohippurate transport by slices of rat renal cortex following in vivo administration of triiodothyronine. Proc Soc Exp Biol Med *131*:513, 1969.
19. Braunlich H: Hormonal control of postnatal development of renal tubular transport of weak organic acids. Pediatr Nephrol *2*:151, 1988.
20. Stopp M, Braunlich H: Kinetics of *p*-aminohippurate transport in renal cortical slices from neonatal and adult rats. Biochem Pharmacol *26*:1809, 1977.
21. Stopp M, Braunlich H: *p*-Aminohippurate (PAH) transport and Na-K-ATPase activity in rat renal cortical slices during postnatal maturation and drug induced stimulation. Biochem Pharmacol *32*:3675, 1983.
22. Schwartz GJ, et al: *p*-Aminohippurate transport in the proximal straight tubule: development and substrate stimulation. Pediatr Res *12*:793, 1978.
23. Hook JB, Hewitt WR: Development of mechanisms for drug excretion. Am J Med *62*:497, 1977.
24. Schwartz GJ, et al: Subtherapeutic dicloxacillin levels in a neonate: possible mechanisms. J Pediatr *89*:310, 1976.
25. Kahn AM, Weinman EJ: Urate transport in the proximal tubule: in vivo and vesicle studies. Am J Physiol *249*:F789, 1985.
26. Enomoto A, et al: Molecular identification of a renal urate anion exchanger that regulates blood urate levels. Nature *417*:447, 2002.
27. Passwell JH, et al: Fractional excretion of uric acid in infancy and childhood: index of tubular maturation. Arch Dis Child *49*:878, 1974.
28. Stapleton FB: Renal uric acid clearance in human neonates. J Pediatr *103*:290, 1983.
29. Stapleton FB, Arant BS: Ontogeny of renal uric acid excretion in the mongrel puppy. Pediatr Res *15*:1513, 1981.

Michael A. Linshaw

Concentration and Dilution of the Urine

PHYSIOLOGY OF THE URINARY CONCENTRATING MECHANISM

The ability to concentrate and dilute the urine greatly expands our range of habitable environments. To accomplish this, the mammalian kidney must deliver sufficient solute to the medulla, establish a solute gradient that increases from cortex to papilla, preserve the gradient despite its tendency to dissipate from continuous flow of blood, and stimulate or suppress reabsorption of water as needed. A solute gradient can develop because membranes of tubule segments have varying solute permeability characteristics. Once a solute gradient is established, water movement from tubule lumen toward the interstitial gradient depends largely on the tubular response to antidiuretic hormone (ADH, vasopressin) and the anatomic integrity of the tubulovascular structures (Fig. 135-1). Since fluid is reabsorbed isotonically in proximal tubules and is not concentrated in distal convoluted tubules, major steps in the concentrating process involve events occurring in the loops of Henle and collecting tubules. A vital site of active salt transport occurs at the thick ascending loop of Henle; other nephron segments move solute and water passively, thereby facilitating conservation of energy. The actual process of urinary concentration requires the presence of ADH and occurs in collecting ducts where water is avidly reabsorbed down an osmolar gradient generated initially by active salt reabsorption in the thick ascending limb of Henle. Good reviews with detailed discussion and extensive references on the urinary concentrating mechanism are available.[1]

Development of the Medullary Gradient

Several processes illustrated in Figure 135-2 occur simultaneously, but it is convenient to start a discussion of the concentrating mechanism at the thick ascending limb of Henle in the outer medulla.[2-4] This segment has a very low hydraulic conductivity, but it can reabsorb NaCl in the relative absence of water (reabsorbs hypertonic NaCl). The result is dilution of fluid remaining in the tubular lumen and an increase in the interstitial concentration of NaCl surrounding the thick limbs. Isotonic fluid from the proximal tubule enters the descending loop of Henle at the level of the outer medulla and is exposed to the increased interstitial osmolality. Descending loop segments have a high hydraulic conductivity, but a low sodium permeability. As a consequence, water in the descending limb moves osmotically into the interstitium, and fluid in the lumen of this segment becomes more concentrated.

Urine, flowing through the thick ascending limb, becomes progressively dilute by virtue of the relative impermeability of this segment to water and then enters the distal convoluted tubule, a cortical segment in which water and salt reabsorption and equilibration with blood produce a largely isotonic urine entering the outer medullary collecting duct. In a hypertonic outer medulla, water is osmotically removed from the tubule lumen, and solutes in the collecting duct become increasingly concentrated. Urea movement in distal tubules is limited, but water reabsorption is substantial, so cortical collecting tubules receive urine with a high urea concentration. This segment has low urea permeability both in the presence and absence of ADH, so a high

urea concentration is maintained in urine entering the outer medullary collecting duct. The outer medullary collecting duct has a low permeability to sodium and urea and is not thought to transport NaCl actively. This segment probably does not contribute to the high interstitial salt content, but its water permeability is high in the presence of ADH.

Vasopressin also stimulates NaCl reabsorption by the medullary thick ascending limb, thereby increasing NaCl content in the outer medullary interstitium.[5-7] This latter step may help counteract the dilution of interstitial NaCl that follows when ADH induces water reabsorption from the outer medullary collecting duct. The net effect of ADH is to increase the osmotic driving force and subsequent reabsorption of water as urine from the collecting tubule traverses the outer medulla. The high water and relatively low urea permeability cause urea to become a dominant solute in the outer medullary collecting duct. The outer medullary interstitium contains relatively little urea, but a significant amount of NaCl reabsorbed from the ascending thick limb. A high luminal urea concentration can drive water toward the tubule lumen. Conversely, a high interstitial NaCl concentration can drive luminal fluid to the interstitium.

Although osmolality is equal across the collecting duct epithelium, the net driving force favors water reabsorption from the lumen because NaCl has a higher reflection coefficient than does urea and exerts a more effective osmotic pressure.[8] This further increases urea concentration in urine entering the inner medullary collecting duct. In contrast to the more proximal collecting duct, the inner medullary collecting duct is permeable to urea in the presence of ADH.[6,7] Vasopressin also increases the permeability of this segment to water, although urea and water may traverse different channels.[9]

Urea diffuses down a chemical gradient to enter the medullary interstitium. Urea can also enter the descending limb, and its concentration actually rises in this segment. Accumulation of urea in the interstitium provides an osmotic driving force that further abstracts water from medullary portions of the descending loop. This increases the luminal concentration of NaCl and urea. The water leaving the descending loop dilutes interstitial NaCl. When urine turns the bend of the loop and enters the thin ascending limb of Henle, the high NaCl concentration in this segment is exposed to an interstitium of similar osmolality but lower NaCl concentration; the remainder of the osmolar concentration is composed mainly of urea. The thin ascending limb has a low hydraulic conductivity, a high NaCl permeability, and a moderate permeability to urea;[10] NaCl can thereby diffuse down its concentration gradient into the interstitium while water tends to remain in the lumen.

The urine begins to become progressively less concentrated, and NaCl accumulates in the interstitium. The presence of this added interstitial NaCl abstracts more water from urine in the inner medullary collecting duct as this segment courses through the interstitium, a step that further concentrates the final urine. In addition, urea can re-enter the lumen of thin ascending limbs to recycle back to the collecting tubule.

While the hypertonic medulla provides the driving force for water reabsorption and urinary concentration, it is noteworthy that cells in the renal medulla are under considerable osmolar stress from the hyperosmolar state. The major solutes are urea

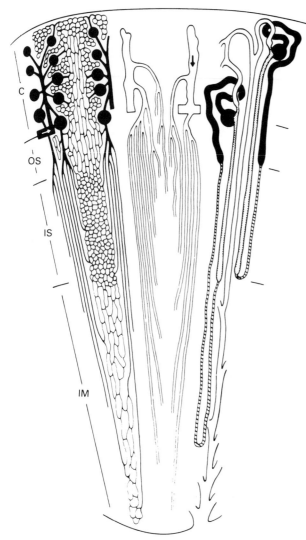

Figure 135–1. Anatomy of tubules and blood vessels and relationship of superficial and deep nephrons. C = cortex; OS = outer stripe; IS = inner stripe; IM = inner medulla. (From Zimmerhackl BL, et al: Kidney Int *31*:641, 1987.)

and salt, the latter capable of damaging cellular DNA and causing cell death when salt concentration is sufficiently high. The medullary cells adapt by synthesizing and accumulating relatively nonpermeant organic solutes. A regulatory protein, tonicity-responsive enhancer binding protein, stimulates genes to produce proteins that transport or synthesize the protective organic osmolytes.[11,12]

Role of Short-Loop Nephrons and Urea

Recycling of urea (to maintain a high medullary urea content) is critical for maximal efficiency of the concentrating process and is facilitated by short-looped nephrons that do not descend deep into the inner medulla.[13,14] These nephrons reabsorb a large portion of filtrate, reducing the volume of fluid and solute that needs to be concentrated. Short-looped nephrons also exhibit permeability and anatomic characteristics that place them in good position to receive urea and facilitate its recycling to the inner medulla.[5] For example, in the rat, urea permeability of thin limbs is greater in short-looped than in long-looped nephrons. Moreover, in contrast to long-looped nephrons, short-looped thin descending limbs run within vascular bundles and are closely

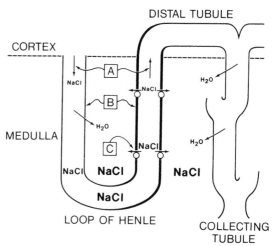

Figure 135–2. The countercurrent movement of water and solutes between the loops of Henle and the collecting tubule. Heavier lines of the ascending thin limb in the inner medulla and of the ascending thick limb in the outer medulla depict impermeability to water. NaCl is actively reabsorbed from the thick limb, diluting urine and increasing osmolality of the outer medulla (1). Water reabsorption continues in the distal tubule and the cortical and outer medullary collecting duct, leading to increased urea concentration (2). Water and urea are reabsorbed from the inner medullary collecting duct (3). Urea accumulates in the interstitium, osmotically abstracts water from the descending limb, and allows NaCl concentration (A) in descending limb fluid to increase and (B) in interstitium to decrease (4). The thin ascending limb is permeable to NaCl and receives fluid rich in NaCl. NaCl enters the interstitium down its concentration gradient, and urine becomes hypo-osmotic to the surrounding interstitium (5). See text for details. (Reprinted by permission of the New England Journal of Medicine, *295*:1059, 1976.)

apposed to vasa rectae that ascend from the inner medulla and contain blood with increased amounts of urea.

The recycling of urea is thought to be accomplished through three major routes (Fig. 135–3). First, urea in the ascending thin limb can remain in the tubule lumen, travel through the distal nephron to the collecting ducts, and then recycle to the interstitium. Second, urea in thin ascending limbs can reach the thick ascending limb, a segment that, in the outer medulla, is permeable to urea and is in close relationship to proximal straight tubules (and therefore descending limbs) of both long- and short-loop nephrons. At this site, urea can return to the inner medulla directly via proximal straight tubules and descending limbs of long-loop nephrons, or it can cycle through loops and collecting ducts of short nephrons to re-enter the medulla. Third, urea can leave the inner medullary interstitium through ascending vasa rectae and re-enter descending limbs of short-looped nephrons. This urea can similarly be carried back through superficial distal nephrons and transported to collecting ducts in the inner medulla.

Urea transfer from vasa rectae to short nephron descending limbs is likely facilitated by the anatomic proximity of these structures in vascular bundles of the inner stripe of the outer medulla. The solute delivered to deep thin ascending limbs of the inner medulla can recycle to maintain a continued presence of deep medullary solute. The solute helps concentrate fluid in the descending limbs of long-looped nephrons and is available to enhance movement of water from the collecting duct before the urine reaches the renal pelvis and ureter. The importance of urea transport in this process is underscored by the presence of urea

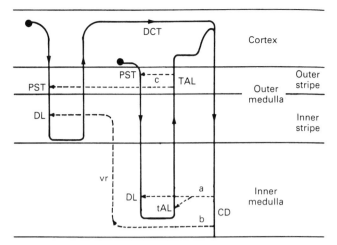

Figure 135–3. Urea recycling pathways in mammalian kidney. Short-looped nephron *(left)* and long-looped nephron *(right)* are depicted by solid lines. Urea transfer between segments at sites a, b, and c is indicated by *dashed arrows*. See text for details. PST = proximal straight tubule; DL = descending limb; AL = thin ascending limb; TAL = thick ascending limb; DCT = distal convoluted tubule; CD = collecting duct; vr = vasa recta. (Reprinted by permission of the New England Journal of Medicine, *31*:629, 1987.)

transporters located in endothelial cells of medullary vasa rectae[15] and the ability of ADH to induce insertion of urea transporters in the luminal membrane of the inner medullary collecting duct.[16,17]

The role of urea is complex. Urea had been thought to cross cell membranes solely by passive diffusion, but rapid urea transport rates in some tissues suggested a facilitative transport mechanism. Several urea transporters (UTs) have been identified in renal tissue that can facilitate transmembrane movement of urea. These transporters may serve different functions. For example, UT-A genes express medullary proteins in inner medullary collecting ducts and thin descending limbs of Henle. These transporters can help generate the hypertonic medulla. Thirsting increases levels of UT-A2 protein, a response mediated by ADH. Rapid movement of urea actually may serve to dissipate a transmembrane osmotic urea gradient.[18-20] By contrast, the UT-B1 gene produces a transporter protein located in endothelial cells of medullary descending vasa recta that allows urea leaving the ascending vasa recta to re-enter the descending vasa recta, become "trapped" in the medulla, and maintain a high medullary urea concentration. It is interesting that the UT-B1 transporter protein is down-regulated by ADH. This may represent a metabolic adaptation to reduce the need for urea transport and allow for reduced urea synthesis in descending medullary vasa recta endothelial cells. It could serve either to favor nitric oxide over urea synthesis (for vasodilation and improved nutrient delivery) or to limit urea production in endothelial cells when a very high inner medullary content of urea is already present.[21,22]

Halperin and colleagues[23] provided insight about urea as an effective osmole for water transfer in the inner medulla. Only solutes with a concentration difference can affect water movement across a semipermeable membrane. ADH increases water and urea permeability in inner medullary collecting ducts. If urea is highly permeant across this membrane, urea concentration equilibrates and adds to final urine osmolality, but induces little increase in urine flow. In one set of experiments, subjects were either fasted or placed on a normal diet and then water-depleted. Those on a regular diet excreted largely urea and NaCl as their nonurea urinary osmoles. Fasted subjects excreted less urea, and their nonurea osmoles were largely NH_4^+ and β-hydroxybutyrate,

not NaCl. Their urea excretion rate and total urine osmolality were lower, but both groups had similar nonurea osmolality and urine flow rates. Therefore, urine flow was related mainly to nonurea osmolar load. Urea did not act as an effective osmole, inducing more water excretion as long as the nonurea osmolar load was similar.

When water-deprived subjects on a normal diet received a urea load, urine flow rate nearly doubled, and rates of excretion of both urea and nonurea osmoles increased. The total urine osmolality was unchanged since a decrease in nonurea osmolality (diluted by increased urine flow) accompanied the increase in urea osmolality generated by the urea load. Therefore, when mainly NaCl was excreted as nonurea solute, urea acted as an effective osmole and induced an osmotic diuresis. The investigators concluded that at low or modest excretion rates of urea, this solute equilibrates between collecting duct and interstitium so that urea exerts no significant osmotic effect and thus no increase in urine flow. Once a urea load is sufficiently large, it becomes an effective osmotic agent, increasing urine flow to help remove excess urea. Were urea not highly permeable, it would remain in the collecting duct lumen (obligate water excretion) and blunt the ability of the kidney to lower water excretion in times of water depletion. In addition, as relatively impermeant nonurea solutes, NH_4^+ and β-hydroxybutyrate ensure a minimal urine flow even during chronic fasting, reducing the risk for hyperkalemia and formation of calculi.[23]

In further studies,[24] human subjects on a regular diet were water deprived, given vasopressin, and then given hydrochlorothiazide to increase the proportion of urinary electrolytes comprising total urinary osmoles. Following the diuretic, the proportion of urea osmoles in urine dropped from about 50% to about 20% of total urinary osmoles. When these subjects, now excreting a high proportion of nonurea osmoles, also received a urea load, there was an increase in urea concentration, no change in nonurea osmolality or nonurea excretion rate, and no change in urine flow rate. By not increasing urinary flow, urea acted as an ineffective, highly permeant osmole. Under a different protocol, subjects received furosemide to induce negative NaCl balance and were placed on a low-salt diet to generate an electrolyte-poor urine. Subjects were then water deprived and given a urea load. With a low nonurea (electrolyte) osmolality, the urea load now induced a marked increase in urine flow rate and a decrease in nonurea osmolality, but no change in total urine osmolality. In this setting, urea acted as an effective, less permeant osmole.

Rats behaved similarly. When rat papillary tip and urine solute content were compared, total as well as urea and nonurea osmolalities were similar when urine had a high proportion of urinary electrolyte osmoles, indicating equilibration of urea and nonurea solutes between papillary interstitium and urine. By contrast, when rats were electrolyte deprived on a low-salt diet and given a urea load, urea concentration was higher in urine than in interstitium, nonurea (electrolyte) concentration was higher in the interstitium, and the total omolalities were similar. Urea now acted as a relatively impermeant osmole and did not equilibrate across the interstitium.

The importance of this finding is apparent when considering that kidneys must reduce urine volume when water conservation is needed (dehydration) without reducing volume so much as to increase the risk for hyperkalemia or stone formation. In the setting of volume depletion and low renal electrolyte excretion, urea becomes less permeant and obligates water, maintaining urine flow to more than severe oliguria. In the setting of adequate urinary electrolytes, the kidney excretes urea (main protein metabolic product) without increasing the minimum urine volume needed to excrete other solutes. This is accomplished because urea becomes more permeant, equilibrates across the medullary interstitium, and thereby is excreted without obligating more water. It is unclear how the kidney alters urea permeability in these situations, but the mechanism may involve a change in the function or number of urea transporters.

Role of Vasa Rectae

Vasa rectae are blood vessels coursing through the interstitium. They provide substrate for and remove end products of metabolic reactions. They also remove solute and fluid reabsorbed by tubules. The vessels are very permeable to solutes and water and have close countercurrent anatomic proximity to tubules. If the vessels coursed through the medullary interstitium only once, they would remove reabsorbed urea and NaCl, depleting the interstitium of solutes and compromising the solute gradient. To avoid this, vasa rectae descend into the medulla to varying degrees, break up into small capillaries that course through localized areas of interstitium, and rejoin to form ascending vasa rectae that move toward the cortex (Fig. 135–4). Descending and ascending vasa rectae are situated adjacently in vascular bundles

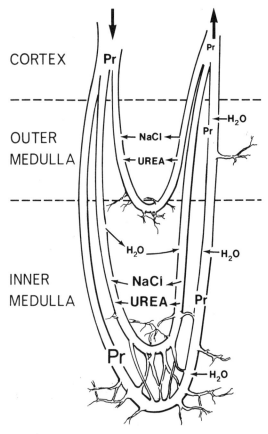

Figure 135–4. Countercurrent exchange in vasa recta. Medullary circulation includes network of interconnecting vessels and main thoroughfares. Vessels are freely permeable to NaCl, urea, and water. Type size denotes solute concentration relative to its location in medulla but not relative to concentration of another solute. Loops of Henle and collecting ducts are responsible for increasing concentration of interstitial NaCl and urea. Solutes can enter descending vasa recta and leave ascending vasa recta to remain trapped in medulla. As water leaves descending vasa recta, protein concentration increases. High osmotic and oncotic pressures in ascending vasa recta enhance capillary fluid uptake, returning water, reabsorbed from tubules, to general circulation. Therefore, vasa rectae trap solute and remove water, preserving hyperosmolality of the renal medulla. Pr = plasma protein. (Reprinted by permission of the New England Journal of Medicine, *295*:1059, 1976.)

and are poised to exchange water and solutes down their concentration gradients.[14, 25] Accordingly, NaCl, found in high concentration in ascending vasa rectae, can enter descending vasa rectae that contain fluid of lower solute concentration, while water can move in the opposite direction. As a result, fluid in the descending vessel penetrates deep in the medulla and carries a high solute concentration close to that in the interstitium. The driving force for passive loss of this solute from interstitium to vessels is thereby minimized. Part of the vascular bundle may include descending limbs of short-loop nephrons. This segment can take up solute from ascending vasa rectae and recycle it to collecting ducts traversing the deep medulla, where solute and water are further reabsorbed.

Role of the Renal Pelvis

The renal pelvis may contribute to urinary concentration.[26] Epithelium covering the inner medulla and papilla and facing the pelvic space is similar to that of papillary collecting ducts. During water diuresis, these cells are closely apposed and intercellular spaces are narrow. During antidiuresis, individual cells are more distinct, and intercellular spaces are widely dilated. This may reflect enhanced transepithelial movement of fluid.[27] Pelvic extensions in some species allow the urinary space to surround vascular bundles and much of the papillae and may reach the cortex.[13] Increased urine concentration has been related to an increase in contact surface area between papilla and pelvic urine.[27, 28] Moreover, an intact renal pelvis may be necessary to produce a maximally concentrated urine. If one excises the ureter to expose the renal papilla of a rat, urine osmolality at the papillary tip drops sharply by nearly 40%.[29] Urine in the renal pelvis circulating around the papillae and inner medulla may reach an area in the medullary interstitium where urea concentration is less than that in the urine. Urea could then recycle from pelvic urine to the medullary interstitium and help maintain a high medullary urea concentration gradient, enhancing abstraction of water from thin descending limbs of Henle. In this regard, the concentration of urea in fluid bathing the papilla, rather than the total osmolality, seems to be a critical factor in determining the final urine concentration. If the papilla is bathed with solutions of varying osmolality and urea concentration, the osmolality of urine from the papillary tip increases when the urea bath concentration is increased, but not necessarily when the bath osmolality is altered.[30] This hypothesis remains uncertain. Other investigators have not found significant urea reabsorption across this epithelium. In addition, not all rodents show a relation between extensions of renal pelvis and fornices around their papillae and the ability to maximally concentrate urine.[26]

Confusion about the impact of urine flow and pelvic reflux on papillary function is evident from some of the following considerations. Once urine leaves the papillary tip, it can descend the ureter, reflux slightly to surround a small portion of the papillary tip, or reflux fully over the entire fornices and pelvic extensions and cover more of the medulla in which solute and water exchange may occur. Full retrograde flow of urine over the entire papillary surface and up toward the outer medulla occurs with bladder and retrograde ureteric contractions. It can be stimulated by increasing hydrostatic pressure in the pelvis by as little as 1 cm H_2O. When the renal pelvis is removed, urine flow is nonpulsatile and continuous, a state not associated with full pelvic reflux. In contrast, when the renal pelvis is intact and performs its contractile or pulsatile action, urine flow in terminal collecting ducts is intermittent rather than continuous. During antidiuresis, when urine flow is slow and urine becomes highly concentrated, full pelvic refluxes also do not occur, even with an intact pelvis. Therefore, the importance of an intact renal pelvis to an efficient urinary concentrating ability may be related more to the contractile nature of the pelvis than to the actual degree of reflux. During a peristaltic contraction, a urine bolus through the terminal papillary collecting duct is seen to enter the renal pelvis quickly, following which urine flow ceases and collecting ducts become empty and remain collapsed for 95% of the time. When urine flow rates are slow, the velocity of a urine bolus is rapid, and the contact time between urine and epithelium at a site about 1 mm from the papillary tip is brief. At higher rates of urine flow, the urine bolus leaves the papillary tip more slowly, and there is actually a greater contact time between urine and papillary epithelium. Therefore, during antidiuresis, when urine flow is slow and urine becomes highly concentrated, the urine is in contact with the reabsorbing epithelium for a shorter time, and retrograde flow of pelvic urine, rich in urea, is an uncommon event.[26, 31-33]

Schmidt-Nielsen and colleagues proposed that during antidiuresis, urinary concentration is augmented by peristaltic action of the renal pelvis that causes intermittent flow of urine and helps urine equilibrate with the hypertonic papillary interstitium.[26, 31-33] The relatively small "tip" reflux in an antidiuretic state, coupled with the small area occupied by the papillary tip and the short contact time of urine with papillary epithelium, might lead one to conclude that solute and water exchange at this site are rather limited. More important, other papillary structures are also affected by the milking, contractile action of the renal pelvis. When the pelvis contracts and constricts the papilla, blood flow in the vasa rectae stops. This may reduce medullary solute washout by allowing more complete solute equilibration between ascending vasa rectae and interstitium. Flow in the loops of Henle is also slowed. This could help accumulate interstitial solute. Therefore, without full reflux, pelvic contraction may alter flow of solute in papillary structures to facilitate the increase in the interstitial solute gradient.[26, 31-33]

Role of Aquaporins

Aquaporins are proteins that traverse the cell membrane lipid bilayer. They appear to represent molecular water-transporting channels and are expressed in a wide variety of tissues.[34-37] Several reviews are available for the interested reader.[38-46] The first water channel protein to be identified, originally named CHIP-28 for the channel-forming integral protein, 28 kDa, was found to be abundant in red blood cells and proximal renal tubules. These tissues have high water permeability and facilitate the constitutive movement of water down an osmotic gradient. To determine whether this protein behaved as a water channel, investigators employed *Xenopus* oocytes, which can survive in fresh water owing to their very low water permeability. When complementary RNA of CHIP-28 was expressed in these oocytes, a dramatic increase in membrane water permeability was observed. The membranes behaved as though they contained water channels. This observation was confirmed by reconstituting the purified protein into proteoliposomes and demonstrating a dramatic increase in osmotic water permeability.[46-48] Seven aquaporins now identified in kidney tissue appear to have specific cellular localization.[42] Some features of aquaporins 1 to 4 are summarized in Table 135-1. Little is known yet about aquaporins 6 to 8.

Aquaporin-1 is found in renal proximal tubules, short- and long-loop thin descending limbs of Henle, and nonfenestrated endothelium of descending vasa rectae. It is not found in other tubule segments, including collecting ducts, or in ascending vasa rectae. These membranes have high osmotic water permeabilities. In nephron segments, this protein is identified in both apical and basolateral membranes, including both basal and lateral infoldings, but not to any substantial degree in cytoplasmic vesicle and vacuole membranes. Accordingly, aquaporin-1 is poised to facilitate transcellular water movement in segments responsible for reabsorbing a major portion of the glomerular filtrate, but it does not appear to require hormonal regulation and therefore is not the ADH-sensitive water channel.[49-51] This protein is also abundant in red blood cells, where it is thought to increase membrane permeability. Although individuals without functional CHIP water channels do not appear to have clinical abnormalities, such as polyuria,[52] rare individuals lacking aquaporin-1 have a urinary concentrating defect in response to ADH or to water deprivation.[53] The role of aquaporin-1 in maintaining urinary concentrating ability is appreciated from studies of transgenic knockout mice lacking aquaporin-1. These mice are polyuric and do not tolerate water deprivation.[54] Moreover, perfused proximal tubules[55] as well as descending thin limbs[56] from such mice have reduced osmotic water permeability. Thus

TABLE 135-1

Characteristics of Aquaporins Found in Kidney Tissue

Genetic Designation	Renal Localization	Proposed Physiologic Role
Aquaporin-1	Proximal tubule S1, S2, S3 segments of short-and long-looped nephrons Descending limb of Henle Nonfenestrated descending vasa rectae Limited in vesicles and vacuoles Present in both apical and basolateral membranes (basal and lateral aspects)	Major transmembrane pathway for H_2O flow, including entry and exit sites Not under hormonal control
Aquaporin-2	Outer and inner medullary collecting duct Primarily apical membrane and intracellular vesicles	The vasopressin-regulated H_2O channel. ADH induces movement of an intracellular vesicle pool of H_2O channels to the apical membrane
Aquaporin-3	Collecting duct principal cells in cortex and medulla; strongest medullary label is at base, not tip, of papilla Mainly in lateral and basolateral infoldings, not in basal aspect, of basolateral plasma membrane Virtually absent from apical membrane; minimally found in intracellular vesicles	Major exit site for osmotically driven H_2O transport; not regulated through vesicular trafficking via ADH; may provide for small nonelectrolyte solute movement
Aquaporin-4	Inner medullary collecting duct principal cells, especially proximal two-thirds of segment; very little in cortex and outer medulla Distributed roughly equally in basal and lateral domains of basolateral plasma membrane, and not in intracellular vesicles	Basolateral exit site of cellular H_2O transport of inner medullary collecting ducts

aquaporin-1 is necessary for maximal concentrating ability. This is likely related to the need for rapid equilibration of water across the thin descending limb of Henle in helping establish the countercurrent multiplication process.

Aquaporin-2 appears to be the ADH-regulated water channel and mediates the short-term renal response to the hormone. This conclusion is supported by the following cumulative observations. Vasopressin binds to a basolateral membrane receptor and initiates a cAMP-mediated chain of signaling events leading to insertion of water channels and increased osmotic water permeability of the collecting duct apical membrane.[57,58] Aquaporin-2 protein is present primarily in cytoplasmic vesicles and in apical plasma membranes of collecting duct principal cells. There is also some staining of basolateral plasma membranes of inner medullary collecting duct principal cells.[42] When expressed in *Xenopus* oocytes, aquaporin-2 induces a dramatic increase in osmotic water permeability.[59] In the water-loaded state, staining for this protein is more prominent in cytoplasmic vesicles. After stimulation by ADH, apical membrane staining for aquaporin-2 intensifies, but it decreases in the subapical vesicles (i.e., aquaporin-2 redistributes from vesicles to membrane).[60, 61] That there is a reservoir of cellular aquaporin-2 protein capable of actually recycling between intracellular cytoplasmic vesicles and the plasma membrane is suggested from studies using LLC-PK1 epithelial cells.[62] Despite inhibition of protein synthesis, aquaporin-2 staining was primarily localized to intracellular vesicles in nonstimulated cells and quickly redistributed (within 10 minutes) to the plasma membrane after exposure to ADH. The pattern was reversible on removal of ADH.

There is also evidence that aquaporin-2 plays a major role in the long-term adaptation to pathophysiologic stimuli known to alter urinary concentrating ability. For example, lithium, a drug used in affective disorders, induces an ADH-resistant concentrating defect characterized by a down-regulation of aquaporin-2 expression in rat inner medullary membranes that coincides with the development of polyuria.[63,64] The ADH-resistant urinary concentrating defect occurring after release of bilaterally obstructed ureters is also associated with a marked down-regulation of inner medullary aquaporin-2 expression that correlates with polyuria. In addition, the slow recovery is marked by persistence of decreased aquaporin-2 expression.[65]

Chronic hypokalemia may lead to ADH-resistant nephrogenic diabetes insipidus. When hypokalemia was induced by potassium deprivation for 11 days, polyuria correlated with down-regulation of aquaporin-2 in both the cortex and inner medulla of rat kidneys. Polyuria and aquaporin-2 expression corrected within a week of potassium repletion.[65] Hypercalcemia is another electrolyte disorder in which a concentrating defect and polyuria have been associated with down-regulation of aquaporin-2.[66, 67] Thirsting increases expression of aquaporin-2 in rat collecting ducts, and in Brattleboro rats, a model of central diabetes insipidus, expression of aquaporin-2 in collecting ducts is reduced in the basal state and is significantly increased upon exposure to ADH.[68,69] The decreased urinary concentrating ability associated with protein-depleted or malnourished subjects is thought to relate to a decrease in deep medullary urea content. However, rats kept on a low-protein diet for 2 weeks, without malnutrition, demonstrate decreased maximal urine osmolality after water deprivation and reduction in ADH-stimulated osmotic water permeability, as well as expression of aquaporin-2 protein in terminal portions of the inner medullary collecting ducts.[70]

These examples of limitations in urinary concentrating ability associated with long-term alterations in aquaporin-2 are of particular interest considering the presence of aquaporins in fetal and neonatal renal tissues (see later). Moreover, aquaporin-2 appears to be necessary for ADH-dependent concentration of urine in humans, as evidenced by a patient with autosomal recessive nephrogenic diabetes insipidus who had two mutations in

the gene encoding aquaporin-2. Expression of the defective proteins in *Xenopus* oocytes showed nonfunctional water channel proteins that failed to increase osmotic water permeability.[71] Such abnormalities may become definable by analyzing urine from such patients.[72, 73] Tsukahara and colleagues reported urinary excretion of aquaporin-2 in premature and term infants.[74] Levels were lower than in adults and correlated with urinary osmolality and ADH, suggesting that early in life (within the first 4 days) aquaporin channels contribute to urinary concentrating in the newborn infant.[74]

In some studies, microdissected arcade segments (branched tubule segments that connect distal convoluted tubules of deep and midcortical nephrons to cortical collecting ducts) were found to express both aquaporin-2 and the V2 ADH receptor protein. Staining of aquaporin-2 was not quite as intense as in cortical collecting ducts but nevertheless was present in large amounts and also was up-regulated in segments dissected from animals that had been thirsted. This indicates that the tubule arcades represent another site of water reabsorption stimulated by water deprivation and probably regulated by ADH.[75] This finding is of interest because extensive water reabsorption in these segments, which are present in the renal cortex, will foster absorption of large amounts of water in the cortex. Water not reclaimed in the cortical vascular circulation but delivered to the deeper medulla might dilute the medullary interstitium and impair maximal concentrating ability.

Aquaporin-3 is expressed along the connecting tubule and entire length of the collecting duct (in principal cells) from the cortex and the outer and inner medulla, especially the base, rather than the tip, of the inner medulla.[76, 77] The protein is found primarily in lateral and basal infoldings of the basolateral membrane, not the basal portion of the membrane. Labeling is virtually absent from the apical plasma membrane and is modest for intracellular cytoplasmic vesicles. Limited labeling of this protein in cytoplasmic vesicles suggests aquaporin-3 does not regulate short-term H_2O movement by vesicular trafficking. However, both water restriction for 48 hours and chronic ADH infusion for 5 days in rats increase expression of aquaporin-3, suggesting that this protein is under long-term influence of ADH and therefore integrally involved in urinary concentration.[78] Moreover, experiments have shown that transgenic knockout mice lacking aquaporin-3 have a concentrating defect and polyuria.[79] Aquaporin-3 also appears to conduct small, nonelectrolyte solutes such as urea.[80]

Aquaporin-4 expression is found primarily in inner medullary collecting duct principal cells, not in the cortex or outer medulla. It is more prominent in the inner medullary base than in the papillary tip and is found in basolateral (both basal and lateral domains) rather than apical membranes. Very little staining is found in intracellular vesicles. When rats were either water restricted for 48 hours or infused chronically over 5 days with ADH, there was no increase in expression of aquaporin-4 over a baseline water-loaded state.[77, 78] These findings are consistent with a role for aquaporin-4 as a basolateral exit pathway for transcellular movement of water in the inner medulla—perhaps in response to osmotic gradients, but not in response to secretion of ADH. The role of aquaporin-4 has been further assessed in transgenic knockout mice lacking aquaporin-4. Such mice had a mild urinary concentrating defect[81] and their perfused inner medullary collecting ducts had reduced ADH-stimulated osmotic water permeability.[82]

Three other aquaporins have been identified in kidney tissue, but their physiologic roles are unclear.[42] Aquaporin-6 is expressed in collecting duct intercalated cells from cortex to inner medulla. The protein appears to be present in intracellular vesicles, not plasma membranes, and may represent an intracellular water and ion channel.[83] Aquaporin-7 is present in the proximal tubular brush border, particularly in the S3 segment,[42] and aquaporin-8 is found in proximal tubule and collecting duct cells as well as other tissues.[84]

Role of Chloride Channels

Rapid abstraction of NaCl down its concentration gradient occurs in medullary thin ascending limbs and is an integral part of the countercurrent multiplication process. This segment is particularly permeant to chloride. Chloride channels would be poised to facilitate transmembrane movement of solute and, in fact, such channels (e.g., ClC-K1) have been identified in the inner medullary thin ascending limbs of Henle in rat kidney. The channel was localized to both apical and basolateral membranes in one study[85] and primarily on the basolateral membrane in another.[86] The channel was not observed in the descending medullary thin limb, a segment that largely abstracts water, rather than NaCl. Although this channel is also found in other, more distal segments in both cortex and medulla, its location in the thin ascending limb underscores its role in concentrating and diluting the urine. In this regard, dehydration was shown to increase expression of the ClC-K1 channel in cortical and medullary segments. Moreover, knockout mice deleted of ClC-K1 showed clinical nephrogenic diabetes insipidus, a defect that was attributed to impaired generation of inner medullary hypertonicity rather than decreased collecting duct water permeability.[87,88] The role of chloride channels in urinary concentration has recently been reviewed.[89]

To summarize, as a result of the countercurrent relationship of loops of Henle, vasa rectae, and proximal straight and collecting tubules, several cycles of solute transfer appear to take place more or less simultaneously. At all levels of the medulla (outer and inner stripes of the outer medulla as well as the inner medulla), but particularly in the inner stripe, in which the vessels located within the vascular bundle are separated only by a thin layer of interstitium, solute has the potential to leave ascending vasa rectae and enter descending vasa rectae. Some of this solute can be taken up by descending loops of Henle from short-loop nephrons that are also within the bundle. This solute can ascend to the cortex and then move to collecting tubules. When deep in the medulla, the solute can be transferred to ascending vasa rectae or to ascending loops of Henle and can then re-enter the descending loop of Henle to recycle in the medulla. In the outer stripe of the outer medulla, fluid in the ascending loop, as well as the ascending vasa recta, may also be able to enter the proximal straight tubules of short- and long-looped nephrons. These relationships provide an ongoing, if complex, transfer of solute between vessels and tubule segments to maintain sodium chloride and urea gradients in the medulla, allowing extraction of water from collecting ducts when there is need to concentrate the urine. Urine leaving the renal papillary collecting ducts enters the renal pelvis and may be able to circulate in the pelvic spaces to bathe portions of the outer medulla. There is then potential for urea to recycle back to the medulla and contribute further to urinary concentration. Functional water channels appear to be amply present in both apical and basolateral membranes and are neatly poised to reclaim water by processes that are dependent on, as well as independent of, ADH.

URINARY CONCENTRATION IN THE FETUS

The placenta, not the kidneys, seems to maintain normal extracellular salt concentration *in utero*, and there is little practical need for the fetus to concentrate or dilute urine during pregnancy. However, kidneys may play a homeostatic role under conditions of fetal stress, and survival of premature infants 24 to 26 weeks of age must depend on kidneys deprived of 3 to 4 months of anatomic and functional *in utero* development. Such

infants, fetal in some of their functions, require special attention to their fluid and electrolyte needs. Information on human fetal renal tubular reabsorption of water and response to ADH is limited. Most information comes from animals in which chronic catheters are inserted. Fetal metabolism, ontogeny, and ADH secretion are conveniently studied in the third trimester of sheep. This model is similar to humans, as both placentas are impermeant to ADH, so that fetal blood ADH levels reflect fetal production.[90] To maximally concentrate urine, ADH must be synthesized, released to the circulation, and carried to collecting tubules, which must respond to the hormone. Loops of Henle, vasa rectae, and tubules must have established the necessary anatomic relationship. Fetal urine, in a variety of species, is usually hypotonic to plasma.[91-97] This observation led to the conclusion that fetal kidneys could not concentrate urine, perhaps because ADH is either unavailable or the fetus is unresponsive to it. That such is not the case is evident from the following considerations.

Maturation of Fetal Water Reabsorption

There is a slight increase in urinary concentration during fetal development.[96,98] At a time when plasma solute concentrations are stable, fetal sheep late in gestation (>130 days of a normal 145-day gestation) have a urine osmolality significantly higher than that in younger fetuses of less than 130 days. Both urea and nonurea urinary solutes are seen to increase, but whereas some investigators[99,100] find that intrarenal urea and salt gradients are present in fetal lamb medulla by midgestation (Fig. 135-5), the actual contribution of urea to total urinary osmolality is relatively small (Fig. 135-6). During late gestation, urine flow rates decrease, but osmolar clearance remains unchanged. Therefore, free water clearance, defined as urine flow rate minus osmolar clearance, is reduced, indicating that free water is more effectively separated (reabsorbed) from solute in the older fetal kidney.[98] Although the degree of urinary concentration in late gestation is unimpressive, the increase in water reabsorption is consistent with a heightened response to endogenous levels of ADH in the older fetus.

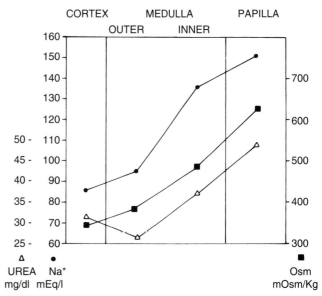

Figure 135–5. Intrarenal solute gradients in fetal lambs at midgestation. (From Moore ES, et al: *In* Spitzer A [ed]: The Kidney During Development: Morphology and Function. New York, Masson, 1982, pp 223-231.)

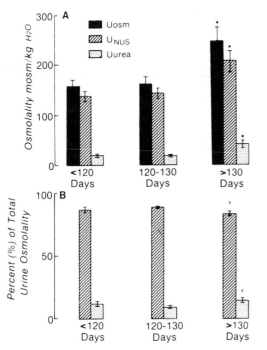

Figure 135–6. Comparison of fetal urine at different gestational ages in lambs.*$p < .05$ and †$p, < .02$ when fetuses 130 days old are compared with other groups. *A,* Urine composition and osmolality. *B,* Percentage of total urine osmolality contributed by urea and nonurea solute. Uosm = urine osmolality; U_{NUS} = urine nonurea solute; Uurea = urine urea. (From Robillard JE, et al: Pediatr Res *13*:1172, 1979.)

Availability of and Responsiveness to Vasopressin

Although fetal pituitary content at term is much lower than that of the adult, ADH has been identified in the human pituitary by the 12th week of gestation, with a demonstrable increase over ensuing weeks.[101-103] Neurosecretory granules and material are found in hypothalamic nuclei, the hypothalamohypophysial tract, and the infundibular process of the neurohypophysis by 16 weeks' gestation in the human fetus.[104] Clearly, ADH is available at an early fetal age. Vasopressin mediates its tubular effect on water permeability by stimulating the generation of cAMP.[105-107] Compared with adults, fetal ADH causes a smaller increase in cAMP from renal medullary tissue obtained from the early fetus.[108-111] To achieve osmotic equilibrium (i.e., osmolality ~300 mOsm/kg H_2O), the fetal kidney needs higher plasma levels of ADH (~5 μU/ml) than the adult, who requires only ~0.7 μU/ml. Moreover, maximal urine osmolality is achieved in both the fetus and adult at similar plasma levels of ADH, 4 to 6 μU/ml, but adult urine is much more concentrated.[98] Therefore, the fetal nephron appears to be less sensitive than the adult to vasopressin.

Exogenous Vasopressin. The fetus responds to exogenous ADH by increasing urine osmolality,[112] a response linearly related to age over the third trimester of the fetal ewe[113, 114] (Fig. 135–7). The human fetal nephron responds to ADH as shown in an isolated, perfused human medullary collecting duct obtained from a 5.5-month male abortus with trisomy D.[115] This tubule increased transmembrane water flow from 2.1 to 12.0 μl/ cm²/Osm/min on exposure to peritubular ADH. Cells swelled with conspicuous dilation of intercellular spaces, indicating outward net flow of water through intercellular spaces and through cell membranes. Thus, collecting duct receptors to ADH are well developed functionally in prenatal life.

Endogenous Vasopressin. In addition to the availability of ADH and tubular reactivity to the hormone, the fetus responds to osmotic, nonosmotic, and volume stimuli (hypertonic saline,

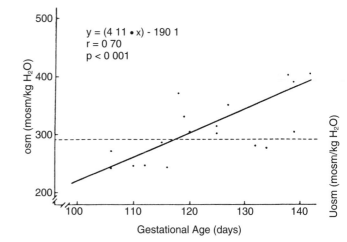

Figure 135–7. The relationship between gestational age and urine osmolality in fetal lambs during an infusion of vasopressin, 600 μU/min/kg. *The horizontal dotted line* represents mean plasma osmolality (291 mOsm/kg) during infusion of vasopressin. (From Robillard JE, Weitzman RE: Am J Physiol *238*:F407, 1980.)

hypoxia, hemorrhage, furosemide, and dehydration) by a prompt increase in endogenous plasma levels of ADH.[116-121] Infusing hypertonic saline into a fetus causes an increased level of plasma ADH that closely relates to plasma osmolality.[96, 98, 120] Fetal infusion of hypertonic saline increases fetal urine osmolality and decreases fetal urine flow rate. This response can be blocked by an ADH antagonist.[122] When water deprivation is imposed on a pregnant ewe, the older fetus, compared with the young fetus, has a higher plasma ADH level for a given plasma osmolality and, for a given plasma ADH level, the older fetus has a greater reduction in urinary water clearance.[116, 118] When varying degrees of hemorrhage are induced in lamb fetuses during the third trimester of pregnancy, plasma ADH levels increase nearly 50-fold and correlate with the degree of blood removed.[123] In late gestation, more than 130 days, a hypoxic stimulus causes fetal plasma ADH levels to rise, which are accompanied by an increase in urine osmolality and a decrease in water clearance without change in osmolar clearance. This response occurs in nearly all (9 of 10) near-term fetuses of over 130 days and about half (5 of 9) of young fetuses of less than 120 days.[98, 118, 124] Therefore, fetal hypoxemia induces antidiuresis, particularly in a near-term fetus.

It appears, then, that in a fetus during the last trimester, volume, osmotic, and nonosmotic receptors for production and release of ADH are functional, ADH is available, and tissue response to the hormone is intact. Other factors may contribute more to limited concentrating ability. Loops of Henle are short,[125, 126] and salt reabsorption in thick ascending limbs is limited in early life.[127] Total cortical flow exceeds that to the medulla, but blood flow/nephron is proportionately greater in the medulla than in the outer cortex in early development.[128-130] These factors tend to limit the efficiency with which a medullary osmotic gradient can be generated and maintained in fetal kidneys. Regardless of quantitative limitations on urinary concentration, a mature fetus or a premature infant is establishing means to tolerate stresses that may alter the osmolality or volume of its fluid environment.

Other Effects of Vasopressin

Vasopressin receptors are found in mesangial cells, aortic smooth muscle, liver, brain, and anterior pituitary. Thus ADH has other potential roles,[131] including (1) blood pressure control by effects on vasculature and baroreceptor reflexes, (2) platelet aggregation, (3) regulation of Factor VIII and von Willebrand factor, (4) release of adrenocorticotropic hormone, (5) glomerular mesangial cell contraction with some control of filtration, (6) synthesis of prostaglandins, and (7) control of/effects on hepatic metabolism by stimulating gluconeogenesis and exerting a glycogenolytic effect on hepatocytes. Some of the responses require high ADH concentration and may be more of pharmacologic interest.

Vasopressin may influence fetal water and electrolyte balance in ways separate from its effect on the kidney. Vasopressin appears to exert some control over fetal osmolar homeostasis through an effect on the placenta.[101] An osmolar gradient, generated by infusing hypertonic saline or mannitol into the mother,[101,118,132] favors transfer of fluid from fetus to mother, and water leaves the fetus to enter the maternal circulation. In the presence of hypertonic saline, neither sodium nor ADH appears to cross the placenta, but fetal serum sodium and plasma ADH increase and fetal ADH levels exceed those in the mother. Infusing hypertonic saline into the mother causes net water flux from the fetus to the maternal fluid compartment, inducing fetal water loss and increased fetal secretion of ADH. This effect is blunted if the fetus is given an ADH infusion. Similarly, mannitol infused into the mother does not cross the placenta but induces sufficient fetal water flow to raise fetal serum osmolality. Infusing ADH into the fetus blunts this response and may even drop fetal and slightly raise maternal osmolality. Therefore, fetal ADH can induce transplacental water flow and cause a net gain of fetal water by inhibiting fetal to maternal water flow despite a hyperosmolar stimulus sufficient to move water from the fetus to the mother.

Vasopressin may help regulate the volume of amniotic fluid by its direct effect on urine flow and its regulatory effect on lung fluid production.[133] Vasopressin also affects fetal cardiovascular homeostasis.[134,135] Vasopressin infusion into a sheep fetus slows heart rate and raises blood pressure within 4 to 5 minutes. Vasopressin also causes redistribution of blood flow so that the proportion of cardiac output to gastrointestinal and peripheral circulation drops, and the percentage of cardiac output to umbilical-placental, cerebral, and myocardial circulations increases. These changes are similar to those following hypoxia and suggest that ADH release helps support the fetal cardiovascular response to stress. Moreover, fetal hemorrhage drops blood pressure, but ADH provides some protection; the fall in pressure is less, and the time for fetal blood pressure recovery toward normal after hemorrhage is shorter in the presence of the hormone.

Aquaporins

Aquaporin-1 expression was shown to increase dramatically (~sevenfold) from 60 to 140 days of gestation in the ovine fetus, reaching adult levels by 6 weeks of postnatal age. This correlates with the maturational changes occurring in the kidney. Although nephrogenesis is complete by birth in the ovine fetus, there is a marked increase in postnatal GFR and considerable tubular growth. This relates to the need for an increased capability for Na and water reabsorption and the need for functional and abundant water channels in portions of the nephron where a large amount of filtrate is absorbed.[136] There is very limited expression of aquaporin-2 early in gestation in the ovine fetus. None was detected in 40-day-old or younger fetuses. It was present in low levels at 64 days, and expression increased from 80 through 140 days of gestation and much further by adulthood. The increased expression of aquaporin-2 during gestation correlates with the heightened sensitivity of the older fetal kidney to ADH in achieving a concentrated urine. It is emphasized that this process is physiologic. The purpose of fetal urine is mainly to provide an adequate volume of amniotic fluid. Maximal concentrating ability is not needed. ADH and aquaporin-2 expression are poised low enough to allow continued excretion of high volumes of dilute urine in the fetal kidney.[137]

In summary, fetal renal concentrating ability increases with gestation, but actual concentrating capacity is small, and the impact of ADH on urine concentration is relatively unimportant. Adult and immature subjects differ in tissue sensitivity to ADH, generation of cAMP, and tubule permeability to salt and urea. However, ADH is present early in gestation, nephrons respond to the hormone, and volume and osmotic responses for ADH release appear to function in the last trimester of pregnancy in the fetal lamb. Therefore, the absence of or nonresponsiveness to ADH does not explain limited concentrating ability in the premature or term neonate. A more likely explanation is inadequate generation and maintenance of a hypertonic medulla. ADH under adverse circumstances helps alter electrolyte and water transfer across the placenta, maintain adequate blood pressure, and redistribute circulating blood volume, all of which would help stabilize fetal circulation. The response to exogenous ADH and to adverse stimuli for release of ADH both mature with advancing age. Therefore, although kidneys are not needed to maintain electrolyte balance *in utero*, fetal kidneys respond to hypoxemia, asphyxia, and volume depletion and probably contribute to electrolyte, volume, osmolar, and blood pressure homeostasis. In late gestation, amniotic fluid is regulated through fetal urine and lung fluid. Accordingly, fetal kidneys and ADH may be important for normal fetal and lung development.

URINARY CONCENTRATION IN THE NEONATE

In practical terms, low neonatal concentrating capacity is of little importance unless the infant is given insufficient water to compensate for dietary solute load and high rate of insensible water loss. A low concentrating ability makes the infant more vulnerable to extrarenal water depletion, as occurs in diarrhea, febrile states, and excessive insensible skin loss. Water needs of premature infants are even greater because of higher skin losses, but the higher water intake needed to offset these losses must be provided with care to prevent overhydration since the ability to excrete a water load is limited by a very low GFR until ~34 weeks' gestation. In general, 100 to 160 ml/kg/day of water can be given to infants without major concern for dehydration or fluid overload.

Neonatal Urinary Concentrating Capacity

In the presence of ADH, human newborn infants produce a urine that is only modestly more concentrated than plasma and much less concentrated than that in the adult.[138-143] Svenningsen and Aronson gave 10 µg of 1-deamino-(8-D-arginine)-vasopressin (DDAVP) to 20 healthy term and preterm infants (30 to 35 weeks' gestational age) and found that by 4 to 6 weeks of age, their mean maximal urinary concentrating capacity was only 565 and 524 mOsm/kg, respectively, although some infants concentrated urine to greater than 600 mOsm/kg.[142] Pratt and Snyderman found that premature infants, 11 to 23 days of age, ingesting evaporated milk and small amounts of water, concentrated their urines to a maximal osmolality of 637 to 985 mOsm/kg.[141] Calcagno and co-workers found maximal urine osmolality to range from 588 to 648 mOsm/kg in five premature infants 5 to 25 days of age after 12 to 18 hours of water restriction.[138]

The dramatic maturation in concentrating ability is appreciated from data in a larger group of children reported nearly 40 years ago.[140] Urine osmolality exceeded 600 mOsm/kg within a week of life, was greater than 1000 mOsm/kg by 1 to 2 months, and was over 1100 mOsm/kg by 1 year (Table 135-2). Children reached the adult level of maximal urine concentrating ability, 1300 to 1400 mOsm/kg by 2 years of age.[144] These values are comparable to the concentrating ability of a group of children 2 to 16 years of age reported by Edelmann and colleagues.[145] After nearly 20 hours of standardized water deprivation, these children concentrated urine to a mean osmolality of 1089 mOsm/kg (range, 873 to 1305 mOsm/kg), with little change occurring beyond 2 years of age. Clearly, with a urine osmolality

TABLE 135-2

Average Maximal Urine Osmolality in 212 Children 3 Days to 18 Years of Age

Age	Maximal Urine Osmolality (mOsm/kg)
Third day	515
Sixth day	663
First month (10–30 days)	896
1–2 months	1054
End of first year	1118
Puberty (14–18 years)	1362

Data from reference 140.

TABLE 135-3

Comparison of Baseline Characteristics of Newborn (3–5 Days) and Adult Rabbit Cortical Collecting Tubules

Characteristic	Neonate	Adult
Net sodium flux (pEq/mm/min)	-83.9 ± 21.3 (19)	-1.4 ± 25.3 (8)
Water absorption (nl/mm/min)	0.35 ± 0.13 (19)	0.12 ± 0.11 (8)
Transepithelial voltage (mV)	-0.1 ± 0.3 (32)	-2.8 ± 0.6 (10)
Transepithelial electrical resistance ($\Omega \cdot cm^2$)	83.2 ± 11.6 (10)	220.6 ± 55 (6)

Values: $M \pm SE$; (n); with bath to lumen sodium gradient (142.5 versus 100 mEq Na/l), adults maintained gradient, but neonates showed net luminal entry of Na; PD of newborn tubules similar to zero; with perfusate hypotonic to bath, water reabsorption in adult tubules similar to zero.
Data from Reyes JL, et al: Biol Neonate 51:212, 1987.

of 1000 mOsm/kg, the 1- to 2-month-old infant is well protected from transient mild to moderate reductions in water intake. In fact, a non–highly concentrated urine of 600 to 700 mOsm/kg is adequate for physiologic needs of the neonate and would even be adequate for an adult under most clinical circumstances. Physiologic and anatomic factors contributing to a low neonatal renal concentrating capacity are summarized next.

Factors Limiting Concentrating Ability in the Neonate

Physiologic Considerations

Fluid Transport in Superficial Nephrons. Micropuncture studies reveal a maturation in water and solute transport in loops of Henle from superficial nephrons.[127,146-148] For example, in the rat,[148] the TF/P (tubular fluid to plasma) inulin ratio of fluid distal to the loop (a measure of water reabsorption) increased from 13 through 39 days of age, a time when there was no change in the fraction of filtered water remaining at the end of the proximal tubule. Therefore, the rise in TF/P inulin ratio was due to increased water reabsorption along the loop. This increase in water reabsorption does not necessarily reflect greater water reabsorption in the thick ascending limb. It may relate to increased water reabsorption from the descending limb as this segment courses through the increasingly hypertonic outer medulla. In the final urine, inulin concentration increased by a factor of 5 during this time interval, indicating increased water reabsorption along the collecting ducts. In addition, the osmolality of the final urine increased from 700 to 1500 mOsm/kg. A rise in fractional reabsorption of sodium and chloride occurred along the loop. Furthermore, the potential diluting ability was also enhanced, as shown by a drop in sodium and chloride concentrations in early distal tubule fluid.

Ascending Thin Limb. Urinary concentration requires (1) a countercurrent multiplication process allowing the medullary interstitium to become progressively hypertonic, and (2) the osmotic equilibration of medullary collecting duct fluid with the hypertonic medullary interstitium. To accomplish this, cells require a variety of channels and transporters. The ascending thin limb of Henle is highly permeable to chloride, likely related to its chloride channel ClC-K1. By facilitating efflux of NaCl to the interstitium, salt can osmotically induce movement of collecting duct water to the interstitium and increase the osmolality of collecting duct fluid. Failure to express this channel causes diabetes insipidus in the mouse.[87] Kobayashi and colleagues related concentrating ability in the rat to expression of this channel.[149] Maturation of the channel and the thin ascending limb correlated with an increase in concentrating ability. After dehydration, urine osmolality remained low until postnatal day 19. Concentrating ability then increased rapidly, with a marked increase by day 21.

The chloride channel was first noted near the papillary tip on day 5, increased by day 14, and was actually comparable to that

of the adult by day 19. Its expression during development coincided with the increase in concentrating ability. Aquaporin-1 was present in inner medullary tubules by postnatal day 1, but its expression was weak. It increased to reach adult levels by day 14. Aquaporin-2 was present in the premature kidney throughout the inner medullary collecting duct, and its pattern did not change with maturation. Therefore, water channels were present to allow for urinary concentration by water abstraction, and chloride channels matured to facilitate solute movement from the medullary ascending thin limb to interstitium to help establish and maintain a medullary gradient.

Fluid Transport in Collecting Tubules. The adult collecting tubule is a "tight" epithelium with high transepithelial electrical resistance and a low rate of reabsorbed sodium backfluxing to the lumen. Basal permeability to water is low, and the epithelial cells can maintain transepithelial osmotic and sodium gradients. By contrast, newborn rabbit (3 to 5 days of age) collecting tubules allow substantially more sodium backflux to the tubule lumen and have a lower transepithelial voltage and electrical resistance (Table 135-3). Therefore, the newborn collecting tubule may be unable to maintain an adequate sodium (osmolar) gradient and, consequently, be unable to build a driving force to abstract water efficiently from more distal parts of the nephron.[150]

Urea. It is curious that a urinary waste product performs a homeostatic function. The importance of urea to mammalian urinary concentration was recognized nearly 70 years ago when Gamble and coworkers[151] noted that adult rats fed urea excreted a more concentrated urine than rats fed a nonurea diet made equimolar by adding inorganic solutes. High-protein diets and urea loads increase urine concentration in the human adult.[152] Urea, a protein metabolic waste product, normally represents ~50% of the solute in maximally concentrated urine, but this is not the case in the neonate. Infants and adults have similar urinary content of nonurea (electrolyte) solute, but the urinary urea solute content of the infant is distinctly lower. Most of the increase in concentrating capacity occurs after birth and can be augmented by dietary alterations.[153,154]

Edelmann and colleagues[145] determined maximal urine concentrating ability in nine full-term and premature infants (7 to 39 days of age) who had been placed on diets varying in protein. Prior to a protein load, concentrating ability in infants was about half that of adults. When given a high-protein diet or a urea load, infants increased their maximal urine osmolality independent of fluid intake or urine output (Table 135-4). The low neonatal concentrating ability seemed to reflect the type of solute available to the renal medulla rather than an intrinsic problem with the newborn kidney. It was postulated that since the infant is in a

TABLE 135-4

Effect of High Protein Intake on Maximal Urine Concentration

	Protein Intake (g/kg)	Fluid Intake (ml/kg)	BUN (mg/dl)	Urine Osmolality (mOsm/kg)
Group 1	8.75	115	29	931
	2.3	215	9	571
Group 2	8.4	172	26	844
	2.4	164	9	657

Group 1 included four infants 13 to 38 days old, birth weight 1840 to 2800 g, first on high-protein–low-fluid intake, then on low-protein–high-fluid intake. Group 2 included five infants 7 to 32 days of age, birth weight 1980 to 3620 g, first on high-protein then low-protein diet without altering fluid intake.
BUN = blood urea nitrogen.
Data from reference 145.

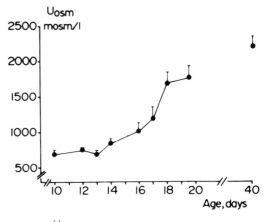

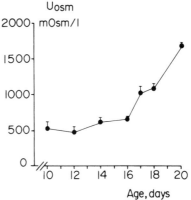

Figure 135-8. Effect of weaning on maturation of concentrating capacity (urine osmolality) after 24 hours of water and food deprivation in rats. Values are M ± SE. *Top,* Normally weaned rats with free access to food. *Bottom,* Unweaned rats fed only breast milk. Urinary concentration was unaffected by weaning. (From Rane S, et al: Pediatr Res *19*:472, 1985.)

highly anabolic state, concentrating ability was limited by the efficient use of protein, which would tend to minimize the amount of urea available to build up a medullary gradient. However, despite the high-protein diet, urine osmolality still did not reach adult levels, and the levels actually reached required an extremely high protein intake (i.e., >8 g/kg) and a very high blood urea nitrogen ranging to 45 mg/dl.

It is evident from other studies as well that urinary concentrating ability does not depend on diet alone.[155-158] Rats are weaned and accordingly change their diet during the third week of life when concentrating capacity is increasing sharply. Rane and co-workers[158] found that maximal concentrating ability increased during the third week both in rats who were normally weaned and in those who continued to nurse, indicating that the improvement in concentrating ability was independent of dietary composition or protein content (Fig. 135-8). There was also no concomitant change in the serum level of ADH. Therefore, the maturational effect is intrarenal. Rather than simply an insufficient urea content, the low level of neonatal urinary concentration is more likely related to some difference in the manner in which urea is handled by the kidney. Although the gradual increase in urea synthetic function that occurs during the neonatal period might contribute in part to the progressive increase in concentrating ability,[159] the search for other physiologic as well as anatomic limitations on neonatal concentrating ability has continued.

Response to Vasopressin. Vasopressin attaches to receptors on basolateral membranes of collecting tubule cells, but its permeability effect is at the apical membrane. In responsive cells, ADH-receptor interaction stimulates adenylate cyclase to form cyclic adenosine monophosphate (cAMP) from adenosine triphosphate (ATP). The cAMP binds a protein kinase that catalyzes phosphorylation of apical membrane proteins. Cytoplasmic tubular structures are present in resting cells. In the presence of ADH, these structures, containing small particles or aggregates, fuse with the apical membrane. The particles represent water channels (membrane proteins) that promote transmembrane osmotic water movement. This requires an intact cytoskeleton; disassembling microtubules interferes with the cellular response to ADH.[160, 161] The newborn lamb responds to stimuli such as hypertonic saline, water loading, furosemide, dehydration, and blood loss (Table 135-5),[120, 162] by appropriately elevating or suppressing ADH levels. The human newborn infant responds to hypertonic saline.[163] Human neonatal concentrating capacity remains limited even in the presence of elevated plasma ADH levels typical of the immediate newborn period in term and preterm infants.[101, 164-167] Clearly, lack of ADH does not explain a gross reduction in neonatal concentrating ability. Nonetheless, investigators still consider that the neonatal ADH-renal axis may be inadequate since, in the immediate newborn period of the rat,

urinary osmolality is lower than papillary tip osmolality, and hormone levels in young animals are further increased (to levels comparable to that of older animals) in response to dehydration. Rather than an insufficient circulating level of ADH, the limited newborn concentrating ability may reflect decreased responsiveness to the hormone or a decreased number of ADH receptors.

Supporting this hypothesis, Schlondorff and co-workers, studying isolated cortical collecting tubules of 10- to 12-day-old and adult rabbits, found that in the newborn rabbit, basal adenylate cyclase activity was considerably lower and stimulation of adenylate cyclase activity by ADH was much less than in the adult. The adult basal level of adenylate cyclase was 2.5 times that of the newborn rabbit. After stimulation with ADH, adult levels increased 10-fold in contrast to the 2.5-fold increase observed in newborn tubules.[110, 111] In isolated rat collecting tubules, Imbert-Teboul and colleagues reported a blunted ability of ADH to stimulate adenylate cyclase in the neonate (Table 135-6).[108] They found an initial increase in ADH-dependent adenylate cyclase over the first week of life, a plateau of activity from days 7 to 14, and a second period of increase in enzyme activity after day 14. Adult levels were reached by day 35.[108] However, the period of greatest increase in activity corresponded to a time when Edwards and group observed the sharpest increase in concentrating ability.[156] In studies of the ontogenetic development of ADH receptors, Rajerison and co-workers found a progressive increase in ADH stimulation of medullary adenylate cyclase in animals over a 2- to 46-day period with a concomitant, although

TABLE 135-5

Concentrations of Vasopressin in Newborn Lambs

	Plasma Vasopressin (μU/ml)	
Condition	Baseline Values	Peak Values
Hypertonic saline (10 mEq/kg; n, 11)	2.9 ± 0.7	22.2 ± 9
Phlebotomy (10 ml/kg; n, 10)	1.9 ± 0.4	72.0 ± 40
Dehydration (18 h; n,9)	0.6 ± 0.1	4.8 ± 1.8
Water loading (100 ml/kg; n,7)	3.4 ± 1.2	1.1 ± 0.3

Plasma vasopressin levels in newborn lambs (1–7 weeks) change appropriately with above stimuli. Values are M ± SE; p < .05 for all peak versus baseline values.
Data from reference 2.

TABLE 135-6

Postnatal Maturation of Vasopressin-Dependent Adenylate Cyclase in Rat Medullary Collecting Tubules

Age (days)	Δ cAMP Formed in Collecting Tubule (fmol/mm/30 min)
3 (n, 4)	203 ± 50 (28)
28 (n, 3)	536 ± 56 (75)
60 (adult; n, 6)	719 ± 68

Values (stimulated minus basal adenylate cyclase activity) are M ± SE; response to 1 μM vasopressin of immature rat as percentage of the response of cAMP formed in adult rat tubules given in parentheses. Note progressive sensitivity of tubule cAMP stimulation by vasopressin.
Adapted from Imbert-Teboul M, et al: Am J Physiol 247: F316, 1984.

slightly earlier, development of ADH binding capacity.[109, 168, 169] Vasopressin binding rapidly increased after birth so that the 3- to 4-week-old rat had a capacity to bind ADH to kidney medullo-papillary membranes that was similar to that of the adult.[109,168,169] These findings suggest that the cAMP system or the binding properties or response to ADH are immature in the neonate.

In more recent studies, immature, isolated, perfused cortical collecting ducts were shown to have basal osmotic water permeability similar to mature tubules. However, the increase in water permeability after exposure to ADH was considerably less than that observed in adult tubules. The blunted response of immature tubules to ADH could not be abolished by exposing tubules to the stimulating effect of cAMP or to the inhibition of prostaglandin synthesis by indomethacin. The investigators concluded that in addition to any impairment in ADH-stimulated cAMP generation or antagonism of cAMP by prostaglandins,

there is likely a more distal pathway disruption, perhaps at the level of the basolateral membrane.[170]

Sulyok[171] suggested that the response of a premature infant kidney to ADH may become blunted by the presence of hyponatremia, a state that may occur in the first few weeks of life. Premature infants with late hyponatremia show an *increase* in ADH excretion with age, even though their serum sodium levels and osmolality fall and their urine osmolality *diminishes* as urine flow rate increases. Renal salt wasting and hyponatremia may hinder establishment of an intrarenal salt gradient at a time when salt, rather than urea, would be the primary medullary solute. Although there might be a delay in maturation of concentrating ability, a blunted response to ADH could minimize the retention of excess water and may thereby serve to limit the severity of the hyponatremia. The late development of hyponatremia in premature infants can be prevented by administration of supplemental NaCl. Such infants have increased sodium excretion, but nevertheless are in positive sodium balance and their ADH secretion is increased. The salt supplement appears to enhance ADH secretion with resultant retention of water, although in proportion to salt retention, as serum sodium remains relatively constant.[172]

Aquaporins. Aquaporin-1 is present in rat renal proximal tubules and thin descending limbs of Henle and is expressed in these tissues shortly before birth. However, the amount of renal aquaporin-1 messenger RNA is small in the kidney prior to and shortly after birth. Significant expression of aquaporin-1 does not occur until after birth.[173] Peak levels appear around 3 weeks of postnatal age. It is present in both apical and basolateral membranes in an equivalent staining intensity, suggesting that this protein appears simultaneously in both membranes.[174, 175] Betamethasone stimulates a significant, modest induction of aquaporin-1 in neonatal rat kidneys 4 days of age. Adult rats showed no such response.[34] By contrast, aquaporin-1 was detected by immunohistochemical staining techniques in the human fetus at 14 weeks' gestation in a newly developing proximal tubule, and by 17 weeks staining was evident in both developing proximal tubules and in newly forming thin limbs from the outer cortex. By 24 weeks, staining was noted in thin limbs of the medulla. At 1 month of postnatal age, aquaporin-1 immunostaining was prominent over apical and basolateral membranes of proximal tubules and thin descending limbs of Henle.[176] This finding correlates with differences in concentrating ability; the human kidney concentrates urine at birth, and concentrating ability approaches that of the adult by 1 to 2 months (see earlier), whereas the rat concentrates urine primarily at the time of weaning.[158]

In other studies, aquaporin-1 was observed as early as 12 weeks' gestation in the human fetus, although not at 8 weeks, and was shown to increase steadily to reach 47% of adult levels at birth and 79% of adult levels by 15 months of postnatal age.[177] This

Figure 135–9. Immunohistochemical staining to localize aquaporin-1 and aquaporin-2 during human nephrogenesis. **A,** Positive staining for aquaporin-1 is restricted to a developing proximal tubule in the inner cortex of a 13-week human fetal kidney. Adjacent ureteric buds (u) and immature glomeruli (g) are unstained. No membrane polarity is localized. **B,** Staining for aquaporin-2 is positive in a branching ureteric bud and localized to the apical membrane in the inner cortex of a 13-week human fetal kidney. Glomeruli (g) and immature proximal tubules (p) are unstained. **C,** Positive staining for aquaporin-1 in a 15-week human fetal kidney. Staining is present for juxtaglomerular proximal tubules extending to the medulla, where an early descending thin limb of Henle is stained *(inset)*; apical membranes are stained in proximal tubules *(arrows)* and thin descending limbs *(inset arrowhead)*. Glomeruli (g), ureteric buds (u), and collecting ducts (cd) are unstained. **D,** Positive staining for aquaporin-2 is restricted to the apical membrane region of medullary collecting ducts in an 18-week human fetal kidney. **E** and **F,** Sections from the cortex of a 24-week human fetal kidney. In **E,** staining for aquaporin-1 is positive in the apical membrane of proximal tubule cells (p). Collecting ducts (cd) are unstained. In **F,** staining for aquaporin-2 is positive in collecting ducts (cd) and not in proximal tubule cells (p). Minimal glomerular (g) staining for aquaporin-1 and basolateral collecting duct staining for aquaporin-2 were nonspecific. **G,** Cortex of an 18-week human fetal kidney shows no aquaporin-1 staining in proximal tubules (p) when tissue is incubated with preimmune serum for aquaporin-1. **H,** Inner cortex of a 14-week human fetal kidney shows no ureteric bud (u) staining when tissue is incubated with preimmune serum for aquaporin-2. See reference 177 for details. (From Devuyst O, et al: Am J Physiol 271 [Renal Fluid Electrolyte Physiol 40]:F169, 1996.)

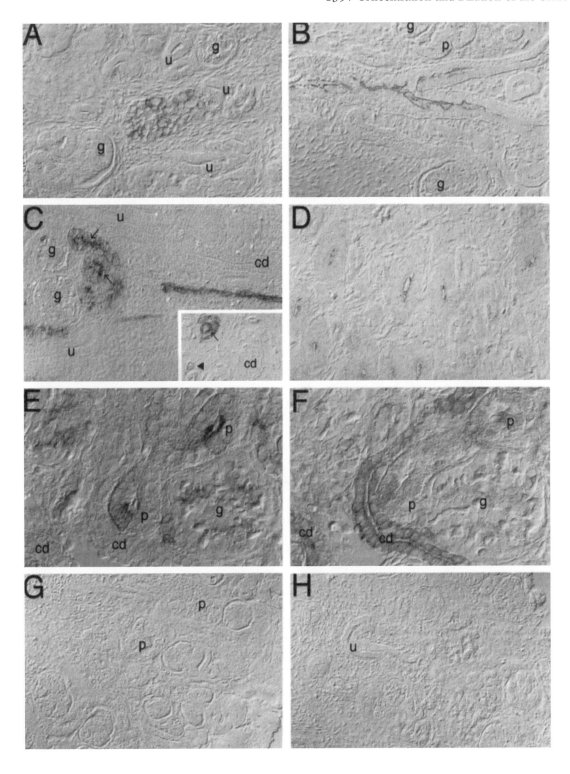

coincides approximately to the age when urine concentrating ability reaches adult values (see Table 135-2). In this study, aquaporin-1 was initially localized to newly forming proximal tubular structures in the inner cortex. S-shaped bodies, glomeruli, and tubular structures of ureteric bud origin were not stained for aquaporin-1. By 15 to 20 weeks, proximal tubular structures in the cortex were better differentiated, and staining could be seen to localize mainly in the apical membrane of polarized epithelial cells to include proximal tubules and thin descending limbs of Henle. Basolateral staining, evident in proximal tubules and thin descend-

ing limbs in adult kidneys, was not clearly defined in the fetal kidneys, even at 24 weeks (Fig. 135-9).[177]

As mentioned earlier, aquaporin-1 is poised to facilitate reabsorption of very large amounts of water in proximal tubules and development of the countercurrent multiplication process by allowing rapid movement of water across thin descending limbs. Whereas osmotic water permeability of neonatal proximal tubules is higher than that of adults, osmotic permeability of brush-border membrane vesicles in neonates is lower. Quigley and colleagues[178] reported that in rabbit proximal tubular basolateral membrane vesicles, both expression of aquaporin-1 protein and osmotic water permeability were lower in neonates than in adults, while solute permeability (NaCl, NaHCO₃) was similar. They concluded that the higher neonatal transepithelial osmotic permeability in the neonate is not related to increased water movement across water channels.

Aquaporin-1 is also present in descending vasa rectae of adult kidneys. However, there is an interesting pattern of distribution of this protein in the developing rat kidney.[179] Aquaporin-1 was found throughout the arterial vascular tree of fetal and neonatal kidneys from 17 days' gestation to 7 days of postnatal age. Over the next week expression regressed, becoming limited to descending vasa rectae. After about 3 weeks of age, aquaporin-1 also appeared in lymphatic vessels. This persisted in adults. The investigators suggest that the transient developmental expression may relate to fluid equilibrium in the developing kidney, or perhaps to a role in regulating fetal growth or branching of the vascular tree.

Aquaporin-2 protein and aquaporin-2 messenger RNA have been reported in rats to increase over 10 to 40 days of life and particularly over the weaning period from 15 to 20 days of life, a period of time when urinary concentrating ability dramatically increases. When rats were exposed to a single injection of beta-methasone, known to accelerate maturation in other organs, there was an increase in renal medullary aquaporin-2 protein and messenger RNA as well as in urine osmolality.[180] In studies of aquaporin expression during human nephrogenesis, aquaporin-2 was seen by the 12th week of gestation, but not at 8 weeks. In contrast to aquaporin-1, aquaporin-2 was found only in structures derived from the ureteric bud. For example, in a 13-week fetal human kidney, aquaporin-2 stained in apical cell membranes in the collecting system and branching ureteric bud as it extended from the medulla toward the cortex. Comma- and S-shaped bodies, glomeruli, and proximal tubular structures did not stain for aquaporin-2, and this pattern continued throughout development. Therefore, it was evident from early in gestation that aquaporin-1 staining was limited to proximal segments and thin descending limbs, whereas aquaporin-2 was exclusively found in ureteric bud–derived cortical and medullary collecting duct segments (see Fig. 135–9).[177]

Bonilla-Felix and Jiang[181] found that aquaporin-2 expression was reduced in immature rats compared with adults. There was a close relation between aquaporin-2 expression and urinary osmolality on *ad libitum* fluid intake. However, while immature rats increased their aquaporin-2 content following stimulation with both dehydration and ADH, there was not a concurrent equal increase in concentrating ability. Immature rats did show an ability to translocate aquaporin-2 from intracellular vesicles (during water loading) to plasma membranes (during dehydration or treatment with ADH). Thus, although aquaporin-2 expression and trafficking were present in immature kidneys, concentrating ability was still limited.

Baum and colleagues[182] found expression of aquaporin-2 (apical membrane) and aquaporin-3 (basolateral membrane) in rat epithelial cells derived from ureteric bud and collecting ducts. Expression was detected as early as 16 to 18 days' gestation. They also found expression of both aquaporins in comparable membranes of collecting ducts in human 3-day-old and adult kidneys. The rat kidneys showed little change in aquaporin expression over the first 3 days of life, but showed a dramatic (2.5-fold) increase in aquaporin-2 messenger RNA by 10 to 14 days of life. Given the presence of fetal and neonatal aquaporins, delay in maturation of maximal concentrating ability in neonates is not related to a simple lack of water channels. However, the importance of functional aquaporin-2 protein in neonates was illustrated in an aquaporin-2 knock-in mouse model of recessive diabetes insipidus. Gene replacement caused a mutant protein leading to death within about 6 days of life without supplemental fluid.[183]

Prostaglandins. Prostaglandins, synthesized in renal medullary interstitial and collecting duct cells, are thought to regulate medullary functions such as blood flow, sodium chloride transport, and water reabsorption. Accordingly, prostaglandins could play a role in urinary concentration.[184, 185] In experimental animals, prostaglandin E₂ (PGE₂) was found to inhibit sodium chloride transport in the medullary thick ascending limb.[186] PGE₂ antagonizes ADH-mediated water flow across the collecting tubule and bladder,[4] inhibits urea flux across toad bladder epithelium, and decreases urea reabsorption in the rat collecting tubule.[187, 188] PGE₂ also can induce renal vasodilation and increase medullary blood flow.[44] These effects tend to wash out a medullary osmolar gradient and decrease maximal concentrating capacity. In fact, prostaglandins reduce the corticomedullary osmotic gradient and the medullary solute (salt and urea) content,[189] thereby reducing the driving force for water reabsorption. It has been suggested that increased prostaglandin synthesis in fetal and neonatal kidneys and blood vessels may interfere with neonatal concentrating ability.[190–192] However, the relationship between prostaglandin excretion and maturation of renal function is not firmly established,[193] and a role of prostaglandins becomes clouded when one recognizes that prostaglandin excretion increases with age. Benzoni and co-workers[194] noted that urinary excretion of PGE increased over the first 24 months of life and correlated linearly with urine osmolality. Although this period is precisely when urinary concentrating ability shows the most dramatic degree of maturation, a clear cause and effect relationship was not established.

Perhaps any limiting effect of prostaglandins on the neonatal concentrating ability is largely masked by the relentless maturation of the many other factors that come to bear on the concentrating process. Nevertheless, studies using molecular biologic techniques are of interest. At least three different receptors for PGE₂ have been identified. These activate different intracellular signaling mechanisms, and the EP3 receptor, which is coupled to an inhibitory guanine nucleotide-binding G protein, inhibits generation of cAMP when stimulated by PGE₂. Immature collecting ducts have decreased generation of cAMP when stimulated by ADH. This response is mediated by prostaglandin, probably by activating the inhibitory G protein.[195] Receptor mRNA expression was found primarily in the distal nephron, i.e., in medullary thick ascending limbs as well as cortical and inner medullary collecting ducts. During development, rabbit kidney expression for the EP3 receptor mRNA increased to a maximum at 2 weeks of postnatal age and then decreased to reach adult levels by 8 to 10 weeks of postnatal age.[196] This finding lends credence to the idea that part of the blunted concentrating ability in maturation relates to increased expression of an inhibitory receptor stimulated by PGE₂ that blunts the ability of ADH to stimulate cAMP in collecting ducts.

Renin-Angiotensin System. It has become clear that the renin-angiotensin axis must be intact during nephrogenesis for normal development of urinary concentration. Profound adverse effects on adult renal function occur when the angiotensin-converting enzyme inhibitor enalopril or the angiotensin II type 1 receptor antagonist losartan is given early in neonatal life during nephrogenesis. For example, use of these agents in neonatal rats and piglets causes irreversible histologic changes, including chronic interstitial inflammation and fibrosis, renal vascular changes involving interlobular arteries, and, most particularly, profound papillary necrosis. Functionally, as adults, such animals show polyuria and a decreased urinary concentrating ability. There is variable effect on other functions. Proximal tubular fluid reabsorption is reduced, whereas glucose reabsorption, urinary acid excretion and acidifying ability, glomerular filtration, and renal blood flow are largely unaffected.[197–201] The most critical period for renal vulnerability for adverse effects appears to be the first 13 days of life in the rat, coinciding with the duration of

TABLE 135–7

Comparison of Sodium and Urea Content in the Cortex and Papilla of Maturing Rabbits

Age	Sodium (mEq/l Tissue Water)			Urea (mm/l Tissue Water)		
	Cortex	Papilla	P/C	Cortex	Papilla	P/C
Newborn (9)	61	137	2.2	24	115	4.8
5 days (3)	63	211	3.3	45	319	7.1
13 days (4)	57	345	6.1	25	345	13.8
28 days (3)	64	340	5.3	22	367	16.7
42 days (2)	68	477	7.0	23	488	26.6
Adult (1)	64	560	8.7	14	512	36.6

P/C is papilla/cortex ratio. Animals were food- and fluid-deprived and given intramuscular pitressin 18 hours before sacrifice. By 6 weeks, values approach those of the adult. Number in parentheses is number of animals.
Reprinted by permission of the publishers from DEVELOPMENTAL NEPHROLOGY by Wallace W. McCrory, M.D. Cambridge, Ma, Harvard University Press. © 1972 by the President and Fellows of Harvard College.

continued postnatal nephrogenesis.[198] Of interest, histologic and functional abnormalities were normalized in enalopril-treated rats when they were concomitantly treated with insulin-like growth factor-I, another renal growth-promoting factor.[202] In functional studies, decreased urine concentrating ability was associated with a decrease in negative water clearance (T_cH_2O), medullary tissue osmolality, Na and urea concentration, and density of inner medullary aquaporin-2. Since density of aquaporin-2 is higher in the proximal one-third than the more distal two-thirds of the inner medullary collecting duct located mainly in the papilla, it would seem that the decreased concentrating ability is not wholly due to papillary atrophy.[200]

Anatomic Considerations

Loops of Henle of Deep Nephrons. Maximal concentrating ability directly correlates with the lengths of long loops of Henle as they descend into the medulla. Species able to develop highly concentrated urine tend to have both longer loops of Henle and a greater proportion of nephrons that send their loops deep into the medulla.[13] In the newborn infant, the length of loops and the renal papillae are relatively short, but they increase during maturation.[125] In newborn rabbit, the inner medulla and papilla are underdeveloped, but over the first week of postnatal life the medulla becomes larger and the papillae become longer. Maximal concentrating ability in the rabbit increases from an osmolality of 600 mOsm/kg at birth to about 2000 mOsm/kg by 3 weeks of age. When osmotic solute gradients in the papilla are measured during development, sodium and urea concentrations are seen to increase gradually and roughly in parallel to approach adult levels by 6 weeks of age (Table 135–7).[144] Improved concentrating ability during development, therefore, might reflect the development of these anatomic parameters. However, Rane and colleagues,[158] evaluating the role of steroid hormones in the development of the concentrating mechanism in rats, observed an increase in urine osmolality and papillary tissue sodium and urea content from day 16 to day 20 that was temporally related to an increase in serum corticosterone. The increased concentrating ability was augmented by treating rats with exogenous glucocorticoids (betamethasone) and prevented by adrenalectomy. However, the length of the papilla, i.e., length of long loops of Henle, was not affected by adrenalectomy, indicating that the growth of long loops of deep nephrons contributed little to maturation of concentrating ability during this time. Perhaps glucocorticoids can modulate enzyme systems that help augment maturation of the hypertonic medullary gradient and the urinary concentrating mechanism.

Loops of Henle of Short Nephrons. Long loops of juxtamedullary nephrons help determine the degree to which urine can be concentrated, but the shorter loops of superficial nephrons also play a pivotal role.[13, 156] These nephrons allow accumulation of urea in the inner medulla by (1) increasing the load and concentration of urea delivered to medullary collecting ducts, and (2) recycling urea to minimize its loss from the medulla. Were interstitial urea to enter long loops and vasa rectae and leave the medulla, the medullary urea gradient would become depleted. By entering descending limbs of superficial nephrons, urea can recycle to the medulla and maintain the gradient. In fact, the descending limbs of short loops of superficial nephrons, not long loops of deep nephrons, are the ones that accompany vascular bundles of the inner stripe of the outer medulla.

Edwards and colleagues[156] clarified the role of short-looped nephrons in maturation of the concentrating mechanism (Fig. 135–10). In the rat, about 40% to 50% of total solute in the adult papillary interstitium is urea. During nephrogenesis, superficial nephrons are the least mature and the last to develop. Their entrance or elongation into the deeper cortical and outer medullary portion of the kidney coincides with improvement in concentrating ability. During the first 16 days of life, the length of the corticopapillary gradient increased 3.4-fold and the superficial nephrons elongated markedly so that they came to cross more than 70% of the outer medulla. During this time, urinary osmolality increased following a period of water deprivation. Once maximal penetration of superficial loops to the outer medulla had occurred, urinary concentrating ability increased even more sharply, coincident with a marked increase in papillary tip osmolality and an increase in the proportion of the papillary solute composed of urea. It should be re-emphasized that the bulk of filtered fluid is reabsorbed in the cortex. This decreases the amount of fluid delivered to the collecting ducts. Therefore, deeper tissues are not faced with the need to reabsorb so much water that the medullary solute gradient would be diluted and dissipated. The arcade segments in the renal cortex appear to play an important role in this regard (see later).

The ability to use urea to enhance urinary concentration matures over the first 3 weeks of life in rabbits and rats.[203, 204] For example, Trimble[204] found that an acute exogenous nondiuretic urea load given subcutaneously had no effect on urinary concentrating ability in rats 10 days of age, but it increased the medullary urea content and maximal concentrating ability in rats 20 days of age (Table 135–8). During this time, developmental changes occur in the length of the corticopapillary gradient and the length of superficial loops so that they penetrate well into the outer medulla. In addition, complex vascular bundles appear in the outer medulla, and the diluting capacity of superficial loops of Henle improves.

Zink and Horster[127] found that in young rats up to 15 days of age on a high-salt diet, fluid from the early distal tubule was isotonic with plasma and contained primarily NaCl as the solute. However, in rats 4 to 5 weeks of age, the early distal tubular fluid became hypotonic and contained a much smaller proportion of total solute as NaCl. Therefore, the loop more efficiently

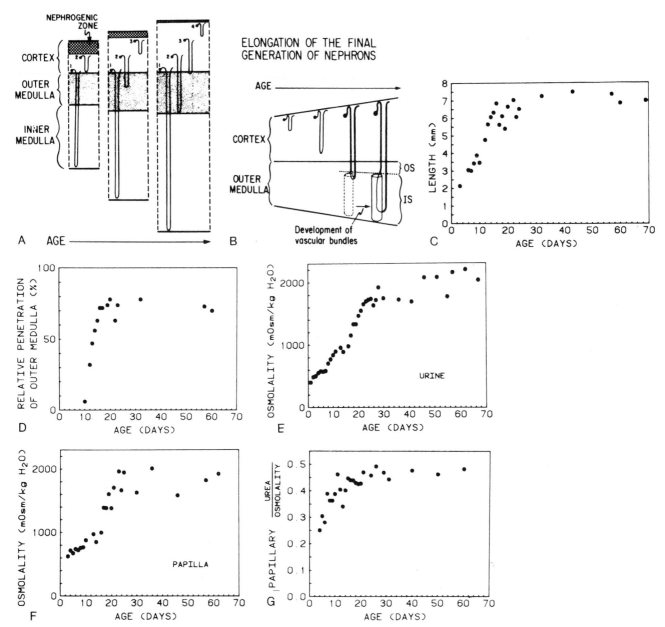

Figure 135–10. These figures depict anatomic maturation of superficial and deep nephrons, penetration of short-looped nephrons toward outer medulla, and maturation of concentrating ability. **A,** Simplified scheme of nephrogenesis in the rat. Numbers refer to successive generations of nephrons. **B,** Diagrammatic representation of elongation of the loop of Henle belonging to a surface nephron. In the rat, the vascular bundles are recognizable at 20 days of age but not at 10 days. The descending limbs of superficial loops become incorporated with these structures. OS = outer stripe; IS = inner stripe. **C,** Length of the corticopapillary gradient as a function of age in the rat (*N* = 28). Each point represents a single animal except for days 13, 15, and 18 (two rats each) and day 14 (three rats), for which averages are shown. **D,** Penetration of outer medulla by superficial loops of Henle. Each point represents a single animal except for day 13 (two rats) and day 14 (three rats). An average of three loops per rat was examined. **E,** Urinary osmolality, following 8 hours of dehydration, as a function of age in the rat (*N* = 138). Each point represents the average value for one to eight rats (mean rats). **F,** Osmolality of the papillary tip, following 8 hours of dehydration, as a function of age in the rat (*N* = 56). Each point represents the average value for one to five rats (mean = 2.3 rats). **G,** Fraction of total papillary osmolality contributed by urea as a function of age in 67 rats dehydrated for 18 hours. Length of corticopapillary gradient increases with age, particularly over the first 16 days, corresponding to time of most marked elongation of superficial loops. Urine and papillary tip osmolality increase primarily over the first 3.5 weeks and most steeply after approximately day 16. The proportion of urea composing papillary osmolality increases until adult proportions are reached by approximately 15 to 20 days. (From Edwards BR, et al: *In* Spitzer A [ed]: The Kidney During Development: Morphology and Function. New York, Masson, 1982, pp 223–240.)

TABLE 135-8

Urine Concentrating Capacity in Rats 10 to 20 Days of Age

	Maximal Urinary Osmolality (mOsm/kg)		Urine (Urea) (mM)		Urine/Plasma Osmolar Ratio	
	10 day	*20 day*	*10 day*	*20 day*	*10 day*	*20 day*
Control	938 ± 28	1449 ± 71	469 ± 23	774 ± 49	3.3 ± 0.1	4.8 ± 0.2
Urea load	907 ± 29	1716 ± 59	482 ± 27	1049 ± 70	3.1 ± 0.1	5.5 ± 0.3

Adapted from Trimble ME: Am J Physiol *219*:1089, 1970.

reabsorbed NaCl without water. In other studies, Horster reported a maturational increase in NaCl reabsorption in rabbit cortical thick ascending limbs.[146,147] These factors help accumulate urea in the medulla. Edwards, in fact, found that the urea contribution to rat papillary osmolality increased sharply over the first 2 to 3 weeks of life, but thereafter further increases in papillary osmolality were associated with proportional increases in urea and nonurea solute.[156] Therefore, urea accumulated in the papilla coincident with an increased activity of sodium absorption in the loop of Henle and a rearrangement of nephrons so that superficial nephron loops came to penetrate the outer medulla.

Renal Inner Medullary Tubule Organization. Liu and colleagues[205] analyzed organization and function of inner medullary tubules during development in isolated perfused tubules from rat kidneys. In thin descending limbs, hydraulic water conductivity was absent on day 1, appeared by day 4, but remained low until day 14 of life. This segment was impermeable to water early in life. Diffusional water permeability of thin ascending limbs was low from day 1 to adulthood, emphasizing low water permeability of this segment. Basal water permeability remained low in inner medullary collecting ducts to adulthood. Water permeability was mildly enhanced by vasopressin in this segment early in life, but remained low and only reached adult levels by day 14 (Fig. 135-11). Therefore, there was little water reabsorption from these segments early in life.

Urea permeability was low in thin descending limbs throughout development and adulthood. In thin ascending limbs, urea permeability was low, but reached two-thirds of adult value by day 14. In the inner medullary collecting duct, basal urea permeability was negligible until day 7 and remained low into adulthood. Vasopressin induced little increase in urea permeability in this segment until day 14, though this value was still less than a third that of the adult (Fig. 135-12). Expression of the urea transporter UT-A1 was not apparent until the late neonatal period. Therefore, urea transport contributed little to neonatal urinary concentration. The chloride channel ClC-K1 was expressed in thin ascending limbs from day 1 through adulthood, but it was functionally absent early in life since there was no appreciable chloride permeability via this channel. The Na-K-Cl2 co-transporter CCC2 was prominent in the thin ascending limb early in life, similar to that in the thick ascending limb, but it regressed in the thin limb by adulthood to be replaced functionally by the chloride channel. In addition, early in life, transepithelial voltages in the thin ascending limb could be inhibited by bumetanide (inhibitor of the Na-K-Cl2 co-transporter in the thick ascending limb) and ouabain (inhibitor of the Na pump), and transepithelial voltages in the inner medullary collecting duct could be inhibited by amiloride (inhibitor of Na channel and active electrogenic Na reabsorption). These results indicate capability for active NaCl reabsorption in the thin ascending limb early in life, in contrast to its passive reabsorption in this segment in adults. Aquaporin-1 was observed by day 4 in thin descending limbs, persisting into adulthood, and aquaporin-2 was present throughout development. These findings, taken with others, indicate that

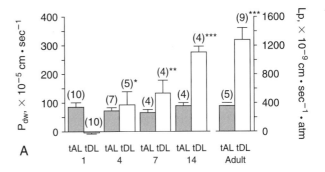

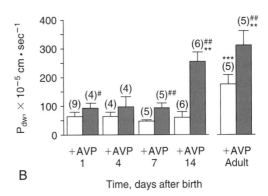

Figure 135-11. Maturational changes in water transport. **A,** Water permeability (P_{dw}) was constant and low through adulthood in thin ascending limb (tAL), emphasizing its impermeability, and remained low in thin descending limb (tDL) until day 14, indicating low water permeability during the neonatal period. **B,** In the inner medullary collecting duct, basal water permeability (*clear bar*) remained low until adulthood. Vasopressin 1 nmol/l (*hatched bar*) stimulated water transport only modestly in the early neonatal period, but did not reach adult levels until day 14. *$p < .05$; **$p < .01$; ***$p < .0001$ vs. day 1; #$p < .05$; ##$p < .01$ vs. baseline. Number in parentheses indicates number of tubules examined. (From Liu W, et al: Kidney Int *60*:680, 2001.)

water channels became poised to support water transfer once other medullary relationships are in place.

The investigators concluded that there is a fundamentally different organization of the inner medulla between neonates and adults (Fig. 135-13). Transiently early in life, the inner medulla is characterized by active reabsorption and accumulation of NaCl. Compared with that of the adult, the thin descending limb is much less permeant to water. Since the thin ascending limb remains impermeant to water, the neonatal inner medulla is poised to reabsorb NaCl actively without water transfer, allowing urinary dilution early in life. At the same time, the inner medullary collecting duct is not geared to recycle urea. Subsequently, tubular transport properties appear that include increased thin

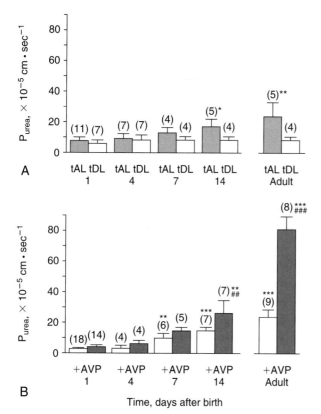

Figure 135–12. Maturational changes in urea permeability. **A,** Urea permeability (P_{urea}) was low through adulthood in thin descending limb (tDL) and gradually increased in thin ascending limb (tAL), approaching adult values only by day 14. **B,** In the inner medullary collecting duct, basal urea permeability increased by day 7 and increased only mildly thereafter. Vasopressin (AVP) stimulated urea transport by day 14, but the value was considerably less than that of the adult. Number in parentheses indicates number of tubules examined. $*p < .05$; $**p < .01$; $***p < .0001$ vs. day 1; $^{\#\#}p < .01$; $^{\#\#\#}p < .0001$ vs. baseline. (From Liu W, et al: Kidney Int *60*:680, 2001.)

descending limb water permeability, passive NaCl reabsorption in the thin ascending limb with functional maturation of a chloride channel, and increased urea permeability and responsiveness to vasopressin. Efficient urinary concentration requires that these properties be in place.

Renal Blood Flow. In the adult kidney, about 90% of blood flows through the cortex only, about 10% perfuses the outer medulla, and about 1% to 2% reaches the inner medulla and papilla. This arrangement helps preserve the osmotic gradient established by the countercurrent mechanism. Rapid flow through the medulla tends to dissipate it. Neonatal renal blood flow is proportionately greater to deeper medullary regions of the kidney, and glomerular blood flow is greater in deep than in superficial nephrons.[128-130] After birth, renal vascular resistance drops more than resistance in systemic vessels, cardiac output and surface area increase briskly, and renal blood flow rises. Increases in single-nephron blood flow are proportionally greater in outer than in deep cortical nephrons. A relatively greater medullary flow in neonatal kidneys may delay establishing the corticomedullary gradient.

Renal Pelvis. The renal pelvis in the newborn animal is relatively narrow and does not extend too far into the body of the kidney. As the animal matures, secondary fornices and outpouchings of the renal pelvis come to extend well toward the renal cortex (Fig. 135–14) so that urine in the pelvis will bathe a

greater part of the papilla.[144, 204] As mentioned previously, this pelvic maturation may facilitate recycling of urea from pelvic urine back to medullary interstitium to further increase both interstitial solute concentration and final urine osmolality. It is of interest that ADH appears to have some impact on the growth of the renal medulla and renal pelvis. In young growing lambs, treatment with ADH (DDAVP) for 13 weeks starting at 2 weeks of life induced an increase in the size of the renal medulla, especially the outer medulla, and the surface area of the renal pelvis. Ruminants have particularly well-developed renal pelvic fornices in their outer medulla. This is the area where dimensions were most impressively enlarged by vasopressin. Therefore, the outer medulla may play a particularly important role in the reabsorption and recycling of urea in these animals.[206] Nevertheless, the role of this whole process in maturation of the urinary concentrating mechanism remains speculative at this point.

In summary, the low urinary concentrating capacity of newborn mammals is related to a variety of anatomic and functional factors. The loops of Henle are relatively short, the transport properties of the thick ascending limb of Henle are immature, and there is an insufficient number of loops of Henle from more superficial nephrons that penetrate deeper into the cortex and outer medulla. Renal blood flow to deeper juxtamedullary nephrons is proportionally greater in the newborn than in the adult. Enhanced prostaglandin production has the potential to reduce salt, water, and urea transport at critical sites and to increase medullary blood flow. These factors may all contribute to the smaller medullary gradient and the lower medullary urea content found in the newborn. Neonatal collecting duct cells have decreased responsiveness to ADH and limited ability to maintain a transepithelial sodium (osmolar) gradient. Pelvic spaces surrounding papillae are narrower and more extensive in adults. This latter anatomic difference may contribute to a low concentrating ability during maturation, since urine bathing the papillae may enhance urine and papillary osmolality. Aquaporin-1 may also limit neonatal concentrating ability, since the amount of this protein is decreased in the human kidney at birth and increases gradually to approach adult levels at a time when the young kidney concentrates urine nearly as well as the adult. Less likely to play a role is aquaporin-2, since this protein is not only present in utero at 20 weeks' gestation, but also must be functional as evidenced by the response of the isolated human fetal medullary collecting tubule of similar gestational age to vasopressin.

PHYSIOLOGY OF THE URINARY DILUTING MECHANISM

Urinary dilution is thought to have developed when our primitive ancestors left the briny seas for more freshwater habitats. In so doing, they were forced to evolve mechanisms that could separate water from solute to preserve needed solute, eliminate imbibed excess water, and avoid fatal dilution of body fluids. It was considerably later in evolution when creatures had to develop a renal concentrating system to retain water as they traveled from one water locale to another.[207] Diluting capacity is considerable in the human adult, who can excrete about 10% to 12% of the filtered load or about 14 to 17 l of water/day if the GFR is 100 ml/minute. More water can be excreted with higher rates of filtration. In terms of absolute volume, this capacity is considerably more limited in the infant, although the young subject can excrete ~15%, and perhaps even more, of the filtered load.

Our ability to dilute urine and remove excess water is more efficient than our ability to concentrate urine and retain needed water. For example, suppose a 70-kg subject has a serum osmolality of 300 mOsm/kg and a daily renal solute excretory load of 600 mOsm. If urine osmolality is 300 mOsm/kg and the 600 mOsm solute load is excreted in 2 l of water, the subject is in water balance because the urine is isotonic to plasma and the

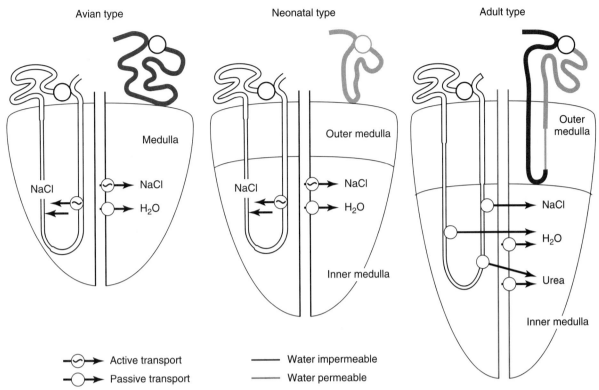

Figure 135–13. Comparison of neonatal and adult renal medullary tubule organization. In the neonatal kidney, only long-looped nephrons penetrate the medulla, and the medulla has essentially no water movement in loops of Henle. Medullary NaCl accumulates by active transport in the thin ascending limb and there is amiloride-sensitive Na reabsorption in the inner medullary collecting duct. During maturation, cortical loops come to penetrate the outer medulla. In addition, NaCl reabsorption becomes passive in thin ascending limb, collecting duct amiloride-sensitive Na reabsorption disappears, the thin descending limb becomes water permeant, and urea permeability in the inner medullary collecting duct becomes highly sensitive to vasopressin. Neonatal tubule organization is likened to the avian kidney. Delayed maturation of neonatal concentrating ability is related to a more "primitive" tubule organization early in life. (From Liu W, et al: Kidney Int *60*:680, 2001.)

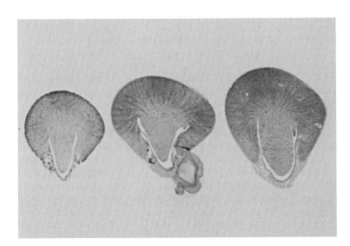

Figure 135–14. Cross-section showing gross structure of kidney and renal pelvis. In a 3-day-old rat *(left)*, specialized fornices, evaginations of pelvic space, are absent and the pelvis is of the simple type. In a 10-day-old rat *(center)*, specialized fornices are just beginning to appear, and by 20 days of age *(right)*, fornices are well developed and extend into kidney tissue between the cortex and outer zone (×7). (From Trimble ME: Am J Physiol *219*:1089, 1970.)

kidney has neither to concentrate nor dilute the urine to maintain a normal serum sodium level. If the subject is water deprived, urine osmolality can increase to a maximum of about 1200 mOsm/kg. At this urine concentration, 500 ml of water is needed to excrete the 600-mOsm solute load. Stated another way, of the 2 l of water/day needed to excrete this solute isotonically, a maximum of about 1500 ml of water/day can be retained to maintain normal serum osmolality; however, 600 mOsm cannot be concentrated in a volume of less than 500 ml. If the subject is water loaded, excess water can be excreted by reducing urine osmolality to a minimum of about 50 mOsm/kg. In this case, the kidney can excrete the 600 mOsm of solute in a urine volume of 12 l and remove 10 l of "pure" water in the process to maintain a normal serum sodium level.

In this example, renal diluting capacity (10 l water) is nearly sevenfold the concentrating capacity (1.5 l water) in terms of actual volume of water handled to maintain osmolar balance. This translates to a 24-fold increase in urine osmolality and urine volume when the urine changes from maximally dilute (osmolality 50 mOsm/kg–volume 12,000 ml) to maximally concentrated (osmolality, 1200 mOsm/kg; volume, 500 ml). Renal excretory solute loads in children usually range from 10 to 40 mOsm/100 calories expended. Urine volume required to excrete this solute varies with diet and availability of water.[208] Ingested water enters the total body water compartment where it is partly incorporated into new cells during growth. Extra water is eliminated by insensible losses and urine output, the latter allowing removal of the renal excretory solute load. A net excess or deficit of water leads to alterations in electrolyte balance.

When water intake is sufficient to lower serum osmolality by about 1% (about 3 mOsm/kg), ADH secretion is suppressed. Solute reabsorption continues in the thick ascending limb, distal nephron, collecting tubule, and collecting duct. The latter segments become less permeable to water when ADH is absent. As a consequence, fluid traversing the distal nephron and entering the medulla becomes progressively dilute. Since water remains in the tubule lumen, urea concentration is reduced, and a major urea concentration difference between collecting duct fluid and interstitium will fail to develop. Since urea permeability in the medullary collecting duct is also decreased in the absence of ADH, urea entering this segment will be more easily excreted. The overall effect is that urea tends to be eliminated from, rather than recycled in, the medullary system. Interstitial as well as urinary urea concentrations decrease, whereas total urea excretion actually increases, but in a larger volume of water.

Reduced tubule permeability to water and continued reabsorption of solute in more distal parts of the nephron might be expected to increase interstitial solute concentrations. However, interstitial solute concentrations are actually reduced compared with the antidiuretic state. It is likely that the water gradient from lumen to interstitium at the medullary collecting duct is high enough to overcome the low water permeability induced by lack of ADH. As a result, reabsorption of water in medullary collecting ducts is actually greater, not less, during water diuresis. Perhaps as much as half the water delivered to collecting ducts backdiffuses into the interstitium, but NaCl is sufficiently reabsorbed along this segment so that the urine actually becomes more dilute.[4, 209]

There is another factor of potential importance to urinary dilution and water excretion.[26] The renal pelvis has contractile properties and can induce reflux of urine around the renal papilla and medulla. Full retrograde pelvic reflux is not typical of the antidiuretic state, but exposure of medullary structures to urine occurs much more often with the high flow rates associated with dilute urine. Urine refluxing into the fornices may actually reduce the amount of urea in the renal medulla (Fig. 135–15). Accordingly, full pelvic reflux may help eliminate a fluid load. Investigators have noted a lack of clear correlation between concentrating ability and size and complexity of pelvic extensions, but there is a correlation between the size of pelvic extensions and the need to excrete a water load. Animals living in arid areas and requiring no drinking water exhibit a high urinary concentrating ability but have difficulty excreting a water load rapidly enough to avoid water intoxication and possible death. Such animals do not have large pelvic fornices. Animals that tolerate dehydration but periodically need water must be able to eliminate water reasonably rapidly and tend to have large pelvic extensions. There is experimental evidence that during antidiuresis water exchanges across the pelvic epithelium and hypotonic fluid can be added to pelvic urine from the medulla to enhance papillary osmolality.[210] Although it has not been directly studied, one might similarly predict that during water diuresis, water from dilute urine could enter the medulla from pelvic extensions and dilute the medullary interstitium, facilitating excretion of water.

Fluid along the proximal tubule is reabsorbed isotonically and does not directly add to urinary dilution. However, the amount of fluid reabsorbed at this site determines, to a major extent, the volume of dilute urine that can later be formed. A drop in filtration rate or an increase in proximal tubular reabsorption allows less fluid to arrive at the diluting site and therefore will limit the actual amount of water excretion. Some segment must be

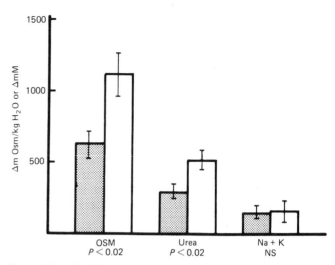

Figure 135–15. Effect of full pelvic refluxes during rising urine flow on solute concentrations in hamsters. Urine flow was increased to a rate just below that needed to cause full pelvic reflux. Refluxes were then mechanically induced for 20 minutes in experimental kidney *(filled bar)*. The other kidney served as a control. Values (mean ± SE) are difference in osmolality (mOsm/kg H_2O), urea (mM), and Na + K (mM) concentrations between renal papilla and refluxing or nonrefluxing kidney. (From Schmidt-Nielsen B: Kidney Int *31*:621, 1987.)

capable of reabsorbing solute in excess of water to allow luminal fluid to become dilute. This process occurs along the entire length of the ascending limb of Henle, especially along its thick portion. Any problem in solute reabsorption along this site will effectively prevent excretion of dilute urine. Once urine passes into the distal nephron, in which solute reabsorption continues, water must remain largely in the lumen. Vasopressin determines the degree to which water will be reabsorbed, since the water permeability of collecting duct epithelium depends on the presence of this hormone.

It becomes apparent, then, that to dilute urine, three fundamental conditions must be met. First, a sufficient amount of filtrate must escape reabsorption along the proximal tubule and reach the diluting segment (ascending loop of Henle) to deliver a sufficient amount of potential pure water. Second, this segment must be able to reclaim NaCl and separate reabsorbed solute from water so that urine becomes dilute (water stays in the lumen for excretion). Third, as solute continues to be reabsorbed from more distal sites, further diluting the urine, the ADH-sensitive nephron segments must be able to eliminate the excess water (these segments must not be exposed to secreted ADH and thereby forced to reclaim free water). Accordingly, urinary dilution results from the active reabsorption of NaCl along the thick ascending limb of Henle and the continued reabsorption of solute along more distal nephron segments, in concert with a disproportionate reduction in reabsorption of water. Absence of any of these factors may lead to a defect in urinary dilution.

Urinary Dilution in the Fetus

The human kidney can dilute urine early in fetal life.[144] Urine voided at birth, i.e., formed *in utero*, is hypotonic compared with the infant's serum. In contrast, maternal urine osmolality is five-fold more concentrated than that of the infant. Urine voided during the first 24 hours after birth becomes more concentrated than serum but still has an osmolality less than half that of the mother's urine.[211] Therefore, the fetal kidney behaves as though it is trying to excrete a water load, whereas the newborn kidney seems to be stimulated to retain water. Amniotic fluid is hypotonic, particularly toward the end of pregnancy. A term fetus ingests substantial amounts of dilute amniotic fluid (~5 ml/kg/hr).[212] This value is similar to the estimated urine flow rate of 5 ml/kg/hr in primates[93] and is close to the amount of breast milk ingested per day by a healthy newborn infant. A need to excrete this fluid load would account for dilution of fetal urine. Since infants often are not given oral fluid immediately after birth, subsequent concentration of urine represents another appropriate response.[144]

Urinary Dilution in the Neonate

One might expect that limitations in concentrating ability would enable an infant to excrete water more easily and protect itself from water intoxication. However, despite effective urinary dilution, there are limitations to water excretion early in life.[213, 214] Low GFR limits the volume of water that can be excreted. A reduced ability to separate solute from water along the immature ascending limb may further limit the amount of free water cleared from this segment,[127, 146, 147] but this factor is probably of limited importance beyond a few weeks of age. In fact, urine from infants can be maximally diluted to an osmolality of about 50 mOsm/kg,[215-217] a value comparable to that in older children and adults. Although data were not strictly limited to neonates, Rodriquez-Soriano and associates[216] found that at periods of maximal free water clearance, urine osmolality in infants dropped to 52 mOsm/kg on average, and urine flow rates reached nearly 23 ml/dl of glomerular filtration. These infants and children effectively eliminated a water load with minimal impact on serum sodium and osmolality. In this study, fractional delivery of sodium to the distal nephron was high, indicating decreased proximal tubular salt reabsorption. However, reabsorption of salt along diluting segments of the distal nephron increased, indicating that enhanced distal reabsorption compensated for decreased proximal reabsorption. In general, the youngest infants tended to have high rates of delivery of sodium to the distal nephron, but they also had high rates of distal tubular sodium reabsorption. Clearly, at a young age, diluting segments have the potential to reabsorb solute avidly, and ADH-sensitive segments can be inhibited effectively from reabsorbing excess water. The primary limitation in neonatal water excretion, therefore, falls largely on the low rates of filtration.

The rapidity of maturation of an infant's ability to excrete an acute water load was illustrated by Ames.[218] In this study, premature and term infants of different postnatal ages received 30 ml/kg of either an oral water load or an intravenous 2.5% dextrose solution load. Water excretion was initially quite low (Fig. 135–16). On average, infants in the first 24 hours of life excreted only 10% to 15% of the fluid load over 2 to 3 hours, with only a mild increase by 3 days of age. However, the ability to excrete the water load improved quickly. Infants 8 to 14 days of age excreted about 60% of the load, and most infants older than 15 days (and all infants older than 30 days) excreted the total fluid load within 2 hours. One premature infant of birth weight 1.2 kg excreted 50% of an infused fluid load by the fourth day of life and excreted 100% by 12 days of age. Infants older than 7 days of age effectively reduced urine specific gravity to 1.002. The increasing ability to excrete the water was associated with a higher GFR. This finding is consistent with the notion that the low GFR limits the absolute amount of water that can be excreted.

Calcagno and co-workers[138] found that 60 minutes after an acute water load, a 1.6-kg, 23-day-old premature infant was able to increase urine flow to 8.3 ml/min/1.73 m² (compared with 12 to 14 ml/min/1.73 m² in the adult) and to decrease urine osmolality to 50 mOsm/kg. In the study by Barnett and coworkers,[215] five premature infants were given a 40-ml/kg oral water load.

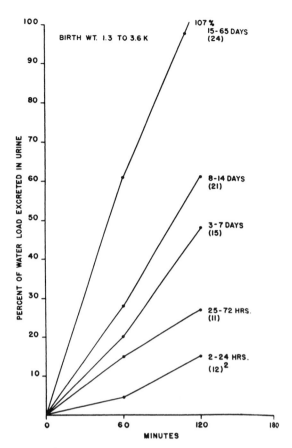

Figure 135–16. Comparison of ability to excrete water load by infants of various ages after intravenous administration of 2.5% glucose, 30 ml/kg body weight given at –10 to 0 minutes. Number in parentheses is number of infants per group. (Reproduced by permission of Pediatrics *12*:272, 1953.)

Urine osmolality dropped to 41 to 63 mOsm/kg. Although their urine flow rates after an hour were, in general, only about half that of adults, one 36-day-old premature infant not only diluted the urine maximally, but also had a urine flow rate fully comparable to that of the adult. Clearly, there is a fairly rapid postnatal maturation of this particular function.

It should be noted that while ability to excrete an acute water load matures quickly, a sustained water load is more difficult to excrete in infants who have a low GFR and a limited ability to reabsorb solute along the distal nephron.[217] Fortunately, GFR matures relatively early in life and allows efficient elimination of a sustained water load. This is illustrated by a 6.5-kg, 2-month-old infant who had been given water whenever he became fretful. He ingested up to 2100 ml/day, developed polyuria, excreted urine with an osmolality of 42 mOsm/kg, and had only mild hyponatremia. His free water clearance was nearly 11 ml/min/dl of glomerular filtration.[219] In the acutely or chronically water-loaded state, ADH is suppressed. Aquaporin-2 staining is more prominent in cytoplasmic vesicles and less so in the apical membrane of collecting ducts. Since aquaporin-2 is thought to be the actual ADH-sensitive water channel, excretion of a water load is likely made possible largely by acutely removing or more chronically down-regulating water channels from the membrane, thereby reducing apical membrane water reabsorption.[60, 61, 78] Recovery from the down-regulation of apical membrane water channels will take time, since this protein up-regulates its production and membrane content in response to subsequent water restriction.

CONCLUSION

In summary, diluting function depends on the ability to deliver adequate quantities of filtrate to nephron segments that can separate solute from water. More distal segments must be relatively water impermeant. Infants can maximally dilute their urine at an early age. Their ability to excrete an acute water load matures within a few weeks of birth. Limited excretion of a sustained water load likely relates to the very low GFR typical of this age. However, moderately large amounts of ingested water can be effectively eliminated even in relatively young infants. Diluting capacity is quantitatively greater than concentrating capacity and tends to mature at an earlier age. The range of these functions is such that infants, even those of very low birth weight, tolerate a large range of fluid intake without having to sustain major alterations to their fluid and electrolyte stability. It is interesting that the staple infant food, breast milk, is dilute with a low renal solute load. The infant kidney must soon become adept at excreting a water load, an important adaptation if extra "free" water is ingested. The delay in maturation of urinary concentration for several months becomes less critical in the healthy infant because there is generally a delay in introducing foods of greater solute content till later in infancy.

REFERENCES

1. De Rouffignac C, Jamison RL (guest editors): The urinary concentrating mechanism. Kidney Int. 31:501, 1987.
2. Jamison RL, Maffly RH: The urinary concentrating mechanism. N Engl J Med 295:1059, 1976.
3. Kokko JP, Rector FC Jr: Countercurrent multiplication system without active transport in inner medulla. Kidney Int. 2:214, 1972.
4. Roy DR, Jamison RL: Countercurrent system and its regulation. In Seldin D, Giebisch G, (eds): The Kidney: Physiology and Pathophysiology. New York, Raven Press, 1985, pp 903–932.
5. Hebert SC, et al: The medullary thick limb: function and modulation of the single-effect multiplier. Kidney Int 31:580, 1987.
6. Knepper MA, Roch-Ramel F: Pathways of urea transport in the mammalian kidney. Kidney Int 31:629, 1987.
7. Kokko JP: The role of the collecting duct in urinary concentration. Kidney Int 31:606, 1987.
8. Sanjana VM, et al: Water extraction from the inner medullary collecting tubule system: a role for urea. Kidney Int 10:139, 1976.
9. Knepper MA, et al: Independence of urea and water transport in rat inner medullary collecting duct. Am J Physiol 256 (Renal Fluid Electrolyte Physiol 25):F610, 1989.
10. Imai M, et al: Function of thin loops of Henle. Kidney Int. 31:565, 1987.
11. Woo SK, Kwon HM: Adaptation of kidney medulla to hypertonicity: role of the transcription factor TonEBP. Int Rev Cytol 215:189, 2002.
12. Woo SK, et al: TonEBP/NFAT5 stimulates transcription of HSP70 in response to hypertonicity. Mol Cell Biol 22:5753, 2002.
13. Jamison RL: Short and long loop nephrons. Kidney Int 31:597, 1987.
14. Lemley KV, Kriz W: Cycles and separations: the histotopography of the urinary concentrating process. Kidney Int 31:538, 1987.
15. Xu Y, et al: Endothelial cells of the kidney vasa recta express the urea transporter. Kidney Int 51:138, 1997.
16. Smith CP, et al: Cloning and regulation of expression of the rat kidney urea transporter (rUT2). J Clin Invest 96:1556, 1995.
17. You G, et al: Expression cloning and characterization of the vasopressin-regulated urea transporter. Nature 365:844, 1993.
18. Bagnasco SM, et al: Cloning and characterization of the human urea transporter UT-A1 and mapping of the human Slc14a2 gene. Am J Physiol Renal Physiol 281:F400, 2001.
19. Fenton RA, et al: Structure and characterization of the mouse UT-A gene (Slc14a2). Am J Physiol Renal Physiol 282:F630, 2002.
20. Shayakul C, et al: Long-term regulation of urea transporter expression by vasopressin in Brattleboro rats. Am J Physiol Renal Physiol 278:F620, 2000.
21. Timmer RT, et al: Localization of the urea transporter UT-B protein in human and rat erythrocytes and tissues. Am J Physiol Renal Physiol 281:C1318, 2001.
22. Trinh-Treng-Tan MM, et al: UT-B1 proteins in rat: tissue distribution and regulation by antidiuretic hormone in kidney. Am J Physiol Renal Physiol 283:F912, 2002.
23. Soroka SD, et al: Minimum urine flow rate during water deprivation: importance of the nonurea versus total osmolality in the inner medulla. J Am Soc Nephrol 8:880, 1997.
24. Gowrishankar M, et al: Minimum urine flow rate during water deprivation: importance of the permeability of urea in the inner medulla. J Am Soc Nephrol 53:159, 1998.

25. Zimmerhackl BL, et al: The medullary microcirculation. Kidney Int 31:641, 1987.
26. Schmidt-Nielsen B: The renal pelvis. Kidney Int 31:621, 1987.
27. Bonventre JV, et al: Renal papillary epithelial morphology in antidiuresis and water diuresis. Am J Physiol 235 (Renal Fluid Electrolyte Physiol 4):F69, 1978.
28. Pfeiffer EW: Comparative anatomical observations of the mammalian renal pelvis and medulla. J Anat 102:321, 1968.
29. Oliver RE, et al: Urinary concentration in the papillary collecting duct of the rat. J Clin Invest 69:157, 1982.
30. Bonventre JV, et al: Effect of urea concentration of pelvic fluid on renal concentrating ability. Am J Physiol 239 (Renal Fluid Electrolyte Physiol 8):F609, 1980.
31. Reinking LN, Schmidt-Nielsen B: Peristaltic flow of urine in the renal papillary collecting ducts of hamsters. Kidney Int 20:55, 1981.
32. Schmidt-Nielsen B, et al: Occurrence of renal pelvic refluxes during rising urine flow rate in rats and hamsters. Kidney Int. 18:419, 1980.
33. Schmidt-Nielsen B, Reinking LN: Morphometry and fluid reabsorption during peristaltic flow in hamster renal papillary collecting ducts. Kidney Int 20:789, 1981.
34. King LS, et al: Aquaporin-1 water channel protein in lung. Ontogeny, steroid-induced expression, and distribution in rat. J Clin Invest 97:2183, 1996.
35. King LS, et al: Aquaporins in health and disease. Mol Med Today 6:60, 2000.
36. Nielsen S, et al: Distribution of the aquaporin CHIP in secretory and resorptive epithelia and capillary endothelia. Proc Natl Acad Sci U S A 90:7275, 1993.
37. Nielsen S, et al: CHIP28 water channels are localized in constitutively water-permeable segments of the nephron. J Cell Biol 120:371, 1993.
38. Klussmann E, et al: The mechanisms of aquaporin control in the renal collecting duct. Rev Physiol Biochem Pharmacol 141:33, 2000.
39. Knepper MA, et al: Renal aquaporins. Kidney Int 49:1712, 1996.
40. Marples D, et al: Long-term regulation of aquaporins in the kidney. Am J Physiol (Renal Fluid Electrolyte Physiol) 276:F331, 1999.
41. Nielsen S, Agre P: The aquaporin family of water channels in kidney. Kidney Int 48:1057, 1995.
42. Nielsen S, et al: Aquaporins in the kidney: from molecules to medicine. Physiol Rev 82:205, 2002.
43. Nielsen S, et al: Physiology and pathophysiology of renal aquaporins. J Am Soc Nephrol 10:647, 1999.
44. Nielsen S, et al: The aquaporin family of water channels in kidney: an update on physiology and pathophysiology of aquaporin-2. Kidney Int 49:1718, 1996.
45. Sasaki S, et al: Water channels in the kidney collecting duct. Kidney Int 48:1082, 1995.
46. Verkman AS, Mitra AK: Structure and function of aquaporin water channels. Am J Physiol (Renal Fluid Electrolyte Physiol) 278:F13, 2000.
47. Preston GM, et al: Appearance of water channels in Xenopus oocytes expressing red cell CHIP 28 protein. Science 256:385, 1992.
48. Zeidel ML, et al: Reconstitution of functional water channels in liposomes containing purified red cell CHIP28 protein. Biochemistry 31:7436, 1992.
49. Agre P, et al: Aquaporin CHIP: the archetypal molecular water channel. Am J Physiol 265 (Renal Fluid Electrolyte Physiol 34):F463, 1993.
50. Maeda Y, et al: Quantification of aquaporin-CHIP water channel protein in microdissected renal tubules by fluorescence-based ELISA. J Clin Invest 95:422, 1995.
51. Nielsen S, et al: Aquaporin-1 water channels in short and long loop descending thin limbs and in descending vasa recta in rat kidney. Am J Physiol 268 (Renal Fluid Electrolyte Physiol 37):F1023, 1995.
52. Preston GM, et al: Mutations in aquaporin-1 in phenotypically normal humans without functional CHIP water channels. Science 265:1585, 1994.
53. King LS, et al: Brief report: defective urinary concentrating ability due to a complete deficiency of aquaporin-1. N Engl J Med 345:175, 2001.
54. Ma T, et al: Severely impaired urinary concentrating ability in transgenic mice lacking aquaporin-1 water channels. J Biol Chem 273:4296, 1998.
55. Schnermann J, et al: Defective proximal tubular fluid reabsorption in transgenic aquaporin-1 null mice. Proc Natl Acad Sci U S A 95:9660, 1998.
56. Chou CL, et al: Reduced water permeability and altered ultrastructure in thin descending limb of Henle in aquaporin-1 null mice. J Clin Invest 103:491, 1999.
57. Brown D: Membrane recycling and epithelial cell function. Am J Physiol 256 (Renal Fluid Electrolyte Physiol 25):F1, 1989.
58. Harris HWJ, et al: Current understanding of the cellular biology and molecular structure of the antidiuretic hormone–stimulated water transport pathway. J Clin Invest 88:1, 1991.
59. Fushimi K, et al: Cloning and expression of apical membrane water channel of rat kidney collecting tubule. Nature 361:549, 1993.
60. Marples D, et al: Redistribution of aquaporin-2 water channels induced by vasopressin in rat kidney inner medullary collecting duct. Am J Physiol 269 (Cell Physiol 38):C655, 1995.
61. Nielsen S, et al: Vasopressin increases water permeability of kidney collecting duct by inducing translocation of aquaporin-CD water channels to plasma membrane. Proc Natl Acad Sci U S A 92:1013, 1995.
62. Katsura T, et al: Direct demonstration of aquaporin-2 water channel recycling in stably transfected LLC-PK1 epithelial cells. Am J Physiol 270 (Renal Fluid Electrolyte Physiol 39):F548, 1996.
63. Marples D, et al: Lithium-induced downregulation of aquaporin-2 water channel expression in rat kidney medulla. J Clin Invest 95:1838, 1995.
64. Frokiaer J, et al: Bilateral ureteral obstruction downregulates expression of vasopressin-sensitive AQP-2 water channel in rat kidney. Am J Physiol 270 (Renal Electrolyte Physiol 39):F657, 1996.

65. Marples D, et al: Hypokalemia-induced downregulation of aquaporin-2 water channel expression in rat kidney medulla and cortex. J Clin Invest 97:1960, 1996.

66. Earm JH, et al: Decreased aquaporin-2 expression and apical plasma membrane delivery in kidney collecting ducts of polyuric hypercalcemic rats. J Am Soc Nephrol 9:2181, 1998.

67. Sands JM, et al: Vasopressin-elicited water and urea permeabilities are altered in IMCD in hypercalcemic rats. Am J Physiol Renal Physiol 274:F978, 1998.

68. DiGiovanni SR, et al: Regulation of collecting duct water channel expression by vasopressin in Brattleboro rat. Proc Natl Acad Sci U S A 91:8984, 1994.

69. Nielsen S, et al: Cellular and subcellular immunolocalization of vasopressin-regulated water channel in rat kidney. Proc Natl Acad Sci U S A 90:11663, 1993.

70. Sands JM, et al: Changes in aquaporin-2 protein contribute to the urine concentrating defect in rats fed a low-protein diet. J Clin Invest 97:2807, 1996.

71. Deen PMT, et al: Requirement of human renal water channel aquaporin-2 for vasopressin-dependent concentration of urine. Science 264:92, 1994.

72. Deen PMT, et al: Urinary content of aquaporin 1 and 2 in nephrogenic diabetes insipidus. J Am Soc Nephrol 7:836, 1996.

73. Elliot S, et al: Urinary excretion of aquaporin-2 in humans: a potential marker of collecting duct responsiveness to vasopressin. J Am Soc Nephrol 7:403, 1996.

74. Tsukahara H, et al: Renal water channel expression in newborns: measurement of urinary excretion of aquaporin-2. Metabolism 47:1344, 1998.

75. Kishore BK, et al: Rat renal arcade segment expresses vasopressin-regulated water channel and vasopressin V2 receptor. J Clin Invest 97:2763, 1996.

76. Ecelbarger CA, et al: Aquaporin-3 water channel localization and regulation in rat kidney. Am J Physiol 269 (Renal Fluid Electrolyte Physiol 38):F663, 1995.

77. Terris J, et al: Distribution of aquaporin-4 water channel expression within rat kidney. Am J Physiol 269 (Renal Fluid Electrolyte Physiol 38):F775, 1995.

78. Terris J, et al: Long-term regulation of four renal aquaporins in rats. Am J Physiol 271 (Renal Fluid Electrolyte Physiol 40):F414, 1996.

79. Ma T, et al: Nephrogenic diabetes insipidus in mice lacking aquaporin-3 water channels. Proc Natl Acad Sci U S A 97:4386, 2000.

80. Echevarria M, et al: Cloning and expression of AQP-3 a water channel from the medullary collecting duct of rat kidney. Proc Natl Acad Sci U S A 91:10997, 1994.

81. Ma T, et al: Generation and phenotype of a transgenic knockout mouse lacking the mercurial-insensitive water channel aquaporin-4. J Clin Invest 100:957, 1997.

82. Chou CL, et al: Fourfold reduction of water permeability in inner medullary collecting duct of aquaporin-4 knockout mice. Am J Physiol (Cell Physiol) 274:C549, 1998.

83. Yasui M, et al: Aquaporin-6: an intracellular vesicle water channel protein in renal epithelia. Proc Natl Acad Sci U S A 96:5808, 1999.

84. Elkjaer ML, et al: Immunolocalization of aquaporin-8 in rat kidney, liver, testis, epididymis, jejunum, colon, principal bronchi and salivary glands. Am J Physiol (Renal Physiol) 281:F1047, 2001.

85. Uchida S, et al: Localization and functional characterization of rat kidney-specific chloride channel, ClC-K1. J Clin Invest 95:104, 1995.

86. Vandewalle A, et al: Localization and induction by dehydration of ClC-K chloride channels in the rat kidney. Am J Physiol 272 (Renal Physiol 41):F678, 1997.

87. Akizuki N, et al: Impaired solute accumulation in inner medulla of Clcnk1-/- mice kidney. Am J Physiol Renal Physiol 280:F79, 2001.

88. Matsumura Y, et al: Overt nephrogenic diabetes insipidus in mice lacking the CLC-K1 chloride channel. Nat Genet 21:95, 1999.

89. Devuyst O, Guggino WB: Chloride channels in the kidney: lessons learned from knockout animals. Am J Physiol Renal Physiol 283:F1176, 2002.

90. Stegner H, et al: Permeability of the sheep placenta to 125I-arginine vasopressin. Dev Pharmacol Ther 7:140, 1984.

91. Alexander DP, Nixon DA: The foetal kidney. Br Med Bull 17:112, 1961.

92. Alexander DP, et al: Gestational variations in the composition of the foetal fluids and foetal urine in the sheep. J Physiol (Lond) 140:1, 1958.

93. Chez RA, et al: Renal function in the intrauterine primate fetus. I. Experimental technique; rate of formation and chemical composition of urine. Am J Obstet Gynecol 90:128, 1964.

94. McCance RA, Stanier MW: The function of the metanephros of foetal rabbits and pigs. J Physiol (Lond) 151:479, 1960.

95. Merlet-Benichou C, deRouffignac C: Renal clearance studies in fetal and young guinea pigs: effect of salt loading. Am J Physiol 232:F178, 1977.

96. Robillard JE, et al: Developmental aspects of renal tubular reabsorption of water in the lamb fetus. Pediatr Res 13:1172, 1979.

97. Smith FG, et al: Studies of renal function in the intact fetal lamb. Am J Obstet Gynecol 96:240, 1966.

98. Robillard JE, et al: Developmental aspects of renal tubular reabsorption of water and fetal renal response to arginine vasopressin. In Spitzer A (ed): The Kidney During Development; Morphology and Function. New York, Masson, 1982, pp 205-213.

99. Moore ES, et al: Ontogeny of intrarenal solute gradients in fetal life. In Spitzer A (ed): The Kidney During Development; Morphology and Function. New York, Masson, 1982, pp 223-231.

100. Stanier MW: Development of intra-renal solute gradients in foetal and post-natal life. Pfluegers Arch 336:263, 1972.

101. Leake RD, Fisher DA: Ontogeny of vasopressin in man. In Czernichow P, Robinson AG, (eds): Diabetes Insipidus in Man, Vol 13. Basel, S Karger, 1985, pp 42-51.

102. Levina SE: Endocrine features in development of human hypothalamus, hypophysis, and placenta. Gen Comp Endocrinol 11:151, 1968.

103. Skowsky WR, Fisher DA: Fetal neurohypophyseal arginine vasopressin and arginine vasotocin in man and sheep. Pediatr Res 11:627, 1977.

104. Rinne UK: Maturation of human hypothalamic neurosecretion. Biol Neonate 4:351, 1962.

105. Ausiello DA, et al: Vasopressin signaling in kidney cells. Kidney Int 31:521, 1987.

106. Dousa TP, Valtin H: Cellular actions of vasopressin in the mammalian kidney. Kidney Int 10:46, 1976.

107. Morel F, et al: Receptors to vasopressin and other hormones in the mammalian kidney. Kidney Int 31:512, 1987.

108. Imbert-Teboul M, et al: Ontogenesis of hormone-dependent adenylate cyclase in isolated rat nephron segments. Am J Physiol 247 (Renal Fluid Electrolyte Physiol 16):F316, 1984.

109. Rajerison RM, et al: Ontogenic development of antidiuretic hormone receptors in rat kidney: comparison of hormonal binding and adenylate cyclase activation. Mol Cell Endocrinol 4:271, 1976.

110. Schlondorff D, et al: Vasopressin activation of adenylate cyclase in isolated collecting tubules of newborn rabbits. In Spitzer A (ed): The Kidney During Development; Morphology and Function. New York, Masson, 1982, pp 257-262.

111. Schlondorff D, et al: Vasopressin responsiveness of renal adenylate cyclase in newborn rats and rabbits. Am J Physiol 234:F16, 1978.

112. Lingwood B, et al: The effects of antidiuretic hormone on urine flow and composition in the chronically-cannulated ovine fetus. Q J Exp Physiol 63:315, 1978.

113. Robillard JE, Weitzman RE: Developmental aspects of the fetal renal response to exogenous arginine vasopressin. Am J Physiol 238:F407, 1980.

114. Wintour EM, et al: Regulation of urine osmolality in fetal sheep. Q J Exp Physiol 67:427, 1982.

115. Abramow M, Dratwa M: Effect of vasopressin on the isolated human collecting duct. Nature 250:492, 1974.

116. Bell RJ, et al: Gestation-dependent aspects of the response of the ovine fetus to the osmotic stress induced by maternal water deprivation. Q J Exp Physiol 69:187, 1984.

117. Fisher DA, et al: Maturation of the vasopressin secretion control mechanism in the fetus and newborn. In Spitzer A (ed): The Kidney During Development; Morphology and Function. New York, Masson, 1982, pp 215-221.

118. Leake RD, et al: Maternal fetal osmolar homeostasis: fetal posterior pituitary autonomy. Pediatr Res 13:841, 1979.

119. Robillard JE, et al: Developmental aspects of the renal response to hypoxemia in the lamb fetus. Circ Res 48:128, 1981.

120. Siegel SR, et al: Effects of furosemide and acute salt loading on vasopressin and renin secretion in the fetal lamb. Pediatr Res 14:869, 1980.

121. Weitzman RE, et al: Arginine vasopressin response to an osmotic stimulus in the fetal sheep. Pediatr Res 12:35, 1978.

122. Wood LL, et al: Role of arginine vasopressin in the fetal response to hypertonicity. Am J Physiol 251 (Renal Fluid Electrolyte Physiol 20):F156, 1986.

123. Robillard JE, et al: The dynamics of vasopressin release and blood volume regulation during fetal hemorrhage in the lamb fetus. Pediatr Res 13:606, 1979.

124. Walker DW: Effect of hypoxia on glomerular filtration rate, urine flow and urine composition in chronically catheterized foetal lambs. J Physiol (Lond) 272:15P, 1977.

125. Osathanondh V, Potter EL: Development of human kidney as shown by microdissection. IV. Development of tubular portions of nephrons. Arch Pathol 82:391, 1966.

126. Speller AM, Moffat DB: Tubulo-vascular relationships in the developing kidney. J Anat 123:487, 1977.

127. Zink H, Horster M: Maturation of diluting capacity in loop of Henle of rat superficial nephrons. Am J Physiol 233:F519, 1977.

128. Aschinberg LC, et al: Neonatal changes in renal blood flow distribution in puppies. Am J Physiol 228:1453, 1975.

129. Jose PA: Intrarenal blood flow distribution in canine puppies. Pediatr Res 5:335, 1971.

130. Olbing H, et al: Postnatal changes in renal glomerular blood flow distribution in puppies. J Clin Invest 52:2885, 1973.

131. Jard S: Vasopressin receptors. In Czernichow P, Robinson AG (eds): Diabetes Insipidus in Man, Vol. 13, Basel, S Karger, 1985, pp 89-104.

132. Leake RD, et al: Arginine vasopressin and arginine vasotocin inhibit ovine fetal/maternal water transfer. Pediatr Res 17:583, 1983.

133. Perks AM, Cassin S: The effects of arginine vasopressin and other factors on the production of lung fluid in fetal goats. Chest (Suppl) 81:63, 1982.

134. Iwamoto HS, et al: Hemodynamic responses of the sheep fetus to vasopressin infusion. Circ Res 44:430, 1979.

135. Kelly RT, et al: Vasopressin is important for restoring cardiovascular homeostasis in fetal lambs subjected to hemorrhage. Am J Obstet Gynecol 146:807, 1983.

136. Wintour EM, et al: Ovine AQP1: cDNA cloning, ontogeny, and control of renal gene expression. Pediatr Nephrol 12:545, 1998.

137. Butkus A, et al: Ovine aquaporin-2: cDNA cloning, ontogeny and control of renal gene expression. Pediatr Nephrol 13:379, 1999.

138. Calcagno PL, et al: Studies on the renal concentrating and diluting mechanisms in the premature infant. J Clin Invest 33:91, 1954.

139. Janovsky M, et al: Antidiuretic activity in the plasma of human infants after a load of sodium chloride. Acta Paediatr Scand 54:543, 1965.

140. Polacek E, et al: The osmotic concentrating ability in healthy infants and children. Arch Dis Child 40:291, 1965.

141. Pratt EL, Snyderman SE: Renal water requirement of infants fed evaporated milk with and without added carbohydrates. Pediatrics 11:65, 1953.

142. Svenningsen NW, Aronson AS: Postnatal development of renal concentration capacity as estimated by DDAVP-test in normal and asphyxiated neonates. Biol Neonate 25:230, 1974.

143. Winberg J: Determination of renal concentration capacity in infants and children without renal disease. Acta Paediatr Scand 48:318, 1959.

144. McCrory WW: Developmental Nephrology. Cambridge, MA, Harvard University Press, 1972.

145. Edelmann CM Jr, et al: A standardized test of renal concentrating capacity in children. Am J Dis Child 114:639, 1967.

146. Horster M: Loop of Henle functional differentiation: in vitro perfusion of the isolated thick ascending segment. Pfluegers Arch 378:15, 1978.

147. Horster MF: Cellular determinants of extracellular osmotic homeostasis in nephron ontogeny. In Spitzer A (ed): The Kidney During Development; Morphology and Function. New York, Masson, 1982, pp 241–248.

148. Lelievre-Pegorier M, et al: Developmental pattern of water and electrolyte transport in rat superficial nephrons. Am J Physiol 245 (Renal Fluid Electrolyte 14):F15, 1983.

149. Kobayashi K, et al: Developmental expression of CLC-K1 in the postnatal rat kidney. Histochem Cell Biol 116:49, 2001.

150. Reyes JL, et al: Net sodium and water movements in the newborn rabbit collecting tubule: lack of modifications by indomethacin. Biol Neonate 51:212, 1987.

151. Gamble JL, et al: An economy of water in renal function referable to urea. Am J Physiol 109:139, 1934.

152. Epstein FH, et al: The effect of feeding protein and urea on the renal concentrating process. J Clin Invest 36:635, 1957.

153. Edelmann CM Jr, et al: Effect of urea on concentration of urinary nonurea solute in premature infants. J Appl Physiol 21:1021, 1966.

154. Edelmann CM Jr, et al: Renal concentrating mechanisms in newborn infants. Effect of dietary protein and water content, role of urea, and responsiveness to antidiuretic hormone. J Clin Invest 39:1062, 1960.

155. Boss JMN, et al: The structure of the kidney in relation to age and diet in white rats during the weaning period. J Physiol (Lond) 168:196, 1963.

156. Edwards BR, et al: Postnatal development of urinary concentrating ability in rats: changes in renal anatomy and neurohypophysial hormones. In Spitzer A (ed): The Kidney During Development; Morphology and Function. New York, Masson, 1982, pp 223–240.

157. Falk G: Maturation of renal function in infant rats. Am J Physiol 181:157, 1955.

158. Rane S, et al: Development of urinary concentrating capacity in weaning rats. Pediatr Res 19:472, 1985.

159. Boehm G, et al: Development of urea-synthesizing capacity in preterm infants during the first weeks of life. Biol Neonate 59:1, 1991.

160. Handler JS: Antidiuretic hormone moves membranes. Am J Physiol 255 (Renal Fluid Electrolyte Physiol 24):F375, 1988.

161. Hays RM, et al: Effects of antidiuretic hormone on the collecting duct. Kidney Int 31:530, 1987.

162. Leake RD, et al: Control of vasopressin secretion in the newborn lamb. Pediatr Res 13:257, 1979.

163. Fisher DA, et al: Studies of control water balance in the newborn. Am J Dis Child 106:137, 1963.

164. Chard T, et al: Release of oxytocin and vasopressin by the human foetus during labor. Nature (Lond) 234:352, 1971.

165. DeVane GW, Porter JC: An apparent stress-induced release of arginine vasopressin by human neonates. J Clin Endocrinol Metab 51:1412, 1980.

166. Hadeed AJ, et al: Possible mechanisms of high blood levels of vasopressin during the neonatal period. J Pediatr 94:805, 1979.

167. Pohjavuori M, Fyhrquist F: Hemodynamic significance of vasopressin in the newborn infant. J Pediatr 97:462, 1980.

168. Bockaert J, et al: Modulation of the coupling function relating occupancy of neurohypophyseal hormone receptors to adenylate cyclase activation. In Beers RF Jr, Bassett EG (eds): Cell Membrane Receptors for Viruses, Antigens, Antibodies, Polypeptide Hormones, and Small Molecules, Vol 9. New York, Raven Press, 1976, pp 354–377.

169. Rajerison RM, et al: Ontogenic development of kidney and liver vasopressin receptors. In Spitzer A (ed): The Kidney During Development; Morphology and Function. New York, Masson, 1982, pp 249–256.

170. Bonilla-Felix M, et al: Water transport in the immature rabbit collecting duct. Pediatr Nephrol 13:103, 1999.

171. Sulyok E: Renal response to vasopressin in premature infants: what is new? Biol Neonate 53:212, 1988.

172. Sulyok E, et al: Influence of NaCl supplementation on vasopressin secretion and water excretion in premature infants. Biol Neonate 64:201, 1993.

173. Yamamoto T, et al: Expression of AQP family in rat kidneys during development and maturation. Am J Physiol (Renal Physiol) 272:F198, 1996.

174. Bondy C, et al: Developmental gene expression and tissue distribution of the CHIP 28 water-channel protein. Proc Natl Acad Sci U S A 90:4500, 1993.

175. Smith BL, et al: Concurrent expression of erythroid and renal aquaporin CHIP and appearance of water channel activity in perinatal rats. J Clin Invest 92:2035, 1993.

176. Agre P, et al: Human red cell aquaporin Chip. II. Expression during normal fetal development and in a novel form of congenital dyserythropoietic anemia. J Clin Invest 94:1050, 1996.

177. Devuyst O, et al: Expression of aquaporins-1 and -2 during nephrogenesis and in autosomal dominant polycystic kidney disease. Am J Physiol 271 (Renal Fluid Electrolyte Physiol 40):F169, 1996.

178. Quigley R, et al: Maturational changes in rabbit renal basolateral membrane vesicle osmotic water permeability. J Membr Biol 174:53, 2000.

179. Kim J, et al: Developmental expression of aquaporin-1 in the rat renal vasculature. Am J Physiol (Renal Physiol) 276:F498, 1999.

180. Yasui M, et al: Development of urinary concentrating capacity: role of aquaporin-2. Am J Physiol 271 (Renal Fluid Electrolyte Physiol 40):F461, 1996.

181. Bonilla-Felix M, Jiang W: Aquaporin-2 in the immature rat: expression, regulation, and trafficking. J Am Soc Nephrol 8:1502, 1997.

182. Baum MA, et al: The perinatal expression of aquaporin-2 and aquaporin-3 in developing kidney. Pediatr Res 43:783, 1998.

183. Yang B, et al: Neonatal mortality in an aquaporin-2 knock-in mouse of recessive nephrogenic diabetes insipidus. J Biol Chem 274:2775, 2001.

184. Berl T, et al: Prostaglandin synthesis inhibition and the action of vasopressin: studies in man and rat. Am J Physiol 232 (Renal Fluid Electrolyte Physiol 1):F529, 1977.

185. Dunn MJ: Renal prostaglandins. In Dunn MJ (ed): Renal Endocrinology. Baltimore, Williams and Wilkins, 1983, pp 1–74.

186. Stokes JB: Effect of prostaglandin E2 on chloride transport across the rabbit thick ascending limb of Henle. J Clin Invest 64:495, 1979.

187. Roman RJ, Lechene C: Prostaglandin E2 and F2a reduces urea reabsorption from the rat collecting duct. Am J Physiol 241 (Renal Fluid Electrolyte Physiol 9):F53, 1981.

188. Zook TE, Strandhoy JW: Inhibition of ADH-enhanced transepithelial urea and water movement by prostaglandins. Prostaglandins 20:1, 1980.

189. Shimizu K, et al: Free water excretion and washout of renal medullary urea by prostaglandin E1. Jpn Heart J 10:437, 1969.

190. Arant BS Jr: Postnatal development of renal function during the first year of life. Pediatr Nephrol 1:308, 1987.

191. Matson JR, et al: Effects of inhibition of prostaglandin synthesis on fetal renal function. Kidney Int 20:621, 1981.

192. Walker D, Mitchell MD: Prostaglandins in the urine of foetal lambs. Nature (Lond) 271:161, 1978.

193. Robillard JE, Nakamura KT: Hormonal regulation of renal function during development. Biol Neonate 53:201, 1988.

194. Benzoni D, et al: Urinary excretion of prostaglandins and electrolytes in developing children. Kidney Int 20:386, 1981.

195. Bonilla-Felix M, John-Phillip C: Prostaglandins mediate the defect in AVP-stimulated cAMP generation in immature collecting duct. Am J Physiol 267 (Renal Fluid Electrolyte Physiol 36):F44, 1994.

196. Bonilla-Felix M, Jiang W: Expression and localization of prostaglandin EP3 receptor mRNA in the immature rabbit kidney. Am J Physiol 271 (Renal Fluid Electrolyte Physiol 40):F30, 1996.

197. Guron G, et al: Urinary acidification and net acid excretion in adult rats treated neonatally with enalopril. Am J Physiol Regul Integr Comp Physiol 274:R1718, 1998.

198. Guron G, et al: Postnatal time frame for renal vulnerability to enalopril in rats. J Am Soc Nephrol 10:1550, 1999.

199. Guron G, et al: Proximal tubular function in adult rats treated neonatally with enalopril. Acta Physiol Scand 164:99, 1998.

200. Guron G, et al: Mechanisms of impaired urinary concentrating ability in adult rats treated neonatally with enalopril. Acta Physiol Scand 165:103, 1999.

201. Guron G, et al: Angiotensin-converting enzyme inhibition in piglets induces persistent renal abnormalities. Clin Exp Pharmacol Physiol 25:88, 1998.

202. Nilsson AB, et al: IGF-I treatment attenuates renal abnormalities induced by neonatal ACE inhibition. Am J Physiol Regul Integr Comp Physiol 279:R1050, 2000.

203. Forrest JN Jr, Stanier MW: Kidney composition and renal concentration ability in young rabbits. J Physiol (Lond) 187:1, 1966.

204. Trimble ME: Renal response to solute loading in infant rats: relation to anatomical development. Am J Physiol 219:1089, 1970.

205. Liu W, et al: "Avian-type" renal medullary tubule organization causes immaturity of urine-concentrating ability in neonates. Kidney Int 60:680, 2001.

206. Bizub V, Leng L: The effect of the long-term administration of vasopressin on the development of the kidneys of growing lambs. Res Vet Sci 62:189, 1997.

207. Smith HW: From Fish to Philosopher. New York, Doubleday, 1961.

208. Winters RW: Principles of Pediatric Fluid Therapy, 2nd ed. Boston, Little, Brown and Co, 1982, pp 69–71.

209. Knepper MA, Rector FC Jr: Urine concentration and dilution. In Brenner BM (ed): The Kidney, 5th ed. Philadelphia, WB Saunders, 1996, pp 532–570.

210. Bargman J, et al: Examination of transepithelial exchange in water and solute in the rat renal pelvis. J Clin Invest 74:1860, 1984.

211. McCance RA, Widdowson EM: Renal function before birth. Proc R Soc (Biol) *141*:488, 1953.
212. Pritchard JA: Deglutition by normal and anencephalic fetuses. Obstet Gynecol *25*:289, 1965.
213. Edelmann CM Jr, Barnett HL: Role of the kidney in water metabolism in young infants. J Pediatr *56*:154, 1960.
214. Heller H: The water metabolism of newborn infants and animals. Arch Dis Child *26*:195, 1951.
215. Barnett HL, et al: Renal water excretion in premature infants. J Clin Invest *31*:1069, 1952.

216. Rodriquez-Soriano J, et al: Renal handling of water and sodium in infancy and childhood: a study using clearance methods during hypotonic saline diuresis. Kidney Int *20*:700, 1981.
217. Rosenfeld WN, et al: Water intoxication: a complication of nebulization with nasal CPAP. J Pediatr *80*:113, 1976.
218. Ames RG: Urinary water excretion and neurohypophysial function in full-term and premature infants shortly after birth. Pediatrics *12*:272, 1953.
219. Linshaw MA, et al: Infantile psychogenic water drinking. J Pediatr *85*:520, 1974.

136

Eileen D. Brewer

Urinary Acidification

The mature kidney plays an important role in the regulation of normal acid-base balance and provides secondary compensation for primary respiratory acidosis or alkalosis. The kidney accomplishes these functions through reabsorption of filtered bicarbonate (HCO_3^-) and excretion of hydrogen ion (H^+) as ammonium (NH_4^+) and titratable acid, all of which are mediated by renal tubular H^+ secretion.[1-3] The resultant urinary pH is usually acidic (<7.4) with respect to blood pH.

Urinary acidification has been studied infrequently in human neonates. Some of the current knowledge has come from actual studies of newborn infants, but much more information has come from studies of fetal and newborn animals, which may not be directly applicable to human infants. Studies of preterm infants, especially those of extremely low birth weight (gestational age < 29 weeks), have helped to clarify our knowledge,[4,5] but more studies are needed. Understanding developmental changes in the fetus and neonate first requires an understanding of current concepts of acid-base physiology in the mature kidney.

TUBULAR REABSORPTION OF FILTERED BICARBONATE IN THE MATURE KIDNEY

Buffering of strong acids is divided about equally between HCO_3^- and non-HCO_3^- buffers (hemoglobin, plasma and intracellular proteins, and phosphate).[6] The most important extracellular fluid (ECF) buffer is HCO_3^-, which is filtered almost completely by the glomerulus and is reclaimed by reabsorption in the renal tubule to maintain a normal ECF HCO_3^- concentration. In the proximal tubule and the thick ascending limb of Henle, reabsorption is mediated by equimolar secretion of H^+ into the tubular lumen via an electroneutral sodium (Na^+)/H^+ exchanger (NHE), specifically isoform NHE-3 as determined by molecular cloning studies,[1,2,7] and to a lesser extent by vacuolar H^+-adenosine triphosphatase (ATPase).[1-3,6] Both NHE and H^+-ATPase are located in the luminal (apical) membrane of these renal tubular cells. Na^+ exchange for H^+ is driven by a downhill Na^+ concentration gradient from lumen to cytoplasm that is maintained by active cellular extrusion of Na^+ at the basolateral surface mediated by Na^+, potassium (K^+)-ATPase within the membrane.

H^+ secretion in the distal tubule occurs by a different mechanism within the intercalated cells of the cortical and medullary collecting duct segments.[1,3,6] Intercalated cells are interspersed among principal cells and in the mature kidney account for about one-third of the tubular cells in the cortical and outer medullary collecting duct and less than 10% in the inner medullary collecting duct. In α-intercalated cells, H^+ secretion is mediated by translocating H^+-ATPase and H^+,K^+-ATPase in the apical membrane.[1,6] Vacuolar H^+-ATPase is also present in a specialized tubulovesicular system in the apical pole cytoplasm and may be important for acute response to acidosis.[8] A second type of intercalated cells, the β-Intercalated cells, located only in the cortical collecting duct, do not secrete H^+ but secrete small amounts of HCO_3^- in exchange for chloride (Cl^-) at the apical membrane and extrude H^+ across the basolateral membrane with H^+-ATPase. β-Intercalated cells may be more important for renal compensation during chronic metabolic alkalosis.[2,6] Acid loading can stimulate a change from β-type to α-type intercalated cells and to a redistribution of vacuolar H^+-ATPase from the tubulovesicular system to the apical membrane itself in α-type cells.[2,6,8] In the cortical collecting duct, principal cells adjacent to α-intercalated cells mediate Na^+ reabsorption, which creates lumen negativity favorable for luminal H^+ secretion into that segment by H^+-ATPase and H^+,K^+-ATPase activity.[1,6] The rate of H^+ secretion may be increased by various factors, including avid renal tubular Na^+ reabsorption, increased luminal HCO_3^- concentration and luminal fluid flow rate, angiotensin II, K^+ depletion, and aldosterone; the rate may be decreased by ECF volume expansion and parathyroid hormone.[1-3,6]

H^+ secreted into the tubular lumen along the nephron combines with filtered HCO_3^- to form carbonic acid (H_2CO_3), which then dissociates to water (H_2O) and carbon dioxide (CO_2). CO_2 diffuses easily across tubular membranes into the renal tubular cells, where cytosolic carbonic anhydrase isoenzyme II activity catalyzes the conversion of CO_2 and H_2O to yield H^+ and HCO_3^-.[2,3,6] HCO_3^- then exits the cell across the basolateral membrane via either of two transport systems, an electrogenic Na^+-$3HCO_3^-$ co-transporter (primarily proximal tubule and loop of Henle) or a Cl^-/HCO_3^- exchanger (primarily distal collecting duct), and returns to the blood in the peritubular capillaries.[2,6] Excess intracellular Cl^- recycles back to the peritubular space through conductive Cl^- channels across the basolateral membrane.[1,2,6] H^+ is secreted again into the tubular lumen to help reclaim more filtered HCO_3^- by the same process.

In the proximal tubule, where 75 to 85% of HCO_3^- reabsorption occurs, carbonic anhydrase isoenzyme IV is present in the luminal brush-border membrane to catalyze the rapid dissociation of H_2CO_3 to H_2O and CO_2, thereby minimizing the luminal concentrations of H_2CO_3 and H^+ and facilitating H^+ secretion.[2,6] The proximal tubule thus has a high capacity for H^+ secretion and HCO_3^- reabsorption. When luminal carbonic anhydrase IV is inhibited by acetazolamide, H+ secretion and HCO3- reabsorption are notably diminished.[2, 6] Proximal tubular reabsorption of HCO3- is also decreased by expansion of ECF or effective arterial blood volume.[9]

The filtered HCO3- not reabsorbed proximally can be reclaimed partially or completely in the distal tubule, primarily in the collecting duct.[1,3,6] When distally delivered HCO3- is entirely reabsorbed, luminal fluid pH falls to less than 6.4, and secreted H+ can combine with ammonia (NH_3) or sodium phosphate (Na_2HPO_4), to be excreted in the urine as NH_4^+ or titratable acid (NaH_2PO_4).[3] Substantial trapping of H+ by NH_3 occurs in the lumen of the inner medullary collecting duct, where urine pH is lowest and NH_3 concentration is greatest.[3,6] Aldosterone directly enhances distal tubular secretion of H+, both by direct stimulation of H+-ATPase in α-intercalated cells and by stimulation of Na+ reabsorption by the adjacent principal cells.[3, 6] Carbonic anhydrase is not present in the brush-border membranes of the distal tubule, so the capacity of the distal tubule to reabsorb HCO3- is much less than that of the proximal tubule. Hence, a relatively small increase in distal delivery of HCO3-, such as that occurring with ECF or effective arterial blood volume expansion, may exceed the reabsorptive capacity of the distal tubule, increase tubular fluid pH and thereby limit H+ excretion as NH_4^+ or NaH_2PO_4, and result in a urinary pH greater than or equal to 6.4.

RENAL BICARBONATE THRESHOLD

The renal HCO3- threshold, which has been measured frequently in studies of renal acidification in neonates,[10-13] is defined as the plasma HCO3- concentration at which HCO3- is no longer completely reabsorbed in the renal tubule and begins to appear in significant amounts in the urine. The HCO3- threshold does not necessarily characterize the intrinsic renal tubular capacity for HCO3- reabsorption, because it is significantly altered by ECF volume status.[8, 14] When ECF volume contraction is maintained during HCO3- loading, the HCO3- threshold is increased, even in neonatal animals.[15] When ECF volume is expanded during HCO3- loading, the HCO3- threshold becomes apparent at a plasma HCO3- concentration of less than 24 mEq/l, but when ECF volume expansion is minimized or prevented, the threshold may not be reached until the plasma HCO3- concentration exceeds 27 mEq/l. Thus, alterations in the renal HCO3- threshold may reflect the effects of ECF volume status on renal tubular HCO3- reabsorption rather than the intrinsic properties or maturity of the renal tubular cells.

URINARY EXCRETION OF HYDROGEN ION BY THE MATURE KIDNEY

Normal metabolism generates H+ in the form of volatile and fixed acids, which must be excreted to prevent acidosis.[16] Volatile acid, primarily H_2CO_3, is excreted by the lungs as CO_2. The fixed acids, which include lactic acid, ketoacids, sulfuric acid, and phosphoric acid, are initially buffered by extracellular buffers, including HCO3-, which must later be regenerated by the kidneys through excretion of H+ in the urine as NH_4^+ and NaH_2PO_4. NH_3 is produced in the kidney principally by metabolism of glutamine by glutaminase and phosphoenolpyruvate carboxykinase in the proximal tubule.[3, 6] The NH_3 generated there freely diffuses into the luminal fluid and traverses to the loop of Henle, where it is subsequently reabsorbed from the relatively alkaline fluid and is then secreted into acidic fluid (pH < 6.4) within the collecting duct.[1, 3, 6] There NH_3 reacts with secreted H+ and is entrapped as NH_4^+ for excretion in the urine. NaH_2PO_4 is derived from filtered Na_2HPO_4, which escapes proximal tubular reabsorption and is delivered to the distal nephron, where it reacts with secreted H+ to be excreted as NaH_2PO_4.[6]

NET ACID EXCRETION

The quantity of H+ excreted as NH_4^+ and NaH_2PO_4 minus any excreted HCO3- (normally a negligible amount) is the net acid excretion.[3,6, 16, 17] Net acid excretion accounts for 3% or less of the H+ secretion by the renal tubule. The primary importance of tubular H+ secretion is to facilitate HCO3- reabsorption and reclamation. Urinary pH itself is not a good indicator of net acid excretion because the pH does not reflect the amount of buffering capacity available as NH_3 and Na_2HPO_4. More H+ can be excreted in urine with excess buffers and a slightly higher pH.

DEVELOPMENTAL ASPECTS OF URINARY ACIDIFICATION

In the human fetus, nephronogenesis is not complete until 34 to 36 weeks' gestation.[14] Functioning renal tubules can be identified by 9 weeks of gestation.[14] During fetal life, H+ is removed primarily through the placenta for excretion by maternal organs,[7] so renal acidification is not important until birth. Exactly when renal acidification mechanisms become functionally active and reach maturity in the developing human kidney is not known. In fetal lambs, urinary pH is always lower than plasma pH, a finding indicating the ability of the developing fetal renal tubule to establish a concentration gradient for H+.[7] Carbonic anhydrase is present in the human fetal kidney in late gestation,[7] and it increases with gestational age,[18] perhaps explaining in part the observed increase of renal HCO3- reabsorption with gestational age.

DEVELOPMENTAL ASPECTS OF URINARY EXCRETION OF HYDROGEN ION

The renal tubular mechanisms for net acid excretion may already be mature in the last-trimester fetal kidney. Although net acid excretion per unit body weight is reduced in near-term fetal lambs compared with nonpregnant ewes, the fetus responds appropriately to acid loading by increasing urinary excretion of both NH_4^+ and NaH_2PO_4 and by lowering urinary pH.[7]

Term infants are able to respond appropriately to an NH_4Cl load within the first month of life[10, 12]; however, it is uncertain whether preterm infants have the same capacity. Svenningsen[12] reported that net acid excretion in NH_4Cl-loaded preterm infants (gestational ages 29 to 36 weeks, birth weights 1300 to 2470 g) was not comparable to that of term infants until after the third week of life. Schwartz and co-workers[11] found that preterm infants (birth weights 1630 ± 250 g) were able to acidify their urine to less than 5.5 and to excrete NH_4^+ and NaH_2PO_4 appropriately during an NH_4Cl-loading test performed just before hospital discharge at least 3 weeks after birth. Unfortunately, Schwartz and colleagues gave no estimates of gestational age at birth or postconceptual age at the time of the NH_4Cl loading to allow comparison with the data of Svenningsen. Kalhoff and associates[4] evaluated urinary pH in a large number of premature infants (83 weighing 1.5 to 2.4 kg and 87 weighing 1.0 to 1.4 kg; no gestational ages given). In approximately one-third of infants in each group, urinary pH values spontaneously decreased to less than 5.4 by the third to fourth weeks of postnatal life, a finding indicating maximal stimulation of tubular H+ secretion. At the same time that urinary pH was low, however, capillary blood pH and base excess showed mild metabolic acidosis, a finding suggesting inadequate net acid excretion, possibly as a result of immaturity of the renal tubule for ammoniagenesis or decreased availability of phosphate (especially low in breast-fed infants).[17] Unfortunately, net acid excretion was not measured. More studies of preterm infants of different gestational ages, especially those less than 29 weeks' gestation and at different postconceptual ages, are needed to evaluate the postnatal development of renal tubular H^+ excretion and the capacity for net acid excretion.

DEVELOPMENTAL ASPECTS OF BICARBONATE REABSORPTION

The normal range for plasma HCO_3^- concentration has been reported to be lower for preterm infants (16 to 20 mEq/l) and term infants (19 to 21 mEq/l) than for children and adults (24 to 28 mEq/l).[10,11] Whether this relative acidosis results from physiologic factors alone or from immaturity of the renal tubule, or both, is still not certain.[3,6,14,19] During the first few weeks of life, the wide range of low but normal values of plasma HCO_3^- concentration is the most likely explanation for the designation in the past of late metabolic acidosis in otherwise healthy preterm infants with values of plasma HCO_3^- concentration in the acidotic range for children or adults.[11,17,20,21]

The renal HCO_3^- threshold measured in term and preterm infants in studies reported before 1980 was found to be low compared with older children and adults.[10-12] These studies were done before our current understanding of the obligatory need for neonatal diuresis of excess ECF in the first week after birth.[5,14] Excess fluid and Na^+ administered during obligatory diuresis may perpetuate ECF volume expansion. ECF volume expansion, which is a major determinant of the HCO_3^- threshold regardless of the acid-base status of the infant, may account in part for the reduced HCO_3^- threshold measured in the classic studies. The likelihood that ECF volume status contributes importantly to the apparently low renal HCO_3^- threshold is suggested by studies of fetal lambs[22] and neonatal puppies.[15] During HCO_3^- loading in fetal and neonatal animals in which the ECF space is volume contracted, the HCO_3^- threshold and tubular reabsorption of HCO_3^- increase, and the urinary pH becomes more acidic. Conversely, in neonatal puppies with ECF volume expansion, the HCO_3^- threshold and tubular reabsorption of HCO_3^- decrease. These findings suggest that the renal tubule in the fetus and neonate can increase its HCO_3^- reabsorption appropriately when stimulated by volume contraction, and, conversely, a reduced HCO_3^- threshold may be, at least in part, a physiologic phenomenon caused by an expanded state of ECF volume.

The ECF volume of the human fetus and newborn at birth is normally 40 to 60% of body weight, and it decreases to less than 30% after birth.[14] The usual ECF volume expansion of the fetus and newborn probably results in depressed proximal tubular HCO_3^- reabsorption, increased delivery of HCO_3^- to the distal nephron, and an alkaline urinary pH. After birth, when obligatory diuresis of excess ECF is complete and ECF volume is contracted, renal tubular HCO_3^- reabsorption increases, and urinary pH can become more acidic. These phenomena were confirmed in studies of extremely low birth weight infants. Ramiro-Tolentino and colleagues[5] studied 22 preterm infants (23 to 29 weeks' gestation; birth weight 540 to 982 g) during the first 5 days of life. Intravenous fluid and electrolyte therapy were carefully controlled to allow body weight loss between 1 and 4% per day during obligatory diuresis and to maintain serum Na^+ concentrations between 130 and 145 mEq/l, serum K^+ concentrations between 4 and 6 mEq/l, and plasma HCO_3^- concentrations between 18 and 22 mEq/l. When diuresis began at about 24 hours after birth, measured glomerular filtration rate and filtered load of HCO_3^- increased, and so did urinary HCO_3^- excretion. After diuresis, when ECF was contracted and glomerular filtration rate was only slightly decreased, urinary HCO_3^- excretion markedly dropped, and cumulative HCO_3^- balance became positive. If prescribed fluid therapy had continued to supply an excess of salt and water during the period of diuresis and ECF volume expansion had persisted, these infants may have developed relative metabolic acidosis caused

by continued depression of renal tubular reabsorption of HCO_3^-.[14]

Immaturity of tubular function may also play a role in the expression of a lowered plasma HCO_3^- threshold in the neonate. Histochemical and biochemical analyses of human fetal kidney tissue suggest that carbonic anhydrase is present in sufficient amounts to allow normal reabsorption of HCO_3^- at 24 to 26 weeks' gestation in fully formed medullary nephrons but not in immature nephrons in the more cortical nephrogenic areas.[23] In preterm infants born at less than 36 weeks' gestation, when nephrogenesis is not yet complete, heterogeneity of nephronal development could contribute to a reduced overall capacity to reabsorb HCO_3^-. In studies of renal tubule segments from infant rats, Karashima and associates[24] found carbonic anhydrase II activity of 1-week-old rats to be only 14% of adult values, increasing to 40% at 3 weeks and 97% by 7 weeks.

Direct studies of tubular HCO_3^- reabsorption[25] and NHE activity[19] in isolated proximal tubular segments of neonatal rabbits suggest that postnatal maturation of the proximal tubule may be important in the development of HCO_3^- reabsorptive capacity, which abruptly and markedly increases after the fourth week of life in this model. A similar abrupt and marked increase in tubular reabsorptive capacity occurs 3 weeks after birth in the proximal tubule of newborn guinea pigs.[26] Nephronogenesis is complete before birth in guinea pigs but not until 4 weeks after birth in rabbits, so neonatal guinea pig kidneys are more comparable to those of term infants, and neonatal rabbit kidneys compare more favorably with those of preterm infants. In both experimental models, the abrupt increase in reabsorption has been associated with a concomitant marked increase in the basolateral membrane surface area of the proximal tubule. Studies of rat proximal tubules also demonstrate a maturational increase from neonate to adult in NHE activity, which is associated with an increase in NHE-3 gene expression.[27]

Increased production of glucocorticoids may play an important role in promoting postnatal maturation of proximal tubule acidification.[19] Administration of exogenous glucocorticoids to neonatal rabbits has been shown to increase markedly proximal tubular NHE and Na^+,K^+-ATPase activity measured *in vitro*.[19] In studies of preterm extremely low birth weight infants, however, urinary HCO_3^- excretion in the first week of life was the same whether infants had received antenatal glucocorticoids or not.[5] More studies in human infants are needed to determine the importance of postnatal renal tubular maturation for HCO_3^- reabsorption during the first few weeks of life.

NEONATAL METABOLIC COMPENSATION FOR RESPIRATORY ACIDOSIS OR ALKALOSIS

If the lungs are diseased and alveolar ventilation is ineffective, as occurs in infants with respiratory distress syndrome or bronchopulmonary dysplasia, CO_2 is retained, blood CO_2 tension rises, and respiratory acidosis occurs. Retained CO_2 is buffered initially by intracellular proteins, phosphates, and plasma hemoglobin.[28] Within 12 to 24 hours of the onset of respiratory acidosis in adults, renal metabolic compensation begins to occur and is not complete for 3 to 5 days. The kidneys attempt to return blood pH toward normal by excreting H^+ in the urine as NH_4^+ and NaH_2PO_4 and by reclaiming filtered HCO_3^-.

Hyperventilation, whether disease related or iatrogenic, leads to respiratory alkalosis. The initial reduction in blood CO_2 tension is acutely titrated by intracellular buffers.[28] In adults, renal metabolic compensation for respiratory alkalosis begins within hours and is complete within 1 to 2 days. Renal compensation is characterized by excretion of HCO_3^- in the urine, by alkaline urinary pH, and by decreased excretion of NH_4^+ and NaH_2PO_4.

Maturation of the ability to compensate for respiratory acid-base disorders has not been carefully studied in the developing kidney. A study in 5- to 12-day-old rabbits[29] suggested that metabolic compensation for acute hypercapnia and hypocapnia is intact. Studies in human infants are needed to elucidate further this aspect of renal acidification.

REFERENCES

1. Alpern RJ, et al: Renal acidification mechanisms. *In* Brenner BM (ed): Brenner & Rector's: The Kidney, 6th ed. Philadelphia, WB Saunders, 2000, pp 455-519.
2. Jones DP, Chesney RW: Tubular function. *In* Barratt TM, et al (eds): Pediatric Nephrology, 4th ed. Baltimore, Williams & Wilkins, 1999, pp 59-82.
3. Herrin JT: Renal tubular acidosis. *In* Barratt TM, et al (eds): Pediatric Nephrology, 4th ed. Baltimore, Williams & Wilkins, 1999, pp 565-581.
4. Kalhoff H, et al: Decreased growth rate of low-birth-weight infants with prolonged maximum renal acid stimulation. Acta Paediatr 82:522, 1993.
5. Ramiro-Tolentino SB, et al: Renal bicarbonate excretion in extremely low birth weight infants. Pediatrics 98:256, 1996.
6. Schwartz GJ: Potassium and acid-base. *In* Barratt TM, et al (eds): Pediatric Nephrology, 4th ed. Baltimore, Williams & Wilkins, 1999, pp 162-189.
7. Robillard JE, et al: Renal function during fetal life. *In* Barratt TM, et al (eds): Pediatric Nephrology, 4th ed. Baltimore, Williams & Wilkins, 1999, pp 21-37.
8. Gluck SL, et al: Distal urinary acidification from Homer Smith to the present. Kidney Int 49:1660, 1996.
9. Purkerson ML, et al: On the influence of extracellular fluid volume expansion on bicarbonate reabsorption in the rat. J Clin Invest 48:1754, 1969.
10. Edelmann CM Jr, et al: Renal bicarbonate reabsorption and hydrogen ion excretion in normal infants. J Clin Invest 46:1309, 1967.
11. Schwartz GJ, et al: Late metabolic acidosis: a reassessment of the definition. J Pediatr 95:102, 1979.
12. Svenningsen NW: Renal acid-base titration studies in infants with and without metabolic acidosis in the post-neonatal period. Pediatr Res 8:659, 1974.
13. Tudvad F, et al: Renal response of premature infants to administration of bicarbonate and potassium. Pediatrics 13:4, 1954.
14. Arant BS Jr: Renal and genitourinary diseases: considerations of normal development. *In* McMillan JA, et al (eds): Oski's Principles and Practice of Pediatrics, 3rd ed. Philadelphia, JB Lippincott, 1999, pp 336-345.
15. Moore ES, et al: Renal reabsorption of bicarbonate in puppies: effect of extracellular volume contraction on the renal threshold for bicarbonate. Pediatr Res 6:859, 1972.
16. Masoro EJ: An overview of hydrogen ion regulation. Arch Intern Med 142:1019, 1982.
17. Manz F, et al: Renal acid excretion in early infancy. Pediatr Nephrol 11:231, 1997.
18. Arant BS Jr: Postnatal development of renal function during the first year of life. Pediatr Nephrol 1:308, 1987.
19. Baum M, Quigley R: Ontogeny of proximal tubule acidification. Kidney Int 48:1697, 1995.
20. Kildeberg P: Disturbances of hydrogen ion balance occurring in premature infants. II. Late metabolic acidosis. Acta Paediatr 53:517, 1964.
21. Radde IC, et al: Growth and mineral metabolism in very low birth weight infants. I. Comparison of the effects of two modes of $NaHCO_3$ treatment of late metabolic acidosis. Pediatr Res 9:564, 1975.
22. Robillard JE, et al: Influence of fetal extracellular volume contraction on renal reabsorption of bicarbonate in fetal lambs. Pediatr Res 11:649, 1977.
23. Lonnerholm G, Wistrand PJ: Carbonic anhydrase in the human fetal kidney. Pediatr Res 17:390, 1983.
24. Karashima S, et al: Developmental changes in carbonic anhydrase II in the rat kidney. Pediatr Nephrol 12:263, 1998.
25. Schwartz GJ, Evan AP: Development of solute transport in rabbit proximal tubule. I. HCO_3^- and glucose absorption. Am J Physiol 245:F382, 1983.
26. Welling LW, et al: Correlation of structure and function in developing proximal tubule of guinea pig. Am J Physiol 256:F13, 1989.
27. Shah M, et al: Ontogeny of Na^+/H^+ antiporter activity in rat proximal convoluted tubules. Pediatr Res 48:206, 2000.
28. Brewer ED: Acid-base disorders. Pediatr Clin North Am 33:429, 1990.
29. Heijden AJVD, Guignard JP: Bicarbonate reabsorption by the kidney of the newborn rabbit. Am J Physiol 256:F29, 1989.

137

Robert L. Chevalier

Response to Nephron Loss in Early Development

OVERVIEW

The developing kidney depends on a complex program of morphogenesis resulting in a delicate balance of growth and differentiation. Numerous factors can interfere with this process in either fetal or neonatal life. The resulting nephron deficit, in turn, leads to adaptive responses that have short-term and long-term consequences. This chapter reviews the causes and consequences of nephron loss, with emphasis on the unique features that increase the vulnerability of the developing kidney.

EXPERIMENTAL STUDIES

Short-Term Reduction in Renal Mass

Immediate Functional Response

Using an electromagnetic flow probe, which allows sensitive measurement of renal blood flow immediately after uninephrectomy, a 30% increase in flow to the remaining kidney was demonstrated in the dog.[1] Similarly, a significant increase was found 30 minutes after contralateral nephrectomy in the young or adult rat.[2] Glomerular filtration rate (GFR) may not increase until 1 or more hours after uninephrectomy,[3] and the increase appears to occur predominantly in superficial nephrons.[4]

As described by Peters in 1963,[5] short-term reduction in renal mass results in a prompt increase in urine flow and cation excretion, which may be regarded as "compensatory adaptation," in contrast to "compensatory hyperfunction," which develops later.

The immediate responses, which have not been studied in early development, are presumably mediated by neural reflexes or humoral factors such as prostaglandins.[6,7]

Long-Term Reduction in Renal Mass

Renal Mass and the Number of Nephrons

Renal growth occurs as a result of normal development or in response to a reduction in renal mass. It is therefore not surprising that the compensatory increase in renal mass after nephron loss is proportionately greater in the newborn than in the adult rat or guinea pig.[8-10] Although additional nephrons are not formed as a result of compensatory renal growth postnatally in the rat,[11, 12] uninephrectomy in the fetal sheep results in a 45% increase in the number of nephrons.[13] In the postnatal development of the guinea pig, there is a recruitment of perfused glomeruli during the first few weeks of life, although there is no actual nephrogenesis after birth.[14] In animals subjected to uninephrectomy at birth, the timing of recruitment of nonperfused glomeruli is accelerated.[14] Glomerular volume, conversely, increases during normal maturation, and uninephrectomy at birth causes a 50% increment over normal growth.[15] Basement membrane surface area and mesangial matrix increase severalfold during normal postnatal growth of the rat, and uninephrectomy in the young animal results in an additional increment in both glomerular components.[15] Despite a significant increase in glomerular volume, both normal growth and compensatory

TABLE 137-1
Causes of Reduced Nephron Number

Developmental factors
    Renal maldevelopment, including obstructive nephropathy
    Intrauterine growth retardation
    Maternal diabetes
Nutritional factors
    Reduced maternal protein intake
    Reduced maternal vitamin A intake
    Reduced fetal potassium inatake
Toxic/iatrogenic influences
    Maternal glucocorticoids
    Maternal aminoglycosides
    Maternal β-lactam antibiotics

renal growth are primarily the result of an increase in proximal tubular mass.[16, 17]

Data have suggested that the complement of nephrons at birth may influence the development of hypertension or renal dysfunction in adulthood.[18] It is now recognized that there is considerable variation in the number of nephrons in physiologically normal subjects.[19] There is a linear relationship between the number of glomeruli and birth weight in humans.[20] Moreover, there appears to be an overall negative correlation between the number of nephrons at birth and blood pressure in adulthood, a finding suggesting that conservation of nephrons is particularly important in early life.[21] These observations have spurred interest in the determinants of nephron number. There are at least three broad categories of factors contributing to the eventual number of nephrons in the metanephric kidney: developmental factors, nutritional factors, and toxic or iatrogenic influences (Table 137–1). Early human fetal urinary tract obstruction results in a reduced number of nephrons, and the number of glomeruli can be related to the time of developmental arrest.[22] In several animal models, ureteral obstruction also results in reduced glomerular number,[23-25] and ureteral obstruction in the neonatal rat impairs nephrogenesis in direct proportion to the duration of obstruction.[26] Fetal rats whose mothers' uterine artery has been ligated grow poorly and have reduced nephron number,[27] whereas infants with intrauterine growth retardation are born with fewer nephrons than those whose birth weight is appropriate for gestational age.[28] Infants of diabetic mothers have an increased incidence of congenital malformations, and maternal hyperglycemia in rats leads to nephron deficit.[29] Reduced maternal protein intake leads to reduced nephron number in experimental animals,[27] and intrauterine malnutrition in aborigines is associated with low birth weight and impaired nephrogenesis.[30] In a provocative study, mild vitamin A deficiency was shown to lead to inborn nephron deficit in the rat: there is a linear relationship between maternal plasma retinol levels and the number of glomeruli in the fetus.[31] This study suggests that small variations in maternal nutritional status may have significant implications for the ultimate complement of nephrons. The electrolyte environment may also play a significant role: fetal mouse kidneys grown *in vitro* exhibited impaired nephrogenesis when potassium concentration was reduced.[32] Finally, maternal exposure to medications, such as glucocorticoids, aminoglycosides, or β-lactam antibiotics, may impair nephrogenesis.[33-35] Administration of specific growth factors may also alter nephrogenesis in developing kidneys *in vivo* or *in vitro*: transforming growth factor-β₁ impairs nephrogenesis, whereas insulin-like growth factor I (IGF-I) stimulates nephrogenesis.[36, 37]

Renal Hemodynamics

The hemodynamic response to nephron loss is proportional to the amount of renal mass removed. Thus, uninephrectomy in the rat

doubles glomerular blood flow, but removal of 75% of renal mass increases flow more than threefold 2 to 3 weeks later.[38] In 8-week-old dogs subjected to 75% nephrectomy at birth, renal plasma flow was not different from that of control littermates; however, flow in 14-week-old dogs studied 6 weeks after 75% renal ablation was 50% less than that in controls.[39] This study indicates that hemodynamic adaptation to nephron loss is more complete in early development than in later life. Similar to the dog, reduction in renal mass in the neonatal guinea pig caused a marked increase in renal blood flow throughout the renal cortex.[40]

A potentially important difference in the hemodynamic response to nephron loss in early compared with later development has been shown for autoregulation of renal blood flow, whereby flow is maintained constant during changes in renal perfusion pressure. Uninephrectomy in the adult rat causes renal vasodilation at reduced as well as normal perfusion pressure; however, uninephrectomy in the neonatal rat increased renal blood flow only at normal, but not at reduced, arterial pressure.[41] Thus, autoregulation is reset to higher flows in the uninephrectomized adult but is impaired in the newborn rat with a single kidney.[41] The neonate with reduced renal mass may therefore be more susceptible to ischemic renal damage than the adult. Another difference between the response to uninephrectomy in neonates compared with adults relates to the development of hypertension: uninephrectomy in the neonatal rat leads to salt-sensitive hypertension in adulthood,[42] and this, in turn, leads to glomerular damage.[43]

Because of the critical dependence of the fetal and neonatal glomerular capillary pressure on angiotensin-mediated efferent arteriolar constriction, the fetus and neonate are particularly susceptible to a marked reduction in GFR after exposure to angiotensin-converting enzyme inhibitors.[44] Both the potency and duration of action of captopril are significantly greater in neonates than in older children.[45] After a reduction in renal mass, the remaining hyperfiltering immature nephrons are even more susceptible to the action of angiotensin-converting enzyme inhibitors, which can induce renal failure and further nephron injury.

Unlike in the adult rat, in which filtration fraction is reduced as a result of uninephrectomy,[46] filtration fraction remains normal after uninephrectomy in the neonatal guinea pig.[40] Because the compensatory increase in GFR in superficial nephrons of guinea pigs uninephrectomized at birth is proportionately greater than that of deeper nephrons,[47] the normal centrifugal pattern of renal functional development may be accelerated by nephron loss at birth. In contrast, reduction in renal mass later in life results in a uniform increase in GFR throughout the cortex.[48, 49] Unlike the increase in superficial nephron GFR resulting from normal growth of the guinea pig in the first month of life, the compensatory increase in the uninephrectomized neonatal animal is caused in part by a 30% increase in effective filtration pressure.[50] Therefore, it appears that the functional response to nephron loss in the neonate is caused by a combination of acceleration and amplification of normal renal development, as well as by specific adaptive changes resulting from the stimulus of nephron loss.

Stimuli for Compensatory Renal Growth

Numerous studies indicate that reduction in renal mass results in release of renotropic factors or suppression of inhibitors of renal growth.[51] Although blood-borne renotropins are probably not released from the kidneys themselves,[52] renal tissue factors may be necessary to activate the humoral compounds.[53] The enhanced compensatory renal hypertrophy observed in the neonate may relate to differences in tissue factors. In this regard, kidneys of adult rats and mice have been found to contain a renal growth inhibitory factor, although none was found in neonatal kidneys.[54] The initial phase of compensatory renal growth after unilateral nephrectomy in immature rats is independent of growth hormone secretion, but it is associated with an increase in IGF-I and IGF-I–receptor gene expression.[55, 56]

In addition to reduction in functional renal mass, numerous compounds have been shown to stimulate renal growth, including sodium, ammonium chloride, folic acid, thyroxine, growth hormone, and mineralocorticoids.[57] One stimulus to renal hypertrophy and hyperfunction that has generated much interest is increased dietary protein intake. Increased protein intake can enhance compensatory renal hypertrophy.[58, 59] However, the RNA/protein ratio and DNA content of the remaining kidney are increased as a result of uninephrectomy, but not with increased dietary protein.[60] Thus, the additive effect of dietary protein is probably the result of a separate mechanism rather than being an amplification of the normal hypertrophic response. Although angiotensin II has been shown to act as a renal growth factor, compensatory renal growth in neonatal mice subjected to unilateral ureteral obstruction is not impaired in animals lacking functional angiotensinogen genes.[61] Perhaps as important as what *stimulates* compensatory renal growth is what *limits* compensatory renal growth. Mice lacking the gene for p21 (cyclin-dependent kinase inhibitor) do not develop progressive renal insufficiency after renal ablation.[62] A shift from renal cellular hypertrophy to proliferation in these mutants may underlie the protective effect.[63]

Adaptation Versus Maladaptation

As described earlier, structural and functional adaptations appear to be more "complete" after reduction of renal mass in the neonate compared with adaptation that follows nephron loss later in life. However, increased intraglomerular pressure and blood flow, and consequent hyperfiltration, may lead to progressive glomerular injury, a maladaptive response.[64, 65] The mechanisms responsible for this process remain incompletely understood, but they include increased filtration of protein and other macromolecules that are taken up by mesangial cells, which are thereby damaged.[66, 65] Proteinuria also leads to injury to the renal tubules and interstitium. Proteinuria can lead to apoptosis of tubular cells[67] and to the development of interstitial fibrosis.[68] Uninephrectomy in the neonatal rat has been shown to result in greater proteinuria and glomerular sclerosis of the remaining kidney than occur after uninephrectomy in the adult.[69,70] In 1927, Moise and Smith[59] showed that a high-protein diet increased the severity of glomerulosclerosis in the uninephrectomized rat, and more recent studies have shown that protein restriction can prevent development of lesions in remnant nephrons.[64] Increased protein intake in the young rat can stimulate kidney growth by promoting cell proliferation, as well as by increasing the GFR.[71] Studies of young rats undergoing unilateral nephrectomy revealed that survival was significantly reduced in animals receiving a high-protein diet compared with a low-protein diet.[72] Moreover, this was preceded by an increase in urinary protein excretion.[73] These data have disturbing implications for neonates with nephron loss, because a more vigorous early adaptive response in remaining renal tissue may lead to progressive renal insufficiency during development. However, attempts to slow the progression by restricting protein in infancy carry the risks of protein malnutrition and impairment of normal somatic growth.

Compensatory Renal Adaptation in the Fetus

Until recently, experimental evidence of compensatory renal growth in the fetus had not been clearly established. Peters and colleagues[74] induced unilateral ureteral occlusion in the fetal lamb at midtrimester and observed a significant increase in contralateral kidney weight within 2 weeks that became maximal by 1 month (50% increase). Although the increase in renal mass in this study was not associated with an increase in the total number of nephrons, ovine fetal uninephrectomy resulted in a 45% increase in the number of nephrons, but a lower glomerular volume.[13] Because the placenta provides the excretory function for the fetus, the results of this study indicate that an increased excretory or homeostatic burden on the kidney is not required to initiate compensatory growth. Rather, alterations in growth factors or inhibitors presumably modulate the prenatal changes.

CLINICAL ASPECTS OF RENAL RESPONSE TO NEPHRON LOSS

Because of the relatively small numbers and heterogeneity of patients with lesions resulting in nephron loss during early development, clinical data are sparse. However, in general, the results of studies addressing this problem are consistent with the experimental findings discussed earlier. Thus, compensatory renal hypertrophy after uninephrectomy appears to be proportionately greater the younger the age at the time of nephrectomy.[75] If nephrectomy is delayed beyond the first year of life, however, a significant effect of age on the compensatory response may be difficult to demonstrate.[76,77]

Prenatal Nephron Loss

Unilateral Multicystic Kidney and Renal Agenesis

Most nephron loss in the neonate results from fetal renal maldevelopment. Unilateral multicystic renal dysplasia results in a nonfunctional kidney early in gestation, and therefore it affords an opportunity to study the adaptation by the remaining kidney. An autopsy study of 20 human fetuses with a unilateral kidney revealed a significant increase in the proportional weight of the single kidney.[78] These findings are corroborated by two prenatal ultrasound studies of fetuses with unilateral renal agenesis or multicystic kidney. In both reports, the single functioning kidneys were significantly longer than those in the control patients.[79, 80] Sonography permits serial measurement of renal size in the fetus, such that renal growth can be compared with normal ranges and followed beyond birth. Such "tracking" of renal size may be clinically useful in monitoring the function of an abnormal contralateral kidney in infants with two functioning kidneys. An exaggerated rate of increase in renal size has been correlated with contralateral renal function that contributes less than 15% of total function.[81]

In infants born with unilateral renal agenesis, renal volume increases to 188% of that of a single normal kidney during postnatal development.[76] Consistent with the hypothesis that hypertrophy and prolonged hyperfiltration by remnant glomeruli lead to progressive renal injury, patients with unilateral renal agenesis may develop focal glomerular sclerosis and renal insufficiency in adulthood.[82-84]

Renal Hypoplasia and Dysplasia

Because of the wide variation in functional nephron loss resulting from renal hypoplasia and dysplasia, it has been difficult systematically to examine the adaptation of remaining nephrons in these disorders. However, in oligomeganephronia, a rare form of congenital renal hypoplasia, infants are born with less than 25% of the normal nephron number.[85] Presumably, because of the severity of nephron loss, compensatory hypertrophy is pushed to its limits, resulting in glomerular volumes that are severalfold greater than normal.[82] This disorder is associated with the eventual development of focal glomerular sclerosis.[82, 85]

Congenital Hydronephrosis

Along with renal hypoplasia or dysplasia, congenital urinary tract obstruction accounts for most cases of nephron loss in the neonate. Complete ureteral obstruction (atresia) early in gestation results in multicystic dysplasia and a nonfunctional kidney.[86] However, most forms of hydronephrosis in the neonate result from incomplete obstruction of the urinary tract or vesicoureteral reflux. Severe bladder obstruction resulting from posterior urethral valves can cause renal maldevelopment *in utero*, such that adaptive renal growth is impaired despite either prenatal or postnatal relief of obstruction.[87, 88] Unilateral ureteropelvic junction obstruction, conversely, may be relatively mild *in utero*, such that most renal damage occurs postnatally unless the obstruction is relieved.[89] Severe vesicoureteral reflux can eventually lead to glomerulosclerosis, proteinuria, and renal insufficiency if both kidneys are involved.[90]

Postnatal Adaptation to Nephron Loss

In cases of unilateral loss of nephrons (or more severe impairment of one kidney than the other), the contralateral kidney generally compensates accordingly. This phenomenon, first called *renal counterbalance* by Hinman,[91] appears to be exaggerated in early development.[92, 93] The postnatal hypertrophic response of the less impaired kidney can be further compromised by the presence of vesicoureteral reflux[94] or infection.[95] As in experimental studies,[38] the hypertrophic response by the intact kidney is dependent on the proportion of nephron loss that is caused by scarring of the affected kidney.[96] Adaptation by remaining nephrons can also be influenced by iatrogenic factors such as radiation or chemotherapy, which may impair compensatory hypertrophy to a greater extent in patients younger than 2 years of age than in older patients.[97]

Silber[98] found that kidneys transplanted from adults to children did not hypertrophy, but those transplanted from children to adults enlarged significantly. As would have been predicted from the magnitude and rapidity of the renal adaptive response, early development of focal glomerulosclerosis has been reported in adult recipients of kidneys from anencephalic donor fetuses.[99] Moreover, compared with kidneys from adult donors, kidneys from pediatric donors younger than 6 years of age develop far more glomerulosclerosis, proteinuria, and decreased GFR 1 year after transplantation into adult recipients.[100] These findings underscore the unique susceptibility of the immature kidney to the long-term deleterious consequences of nephron loss.

Prediction of Ultimate Renal Function

A major problem confronting the physician caring for the infant with reduced functioning renal mass is the lack of a reliable means of predicting the ultimate compensatory renal adaptation: Will the infant require dialysis or renal transplantation and, if so, when? As described earlier, normal development and compensatory renal development are interdependent and are significantly influenced by the cause of nephron loss, the proportion of intact nephrons remaining, and the presence of factors that impair the adaptive process. It is becoming increasingly clear that many of the currently available data reflect an insufficient follow-up period. Thus, although unilateral renal agenesis was previously thought to represent a benign condition, the deleterious consequences may not appear until late adulthood. Nevertheless, it is still reasonable to predict that an infant with a single normal kidney can have a relatively normal life expectancy, particularly if dietary protein intake is not excessive. In the neonatal period, it may be difficult to demonstrate that a single functioning kidney is entirely normal, particularly if the contralateral kidney is multicystic.[4] Because nephrogenesis is not complete until the 34th week, preterm infants with nephron loss may have a slower increase in renal mass and function than term infants. Moreover, because even an abnormal kidney undergoes accelerated growth at the time of the pubertal growth

spurt,[96] the patient with limited renal reserve may not manifest significant renal insufficiency until adolescence.[101]

Adults subjected to partial removal of a solitary kidney (after contralateral nephrectomy for renal cancer) are at increased risk of proteinuria, glomerulopathy, and progressive renal failure.[102] Twenty-five to 30% of patients undergoing unilateral nephrectomy in childhood (mean age, 7 years) developed proteinuria and renal insufficiency after a median follow-up of 25 years.[103] The infant with a GFR of less than 50% of normal for age at the time of diagnosis is even more likely to experience progressive renal insufficiency.[101, 104] Although infants with posterior urethral valves and a serum creatinine concentration less than 0.8 mg/dl during the first 12 months of life are likely to maintain adequate renal function for several years,[105] acceleration of the rate of renal deterioration may increase at adolescence or during adulthood. As discussed earlier, certain conditions are associated with impairment of nephrogenesis (see Table 137–1), which may predispose patients to hypertension, proteinuria, and renal insufficiency in adulthood.[18]

Until more comprehensive predictive data are available, the most prudent approach to follow-up of the neonate with nephron loss from any cause is periodic measurement of somatic and renal growth (by ultrasonography), GFR (by serum creatinine concentration), and urine protein excretion (by urine protein/creatinine ratio). Blood pressure, urinalysis, and serum calcium, phosphorus, and total carbon dioxide concentrations should be monitored, and urine should be cultured periodically in high-risk patients. By continuous tracking of these parameters, the natural history of adaptation to congenital nephron loss may be clarified, and ultimate renal adaptation can be optimized for each patient. It appears that the progression of renal disease may be slowed by the judicious use of inhibition of intrarenal angiotensin II, either by using an angiotensin-converting enzyme inhibitor or an angiotensin receptor blocker.[106] In addition to controlling hypertension, experimental studies have shown a salutary effect of angiotensin inhibition on proteinuria and the development of interstitial fibrosis. As noted earlier, because angiotensin II is necessary for normal renal development and for maintaining renal hemodynamics perinatally, inhibition of angiotensin should be avoided if possible during the perinatal and neonatal periods. Patients with a reduced number of nephrons should also avoid the use of nonsteroidal antiinflammatory drugs, in view of the vasoconstrictor effects of these agents. The combination of improved perinatal or neonatal evaluation and management, as well as seamless longitudinal follow-up by the pediatrician and internist, should lead to optimal preservation of renal function in infants born with a reduction in renal mass.

REFERENCES

1. Krohn AG, et al: Compensatory renal hypertrophy: the role of immediate vascular changes in its production. J Urol *103*:564, 1970.
2. Chevalier RL, Kaiser DL: Effects of acute uninephrectomy and age on renal blood flow autoregulation in the rat. Am J Physiol *249*:F672, 1985.
3. Provoost AP, Molenaar JC: Changes in the glomerular filtration rate after unilateral nephrectomy in rats. Pflugers Arch *385*:161, 1980.
4. De Klerk DP, et al: Multicystic dysplastic kidney. J Urol *118*:306, 1977.
5. Peters G: Compensatory adaptation of renal functions in the unanesthetized rat. Am J Physiol *205*:1042, 1963.
6. Hartupee DA, Weidner WJ: Influence of indomethacin on cation excretion after acute unilateral nephrectomy in dogs. Prostaglandins Med *5*:243, 1980.
7. Ribstein J, Humphreys MH: Renal nerves and cation excretion after acute reduction in functioning renal mass in the rat. Am J Physiol *246*:F260, 1984.
8. Dicker SE, Shirley DG: Compensatory renal growth after unilateral nephrectomy in the newborn rat. J Physiol (Lond) *228*:193, 1973.
9. Hayslett JP: Functional adaptation to reduction in renal mass. Physiol Rev *59*:137, 1979.
10. Shirley DG: Developmental and compensatory renal growth in the guinea pig. Biol Neonate *30*:169, 1976.
11. Kaufman JM, et al: Age-dependent characteristics of compensatory renal growth. Kidney Int *8*:21, 1975.

12. Larsson L, et al: Effect of normal development on compensatory renal growth. Kidney Int *18*:29, 1980.
13. Douglas-Denton R, et al: Compensatory renal growth after unilateral nephrectomy in the ovine fetus. J Am Soc Nephrol *13*:406, 2002.
14. Chevalier RL: Glomerular number and perfusion during normal and compensatory renal growth in the guinea pig. Pediatr Res *16*:436, 1982.
15. Olivetti G, et al: Morphometry of the renal corpuscle during postnatal growth and compensatory hypertrophy. Kidney Int *17*:438, 1980.
16. Hayslett JP, et al: Functional correlates of compensatory renal hypertrophy. J Clin Invest *47*:774, 1968.
17. Horster M, et al: Intracortical distribution of number and volume of glomeruli during postnatal maturation in the dog. J Clin Invest *50*:796, 1971.
18. Brenner BM, Mackenzie HS: Nephron mass as a risk factor for progression of renal disease. Kidney Int Suppl *63*:S124, 1997.
19. Clark AT, Bertram JF: Molecular regulation of nephron endowment. Am J Physiol Renal Physiol *276*:F485, 1999.
20. Manalich R, et al: Relationship between weight at birth and the number and size of renal glomeruli in humans: a histomorphometric study. Kidney Int *58*:770, 2000.
21. Barker DJP: Fetal undernutrition and adult hypertension. *1*:587, 1999.
22. Gasser B, et al: A quantitative study of normal nephrogenesis in the human fetus: its implication in the natural history of kidney changes due to low obstructive uropathies. Fetal Diagn Ther *8*:371, 1993.
23. Peters CA, et al: The response of the fetal kidney to obstruction. J Urol *148*:503, 1992.
24. Liapis H, et al: Effects of experimental ureteral obstruction on platelet-derived growth factor-A and type I procollagen expression in fetal metanephric kidneys. Pediatr Nephrol *8*:548, 1994.
25. McVary KT, Maizels M: Urinary obstruction reduces glomerulogenesis in the developing kidney: a model in the rabbit. J Urol *142*:646, 1989.
26. Chevalier RL, et al: Recovery from release of ureteral obstruction in the rat: relationship to nephrogenesis. Kidney Int *61*:2033, 2002.
27. Merlet-Benichou C, et al: Intrauterine growth retardation leads to a permanent nephron deficit in the rat. Pediatr Nephrol *8*:175, 1994.
28. Hinchliffe SA, et al: The effect of intrauterine growth retardation on the development of renal nephrons. Br J Obstet Gynaecol *99*:296, 1992.
29. Amri R, et al: Adverse effects of hyperglycemia on kidney development in rats: in vivo and in vitro studies. Diabetes *48*:2240, 1999.
30. Hoy WE, et al: A new interpretation of the Barker hypothesis: low birthweight and susceptibility to renal disease. Kidney Int *56*:1072, 1999.
31. Lelievre-Pegorier M, et al: Mild vitamin A deficiency leads to inborn nephron deficit in the rat. Kidney Int *54*:1455, 1998.
32. Crocker JFS, Vernier RL: Fetal kidney in organ culture: abnormalities of development induced by decreased amounts of potassium. Science *169*:485, 1970.
33. Ortiz LA, et al: Effect of prenatal dexamethasone on rat renal development. Kidney Int *59*:1663, 2000.
34. Gilbert T, et al: Long-term effects of mild oligonephronia induced in utero by gentamicin in the rat. Pediatr Res *30*:450, 1991.
35. Nathanson S, et al: In utero and in vitro exposure to beta-lactams impair kidney development in the rat. J Am Soc Nephrol *11*:874, 2002.
36. Clark AT, et al: In vitro studies on the roles of transforming growth factor-pi in rat metanephric development. Kidney Int *59*:1641, 2001.
37. Doublier S, et al: Overexpression of human insulin-like growth factor binding protein-1 in the mouse leads to nephron deficit. Pediatr Res *49*:660, 2001.
38. Kaufman JM, et al: Functional and hemodynamic adaptation to progressive renal ablation. Circ Res *36*:286, 1975.
39. Aschinberg LC, et al: The influence of age on the response to renal parenchymal loss. Yale J Biol Med *51*:341, 1978.
40. Chevalier RL: Hemodynamic adaptation to reduced renal mass in early postnatal development. Pediatr Res *17*:620, 1983.
41. Chevalier RL, Kaiser DL: Autoregulation of renal blood flow in the rat: effects of growth and uninephrectomy. Am J Physiol *244*:F483, 1983.
42. Woods LL: Neonatal uninephrectomy causes hypertension in adult rats. Am J Physiol *276*:R974, 1999.
43. Woods LL: Hypertension after neonatal uninephrectomy in rats precedes glomerular damage. Hypertension *38*:337, 2001.
44. Martin RA, et al: Effect of ACE inhibition on the fetal kidney: decreased renal blood flow. Teratology *46*:317, 1992.
45. O'Dea RF, et al: Treatment of neonatal hypertension with captopril. J Pediatr *113*:403, 1988.
46. Lopez-Novoa JM, et al: Functional compensatory changes after unilateral nephrectomy in rats. Ren Physiol *5*:76, 1982.
47. Chevalier RL: Functional adaptation to reduced renal mass in early development. Am J Physiol *242*:F190, 1982.
48. Buerkert J, et al: Response of deep nephrons and the terminal collecting duct to a reduction in renal mass. Am J Physiol *236*:F454, 1979.
49. Carriere S, Brunette MG: Compensatory renal hypertrophy in dogs: single nephron glomerular filtration rate. Can J Physiol Pharmacol *55*:105, 1977.
50. Chevalier RL: Reduced renal mass in early postnatal development: glomerular dynamics in the guinea pig. Biol Neonate *44*:158, 1983.
51. Austin H, et al: Humoral regulation of renal growth. Nephron *27*:163, 1981.
52. Harris RH, et al: Renotrophic factors in urine. Kidney Int *23*:616, 1983.
53. Preuss HG, Goldin H: A renotropic system in rats. J Clin Invest *57*:94, 1976.
54. Dicker SE, Morris C: Renal control of kidney growth. J Physiol (Lond) *241*:20P, 1974.
55. Mulroney SE, et al: Renal IGF-1 mRNA levels are enhanced following unilateral nephrectomy in immature but not adult rats. Endocrinology *128*:2660, 1991.
56. Mulroney SE, et al: Effect of a growth hormone-releasing factor antagonist on compensatory renal growth, insulin-like growth factor-I (IGF-I), and IGF-I receptor gene expression after unilateral nephrectomy in immature rats. Endocrinology *130*:2697, 1992.
57. Goss RJ, Dittmer JE: Compensatory renal hypertrophy: problems and prospects. *In* Nowinsky WW, Goss RJ (eds): Compensatory Renal Hypertrophy. New York, Academic Press, 1969, pp 299–307.
58. Dicker SE, Shirley DG: Mechanism of compensatory renal hypertrophy. J Physiol (Lond) *219*:507, 1971.
59. Moise TS, Smith AH: The effect of high protein diet on the kidneys: an experimental study. Arch Pathol *4*:530, 1927.
60. Halliburton IW: The effect of unilateral nephrectomy and of diet on the composition of the kidney. *In* Nowinsky WW, Goss RJ (eds): Compensatory Renal Hypertrophy. New York, Academic Press, 1969, pp 101–130.
61. Fern RJ, et al: Reduced angiotensinogen expression attenuates renal interstitial fibrosis in obstructive nephropathy in mice. J Clin Invest *103*:39, 1999.
62. Megyesi J, et al: The lack of a functional p21(WAF1/CIP1) gene ameliorates progression to chronic renal failure. Proc Natl Acad Sci U S A *96*:10830, 1999.
63. Al-Awqati Q, Preisig PA: Size does matter: will knockout of p21[WAF1/CIP1] save the kidney by limiting compensatory renal growth? Proc Natl Acad Sci U S A *96*:10551, 1999.
64. Hostetter TH, et al: Hyperfiltration in remnant nephrons: a potentially adverse response to renal ablation. Am J Physiol *241*:F85, 1981.
65. Olson JL, et al: Altered glomerular permselectivity and progressive sclerosis following extreme ablation of renal mass. Kidney Int *22*:112, 1982.
66. Grond J, et al: Mesangial function and glomerular sclerosis in rats after unilateral nephrectomy. Kidney Int *22*:338, 1982.
67. Thomas ME, et al: Proteinuria induces tubular cell turnover: a potential mechanism for tubular atrophy. Kidney Int *55*:890, 1999.
68. Palmer BF: The renal tubule in the progression of chronic renal failure. J Invest Med *45*:346, 1997.
69. Celsi G, et al: Development of focal glomerulosclerosis after unilateral nephrectomy in infant rats. Pediatr Nephrol *1*:290, 1987.
70. Okuda S, et al: Influence of age on deterioration of the remnant kidney in uninephrectomized rats. Clin Sci *72*:571, 1987.
71. Jakobsson B, et al: Influence of different protein intake on renal growth in young rats. Acta Paediatr Scand *76*:293, 1987.
72. Provoost AP, et al: Effect of protein intake on lifelong changes in renal function of rats unilaterally nephrectomized at young age. J Lab Clin Med *114*:19, 1989.
73. Baudoin P, Provoost AP: Effects of age at the time of unilateral nephrectomy and dietary protein on long-term renal function in rats. Pediatr Nephrol *7*:536, 1993.
74. Peters CA, et al: Fetal compensatory renal growth due to unilateral ureteral obstruction. J Urol *150*:597, 1993.
75. Aperia A, et al: Renal growth and function in patients nephrectomized in childhood. Acta Paediatr Scand *66*:185, 1977.
76. Dinkel E, et al: Renal growth in patients nephrectomized for Wilms tumour as compared to renal agenesis. Eur J Pediatr *147*:54, 1988.
77. Robitaille P, et al: Long-term follow-up of patients who underwent unilateral nephrectomy in childhood. Lancet *1*:1297, 1985.
78. Hartshorne N, et al: Compensatory renal growth in human fetuses with unilateral renal agenesis. Teratology *44*:7, 1991.
79. Glazebrook KN, et al: Prenatal compensatory renal growth: documentation with US. Radiology *189*:733, 1993.
80. Mandell J, et al: Human fetal compensatory renal growth. J Urol *150*:790, 1993.
81. O'Sullivan DC, et al: Compensatory hypertrophy effectively assesses the degree of impaired renal function in unilateral renal disease. Br J Urol *69*:346, 1992.
82. Bhathena DB, et al: Focal sclerosis of hypertrophied glomeruli in solitary functioning kidneys of humans. Am J Kidney Dis *5*:226, 1985.
83. Kiprov DD, et al: Focal and segmental glomerulosclerosis and proteinuria associated with unilateral renal agenesis. Lab Invest *46*:275, 1982.
84. Wikstad I, et al: Kidney function in adults born with unilateral renal agenesis or nephrectomized in childhood. Pediatr Nephrol *2*:177, 1988.
85. Elema JD: Is one kidney sufficient? Kidney Int *9*:308, 1976.
86. Griscom NT, et al: Pelvoinfundibular atresia: the usual form of multicystic kidney—44 unilateral and two bilateral cases. Semin Roentgenol *10*:125, 1975.
87. Harrison MR, et al: Correction of congenital hydronephrosis in utero. II. Decompression reverses the effects of obstruction on the fetal lung and urinary tract. J Pediatr Surg *17*:965, 1982.
88. Nakayama DK, et al: Prognosis of posterior urethral valves presenting at birth. J Pediatr Surg *21*:43, 1986.
89. King LR, et al: The case for immediate pyeloplasty in the neonate with ureteropelvic junction obstruction. J Urol *132*:725, 1984.
90. Torres VE, et al: The progression of vesicoureteral reflux nephropathy. Ann Intern Med *92*:776, 1980.
91. Hinman F: Renal counterbalance: an experimental and clinical study with reference to the significance of disuse atrophy. J Urol *9*:289, 1923.
92. Miller M, Mortensson W: Size of the unaffected kidney in children with unilateral hydronephrosis. Acta Radiol Diagn *21*:275, 1980.

93. Taki M, et al: Impact of age on effects of ureteral obstruction on renal function. Kidney Int 24:602, 1983.
94. Wilton P, et al: Compensatory hypertrophy in children with unilateral renal disease. Acta Paediatr Scand 69:83, 1980.
95. Hellstrom M, et al: Renal growth after neonatal urinary tract infection. Pediatr Nephrol 1:269, 1987.
96. Claesson I, et al: Compensatory kidney growth in children with urinary tract infection and unilateral renal scarring: an epidemiologic study. Kidney Int 20:759, 1981.
97. Luttenegger TJ, et al: Compensatory renal hypertrophy after treatment for Wilms' tumor. AJR Am J Roentgenol 125:348, 1975.
98. Silber SJ: Renal transplantation between adults and children: differences in renal growth. JAMA 228:1143, 1974.
99. Leunissen KML, et al: Focal glomerulosclerosis in neonatal kidney grafts. Lancet 2:1019, 1987.
100. Hayes JM, et al: The development of proteinuria and focal-segmental glomerulosclerosis in recipients of pediatric donor kidneys. Transplantation 52:813, 1991.
101. Scott JES: Management of congenital posterior urethral valves. Brit J Urol 57:71, 1985.
102. Novick AC, et al: Long-term follow-up after partial removal of a solitary kidney. N Engl J Med 325:1058, 1991.
103. Argueso LR, et al: Prognosis of children with solitary kidney after unilateral nephrectomy. J Urol 148:747, 1992.
104. Mathieu H, et al: Long-term outcome of children with malformative uropathies. Int J Pediatr Nephrol 6:3, 1985.
105. Warshaw BL, et al: Prognostic features in infants with obstructive uropathy due to posterior urethral valves. J Urol 133:240, 1985.
106. Hebert LA, et al: Renoprotection: one or many therapies? Kidney Int 59:1211, 2001.

138

Tracy E. Hunley and Valentina Kon

Pathophysiology of Acute Renal Failure in the Neonatal Period

PATHOPHYSIOLOGIC MECHANISMS OF ACUTE RENAL FAILURE

Acute renal failure (ARF) is the precipitous development of azotemia resulting from a depressed rate of glomerular filtration. Specific causes of ARF have conventionally been classified into prerenal, renal, or postrenal, thereby localizing the primary site of the disorder. *Prerenal failure* describes a process whereby a disorder in the systemic circulation causes renal hypoperfusion, and it reflects contraction of the intravascular volume or cardiac pump failure, or both. The implication of this disorder is that correction of the underlying disturbance, with volume repletion or improvement in cardiac function, or both, will restore glomerular filtration. When correction of the circulatory impairment does not restore a normal level of filtration, development of renal parenchymal damage and transition to *intrinsic renal failure* are implied. An important subset of intrinsic renal failure is *acute tubular necrosis*. Although necrosis is not always evident histologically, the term connotes a clinical syndrome that results from ischemia and excludes prerenal and postrenal failure, as well as intrinsic renal damage resulting from vascular, glomerular, or interstitial lesions. *Postrenal failure* refers to obstruction of urine flow by a bilateral lesion or a site within the bladder or urethra. An important example of the latter in the neonate is posterior urethral valves.

The final common pathway that underlies ARF, regardless of the cause or primary site of injury, is a fall in the glomerular filtration rate (GFR), which becomes inadequate to eliminate metabolic waste products. The total GFR in both kidneys depends on the number of filtering nephrons and the GFR in each individual nephron. Thus, reduction in the total kidney GFR may result from a loss of a number of filtering nephron units or a decrease in the rate of filtration in individual nephrons. However, unless the cause of ARF is trauma, surgery, or thrombus involving circumscribed areas of the kidney, a reduction in nephron numbers ordinarily does not contribute to the decreased GFR in ARF in neonates. This finding is in contrast to the pattern in chronic renal failure, in which functional internephron heterogeneity predominates so some nephrons are severely damaged, or even completely nonfunctional, whereas others attain normal (or increased) function. Some studies have revealed considerable variability in nephron number among physiologically normal individuals.[1] Although it is not known whether such variability in the complement of nephrons affects the occurrence or severity of acute injury, it appears to have profound impact on the consequence of the acute injury (see later).

Certain nephron populations may be at greater risk of damage. In experimental studies of adult animals, deeper nephrons sustain greater injury after ischemia than do superficial cortical nephrons, and the deeper medullary region of the kidney appears metabolically at greater risk of ischemic damage.[2, 3] These observations may be relevant in the premature infant whose renal development normally proceeds in a centrifugal manner and continues through the 36th week of gestation.[4,5] It is possible, therefore, that renal injury in an extremely premature baby would occur in the deeper, perhaps more vulnerable, areas of the kidney before the relatively more resistant cortical nephrons have developed. This is an especially pivotal locus with respect to nephron generation, and injury at this site may have additional adverse implications in limiting the number and integrity of future nephrons. Conversely, reparative processes, which involve growth factors acting as mitogens and morphogens, may repair injured nephrons and encourage nephrogenesis. Indeed, recovery of renal function in a premature baby after renal insult likely represents both healing of injured nephrons and acquisition of new nephrons. How such injury occurring in premature babies affects the ultimate number of nephrons is currently unknown. There is no evidence, however, that premature babies who sustain renal injury acquire more than the usual complement of 1 million nephrons contained in normal kidneys. Further, once formation of new nephrons is completed (by 36 weeks' gestational age), recovery from renal injury does not reflect new nephrogenesis, even after extensive loss of renal parenchyma.

Not only are certain nephron populations at greater risk of damage, but also certain nephron segments, particularly those located in the outer medulla, appear especially susceptible to injury. Thus, the straight segment of the proximal tubule (S3 segment) and the medullary thick ascending limb demonstrate heightened susceptibility to ischemic and nephrotoxic injuries.[6] This susceptibility relates to low oxygen tension in this region, limited capacity to achieve anaerobic respiration, and high work-

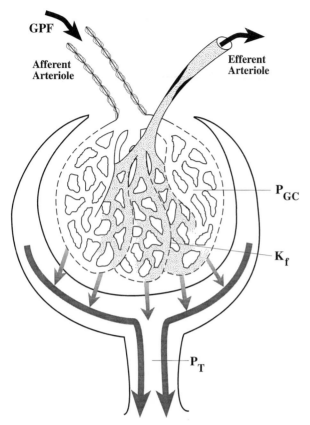

GPF

Afferent Arteriole

Efferent Arteriole

P_{GC}

K_f

P_T

Figure 138–1. Schematic presentation of the glomerular filtration process. Glomerular filtration is determined by the rate of glomerular plasma flow (GPF) entering the afferent arteriole; hydraulic pressure within the glomerular capillary (P_{GC}) minus hydraulic pressure in proximal tubule (P_T); glomerular capillary ultrafiltration coefficient (K_f), which describes the permeability properties of the glomerular capillary membrane. (Adapted from Winkler D, et al: Kidney Int *39:*S2, 1991.)

load in these segments.[6,7] One can postulate that fetal hemoglobin, with its characteristically higher oxygen affinity, may be less able to deliver oxygen to the deep nephrons than adult hemoglobin. This may contribute to the disproportionately high rate of ARF occurring in neonates as compared with older children. Impairment of oxygen delivery to the susceptible outer medullary region has been linked to endothelial injury together with leukocyte activation that physically impedes blood flow.[8] The endothelial injury, in turn, is related to reactive oxygen species, whereas leukocyte infiltration has been related to adhesion molecules, such as selectins and integrins as well as inflammatory cytokines such as interleukin-1 and tumor necrosis factor-α.[8-10] It is postulated that this medullary congestion is pivotal to the central pathologic lesion of ARF, namely, tubular injury.[10]

As noted earlier, regardless of the origin or primary site of injury, the decrease in whole-kidney GFR in ARF reflects a decreased rate of glomerular filtration in individual nephrons. It is useful, therefore, to review the conceptual factors determining single-nephron GFR (SNGFR), along with pertinent clinical examples as well as molecular studies that illustrate their individual roles in decreasing the GFR. Reduction in the SNGFR in ARF can be attributed to changes in one or more of the following parameters (Fig. 138–1)[11]: (1) the rate of glomerular plasma flow; (2) glomerular transcapillary hydraulic pressure difference (the pressure within the glomerular capillary bed favoring

ultrafiltration of fluid minus the pressure in the proximal tubule opposing ultrafiltration); (3) systemic plasma colloid osmotic pressure; and (4) permeability properties of glomerular capillaries. Although perturbations in these parameters can describe any type of ARF,[11-13] this discussion focuses primarily on the pathopsychological mechanisms in intrinsic ARF.

Plasma Flow Rate

A decreased glomerular plasma flow rate is seen in systemic circulatory impairment (prerenal failure) and may continue even after systemic and circulatory impairments are apparently restored (intrinsic renal failure). This hypoperfusion reflects enhanced vasoconstriction of the renal vasculature.[14,15] Increasing renal blood flow by volume expansion or administration of vasodilators before or soon after the onset of renal failure can prevent or ameliorate the development of certain human and experimental ARF. Until recently, most treatments designed to increase filtration by increasing renal blood flow failed once renal failure was established. Several agents, however, have been shown to increase renal blood flow with resultant improvement in GFR, even in well-established ARF in animal models and in humans. These agents include atrial natriuretic peptide, insulin-like growth factor I, hepatic growth factor, α-melanocyte-stimulating hormone, osteogenic protein-1, and antagonists of adenosine or endothelin.[16-24] Decreased blood flow, however, does not typify all cases of ARF. Therefore, attempts to increase renal blood flow in this setting would not be expected to be universally successful. The clinical implications of these observations are that trials of volume infusion and vasodilators may be useful in the prevention and treatment of ARF, especially in the early stages. However, these maneuvers carry the risks of systemic vasodilation and hypotension that could worsen renal perfusion, as well as volume overload and congestive heart failure once the transition has been made to established renal failure.

Despite the near-normal renal plasma flow observed in many forms of clinical and experimental ARF, there is accumulating evidence that the vascular responsiveness of the kidney is impaired and may contribute to hypofiltration under certain circumstances. The ability of the renal vasculature of healthy persons to vasodilate and vasoconstrict is the basis for maintaining remarkably constant levels of renal blood flow and glomerular filtration in the presence of sudden changes in systemic pressure, that is, *renal autoregulation*.[25] For example, decreasing renal perfusion pressure causes the preglomerular, afferent arteriole to vasodilate and the postglomerular, efferent arteriole to constrict (see Fig. 138–1). The sum total consists of a decrease in total renal vascular resistance and preservation of renal blood flow. In contrast, blood flow autoregulation appears to be impaired in ARF, so decreasing renal perfusion pressure increases renal vascular resistance and decreases renal blood flow, and this may be sufficient to cause hypofiltration.[26-30] This is important because even minimal (not hypotensive) decreases in systemic blood pressure may cause additional renal ischemia and may perpetuate hypofiltration or even parenchymal renal damage in the already injured kidney.[27] These observations underscore that seemingly normal values of renal blood flow belie the abnormal autoregulation of injured kidneys.

At first glance, newborn babies seem to be at risk of hypoperfusion. When compared with adults, normal newborns have a low level of renal plasma flow, and their systemic blood pressure is less than the lower limits for autoregulation in adults (80 to 90 mm Hg). However, normal young animals autoregulate blood flow efficiently at the lower prevailing systemic blood pressure.[29-31] By contrast, young animals that undergo removal of one kidney demonstrate impairment in renal blood flow autoregulation immediately after uninephrectomy, and this impairment persists for at least 4 to 5 weeks.[31] Furthermore, young umnephrectomized animals that are also volume-contracted have a higher renal vascular resistance and lower renal blood flow over a range of decreasing renal perfusion pressures when compared with saline-infused animals. Thus, renal injury and neonatal volume status determine the effectiveness of renal blood flow autoregulation in the setting of ARF. The clinical implication is that volume depletion negatively affects this protective autoregulatory mechanism and makes the infant more susceptible to developing and propagating ARF.

Glomerular Transcapillary Hydraulic Pressure Difference

Glomerular capillary hydraulic pressure favors glomerular filtration. It is opposed by pressure in the proximal tubule (see Fig. 138-1). Although both these pressures are fairly stable under normal circumstances, the pathophysiologic processes of ARF can affect either or both by several mechanisms. Decreased renal perfusion pressure normally causes a selective increase in the postglomerular, efferent arteriolar resistance, thereby maintaining intraglomerular capillary pressure, which contributes to constancy in GFR. When the systemic blood pressure falls to less than the autoregulatory range, glomerular capillary pressure, renal plasma flow, and the GFR follow the fall in systemic blood pressure.[25] Thus, in circulatory collapse, as may precede the development of ARF, the autoregulatory response of the renal vasculature is exceeded, and severe hypofiltration may result. In addition to profound hypotension, which overwhelms the normal autoregulatory mechanisms, under certain conditions even relatively modest systemic hypotension is associated with apparent ineffective autoregulation and a decrease in the GFR. As noted earlier, in animals with volume depletion or congestive heart failure, a 30% decrease in renal perfusion pressure (which did not affect GFR in normal rats) caused a more than 25% fall in the GFR.[32] The impaired ability to preserve the GFR in the presence of reduced renal perfusion pressure in both conditions was, at least in part, the result of a fall in the glomerular capillary pressure, which, in turn, reflected an inadequate vasoconstrictive response within the efferent arterioles.

As noted earlier, afferent arteriolar dilation and renal blood flow adjust to decreasing renal perfusion pressure in adult and immature animals. However, one study found that although decreasing the renal perfusion pressure by about 30% from baseline was accompanied by a minimal fall in the GFR in adult rats, in young rats the GFR plummeted by more than 80%.[29] Micropuncture experiments revealed that the profound hypofiltration in young rats largely reflected decreased glomerular capillary pressure. Because angiotensin II (AII) is known to vasoconstrict the efferent arteriole and to maintain glomerular capillary pressure, it is thought to have an important role in autoregulation of the GFR. A similar degree of water deprivation causes a greater increase in plasma renin activity in adult animals than in immature ones, and a higher dose of exogenous AII is required in immature than in adult animals to cause a similar increase in glomerular capillary pressure.[29] Taken together, young animals have limited ability to activate at least one vasoconstrictor system, namely, AII, and the immature efferent arteriole may have limited responsiveness to AII. Thus, even in the presence of afferent vasodilation after decreasing renal perfusion pressure, young animals may develop hypofiltration. These observations provide a mechanism for dissociation between renal blood flow and the GFR in that dilation in the afferent arteriole without sufficient vasoconstriction in the efferent arteriole is insufficient to maintain a transcapillary pressure that promotes glomerular filtration. Of the two currently recognized receptors for AII, AT1 and AT2, the AT1 is most abundantly expressed and transduces the bulk of the recognized actions of AII including efferent arteriolar constriction.[33,34] Glomerular AII hyporesponsiveness in the neonatal kidney does not appear to reflect inade-

quate AT1 receptor density, because kidney AT1 expression peaks postnatally at twice the adult level.[35] Further, AII availability is also maximized, reflecting an abundance of renal angiotensin-converting enzyme that increases postnatally such that within 2 weeks of birth it surpasses adult levels, as does circulating angiotensin-converting enzyme.[36] Moreover, renin production in neonates is robust and extends beyond the juxtaglomerular apparatus to include more proximal segments of the renal arterial tree.[37] Angiotensinogen also undergoes a dramatic postnatal increase in liver expression before decreasing and settling to the adult level.[38] Overall, the receptors as well as the enzymes required for production of the mature AII ligand are exuberantly expressed in the neonatal kidney. The observed hyporesponsiveness of the neonatal kidney therefore appears to reflect inadequate postnatal maturation of postreceptor processes. It is possible, however, that the blunted vasoconstriction of the neonatal efferent arteriole in response to AII reflects the vasodilatory contribution of the AT2 receptor. This may occur though a direct effect of the AT2 receptor or though AT2-mediated stimulation of nitric oxide and bradykinin.[39]

The transcapillary hydraulic pressure difference includes not only the hydraulic pressure within the glomerular capillaries but also the opposing pressure in the tubules. Tubular injury is an important component in the pathophysiology of ARF.[6-14] Studies have clarified the cellular and molecular events that underlie the tubular injury. Under normal conditions, tubular epithelial cell function depends on maintenance of defined apical and basolateral membranes with distinct protein populations. One such class of protein consists of the *integrins,* which are membrane-spanning glycoproteins located on the basolateral surface. Integrins interact with the intracellular cytoskeleton as well as the extracellular matrix, and they mediate tubular cell adhesion.[40] Renal ischemia and subsequent ATP depletion induce redistribution of integrins to the apical surface and cause the actin cytoskeleton to move from its normal circumferential position to a perinuclear location. These injury-induced changes culminate in cellular rounding, retraction, and detachment from the basement membrane. Moreover, redistribution of integrins to the apical surface in the detached cells may contribute to aggregation of these cells within the tubular lumen. This may, in turn, contribute to tubule obstruction, increased intratubular pressure, and decreasing transcapillary pressure. Indeed, infusion of the tripeptide arginine–glycine–aspartic acid that interferes with integrin adhesion mechanisms has been shown to abolish tubule obstruction and to improve renal function.[41] Noteworthy are the observations that intratubular material contains not only cellular debris but also viable cells. Thus, viable cells have been recovered from the urine of patients with ARF, a finding implying lethal cellular injury as well as disturbance in mechanisms of normal cellular adhesion as underlying tubule pathophysiology in ARF.[42] Ischemia induces redistribution of another protein—sodium, potassium, adenosine triphosphatase (Na$^+$,K$^+$-ATPase), which is normally localized to the basolateral side of the epithelial cells and reverses its normal function of sodium reabsorption.[43] This may, at least in part, be responsible for the increased urinary sodium excretion observed in ARF. Additionally, increased distal sodium delivery may stimulate vasoactive substances that decrease renal blood flow through the tubuloglomerular feedback mechanism.

In addition to direct feedback mechanisms that affect the glomerular hemodynamics, tubular injury also interrupts structural integrity, and this allows creatinine and other markers of glomerular filtration to permeate the tubules and return into the circulation (i.e., backleak) (Fig. 138-2). As noted earlier, disruption of the junctional complexes affects not only the epithelial cell polarity but also tubular permeability. Histologic and functional data in human and experimental ARF support a disruption in the integrity of tubular epithelium and the presence of

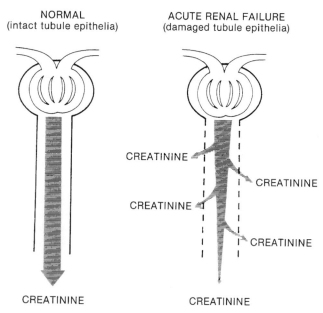

NORMAL
(intact tubule epithelia)

ACUTE RENAL FAILURE
(damaged tubule epithelia)

CREATININE

CREATININE

CREATININE

CREATININE

CREATININE

CREATININE

Figure 138–2. Role of backleak in reduced glomerular filtration rate (GFR) in acute renal failure (ARF). Disruption in the integrity of the tubule epithelium permits return into the circulation of creatinine and other GFR markers, which underestimates true GFR. (From Kon V, Ichikawa I: J Pediatr *105:*351, 1984.)

backleak.[44-46] Loss of junctional complexes that encompass tight junctions, adherent junctions, desmosomes, and gap junctions are especially relevant to backleak. At least in part, tyrosine phosphorylation of proteins within adherent junctions alters paracellular permeability and likely contributes to backleak.[47] By reducing the clearance of GFR markers, as well as metabolic waste products, backleak contributes to the high levels of creatinine in the circulation and maintenance of azotemia in ARF. Currently, no data are available regarding the extent to which backleak contributes to elevated serum creatinine and an apparent decrease in the GFR in ARF.

Plasma Colloid Osmotic Pressure

Theoretically, an increase in systemic plasma colloid osmotic pressure, which opposes filtration, will decrease the GFR. However, newborn infants normally have lower levels of plasma protein (6.5 mg/dl in term babies versus 7.5 mg/dl in adults), which tend to increase the GFR. Furthermore, hyperoncotic states (e.g., dysproteinemia) are almost unheard of in neonates, and even severe dehydration-induced hemoconcentration that occurs in neonates is unlikely to be accompanied by changes in plasma colloid osmotic pressure sufficient to change the GFR.[48]

Glomerular Capillary Ultrafiltration Coefficient

In addition to alterations in the pressures and flows already described, changes in the glomerular membrane properties themselves can contribute to the depressed level of glomerular filtration in ARF. The glomerular capillary ultrafiltration coefficient (K_f) encompasses the capillary surface area available for filtration and the permeability property of the capillaries themselves. Although technical advances have permitted study of this parameter in numerous experimental diseases, difficulties relating to the size and accessibility for direct glomerular measurements in immature animals are evidenced by the paucity of information on K_f in ARF in neonates. It is known that K_f is low

in immature animals and increases with maturation.[5] One experimental study also suggested that a decrease in this parameter may lower the SNGFR to a greater extent in immature than in adult animals.[49] The study showed that despite lower amounts of antiglomerular basement membrane antibody binding in young rats, the degree of reduction in the SNGFR was greater when compared with adults. Entities causing inflammatory, proliferative, and microangiopathic changes in glomerular capillaries, which are expected to decrease glomerular capillary permeability, are distinctly unusual causes of ARF in the neonate. Renal ischemia and nephrotoxins are the most frequent pathogenic factors. In these conditions, glomeruli are, morphologically, relatively spared.[46] However, because of our lack of knowledge regarding the primary site determining the impedance to the filtrate, it remains unclear whether subtle morphologic changes noted in some forms of human and experimental ARF, that is, reduction in endothelial fenestrae, indicate decreased glomerular capillary permeability. Moreover, changes in the permeability of glomerular capillaries do not necessarily require fixed structural alterations in glomerular anatomy. Instead, a decrease in K_f may occur by hormonal autacoid (AII, vasopressin, prostaglandins, leukotrienes, endothelins) regulation of contractile cells within the glomerulus, which modulates the capillary area available for filtration.[48]

CAUSES OF ACUTE RENAL FAILURE

Improved supportive care and survival of extremely premature and sick babies have led to an increased incidence and recognition of ARF in neonates. The incidence of ARF in the neonatal period has been estimated to range from 1 to 23%.[50-55] In one study, 8% of babies in neonatal intensive care units experienced ARF.[50] Although the incidence of ARF in children overall is less than that in adults, the incidence in infants actually surpasses that in adults.[53] Moreover, the incidence of neonatal ARF may well be underestimated because nonoliguric ARF may go unrecognized but may be an important entity in neonates. ARF in the neonatal period may have numerous causes (Table 138-1). As in older children and adults, prerenal failure is the most common type. In a study by Norman and Asadi,[50] 72% of ARF was prerenal. Asphyxia is reported to be a frequent precipitating factor in ARF, cited as the cause of 4 to 70% of cases of ARF.[50-55] Intrinsic renal failure occurs with asphyxia when hypoxia is prolonged, and it may range from prerenal failure to ATN to cortical necrosis. Earlier reports suggested that congenital renal diseases such as dysplasia and hypoplasia were responsible for 10 to 30% of intrinsic ARF cases. However, more recent observations indicate that congenital heart disease has become the primary underlying condition associated with ARF. Thus, among neonates requiring dialysis, nearly two-thirds have congenital cardiac abnormalities.[53] In view of the advances in the care of critically ill infants, it is anticipated that this percentage will increase. Other disorders causing intrinsic neonatal ARF are sepsis and vascular disorders such as renal artery or renal vein thrombosis. Prothrombotic mutations may contribute to the development of neonatal renal thromboses.[56, 57] Nephrotoxicity resulting from aminoglycosides or indomethacin is also common. Notably, such renal dysfunction may occur even in the infant whose mother receives such agents before delivery.[58, 59] Angiotensin-converting enzyme inhibition has become the mainstay of medical treatment in hypertensive, cardiovascular, and renal disorders. This approach has led to the recognition of functional and structural abnormalities in infants of mothers treated with angiotensin-converting enzyme inhibitors. Half of such infants have been observed to have oligohydramnios, hypotension, and anuria that is associated with a 25% mortality.[60-62] Postrenal failure is an important but rarer cause of renal failure in newborns. In a study by Ellis and Arnold,[63] about 7% of neonates with ARF had postrenal failure.

TABLE 138-1
Causes of Acute Renal Failure in Neonates

Prenal
- Hypovolemia or renal hypoperfusion
- Asphyxia
- Respiratory distress syndrome (RDS)
- Dehydration
- Hemorrhage (maternal antepartum, twin-to-twin transfusion, intraventricular bleeding, hemolytic disease)
- Sepsis
- Cardiac disease (patent ductus arteriosus, aortic coarctation)
- Polycythemia (hyperviscosity)
- Indomethacin

Renal
- Acute tubular necrosis (ATN)
- Persistent prerenal disturbances
- Nephrotoxins (nephrotoxic antibiotics, e.g., aminoglycosides, contrast agents angiotensin-converting enzyme [ACE] inhibitors)
- Myoglobinuria, hemoglobinuria, hyperuricemia
- Vascular disorders (renal vein thrombosis, renal artery thrombosis, aortic thrombosis, disseminated intravascular coagulation)
- Congenital renal anomaly (dysplasia, hypoplasia, polycystic kidney, agenesis)
- Pyelonephritis
- Transient acute renal failure of the neonate
- Maternal etiology (gentamicin, indomethacin, ACE inhibitors, paraproteinemia[75])

Postrenal
- Congenital anomaly (ureteral or urethral obstruction, neurogenic bladder, megacystis-megaureter)
- Obstruction secondary to circumcision
- Renal candidiasis[76]
- Calculi
- Neurogenic bladder

PROGNOSIS

The prognosis of ARF in neonates depends on the primary cause. As in other age groups, prerenal failure tends to have a better prognosis because, by definition, restoration of circulatory function restores the glomerular filtration unless the cause of prerenal ARF is a primary cardiac abnormality. Intrinsic renal failure has been associated with high mortality, ranging from 20 to 75%, with survival relating to the reversibility of the underlying condition (hypoxia, shock, infection, cardiac failure). Among neonates with ARF requiring dialysis, the reported overall mortality rate was 50%.[53] The underlying condition had a remarkable effect on mortality. Infants with ARF requiring dialysis in the setting of congenital heart disease had a mortality rate approaching 60%, whereas infants with ARF without a cardiac condition had a mortality rate of less than 30%.[53] The deleterious effect of congenital heart defect holds true regardless of whether dialysis is necessary.[64] Birth weight, Apgar scores, age at diagnosis, fractional sodium excretion, pulmonary function, and peak creatinine or blood urea nitrogen values do not affect the prognosis.[51] Lack of oliguria and the presence of identifiable renal uptake of radionucleotide are reported to be good prognostic signs.[51] The composite of several individual variables, including hypotension, mechanical ventilation, dialysis, and blood urea nitrogen have been reported to predict pediatric mortality with ARF.[65] Many survivors have chronically impaired renal function and renal growth. In one study, residual damage, such as chronic renal failure, hypertension, and growth retardation, occurred in 36% of patients with ARF caused by asphyxia, vascular thrombosis, hypotension, and toxins.[52] Indeed, one report documented a poor long-term renal outcome in full-term neonates with ARF who did not require dialysis. At 6.5- to 19-year follow-up, two-

thirds of these children had renal insufficiency, hypertension, or even end-stage renal failure. These observations underscore the need for caution in assigning prognosis to infants with neonatal ARF.[54]

More recently, another risk factor for residual damage was suggested. Observations indicate considerable interindividual variability in the complement of nephrons, and this has profound consequences for progressive renal damage after any number of injuries that may include ARF in the neonatal period. Thus far, low birth weight, especially fetal growth retardation, vitamin A deficiency, drugs such as gentamicin, aminopenicillins, cyclosporine, and glucocorticoids, and metabolic disorders such as hyperglycemia have all been shown to cause a significant nephron deficit.[1, 66-72] The relevance of these findings stems from observations that even a modest decrease in nephron number predisposes the kidneys to chronic renal dysfunction as well as hypertension.[1, 73, 74] Thus, although it is currently unknown whether neonates with fewer nephrons are more susceptible to ARF or more severe ARF, they may well have an increased incidence of persistent urinary abnormalities, residual renal damage, and hypertension after neonatal ARF.

REFERENCES

1. Merlet-Benichou C, et al: Nephron number: variability is the rule. Causes and consequences. Lab Invest 79:515, 1999.
2. Mason J, et al: Role of the medullary perfusion defect in the pathogenesis of ischemic renal failure. Kidney Int 26:283, 1984.
3. Brezis M, et al: Renal ischemia: a new perspective. Kidney Int 26:375, 1984.
4. Potter EL, Craig JM: Kidneys, ureters, urinary bladder and urethra. In Potter EL (ed): Pathology of the Fetus and the Infant, 3rd ed. Chicago, Year Book Medical Publishers, 1975.
5. Yared A, Ichikawa I: Postnatal development of glomerular filtration. In: Fetal and Neonatal Physiology, 2nd ed. Philadelphia, WB Saunders, 1998.
6. Brezis M, Rosen S: Mechanisms of disease: hypoxia of the renal medulla—its implications for disease. N Engl J Med 332:647, 1995.
7. Siegel NJ, et al: Renal cell injury: metabolic and structural alterations. Pediatr Res 30:129, 1994.
8. Bonventre JV: Mechanisms of ischemic acute renal failure. Kidney Int 43:1160, 1993.
9. Andreoli SP: Reactive oxygen molecules, oxidant injury and renal disease. Pediatr Nephrol 5:733, 1991.
10. Sheridan AM, Bonventre J: Cell biology and molecular mechanisms of injury in ischemic acute renal failure. Curr Opin Nephrol Hypertens 9:427, 2000.
11. Kon V, Ichikawa I: Research seminar: physiology of acute renal failure. J Pediatr 105:351, 1984.
12. Chevalier RL: Molecular and cellular pathophysiology of obstructive nephropathy. Pediatr Nephrol 13:612, 1999.
13. Badr KF, Ichikawa I: Prerenal failure: a deleterious shift from renal compensation to decompensation. N Engl J Med 319:623, 1988.
14. Hostetter TH, Brenner BM: Renal circulatory and nephron function in experimental acute renal failure. In Brenner BM, Lazarus JM (eds): Acute Renal Failure, 2nd ed. New York, Churchill Livingstone, 1988, p 67.
15. Madias NE, et al: Postischemic acute renal failure. In Brenner BM, Lazarus JM (eds): Acute Renal Failure, 2nd ed. New York, Churchill Livingstone, 1988, p 251.
16. Rahman SN, et al: Effects of atrial natriuretic peptide in clinical acute renal failure. Kidney Int 45:1731, 1994.
17. Sward K, et al: Long-term infusion of atrial natriuretic peptide (ANP) improves renal blood flow and glomerular filtration rate in clinical acute renal failure. Acta Anaesthesiol Scand 45:536, 2001.
18. Allgren R, et al: Anaritide in acute tubular necrosis. N Engl J Med 336:282, 1997.
19. Hammerman MR, Miller SB: Therapeutic use of growth factors in renal failure. J Am Soc Nephrol 5:1, 1994.
20. Chiao H, et al: α-Melanocyte-stimulating hormone protects against renal injury after ischemia in mice and rats. J Clin Invest 99:1165, 1997.
21. Vukicevic S, et al: Osteogenic protein-1 (bone morphogenetic protein-7) reduces severity of injury after ischemic acute renal failure in rat. J Clin Invest 102:202, 1998.
22. Okusa MD, et al: Enhanced protection from renal ischemia: reperfusion injury with A2A-adenosine receptor activation and PDE 4 inhibition. Kidney Int 59:2114, 2001.
23. Kon V, et al: Glomerular actions of endothelin in vivo. J Clin Invest 83:1762, 1989.
24. Gellai M, et al: Reversal of postischemic acute renal failure with a selective endothelin A receptor antagonist in the rat. J Clin Invest 93:900, 1994.
25. Robertson CR, et al: Dynamics of glomerular ultrafiltration in the rat. III. Hemodynamics and autoregulation. Am J Physiol 223:1191, 1972.

26. Adams PL, et al: Impaired renal blood flow autoregulation in ischemic acute renal failure. Kidney Int *18*:68, 1980.

27. Solez K, et al: The morphology of "acute tubular necrosis" in man: analysis of 57 renal biopsies and comparison with the glycerol model. Medicine (Baltimore) *58*:362, 1979.

28. Kelleher SP, et al: Effect of hemorrhagic reduction in blood pressure on recovery from acute renal failure. Kidney Int *31*:725, 1987.

29. Yared A, Yoshioka T: Uncoupling of the autoregulation of renal blood flow and glomerular filtration rate in immature rats: role of the renin-angiotensin system. Kidney Int *33*:414, 1988.

30. Robillard JE, et al: Renal hemodynamics and functional adjustments to postnatal life. Semin Perinatol *12*:143, 1988.

31. Chevalier RL, Kaiser DL: Effects of acute uninephrectomy and age on renal blood flow autoregulation in the rat. Am J Physiol *249*:F672, 1985.

32. Yoshioka T, et al: Impaired preservation of glomerular filtration during hypotension in rats with pre-existing renal hypoperfusion. Am J Physiol *256*:F314, 1989.

33. Kakuchi J, et al: Developmental expression of renal angiotensin II receptor genes in the mouse. Kidney Int *47*:140, 1995.

34. Harris JM, Gomez RA: Renin-angiotensin system genes in kidney development. Microsc Res Tech *39*:211, 1997.

35. Tufro-McReddie A, et al: Ontogeny of type 1 angiotensin II receptor gene expression in the rat. J Clin Invest *91*:530, 1993.

36. Yosipiv IV, El-Dahr SS: Developmental biology of angiotensin-converting enzyme. Pediatr Nephrol *12*:72, 1998.

37. Gomez RA: Distribution of renin mRNA and its protein in the developing kidney. Am J Physiol *257*:F850, 1989.

38. Gomez RA, et al: Fetal expression of the angiotensinogen gene. Endocrinology *123*:2298, 1988.

39. Carey R, et al: Role of the angiotensin type 2 receptor in the regulation of blood pressure and renal function. Hypertension *35*:155, 2000.

40. Goligorsky MS, et al: Integrin receptors in renal tubule epithelium: new insights into pathophysiology of acute renal failure. Am J Physiol *264*:F1, 1993.

41. Goligorsky M, et al: Therapeutic potential of RGD peptides in acute renal injury. Kidney Int *51*:1487, 1997.

42. Racusen LC, et al: Dissociation of tubule cell detachment and tubule cell death in clinical and experimental "acute tubular necrosis." Lab Invest *64*:546, 1991.

43. Fish EM, Molitoris BA: Alteration in epithelial polarity and the pathogenesis of disease states. N Engl J Med *330*:1580, 1994.

44. Fanning AS, et al: Transmembrane protein in the tight junction barrier. J Am Soc Nephrol *10*:1337, 1999.

45. Myers BD, et al: Transtubular leakage of glomerular filtrate in human acute renal failure. Am J Physiol *237*:F319, 1979.

46. Kreisberg JI, Venkatachalam MA: Morphologic factors in acute renal failure. *In* Brenner BM, Lazarus JM (eds): Acute Renal Failure, 2nd ed. New York, Churchill Livingstone, 1988, p 45.

47. Schwartz JH, et al: ATP depletion increases tyrosine phosphorylation of β-catenin and plakoglobin in renal tubular cells. J Am Soc Nephrol *10*:2297, 1999.

48. Maddox DA, Brenner BM: Glomerular ultrafiltration. *In* Brenner BM (ed): The Kidney, 6th ed. Philadelphia, WB Saunders, 2000, p 319.

49. Yared A, et al: Effect of diet, age and sex on the renal response to immune injury in the rat. Kidney Int *33*:561, 1988.

50. Norman ME, Asadi FK: A prospective study of acute renal failure in the newborn infant. Pediatrics *63*:475, 1979.

51. Chevalier RL, et al: Prognostic factors in neonatal acute renal failure. Pediatrics *74*:265, 1984.

52. Stapleton FB, et al: Acute renal failure in neonates: incidence, etiology and outcome. Pediatr Nephrol *1*:314, 1987.

53. Moghal NE, et al: A review of acute renal failure in children: incidence, etiology and outcome. Clin Nephrol *49*:91, 1998.

54. Polito C, et al: Long-term prognosis of acute renal failure in the full-term neonate. Clin Pediatr *37*:381, 1998.

55. Toth-Heyn P, et al: The stressed neonatal kidney: from pathophysiology to clinical management of neonatal vasomotor nephropathy. Pediatr Nephrol *14*:227, 2000.

56. Giordano P, et al: Renal vein thrombosis in a newborn with prothrombotic genetic risk factors. J Perinat Med *29*:163, 2001.

57. Leret N, et al: Neonatal renal vein thrombosis in a heterozygous carrier of both factor V Leiden and prothrombin mutations. Arch Pediatr *8*:1222, 2001.

58. Pomeranz A, et al: Acute renal failure in the neonate induced by the administration of indomethacin as a tocolytic agent. Nephrol Dial Transplant *11*:1139, 1996.

59. Gouyon JB, et al: Neonatal kidney insufficiency and intrauterine exposure to ketoprofen. Arch Fr Pediatr *48*:347, 1997.

60. Shotan A, et al: Risks of angiotensin-converting enzyme inhibition during pregnancy: experimental and clinical evidence, potential mechanisms, and recommendations for use. Am J Med *96*:451, 1994.

61. Kreft-Jais C, et al: Angiotensin-converting enzyme inhibitors during pregnancy: a survey of 22 patients given captopril and nine given enalapril. Br J Obstet Gynaecol *74*:371, 1989.

62. Sedman AB, et al: Recognition and management of angiotensin converting enzyme inhibitor fetopathy. Pediatr Nephrol *9*:382, 1995.

63. Ellis EN, Arnold WC: Use of urinary indexes in renal failure in the newborn. Am J Dis Child *136*:615, 1982.

64. Hentschel R, et al: Renal insufficiency in the neonatal period. Clin Nephrol *46*:54, 1996.

65. Gallego N, et al: Prognosis of patients with acute renal failure without cardiopathy. Arch Dis Child *84*:258, 2001.

66. Hinchliffe SA, et al: The effect of intrauterine growth retardation on the development of renal nephrons. Br J Obstet Gynaecol *99*:296, 1992.

67. Vilar J, et al: Metanephros organogenesis is highly stimulated by vitamin A derivatives in organ culture. Kidney Int *49*:1478, 1996.

68. Lelievre-Pegorier M, et al: Mild vitamin A deficiency leads to inborn nephron deficit in the rat. Kidney Int *54*:1455, 1998.

69. Fernandez H, et al: Fetal levels of tobramycin following maternal administration. Obstet Gynecol *76*:992, 1990.

70. Amri K, et al: Adverse effects of hyperglycemia on kidney development in rats: in vivo and in vitro studies. Diabetes *48*:2240, 1999.

71. Leroy B, et al: Intrauterine growth retardation (IUGR) and nephron deficit: preliminary study in man. Pediatr Nephrol *16*:3, 1992.

72. Merlet-Benichou C, et al: Rat metanephric organ culture in terato-embryology. Cell Biol Toxicol *12*:305, 1996.

73. Brenner BM, Chertow GM: Congenital oligonephropathy: an inborn cause of adult hypertension and progressive renal injury? Curr Opin Nephrol Hypertens *2*:69, 1993.

74. Barker DJ, et al: Growth in utero, blood pressure in childhood and adult life, and mortality from cardiovascular disease. BMJ *298*:564, 1989.

75. Dolfin T, et al: Acute renal failure in a neonate caused by the transplacental transfer of a nephrotoxic paraprotein: successful resolution by exchange transfusion. Am J Kidney Dis *34*:1129, 1999.

76. Hari P, et al: Neonatal renal failure due to obstructive candidal bezoars. Pediatr Nephrol *11*:497, 1997.

SECTION XVII

Fluid and Electrolyte Metabolism

139

Robert A. Brace

Fluid Distribution in the Fetus and Neonate

Fluid within the fetus and neonate is distributed among three major fluid spaces: plasma, interstitial fluid, and cellular fluid. In relationship to body weight, the amount of fluid in each of these three compartments is dramatically different in the fetus and newborn than in the adult. This implies that during the perinatal period, the associated volume regulatory mechanisms are functioning at a level that is unique in comparison with that in later life. In addition, the amniotic fluid that surrounds the fetus is often considered to be an extension of the fetal extracellular space, again suggesting unique volume regulatory mechanisms before birth. The purpose of this chapter is to review and discuss the regulation of fluid distribution between the plasma and interstitial fluids in the fetus and newborn, as well as to discuss the role of the lymphatic system and the capillary membrane in mediating and maintaining this distribution. Because the regulation of plasma volume is largely a consequence of blood volume regulation, plasma volume in the perinatal period has of necessity been related to fetal and neonatal blood volume.

DISTRIBUTION OF FLUIDS IN THE FETUS AND NEONATE

Total Body Fluids

In 1961, Friis-Hansen[1] reported the developmental changes in the relative fluid volumes in humans from the early fetal period through adulthood. As shown in Figure 139-1, in the early fetal period, approximately 95% of the fetus is water. The proportion of total body weight that is water gradually decreases throughout the fetal period to reach 80% at 8-months' gestation and 75% water at term. Although it was once thought that the amount of water in the newborn infant varied with mode of delivery, studies suggest that normal infants born vaginally or by cesarean section average 75% water, irrespective of mode of delivery.[2]

Concurrent with the decline in total body water content during fetal life, there are major changes in the distribution of fluid, that is, the percentage of the body that is extracellular fluid sharply decreases, whereas there is a more gradual rise in the percentage of the body fluid that resides within the cells. These changes appear to be attributable to the combined effects of an increase in cell density, deposition of ground substance in the extracellular matrix, and deposition of body fat late in the fetal period.

This changing distribution of fluid continues throughout the neonatal period. As shown in Figure 139-1, there is a continued decrease in total body water content until approximately 9 months of age when it reaches 62%. Simultaneously, at about 2-months' postnatal life, the cellular water content reaches its maximum value of 43% and the extracellular fluid volume declines to 30% of body weight. Thereafter, both the cellular and extracellular fluid volumes decrease with time in relationship to body weight.

The amount of fluid within the body during development as well as its distribution between extracellular and intracellular sites varies among species. Figure 139-2 compares total body water content in human, guinea pig, and sheep fetuses. The decrease in water content in the human compared with the sheep fetus late in the fetal period may be attributable to the large amount of fat accretion in the human fetus during the last 2 months of gestation; the sheep fetus deposits very little body fat. The difference between the guinea pig fetus and the others cannot be attributed to fat deposition because there is relatively little fat deposition in the term fetal guinea pig. In addition, these differences cannot be explained on the basis of maturity at birth because both the sheep and guinea pig are mature and able to walk shortly after birth.

Blood, Plasma, and Red Blood Cell Volumes

Although few studies have estimated blood or plasma volumes in the human fetus before delivery, many studies have determined these volumes in fetal animals as well as in human and animal newborns. Reported values for the fetus and newborn of several species are shown in Table 139-1 and Table 139-2, respectively. These data should be interpreted cautiously because there is the potential for major methodologic errors with most determinations of volume. Nonetheless, it is clear that the volume of blood circulating in the fetus is considerably greater than that in the newborn, largely because roughly one-third of the fetal blood volume is contained in the cord and fetal side of the placenta.[3,4] In addition to this difference, it is clear that the neonate has a significantly higher blood volume than the adult. As illustrated in Table 139-3, the ratio of newborn to adult blood volume is greater than unity in all species.

Plasma and Interstitial Fluid Volumes

The extracellular fluid compartment described earlier is functionally divided into two major spaces: (1) the plasma and (2) the interstitial fluid space. There is little known about which factors regulate the distribution of fluid between the plasma and

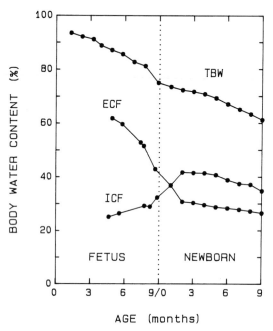

Figure 139–1. Total body water (TBW) content and fluid distribution between intracellular fluid (ICF) and extracellular fluid (ECF) compartments in humans during the fetal and neonatal periods and during the first 9 months after birth. (Data are averaged values from Friis-Hansen.[1])

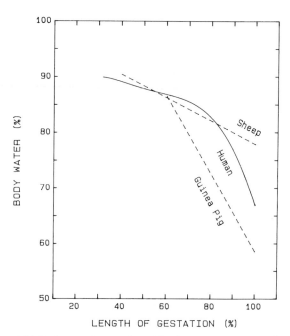

Figure 139–2. Comparisons of total body water content in fetal humans, guinea pigs, and sheep. (Lines are smoothed data from Battaglia and Meschia.[76])

TABLE 139-1

Blood, Red Blood Cell (RBC), and Plasma Volumes in Fetuses (ml/kg)

Blood Volume (ml/kg)	Plasma Volume (ml/kg)	RBC Volume (ml/kg)	Species	Age	References
162*			Human	16–22 wk	77
105†			Human	Term	41
101‡			Human	18–31 wk	78
142*	82*	60*	Sheep	67–145 d	3
110.3*	86.9*	33.7†	Sheep	125–137 d	5
120.2§			Sheep	125–137 d	5
113.3†			Sheep	124–136 d	59
110.1†			Sheep	130 d	67
116†			Sheep	121–138 d	79
	97*		Sheep	105–144 d	80
156.1*			Sheep	112–146 d	54
134.7§	89.9†	44.8†	Sheep	112–146 d	54
113.3†			Sheep	112–146 d	54

* Determined with plasma label.
† Determined with red blood cell label.
‡ Determined from hematocrit changes during packed cell transfusions.
§ Determined with red blood cell plus plasma label.

interstitial spaces in normal human fetuses because measurements in live fetuses have been made only in experimental animals. In late-gestation fetal sheep, the best estimate for plasma volume is 76 ml/kg,[5] although considerably higher volumes have been observed when less stringent techniques for measurement have been used (see Table 139-1). Interstitial volume has been estimated to average three times this volume, or 235 to 240 ml/kg of body weight.[6, 7] The extent to which these vary with gestational age is unclear, although the plasma volume in fetal sheep (76 ml/kg) is independent of fetal weight over the range of 1 to 4 kg.[5] It should be noted that the ratio of interstitial fluid volume to plasma volume in the sheep fetus (3:1) is similar to that which occurs in the adult. This ratio can be misleading

because, as noted earlier, roughly 30% of the plasma that circulates in the fetus is located outside the fetal body (i.e., in the umbilical cord and placenta). When corrected for this, the ratio of interstitial to plasma volume becomes 4.4:1 in the fetus. This ratio clearly indicates that the interstitial space of the fetus is expanded relative to the adult. The elevated interstitial volume is consistent with the observation that interstitial compliance in the ovine fetus is roughly 10 times that observed in the adult.[6] Furthermore, if one assumes that the weight-normalized fetal plasma volume does not vary with fetal weight,[5] this suggests that the large decrease in fetal extracellular fluid volume with advancing gestational age (see Fig. 139-1) is due to a reduction in interstitial fluid volume rather than plasma volume.

TABLE 139-2

Blood, Plasma, and Red Blood Cell (RBC) Volumes in Newborns (ml/kg)*

Blood Volume (ml/kg)	Plasma Volume (ml/kg)	RBC Volume (ml/kg)	Species	Age	References
100†	62†	37.7†	Human	0-1 d	58
84.7‡	41†	41§	Human	0-1 d	38
76.9†	42.7†	34.6†	Human	0 d	39
78†	46†	32†	Human	0 d	40
80.8§			Sheep	0.3-10 d	79
104‡	72.4†	31.6§	Sheep	0 d	54
100.3†	69.4†	30.9†	Sheep	0 d	81
81.5‡	54†	27.4§	Sheep	1-3 wk	9
87‡	66†	22§	Dog	6-14 d	82
97‡	73†	24§	Pig	1-14 d	83

* Human data exclude cord stripping and late cord clamping.
† Determined with plasma label.
‡ Determined with red blood cell plus plasma label.
§ Determined with red blood cell label.

TABLE 139-3

Comparisons of Blood Volumes in Newborns and Adults

| Blood Volume (ml/kg) | | | | Plasma/Red | |
Newborn	Adult	Ratio*	Species	Blood Cell Label	References
67.4	37.6		Rabbit		61
	56.4	1.43	Rabbit	Both	20
90.2			Pig	Both	84
67.3	45	1.75	Pig	Red blood cell	85
73	68	1.22	Cat		61
80.8			Sheep	Red blood cell	79
82.3			Sheep	Red blood cell	101
	61.1		Sheep	Red blood cell	87
	56.5		Sheep		88
	58.0	1.39	Sheep	Plasma	20
84.7			Human	Both	38
78			Human†		40
77			Human†		39
95			Human	Plasma	72
	71.9	1.16	Human	Plasma	20

* Calculated as average neonatal volume/average adult volume for each species.
† Early cord clamp.

Although plasma and interstitial fluid volumes have not been measured in human fetuses, it is clear that aberrations in the volume of fluid in these two compartments are associated with a variety of disease states. For example, gross fetal edema (i.e., hydrops fetalis) is often associated with severe erythroblastosis. The hydropic fetus can be more than twice normal body weight owing to excess fluid within its interstitial compartment. In a review of hydrops fetalis, Hansen and Gest[8] concluded that under several conditions, an elevated capillary pressure within the fetal body may be a causative factor in promoting edema formation. However, there must also be simultaneous fluid retention by the fetal kidneys and/or excess fluid transfer across the placenta from the maternal circulation. It remains unclear what simultaneously promotes these conditions.

Although there are a great number of studies that have measured plasma volumes in the newborn, there are surprisingly few studies that have simultaneously measured plasma and interstitial fluid volumes. In the human, data from different studies[9, 10] have yielded an average plasma volume of approximately 40 to 50 ml/kg (see Table 139-2), and other studies have found extracellular fluid volume to average 397 ml/kg.[9] The difference between these numbers (350 ml/kg) represents interstitial fluid volume. The interstitial to plasma volume ratio calculated from

these numbers is 7.6:1. In contrast, the plasma and interstitial volumes in 1- to 3-week-old lambs have been reported to be 54 and 283 ml/kg, respectively.[9] This ratio (5.2:1) is significantly lower than that calculated for the human newborn infant. Furthermore, in anesthetized newborn puppies, the plasma volume is 82 ml/kg, and the interstitial volume is 172 ml/kg.[11] This ratio (2.1:1) is also considerably lower than the value already quoted for the human neonate and is even lower than the ratio observed for the ovine neonate, suggesting that there may be considerable differences in the ratio of plasma to interstitial fluid volumes in the newborns of different species. Some of these discrepancies appear to be related to differences in hematocrit at birth. For example, the high hematocrit of human neonates is associated with a low plasma volume, which, in turn, elevates the ratio of interstitial to plasma volume. In comparison, the much lower hematocrit in lambs produces a lower interstitial fluid to plasma volume ratio. Furthermore, methodologic errors may significantly contribute to those interstudy differences.

Lymph and Lymph Flow

The volume of fluid within the lymphatic system is small and averages only 1 ml/kg body weight in adult dogs as estimated from lymph flow dynamics.[12] An estimate of lymphatic volume in the fetus or neonate has not been made. However, it is reasonable to speculate that there are developmental changes in lymphatic volume.[13]

There are a few estimates of lymph flow in developing animals that allow comparison with adult values. It has been known for more than 60 years that lymph flow from subcutaneous tissue in anesthetized puppies is about twice that observed in adult dogs when expressed in relation to body weight.[14] Furthermore, lymph flow from the lungs is higher in anesthetized newborn lambs and puppies than in their adult counterparts.[15, 16] Other studies in unanesthetized newborn lambs have also demonstrated higher pulmonary lymph flow rates.[17, 18] These observations support the concept that the local as well as whole body lymph flow rates (in relation to body weight) are significantly greater in the neonatal period than later in life. The increased lymphatic flow during the neonatal period is probably indicative of the elevated interstitial volume in the neonate in relation to the adult.

In the fetus, lymph flow rates (relative to weight) appear to be greater than in the newborn. For example, in anesthetized fetal sheep, rate of pulmonary lymph flow in the right thoracic duct is higher than in newborn lambs or adult sheep.[15] However, in older studies in anesthetized animals, fetal left thoracic duct flow (0.08 ml/minute per kg) was roughly comparable with adult flow rates.[19, 20] It should be emphasized, however, that those studies were confounded by an extremely high resistance to flow in the long small-diameter catheters that were used. In studies in unanesthetized fetal sheep, thoracic duct lymph flow averaged .25 ml/minute/kg when low-resistance catheters were used and the lymph was returned to the fetal circulation.[21] Thus, basal lymph flow rates in the fetus are substantially higher than those in the adult and may be considerably higher than in the newborn. However, the puppies and many of the neonatal lambs described earlier were anesthetized and anesthesia has been reported to reduce lymph flow rates.[22]

Even though lymph flow rates in the fetus and neonate are higher than those in the adult, the concentration of protein in the thoracic duct lymph displays an apparently uniform relationship to the plasma protein concentration. For example, under resting conditions, the thoracic duct lymph protein concentration averages roughly 50 to 75% of the plasma concentration in the fetus, newborn, and adult. This does not mean that the concentrations are the same, because fetal plasma protein concentrations increase during gestation and average a little more than half of adult values before labor and delivery (although there are species-related differences).[23, 24] Neonatal concentrations are closer to adult concentrations and depend on the amount of placental transfusion that occurs at the time of delivery as well as on gastrointestinal uptake of proteins ingested in milk by newborn animals such as lambs.

It is now becoming clear that there are major developmental differences in the functional ability of the lymphatic system to pump fluid from the interstitial spaces back into the circulation. These differences are illustrated by the lymph flow function curves in Figure 139–3. To interpret these curves, it should be recalled that normal outflow pressure for the lymphatic system is venous pressure. In Figure 139–3, it can be seen that at low venous pressures, the lymph flow rate is greater in the fetus than in the adult. Although there is a developmental increase in venous pressure in the ovine fetus,[25] in the near-term fetus venous pressure is the same as in the adult and averages 3 to 4 mm Hg. Thus, normal venous pressure in the fetus does not appear to be an impediment to basal lymph flow, but any increase in venous pressure is likely to reduce the lymph flow rate.[26, 27] In contrast, venous pressure in the adult must be increased to values significantly greater than normal before lymph flow begins to decrease with increasing outflow

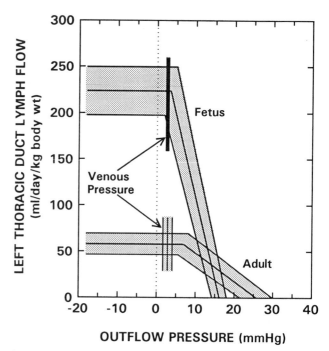

Figure 139–3. Comparisons of lymph flow function curves for the left thoracic lymph duct in unanesthetized fetal and adult sheep. Stippled area covers means 2 SEs. Outflow pressure varied independently of venous pressure and was corrected for catheter resistance. (Data from references.[26,28])

pressure.[28] Furthermore, lymph flow stops in the fetus when venous pressure is elevated to only 16 mm Hg,[26] whereas venous pressure must be increased to 26 mm Hg before thoracic duct lymph flow is inhibited in adult sheep.[28]

Special Fluid Compartments

There are additional fluid spaces that must be considered to understand the regulation of plasma and interstitial volumes during the perinatal period. Before birth, the developing lungs are filled with fluid rather than with gas as in later life. This fluid is formed by an active secretion of chloride ions into the alveolar spaces, resulting in a progressive accumulation of fluid in the lungs as gestation progresses. The secretion of lung fluid is far in excess of that needed for volume expansion of the lungs, so the excess lung fluid exits through the trachea. Rather than a gradual egress, fluid appears to flow out of the trachea in bouts and either is swallowed or enters the amniotic fluid.[29] In fetal lambs, the tracheal flow rate averages 4.4 ml/kg per hour during the latter half of gestation,[29-31] and in a 24-hour period, this volume represents approximately 10 to 15% of body weight. The volume of fluid that resides in the airways during the fetal period depends on the developmental stage of the lungs. Volume is very low early in gestation and increases rapidly with the accelerated lung growth that occurs late in gestation. At term gestation in fetal lambs, lung liquid volume averages 45 ml/kg of body weight,[29] or slightly more than one-half of the plasma volume. This large volume suggests that lung liquid may be a potential source of fluid to the fetus; however, it is not certain how easily fetal lung fluid can be transferred to the circulation.

The stomach may also be a major fluid reservoir in the fetus and neonate. Swallowing during the perinatal period is episodic, and the volume of fluid swallowed in one event may be as large as 100 to 200 ml, which is roughly equal to 3 to 5% of body weight.

FLUID CHANGES IN THE IMMEDIATE PERINATAL PERIOD

Prelabor Changes

Several observations collectively suggest that the fetus undergoes significant changes in its fluid status during the last few days, hours, and minutes before delivery. Studies have shown that the lungs begin to dry out several days before delivery,[29, 32] in large part because the amount of fluid secreted by the lungs gradually decreases.[30] The decrement in fetal lung fluid secretion may be mediated by changes in plasma catecholamine, vasopressin, or cortisol concentrations, or all three.[29,30,33,34] There are also relatively large increases in arterial pressure (20%) in fetal lambs during the last few days before delivery.[35] If this pressure were transmitted to the capillaries, it would exert a major effect on the transcapillary distribution of fluid and perhaps protein.

Changes During Labor and Delivery

In fetal sheep, the hematocrit increases by an average of 13% at 15 minutes before delivery compared with that 1 hour before delivery.[35] Because fetal sheep do not have a releasable pool of noncirculating red blood cells (RBCs),[5] this increase in hematocrit represents a loss of plasma from the circulation and a decrease in blood volume. The extent of this loss is inversely proportional to the hematocrit changes (i.e., blood volume is reduced to 88% of the prelabor volume). This 12% decrease in blood volume corresponds to an 18% decrease in circulating plasma volume. Immediately after delivery, the hematocrit increases further by 9%, reflecting an additional decrease in circulating plasma and blood volumes, as a result of a loss of fluid from the plasma compartment.

This decrease in circulating fetal plasma and blood volumes during labor and delivery in animal models is consistent with studies in humans. The umbilical vein hematocrit averages 44% in infants delivered by elective cesarean section without labor[36] and 51% immediately after delivery if labor has occurred.[37-41] Assuming that RBCs are not released into the circulation with labor, this ratio of 44:51 demonstrates that the circulating blood volume is reduced by 14%. This corresponds to a reduction in plasma volume of 25%.

Thus, blood volume decreases in both human and animal fetuses during labor. Further decreases occur during vaginal delivery owing to a loss of plasma from the circulation. In fetal sheep, this loss of fluid occurs largely across fetal body capillaries rather than across the placenta because the fetal body capillaries have a filtration capacity (i.e., capillary filtration coefficient) approximately 100 times that of the placenta.[6] The loss of plasma during labor and delivery in the human fetus most likely occurs by the same pathway, although the capillary filtration capacity of the body relative to the placenta has not been estimated in the human fetus or newborn.

The mechanisms that mediate the loss of plasma during labor and delivery are multifactorial. Mild, nonlabor uterine contractions cause a direct compression or transformational change of the fetus.[42] As during a Valsalva maneuver, this elevates fetal vascular pressures, reducing circulating blood volume of 2 to 4%.[5, 43] Stronger uterine contractions during labor would be expected to result in even greater reductions in fetal blood volumes and hence in plasma volumes. Furthermore, mild hypoxia reduces circulating blood volume in fetal sheep, resulting from a loss of plasma volume into the interstitial space.[44,45] More severe hypoxia causes a greater reduction in plasma volume and is associated with elevations in arterial and venous pressures.[44,45] The placenta may also contribute to the reduction in fetal blood volume during labor and delivery in that severe hypoxia may produce an *in utero* translocation of fetal blood out of the placenta and into the fetal body.[46] As noted earlier, this leads to a rise in capillary pressure and the transcapillary filtration of fluid out of the fetal circulation. Mechanisms other than hypoxia may also be involved in the reduction of plasma volume during labor. For example, during the last few days before delivery, in fetal sheep, there is a sharp rise in arterial pressure, even though arterial oxygen tension does not change.[35] Additionally, there are major changes in the plasma concentrations of many vasoactive hormones during labor and delivery. Although the effects of only a few hormones have been investigated, arginine vasopressin,[47] norepinephrine, cortisol,[48] and atrial natriuretic factor[7, 16, 49, 50] have the ability to reduce the circulating blood volume and plasma volume when acutely infused into the circulation of fetal sheep at low to moderate rates. The umbilical cord concentrations of each of these hormones are elevated following vaginal delivery in humans, suggesting that these hormones may indeed play a role in mediating the shift of fluid from the plasma into the interstitial compartment at the time of labor and delivery.

Effects of Placental Transfusion on Neonatal Volumes

The single most important factor that affects blood volume and hence plasma volume in the newborn during the first few days of life is the extent of the placental transfusion that occurs at the time of delivery.[37, 38, 40, 41] If the umbilical cord is clamped immediately at the time of delivery, the hematocrit in the newborn infant averages 48 to 51% and is stable over a period of days.[37, 38, 40, 41] However, if the cord is not clamped immediately and the newborn infant is positioned at or below the level of the placenta, the placenta gradually transfuses the neonate with blood, which reaches a maximum of 75 to 100 ml at 3 to 4 minutes after delivery.[37, 40, 41] This placental transfusion of 25 to 50 ml/kg represents an increase in RBC and blood volumes within the neonate of 50%[40] and may have adverse effects.[37, 40, 41, 51] There has been a suggestion, however, that placental transfusion may reduce the incidence of respiratory distress syndrome following cesarean delivery.[52] With delayed cord clamping, the hematocrit gradually increases over 30 minutes to 2 hours to average 60 to 65%, or higher if the cords are stripped.[37, 40, 41] This increase in hematocrit is due to a loss of plasma from the circulation. Further increases in hematocrit occur over the next 2 hours as a total of 30 ml/kg of plasma is lost from the circulation during the first 4 hours of life in infants with late cord clamping. This reduction in plasma volume is due largely to a shift of fluid from the plasma into the interstitial space, although urine flow is elevated as well.[41]

Neonatal Weight Loss

It is well recognized that normal, healthy, human newborns lose an average of 5 to 10% of their body weight during the first week of life, and premature infants may lose even more of their body weight. Although it is clear that this weight loss is due largely to a loss of fluid, data are conflicting whether the lost fluid originates from the cellular or extracellular space or both. In one review, Coulter[53] evaluated relevant data and suggested that it is primarily cellular rather than extracellular fluid that is lost during the first week of life in the newborn. Coulter hypothesized that prolactin may mediate fluid loss by translocating sodium ions out of a cellular sodium pool present in the newborn. This theory needs further exploration.

REGULATION OF PLASMA AND INTERSTITIAL VOLUMES

The detailed mechanisms that determine the distribution of fluid between the plasma and interstitial compartments in the fetus and neonate are far from completely understood. As background, it is important to recognize two facts: first, it is blood volume and not plasma volume that is regulated in the fetus and neonate, just as occurs in the adult. In other words, one of the major determinants of plasma loss across the body capillaries is the hydrostatic pressure of the blood as it circulates, which, in turn, depends on total blood volume rather than plasma volume. This rationale dictates that on a short-term basis, the interstitium is largely a volume reservoir for the vascular compartment. Second, our understanding of the fluid volume regulatory mechanisms depends on the accuracy of methods used for measuring the plasma and interstitial fluid volumes. As discussed later in this chapter, much of our lack of understanding of the distribution between the plasma and interstitial spaces relates to the fact that the methods used for measuring these volumes are somewhat inaccurate.

Although the exact details of the mechanisms that regulate plasma-interstitial compartment distributions are not well understood, the problem is conceptually simple. Fluid leaves the plasma and enters the interstitium because of the combined effects of hydrostatic and osmotic pressure gradients at the capillary membrane. The lymphatic system counterbalances this egress by pumping interstitial fluid through the lymphatic vessels back to the circulation. Thus, in the steady state, the balance between plasma and interstitial fluid is simply determined by the relationship between capillary filtration and lymph flow rate. Unfortunately, at present we understand neither the regulation of lymphatic function nor the regulation of capillary fluid movements during the perinatal period. The most elegant studies to date have been of fluid balance in the lung during the perinatal transition to air breathing.[17, 29, 33, 39] Because little else has been explored in detail, we must resort to descriptive studies in hopes of providing insight into the fluid regulatory mechanisms.

Measurement of Blood, Plasma, and Interstitial Fluid Volumes

It is difficult if not impossible to measure blood, plasma, or interstitial fluid volumes in the fetus and newborn (as well as in the adult) accurately. Interstitial fluid volume can be calculated as the difference between extracellular fluid volume and plasma volume. However, measurement of each of these volumes is subject to considerable error. Extracellular volume has been measured as the volume of distribution of a variety of labels injected into the circulation. Some of the labels (such as radioactive sodium ion) enter the cells or are metabolized and thus overestimate volume, but others (e.g., sucrose) may not penetrate the entire extracellular volume and thus underestimate volume. Bromide space is one of the more widely used extracellular fluid markers in the newborn,[9, 53] but this label may not be adequate in the fetus because of transplacental losses.[9] In addition, bromide may have a considerable intracellular distribution during the fetal and neonatal periods.[53]

Plasma volumes are measured as the dilutional space of labeled high molecular weight substances (such as dye- or radio-labeled albumin or plasma proteins) following injection into the circulation. These measurements frequently are corrected for loss of the label from the circulation by extrapolating the concentration-time curve backward to the time of injection. Even with this correction, plasma volume measurements are subject to large errors for two major reasons:

1. All plasma labels are rapidly lost from the circulation through the capillary membranes of organs, such as the liver, which have high permeabilities even to high molecular weight substances. Extrapolating back to the time of injection does not correct for this loss because it is too rapid to be detected.
2. Most labels such as radioisotopes or dyes are not completely bound to the plasma proteins when injected into the circulation. The unbound labels are rapidly lost from the circulation and again lead to a considerable overestimation of plasma volume.

TABLE 139-4

Estimates of the Whole Body to Large Vessel Hematocrit Ratio

Fetus	Neonate	Adult	Species	References
0.839			Rabbit	89
0.832			Sheep	54
0.980*			Sheep	5
	0.80		Sheep	9
	0.71		Sheep	101
	0.80		Dog	82
	0.84		Pig	83
	0.84		Pig	84
	0.87		Human	40
	0.893		Human	90
	0.86		Human	84
	0.89		Human	37
	0.868	0.868	Human	38
		0.756	Pig	85
		0.96*	Sheep	56
		0.81	Sheep	91
		0.938*	Dog	55

* Special efforts to reduce or correct for loss of plasma label.

The errors in plasma volume measurement produce major errors in blood volume determinations as well. These can be evaluated from estimation of the whole body to large vessel (WB/LV) hematocrit ratio. This ratio is calculated as the blood volume determined using labeled RBCs (indicator dilution techniques) divided by the blood volume as determined by the sum of RBC plus plasma volumes (double indicator dilution techniques). Table 139–4 lists reported values for WB/LV hematocrit ratios. To explore the errors inherent in blood volume determinations one should consider measurements made in fetal sheep. Creasy and colleagues[54] have demonstrated that blood volume as determined with ^{51}Cr-labeled RBCs averages 113.3 ml/kg in fetal sheep. In contrast, when ^{125}I-labeled albumin is used to estimate blood volume, it averages 156.1 ml/kg, and when the double indicator dilution technique is employed, blood volume averages 134.7 ml/kg. Therefore, the WB/LV hematocrit ratio equals 113.3:134.7, or .841. The reasons for these differences in blood volume determinations are twofold: physiologic differences and measurement error. From a physiologic viewpoint, it is well established that because of rheologic factors, the hematocrit of the blood within the capillaries of the body (or within small-diameter glass tubes) is less than that in larger blood vessels. The reduction in hematocrit occurs in blood vessels smaller than 100 µm in diameter, and it has been estimated that capillary blood averages a hematocrit that is 75% of the large vessel hematocrit. The net effect is to lower the average hematocrit within the body as a whole in relationship to that measured in blood sampled from large vessels such as the veins. To overcome this problem, most investigators have advocated the use of double indicator dilution techniques to measure plasma and RBC volumes separately. These values are then summed to obtain blood volume. Many investigators use a single label to estimate either plasma or RBC volume and then use the WB/LV hematocrit ratio to calculate total blood volume. Studies in the neonate as well as in the adult have reported values of 0.70 to 0.90 for the WB/LV hematocrit ratio (see Table 139–4). However, from a mechanistic viewpoint, it has been estimated that less than 10% of the blood in the body is in the systemic capillaries. If the hematocrit in capillaries is reduced by 25% compared with that of the large vessels as noted earlier, the whole body to large vessel hematocrit ratio should average 0.975 and not 0.70 to 0.90 as has been widely reported. Thus, the difference between 0.70 to 0.90 and 0.975 is likely to be a measurement artifact created by loss of the plasma label from the circulation.

If the preceding assumptions are true, reducing the amount of unbound label as well as using higher molecular weight substances for plasma labels should lead to a higher and thus more accurate estimate of the whole body to large vessel hematocrit ratio. In fact, early attempts in adults to reduce the amount of unbound dye did increase the WB/LV hematocrit ratio from 0.8 to 0.85. Similarly, as the use of radiolabeled albumin increased, careful attempts to reduce the unbound ^{125}I led to an increase in the whole body to large vessel hematocrit ratio from 0.85 to 0.9. Furthermore, use of radiolabeled fibrinogen, which has a higher molecular weight than albumin, increased the ratio to 0.938.[55] The largest molecule used as a plasma label thus far has been radiolabeled gamma-globulin, and it has generated a ratio of 0.96.[56] In addition, γ-globulin is rapidly lost into the interstitial space of the liver, so the ratio of 0.96 is still an underestimate. Thus, it is clear that the widely reported values for the WB/LV hematocrit ratio of 0.7:0.9 are simply measurement artifacts because the whole body to large vessel hematocrit ratio lies somewhere between 0.96 and 1.0.

The adequacy of methods for measuring blood and plasma volumes has been explored in the unanesthetized sheep fetus. Blood volume as determined with labeled RBCs was 110.3 ml/kg.[5] Sampling at 1-minute intervals with careful extrapolation of the radiolabeled albumin and fibrinogen to the time of injection yielded a double indicator dilution estimate for fetal blood volume of 120.6 ml/kg[5] and a WB/LV hematocrit ratio of 110.3:120.6, or 0.915. An additional correction for the rapid loss of the labels into the liver interstitium reduced the double indicator estimate of volume to 112.5 ml/kg and produced a ratio of 110.3:112.5 or 0.98. This represents a best estimate of the whole body to large vessel hematocrit ratio in the fetal sheep.

The major importance of this observation is that it demonstrates that a RBC label produces a more accurate as well as a more precise estimate of blood volume in the fetus than does the double indicator dilution technique, which measures RBC and plasma volumes separately. This finding is also important because it shows that the most accurate estimate of plasma volume is obtained by measuring blood volume with a RBC label and then multiplying by one minus the fractional large vessel hematocrit. This is true because the whole body to large vessel hematocrit ratio is much closer to unity than has been recognized. In contrast, Wright and associates[57] concluded that use of a constant for the whole body to large vessel hematocrit ratio should be abandoned and that plasma and RBC volumes should be measured separately. However, their suggestion fails to take into account the inadequacies of the commonly used plasma labels as discussed earlier and as seen by the disparity of values in Table 139-4. Thus, given the present state of the art, a RBC label provides the best estimates of plasma, RBC, and blood volumes provided that errors due to unbound labels are minimized.

Volumes Under Steady-State Conditions

The relationship between blood and plasma volumes in the neonate has been explored in several studies. Neonates with high blood volumes (weight normalized) also have high RBC volumes but decreased plasma volumes.[38, 58] The weight-normalized RBC volume also increases with venous hematocrit, whereas plasma volume varies inversely with hematocrit.[38, 58]

The relationships among plasma volume, RBC volume, and blood volume have not been explored in the human fetus. In chronically catheterized fetal sheep under resting conditions, plasma, RBC, and blood volumes averaged 75, 36, and 111 ml/kg, respectively, and these were independent of fetal weight over the range of 1 to 4 kg.[59] However, as seen in Figure 139-4, fetuses with a high weight-normalized blood volume have a significantly higher plasma volume as well as a higher RBC volume. The cause of the increased plasma volume cannot be easily explained (e.g., plasma volume is not statistically related to

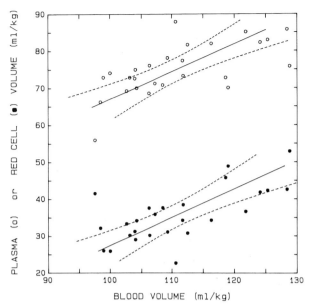

Figure 139–4. Relationship between resting weight normalized blood, plasma, and red blood cell volumes in chronically catheterized fetal sheep. Solid lines are regression lines and dashed lines 95% confidence intervals about regression line. *Top*, Y .744 7.4 (r = 0.649; p = .0003); *Bottom*, Y .767 49.3 (r = 0.674; p = .0002). (Data from Brace[5] and from Brace.[59])

plasma protein concentration). Multivariate regression analysis has demonstrated that plasma volume is positively related to arterial pH and heart rate and negatively related to mean arterial pressure (p = .0009). The negative relationship between plasma volume and arterial pressure makes sense if the elevated arterial pressure is at least partially transmitted to the capillaries. The positive relationships among plasma volume, pH, and heart rate obviously are not direct cause-and-effect relationships. Instead, these data suggest that there is a common, yet unknown factor or factors that favor(s) a high plasma volume and at the same time a high pH and heart rate.

As in the human infant, plasma volume in the ovine fetus under resting conditions is negatively related to large vessel hematocrit. Similarly, RBC volume in the ovine fetus is positively related to hematocrit (Fig. 139-5). This suggests that the relationships between blood volume, RBC volume, plasma volume, and hematocrit that have been observed in the human neonate also occur in the ovine fetus and thus probably exist in the human fetus *in utero*. They are not simply the consequence of varying degrees of placental transfusion at birth.

Responses to Hemorrhage

In adults of several species, including humans, dogs, rats, cats, and sheep, 24 to 48 hours are required for blood volume to return to normal following a loss of blood.[60] This restoration of volume occurs as plasma volume returns to or rises above normal, whereas RBC volume remains reduced. The time required for full volume restoration after hemorrhage in the fetus or neonate may be quite different from that in the adult. Mott[61, 62] found that neonatal kittens and rabbits were better able to tolerate blood loss than adults were, in that more blood had to be removed before arterial pressure fell. This was attributed to a more rapid mobilization of interstitial fluid in the young animals. It was also shown that fetal sheep restore twice the volume within 30 minutes after rapid hemorrhage than the adult.[63] The ovine fetus also restores its blood volume to normal within 3 to 4 hours after a 30% hemorrhage over 2 hours,[64] that is, the posthemorrhage restitution of blood volume in the ovine fetus

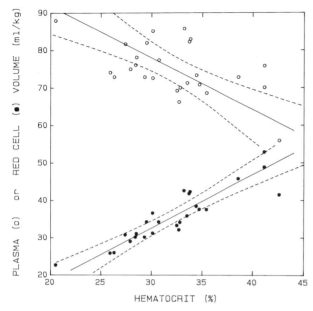

Figure 139–5. Relationship between resting weight normalized red blood cell volume, plasma volume, and hematocrit in chronically catheterized fetal sheep. *Top,* Y 119.4 1.381 ($r = .534; p = .005$); *Bottom,* Y 10 1.423 ($r = .901, p < 10^6$). (Data from Brace[5] and from Brace.[59])

occurs in one-tenth the time required in the adult.[60] This rapid restoration is mediated by a translocation of fluid and protein from the interstitial space into the vascular space but does not appear to be attributable to a net movement of fluid across the placenta.[65] In the first week of life, lambs also rapidly restore their blood volume to normal after hemorrhage.[66] The human newborn probably can restore its blood volume to normal after hemorrhage more rapidly than the adult, but this has yet to be documented.

Responses to Volume Loading

Rapid intravascular infusions of isotonic solutions, such as saline or Ringer lactate, expand blood volume by only a fraction of the infused volume owing largely to a loss of the infused fluid into the interstitial spaces. When adults of several species received intravascular infusions of isotonic crystalloidal solutions, intravascular retention averaged 20 to 50% of the infused volumes 30 to 60 minutes after rapid infusion. In the unanesthetized ovine fetus, similar infusions increased blood volume by only 6 to 7% of the infused volume.[67] This is quite different from the response in anesthetized newborn sheep, in that intravascular retention was similar to that of the adult and averaged 30 or 40% following intravascular saline infusions.[68] The reduced intravascular retention of crystalloid during fetal life is due largely to a high interstitial compliance/vascular compliance ratio as well as a higher capillary filtration coefficient.[6] The increased capillary filtration coefficient permits very rapid fluid movements across the capillary membrane, and the high interstitial to vascular compliance ratio allows for extensive fluid movements.

As might be expected, the plasma and interstitial protein concentrations are affected differently in the fetus than in the adult following volume expansion with crystalloid. In the fetus, the lymph/plasma protein concentration ratio decreases following volume expansion,[69] whereas this protein concentration ratio increases transiently in adult animals[12] and newborn sheep.[68]

The reduced intravascular retention of fluid in the fetus compared with that of the adult may also be a primary factor in determining the urine flow responses to volume loading. It is well established that following volume loading, normal adults will excrete the entire volume load through their kidneys over a period of several hours. Newborns of several species, including human and ovine, have a reduced capacity to excrete volume loads. This reduced excretory capacity can, in part, be attributed to the reduced intravascular retention,[70] that is, with high intravascular retention in the adult, plasma renin activity and plasma concentrations of arginine vasopressin and atrial natriuretic factor all change in a direction appropriate for elevating urine flow. In the ovine fetus with a low intravascular retention, plasma arginine vasopressin and renin activity are unchanged, and atrial natriuretic factor undergoes only a transient increase.[70] Thus, fetal urine flow rapidly returns to normal following rapid vascular volume expansion because the hormonal stimuli that promote urinary output are not maintained.[70] It has yet to be documented whether this is indeed the mechanism responsible for the diminished response to volume loading in human newborn infants.

Responses to Hypoxia

Newborns with a history of fetal distress and birth asphyxia have elevated blood and plasma volumes similar to those of normal infants with late cord clamping, even though the cord is clamped immediately after birth.[10] These observations suggest that prenatal hypoxia or asphyxia induces a placental transfusion before delivery. This is consistent with the observation that acute hypoxia promotes a translocation of fetal blood out of the placenta in sheep.[46] In addition, Yao and colleagues[71] have shown that 10 to 20 minutes of hypoxia immediately before delivery in sheep elevates plasma, RBC, and blood volumes in the newborn compared with lambs with early cord clamping. Linderkamp and co-workers[72] also observed that intrauterine hypoxia is associated with an elevated RBC volume in the newborn but that acute, intrapartum asphyxia is not associated with a predelivery placental transfusion. Thus, there is ample evidence supporting the concept that prenatal hypoxia causes a partial placental transfusion *in utero*, but its time course, exact extent, and reversibility are unclear.

It has been known for several years that hypoxia reduces blood volume in the human fetus owing to a loss of plasma and proteins from the circulation,[51] but the causes of the reduced volume have not been explained. In the ovine fetus, this reduction in blood volume occurs rapidly and is linearly related to the reduction in arterial oxygen tension[44, 45] (there is a 1% decrease in blood volume for each 1 mm Hg decrease in arterial PO_2). The loss of plasma is undoubtedly due to an elevation of capillary pressure within the fetal body. This phenomenon occurs with no changes in fetal arterial or venous pressure during mild hypoxia (presumably owing to vasodilation in selected organs) and is accompanied by increases in arterial and venous pressures with moderate to severe hypoxia.[45]

ROLE OF LYMPHATICS AND CAPILLARY MEMBRANE

In principle, it is clear that the distribution of fluid between the plasma and interstitial compartments depends on the balance between lymphatic function and capillary permeability. In the ovine fetus, the lymph/plasma protein concentration ratio decreases following volume expansion, whereas the ratio increases transiently in the newborn lamb and in adults of several species. This difference is due largely to developmental differences in the capillary permeability characteristics. However, very little is known about either capillary permeability or lymphatic function during the fetal or neonatal period. There are suggestions that fluid and protein may cross the capillaries of the human fetus and newborn more readily than in the adult.[10] Studies in the sheep support this hypothesis in that the capillaries within the body of the ovine fetus have a filtration coefficient five times that of adult values[6] and a permeability for plasma proteins 15 times that in the adult.[18] Capillary permeability to plasma proteins in the lungs may be the same in near-term fetal and neonatal sheep.[17] Although no similar estimates exist for other species, including humans, these values clearly show that there are developmental changes in the capillary permeability characteristics.

Figure 139-3 demonstrates that there are major differences in basal lymphatic function between the fetus and adult; however, there is little else known about the fetal or neonatal lymphatic system except that both fetal and newborn sheep undergo an increase in left thoracic duct lymph flow following vascular volume expansion.[68,69] Studies in the ovine fetus[73-75] have found that angiotensin II augments left thoracic duct lymph flow and atrial natriuretic factor suppresses lymph flow. Extensive vascular volume loading increases the lymph flow rate to a maximum of 3.5 times normal, and draining the thoracic duct externally causes a rapid fall in fetal blood volume of 10% within 2 to 3 hours. No comparable studies of whole body (i.e., left thoracic duct) lymph flow rates during the newborn period have been conducted. We need to know much more about regulation of lymphatic function by the endocrine and autonomic nervous systems to begin to relate volume distributions in the fetus and neonate to functioning of the lymphatic system.

ROLE OF THE PLACENTA

The question of how the growing fetus acquires water from its mother has long fascinated obstetrician and basic scientist alike. This question is important because excess fetal water may produce hydrops fetalis or polyhydramnios or both, whereas insufficient water may result in fetal growth retardation or oligohydramnios. With an estimated 20% of the water in the human conceptus (fetus, placenta, and amniotic sac) at term produced as a byproduct of metabolism,[92] most fetal water must be acquired transplacentally by either hydrostatic or osmotic forces, the only two theoretical possibilities. Although computer modeling has suggested that osmotic forces may be the dominant force that determines transplacental water movement,[93] there exists little practical understanding. For animals with relatively low placental permeabilities such as the sheep, it was suggested[94] that transplacental acquisition of sodium and chloride limits fetal water acquisition and hence fetal growth. However, intravascular infusion of large amounts of concentrated NaCl into fetal sheep did not result in fetal water accumulation as predicted but instead resulted in the transfer of all of the infused sodium and chloride across the placenta to the mother either against or in the absence of chemical concentration gradients.[95] The intravascular infusion of large volumes of physiologic crystalloid solutions in fetal sheep similarly resulted in the transfer of large amounts of water and solute across the placenta to the mother.[96] These observations suggest that a normal fetus can protect itself against both volume and salt overloads by rapid transfer of excess to the mother.

The role of the mother and her hydration status on fetal water accumulation is similarly not well understood. Prolonged water deprivation has long been know to result in reduced amniotic fluid volumes but is it not known whether the primary forces that deprive the fetus of water are osmotic or hydrostatic. In women with reduced amniotic fluid volumes and perhaps in humans with normal amniotic fluid volumes, the ingestion of 2 L of water may be followed by a significant increase in the amniotic fluid index over a few hours.[97,98,99] This increase in amniotic fluid volume appears to be due a cascade induced by a reduced

maternal osmolality that increases transplacental movement of water to the fetus with an associated fetal diuresis.[100]

The role played by the filtration and transport characteristics of the placenta in determining fluid balance in the conceptus is essentially unexplored as is the associated molecular regulatory mechanisms. Although water channels are just beginning to be identified in the placenta, it is not known what role they play, or whether abnormalities in either their type or number are associated with fetal water diseases.

ACKNOWLEDGMENTS

This work was supported in part by Grants HD20295, HD35890 and HD33054 from the National Institute of Child Health and Human Development.

REFERENCES

1. Friis-Hansen B: Body water compartments in children: changes during growth and related changes in body composition. Pediatrics 28:169, 1961.
2. Cheek DB, et al: Hydration in the first 24 h of postnatal life in normal infants born vaginally or by caesarean section. Early Hum Dev 7:323, 1982.
3. Barcroft J, Kennedy JA: The distribution of blood between the foetus and the placenta in sheep. J Physiol 95:173, 1939.
4. Yao AC, et al: Distribution of blood between infant and placenta after birth. Lancet 2:871, 1969.
5. Brace RA: Blood volume and its measurement in the chronically catheterized sheep fetus. Am J Physiol 244:H487, 1983.
6. Brace RA, Gold PS: Fetal whole-body interstitial compliance, vascular compliance, and capillary filtration coefficient. Am J Physiol 247:R800, 1984.
7. Brace RA, Cheung CY: Cardiovascular and fluid responses to atrial natriuretic factor in sheep fetus. Am J Physiol 253:R561, 1987.
8. Hansen TN, Gest AL: Hydrops fetalis. In Brace RA, et al (eds): Fetal and Neonatal Body Fluids: The Scientific Basis for Clinical Practice. Ithaca, NY, Perinatology Press, 1989.
9. Longo LD, et al: The interrelations of blood and extracellular fluid volumes and cardiac output in the newborn lamb. In Longo LD, Reneau DD (eds): Fetal and Newborn Cardiovascular Physiology. New York, Garland STPM Press, 1978, pp 345–367.
10. Yao AC, Lind J: Blood volume in the asphyxiated term neonate. Biol Neonate 21:199, 1972.
11. Horton JW, Coln D: Cardiovascular function and fluid compartments in newborn canine hemorrhagic shock. Am J Physiol 248:R724, 1985.
12. Brace RA, Power GG: Thoracic duct lymph flow and protein flux dynamics: Responses to intravascular saline. Am J Physiol 240:R282, 1981.
13. Yoffey JM, Courtice FC: Lymphatics, Lymph and the Lymphomyeloid Complex. New York, Academic Press, 1970.
14. Holman R: The flow and protein content of subcutaneous lymph in dogs of different ages. Am J Physiol 118:354, 1937.
15. Boston RW, et al: Lymph flow and clearance of liquid from the lungs of the foetal lamb. Lancet 2:473, 1965.
16. Shine P, et al: Action of atrial natriuretic peptide in the immature ovine kidney. Pediatr Res 22:11, 1987.
17. Bland RD, et al: Lung lymph flow and protein flux in unanesthetized fetal and newborn lambs. Fed Proc 39:280, 1980.
18. Gold PS, Brace RA: Fetal whole-body permeability-surface area product and reflection coefficient for plasma proteins. Microvasc Res 36:262, 1988.
19. Pearson LD, et al: Lymphopoiesis and lymphocyte recirculation in the sheep fetus. J Exp Med 143:167, 1976.
20. Smeaton TC, et al: Techniques for the long-term collection of lymph from the unanaesthetized foetal lamb in utero. Aust J Exp Biol Med Sci 47:565, 1969.
21. Brace RA: Thoracic duct lymph flow and its measurement in chronically catheterized sheep fetus. Am J Physiol 256:H16, 1989.
22. Schad H, Brechttelsbauer H: Thoracic duct lymph flow and composition in conscious dogs and the influence of anaesthesia and passive limb movement. Pfluger Arch 371:25, 1977.
23. Brace RA: Fetal blood volume, extracellular fluid, and lymphatic function. In Brace RA, et al (eds): Fetal and Neonatal Body Fluids: The Scientific Basis for Clinical Practice. Ithaca, NY, Perinatology Press, 1989.
24. Brace RA, Christian JL: Transcapillary Starling pressures in the fetus, newborn, adult, and pregnant adult. Am J Physiol 240:H843, 1981.
25. Brace RA: Ovine fetal cardiovascular responses to packed red blood cell transfusions. Am J Obstet Gynecol 161:1367, 1989.
26. Brace RA: Effects of outflow pressure on fetal lymph flow. Am J Obstet Gynecol 160:494, 1989.
27. Gest AL, et al: The effect of outflow pressure upon thoracic duct lymph flow rate in fetal sheep. Pediatr Res 32:585, 1992.
28. Brace RA, Valenzuela GJ: Effects of outflow pressure and vascular volume loading on thoracic duct lymph flow in adult sheep. Am J Physiol 258:R240, 1990.
29. Harding R: Fetal lung fluid. In Brace RA, et al (eds): Fetal and Neonatal Body Fluids: The Scientific Basis for Clinical Practice. Ithaca, NY, Perinatology Press, 1989.

30. Kitterman JA, et al: Tracheal fluid in fetal lambs: Spontaneous decrease prior to birth. J Appl Physiol 47:985, 1979.
31. Mescher EJ, et al: Ontogeny of tracheal fluid, pulmonary surfactant, and plasma corticoids in the fetal lamb. J Appl Physiol 39:1017, 1975.
32. Maloney JE: Preparation of the respiratory system for the early neonatal period. J Dev Physiol 6:21, 1984.
33. Bland RD, et al: Clearance of liquid from lungs of newborn rabbits. J Appl Physiol 49:171, 1980.
34. Perks AM, Cassin S: The effects of arginine vasopressin and other factors on the production of lung fluid in fetal goats. Chest 81s:63s, 1982.
35. Comline RS, Silver M: The composition of foetal and maternal blood during parturition in the ewe. J Physiol 222:233, 1972.
36. Teramo KA, et al: Amniotic fluid erythropoietin correlates with umbilical plasma erythropoietin in normal and abnormal pregnancy. Obstet Gynecol 69:710, 1987.
37. Linderkamp O: Placental transfusion: determinants and effects. Clin Perinatol 9:559, 1982.
38. Mollison PL, et al: Red cell and plasma volume in newborn infants. Arch Dis Child 25:242, 1950.
39. Oh W, et al: Further study of neonatal blood volume in relation to placental transfusion. Ann Paediatr 207:147, 1966.
40. Usher R, et al: The blood volume of the newborn infant and placental transfusion. Acta Paediatr 52:497, 1963.
41. Yao AC, Lind J: Placental transfusion. Am J Dis Child 127:128, 1974.
42. Shields LE, Brace RA: Fetal vascular pressure responses to non-labor uterine contractions: dependency on amniotic fluid volume in the ovine fetus. Am J Obstet Gynecol 171:84, 1994.
43. Brace RA, Brittingham DS: Fetal vascular pressure and heart rate responses to nonlabor uterine contractions. Am J Physiol 251:R409, 1986.
44. Brace RA: Fetal blood volume responses to acute fetal hypoxia. Am J Obstet Gynecol 155:889, 1986.
45. Brace RA, Cheung CY: Role of catecholamines in mediating fetal blood volume decrease during acute hypoxia. Am J Physiol 253:H927, 1987.
46. Oh W, et al: Placenta to lamb fetus transfusion in utero during acute hypoxia. Am J Obstet Gynecol 122:316, 1975.
47. Tomita H, et al: Vasopressin dose-response effects on fetal vascular pressures, heart rate, and blood volume. Am J Physiol 249:H974, 1985.
48. Wood CE, et al: Fetal heart rate, arterial pressure, and blood volume responses to cortisol infusion. Am J Physiol 253:R904, 1987.
49. Brace RA, et al: Fetal cardiovascular, endocrine, and fluid responses to atrial natriuretic factor infusion. Am J Physiol 257:R580, 1989.
50. Robillard JE, et al: Ontogeny of the renal response to natriuretic peptide in the sheep. Am J Physiol 254:F634, 1988.
51. Towell ME: Blood volume of the fetus and the newborn infant. In Goodwin JW, et al (eds): Perinatal Medicine: The Basic Science Underlying Clinical Practice. Baltimore, Williams & Wilkins, 1976, pp 209–222.
52. Peltonen T: Placental transfusion-Advantage and disadvantage. Eur J Pediatr 137:141, 1981.
53. Coulter DM: Postnatal fluid and electrolyte changes and clinical implications. In Brace RA, et al (eds): Fetal and Neonatal Body Fluids: The Scientific Basis for Clinical Practice. Ithaca, NY, Perinatology Press, 1989.
54. Creasy RK, et al: Determination of fetal, placental and neonatal blood volumes in the sheep. Circ Res 27:407, 1970.
55. Baker CH: Cr51-labeled red cell, I-131-fibrinogen, and T-1824 dilution spaces. Am J Physiol 204:176, 1963.
56. Boyd GW: The reproducibility and accuracy of plasma volume estimation in the sheep with both 1311 gamma globulin and Evan's blue. Aust J Exp Biol Med Sci 45:51, 1967.
57. Wright RR, et al: Blood volume. Semin Nucl Med 5:63, 1975.
58. Brans YW, et al: Neonatal polycythemia: II. Plasma, blood, and red cell volume estimates in relation to hematocrit levels and quality of intrauterine growth. Pediatrics 68:175, 1981.
59. Brace RA: Blood volume in the fetus and methods for its measurement. In Nathanielsz PW (ed): Animal Models in Fetal Medicine. Ithaca, NY, Perinatology Press, 1984, pp 19–36.
60. Grimes JM, et al: Blood volume restitution after hemorrhage in adult sheep. Am J Physiol 253:R541, 1987.
61. Mott JC: Haemorrhage as a test of the function of the cardiovascular system in rabbits of different ages. J Physiol 181:728, 1965.
62. Mott JC: The effect of haemorrhage on haemoglobin concentration, blood volume and arterial pressure in kittens and cats. J Physiol 194:659, 1968.
63. Brace RA: Fetal blood volume responses to acute fetal hemorrhage. Circ Res 52:730, 1983.
64. Brace RA, Cheung CY: Fetal cardiovascular and endocrine responses to prolonged fetal hemorrhage. Am J Physiol 251:R417, 1986.
65. Brace RA: Mechanisms of fetal blood volume restoration after slow fetal hemorrhage. Am J Physiol 256:R1040, 1989.
66. Block SM, et al: Blood volume restitution after hemorrhage in the newborn lamb. Am J Physiol 257:R647, 1989.

67. Brace RA: Fetal blood volume responses to intravenous saline solution and dextran. Am J Obstet Gynecol 147:777, 1983.
68. Harake B, Power GG: Thoracic duct lymph flow: a comparative study in newborn and adult sheep. J Dev Physiol 8:87, 1986.
69. Brace RA: Fetal thoracic duct lymph flow response to intravascular saline infusion. Am J Physiol 254:R1007, 1988.
70. Brace RA, et al: Fetal and adult urine flow and ANF responses to vascular volume expansion. Am J Physiol 255:R846, 1988.
71. Yao AC, et al: Effect of prenatally induced hypoxia on blood volume of newborn lambs. Life Sci 2:931, 1978.
72. Linderkamp O, et al: The effect of intra-partum and intrauterine asphyxia on placental transfusion in premature and full-term infants. Eur J Pediatr 127:91, 1978.
73. Brace RA: Maximal lymph flow in the ovine fetus. Am J Obstet Gynecol 169:1487, 1993.
74. Brace RA: Blood volume response to drainage of left thoracic duct lymph in the ovine fetus. Am J Physiol 266:R709, 1994.
75. Brace RA, Andres RL: Left thoracic duct lymph flow responses to angiotensin II or atrial natriuretic factor infusion in the ovine fetus. Am J Obstet Gynecol 165:1607, 1991.
76. Battaglia FC, Meschia G: An introduction to fetal physiology. Orlando, FL, Academic Press, 1986.
77. Morris JA, et al: Measurement of fetoplacental blood volume in the human previable fetus. Am J Obstet Gynecol 118:927, 1974.
78. Nicolaides KH, et al: Measurement of human fetoplacental blood volume in erythroblastosis fetalis. Am J Obstet Gynecol 157:50, 1987.
79. Broughton-Pipkin F, Kirkpatrick SML: The blood volumes of fetal and newborn sheep. Q J Exp Physiol 58:181, 1973.
80. Caton D, et al: The circulating plasma volume of the foetal lamb as an index of its weight and rate of weight gain (g/day) in the last third of gestation. Q J Exp Physiol 60:45, 1975.
81. Creasy RK, et al: Effect of ventilation on transfer of blood from placenta to neonate. Am J Physiol 222:186, 1972.
82. Leblanc MH, Pate K: Effect of polycythemia on vascular volume in the newborn dog. Am J Physiol 246:H830, 1984.
83. Linderkamp O, et al: Blood volume and hematocrit in various organs in newborn piglets. Pediatr Res 14:1324, 1980.
84. Linderkamp O, et al: Blood volume in newborn piglets: Effects of time of natural cord rupture, intra-uterine growth retardation, asphyxia, and prostaglandin-induced prematurity. Pediatr Res 15:53, 1981.
85. Hannon JP, et al: Splenic red cell sequestration and blood volume measurement in conscious pigs. Am J Physiol 248:R293, 1985.
86. Taylor PM, et al: Clearances of plasma proteins from pulmonary vascular beds of adult dogs and pups. Am J Physiol 213:441, 1967.
87. Ueda S, et al: Estrogen effects on plasma volume, arterial blood pressure, interstitial space, plasma proteins, and blood viscosity in sheep. Am J Obstet Gynecol 155:195, 1986.
88. Nakayama S, et al: Small-volume resuscitation with hypertonic saline (2400 mosm/liter) during hemorrhagic shock. Circ Shock 13:149, 1984.
89. Newcomb SL, Power GG: Hematocrit of the fetal rabbit placenta. Am J Physiol 229:1393, 1975.
90. Linderkamp O, et al: Accuracy of blood volume estimations in critically ill children using 125I-labelled albumin and 51Cr-labelled red cells. Eur J Pediatr 125:143, 1977.
91. Hodgetts VE: The dynamic red cell storage function of the spleen in sheep. Aust J Exp Biol 39:187, 1961.
92. Power GG, et al: Water transfer across the placenta: hydrostatic and osmotic forces and the control of fetal cardiac output. pp. 317–344 In Longo, LD, Reneau DD (eds): Fetal and Newborn Cardiovascular Physiology. Vol 1. New York, Garland Press, 1978.
93. Wilbur WJ, et al: Water exchange in the placenta a mathematical model. Am J Physiol 235:R181, 1978.
94. Faber JJ, Anderson DF: Model study of placental water transfer and causes of fetal water disease in sheep. Am J Physiol 258:R1257, 1990.
95. Powell TL, Brace RA: Fetal fluid responses to long-term 5 M NaCl infusion: where does all the salt go? Am J Physiol 261:R412, 1991.
96. Brace RA: Fetal blood volume, urine flow, swallowing, and amniotic fluid volume responses to long-term intravascular infusions of saline. Am J Obstet Gynecol 161:1049, 1989.
97. Kilpatrick SJ, et al: Maternal hydration increases amniotic fluid index. Obstet Gynecol 78:1098, 1991.
98. Kilpatrick SJ: Therapeutic interventions for oligohydramnios: amnioinfusion and maternal hydration. Clin Obstet Gynecol. 40:328, 1997.
99. Heilmann L, et al: Acute maternal hydration in third-trimester oligohydramnios. Am J Obstet Gynecol 175:237, 1996.
100. Doi S, et al: Effect of maternal hydration on oligohydramnios: a comparison of three volume expansion methods. Obstet Gynecol. 92:525, 1998.
101. Stankewytsch-Janusch B, et al: Measurement of blood volume in fetal and neonatal sheep using red blood cels labelled with 99m technetium. J Dev Physiol 3:245, 1981.

140

Fetal and Neonatal Body Water Compartment Volumes with Reference to Growth and Development

Water is the most abundant component of the body and is the solvent in which all metabolic reactions occur. Body water exists in compartments with diverse solute compositions that are separated by semipermeable lipid membranes. Thus, although there are recognizable anatomic boundaries, physiologically these compartments are interconnected.

COMPARTMENTATION OF BODY WATER

Total body water (TBW) includes water both inside and outside of cells and water normally present in the nasorespiratory, gastrointestinal, and genitourinary systems. TBW can be theoretically divided into two main compartments (Figure 140-1). The *anatomic extracellular water* (ECW) includes all water external to cell membranes. *Intracellular water* (ICW) includes all water within cell membranes and constitutes the medium in which chemical reactions of cell metabolism occur. This compartment is heterogeneous and discontinuous; the interior of each cell is separated from the ECW and from the interior of other cells by the semipermeable cell membrane.

The anatomic ECW is functionally subdivided into *physiologic ECW* and *transcellular water*. The physiologic ECW is the portion of the anatomic ECW whose volume is accessible to direct measurement. It constitutes the medium through which all metabolic exchange occurs; it includes *plasma* (intravascular water) and *interstitial fluid* (ISF). The ISF is the fluid that directly bathes the cells of the body. It is the ECW into which ions and small molecules diffuse freely from plasma. The composition of the physiologic ECF is fairly uniform throughout the body. In addition, there are potential spaces in the body (pericardial, pleural, peritoneal, and synovial) that are normally empty except for a few milliliters of viscous lubricating fluid and are considered to be part of the ISF compartment. Transcellular water includes water in extracellular compartments enclosed by an epithelial membrane, the volume and composition of which are determined by the cellular activity of that membrane. These heterogeneous compartments include the aqueous humor in the eye, the cerebrospinal fluid, and water within the nasorespiratory, gastrointestinal, and genitourinary systems. The volume of the transcellular water portion of the anatomic ECW is not included in conventional measurements of ECW.

ESTIMATION OF BODY WATER COMPARTMENT MASSES AND VOLUMES

All *in vivo* methods used to measure the mass or volume of body water compartments are of limited accuracy and precision. Accuracy of measurement is limited by the degree to which the assumptions on which methods are based are true. Precision is limited by biologic variability (body water compartment volumes may vary during the course of a day) and analytical error. Body water compartment volumes cannot be measured with a precision much greater than 2 to 5% in the healthy adult.[1-5] Therefore, these techniques are better suited to estimate average body water compartment volumes in groups of subjects rather those of individual persons. Sutcliff[6] and Ellis[7] have published in-depth reviews of the techniques discussed in the following subsections.

Total Body Water

Desiccation

With this method, TBW is calculated as the difference in body mass before and after whole body desiccation to a constant mass at 100°C. Although it is most accurate, this technique is obviously not applicable to *in vivo* studies.

Densitometry

Fat has a much lower density (0.92) than lean body mass (LBM; 1.10). Therefore, the proportion of body mass that is fat can be determined from whole body density by underwater weighing, as follows:

$$(4.570 \,/\, \text{whole body density}) - 4.142.$$

Whole body density must be corrected for air in the lungs and the gastrointestinal tract. The error in measurement of the former is the major source of analytical error with this method. LBM is calculated as the difference between total body mass and fat mass. This technique assumes that the density of fat and LBM are constant. This is more true for fat than for LBM, even in adults.[8-12] TBW mass can then be calculated from LBM, assuming that TBW is a constant 73.2% of the latter. This is a reasonable assumption for healthy young white adults. However, for samples of very young or old persons or of persons of different ethnicity or with disease states, the proportion is not a constant, only an average value that is population specific. This technique is not applicable to the fetus, newborn, and infant because the density of LBM increases during development, the proportion of LBM that is water decreases during development, and substantial subject cooperation is required. Determination of body density by air-displacement plethysmography obviates the last limitation, but not the others.

Indicator Dilution Method

This method is based on *Fick's principle*: if a known amount of a solute (indicator) is administered to a subject and limited to and distributed evenly throughout a body water compartment, then the volume of the compartment can be calculated as the quotient of the amount administered and the concentration of the indicator in body water within the compartment of interest. The ideal indicator is (1) nontoxic; (2) limited to and evenly distributed throughout the body water compartment; (3) not lost from the body during the time necessary for the indicator to distribute throughout the compartment evenly; (4) metabolically inert; and (5) with a concentration that is easily, precisely, and accurately measurable in small volumes of body fluid. No ideal indicators exist for measurement of any body water compartment volumes. Figure 140-2 is a schematic diagram of the volumes of distribution of indicators used to estimate body water compartment volumes. Most are excreted in the urine, are metabolized, or exchange with components of body solids.

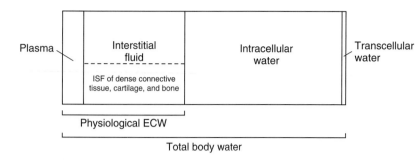

Figure 140–1. Body water compartments. The anatomic extracellular water (ECW) compartment includes the physiologic extracellular water compartment and the transcellular water compartment. ISF, interstitial fluid. (From Lorenz JM, Kleinman LI: Physiology and pathophysiology of body water and electrolytes. *In* Kaplan L, Pesce A [eds]: Clinical Chemistry, 4th ed. St. Louis, CV Mosby, 2003.)

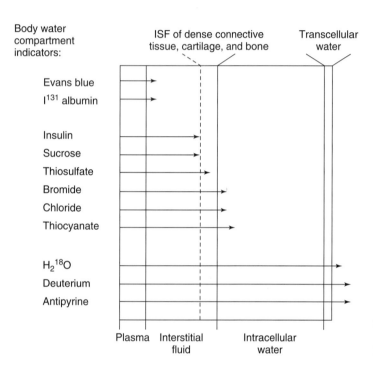

Figure 140–2. Apparent volumes of distribution of indicators used to estimate body water compartment volumes. ISF, interstitial fluid.

All these properties will lead to overestimation of the volume of the body compartment, if corrections are not made. Depending on how the indicator is "lost" from the compartment, the rate of this loss, and the time required for the indicator to distribute evenly throughout a body water compartment, two methods are used to determine an indicator's volume of distribution: the plateau method and the back-extrapolation method. Assumptions implicit in both methods are not strictly valid. Therefore, the volume of distribution with the former method is greater than the true volume of the body water compartment, and with the latter it is less than the true volume of the body water compartment.[13]

Antipyrine, deuterium, and 18O-labeled water are used as indicators of ECW volume. Antipyrine is less difficult to analyze than isotopes of water, but it is relatively rapidly metabolized. In addition, approximately 10% is protein bound. With the use of the back-extrapolation method to correct for metabolism, the latter results in an apparent volume of distribution less than true TBW volume.[14] Measurement of isotopes of water requires elaborate equipment. Moreover, the volume of distribution of hydrogen water isotopes is approximately 4% higher than TBW measured by desiccation, as a result of exchange of nonaqueous exchangeable hydrogen atoms, mainly on carboxyl and hydroxyl groups.[15] $H_2{}^{18}O$ also exchanges with nonaqueous exchangeable oxygen atoms, but to a lesser extent—its volume of distribution is approximately 1% greater than TBW volume.[16, 17]

Bioelectrical Impedance Analysis

Total body bioelectrical impedance analysis (BIA) is a frequently used bedside method of estimating TBW mass.[18-20] The method is based on the assumptions that only water can conduct electricity within the body and that the body is a homogeneous, perfect cylinder with a uniform cross-sectional area. Bioelectrical impedance is determined by measuring the voltage drop when a small electrical current (800 µA) is applied across the skin of the subject at a frequency capable of penetrating cell membranes (usually 50 kHz). The impedance is composed of two components: the resistance and the reactance. The magnitude of the resistance component seems to be well correlated with the volumes of distribution of tritiated water and deuterium.[5, 21-23] TBW is calculated from resistance using a regression equation that includes at least some anthropometric index of total body volume. This equation must be derived for the population of interest using TBW volume determined by a reference standard. The advantages of this technique are that it is noninvasive, safe, and rapid, and the equipment is portable and inexpensive. Measurement of TBW using BIA has been reported to compare favorably with the volume of distribution of $H_2{}^{18}O$ in neonates.[24-27] However, there is considerable variation in the regression equations used to predict TBW among these studies. It is unclear whether this variation is the result of electrode position,[28] postnatal age,[24] gestational age, birth weight, or possibly other factors. Thus, the major limitation of this technique is that the regression equations do not provide accurate estimates in populations other than those in which they were derived. Therefore, prediction equations should be validated in or derived for each sample in which they are used. Validation consists of comparison with a reference method.

Total Body Electrical Conductivity

Total body electrical conductivity (TOBEC) is an alternate bioelectrical technique for estimating TBW. Eddy currents are induced in the conductive tissues of the body by placing the patient in a coil that generates a time-varying electromagnetic field. These eddy currents, in turn, change the impedance of the coil. The difference of the impedance with the coil empty and the coil with the body in place is the TOBEC number. The latter is proportional to the conducting volume of the body, that is, to TBW. Estimation of TBW volume requires a regression equation, which (as with BIA) must be derived using a reference standard. An instrument is available for infants. Furthermore, the TOBEC number has been shown to correlate well with the volume of distribution of $H_2^{18}O$ in healthy infants,[29] and a regression equation has been derived for healthy infants 2 to 12 weeks of age.[30] Limitations of this technique are that the regression equation may not provide accurate estimates in populations other than that from which it was derived.[31] The technique is applicable only to neonates who do not require support that would preclude safely placing them in the instrument, and the instrument is expensive and not portable.

Extracellular Water

Total Body Chloride

Total body chloride content, measured by neutron activation *in vivo*[32] or analysis of total body ash content, has been used to estimate the ECW volume. ECW is calculated as the quotient of total body chloride content and ECF chloride concentration, assuming that all body chloride is extracellular and is uniformly distributed throughout the ECW compartment. However, there is intracellular chloride, principally in red blood cells. Moreover, the apparatus required for neutron activation analysis is expensive, is difficult to calibrate, and requires irradiation. The last feature precludes the use of this method in infants and children.

Indicator Dilution

Inulin, sucrose, thiosulfate, and bromide are commonly used indicators to estimate ECW volume in neonates, infants, children, and adults. No indicator used to estimate ECW volumes is uniformly distributed throughout and limited to these compartments. As illustrated in Figure 140-2, the volume measured depends on the degree to which the indicator leaks into cells or penetrates the ISF of dense connective tissue. Under normal circumstances, ISF does not behave as a simple aqueous solution. Solutes do not penetrate as easily into the ISF of dense connective tissue, cartilage, or bone. Therefore, when one uses indicators to estimate ECW volume, it is more correct to refer to the value of the indicator's *volume of distribution*. Correction of the volume of distribution of ECW indicators for volume of protein in plasma and (in the case of indicators that exist in solution as ions) for the Donnan equilibrium is required when the concentration of the indicator is measured in the plasma.[33]

The proportion of ECW contained in the ISF of dense connective tissue is lower in infants than in children and lower in children than in adults. Therefore, differences between the physiologic ECW volume and the volumes of distribution of indicators for which diffusion into connective tissue ISF is limited (inulin, sucrose, thiosulfate) are less in the neonate than in the adult, and these differences increase during development.

Bromide penetrates connective tissue ISF well, but it is not completely limited to the ECW compartment; it diffuses to some extent into ICW. It does not cross the blood-brain barrier, and because the ECF is 6% of ECW volume in newborns compared with 1% in adults, the difference between the physiologic ECW volume and the volume of distribution of bromide is greater in the newborn than in the adult.

Multiple-Frequency Bioelectrical Impedance Analysis

BIA can also be used to estimate ECW volume. Theoretically, the most appropriate measure of ECW volume is given by impedance measure at zero frequency. However, measurement of impedance at zero frequency is not practical. Measurement of impedance over a range of frequencies allows resistance and reactance to be determined at each frequency. Reactance is then plotted against resistance, and the theoretical value of resistance at zero frequency is obtained by extrapolation of the curve to zero frequency. Measurement of TBW using multiple-frequency BIA analysis has been reported to compare favorably with the corrected bromide space in adults[5] and in preterm and term neonates.[34]

Plasma Water

Plasma water volume can be more accurately measured than ECW volume. Evans blue and iodine-131–labeled serum albumin are commonly used indicators to estimate plasma volume. Both are evenly distributed throughout the plasma water compartment, but both leak into from the plasma water into the ISF compartment during the time required for distribution to occur. The rate of loss of these two indicators and their volumes of distributions are similar in the adult[35, 36] and in the newborn.[37] However, the rate of loss is three- to fourfold greater in the newborn in the first day of life than in the adult—0.2 to 0.5% of the injected dose per minute.[37-39] Failure to correct for loss of the injected dose during the period necessary for even distribution throughout the plasma water compartment using the back-extrapolation method results in an apparent volume distribution greater that true plasma volume.

Interstitial Fluid

ISF volume cannot be directly measured. It is calculated as the difference between ECW volume and plasma water volume. Therefore, its value depends on techniques used to estimate ECW and plasma water volumes and is subject to the errors of both techniques.

Intracellular Water

The volume of the ICW compartment is usually calculated as the difference between TBW volume and ECW volume. Therefore, its value depends on techniques used to estimate TBW and ECW volumes and is subject to the errors of both techniques.

MATURATIONAL CHANGES IN BODY WATER COMPARTMENT VOLUMES

TBW is 65% of body weight in average men and 55% of body weight in women. This difference between men and women is largely the result of differences in body fat. As a percentage of total body weight, TBW varies inversely with body fat content, from approximately 70% in very thin persons to 50% in very obese persons.

When the volume of distribution of thiosulfate is used to estimate the physiologic ECW volume, it is approximately 20% of body mass and one-third of TBW volume in the average adult. Plasma volume is 5% of body mass. ISF volume is approximately 15% of body weight and one-fourth of TBW. ICW water, calculated as the difference between the TBW and ECW mass, is equal to 40% of body weight and two-thirds of TBW in the average adult. ICW mass calculated in this manner includes transcellular water, which has been estimated to be 1 to 3% of body weight.

The fraction of body mass that is water and the distribution of body water between the ECW and ICW do not remain constant during growth. Figure 140-3 is a compilation of body water compartment estimations from the literature. Variability among study subjects,[40] differences in the methods used to estimate body water compartment volume, and the cross-sectional nature of the data all contribute to the variability at a given age. TBW

expressed as a percentage of body mass gradually decreases during gestation and early childhood from approximately 90% during the first trimester to approximately 80% at 26 weeks of gestation to approximately 75% at term, and it reaches a value approximating that in the adult by about 3 years of age. This change results from an increased accretion of body solids (protein, fat, and minerals) relative to water during development.[41-43] During this time, ECW (expressed as a percentage of body weight) decreases and ICW (expressed as a percentage of body weight) increases. Thus, ECW becomes a lesser and ICW a greater proportion of TBW. ECW decreases from more than 50%

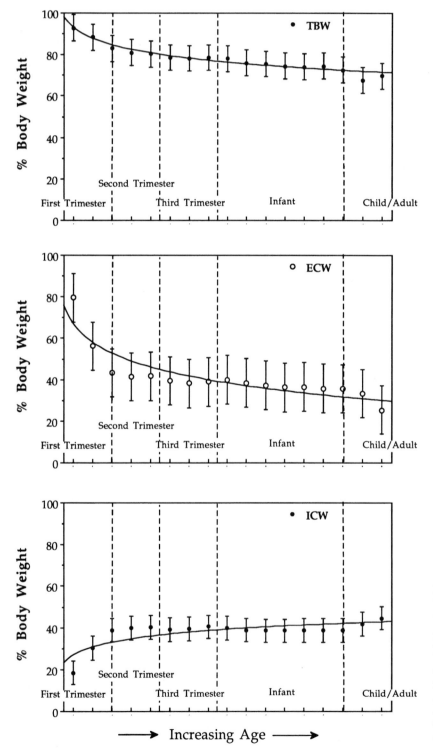

Figure 140–3. Change in body water and distribution with age. *Points* are means; *error bars* are standard deviations. Curves were fitted logarithmically. ECW = extracellular water; ICW = intracellular water; TBW = total body water. (From Costarino AR Jr, Brans YW: Fetal and neonatal body fluid composition with reference to growth and development. *In* Polin RA, Fox WW [eds]: Fetal and Neonatal Physiology, 2nd ed. Philadelphia, WB Saunders Co, 1998. Based on data from references 42, 43, 45, 63, and 71-84.)

of body mass during the first trimester to approximately 45% at 26 weeks to 40% at term, and it reaches a value approximating that in the adult by 3 years of age. This decrease is the result of decrease in the proportion of body mass that is ISF during development, because plasma volume remains constant at 4 to 5% of body weight throughout life. This relative decrease in ECW and the increase in ICW during development are the result of changes in the proportions that various tissues contribute to total body weight (the proportion of water that is extracellular and intracellular differs among tissues) and changes in the proportion of water that is extracellular and intracellular within given tissues during development.[42] Of course, the absolute volumes of TBW, ECW, ICW, and plasma all increase with growth.

POSTNATAL CHANGES IN BODY FLUID COMPARTMENTS

Independent of the gradual changes in the proportion of body weight that is water and the changes in the proportions of TBW contributed by the ECW and ICW compartments during development, there is an abrupt and absolute decrease in TBW volume in the first few days after birth. What proportion of this decrease in TBW is ECW and what proportion is ICW are controversial, but the best evidence is that a disproportionate loss of water occurs from the ECW compartment in appropriate for gestational age (AGA) very low birth weight infants (Fig. 140–4).[40, 44-47] This decrease in ECW volume is the result of decrease in ISF volume, without change in plasma volume.[46] Decreases in plasma volume during the first hours of life in early studies in term and preterm newborns[39, 48-52] were a physiologic response to placental transfusion as the result of the then prevalent practice of delaying cord clamping.

Although physiologic correlates of the postnatal diuresis and natriuresis have been described,[53-59] the *reason* is unknown. The disproportionate decrease in ISF precludes ascribing this decrease solely to catabolism. That it is physiologic is suggested by certain observations. First, relatively large differences in water and caloric intake are required to moderate this weight loss.[60-62] Furthermore, higher caloric intake has been correlated with less postnatal weight loss, but no difference in the magnitude of ECW contraction.[47] Moreover, increases in ICW and body solids *per kilogram of body weight*, but not in ECW *per kilogram body weight*, occur with subsequent weight gain.[40,63] Fluid and sodium intakes high enough to prevent this decrease in ECW volume[64] have been associated with increased morbidity in premature newborns.[62,65,66]

Data are more limited for term and small for gestational age (SGA) infants. There are no studies of ECW volume before and after postnatal weight loss. In the single study of the change in TBW with postnatal weight loss in AGA term infants, no change in the proportion of body weight that was water was associated with postnatal weight loss, consistent with proportionate decreases in TBW and total body solids.[67] Bauer and colleagues[68] observed a decrease in body weight and TBW during the first week of life in preterm AGA infants (mean gestational age 31 weeks), but no change in body weight or TBW in weight-matched SGA infants (mean gestational age 35 weeks). Van der Wagen and associates[69] found that the proportion of TBW and total body solids remained constant during the period of postnatal weight loss and subsequent weight gain in SGA infants with a mean gestational age of 35.7 weeks. These studies suggest that postnatal weight loss, if it occurs, is the result of catabolism rather than reduction in ECW volume in the term and SGA infant. Conversely, Singhi and colleagues[70] found that nearly 90% of the decrease in TBW was the result of a decrease in ECW in both preterm AGA and gestational age-matched SGA infants. The reason for this difference between the studies of Bauer and associates[68] and van der Wagen and colleagues[69] and that of Singh and associates[70] in SGA infants may be that the SGA infants in the first two studies were closer to term, whereas the SGA infants in the latter study were more preterm. Taken together, these data could be interpreted to be consistent with postnatal weight loss as the result of decrease in ECW in more premature infants and the result of catabolism in near-term infants, regardless of appropriateness for growth.

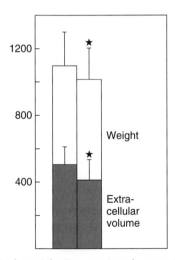

Figure 140–4. Body weight (in grams) and extracellular water volume (volume of distribution of sucrose, in milliliters) in 13 preterm appropriate for gestational age infants within the first 12 hours of life (*left bars*) and when postnatal weight loss exceeded 5% (*right bars; average age, 84 hours*). *Error bars* are standard deviations. (*p* ⋆< .001 versus respective values within the first 12 hours of life.) Mean weight loss was the same as the mean decrease in extracellular water volume. (Adapted from Bauer K, Versmold H: Postnatal weight loss in preterm neonates < 1599 g is due to isotonic dehydration of the extracellular volume. Acta Paediatr Scand Suppl *360*:37, 1989.)

REFERENCES

1. Mather K, et al: The precision of plasma volume determinations with the Evans blue method. Br J Exp Pathol *28*:12, 1947.
2. von Porat BTD: Blood volume determinations with Evans blue dye. Acta Med Scand Suppl *256*:1, 1951.
3. Haxhe JJ: La composition corporelle normale. Paris, Librairie Maloine, 1963.
4. Price WF, et al: Reproducibility of body composition measurements. J Lab Clin Med *74*:557, 1969.
5. Patel RV, et al: Estimation of total body extracellular water using single and multiple frequency bioimpedance. Ann Pharmacother *28*:565, 1994.
6. Sutcliff JF: A review on in vivo experimental methods to determine the composition of the human body. Phys Med Biol *41*:791, 1996.
7. Ellis KJ: Human body composition: in vivo methods. Physiol Rev *80*:649, 2000.
8. Fidanza FA, et al: Density of fat in man and other animals. J Appl Physiol *6*:252, 1953.
9. Martin AD, et al: Adipose density, estimated adipose lipid fraction and whole body adiposity in male cadavers. Int J Obesity *18*:73, 1962.
10. Schutte JE, et al: Density of lean body mass is greater in blacks than whites. J Appl Physiol *56*:1647, 1984.
11. Heymsfield SBJ, et al: Chemical determination of human body density in vivo: relevance to hydrodensity. Am J Clin Nutr *50*:1282, 1989.
12. Cote KD, Adams WC: Effect of bone density on body composition estimates in young adult black and white women. Med Sci Sports *25*:290, 1993.
13. Davies PSW, Wells JCK: Calculation of total body water in infancy. Eur J Nutr *48*:490, 1994.
14. Soberman R, et al: The use of antipyrine in the measurement of total body water in man. J Biol Chem *79*:31, 1947.
15. Sheng HP, Huggins RA: A review of body composition studies with emphasis on total body water and fat. Am J Clin Nutri *32*:630, 1979.
16. Schoeller DA, et al: Total body water measurement in humans with ^{2}H and ^{18}O labeled water. Am J Clin Nutr *33*:2686, 1980.
17. Racette SB, et al: Relative dilution spaces of ^{2}H and ^{18}O labeled water in humans. Am J Physiol *267*:E585, 1994.

18. National Institutes of Health Technology Assessment: Conference statement. Am J Clin Nutr 64(Suppl 3):524S, 1994.

19. Schoeller DA: Bioelectrical impedance analysis for measurement of human body composition: where do we stand and what is the next step. Nutrition 12:760, 1996.

20. Ellis KJ, et al: Bioelectrical impedance methods in clinical research: a follow-up to the NIH technology assessment conference. Nutrition 15:874, 1999.

21. Hoffer EC, et al: Correlation of whole-body impedance with total body water volume. J Appl Physiol 27:531, 1969.

22. Lukaski HC, et al: Assessment of fat free mass using bioelectrical impedance measurements in the human body. Am J Clin Nutr 41:810, 1985.

23. Kushner RF, Schoeller DA: Estimation of total body water by bioelectrical impedance analysis. Am J Clin Nutr 44:417, 1986.

24. Mayfield SR, et al: Body composition of low-birth-weight infants determined by using bioelectrical resistance and reactance. Am J Clin Nutr 54:296, 1991.

25. Wilson DC, et al: Total body water measurement by bioelectrical impedance in the extremely low birth weight infant. Basic Life Sci 60:185, 1993.

26. Tang W, et al: Assessment of total body water using bioelectrical impedance analysis in neonates receiving intensive care. Arch Dis Child 77:F123, 1997.

27. Raghavan CV, et al: Estimation of total body water in very-low-birth-weight infants by anthropometry with and without bioelectrical impedance and H_2O^{18}. Am J Clin Nutr 68:668, 1998.

28. Gartner A, et al: Importance of electrode position in bioelectrical impedance analysis. Am J Clin Nutr 56:1067, 1992.

29. Klish WJ, et al: The bioelectrical measurement of body composition during infancy. Hum Biol 59:319, 1987.

30. Fiorotto ML, et al: Fat-free bass and total body water of infants estimated from total body electrical conductivity measurements. Pediatr Res 22:417, 1987.

31. Fiorotto ML, et al: Total body water electrical conductivity measurements: an evaluation of current instrumentation for infants. Pediatr Res 37:84, 1995.

32. Cohn SH: In vivo neutron activation analysis: state of the art and future prospects. Med Phys 8:145, 1981.

33. Bell EF, et al: Errors in bromide space correction (letter). Pediatr Res 18:392, 1984.

34. Lingwood BE, et al: Measurement of extracellular fluid volume in the neonate using multiple frequency bio-impedance analysis. Physiol Meas 21:251, 2000.

35. Reeve EB: The contribution of I^{131} labeled proteins to measurement of blood volume. Ann NY Acad Med 70:137, 1957.

36. Franks JJ, Zigga F: Simultaneous measurement of plasma volume in man with T-1824 and an improved I^{131} albumin method. J Appl Physiol 13:299, 1958.

37. Parving HH, et al: Simultaneous determination of plasma volume and transcapillary escape rate with I^{131} labeled albumin and T-1824 in the newborn. Acta Paediatr Scand 62:248, 1973.

38. Steele MW: Plasma volume changes in the neonate. Arch Dis Child 103:42, 1962.

39. Cassady G: Plasma volume studies in low birth weight babies. Pediatrics 38:1029, 1966.

40. Singhi S, et al: Composition of postnatal weight loss and subsequent weight gain in preterm infants. Indian J Med Res 101:157, 1995.

41. Iob V, Swanson WW: Mineral growth of the human fetus. Am J Dis Child 47:302, 1934.

42. Widdowson EM, Spray CM: Chemical development in utero. Arch Dis Child 26:205, 1951.

43. Jirasek JE, et al: Water and nitrogen content of the body of young human embryos. Am J Obstet Gynecol 96:868, 1966.

44. Bauer K, Versmold H: Postnatal weight loss in preterm neonates < 1599 g is due to isotonic dehydration of the extracellular volume. Acta Paediatr Scand Suppl 360:37, 1989.

45. Shaffer SG, et al: Postnatal changes in total body water and extracellular volume in preterm infants with respiratory distress syndrome. J Pediatr 109:509, 1986.

46. Bauer K, et al: Postnatal weight loss in ventilated premature infants below 1500 g: significance of renal and extrarenal fluid loss. Monatsschr Kinderheilkd 139:452, 1991.

47. Heimler R, et al: Relationship between nutrition, weight change, and fluid compartments in preterm infants during the first week of life. J Pediatr 122:110, 1993.

48. Mollison PL, et al: Red cell and plasma volume in newborn infants. Am J Dis Child 25:242, 1950.

49. Gairdner D, et al: The shift of fluid from the vascular compartment immediately after birth. Arch Dis Child 33:489, 1958.

50. Clark ACL, Gairdner D: Postnatal plasma shift in preterm infants. Arch Dis Child 35:352, 1960.

51. Lind J: Physiological adaptation to the placental transfusion. Can Med Assoc J 93:1091, 1965.

52. Ingomar CJ, et al: The transcapillary escape of t-1824 in healthy newborn infants: the influence of the placental transfusion. Acta Paediatr Scand 62:617, 1973.

53. Costarino At, et al: Renal adaptation to extrauterine life in patients with respiratory distress syndrome. Am J Dis Child 139:1060, 1985.

54. Kojima T, et al: Plasma atrial natriuretic factor and spontaneous diuresis in sick neonates. Arch Dis Child 62:667, 1987.

55. Tulassay T, et al: Atrial natriuretic peptide abd extracellular volume contraction after birth. Acta Paediatr Scand 76:444, 1987.

56. Bidiwala KS, et al: Renal function correlates of postnatal diuresis in preterm infants. Pediatrics 82:50, 1988.

57. Kojima T, et al: Effect of atrial natriuretic factor (ANF) on water homeostasis of the neonate. Early Hum Dev 29:161, 1992.

58. Lorenz JM, et al: Phases of fluid and electrolyte homeostasis in the extremely low birth weight infant. Pediatrics 96:484, 1995.

59. Modi N, et al: Postnatal weight loss and contraction of the extracellular compartment is triggered by atrial natriuretic peptide. Early Hum Dev 59:201, 2000.

60. Lorenz JM, et al: Water balance in very low birth weight infants: relationship to water and sodium intake and effect on outcome. J Pediatr 101:423, 1982.

61. Shaffer SG, Meade VM: Sodium balance and extracellular volume regulation in very low birth weight infants. J Pediatr 115:285, 1989.

62. Hartnoll G, et al: Randomized controlled trial of postnatal sodium supplementation on body composition in 25 to 30 week gestation age infants. Arch Dis Child 82:F24, 2000.

63. Shaffer SG, et al: Extracellular fluid volume changes in very low birth weight infants during the first 2 postnatal months. J Pediatr 111:124, 1987.

64. Stonestreet BS, et al: Renal response in low-birth-weight neonates: results of prolonged intake of two different amounts of fluid and sodium. Am J Dis Child 137:215, 1983.

65. Bell EF, et al: Effect of fluid administration on the development of symptomatic patent ductus arteriosus and congestive heart failure in premature infants. N Engl J Med 302:598, 1980.

66. Bell EF, et al: High-volume intake predisposes premature infants to necrotizing enterocolitis (letter). Lancet 2:90, 1979.

67. Rodriguez G, et al: Changes in body composition during the initial hours of life in breast-fed healthy term infants. Biol Neonate 77:12, 2000.

68. Bauer K, et al: Effect of intrauterine growth retardation on postnatal weight change in preterm infants. J Pediatr 123:301, 1993.

69. Van der Wagen A, et al: Composition of postnatal weight loss and subsequent weight gain in small for dates newborn infants. Acta Paediatr Scand 74:57, 1985.

70. Singhi S, et al: Effects of intrauterine growth retardation on postnatal changes in body composition of preterm infants. Indian J Med Res 102:275, 1995.

71. Flexner LB, et al: The estimation of extracellular and total body water in the newborn human infant with radioactive sodium and deuterium oxide. J Pediatr 30:413, 1947.

72. Friis-Hansen BJ, et al: Total body water in children. Pediatrics 7:321, 1951.

73. Perley A, et al: Determination of sodium "space" in infants, children, and adults. J Pediatr 38:299, 1951.

74. Ely RS, Sutow WW: Growth of thiocyanate space in infancy and childhood. Pediatrics 10:115, 1952.

75. Christian JR, et al: Total body water and exchangeable sodium in normal full-term infants. Am J Dis Child 92:325, 1956.

76. Finley SC, Hare RS: Bromide space in infants and children. Am J Dis Child 98:749, 1959.

77. Fink CW, Cheek DB: The corrected bromide space in (extracellular volume) in the newborn. Pediatrics 26:397, 1960.

78. Cheek DB: Extracellular volume: its structure and measurements and the influences of age and disease. J Pediatr 58:103, 1961.

79. Cheek DB, et al: Further observation on the corrected bromide space of the neonate and investigation of water electrolyte status in infants born of diabetic mothers. Pediatrics 28:861, 1961.

80. Clapp WM, et al: Body water compartments in the premature infant with special reference to the effects of the respiratory distress syndrome and of maternal diabetes and toxemia. Pediatrics 29:883, 1962.

81. Cassady G: Bromide space studies in infants of low birth weight. Pediatr Res 4:14, 1970.

82. Cassady G, Milstead RR: Antipyrine space studies and cell water estimates in infants of low birth weight. Pediatr Res 5:673, 1971.

83. Brans YW, Cassady G: Fetal nutrition and body composition. In Ghadimi H (ed): Total Parenteral Nutrition: Premises and Promises. New York, John Wiley & Sons, 1975, pp 301–333.

84. van der Wagen A, et al: Body water compartments and dry body weight in small-for-dates (SFD) and appropriate-for-dates (AFD) newborn infants at birth. Pediatr Res 17:340A, 1983.

85. Bauer K, et al: Body composition, nutrition, and fluid balance during the first two weeks of life in preterm neonates weighing less than 1500 grams. J Pediatr 118:615, 1991.

David P. Carlton

Pathophysiology of Edema

GENERAL CONSIDERATIONS

Edema is the clinical term used to describe excessive fluid accumulation in the adventitial tissue spaces of the body. Excess fluid accumulation results when the rate of transvascular fluid filtration from the microcirculation is exceeded by the rate of fluid clearance from the interstitial space by lymphatics. Postnatally, edema occurs in the neonate in association with a variety of conditions, including respiratory failure, sepsis, and renal failure. Underlying all circumstances in which there is edema, a disturbance in the normal balance of total body salt and water is present, whether this occurs as a primary (e.g., anuria) or secondary (e.g., retention of fluid to preserve circulating volume) event.[1] Although renal or hormonal abnormalities are not responsible for edema formation, nearly all conditions associated with edema have disturbances in these systems. The resolution of edema ultimately occurs when normal renal and hormonal control of fluid and salt balance is established.

Total body fluid dynamics are not constant during development.[2] Early in gestation, total body water content is approximately 95% of total body weight, decreasing to approximately 75% of body weight at term, and then to near 60% of body weight by the end of the first year after birth. The fraction of total body water that comprises interstitial fluid declines during fetal development.

TRANSVASCULAR FLUID FILTRATION

Fluid movement across the endothelium is driven by forces that regulate fluid flux across a semipermeable membrane.[3] These forces are the hydrostatic and protein osmotic, or oncotic, pressures of the intravascular and interstitial spaces. The ostensibly quantitative expression of how these forces influence fluid filtration is shown in the equation.

$$J_v = K \{(P_{mv} - P_i) - \sigma(\pi_{mv} - \pi_i)\} \qquad (1)$$

where J_v represents net transvascular fluid flow, K is a coefficient that accounts for the permeability of the barrier and surface area for filtration, σ is the reflection coefficient of the barrier to protein, P_{mv} and P_i are the hydrostatic pressures of the microvascular compartment and interstitium, respectively, and π_{mv} and π_i are the osmotic pressures generated by the protein in the microvascular and interstitial spaces, respectively. For a barrier that is completely impermeable to protein, σ would assume the value of 1, and for a barrier across which protein flows without restriction, σ would assume the value of 0. The most complete analysis of fluid filtration across the endothelium would include values for σ that are specific for each plasma protein.

Countless attempts have been made to quantify each of the variables in Equation 1 for different organs in animals and in man. All experimental approaches involve assumptions about the validity of the values measured and thus all values so measured lack a sense of finality, particularly in the fetus and newborn.[4,5]

In most tissue spaces in the body, under most circumstances, J_v is greater than 0. That is, the sum of forces regulating fluid filtration result in a net movement of fluid out of the microcirculation.[6] It is important to recognize, however, that fluid filtration processes are dynamic and at any one time, in any specific section of the microcirculation, filtration forces may not result in

fluid moving into the interstitium, even though the net J_v of the tissue or organ is greater than 0. For instance, the clearance of alveolar liquid from the lung that occurs after birth takes place predominantly across the microcirculation and not by lymphatic channels.[7]

Intravascular pressure in the microcirculation, P_{mv}, can be measured by direct techniques using micropuncture and by indirect techniques using isogravimetric approaches.[8] It is unlikely that intravascular pressure remains constant across the entire fluid-exchanging surface, because resistance to flow along the vessel will result in a drop in pressure. Therefore, P_{mv} is understood to be the net hydrostatic force for the surface area involved in fluid exchange, even if the hydrostatic pressure at the arterial end of the vessel might result in fluid filtration and hydrostatic pressure at the venous end might result in fluid reabsorption.

P_{mv} is influenced by the relative vascular resistances in the circulation before and after the fluid-exchanging regions.[9] An increase in upstream resistance or a decrease in downstream resistance will reduce P_{mv} and reduce fluid filtration. A decrease in upstream resistance or an increase in downstream resistance will have the opposite effect on fluid filtration. The importance of considering the profile of vascular resistance distribution is that the effect of a change in arterial pressure on fluid filtration cannot be predicted with certainty. The redistribution of vascular resistance in response to an intervention or a change in condition ultimately will determine whether transvascular fluid filtration is affected, and because resistance cannot be assessed clinically, the ability to predict whether a change in transvascular filtration will occur is difficult. For instance, alveolar hypoxia increases pulmonary arterial pressure in both adults and neonates, but alveolar hypoxia affects transvascular fluid filtration only in the newborn lung.[10,12]

Interstitial pressure, P_i, has been assessed by several different techniques, including porous capsule embedment, direct micropuncture, and cotton wick insertion into the tissue space.[8] It is not possible to assign a general value to P_i because it assumes different values depending on the tissue bed under study. Values that exceed atmospheric pressure and those that are subatmospheric have been measured.[13] Although P_i usually assumes a value near 0 mm Hg, changes in interstitial pressure in response to physiologic disturbances can be dramatic. For example, in tissue that has suffered thermal trauma, P_i may decrease manyfold over baseline values, thus, in part, accounting for the rapid accumulation of interstitial fluid seen with burn injuries.[14] The molecular mechanisms underlying control of interstitial pressure are not clear, but the binding of collagen molecules on the surface of adventitial cells may play a role, because antibodies to the β_1-integrin lowers interstitial pressure and prompts edema formation.[15]

Microvascular protein osmotic pressure, π_{mv}, has been the focus of investigation and clinical study in order to understand better whether changing this value can improve total body fluid balance.[16,17] In the strictest analysis, π_{mv} should be measured for each plasma protein constituent along with the corresponding σ, but like the aforementioned P_{mv}, a net value of osmotic pressure generated by the sum of plasma proteins suffices to account qualitatively for the relative importance of plasma oncotic pressure to transvascular fluid filtration. The value of transvascular differences in protein osmotic pressure as an important feature of transvascular fluid filtration is highlighted by recognizing that the osmotic force of all components of the extracellular fluid is on the order of 5000 to 6000 mm Hg, but because these components pass unimpeded across the endothelial barrier of the microcirculation (that is, they have a reflection coefficient of 0), they exert no influence on fluid flux.[18] Because plasma proteins do not move with complete freedom across the circulation, they have a significant effect on fluid filtration, despite an osmotic pressure in plasma in the range of 10 to 20 mm Hg.

Interstitial protein osmotic pressure, π_i, has been measured by direct micropuncture techniques, implanted tissue capsules, and absorbent materials placed within the tissue space.[8,18] In vivo measurements of π_i have relied on collection of lymph from organs of interest, with the assumption that protein concentration of lymph is equivalent to that of interstitial fluid (likely a safe assumption under steady-state conditions when lymph is collected from afferent lymphatics).

The membrane parameter, σ, represents the sieving ability of a semipermeable membrane for protein. High values of σ imply that osmotic pressure differences across the vascular barrier will exert a greater effect on fluid flux than will lower values of σ. One can measure σ in vitro as the ratio between the measured and expected osmotic pressure generated by the protein of interest. Furthermore the value of this coefficient can be estimated in vivo from experiments in which transvascular fluid filtration is maximized (i.e., under conditions in which protein flow is nearly all convective).

Equation 1 describes the driving forces for transvascular fluid movement, but a different mathematical relationship exists for describing transvascular protein movement. This relationship contains two components, one describing flow of protein as a result of convective movement:

$$J_s = (1 - \sigma)P\,J_v$$

where J_s is transvascular protein flow, σ is the protein reflection coefficient, P is the concentration of protein in the vasculature, and J_v represents net transvascular fluid movement. The second relationship describes the flow of protein as a result of diffusion:

$$J_s = K(P - L)$$

where K is the product of the permeability and surface area of the microcirculation, and P and L represent the concentration of protein in the vasculature and lymph (interstitium), respectively. Combining these two equations yields the equation that describes net total transvascular protein movement:

$$J_s = (1 - \sigma)P\,J_v + K(P - L)$$

Under steady-state conditions, lymph will contain all the transvascular protein filtered if no metabolism occurs in the interstitium, and thus J_s reduces to LJ_v. In this analysis, J_v is equal to lymph flow and L is equal to lymph protein concentration. Rearranging the above equation, simplifying it, and setting up experimental conditions in which lymph flow is maximized yields the equation $\sigma = 1 - L/P$.[19] When measured experimentally, σ is well over 0.5 in most tissue beds and usually in the range of 0.75 to 0.90, even in the neonate[20] Capillary beds that contain fenestrations, as in the liver, represent little restriction to transvascular protein movement, and under such conditions σ would be low. On the other hand, capillaries in other vascular beds contain few, if any, discontinuous regions, and σ under these circumstances would be closer to 1. The closer σ is to unity, the greater the influence of plasma proteins on fluid filtration.[19]

The lower the value of σ, the less able are proteins to generate a force-counteracting fluid filtration. This arises for two reasons. First, with a less restrictive barrier, π_i increases numerically toward π_{mv} because the sieving quality of the membrane is diminished. Second, any difference between π_{mv} and π_i is minimized as σ decreases. Thus, under conditions in which the vascular barrier is injured, allowing a greater degree of protein leak, administration of protein intravenously to augment vascular protein osmotic pressure and reduce edema formation theoretically should have little, if any, effect. The administration of protein to affect fluid balance in some other fashion (for example, on barrier function per se or to provide other favorable effects unrelated to fluid balance (for instance, to maintain plasma drug-binding) may subserve some clinical benefit, but such a rationale would be independent of the presumed advantage of an increase in microvascular protein osmotic pressure on transvascular fluid filtration.

Finally, the coefficient K represents the product of barrier hydraulic conductivity and the surface area available for fluid filtration.[16] These two components of K are difficult to separate experimentally. Hydraulic conductivity itself is a function predominantly of the density of the pathways for liquid and solute movement and is not necessarily a measure of protein permeability. That is, more pathways, or pores, for solute and liquid exchange might exist under different conditions without the individual pathways being more permeable. Thus, changes in K may occur with true alterations in liquid and solute permeability (that is, pathways that allow passage of larger proteins), but changes in K may occur simply with an alteration in the density of pathways for liquid and solute movement or with changes in surface area for filtration, as would occur when unperfused capillaries are filled.

Consideration of Equation 1 allows several general statements about fluid filtration under normal conditions during steady-state.[19] First, because there is always some degree of sieving across the microvascular barrier, the protein concentration in the interstitium will be less than that in the vascular space. This difference in protein concentration yields a difference in protein osmotic pressures that is subtracted from the hydrostatic pressure difference term. In this sense, protein osmotic pressure attempts to balance the "edema-promoting" effect of microvascular hydrostatic pressure. Second, because there is net transvascular fluid filtration out of the circulation, the hydrostatic pressure difference term in Equation 1 must exceed the difference in osmotic pressure term when total body fluid balance is under consideration. There is no experimental evidence indicating the presence of net "active" transport of water and solute across the endothelium that would influence transvascular fluid flux.

Although the concepts expressed in Equation 1 serve physiologists and clinicians well when considering fluid balance in a general sense, the equation does not always allow a precise calculation of the change in fluid filtration (J_v) when one variable in the equation changes. This arises because a change in one of the variables in Equation 1 usually results in a change in one of the other variables, even if such a change is unexpected. For instance, under conditions in which microvascular hydrostatic pressure is increased, one might assume that transvascular flow will increase by an amount that can be arrived at arithmetically from Equation 1. When P_{mv} increases in the presence of a stable vascular barrier, J_v will increase, but as it does, interstitial protein concentration will decrease. This occurs because the driving force for liquid exceeds the bulk flow of protein across the barrier since σ is greater than 0 for protein; there is no sieving of water. When interstitial protein concentration is reduced, the protein osmotic pressure difference between the vascular and interstitial spaces increases. Thus from Equation 1, J_v will increase in response to an increase in P_{mv}, but as ($\pi_{mv} - \pi_i$) becomes larger, J_v will assume a new steady-state value that will be less than that predicted by the increase in P_{mv} alone. Additionally, if excess fluid expands the interstitium, interstitial pressure will increase to some extent, although the magnitude of this change is not predictable because tissue space compliance is not linear in the presence of increasing interstitial edema. This increase in tissue hydrostatic pressure will also act to slow transvascular fluid movement. Changes that occur in driving forces for filtration that counteract the change in the "edema-promoting" variable are referred to as the "edema safety factors." The implication of the edema safety factors is that increases in transvascular filtration are blunted because of the countervailing changes seen in other variables in Equation 1.[8,16,18,19]

LYMPH FLOW MODULATION OF EDEMA

An increase in interstitial fluid volume can be conceptually understood as an inability of the lymphatic system to remove fluid at the same rate as has been filtered across the microcirculation. Lymphatics are present in most, but not all, tissue beds.[19] The brain, specific areas of the eye, and bone marrow are examples of organs that do not contain lymphatics. With regard to fluid balance, lymphatics serve to transport not only water but also proteins back into the circulation. Without the return of protein to the circulation, protein concentration differences between the interstitium and circulation would narrow. Lymphatics are located primarily in loose connective tissue spaces and appear to end bluntly. Like blood vessel capillaries, there is no smooth muscle around the smallest terminal lymphatics, but actin filaments have been observed in lymphatic endothelium, suggesting that the initial lymphatics may possess contractile properties. As the lymphatic vasculature is traced centrally, valves appear, and smooth muscle cells surrounding the lymphatics are more consistently observed. Lymphatics ultimately drain into the central circulation through the thoracic and right lymphatic ducts. The movement of interstitial fluid from the tissue space into the terminal lymphatics requires a driving force. Experimental evidence points to the importance of both interstitial pressure and interstitial volume in modulating lymph flow. However, an increase in interstitial pressure alone, in the absence of a change in interstitial volume, would be unlikely to result in a hydrostatic pressure gradient sufficient to account for lymphatic filling. It is the combination of anchoring filaments attached to the external wall of the lymphatics and an increase in interstitial volume that results in a pressure gradient sufficient to account for initial lymphatic filling.[18,19]

Lymph drainage is not constant but rather varies with changes in filtration driving force.[16] Thus, lymph drainage can also be considered an edema safety factor. Interstitial pressure is closely associated with lymph flow, but the relationship between interstitial pressure and lymph flow is not linear over all tissue pressures. Although an association exists between interstitial pressure and lymph flow, other factors also influence lymphatic clearance. One of the most important is the presence of valves within the lymphatics that provide directionality to flow.[19] Valves also reduce the direct influence of downstream outflow pressure on transendothelial fluid movement into the terminal lymphatics. Lymph is propelled centrally by extrinsic and intrinsic factors. Extrinsic forces include both passive and active muscular movement. Intrinsic forces are those associated with spontaneous lymph vessel contraction and relaxation. Motion associated with respiration and with blood vessel pulsation also contributes to lymphatic movement.

Effect of Outflow Pressure on Lymphatic Drainage

Lymph from large collecting vessels ultimately drains into the central circulation. If lymph drainage is obstructed, interstitial tissue volume increases and edema becomes obvious, implying that outflow pressure is an important variable influencing the effectiveness of lymph drainage.[21] Because the outflow pressure for the thoracic duct is the central venous circulation, an increase in central venous pressure should be an important

factor influencing lymph drainage. Experimental evidence from fetal and adult animals confirms this supposition.[22-24]

MOVEMENT OF PROTEIN ACROSS THE MICROVASCULAR BARRIER

The specific site of fluid and protein transfer along the circulation is likely variable within an organ and among tissues. Venules, arterioles, and capillaries may each contribute to transvascular fluid filtration. Molecular size plays a role in transvascular filtration, with ease of transport into the interstitium being inversely proportional to size.[17] Proteins cross the endothelium through channels or pores and by transcytosis, but the magnitude of each to total transvascular protein movement is debated.[25] The importance of protein movement through pores of various sizes in the vascular barrier is highlighted by studies that show that protein moves into the interstitium closely linked to the flow of liquid, that is, moving by convection or bulk flow. In the lung, inhibitors of transcytosis do not significantly decrease transvascular protein transport, casting doubt on the importance of transcytosis as an important pathway for transvascular protein movement involved in fluid balance.[26]

The morphologic basis for an increase in microvascular permeability is not completely resolved. Under some conditions, gaps between endothelial cells can be seen microscopically, but this is not a consistent observation.[25] Intercellular proteins between endothelial cells are linked to actin and other intracellular structures that are thought to regulate microvascular protein permeability by rearrangement of the cytoskeleton. Cellular contraction is thought to be the means by which intercellular gaps are formed and thus permeability regulated.[27]

Like studies examining the morphologic basis for permeability changes, the molecular basis for changes in permeability is incompletely understood.[28-30] Clinically, inflammatory processes are frequently associated with changes in permeability. The molecular initiation of permeability occurs, at least in a number of circumstances, as a result of calcium-dependent events. Calcium entry appears to be regulated, at least in part, by potassium modulation of transmembrane potential and not through voltage-regulated calcium channels. An increase in intracellular calcium is thought to promote myosin light chain phosphorylation by kinases and thus initiate contraction. Although mediator-induced changes in cytosolic calcium concentration are common, the fact that intracellular calcium may be influenced by novel means is shown by experiments in which surface molecules not thought to be receptors for the typical inflammatory ligands influence vascular permeability. A well-studied example is the ligation of the luminal surface integrin, $\alpha_v\beta_3$, on the microvasculature.[31] Another effect of an increase in intracellular calcium is the modulation of nitric oxide synthesis and the generation of cyclic guanosine monophosphate (cGMP). These mediators are known to affect vascular permeability, but the mechanism by which this occurs is unclear. Their effect may be indirect, perhaps by modulating the concentration of intracellular cyclic adenosine monophosphate (cAMP). cAMP blunts cell contraction and myosin light chain phosphorylation, but it also may influence the expression of molecules important in intercellular binding and thus limit the ability of the cytoskeleton to influence permeability.[25]

SPECIFIC CLINICAL CONSIDERATIONS: CHANGES IN TRANSVASCULAR FLUID FILTRATION WITH INTRAVENOUS PROTEIN INFUSIONS

Intravenous infusion of solutions containing protein or dextran are frequently administered to patients with edema to increase plasma protein osmotic pressure, in the expectation that transvascular fluid filtration will be less after the plasma protein concentration is increased. Experiments that address this issue show that infusing albumin in sufficient quantities to increase plasma albumin concentration by as much as 20%, or infusing dextran in sufficient quantity to increase plasma osmotic pressure by more that twofold, have little effect on steady-state lymph flow.[32,33] However, if microvascular hydrostatic pressure is then increased, the additional plasma osmotic pressure blunts the expected increase in transvascular fluid filtration. The explanation for this response is not completely forthcoming, but likely results from changes in hydraulic conductivity and from changes in the distribution of vascular resistance, resulting in changes in effective P_{mv}.

Experiments evaluating hypoproteinemia in the neonate predictably show that lymph flow increases when protein is removed from the circulation.[20,34] The explanations for this response are conflicting, but at least in the newborn lamb increases appear to result from a decrease in transvascular protein osmotic pressure difference and an increase in vessel hydraulic conductivity, but not from an increase in protein permeability. Whether albumin plays some role in maintaining the health of the barrier wall is uncertain. In vitro information suggests that albumin per se favorably influences the endothelial barrier.[35]

The preceding discussion examines the issue of plasma proteins and fluid balance in the context of a normally permeable microvascular barrier. When barrier integrity is compromised, the movement of protein is less restricted, the reflection coefficient is reduced, and any effect of protein osmotic pressure on fluid movement is minimized. Consistent with this theoretical analysis, experiments in which the lung microvasculature has been injured show no change in fluid movement out of the pulmonary circulation with the infusion of albumin.[36] Thus, any favorable effect of plasma protein osmotic pressure on transvascular fluid balance depends on the extent to which the endothelial barrier remains intact.

SPECIAL CONSIDERATIONS OF EDEMA IN THE FETUS

An edematous fetus, regardless of the etiology of the edema, is labeled with the diagnosis of hydrops fetalis. Over 100 different medical illnesses or conditions are associated with hydrops, but the pathophysiologic link between the condition and edema formation is not clear in many of these patients.[37] Approximately 75% of the cases of nonimmune hydrops in the United States occur in association with an identifiable disorder, and in the remainder the condition is labeled idiopathic.[38]

PROPOSED MECHANISMS OF EDEMA FORMATION IN PATIENTS WITH HYDROPS

From the foregoing discussion, it is seen that edema may form if the driving forces for fluid filtration or vascular permeability increase without a concomitant increase in lymphatic drainage. Although disturbances in microvascular permeability could be relevant in explaining some cases of fetal hydrops, there is no evidence at this time that vascular protein permeability is significantly different, at least in the lung; in the fetus, neonate, or adult; or between hydropic and nonhydropic fetuses.[7,39,40]

A variety of hypotheses might explain the pathophysiology of hydrops, but one that is most compatible with the current experimental evidence is that elevation of central venous pressure is a critical element in the pathogenesis of fetal edema. Conditions that elevate central venous pressure are common in hydropic infants and thus provide a compelling clinical link for this hypothesis. An elevation in central venous pressure will increase microvascular pressure upstream and thus enhance

transvascular fluid movement. An increase in central venous pressure also will impair lymphatic drainage into the central circulation and thus increase interstitial fluid volume. If lymphatic drainage is completely interrupted (an "infinite" central venous pressure), the fetus becomes hydropic.[21] In experiments designed to evaluate more modest effects of disturbances in central venous pressure on lymph drainage, thoracic duct lymph flow was found to be inversely proportional and linearly related to outflow pressure. In these studies, increasing central venous pressure by only 5 mm Hg impaired by nearly 50% the rate of lymph drainage.[24]

A helpful model that clarifies total body fluid dynamics in the presence of elevated central venous pressure is the fetal lamb that undergoes rapid atrial pacing. When fetal sheep are paced at rates of 300 to 320/min, central venous pressure nearly doubles, without changes in systemic arterial pressure, plasma albumin concentration, or vascular protein permeability.[41,42] Fetal edema occurs quickly, sometimes within 12 to 24 hours, indicating excessive transvascular fluid filtration, impaired lymphatic clearance, or both. Thoracic duct lymph flow increases by nearly 50% when measured at an outflow pressure equivalent to central venous pressure under baseline conditions, but when measured at the central venous pressure induced by pacing, lymph flow is significantly reduced. Thus, in conditions that increase central venous pressure, hydrops may be caused, or at least aggravated, by two distinct mechanisms: increased transvascular fluid entry and impaired interstitial fluid clearance.

Anemia is another human fetal condition often associated with hydrops. Exchange transfusion in fetal lambs sufficient to reduce hematocrit from 32% to 12% produces hydrops, but only if the anemia is associated with an increase in central venous pressure.[43] Whether edema develops may depend to a large extent on whether lymph drainage can accommodate the increase in fluid filtration.

In newborn sheep made hypoproteinemic, plasma protein osmotic pressure is reduced and transvascular fluid filtration increases, but no increase in interstitial fluid volume occurs, at least in the lung, because lymph flow increases to match transvascular filtration.[20,34] Likewise, in fetal sheep, simply lowering plasma protein oncotic pressure by removing protein from the circulation has no effect on total body water.[44] The lack of effect of hypoproteinemia on edema formation is likely a result of increased lymphatic drainage back into the central circulation. In isolated fetal hypoproteinemia, central venous pressure does not increase, and thus there is no impediment to lymph drainage back into the central circulation. The increase in fetal lymph flow is likely on the order of approximately 40%, similar to that seen in newborn lambs made hypoproteinemic.[20,34] Because fetal lymph flow can increase two- to fourfold over baseline values, increases in transvascular filtration prompted by hypoproteinemia can be easily accommodated by increases in fetal lymph flow.

REFERENCES

1. Witte CL, Witte MH: On the causation of edema: a lymphologic perspective. Perspect Biol Med 41:86, 1997.
2. Simpson J, Stephenson T: Regulation of extracellular fluid volume in neonates. Early Hum Dev 34:179, 1993.
3. Joles JA, et al: Plasma volume regulation: defenses against edema formation (with special emphasis on hypoproteinemia). Am J Nephrol 13:399, 1993.
4. Gold PS, Brace RA: Fetal whole-body permeability—surface area product and reflection coefficient for plasma proteins. Microvasc Res 36:262, 1988.
5. Brace RA, Gold PS: Fetal whole-body interstitial compliance, vascular compliance, and capillary filtration coefficient. Am J Physiol 247:R800, 1984.
6. Nicoll PA, Taylor AE: Lymph formation and flow. Annu Rev Physiol 39:73, 1977.
7. Bland RD, et al: Lung fluid balance in lambs before and after birth. J Appl Physiol 53:992, 1982.
8. Taylor AE: Capillary fluid filtration. Starling forces and lymph flow. Circ Res 49:557, 1981.

9. Cope DK, et al: Pulmonary capillary pressure: a review. Crit Care Med 20:1043, 1992.
10. Bland RD, et al: Lung fluid balance in hypoxic, awake newborn lambs and mature sheep. Biol Neonate 38:221, 1980.
11. Bressack MA, Bland RD: Alveolar hypoxia increases lung fluid filtration in unanesthetized newborn lambs. Circ Res 46:111, 1980.
12. Bland RD, et al: Effects of alveolar hypoxia on lung fluid and protein transport in unanesthetized sheep. Circ Res 40:269, 1977.
13. Reed RK, et al: Control of interstitial fluid pressure: role of beta$_1$-integrins. Semin Nephrol 21:222, 2001.
14. Lund T, et al: Acute postburn edema: role of strongly negative interstitial fluid pressure. Am J Physiol 255:H1069, 1988.
15. Reed RK, et al: Blockade of beta$_1$-integrins in skin causes edema through lowering of interstitial fluid pressure. Circ Res 71:978, 1992.
16. Taylor AE: The lymphatic edema safety factor: the role of edema-dependent lymphatic factors (EDLF). Lymphology 23:111, 1990.
17. Renkin EM: Some consequences of capillary permeability to macromolecules: Starling's hypothesis reconsidered. Am J Physiol 250:H706, 1986.
18. Aukland K, Nicolaysen G: Interstitial fluid volume: local regulatory mechanisms. Physiol Rev 61:556, 1981.
19. Aukland K, Reed RK: Interstitial-lymphatic mechanisms in the control of extracellular fluid volume. Physiol Rev 73:1, 1993.
20. Hazinski TA, et al: Effect of hypoproteinemia on lung fluid balance in awake newborn lambs. J Appl Physiol 61:1139, 1986.
21. Andres RL, Brace RA: The development of hydrops fetalis in the ovine fetus after lymphatic ligation or lymphatic excision. Am J Obstet Gynecol 162:1331, 1990.
22. Laine GA, et al: Effect of systemic venous pressure elevation on lymph flow and lung edema formation. J Appl Physiol 61:1634, 1986.
23. Brace RA: Effects of outflow pressure on fetal lymph flow. Am J Obstet Gynecol 160:494, 1989.
24. Gest AL, et al: The effect of outflow pressure upon thoracic duct lymph flow rate in fetal sheep. Pediatr Res 32:585, 1992.
25. Michel CC, Curry FE: Microvascular permeability. Physiol Rev 79:703, 1999.
26. Rippe B, Taylor A: NEM and filipin increase albumin transport in lung microvessels. Am J Physiol Heart Circ Physiol 280:H34, 2001.
27. Dudek SM, Garcia JG: Cytoskeletal regulation of pulmonary vascular permeability. J Appl Physiol 91:1487, 2001.
28. Lum H, Malik AB: Mechanisms of increased endothelial permeability. Can J Physiol Pharmacol 74:787, 1996.
29. Lum H, Malik AB: Regulation of vascular endothelial barrier function. Am J Physiol 267:L223, 1994.
30. Stevens T, et al: Mechanisms regulating endothelial cell barrier function. Am J Physiol Lung Cell Mol Physiol 279:L419, 2000.
31. Tsukada H, et al: Ligation of endothelial alpha$_v$ beta$_3$ integrin increases capillary hydraulic conductivity of rat lung. Circ Res 77:651, 1995.
32. Wareing TH, et al: Increased plasma oncotic pressure inhibits pulmonary fluid transport when pulmonary pressures are elevated. J Surg Res 46:29, 1989.
33. Demling RH, et al: Effect of albumin infusion on pulmonary microvascular fluid and protein transport. J Surg Res 27:321, 1979.
34. Cummings JJ, et al: Hypoproteinemia slows lung liquid clearance in young lambs. J Appl Physiol 74:153, 1993.
35. Schneeberger EE, Hamelin M: Interaction of serum proteins with lung endothelial glycocalyx: its effect on endothelial permeability. Am J Physiol 247:H206, 1984.
36. Nanjo S, et al: Concentrated albumin does not affect lung edema formation after acid instillation in the dog. Am Rev Respir Dis 128:884, 1983.
37. Jones DC: Nonimmune fetal hydrops: diagnosis and obstetrical management. Semin Perinatol 19:447, 1995.
38. Carlton DP, et al: Nonimmune hydrops fetalis: a multidisciplinary approach. Clin Perinatol 16:839, 1989.
39. Carlton DP, et al: Lung vascular protein permeability in preterm fetal and mature newborn sheep. J Appl Physiol 77:782, 1994.
40. Phibbs RH, et al: Cardiorespiratory status of erythroblastotic newborn infants. II. Blood volume, hematocrit, and serum albumin concentration in relation to hydrops fetalis. Pediatrics 53:13, 1974.
41. Gest AL, et al: Thoracic duct lymph flow in fetal sheep with increased venous pressure from electrically induced tachycardia. Biol Neonate 64:325, 1993.
42. Gest AL, et al: Atrial tachycardia causes hydrops in fetal lambs. Am J Physiol 258:H1159, 1990.
43. Blair DK, et al: Hydrops in fetal sheep from rapid induction of anemia. Pediatr Res 35:560, 1994.
44. Moise AA, et al: Reduction in plasma protein does not affect body water content in fetal sheep. Pediatr Res 29:623, 1991.

Philippe S. Friedlich and Istvan Seri

142 Regulation of Acid-Base Balance in the Fetus and Neonate

Most of the existing information on the regulation of acid-base homeostasis in mammals and humans was obtained from studies in adult subjects. With the current revolution in micromethodology and advances in understanding of developmental physiology and molecular biology, however, data have been accumulating on fetal and neonatal regulation of acid-base balance.

In general, acid-base homeostasis is tightly regulated by extracellular and intracellular buffer systems and respiratory and renal compensatory mechanisms of the organism. The normal range of hydrogen (H^+) ion concentration in the extracellular fluid is 35 to 45 mEq/L, corresponding to a pH of 7.35 to 7.45. Under physiologic circumstances, volatile and fixed acids generated by normal metabolism are excreted, and the pH remains stable.[1] Volatile carbonic acid is produced in the largest amounts, and it is readily excreted by the lungs in the form of carbon dioxide. Fixed acids, which include lactic acid, ketoacids, phosphoric acid, and sulfuric acid, are buffered principally by extracellular bicarbonate. The bicarbonate used in this process is then regenerated by the kidneys in a series of transmembrane transport processes resulting in the excretion of H^+ ions in the form of titratable acids and ammonium.

EXTRACELLULAR BUFFER SYSTEM

Using various acid-base pairs, the extracellular buffer system responds immediately to alterations in pH in a fashion represented by the *Henderson-Hasselbalch equation*. The carbonic acid–bicarbonate system is the most important component of this buffer system. Because the *isohydric principle*[2] allows one to follow the changes in the concentrations of a single acid-base pair as an indicator of acid-base homeostasis for the entire system, serial measurements of the carbonic acid–bicarbonate buffer system have been used to describe accurately the changes in both experimental and clinical settings.

INTRACELLULAR BUFFER SYSTEM

The most important components of the intracellular buffer system are the hemoglobin and intracellular proteins and phosphates acting as an intracellular H^+ sink and reservoir attached to the extracellular buffers. This system provides buffering at a slower rate compared with extracellular buffers and requires several hours to reach maximum capacity.[3]

RESPIRATORY COMPENSATORY MECHANISM

Because of the open nature of the carbonic acid–bicarbonate system, normal gas exchange in the lungs serves as an immediate regulator of acid-base homeostasis by maintaining a normal arterial carbon dioxide tension, thus eliminating the excess carbon dioxide generated by an acid load. Activation of the respiratory compensatory mechanism is necessary, however, to return pH closer to normal. Full activation of this system occurs only a few hours after the development of metabolic acidosis, because (1) the movement of bicarbonate across the blood-brain barrier is regulated by active transport mechanisms,[4] and (2) the central respiratory drive is triggered by low steady-state values of the cerebrospinal fluid and not by the plasma bicarbonate.[5] Because carbon dioxide moves freely across the blood-brain barrier,[5] cerebrospinal fluid and cerebral interstitial fluid H+ ion concentrations are altered more rapidly by respiratory acidosis, leading to an immediate activation of the respiratory compensatory mechanism in such cases.

RENAL COMPENSATORY MECHANISM

By altering renal H+ excretion, renal compensation is the ultimate mechanism to adjust H+ content in the body.[6] This system, however, requires hours to 2 to 3 days for a full response.

REGULATION OF ACID-BASE BALANCE IN THE FETUS

Fetal Extracellular Buffer System

The fetus has an intact extracellular buffer system. The carbonic acid–bicarbonate buffer system is especially important because it contains a volatile element, carbon dioxide gas. For the fetus, the placenta is the organ of respiration, and it quickly eliminates excess carbon dioxide generated by the development of fetal metabolic acidosis, provided placental function, uterine and umbilical blood flows, and maternal respiratory status are uncompromised.[7]

Fetal Intracellular Buffer System

Although the fetus has a significantly smaller intracellular compartment compared with the child or adult, its intracellular buffering capacity is still considerably larger than the extracellular capacity.[7]

Fetal Respiratory and Renal Compensatory Mechanisms

The respiratory and renal compensatory mechanisms of the fetus are limited by its level of maturity and by the surrounding maternal environment. The placentomaternal unit performs most of the effective compensatory functions.[7] However, the fetal kidney has the ability to contribute to the maintenance of fetal acid-base balance. For instance, ammonium excretion and hence generation of bicarbonate as well as sodium excretion have been documented to increase during the recovery period from hypocapnic hypoxia in fetal sheep.[8]

Fetal Metabolic Acidosis

The most frequent cause of fetal metabolic acidosis is fetal hypoxemia, owing to abnormalities of uteroplacental function or blood flow, or both. Primary maternal hypoxemia or maternal metabolic acidosis secondary to maternal diabetes mellitus, sepsis, or renal tubular abnormalities is an unusual cause of fetal metabolic acidosis. During the course of fetal hypoxemia, metabolism becomes anaerobic, and large quantities of lactic acid accumulate. H+ ions are buffered by the extracellular and intracellular buffering systems, and pH drops as plasma bicarbonate decreases. Because of the unhindered diffusion of carbon dioxide through the placenta,[9] restoration of fetal pH toward normal initially occurs through elimination of the volatile element of the carbonic acid–bicarbonate system by the maternal lungs. Lactate and other fixed acids cross the placenta more slowly,[7] however, so that effective maternal renal compensation of fetal metabolic acidosis is delayed. If fetal oxygenation improves, the products of anaerobic metabolism are also metabolized by the fetus.

Although metabolic acidosis stimulates fetal breathing movements,[10] the respiratory control system in the fetus is much less sensitive to changes in pH than after birth.[11] There is no physiologic significance, however, to this compensatory mechanism *in utero*.

Several lines of evidence indicate that the fetal kidney is able to excrete acid[12-14] and organic acids,[15] as well as to generate more bicarbonate.[16] Studies in fetal sheep have found age-dependent increases in glomerular filtration rate (GFR), urinary titratable acid, ammonium, and net acid excretion.[12] Furthermore, a positive relationship has been demonstrated between changes in GFR and bicarbonate, sodium, and chloride excretion.[12, 13] The fetal kidney, however, has a developmentally regulated limited ability to adapt to changes in fetal acid-base balance. In fetal sheep, in response to metabolic acidosis induced by the infusion of hydrochloric acid, blood pressure increases, whereas the GFR does not change. Urinary titratable acid, ammonium, and net acid excretion increase without significant changes in renal bicarbonate absorption.[14] Evidence also suggests that the fetal kidney has the ability to increase bicarbonate reabsorption, at least during periods of volume depletion.[16] With regard to the human fetus, only limited information is available concerning renal acidification.[17] The physiologic importance of these adaptive fetal renal responses, however, is limited when compared with responses in the postnatal period because the acid load excreted in the fetal urine remains within the immediate fetal environment and still has to be eliminated by the placenta or metabolized by the fetus.

Fetal Respiratory Acidosis

Fetal respiratory acidosis develops when prolonged maternal hypoventilation results from maternal asthma, airway obstruction, narcotic overdosing, maternal anesthesia, and magnesium sulfate toxicity. Fetal breathing movements increase, and the fetal kidney exerts a maturation-dependent limited response by reclaiming more bicarbonate in an attempt to restore the 20:1 ratio of bicarbonate to carbonic acid and thus increase the pH toward normal.[7] Obviously, the renal compensation has only limited physiologic significance for the fetus in cases of respiratory acidosis.

Fetal Metabolic Alkalosis

Metabolic alkalosis rarely affects the fetus, but it may occur in hyperemesis gravidarum. As a result of the significant hydrogen chloride losses in this condition, bicarbonate is retained by the mother to maintain anionic balance with sodium in the serum. Because bicarbonate is transported slowly across the placenta, the development of fetal metabolic alkalosis lags behind that of the mother. Maternal hypoventilation (as compensation for the metabolic alkalosis) tends to restore normal pH in the fetus as a result of the rapid movement of carbon dioxide across the placenta.

Fetal Respiratory Alkalosis

The *physiologic hyperventilation* of the pregnant woman causes a compensatory decrease in her serum bicarbonate concentration to approximately 22 mM.[7] Acute hyperventilation, however, may lead to the development of fetal metabolic acidosis because it induces uterine vasoconstriction.[18] In such cases, restoration of maternal carbon dioxide levels rapidly corrects both the abnormal uterine blood flow and the acid-base abnormality in the fetus.

REGULATION OF ACID-BASE BALANCE IN THE NEONATE

The neonate continues to undergo maturation of the overall adaptive responses to changes in acid-base homeostasis. Available information suggests that an abrupt increase in the sensitivity of the central respiratory control system to pH changes occurs at the time of delivery, and regulation of acid-base balance becomes tighter postnatally compared with that in the fetus.[11] The cellular mechanism responsible for the increased sensitivity of the acid-base balance regulation system is not known.

Neonatal Extracellular and Intracellular Buffer Systems

The neonate has well-functioning extracellular and intracellular buffering systems. Postnatally, the gradual increase in the intracellular compartment further enhances the overall buffering capacity.

Neonatal Respiratory Compensatory Mechanism

With postpartum establishment of the functional residual capacity, the neonate's lungs become the end-organ of the respiratory compensatory mechanism to changes in acid-base balance. Respiratory acidosis induces immediate increases in ventilation because carbon dioxide diffuses freely across the blood-brain barrier.[5] In the case of metabolic acidosis, however, full respiratory compensation is delayed for a few hours until cerebrospinal fluid and cerebral interstitial bicarbonate completely equilibrate with plasma bicarbonate.[4]

The effectiveness of respiratory compensation depends on the maturity of the central respiratory control system and pulmonary function. Because central respiratory control is sensitive to changes in cerebral interstitial pH in the neonate,[4, 11] the effectiveness of the postnatal respiratory response depends mainly on pulmonary function. Therefore, neonates with parenchymal lung disease have a limited ability to increase ventilation in response to metabolic acidosis.

Neonatal Renal Compensatory Mechanism

As mentioned earlier, by regulating bicarbonate and acid secretion in response to changes in extracellular pH, renal compensation is the ultimate mechanism to adjust the H+ content of the body. Although full activation of this system usually requires 2 to 3 days, alterations in renal acidification may be seen as early as a few hours after the development of acid-base disturbance.

The renal compensatory mechanisms of the neonate are immature and result in a developmentally regulated decreased ability to maintain acid-base balance.[19, 20] Both renal microhemodynamic and tubular epithelial factors play a role in the limited renal compensatory capacity of the newborn.

Renal blood flow significantly increases after the immediate postnatal period, and the vasodilatory mechanisms appear to be functionally mature as early as the 24th week of gestation.[21] GFR is also very low in the immediate postnatal period, and it increases as a function of both gestational and postnatal age.[22, 23] The low GFR is one of the most important factors limiting the ability of the preterm and term infant to handle an acid load adequately.[19, 20] Net renal acid excretion also depends on several gestational and postnatal age dependent tubular epithelial functions.[20, 24] Under physiologic conditions in the proximal tubule, four transport mechanisms regulate active acid extrusion and transepithelial bicarbonate reabsorption: the H+-ATPase, the electrogenic sodium/bicarbonate ($Na^+/3HCO_3^-$) co-transporter, the sodium, potassium-adenosine triphosphatase (Na,K+-ATPase)–driven secondary active Na^+/H^+ antiporter, and the Na,K+-ATPase–driven tertiary active Na+-coupled organic ion transporter.[24] Because approximately 85 to 90% of the filtered bicarbonate is reabsorbed in the proximal tubule,[20, 24] the function of these proximal tubular transporters essentially determines the renal threshold for bicarbonate reabsorption. The bicarbonate threshold is 18 mEq/L in the premature infant and 21 mEq/L in the full-term infant, and it reaches adult levels (24 to 26 mEq/L) only after the first year of life.[25, 26] In the extremely premature neonate, however, the renal bicarbonate threshold may be as low as 14 mEq/L. Because renal carbonic anhydrase is present and active during fetal life,[27] and because its activity is similar in the 26-week-old extremely immature neonate to that of the adult,[28] a developmentally regulated immaturity of the expression, molecular structure, membrane assembly, or second-messenger and third-messenger function of the previously described proximal tubular transporters is most likely responsible for the low bicarbonate threshold during early development. Indeed, both the activity and the hormonal responsiveness of the proximal tubular Na^+,K+-ATPase are decreased in younger rather than older animals.[29]

Medications used in the treatment of critically ill neonates may also affect proximal tubular bicarbonate reabsorption. For example, dopamine administration may potentially decrease the low bicarbonate threshold of the neonate,[30] because the drug inhibits activity of the proximal tubular Na^+/H^+ antiporter.[31] Carbonic anhydrase inhibitors also decrease proximal tubular bicarbonate reabsorption by limiting bicarbonate formation and H+ ion availability for the Na^+/H^+ countertransporter. Furosemide acts on several transport proteins along the nephron, and it directly increases urinary excretion of titratable acids and ammonium.[32]

Under physiologic circumstances, the distal nephron reabsorbs the remaining 10 to 15% of filtered bicarbonate through transport mechanisms similar to those of the proximal tubule.[24] An important difference between proximal and distal tubular bicarbonate reabsorption is the absence of the carbonic anhydrase enzyme in the distal tubule.[24] Net H+ ion secretion in the distal nephron continues even after the reabsorption of virtually all bicarbonate through active H+ secretion and the ability of the distal tubular epithelium to maintain large transepithelial concentration gradients for H+ and bicarbonate.[24] Among the endocrine factors influencing distal tubular acidification, aldosterone is one of the most important hormones.[24] By affecting the function of several different transport mechanisms, aldosterone stimulates net H+ ion excretion in the distal nephron. The distal nephron of the premature neonate, however, has a developmentally regulated relative insensitivity to aldosterone.[26, 33]

The secreted H+ ions are excreted in the urine in the form of titratable acids (phosphate and sulfate salts) and as ammonium salts, which are formed by the combination of H+ with ammonia.[24] Because the major constituent of titratable acid in the urine is phosphoric acid, drugs that decrease proximal tubular phosphate reabsorption and thus increase the delivery of phosphate to the distal nephron may increase the renal acidification capacity of the neonate. Indeed, by inhibiting proximal tubular phosphate reabsorption, dopamine has been shown to increase the excretion of titratable acids in preterm infants.[34]

Urinary excretion of titratable acid and ammonium increases as a function of gestational and postnatal age.[20] However, because the ability to acidify the urine effectively is acquired by the age of 1 month even in very premature infants, distal tubular H+ ion secretion appears to be inducible independent of the gestational age of the infant.[35]

Neonatal Metabolic Acidosis

The most frequent causes of increased anion-gap metabolic acidosis in the neonate are as follows: hypoxemia or ischemia secondary to perinatal asphyxia; severe lung disease; volume depletion; vasoregulatory disturbances; and myocardial dysfunction caused by immaturity, sepsis, or asphyxia. Severe metabolic acidosis caused by a neonatal metabolic disorder is rare but should always be considered. As discussed earlier, preterm neonates frequently present with a mild to moderate normal anion-gap acidosis, which is almost always the consequence of the low renal bicarbonate threshold of the premature kidney.[20, 25, 26] However, the use of carbonic anhydrase inhibitors and parenteral alimentation, as well as the maturation-related decreased sensitivity to aldosterone, may also contribute to the development of normal anion-gap acidosis in the neonate.[2,26,33]

In metabolic acidosis caused by the accumulation of lactic acid, H^+ ions are buffered by the extracellular and intracellular buffering systems; pH drops as the plasma bicarbonate concentration decreases. Restoration of pH toward normal initially occurs through elimination of the volatile element of the carbonic acid–bicarbonate system by the lungs. This process, however, may be severely compromised in the sick preterm and term neonate with parenchymal lung disease. As described earlier, the renal compensatory mechanisms are also less effective because of the developmentally regulated immaturity of renal function in the neonate. The main elements of the response of the neonatal kidney to metabolic acidosis in the immediate postnatal period are the attenuated increases in GFR, proximal tubular bicarbonate reabsorption, and distal tubular net acid secretion. A significant improvement in the overall renal response, however, occurs after the first month of life even in the premature infant.[20]

Neonatal Respiratory Acidosis

In the clinical setting, neonatal respiratory acidosis develops most frequently in preterm infants with respiratory distress syndrome. Although stimulation of the central respiratory center by the elevated interstitial carbon dioxide immediately increases respiratory rate and depth, carbon dioxide elimination by the lungs is usually limited because of immaturity and parenchymal disease. The kidneys reclaim more bicarbonate in response to respiratory acidosis. However, renal compensation is limited by the developmentally regulated immaturity of proximal and distal tubular functions, especially during the first few weeks of life.

Neonatal Metabolic Alkalosis

Metabolic alkalosis most frequently develops in the preterm neonate who receives prolonged diuretic treatment for bronchopulmonary dysplasia. The respiratory response is a decrease in the rate and depth of breathing to increase carbon dioxide retention. This response may not be effective if the intubated neonate is relatively overventilated with the mechanical ventilator. In response to a metabolic alkalosis, urinary bicarbonate reabsorption and distal tubular net acid excretion fall, resulting in a return of the extracellular pH toward normal.

Neonatal Respiratory Alkalosis

Neonatal respiratory alkalosis occurs most frequently secondary to fever and iatrogenic hyperventilation of the intubated preterm and term infant. Rarely, respiratory alkalosis may be the presenting sign of a urea cycle disorder during the first days of life because rising ammonia levels may initially stimulate the central respiratory center. Renal compensation plays an important, although limited, role in cases of respiratory alkalosis in the neonate.

SUMMARY

The fetus and the neonate exhibit a limited ability to maintain and regulate acid-base homeostasis. Regardless of the state of maturity, however, an abrupt increase in the sensitivity of acid-base regulation occurs with delivery. The mechanisms for this accelerated maturation are unclear.

REFERENCES

1. Masoro EJ: An overview of hydrogen ion regulation. Arch Intern Med 142:1019, 1982.
2. Brewer ED: Disorders of acid-base balance. Pediatr Clin North Am 37:429, 1990.
3. Kaehny WD: Pathogenesis and management of respiratory and mixed acid-base disorders. In Schrier RW (ed): Renal and Electrolyte Disorders, 3rd ed. Boston, Little, Brown and Co, 1986, p 187.
4. Vogh BP, Maren TH: Sodium, chloride, and bicarbonate movement from plasma to cerebrospinal fluid in cats. Am J Physiol 228:673, 1975.
5. Sorensen SC: The chemical control of ventilation. Acta Physiol Scand Suppl 361:1, 1971.
6. Gennari FJ, Maddox DA: Renal regulation of acid-base homeostasis. In Seldim DW, Cicbisch G (eds): The Kidney: Physiology and Pathophysiology, 2nd ed. New York, Raven Press, 1992, pp 2695–2732.
7. Blechner JN: Maternal-fetal acid-base, physiology. Clin Obstet Gynecol 36:3, 1993.
8. Gibson K, et al: Renal acid-base and sodium handling in hypoxia and subsequent mild metabolic acidosis in foetal sheep. Clin Exp Pharmacol Physiol 27:67, 2000.
9. Blechner JN, et al: A study of the acid-base balance of fetal sheep and goats. Q J Exp Physiol 45:60, 1960.
10. Molteni RA, et al: Induction of fetal breathing by metabolic acidemia and its effect on blood flow to the respiratory muscles. Am J Obstet Gynecol 136:609, 1980.
11. Jansen A, Shernick V: Fetal breathing and development of control of breathing. J Appl Physiol 70:143, 1991.
12. Kesby GJ, Lumbers ER: Factors affecting renal handling of sodium, hydrogen ions, and bicarbonate in the fetus. Am J Physiol 251:F226, 1986.
13. Hill KJ, Lumbers ER: Renal function in adult and fetal sheep. Dev Physiol 10:149, 1988.
14. Kesby GJ, Lumbers ER: The effects of metabolic acidosis on renal function of fetal sheep. J Physiol (Lond) 396:65, 1988.
15. Elbourne I, et al: The secretion of organic acids and bases by the ovine fetal kidney. Exp Physiol 75:211, 1990.
16. Robillard JE, et al: Influence of fetal extracellular volume contraction on renal reabsorption of bicarbonate in fetal lambs. Pediatr Res 11:649, 1977.
17. Blechner JN, et al: Effects of maternal metabolic acidosis on the human fetus and newborn infant. Am J Obstet Gynecol 9:46, 1967.
18. Moya F, et al: Influence of maternal hypoventilation on the newborn infant. Am J Obstet Gynecol 91:76, 1965.
19. Guignard JP, John EG: Renal function in the tiny premature infant. Clin Perinatol 13:377, 1986.
20. Jones DP, Chesney RW: Development of tubular function. Clin Perinatol 19:33, 1992.
21. Seri I, et al: Regional hemodynamic effects of dopamine in the sick preterm infant. J Pediatr 133:728, 1998.
22. Fawer CL, et al: Maturation of renal function in full-term and premature neonates. Helv Paediatr Acta 34:11, 1979.
23. Guignard JP, et al: Glomerular filtration rate in the first three weeks of life. J Pediatr 87:268, 1975.
24. Hamm LL, Alpern RJ: Cellular mechanisms of renal tubular acidification. In Seldin DW, Giebisch G (eds): The Kidney: Physiology and Pathophysiology, 2nd ed. New York, Raven Press, 1992, pp 2581–2626.
25. Avner ED, et al: Normal neonates and the maturational development of homeostatic mechanisms. In Ichikawa I (ed): Pediatric Textbook of Fluids and Electrolytes. Baltimore, Williams & Wilkins, 1990, pp 107–118.
26. Sulyok E, et al: Relationship between maturity, electrolyte balance and the function of the renin-angiotensin-aldosterone system in newborn infants. Biol Neonate 35:60, 1979.
27. Robillard JP, et al: In vivo demonstration of renal carbonic anhydrase activity in the fetal lamb. Biol Neonate 34:253, 1978.
28. Lonnerholm C, Wistrand PJ: Carbonic anhydrase in the human fetal kidney. Pediatr Res 17:390, 1983.
29. Fryckstedt J, et al: The effect of dopamine on adenylate cyclase and Na^+,K^+-ATPase activity in the developing rat renal cortical and medullary tubule cells. Pediatr Res 34:308, 1993.
30. Seri I: Cardiovascular, renal, and endocrine actions of dopamine in neonates and children. J Pediatr 126:333, 1995.
31. Felder CC, et al: Dopamine inhibits Na^+/H^+ exchanger activity in renal BBMV by stimulation of adenylate cyclase. Am J Physiol 259:F297, 1990.
32. Hropot M, et al: Tubular action of diuretics: distal effects on electrolyte transport and acidification. Kidney Int 28:477, 1985.
33. Stephenson G, et al: Ontogeny of renal mineralocorticoid receptors and urinary electrolyte responses in the rat. Am J Physiol 247:F665, 1984.
34. Seri I, et al: Effects of low-dose dopamine on cardiovascular and renal functions, cerebral blood flow, and plasma catecholamine levels in sick preterm neonates. Pediatr Res 34:742, 1993.
35. Stonestreet BS, et al: Renal function of low birth weight infants with hyperglycemia and glucosuria produced by glucose infusions. Pediatrics 66:561, 1980.

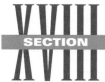

Developmental Hematopoiesis

Mervin C. Yoder

143 Biology of Stem Cells and Stem Cell Transplantation

Increasing attention has been focused on the biology of stem cells. The isolation of human embryonic stem (ES) cells has fueled speculation that these cells may be useful in the repair and regeneration of tissues and organs for a host of patient disorders. At present, much basic and translational research will be required to achieve the widely publicized therapeutic claims. It has become clear that the controlled differentiation of stem cells into specialized mature cells, the expansion of stem cells *in vitro* with retention of multipotentiality, and the best source of stem cells for a particular therapeutic application all remain to be determined.

This chapter introduces the reader to the broad field of stem cell biology. Stem cell terminology and discussion of the general categories of stem cells are presented first. Discussion of selected aspects of murine ES cell biology serves as an introduction to human ES cells. An overview of the biology of adult stem cell populations summarizes the chapter.

DEFINITION OF STEM CELLS AND STEM CELL TERMINOLOGY

The human body is composed of more than 200 different cell populations that are assimilated into multiple specialized tissues and organs of diverse functions. All these cells are ultimately derived from the "mother" of all stem cells, the fertilized oocyte. Whereas many tissues and organs are fully formed and the cell populations comprising these tissues are stable postnatally, other organs (e.g, blood, skin, and intestine) depend on a continuous influx of new cells to maintain tissue homeostasis throughout adult life. Thus, not only are stem cells required for the initiation of embryo formation, but also they are critical for homeostasis of the adult organism.

Stem cells are defined as cells possessing the capacity to self-renew (cell division giving rise to at least one cell retaining all the properties of the parent cell) and the ability to proliferate and differentiate into one or all of the more than 200 cell types comprising the fully formed body.[1] The fertilized oocyte or zygote is a *totipotent cell* that can form all the cells of all tissues and organs that form an embryo. *Pluripotent stem cells* are defined as cells that can give rise to cells developing from all three embryonic germ layers: endoderm, ectoderm, and mesoderm. The primary difference between pluripotent and totipotent cells is the ability of the latter to give rise to trophectoderm cells that form the placenta. *Bipotent and unipotent progenitor cells* give rise to cells derived from two or one of the germ layers, respectively.

Stem cells may be generally divided into ES and adult stem cell groups. ES cells are derived from the inner cell mass of the mammalian blastocyst.[2,3] When the inner cell mass cells are dispersed into preestablished cultures of murine embryonic fibroblasts, the resulting clones of proliferating cells are called *ES cells*. ES cells do not exist *in vivo*, but they develop *in vitro* from the cultured inner cell mass cells of the blastocyst. ES cells are pluripotent and display unlimited proliferative potential *in vitro* in the presence of embryonic fibroblasts. Murine ES cells can be maintained in the absence of the feeder layers when they are fed high concentrations of leukemia inhibitory factor (LIF).[4] Murine ES cells maintained under these conditions *in vitro* retain the potential to form a complete embryo when they are injected into a recipient blastocyst and are implanted in the womb of a pseudopregnant dam.

A second form of stem cells derived from the embryo can be isolated from the developing gonads of fetal mammals.[5, 6] Recovery of developing murine gonads, dispersion of the germ cells onto a layer of embryonic fibroblasts *in vitro*, and passage of the resulting colonies lead to the isolation of *embryonic germ (EG) cells*. EG cells are also pluripotent, exhibit high proliferative potential, and must be maintained in culture similar to ES cells. ES and EG cells display similar capacities for differentiation into a variety of differentiated cell types *in vitro*.

Stem cells are said to differentiate when they divide, and at least one of the progeny commits to the activation of a new gene expression pattern or inactivation of the genes maintaining the stem cell state. These genetic changes cause the cells to take on new properties characteristic of mature cells of a particular tissue or organ. Once the ES or EG cells begin the commitment process to differentiate into a mature cell type, it is probably not possible for these cells to reacquire the pluripotentiality that is characteristic of a self-renewing ES or EG cell.

Adult stem cells are cells residing in tissues and organs that maintain homeostasis by repleting cells lost to cellular senescence, disease, or injury. The most widely recognized organs with stem cells include bone marrow, skin, intestine, and liver. However, the brain, cornea, retina, skeletal muscle, and dental pulp also contain renewable stem cells. Adult stem cells are also called *somatic stem cells* to distinguish them from the germ cells of the adult organism. Adult stem cells in general fail to display the *in vitro* proliferative potential of ES or EG cells, although these cells obviously self-renew for the life of the organism (or we would run out of blood, and intestinal villi, and skin, and so on). In general, adult stem cells display tissue-specific characteristics and differentiate into progeny specialized for the tissue or organ within which they reside. This fundamental tenet of biology is reflected in the clinical use of stem cells. Thus, when a patient needs a bone marrow transplant, hematopoietic stem cells are transplanted as the donor tissue and not stem cells derived from another organ.

Some adult stem cell populations have been demonstrated to give rise to progeny *in vitro* and *in vivo* that are not normally derived from that type of stem cell. For example, some bone marrow cells have been found to differentiate into cardiomyocytes in mice after experimentally induced myocardial ischemia.[7] This ability of an adult stem cell of one tissue to generate mature cells of another tissue type has been called *stem cell plasticity*. This is a relatively new concept and is not yet mechanistically understood. Evidence suggests that stem cell plasticity is a rare event, and it is unclear whether this phenomenon normally occurs to maintain homeostasis.[8]

A feature of most adult stem cells is the production of a variety of progenitor cell populations with varying levels of proliferative potential. For example, hematopoietic stem cell proliferation may cause one daughter cell to retain stem cell potential (self-renewal) but the other daughter cell to become a progenitor cell. The progenitor cell may retain the ability to proliferate into additional progenitor daughter cells, but it cannot regain the potential to recreate itself (self-renew). In a stepwise hierarchical fashion, progenitor cells become more committed to mature cell differentiation with each subsequent division and progressively lose proliferative potential.

ES, EG, or adult stem cells may or may not be clonally derived. *Clonality* is defined when all the cells in a population can be demonstrated to be the progeny of a single initiating stem cell. Several clonal human ES cell lines have been created.[9] Obtaining a clone of adult stem cells has been more difficult. Methods to isolate adult stem cells generally result in a mixture of stem and progenitor cells. This is an important point when considering the question of stem cell plasticity. As discussed later, the term *stem cell plasticity* should be reserved for those instances when it is clear that a single stem cell derived from one tissue can be demonstrated to give rise to a clone of progeny of another tissue.

EMBRYONIC STEM CELLS

Murine Cells

Isolation

Efforts to isolate murine cells with pluripotent properties began in the 1950s. Leroy Stevens observed that male mice of the 129 strain developed testicular teratomas, and cells from these tumors could be transplanted with recurrence of the teratoma.[10] Further studies revealed that fetal germs cells (derived from 129 strain of mice) implanted in the testicle could also give rise to teratocarcinoma formation. However, the most profound insight provided by these studies was that cells isolated from the inner cell mass of murine blastocysts also gave rise to teratocarcinomas on transplantation. Stevens called these cells *pluripotent ES cells*, the first such designation of inner cell mass–derived cells as ES cells.[11] However, the injected embryonic cells gave rise to carcinomas as well as teratomas in this model and became known as embryo carcinoma (EC) cells.

Two independent groups of investigators reported in 1981 that cells from the inner cell mass of the murine blastocyst could be maintained *in vitro* in a pluripotent state under defined conditions that in some cases included addition of conditioned medium from cultured teratocarcinoma cells.[3, 12] Growth of the cells from the inner cell mass required a co-culture system using preestablished murine embryonic fibroblast feeder monolayers. LIF was identified as the factor secreted by the embryonic fibroblast that was required to retain ES cells with high proliferative potential and to maintain pluripotency *in vitro*.[4] ES cells can be

maintained indefinitely without chromosomal aberrations under these culture conditions and contribute to the formation of extraembryonic, fetal, and germ cell lineages on reintroduction into donor blastocysts and transfer into the fallopian tubes of pseudopregnant female mice.

Maintenance of Self-Renewal

The molecular mechanisms that maintain ES cells in a self-renewal state are not clearly delineated. It is clear, however, that signals generated during LIF binding to the cell surface LIF receptor are sufficient to maintain pluripotency.[13] LIF binding to a cell surface heterodimeric receptor results in activation of numerous molecules including nonreceptor tyrosine kinases. These kinases subsequently activate nuclear transcription factors including signal transducer and activator of transcription 3 (STAT3). STAT3 activation alone is sufficient to maintain murine ES cells in a self-renewal state with inhibition of cellular differentiation.[14] STAT3 proliferative effects on ES cells can be blocked by activation of the extracellular regulated kinase (Erk) pathway. A balance between the differentiating effects of Erk kinase activation and the proliferative effects of STAT3 activation appears to play a key role in determining whether ES cells are maintained in a pluripotent state.[15]

Another hallmark of pluripotent ES cell homeostasis is expression of the nuclear transcription factor Oct-4. This factor is present in the mouse zygote and is required for normal formation of the blastocyst and maintenance of the pluripotent state of the inner cell mass and is also highly expressed in germ cells. Evidence to date implicates specific control of the level of Oct-4 expression for maintaining the pluripotent state.[16] Overexpression of Oct-4 in ES cells leads to differentiation of the cells along the endoderm and mesoderm lineages, and diminished expression inhibits trophectoderm formation. To date, only a few of the target genes regulated by Oct-4 have been identified; transcription of some is inhibited and of others is increased by Oct-4 binding to target sequences in these genes. In general, the current theory is that Oct-4 may prevent expression of those genes required for ES cell differentiation.

In Vitro Differentiation

The ability to culture pluripotent cells *in vitro* has permitted novel insights and greater accessibility into gene expression and cellular differentiation pathways than previously available during attempts to study the murine post-implantation embryo *in situ*. Removal of LIF from the culture medium initiates murine ES cell differentiation. Plating LIF-deprived ES cells on nonadhesive culture plates or semisolid medium (methylcellulose) or placing ES cells into suspended drops of culture medium induces the cells to form spherical structures called *embryoid bodies* (EBs).[17] Within the EB, cells derived from the embryonic germ layers develop with relationships similar to those of the developing embryo—embryonic endoderm on the exterior of the EB and mesoderm and ectoderm on the interior surrounding a fluid-filled cavity (yolk sac–like). ES cells present in the EBs differentiate into multiple mature cell types including neurons, pancreatic cells, blood cells, endothelial cells, cardiomyocytes, skeletal muscle cells, adipocytes, and numerous other cells.[18] By extrapolation, the ability of murine ES cells to proliferate extensively *in vitro* and to differentiate into specific cell types underlies the current enthusiasm for studying human ES cells as a future means to create mature cells to replace aged or damaged cells in human patients.

Human Cells

Isolation and Characterization

The isolation and characterization of human ES cells were reported in 1998.[2] In this study, infertile couples donated cleavage-stage human embryos, after informed consent and institutional review board approval of the study. From the 36 donor embryos, 20 were successfully grown to the blastocyst stage (day 5 after fertilization), immunosurgery was then performed to remove the trophoblast cells, and inner cell mass cells were plated on murine fibroblast feeder cell layers (similar to derivation of murine ES cells). Five ES cell lines from five separate embryos were derived, and each continuously proliferated for 6 months, and all were successfully cryopreserved. The karyotype of the ES cells was normal; three lines were female and two were male. The murine fibroblast monolayer was required to prevent the ES cells from differentiating. However, when the ES cells were allowed to overgrow and "pile up" on the feeder layers, the ES cells also underwent differentiation. Addition of human LIF to the human ES cells plated in the absence of mouse feeder layers failed to maintain ES cell pluripotency and growth. Therefore, one early notable difference between murine and human ES cells was the inability of LIF to maintain ES cell pluripotency in the human cells.

The morphology of human ES cells is similar to murine ES cells. Both demonstrate a high nuclear/cytoplasmic ratio with prominent nucleoli. Human ES cells form colonies *in vitro* that are not as compact as murine ES cells but are similar to rhesus monkey ES cells. Human ES cells express the cell surface markers SSEA-3 and alkaline phosphatase. Oct-4 expression is high, consistent with the self-renewal potential of these cells. Like murine ES cells, human ES cells express high levels of telomerase, an enzyme that lengthens telomeres that normally shorten with each cell division. Telomere length maintenance is a property of self-renewing stem cells and some cancer cells.

The most favored test of human ES cell pluripotency is injection of the cells into immunocompromised mice and observation for development of subcutaneous teratomas.[2] Analysis of the tissue in the teratomas has demonstrated that derivatives of all three embryonic germ layers are present. Two cloned human ES cell lines were derived from one of the original ES cell lines.[9] The cloned human ES cells formed teratomas *in vivo* similar to the original ES cell population. This result confirms that the progeny of a single human ES cell retains pluripotency, even though these cells have been passaged extensively *in vitro*.

In Vitro Differentiation

Advances in the *in vitro* differentiation of human ES cells into specific lineages have been reported.[19,20] The addition of retinoic acid and nerve growth factor to cultured human ES cells was reported to enhance neuronal cell differentiation significantly. The differentiated cells demonstrated extensive outgrowth of neuronal processes and expression of neuron-specific molecules. Co-culture of human ES cells with murine bone marrow or yolk sac cell lines induced hematopoietic differentiation *in vitro*.[21] The ES cell–derived hematopoietic cells expressed known human hematopoietic cell surface antigens and transcription factors. When they were plated in colony-forming cell assay cultures containing hematopoietic growth factors, numerous hematopoietic progenitor populations were identified. Hematopoietic cell maturation appeared to be normal. Finally, plating of human ES cells in conditions that promote EB formation resulted in spontaneous contractions in 8.1% of the EBs.[22] Cells from the areas of spontaneous contractions expressed cardiac-specific proteins and mRNA for cardiac-specific transcription factors, and they displayed morphologic evidence of sarcomeric organization and intercalated disk formation connecting adjacent cells. In addition, the ES cell–derived cells exhibited cardiomyocyte-like calcium ion transients that were synchronous with the recorded contractions and responded to both positive and negative chronotropic agents. These data suggest that human ES cells can be differentiated into neurons, hematopoietic cells, and cardiomyocytes *in vitro*. At present, it is unknown whether these cells would function *in vivo*, a critical experimental hurdle for which new transplantation models may be required.

Potential Uses

ES cells may hold the potential for replacing cells and tissues lost to a variety of devastating illnesses. Neurologic diseases, diabetes, heart failure, end-stage kidney disease, and liver failure are a few areas in which availability of a replenishable source of cells and tissues may provide new therapeutic alternatives. In addition, ES cells differentiated into certain tissues may serve as a powerful *in vitro* screening method for new pharmacologic agents, teratogens, and environmental toxins. However, to achieve these breakthroughs, much research is required to address the following questions: (1) What mechanisms maintain ES cells in a pluripotent state? (2) What cellular and molecular signals are required to activate ES cells to begin differentiating into a single specialized cell type? (3) Are ES cells homogeneous or heterogeneous? (4) Do all ES cells pass through a progenitor stage during the process of cellular differentiation? (5) What stage of differentiation of ES cells will be most optimal for transplantation? (6) How will differences in transplantation antigens between the ES cell–derived transplantable tissue and the host be overcome?

ADULT STEM CELLS

Hematopoietic Stem Cells: Murine Cells

Isolation

More information is known about the hematopoietic stem cell than any other stem cell population. In fact, hematopoietic stem cells currently represent the only stem cell population used as a standard therapy in human patients. The mouse has been an invaluable tool in the search for the hematopoietic stem cell that began nearly 50 years ago.

Whole body irradiation was noted to depress hematopoiesis and cause life-threatening pancytopenia (a condition in which all blood types are diminished in number in the bloodstream) in exposed mice. However, animals could be protected from radiation-induced hematopoietic impairment if the spleen of the irradiated animal was shielded from the radiation beam or if hematopoietic cells from another mouse were infused into the radiation-exposed animal.[23,24] Confirmation that blood cells and not plasma conferred radiation protection was reported soon after.[25] In 1961, Till and McCulloch[26] provided evidence that a single blood cell precursor (colony-forming unit–spleen cell) present in the bone marrow could be identified *in vivo* by intravenously injecting the donor marrow cells into a lethally irradiated recipient animal and examining the host spleen for blood cell containing colonies 8 to 12 days later. This experimental method advanced the study of blood cell production by supporting the concept of a transplantable hematopoietic precursor population that could produce numerous progeny *in vivo* and led the way to identification of hematopoietic stem cells.

Several assays of stem cell function have been developed. The current standard is to measure stem cell function by transplanting donor test cells into a lethally irradiated mouse and then documenting that donor-derived cells have replaced host blood cell lineages over a prolonged period (>4 months).[27] Analysis for donor derived cells in the host requires distinction of the exogenous and endogenous cells. Male-to-female mismatch transplants, use of congenic mouse strains that differ at one or two genetic loci, use of gene transfer to mark the donor cells, or application of fluorescent labeling dyes to the donor cells have all been successfully used to identify donor cells in the host. As a surrogate for the *in vivo* analysis of stem cell function, several *in vitro* assays whereby hematopoietic stem cells are co-cultured with stromal cells and the co-cultures are examined for prolonged production of colony-forming cells *in vitro* have been reported. A good correlation between the *in vitro* assays and *in vivo* repopulating activity has been reported when identifying stem cell activity in adult murine bone marrow cells.[28]

In mice, hematopoietic stem cell repopulating activity appears to be conferred by two populations of cells.[29] Some transplanted cells demonstrate the capacity to reconstitute the bloodstream of the irradiated host for several months and rescue the animal from pancytopenia. However, these short-term repopulating cells do not continue to produce circulating blood cell progeny after 3 to 4 months, and the bone marrow of animals reconstituted with these cells is devoid of donor stem cells that are capable of repopulating the hematopoietic system of a secondary recipient mouse on transplantation. However, long-term repopulating hematopoietic stem cells continue to produce hematopoietic progeny for the life of the primary recipient, and bone marrow from the primary recipient animal is capable of repopulating secondary recipient mice. Only recently have these two populations and even more committed progenitor cell populations been identifiable and amenable to isolation and study.[30]

Various techniques have been used to isolate hematopoietic stem cells. Stem cells can be separated from more committed cells using velocity sedimentation, adhesion, or exposure to chemotherapeutic agents. One useful method for isolating hematopoietic stem cells from mice takes advantage of the finding that stem cells express a variety of proteins and carbohydrates on their cell surface, some which appear to be hematopoietic specific. If monoclonal antibodies to these cell surface proteins are labeled with fluorescence-emitting molecules, the stem cells with bound antibodies may be analyzed and isolated by flow cytometry.[31] In the mouse, expression of antigens such as stem cell antigen-1 (Sca-1), c-Kit, CD34, CD38, CD43, CD44, CD45, Thy-1, and AC133, high expression of the ABCG2 transporter protein, and low expression of RNA- or DNA-binding dyes enrich for hematopoietic stem cells.[32] Stem cells do not express markers that are commonly expressed by myeloid and lymphoid lineages (lin) and therefore are described as lin⁻. Using multiparameter sorting, murine hematopoietic stem cells have been reportedly purified to homogeneity.[33, 34]

Characterization

The site of hematopoietic stem cell residence changes during murine ontogeny.[35] Hematopoietic cells first appear in the yolk sac on embryonic day 7.0 (E7.0). Although the immediate precursor of the first hematopoietic progenitor cells has not yet been identified, hematopoietic cells are known to emerge from the mesoderm cells that emigrate into the yolk sac after migrating away from the primitive streak during gastrulation. Stem cell activity has been identifiable in the yolk sac as early as E9.0 but only if the donor cells are infused into sublethally myeloablated newborn mice.[36] The first stem cells to repopulate lethally irradiated adult mice appear in the region of the developing gonads, mesonephros, and aorta on E10.[37] Stem cell activity is present in the fetal liver on E11.0 and subsequently is found in the blood, spleen, and marrow just before and after birth. The liver becomes significantly depleted of hematopoietic stem cells after 2 weeks of life, although stem cell activity can be identified in circulating blood and thus all organs in the adult mouse.[38] The spleen and marrow compartments are lifelong sites of hematopoietic stem cell production in the mouse. A direct comparison of hematopoietic repopulating ability of stem cells from each of these sites has not been conducted; however, fetal liver hematopoietic stem cell repopulating ability is nearly twofold greater than that of marrow-derived hematopoietic stem cells.

Murine hematopoietic stem cells are estimated to be present at a frequency of 1 per 10,000 to 1 per 100,000 bone marrow cells. The hematopoietic stem cells with the greatest repopulating potential in adult mice are characterized by preferential

existence in a quiescent state.[39] Most of these cells are arrested in the G_0 stage of the cell cycle. Two estimates of the turnover of the stem cell pool have been reported. Young adult mice were reported to have 8% of the stem cell pool randomly enter the cell cycle daily.[40] Using another method of analysis, hematopoietic stem cells were estimated to display a half-life (the time required for 50% of the cells to divide) of approximately 19 days.[41] Of interest, commitment of hematopoietic stem cells to the progenitor compartment results in an increase in the frequency of cells in cycle. One estimate of the total number of cell divisions required to produce a mature blood cell from an initiating hematopoietic stem cell ranges from 17 to 19.5 or an overall net amplification of between approximately 170,000- to 720,000-fold.[42]

The behavior of hematopoietic stem cells can be allocated into four general activities in the marrow environment: self-renewal, differentiation, migration, and apoptosis. Each of these activities is briefly discussed. The mechanisms that regulate the overall activity state of the marrow stem cell population remain elusive.

Self-Renewal Ability

Self-renewal divisions are difficult to prove *in vitro*. Such events clearly occur *in vivo* on bone marrow transplantation when the stem cell must not only repopulate all the mature blood cell lineages but also expand the stem cell pool to normal levels. Coculture of hematopoietic stem cells with certain hematopoietic stromal cells *in vitro* has permitted documentation of self-renewal divisions, as evidenced by maintenance or slight expansion of repopulating activity on transplantation.[43, 44] Certain growth factors (stem cell factor, LIF, and thrombopoietin) appear capable of stimulating hematopoietic stem cells to undergo limited self-renewal division *in vitro*.[45] Overexpression of the transcription factor HOXB4 permits extensive proliferation of hematopoietic stem cells *in vivo* and *in vitro*, with retention of repopulating ability inferring numerous self-renewal divisions.[46] Novel approaches such as identifying specific genes that are expressed in different populations of stem cells with differing repopulating potentials may provide new insights into the mechanisms regulating hematopoietic stem cell self-renewal.[47]

Differentiation

The stem cell theory of hematopoiesis states that the hematopoietic system can be viewed as being composed of a continuum of functionally distinct hematopoietic cell compartments. Once the commitment decision is made by a dividing stem cell, the progenitor cell gives rise to progressively more lineage committed hematopoietic progenitor cells and eventually mature blood cells. It remains unclear whether the commitment process occurs randomly (stochastic theory) or is deterministic (controlled by growth factors or other factors released into each specific microenvironment in which the stem cells reside). Nevertheless, evidence suggests that progenitor cells in each functional compartment express distinct combinations of cell surface markers that permit isolation and determination of the stage of hematopoietic commitment of these cells.[30]

Migration

Migration of hematopoietic stem cells through the circulation into developing organs is a hallmark of early fetal and neonatal hematopoiesis. Evidence confirms that hematopoietic stem cell migration throughout the systemic circulation is a consistent feature even in adult mice.[38] At present, it is unclear whether certain organ vascular beds sequester the circulating stem cells or whether the stem cells are randomly distributed throughout the systemic circulation. Progress has been made in identifying strategies to mobilize large concentration of stem cells into the circulation using growth factors and chemotherapeutic agents; however, the mechanisms regulating the constitutive release, circulation, and reentry of stem cells into the marrow compartment remain elusive.[48]

Apoptosis

The size of the hematopoietic stem cell pool remains relatively constant. One mechanism to regulate pool size is to control the rate of stem cell division tightly (see earlier). A backup mechanism is to stimulate apoptosis of stem cells if excessive numbers are produced. Evidence that apoptosis is an active component of normal hematopoietic stem cell homeostasis is derived from experiments in which overexpression of the anti-apoptotic protein Bcl-2 results in significant expansion of the total hematopoietic stem cell pool in transgenic mice.[49] Hematopoietic stem cells readily undergo apoptosis *in vitro* if they are not supplied with appropriate growth factors, serum, or hematopoietic stromal cells for co-culture.

Human Cells

Isolation

Identification of the human hematopoietic stem cell has relied heavily on correlations between murine and human *in vitro* hematopoietic colony-forming cell assays and murine transplantation experiments. Correlative data have also been obtained from canine and nonhuman primate transplantation models. Several xenotransplantation models in which human hematopoietic stem cells are infused into immunodeficient mice or preimmune fetal sheep *in utero* have permitted identification of cells with properties of human hematopoietic stem cells.[50, 51] However, the current standard for defining stem cell activity ultimately must rely on effective engraftment and repopulation of a human patient with the test cells.

The history of hematopoietic stem cell transplantation in human patients spans less than 50 years.[52] E. Donnall Thomas and colleagues[53] reported that careful filtering of human marrow to remove fat and bone particles allowed large amounts of marrow to be infused into patients, although with little clinical improvement. Many unsuccessful reports followed these early transplantation attempts and led to several decades of intense research in animal models, to understand better the complex biologic and immunologic barriers that needed to be overcome including graft-versus-host disease (GVHD), histocompatibility mismatch, and finding alternatives to total body irradiation as a pretransplant conditioning method.[52] Improvements in all aspects of clinical transplantation have resulted in a growing number of transplant recipients; more than 18,000 patients received a bone marrow transplant in the year 2000.

While the scientific foundation for effective clinical transplantation was being investigated, advances in the culture of marrow cells led to identification of human hematopoietic progenitor cells.[32] As in the mouse, human hematopoietic stem and progenitor cells can be isolated using monoclonal antibodies and flow cytometry. CD34 is an antigen expressed by most hematopoietic stem and progenitor cells, although endothelial cells also express this antigen. Some hematopoietic stem cells do not express CD34, and it is unclear whether these cells are the precursors for the CD34-expressing population. Some patients transplanted with CD34-expressing bone marrow cells have demonstrated multilineage engraftment more than 7 years after the procedure, a finding indicating that the CD34+ cells possess long-term repopulating ability. Other antigens expressed by the human hematopoietic stem cell population include c-Kit, Thy-1, CD133, and the ABCG2 transporter protein. The presence of this transporter protein results in rapid efflux of many different molecules including certain DNA dyes, thus allowing for selection of DNA dye low-staining stem cells referred to as a *side-population profile* on the flow cytometer.

When bone marrow cells are first depleted of all cells expressing mature blood cell lineage markers (lin) and are then selected for CD34 expression (CD34+lin-), the frequency of hematopoietic stem cells in the enriched population ranges from 1 per 200 to 1 per 500.[54] As noted earlier, analysis of human hematopoietic stem cell number and function is often inferred from experiments performed *in vitro* or from *in vivo* xenotransplantation assays. Plating of human marrow cells in colony-forming assays (to enumerate progenitor cell activity) or in co-culture with stromal cells to evaluate the proliferative potential of the cells may reflect the population of cells that retains the most potential. Intravenous administration of human hematopoietic cells into immunocompromised mice or the preimmune sheep fetus permitted assay of the ability of the human hematopoietic stem and progenitor cells to home to the marrow compartment and to produce committed progenitor and mature cells *in vivo*.[55] Although these types of stem cell transplantation models clearly have limitations, no better surrogate for human clinical transplantation currently exists.

Characterization

The site of human hematopoietic cell production also varies during *in utero* development. Although the exact site of origin of human hematopoietic stem cells remains elusive, evidence suggests that the intra-aortic clusters of cells identified in the month-old embryo may be one of the first sites composed of hematopoietic stem and progenitor cells.[56] The human fetal liver is a prominent site of hematopoiesis for much of the pregnancy. Circulating hematopoietic cells that engraft in immunocompromised mice have been identified in the second trimester. Umbilical cord blood is enriched in hematopoietic stem and progenitor cells; preterm infant cord blood is more enriched for these cells than cord blood derived from full-term infants. Umbilical cord blood cells engraft 10- to 50-fold better than adult marrow hematopoietic cells on transplantation into immunocompromised mice.[57] Cord blood hematopoietic cells have higher proliferative potential *in vitro* than adult marrow progenitor cells. No direct comparison of the hematopoietic repopulating ability of marrow cells isolated from young versus old subjects has been performed to date.

Administration of granulocyte colony-stimulating factor to human subjects results in mobilization of hematopoietic stem and progenitor cells into the systemic circulation. Combining granulocyte colony-stimulating factor administration with leukopheresis permits isolation of an enriched population of peripheral blood transplantable cells. Stem cell mobilization has become a preferred method for isolating cells for clinical transplants because of the increased numbers of cells recovered and the earlier neutrophil and platelet recovery in the conditioned patient.[32]

Human hematopoietic stem cells are difficult to maintain in culture. Most methods developed for expansion of hematopoietic cells *ex vivo* have resulted in large increases in the number of committed progenitor cells with loss of the stem cells. This is particularly true for culture conditions relying solely on combinations of recombinant growth factors to induce the cellular proliferation. The addition of extracellular proteins or certain endothelial or stromal cell lines appears to improve the *ex vivo* maintenance of the most primitive hematopoietic progenitor and stem cells while inducing overall cellular expansion.[58, 59]

Therapy for Human Clinical Disorders

Bone marrow transplantation is a potentially useful therapy for various cancers of the blood including acute lymphoblastic and myeloblastic leukemia, chronic myelogenous leukemia, Hodgkin disease, multiple myeloma, and non-Hodgkin lymphoma.[32] Transplantation can be performed using autologous (patient's own) cells or allogeneic (another person's) cells. Cells from the bone marrow or mobilized cells in the peripheral blood can be used for either type of transplant. Although autologous cells can be transplanted without concern for whether the cells will be rejected or induce GVHD, these cells may harbor the very transformed cells that the patient is receiving chemotherapy to eradicate. The use of flow cytometry to isolate hematopoietic stem cells can provide graft cells free of detectable tumor cells.

Allogeneic grafts for hematopoietic reconstitution in patients with cancer are rational because these donor cells are not contaminated with the cancer cells. However, both bone marrow and mobilized peripheral blood grafts contain T lymphocytes that will recognize host tissues as foreign on transplantation and will induce GVHD unless the host and donor share the same histocompatibility antigens (human leukocyte antigens [HLA]). HLA typing of the donor and host are routine, to obtain the best possible match. Because of the polymorphic nature of HLA genes, the probability of a match between a host and a sibling is only 25%.

In certain circumstances, the provision of donor-derived T cells in a HLA-matched allogeneic graft may cause a graft-versus-leukemia response and may actually help to kill the transformed cells in the patient. In fact, once transplanted cells have engrafted and the patient has recovered from any GVHD, peripheral blood lymphocytes from the graft donor can be recovered and infused into the patient to provide a stronger graft-versus-leukemia effect. This strategy has been used successfully in patients with chronic myelogenous leukemia.[52]

Allogeneic grafts are useful in the treatment of inherited blood disorders. Aplastic anemia, β-thalassemia, Blackfan-Diamond syndrome, sickle cell anemia, severe combined immunodeficiency, X-linked lymphoproliferative syndrome, and Wiskott-Aldrich syndrome are some of the candidate diseases for this therapy.[52] Single-gene metabolic defects such as Hunter syndrome and Hurler syndrome and certain forms of osteopetrosis are also amenable to bone marrow transplantation.

Umbilical cord blood is becoming a favored graft source when lack of a suitable HLA-matched donor is available. Mismatched umbilical cord blood appears to engraft with less GVHD in pediatric or adult patients when compared with partial mismatched marrow or peripheral blood grafts. The primary concern for using umbilical cord blood as a source of donor cells is that the number of hematopoietic stem cells in the cord blood sample may be limiting for large adult subjects. Efforts to expand the hematopoietic stem and progenitor cells in cord blood samples remain experimental (see earlier).

Improvements in gene transfer technology have resulted in the first examples of clinical cure of patients using autologous hematopoietic stem cells corrected by gene transfer. Four patients with immunodeficiency were successfully cured with restoration of circulating lymphocytes after transplantation of autologous stem cells corrected by retroviral gene therapy.[60] Additional progress in the use of lentiviral vectors to infect hematopoietic stem cells and the reported cure of murine forms of β-thalassemia after transplantation with human β-globin–expressing blood cells hold promise for human clinical trials.[61]

Neural Stem Cells

The central nervous system (CNS) is composed of hundreds of different types of neurons, astrocytes, and oligodendrocytes. Although the CNS is susceptible to the same environmental, genetic, metabolic, and infectious stressors as other tissues in the body, the neuronal cell types were thought to differ from cells in other organs in being completely postmitotic. However, numerous studies since the early 1990s provided compelling evidence that neurogenesis occurs in the adult brain, and cells are being continuously generated in some portions of the adult CNS.[62]

Furthermore, more recent techniques have permitted isolation of the neural stem cells (NSCs), and methods to expand, differentiate, and transplant these cells are being developed. Such rapid progress has been exceeded only by the growing hope of anticipated benefits generated by families of patients and patients suffering from CNS disorders.

Neurogenesis in the adult brain occurs in primarily two areas: the dentate gyrus (DG) of the hippocampus and the olfactory bulb (OB) in humans, rodents, and nonhuman primates.[63] The *neural progenitor cells* (NPCs) that give rise to the new neurons in the DG of the hippocampus are derived from the subgranular zone of the DG. The neuronal progeny and glial progeny of the NPC are formed in the granular layer of the DG after migration of the NPC into this layer. Functional connections with other neurons in the hippocampus are established in as few as 4 to 10 days after neuronal differentiation is initiated in the NPC progeny. NPCs that seed the OB are derived from the anterior part of the subventricular zone (layer of cells beneath the ependymal lining cells of the lateral ventricles).[64] Migration of the NPCs from the subventricular zone to the OB occurs through a rostromigratory stream composed of specialized astrocytes. Cell-to-cell communication between the NPC and the astrocytes is mediated by secreted glycoproteins on the surface of the NPC. Disruption of these important cellular interactions results in diminished NPC migration and a reduction in the size and organization of the OB.

Like the hematopoietic system, the neuropoietic system is a hierarchy with fully mature cells composing the base and NSC composing the apex of the pyramid. NSCs give rise to NPCs, which give rise to unipotent committed neural or glial progenitors. Unlike the hematopoietic system, little is known of the kinetics of neuronal turnover. Young rats appear to generate 9000 new neurons daily in the DG or about 0.1% of the total granule cell population.[65] Another estimate suggests that one new neuron is generated daily for every 2000 existing neurons in the mouse. Whereas neurogenesis (and the presence of NSCs) persists throughout adulthood in mammals in the DG and OB, the rate of neurogenesis diminishes with age.

Like other adult stem cells, NSCs are defined as CNS cells that can give rise to themselves in a self-replicating way and also can give rise to neurons, astrocytes, and oligodendrocytes. *In vitro* assays of neurosphere formation have proved useful in identifying the clonal proliferative behavior consistent with NSC. The standard method for isolating NSCs begins with dissecting tissue from a region in a fetal or adult brain known to harbor NSCs.[62] The tissue is disaggregated, and cells are plated in the presence of growth factors, such as epidermal growth factor (EGF) or fibroblast growth factor 2. NSCs present in the cultured tissue spontaneously form spherical structures. These neurospheres are highly proliferative and can be expanded into large numbers of cells. By withdrawing epidermal growth factor or fibroblast growth factor 2 or adding other morphogens, NSCs can be differentiated into specific cell types *in vitro* or can be transplanted *in vivo*, where the NSCs become incorporated into various central and peripheral nervous system cell types.[63]

NSCs have been difficult to isolate directly from CNS tissue. Successes in using specific monoclonal antibodies and flow cytometry have led to reports of NSC isolation from human fetal spinal cord and CNS tissue. These human NSCs express the cell surface AC133 antigen but not CD34 or CD45.[66] Single sorted cells were capable of initiating neurosphere cultures and could be recloned with retained neurosphere potential. Other similar enrichments of NSCs have been reported in rats and mice using both positive and negative selection strategies.[64] These techniques will permit rapid progress in understanding the growth and expansion requirements of NSCs and will permit comparisons of the molecular regulation of NSC self-renewal with other adult stem cell populations.

Although a detailed study of the biology of NSCs will require considerable time, use of neural tissue for human clinical transplantation has already proved feasible. What types of grafts will be the most desirable? Human fetal CNS tissue has proved effective in providing symptomatic relief in patients with Parkinson disease; however, technical and ethical issues may preclude provision of sufficient numbers of cells for wide application.[64] NSCs cultured to large cell concentrations would appear to be an ideal source of cells. Whether the NSCs isolated from fetal CNS tissue or adult tissue display similar *in vivo* repopulating ability has not been directly tested. The report of isolation of NPCs from postmortem human OB, DG, and the subventricular zone of the forebrain suggests another potential source of transplantable NPCs.[67] Finally, ES cells can be differentiated into numerous neuronal cell types and may serve as a source of cells for repair of CNS damage.

Hepatic Stem Cells

The murine liver is formed by migration of foregut endoderm cells into the septum transversum on E8.5. Interactions between the endoderm cells and both cardiac mesenchymal and endothelial cells are critical for liver formation.[68] The foregut-derived cells begin expressing α-fetoprotein on E9.0 and albumin soon after. Further differentiation into hepatoblast cells occurs over the next 24 hours. Several days later (E12), the bipotent hepatoblast cells begin to proliferate rapidly as they differentiate into hepatocytes and cholangiocytes (biliary tract precursors). Distinct patterns of gene expression along the primary cellular lineages in the liver are demonstrable from E16 onward.[69] The basic lobular structure of the liver is not fully formed until several weeks after birth. One interesting feature of liver development is the inverse relationship between the level of hematopoiesis in the rodent fetal liver and the synthetic, metabolic, and enzymatic functions of the organ. As the liver function rapidly increases over the first 2 weeks of life postnatally, the hematopoietic function of the liver diminishes.

The regenerative capacity of the mature liver is unique among solid organs.[70] Up to two-thirds of the fully mature rodent liver may be resected, and within 1 to 2 weeks, compensatory growth and restoration of cellular numbers and function by the remaining cells have occurred. Technically, the lost structures in the resected liver are not replaced or regenerated; instead, the remaining liver simply expands to the original mass of the organ. Surprisingly, this liver expansion results from proliferation of 70 to 90% of the hepatocytes in the unresected portion undergoing proliferation. It has been estimated that the proliferative capacity of adult hepatocytes is sufficient to repopulate up to two-thirds liver resection without the need to recruit progeny from liver stem or progenitor cell populations. To date, the mechanisms regulating the overall mass and turnover of liver parenchymal cells remain obscure.

There are certain experimental circumstances in which recruitment of hepatocytes from precursors can be demonstrated. In each case, proliferation and differentiation of the hepatic stem and progenitor cells can be induced only if there is a concomitant block in the proliferative ability of mature hepatocytes.[70] Thus, treatment of rodents with irradiation, carcinogens (ethionine, 2-acetylaminofluorene, and 3-methyl-4-dimethylaminobenzene), RNA and protein synthesis inhibitors (D-galactosamine), and DNA alkylating agents (retrosine) has been used to demonstrate appearance of a proliferative population of epithelial cells called *oval cells* in the periportal region.[70] Oval cells initially proliferate in the canals of Hering (luminal channels linking the hepatocyte canalicular system to the biliary tree) and then differentiate into hepatocytes and bile duct cells in mice and rats treated with the aforementioned injurious agents.[71] The finding that differentiating oval cells recapitulate

hepatocyte and bile duct gene expression patterns in a sequence similar to that seen during embryonic liver development strengthens the evidence that oval cells serve as a stem cell population for the liver.

Proof that oval cells repopulate the liver requires *in vivo* transplantation data. Limited hepatocyte and bile duct repopulation occurs in normal adult mice transplanted with oval cells isolated from D-galactosamine–treated rodents.[70] When the recipient animals underwent two-thirds partial hepatectomy alone, oval cell engraftment was observed, but proliferation was again limited. High levels of engraftment were observed only when the cells were transplanted into mice with an ongoing liver injury (inherited metabolic defect). In contrast, transplantation of oval cells from E12 to E16 rat fetal livers into normal adult hosts led to long-term engraftment of both hepatocytes and bile duct cells in up to 10% of the normal adult recipient liver. Whether this represents a difference in mouse and rat biology or young versus older donor oval cells remains to be determined.

Specific reagents to isolate hepatic stem and progenitor cells remain elusive. Suzuki and associates[72] used monoclonal antibodies and flow cytometry to isolate murine fetal liver progenitor cells expressing the α_6 integrin and the β_1 integrin. Fetal liver hematopoietic progenitor cells do not express this combination of integrins. In addition, the murine fetal liver progenitor cells did not express c-Kit, a tyrosine kinase receptor that is expressed by fetal liver hematopoietic stem cells. Some evidence has been presented that the pancreas possesses cells capable of differentiating into hepatocytes. Putative hepatic stem and progenitor cell populations from human liver and bone marrow have also been reported.[73] More controversial are several reports that bone marrow or hematopoietic stem cells possess the capacity to differentiate into hepatocytes and bile duct cells *in vivo* (see the later discussion of stem cell plasticity).[34,74]

In sum, the rodent liver possesses remarkable regenerative ability. Mature hepatocytes may be induced to proliferate and compensate for up to a loss of two-thirds of a mature liver. When the mature hepatocytes are inhibited in their proliferation, oval cells proliferate and differentiate to produce hepatocytes and bile duct cells. Whether oval cells or other stem cell populations participate in maintaining the hepatic parenchyma during homeostasis or participate in restoring normal hepatocyte numbers during liver regeneration remains to be determined.

Other Epithelial Stem Cells

Skin, hair follicles, and intestinal villi are all examples of tissues that must undergo rapid and continual self-renewal. The outer layer of human epidermis is sloughed, with continued replacement by differentiating cells moving upward from a basal layer in the dermis.[75] Cells in the basal layer display slow but persistent cell division. Within this layer are epidermal stem cells and transient amplifying cells (progenitors). Given that the human epidermal layer completely turns over every 2 weeks and that transient amplifying basal cells divide only three to six times before differentiating into epidermal cells, the self-renewal capacity of the epidermal stem cells is astounding.[76]

Hair follicles are composed of an outer root sheath that is contiguous with the epidermis, an inner root sheath, and the hair shaft.[77] Proliferating cells that give rise to the inner root sheath and the hair shaft are located at the base of the follicle and compose the dermal papilla. In human adult skin, the proliferative capacity of the dermal papilla cells is cyclically exhausted, and the lower segment of the hair follicle regresses upward toward the permanent epithelial portion of the follicle called the *bulge*. Follicle stem cells reside in the bulge and can regenerate the dermal papilla on receiving appropriate signals.[77] These follicle stem cells are also capable of regenerating epidermis and play an important role in the repair of wounds and burns to the epidermal layer. *In vitro,* a single human follicle stem cell can generate 1.7×10^{38} progeny, more epidermal cells than required to cover the surface of an adult human.[1]

The architecture of the small and large intestinal lining is unique, with extensive folding of the epithelial cells to form crypts and fingerlike projections called *villi*.[78] Such an arrangement increases the overall surface area of the intestinal lumen to permit maximal interaction of ingested nutrients with the epithelial cells for efficient absorption. As in the epidermis, newly formed cells move in a polarized fashion as a column of cells from the lower part of the crypt upward to an adjacent villus, where migration occurs along the villus until the cells are shed at the villus tip. The absorptive functions of the cells occur during the migration from the base to the tip of the villus. The entire migratory passage from newly formed cell in the crypt to sloughed cell at the villus tip is thought to occur within 5 to 7 days.[79] In both the small and large intestine, villi are composed of enterocytes, mucus-secreting goblet cells, and peptide hormone–secreting enteroendocrine cells. An additional cell called *the Paneth cell* is present in small intestinal villi. Paneth cells participate in innate immune defense of the gut by sensing pathogenic microbes and secreting microbicidal peptides.

The unique architecture and migratory route of the epithelial cells permit specific identification of the position of each cell during maturation. In the mouse, each adult intestinal crypt is thought to contain four to six stem cells, each giving rise to dividing transit cells. These cells give rise to up to six generations of daughter cells that form the 250 cells composing the mature villus.[80] During the lifetime of a mouse, intestinal epithelial stem cells in each crypt produce 3.3×10^5 cells, a finding suggesting that each stem cell may undergo a thousand cell divisions. In humans, the number of stem cell divisions may equal up to 5000.[79]

Multipotent Adult Progenitor Cells

A novel population of stem cells has been identified in adult rat, mouse, and human subjects.[81] These cells, called *multipotent adult stem cells* (MAPCs), are derived *in vitro* and co-purify with mesenchymal stem cells from the bone marrow compartment. Novel properties of these cells include nearly unlimited proliferative potential, expression of high levels of telomerase, low but detectable Oct-4 expression, requirement for LIF to maintain pluripotency for murine but not human MAPCs, and the ability of single MAPC to contribute to nearly all tissues of a mouse when it is injected into a blastocyst. Clones of MAPC have been differentiated *in vitro* into endothelial cells, neuronal cells, and hepatocytes in large cell numbers.[81] Such properties are highly reminiscent of human and murine ES cell behavior.

STEM CELL PLASTICITY

The term *stem cell plasticity* has emerged to explain a large number of reports in which somatic or adult stem cells from one tissue have apparently "transdifferentiated" or "dedifferentiated" to produce progeny of another tissue. Some examples include bone marrow cells that become cardiomyocytes, NSCs that give rise to all tissues in an embryo, hematopoietic cells that turn into hepatocytes, endothelial cells, epithelial cells, and neurons, and skeletal muscle cells that turn into hematopoietic cells, adipocytes, osteoblasts, and chondrocytes.[8, 82-84] These results have caused scientists to reconsider the embryologic dogma that cellular commitment to a particular germ layer during gastrulation is irreversible and that progeny of the germ layers is restricted to particular organs and tissues. A corollary tenet is that somatic stem cells of one tissue are restricted to giving rise to mature progeny of that same tissue and of none other.

How can one be sure that stem cell plasticity is actually occurring? These studies can be difficult to interpret. Evidence indicates that, under some experimental conditions, test cells may be fusing with host cells on mixing, and apparent instances of stem cell plasticity could be explained by cell fusion events.[85] Results of other examples of stem cell plasticity could be explained by rare unexplained transdifferentiation events that have a low probability of occurring under normal conditions. In some instances, cells may appear to be contributing to a particular tissue or cell type, but no evidence was provided that the cells functionally participated in the normal homeostasis of that tissue or organ.

Some suggested guidelines for strict proof of stem cell plasticity have been published.[83, 85] Proof of plasticity should include some form of clonal analysis. All the progeny derived from a single stem cell should give rise not only to the "unexpected" result but also to the "expected" outcome. Therefore, hematopoietic stem cell transplantation should lead to clonal hematopoietic reconstitution in the host animal as well as whatever other tissue is found to be derived from the transplant (e.g., clonal liver, heart, or muscle cells). The clonal-derived donor cells should be functionally incorporated into the organ or tissue being examined. The incorporated donor cells should compose a robust portion of the organ and should persist for the expected life span of the normal cells of that organ or tissue. Finally, the clonal-derived donor cells that have differentiated into an "unexpected" mature cell type should be demonstrated to contain a normal complement of chromosomes to rule out a cell fusion event. Use of these strict criteria will permit a more critical examination of the phenomenon of stem cell plasticity.

REFERENCES

1. Fuchs E, Segre J: Stem cells: a new lease on life. Cell *100*:143, 2000.
2. Thomson JA, et al: Embryonic stem cell lines derived from human blastocysts. Science *282*:1145, 1998.
3. Martin G: Isolation of a pluripotent cell line from early mouse embryos cultured in medium conditioned by teratocarcinoma stem cells. Proc Natl Acad Sci U S A *78*:7634, 1981.
4. Williams R, et al: Myeloid leukemia inhibitory factor maintains the developmental potential of embryonic stem cells. Nature *336*:684, 1988.
5. Matsui Y, et al: Derivation of pluripotential embryonic stem cells from murine primordial germ cells in culture. Cell *70*:841, 1992.
6. Shamblott M, et al: Derivation of pluripotent stem cells from cultured human primordial germ cells. Proc Natl Acad Sci U S A *95*:13726, 1998.
7. Orlic D, et al: Bone marrow cells regenerate infarcted myocardium. Nature *410*:701, 2001.
8. Wagers A, et al: Little evidence for developmental plasticity of adult hematopoietic stem cells. Science *5*:5, 2002.
9. Amit M, et al: Clonally derived human embryonic stem cell lines maintain pluripotency and proliferative potential for prolonged periods of culture. Dev Biol *227*:271, 2000.
10. Stevens L: Studies on transplantable testicular teratomas of strain 129 mice. J Natl Cancer Inst *20*:1257, 1958.
11. Stevens L: The development of transplantable teratocarcinomas from intratesticular grafts of pre- and postimplantation mouse embryos. Dev Biol *21*:364, 1970.
12. Evans M, Kaufman M: Establishment in culture of pluripotential cells from mouse embryos. Nature *292*:145, 1981.
13. Burdon T, et al: Signaling mechanisms regulating self-renewal and differentiation of pluripotent embryonic stem cells. Cells Tissues Organs *165*:131, 1999.
14. Matsuda T, et al: STAT3 activation is sufficient to maintain an undifferentiated state of mouse embryonic stem cells. EMBO J *2*:4261, 1999.
15. Burdon T, et al: Suppression of SHP-2 and ERK signalling promotes self-renewal of mouse embryonic stem cells. Dev Biol *210*:30, 1999.
16. Pesce M, et al: Lessons of totipotency from embryonic stem cells. Cells Tissues Organs *165*:144, 1999.
17. O'Shea K: Embryonic stem cell models of development. Anat Rec *257*:32, 1999.
18. Weiss M, Orkin S: *In vitro* differentiation of murine embryonic stem cells. J Clin Invest *97*:591, 1996.
19. Odorico J, et al: Multilineage differentiation of human embryonic stem cell lines. Stem Cells *19*:193, 2001.
20. Reubinoff B, et al: Embryonic stem cell lines from human blastocysts: somatic differentiation *in vitro*. Nat Biotech *18*:399, 2000.
21. Kaufman D, et al: Hematopoietic colony-forming cells derived from human embryonic stem cells. Proc Natl Acad Sci U S A *98*:10716, 2001.

22. Kehat I, et al: Human embryonic stem cells can differentiate into myocytes with structural and functional properties of cardiomyocytes. J Clin Invest *108*:407, 2001.
23. Jacobson L, et al: The effect of spleen protection on mortality following X-irradiation. J Lab Clin Med *34*:1538, 1949.
24. Lorenz E, et al: Modification of irradiation injury in mice and guinea pigs by bone marrow injections. J Natl Cancer Inst *12*:197, 1951.
25. Ford C, et al: Cytological identification of radiation-chimaeras. Nature *177*:452, 1956.
26. Till J, McCulloch E: A direct measurement of the radiation sensitivity of normal mouse bone marrow cells. Radiat Res *14*:213, 1961.
27. Orlic D, Bodine D: What defines a pluripotent hematopoietic stem cell (PHSC): will the real PHSC please stand up! Blood *84*:3991, 1994.
28. Ploemacher R, et al: Use of limiting-dilution type long-term marrow cultures in frequency analysis of marrow-repopulating and spleen colony-forming hematopoietic stem cells in the mouse. Blood *78*:2527, 1991.
29. Morrison S, Weissman I: The long-term repopulating subset of hematopoietic stem cells is deterministic and isolatable by phenotype. Immunity *1*:661, 1994.
30. Nakorn T, et al: Myeloerythroid-restricted progenitors are sufficient to confer radioprotection and provide the majority of day 8 CFU-S. J Clin Invest *109*:1579, 2002.
31. Spangrude G, et al: Purification and characterization of mouse hematopoietic stem cells. Science *241*:58, 1988.
32. Verfaillie C: Hematopoietic stem cells for transplantation. Nat Immun *3*:314, 2002.
33. Osawa M, et al: Long-term lymphohematopoietic reconstitution by a single CD34-low/negative hematopoietic stem cell. Science *273*:242, 1996.
34. Krause DS, et al: Multi-organ, multi-lineage engraftment by a single bone marrow-derived stem cell. Cell *105*:369, 2001.
35. Palis J, Yoder M: Yolk sac hematopoiesis: the first blood cells of mouse and man. Exp Hematol *29*:927, 2001.
36. Yoder MC, et al: Characterization of definitive lymphohematopoietic stem cells in the day 9 murine yolk sac. Immunity *7*:335, 1997.
37. Muller A, et al: Development of hematopoietic stem cell activity in the mouse embryo. Immunity *1*:291, 1994.
38. Wright D, et al: Physiological migration of hematopoietic stem and progenitor cells. Science *294*:1933, 2001.
39. Cheng T, et al: Hematopoietic stem cell quiescence maintained by p21$^{cip1/waf1}$. Science *287*:1804, 2000.
40. Cheshier SH, et al: *In vivo* proliferation and cell cycle kinetics of long-term self-renewing hematopoietic stem cells. Proc Natl Acad Sci U S A *96*:3120, 1999.
41. Bradford G, et al: Quiescence, cycling, and turnover in the primitive hematopoietic stem cell compartment. Exp Hematol *25*:445, 1997.
42. MacKey M: Cell kinetic status of haematopoietic stem cells. Cell Prolif *34*:71, 2001.
43. Fraser C, et al: Proliferation of totipotent hematopoietic stem cells *in vitro* with retention of long-term competitive *in vivo* reconstituting ability. Proc Natl Acad Sci U S A *89*:1968, 1992.
44. Moore KA, et al: *In vitro* maintenance of highly purified, transplantable hematopoietic stem cells. Blood *89*:4337, 1997.
45. Sitnicka E, et al: The effect of thrombopoietin on the proliferation and differentiation of murine hematopoietic stem cells. Blood *87*:2, 1996.
46. Antonchuk J, et al: HOXB4-Induced expansion of adult hematopoietic stem cells *ex vivo*. Cell *109*:39, 2002.
47. Phillips PL, et al: The genetic program of hematopoietic stem cells. Science *288*:1635, 2000.
48. Lapidot T, Petit I: Current understanding of stem cell mobilization. Exp Hematol *30*:973, 2002.
49. Domen J, Weissman IL: Hematopoietic stem cells need two signals to prevent apoptosis; BCL-2 can provide one of these, Kitl/c-Kit signaling the other. J Exp Med *192*:1707, 2000.
50. Dick J, et al: Assay of human cells by repopulation of NOD/SCID mice. Stem Cells *15*:199, 1997.
51. Civin C, et al: Sustained, retransplantable, multilineage engraftment of highly purified adult human bone marrow stem cells *in vivo*. Blood *88*:4102, 1996.
52. Little M-T, Storb R: History of haematopoietic stem-cell transplantation. Nat Rev Cancer *2*:231, 2002.
53. Thomas E, et al: Intravenous infusion of bone marrow in patients receiving radiation and chemotherapy. N Engl J Med *257*:491, 1957.
54. Uchida N, et al: Transplantable hematopoietic stem cells in human fetal liver have a CD34+ side population (SP) phenotype. J Clin Invest *108*:1071, 2001.
55. Dao MA, et al: Animal xenograft models for evaluation of gene transfer into human hematopoietic stem cells. Curr Opin Mol Ther *1*:553, 1999.
56. Tavian M, et al: The human embryo, but not its yolk sac, generates lympho-myeloid stem cells: mapping multipotent hematopoietic cell fate in intraembryonic mesoderm. Immunity *15*:487, 2001.
57. Holyoake TL, et al: Functional differences between transplantable human hematopoietic stem cells from fetal liver, cord blood, and adult marrow. Exp Hematol *27*:1418, 1999.
58. Prosper F, Verfaillie CM: Regulation of hematopoiesis through adhesion receptors. J Leukoc Biol *69*:307, 2001.
59. Brandt J, et al: Bone marrow repopulation by human marrow stem cells after long-term expansion culture on a porcine endothelial cell line. Exp Hematol *26*:950, 1998.
60. Fischer A, et al: Gene therapy for human severe combined immunodeficiencies. Immunity *15*:1, 2001.
61. Sadelain M: Globin gene transfer for the treatment of severe hemoglobinopathies: a paradigm for stem cell-based gene therapy. J Gene Med *4*:113, 2002.
62. Gage F: Mammalian neural stem cells. Science *287*:1433, 2000.
63. Taupin P, Gage F: Adult neurogenesis and neural stem cells of the central nervous system in mammals. J Neurosci Res *69*:745, 2002.
64. Okano H: Stem cell biology of the central nervous system. J Neurosci Res *69*:698, 2002.
65. Cameron H, McKay R: Adult neurogenesis produces a large pool of new granule cells in the dentate gyrus. J Comp Neurol *435*:406, 2001.
66. Uchida N, et al: Direct isolation of human central nervous system stem cells. Proc Natl Acad Sci U S A *97*:14720, 2000.
67. Palmer T, et al: Cell culture: progenitor cells from human brain after death. Nature *411*:42, 2001.
68. Matsumoto K, et al: Liver organogenesis promoted by endothelial cells prior to vascular function. Science *294*:559, 2001.
69. Zaret K: Molecular genetics of early liver development. Annu Rev Physiol *58*:231, 1996.
70. Shafritz D, Dabeva M: Liver stem cells and model systems for liver repopulation. J Hepatol *36*:552, 2002.
71. Farber E: Similarities of the sequence of the early histological changes induced in the liver of the rat by ethionine, 2-adetylaminofluorene, and 3-methyl-4-dimethylaminoazobenzene. Cancer Res *16*:142, 1956.
72. Suzuki A, et al: Flow cytometric separation and enrichment of hepatic progenitor cells in the developing mouse liver. Hepatology *32*:1230, 2000.
73. Danet G, et al: C1qRp defines a new human stem cell population with hematopoietic and hepatic potential. Proc Natl Acad Sci U S A *99*:10441, 2002.
74. Peterson BE, et al: Bone marrow as a potential source of hepatic oval cells. Science *284*:1168, 1999.
75. Toma J, et al: Isolation of multipotent adult stem cells from the dermis of mammalian skin. Nat Cell Biol *3*:778, 2001.
76. Slack J: Stem cells in epithelial tissues. Science *287*:1431, 2000.
77. Oshima H, et al: Morphogenesis and renewal of hair follicles from adult multipotent stem cells. Cell *104*:233, 2001.
78. Potten CS, et al: The intestinal epithelial stem cell: the mucosal governor. Int J Exp Pathol *78*:219, 1997.
79. Bach SP, et al: Stem cells: the intestinal stem cell as a paradigm. Carinogenesis *21*:469, 2000.
80. Booth C, Potten CS: Gut instincts: thoughts on intestinal epithelial stem cells. J Clin Invest *105*:1493, 2000.
81. Jiang Y, et al: Pluripotency of mesenchymal stem cells derived from adult marrow. Nature *418*:41, 2002.
82. Wulf G, et al: Somatic stem cell plasticity: current evidence and emerging concepts. Exp Hematol *29*:1361, 2001.
83. Anderson D, et al: Can stem cells cross lineage boundaries? Nat Med *7*:393, 2001.
84. Orkin S: Stem cell alchemy. Nat Med *6*:1212, 2000.
85. Lemischka I: A few thoughts about the plasticity of stem cells. Exp Hematol *30*:848, 2002.

Mervin C. Yoder and Kurt R. Schibler

144
Developmental Biology of the Hematopoietic Growth Factors

HEMATOPOIESIS

Hematopoiesis may be defined as the process of blood cell production. Although it is highly variable, all blood cells have a finite life span. For example, red blood cells circulate for 120 days, platelets for nearly 10 days, and neutrophils for only about 6 hours.[1] Under normal conditions, blood cells are replenished at a constant pace that maintains the concentrations of circulating cells within a narrow range and effectively masks the magnitude and complexity of the process. Approximately 200 billion red blood cells and 70 billion neutrophils must be released into the circulation and replace the damaged and senescent cells on a daily basis in the 70-kg adult. The mechanisms regulating the precise number of circulating blood cells in each lineage and the turnover of each cell lineage remain elusive, although the concentrations of some hematopoietic growth factors appear to play a direct role in this process.[2]

Development of *in vitro* methods for the culture of hematopoietic cells has permitted analysis of the effects of soluble and membrane-bound growth factors on the survival, proliferation, and differentiation of hematopoietic stem and progenitor cells. Numerous growth factors have been characterized at the protein and nucleic acid level. The goal of this chapter is to review basic concepts of hematopoiesis and to provide an overview of some of the growth factors and their cognate receptors that are critical for normal hematopoiesis. Basic concepts of ligand-receptor interactions and initiation of intracellular signaling pathways are reviewed. We also highlight differences in growth factor responsiveness of hematopoietic cells during *in utero* and postnatal development.

STEM AND PROGENITOR CELLS

Background

The hematopoietic system may be characterized as a hierarchy of cell intermediates progressing from the primitive stem cell to mature cells of each of the eight specific blood cell lineages (Fig. 144-1). A single stem cell can sustain the entire hematopoietic system for the lifetime of a mouse under certain experimental systems.[3,4] Stem cells generally exist in a quiescent state, but 8% of the stem cell pool is renewed daily in young mice.[5] Some of the daughter cells of the stem cell divisions may commit to differentiate and may become more highly proliferative multipotent progenitor cells. These cells, in turn, give rise to more proliferative bipotent progenitor cells that eventually produce unilineage committed progenitor cells (see Fig. 144-1). The total cellular amplification that occurs from the time of a single stem cell division to production of a mature blood cell is estimated to be 720,000-fold as a result of at least 17 cell divisions.[6]

Hematopoietic Stem Cells

Analysis of hematopoietic stem cell function has been most reliably understood from the standpoint of functional reconstitution of the hematopoietic system of a lethally irradiated host. In the mouse, multilineage reconstitution of hematopoiesis in a lethally irradiated recipient for more than 4 to 6 months after transplantation constitutes the full definition of a hematopoietic stem cell.[7] In the human system, such experimental proof cannot be undertaken in patients. However, in practical terms, hematopoietic stem cell function has long been demonstrated in those patients who have undergone bone marrow transplantation using allogeneic donor bone marrow, umbilical cord blood, autologous marrow, or mobilized peripheral blood.[8] Both *in vitro* and *in vivo* experimental systems have been developed to test for human hematopoietic stem cell function.

In vitro systems for culture of hematopoietic stem cells can be divided into stromal-dependent and stromal-independent systems. Preplating of stromal cells onto culture dishes followed by addition of hematopoietic stem cells (with or without growth factors) to establish a co-culture can result in retention of hematopoietic stem cell function *ex vivo* and, in some cases, expansion of stem cell function.[9-14] Transplantable activity can also be maintained in stromal-independent cultures in the presence of interleukin-6 (IL-6) and IL-11 plus stem cell factor (SCF), flt-3 ligand, thrombopoietin (Tpo), or leukemia inhibitory factor.[15,16]

Several xenotransplantation models have been developed to assess human hematopoietic stem cell function *in vivo*. First, human cells can be transplanted and will engraft in the marrow of immunocompromised mice.[17, 18] The extent of human hematopoietic stem cell expansion and differentiation can be then examined in the marrow of the transplanted mice. Implantation of human fetal thymic and bone fragments into the immunocompromised mice (producing human hematopoietic microenvironments in the mouse) permits a more detailed analysis of human stem cell differentiation into lymphocyte and erythroid populations.[19] Finally, human hematopoietic stem cells engraft in the marrow of fetal sheep *in utero* and produce human hematopoietic progeny long term in the sheep postnatally.[20,21]

Understanding the innate properties of hematopoietic stem cells has been advanced through the development of techniques to isolate and characterize murine cell populations (using the foregoing assays).[3,4,22] Human hematopoietic stem cells have also been isolated via the use of monoclonal antibodies and flow cytometry and are characterized by expression of the cell-surface antigens AC133, CD34, Thy-1 (low level), rhodamine-123 (low level), and Hoechst 33342 (low level), but not CD33, CD38, human leukocyte antigen (HLA)–DR, and antigens expressed by mature cells of each lineage.[23-25] An alternative *in vitro* strategy uses a combination of antimetabolite treatment and addition of growth factors to enrich for human hematopoietic stem cells.[26]

Substantial evidence supports the hypothesis that the stem cell population resides in a dormant state with respect to the cell cycle. At any given time, only a few stem cells enter the cell cycle, undergo clonal expansion, and supply all the hematopoietic cells to maintain homeostasis. Prolonged residence in the G_0 or the noncycling state is thought to permit sufficient time to repair damaged DNA that may have accumulated during previous cell divisions and to diminish the chance of a clonal proliferative abnormality.

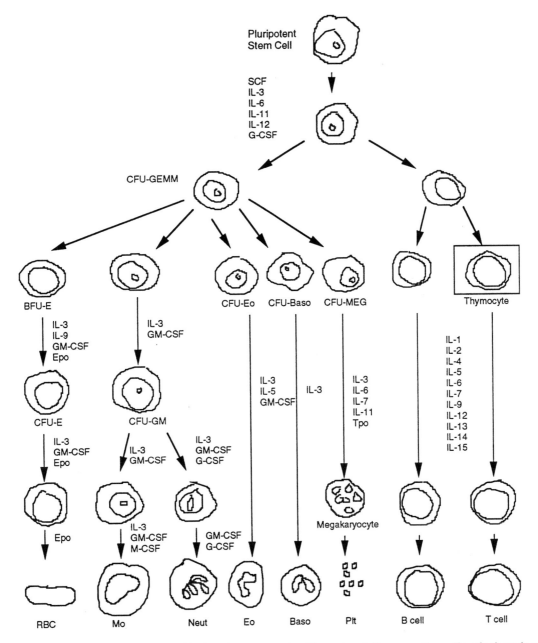

Figure 144–1. Pluripotent hematopoietic stem cells give rise to committed hematopoietic progenitor cells, which undergo clonal expansion and differentiation under the permissive support of hematopoietic growth factors. In the absence of growth factors, committed progenitor cells undergo apoptosis (not shown). This illustration depicts hematopoietic growth factors required for proliferation and differentiation of committed eosinophils (Eo), basophils (Baso), and platelets (Plt). Also shown are hematopoietic growth factors (see text for details) that support maturation of a committed lymphohematopoietic progenitor into B cells and T cells.

Hematopoietic Progenitor Cells

The discovery of *in vitro* culture systems to examine hematopoietic progenitor cell formation as isolated colonies has enabled study of the categorization, functional analysis, and growth factor requirements of the various hematopoietic progenitor cells.[27, 28] Figure 144-1 schematically depicts the hierarchy of hematopoiesis from the stem cell to mature blood cells of each lineage. Growth factors required to support clonal expansion and differentiation of the various hematopoietic lineages are represented. In general, the hierarchy can be divided into myeloid and lymphoid pathways. Progenitor cells that form colonies containing neutrophils, ery-

throcytes, macrophages, and megakaryocytes (colony-forming unit–granulocyte, erythrocyte, megakaryocyte, macrophage [CFU-GEMM]) reside at the pinnacle of the myeloid pathway. These multipotent progenitors no longer possess the self-renewal properties of the stem cell, but they are referred to as a primitive progenitor based on the capacity of these cells to give rise to progeny of multiple lineages. These cells are also highly proliferative and give rise to numerous progeny of more committed progenitors. As the progenitor cells become more committed to a particular lineage, one can begin to identify certain combinations of growth factors that appear to be required for the survival, proliferation, and full maturation of those cells.

The number of hematopoietic growth factors and cytokines that have been identified and characterized (and the genes cloned) is growing rapidly. Table 144-1 is a partial list of the growth factors, their molecular masses, genomic location, and known target cell populations. Although these factors exhibit either stimulatory or inhibitory functions when they are evaluated in culture as single agents, most exhibit more complex actions when they are tested in combinations with other growth factors. Many hematopoietic growth factors have functions that extend outside the hematopoietic system. IL-6 regulates certain aspects of immunologic, neuroendocrine, hepatic, and renal functions.[29] Furthermore, several hematopoietic growth factors are known to orchestrate functions affecting cells at different stages of hematopoietic differentiation. For example, injection of granulocyte colony-stimulating factor (G-CSF) into murine and human subjects triggers cycling of stem cells and mobilization into the systemic circulation, but it participates in a very specific way to support the proliferation and maturation of lineage-committed neutrophilic progenitor cells.[30]

HEMATOPOIETIC MICROENVIRONMENT

Ontogeny of Hematopoiesis

Hematopoiesis is tissue specific and developmentally regulated. The first blood cells to appear in the murine and human embryo are formed in the extraembryonic yolk sac. Within 72 hours in the mouse, and 4 to 6 weeks in the human, blood cells are beginning to be formed in the liver.[31] The liver predominates as the site of hematopoiesis until 3 to 4 days before birth in the mouse, when circulating cells seed the spleen and bone marrow compartments. After birth, the liver diminishes in hematopoietic cell production and no longer serves as a primary hematopoietic site by 2 to 3 weeks of age, whereas the spleen and marrow serve as lifelong sites of blood cell production.[32]

Yolk Sac

The first cells to form in the yolk sac are unique products of this organ and are called *primitive erythroblasts*. These are large red blood cells that express embryonic hemoglobin molecules and retain their nucleus even as circulating blood cells.[33] Primitive erythroblast progenitor cells are first identifiable on embryonic day 7.0 and are no longer detectable in the yolk sac by day 9.0. The primitive erythroblasts formed retain the ability to proliferate, and a rapid expansion in cell number occurs over a 48-hour period. The only other mature blood cells formed during this time include macrophages and a rare number of megakaryocytes.

Yolk sac hematopoiesis is not restricted to the formation of primitive erythroblasts. Evidence indicates that large numbers of definitive hematopoietic progenitor cells are also formed in the yolk sac, but they do not mature in this organ.[34,35] Circumstantial evidence suggests that the definitive progenitor cells (so called

---

TABLE 144-1

Hematopoietic Growth Factors

Factor	Molecular Mass (kDa)	Chromosomal Location	Target Cell
Stem cell factor	28–35	12q4.3–12	All hematopoietic progenitors
Erythropoietin	34–39	7q11–22	CFU-E, mature BFU-E, fetal BFU-E
Thrombopoietin	35	3q26–27	CFU-MEG, megakaryocytes
Granulocyte-macrophage colony-stimulating factor	18–30	5q23–31	CFU-GM, CFU-MIX, BFU-E, CFU-GEMM, macrophage, neutrophil
Granulocyte colony-stimulating factor	20	17q11.2–21	CFU-G, neutrophil, CFU-GM, CFU-MIX, CFU-GEMM, BFU-E
Macrophage colony-stimulating factor	70–90 (dimer)	5q33.1	CFU-M, CFU-GM, macrophage, placenta
Interleukin-1	17	(beta) 2q13–21	Hepatocytes, endothelial cells
		(alpha) 2q13	Osteoclast, neutrophil, macrophage, TH2 lymphocyte
Interleukin-2	15.5	4q26–27	T lymphocyte, cytotoxic lymphocyte
Interleukin-3	15–30	5q23–31	CFU-GEMM, CFU-MIX, CFU-MEG, CFU-GM, BFU-E, cytotoxic lymphocyte, macrophage
Interleukin-4	16–20	5q31	T lymphocyte, B lymphocyte
Interleukin-5	46 (dimer)	5q31	CFU-Eo, B lymphocyte
Interleukin-6	19–21	7p15	CFU-GEMM, CFU-MIX, T lymphocyte, B lymphocyte, fetal CFU-GM, fetal BFU-E, macrophage, hepatocyte, neural cell
Interleukin-7	25	8q12–13	B lymphocyte
Interleukin-8	8–10	4	Neutrophil, endothelial cell, T lymphocyte
Interleukin-9	16	5q31–32	BFU-E, CFU-GEMM, CFU-MIX, fetal CFU-GM
Interleukin-10	35–40	1	T lymphocyte, B lymphocyte, mast cell
Interleukin-11	20	19q13.3–13.4	CFU-GEMM, CFU-MIX, fetal BFU-E
Interleukin-12	70–75 (dimer)	—	T lymphocyte
Interleukin-13	9	5q23–31	Pre-B lymphocyte, macrophage
Interleukin-14	53	—	B lymphocyte
Interleukin-15	14–15	—	B lymphocyte, T lymphocyte, cytotoxic lymphocyte
Interleukin-γ	15–45	12	CFU-GEMM, CFU-GM, BFU-E macrophage
Macrophage inflammatory protein-1α	8–10	17q11–21	CFU-GEMM, CFU-E, BFU-E, macrophage, neutrophil, T lymphocyte
Transforming growth factor-β	25	19	CFU-GEMM, CFU-MIX
Tumor necrosis factor-α	17	6p23	CFU-E, macrophage, T lymphocyte, cytotoxic lymphocyte

BFU-E = burst-forming unit, erythroid; CFU-E = colony-forming unit, erythroid; CFU-G = CFU granulocyte; CFU-GM = CFU, granulocyte-macrophage; CFU-GEMM = CFU, granulocyte-erythrocyte-megakaryocyte-macrophage; CFU-MEG = CFU, megakaryocyte.

because these cells are like progenitors formed in the liver and marrow) enter the circulation, migrate via the bloodstream to the developing liver, enter the liver, and complete the differentiation process to mature blood cells.

Aorta-Gonad-Mesonephros Region

Hematopoietic cells are also formed in the embryo in sites other than the yolk sac and liver early in embryogenesis. There is an anatomic site in which the primordial germ cells coalesce to form the nascent gonads and the mesonephros forms called the *aorta-gonad-mesonephros* region. Along the ventral wall of the aorta in this region, one can observe clusters of hematopoietic cells that appear to emerge from the endothelium.[36] Evidence suggests that this region may be the site of the first hematopoietic stem cells to emerge in the murine and human embryo.[36] Similar clusters of hematopoietic cells have also been identified in the vitelline and umbilical arteries and in the yolk sac, where stem cell activity can also be demonstrated to exist.[37] Apparently, the hematopoietic stem and progenitor cells formed in the aorta-gonad-mesonephros region do not mature in this site but must also migrate to other organs, such as the liver, to differentiate into mature cells.[38]

Fetal Liver

As the principal site of hematopoiesis shifts to the fetal liver in the fifth to eighth week of human gestation, the total content of hematopoietic progenitor cells increases 10- to 100-fold compared with the yolk sac. As in the yolk sac, erythropoiesis continues to predominate over granulocyte production.[39] In fact, the concentration of CFU-GM may even decrease during the transition of hematopoiesis from yolk sac to fetal liver. It remains unclear whether this paucity of granulocytic differentiation is secondary to diminished hepatic production of granulocytic growth factors or results from insensitivity of the fetal liver CFU-GM to granulopoietic factors.

Bone Marrow

The transition of human hematopoiesis from the liver to the bone marrow occurs over the third trimester of intrauterine life. The microenvironment in the bone marrow has been well defined anatomically and is known to consist of osteoblasts, barrier cells, endothelial cells, macrophages, fibroblast cells, mesenchymal stem cells, and adipocytes.[40, 41] Barrier cells are the major component of the stroma.[42] These fibroblast-like cells are located around the venous sinuses and form a sheath around the abluminal surface of the endothelium. Some barrier cells are interspersed within the hematopoietic elements in the marrow and extend cell processes that interact with the maturing hematopoietic cells. Macrophages constitute a second major cell type in the microenvironment. These cells are particularly important for erythrocyte maturation because macrophages engulf the extruded nuclei of the maturing red cells. Macrophages also secrete growth factors that promote progenitor cell survival and maturation. Adipocytes and endothelial cells provide supportive roles to the maturing hematopoietic elements, but they may also directly modulate progenitor cell function via secretion of cytokines and growth factors.

GROWTH FACTOR EFFECTS ON STEM AND PROGENITOR CELLS

Factors Influencing Hematopoietic Stem Cells

Certain growth factors are required for primitive hematopoietic stem cells to survive in a quiescent state, whereas others trigger cycling of progenitors once committed to a differentiation pathway. Some data suggest that G-CSF, IL-3, and SCF may act as survival factors for murine hematopoietic stem cells *in vitro*.[43,44] Other studies, using enriched murine bone marrow progenitor

cells, demonstrated that IL-3 and SCF, but not G-CSF, supported survival of G_0 progenitors.[45] Studies by Leary and colleagues[46, 47] demonstrated that IL-3 and granulocyte-macrophage CSF (GM-CSF) maintain survival of human primitive progenitors in G_0 phase, whereas IL-6, IL-11, and G-CSF do not promote survival of these dormant progenitors *in vitro*.[47]

Several factors have been identified that appear to be involved in triggering division of dormant hematopoietic stem cells. IL-1 and IL-3 have been shown to act synergistically in supporting proliferation of murine hematopoietic stem cells.[48, 49] Mapping studies of murine blast cell colony formation demonstrated that IL-6, IL-11, IL-12, G-CSF, and SCF act synergistically in support of colony formation from quiescent progenitors.[50-54] Similarly, synergism between IL-1 and IL-3 has been demonstrated in cultures enriched for human marrow progenitor cells.[55]

Factors Affecting Multipotent Progenitor Cells

Intermediate-acting, lineage-nonspecific factors include IL-3, IL-4, and GM-CSF. These factors support proliferation of pluripotent progenitors, but only after they have emerged from quiescence. Suda and colleagues[56] observed that, in the presence of IL-3, murine multipotent progenitors developed into blast cell colonies in an asynchronous manner over several days. When the addition of IL-3 was delayed, however, decreased numbers of multipotent colonies developed, and they continued to develop in an asynchronous manner.[56] Thus, IL-3 does not trigger cycling, but it supports proliferation of multipotential progenitors. IL-3 as a single agent does not appear to support terminal differentiation of hematopoietic cells. In fact, in both murine and human models of hematopoiesis, progenitors lose their responsiveness to IL-3 as they differentiate.

Although GM-CSF was first characterized as a lineage-specific factor supporting the granulocyte-macrophage cell lineage, subsequent studies placed it as an intermediate factor.[57] In murine culture systems, GM-CSF supports mitosis in multipotential cells. In human studies, the functions of GM-CSF and IL-3 overlap significantly.[58]

IL-4 also is included in the family of non–lineage-specific factors.[59] It acts in combination with lineage-specific factors, such as erythropoietin (Epo), to support proliferation of murine multilineage colonies *in vitro*.

Lineage-Specific Factors

This subgroup of lineage-specific factors supports proliferation and maturation of committed progenitors. Members of this group include Epo, G-CSF, IL-5, macrophage CSF (M-CSF), and Tpo. Epo is a physiologic regulator of erythropoiesis.[60] IL-5 and M-CSF are believed to be specific for eosinophils and macrophage/monocyte progenitors.[61,62] Tpo and G-CSF specifically support maturation of megakaryocytic and neutrophilic committed progenitors, respectively; however, these factors also directly stimulate hematopoietic stem cells.[63,64]

Inhibitory Factors

Several cytokines have been demonstrated to inhibit hematopoiesis. These include interferons (IFNs), macrophage inflammatory peptide-1 (MIP-2), tumor necrosis factor-α (TNA-α), and transforming growth factor-β (TGF-β).[65-67] MIP-1 is reported to inhibit proliferation of primitive hematopoietic progenitors.[68]

RECEPTORS

Cytokine Receptor Families

Hematopoietic growth factor receptors have been categorized (based on similarities in extracellular genetic characteristics) into several families of receptors (Fig. 144–2).[69-71] Some receptors contain structural domains characteristic of two or three subgroups within the cytokine superfamily of receptors. For instance, the receptors for IL-1, IL-6, SCF (c-*kit*), and M-CSF (c-*fms*) contain extracellular immunoglobulin-like domains, placing them in the immunoglobulin superfamily. IL-1 receptors are distinct from other Type I cytokine receptors such as IL-6R because they lack the WS motif, fibronectin-like domains, and conserved cysteine residues. The receptors for SCF and M-CSF differ from other hematopoietic growth factor receptors in that they contain intrinsic intracellular protein tyrosine kinase motifs that are involved in signal transduction. The IL-2Rβc, IL-3Rα, IL-3Rβc, IL-4Rα, Il-5Rα, IL-6Rα, IL-6Rβc (gp130), IL-7Rα, IL-9Rα, IL-12Rβ, EpoR, G-CSFR, and GM-CSFR belong to the Type I family of receptors and share several highly conserved protein motifs.[72-79] The structural similarities among these conserved regions suggest that members of this receptor family evolved from a common ancestral gene. Other cytokine receptors include the IFN group (IFNR Type 1, IFNRα Type II, IFN-β Type II, and IL-10R), which possess a common binding domain characterized by cysteine pairs at both the amino-terminal and the carboxyl-terminal, and the TNF group (TNFR Type I and Type II), which contain several cysteine-rich domains.[80] The IL-8 receptor belongs to still another family of receptors, the chemokine family. Structurally, it differs markedly from other cytokines because it contains seven transmembrane domains.[81,82]

Although cytokine receptors are clearly evolutionarily related, their intracellular domains exhibit little homology.[83] Furthermore, there is a conspicuous lack of protein kinase–related sequences in most family members even though ligand-receptor interaction triggers a cascade of tyrosine phosphorylation within target cells.[84] Moreover, although cytokine receptor family members do not belong to the protein kinase family, they use protein kinase activity to propagate their intracellular signals.

The finding that intracellular domains of cytokine receptors lack sequences known to be important in signal transduction suggested that associated molecules must be responsible for propagating the signal intracellularly. Cytokine receptors can be subdivided into two distinct groups based on the mechanism by which they associate to transduce their signal. One group of receptors forms homodimers for signal transduction (e.g., Epo), and the second group consists of receptors that require two distinct subunits to produce effective high-affinity ligand binding and signal transduction.[85] The βc chains are shared by several receptors in this family. For instance, the IL-3Rβc forms heterodimers with IL-5R and GM-CSFR after ligand binding to form a high-affinity interaction that is capable of propagating intracellular signals. Similarly, the IL-6Rβc (gp130) chain is shared with IL-11R, and the IL-2γc chain is shared with IL-4R, IL-7R, IL-9R, and IL-15R (Fig. 144–3).[86]

Soluble Growth Factors and Growth Factor Receptors

Growth factor regulation at the level of the receptor occurs by several distinct mechanisms. First, receptors may be restricted to specific cell types. Second, receptor number on the membrane surface may differ because of varying receptor mRNA expression, receptor degradation, or internalization. Third, receptor affinity may be modified by other membrane proteins or by availability of shared common receptor chains. Finally, membrane-bound receptors may be cleaved to soluble forms or, alternatively, secreted directly as soluble receptors. Table 144–2

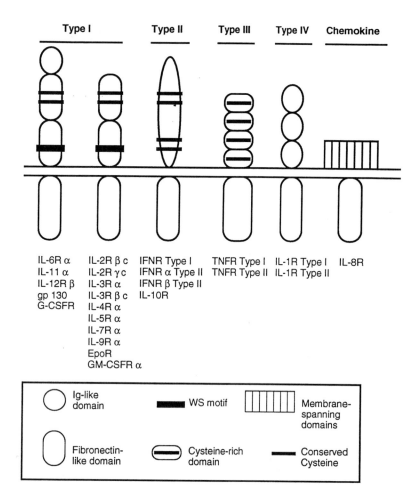

Figure 144–2. Cytokine receptors have been grouped into related families based on presence of conserved structural elements in their extracellular domains. Type 1 receptors (including interleukin-2 [IL-2], IL-3, IL-4, IL-5, IL-6, IL-7, IL-9, IL-11, IL-12, granulocyte colony-stimulating factor [G-CSF], granulocyte-macrophage CSF [GM-CSF], and erythropoietin [Epo] receptor chains) are characterized by the presence of fibronectin-like domains, conserved cysteine residues, and the WS motif (a highly conserved region containing a tryptophan-serine-1 amino acid–tryptophan-serine motif). Type II receptors, which possess several conserved cysteine residues, include the interferon-α (IFN-α), IFN-β, IFN-γ, and IL-10 receptors. Type III receptors include two varieties of tumor necrosis factor (TNF) receptors (Types I and II), which are characterized by repeated cysteine-rich domains. The IL-1 receptors are characteristic of Type IV class of receptors (immunoglobulin superfamily receptors). Several members of the Type I family also include immunoglobulin-like domains (IL-6Rα, IL-11Rα, IL-12Rβ, G-CSFR, and gp130). The IL-8 receptor differs from other receptors because it includes seven transmembrane domains. This structure is characteristic of the chemokine receptors.

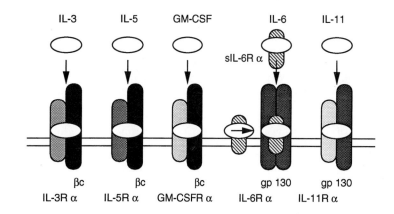

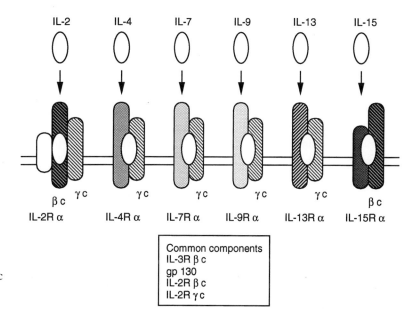

Figure 144–3. Cytokines and hematopoietic growth factors bind to their specific α-chain receptors to form low-affinity complexes that do not initiate signal transduction. Subsequently, they form high-affinity complexes capable of signal transduction by interacting with other α-chains to form homodimers as with Epo (not shown) or by interacting with common chains (interleukin-2Rβc [IL-2Rβc], IL-2Rγc, IL-3Rβc, and gp130) to form heterodimeric complexes. GM-CSFR = granulocyte-macrophage CSF receptor.

TABLE 144-2

Soluble Cytokine Receptors

Soluble Receptor	Molecular Weight (kDa)	Site of Detection	Possible Function
sIL-1RI			
sIL-1RII	45	Serum	IL-1 scavenger
sIL-2Rα	43	Not detected	
sIL-2Rβ		Not detected	
sIL-4R	30–40	Serum	IL-4 carrier/depot
sIL-5R		Not detected	
sIL-6Rα	50–60	Serum/urine	Complex of IL-6 and IL-6R acts as agonist
sIL-6Rβ	90–100	Serum	IL-6, IL-11 antagonist
sIL-7R		Not detected	
sIL-9R		Not detected	
sG-SCFR		Not detected	
sGM-CSFR		Not detected	
TNFR I	28	Plasma	Protects against proteolysis
TNFR II	32	Plasma, ascites, synovial fluid	Protects against proteolysis

G-SCFR = granulocyte stem cell factor receptor; GM-SCFR = granulocyte-macrophage SCFR; IL = interleukin; s = soluble; TNFR = tumor necrosis factor receptor.

is a partial list of known soluble receptors and their recognized functions. Two mechanisms responsible for generation of soluble receptors are differential splicing of the receptor pre-mRNA (which results in formation of receptors lacking the transmembrane portion of the receptor molecule) and proteolytic cleavage of the membrane-bound form (releasing the extracellular portion of the molecule).[87]

The actual physiologic role of the soluble receptors depends on the relative concentrations of growth factor–receptor complexes, the individual components, and their dissociation constants. In the case of IL-6, circulating levels are generally 10 pg/mL or less in normal individuals, whereas the soluble receptor concentrations are approximately 70 ng/mL.[88,89] With a dissociation constant of 1×10^{-9} mol, all IL-6 in the serum should be present in complexes with soluble receptors. Therefore, it would be anticipated that this interaction would antagonize the effects of IL-6. In fact, studies by Narazaki and colleagues[90] demonstrated antagonist activity in complexes of IL-6, IL-6R, and gp130. In contrast, *in vitro* studies suggest that soluble IL-6 receptor complexes may propagate an agonist IL-6 effect on cells not expressing the IL-6R subunit but expressing the gp130 chain.[91,92] Thus, IL-6 and IL-6 receptors shed from one cell type could alter ligand binding and act on a cell type not expressing IL-6R but expressing gp130. Such interactions have been documented in hepatoma cell lines and in hematopoietic cells.[93,94]

SIGNAL TRANSDUCTION

Tyrosine kinase–based signaling can be initiated both by receptors possessing intrinsic tyrosine kinase and by receptors lacking an intrinsic tyrosine kinase. Hematopoietic growth factors possessing intrinsic tyrosine kinase activity include SCF and M-CSF. Factors such as GM-CSF and the interleukins lack intrinsic catalytic activity, but they trigger signaling activity through cytoplasmic tyrosine kinases. The carboxyl-terminal portion of these receptors, although lacking motifs involved in known catalytic activity such as the protein tyrosine kinase domains, contains highly conserved motifs in the intracellular membrane proximal region.[95-97] These structures are instrumental in triggering downstream signaling events.

Common features of the intracellular signal transduction mechanism of cytokine receptors are noteworthy. First, ligand binding to monomeric forms of these receptors alone is generally insufficient to initiate signal transduction; however, once specific ligand binding has occurred, the receptors are capable of forming homodimers or heterodimers that initiate signal transduction.[98] Second, several receptor subunits are shared with other hematopoietic growth factors.[99] Third, on binding of the specific ligand and dimerization of the receptor subunits, autophosphorylation and transphosphorylation can occur, and they initiate a cascade of tyrosine phosphorylation of sites intrinsic to the intracellular portions of the receptors and also on nonreceptor protein tyrosine kinase molecules associated with the intracellular domains of the cytokine receptors. Signal transducing proteins containing *Src* homology 2 (SH2) domains associate with the phosphotyrosine residues on the activated receptor and activated nonreceptor protein tyrosine kinases and, in turn, are activated and propagate the signal downstream.[100] This interaction affords another level of specificity on biologic actions of cytokines as each particular receptor interacts with its own specific subset of SH2-containing proteins.[101] The key features of the signal transduction process are illustrated in Figure 144–4.

Several families of nonreceptor protein tyrosine kinases have been isolated and have been implicated in cytokine signal transduction. These include molecules in the Src family, the Syk-ZAP70 family, the Btk-Tec family, and the Janus kinase (JAK) family.[95] The mechanisms by which these factors mediate downstream events have not been fully defined; however, the interactions between the JAK and Src proteins and several downstream factors have been partially characterized.

JAK Protein Tyrosine Kinases

One family of protein tyrosine kinases recognized to be involved in cytokine signaling is the JAK family. Early clues implicating the involvement of a receptor-associated tyrosine kinase was drawn

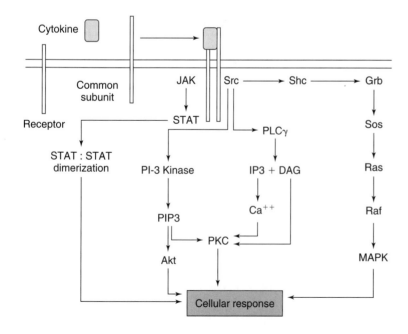

Figure 144–4. Transduction of external signals across the cell membrane is accomplished by binding of a cytokine with its specific receptor. The receptor then forms dimers with a common receptor chain to form a high-affinity complex. This association initiates a cascade of tyrosine phosphorylation both on the intracellular domains on the receptor itself and on receptor-associated tyrosine kinase molecules. One family of nonreceptor tyrosine kinases is the JAK proteins. The phosphorylation events lead to docking of STAT proteins. These interactions lead to phosphorylation and dimerization of STAT proteins, nuclear translocation, and transcription of cellular response genes. Receptor phosphorylation can activate other receptor-associated tyrosine protein kinases such as Src. Activation of Src triggers activation of phosphatidylinositol 3-kinase (PI-3 kinase) and phospholipase Cγ (PLCγ). Tyrosine kinases also trigger activation of the serine threonine kinase Raf through the coupled proteins Shc and Grb, the nucleotide exchange factor Sos, and the small G-protein Ras. Raf activates mitogen-activated protein kinase (MAPK) to regulate cellular responses.

from the observation that purified growth hormone receptor exhibited kinase activity.[102] Members of the JAK family were isolated by polymerase chain reaction technology using degenerate primers based on a conserved catalytic domain.[103] Evidence pointing to the role of this family of proteins in cytokine signaling was provided by genetic complementation studies in a cell line defective in Type I IFN signaling.[104] This mutant line was rescued by transfection of these cells with genomic DNA encoding Tyk2, a member of this kinase family. Similar studies on IFN-γ provided evidence for Jak1 and Tyk2 in type I receptor signaling and Jak1 and Jak2 in the IFN Type II signaling mechanism.[105] The JAK family of protein tyrosine kinases has been found to be a critical component in signaling through certain cytokine receptors including IL-2R, IL-3R, IL-4R, IL-5R, IL-6Rβc (gp130), IL-7R, IL-12R, and EpoR.[106] Each receptor appears to associate with distinct members of the JAK family. For instance, IL-2R associates with Jak1 and Jak3, whereas the EpoR associates only with Jak2.[106] A restrictive interaction of the cytokine receptor intracellular domains with specific signal transduction elements, such as Jak protein kinases, is one mechanism regulating the specificity of growth factor action.

Dimerization of the cytokine receptor induced by ligand brings Jak proteins in proximity with each other, resulting in cross-phosphorylation.[106] This interaction is somewhat restrictive because Jak1 and Jak3 always bind in conjunction with other family members, whereas Jak2 binds to receptors alone.[95] Thus, Jak2 molecules are capable of cross-phophorylating each other, whereas the other Jak proteins appear to require interaction with related family members to effect optimal activation.[95] The observation that patterns of Jak protein phosphorylation are distinct in different cell lines may provide insight into the functional pleiotropism of cytokines.[106, 107]

The Jak proteins appear to associate with the box 1 motif in the membrane proximal portion of cytokine receptors. This region exhibits a high degree of sequence conservation.[108] Presence of the box 1 motif is critical in the mitogenic response to several cytokines.[109] Although the downstream signal propagating events that follow Jak protein phosphorylation are not fully understood, its role in activation of one family of latent transcription factors, called STATs (signal transducers and activators of transcription), has been characterized. In addition, the phosphorylation of cytokine receptors by Jak proteins potentiates the interaction between the receptor complex and other signal transducing molecules such as those containing SH2 regions.[110] STAT proteins, present in the cytoplasm, become activated on interaction with activated Jak proteins. The phosphorylated Stat proteins form homodimers or heterodimers with peptides containing SH2 domains; these dimers are subsequently transported to the nucleus, where they function as transcription factors.[107-110]

SRC Protein Tyrosine Kinases

Src is the prototype for a family of tyrosine kinases that includes at least nine members: Src, Fyn, Yes, Lyn, Hck, Fgr, Lck, Blh, and Yrk.[111] All Src members contain a site near the N-terminus signaling for myristylation, and in many cases for palmitoylation, which direct the association of these proteins with cellular membranes. C-terminal to this region is the Src homology 3 (SH3) domain that promotes protein-protein interactions with proteins exhibiting left-handed polyproline Type II helices.[112,113] The next adjacent domain toward the C-terminus is the Src homology 2 (SH2) domain. The SH2 domain is the binding site for phospho-tyrosine-containing proteins. This domain is frequently found in phospholipase Cγ, phosphatidylinositol-3-kinase, Shc, and STAT proteins, which are involved in tyrosine kinase–based signal transduction.[101, 112] The SH2 domains of Src kinases mediate interactions of these proteins with receptor-type protein tyrosine kinases and with protein substrates. C-terminal to the SH2

domain is the catalytic domain. Phosphorylation of Tyr416 in the catalytic domain is required for optimal activity. In addition, the presence of a conserved tyrosine (Tyr527) in the C-terminal tail region is essential for the phosphorylation-based activity characteristic of Src tyrosine kinases. Multiple Src family members have been observed in hematopoietic cells; however, it is not known to what extent selective roles exist for each Src family member or whether there is redundancy in Src-based signal transduction.

Downstream Signaling Mechanisms

Members of the Ras guanosine triphosphatase (GTPase) superfamily modulate many signal transduction pathways. These proteins are low molecular weight GTP-binding proteins that act as molecular switches in regulating many different signaling pathways in virtually all cells.[113] Approximately 60 Ras family members have been identified to date in mammalian cells. GTPases exist in an inactive (guanosine diphosphate [GDP]–bound) and an active (GTP-bound) conformation. Guanine nucleotide exchange factors catalyze the release of GDP and allow GTP to bind. In the active, GTP-bound state, Ras interacts with target proteins to promote a cellular response. An intrinsic GTPase activity, catalyzed further by GTPase-activating proteins, returns Ras GTPase to its inactive, GDP-bound state Figure 144–5.

Striking features of the Ras superfamily include (1) the diversity of membrane receptors and upstream regulators that can activate these GTPases, (2) the diversity of cellular targets that can interact with an individual GTPase, and (3) the extensive cross-talk that exists among GTPase-regulated signal transduction pathways.[113] Numerous examples of the coordinated activation and functional cooperation between Ras superfamily members at the molecular and cellular level have been described in animal cells. The best characterized of these functions are cell proliferation, gene expression, and actin-based cell motility.

Cell-cycle progression depends on cyclin-dependent protein kinases whose activity vacillates periodically during growth and division of cells.[114] The critical role for Ras in cell-cycle progression was suggested by experiments in which Ras activity was disrupted by microinjection of anti-Ras neutralizing antibodies or by expression of a dominant mutant interfering with endogenous Ras expression. These manipulations prevented mitogen-induced progression through G_1 and entry into S phase of the cell cycle. More recent studies have determined that the proliferative effects of Ras are dependent on signaling input from other Ras family members, Rho and Rac (Fig. 144–6).[108, 115]

The link between Ras superfamily GTPase activity and hematopoietic growth factor–induced proliferation and differentiation has been elucidated through in vitro and in vivo experiments. Ras-related GTPase, *Rac1*, overexpression enhanced the proliferative signal provided by GM-CSF in cultured cells.[116] Expression of a dominant negative ras mutant (rasT17N) partially suppressed proliferation of cultured cells in response to GM-CSF. Studies to delineate M-CSF and GM-CSF receptor activation revealed differential modulation of the macrophage scavenger receptor A through the Ras signaling pathway (Fig. 144–7).[117]

The role of neurofibromin, the protein encoded by the *NF1* tumor suppressor gene, in Ras signaling and hematopoietic cell proliferation has been examined in vitro and in vivo using the genetic approach. Humans and animals with mutations in *NF1* are predisposed to juvenile myelomonocytic leukemia (JMML). A hallmark of both human JMML cells and murine Nf1-deficient myeloid progenitors is a selective hypersensitivity to GM-CSF.[118] Whereas homozygous NF1-mutant (Nf1-/-) embryos die *in utero*, adoptively transferred Nf1-/- fetal liver cells consistently induce JMML-like disorder in irradiated recipients.[119] GM-CSF appears to play a central role in establishing and maintaining this phenotype *in vivo*.[120] Primary Nf1-/- hematopoietic cells exhibit constitutive activation of the Ras-Raf-MAP kinase signaling

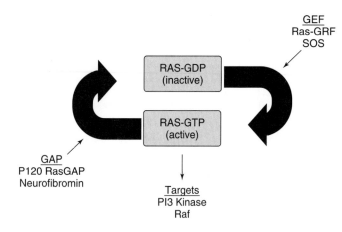

Figure 144–5. Ras interacts with multiple guanine nucleotide exchange factors (GEF), guanosine triphosphatase–activating proteins (GAP), and target proteins. The figure shows only a few examples of many interacting proteins identified to date. GDP = guanosine diphosphate.

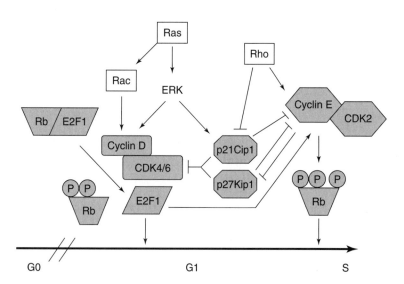

Figure 144–6. Influence of Ras and Ras family members Rho and Rac on cell-cycle progression. Cell-cycle regulatory proteins targeted by Ras, Rho, and Rac signal transduction pathways are shown. Cyclin D is a major target for Ras and Rac, whereas Rho acts primarily downstream of the CDK inhibitors p21Cip1 and p27Kip1. Rac and Ras act synergistically to activate cyclin-dependent kinase 4 (CDK4) and CDK6 through mechanisms to induce cyclin D transcription and assembly of cyclinD-CDK4/6 complexes at an early stage of G_1. The principal activity of these complexes is to phosphorylate Rb protein and thus allow activation of E2F transcription factors that regulate genes required for the G_1/S transition. Under circumstances in which Ras expression leads to cell-cycle arrest caused by induction of p21Cip1, Rho can suppress the induction of p21Cip1, thus enabling Ras to stimulate cell-cycle progression. Rho also regulates cell-cycle progression by inducing degradation of the CDK inhibitor p27Kip1 through cyclin E/CDK2 activity. ERK = extracellular regulated kinase.

pathway and enhanced cell proliferation in response to SCF and IL-3 or GM-CSF.[119]

PLEIOTROPY AND REDUNDANCY OF CYTOKINE FUNCTION

Regulation of hematopoietic growth factors clearly occurs on many levels, including production (quantity and location), interaction with other factors, receptors (location, cell type, soluble versus membrane bound), and signal transduction mechanisms. *Pleiotropy* describes the property in which cytokines exhibit many different effects on various tissue and cell types. *Redundancy* refers to the property of cytokines in which two or more factors mediate similar biologic effects on the same cell type.

A cytokine designated IL-11 was cloned in 1990, based on its capacity to produce a mitogenic activity for the IL-6–dependent cell line T1165.[121] Even though IL-11 is not similar in structure to IL-6, the two cytokines exhibit certain similarities in their spectrum of biologic activities, as shown in Table 144–3.[122,123] IL-6 and IL-11 have been shown to share the common signal transduction element, gp130.[124] Moreover, several cytokines share common chains to form heterodimers to effect signal transduction. The redundancy in function of several of these cytokines may, in part, be attributed to downstream actions of shared receptors.

Redundancy of cytokine function is not solely the result of shared receptor signal transduction elements. M-CSF and GM-CSF are both responsible for various aspects of macrophage differentiation and function. Although they do not share receptors, activation of M-CSF and GM-CSF receptors results in expression of

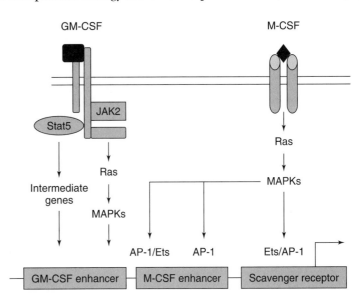

Figure 144–7. Mechanism for transcriptional control of scavenger receptor A (SR-A) by granulocyte-macrophage CSF (GM-CSF) and macrophage-CSF (M-CSF). Activation of SR-A by GM-CSF is dependent on a distinct enhancer element located upstream of the M-CSF–dependent enhancer. The GM-CSF enhancer is occupied by constitutively expressed transcription factors that, on regulation by Ras, activate immediate to early transcriptional responses. Sustained expression of SR-A in response to GM-CSF may be directed in part by transcription factors that are targets of STAT5.A M-CSF. These transcription factors are targets of a Ras-dependent mitogen-activated protein kinase (MAPK) cascade that controls their level of expression and activities. AP-1 = activator protein-1; Ets = e twenty-six specific.

TABLE 144–3

Comparison of Interleukin-6 and Interleukin-11

Characteristic	Interleukin-6	Interleukin-11
Molecular weight (kDa)	26	23
Sequence homology	No	No
Glycosylated	Yes	No
Hematopoietic progenitor proliferation	Yes	Yes
B-lymphocyte differentiation	Yes	Yes
Thrombopoiesis	Yes	Yes
Synthesis of acute phase reactants	Yes	Yes
Erythropoiesis	No	Yes
T-lymphocyte proliferation	Yes	No

the macrophage scavenger receptor A. Both receptors use components of the Ras signal transduction pathway to effect this response. However, M-CSF exerts its action by engaging the M-CSF–dependent enhancer recognized by activator protein-1 and cooperating Ets domain transcription factors, whereas activation of scavenger receptor A by GM-CSF is dependent on a distinct enhancer located immediately upstream of the M-CSF enhancer (see Fig. 144–7).[117]

MATERNAL AND PLACENTAL PRODUCTION OF GROWTH FACTORS

Placental Production of Hematopoietic Growth Factors

The precise role and significance of growth factor production by placental tissues in maintenance of viable pregnancy and in the labor process are far from complete; however, it is likely that they are involved in two distinct regulatory processes: the neutralization of the immune response against the fetus and the provision of an environment conducive to the maturation and differentiation of the fetus.[125] From the immunologic standpoint, pregnancy has been likened (in the borrowed terms of transplant immunology) to the presence of a fetal allograft. Furthermore, the aggressive nature of the implantation events has to some investigators appeared to be similar to tumor inva-

sion. Although there are certain similarities, the immunology of pregnancy exhibits unique features.

The components required to mount an immune response against the fetopaternal antigens are present in the maternal desidua. In addition to foreign antigen, antigen-presenting cells and effector cell are present. Despite this milieu, there appear to be several mechanisms that abrogate the T-cell–mediated immune response at the fetomaternal interface. Although the mature T cells and natural killer (NK) cells are capable of migrating to the desidua and recognizing foreign antigen, they do not express their cytotoxic effects in this microenvironment. Certain mechanisms appear to act in concert to inhibit T-cell proliferation and cytotoxicity. First, the decidua produces large quantities of prostaglandin E_2 during the first trimester.[126] Prostaglandin E_2 has been shown to down-regulate T-cell activation and IL-2 production. Second, the steroid hormones, which provide functions essential for maintenance of pregnancy, also exert significant immunologic functions. For instance, dihydroepiandrosterone (DHEA) dramatically enhances the production of IL-2 by stimulated lymphocytes. During pregnancy, DHEA levels decrease by approximately 50% because of rapid conversion of DHEA to estriol and other estrogen metabolites. Estrogens indirectly inhibit IL-2 production and accentuate IL-4 production through potentiation of the activity of 1,25-dihydroxyvitamin D_3. IL-4 effects a T-helper 2–type response that down-regulates cell-mediated cytotoxicity and phagocytic functions and favors humoral immunity.

Although the adaptive immune system appears to be inhibited by the physiologic alterations in the uterus during pregnancy, cells within the fetomaternal interface produce several hematopoietic growth factors. Among these are IL-1, IL-4, IL-6, IL-8, GM-CSF, M-CSF, TGF-β, and TNF. Production of these factors during gestation appears to be tightly regulated and to follow a specific sequence of expression. These cytokines can exhibit dichotomous functions. For instance, expressed at the proper time, concentration, and location, growth factors may promote trophoblast growth, whereas if they are expressed in abnormal amounts or sites, they may have pathophysiologic actions such as facilitating the onset of preterm labor.

Transport of Factors Across the Placenta

Studies in sheep have demonstrated that no transplacental transfer of Epo occurs.[127] Moreover, *in vitro* studies of Epo transport across the perfused human placenta provide evidence that Epo does not cross the placenta. However, no studies have been published to address whether the transplacental transfer of Epo occurs *in vivo* in humans.[128]

Studies in rats demonstrated that G-CSF (at least in small quantities) can cross from the maternal to the fetal circulation.[129] Although transfer appears to be meager, in one animal study it was sufficient to improve survival of rat pups subsequently exposed to group B streptococci.[130] Administration of recombinant G-CSF to humans resulted in transplacental passage of G-CSF in an amount capable of stimulating fetal granulopoiesis.[131] The mechanism underlying this transfer is uncertain, but it does not require an intact G-CSF receptor.[132] The physiologic relevance of transplacental passage of maternally derived hematopoietic cytokines remains to be delineated.

DEVELOPMENTAL ASPECTS OF INTERACTION BETWEEN HEMATOPOIETIC GROWTH FACTORS AND HEMATOPOIETIC PROGENITORS

Developmental Differences Between Adult and Fetal Progenitors

Developmental differences have been identified among hematopoietic progenitors from various sources. For instance, several differences exist between fetal liver–derived and adult bone marrow–derived progenitors. Fetal liver progenitors exhibit a rapid cycling rate, rapidly expanding pool size, accelerated *in vitro* maturation time, increased sensitivity to Epo, and decreased sensitivity to GM-CSF compared with adult marrow progenitors.[133] Furthermore, circulating hematopoietic progenitor cells derived from umbilical cord blood differ from those derived from adult human bone marrow in that a subset of cord blood progenitors grows in methylcellulose cultures in the absence of added growth factors. Hematopoietic progenitors obtained from fetal subjects also differ from those obtained from adults. For instance, Roodman and colleagues observed that by including dexamethasone with cultures of human fetal progenitors, fewer erythroid colonies and fewer normoblasts per colony developed. These reductions were not observed when progenitors from adults were subjected to the same conditions.[134] In addition, Christensen and colleagues observed that high concentrations of Epo *in vitro* resulted in a dose-dependent downmodulation of neutrophil production from fetal, but not from adult, CFU-GM.[135] A third difference between fetal and adult progenitors was observed by Emerson and associates[136] and by Valtieri and colleagues,[137] who reported that Epo alone induced erythroid burst formation from embryonic and fetal burst-forming units, erythroid (BFU-E), whereas BFU-E of adult origin required GM-CSF or IL-3 in addition to Epo. A fourth difference is that some fetal progenitors undergo clonogenic maturation in the absence of added growth factors or when they are stimulated with factors such as IL-11 that, as single agents, do not support maturation of progenitors from adults.[123, 138] Other studies suggest that the progenitor cells or their progeny express growth factors, IL-3, and GM-CSF, and thus support clonal expansion in an autocrine or paracrine fashion.[139]

Experiments to delineate the effects of hematopoietic growth factors on fetal hematopoietic progenitor cells have demonstrated differences in the actions of these factors on fetal versus adult progenitors. For instance, the presence of early-acting factors (IL-6 and SCF) initiates clonal expansion *in vitro* in the absence of other growth factors added to the culture. In addition, IL-11 enhances cycling of both committed multipotential and lineage-specific colonies from cord blood, but it does not induce cycling of adult progenitors derived from bone marrow.[123, 138–140]

Effects of Hematopoietic Growth Factors on Nonhematopoietic Tissues During Embryonic and Fetal Development

SCF appears to have a critical role in embryonic and fetal hematopoietic development. Schmitt and colleagues observed that SCF and c-*kit* were among the factors expressed in undifferentiated embryonic murine stem cells.[141] The importance of SCF and its interaction with the c-*kit* receptor during early development are illustrated by murine strains with mutations at the (W) locus encoding the c-*kit* product, and mice with the mutation of the (Sl) locus encoding SCF protein.[142, 143] Both strains exhibit pleotropic developmental defects, not only in hematopoiesis, but also in gametogenesis and melanogenesis.

The utilization of homologous recombination to generate transgenic mouse models with deletion of specific growth factors has shed light on the role of these factors during development and their relative importance in normal hematopoietic homeostasis. The GM-CSF knock-out mouse illustrates this point well.[144] It was expected that a mouse homozygous for defective GM-CSF alleles would exhibit defects in hematopoietic development. Such is not the case, because these mice do not exhibit detectable hematopoietic defects. Rather unexpectedly, they develop a form of alveolar proteinosis. Whether the pathophysiology observed in this defect results from defective alveolar macrophage function, pulmonary epithelial function, or a combination of both is unclear.

Mice deficient in both GM-CSF and M-CSF gene products (genotype GM$^{-/-}$M$^{-/-}$) have been generated by interbreeding GM-CSF–deficient mice with M-CSF–deficient osteopetrotic mice.[145] These mice exhibit coexistent features of both deficiency states, yet they still have circulating monocytes and phagocytic tissue macrophages. This would indicate that factors other than GM-CSF and M-CSF are capable of supporting macrophage lineage differentiation. These mice (like the GM-CSF–deficient mice) exhibit a form of chronic lung disease that is more severe than that of GM-CSF deficiency alone, a finding implicating M-CSF in modulating the pulmonary disease associated with GM-CSF deficiency *in vivo*.

Several hematopoietic growth factors including Epo, G-CSF, GM-CSF, IL-6, IL-8, IL-11, Tpo, and their respective receptors have been identified in nonhematopoietic tissues of the human fetus and neonate. Epo receptor has been identified in murine cell lines of neuronal origin, in cultured murine embryonic neurons, and in the brain and spinal cord of rodents.[146,147] The presence of Epo was also identified in the cerebrospinal fluid of normal and preterm infants.[148] Subsequently, Epo and its receptor were identified in the central nervous system of human fetuses as early as 5 to 6 weeks after conception.[149] The expression of Epo and Epo receptor mRNA in the spinal cord remained relatively constant from 7 to 16 weeks' gestation, whereas they both increased in the brain as gestation progressed. By immunohistochemical analysis, Epo and Epo receptor are localized to the periventricular germinal zone at 5 to 6 weeks' gestation.[150] By late gestation, Epo and Epo receptor localization has diverged; Epo is localized primarily in neurons, and Epo receptor reactivity is localized most prominently in astrocytes. *In vitro* studies of neuronal cell lines subjected to hypoxic conditions and glutamate-induced injury demonstrated a protective effect of Epo.[147, 149] *In vivo* studies in animals also demonstrated a protective effect of Epo in ischemic brain injury models.[151,152] The role these hematopoietic factors play in neurodevelopment and homeostasis remains to be identified.

G-CSF and G-CSF receptor are present in virtually all organs between 8 and 24 weeks' gestation.[153,154] Their distribution in the intestine and kidney changes with progression of gestation. In preterm and term neonates, G-CSF protein concentration has been examined. GM-CSF protein and mRNA are detected during human fetal development in the lung, spleen, adrenal gland, and neuronal tissue.[155] The cell types expressing GM-CSF include macrophages, neurons, and glial cells.

IL-11 is a hematopoietic growth factor that also affects non-hematopoietic tissues. IL-11 is produced by alveolar and bronchial epithelial cells in large amounts and may play a significant role in pulmonary inflammation. Additionally, both IL-11 and its receptor are expressed in epithelial cells of the gastrointestinal tract.[156] IL-11 interacts with gastrointestinal epithelial cells and reversibly inhibits proliferation of intestinal crypt stem cell lines. This activity may play a role in normal intestinal growth and in resistance to injury. IL-11 has been evaluated for its protective effects in several models of gastrointestinal disease, including acute chemical-induced colitis and chronic inflammatory bowel disease in transgenic animals expressing human HLA-B27 and β_2-microglobulin.[157] IL-11 has also been used to ameliorate damage in a model of ischemic bowel injury, a murine burn model, and a rat model of short bowel syndrome.[158-160] IL-11 administration increased survival rates and decreased bacterial translocation in these models.

DEVELOPMENTAL DIFFERENCES IN PRODUCTION OF CYTOKINES BY MATURE EFFECTOR CELLS

Some cytokines regulating pivotal functions required for activation of immune effector cells are synthesized in diminished quantities by human neonates compared with adults. Production of IFN-γ and of IL-6 is decreased by circulating leukocytes derived from neonates compared with adults.[161-163] The role of these factors in the immune response to certain bacterial and viral pathogens is underscored by experiments involving IFN-γ– and IL-6–deficient mice generated by homologous recombination and by studies using neutralizing antibodies to these factors.[163-166] IFN-γ–deficient mice manifest severely impaired defenses against both bacterial and viral pathogens. IL-6–deficient mice exhibit defective cytolytic activity of T cells in response to viral infections and diminished capacity to recruit immune cells to sites of infection after experimental bacterial inoculation. The mechanism underlying these developmental defects has not been fully defined; however, diminished production of IL-12 by antigen-presenting cells may contribute to diminished IFN-γ responses. Investigations of neonatal monocyte-derived dendritic cells revealed a selective defect in IL-12 synthesis at the protein and mRNA level in response to lipopolysaccharide, CD40 ligation, or polynucleotides.[167] Moreover, these investigators found that neonatal dendritic cells were less effective than adult dendritic cells in stimulating IFN-γ production by allogeneic adult T cells. This deficit was corrected with addition of recombinant IL-12. Deficiencies in production of these factors could account for impairment in certain aspects of host defenses observed in the newborn period.

Two hematopoietic growth factors, GM-CSF and G-CSF, which exhibit significant effects on myeloid clonal expansion and differentiation, are also produced in diminished quantities by neonatal blood mononuclear cells compared with adult cells.[168, 169] Although GM-CSF receptor numbers and binding affinity appear to be similar between adult and neonatal blood mononuclear cells, GM-CSF gene expression by these cells is clearly lower in cells derived from term neonates. Similarly, monocytes from term human neonates produce significantly lower quantities of G-CSF *in vitro* than cells derived from adults. Furthermore, developmental dysregulation of G-CSF expression appears to be more pronounced in cells of preterm neonates. Studies in mice demonstrate similar decreases in expression of IL-6 and G-CSF *in vivo*.[163] Diminished production of GM-CSF by phytohemagglutinin- and phorbol myristate acetate–stimulated newborn mononuclear cells compared with adult mononuclear cells is secondary to posttranslational regulation of mRNA stability. The precise molec-

ular mechanisms responsible for the differences in regulation of G-CSF between neonates and adults have not been delineated; however, currently available data support a posttranscriptional mechanism.[170]

REFERENCES

1. Sieff C, Williams D: Hematopoiesis. *In* Handin R, et al (eds): Blood: Principles and Practice of Hematology. Philadelphia, JB Lippincott, 1995, pp 171–224.
2. Wendling F, et al: c-Mpl ligand is a humoral regulator of megakaryocytopoiesis. Nature *369*:571, 1994.
3. Jordan C, Lemischka I: Clonal and systemic analysis of long-term hematopoiesis in the mouse. Genes Dev *4*:220, 1990.
4. Osawa M, et al: Long-term lymphohematopoietic reconstitution by a single CD34-low/negative hematopoietic stem cell. Science *273*:242, 1996.
5. Cheshier SH, et al: In vivo proliferation and cell cycle kinetics of long-term self- renewing hematopoietic stem cells. Proc Natl Acad Sci U S A *96*:3120, 1999.
6. MacKey M: Cell kinetic status of haematopoietic stem cells. Cell Prolif *34*:71, 2001.
7. Orlic D, Bodine D. What defines a pluripotent hematopoietic stem cell (PHSC): will the real PHSC please stand up! Blood *84*:3991, 1994.
8. Little M-T, Storb R: History of haematopoietic stem-cell transplantation. Nat Rev Cancer *2*:231, 2002.
9. Hirayama F, et al: Differentiation in culture of murine primitive lymphohematopoietic progenitors toward T-cell lineage. Blood *93*:4187, 1999.
10. Trevisan M, et al: Cycle initiation and colony formation in culture by murine marrow cells with long-term reconstituting potential in vivo. Blood *88*:4149, 1996.
11. Fraser C, et al: Expansion in vitro of retrovirally marked totipotent hematopoietic stem cells. Blood *76*:1071, 1990.
12. Fraser C, et al: Proliferation of totipotent hematopoietic stem cells in vitro with retention of long-term competitive in vivo reconstituting ability. Proc Natl Acad Sci U S A *89*:1968, 1992.
13. Wineman J, et al: Maintenance of high levels of pluripotent hematopoietic stem cells in vitro: effect of stromal cells and c-kit. Blood *81*:365, 1993.
14. Moore KA, et al: In vitro maintenance of highly purified, transplantable hematopoietic stem cells. Blood *89*:4337, 1997.
15. Matsunaga T, et al: Thrombopoietin promotes the survival of murine hematopoietic long-term reconstituting cells: comparison with the effects of flt3/flk-2 ligand and interleukin-6. Blood *92*:452 1998.
16. Miller C, Eaves C: Expansion in vitro of adult murine hematopoietic stem cells with transplantable lympho-myeloid reconstituting ability. Proc Natl Acad Sci U S A *94*:13648, 1997.
17. Bhatia M, et al: Purification of primitive human hematopoietic cells capable of repopulating immune-deficient mice. Proc Natl Acad Sci U S A *94*:5320, 1997.
18. Dick J, et al: Assay of human cells by repopulation of NOD/SCID mice. Stem Cells *15*:199, 1997.
19. Namikawa R, et al: Long-term human hematopoiesis in the SCID-hu mouse. J Exp Med *172*:1055, 1990.
20. Zanjani E, et al: Long-term repopulating ability of xenogenic transplanted human fetal liver hematopoietic stem cells in sheep. J Clin Invest *93*:1051, 1994.
21. Civin C, et al: Sustained, retransplantable, multilineage engraftment of highly purified adult human bone marrow stem cells in vivo. Blood *88*:4102, 1996.
22. Spangrude G, et al: Mouse hematopoietic stem cells. Blood *78*:1395, 1992.
23. Baum C, et al: Isolation of a candidate human hematopoietic stem-cell population. Proc Natl Acad Sci U S A *89*:2804, 1992.
24. Verfaillie C: Hematopoietic stem cells for transplantation. Nat Immun *3*:314, 2002.
25. Uchida N, et al: Transplantable hematopoietic stem cells in human fetal liver have a CD34+ side population (SP) phenotype. J Clin Invest *108*:1071, 2001.
26. Beradi A, et al: Functional isolation and characterization of human hematopoietic stem cells. Science *267*:104, 1995.
27. Pluznik D, Sachs: The cloning of normal "mast" cells in tissue culture. J Cell Comp Physiol *66*:319, 1965.
28. Bradley T, Metcalf D: The growth of mouse bone marrow cells in vitro. Aust J Exp Biol Med Sci *44*:287, 1966.
29. Kishimoto T, et al: Cytokine signal transduction. Cell *76*:253, 1994.
30. Welte K, et al: Filgrastim (r-metHuG-CSF): the first 10 years. Blood *88*:1907, 1996.
31. Palis J, Yoder M. Yolk sac hematopoiesis: the first blood cells of mouse and man. Exp Hematol *29*:927, 2001.
32. Zon L: Developmental biology of hematopoiesis. Blood *86*:2876, 1995.
33. Yoder M, Palis J: Ventral (yolk sac) hematopoiesis in the mouse. *In* Zon L (ed): Hematopoiesis. Oxford, Oxford University Press, 2001, p 180.
34. Palis J, et al: Development of erythroid and myeloid progenitors in the yolk sac and embryo proper of the mouse. Development *126*:5073, 1999.
35. Palis J, et al: Spatial and temporal emergence of high proliferative potential hematopoietic precursors during murine embryogenesis. Proc Natl Acad Sci U S A *98*:4528, 2001.

36. Tavian M, et al: The human embryo, but not its yolk sac, generates lympho-myeloid stem cells: mapping multipotent hematopoietic cell fate in intra-embryonic mesoderm. Immunity 15:487, 2001.

37. North T, et al: Cbfa2 is required for the formation of intra-aortic hematopoietic clusters. Development 126:2563, 1999.

38. Godin I, et al: Stem cell emergence and hematopoietic activity are incompatible in mouse intraembryonic sites. J Exp Med 190:43, 1999.

39. Migliaccio A, Migliaccio G: Human embryonic hemopoiesis: control mechanisms underlying progenitor differentiation in vitro. Develop Biol 125:127, 1988.

40. Allen T, et al: Marrow biology and stem cells. In Dexter T, et al (eds): Colony-Stimulating Factors: Molecular and Cellular Biology. New York, Marcel Dekker, 1990, p 1.

41. Campbell A, Wicha MS: Extracellular matrix and the hematopoietic microenvironment. J Lab Clin Med 112:140, 1988.

42. Weiss L, Geduldig U: Barrier cells: stromal regulation of hematopoiesis and blood cell release in normal and stressed murine bone marrow. Blood 78:9750, 1991.

43. Bodine DM, et al: Effects of hematopoietic growth factors on the survival of primitive stem cells in liquid suspension culture. Blood 78:914, 1991.

44. Itoh Y, et al: Interleukin-3 and granulocyte colony-stimulating factor as survival factors in murine hematopoietic stem cells in vitro. Int J Hematol 55:139, 1992.

45. Katayama N, et al: Growth factor requirement for survival in cell cycle dormancy of primitive murine lymphohematopoietic progenitors. Blood 81:610, 1993.

46. Leary AG, et al: Survival of hematopoietic progenitors in G0 does not require early hematopoietic regulators. Proc Natl Acad Sci U S A 86:4535, 1989.

47. Leary AG, et al: Growth factor requirements for survival in G0 and entry into cell cycle of primitive human hematopoiesis progenitors. Proc Natl Acad Sci U S A 89:4013, 1992.

48. Jubinsky PT, Stanley ER: Purification of hemopoietin 1: a multi-lineage hematopoietic growth factor. Proc Natl Acad Sci U S A 82:2764, 1985.

49. Mochizuki DY, et al: Interleukin-1 regulates hematopoietic activity, a role previously ascribed to hemopoietin 1. Proc Natl Acad Sci U S A 84:5267, 1987.

50. Ikebuchi K, et al: Interleukin-6 enhancement of interleukin-3-dependent proliferation of multipotential hematopoietic progenitors. Proc Natl Acad Sci U S A 84:9035, 1987.

51. Ikebuchi K, et al: Granulocyte colony-stimulating factor enhances interleukin-3-dependent proliferation of multi-potential hematopoietic progenitors. Proc Natl Acad Sci U S A 85:3445, 1988.

52. Musashi K, et al: Direct and synergistic effects of interleukin-11 on murine hematopoiesis in culture. Proc Natl Acad Sci U S A 88:765, 1991.

53. Tsuji K, et al: Enhancement of murine blast cell colony formation in culture by recombinant rat stem cell factor (rrSCF), ligand for c-kit. Blood 78:1223, 1991.

54. Hirayama F, et al: Synergistic interaction between interleukin-12 (natural killer cell stimulatory factor, cytotoxic lymphocyte maturation factor) and steel factor in support of proliferation of murine lymphohemopoietic progenitors in culture. J Cell Biochem 17B:225, 1993.

55. Srour EF, et al: Relationship between cytokine-dependent cell cycle progression and MHC class II antigen expression by human CD34+ HLA-DR-bone marrow cells. J Immunol 148:815, 1992.

56. Suda T, et al: Permissive role of interleukin-3 in proliferation and differentiation of multipotential hematopoietic progenitor in culture. J Cell Physiol 124:182, 1985.

57. Metcalf D, et al: Direct stimulation by purified GM-CSF of the proliferation of multipotential and erythroid precursors. Blood 55:138, 1980.

58. Sieff CA, et al: Human recombinant granulocyte-macrophage colony-stimulating factor: a multilineage hemopoietin. Science 230:1171, 1985.

59. Peschel C, et al: Effects of B cell stimulatory factor 1/interleukin-4 on hematopoietic progenitor cells. Blood 70:254, 1985.

60. Jacobs K, et al: Isolation and characterization of genomic and cDNA clones of human erythropoietin. Nature 313:806, 1985.

61. Sanderson CJ: Interleukin-5, eosinophils, and disease. Blood 79:3101, 1989.

62. Ralph P, et al: Biological properties and molecular biology of the human macrophage growth factor, CSF-1. Immunobiology 172:194, 1986.

63. Demetri GD, Griffin JD: Granulocyte colony-stimulating factor and its receptor. Blood 78:2791, 1991.

64. Kaushansky K: Thrombopoietin and the hematopoietic stem cell. Blood 92:1, 1998.

65. Akahane K, et al: Effects of recombinant human tumor necrosis factor (rhTNF) on normal human and mouse hematopoietic progenitor cells. Int J Cell Cloning 5:16, 1987.

66. Cashman JD, et al: Mechanisms that regulate the cell cycle status of very primitive hematopoietic cells in long-term human marrow cultures. I. Stimulatory role of a variety of mesenchymal cell activators and inhibitory role of TGF-β. Blood 75:96, 1990.

67. McNiece IK, et al: Transforming growth factor-b inhibits the action of stem cell factor on mouse and human hematopoietic progenitors. Int J Cell Cloning 10:80, 1992.

68. Broxmeyer HE, et al: Enhancing and suppressing effects of recombinant murine macrophage inflammatory proteins on colony formation in vitro by bone marrow myeloid progenitor cells. Blood 76:1110, 1992.

69. Foxwell BMJ, et al: Cytokine receptors: structure and signal transaduction. Clin Exp Immunol 90:161, 1992.

70. Sims JE, et al: cDNA expression cloning of the IL-1 receptor, a member of the immunoglobulin superfamily. Science 241:585, 1988.

71. Yamasaki K, et al: Cloning and expression of the human interleukin-6 (BSF-2/IFN beta 2) receptor. Science 241:825, 1988.

72. Bazon JF: Growth hormone, prolactin, erythropoietin, and IL-6 receptors, and the p75 IL-2 receptor β-chain. Biochem Biophys Res Commun 164:788, 1989.

73. Gearing DP, et al: Expression cloning of a receptor for human granulocyte-macrophage colony-stimulating factor. EMBO J 8:3667, 1989.

74. Itoh N, et al: Cloning of an interleukin-3 receptor gene: a member of a distinct receptor gene family. Science 247:324, 1990.

75. Idzerda RL, et al: Human interleukin 4 receptor confers biological responsiveness and defines a novel receptor superfamily. J Exp Med 171:861, 1990.

76. Goodwin RG, et al: Cloning of the human and murine interleukin-7 receptors: demonstration of a soluble form and homology to a new receptor superfamily. Cell 60:941, 1990.

77. Fukunaga R, et al: Expression cloning of a receptor for murine granulocyte colony-stimulating factor. Cell 61:341, 1990.

78. Renauld JC, et al: Interleukin-9 and its receptor: involvement in mast cell differentiation and T cell oncogenesis. J Leukoc Biol 57:353, 1995.

79. Bacon CM, et al: Interleukin-12 (L-12) induces tyrosine phosphorylation of JAK2 and TYK2: differential use of Janus family tyrosine kinases by IL-2 and IL-12. J Exp Med 181:399, 1995.

80. Langer JA, Pestka S: Interferon receptors. Immunol Today 9:393, 1988.

81. Suzuki H, et al: The N terminus of the interleukin-8 (IL8) receptor confers high affinity binding to human IL-8. J Biol Chem 269:18263, 1994.

82. Clore GM, Gronenborn AM: Three dimensional structure of the αβ chemokines. FASEB J 9:47, 1995.

83. Davies DR, Wlodawer A: Cytokines and their receptor complexes. FASEB J 9:50, 1995.

84. Taniguchi T: Cytokine signaling through nonreceptor protein tyrosine kinases. Science 268:251, 1995.

85. Wilks AF, Harpur AG: Cytokine signal transduction and the JAK family of protein tyrosine kinases. Bioessays 16:313, 1994.

86. Kishimpoto T, et al: Interleukin-6 and its receptor: a paradigm for cytokines. Science 258:593, 1992.

87. Rose-John S, Heinrich PC: Soluble receptors for cytokines and growth factors: generation and biological function. Biochem J 300:281, 1994.

88. Nijsten MWN, et al: Serum levels of interleukin-6 and acute phase responses. Lancet 2:921, 1987.

89. Honda M, et al: Human soluble IL-6 receptor: its detection and enhanced release by HIV infection. J Immunol 148:2175, 1992.

90. Narazaki M, et al: Soluble forms of the interleukin-6 signal-transducing receptor component gp130 in human serum possessing a potential to inhibit signals through membrane-anchored gp130. Blood 82:1120, 1993.

91. Taga T, et al: Interleukin-6 triggers the association of its receptor with a possible signal transducer, gp130. Cell 58:573, 1989.

92. Hibi M, et al: Molecular cloning and expression of an IL-6 signal transducer, gp130. Cell 63:1149, 1990.

93. Mackiewicz A, et al: Complex of soluble human IL-6-receptor/IL-6 up-regulates expression of acute-phase proteins. J Immunol 149:2021, 1992.

94. Peters M, et al: Interleukin-6 and soluble interleukin-6 receptor: direct stimulation of gp130 and hematopoiesis. Blood 92:3495, 1998.

95. Taniguchi T: Cytokine signaling through nonreceptor protein tyrosine kinases. Science 268:251, 1995.

96. Ullrich A, Schlessinger J: Signal transduction by receptors with tyrosine kinase activity. Cell 61:203, 1990.

97. Heldin CH: Dimerization of cell surface receptors in signal transduction. Cell 80:213, 1995.

98. Davies DR, Wlodawer A: Cytokines and their receptor complexes. FASEB J 9:50, 1995.

99. Nicola NA, Metcalf D: Subunit promiscuity among hemopoietic growth factor receptors. Cell 67:1, 1991.

100. Koch CA, et al: SH2 and SH3 domains: elements that control interactions of cytoplasmic signaling proteins. Science 252:668, 1991.

101. Songyan Z, et al: SH2 domains recognize specific phosphopeptide sequences. Cell 72:767, 1993.

102. Carter-Su C, et al: Phosphorylation of highly purified growth hormone receptors by a growth hormone receptor-associated tyrosine kinase. J Biol Chem 264:18654, 1989.

103. Wilks AF: Two putative protein-tyrosine kinases identified by application of the polymerase chain reaction. Proc Natl Acad Sci U S A 86:1603, 1989.

104. Velazque L, et al: A protein tyrosine kinase in the interferon alpha/beta signaling pathway. Cell 70:313, 1992.

105. Watling D, et al: Complementation by the protein tyrosine kinase JAK2 of a mutant cell line defective in the interferon-gamma signal transduction pathway. Nature 366:166, 1993.

106. Ihle JN, et al: Signaling by the cytokine receptor superfamily: JAKs and STATs. Trends Biochem Sci 19:222, 1994.

107. Ihle JN, Kerr IM: Jaks and Stats in signaling by the cytokine receptor superfamily. Trends Genet 11:69, 1995.

108. O'Neal KD, Yu-Lee Y: The proline-rich motif (PRM): a novel feature of the cytokine/hematopoietin receptor superfamily. Lymphokine Cytokine Res 12:309, 1993.

109. D'Andre AD, et al: The cytoplasmic region of the erythropoietin receptor contains non-overlapping positive and negative regulatory domains. Mol Cell Biol 11:1980, 1991.

110. Darnell JE Jr, et al: Jak-STAT pathways and transcriptional activation in response to IFNs and other extracellular signaling proteins. Science 264:1415, 1994.
111. Superti-Furga G: Regulation of the Src protein kinases. FEBS Lett 369:62, 1995.
112. Pawson T: Protein modules and signalling networks. Nature 373:573, 1995.
113. Bar-Sagi D, Hall A: Ras and Rho GTPases: a family reunion. Cell 103:227, 2000.
114. Sherr CJ: Cancer cell cycles. Science 274:672, 1996.
115. Kerkhoff E, Rapp UR: Cell cycle targets of Ras/Raf signalling. Oncogene 17:1457, 1998.
116. Burstein ES, et al: The ras-related GTPase rac1 regulates a proliferative pathway selectively utilized by G-protein coupled receptors. Oncogene 17:1617, 1998.
117. Guide F, et al: Differential utilization of Ras signaling pathways by macrophage colony-stimulating factor (CSF) and granulocyte-macrophage CSF receptors during macrophage differentiation. Mol Cell Biol 18:3851, 1998.
118. Emanuel PD, et al: The role of monocyte-derived hemopoietic growth factors in the regulation of myeloproliferation in juvenile chronic myelogenous leukemia. Exp Hematol 19:1017, 1991.
119. Zhang YY, et al: Nf1 regulates hematopoietic progenitor cell growth and ras signaling in response to multiple cytokines. J Exp Med 187:1893, 1998.
120. Birnbaum RA, et al: Nf1 and GMcsf interact in myeloid leukemogenesis. Mol Cell 5:189, 2000.
121. Paul SR, et al: Molecular cloning of a cDNA encoding interleukin 11, a stromal cell-derived hematopoietic cytokine. Proc Natl Acad Sci U S A 87:7512, 1990.
122. Du XX, Williams DA: Interleukin-11: a multifunctional growth factor derived from the hematopoietic microenvironment. Blood 83:2023, 1994.
123. Schibler KR, et al: Effect of interleukin-11 on cycling status and clonogenic maturation of fetal and adult hematopoietic progenitors. Blood 80:900, 1992.
124. Yin T, et al: Involvement of IL-6 signal transducer gp130 in IL-11–mediated signal transduction. J Immunol 151:2555, 1993.
125. Mitchel MD, et al: Cytokine networking in the placenta. Placenta 14:249, 1993.
126. Parhar RS, et al: PGE2-mediated immunosuppression by first trimester human decidual cells blocks activation of maternal leukocytes in the decidua with potential anti-trophoblast activity. Cell Immunol 120:61,1989.
127. Zanjani ED, et al: Erythropoietin does not cross the placenta into the fetus. Pathobiology 61:211, 1993.
128. Malek A, et al: Lack of transport of erythropoietin across the human placenta as studied by an in vitro perfusion system. Pflugers Arch 427:157, 1994.
129. Medlock ES, et al: Granulocyte colony-stimulating factor crosses the placenta and stimulates fetal rat granulopoiesis. Blood 81:9, 1993.
130. Novales JS, et al: Maternal administration of granulocyte colony-stimulating factor improves neonatal rat survival after a lethal group B streptococcal infection. Blood 81:923, 1993.
131. Calhoun DA, et al: Granulocyte colony-stimulating factor in preterm and term pregnancy, parturition, and intra-amniotic infection. Obstet Gynecol 97:229, 2001.
132. Calhoun DA, et al: Transfer of recombinant human granulocyte colony stimulating factor (rhG-CSF) from the maternal to the fetal circulation is not dependent upon a functional G-CSF-receptor. Placenta 22:609, 2001.
133. Migliaccio AR, Migliaccio G: Human embryonic hemopoiesis: control mechanisms underlying progenitor differentiation in vitro. Dev Biol 125:127, 1988.
134. Roodman GD, et al: Effects of dexamethasone on erythroid colony and burst formation from human fetal liver and adult marrow. Br J Haematol 53:62, 1983.
135. Christensen RD, et al: Down-modulation of neutrophil production by erythropoietin in human hematopoietic clones. Blood 74:817, 1989.
136. Emerson SG, et al: Developmental regulation of erythropoiesis by hematopoietic growth factors: analysis on populations of BFU-E from bone marrow, peripheral blood, and fetal liver. Blood 74:49, 1989.
137. Valtieri M, et al: Erythropoietin alone induces erythroid burst formation by human embryonic but not adult BFU-E in unicellular serum-free culture. Blood 74:460, 1989.
138. Gardner JD, et al: Effects of interleukin-6 on fetal hematopoietic progenitors. Blood 75:2150, 1990.
139. Schibler KR, et al:, Possible mechanisms accounting for the growth factor independence of hematopoietic progenitors from umbilical cord blood. Blood 84:3679, 1994.
140. Schibler KR, et al: Effect of recombinant stem cell factor on clonogenic maturation and cycle status of human fetal hematopoietic progenitors. Pediatr Res 35:303, 1994.
141. Schmitt RM, et al: Hematopoietic development of embryonic stem cells in vitro: cytokine and receptor gene expression. Genes Dev 5:728, 1991.
142. Zsebo KM, et al: Stem cell factor is encoded at the Sl locus of the mouse and is the ligand for the c-kit tyrosine kinase receptor. Cell 63:213, 1990.
143. Chabo, B, et al: The proto-oncogene c-kit encoding a transmembrane tyrosine kinase receptor maps to the mouse W locus. Nature 335:88, 1988.
144. Dranof G, et al: Involvement of granulocyte-macrophage colony-stimulating factor in pulmonary homeostasis. Science 264:713, 1994.
145. Lieschke GJ, et al: Mice lacking both macrophage- and granulocyte-macrophage colony-stimulating factor have macrophages and coexistent osteopetrosis and severe lung disease. Blood 84:27, 1994.
146. Masuda S, et al: Functional erythropoietin receptor of the cells with neural characteristics: comparison with receptor properties of erythroid cells. J Biol Chem 268:11208, 1993.
147. Morishita E, et al: Erythropoietin receptor is expressed in rat hippocampal and cerebral cortical neurons, and erythropoietin prevents in vitro glutamate-induced neuronal death. Neuroscience 76:105, 1997.
148. Li Y, et al: Erythropoietin receptors are expressed in the central nervous system of mid-trimester human fetuses. Pediatr Res 40:376, 1996.
149. Juul SE, et al: Erythropoietin and erythropoietin receptor in the developing human central nervous system. Pediatr Res 43:40, 1998.
150. Juul SE, et al: Immunohistochemical localization of erythropoietin and its receptor in the developing human brain. Pediatr Dev Pathol 2:148, 1999.
151. Brines ML, et al: Erythropoietin crosses the blood-brain barrier to protect against experimental brain injury. Proc Natl Acad Sci U S A 97:10526, 2000.
152. Sakanak M, et al: In vivo evidence that erythropoietin protects neurons from ischemic damage. Proc Natl Acad Sci U S A 95:4635, 1998.
153. Slayton WB, et al: Hematopoiesis in the liver and marrow of human fetuses at 5 to 16 weeks postconception: quantitative assessment of macrophage and neutrophil populations. Pediatr Res 43:774, 1998.
154. Calhoun DA, et al: Distribution of granulocyte colony-stimulating factor (G-CSF) and G-CSF–receptor mRNA and protein in the human fetus. Pediatr Res 46:333, 1999.
155. Dame JB, et al: The distribution of granulocyte-macrophage colony-stimulating factor and its receptor in the developing human fetus. Pediatr Res 46:358, 1999.
156. Du XX, et al: A bone marrow stromal-derived growth factor, interleukin-11, stimulates recovery of small intestinal mucosal cells after cytoablative therapy. Blood 83:33, 1994.
157. Keith JC, Jr, et al: IL-11, a pleiotropic cytokine: exciting new effects of IL-11 on gastrointestinal mucosal biology. Stem Cells 12:89, 1994.
158. Du X, et al: Protective effects of interleukin-11 in a murine model of ischemic bowel necrosis. Am J Physiol 272:G545, 1997.
159. Schindel D, et al: Interleukin-11 improves survival and reduces bacterial translocation and bone marrow suppression in burned mice. J Pediatr Surg 32:312, 1997.
160. Liu Q, et al: Trophic effects of interleukin-11 in rats with experimental short bowel syndrome. J Pediatr Surg 31:1047, 1996.
161. Bryson YJ, et al: Deficiency of immune interferon production by leukocytes of normal newborns. Cell Immunol 55:191, 1980.
162. Schibler KR, et al: Defective production of interleukin-6 by monocytes: a mechanism underlying several host defense deficiencies of neonates. Pediatr Res 31:18, 1992.
163. Liechty KW, et al: The failure of newborn mice infected with Escherichia coli to accelerate neutrophil production correlates with their failure to increase transcripts for granulocyte colony-stimulating factor and interleukin-6. Biol Neonate 64:331, 1993.
164. Huang S, et al: Immune response in mice that lack the interferon-gamma receptor. Science 259:1742, 1993.
165. Dalton DK, et al: Multiple defects of immune cell function in mice with disrupted interferon-gamma genes. Science 259:1739, 1993.
166. Buchmeier NA, Schreiber RD: Requirement of interferon-gamma for resolution of Listeria monocytogenes infection. Proc Natl Acad Sci U S A 82:7404, 1985.
167. Goriely S, et al: Deficient IL-12(p35) gene expression by dendritic cells derived from neonatal monocytes. J Immunol 166:2141, 2001.
168. Cairo MS, et al: Decreased stimulated GM-CSF production and GM-CSF gene expression but normal numbers of GM-CSF receptors in human term newborns compared with adults. Pediatr Res 30:362, 1991.
169. Schibler, KR, et al: Production of granulocyte colony-stimulating factor in vitro by monocytes from preterm and term neonates. Blood 82:2478, 1993.
170. Lee SM, et al: Transcriptional rates of granulocyte-macrophage colony-stimulating factor, granulocyte colony-stimulating factor, interleukin-3, and macrophage colony-stimulating factor genes in activated cord versus adult mononuclear cells: alteration in cytokine expression may be secondary to posttranscriptional instability. Pediatr Res 34:560, 1993.

145 Developmental Granulocytopoiesis

FETAL GRANULOCYTE PROGENITORS

The mammalian embryonic circulation is first supplied with blood cells derived from the extraembryonic mesoderm of the yolk sac.[1] As the embryo develops, hematopoiesis switches to the liver and then to the bone marrow, which supplies the adult multilineage blood system. Previously, it was thought that these hematopoietic organs were seeded by yolk sac–derived hematopoietic stem cells. However, there is now considerable debate that, in addition to the yolk sac hematopoietic stem cells (which may be a transient embryonic population), the definitive stem cells may also arise from a distinct, aorta-gonad-mesonephros region within the embryonic splanchnopleuric mesoderm. Although the origin of hematopoietic stem cells is not clearly known in the human embryo, these cells are restricted spatially to the ventral aspect of the dorsal aorta in the preumbilical aorta-gonad-mesonephros region around the anterior limb bud level, and they are observed between 30 and 37 days of gestation. These cells are closely associated with the endothelial cells lining the dorsal aorta, although it remains somewhat unclear whether they are derived *in situ* from a common hemangioblast precursor or arise from a separate population and migrate to this site.

Yolk sac hematopoiesis continues from the 3rd through the 8th to 10th week after conception. There is some overlap, therefore, with hematopoiesis in the liver, which begins about the 5th week and continues through at least 20 to 24 weeks. In the marrow, however, hematopoiesis starts only in the 11th week and overlaps with the liver during the mid-trimester.[2] Committed granulocytic progenitors first appear in the clavicular marrow in the 11th week, and mature neutrophils can be observed from the 14th week onward (mature neutrophils are not identifiable) in the liver, although neutrophil progenitors are abundant.[3]

Hematopoietic progenitor cells can be grown in semisolid media *in vitro*. Pluznick and Sachs,[4] and Bradley and Metcalf,[5] termed the progenitor cell that, in culture, develops into a colony of hemic cells a *colony-forming unit* (CFU). It was observed that when cultured in appropriate conditions, certain CFUs gave rise to clones containing a mixture of many varieties of blood cells, including macrophages, monocytes, neutrophils, and erythrocytes. These CFUs were referred to as *CFU-MIX* or, if the colony contained granulocytes, erythrocytes, megakaryocytes, and macrophages, *CFU-GEMM*. Thus, CFU-MIX and CFU-GEMM are, by definition, pluripotent progenitors because they have the capacity to generate cells of several types. Other CFUs were noted to give rise to colonies consisting exclusively of only one or two varieties of blood cells. Those that developed into colonies containing only neutrophils were termed *CFU-G* (granulocyte), and those that developed into colonies containing only macrophages or monocytes were termed *CFU-M* (macrophages or monocytes). Those that gave rise to colonies containing neutrophils plus macrophages or monocytes (or both) were termed *CFU-GM*, and those that gave rise to colonies containing only megakaryocytes were termed *CFU-Meg*.[6] Other progenitors develop into colonies of normoblasts. These progenitors can be divided into two classes, depending on whether they are relatively primitive or differentiated. Those that are more primitive, closely related to CFU-MIX, give rise to a large burst of normoblasts in culture and are termed *burst-forming units–erythroid (BFU-E)*. Erythroid progenitors that are more mature

and thus more closely related to the pronormoblast give rise to a smaller clone of normoblasts in culture and are termed *colony-forming units–erythroid (CFU-E)*. This chapter focuses only on the varieties of hematopoietic progenitors that appear to be relevant to the granulocytopoiesis. The transcriptional mechanisms underlying this process of lineage commitment and progression are now beginning to be understood. Early granulocytopoiesis seems to need the C/EBPα, PU.1, RAR, CBF, and c-Myb transcription factors, whereas terminal neutrophil differentiation depends on C/EBPε, PU.1, Sp1, CDP, and HoxA10. Orchestration of the myeloid developmental program is achieved via cooperative gene regulation, synergistic and inhibitory protein-protein interaction, promotor autoregulation and cross-regulation, regulation of factor levels, and induction of cell cycle arrest. A detailed review of these regulatory processes is available elsewhere.[7]

Umbilical cord blood and fetal blood sampled *in utero* have a 10- to 50-fold higher concentration of CFU-GM than does the blood of adults.[8] This finding has also been noted in rats, and yet when the total body content of CFU-GM is quantified (the sum of all CFU-GM in the blood, bone marrow, liver, and spleen), newborn rats actually have less than 20% of the CFU-GM/g body weight observed in adult animals.[9] Similar findings are reported for CFU-MIX in rats.[10] It is unclear whether the total body content of neutrophil progenitors in human preterm or term neonates is significantly less than that observed in adult subjects. There is indirect evidence from studies on plasma concentration of soluble FcRIII (sCD16), however, that the total neutrophil cell mass in human neonates born before 32 weeks' gestation may only be about one-fourth of that of adult subjects. sCD16 is derived from apoptotic neutrophils, and its concentration in plasma reflects the total body neutrophil mass as well as overall production of neutrophils in the bone marrow. In contrast to the low values observed in preterm neonates, term infants have plasma sCD16 concentrations and (by implication) neutrophil stores within the normal adult range. The low sCD16 levels of premature infants reach adult values by the fourth postnatal week.[11]

Studies using uptake of tritiated thymidine indicate that the population of CFU-GM obtained from human fetuses has a high proportion of actively cycling cells.[8] Active cycling of CFU-GM appears to be one of the mechanisms employed for increasing neutrophil production. The reasons for the rapid baseline rate of neutrophil production in the midtrimester fetus include the following:

1. Neutrophil production begins relatively late in human gestation (14 to 16 weeks), and the neutrophil reserve pool size is extremely small during the mid-trimester. To build a sizable neutrophil reserve pool in preparation for birth, a rapid rate of neutrophil production is needed.
2. The fetus is growing rapidly, and, therefore, in contrast to the adult, a rapid rate of neutrophil production is needed just to maintain a neutrophil reserve of a certain size per gram of body weight.

Basic differences in hematopoietic progenitors of fetal versus adult origin have been postulated. For instance, Emerson and colleagues,[12] Valtieri and colleagues,[13] and Holbrook and colleagues[14] observed that fetal BFU-E undergoes clonal maturation in the presence of erythropoietin alone, whereas BFU-E of adult origin requires other factors, such as granulocyte-macrophage colony-stimulating factor (GM-CSF), interleukin-3 (IL-3), or IL-9, in addition to erythropoietin. Gardner and colleagues[15] and Schibler and colleagues[16] reported a similar phenomenon for fetal CFU-GM. Gardner and colleagues[15] observed that a fraction of fetal CFU-GM underwent clonal maturation *in vitro* when IL-6 alone was included in the tissue culture dishes, whereas CFU-GM from adults required other factors as well. Schibler and colleagues[16] reported a similar finding with IL-11. Some of this apparent difference between fetal and adult hematopoietic progenitors may, in fact, be explained by environmental differences rather than by differences intrinsic to the progenitors. An example of this was shown by Schibler and co-workers,[17] who observed transcripts for GM-CSF and IL-3 in fetal but not adult CD34+ progenitors. They concluded that the "growth factor independence" observed in fetal hematopoietic progenitors was the result of generation of factors such as GM-CSF and IL-3 in the culture dishes. The growth factor independence of fetal progenitors has been ablated experimentally by adding neutralizing anti–GM-CSF and anti–IL-3 antibodies to the culture dish.

Limited studies have sought to assess differences in responsiveness of fetal versus adult granulocytopoietic progenitors to the recombinant hematopoietic growth factors granulocyte colony-stimulating factor (G-CSF) and GM-CSF. Thus far, no significant differences have been observed.[18,19]

FETAL HEMATOPOIETIC MICROENVIRONMENT

Fetal hepatic hematopoiesis is characterized by a predominance of erythropoiesis, whereas the fetal bone marrow has a predominance of granulocytopoiesis.[19-23] The progenitors populating both organs, however, are capable of both erythropoiesis and granulocytopoiesis when they are cultured *in vitro*.[19,24-28] Thus, it appears to be the local microenvironment that determines the commitment of fetal hematopoietic progenitors to erythropoiesis or granulocytopoiesis (Fig. 145–1).

Cellular elements, growth factors, and the extracellular matrix (ECM) compose the hematopoietic microenvironment. The cellular elements consist primarily of macrophages, reticular cells, adipocytes, and endothelial cells. Collagen and various glycoproteins, such as hemonectin and fibronectin, constitute the ECM.[29]

The cellular elements of the hematopoietic system have specific roles within the hepatic and bone marrow microenvironment (Fig. 145–2). Macrophages appear to be associated more with erythropoiesis than with granulocyte production. Weiss[30] demonstrated that the macrophage-like cells of the microenvironment have long branching processes encircling erythroblasts. Similarly, *in vitro* erythroid colonies generally develop around a nesting macrophage.[31] Macrophages and hepatocytes are both closely associated with erythroid development in the fetal liver.[32] Granulocytes are associated with the reticular cells of the marrow microenvironment.[33, 34] These cells have fibroblast-like functions. They also seem to be the cells that lay down the meshwork of the bone marrow microenvironment. The reticular cells also possess specific glycoproteins that selectively bind progenitor cells. As these cells mature, they lose their binding sites for adhesive molecules and are released into circulation.

Differences in the fetal versus adult hematopoietic microenvironment may be based, in part, on differences in the stromal cell populations. Bethel and colleagues[33] assessed this possibility by obtaining fetal liver, fetal marrow, and adult marrow as sources of microenvironmental stroma. They observed no differences in the cellular elements from the three sources and on that basis speculated that differences in the stroma of a fetus versus an adult did not result from differences in the cellular portion of the hematopoietic microenvironment.

The studies of Chen and Weiss[35] demonstrated that vertebral bone marrow first exhibits infiltration by vessels, which is then followed by macrophages and fibroblast or reticular cells that form the meshwork of the microenvironment. Hematopoietic cells nest in this meshwork, and hematopoiesis develops. Weiss[30] wrote that the mechanisms "learned" during embryogenesis control hematopoiesis from embryo to adult.

ECM components also bind to growth factors produced by stromal cells, thus providing higher local concentrations. For example, heparan-sulfated proteoglycans can bind to tumor growth factor-β, basic fibroblast growth factor, IL-3, GM-CSF, and IL-7. Osteonectin can immobilize platelet-derived growth factor. In addition, ECM can bind to cell surface glycoproteins. Fibronectin, collagens, and laminin are ligands for integrins, which not only control anchorage, spreading, and migration of hematopoietic cells but are also involved in various intracellular signaling cascades. Hyaluronan is a ligand of CD44 and, in several systems, facilitates cell-to-cell adhesion and cell migration.[36]

Collagens I, III, and IV have been found in the adherent cell layer of long-term marrow cultures.[37-39] The specific role of collagen has not been defined, but Zuckerman and colleagues,[40] using a murine long-term bone marrow culture system and a proline analogue *cis*-4-hydroxyproline to inhibit collagen synthesis, demonstrated that collagen is important in long-term cultures. Using various concentrations of *cis*-4-hydroxyproline, these investigators documented decreased cellularity of adherent cell layers in the presence of *cis*-4-hydroxyproline, decreased

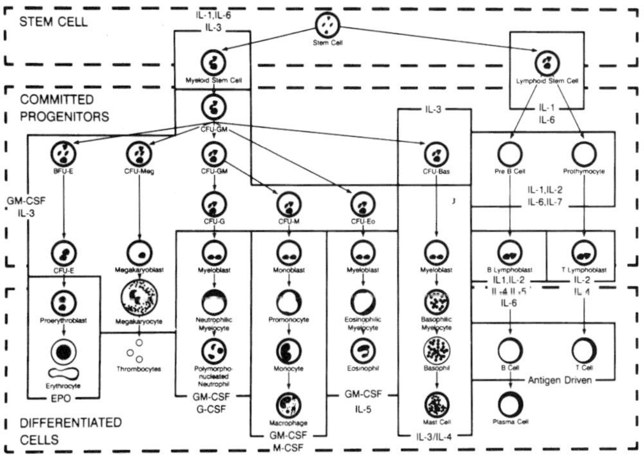

Figure 145–1. Hematopoietic development and regulation of myeloid committed progenitors.

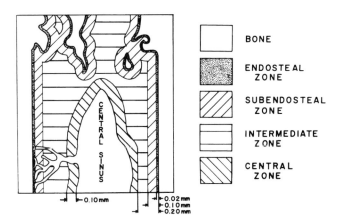

Figure 145–2. Scale drawing of the stereologic zones used for the determination of hematopoietic colony cell distribution. (From Lambersen, Weiss L: Blood 63:287, 1984).

synthesis of collagen, and decreased hematopoietic growth. Biochemically, there was decreased synthesis of collagen but not of other proteins.

Proteoglycans are also important in hematopoiesis. Polycythemia, which suppresses erythropoiesis, has been shown in mice to be associated with an increased bone marrow content of sulfated glycosaminoglycans.[41] Similarly, proteoglycans are increased in the marrow of starved animals (in which hematopoiesis is disturbed),[42] and chondroitin sulfate and hyaluronic acid are increased in the bone marrow of SI/SI[d] mice, which have a defective marrow microenvironment.[43-45] In contrast, Spooncer and colleagues[46] demonstrated that stimulation of glycosaminoglycan synthesis with β-D-xylosides promotes hematopoietic proliferation.

Proteoglycans and glycosaminoglycans may play a role in cell adhesion to the ECM. Del Rosso and co-workers[47] showed that mature granulocytes did not normally adhere to the ECM, but when they were treated with haluronidase, 60% adhered. Treatment of stroma with heparitinase reduced adhesion of immature marrow granulocytes to the stroma. Glycosaminoglycans may function indirectly to stimulate hematopoiesis. Gordon and colleagues[48] showed that glycosaminoglycans from the bone marrow stromal layer were capable of trapping GM-CSF. Extraction with 2 mol/L sodium chloride removed the colony-stimulating activity from the stromal layer. Fibronectin did not trap GM-CSF, and glycosaminoglycans from fetal liver adherent cells were not able to trap GM-CSF. Thus, different proteoglycans or glycosaminoglycans may have different roles in hematopoiesis. They may stimulate or inhibit hematopoiesis or may select myelopoiesis over erythropoiesis.

Fibronectin has been demonstrated in the adherent cell layer of long-term marrow cultures.[37] Sorrell[49] demonstrated fibronectin in the bone marrow microenvironment of embryonic chicks with the use of immunohistochemical techniques. Erythroid cells have fibronectin receptors, which they lose as the cells mature, a finding suggesting that fibronectin may also be involved in the release of cells from the bone marrow.[50] Studies demonstrated that various fibronectin fragments consisting of the cell-binding domain or CS1 portion augment clonogenic growth of hematopoietic stem and progenitor cells in vitro.[51]

Tsai and colleagues[52] developed an in vitro colony assay on coverslips that required no growth factors other than erythropoietin. The coverslips had a layer of adherent cells derived from a fetal hepatic cell line, and fibronectin was present within these cells. Using partially purified mononuclear cells from bone marrow, these investigators studied the differential binding of CFU-GM and BFU-E to the coverslip system. In this system, developing colonies were primarily erythroid. BFU-E preferentially bound to the adherent cell layer, whereas CFU-GM did not develop despite the addition of a source of GM-CSF. Rabbit antifibronectin serum blocked the binding of BFU-E. A monoclonal antibody to the cell-binding domain of fibronectin was also able to inhibit BFU-E binding to the adherent cell layer. A different glycoprotein was isolated from bone marrow ECM by Campbell and co-workers.[53] It was a 6-kDa molecular weight protein, and strikingly, 90% of the cells binding to this protein were granulocytic. From these studies emerged a model of hematopoietic control at the ECM level involving cell-to-cell and matrix interaction.

Hemonectin, a component of the bone marrow ECM, is a lineage-specific and an organ-specific attachment molecule for cells of the granulocytic lineage. Tsai and colleagues[52] used an affinity-purified polyclonal antibody to purify hemonectin as a probe for developing granulocytopoietic organs. They observed that hemonectin was coordinately expressed in those tissues that supported hematopoiesis in the mouse. However, they also observed hemonectin expression in other tissues, such as skin and capillary endothelium, a finding suggesting

that this molecule has other developmental nongranulocytopoietic functions.

NEUTROPHIL PROLIFERATIVE AND STORAGE POOLS

Myeloblasts, promyelocytes, and myelocytes all have the capacity for cell division, and thus they are collectively termed the *mitotic compartment* or the *neutrophil proliferative pool* (NPP). As neutrophils mature, their capacity to undergo cell division is lost. Thus, metamyelocytes, band neutrophils, and segmented neutrophils are collectively termed the *postmitotic compartment*, the *maturation compartment*, or the *neutrophil storage pool* (NSP). Studies in fetal and newborn rodents indicate that the liver and spleen, similar to the bone marrow, house a significant fraction of the NPP and NSP.[9, 54] In contrast, studies using human mid-trimester aborted fetuses indicate that the liver and spleen are not sites for neutrophil production or storage.[19]

Studies in adult humans and dogs indicate that, under steady-state conditions, four to five cell divisions occur among cells of the NPP.[55] Similar studies have not been reported for children or neonates. In adult humans, studies using tritiated thymidine incorporation and 32P-deoxyfluoridine (DF-^{32}P) labeling indicate that the NPP contains about 2×10^9 cells/kg body weight and the NSP contains about 6×10^9 cells/kg.[56] Adult rats also have an NSP that contains about 6×10^9 cells/kg; however, no neutrophils at all are observed before about 14 days of gestation. By 19 days of gestation (term = 21 days), the rat has an NSP of 0.9×10^9 cells/kg, and by term, the NSP has increased to 1.2×10^9 cells/kg (Fig. 145–3).[54] Although the size of the NSP has not been precisely quantified in human neonates, it appears from preliminary studies of aborted human fetuses that no neutrophils are present before 14 weeks' gestation and the number per kilogram body weight at 22 to 24 weeks' gestation is probably far fewer that at term.[19] It also appears that, in contrast to rodents, granulocytopoiesis in the human fetus takes place almost exclusively in the bone marrow.[19] Although the spleen contains CFU-GM, these appear to be within the blood that is circulating through the spleen and not part of granulocytopoiesis within the spleen. Histologic sections of fetal spleen fail to show nests of granulocytopoietic activity, and RNA extracted from fetal spleen fails to reveal transcripts for neutrophil-specific growth factors. Similarly, differential cell counts, histologic section, and RNA studies of human fetal liver reveal little, if any, granulocytopoiesis in that organ. Moreover, the fetal liver *in vivo* does not exhibit nests of granulocytopoiesis and contains undetectably low concentrations of G-CSF mRNA, even though it houses CFU-GM capable of generating clones of neutrophils *in vitro*. Thus, the spleen and liver contain granulocyte progenitors, but they are probably not normally active sites of granulocytopoiesis in the normal human fetus.

CIRCULATING AND MARGINATED BLOOD NEUTROPHIL POOLS

Neutrophils flow from the NSP into the blood, where they distribute into the circulating neutrophil and the marginal neutrophil pools. Neutrophils in these two pools are in equilibrium, and an approximately equal number of neutrophils populates each pool. In physiologically normal adult humans, the total blood neutrophil pool contains about 0.6×10^9 cells/kg body weight; about one-half of those cells (0.3×10^9 cells/kg) are found in the circulating pool.[56]

The ratio of band neutrophils to segmented neutrophils is much higher in the marrow than in the blood. On that basis, it is likely that a selective release of segmented neutrophils occurs from the NSP. The mechanisms controlling that release, however, are only partly understood. Clearly, G-CSF can induce release of cells from the NSP,[57] as illustrated by the G-CSF–deficient mice

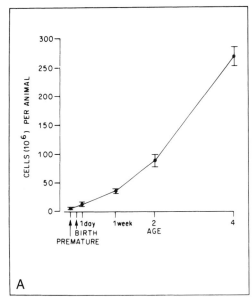
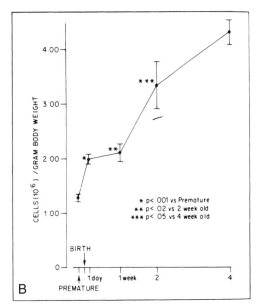

Figure 145–3. A, Neutrophil storage pool size at various ages in the developing rat. Each point represents the mean of 8 to 12 animals ± SE. **B,** Neutrophil storage pool size per gram of body weight at various stages in the developing rat. Each point represents the mean of 8 to 12 animals ± SE. (From Erdmann SH, et al: Biol Neonate *41*:132, 1982; S Karger AG, Basel.)

produced by Lieschke and colleagues.[58] Hydrocortisone and many related corticosteroids can also induce release of neutrophils from the NSP into the blood.[56] Some evidence exists that a factor derived from the activation of C3 can induce NSP release as well.[59]

Rapid movement of neutrophils from the marginated pool into the circulating pool follows the administration of epinephrine.[56] The neutrophilia thus produced is observed for 30 to 45 minutes. No change in differential cell count accompanies the demargination; thus, the proportion of segmented neutrophils is the same in the marginated and circulating neutrophil pools. The opposite movement of neutrophils, from the circulating pool to the marginated pool, occurs for 1 to 2 hours after the experimental intravenous administration of endotoxin. Newborn infants with strenuous crying can experience neutrophil demargination and as much as double their blood neutrophil concentration within 3 to 5 minutes.[60] A mild demarginating response is also reported to occur in preterm infants after red cell transfusions.[61]

The half-life of neutrophils in the blood of adult humans, measured by autologous DF-^{32}P labeling, is only about 6.3 hours,[62] and this finding agrees closely with other studies that have used ^{3}H-thymidine (7.4 hours).[63] Similar studies on the half-life of neutrophils from human fetal subjects have not been reported. Preliminary *in vitro* studies on cord blood neutrophils, however, do suggest a lower rate of spontaneous apoptosis as compared with adult cells. The significance of these findings remains to be seen, because information on other determinants of neutrophil life-span in the tissues is scant. It is likely that neutrophils leave the blood and enter the tissues randomly, rather than according to their age, as is the case for erythrocytes and platelets. This theory is supported by the observation that transfused, labeled neutrophils appear in the blood and saliva simultaneously.[56]

After their short time in the blood, neutrophils move through vessel walls to enter the tissues. Within minutes of development of a local site of tissue damage or infection, adherence of neutrophils to the endothelium and their subsequent migration into the tissues can be observed. Studies on fetal sheep show that after intra-amniotic exposure to endotoxin, the number of circulating neutrophils initially decreases by 4 hours because

TABLE 145–1

Fetal White Blood Cell and Neutrophil Counts

Gestational Age (wk)	White Blood Cells ($\times 10^3$/mm³)	Neutrophils (%)
18–20	4.2	5 ± 2
21–22	4.19	5.5 ± 3.5
23–25	3.95	7.5 ± 4.5
26–30	4.44	8.5 ± 2.5

Data from refs. 136–138, 140.

of egress into the tissues, and this is followed by a gradual endotoxin-dose dependent increase over the next 6 days.[64] After the initial adherence of the neutrophil to an endothelial cell, it projects pseudopodia and forces a passageway between endothelial cells.[65] The length of time that neutrophils spend in the tissues and their fate there are not completely clear. Labeled neutrophils are found in saliva, although they are not found in the salivary ducts.[56] This is presumably the result of migration of neutrophils into the gingiva. Some loss of neutrophils into the urine has also been observed in normal subjects. Neutrophils are also removed during passage through the lungs, liver, spleen, and gastrointestinal tract.[56] Clearly, not all neutrophils are used by encountering infectious organisms because the size of the marrow and blood neutrophil pools is essentially the same in germ-free and normal mice.[66]

Multiple studies have looked at the normal range of circulating neutrophil concentrations during gestation. The percentage of neutrophils in early gestation is on the order of 5% (Table 145–1). As gestation progresses, the percentage of neutrophils rises slowly. In samples obtained by hysterotomy at 26 to 30 weeks' gestation, neutrophils constitute 8.5% of the leukocytes in blood or only about 350/μL.[67] Postnatal samples of both premature and full-term infants, however, have revealed much higher values. Playfair and associates[68] studied blood counts from 137 fetuses. Ninety-six samples were obtained from pregnancies terminated by hysterotomies, and 41 were obtained

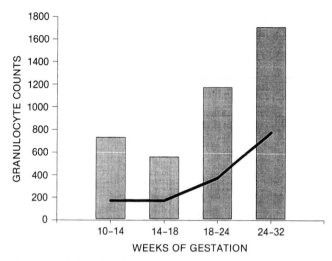

Figure 145–4. Mean and range of neutrophil counts at 10 to 14, 14 to 18, 18 to 24, and 24 to 32 weeks of gestational age. (From Thomas DB, Yoffey JM: Br J Haematol 8:290, 1962.)

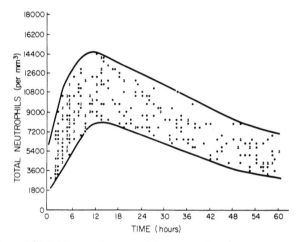

Figure 145–5. The total neutrophil count reference range in the first 60 hours of life. (From Manroe BL, et al: J Pediatr 95:89, 1979.)

from fetuses aborted vaginally. Neonates delivered vaginally had neutrophil counts that were much higher than those delivered operatively. Neutrophil counts may also be higher for up to 3 days in preterm infants after antenatal maternal administration of betamethasone when the drug is administered close to delivery.[69]

The neutrophil count rises progressively to term. There is a doubling of the absolute neutrophil count from 14 to 18 weeks' gestation and a fourfold increase by 24 to 32 weeks' gestation (Fig. 145–4).[70] At birth, the neutrophil count is much higher. Manroe and co-workers[71] published a detailed study of neutrophil counts in normal newborns (38.9±2.4 weeks' gestation) obtained during the 28 days after birth. Peak neutrophil counts occurred between 12 and 24 hours postnatally (Fig. 145–5). At that time, the 95% confidence limit for neutrophil count ranged from a low of 7800 to a high of 14,500 cells/µL. The neutrophil count then decreased, achieving a stable lower value of 1750 by 72 hours of life. The stable upper limit of the next 28 days was not achieved until 6.6 days of age.

Mouzinho and colleagues[72] revised the reference ranges for blood neutrophil concentrations in very low birth weight infants. Serial counts (n = 1788) were obtained prospectively

between birth and 28 days of age from 63 normal infants of 29.9±2.3 weeks' gestation. No difference in the upper limit of normal (neutrophilia) was observed between those very low birth weight infants and the group of more mature infants reported in 1979. Concentrations of neutrophils greater than 14,000/µL at 12 hours of life and greater than 9000/µL after 48 hours defined neutrophilia. The very low birth weight infants, however, exhibited a wider range of counts, encompassing substantially lower values compared with mature infants, with neutropenia defined as a concentration less than 2000/µL at 12 hours of life and less than 100/µL after 48 hours. Lower counts in healthy very low birth weight infants were also reported by Prober and colleagues.[73] In a study[74] examining the reference ranges in very low birth weight infants with infections, the figures from Manroe and colleagues were observed to provide greater sensitivity, although the revised ranges of Mouzinho and co-workers were more specific when neonates with early-onset group B streptococcal infection were compared with a matched control group. The ratio of immature neutrophils to total neutrophil cells in reasonably healthy premature infants, however, exhibits a relatively narrow range.[71-73,75-77] This ratio has been proposed to represent a good discriminating parameter for neonatal infection.

NEUTROPHIL ANTIGENS IN THE FETUS

The expression of specific granulocyte antigens was reviewed by McCullough.[78] In 1926, Doan[79] observed that serum from some patients agglutinated leukocytes. Although techniques for measuring leukoagglutinins have improved over the years, the field of recognition of granulocyte antigens has been plagued by an inherent tendency of granulocytes to agglutinate. Neutrophil-specific antigens were initially discovered by Lalezari and Radel[80] while they were studying neonatal neutropenia. Numerous other antigens have been added subsequently, and they can be broadly classified into three subgroups: (1) antigens with expression limited to granulocytes (e.g., NA, NB, NC, ND, NE, HGA-3, and LAN), (2) antigens that can also be detected on other cell types (e.g., HGA-1, Mart, and Ond), and (3) antigens distributed throughout the body (e.g., the human leukocyte antigen [HLA] system). In the original nomenclature, the letter *N* stood for neutrophil-specific antigen followed by a capital letter designating a specific gene locus and a number designating a certain allele at that locus. As is apparent from the foregoing list, a number of antigens described later did not follow this convention, and the subsequent molecular characterization of the antigens showed that some of these were actually identical to each other.

A newer nomenclature proposed by the Granulocyte Antigen Working Party of the International Society of Blood Transfusion attempted to address these anomalies.[81] It named the well-defined granulocyte alloantigens HNA, which stands for human neutrophil alloantigen. Glycoprotein location of the antigen is coded by a number (e.g., location on Fcγ receptor IIIb is denoted HNA-1). Different polymorphisms of the same glycoprotein are designated alphabetically, in order of the date of publication (HNA-1a, HNA-1b, and so on). The genes coding for glycoproteins are named according to the guidelines of the International Workshop on Human Gene Mapping (e.g., Fcγ receptor IIIb is abbreviated to FCGR3B). The allelic variants of the gene are then designated with Arabic numerals and are separated from the gene designation by an asterisk (e.g., FCGR3B*1). For the naming of newly detected antigens, the use of acronyms is permitted until their eventual inclusion in this system.

The HNA system currently comprises seven antigens that are assigned to five glycoproteins (Table 145–2). This classification does not include NB2, NC1, ND1, NE1, SAR, LAN, LEA, CN1, and RED antigens. NB2 is not the antithetical antigen to NB1, and it may in fact be identical to 9a. NC1 seems to be identical to NA2.

TABLE 145-2

Human Neutrophil Antigens (HNA)

Antigen	Location	Polymorphisms	Older Terminology	Allelic Variants
HNA-1	Fc γRIIIb	HNA-1a	NA1	FCGR3B*1
		HNA-1b	NA2	FCGR3B*2
		HNA-1c	SH	FCGR3B*3
HNA-2	GP 50	HNA-2a	NB1	—
HNA-3	GP 70–95	HNA-3a	5b	—
HNA-4	CD11b (MAC-1)	HNA-4a	MART	CD11B*1
HNA-5	CD-11A(LFA-1)	HNA-5a	OND	CD11A*1

From Bux J: Vox Sang *78*(Suppl 2): 125, 2000.

ND1 and NE1 are solitary representatives of other presumed systems that have been associated with autoimmune neutropenia, but specific antisera against these two antigens are no longer available, and hence testing is not possible. The other antigens are still being characterized. A detailed description of individual antigens can be found elsewhere.[82]

Neutrophil-specific antigens have been identified on mature adult neutrophils, myeloid precursors, and cord blood neutrophils. The other antigens seen on the neutrophils include those of the HLA system and the red cell antigens. Class I HLA antigens (HLA-A, HLA-B, and HLA-C) are seen on neutrophils and their precursors in the bone marrow, although it is not known whether these are intrinsic or are passively absorbed from the plasma. Class II HLA antigens have not been described on neutrophils, but they are present on immature granulocytes. Red cell antigen groups expressed on neutrophils include the polylactosaminyl glycolipids bearing Ii, Le[x], and P systems. Although the antigens of the ABO systems were initially reported to be present, subsequent investigations provided evidence to the contrary. Similarly, the MN, Rh, Kidd, Duffy, Kell, and Kx antigen systems are not present on the surface of granulocytes.

Neutrophil antigens inherited from fathers but not present in mothers may cause an antibody response during gestation. Antineutrophil antibody can cross the placenta to the fetal circulation and can cause severe neutropenia in the fetus and newborn infant. Many different antigenic targets, including HNA-1, HNA-2, and HNA-3, NC1, SH, SAR, LAN, LEA, CN1, and possibly, HLA, have been identified in alloimmune neutropenia. In the United States, one-half of all the cases of alloimmune neutropenia are mediated by antibodies that bind to HNA-1a, HNA-1b, or HNA-2a antigens. Estimates of the frequency of alloimmune neutropenia vary from 0.2 to 20%, although the incidence of granulocyte-specific antibodies is likely to be higher. Although self-limited, alloimmune neutropenia can be associated with serious infections and death.[83] A mortality as high as 5% has been reported. Antineutrophil antibodies may also develop as an isolated autoimmune phenomenon, and they may be seen even in premature neonates.

The etiologic reasons for autoimmune neutropenia of infancy are not exactly known, but associations with parvovirus B19 infection and β-lactam antibiotics have been reported. Suggested mechanisms include development of cross-reacting antibodies resulting from molecular mimicry, changes in endogenous antigens, enhanced HLA expression, or loss of suppression of clones of self-reacting lymphocytes. HNA-1a (NA1) autoimmunization has been linked with HLA DR2, a finding indicating the involvement of immune response genes. However, the occurrence of autoimmune neutropenia of infancy in only one of monozygotic twins suggests that genetics may not be the sole responsible factor. As in alloimmune neutropenia, these infants also present with minor infections such as otitis media, respiratory tract infections, gastroenteritis, or cellulitis, or they may be diagnosed only by chance after the detection of neutropenia. Autoimmune neutropenia of infancy is a self-limiting disorder, with a median duration of approximately 30 months (range, 6 to 60 months), and 95% of patients recover by 4 years of age. Neutropenia, in rare instances, may also be seen in newborn infants born to mothers with autoimmune neutropenia, owing to transplacental passage of her antineutrophil autoantibodies. A review of these disorders can be found elsewhere.[84]

The therapy for immune-mediated neutropenias in neonates is supportive, and a prompt clinical response can usually be obtained with the use of recombinant hematopoietic growth factors such as the G-CSF. Antibiotic prophylaxis has not been shown to be effective. Exchange transfusion has been suggested as a way to lower the antibody titer, but this therapy has not been subjected to adequate testing. Steroid therapy has not been shown to be effective. These disorders are self-limited, but infection must be treated promptly.

ACCELERATING NEUTROPHIL PRODUCTION IN THE FETUS AND NEONATE

In the near-term and term rat, neutrophil production occurs at such a marked pace that significant further increases in neutrophil production may not be possible.[9, 85] At 14 days' gestation (term is ~21 days), no neutrophils whatsoever are observed in the fetal rat liver, marrow, spleen, or blood. The remarkably rapid development of neutrophils just before and after birth result in a total body sum of neutrophils of 1.2×10^6/g at birth and 5×10^6/g by 4 weeks of life.[53] To achieve this, granulocyte progenitors appear to be cycling at near-maximal capacity,[9, 85] Indeed, during the experimental infection of newborn rats, cycling of granulocyte progenitors does not appear to increase beyond that observed in the baseline, noninfected state.

In adult mice, inoculation with *Escherichia coli* results in a rapid, marked acceleration of neutrophil production.[86] This increase is preceded by an increase in G-CSF transcripts within hematopoietic and nonhematopoietic organs (particularly in the lungs). Mice who lack the G-CSF gene (because of homologous recombination knock-out experiments) fail to accelerate neutrophil production during bacterial infection and have an extremely high mortality rate from infection.[58] In contrast to adult mice, newborn mice inoculated with *E. coli* fail to develop a marked increase in G-CSF transcripts in hematopoietic or nonhematopoietic organs, fail to accelerate neutrophil production, and have a high mortality rate from infection.[86] Thus, the capacity of newborn mice to accelerate neutrophil production during infection appears to be limited in at least two ways: by an already rapid rate of production in the noninfected state and by lack of prompt production of G-CSF after bacterial inoculation.

It is not clear to what extent the observations on neutrophil production during infection made in rodents apply to human neonates.[87] Although certain parallels are likely, it does not

TABLE 145-3

Peripartum Complications Found to Have a Significant Effect on Neutrophil Values

Complications	Total Infants	Normal Infants	Neutropenia	Neutrophilia
Maternal hypertension	70	12 (17%)*	53 (76%)	0
Periventricular hemorrhage	13	0	8 (62%)	3 (23%)
Asphyxia	7	0	1 (14%)	2 (10%)
Reticulocytosis	20	3 (15%)	5 (25%)	2 (10%)
Hemolytic disease	86	23 (27%)	0	40 (47%)
Asymptomatic hypoglycemia	16	0	0	7 (44%)
Intrapartum oxytocin	22	0	0	6 (27%)
Maternal fever only	48	0	0	22 (46%)
Postoperative	10	0	0	10 (100%)
Stressful labor†	21	1	0	14 (67%)
Seizures‡	7	0	0	5 (71%)
Pneumothorax	5	0	0	4 (80%)
Meconium aspiration syndrome	9	0	0	7 (78%)

* The percentage of affected infants shown in parentheses. With each complication, $p < .01$ by one-tail test.
† Included are labor ≥ 18 h, midforceps rotation, breech extraction, and ≤ 10 min second stage of labor.
‡ This is not associated with hypoglycemia, intracranial hemorrhage, or asphyxia.
Adapted from Stockman JA, et al: J Pediatr *105*:786, 1984.

appear that neutrophil production in the noninfected human fetus is maximal, and human neonates do appear capable of generating G-CSF during an infectious challenge, although perhaps not as responsively as adults (Table 145-3). For example, during chorioamnionitis, maternal and fetal blood concentrations of G-CSF increase from their baseline low levels (generally <5 pg/mL) to 2000 to 4000 g/mL.[88] The concordance of maternal and fetal G-CSF blood concentrations during chorioamnionitis has led to the speculation that G-CSF produced in tissues of maternal origin (e.g., decidual macrophages) crosses from the maternal to the fetal circulation.[88] This hypothesis is supported by the finding that, during chorioamnionitis, low concentrations of G-CSF mRNA transcripts are found in the fetal blood, but high concentrations are present in the mother's blood.[88] Stallmach and Karolyi[89] observed that during chorioamnionitis granulocyte production increases in the fetus, in fact, expanding to sites in the liver and spleen that do not normally contain granulocytopoietic activity. Thus, granulocytopoiesis in the human fetus is clearly capable of increasing to more than the baseline, noninfected rate. However, in neonates with sepsis-induced neutropenia, serum and urine G-CSF concentrations are significantly higher than those with low neutrophil counts from other causes. These findings suggest that the G-CSF receptors may already be saturated in neonates with sepsis-induced neutropenia, and they raise the possibility that recombinant G-CSF (rG-CSF) therapy may not be highly effective in these patients.[90]

If transplacental passage of G-CSF from the mother to the fetus occurs during chorioamnionitis, it is likely that rG-CSF administered before delivery would also cross from the maternal to the fetal circulation. This possibility was tested in a pregnant rat model by Medlock and colleagues[91] and by Novales and colleagues.[92] They observed that a single dose (50 µg/kg) of G-CSF given to pregnant rats 1 day before delivery resulted in maternal peak G-CSF serum concentrations of 1200 ng/mL and fetal peak serum concentrations of 1.5 ng/mL. Despite the relatively low apparent transplacental passage, this concentration of G-CSF in the fetal rats constituted a significant increase above their normally undetectable baseline G-CSF concentrations. Moreover, the increase in G-CSF concentrations was sufficient to stimulate fetal neutrophil production, elevate blood neutrophil concentrations, and improve the outcome of pups that were subsequently inoculated with group B streptococci. Calhoun and associates[93] performed a human counterpart study, by administering rG-CSF (one dose of 25 µg/kg) to 11 women about to deliver an extremely preterm neonate. As in the rat model, transplacental

passage of a small quantity of G-CSF was detected, and in those infants born 24 to 72 hours after maternal treatment, neutrophilia of 5 to 7 days' duration was observed. It is not clear, however, whether human fetuses may derive benefit from antenatal rG-CSF treatment in the same manner as was shown in the pregnant rat model.

Several clinical trials have tested the hypothesis that rG-CSF administration to neonates with sepsis will alleviate neutropenia and reduce mortality. Gillan and colleagues[94] reported a dose-dependent biologic effect of rG-CSF in human neonates. They studied 42 neonates who had presumed bacterial infection during their first 3 days of life who were randomized to receive a placebo or 1.0, 5.0, 10.0, or 20.0 µg rG-CSF/kg body weight/day for 3 consecutive days. A significant, dose-dependent increase in blood neutrophil concentrations was observed, and a dose-dependent increase in the size of the marrow neutrophil reserve was also seen. Neutrophil C3bi expression was significantly increased 24 hours after starting at least 10 µg/kg. The rG-CSF doses were well tolerated in all infants. Since then, the efficacy of rG-CSF in neonatal sepsis has been examined by Schibler,[95] Bedford-Russell,[96] Miura,[97] Barak,[98] and Kocherlakota and their colleagues.[99] In a meta-analysis based on these studies, 73 rG-CSF recipients had a lower mortality than 82 controls.[100] However, when the nonrandomized studies were excluded, the analysis did not remain statistically adequate. Makhlouf[101] and La Gamma[102] also reported successful use of rG-CSF to treat neutropenia in neonates delivered to women with pregnancy-induced hypertension. rG-CSF therapy is generally well tolerated in neonates, although reductions in platelet counts have been reported. However, it is unclear whether the thrombocytopenia is caused by rG-CSF administration or by the underlying sepsis. With longer-term rG-CSF therapy, greater vigilance is needed in view of reports of leukemic transformation (described in a child with Kostmann syndrome),[103] anti-GCSF antibodies, and osteopenia.

Recombinant GM-CSF (rGM-CSF) has been given to a limited number of human neonates. Cairo and associates[104] administered either placebo or 5.0 or 10.0 µg rGM-CSF/kg/day to 20 neonates. Very low birth weight infants (<1500 g) began treatment in the first 72 hours of life and received daily treatments for 7 days. Within 48 hours of beginning the drug, significant dose-dependent increases in circulating neutrophil and monocyte concentrations were observed. Tibial marrow aspirates revealed an increase in neutrophil reserves, and neutrophil C3bi receptor expression was increased within 24 hours of beginning treatment. Bilgin and co-workers,[105] in a prospective, randomized study, administered rGM-CSF to 30 patients for 7 consecutive days. Twenty-five patients from the rGM-CSF group and 24 from the conventionally treated group had early-onset sepsis, and the remaining 11 patients had late-onset sepsis. The rGM-CSF treated group showed significantly higher absolute neutrophil counts and a lower mortality rate.

rGM-CSF has also been evaluated as prophylaxis against noso-comial infections in very low birth weight infants. Carr and colleagues[106] administered 10 μg/kg rGM-CSF to 75 noninfected newborn infants less than 32 weeks' gestation, initiated within the first 72 hours, for 5 days. Prophylactic GM-CSF therapy abolished neutropenia in treated infants, including those with and without sepsis, during a 4-week period after study entry. Although the rGM-CSF recipients had fewer symptomatic, blood culture–positive episodes than controls, the difference did not reach statistical significance. Similar results were obtained in a large, randomized, placebo-controlled trial in 264 very low birth weight neonates weighing less than 1000 g. rGM-CSF was administered prophylactically at a daily dosage of 8 μg/kg for the first 7 days and then every other day for 21 days. The treated infants had higher absolute neutrophil counts, but the incidence of confirmed noso-comial infection did not differ from that in controls.[107]

The benefits and risks of recombinant myeloid growth factor therapy for conditions in the fetus and newborn infant are still being defined. Despite evidence of benefit from animal studies and promising clinical trials, the evidence currently available is insufficient to support the routine use of rG-CSF or rGM-CSF in neonatal sepsis.[108] Further studies are needed (particularly in high-risk neonatal subgroups with sepsis) because preliminary evidence suggests that such an approach may be more effective. The newer, longer-acting polyethylene glycol–conjugated or gly-cosylated forms of G-CSF also hold promise as viable therapeutic alternatives.

REFERENCES

1. Palis J, Yoder MC: Yolk sac hematopoiesis: the first blood cells of mouse and man. Exp Hematol 29:927, 2001.
2. Slayton WB, et al: The first-appearance of neutrophils in the human fetal bone marrow cavity. Early Hum Dev 53:129, 1998.
3. Slayton WB, et al: Hematopoiesis in the liver and marrow of human fetuses at 5 to 16 weeks postconception: quantitative assessment of macrophage and neutrophil populations. Pediatr Res 43:774, 1998.
4. Pluznick DH, Sachs L: The cloning of normal mast cells in tissue culture. J Cell Physiol 66:319, 1965.
5. Bradley TR, Metcalf D: The growth of mouse bone marrow cells in vitro. Aust J Exp Biol Med Sci 46:335, 1968.
6. Rothstein G: Origin and development of the blood and blood-forming tissues. In Lee GR, et al (eds): Wintrobe's Clinical Hematology, 9th ed. Philadelphia, Lea & Febiger, 1993, pp 50–51.
7. Friedman AD: Transcriptional regulation of granulocyte and monocyte development. Oncogene 21:3377, 2002.
8. Christensen RD, et al: Granulocyte-macrophage progenitor cells in term and preterm neonates. J Pediatr 109:1047, 1986.
9. Christensen RD, Rothstein G: Pre- and postnatal development of granulocytic stem cells in the rat. Pediatr Res 18:599, 1984.
10. Christensen RD: Circulating pluripotent hematopoietic progenitor cells in neonates. J Pediatr 110:623, 1987.
11. Carr R, Huizinga TW: Low soluble FcRIII receptor demonstrates reduced neutrophil reserves in preterm neonates. Arch Dis Child Fetal Neonatal Ed 83:F160, 2000.
12. Emerson SG, et al: Developmental regulation of erythropoiesis by hematopoietic growth factors: analysis on populations of BFU-E from bone marrow, peripheral blood and fetal liver. Blood 74:49, 1989.
13. Valtieri M, et al: Erythropoietin alone induces erythroid burst formation by human embryonic but not adult BFU-E in unicellular serum-free culture. Blood 74:460, 1989.
14. Holbrook ST, et al: Effect of interleukin-9 on clonogenic maturation and cell-cycle status of fetal and adult hematopoietic progenitors. Blood 77:2129, 1991.
15. Gardner JD, et al: Effects of interleukin-6 on fetal hematopoietic progenitors. Blood 75:2150, 1990.
16. Schibler KR: Effect of interleukin-11 on cycling status and clonogenic maturation of fetal and adult hematopoietic progenitors. Blood 80:900, 1992.
17. Schibler KR, et al: Possible mechanisms accounting for the growth factor independence of hematopoietic progenitors from umbilical cord blood. Blood 84:3679, 1994.
18. Schibler KR, et al: Production of granulocyte colony-stimulating factor in vitro by monocytes from preterm and term neonates. Blood 82:2478, 1993.
19. Ohls RK, et al: Neutrophil pool sizes and granulocyte colony-stimulating factor production in human mid-trimester fetuses. Pediatr Res 37:806, 1995.
20. Gilmour JR: Normal haemopoiesis in intra-uterine and neonatal life. J Pathol 52:25, 1984.
21. Kelemen E, et al: Atlas of Human Hemopoietic Development. Berlin, Springer-Verlag, 1979.
22. Moore MAS, Metcalf D: Ontogeny of the haemopoietic system: yolk sac origin of in vivo and in vitro colony forming cells in the developing mouse embryo. Br J Haematol 18:279, 1970.
23. Hann IM, et al: Development of pluripotent hematopoietic progenitor cells in the human fetus. Blood 62:118, 1983.
24. Toksoz D, Brown G: Maintenance of granulocyte-monocyte progenitor cells in liquid cultures of human foetal liver. J Cell Physiol 119:227, 1984.
25. Cappelini MD, et al: Fetal liver: Erythropoiesis in vivo, sustained granulopoiesis in vitro. In Gale R, et al (eds): Fetal liver transplantation. New York, Alan R Liss, 1985, pp 113–119.
26. Slaper-Cortenbach I, et al: Different stimulative effects of human bone marrow and fetal liver stromal cells on erythropoiesis in long-term culture. Blood 69:135, 1987.
27. Barak Y, et al: Regulation of in vitro granulopoiesis by human fetal liver stromal cells. In Gale R, et al (eds): Fetal liver transplantation. New York, Alan R Liss, 1985, 157–165.
28. Anckaert MA, Symann M: In vivo induction of granulopoiesis in visceral yolk-sac cells by foetal hepatic factors. J Embryol Exp Morphol 73:87, 1983.
29. Campbell AD, Wicha MS: Extracellular matrix and the hematopoietic microenvironment. J Lab Clin Med 112:140, 1988.
30. Weiss L: The hematopoietic microenvironment of the bone marrow: an ultra-structural study of the stroma in rats. Anat Rec 186:161, 1976.
31. Gordon LI, et al: Regulation of erythroid colony formation by bone marrow macrophages. Blood 55:1047, 1980.
32. Allen TD, Dexter TM: The essential cells of the hemopoietic microenvironment. Exp Hematol 12:517, 1984.
33. Bethel CA, et al: Stromal microenvironment of human fetal hematopoiesis: in vitro morphologic studies. Pathobiology 62:99, 1994.
34. Westen H, Bainton DF: Association of alkaline-phosphatase–positive reticulum cells in bone marrow with granulocytic precursors. J Exp Med 150:919, 1979.
35. Chen LT, Weiss L: The development of vertebral bone marrow of human fetuses. Blood 46:389, 1975.
36. Whetton AD, Spooncer E: Role of cytokines and extracellular matrix in the regulation of hematopoietic stem cells. Curr Opin Cell Biol 10:721, 1998.
37. Zuckerman KS, Wicha MS: Extracellular matrix production by the adherent cells of long-term murine bone marrow cultures. Blood 61:540, 1983.
38. Bentley SA, et al: Phagocytic properties of bone marrow fibroblasts. Exp Hematol 9:313, 1981.
39. Bentley SA: Collagen synthesis by bone marrow stromal cells: a quantitative study. Br J Haematol 50:491, 1982.
40. Zuckerman KS, et al: Inhibition of collagen deposition in the extracellular matrix prevents the establishment of a stroma supportive of hematopoiesis in long-term murine bone marrow cultures. J Clin Invest 75:970, 1985.
41. Nordegraaf EM, et al: Studies of hematopoietic microenvironments. IV. Changes in glycosaminoglycan content of murine spleen in relation to hematological parameters following induction of anemia or polycythemia. Haematologica 66:409, 1981.
42. Pearson HA: Marrow hypoplasia in anorexia nervosa. J Pediatr 71:211, 1967.
43. Tavassoli M, et al: Gelatinous transformation of bone marrow in prolonged self-induced starvation. Scand J Haematol 16:311, 1976.
44. McCuskey RS, Meineke HA: Studies of the hematopoietic microenvironment. III. Differences in the splenic microvascular system and stroma between SL-SL d and W-W v anemic mice. Am J Anat 137:187, 1973.
45. Schrock LM, et al: Differences in concentration of acid mucopolysaccharides between spleens of normal and polycythemic CF1 mice. Proc Soc Exp Biol Med 144:593, 1973.
46. Spooncer E, et al: Regulation of haemopoiesis in long-term bone marrow cultures. IV. Glycosaminoglycan synthesis and the stimulation of haemopoieisis by beta-D-xylosides. J Cell Biol 96:510, 1983.
47. Del Rosso M, et al: Involvement of glycosaminoglycans in detachment of early myeloid precursors from bone-marrow stromal cells. Biochim Biophys Acta 676:129, 1981.
48. Gordon MY, et al: Compartmentalization of a haematopoietic growth factor (GM-CSF) by glycosaminoglycans in the bone marrow microenvironment. Nature 326:403, 1987.
49. Sorrell JM: Ultrastructural localization of fibronectin in bone marrow of the embryonic chick and its relationship to granulopoiesis. Cell Tissue Res 252:565, 1988.
50. Patel VP, et al: Mammalian reticulocytes lose adhesion to fibronectin during maturation to erythrocytes. Proc Natl Acad Sci U S A 82:440, 1985.
51. Yokota T, et al: Growth-supporting activities of fibronectin on hematopoietic stem/progenitor cells in vitro and in vivo: structural requirement for fibronectin activities of CS1 and cell-binding domains. Blood 91:3263, 1998.

52. Tsai S, et al: Differential binding of erythroid and myeloid progenitors to fibroblasts and fibronectin. Blood *69*:1587, 1987.
53. Campbell AD, et al: Haemonectin, a bone marrow adhesion protein specific for cells of granulocyte lineage. Nature *329*:744, 1987.
54. Erdman SH, et al: Supply and release of storage neutrophils. A developmental study. Biol Neonate *41*:132, 1982.
55. Warner HR, Athens JW: An analysis of granulocyte kinetics in blood and bone marrow. Ann NY Acad Sci *113*:523, 1964.
56. Athens JW. Granulocytes-neutrophils. *In* Lee GR, et al (eds): Wintrobe's Clinical Hematology, 9th ed. Philadelphia, Lea & Febiger, 1993.
57. Cairo MS: Review of G-CSF and GM-CSF. Effects on neonatal neutrophil kinetics. Am J Pediatr Hematol Oncol *11*:238, 1989.
58. Lieschke GJ, et al: Mice lacking granulocyte colony-stimulating factor have chronic neutropenia, granulocyte and macrophage progenitor cell deficiency, and impaired neutrophil mobilization. Blood *84*:1737, 1994.
59. Rother K: Leukocyte mobilizing factor: a new biological activity derived from the third component of complement. Eur J Immunol *2*:550, 1972.
60. Christensen RD, Rothstein G: Pitfalls in the interpretation of leukocyte counts of newborn infants. Am J Clin Pathol *72*:608, 1979.
61. Wright IM, Skinner AM: Post-transfusion white cell count in the sick preterm neonate. J Paediatr Child Health *37*:44, 2001.
62. Bishop CR, et al: Leukokinetic studies. XIV. Blood neutrophil kinetics in chronic, steady-state neutropenia. J Clin Invest *50*:1678, 1971.
63. Dancey JT, et al: Neutrophil kinetics in man. J Clin Invest *58*:705, 1976.
64. Nitsos I, et al: Fetal responses to intra-amniotic endotoxin in sheep. J Soc Gynecol Invest *9*:80, 2002.
65. Anderson DC, Springer TA: Leukocyte adhesion deficiency: an inherited defect in the Mac-1, LFA-1, and p150,95 glycoproteins. Annu Rev Med *38*:175, 1987.
66. Boggs DR, et al: Granulocytopoiesis in germfree mice. Proc Soc Exp Biol Med *125*:325, 1967.
67. Forestier F, et al: Hematological values of 163 normal fetuses between 18 and 30 weeks of gestation. Pediatr Res *20*:342, 1986.
68. Playfair JHL, et al: The leukocytes of peripheral blood in the human foetus. Br J Haematol *9*:336, 1963.
69. Barak M, et al: Total leukocyte and neutrophil count changes associated with antenatal betamethasone administration in premature infants. Acta Paediatr *81*:760, 1992.
70. Thomas DB, Yoffey JM: Human fetal hematopoiesis: I. the cellular composition of foetal blood. Br J Haematol *8*:290, 1962.
71. Manroe BL, et al: The neonatal blood count in health and disease. I. Reference values for neutrophilic cells. J Pediatr *95*:89, 1979.
72. Mouzinho A, et al: Revised reference ranges for circulating neutrophils in very-low-birth-weight neonates. Pediatrics *94*:76, 1994.
73. Prober CG, et al: The white cell ratio in the very low birth weight infant. Clin Pediatr *18*:481, 1979.
74. Engle WD, et al: Circulating neutrophils in septic preterm neonates: comparison of two reference ranges. Pediatrics *99*:E10, 1997.
75. Christensen RD, et al: The leukocyte left shift in clinical and experimental neonatal sepsis. J Pediatr *98*:101, 1981.
76. Spector SA, et al: Study of the usefulness of clinical and hematologic findings in the diagnosis of neonatal bacterial infections. Clin Pediatr *20*:385, 1981
77. Rodwell RL, et al: Early diagnosis of neonatal sepsis using a hematologic scoring system. J Pediatr *112*:761, 1988.
78. McCullough J: Granulocyte antigen systems and antibodies and their clinical significance. Hum Pathol *14*:228, 1983.
79. Doan CA: The recognition of a biologic differentiation in the white blood cells. JAMA *86*:1593, 1926.
80. Lalezari P, Radel E: Neutrophil-specific antigens: immunology and clinical significance. Semin Hematol *11*:281, 1974.
81. ISBT Granulocyte Antigen Working Party: Nomenclature of granulocyte alloantigens. Vox Sang *77*:251, 1999.
82. Bux J: Molecular nature of granulocyte antigens. Transfusion Clin Biol *8*:242, 2001.
83. Levine DH, Madyastha PR: Isoimmune neonatal neutropenia. Am J Perinatol *3*:231, 1986.
84. Maheshwari A, et al: Immune neutropenia in the neonate. Adv Pediatr *49*:317, 2002.
85. Christensen RD, et al: Granulocytic stem cell (CFUc) proliferation in experimental group B streptococcal sepsis. Pediatr Res *17*:278, 1983.
86. Liechty KW, et al: The failure of newborn mice infected with Escherichia coli to accelerate neutrophil production correlates with their failure to increase transcripts for granulocyte colony-stimulating factor and interleukin-6. Biol Neonate *64*:331, 1993.
87. Koenig JM, et al: Cell cycle status of CD34+ cells in human fetal bone marrow. Early Hum Dev *65*:159, 2001.
88. Li Y, et al: Maternal and umbilical serum concentrations of granulocyte colony-stimulating factor and its messenger RNA during clinical chorioamnionitis. Obstet Gynecol *86*:428, 1995.
89. Stallmach T, Karolyi L: Augmentation of fetal granulopoiesis with chorioamnionitis during the second trimester of gestation. Hum Pathol *25*:244, 1994.
90. Calhoun DA, et al: Granulocyte colony-stimulating factor serum and urine concentrations in neutropenic neonates before and after intravenous administration of recombinant granulocyte colony-stimulating factor. Pediatrics *105*:392, 2000.
91. Medlock ES, et al: Granulocyte colony-stimulating factor crosses the placenta and stimulates fetal rat granulopoiesis. Blood *81*:916, 1993.
92. Novales JS, et al: Maternal administration of granulocyte colony-stimulating factor improves neonatal rat survival after a lethal group B streptococcal infection. Blood *81*:923, 1993.
93. Calhoun DA, et al: Transplacental passage of recombinant human granulocyte colony-stimulating factor in women with an imminent preterm delivery. Am J Obstet Gynecol *174*:1306, 1996.
94. Gillan ER, et al: A randomized, placebo-controlled trial of recombinant human granulocyte colony-stimulating factor administration in newborn infants with presumed sepsis: significant induction of peripheral and bone marrow neutrophilia. Blood *84*:1427, 1994.
95. Schibler KR, et al: A randomized, placebo-controlled trial of granulocyte colony-stimulating factor administration to newborn infants with neutropenia and clinical signs of early-onset sepsis. Pediatrics *102*:6, 1998.
96. Bedford-Russell AR, et al: A trial of recombinant human granulocyte colony stimulating factor for the treatment of very low birthweight infants with presumed sepsis and neutropenia. Arch Dis Child Fetal Neonatal Ed *84*:F172, 2001.
97. Miura E, et al: A randomized, double-masked, placebo-controlled trial of recombinant granulocyte colony-stimulating factor administration to preterm infants with the clinical diagnosis of early-onset sepsis. Pediatrics *107*:30, 2001.
98. Barak Y, et al: The in vivo effect of recombinant human granulocyte-colony stimulating factor in neutropenic neonates with sepsis. Eur J Pediatr *156*:643, 1997.
99. Kocherlakota P, La Gamma EF: Human granulocyte colony-stimulating factor may improve outcome attributable to neonatal sepsis complicated by neutropenia. Pediatrics *100*:E6, 1997.
100. Bernstein HM, et al: Administration of recombinant granulocyte colony-stimulating factor to neonates with septicemia: a meta-analysis. J Pediatr *138*:917, 2001.
101. Makhlouf RA, et al: Administration of granulocyte colony-stimulating factor to neutropenic low birth weight infants of mothers with preeclampsia. J Pediatr *126*:454, 1995.
102. La Gamma EF, et al: Effect of granulocyte colony-stimulating factor on preeclampsia-associated neonatal neutropenia. J Pediatr *126*:457, 1995.
103. Weinblatt ME, et al: Transformation of congenital neutropenia into monosomy 7 and acute nonlymphoblastic leukemia in a child treated with granulocyte colony-stimulating factor. J Pediatr *126*:263, 1995.
104. Cairo MS, et al: Results of a phase I/II trial of recombinant human granulocyte-macrophage colony-stimulating factor in very low birthweight neonates: significant induction of circulatory neutrophils, monocytes, platelets, and bone marrow neutrophils. Blood *86*:2509, 1995.
105. Bilgin K, et al: A randomized trial of granulocyte-macrophage colony-stimulating factor in neonates with sepsis and neutropenia. Pediatrics *107*:36, 2001.
106. Carr R, et al: A randomized, controlled trial of prophylactic granulocyte-macrophage colony-stimulating factor in human newborns less than 32 weeks gestation. Pediatrics *103*:796, 1999.
107. Cairo MS, et al: A randomized, double-blind, placebo-controlled trial of prophylactic recombinant human granulocyte-macrophage colony-stimulating factor to reduce nosocomial infections in very low birth weight neonates. J Pediatr *134*:64, 1999.
108. Calhoun DA, et al: Consistent approaches to procedures and practices in neonatal hematology. Clin Perinatol *27*:733, 2000.

Robin K. Ohls

Developmental Erythropoiesis

ERYTHROCYTE KINETICS

Sites and Stages of Fetal Red Blood Cell Production

Extraembryonic Erythropoiesis

Extraembryonic erythropoiesis begins in the fetal yolk sac by 14 days' gestation.[1, 2] Small nests of nucleated blood cells are present in the mesenchymal and endodermal layers of the yolk sac.[3] These red blood cells, or hematocytoblasts, are the product of primitive megaloblastic erythropoiesis, and they differ from erythrocytes formed later in gestation when definitive normoblastic erythropoiesis occurs. Primitive erythroblasts are nucleated, macrocytic, and 20 to 25 μm in diameter. They are characterized by a mean cell volume (MCV) of more than 180 fl, and they have a characteristic fine nuclear chromatin pattern and a polychromatophilic cytoplasm containing abundant hemoglobin.[1, 3] Red blood cells enter the embryonic circulation at 3 to 4 weeks' gestation, coincident with joining of the vitelline and umbilical circulations.[4]

Intraembryonic Erythropoiesis

Definitive normoblastic erythropoiesis of the fetus begins in the liver during the early first trimester. By 6 to 8 weeks' gestation, the liver replaces the yolk sac as the primary site of red blood cell production, and by 10 to 12 weeks' gestation, extraembryonic erythropoiesis has essentially ceased. Red blood cell production occurs in the liver throughout the remainder of gestation, although production begins to diminish during the second trimester as bone marrow erythropoiesis increases (Fig. 146–1). Erythroblasts are first noted in the marrow at 8 to 9 weeks' gestation.[2] By the end of the third trimester, almost all erythropoiesis is taking place in the bone marrow, although residual erythropoiesis may continue in the liver, and it may be found in other sites. In rodents, the spleen is also a site of erythropoiesis before the onset of marrow red blood cell production. As with the liver, this site ceases production shortly after birth.[5] It is unclear whether the spleen contributes to erythropoiesis in the human fetus. Although erythroid precursors have been identified as early as 6 to 7 weeks' gestation in human splenic tissue,[6] it is not clear whether such cells are actually developing within splenic tissue or whether they are simply part of the circulation.[7]

Ontogeny of Stem Cells

Red blood cell precursors in the yolk sac are extremely primitive cells, and they may either disappear or seed other areas where erythropoiesis later becomes prominent. Various theories have evolved regarding the origin of stem cells in erythropoiesis. One theory, known as the *unicentric theory*, proposes that all hematopoietic stem cells originate from the yolk sac, then migrate from one hematopoietic site to another. Moore and Metcalf[8] demonstrated circulating pluripotent stem cells in the peripheral blood just before the development of liver erythropoiesis. They suggested that the development of intraembryonic hematopoiesis requires an intact yolk sac, and migration of stem cells from the yolk sac to hematopoietic tissue is necessary for the development of intraembryonic hematopoiesis. The development of other organ systems via migration of cells (such as neural crest tissue) gives credence to this theory.

A second theory, known as the *multicentric theory*, suggests that a new clonal formation of hematopoietic stem cells occurs at different sites of hematopoiesis during fetal development. Yolk sac cells are capable of producing granulocytic, megakaryocytic, and erythroid colonies when transplanted into adult irradiated recipients and in conditioned newborn recipients,[8, 9] a finding that supports the view that fetal stem cells possess the capacity to be pluripotent and their differentiation is controlled by microenvironmental factors. The relationship among embryonic hematopoietic stem cells, hematopoietic growth factors, and their associated progenitors remains to be determined.

Marrow, Liver, and Blood Differentials

Table 146–1 describes the differential counts in fetal liver, marrow, and circulating blood according to gestational age.[10-13] The liver of the mid-trimester human fetus is the major erythroid organ, with a myeloid/erythroid ratio ranging from 0.07 at 14 to 17 weeks' gestation to 0.2 at 21 to 24 weeks' gestation.[10] By 24 weeks, the composition of the fetal bone marrow begins to resemble that of adult marrow, differing by the presence of a large number of stromal elements, the absence of plasma cells and lymph follicles, and an overall increased cellularity in the fetal marrow. Unlike in adult marrow, large fat cells are not present in fetal bone marrow. Between 18 and 22 weeks' gestation, the mitotic index of the fetal bone marrow becomes virtually identical to that of adult bone marrow. The fetal bone marrow myeloid/erythroid ratio starts to exceed the normal adult bone marrow ratio (1.5±0.4) early in mid-gestation and remains elevated even at the time of birth.

Progenitor Cell Concentrations

Studies of bone marrow cells in tissue culture have identified specific committed red blood cell precursors, termed *erythroid progenitors*,[14-17] based on their characteristic growth *in vitro*. When bone marrow cells are placed in semisolid media culture systems for 5 to 7 days, an erythropoietin (Epo)-sensitive erythroid progenitor cell, termed *colony-forming unit-erythroid* (CFU-E), clonally matures into a single cluster containing 30 to 100 normoblasts (Fig. 146–2). An erythroid-specific progenitor that is less well differentiated than a CFU-E (and, therefore, a more primitive cell) is termed a *burst-forming unit-erythroid* (BFU-E). Twelve to 14 days after bone marrow cells are placed in culture, a BFU-E develops into a large, multicentered colony of normoblasts, in which each center contains 200 to 10,000 normoblasts. Finally, the most primitive erythroid progenitor cell identifiable through *in vitro* culture is termed a *colony-forming unit-granulocyte, erythrocyte, macrophage, megakaryocyte* (CFU-GEMM, or CFU-MIX). Twelve to 14 days after marrow cells are placed in culture, this multipotent progenitor develops into a mixed colony of both normoblast clusters and granulocyte-macrophage clusters.

The ability of an organ to produce red blood cells is based on the number of progenitor cells it contains, as well as the growth factors stimulating those cells to proliferate. Determination of erythroid progenitor numbers obtained from cell suspensions of liver, marrow, spleen, and blood of mid-trimester human fetuses (Table 146–2) showed twice the number of multipotent progenitors and erythroid progenitors in the fetal liver compared with marrow.[7,10,11] Erythroid progenitors from fetal liver also appeared

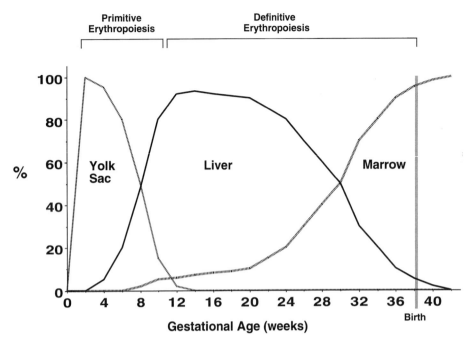

Figure 146–1. Sites and stages of fetal erythropoiesis. Primitive erythropoiesis begins in the yolk sac at 2 to 3 weeks after conception. By the end of the first trimester, the liver has become the main erythroid organ. The liver is the primary source of red blood cells during the second trimester, and the bone marrow is the primary source of red blood cells during the last trimester.

to be more sensitive to Epo (the primary erythroid growth factor) than were progenitors from fetal marrow. Progenitor cell concentrations in the spleen were nearly identical to concentrations in the circulation.[7,11] Whether the progenitors isolated from liver and marrow represent different subpopulations of progenitors (e.g., populations that express different erythroid growth factor receptors, different receptor numbers, different receptor affinity, or different cycling rates) remains to be determined.

Regulation of Erythropoiesis

Erythropoietic regulation in the human fetus differs markedly from that in the adult. In the adult, erythropoietic regulation primarily involves maintaining the red blood cell mass. In contrast, constant and dramatic changes characterize erythropoiesis in the embryo and fetus. The incredible rate of somatic growth and the resultant need constantly to increase the fetal red blood cell mass necessitate an extraordinary erythropoietic effort. Moreover, the relatively low oxygen tensions but high metabolic rates of fetal tissues require a system of oxygen delivery that differs significantly from the adult system.

Erythroid Growth Factors

The production of erythrocytes, from pluripotent stem cell to mature red blood cell, is governed by various growth factors. These erythropoietic growth factors are produced by accessory cells such as liver macrophages and marrow stromal cells, and they stimulate maturation, growth, and differentiation at various stages of red blood cell production. The progenitors involved in red blood cell production and the factors that stimulate their cellular maturation are depicted in Figure 146–2. Although these growth factors all facilitate production of red blood cells, none plays a more important regulatory role than Epo. Epo is a 30- to 39-kDa glycoprotein that binds to specific receptors on the surface of erythroid precursors and stimulates their differentiation and clonal maturation into mature erythrocytes.[18,19] The gene for Epo is located on chromosome 7q 21-22.[20] In the human fetus, Epo is produced principally by cells of monocyte/macrophage

origin residing in the liver. Postnatally, Epo is produced almost exclusively by peritubular cells of the kidney.

Other growth factors besides Epo play a role in the differentiation and clonal expansion of erythroid progenitors. These include granulocyte-macrophage colony-stimulating factor (GM-CSF),[14] stem cell factor (SCF, also known as c-kit ligand or steel factor),[21] and interleukin-3 (IL-3), IL-6, and IL-9.[22-24] Thrombopoietin, a growth factor involved in platelet production whose receptor is similar in structure to the Epo receptor, also stimulates erythroid colony formation.[25] IL-3 and GM-CSF were the first growth factors noted to have erythroid-stimulating properties, initially described as "burst-promoting activity." In combination with Epo, these factors synergistically stimulate differentiation and proliferation of BFUs-E and CFUs-GEMM.

SCF is a multipotent growth factor that, in combination with other factors, supports clonal maturation of hematopoietic progenitors. Murine studies indicate that SCF may be expressed during embryogenesis, thereby affecting embryonic and fetal erythropoiesis. *In vitro* studies show that SCF alone stimulates clonal maturation of fetal (but not adult) multipotent progenitors. Erythroid progenitors isolated from term cord blood are more responsive to SCF, alone and in synergism with GM-CSF and IL-3, than adult marrow progenitors.[21]

Term circulating erythroid progenitors are also more sensitive to IL-6 and IL-9 than are adult progenitors.[23] IL-6 is a multifunctional, 22- to 26-kDa glycoprotein cytokine involved in B-cell stimulation and immunoglobulin production, acute phase reactions, and induction of hematopoietic progenitors from a noncycling (G$_0$) phase into an active cycling (S) phase. IL-6 alone supports clonogenic maturation of newborn cord blood BFUs-E and CFUs-GEMM and induces progenitor cell cycling.[23] IL-9 is also a multipotent cytokine and is similar to IL-6 in its ability to stimulate primitive erythroid progenitors and multipotent progenitors isolated from cord blood.[24]

Unique Features of Fetal Progenitors

Fetal erythroid progenitors respond in a slightly different fashion than do adult erythroid progenitors. In addition to the features

TABLE 146-1

Differential Counts in Liver, Marrow, and Blood During Gestation

A. Differential Counts (in Percentages ± SD) of Liver Cell Suspensions from Fetuses at 14 to 24 Weeks' Gestation

Cells	Gestation (wk)		
	14–17 (n = 5)	18–20 (n = 7)	21–24 (n = 8)
Normoblast			
Pronormoblast	3.1 ± 1.4	3.4 ± 1.0	2.9 ± 1.8
Basophilic	18.4 ± 7.6	13.7 ± 1.6	13.7 ± 4.7
Polychromatophilic	57.5 ± 12.6	55.3 ± 7.5	51.1 ± 5.5
Orthochromic	13.9 ± 5.2	15.9 ± 3.7	14.2 ± 5.0
Total erythroid	9.3 ± 6.3	87.8 ± 4.8	81.9 ± 5.0
Neutrophil			
Promyelocyte	0 ± 0	0.2 ± 0.2*	1.2 ± 0.4*†
Myelocyte	0 ± 0	0 ± 0	0.2 ± 0.2*†
Metamyelocyte	0 ± 0	0 ± 0	0 ± 0
Band	0 ± 0	0 ± 0	0 ± 0
Segmented	0 ± 0	0 ± 0	0 ± 0
Total neutrophils	0 ± 0	0.2 ± 0.2	1.4 ± 0.5*†
Undifferentiated blast	0.5 ± 0.6	3.1 ± 1.8*	2.2 ± 0.7*
Macrophage	0.5 ± 0.6	1.2 ± 4.0*	1.3 ± 5.0
Lymphocyte	5.4 ± 2.6	3.9 ± 3.6	11.3 ± 4.2*†
Eosinophil	0 ± 0	0 ± 0	0 ± 0
Other‡	0.8 ± 0.8	3.4 ± 2.4	1.9 ± 2.4

* $p < .05$ vs. 14–17 wk.
† $p < .05$ vs. 18–20 wk.
‡ Hepatocyte, megakaryocyte, or cell of undetermined origin.

B. Differential Counts (in Percentages ± SD) of Marrow Cell Suspensions from Fetuses at 14 to 24 Weeks' Gestation

Cells	Gestation (wk)		
	14–17 (n = 6)	18–20 (n = 6)	21–24 (n = 8)
Normoblast			
Pronormoblast	0.3 ± 0.2*	1.1 ± 0.4*	0.5 ± 0.2*
Basophilic	1.4 ± 0.6*	3.1 ± 0.8*	1.7 ± 1.0*
Polychromatophilic	9.2 ± 5.0*	12.9 ± 6.2*	12.3 ± 5.2*
Orthochromic	12.1 ± 11.1	20.7 ± 12.2	8.1 ± 4.4
Total erythroid	23.0 ± 13.3*	37.8 ± 16.8*	22.6 ± 9.0*
Neutrophil			
Promyelocyte	5.9 ± 2.9*	5.8 ± 2.6*	5.0 ± 1.7*
Myelocyte	2.7 ± 1.4*	3.4 ± 1.6*	2.1 ± 1.0*
Metamyelocyte	2.1 ± 1.0*	2.5 ± 1.8*	1.7 ± 1.0*
Band	3.1 ± 1.8*	3.2 ± 2.7*	1.6 ± 1.2*
Segmented	1.2 ± 1.3*	1.1 ± 1.3*	0.4 ± 0.2*
Total neutrophils	13.8 ± 6.1*	16.1 ± 8.0*	10.7 ± 5.0*
Undifferentiated blast	8.9 ± 12.4*	11.4 ± 5.4*	11.6 ± 3.6*
Macrophage	5.4 ± 3.8*	4.2 ± 2.4*	3.1 ± 1.6*
Lymphocyte	35.3 ± 15.8*	28.8 ± 8.0*	50.3 ± 6.8*
Eosinophil	0.5 ± 0.6	1.1 ± 1.2	1.2 ± 0.8*
Other†	0.8 ± 0.4	0.5 ± 0.4	0.4 ± 0.2

* $p < .05$ vs. fetal liver.
† Megakaryocyte, or cell of undetermined origin.

C. Differential Counts (in Percentages ± SD) of Cord Blood Samples from Fetuses at 18 to 29 Weeks' Gestation

Cells	Gestation (wk)		
	18–21 (n = 186)	22–25 (n = 230)	26–29 (n = 144)
Normoblast (%WBCs)	45.0 ± 86.0	21.0 ± 23.0	21.0 ± 67.0
Basophilic	0.5 ± 1.0	0.5 ± 1.0	0.5 ± 1.0
Neutrophil	6.0 ± 4.0	6.5 ± 3.5	8.5 ± 4.0
Lymphocyte	88.0 ± 7.0	87.0 ± 6.0	85.0 ± 6.0
Eosinophil	2.0 ± 3.0	3.0 ± 3.0	4.0 ± 3.0
Monocyte	3.5 ± 2.0	3.0 ± 2.5	3.0 ± 2.5

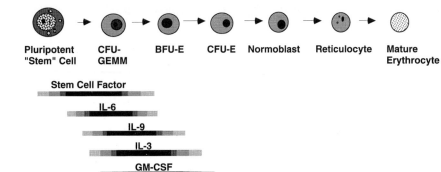

Figure 146–2. Erythropoietic progenitors and the growth factors influencing erythropoiesis. BFU-E = erythroid burst-forming unit; CFU-E = erythroid colony-forming unit; CFU-GEMM = colony-forming unit–granulocyte, erythrocyte, macrophage, and megakaryocyte; Epo = erythropoietin; GM-CSF = granulocyte-macrophage colony-stimulating factor; IL = interleukin.

TABLE 146–2

Progenitor Cell Concentrations per 5×10^3 Plated Cells

	CFU-MIX	BFU-E
Liver	12.7 ± 2.1	20.7 ± 3.1
Marrow	$6.7 \pm 1.4^*$	$9.3 \pm 2.7^*$
Spleen	$4.2 \pm 2.7^*$	$5.9 \pm 3.7^*$
Blood	—	$8.0 \pm 5.4^*$

$^* p < .05$ versus liver.
BFU-E = burst-forming unit–erythroid; CFU-MIX = colony-forming unit–granulocyte, erythrocyte, macrophage, megakaryocyte.

noted earlier, fetal progenitors appear more sensitive than adult erythroid progenitors to Epo.[26] Specifically, BFUs-E of fetal origin develop more rapidly into erythroid colonies, and the colonies generally contain significantly more normoblasts. In addition, BFUs-E from adult bone marrow require a combination of Epo plus another factor, such as IL-3 or GM-CSF, to mature clonally; however, many fetal BFUs-E mature in the presence of Epo alone.[27] Studies have shown that fetal clones produce GM-CSF and IL-3, which may explain their unique capability for growth factor independence and autostimulation.[28]

Control of Erythropoietin Production

Erythropoiesis *in utero* is controlled by erythroid growth factors produced by the fetus, not the mother. Epo is the primary regulator of erythropoiesis in adults and appears to be the controlling factor for fetal erythropoiesis, especially during late gestation. Epo does not cross the placenta in humans,[29, 30] monkeys,[30] or sheep,[31] although it has been reported to do so in mice.[32] In the mouse, suppression of maternal erythropoiesis by hypertransfusion does not suppress fetal erythropoiesis.[33] In humans, stimulation of maternal Epo production does not result in stimulation of fetal red cell production.[34]

The exact mechanism regulating the expression of Epo is unknown, but it is thought to be controlled by an oxygen-sensing mechanism in the liver and kidney.[35] It is known that both hypoxia and anemia stimulate erythropoiesis by stimulating mRNA transcription and Epo protein production.[36] Promoter and enhancer elements within the Epo gene are responsive to hypoxia, as well as to cobalt exposure *in vitro*.[37] The liver-sensing mechanism has a decreased sensitivity to hypoxia, producing one-tenth the amount of Epo in response to comparable stimuli in the kidney.[38, 39] The liver also appears to require more prolonged hypoxia to achieve an Epo response.[40, 41] Other hormones or factors have been shown to enhance Epo production or its effects, either *in vivo* or *in vitro*.[42, 43] These factors include testosterone,[44] estrogen,[45] thyroid hormone,[46] prostaglandins,[47] vitamin E,[48] and lipoproteins.[49]

It is not known what factors regulate the switch of Epo production from the liver to the kidney. It appears that renal production of Epo is not necessary for normal fetal erythropoiesis.[50] The lack of renal contribution to Epo production is illustrated by the normal serum Epo concentrations and normal hematocrits of anephric fetuses.[51] In the sheep, Epo production in both the liver and the kidney is highest at 60 days' gestation (term being 140 days).[52] Epo production in the fetal liver decreases by 90 days' gestation; however, increased renal production of Epo continues until 130 days' gestation, when production falls to levels seen in adult sheep.

Studies in human fetal and neonatal kidney obtained from postmortem specimens also report measurable quantities of Epo mRNA,[53] and quantitative mRNA studies in mid-trimester human fetuses reveal that the fetal kidney produces approximately 5% of the amount of Epo message that the fetal liver produces during the second trimester.[54] Thus, it appears that regulation of Epo gene transcription differs between liver and kidney *in utero*.

Epo levels have been measured in cord blood during the third trimester, and these levels gradually increase throughout later development.[55-57] From Epo measurements made in cord blood from infants of laboring and nonlaboring mothers[58] and from infants undergoing labor stress,[59-61] it seems that individual cord Epo levels primarily reflect hypoxic stress during labor and delivery. Serum Epo concentrations at birth normally range from 5 to 100 mU/mL. For comparison, serum Epo concentrations in anemic, nonuremic adults may be as high as 300 to 400 mU/mL.[62]

Red Blood Cell Indices in the Fetus and Neonate

Red Blood Cell Concentrations and Hematocrit

Red blood cell indices change during gestation and continue to change through the first year of life. Circulating red blood cell concentrations gradually increase during the second trimester, from $2.85 \pm 0.36 \times 10^6/\mu L$ at 18 to 21 weeks to $3.82 \pm 0.64 \times 10^6/\mu L$ at 30 weeks (Table 146–3).[11] At term, circulating red blood cell concentrations range from 5.0 to $5.5 \times 10^6/\mu L$.[63] In parallel with increasing red blood cell concentrations, hematocrit values increase from 30 to 40% during the second trimester and continue to increase to term values over the latter part of the third trimester. Term hematocrit values range from 50 to 63%, with some variability noted because of delayed clamping of the umbilical cord.[64] Values are also dependent on the sampling site. Capillary hemoglobin concentrations measure as much as 3.5 g/dL higher than venous samples.[65]

Hemoglobin

The hemoglobin concentration gradually rises during gestation.[66] At 10 weeks' gestation, the average hemoglobin concentration is approximately 9 g/dL.[67] By 22 to 24 weeks' gestation, fetal hemoglobin values reach 11 to 12 g/dL, and by 30 weeks, the hemoglo-

TABLE 146-3

Red Blood Cell Indices During Gestation

Week of Gestation	White Blood Cells* ($\times 10^9$/L)	Total White Blood Cell Count ($\times 10^9$/L)	Platelets ($\times 10^9$/L)	Red Blood Cells ($\times 10^{12}$/L)	Hemoglobin (g/dL)	Hematocrit (%)	Mean Corpuscular volume (fl)
18–21 (n = 760)	4.68 ± 2.96	2.57 ± 0.42	234 ± 57	2.85 ± 0.36	11.69 ± 1.27	37.3 ± 4.3	131.1 ± 11.0
22–25 (n = 1200)	4.72 ± 2.82	3.73 ± 2.17	247 ± 59	3.09 ± 0.34	12.2 ± 1.6	38.6 ± 3.9	125.1 ± 7.8
26–29 (n = 460)	5.16 ± 2.53	4.08 ± 0.84	242 ± 69	3.46 ± 0.41	12.91 ± 1.38	40.9 ± 4.4	118.5 ± 8.0
>30 (n = 440)	7.71 ± 4.99	6.40 ± 2.99	232 ± 87	3.82 ± 0.64	13.64 ± 2.21	43.6 ± 7.2	114.4 ± 9.3

* Including nomoblasts.
From Forestier F, et al: Blood 77:2360, 1991.

TABLE 146-4

Expected Hemoglobin Values (g/dL) in Low Birth Weight Infants

Birth Weight (g)	Age (wk)				
	2	*4*	*6*	*8*	*10*
800–1000	16.0 (14.8–17.2)	10.0 (6.8–13.2)	8.7 (7.0–10.2)	8.0 (7.1–9.8)	8.0 (6.9–10.2)
1001–1200	16.4 (14.1–18.7)	12.8 (7.8–15.3)	10.5 (7.2–12.3)	9.1 (7.8–10.4)	8.5 (7.0–10.0)
1201–1400	16.2 (13.6–18.8)	13.4 (8.8–16.2)	10.9 (8.5–13.3)	9.9 (8.0–11.8)	9.8 (8.4–11.3)
1401–1500	15.6 (13.4–17.8)	11.7 (9.7–13.7)	10.5 (9.1–11.9)	9.8 (8.4–12.0)	9.9 (8.4–11.4)
1501–2000	15.6 (13.5–17.7)	11.0 (9.6–14.0)	9.6 (8.8–11.5)	9.8 (8.4–12.1)	10.1 (8.6–11.8)

Reprinted by permission of the New England Journal of Medicine, *292*:887, 1975.

bin concentrations are 13 to 14 g/dL.[11] Premature male infants reach term cord hemoglobin values earlier than premature female infants,[68] possibly because of the erythropoietic effects of testosterone.[45] Hemoglobin concentrations are relatively constant over the last 6 to 8 weeks of gestation, and at term the average hemoglobin concentration is approximately 16 to 17 g/dL.[69-71] At birth, there may be a 1- to 2-g/dL rise in hemoglobin as a result of transfusion of placental blood at delivery.[72] An increase in hemoglobin by 2 hours of postnatal life occurs in most infants, resulting from a decrease in plasma volume. By 8 to 12 hours of life, the hemoglobin concentration achieves a relatively constant level. Red blood cell production decreases significantly at birth, so by the end of the first postnatal week, hemoglobin concentrations gradually decline.[64] The decrease in red blood cell production after birth is predominantly the result of the increased availability of oxygen in the extrauterine environment, which greatly reduces Epo production and endogenous erythropoiesis. The continued fall in hemoglobin concentration over the next several weeks results from (1) decreased red blood cell production, (2) a shortened red blood cell life span of the fetal erythrocyte, and (3) plasma dilution and an increase in blood volume related to growth. The nadir of hemoglobin concentration in full-term infants is seen at approximately 8 weeks, with an average hemoglobin concentration of 11.2 g/dL.[63,67] This value gradually rises so that, by 6 months, the average term infant has a hemoglobin concentration of 12.1 g/dL. Altitude may have a modest effect on the postnatal changes in hemoglobin concentration. Infants living at 1600 meters had higher hemoglobin concentrations (by 0.4 g/dL) by 6 months of age than infants living at sea level.[73,74]

The average decline in the hemoglobin of preterm infants weighing less than 1500 g is remarkably different from that of term infants. This is partly because of phlebotomy losses that invariably occur in preterm infants, as well as the effects of transfusions on endogenous erythropoiesis. Such infants reach a nadir of hemoglobin, which averages 8 g/dL at 4 to 8 weeks of age.[75] Tables 146-4 and 146-5 demonstrate relationships among birth weight, chronologic age, and red blood cell indices in term and preterm infants.[63,67,74-78]

These data do not always apply to infants born small for gestational age, in whom placental insufficiency and secondary polycythemia are common.[72,79] Infants of diabetic mothers, infants of smoking mothers, and infants born at higher altitudes also tend to have higher hemoglobin concentrations at birth.[73,80,81] In growth-restricted infants born to hypertensive mothers, the blood supply to the placenta and the capacity to deliver oxygen to the fetus are diminished. Accelerated erythropoiesis is thought to be part of a compensating mechanism designed to raise oxygen-carrying capacity to maintain an adequate supply to the fetus. In infants of diabetic mothers, increased metabolic demands of the fetus (resulting from increased glucose availability) may account for the higher fetal oxygen needs and the compensatory increase in hemoglobin concentration by the fetus. The increased red blood cell mass in infants of diabetic mothers is not thought to result from higher maternal levels of hemoglobin A_{1c} (a high-affinity hemoglobin capable of decreasing the oxygen transferred to the fetus). In smoking mothers, the increase in fetal carbon monoxide and the subsequent decrease in oxygen available from hemoglobin are the likely causes of the compensatory increase in hemoglobin levels in the fetus.

Mean Cell Volume

The size of the red blood cell gradually decreases during development. The MCV is more than 180 fl in the embryo, falls to 130 fl by midgestation, and decreases to 115 fl by the end of pregnancy. By 1 year of age, the MCV reaches an average of 82 fl.[77] Similar to cells of other organs in the infant born prematurely, the MCV of preterm infants declines quickly after birth, and the postpartum changes in MCV appear to be related to chronologic age rather than postconceptional age.[76] The mean corpuscular hemoglobin concentrations remain relatively constant, and the value for mean corpuscular hemoglobin decreases slightly.[81]

TABLE 146-5

Postnatal Changes in Red Blood Cell Indices in Term Infants*

RBC Indices	Birth (cord blood)	Days		Weeks			Months					
		1	3	1	2	4	2	3	4	6	9	12
Hemoglobin (g/dL)	16.5 (13.0)	18.5 (14.5)	18.6 (16.5)	17.5 (13.5)	16.6 (13.4)	13.9 (10.7)	11.2 (9.4)	11.5 (9.5)	12.2 (10.3)	12.6 (11.1)	12.7 (11.4)	12.7 (11.3)
Hematocrit (%)	51 (42)	56 (45)	55 (42)	54 (41)	53 (33)	44 (28)	35 (29)	35 (32)	38 (31)	36 (32)	36 (33)	37
Red blood cells (× 10^{12}/L)	4.7 (3.9)	5.3 (4.0)	5.6 (3.9)	5.1 (3.9)	4.9 (3.3)	4.3 (3.1)	3.7 (3.1)	3.8 (3.5)	4.3 (3.9)	4.7 (4.0)	4.7 (4.1)	4.7
Mean corpuscular volume (fl)	108 (98)	108 (95)	110 (104)	107 (88)	105 (88)	101 (91)	95 (84)	91 (74)	87 (76)	76 (68)	78 (70)	78 (71)
MCH (pg)	34 (31)	34 (31)	36.7	34 (28)	33.6 (30.0)	32.5 (29)	30.4 (27)	30 (25)	28.6 (25)	26.8 (24)	27.3 (25)	26.8 (24)
MCHC (g/dL)	33 (30)	33 (29)	33.1	33 (28)	31.4 (28.1)	31.8 (28.1)	31.8 (28.3)	33 (30)	32.7 (28.8)	35 (32.7)	34.9 (32.4)	34.3 (32.1)

* Values represent means (values in parentheses are –2SD).
MCH = mean corpuscular hemoglobin; MCHC = MCH concentration.
Data from Saarinen UM, Siimes MA: Developmental changes in red blood cell counts and indices of infants after exclusion of iron deficiency by laboratory criteria and continuous iron supplementation. J Pediatr 78:1978; and Dallman PR: In Rudolph A (ed): Pediatrics, 16th ed. New York, Appleton-Century-Crofts, 1977, p 1111.

Blood Volume

The placenta and umbilical cord contain 75 to 125 mL of blood at term, or approximately one-fourth to one-third of the fetal blood volume.[63] Umbilical arteries constrict shortly after birth, but the umbilical vein remains dilated, and blood flows in the direction of gravity. Infants held below the level of the placenta can receive half of the placental blood volume (30 to 50 mL) in 1 minute. Conversely, infants held above the placenta can lose 20 to 30 mL of blood back into the placenta per minute.[82] The blood volume of infants with early cord clamping averages 72 mL/kg, and the volume of infants with delayed cord clamping averages 93 mL/kg. Preterm infants have slightly larger blood volumes (89 to 105 mL/kg), owing to an increased plasma volume. By 1 month of age, blood volumes in term infants average 73 to 77 mL/kg.

Fetomaternal Red Blood Cell Transfer

Maternal and fetal circulating cells may, at varying times, cross the placental barrier. Fetal contamination of the maternal circulation can occur before delivery, as evidenced by studies of maternal blood group immunization. About 50 to 75% of pregnancies are associated with some degree of fetomaternal transfer of blood. This event is uncommon in the first trimester (3%). Volumes of fetal transplacental transfer are relatively small, usually on the order of 0.01 to 0.1 mL, but on occasion they may be much greater. About one pregnancy in 400 is associated with fetal transplacental bleeding of 30 mL or greater, and about one pregnancy in 2000 is associated with a potential fetal transplacental hemorrhage of 100 mL or more.[83] The overall risk of Rh immunization occurring in an Rh-incompatible pregnancy is 16% if the fetus is Rh positive and ABO compatible with its mother. This risk is 1.5% if the fetus is Rh positive and ABO incompatible. Fetal transfer of cells to the mother occurs during abortions as well (about a 2% incidence of such transfer with spontaneous abortion and a 4 to 5% rate if induced).[84] Because fetal hemoglobin is resistant to acid elution, cells containing fetal hemoglobin can be distinguished from cells containing hemoglobin A. The Kleihauer Betke stain of peripheral maternal blood uses this characteristic of fetal hemoglobin to detect fetal cells in the maternal circulation,[85] although results from mothers with increased fetal hemoglobin synthesis (i.e., sickle cell disease,

thalassemia, and hereditary persistence of fetal hemoglobin) are not reliable. Diagnosis of fetomaternal hemorrhage may also be missed when the mother and infant are ABO incompatible. In these cases, the fetal cells are rapidly cleared from the maternal circulation by maternal anti-A or anti-B antibodies.

ERYTHROCYTE BIOCHEMISTRY

Hemoglobin Synthesis

During fetal erythropoiesis, an orderly evolution of the production of different hemoglobins occurs. Eight globin genes direct the synthesis of six different polypeptide chains, designated α, β, γ, δ, ϵ, and ζ. These globin chains combine in the developing erythroblast to form seven different hemoglobin tetramers: hemoglobin Gower 1 (ζ_2-ϵ_2), hemoglobin Gower 2 (α_2-ϵ_2), hemoglobin Portland (ζ_2-γ_2), fetal hemoglobin (α_2-γ_2), and two types of adult hemoglobin (α_2-β_2, known as hemoglobin A, and α_2-δ_2, known as hemoglobin A_2).

Globin Genes

The globin genes are organized into two clusters (Fig. 146-3). The α-like genes are located along a 20-kB distal segment of the short arm of chromosome 16. The cluster contains three functional genes (α_1, α_2, and ζ_2), three pseudogenes (evolutionary remnants of genes that are not expressed because of inactivating mutations that prevent production of a functional globin protein), and one gene of undetermined function (a globinlike gene without inactivating mutations). The β-like gene cluster is located along a 60-kB segment of the short arm of chromosome 11, and it contains five functional genes (β, δ, $^A\gamma$, $^G\gamma$, and ϵ) and one pseudogene. Within each complex, the genes are all in the same 5'-3' orientation, and they are arranged in the order in which they are expressed during development.[86]

The α genes are duplicated in humans. Each α gene is approximately 4 kB long, interrupted by two small nonhomologous regions. Within each gene are intervening sequences (introns) that do not code for any protein structure, although the entire gene is transcribed into mRNA. The exons and first introns of the two α-globin genes have identical sequences, but the second intron of α_1 is nine bases longer and differs by three bases from

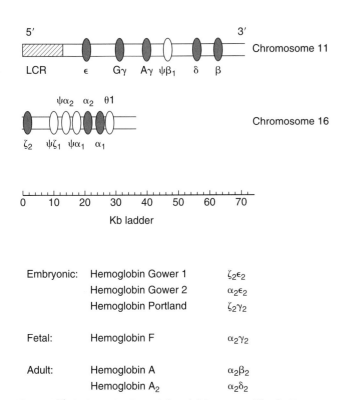

Figure 146–3. Organization of the globin genes. The *bottom line* reflects the scale in kilobases (kB). Transcription of mRNA takes place from the 5′ to the 3′ end, and for both chromosomes the genes are arranged in order of their developmental activation. The *upper segment* represents the β-like globin genes on the short arm of chromosome 11 and the lower segment, the α-like genes on the distal short arm of chromosome 16. Regions of the gene that code for primary globin proteins are shown as *shaded ovals*, and regions that code for pseudogenes (ψ-nonexpressed remnants with certain inactivating mutations that prevent transcription and translation into functional globin protein) are shown as *open ovals*. θ1 is a globinlike gene without inactivating mutations. The locus control region (LCR) is shown as a *hatched segment*. The composition of embryonic, fetal, and adult hemoglobins is listed.

that of the α2 gene. Despite the high degree of similarity or *homology* between these two genes, the sequences diverge in the 3′ untranslated regions, 13 bases beyond the TAA stop codon. Because of these sequence differences, the relative output of the two genes can be measured. α2 mRNA is produced two to three times more abundantly than α1 in fetal liver and marrow and in fetal and adult erythrocytes.[86]

The ζ gene appears critical to normal fetal development. In a murine model, both α- and ζ-gene expression can be measured from the onset of erythropoiesis in the yolk sac.[87] In addition, expression of both genes occurs concomitantly within the same cells. ζ-Gene expression occurs predominantly through the first 6 to 8 weeks of gestation, although minute quantities of ζ-globin can be measured in fetal and neonatal red cells.[88]

Like the α1 and α2 genes, the $^G\gamma$ and $^A\gamma$ genes appear to be virtually identical over a span of 1.5 kB, suggesting a mechanism for gene matching during evolution. Amino acid sequencing of normal cord blood has shown that either glycine ($^G\gamma$) or alanine ($^A\gamma$) is present at the 136 position in the γ-chain.[89] Short chain organic acids, such as butyrate and acetate, increase γ-gene promoter activity. This activity can be enhanced even further by incorporation of sections of the β-gene locus control region.[90,91]

The β-globin gene cluster occupies a region of approximately 17 kB on the short arm of chromosome 11.[92] Each of its constituent genes, their flanking regions, and large stretches of the regions between them have been sequenced. Studies suggest that the transcription factor NF-E1 regulates increased β-globin gene expression during erythroid maturation. Deletion of the NF-E1 binding site in the upstream segment of the β-globin promoter blocks induction of transcription in murine leukemia cells.[93]

δ-Globin gene expression occurs early at the erythroid progenitor stage. By the reticulocyte stage, no δ-globin mRNA synthesis can be detected. The δ-globin gene promoter functions at a much lower level than the β-globin gene promoter, resulting in significantly lower levels of δ-globin mRNA production. Evidence suggests the presence of a globin promoter–specific silencer element located upstream of the δ-globin gene.[94] Moreover, δ-globin mRNA is less stable than β-globin mRNA, which likely accounts for the early cessation of δ-globin synthesis and the low levels of hemoglobin A2 compared with hemoglobin A1.

The ε gene is located 5′ of the other β-like genes, and it is expressed during embryonic development. The ε gene is similar in sequence to the γ genes. A silencing element of the promoter region may be responsible for inactivating gene expression after the embryonic stage.[95] The only known mutation that results in persistent expression of this globin gene occurs in trisomy 13, in which there is a delay in the switch from ε- to γ-globin production.[96]

Globin Chain Synthesis

It has been possible to analyze the patterns of globin chain production at early ages of embryonic development during the transition from yolk sac (primitive) to hepatic (definitive) erythropoiesis. It is unknown why primitive erythroid progenitors programmed to produce one type of hemoglobin, such as Gower 1, give way to definitive progenitors programmed to produce a different type of hemoglobin, such as fetal hemoglobin. Quantification of globin gene synthesis reflects production by numerous red blood cells, and production of a specific hemoglobin is usually reported as a percentage of the total hemoglobin measured. Studies evaluating hemoglobin production by erythroid colonies in culture, however, show that individual cells in a colony produce predominantly one type of hemoglobin.[97]

During the fourth to fifth week, the main globin chains synthesized are ζ, δ, and ε chains (Fig. 146–4). During the sixth to seventh week, α, δ, ε, $^G\gamma$, and $^A\gamma$ chains are produced in the remaining primitive erythroblasts, and α, ε, $^G\gamma$, and $^A\gamma$ chains are produced in definitive erythrocytes. By the seventh to eighth week, ε- and ζ-chain synthesis is no longer detectable, and the main globin chains produced are α, $^G\gamma$, and $^A\gamma$. β-Chain production is just barely detectable at this time and gradually increases, so by 10 weeks, it makes up 10% of total non–α-chain production.[98] As soon as β-chain production occurs, genetic disorders associated with β-chain synthetic or structural abnormalities may be detected *in utero*, a finding suggesting an asynchronous transition from ζ- to α- as compared with ε- to γ-chain production, with the ζ-α switch occurring slightly earlier.[99]

From the 10th to about the 33rd week of gestation, the main globin chains synthesized are α, $^G\gamma$, $^A\gamma$, and β. Assessment of the output of the two linked α-globin genes by mRNA analysis suggests that they are expressed in the ratio of α2/α1, ranging from 1.5 to 3.0/1 throughout fetal life. This does not appear to change during development and is the same as that observed in normal adults. The relative rates of $^G\gamma$-chain and $^A\gamma$-chain production are also constant throughout fetal life at a $^G\gamma/^A\gamma$ ratio of approximately 3:1.[89] It is not known whether these pairs of genes are initially activated at this ratio; however, this production ratio is reached early in development.

Somewhere between the 32nd and 36th weeks of gestation, the relative rate of β-chain synthesis increases and that of γ-chain

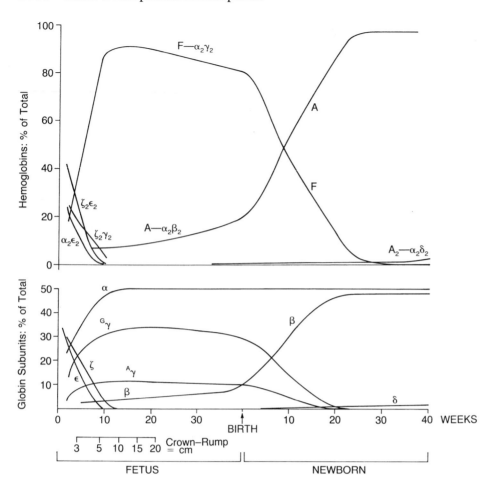

Figure 146–4. Changes in hemoglobin tetramers (*top*) and in globin subunits (*bottom*) during human development from embryo to early infancy. (From Bunn HF, Forget BG: Hemoglobin: Molecular, Genetic and Clinical Aspects. Philadelphia, WB Saunders Co, 1986, p 68.)

production declines, so at birth, β-chain synthesis makes up approximately 50% of non-α-chain synthesis. It is generally held that the transition from fetal to adult erythropoiesis starts at 30 to 36 weeks after conception, but the rate of the transition has been controversial.[98] A gradual transition from fetal to adult hemoglobin synthesis occurs, starting in the first trimester.[99, 100] Considerable variation among infants occurs, however, because many infants show prolonged dependence on fetal hemoglobin. After birth, the level of γ-chain production steadily declines and that of β-chain production increases, so by the end of the first year, γ-chain synthesis reaches the low level characteristic of adult life. The normal range of postnatal fetal hemoglobin production may be seen in Figure 146–5. Over the first few months of life, the $^G\gamma/^A\gamma$ ratio changes from 3:1 to 2:3, although this ratio is variable in adults.[101-103]

δ-Chain production has been observed as early as 32 weeks. δ-Gene activation lags behind β-gene activation, so the adult β/δ synthesis ratio is not reached until 4 to 6 months after birth.

Hemoglobin Production

Developmental changes in the production of the various hemoglobins are noted in Figure 146-4. Before the onset of other chain formation, unpaired globin chains may form tetramers, resulting in the presence of ε_4.[104] Almost immediately thereafter, α- and ζ-chain production begins, and hemoglobins Gower 1 ($\zeta_2\varepsilon_2$), Gower 2 ($\alpha_2\varepsilon_2$), and Portland ($\zeta_2\gamma_2$) are formed.[105] By 5 to 6 weeks' gestation, hemoglobins Gower 1 and Gower 2 constitute 42 and 24% of the total hemoglobin, respectively, with fetal hemoglobin (α_2-γ_2) making up the remainder. By 14 to 16 weeks, hemoglobin F constitutes 50% of the total hemoglobin, and by 20 weeks, it forms more than 90% of the hemoglobin.[106,107] Small quantities of hemoglobin A (α_2-β_2) are found, beginning at 6 to

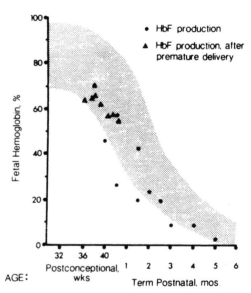

Figure 146–5. Postnatal changes in percentage fetal hemoglobin (HbF) (*shaded area*).[60-64] The *triangles* represent postnatal production by reticulocytes in premature infants, and the *dots* represent cord and postnatal reticulocyte production in term infants. The percentage of HbF present reflects HbF production over the previous weeks, whereas rate of HbF production is a result of the current proportion of HbF produced by reticulocytes present and is thus lower as the HbF-to-HbA switch progresses. (From Brown MS: *In* Stockman JA, Pochedly C [eds]: Developmental and Neonatal Hematology. New York, Raven Press, 1988, p 258.)

8 weeks' gestation. The increase in β-chain production occurring between 12 and 20 weeks' gestation accounts for the sudden rise in hemoglobin A found at the end of the first trimester of pregnancy. Tetramers of γ chains (γ_4, or hemoglobin Barts) and β-chains (β_4, or hemoglobin H) can be found in conditions in which α-chain synthesis is impaired or absent, such as the α-thalassemia syndromes.

Fetal hemoglobin is easily distinguished immunologically and biochemically from adult hemoglobin. The most significant physiologic characteristic of fetal hemoglobin is the decreased interaction with 2,3-diphosphoglycerate (2,3-DPG). 2,3-DPG binds to deoxyhemoglobin in a cavity between the β-chains and stabilizes the deoxy form of hemoglobin, resulting in a reduced hemoglobin-oxygen affinity. 2,3-DPG binds less effectively to the γ-globin chains, because of the differing amino acid sequence in the non-α-chain. Consequently, 2,3-DPG does not reduce the oxygen affinity of hemoglobin F as much as that of hemoglobin A.

Other differences in physical properties exist between fetal and adult hemoglobin. Hemoglobin F is more soluble in strong phosphate buffers than hemoglobin A.[85] Hemoglobin F is oxidized to methemoglobin more easily than hemoglobin A, and it has a considerably greater affinity for oxygen than adult hemoglobin as a result of differences in binding to 2,3-DPG. Fetal hemoglobin is resistant to acid elution, which allows differentiation of cells containing fetal hemoglobin from cells containing hemoglobin A.[85]

$^G\gamma$-Chains represent 70 to 80% of the total γ-chains in the blood of the fetus and newborn. This fraction falls to about 40% by 5 months of age. This unique difference in $^G\gamma$-chain production found in the fetus helps to distinguish fetal hematopoiesis from that found in later life. Under stress, the older infant and adult revert to this intrauterine form of fetal hemoglobin structure. This often occurs in leukemic states in children and adults, and in other conditions as well.[108, 109] The delay in the switch of fetal hemoglobin to hemoglobin A has been noted in conditions of maternal hypoxia,[110] in infants small for gestational age,[111] and in infants of diabetic mothers.[112, 113] Elevated levels of fetal hemoglobin may have protective effects in some disease states: One study suggests that a high level of fetal hemoglobin in sickle cell patients may be a predictor of increased adult life expectancy.[114]

The postpartum decline of fetal hemoglobin production and of the intercellular distribution of fetal and adult hemoglobins has been extensively examined over the first few months of life. Immediately after birth, there is a brief rise in hemoglobin F, followed by a steady decline (see Fig. 146–5). Studies of the intercellular distribution of hemoglobin F, using the relatively insensitive acid-elution technique, have shown that over the first few months of life the distribution of hemoglobin F is quite heterogeneous. At 3 months, the distribution of hemoglobin F becomes bimodal, with populations of cells that contain acid-resistant hemoglobin F and populations of adult "ghost" cells. These observations have suggested that fetal hemoglobin-containing cells are replaced by a population of cells containing adult hemoglobin during the early postnatal period.

Profound changes occur in the rates of red blood cell production immediately before birth and during the first few months after birth. On a body-weight basis, red blood cell production during the latter months of gestation is extremely high compared with that in adult life. Immediately after birth, erythropoiesis is considerably reduced, presumably as an adaptation to the extrauterine environment, and red blood cell production occurs at a low level for the first few weeks of life. It is clear from globin-chain synthetic studies that there is a steady and linear decline in γ-chain synthesis during the period of reduced neonatal erythropoiesis. Newly synthesized red blood cells appearing in the circulation when erythropoiesis resumes contain predominantly adult hemoglobin. These observations may explain the short plateau in the proportion of fetal hemoglobin (but not absolute levels) after birth and the appearance of predominantly adult hemoglobin–containing cells during the second and third months of life. These findings, together with the results of analyses of the intercellular distribution of fetal and adult hemoglobin by sensitive immunologic methods, suggest, although they do not prove, that the transition from fetal to adult hemoglobin production occurs in the same erythrocyte population. This conclusion is also consistent with the patterns of fetal and β-chain production in red cell colonies grown from neonatal blood.[115]

Studies show that the type of globin chains produced at different stages of development are not closely related to the site of erythropoiesis. It appears that ζ- and ε-chains are synthesized in both primitive and definitive cell lines. Moreover, the switch from γ- to β-chain production occurs synchronously throughout the liver and bone marrow during the later stages of fetal development. The transition from γ- to β-chain synthesis is most closely related to postconceptional age and not chronologic age.[108] Thus, premature infants continue to synthesize relatively large quantities of γ-chains (and fetal hemoglobin) until 40 weeks' gestation.

Erythrocyte Metabolism

The mature red blood cell differs from other cells in the body in that it has no nucleus; it consequently lacks the ability to engage in *de novo* protein synthesis. It has no mitochondria or ribosomes, no nucleic acid or deoxyribonucleic acid synthesis, no Krebs cycle of intermediary metabolism, and no electron transport system for oxidative phosphorylation. Thus, cellular metabolism is dependent on a limited supply of preexisting enzymes. These enzymes, coenzymes, and the substrates of glucose metabolism interact with hemoglobin and the red blood cell membrane to perform all the primary functions of the red blood cell, the most important being oxygen transport.

Important functions of red blood cell metabolism include maintaining adequate amounts of energy in the form of adenosine triphosphate (ATP), producing reducing substances to act as antioxidants, and maintaining appropriate amounts of red blood cell 2,3-DPG to assist in the modulation of hemoglobin's oxygen affinity. Energy metabolism is largely a function of the Embden-Meyerhof pathway. This pathway also regulates the quantity of red blood cell 2,3-DPG within the cell. The pentose phosphate pathway, among other functions, has a vital role in the production of reducing substances such as reduced nicotinamide adenine dinucleotide phosphate ($NADPH_2$). Table 146–6 lists the various metabolic characteristics of neonatal erythrocytes. A few of the variations seen in comparison with adult red blood cells are clinically significant in that they affect the life span of neonatal red blood cells.

Glycolysis

Red blood cells need a constant supply of carbohydrate to maintain adequate levels of ATP. Although glucose is the preferred carbohydrate, the red blood cell metabolizes fructose or mannose almost as readily. Galactose is metabolized much more slowly. Intracellular glucose concentrations equilibrate immediately with changes in plasma glucose concentrations. Glucose enters the human erythrocyte by facilitated transfer, and it is either converted to glucose-6-phosphate or reduced to its polyol derivative, sorbitol, which is then converted to fructose (Fig. 146–6).[116] Once formed, glucose-6-phosphate is metabolized by one of three pathways. The Embden-Meyerhof pathway converts glucose-6-phosphate to lactate or pyruvate and in the process generates ATP. Metabolism by way of the pentose phosphate pathway produces reduced intermediates and a phosphorylated pentose sugar (ribulose-5-P). This sugar ultimately returns to the Embden-Meyerhof pathway. Finally, glucose-6-phosphate may be converted to glucose-1-phosphate and then to glycogen, although less than 1% of glucose is metabolized to glycogen within the red blood cell.[117]

TABLE 146-6

Metabolic Characteristics of the Erythrocytes of the Newborn

Carbohydrate Metabolism

Glucose consumption increased
Galactose more completely utilized as substrate both under normal
    circumstances and for methemoglobin reduction*
Decreased activity of sorbitol pathway*
Decreased triokinase activity*

Glycolytic Enzymes

Increased activity of hexokinase, phosphoglucose isomerase,* aldolase,
    glyceraldehyde-3-phosphate dehydrogenase,* phosphoglycerate
    kinase,* phosphoglycerate mutase, enolase,* pyruvate kinase, lactate
    dehydrogenase, glucose-6-phosphate dehydrogenase, 6-
    phosphogluconic dehydrogenase, galactokinase, and galactose-
    1-phosphate uridyltransferase
Decreased activity of phosphofructokinase*
Distribution of hexokinase isoenzymes differs from that of adults*

Nonglycolytic Enzymes

Increased activity of glutamic oxaloacetic transaminase and glutathione
    reductase
Decreased activity of NADP-dependent methemoglobin reductase,*
    catalase,* glutathione peroxidase, carbonic anhydrase,* adenylate
    kinase,* and glutathione synthetase*
Presence of α-glycerol-3-phosphate dehydrogenase*

Adenosine Triphosphate (ATP) and Phosphate Metabolism

Decreased phosphate uptake,* slower incorporation into ATP and
    2,3-diphosphoglycerate*
Accelerated decline of 2,3-diphosphoglycerate into red blood cell
    incubation*
Increased ATP levels
Accelerated decline of ATP during brief incubation

Storage Characteristics

Increased potassium efflux and greater degrees of hemolysis during
    short periods of storage
More rapid assumption of altered morphologic forms on storage or
    incubation*

Membrane

Decreased ouabain-sensitive ATPase*
Decreased potassium influx*
Decreased permeability to glycerol and thiourea*
Decreased membrane filterability*
Increased sphingomyelin, decreased lecithin content of stromal
    phospholipids
Decreased content of linoleic acid*
Increase in lipid phosphorus and cholesterol per cell
Greater affinity for glucose*

Other

Increased methemoglobin content*
Increased affinity of hemoglobin for oxygen*
Glutathione instability*
Increased tendency for Heinz body formation in presence of oxidant
    compounds*

* Appears to be a unique characteristic of the newborn's erythrocytes and not
merely a function of the presence of young red cells.
From Oski FA, Naiman JL: Hematologic Problems in the Newborn, 3rd ed.
Philadelphia, WB Saunders Co, 1982, p 107.

Embden-Meyerhof Pathway

At least 90% of glucose is metabolized via the Embden-Meyerhof pathway.[118, 119] Two moles of ATP are produced for every mole of glucose catabolized, yielding two moles of lactic acid. This potential for the production of ATP is not fully achieved because approximately 20% of metabolized glucose traverses the 2,3-DPG cycle, thus bypassing one of the kinase steps, which is a site of ATP generation.[120]

The Embden-Meyerhof pathway has several unique characteristics with respect to fetal and newborn cells. These cells consume greater quantities of glucose than do the red blood cells of adults.[121] Galactose metabolism in the newborn red blood cell also differs.[122] Galactokinase activity is three times greater in the erythrocytes of newborns, and these cells consume galactose more rapidly than do those of the adult. The glycolytic enzymes phosphoglycerate kinase and enolase are much more active in the cells of the fetus and newborn infant than would be anticipated from their young cell age.[123, 124] In contrast, the activity of phosphofructokinase (a rate-controlling enzyme in glycolysis) is lower than normal in the erythrocytes from newborn infants.[123, 125, 126] Developmental changes in the activities of these three enzymes toward normal adult values during the first year of life appear to be independent of red blood cell age and reflect a transition from fetal to adult erythropoiesis. The decreased phosphofructokinase activity of fetal cells may be a consequence of accelerated decay of an unstable enzyme. The relative deficiency of this enzyme appears to result in alterations in glucose metabolism, and it could be functionally significant. Several of the other enzymes of the Embden-Meyerhof pathway have shown differences in the staining intensity of certain isoenzyme zones as compared with adult controls, although the significance of this observation is not known.

The ATP generated via the Embden-Meyerhof pathway is necessary for the maintenance of the normal biconcave shape of the erythrocyte.[127] It is also necessary for pyrimidine nucleotide synthesis, completion of purine nucleotide synthesis and glutathione synthesis,[128] incorporation of fatty acids into membrane phospholipids,[129] active cation transport,[126] and the initial step in the phosphorylation of glucose by the hexokinase enzyme. Not all these synthesizing functions are important in the mature red blood cell, which lacks a nucleus. However, loss of red blood cell ATP produces a marked decrease in red blood cell deformability. As the cell ages, ATP levels fall, and older cells have lower glucose utilization, greater osmotic fragility on incubation, lower membrane lipid content, lower potassium concentration, and greater sodium concentration. They are less deformable and have a shorter red blood cell life span. The red blood cells of term and preterm infants, when studied in the first several days of life, contain higher levels of ATP than do cells from adults.[130, 131] The small premature infant has even higher ATP levels.[130]

Newborn red blood cells seem to demonstrate a transient immaturity in their metabolism. This results in a slower uptake of phosphorus, a delayed incorporation into 2,3-DPG, and a marked decline in 2,3-DPG, as well as ATP, during short periods of incubation *in vitro*. The precise reason for this relatively transient immaturity is not known, but it may explain why the newborn red blood cell loses potassium at an accelerated rate and undergoes marked morphologic alteration during short incubations *in vitro*.

Pentose Phosphate Pathway

Glucose-6-phosphate undergoes oxidative decarboxylation through the pentose phosphate pathway (Fig. 146-7), consuming oxygen and producing carbon dioxide. The pentose pathway requires NADP as a cofactor. In the first step, oxidation of glucose-6-phosphate to 6-phosphogluconolactone is catabolized by glucose-6-phosphate dehydrogenase, generating $NADPH_2$. This step is followed by enzymatic hydrolysis of 6-phosphogluconolactone to 6-phosphogluconate, which is then oxidized in the presence of 6-phosphogluconic dehydrogenase to ribulose-5-phosphate with the production of carbon dioxide. Approximately 3 to 10% of all glucose metabolized by the cell is cycled through the pentose pathway. Hypoxia and acidosis increase the proportion of glucose metabolism shunted through this pathway.

The pentose phosphate shunt results in the production of two important products, ribose-5-phosphate and $NADPH_2$. Ribose-5-

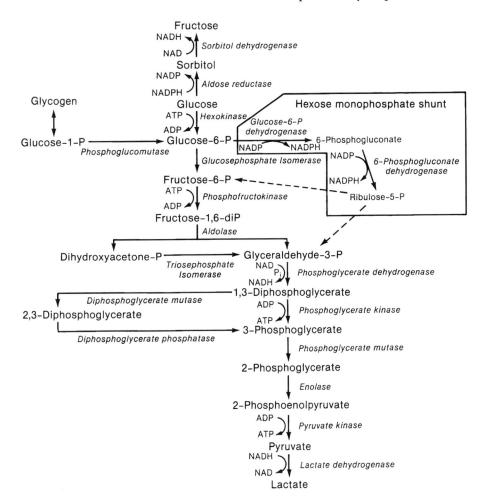

Figure 146–6. Pathways of red blood cell glucose metabolism. See text for details.

phosphate is a vital constituent of the pyridine nucleotides, NAD and NADP, and the purine nucleotides, adenosine diphosphate (ADP) and ATP. There is no pathway for *de novo* purine formation inside the red blood cell; however, the mature red blood cell does retain the ability for pyridine nucleotide formation. NADPH₂ is critical for preservation of cell integrity because it is necessary for methemoglobin reduction, the reduction of glutathione, and the stabilization of certain enzymes.[132] NADPH₂ serves as a hydrogen donor in the presence of the enzyme glutathione reductase, resulting in reduction of glutathione. Reduced glutathione ultimately serves as a substrate for the enzyme glutathione peroxidase, which is responsible for the detoxification of hydrogen peroxide. Hydrogen peroxide is a byproduct of the conversion of oxyhemoglobin to methemoglobin, which is a naturally occurring reaction inside the red blood cell in the presence of oxidative stress. The absence of NADPH₂ (or anything that interferes with the production of reduced glutathione), the synthesis of glutathione, or the inability to detoxify hydrogen peroxide severely impairs the viability of the red blood cell.

The pentose phosphate pathway in the newborn red cell differs from that in the adult red blood cell. Two enzymes of the pentose pathway, glucose-6-phosphate dehydrogenase and 6-phosphogluconic acid dehydrogenase, are active at levels higher than those seen in adult red blood cells.[133] Carbon dioxide production by erythrocytes of term and preterm infants is equal to or greater than that seen in red blood cells of adults.

Although there are suggestions that the pentose phosphate pathway activity in the newborn is normal, there is also evidence that newborn infants are more susceptible to oxidant-induced injury, leading to glutathione instability, Heinz body formation, and

the development of methemoglobinemia.[134, 135] This oxidant vulnerability may be caused by factors unrelated to the pentose phosphate pathway. For example, the red blood cell membrane in the fetus and newborn may have a decreased number of membrane sulfhydrol groups, making these cells more susceptible than mature red cells to Heinz body formation.[135] Additionally, NADPH-methemoglobin reductase activity is decreased in neonatal red cells, and the plasma of newborn infants appears to have a diminished antioxidant capacity.[136] The precise mechanisms surrounding the newborn red blood cell vulnerability to oxidant injury are not known. Fetal and newborn red blood cells have diminished glutathione peroxidase, which may render the cells more vulnerable to hydrogen peroxide-induced oxidant injury. In addition, the newborn red blood cell may have a diminished capacity for handling other activated oxygen radicals, such as singlet oxygen and the superoxide radical.[137] The latter is converted to hydrogen peroxide in the presence of the enzyme superoxide dismutase. Superoxide dismutase levels vary widely between infants. Diminished activity of the superoxide dismutase enzyme could result in accumulation of superoxide radicals. Free radicals generally are detoxified by antioxidants such as α-tocopherol (vitamin E). However, if (as has been described in some infants) superoxide dismutase levels are increased, the hydrogen peroxide presented to reduced glutathione may not be adequately detoxified.[138] Therefore, a delicate balance appears to exist between enzymes involved in production and detoxification of free radicals and oxidative intermediates. The use of inhaled nitric oxide as treatment for pulmonary hypertension in sick neonates may affect this balance, and further studies are required to determine its impact on oxidant injury beyond an increase in methemoglobin formation.

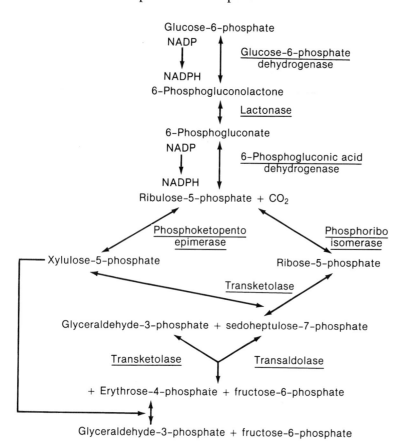

Figure 146–7. The pentose phosphate pathway. See text for details.

2,3-Diphosphoglycerate Metabolism

The affinity of a hemoglobin solution for oxygen can be decreased by interaction with certain organic phosphates.[139] Among the organic phosphates tested, 2,3-DPG and ATP are the most effective in lowering oxygen affinity. The highly charged anion 2,3-DPG binds to deoxyhemoglobin but not to oxyhemoglobin. Various conditions increase the amount of 2,3-DPG present within the red blood cell, as regulated in the Embden-Meyerhof pathway. Once formed, 2,3-DPG binds reversibly to 1 mol of deoxyhemoglobin tetramer under physiologic conditions of solute concentration and pH. Fetal deoxyhemoglobin does not possess as great an affinity for 2,3-DPG as does adult deoxyhemoglobin, and therefore it cannot bind 2,3-DPG to the same degree as adult hemoglobin. Thus, the fetal leftward shifted hemoglobin oxygen dissociation curve is not easily modulated in the presence of 2,3-DPG. The half-saturation pressure (P_{50}) value of fetal blood is 19 to 21 mm Hg, some 6 to 8 mm Hg lower than that of adult blood. As the fetal hemoglobin concentration declines, however, there is a marked rightward shift in the hemoglobin oxygen equilibrium curve (Fig. 146-8). The percentage of adult hemoglobin and the red cell 2,3-DPG content alter the position of the hemoglobin oxygen dissociation curve. Infants with a greater proportion of adult hemoglobin but less 2,3-DPG may have the same P_{50} as those with increased quantities of fetal hemoglobin but a high red cell 2,3-DPG content.

ERYTHROCYTE PHYSIOLOGY

Physical Properties of Neonatal Erythrocytes

The fetal and neonatal red blood cell differs from the mature red blood cell of the older infant, child, and adult in various ways. Specific characteristics of fetal red blood cells include a short-

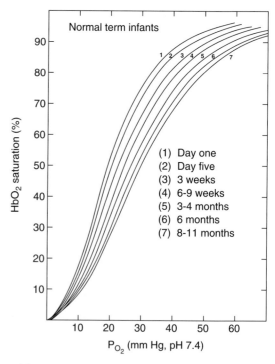

Figure 146–8. Oxygen equilibrium curve of blood from full-term infants at different postnatal ages. The oxygen half-saturation pressure of hemoglobin (P_{50}) on day 1 is 19.4±1.8 mm Hg and has shifted to 30.3±0.7 mm Hg at age 11 months (normal adult, 27.0±1.1 mm Hg). (From Oski FA, Naiman JL: Hematologic Problems in the Newborn, 3rd ed. Philadelphia, WB Saunders Co, 1982, p 250.)

ened life span, macrocytosis, high fetal hemoglobin content with a $^G\gamma/^A\gamma$ ratio of 3:1, the presence of i antigen,[140] and low carbonic anhydrase enzyme activity.[141]

Life Span

The differences in physical properties of red blood cells derived from term and preterm infants may in part account for the decreased life span of neonatal red blood cells within the circulation. The average life span for a neonatal red blood cell is 60 to 90 days,[142] approximately one-half to two-thirds that of an adult red blood cell. When neonatal red blood cells are transfused into adults, they exhibit a shortened life span, owing to alterations intrinsic to the neonatal red blood cell.[143] In contrast, cells transfused from adult donors appear to survive normally in newborns.[143] With increasing degrees of prematurity, remarkably shorter red cell life spans (35 to 50 days) are found. Fetal studies using [14C]cyanate-labeled red cells in sheep revealed an average red cell life span of 63.6±5.8 days.[144] The mean red cell life span increased linearly from 35 to 107 days as the fetal age increased from 97 days (mid-gestation) to 136 days (term).

The shortened red blood cell life span of the preterm and term neonate may be explained by some of the characteristics specific to newborn cells, namely, a rapid decline in intracellular enzyme activity and ATP,[145] loss of membrane surface area by internalization of membrane lipids, decreased levels of intracellular carnitine,[146] increased susceptibility of membrane lipids and protein to peroxidation,[147] and increased mechanical fragility resulting from increased membrane deformability.[148]

Size

Red blood cell dimensions change markedly during fetal and neonatal development. Early in embryogenesis, cell diameters range from 20 to 25 μm, and the MCV averages 150 to 180 fl.[1] During fetal development, red cells gradually decrease in size and volume (see Table 146-3); at birth, the average cell is 8 to 10 μm in diameter, with an MCV between 108 and 118 fl. Over the first year of life, red blood cells continue to diminish in size, and at 1 year of life, they resemble adult red blood cells (see Table 146-5).

Shape and Deformability

Just as there is variation in the size of newborn red blood cells, there is variation in shape. Irregularly shaped cells are present in much greater numbers in the peripheral blood of newborn infants than in that of adults.[149] Target cells, acanthocytes, puckered immature erythrocytes, and other irregular projections may normally be found. For example, a greater percentage of neonatal red blood cells has membrane surface pits, which are most likely the sites of formation of endocytic vacuoles. In normal adults, 2.6% of erythrocytes appear to have surface pits or craters varying in size from 0.2 to 0.5 μm in diameter, demonstrated by interference-contrast microscopy.[150] In contrast, pits can be found in almost half of the erythrocytes of preterm infants and in one fourth of the erythrocytes of term infants.

Red blood cell deformability is principally governed by three factors: the surface-area/volume relationship of the red blood cell, the viscosity of the cytoplasm of the cell, and intrinsic red blood cell membrane rigidity.[148] The deformability of erythrocytes is important for several reasons. First, red blood cell deformability appears to be an important determinant of red blood cell life span *in vivo*. The removal of a red blood cell from the circulation is thought to be a consequence of declining deformability, making the red blood cell susceptible to sequestration in the spleen and other organs, where it must negotiate extraordinarily narrow passages. Second, red blood cell deformability directly influences blood flow in the peripheral circulation. Third, red blood cell deformability affects whole blood viscosity, which, in turn, affects peripheral vascular resistance and cardiac work load.[151]

Neonatal red blood cells with the greatest density (representing the oldest cells in the circulation) lose more volume than adult red blood cells, have a higher mean corpuscular hemoglobin concentration, and are less deformable than the oldest red blood cells seen in adults. This suggests an accelerated decrease in deformability of aging red blood cells related to a more pronounced increase in the mean corpuscular hemoglobin concentration, the principal determinant of the internal viscosity of the red blood cell. Neonatal red blood cell membranes deform more readily to a given shear force than do adult red blood cell membranes, resulting in greater susceptibility of neonatal cell membranes to yield and fragment.[151] These mechanical properties may lead to accelerated membrane loss and a decreased life span.

Surface Charge

The surface charge of newborn red blood cells is more negative than that of adult red blood cells. The negative charge at the red blood cell surface is largely responsible for the electrophoretic mobility of the cell, and it appears to reflect the sialic acid content of the red blood cell membrane.[152,153] Proteases expose more negative sites on neonatal red blood cells than on adult red blood cells and increase the electrophoretic mobility to a greater degree.[154] The sialic acid content of the newborn infant's erythrocyte membrane shows a gradual but significant decrease in the first several weeks of life.[155] Most studies, however, have shown that the electrophoretic mobility of the neonatal cell is similar to that of the adult cell.[153] The more negative surface charge of the neonatal red blood cell membrane is one of the many characteristics that results in a decreased sedimentation rate in newborns.[156]

Osmotic Fragility

The osmotic fragility of red blood cells is a composite index of their shape, hydration, and, within certain limitations, proneness to *in vivo* destruction.[148,157] Preterm and term infants have an increased osmotic resistance.[158,159] The osmotic fragility of neonatal cells begins to revert toward adult values shortly after birth, and osmotic resistance reaches adult values by 4 to 6 weeks of age. There is no known advantage to the increased osmotic resistance seen in the neonatal red blood cell. However, studies of osmotic fragility in neonates have practical implications. It has been suggested that the diagnostic criteria for hereditary spherocytosis used in adults and older children are unreliable in newborn infants. For example, spherocytes are not regularly seen in all infants with hereditary spherocytosis. Indeed, spherocytes may be frequently found in ABO incompatibility. When one is performing an osmotic fragility test, a neonatal osmotic fragility curve must be used rather than an adult curve.[160] This underscores the need for calculating an osmotic fragility curve for newborn infants in whom a diagnosis of hereditary spherocytosis is considered.

Surface Receptors and Antigens

The neonatal red blood cell differs from the adult red blood cell in its ability to bind various substances. For example, the neonatal red blood cell binds more insulin than the adult red blood cell because of the presence of greater numbers of insulin receptors per cell.[161,162] Newborn red blood cells also have approximately 2.5 times the number of digoxin receptors, in comparison with adult red blood cells,[163] and as a consequence they have erythrocyte/plasma digoxin ratios three times those of adults. This may explain the greater tolerance of newborns who are receiving maintenance digoxin therapy.

Another unique characteristic of the fetal red blood cell is the manifestation of the i antigen on the cell surface (adult red blood cells express I antigen). Membrane i antigen is a carbohydrate moiety located on protein membrane band 3, which, during development, is converted from a linear polylactosamine to a branched carbohydrate chain of *N*-acetyl lactosamine units.[140] Red blood cells bearing the i antigen are usually not detectable by the first year of age. It has been suggested that the switch from fetal to adult hemoglobin and the transformation of i antigen expression that occur during the first year of life are governed by a common control mechanism; therefore, the presence of i antigen can serve as a marker of fetal hematopoiesis.

Red blood cell antigens in the ABO, MN, Rh, Kell, Duffy, and Vel systems are well developed in early intrauterine life.[164] They are easily demonstrated in the fifth to seventh gestational weeks and remain constant through the remainder of intrauterine development. Other antigens, such as the Lutheran and XgA systems, develop more slowly but are present at birth. Lewis antigens are lacking in the newborn. By approximately 2 years of age, the child's red blood cell and plasma antigens have developed a pattern that is seen throughout the remainder of life.[165]

Although A and B antigens are present early *in utero*, A and B isoagglutinin production occurs much later.[166] By 30 to 34 weeks' gestation, however, about 50% of infants have some measurable anti-A or anti-B antibodies. The fetal production of such antibodies is not related to maternal ABO blood type. Intrauterine exposure to gram-negative organisms, whose antigens are chemically related to those of blood groups A and B, is a potent stimulus for the development of these antibodies. Isohemagglutinin antibodies ultimately are demonstrable in normal infants by 6 months of age and approach adult values at 2 years of age. Low to absent titers after this time are suggestive of immune deficiency.[167]

Oxygen Transport

At no other time of life are the mechanisms controlling oxygen transport more complicated than *in utero* and during the immediate postpartum period. During prenatal life, the fetal arterial oxygen tension (P_{O_2}) is approximately 30 mm Hg, and the venous P_{O_2} is approximately 15 mm Hg (Fig. 146-9). This low P_{O_2} contributes to the development of relative polycythemia in the fetus. After birth, numerous factors affect oxygenation, including the inspired gas mixture, pulmonary function, the arterial oxygen dissociation curve, and the ability to extract oxygen at the tissue level.[168, 169] It has been speculated that the actual amount of oxygen released to tissues may be greater *in utero*, given the characteristics of the hemoglobin-oxygen dissociation curve (Fig. 146-10).

If pulmonary function is normal, there will be a rise in the P_{O_2} of pulmonary blood in adults and neonates, from the 40 mm Hg

of pulmonary arterial blood to the 100 mm Hg of pulmonary venous blood. Because of the shape of the hemoglobin-oxygen dissociation curve, these P_{O_2} values permit 95% saturation of hemoglobin by oxygen. Further increases in P_{O_2} produce little additional rise in saturation. In the normal adult (see Fig. 146-9), approximately 50% of hemoglobin will be saturated with oxygen

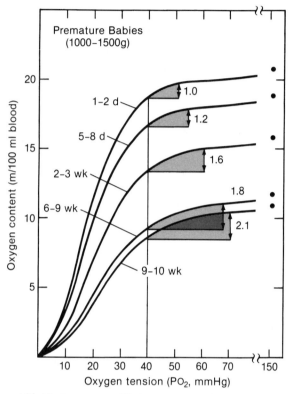

Figure 146–10. Oxygen equilibrium curves of blood from premature infants (1001 to 1500 g) at different postnatal ages. The *double arrows* represent the oxygen unloading capacity between a given arterial and venous oxygen tension. Points corresponding to 150 mm Hg on the abscissa are the oxygen capacities. Each curve represents the mean value of the infants studied in each group. (From Delivoria-Papadopoulos M, et al: Pediatr Res 5:235, 1971.)

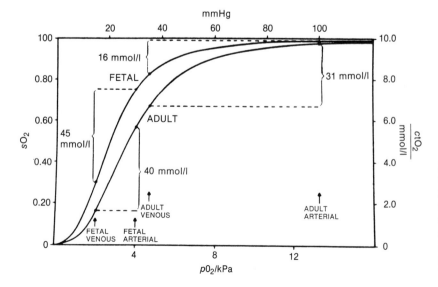

Figure 146–9. Differences in the hemoglobin oxygen dissociation curve between the newborn and the adult. This figure demonstrates the effects of these differences on oxygen tension (ctO_2) and oxygen saturation (sO_2). (From Stockman JA: Fetal hematology. *In* Eden RD, Boehm J [eds]: Assessment and Care of the Fetus. Norwalk, CT, Appleton & Lange, 1989, p 124.)

when the P_{O_2} has fallen to 27 mm Hg (P_{50} = 27). In situations in which the hemoglobin-oxygen dissociation curve has shifted to the right, the affinity of hemoglobin for oxygen is reduced. Thus, at any given P_{O_2}, more oxygen is released to tissues. Conversely, if the curve is shifted to the left, the affinity of hemoglobin for oxygen is increased. Thus, at any given P_{O_2}, less oxygen is released to the tissues.

Certain factors are known to alter hemoglobin's affinity for oxygen (Table 146-7). The most important of these are the fetal hemoglobin concentration and the red cell 2,3-DPG content. The level of red blood cell 2,3-DPG gradually increases with gestation. At term, the concentration of red blood cell 2,3-DPG is similar to that of adults. By the end of the first week of life, the 2,3-DPG levels are considerably higher than they are at birth. After the first week, red blood cell 2,3-DPG levels remain relatively unchanged for the next 6 months. In term infants, the hemoglobin-oxygen dissociation curve gradually shifts to the right, and by 4 to 6 months of age, the P_{50} values approximate those of the adult.

The situation is somewhat different in preterm infants. Fetal hemoglobin synthesis is still quite active; therefore, increases in P_{50} seen in term infants as a result of the switch from fetal to adult hemoglobin do not occur. The red blood cell 2,3-DPG concentrations are slightly lower in preterm infants as well.[78] These concentrations can be increased with the use of Epo, thereby shifting the oxygen dissociation curve to the right.[170]

A precise relationship between the decrease in oxygen affinity of a neonate's blood and the progressive decline in the concentration of fetal hemoglobin does not exist.[169] Rather, changes in P_{50} reflect the interplay between the levels of red blood cell 2,3-DPG, the decline in fetal hemoglobin, and the subsequent increase in hemoglobin A. A unifying concept has emerged consisting of a "functioning 2,3-DPG fraction,"[78] which determines how well hemoglobin is able to release oxygen to tissues. The functioning 2,3-DPG fraction (expressed as millimicromoles per milliliter of red blood cells) is calculated by multiplying the red blood cell 2,3-DPG content by the percentage of adult hemoglobin:[75]

$$[2,3\text{-DPG}]_{functional} = [2,3\text{-DPG}]_{observed} \times [100 - \% \text{ hemoglobin F}]$$

If P_{50} cannot be measured directly, it may be calculated from the following equation[75] after determining the functioning 2,3-DPG fraction:

$$P_{50} = 18.4 + 0.0016 \, [2,3\text{-DPG}]_{functional}$$

Table 146-8 illustrates the expected changes in hemoglobin concentration, 2,3-DPG, functional 2,3-DPG fraction, and P_{50} during the first 3 months of life in low birth weight infants. In low birth weight infants, the amount of oxygen released by hemoglobin can be determined (based on unloading from a normal arterial P_{O_2} adjusted for age to an arbitrary central venous P_{O_2} of 40 mm Hg).[75] Although oxygen-carrying capacity (hemoglobin concentration × percentage of oxygen saturation × 1.36 mL oxygen/g of hemoglobin) decreases over the first few months of life as a consequence of a decline in hemoglobin concentration, the amount of oxygen capable of being delivered to tissues actually increases. For example, a newborn weighing 1000 g with a hemoglobin concentration of 15 g/dL, a P_{50} of 19, and a central venous P_{O_2} of 40 mm Hg will unload 1 mL of oxygen to tissues for every 100 mL of blood that passes through the capillary bed. At 10 weeks of age, the P_{50} has shifted to the right and is now 24 mm Hg. This same infant will now deliver 2.1 mL of oxygen per 100 mL of blood, even though the hemoglobin has declined to 8 g/dL (see Fig. 146-10).

These calculations emphasize the importance of understanding an infant's ability to deliver oxygen to tissues when determining whether to administer an erythrocyte transfusion. The

TABLE 146-7

Factors Affecting Hemoglobin-Oxygen Affinity

Increased red blood cell 2,3-DPG, increased P_{50}
  Adaptation to high altitude
  Hypoxemia associated with chronic pulmonary disease
  Hypoxemia associated with cyanotic heart disease
  Anemia
    Secondary to iron deficiency
    Secondary to chronic renal disease
    Caused by sickle cell anemia
  Decreased red blood cell mass
  Chronic liver disease
  Hyperthyroidism
  Red cell pyruvate kinase deficiency
Decreased red blood cell 2,3-DPG, decreased P_{50}
  Septic shock
  Severe acidosis
  Following massive transfusions of stored blood
  Neonatal respiratory distress syndrome
Increased P_{50}, no consistent alteration in red blood cell DPG
  Abnormal hemoglobins (Kansas, Seattle, Hammersmith, Tacoma, E)
  Vigorous exercise
Decreased P_{50}, no consistent alteration in red blood cell DPG
  Abnormal hemoglobins (Kempsey, Chesapeake, J. Capetown, Yakima, Rainier).

DPG = diphosphoglycerate.

decision to transfuse should not be based on hemoglobin concentration alone. Transfusions significantly affect an infant's endogenous erythropoiesis. For infants who undergo exchange transfusion or multiple transfusions, both Epo concentrations and reticulocyte counts are lower at any given hemoglobin concentration (Fig. 146-11).[75,171]

It is often assumed that oxygen delivery is decreased in newborns because of the presence of high-affinity hemoglobin. In fact, a leftward shift in the hemoglobin-oxygen dissociation curve resulting from high levels of fetal hemoglobin may better maintain oxygen delivery during episodes of severe hypoxemia. Figure 146-12 illustrates the arterial P_{O_2} below which shifts to the right in the neonatal oxygen dissociation curve are no longer advantageous. The gas tension at which this occurs is known as the *cross-over* P_{O_2}.[172] The cross-over P_{O_2} is dependent on how low the venous P_{O_2} falls before oxygen delivery ceases.[173] Wimberley[173] calculated that if the arterial P_{O_2} fell to less than 32 mm Hg, and if the venous P_{O_2} fell to 10 mm Hg (a value found in the cerebral venous blood of some sick newborns), the infant would achieve better oxygen delivery with a fetal oxygen dissociation curve than with an adult curve. Conversely, if arterial P_{O_2} can be maintained at a higher value, better oxygen delivery would exist if the oxygen dissociation curve were shifted to the right.

In neonates with hypoxemia (e.g., infants with cyanotic congenital heart disease), a shift to the right (a higher P_{50}) in the hemoglobin-oxygen dissociation curve tends to lower the arterial and venous oxygen saturation at any given P_{O_2}. It has been documented that if arterial hypoxemia results from right-to-left shunting, shifts to the right in the oxygen dissociation curve always tend to increase the arterial-venous oxygen difference and thus improve oxygen delivery.[174]

After intrauterine transfusion, infants have oxygen-unloading properties characteristic of those of adult blood. Despite the decrease in oxygen affinity that accompanies intrauterine transfusion, no deleterious effects of this procedure with respect to oxygen uptake by the fetus have been documented.[175] The physiologic significance of manipulating the hemoglobin-oxygen affinity of fetuses remains to be determined.

TABLE 146-8
Changes in Hemoglobin Concentration, Hematocrit, and Other Markers of Oxygen Delivery During the First 3 Months of Life in Low Birth Weight Infants

Age	Total Hemoglobin Blood (g/dL)	Hematocrit (%)	MCHC (%)	O₂ Capacity Blood (mL/dL)	P₅₀ at pH 7.40 (mm Hg)	2,3-Diphosphoglycerate (mμmol/mL) RBC	Fetal Hemoglobin (% of Total)	FFDPG (mμmol/mL)
Group I (<1000 g)*								
2 wk	17.2	47.0	36.6	23.9	18.0	6255	83.0	1002
4 wk	8.5	26.0	32.7	11.8	15.0	3923	81.0	761
9 wk	7.2	22.0	32.7	10.0	15.0	4636	87.1	974
11 wk	7.7	22.5	34.2	10.7	17.0	5867	78.0	1290
Group II (1001–1500 g)								
1–2 d	15.1 ±1.3†	45.7 ±3.7	33.0 ±0.7	21.0 ±1.8	18.0 ±1.7	4124 ±1562	86.6 ±3.1	580 ±287
5–8 d	13.4 ±1.1	41.4 ±3.2	33.5 ±2.9	18.7 ±1.5	18.9 ±3.0	4501 ±1919	84.4 ±3.8	903 ±689
2–3 wk	12.6 ±3.1	33.6 ±6.0	34.2 ±1.1	15.9 ±3.1	21.2 ±1.9	5721 ±1375	83.3 ±5.1	1119 ±557
4–5 wk	8.8 ±0.9	25.3 ±1.8	34.9 ±1.7	12.3 ±1.3	20.5 ±1.7	6095 ±2081	85.2 ±2.3	931 ±456
6–9 wk	9.1 ±1.7	24.5 ±5.8	35.1 ±2.2	11.8 ±2.4	23.4 ±1.1	8734 ±1834	77.2 ±1.9	1995 ±480
9–10 wk‡	8.2 ±0.7	24.0 ±1.7	34.0	11.1	24.0	9000	77.0	2070
Group III (1501–2000 g)								
1–2 d	16.1 ±0.9	47.8 ±1.9	33.7 ±1.9	22.4 ±1.2	19.3 ±0.9	4475 ±1174	87.2 ±3.6	703 ±331
5–8 d	16.8 ±3.3	48.5 ±10.0	34.7 ±0.5	25.3 ±4.7	19.8 ±1.3	5489 ±1428	79.4 ±5.0	1056 ±590
2–3 wk	13.6 ±3.0	40.4 ±9.8	34.4 ±1.5	18.8 ±4.0	21.3 ±1.8	6002 ±998	80.6 ±5.8	1184 ±329
4–5 wk	11.2 ±2.8	31.9 ±9.9	35.5 ±2.2	15.5 ±3.8	20.8 ±1.6	5841 ±839	75.8 ±7.8	1569 ±577
6–9 wk	8.0 ±0.7	22.1 ±1.7	35.9 ±0.7	11.1 ±1.0	24.0 ±0.9	7290 ±634	67.5 ±6.2	2457 ±575
Group IV (2001–2500 g)								
1–2 d	15.9 ±0.9	46.2 ±5.8	35.8 ±1.9	21.9 ±1.5	20.2 ±1.6	5306 ±1075	76.8 ±5.43	1258 ±392
5–8 d	15.6 ±1.7	47.0 ±5.0	34.2 ±1.1	21.5 ±2.4	21.3 ±3.3	6417 ±1527	77.7 ±6.3	1457 ±603
2–3 wk	12.3 ±1.1	35.1 ±3.2	34.9 ±0.5	17.1 ±1.5	22.0 ±1.3	7145 ±1737	76.9 ±4.7	1666 ±472
6–9 wk‡	14.0	44.0	34.0	19.5	25.5	7100	43.0	3212

* Only one patient.
† Values are given as mean ± *SD*.
‡ Fewer than five infants.

From Delivoria-Papadopoulos M, et al: Pediatr Res 5: 235, 1971.
FFDPG = functioning fraction of 2,3-diphosphoglycerate; MCHC = mean corpuscular hemoglobin concentration.

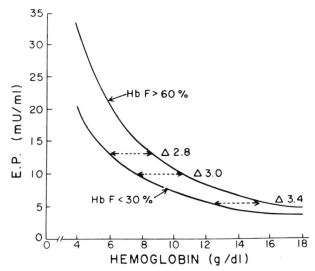

Figure 146–11. In infants born prematurely who have been exchange transfused or multiply transfused (fetal hemoglobin [Hb F] <30%), the hemoglobin concentration may fall several grams per deciliter before resumption of erythropoietin production (E.P.). (Reprinted by permission of The New England Journal of Medicine, *296*:647, 1977.)

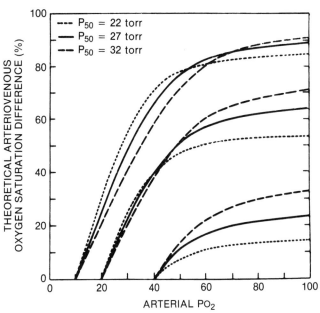

Figure 146–12. The effect of arterial partial pressure of oxygen (Po_2) on theoretical arteriovenous oxygen content difference when venous Po_2 is 40 mm Hg (*lower* set of curves), 20 mm Hg (*middle* set of curves), or 10 mm Hg (*upper* set of curves) at varying P_{50} values. P_{50} = oxygen half-saturation pressure of hemoglobin. (From Woodson RD: Crit Care Med 7:368, 1979. © Williams & Wilkins, 1979.)

HYPOPROLIFERATIVE ANEMIAS

Physiologic and Pathologic Anemia in Neonates

A gradual decrease in hemoglobin concentration occurs over the first 2 to 3 months of life in term and preterm infants. The hemoglobin concentration remains stable over the next several weeks and then slowly rises. In term infants, the fall in red cell production after birth is the result of improved oxygenation and occurs as a natural adaptation to extrauterine life. Because of this, the decrease in hemoglobin concentration has been termed a *physiologic nadir*, rather than true anemia. However, in preterm infants, adaptive mechanisms may not be complete. Preterm infants generally have a drop in hemoglobin to lower values than those seen in term infants, and the nadir varies with the degree of prematurity. Table 146-4 illustrates the decline in hemoglobin concentration based on birth weight and gestational age. Hemoglobin values as low as 7 g/dL are common in preterm infants who have not undergone phlebotomies.[76,176]

Assessing the factors that characterize oxygen supply and oxygen demand has provided insight into the adaptive changes occurring in preterm infants in response to low hemoglobin concentrations. In preterm infants, a low central venous Po_2 correlates with a mild increase in Epo production (Fig. 146-13).[177] The decline in central venous Po_2 appears to be a sensitive indicator of the presence of anemia, representing the integration of variables that determine oxygen supply and demand: hemoglobin concentration, red cell–oxygen affinity, intravascular volume, oxygen consumption, heart rate, cardiac stroke volume, and arterial oxygenation. The hemoglobin concentration is only one of many important variables ensuring adequate oxygen delivery in both term and preterm infants.[169]

Anemia of Prematurity

Characteristics. Despite the slight increase in Epo production that occurs in response to declining central venous Po_2 values, Epo concentrations in preterm infants are still significantly low, given the degree of anemia.[62,177-179] This anemia, termed the *anemia of prematurity,* affects infants born at less than 32 weeks' gestation, and it is the most common anemia encountered in the neonatal period. It is a normocytic, normochromic

anemia, generally associated with hemoglobin concentrations less than 10 g/dL and low reticulocyte counts. Some infants may be asymptomatic, whereas others demonstrate signs of anemia that are alleviated by transfusion. These signs traditionally include tachycardia, increased episodes of apnea and bradycardia, poor weight gain, an increased oxygen requirement, and elevated serum lactate concentrations that decrease after transfusion.[180-183]

Anemia of prematurity was first described by Schulman,[184] who divided the anemia into three phases. *Early anemia* was marked by an initial fall in hemoglobin concentration. The second, or *intermediate*, phase was characterized by maintenance of low hemoglobin concentrations. The third phase, *late anemia of prematurity*, resulted in hemoglobin concentrations that continued to fall, despite symptoms of anemia. The anemia of prematurity usually resolved spontaneously by 3 to 6 months of life.

Although much information has accumulated since the 1970s, the mechanisms responsible for the anemia of prematurity remain poorly defined. Shortened erythrocyte survival,[185] hemodilution associated with a rapidly increasing body mass,[186] and the transition from fetal to adult hemoglobin[78] have all been implicated. Despite diminished available oxygen to tissues[75,178] and the appearance of signs of anemia,[179] serum Epo concentrations remain low.[179] However, erythroid progenitors are highly sensitive to Epo,[187,188] and concentrations of other erythropoietic growth factors, including IL-3 and GM-CSF, appear to be normal.[189]

Infants born prematurely lack a normal response to anemia and fail to increase Epo production despite an apparent need for improved tissue oxygenation.[190] This occurs regardless of the cause of anemia, whether it is the early anemia of phlebotomy loss or the later anemia of prematurity. Possible molecular and cellular mechanisms responsible for this lack of responsiveness include defects in transferring the hypoxic signal to the nucleus, diminished or defective binding of transcription factors to the promoter or enhancer regions of the gene, decreased production or stability of the transcriptional factors, decreased production

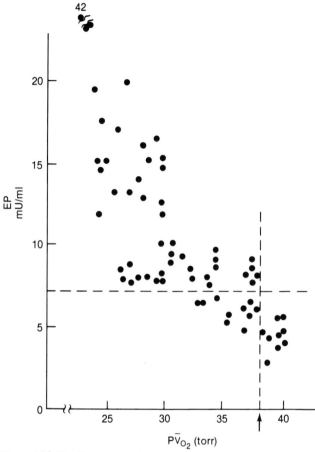

Figure 146–13. Changes in plasma erythropoietin concentrations in response to declines in central venous oxygen tension (Pv$_{O2}$) in preterm neonates. The *arrow* represents the position of 38 mm Hg, which for the purposes of this figure is the lower limit of normal for Pv$_{O2}$. The *horizontal dashed line* is the upper limit of normal for erythropoietin, taking Pv$_{O2}$ 38 mm Hg or higher as normal. EP = erythropoietin production. (From Stockman JA, et al: J Pediatr *105*:786, 1984.)

or stability of Epo mRNA, diminished or unstable protein production, or increased production of counterregulatory proteins such as IL-1 or tumor necrosis factor. The inability of the kidney or liver in the premature infant to produce Epo mRNA with magnitude equal to that seen in the fetus may also involve a developmental delay in expression of transcriptional factors responsible for increasing Epo production. Because Epo produced by the liver is indistinguishable from that produced by the kidney, it is unknown whether preterm infants rely on Epo produced by the liver, the kidney, or a combination of the two. However, macrophages from preterm infants generate Epo mRNA and protein as effectively as do those from term infants and adults.[191] The anemia of prematurity likely involves a delay in shifting the anatomic site of Epo from prenatal to postnatal sites of production.

Clinical Trials. Multiple clinical studies have been performed evaluating Epo administration administered to preterm infants.[192, 193] Randomized, controlled studies using Epo doses of more than 500 U/kg/week are summarized in Table 146–9.[194-202] In the first randomized multicenter trial published, Maier and the European Epo Study Group[194] evaluated the effect of Epo on the need for transfusions in preterm infants weighing 750 to 1499 g. Infants who were not receiving mechanical ventilation were randomized on day 3 of life to receive Epo or no treatment. A total

of 241 infants were evaluated, 177 of whom completed the study according to protocol. Epo recipients received fewer transfusions (1.2 versus 0.8) and had a greater success rate (defined as maintaining hematocrit of more than 32% without transfusions) than did placebo recipients.

Shannon and the United States Study Group[196] evaluated Epo to treat the anemia of prematurity. Infants of 1250 g birth weight or less and less than 31 weeks' gestation were randomized to receive Epo (100 U/kg) or placebo, administered subcutaneously, 5 days a week, for a total of 6 weeks. Infants were receiving enteral feedings of at least 60 kcal/kg/day, had hematocrit values lower than 40%, and had minimal phlebotomy losses at the time of study entry. Infants in both groups received oral iron and vitamin E supplementation, and uniform transfusion criteria were followed by all participating centers. Infants were 24 days of age at the beginning of the study, and they had received an average of 3.5 transfusions before study entry. Epo recipients required a lower number (1.1 versus 1.6) and smaller volume of transfusions (16 mL/patient versus 24 mL/patient) than did placebo recipients, and no adverse effects were noted.

Our laboratory evaluated the efficacy and cost effectiveness of treating very low birth weight infants with Epo for 2 weeks, starting in the first 2 days of life.[197] Epo recipients received a lower number and smaller volume of transfusions than did the placebo recipients (0.2 versus 1.4 transfusions per patient). When compared with other infants in the intensive care unit who met all study eligibility criteria, the placebo recipients were given fewer transfusions than infants who were not in the study (2.8 transfusions per patient during the same period). This finding was also noted by Bifano and colleagues,[203] who observed that instituting standardized transfusion guidelines decreased the transfusion requirements of very low birth weight infants.

In the Argentina multicenter trial,[200] Donato and colleagues randomized infants weighing less than 1250 g to early (250 U/kg five times a week intravenously for 2 weeks, then 250 U/kg three times a week subcutaneously for 6 weeks) versus late Epo (placebo for 2 weeks, then 250 U/kg three times a week subcutaneously for 6 weeks). These investigators concluded that, although there was no difference in total number of transfusions between the early and late groups, infants weighing less than 800 g with a phlebotomy loss of more than 30 mL/kg (the early Epo group) appeared to benefit; however, the benefit was noted only after 2 weeks of therapy. A similar delay in response was seen in extremely low birth weight infants in the National Institute of Child Health and Human Development Network study,[201] which showed a benefit to Epo treatment after 8 weeks.

Maier and colleagues also compared early administration of Epo (from the first week for 9 weeks) with late Epo (from the fourth week for 6 weeks) in infants weighing less than 1000 g.[202] These investigators included a control group that did not receive Epo. As in their previous studies, the authors measured rate of "success," defined by no transfusions and a hematocrit value that never fell to less than 30%. The success rate of early Epo was threefold greater than in controls: 13% in the early Epo group, 11% in the late Epo group, and 4% in controls. These investigators reported more than twice the "success" rate (27.6%) in the same size infants using a similar dose, dosing schedule, transfusion criteria, and study protocol in one of their previous studies.[199]

Pharmacokinetics. Pharmacokinetic studies in newborn monkeys and sheep indicate that neonates have a larger volume of distribution and a faster elimination of Epo,[204, 205] necessitating the use of higher doses than are required for adults.[206] These pharmacokinetic differences apply to preterm infants as well.[207, 208] Although various Epo doses and dosing schedules have been evaluated in preterm infants (see Table 146-9), the erythrokinetics of Epo (the interaction between erythroid progenitors and their growth factors) in preterm infants are unknown. Brown and associates[209] compared two dosing schedules in preterm

TABLE 146-9

Randomized Studies of Erythropoietin in Preterm Infants*

References	Population	Erythropoietin Dose and Schedule (Number of Patients)	Iron Supplementation	Transfusions per Patient (or % Success)	Volume Transfused
Maier et al, 2002 (202)	219 infants 500–999 g	250 U/kg 3×/wk IV/SC starting wk 1 (74)	3 mg/kg/d orally	13%†	0.4 mL/kg/d†
		250 U/kg 3×/wk IV/SC starting wk 4 (74)	Adjusted to transferrin saturation	11%	0.5 mL/kg/d
		Controls (71)		4%	0.7 mL/kg/d
Ohls et al, 2001 (201)	172 infants 401–1000 g	400 U/kg/3×/wk IV/SC to 36 wk PCA (87)	Erythropoietin: 5 mg/kg/wk IV	4.3±3.6	80±53 mL/kg†
		Placebo (85)	Placebo: 1 mg/kg/wk IV	5.2±4.2	95±63 mL/kg
	118 infants 1001–1250 g	400 U/kg/3×/wk IV/SC to 36 wk PCA (59)	Both: 6 mg/kg/d orally	1.0±1.6	39±26 mL/kg
		Placebo (59)	Adjusted to ferritin	1.1±1.6	35±24 mL/kg
Donato et al, 2000 (200)	114 infants ≤1250 g	1250 U/kg/wk × 2 wk, then 750 U/kg/wk (57)	Both: 6 mg/kg/d orally	3.4±1.1	51±35 mL/kg
		Placebo × 2 wk, then 750 U/kg/wk (57)		5.4±3.7	84±54 mL/kg
Maier et al, 1998 (199)	184 infants <1000 g	250 U/kg SC 3×/wk, to 38 wk PCA (93)	3 mg/kg/d orally	30%	12.9 mL/pt
		500 U/kg SC 3×/wk, to 38 wk PCA (91)	Adjusted to transferrin saturation	28%	10.5 mL/pt
Ohls et al, 1997 (198)	28 infants ≤750 g	200 U/kg/d IV for 14 d (15)	Both: 1 mg/kg/d IV	4.7±0.7†	70±11 mL/kg†
		Placebo (13)	Both: 6 mg/kg/d orally	7.5±1.1	112±17 mL/kg
Ohls et al, 1995 (197)	20 infants ≤1500 g	200 U/kg IV d for 14 d (10)	Both: 3–6 mg/kg/d orally	0.2±0.1†	2.7 mL/kg†
		Placebo (10)		1.4±0.4	22.3 mL/kg
Shannon et al, 1995 (196)	157 infants ≤1250 g	100 U/kg SC 5×/wk for 6 wk (77)	Both: 3–6 mg/kg/d orally	1.1±1.5†	17±23 mL/pt
		Placebo (80)	Adjusted to ferritin	1.6±1.7	24±26 mL/pt
Meyer et al, 1994 (195)	80 infants <32 wk	200 U/kg SC 3×/wk for 6 wk (40)	3 mg/kg/d orally	7 total†	148 mL total†
		Placebo (40)	Adjusted to ferritin	21 total	438 mL total
Maier et al, 1994 (194)	241 infants 750–1499 g	250 U/kg SC 3×/wk, DOL 3 to 42 (121)	Both: 2–6 mg/kg/d orally	0.87†	0.09 mL/kg/d†
		Controls (120)	Adjusted to ferritin	1.25	0.41 mL/kg/d

* Using ≥500 U erythropoietin/kg/wk

† $p < .05$ vs control or placebo.

DOL = day of life; PCA = postconceptional age.

infants: 100 U/kg five times a week versus 250 U/kg twice a week. These investigators reported that the more frequent dosing schedule appeared more effective in stimulating erythropoiesis, although there were no differences in transfusion requirements between the two dosing schedules. In a study during which Epo was given continuously over 24 hours to preterm infants for 10 days (versus a daily subcutaneous injection), Epo concentrations and reticulocyte responses were similar in both groups.[208] Peak concentrations in both groups declined from day 3 to day 10.

The route of administration also influences the effectiveness of Epo. Rapid intravenous administration of Epo generates peak serum concentrations that far exceed physiologic concentrations.[210] This may result in wasted drug via increased renal excretion or binding to nonerythropoietic receptors. Dosing strategies that achieve lower peak serum concentrations over a more prolonged period may be more effective. It appears that doses in the range of 500 to 1400 U/kg/week, administered subcutaneously every day or every other day, result in an adequate clinical response.

Side Effects of Treatment. Side effects in neonates receiving Epo have been rare. A side effect unique to neonates, transient neutropenia, was noted in early studies.[211-213] The neutropenia was not associated with depletion of either neutrophil reserves or colony-forming unit–granulocyte-macrophage concentrations, but it appeared to involve reduced production of neutrophils from granulocytic progenitors;[214,215] it resolved after discontinuation of the Epo. The cause may involve depletion of the total number of progenitors in slightly older preterm infants, or it may involve down-modulation of granulocyte-CSF receptors on pluripotent progenitors. In animal studies, neutropenia occurs in newborns after administration of very high doses of recombinant Epo as a result of decreased production of neutrophils from progenitors.[214]

Neutropenia was not reported in any of the Epo trials evaluating administration to preterm infants starting in the first days of life. In addition, Epo recipients did not experience any increase in morbidity or adverse outcome measures when compared with the placebo recipients. Early studies reported a decreased incidence of symptomatic patent ductus arteriosus,[195,197] possibly as a result of interactions between Epo and endothelin production.[216] Later studies have not shown a statistical effect of Epo on the incidence of symptomatic patent ductus arteriosus.[200-202] In the clinical trial by Emmerson and colleagues,[217] two infants in the Epo-treated group died of sudden infant death syndrome. Meyer and associates[195] also reported one late death ascribed to this syndrome. No other studies reported this association, and follow-up studies did not reveal an association between sudden infant death syndrome and Epo administration.[218]

Overall, the side effects of Epo administration in preterm infants have been minimal compared with those reported in adults (hypertension, bone pain, rash, and, rarely, seizures). None of these effects were reported in preterm infants involved in clinical trials. Moreover, no studies have reported differences between placebo and Epo recipients in the incidence of neonatal morbidities such as chronic lung disease, intraventricular hemorrhage, necrotizing enterocolitis, retinopathy of prematurity, or late-onset sepsis. Although long-term follow-up studies are few, it appears that the administration of Epo has no adverse effect on developmental outcome or growth, measured at 18 to 22 months.[218] However, as with many new therapies, reports of adverse effects invariably surface as use of the drug increases. Casadevall and colleagues[219] reported a series of 13 patients receiving Epo in whom aplastic anemia developed as a result of the production of anti-Epo antibodies. Similar occurrences have not been reported in infants; however, careful observation must continue when a new drug is evaluated in neonatal populations.

Advances in molecular biology have led to the creation of recombinant proteins that have been biologically altered to improve their pharmacokinetics.[220] Long-acting erythropoietic proteins such as ARA-NESP (novel erythropoietic stimulating protein, or Darbepoietin, manufactured by Amgen) are being studied in adults and may be beneficial in the neonatal population, especially if fewer subcutaneous doses could be administered with the same efficacy and negligible side effects.

Nutritional Supplementation. Iron has been administered both parenterally and enterally in published studies. Carnielli and colleagues reported no adverse effects of intravenous iron,[221] using doses of 20 mg/kg once a week. These infants also received vitamin E, 10 mg/kg intramuscularly twice a week. This dose of intravenous iron, although not the standard dose or typical route of administration in the United States, may have improved iron availability and resulted in a greater and more prolonged erythropoietic response than that seen in other studies. Friel and colleagues[222] reported iron accretion rates of preterm infants (not receiving Epo) of 1000 μg/kg/day.[222] Multicenter trials using intravenous iron at doses of 1 to 5 mg/kg/week have shown no adverse effects while achieving adequate iron status,[198,201,223] and no long-term oxidant effects have been reported after low-dose parenteral iron infusion.[224]

Oral iron supplementation has ranged from 2 to 40 mg/kg/day. Studies evaluating the oxidant effects of infant formulas and oral iron[172] showed increased erythrocyte lysis associated with formulas containing greater amounts of iron and polyunsaturated fatty acids. These effects resolved with the addition of vitamin E. Functional iron deficiency has frequently been reported in pediatric and adult patients receiving Epo, and it likely limited the success of some of the early Epo trials in preterm infants. Studies evaluating iron stores in Epo recipients[194,195] noted increased iron requirements in infants receiving Epo, as evidenced by diminished ferritin concentrations and elevated numbers of hypochromic red blood cells, despite iron doses of 6 mg/kg/day. Infants receiving Epo are likely at greater risk of iron deficiency than for iron overload and increased oxidant stress. However, further evaluation is required to determine the optimal dose and most effective route of administration of iron in preterm infants receiving Epo.

Vitamin E is an antioxidant, inhibiting peroxidation of polyunsaturated fatty acids in the lipid bilayers of all cell membranes. Vitamin E requirements may be increased secondary to increased iron supplementation, because iron promotes oxidation of polyunsaturated fatty acids. Pathak and colleagues[225] evaluated high-dose vitamin E in preterm infants receiving Epo and showed no benefit to doses of 50 IU/kg/day over standard nutritional supplements. Further study is needed to determine the optimal dose of vitamin E in preterm infants receiving Epo.

Other Erythropoietin-Responsive Anemias in the Newborn Period

Late Anemia of Rh Disease. Infants with Rh hemolytic disease often have an early (congenital) anemia caused by ongoing, antibody-mediated hemolysis, and they can develop late (age 1 to 3 months) anemia resulting from diminished erythrocyte production. The incidence of late anemia appears to be much higher in infants who receive intrauterine transfusions.[226] This anemia is characterized by low serum concentrations of Epo, but erythroid progenitors that remain highly responsive to recombinant Epo *in vitro.*[227] Infants with the late anemia of Rh hemolytic disease routinely receive transfusions until their anemia spontaneously resolves, generally by the third or fourth month of life. During the period of decreased circulating antibody synthesis and delayed endogenous Epo production, administration of exogenous Epo may serve as an alternative to erythrocyte transfusion. In centers in which infants are hospitalized for transfusions, Epo administration may also diminish or eliminate the need for hospitalization because Epo can be given in an outpatient setting. Preliminary studies have evaluated the use of recombinant Epo as treatment for the late anemia of Rh hemolytic disease, and they have shown it to be effective in stimulating reticulocyte production and increasing hematocrit.[228,229]

Anemia of Bronchopulmonary Dysplasia. Alverson and associates[230] observed the development of anemia in patients with bronchopulmonary dysplasia (BPD) and reported that repeat transfusions are generally required for management of anemia. Christensen and colleagues[231] subsequently characterized the anemia of BPD as normocytic, normochromic, hyporegenerative anemia, with marrow normoblast iron stains that are distinct from those observed in both the anemia of chronic disorders and the anemia of prematurity. Patients with the anemia of BPD differed from infants with the anemia of prematurity in that not all of the patients with the anemia of BPD were born prematurely, and their average age was older than that usually seen in anemia of prematurity. Preliminary results show Epo to be effective as treatment for the anemia of BPD.[232] Further study is ongoing to determine the explanation for reduced Epo production in patients with BPD, including the evaluation of factors that could create a relatively Epo-resistant environment, such as IL-1, tumor necrosis factor, and interferon-γ.

Anemia in Neonates with Congenital Heart Disease. In an attempt to decrease transfusion requirements and possibly decrease the incidence of graft rejection, infants with congenital heart disease awaiting transplantation received daily Epo (200 U/kg/day).[233] These infants showed a significant increase in hematocrit and decreased transfusion requirements. Although case reports of infants undergoing open heart surgery exist,[234] randomized controlled trials evaluating the use of Epo to decrease transfusion requirements of newborns with congenital heart disease should be completed before its widespread use in this population.

Anemia in Neonates with Congenital Anomalies Requiring Surgery. Many adult studies have been performed evaluating the use of Epo as an adjuvant to transfusion before surgery. Pediatric studies are limited. Neonates who are born with problems that require surgical repair, such as omphalocele, gastroschisis, meningomyelocele, congenital diaphragmatic hernias, and craniofacial abnormalities often undergo surgery during the period of physiologic anemia. These infants are hospitalized and undergo blood loss through phlebotomy, the surgery itself, and postoperative care. As a result, the physiologic anemia is exacerbated, and hemoglobin concentrations may drop to such a low level that transfusions are given. Although pilot studies on the use of Epo in these populations have shown promise,[235] randomized studies are required to determine whether these infants will respond to Epo administration by increasing erythropoiesis.

In addition to neonates who require surgery, other neonatal populations may benefit from Epo therapy. As in adults, Epo has been used successfully to treat anemia in newborns with end-stage renal disease.[236] In addition, infants with ABO incompatibility,[237] hemolytic disease from Kell antibody,[238] and hereditary spherocytosis[239] have been treated with Epo. Further studies are required in these populations to determine whether treatment with Epo is beneficial and does not cause further harm through increased hemolysis and hyperbilirubinemia.

It could be argued that, given the risks of transfusion, such as transmission of hepatitis, cytomegalovirus, and human immunodeficiency virus, as well as the possible development of graft-versus-host disease,[240] treatment of anemic neonates using recombinant Epo could be cost effective. It is likely that Epo administration, in combination with the development of more rigorous and standardized transfusion criteria and the diminished volume of blood lost through phlebotomy, will have the greatest impact in decreasing transfusion requirements in term and preterm infants. Regardless of treatment strategy, a critical understanding of the physiologic influences affecting oxygen delivery in term and preterm infants is required before altering the hematocrit, through either the administration of an erythrocyte transfusion or the administration of Epo.

ACKNOWLEDGMENT

Parts of this chapter were adapted from sections of Chapter 134 of the first edition of this book by James A. Stockman III and Pedro A. DeAlarcon.

REFERENCES

1. Keleman E, et al: Atlas of Human Hemopoietic Development. Atlas of Human Hematopoietic Tissue. New York, Springer-Verlag, 1979, pp 1–261.
2. Gilmore JR: Normal hematopoiesis in intra-uterine and neonatal life. J Pathol Bacteriol 52:25, 1941
3. Takashina T: Haemopoiesis in the human yolk sac. J Anat 151:125, 1987.
4. Moore KL: The Developing Human: Clinically Oriented Embryology, 4th ed. Philadelphia, WB Saunders Co, 1988.
5. Wood WG: Hemoglobin synthesis during fetal development. Br Med Bull 32:282, 1976.
6. Dgaldetti M: Hematopoietic events in human embryonic spleens at early gestational ages. Biol Neonate 36:133, 1979.
7. Calhoun DA, et al: Assessment of the contribution of the spleen to granulocytopoiesis and erythropoiesis of the mid-gestation human fetus. Early Hum Dev 46:217, 1996.
8. Moore MAS, Metcalf D: Ontogeny of the hematopoietic system: Yolk sac origin of in vivo and in vitro colony forming cells in the developing mouse embryo. Br J Haematol 18:279, 1970.
9. Yoder M, Hiatt K: Engraftment of embryonic hematopoietic cells in conditioned newborn recipients. Blood. 89:2176, 1997
10. Ohls RK, et al: Neutrophil pool sizes and granulocyte colony-stimulating factor production in human mid-trimester fetuses. Pediatr Res 37:806, 1995.
11. Forestier F, et al: Developmental hematopoiesis in normal human fetal blood. Blood 77:2360, 1991.
12. Rosse C, et al: Bone marrow cell populations of normal infants: the predominance of lymphocytes. J Lab Clin Med 89:1225, 1977.
13. Carbonell F, et al: Cellular composition of human fetal bone marrow. Acta Anat 113:371, 1982.
14. Sieff CA, et al: Dependence of highly enriched human bone marrow progenitors on hematopoietic growth factors and their response to recombinant erythropoietin. J Clin Invest 77:74, 1986.
15. Lipton JM, et al: Response of three classes of human erythroid progenitors to the absence of erythropoietin in vitro as a measure of progenitor maturity. Exp Hematol 9:1035, 1981.
16. Golde DW, Takaku F (eds): Hematopoietic Stem Cells. New York, Marcel Dekker, 1985, pp 20–43.
17. Heath DS, et al: Separation of the erythropoietin-responsive progenitors BFU-E and CFU-E in mouse bone marrow by unit gravity sedimentation. Blood 47:777, 1976.
18. Spivak JL: The mechanism of action of erythropoietin. Int J Cell Cloning 4:139, 1986.
19. Dessypris EN, et al: Effects of recombinant erythropoietin on the concentration and cycling status of human marrow hematopoietic progenitor cells in vivo. Blood 72:2060, 1988.
20. Jacobs K, et al: Isolation and characterization of genomic and cDNA clones of human erythropoietin. Nature 313:806, 1985.
21. Schibler KS, et al: Effect of recombinant stem cell factor on clonogenic maturation and cycle status of human fetal hematopoietic progenitors. Pediatr Res 35:303, 1994.
22. Umemura T, et al: The mechanism of expansion of late erythroid progenitors during erythroid regeneration: target cells and effects of erythropoietin and interleukin-3. Blood 73:1993, 1989.
23. Gardner JD, et al: Effects of interleukin-6 on fetal hematopoietic progenitors. Blood 75:2150, 1990.
24. Holbrook ST, et al: Effect of interleukin-9 on clonogenic maturation and cell-cycle status of fetal and adult hematopoietic progenitors. Blood 77:2129, 1991.
25. Kaushansky K, et al: Do the preclinical effects of thrombopoietin correlate with its in vitro properties? Stem Cells 14(Suppl 1):108, 1996.
26. Emerson SG, et al: Developmental regulation of erythropoiesis by hematopoietic growth factors: analysis on populations of BFU-E from bone marrow, peripheral blood, and fetal liver. Blood 74:49, 1989.
27. Valtieri M, et al: Erythropoietin alone induces erythroid burst formation by human embryonic but not adult BFU-E in unicellular serum-free culture. Blood 74:460, 1989.
28. Schibler KR, et al: Possible mechanisms accounting for the growth factor independence of hematopoietic progenitors from umbilical cord blood. Blood 84:3679, 1994.
29. Zanjani ED, et al: Erythropoietin does not cross the placenta into the fetus. Pathobiology 61:211, 1993.
30. Malek A, et al: Lack of transport of erythropoietin across the human placenta as studied by an in vitro perfusion system. Pflugers Arch 427:157, 1994.

31. Widness JA, et al: Lack of maternal to fetal transfer of ^{125}I-erythropoietin in sheep. J Dev Physiol 15:139, 1991.
32. Koury MJ, et al: Erythropoietin messenger RNA levels in developing mice and the transfer of ^{125}I-erythropoietin by the placenta. J Clin Invest 82:154, 1988.
33. Jacobsen LO, et al: The effect of transfusion-induced polycythemia in the mother of the fetus. Blood 14:694, 1959.
34. Matoth Y, Zaizov R: Regulation of erythropoiesis in the fetal rat. In Proceedings of the Tel Aviv University Conference on Erythropoiesis. Petak Tikva, ed. New York, Academic Press, 1970, p 24.
35. Goldberg MA, et al: Regulation of the erythropoietin gene: Evidence that the oxygen sensor is a heme protein. Science 242:524, 1988.
36. Peschle C, et al: Erythropoietin production by the liver in fetal-neonatal life. Life Sci 17:1325, 1975.
37. Imagawa S, et al: Regulatory elements of the erythropoietin gene. Blood 77:278, 1991.
38. Fried W: The liver as a source of extrarenal erythropoietin production. Blood 40:671, 1972.
39. Erslev AJ, et al: Renal and extrarenal erythropoietin production in anemic rats. Br J Haematol 45:65, 1980.
40. Naughton VA, et al: Hepatic and renal erythropoietin production during various intervals of short-term hypoxia. J Med 15:45, 1984.
41. Beru N, et al: Expression of erythropoietin gene. Mol Cell Biol 25:71, 1986.
42. Arnaud S, Blanchet JP: Mouse serum enables CFU-E to grow under physiologic concentration of erythropoietin in vitro. Exp Hematol 14:143, 1986.
43. DeWitte T, et al: Influence of peripheral blood admixture on the number of hematopoietic progenitor cells (CFU-GM and BFU-E) in human bone marrow aspirates. Acta Haematol 70:74, 1985.
44. Zanjani ED, Banisadre M: Hormonal stimulation of erythropoietin production and erythropoiesis in anephric sheep fetuses. J Clin Invest 64:1181, 1979.
45. Udupa KB, et al: In vitro culture of proerythroblasts: Characterization of proliferative response to erythropoietin and steroids. Br J Haematol 62:705, 1986.
46. Zanjani ED, et al: Effects of thyroid hormone on erythropoiesis and the switch from fetal to adult hemoglobin synthesis in fetal sheep. In Stamatoyannopoulos G, Nienhuis AW (eds): Cellular and Molecular Regulation of Hemoglobin Switching. New York, Grune & Stratton, 1979, pp 169–178.
47. Datta MC: Prostaglandin E_2 mediated effects on synthesis of fetal and adult hemoglobin in blood erythroid bursts. Prostaglandins 29:561, 1985.
48. Drake JR, Fitch CD: Status of vitamin E as an erythropoietic factor. Am J Clin Nutr 33:2386, 1980.
49. Konwalinka G, et al: Effect of human plasma lipoproteins on the erythropoietic progenitor cells in serum-free cultures. Blut 52:191, 1986.
50. Zanjani ED, et al: Liver as primary site of erythropoietin formation in the fetus. J Lab Clin Med 89:640, 1977.
51. Widness JA, et al: Erythropoietin levels and erythropoiesis at birth in infants with Potter's syndrome. J Pediatr 117:155, 1990.
52. Lim GB, et al: Ontogeny of erythropoietin gene expression in the sheep fetus: Effect of dexamethasone at 60 days gestation. Blood 83:460, 1994.
53. Dame C, et al: Erythropoietin mRNA expression in human fetal and neonatal tissue. Blood 92:3218, 1998.
54. Ohls RK: Erythropoietin and hypoxia inducible factor-1 expression in the mid-trimester human fetus. Acta Paediatr 91:27, 2002.
55. Halvorsen S, Finne PH: Erythropoietin production in the human fetus and newborn. Ann NY Acad Sci 149:576, 1968.
56. Meberg A: Hemoglobin concentration and erythropoietin levels inappropriate in small for gestational age infants. Scand J Haematol 24:162, 1980.
57. Thomas RM, et al: Erythropoietin in cord blood hemoglobin and the regulation of fetal erythropoiesis. Br J Obstet Gynaecol 90:795, 1983.
58. Widness JA, et al: Increased immunoreactive erythropoietin in cord blood after labor. Am J Obstet Gynecol 148:194, 1984.
59. Stevenson DK, et al: Increased immunoreactive erythropoietin in cord blood and neonatal bilirubin production in normal term infants after labor. Obstet Gynecol 67:69, 1986.
60. Finne PH: Erythropoietin levels in cord blood as an indicator of intrauterine hypoxia. Acta Paediatr Scand 55:478, 1986.
61. Widness JA, et al: Correlation of the interpretation of fetal heart rate records with cord plasma erythropoietin levels. Br J Obstet Gynaecol 92:326, 1985.
62. Erslev AJ: Erythropoietin titers in anemic, nonuremic patients. J Lab Clin Med 109:429, 1987.
63. Oski FA: The erythrocyte and its disorders. In Oski FA, Nathan DG (eds): Hematology of Infancy and Childhood. Philadelphia, WB Saunders Co, 1993, pp 18–43.
64. Usher R, et al: The blood volume of a newborn infant and placental transfusion. Acta Paediatr Scand 52:497, 1963.
65. Oettinger L Jr, Mills WB: Simultaneous capillary and venous hemoglobin determinations in newborn infants. J Pediatr 35:362, 1949.
66. Bratteby L: Studies on the erythro-kinetics in infancy: red cell volume of newborn infants in relation to gestational age. Acta Paediatr Scand 57:132, 1968.
67. Walker J, Turnbull EPN: Hemoglobin and red cells in the human fetus and the relation to oxygen content of the blood of the vessels of the umbilical cord. Lancet 2:312, 1953.
68. Burman D, Morris AF: Cord hemoglobin and low birth weight infants. Arch Dis Child 49:382, 1974.
69. Marks J, et al: Blood formation in infancy. III. Cord blood. Arch Dis Child 30:117, 1955.
70. Guest GM, Brown EW: Erythrocytes and hemoglobin of the blood in infancy and childhood. III. Factors in variability, statistical studies. Am J Dis Child 93:486, 1957.
71. Mollison PL, et al: Red cell and plasma volume in newborn infants. Arch Dis Child 25:242, 1950.
72. Humbert JR, et al: Polycythemia in small for gestational age infants. J Pediatr 75:812, 1969.
73. Moore LG, et al: Increased incidence of neonatal hyperbilirubinemia at 3100 m in Colorado. Am J Dis Child 138:158, 1984.
74. Brown MS: Fetal and neonatal erythropoiesis. In Stockman JA, Pochedly C (eds): Developmental and Neonatal Hematology. New York, Raven Press, 1988.
75. Stockman JA, et al: The anemia of prematurity: factors governing the erythropoietin response. N Engl J Med 296:647, 1977.
76. Stockman JA, Oski FA: Red blood cell values in low birth weight infants during the first seven weeks of life. Am J Dis Child 134:945, 1980.
77. Grauel EL, et al: Separation and characterization of red blood cells from newborns and infants during the first trimenon of life using a dextran density gradient, mean corpuscular volume and mean cellular hemoglobin concentration. Acta Haematol 67:102, 1982.
78. Delivoria-Papadopoulos M, et al: Postnatal changes in oxygen transport of term, preterm and sick infants: the role of red cell 2,3 diphosphoglycerate in adult hemoglobin. Pediatr Res 5:235, 1971.
79. Hakanson DO, Oh W: Hyperviscosity in the small for gestational age infant. Pediatr Res 11:472A, 1977.
80. Bureau MA, et al: Maternal cigarette smoking and fetal oxygen transport: a study of P_{50}, 2,3-diphosphoglycerate, total hemoglobin, hematocrit, and type F hemoglobin in fetal blood. Pediatrics 2:22, 1983.
81. Matoth Y, et al: Postnatal changes in some red cell parameters. Acta Paediatr Scand 60:317, 1971.
82. Oh W, Lind J: Venous and capillary hematocrit in newborn infants and placental transfusion. Acta Paediatr Scand 55:38, 1966.
83. Scott JR, Warenski JC: Tests to detect and quantitate fetal maternal bleeding. Clin Obstet Gynecol 25:277, 1982.
84. Bowman JM: Maternal blood group immunization. In Eden RD, Boehm FH (eds): Assessment and Care of the Fetus. Physiologic, Clinical and Medicolegal Principles. Norwalk, CT, Appleton & Lange, 1989, pp 749–772.
85. Kleihauer E, et al: Demonstration of fetal hemoglobin in the erythrocytes of the blood of a newborn. Klin Wochenschr 35:637, 1957.
86. Weatherall DJ, et al: The developmental genetics of human hemoglobin. In Stamatoyannopoulos G, Nienhuis AW (eds): Experimental Approaches for the Study of Hemoglobin Switching. New York, Alan R Liss, 1985, pp 3–25.
87. Leder A, et al: In situ hybridization reveals co-expression of embryonic and adult alpha-globin genes in the earliest murine erythrocyte progenitors. Development 116:1041, 1992.
88. Chui DH, et al: Human embryonic zeta-globin chains in fetal and newborn blood. Blood 74:1409, 1989.
89. Malala B, et al: A study of the switch of fetal hemoglobin and newborn erythrocytes fractionated by density gradient. Hemoglobin 7:567, 1983.
90. Safaya S, et al: Augmentation of gamma-globin gene promoter activity by carboxylic acids and components of the human beta-globin locus control region. Blood 84:3929, 1994.
91. Stamatoyannopoulos G, et al: Fetal hemoglobin induction by acetate, a product of butyrate catabolism. Blood 84:3198, 1994.
92. Wood WG, Weatherall DJ: Developmental genetics of the human hemoglobins. Biochem J 215:1, 1983.
93. deBoer E, et al: The human beta-globin promoter: nuclear protein factors and erythroid specific induction of transcription. EMBO J 7:4203, 1988.
94. Vitale M, et al: Evidence for a globin promoter-specific silencer element located upstream of the human delta-globin gene. Biochem Biophys Res Commun 204:413, 1994.
95. Cao S-X, et al: Identification of a transcriptional silencer in the 5' flanking region of the human epsilon-globin gene. Proc Natl Acad Sci U S A 86:5306, 1989.
96. Huehns ER, et al: Developmental hemoglobin anomalies in a chromosomal triplication: D1 trisomy syndrome. Proc Natl Acad Sci U S A 51:89, 1964.
97. Papayannopoulou T, et al: Asynchronous synthesis of HbF and HbA during erythroblast maturation. II. Studies of G gamma, A gamma, and beta chain synthesis in individual erythroid clones from neonatal and adult BFU-E cultures. Blood 57:531, 1981.
98. Kleihauer E: The hemoglobins. In Stave U (ed): Physiology of the Perinatal Period, Vol 1. New York, Appleton-Century-Crofts, 1970, p 255.
99. Peschle C, et al: Hemoglobin switching in the human embryos: a synchrony of the zeta to alpha and epsilon to gamma-globin genes in primitive and definitive erythropoietic lineage. Nature 313:235, 1985.
100. Phillips HM, et al: Definitive estimate of the rate of hemoglobin switching: measurement of percent hemoglobin F in neonatal erythrocytes. Pediatr Res 23:595, 1988.
101. Schröeder WA, et al: Worldwide occurrence of nonallelic genes for the gamma-chain of human foetal haemoglobin in newborns. Nature 240:273, 1972.
102. Schröeder WA, et al: Postnatal changes in chemical heterogeneity of human fetal hemoglobin. Pediatr Res 5:473, 1971.

103. Schröeder WA, Huisman THJ: Human gamma-chains: structural features. *In* Stamatoyannopoulos G, Nienhuis AW (eds): Cellular and Molecular Regulation of Hemoglobin Switching. New York, Grune & Stratton, 1979, pp 29–45.

104. Szelengi JG, Holland SR: Studies on the structure of human embryonic hemoglobin. Acta Biochim Biophys Acad Sci Hung 4:47, 1969.

105. Hecht F, et al: Predominance of hemoglobin Gower 1 in early human embryonic development. Science 152:91, 1966.

106. Huehns ER, et al: Human embryonic hemoglobins. Symp Quant Biol 29:327, 1964.

107. Heizman THJ, et al: Further studies of the postnatal change in chemical heterogeneity of human fetal hemoglobin in several abnormal conditions. Pediatr Res 9:1, 1975.

108. Bard H, et al: The reactivation of fetal hemoglobin synthesis during anemia of prematurity. Pediar Res 36:253, 1994.

109. Bard H, et al: Hypoxemia and increased fetal hemoglobin synthesis. J Pediatr 124:941, 1994.

110. Bromberg YM, et al: The effect of maternal anoxaemia on the foetal hemoglobin. J Obstet Gynaecol 63:875, 1956.

111. Bard H: The effect of placental insufficiency on fetal hemoglobin and adult hemoglobin synthesis. Am J Obstet Gynecol 120:67, 1974.

112. Bard H, Prosmanne J: Relative rates of fetal hemoglobin and adult hemoglobin synthesis in the cord blood of infants of insulin-dependent diabetic mothers. Pediatrics 75:1143, 1985.

113. Perrine SP, et al: Delay in fetal hemoglobin switch in infants of diabetic mothers. N Engl J Med 312:334, 1985.

114. Platt OS, et al: Mortality in sickle cell disease. Life expectancy and risk factors for early death. N Engl J Med 330:1639, 1994.

115. Peschle C, Condorelli M: Regulation of fetal and adult erythropoiesis. *In* Congenital Disorders of Erythropoiesis, Vol 37. Amsterdam, Ciba Foundation, 1976, p 25.

116. Travis SF, et al: Metabolic alterations in the human erythrocyte produced by increases in glucose concentration. The role of the polyol pathway. J Clin Invest 50:2104, 1971.

117. Moses SW, et al: Glucose and glycogen metabolism in erythrocytes from normal and glycogen storage III subjects. J Clin Invest 47:1343, 1968.

118. Murphy JR: Erythrocyte metabolism. II. Glucose metabolism and pathways. J Lab Clin Med 55:286, 1960.

119. Oski FA: Red cell metabolism in the preterm infant. II. The pentose phosphate pathway. Pediatrics 39:689, 1967.

120. Gerlach E, et al: Metabolism of 2,3 diphosphoglycerate in the red blood cells under various experimental conditions. *In* Brewer G (ed): Red Cell Metabolism and Function. New York, Plenum Press, 1970, p 155.

121. Oski FA, Naiman JL: Red cell metabolism in the premature infant. I. Adenosine triphosphate levels, adenosine triphosphate stability, and glucose consumption. Pediatrics 36:104, 1965.

122. Ng WG, et al: Galactokinase activity in human erythrocytes of individuals at different ages. J Lab Clin Med 66:115, 1965.

123. Travis SF, et al: Red cell metabolic alterations and postnatal life in term infants: glycolytic enzymes and glucose-6-phosphate dehydrogenase. Pediatr Res 14:1349, 1980.

124. Conrad PM, et al: Enzymatic activities and glutathione content of erythrocytes in the newborn: comparison with red cells of older subjects and those with comparable reticulocytosis. Acta Haematol 48:193, 1972.

125. Gross RT, Schroeder EAR: The relationship of triphosphopyridine nucleotide content to abnormalities in the erythrocytes of preterm infants. J Pediatr 63:823, 1963.

126. Whittam R: Transport and Diffusion of Red Blood Cells. London, Edward Arnold, 1964, p 192.

127. Nakao M, et al: Adenosine triphosphate in the shape of erythrocytes. J Biochem 49:487, 1961.

128. Koj A: Biosynthesis of glutathione in human blood. Acta Biochem Biol 9:11, 1962.

129. Oliveira MM, Vaughan M: Incorporation of fatty acids into phospholipids of erythrocyte membranes. J Lipid Res 5:156, 1964.

130. Stave U, Cara J: Adenosinophosphate in Blut Frühgeborener. Biol Neonate 3:160, 1961.

131. DeLuca C, et al: Simultaneous multiple-column chromatography: its application to the separation of the adenine nucleotides of human erythrocytes. Anal Biochem 4:39, 1962.

132. Huennekens FM, et al: Electron transport sequence of methemoglobin reductase. Ann NY Acad Sci 75:167, 1958.

133. Gross RT, Hurwitz RE: The pentose phosphate pathway in human erythrocytes: relationship between the age of the subject and enzyme activity. Pediatrics 22:453, 1958.

134. Schröter W, Tillman W: Heinz body susceptibility of red cells and exchange transfusion. Acta Haematol 49:74, 1973.

135. Tillman W, et al: The formation of Heinz bodies in ghosts of human erythrocytes of adults and newborn infants. Clin Wochenschr 51:201, 1973.

136. Stockman JA, Clark DA: Diminished antioxidant activity of newborn infants. Pediatr Res 15:684, 1981.

137. Carrell RW, Winterbourn CC: Activated oxygen and hemolysis. Br J Haematol 30:259, 1975.

138. Stockman JA: Newborn red cells, the nature of oxidant injury. Pediatr Res 11:41, 1977.

139. Benesch R, et al: Reciprocal binding of oxygen and diphosphoglycerate by human hemoglobin. Proc Natl Acad Sci U S A 59:526, 1968.

140. Childs RA, et al: Blood group I activity associated with band 3, the major intrinsic membrane protein of human erythrocytes. Biochem J 173:333, 1978.

141. Alter B: Fetal erythropoiesis in bone marrow failure syndromes. *In* Stamatoyannopoulos G, Nienhuis AW (eds): Cellular and Molecular Regulation of Hemoglobin Switching. New York, Grune & Stratton, 1979, pp 87–105.

142. Wranne L: Studies on erythrokinetics in infancy. Acta Paediatr Scand 56:381, 1967.

143. Mollison PL: The survival of transfused erythrocytes in hemolytic disease of the newborn. Arch Dis Child 18:161, 1943.

144. Brace RA, et al: Red blood cell life span in the ovine fetus. Am J Physiol 279:R1196, 2000.

145. Komazawa M, Oski FA: Biochemical characteristics of "young" and "old" erythrocytes of the newborn infant. J Pediatr 87:102, 1975.

146. Schmidt-Sommerfield E, Penn D: Carnitine and total parenteral nutrition of the neonate. Biol Neonate 58:81, 1990.

147. Bracci R, et al: Changes in erythrocyte properties during the first hours of life: electron spin resonance of reacting sulfhydryl groups. Pediatr Res 24:391, 1988.

148. Bohler T, et al: Mechanical fragility of erythrocyte membrane in neonates and adults. Pediatr Res 32:92, 1992.

149. Zipursky A, et al: The erythrocyte differential count in newborn infants. Am J Pediatr Hematol Oncol 5:45, 1983.

150. Holyrode CP, et al: The "pocked" erythrocyte. N Engl J Med 281:516, 1969.

151. Linderkamp O, et al: Blood viscosity and optimal hematocrit in preterm and full-term neonates in 50- to 500-μm tubes. Pediatr Res 32:97, 1992.

152. Cook GMW, et al: Sialic acids and the electrokinetic charge of the human erythrocyte. Nature 191:45, 1961.

153. Eylar EH, et al: The contribution of sialic acid to the surface charge of the erythrocyte. J Biol Chem 237:1992, 1962.

154. Kosztolany G, Jobst K: Electrokinetic analysis of the fetal erythrocyte membrane after trypsin digestion. Pediatr Res 14:138, 1980.

155. Calatroni A, et al: Erythrocyte membrane sialic acid in newborn infants. Acta Haematol 71:198, 1984.

156. Adler SM, Denton RL: The erythrocyte sedimentation rate in the newborn. J Pediatr 86:942, 1975.

157. Linderkamp O, Meiselman HJ: Geometric and membrane mechanical properties of density separated human red cells. Blood 59:1121, 1982.

158. Goldblume A, Gotlieb R: Icterus neonatorum. Am J Dis Child 38:57, 1929.

159. Wheh TR, et al: Studies on newborns. Am J Med Sci 198:646, 1939.

160. Schröter W, Kahsnitz E: Diagnosis of hereditary spherocytosis in newborn infants. J Pediatr 103:460, 1983.

161. Hendricks S, et al: Insulin binding to erythrocytes of normal infants, children and adults: variation with age and sex. J Clin Endocrinol Metab 52:969, 1981.

162. Herzberg VL, et al: Insulin receptor binding to cord blood erythrocytes of varying gestational age and composition with adult values. Pediatr Res 14:4, 1980.

163. Kearin M, et al: Digoxin receptors in neonates: an explanation of less sensitivity to digoxin in adults. Clin Pharmacol Ther 28:346, 1980.

164. Toivanen B, Hirvonen T: Iso- and heteroagglutinins in human fetal and neonatal sera. Scand J Haematol 6:42, 1969.

165. Marsh WL, Allen FH: Erythrocyte blood groups in humans. *In* Nathan DG, Oski FA (eds): Hematology of Infancy and Childhood, 3rd ed. Philadelphia, WB Saunders Co, 1987, pp 1497–1521.

166. Thomaidis T, et al: Natural isohemagglutinin production by the fetus. J Pediatr 74:39, 1969.

167. Gartner OT, et al: Anti-A and anti-B antibodies in children. JAMA 201:206, 1967.

168. Stockman JA: Anemia of prematurity. Clin Perinatol 4:239, 1977.

169. Stockman JA: Anemia of prematurity: current concepts in the issue of when to transfuse. Pediatr Clin North Am 33:111, 1986.

170. Soubasi V, et al: Use of erythropoietin and its effects on blood lactate and 2,3-diphosphoglycerate in premature neonates. Biol Neonate 78:281, 2000.

171. Oski FA, Stockman JA: Anaemia in early infancy. Br J Haematol 27:195, 1974.

172. Aberman RA: Cross over PO_2, a measure of the variable effect of increased P_{50} on mixed venous PO_2. Am Rev Respir Dis 115:173, 1977.

173. Wimberley PD: Fetal hemoglobin, 2,3-diphosphoglycerate and oxygen transport in the newborn premature infant. Scand J Clin Lab Invest Suppl 161:1, 1982.

174. Rossoff L, et al: Changes in blood P_{50}: effects on oxygen delivery when arterial hypoxemia is due to shunting. Chest 77:142, 1980.

175. Novy MJ, et al: Changes in umbilical-cord blood oxygen affinity after intrauterine transfusions for erythroblastosis. N Engl J Med 285:589, 1971.

176. Williams ML, et al: Role of dietary iron and fat in vitamin E deficiency anemia of infancy. N Engl J Med 292:887, 1975.

177. Stockman JA, et al: Anemia of prematurity: determinants of the erythropoietin response. J Pediatr 105:786, 1984.

178. Ohls RK: Evaluation and treatment of anemia in the neonate. *In* Christensen RD (ed): Hematologic Problems in the Neonate. Philadelphia, WB Saunders Company, 2000.

179. Brown MS, et al: Decreased response of plasma immunoreactive erythropoietin to "available oxygen" in anemia of prematurity. J Pediatr 105:793, 1984.

180. Ross MP, et al: A randomized trial to develop criteria for administering erythrocyte transfusions to anemic preterm infants 1 to 3 months of age. J Perinatol 9:246, 1989.

181. Bifano EM, et al: Relationship between determinants of oxygen delivery and respiratory abnormalities in preterm infants with anemia. J Pediatr 120:292, 1992.

182. Keyes WG, et al: Assessing the need for transfusion of premature infants and the role of hematocrit, clinical signs, and erythropoietin level. Pediatrics 84:412, 1989.

183. Izraeli S, et al: Lactic acid as a predictor for erythrocyte transfusion in healthy preterm infants with the anemia of prematurity. J Pediatr 122:629, 1993.

184. Schulman I: The anemia of prematurity. J Pediatr 54:663, 1959.

185. Pearson HA: Life-span of the fetal red blood cell. J Pediatr 70:166, 1967.

186. Bratteby LE: Studies on erythrokinetics in infants. IX. Prediction of red cell volume from venous haematocrit in early infancy. Acta Pediatr Scand 7:125, 1968.

187. Shannon KM, et al: Circulating erythroid progenitors in the anemia of prematurity. N Engl J Med 31:728, 1987.

188. Rhondeau SM, et al: Responsiveness to recombinant human erythropoietin of marrow erythroid progenitors from infants with the "anemia of prematurity." J Pediatr 12:935, 1988.

189. Ohls RK, et al: Erythroid "burst promoting activity" in the serum of patients with the anemia of prematurity. J Pediatr 116:786, 1990.

190. Ohls RK et al: Serum erythropoietin concentrations fail to increase following significant phlebotomy losses in ill, preterm infants. J Perinatol 17:465, 1997.

191. Ohls RK, et al: Erythropoietin production by preterm macrophages: implications regarding the anemia of prematurity. Pediatr Res 35:169, 1994.

192. Ohls RK: The use of erythropoietin in neonates. Clin Perinatol 3:681, 2000.

193. Ohls RK. Human recombinant erythropoietin in the prevention and treatment of anemia of prematurity. Pediatr Drugs 4:111, 2002.

194. Maier RF, et al: The effect of epoetin beta (recombinant human erythropoietin) on the need for transfusion in very low birth weight infants. N Engl J Med 330:1173, 1994.

195. Meyer MP, et al: Recombinant human erythropoietin in the treatment of the anemia of prematurity: results of a double-blind, placebo-controlled study. Pediatrics 93:918, 1994.

196. Shannon KM, et al: Recombinant human erythropoietin stimulates erythropoiesis and reduces erythrocyte transfusions in very low birth weight preterm infants. Pediatrics 95:1, 1995.

197. Ohls RK, et al: Efficacy and cost analysis of treating very low birth weight infants with erythropoietin during their first two weeks of life: a randomized, placebo controlled trial. J Pediatr 126:421, 1995.

198. Ohls RK, et al: The effect of erythropoietin on the transfusion requirements of preterm infants ≤750 grams: a randomized, double-blind, placebo-controlled study. J Pediatr 131:66, 1997.

199. Maier RF, et al: High- versus low-dose erythropoietin in extremely low birth weight infants. J Pediatr 132:866, 1998.

200. Donato H, et al: Effect of early versus late recombinant human erythropoietin on transfusion requirements in premature infants: results of randomized, placebo-controlled, multicenter trial. Pediatrics 105:1066, 2000.

201. Ohls RK, et al: Effects of early erythropoietin therapy on the transfusion requirements of preterm infants below 1250 grams birthweight: a multicenter, randomized controlled trial. Pediatrics 108:934, 2001.

202. Maier RF, et al: Early treatment with erythropoietin beta ameliorates anemia and reduces transfusion requirements in infants with birth weights below 1000 grams. J Pediatr 140:7, 2002.

203. Bifano EM, et al: Impact of transfusion guidelines on transfusion practices in premature infants. Pediatrics 35:216A, 1994.

204. George JW, et al: Age-related differences in erythropoietic response to recombinant human erythropoietin: comparison in adult and infant Rhesus monkeys. Pediatr Res 28:567, 1990.

205. Widness JA, et al: Developmental changes in erythropoietin (Ep) pharmacokinetics in fetal and neonatal sheep. Pediatr Res 28:284, 1990.

206. Eschbach JW, et al: Correction of the anemia of end stage renal disease with recombinant human erythropoietin. N Engl J Med 310:73, 1987.

207. Brown MS, et al: Single-dose pharmacokinetics of recombinant human erythropoietin in preterm infants after intravenous and subcutaneous administration. J Pediatr 122:655, 1993.

208. Ohls RK, et al: Pharmacokinetics and effectiveness of recombinant erythropoietin administered to preterm infants by continuous infusion in parenteral nutrition solution. J Pediatr 128:518, 1996.

209. Brown KE, Keith JF. Comparison between two and five doses a week of recombinant human erythropoietin for anemia of prematurity: a randomized trial. Pediatrics 104:210, 1999.

210. Cogar AA, et al: Endothelin concentrations in preterm infants treated with human recombinant erythropoietin. Bio Neonate 77:105, 2000.

211. Halperin DS, et al: Effects of recombinant human erythropoietin in infants with the anemia of prematurity: a pilot study. J Pediatr 116:779, 1990.

212. Ohls RK, Christensen RD: Recombinant erythropoietin compared with erythrocyte transfusion in the treatment of anemia of prematurity. J Pediatr 119:781, 1991.

213. Beck D, et al: Weekly intravenous administration of recombinant human erythropoietin in infants with the anaemia of prematurity. Eur J Pediatr 150:767, 1991.

214. Christensen RD, et al: Administration of erythropoietin to newborn rats results in diminished neutrophil production. Blood 78:1241, 1991.

215. Christensen RD, Rothstein G: Erythropoietin affects the maturation pattern of fetal G-CSF-responsive progenitors. Am J Hematol 39:108, 1992.

216. Katoh K, et al: Direct evidence for erythropoietin-induced release of endothelin from peripheral vascular tissue. Life Sci 54:253, 1994.

217. Emmerson AJB, et al: Double blind trial of recombinant erythropoietin in preterm infants. Arch Dis Child 68:291, 1993.

218. Ehrenkranz R, et al: Neurodevelopmental outcome and growth at 18-22 months in extremely low birth weight infants treated with early erythropoietin and iron. Pediatr Res 51:291A, 2002.

219. Casadevall N, et al: Pure red-cell aplasia and antierythropoietin antibodies in patients treated with recombinant erythropoietin. N Engl J Med 346:469, 2002.

220. Egrie JC: Development and characterization of novel erythropoiesis stimulating protein (NESP). Br J Cancer 84(Suppl 1):3, 2001.

221. Carnielli V, et al: Effect of high doses of human recombinant erythropoietin on the need for blood transfusions in preterm infants. J Pediatr 121:98, 1992.

222. Friel JK, et al: Intravenous iron administration to very-low-birth-weight newborns receiving total and partial parenteral nutrition. JPEN J Parenter Enteral Nutr 19:114, 1995.

223. Meyer MP, et al: A comparison of oral and intravenous iron supplementation in preterm infants receiving recombinant erythropoietin. J Pediatr 129:258, 1996.

224. Pollak A, et al: Effect of intravenous iron supplementation on erythropoiesis in erythropoietin-treated premature infants. Pediatrics 107:78, 2001.

225. Pathak A et al: Role of vitamin E in the treatment of anemia of prematurity. Arch Dis Child in press, 2003.

226. Millard DD, et al: Effects of intravascular, intrauterine transfusion on prenatal and postnatal hemolysis and erythropoiesis in severe fetal isoimmunization. J Pediatr 117:447, 1990.

227. Koenig JM, et al: Late hyporegenerative anemia in Rh hemolytic disease. J Pediatr 115:315, 1989.

228. Ohls RK, et al: Recombinant erythropoietin as treatment for the late hyporegenerative anemia of Rh hemolytic disease. Pediatrics 90:678, 1992.

229. Scaradavou A, et al: Suppression of erythropoiesis by intrauterine transfusions in hemolytic disease of the newborn: use of erythropoietin to treat the late anemia. J Pediatr 123:279, 1993.

230. Alverson DC, et al: Effect of booster blood transfusions on oxygen utilization in infants with bronchopulmonary dysplasia. J Pediatr 113:722, 1988.

231. Christensen RD, et al: Evaluation of the mechanism causing anemia in infants with bronchopulmonary dysplasia. J Pediatr 120:593, 1992.

232. Ohls RK, et al: A randomized, placebo-controlled trial of recombinant erythropoietin as treatment for the anemia of bronchopulmonary dysplasia. J Pediatr 123:996, 1993.

233. Shaddy RE, et al: Epoetin alpha therapy in infants awaiting heart transplantation. Arch Pediatr Adolesc Med 149:322, 1995.

234. Alexi-Meskishvili V, et al: Correction of cor triatriatum sinistrum in a Jehovah's Witness infant. Eur J Cardiothorac Surg 18:724, 2000.

235. Fearon JA, Weinthal J: The use of recombinant erythropoietin in the reduction of blood transfusion rates in craniosynostosis repair in infants and children. Plast Reconstr Surg 109:2190, 2002.

236. Kling PJ, et al: Pharmacokinetics and pharmacodynamics of erythropoietin therapy in an infant with renal failure. J Pediatr 121:822, 1992.

237. Lakatos L, et al: "Bloodless" treatment of a Jehovah's Witness infant with ABO hemolytic disease. J Perinatol 19:530, 1999.

238. Dhodapkar KM, Blei F: Treatment of hemolytic disease of the newborn caused by anti-Kell antibody with recombinant erythropoietin. J Pediatr Hematol Oncol 1:69, 2001.

239. Tchernia G, et al: Recombinant erythropoietin therapy as an alternative to blood transfusions in infants with hereditary spherocytosis. Hematol J 1:146, 2000.

240. DePalma L, Luban NLC: Blood component therapy in the perinatal period: guidelines and recommendations. Semin Perinatol 14:403, 1990.

Thomas A. Olson

147

Developmental Megakaryocytopoiesis in Fetal and Neonatal Physiology

BACKGROUND

Megakaryocytes, among the rarest and most physically unusual hematopoietic cells in the human bone marrow, comprise 0.02 to 0.1% of the total nucleated marrow cells.[1,2] Megakaryocytes are distinct from other hematopoietic cells in that they undergo endoreduplication and attain great size (>40 μm) and increased ploidy classes (≤128 N).[3] In theory, increased cell DNA production and increased megakaryocyte size will lead to increased platelet production.[2-5] Although we were initially hampered by the low frequency and intrinsic fragility of megakaryocytes, our understanding of megakaryocytopoiesis increased as a result of two significant scientific advances. First, newer culture methods yielded increased numbers and increased purity of megakaryocytes that allowed the application of molecular biology and flow cytometry techniques to study megakaryocytopoiesis. Second, thrombopoietin (TPO), the most important cytokine regulating megakaryocytopoiesis, was cloned in 1994. Although our understanding of cellular and molecular biology of megakaryocytopoiesis has increased, few data are available on developmental or fetal megakaryocytopoiesis. The complex process of megakaryocytopoiesis is summarized before the known patterns of fetal megakaryocytopoiesis are described.

MEGAKARYOCYTOPOIESIS

The rate of platelet production depends on the proliferation of megakaryocyte progenitors, differentiation into megakaryocytes, development of megakaryocytes into larger, mature megakaryocytes, and, finally, shedding of platelets (Fig. 147-1).[3,6] The criteria that differentiate all stages of megakaryocytopoiesis are not clear. There is considerable overlap between each stage, and this applies to all classification schemes.

Progenitors

The earliest identifiable megakaryocyte progenitor is the burst-forming unit, megakaryocyte (BFU-MK). A later progenitor has been designated colony-forming unit, megakaryocyte (CFU-MK). Human BFU-MK have been identified and characterized.[7,8] BFU-MK consist of foci of cells containing 100 to 500 cells per foci. They are seen later in culture than CFU-MK, a situation similar to erythrocyte progenitors. Both BFU-MK and CFU-MK have proliferative potential. Immunologic phenotyping showed that CFU-MK express CD34+ and human leukocyte antigen (HLA)-DR, whereas BFU-MK express only CD34+ (Fig. 147-2). Later, as megakaryocytes mature, HLA-DR expression is lost.[9] CFU-MK are more plentiful in the marrow and were the first to be quantified in clonal assay systems that used immunologic staining of megakaryocyte colonies.[10,11] Circulating peripheral blood contains more BFU-MK than CFU-MK.[12] Immunologic markers have been identified for different stages of megakaryocyte development (see Fig. 147-2).[9,13,14] Expression of CD34+ on cells of the megakaryocytic lineage correlates with the appearance of platelet glycoproteins (GPs).[15] Although it is known that megakaryocyte progenitors express CD34+, the timing of the loss

of CD34+ expression is unknown. Pluripotent stem cells do not express GPIIb,[16] but GPIIa (CD61) and the GPIIb/IIIa complex (CD41) probably appear at the CFU-MK stage and continue on mature megakaryocytes (see Fig. 147-2).

Transitional Cells

A uniquely megakaryocytic process is polyploidization. BFU-MK and CFU-MK are typically of 2 to 4 N ploidy classes. The proliferative potential slows, and transitional cells develop, with low proliferative potential and increased ploidy (4 to 8 N). These cells are difficult to identify morphologically. Immunologic studies have suggested that transitional cells (precursors) express both CD34 and CD61 (GPIIIa) and retain proliferative capabilities.[15] One transitional cell may be a megakaryoblast, the earliest cell of the megakaryocyte lineage that can be identified with the platelet peroxidase reaction.[17] During this phase, the cells begin to accumulate various α-granule proteins: platelet factor 4 (PF4), thrombospondin, β-thromboglobulin, von Willebrand factor, and platelet GPIb, the von Willebrand factor receptor,[18] which can later be detected on megakaryocytes (see Fig. 147-2).[9,13,19-21]

Megakaryocytes

Megakaryocytes lose the ability to proliferate and continue to differentiate. The process of differentiation has been examined on many levels. Both cytoplasmic differentiation and nuclear differentiation proceed. Morphologic classifications have centered on size, maturation stage, and ploidy distribution. Generally accepted megakaryocytic maturation characteristics have been described (Table 147-1).[22] There is circumstantial evidence that platelet production is closely related to megakaryocyte size.[2,5] Maturation stages and ploidy classes are also related to size.[1,23] A large Stage III megakaryocyte may produce up to 6000 platelets.[24] Nuclear differentiation is marked by *endoreduplication* (endomitosis), a process in which the ploidy of the cell increases without cellular division. Endoreduplication can be measured on stained individual cells in a cytospin, in a colony, or by flow cytometry.[1,25-28] In cytospins of adult marrow, the 16 N ploidy class predominates.[3,28] Eventually, as platelets are released, the megakaryocyte becomes smaller, and multiple nuclear lobes coalesce into a compact nucleus.[18]

Morphologic classification is often difficult. Megakaryoblasts and Stage I and II megakaryocytes are often missed on microscopic examination. Other criteria have been established for differentiation, including the development of surface GPs and the appearance of specific granules.[9,19] Both GPIIIa and GPIIb/IIIa appear on very early megakaryocytes. The sequential evolution of other GPs includes the later appearance of GPIb (CD42b) and then GPIV (CD36) on mature megakaryocytes (see Fig. 147-2).[13,29,30] The GPIb-V-IX (CD42) complex has been identified on late megakaryocytes.[31] Many platelet surface antigens actually function as protein receptors and are members of the integrin families. The development of the demarcation system and of α-granules has been documented by electron microscopy. Contents of the α-granules such as fibrinogen,

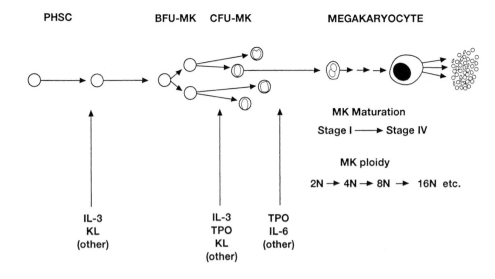

PHSC   BFU-MK   CFU-MK   MEGAKARYOCYTE

MK Maturation

Stage I ⟶ Stage IV

MK ploidy

2N → 4N → 8N → 16N etc.

IL-3   IL-3   TPO
KL   TPO   IL-6
(other)   KL   (other)
               (other)

Figure 147–1. Simplified scheme of megakaryocyte (MK) development. Many growth factors probably influence megakaryocytopoiesis at each stage. In some studies, the synergistic effect of interleukin-3 (IL-3) and thrombopoietin (TPO) was demonstrated. IL-3 seems to be essential for early megakaryocyte proliferation (especially fetal) from pluripotent hematopoietic stem cell (PHSC) through colony-forming unit, megakaryocyte (CFU-MK). Although many factors affect megakaryocyte maturation, TPO is probably the primary stimulant. BFU = burst-forming unit.

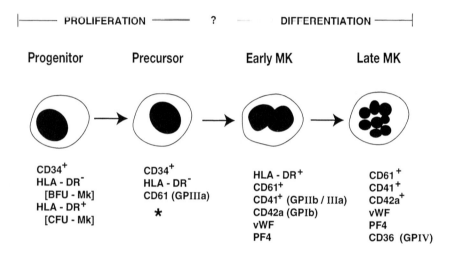

├── PROLIFERATION ── ? ── DIFFERENTIATION ──┤

Progenitor   **Precursor**   **Early MK**   **Late MK**

CD34⁺   CD34⁺   HLA - DR⁺   CD61⁺
HLA - DR⁻   HLA - DR⁻   CD61⁺   CD41⁺
[BFU - Mk]   CD61 (GPIIIa)   CD41⁺ (GPIIb / IIIa)   CD42a⁺
HLA - DR⁺   CD42a (GPIb)   vWF
[CFU - Mk]   *   vWF   PF4
                                      PF4   CD36 (GPIV)

Figure 147–2. Immunologic classification of megakaryocyte (MK) development. Burst-forming unit, megakaryocyte (BFU-MK) and colony-forming unit, megakaryocyte (CFU-MK) are considered progenitor cells. CFU-MK may transition into a precursor cell that still retains proliferative potential. Fragmentary data on various stages of megakaryocyte differentiation suggest a chronologic appearance of specific platelet glycoproteins (GP) and other platelet antigens such as von Willebrand factor (vWf) and platelet factor 4 (PF4). The *asterisk* indicates that megakaryocyte antigens CD41 (GPIIb/IIIa) and CD41a (GPIIb) may be expressed on an earlier cell of the megakaryocyte lineage that retains proliferative capacity.

TABLE 147-1

Cytologic Characteristics of Megakaryocyte Maturation States and Nuclear:Cytoplasmic Ratios at Each State (Much of the Size Variation for Each Stage Is Related to Ploidy Level)

Stage	Nuclear Morphology	Cytoplasmic Staining (Wright-Giemsa)	Approximate Size Range	Demarcation Membranes	Granules	Suggested Name
I	Compact (lobed)	Basophilic	6–24 μm	Present by electron microscopy	Few present by electron microscopy	Megakaryoblast
II	Horseshoe	Pink center	10–30 μm	Proliferating to center of cell	Starting to increase	Promegakaryocyte
III	Multilobed	Increasingly more pink than blue	16–56 μm	Extensive but asymmetric	Great numbers	Granular megakaryocyte
IV	Compact but highly lobulated	Eosinophilic	20–50 μm	Evenly distributed	Organized into platelet fields	Mature megakaryocyte

Modified from Williams N, Levine RF. Br J Haematol 52:173, 1991.

thrombospondin, and von Willebrand factor correlate with megakaryocyte maturation.[13, 19, 21] Fibrinogen appears late in megakaryocyte maturation.

Cytokine Effects on Megakaryocytopoiesis

In the past, many investigators suggested that two different growth factors were responsible for proliferation of megakary-

ocyte progenitors and maturation of megakaryocytes. These putative factors, although not isolated, were called megakaryocyte colony-stimulating activity or factor (MK-CSA or MK-CSF) and TPO. MK-CSA was the primary stimulant of proliferation, and TPO furthered maturation into large megakaryocytes and led to increased platelet production.

CFU-MK proliferation was noted in the presence of serum from patients with aplastic anemia.[10, 11, 32] The numbers of CFU-MK

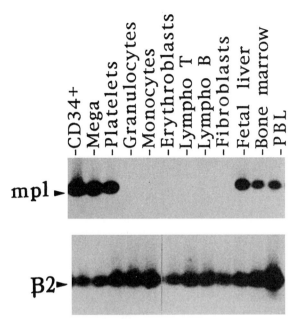

Figure 147–3. Expression of *c-mpl* and β_2-macroglobulin (β2) in normal purified hematopoietic cell populations and total tissues. Reverse transcriptase polymerase chain reaction was performed on 100-ng total RNA, except for the CD34+ population, in which total RNA was extracted from a pellet containing 1×10^5 cells. Autoradiographs were exposed for 6 hours at $-80°C$ with intensifying screens. PBL = peripheral blood lymphocytes. (From Wendling F, et al (eds). Molecular Biology of Haematopoeisis, Vol 3. 1994. Andover, UK, Intercept. Copyright © 1994, reprinted by permission of Intercept Ltd, Andover, UK.)

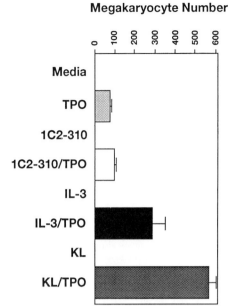

Figure 147–4. AA+ Sca+ stem cells were isolated and cultured in suspension with the addition of the following growth factors: thrombopoietin (TPO) alone, TPO and IC2-310, TPO and kit ligand (KL), and TPO and interleukin-3 (IL-3). (Original magnification ×40.) Suspension cultures were performed as described, and cells were harvested after 6 days. Cytospins of the resultant cells were performed and were stained using Wright-Giemsa and Megacolor. Mature megakaryocytes were counted from the Megacolor slides. (From Ziegler FC, et al. Blood *84*:4048, 1994.)

grown with this serum factor was inversely related to the marrow megakaryocyte mass, and it has been suggested that a proliferative megakaryocyte factor is not induced until marrow megaryocyte mass is depleted.[33] This serum factor was later referred to as MK-CSF after several enrichment steps.[34] Significant levels of MK-CSA were found in sera from experimentally radiated animals.[35-38] MK-CSA was also described in both the urine and sera of patients undergoing bone marrow transplantation.[39, 40] This effect was seen immediately after the start of ablation, before the platelet counts fell, a finding indicating that an early effect on marrow megakaryocytes may be involved.

If marrow aplasia were necessary for stimulation of a proliferative factor, what would be the effect of thrombocytopenia? A factor, named "thrombopoietin,"[41] had long been proposed as important to the regulation of megakaryocytopoiesis. Characteristics assigned to this theoretical factor included the ability to (1) increase megakaryocyte number and size, (2) increase endomitosis and ploidy, and (3) increase megakaryocyte cytoplasmic maturation. Many investigators attempted to isolate this factor, without success.

The murine myeloproliferative virus contains a cellular oncogene, v-*mpl*, that has structural similarities to the cytokine receptor superfamily.[42] The murine *mpl* was shown to have effect on cellular proliferation in association with interleukin-3 (IL-3) and other cytokines.[43, 44] The human homologue, c-*mpl*, was cloned and was confirmed as a member of the hematopoietin receptor superfamily.[45, 46] c-*mpl* expression was identified using reverse transcriptase polymerase chain reaction, in unseparated fetal liver, adult bone marrow, CD34+ cells, megakaryocytes, and platelets (Fig. 147–3).[47] No expression was detected in erythrocytes, neutrophils, monocytes, and lymphocytes. The investigators postulated that c-*mpl* was a receptor, specific to the

megakaryocyte lineage. Antisense oligonucleotides to *c-mpl* were constructed and inhibited megakaryocytopoiesis *in vitro* without affecting colony growth of other lineages.[48] Five groups of investigators isolated and cloned this ligand.[49-53] The ligand bound to the *c-mpl* receptor,[48] and the *c-mpl* receptor was expressed in the megakaryocyte lineage from progenitor (CD34+ GPIIIa+) to platelets.[54] The name *thrombopoietin* was given to the *c-mpl* ligand at a National Institutes of Health Workshop on Megakaryocytopoiesis and Platelet Production in August 1994. A PEGylated product was called megakaryocyte growth and development factor (MGDF).[49] The human TPO cDNA sequence predicts a protein of 332 amino acids. The TPO gene was localized to human chromosome 3q27-28, which is of great interest because this area has been linked with thrombocytosis in acute nonlymphocytic leukemia.[55-57] Expression of the TPO gene has been highest in liver.[49-51] TPO expression has been identified in the kidney, spleen, and bone marrow.[58]

TPO is, in fact, a proliferative factor (MK-CSF). Addition of human TPO to murine fetal liver or marrow cultures results in significant megakaryocytopoiesis with both proliferation and differentiation (Fig. 147–4).[59] IL-3 and stem cell factor (SCF) enhances the effect. In murine suspension cultures, TPO increases CFU-MK growth and megakaryocyte ploidy.[60] However, in humans, TPO is primarily involved in proliferation because it does not increase ploidy.[61] The highest proliferative rates occur with IL-3 and TPO. MGDF also supports human megakaryocyte proliferation *in vitro*.[49] Experiments in *c-mpl* deficient transgenic mice demonstrated decreased platelet counts and greatly decreased marrow megakaryocytes,[62] but the mice were healthy and viable. However, when the transcription factor NF-E2 was disrupted in an embryonic stem cell, transgenic mice had marrow megakaryocytes but no platelets. The megakaryocytes were abnormal, and the mice died,[63,64] findings suggesting that other factors are also involved in megakaryocytopoiesis. GATA-1 mice have increased numbers of megakaryocytes, but the megakaryocytes are small and immature.[65] Nichols and colleagues reported one patient with dysfunctional GATA-1 and abnormal platelet formation.[66]

Although TPO is primarily involved with megakaryocytopoiesis, it is not lineage specific. TPO helps to maintain pluripotent stem cells (CD34+) and proliferation of erythroid and granulocyte progenitors.[67,68] The regulation of TPO production in the liver is linked to megakaryocyte mass. Excess TPO binds to c-*mpl* expressed on platelets and megakaryocytes.[69,70] There are reports that bone marrow expression of TPO may respond to thrombocytopenia.[70] PF4, thrombospondin, and transforming growth factor-β (TGF-β) suppress TPO mRNA expression.[71]

Many other growth factors affect megakaryocyte colony growth *in vitro*. Granulocyte-macrophage CSF (GM-CSF) and IL-3 stimulate megakaryocytopoiesis alone or in combination.[34,72,73] Both IL-3 and GM-CSF induce CFU-MK growth, although maximal doses of IL-3 induce more colony growth. The combination is additive. A synergistic effect of IL-3 and GM-CSF has also been documented.[73] Other studies demonstrated that the number of cells per colony, and proliferative rate, also increased in the presence of either IL-3 or GM-CSF.[34] Soluble human kit ligand or SCF, the product of the c-*kit* oncogene, increases proliferation of CFU-MK and mature megakaryocytes.[74] Briddell and associates reported a synergistic effect of SCF with IL-3 or GM-CSF on human megakaryocytopoiesis *in vitro*.[75] SCF augmented CFU-MK proliferation with either IL-3 or GM-CSF, but augmentation of BFU-MK was seen only with IL-3. These data suggest that cytokines may interact at various developmental stages. IL-6 affects megakaryocytopoiesis *in vitro* and megakaryocyte maturation in particular.[76,75,72,77] IL-6 promotes CFU-MK proliferation of *in vitro* human marrow cultures, although the effect is less than seen with IL-3 or GM-CSF.[76] This effect is inhibited by TGF-β. Mei and Burstein demonstrated maturational effects of IL-6 on megakaryocytes in long-term murine marrow cultures.[78] High IL-6 bioactivity in the first 2 weeks of culture correlated with large higher-ploidy megakaryocytes. The effect was blocked by the addition of anti–IL-6 neutralizing antibody. The IL-6 receptor has been identified on megakaryocytes by *in situ* hybridization techniques, and the administration of IL-6 to suspension cultures increases ploidy.[79] In nonhuman primates, recombinant human IL-6 has been shown to effect megakaryocytopoiesis *in vivo*.[80-82] Recombinant IL-6 (5 to 80 μg/kg/day), injected twice daily for 14 days, caused dose-related increases in platelets and a shift to larger megakaryocytes in the bone marrow, findings indicating a maturational effect. Furthermore, modal ploidy increased from 16 to 64 N.[80] In a clinical Phase I/II study, recombinant human IL-6 was administered to 20 patients with cancer.[83] Doses of 0.5 to 20 μg/kg/day were used. Increases in platelet counts were noted at doses higher than 1 μg/kg/day. Side effects included fever, headache, myalgia, and erythema. At doses higher than 2.5 μg/kg, nausea, elevated liver enzymes, and anemia were noted. Although useful, IL-6 has sufficiently severe side effects to make its use in neonates problematic.

Megakaryocyte proliferation, endoreduplication, and maturation can be studied in suspension culture with flow cytometry.[84] Plasma from patients with aplastic anemia increased both proliferation and endoreduplication. IL-3 had a proliferative effect but did not induce endoreduplication, and it even suppressed endoreduplication when it was co-cultured with plasma from patients with aplastic anemia.

IL-11 increases megakaryocyte proliferation *in vitro* with IL-3, but not alone.[85] IL-11 has been released for clinical use. It has been shown to stimulate megakaryocytopoiesis in adults and children.[86-88] However, IL-11 must be administered daily for long periods and is associated with significant flulike symptoms and edema that limit its use. *In vitro* studies of the effect of recombinant human erythropoietin (rhEPO) on human megakaryocytopoiesis have been equivocal. Megakaryocyte progenitors were not increased in the presence of rhEPO alone,[72,73,76,89] but rhEPO augmented CFU-MK growth induced by other cytokines such as IL-3 or GM-CSF. In an *in vivo* study, high doses of rhEPO increased platelet counts within 2 days.[90] However, the long-term administration of rhEPO for 7 days led to a decrease in megakaryocytopoiesis and decreased platelet counts.[91] Simultaneously, mice that were recovering from experimentally induced thrombocytopenia had increased platelet counts and decreased hematocrits. The authors suggested that competition between the stem cells of the erythrocyte and megakaryocyte lineages was the cause. Cytokines that inhibit *in vitro* megakaryocytopoiesis include TGF-β, PF4, and the interferons.[92-95] The effect of TGF-β is predominantly anti–IL-3.[96]

FETAL AND NEONATAL MEGAKARYOPOIESIS

Fetal and Neonatal Megakaryocytes

The yolk sac appears to be the first site for fetal hematopoiesis.[97] Megakaryocytes have been noted in the yolk sac by 5 weeks' gestation,[98] and the first platelets appear in the circulation at 8 to 9 weeks' gestation.[99,100] The transition to hepatic hematopoiesis may involve migration of stem cells from the yolk sac to the liver.[101] Bleyer and colleagues documented that platelets could be found in fetuses at 10 to 12 weeks' gestation and megakaryocytes in liver and spleen tissue by 10 weeks' gestation.[102] As hematopoiesis switches to the liver, two populations of megakaryocytes are seen: early megakaryoblasts and promegakaryocytes.[103] Every stage of megakaryocyte development can be documented in the liver phase, although all cells are smaller than adult megakaryocytes.[104-107] Fetal bone marrow hematopoiesis has been documented as early as the 11th week of gestation, and megakaryocytes constitute 0.58% of the nucleated cells (this percentage increases to 1.2% by week 22).[108] By the 18th week, in fetal bone marrow, hematopoiesis is well established.[107,109-112] Izumi and Graeve and De Alarcon reported that newborn megakaryocytes are substantially smaller than adult megakaryocytes, and megakaryocyte size increases with gestational age (Table 147-2). There are also fewer Stage IV megakaryocytes seen in the fetal bone marrow (Table 147-3).

Adult-size megakaryocytes appear by 2 years of age, although insufficient data exist on children from birth to 1 year of age, owing to the lack of normal marrow specimens. These experiments were conducted on necropsy material, which can be associated with artifact. However, the results were confirmed on circulating cord blood megakaryocytes (Table 147-4). Megakaryocytes elutriated from umbilical venous cord blood are increased in number, but they are significantly smaller than adult circulating megakaryocytes.[37] Cord blood megakaryocytes also differ morphologically from similar-stage adult megakaryocytes, and micromegakaryocytes have been observed in cord blood (Fig. 147-5). Flow cytometry and immunogold silver staining have been used to characterize presumed megakaryocyte precursors in cord blood.[113] Approximately 2% (identified by immunogold silver) or 4% (fluorescence-activated cell sorter) of cord blood mononuclear cells express GPIIb/IIIA. Thoma and associates investigated the expression of other antigens coexpressed on cord blood CD34+ cells by flow cytometry and cDNA polymerase chain reaction.[114] CD61+ expression was noted on 5% of the circulating CD34+ cells. Care must be taken to remove platelets, which adhere to other mononuclear cells and yield falsely high CD61 expression. Platelets seen in early gestational fetuses appear to be larger with fewer granules, indicating less maturity.[102] Because fetal and neonatal megakaryo-

TABLE 147-2

Mean (SD) Diameter of Megakaryocytes* in Biopsy Specimens

Stage	Fetal (μm)	Adult (μm)	p Value
I	12.2 (1.2)	15.2 (3.9)	.2
II	15.8 (1.1)	22.4 (2.4)	.003
III	20.7 (4.9)	29.2 (1.3)	<.001
IV	22.6 (5.4)	29.3 (2.4)	<.001
Total	15.2 (1.4)	20.6 (4.1)	.04

* Megakaryocytes identified by staining with anti-glycoprotein IIb antibody.
Modified from Graeve JLA, de Alarcon PA. Arch Dis Child *64*:483, 1989.

TABLE 147-3

Percentage Distribution of Megakaryocytes* by Age

Stage	Fetal (%)	Adult (%)	p value
I	50	49	.7
II	28	22	.004
III	14	13	.3
IV	8	16	<.001
Total	100	100	<.001

* Megakaryocytes identified by staining with anti anti-glycoprotein IIb antibody.
Modified from Graeve JLA, de Alarcon PA. Arch Dis Child *64*:483, 1989.

TABLE 147-4

Characteristics of Circulating Adult Central Venous Blood and Neonatal Venous Cord Blood Megakaryocytes

	Intact	Naked Nuclei	Cytoplasm Fragments
Adult aortic blood (n = 20)			
Number* cells/mL	0.5 ± 0.7	6.8 ± 5.7	3.4 ± 2.7
Size† μm	26.8 ± 5.1	19.8 ± 2.3	20.7 ± 4.5
Venous cord blood (n = 8)			
Number* cells/mL	30.1 ± 16.5	209 ± 79.4	23.0 ± 8.9
Size† μm	21.5 ± 1.9	16.2 ± 1.6	18.5 ± 2.9

* Number of megakaryocytes are expressed cells/mL original sample (mean ± SD). In all all three categories (intact, naked nuclei, cytoplasm fragments) cord blood numbers are significantly higher compared with adult blood (*p* < .001, student's *t*-test).
† Two hundred forty intact megakaryocytes from 8 cord blood specimens were sized. One hundred intact adult megakaryocytes from 15 specimens were sized (5 specimens had no intact megakaryocytes). Cord blood intact megakaryocytes were smaller than adult megakaryocytes (*p* < .002, student's *t*-test).
From Olson TA, et al. Am J Pediatr Hematol Oncol *14*:246, 1992.

cytes are smaller than adult megakaryocytes, the release of fewer platelets per cell may be expected. Yet adult platelet count values are seen early in gestation.[115, 116] Platelet numbers are probably maintained by increased proliferation of fetal megakaryocyte progenitors.

Fetal Megakaryocyte Progenitors

The study of fetal megakaryocytopoiesis is intrinsically difficult because of the low frequency of megakaryocytes in fetal bone marrow and the limited availability of neonatal bone marrow specimens. Hegyi and associates obtained megakaryocytes from suspension cultures of fetal liver mononuclear cells.[117] Fetal megakaryocytes were smaller and had a lower mean ploidy class (4 N) than megakaryocytes from adult marrow cultures. Megakaryocyte progenitors can readily be obtained from cord blood.[118] Cord blood CFU-MK have characteristics, distinct from adult CFU-MK. Plasma clot culture and immunostaining can be used to identify CFU-MK in cord blood. Both adult and cord blood plasma clot cultures showed similar responses to stimulation with postirradiated aplastic canine serum (PICS) in terms of the number of CFU-MK per mononuclear cells plated. However, cord blood CFU-MK contained more cells than adult colonies at all dose levels.[37] Zauli and colleagues collected fetal blood from 18- to 22-week fetuses via umbilical vein sampling for medical reasons.[119] CD34+-enriched populations were obtained, and fibrin clot assays were done. Differences in cells per colony in cord blood and adult marrow were observed only with BFU-MK (not CFU-MK). Fetal BFU-MK contained up to 500 cells per colony. Fetal BFU-MK were more plentiful than fetal CFU-MK, and both appeared earlier in culture than did adult BFU-MK and CFU-MK. HLA-DR was expressed on fetal megakaryocyte pro-

genitors, and the treatment of cultures with anti–HLA-DR antibody eliminated cord blood CFU-MK growth, but it had only a minimal effect on BFU-MK proliferation. IL-3 alone, but not IL-6, supported progenitor proliferation. The responses of cord blood and adult marrow CFU-MK and BFU-MK to IL-3, IL-6, SCF, and PICS have also been compared.[38, 120] IL-3 stimulates the growth of more megakaryocyte progenitors in fetal cord blood cultures than in adult cultures. However, the stimulation of BFU-MK was not increased in 34-week gestation samples. IL-6 and IL-3 also produced a response in cord blood megakaryocytes that was gestationally related. The most potent stimulator, PICS-J (contains TPO), induced the most colonies and the highest cellularity within these colonies. Spontaneous megakaryocytopoiesis (without cytokine stimulation) was noted before 35 weeks' gestation. Clapp and associates described a similar gestational age-related decrease for other committed progenitors.[121] Imai and colleagues reported that IL-6 and IL-3 had a synergistic effect on CFU-MK proliferation in cord blood mononuclear cell cultures.[122] The response was dose related, peaking at 40 mg/mL, and was abrogated by neutralizing anti–IL-6 antibody. Colonies grown with IL-3 and IL-6 contained more cells per colony and larger megakaryocytes. Replanting experiments were done, by plucking individual colonies grown with IL-3 on day 9. Cells were then incubated with IL-3 or IL-6 for 2 days (3 days for ploidy). The megakaryocytes stimulated with IL-6 were significantly larger and of higher ploidy classes than those cultured without IL-6. This effect was blocked by anti–IL-6 antibody. The authors suggested that this demonstrated the ability of IL-6 to support differentiation of cord blood megakaryocytes in an *in vitro* system.

Several newer culture systems, which emphasize quantitation of small samples, have been developed to aid in the study of fetal megakaryocytopoiesis. Increased numbers of both BFU-MK (414±61 versus 151±18) and CFU-MK (2444±337 versus 869±64) per milliliter of preterm versus term cord blood were observed using a miniaturized culture system.[123] Warren and colleagues used a suspension culture method and enzyme-linked immunosorbent assay to identify and more accurately quantitate cord blood megakaryocyte growth in response to cytokines (IL-6, IL-3, leukemia inhibitory factor, kit ligand, and GM-CSF).[124] IL-3 produced a strong GPIIIb/IIIa signal in this assay, and other cytokines were additive.

After the identification of TPO as the primary regulator of megakaryocytopoiesis, many studies were done using cord blood cells. Sola and associates reported that cord blood TPO levels (enzyme-linked immunosorbent assay) were higher than adult plasma TPO levels. The levels did not correlate with gestational age or platelet counts.[125] The distributions of TPO and c-*mpl*, as detected by reverse transcriptase polymerase chain reaction, were similar to those seen in adults. Cord blood mean TPO levels ranged from 76 to 191 pg/mL.[125-131] Ishiguro and associates described a gradual decline of TPO levels throughout childhood.[131] In neonates with thrombocytopenia, there was no correlation between TPO levels and the degree of thrombocytopenia.

Initial studies reported similar responses to TPO, whether cord blood, peripheral blood, or bone marrow stem cells were cultured.[126, 126, 132] However, several investigators described a more proliferative megakaryocyte progenitor in cord blood compared with adult bone marrow.[133, 134] Using suspension cultures, Mwamtemi and colleagues demonstrated that cord blood CD34+ cells generated significantly more megakaryocytes than adult bone marrow CD34+ cells.[134] Other lineages were also stimulated by TPO.

Sola and associates compared the effects of TPO on neonatal (anterior iliac crest) and adult bone marrow stem cells.[133] Marrow cultures from either thrombocytopenic or nonthrombocytopenic neonates yielded three times more megakaryocyte colonies that adult marrow cultures. These neonatal colonies also contained more cells. Although TPO-induced proliferation of megakaryocyte progenitors is superior in cultures of cord blood CD34+ cells compared with adult CD34+ cells, the number of mature megakaryocytes produced is higher in adult marrow.[135] However, TPO may lead to increased CFU-MK proliferation but not megakaryocyte maturation. Ryu and colleagues reported that after an initial increase in CFU-MK proliferation, the cells proceeded to apoptosis.[136]

SITE OF PLATELET PRODUCTION

Although the regulation of megakaryocytopoiesis is not well understood, even less information is known on the mechanism of platelet release from megakaryocytes. Several theories exist. Investigators have proposed that protoplatelets are formed that "bud" off into platelets.[137,138] This process is believed to occur in

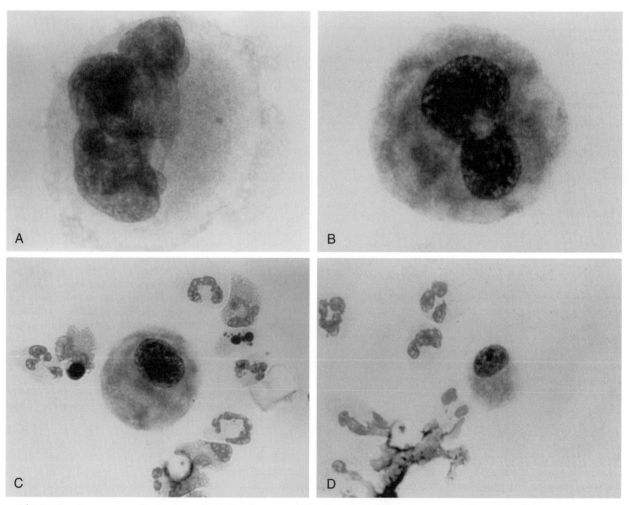

Figure 147-5. Megakaryocytes obtained by elutriation from cord blood and adult bone marrow. **A,** Stage III adult marrow megakaryocyte with multilobed nuclear development (46 μm). **B,** Stage III cord blood megakaryocyte with less nuclear development (44 μm). **C,** Stage IV cord blood megakaryocyte (32 μm). **D,** Cord blood micromegakaryocyte (18 μm).

the marrow and other organs,[139] and it has been described *in vitro*.[140] Another theory links platelet release to mechanical forces. The presence of circulating megakaryocytes has previously been documented,[141, 142] and the lung contains more megakaryocytes than any organ other than bone marrow.[143, 144] Levine and colleagues noted that more than 10 times the number of intact megakaryocytes entered the lung than exited.[24] Whereas large megakaryocytes were seen in the pulmonary artery circulation, only smaller megakaryocytes or fragments were seen in aortic blood. Megakaryocyte numbers and sizes were used to calculate the steady-state platelet production and estimated that 134.8×10^9 platelets may be produced daily by this method in the lungs. Platelet release in the lung by shear forces has been proposed.[24, 142] Circulating megakaryocytes have also been seen in the placental circulation.[37, 145-147] If platelet release in the lungs contributes to platelet production, perhaps the same mechanism occurs in the placenta, which is part of the fetal respiratory unit.

NEONATAL THROMBOCYTOPENIA

Platelet Counts

Platelets are produced very early in the fetus, and platelet counts rise in a linear fashion.[148, 149] In term infants, platelet counts are equivalent to those in older children and adults.[150, 151] Platelet counts similar to adult levels are achieved very early in gestation, with a mean platelet count of 208,000/mm³ in 17- to 20-week gestation fetuses.[116] Sell and Corrigan reviewed the development of clotting factors, including platelets in infants of various gestational ages.[115] Figure 147-6 shows the platelet count distribution for four gestational age groups. Platelet counts reach adult levels by 27 weeks' gestation. Forestier and associates documented adult platelet count values by 18 weeks' gestation.[149] Other studies also confirmed normal (adult) values in preterm infants, although it is difficult to determine the gestational ages because divisions were set by infant size (Table 147-5).[150, 152] In these studies, platelet counts lower than 100,000/mm³ were uncommon, and counts less than 50,000/mm³ were usually associated with some clinical abnormality. The platelet counts rose for several weeks after delivery.

Thrombocytopenia is a frequent problem in newborns admitted to neonatal intensive care units. An excellent summary of thrombocytopenia was completed by Sola and colleagues.[133] Newborns differ from adults in that severe morbidity is associated with thrombocytopenia. Infants who weigh less than 1500 g are particularly susceptible to neonatal complications compared with larger infants.[153] In thrombocytopenic patients who weigh less than 1500 g, the incidence of intraventricular hemorrhage (by ultrasound) is 30% higher than in nonthrombocytopenic preterm

infants (Fig. 147-7). Thrombocytopenic infants also have more sequelae. Thrombocytopenia is common in patients admitted to the intensive care nursery. Castle and associates reported a 22% incidence of thrombocytopenia in consecutive admissions to the neonatal intensive care unit.[154] The nadir of thrombocytopenia occurred at 4 days of age and resolved by 10 days of age. Although platelet destruction is one possible mechanism of thrombocytopenia, it does not explain the prolonged periods of thrombocytopenia in these infants. There are many causes of neonatal thrombocytopenia, and guidelines as described by Cohen and Baglin may be useful to the clinician (Fig. 147-8).[155] Hohlfeld and colleagues retrospectively studied 5194 consecutive fetal blood samplings[156] and analyzed the incidence and causes of thrombocytopenia in these infants. Thrombocytopenia was found in 247 fetuses, and the most common causes were infectious disease (28%), immune disorders (18%), and chromosomal anomalies (17%). Other causes were nonchromosomal abnormalities (13%), growth retardation (6%), Rh disease (4%), and gestational thrombocytopenia (2%). Castle and associates reported a shift toward immune causes of thrombocytopenia in infants admitted to the neonatal intensive care unit (Fig. 147-9).[154]

Maternal Causes

Maternal thrombocytopenia is frequently a concern for both obstetricians and neonatologists. The relation of maternal

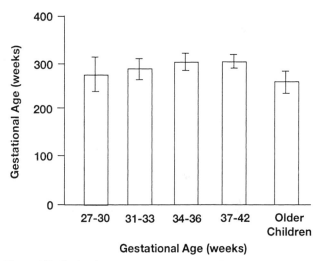

Figure 147-6. Platelet counts in normal newborn infants according to gestational age. (From Sell EJ, Corrigan JJ. J Pediatr *82*:1030, 1973.)

TABLE 147-5

Comparison of Venous Platelet Counts in Low Birth Weight Infants According to Birth Weight

	1700–2500 g			Under 1700 g		
Day	Number of Infants	Mean/mm³	Range 000 s/mm³	Number of Infants	Mean/mm³	Range 000 s/mm³
1	40	202,000	80-356	20	205,000	102-292
3	29	211,000	130-335	18	201,000	61-315
5	9	245,000	100-502	5	211,000	112-345
7	36	319,000	124-678	16	320,000	164-510
10	27	406,000	245-680	13	385,000	172-609
14	33	408,000	262-670	17	343,000	147-460
21	31	403,000	259-720	16	384,000	201-470
28	23	357,000	212-625	17	421,000	278-600

From Appleyard WJ, Brinton A. Biol Neonat *17*:5, 1971, S. Karger AG, Basel, Switzerland.

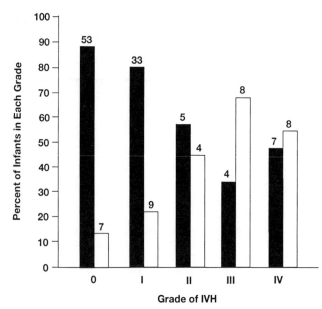

Figure 147–7. Relation between grade of intraventricular hemorrhage (IVH) and proportion of thrombocytopenic (n = 36, *light bars*) and nonthrombocytopenic (n = 102, *dark bars*) infants weighing less than 1500 g who were admitted to an intensive care unit with ultrasound examination performed. The percentage of thrombocytopenic infants with IVH increases as the grade of IVH increases. (From Andrew M, et al. J Pediatr *110*:462, 1987.)

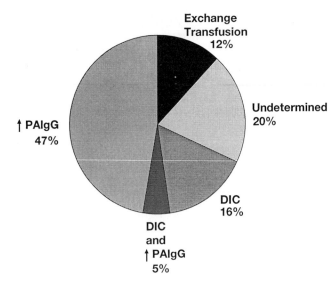

Figure 147–9. Mechanisms responsible for thrombocytopenia in 97 consecutive infants with platelet count less than $100 \times 10^9/L$. The mechanism can be identified in 80% of infants. DIC = disseminated intravascular coagulation; PAIgG = platelet-associated immunoglobulin G. (From Castle V, et al. J Pediatr *108*:753, 1986.)

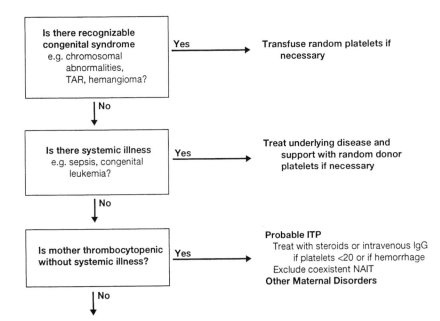

Figure 147–8. Scheme for the clinical evaluation of neonatal thrombocytopenia. ITP = immune thrombocytopenic purpura; NAIT = neonatal alloimmune thrombocytopenia; TAR = thrombocytopenia–absent radius syndrome. (Modified from Cohen DL, Boglin TP. Arch Dis Child *72*:F73, 1995.)

thrombocytopenia to the incidence of neonatal thrombocytopenia may determine obstetric management. Causes of pregnancy-associated thrombocytopenia reviewed by McCrae and associates[157] are shown in Table 147-6. The most common disorder is maternal idiopathic thrombocytopenic purpura (ITP). Thrombocytopenia (platelet count <50,000/mm³) is found in 15 to 65% of infants born to mothers with ITP.[158-161] The management of this condition is difficult, especially given that maternal and fetal platelet counts do not correlate well.[159, 161] If incidental maternal thrombocytopenia is present, only obstetric considerations should be considered. With ITP, however, the decisions are not as clear. One study suggested that the absence of a history of ITP, or nega-

TABLE 147-6

Causes of Maternal Thrombocytopenia

Immune thrombocytopenic purpura
Preeclampsia
Hemolysis, elevated liver function tests, low platelets (HELLP syndrome)
Thrombotic thrombocytopenic purpura
Hemolytic uremic syndrome
Miscellaneous conditions

Modified from McCrae KR, et al. Blood *80*:2607, 1992.

TABLE 147-7

Possible Causes of Thrombocytopenia in Sick Newborns

Infection	Small for gestational age
Viral	Necrotizing enterocolitis
Bacterial	Polycythemia
Protozoal	Cold injury
Mycotic	Rh disease
Asphyxia	Hyperbilirubinemia
Aspiration	Phototherapy
Pulmonary hypotension	Cardiac thrombosis
Respiratory distress syndrome	Diffuse intravascular coagulation

From de Alarcon PA. *In* Stockman JA, Pochedly C (eds). Developmental and Neonatal Hematology. New York, Raven Press, 1988, p 121.

tive maternal circulating antibodies, indicated a low risk to the fetus.[160] In 61 infants born to mothers with ITP, there were only 3 with platelet counts less than 50,000/mm³ and no morbidity or mortality.[158] In another study, percutaneous umbilical blood samplings were done on 21 women with ITP; only 5 infants had a platelet count less than 150,000/mm³, and only 1 infant had a platelet count lower than 50,000/mm³ (20,000/mm³).[162] Some investigators recommend fetal blood sampling when maternal platelet counts are less than 75,000/mm³.[162, 157] Infants with platelet counts lower than 50,000/mm³ may be considered for delivery by cesarean section. Infants born to mothers with preeclampsia and HELLP (hemolysis, elevated liver enzymes, and low platelet count) syndrome can also develop thrombocytopenia, although the incidence is low.[163, 164] Thrombocytopenia usually develops after birth and is associated with sepsis and respiratory distress syndrome. Burrows and Kelton followed mothers who were found to have incidental thrombocytopenia.[165] Only 45 of the infants born to these mothers had thrombocytopenia, and no infant developed a platelet count lower than 100,000/mm³. This finding was confirmed in a larger study,[160] and the term *gestational thrombocytopenia* has been applied.[166] It is important to treat the patient and not the platelet count, because gestational thrombocytopenia is not associated with neonatal morbidity.

Neonatal Alloimmune Thrombocytopenia

Immune thrombocytopenia should be considered in any well infant without obvious malformations. Neonatal alloimmune thrombocytopenia (NAIT) differs from passive transmission of antiplatelet antibodies in maternal ITP. There is a significant incidence of intracranial hemorrhage (30%).[167] The most common cause of NAIT is alloantibodies against PL^{A1}. However, incompatibilities against many platelet antigens have been described.[168,169] These antigens are now designated HPA-1 (PL^{A1}), with a and b indicating the different alleles. HPA-1b represents the typing of a PL^{A1-} mother. HPA antigen distribution may be related to race. Many patients who are severely affected by NAIT do not have detectable antibodies. Platelet antigens can be typed serologically or by DNA analysis. This is especially important for families who want other children.[170] NAIT can occur in first-born infants, and recurrences in siblings are common.[171] Treatment should be considered in severely affected infants, whose platelet counts are less than 50,000/mm³. The affected infants do not usually respond to random donor platelet transfusion, but platelet counts increase after a transfusion with maternal platelets. Maternal platelet transfusions may be needed for several weeks.[172] High-dose intravenous immunoglobulin (IVIgG) (2 g/kg) has been reported to raise platelet counts to at least twice the baseline level in 48 hours.[173] Bussel, of the New York Weill Cornell Medical Center, uses methylprednisolone 1 mg/kg/day and IVIgG 1 g/kg/day, until the platelet count rises. Retreatment is occasionally required.[169] Subsequent pregnancies can also be managed to limit the risk of fetal bleeding.[174,175] Treatments include (1) administration of high-dose IVIgG or steroids to mothers and (2) intrauterine platelet transfusions. In a study by Bussel and associates,[174] the adminis-

tration of IVIgG (with or without steroids) to mothers who had previously delivered an infant with a platelet count lower than 30,000/mm³ increased platelet counts by an average of 75,000± 62,000/mm³. No infants had intracranial hemorrhage.

Infection

Most of the infants with immune platelet disorders appear well. Sick infants should be investigated for an underlying cause (Table 147-7).[112] Infections have been associated with the development of thrombocytopenia. Platelet counts less than 150,000/mm³ were noted in 77% of patients with gram-positive septicemia and in 55% of the patients with gram-negative septicemia.[176] In a small series of neonates with septicemia, 16 of 21 culture-positive neonates had platelet counts lower than 100,000/mm³.[177] Increased platelet-associated immunoglobulin G (PAIgG) has been observed in both bacterial and viral neonatal infections.[178, 179] Most infants with disseminated intravascular coagulation are thrombocytopenic,[180] and sepsis has been associated with decreased megakaryocyte production in the marrow.[181] In all cases, treatment should be directed at the underlying infection; platelet transfusions should begin as needed.

Congenital infections are also associated with neonatal thrombocytopenia.[182-184] Congenital cytomegalovirus (CMV) infections are associated with hematologic abnormalities,[185] and thrombocytopenia is present in both congenital and acquired CMV infections.[186, 187] In murine CMV infections, there is evidence that thrombocytopenia may be caused by direct marrow suppression.[188] Chesney and associates documented CMV inclusion bodies in the marrow megakaryocytes of a boy congenitally infected with CMV. At birth, the platelet count was 48,000/mm³ and increased to 100,000/mm³ by age 4 years (the time of the marrow).[189] The megakaryocyte numbers appeared normal, but megakaryocytes were vacuolated, a finding indicating a direct effect on marrow megakaryocytes. Fetal blood sampling has been used to detect severe thrombocytopenia in the fetuses of mothers with active CMV infections.[190] In mothers infected with *Toxoplasmosis gondii* during pregnancy, 12 of 39 infected infants had low platelet counts.[191] Small for gestational age infants often have low platelet and white blood cell counts.[192] Cox and colleagues[193] studied 24 cases of idiopathic growth retardation with percutaneous umbilical blood sampling, and although thrombocytopenia was not common, platelet counts below the mean were associated with a poor clinical outcome. The cause of thrombocytopenia is not known; however, it has been suggested that there is a lack of increased TPO production.[127]

Congenital Thrombocytopenia

The failure of megakaryocyte production is not a usual clinical finding in the pediatric population. More commonly, platelet production defects result from marrow damage either from malignant infiltration or from aplasia. These conditions can occur but are rare in the neonatal period. Many syndromes that are associated with thrombocytopenia are characterized by other clinical features that can be identified in the neonatal period. Thrombocytopenia is not usually noted. Several inherited disorders are associated with thrombocytopenia and other clinical features. Wiscott-Aldrich syndrome is an X-linked disease with microplatelets and immunodeficiency.[194, 195] Epstein syndrome, an autosomal dominant disorder with renal disease and deafness, is associated with thrombocytopenia.[196, 197] The presence of thrombocytopenia is variable in May-Hegglin anomaly, a disorder of white blood cell inclusion bodies.[198, 199] The platelets in May-Hegglin anomaly are remarkable for their large (>7 µm) size.[200-202] Familial thrombocytopenia without any associated clinical abnormalities (Bernard-Soulier syndrome, Gray-platelet syndrome, and Montreal platelet syndrome) has been reported.[203-205]

Other reports of isolated familial thrombocytopenia have been summarized by Olson and colleagues.[37] Savoia and associates described a large Italian family with autosomal dominant thrombocytopenia.[206] The disease has been mapped to chromosome 10p. Another similar family has been reported.[207] These patients had decreased dysmature megakaryocytes, with slightly elevated TPO levels. This finding contrasted with a family reported by van den Oudenrijn, with normal TPO level and increased number of dysmorphic megakaryocytes.[208]

The most easily recognized neonatal syndrome with thrombocytopenia is the thrombocytopenia–absent radius syndrome (TAR), an autosomal recessive disorder.[209-211] In one study, the lack of megakaryocyte progenitors at birth was noted.[212] More recently, de Alarcon and colleagues cultured CFU-MK from an infant with TAR, but the colonies and the megakaryocytes were abnormal.[213] The colonies contained more cells than control colonies, and the cells were small. Megakaryocytes obtained from the marrow were also small and of lower ploidy classes than control megakaryocytes. One proposed explanation was a defect in the TPO effect. Ballmaier and associates reported that a patient with TAR had elevated TPO levels and normal expression of c-*mpl* on platelets and megakaryocytes.[214] These investigators postulated that thrombocytopenia in TAR may be related to a signal transduction defect because CFUs-MK did not respond to TPO. The association of thrombocytopenia and absent radius has also been seen in trisomy 18.[215] However, the radius may be normal, and thrombocytopenia may still be present.[216] Congenital amegakaryocytic thrombocytopenia (CAMT) may present with neonatal thrombocytopenia. However, platelet counts may be normal at birth. It is probably an intrinsic stem cell defect[217] that progresses over several years to aplastic anemia. Patients with CAMT have been shown to have point mutation in or a deletion in the cooling region of c-*mpl*. This finding suggests that the defect in CAMT may be at the receptor level.[218] All patients with CAMT have high TPO levels, low glycocalicin levels, and no megakaryocytes, whereas patients with Wiscott-Aldrich syndrome have normal TPO, glycocalicin levels and megakaryocyte numbers.

REFERENCES

1. Levine RF, Bunn PA Jr, Hazzard KC, Schlam ML. Flow cytometric analysis of megakaryocyte ploidy: comparison with Feulgen microdensitometry and discovery that 8N is the predominant ploidy class in guinea pig and monkey marrow. *Blood.* 1980;56:210–217.
2. Harker LA. Kinetics of thrombopoiesis. *J Clin Invest.* 1968;94:458–469.
3. Levine RF. Isolation and characterization of normal human megakaryocytes. *Br J Haematol.* 1980;45:487–497.
4. Williams N, Levine RF. The origin, development and regulation of megakaryocytes. *Br J Haematol.* 1982;52:173–180.
5. Harker LA, Finch CA. Thrombokinetics in man. *J Clin Invest.* 1969;48:963–974.
6. Williams N, McDonald TP, Rabellino EM. Maturation and regulation of megakaryocytopoiesis. *Blood Cells.* 1979;5:43–55.
7. Briddell RA, Brandt JE, Straneva JE, Srour EF, Hoffman R. Characterization of the human burst-forming unit-megakaryocyte. *Blood.* 1989;74:145–151.
8. Briddell RA, Hoffman R. Cytokine regulation of the human burst-forming unit-megakaryocyte. *Blood.* 1990;76:516–522.
9. Vainchenker W, Kieffer N. Human megakaryocytopoiesis: in vitro regulation and characterization of megakaryocytic precursor cells by differentiation markers. *Blood Rev.* 1988;2:102–107.
10. Mazur EM, Hoffman R, Bruno E. Regulation of human megakaryocytopoiesis: an in vito analysis. *J Clin Invest.* 1981;68:733–741.
11. Hoffman R, Mazur E, Bruno E, Floyd V. Assay of an activity in the serum of patients with disorders of thrombopoiesis that stimulates formation of megakaryocytic colonies. *N Engl J Med.* 1981;305:533–538.
12. Zauli G, Vitale L, Brunelli MA, Bagnara GP. Prevalence of the primitive megakaryocyte progenitors (BFU-meg) in adult human peripheral blood. *Exp Hematol.* 1992;20:850–854.
13. Vinci G, Tabilio A, Deschamps JF, et al. Immunological study of in vitro maturation of human megakaryocytes. *Br J Haematol.* 1984;56:589–605.
14. Levene RB, Lamaziere JM, Broxmeyer HE, Lu L, Rabellino EM. Human megakaryocytes. V. Changes in the phenotypic profile of differentiating megakaryocytes. *J Exp Med.* 1985;161:457–474.
15. Debili N, Issaad C, Masse JM, et al. Expression of CD34 and platelet glycoproteins during human megakaryocytic differentiation. *Blood.* 1992;80:3022–3035.
16. Molla A, Andrieux A, Chapel A, Schweitzer A, Berthier R, Marguerie G. Lack of transcription and expression of the alpha IIb integrin in human early haematopoietic stem cells. *Br J Haematol.* 1992;82:635–639.
17. Breton-Gorius J, Guichard J. Ultrastructural localization of peroxidase activity in human platelets and megakaryocytes. *Am J Pathol.* 1972;66:277–293.
18. Williams N, Eger RR, Jackson HM, Nelson DJ. Two-factor requirement for murine megakaryocyte colony formation. *J Cell Physiol.* 1982;110:101–104.
19. Cramer EM, Savidge GF, Vainchenker W, et al. Alpha-granule pool of glycoprotein IIb-IIIa in normal and pathologic platelets and megakaryocytes. *Blood.* 1990;75:1220–1227.
20. Rabellino EM, Levene RB, Leung LL, Nachman RL. Human megakaryocytes. II. Expression of platelet proteins in early marrow megakaryocytes. *J Exp Med.* 1981;154:88–100.
21. Cramer EM, Debili N, Martin JF, et al. Uncoordinated expression of fibrinogen compared with thrombospondin and von Willebrand factor in maturing human megakaryocytes. *Blood.* 1989;73:1123–1129.
22. Levine RF, Williams N, Levin J, Evatt BL. Megakaryocyte development and function. *In* Proceedings of the Conference on Megakaryocyte Development and Function. 1986. New York, Alan R. Liss.
23. Levine RF, Hazzard KC, Lamberg JD. The significance of megakaryocyte size. *Blood.* 1982;60:1122–1131.
24. Levine RF, Eldor A, Shoff PK, Kirwin S, Tenza D, Cramer EM. Circulating megakaryocytes: delivery of large numbers of intact, mature megakaryocytes to the lungs. *Eur J Haematol.* 1993;51:233–246.
25. Arriaga M, South K, Cohen JL, Mazur EM. Interrelationship between mitosis and endomitosis in cultures of human megakaryocyte progenitor cells. *Blood.* 1987;69:486–492.
26. Levin J, Levin FC, Penington DG, Metcalf D. Measurement of ploidy distribution in megakaryocyte colonies obtained from culture: with studies of the effects of thrombocytopenia. *Blood.* 1981;57:287–297.
27. Kuter DJ, Rosenberg RD. Regulation of megakaryocyte ploidy in vivo in the rat. *Blood.* 1990;75:74–81.
28. Tomer A, Friese P, Conklin R, et al. Flow cytometric analysis of megakaryocytes from patients with abnormal platelet counts. *Blood.* 1989;74:594–601.
29. Breton-Gorius J, Vainchenker W. Immunological and cytochemical characterization of megakaryocytic lineage leukemia. *Prog Clin Biol Res.* 1986;215:301–317.
30. Duperray A, Berthier R, Chagnon E, et al. Biosynthesis and processing of platelet GPIIb-IIIa in human megakaryocytes. *J Cell Biol.* 1987;104:1665–1673.
31. Lepage A, Leboeuf M, Cazenave JP, de la SC, Lanza F, Uzan G. The alpha(IIb)beta(3) integrin and GPIb-V-IX complex identify distinct stages in the maturation of CD34(+) cord blood cells to megakaryocytes. *Blood.* 2000;96:4169–4177.
32. Mazur EM, Hoffman R, Chasis J, Marchesi S, Bruno E. Immunofluorescent identification of human megakaryocyte colonies using an antiplatelet glycoprotein antiserum. *Blood.* 1981;57:277–286.
33. Mazur EM, de Alarcon P, South K, Miceli L. Human serum megakaryocyte colony-stimulating activity increases in response to intensive cytotoxic chemotherapy. *Exp Hematol.* 1984;12:624–628.
34. Hoffman R, Yang HH, Bruno E, Straneva JE. Purification and partial characterization of a megakaryocyte colony-stimulating factor from human plasma. *J Clin Invest.* 1985;75:1174–1182.
35. Miura M, Jackson CW, Steward SA. Increase in circulating megakaryocyte growth-promoting activity (Meg-GPA) following sublethal irradiation is not related to decreased platelets. *Exp Hematol.* 1988;16:139–144.
36. Mazur EM, South K. Human megakaryocyte colony-stimulating factor in sera from aplastic dogs: partial purification, characterization, and determination of hematopoietic cell lineage specificity. *Exp Hematol.* 1985;13:1164–1172.
37. Olson TA, Levine RF, Mazur EM, Wright DG, Salvado AJ. Megakaryocytes and megakaryocyte progenitors in human cord blood. *Am J Pediatr Hematol Oncol.* 1992;14:241–247.

38. Deutsch VR, Olson TA, Nagler A, Slavin S, Levine RF, Eldor A. The response of cord blood megakaryocyte progenitors to IL-3, IL-6 and aplastic canine serum varies with gestational age. *Br J Haematol.* 1995;89:8-16.

39. de Alarcon PA, Schmieder JA, Gingrich R, Klugman MP. Pattern of response of megakaryocyte colony-stimulating activity in the serum of patients undergoing bone marrow transplantation. *Exp Hematol.* 1988;16:316-319.

40. Fauser AA, Kanz L, Spurll GM, Lohr GW. Megakaryocytic colony-stimulating activity in patients receiving a marrow transplant during hematopoietic reconstitution. *Transplantation.* 1988;46:543-548.

41. Kelemen E, Cserhati I, Tanos B. Demonstration and some properties of human thrombopoietin in thrombocythemic sera. *Am J Pediatr Hematol Oncol.* 1958;20:350-355.

42. Souyri M, Vigon I, Penciolelli JF, Heard JM, Tambourin P, Wendling F. A putative truncated cytokine receptor gene transduced by the myeloproliferative leukemia virus immortalizes hematopoietic progenitors. *Cell.* 1990;63:1137-1147.

43. Vigon I, Florindo C, Fichelson S, et al. Characterization of the murine Mpl proto-oncogene, a member of the hematopoietic cytokine receptor family: molecular cloning, chromosomal location and evidence for a function in cell growth. *Oncogene.* 1993;8:2607-2615.

44. Skoda RC, Seldin DC, Chiang MK, Peichel CL, Vogt TF, Leder P. Murine c-mpl: a member of the hematopoietic growth factor receptor superfamily that transduces a proliferative signal. *EMBO J.* 1993;12:2645-2653.

45. Vigon I, Mornon JP, Cocault L, et al. Molecular cloning and characterization of MPL, the human homolog of the v-*mpl* oncogene: identification of a member of the hematopoietic growth factor receptor superfamily. *Proc Natl Acad Sci U S A.* 1992;89:5640-5644.

46. Mignotte V, Vigon I, Boucher dC, Romeo PH, Lemarchandel V, Chretien S. Structure and transcription of the human c-mpl gene (MPL). *Genomics.* 1994;20:5-12.

47. Methia N, Louache F, Vainchenker W, Wendling F. Oligodeoxynucleotides antisense to the proto-oncogene c-mpl specifically inhibit in vitro megakaryocytopoiesis. *Blood.* 1993;82:1395-1401.

48. Wendling F, Maraskovsky E, Debili N, et al. cMpl ligand is a humoral regulator of megakaryocytopoiesis. *Nature.* 1994;369:571-574.

49. Bartley TD, Bogenberger J, Hunt P, et al. Identification and cloning of a megakaryocyte growth and development factor that is a ligand for the cytokine receptor Mpl. *Cell.* 1994;77:1117-1124.

50. Lok S, Kaushansky K, Holly RD, et al. Cloning and expression of murine thrombopoietin cDNA and stimulation of platelet production in vivo. *Nature.* 1994;369:565-568.

51. de Sauvage FJ, Hass PE, Spencer SD, et al. Stimulation of megakaryocytopoiesis and thrombopoiesis by the c-Mpl ligand. *Nature.* 1994;369:533-538.

52. Kuter DJ, Beeler DL, Rosenberg RD. The purification of megapoietin: a physiological regulator of megakaryocyte growth and platelet production. *Proc Natl Acad Sci U S A.* 1994;91:11104-8.

53. Miyazaki,H, Kato T, Ogami K, Iwamatsu A, Shimada Y, et.al. Isolation and cloning of a novel human thrombopoietic factor (abstract). *Exp Hematol.* 1994;22:838.

54. Debili N, Wendling F, Cosman D, et al. The Mpl receptor is expressed in the megakaryocytic lineage from late progenitors to platelets. *Blood.* 1995;85:391-401.

55. Rowley JD, Potter D. Chromosomal banding patterns in acute nonlymphocytic leukemia. *Blood.* 1976;47:705-721.

56. Pintado T, Ferro MT, San Ramon C, Mayayo M, Larana JG. Clinical correlations for the 3q21;q26 cytogenic anomaly. *Cancer.* 1985;55:535.

57. Bernstein R, Pinto MR, Behr A, Mendelow B. Chromosome 3 abnormalities in acute nonlymphocytic leukemia (ANLL) with abnormal thrombopoiesis: report of three patients with a "new" inversion anomaly and a further case of homologous translocation. *Blood.* 1982;60:613-617.

58. Sungaran R, Markovic B, Chong BH. Localization and regulation of thrombopoietin mRNa expression in human kidney, liver, bone marrow, and spleen using in situ hybridization. *Blood.* 1997;89:101-107.

59. Zeigler FC, de Sauvage F, Widmer HR, et al. In vitro megakaryocytopoietic and thrombopoietic activity of c-*mpl* ligand (TPO) on purified murine hematopoietic stem cells. *Blood.* 1994;84:4045-4052.

60. Kaushansky K, Lok S, Holly RD, et al. Promotion of megakaryocyte progenitor expansion and differentiation by the c-*mpl* ligand thrombopoietin. *Nature.* 1994;369:568-571.

61. Schipper LF, Brand A, Reniers NC, Melief CJ, Willemze R, Fibbe WE. Effects of thrombopoietin on the proliferation and differentiation of primitive and mature haemopoietic progenitor cells in cord blood. *Br J Haematol.* 1998;101:425-435.

62. Gurney AL, Carver-Moore K, de Sauvage FJ, Moore MW. Thrombocytopenia in c-*mpl*-deficient mice. *Science.* 1994;265:1445-1447.

63. Shivdasani,RA, Rosenblatt MF, Zucker-Franklin D, et al. Transcription factor NF-E2 is required for platelet formation independent of the actions of thrombopoietin/MGDF in megakaryocyte development (abstract). *Blood.* 1995;84:110.

64. Shivdasani RA, Fielder P, Keller GA, Orkin SH, de Sauvage FJ. Regulation of the serum concentration of thrombopoietin in thrombocytopenic NF-E2 knockout mice. *Blood.* 1997;90:1821-1827.

65. Vyas P, Ault K, Jackson CW, Orkin SH, Shivdasani RA. Consequences of GATA-1 deficiency in megakaryocytes and platelets. *Blood.* 1999;93:2867-2875.

66. Nichols KE, Crispino JD, Poncz M, et al. Familial dyserythropoietic anaemia and thrombocytopenia due to an inherited mutation in GATA1. *Nat Genet.* 2000;24:266-270.

67. Solar GP, Kerr WG, Zeigler FC, et al. Role of c-mpl in early hematopoiesis. *Blood.* 1998;92:4-10.

68. Ritchie A, Vadhan-Raj S, Broxmeyer HE. Thrombopoietin suppresses apoptosis and behaves as a survival factor for the human growth factor–dependent cell line, M07e. *Stem Cells.* 1996;14:330-336.

69. Kuter DJ, Rosenberg RD. The reciprocal relationship of thrombopoietin (c-*mpl* ligand) to changes in the platelet mass during busulfan-induced thrombocytopenia in the rabbit. *Blood.* 1995;85:2720-2730.

70. Nagata Y, Shozaki Y, Nagahisa H, Nagasawa T, Abe T, Todokoro K. Serum thrombopoietin level is not regulated by transcription but by the total counts of both megakaryocytes and platelets during thrombocytopenia and thrombocytosis. *Thromb Haemost.* 1997;77:808-814.

71. Sungaran R, Chisholm OT, Markovic B, Khachigian LM, Tanaka Y, Chong BH. The role of platelet alpha-granular proteins in the regulation of thrombopoietin messenger RNA expression in human bone marrow stromal cells. *Blood.* 2000;95:3094-3101.

72. Lu L, Briddell RA, Graham CD, Brandt JE, Bruno E, Hoffman R. Effect of recombinant and purified human haematopoietic growth factors on in vitro colony formation by enriched populations of human megakaryocyte progenitor cells. *Br J Haematol.* 1988;70:149-156.

73. Teramura M, Katahira J, Hoshino S, Motoji T, Oshimi K, Mizoguchi H. Effect of recombinant hemopoietic growth factors on human megakaryocyte colony formation in serum-free cultures. *Exp Hematol.* 1989;17:1011-1016.

74. Avraham H, Vannier E, Cowley S, et al. Effects of the stem cell factor, c-*kit* ligand, on human megakaryocytic cells. *Blood.* 1992;79:365-371.

75. Briddell RA, Bruno E, Cooper RJ, Brandt JE, Hoffman R. Effect of c-*kit* ligand on in vitro human megakaryocytopoiesis. *Blood.* 1991;78:2854-2859.

76. Bruno E, Hoffman R. Effect of interleukin 6 on in vitro human megakaryocytopoiesis: its interaction with other cytokines. *Exp Hematol.* 1989;17:1038-1043.

77. Ishibashi T, Kimura H, Uchida T, Kariyone S, Friese P, Burstein SA. Human interleukin 6 is a direct promoter of maturation of megakaryocytes in vitro. *Proc Natl Acad Sci U S A.* 1989;86:5953-5957.

78. Mei RL, Burstein SA. Megakaryocytic maturation in murine long-term bone marrow culture: role of interleukin-6. *Blood.* 1991;78:1438-1447.

79. Navarro S, Debili N, Le Couedic JP, et al. Interleukin-6 and its receptor are expressed by human megakaryocytes: in vitro effects on proliferation and endoreplication. *Blood.* 1991;77:461-471.

80. Stahl CP, Zucker-Franklin D, Evatt BL, Winton EF. Effects of human interleukin-6 on megakaryocyte development and thrombocytopoiesis in primates. *Blood.* 1991;78:1467-1475.

81. Asano S, Okano A, Ozawa K, et al. In vivo effects of recombinant human interleukin-6 in primates: stimulated production of platelets. *Blood.* 1990;75:1602-1605.

82. Zeidler C, Kanz L, Hurkuck F, et al. In vivo effects of interleukin-6 on thrombopoiesis in healthy and irradiated primates. *Blood.* 1992;80:2740-2745.

83. van Gameren MM, Willemse PH, Mulder NH, et al. Effects of recombinant human interleukin-6 in cancer patients: a phase I-II study. *Blood.* 1994;84:1434-1441.

84. Debili N, Hegyi E, Navarro S, et al. In vitro effects of hematopoietic growth factors on the proliferation, endoreplication, and maturation of human megakaryocytes. *Blood.* 1991;77:2326-2338.

85. Bruno E, Briddell RA, Cooper RJ, Hoffman R. Effects of recombinant interleukin 11 on human megakaryocyte progenitor cells. *Exp Hematol.* 1991;19:378-381.

86. Cairo,MS, kirov II, Goldman S, et al. Recombinant human interleukin-11 enhances recovery following ICE chemotherapy in children with solid tumors or lymphoma: analysis of hematopoietic responses, cytokine induction, pharmacokinetics and stem cell mobilization (abstract). Proc ASCO 1998;17.

87. Tepler I, Elias L, Smith JW, et al. A randomized placebo-controlled trial of recombinant human interleukin- 11 in cancer patients with severe thrombocytopenia due to chemotherapy. *Blood.* 1996;87:3607-3614.

88. Isaacs C, Robert NJ, Bailey FA, et al. Randomized placebo-controlled study of recombinant human interleukin-11 to prevent chemotherapy-induced thrombocytopenia in patients with breast cancer receiving dose-intensive cyclophosphamide and doxorubicin. *J Clin Oncol.* 1997;15:3368-3377.

89. Bruno E, Briddell R, Hoffman R. Effect of recombinant and purified hematopoietic growth factors on human megakaryocyte colony formation. *Exp Hematol.* 1988;16:371-377.

90. McDonald TP, Cottrell MB, Clift RE, Cullen WC, Lin FK. High doses of recombinant erythropoietin stimulate platelet production in mice. *Exp Hematol* 1987;15:719-721.

91. McDonald TP. Thrombopoietin. Its biology, clinical aspects, and possibilities. *Am J Pediatr Hematol Oncol.* 1992;14:8-21.

92. Han ZC, Bellucci S, Tenza D, Caen JP. Negative regulation of human megakaryocytopoiesis by human platelet factor 4 and beta thromboglobulin: comparative analysis in bone marrow cultures from normal individuals and patients with essential thrombocythaemia and immune thrombocytopenic purpura. *Br J Haematol.* 1990;74:395-401.

93. Kuter DJ, Gminski DM, Rosenberg RD. Transforming growth factor beta inhibits megakaryocyte growth and endomitosis. *Blood.* 1992;79:619-626.

94. Gewirtz AM, Calabretta B, Rucinski B, Niewiarowski S, Xu WY. Inhibition of human megakaryocytopoiesis in vitro by platelet factor 4 (PF4) and a synthetic COOH-terminal PF4 peptide. *J Clin Invest.* 1989;83:1477-1486.

95. Griffin CG, Grant BW. Effects of recombinant interferons on human megakaryocyte growth. *Exp Hematol.* 1990;18:1013-1018.

96. Han ZC, Bellucci S, Wan HY, Caen JP. New insights into the regulation of megakaryocytopoiesis by haematopoietic and fibroblastic growth factors and transforming growth factor beta 1. *Br J Haematol.* 1992;81:1-5.

97. Moore MA, Metcalf D. Ontogeny of the haemopoietic system: yolk sac origin of in vivo and in vitro colony forming cells in the developing mouse embryo. *Br J Haematol.* 1970;18:279-296.

98. Fukuda T. Fetal hemopoiesis. II. Electron microscopic studies on human hepatic hemopoiesis. *Virchows Arch B Cell Pathol.* 1974;16:249-270.

99. Yoffey JM. The stem cell problem in the fetal and neonatal erythropoiesis. *Isr J Med Sci.* 1962;7:825.

100. Yoffey JM, Thomas DB. The development of bone marrow in the suman fetus. *J Anat.* 1964;98:463.

101. Migliaccio G, Migliaccio AR, Petti S, et al. Human embryonic hemopoiesis: kinetics of progenitors and precursors underlying the yolk sac–liver transition. *J Clin Invest.* 1986;78:51-60.

102. Bleyer WA, Hakami N, Shepard TH. The development of hemostasis in the human fetus and newborn infant. *J Pediatr.* 1971;79:838-853.

103. Emura I, Sekiya M, Ohnishi Y. Two types of immature megakaryocytic series in the human fetal liver. *Arch Histol Jpn.* 1983;46:103-114.

104. Enzan H, Takahashi H, Kawakami M, Yamashita S, Ohkita T, Yamamoto M. Light and electron microscopic observations of hepatic hematopoiesis of human fetuses. II. Megakaryocytopoiesis. *Acta Pathol Jpn.* 1980;30:937-954.

105. Daimon T, David H. An automatic image analysis of megakaryocytes in fetal liver and adult bone marrow. *Z Mikrosk Anat Forsch.* 1982;96:454-460.

106. Kelemen E. Small megakaryocytes in human embryonic liver. *Blooc Cells.* 1979;5:101-102.

107. Izumi T, Kawakami M, Enzan H, Ohkita T. The size of megakaryocytes in human fetal, infantile and adult hematopoiesis. *Hiroshima J Med Sci.* 1983;32:257-260.

108. Carbonell F, Calvo W, Fliedner TM. Cellular composition of human fetal bone marrow. Histologic study in methacrylate sections. *Acta Anat (Basel).* 1982;113:371-375.

109. Thomas DB, Yoffey JM. Human fetal heamatopoiesis I. The cellular composition of fetal blood. *Br J Haematol.* 1962;8:290.

110. Izumi T. Morphometric studies of megakaryocytes in human and rat fetal, infantile and adult hematopoiesis. I. Observations on human fetuses and blood dyscrasias. *Hiroshima J Med Sci.* 1987;36:25-30.

111. Graeve JLA, de Alarcon PA. Megakaryocytopoiesis in the human fetus. *Arch Dis Child.* 1989;64:481-484.

112. de Alarcon PA. Thrombopoiesis in the fetus and newborn. In Stockman JA, Pochedly C, eds. Developmental and Neonatal Hematology. New York: Raven Press, 1988;103.

113. Zucker-Franklin D, Yang JS, Grusky G. Characterization of glycoprotein IIb/IIIa-positive cells in human umbilical cord blood: their potential usefulness as megakaryocyte progenitors. *Blood.* 1992;79:347-355.

114. Thoma SJ, Lamping CP, Ziegler BL. Phenotype analysis of hematopoietic CD34+ cell populations derived from human umbilical cord blood using flow cytometry and cDNA-polymerase chain reaction. *Blood.* 1994;83:2103-2114.

115. Sell EJ, Corrigan JJ Jr. Platelet counts, fibrinogen concentrations, and factor V and factor VIII levels in healthy infants according to gestational age. *J Pediatr.* 1973;82:1028-1032.

116. Holmberg L, Gustavii B, Jonsson A. A prenatal study of fetal platelet count and size with application to fetus at risk for Wiskott-Aldrich syndrome. *J Pediatr.* 1983;102:773-776.

117. Hegyi E, Nakazawa M, Debili N, et al. Developmental changes in human megakaryocyte ploidy. *Exp Hematol.* 1991;19:87-94.

118. Vainchenker W, Guichard J, Breton-Gorius J. Growth of human megakaryocyte colonies in culture from fetal, neonatal, and adult peripheral blood cells: ultrastructural analysis. *Blood Cells.* 1979;5:25-42.

119. Zauli G, Valvassori L, Capitani S. Presence and characteristics of circulating megakaryocyte progenitor cells in human fetal blood. *Blood.* 1993;81:385-390.

120. Deutsch VR, Eldor A, Olson T, Barak V, Pick M, Nagler A. Stem cell factor (SCF) synergizes with megakaryocyte colony stimulating activity in post-irradiated aplastic plasma in stimulating human megakaryocytopoiesis. *Med Oncol.* 1996;13:31-42.

121. Clapp DW, Baley JE, Gerson SL. Gestational age-dependent changes in circulating hematopoietic stem cells in newborn infants. *J Lab Clin Med.* 1989;113:422-427.

122. Imai T, Koike K, Kubo T, et al. Interleukin-6 supports human megakaryocytic proliferation and differentiation in vitro. *Blood.* 1991;78:1969-1974.

123. Murray NA, Roberts IA. Circulating megakaryocytes and their progenitors (BFU-MK and CFU-MK) in term and pre-term neonates. *Br J Haematol.* 1995;89:41-46.

124. Warren MK, Guertin M, Rudzinski I, Seidman MM. A new culture and quantitation system for megakaryocyte growth using cord blood CD34+ cells and the GPIIb/IIIa marker. *Exp Hematol.* 1993;21:1473-1479.

125. Sola MC, Juul SE, Meng YG, et al. Thrombopoietin (Tpo) in the fetus and neonate: Tpo concentrations in preterm and term neonates, and organ distribution of Tpo and its receptor (*c-mpl*) during human fetal development. *Early Hum Dev.* 1999;53:239-250.

126. Murray NA, Watts TL, Roberts IA. Endogenous thrombopoietin levels and effect of recombinant human thrombopoietin on megakaryocyte precursors in term and preterm babies. *Pediatr Res.* 1998;43:148-151.

127. Watts TL, Murray NA, Roberts IA. Thrombopoietin has a primary role in the regulation of platelet production in preterm babies. *Pediatr Res.* 1999;46:28-32.

128. Walka MM, Sonntag J, Dudenhausen JW, Obladen M. Thrombopoietin concentration in umbilical cord blood of healthy term newborns is higher than in adult controls. *Biol Neonate.* 1999;75:54-58.

129. Albert TS, Meng YG, Simms P, Cohen RL, Phibbs RH. Thrombopoietin in the thrombocytopenic term and preterm newborn. *Pediatrics.* 2000;105:1286-1291.

130. Sola MC, Calhoun DA, Hutson AD, Christensen RD. Plasma thrombopoietin concentrations in thrombocytopenic and non-thrombocytopenic patients in a neonatal intensive care unit. *Br J Haematol.* 1999;104:90-92.

131. Ishiguro A, Nakahata T, Matsubara K, et al. Age-related changes in thrombopoietin in children: reference interval for serum thrombopoietin levels. *Br J Haematol.* 1999;106:884-888.

132. Nishihira H, Toyoda Y, Miyazaki H, Kigasawa H, Ohsaki E. Growth of macroscopic human megakaryocyte colonies from cord blood in culture with recombinant human thrombopoietin (*c-mpl* ligand) and the effects of gestational age on frequency of colonies. *Br J Haematol.* 1996;92:23-28.

133. Sola MC, Del Vecchio A, Rimsza LM. Evaluation and treatment of thrombocytopenia in the neonatal intensive care unit. *Clin Perinatol.* 2000;27:655-679.

134. Mwamtemi HH, Higuchi T, Sawai N, Hidaka E, Koike K. Quantitative and qualitative differences in thrombopoietin-dependent hematopoietic progenitor development between cord blood and bone marrow. *Transplantation.* 2000;69:1645-54.

135. Miyazaki R, Ogata H, Iguchi T, et al. Comparative analyses of megakaryocytes derived from cord blood and bone marrow. *Br J Haematol.* 2000;108:602-609.

136. Ryu KH, Chun S, Carbonierre S, et al. Apoptosis and megakaryocytic differentiation during ex vivo expansion of human cord blood CD34+ cells using thrombopoietin. *Br J Haematol.* 2001;113:470-478.

137. Tavassoli M. Megakaryocyte-platelet axis and the process of platelet formation and release. *Blood.* 1980;55:537-545.

138. Tong M, Seth P, Penington DG. Proplatelets and stress platelets. *Blood.* 1987;69:522-528.

139. Radley JM, Haller CJ. Fate of senescent megakaryocytes in the bone marrow. *Br J Haematol.* 1983;53:277-287.

140. Choi ES, Nichol JL, Hokom MM, Hornkohl AC, Hunt P. Platelets generated in vitro from proplatelet-displaying human megakaryocytes are functional. *Blood.* 1995;85:402-413.

141. Oelhafen H. Über Knochenmarkriesen Zellen in stromenden Blut. *Floia Haemtol.* 1914;18:171-181.

142. Kaufman RM, Airo R, Pollack S, Crosby WH. Circulating megakaryocytes and platelet release in the lung. *Blood.* 1965;26:720-731.

143. Sharnoff JG, Kim ES. Evaluation of pulmonary megakaryocytes. *J Pathol.* 1958;66:176-182.

144. Scott GB. Circulating megakaryocytes. *Histopathology.* 1982;6:467-475.

145. Woods MJ, Landon CR, Greaves M, Trowbridge EA. The placenta: a site of platelet production? *Platelets.* 1992;3:211-215.

146. Johnson CA, Human DG, Sacks RT, Mills AE. Circulating megakaryocytes and platelet production in children with congenital cardiac defects undergoing cardiac catheterisation. *S Afr Med J.* 1988;73:578-580.

147. Pedersen NT, Petersen S, Greulich L. Megakaryocytes in the foetal circulation and in cubital venous blood in the mother before and after delivery. *Scand J Haematol.* 1980;25:5-11.

148. Van den Hof MC, Nicolaides KH. Platelet count in normal, small, and anemic fetuses. *Am J Obstet Gynecol.* 1990;162:735-739.

149. Forestier F, Daffos F, Catherine N, Renard M, Andreux JP. Developmental hematopoiesis in normal human fetal blood. *Blood.* 1991;77:2360-2363.

150. Ablin AR, Kushner JH, Murphy A, Zippin C. Platelet enumeration in the neonatal period. *Pediatrics.* 1961;822-824.

151. Effiong CE, Usanga EA, Mellits ED. Platelet counts in healthy full-term nigerian neonates. *Trop Geogr Med.* 1976;28:323-328.

152. Appleyard WJ, Brinton A. Venous platelet counts in low birth weight infants. *Biol Neonate.* 1971;17:30-34.

153. Andrew M, Castle V, Saigal S, Carter C, Kelton JG. Clinical impact of neonatal thrombocytopenia. *J Pediatr.* 1987;110:457-464.

154. Castle V, Andrew M, Kelton J, Giron D, Johnston M, Carter C. Frequency and mechanism of neonatal thrombocytopenia. *J Pediatr.* 1986;108:749-755.

155. Cohen DL, Baglin TP. Assessment and management of immune thrombocytopenia in pregnancy and in neonates. *Arch Dis Child.* 1995;72:F71-F76.

156. Hohlfeld P, Forestier F, Kaplan C, Tissot JD, Daffos F. Fetal thrombocytopenia: a retrospective survey of 5,194 fetal blood samplings. *Blood.* 1994;84:1851-1856.

157. McCrae KR, Samuels P, Schreiber AD. Pregnancy-associated thrombocytopenia: pathogenesis and management. *Blood.* 1992;80:2697-2714.

158. Burrows RF, Kelton JG. Low fetal risks in pregnancies associated with idiopathic thrombocytopenic purpura. *Am J Obstet Gynecol.* 1990;163:1147-1150.

159. Kaplan C, Daffos F, Forestier F, et al. Fetal platelet counts in thrombocytopenic pregnancy. *Lancet.* 1990;336:979–982.
160. Samuels P, Bussel JB, Braitman LE, et al. Estimation of the risk of thrombocytopenia in the offspring of pregnant women with presumed immune thrombocytopenic purpura. *N Engl J Med.* 1990;323:229–235.
161. Scott JR, Rote NS, Cruikshank DP. Antiplatelet antibodies and platelet counts in pregnancies complicated by autoimmune thrombocytopenic purpura. *Am J Obstet Gynecol.* 1983;145:932–939.
162. Moise KJ Jr, Carpenter RJ Jr, Cotton DB, Wasserstrum N, Kirshon B, Cano L. Percutaneous umbilical cord blood sampling in the evaluation of fetal platelet counts in pregnant patients with autoimmune thrombocytopenia purpura. *Obstet Gynecol.* 1988;72:346–350.
163. Kleckner HB, Giles HR, Corrigan JJ Jr. The association of maternal and neonatal thrombocytopenia in high-risk pregnancies. *Am J Obstet Gynecol.* 1977;128:235–238.
164. Brazy JE, Grimm JK, Little VA. Neonatal manifestations of severe maternal hypertension occurring before the thirty-sixth week of pregnancy. *J Pediatr.* 1982;100:265–271.
165. Burrows RF, Kelton JG. Incidentally detected thrombocytopenia in healthy mothers and their infants. *N Engl J Med.* 1988;319:142–145.
166. Aster RH. "Gestational" thrombocytopenia: a plea for conservative management. *N Engl J Med.* 1990;323:264–266.
167. Naidu S. Central nervous system lesions in neonatal isoimmune thrombocytopenia. *Arch Neurol.* 1983;40:552–554.
168. dem Borne AE, van Leeuwen EF, von Riesz LE, van Boxtel CJ, Engelfriet CP. Neonatal alloimmune thrombocytopenia: detection and characterization of the responsible antibodies by the platelet immunofluorescence test. *Blood.* 1981;57:649–656.
169. Bussel JB. Alloimmune thrombocytopenia in the fetus and newborn. *Semin Thromb Hemost.* 2001;27:245–252.
170. McFarland JG, Aster RH, Bussel JB, Gianopoulos JG, Derbes RS, Newman PJ. Prenatal diagnosis of neonatal alloimmune thrombocytopenia using allele-specific oligonucleotide probes. *Blood.* 1991;78:2276–2282.
171. Flug F, Karpatkin M, Karpatkin S. Should all pregnant women be tested for their platelet PLA (Zw, HPA-1) phenotype? *Br J Haematol.* 1994;86:1–5.
172. McIntosh S, O'Brien RT, Schwartz AD, Pearson HA. Neonatal isoimmune purpura: response to platelet infusions. *J Pediatr.* 1973;82:1020–1027.
173. Blanchette V, Andrew M, Perlman M, Ling E, Ballin A. Neonatal autoimmune thrombocytopenia: role of high-dose intravenous immunoglobulin G therapy. *Blut.* 1989;59:139–144.
174. Bussel JB, Berkowitz RL, McFarland JG, Lynch L, Chitkara U. Antenatal treatment of neonatal alloimmune thrombocytopenia. *N Engl J Med.* 1988;319:1374–1378.
175. Lynch L, Bussel JB, McFarland JG, Chitkara U, Berkowitz RL. Antenatal treatment of alloimmune thrombocytopenia. *Obstet Gynecol.* 1992;80:67–71.
176. Corrigan JJ Jr. Thrombocytopenia: a laboratory sign of septicemia in infants and children. *J Pediatr.* 1974;85:219–221.
177. Modanlou HD, Ortiz OB. Thrombocytopenia in neonatal infection. *Clin Pediatr (Phila).* 1981;20:402–407.
178. Tate DY, Carlton GT, Johnson D, et al. Immune thrombocytopenia in severe neonatal infections. *J Pediatr.* 1981;98:449–453.
179. Kelton JG, Neame PB, Gauldie J, Hirsh J. Elevated platelet-associated IgG in the thrombocytopenia of septicemia. *N Engl J Med.* 1979;300:760–764.
180. Corrigan JJ, Ray WL, May N. Changes in the blood coagulation system associated with septicemia. *N Engl J Med.* 1968;279:841.
181. Bonnet-Gajdos M, Navarro J, Roy C. Transitory insufficiency of megacaryocytes and erythroblasts during bacterial infections in babies. *Nouv Rev Fr Hematol.* 1974;14:671–675.
182. Cooper LZ, Green RH, Krugman S, Giles JP, Mirick GS. Neonatal thrombocytopenic purpura and other manifestations of rubella contracted in utero. *Am J Dis Child.* 1965;110:416–427.
183. Scott S, Reimers HJ, Chernesky MA, et al. Effect of viruses on platelet aggregation and platelet survival in rabbits. *Blood.* 1978;52:47–55.
184. Chesney PJ, Shahidi NT. Acute viral-induced thrombocytopenia: a review of human disease, animal models and in vitro studies. *In* Acquired Bleeding Disorders in Children. New York: Masson Publishing, 1981;65.
185. Jamsjaw HB. Congenital and acquired cytomegalovirus infection. *Pediatr Clin North Am.* 1966;13:279–293.
186. Fiala M, Kattlove H. Letter: Cytomegalovirus mononucleosis with severe thrombocytopenia. *Ann Intern Med.* 1973;79:450–451.
187. Harris AI, Meyer RJ, Brody EA. Letter: Cytomegalovirus-induced thrombocytopenia and hemolysis in an adult. *Ann Intern Med.* 1975;83:670–671.
188. Osborn JE, Shahidi NT. Thrombocytopenia in murine cytomegalovirus infection. *J Lab Clin Med.* 1973;81:53–63.
189. Chesney PJ, Taher A, Gilbert EM, Shahidi NT. Intranuclear inclusions in megakaryocytes in congenital cytomegalovirus infection. *J Pediatr.* 1978;92:957–958.

190. Hohlfeld P, Vial Y, Maillard-Brignon C, Vaudaux B, Fawer CL. Cytomegalovirus fetal infection: prenatal diagnosis. *Obstet Gynecol.* 1991;78:615–618.
191. Daffos F, Forestier F, Capella-Pavlovsky M, et al. Prenatal management of 746 pregnancies at risk for congenital toxoplasmosis. *N Engl J Med.* 1988;318:271–275.
192. Philip AG, Tito AM. Increased nucleated red blood cell counts in small for gestational age infants with very low birth weight. *Am J Dis Child.* 1989;143:164–169.
193. Cox WL, Daffos F, Forestier F, et al. Physiology and management of intrauterine growth retardation: a biologic approach with fetal blood sampling. *Am J Obstet Gynecol.* 1988;159:36–41.
194. Wolff JA, Bertucio M. Sex-linked genetic syndrome in a negro family manifested by thrombocytopenia, eczema, bloody diarrhea, recurrent infections, anemia and epistaxis. *Am J Dis Child.* 1957;93:74.
195. Grottum KA, Hovig T, Holmsen H, Abrahamsen AF, Jeremic M, Seip M. Wiskott-Aldrich syndrome: qualitative platelet defects and short platelet survival. *Br J Haematol.* 1969;17:373–388.
196. Epstein CJ, Sahud MA, Piel CF, et al. Hereditary macrothrombocytopathia, nephritis and deafness. *Am J Med.* 1972;52:299–310.
197. Parsa KP, Lee DB, Zamboni L, Glassock RJ. Hereditary nephritis, deafness and abnormal thrombopoiesis: study of a new kindred. *Am J Med.* 1976;60:665–672.
198. Godwin HA, Ginsburg AD. May-Hegglin anomaly: a defect in megakaryocyte fragmentation? *Br J Haematol.* 1974;29:117–128.
199. Burns ER. Platelet studies in the pathogenesis of thrombocytopenia in May-Hegglin anomaly. *Am J Pediatr Hematol Oncol.* 1991;13:431–436.
200. Lusher JM, Schneider J, Mizukami I, Evans RK. The May-Hegglin anomaly: platelet function, ultrastructure and chromosome studies. *Blood.* 1968;32:950–961.
201. Rosenberg T, Arad E, Pillar T, Gidron E. May-Hegglin anomaly. *Isr J Med Sci.* 1971;7:1073–1078.
202. Greinacher A, Mueller-Eckhardt C. Hereditary types of thrombocytopenia with giant platelets and inclusion bodies in the leukocytes. *Blut.* 1990;60:53–60.
203. Bernard J, Soulier JP. Sur une nouvelle variété de dystrophie thrombocytaire hemorragipare congenitale. *Sem Hop Paris.* 1948;24:3217–3223.
204. Reccuglia G. Gray platelet syndrome: a variety of qualitative platelet disorders. *Am J Med.* 1971;51:818–828.
205. Lacombe M, d'Angelo G. Etude sur une thrombopathie familiale. *Nouv Rev Fr.* 1963;3:611–614.
206. Savoia A, Del Vecchio M, Totaro A, et al. An autosomal dominant thrombocytopenia gene maps to chromosomal region 10p. *Am J Hum Genet.* 1999;65:1401–1405.
207. Drachman JG, Jarvik GP, Mehaffey MG. Autosomal dominant thrombocytopenia: incomplete megakaryocyte differentiation and linkage to human chromosome 10. *Blood.* 2000;96:118–125.
208. van den OS, Bruin M, Folman CC, Bussel J, de Haas M, dem Borne AE. Three parameters, plasma thrombopoietin levels, plasma glycocalicin levels and megakaryocyte culture, distinguish between different causes of congenital thrombocytopenia. *Br J Haematol.* 2002;117:390–398.
209. Day HJ, Holmsen H. Platelet adenine nucleotide "storage pool deficiency" in thrombocytopenic absent radii syndrome. *JAMA.* 1972;221:1053–1054.
210. Hedberg VA, Lipton JM. Thrombocytopenia with absent radii: a review of 100 cases. *Am J Pediatr Hematol Oncol.* 1988;10:51–64.
211. Hall JG, Levin J, Kuhn JP, Ottenheimer EJ, van Berkum KA, McKusick VA. Thrombocytopenia with absent radius (TAR). *Medicine (Baltimore).* 1969;48:411–439.
212. Homans AC, Cohen JL, Mazur EM. Defective megakaryocytopoiesis in the syndrome of thrombocytopenia with absent radii. *Br J Haematol.* 1988;70:205–210.
213. de Alarcon PA, Graeve JA, Levine RF, McDonald TP, Beal DW. Thrombocytopenia and absent radii syndrome: defective megakaryocytopoiesis-thrombocytopoiesis. *Am J Pediatr Hematol Oncol.* 1991;13:77–83.
214. Ballmaier M, Schulze H, Strauss G, et al. Thrombopoietin in patients with congenital thrombocytopenia and absent radii: elevated serum levels, normal receptor expression, but defective reactivity to thrombopoietin. *Blood.* 1997;90:612–619.
215. Rabinowitz JG, Moseley JE, Mitty HA, Hirschhorn K. Trisomy 18, esophageal atresia, anomalies of the radius, and congenital hypoplastic thrombocytopenia. *Radiology.* 1967;89:488–491.
216. Markenson AL, Hilgartner MW, Miller DR. Transient thrombocytopenia in 18-trisomy (letter). *J Pediatr.* 1975;87:834–835.
217. Freedman MH, Estrov Z. Congenital amegakaryocytic thrombocytopenia: an intrinsic hematopoietic stem cell defect. *Am J Pediatr Hematol Oncol.* 1990;12:225–230.
218. van den OS, Bruin M, Folman CC, et al. Mutations in the thrombopoietin receptor, Mpl, in children with congenital amegakaryocytic thrombocytopenia. *Br J Haematol.* 2000;110:441–448.

XIX

Hemostasis

148

Paul Monagle* and J. Nathan Hagstrom

Developmental Hemostasis

Hemostasis is a dynamic, evolving process that is age dependent and begins *in utero*. Although evolving, the hemostatic system in healthy fetuses and infants must be considered physiologic. Because the hemostatic system is dynamic, multiple reference ranges reflecting the gestational age and postnatal age of infants are necessary.[1] The evaluation of newborn infants for hemorrhagic or thrombotic complications presents unique problems that are not encountered in older children and adults. For example, physiologic levels of many coagulation proteins in neonates are low, and this makes the diagnoses of some inherited and acquired hemostatic problems difficult to establish. An understanding of developmental hemostasis in the broadest sense optimizes the prevention, diagnoses, and treatment of hemostatic problems during childhood and undoubtedly provides new insights into the pathophysiology of hemorrhagic and thrombotic complications for all ages.

THE COAGULATION SYSTEM

Our understanding of hemostatic physiology in neonates and infants is deficient when compared with our knowledge of this subject in adults. The reasons for this deficit are several: in neonates and infants, multiple reference ranges are required because these patients have rapidly evolving systems;[1-4] blood sampling in the young is technically difficult; only small blood samples can be obtained; microtechniques are required;[5] and greater variability in plasma concentrations of coagulation proteins necessitates the use of large patient numbers to establish normative data.

Coagulation proteins are independently synthesized by the fetus and do not cross the placenta.[6-18] By 10 weeks' gestational age, plasma concentrations of most coagulation proteins are measurable, and they continue to increase gradually in parallel with the gestational age. Samples obtained during fetoscopy provide the best assessment of normal values for fetuses, and by extrapolation, very premature infants (Tables 148-1 and 148-2).[19] True reference ranges for extremely premature infants are not available because the majority of these infants have postnatal complications. Tables 148-3 to 148-6[1-3] provide reference ranges for coagulation proteins, inhibitors of coagulation, and components of the fibrinolytic system for premature (30 to 36 weeks' gestational age) and full-term infants on day 1 of life, as well as longitudinally over the first 6 months of life. Tables 148-7 to 148-9[20] provide similar data for older children.

The variable results for coagulation screening tests reflect the use of cord blood samples rather than samples from infants or differing ethnic populations, or the use of different reagents.[21,22] Variation in prothrombin time (PT) results can be minimized by reporting the PT as an *international normalized ratio* (INR).[23] The INR is calculated as the patient PT/control PT to the power of the *international sensitivity index* (ISI). The ISI corrects for the large variation in sensitivity of thromboplastin reagents to plasma concentrations of coagulation proteins. Unfortunately, there is no such standardization for activated partial thromboplastin times (APTT). Reference ranges for APTTs will differ with each different reagent and analyzer system, often significantly. Table 148-10 shows the variability in APTT reference ranges using the same patient samples, but with different APTT reagents.[24] The thrombin-clotting time performed in the absence of calcium is prolonged because of the presence of the "fetal" form of fibrinogen at birth.[1-3] For Tables 148-3 and 148-4, the thrombin-clotting time was measured in the presence of calcium, so that abnormal values secondary to the presence of heparin, as well as low levels of fibrinogen, could be detected.

Coagulant Proteins

The vitamin K–dependent factors are the most extensively studied group of factors in infants, reflecting the clinical significance of hemorrhagic disease of the newborn (HDN).[25-27] Physiologically low levels of factors (F)II, FVII, FIX, and FX in Tables 148-3 and 148-4 are similar to those in other reports[1-3, 28-38] and were measured in infants who received vitamin K prophylaxis at birth. The levels of the VK-dependent factors and the contact factors (FXI, FXII, prekallikrein, and high molecular weight kininogen) gradually increase to values approaching adult levels by 6 months of life.[1-3] The prolonged activated partial thromboplastin time (APTT) during the first months of life is in large part due to the low levels of the contact factors.[39]

Plasma levels of fibrinogen, FV, FVIII, and FXIII, and vWf are not decreased at birth (Tables 148-3 and 148-4). Fibrinogen levels continue to increase after birth.[40] Plasma levels of FVIII are skewed toward the high measurements, necessitating an adjustment of the lower limit of normal (Tables 148-3 and 148-4). Levels of both vWf and high molecular weight multimers are increased at birth and for the first 3 months of life.[1]

Potential mechanisms for the developmental differences in plasma protein levels include reduced production of coagulation factors. Messenger ribonucleic acid (mRNA) levels have been measured for FVII, FVIII, FIX, and FX, fibrinogen, AT, and protein C in hepatocytes from 5- to 10-week-old human embryos and fetuses and in those from adults. Embryonic-fetal transcripts and adult mRNAs are similar in size; and the nucleotide sequences of mRNA for factors IX and X were identical.[41, 42] However, the expression of mRNA was variable, with adult values existing for some coagulation proteins but decreased expression for others.

* Dr. Monagle is supported by a research fellowship from the Murdoch Children's Research Institute.

TABLE 148-1

Coagulation Screening Tests and Coagulation Factor Levels in Fetuses, Full-Term Infants, and Adults

Parameter	Fetuses (Weeks of Gestation)			Neonates	Adults
	19–23 (n=20)	*24–29 (n=22)*	*30–38 (n=22)*	*(n=60)*	*(n=40)*
PT (sec)	32.5 (19–45)	32.2 (19–44)†	22.6 (16–30)†	16.7 (12.0–23.5)*	13.5 (11.4–14.0)
PT (INR)	6.4 (1.7–11.1)	6.2 (2.1–10.6)†	3.0 (1.5–5.0)*	1.7 (0.9–2.7)*	1.1 (0.8–1.2)
APTT (sec)	168.8 (83–250)	154.0 (87–210)†	104.8 (76–128)†	44.3 (35–52)*	33.0 (25–39)
TCT (sec)	34.2 (24–44)*	26.2 (24–28)	21.4 (17.0–23.3)	20.4 (15.2–25.0)†	14.0 (12–16)
Factor I (g/l) von Clauss	0.85 (0.57–1.50)	1.12 (0.65–1.65)	1.35 (1.25–1.65)	1.68 (0.95–2.45)†	3.0 (1.78–4.50)
I Ag (g/l)	1.08 (0.75–1.50)	1.93 (1.56–2.40)	1.94 (1.30–2.40)	2.65 (1.68–3.60)†	3.5 (2.50–5.20)
IIc (%)	16.9 (10–24)	19.9 (11–30)*	27.9 (15–50)†	43.5 (27–64)†	98.7 (70–125)
VIIc (%)	27.4 (17–37)	33.8 (18–48)*	45.9 (31–62)	52.5 (28–78)†	101.3 (68–130)
IXc (%)	10.1 (6–14)	9.9 (5–15)	12.3 (5–24)†	31.8 (15–50)†	104.8 (70–142)
Xc (%)	20.5 (14–29)	24.9 (16–35)	28.0 (16–36)†	39.6 (21–65)†	99.2 (75–125)
Vc (%)	32.1 (21–44)	36.8 (25–50)	48.9 (23–70)†	89.9 (50–140)	99.8 (65–140)
VIIIc (%)	34.5 (18–50)	35.5 (20–52)	50.1 (27–78)†	94.3 (38–150)	101.8 (55–170)
XIc (%)	13.2 (8–19)	12.1 (6–22)	14.8 (6–26)†	37.2 (13–62)†	100.2 (70–135)
XIIc (%)	14.9 (6–25)	22.7 (6–40)	25.8 (11–50)†	69.8 (25–105)†	101.4 (65–144)
PK (%)	12.8 (8–19)	15.4 (8–26)	18.1 (8–28)†	35.4 (21–53)†	99.8 (65–135)
HMWK (%)	15.4 (10–22)	19.3 (10–26)	23.6 (12–34)†	38.9 (28–53)†	98.8 (68–135)

Values are the mean, followed in parentheses by the lower and upper boundaries, including 95% of the population.
*p <.05; †p <.01.
Ag = antigen; APTT = activated partial thromboplastin time; HMWK = high molecular weight kininogen; INR = international normalized ratio; n = number;
PK = prekallikrein; PT = prothrombin time; TCT = thrombin-clotting time.
From Reverdiau-Moalic P, et al: Blood *88*:900, 1996.

TABLE 148-2

Blood Coagulation Inhibitor Levels in Fetuses, Full-Term Infants, and Adults

Parameter	Fetuses (Weeks of Gestation)			Neonates	Adults
	19–23 (n=20)‡	*24–29 (n=22)*	*30–38 (n=22)*	*(n=60)*	*(n=40)*
AT (%)	20.2 (12–31)*	30.0 (20–39)	37.1 (24–55)†	59.4 (42–80)†	99.8 (65–130)
HCII (%)	10.3 (6–16)	12.9 (5.5–20)	21.1 (11–33)†	52.1 (19–99)†	101.4 (70–128)
TFPI (%)‡	21.0 (16.0–29.2)	20.6 (13.4–33.2)	20.7 (10.4–31.5)†	38.1 (22.7–55.8)†	73.0 (50.9–90.1)
PC Ag (%)	9.5 (6–14)	12.1 (8–16)	15.9 (8–30)†	32.5 (21–47)†	100.8 (68–125)
PC Act (%)	9.6 (7–13)	10.4 (8–13)	14.1 (8–18)*	28.2 (14–42)†	98.8 (68–125)
Total PS (%)	15.1 (11–21)	17.4 (14–25)	21.0 (15–30)†	38.5 (22–55)†	99.6 (72–118)
Free PS (%)	21.7 (13–32)	27.9 (19–40)	27.0 (18–40)†	49.3 (33–67)†	98.7 (72–128)
Ratio of Free PS: Total PS	0.82 (0.75–0.92)	0.83 (0.76–0.95)	0.79 (0.70–0.89)†	0.64 (0.59–0.98)†	0.41 (0.38–0.43)
C4b-BP (%)	1.8 (0–6)	6.1 (0–12.5)	9.3 (5–14)	18.6 (3–40)†	100.3 (70–124)

Values are the mean, followed in parentheses by the lower and upper boundaries, including 95% of the population.
* p<.05.
† p<.01.
‡ Twenty samples were assayed for each group but only 10 for 19–23-week-old fetuses.
AT = antithrombin; HCII = heparin cofactor II; TFPI = tissue factor pathway inhibitor; PC = protein C; PS = protein S; Ag = antigen; Act = activity.
From Reverdiau-Moalic P, et al: Blood *88*:900, 1996.

Similar concentrations of prothrombin mRNA were found in the livers of newborn and adult rabbits;[43] another study reported lower prothrombin mRNA concentrations in sheep. In addition, increased clearance of plasma proteins may be significant. Fibrinogen, whether of fetal or adult origin, is cleared more rapidly in newborn lambs than it is in sheep.[44] Similarly, clearance of fibrinogen is accelerated in premature infants with or without RDS.[45] An increased basal metabolic rate in the young probably contributes to the accelerated clearance of proteins.[46]

Differences in function and structure of fetal versus adult fibrinogen have been recognized for a number of years.[47] These differences have been primarily attributed to an increased sialic acid content of the fetal fibrinogen.[48]

Regulation of Thrombin

Thrombin regulation is both delayed and decreased in newborn plasma compared with adult plasma, and similar to plasmas from

adults receiving therapeutic doses of warfarin or heparin.[49] Thrombin generation in newborn plasma is further decreased in the presence of endothelial cell surfaces, but not to the same extent as adult plasma.[50] The amount of thrombin generated is directly proportional to the prothrombin concentration,[51] whereas the rate of thrombin generation reflects the concentration of other procoagulants.

Thrombin is directly inhibited by antithrombin (AT), heparin cofactor II (HCII), and α_2-macroglobulin (α_2M). In addition, a circulating physiologic anticoagulant in cord blood has properties similar to those of dermatan sulfate.[52] The fetal proteoglycan is present in plasma in concentrations of 0.29 µg/mL, has a molecular weight of 150,000 kd, and catalyzes thrombin inhibition by means of the natural inhibitor HCII. The fetal anticoagulant also is present in plasmas from pregnant women and is produced by the placenta.[53] The length of time that the fetal anticoagulant circulates in neonates is not known. Alpha$_2$-macroglobulin is a more important inhibitor of thrombin in plasmas from neonates than it

Text continued on page 1442

TABLE 148-3
Reference Values for Coagulation Tests in Healthy Premature Infants (30–36 Weeks' Gestation) During the First 6 Months of Life

	Day 1		Day 5		Day 30		Day 90		Day 180		Adults	
	M	B	M	B	M	B	M	B	M	B	M	B
PT (sec)	13.0 (10.6–16.2)*		12.5 (10.0–15.3)*		11.8 (10.0–13.6)*		12.3 (10.0–14.6)		12.5 (10.0–15.0)*		12.4 (10.8–13.9)	
INR	1.0 (0.61–1.70)		0.91 (0.53–1.48)		0.79 (0.53–1.11)		0.88 (0.53–1.32)		0.91 (0.53–1.48)		0.89 (0.64–1.17)	
APTT (sec)	53.6 (27.5–79.4)†		50.5 (26.9–74.1)		44.7 (26.9–62.5)		39.5 (28.3–50.7)		37.5 (27.2–53.3)		33.5 (26.6–40.3)	
TCT (sec)	24.8 (19.2–30.4)		24.1 (18.8–29.4)*		24.4 (18.8–29.9)		25.1 (19.4–30.8)		25.2 (18.9–31.5)		25.0 (19.7–30.3)	
Fibrinogen (g/l)	2.43 (1.50–3.73)*†		2.80 (1.60–4.18)*†		2.54 (1.50–4.14)		2.46 (1.50–3.52)		2.28 (1.50–3.60)		2.78 (1.56–4.00)	
II (U/ml)	0.45 (0.20–0.77)		0.57 (0.29–0.85)†		0.57 (0.36–0.95)		0.68 (0.30–1.06)		0.87 (0.51–1.23)		1.08 (0.70–1.46)	
V (U/ml)	0.88 (0.41–1.44)*†		1.00 (0.46–1.54)*		1.02 (0.48–1.56)*		0.99 (0.59–1.39)		1.02 (0.58–1.46)*		1.06 (0.62–1.50)	
VII (U/ml)	0.67 (0.21–1.13)		0.84 (0.30–1.38)		0.83 (0.21–1.45)		0.87 (0.31–1.43)		0.99 (0.47–1.51)*		1.05 (0.67–1.43)	
VIII (U/ml)	1.11 (0.50–2.13)		1.15 (0.53–2.05)*†		1.11 (0.50–1.99)		1.06 (0.58–1.88)*†		0.99 (0.50–1.87)*†		0.99 (0.50–1.49)	
vWF (U/ml)	1.36 (0.78–2.10)		1.33 (0.72–2.19)		1.36 (0.66–2.16)		1.12 (0.75–1.84)*†		0.98 (0.54–1.58)*		0.92 (0.50–1.58)*	
IX (U/ml)	0.35 (0.19–0.65)†		0.42 (0.14–0.74)†		0.44 (0.13–0.80)		0.59 (0.25–0.93)		0.81 (0.50–1.20)		1.09 (0.55–1.63)	
X (U/ml)	0.41 (0.11–0.71)		0.51 (0.19–0.83)		0.56 (0.20–0.92)		0.67 (0.35–0.99)		0.77 (0.35–1.19)		1.06 (0.70–1.52)	
XI (U/ml)	0.30 (0.08–0.52)†		0.41 (0.13–0.69)†		0.43 (0.15–0.71)†		0.59 (0.25–0.93)*		0.78 (0.46–1.10)		0.97 (0.67–1.27)	
XII (U/ml)	0.38 (0.10–0.66)†		0.39 (0.09–0.69)†		0.43 (0.11–0.75)		0.61 (0.15–1.07)		0.82 (0.22–1.42)		1.08 (0.52–1.64)	
PK (U/ml)	0.33 (0.09–0.57)		0.45 (0.25–0.75)		0.59 (0.31–0.87)		0.79 (0.37–1.21)		0.78 (0.40–1.16)		1.12 (0.62–1.62)	
HK (U/ml)	0.49 (0.09–0.89)		0.62 (0.24–1.00)†		0.64 (0.16–1.12)†		0.78 (0.32–1.24)		0.83 (0.41–1.25)*		0.92 (0.50–1.36)	
XIIIa (U/ml)	0.70 (0.32–1.08)		1.01 (0.57–1.45)*		0.99 (0.51–1.47)*		1.13 (0.71–1.55)*		1.13 (0.65–1.61)*		1.05 (0.55–1.55)	
XIIIb (U/ml)	0.81 (0.35–1.27)		1.10 (0.68–1.58)*		1.07 (0.57–1.57)*		1.21 (0.75–1.67)		1.15 (0.67–1.63)		0.97 (0.57–1.37)	

All factors except fibrinogen are expressed as units per milliliter (U/ml) in which pooled plasma contains 1.0 U/ml. All values are given as a mean (M) followed by the lower and upper boundaries encompassing 95% of the population (B). Between 40 and 96 samples were assayed for each value for the neonate. Some measurements were skewed due to a disproportionate number cf high values. The lower limit which excludes the lower 2.5% of the population, has been given (B).

* $p < .05$; † $p < .01$.

PT = prothrombin time; INR = international normalized ratio; APTT, activated partial thromboplastin time; TCT = thrombin-clotting time; vWF = von Willebrand factor; PK = prekallikrein; HG = high molecular weight kininogen.

From Andrew M, et al: Blood 72:1651, 1988.

TABLE 148–4

Reference Values for Coagulation Tests in Healthy Full-Term Infants During the First 6 Months of Life

	Day 1		Day 5		Day 30		Day 90		Day 180		Adults	
	M	B	M	B	M	B	M	B	M	B	M	B
PT (sec)	13.0 (10.1–15.9)*		12.4 (10.0–15.3)*		11.8 (10.0–14.3)*		11.9 (10.0–14.2)*		12.3 (10.7–13.9)*		12.4 (10.8–13.9)	
INR	1.00 (0.53–1.62)		0.89 (0.53–1.48)		0.79 (0.53–1.26)		0.81 (0.53–1.26)		0.88 (0.61–1.17)		0.89 (0.64–1.17)	
APTT (sec)	42.9 (31.3–54.5)		42.6 (25.4–59.8)		40.4 (32.0–55.2)		37.1 (29.0–50.1)*		35.5 (28.1–42.9)*		33.5 (26.6–40.3)	
TCT (sec)	23.5 (19.0–28.3)*		23.1 (18.0–29.2)		24.3 (19.4–29.2)*		25.1 (20.5–29.7)*		25.5 (19.8–31.2)*		25.0 (19.7–30.3)	
Fibrinogen (g/l)	2.83 (1.67–3.99)*		3.12 (1.62–4.62)*		2.70 (1.62–3.78)*		2.43 (1.50–3.79)*		2.51 (1.50–3.87)*		2.78 (1.56–4.00)	
II (U/ml)	0.48 (0.26–0.70)		0.63 (0.33–0.93)		0.68 (0.34–1.02)		0.75 (0.45–1.05)		0.88 (0.60–1.16)		1.08 (0.70–1.46)	
V (U/ml)	0.72 (0.34–1.08)		0.95 (0.45–1.45)		0.98 (0.62–1.34)		0.90 (0.48–1.32)		0.91 (0.55–1.27)		1.06 (0.62–1.50)	
VII (U/ml)	0.66 (0.28–1.04)		0.89 (0.35–1.43)		0.90 (0.42–1.38)		0.91 (0.39–1.43)		0.87 (0.47–1.27)		1.05 (0.67–1.43)	
VIII (U/ml)	1.00 (0.50–1.78)*		0.88 (0.50–1.54)*		0.91 (0.50–1.57)*		0.79 (0.50–1.25)*		0.73 (0.50–1.09)		0.99 (0.50–1.49)	
vWF (U/ml)	1.53 (0.50–2.87)		1.40 (0.50–2.54)		1.28 (0.50–2.46)		1.18 (0.50–2.06)		1.07 (0.50–1.97)		0.92 (0.50–1.58)	
IX (U/ml)	0.53 (0.15–0.91)		0.53 (0.15–0.91)		0.51 (0.21–0.81)		0.67 (0.21–1.13)		0.86 (0.36–1.36)		1.09 (0.55–1.63)	
X (U/ml)	0.40 (0.12–0.68)		0.49 (0.19–0.79)		0.59 (0.31–0.87)		0.71 (0.35–1.07)		0.78 (0.38–1.18)		1.06 (0.70–1.52)	
XI (U/ml)	0.38 (0.10–0.66)		0.55 (0.23–0.87)		0.53 (0.27–0.79)		0.69 (0.41–0.97)		0.86 (0.49–1.34)		0.97 (0.67–1.27)	
XII (U/ml)	0.53 (0.13–0.93)		0.47 (0.11–0.83)		0.49 (0.17–0.81)		0.67 (0.25–1.09)		0.77 (0.39–1.15)		1.08 (0.52–1.64)	
PK (U/ml)	0.37 (0.18–0.69)		0.48 (0.20–0.76)		0.57 (0.23–0.91)		0.73 (0.41–1.05)		0.86 (0.56–1.16)		1.12 (0.62–1.62)	
HMWK (U/ml)	0.54 (0.06–1.02)		0.74 (0.16–1.32)		0.77 (0.33–1.21)		0.82 (0.30–1.46)*		0.82 (0.36–1.28)*		0.92 (0.50–1.36)	
XIII$_a$ (U/ml)	0.79 (0.27–1.31)		0.94 (0.44–1.44)*		0.93 (0.39–1.47)*		1.04 (0.36–1.72)*		1.04 (0.46–1.62)*		1.05 (0.55–1.55)	
XIII$_b$ (U/ml)	0.76 (0.30–1.22)		1.06 (0.32–1.80)		1.11 (0.39–1.73)*		1.16 (0.48–1.84)*		1.10 (0.50–1.70)*		0.97 (0.57–1.37)	

All factors except fibrinogen are expressed as units per milliliter (U/ml) where pooled plasma contains 1.0 U/ml. All values are expressed as mean (M) followed by the lower and upper boundaries encompassing 95% of the population (B). Between 40 and 77 samples were assayed for each value for the neonate. Some measurements were skewed due to a disproportionate number of high values. The lower limit, which excludes the lower 2.5% of the population, has been given.

* Values that are indistinguishable from those of the adult.

Abbreviations given in Table 148–3.

From Andrew M, et al: Blood 70:165, 1987.

TABLE 148-5

Reference Values for the Inhibitors of Coagulation in Healthy Full-Term Infants During the First 6 Months of Life

	Day 1		Day 5		Day 30		Day 90		Day 180		Adults	
	M	B	M	B	M	B	M	B	M	B	M	B
AT (U/ml)	0.63 (0.39-0.87)†		0.67 (0.41-0.93)		0.78 (0.48-1.08)		0.97 (0.73-1.21)*		1.04 (0.84-1.24)*		1.05 (0.79-1.31)	
₂M (U/ml)	1.39 (0.95-1.83)		1.48 (0.98-1.98)		1.50 (1.06-1.94)		1.76 (1.26-2.26)		1.91 (1.49-2.33)		0.86 (0.52-1.20)	
C₁E-INH (U/ml)	0.72 (0.36-1.08)		0.90 (0.60-1.20)*		0.89 (0.47-1.31)		1.15 (0.71-1.59)		1.41 (0.89-1.93)		1.01 (0.71-1.31)	
₁AT (U/ml)	0.93 (0.49-1.37)*		0.89 (0.49-1.29)*		0.62 (0.36-0.88)		0.72 (0.42-1.02)		0.77 (0.47-1.07)		0.93 (0.55-1.31)	
HCII (U/ml)	0.43 (0.10-0.93)		0.48 (0.00-0.96)		0.47 (0.10-0.87)		0.72 (0.10-1.46)		1.20 (0.50-1.90)		0.96 (0.66-1.26)	
Protein C (U/ml)	0.35 (0.17-0.53)		0.42 (0.20-0.64)		0.43 (0.21-0.65)		0.54 (0.28-0.80)		0.59 (0.37-0.81)		0.96 (0.64-1.28)	
Protein S (U/ml)	0.36 (0.12-0.60)		0.50 (0.22-0.78)		0.63 (0.33-0.93)		0.86 (0.54-1.18)*		0.87 (0.55-1.19)*		0.92 (0.60-1.24)	

In Healthy Premature Infants (30 to 36 Weeks' Gestation) During the First 6 Months of Life

	Day 1		Day 5		Day 30		Day 90		Day 180		Adults	
	M	B	M	B	M	B	M	B	M	B	M	B
AT (U/ml)	0.38 (0.14-0.62)†		0.56 (0.30-0.82)		0.59 (0.37-0.81)†		0.83 (0.45-1.21)†		0.90 (0.52-1.28)†		1.05 (0.79-1.31)	
₂M (U/ml)	1.10 (0.56-1.82)†		1.25 (0.71-1.77)		1.38 (0.72-2.04)		1.80 (1.20-2.66)		2.09 (1.10-3.21)		0.86 (0.52-1.20)	
C₁E-INH (U/ml)	0.65 (0.31-0.99)		0.83 (0.45-1.21)		0.74 (0.40-1.24)†		1.14 (0.60-1.68)*		1.40 (0.96-2.04)		1.01 (0.71-1.31)	
₁AT (U/ml)	0.90 (0.36-1.44)*		0.94 (0.42-1.46)*		0.76 (0.38-1.12)†		0.81 (0.49-1.13)*†		0.82 (0.48-1.16)*		0.93 (0.55-1.31)	
HCII (U/ml)	0.32 (0.10-0.60)†		0.34 (0.10-0.69)		0.43 (0.15-0.71)		0.61 (0.20-1.11)		0.89 (0.45-1.40)*†		0.96 (0.66-1.26)	
Protein C (U/ml)	0.28 (0.12-0.44)†		0.31 (0.11-0.51)		0.37 (0.15-0.59)†		0.45 (0.23-0.67)†		0.57 (0.31-0.83)		0.96 (0.64-1.28)	
Protein S (U/ml)	0.26 (0.14-0.38)†		0.37 (0.13-0.61)		0.56 (0.22-0.90)		0.76 (0.40-1.12)†		0.82 (0.44-1.20)		0.92 (0.60-1.24)	

All values are expressed in units per milliliter (U/ml), in which pooled plasma contains 1.0 U/ml. All values are given as a mean (M) followed by the lower and upper boundaries encompassing 95% of the population (B). Between 40 and 75 samples were assayed for each value for the neonate. Some measurements were skewed due to a disproportionate number of high values. The lower limit, which excludes the lower 2.5% of the population, has been given (B).

* Values that are indistinguishable from those of the adult.† Values different from those of full-term infants.

AT = antithrombin; ₂M = ₂ = macroglobulin; C₁ = EINH = C₁ = esterase inhibitor; ₁AT = antitrypsin; HCII = heparin cofactor II.
From Andrew M. et al: Am J Pediatr Hematol Oncol *12*:95, 1990.

TABLE 148-6

Reference Values for the Components of the Fibrinolytic System in Healthy Full-Term Infants During the First 6 Months of Life

	Day 1		Day 5		Day 30		Day 90		Day 180		Adults	
	M	*B*	*M*	*B*	*M*	*B*	*M*	*B*	*M*	*B*	*M*	*B*
Plasminogen (U/ml)	1.95 (1.25–2.65)		2.17 (1.41–2.93)		1.98 (1.26–2.70)		2.48 (1.74–3.22)		3.01 (2.21–3.81)		3.36 (2.48–4.24)	
TPA (ng/ml)	9.6 (5.0–18.9)		5.6 (4.0–10.0)*		4.1 (1.0–6.0)*		2.1 (1.0–5.0)*		2.8 (1.0–6.0)*		4.9 (1.4–8.4)	
$_2$AP (U/ml)	0.85 (0.55–1.15)		1.00 (0.70–1.30)*		1.00 (0.76–1.24)*		1.08 (0.76–1.40)*		1.11 (0.83–1.39)*		1.02 (0.68–1.36)	
PAI-1 (U/ml)	6.4 (2.0–15.1)		2.3 (0.0–8.1)*		3.4 (0.0–8.8)*		7.2 (1.0–15.3)		8.1 (6.0–13.0)		3.6 (0.0–11.0)	

In Healthy Premature Infants (30 to 36 Weeks' Gestation) During the First 6 Months of Life

	Day 1		Day 5		Day 30		Day 90		Day 180		Adults	
Plasminogen (U/ml)	1.70 (1.12–2.48)†		1.91 (1.21–2.61)+		1.81 (1.09–2.53)		2.38 (1.58–3.18)		2.75 (1.91–3.59)+		3.36 (2.48–4.24)	
TPA (ng/ml)	8.48 (3.00–16.70)		3.97 (2.00–6.93)*		4.13 (2.00–7.79)*		3.31 (2.00–5.07)*		3.48 (2.00–5.85)*		4.96 (1.46–8.46)	
$_2$AP (U/ml)	0.78 (0.40–1.16)		0.81 (0.49–1.13)†		0.89 (0.55–1.23)†		1.06 (0.64–1.48)*		1.15 (0.77–1.53)		1.02 (0.68–1.36)	
PAI-1 (U/ml)	5.4 (0.0–12.2)*†		2.5 (0.0–7.1)*		4.3 (0.0–10.9)*		4.8 (1.0–11.8)*†		4.9 (1.0–10.2)*†		3.6 (0.0–11.0)	

For $_2$AP, values are expressed as units per milliliter (U/ml) in which pooled plasma contains 1.0 U/ml. Plasminogen units are those recommended by the Committee on Thrombolytic Agents. Values for TPA are given as nanograms per milliliter. Values for PAI-1 are given as units per ml where one unit of PAI-1 activity is defined as the amount of PAI-1 that inhibits one international unit of human single-chain TPA. All values are given as a mean (M) followed by the lower and upper boundaries encompassing 95% of the population (B).
* Values that are indistinguishable from those of the adult.
† Values that are different from those of the full-term infant. TPA, tissue plasminogen activator; $_2$-antiplasmin; PAI-1 = plasminogen activator inhibitor-1.
From Andrew M, et al: Am J Pediatr Hematol Oncol *12*:95, 1990.

TABLE 148-7

Reference Values for Coagulation Tests in Healthy Children Ages 1 to 16 Years Compared with Adults

	1 to 5 y		6 to 10 y		11 to 16 y		Adults	
	M	**B**	**M**	**B**	**M**	**B**	**M**	**B**
PT (sec)	11 (10.6–11.4)		11.1 (10.1–12.1)		11.2 (10.2–12.0)		12 (11.0–14.0)	
INR	1.0 (0.96–1.04)		1.01 (0.91–1.11)		1.02 (0.93–1.10)		1.10 (1.0–1.3)	
APTT (sec)	30 (24–36)		31 (26–36)		32 (26–37)		33 (27–40)	
Fibrinogen (g/l)	2.76 (1.70–4.05)		2.79 (1.57–4.0)		3.0 (1.54–4.48)		2.78 (1.56–4.0)	
Bleeding Time (min)	6 (2.5–10)*		7 (2.5–13)*		5 (3–8)*		4 (1–7)	
Fll (U/ml)	0.94 (0.71–1.16)*		0.88 (0.67–1.07)		0.83 (0.61–1.04)*		1.08 (0.70–1.46)	
FV (U/ml)	1.03 (0.79–1.27)		0.90 (0.63–1.16)*		0.77 (0.55–0.99)*		1.06 (0.62–1.50)	
FVII (U/ml)	0.82 (0.55–1.16)		0.85 (0.52–1.20)		0.83 (0.58–1.15)*		1.05 (0.67–1.43)	
FVIII (U/ml)	0.90 (0.59–1.42)		0.95 (0.58–1.32)		0.92 (0.53–1.31)		0.99 (0.50–1.49)	
vWF (U/ml)	0.82 (0.60–1.20)		0.95 (0.44–1.44)		1.00 (0.46–1.53)		0.92 (0.50–1.58)	
FIX (U/ml)	0.73 (0.47–1.04)		0.75 (0.63–0.89)*		0.82 (0.59–1.22)*		1.09 (0.55–1.63)	
FX (U/ml)	0.88 (0.58–1.16)		0.75 (0.55–1.01)*		0.79 (0.50–1.17)*		1.06 (0.70–1.52)	
FXI (U/ml)	0.97 (0.56–1.50)		0.86 (0.52–1.20)		0.74 (0.50–0.97)		0.97 (0.67–1.27)	
FXII (U/ml)	0.93 (0.64–1.29)		0.92 (0.60–1.40)		0.81 (0.34–1.37)*		1.08 (0.52–1.64)	
PK (U/ml)	0.95 (0.65–1.30)		0.99 (0.66–1.31)		0.99 (0.53–1.45)		1.12 (0.62–1.62)	
HMWK (U/ml)	0.98 (0.64–1.32)		0.93 (0.60–1.30)		0.91 (0.63–1.19)		0.92 (0.50–1.36)	
FXIIIa (U/ml)	1.08 (0.72–1.43)		1.09 (0.65–1.51)*		0.99 (0.57–1.40)		1.05 (0.55–1.55)	
FXIIIs (U/ml)	1.13 (0.69–1.56)		1.16 (0.77–1.54)*		1.02 (0.60–1.43)		0.97 (0.57–1.37)	

All factors except fibrinogen are expressed as units/ml (U/ml), in which pooled plasma contains 1.0 U/ml. All data are expressed as the mean (M), followed by the upper and lower boundaries encompassing 95% of the population (B). Between 20 and 50 samples were assayed for each value for each age group. Some measurements were skewed due to a disproportionate number of high values. The lower limit, which excludes the lower 2.5% of the population, has been given.
* Values that are significantly different from those of adults.
PT = prothrombin time; INR = international normalized ratio; APTT = activated partial thromboplastin time; F = factor; vWF = von Willebrand factor; PK = prekallikrein; HMWK = high molecular weight kininogen.
From Andrew M, et al: Blood *80*:1998, 1992.

TABLE 148-8

Reference Values for the Inhibitors of Coagulation in Healthy Children Ages 1 to 16 Years Compared with Adults

	1 to 5 yr		6 to 10 yr		11 to 16 yr		Adults	
	M	**B**	**M**	**B**	**M**	**B**	**M**	**B**
AT (U/ml)	1.11 (0.82–1.39)		1.11 (0.90–1.31)		1.05 (0.77–1.32)		1.0 (0.74–1.26)	
₂M (U/ml)	1.69 (1.14–2.23)		1.69 (1.28–2.09)*		1.56 (0.98–2.12)		0.86 (0.52–1.20)	
C1E-INH (U/ml)	1.35 (0.85–1.83)*		1.14 (0.88–1.54)		1.03 (0.68–1.50)		1.0 (0.71–1.31)	
₁AT (U/ml)	0.93 (0.39–1.47)		1.00 (0.69–1.30)		1.01 (0.65–1.37)		0.93 (0.55–1.30)	
HCII (U/ml)	0.88 (0.48–1.28)*		0.86 (0.40–1.32)*		0.91 (0.53–1.29)*		1.08 (0.66–1.26)	
Protein C (U/ml)	0.66 (0.40–0.92)*		0.69 (0.45–0.93)*		0.83 (0.55–1.11)*		0.96 (0.64–1.28)	
Protein S								
Total (U/ml)	0.86 (0.54–1.18)		0.78 (0.41–1.14)		0.72 (0.52–0.92)		0.81 (0.60–1.13)	
Free (U/ml)	0.45 (0.21–0.69)		0.42 (0.22–0.62)		0.38 (0.26–0.55)		0.45 (0.27–0.61)	

All values are expressed in units per milliliter (U/ml), in which for all factors pooled plasma contains 1.0 U/ml, with the exception of free protein S, which contains a mean of 0.4 U/ml. All values are given as a mean (M), followed by the lower and upper boundaries encompassing 95% of the population (B). Between 20 and 30 samples were assayed for each value for each age group. Some measurements were skewed due to a disproportionate number of high values. The lower limits, which excludes the lower 2.5% of the population, have been given.
* Values that are significantly different from those of adults.
Abbreviations given in Table 148-5.
From Andrew M, et al: Blood *80*: 1998,1992.

TABLE 148-9

Reference Values for the Fibrinolytic System in Healthy Children Ages 1 to 16 Years Compared with Adults

	1 to 5 y		6 to 10 y		11 to 16 y		Adults	
	M	*B*	*M*	*B*	*M*	*B*	*M*	*B*
Plasminogen (U/ml)	0.98 (0.78-1.18)		0.92 (0.75-1.08)		0.86 (0.68-1.03)*		0.99 (0.77-1.22)	
TPA (ng/ml)	2.15 (1.0-4.5)*		2.42 (1.0-5.0)*		2.16 (1.0-4.0)*		4.90 (1.40-8.40)	
$_2$AP (U/ml)	1.05 (0.93-1.17)		0.99 (0.89-1.10)		0.98 (0.78-1.18)		1.02 (0.68-1.36)	
PAI-1 (U/ml)	5.42 (1.0-10.0)		6.79 (2.0-12.0)*		6.07 (2.0-10.0)		3.60 (0-11.0)	

For $_2$AP, values are expressed as units per ml (U/ml), in which pooled plasma contains 1.0 U/ml. Values for TPA are given as nanograms per ml (ng/ml). Values for PAI-1 are given as units/ml, in which 1 unit of PAI-1 activity is defined as the amount of PAI-1 that inhibits one international unit of human single-chain TPA. All values are given as mean (M), followed by the lower and upper boundaries encompassing 95% of the population (B).
* Values that are significantly different.
TPA = tissue plasminogen activator; $_2$AP = alpha$_2$-antiplasmin; PAI-1 = plasminogen activator inhibitor-1.
from Andrew M, et al: Blood *80*:1998, 1992.

TABLE 148-10

APTT Results Obtained Using Different APTT Reagents on a STA-Compact Automated Coagulation Analyzer (Diagnostica STAGO)

	Population Tested	
Reagent Used	*Children 1–10 y* *Mean (95% Population)*	*Adults* *Mean (95% Population)*
PTT-A (Diagnostica STAGO)	38.1 (31.3-44.1)	33.2 (28.1-38.2)
CK-Prest (Diagnostica STAGO)	33.0 (28.7-37.5)	29.1 (24.9-31.5)
Actin FSL (Dade Behring)	37.2 (27.8-43.9)	30.8 (24.1-34.4)
Platelin L (Organon Teknika)	38.0 (28.2-45.0)	31.3 (25.2-35.4)

---

is in plasmas from adults.[54,55] Alpha$_2$-macroglobulin compensates, in part, for the low levels of AT in neonates, even in the presence of endothelial cell surfaces. AT survival times are shorter in healthy infants requiring exchange transfusion than they are in adults.[56] Despite these differences, the rate of inhibition of thrombin is still slower in newborn infants than it is in adults.

Whether the overall activity of the protein C/protein S system varies with age is unknown. However, at birth, plasma concentrations of protein C are very low, and they remain decreased during the first 6 months of life.[1,2] Protein C in neonatal plasma has a twofold increase in single-chain form, compared with the double-chain form that is prominent in adults.[57,58] Animal data suggest that fetal protein C has increased glycosylation compared with that of adults. Despite these changes, there is no evidence that protein C is functionally different in neonates. Although total amounts of protein S are decreased at birth, functional activity is similar to that in the adult because protein S is completely present in the free, active form due to the absence of C4 binding protein.[59,60] Furthermore, the interaction of protein S with activated protein C in newborn plasma may be regulated by the increased levels of α_2M.[61] Plasma concentrations of thrombomodulin are increased in early childhood, decreasing to adult values by the late teenage years; however, the influence of age on endothelial cell expression of thrombomodulin has not been determined.[62-66]

Total tissue factor pathway inhibitor (TFPI) levels in newborn infants are reported as being similar to levels in older children or adults. Free TFPI is reported as being significantly lower in neonates.[67]

The capacity of newborn fibrin clots to bind thrombin has been assessed through the measurement of fibrinopeptide A (FPA) production. Cord plasma clots generate significantly less FPA than do adult plasma clots because of the decreased

plasma concentrations of prothrombin in cord plasma.[68] This observation suggests that thrombi in newborn infants may not have the same propensity to propagate as do thrombi in adult patients.

THE FIBRINOLYTIC SYSTEM

Although plasmin is generated and inhibited similarly in infants and adults, important differences do exist.[2] In neonates, plasminogen levels are only 50% of adult values, α_2-antiplasmin (α_2AP) levels are 80% of adult values, and plasma concentrations of plasminogen activator inhibitor-1 (PAI-1) and tissue plasminogen activator (TPA) are significantly greater than adult levels.[1-3, 28-36,38,69-71] Increased levels of TPA and PAI-1 on day 1 of life are in marked contrast to values from cord blood, in which concentrations of these two proteins are significantly lower than they are in adults.[38,68,69] The discrepancy between newborn and cord plasma concentrations of TPA and PAI-1 can be explained by the enhanced release of TPA and PAI-1 from the endothelium shortly following birth. PAI-2 levels are detectable in cord blood but are significantly lower than they are in pregnant women.[72] Plasminogen, like fibrinogen, has a fetal form. Fetal plasminogen exists in two glycoforms that have increased amounts of mannose and sialic acid.[73] The enzymatic activity of "fetal plasmin," as well as its binding to cellular receptors for fetal plasminogen, are decreased.

Short whole-blood clotting times, short euglobulin lysis times (ELTs) and increased plasma concentrations of the Bβ15-42 fibrin-related peptides all suggest that the fibrinolytic system is activated at birth.[1,71] At the same time, the capacity of the fetal fibrinolytic system to generate plasmin in response to stimulation by a thrombolytic agent is decreased when compared with that of adults; this reflects low levels of plasminogen.[74]

TABLE 148-11

Pre- and Postocclusion Results of Euglobulin Lysis Time (ELT) Expressed as Mean (± 95% CI)

ELT (h)	Children		Adults		
	Female	*Male*	*Female*	*Male*	*P*-value
Preocclusion	5.2 (0.30)	4.7 (0.50)	4.2 (0.80)	4.8 (0.60)	NS*
Postocclusion	3.0 (0.50)†	3.2 (0.60)†	1.7 (0.80)	2.0 (0.60)	*p* = .002†

Analyzed by one-way analysis of variance. *Not significant; †adolescents had significantly longer ELT postocclusion results when compared with adults. There was no effect of gender.
CI = confidence interval.

The fibrinolytic response to venous occlusion stress testing in healthy adolescents has been compared with the response in healthy adults[75, 76] Healthy adolescents (13 to 18 years) from a school population and normal adults were recruited. Pre- and postvenous occlusion blood samples were collected by means of standard techniques. Adolescents had significantly decreased tPA antigen levels and increased PAI-1 activity levels after venous occlusion, resulting in significantly prolonged ELTs (Table 148-11). The age-related differences in fibrinolytic responses to venous occlusion of younger children, and the significance of these differences on the pathophysiology of clinical hemostatic disorders in children, require further studies.

PLATELETS

Classic platelet studies in newborn infants are inhibited by sample volume requirements. Flow cytometry is useful because of the small sample volume required for extensive platelet function studies. Differences in sample timing, method of collection, and concentrations and compositions of platelet agonists likely contribute to apparently conflicting reports on cord platelet function.

Megakaryocytopoiesis has been difficult to study in the fetus and neonate because of the intrinsic low level of megakaryocyte production in the marrow and the lack of availability of marrow samples to study. Using microassay techniques, Murray and Roberts have shown that megakaryocytopoiesis is likely increased at 24 to 36 weeks' gestation versus full-term.[77] Platelets appear at 5 weeks postconception, and megakaryocytes appear in the liver at 8 weeks. Fetal and neonatal megakaryocytes are smaller than adult megakaryocytes.[78]

Megakaryocytes

Cord blood of preterm babies has increased numbers of all megakaryocyte precursors compared with term infants. Term infants have increased circulating megakaryocyte progenitor numbers at birth correlated with platelet numbers, compared with adults.[79] The magnitude of cord blood megakaryocyte progenitors' proliferative and maturational responses to cytokines is related to developmental age.[77] Reticulated platelet counts are reported as similar to adult levels in healthy neonates greater than 30 weeks' gestational age (GA) and increased in neonates younger than 30 weeks' GA,[80] although another study reports reduced reticulated platelet counts in neonates of all GAs compared with adults.[81] There is no information on developmental differences of megakaryocyte and platelet precursors during childhood.

Platelets in Cord Blood

Platelet counts and mean platelet volumes in neonates are similar to those in adults, with values of 150,000 to 450,000 × 10⁹/L and 7 to 9 fL, respectively.[82-89a] Platelet counts in fetuses between 18 and 30 weeks' GA also fall within the adult range, with the average value being 250×10^9/L.[90] Platelet survival has not been measured in healthy infants. Electron microscopy studies on cord platelets have demonstrated normal numbers of granules; however, serotonin and adenosine diphosphate (ADP), which are stored in dense granules, are present at concentrations that are less than 50% of adult values. Flow cytometry studies in whole blood without added agonists show that there are no significant differences between neonates and adults in platelet binding of monoclonal antibodies for glycoprotein (GP) Ib or P-selectin; however, GP IIb/IIIa is significantly reduced.[91,92] Platelet adhesion at birth has not been assessed with sensitive and reproducible assays; this may explain the conflicting *in vitro* results given in the literature.[93,94] GP Ib is present on fetal platelet membranes in adult quantities.[95]

Both the plasma concentrations of von Willebrand factor (vWF) and the proportion of high molecular weight multimers (and therefore more active forms) of vWF are increased in neonates.[96, 97] The cord multimeric pattern of vWF appears similar to the forms released by endothelial cells. This may be explained by the recent finding that newborn plasma has little if any detectable vWF cleaving protease.[98,99] The quantitative and qualitative differences in vWF at birth are likely responsible for the enhanced cord platelet agglutination to low concentrations of ristocetin[100,101] and contribute to the short bleeding time in neonates.[102-104] Glycoprotein IIb/IIIa complexes are expressed on platelet membranes early in gestation;[105] however, the capacity of cord platelets to aggregate following exposure to a variety of agonists has been variable, with some observations being more consistent than others. Recently, differences between cord blood of premature versus full-term infants have been described, with reduced aggregation in preterm infants.[106]

Epinephrine-induced aggregation of cord platelets is consistently decreased when compared with that of adult platelets because of the decreased availability of α-adrenergic receptors.[107-114] Ristocetin-induced agglutination of cord platelets is consistently increased compared with that of adult platelets, likely because of quantitative and qualitative increases in the level of vWF. Aggregation of cord platelets induced by ADP, collagen, thrombin, and arachidonic acid is variable and may be moderately decreased or similar to that of adult platelets.[115-117] There is reduced thromboxane A₂ production in neonates, despite normal receptor binding, suggesting a postreceptor signal transduction problem.[118]

Inositol phosphate production and protein phosphorylation are normal, as is production of arachidonic acid and its metabolites.[119] In fact, cord platelets release more arachidonic acid than adult platelets in response to stimulation by thrombin.[120] This increased release may be due to the greater reactivity of platelet membranes induced by low levels of vitamin E.[121, 122] Agonist receptors, with the exception of the α-adrenergic receptor discussed previously, do not appear to be decreased in number. Despite a poor response to collagen stimulation, cord platelets have normal numbers of the collagen receptor GP Ia/IIa present in platelet membranes.[123] Coupling of agonist receptors to phospholipases may be the site of this transient activation defect in response to collagen.[124]

Platelet Function in Neonates

A few studies have assessed aggregation of newborn platelets obtained during the first few days of life; other studies have evaluated platelets of older neonates.[125] Improved platelet aggregation was seen in newborn platelets drawn 2 hours after birth, with normalization of platelet aggregation at 48 hours. Studies using whole-blood flow cytometry show that, compared with adult platelets, neonatal platelets are hyporeactive to thrombin, a combination of ADP and epinephrine, and a thromboxane A_2 analogue.[126-129] The clinical significance of these observations remains unknown.

Bleeding Time

Measurement of the bleeding time is currently the best *in vivo* test of platelet interaction with the vessel wall.[130] Bleeding times in infants during the first week of life are significantly shorter than those in adults.[131] Several mechanisms contribute to this enhanced platelet/vessel wall interaction, including higher plasma concentrations of vWF,[1–3] enhanced function of vWF due to a disproportional increase in the high molecular weight multimeric forms,[132,133] active multimers, large red cells, and high hematocrits.[134,135] The significance of mild platelet aggregation defects in cord platelets is uncertain when bleeding times in neonates are shorter than those in adults. Although automated bleeding time devices modified for newborn infants and children are available and have been standardized, the test remains difficult to reproduce in clinical laboratories.[136]

The platelet function analyzer (PFA)-100 system provides an *in vitro* method of assessing primary platelet-related hemostasis by measuring the time (closure time, or CT) taken for a platelet plug to occlude a microscopic aperture cut into a membrane coated with collagen and either adrenaline or ADP. The PFA-100 system is ideal for neonates because of the small volume required and the rapidity of testing. Normal ranges for the CT of children are similar to those of adults. Newborn infants have shorter CTs that are not influenced by red or white cells.[137-141] The ease of the PFA-100 system and the associated difficulties in performing skin bleeding times have reduced the clinical utility of skin bleeding times. Further studies are required to determine the optimal method of assessing primary hemostasis in neonates and children.

Activation During the Birth Process

There is strong evidence that platelets are activated during the birth process. Cord plasma levels of thromboxane B_2, β-thromboglobulin, and platelet factor-4 are increased, the granular content of cord platelets is decreased, and epinephrine receptor availability is reduced, perhaps secondary to occupation.[142-144] The mechanisms of activation are likely multifactorial and include thermal changes, hypoxia, acidosis, adrenergic stimulation, and the thrombogenic effects of amniotic fluid. Activation of the coagulation system may provide an explanation for the paradox that one-stage coagulation times are prolonged in the neonate but that various measures of whole-blood clotting duration are shortened compared with those in the adult.[145]

BLOOD VESSEL WALL

The vessel wall profoundly influences hemostasis due to the procoagulant and anticoagulant properties of endothelial cells and extracellular matrix components. Each of these properties is significantly influenced by age. One of the anticoagulant properties of endothelial cell surfaces is mediated by lipoxygenase and cyclooxygenase metabolites of unsaturated fatty acids.

Prostaglandin I_2 (PGI_2) production from cord vessels exceeds that of vessels from adults.[146] In a rabbit venous model, there is a significant increase in glycosaminoglycans (GAGs) by mass in inferior vena cavas (IVCs) from pups compared with adult rabbits. The antithrombin (AT)-mediated anticoagulant activity of IVC GAGs, especially heparin sulfate, is increased in pups compared with adult rabbits.[147] In a rabbit arterial model, total proteoglycan, chrondroitin sulfate, and heparin sulfate content are increased in the intima and media of aortas from pups compared with adult rabbits. AT activity in aortas of pups, due to heparin sulfate GAGs, is also increased.[148] The increased GAG-mediated vessel wall AT activity in pups compared with adult rabbits suggests that young blood vessels may have greater antithrombotic potential.

When measured directly, thrombin generation in cord plasma is decreased in the presence of human umbilical endothelial cells compared with plastic owing to cell surface promotion of AT inhibition of thrombin.[149] Soluble levels of endothelial cell adhesion molecules and selectins are also age dependent, suggesting developmental differences in endothelial cell expression and secretion of these molecules.[150]

Nitric oxide (NO), or EDRF, is a labile humeral agent that modulates vascular tone in fetal and postnatal lungs and contributes to the normal decline in pulmonary vascular resistance at birth. NO is a potent inhibitor of platelet adhesion, aggregation and stimulates disaggregation of platelet aggregates. NO likely interacts with PGI_2 and other metabolites of the lipoxygenase pathway to modulate platelet function in a synergistic manner.[151]

It has been observed in sheep that vessel wall thickness increases in the perinatal period.[152] This is likely in response to increases in stress per vessel internal diameter. Contractility also increases with fetal development.[153] The endothelial cells of fetal vessels are larger and less uniform and protrude into the lumen.[154]

ANIMAL MODELS OF COAGULATION

Animal models have been used to increase our understanding of developmental hemostasis.[155] The lamb has been the most frequently used model. Both the pig and sheep have similar vascular and hemostatic physiologies to that of humans. The newborn dog has been used as a model of intraventricular hemorrhage.[156]

Using targeted manipulations of the mouse genome, murine models of deficiencies in virutally every protein involved in hemostasis have been created. The information learned from these models has increased our understanding of the role of these proteins in fetal development.[157]

The tissue factor–factor VII complex, formed when the subendothelial surface is exposed by injury, activates factors X and IX and initiates coagulation. Tissue factor deficiency has never been described in humans, indicating its essential function in hemostasis. The absence of tissue factor expression leads to embryonic lethality by days 8.5 to 10.5 in the mouse.[158] Pools of red blood cells can be seen in the yolk sac of these mice embryos.[159] Most interesting was that these embryos lacked the large vitelline vessels that connect the yolk sac and embryonic vasculature, and no blood flow was seen in the yolk sac vessels.[160] Thus, tissue factor is essential for vascular development and integrity during embryonic development. In contrast to tissue factor null mice, factor VII–deficient mice survived to term, but the majority died in the first 24 hours from intra-abdominal hemorrhage, and the remaining died in the first 3 to 4 weeks of life.[161]

ANGIOGENESIS

Serum levels of the angiogenic factors angiogenin, basic fibroblast growth factor (bFGF), and vascular endothelial growth factor (VEGF) change soon after birth.[162] When sera from healthy full-term infants at birth, day 1, and day 4 postpartum and sera from their mothers were analyzed by enzyme immunoassays for angiogenin, bFGF, and VEGF, significant differences were seen, which were thought to be primarily from the presence, then absence, of the placenta. It is known that the placenta produces an angiogenin inhibitor. bFGF and VEGF maternal levels were lower than fetal and neonatal ones. Neonatal bFGF levels did not differ from fetal levels. VEGF levels increased in neonatal serum. Angiogenesis has been shown to be important for alveolarization in the fetal and neonatal lung.[163] Studying angiogenesis in the fetal and neonatal lung may lead to therapeutic strategies.

SUMMARY

The vascular and hemostatic systems of the fetus and neonate are continually evolving. One must take this into consideration when evaluating these systems for dysfunction. Adult normative data do not apply to the fetus or neonate. Although different in content and structure, these systems should be considered physiologically in the fetus and neonate. This is an important consideration when determining and monitoring therapeutic intervention.

REFERENCES

1. Andrew M, et al: Development of the hemostatic system in the neonate and young infant. Am J Pediatr Hematol Oncol 12:95, 1990.
2. Andrew M, et al: Development of the human coagulation system in the full-term infant. Blood 70:165, 1987.
3. Andrew M, et al: Development of the human coagulation system in the healthy premature infant. Blood 72:1651, 1988.
4. Sanford HN, et al: The substances involved in the coagulation of the blood of the newborn. Am J Dis Child 43:58, 1932.
5. Johnston M, Zipursky A: Microtechnology for the study of the blood coagulation system in newborn infants. Can J Med Tech 42:159, 1980.
6. Forestier F, et al: Hematological values of 163 normal fetuses between 18 and 30 weeks of gestation. Pediatr Res 20:342, 1986.
7. Cade JF, et al: Placental barrier to coagulation factors: its relevance to the coagulation defect at birth and to haemorrhage in the newborn. BMJ 2:281, 1969.
8. Kisker CT, et al: Development of blood coagulation—a fetal lamb model. Pediatr Res 15:1045, 1981.
9. Andrew M, et al: Fetal lamb coagulation system during normal birth. Am J Hematol 28:116, 1988.
10. Holmberg L, et al: Coagulation in the human fetus. Comparison with term newborn infants. J Pediatr 85:860, 1974.
11. Jensen AH, et al: Evolution of blood clotting factor levels in premature infants during the first 10 days of life: a study of 96 cases with comparison between clinical status and blood clotting factor levels. Pediatr Res 7:638, 1973.
12. Mibashan RS, et al: Plasma assay of fetal factors VIIIC and IX for prenatal diagnosis of haemophilia. Lancet 1:1309, 1979.
13. Forestier F, et al: The assessment of fetal blood samples. Am J Obstet Gynecol 158:1184, 1988.
14. Forestier F, et al: Vitamin K dependent proteins in fetal hemostasis at mid trimester of pregnancy. Thromb Haemost 53:401, 1985.
15. Forestier F, et al: Prenatal diagnosis of hemophilia by fetal blood sampling under ultrasound guidance. Haemostasis 16:346, 1986.
16. Toulon P, et al: Antithrombin III (ATIII) and heparin cofactor II (HCII) in normal human fetuses (21st–27th week) [letter]. Thromb Haemost 56:237, 1986.
17. Barnard DR, et al: Coagulation studies in extremely premature infants. Pediatr Res 13:1330, 1979.
18. Nossel HL, et al: A study of coagulation factor levels in women during labour and in their newborn infants. Thromb Diath Haemorrh 16:185, 1966.
19. Reverdiau-Moalic P, et al: Evolution of blood coagulation activators and inhibitors in the healthy human fetus. Blood 88:900, 1996.
20. Andrew M, et al: Maturation of the hemostatic system during childhood. Blood 80:1998, 1992.
21. Hirsh J, et al: Advances in antithrombotic therapy. In Hoffbrand AV (ed): Recent Advances in Hematology. New York, Churchill Livingstone, 1985, pp 333–367.
22. Koepke JA: Partial thromboplastin time test—proposed performance guidelines. ICSH Panel on the PTT. Thromb Haemost 55:143, 1986.
23. Hirsh J: Oral anticoagulant drugs [see comments]. N Engl J Med 324:1865, 1991.
24. Monagle P, et al: The importance of age-appropriate haemostasis reference ranges (abstract). Blood 100:94, 2002.
25. Townsend CW: The haemorrhagic disease of the newborn. Arch Pediatr 11:559, 1894.
26. Dam H, et al: K-avitaminose hos spaede born som aarag til hemorrhagisk diathese. Ugesk Laeger 101:896, 1939.
27. Brinkhous KM, et al: Plasma prothrombin level in normal infancy and in hemorrhagic disease of the newborn (abstract). Am J Med Sci 193:475, 1937.
28. Bleyer WA, et al: The development of hemostasis in the human fetus and newborn infant. J Pediatr 79:838, 1971.
29. Hathaway WE, Bonnar J: Bleeding disorders in the newborn infant. In Oliver TK Jr (ed): Perinatal Coagulation; Monographs in Neonatology. New York, Grune and Stratton, 1978, pp. 115–169.
30. Gross S, Melhorn D: Exchange transfusion with citrated whole blood for disseminated intravascular coagulation. J Pediatr 78:415, 1971.
31. Buchanan GR: Coagulation disorders in the neonate. Pediatr Clin North Am 33:203, 1986.
32. Montgomery RR, et al: Newborn haemostasis. Clin Haematol 14:443, 1985.
33. Gibson B: Neonatal haemostasis. Arch Dis Child 64:503, 1989.
34. Gobel U, et al: Etiopathology and classification of acquired coagulation disorders in the newborn infant. Klin Wochenschr 57:81, 1979.
35. McDonald MM, Hathaway WE: Neonatal hemorrhage and thrombosis. Semin Perinatol 7:213, 1983.
36. Stothers J, et al: Neonatal coagulation (letter). Lancet 1:408, 1975.
37. Bahakim H, et al: Coagulation parameters in maternal and cord blood at delivery. Ann Saud Med 10:149, 1990.
38. Aballi AJ, de Lamerens S: Coagulation changes in the neonatal period and in early infancy. Pediatr Clin North Am 9:785, 1962.
39. Andrew M, Karpatkin M: A simple screening test for evaluating prolonged partial thromboplastin times in newborn infants. J Pediatr 101:610, 1982.
40. Zipursky A, Jaber HM: The haematology of bacterial infection in newborn infants. Clin Haematol 7:175, 1978.
41. Kisker CT, et al: Measurement of prothrombin mRNA during gestation and early neonatal development. J Lab Clin Med 112:407, 1988.
42. Hassan HJ, et al: Blood coagulation factors in human embryonic-fetal development: preferential expression of the FVII/tissue factor pathway. Blood 76:1158, 1990.
43. Karpatkin M, et al: Prothrombin expression in the adult and fetal rabbit liver. Pediatr Res 30:266, 1991.
44. Andrew M, et al: Fibrinogen has a rapid turnover in the healthy newborn lamb. Pediatr Res 23:249–252, 1988.
45. Karitzky D, et al: Fibrinogen turnover in the premature infant with and without idiopathic respiratory distress syndrome. Acta Paediatr Scand 60:465, 1971.
46. Schmidt B, et al: Plasma elimination of antithrombin III (heparin cofactor activity) is accelerated in term newborn infants. Eur J Pediatr 141:225, 1984.
47. Witt I: Evidence for the existence of foetal fibrinogen. Thromb Diath Haemorrh 22:101–109, 1969.
48. Francis JL, Armstrong DJ: Sialic acid and enzymatic desialation of cord blood fibrinogen. Haemostasis 11:223, 1982.
49. Schmidt B, et al: Anticoagulant effects of heparin in neonatal plasma. Pediatr Res 25:405, 1989.
50. Xu L, et al: Thrombin generation in newborn and adult plasma in the presence of an endothelial surface (abstract). Thromb Haemost 65:1230, 1991.
51. Andrew M, et al: Thrombin generation in newborn plasma is critically dependent on the concentration of prothrombin. Thromb Haemost 63:27, 1990.
52. Andrew M, et al: An anticoagulant dermatan sulfate proteoglycan circulates in the pregnant woman and her fetus. J Clin Invest 89:321, 1992.
53. Delorme MA, et al: Anticoagulant dermatan sulfate proteoglycan (decorin) in the term human placenta. Thromb Res 90:147, 1998.
54. Schmidt B, et al: Alpha-2-macroglobulin is an important progressive inhibitor of thrombin in neonatal and infant plasma. Thromb Haemost 62:1074, 1989.
55. Levine JJ, et al: Elevated levels of alpha-macroglobulin-protease complexes in infants. Biol Neonate 51:149, 1987.
56. Schmidt B, et al: Plasma elimination of antithrombin III (heparin cofactor activity) is accelerated in term newborn infants. Eur J Pediatr 141:225, 1984.
57. Greffe BS, et al: Neonatal protein C: molecular composition and distribution in normal term infants. Thromb Res 56:91, 1989.
58. Manco-Johnson MJ, et al: Identification of a unique form of protein C in the ovine fetus: developmentally linked transition to the adult form. Pediatr Res 37:365, 1995.
59. Moalic P, et al: Levels and plasma distribution of free and C4b-BP-bound protein S in human fetuses and full-term newborns. Thromb Res 49:471, 1988.
60. Schwarz HP, et al: Low total protein S antigen but high protein S activity due to decreased C4b-binding protein in neonates. Blood 71:562, 1988.
61. Cvirn G, et al: Efficacy of the anticoagulant action of protein S is regulated by the alpha-2-macroglobulin level in cord and adult plasma (abstract). Thromb Haemost Suppl:P282, 2001.
62. Knofler R, et al: Molecular markers of the endothelium, the coagulation and the fibrinolytic systems in healthy newborns. Semin Thromb Hemost 24:453, 1998.
63. Yurdakok M, et al: Plasma thrombomodulin levels in early respiratory distress syndrome. Turk J Pediatr 40:85, 1998.
64. Distefano G, et al: Thrombomodulin serum levels in ventilated preterm babies with respiratory distress syndrome. Eur J Pediatr 157:327, 1998.
65. Yurdakok M, Yigit S: Plasma thrombomodulin, plasminogen activator and plasminogen activator inhibitor levels in preterm infants with or without respiratory distress syndrome [letter; comment]. Acta Paediatr 86:1022, 1997.
66. Nako Y, et al: Plasma thrombomodulin level in very low birthweight infants at birth. Acta Paediatr 86:1105, 1997.

67. Van Dreden P, et al: Tissue factor pathway inhibitor in infants and children (abstract). Thromb Haemost *Suppl*:P2134, 2001.
68. Patel P, et al: Decreased thrombin activity of fibrin clots prepared in cord plasma compared with adult plasma. Pediatr Res *39*:826, 1996.
69. Corrigan JJ Jr: Neonatal thrombosis and the thrombolytic system: pathophysiology and therapy. Am J Pediatr Hematol Oncol *10*:83, 1988.
70. Corrigan JJ Jr, et al: Newborn's fibrinolytic mechanism: components and plasmin generation. Am J Hematol *32*:273, 1989.
71. Kolindewala JK, et al: Blood fibrinolytic activity in neonates: effect of period of gestation, birth weight, anoxia and sepsis. Indian Pediatr *24*:1029, 1987.
72. Lecander I, Astedt B: Specific plasminogen activator inhibitor of placental type PAI 2 occurring in amniotic fluid and cord blood. J Lab Clin Med *110*:602, 1987.
73. Edelberg JM, et al: Neonatal plasminogen displays altered cell surface binding and activation kinetics. Correlation with increased glycosylation of the protein. J Clin Invest *86*:107, 1990.
74. Andrew M, et al: Fibrin clot lysis by thrombolytic agents is impaired in newborns due to a low plasminogen concentration. Thromb Haemost *68*:325, 1992.
75. Monagle P, et al: The fibrinolytic system in adolescents: response to venous occlusion stress tests. Pediatr Res *53*:333, 2003.
76. Monagle P, et al: The fibrinolytic system in adolescents: response to venous occlusion stress tests. Pediatr Res *53*:333, 2003.
77. Murray NA, Roberts IAG: Circulating megakaryocytes and their progenitors (BFU-MK and CFU-MK) in term and pre-term neonates. Br J Haemotol *89*:41, 1995.
78. Allen Graeve JL, de Alarcon PA: Megakaryocytopoiesis in the human fetus. Arch Dis Child *64*:481, 1989.
79. Deutsch VR, et al: The response of cord blood megakaryocyte progenitors to IL-3, IL-6 and aplastic canine serum varies with gestational age. Br J Haematol *89*:8, 1995.
80. Peterec SM, et al: Reticulated platelet values in normal and thrombocytopenic neonates. J Pediatr *129*:269, 1996.
81. Joseph MA, et al: Flow cytometry of neonatal platelet RNA. J Pediatr Hematol Oncol *18*:277, 1996.
82. Aballi AJ, de Lamerens S: Coagulation changes in the neonatal period and in early infancy. Pediatr Clin North Am *9*:785, 1962.
83. Andrew M, Kelton J: Neonatal thrombocytopenia. Clin Perinatol *11*:359, 1984.
84. Pearson HA, McIntosh S: Neonatal thrombocytopenia. Clin Haematol *7*:111, 1978.
85. Gill FM: Thrombocytopenia in the newborn. Semin Perinatol *7*:201, 1983.
86. Mehta P, et al: Thrombocytopenia in the high-risk infant. J Pediatr *97*:791, 1980.
87. Castle V, et al: Frequency and mechanism of neonatal thrombocytopenia. J Pediatr *108*:749, 1986.
88. Beverley DW, et al: "Normal" haemostasis parameters: a study in a well-defined inborn population of preterm infants. Early Hum Dev *9*:249, 1984.
89. Kipper SL, Sieger L: Whole blood platelet volumes in newborn infants. J Pediatr *101*:763, 1982.
89a. Arad ID, et al: The mean platelet volume (MPV) in the neonatal period. Am J Perinatol *3*:1, 1986.
90. Forestier F, et al: Hematological values of 163 normal fetuses between 18 and 30 weeks of gestation. Pediatr Res *20*:342, 1986.
91. Rajasekhar D, et al: Neonatal platelets are less reactive than adult platelets to physiological agonists in whole blood. Thromb Haemost *72*:957, 1994.
92. Hurtaud-Roux MF, et al: Quantification of the major integrins and P-selectin in neonatal platelets by flow cytometry (abstract). Thromb Haemost *Suppl*:P284, 2001.
93. Mull MM, Hathaway WE: Altered platelet function in newborns. Pediatr Res *4*:229, 1970.
94. Whaun JM, et al: Effect of prenatal drug administration on maternal and neonatal platelet aggregation and PF4 release. Haemostasis *9*:226, 1980.
95. Gruel Y, et al: Determination of platelet antigens and glycoproteins in the human fetus. Blood *68*:488, 1986.
96. Katz JA, et al: Relationship between human development and disappearance of unusually large von Willebrand factor multimers from plasma. Blood, *73*:1851, 1989.
97. Weinstein MJ, et al: Fetal and neonatal von Willebrand factor (vWF) is unusually large and similar to the vWF in patients with thrombotic thrombocytopenic purpura. Br J Haematol *72*:68, 1989.
98. Takahashi Y, et al: Plasma von Willebrand factor–cleaving protease is low in newborns (abstract). Thromb Haemost *Suppl*:P285, 2001.
99. Katz JA, et al: Relationship between human development and disappearance of unusually large von Willebrand factor multimers from plasma. Blood *73*:1851, 1989.
100. Weinstein MJ, et al: Fetal and neonatal von Willebrand factor (vWF) is unusually large and similar to the vWF in patients with thrombotic thrombocytopenic purpura. Br J Haematol *72*:68, 1989.
101. Ts'ao CH, et al: Function and ultrastructure of platelets of neonates: enhanced ristocetin aggregation of neonatal platelets. Br J Haematol *32*:225, 1976.
102. Harker LA, Slichter SJ: The bleeding time as a screening test for evaluation of platelet function. N Engl J Med *287*:155, 1972.
103. Feusner JH: Normal and abnormal bleeding times in neonates and young children utilizing a fully standardized template technic. Am J Clin Pathol *74*:73, 1980.
104. Mull MM, Hathaway WE: Altered platelet function in newborns. Pediatr Res *4*:229, 1970.
105. Gruel Y, et al: Determination of platelet antigens and glycoproteins in the human fetus. Blood *68*:488, 1986.
106. Ucar T, et al: Platelet functions in preterm and term newborns (abstract). Thromb Haemost *Suppl*:CD3398, 2001.
107. Stuart MJ, et al: Differences in thromboxane production between neonatal and adult platelets in response to arachidonic acid and epinephrine. Pediatr Res *18*:823, 1984.
108. Corby DG, O'Barr TP: Decreased alpha-adrenergic receptors in newborn platelets: cause of abnormal response to epinephrine. Dev Pharmacol Ther *2*:215, 1981.
109. Barradas MA, et al: An investigation of maternal and neonatal platelet function. Biol Res Pregnancy Perinatol *7*:60, 1986.
110. Gader AM, et al: Dose-response aggregometry in maternal/neonatal platelets. Thromb Haemost *60*:314, 1988.
111. Hicsonmez G, Prozorova-Zamani V: Platelet aggregation in neonates with hyperbilirubinaemia. Scand J Haematol *24*:67, 1980.
112. Alebouyeh M, et al: The effect of 5-hydroxytryptamine and epinephrine on newborn platelets. Eur J Pediatr *128*:163, 1978.
113. Sadowitz PD, et al: Decreased plasma arachidonic acid binding capacity in neonates. Biol Neonate *51*:305, 1987.
114. Landolfi R, et al: Placental-derived PGI2 inhibits cord blood platelet function. Haematologica *73*:207, 1988.
115. Ahlsten G, et al: Arachidonic acid-induced aggregation of platelets from human cord blood compared with platelets from adults. Biol Neonate *47*:199, 1985.
116. Andrews NP, et al: Blood platelet behaviour in mothers and neonates. Thromb Haemost *53*:428, 1985.
117. Israels SJ, et al: Deficient collagen-induced activation in the newborn platelet. Pediatr Res *27*:337, 1990.
118. Israels SJ, et al: Contractile activity of neonatal platelets. Pediatr Res *21*:293, 1987.
119. Israels SJ, et al: Deficient collagen-induced activation in the newborn platelet. Pediatr Res *27*:337, 1990.
120. Stuart MJ, et al: Differences in thromboxane production between neonatal and adult platelets in response to arachidonic acid and epinephrine. Pediatr Res *18*:823, 1984.
121. Stuart MJ, Dusse J: In vitro comparison of the efficacy of cyclooxygenase inhibitors on the adult versus neonatal platelet. Biol Neonate *47*:265, 1985.
122. Stuart MJ, Oski FA: Vitamin E and platelet function. Am J Pediatr Hematol Oncol *1*:77, 1979.
123. Gruel Y, et al: Determination of platelet antigens and glycoproteins in the human fetus. Blood *68*:488, 1986.
124. Corby DG, O'Barr TP: Neonatal platelet function: a membrane-related phenomenon? Haemostasis *10*:177, 1981.
125. Landolfi R, et al: Placental-derived PGI2 inhibits cord blood platelet function. Haematologica *73*:207, 1988.
126. Stuart MJ, et al: Differences in thromboxane production between neonatal and adult platelets in response to arachidonic acid and epinephrine. Pediatr Res *18*:823, 1984.
127. Corby DG, O'Barr TP: Decreased alpha-adrenergic receptors in newborn platelets: cause of abnormal response to epinephrine. Dev Pharmacol Ther *2*:215, 1981.
128. Alebouyeh M, et al: The effect of 5-hydroxytryptamine and epinephrine on newborn platelets. Eur J Pediatr *128*:163, 1978.
129. Jones CR, et al: Maternal and fetal platelet responses and adrenoceptor binding characteristics. Thromb Haemost *53*:95, 1985.
130. Harker LA, Slichter SJ: The bleeding time as a screening test for evaluation of platelet function. N Engl J Med *287*:155, 1972.
131. Feusner JH: Normal and abnormal bleeding times in neonates and young children utilizing a fully standardized template technic. Am J Clin Pathol *74*:73, 1980.
132. Katz JA, et al: Relationship between human development and disappearance of unusually large von Willebrand factor multimers from plasma. Blood *73*:1851, 1989.
133. Weinstein MJ, et al: Fetal and neonatal von Willebrand factor (vWF) is unusually large and similar to the vWF in patients with thrombotic thrombocytopenic purpura. Br J Haematol *72*:68, 1989.
134. Aarts PA, et al: Red blood cell size is important for adherence of blood platelets to artery subendothelium. Blood *62*:214, 1983.
135. Fernandez F, et al: Low hematocrit and prolonged bleeding time in uraemic patients: effect of red cell transfusions. Br J Haematol *59*:139, 1985.
136. Widdershoven J, et al: Biochemical vitamin K deficiency in early infancy: diagnostic limitation of conventional coagulation tests. Helv Paediatr Acta *41*:195, 1986.
137. Carcao MD, et al: The platelet function analyzer (PFA-100): a novel in vitro system for evaluation of primary haemostasis in children. Br J Haematol *101*:70, 1998.
138. Roschitz B, et al: Shorter PFA-100 closure time in neonates than in adults is not caused by high red or white blood cell counts but depends on platelets and von Willebrand factor (abstract). Thromb Haemost *Suppl*:P280, 2001.
139. Slavec B, Benedik DM: The platelet function analyzer (PFA-100): a novel system for evaluation of primary haemostasis (abstract). Thromb Haemost *Suppl*:CD3310, 2001.

140. Harrison P, et al: Performance of the PFA-100R as a potential screening tool for platelet dysfunction (abstract). Thromb Haemost *Suppl*:P376, 2001.
141. Burgess CA, et al: An evaluation of the usefulness of the PFA-100 device in 60 consecutive paediatric patients referred for investigation of potential haemostatic disorders (abstract). Thromb Haemost *Suppl*:P378, 2001.
142. Suarez CR, et al: Neonatal and maternal hemostasis: value of molecular markers in the assessment of hemostatic status. Semin Thromb Hemost *10*:280, 1984.
143. Kaplan KL, Owen J: Plasma levels of beta-thromboglobulin and platelet factor 4 as indices of platelet activation in vivo. Blood *57*:199, 1981.
144. Suarez CR, et al: Neonatal and maternal platelets: activation at time of birth. Am J Hematol *29*:18, 1988.
145. Mull MM, Hathaway WE: Altered platelet function in newborns. Pediatr Res *4*:229, 1970.
146. Jacqz EM, et al: Prostacyclin concentrations in cord blood and in the newborn. Pediatrics *76*:954, 1985.
147. Nitschmann E, et al: Morphological and biochemical features affecting the antithrombotic properties of the inferior vena cava in adult rabbits and rabbit pups. Pediatr Res *43*:62, 1998.
148. Nitschmann E, et al: Morphological and biochemical features affecting the antithrombotic properties of the aorta in adult rabbits and rabbit pups. Thromb Haemost *79*:1034, 1998.
149. Ling Xu, et al: Alpha 2-macroglobulin remains as important as antithrombin III for thrombin regulation in cord plasma in the presence of endothelial cell surfaces. Pediatr Res *37*:373, 1995.
150. Nash MC, et al: Normal levels of soluble E selectin, soluble intercellular adhesion molecule 1 (sICAM-1), and soluble vascular adhesion molecule (sVCAM-1) decrease with age. Clin Exp Immunol *103*:167, 1996.
151. Cheung PY, et al: Nitric oxide and platelet function: implications for neonatology. Semin Perinatol *21*:409, 1997.
152. Pearce WJ, Longo LD: Developmental aspects of endothelial function. Semin Perinatol *15*:40, 1991.
153. Cox RH, et al: Mechanics and electrolyte composition of arterial smooth muscle in developing dogs. Am J Physiol *231*:77, 1976.
154. Cayette AJ, et al: Morphological and smooth muscle phenotypic changes in fetal rabbit aorta during early development. Basic Res Cardiol *84*:259, 1989.
155. Kisker CT: The animal models for hemorrhage and thrombosis in the neonate. Thromb Haemostas *57*:118, 1987.
156. Goddard J, et al: Intraventricular hemorrhage—an animal model. Biol Neonate *37*:39, 1980.
157. Hogan KA, et al: Mouse models in coagulation. Thromb Haemost *87*:563, 2002.
158. Bugge TH, et al: Fetal embryonic bleeding events in mice lacking tissue factor, the cell-associated initiator of blood coagulation. Proc Natl Acad Sci U S A *93*:6258, 1996.
159. Toomey JR, et al: Targeted disruption of the murine tissue factor gene results in embryonic lethality. Blood *88*:1583, 1996.
160. Carmeliet P, et al: Role of tissue factor in embryonic blood vessel development. Nature *383*:73, 1996.
161. Rosen ED, et al: Mice lacking factor VII develop normally but suffer fatal perinatal bleeding. Nature *390*:290, 1997.
162. Malamitsi-Puchner A, et al: Angiogenic factors in the perinatal period: diversity in biological functions reflected in their serum concentrations soon after birth. Ann N Y Acad Sci *900*:169, 2000.
163. Muratore CS, et al: Stretch-induced upregulation of VEGF gene expression in murine pulmonary culture: a role for angiogenesis in lung development. J Pediatr Surg *35*:906, 2000.

J. Nathan Hagstrom

149 Pathophysiology of Bleeding Disorders in the Newborn

NORMAL HEMOSTASIS

The primary function of hemostasis is to prevent hemorrhage at sites of vascular injury. Since the early 1990s, it has become clear that components of the hemostatic system also play major roles in vascular development and participate in inflammation and tissue repair. Traditionally, hemostasis has been conceptualized as a series of steps, or a cascade.[1, 2] The elucidation of the role of Factor VII and tissue factor in the activation of both Factors X and IX[3] and the discovery of tissue factor pathway inhibitor[4] gave rise to a revised model of hemostasis and explained, in part, why severe deficiencies in Factors VIII and IX result in such severe bleeding diatheses.[5] Further elucidation of this system has shown that the process of hemostasis is very complex and includes contributions from the following compartments: (1) the surrounding smooth muscle of the vasculature providing vasconstriction, which is in part mediated by prostaglandins and nitric oxide; (2) the surrounding connective tissue providing tissue factor expression, as well as binding sites for platelets, von Willebrand Factor (vWF), vitronectin, and other proteins; (3) the endothelium, which produces various secreted proteins and cell-membrane surface and integrated proteins; (4) platelets, which contain various proteins and molecules contained in granules that play critical roles in blood hemostasis; (5) other circulating cells of the blood (i.e., red cells and white cells); and finally (6) the plasma-based proteins that provide the regulated generation of thrombin, which enzymatically forms the fibrin clot.[6]

When there is vascular injury, multiple pathways are activated that interact through complex positive and negative feedback loops to cease blood loss while maintaining tissue perfusion. The critical step is thrombin generation, which produces fibrin deposition and activates platelets at the site of injury. With injury, tissue factor is exposed, initiating coagulation. In addition, injury exposes subendothelial collagen and results in platelet adhesion, which is mediated in part by vWF. *Thrombin generation* is the rate-limiting step in hemostasis and is regulated by the inhibition of activated procoagulants by antithrombin and the protein C pathways. *Thrombus formation* is contained by fibrinolysis, with the chief enzyme being plasmin, which is formed from plasminogen by tissue plasminogen activator or urokinase.

When vascular injury has occurred, the first step in hemostasis is vasoconstriction, with the intent to decrease blood flow into the injured blood vessel, thus minimizing blood loss. This vasoconstriction is mediated by multiple factors including prostaglandins and nitric oxide. The second step is platelet adhesion, followed by platelet aggregation; this is referred to as *primary hemostasis*. Thrombocytopenia is often present in ill neonates and potentially impairs primary hemostasis.[7] Data are accumulating that suggest that neonatal platelets are hyporeactive.[8, 9] Neonates normally have increased levels of vWF compared with adults, and this may help to offset the decreased platelet capacity.[10] In addition, the increased hematocrit may also contribute to reduced bleeding with vascular injury because of the greater viscosity.[11]

Levels of coagulation proteins differ in the neonate compared with the adult. Vitamin K–dependent procoagulant (prothrombin and Factors VII, IX, and X) levels are normally lower in neonates compared with children, and children have slightly lower levels compared with adults.[12] The functional levels of these proteins are reduced by warfarin therapy and are especially sensitive to mild liver dysfunction or dietary vitamin K deficiency. Levels of the cofactors (Factors VIII and V) are similar to those in adults. Factor VIII is an acute phase reactant that is often elevated in the neonate. Persistently elevated levels of Factor VIII have been associated with thromboembolic disease.[13,14] Contact factors (Factors XI and XII, high molecular weight kininogen and prekallikrein) are lower in neonates compared with children and adults.[15] *In vitro* studies have shown that thrombin generation in neonatal plasma is decreased compared with adult plasma.[16] A computer model of neonatal hemostasis suggests that thrombin generation *in vivo* should be essentially normal because the low levels of procoagulants are balanced by the low levels of anticoagulants.[17] However, α-macroglobulin levels are increased in the neonate, thereby possibly tipping the balance in favor of decreased thrombin generation.[18] Nevertheless, bleeding is uncommon in the newborn despite significant stress during delivery, a finding suggesting that hemostasis is physiologically balanced in the newborn.

EVALUATION OF THE NEONATE WITH ABNORMAL BLEEDING

Careful collection and synthesis of clinical and laboratory data are imperative when evaluating bleeding in the newborn. The first step is to determine whether the bleeding is abnormal and whether it is a localized or systemic phenomenon. Abnormal bleeding may be related more to the injury itself and may reflect local failure of hemostasis, rather than a systemic flaw in the hemostatic system. Furthermore, what is perceived to be abnormal bleeding may not be abnormal at all, or it may not even be bleeding at all. Maternal blood swallowed at the time of delivery may, to an observer, look like the result of bleeding in the neonate, when in fact no bleeding has occurred. In addition, bruising may occur at the time of delivery that may appear to be outside the norm, but this may be more a product of the position and forces during labor than an abnormality in hemostasis. Bleeding may occur as a result of local invasion of a vascular structure from infection or neoplasia. Vascular anomalies and malformations are prone to localized bleeding.

Once it has been determined that hemostasis may be abnormal and thus requires scrutinizing, one must perform a screening battery of tests, choosing carefully from a wide array of laboratory tools. The sensitivity and specificity of these various tools are less than ideal, especially in the neonate. Abnormal hemostasis may be present, and yet our current laboratory techniques may be inadequate to ascertain the precise abnormality. Nonetheless, the tests available can be useful in most cases (Fig. 149–1).

Clinical Laboratory Evaluation

Microtechniques for maximizing the use of the smaller amounts of plasma obtained from the fetus and newborn have been described.[19] However, most laboratories do not use these techniques on a routine basis. The following tests are used to evaluate hemostasis:

1. Platelet count, mean platelet volume, and platelet morphology: The normal range for the platelet count and the mean platelet volume in the newborn are similar to those in adults.[20] A peripheral smear should always be reviewed to confirm thrombocytopenia because platelet clumping may give falsely low values. Blood sampled from neonates often contains thrombin as a result of early activation of coagulation from either heel stick (tissue injury) or difficult venipuncture (slow draw). Thrombin is a potent platelet agonist, and a small amount of thrombin in the sample could cause platelet clumping. The presence of large platelets may indicate one of the inherited thrombocytopenias associated with large platelets, such as Bernard-Soulier disease or May-Hegglin anomaly, or increased destruction with increased production of new, large platelets.

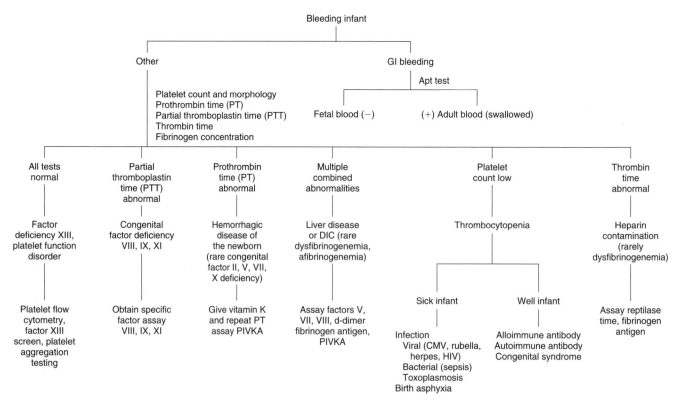

Figure 149–1. Flow diagram for evaluation of a bleeding newborn.

2. Bleeding time: The bleeding time lacks sensitivity and specificity for predicting risk of bleeding. It has limited practical use in neonates. The bleeding time can be difficult to perform with any meaningful accuracy or precision. The bleeding time can be shortened in the neonate because of the large red cell size[21] and the increased amount of vWF.[22, 23] However, platelet function in the neonate is probably decreased compared with older children and adults, as seen in studies using flow cytometry.[24] Therefore, the sensitivity and specificity of the bleeding time are especially poor in the neonate. The ability to predict risk of bleeding with this test is marginal. The bleeding time is discussed again in the section on qualitative platelet disorders.

3. PFA-100: This is a method for measuring an *in vitro* "bleeding time" on a small volume of whole blood.[25, 26] As blood is passed through an aperture lined with collagen/adenosine diphosphate or collagen/epinephrine, a platelet plug forms, obstructing blood flow, which results in a closure time. The hematocrit and leukocyte count are inversely correlated with the closure time. PFA-100 is very sensitive to even mild thrombocytopenia.[23] Its clinical usefulness in newborns is unknown.

4. Platelet aggregation testing: Because of the volume of blood required for platelet aggregation testing on platelet-rich plasma in response to agonists, this type of testing is rarely done during the newborn period. However, whole blood platelet aggregation testing is now widely available, and protocols exist that use small amounts of blood, therefore making platelet aggregation testing in neonates possible.[27]

5. Platelet flow cytometry: This has been used to measure platelet reactivity.[24] Flow cytometry techniques can be used to measure platelet function as well.[28]

6. vWF assays: vWF levels are elevated in neonates compared with adults. Severe vWF deficiency is uncommon, but it should be considered in someone with mild to moderate Factor VIII deficiency who has significant mucocutaneous bleeding.

7. Prothrombin time (PT): The PT is performed by adding an excess of tissue factor and calcium, and it does not reflect normal physiology; nonetheless, it can be useful in assessing hemostasis. The PT is elevated in the neonate compared with adults with a wider range of normal. However, it remains useful for assessing liver disease and disseminated intravascular coagulation (DIC). The PT is especially sensitive to deficiencies in Factors VII and II. It may also be elevated in combined mild factor deficiencies involving Factors II, VII, and X, which may be seen in mild liver dysfunction, mild vitamin K deficiency, or early DIC. The PT is less sensitive to heparin and to the presence of a lupus anticoagulant compared with the activated partial thromboplastin time (aPTT), but the PT can be prolonged when these two substances are present in high concentrations.

8. aPTT: The aPTT is performed by activating the contact system, which is not essential for maintaining hemostasis *in vivo*, and therefore does not reflect true physiology. Despite this, the PTT remains useful for detecting deficiencies in Factors VIII, IX, XI and vWF. With the PT, the aPTT assists in evaluating the common pathway (Factors II, V, X, and fibrinogen). Elevations in the PTT may be related to heparin , the presence of a lupus anticoagulant, a factor deficiency, or factor inhibitor. In the neonate, the PTT is significantly elevated and has a wide normal range. This limits its use as a tool for assessing hemostasis in the neonate.

9. Thrombin time: The thrombin time is elevated in hypofibrinogenemia and is very sensitive to the presence of heparin; therefore, it is a rapid way to screen for heparin contamination in samples drawn from a central venous catheter. The thrombin time is essentially normal in the neonate. Therefore, it can be a useful tool. Subtle fibrinogen dysfunction may be present in the neonate as a result of increased sialic acid content.[29] However, there is no evidence that this subtle difference in structure and function is clinically relevant. The reptilase time can be useful in evaluating for dysfunctional fibrinogen and is not affected by heparin.

10. Factor assays: These tests are performed by adding diluted plasma to factor deficient plasma and then performing a PT- or PTT-based clotting assay. The results are compared with a standard curve. Factor assays are helpful when evaluating an elevated PT or PTT.

11. Factor XIII deficiency screen: This test is performed using the urea clot solubility test. Severe deficiency must be present for this screening test to be positive. A quantitative test for Factor XIII is not commercially available.

12. Thromboelastogram: The Sonolcot analyzer has been used to assess whole blood clotting *in vitro*. Specifically, it has been used to assist in determining hypocoagulability or hypercoagulability for the purpose of determining transfusion parameters and concentration of heparin in fluids running through indwelling catheters. However, no data are available to validate its use in neonates. There are few published reports using the thromboelastogram in neonates.[30]

Limitations of the Clinical Laboratory

Hathaway described the limitations of blood sampling in the neonate for the purposes of assessing coagulation.[31] The volume of blood available for testing is limited in the newborn and fetus. Therefore, careful consideration must be given to which tests are performed, prioritizing the tests using clinical, laboratory, and epidemiologic data. The dynamic nature of the developing neonatal hemostatic system makes interpretation of certain coagulation tests difficult. For example, the vitamin K–dependent proteins (Factors II, VII, IX, and X and proteins C and S) are low in the fetus and newborn, with a wide range of normal values. In addition, the levels of these factors increase with time after birth.

Methods for collecting and processing the blood sample to be analyzed will affect the result of the assay performed. Blood is often collected from indwelling catheters. Plasma samples drawn from an indwelling catheter may contain heparin and therefore give erroneous results for clotting-based tests.[32] It is recommended that, when drawing samples from catheters, a validated "discard" volume protocol be used or the sample be treated with heparinase I (Hepzyme) before performing any clotting-based assays. Samples drawn for the purposes of monitoring heparin therapy or for measuring heparin levels may need to be drawn peripherally. Venipuncture is technically difficult in newborns, and often an adequate amount of free-flowing blood cannot be obtained. The tissue injury that occurs with difficult venipunctures can introduce tissue factor into the specimen. The actual amount of plasma collected depends on the hematocrit, which is significantly increased in newborns (Fig. 149–2). The higher the hematocrit, the higher are the chances that the sodium citrate anticoagulant will interfere with the clotting-based assays. The amount of anticoagulant should be corrected for the higher hematocrits in newborns, which decreases the yield of plasma making the standard 1:10 ratio of citrate to whole blood excessive. The appropriate adjustment of anticoagulant to maintain a proper ratio has been described.[33] In certain instances, blood samples are taken from the umbilical cord at the time of delivery. This is best achieved by double clamping a segment of the cord and obtaining the specimen immediately after delivery. The blood in the umbilical cord often shows signs of thrombin generation and platelet activation, which likely occurred after delivery and thus does not reflect *in vivo* activation. This activation can affect the results of clotting-based assays.

Assessing the Risk of Hemorrhagic Complications

Many tests are available for evaluating hemostasis (see earlier). However, no one test can accurately characterize a patient's risk of bleeding. To assess the risk of bleeding fully, one must consider the pertinent clinical history, physical examination findings, and laboratory results together. In the neonate, the presence of conditions such as prematurity, sepsis, and asphyxia may increase the risk of bleeding. Liver dysfunction, malnutrition, renal insufficiency, and cholestasis can be associated with bleeding complications. Certain fungal and bacterial infections can be associated with severe bleeding secondary to invasion of blood vessels (e.g., aspergillosis, *Pseudomonas* infection).

Initially, a complete blood count with platelet count, PT, aPTT, and thrombin time are performed. However, these screening tests will not detect Factor XIII deficiency, α_2-antiplasmin deficiency, plasminogen activator inhibitor-1 deficiency, collagen vascular disorders such as Ehlers-Danlos syndrome, or most qualitative platelet disorders. Fortunately, most of these inherited bleeding disorders are extremely rare. Given the many factors that can affect the foregoing screening tests, the results must be interpreted in the context of the clinical history and condition of the infant (Table 149-1). There are multiple treatment options for the bleeding neonate, which can be targeted to specific abnormalities in hemostasis (Table 149-2). However, there are times when empiric therapy needs to be initiated before a definitive diagnosis can be made. Plasma, platelets, and Novoseven (recombinant Factor VIIa) are useful for empiric therapy.

INHERITED COAGULATION FACTOR DEFICIENCIES

Hemophilia

An isolated elevation in the aPTT in an otherwise well neonate with symptoms and signs of bleeding may be indicative of hemophilia. There are three types of hemophilia: A (Factor VIII deficiency), B (Factor IX deficiency), and C (Factor XI deficiency). Hemophilia A has an incidence of 1 per 5000 live births, which is six times more prevalent than the incidence of hemophilia B, at 1 per 30,000 live births.[34] Hemophilia C is even less common, with an incidence of 1 per 1 million births.[34] A family history of bleeding is present in 50 to 75% of boys diagnosed with hemophilia. A diagnosis of severe hemophilia can be made from cord blood if it is collected and placed into anticoagulant quickly after delivery. The diagnosis can also be made prenatally with percutaneous cord blood sampling,[35] but this carries substantial risk, and the empiric administration of recombinant factor concentrate is necessary. Carrier testing is best done using DNA analysis techniques. Factor levels in carriers vary considerably and are often normal. Prenatal testing can be done by using polymerase chain reaction techniques for restriction fragment length polymorphisms or sequencing for a known mutation using DNA obtained from chorionic villous sampling or amniocentesis.

The genes for Factors VIII and IX are found on the X chromosome, and the gene for Factor XI is found on chromosome 4. Factor VIII is a large glycoprotein that, when activated by thrombin, becomes a cofactor for activated Factor IX (FIXa). This complex activates Factor X, which then converts prothrombin to thrombin.[36] Factor XI,, after undergoing cleavage by thrombin, activates Factor IX.

A male infant with abnormal bleeding who has an elevated PTT, a normal platelet count, a normal PT time, and a normal thrombin time should be evaluated for Factor VIII deficiency (hemophilia A) or Factor IX deficiency (hemophilia B). Because both hemophilia A

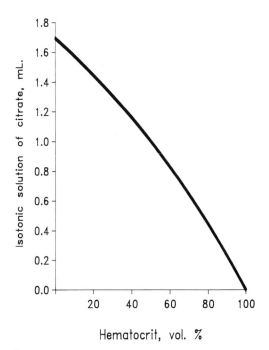

Figure 149-2. Nomogram for the amount of anticoagulant to add based on the hematocrit to achieve a constant ratio of anticoagulant to plasma. (Data from Risau W: Embryonic angiogenesis factors. Pharmacotherapy *51*:371, 1991.)

and B are X-linked, both are extremely uncommon in female infants. However, cases of hemophilia A and B, including severe deficiencies, have been described in phenotypical females. Factor XI deficiency, an autosomal recessive disorder, is a less severe bleeding disorder, but it should still be considered in any neonate with abnormal bleeding who has an isolated elevated PTT.[37]

In a large retrospective review of 192 patients with Factor VIII or IX deficiency, only 9 infants experienced significant bleeding during the first week of life.[38] Schulman found that less than half the infants with severe Factor VIII or IX deficiency had hemorrhagic symptoms during the first week of life, and fewer than 10% of patients with mild hemophilia had bleeding.[39]

Bleeding associated with circumcision is common in boys with hemophilia. In one series, 30 of 94 infants with hemophilia A or B had bleeding associated with circumcision.[40] In 20 patients with severe hemophilia, 10 had bleeding after circumcision, and of 16 with mild or moderate hemophilia, 2 had bleeding with circumcision.[41]

Intracranial hemorrhage (ICH) is rare in neonates with hemophilia. In a survey of German hemophilia treatment centers, 30 of 744 male patients with hemophilia (4.0%) were reported to have had ICH as neonates.[42] There was no significant difference in the prevalence of ICH in those patients with hemophilia A versus B (3.5% versus 6.3%). Bleeding was diagnosed within 1 week of birth in 11 of 27 patients (41%). The most important factor was trauma (17 of 30 = 57%), either during birth (9 of 30 = 30%) or later in life (8 of 30 = 27%). Seizures were common, occurring in 19 of 30 patients (63%). A review by Kulkarni and Lusher[43] found 102 newborns with hemophilia and ICH described in 33 publications.[44] The cumulative incidence of ICH and extracranial hemorrhage was 3.58% in five studies that reported the total newborn population or examined birth records.

The proper perinatal management of a pregnancy suspected of being or known to be affected by hemophilia has not been evaluated in a prospective randomized trial. Practice varies considerably.[45] Cesarean section is not recommended for the purposes of preventing ICH hemorrhage.[46,47]

TABLE 149-1

Test Interpretation for Bleeding Disorders

	Screening Tests			Differential Diagnosis	
Platelet Count	Prothrombin Time	*Partial Thromboplastin Time*	*Thrombin Time*	*Ill-Appearing Neonate*	*Healthy Neonate*
Normal	Normal	Normal	Normal	Localized failure of hemostasis	Rare inherited bleeding disorder
Decreased	Normal	Normal	Normal	Mild DIC, thrombosis, (see Table 149-4)	Maternal immune thrombocytopenic purpura, alloimmune thrombocytopenia (see Table 149-4)
Normal	Increased	Normal	Normal	Mild liver dysfunction, Mild DIC	Mild vitamin K deficiency, mild DIC
Normal	Normal	Increased	Normal	Mild DIC	Factor VIII, IX, or XI deficiency
Normal	Normal	Normal	Increased	Mild DIC, heparin contamination	Mild hypofibrinogenemia, Dysfibrinogenemia
Normal	Increased	Increased	Increased	DIC, Liver failure	Severe hypofibrinogenemia
Normal	Increased	Increased	Normal	DIC, Liver failure	Severe vitamin K deficiency, Factor II, X, or V deficiency
Decreased	Increased	Increased	Increased	DIC, Liver failure	

DIC = disseminated intravascular coagulation.

TABLE 149-2

Treatment of Bleeding Disorders

	Dose According to Severity of Bleeding		
Treatment	*Mild*	*Moderate*	*Severe*
Platelets	0.1 U/kg	0.2 U/kg	Continuous infusion
Plasma (fresh frozen)	10-20 ml/kg x1	10-20 cc/kg q6h	Continuous infusion
Cryoprecipitate	1 bag	1 bag	1 bag
Aminocaproic acid	100 mg/kg IV/PO	100 mg/kg q6h	Continuous infusion
Desmopressin	0.3 µg/kg		
Novoseven		10-60 µg/kg	60-90 µg/kg q2h (higher doses have been used)
Prothrombin complex concentrates			50 U/kg
Vitamin K$_1$	1-2.5 mg PO QD	1-5 mg SC (0.1 mg/kg)	1-5 mg IV (0.1 mg/kg)
Protamine		1 mg for every 100 U of heparin	
Aprotinin			4 mg/kg

The severity of bleeding and thus the age of onset of symptoms are variable among patients with severe hemophilia. This is in part the result of other genetic modifying factors, such as common prothrombotic polymorphisms.[48] However, the reason that more bleeding complications do not occur in neonates with hemophilia during the birthing process is not entirely clear.

Inhibitor (antibody) formation to the missing factor is one of the most serious complications of hemophilia. Inhibitors can develop in the newborn period after exposure to factor concentrate, but this is unusual.[49] Acquired Factor VIII deficiency can occur during pregnancy associated with the development of autoantibodies to Factor VIII. These autoantibodies can cross the placenta and can result in acquired hemophilia in the newborn.[50]

Once a neonate has been identified as having hemophilia, it is recommended that an ultrasound examination of the head be performed before discharge. Circumcision is not recommended.[47]

Factor replacement therapy should be carried out with recombinant product if available. Plasma-derived monoclonal purified viral inactivated product is a safe alternative. Plasma should be used only if factor concentrates are not available (Table 149-3).

Deficiencies in Factors II, V, and X

Severe deficiencies in Factors II, V, and X have been well described and may present in the neonatal period. Increases in both the PT and PTT is present in all three of these factor deficiencies. Inherited combined factor deficiencies have also been described that result in this laboratory profile (see later). The thrombin time is normal in these rare factor deficiencies.

Severe Factor V deficiency may present in the perinatal period with ICH.[51] Soft tissue and umbilical stump bleeding may also occur. I have a patient who presented as an infant with severe

TABLE 149-3

Treatment of Hemophilia and Related Disorders

Clinical Disorder	Hemostatic Test	Treatment
Hemophilia A (Factor VIII deficiency)	↑ PTT, ↓ Factor VIII	Recombinant Factor VIII (Refacto, Helixate FS, Kogenate FS, Recombinate)
Hemophilia B (Factor IX deficiency)	↑ PTT, ↓ Factor IX	Recombinant Factor IX (Benefix)
Hemophilia C (Factor XI deficiency)	↑ PTT, ↓ Factor XI	FFP (plasma)
Factor VII deficiency	↑ PT, ↓ Factor VII	Novoseven (recombinant Factor VIIa)
Other rare inherited factor deficiencies		FFP (plasma)
Factor XIII deficiency	Urea clot solubility test or Factor XIII screen abnormal	Cryoprecipitate, FFP, Fibrogammin
Hypofibrinogenemia	↑ TT, ↓ Fibrinogen	Cryoprecipitate
Severe thrombocytopenia	↓ Platelet count	Platelet transfusion. If no response, consider using aminocaproic acid, desmopressin, or Novoseven (rFVIIa)
Liver dysfunction	↑PT, ±↑PTT, ↓Factors II, V, VII, IX, and X	FFP. Novoseven. Platelet transfusions
Vitamin K deficiency	↑PT, ± ↑PTT, ↓Factors II, VII, IX, and X	Vitamin K, prothrombin complex concentrate (Autoplex, FEIBA), FFP
Disseminated intravascular coagulation	↑PT, ↑PTT, ↑TT, ↑D-dimers, Factors II, V, VII, VIII, IX, and X, fibrinogen	FFP, platelet transfusion, cryoprecipitate, Novoseven, heparin, antithrombin (Thrombate), APC (recombinant activated protein C)

FFP = fresh frozen plasma; PT = prothrombin time; PTT = partial thromboplastin time; TT = thrombin time.

paraspinal and epidural bleeding with spinal cord compression after a lumbar puncture. Plasma transfusions are the primary treatment for severe Factor V deficiency.[52] Platelet transfusions may also be helpful in cases of refractory bleeding.

Severe Factor II deficiency may present in the neonatal period with ICH or gastrointestinal bleeding.[53, 54] Treatment options include prothrombin complex concentrates and plasma.

Severe Factor X deficiency may also present with ICH as well as umbilical stump and gastrointestinal bleeding.[55,56] Plasma and prothrombin complex concentrates may also be used for this factor deficiency.

Factor XIII Deficiency

Factor XIII deficiency is extremely rare but can present as severe bleeding in the neonatal period. Umbilical stump bleeding is common.[57] Poor wound healing is a feature of Factor XIII deficiency.[58] ICH is more common in severe Factor XIII deficiency than other factor deficiencies.[59] Factor XIII is a plasma transglutaminase, which cross-links fibrin. Various missense and nonsense mutations, and deletions or insertions with or without out-of-frame shift or premature termination and splicing abnormalities have been identified in the genes for A and B subunits in Factor XIII deficiency.[60] The most common test available to screen for Factor XIII deficiency is the urea clot solubility test. The PT, aPTT, thrombin time, and fibrinogen are all normal in this disease.

Other Inherited Bleeding Disorders

The most common human bleeding disorder described is von Willebrand disease (vWD), and it has been reviewed in the literature.[61] There are three major types—1, 2, and 3—with type 1 by far the most common. It is unusual for type 1 or type 2 vWD to present in the neonatal period. However, type 3 vWD may present with mucocutaneous bleeding. This type of vWD is associated with mild to moderate Factor VIII deficiency and complete absence of vWF. To evaluate for vWD, the following tests should be performed: Factor VIII activity, vWF antigen, vWF ristocetin cofactor activity, and vWF multimers.

Inherited deficiencies of plasminogen activator inhibitor-1,[62] α_2-antiplasmin,[63] and Factor VII[64] are autosomal recessive and extremely rare but can result in severe bleeding. ICH in the newborn period has been reported in severe Factor VII deficiency.[64, 65] The PT is significantly elevated in severe Factor VII deficiency, and the PTT is normal. Plasminogen activator inhibitor-1 and α_2-antiplasmin deficiencies can be screened for by using the euglobulin clot lysis time.[62] The PT, aPTT, and thrombin time are normal in these rare factor deficiencies. Severe deficiencies of prekallikrein, high molecular weight kininogen, and Factor XII do not result in bleeding.

Combined Factor Deficiencies

Combined deficiency of Factors V and VIII resulting from an autosomal recessive defect in the ERGIC-53 protein[66] has been well described and results in a severe bleeding diathesis.[67] Combined deficiency of the vitamin K–dependent factors has been described,[68] and in most cases the combined deficiency is the result of a defect in the γ-carboxylation of the glutamic acid residues in the amino-terminal portion of the peptide. Mutations in the carboxylase gene have been linked to defects in carboxylation.[69, 70]

VITAMIN K–DEFICIENCY BLEEDING

Severe vitamin K deficiency is present in a significant number of newborns at the time of birth.[71] This is true whether one uses vitamin K levels measured in cord plasma[72] or levels of proteins induced in the absence of vitamin K[73] as the measure of vitamin K deficiency. Vitamin K is necessary for the production of functional key coagulation proteins: procoagulant Factors II, VII, IX, and X and protein Z and anticoagulant proteins C and S. Without vitamin K supplementation at birth, this severe vitamin K deficiency can worsen, especially in breast-fed infants, resulting in bleeding that can be life threatening. The bleeding usually manifests itself 2 to 5 days after birth. The most common site of bleeding is the gastrointestinal tract. This has been referred to as *classic hemorrhagic disease of the newborn* and was first described by Townsend in 1894, who hypothesized that there was an infectious cause and prescribed cow's milk to affected babies with a positive therapeutic response in some patients.[74] The preferred terminology is now *vitamin K–deficiency bleeding*. Professor Sutor proposed a clear and concise definition of this condition in 1995.[75] His definition was endorsed by the International Society on Thrombosis and Haemostasis Pediatric/Perinatal Subcommittee in 1999.[76]

Henrik von Dam and colleagues discovered vitamin K[77] and linked it to hemorrhagic disease of the newborn.[78] As a medical student, he observed subcutaneous and intraperitoneal hemorrhage in chicks fed a fat-free diet.[79] He hypothesized that there was a fat-soluble substance critical for coagulation, which he coined vitamin K. He later linked this vitamin K deficiency to reduced prothrombin activity.[80] Brinkhous and associates showed that hemorrhagic disease of the newborn was associated with a prothrombin level of less than 5%.[81] In a bleeding infant, a prolonged PT, together with a normal fibrinogen level and platelet count, is almost diagnostic of vitamin K–deficiency bleeding; rapid correction of the PT and cessation of bleeding after vitamin K administration are confirmative. The PTT is always elevated in clinically significant vitamin K deficiency and should also correct with administration of vitamin K.

In 1952, von Dam described classic hemorrhagic disease of the newborn in a large study involving 33,000 neonates. He demonstrated that hypoprothrombinemia in newborns was linked to vitamin K deficiency and breast-feeding and was most common on the second to third day of life.[82] There are early and late forms of vitamin K deficiency that are usually associated with underlying maternal or infant factors. Lane and Hathaway described three distinct syndromes associated with vitamin K deficiency in the neonate.[83] *Early hemorrhagic disease of the newborn* occurs in the first 24 hours of life in infants born to mothers taking medications that interfere with vitamin K function such as phenytoin or warfarin. Early hemorrhagic disease can be severe, and ICH is not uncommon. *Classic hemorrhagic disease of the newborn* presents on average around 1 to 7 days of age. With this form, mucocutaneous bleeding is the most common manifestation. *Late hemorrhagic disease of the newborn* occurs at 1 week to 12 months of age, with ICH a common manifestation.[75]

Cord blood levels of vitamin K_1 are significantly lower than maternal levels.[84, 85] This finding suggests an active barrier to vitamin K transport across the placenta. It has been proposed that vitamin K may be harmful to the fetus and that evolution has provided a significant barrier to it to reduce levels in the fetus. This relative vitamin K deficiency in the fetus does not explain why vitamin K–dependent factors are low. Proteins induced by vitamin K absence are found in minimal concentrations, or are totally absent, even in low birth weight infants.[86-88] This would suggest that perhaps the fetus is not functionally vitamin K deficient. In fact, vitamin K levels in neonates do not appear to correlate with the presence of proteins induced by vitamin K.[88] Some evidence suggests that hepatic cycling of vitamin K may be inefficient late in gestation.[88]

The extremely low levels of vitamin K in cord blood and the large gradient that exists across the placental barrier suggest that vitamin K may be toxic to the fetus. One explanation is that vitamin K increases phase I metabolism of xenobiotics such as benzopyrene creating benzopyrene/DNA adducts that damage DNA.[89] A study by Israels and colleagues showed that vitamin K could promote chromosomal damage in the developing fetus.[90] Cornelissen and associates could not demonstrate such an effect.[91] Data from Great Britain suggested that the use of large doses of parenteral vitamin K in the newborn increased the risk of childhood leukemia.[92] A large retrospective epidemiologic study performed in the United States failed to show a strong link between vitamin K supplementation in the newborn and childhood leukemia.[93] Nonetheless, a small increase in the risk of leukemia from parenteral vitamin K is difficult to disprove.[94]

Vitamin K_1, a phylloquinone, is the only homologue of vitamin K synthesized by plants. The vitamin K_2 homologues, known as menaquinones, are synthesized by bacteria commonly found in the intestinal tract (Fig. 149-3). These homologues contain unsaturated side chains differing in the number of isoprenyl units. The structural differences in these homologues are depicted in Figure 149-3. Vitamin K is a fat-soluble vitamin and may be malabsorbed if there is liver or pancreatic dysfunction.

Vitamin K is necessary for the posttranslational modifications of procoagulants Factors II, VII, IX, and X and protein Z and the anticoagulants proteins C and S.[95] Protein Z is also involved in coagulation, because its function seems to be the fixation of thrombin to the site of injury.[96] Vitamin K is a cofactor for γ-glutamylcarboxylase, an endoplasmic enzyme involved in the posttranslational carboxylation of glutamate residues into γ-carboxyglutamate (Gla) (Fig. 149-4).[97] Vitamin K hydroquinone forms the active coenzyme, the oxidation of which into vitamin

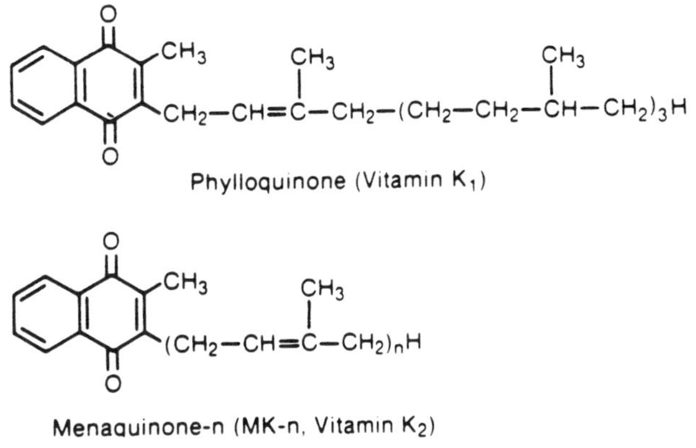

Figure 149–3. Structure of phylloquinone (vitamin K_1) and the menaquinones (vitamin K_2).

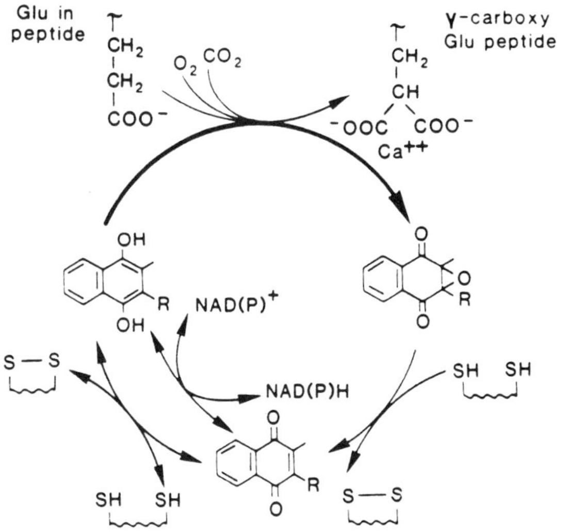

Figure 149–4. Vitamin K metabolism in rat liver microsomes. In addition to the carboxylase/epoxidase system, liver microsomes contain a dithiol-linked quinone reductase and at least two NAD(P)H-linked quinone reductases. It is likely that the two dithiol-linked reductase activities represent the same enzyme or that they share a common subunit. These two activities are strongly inhibited by the 4-hydroxycoumarin anticoagulants. (From Bovill EG, Mann KG: Adv Exp Med Biol *214*:17, 1987.)

K 2,3-epoxide provides the energy to drive the carboxylation reaction.[98] Stenflo was the first to show the presence of Gla residues near the amino terminus of bovine prothrombin.[99] These Gla residues are necessary for proper interaction with calcium and phospholipid surfaces.[100] Vitamin K–dependent coagulation proteins with reduced Gla residues do not undergo the confirmational change on binding of calcium necessary to facilitate binding to a phospholipid surface. Radiograph crystal structure analysis and two-dimensional nuclear magnetic resonance spectroscopy have shown that binding of calcium ions to normal Gla domains causes the coagulation factors to undergo structural changes leading to internalization of the Gla-calcium ion complex in the core of the protein and exposure of the phospholipid-binding domain.[101]

Prevention of hemorrhagic disease of the newborn with prophylactic vitamin K administration shortly after birth has been recommended by the American Academy of Pediatrics since 1961.[102] The most widely used regimen is to administer intramuscular vitamin K_1 shortly after birth at a dose of 1 mg; 0.5 mg is also used. Oral supplementation has also been extensively used in Europe and Japan. However, oral supplementation has not been protective against late hemorrhagic disease of infancy. The pharmacokinetics of vitamin K_1 is markedly different when it is given intramuscularly versus orally, with levels after an oral dose falling to baseline much sooner than after an intramuscular dose.[103, 104] Daily oral supplementation of 25 μg of vitamin K after a 1-mg dose at birth in breast-fed infants is probably equivalent to the single parenteral administration at birth.[105] Maternal supplementation has also been explored as an option for preventing vitamin K–deficiency bleeding in the infant.[106] Vitamin K_1 supplementation is not associated with a hypercoagulable state and therefore is safe in pregnant and postpartum women.[104]

LIVER DISEASE

Coagulopathy may be associated with liver disease. Liver dysfunction is associated with a decrease in the production of many proteins, including proteins involved in coagulation. The levels of both procoagulants and anticoagulants may be reduced, creating an imbalance that could result in either a bleeding diathesis or a prothrombotic state. The vitamin K–dependent factors are significantly reduced and are among the first to be affected in acute liver failure. Thus, elevation in the PT is often the first evidence of liver dysfunction. Because Factor VII has a short half-life of approximately 6 hours, its levels drop quickly after the onset of acute hepatic damage. However, the vitamin K factors are lower in the neonate compared with the adult, and the normal range is rather wide. Therefore, it may be more useful to rely on other factor levels to determine hepatic synthetic capacity.

The measurements of Factors V and VIII are helpful in the evaluation of liver disease. The level of Factor V in the neonate is equivalent to that of the adult. Factor V is synthesized by the liver and is not dependent on vitamin K. Therefore, in the absence of DIC, low Factor V levels could be indicative of poor hepatic function. Factor VIII levels are also equivalent to adult levels, and its synthesis is also not dependent on vitamin K. However, it is primarily synthesized by the endothelial cell and is not decreased in liver failure. Thus, in the presence of decreased Factor V activity, decreased Factor VIII activity suggests consumption, whereas a normal Factor VIII level suggests diminished production of Factor V by the liver.

Fibrinogen is one of the last proteins to be reduced in liver failure. It is also reduced in DIC. Because the degradation products of fibrin and fibrinogen are cleared by the liver, the D-dimer and fibrin split products may be elevated in liver disease in the absence of DIC.

Cholestatic liver disease can lead to vitamin K deficiency, which may result in a hemorrhagic diathesis. However, with the nearly universal employment of parenteral vitamin K supplementation at birth, this complication of cholestatic liver disease is unusual in the first month of life.

Hereditary tyrosinemia presenting during early infancy can be associated with significant coagulopathy in the absence of overt signs of liver disease.[107] Tyrosinemia type 1 is an inherited metabolic disorder attributable to deficiency of fumarylacetoacetate hydrolase, a terminal enzyme in the degradation pathway of tyrosine. Hemophagocytic lymphohistiocytosis or familial erythrophagocytic lymphohistiocytic syndrome may present in early infancy and is associated with coagulopathy, with hypofibrinogenemia a consistent finding.

Mild to moderate thrombocytopenia may be seen in liver disease as a result of hypersplenism.[108, 109] In addition, platelet dysfunction has been described in liver disease.[110-112]

The perinatal form of acute liver failure may be secondary to perinatally acquired viral infections, including infections with echovirus, herpesvirus, and various enterovirus subtypes. Liver injury that begins *in utero* may present in the neonatal period as chronic hepatic insufficiency, for which there may be little evidence of acute liver injury at the time of birth. The findings of coagulopathy and hyperbilirubinemia in an infant with hypoalbuminemia, ascites, or splenomegaly should suggest to the clinician hepatic failure, with neonatal hemochromatosis as a commonly recognized cause.[113]

INTRACRANIAL HEMORRHAGE

Many different pathophysiologic processes can lead to ICH in the neonate. Intraventricular hemorrhage (IVH) seen in the premature infant is the result of a complex interaction of multiple factors, including local and systemic vascular factors, brain tissue milieu, and hemostatic factors. ICH in the full-term infant may be related to an underlying bleeding disorder, but it may also be a hemorrhagic transformation of an ischemic infarct from thromboembolic disease. In addition, ICH may result from vascular malformations or trauma.

Compromised hemostasis has been proposed as a contributing factor in intraventicular hemorrhage of prematurity. In infants weighing less than 1500 g, the incidence, severity, and adverse neurologic sequelae of ICH are increased in infants with platelet counts of fewer than 100,000 μL than in an age-, weight-, and disease-matched cohort.[114] McDonald and colleagues observed hypofibrinogenemia, thrombocytopenia, or prolonged clotting time in 11 of 15 infants with IVH and in only 5 of 35 with no IVH.[115]

Poorly controlled cerebral circulation, perhaps caused by excessive production of nitric oxide, has been suggested as a contributing factor to IVH in the premature neonate. Van Bel and associates[116] hypothesized that increased plasma levels of cyclic guanosine monophosphate (cGMP) resulting in endogenous vasodilatory nitric oxide production contributed to IVH. In 83 consecutively admitted preterm neonates, nitric oxide production was assessed by measuring serial plasma cGMP levels. Serial cranial ultrasound investigations were also performed. The investigators showed that 60 neonates (72%) had no IVH, 18 neonates (22%) had mild to moderate IVH, and 5 neonates (6%) had severe IVH. At 48 and 72 hours of age, cGMP levels of infants with severe IVH were significantly higher than those of infants with no or only mild IVH. Thus, increased cGMP levels are associated with the development of IVH, and vasodilatory nitric oxide–induced impairment of cerebral autoregulation is part of the pathophysiology that leads to IVH.[116] The use of heparin to maintain the patency of indwelling catheters does not appear to increase the risk of ICH in premature infants.[117]

Hemorrhage is a frequent and often serious complication associated with the use of extracorporeal membrane oxygenation (ECMO).[118] ICH is common[119] and can lead to significant long-term morbidity.[120] McManus and associates demonstrated that critically ill infants receiving ECMO often have extensive coagulation factor deficiencies that persist despite using plasma in the priming protocol.[121] In one study, infants treated with ECMO who had ICH required more frequent platelet transfusions and had difficulty maintaining activated clotting times within a normal range.[122]

The origin of IVH may include initially venous infarction followed by hemorrhagic transformation. In a study of 22 infants (gestational age, 24.3 to 39.9 weeks; median, 28.0 weeks) with Grades II to IV IVH, four (18%) were heterozygous for Factor V Leiden versus 3% of a control group without IVH. The odds ratio for being heterozygous for Factor V Leiden for patients with IVH was 5.9 (95% CI, 1.7 to 20.3) and for patients without IVH was 0.9 (95% CI, 0.1 to 7.6).[123]

Cerebellar hemorrhage has been reported in neonates with organic acidemias.[124] Methylmalonic, propionic, and isovaleric acidemias have all been associated with ICH resulting in death.

QUALITATIVE PLATELET DISORDERS

Qualitative platelet disorders that result in severe bleeding are rare. The two most notable inherited qualitative platelet disorders are Bernard-Soulier syndrome and Glanzmann thrombasthenia. They are the most severe of the qualitative platelet disorders and have been described both clinically and on a molecular level.[125] Although it is rare for an inherited qualitative platelet disorder to present in the neonatal period, it is important to consider these disorders if a neonate is having mucocutaneous bleeding but has a normal platelet count and a normal coagulation screening profile. Certain medical conditions and therapeutic agents may result in altered platelet function. Maternal low-dose aspirin used in high-risk pregnancies does not appear to alter fetal platelet function significantly.[126] However, there have been cases of severe hemorrhage in neonates born to mothers taking aspirin.[127] Nitric oxide has been shown to inhibit platelet adhesion, aggregation, and stimulate disaggregation of preformed platelet aggregates. An inhibition of platelet function, resulting in a prolonged bleeding time, has been shown in adults receiving inhaled nitric oxide. It has been recommended that careful attention be given to maintaining an adequate hemostasis profile in neonates receiving nitric oxide.[128]

The bleeding time has been used for years as a tool to screen for platelet dysfunction.[129] Unfortunately, its poor sensitivity and specificity, coupled with its poor reproducibility and labor-intensive methodology, requiring experienced and specially trained personnel have made it an impractical tool in the clinical setting.[130, 131] An elevated bleeding time does not offer any more information than good clinical suspicion. The bleeding time has been used in neonates extensively, but no data have been produced that support its regular use in the neonatal population. An abnormal bleeding time neither offers the clinician a specific diagnosis nor suggests the appropriate treatment. No data suggest that an elevated bleeding time in the neonate predicts the risk of bleeding. Nevertheless, the neonatologist must be prepared to confront the rare case of a qualitative platelet disorder in the neonate. The observation that a standard small heel incision done for the purpose of obtaining a capillary sample bleeds excessively should suggest that perhaps a bleeding disorder is present. If the complete blood count and coagulation screening tests are normal, then an evaluation for a qualitative platelet disorder should be considered. The various tools available include platelet morphology, platelet aggregation studies, flow cytometry, and electron microscopy. Platelet aggregation is likely to be the most useful of these tests, but is technically challenging to do in the neonate, and there are few data available to evaluate its use in this patient population.

THROMBOCYTOPENIA

Thrombocytopenia is uncommon in the well neonate. In one study, thrombocytopenia was detected in 64 of 9142 consecutive cord blood samples of neonates born to mothers without thrombocytopenia, for a prevalence of 0.7%.[132] In a similar study that did not exclude mothers with a history of thrombocytopenia, the prevalence was 0.9%.[133] In the largest study to date of platelet counts on consecutive cord blood samples, the prevalence of signficant thrombocytopenia (platelet count <50,000) was 0.12%.[134]

Bleeding from thrombocytopenia is uncommon in the neonate. Even with severe thrombocytopenia, serious bleeding usually does not occur. Nevertheless, thrombocytopenia is frequently encountered in neonates admitted to the neonatal intensive care unit because of the universal use of the complete blood count to screen for disease. Severe thrombocytopenia is rare in the newborn, but mild to moderate thrombocytopenia is common in the ill neonate. Castle and colleagues found that thrombocytopenia developed in 22% of 802 consecutive infants admitted to an intensive care unit.[135] Mehta and associates found that 80% of sick full-term infants had thrombocytopenia, compared with only 22% of healthy newborns.[136]

Mild thrombocytopenia (platelet count of 50,000 to 150,000) is likely to be a secondary phenomenon associated with an underlying illness such as infection, thrombosis, maternal hypertension, or asphyxia. Severe thrombocytopenia is more likely to be associated with a primary disorder of platelet quantity. However, severe thrombocytopenia can be seen in sepsis and thrombosis.

The differential diagnosis of thrombocytopenia in the neonate can be found in Table 149-4. Most of these disorders can be classified by mechanism: increased consumption, decreased production, and sequestration.[137] However, direct proof linking one of these mechanisms to the various secondary thrombocytopenias is somewhat lacking. Often, a combination of these mechanisms may be present. Blanchette and Rand recommended an approach to thrombocytopenia in the neonate (see Fig. 149-1).[138]

Mehta and associates performed a large study that showed the prevalence of thrombocytopenia in neonates admitted to the neonatal intensive care unit to be 35%.[136] These investigators were able to determine a cause in 60% of those patients. They concluded, based on minimal changes in the mean platelet volumes in the majority of patients and decreased megakaryocytes in the bone marrow of 14 of their subjects at autopsy, that poor production contributes significantly to thrombocytopenia in this population. However, in a large series, thrombocytopenia in the sick neonate was concluded to be secondary to increased platelet destruction, as evidenced by decreased indium-111 oxide–labeled platelet survival, increased mean platelet volume, normal or increased numbers of bone marrow megakaryocytes, and decreased survival of transfused platelets.[135]

Primary Thrombocytopenias

The most common primary thrombocytopenia to be diagnosed in the delivery room, even before a platelet count has been measured, is thrombocytopenia–absent radius syndrome (TAR syndrome). In TAR syndrome, the thrombocytopenia is present at birth and is associated with skeletal anomalies of the radius but not the thumb.[139] The thrombocytopenia is most pronounced in the neonatal period and early infancy, and it tends to improve during the first year of life.[140] A leukemoid reaction may be present at times, especially in early infancy. Homans and colleagues demonstrated, using *in vitro* studies, that the megakaryocyte progenitor cell is defective in patients with TAR syndrome, with elevated levels of plasma thrombopoietic activity presumed to be thrombopoietin.[141]

TABLE 149-4

Differential Diagnosis of Thrombocytopenia

Well Infant

Increased Consumption	Decreased Production	Mixed
Neonatal alloimmune thrombocytopenia	Thrombocytopenia–absent radius syndrome	Maternal preeclampsia
Maternal autoimmune thrombocytopenia	Fanconi anemia	Giant platelet syndromes
Phototherapy	Wiskott-Aldrich syndrome	May-Hegglin anomaly
Type 2B von Willebrand disease	X-linked thrombocytopenia	Bernard-Soulier syndrome
	Congenital amegakaryocytic thrombocytopenia	Maternal drugs
	Alport syndrome	
	Congenital aplastic anemia	

Sick Infant

Increased Consumption	Decreased Production	Mixed
Thrombosis	Metabolic disorders	Cytomegalovirus infection
Kasabach-Merritt syndrome	Neoplasia (leukemia)	Herpesvirus infection
Disseminated intravascular coagulation	Paris-Trousseau with dysmegakaryopoietic	Rubella
Exchange transfusion	thrombocytopenia, giant platelet (α-granules,	HIV infection
Meconium aspiration syndrome	and chromosome 11q23 deletion	Sepsis
Severe birth trauma	Trisomies 13, 18, and 21	Toxoplasmosis
Hypersplenism		Birth asphyxia
Extra corporeal membrane oxygenation		Liver disease
		Erythroblastosis
		Polycythemia
		Neuroblastoma

A rare congenital defect in platelet production that may not be apparent at birth is congenital amegakaryocytic thrombocytopenia. Patients with this disorder have thrombocytopenia at an early age, but they may not have other physical anomalies. These patients often show evidence of a broader hematopoietic stem cell defect, as indicated by the presence of red cell macrocytosis and by the tendency for pancytopenia to develop in some later in life.[142]

Fanconi anemia is a rare, autosomal recessive disease characterized by multiple congenital abnormalities, bone marrow failure, and cancer susceptibility.[143] Patients with Fanconi anemia develop macrocytosis and pancytopenia, usually during the first decade of life. Deficiencies in platelets or red blood cells usually precede the leukopenia. The patients have "fetal-like" erythropoiesis, with increased antigen and hemoglobin F, and they generally have high serum erythropoietin levels. The progression to pancytopenia is variable, and presentation in the newborn period is unusual. Most patients with Fanconi anemia who are diagnosed as neonates present with congenital anomalies that trigger the evaluation.

Several uncommon disorders of platelet production or function may present with thrombocytopenia and giant platelets. The Bernard-Soulier syndrome is characterized by mild thrombocytopenia, large platelets, and a qualitative platelet defect caused by the absence of the GPIb/IX complex. Other giant platelet disorders are characterized by the association of thrombocytopenia with neutrophil inclusions; these include the May-Hegglin, Fechtner, and Sebastian anomalies.[144]

Wiskott-Aldrich syndrome is an X-linked disease characterized by thrombocytopenia with small platelets, eczema, recurrent infections, autoimmune disorders, and an increased incidence of hematopoietic malignancies. The identification of the responsible gene, *WASP* (Wiskott-Aldrich syndrome protein), revealed clinical heterogeneity of the syndrome and showed that X-linked thrombocytopenia without immunodeficiency is also caused by mutations of *WASP*.[145]

Secondary Thrombocytopenias

Thrombocytopenia is commonly encountered in sepsis, viral and bacterial infections, thrombosis, severe respiratory distress syndrome, asphyxia, maternal preeclampsia, hypothermia, erythroblastosis, meconium aspiration syndrome, phototherapy, and conditions that cause DIC. There is indirect evidence to suggest that immune- and nonimmune-mediated increased consumption and decreased production of platelets contribute to secondary thrombocytopenia in the neonate. A combination of these factors may be present in any one disease process. Using isotope labeling of transfused platelets, Castle and colleagues were able to demonstrate that in most infants (10 of 11 studied), platelet survival was significantly reduced.[135] The mechanism of thrombocytopenia in birth trauma, hypoxia, and acidosis is not clear; it may in part be secondary to an increased sensitivity of fetal megakaryocytes to hypoxic injury.[146]

Thrombocytopenia has been associated with sepsis in 50 to 60% of cases, but it may not always be associated with other evidence for DIC.[147-149] Thrombocytopenia usually appears within 48 hours of the onset of infection and can be severe, but it is not often complicated by severe bleeding.[148] Although platelet-associated antibodies can be seen in adults and infants with various types of infection,[150,151] there is no substantial proof that these antibodies are specific for a platelet surface antigen or they are responsible for the thrombocytopenia. In infants with sepsis, hypotension is a risk factor for developing thrombocytopenia.[151] An interesting disease process that may result in DIC is Kasabach-Merritt syndrome, in which consumptive thrombocytopenia and coagulopathy are associated with giant hemangiomas.[152]

Prolonged perinatal hypoxia associated with birth asphyxia has been associated with thrombocytopenia. In the study by Castle and associates,[135] 70% of sick infants with platelet counts lower than 100,000/μL had Apgar scores of 7 or lower. The mechanism is unclear but is likely multifactorial, with both decreased production and increased consumption contributing.

Studies in mice supported this notion.[153] Necrotizing enterocolitis is associated with thrombocytopenia,[154] and fungal infections are also commonly associated with thrombocytopenia.

Certain genetic disorders have been associated with thrombocytopenia. Among the metabolic disorders associated with thrombocytopenia are isovaleric acidemia, methylmalonic acidemia, holocarboxylase deficiency, ketotic hyperglycinemia, Pearson syndrome, and Kearns-Sayer syndrome. Trisomies 13, 18, and 21 have been associated with isolated thrombocytopenia in the neonatal period.[155,156]

Congenital neoplasia may result in thrombocytopenia because of infiltration of the bone marrow. Congenital leukemias are often of the myeloid or undifferentiated phenotype, but lymphoblastic leukemia may also be congenital. Solid tumor malignancies, particularly neuroblastoma, occasionally present during the newborn period.

Infants with trisomy 21 may be born with congenital leukemia characterized by hepatosplenomegaly and often associated with thrombocytopenia. The blasts are usually megakaryocytic or have both megakaryocyte and erythroid features. Although this leukemia has the biologic characteristics of a true malignancy, it resolves without treatment over several months in nearly all cases. Infants with Down syndrome who have this transient congenital leukemia are more prone to true leukemia 1 to 2 years later.[157]

Autoimmune Thrombocytopenia

Autoimmune thrombocytopenia is the most common cause of severe thrombocytopenia in the otherwise healthy newborn. The antiplatelet antibodies associated with autoimmune thrombocytopenia, whether alloimmune or autoimmune, are of the IgG class, are produced by the mother and cross the placenta, and generally have a finite life span in the circulation of the infant, usually a matter of weeks to a month.

Maternal immune thrombocytopenic purpura may result in fetal and neonatal thrombocytopenia. However, most neonates born to mothers with immune thrombocytopenic purpura do not have thrombocytopenia. In those who do have thrombocytopenia, clinically significant bleeding hardly ever occurs. Several large studies totaling more than 300 women with immune thrombocytopenic purpura showed that only 10 to 15% of infants have platelet counts of less than 100,000 μL, with about half of those having platelet counts of less than 50,000 μL.[158,159] In two studies of pregnancy outcomes in maternal immune thrombocytopenic purpura, none of the infants suffered a serious hemorrhage.[160,161]

Neonatal Alloimmune Thrombocytopenia

Neonatal alloimmune thrombocytopenia (NAIT) occurs when an antigen is present on the fetal platelets but is not present on maternal platelets.[162] On exposure to fetal platelets, the mother develops antiplatelet antibodies, which are specific for the fetal platelets. The antibodies cross the placenta and attach to the antigen on fetal platelets, which are then removed from circulation by the reticuloendothelial system of the fetus. In almost all cases of NAIT, the human platelet antigen (HPA) system is involved. In whites, 80 to 90% of cases of NAIT are the result of fetomaternal HPA-1 incompatibility.[163] However, other antigens may be involved. The second most common antigen to be involved in whites is HPA-5b.[164] In Asians, the most common antigen involved is HPA-4.[165] The HPA-3a antigen may also be involved.[166]

NAIT is not commonly diagnosed despite the severe thrombocytopenia that can occur and the large number of HPA-1a-negative women who become pregnant every year. The estimated prevalence of homozygosity for HPA-1b in whites is 2%.[167]

This would predict that NAIT would occur in 1 of 50 pregnancies. However, NAIT occurs in only 1 out of 1000 to 2000 pregnancies and therefore only occurs in 1 in 20 to 40 incompatible pregnancies.[168] In a large study of platelet counts on 9142 consecutive cord blood samples, of the 64 neonates with thrombocytopenia, 6 had NAIT confirmed by serologic testing, for an overall incidence of NAIT of 0.06% or 1 in 1800 births.[132] In the study by Uhrynowska and colleagues, of the 64 neonates with thrombocytopenia, 6 had NAIT confirmed by serologic testing, for an overall incidence of NAIT of 0.06% or 1 in 1800 births.[132]

Because prenatal screening for platelet alloantibodies is not routinely performed and 20 to 60% of diagnosed cases of NAIT are born to primiparous women, the typical presentation is a well newborn with petechiae and purpura with unexpected severe thrombocytopenia.[169] The most severe complication of NAIT is ICH, which results in significant morbidity and mortality rates.[170] Severe internal bleeding may occur as well. The frequency of life-threatening bleeding is nearly 50%.[164] The history of a sibling with ICH is the best predictor of severe thrombocytopenia and risk of serious bleeding.[171]

Percutaneous umbilical cord sampling (PUBS) allows for fetal platelet count measurements and *in utero* platelet transfusions.[172] For severe NAIT, weekly *in utero* platelet transfusions have been used.[173] The goal is to maintain the platelet count at greater than 20,000 because ICH is rare at levels higher than this.[174] Various treatment strategies have been used in NAIT with the goal of preventing ICH and avoiding the need for percutaneous umbilical cord sampling and *in utero* platelet transfusions. In most protocols, pregnancies are categorized by risk. Bussel and associates used prenatal administration of intravenous immunoglobulin to the mother, with positive responses in most patients.[175,176] Another group used similar strategies to devise a less invasive approach that minimizes the number of percutaneous umbilical cord samplings.[177]

REFERENCES

1. Davie EW, Ratnoff OD: Waterfall sequence for intrinsic blood clotting. Science 145:1310, 1964.
2. MacFarlane RG: An enzyme cascade in the blood clotting mechanism, and its function as a biochemical amplifier. Nature 202:498, 1964.
3. Osterud B, Rapaport SI: Activation of factor IX by the reaction product of tissue factor and factor VII: additional pathway for initiating blood coagulation. Proc Natl Acad Sci USA 74:5260, 1977.
4. Broze GJ Jr: Tissue factor pathway inhibitor. Thromb Haemost 74:90, 1995.
5. Luchtman-Jones L, Broze GJ Jr: The current status of coagulation. Ann Med 27:47, 1995.
6. Colman RW, et al: Overview of hemostasis. In Colman RW, et al (eds): Hemostasis and Thrombosis. Philadelphia, JB Lippincott, 2001, pp 3–16.
7. Castle V, et al: Frequency and mechanism of neonatal thrombocytopenia. J Pediatr 108:749, 1986.
8. Rajasekhar D, et al: Neonatal platelets are less reactive than adult platelets to physiological agonists in whole blood. Thromb Haemost 72:957, 1994.
9. Rajasekhar D, et al: Platelet hyporeactivity in very low birth weight neonates. Thromb Haemost 77:1002, 1997.
10. Stuart MJ: Platelet function in the neonate. Am J Pediatr Hematol Oncol 1:227, 1974.
11. Del Vecchio A: Use of the bleeding time in the neonatal intensive care unit. Acta Paediatr Suppl 91:82, 2002.
12. Andrew M: Developmental hemostasis: relevance to thromboembolic complications in pediatric patients. Thromb Haemost 74:415, 1995.
13. Koster T, et al: Role of clotting factor VIII in effect of von Willebrand factor on occurrence of deep-vein thrombosis. Lancet 345:152, 1995.
14. Rosendaal FR: High levels of factor VIII and venous thrombosis. Thromb Haemost 83:1, 2000.
15. Andrew M, et al: Factors XI and XII and prekallikrein in sick and healthy premature infants. N Engl J Med 305:1130, 1981.
16. Andrew M, et al: Thrombin regulation in children differs from adults in the absence and presence of heparin. Thromb Haemost 72:836, 1994.
17. Butenas S, et al: Tissue factor-initiated thrombin generation in the newborn. Blood 100:488a, 2002.
18. Mitchell L, et al: Alpha-2-macroglobulin may provide protection from thromboembolic events in antithrombin III deficient children. Blood 78:2299, 1991.

19. Johnston M, Zipursky A: Microtechnology for the study of the blood coagulation system in newborn infants. Can J Med Technol 42:159,1980.
20. Arad JD, et al: The mean platelet volume in the neonatal period. Am J Perinatol 3:1, 1986.
21. Aarts PA, et al: Red blood cell size is important for adherence of blood platelets to artery subendothelium. Blood 62:214, 1983.
22. Katz JA, et al: Relationship between human development and disappearance of unusually large von Willebrand factor multimers from plasma. Blood 73:1851, 1989.
23. Roschitz B, et al: Shorter PFA-100 closure times in neonates than in adults: role of red cells, white cells, platelets and von Willebrand factor. Acta Paediatr 90:664, 2001.
24. Knofler R, et al: Platelet function tests in childhood: measuring aggregation and release reaction in whole blood. Semin Thromb Hemost 24:513, 1998.
25. Michelson AD: Platelet activation by thrombin can be directly measured in whole blood through the use of the peptide GPRP and flow cytometry: methods and clinical applications. Blood Coagul Fibrinolysis 5:121, 1994.
26. Israels SJ: Evaluation of primary hemostasis in neonates with a new in vitro platelet function analyzer. J Pediatr 138:116, 2001.
27. Carcao MD, et al: The Platelet Function Analyzer (PFA-100): a novel in-vitro system for evaluation of primary haemostasis in children. Br J Haematol 101:70, 1998.
28. Rinder HM: Platelet function testing by flow cytometry. Clin Lab Sci 11:365, 1998.
29. Andrew M, et al: Development of the human coagulation system in the full-term infant. Blood 70:165, 1987.
30. Suzuki S, Wake N, Yoshiaki K. New neonatal problems of blood coagulation and fibrinolysis. I. The change of plasmin inhibitor levels in the newborn infant. J Perinat Med 4:213, 1976.
31. Hathaway WE: Coagulation problems in a newborn infant. Pediatr Clin North Am 17:929, 1970.
32. Pzapek E: Iatrogenic prolonged aPTT: a nondisease state. JAMA 227:1304, 1974.
33. Hellum AJ: The assay of platelet adhesiveness. Scand J Clin Lab Invest 12 (Suppl 51):18, 1960.
34. Arun B, Kessler C: Clinical manifestations and therapy of the hemophilias. In Colman RW, et al (eds): Hemostasis and Thrombosis: Basic Principles and Clinical Practice. Philadelphia, Lippincott Williams & Wilkins, 2001, p 815.
35. Daffos F, et al: Prenatal diagnosis and management of bleeding disorders with fetal blood sampling. Am J Obstet Gynecol 158:939, 1988.
36. Kaufman RJ, Pipe SW: Regulation of factor VIII expression and activity by von Willebrand factor. Thromb Haemost 82:201, 1999.
37. Kitchens CS: Factor XI: a review of its biochemistry and deficiency. Semin Thromb Hemost 17:55, 1991.
38. Baehner RL, Strauss HS: Hemophilia in the first year of life. N Engl J Med 275:524, 1966.
39. Schulman I: Pediatric aspects of the mild hemophilias. Med Clin North Am 46:93, 1962.
40. Hartmann JR, Diamond LK: Hemophilia and related hemorrhagic disorders. Practitioner 178:179, 1957.
41. Strauss H: Clinical pathological conference. J Pediatr 66:443, 1965.
42. Klinge J, et al: Prevalence and outcome of intracranial haemorrhage in haemophiliacs: a survey of the paediatric group of the German Society of Thrombosis and Haemostasis (GTH). Eur J Pediatr 158(Suppl 3):S162, 1999.
43. Kulkarni R, Lusher JM: Intracranial and extracranial hemorrhages in newborns with hemophilia: a review of the literature. J Pediatr Hematol Oncol 21:289, 1999.
44. Johnston M, Zipursky A: Microtechnology for the study of the blood coagulation system in newborn infants. Can J Med Technol 42:159, 1980.
45. Kulkarni R, et al: Current practices regarding newborn intracranial haemorrhage and obstetrical care and mode of delivery of pregnant haemophilia carriers: a survey of obstetricians, neonatologists and haematologists in the United States, on behalf of the National Hemophilia Foundation's Medical and Scientific Advisory Council. Haemophilia 5:410, 1999.
46. Ljung R, et al: Normal vaginal delivery is to be recommended for haemophilia carrier gravidae. Acta Paediatr 83:609, 1994.
47. Kulkarni R, Lusher J: Perinatal management of newborns with haemophilia. Br J Haematol 112:264, 2001.
48. Escuriola Ettingshausen C, et al: Symptomatic onset of severe hemophilia A in childhood is dependent on the presence of prothrombotic risk factors. Thromb Haemost 85:218, 2001.
49. Haya S, et al: Development of a factor VIII inhibitor in a newborn hemophiliac. Haemophilia 4:755, 1998.
50. Ries M, et al: Severe intracranial hemorrhage in a newborn infant with transplacental transfer of an acquired factor VII:C inhibitor. J Pediatr 127:649, 1995.
51. Whitelaw A, et al: Factor V deficiency and antenatal intraventricular haemorrhage. Arch Dis Child 59:997, 1984.
52. Rush B, Ellis H: The treatment of patients with factor V deficiency. Thromb Diath Haemorrh 14:74, 1965.
53. Gill FM, et al: Severe congenital hypoprothrombinemia. J Pediatr 93:264, 1978.
54. Viola L, et al: Intracranial hemorrhage in congenital factor II deficiency. Pediatr Med Chir 17:593, 1995.
55. Machin SJ, et al: Factor X deficiency in the neonatal period. Arch Dis Child 55:406, 1980.
56. Sandler E, Gross S: Prevention of recurrent intracranial hemorrhage in a factor X–deficient infant. Am J Pediatr Hematol Oncol 14:163, 1992.
57. Fisher S, et al: Factor XIII deficiency with severe hemorrhagic diathesis. Blood 28:34, 1966.
58. Anwar R, Miloszewski KJ: Factor XIII deficiency. Br J Haematol 107:468, 1999.
59. Abbondanzo SL, et al: Intracranial hemorrhage in congenital deficiency of factor XIII. Am J Pediatr Hematol Oncol 10:65, 1988.
60. Ichinose A: Physiopathology and regulation of factor XIII. Thromb Haemost 86:57, 2001.
61. Werner EJ: von Willebrand disease in children and adolescents. Pediatr Clin North Am 43:683, 1996.
62. Minowa H, et al: Four cases of bleeding diathesis in children due to congenital plasminogen activator inhibitor-1 deficiency. Haemostasis 29:286, 1999.
63. Griffin GC, et al: Alpha 2-antiplasmin deficiency: an overlooked cause of hemorrhage. Am J Pediatr Hematol Oncol 15:328, 1993.
64. Ariffin H, Lin HP: Neonatal intracranial haemorrhage secondary to congenital factor VII deficiency: two case reports. Am J Hematol 54:263, 1997.
65. Matthay KK, et al: Intracranial hemorrhage in congenital factor VII deficiency. J Pediatr 94:413, 1979.
66. Nichols WC, et al: Mutations in the ER-Golgi intermediate compartment protein ERGIC-53 cause combined deficiency of coagulation factors V and VIII. Cell 93:61, 1998.
67. Seligsohn U, et al: Combined factor V and factor VIII deficiency among non-Ashkenazi Jews. N Engl J Med 307:1191, 1982.
68. Chung KS, et al: Congenital deficiency of blood clotting factors II, VII, IX, and X. Blood 53:776, 1979.
69. Brenner B: Hereditary deficiency of vitamin K-dependent coagulation factors. Thromb Haemost 84:935, 2000.
70. Brenner B, et al: A missense mutation in gamma-glutamyl carboxylase gene causes combined deficiency of all vitamin K-dependent blood coagulation factors. Blood 92:4554, 1998.
71. Lane PA, Hathaway WE: Vitamin K in infancy. J Pediatr 106:351, 1985.
72. Shearer MJ, et al: Plasma vitamin K1 in mothers and their newborn babies. Lancet 28;2:460, 1982.
73. Shapiro AD: Vitamin K deficiency in the newborn infant: prevalence and perinatal risk factors. J Pediatr 109:675, 1986.
74. Townsend CW: The hemorrhagic disease of the newborn. Arch Pediatr 11:559, 1894.
75. Sutor A: Vitamin K deficiency bleeding in infants and children. Semin Thromb Hemostast 21:317, 1995.
76. Sutor AH, et al: Vitamin K deficiency bleeding (VKDB) in infancy: ISTH Pediatric/Perinatal Subcommittee, International Society on Thrombosis and Haemostasis. Thromb Haemost 81:456, 1999.
77. von Dam H, et al: Cholesterinstoffwechsel in Huhnereirn und Huhnchen. Biochem Z 215:475, 1929.
78. von Dam H, et al: The relation of vitamin K deficiency to hemorrhagic disease of the newborn. Adv Pediatr 5:129, 1952.
79. von Dam H: Cholesterinstoffwechsel in Huhnereirn und Huhnchen. Biochem Z 215:475, 1929.
80. von Dam H, et al: CLV. Studies on the mode of vitamin K. Biochem J 30:1075, 1936.
81. Brinkhous KM, et al: Plasma prothrombin level in normal infancy, and in hemorrhagic disease of the newborn. Am J Med Sci 193:475, 1937.
82. van Dam H, et al: The relation of vitamin K deficiency to hemorrhagic disease of the newborn. Adv Pediatr 5:129, 1952.
83. Lane PA, Hathaway WE: Vitamin K in infancy. J Pediatr 106:351, 1985.
84. Pietersma-de Bruyn ALJM, van Haard PMM: Vitamin K1 in the newborn. Clin Chim Acta 150:95, 1985.
85. Greer FR, et al: Vitamin K1 (phylloquinone) and vitamin K2 (menaquinone) status in newborns during the first week of life. Pediatrics 81:137, 1988.
86. Corrigan JJ, Kyre JJ: Factor II levels in cord blood: Correlation of coagulant activity with immunoreactive protein. J Pediatr 97:979, 1980.
87. van Doorm JM, Hemker HC: Vitamin K deficiency in the newborn. Lancet 2:708, 1977.
88. Bovill EG, et al: Vitamin K1 metabolism and the production of des-carboxy prothrombin and protein C in the term and premature neonate. Blood 81:77, 1993.
89. Israels LG, Israels ED: Observations on vitamin K deficiency in the fetus and newborn: has nature made a mistake? Semin Thromb Hemost 21:357, 1995.
90. Israels LG, et al: Vitamin K1 increases sister chromatid exchange in vitro in human leukocytes and in vivo in fetal sheep cells: a possible role for "vitamin K deficiency" in the fetus. Pediatr Res 22:405, 1987.
91. Cornelissen M, et al: Analysis of chromosome aberrations and sister chromatid exchanges in peripheral blood lymphocytes of newborns after vitamin K prophylaxis at birth. Pediatr Res 30:550, 1991.
92. Golding J, et al: Factors associated with childhood cancer in a national cohort study. Br J Cancer 62:304, 1990.
93. Klebanoff MA, et al: The risk of childhood cancer after neonatal exposure to vitamin K. N Engl J Med 329:905, 1993.
94. Passmore SJ, et al: Case-control studies of relation between childhood cancer and neonatal vitamin K administration. BMJ 316:178, 1998.
95. Vermeer C, Schurgers LJ: A comprehensive review of vitamin K and vitamin K antagonists. Hematol Oncol Clin North Am 14:339, 2000.

96. Hogg PJ, Stenflo J: Interaction of vitamin K-dependent protein Z with thrombin: consequences for the amidolytic activity of thrombin and the interaction of thrombin with phospholipid vesicles. J Biol Chem 266:10953, 1991.
97. Furie B, et al: Vitamin K-dependent biosynthesis of gamma-carboxyglutamic acid. Blood 93:1798, 1999.
98. Vermeer C: Gamma-carboxyglutamate-containing proteins and the vitamin K-dependent carboxylase. Biochem J 266:625, 1990.
99. Stenflo J, et al: Vitamin K dependent modifications of glutamic acid residues in prothrombin. Proc Natl Acad Sci USA 71:2730, 1974.
100. Davie EW: Biochemical and molecular aspects of the coagulation cascade. Thromb Haemost 74:1, 1995.
101. Li L, et al: Refinement of the NMR resolution structure of the gamma-carboxyglutamic acid domain of coagulation factor IX using molecular dynamics simulation with initial Ca2+ positions determined by a genetic algorithm. Biochemistry 36:2132, 1997.
102. American Academy of Pediatrics, Committee on Nutrition: Vitamin K compounds and their water soluble analogues: use in therapy and prophylaxis in pediatrics. Pediatrics 28:501, 1961.
103. McNinch AW, et al: Plasma concentrations after oral or intramuscular vitamin K1 in neonates. Arch Dis Child 60:814, 1985.
104. Hagstrom JN, et al: The pharmacokinetics and lipoprotein fraction distribution of intramuscular vs. oral vitamin K1 supplementation in women of childbearing age: effects on hemostasis. Thromb Haemost 74:1486, 1995.
105. Cornelissen M, et al: Prevention of vitamin K deficiency bleeding: efficacy of different multiple oral dose schedules of vitamin K. Eur J Pediatr 156:126, 1997.
106. Greer FR, et al: Improving the vitamin K status of breastfeeding infants with maternal vitamin K supplements. Pediatrics 99:88, 1997.
107. Croffie JM, et al: Tyrosinemia type 1 should be suspected in infants with severe coagulopathy even in the absence of other signs of liver failure. Pediatrics 103:675, 1999.
108. Aster RH: Pooling of platelets in the spleen: role in the pathogenesis of "hypersplenic" thrombocytopenia. J Clin Invest 45:645, 1966.
109. Stein, SF, Harker LA: Kinetic and functional studies of platelets, fibrinogen, and plasminogen in patients with hepatic cirrhosis. J Lab Clin Med 99:217, 1982.
110. Breedin von K: Hamorrhagische Diathesen bei Lebererkrankungen unter besonderer Berucksichtigung der Thrombocytenfunction. Acta Haematol (Basel) 27:1, 1962.
111. Rubin MH, et al: Abnormal platelet function and ultrastructure in fulminant hepatic failure. Q J Med 46:339, 1977.
112. Weston MJ, et al: Platelet function in fulminant hepatic failure and effect of charcoal haemoperfusion. Gut 18:897, 1977.
113. Vohra P, et al: Neonatal hemochromatosis: the importance of early recognition of liver failure. J Pediatr 136:537, 2000.
114. Andrew M, et al: Clinical impact of neonatal thrombocytopenia. J Pediatr 110:457, 1987.
115. McDonald M, et al: Role of coagulopathy in newborn intracranial hemorrhage. Pediatrics 1984; 74:26-31.
116. van Bel F, et al: Plasma guanosine 3',5'-cyclic monophosphate and severity of peri/intraventricular haemorrhage in the preterm newborn. Acta Paediatr 91:434, 2002.
117. Chang GY, et al: Heparin and the risk of intraventricular hemorrhage in premature infants. J Pediatr 131:362, 1997.
118. Sell LL, et al: Hemorrhagic complications during extracorporeal membrane oxygenation: prevention and treatment. J Pediatr Surg 21:1087, 1986.
119. Cilley RE, et al: Intracranial hemorrhage during extracorporeal membrane oxygenation in neonates. Pediatrics 78:699, 1986.
120. Glass P, et al: Morbidity for survivors of extracorporeal membrane oxygenation: neurodevelopmental outcome at 1 year of age. Pediatrics 83:72, 1989.
121. McManus ML, et al: Coagulation factor deficiencies during initiation of extracorporeal membrane oxygenation. J Pediatr 126:900, 1995.
122. Dela Cruz TV, et al: Risk factors for intracranial hemorrhage in the extracorporeal membrane oxygenation patient. J Perinatol 17:18, 1997.
123. Petaja J, et al: Increased risk of intraventricular hemorrhage in preterm infants with thrombophilia. Pediatr Res 49:643, 2001.
124. Dave P, et al: Cerebellar hemorrhage complicating methylmalonic and propionic acidemia. Arch Neurol 41:1293, 1984.
125. Nurden AT, George JN: Inherited abnormalities of the platelet membrane: Glanzmann thromboasthenia, Bernard-Soulier syndrome, and other disorders. In Colman RW, et al (eds): Hemostasis and Thrombosis: Basic Principles and Clinical Practice. Philadelphia, Lippincott Williams & Wilkins, 2001, pp 921-944.
126. Dasari R, et al: Effect of maternal low dose aspirin on neonatal platelet function. Indian Pediatr 35:507, 1998.
127. Sasidharan CK, et al: Fetal intracranial hemorrhage due to antenatal low dose aspirin intake. Indian J Pediatr 68:1071, 2001.
128. Cheung PY, et al: Nitric oxide and platelet function: implications for neonatology. Semin Perinatol 21:409, 1997.
129. Harker LA, Slichter SJ: The bleeding time as a screening test for the evaluation of platelet function. N Engl J Med 287:155, 1972.
130. Peterson P, et al: The preoperative bleeding time test lacks clinical benefit: College of American Pathologists' and American Society of Clinical Pathologists' position article. Arch Surg 133:134, 1998.
131. De Caterina R, et al: Bleeding time and bleeding: an analysis of the relationship of the bleeding time test with parameters of surgical bleeding. Blood 84:3363, 1994.

132. Uhrynowska M, et al: Neonatal thrombocytopenia: incidence, serological and clinical observations. Am J Perinatol 14:415, 1997.
133. Dreyfus M, et al: Frequency of immune thrombocytopenia in newborns: a prospective study. Blood 89:4402, 1997.
134. Burrows R, Kelton J: Fetal thrombocytopenia and its relation to maternal thrombocytopenia. N Engl J Med 329:1463, 1993.
135. Castle VP, et al: Frequency and mechanism of neonatal thrombocytopenia. J Pediatr 108:749, 1986.
136. Mehta P, et al: Thrombocytopenia in the high-risk infant. J Pediatr 97:791, 1980.
137. Homans A: Thrombocytopenia in the neonate. Pediatr Clin North Am 43:737, 1996.
138. Blanchette VS, Rand ML: Platelet disorders in newborn infants: diagnosis and management. Semin Perinatol 21:53, 1997.
139. Hall J, et al: Thrombocytopenia with absent radius (TAR). Medicine (Baltimore) 48:411, 1969 .
140. Hedberg V, Lipton J: Thrombocytopenia with absent radii. Am J Pediatr Hematol Oncol 10:51, 1988.
141. Homans A: Defective megakaryocytopoiesis in the syndrome of thrombocytopenia with absent radii. Br J Haematol 70:205, 1988.
142. Freedman M, Estrov Z: Congenital amegakaryocytic thrombocytopenia: an intrinsic hematopoietic stem cell defect. Am J Pediatr Hematol Oncol 12:225, 1990.
143. Kupfer GM, et al: Molecular biology of Fanconi anemia. Hematol Oncol Clin North Am 11:1045, 1997.
144. Greinacher A, Mueller-Eckhardt C: Hereditary types of thrombocytopenia with giant platelets and inclusion bodies in the leukocytes. Blut 60:53, 1990.
145. Sullivan K, et al: A multiinstitutional survey of the Wiskott-Aldrich syndrome. J Pediatr 125:876, 1994.
146. Bussel JB: Thrombocytopenia in newborns, infants, and children. Pediatr Ann 19:181, 1990.
147. Corrigan JJ Jr: Thrombocytopenia: a laboratory sign of septicemia in infants and children. J Pediatr 85:219, 1974.
148. Zipursky A, Jaber HM: The haematology of bacterial infection in newborn infants. Clin Haematol 7:175, 1978.
149. Modanlou HD, Ortiz OB: Thrombocytopenia in neonatal infection. Clin Pediatr 20:402, 1981.
150. Kelton JG, et al: Elevated platelet-associated IgG in the thrombocytopenia of septicemia. N Engl J Med 300:760, 1979.
151. Tate DY, et al: Immune thrombocytopenia in severe neonatal infections. J Pediatr 98:449, 1981.
152. Kasabach H, Merritt K: Capillary hemangioma with extensive purpura. Am J Dis Child 59:1063, 1940.
153. Birks JW, et al: Hypoxia-induced thrombocytopenia in mice. J Lab Clin Med 86:230, 1975.
154. Hutter JJ, et al: Hematologic abnormalities in severe neonatal necrotizing enterocolitis. J Pediatr 88:1026, 1976.
155. Hord JD, et al: Thrombocytopenia in neonates with trisomy 21. Arch Pediatr Adolesc Med 149:824, 1995.
156. Markenson AL, et al: Transient thrombocytopenia in 18-trisomy (letter). J Pediatr 87:834, 1975.
157. Homans A, et al: Transient abnormal myelopoiesis of infancy associated with trisomy 21. Am J Pediatr Hematol Oncol 15:392, 1993.
158. Burrows R, Kelton J: Fetal thrombocytopenia and its relation to maternal thrombocytopenia. N Engl J Med 329:1463, 1993.
159. McCrae K, et al: Pregnancy-associated thrombocytopenia: Pathogenesis and management. Blood 80:2697, 1992.
160. Burrows R, Kelton J: Low fetal risk in pregnancies associated with idiopathic thrombocytopenic purpura. Am J Obstet Gynecol 163:1147, 1990.
161. Cook R, et al: Immune thrombocytopenic purpura in pregnancy: a reappraisal of management. Obstet Gynecol 78:578, 1991.
162. Bussel JB: Alloimmune thrombocytopenia in the fetus and newborn. Semin Thromb Hemost 27:245, 2001.
163. Kaplan C, et al: Fetal and neonatal alloimmune thrombocytopenia: current trends in diagnosis and therapy. Transfus Med 2:265, 1992.
164. Meuller-Eckhardt C, et al: 348 cases of suspected neonatal alloimmune thrombocytopenia. Lancet 2:363, 1989.
165. Tanaka S, et al: Gene frequencies of human platelet antigens on glycoprotein IIIa in Japanese. Transfusion 36:813, 1996.
166. Glade-Bender J, et al: Anti-HPA-3A induces severe neonatal alloimmune thrombocytopenia. J Pediatr 138:862, 2001.
167. Ahya R, et al: Fetomaternal alloimmune thrombocytopenia. Transfus Apheresis Sci 25:139, 2001.
168. Flug F, et al: Should all pregnant women be tested for their platelet PLA (Zw, HPA-1) phenotype? Br J Haematol 86:1, 1994.
169. Kickler TS: Neonatal alloimmune thrombocytopenia. Clin Lab Med 12:577, 1995.
170. Sharif U, Kuban K: Prenatal intracranial hemorrhage and neurologic complications in alloimmune thrombocytopenia. J Child Neurol 16:838, 2001.
171. Bussel JB, et al: Fetal alloimmune thrombocytopenia. N Engl J Med 337:22, 1997.
172. Kaplan C, et al: Management of alloimmune thrombocytopenia: antenatal diagnosis and in utero transfusion of maternal platelets. Blood 72:340, 1988.
173. Nicolini U, et al: In-utero platelet transfusion for alloimmune thrombocytopenia. Lancet 2:506, 1988.

174. Bussel JB, et al: Recommendations for the evaluation and treatment of neonatal autoimmune and alloimmune thrombocytopenia: the Working Party on Neonatal Immune Thrombocytopenia of the Neonatal Hemostasis Subcommittee of the Scientific and Standardization Committee of the ISTH. Thromb Haemost 65:631, 1991.
175. Bussel JB, et al: Antenatal treatment of neonatal alloimmune thrombocytopenia. N Engl J Med 319:1374, 1988.

176. Bussel JB, et al: Antenatal management of alloimmune thrombocytopenia with intravenous gamma-globulin: a randomized trial of the addition of low-dose steroid to intravenous gamma-globulin. Am J Obstet Gynecol 174:1414, 1996.
177. Radder CM, et al: A less invasive treatment strategy to prevent intracranial hemorrhage in fetal and neonatal alloimmune thrombocytopenia. Am J Obstet Gynecol 185:683, 2001.

150

Marilyn J. Manco-Johnson

Pathophysiology of Neonatal Disseminated Intravascular Coagulation and Thrombosis

DISSEMINATED INTRAVASCULAR COAGULATION IN THE NEONATE

Substantial discoveries have been made in basic molecular and biochemical mechanisms of coagulation. These findings alter former concepts regarding normal physiology of clotting activation and regulation and provide insights into the pathophysiology of disseminated intravascular coagulation (DIC) and thrombosis. Even though data for many newly described components of coagulation have not been determined for newborn infants, it is likely that current models of adult coagulation will inform our understanding of DIC and thrombosis during the neonatal period. Pediatricians and neonatalogists cannot interpret coagulation studies in newborn infants without a comprehensive and cohesive conceptual framework. To place current data regarding neonatal DIC and thrombosis within newer paradigms of hemostasis and inflammation, the first part of this chapter has two parallel discussions: the first describes a new cell-based system of coagulation activation and regulation that integrates regulation of coagulation activation and inflammation in adults, and the second describes data derived in newborn infants with DIC and thrombosis and relates results to emerging patterns determined in adults.

Pathophysiology of Disseminated Intravascular Coagulation

DIC is a syndrome of systemic activation of blood clotting leading to depletion of platelets and fibrinogen as well as other coagulation proteins.[1] This failure of coagulation regulatory mechanisms results in a clinical presentation of hemorrhage, thrombosis, or the paradoxical coexistence of both bleeding and clotting.[2] Key to current concepts of DIC is cellular activation as the initiator of host defense.[3-9] In the sepsis paradigm, endotoxin activation of phagocytic cells results in expression of the inflammatory response, a physiologic protective pathway that results in containment of a homeostatic threat, healing, and host survival. The inflammatory response, when initiated locally, is protective. When the inflammatory response becomes systemic and dysregulated, a series of reactions is initiated that results in a spectrum of cell injury, dysfunction, and death and that progresses from the systemic inflammatory response syndrome (SIRS) to the multiple organ dysfunction syndrome.[10] Clinically, DIC occurs in settings of severe hypoxia with acidosis,[11] inadequate cardiac output with poor perfusion,[12] major trauma,[13] malignancy,[14] obstetric complications,[6] and bacterial, viral, and fungal sepsis.[3, 4, 15, 16] Sepsis is the classic disease provoking the

SIRS and, potentially, resulting in DIC.[17, 18] The target cells responding to an inflammatory trigger include monocytes, macrophages, neutrophils, platelets, and endothelial cells.[4, 5, 7, 8, 16] These cells form the reticuloendothelial (RE) system, which is an important organ system in host defense. Cellular events leading to the physiologic inflammatory response or pathologic DIC include the following:

1. Cellular activation through specific cell receptors resulting in the expression of inflammatory cytokines and adhesive molecules
2. Coagulation activation
3. Consumption of physiologic inhibitors of coagulation
4. Cell signaling leading to up-regulation of further synthesis and release of inflammatory cytokines, adhesive molecules, and procoagulant and antifibrinolytic proteins
5. Increased vascular permeability, extracellular inflammation, fibrin deposition, and cell damage
6. Fibrinolytic inhibition
7. Consumptive coagulopathy and multiple organ failure

Figure 150–1 displays current concepts of phases of cell-based coagulation including thrombin initiation, amplification, and propagation as well as fibrin clot formation.[19] Figure 150–2 shows

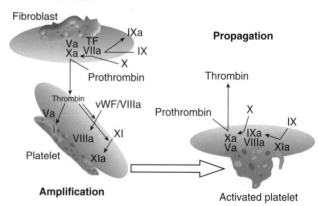

Figure 150–1. A cell-based model of coagulation. The three phases of coagulation occur on different cell surfaces: initiation on the tissue factor-bearing cell, amplification on the platelet as it becomes activated, and propagation on the activated platelet surface. (From Hoffman M, Monroe DM III. 2001 Thromb Haemost 85:958–965.)

NORMAL FUNCTION

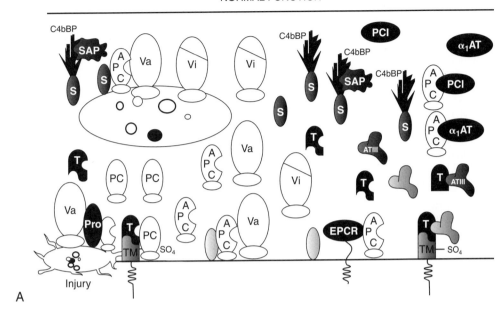

A   Injury

AFTER INFLAMMATION

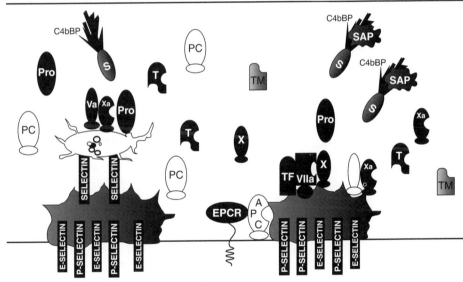

B

Figure 150–2. Coagulation regulation during normal (A) and inflammatory (B) states. A, The protein C anticoagulant pathway under normal conditions. Vascular injury initiates prothrombin (Pro) activation, which results in thrombin (T) formation. Prothrombin activation involves complex formation between Factor Va (Va) and Factor Xa (Xa). Thrombin then binds to thrombomodulin (TM) on the lumen of the endothelium, illustrated by the *heavy line*, and the thrombin-TM complex converts protein C (PC) to activated protein C (APC). Thrombin bound to TM can be inactivated very rapidly by antithrombin III (ATIII), at which time the thrombin–antithrombin III complex rapidly dissociates. APC then binds to protein S (S) on cellular surfaces. The APC-protein S complex then converts factor Va to an inactive complex (Vi), illustrated by the *slash* through the larger part of the two-subunit factor Va molecule. Protein C and APC interact with an endothelial cell protein C receptor (EPCR). This may concentrate the zymogen and enzyme near the cell surface and facilitate the function of the pathway, but this is yet to be shown directly. Protein S circulates in complex with C4bBP, which may, in turn, bind serum amyloid protein (SAP). APC is inhibited by forming complexes with the protein C inhibitor (PCI), α_1-antitrypsin (α_1AT), or α_2-macroglobulin (not shown). **B,** The influence of inflammation on coagulation and the protein C pathway. Inflammation triggers binding of neutrophils and monocytes to the endothelium by inducible adhesion receptors including the selectins. Activated platelets can bind to adherent neutrophils via selectins and potentially provide surfaces on which coagulation can be propagated by interaction with the prothrombin activation complex (Xa-Va). The monocytes can express tissue factor (TF) and bind Factor VIIa to initiate coagulation. Activated monocytes release cytokines that down-regulate TM biosynthesis. The neutrophil proteases can cleave TM from the vessel surface resulting in elevated levels of circulating TM. Inflammation often decreases the level of circulating free protein S (S), and the protein S that is present is often found primarily in complex with C4bBP and thus in a form that cannot support anticoagulant activity. C4bBP complexes with SAP. Although EPCR is down-regulated by tumor necrosis factor (TNF) in endothelial cell culture, it is shown here in complex with APC, based on the assumption that this complex may be involved in regulating inflammation. The net result of these changes is to produce a hypercoagulable state. (Modified from Arterioscler Thromb *12*:135–145, 1992 © American Heart Association; and redrawn from Esmon CT, Fukudome K. 1995 Semin Cell Biol 6:259–268.)

protective anticoagulant mechanisms during normal as well as inflammatory states.[5] Figure 150-3 depicts interactions of coagulation and inflammation through cell-signaling events.[17]

Cellular Activation

Endotoxin binds to monocytes and macrophages, forms complexes with cell-surface receptors, and thus triggers extracellular clotting as well as intracellular signaling. These processes result in a complex series of events favoring hypercoagulability and the acute inflammatory response. Lipopolysaccharide (LPS), the cell-stimulatory component of endotoxin secreted by gram-negative bacteria, is bound in plasma to a binding protein. The LPS-binding protein complex docks through the CD14 receptor to a Toll-like receptor 4 (TLR4).[20] An additional surface receptor (MD2) may be involved in this complex.[20] Formation of the LPS/LPS binding protein/MD2/TLR4 complex initiates intracellular signal transduction events.[3, 4, 20-23] An analogous receptor exists for signaling initiated by gram-positive bacteria and is called the Toll-like receptor 2 (TLR2).[4] Intracellular calcium is mobilized. Subsequently, intracellular $\kappa\beta$ (I$\kappa\beta$) is activated, and nuclear factor-$\kappa\beta$ is translocated into the nucleus, where it binds to DNA, acts as a transcriptional factor, and up-regulates synthesis and release of inflammatory cytokines (interleukin-1 [IL-1], IL-6, and IL-8) and adhesive molecules, P-selectin, S-selectin, intercellular adhesive molecule 1, and vascular endothelial growth factor.[16,24] Alterations in the pattern of protein transcription result in the acute phase reaction in which synthesis and secretion of certain proteins, including fibrinogen, Factor VIII, plasminogen activator inhibitor 1 (PAI-1), C4b-binding protein, α_1-antitrypsin, and C-reactive protein are increased, whereas others, including protein C, protein S, antithrombin (AT), and albumin, are decreased.[24-26] Increased nitric oxide is produced during DIC and results in vasodilatation and hypotension.[16, 25] Activation of monocytes causes release of macrophage inhibitor factor, a chemoattractant molecule, as well as expression of surface adhesive proteins.[27] Adhesive molecules promote the activation and incorporation of platelets and neutrophils that express tissue factor (TF) at the site of inflammation.[28, 29] Activation of endothelial cells, platelets, and leukocytes in the inflammatory process results in local tissue damage as well as systemic activation of coagulation.

Coagulation Activation

TF expression is induced by LPS, tissue hypoxia, and inflammatory cytokines, particularly IL-1α, IL-1β, and tumor necrosis factor-α (TNF-α).[24, 30] TF is a 47-kDa transmembrane glycoprotein that binds coagulation Factor VII and activated Factor VII (VIIa) and rapidly promotes the activation of Factor VII to VIIa.[19, 31] The Factor VIIa/TF complex activates Factor X to Factor Xa. The Factor VIIa/TF complex additionally activates Factor Xa through its activation of Factor IXa. The generation of trace amounts of Factor Xa and thrombin activates additional platelets, monocytes, and macrophages as well as coagulation co-Factors Va and VIIIa.[19] Activated cell surfaces provide the procoagulant surface for subsequent augmentation of coagulation through rapid generation of Factor Xa via Factors XIa, VIIIa, and IXa. After activation, Factor Xa, in complex with co-Factor Va, cleaves zymogen prothrombin to thrombin. The final result of coagulation activation is formation of fibrin by thrombin cleavage of small peptides from the Aα and Bβ chains of fibrinogen.[32] Fibrin monomers rapidly polymerize and become stably cross-linked through transamidation mediated by thrombin-activated Factor XIII.[32] Fibrin is a potent promoter of further cellular activations as well as of fibrinolysis.[33] Cell-based activation of coagulation promotes dissemination of thrombin generation leading to DIC.

Consumption of Coagulation Inhibitors

Coagulation is regulated by four major inhibitory proteins and several minor inhibitors. First, TF, when in a ternary complex with Factors VIIa and Xa, is inhibited by the tissue factor pathway inhibitor (TFPI).[34] Second, AT is the major inhibitor of the serine proteases, including Factors XIIa, XIa, IXa, Xa, and thrombin as well as kallikrein.[35] AT inactivation is catalyzed by heparin-like molecules on the endothelium, including heparin sulfate. Factor VIIa is weakly inhibited by AT. Additional minor inhibitors of thrombin include heparin cofactor and α_2-macroglobulin. Third, thrombin binds to a cellular thrombin receptor, thrombomodulin (TM).[36] Complexes of thrombin with TM lose their procoagulant functions in activation of cofactors V and VIII, platelet activation and fibrin cleavage. The thrombin/TM complex functions to activate protein C and the procarboxypeptidase B (also called the thrombin activatable fibrinolytic inhibitor, TAFI). The endothelial protein C receptor (EPCR) additionally promotes protein C activation.[37,38] Protein S is a cofactor for activated protein C (APC). Protein S bound to platelet or endothelial cell membranes is able to accelerate the APC-mediated neutralization of Factors Va and VIIIa by a value of at least 10,000.[39] The APC cofactor activity of protein S is modified by its binding in plasma to the binding protein of the C4b component of complement (C4b-bp). Activated protein C (APC) is a pivotal regulatory protein that, in complex with its cofactor, protein S, down-regulates coagulation by neutralizing inactivated factors Va and VIIIa, thus dampening the augmentation phase of coagulation.[5,17] APC also promotes fibrinolysis by decreasing thrombin available to activate TAFI and by binding the plasminogen activator inhibitor (PAI-1), and thus allowing increased functional tissue plasminogen activator (TPA); both of these effects limit fibrinolytic inhibition and thereby increase fibrinolytic activity.[17] Fourth, fibrin binds thrombin and serves as a major physiologic inhibitor of thrombin.[33,40] During the inflammatory response, synthesis and release of protein S are decreased while C4b-bp is increased; these changes serve to decrease the effectiveness of the protein C system during the inflammatory response.[5] Acquired deficiencies and dysfunctions of coagulation regulatory proteins are regularly found in patients with DIC and may provide a target for therapeutic intervention.[41]

Cell Signaling

Several cell receptors are proteolytically activated by a subclass of G-protein coupled receptors called protease activated receptors (PARs).[42] Cleavage of four PARs (PAR1 through PAR4) by TF, thrombin, or factor Xa results in cellular adhesion, cleavage of cellular TM with generation of a truncated, soluble TM molecule in the plasma, and secretion of the von Willebrand factor (vWF), TPA, and PAI-1.[16, 42-46] After an initial wave of augmented fibrinolysis, there is a protracted fibrinolytic inhibition.[47] Recent evidence supports that APC (but not zymogen protein C), possibly in concert with EPCR, initiates signaling to the nucleus or is translocated from the cell membrane to the nucleus where it may bind directly to DNA and act as a transcriptional factor to decrease the synthesis and release of inflammatory cytokines, as well as acute phase proteins.[17,48] By this mechanism, APC provides a direct molecular and biochemical link between regulation of coagulation and inflammation, supporting the clinical association of these two processes and again, offering potentials for therapeutic intervention.

Vascular Permeability and Tissue Damage

Nitric oxide released during DIC causes vasodilatation and hypotension.[16] Activation of the contact factors XII and prekallikrein leads to the generation of kallikrein and bradykinin, causing increased vascular permeability and capillary leak syn-

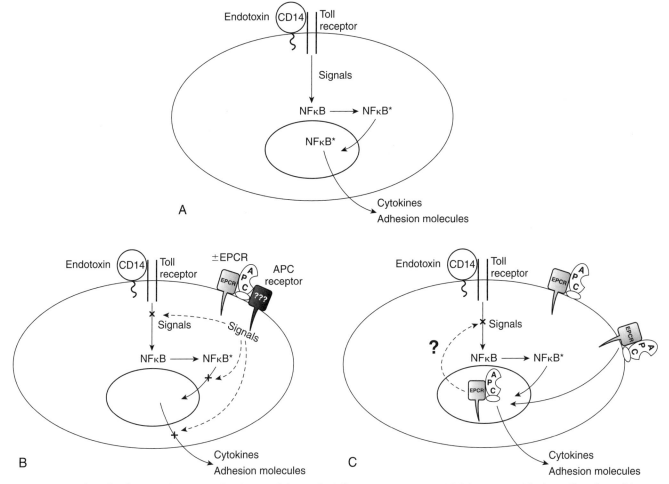

Figure 150–3. The role of activated protein C (APC) in modulating the inflammatory response. APC interacts with the cell surface either through EPCR or directly with a distinct APC receptor. This interaction generates signals that block nuclear factor (NF)-κB nuclear translocation. Alternatively, the endothelial cell protein C receptor (EPCR)–APC complex undergoes nuclear translocation, which, in turn, generates new gene products that may modulate this process. (Redrawn from Esmon CT. 2001 Crit Care Med *29*[Supplement]:S48–S52.)

drome.[11,16,32,35] Neutrophils, macrophages, monocytes and platelets are allowed access to subendothelial tissues where secreted neutrophil enzymes including elastase, inflammatory cytokines, particularly IL-6 and IL-8, coagulation activation and fibrin deposition lead to oxidative damage, local tissue hypoxia and tissue ischemia.[7,10,11,16,25,28] Physiologically these processes serve to localize the inflammatory response to the site of an offending physical or infectious insult, protecting the remainder of the host. If unchecked, these processes lead from local inflammation through the SIRS and culminate in the multiple organ dysfunction syndrome. Finally, overwhelming consumption of clotting proteins and platelets results in disseminated thrombosis and hemorrhage. Pathophysiologic processes similar to those described for sepsis have been documented in hypoxia, adult respiratory distress syndrome (RDS), obstetric complications, cancer, massive trauma, and burns.[6,11-14,41]

Suppression of Fibrinolysis

Markers of plasmin activation are routinely detected in DIC, and their absence has a high negative predictive value.[49,50] However, an acquired decrease in fibrinolytic potential can be determined

and portends a poor outcome in patients with DIC.[13,24,47,48] TAFI activity and antigen concentrations are reduced in patients with DIC.[51]

Consumptive Coagulopathy and Multiple Organ Failure

Current concepts of DIC emphasize the excess generation of thrombin in its pathophysiology. The nomenclature *overt DIC* is given to uncompensated DIC with the classic findings of low fibrinogen with prolonged prothrombin time (PT) and activated partial thromboplastin time (aPTT) and clinical bleeding.[1] A newer concept of *nonovert* or *compensated DIC* is applied to patients with laboratory evidence of elevated markers of thrombin and plasmin activation with high or normal plasma concentrations of fibrinogen, in whom screening PT and aPTT can be normal or slightly prolonged.[1,52,53] SIRS with elevated acute phase proteins including fibrinogen may be associated with nonovert DIC and has been found primarily in patients with sepsis and solid organ malignant disease.[50] Adults with nonovert DIC have evidence of persistent endothelial cell injury and an increased risk of multiple organ failure and death.

Pathophysiology of Neonatal Disseminated Intravascular Coagulation

Neonatal DIC always presents in infants with predisposing medical conditions, as shown in Table 150–1. Blood and tissue abnormalities in DIC are variable and depend on the rate and amount of thrombin generated within the circulation as well as the body's capacity to resist thrombin generation. Physiologic homeostatic mechanisms to resist DIC include the ability of the RE system to clear activated enzyme complexes, the capacity of the inhibitory proteins to neutralize potent coagulation enzymes, the activation of fibrinolysis to clear intravascular fibrin strands, and the rate of production of both platelets and clotting factors to replenish blood levels. DIC reflects a failure of the regulatory system of coagulation. As noted later, each regulatory component is defective in the neonate, and this may contribute to the apparent increased susceptibility of the newborn to consumptive coagulopathies.

Newer models of coagulation activation emphasize the role of TF as the most clinically relevant activator of coagulation. TF (see earlier) is a transmembrane protein that, along with its inhibitor TFPI, is widely expressed on ectodermal and endodermal cell surfaces by early embryonic gestation, in which it probably acts through cell signaling in tissue differentiation and proliferation.[54-56] Reports in adults have demonstrated that soluble TF in plasma is functionally active in promoting Factor X activation, and elevated plasma TF in excess of TFPI conveys a poor prognosis in sepsis.[41,57] Evidence that umbilical cord blood leukocytes expressed increased TF activity in comparison with adult cells was first reported by Rivers and Hathaway in 1975, and monocytes were identified as the primary source of TF activity.[58, 59] Grabowski and colleagues, employing a model of whole blood flowing through human term umbilical veins, determined that IL-1–stimulated neonatal endothelial cells exhibit increased TF activity in comparison with adult saphenous vein cells.[60] Grabowski and associates further showed that increased TF activity was posttranslational because it was not accompanied by increased expression of TF mRNA. Streif and colleagues showed an increased rate, but not amount, of thrombin generation in cord plasma of human preterm infants.[61] Accelerated thrombin generation in the study by Streif and associates was related to increased plasma TF activity *in vivo* because pretreatment of cord plasma with an antibody to TF abolished the effect.[61] Enhanced expression of TF activity is likely to play an important role in the increased susceptibility of the near-term

fetus and neonate to DIC and could theoretically pose a risk of DIC in response to coagulant therapy with activated Factor VII.

Activation of trace concentrations of thrombin results in activation of platelets, on whose surface coagulation complexes rapidly assemble. Factors VIIIa and Va play critical roles in amplification of early thrombin generation on the surface of activated platelets. Both Factors VIII and V achieve plasma concentrations within the adult normal range by term birth, in contrast to vitamin K–dependent and contact procoagulant proteins, which show protracted developmental delays.[62, 63] Healthy term and preterm infants exhibit plasma fibrinogen concentration and platelet counts within the adult normal range.[62-64] However, in spite of increased TF expression, accelerated thrombin generation rate, and levels of co-Factors V and VIII as well as fibrinogen and platelets within the adult normal ranges, thrombin generation capacity is decreased in the cord blood plasma and is limited by low plasma concentrations of prothrombin.[65]

vWF forms ultralarge multimers in fetal plasma that persist up to 1 month postnatally.[66] These very large vWF multimers, similar to those found in thrombotic thrombocytopenia purpura, facilitate enhanced platelet-vessel interactions in the newborn infant and likely facilitate platelet activation and consumption.[67, 68] In addition, the vWF cleaving protease is decreased in neonatal plasma.[69]

AT (previously called antithrombin III) is the primary physiologic inhibitor of thrombin. Levels of AT in well term and preterm infants are 60 and 40% of normal adult levels, respectively.[62-64] These diminished levels of AT appear adequate to inhibit the reduced amounts of thrombin that potentially could be generated from newborn plasma owing to the proportionately decreased level of prothrombin, and they appear to be adequate to inhibit levels of thrombin that potentially could be generated from neonatal levels of prothrombin.[70] In addition, heparin-like molecules have been detected in cord blood plasma in concentrations exceeding those found in healthy adults.[71, 72] However, the sick infant is prone to acquired decreases in AT plasma concentration and protein function that may contribute to the pathophysiology and severity of neonatal DIC.[73-75]

Protein C is a late-developing coagulation protein. The lower limit of normal in healthy term infants is 25 U/dL; protein C levels of less than 10 U/dL are also seen occasionally in preterm infants who have no evidence of DIC.[62,64,76] However, low levels of protein C in the neonate may be inadequate to neutralize Factors Va and VIIIa, which could be generated during DIC. After activation, protein C is inhibited by certain proteins, including protein C inhibitor, α_1-antitrypsin, and α_2-macroglobulin. Plasma concentrations of protein C inhibitors are at or higher than the adult normal range by term gestation.[62, 77] Although protein S levels are decreased at birth, the physiologically low levels of C4b-bp in healthy infants serve to increase the functional unbound or "free" protein S.[78] Elevations in C4b-bp with decreases in free protein S have been described in infants with sepsis similar to adults with inflammation.[79]

In spite of decreased concentration and activity of plasminogen in cord blood plasma and increased PAI-1, the fibrinolytic potential of neonatal plasma, as reflected in the euglobulin clot lysis time, is shorter than the normal adult value in cord plasma.[80-84] Neonates with RDS show signs of increased activation of both coagulation and fibrinolysis, as evidenced by increased plasma concentrations of markers of thrombin and plasmin generation.[79,85-87] However, a postnatal decrease in fibrinolytic capacity is regularly found in infants with severe RDS and heralds a poor prognosis.[88,89] At postmortem examination, preterm infants who die of RDS are noted to have diffuse fibrin deposition in the lungs, liver, kidneys, and other organs. Large-vessel thromboses that were not clinically suspected *in vivo* are common. Although exhaustion of fibrinolytic potential is suspected in sick preterm infants with DIC, the exact cause of decreased fibrinolysis in sick preterm infants is unknown.

TABLE 150-1

Clinical Conditions Associated with Disseminated Intravascular Coagulation in Newborn Infants

Severe hypoxia with acidosis (severe respiratory distress syndrome)
Cardiac failure with poor perfusion
Sepsis
    Bacterial: gram-negative organisms, especially
    Viral: rubella, herpes, cytomegalovirus, enteroviruses
    Fungal: *Candida*
Massive thrombosis
Tissue necrosis
Liver disease (severe)
Vascular malformations: Kasabach-Merritt, arteriovenous malformations
    Chorangiomatous malformation of the placenta
Thrombophilia: homozygous or multiple mutation
Massive hemolysis
Lactic acidosis
Obstetric complications: chorioamnionitis, abruptio placentae, placental
    accreta, fetal demise of one twin, preeclampsia

Decreased fibrinolysis has been determined in adults with severe DIC.

Activated coagulation products such as complexes of TF with Factor VIIa, thrombin, Factor Xa, and plasmin generated during DIC are complexed to their inhibitors and are cleared through the RE system, primarily the liver and spleen. Fibrin(ogen) degradation products such as fibrin monomer, the X, Y, D, and E fragments formed by plasmin action on either fibrinogen or fibrin, or the D-dimer fragment of cross-linked fibrin act as inhibitors of both plasma and platelet clotting until they, too, are removed by the RE system. There is evidence that the neonate is functionally hyposplenic.[90] Decreased splenic function in neonates with DIC could delay the clearance of activators or trigger intravascular clotting as well as diminish clearance of fibrin(ogen) degradation products. Blood flow is important in transporting these activation products from the site of generation to the RE system for clearance. Fibrin generated within small vessels during DIC impairs the circulation and slows the body's efforts to restore homeostasis. Polycythemia and shock, which frequently coexist in the stressed term infant, further impede the circulation and compound delayed clearance by the liver and spleen.

Thrombocytopenia and hypofibrinogenemia are common in many neonatal conditions, including RDS, bacterial and viral sepsis, and necrotizing enterocolitis. Survival studies employing labeled platelets and fibrinogen suggest a shortened half-life in sick infants with plasma levels maintained by increased production in some babies.[91-93] Results of studies by Feusner and colleagues suggest that the least mature babies may be at greatest risk of peripheral depletion because of a decreased ability to increase production.[91]

Coagulation Findings

The diagnosis of DIC requires, first and foremost, the presence of an underlying disorder known to be associated with consumptive coagulopathy. Clinical hemorrhage and thrombosis add to the assessment of DIC. Diagnostic laboratory criteria for DIC in adults, as adopted by the International Society for Thrombosis and Haemostasis (ISTH), include assay of PT, fibrinogen, platelet count, and determination of fibrin(ogen) degradation products in addition to the clinical criteria.[2] Various molecular species of fibrin, including soluble fibrin monomer, are found in DIC. Accordingly, multiple assays have been developed to detect fibrin, but none have been universally adopted.[49,94-96] Adult laboratory criteria cannot be directly applied to investigations in sick newborn infants, however, because physiologic neonatal values differ from those in adults. Although no laboratory criteria for neonatal DIC have been validated to date, a diagnostic panel is displayed in Table 150-2.

In a series of 100 children with DIC including 45 neonates, bleeding was found in 60%, and thrombosis was diagnosed in 20%; the overall fatality rate was 42%.[97] Bleeding symptoms are frequent in infants with overt DIC and are associated with a platelet count of less than 100,000/μL, a fibrinogen value of less

than 100 mg/dL, and a decrease in Factor V severe enough to prolong the PT. A simple but helpful screening panel includes the platelet count, fibrinogen level, D-dimer assay of cross-linked fibrin, and PT. These tests can all be performed on capillary blood specimens and give an estimate both of ongoing activation and of acute hemorrhagic potential. Low Factor VII activity may be helpful to support a diagnosis of severe liver disease, and assays of protein C and protein S are necessary in infants with purpura fulminans. Other specific factor assays add confirmatory information but neither increase diagnostic sensitivity nor aid clinical management.

Markers of thrombin and plasmin activation (thrombin-AT and plasmin-antiplasmin complexes, respectively) are frequently elevated in sick infants, a finding suggesting that activation of coagulation and fibrinolysis indicative of nonovert DIC is common in the neonate.[85-87] Fibrinogen consumption is more common in infants with severe hypoxia, whereas thrombocytopenia is a sensitive indicator of sepsis.[85]

In DIC, intravascular deposition of fibrin results in microangiopathic hemolytic anemia by trapping and shearing circulating red cells. Damaged red blood cells are subsequently remolded or are removed from the circulation by the spleen. The blood count reflects a drop in hemoglobin concentration, and examination of the peripheral smear reveals abnormal red cell morphology including acanthocytes, schizocytes, and spherocytes. An increase in polychromatophilic and nucleated red cells is often seen. If sepsis occurs, severe neutropenia is often present, with an increase in immature neutrophils.

Therapy of Neonatal Disseminated Intravascular Coagulation

Definitive therapy for DIC requires reversal of the trigger for coagulation activation. Supportive care for neonates with DIC employing adequate ventilation, volume expansion, and antibiotics, as indicated, is reflected in improved coagulation screening tests within 24 hours. DIC in infants with RDS or sepsis usually resolves within 72 hours. Resolution of thrombocytopenia may require 2 to 4 additional days.

In addition to supportive care, various strategies have been attempted in adult clinical trials specifically to target key proteins altered by the pathophysiologic process. Animal models of sepsis have demonstrated resolution of DIC and improvement in mortality rates using replacement therapy with AT, APC, and TFPI.[98] Human clinical trials have shown significant reduction of mortality in severe sepsis using recombinant APC (drotrecogen alfa).[99] Replacement of zymogen protein C preliminarily appears less effective in sepsis-associated DIC.[100] Therapy with an anti–TNF monoclonal antibody showed a small but significant decrease in mortality.[101]

Table 150-3 displays results of randomized clinical trials for DIC in neonates. Four randomized clinical trials employing coagulation replacement therapy for DIC failed to show improved survival after administration of blood component therapy.[102-105] Taylor's experiments demonstrated a persistence of altered inflammation beyond the duration of perturbed coagulation in a sepsis model of DIC.[53] These experiments may explain the failure of coagulation therapies to alter overall mortality rates in DIC. The ability of APC, but not zymogen protein C, to down-regulate the inflammatory response may explain its success in treatment of DIC in adults and children.[100] Trials employing APC showed a trend toward increased bleeding toxicity in treated patients that could pose a significant disadvantage in preterm infants at risk for intracranial hemorrhage.

Infants with bleeding may be supported with infusions of fresh frozen plasma (10 to 20 mL/kg) and single-donor platelets (10 mL/kg) every 12 to 24 hours. Cryoprecipitate (10 mL/kg)

TABLE 150-2

Diagnosis of Disseminated Intravascular Coagulation in Newborn Infants

An underlying abnormality known to predispose to disseminated
  intravascular coagulation
Prolonged prothrombin time
Decreased fibrinogen
Decreased platelet count
Increased D-dimer or other marker of fibrin(ogen) degradation
Possible clinical bleeding and/or thrombosis

TABLE 150-3

Randomized Clinical Trials for Neonatal Disseminated Intravascular Coagulation

Author	Treatment 1	Treatment 2	Control	Outcome
Gross and Filston, 1982	Exchange transfusion (N = 11)	Fresh frozen plasma and platelets N = 11	Standard therapy (N = 11)	Mortality: no difference Coagulopathy: no difference
Andrew et al, 1993	Platelet transfusion; 10 ml/kg plus standard therapy (N = 78)		Standard therapy (N = 74)	Mortality: no difference Intracranial hemorrhage: no difference Bleeding time shortened in treated group; platelet count higher in treated group
Gobel et al, 1980	Standard heparin (N = 20)		Placebo (N = 20)	Mortality: no difference Coagulopathy resolved more rapidly with heparin
Schmidt et al, 1998	Antithrombin 100 U/kg load; 50 U/kg q6h × 48 h (N = 61)		Placebo (N = 61)	Mortality, days ventilated: increased with antithrombin F 1+2 decreased more rapidly with antithrombin

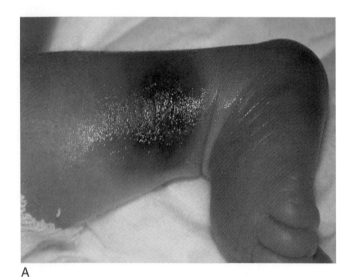
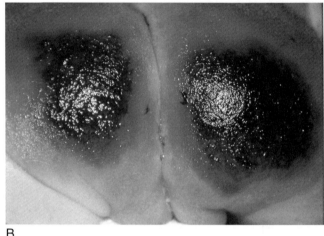

Figure 150–4. Purpura fulminans caused by compound heterozygous protein C deficiency. Black and indurated areas of skin necrosis with central bullae and peripheral erythema, typical of severe protein C deficiency, are seen on the ankle (**A**) and buttocks (**B**) in a 2-day-old affected infant.

may be infused to increase fibrinogen. The clinical goal in a sick infant with bleeding is to maintain the fibrinogen higher than 100 mg/dL, the platelet count greater than 50,000/μL, and the INR lower than 1.5. Rapid consumption of replaced blood proteins and platelets may be temporarily slowed by exchange transfusion using packed red cells and fresh frozen plasma, as well as by low-dose standard heparin (SH) (10 U/kg/hour). Coagulation therapies are useful to support the infant with DIC long enough to allow specific therapy to remove the trigger for DIC. If cardiovascular function is not normalized during several days of support, multiple organ failure generally ensues, signaling a progressive downward spiral terminating in death.

NEONATAL PURPURA FULMINANS

Neonatal purpura fulminans is a unique syndrome that presents a few hours to a few days after birth.[106-108] Red serpiginous skin lesions classically appear on the scalp, the buttocks, and the dependent surfaces of the lower extremities and trunk, as shown in Figure 150-4. The upper extremities are usually spared. The lesions quickly become indurated and black, and they form an eschar. Lesions of purpura fulminans may heal with extensive scarring and may require skin grafting. Histologic evaluation of the lesions reveals thrombi in the capillaries and venules of the skin and soft tissues. Most infants with purpura fulminans have been noted to have vitreal hemorrhage, apparently caused by bleeding into thrombosed primary vitreal veins *in utero,* with blindness as the usual sequela.[109-111] Additionally, many affected infants have been found to suffer renal vein thrombosis or cerebral infarcts *in utero.*[107,112] The outcomes of fetal cerebral infarcts range from none to severe motor and cognitive deficits.

Purpura fulminans is caused by a severe deficiency of protein C or protein S.[106, 107, 112-124] One case report described purpura fulminans in an infant with homozygous Factor V Leiden.[125] However, considering the frequency of the Factor V Leiden mutation in the white population (5 to 8% heterozygosity), purpura fulminans with Factor V Leiden is very rare. Genetic mutations causing severe deficiency of protein C or protein S are heterogeneous and include large and small deletions, frameshift mutations, missense mutations, nonsense mutations, amino acid substitutions, and generation of a stop codon signal.[113-120, 123, 124] Most neonates with purpura fulminans are found to have compound heterozygous defects unless these children are the product of consanguinity. Most parents of infants with neonatal purpura fulminans have a heterozygous deficiency, but most have not had thrombosis. In older infants and children, purpura fulminans may develop with severe bacterial infections, especially meningococcus,[126] and after certain viral infections, most

TABLE 150-4
Laboratory Testing for Thrombophilia in Neonates

Level I
Infant
  Complete blood count and platelets
  Antithrombin activity
  Protein C activity
  Protein S, free and total, immunologic
  Activated protein C resistance (functional) and/or Factor V Leiden
    (polymerase chain reaction)
  Prothrombin 20210 by polymerase chain reaction
  Fasting homocysteine and/or MTHFR C677T (*C677T*)
Maternal
  Lipoprotein (a)
  Lupus anticoagulant
  Anticardiolipin antibody, anti-β2GP1 antibody

Level II
  Euglobulin clot lysis time
  Plasminogen
  Dysfibrinogenemia: thrombin time, reptilase time, fibrinogen activity,
    antigen and crossed immunoelectrophoresis, fibrin degradation
    products
  Heparin cofactor II

TABLE 150-5
Clinical Conditions Associated with Thrombosis in Neonates

Indwelling catheters
Low blood flow, shock
Infection
Thrombophilia, especially multiple gene mutations
Polycythemia, hyperviscosity
Dehydration
Maternal antiphospholipid antibodies
Maternal diabetes mellitus

classically varicella.[127] Rarely, purpura fulminans can be caused by acquired severe inhibitory protein deficiency in the newborn infant.[128]

A few neonates with heterozygous deficiencies of protein C or protein S have been reported to present with large vessel thrombosis, usually with multiple thrombolytic traits.[112] DIC may be present, but frank purpura fulminans is not a typical feature of infants with more than trace plasma concentrations of protein C or protein S.

Coagulation Findings

Immediately after birth and early in the course of purpura fulminans, screening coagulation assays may be normal or nearly normal for age. Quickly, however, typical findings of DIC occur, with decreased fibrinogen and platelet count and prolongations in the aPTT and PT. Assays of coagulation regulatory proteins, protein C, protein S, and AT often reflect decreases consistent with consumption. However, in severe genetic deficiencies, the affected protein is undetectable or nearly undetectable. The value of assaying regulatory proteins in the setting of neonatal purpura fulminans is to determine the one protein that is absent or nearly absent compared with moderate decreases in the other proteins. Infants with deficiencies in plasma concentration of multiple regulatory proteins should be restudied after complete resolutions of purpura fulminans, DIC, or thrombosis (ideally at 6 to 12 months), to confirm the presence and severity of a genetic deficiency. A complete thrombophilia evaluation should be performed because multiple thrombophilic traits are not rare. Table 150-4 displays thrombophilia testing for children as recommended by the Pediatric Subcommittee of the ISTH.[129] Genetic sequencing is used routinely to confirm the diagnosis and to provide carrier and prenatal testing.

Therapy

Before initiating therapy for neonatal purpura fulminans, it is imperative to collect and process diagnostic blood samples adequate in quality and quantity. Peripheral venous samples are optimal for coagulation studies. However, venipuncture is not always successful in a critically ill neonate. Capillary samples collected directly into citrate anticoagulant are adequate to exclude a severe genetic deficiency of protein C or protein S; sampling from indwelling vascular lines is adequate after clearing the line of at least five times the volume in the length of tubing. After samples have been collected to evaluate neonatal purpura fulminans, therapy should be promptly initiated with infusions of fresh frozen plasma (10 mL/kg every 8 to 12 hours).[107] Infants with severe deficiencies of protein C have been successfully treated with a human plasma–derived, highly purified, virally inactivated protein C concentrate that is licensed in Europe and is available for compassionate use in North America.[130] Recombinant APC has been successfully used to treat a newborn infant with purpura fulminans secondary to homozygous protein C deficiency.[120] Human plasma–derived, highly purified, virally inactivated concentrates of AT are licensed in the United States and have been used in the treatment of neonates and children.[131] Affected infants have been maintained long term on protein C concentrate replacement, low molecular weight heparin (LMWH), and very early institution of oral anticoagulant therapy with warfarin.[107, 130, 132] In choosing these therapeutic options, the clinician must weigh the risks of protein replacement (primarily thrombotic and infectious risks of central venous access devices in addition to viral safety) against the risks of oral anticoagulation (difficulty in maintaining stable anticoagulation and bleeding complications) and LMWH (potential decrease in bone density, lipodystrophy, subcutaneous hematomas, and bleeding complications). Almost all children with severe deficiencies of protein C or protein S are ultimately managed with long-term oral anticoagulation.

NEONATAL THROMBOSIS

Neonatal thrombosis is characterized by an increased incidence in the neonate, a predilection for major vessels, and frequent involvement of the arterial circulation. Since the early 1990s, substantial progress has been made regarding genetic and acquired risk factors for neonatal thrombosis. Despite the continued lack of any randomized clinical trials for neonates with thrombi, data are emerging to guide effective therapy.

Pathophysiology

The prevalence of symptomatic thrombosis in neonates has been estimated at 2.4 per 1000 neonatal intensive care unit admissions in a Canadian series compared with 5.1 per 100,000 births in a German registry.[133, 134] Thrombi can be caused by abnormalities of blood vessels, abnormalities of blood flow, or abnormalities of the blood itself. Clinical conditions associated with thrombosis in the newborn infant are displayed in Table 150-5.

Vascular injury incurred by catheterization is the most important cause of arterial and venous thromboses in infants. Catheters were implicated in approximately 90% of cases of neonatal thrombosis in two large national registries.[133, 134] Using current catheters and insertion techniques, the most important predictors for catheter-related-thrombosis are small size of the infant (and catheterized vessel), longer duration of catheter use,[135,136] composition of infused materials,[136] and sepsis.[133] Early studies of neonatal catheter-related thrombosis implicated catheter composition,[137] construction,[138] and placement site.[139]

The dynamics of altered blood flow are important in the pathogenesis of neonatal thrombosis. The stressed newborn infant is especially susceptible to decreased cardiac output and poor perfusion as a result of hypoxia, hypoglycemia, hypovolemia, or infection. Venous thrombi resulting from episodes of diminished blood flow in the neonate have a definite predilection for renal and central nervous system veins. Neonatal renal vein thrombosis is generally initiated as small vessel disease of the intrarenal vessels that is propagated centrally along the venous system. Thrombosis may be found in the main renal vein and less commonly in the inferior vena cava or may be absent from either. Although generally asymmetric, this is usually a bilateral disease affecting both kidneys to some degree.[140] Neonatal renal venous thrombosis leads to irreversible kidney damage in most affected infants, regardless of antithrombotic therapy.[141,142] Risk factors for renal vein thrombosis include diabetic gestation, hyperviscosity, asphyxia, and shock.

Neonatal venous thromboses also involve the cerebral sinuses in increased frequency; half of all childhood cerebral venous thromboses occurs during the neonatal period.[143] Results of several pathologic studies have suggested that neonatal germinal matrix hemorrhage originates in areas of venous infarction and follows episodes of low flow.[144]

The neonate with critically altered blood flow is also at risk of arterial thrombosis. Spontaneous occlusions of the aorta, renal arteries, mesenteric arteries, and middle cerebral arteries follow episodes of shock and poor perfusion. The incidence of symptomatic ischemic stroke in neonates has been reported at 1.35 per 100,000 live births.[145] Half of the children in this German registry had acquired risk factors including asphyxia, sepsis, and patent foramen ovale.[145] Necrotizing enterocolitis is a vasoocclusive disease that may be related to umbilical artery catheterization in the very low birth weight infant.[146]

Several features of the unique neonatal hemostatic system, many of which are described earlier, foster thrombogenesis. Primary hemostasis is accelerated in the neonate by higher hematocrit and increased platelet-vessel interactions. The hematocrit of the term infant (normal range, 40 to 60%) is relatively polycythemic as compared with the adult. As the hematocrit is elevated above 65%, infants show an increased tendency for diminished blood flow, especially in the hepatic, cerebral, renal, and mesenteric circulations.[147] Neonatal hyperviscosity is almost always caused by an increase in red blood cells. Circulatory impairment in association with white blood cell counts of greater than 100,000 is rare but may be seen in neonatal leukemia.

Despite diminished platelet aggregation function, closure times using the platelet function analyzer (PFA-100) are shorter in healthy neonates than in adult controls.[68,148,149] Platelet thromboxane A_2 is increased relative to prostacyclin in infants of diabetic mothers, a patient group at increased risk of thrombosis.[150,151] In addition to TF exposure by endothelial damage caused by catheters, stimulated neonatal monocytes and endothelial cells generate increased TF activity compared with adult cells, as noted earlier.[58-60] Plasma concentrations of regulatory proteins AT and protein C, which are physiologically low in healthy preterm infants, are further depressed in infants with RDS and may contribute to a thrombotic tendency.[63,64,70,73-76]

As noted earlier, the neonatal fibrinolytic system differs in many respects from that of the adult. After a brief period of activation during labor and delivery, neonatal fibrinolysis is decreased with a relative excess of PAI-1 compared with tPA.[64] Plasma concentrations of the fibrinolytic zymogen plasminogen are low.[64,78-80,83] A fetal form of plasminogen exists with decreased specific activity of the active site.[81,82] However, increased neonatal fibrinolysis is favored by other characteristics of neonatal fibrinolysis. Histidine-rich glycoprotein is low in neonatal plasma, which renders most of the plasminogen to a more activatable form.[80] Fetal plasminogen can be activated by lower concentrations of tPA compared with the adult molecule.[84] Finally, fetal plasmin is more slowly inactivated by α_2-antiplasmin.[82]

Massive thromboses may occur in infants of mothers with antiphospholipid antibodies.[152,153] Maternal testing for the lupus anticoagulant and anticardiolipin antibody should be performed to exclude this diagnosis.

Thrombophilia describes a constitutional predisposition to thrombosis. Thrombophilia is caused by many genetic mutations resulting in increased thrombin generation, decreased thrombin regulation, or decreased fibrinolysis.[154-156] The role of thrombophilia in fetal and neonatal thromboses, as well as adverse pregnancy outcome, has received much attention. Data linking thrombophilia to neonatal thrombosis have been summarized.[157,158] The most common thrombophilic mutations are the Factor V Leiden mutation, a point mutation in the Factor V molecule that prevents inactivation of Va by APC, and the prothrombin 20210 mutation, which results in a moderate increase in plasma prothrombin concentration. The prevalence of Factor V Leiden and prothrombin 20210 in whites is 5 to 8% and 1 to 2%, respectively. These genes are not found generally in Asia or Africa but have been reported in low frequency in Mexican mestizos.[159] Neonates with arterial and venous thrombi, including central nervous system thrombi, have an increased prevalence of Factor V Leiden.[160,161] Neonates with central nervous system thrombi, both arterial and venous, have an increased prevalence of prothrombin 20210.[162] Mutations in the genes for AT, protein C, and protein S are less common but more heterogeneous; neonates have presented with thrombosis in association with heterozygous deficiencies of AT and protein C.[163,164] Infants with homozygous deficiency of cystathionine β-synthase have markedly elevated levels of plasma homocysteine and an increased incidence of arterial and venous thrombi.[165] Moderate elevations of homocysteine associated with the thermolabile polymorphism of the *MTHFR* gene contribute a modest increase in thrombosis risk.[166] Infants with multiple thrombophilic gene mutations are at increased risk of symptomatic thrombosis as well as thrombus recurrence.[112,167] Elevations in the genetically determined lipoprotein carrier, Lp(a), have been linked to venous thrombosis in pediatric patients, including neonates, by German investigators; however, this finding has not yet been confirmed in other populations.[168] Neonatal intracranial hemorrhage originates from venous thrombi in the germinal matrix of the choroids plexus.[144] Preterm infants with intracranial hemorrhage have been found to have an increased risk for thrombophilia.[169] Attention has been focused on the relationship of maternal antiphospholipid antibodies as well as maternal and fetal thrombophilic genes in the pathogenesis of various adverse pregnancy outcomes including fetal demise, intrauterine growth retardation, preeclampsia, and placental abruption. Evidence to date suggests a relationship between thrombophilia and adverse pregnancy outcome, although the disorders appear to be multifactorial, and more data are needed.[170-173]

Coagulation Testing

Recommendations for testing infants with thrombosis for thrombophilia, adopted by the Perinatal and Pediatric Subcommittee of the ISTH, are shown in Table 150-4. A complete blood count should be performed on every infant with thrombosis. Hyperviscosity caused by increased red cells, white cells, or platelets should be excluded. The neonate is far more likely than the adult to exhibit consumptive coagulopathy as a result of major vessel thrombosis. Thrombocytopenia, hypofibrinogenemia, and acquired depletions of AT, protein C, and plasminogen are often seen with large aortic thromboses. D-dimer is usually positive. These findings are nonspecific and corroborate, but do not confirm, ongoing thrombosis.

Spontaneous thrombosis in otherwise well term neonates is very uncommon. Most infants with thrombosis have underlying triggering or predisposing conditions including catheters, infection, inflammation, surgery, gestational diabetes, and diminished blood flow.[133] However, severe genetic deficiencies of protein C, protein S, and Factor V Leiden, as well as combined thrombophilic gene mutations, have been associated with unprovoked thrombi in newborn infants.[112,167] Baseline screening tests of PT, fibrinogen, platelet count, and D-dimer or other markers of fibrinolysis, as shown in Table 150-2, are important to assess the need for coagulation support during antithrombotic therapy, to minimize bleeding risk. AT concentration may be determined in infants who are resistant to the anticoagulant effects of standard LMWH. Plasminogen should be determined in infants who do not exhibit fibrin degradation in association with thrombolytic therapy. Immediate diagnosis of severe genetic deficiencies of AT, protein C, and protein S should be made when replacement therapy may be critical for patient care. Determinations of Factor V Leiden and the prothrombin 20210 mutations by polymerase chain reaction technique are valid at any time. Diagnoses of heterozygous thrombophilic traits (using functional assays for coagulation proteins) are best delayed until the infant is 6 months of age or older.

Several issues related to thrombophilia screening are currently unresolved. The contribution of thrombophilic genes to the pathogenesis of thrombosis in sick, preterm infants with catheter-related thrombi is not yet clear, and no definitive recommendations can be made at this time regarding routine evaluation of infants with neonatal catheter-related thrombi for thrombophilia. The current development of multiple large registries of neonatal thrombosis will facilitate collection of data regarding testing and management of newborn infants with thrombosis. Likewise, the value of routine thrombophilia testing in women with adverse pregnancy outcomes has not been determined. Early evidence suggests that, although these gene mutations appear to play an etiologic role in adverse pregnancy outcome, the clinical syndromes are multifactorial, and thrombophilia is unlikely to explain all affected cases. Firm recommendations for testing cannot be made at this time. However, until definitive information is available, obstetric recommendations call for thrombophilia testing in women who have suffered three or more first trimester losses, two or more first and second trimester losses, or one unexplained third trimester or neonatal death.

Therapy

There are no prospective randomized, controlled trials of therapy for neonatal thrombosis on which to base therapeutic deci-

sions. The relative rarity of these lesions, the heterogeneity of the clinical presentations, and the frequent instability of the affected infant severely hamper clinical research efforts. Despite these limitations, infants with life- or limb-threatening or progressive thrombosis require therapy. Bleeding complications of antithrombotic therapy are less than 10% if care is taken to observe specific contraindications to anticoagulant and thrombolytic therapy, as shown in Table 150-6. The risk of hemorrhage during anticoagulant therapy with heparin, either SH or LMWH, is lower than that associated with thrombolysis. Infants with a history of asphyxia, central nervous system infarction or hemorrhage, or extreme prematurity are at highest risk of intracranial hemorrhage with antithrombotic therapy.

Heparins, both SH and LMWH, require binding to AT to express activity. Plasma concentration of AT is low in the newborn infant. The volume of distribution and the clearance of heparins are accelerated in the neonate, especially the term infant.[174] With low AT and accelerated pharmacokinetics, the newborn infant requires higher heparin dosing compared with older children and adults. Increased heparin sensitivity is rarely seen in neonates and is usually confined to extremely preterm infants. The aPTT cannot be reliably used as an indicator of heparin effect in neonatal plasma because of the physiologically low concentrations of contact factors that prolong the aPTT. Instead, an anti-Factor Xa activity assay should be used. Carefully collected capillary samples are adequate for heparin assays. Limited pharmacokinetic data for SH and LMWH are available for newborn infants.[175-177] Dosing recommendations in Table 150-7 are based on these studies. Term infants, particularly infants of diabetic mothers, can require enormous doses of SH to achieve a therapeutic plasma level, exceeding 50 U/kg/hour. Infusions of AT concentrate may increase heparin sensitivity in these infants. Heparin-induced thrombocytopenia has been documented in newborn infants.[178,179] Although it is uncommon, heparin-induced thrombocytopenia should be considered in an infant with prior heparin exposure who manifests thrombocytopenia or decreasing platelet count, thrombus presentation, or thrombus progression while receiving heparin anticoagulation.

Duration of anticoagulant therapy in neonates has been derived empirically. Arterial thrombi can be treated for 7 to 14 days, and venous thrombi can be treated for 4 to 6 weeks. The newborn infant appears to have a lower rate of thrombus recurrence compared with adults after discontinuation of anticoagulation; for this reason, long-term anticoagulation is not often administered. Efficacy of anticoagulation therapy can be judged only by careful prospective outcome studies; to date, such data are not available.

Thrombolytic therapy has been increasingly applied to treatment of newborn infants with thrombi, with a large degree of success. Experience with thrombolysis of arterial and venous thrombi in neonates compared with results in older children has been summarized; recommendations for tPA thrombolysis, as adopted by the Perinatal and Pediatric Subcommittee of the

---

TABLE 150-6

Contraindications for Antithrombotic Therapies in Neonates

Therapeutic Anticoagulation	Thrombolytic Therapy
Active bleeding	Active bleeding
Major surgery within 72 h*	Major surgery within 10 d
Intracranial hemorrhage within 72 h*	Intracranial hemorrhage within 10 d
Invasive procedures within 72 h*	Major asphyxial event within 7 d
Platelet count < 50,000/μl	Invasive procedures within 72 h
Fibrinogen < 100 mg/dl	Seizures within 48 h
	Platelet count < 50,000/μl
	Fibrinogen < 100 mg/dl

* Anticoagulate with caution

TABLE 150–7

Recommendations for Starting Doses of Antithrombotic Therapy in Neonates

Drug and Dose	Term	Preterm	Monitoring
Unfractionated heparin			
Bolus	100 U/kg	50 U/kg	
Continuous infusion	30 U/kg	20–25 U/kg	Anti-Xa 0.3–0.7 U/ml
Low molecular weight heparin			
Enoxaparin subcutaneously q12h	1.5 mg/kg	1.5 mg/kg	Anti-Xa 0.5–1.0 U/ml
Dalteparin subcutaneously q24h	150 U/kg	150 U/kg	Anti-Xa 0.5–1.0 U/ml
tPA thrombolysis			
Low dose, especially for venous thrombi	0.06–0.12 mg/kg/h for 48 h		Clot lysis by imaging
High dose, especially for arterial thrombi	0.1–0.5 mg/kg/h for 3–12 h		Clot lysis by imaging
tPA is given by continuous infusion, without a load, with no dose-adjustment for gestational age			

tPA = tissue-type plasminogen activator.

TABLE 150–8

Recommendations for Coagulation Support for Neonates with Disseminated Intravascular Coagulation or Thrombosis

Component	Dose	Indication
Cryoprecipitate	10–15 ml/kg	Fibrinogen < 50 mg/dl;
Fresh frozen plasma	10–15 ml/kg	Plasminogen < 30 U/dl with thrombolysis; prothrombin time prolongation
Platelet concentrate	10 ml/kg	Platelets < 50,000/μl
Antithrombin	100 U/kg	Severe heparin insensitivity; disseminated intravascular coagulation refractory to transfusion support

ISTH, are shown in Table 150–7.[180] In general, the neonate requires a higher dose of tPA compared with older infants and children.[181] Although the rate of clot lysis is 75% for arterial clots and 50% with venous thrombi, it is less than reported outcomes in older infants and children.[180] Careful patient selection and monitoring are essential. Local delivery of tPA using catheters directed into the thrombus offers the potential of a higher local concentration of tPA and enhanced thrombolytic effect, but it was not shown to convey a practical advantage in a comprehensive cohort of neonates and children treated with tPA.[181] Before removing a central vascular catheter associated with a neonatal thrombosis, it is useful to evaluate whether that catheter may be used to instill thombolytic agents directly into the clot. Renal vein thrombosis is associated with a very high rate of segmental or cortical atrophy after supportive care or heparin anticoagulation. Combined therapy with anticoagulation and thrombolysis offers the best opportunity for preserved organ function.[142, 182]

Before initiating anticoagulant or fibrinolytic therapy in the neonate, it is critical to confirm hemostatic concentrations of fibrinogen (100 mg/dL) and platelets (50,000/μL) and to support the patient with blood product replacement if necessary. Cranial sonography should be performed in all preterm infants before anticoagulant or fibrinolytic therapy, to exclude intracranial hemorrhage. Recommendations for coagulation support are given in Table 150–8.

REFERENCES

1. Taylor FB Jr, Toh C-H, Hoots WK, Wada H, Levi M. 2001 Towards definition, clinical and laboratory criteria, and a scoring system for disseminated intravascular coagulation: on behalf of the Scientific Subcommittee on Disseminated Intravascular Coagulation (DIC) of the International Society on Thrombosis and Haemostasis (ISTH). Thromb Haemost 86:1327–1330
2. Levi M, de Jonge E, van der Poll T, ten Cate H. 2001 Advances in the understanding of the pathogenetic pathways of disseminated intravascular coagulation result in more insight in the clinical picture and better management strategies. Semin Thromb Hemost 27(6):569–575
3. Beutler B, Poltorak A. 2001 Sepsis and evolution of the innate immune response. Crit Care Med 29[Supplement]:S2–S7
4. Aderem A. 2001 Role of Toll-like receptors in inflammatory response in macrophages. Crit Care Med 29[Supplement]:S16–S18
5. Esmon CT, Fukudome K. 1995 Cellular regulation of the protein C pathway. Semin Cell Biol 6(5):259–268
6. Osterud B, Bjorklid E. 2001 The tissue factor pathway in disseminated intravascular coagulation. Semin Thromb Hemost 27(6):605–617
7. Hack CE, Zeerleder S. 2001 The endothelium in sepsis: source of and a target for inflammation. Crit Care Med 29[Supplement]:S21–S27
8. Nieuwland R, Berckmans RJ, McGregor S, Böing AN, Romjin FPHTM, Westendorp RGJ, Hack CE, Sturk A. 2000 Cellular origin and procoagulant properties of microparticles in meningococcal sepsis. Blood 95(3):930–935
9. Faust SN, Levin M, Harrison OB, Goldin RD, Lockhart MS, Kondaveeti S, Laszik Z, Esmon CT, Heyderman RS. 2001 Dysfunction of endothelial protein C activation in severe meningococcal sepsis. N Engl J Med 345(6):408–416
10. Marshall JC. 2001 Inflammation, coagulopathy, and the pathogenesis of multiple organ dysfunction syndrome. Crit Care Med 29[Supplement]:S99–S106
11. ten Cate H, Schoenmakers SHHF, Franco R, Timmerman JJ, Groot AP, Spek CA, Reitsma PH. 2001 Microvascular coagulopathy and disseminated intravascular coagulation Crit Care Med 29[Supplement]:S95–S98
12. Inglis TC, Breeze GR, Stuart J, Abrams LD, Roberts KD. 1975 Excess intravascular coagulation complicating low cardiac output. J Clin Pathol 28(1):1–7
13. Gando S. 2001 Disseminated intravascular coagulation in trauma patients. Semin Thromb Hemost 27(6):585–592
14. Maiolo A, Tua A, Grignani G. 2002 Hemostasis and cancer: tumor cells induce the expression of tissue factor-like procoagulant activity on endothelial cells. Haematologica 87(6):624–628
15. de Kleijn ED, Hazelzet JA, Kornelisse RF, de Groot R. 1998 Pathophysiology of meningococcal sepsis in children. Eur J Pediatr 157:869–880
16. Vallet B, Wiel E. 2001 Endothelial cell dysfunction and coagulation. Crit Care Med 29[Supplement]:S36–S41
17. Esmon CT. 2001 Protein C anticoagulant pathway and its role in controlling microvascular thrombosis and inflammation. Crit Care Med 29[7 Supplement]:S48–S52
18. Faust SN, Heyderman RS, Levin M. 2001 Coagulation in severe sepsis: a central role for thrombomodulin and activated protein C. Crit Care Med 29[Supplement]:S62–S68
19. Hoffman M, Monroe DM III. 2001 A cell-based model of hemostasis. Thromb Haemost 85(6):958–965
20. Ulevitch RJ. 2001 New therapeutic targets revealed through investigations of innate immunity. Crit Care Med 29[Supplement]:S8–S12
21. Petersen LC, Freskgard P, Ezban M. 2000 Tissue factor-dependent factor VIIa signaling. Trends Cardiovasc Med 10(2):47–52
22. Asakura H, Suga Y, Aoshima K, Ontachi Y, Mizutani T, Kato M, Saito M, Morishita E, Yamazaki M, Takami A, Miyamoto K, Nakao S. 2002 Marked difference in pathophysiology between tissue factor-and lipopolysaccharide-induced disseminated intravascular coagulation models in rats. Crit Care Med 30(1):161–164

23. Xuereb JM, Sie P, Boneu B, Constans J. 2000 Inhibition of tissue factor synthesis by disruption of ERK kinase and PKC signaling pathways in human vascular SMCs. Thromb Haemost 84(1):129-136
24. van der Poll T, de Jonge E, Levi M. 2001 Regulatory role of cytokines in disseminated intravascular coagulation. Semin Thromb Hemost 27(6):639-651
25. Dhainaut, J-F, Marin N, Mignon A, Vinsonneau C. 2001 Hepatic response to sepsis: interaction between coagulation and inflammatory processes. Crit Care Med 29[Supplement]:S42-S47
26. Kerr R, Stirling D, Ludlam CA. 2001 Interleukin 6 and haemostasis. Br J Haematol 115(1):3-12
27. Froidevaux C, Roger T, Martin C, Glauser MP, Calandra T. 2001 Macrophage migration inhibitory factor and innate immune responses to bacterial infections. Crit Care Med 29[Supplement]:S13-S15
28. McEver RP. 2001 Adhesive interactions of leukocytes, platelets, and the vessel wall during hemostasis and inflammation. Thromb Haemost 86(3):746-756
29. Bouchard BA, Tracy PB. 2001 Platelets, leukocytes, and coagulation. Curr Opin Hematol 8(5):263-269
30. Rapaport SI, Rao LV. 1995 The tissue factor pathway: how it has become a "prima ballerina." Thromb Haemost 74(1):7-17
31. Peppelenbosch MP, Versteeg HH. 2001 Cell biology of tissue factor, an unusual member of the cytokine receptor family. Trends Cardiovasc Med 11(8):335-339
32. Sidelmann JJ, Gram J, Jespersen J, Kluft C. 2000 Fibrin clot formation and lysis: basic mechanisms. Semin Thromb Hemost 26(6):605-618
33. Mosesson MW, Siebenlist KR, Meh DA. 2001 The structure and biological features of fibrinogen and fibrin. Ann NY Acad Sci 936:11-30
34. Bajaj MS, Birktoft JJ, Steer SA, Bajaj SP. 2001 Structure and biology of tissue factor pathway inhibitor. Thromb Haemost 86(4):959-972
35. Opal SM, Kessler CM, Roemisch J, Knaub S. 2002 Antithrombin, heparin, and heparan sulfate. Crit Care Med 30[Supplement]:S325-S331
36. Wu KK, Matijevic-Aleksic N. 2000 Thrombomodulin: a linker of coagulation and fibrinolysis and predictor of risk of arterial thrombosis. Ann Med 32[Supplement 1]:73-77
37. Esmon CT. 2000 The endothelial cell protein C receptor. Thromb Haemost 83(5):639-643
38. Fukudome K, Ye X, Tsuneyoshi N, Tokunaga O, Sugawara K, Mizokami H, Kimoto M. 1998 Activation mechanism of anticoagulant protein C in large blood vessels involving the endothelial cell protein C receptor. J Exp Med 187(7):1029-1035
39. Clouse LH, Comp PC. 1986 The regulation of hemostasis: the protein C system. N Engl J Med 314(20):1298-1304
40. de Bosch NB, Mosesson MW, Ruiz-Saez A, Echenagucia M, Rodriguez-Lemoin A. 2002 Inhibition of thrombin generation in plasma by fibrin formation (antithrombin I). Thromb Haemost 88(2):253-258
41. Levi M, de Jonge E, van der Poll T. 2001 Rationale for restoration of physiological anticoagulant pathways in patients with sepsis and disseminated intravascular coagulation. Crit Care Med 29[Supplement]: S90-S94
42. Schmidlin F, Bunnett NW. 2001 Protease-activated receptors: how proteases signal to cells. Curr Opin Pharmacol 1(6):575-582
43. Riewald M, Ruf W. 2002 Orchestration of coagulation protease signaling by tissue factor. Trends Cardiovasc Med 12:149-154
44. Versteeg HH, Peppelenbosch MP, Spek CA. 2001 The pleiotropic effects of tissue factor: a possible role for factor VIIa-induced intracellular signaling? Thromb Haemost 86(6):1353-1359
45. Sambrano GR, Weiss EJ, Zheng YW, Huang W, Coughlin SR. 2001 Role of thrombin signaling in platelets in haemostasis and thrombosis. Nature 413(6851):74-78
46. Leadley RJ Jr, Chi L, Porcari AR. 2001 Non-hemostatic activity of coagulation factor Xa: potential implications for various diseases. Curr Opin Pharmacol 1(2):169-175
47. Hack CE. 2001 Fibrinolysis in disseminated intravascular coagulation. Semin Thromb Hemost 27(6):633-638
48. Grinnell BW, Joyce D. 2001 Recombinant human activated protein C: a system modulator of vascular function for treatment of severe sepsis. Crit Care Med 29[Supplement]: S53-S61
49. Horan JT, Francis CW. 2001 Fibrin degradation products, fibrin monomer and soluble fibrin in disseminated intravascular coagulation. Semin Thromb Hemost 27(6):657-666
50. Watanabe R, Wada H, Miura Y, Murata Y, Watanabe Y, Sakakura M, Okugawa Y, Nakasaki T, Mori Y, Nishikawa M, Gabazza EC, Shiku H, Nobori T. 2001 Plasma levels of total plasminogen activator inhibitor-1 (PAI-1) and tPA/PAI-1 complex in patients with disseminated intravascular coagulation and thrombotic thrombocytopenic purpura. Clin Appl Thromb Hemost 7(3):229-233
51. Watanabe R, Wada H, Watanabe Y, Sakakura M, Nakasaki T, Mori Y, Nishikawa M, Gabazza EC, Nobori T, Shiku H. 2001 Activity and antigen levels of thrombin-activatable fibrinolysis inhibitor in plasma of patients with disseminated intravascular coagulation. Thromb Res 104(1):1-6
52. Wada H, Yamamuro M, Inoue A, Shiku H, Sakuragawa N, Redl H, Peer G, Taylor FB Jr. 2001 Comparison of the responses of global tests of coagulation with molecular markers of neutrophil, endothelial, and hemostatic system perturbation in the baboon model of E. coli sepsis: toward a distinction between uncompensated overt DIC and compensated non-overt DIC. Thromb Haemost 86(6):1489-1494
53. Taylor FB Jr. 2001 Staging of the pathophysiologic responses of the primate microvasculature to Escherichia coli and endotoxin: examination of the ele-

54. Luther T, Flossel C, Mackman N, Bierhaus A, Kasper M, Albrecht S, Sage EH, Iruela-Arispe L, Grossmann H, Strohlein A, Zhang Y, Nawroth PP, Carmeliet P, Loskutoff DJ, Muller M. 1996 Tissue factor expression during human and mouse development. Am J Pathol 149(1):101-113
55. Parry GCN, Mackman N. 2000 Mouse embryogenesis requires the tissue factor extracellular domain but not the cytoplasmic domain. J Clin Invest 105(11):1547-1554
56. Edstrom CS, Calhoun DA, Christensen RD. 2000 Expression of tissue factor pathway inhibitor in human fetal and placental tissues. Early Hum Dev 59(2):77-84
57. Giesen PLA, Rauch U, Bohrmann B, Kling D, Roqué M, Fallon JT, Badimon JJ, Himber J, Riederer MA, Nemerson Y. 1999 Blood-borne tissue factor: another view of thrombosis. Proc Natl Acad Sci USA 96: 2311-2315
58. Rivers RP, Hathaway WE. 1975 Studies on tissue factor activity and production by leukocytes of human umbilical cord and adult origin. Pediatr Res 9(4):167-171
59. Rivers RP, Hathaway WE, Weston WL. 1975 The endotoxin-induced coagulant activity of human monocytes. Br J Haematol 30(3):311-316
60. Grabowski EF, Carter CA, Tsukurov O, Conroy N, Hsu CY, Abbott WM, Ingelfinger JR, Orkin RW. 2000 Comparison of human umbilical vein and adult saphenous vein endothelial cells: implications for newborn hemostasis and for laboratory models of endothelial cell function. J Pediatr Hematol Oncol 22(3):266-268
61. Streif W, Paes B, Berry L, Andrew M, Andreasen RB, Chan AKC. 2000 Influence of exogenous factor VIIa on thrombin generation in cord plasma of full-term and pre-term newborns. Blood Coagul Fibrinolysis 11:349-357
62. Andrew M, Paes B, Milner R, Johnston M, Mitchell L, Tollefsen DM, Powers P. 1987 Development of the human coagulation system in the fullterm infant. Blood 70(1):165-172
63. Barnard DR, Simmons MA, Hathaway WE. 1979 Coagulation studies in extremely premature infants. Pediatr Res 13(12):1330-1335
64. Andrew M, Paes B, Milner R, Johnston M, Mitchell L, Tollefsen DM, Castle V, Powers P. 1988 Development of the human coagulation system in the healthy premature infant. Blood 72(5):1651-1657
65. Patel P, Weitz J, Brooker LA, Paes B, Mitchell L, Andrew M. 1996 Decreased thrombin activity of fibrin clots prepared in cord plasma compared with adult plasma. Pediatr Res 39(5):826-830
66. Katz JA, Moake JL, McPherson PD, Weinstein MJ, Moise KJ, Carpenter RJ, Sala DJ. 1989 Relationship between human development and disappearance of unusually large von Willebrand factor multimers from plasma. Blood 73(7):1851-1858
67. Shenkman B, Linder N, Savion N, Tamarin I, Dardik R, Kennet G, German B, Varon D. 1999 Increased neonatal platelet deposition on subendothelium under flow conditions: the role of plasma von Willebrand factor. Pediatr Res 45(2):270-275
68. Carcao MD, Blanchette VS, Dean JA, He L, Kern MA, Stain AM, Sparling CR, Stephens D, Ryan G, Freedman J, Rand ML. 1998 The platelet function analyzer (PFA-100): a novel in-vitro system for evaluation of primary haemostasis in children. Br J Haematol 101(1):70-73
69. Mannucci PM, Canciani MT, Forza I, Lussana F, Lattuada A, Rossi E. 2001 Changes in health and disease of the metalloprotease that cleaves von Willebrand factor. Blood 98(9):2730-2735
70. McDonald MM, Hathaway WE, Reeve EB, Leonard BD. 1982 Biochemical and functional study of antithrombin III in newborn infants. Thromb Haemost 47(1):56-58
71. Xiao H, Miller SJ, Bang NU, Faulk WP. 1999 Protein-bound heparin/heparan sulfates in human adult and umbilical cord plasma. Haemostasis 29(4):237-246
72. Andrew M, Mitchell L, Berry L, Paes B, Delorme M, Ofosu F, Burrows R, Khambalia B. 1992 An anticoagulant dermatan sulphate proteoglycan circulates in the pregnant woman and her fetus. J Clin Invest 89(1):321-326
73. McDonald MM, Johnson ML, Rumack CM, Koops BL, Guggenheim MA, Babb C, Hathaway WE. 1984 Role of coagulopathy in newborn intracranial hemorrhage. Pediatrics 74(1):26-31
74. Peters M, Ten Cate JW, Breederveld C, De Leeuw R, Emeis J, Koppe J. 1984 Low antithrombin III levels in neonates with idiopathic respiratory distress syndrome: poor prognosis. Pediatr Res 18(3):273-276
75. Andrew M, Massicotte-Nolan P, Mitchell L, Cassidy K. 1985 Dysfunctional antithrombin III in sick premature infants. Pediatr Res 19(2):237-239
76. Manco-Johnson MJ, Abshire TC, Jacobson LJ, Marlar RA. 1991 Severe neonatal protein C deficiency: prevalence and thrombotic risk. J Pediatr 119(5): 793-798
77. Suzuki K. 1993 Protein C inhibitor. Methods Enzymol 222:385-399
78. Reverdiau-Moalic P, Delahousse B, Body G, Bardos P, Leroy J, Gruel Y. 1996 Evolution of blood coagulation activators and inhibitors in the healthy human fetus. Blood 88(3):900-906
79. Roman J, Velasco F, Fernandez F, Fernandez M, Villalba R, Rubio V, Vicente A, Torres A. 1993 Coagulation, fibrinolytic and kallikrein systems in neonates with uncomplicated sepsis and septic shock. Haemostasis 23(3):142-148
80. Corrigan JJ Jr, Jeter MA. 1990 Histidine-rich glycoprotein and plasminogen plasma levels in term and preterm newborns. Am J Dis Child 144(7): 825-828
81. Benavent A, Estelles A, Aznar J, Martinez-Sales V, Gilabert J, Fornas E. 1984 Dysfunctional plasminogen in full term newborn: study of active site of plasmin. Thromb Haemost 51(1):67-70

82. Ries M. 1997 Molecular and functional properties of fetal plasminogen and its possible influence on clot lysis in the neonatal period. Semin Thromb Hemost 23(3):247-252

83. Hathaway WE, Mahasandana C, Makowski EL. 1975 Cord blood coagulation studies in infants of high-risk pregnant women. Am J Obstet Gynecol 121:51-57

84. Trusen B, Ries M, Zenker M, Rauh M, Beinder E, Keuper H, Harms D. 1998 Whole blood clot lysis in newborns nad adults after adding different concentrations of recombinant tissue plasminogen activator (RTPA). Semin Thromb Haemost 24(6):599-604

85. Aronis S, Platokouki H, Photopoulos S, Adamtziki E, Xanthou M. 1998 Indications of coagulation and/or fibrinolytic system activation in healthy and sick very-low-birth-weight neonates. Biol Neonate 74(5):337-344

86. Suzuki S, Morishita S. 1998 Hypercoagulability and DIC in high-risk infants. Semin Thromb Hemost 24(5):463-466

87. Schmidt B, Vegh P, Johnston M, Andrew M, Weitz J. 1993 Do coagulation screening tests detect increased generation of thrombin and plasmin in sick newborn infants? Thromb Haemost 69(5):418-421

88. Markarian M, Githens JH, Rosenblut E, Fernandez F, Jackson JJ, Bannon AE, Lindley A, Lubchenco LO, Martorell R. 1971 Hyercoagulability in premature infants with special reference to the respiratory distress syndrome and hemorrhage. I. Coagulation studies. Biol Neonate 17:84-97

89. Brus F, Oetomo SB, Schieving J, Groothuis E, Okken A, van Oeveren W. 1999 Increased tissue-type plasminogen activator antigen release is not accompanied by increased systemic fibrinolytic activity in severe neonatal respiratory distress syndrome. Pediatr Res 45(4):588-594

90. Aoki S, Hata T, Kitao M. 1992 Ultrasonographic assessment of fetal and neonatal spleen. Am J Perinatol 9(5-6):361-367

91. Feusner JH, Slichter SJ, Harker LA. 1983 Acquired haemostatic defects in the ill newborn. Br J Haematol 53(1):73-84

92. Karitzky D, Kleine N, Pringsheim W, Kunzer W. 1971 Fibrinogen turnover in the premature infant with and without idiopathic respiratory distress syndrome. Acta Paediatr Scand 60:465-470

93. Castle V, Coates G, Kelton J, Andrew M. 1987 In-oxine platelet survivals in thrombocytopenic infants. Blood 70(3):652-656

94. Gaffney PJ. 2001 Fibrin degradation products. A review of structures found in vitro and in vivo. Ann NY Acad Sci 936:594-610

95. Dempfle C-E. 1999 The use of soluble fibrin in evaluating the acute and chronic hypercoagulable state. Thromb Haemost 82(2):673-683

96. Boisclair MD, Ireland H, Lane DA. 1990 Assessment of hypercoagulable states by measurement of activation fragments and peptides. Blood Rev 4(1):25-40

97. Chuansumrit A, Hotrakitya S, Sirinavin S, Supapanachart S, Khowsathit P, Chantarojanasiri T, Phuapradit P, Hathirat P. 1999 Disseminated intravascular coagulation findings in 100 patients. J Med Assoc Thai 82[Supplement 1]:S63—S68

98. de Jonge E, van der Poll T, Kesecioglu J, Levi M. 2001 Anticoagulant factor concentrates in disseminated intravascular coagulation: rationale for use and clinical experience. Semin Thromb Hemost 27(6):667-674

99. Bernard GR, Vincent J-L, Laterre P-F, LaRosa SP, Dhainaut J-F, Lopez-Rodriguez A, Steingrub JS, Garber GE, Helterbrand JD, Ely EW, Fisher CJ Jr. 2001 Efficacy and safety of recombinant human activated protein C for severe sepsis. N Engl J Med 344(10):699-709

100. Yan SB, Dhainaut J-F. 2001 Activated protein C versus protein C in severe sepsis. Crit Care Med 29[Supplement]:S69-S74

101. Reinhart K, Karzai W. 2001 Anti-tumor necrosis factor therapy in sepsis: update on clinical trials and lessons learned. Crit Care Med 29[Supplement]:S121-S125

102. Gross SJ, Filston HC, Anderson JC. 1982 Controlled study of treatment for disseminated intravascular coagulation in the neonate. J Pediatr 100(3):445-448

103. Andrew M, Vegh P, Caco C, Kirpalani H, Jefferies A, Ohlsson A, Watts J, Saigal S, Milner R, Wang E. 1993 A randomized, controlled trial of platelet transfusion in thrombocytopenic premature infants. J Pediatr 123(2):285-291

104. Gobel U, von Voss JH, Jurgens H, Petrich C, Pothmann R, Sprock I, Lemburg P. 1980 Efficiency of heparin in the treatment of newborn infants with respiratory distress syndrome and disseminated intravascular coagulation. Eur J Pediatr 133(1):47-49

105. Schmidt B, Gillie P, Mitchell L, Andrew M, Caco C, Roberts R. 1998 A placebo-controlled randomized trial of antithrombin therapy in neonatal respiratory distress syndrome. Am J Respir Crit Care Med 158:470-476

106. Sills RH, Marlar RA, Montgomery RR, Deshpande GN, Humbert JR. 1984 Severe homozygous protein C deficiency. J Pediatr 105(3):409-413

107. Hartman KR, Manco-Johnson MJ, Rawlings JS, Bower DJ, Marlar RA. 1989 Homozygous protein C deficiency: early treatment with warfarin. Am J Pediatr Hematol Oncol 11(4):395-401

108. Mahasandana C, Suvatte V, Marlar RA, Manco-Johnson MJ, Jacobson LJ, Hathaway WE. 1990 Neonatal purpura fulminans associated with homozygous protein S deficiency. Lancet 335(8680):61-62

109. Cassels-Brown A, Minford AM, Chatfield SL, Bradbury JA. 1994 Ophthalmic manifestations of neonatal protein C deficiency. Br J Ophthalmol 78(6):486-487

110. Hattenbach LO, Beeg T, Kreuz W, Zubcov A. 1999 Ophthalmic manifestations of congenital protein C deficiency. J AAPOS 3(3):188-190

111. Mintz-Hittner HA, Miyashiro MJ, Knight-Nanan DM, O'Malley RE, Marlar RA. 1999 Vitreoretinal findings similar to retinopathy of prematurity in infants

112. Formstone CJ, Hallam PJ, Tuddenham EG, Voke J, Layton M, Nicolaides K, Hann IM, Cooper DN. 1996 Severe perinatal thrombosis in double and triple heterozygous offspring of a family segregating two independent protein S mutations and a protein C mutation. Blood 87(9):3731-3737

113. Aiach M, Gandrille S. 1996 Molecular basis for protein C hereditary deficiency. Haemostasis 26[Supplement 4]:9-19

114. Millar DS, Johansen B, Berntorp E, Minford A, Bolton-Maggs P, Wensley R, Kakkar V, Schulman S, Torres A, Bosch N, Cooper DN. 2000 Molecular genetic analysis of severe protein C deficiency. Hum Genet 106(6):646-653

115. Ido M, Ohiwa M, Hayashi T, Nishioka J, Hatada T, Watanabe Y, Wada H, Shirakawa S, Suzuki K. 1993 A compound heterozygous protein C deficiency with a single nucleotide G deletion encoding Gly-381 and an amino acid substitution of Lys for Gla-26. Thromb Haemost 70(4):636-641

116. Soria JM, Brito D, Barceló J, Fontcuberta J, Botero L, Maldonado J, Estivill X, Sala N. 1994 Severe homozygous protein C deficiency: identification of a splice site missense mutation (184, Q-*bgH) in exon 7 of the protein C gene. Thromb Haemost 72(1):65-69

117. Millar DS, Allgrove J, Rodeck C, Kakkar VV, Cooper DN. 1994 A homozygous deletion/insertion mutation in the protein C (PROC) gene causing neonatal purpura fulminans: prenatal diagnosis in an at-risk pregnancy. Blood Coagul Fibrinolysis 5(4):647-649

118. Witt I Beck K, Seydewitz HH, Tasangil C, Schenck W. 1994 A novel homozygous missense mutation (Val 325-*bgAla) in the protein C gene causing neonatal purpura fulminans. Blood Coagul Fibrinolysis 5(4):651-653

119. Soria JM, Morell M, Jimenez-Astorga C, Estivill X, Sala N. 1995 Severe type I protein C deficiency in a compound heterozygote for Y124C and Q132X mutations in exon 6 of the PROC gene. Thromb Haemost 74(5):1215-1220

120. Nakayama T, Matsushita T, Hidano H, Suzuki C, Hamaguchi M, Kojima T, Saito H. 2000 A case of purpura fulminans is caused by homozygous delta8857 mutation (protein C-nagoya) and successfully treated with activated protein C concentrate. Br J Haematol 110(3):727-730

121. Wermes C, Bergmann F, Reller B, Sykora KW. 1999 Severe protein C deficiency and aseptic osteonecrosis of the hip joint: a case report. Eur J Pediatr 158[Supplement 3]:S159-S161

122. Ezer U, Misirlioglu ED, Colba V, Ogoz E, Kurt C. 2001 Neonatal purpura fulminans due to homozygous protein C deficiency. Pediatr Hematol Oncol 18(7):453-8

123. Pung-amritt P, Poort SR, Vos HL, Bertina RM, Mahasandana C, Tanphaichitr VS, Veerakul G, Kankirawatana S, Suvatte V. 1999 Compound heterozygosity for one novel and one recurrent mutation in a Thai patient with severe protein S deficiency. Thromb Haemost 81(2):189-192

124. Tsuda H, Urata M, Tsuda T, Wakiyama M, Iida H, Nakahara M, Kinoshita S, Hamasaki N. 2002 Four missense mutations identified in the protein S gene of thrombosis patients with protein S deficiency: effects on secretion and anticoagulant activity of protein S. Thromb Res 105(3):233-239

125. Pipe SW, Schmaier AH, Nichols WC, Ginsburg D, Bozynski ME, Castle VP. 1996 Neonatal purpura fulminans in association with factor V R506Q mutation. J Pediatr 128(5):706-709

126. Rivard GE, David M, Farrell C, Schwarz HP. 1995 Treatment of purpura fulminans in meningococcemia with protein C concentrate. J Pediatr 126(4):646-652

127. Manco-Johnson MJ, Nuss R, Key N, Moertel C, Jacobson L, Meech S, Weinberg A, Lefkowitz J. 1996 Lupus anticoagulant and protein S deficiency in children with postvaricella purpura fulminans or thrombosis. J Pediatr 128:319-323

128. Chuansumrit A, Hotrakitya S, Kruavit A. 1996 Severe acquired neonatal purpura fulminans. Clin Pediatr 35(7):373-376

129. Manco-Johnson MJ, Grabowski EF, Hellgreen M, Kemahli AS, Massicotte MP, Muntean W, Peters M, Nowak-Göttl U. 2002 Laboratory testing for thrombophilia in pediatric patients: on behalf of the Subcommittee for Perinatal and Pediatric Thrombosis of the Scientific and Standardization Committee of the International Society of Thrombosis and Haemostasis (ISTH) Thromb Haemost 88:155-156

130. Dreyfus M, Masterson M, David M, Rivard GE, Muller F-M, Kreuz W, Beeg T, Minford A, Allgrove J, Cohen JD, Christoph J, Bergmann F, Mitchell VE, Haworth C, Nelson K, Schwarz HP. 1995 Replacement therapy with a monoclonal antibody purified protein C concentrate in newborns with severe congenital protein C deficiency. Semin Thromb Hemost 21(4):371-381

131. Kreuz WD, Schneider W, Nowak-Göttl U. 1999 Treatment of consumption coagulopathy with antithrombin concentrate in children with acquired antithrombin deficiency: a feasibility pilot study. Eur J Pediatr 158[Supplement 3]:S187-S191

132. Monagle P, Andrew M, Halton J, Marlar R, Jardine L, Vegh P, Johnston M, Webber C, Massicotte MP. 1998 Homozygous protein C deficiency: description of a new mutation and successful treatment with low molecular weight heparin. Thromb Haemost 79(4):756-761

133. Schmidt B, Andrew M. 1995 Neonatal thrombosis: report of a prospective Canadian and international registry. Pediatrics 96(5):939-943

134. van Ommen CH, Heijboer H, Buller HR, Hirasing RA, Heijmans HS, Peters M. 2001 Venous thromboembolism in childhood: a prospective two-year registry in the Netherlands. J Pediatr 139(5):676-681

135. Salonvaara M, Riikonen P, Kekomaki R, Heinonen K. 1999 Clinically symptomatic central venous catheter-related deep venous thrombosis in newborns. Acta Paediatr 88(6):642-646

136. Kim JH, Lee YS, Kim SH, Lee SK, Lim MK, Kim HS. 2001 Does umbilical vein catheterization lead to portal venous thrombosis? Prospective US evaluation in 100 neonates. Radiology 219(3):645-650

137. Kido DK, Paulin S, Alenghat JA, Waternaux C, Riley WD. 1982 Thrombogenicity of heparin- and non-heparin-coated catheters: clinical trial. AJR Am J Roentgenol 139(5):957-961

138. Hecker JF. 1981 Thrombogenicity of tips of umbilical catheters. Pediatrics 67(4):467-471

139. Mokrohisky ST, Levine RL, Blumhagen JD, Wesenberg RL, Simmons MA. 1978 Low positioning of umbilical-artery catheters increases associated complications in newborn infants. N Engl J Med 299(11):561-564

140. McDonald P, Tarar R, Gilday D, Reilly BJ. 1974 Some radiologic observations in renal vein thrombosis. Am J Roentgenol Radium Ther Nucl Med 120(2):368-388

141. Bokenkamp A, von Kries R, Nowak-Gottl U, Gobel U, Hoyer PF. 2000 Neontal renal venous thrombosis in Germany between 1992 and 1994: epidemiology, treatment and outcome. Eur J Pediatr 159:44-48

142. Nuss R, Hays T, Manco-Johnson M. 1994 Efficacy and safety of heparin anticoagulation for neonatal renal vein thrombosis. Am J Pediatr Hematol Oncol 16(2):127-131

143. deVeber G, Andrew M, Adams C, Bjornson B, Booth F, Buckley DJ, Camfield CS, David M, Humphreys P, Langevin P, MacDonald EA, Meaney B, Shevell M, Sinclair DB, Yager J, Gillett J. 2001 Cerebral sinovenous thrombosis in children. N Engl J Med 345(6):417-423

144. Volpe JJ. 1989 Intraventricular hemorrhage in the premature infant-current concepts. I. Ann Neurol 25(1):3-11

145. Gunther G, Junker R, Sträter R, Schobess R, Kurnik K, Heller C, Kosch A, Nowak-Göttl U. 2000 Symptomatic ischemic stroke in full-term neonates: role of acquired and genetic prothrombotic risk factors. Stroke 31:2437-2441

146. Rand T, Weninger M, Kohlhauser C, Bischof S, Heinz-Peer G, Trattnig S, Popow C, Salzer HR. 1996 Effects of umbilical arterial catheterization on mesenteric hemodynamics. Pediatr Radiol 26(7):435-438

147. Gross GP, Hathaway WE, McGaughey HR. 1973 Hyperviscosity in the neonate. J Pediatr 82(6):1004-1012.

148. Borzini P, Lazzaro A, Mazzucco L, Papili F. 2001 The in-vitro bleeding time for the screening of platelet function in the newborn: assessment of a normal reference range. Eur J Pediatr 160(3):199-200

149. Knofler R, Weissbach G, Kuhlisch E. 1998 Platelet function tests in childhood: measuring aggregation and release reaction in whole blood. Semin Thromb Hemost 24(6):513-521

150. Stuart MJ, Elrad H, Graeber JE, Hakanson DO, Sunderji SG, Barvinchak MK. 1979 Increased synthesis of prostaglandin endoperoxides and platelet hyperfunction in infants of mothers with diabetes mellitus. J Lab Clin Med 94(1):12-26.

151. Stuart MJ, Sunderji SG, Allen JB. 1981 Decreased prostacylin production in the infant of the diabetic mother. J Lab Clin Med 98(3):412-416

152. Sheridan-Pereira M, Porreco RP, Hays T, Burke MS. 1988 Neonatal aortic thrombosis associated with the lupus anticoagulant. Obstet Gynecol 71(6):1016-1018

153. Finazzi G, Cortelazzo S, Viero P, Galli M, Barbui T. 1987 Maternal lupus anticoagulant and fatal neonatal thrombosis. Thromb Haemost 57(2):238

154. Reitsma PH. 2000 Genetic heterogeneity in hereditary thrombophilia. Haemostasis 30 [Supplement 2]:1-10

155. Rosendaal FR. 1997 Thrombosis in the young: epidemiology and risk factors. A focus on venous thrombosis. Thromb Haemost 78(1):1-6

156. Manco-Johnson MJ. 1997 Disorders of hemostasis in childhood: risk factors for venous thromboembolism. Thromb Haemost 78(1):710-714

157. Manco-Johnson MJ, Nuss R. 2001 Thrombophilia in the infant and child. Adv Pediatr 48:363-384.

158. Nowak-Göttl U, Kosch A, Schlegel N, Salem M, Manco-Johnson M. 2002 Thromboembolism in children. Curr Opin Hematol 9:448-453

159. Ruiz-Arguelles GJ, Garces-Eisele J, Reyes-Nunez V, Ramirez-Cisneros FJ. 2001 Primary thrombophilia in Mexico. II. Factor V G1691A (Leiden), prothrombin G20210A, and methylenetetrahydrofolate reductase C677T polymorphism in thrombophilic Mexican mestizos. Am J Hematol 66(1):28-31

160. Hagstrom JN, Walter J, Bluebond-Langner R, Amatniek JC, Manno CS, High KA. 1998 Prevalence of the factor V Leiden mutation in children and neonates with thromboembolic disease. J Pediatr 133(6):777-781

161. Günther G, Junker R, Sträter R, Schobess R, Kurnik K, Kosch A, Nowak-Göttl U, Childhood Stroke Study Group. 2000 Symptomatic ischemic stroke in full-term neonates: role of acquired and genetic prothrombotic risk factors. Stroke 31(10):2437-2441

162. Young G, Manco-Johnson M, Gill JC, DiMichele DM, Tarantino MD, Abshire T, Nugent DJ. 2003 Clinical manifestations of the prothrombin G20210A mutation in children: a pediatric coagulation consortium study. J Thromb Haemost 1(5): 958-962.

163. Ambruso DR, Jacobson LJ, Hathaway WE. 1980 Inherited antithrombin III deficiency and cerebral thrombosis in a child. Pediatrics 65(1):125-131

164. Gould RJ, Black K, Pavlakis SG. 1996 Neonatal cerebral arterial thrombosis: protein C deficiency. J Child Neurol 11(3):250-252

165. Yap S, Boers GH, Wilcken B, Wilcken DE, Brenton DP, Lee PJ, Walter JH, Howard PM, Naughten ER. 2001 Vascular outcome in patients with homocystinuria due to cystathionine β-synthase deficiency. Thromb Vasc Biol 21(12): 2080-2085

166. Coppola A, Davi G, De Stefano V, Mancini FP, Cerbone AM, Di Minno G. 2000 Homocysteine, coagulation, platelet function, and thrombosis. Semin Thromb Hemost 26(3):243-254

167. Nowak-Göttl U, Junker R, Kreuz W, von Eckardstein A, Kosch A, Nohe N, Schobess R, Ehrenforth S, Childhood Thrombophilia Study Group. 2001 Risk of recurrent venous thrombosis in children with combined prothrombotic risk factors. Blood 97(4):858-862

168. von Depka M, Nowak-Göttl U, Eisert R, Dieterich C, Barthels M, Scharrer I, Ganser A, Ehrenforth S. 2000 Increased lipoprotein (a) levels as an independent risk factor for venous thromboembolism. Blood 2000 96(10): 3364-3368

169. Petäjä J, Hiltunen L, Fellman V. 2001 Increased risk of intraventricular hemorrhage in preterm infants with thrombophilia. Pediatr Res 49(5):643-646

170. Alfirevic Z, Roberts D, Martlew V. 2002 How strong is the association between maternal thrombophilia and adverse pregnancy outcome? A systematic review. Eur J Obstet Gynecol Reprod Biol 101(1):6-14

171. Gris JC, Quere I, Monpeyroux F, Mercier E, Ripart-Neveu S, Tailland ML, Hoffet M, Berlan J, Daures JP, Mares P. 1999 Case-control study of the frequency of thrombophilic disorders in couples with late foetal loss and no thrombotic antecedent: the Nimes Obstetricians and Haematologists Study 5 (NOHA5). Thromb Haemost 81(6):891-899

172. Verspyck E, Le CD, Goffinet F, Tron F, Marpeau L, Borg JY. 2002 Thrombophilia and immunologic disorders in pregnancies as risk factors for small for gestational age infants. Br J Obstet Gynaecol 109(1):28-33

173. von Kries R, Junker R, Oberle D, Kosch A, Nowak-Gotti U. 2001 Foetal growth restriction in children with prothrombotic risk factors. Thromb Haemost 86(4):1012-1016

174. McDonald MM, Jacobson LJ, Hay WW JR, Hathaway WE. 1981 Heparin clearance in the newborn. Pediatr Res 15(7):1015-1018

175. McDonald MM, Hathaway WE. 1982 Anticoagulant therapy by continuous heparinization in newborn and older infants. J Pediatr 101(3):451-457

176. Massicotte P, Adams M, Marzinotto V, Brooker LA, Andrew M. 1996 Low molecular weight heparin in pediatric patients with thrombotic disease: a dose finding study. J Pediatr 128(3):313-318

177. Punzalan RC, Hillery CA, Montgomery RR, Scott CA, Gill JC. 2000 Low-molecular-weight heparin in thrombotic disease in children and adolescents. J Pediatr Hematol Oncol 22(2):137-142

178. Severin T, Sutor AH. 2001 Heparin-induced thrombocytopenia in pediatrics. Semin Thromb Hemost 27(3):293-299

179. Spadone D, Clark F, James E, Laster J, Hoch J, Silver D. 1992 Heparin-induced thrombocytopenia in the newborn. J Vasc Surg 15(2):306-311

180. Manco-Johnson MJ, Grabowski EF, Hellgren M, Kemahli AS, Massicotte MP, Muntean W, Peters M, Schlegel N, Wang M, Nowak-Göttl U. 2002 Recommendations for tPA thrombolysis in children: on behalf of the Scientific Subcommittee on Perinatal and Pediatric Haemostasis of the Scientific and Standardization Committee of the International Society of Thrombosis and Haemostasis. Thromb Haemost 88(1):157-158

181. Wang M, Hays T, Balasa V, Bagatell R, Gruppo R, Grabowski EF, Valentino LA, Tsao-Wu G, Manco-Johnson MJ. 2003 Low-dose tissue plasminogen activator thrombolysis in children. J Pediatr Hematol Oncol 25(5):379-386

182. Bokenkamp A, von Kries R, Nowak-Gottl U, Gobel U, Hoyer PF. 2000 Neonatal renal venous thrombosis in Germany between 1992 and 1994: epidemiology, treatment and outcome. Eur J Pediatr 159(1-2):44-48

Developmental Immunobiology

151

Timothy R. La Pine and Harry R. Hill

Host Defense Mechanisms Against Bacteria

This chapter provides an overview of host defense mechanisms against bacterial infections. Bacterial sepsis is a major contributor to neonatal mortality and morbidity. The incidence of sepsis in the first month of life ranges from 1 to as high as 10 cases per thousand live births.[1] In certain geographic areas, this rate may be significantly higher.[2] Bacterial sepsis occurs more frequently in preterm infants and when there have been maternal complications, such as premature rupture of membranes or intrapartum infections.[1,2] Although advancements in maternal medical management and neonatal intensive care have decreased infant mortality and morbidity, prolonged hospitalization and invasive procedures have contributed to an increased incidence of certain bacterial infections. In spite of the development of potent antimicrobial agents, the mortality rate associated with neonatal bacterial sepsis ranges from 5 to 15%.[1,2] Furthermore, the compromised nature of a developing neonate's host defense system allows for bacterial dissemination from intravascular to extravascular sites, including the meninges, lungs, and bones. The morbidity from these secondary infections is high.[3,4]

The unique predisposition of the human neonate to bacterial infections is attributed to defects in both innate and acquired immune responses. The innate, or natural, immune response is nonspecific and not influenced by prior antigen interactions. Various physical (e.g., skin, cilia, mucus) and biochemical barriers (e.g., gastric acid, lysozyme, surfactant proteins), as well as phagocytic cells (e.g., granulocytes and macrophages) and the plasma factors (e.g., acute-phase reactants, the complement system, the coagulation cascade, and pattern recognition receptors) comprise innate immune responses. The acquired, or adaptive, immune response is specific. It is characterized by direct immune responsiveness as a result of an initial antigen exposure, with a memory, or anamnestic, response on antigen re-exposure. Acquired immune responses include humoral immunity involving immunoglobulin production by B lymphocytes and cellular immunity mediated by T lymphocytes and associated factors (e.g., natural killer cells, cytokines, and interleukins). Neonatal immune development is discussed in depth in other chapters within this section; here we highlight deficiencies of this development in host defense against bacterial infections.

THE CHANGING NATURE OF NEONATAL BACTERIAL INFECTIONS

Group A streptococci and other gram-positive organisms often were the etiologic agents of newborn bacterial sepsis prior to the introduction of antibiotics. Later, after penicillins and sulfonamides were introduced in the 1940s, gram-negative organisms such as *Escherichia coli*, *Klebsiella pneumoniae*, and *Pseudomonas aeruginosa* became prominent.[5] Since the mid-1960s, group B streptococcal infections have become the most common infections in neonates throughout the United States and in other developed countries.[1,6] It is interesting that this organism has not played a major role in neonatal sepsis in many developing countries such as Mexico, India, and Thailand, where *Klebsiella* and *E. coli* are still the predominant pathogens.[2] The reasons for this are not clear. Infants generally acquire group B streptococcal infections by vertical transmission from the birth canal of a colonized mother. The low rates of invasive neonatal group B streptococcal disease in developing countries may reflect low maternal colonization rates, less virulent strains of group B streptococci bacteria, or high levels of transplacental acquired antibody.

While group B streptococci and *E. coli* together account for over 70% of serious bacterial infections in neonates, their distribution is changing.[2] Antibiotics are increasingly used perinatally to reduce the risk of neonatal group B streptococcal infection during premature labor and premature rupture of the membranes. There is concern that this increased use of antibiotics may result in a change in the spectrum of organisms and their susceptibility to antibiotics. Stoll and associates,[7] in a multicenter trial evaluating the etiology of early-onset neonatal sepsis among infants weighing less than 1500 g, found an increased prevalence of *E. coli* sepsis and a marked reduction in group B streptococcal sepsis between 1998 and 2000 when compared with an earlier cohort born between 1991 and 1993. Furthermore, 85% of the *E. coli* isolates were resistant to ampicillin. The mothers who received intrapartum ampicillin for group B streptococcal carriage were more likely to have infants with ampicillin-resistant *E. coli* infections. Antibiotic use can change the spectrum of neonatal bacterial infections and increase the prevalence of antibiotic-resistant organisms.

Staphylococci are a major cause of nosocomial neonatal bacteremia and sepsis in intensive care nurseries. Noel and Edelson[8] identified 23 cases of clinically significant neonatal ICU *Staphylococcus epidermidis* infections during a 17-month period. Ten of these episodes were associated with colonized indwelling catheters. Staphylococci have surface proteins that mediate their attachment to intravascular devices and other foreign bodies in addition to damaged endothelial cells. Once this surface attachment takes place, phagocytosis by neutrophils is inhibited, as is antibiotic penetration, and a nidus for infection is established. Infections with staphylococcal species are of particular concern in the extremely low birth weight infants requiring indwelling catheters.

Other organisms such as *Listeria monocytogenes*, *Haemophilus influenzae*, *Neisseria meningitidis*, and groups C, D, and G streptococci also can cause serious neonatal infection.[3] Anaerobic organisms additionally may be isolated alone or in combination with aerobes from septic neonates.

Campylobacter fetus, jejuni, and *coli* also have been implicated in premature delivery and associated with fetal and neonatal infection and mortality.[9]

THE COMPONENTS OF INNATE HOST DEFENSE

The innate, or natural, immune system provides host protection against microbial invasion without the need for prior exposure to that microbe. The innate immune system developed first phylogenetically, appearing in all multicellular organisms, including plants, insects, and animals, and is the first line of defense against invasive pathogens.[10,11] It is active before the acquired immune responses and does not change or amplify upon pathogen re-exposure. The activities of innate immunity are both rapid, to prevent early microbial invasion, and nonspecific, to protect against multiple pathogens of diverse nature. Cells of the innate immune system contribute to antigen processing and presentation as well.[10]

Epithelial Cells, Normal Bacterial Flora, and Mucosal Barriers

Integrity of the skin and the epithelial surfaces of the respiratory and gastrointestinal tracts serves to impede microbe ingress physically. Premature infants with incomplete skin epithelization who require indwelling catheters are predisposed to bacterial infections, particularly with staphylococcal species. Damage to the respiratory epithelium with ventilation and oxygenation can predispose neonates to pneumonias. Similarly, immaturity of innate immune responses in the developing gastrointestinal tract predispose preterm infants to necrotizing enterocolitis and other intestinal infections, all of which can lead to invasive bacterial infections.

Normal microbial flora contribute to innate host defense at epithelial and mucosal surfaces. Humans are colonized with a variety of microorganisms that suppress the overgrowth of pathogenic microbes. Normal flora produce bacteriocins and other antimicrobial agents that suppress the growth of invasive pathogens.[12] Alteration of the flora by antimicrobial therapy may result in the emergence of invasive pathogens.

The moisture content or type of epithelial cell surface may predispose the host to colonization with pathogens. Circumcision decreases the incidence of urinary tract infections.[13,14] Uncircumcised infants are more likely to harbor *E. coli* and *Proteus mirabilis* in the urethral meatus and periurethral area than circumcised boys.[15,16] Fimbriated *E. coli* adhere better to the moist inner surface of the foreskin than to the outer keratinized surface.[17]

To produce invasive infection, group B streptococci (GBS) must first broach the mucosal barrier. Adherence of GBS to mucosal epithelial cells is a critical step for both maternal colonization and invasion of the neonatal respiratory tract. Adhesins are surface molecules on bacteria that facilitate binding to host eukaryotic cells. Lipoteichoic acid and surface proteins facilitate GBS binding to epithelial cells.[18-21] The greater adherence of type III GBS to neonatal respiratory epithelium facilitates its colonization and predominance in early-onset neonatal sepsis. The physical disruption of the epithelial cell surface, however, may not be required for GBS invasion. GBS can transgress intact cultured respiratory epithelial cells via actin microfilament-dependent processes.[22]

Innate immunity in the respiratory tract includes the cilia of the nasal mucosa and the passageways of the upper airways, bronchi, and bronchioles. Cilia present on respiratory epithelium serve to impede respiratory invasion of microbial pathogens and remove or expel them.[23] Abnormalities, such as those seen in Kartagener syndrome, underscore the role of cilia in innate host defense. These patients suffer chronic bronchitis and bron-chiectasis because of a defect in ciliary rods that results in immotile cilia. Patients with tracheotomies, or requiring prolonged ventilation, are predisposed to pulmonary infections as a result of the breakdown of epithelial immune integrity in the nasopharynx, glottis, trachea, and lung.

Mucin glycoproteins contribute to airway surface fluid. They provide viscosity and physically impede microbe invasion.[24,25] The genes for the mucin glycoproteins, MUC2 and MUC5A, are up-regulated by lipopolysaccharide and by gram-positive and gram-negative bacteria.[26] These glycoproteins do not possess antimicrobial activity, but provide a milieu for immune defense. The airway surface fluid contains a variety of antimicrobial proteins, such as lysozyme, lactoferrin, and defensins, as well as reactive oxygen and nitrogen species.[25,27,28] Other inflammatory cells of the respiratory tract include macrophages, neutrophils, mast cells, and natural killer cells. The cytokines produced by these cells and the respiratory epithelium also contribute to the antimicrobial activity of airway surface fluid.

The salt or fluid content at the airway surface may protect against microbial invasion. The high salt content or the decreased airway fluid observed in cystic fibrosis patients, may inhibit normal airway antibacterial activities and contribute to the persistent bacterial colonization and chronic infections seen in these patients.[27,29]

Growth factors and cytokines within the amniotic fluid contribute to fetal gastric immune development. Pregnancies complicated by oligohydramnios, whether due to premature membrane rupture or congenital abnormalities, are at higher risk for intestinal infections.[30] Transplacentally acquired immunoglobulins and hormones also influence the development of the enteric immune system. Immunoglobulins, particularly IgA, present in breast milk, both promote and provide intestinal mucosal immunity.[31] Within hours after birth, the neonate's intestinal tract is colonized by multiple species of bacteria and some viruses. Premature delivery, systemic infection, diet, and antibiotic exposure can alter enteric flora, resulting in local inflammation or invasive infection.[30]

Cells Involved in Innate Host Defense

The innate immune response involves neutrophils, monocytes, macrophages, and dendritic cells capable of phagocytosis. These cells, along with mast cells, also produce a number of inflammatory mediators, including colony-stimulating factors and a variety of cytokines that have roles in both innate and acquired immune responses.

Neutrophils

Neutrophils are central to neonatal host defense against bacteria. Neutrophils appear after macrophages appear in the human fetus. Scattered neutrophil precursors occur in the liver as early as 5 weeks. Bone marrow neutrophils are first present around 10 to 11 weeks.[32-34] Neutrophils are the first cells to migrate into a local area of microbial invasion and are important components of early innate defense.[35] Activated neutrophils must adhere to and migrate through capillary epithelial cell surfaces, then engulf and destroy invading pathogens. Neonatal neutrophils have profound deficiencies in their ability to perform these functions, which contribute to their increased susceptibility to infection. Bone marrow neutrophil storage pools are also low in neonates, further predisposing them to bacterial infections.[35]

Neutrophils possess individual receptors for complement fragments such as C5a, formylated peptides, leukotriene B$_4$, and chemokines such as IL-8. These receptors initiate intracellular responses through α, β, and γ and guanosine triphosphate-binding proteins, leading to the activation of protein kinase C and the release of intracellular calcium. Activation of these signaling pathways and the binding of inflammatory mediators induce changes in the neutrophil surface charge, membrane potential, iron flux, and membrane fluidity. This interaction upregulates the surface expression of adhesive glycoproteins, such as leukocyte selectin, Sialyl-Lewis X, and the integrins CD11/CD18.[35,36] Sialyl-Lewis X promotes neutrophil-endothelial cell selectin interactions, resulting in the rolling along and tethering to activated endothelial cell surfaces. The integrins Mac-1 (CD11b/18) bind to endothelial cell intracellular adhesion molecule-1 (ICAM 1), contributing to tight neutrophil adhesion at the site of microbial inoculation. Stimulated neonatal neutrophils have defective membrane potential changes, decreased fluidity, and an associated decreased intracellular calcium flux when compared with adult neutrophils.[35,36] Their ability to adhere to endothelial cell surfaces in vitro is also reduced when compared with adult cells.[37]

Neutrophil movement is initiated through G-proteins and calcium binding to calmodulin, which activates the contraction of cytoskeleton actin and myosin filaments. This leads to diapedesis through the epithelial cell surface and chemotaxis toward the inflammatory focus. Movement is partially dependent on interactions between Mac-1 (CD11b/18), as well as the other integrins and the extracellular matrix.[38, 39] When neutrophils arrive at sites of microbial invasion, the cells spread out and upregulate several phagocytic cell surface receptors. These include receptors for the Fc fragment of immunoglobulin, the complement receptors, C3b and iC3b, fibronectin, and other nonspecific receptors of innate immunity.[36] Neonatal neutrophils show impaired directed movement. The possible mechanisms for this include decreased complement receptors, defects in signal transduction resulting in low intracellular calcium responses, impaired cytoskeletal regulation, incomplete receptor up-regulation, and reduced energy metabolism.[37]

Neutrophils ingest pathogens opsonized with natural antibodies, specific antibodies, complement fragments, or nonspecific opsonins such as fibronectin.[40] Pathogens are killed by oxygen-dependent or -independent processes and antimicrobial factors. Phagolysosome fusion permits entry of granule contents into phagocytic vacuoles. Myeloperoxidase from primary or azurophilic granules catalyzes the production of hypochlorite ion from chloride and hydrogen peroxide, which can react with amines to produce toxic chloramines.[23] Neutrophils from stressed or infected neonates have decreased respiratory burst activity on exposure to GBS, *E. coli*, and *S. aureus* when compared with adults.[41,42] Other components of azurophilic granules include the antibacterial activities of the defensins, lysozyme, and bacterial permeability-increasing protein.[43] Neutrophils also produce a number of proinflammatory cytokines, including TNF-α, IL-1β, and IL-6, further activating innate and acquired immune responses.[44]

Monocytes, Macrophages, and Dendritic Cells

Mononuclear phagocytes, monocytes and macrophages, like neutrophils, are recruited to sites of infection. Neonates have diminished influx of monocytes to areas of inflammation. The adhesion of fetal and newborn monocytes is comparable to that of adult monocytes, but they have reduced chemotactic ability.[45-47] Monocytes exhibit considerably less respiratory burst production of hydrogen peroxide and other toxic reactive molecules compared with neutrophils.[48,49] The ability of fetal and neonatal monocytes to kill pathogens including *S. aureus*, *S. epidermidis*, *E. coli*, group B streptococci, and *Candida albicans*, is equal to that of adult monocytes.[50,51]

Monocytes synthesize and secrete numerous products involved in the inflammatory process. These include polypeptide hormones, complement components, cytokines, coagulation factors, enzymes, extracellular matrix proteins, and bioactive oligopeptides and lipids.[52] Certain products, such as the polypeptides IL-1, IFN-α, and tumor necrosis factor alpha, are synthesized in similar concentrations by newborn and adult monocytes.[53-55] Other molecules, including polypeptides such as IFN-γ, IL-8, IL-10, and G-CSF; extracellular matrix proteins such as fibronectin; and bioreactive lipids, such as leukotriene B₄, are synthesized in reduced concentrations by neonatal monocytes.[56-60] The principal function of monocytes in neonatal host defense may be their production of inflammatory mediators. The significance of these differences in host defense is currently under investigation.

Monocytes from developing bone marrow stores are released into the blood stream where they may circulate for extended periods of time. These monocytes may then enter into tissues and differentiate into macrophages.[32-34] Macrophages have been described in the developing yolk sac, lung, and liver long before monocyte bone marrow development has been established. Fetal liver and lung macrophages are capable of self-proliferation.[61-63] Macrophages line the vascular sinusoids of the spleen, liver, and lymph nodes. This strategic placement allows for host defense of pathogens just below the epithelial barriers of the skin and respiratory and gastrointestinal tracts, and at blood-filtering sites. Macrophages alert cells of both innate and acquired immunity to microbial invasion through the release of cytokines and other inflammatory mediators.

Macrophages are avidly phagocytic and can readily kill most pathogens such as *S. pneumoniae*, *H. influenzae*, and *S. aureus*.[23] Some intracellular bacteria, such as *Mycobacteria*, *Nocardia*, and *Legionella* can survive within macrophages. Cytokine stimulation of infected macrophages (e.g., IFN-γ, IL-12, IL-18, and CSFs), is required to kill these pathogens. Deficiency of these cytokines or their receptors can result in infections with these intracellular bacteria.[23]

Macrophages generate several mediators and proteins that contribute to microbial killing. The ligands include arachidonic acid pathway–derived components such as leukotriene B₄. The proteins include lysozyme, lactoferrin, transferrin, and the defensins.[23] Macrophage-derived mediators initiate the inflammatory response and recruit neutrophils. These include the cytokines, TNF-α, IL-1, IL-12, IFN-γ, GM-CSF, G-CSF; the chemokines, chemotactic peptides, IL-8, macrophage inflammatory proteins, macrophage chemotactic peptide, and other related chemokines.[23,64,65]

Dendritic cells are macrophage-like cells that are less phagocytic and less adherent than macrophages. They are notable for their irregular shape with numerous membrane processes. These cells may leave the skin and migrate to afferent lymphatics and regional lymph nodes. Dendritic cells are present throughout the lungs and most organs except the brain. These cells, which ultimately initiate acquired immune responses via T cells, have the ability to migrate through tissues and ingest extracellular microbes by endocytosis.[66,67]

Mast Cells

Mast cells can be activated by IgE or by microbial pathogens.[68] Mast cell interaction with microbes such as *Salmonella typhimurium* and *Schistosoma mansoni* may be opsonin-dependent or mediated by complement fragments including C3b and iC3b.[69,70] Bacteria such as *E. coli* and *K. pneumoniae* may associate with mast cells in an opsonin-independent manner through mast cell pattern receptors.[71-73] The pattern recognition receptor on mast cells for mannose-binding lectin on *E. coli* and other enterobacteria appears to be a mannose-containing receptor molecule.[74] In addition, gram-positive bacteria such as *S. aureus* and streptococci are able to induce mast cell-mediated cytokine release.[71]

Mast cell degranulation can initiate leukocyte recruitment and enhance host defense against microbial invasion.[75,76] Leukocyte recruitment is mediated, in part, by TNF-α stimulation of vascular and bronchial ICAM-1 leading to leukocyte adherence. Histamine up-regulates selectins, which promote leukocyte rolling along and tethering to the endothelial cell surface. Platelet-activating factor may enhance CD-18–dependent leukocyte adhesion.[77] Mast cells may release IL-8, which stimulates neutrophil migration. Mast cells can phagocytize and kill both gram-positive and gram-negative bacteria.[71,72,78] Mast cells can present antigen, in the context of class I or II HLA molecules, to cells of the acquired immune system.[79] Mast cells or their products also play an important role in the defense against parasitic infections.[80]

γδ T Lymphocytes and B-1 Lymphocytes

The late innate response to bacterial, viral, and parasitic infections includes γδ T lymphocyte infiltration and B-1 lymphocyte activation.[81] The γδ T cell receptors recognize glycolipid antigens present on many microbes.[82] Located in the epithelial linings of the skin and gastrointestinal and respiratory tracts, where they proliferate and release cytokines, they are also termed *intraepithelial T lymphocytes*.[83-85] The peritoneal cavity contains B lymphocytes termed B-1 cells.[86] The antigen receptors of these cells, like intraepithelial γδ T cells, have limited diversity.[82,87] B-1 lymphocyte cell receptors bind immunoglobulins, mainly IgM, which are reactive with common microbial antigens, such as lipopolysaccharide and phosphorylcholine. B-1 lymphocytes produce natural antibodies specific for a variety of microbes present at epithelial cell surfaces.

Natural Opsonins

Nonspecific opsonins contribute to the innate immune responses before specific opsonic antibody can be generated. These natural opsonins include natural antibodies, complement fragments, and fibronectin.

Natural Antibodies

Natural antibodies are antibodies present in normal sera; they are not the result of antigen stimulation.[88] They may be self- or autoreactive, or reactive against a variety of bacterial, viral, and fungal pathogens.[89,90] Natural antibodies are mainly the products of B-1 lymphocytes that develop in the fetus and neonate.[86] Natural antibodies serve as a second line of defense, after an organism has breached the epithelial or mucosal barrier. Most natural antibodies are IgM and activate the complement system, but they may be IgG and IgA. They bind to repeating moieties of polysaccharides.[91,92] Since many microorganisms share structural polysaccharides and phospholipids, natural antibodies protect against a wide variety of pathogens. Mice lacking natural antibody have enhanced susceptibility to bacterial peritonitis, reduced cytokine expression, particularly TNF-α, and higher mortality rates from infection.[90,93,94]

Complement

The complement system is part of the innate immune system that defends against initial pathogen invasion. Complement is composed of two pathways: the classic pathway and the alternative pathway. It has three main physiologic effects: (1) bridging the innate and acquired immune responses, (2) defense against pyogenic bacterial infections, and, (3) disposing of immune complexes and the products of inflammatory injury. The complement system is made up of a series of more than 30 plasma and regulatory membrane proteins. Genes for several of the complement components are found within the major histocompatibility complex class III region on chromosome 6. Complement functions include (1) amplification of leukocyte-associated inflammatory responses, (2) anaphylactoid responses through stimulation of histamine release, (3) chemoattraction and activation of neutrophils and macrophages, (4) opsonization of foreign microbes and antigens, and (5) cytolysis of target cell membranes.[95]

The classic complement pathway is triggered primarily by antigen-antibody complexes or aggregated IgM or IgG. Natural IgM and IgG antibodies can trigger the complement system, resulting in classic pathway activation and formation of the inflammatory components C3a and C5a, and opsonic fragments C3b and iC3b.[96] Mannose-binding protein activates the classic complement pathway.[97]

The alternative complement pathway is triggered by complex polysaccharides, lipopolysaccharides, bacterial cell wall components, aggregated IgA and IgE, and yeast. Phagocytic cells have receptors for C3b (CR1) and iC3b (CR3 and CR4) that allow them to ingest, process, and kill pathogens.[82] C1q-coated particles can be ingested by macrophages. The terminal complement components C5 to C9 can lyse some bacteria, notably *Neisseria* species and *E. coli*.[95,98]

The major effects of complement components include anaphylotoxic (C3a and C5a), opsonic (C3bi and C3b), chemotactic (C5a), and cytolytic activity (membrane attack complex, C5 to C9). Deficiency of the early components of the classic pathway results in a high incidence of collagen vascular–like and lupus-like disease, including arthritis, skin rash, and glomerulonephritis (C1q, C1r, C1s, C4, or C2 deficiency), and some patients may have recurrent infection, usually with *S. pneumoniae*.[95,98] Patients with deficiency of C3 usually have pyogenic infections because both the classic and alternative pathways are impaired. Patients with late complement deficiencies have recurrent infections with *N. meningitidis* or *N. gonorrhoeae*.[98]

The production and function of complement proteins is quantatively and qualitatively different in the neonate compared with adults. Complement protein synthesis in the developing human fetus occurs between 8 and 19 weeks' gestational age. The synthesis of C4, C2, and C3 occurs in the liver between 8 and 14 weeks, and functionally active C5 can be detected in fetal lungs and liver as early as 8 to 9 gestational weeks. Complement proteins are produced in decreased quantity with decreased functional activity, depending on the gestational age of the fetus.[95] Few, if any, of the maternal complement components cross the placenta to the developing fetus. Results of studies done in preterm and term infants compared with adults show that preterm and term infants are markedly deficient in complement components, especially C9 and factor B of the alternative pathway.[99,100] Neonatal serum complement opsonic activity and/or chemotactic activity has been studied with strains of *E. coli*, staphylococcus, and group B streptococcus. Neonates and especially preterm infants have deficiencies in complement opsonic activity critical to bacterial host defense.[95] In addition, the cellular and humoral factors required for the activation of complement are also deficient in neonates. Most neonates have low levels of IgM because there is no maternal passage of this immunoglobulin and little production in the developing fetus. Because many antibodies against bacteria are of the IgM class, opsonization and subsequent bacterial killing are reduced in newborn infants because of insufficient IgM to activate the classic pathway of complement.[95]

Fibronectin

Fibronectin is a high molecular weight glycoprotein (440 kD), which participates in a number of complex processes, including hemostasis, wound healing, cell migration and differentiation, and phagocytosis.[101]

Fibronectin (Fn) binds to organisms such as *S. aureus*, *S. epidermidis*, and *Streptococcus pyogenes* to promote their interactions with phagocytic cells, including macrophages and neutrophils.[102-104] Fn enhances the binding of *S. aureus* to neutrophils and their subsequent ingestion when activated by inflammatory mediators.[105] Fn increases the uptake of antibody-coated group B streptococci by human neutrophils and enhances survival of neonatal rats infected with these organisms.[106] Similar observations have been made utilizing macrophages.[107] Yang and associates[104] also found that Fn increases the respiratory burst activity, phagocytosis, and intracellular killing of *S. aureus* and *S. epidermidis* by human neutrophils in the absence of antibody, probably through functional binding of organisms to Fn receptors on phagocytic cells. In contrast, group B streptococci and *E. coli* uptake and killing are enhanced by Fn but only in the presence of opsonic antibody.[106] Binding of Fn to its receptor on neutrophils, monocytes, or macrophages enhances the respiratory burst activity, alters actin polymerization, and promotes the release of TNF-α.[108,109] Reduced levels of plasma fibronectin are seen in normal newborn infants, neonates with respiratory distress, perinatal asphyxia and sepsis, as well as patients with severe trauma, septic shock, or severe burns.[101,106,110–117]

Pathogen-Associated Receptors

Pattern recognition receptors are expressed on most effector cells of the innate immune system, including mast cells, macrophages, dendritic cells, and B-1 cells. They recognize specific pathogen-associated molecular patterns present on many microbes. They are secreted into the plasma or tissue fluid or contained intracellularly as cytoplasmic proteins.[10,118]

Collectins

The collectins are a family of pattern recognition receptors (PPR), including mannose-binding protein and surfactant proteins A and D, which contain collagen and lectin domains and share biologic activities.[10,119,120]

Mannose-binding protein (MBP) is probably the best characterized of the PRR collectins.[121] It binds to carbohydrate structures on gram-positive and gram-negative bacteria, yeast, parasites, and some viruses.[122] MBP is encoded on chromosome 10.[121] Microbial pathogens bound by MBP in the blood or tissue fluid are then opsonized and phagocytized or lysed by the complement system.[10] Deficiency of MBP is a disorder associated with increased susceptibility to bacterial, fungal, and viral infections, usually beginning early in life prior to the maturation of acquired immune responses.[121,123,124] These patients usually suffer from recurrent upper respiratory infections, otitis media, chronic diarrhea of infancy, and failure to thrive within the first year of life.[123,124] Deficiency of MBP also may contribute to the severity and progression of infection beyond infancy because of abnormal interaction of MBP with the complement system.[123]

Surfactant is a mixture of proteins and lipids that promotes normal respiratory function and enhances lung host defense.[119,125] Two surfactant proteins, SP-A and SP-D, belong to the collectin family of pattern recognition receptors. These are products of alveolar type II cells during the latter stages of pregnancy.

LaForce and colleagues,[126] initially reported that surfactant improves macrophage killing of *S. aureus*. SP-A and SP-D bind to certain bacteria, viruses, yeast, and fungi to promote their attachment to phagocytic cells via Fc receptors of immunoglobulin and complement receptors, which facilitates their elimination.[119,127] SP-A and SP-D bind to gram-positive and gram-negative bacteria, *Pneumocystis carinii*, fungi such as *Aspergillus*, yeast including *Cryptococcus neoformans*, bacteria such as *H. influenzae*, as well as Herpes simplex virus, *Mycobacterium tuberculosis*, and *Mycoplasma pulmonis*.[128–138] SP-A and especially SP-D promote the formation of microbe aggregates that may enhance their mucociliary clearance.[125]

The surfactant collectins stimulate neutrophil and macrophage chemotaxis, actin polymerization, respiratory burst activity, and nitric oxide production. SP-A knockout mice cannot kill mycoplasma via nitric oxide–dependent mechanisms. They also have abnormalities in neutrophil recruitment, production of toxic oxygen and nitrogen intermediates, and defective phagocytosis.[119] These knockout mice develop disseminated group B streptococci infection following intratracheal inoculation and have diminished clearance of *S. aureus* and *Pseudomonas aeruginosa*.[139–141]

SP-A and SP-D bind lipopolysaccharide (LPS) from organisms such as *E. coli*, *K. pneumoniae*, and *P. aeruginosa*, SP-A and LPS subsequently bind to macrophages via CD14 dependent and independent mechanisms, increasing TNF-α release.[128,142] SP-A and SP-D function by clumping pathogens and promoting adherence to inflammatory cells.[119,143] Furthermore, they may down-regulate T cells and their cytokine responses and suppress the response to inhaled allergens.[144,145]

Deficiencies of surfactant are observed in premature infants and patients with cystic fibrosis, respiratory syncytial virus infection, and adult respiratory distress syndrome. Reduced SP-D opsonization has been observed in diabetic mice because of competition by free glucose for SP-D binding sites.[119]

Selectins

Selectins are a family of adhesion molecules that facilitate neutrophil rolling along and tethering to the vascular endothelium. Selectins include leukocyte selectin (L-selectin) endothelial selectin (E-selectin) and platelet selectin (P-selectin), which have lectin-like domains.[146] L-selectin binds lipid-linked galactose with sulfate residues. P-selectin binds sulfotyrosine, and E-selectin binds fuco-oligosaccharides present on leukocytes, epithelial cells, and some tumor cells.[120] Deficiency of L-selectin results in leukocyte adhesion deficiency type II and is associated with decreased leukocyte infiltration, resulting in a poor inflammatory response along with associated neurologic and developmental abnormalities due to impaired fucose metabolism.[147]

Bacterial Lipopolysaccharide

Bacterial lipopolysaccharide (LPS) is a virulence factor of gram-negative bacteria. It is a powerful cellular activator and promotes cytokine release from neutrophils, macrophages, and other cells of the innate immune response. The polysaccharide groups of LPS vary considerably from species to species, and even between strains of the same species, permitting bacteria such as *E. coli* to be serotyped. The lipid moiety of LPS is generally highly conserved.[10,82]

The primary cellular receptor for LPS is CD14, a glycosylphosphatidylinositol-linked protein.[25] CD14 was first identified on phagocytic cells but also occurs on many other cells. Binding of LPS to CD14 is markedly potentiated by lipopolysaccharide binding protein (LBP), a normal component of the serum. Binding of LPS to LBP enhances effector cell responsiveness to LPS, promoting cellular activation and cytokine release.[10]

Bacterial Permeability–Increasing Factor

Bacterial permeability–increasing factor (BPI) is a 55-kD pattern recognition receptor present in neutrophil granules, which contain two domains, one of which binds with LPS to increase membrane permeability and lysis of gram-negative bacteria, whereas the other promotes opsonization.[10] Neutrophil BPI functions in concert with defensins and the membrane attack complex of complement to cause bacterial lysis. Neonates have reduced release and activity of BPI, perhaps contributing to their enhanced susceptibility to gram-negative bacterial infections.[148]

Natural Antimicrobial Agents

Antimicrobial peptides, first described in insects in 1981,[149] have now been found in all multicellular organisms, including, plants, insects, and humans.[10] The most important antimicrobial peptides in humans are the α and β defensins. They are contained in the primary, or azurophilic, granules and in secondary, or specific, granules of phagocytic cells.

Defensins

The defensins are strongly cationic, single chain peptides with molecular weights of between 3 and 4.5 kD. Defensins make up 50% of the protein content of the neutrophil primary granules.[23,150] These are divided into α and β defensins. These peptides possess antimicrobial activity against gram-positive and gram-negative bacteria, fungi, mycobacteria, and some viruses. The defensins create voltage-sensitive pores in microbial membranes, resulting in lysis. Humans have six human alpha defensins (HD1 to 6) and two human beta defensins (HBD-1 and HBD-2).[150]

The α defensins, HD 1 to 6, are made primarily by neutrophils and compose 30 to 50% of the primary granule content.[151] Defensins are present after neutrophil degranulation induced by LPS, IL-8, C5a, and other stimuli. They are also found on the epithelial surfaces of the bronchi and in bronchial lavage fluid of patients with various types of inflammatory lung injury. The antimicrobial activity of defensins is inhibited by high salt content, which may contribute to the decreased microbial activity of lung surface fluid in cystic fibrosis patients.[152]

The β defensins are produced by epithelial cells of the respiratory and gastrointestinal tracts.[12,153] HBD-1 is expressed constitutively by epithelial cells in the bronchi and intestine, whereas HBD-2 synthesis is up-regulated by inflammatory stimuli, including LPS, TNFα bacterial infection, and injury. Thus, HBD-1 acts to kill organisms in the absence of inflammation, whereas HBD-2 acts primarily as part of the inflammatory process. In inflammatory lung disease both α HD 1 to 6 defensins and β HBD-2 may be increased significantly, perhaps contributing to airway inflammation.[23]

Lysozyme and Myeloperoxidase

Lysozyme, present in primary and secondary granules of neutrophils, is an antimicrobial component present in inflammatory exudates, nasal secretions, and alveolar surface fluid.[25] Lysozyme is a small cationic enzyme that hydrolyzes glycosidic bonds that disrupt the peptidoglycan structural components of some gram-positive bacterial cell walls. Lysozyme can be present in airway surface fluid, where it may be an important component of the innate defense system.[27,28]

Myeloperoxidase is the most abundant enzyme in the primary granules of phagocytes. It catalyzes the reaction between chloride and hydrogen peroxide to form hypochlorite ion, a potent microbicidal agent of the respiratory burst. Bacterial killing takes almost twice as long if this enzyme is missing.[35]

THE COMPONENTS OF ADAPTIVE HOST DEFENSE

The hallmark of acquired, or adaptive, immunity is its specificity for structurally distinct antigens and memory of prior exposure. T and B lymphocytes orchestrate the cellular and humoral immune responses of acquired host defense. Acquired immune responses are the last to develop phylogenetically and the last to mature developmentally; they require close cooperation between cellular elements of the innate immune system and the T and B lymphocytes.[10,154]

T Lymphocytes

The major functions of the T-lymphocyte system are in host defense against intracellular pathogens (fungus, viruses, protozoa, and intracellular bacteria such as mycobacteria and *Listeria* species). T lymphocytes play a limited protective role against pyogenic bacteria like group B streptococci. The T-lymphocyte system also functions in tumor surveillance, delayed hypersensitivity reactions, and graft-versus-host disease.[155-157]

Thymus-dependent T cells are derived from pluripotent lymphopoietic stem cells residing in developing bone marrow stores. As early as the eighth gestational week, immature T cells infiltrate the thymus, where they differentiate and mature under the influences of thymic humoral factors, before migrating to specific lymphoid tissues. During their intrathymic migration, T cells develop specific outer membrane–bound glycoproteins at different stages. Most of the mature T cells express T-cell antigen receptors as well as CD3 membrane glycoproteins. Nearly 70% of the T cells also express the CD4 membrane glycoproteins, the helper-inducer T-cell marker. The remaining 30% express the CD8 membrane glycoproteins, the cytotoxic-suppressor T-cell marker. The CD4 and CD8 membrane glycoproteins typically are not presented on the same mature T cell and serve as functional markers of helper-inducer and cytotoxic-suppressor T-cell populations in the peripheral blood or tissues.

The T-lymphocyte system orchestrates pathogen annihilation through antigen-dependent cellular interaction. Antigen-presenting cells, mainly the monocytes and macrophages, produce soluble antigen and present it in combination with HLA class II antigens on their cell surfaces. Thymus-dependent CD4 helper-inducer T cells recognize and bind to this altered antigen HLA class II complex through the antigen-specific T-cell receptors. During this process, the cytokines interleukin 1 (IL-1) and tumor necrosis factor alpha (TNFα) are released from the antigen-presenting cells. The binding of free IL-1 to its receptor on helper-inducer T-cell surfaces initiates T-cell activation. Once activated, the CD4 helper-inducer T cells produce interleukin-2 (IL-2), which functions as a T-cell promoter causing the T cells to proliferate and release a number of other cytokines. This initiates a cascade of events that serves to amplify and regulate the immune response with the cooperation and recruitment of many other cell types. IL-2 also interacts directly with CD8 cytotoxic-suppressor T cells that bind viral antigens present on the surface of infected cells, resulting in cellular destruction.[155]

At birth, T-cell immunity is immature compared with that of the adult, in part because of the lack of exposure of the fetal immune system to foreign antigens and decreased cytokine production. Neonatal T cells provide ineffective signals to B cells as a result of developmental defects in local cytokine production and cell-cell interaction. Any defect in T-cell immunity is also associated with variable degrees of B-cell deficiency because most of the maturation, differentiation, and activation processes of B cells require T-cell help.[155,156] The most severe form of immunodeficiency is the syndrome of severe combined immunodeficiency. This immunodeficiency category includes a spectrum of X-linked, autosomal recessive, and sporadic genetic defects characterized by the inability to mount a normal T-lymphocyte and B-lymphocyte immunity. Patients usually suffer from failure to thrive, persistent oral candidiasis, recurrent diarrhea, and pneumonia, usually interstitial and often caused by *Pneumocystis carinii*, in the first months of life.[157]

In response to microbial invasion, most cells of the innate and acquired immune system produce cytokines, which function in autocrine, paracrine, and endocrine fashions. Macrophages, natural killer cells, neutrophils, mast cells, and γδ T cells produce cytokines critical in the early response to microbial invasion. Antigen-activated T and B lymphocytes also produce cytokines that can activate, or recruit, effector cells of the innate immune system. Lymphocytes, macrophages, and stromal cells of the bone marrow produce colony-stimulating factors that promote the growth and differentiation of immature leukocytes.[82,158] The placenta also produces cytokines in response to infection. Levels of cytokines, including granulocyte colony–stimulating factor (G-CSF), granulocyte-macrophage colony–stimulating factor (GM-CSF), TNF-α IL-1, IL-6, and IL-8, are increased 10-fold in the amniotic fluid of mothers with chorioamnionitis.[159] We will consider select cytokines that mediate host defense to bacteria—notably, tumor necrosis factor, interleukins (IL-1, IL-6, IL-8, IL-11,

IL-12, and IL-18), interferons (IFN-α and IFN-γ), and colony-stimulating factors (G-CSF, M-CSF, and GM-CSF),

Tumor Necrosis Factor

Tumor necrosis factor-alpha (TNF-α) and tumor necrosis factor-beta (TNF-β) are structurally related. They bind to the same receptors with equal affinity and elicit similar biologic effects.[82] TNF-α is primarily the product of macrophages and other antigen presenting cells, natural killer cells, and activated mast cells of the innate immune system, but it can also be produced by antigen-activated T cells. TNF-β is synthesized by T lymphocytes.[160-165]

TNF-α is the cytokine responsible for the host response to gram-negative bacterial infections and specifically to LPS, as well as to gram-positive bacteria.[164,166-168] Along with IL-1, TNF-α is a principal mediator of septic shock. TNF-α activates neutrophils, stimulates their adhesion to vascular endothelial cells, and induces their production of toxic oxygen products.[23,169-172] If TNF-α production is excessive, these toxic oxygen products damage endothelial cells and cause fluid leak, hypovolemia, and depressed cardiac contractility leading to septic shock. TNF-α production is primarily induced by (1) gram-positive bacteria and their products, including peptidoglycans, lipoteichoic acids, and pyogenic exotoxins[173-176]; (2) nonspecific mediators such as fibronectin, C5a, and surfactant proteins[109,177-179]; and (3) lactic acid, which is elevated in septic shock.[180]

TNF-α knockout mice, or normal mice pretreated with anti-TNF-α monoclonal antibody, have increased susceptibility to bacterial infection and a decreased occurrence of septic shock. In vitro, human mononuclear cells stimulated by group B streptococci (GBS) first generate TNF-α followed by IL-1, IL-6, IL-8, and IFN-γ.[176,181] In experimental models of group B streptococci, anti-TNF-α monoclonal antibody therapy, administered early during infection, improves survival, probably by limiting cytokine-mediated septic shock.[182]

Interleukins

Interleukin-1. IL-1 is produced predominantly by macrophages and macrophage-like cells but also by endothelial and epithelial cells. There are two forms of IL-1, IL-α and IL-β, encoded by two separate genes, which bind to the same IL-1 receptors. Two IL-1 receptors bind to the two forms of IL-1 with different affinities. They are distributed on a variety of cells in different concentrations throughout the body.[82]

During development, IL-1 production by fetal macrophages in response to LPS up-regulates G-CSF production by monocytes from the bone marrow and liver of human fetuses.[183] During inflammation, IL-1 up-regulates the expression of endothelial adhesive glycoproteins, such as ICAM-1, promoting neutrophil attachment.[184] IL-1 also promotes IL-6, IL-8, and other chemokine production by macrophages. IL-1, along with TNF-α, induces prostaglandin E_2 production in the hypothalamus, raising the body's temperature. IL-1, TNF-α, and IL-6 cause production and release of acute-phase reactants by the liver, including alpha-1 antitrypsin, haptoglobin, C-reactive protein, serum amyloid P protein, complement components, and fibrinogen.[185]

Interleukin-6. IL-6 supports hematopoietic progenitor growth, promotes T and B cell function, and mediates some acute-phase responses of inflammation. Interleukin-6 is produced mainly by macrophages and mononuclear cells, but also by fibroblasts and endothelial cells. IL-6 is secreted in response to both TNF-α and IL-1, as well as microbes and their products.[82,158] Following cellular activation, IL-1 and TNF-α production occurs, followed by IL-6 synthesis. IL-6 does not activate neutrophils or induce cytotoxicity, but it does increase the production of acute-phase reactants. IL-6 promotes the growth of B cells, stimulates antibody production, and enhances T-cell proliferation. IL-6 also enhances the activity of hematopoietic growth factors such as granulocyte and macrophage colony–stimulating factors, thus playing a role in both innate and acquired immunity.[186] IL-6–deficient mice

have increased mortality associated with bacterial infections because of impairment of neutrophil and macrophage responses.[187]

Interleukin-8. IL-8 is a member of the chemokine family that attracts neutrophils to sites of inflammation and plays an important role in host defense against bacterial infections.[188] IL-8 is produced by fetal thymic epithelial cells, and its in vitro production is increased by IL-1. IL-8 is present in the cord blood of babies born with chorioamnionitis. Its expression is decreased in babies of mothers receiving steroids to induce fetal lung maturation.[189] IL-8 is a major factor in recruitment of neutrophils to the lung in bacterial pneumonia.[64,190]

Interleukin-11. IL-11 was initially characterized as a hematopoietic cytokine with thrombopoietic activity. It is expressed in the central nervous system and the gastrointestinal tract. The hematopoietic actions of IL-11 include the stimulation and proliferation of primitive stem cells. It acts in synergy with other cytokines to support the proliferation and differentiation of all lineages of hematopoietic stem cells.[191-193]

IL-11 has been used effectively in animal models of sepsis and septic shock. Neonatal rats pretreated with IL-11 and then exposed to group B streptococci demonstrated a significant reduction in mortality.[194] There are gastrointestinal protective effects of IL-11 as well. IL-11 administration in animal models of chemical-induced acute colitis and ischemic bowel disease results in significant increases in survival.[195-197] Decreased translocation of enteric bacteria is observed in the IL-11–treated animals. Phase I/II trials of IL-11 in patients with Crohn disease have been completed, and studies of IL-11 administration for the prevention or treatment of necrotizing enterocolitis in neonates is under consideration.[198]

Interleukin-12. Mononuclear cell production of IL-12 is an important component of the early response to microbial infection.[199] While monocytes and macrophages are the main source of IL-12, other cells, including B cells, also can produce IL-12.[200,201] IL-12 induces interferon gamma (IFN-γ) production by T cells and NK cells and promotes cellular cytotoxicity and lymphocyte proliferation. It is down-regulated by IL-10.[202] IL-12 can be induced by exposure of mononuclear cells to microbes or their products, including *S. aureus*, group B streptococci, and LPS.[202-206] The IL-12 receptor, composed of β1 and β2 subunits, binds IL-12 with high affinity.[206]

Decreased transcription and secretion of IL-12 and decreased IFN-γ production by newborn mononuclear cells suggest an abnormality within the IL-12/IFN-γ pathway. In vitro studies suggest that IL-12 can partially correct the IFN-γ deficiency.[203] IL-12 administration to neonatal mice with group B streptococcal infection significantly improves their survival.[207] The IL-12/IFN-γ pathway is also suppressed in older patients with critical infections.[208] Hyper-IgE patients have defective synthesis of IFN-γ in response to exposure to staphylococci and candida, suggesting an abnormality in the IL-12/IFN-γ pathway in these patients as well.[209]

Interleukin-18. IL-18 is produced by monocytes, macrophages, osteoclasts, and keratinocytes and stimulates the production of IFN-γ. Its structure is similar to that of IL-1, and its receptor is also closely related to the IL-1 receptor.[210] IL-18 stimulates IFN-γ production using a different transcription promoter than that used by IL-12, but IL-12 and IL-18 act synergistically to enhance IFN-γ production in response to microbes and their products. IL-18 knockout mice do not have a complete deficiency of IFN-γ.[211-213]

Stimulation of NK cells with IL-18 markedly enhances their cytotoxic activity.[214,215] IL-18 knockout mice have decreased but not eliminated NK activity.[211] IL-18 stimulates CD4+ T cells and B cells to produce cytokines and antibodies. It also stimulates IL-8 production by mononuclear cells and IFN-γ production by NK cells.[216] Decreased IL-18 production in cord blood mononuclear cells exposed to group B streptococci, along with their deficiency in IL-12 production, contributes to inadequate IFN-γ production and increased susceptibility to group B streptococci and other infections.[217]

Interferons

The interferons (IFNs) are cytokines between 18 and 20 kD produced by a variety of cells that function in both innate and acquired immunity. Interferons are divided into type I interferons, which includes IFN-α and IFN-β and type II, or immune IFN-γ. The type I interferons share a common receptor, induce similar responses, and are encoded on chromosome 9p21 by a cluster of intronless genes. Type II interferon, IFN-γ, has a distinct receptor separate from that of IFN-α and β. IFN-γ is also structurally distinct from the type I interferons and is encoded on chromosome 12p24.[82,158]

IFN-α is the product of mononuclear phagocytes and has been known as leukocyte IFN, whereas IFN-β is produced by fibroblasts and is known as fibroblast IFN. The major stimulus for type I IFN production is a viral infection. In addition, both type I IFNs are stimulated by the acquired immune response to antigens, in response to T-cell–derived factors.[82]

Interferon-γ is a 20- to 25-kD glycoprotein encoded by a single gene on chromosome 12p24.[218,219] It is produced by CD4+ and CD8+ T cells and by NK cells and is a component of both the acquired and innate immune systems. T-cell IFN-γ production occurs following antigen stimulation in the presence of IL-2, IL-12 and IL-18. IFN-γ also has antiviral and antiproliferative activity and up-regulates both class I and class II HLA molecule expression.[219]

Activated macrophages can generate cytokines (IL-12, IL-15, and IL-18) that induce NK cell activation and IFN-γ production, and enhance macrophage antibacterial activity. IFN-γ activates mononuclear phagocytes and neutrophils, resulting in enhanced killing of phagocytized microbes and intracellular pathogens, such as *Mycobacteria* and *Listeria*. Patients with defects in IFN-γ receptors suffer severe infections with *Mycobacteria* and related pathogens.[220,221]

Neonates have a deficiency in the transcription and production of IFN-γ.[203,222,223] In vitro administration of IFN-γ enhances the chemotactic activity of newborn neutrophils.[218,219] IFN-γ is also decreased in the hyperimmunoglobulinemia-E syndrome.[224,225] Borges and associates[209] showed that mononuclear cells of these patients have decreased IFN-γ responses to staphylococci. In vitro incubation of their neutrophils with recombinant human IFN-γ significantly improves their chemotactic responsiveness.[219,226] IFN-γ administration to hyper-IgE patients increased neutrophil responsiveness, improved eczema, and decreased respiratory symptoms.[227] IFN-γ lowers the incidence of serious infections in patients with chronic granulomatous disease without demonstrating an effect on their neutrophil respiratory burst.[228]

Colony-Stimulating Factors

The production and function of neutrophils and macrophages is regulated, in part, by colony-stimulating factors.[229,230] Granulocyte-macrophage colony-stimulating factor (GM-CSF) is a 14- to 35-kD glycoprotein encoded on chromosome 5q23–31 that stimulates production of neutrophils, macrophages, and eosinophils.[158,231] Granulocyte colony–stimulating factor (G-CSF) is an 18- to 22-kD glycoprotein encoded on chromosome 17q11–21 that stimulates neutrophil production. Macrophage colony–stimulating factor (M-CSF) is a 21-to 40-kD glycoprotein encoded on chromosome 5q23–31 that stimulates monocyte production.[158]

GM-CSF is produced by activated T cells and mononuclear phagocytes, vascular endothelial cells, and fibroblasts. It promotes the growth and differentiation of monocytes, macrophages, and neutrophils and, to a lesser extent, platelets and progenitor red blood cells. It activates macrophages in much the same fashion as

IFN-γ. GM-CSF is produced by macrophages, fibroblasts, and endothelial cells at inflammatory focuses but is not present in the circulation.[158]

G-CSF is also produced by macrophages, fibroblasts, and endothelial cells and is present in low concentrations in the bloodstream. Microbes and their products and cytokines, such as TNF-α and IL-1β, stimulate the production of G-CSF.[23] G-CSF acts on neutrophil progenitors to produce neutrophil maturation and release from the marrow. It also activates and enhances the function of neutrophils and macrophages.[158,232-234] G-CSF regulates neutrophil adhesion molecule expression, and also neutrophil adhesion, chemotaxis, respiratory burst activity, phagocytosis, and intracellular microbial killing.[235-237] Pulmonary or systemic infection stimulates the production of G-CSF in the blood, with resultant neutrophilia and enhanced inflammatory response.[238,239]

Monocytes and mononuclear cells from human neonates produce G-CSF and GM-CSF in reduced amounts, compared with adults, in response to inflammatory agents in vitro. Preterm infants have even further reduction in G-CSF and GM-CSF production than do term infants. These deficiencies contribute to the diminished neonatal neutrophil storage pool. Plasma concentrations of G-CSF are low in the preterm infant and in newborns with neutropenia and sepsis. Clinical trials are underway to define the efficacy of G-CSF and GM-CSF in preterm infants and infected neonates.[37]

Natural Killer Cells

Natural killer (NK) cells are non-B, non-T cells lacking surface immunoglobulins and T-cell antigen receptors that are essential components of the acquired immune system.[240] NK cells appear in the human liver as early as 5 weeks postconception and increase in numbers and functional ability as development progresses. At birth, however, NK function is low compared with adult cells.[240-241]

NK cells release a variety of cytokines, including TNF-α, TNF-β, IFN-γ, GM-CSF, and colony-stimulating factor 1 (CSF-1).[242] Several cytokines enhance NK activity, notably IL-2, IL-12, IL-15, IFN-α, IFN-β, and IFN-γ. Natural killer cells also appear to be important in protection against intracellular infections such as *L. monocytogenes* and *Toxoplasma gondii*.[243-245] These pathogens induce macrophages to secrete the NK cell–activating cytokines IL-12 and IL-15, which induce NK cells to produce IFN-γ. This NK cell–derived IFN-γ then stimulates macrophages to kill these intracellular pathogens. The newborn infant has depressed NK cell activity, which might contribute to the susceptibility to these pathogens as well as to other bacteria and viruses.[246,247]

B Lymphocytes

The neonatal ability to produce antibodies is quantitatively and qualitatively different than that of adults. The B-lymphocytic system is derived from stem cells residing in bone marrow stores. These stem cells produce cytoplasmic IgM heavy chains and become pre-B cells as early as 10 weeks' gestation. Pre-B cells continue to differentiate to become mature surface IgM, or IgM- and IgD-bearing B cells, which seed peripheral lymphoid tissues via the circulation. Upon stimulation, IgM-bearing B cells may undergo class switching to IgG-, IgA-, or IgE-bearing B cells. These B cells can then differentiate into immunoglobulin-secreting plasma cells with the help of T cells and T-cell–derived cytokines. Some of the B cells further differentiate into small memory B cells.[248]

The major function of B lymphocytes is to produce antibodies to the protein and carbohydrate antigens present on microorganisms, toxins, or other potentially harmful antigenic substances. These antibodies are classified into nine different immunoglobulin isotypes, including IgM, IgG1, IgG2, IgG3, IgG4, and IgA1, IgA2, IgE, and IgD. The IgM antibodies are made first and are the most effective and efficient in activating the classic complement system. IgM antibodies do not cross the placenta, thus, the presence of IgM in the newborn infant may suggest congenital infection.[248,249]

The IgG antibodies, which represent 75% of serum immunoglobulin, are the only immunoglobulin class maternal antibodies that are transplacentally passed; they provide the developing infant with passive immunity. Passively acquired IgG has a half-life of approximately 20 days. All IgG subclasses cross the placenta. At birth, newborn IgG concentrations actually exceed maternal IgG levels, but they immediately begin to decrease until a nadir (400 mg/dL) is reached at 3 to 4 months of age in term infants. The IgG1 subclass represents approximately 70% of IgG and usually contains antiprotein antibody that also activates complement. The IgG2 subclass represents 20% of IgG and usually contains an antipolysaccharide antibody. The ability to produce antibodies to protein and carbohydrate antigens is different during the first 2 years of life. An infant's ability to produce IgG1 protein antibodies in the first few months of life is similar to that of adults. Their ability to produce IgG2 antibodies to polysaccharide antigens, however, is much lower, and effective antibody concentrations are not reached until after 2 years of age. Thus, children less than 2 years of age are predisposed to infections by polysaccharide-coated organisms (e.g., *H. influenzae*, pneumococcus, meningococcus). The IgG3 subclass represents 6% of IgG and usually contains antiviral protein antibody.[248,249]

Decreased passage of maternal antibody is suspected to be a major determinant in neonatal infections with group B streptococci and *E. coli*, especially in premature infants. Before 32 weeks of gestation, the developing neonate's IgG concentrations are less than 50% of maternal values. Neonates with deficiency of type-specific antibody to the type III polysaccharide of GBS or the K-1 capsule of *E. coli*, whether due to inadequate maternal stores or decreased maternal antibody transport are predisposed to GBS and *E. coli* infections.[250]

IgA antibodies are selectively transported across mucous membranes by secretory piece. These IgA antibodies prevent the attachment of microorganisms, absorb harmful antigens from mucous membranes, and are present in human breast milk. Secretory IgA is undetectable in the mucosal secretions at birth and first appear between 1 week and 2 months of age. It has been suggested that decreased levels of secretory IgA may predispose the developing neonate to colonization with pathogenic type III GBS.[251,252]

The IgE antibodies are found on mast cells and basophils and are primarily responsible for allergic reactions, protection against parasites, and anaphylaxis. The IgD antibodies serve as early antigen receptors on B cells; their role in host defense is currently under investigation.[248]

REFERENCES

1. Baker CJ: Group B streptococcal infections. *In* Stoll BJ, Weisman LE (eds): Infections in Perinatology. Clin Perinatol *24*:59, 1997.
2. Stoll BJ: The global impact of neonatal infection. *In* Stoll BJ, Weisman LE (eds): Infections in Perinatology. Clin Perinatol *24*:1, 1997.
3. Hill HR: Diagnosis and treatment of sepsis in the neonate. *In* Root RK, Sand MA (eds): Septic Shock: Contemporary Topics in Infectious Diseases. New York, Churchill Livingstone, 1985, pp 219–232.
4. Santos JI, Hill HR: Bacterial infections in the neonate. *In* Wedgwood RJ, et al. (eds): Infections in Children. Philadelphia, Harper and Row, 1982, pp 179–202.
5. Starr SE: Antimicrobial therapy of bacterial sepsis in the newborn infant. J Pediatr *106*:1043, 1985.
6. Hill HR: Group B streptococcal infections. *In* Holmes KK, et al. (eds): Sexually Transmitted Diseases. New York, McGraw Hill, 1984, pp 397–407.
7. Stoll BJ, et al: Changes in pathogens causing early-onset sepsis in very-low-birth-weight infants. N Engl J Med *347*:240, 2002.
8. Noel GJ, Edelson PJ: *Staphylococcus epidermidis* bacteremia in neonates: further observations and the occurrence of focal infection. Peditrics *74*:832, 1984.
9. Simor AE, et al: Abortion and perinatal sepsis associated with *Campylobacter* infection. Rev Infect Dis *8*:397, 1986.
10. Hoffman JA, et al: Phylogenetic perspectives in innate immunity. Science *284*:1313, 1999.
11. Qureshi ST, et al: Comparative genomics and host resistance against infectious diseases. Emerg Infect Dis *5*:36, 1999.
12. Boman HG: Innate immunity and the normal microflora. Immunol Rev *173*:5, 2000.
13. Schoen EJ, et al: Newborn circumcision decreases incidence and costs of urinary tract infections during the first year of life. Pediatrics *105*:789, 2000.
14. Wiswell TE: The prepuce, urinary tract infections, and the consequences. Comment Pediatr *105*:860, 2000.
15. Wiswell TE, et al: Effect of circumcision status on periurethral bacterial flora during the first year of life. J Pediatr *113*:442, 1988.
16. Glennon J, et al: Circumcision and periurethral carriage of *Proteus mirabilis* in boys. Arch Dis Child *63*:556, 1988.
17. Fussell EN, et al: Adherence of bacteria to human foreskins. J Urol *140*:997, 1988.
18. Nealon TJ, Mattingly SJ: Role of cellular lipoteichoic acids in mediating adherence of serotype III strains of group B streptococci to human embryonic, fetal, and adult epithelial cells. Infect Immun *43*:523, 1984.
19. Cox F, et al: Prevention of group B streptococcal colonization and bacteremia in neonatal mice with topical vaginal inhibitors. J Infect Dis *167*:1118, 1993.
20. Miyazaki S, et al: Adherence of *Streptococcus agalactiae* to synchronously growing human cell monolayers without lipoteichoic acid and involvement. Infect Immun *56*:505, 1988.
21. Tamura GS, et al: Adherence of group B streptococci to cultured epithelial cells: roles of environmental factors and bacterial surface components. Infect Immun *62*:2450, 1994.
22. Rubens CE, et al: Respiratory epithelial cell invasion by group B streptococci. Infect Immun *60*:5157, 1992.
23. Zhang P, et al: Innate immunity and pulmonary host defense. Immunol Rev *173*:39, 2000.
24. Rose MC: Mucins: structure, function, and role in pulmonary diseases. Am J Physiol *263*:L413-429, 1992.
25. Diamond G, et al: The innate immune responses of the respiratory epithelium. Immunol Rev *173*:27, 2000.
26. Dohrman A, et al: Mucin gene (MUC 2 and MUC 5AC) upregulation by grampositive and gram-negative bacteria. Biochim Biophys Acta *1406*:251, 1998.
27. Travis SM, et al: Activity of abundant antimicrobials of the human airway. Am J Respir Cell Mol Biol *20*:872, 1999.
28. Harbitz O, et al: Lysozyme and lactoferrin in sputum from patients with chronic obstructive lung disease. Eur J Respir Dis *65*:512, 1984.
29. McCray PB Jr, et al: Efficient killing of inhaled bacterial in DeltaF508 mice: role of airway surface liquid composition. Am J Physiol *277*:L183, 1999.
30. Srivastava MD, Walker WA: The development of the mucosal immune system in the sick neonate. *In* Bellanti JA, et al: (eds): Neonatal Hematology and Immunology III. New York, Elsevier Science 1997, pp 115–120.
31. Siafakas C, et al: Breast milk cells and their interaction with intestinal mucosa. *In* Bellanti JA, et al. (eds): Neonatal Hematology and Immunology III. New York, Elsevier Science, 1997, pp 121–126.
32. Kelemen E, et al: Atlas of Human Hemopoietic Development. New York, Springer-Verlag, 1979.
33. Kelemen E, Janossa M: Macrophages are the first differentiated blood cells formed in human embryonic liver. Exp Hematol *8*:996, 1980.
34. Slayton WB, et al: Hematopoiesis in the liver and marrow of human fetuses at 5 to 16 weeks' postconception: quantitative assessment of macrophage and neutrophil populations. Pediatr Res *43*:774, 1998.
35. Yang KD, et al: Phagocytic system. *In* Ochs HD, et al. (eds): Primary Immunodeficiency Diseases. A Molecular and Genetic Approach. New York, Oxford University Press, 1999, pp 82–96.
36. Hill HR: Biochemical, structural, and functional abnormalities of polymorphonuclear leukocytes in the neonate. Pediatr Research *22*:375, 1987.
37. Schibler K: Leukocyte development and disorders during the neonatal period. *In* Christensen R (ed): Hematologic Problems of the Neonate. Philadelphia, WB Saunders, 2000, pp 311–342.
38. Bohnsack JF: CD11/CD18-independent neutrophil adherence to laminin is mediated by integrin VLA-6. Blood *79*:1545, 1992.
39. Bohnsack JF, Zhou X: Divalent cation substitution reveals CD18- and very late antigen-dependent pathways that mediate human neutrophil adherence to fibronectin. J Immunol *149*:1340, 1992.
40. Gresham HD, et al: Pertussis toxin and cholera toxin modulation of human neutrophil Fc-receptor–mediated phagocytosis. J Cell Biol *103*:215A, 1986.
41. Wright WC, et al: Decreased bactericidal activity of leukocytes of stressed newborn infants. Pediatrics *56*:579, 1975.
42. Shigeoka AO, et al: Functional analysis of neutrophil granulocytes from healthy, infected, and stressed neonates. J Pediatr *95*:454, 1979.
43. Borregaard N, Cowland JB: Granules of the human neutrophilic polymorphonuclear leukocyte. Blood *89*:3503, 1997.
44. Xing X, et al: Cytokine expression by neutrophils and macrophages in vivo: endotoxin induces tumor necrosis factor-α, macrophage inflammatory

protein-2, interleukin-1β, and interleukin-6 but not RANTES or transforming growth factor-β1 mRNA expression in acute lung inflammation. Am J Respir Cell Mol Biol 10:148, 1994.

45. Marodi L, et al: Chemotactic and random movement of human newborn monocytes. Eur J Pediatr 135:73, 1980.
46. Klein RB, et al: Decreased mononuclear and polymorphonuclear chemotaxis in human newborns, infants, and young children. Pediatrics 60:467, 1977.
47. Roth P, Polin RA: Adherence of human newborn infants' monocytes to matrix-bound fibronectin. J Pediatr 121:285, 1992.
48. Nathan CF, Tsunawaki S: Secretion of toxic oxygen products by macrophages: regulatory cytokines and their effects on the oxidase. Ciba Found Symp 118:211, 1986.
49. Reiss M, Roos D: Differences in oxygen metabolism of phagocytosing monocytes and neutrophils. J Clin Invest 61:480, 1978.
50. Speer CP, Johnston RB Jr: Phagocyte function. In Ogra PL (ed): Neonatal Infections: Nutritional and Immunological Interactions. Orlando, FL, Grune & Stratton, 1984, pp 21–36.
51. D'Ambola JB, et al: Human and rabbit newborn lung macrophages have reduced anti-Candida activity. Pediatr Res 68:285, 1988.
52. Nathan CF: Secretory products of macrophages. J Clin Invest 1987:319, 1987.
53. Bessler H, et al: Production of interleukin-1 by mononuclear cells of newborns and their mothers. Clin Exp Immunol 68:655, 1987.
54. Wilson CB: Immunologic basis for increased susceptibility of the neonate to infection. J Pediatr 108:1, 1986.
55. Weatherstone KB, Rich EA: Tumor necrosis factor/cachectin and interleukin-1 expression in cord blood monocytes from term and preterm neonates. Pediatr Res 25:342, 1989.
56. Bryson YJ, et al: Deficiency of immune interferon production by leukocytes of normal newborns. Cell Immunol 55:191, 1980.
57. Rowen JL, et al: Group B streptococci elicit leukotriene B$_4$ and interleukin-8 from human monocytes: neonates exhibit a diminished response. J Infect Dis 712:420, 1995.
58. Schibler KR, et al: Diminished transcription of interleukin-8 by monocytes from preterm neonates. J Leukoc Biol 53:399, 1993.
59. Le T, et al: Regulation of interleukin-10 gene expression: possible mechanisms accounting for its up-regulation and for maturational differences in its expression by blood mononuclear cells. Blood 89:4112, 1997.
60. Schibler KR, et al: Production of granulocyte colony–stimulating factor by monocytes from preterm and term neonates. Blood 82:2478, 1993.
61. Van Furth R: Cellular biology of pulmonary macrophages. Int Arch Allergy Appl Immunol 76:21, 1985.
62. Sorokin SP, et al: CFU-rAM, the origin of lung macrophages, and the macrophage lineage. Am J Physiol 263:L299, 1992.
63. Naito M, et al: Development, differentiations, and maturation of macrophages in the fetal mouse liver. J Leukoc Biol 48:27, 1990.
64. Standiford TJ, et al: Expression and regulation of chemokines in bacterial pneumonia. J Leukoc Biol 59:24, 1996.
65. Sibille Y, Reynolds HY: Macrophages and polymorphonuclear neutrophils in lung defense and injury. Am Rev Respir Dis 141:471, 1990.
66. Hart DN: Dendritic cells: unique leukocyte populations which control the primary immune response. Blood 90:3245, 1997.
67. Steinman RM, Cohn ZA: Identification of a novel cell type in peripheral lymphoid organs of mice. I. Morphology, quantitation, and tissue distribution. J Exp Med 137:1142, 1993.
68. Mekori YA, Metcalfe DD: Mast cells in innate immunity. Immunol Rev 173:131, 2000.
69. Sher A: Complement-dependent adherence of mast cells to schistosomula. Nature 263:334, 1976.
70. Sher A, et al: Complement receptors promote the phagocytosis of bacteria by rat peritoneal mast cells. Lab Invest 41:490, 1979.
71. Arock M, et al: Phagocytic and tumor necrosis factor-α response of human mast cells following exposure to gram-negative and gram positive bacteria. Infect Immun 66:6030, 1998.
72. Malaviya R, et al: Mast cell phagocytosis of FimH-expressing enterobacteria. J Immunol 152:1907, 1994.
73. Bidri M, et al: Evidence for direct interaction between mast cells and Leishmania parasites. Parasite Immunol 19:475, 1997.
74. Malaviya R, et al: The mast cell tumor necrosis factor-α response to FimH-expressing E. coli is mediated by the glycosylphosphatidylinositol-anchored molecule CD48. Proc Natl Acad Sci U S A 96:8110, 1999.
75. Malaviya R, et al: Mast cell modulation of neutrophil influx and bacterial clearance at sites of infection through TNF-alpha. Nature 381:77, 1996.
76. Echtenacher B, et al: Critical protective role of mast cells in a model of acute septic peritonitis. Nature 381:75, 1996.
77. Gaboury JP, et al: Mechanisms underlying acute mast cell–induced leukocyte rolling and adhesion in vivo. J Immunol 154:804, 1995.
78. Abraham SN, Arock M: Mast cell and basophils in innate immunity. Semin Immunol 10:373, 1998.
79. Mecheri S, David B: Unravelling the mast cell dilemma: culprit or victim of its generosity? Immunol Today 18:212, 1997.
80. Metcalfe DD, et al: Mast cells. Physiol Rev 77:1033, 1997.
81. Born W, et al: Immunoregulatory functions of γδ T cells. Adv Immunol 71:77, 1999.
82. Abbas AK, et al: Innate immunity. In Abbas AK, et al (eds): Cellular and Molecular Immunology, 4th ed. Philadelphia, WB Saunders, 2000, pp 270–290.

83. Munk ME, et al: In vitro activation of human γδ T cells by bacteria: evidence for specific interleukin secretion and target cell lysis. Curr Top Microbiol Immunol 173:159, 1991.
84. Kabelitz D, et al: A large fraction of human peripheral blood γδ T cells is activated by Mycobacterium tuberculosis but not by its 65-kDa heat shock protein. J Exp Med 171:667, 1990.
85. Carding SR, Egan PJ: The importance of γδ T cells in the resolution of pathogen-induced inflammatory immune responses. Immunol Rev 173:98, 2000.
86. Hardy RR, Hayakawa K: CD5 B cells, a fetal B cell lineage. Adv Immunol 55:297, 1994.
87. Gommerman JL, Carroll MC: Negative selection of B lymphocytes: a novel role for innate immunity. Immunol Rev 173:120, 2000.
88. Boyden SV: Natural antibodies and the immune response. Adv Immunol 5:1, 1966.
89. Avrameas S, Ternynck T: The natural autoantibodies system: between hypotheses and facts. Mol Immunol 30:1133, 1993.
90. Ochsenbein AF, et al: Control of early viral and bacterial distribution and disease by natural antibodies. Science 286:2156, 1999.
91. Yancopoulos GD, et al: Preferential utilization of the most J$_H$-proximal V$_H$ gene segments in pre-B-cell lines. Nature 311:727, 1984.
92. Feeney AJ: Lack of N regions in fetal and neonatal mouse immunoglobulin V-D-J junctional sequences. J Exp Med 172:1377, 1990.
93. Boes M, et al: A critical role of natural immunoglobulin M in immediate defense against systemic bacterial infection. J Exp Med 188:2381, 1998.
94. Mirilas P, et al: Natural antibodies in childhood: development, individual stability, and injury effect indicate a contribution to immune memory. J Clin Immunol 19:109, 1999.
95. La Pine TR, Hill HR: Complement disorders. In Osborn L, et al (eds): Comprehensive Pediatrics. St. Louis, Harcourt Health Sciences (in press).
96. Johnston RB Jr: The complement system in host defense and inflammation: the cutting edges of a double-edged sword. Pediatr Infect Dis J 12:933, 1993.
97. Schweinle JE, et al: Human mannose-binding protein activates the alternative complement pathway and enhances serum bactericidal activity on a mannose-rich isolate of Salmonella. J Clin Invest 84:1821, 1989.
98. Figueroa JE, Densen P: Infectious diseases associated with complement deficiencies. Clin Microbiol Rev 4:359, 1991.
99. Hill HR, et al: Evaluation of nonspecific (alternative pathway) opsonic activity by neutrophil chemiluminescence. Int Arch Allergy Appl Immunol 53:490, 1977.
100. Lassiter HA, et al: Complement factor 9 deficiency in serum of human neonates. J Infect Dis 166:53, 1992.
101. Yang KD, et al: Fibronectin in host defense: implications in the diagnosis, prophylaxis and therapy of infectious diseases. Pediatr Infect Dis J 12:234, 1993.
102. Proctor RA, et al: Fibronectin mediates attachment of Staphylococcus aureus to human neutrophils. Blood 59:681, 1982.
103. Simpson WA, et al: Fibronectin-mediated binding of group A streptococci to human polymorphonuclear leukocytes. Infect Immun 805–810:37:805, 1982.
104. Yang KD, et al: Effects of fibronectin on the interaction of polymorphonuclear leukocytes with unopsonized and antibody-opsonized bacteria. J Infect Dis 158:823, 1988.
105. Proctor RA: Fibronectin: an enhancer of phagocyte function. Rev Infect Dis 9:S412, 1987.
106. Hill HR, et al: Mechanism of fibronectin enhancement of group B streptococcal phagocytosis by human neutrophils and culture-derived macrophages. Infect Immun 61:2334, 1993.
107. Jacobs RF, et al: Phagocytosis of type III group B streptococci by neonatal monocytes: enhancement by fibronectin and gammaglobulin. J Infect Dis 152:695, 1985.
108. Yang KD, et al: Effects of fibronectin on actin organization and respiratory burst activity in neutrophils, monocytes, and macrophages. J Cell Physiol 158:347, 1994.
109. Peat EB, et al: Effects of fibronectin and group B streptococci on tumour necrosis factor-α production by human culture-derived macrophages. Immunology 84:440, 1995.
110. Hill HR, et al: Fibronectin deficiency: a correctable defect in the neonate's host defense mechanism. Pediatr Res 17:25A, 1983.
111. Barnard DR, Arthur MM: Fibronectin (cold insoluble globulin) in the neonate. J Pediatr 102:453, 1983.
112. Akiyama SK, Yamada KM: Fibronectin in disease. In Wagner B, Kaufman N (eds): Connective Tissue Diseases. Baltimore, Williams & Wilkins, 1983, pp 55–96.
113. Saba TM, et al: Cryoprecipitate reversal of opsonic alpha$_2$ surface-binding glycoprotein deficiency in septic surgical and trauma patients. Science 201:622, 1978.
114. Lanser ME, et al: Opsonic glycoprotein (plasma fibronectin) levels after burn injury. Relationship to extent of burn and development of sepsis. Ann Surg 192:776, 1980.
115. Yoder MC, et al: Plasma fibronectin in healthy newborn infants, respiratory distress syndrome and perinatal asphyxia. J Pediatr 102:777, 1983.
116. Ganrot PO: Variation of the concentration of some plasma proteins in normal adults, in pregnant women and in newborns. Scand J Clin Lab Invest 124:83, 1972.
117. Gerdes JS, et al: Decreased plasma fibronectin in neonatal sepsis. Pediatrics 72:877, 1983.
118. Medzhitov R, Janeway C Jr: Innate immunity. N Engl J Med 343:338, 2000.

119. Lawson PR, Reid KBM: The roles of surfactant proteins A and D innate immunity. Immunol Rev 173:66, 2000.

120. Feizi T: Carbohydrate-mediated recognition systems in innate immunity. Immunol Rev 173:79, 2000.

121. Turner MW: Mannose-binding lectin: the pluripotent molecule of the innate immune system. Immunol Today 17:532, 1996.

122. Epstein J, et al: The collectins in innate immunity. Curr Opin Immunol 8:29, 1996.

123. Super M, et al: Association of low levels of mannan-binding protein with a common defect of opsonization. Lancet 2:1236, 1989.

124. Sumiya M, et al: Molecular basis of opsonic defect in immunodeficient children. Lancet 337:1569, 1991.

125. Crouch EC: Modulation of host-bacterial interactions by collectins. Am J Respir Cell Mol Biol 21:558, 1999.

126. LaForce FM, et al: Inactivation of staphylococci by alveolar macrophages with preliminary observations on the importance of alveolar lining material. Am Rev Respir Dis 108:784, 1973.

127. Geertsma MF, et al: Binding of surfactant protein A to C1q receptors mediates phagocytosis of Staphylococcus aureus by monocytes. Am J Physiol 267:L578, 1994.

128. Stamme C, Wright JR: Surfactant protein A enhances the binding and deacylation of E. coli LPS by alveolar macrophages. Am J Physiol 276:L540, 1999.

129. Zimmerman PE, et al: 120-kD surface glycoprotein of Pneumocystis carinii is a ligand for surfactant protein A. J Clin Invest 89:143, 1992.

130. Tino MJ, Wright JR: Surfactant protein A stimulates phagocytosis of specific pulmonary pathogens by alveolar macrophages. Am J Physiol 270:L677, 1996.

131. McNeely TB, Coonrod JD: Aggregation and opsonization of type A but not type B Hemophilus influenzae by surfactant protein A. Am J Respir Cell Mol Biol 11:114, 1994.

132. Schelenz S, et al: Binding of host collectins to the pathogenic yeast Cryptococcus neoformans: human surfactant protein D acts as an agglutinin for acapsular yeast cells. Infect Immun 63:3360, 1995.

133. Kabha K, et al: SP-A enhances phagocytosis of Klebsiella by interaction with capsular polysaccharides and alveolar macrophages. Am J Physiol 272:L344, 1997.

134. O'Riordan DM, et al: Surfactant protein D interacts with Pneumocystis carinii and mediates organism adherence to alveolar macrophages. J Clin Invest 95:2699, 1995.

135. Van Iwaarden JF, et al: Binding of surfactant protein A (SP-A) to herpes simplex virus type 1–infected cells is mediated by the carbohydrate moiety of SP-A. J Biol Chem 267:25039, 1992.

136. Gaynor CD, et al: Pulmonary surfactant protein A mediates enhanced phagocytosis of Mycobacterium tuberculosis by a direct interaction with human macrophages. J Immunol 155:5343, 1995.

137. Madan T, et al: Binding of pulmonary surfactant proteins A and D to Aspergillus fumigatus conidia enhances phagocytosis and killing by human neutrophils and alveolar macrophages. Infect Immun 65:3171, 1997.

138. Hickman-Davis JM, et al: Surfactant protein A mediates mycoplasmacidal activity of alveolar macrophages. Am J Physiol 274:L270, 1998.

139. LeVine AM, et al: Surfactant protein A–deficient mice are susceptible to group B streptococcal infection. J Immunol 158:4336, 1997.

140. LeVine AM, et al: Surfactant protein-A–deficient mice are susceptible to Pseudomonas aeruginosa infection. Am J Respir Cell Mol Biol 19:700, 1998.

141. LeVine AM, et al: Surfactant protein-A binds group B streptococcus enhancing phagocytosis and clearance from lungs of surfactant protein-A–deficient mice. Am J Respir Cell Mol Biol 20:279, 1999.

142. Sano H, et al: Pulmonary surfactant protein A modulates the cellular response to smooth and rough lipopolysaccharides by interaction with CD14. J Immunol 163:387, 1999.

143. Acton S, et al: The collagenous domains of macrophage scavenger receptors and complement component C1q mediate their similar but not identical, binding specificities for polyanionic ligands. J Biol Chem 268:3530, 1993.

144. Madan T, et al: Lung surfactant proteins A and D can inhibit specific IgE binding to the allergens of Aspergillus fumigatus and block allergen-induced histamine release from human basophils. Clin Exp Immunol 110:241, 1997.

145. Wang JY, et al: Inhibitory effect of pulmonary surfactant proteins A and D on allergen-induced lymphocyte proliferation and histamine release in children with asthma. Am J Respir Crit Care Med 158:510, 1998.

146. Bevilacqua MP, Nelson RM: Selectins. J Clin Invest 91:379, 1993.

147. Phillips ML: Neutrophil adhesion in leukocyte adhesion deficiency syndrome type 2. J Clin Invest 96:2898, 1995.

148. Levy O, et al: Impaired innate immunity in the newborn: newborn neutrophils are deficient in bactericidal/permeability-increasing protein. Pediatrics 104:1327, 1999.

149. Steiner H, et al: Sequence and specificity of two antibacterial proteins involved in insect immunity. Nature 292:246, 1981.

150. Ganz T, Weiss J: Antimicrobial peptides of phagocytes and epithelia. Semin Hematol 34:343, 1997.

151. Harwig SSL, et al: Neutrophil defensins: purification, characterization and antimicrobial testing. Methods Enzymol 236:160, 1994.

152. Goldman MJ, et al: Human β-defensin-1 is a salt-sensitive antibiotic in lung that is inactivated in cystic fibrosis. Cell 88:553, 1997.

153. Selsted ME, Ouellette AJ: Defensins in granules and non-phagocytic cells. Trends Cell Biol 5:114, 1995.

154. Dudley DJ, Wiedmeier S: The ontogeny of the immune response: perinatal perspectives. Semin Perinatol 184-195:15:184, 1991.

155. Haynes BF, et al: Early events in human T cell ontogeny: phenotypic characterization and immunohistologic localization of T cell precursors in early human fetal tissues. J Exp Med 168:1061, 1988.

156. Kingsley G, et al: Correlation of immunoregulatory function with cell phenotype in cord blood lymphocytes. Clin Exp Immunol 73:40, 1988.

157. Shyur SD, Hill HR: Recent advances in the genetics of primary immunodeficiency syndromes. J Pediatr 129:8, 1996.

158. La Pine TR, Hill HR: Immunomodifiers applicable to the prevention and management of infectious diseases in children. In Arnoff SC (ed.): Advances in Pediatric Infectious Diseases, Vol 9. St Louis, Mosby–Year Book, 1994, pp 37–58.

159. Stallmach T, et al: Cytokine production and visualized effects in the feto-maternal unit: quantitative and topographic data on cytokines during intrauterine disease. Lab Invest. 73:384, 1995.

160. Carswell EA, et al: An endotoxin-induced serum factor that causes necrosis of tumors. Proc Nat Acad Sci USA 72:3666, 1975.

161. Haranaka K, et al: Antitumor activity of murine tumor necrosis factor (TNF) against transplanted murine tumors and heterotransplanted human tumors in nude mice. Int J Cancer 34:263, 1984.

162. Old LJ: Tumor necrosis factor (TNF). Science 230:630, 1985.

163. Beutler B, et al: Purification of cachectin, a lipoprotein lipase–suppressing hormone secreted by endotoxin–induced RAW 264.7 cells. J Exp Med 161:984, 1985.

164. Kawakami M, Cerami A: Studies of endotoxin-induced decrease in lipoprotein lipase activity. J Exp Med 154:631, 1981.

165. Beutler B, Cerami A: Cachectin and tumour necrosis factor as two sides of the same biological coin. Nature 320:584, 1986.

166. Movat HZ: Tumor necrosis factor and interleukin-1: role in acute inflammation and microvascular injury. J Lab Clin Med 110:668, 1987.

167. Movat HZ, et al: Acute inflammation in gram-negative infection: endotoxin, interleukin-1, tumor necrosis factor, and neutrophils. Fed Proc 46:97, 1987.

168. Tracey KJ, et al: Cachectin: a hormone that triggers acute shock and chronic cachexia. J Infect Dis 157:413, 1988.

169. Salyer JL, et al: Mechanisms of tumor necrosis factor-alpha alteration of PMN adhesion and migration. Am J Pathol 136:831, 1990.

170. Koivuranta-Vaara P, et al: Bacterial-lipopolysaccharide–induced release of lactoferrin from human polymorphonuclear leukocytes: role of monocyte-derived tumor necrosis factor α. Infect Immun 55:2956, 1987.

171. Berkow RL, et al: Enhancement of neutrophil superoxide production by preincubation with recombinant human tumor necrosis factor. J Immunol 139:3783, 1987.

172. Tsujimoto M, et al: Tumor necrosis factor provokes superoxide anion generation from neutrophils. Biochem Biophys Res Commun 137:1094, 1986.

173. Fast DJ, et al: Toxic shock syndrome–associated staphylococcal and streptococcal pyogenic exotoxins are potent inducers of tumor necrosis factor production. Infect Immun 57:291, 1989.

174. Mancuso G, et al: Induction of tumor necrosis factor alpha by the group and type-specific polysaccharides form type III group B streptococci. Infect Immun 62:2748, 1994.

175. Vallejo JG, et al: Roles of the bacterial cell wall and capsule in induction of tumor necrosis factor alpha by type III group B streptococci. Infect Immun 64:5042, 1996.

176. Williams PA, et al: Production of tumor necrosis factor by human cells in vitro and in vivo, induced by group B streptococci. J Pediatr 123:292, 1993.

177. Okusawa S, et al: C5a stimulates secretion of tumor necrosis factor from human mononuclear cells in vitro. J Exp Med 168:443, 1988.

178. Schindler R, et al: Recombinant C5a stimulates transcription rather than translation of interleukin-1 (IL-1) and tumor necrosis factor: translational signal provided by lipopolysaccharide or IL-1 itself. Blood 76:1631, 1990.

179. Kremlev SG, Phelps DS: Surfactant protein A stimulation of inflammatory cytokine and immunoglobulin production. Am J Physiol 267:L712, 1994.

180. Steele PM, et al: The effect of lactic acid on mononuclear cell secretion of proinflammatory cytokines in response to group B streptococci. J Infect Dis 177:1418, 1998.

181. Kwak DJ, et al: Intracellular and extracellular cytokine production by human mixed mononuclear cells in response to group B streptococci. Infect Immunity 68:320, 2000.

182. Teti G, et al: Cytokine appearance and effects of anti-tumor necrosis factor alpha antibodies in a neonatal rat model of group B streptococcal infection. Infect Immun 61:227, 1993.

183. Wood GW, Greenwood JH: Murine CD4- CD8- thymocytes are stimulated by interleukin-2 to proliferate in vitro in chemically defined medium. Thymus 18:15, 1991.

184. Bevilacqua MP, et al: Interleukin-1 acts on cultured human vascular endothelium to increase the adhesion of polymorphonuclear leukocytes, monocytes, and related cell lines. J Clin Invest 76:2003, 1985.

185. Cannon JG, et al: Circulating interleukin-1 and tumor necrosis factor in septic shock and experimental endotoxin fever. J Infect Dis 161:79, 1990.

186. Liechty KW, et al: Production of interleukin-6 by fetal and maternal cells in vivo during intraamniotic infection and in vitro after stimulation with interleukin-1. Pediatr Res 29:1, 1991.

187. Romani L, et al: Impaired neutrophil response and CD4+T helper cell 1 development in interleukin-6-deficient mice infected with Candida albicans. J Exp Med 183:1345, 1996.

188. Baggiolini M, et al: Interleukin-8 and related chemotactic cytokines—CXC and CC chemokines. Adv Immunol 55:97, 1994.

189. Shimoya K, et al: Interleukin-8 in cord sera: a sensitive and specific marker for the detection of preterm chorioamnionitis. J Infect Dis 165:957, 1992.

190. Greenberger MJ, et al: Neutralization of macrophage inflammatory protein-2 attenuates, neutrophil recruitment and bacterial clearance in murine *Klebsiella* pneumonia. J Infect Dis 173:159, 1996.

191. Du X, Williams DA: Interleukin-11: review of molecular, cell biology, and clinical use. Blood 89:3897, 1997.

192. van de Ven C, et al: IL-11 in combination with SLF and G-CSF or GM-CSF significantly increases expansion of isolated CD34⁻ cell populations from cord blood versus adult bone marrow. Exp Hematol 23:1289, 1995.

193. Lemoli RM, et al: Interleukin-11 stimulates proliferation of human hematopoietic CD34⁻ and CD34⁻ CD33⁻DR⁻ cells and synergizes with stem cell factor, interleukin-3, and granulocyte-macrophage colony–stimulating factor. Exp Hematol 21:1668, 1993.

194. Chang M, et al: Role of interleukin-11 (IL-11) during experimental group B streptococcal (GBS) sepsis in rats: prophylactic use of IL-11 improves survival and enhances platelet recovery (abstract). Blood 84:477, 1994.

195. Keith JC Jr, et al: IL-11, a pleiotropic cytokine: exciting new effects of IL-11 on gastrointestinal mucosal biology. Stem Cells 12:79, 1994.

196. Du X, et al: The protective effects of interleukin-11 (IL-11) in a murine model of ischemic bowel necrosis. Am J Physiol 272:543, 1997.

197. Schindel D, et al: Interleukin-11 improves survival and reduces bacterial translocation and bone marrow suppression in burned mice. J Pediatr Surg 32:312, 1997.

198. Bank I, et al: Safety and activity evaluation of rhIL-11 in subjects with active Crohn's disease. Shock 7:520, 1997.

199. Trinchieri G: Interleukin-12: a proinflammatory cytokine with immunoregulatory functions that bridge innate resistance and antigen-specific adaptive immunity. Annu Rev Immunol 13:25, 1995.

200. Kobayashi M, et al: Identification and purification of natural killer cell stimulatory factor (NKSF), a cytokine with multiple biologic effects on human lymphocytes. J Exp Med 170:827, 1989.

201. D'Andrea A, et al: Production of natural killer cell stimulatory factor (NKSF/IL-12) by peripheral blood mononuclear cells. J Exp Med 176:1387, 1992.

202. Aste-Amezaga M, et al: Molecular mechanisms of the induction of IL-12 and its inhibition by IL-10. J Immunol 160:5936, 1998.

203. Joyner JL, et al: Interleukin-12 increases IFN-γ production by cord and adult blood mononuclear cells in response to group B streptococci. Pediatr Res 47:333A, 2000.

204. Snijders A, et al: Regulation of bioactive IL-12 production in lipopolysaccharide-stimulated human monocytes is determined by the expression of the p35 subunit. J Immunol 156:1207, 1996.

205. Cenci E, et al: IFN-γ is required for IL-12 responsiveness in mice with *Candida albicans* infection. J Immunol 161:3543, 1998.

206. Presky DH, et al: A functional interleukin-12 receptor complex is composed of two beta-type cytokine receptor subunits. Proc Natl Acad Sci U S A 93:14002, 1996.

207. Mancuso G, et al: Role of interleukin-12 in experimental neonatal sepsis caused by group B streptococci. Infect Immun 65:373, 1997.

208. Ertel W, et al: Inhibition of the immune system stimulating interleukin-12 interferon-γ pathway during critical illness. Blood 89:1612, 1997.

209. Borges WG, et al: Defective interleukin-12/interferon-γ pathway in patients with hyperimmunoglobulinemia E syndrome. J Pediatr 136:176, 2000.

210. Dinarello CA: IL-18: A Th1-inducing, proinflammatory cytokine and new member of the IL-1 family. J Allergy Clin Immunol 103:11, 1999.

211. Takeda K, et al: Defective NK cell activity and Th1 response in IL-18—deficient mice. Immunity 8:383, 1998.

212. Gu Y, et al: Activation of interferon-γ inducing factor mediated by interleukin-1β converting enzyme. Science 275:206, 1997.

213. Ghayur T, et al: Caspase-1 processes IFN-γ-inducing factor and regulates LPS-induced IFN-γ production. Nature 386:619, 1997.

214. Okamura H, et al: Cloning of a new cytokine that induces interferon-γ. Nature 378:88, 1995.

215. Ushio S, et al: Cloning of the cDNA for human IFN-γ-inducing factor, expression in *Escherichia coli*, and studies on the biologic activities of the protein. J Immunol 156:4274, 1996.

216. Puren AJ, et al: Interleukin-18 (IFN-γ-inducing factor) induces IL-1β and IL-8 via TNF-α production from non-CD14+ human blood mononuclear cells. J Clin Invest 101:711, 1998.

217. La Pine TR, et al: Defective production of IL-18 and IL-12 by cord blood mononuclear cells influences the Th-1 IFN-γ response to group B streptococci. Pediatr Res 54:276, 2003.

218. Hill HR, et al: Human recombinant interferon γ enhances neonatal polymorphonuclear leukocyte activation and movement, and increases free intracellular calcium. J Exp Med 173:767, 1991.

219. Hill HR: Modulation of host defenses with interferon-γ in pediatrics. J Infect Dis 167:S23, 1993.

220. Dorman SE, Holland SM: Interferon-gamma and interleukin-12 pathway defects and human disease. Cytokine Growth Factor Rev 11:321, 2000.

221. Holland SM: Treatment of infections in the patient with Mendelian susceptibility to mycobacterial infection. Microbes Infect 2:1579, 2000.

222. Bryson YJ, et al: Deficiency of immune interferon production by leukocytes of normal newborns. Cell Immunol 55:191, 1980.

223. Wilson CB, et al: Decreased production of interferon-gamma by human neonatal cells: intrinsic and regulatory deficiencies. J Clin Invest 77:860, 1986.

224. Davis SD, et al: Job's syndrome: recurrent "cold" staphylococcal abscesses. Lancet 1:1013, 1966.

225. Del Prete G, et al: Defective in vitro production of γ-interferon and tumor necrosis factor-α by circulating T cells from patients with the hyper-immunoglobulin E syndrome. J Clin Invest 84:1830, 1989.

226. Jeppson JD, et al: Use of recombinant human interferon gamma to enhance neutrophil chemotactic responses in Job syndrome of hyper-immunoglobulin E and recurrent infections. J Pediatr 118:383, 1991.

227. Petrak BA, et al: Recombinant human interferon gamma treatment of patients with Job's syndrome of hyperimmunoglobulin E and recurrent infections. Clin Res 42:1A, 1994.

228. International Chronic Granulomatous Disease Cooperative Study Group: A controlled trial of interferon gamma to prevent infection in chronic granulomatous disease. N Engl J Med 324:509, 1991.

229. Clark SC, Kamen R: The human hematopoietic colony-stimulating factors. Science 236:1229, 1987.

230. Groopman JE, et al: Recombinant alpha-2 interferon therapy for Kaposi's sarcoma associated with acquired immunodeficiency syndrome. Ann Intern Med 100:671, 1984.

231. Lau AS, et al: Biology and therapeutic uses of myeloid hematopoietic growth factors and interferons. Pediatr Infect Dis J 15:563, 1996.

232. Wolach B, et al: Effect of granulocyte and granulocyte macrophage colony stimulating factors (G-CSF and GM-CSF) on neonatal neutrophil functions. Pediatr Res 48:369, 2000.

233. Vadhan-Raj S, et al: Stimulation of myelopoiesis in patients with aplastic anemia by recombinant human granulocyte-macrophage colony–stimulating factor. N Engl J Med 319:1628, 1988.

234. Campbell JR, Edwards MS: Cytokines enhance opsonophagocytosis of type III group B streptococcus. J Perinatol 20:225, 2000.

235. Roilides E, et al: Granulocyte colony–stimulating factor enhances the phagocytic and bactericidal activity of normal and defective human neutrophils. J Infect Dis 163:579, 1991.

236. Zhang P, et al: Enhancement of peritoneal leukocyte function by granulocyte colony–stimulating factor in rats with abdominal sepsis. Crit Care Med 26:315, 1998.

237. Sullivan GW, et al: The effect of three human recombinant hematopoietic growth factors (granulocyte-macrophage colony–stimulating factor, granulocyte colony–stimulating factor, and interleukin-3) on phagocyte oxidative activity. Blood 81:1863, 1993.

238. Pauksen K, et al: Serum levels of granulocyte colony–stimulating factor (G-CSF) in bacterial and viral infections, and in atypical pneumonia. Br J Haematol 88:256, 1994.

239. Kawakami M, et al: Levels of serum granulocyte colony–stimulating factor in patients with infections. Blood 76:1962, 1990.

240. Whiteside TL, Herberman RB: Role of human natural killer cells in health and disease. Clin Diagn Lab Immunol 1:125, 1994.

241. Whiteside TL, Herberman RB: The role of natural killer cells in human disease. Clin Immunol Immunopathol 53:1, 1989.

242. Seaman WE: Natural killer cells. *In* Rich RR, et al (eds): Clinical Immunology: Principles and Practice. St. Louis, Mosby, 1996, pp 282–289.

243. Bancroft GJ, et al: Natural immunity: a T-cell-independent pathway of macrophage activation, defined in the scid mouse. Immunol Rev 124:5, 1991.

244. Tripp CS, et al: Interleukin-12 and tumor necrosis factor alpha are costimulators of interferon gamma production by natural killer cells in severe combined immunodeficiency mice with listeriosis, and interleukin-10 is a physiologic antagonist. Proc Natl Acad Sci U S A 90:3725, 1993.

245. Gazzinelli RT, et al: Interleukin-12 is required for the T-lymphocyte-independent induction of interferon gamma by an intracellular parasite and induces resistance in T cell-deficient hosts. Proc Natl Acad Sci U S A 90:6115, 1993.

246. Ching C, Lopez C: Natural killing of herpes simplex virus type 1—infected target cells: normal human responses and influence of antiviral antibody. Infect Immun 26:49, 1979.

247. Kohl S: Interferon induction of natural killer cytotoxicity in human neonates. J Pediatr 98:379, 1981.

248. van Furth R, et al: The immunologic development of the human fetus. J Exp Med 122:1173, 1965.

249. Cates KL, et al: The premature infant as a compromised host. Curr Prob Pediatr 13:1, 1983.

250. La Pine R, Hill HR: Monoclonal antibodies. Semin Pediatr Infect Dis 12:64, 2001.

251. Burgio GR, et al: Ontogeny of secretory immunity: levels of secretory IgA and natural antibodies in saliva. Pediatr Res 14:1111, 1980.

252. Mellander L, et al: Secretory IgA antibody response against *Escherichia coli* antigens in infants in relation to exposure. J Pediatr 107:430, 1985.

152 Host Defense Mechanisms Against Fungi

Fungal infections are commonly classified as either endemic or opportunistic.[1] An *endemic fungal infection* may occur in anyone living in a geographic area that is the natural habitat of that fungus. Histoplasmosis, coccidioidomycosis, and blastomycosis, which are usually acquired by inhalation, are examples. Although exposure to endemic fungi may be possible in the newborn period, it is unlikely under normal circumstances. Therefore, we do not discuss mechanisms of resisting these organisms, but rather focus on resistance to opportunistic fungi.

Opportunistic fungal infections occur primarily in immunocompromised persons.[2] Extensive investigation of host defense mechanisms in the newborn has indicated that multiple systems are partially compromised, or blunted, and it is probably this combination of partial deficiencies that places the newborn at risk.[3] Among the opportunistic fungi, *Candida* species stand out as particularly threatening to the newly born baby.[4-8] Although our understanding of how the host resists fungal infection is incomplete, host-*Candida* interactions have been relatively well studied. For these reasons, this chapter focuses primarily on *Candida:* what is known about how humans resist its infection, what mechanisms of host defense may be predicted to play a role, and how these may be involved in defending the newborn against candidal infection. The use of "may be" here is meant to indicate that few data directly relate current knowledge of antifungal defense mechanisms to their expression or disruption in human newborns.

Perineal and oral thrush caused by *Candida* species is common in otherwise normal neonates. In neonatal intensive care units, the newborn is at risk of more serious systemic disease, and since the 1980s, the incidence of candidemia in these units has increased.[4-6] *C. albicans* remains the most common cause of neonatal candidiasis, but other species such as *C. parapsilosis* and *C. glabrata* are also frequent causes of invasive neonatal infection, especially in low birth weight infants.[8,9] The frequency of serious candidal disease in newborns may be attributed to technical improvement of medical practices and intensive care measures combined with the newborn's blunted capacity to fight infection.[3,4,10] The prominence of neonatal candidal infections and the difficulties in diagnosis and treatment of invasive candidiasis emphasize the importance of acquiring a better understanding of the mechanisms by which this genus causes infection in newborns.

This chapter is divided into (1) a discussion of antifungal defense mechanisms believed to be active at body surfaces and how these may be related to mucocutaneous candidiasis and (2) a review of those mechanisms expected to defend the newborn against systemic candidal infection. In discussing both forms of candidiasis, we use the experience in patients with primary immunodeficiency disease with fungal infections as a guide to understanding basic host-fungal interactions and how these may be expressed in newborn babies.

DEFENSE AGAINST MUCOCUTANEOUS CANDIDIASIS

Candida Virulence Factors and Surface Host Defense

Candida species cause a broad range of mucocutaneous infections involving the skin and mucous membranes.[10,11] *C. albicans* is part of the common commensal microbial flora of the oral cavity and the gastrointestinal and genitourinary tracts of healthy humans. Candidal vulvovaginitis occurs commonly in most women during pregnancy, and the body surfaces of newborns are colonized at birth. Overgrowth of these colonizing *Candida* organisms may lead to mucosal or cutaneous candidiasis characterized by local signs of infection and visible white patches. Transformation from the yeast phase to the filamentous form (pseudohyphae, hyphae, and germ tubes) appears to be essential for candidal pathogenicity.[12] Adhesins on blastospores and hyphae of *C. albicans*, like integrins on human leukocytes, can recognize arginine-glycine-aspartic acid (RGD) sequences on epithelial cells and several extracellular matrix proteins.[13] The *Candida* gene *INT1* encodes an adhesin, INT1p, that recognizes the RGD-containing proteins and promotes the growth of filaments. This candidal adhesin is homologous to mammalian integrins and itself contains an RGD site that may be recognized by integrins on human cells, thus facilitating further the adhesion of *Candida* to the cell surface.[13] These findings provide at least a partial explanation for the symbiosis of *Candida* with humans and to the tropism of these fungi to intestinal and mucosal epithelium.

On the host side, secretory antibody (especially of the immunoglobulin A [IgA] class), the mucous layer, and cilia act to prevent adhesion to mucosal surfaces, and various antimicrobial agents protect both the skin and the mucosae. These mechanisms have the potential to prevent the penetration of commensal fungi such as *Candida*. Demonstration that peptides with broad and potent antimicrobial properties—the magainins—exist in frog skin proved this principle.[14] These cationic peptides bind to anionic components of the microbial membrane and form pores that permeabilize the cell. Subsequently, two major classes of cationic antimicrobial polypeptides were described in human skin and epithelia: the β-defensins[15] and the cathelicidins.[16] Both polypeptides can kill fungi. An additional peptide, dermicidin, which is secreted in sweat, can also kill fungi.[17] Nasal and lung secretions contain the antimicrobial polypeptide constituents lysozyme, lactoferrin, and secretory leukoprotease inhibitor, as well as neutrophil and epithelial defensins.[18] The experiments of nature represented by absent function of these proteins have not yet been detected, and the precise role of these surface agents in defense against fungal (or any) infection is not yet clear.

Lessons from Primary and Acquired Immunodeficiency Disorders

Neonatal deficiency of T-cell–mediated immunity may play a part in the frequent mucocutaneous candidal infections in newborns. Persistent mucosal candidiasis and oropharyngeal thrush are common complications of primary T-cell deficiencies such as DiGeorge syndrome and combined immunodeficiency disease.[19] Patients with autoimmune polyendocrinopathy-candidiasis-ectodermal dystrophy syndrome, chronic mucocutaneous candidiasis, and hyper-IgE syndrome, all of which are characterized by subtle, nonlethal defects in T lymphocytes, have protracted candidal infections of the mucous membranes, nails, and skin.[11,19,20] These patients, however, are no more susceptible to life-threatening, generalized candidiasis than are immunocompetent persons. Mice with CD4+ T-cell deficiency are also naturally susceptible to mucosal candidiasis.[21]

Oral and gastrointestinal candidiasis is a common manifestation of human immunodeficiency virus infection, and esophageal candidiasis is one of the diagnostic criteria of the acquired immunodeficiency syndrome (AIDS).[22] Disseminated candidiasis is much less frequent in patients with AIDS than in immunosuppressed patients without AIDS, and it occurs only in end-stage disease when other immune functions are also severely impaired. Oral or esophageal candidiasis associated with AIDS is generally not considered to be caused by the presence of a unique or particularly virulent strain but is likely the consequence of a defect in T-cell–mediated host defense.[22] An adequate number of functioning T cells is required for the development of a normal secretory immune response to *Candida*, and T cells seem to play a critical role in stimulating the differentiation of IgA-positive B lymphocytes into plasma cells that produce secretory IgA.[23]

Taken together, these observations support the concept that partial (selective) T-cell deficiency is responsible for the development of mucosal candidiasis in a variety of conditions, including chronic mucocutaneous candidiasis, secretory IgA deficiency, AIDS, and, perhaps, the newborn state. This concept is further supported by the observation in mice that recovery from oropharyngeal infection with *C. albicans* depends largely on CD4+ T-cell augmentation of monocyte and neutrophil functions through activity of Th1-type cytokines such as interleukin-12 (IL-12), and interferon-γ (IFN-γ).[24]

Deficient T-Cell–Mediated Immunity in Newborns

Neonatal T-cell responses are compromised at several steps including deficient production of cytokines by CD4+ T cells. Deficiency in IFN-γ production by neonatal T cells has been well documented.[25-27] IFN-γ deficiency in neonates may be attributed to lymphocyte immaturity and also to decreased production of IL-12 by cord blood mixed mononuclear cells.[27, 28] In addition, diminished production of IL-12 by cord-derived dendritic cells has also been reported.[29] These studies suggest that neonatal T cells, mononuclear phagocytes, and dendritic cells do not mount a normally vigorous Th1 response. This apparent down-regulation of Th1 responses in human neonates may be responsible, at least in part, for the developmental immaturity of the immune system on mucosal surfaces[30] and the susceptibility of newborns to oropharyngeal candidiasis.

DEFENSE AGAINST INVASIVE CANDIDIASIS

Invasive candidal disease may arise from translocation of the gut flora, and it may be propagated by the ability of *Candida* to adhere to nonbiologic materials such as intravenous catheters.[31-34] The use of heparin to prevent blood clot formation in newborns with intravascular catheters may accidentally trigger invasive candidal disease by transforming yeasts into life-threatening pathogens. Heparin, in concentrations equivalent to those in intravascular catheters, appears to facilitate the cleavage of the *C. albicans* surface adhesion protein INT1p, with release of a cleavage product that acts as a superantigen capable of activating T lymphocytes and stimulating release of inflammatory cytokines.[35]

Once in the bloodstream, *Candida* organisms are able to adhere to the vascular endothelium. INT1p appears to play an essential role in both adhesion and development of filamentous forms.[13] Administration of broad-spectrum antibiotics and glucocorticoids, risk factors for disseminated candidiasis in newborns, accentuated the pathogenetic capacity of INT1p in mice inoculated with *C. albicans* by mouth.[4]

Pulmonary surfactant protein-D has been implicated in host defense against *C. albicans* in alveolar compartments of the lung.[36] Surfactant protein-D may facilitate mucociliary clearance by agglutinating *C. albicans* into large complexes and may

decrease hyphal outgrowth. Decreased concentration of surfactant protein-D in neonates or alteration in levels of this protein as a result of lung disease and mechanical ventilation could disrupt local host defense and could contribute to the development of pulmonary candidal infection.

Pseudomonas aeruginosa can form a dense biofilm on *C. albicans* filaments and can kill the fungi.[37] This example of a bacterial antifungal suppressive mechanism emphasizes the risk of *Candida* infection posed by the administration of broad-spectrum antibiotic therapy.

Role of Phagocytes in Protection Against Invasive Candidiasis

Phagocytic cells are an essential defense against infections by *Candida* and other fungi. Patients with chronic granulomatous disease, whose phagocytes cannot convert oxygen to toxic oxidants, and patients with primary or secondary neutropenia have increased susceptibility to infections by *C. albicans* and other fungi. This predisposition exists in the absence of antibiotic or corticosteroid therapy, depressed cell-mediated immunity, or intravenous lines.[38-41] A few patients with complete deficiency of myeloperoxidase and diabetes mellitus have sustained systemic candidiasis,[42] and phagocytes from myeloperoxidase-deficient patients have an impaired ability to kill ingested *C. albicans*.[42, 43] These observations suggest that hydrogen peroxide–dependent microbicidal mechanisms are of critical importance in the phagocytic killing of *Candida*.

In vitro studies have suggested that antibody-mediated immunity can protect against invasive candidal disease.[44-46] We have found that optimal phagocytosis of *Candida* species by human mononuclear phagocytes requires opsonization by human serum, a finding that supports this hypothesis.[47] However, there are no clinical observations to suggest that patients with immunodeficiency disorders other than quantitative or functional phagocytic cell defects suffer increased susceptibility to invasive candidiasis. Patients with X-linked agammaglobulinemia or other severe hypogammaglobulinemias do not exhibit increased susceptibility to either mucocutaneous or invasive candidal infections. In such patients, T cells, NK cells, and antimicrobial peptides may suppress *Candida* at the surface, and macrophages and keratinocytes, which phagocytose and kill candidal yeasts through the mannose receptor,[47, 48] may protect without the need for antibody opsonization.

Deficient Anticandidal Activities of Neonatal Monocytes and Macrophages

In one report, the extent of phagocytosis and killing of serum-opsonized *Candida* by resident monocytes and monocyte-derived macrophages were comparable in newborns and adults.[49] In the absence of serum, ingestion and killing by cord and adult cells were reduced by half but still equivalent, and mannan inhibited ingestion of unopsonized *Candida* by macrophages in a concentration-dependent manner, a finding suggesting a role for the mannose receptor. However, exposure of cord and adult macrophages to IFN-γ gave quantitatively different results in *Candida* killing, as well as in release of superoxide anion. Maximal increase in these functions with adult macrophages was achieved with 100 U/mL IFN-γ. No enhancement with cord macrophages could be detected after treatment with 100 U/mL, and at 500 U/mL there was still significantly lower killing and superoxide release by cord macrophages compared with adult cells.[49] A similar blunted response of cord macrophages to activation by IFN-γ and increased killing was found using group B streptococci as the target organism.[50] The number and binding capacity of IFN-γ receptors were greater on newborn than on adult mononuclear phagocytes.[49] These data suggest that neonatal macrophages have a normal capacity to ingest and kill both opsonized and unopsonized *Candida* organisms but cannot be fully activated by IFN-γ, a finding that could not be attributed to lower expression of IFN-γ receptors on neonatal cells.[49]

Could the decreased activation of cord macrophages by IFN-γ result from defective signal transduction? In response to IFN-γ, there was significantly decreased phosphorylation of signal transducer and activator of transcription-1 (STAT-1) in neonatal monocytes and macrophages.[51] The STAT family consists of a group of key signaling molecules linking cytokine binding to macrophage proinflammatory responses. These proteins are phosphorylated by Janus kinases that are activated by the binding of IFN-γ to its receptors. Expression of STAT-1 protein was equivalent in cord and adult monocytes and macrophages, but STAT-1 phosphorylation was deficient in cord cells.[51] Thus, it is possible that the decreased capacity of cord macrophages to be activated is the result of defective signal transduction; this defect remains to be defined.

Intracellular parasites have evolved various mechanisms to evade phagocytic killing by macrophages. *Candida* yeasts have a thick glycoprotein cell wall composed of mannoprotein and covalently linked chitin-glucan components that is highly resistant to lysosomal enzymes.[52] Phagocytosis of *C. albicans* by mouse macrophages reportedly induces rapid fusion of the phagolysosome membrane with late endosomes and lysosomes.[53] The ensuing acidification of the phagolysosome promotes germ tube formation, which leads to distention of the phagocyte's membranes and eventual escape of the organism.

Ingestion of *Candida* by macrophages can induce genes of the organism's glyoxylate cycle, a metabolic pathway by which two-carbon compounds are assimilated into the tricarboxylic acid cycle.[54] In *C. albicans* that were isolated from phagolysosomes of macrophages, the principal enzymes of the glyoxylate cycle, isocitrate lyase-1 and malate synthase, are up-regulated. *C. albicans* mutants lacking isocitrate lyase-1 were markedly less virulent in mice than wild-type *Candida*.[54] These findings demonstrate the significance of the glyoxylate cycle to candidal virulence and point to the complexity of the host-parasite interactions that have the potential to influence the outcome of invasive candidal disease.

REFERENCES

1. Pfaller MA: Epidemiology and control of fungal infections. Clin Infect Dis 19(Suppl 1):S8, 1994.
2. Levitz SM: Overview of host defenses in fungal infections. Clin Infect Dis 14(Suppl 1):S37, 1992.
3. Johnston RB Jr: Function and cell biology of neutrophils and mononuclear phagocytes in the newborn infant. Vaccine 16:1363, 1998.
4. Bendel CM, et al: Cecal colonization and systemic spread of *Candida albicans* in mice treated with antibiotics and dexamethasone. Pediatr Res 51:290, 2002.
5. Johnson DE, et al: Systemic candidiasis in very low-birth-weight infants (less than 1,500 grams). Pediatrics 73:138, 1984.
6. Baley JE, et al: Disseminated fungal infections in very low-birth-weight infants: clinical manifestations and epidemiology. Pediatrics 73:144, 1984.
7. Greenough A: Neonatal infections. Curr Opin Pediatr 8:6, 1996.
8. Benjamin DK Jr, et al: When to expect fungal infections in neonates: a clinical comparison of *Candida albicans* and *Candida parapsilosis* fungemia with coagulase-negative staphylococcal bacteremia. Pediatrics 106:712, 2000.
9. Fairchild KD, et al: Neonatal *Candida glabrata* sepsis: clinical and laboratory features compared with other *Candida* species. Pediatr Infect Dis J 21:39, 2002.
10. Maródi L: Local and systemic host defense mechanisms against *Candida*: immunopathology of candidal infections. Pediatr Infect Dis J 16:795, 1997.
11. Kirkpatrick CH: Chronic mucocutaneous candidiasis. Pediatr Infect Dis J 20:197, 2001.
12. Lo HJ, et al: Nonfilamentous *C. albicans* mutants are avirulent. Cell 90:939, 1997.
13. Hostetter MK: RGD-mediated adhesion in fungal pathogens of humans, plants and insects. Curr Opin Microbiol 3:344, 2000.
14. Zasloff M: Magainins, a class of antimicrobial peptides from Xenopus skin: isolation, characterization of two active forms, and partial cDNA sequence of a precursor. Proc Natl Acad Sci USA 84:5449, 1987.
15. Harder J, et al: A peptide antibiotic from human skin. Nature 387:861, 1997.
16. Frohm NM, et al: The human cationic antimicrobial protein (hCAP18), a peptide antibiotic, is widely expressed in human squamous epithelia and colocalizes with interleukin-6. Infect Immun 67:2561, 1999.
17. Schittek B, et al: Dermicidin: a novel human antibiotic peptide secreted by sweat glands. Nat Immunol 2:1133, 2001.
18. Ganz T: Antimicrobial polypeptides in host defense of the respiratory tract. J Clin Invest 109:693, 2002.
19. Shyur S-D, Hill HR: Immunodeficiency in the 1990s. Pediatr Infect Dis J 10:595, 1991.
20. Grimbacher B, et al: Hyper-IgE syndrome with recurrent infections: an autosomal dominant multisystem disorder. N Engl J Med 340:692, 1999.
21. Cantorna MT, Balish E: Role of CD4+ lymphocytes in resistance to mucosal candidiasis. Infect Immun 59:2447, 1991.
22. Whelan WL, et al: *Candida albicans* in patients with the acquired immunodeficiency syndrome: absence of a novel hypervirulent strain. J Infect Dis 162:513, 1990.
23. McGhee JR, et al: Regulation of IgA synthesis and immune response by T cells and interleukins. J Clin Immunol 9:175, 1989.
24. Farah CS, et al: T cells augment monocyte and neutrophil function in host resistance against oropharyngeal candidiasis. Infect Immun 69:6110, 2001.
25. Bryson YJ, et al: Deficiency of immune interferon production by leukocytes of normal newborns. Cell Immunol 55:191, 1980.
26. Wilson CB, et al: Decreased production of interferon gamma by human neonatal cells. J Clin Invest 77:860, 1986.
27. Joyner JL, et al: Effects of group B streptococci on cord and adult mononuclear cell interleukin-12 and interferon-γ mRNA accumulation and protein secretion. J Infect Dis 182:974, 2000.
28. Lee SM, et al: Decreased interleukin-12 from activated cord versus adult peripheral blood mononuclear cells and upregulation of interferon-γ, natural killer, and lymphokine-activated killer activity by IL-12 in cord blood mononuclear cells. Blood 88:945, 1996.
29. Langrish CL, et al: Neonatal dendritic cells are intrinsically biased against Th-1 immune response. Clin Exp Immunol 128:118, 2002.
30. Maródi L: Down-regulation of Th1 responses in human neonates. Clin Exp Immunol 128:1, 2002.
31. Klotz SA, et al: Factors governing adherence of *Candida* species to plastic surfaces. Infect Immun 55:97, 1985.
32. Rotrosen D, et al: Adherence of *Candida* species to host tissues and plastic surfaces. Rev Infect Dis 8:73, 1986.
33. Scherer S, Stevens DA: *Candida albicans* dispersed, repeated gene family and its epidemiological applications. Proc Natl Acad Sci USA 85:1452, 1988.
34. Fox BC, et al: The use of a DNA probe for epidemiological studies of candidiasis in immunocompromised hosts. J Infect Dis 159:488, 1989.
35. Stephenson J: Can a common medical practice transform *Candida* infections from benign to deadly? JAMA 286:2531, 2001.
36. Van Rozendaal BA, et al: Role of pulmonary surfactant protein D in innate defense against *Candida albicans*. J Infect Dis 182:917, 2000.
37. Hogan DA, Kolter R: *Pseudomonas-Candida* interactions: an ecological role for virulence factors. Science 296:2229, 2002.
38. Johnston RB Jr, Newman SL: Chronic granulomatous disease. Pediatr Clin North Am 24:365, 1977.
39. Winkelstein JA, et al: Chronic granulomatous disease: report on a national registry of 368 patients. Medicine (Baltimore) 79:155, 2000.
40. Rex JH, et al: Practice guidelines for the treatment of candidiasis. Clin Infect Dis 30:662, 2000.
41. Cohen MS, et al: Fungal infection in chronic granulomatous disease. Am J Med 71:59, 1981.
42. Lehrer RI, Cline MJ: Leukocyte myeloperoxidase deficiency and disseminated candidiasis: the role of myeloperoxidase in resistance to candida infection. J Clin Invest 2:135, 1969.
43. Nauseef WM: Myeloperoxidase deficiency. Hematol Oncol Clin North Am 2:135, 1988.
44. Matthews R, et al: *Candida* and AIDS: evidence for protective antibody. Lancet 2:263, 1988.
45. Han Y, Cutler JE: Antibody response that protects against disseminated candidiasis. Infect Immun 63:2714, 1995.
46. Han Y, et al: Biochemical characterization of *Candida albicans* epitopes that can elicit protective and nonprotective antibodies. Infect Immun 65:4100, 1997.
47. Maródi L, et al: Mechanisms of host defense against *Candida* species. I. Phagocytosis by monocytes and monocyte-derived macrophages. J Immunol 146:2783, 1991.
48. Szolnoky G, et al: A mannose-binding receptor is expressed on human keratinocytes and mediates killing of *Candida albicans*. J Invest Dermatol 117:205, 2001.
49. Maródi L, et al: Candidacidal mechanisms in the human neonate: impaired IFN-γ activation of macrophages in newborn infants. J Immunol 153:5643, 1994.
50. Maródi L, et al: Survival of group B *Streptococcus* type III in mononuclear phagocytes: differential regulation of bacterial killing in cord macrophages by human recombinant gamma interferon and granulocyte-macrophage colony-stimulating factor. Infect Immun 68:2167, 2000.
51. Maródi L, et al: Cytokine receptor signaling in neonatal macrophages: defective STAT-1 phosphorylation in response to stimulation with IFN-γ. Clin Exp Immunol 126:456, 2001.
52. Marquis G, et al: Histochemical and immunochemical study of the fate of *Candida albicans* inside human neutrophil phagolysosomes. J Leukoc Biol 50:587, 1991.
53. Káposzta R, et al: Rapid recruitment of late endosomes and lysosomes in mouse macrophages ingesting *Candida albicans*. J Cell Sci 112:3237, 1999.
54. Lorenz MC, Fink GR: The glyoxylate cycle is required for fungal virulence. Nature 412:83, 2001.

153
Host Defense Mechanisms Against Viruses

OVERVIEW OF INNATE AND ADAPTIVE ANTIVIRAL IMMUNITY

Viral host defense mechanisms of vertebrates depend on a combination of innate and adaptive immune mechanisms that are highly interlinked. Key innate immune mechanisms include antiviral and proinflammatory cytokines, such as type I interferon (IFN), IFN-γ, and tumor necrosis factor (TNF)-α, which have pleiotropic immunoregulatory effects and multiple potential cellular sources, including mononuclear phagocytes, dendritic cells, and natural killer (NK) cells. Dendritic cells are key for initiating the adaptive immune response and efficiently take up viral material in various forms, such as necrotic or apoptotic cellular debris. For some viral pathogens, such as human immunodeficiency virus (HIV), dendritic cells also may be directly infected. Dendritic cells process viral proteins and present these in the form of peptides bound to class I (HLA-A, -B, and -C in humans) and class II (HLA-DR, -DP, and -DQ in humans) major histocompatibility complex (MHC) molecules for activation of CD8 and CD4 T cells, respectively.

As a result of clonal expansion and differentiation, viral-specific CD8 and CD4 effector T cells are generated that carry out direct and indirect antiviral immune functions. CD4 T cells provide key help to B cells for the production of antiviral antibodies, and to CD8 T cells, which are a major source of cytokines with antiviral activity, and in some cases may also play a role in cell-mediated cytotoxicity. Effector CD8 T cells are the key cells involved with the clearance of virally infected cells from infected tissues by cell-mediated cytotoxicity, which is triggered when their T cell receptors (TCR) recognize viral peptide/class I MHC complexes on the surfaces of target cells. B cells provide antiviral antibody that can neutralize viral attachment and entry into cells. Viruses, particularly those of the herpesvirus group, can block antigen presentation and may down-regulate the overall level of class I MHC expression on the cell, potentially thwarting CD8 T cell recognition. As a countermeasure, NK cells recognize and immediately kill cells with reduced class I MHC expression, providing innate and early protection against viral infection prior to the appearance of differentiated T cells and B cells. NK cell–mediated killing is also augmented by viral-specific antibody produced by B cells, a further example of the linkage of innate and adaptive immunity. Unlike innate immune mechanisms, T cell– and B cell–specific viral immunity persists for years or for a lifetime.

Host Defense Against Herpes Simplex Virus as a Prototype of Neonatal Antiviral Mechanisms

The neonate is at risk for severe or rapidly progressive infection with certain viruses, most notably herpesviruses (herpes simplex virus, HSV-1, HSV-2), HIV, and enteroviruses. Another herpesvirus, cytomegalovirus (CMV), often causes severe disease in the premature neonate and is the major viral cause of congenital sensorineural deafness. Because viruses replicate intracellularly, mechanisms that control or block infection within cells, spread of virus from cell to cell, or both, are the most critical for effective host defense. Antibody and complement may also modify viral expression, especially by preventing spread of virus into the central nervous system (CNS), but cellular immune responses are the most central for control of viral replication and the elimination of virally infected cells.

This discussion focuses on host defenses operative against HSV-1 and HSV-2, both of which cause strikingly more severe primary disease in the neonate than in the immunocompetent adult.[1] For most of this discussion, HSV-1 and HSV-2 are collectively referred to as HSV, because these two viruses are very closely related and, in most instances, have very similar pathogenic properties. Studies of human immune responses to CMV and of murine immunity to HSV and murine CMV are also included. Although outside the scope of this chapter, the topic of innate and adaptive human fetal and neonatal immune function has recently been comprehensively reviewed.[2]

Herpesvirus Biology

HSV-1 and HSV-2 are two of eight herpesviruses that have been isolated, to date, from humans (the others include CMV, varicella-zoster virus [VZV], Epstein-Barr virus [EBV], and human herpesviruses [HHV] 6 through 8). HSV is an enveloped virus surrounded by a lipid bilayer derived from the host cell. It has a large DNA genome of approximately 150 kilobases contained within an inner core lined by capsid protein. HSV entry into the cell involves attachment of the virus via its gC and gB envelope glycoproteins with cell surface proteoglycans, such as heparan sulfate. This is followed by a second step in which the gD glycoprotein interacts with the HveB, HveC, or HigR co-receptor molecules. These co-receptors, also known as nectins, are members of the immunoglobulin superfamily. They are involved in intercellular adhesion and are widely expressed.[3] Herpesvirus entry mediator (HVEM) (TNF receptor superfamily member 14), which is expressed mainly by lymphocytes and is a member of the TNF receptor family, also may be used as a co-receptor. The final step in cell entry involves fusion with the host cell plasma membrane and involves the HSV glycoproteins gD, gB, and the gH-gL heterodimer. The HSV genome encodes more than 75 proteins,[4] including a large number of enzymes involved in nucleic acid metabolism, some of which are targets for antiviral therapy (e.g., thymidine kinase). Synthesis of the HSV DNA genome, as well as its assembly with capsid proteins, occurs in the nucleus. The production of HSV progeny results in the irreversible destruction of the host cell, resulting in viral release. Despite this lytic effect, a substantial proportion of both primary HSV-1 and HSV-2 infections are asymptomatic.[5]

Following recovery from acute infection, HSV typically persists for life in humans, due to a latent state established in neurons, such as those of the trigeminal ganglion. In cells containing latent virus, the viral genome is in a circular configuration and associated with histone proteins. The latency-reactivation cycle can be divided into three major steps of latency establishment, latency maintenance, and reactivation.[6] During latency there is prominent expression of a single viral gene, the latency-associated transcript (LAT). LAT appears to be important but not absolutely required for establishment of latency, as well as for maintaining the viability of HSV-infected neutrons by inhibiting apoptosis.[7, 8] It remains controversial whether the regulatory effects of LAT on latency are mediated at the RNA level or require LAT mRNA translation into protein.

INNATE ANTIVIRAL IMMUNITY

The antiviral immune response generally can be divided into an early, nonspecific phase (typically the first 5 to 7 days in HSV infection) involving innate immune mechanisms. This is followed by a later antigen-specific phase involving adaptive immunity by T and B cells.[9] The early phase is critical, as infection either may be successfully contained or, alternatively, may disseminate throughout the host. Interferons, cytokines, chemokines, and surfactant proteins that are exclusively or mainly produced by cell types other than T cells will be discussed as part of innate antiviral mechanisms, followed by a brief overview of cellular innate immune mechanisms.

Type I Interferons and Their Cellular Sources

Interferons (IFNs) can be divided into type I IFN, which includes a group of highly similar IFN-α proteins (encoded by a cluster of genes on chromosome 9p) and IFN-β, and type II IFN, which consists of a single molecular species, IFN-γ.[10] The proteins comprising type I IFN utilize a common type I interferon receptor that is widely expressed and is a heterodimer consisting of IFN-α receptor 1 and IFN-α receptor 2 subunits. IFN-γ, binds to a distinct heterodimeric receptor consisting of IFN-γ receptor 1 and IFN-γ receptor 2 units.

Viral infection of cells results in phosphorylation of cytoplasmic interferon regulatory factor (IRF)-3, which then translocates to the nucleus and associates with transcriptional co-activators to promote the transcription of IFN-α and IFN-β.[11] Double-stranded RNA, which is a component of the life cycle of many RNA viruses, or its mimic, poly I/C, is able to activate Toll-like receptor (TLR)-3[12] and type I IFN gene transcription.[13] IFN-β is made mainly by nonhematopoietic cell types, such as fibroblasts, in response to viral infection, whereas IFN-α is produced in particularly high levels by plasmacytoid dendritic cells, which belong to the DC2 cell lineage.[14-16] Plasmacytoid dendritic cells have a distinct cell surface phenotype from myeloid dendritic cells that includes high levels of the IL-3 receptor (CD123) and CD4 and low or undetectable amounts of CD11c and immunoglobulin-like transcript receptor (ILT)-1.[17]

Viruses such as HSV and influenza trigger high levels of type I IFN secretion by plasmacytoid dendritic cells, but the precise recognition mechanism remains unclear. Recognition of the HSV viral genome by TLR-9 is one possibility. The HSV genome consists of double-stranded DNA that is unmethylated at CpG dinucleotide residues. TLR-9 preferentially recognizes pathogen-derived DNA containing unmethylated CpG residues rather than host DNA, in which these residues are predominantly methylated.[13] Consistent with this possible recognition mechanism for HSV, human plasmacytoid dendritic cells express very high levels of TLR-9 compared with other dendritic cell populations, such as most myeloid dendritic cells.[18] The secretion of high levels of IFN-α by plasmacytoid dendritic cells likely results in a systemic antiviral state, as receptors for type I interferons are essentially ubiquitous. Exposure of secondary lymphoid tissue to IFN-α may also enhance local adaptive immune responses.[19]

Type I interferons mediate their effect by engaging the type I IFN receptor and activating the Tyk-2 and Jak-1 tyrosine kinases associated with cytoplasmic tails of the receptor components, which results in tyrosine phosphorylation of signal transducer and transcriptional activator (STAT) proteins including STAT-1 and STAT-2. STAT-1 and STAT-2 form with p48 (IRF-9), a heterotrimeric complex known as ISGF3, that binds to ISRE (IFN-stimulated response elements) of DNA and influences the transcription of a distinct group of genes.[20] These include the gene for IRF-7, which amplifies type I IFN production if viruses infect cells that previously have been exposed to type I IFN.[11] Tyrosine-

phosphorylated STAT-1 also can homodimerize and bind to GAS (gamma-interferon-activating sequences).[10] Since STAT-1 but not other STATs is tyrosine phosphorylated by IFN-γ binding to its specific receptor,[10] there is the potential for type I IFN to induce genes that are characteristic of IFN-γ responses, but not vice-versa.

Patients who have genetic defects in STAT-1 that compromise the GAS pathway but not the interferon-stimulated response element (ISRE) pathway of gene regulation, are not prone to severe viral infections.[21] This point argues that the regulation of the GAS pathway by type I interferons, and the induction of certain gene products such as IRF-1,[11] are dispensable for antiviral immunity in humans. In contrast, complete lack of STAT-1 function and, as a result, loss of the ISRE-mediated pathway of signal transduction in humans resulted in recurrent HSV-1 encephalitis and death.[22] The critical importance of the ISRE pathway is also supported by the observation that mice genetically deficient in the type I interferon receptor are highly susceptible to HSV.[23]

Substantial amounts of type I IFN are found in the tissues of HSV-infected animals and humans.[24, 25] Although HSV efficiently induces the secretion of type I IFN, the virus is relatively resistant to their antiviral effects. This may account for the limited ability of type I interferons to treat recurrences of established HSV infections, such as of the eye. HSV resistance to interferon may be explained partially by its ICP34.5 protein, which prevents the normal shut-off of host cell protein synthesis in response to IFN-α by a complex mechanism.[23] HSV infection of certain cell types also may inhibit type I IFN-mediated activation of the JAK/STAT pathway.[26] In contrast, a combination of type I IFN and IFN-γ may be highly effective in the control of HSV infection, at least in mice,[27] suggesting that cellular sources of IFN-γ *in vivo* (Th1 CD4 T cells, CD8 T cells, gamma/delta T cells, NK cells, or NK T cells) may play an important role in host defense against HSV by acting in concert with type I IFN.

Cytokines

IL-1 and IL-18

Interleukin-1 (IL-1) is induced at sites of HSV infection inflammation, such as the cornea, and may contribute to pathogenic inflammation.[28] It is produced by many cell sources, including activated mononuclear phagocytes. Recombinant IL-1-α administered to neonatal mice also can enhance survival,[29] but the role of endogenously produced IL-1 in the control of HSV infections is unclear. IL-18 is an IL-1 family member that is also produced by activated mononuclear phagocytes; it is a potent inducer of IFN-γ production by T cells and NK cells. IL-18 administration to mice, including those lacking both T and B cell immunity, provides substantial protection against systemic HSV infection.[30] In wild-type mice, this protective effect depends largely on IFN-γ but not on NK cells.[30] Mice genetically deficient in IL-18 also die earlier and have increased viral load compared with wild-type mice after a lethal intravaginal challenge with HSV.[31] The production of IL-18 during human HSV infection remains to be characterized.

IL-12 and IL-23

IL-12 and IL-23 are heterodimeric cytokines that share a common p40 subunit and have distinct p35 and p19 subunits, respectively. The IL-12 receptor on cells consists of an IL-12Rβ1 and IL-12Rβ2 chain, whereas the IL-23 receptor consists of an IL-12Rβ1 and IL-23R subunit. IL-12, and likely IL-23, have multiple potentially important antiviral host effects, such as promoting CD4 and CD8 T cell proliferation and cytolytic function and augmenting NK cell activity. IL-12 is produced by myeloid dendritic cells and by plasmacytoid dendritic cells, including after their exposure to HSV. Mononuclear phagocytes also produce IL-12 in response to

HSV infection *in vitro*, and this appears to require intermediary synthesis of viral and host proteins and transcriptional activation by NF-κB/Rel proteins.[32] HSV corneal infection has also been reported to induce IL-12 p40 mRNA by neutrophils,[33] but it is unclear whether these cells produce functional IL-12 and/or IL-23 protein. IL-23 transcripts have been detected in the ganglia of HSV-1 infected mice, but the cellular source has not been defined.[34]

IL-12 and IL-23 are important for directing the differentiation of naive CD4 T cells into Th1 immune effectors that secrete high levels of IFN-γ in response to TCR stimulation.[35,36] They also can directly induce NK cells and effector T cells to produce IFN-γ. The production of IL-12 by plasmacytoid dendritic cells after their exposure to HSV may skew the immune response to HSV toward a Th1 outcome. In addition, type I IFN also favors Th1 differentiation, most likely by increasing expression of the IL-12Rβ2 receptor on activated T cells.[37] Together, these mechanisms may account for the predominance of IFN-γ-producing effector and memory CD4 T cells following most viral infections, such as with herpesviruses.[38,39]

Nevertheless, the role of IL-12 and IL-23 in the control of HSV infection and other herpesviruses remains unclear. Mice lacking both IL-12 and IL-23 owing to a gene disruption of the common p40 subunit die more rapidly than wild-type mice do after a lethal challenge with HSV.[31] However, we recently identified a 6-year-old boy with complete IL-12Rβ1 chain deficiency and an absence of detectable CD4 Th1 cells.[40] This boy did not have any history of increased severity of viral infections, and such a predisposition has not been reported in recent series of other patients with this disorder or with p40 deficiency.[41] Regardless of their role in primary control of HSV, IL-12 and IL-23 may contribute to inflammatory corneal scarring of HSV infection,[42] suggesting a deleterious impact in cases of established infection.

HSV can infect myeloid dendritic cells and down-regulate their production of IL-12 *in vitro*.[43] However, these infected cells also secrete products that may prime neighboring uninfected dendritic cells for enhanced IL-12 production. HSV-infected epithelial cells also appear to secrete factors that result in the induction of IL-12 by inflammatory leukocytes.[44] These secreted factors have not been identified.

IL-15

IL-15 is a relative of IL-2, which binds to a receptor consisting of a unique IL-15 receptor alpha chain in conjunction with an IL-2 receptor beta chain and a common gamma chain, two components that are also part of the IL-2 receptor. In contrast to IL-2, IL-15 is not produced by T cells but by other cell types, especially bone marrow stromal cells and activated mononuclear phagocytes. IL-15 appears to be key for NK cell development and for the generation and maintenance of memory T cells, particularly those of the CD8 subset. IL-15 is also a potent activator of NK cells for enhanced cytotoxicity against most herpesviruses, including HSV.[45] Exposure of human peripheral blood mononuclear cells to HSV also up-regulates NK cytotoxic activity by an IL-15-dependent mechanism.[46] Infection of mice results in a rapid and substantial increase in serum levels of IL-15, peaking at approximately 3 days postinfection,[47] suggesting a role in the early innate immune response. IL-15 administration is also protective to wild-type mice given an otherwise lethal dose of HSV.[47] Mice lacking the IL-2 receptor beta chain are highly susceptible to systemic infection with HSV, but the individual contribution of IL-15 versus IL-2 in providing protection remains to be determined.

Chemokines

Chemokines secreted by mononuclear phagocytes and dendritic cells, as well as nonhematopoietic cells, play an important role in the recruitment of NK cells and subsequently T cells to sites of infection and in maintaining inflammation. In the case of herpes keratitis, the production of the CC chemokine MIP-1α contributes to inflammatory disease but does not influence viral replication.[48] The CXC chemokine IL-8, which is a potent neutrophil chemoattractant, is produced by corneal keratocytes[49] and possibly by corneal epithelial cells,[50] and this likely accounts for the prominence of neutrophils in HSV keratitis.

Elevated CSF levels of the CC chemokines, MCP-1, MIP-1α, and RANTES, and of IL-8 have also been documented in cases of human HSV encephalitis,[51] suggesting their role in CNS inflammation. CSF mononuclear phagocytes, such as macrophages or microglia, are likely sources of at least a portion of these chemokines, an idea supported by the ability of microglia or macrophages infected by HSV to produce chemokines, such as RANTES.[52,53] In addition to their proinflammatory role, certain chemokines potentially may skew the outcome of the adaptive immune response to viral infection. For example, MCP-1 is produced in the cerebrospinal fluid (CSF) of experimental infection of mice with HSV-2. This appears to result in decreased survival compared with mice in which this chemokine is neutralized.[54] MCP-1 appears to skew the CD4 T cell response toward a nonprotective Th2 (IL-4, IL-5, and IL-13 predominant) response rather than a protective Th1 response. This is consistent with earlier studies that found that administration of relatively small doses of IL-4 in an HSV-1 encephalitis mouse model increased disease severity.[55]

Surfactant Proteins

Surfactant proteins (SP)-A and SP-D are members of the collectin family and are synthesized by type II alveolar epithelial cells, lung epithelial Clara cells, and certain extrapulmonary cell types.[56] An *in vivo* role for these proteins in modulating viral infection has been revealed in mice with selective gene disruptions: Mice lacking SP-A have an increased viral load after challenge with respiratory syncytial virus (RSV), and this is associated with increased neutrophil inflammation of the lung and production of proinflammatory cytokines.[57] Many of the conditions that predispose to severe RSV infection, including prematurity and bronchopulmonary dysplasia, are associated with decreased SP-A expression by the lung, and it is plausible that these decreases could contribute to disease severity. SP-A also appears to be important for limiting the inflammatory response to influenza A infection,[58] although the mechanism (antiviral versus anti-inflammatory effect) remains controversial. SP-A can also bind to HSV-1, and CMV promotes their uptake by rodent alveolar macrophages,[59-61] but the importance of this *in vivo* has not been studied. SP-D binds *in vitro* to influenza A virus via its hemagglutinin molecule and can promote internalization of the virus by neutrophils. Mice lacking SP-D have reduced influenza A viral clearance, and this is also associated with increased neutrophil inflammation and expression of proinflammatory cytokines. Although this suggests a role for SP-D in viral clearance, mice lacking SP-D also have perturbed surfactant homeostasis and alveolar macrophage function, which could contribute to the phenotype of infection by mechanisms other than decreased SP-D–mediated clearance of virus.[62]

Innate Cellular Mechanisms

Mononuclear Phagocytes and Inducible Nitric Oxide Synthase

Mononuclear phagocytes are widely distributed in the tissues as macrophages and are likely to play an important role in the local containment of HSV infection until adaptive immune responses can come into play. After intraperitoneal injection of HSV or murine CMV into mice, viral containment appears to involve macrophages that are activated by TNF-α and IFN-γ.[63] A similar role for TNF-α and IFN-γ in containment of HSV-1 corneal infection also has been described: After corneal infection, the virus replicates briefly in the trigeminal ganglion, reaching peak levels by about 3 to 5 days postinoculation. During this peak level of viral replication, macrophages appear to be the predominant cell type and produce TNF-α *in situ*. In addition to macrophages, T cells expressing gamma/delta TCR (gamma/delta-T cells), a cell type that is also described in a separate section later, are present and produce IFN-γ.

Macrophages and gamma/delta T cells and the cytokines these two cell types produce may provide important antiviral activity by several mechanisms. TNF-α has direct anti-HSV effects, particularly in combination with IFN-γ,[64] and these two cytokines may also synergize to increase expression of leukocyte adhesion molecules and inducible nitric oxide synthase (iNOS) expression by mononuclear phagocytes. HSV infection of mononuclear phagocytes also synergizes with IFN-γ for promoting expression of iNOS,[65] which has anti-HSV effects *in vitro*,[66] and for production of TNF-α.[67] Systemic depletion of mononuclear phagocytes (by administration of liposomes containing dichloromethylene diphosphonate) or of gamma/delta T cells, or inhibition of TNF-α, IFN-γ, or iNOS activity in the HSV corneal infection model, results in increased HSV-1 replication within the ganglion.[68, 69] These complex interactions illustrate the importance of these cellular and cytokine components in local antiviral host defense. In addition, similar macrophage depletion studies have shown that macrophages also restrict HSV growth in the cornea.[70]

An antiviral role for iNOS is also suggested by the increased susceptibility of mice with complete genetic deficiency of iNOS to HSV infection via footpad injection. These mice also develop exaggerated Th1 responses, indicating that iNOS may have key antiviral effects, as well as inhibitory effects on Th1 differentiation.[71] However, innate antiviral immune mechanisms mediated by mononuclear phagocytes, such as iNOS induction, may not necessarily be beneficial in all contexts of HSV infection. In a murine model of HSV pneumonia, inhibition of iNOS activity, which is increased following viral infection, markedly reduced pulmonary inflammation and improved survival, despite increases in the lung tissue HSV viral titer.[72] Inhibition of iNOS activity was also beneficial in experimental HSV-1 encephalitis of rats, and in this study was not associated with increased viral load.[73]

Mononuclear phagocytes may not only have antiviral effects but also serve as targets of infection with viruses, such as HSV. Older studies suggested that HSV infection is usually nonpermissive and does not result in viral replication, but infection may result in apoptosis.[74] This could limit antiviral immune mechanisms, such as cytokine production. Differentiation of monocytes into macrophage-like cells *in vitro* results in increased permissiveness for infection.[75,76] HSV of monocytes undergoing such *in vitro* differentiation may also block this process.[77] However, the relevance of these observations to natural tissue macrophages and their generation *in vivo* from monocyte precursors is unknown.

Myeloid Dendritic Cells

Myeloid dendritic cells act as the sentinels of the immune system and are the key cells in activating naive T cells and initiating the adaptive immune response. Those myeloid dendritic cells of the skin and of the interstitial area of solid organs, such as heart and kidney, are highly effective in uptake of antigen in soluble or particulate form.[78] They express CD11c and ILT1[79] and high levels of CD83 but are lineage (Lin) negative, i.e., they lack expression of markers characteristic of other cell lineages, such as T cells, B cells, NK cells, and granulocytes.[80] Myeloid dendritic cells also have been referred to as DC1 cells,[81] in contrast to DC2 cells, which include plasmacytoid dendritic cells.

Myeloid dendritic cells have prominent dendrite-like cytoplasmic protrusions and express high levels of molecules involved in antigen presentation to T cells, including class I and class II MHC

molecules. Exposure of immature DC1 cells to inflammatory stimuli results in cessation of antigen uptake and a maturation process in which previously internalized antigen is processed and displayed, and up-regulation of the CCR7 chemokine receptor occurs. CCR7 expression facilitates the migration of these cells via lymphatics to T cell-dependent areas of secondary lymphoid organs that express CCR7 ligands.[82]

Myeloid dendritic cell maturation and migration can be triggered by a variety of pathogen-derived products that bind to Toll-like receptors (TLRs). These include double-stranded RNA binding via TLR-3 and LPS binding via TLR-4.[83] Maturation is also induced by engagement of CD40 on the dendritic cell surface by CD40-ligand (CD154), a molecule that is expressed at particularly high levels by activated CD4 T cells. Mature myeloid dendritic cells express high levels of molecules for T cell co-stimulation, such as CD80 and CD86, and are highly efficient for presenting antigen and activating naive CD4 and CD8 T cells.[79] Dendritic cells also have an important influence on whether naive CD4 T cells differentiate into Th1 (capable of producing IFN-γ but not IL-4, IL-5, or IL-13) or Th2 (capable of producing IL-4, IL-5, or IL-13 but not IFN-γ) effector cell populations.

The *in vivo* role of dendritic cells in the control of viral infections is only now being unraveled. A recent study using the HSV-2 vaginal infection model in mice has demonstrated the importance of vaginal submucosal dendritic cells in viral antigen presentation to T cells in the draining lymph nodes.[84] Only this cell population and not Langerhans cells (myeloid dendritic cells of the dermis) and not other antigen-presenting cell (APC) populations, such as B cells or macrophages, was capable of activating HSV-specific T cells.[84] Determining the role of particular dendritic cell populations in presenting HSV antigens at other tissue sites of infection will be important for understanding the initiation of the adaptive immune response against the virus.

Culturing blood monocytes with IL-4 and GM-CSF results in their acquiring features of immature dendritic cells. These monocyte-derived dendritic cells (MDDC) have a high capacity for antigen uptake, a low capacity for antigen processing, and low levels of expression of T cell co-stimulatory molecules. They acquire mature features, such as an increased capacity for antigen processing and presentation and increased expression of co-stimulatory molecules and CD83, if treated with proinflammatory stimuli, such as TNF-α. MDDC have been widely used as a convenient model for myeloid dendritic cells, although a caveat is that these two cell populations have not been systematically compared for their gene and protein expression profiles. HSV can efficiently infect both mature and immature MDDC,[17,85] and is able to replicate in immature, but not mature, MDDC. HSV infection of MDDC also results in decreased expression of key co-stimulatory molecules and adhesion molecules[86] and may also hamper their maturation program. This inhibition of maturation is dependent on expression of the HSV virion host shut-off protein,[85] which generally destabilizes mRNA in infected cells and favors the translation of rapidly produced viral mRNA over more slowly synthesized host transcripts. HSV infection of mature MDDC also has been shown to down-regulate expression of CD83 by interfering with nuclear export of CD83 mRNA;[87] this is associated with a decreased capacity of these cells to activate T cells *in vitro*.[88] Finally, HSV infection of purified dendritic cells from adult humans stimulates them to secrete IFN-α and IL-1, but not to secrete IL-12 or express increased amounts of CD80 or CD86.[89] Together, these results suggest that dendritic cells are not effectively activated by HSV infection, and that, instead, they may be direct cellular targets of HSV-mediated immunosuppression. Nevertheless, the relevance of these *in vitro* observations remains unclear. For example, mouse models have not demonstrated detectable *in vivo* infection of dendritic cells, based on absence of viral DNA in the draining lymph nodes, after either infection of the footpad[90] or vagina.[84]

NK Cells

NK cells are bone marrow–derived lymphocytes that lack the antigen-specific TCRs or immunoglobulins that are characteristic of T and B cells, respectively. They are relatively large cells with granular contents (hence their earlier designation of large granular lymphocytes), and they provide protection mainly in the form of cell-mediated cytotoxicity of virally infected target cells by a mechanism that is not antigen-specific. NK cell killing and, as discussed later, T cell–mediated cytotoxicity, are mainly mediated by perforin/granzyme or fas-ligand–dependent mechanisms. But in contrast to T cell–mediated cytotoxicity, NK cells are able to lyse virally infected or tumor target cells in a non-MHC-restricted manner and without prior sensitization.[91]

NK cells express a number of inhibitory receptors that (at basal conditions) keep them inactive as killer cells.[91] Activation of NK cells for target cell lysis, termed *natural cytotoxicity*, requires decreased engagement of these inhibitory receptors by self-class I MHC alleles or HLA-E (Fig. 153–1). The two major groups of inhibitory NK receptors are the killer inhibitory receptors (KIRs) and CD94/NKG2A. The KIRs bind to portions of HLA-B and HLA-C molecules located outside the peptide-binding groove recognized by the TCR, whereas CD94/NKG2A binds to HLA-E, a nonclassic and nonvariable MHC molecule that requires hydrophobic leader peptides from HLA-A,-B, and -C for its surface expression. These NK cell receptors help counteract the ability of viruses to decrease surface expression of class I MHC molecules, thereby limiting CD8 T cell–mediated viral clearance. For example, the down-regulation of HLA-C by HSV results in killing by an NK cell clone by its release from inhibition of KIRs.[92] NK cells also express positive activating receptors,[93] such as 2B4 (CD244), NKG2D, NKp30, NKp44, NKp46, and NKR-P1A (CD161), that are important for killing. NKG2D may be activated

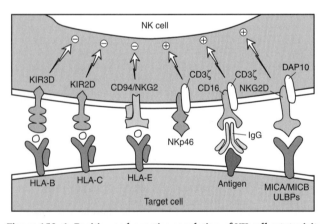

Figure 153–1. Positive and negative regulation of NK cell cytotoxicity by receptor/ligand interactions. NK cell cytotoxicity is inhibited by engagement of killer inhibitory receptors (KIRs) by class I MHC molecules, such as HLA-B and HLA-C. In addition, NK cells are inhibited when CD94/NKG2 complex, a member of the C-type lectin family, on the NK cell is engaged by HLA-E. HLA-E binds hydrophobic leader peptides derived from HLA-A, -B, and -C molecules and requires these for its surface expression. Thus, HLA-E surface expression on a potential target cell indicates its overall production of conventional class I MHC molecules. These inhibitory influences on NK cell cytotoxicity are overcome if viral infection of the target cell results in decreased class I MHC and HLA-E levels. NK cell cytotoxicity is positively regulated by the engagement of NKp46; CD16, which is an Fc receptor for IgG; and NKG2D, which is a receptor for MICA, MICB, and ULBPs. These positive receptors are associated with CD3-ζ (CD16 and NKp46) or with DAP10, which mediates intracellular activation signals.

by binding to MICA/MICB or ULBPs on the target cell; these molecules may be induced by cell stress. Direct activation by viral products is also possible. For example, the Ly49H activating receptor of murine NK cells specifically recognizes a murine CMV-encoded protein, m157.[94] HSV infection of target cells also can disarm NK cell activity, although the precise mechanism is unclear. Other herpesviruses, including CMV, employ a wide variety of strategies to inhibit NK cell–mediated cytotoxicity, indicating the importance of this antiviral mechanism *in vivo*.[95]

NK cells are a particularly important restraint on viral replication and dissemination prior to the appearance of adaptive immune responses mediated by T cells and B cells. This has been demonstrated most clearly in the severity of primary infections with herpesviruses, including HSV, CMV, and VZV, in patients with a selective lack of NK cells.[96] Although the initial disease is severe, these patients are able eventually to clear virus, presumably by T cell–mediated immunity.[40,96]

NK cells may contribute to the control of viral infection by the direct lysis of virally infected cells, as described earlier, or by lysis of virally infected cells via antibody-dependent cellular cytotoxicity (ADCC) (see Fig. 153–1). In the case of ADCC, antibody that recognizes viral proteins on the surface of the infected cell can bind to the NK cell via surface Fc receptors, and enhance NK cell recognition and lysis of infected target cells. NK cells also produce proinflammatory cytokines that increase intrinsic antiviral resistance (e.g., type I IFN) and promote the development of antigen-specific Th1 cell immunity (both type I IFN and IFN-γ). Thus, the NK cell, via these mechanisms, may contribute both to the innate phase and the late phase of control of herpesvirus infections, and be of particular importance in settings in which class I MHC expression is down-regulated and CD8 T cell recognition of infected target cells is hampered.

Infection of mice with HSV also demonstrates the importance of NK cells in the early control of viral infection period. If NK cells are eliminated by injection with specific antiserum concurrent with the administration of virus, the titers of HSV in internal organs and the rate of mortality are both markedly increased, but this treatment has no significant effect if started 5 days after viral challenge.[97] Adoptive transfer studies in immunosuppressed mice demonstrate that significant protection against HSV is provided by NK cells.[98] More detailed study has found that following HSV inoculation into the anterior chamber, NK cells accumulated within the eye by day 5 postinoculation and that depletion of these cells by specific antiserum resulted in spread of the infection to the retina.[99]

Studies with murine CMV also suggest that NK cells are important in the early control of herpesvirus infection,[100] and that IFN-γ produced by NK cells is more important for this protection than is NK cell–mediated cytolytic activity.[101] The production of IFN-γ by NK cells *in vivo* during the early phase of murine CMV infection requires IL-12 and is enhanced by TNF-α, but not type I IFN. In contrast, endogenously produced type I IFN, but not IL-12 or TNF-α, greatly enhances NK cell–mediated cytotoxicity and proliferation.[102] How IFN-γ is protective in early viral infection remains unclear, but it could act directly to limit productive viral infection in cells that are otherwise permissive for infection, such as hepatocytes. There is evidence for such a noncytolytic mechanism of protection of hepatocytes in hepatitis B and hepatitis C infections, particularly via effects mediated by IFN-γ or TNF-α.[103-105]

IFN-γ produced by NK cells also increases class II MHC expression on mononuclear phagocytes *in vivo* and probably other cell types in response to HSV or murine CMV infection,[63] an effect that facilitates antigen presentation to CD4 T cells. Increased IFN-γ during the early phases of T-cell activation and differentiation may also favor the development of T cells with an enriched capacity to secrete Th1-type cytokines. This effect may be mediated by the ability of IFN-γ rapidly to increase expression by

T-cell cells of T-bet, a master regulatory transcription factor that directs Th1 development.[106]

ADAPTIVE ANTIVIRAL IMMUNE MECHANISMS

Adaptive immune responses mediated by HSV antigen-specific T cells and B cells are first detected 5 to 7 days after the onset of primary HSV infection in adult humans, and the peak response is achieved approximately 2 to 3 weeks after infection.[107-109] In virtually all individuals, antigen-specific immunity does not eradicate infection, i.e., achieve sterile immunity, but rather terminates active viral replication and the acute infection. HSV is able to persist in the form of latent virus in neurons, where it may cause recurrent localized disease. Recurrent viral replication may be frequent and, in many cases, asymptomatic.

Antiviral T Cell Immunity—An Overview

T cells play the critical role in resolution of active HSV infection and the maintenance of viral latency.[110,111] Adaptive transfer studies and T cell depletion studies using CD4 or CD8 monoclonal antibodies indicate that both CD4 and CD8 T cells may contribute to clearance of HSV following acute infection in mice, acting, in part, through the production of IFN-γ;[112] in contrast, B cells are not able to provide protection in the absence of T cells.[109,113-115] The importance of T cells in the control of human HSV and other herpesvirus infections is indicated by the increased susceptibility of those with quantitative (purine nucleoside phosphorylase deficiency,[116] late HIV infection) or qualitative T cell and antigen presentation defects (Wiskott-Aldrich syndrome). Murine studies also suggest that CD4 T cells are more important than CD8 T cells in the control of HSV infections of the skin and peripheral nervous system,[113] suggesting that the relative importance of CD4 versus CD8 T cells in antiviral control is tissue-specific. However, the relative importance of CD4 and CD8 T cells in HSV infections in humans is controversial.

CD4 T Cell–Mediated Antiviral Immunity

CD4 T cells appear to play a key role in protection from HSV and have been identified in the circulation[117] and from sites of recurrent human HSV infection, such as the skin,[118,119] cervix,[120] cornea,[121] and retina.[122] Natural infection results in CD4 T cells recognizing peptide epitopes from a variety of HSV proteins, including those of the envelope, tegument, and capsid.[39,123] The following are likely to be important mechanisms, reflecting the central and diverse roles of CD4 T cells in mediating and regulating antigen-specific immunity: First, CD4 T cells may inhibit viral replication directly through the production of IFN-γ, TNF-α and CD40-ligand, each of which has antiviral activity against HSV.[124,125] Second, CD4 T cells appear to be required for the generation and survival of anti-HSV effector CD8 cytolytic T cells in mice.[112,126,127] This effect may be mediated, in part, by the ability of CD4 T cells to prime dendritic cells (and perhaps other antigen-presenting cells) through CD40-ligand.[128,129] Consistent with this, CD4 T cells are not required for the development of CD8 cytolytic T cells if primed dendritic cells are used as the source of antigen-presenting cells.[126] Production of IL-2 by CD4 T cells also may contribute to the expansion and differentiation of cytolytic T cells. Third, and as discussed in more detail later, IFN-γ produced by CD4 T cells may play a central role in overriding HSV ICP47-mediated inhibition of class I MHC expression.[111,130] Fourth, CD4 T cells may lyse cells expressing viral peptides bound to class II MHC.[131] Such cytotoxic CD4 T cells frequently have been isolated from humans after infection with HSV, and they appear to comprise about 30% of the cytotoxic T cells in murine HSV infection.[118,132]

Th1 Cytokine Production

IFN-γ is a key immunoregulatory cytokine that is produced in substantial amounts by CD4 T cells of the Th1 subset, CD8 T cells, gamma/delta T cells, and NK cells. It is a key component in appropriately regulating adaptive and innate cellular mechanisms of antiviral control (Fig. 153–2). Although it is discussed here as part of the CD4 T cell effector mechanisms, these potential cellular sources of this cytokine and their temporal appearance (e.g., NK and gamma/delta T cell-derived IFN-γ production may precede CD4 and CD8 T cell–mediated production), as well as their location, need to be considered when evaluating the importance of IFN-γ *in vivo*. IFN-γ acts to increase the antiviral state of many cell types, such as mononuclear phagocytes. In addition, this cytokine enhances the expression of the class I heavy chain, beta-2-microglobulin, and TAP transporter. These effects on antigens help counteract the negative effects of HSV on class I MHC antigen presentation (which are discussed later), and increase the ability of infected cells to be lysed.[130] CD40-ligand expression by CD4 T cells is also key for the antibody production by B cells and isotype switching.

The HSV-specific CD4 T cell response of humans is characterized by a predominant Th1 response.[133] The differentiation of naive CD4 T cells into Th1 effector cells is favored by production of cytokines, such as IL-12, IL-23, and IL-27,[35] which are induced as part of HSV infection *in vivo*. These cytokines also can directly induce differentiated Th1 cells to produce IFN-γ. HSV infection may also promote Th1 immunity by inducing the production of osteopontin by T cells at an early stage of activation and differentiation. This cytokine may act on antigen-presenting cells (APCs) by interacting with $\beta3$ integrins to maintain IL-12 production and with CD44 to inhibit IL-10 production, thereby favoring a Th1 adaptive immune response.[134] Osteopontin is required for the development of delayed-type hypersensitivity responses

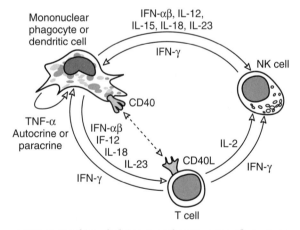

Figure 153–2. Cytokines link innate and antigen-specific immune mechanisms against intracellular pathogens, such as viruses. Activation of T cells by antigen-presenting cells (APCa), such as mononuclear phagocytes or dendritic cells, result in the expression of CD40-ligand (CD154) and the secretion of cytokines, such as IL-2 and IFN-γ. Mononuclear phagocytes are activated by IFN-γ and the engagement of CD40 with increased microbicidal activity. Mononuclear phagocytes produce TNF-α which enhances their microbicidal activity in a paracrine or autocrine manner. Mononuclear phagocytes and dendritic cells also secrete the cytokines IFN-α/β, IL-12, IL-15, IL-18, IL-23, and, likely, IL-27. These cytokines promote Th1 effector cell differentiation and also promote NK cell activation. Activated NK cells, in turn, secrete IFN-γ, which further enhances mononuclear phagocyte activation and Th1 effector cell differentiation.

(characteristic of Th1 immunity) to HSV and HSV-induced corneal inflammation, which is Th1 dependent.[134]

The effect of IFN-γ or IFN-γ receptor gene disruption or of IFN-γ neutralization on HSV infection in wild-type mice has varied, depending on the model and dose of virus employed, but appears to be important in the initial containment of disease following primary infection at most sites, such as the vagina, footpad, skin, and cornea, rather than for maintenance of latency.[115, 124, 135–138] In survivors of infection, the lack of IFN-γ also was associated with increased viral load in the eye or trigeminal ganglion basally[135] and after reactivation by UV irradiation[138] or hyperthermia.[139] It is interesting that greater severity of HSV disease after corneal infection also was observed in mice lacking the IFN-γ receptor compared with those lacking the IFN-γ ligand, even though these animals were of the same genetic background.[140, 141] This raises the possibility of a ligand for the IFN-γ receptor in addition to IFN-γ that contributes to host defense.

Virus-specific Th1 cells are also major sources of TNF-α,[38] which has direct antiviral effects, particularly in conjunction with IFN-γ, and also proinflammatory effects, e.g., by increasing adhesion molecule expression by nonhematopoietic cells, such as endothelium, and production of chemokines. In the case of murine CMV infection, some of these antiviral effects mediated by IFN-γ may be cell type–specific, e.g., operative for mononuclear phagocytes but not fibroblasts, and involve novel mechanisms that are shared with type I IFN.[142] Some of these Th1 cells are also a rich source of IL-17, which is found at sites of HSV infection, such as the cornea. IL-17 may contribute to local inflammation by increasing the production of proinflammatory cytokines and neutrophil chemotactic proteins, such as chemokines.[143]

CD40-Ligand/CD40 Interactions

CD40-ligand (CD154) is a member of the TNF ligand superfamily and is expressed in high amounts on the surface of activated but not resting CD4 T cells (Fig. 153–3). CD40-ligand engages CD40, a molecule expressed by "professional" APCs,[144] including dendritic cells, mononuclear phagocytes, B cells, and possibly CD8 T cells.[145] Engagement of CD40 on dendritic cells is a potent maturation signal and an inducer of IL-12. This engagement also counteracts the inhibitory effect of other cytokines, such as IL-10.[146] The CD40 ligand/CD40 interaction is essential for many events in adaptive immunity, including the generation of memory CD4 T cells of the Th1 type and memory B cells, as well as most immunoglobulin isotype switching.[147]

The role of CD40 ligand in viral host defense appears to vary for the particular pathogen, but in general correlates with the particular requirement for CD4 T cells, indicating that CD4 T cells and CD40 ligand are linked in mediating such help. Mice lacking CD40 ligand, as a result of selective gene disruption or in which CD40 ligand/CD40 interactions were neutralized by monoclonal antibody, have increased CNS infection and paralysis compared with wild-type mice after footpad inoculation with HSV,[148] and this correlated with reductions in CD4 but not CD8 T cell responses. The absence of CD40 ligand/CD40 interactions eliminates most antiviral antibodies and results in severe disease in viral infections in which antibody plays a critical role, e.g., in the dissemination of vesicular stomatitis virus to the central nervous system (CNS). In humans, CD40 ligand also appears to play an important role in the expansion of CD8 T cell recognizing viral peptide antigens, such as from influenza A and HIV-1 proteins, based on an *ex vivo* assay using monocyte-derived dendritic cells as APCs.[149]

Cytolytic CD4 T Cell–Mediated Mechanisms

In humans, a major portion of the cytolytic T cell response to HSV infection may be mediated by CD4 T cells, which recognize peptides bound to class II MHC rather than to class I MHC.[131] Such cytotoxic CD4 T cells have been frequently isolated from humans after infection with HSV and comprise about 30% of the cytotoxic T cells in murine HSV infection. Human CD4 cytotoxic cells can recognize peptides derived from viral glycoproteins found in the HSV lipid envelope,[110, 150, 151] such as gB, gC, and gD,[152] and it is likely that these viral glycoproteins enter into the class II antigen-processing endocytic pathway by first fusing with the host cell membrane.

CD4 T cell–mediated cytotoxicity may contribute to the clearance of HSV infection by lysing infected host cells that bear class II MHC. In humans, CD4 T cell cytolytic activity is probably mainly mediated by secretion of cytotoxins, such as perforin and granzymes, rather than via fas-ligand engagement of fas on target cells.[153] Although class II MHC is normally expressed by APCs, such as B cells, mononuclear phagocytes, and dendritic cells, a wide variety of cell types can express class II MHC and, most cases, present antigen, after exposure to IFN-γ, GM-CSF, or TNF-α.

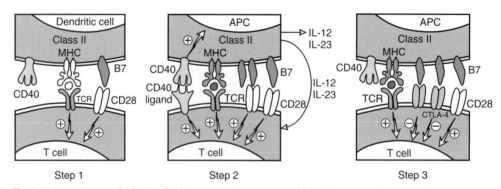

Figure 153–3. T cell–APC interactions early during the immune response to peptide antigens. A class II MHC-restricted response by CD4 T cells is shown as an example. Dendritic cells are probably the most important APC for antigenically naive T cells and constitutively express B7, CD40, and class II MHC molecules on their cell surface. Engagement of the CD4 T cell by antigenic peptide bound to MHC on the dendritic cells, in conjunction with co-stimulation by B7/CD28 interactions, leads to T cell activation (*Step 1*). The activated T cell expresses CD40-ligand on its surface, which engages CD40; this increases B7 expression on the dendritic cell, enhancing T cell co-stimulation (*Step 2*). CD40 engagement also activates the dendritic cells to produce cytokines, such as IL-12 and IL-23. These cytokines, in turn, promote the differentiation of T cells into Th1-type effector cells that produce high levels of IFN-γ and low or undetectable amounts of IL-4. CTLA-4 is expressed on the T cells during the later stages of T cell activation. Engagement of CTLA-4 by B7 molecules on the APC delivers negative signals that help terminate T cell activation (*Step 3*).

These cell types, which include endothelial cells, enterocytes, renal epithelial cells, thyroid epithelial cells, microglia, epidermal keratinocytes, myoblasts, eosinophils, NK cells, and T cells themselves,[2] might then become potential targets for cytotoxic CD4 T cells. However, the importance of CD4 T cell–mediated cytotoxicity in the control of infection has been questioned, given that substantial CD8 T cell responses to HSV are generated in humans, and that HSV-specific CD8 T cells constitute a prominent part of the viral response in tissues such as the skin and cervix.

CD8 T Cell–Mediated Antiviral Immunity

The efficient clearance of most viral infections in which multiple tissues are infected depends on T cell–mediated cytotoxicity, with CD8 T cells typically playing a central role in this process. In adults with chronic infection, HSV-specific CD8 T cells are found mainly at sites of local recurrence of virus, such as the skin adjacent to the genital tract,[118, 154] cervix,[120] and cornea,[155] but are not detectable in the circulation using standard techniques, such as intracellular cytokine staining after stimulation with whole HSV virus.[117]

T cell–mediated cytotoxicity involves two major pathways of killing of cellular targets via either the secretion of perforin and granzymes or via the engagement of fas by fas ligand (Fig. 153–4). In addition to these pathways, other granule proteins, such as granulysin, may also promote apoptosis of infected target cells, such as in VZV infection.[156] CD8 T cells when first activated by antigen are not effective killers, but, under the influence of cytokines such as IL-2 and IL-15, proliferate and differentiate into an effector cell lymphoblast population that efficiently kills. This differentiation includes increased expression of molecules involved in cytotoxicity, such as perforin, granzymes, fas-ligand, and granulysin, as well as an increased capacity to produce cytokines, such as IFN-γ and TNF-α.

Studies using class I MHC/viral peptide tetramers, which allow direct detection of CD8 T cells based on their TCR specificity, have documented that virus-specific CD8 T cells undergo a dramatic expansion *in vivo* during viral infection. In some instances, such as primary EBV infection, more than 40% of circulating CD8 T cells may be reactive with a single viral peptide epitope.[157] Most CD8 effector T cells have a relatively short life span and are probably eliminated by apoptosis following antigen clearance. CD4 T cells may aid directly in the generation of CD8 cytolytic T cells by the production of several cytokines, including IL-2 and IFN-γ. In addition, CD4 T cells may indirectly influence this process by enhancing dendritic cell function via a CD40-ligand/CD40 interaction; dendritic cells, in turn, may then help promote CD8 cytolytic T cell generation by secreting cytokines and engaging co-stimulatory molecules. For persistent viral infections, CD4 T cells also may be required for CD8 effector cells to maintain their cytotoxic function *in vivo*.

The most direct evidence for the importance of CD8 T cells in the control of herpesvirus infections in humans has come from studies showing that the adoptive transfer of donor–derived CD8 T cells against CMV or EBV provides considerable protection of hematopoietic cell transplant recipients from primary infection with these viruses.[158, 159] In animal models, CD8 T cells also appear key in resolving HSV lytic infection of ganglion during primary infection,[160, 161] and in preventing reactivation of virus from latency in sensory neurons;[162] this may involve an IFN-γ-dependent mechanism.[163] Direct recognition of infected ganglion cells by CD8 T cells is likely, as HSV infection induces detectable class I MHC expression by sensory neurons.[164] Noncytolytic mechanisms,[165] such as the production of cytokines with antiviral activity, e.g., IFN-γ,[163] or the secretion of granzyme A,[166] may be key for CD8 T cells to maintain latency and to prevent viral spread. In contrast, cytolytic mechanisms, such as those mediated by perforin, may not be necessary for

control of HSV infection at particular tissue sites, such as the cornea, and may even contribute to inflammatory disease.[167]

Most viral protein antigens recognized by CD8 T cells are derived from cytosolic proteins of the target cells (Fig. 153–5). These can either be synthesized within the cell, e.g., viral regulatory proteins that are not components of the final virion, or enter the cytosol upon viral entry, e.g., viral tegument proteins surrounding the nucleocapsid or the nucleocapsid itself. In either case, these proteins enter into the class I MHC antigen-processing pathway be undergoing degradation into peptides in the proteosome, followed by transport of these peptides into the endoplasmic reticulum by the TAP transporter. In the endoplasmic reticulum, peptides assemble with the class I MHC heavy chain and beta-2-microglobulin, and this trimeric complex is subsequently transported to the cell surface. The presence of class I MHC on virtually all cells allows CD8 T cells to recognize and lyse virus-infected cells in most tissues. Class I MHC is also necessary for the development of CD8 T cells in the thymus by the process of positive selection. It is not surprising that mice that lack class I MHC as a result of selective gene disruption (e.g., mice genetically deficient in beta-2-microglobin or in one of the

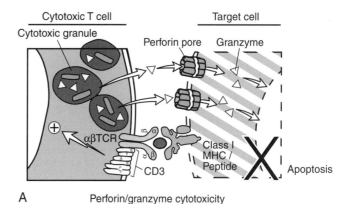

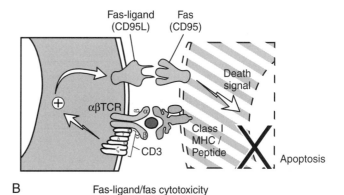

Figure 153–4. Two major mechanisms of antigen-specific class I MHC-restricted T cell–mediated cytotoxicity. Engagement of $\alpha\beta$-TCR of CD8 T cells by antigenic peptide bound to class I MHC on the target cell leads to T cell activation and target cell death. **A,** Cytotoxicity may occur by the extracellular release of the contents of cytotoxic granules from the T cell, including perforins and granzymes. Perforins introduce pores by which granzymes can enter into the target cell, leading to the triggering of apoptosis and cell death. **B,** Activation of T cells results in their surface expression of fas-ligand (CD95L), which engages fas (CD95) on the target cell, resulting in the delivery of the death signal, culminating in apoptosis. Both of these mechanisms are also utilized for killing by NK T cells and by NK cells.

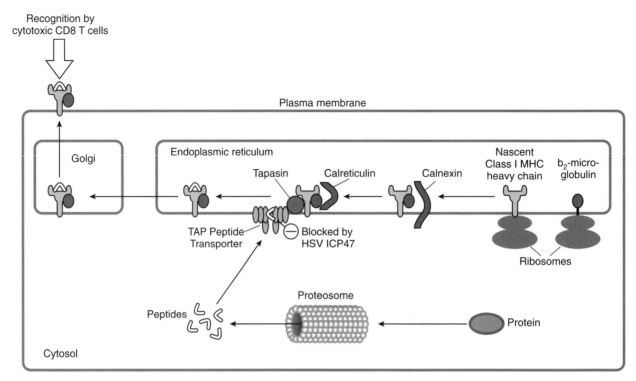

Figure 153–5. The class I MHC pathway of antigen presentation. Foreign peptides that bind to class I MHC are derived predominantly from cytoplasmic proteins. These may be synthesized *de novo* within the cell, such as those encoded by the viral genome and translated from viral mRNA, or those components of the virus that enter the cytosol upon its penetrating the cell. Dendritic cells also have the ability to transfer viral proteins taken up from outside the cell into the class I MHC pathway. Cytoplasmic proteins are degraded by proteosomes into peptides, which then enter into the endoplasmic reticulum via the TAP transporter system. Peptide binding to class I MHC takes place within the endoplasmic reticulum. Nascent class I MHC heavy chains first associate with the beta-2-microglobulin protein, which is an obligatory part of the class I MHC molecule but is not part of the peptide binding groove. The empty class I MHC heavy chain/beta-2-microglobulin complex is chaperoned to the TAP transporter by a series of proteins, including calnexin, calreticulin, and tapasin. Following loading with peptide, the fully mature viral peptide/class I MHC molecule goes to the Golgi and then rapidly to the cell surface where it can be evaluated by CD8 T cells. The TAP transporter is blocked by the HSV ICP47 protein, which is likely to be an important mechanism limiting the efficiency of HSV-specific CD8 T cell immunity in humans.

components of the TAP transporter) are highly susceptible to viral infection. On the other hand, lysis of host cells by CD8 T cells could, in some contexts, be detrimental to the host. For example, CD8 T cells with high levels of direct cytolytic activity are found at sites of focal temporal lobe lesions in mice with experimental HSV encephalitis,[168] and such cytolytic activity, although important in viral clearance, might well contribute to neuronal destruction.

Viral Inhibition of Antigen Presentation and Effect on the T Cell Immune Response

Given the importance of class I MHC-restricted cytotoxicity in the control of viral infection, it is perhaps not surprising that a number of viruses, including HSV and CMV,[169] have evolved mechanisms to inhibit class I MHC antigen presentation. Two gene products of HSV are key in blocking presentation of viral proteins by class I MHC: the viral host shut-off protein, which is present in the viral particle and immediately active after cell entry, and the immediate-early protein ICP47, which is synthesized by the host cell early after infection and binds to human TAP (see Fig. 153–5). The viral host shut-off protein, which is required for viral pathogenicity,[170] results in increased destruction of cellular mRNA and decreased host cell protein synthesis, including class I MHC molecules.[130] This limits CD8 T cell–mediated cytotoxicity of HSV-infected target cells, such as fibroblasts and keratinocytes.[171] The ICP47/TAP interaction blocks

loading of peptides onto class I MHC and transport of peptide/class I MHC complexes to the cell surface.[16, 130, 172–174] Together, these and other virus-mediated mechanisms may limit not only CD8 T cell–mediated cytotoxicity, but the activation and proliferation of antigenically naive CD8 T cells that are necessary for their expansion and acquisition of effective cytotoxic activity. The net effect of these proteins is to mask the recognition of HSV-infected cells by CD8 T cells.

The importance of selective inhibition of class I MHC antigen presentation in the pathogenicity of HSV and CMV has not yet been formally tested *in vivo*, but it is notable that NK cells and HSV antigen-specific CD4 T cells are detected earlier than antigen-specific CD8 T cells in lesions of adult humans with recurrent HSV-2 disease.[118] This has led to the proposal that IFN-γ produced by infiltrating NK and CD4 T cells overrides the inhibitory effects of ICP47 on MHC class I expression,[130, 175] thereby allowing the subsequent eradication of virus by CD8 T cells, which increase in lesions around the time of viral clearance.[111, 118] This possibility is supported by the finding that in patients with acquired immune deficiency syndrome (AIDS), a lower frequency of circulating HSV antigen-specific CD8 CTL precursors is associated with more frequent and severe recurrences of genital disease.[154] HSV-specific CD8 T cells also locally persist at sites of local infection, such as the cervix in cases of genital herpes,[120] and may explain a relative resistance of these patients to reinfection. It is important to note that the finding that the therapeutic administration of donor-derived anti-CMV CD8 cytolytic T cells also provides considerable protection of hematopoietic cell transplant recipients against disease due to CMV, supports the notion that CD8 cytolytic T cells play a key role in host defense to herpesviruses, despite virus-mediated inhibition of MHC class I expression.

The ability to address the role of CD4 versus CD8 T cells in the control of primary HSV infection with the use of murine models is partly compromised by the fact that HSV ICP47 inhibits murine TAP poorly,[172,174] which may explain the greater ease with which anti-HSV CD8 cytolytic T cells have been detected in mice compared with humans.[110,111,118,160,176,177] This species difference also raises a concern that murine models, including those in which human cells are adoptively transferred, may not faithfully replicate the role of a particular immunologic mechanism to control the virus in humans. In addition to HSV ICP47, many other gene products of the virus are dispensable *in vitro*, suggesting an *in vivo* role, such as immunoevasion or immunomodulation. In most cases the function of these gene products is unknown. Thus, we currently lack a complete knowledge of HSV-encoded immunoevasive functions and their function in mice compared with humans, and this is an important caveat when applying the results of murine models to human HSV disease. Nevertheless, it is important that studies in the mouse suggest that CD4 T cells may play the most critical role in protection,[113] although CD8 T cells may contribute, particularly in the nervous system.[124,160,178] This suggests a key role for CD4 T cells even in situations when the virus is less capable of inhibiting CD8 T cell–mediated immunity.

Despite these inhibitory mechanisms, class 1 MHC–restricted human CD8 T cells that can lyse HSV-infected targets can be isolated from HSV-2 lesions of patients with genital disease[111,132] or from the blood of HSV-immune donors.[179,180] The CD8 T cell response in humans appears to be dominated by recognition of HSV proteins that are internal structural components of the virion, such as those of the tegument and nucleocapsid, or those that are rapidly induced upon viral entry, such as certain immediate early genes.[181,182] These proteins apparently can be processed into peptides and presented on class I MHC molecules prior to the inhibitory effect of either the virion host shut-off or TAP-inhibitor proteins. Similarly, immediate-early gene products and tegument and nucleocapsid proteins also may be important targets of the human CD8 T cell response against CMV by being presented to CD8 T cells prior to the onset of multiple mechanisms that interfere with class I MHC antigen presentation. In contrast, viral glycoproteins that are found in the HSV lipid envelope do not appear to be important antigens for class I MHC–restricted responses, probably because they fuse with the host cell membrane and do not enter in the cytoplasm in substantial amounts.[130]

Human CMV also encodes proteins that inhibit class II MHC antigen presentation (reviewed in reference 183). Although specific proteins in HSV have not yet been identified with such activity, they may well exist. Infection of mice with virulent HSV strains results in CNS lesions in which class II MHC expression remains intracellular, thereby avoiding any chance of detection by CD4 T cells.[184]

CD28/CD80–86 Co-Stimulation

In addition to engagement of the αβ-TCR by peptide/class II MHC antigen, full naive T cell activation is thought to require co-stimulation, such as by engagement of CD28 on the T cell by CD80 or CD86 on the APC (see Fig. 153–3). Murine studies indicate that such co-stimulation is critical for the development of an effective adaptive immune response to HSV. CD28/CD80–86 interactions appear critical for paralysis-free survival as well as for the generation of both HSV-specific CD4 and CD8 T cell responses in the footpad injection model.[148] This was demonstrated using mice with selective genetic disruption of CD28, as

well as in normal mice in which CD28/CD80–CD86 interactions were neutralized *in vivo* by administration of CTLA-4-Ig,[148] a soluble molecule that effectively competes with T cell-associated CD28 for CD80–CD86 binding. T cell–expressed CTLA-4 normally acts to down-regulate the later stages of T cell activation (see Fig. 153–3). In an intravaginal HSV murine model, mice lacking both CD80 and CD86 were prone to severe local and disseminated disease and death,[185] and similar to the other study were unable to mount effective CD4 or CD8 T cell responses and had more severe disease and mortality.[186]

Chemotactic and Homing Receptor Expression by Viral Antigen-Specific T Cells

The differential expression of chemokine and homing receptors by T cells is important in their selective trafficking, either to sites where naive T cells may potentially encounter antigen for the first time, such as the spleen and lymph nodes, or to inflamed tissues for effector functions.[82] CCR7 expression by naive T cells allows these cells to recirculate between the blood and uninflamed lymphoid organs, which constitutively express the two major ligands for CCR7, ELC (CCL19), and SLC (CCL21). In general, the down-regulation of CCR7 and up-regulation of other chemokine receptors by effector T cells is important for redirecting these cells from secondary lymphoid tissue to other sites of tissue inflammation where they can carry out their effector functions. This appears to be true for CMV-specific CD4 and CD8 T cell immunity in humans, in that effector functions, such as IFN-γ production and expression of cytolytic proteins, are mainly limited to memory T cells that are CCR7low. Such CCR7low memory T cells have been called effector memory cells. However, the majority of human memory CD4 T cells, as identified by a CD45RAlowCD45R0high CD45 isoform pattern, are CCR7high. These CCR7high memory CD4 T cells lack the capacity to produce Th1- or Th2-type effector cytokines. An analogous CCR7high memory CD8 T cell population also exists with limited effector activity. These CCR7high cells have been called central memory T cells, based on the expectation that their expression of CCR7 would confer a circulation pattern in which they circulate between the blood and central lymphoid organs, such as the lymph node and spleen.[82] Central memory T cells may be intermediates between naive T cells and effector memory T cells, although this is controversial.[82]

In established HSV infection, most recurrences of viral replication occur in keratinocytes found at epithelial sites, such as the skin and genitourinary mucosa. During symptomatic recurrences of virus at these sites, virus-specific CD4 T cells and NK cells may infiltrate by 48 hours after the appearance of lesions. This is followed several days later by virus-specific CD8 T cells, which are associated with viral clearance.[118] Consistent with the importance of CD8 T cell immunity at these local sites of replication, a majority of CD8 T cells that recognize a particular HSV peptide, as assessed by staining with viral peptide/class I MHC tetramers, express CLA (cutaneous lymphocyte-associated antigen).[119] CLA is likely involved in homing of T cells to skin and other tissues that contain keratinocytes, such as the genital tract. It is interesting that these CLA+ HSV-specific CD8 T cells were CCR7high and expressed L-selectin, indicating that they were similar to central memory cells by these criteria, although their expression of perforin or capacity to produce cytokines was not evaluated.

It is likely that HSV-specific T cells that enter sites of viral replication, such as the CNS during HSV encephalitis, utilize a distinct combination of homing and chemotactic receptors to achieve selective trafficking. Based on studies in mice using other neutrotropic viruses, expression of the CCR2 and CCR5 chemokine receptors may allow CD8 T cells to enter into the CNS.[187] Other chemokine and homing receptor combinations are likely to be important for trafficking of HSV-specific T cells to the liver and gastrointestinal tract in cases of disseminated disease.

Gamma/Delta T Cells

Gamma/delta T cells, which express a TCR heterodimer consisting of a gamma (γ) and delta (δ) chain in association with the CD3 complex proteins, are rarer than αβ-T cells in most tissues. A major exception is the intestinal epithelium, where they predominate.[188] Although some gamma/delta TCRs can recognize conventional peptide antigens presented by MHC, most directly recognize three-dimensional nonprotein or protein structures. Gamma/delta T cells, particularly those bearing Vγ2Vδ2 T cell receptors (updated nomenclature) obtained from HSV seropositive donors, can lyse HSV-infected cells in a non-MHC–restricted manner.[189] The ligands on the target cells that activate these T cells remain to be defined. It is interesting that this gamma/delta T cell population is also effective in lysis of target cells infected with vaccinia virus. Because HSV and vaccinia virus are not closely related and are unlikely to share common peptide antigens, this supports the idea that gamma/delta T cells may recognize a host cell–derived molecule that is induced by viral expression, rather than a specific virus-derived antigen.

NK T Cells

A small population of circulating human T cells expresses alpha/beta TCRs, lacks expression of both CD4 and CD8, and expresses NKR-P1A, the human orthologue of the mouse NK1.1 protein. These features, as well as others (such as CD56 and CD57 surface expression, and a dependence on the cytokine IL-15 for their development[190]) are characteristic of NK cells. For this reason, these cells are frequently referred to as NK T cells, or natural T cells. Like murine T cells expressing NK1.1, human NK T cells have a restricted TCR repertoire and mainly recognize antigens presented by the nonclassic MHC molecule CD1d, rather than by class I or class II MHC molecules. These CD1d restricted antigens that can be recognized by NK T cells include certain lipid molecules as well as hydrophobic peptides. NK T cells also have the ability to secrete high levels of IL-4 and IFN-γ and to express death-inducing ligands (fas-ligand and TNF-related apoptosis-inducing ligand [TRAIL]) on their cell surface upon primary stimulation, a capacity not observed with most antigenically naive alpha/beta T cells,[191, 192] suggesting that they could play a role in the early stages of the immune response. NK T cells have been mainly implicated as regulatory cells that limit autoimmune disease.[193] Murine NK T cells also contribute to the control of zosteriform HSV infection,[194] although the antiviral mechanisms involved remain to be defined.

B Cells, Antibody, ADCC, and Complement

Although preexisting antibody, e.g., induced by vaccination, can be effective for preventing the initiation of certain viral infections, antibody probably plays a relatively limited role in the control of viral infections that are established. This probably also applies to human herpesvirus infection, since patients with X-linked agammaglobulinemia, who lack mature B cells and antibody production, are not generally susceptible to these pathogens. However, antibody may serve an auxiliary role in host defense against herpesvirus infection, particularly when cellular components of the response are deficient, such as in the human neonate. Antibody may be important for prevention of dissemination of viral infections to the CNS. This is particularly evident in the case of enteroviral infections, in which agammaglobulinemic or hypogammaglobulinemic patients may develop paralytic poliomyelitis or severe chronic encephalitis with ECHO viruses or coxsackieviruses.[195]

In contrast to these observations for human HSV disease, murine models suggest a more important role of B cells and anti-body in host defense. In the cutaneous HSV model, mice lacking B cells as a result of selective gene targeting have been reported to be markedly more susceptible to infection and to have impaired Th1 responses.[196] This finding of decreased Th1 responses is particularly surprising given the normal T cell immunity observed in humans with X-linked agammaglobulinemia. B cell-deficient mice also have more local inflammation and viremia than do wild-type mice when challenged intravaginally with an attenuated strain.[197] It is interesting that serum from nonimmune, wild-type mice transferred into B cell-deficient mice was found to decrease vaginal HSV shedding, suggesting that natural antibody may inhibit viral replication.[197] Whether such antibody activity is found in the human circulation is unknown.

Human HSV infection results in the induction of antibodies against a diverse set of proteins, including the surface glycoproteins involved in cell attachment and entry.[198] The production of HSV-specific antibodies by B cells is T cell-dependent and also requires the C3 and C4 complement components, as well as the CD21 complement receptor on B cells,[199] which acts as a co-stimulatory molecule. However, if antibody is passively acquired, as in the case of maternal-to-fetal transfer, humoral immunity may exist independently of T cell immunity. Although enveloped viruses, such as herpesviruses, can be lysed by antibody and complement in vitro, this is unlikely to be an important mechanism in vivo because of the high concentrations of antibody required.[200] Under relatively physiologic conditions, IgG and alternative pathway complement components can coat the surfaces of many viruses, including HSV, and effectively neutralize their infectivity, possibly by preventing their attachment or fusion with cell membranes.[200,201] Antibodies can also react with viral proteins found on the surface of infected cells. IgG and complement components can lyse in vitro human cells infected with a number of different viruses, including HSV, influenza, parainfluenza, measles, and mumps.[202-204] However, the importance of complement in viral host defense is uncertain because serious viral infection is not a feature of patients with inherited complement deficiencies[205] or of animals made acutely hypocomplementemic.[206]

A potentially more effective system for the elimination of virus-infected cells by specific antibody is by antibody-dependent cellular cytotoxicity (ADCC).[207] In this system, the killer cell is a nonspecific immune effector, such as a mononuclear phagocyte, NK cell, or polymorphonuclear neutrophil (PMN), which has surface receptors for IgG. NK cells are probably the most efficient effector cells for ADCC.[208] The specificity of cytotoxicity is due to the specific recognition by antibody of viral antigens present on the infected cell surface. In vitro ADCC requires relatively low concentrations of antibody[209] and occurs rapidly (within hours),[207] making it less likely that the virus will have had sufficient time to produce infectious particles. ADCC mediated by all types of effectors is up-regulated by cytokines, such as IFN-γ, type I IFN, IL-12, and IL-15.[210-212] Although in vitro ADCC activity correlates (in some cases) with protection against serious viral infections in humans and in animal models, it remains uncertain to what extent this occurs in vivo.

Part of the apparent limited impact of antibody and complement on HSV infection in humans may reflect viral immunoevasion mechanisms that have hampered antibody effector functions. For example, the HSV gC protein is an inhibitor of the complement cascade, especially via the alternative pathway,[213] and acts by directly binding C3.[214] The gE-gI heterodimer also binds the Fc portion of antibody molecules and ablates their neutralization activity.[215] It is possible that these or other HSV-encoded inhibitory mechanisms that block viral neutralization may not be as effective in mice as in humans, analogous with ICP47 inhibition of TAP. This might account for the striking differences in the effects of genetic ablation of B cells on HSV infection in humans versus mice.

NEONATAL ANTIVIRAL IMMUNE MECHANISMS

HSV infection is severe in term infants infected at the time of parturition, as well as in the uncommon cases when it is acquired *in utero*. Characteristically, HSV infection in neonates spreads rapidly to produce either disseminated or CNS disease. Enterovirus infections are also severe and may be fatal when acquired in the perinatal period; they have a similar propensity for disseminated and CNS disease. Both infections are usually effectively controlled when acquired after 4 weeks of age, suggesting that common developmental limitations in antiviral immunity may be responsible for neonatal vulnerability. This discussion focuses on potential limitations in innate and adaptive cellular immune function of the neonate that may explain the vulnerability to these viral pathogens. Deficiencies in the function of neonatal NK cells and plasmacytoid dendritic cells may contribute to the poor early control of infection by the innate immune response. Neonates also may develop critical antigen-specific T cell responses to the virus too slowly to prevent the virus from producing irreparable tissue injury or death, and this may be due to limitations in the function of myeloid dendritic cells or T cells or both. This discussion mainly focuses on limitations in cellular innate and adaptive antiviral immune mechanisms of the neonate, as these are the best characterized. Neonatal myeloid dendritic cell function is discussed in the context of its serving as a key APC for T cell activation.

Innate Immunity—Cytokines

Little is known of the cytokine production characteristic of the innate immune response during primary HSV infection in neonates. Potential limitations in this must be inferred from *in vitro* studies in which innate immune cells, such as mononuclear phagocytes, are stimulated *in vitro*. The production of cytokines that enhance defenses against intracellular pathogens, by monocytes derived from newborn infants such as TNF-α, is modestly reduced. In an early study, type I IFN production by neonatal lymphocytes and monocytes was equivalent to adult cells for a variety of inducers, including HSV and other viruses.[216] However, a more recent study[217] found that type I IFN production by peripheral blood mononuclear cells and the frequency of IFN-α-producing cells (assayed by the ELISPOT technique) in response to fixed HSV were diminished compared with adults, particularly for prematurely born infants. It is likely that the major cell type that produces type I IFN in this assay is the plasmacytoid dendritic cell, but direct comparisons of type I IFN production by neonatal and adult plasmacytoid dendritic cells at the single cell level have not been reported.

IL-12 and IL-15 production by mononuclear cells (presumably mainly monocytes) from term neonates after stimulation with lipopolysaccharide (LPS) was approximately 25% of that of adult cells.[218, 219] Although this could contribute to the observed reduced HSV-specific Th1 response *in vivo* of neonates, such reduced responses are highly stimulus dependent. For example, neonatal and adult blood mononuclear cells stimulated with *Staphylococcus aureus* or meningococcal outer membrane proteins produce equivalent amounts of IL-12.[218-221] Freshly isolated monocytes from neonates or adults also express similar low levels of CD40,[222] but whether they have similar capacity to produce cytokines in response to CD40-ligand engagement remains unclear. The capacity of neonatal mononuclear phagocytes to produce more recently identified cytokines, such as IL-18, IL-23, and IL-27, is unknown.

NK Cells

In assays using tumor cell targets, such as the K562 erythroleukemia cell line, the cytolytic function of NK cells

increases progressively during fetal life to reach values approximately 50% (a range of 15% to 60% in various studies) of those in adult cells at term.[223-233] Reduced cytotoxic activity by neonatal NK cells has been observed using cord blood obtained from the placentas of vaginal or caesarean section deliveries, or from peripheral blood obtained 2 to 4 days after birth.[234] NK cells from the premature infant also have reduced cytotoxic function compared with those of the term neonate. It is important to note that decreased cytotoxic activity by neonatal NK cells compared with adult cells is also consistently observed with HSV-infected[233, 235, 236] and CMV-infected target cells,[237] but not with HIV-1 infected cells.[238, 239] Paralleling the reduction in natural cytotoxic activity of neonatal cells, ADCC of neonatal mononuclear cells is approximately 50% of that by adult mononuclear cells, including against HSV-infected targets.[239] Decreased ADCC mediated by purified neonatal NK cells appears to be caused, in part, by a defect in the NK cell adhering to target cells.[240]

Unlike adult NK cells, which are predominantly CD56high, most neonatal NK cells are CD56low. This CD56low subset, which is phenotypically immature, has relatively low NK cell activity compared with CD56high cells. However, the molecular basis for reduced activity of the CD56low subset remains poorly defined, as does the mechanism responsible for pathogen-specific differences in neonatal NK cell function.[2] It is clear that reduced neonatal NK cell activity is not determined at the level of the hematopoietic stem cell or later precursor cells of the NK cell lineage, because donor-derived NK cells appear early following cord blood transplantation and mediate robust cytotoxicity via the perforin/granzyme and fas/fas-ligand cytotoxic pathways.[241]

Like their effects on adult NK cells, cytokines such as IL-2, IL-12, IL-15, type I IFN, and IFN-γ can augment the cytolytic activity of neonatal NK cells within a few hours,[242-244] consistent with normal levels of expression of surface receptors for these cytokines.[245] However, neonatal NK cells are less responsive to activation by the combination of IL-12 and IL-15 than are adult NK cells, based on the induction of CD69 surface expression.[246]

Circulating neonatal NK cells also have increased natural cytotoxic activity and ADCC activity on more prolonged incubation (from 18 hours to 3 weeks) with IL-2, IL-12, IL-15, IL-18, or combinations of these to generate LAK (lymphokine-activated killer) cells.[236,239,243,246-254] The generation of neonatal LAK cells from NK cells also increases their surface expression of CD56 due to differentiation of CD56low NK cells into CD56high LAK cells.[251,255] Again, this suggests that the neonatal CD56low NK cell population is a phenotypically and functionally immature NK cell subset that gives rise to a mature CD56high population. Studies in which cytokine-primed NK cells of neonates versus adults have been tested against cell targets infected with HSV or other herpesviruses are few.

Cytokine production by NK cells is another potentially important mechanism of host defense against HSV (see Fig. 153–2). Neonatal NK cells produce IFN-γ as effectively as adult NK cells in response to exogenous IL-2 and HSV[256] or to polyclonal stimulation with ionomycin and phorbal myristate acetate (PMA).[257] Although IL-12–induced production of IFN-γ by neonatal mononuclear cells (most likely NK cells) may be reduced compared with adult cells,[218,242] purified neonatal NK cells produce substantially more IFN-γ than adult NK cells after stimulation with the combination of IL-12 and IL-18.[254] Fewer neonatal NK cells express TNF-α than do adult NK cells following ionomycin and PMA stimulation.[257] However, neonatal NK cell production of these and other cytokines in response to physiologic stimulation, e.g., with HSV-infected cell targets in the absence of exogenous cytokines, is not known.

Reduced NK cell cytolytic activity and cytokine production may be an important contributor to the pathogenesis of neonatal HSV infection, based on a neonatal murine model in which human cells are adoptively transferred. In this model, the age-related maturation of NK cell function parallels the development of resistance to HSV.[9,258] Neonatal mice, which like human neonates are more susceptible to HSV, can be protected by adoptive transfer of human blood mononuclear cells from adults, but not from neonates. Addition of IL-2 augments protection mediated by cells from adults, but not cells from neonates, and protection depends on IFN-γ production by the transferred cells. The failure of human neonatal cells to transfer resistance in this model also can be corrected by the addition of IFN-γ, a cytokine produced poorly by neonatal T cells, as discussed later. This suggests that lack of IFN-γ production may be one important difference between adult and neonatal cells. Whether deficits in NK cell, IFN-γ production, and/or cytotoxicity may contribute to the failure of neonatal mononuclear cells to confer protection in this model is uncertain.

It is important to note that there have been no studies directly comparing NK cell function against HSV targets in neonates versus adults with primary HSV infection, including after-treatment with various immunostimulatory cytokines. Nor have their been measurements of systemic or cell-associated levels of cytokines that could be useful for augmenting NK cell function in this infection. It is also unknown whether neonatal NK cell activity is reduced against enteroviruses, which can cause a similar spectrum of severe disseminated and CNS disease in the neonate, particularly when acquired perinatally or shortly after birth.

CD4 T Cells and Dendritic Cells

Some of the best-documented limitations in neonatal adaptive immunity come from two studies in which T cell responses by neonates and adults with primary HSV infection were compared.[107,259] HSV-specific proliferation of peripheral blood mononuclear cells and production of IFN-γ and TNF-α were all diminished and delayed in the neonates compared with the adults. The neonates did not achieve adult levels of these responses for 3 to 6 weeks after clinical presentation, whereas the adults all developed robust responses by 2 weeks. These studies employed UV-irradiated viral preparations to stimulate peripheral blood mononuclear cells, in which viral proteins are mainly processed by the class II rather than the class I MHC antigen presentation pathway. Therefore, they mainly assayed CD4 and not CD8 T cell function.

These results suggests a profound lag in developing adaptive immunity to the HSV in normal neonates during which viral replication and cell lysis could continue. Because, as discussed earlier, CD4 T cells provide multiple critical effector mechanisms that may be critical for the resolution of HSV infection (including direct antiviral cytokine production and providing help for CD8 T cells and B cell responses), these findings suggest that a lag in T cell immunity may be an important contributor to the tendency of HSV infection to disseminate and to cause prolonged disease in neonates.

It is interesting that we have also observed profoundly reduced CMV-specific CD4 T cell responses, including CMV-specific IFN-γ, IL-2, and CD40-ligand expression, in healthy older infants and young children with postnatally acquired CMV infection.[260] In contrast to HSV infection, these decreased CMV-specific responses persisted for at least a year following viral acquisition. In contrast, the frequency of CMV-specific CD8 T cells in these children was similar to that of adults.[261] These results indicate that developmental limitations in the response to herpesviruses is highly species- and T cell subset–specific. The ontogeny of HSV-specific T cell immunity to primary infection after the neonatal period is not known.

Studies of the responses of neonates and infants to viral vaccines also support the idea that CD4 T cell immunity to viruses may be blunted early in life. Peripheral blood mononuclear cells

from neonates given oral poliovirus vaccine (OPV) at birth and at 1, 2, and 3 months of age had decreased OPV-specific proliferation, IFN-γ production, and IFN-γ-positive cells than immunized (but not reimmunized) adults.[262] In contrast, their antibody titers were higher than those of adults.

The generation of CD4 T effector cells is a complex process, involving antigen presentation by dendritic cells to naive CD4 T cells and multiple steps of T cell clonal expansion and differentiation; compromise of any of these steps could result in limited Th1 immunity. Myeloid dendritic cells are key in promoting naive CD4 T cell differentiation to Th1 effector and memory T cells. Key events promoting Th1 differentiation include the elaboration by dendritic cells of cytokines, such as IL-12, IL-23, and IL-27, and their binding to specific receptors on CD4 T cells.[35] CD40-ligand is expressed by naive CD4 T cells after the T cell recognizes peptide antigen/MHC complexes via the αβ-TCR and receives co-stimulation via CD28 binding to CD80 and CD86 (see Fig. 153–3). The engagement of CD40 on the dendritic cell by CD40-ligand on the T cell enhances the dendritic cell production of these Th1-promoting cytokines and also increases the expression of CD80 and CD86, which helps sustain T cell activation. Humans who are genetically deficient in CD40-ligand[263] or in the ability to respond to IL-12 and IL-23[40] have absent or severely depressed antigen-specific Th1 responses, supporting the validity of this model.

The basis for the delayed development of HSV antigen-specific CD4 T cells in neonates is not known; it could reflect limitations at one or more of the steps just described. Neonates have been reported to have a lower frequency of precursor T cells capable of responding to HSV and CMV.[264] This is unlikely to be due to a limitation in the diversity of the αβ-TCR repertoire[265-267] and more likely reflects intrinsic limitations in T cell function.

In vitro models of activation have shown that neonatal CD4 T cells differ from adult CD4 T cells in tending to become anergic (permanently nonresponsive to antigenic stimuli) unless antigen is presented by primed/mature dendritic cells expressing co-stimulatory molecules and cytokines.[268-271] This anergic tendency may apply to CD4 T cells that are expanded in cases when neonates are infected with bacteria that express superantigen toxins, such as toxic shock syndrome toxin-1.[272]

Limitations in dendritic cell antigen presentation or co-stimulatory function could promote such T cell anergy or a failure of expanded CD4 T cells to acquire Th1 effector activity. Of note, infants between 6 and 12 months of age have lower CD4 T cell–derived IL-2 production in response to tetanus toxoid than do older children and adults.[273] This supports the idea that either antigen-specific memory CD4 T cell generation or function is decreased not only for HSV but more generally during early infancy. *In vitro* studies suggest that reduced class II MHC antigen presentation could contribute to this outcome.[273]

Such limitations might be compounded in HSV infection. In addition to its well-known inhibition of class I MHC antigen presentation, HSV infection of neonatal monocytes,[274] monocyte-derived dendritic cells,[17] or B cells[275] can block the ability of these cells to activate CD4 T cells. Studies using dendritic cell-enriched fractions that contain both myeloid and plasmacytoid dendritic cells also suggest that neonatal dendritic cells overall are less able to activate CD4 T cells.[276,277] However, plasmacytoid dendritic cells make up a greater fraction of circulating dendritic cells in neonates compared with adults, and plasmacytoid dendritic cells are relatively poor in activating T cells.[278] Therefore, studies in which the neonatal and adult function of myeloid dendritic cells are compared are needed to assess accurately developmental limitations in dendritic cell function.

Limitations in neonatal myeloid dendritic cell cytokine production might also limit Th1 immunity to HSV. For example, cord blood monocyte-derived dendritic cells have a low capacity to produce IL-12 in response to either lipopolysaccharide (LPS), engagement of CD40, or treatment with double-stranded RNA [poly (I:C)]; this is apparently due to a selective decrease in mRNA expression of the IL-12 (p35) chain component.[279] Type I IFN, which is produced in particularly high amounts by plasmacytoid dendritic cells, also promotes Th1 differentiation in humans. The capacity of plasmacytoid DC of the neonate to produce type I IFN and IL-12 in response to viral challenge, such as HSV, is not known.

Myeloid dendritic cells derived from immature precursors in neonatal or adult blood can be primed for efficient antigen presentation by engagement of their CD40 molecule by CD40 ligand expressed by activated T cells, or by their exposure to microbial products or inflammatory cytokines induced by these products. Recent observations support the idea that overall myeloid dendritic cell maturity is increased following exposure to microbial products, such as from endogenous bacterial flora. Myeloid dendritic cells from adult mice lacking functional TLR-4, which recognizes LPS and other bacterial products, have reduced levels of expression of co-stimulatory molecules and a capacity to direct T cell activation.[280] Thus, it is possible that the lack of prior exposure to microbes (which occurs in a cumulative manner after birth) could contribute to diminished dendritic cell function and the slow rate at which antigen-specific T cells develop.

CD40-Ligand/CD40 Interactions

Given the importance of CD40 ligands in multiple aspects of the immune response,[147] limitations in CD40 ligand production could contribute to decreased antigen-specific immunity mediated by Th1 effector cells and B cells in the neonate. Initial studies reporting a marked deficiency of CD40-ligand expression by neonatal T cells compared with adult cells used calcium ionophore and phorbol ester stimulation, a combination that maximizes the production of most cytokines but may not accurately mimic physiologic T cell activation.[281-284] Reduced CD40-ligand surface expression by neonatal T cells after activation by a combination of anti-CD3 and anti-CD28 monoclonal antibodies has also been observed by some,[285, 286] but not by others.[287, 288] Using more physiologically relevant stimulation, neonatal CD4 T cells co-cultured with dendritic cells increase their expression of CD40 ligand[289] and induce IL-12 production by dendritic cells.[290] However, we found that CD40 ligand expression by purified neonatal naive CD4 T cells co-cultured with adult allogeneic dendritic cells was substantially less than by adult naive CD4 T cells after 24 to 48 hours of stimulation. This reduced CD40-ligand production was accompanied by reduced IL-12 production (by monocyte-derived dendritic cells) and IFN-γ production (by naive CD4 T cells).[291] This suggests that CD40 ligand surface expression is at least initially more limited for neonatal T cells, but with continued priming *in vitro* this can be overcome. A likely consequence is that the differentiation of naive CD4 T cells into Th1 effector cells by an IL-12–dependent and dendritic cell–dependent process may be delayed.

IFN-γ Production by CD4 T Cells

Antigenically naive CD4 T cells initially have a very limited capacity to express cytokines other than IL-2, whereas distinct subsets of memory CD4 T cells express particular cytokines. Th1 and Th2 cells produce IFN-γ and IL-4, respectively.[292] Thus, the essential absence of memory CD4 T cells in the circulation of neonates accounts for the limited ability of neonatal CD4 T cells to produce IFN-γ compared with adult CD4 T cells.[293] If naive CD4 T cells are activated *in vitro*, they differentiate into effector-like cells that acquire the capacity to produce IFN-γ (Th1 effectors) or IL-4 (Th2 effectors), depending on the conditions used in terms of cytokine milieu and antigen presenting cell populations.[37, 294-296] However, as mentioned earlier, our

studies suggest that neonatal naive CD4 T cells have a decreased capacity to become IFN-γ-producing cells compared with adult naive CD4 T cells in response to short-term (i.e., 24 to 48 hours' duration) stimulation by allogeneic dendritic cells.[291]

This decreased expression of IFN-γ by neonatal CD4 T cells is likely due to several factors. First, neonatal CD4 T cells are less effective than adult naive cells at inducing the co-cultured adult dendritic cells to produce IL-12, a key cytokine for promoting IFN-γ production.[291] Second, as discussed earlier, neonatal antigen presenting cells, such as dendritic cells, may have a decreased capacity to produce IL-12 and related cytokines that are key for Th1 differentiation.[279] It is interesting that this decreased capacity for IL-12 production by mononuclear cells may continue into early childhood, at least for certain stimuli, such as lipopolysaccharide.[297] Third, neonatal naive CD4+ T cells have decreased expression of certain transcription factors that may play a role in the induction of IFN-γ gene expression, such as the NFATc2 protein.[298, 299] Fourth, the greater methylation of DNA of the IFN-γ genetic locus in neonatal T cells also may contribute to a reduced and delayed acquisition of IFN-γ production following activation *in vitro*.[300] Some or all of these mechanisms are likely to contribute to the delay in the appearance of IFN-γ production by antigen-specific CD4 T cells following infection in the neonatal period, such as HSV.

In contrast to the results with dendritic cell allostimulation, neonatal T cells, if polyclonally activated under conditions that favor repeated cell division (strong activation stimuli in common with the provision of exogenous IL-2), acquire the features of fully competent memory/effector cells. These characteristics include a CD45RA^low CD45R0^high surface phenotype, an enhanced ability to be activated by anti-CD2 or anti-CD3 monoclonal antibodies, and an increased capacity to produce cytokines (e.g., IL-4 and IFN-γ).[301-304] This suggests that such approaches *in vivo*, e.g., IL-2 immunotherapy, might similarly enhance neonatal T cell clonal expansion and differentiation.

Cytolytic CD4 T Cells

HSV-specific CD4 T cells with cytolytic activity are readily isolated from adults and may serve as an important source of viral clearance that counteracts viral suppression of class I MHC antigen presentation, e.g., by ICP47 inhibition of the TAP transporter (see Fig. 153–5). CD4 T cell–mediated viral clearance ordinarily would be limited to target cells that express class II MHC, particularly professional antigen-presenting cells. However, an expanded target cell range is possible because class II MHC expression is upregulated on many non-antigen-presenting cell types in response to cytokines, such as IFN-γ (reviewed in reference 2). Thus, it is plausible that CD4 cytolytic T cells play an important role in the resolution of HSV infection in humans. No studies have examined cytolytic activity mediated by neonatal CD4 T cells for HSV or other infections.

CD8 T Cells

There has been great interest recently in the capacity of neonatal CD8 T cells to mediate cytotoxicity and potentiate graft rejection thanks to the growing use of cord blood for hematopoietic cell transplantation, and the possibility that its use reduces the risk of graft-versus-host disease. Early studies of cytotoxicity mediated by neonatal T cells mostly used unfractionated mononuclear cells as a source of killer cells in a variety of nonantigen-specific assays, such as lectin-mediated cytotoxicity or redirected cytotoxicity using CD3 monoclonal antibodies. Reduced cytotoxicity was observed with lectin-activated cord blood lymphocytes, particularly if purified T cells were used.[224,305,306]

CD8 T cells also can be sensitized *in vitro* for cytotoxicity using allogeneic (MHC other than self) stimulator cells, followed by testing for cytotoxic activity against allogeneic target cells. With this approach, most studies have found that neonatal T cells are moderately less effective than adult T cells as cytotoxic effector cells.[247, 307-309] More substantial defects in T cell-mediated cytotoxicity by neonatal T cells after allogeneic priming are observed when no exogenous cytokines are added, such as IL-2.[310, 311] This suggests that this decreased cytolytic activity could be of physiologic significance *in vivo* if there were also limitations in CD4 T cell help. The capacity of neonatal CD8 T cells to become cytolytic effector cells when primed using optimal antigen-presenting cells such as dendritic cells, remains to be determined.

Part of the apparent deficiency of cytolytic activity observed after allogeneic stimulation may reflect the absence of effector and memory CD8 T cells, as identified by their expression of CD45R0 and/or their lack of CD27 and CD28.[312] This would be expected in neonates and fetuses that have not experienced significant congenital or perinatal infections. For example, CD8 effector and memory T cells kill more efficiently than antigenically naive T cells after stimulation with lectin or anti-CD3 monoclonal antibody[313] or after allogeneic sensitization.[314-316]

The mechanism for reduced neonatal T cell–mediated cytotoxicity remains poorly understood. Two studies have found that only a low percentage of neonatal CD8 T cells constitutively express perforin, whereas approximately 30% of adult CD8 T cells contain this protein.[317,318] In contrast, another study found that approximately 30% of neonatal T cells expressed perforin, a frequency similar to that of adult T cells.[319] The capacity of neonatal CD8 T cells to express fas-ligand (CD95L) and to mediate fas-ligand-dependent cytotoxicity in response to priming by alloantigen is also not known.

There are few studies of antigen-specific cytotoxic T cell responses in the fetus, neonate, or young infant, reflecting, in part, the technical difficulties of performing classic cytotoxicity assays, which require HLA-matched or autologous virally infected target cells. The recent development of alternative flow cytometric techniques, such as analyzing perforin content of T cells (identified as viral peptide-specific) based on class I MHC/viral peptide tetramer staining, should facilitate these studies.

Much of the studies of antigen-specific cytotoxicity to date have focused on congenital and perinatal HIV-1 infection. In congenital HIV-1 infection, an expansion of HIV-specific cytotoxic T cells was detected at birth, indicating that fetal T cells were activated by viral antigens.[320] In another case of *in utero* HIV infection, HIV-specific T cell–mediated cytotoxicity was detected at 4 months of age and persisted for several years despite a high HIV viral load.[321] Cytotoxic responses to HIV in perinatally infected infants suggest that, although CD8 T cells capable of mediating cytotoxicity have undergone clonal expansion *in vivo* as early as 4 months of age,[322] their cytotoxicity may be reduced and delayed in appearance compared with that of adults.[323] In many cases, HIV-1-specific cytotoxic lymphocyte responses were not detectable during the first few months of life.[320, 323] When evaluated beyond infancy, cytolytic activity directed to HIV envelope proteins were commonly detected, but cytolytic activity directed against *gag* or *pol* proteins was rarely detected.[324] There was also decreased HIV-specific CD8 T-cell production of IFN-γ by young infants with perinatal HIV infection,[325] and an inability to generate HIV-specific cytotoxic T cells following anti-retroviral therapy.[326] Together, these results suggest that there may be a delay in the development of CD8 T cell–mediated responses compared with adults, and that the nature of the target antigens recognized by neonatal CD8 T cells may be more limited. These developmental limitations in CD8 T cell function may not necessarily be limited to HIV-1, at least in early infancy, because one study of respiratory syncytial virus (RSV)-specific cytotoxicity found that it was more pronounced and frequent in infants 6 to 24 months of age than in younger infants.[327]

HIV-1 infection has a number severely immunosuppressive features that may not apply to most other viral infections. These include impairment of antigen presentation,[328] decreasing thymic T cell output,[329] and promoting T cell apoptosis.[330] It is important to note that these suppressive effects of HIV-1 on cytotoxic responses may be relatively specific for HIV-1, because HIV-infected infants who lack HIV-specific cytotoxic T cells may maintain CD8 T cells against EBV and CMV.[325,326] Whether there is a lag in the acquisition of herpesvirus-specific CD8 T cell responses in neonates and infants (either HIV-infected or uninfected) compared with adults with primary infection, remains unclear. It is interesting to note that some of the inhibitory effects of HIV-1 infection may also occur in HIV-exposed but uninfected infants born to HIV-infected mothers.[329,331]

Co-Stimulation

Neonatal T cells express levels of CD28 similar to those of adult T cells and produce IL-2 and proliferate as well as adult T cells in response to mouse antigen-presenting cells expressing human CD80 or CD86, and to anti-CD3 monoclonal antibody, indicating that CD28-mediated signaling is intact.[332] This is also supported by a study showing that anti-CD28 monoclonal antibody treatment of neonatal T cells markedly augments their ability to produce IL-2 and proliferate in response to anti-CD2 monoclonal antibody.[333] These results do not exclude the possibility that neonatal T cell co-stimulation via CD28 could be limited because of decreased expression of CD80 or CD86 by key antigen-presenting cells, such as neonatal myeloid dendritic cells.

Chemotactic and Homing Receptor Expression

As discussed earlier, the down-regulation of CCR7 and up-regulation of other chemokine receptors by effector T cells is probably important for redirecting these cells from secondary lymphoid tissue to other sites of tissue inflammation where they can carry out their effector functions. This appears to be true for herpesvirus-specific CD4 T cell responses, as we have found that CMV-specific human memory CD4 T cells, which are capable of producing antiviral Th1 cytokines, such as IFN-γ, are essentially all CCR7low cells.[260] This restriction of CMV-specific Th1 effector function to CCR7low cells has been observed with both adults and young children following primary CMV infection but has not been evaluated in cases of congenital or perinatal CMV infection or in cases of HSV infection.

Human neonatal naive T cells differ from those of adults in that they do not increase CXCR3 expression, which favors trafficking to inflamed tissues that have been exposed to IFN-γ, and they decrease CCR7 expression after activation via anti-CD3 and CD28 monoclonal antibodies.[334,335] The CCR7 expressed on neonatal T cells is functional and mediates chemotaxis of these cells in response to CCL19 and CCL21.[336] These results suggest that activated neonatal T cells may be limited in their capacity to traffic to nonlymphoid tissue sites of inflammation and may recirculate between the blood and peripheral lymphoid organs. Neonatal T cells can increase the surface expression of CCR5 by treatment with either mitogen or IL-2[337] or after differentiation *in vitro* in a cytokine milieu that favors Th1 development.[82, 338, 339] Whether CCR5 expression by T cells, which is likely important for their homing to the CNS, is up-regulated in cases of neonatal or postnatal HSV encephalitis is not known.

T Cell Apoptosis

During a typical viral infection, effector T cells, particularly those of the CD8 T cell subset, undergo a marked but transient clonal expansion followed by a rapid decrease in cell numbers once the antigenic stimulus is removed, e.g., by effective viral clearance.

This decrease is due to apoptosis and illustrates the importance of the regulation of apoptosis in appropriate lymphocyte homeostasis. It is also plausible that neonatal T cell–mediated immune responses might be more limited than those of adults because of a greater apoptotic tendency. In support of this possibility, mononuclear cells from cord blood, including naive CD4 T cells, are more prone than those from the adult circulation to undergo spontaneous apoptosis during *in vitro* culture.[333, 340-343] The mechanism is unclear but is most likely not mediated by fas/fas-ligand interactions but other pathways. Similarly, neonatal T cells primed *in vitro* using activating stimuli subsequently become more susceptible to apoptosis than adult cells after restimulation with CD3 monoclonal antibody, yet they remain relatively resistant to fas-induced apoptosis.[344] This increased apoptotic tendency may be mediated by the p55 and p75 TNF-α receptors.[345] Neonatal T cells also express a lower ratio of bcl-2 to bax mRNA and protein compared with adult T cells, both basally and after culture *in vitro*, which may decrease protection from apoptosis.[340, 341, 344] Together, these suggest pro-apoptotic mechanisms by which the clonal expansion of neonatal T cells is limited following activation. They also raise the possibility that exogenous cytokines, such as IL-2, could be used to counteract this apoptotic tendency, because IL-2 treatment *in vitro* blocks TNF-receptor–mediated apoptosis of activated neonatal T cells.[345] Direct comparisons of spontaneous versus activation-induced apoptosis by T cells generated during primary HSV infection, including in newborn infants, has not been reported.

Gamma/Delta T Cells

Based on murine models discussed earlier, gamma/delta T cells may be an important contributor to the early control of HSV infection at sites such as neural ganglia. Although human neonatal gamma/delta T cells proliferate *in vitro* to mycobacterial lipid antigens,[346] they express lower levels of serine esterases than do adult gamma/delta T cells, suggesting that they are less effective cytotoxic cells.[347] Gamma/delta T cell clones derived from cord blood also have a markedly reduced capacity to mediate cytotoxicity against tumor cells extracts.[189] Because these neonatal clones also have lower CD45R0 surface expression than the adult clones, their reduced activity may reflect their antigenic naiveté. Whether the frequency of gamma/delta T cells is increased during primary HSV infection, including in neonates, is not known.

NK T Cells

A recent report indicates a role of NK T cells in the control of HSV-1 infection, although the effector mechanisms involved, e.g., cytokine production or cell-mediated cytotoxicity, remain unclear.[194] Limitations in NK T cell–mediated immunity in neonates could contribute to the severity of HSV infection. First, only small numbers of NK T cells (<1.0% of circulating T cells) are present in the neonatal circulation, but these subsequently increase with ageing.[348] This suggests that NK T cells may either undergo postnatal expansion, e.g., in relation to exposure to a ubiquitous antigen, or that their production by the thymus or at extrathymic sites occurs mainly postnatally. Neonatal NK T cells differ from adult NK T cells in producing only limited amounts of IFN-γ on primary stimulation, indicating functional immaturity.[349] This decreased capacity may be due to mechanisms similar to those for the reduced IFN-γ production by neonatal CD4 T cells, such as decreased levels of the NFATc2 transcription factor or increased methylation of the IFN-γ genetic locus. Neonatal CD56+ T cells constitutively express less perforin than do adult cells.[318] Because the CD56+ T cell population is highly enriched in NK T cells, NK T cell cytotoxicity is probably limited at birth and gradually increases with age. Culturing of neonatal NK T cells

in vitro for several weeks results in acquisition of potent cytotoxic activity against tumor cell targets,[350] indicating that developmental limitations can be overcome following expansion and differentiation. Given these developmental limitations in NK T cell–mediated immunity, it will be of interest to compare the NK T cell immune response in primary HSV infection in neonates and adults.

B Cells, Antibody, ADCC, and Complement

The neonatal IgM response to most protein antigens is intact, and only slightly limited for IgG responses to certain vaccines, such as hepatitis B surface antigen. Nevertheless, there are clear differences between neonates and older infants in the magnitude of the antibody response to most protein neoantigens, but this rapidly resolves following birth. This may be more pronounced in those born prematurely, but, again, it resolves rapidly after the neonatal period. Thus, chronologic (i.e., postnatal) age is more of a determinant of antibody responses to T-dependent antigens than is gestational age. Isotype expression by B cells after immunization with T-dependent antigens is limited by T cell function, such as reduced CD40-ligand production, and intrinsic limitations of B cell maturation and function.[2] These limitations are exaggerated in the fetus.

It is likely that these limitations in response to T-dependent antigens apply to neonatal HSV infection. Assuming that neutralizing or ADCC HSV-specific antibody contributes to the control of primary HSV infection in humans, it is possible that limitations in isotype switching from IgM to IgG or a slower rate of somatic hypermutation of IgG responses could contribute to the severity of neonatal infection. The neonate is also unable to produce antibodies in response to T-independent type II antigens, e.g., the capsular polysaccharides of bacteria. However, this is unlikely to be an important factor in the severity of neonatal HSV infection, because no T-independent type II HSV antigen-specific responses by human B cells have been described.

The neonate is also partially protected from infection by passive maternal IgG antibody, predominantly transferred during the latter third of pregnancy. Fetal IgG concentrations are equal to or higher than maternal concentrations after 34 weeks of gestation, reflecting active transport mechanisms. In newborn infants with gestational age less than 38 weeks, a greater fraction of this maternally derived HSV-specific IgG may enter into the CNS,[351] reflecting a generally less effective blood-brain barrier. Whether this is in sufficient amounts to provide protection from CNS disease is unknown. The risk of transmission of HSV from mother to infant in cases of primary or initial maternal infection is much higher (~35%) than in cases of recurrent maternal infection. This may reflect, in part, lesser amounts of virus in the maternal genital tract in recurrent infection, but it also appears to correlate with HSV type-specific antibody, particularly to glycoprotein G.[352] Kohl[9] has also shown that of HSV-infected infants, those with greater concentrations of ADCC antibody had less severe disease. It is important to note that healthy adults and older children with primary HSV infection, who by definition lack antibody to HSV, do not develop severe disease as do neonates with primary infection. This indicates that the deficits intrinsic to the neonate are the important factors predisposing the neonate to infection. Nevertheless, passively acquired antibody may play a role in decreasing transmission or ameliorating disease severity.

Adjunct Therapy and Vaccination for Herpesvirus Infections

The foregoing studies raise the possibility that neonates could be passively protected by administration of antibody to HSV, particularly antibody that would facilitate ADCC. *In vitro* studies also suggest that antibody, and particularly monoclonal antibodies, potentially could be protective by directly blocking HSV transmission from neurons to epithelial cells.[353] Passive antibody can even provide substantial protection from low inoculum HSV challenge in the absence of both type I IFN signaling and T and B cells; the protective mechanism requires IL-12 and IFN-γ,[354] at least in mice. Human monoclonal antibodies, murine monoclonal antibodies that have been humanized, and specific hyperimmunoglobulin potentially could be employed for this purpose. For example, the phage display technique has been used to select human monoclonal antibodies with an ability effectively to neutralize either HSV-1 or HSV-2 at a relatively low concentration *in vitro*,[355] but it remains to be seen whether this or related antibodies will be efficacious in limiting the extent of primary HSV infection in humans.

The unique capacity of IFN-γ to endow human neonatal blood mononuclear cells with the ability to protect neonatal mice from infection suggests that exogenous IFN-γ may also be a potentially useful means to enhance the human neonate's resistance to HSV. However, in the experimental models described by Kohl,[9] passive immunotherapy must be given before or at the time of infection. This raises the concern that such therapy, if administered once infection is established, may be less effective. In addition, unanticipated fatal toxicity and mortality from administration of IL-12 to adult cancer patients[356] indicates that there is reason to be cautious in using exogenous cytokine therapy in the seriously ill neonate. It should be emphasized again that there is as yet no direct evidence that the initial innate immune response of the neonate to HSV infection is deficient in terms of cytokine production (e.g., for IL-12, TNF-α, and IFN-γ) derived from cells other than T cells. Facilitating the more rapid development of antigen-specific CD4 and CD8 T cells with appropriate effector function might be a more physiologic approach, allowing these cells and the cytokines they produce to localize properly to the sites of infection. Further elucidation of the cellular and molecular mechanisms that underlie the lag in the development of antigen-specific immunity in the neonate in response to HSV may help in devising therapies to overcome these limitations in host defenses.

HSV-2 vaccines employing recombinant glycoproteins, such as glycoprotein B and D in combination[357, 358] or glycoprotein D alone,[359] with various adjuvants have had limited efficacy in preventing infection of those who are HSV-2 seronegative, and in providing substantial clinical benefit to those who are already HSV-2 infected. Although these vaccines have induced high levels of IgG antibodies against the glycoprotein immunogens, these antibodies may not efficiently mediate ADCC.[360] Thus, if ADCC is important in preventing maternal-to-neonatal HSV transmission, these vaccines do not appear to be beneficial in reducing neonatal HSV disease. Further efforts to develop a vaccine that will prevent or at least ameliorate disease in adults and neonates are indicated. Following the failure of the recombinant glycoprotein vaccines, a number of other strategies are being considered, including a replication-defective HSV vaccine, e.g., gD-deficient HSV viruses that can undergo only one round of productive infection, or employing other viruses that are modified by recombinant DNA technology to encode HSV proteins.[39,361] It will also be important to define which immunologic parameters most closely correlate with reduced disease, and with reduced viral shedding in adults as well as children, to help focus on the appropriate goal of vaccination.

REFERENCES

1. Arvin AM, Whitley RJ: Herpes simplex virus infections. *In* Remington JS, Klein JO (eds): Infectious Diseases of the Fetus and Newborn Infant. Philadelphia, WB Saunders, 2001, pp 425–446.
2. Lewis DB, Wilson CB: Developmental immunology and role of host defenses in fetal and neonatal susceptibility to infection. *In* Remington JS, Klein JO (eds): Infectious Diseases of the Fetus and Newborn Infant. Philadelphia, WB Saunders, 2001, pp 25–138.
3. Roizman B, Knipe DM: Herpes simplex viruses and their replication. *In* Knipe DM, Howley PM (eds): Fields Virology. Philadelphia, Lippincott Williams & Wilkins, 2001, pp 2399–2459.
4. Ward PL, Roizman B: Herpes simplex genes: the blueprint of a successful human pathogen. Trends Genet *10*:267, 1994.
5. Langenberg AG, et al: A prospective study of new infections with herpes simplex virus type 1 and type 2. Chiron HSV Vaccine Study Group. N Engl J Med *341*:1432, 1999.
6. Jones C: Herpes simplex virus type 1 and bovine herpesvirus 1 latency. Clin Microbiol Rev *16*:79, 2003.
7. Perng GC, et al: Virus-induced neuronal apoptosis blocked by the herpes simplex virus latency-associated transcript. Science *287*:1500, 2000.
8. Thompson RL, Sawtell NM: Herpes simplex virus type 1 latency–associated transcript gene promotes neuronal survival. J Virol *75*:6660, 2001.
9. Kohl S: The neonatal human's immune response to herpes simplex virus infection: a critical review. Pediatr Infect Dis J *8*:67, 1989.
10. Katze MG, et al: Viruses and interferon: a fight for supremacy. Nat Rev Immunol *2*:675, 2002.
11. Taniguchi T, Takaoka A: The interferon-alpha/beta system in antiviral responses: a multimodal machinery of gene regulation by the IRF family of transcription factors. Curr Opin Immunol *14*:111, 2002.
12. Alexopoulou L, et al: Recognition of double-stranded RNA and activation of NF-kappaB by Toll-like receptor 3. Nature *413*:732, 2001.
13. Yamamoto M, et al: Cutting edge: a novel Toll/IL-1 receptor domain–containing adapter that preferentially activates the IFN-beta promoter in the Toll-like receptor signaling. J Immunol *169*:6668, 2002.
14. Siegal FP, et al: The nature of the principal type 1 interferon-producing cells in human blood. Science *284*:1835, 1999.
15. Kadowaki N, Liu YJ: Natural type I interferon-producing cells as a link between innate and adaptive immunity. Hum Immunol *63*:1126, 2002.
16. Bauer D, Tampe R: Herpes viral proteins blocking the transporter associated with antigen processing TAP—from genes to function and structure. Curr Topics Microbiol Immunol *269*:87, 2002.
17. Salio M, et al: Inhibition of dendritic cell maturation by herpes simplex virus. Eur J Immunol *29*:3245, 1999.
18. Kadowaki N, Liu YJ: Natural type I interferon-producing cells as a link between innate and adaptive immunity. Hum Immunol *63*:1126, 2002.
19. Le Bon A, et al: Type 1 interferons potently enhance humoral immunity and can promote isotype switching by stimulating dendritic cells in vivo. Immunity *14*:461, 2001.
20. Grandvaux N, et al: Transcriptional profiling of interferon regulatory factor 3 target genes: direct involvement in the regulation of interferon-stimulated genes. J Virol *76*:5532, 2002.
21. Dupuis S, et al: Impairment of mycobacterial but not viral immunity by a germline human STAT1 mutation. Science *293*:300, 2001.
22. Dupuis S, et al: Impaired response to interferon-alpha/beta and lethal viral disease in human STAT1 deficiency. Nat Genet *33*:388, 2003.
23. Leib DA, et al: Interferons regulate the phenotype of wild-type and mutant herpes simplex viruses in vivo. J Exp Med *189*:663, 1999.
24. Lebon P, et al: Early intrathecal synthesis of interferon in herpes encephalitis. Biomedicine *31*:267, 1979.
25. Zawatzky R, et al: Experimental infection of inbred mice with herpes simplex virus. III. Comparison between newborn and adult C57BL/6 mice. J Gen Virol *60*:25, 1982.
26. Yokota S, et al: Herpes simplex virus type 1 suppresses the interferon signaling pathway by inhibiting phosphorylation of STATs and janus kinases during an early infection stage. Virology *286*:119, 2001.
27. Sainz B Jr, Halford WP: Alpha/beta interferon and gamma interferon synergize to inhibit the replication of herpes simplex virus type 1. J Virol *76*:11541, 2002.
28. Keadle TL, et al: IL-1 and TNF-alpha are important factors in the pathogenesis of murine recurrent herpetic stromal keratitis. Invest Ophthalmol Vis Sci *41*:96, 2000.
29. Berkowitz C, Becker Y: Recombinant interleukin-1 alpha, interleukin-2 and M-CSF-1 enhance the survival of newborn C57BL/6 mice inoculated intraperitoneally with a lethal dose of herpes simplex virus-1. Arch Virol *124*:83, 1992.
30. Fujioka N, et al: Interleukin-18 protects mice against acute herpes simplex virus type 1 infection. J Virol *73*:2401, 1999.
31. Harandi AM, et al: Interleukin-12 (IL-12) and IL-18 are important in innate defense against genital herpes simplex virus type 2 infection in mice but are not required for the development of acquired gamma interferon–mediated protective immunity. J Virol *75*:6705, 2001.
32. Malmgaard L, et al: Herpes simplex virus type 2 induces secretion of IL-12 by macrophages through a mechanism involving NF-kappaB. J Gen Virol *81*:3011, 2000.
33. Kanangat S, et al: Herpes simplex virus type 1–mediated up-regulation of IL-12 (p40) mRNA expression. Implications in immunopathogenesis and protection. J Immunol *156*:1110, 1996.
34. Broberg EK, et al: Herpes simplex virus type 1 infection induces upregulation of interleukin-23 (p19) mRNA expression in trigeminal ganglia of BALB/c mice. J Interferon Cytokine Res *22*:641, 2002.
35. Trinchieri G: Interleukin-12 and the regulation of innate resistance and adaptive immunity. Nat Rev Immunol *3*:133, 2003.
36. Lankford CS, Frucht DM: A unique role for IL-23 in promoting cellular immunity. J Leukoc Biol *73*:49, 2003.

37. Rogge L, et al: Selective expression of an interleukin-12 receptor component by human T helper 1 cells. J Exp Med *185*:825, 1997.
38. Waldrop SL, et al: Determination of antigen-specific memory/effector CD4 T cell frequencies by flow cytometry: evidence for a novel, antigen-specific homeostatic mechanism in HIV-associated immunodeficiency. J Clin Invest *99*:1739, 1997.
39. Koelle DM, Corey L: Recent progress in herpes simplex virus immunobiology and vaccine research. Clin Microbiol Rev *16*:96, 2003.
40. Cleary AM, et al: Impaired accumulation and function of memory CD4 T cells in human IL-12 receptor beta 1 deficiency. J Immunol *170*:597, 2003.
41. Fieschi C, et al: Low penetrance, broad resistance, and favorable outcome of interleukin-12 receptor beta-1, deficiency: medical and immunological implications. J Exp Med *197*:527, 2003.
42. Osorio Y, et al: Reduced severity of HSV-1–induced corneal scarring in IL-12–deficient mice. Virus Res *90*:317, 2002.
43. Pollara G, et al: Herpes simplex virus infection of dendritic cells: balance among activation, inhibition, and immunity. J Infect Dis *187*:165, 2003.
44. Kumaraguru U, Rouse BT: The IL-12 response to herpes simplex virus is mainly a paracrine response of reactive inflammatory cells. J Leukoc Biol *72*:564, 2002.
45. Gosselin J, et al: Interleukin-15 as an activator of natural killer cell–mediated antiviral response. Blood *94*:4210, 1999.
46. Fawaz LM, et al: Up-regulation of NK cytotoxic activity via IL-15 induction by different viruses: a comparative study. J Immunol *163*:4473, 1999.
47. Tsunobuchi H, et al: A protective role of interleukin-15 in a mouse model for systemic infection with herpes simplex virus. Virology *275*:57, 2000.
48. Tumpey TM, et al: Absence of macrophage inflammatory protein-1alpha prevents the development of blinding herpes stromal keratitis. J Virol *72*:3705, 1998.
49. Oakes JE, et al: Induction of interleukin-8 gene expression is associated with herpes simplex virus infection of human corneal keratocytes but not human corneal epithelial cells. J Virol *67*:4777, 1993.
50. Miyazaki D, et al: Neutrophil chemotaxis induced by corneal epithelial cells after herpes simplex virus type 1 infection. Curr Eye Res *17*:687, 1998.
51. Rosler A, et al: Time course of chemokines in the cerebrospinal fluid and serum during herpes simplex type 1 encephalitis. J Neuro Sci *157*:82, 1998.
52. Lokensgard JR, et al: Glial cell responses to herpesvirus infections: role in defense and immunopathogenesis. J Infect Dis 186 Suppl 2:S171, 2002.
53. Melchjorsen J, et al: Herpes simplex virus selectively induces expression of the CC chemokine RANTES/CCL5 in macrophages through a mechanism dependent on PKR and ICP0. J Virol *76*:2780, 2002.
54. Nakajima H, et al: Monocyte chemoattractant protein-1 enhances HSV-induced encephalomyelitis by stimulating Th2 responses. J Leukoc Biol *70*:374, 2001.
55. Ikemoto K, et al: Small amounts of exogenous IL-4 increase the severity of encephalitis induced in mice by the intranasal infection of herpes simplex virus type 1. J Immunol *155*:1326, 1995.
56. Epstein J, et al: The collectins in innate immunity. Curr Opin Immunol *8*:29, 1996.
57. LeVine AM, et al: Surfactant protein-A enhances respiratory syncytial virus clearance in vivo. J Clin Invest *103*:1015, 1999.
58. LeVine AM, et al: Absence of SP-A modulates innate and adaptive defense responses to pulmonary influenza infection. Am J Physiol *282*:L563, 2002.
59. van Iwaarden JF, et al: Surfactant protein A is opsonin in phagocytosis of herpes simplex virus type 1 by rat alveolar macrophages. Am J Physiol *261*:L204, 1991.
60. van Iwaarden JF, et al: Binding of surfactant protein A (SP-A) to herpes simplex virus type 1-infected cells is mediated by the carbohydrate moiety of SP-A. J Biol Chem *267*:25039, 1992.
61. Weyer C, et al: Surfactant protein A binding to cytomegalovirus proteins enhances virus entry into rat lung cells. Am J Respir Cell Mol Biol *23*:71, 2000.
62. Shepherd VL: Distinct roles for lung collectins in pulmonary host defense. Am J Respir Cell Mol Biol *26*:257, 2002.
63. Heise MT, Virgin HWT: The T-cell–independent role of gamma interferon and tumor necrosis factor alpha in macrophage activation during murine cytomegalovirus and herpes simplex virus infections. J Virol *69*:904, 1995.
64. Feduchi E, et al: Human gamma interferon and tumor necrosis factor exert a synergistic blockade on the replication of herpes simplex virus. J Virol *63*:1354, 1989.
65. Baskin H, et al: Herpes simplex virus type 2 synergizes with interferon-gamma in the induction of nitric oxide production in mouse macrophages through autocrine secretion of tumour necrosis factor-alpha. J Gen Virol *78*:195, 1997.
66. Croen KD: Evidence for antiviral effect of nitric oxide. Inhibition of herpes simplex virus type 1 replication. J Clin Invest *91*:2446, 1993.
67. Paludan SR, Mogensen SC: Virus-cell interactions regulating induction of tumor necrosis factor alpha production in macrophages infected with herpes simplex virus. J Virol *75*:10170, 2001.
68. Sciammas R, et al: T cell receptor-gamma/delta cells protect mice from herpes simplex virus type 1–induced lethal encephalitis. J Exp Med *185*:1969, 1997.
69. Kodukula P, et al: Macrophage control of herpes simplex virus type 1 replication in the peripheral nervous system. J Immunol *162*:2895, 1999.
70. Cheng H, et al: Role of macrophages in restricting herpes simplex virus type 1 growth after ocular infection. Invest Ophthalmol Vis Sci *41*:1402, 2000.
71. MacLean A, et al: Mice lacking inducible nitric-oxide synthase are more susceptible to herpes simplex virus infection despite enhanced Th1 cell responses. J Gen Virol *79*:825, 1998.
72. Adler H, et al: Suppression of herpes simplex virus type 1 (HSV-1)–induced pneumonia in mice by inhibition of inducible nitric oxide synthase (iNOS, NOS2). J Exp Med *185*:1533, 1997.
73. Fujii S, et al: Role of nitric oxide in pathogenesis of herpes simplex virus encephalitis in rats. Virology *256*:203, 1999.
74. Fleck M, et al: Herpes simplex virus type 2 infection induced apoptosis in peritoneal macrophages independent of Fas and tumor necrosis factor-receptor signaling. Viral Immunol *12*:263, 1999.
75. Daniels CA, et al: Abortive and productive infections of human mononuclear phagocytes by type I herpes simplex virus. Am J Pathol *91*:119, 1978.
76. Bruun T, et al: Interaction of herpes simplex virus with mononuclear phagocytes is dependent on the differentiation stage of the cells. APMIS *106*:305, 1998.
77. Bruun T, et al: Herpes simplex virus type 1 inhibits in vitro differentiation and selected functions of human blood-derived monocytes. APMIS *106*:1194, 1998.
78. Mellman I, Steinman RM: Dendritic cells: specialized and regulated antigen processing machines. Cell *106*:255, 2001.
79. Banchereau J, et al: Immunobiology of dendritic cells. Ann Revu Immunol *18*:767, 2000.
80. Steinman RM, Inaba K: Myeloid dendritic cells. J Leukoc Biol *66*:205, 1999.
81. Liu YJ: Dendritic cell subsets and lineages, and their functions in innate and adaptive immunity. Cell *106*:259, 2001.
82. Sallusto F, Lanzavecchia A: Understanding dendritic cell and T-lymphocyte traffic through the analysis of chemokine receptor expression. Immunol Rev *177*:134, 2000.
83. Akira S, et al: Toll-like receptors: critical proteins linking innate and acquired immunity. Nat Immunol *2*:675, 2001.
84. Zhao X, et al: Vaginal submucosal dendritic cells, but not Langerhans cells, induce protective Th1 responses to herpes simplex virus-2. J Exp Med *197*:153, 2003.
85. Samady L, et al: Deletion of the virion host shutoff protein (vhs) from herpes simplex virus (HSV) relieves the viral block to dendritic cell activation: potential of vhs(-) HSV vectors for dendritic cell-mediated immunotherapy. J Virol *77*:3768, 2003.
86. Mikloska Z, et al: Immature monocyte-derived dendritic cells are productively infected with herpes simplex virus type 1. J Virol *75*:5958, 2001.
87. Kruse M, et al: Inhibition of CD83 cell surface expression during dendritic cell maturation by interference with nuclear export of CD83 mRNA. J Exp Med *191*:1581, 2000.
88. Kruse M, et al: Mature dendritic cells infected with herpes simplex virus type 1 exhibit inhibited T-cell stimulatory capacity. J Virol *74*:7127, 2000.
89. Ghanekar S, et al: Cytokine expression by human peripheral blood dendritic cells stimulated in vitro with HIV-1 and herpes simplex virus. J Immunol *157*:4028, 1996.
90. Mueller SN, et al: Rapid cytotoxic T lymphocyte activation occurs in the draining lymph nodes after cutaneous herpes simplex virus infection as a result of early antigen presentation and not the presence of virus. J Exp Med *195*:651, 2002.
91. Miller JS: The biology of natural killer cells in cancer, infection, and pregnancy. Exp Hematol *29*:1157, 2001.
92. Huard B, Fruh K: A role for MHC class I down-regulation in NK cell lysis of herpes virus–infected cells. Eur J of Immunol *30*:509, 2000.
93. Lanier LL: On guard—activating NK cell receptors. Nat Immunol *2*:23, 2001.
94. Vivier E, Biron CA: Immunology. A pathogen receptor on natural killer cells. Science *296*:1248, 2002.
95. Orange JS, et al: Viral evasion of natural killer cells. Nat Immunol *3*:1006, 2002.
96. Biron CA, et al: Severe herpesvirus infections in an adolescent without natural killer cells. N Eng J Med *320*:1731, 1989.
97. Habu S, et al: In vivo significance of NK cell on resistance against virus (HSV-1) infections in mice. J Immunol *133*:2743, 1984.
98. Rager-Zisman B, et al: Role of NK cells in protection of mice against herpes simplex virus-1 infection. J Immunol *138*:884, 1987.
99. Tanigawa M, et al: Natural killer cells prevent direct anterior-to-posterior spread of herpes simplex virus type 1 in the eye. Invest Ophthalmol Vis Sci *41*:132, 2000.
100. Tay CH, et al: NK cell response to viral infections in beta 2-microglobulin-deficient mice. J Immunol *154*:780, 1995.
101. Orange JS, et al: Requirement for natural killer cell–produced interferon gamma in defense against murine cytomegalovirus infection and enhancement of this defense pathway by interleukin-12 administration. J Exp Med *182*:1045, 1995.
102. Orange JS, Biron CA: Characterization of early IL-12, IFN-alpha/beta, and TNF effects on antiviral state and NK cell responses during murine cytomegalovirus infection. J Immunol *156*:4746, 1996.
103. Thimme R, et al: Determinants of viral clearance and persistence during acute hepatitis C virus infection. J Exp Med *194*:1395, 2001.
104. Thimme R, et al: CD8(+) T cells mediate viral clearance and disease pathogenesis during acute hepatitis B virus infection. J Virol *77*:68, 2003.
105. Biermer M, et al: Tumor necrosis factor alpha inhibition of hepatitis B virus replication involves disruption of capsid integrity through activation of NF-kappaB. J Virol *77*:4033, 2003.

106. Ho IC, Glimcher LH: Transcription: tantalizing times for T cells. Cell *109(Suppl)*:S109, 2002.

107. Burchett SK, et al: Diminished interferon-gamma and lymphocyte proliferation in neonatal and postpartum primary herpes simplex virus infection. J Infect Dis *165*:813, 1992.

108. Lafferty WE, et al: Alteration of lymphocyte transformation response to herpes simplex virus infection by acyclovir therapy. Antimicrob Agents Chemother *26*:887, 1984.

109. Whitley RJ: Herpes simplex virus. *In* Knipe DM, Howley PM (eds): Fields Virology, Philadelphia, Lippincott Williams & Wilkins, 2001, pp 2461–2509.

110. Schmid DS, Rouse BT: The role of T cell immunity in control of herpes simplex virus. Curr Topics Microbiol Immunol *179*:57, 1992.

111. Posavad CM, et al: Tipping the scales of herpes simplex virus reactivation: the important responses are local. Nat Med *4*:381, 1998.

112. Smith PM, et al: Control of acute cutaneous herpes simplex virus infection: T cell–mediated viral clearance is dependent upon interferon-gamma (IFN-gamma). Virology *202*:76, 1994.

113. Manickan E, Rouse BT: Roles of different T-cell subsets in control of herpes simplex virus infection determined by using T-cell deficient mouse-models. J Virol *69*:8178, 1995.

114. Milligan GN, Bernstein DI: Analysis of herpes simplex virus–specific T cells in the murine female genital tract following infection with herpes simplex virus type 2. Virology *212*:481, 1995.

115. Milligan GN, Bernstein DI: Interferon-gamma enhances resolution of herpes simplex virus type 2 infection of the murine genital tract. Virology *229*:259, 1997.

116. Rijksen G, et al: A new case of purine nucleotide phosphorylase deficiency: enzymologic, clinical, and immunologic characteristics. Pediatr Res *21*:137, 1987.

117. Asanuma H, et al: Frequencies of memory T cells specific for varicella-zoster virus, herpes simplex virus, and cytomegalovirus by intracellular detection of cytokine expression. J Infect Dis *181*:859, 2000.

118. Koelle DM, et al: Clearance of HSV-2 from recurrent genital lesions correlates with infiltration of HSV-specific cytotoxic T lymphocytes. J Clin Invest *101*:1500, 1998.

119. Koelle DM, et al: Expression of cutaneous lymphocyte-associated antigen by CD8(+) T cells specific for a skin-tropic virus. J Clin Invest *110*:537, 2002.

120. Koelle DM, et al: Antigen-specific T cells localize to the uterine cervix in women with genital herpes simplex virus type 2 infection. J Infect Dis *182*:662, 2000.

121. Koelle DM, et al: Tegument-specific, virus-reactive CD4 T cells localize to the cornea in herpes simplex virus interstitial keratitis in humans. J Virol *74*:10930, 2000.

122. Verjans GM, et al: Intraocular T cells of patients with herpes simplex virus (HSV)-induced acute retinal necrosis recognize HSV tegument proteins VP11/12 and VP13/14. J Infect Dis *182*:923, 2000.

123. Koelle DM, et al: CD4 T-cell responses to herpes simplex virus type 2 major capsid protein VP5: comparison with responses to tegument and envelope glycoproteins. J Virol *74*:11422, 2000.

124. Holterman AX, et al: An important role for major histocompatibility complex class I-restricted T cells, and a limited role for gamma interferon, in protection of mice against lethal herpes simplex virus infection. J Virol *73*:2058, 1999.

125. Ruby J, et al: CD40 ligand has potent antiviral activity. Nature Med *1*:437, 1995.

126. Mercadal CM, et al: Apparent requirement for CD4+ T cells in primary anti-herpes simplex virus cytotoxic T-lymphocyte induction can be overcome by optimal antigen presentation. Viral Immunol *4*:177, 1991.

127. Stohlman SA, et al: CTL effector function within the central nervous system requires CD4+ T cells. J Immunol *160*:2896, 1998.

128. Bennett SRM, et al: Help for the cytotoxic T-cell responses is mediated by CD40 signalling. Nature *393*:478, 1998.

129. Ridge JP, et al: A conditioned dendritic cell can be a temporal bridge between a CD4+ T-helper and a T-killer cell. Nature *393*:474, 1998.

130. Tigges MA, et al: Human herpes simplex virus (HSV)-specific CD8+ CTL clones recognize HSV-2-infected fibroblasts after treatment with IFN-gamma or when virion host shutoff functions are disabled. J Immunol *156*:3901, 1996.

131. Borysiewicz LK, Sissons JG: Cytotoxic T cells and human herpes virus infections. Curr Topics Microbiol Immunol *189*:123, 1994.

132. Koelle DM, et al: Direct recovery of herpes simplex virus (HSV)-specific T lymphocyte clones from recurrent genital HSV-2 lesions. J Infect Dis *169*:956, 1994.

133. Carmack MA, et al: T cell recognition and cytokine production elicited by common and type-specific glycoproteins of herpes simplex virus type 1 and type 2. J Infect Dis *174*:899, 1996.

134. Ashkar S, et al: Eta-1 (osteopontin): an early component of type-1 (cell-mediated) immunity. Science *287*:860, 2000.

135. Lekstrom-Himes JA, et al: Gamma interferon impedes the establishment of herpes simplex virus type 1 latent infection but has no impact on its maintenance or reactivation in mice. J Virol *74*:6680, 2000.

136. Yu Z, et al: Role of interferon-gamma in immunity to herpes simplex virus. J Leukoc Biol *60*:528, 1996.

137. Bouley DM, et al: Characterization of herpes simplex virus type-1 infection and herpetic stromal keratitis development in IFN-gamma knockout mice. J Immunol *155*:3964, 1995.

138. Minami M, et al: Role of IFN-gamma and tumor necrosis factor-alpha in herpes simplex virus type 1 infection. J Interferon Cytokine Res *22*:671, 2002.

139. Cantin E, et al: Role for gamma interferon in control of herpes simplex virus type 1 reactivation. J Virol *73*:3418, 1999.

140. Cantin E, et al: Gamma interferon (IFN-gamma) receptor null-mutant mice are more susceptible to herpes simplex virus type 1 infection than IFN-gamma ligand null-mutant mice. J Virol *73*:5196, 1999.

141. Han X, et al: Gender influences herpes simplex virus type 1 infection in normal and gamma interferon-mutant mice. J Virol *75*:3048, 2001.

142. Presti RM, et al: Novel cell type-specific antiviral mechanism of interferon gamma action in macrophages. J Exp Med *193*:483, 2001.

143. Maertzdorf J, et al: IL-17 expression in human herpetic stromal keratitis: modulatory effects on chemokine production by corneal fibroblasts. J Immunol *169*:5897, 2002.

144. van Kooten C, Banchereau J: CD40-CD40 ligand. J Leukoc Biol *67*:2, 2000.

145. Bourgeois C, et al: A role for CD40 expression on CD8+ T cells in the generation of CD8+ T cell memory. Science *297*:2060, 2002.

146. Brossart P, et al: Tumor necrosis factor alpha and CD40 ligand antagonize the inhibitory effects of interleukin 10 on T-cell stimulatory capacity of dendritic cells. Cancer Res *60*:4485, 2000.

147. Schonbeck U, Libby P: The CD40/CD154 receptor/ligand dyad. Cell Mol Life Sci *58*:4, 2001.

148. Edelmann KH, Wilson CB: Role of CD28/CD80–86 and CD40/CD154 co-stimulatory interactions in host defense to primary herpes simplex virus infection. J Virol *75*:612, 2001.

149. Ostrowski MA, et al: The role of CD4+ T cell help and CD40 ligand in the in vitro expansion of HIV-1-specific memory cytotoxic CD8+ T cell responses. J Immunol *165*:6133, 2000.

150. Schmid DS, Mawle AC: T cell responses to herpes simplex viruses in humans. Rev Infect Dis *13 Suppl 11*:946, 1991.

151. Yasukawa M, Zarling JM: Human cytotoxic T cell clones directed against herpes simplex virus-infected cells. III. Analysis of viral glycoproteins recognized by CTL clones by using recombinant herpes simplex viruses. J Immunol *134*:2679, 1985.

152. Mikloska Z, Cunningham AL: Herpes simplex virus type 1 glycoproteins gB, gC and gD are major targets for CD4 T-lymphocyte cytotoxicity in HLA-DR expressing human epidermal keratinocytes. J Gen Virol *79*:353, 1998.

153. Yasukawa M, et al: Fas-independent cytotoxicity mediated by human CD4+ CTL directed against herpes simplex virus-infected cells. J Immunol *162*:6100, 1999.

154. Posavad CM, et al: Severe genital herpes infections in HIV-infected individuals with impaired herpes simplex virus–specific CD8+ cytotoxic T lymphocyte responses. Proc Natl Acad Sci USA *94*:10289, 1997.

155. Maertzdorf J, et al: Restricted T cell receptor beta-chain variable region protein use by cornea-derived CD4+ and CD8+ herpes simplex virus-specific T cells in patients with herpetic stromal keratitis. J Infect Dis *187*:550, 2003.

156. Hata A, et al: Granulysin blocks replication of varicella-zoster virus and triggers apoptosis of infected cells. Viral Immunol *14*:125, 2001.

157. Callan MFC, et al: Direct visualization of antigen-specific CD8+ T cells during the primary immune response to Epstein-Barr virus in vivo. J Exp Med *187*:1395, 1998.

158. Walter EA, et al: Reconstitution of cellular immunity against cytomegalovirus in recipients of allogeneic bone marrow by transfer of T-cell clones from the donor. N Eng J Med *333*:1038, 1995.

159. Gahn B, et al: Immunotherapy to reconstitute immunity to DNA viruses. Semin Hematol *39*:41, 2002.

160. Simmons A, Tscharke DC: Anti-CD8 impairs clearance of herpes simplex virus from the nervous system: implications for the fate of virally infected neurons. J Exp Med *175*:1337, 1992.

161. Speck P, Simmons A: Precipitous clearance of herpes simplex virus antigens from the peripheral nervous systems of experimentally infected C57BL/10 mice. J Gen Virol *79*:561, 1998.

162. Liu T, et al: CD8(+) T cells can block herpes simplex virus type 1 (HSV-1) reactivation from latency in sensory neurons. J Exp Med *191*:1459, 2000.

163. Liu T, et al: Gamma interferon can prevent herpes simplex virus type 1 reactivation from latency in sensory neurons. J Virol *75*:11178, 2001.

164. Pereira RA, Simmons A: Cell surface expression of H2 antigens on primary sensory neurons in response to acute but not latent herpes simplex virus infection in vivo. J Virol *73*:6484, 1999.

165. Martz E, Gamble SR: How do CTL control virus infections? Evidence for pre-lytic halt of herpes simplex. Viral Immunol *5*:81, 1992.

166. Pereira RA, et al: Granzyme A, a noncytolytic component of CD8(+) cell granules, restricts the spread of herpes simplex virus in the peripheral nervous systems of experimentally infected mice. J Virol *74*:1029, 2000.

167. Chang E, et al: Pathogenesis of herpes simplex virus type 1–induced corneal inflammation in perforin-deficient mice. J Virol *74*:11832, 2000.

168. Hudson SJ, Streilein JW: Functional cytotoxic T cells are associated with focal lesions in the brains of SJL mice with experimental herpes simplex encephalitis. J Immunol *152*:5540, 1994.

169. Ploegh HL: Viral strategies of immune evasion. Science *280*:248, 1998.

170. Smith TJ, et al: Pathogenesis of herpes simplex virus type 2 virion host shutoff (vhs) mutants. J Virol *76*:2054, 2002.

171. Koelle DM, et al: Herpes simplex virus infection of human fibroblasts and keratinocytes inhibits recognition by cloned CD8+ cytotoxic T lymphocytes. J Clin Invest *91*:961, 1993.

172. Ahn K, et al: Molecular mechanism and species specificity of TAP inhibition by herpes simplex virus ICP47. EMBO J *15*:3247, 1996.
173. Hill A, et al: Herpes simplex virus turns off the TAP to evade host immunity. Nature *375*:411, 1995.
174. Tomazin R, et al: Herpes simplex virus type 2 ICP47 inhibits human TAP but not mouse TAP. J Virol *72*:2560, 1998.
175. Mikloska Z, et al: Herpes simplex virus protein targets for CD4 and CD8 lymphocyte cytotoxicity in cultured epidermal keratinocytes treated with interferon-gamma. J Infect Dis *173*:7, 1996.
176. Bonneau RH, et al: Epitope specificity of H-2Kb-restricted, HSV-1-, and HSV-2-cross-reactive cytotoxic T lymphocyte clones. Virology *195*:62, 1993.
177. Cose SC, et al: Characterization of a diverse primary herpes simplex virus type 1 gB-specific cytotoxic T-cell response showing a preferential Vbeta bias. J Virol *69*:5849, 1995.
178. Goldsmith K, et al: Infected cell protein (ICP)47 enhances herpes simplex virus neurovirulence by blocking the CD8+ T cell response. J Exp Med *187*:341, 1998.
179. Torpey DJ, et al: HLA-restricted lysis of herpes simplex virus–infected monocytes and macrophages mediated by CD4+ and CD8+ T lymphocytes. J Immunol *142*:1325, 1989.
180. Tigges MA, et al: Human CD8+ herpes simplex virus–specific cytotoxic T-lymphocyte clones recognize diverse virion protein antigens. J Virol *66*:1622, 1992.
181. Mikloska Z, et al: Monophosphoryl lipid A and QS21 increase CD8 T lymphocyte cytotoxicity to herpes simplex virus-2 infected cell proteins 4 and 27 through IFN-gamma and IL-12 production. J Immunol *164*:5167, 2000.
182. Koelle DM, et al: CD8 CTL from genital herpes simplex lesions: recognition of viral tegument and immediate early proteins and lysis of infected cutaneous cells. J Immunol *166*:4049, 2001.
183. Mocarski ES Jr: Immunomodulation by cytomegaloviruses: manipulative strategies beyond evasion. Trends Microbiol *10*:332, 2002.
184. Lewandowski GA, et al: Interference with major histocompatibility complex class II-restricted antigen presentation in the brain by herpes simplex virus type 1: a possible mechanism of evasion of the immune response. Proc Natl Acad Sci U S A *90*:2005, 1993.
185. Thebeau LG, Morrison LA: B7 co-stimulation plays an important role in protection from herpes simplex virus type 2-mediated pathology. J Virol *76*:2563, 2002.
186. Thebeau LG, Morrison LA: Mechanism of reduced T-cell effector functions and class-switched antibody responses to herpes simplex virus type 2 in the absence of B7 co-stimulation. J Virol *77*:2426, 2003.
187. Nansen A, et al: CCR2+ and CCR5+ CD8+ T cells increase during viral infection and migrate to sites of infection. Eur J Immunol *30*:1797, 2000.
188. Kaufmann SH: Gamma/delta and other unconventional T lymphocytes: what do they see and what do they do? Proc Natl Acad Sci U S A *93*:2272, 1996.
189. Bukowski JF, et al: Recognition and destruction of virus-infected cells by human gamma delta CTL. J Immunol *153*:5133, 1994.
190. Ohteki T, et al: Role for IL-15/IL-15 receptor beta-chain in natural killer 1.1+ T cell receptor–alpha beta+ cell development. J Immunol *159*:5931, 1997.
191. Godfrey DI, et al: NK T cells: facts, functions and fallacies. Immunol Today *21*:573, 2000.
192. Nieda M, et al: TRAIL expression by activated human CD4(+)Valpha24 NK T cells induces in vitro and in vivo apoptosis of human acute myeloid leukemia cells. Blood *97*:2067, 2001.
193. Kronenberg M, Gapin L: The unconventional lifestyle of NK T cells. Nat Rev Immunol *2*:557, 2002.
194. Grubor-Bauk B, et al: Impaired clearance of herpes simplex virus type 1 from mice lacking CD1d or NKT cells expressing the semivariant V alpha 14-J alpha 281 TCR. J Immunol *170*:1430, 2003.
195. Sanna PP, Burton DR: Role of antibodies in controlling viral disease: lessons from experiments of nature and gene knockouts. J Virol *74*:9813, 2000.
196. Deshpande SP, et al: Dual role of B cells in mediating innate and acquired immunity to herpes simplex virus infections. Cell Immunol *202*:79, 2000.
197. Harandi AM, et al: Differential roles of B cells and IFN-gamma-secreting CD4(+) T cells in innate and adaptive immune control of genital herpes simplex virus type 2 infection in mice. J Gen Virol *82*:845, 2001.
198. Westra DF, et al: Natural infection with herpes simplex virus type 1 (HSV-1) induces humoral and T cell responses to the HSV-1 glycoprotein H:L complex. J Gen Virol *81*:2011, 2000.
199. Da Costa XJ, et al: Humoral response to herpes simplex virus is complement-dependent. Proc Natl Acad Sci U S A *96*:12708, 1999.
200. Frank MM: The complement system in host defense and inflammation. Rev Infect Dis *1*:483, 1979.
201. Gollins SW, Porterfield JS: A new mechanism for the neutralization of enveloped viruses by antiviral antibody. Nature *321*:244, 1986.
202. Perrin LH, et al: Mechanism of injury of virus-infected cells by antiviral antibody and complement: participation of IgG, F(ab′)2, and the alternative complement pathway. J Exp Med *143*:1027, 1976.
203. Courtney RJ: Virus-specific components of herpes simplex virus involved in the immune response. *In* Rouse BT, Lopez C (eds): Immunobiology of Herpes Simplex Virus Infection. Boca Raton, FL, CRC Press, 1984, pp 33–44.
204. Sissons JG, Oldstone MB: Antibody-mediated destruction of virus-infected cells. Adv Immunol *29*:209, 1980.
205. Figueroa JE, Densen P: Infectious diseases associated with complement deficiencies. Clin Microbiol Rev *4*:359, 1991.
206. McKendall RR: IgG-mediated viral clearance in experimental infection with herpes simplex virus type 1: role for neutralization and Fc-dependent functions but not C′ cytolysis and C5 chemotaxis. J Infect Dis *151*:464, 1985.
207. Shore SL, et al: Antibody-dependent cell-mediated cytotoxicity to target cells infected with herpes simplex viruses. Adv Exp Med Biol *73*:217, 1976.
208. Kohl S, et al: Human monocyte-macrophage–mediated antibody-dependent cytotoxicity to herpes simplex virus–infected cells. J Immunol *118*:729, 1977.
209. Moller-Larsen A, et al: Cell-mediated cytotoxicity to herpes-infected cells in humans: dependence on antibodies. Infect Immun *16*:43, 1977.
210. Petroni KC, et al: Modulation of human polymorphonuclear leukocyte IgG Fc receptors and Fc receptor–mediated functions by IFN-γ and glucocorticoids. J Immunol *140*:3467, 1988.
211. Lin SJ, et al: Effect of interleukin (IL)-12 and IL-15 on activated natural killer (ANK) and antibody-dependent cellular cytotoxicity (ADCC) in HIV infection. J Clin Immunol *18*:335, 1998.
212. Poaty-Mavoungou V, et al: Enhancement of natural killer cell activation and antibody-dependent cellular cytotoxicity by interferon-alpha and interleukin-12 in vaginal mucosae Sivmac251–infected *Macaca fascicularis*. Viral Immunol *15*:197, 2002.
213. Fries LF, et al: Glycoprotein C of herpes simplex virus 1 is an inhibitor of the complement cascade. J Immunol *137*:1636, 1986.
214. Lubinski J, et al: In vivo role of complement-interacting domains of herpes simplex virus type 1 glycoprotein gC. J Exp Med *190*:1637, 1999.
215. Johnson DC, et al: Herpes simplex virus immunoglobulin G Fc receptor activity depends on a complex of two viral glycoproteins, gE and gI. J Virol *62*:1347, 1988.
216. Ray CG: The ontogeny of interferon production by human leukocytes. J Pediatr *76*:94, 1970.
217. Cederblad B, et al: Deficient herpes simplex virus–induced interferon-alpha production by blood leukocytes of preterm and term newborn infants. Pediatr Res *27*:7, 1990.
218. Lee SM, et al: Decreased interleukin-12 (IL-12) from activated cord versus adult peripheral blood mononuclear cells and upregulation of interferon-gamma, natural killer, and lymphokine-activated killer activity by IL-12 in cord blood mononuclear cells. Blood *88*:945, 1996.
219. Qian JX, et al: Decreased interleukin-15 from activated cord versus adult peripheral blood mononuclear cells and the effect of interleukin-15 in upregulating antitumor immune activity and cytokine production in cord blood. Blood *90*:3106, 1997.
220. Scott ME, et al: High level interleukin-12 production, but diminished interferon-gamma production, by cord blood mononuclear cells. Pediatr Res *41*:547, 1997.
221. Perez-Melgosa M, et al: Carrier-mediated enhancement of cognate T cell help: the basis for enhanced immunogenicity of meningococcal outer membrane protein polysaccharide conjugate vaccine. Eur J Immunol *31*:2373, 2001.
222. Varis I, et al: Expression of HLA-DR, CAM and co-stimulatory molecules on cord blood monocytes. Eur J Haematol *66*:107, 2001.
223. Toivanen P, et al: Development of mitogen responding T cells and natural killer cells in the human fetus. Immunol Rev *57*:89, 1981.
224. Lubens RG, et al: Lectin-dependent T-lymphocyte and natural killer cytotoxic deficiencies in human newborns. Cell Immunol *74*:40, 1982.
225. Tarkkanen J, Saksela E: Umbilical-cord-blood–derived suppressor cells of the human natural killer cell activity are inhibited by interferon. Scand J Immunol *15*:149, 1982.
226. Ueno Y, et al: Differential effects of recombinant human interferon-gamma and interleukin 2 on natural killer cell activity of peripheral blood in early human development. J Immunol *135*:180, 1985.
227. Seki H, et al: Mode of in vitro augmentation of natural killer cell activity by recombinant human interleukin 2: a comparative study of Leu-11+ and Leu-11– cell populations in cord blood and adult peripheral blood. J Immunol *135*:2351, 1985.
228. Baley JE, Schacter BZ: Mechanisms of diminished natural killer cell activity in pregnant women and neonates. J Immunol *134*:3042, 1985.
229. Nair MP, et al: Association of decreased natural and antibody-dependent cellular cytotoxicity and production of natural killer cytotoxic factor and interferon in neonates. Cell Immunol *94*:159, 1985.
230. Kaplan J, et al: Human newborns are deficient in natural killer activity. J Clin Immunol *2*:350, 1982.
231. Sancho L, et al: Two different maturational stages of natural killer lymphocytes in human newborn infants. J Pediatr *119*:446, 1991.
232. McDonald T, et al: Natural killer cell activity in very low birth weight infants. Pediatr Res *31*:376, 1992.
233. Phillips JH, et al: Ontogeny of human natural killer NK cells: fetal NK cells mediate cytolytic function and express cytoplasmic CD3 epsilon,delta proteins. J Exp Med *175*:1055, 1992.
234. Georgeson GD, et al: Natural killer cell cytotoxicity is deficient in newborns with sepsis and recurrent infections. Eur J Pediatr *160*:478, 2001.
235. Cicuttini FM, et al: A novel population of natural killer progenitor cells isolated from human umbilical cord blood. J Immunol *151*:29, 1993.
236. Webb BJ, et al: The lack of NK cytotoxicity associated with fresh HUCB may be due to the presence of soluble HLA in the serum. Cell Immunol *159*:246, 1994.
237. Harrison CJ, Waner JL: Natural killer cell activity in infants and children excreting cytomegalovirus. J Infect Dis *151*:301, 1985.

238. Jenkins M, et al: Natural killer cytotoxicity and antibody-dependent cellular cytotoxicity of human immunodeficiency virus–infected cells by leukocytes from human neonates and adults. Pediatr Res *33*:469, 1993.

239. Merrill JD, et al: Characterization of natural killer and antibody-dependent cellular cytotoxicity of preterm infants against human immunodeficiency virus–infected cells. Pediatr Res *40*:498, 1996.

240. Kohl S, et al: Adhesion defects of antibody-mediated target cell binding of neonatal natural killer cells. Pediatr Res *46*:755, 1999.

241. Brahmi Z, et al: NK cells recover early and mediate cytotoxicity via perforin/granzyme and Fas/FasL pathways in umbilical cord blood recipients. Hum Immunol *62*:782, 2001.

242. Lau AS, et al: Interleukin-12 induces interferon-γ expression and natural killer cytotoxicity in cord blood mononuclear cells. Pediatr Res *39*:150, 1996.

243. Nguyen QH, et al: Interleukin (IL)-15 enhances antibody-dependent cellular cytotoxicity and natural killer activity in neonatal cells. Cell Immunol *185*:83, 1998.

244. Kohl S: Human neonatal natural killer cell cytotoxicity function. Pediatr Infect Dis J *18*:635, 1999.

245. Han P, et al: Phenotypic analysis of functional T-lymphocyte subtypes and natural killer cells in human cord blood: relevance to umbilical cord blood transplantation. Br J Haematol *89*:733, 1995.

246. Lin SJ, et al: The effect of interleukin-12 and interleukin-15 on CD69 expression of T-lymphocytes and natural killer cells from umbilical cord blood. Biol Neonate *78*:181, 2000.

247. Harris DT: In vitro and in vivo assessment of the graft-versus-leukemia activity of cord blood. Bone Marrow Transplant *15*:17, 1995.

248. Keever CA, et al: Characterization of the alloreactivity and anti-leukemia reactivity of cord blood mononuclear cells. Bone Marrow Transplant *15*:407, 1995.

249. Gaddy J, et al: Cord blood natural killer cells are functionally and phenotypically immature but readily respond to interleukin-2 and interleukin-12. J Interferon Cytokine Res *15*:527, 1995.

250. Umemoto M, et al: Two cytotoxic pathways of natural killer cells in human cord blood: implications in cord blood transplantation. Br J Haematol *98*:1037, 1997.

251. Gaddy J, Broxmeyer HE: Cord blood CD16+56– cells with low lytic activity are possible precursors of mature natural killer cells. Cell Immunol *180*:132, 1997.

252. Condiotti R, Nagler A: Effect of interleukin-12 on antitumor activity of human umbilical cord blood and bone marrow cytotoxic cells. Exp Hematol *26*:571, 1998.

253. Lin SJ, et al: Effect of interleukin-15 and Flt3-ligand on natural killer cell expansion and activation: umbilical cord vs. adult peripheral blood mononuclear cells. Pediatr Allergy Immunol *11*:168, 2000.

254. Nomura A, et al: Functional analyses of cord blood natural killer cells and T cells: a distinctive interleukin-18 response. Exp Hematol *29*:1169, 2001.

255. Malygin AM, Timonen T: Non-major histocompatibility complex–restricted killer cells in human cord blood: generation and cytotoxic activity in recombinant interleukin-2–supplemented cultures. Immunology *79*:506, 1993.

256. Hayward AR, et al: Herpes simplex virus–stimulated interferon-gamma production by newborn mononuclear cells. Pediatr Res *20*:398, 1986.

257. Krampera M, et al: Intracellular cytokine profile of cord blood T-, and NK-cells and monocytes. Haematologica *85*:675, 2000.

258. Kohl S: Protection against murine neonatal herpes simplex virus infection by lymphokine-treated human leukocytes. J Immunol *144*:307, 1990.

259. Sullender WM, et al: Humoral and cell-mediated immunity in neonates with herpes simplex virus infection. J Infect Dis *155*:28, 1987.

260. Tu W, et al: Persistent deficiency of CD4 T cell immunity to cytomegalovirus in immunocompetent young children (submitted for publication).

261. Chen S, et al: Antiviral CD8 T cells in the control of primary cytomegalovirus infection in early childhood (submitted for publication).

262. Vekemans J, et al: T cell responses to vaccines in infants: defective interferon-gamma production after oral polio vaccination. Clin Exp Immunol *127*:495, 2002.

263. Jain A, et al: Defects of T-cell effector function and post-thymic maturation in X-linked hyper-IgM syndrome. J Clin Invest *103*:1151, 1999.

264. Hayward AR, et al: Specific immunity after congenital or neonatal infection with cytomegalovirus or herpes simplex virus. J Immunol *133*:2469, 1984.

265. Garderet L, et al: The umbilical cord blood alpha/beta T-cell repertoire: characteristics of a polyclonal and naive but completely formed repertoire. Blood *91*:340, 1998.

266. Kou ZC, et al: T-Cell receptor Vbeta repertoire CDR3 length diversity differs within CD45RA and CD45RO T-cell subsets in healthy and human immunodeficiency virus-infected children. Clin Diagn Lab Immunol *7*:953, 2000.

267. van den Beemed R, et al: Flow cytometric analysis of the Vbeta repertoire in healthy controls. Cytometry *40*:336, 2000.

268. Risdon G, et al: Alloantigen priming induces a state of unresponsiveness in human umbilical cord blood T cells. Proc Natl Acad Sci U S A *92*:2413, 1995.

269. Takahashi N, et al: Evidence for immunologic immaturity of cord blood T cells. Cord blood T cells are susceptible to tolerance induction to in vitro stimulation with a superantigen. J Immunol *155*:5213, 1995.

270. Imanishi K, et al: Post-thymic maturation of migrating human thymic single-positive T cells: thymic CD1a– CD4+ T cells are more susceptible to anergy induction by toxic shock syndrome toxin-1 than cord blood CD4+ T cells. J Immunol *160*:112, 1998.

271. Porcu P, et al: Alloantigen-induced unresponsiveness in cord blood T lymphocytes is associated with defective activation of Ras. Proc Natl Acad Sci U S A *95*:4538, 1998.

272. Takahashi N, et al: Immunopathophysiological aspects of an emerging neonatal infectious disease induced by a bacterial superantigen. J Clin Invest *106*:1409, 2000.

273. Clerici M, et al: Analysis of T helper and antigen-presenting cell functions in cord blood and peripheral blood leukocytes from healthy children of different ages. J Clin Invest *91*:2829, 1993.

274. Hayward AR, et al: Herpes simplex virus interferes with monocyte accessory cell function. J Immunol *150*:190, 1993.

275. Barcy S, Corey L: Herpes simplex inhibits the capacity of lymphoblastoid B cell lines to stimulate CD4+ T cells. J Immunol *166*:6242, 2001.

276. Hunt DW, et al: Studies of human cord blood dendritic cells: evidence for functional immaturity. Blood *84*:4333, 1994.

277. Petty RE, Hunt DW: Neonatal dendritic cells. Vaccine *16*:1378, 1998.

278. Borras FE, et al: Identification of both myeloid CD11c+ and lymphoid CD11c– dendritic cell subsets in cord blood. Br J Haematol *113*:925, 2001.

279. Goriely S, et al: Deficient IL-12 (p35) gene expression by dendritic cells derived from neonatal monocytes. J Immunol *166*:2141, 2001.

280. Dabbagh K, et al: Toll-like receptor 4 is required for optimal development of Th2 immune responses: role of dendritic cells. J Immunol *168*:4524, 2002.

281. Brugnoni D, et al: Ineffective expression of CD40 ligand on cord blood T cells may contribute to poor immunoglobulin production in the newborn. Eur J Immunol *24*:1919, 1994.

282. Fuleihan R, et al: Decreased expression of the ligand for CD40 in newborn lymphocytes. Eur J Immunol *24*:1925, 1994.

283. Durandy A, et al: Undetectable CD40 ligand expression on T cells and low B cell responses to CD40 binding agonists in human newborns. J Immunol *154*:1560, 1995.

284. Nonoyama S, et al: Diminished expression of CD40 ligand by activated neonatal T cells. J Clin Invest *95*:66, 1995.

285. Sato K, et al: Aberrant CD3- and CD28-mediated signaling events in cord blood T cells are associated with dysfunctional regulation of Fas ligand-mediated cytotoxicity. J Immunol *162*:4464, 1999.

286. Jullien P, Lewis DB: Decreased CD154 expression by neonatal CD4 T cells is due to limitations in both proximal and distal T cell activation events (submitted for publication).

287. Splawski JB, et al: CD40 ligand is expressed and functional on activated neonatal T cells. J Immunol *156*:119, 1996.

288. Reen DJ: Activation and functional capacity of human neonatal CD4 T-cells. Vaccine *16*:1401, 1998.

289. Matthews NC, et al: Sustained expression of CD154 (CD40L) and proinflammatory cytokine production by alloantigen-stimulated umbilical cord blood T cells. J Immunol *164*:6206, 2000.

290. Ohshima Y, Delespesse G: T cell–derived IL-4 and dendritic cell–derived IL-12 regulate the lymphokine-producing phenotype of alloantigen-primed naive human CD4 T cells. J Immunol *158*:629, 1997.

291. Chen L, Lewis DB: Reduced CD40 ligand expression by neonatal CD4 T cells after stimulation by allogeneic dendritic cells (submitted for publication).

292. Lewis DB, et al: Restricted production of interleukin 4 by activated human T cells. Proc Natl Acad Sci U S A *85*:9743, 1988.

293. Lewis DB, et al: Cellular and molecular mechanisms for reduced interleukin 4 and interferon-gamma production by neonatal T cells. J Clin Invest *87*:194, 1991.

294. Demeure CE, et al: In vitro maturation of human neonatal CD4 T lymphocytes. II. Cytokines present at priming modulate the development of lymphokine production. J Immunol *152*:4775, 1994.

295. Sornasse T, et al: Differentiation and stability of T helper 1 and 2 cells derived from naive human neonatal CD4+ T cells, analyzed at the single-cell level. J Exp Med *184*:473, 1996.

296. Delespesse G, et al: Maturation of human neonatal CD4+ and CD8+ T lymphocytes into Th1/Th2 effectors. Vaccine *16*:1415, 1998.

297. Upham JW, et al: Development of interleukin-12–producing capacity throughout infancy. Infect Immun *70*:6583, 2002.

298. Kadereit S, et al: Reduced NFAT1 protein expression in human umbilical cord blood T lymphocytes. Blood *94*:3101, 1999.

299. Kiani A, et al: Regulation of interferon-gamma gene expression by nuclear factor of activated T cells. Blood *98*:1480, 2001.

300. White GP, et al: Differential patterns of methylation of the IFN-gamma promoter at CpG and non-CpG sites underlie differences in IFN-gamma gene expression between human neonatal and adult CD45RO– T cells. J Immunol *168*:2820, 2002.

301. Ehlers S, Smith KA: Differentiation of T cell lymphokine gene expression: the in vitro acquisition of T cell memory. J Exp Med *173*:25, 1991.

302. Pirenne H, et al: Comparison of T cell functional changes during childhood with the ontogeny of CDw29 and CD45RA expression on CD4+ T cells. Pediatr Res *32*:81, 1992.

303. Clement LT: Isoforms of the CD45 common leukocyte antigen family: markers for human T-cell differentiation. J Clin Immunol *12*:1, 1992.

304. Hayward A, Cosyns M: Proliferative and cytokine responses by human newborn T cells stimulated with staphylococcal enterotoxin B. Pediatr Res *35*:293, 1994.

305. Campbell AC, et al: Lymphocyte subpopulations in the blood of newborn infants. Clin Exp Immunol *18*:469, 1974.

306. Andersson U, et al: Humoral and cellular immunity in humans studied at the cell level from birth to two years of age. Immunol Rev *57*:1, 1981.
307. Rayfield LS, et al: Development of cell-mediated lympholysis in human foetal blood lymphocytes. Clin Exp Immunol *42*:561, 1980.
308. Granberg C, Hirvonen T: Cell-mediated lympholysis by fetal and neonatal lymphocytes in sheep and man. Cell Immunol *51*:13, 1980.
309. Risdon G, et al: Allogeneic responses of human umbilical cord blood. Blood Cells *20*:566, 1994.
310. Barbey C, et al: Characterisation of the cytotoxic alloresponse of cord blood. Bone Marrow Transplant *22 (Suppl 1)*:S26, 1998.
311. Slavcev A, et al: Alloresponses of cord blood cells in primary mixed lymphocyte cultures. Hum Immunol *63*:155, 2002.
312. Appay V, et al: Memory CD8+ T cells vary in differentiation phenotype in different persistent virus infections. Nat Med *8*:379, 2002.
313. de-Jong R, et al: Human CD8+ T lymphocytes can be divided into CD45RA+ and CD45RO+ cells with different requirements for activation and differentiation. J Immunol *146*:2088, 1991.
314. Akbar AN, et al: Human CD4+CD45RO+ and CD4+CD45RA+ T cells synergize in response to alloantigens. Eur J Immunol *21*:2517, 1991.
315. Mescher MF: Molecular interactions in the activation of effector and precursor cytotoxic T lymphocytes. Immunol Rev *146*:177, 1995.
316. Hamann D, et al: Phenotypic and functional separation of memory and effector human CD8+ T cells. J Exp Med *186*:1407, 1997.
317. Berthou C, et al: Cord blood T lymphocytes lack constitutive perforin expression in contrast to adult peripheral blood T lymphocytes. Blood *85*:1540, 1995.
318. Kogawa K, et al: Perforin expression in cytotoxic lymphocytes from patients with hemophagocytic lymphohistiocytosis and their family members. Blood *99*:61, 2002.
319. Rukavina D, Podack ER: Abundant perforin expression at the maternal-fetal interface: semiallogeneic transplant? Immunol Today *21*:160, 2000.
320. Luzuriaga K, et al: HIV-1-specific cytotoxic T lymphocyte responses in the first year of life. J Immunol *154*:433, 1995.
321. Brander C, et al: Persistent HIV-1-specific CTL clonal expansion despite high viral burden post in utero HIV-1 infection. J Immunol *162*:4796, 1999.
322. Buseyne F, et al: Early HIV-specific cytotoxic T lymphocytes and disease progression in children born to HIV-infected mothers. AIDS Res Hum Retroviruses *14*:1435, 1998.
323. Pikora CA, et al: Early HIV-1 envelope–specific cytotoxic T lymphocyte responses in vertically infected infants. J Exp Med *185*:1153, 1997.
324. Buseyne F, et al: Early HIV-specific cell-mediated cytotoxicity in the peripheral blood from infected children. J Immunol *150*:3569, 1993.
325. Scott ZA, et al: Infrequent detection of HIV-1–specific, but not cytomegalovirus-specific, CD8(+) T cell responses in young HIV-1-infected infants. J Immunol *167*:7134, 2001.
326. Luzuriaga K, et al: Early therapy of vertical human immunodeficiency virus type 1 (HIV-1) infection: control of viral replication and absence of persistent HIV-1–specific immune responses. J Virol *74*:6984, 2000.
327. Chiba Y, et al: Development of cell-mediated cytotoxic immunity to respiratory syncytial virus in human infants following naturally acquired infection. J Med Virol *28*:133, 1989.
328. Stumptner-Cuvelette P, et al: HIV-1 Nef impairs MHC class II antigen presentation and surface expression. Proc Natl Acad Sci U S A *98*:12144, 2001.
329. Nielsen SD, et al: Impaired progenitor cell function in HIV-negative infants of HIV-positive mothers results in decreased thymic output and low CD4 counts. Blood *98*:398, 2001.
330. Badley AD, et al: Mechanisms of HIV-associated lymphocyte apoptosis. Blood *96*:2951, 2000.
331. Chougnet C, et al: Influence of human immunodeficiency virus–infected maternal development of infant interleukin-12 production. J Infect Dis *181*:1590, 2000.
332. Cayabyab M, et al: CD40 preferentially co-stimulates activation of CD4+ T lymphocytes. J Immunol *152*:1523, 1994.
333. Hassan J, Reen DJ: Cord blood CD4+ CD45RA+ T cells achieve a lower magnitude of activation when compared with their adult counterparts. Immunology *90*:397, 1997.
334. Berkowitz RD, et al: CXCR4 and CCR5 expression delineates targets for HIV-1 disruption of T cell differentiation. J Immunol *161*:3702, 1998.
335. Sato K, et al: Chemokine receptor expressions and responsiveness of cord blood T cells. J Immunol *166*:1659, 2001.
336. Christopherson K 2nd, et al: Regulation of naive fetal T-cell migration by the chemokines Exodus-2 and Exodus-3. Immunol Lett *69*:269, 1999.
337. Mo H, et al: Expression patterns of the HIV type 1 coreceptors CCR5 and cells and monocytes from cord and adult blood. AIDS Res Hum Retroviruses *14*:607, 1998.
338. Bonecchi R, et al: Differential expression of chemokine receptors and chemotactic responsiveness of type 1 T helper cells (Th1s) and Th2s. J Exp Med *187*:129, 1998.
339. Fraticelli P, et al: Fractalkine (CX3CL1) as an amplification circuit of polarized Th1 responses. J Clin Invest *107*:1173, 2001.
340. Soares MV, et al: IL-7-dependent extrathymic expansion of CD45RA+ T cells enables preservation of a naive repertoire. J Immunol *161*:5909, 1998.
341. Hassan J, Reen DJ: Human recent thymic emigrants—identification, expansion, and survival characteristics. J Immunol *167*:1970, 2001.
342. El Ghalbzouri A, et al: An in vitro model of allogeneic stimulation of cord blood: induction of Fas independent apoptosis. Hum Immunol *60*:598, 1999.
343. Tu W, et al: Insulin-like growth factor 1 promotes cord blood T cell maturation and inhibits its spontaneous and phytohemagglutinin-induced apoptosis through different mechanisms. J Immunol *165*:1331, 2000.
344. Aggarwal S, et al: Programmed cell death (apoptosis) in cord blood lymphocytes. J Clin Immunol *17*:63, 1997.
345. Yang YC, et al: Tumour necrosis factor-alpha–induced apoptosis in cord blood T lymphocytes: involvement of both tumour necrosis factor receptor types 1 and 2. Br J Haematol *115*:435, 2001.
346. Tsuyuguchi I, et al: Increase of T-cell receptor gamma/delta-bearing T cells in cord blood of newborn babies obtained by in vitro stimulation with mycobacterial cord factor. Infect Immun *59*:3053, 1991.
347. Smith MD, et al: T gamma delta-cell subsets in cord and adult blood. Scand J Immunol *32*:491, 1990.
348. Musha N, et al: Expansion of CD56+ NK T and gamma delta T cells from cord blood of human neonates. Clin Exp Immunol *113*:220, 1998.
349. D'Andrea A, et al: Neonatal invariant Valpha24+ NKT lymphocytes are activated memory cells. Eur J Immunol *30*:1544, 2000.
350. Gansuvd B, et al: Human umbilical cord blood NK T cells kill tumors by multiple cytotoxic mechanisms. Hum Immunol *63*:164, 2002.
351. Osuga T, et al: Transfer of specific IgG and IgG subclasses to herpes simplex virus across the blood-brain barrier and placenta in preterm and term newborns. Acta Paediatrica *81*:792, 1992.
352. Ashley RL, et al: Herpes simplex virus-2 (HSV-2) type-specific antibody correlates of protection in infants exposed to HSV-2 at birth. J Clin Invest *90*:511, 1992.
353. Mikloska Z, et al: Neutralizing antibodies inhibit axonal spread of herpes simplex virus type 1 to epidermal cells in vitro. J Virol *73*:5934, 1999.
354. Vollstedt S, et al: Interleukin-12- and gamma interferon–dependent innate immunity are essential and sufficient for long-term survival of passively immunized mice infected with herpes simplex virus type 1. J Virol *75*:9596, 2001.
355. Burioni R, et al: Recombinant human Fab to glycoprotein D neutralizes infectivity and prevents cell-to-cell transmission of herpes simplex viruses 1 and 2 in vitro. Proc Natl Acad Sci U S A *91*:355, 1994.
356. Cohen J: IL-12 deaths: explanation and a puzzle. Science *270*:908, 1995.
357. Straus SE, et al: Immunotherapy of recurrent genital herpes with recombinant herpes simplex virus type 2 glycoproteins D and B: results of a placebo-controlled vaccine trial. J Infect Dis *176*:1129, 1997.
358. Corey L, et al: Recombinant glycoprotein vaccine for the prevention of genital HSV-2 infection: two randomized controlled trials. Chiron HSV Vaccine Study Group. JAMA *282*:331, 1999.
359. Stanberry LR, et al: Glycoprotein-D-adjuvant vaccine to prevent genital herpes. N Engl J Med *347*:1652, 2002.
360. Kohl S, et al: Limited antibody-dependent cellular cytotoxicity antibody response induced by a herpes simplex virus type 2 subunit vaccine. J Infect Dis *181*:335, 2000.
361. Whitley RJ, Roizman B: Herpes simplex viruses: is a vaccine tenable? J Clin Invest *110*:145, 2002.

154 T-Cell Development

THYMUS AND THE EMBRYOLOGY OF T CELLS

The thymus is the principal and perhaps the only site where T cells develop. It also determines the initial range of potential antigens that can be recognized by the T-cell population in a given individual. The human thymus originates as an epithelial outgrowth from the third and fourth pharyngeal pouches between the sixth and seventh weeks of gestation. It grows caudally into the mediastinum as two elongated structures that fuse at midlevel at about the eighth week of gestation.[1] The process of T-cell differentiation has been studied mainly in rodents. In mice, the epithelial component of the thymus completes migration by day 10 of the 19- to 21-day gestation period, and lymphoid cells appear on day 11.[2] By days 12 to 13, these T-lymphocyte precursors are proliferating, and by day 14, their surface phenotype shows that they have committed to the T-cell lineage. Further maturation of these precursors occurs over the following week, resulting in the development of distinct corticomedullary demarcation by the time of birth. The first wave of differentiation from precursors to mature T cells requires about 7 days in humans as well.

Stem Cells and Colonization of the Thymus

In mammals, lymphocytes, myelocytes, and erythrocytes share a common stem cell. These multipotent precursors are present in the yolk sac during early embryonic life; are subsequently found in the fetal liver; and ultimately locate in the marrow, where they continue to seed the thymus throughout adult life. Hematopoietic stem cells have high levels of CD34 on the cell surface, but they lack lineage-specific antigens such as the lymphocyte-specific CD52 molecule and the CD3, CD4, and CD8 molecules that are restricted in expression primarily to thymocytes and mature T cells. Table 154–1 summarizes the relevant CD antigen designations. The characterization of T-cell precursors has become important in relation to attempts at gene therapy. The least mature precursor cells in the marrow are normally resting and are triggered to divide by stem cell factor (SCF) and interleukin-3 (IL-3).[3] These and other cytokines important in T cell development are shown in Table 154–2. A family of Ikaros proteins, required for the differentiation of lymphoid precursors[4] in the bone marrow and thymus, regulates chromatin remodeling in preparation for commitment to lymphoid lineages. Subsequently, stromal cell–derived cytokines such as interleukin-7 (IL-7) and thymic stromal lymphopoietin (TSLP) signal through the IL-7 receptor complex to enhance proliferation of T-cell precursors and promote rearrangement of the T-cell receptor γ-chain locus (see later).[5] Another subpopulation of thymocytes, which does not rearrange T-cell receptor (TCR) genes, differentiates into natural killer cells following the binding of interleukin-15 to the combined IL-2/IL-15-receptor, signaling via the common γ-chain.[6, 7] Many of these cytokine signals are transmitted through common pathways involving *Janus kinases*[8] (particularly JAK2 and JAK3) and their target *signal transducers and activators of transcription* (STAT3 and STAT5), suggesting that other growth and differentiation factors must modulate the responsiveness of developing precursors to these stereotypical signaling pathways.[9]

Functional thymic epithelium is required for the development of mature T cells.[10] Mice with a single gene defect in thymic epithelial development (known as nude mice because they are also hairless) have few T cells and an impaired ability to reject grafts.[11] Similarly, in humans, deletion of a gene or genes on chromosome 22 that contributes to pharyngeal pouch development causes the DiGeorge syndrome with variable degrees of T-cell deficiency.[12] Actual cell-cell contact between lymphocytes and epithelial cells appears to be required for T-lineage antigens to be expressed because soluble factors derived from thymic epithelial cultures are unable to promote continued T-cell development. Functional T cells, however, are also required for inducing and maintaining the epithelial cells characteristic of the thymic cortex and medulla. Without continued contact between epithelium and developing T cells, the thymus may lose the ability to support full T-cell maturation with time.[13, 14]

Commitment to the T-Cell Lineage

Mouse T-cell precursors begin to express adhesion molecules common to hematopoietic lineages 2 to 3 days after their first appearance in the thymus. The adhesion molecule CD18/CD11a (also known as *leukocyte function associated antigen-1* [LFA-1]) regulates the entry of mature leukocyte populations into sites of inflammation and enhances T-cell activation following antigen stimulation. LFA-1 is expressed on lymphoid precursors shortly after their entry into the thymus and is likely to mediate intercellular interactions that are required for subsequent steps in thymocyte development.[15] Receptors for growth and differentiation factors common to all hematopoietic precursors found in bone marrow (e.g., c-kit [CD117], which binds stem cell factor) are still detectable at this stage as well. Commitment to the lymphoid lineage is demonstrated on a fraction of thymocytes by expression of one form of the lymphocyte-specific IL-2 receptor (CD25[16]) as well as by activation of the enzyme complex (recombinase) that generates functional lymphocyte antigen receptors (see later). Cells from this subset rapidly and selectively begin to activate and express the T-cell-specific antigen receptors. They can efficiently repopulate a recipient thymus with developing T cells in cell transfer experiments. The interactions of IL-2 and other autocrine growth factors with their receptors on thymocytes at this stage of development are likely to be important for the subsequent differentiation of mature T cells and may be the target of pharmacologic intervention (as shown by suppression of mature T-cell production by cyclosporin A[17]).

Generation of Antigen Receptors

T cells are characterized by their specific cell surface receptors for antigens (TCRs). Each antigen receptor is composed of two polypeptide chains with two internal disulfide-linked domains. α-Chains generally pair with β-chains and δ-chains with γ-chains, defining two different populations of T cells in the mature animal.[18] Carboxy-terminal domains include the peptides spanning the cell membrane. Each has 138 to 179 amino acids of relatively invariant sequence, which include a hydrophobic transmembrane section and a short cytoplasmic tail. These are known as the constant (C) regions. The variability in protein sequence among TCR molecules, which allows recognition of a wide array of antigens, is determined by the availability of multiple cassette-like alternative sequences for the amino-terminus of each receptor chain.

TABLE 154-1

CD Antigens and T-cell Development

CD Antigen	Common Name	Present on	Function
CD1		Most nucleated hematopoietic cells	Antigen presentation
CD2			Adhesion, co-stimulation of TCR signals
CD3		T cells	TCR-mediated signal transducer
CD4		MHC class II-restricted T cells	Adhesion, co-stimulation of TCR signals
CD7		Most hematopoietic cells; high on immature cells	Co-stimulation of TCR signals
CD8		MHC class I-restricted T cells	Adhesion, co-stimulation of TCR signals
CD11a	LFA-1 α-chain	Most nucleated hematopoietic cells	Adhesion, co-stimulation of TCR signals
CD18	LFA-1 β-chain	Most nucleated hematopoietic cells	Adhesion, co-stimulation of TCR signals
CD25	High-affinity IL-2 receptor	Immature (CD4-/CD8-) thymocytes, activated mature T cells	Supports proliferation, differentiation
CD28		Mature, activated T cells	Co-stimulation of TCR signals
CD34	Sialomucin	Multipotent bone marrow stem cells	Adhesion
CD40		B cells, monocytes, dendritic cells, endothelial cells	B cell proliferation, Ig class switching
CD45	Leukocyte common antigen	Most hematopoietic cells	Co-stimulation of TCR signals
CD45RA		High on naive T cells	Co-stimulation of TCR signals
CD45R0		High on memory T cells	Co-stimulation of TCR signals
CD52		Most hematopoietic cells	Unknown
CD80	B7-1	Activated B cells, macrophages	CD28 ligand
CD86	B7-2	Activated B cells, macrophages	CD28 ligand
CD117	c-kit	T cell precursors	Proliferation of precursors
CD154	CD40 ligand (CD40L)	Activated T cells	Adhesion, transmission of signal to B cells

TCR, T-cell receptor.

In a process called *rearrangement*, selected variable sequences are moved into close proximity to the C region coding sequences by enzyme-catalyzed excision of the intervening loop of DNA, thus creating a complete gene sequence for each polypeptide chain. Gene rearrangement at the TCR and immunoglobulin loci in lymphocytes is accomplished via a multicomponent recombinase complex, which includes two recently identified gene products known as recombinase-activating genes 1 and 2 (RAG-1, RAG-2).[19] A third component of the complex is encoded by genes that are used in other enzyme-mediated DNA repair systems. Mutations in the recombinase and DNA repair genes impair cell-mediated immunity by inhibiting productive rearrangements in lymphocyte receptor genes as well as repair of radiation-induced DNA strand breaks.[20]

Recombination of TCR genes, similar to that of immunoglobulin genes, follows a well-regulated sequence in the presence of a normal recombinase complex. In the generation of a functional β-chain, gene sequences coding for variable (V), diversity (D), and joining (J, 18 to 20 amino acids) segments are used. In this process, a D region segment is first brought into close proximity to the J-C region by looping out and deleting much of the intervening DNA. The excised DNA persists as a circle in the

TABLE 154-2

Cytokines and T-cell Development

Cytokine	Common Name	Produced by	Function
IL-1β	Interleukin-1 beta	Monocytes, macrophages	Enhanced inflammation; thymocyte proliferation
IL-2	Interleukin-2	Activated CD4+ T cells	T cell proliferation; thymocyte differentiation
IL-3	Interleukin-3	Stromal cells in bone marrow and thymus	TCR-mediated signal transducer
IL-4	Interleukin-4	Activated Th2 cells	B-cell proliferation and antigen presentation; Ig production; switch to IgE
IL-7	Interleukin-7	Stromal cells: bone marrow, thymus; intestinal epithelium	Expansion of lymphoid precursors
IL-10	Interleukin-10	Activated Th2 cells	Suppression of macrophage activation; B-cell proliferation
IL-12	Interleukin-12	Activated macrophages	IFNγ production; macrophage activation
IL-13	Interleukin-13	Activated Th2 cells, activated CD8+ T cells	Similar to IL-4 with additional pro-inflammatory signals for fibroblasts and tissue granulocytes
IL-15	Interleukin-15	Many cell types	Differentiation and proliferation of NK cells, CD8+ T cells
IFNγ	γ-Interferon, Type II interferon	Activated T cells, NK cells	Enhanced antigen presentation, inflammation
SCF	Stem cell factor	Stromal cells: bone marrow, thymus; intestinal epithelium	Proliferation, differentiation of precursor cells
TGFβ	Transforming growth factor beta	Activated regulatory T cells	Suppression of mature T-cell activation; accelerated T-cell development
TSLP	Thymic stromal lymphopoietin	Stromal cells: thymus	Expansion of T-cell precursors; TCR γ-chain rearrangement

TCR, T-cell receptor.

cell and is known as a T-cell receptor excision circle (TREC). The TREC does not replicate in parallel with nuclear DNA, so counting TRECs in blood T cells gives an indirect estimate of T-cell production from the thymus that is also affected by cell division.[21] The rearrangement process that generates the TREC allows for transcriptional activity at the site as well as a commitment to express 1 of 12 potential J regions. A V segment then selected and moved closer to the D-J-C site by a similar process, enhancing transcription rates even further. The mechanisms operating to determine which of the 20 or so V regions and which D or J region is selected for expression are poorly understood but appear to be random. δ-Chains resemble β-chains in having V, D, J, and C segments. α-Chains and γ-chains are somewhat simpler in structure and lack D regions. The rearranged V(D)J segments of TCR chains achieve additional diversity by addition or subtraction of nucleotides at the joints between the V, D, and J segments. This phenomenon appears to result from the properties of the recombinase enzymes in conjunction with an enzyme designated terminal deoxytransferase (Tdt) that is known as *N-segment diversity*. The thymocytes of fetal mice rearrange their β-, γ-, and δ-chain genes[17] at about 13 to 14 days' gestation, and α-chain rearrangement follows 1 to 2 days later. mRNA for α-chains is detectable on day 16 to 17 of gestation, and α-chains are present on the surface of fetal thymocytes on day 17 to 18 so that the appearance of complete γδ heterodimers precedes that of αβ heterodimers by 1 to 2 days. Expression of a rearranged β-chain suppresses further rearrangements of β-chain loci via signaling through a receptor-related tyrosine kinase, p56[lck], in a process known as *allelic exclusion*.[22] Alpha, γ-, and δ-chain gene rearrangements are also largely suppressed following the binding of mature TCR to MHC molecules on the surface of thymic macrophages or epithelial cells. However, a subset of CD8 cells appears to rearrange both α-chain loci, creating a small population of potentially bi-specific cells.

When either pair of receptor genes (αβ or γδ) has been rearranged and transcribed, it is associated on the cell surface with the five polypeptides of the CD3 complex. The cytoplasmic tail of each TCR chain is small, and intracellular signaling leading to the activation of T-cell signaling cascades is actually mediated through the CD3 complex.[23]

Extrathymic T-Cell Development

Most lymphocytes carrying αβ or γδ antigen-specific receptors develop in the thymus and are exported to peripheral lymphoid organs. However, a small number of lymphocytes carrying T-cell surface markers may develop extrathymically. In particular, lymphoid cells may appear within the epithelium of the small and large intestines in the absence of a functioning thymus. Intraepithelial lymphocytes (IEL) in normal adult individuals are composed of both αβ and γδ CD3+ cells. In contrast to their representation in the thymus, γδ cells are more frequent than αβ cells in the intestinal epithelium. Precursors for the γδ subset appear to begin differentiating within lymphoid aggregates associated with epithelial crypts in the small intestine. Cells in these *cryptopatches* express the recombinase-activating genes RAG-1 and RAG-2, as well as the c-kit ligand and the IL-7 receptor.[24] Loss of these early lineage determinants is co-incident with expression of TCR and CD3 signaling molecules on lymphoid cells in these aggregates, suggesting that active T-like differentiation is occurring *in situ*. These cells can develop in athymic nude mice, albeit more slowly than in immunologically normal animals, suggesting that thymus-derived factors are not absolutely required for local development of T-like lymphocytes in the gut. Intestinal immune responses are critical as a first line of defense against intestinal flora and have also been shown to be important in generating tolerance to ubiquitous environmental antigens. However, the importance of local extrathymic T-cell development in perform-

ing these functions is unknown. γδ Subsets found in other epithelial compartments (skin; alveolar and bronchial epithelium) seem to be dependent on thymic output, and there is no evidence for significant extrathymic differentiation of the αβ subset.

CONTROL OF THE T-CELL REPERTOIRE FOR ANTIGEN RECOGNITION

Role of T-Cell Receptor/Major Histocompatibility Complex Interactions in T-Cell Development

B and T cells, despite the similarities in construction of their antigen receptors, interact with antigen in different ways. In generating a response from B cells, immunoglobulin carried on the B-cell surface binds directly to antigen, whether this is free in blood or tissues or part of the surface of a cell or microbe. In contrast, TCR must bind simultaneously to a distinct peptide or glycolipid and a major histocompatibility complex (MHC) molecule of a type found in the animal in which the T cell differentiated. The random selection of variable regions and the N region diversification described previously generate a diverse repertoire of antigen specificities. Estimates of the potential diversity of TCRs that might be achieved by the processes of V(D)J recombination and N region diversification exceed 10^{15} for both αβ and γδ heterodimers.[26] This repertoire is subjected to important selection steps in the thymus. Although the pool of T cells in an animal must have broad diversity to recognize a wide array of foreign antigens, for efficiency it must also be limited to those cells bearing TCR capable of binding to self-MHC. The thymus also selects against T-cell precursors that bind too efficiently to self-MHC, alone or complexed with self-peptides. These two phenomena, known as *positive selection* and *negative selection*, provide the host with a T-cell pool restricted to recognizing foreign antigen bound to cells bearing the self-MHC but tolerant of most molecules (including self-MHC) normally found in the host.

Current models[26] favor the hypothesis that these two processes occur as distinct steps during thymic maturation. Positive selection has been shown to occur via TCR interactions with MHC molecules expressed on thymic cortical epithelial cells during the CD4+/CD8+ (double-positive) stage in thymocyte maturation; the large numbers of developing thymocytes that do not bind self-MHC die in the thymus. TCR/MHC interactions that exceed a threshold level, however, result in additional cell death. This negative selection step is the first level of protection against autoimmunity. Negative selection can be initiated by thymocyte contact with virtually any MHC+ cell in the thymus, suggesting that positive and negative selection may be distinguished not only by the affinity of the TCR/MHC interaction, but also by the requirement for epithelium-derived signals in positive selection.[27]

Expression of Other T-Lineage Specific Molecules

Although antigen specificity and activation signals are determined by the TCR complex, the CD4 and CD8 co-receptors on T cells play a significant role in thymocyte differentiation as well as in the post-thymic activation of mature T cells. These molecules bind to MHC molecules at sites distant from binding sites for the T-cell antigen receptor. CD4 molecules bind to MHC class II molecules (HLA DP, DQ, and DR in humans), which are expressed primarily on cells of hematopoietic origin and participate in generating an immune response. CD8 molecules bind to the MHC class I molecules found on nearly every nucleated cell in the body (HLA A, B, and C). The cells that first arrive in the thymus are negative for CD4 and CD8 cell surface antigens. Maturation of T cells in the thymus is accompanied by sequential expression of these surface proteins, until only a small fraction of thymocytes continue to have the double-negative

(CD4⁻/CD8⁻) phenotype.[28] Thymocytes expressing surface αβ TCR for the first time co-express both CD4 and CD8, enhancing the likelihood of TCR-MHC interactions during the critical steps of positive and negative selection. As thymocytes mature, expression of the CD4 and CD8 molecules generally becomes mutually exclusive. These molecules, therefore, can enhance the TCR-mediated interactions of different functional T cell subsets with selected classes of MHC molecules and different cell types. CD4 and CD8 also participate in modification of intracellular signaling through their links to the protein tyrosine kinase p56^{lck}.

In contrast to mature T cells, the predominant lymphocyte population in the adult murine thymus expresses both CD4 and CD8 surface antigens. The switch from the CD4⁻/CD8⁻ phenotype to CD4⁺/CD8⁺ is probably by way of an immature thymocyte, which has low levels of surface CD3,[29] and a signaling molecule composed of the rearranged TCR β-chain and an invariant α-chain known as *pre-Tα*, which supports proliferation of T-cell precursors that have successfully rearranged a β-chain allele. In mice, this complex is first detectable at 16 days' gestation. CD4⁺/CD8⁺ cells first appear 1 day later, and *in vivo* labeling studies indicate that CD25 is lost immediately before CD4 and CD8 are expressed. Commitment to the CD8 pathway appears to require a specific signal, presumably mediated by binding to a class I MHC molecule. If this signal cannot be transduced, as, for example, in children who lack the Zap70 kinase, no CD8 cells appear in the blood.[30] CD4⁺/CD8⁺ double-positive cells that survive positive and negative selection and that do not become CD8 cells appear to enter a default pathway, becoming CD4 single-positive cells in the blood.[31]

OBSERVATIONS IN HUMANS

T-Cell Phenotypes and Antigen Receptors

T-cell development in the human thymus starts at about 7 weeks' gestation[32] with the entry of precursors with the leukocyte antigens CD7 and CD45 on their surface. These cells mature to express first the CD2[33] co-stimulatory molecule and, around 8.5 weeks of gestation, CD3. By 9.5 weeks of gestation, 32% of the CD3⁺ cells have the β-chain of the TCR in the cytoplasm, and at 10 weeks, many of the cells have α-chain in addition to β-chain in the cytoplasm. The percent of cells expressing the δ-chain of the γδ TCR is highest at 9.5 weeks' gestation (11%) and rapidly diminishes (4% at 10 weeks' and 1% at 12 weeks' gestation). CD1, CD4, and CD8 appear on lymphocytes in the thymus by 10 weeks' gestation, and the high-density CD3 phenotype (associated with mature antigen receptor expression) appears on these cells at about 12 weeks. A population of immature CD7⁺ cells with potential for multiple differentiation pathways is present in cord blood.[34]

The biochemistry of the human T-cell antigen receptor resembles that of mice. The αβ heterodimer is about 90 kDa. The α- and δ-chain genes are on chromosome 14, and the β-chain genes are on chromosome 7. The complete αβ or γδ heterodimer is expressed on the T-cell surface in association with five invariant chains, which constitute CD3.

Some estimate of the time and rate of T-cell export from the human fetal thymus comes from measurement of T cells in the blood and spleen. Occasional CD3⁺ cells are present in blood from the end of the 12th week of gestation, their proportion rising from 20 to 30% at 14 weeks to 50% or more by 22 weeks. Studies suggest that the range of VDJ recombinations that can be made before 14 weeks of gestation is limited.[35,36] The mechanism for limited diversity during fetal life may relate to a limited use of N-region diversification, secondary to low levels of the Tdt enzyme in the thymus. It is interesting that the diversity of the fetal B-cell repertoire is also limited, although a selective preference for certain VH genes appears to be the explanation in this case.[37] If the T-cell diversity data are correct, the fetus may have

much less ability to respond to antigen (or reject foreign grafts) than might be predicted from the presence of CD3 cells in the blood. Much remains to be learned about the range of TCR gene recombinations that can be made at different gestational ages.[38]

Of fetal CD3⁺ cells in blood and spleen, 90 to 96% use αβ heterodimers, and the percentage of γδ receptor-positive cells is between 2 and 8% between 20 and 40 weeks' gestation, which is similar to the frequency found in adults.[39] Fetal T cells resemble adult lymphocytes in expressing either CD4 or CD8 but not both. They appear in blood in parallel with the spleen and liver and increase in proportion to 50% or more between 25 and 30 weeks' gestation (Table 154-3). T cells also appear in the intestinal epithelium and lamina propria by 14 weeks of gestation.[40] Cells carrying γδ TCR populate the epithelium more slowly than αβ TCR+ cells and may arise, in part, from local differentiation rather than exclusively from thymic sources. Gut-associated γδ lymphocytes increase rapidly in the fed neonate,[41] suggesting that local antigenic stimulation may be responsible for the expansion of this population.

By analogy with studies in animals, it seems likely that T cells accumulate in the blood and lymph nodes of fetuses during the second half of gestation, principally as a result of thymic emigration. This view is supported by studies of CD45 isoforms, which distinguish between naive and memory T cells. More than 99% of the lymphocytes in the cord blood of neonates express high molecular weight isoforms of CD45 (CD45RA and CD45RB),[42] in association with the low levels of LFA-1 (CD11a/CD18) and other integrins that characterize the naive phenotype (Table 154-4). When stimulated, the naive cells of newborn infants switch to express the CD45R0 isoform of CD45. This isoform is present on T cells in adult blood that respond to recall antigens. The low number of CD45R0 cells in the blood of healthy term neonates suggests that there is little antigen-driven expansion of T cells before birth. The minor population of memory phenotype cells that does appear during fetal life may be related to autoantigen stimuli (see later).

Functional Responses of Fetal T Cells

In vitro tests indicate that several components of a T-cell response (proliferation to mitogens or to alloantigen in mixed lymphocyte culture, IL-2 production, and the expression of IL-2 receptors) exist from about 12 weeks of gestation. In addition to these ligand-driven proliferative responses, T cells of neonates also can be maintained in culture using a combination of IL-4 and IL-2 or IL-4 and IL-12.[43] Evidence that fetal T cells could make antigen-specific responses comes from their proliferation in mixed lymphocyte culture, together with the generation of antigen-specific cytotoxic cells.[44] Other stimuli, such as staphylococcus enterotoxins and anti-TCR antibodies, tend to elicit lesser responses by neonatal compared with adult cells.[45] This difference, at least in part, is accounted for by the lower proportion of CD45R0 cells in neonates compared with adults,[46]

The maturation of naive cells to the memory cell phenotype most likely follows encounter with antigen presented on a specialized antigen-presenting cell, such as a B lymphocyte or a dendritic cell in a lymph node. Several studies suggest that naive

TABLE 154-3

Summary of T Lymphopoiesis in Human Fetuses

Age in Weeks	Developmental Step
7	Precursors in fetal liver
10	Thymus becomes lymphoid
12	Hassals corpuscles in thymus
12+	T cells appear in blood

TABLE 154–4

Summary of Differences Between Naive and Memory T Cells

Quality	Naive T cells	Memory T cells
Definition	Cell that has not yet been triggered by antigen	Product of antigen-driven clonal expansion
CD45 phenotype	CD45RA+, CD45RB+, CD45R0-	CD45R0+
Other cell surface antigens	LFA-1^{low}	CD2^{high}, LFA1^{high}, LFA3^{high}
Cytokine response to stimulation	IL-2	IL-2, IL-4, IL-10, IL-12, γ-IFN
CD40L response to stimulation	Low	High

T cells that encounter antigen in the absence of co-stimulation enter a pathway that leads to unresponsiveness, also known as *anergy*, which may be temporary or permanent.[47] A polyclonal population of CD4 and CD8 memory phenotype T cells comprising 25% of human fetal spleen cells has high-affinity IL-2 receptors and proliferates in response to exogenous IL-2 but not to CD2 or CD3 antibodies.[48] Some of these cells might be autoreactive T cells destined to become unresponsive, whereas others in the CD4 lineage might be members of a recently identified population of CD25^{high}CD4+ T cells with regulatory properties. Umbilical cord blood likewise contains a population of T cells that is driven to reduced *in vivo* responsiveness following ligation of cell surface CD47.[49]

The production of soluble mediators, or cytokines, by T cells responding to antigen stimulation is essential for host defense.[50] Naive and memory T cells make similar amounts of IL-2, which is required for T-cell proliferation, whereas other cytokines, including IL-4, IL-10, IL-12, and γ-interferon (γ-IFN), are made largely by memory T cells. Consequently, T cells of newborns make little γ-IFN or IL-4, unless they first undergo several cycles of proliferation and maturation[51] or they are cultured with stimulation that persists for several days.[52] These differences are likely to be important because T cells show functional specialization regarding their predominant cytokine production.[53] The cells making IL-4 and IL-10 are described as Th2 cells. These cells have an essential role in promoting B-cell replication and increase the production of IgE isotype antibodies. Th1 cells make mainly γ-IFN, and they promote local inflammatory responses as well as stimulate B cells to make IgG. A third class of Th0 cells can make both γ-IFN and IL-4. The specialization of cells into a Th1 or Th2 phenotype from Th0 cells is determined, in part, by the cytokine environment in which stimulation occurs. The presence of γ-IFN, for example, biases responses toward a Th1 phenotype, whereas IL-4 tends to suppress γ-IFN production and to promote differentiation toward a Th2 phenotype. Human newborn naive cells can mature into those making IL-4 apparently in the absence of preexisting IL-4.[54] IL-13, an important cytokine in the Th2 pathway, is produced by newborns' CD8 T cells even when their production of IL-4, IL-10, and γ-IFN remains low.[55] Different specificities of cytokine receptors on the surface of Th1 and Th2 cells cause them to have different homing patterns in intact animals. Responses to immunization can be markedly altered by deliberate manipulation of the cytokine milieu in which immunizing antigens are presented to the immune system. This strategy may be useful in the design of future vaccines.[56]

The extent of signaling through the TCR-CD3 complex also can be modified by simultaneous interactions of receptor-ligand pairs of *co-stimulatory molecules* on the surface of T cells and antigen-presenting cells. Interaction of CD28 molecules on the T cell surface with its ligands B7-1 and B7-2 on B cells, macrophages, and dendritic cells markedly enhances the proliferation and cytokine production of "naive" T cells in response to specific antigen-MHC complexes. Other surface molecules with co-stimulatory function include LFA-1, the "inducible costimulator" ICOS (another CD28/B7 family member), and tumor necrosis

family members such as OX40. These membrane-bound receptors carry activation signals in their cytoplasmic tails which recruit activating kinases that can amplify intracellular signaling pathways. Other members of the CD28 family of molecules, such as CTLA-4, contain intracytoplasmic inhibitory sequences that can activate a series of intracellular phosphatases with the opposite function. Although CTLA-4 can also bind B7-1 and B7-2 molecules on the surface of antigen-presenting cells, its ligation actively suppresses intracellular TCR signaling in most instances. The balance of positive and negative *co-stimulation* shapes the final T cell repertoire by regulating both clonal expansion and differential cytokine production of the responding T cells. Interruption of these co-stimulatory and regulatory interactions can markedly alter the development of antigen-specific T cell responses. The effectiveness of blocking CD28 interactions with B7-1 and B7-2 in limiting or reversing rejection of allogeneic tissue grafts is currently being explored.[57]

Postnatal Development of Memory T Cells

Naive T cells—the predominant population in human newborn infants—have the TRECs that identify recent thymic emigrants.[58] Their recirculatory pathway takes them through the specialized venules of lymph nodes and other lymphoid tissue to migrate past dendritic cells in the T-dependent areas. The cells that do not encounter antigen leave the node in the efferent lymph and return to the blood stream through the thoracic duct. Naive T cells, whose surface antigen receptors are cross-linked by antigen appropriately expressed with self-MHC, enter a response cycle that is accompanied by expression of a surface receptor for IL-2. Provided that a co-stimulator signal (such as binding of B7-1 or B7-2 to CD28) is present, the T cells themselves release IL-2. This autocrine loop permits cell division of IL-2–dependent cells for as long as the antigen stimulus persists. The development of a useful repertoire of T cells in the circulation is, therefore, best thought of as a consequence of antigenic experience stimulating T-cell proliferation. Specialized dendritic cells (DCs) probably play the principal role in capturing antigens in tissues and at body surfaces and transporting them through lymphatics to the local lymph node. The migration of DCs is regulated by chemokine gradients (particularly CCR7), and their handling of antigen is affected by receptors for bacterial products such as lipopolysaccharides and certain unmethylated dinucleotides.[59] DCs are likely to contribute to the specialization of T cells along Th1 or Th2 pathways (described earlier). B lymphocytes also are important presenters of antigen present in low concentrations that they are able to capture through their cell surface immunoglobulin molecules.

The response of the naive T-cell population to antigen stimulus depends largely on the co-stimulatory environment.[60] Stimulation results in an increase in percentage of CD45R0 cells from less than 5% at birth to 35 to 45% by age 16 years. The increase occurs mainly during the first years of life,[46] and one attribute of memory cells, the production of γ-IFN, is mature around the age of 2 years. The expansion of populations of defined specificities has been documented for only a few antigens. For example, the frequency of lymphocytes in blood responding to varicella zoster virus (VZV) antigen is less than 1:10[6] before immunization or infection.[61] Following a varicella infection, VZV-responsive cells do not appear in the blood for about 10 days. One month into convalescence, the responder cell frequency is about 1:20,000 cells, rising to 1:10,000 after 3 months.[62] VZV is a latent virus, and responder cell frequencies in the range of 1:10,000 to 1:20,000 are maintained through the age of 50 years, when they start to decline. The frequency of T cells with specificity for a nonreplicating antigen, tetanus toxoid, fluctuates directly in relationship to immunization. Before infants receive tetanus toxoid, they have fewer than 1:10[5] cells that respond to this antigen. Six weeks after first immunization, the responder cell frequency is still less than 1:40,000. The course of three injections up to 6 months of age raises the responder cell frequency to 1:10,000 cells, and this falls to less than 1:40,000 1 year later.

Help for B Lymphocytes

B cells that bind antigen through their surface immunoglobulin receptors enter a pathway that leads either to self-destruction by apoptosis[63] or, if a T-cell signal is received, to proliferation and differentiation. The T-cell signal for B-cell proliferation is supplied by cytokines and is mostly delivered at the T/B cell interface in lymph nodes. T cells control the switch from IgM to IgG (isotype switching) as well as proliferation. The switch signal is supplied by binding a 39,000-kDa glycoprotein (termed CD40 ligand, or CD40L) to the CD40 receptor, which is constitutively expressed on the B-cell surface. Resting memory T cells express CD40L within a few hours of a response to antigen, whereas naive T cells take longer to become CD40L positive. *In vitro* experiments suggest that delay in CD40L expression on naive T cells is an important factor limiting the ability of human newborn infants to make antibody responses.[64] Th1 cells help certain IgG responses and IL-4 from Th2-type cells promotes IgA and IgE responses. As noted previously, Th2 cells are most efficiently generated in an environment already containing IL-4 and IL-13.

SUMMARY

T-cell development occurs in multiple discrete steps, beginning with lineage commitment by hematopoietic in the specialized environment of the thymus. Progression through the developmental pathway in the thymus is controlled by soluble cytokine growth factors and cellular interactions between the maturing thymocytes and the local stromal cell compartment. The repertoire of antigen-specific TCRs expressed on mature thymocytes prior to export to the periphery results from both positive and negative selection of receptor specificities generated by random association of variable regions for TCR heterodimers and the addition of N-region diversity through random nucleotide deletions/additions during the recombination events. After export from the thymus, the mature T-cell pool is further shaped by antigen exposure and the local production of cytokines during initial activation and clonal expansion in lymph nodes, spleen, and epithelial structures such as skin and intestine. Although mature T cells are present in significant numbers during the second trimester of pregnancy in humans, a fully mature T-cell population develops slowly after birth in response to antigen exposure.

REFERENCES

1. Goldstein G, Mackay IR: The Human Thymus. London, William Heinemann, 1969, pp 26–27.
2. Moore MAS, Owen JJ: Experimental studies on the development of the thymus. J Exp Med 126:715, 1967.
3. Berardi AC, et al: Functional isolation and characterization of human hematopoietic stem cells. Science 267:104, 1995.
4. Georgopoulos K, et al: The Ikaros gene is required for the development of all lymphoid lineages. Cell 79:143, 1994.
5. Candeias S, et al: Defective T-cell receptor gamma gene rearrangement in interleukin-7 receptor knockout mice. Immunol Letters 57:9, 1997.
6. Sanchez MJ, et al: Identification of a common T/natural killer cell progenitor in human fetal thymus. J Exp Med 180:569, 1994.
7. Carlyle JR, et al: Identification of a novel developmental stage marking lineage commitment of progenitor thymocytes. J Exp Med 186:173, 1997.
8. Igaz P, et al: Biological and clinical significance of the JAK-STAT pathway; lessons from knockout mice. Inflamm Research 50:435, 2001.
9. Spits H, et al: Early stages in the development of human T, natural killer and thymic dendritic cells. Immunol Rev 165:75, 1998.
10. van Ewijk W, et al: Stepwise development of thymic microenvironments in vivo is regulated by thymocyte subsets. Development (Suppl) 127:1583, 2000.
11. Hoyne GF, et al: Notch signalling in the regulation of peripheral immunity. Immunol Rev 182:215; 2001.
12. Carey AH, et al: Localization of 27 DNA markers to the region of human chromosome 22q11-pter deleted in patients with the DiGeorge syndrome and duplicated in the der22 syndrome. Genomics 7:299, 1990.
13. Surh CD, et al: Growth of epithelial cells in the thymic medulla is under the control of mature T cells. J Exp Med 176:611, 1992.
14. Frey JR, et al: Thymus-grafted SCID mice show transient thymopoiesis and limited depletion of V 11+ T cells. J Exp Med 175:1067, 1992.
15. McDuffie M, Golde WT: The accessory molecule, Lgp55, is required for thymocyte maturation. Dev Immunol 3:257, 1994.
16. Moore TA, Zlotnik A: T-cell lineage commitment and cytokine responses of thymic progenitors. Blood 86:1850, 1995.
17. Gao E-K, et al: Abnormal differentiation of thymocytes in mice treated with cyclosporin A. Nature 336:176, 1988.
18. Pardoll DM, et al: Differential expression of two different T cell receptors during thymocyte development. Nature 326:79, 1987.
19. Oettinger MA, et al: RAG-1 and RAG-2, adjacent genes that synergistically activate V(D)J recombination. Science 248:1517, 1990.
20. Banga SS, et al: Complementation of V(D)J recombination defect and x-ray sensitivity of scid mouse cells by human chromosome 8. Mutat Res 315:239, 1994.
21. Ye P, Kirschner DE: Reevaluation of T cell receptor excision circles as a measure of human recent thymic emigrants. J Immunol 168:4968, 2002.
22. Anderson SJ, et al: Protein tyrosine kinase p56lck controls allelic exclusion of T-cell receptor beta-chain genes. Nature 365:552, 1993.
23. Griesser H, Mak TW: The T-cell receptor—structure, function, and clinical application. Hematol Pathol 8:1, 1994.
24. Lambolez F, et al: Characterization of T cell differentiation in the murine gut. J Exp Med 195:437, 2002.
25. Rothenberg EV, et al: Molecular indices of functional competence in developing T cells. Immunol Rev 104:29, 1988.
26. Robey E, Fowlkes BJ: Selective events in T cell development. Annu Rev Immunol 12:657, 1994.
27. Fowlkes BJ, Schweighoffer E: Positive selection of T cells. Curr Opin Immunol 7:188, 1995.
28. von Boehmer H: Positive selection of lymphocytes. Cell 76:218, 1994.
29. Levelt CN, et al: Restoration of early thymocyte differentiation in T-cell receptor β-chain–deficient mutant mice by transmembrane signalling through CD3 epsilon. Proc Natl Acad Sci 90:11401, 1993.
30. Chan AC, et al: ZAP-70 deficiency in an autosomal recessive form of severe combined immunodeficiency. Science 264:1599, 1994.
31. Suzuki H, et al: Asymmetric signalling requirement for thymocyte commitment to the CD4+ versus CD8+ T cell lineages: a new perspective on thymic commitment and selection. Immunity 2:413, 1995.
32. Royo C, et al: Ontogeny of T lymphocyte differentiation in the human fetus: acquisition of phenotype and functions. Thymus 10:57, 1987.
33. Hayes BF, et al: Early events in human T cell ontogeny: phenotypic characterization and immunohistologic localization of T cell precursors in early human fetal tissues. J Exp Med 168:1061, 1988.
34. Hao QL, et al: Identification of a novel, human multilymphoid progenitor in cord blood. Blood 97:3683, 2001.
35. Raaphorst FM, et al: Non-random employment of Vβ6 gene elements and conserved amino acid usage profiles in CDR3 regions of human fetal and adult TCR β chain rearrangements. Int Immunol 6:1, 1994.
36. Krangel MS, et al: A distinct wave of human γ/δ lymphocytes in early fetal thymus: evidence for controlled gene rearrangement and cytokine production. J Exp Med 172:847, 1990.
37. Pascual V, et al: Analysis of Ig H chain gene segment utilization in human fetal liver: revisiting the "proximal utilization hypothesis." J Immunol 151:4164, 1993.
38. Schultz C, et al: Maturational changes of lymphocyte surface antigens in human blood: comparison between fetuses, neonates and adults. Biol Neonate 78:77, 2000.
39. Lobach DF, et al: Human T cell antigen expression during the early stages of fetal thymic maturation. J Immunol 135:1752, 1985.
40. Machado CS, et al: Assessment of gut intraepithelial lymphocytes during late gestation and the neonatal period. Biol Neonate 66:324, 1994.

41. Spencer J, et al: Heterogeneity in intraepithelial lymphocyte subpopulations in fetal and postnatal human small intestine. J Pediatr Gastroenterol Nutr 9:173, 1989.
42. Bofill M, et al: Immature CD45RA^{low}R0^{low} T cells in the human cord blood: 1. antecedents of CD45RA+ unprimed T cells. J Immunol 152:5613, 1994.
43. Wu CY, et al: In vitro maturation of human neonatal CD4 T lymphocytes. I. Induction of IL-4–producing cells after long-term culture in the presence of IL-4 plus either IL-2 or IL-12. J Immunol 152:1141, 1994.
44. Rayfield LS, et al: Development of cell-mediated lympholysis in human foetal blood lymphocytes. Clin Exp Immunol 42:561, 1980.
45. Horgan KJ, et al: Hyporesponsiveness of naive (CD45RA) human T cells to multiple receptor-mediated stimuli but augmentation of responses by co-stimuli. Eur J Immunol 20:1111, 1990.
46. Hayward AR, et al: Ontogeny of expression of UCHL1 on TCD1 and TCR-delta positive T cells. Eur J Immunol 19:771, 1989.
47. Durie FH, et al: The role of CD40 in the regulation of humoral and cell-mediated immunity. Immunol Today 15:406, 1994.
48. Byrne JA, et al: A novel subpopulation of primed T cells in the human fetus. J Immunol 152:3098, 1994.
49. Avice MN, et al: Role of CD47 in the induction of human naive T cell anergy. J Immunol 167:2459, 2001.
50. Leonard WJ: Cytokines and immunodeficiency diseases. Nature Rev Immunol 1:200, 2001.
51. Ehlers S, Smith KA: Differentiation of T cell lymphokine expression: the in vitro acquisition of T cell memory. J Exp Med 173:25, 1991.
52. Hayward AM, Cosyns M: Proliferative and cytokine responses by human newborn T cells stimulated with staphylococcal enterotoxin B. Pediatr Res 35:293, 1994.
53. Mosmann TR, Coffman RL: Th1 and Th2 cells: different patterns of lymphokine secretion lead to different functional properties. Annu Rev Immunol 7:145, 1989.
54. Kalinski P, et al: Functional maturation of human naive T helper cells in the absence of accessory cells: generation of IL-4 producing T cells does not require exogenous IL4. J Immunol 154:3753, 1995.
55. Ribeiro-do-Couto LM, et al: High IL-13 production by human neonatal T cells: neonate immune system regulator? Eur J Immunol 31:3394, 2001.
56. Silva RA, et al: Evaluation of IL-12 in immunotherapy and vaccine design in experimental Mycobacterium avium infections. J Immunol 161:5578, 1998.
57. Jacobsohn DA, Vogelsang GB: Novel pharmacotherapeutic approaches to prevention and treatment of GVHD. Drugs 62:879, 2002.
58. Hassan J, Reen DJ: Human recent thymic emigrants—identification, expansion, and survival characteristics. J Immunol 167:1970, 2001.
59. Krieg AM: CpG motifs in bacterial DNA and their immune effects. Annu Rev Immunol 20:709, 2002.
60. Fadel S, Sarzotti M: Cellular immune responses in neonates. Int Rev Immunol 19:173, 2000.
61. Chilmonczyk B, et al: Characterization of the newborn response to herpes virus antigens. J Immunol 134:4184, 1985.
62. Rotbart HA, et al: Immune responses to varicella zoster virus infections in healthy children. J Infect Dis 167:195, 1993.
63. Punnonen J, et al: Induction of isotype switching and Ig production by CD5+ and CD10+ human fetal B cells. J Immunol 148:3398, 1992.
64. Brugnoni D, et al: Ontogeny of CD40L expression by activated peripheral blood lymphocytes in humans. Immunol Lett 49:27, 1996.

155

James E. Crowe, Jr., Joern-Hendrik Weitkamp, and John V. Williams

B-Cell Development

ORIGIN OF B CELLS: OVERVIEW

The ontogeny of B cells has long held interest for developmental biologists and immunologists because these cells offer a tractable system to study the mechanisms that control development of cells from the earliest stages of fetal life through adulthood. B cells are readily accessible (from blood or many solid organs), can be manipulated *in vitro*, and can be transferred from one experimental animal to another. Although B cells provide a critical arm of host defense, strictly speaking they are not required for the survival of the organism, a fact that has allowed investigators to generate mice with directed defects in lymphoid development. B-cell development is a multistage differentiation process that ends with the generation of antibody-secreting plasma cells.

ANATOMIC SITES OF B-CELL GENERATION

The successive sites of B-cell development in humans and other mammals are the omentum and liver in early fetal life and the bone marrow after birth.[1, 2] The primary B-cell population is continuously renewed throughout life. Bone marrow stromal factors are important to early lymphopoiesis. The earliest cells to emerge after commitment to the B lineage require appropriate molecules produced by stromal cells for survival and proliferation. The environmental factors necessary for the earliest stages of B lymphopoiesis are not well defined; however, stromal cell–derived factor-1/pre-B-cell growth-stimulating factor (SDF-1/PBSF), a member of a family of chemokines, and its primary receptor, CXCR4, appear to play central roles in the early survival of B-lineage cells.[3] Cytokines produced by stromal cells in the microenvironment and their receptors, such as interleukin-7 (IL-7) and the IL-7 receptor, are essential for B lymphopoiesis in animals.

COMMITMENT TO THE B-CELL LINEAGE

B-cell development occurs in discontinuous steps, progressing through checkpoints controlled by the relative level of numerous transcription factors and surface receptors. These complex interactions of transcriptional programs work through balanced control mechanisms rather than simple "on/off" signals. Lymphocytes derive from pluripotent hematopoietic stem cells (HSCs) that reside in the bone marrow. The first HSCs generated in the embryo differentiate without self-renewal, but HSCs are self-renewing in adults. Therefore, a few HSCs can reconstitute the entire hematopoietic system, a characteristic that is being exploited for therapeutic purposes. Adult HSCs generate common lymphoid progenitors (CLPs) in the bone marrow, where they undergo B-cell commitment and maturation in response to inductive signals. HSCs differentiate into progenitors with more restricted lineage potential that yield all the blood cell lineages through a series of highly regulated lineage commitment events. Down-regulation of genes associated with the stem cell state and the concomitant activation of lineage-restricted genes result in the observed change in broad potential of HSCs to the restricted potential of CLPs. Investigations suggest that commitment to T-cell and B-cell lineages may occur, not through a single CLP, but instead through myeloid/T and myeloid/B bipotential stages, respectively.[4] The T-cell/B-cell fate decision is determined by the relative activity of opposing transcription factors such as Notch-1, Deltex, and Lunatic-Fringe.[5-7] B-cell development occurs as a default pathway in the absence of Notch-1 signaling. This concept of molecular control of development through finely regulated opposing transcriptional control programs appears to be common throughout early and late B-cell development. Studies have identified particular factors that regulate differentiation of HSCs into B-cell progenitors, such as PU.1 and Ikaros, or further differentiation of these progenitors into mature B cells, such as nuclear factor-κB, E2A, early B-cell factor, and B-cell lineage–specific activator (BSAP, encoded by Pax5). Mice with disruptions of λ5, Pax5, recombinase-activating (RAG) genes 1 and 2, or the immunoglobulin-α (Igα) and Igβ heterodimeric signaling unit genes have greatly reduced production of B cells,[8] findings indicating that these proteins play an important role in the differentiation of these cells.[9,10]

POSTCOMMITMENT DEVELOPMENT

After B-cell lineage commitment, two major phases of B-cell development have been defined: (1) early development, which is independent of antigenic stimulation; and (2) late development, induced by T-cell help and antigen. Discrete steps in early B-cell generation can be identified by differential expression of proteins on the surface or in the cytoplasm of B cells. B cells initially derive from the CLP cell population, which gives rise to progenitor B cells (pro–B cells) that are dividing and have begun to rearrange Ig heavy chain genes. The cells also begin at this stage to express the enzyme terminal deoxynucleotidyltransferase, which adds nontemplated (N) sequences at the junctions of the VDJ genes being recombined to form the rearranged antibody gene. All B cells from the pro–B-cell stage onward express the surface marker CD19. Production of heavy chain in the cell cytoplasm indicates successful rearrangement and marks the transition from the pro–B-cell stage to the pre–B-cell stage. The pre–B-cell receptor comprising the μ heavy chain/surrogate light chain complex is formed at that stage. Rearrangement of light chain genes usually occurs after heavy chain rearrangement. Synthesis of intact light chain permits efficient assembly and transfer of monomeric IgM and IgD molecules to the cell surface. The disappearance of the pre–B-cell receptor and the expression of cell-surface Ig receptor indicate the transition from pre–B cells to immature B cells (Fig. 155–1).

Mature B cells that undergo DNA recombination in the variable region genes are selected by low-avidity interactions between the B-cell receptor and self-antigens, and then they leave the bone marrow.[11] Functional heterogeneity appears within the peripheral mature B-cell population. Two types of transitional mature B-cell precursors have been described in the spleen. Newly formed B cells in the spleen that are recent immigrants from the bone marrow are sometimes referred to as Type 1 (T1) transitional B cells, and these can develop into Type 2 (T2) transitional B cells in the spleen. In the spleen, immature transitional B cells can further differentiate into follicular B and marginal zone B cells, which are distinguished by the level of expression of surface markers such as CD21 and CD23. Follicular B cells respond to thymus-dependent antigens and proliferate extensively to form germinal centers (GCs), in which somatic hypermutation and class switch recombination take place. The function of marginal zone B cells is under investigation.

The final stages of B-cell differentiation are initiated by the binding of antigen and usually require helper signals from activated T cells. Appropriately stimulated B cells proliferate and differentiate to form either memory cells or antibody-secreting plasma cells. Only a few of the B cells generated during the first stages of development survive to encounter antigens and complete their differentiation. Most of the cells are believed to undergo apoptosis (programmed cell death). Both soluble and contact factors promote persistence of particular B-cell clones. B-cell receptor interactions with antigens are not all-or-none events. Murine studies demonstrated that the strength of B-cell receptor signaling influences both the selection of cells during ontogeny and later antigen-specific responses. Soluble factors play a critical role in the rescue of cells from apoptosis. The principal factor for this process is B-cell activating factor (BAFF), a member of the family of tumor necrosis factor (TNF) ligands. BAFF is produced by cells of the myeloid lineage, such as monocytes and dendritic cells, and also by some T cells.[12,13] BAFF binds to three members of the family of TNF receptors: BAFF receptor, TACI (the transmembrane activator and CAML-interactor), and the B-cell maturation antigen.[14] APRIL is another TNF-like ligand that binds these receptors. These factors appear to regulate the fate of the mature pool of peripheral B cells. Immature B cells can also be rescued from apoptosis in numerous BAFF-independent ways via stimulation of Toll-like receptors by substances such as bacterial lipopolysaccharide, lipoprotein, or polysaccharides.

GERMINAL CENTERS

Affinity maturation during the humoral immune response to T-cell–dependent antigens occurs in GCs.[15,16] GCs are specialized environments in the B-cell follicle that facilitate the induction of somatic hypermutations and extensive proliferation of B cells.[17,18] GCs provide a specialized milieu in which extremely high rates of B-cell division enable rapid accumulation of cells with somatic hypermutations that can be selected for high affinity. Antigen is stored in this environment in the form of immune complexes on potent antigen-presenting cells called follicular dendritic cells. Antigen is required for a GC reaction, because B cells that have new mutations must still bind antigen to be rescued from apoptosis.[19] Such interactions with antigen result in the selection of high-affinity B cells, which, in turn, interact with GC T cells and increase their likelihood of survival.[20,21]

The molecular basis for B- and T-cell interactions is an area of intense study. Binding of CD40 ligand (CD40L or CD154), which is expressed on activated helper T lymphocytes, to its receptor CD40, which is expressed on B cells, is essential for thymus-dependent antibody responses. This receptor-ligand engagement stimulates expansion of B-cell clones, GC formation, production of memory B cells, antibody isotype switching, affinity maturation, and the generation of long-lived plasma cells. The mechanism underlying these effects is that oligomerization of CD40 by

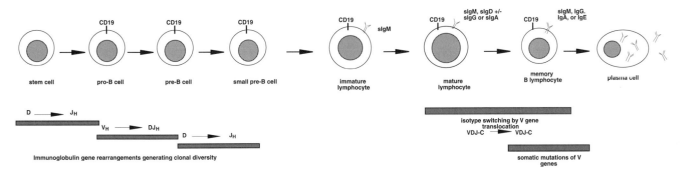

Figure 155–1. Transition from stem cell to plasma cell.

CD154 induces cytoplasmic signaling via recruitment of TNF receptor (TNFR)–associated factors (TRAFs) 1, 2, 3, 5, and 6 to specific domains in the cytoplasmic tail of CD40. These adapter molecules activate serine and threonine kinases that couple the receptor complex to downstream signaling cascades. Therefore, TRAFs appear to control the process of antigen-induced B-cell differentiation *in vivo*.

PLASMA CELL DIFFERENTIATION

Activated dividing cells termed plasmablasts residing in extrafollicular regions become terminally differentiated, nondividing cells called plasma cells, which have a life span of a few days to several months. As in earlier stages of B-cell differentiation, the relative activity of transcriptional factors controls the final differentiation to plasma cells. Three key transcription factors involved in plasma cell development have been identified: B-lymphocyte–induced maturation protein 1 (Blimp-1),[22, 23] interferon-regulatory factor 4,[24] and X box-binding protein 1.[25] Plasma cell differentiation can be distinguished by changes in cell morphology and surface proteins, associated with an increase in the amount of rough endoplasmic reticulum, the number of secretory vacuoles, and the amounts of Ig heavy and light chain mRNA.[26] Two characteristic surface molecules, the proteoglycan syndecan-1, which recognizes extracellular matrix and growth factors, and the chemokine receptor CXCR4, are expressed at high levels in plasma cells. Many other integrin family molecules involved in GC trafficking are decreased in plasma cells, resulting in the movement of these cells from the follicles to other locations, including the bone marrow.

B-CELL RECEPTOR DIVERSITY

Ig genes are organized in three families that encode heavy chains, κ light chains, and λ light chains. Each gene family represents groups of V and J genes (light chains) or V, D, and J genes (heavy chains) upstream from the genes of the constant (C) region. V, D, and J genes encode the antigen-binding site, whereas C genes determine the antibody class and light chain type. The heavy chain cluster is located on chromosome 14; the κ light chain cluster is on chromosome 2, and the λ light chain cluster is on chromosome 22. The heavy chain locus contains 123 V_H gene segments grouped into seven families,[27] and there are numerous D_H genes, six J_H genes, and nine functional C_H genes (μ, δ, γ3, γ1, α1, γ2, γ4, ε, α2). Forty-four or 51 of the V_H genes are functional, the difference depending on whether an insertion/deletion polymorphic region is present.[27, 28] Certain V_H segments are preferentially rearranged in both in-frame and out-of-frame rearrangements, even during the earliest recombination events in pro-B cells, before expression of functional antibody.[29] Some V_H-dependent mechanisms probably influence overrepresentation of certain V_H genes at these early stages during B-cell development. Mechanisms for this bias are not fully defined, but they may include accessibility to the recombinase or the nature of the recombination signal sequence. Most of the fetal V_H genes of mice map close to the D locus, a finding that suggests a location-dependent mechanism for V_H readout.[30] The human fetal repertoire is similarly restricted, but the expressed genes are scattered throughout the locus, thus making the positional hypothesis less likely.[31-34]

Functional Ig genes are formed by sequential DNA rearrangements mediated by the highly specialized RAG1/RAG2 recombinase enzyme complex that recognizes conserved signal sequences flanking the coding segments to be joined.[35] The recombinase splices, for example, a D gene to a J gene. This complex assembles antigen-receptor genes by V(D)J recombination. RAG1 and RAG2 act together to initiate the reaction by cleaving DNA. The enzyme complex has other activities and probably multiple roles in V(D)J recombination, such as holding broken DNA ends together, rejoining DNA fragments, performing transposition, and opening hairpin structures. The precise location of splice junctions in coding joints is variable. Additional nucleotides may be added or removed through the action of deoxynucleotidyltransferase isoforms to generate N diversity. This imprecision in the formation of coding joints increases diversity in the antigen-binding site but also generates many sequences that are not functional.

V(D)J rearrangements proceed in a controlled order, usually beginning with D-J gene splicing in the heavy chain locus,[36] followed by translocation of a V gene. The cell makes the transition from pro-B to pre-B by initiating synthesis of μ chain.[37] Nascent μ chains combine in the endoplasmic reticulum with a surrogate light chain, the product of two pre-B-cell genes called λ5 (mouse) or 14.1 (human) and V_{pre-B}. The complex of μ and surrogate light chain is transported to the cell surface.[38] Although a surrogate light chain is produced in pro-B as well as pre-B cells, it is expressed on the surface of only the most mature pre-B cells.[10] Light chain rearrangement usually follows productive heavy chain rearrangement but can occur independently.[39] κ chains are generally rearranged before λ chains, and about two-thirds of the peripheral blood repertoire uses κ chains. Usually, a functional rearrangement at a particular locus inhibits further rearrangements at that locus, resulting in the characteristic *allelic exclusion* of the polypeptides of lymphocyte receptors. The result is that each newly generated B cell expresses a single unique receptor, but the population of B cells in an individual contains many different receptor specificities.

ONTOGENY OF V-GENE EXPRESSION

The fetal repertoire of expressed V-genes is restricted in some respects. There is less junctional diversity at V(D)J splice sites in fetal heavy chains than in neonatal heavy chains, a finding apparently reflecting a developmental delay in expression of deoxynucleotidyltransferase.[40] Splice junctions are located in the principal region of antigen contact, the heavy chain complementarity determining region 3 (CDR3). Therefore, lack of junctional diversity can significantly restrict structural diversity of the antigen binding site. The neonatal repertoire is substantially more diverse than that of the fetus, and it more closely resembles the adult repertoire because it contains a broader spectrum of V, D, and J genes, somatic hypermutations, and longer CDR3 regions, owing to greater N-region diversity.[41, 42] Preferential rearrangement of certain V_H genes has been demonstrated using cDNA from fetal liver,[31,32,43-45] adult bone marrow,[42, 46] and adult peripheral blood cells.[47] Narrow antigen-specific repertoires with preferred V_H regions have been identified in human responses to the polysaccharide antigens of *Haemophilus influenzae* type B, *Streptococcus pneumoniae*, and the yeast *Cryptococcus neoformans*. Antibody responses to these antigens are T-cell independent. These studies suggest that, for simple antigens with a limited diversity of structure, the number of structurally ideal antibody combining sites in the germline is limited. Additional V-gene biases are observed in special populations of humans such as fetuses and the elderly. V_H region biases that change with age may contribute to impaired functional antibody responses to infection and immunization. We have shown that virus protein-specific repertoires of infants are remarkably similar to those used by adults to the same antigen.

CD5+ B CELLS

There have been many studies of B cells that express CD5, an adhesion and cell-surface signaling molecule expressed on a subpopulation of adult B cells and on all T cells. B cells that develop earliest in ontogeny bear CD5, and it is thought that these cells may represent a distinctive peripheral B-cell population, enriched for natural autoreactive specificities that appear to be encoded by particular germline V_H/V_L combinations. These cells have been associated with the production of polyreactive autoantibodies,[48] and they are present in relatively high proportions during fetal life. In the mouse, a similar class of cells expressing CD5 (termed B-1a cells) is found in abundance in the peritoneal cavity and has been intensively studied. These long-lived cells frequently produce antibodies that are encoded by unmutated germline Ig genes and that react with autoantigens or bacterial carbohydrates such as pneumococcal phosphatidylcholine.[49] The developmental origin of these cells and the role of these cells in human autoimmunity or specific immune responses to foreign pathogens are not clear at this time.

DIVERSIFICATION AFTER V(D)J RECOMBINATION

B cells use three distinct processes that are not found in T cells to enhance receptor diversity of Ig genes further after recombination: class switch recombination, somatic hypermutation, and gene conversion. Class switch recombination replaces the constant region of the Ig heavy chain gene, whereas somatic hypermutation and gene conversion alter the heavy and light chain variable-region exons. Somatic hypermutation is triggered by antigen and forms the basis of the process of affinity maturation. The molecular mechanism of somatic hypermutation is under intense investigation. DNA strand breaks, the critical initial step in somatic hypermutation, are tightly associated with the reaction. Studies have revealed many *cis*-acting elements within the Ig locus that are required for hypermutation. These include an intronic enhancer and the V-region promoter, although the Ig promoter itself is not necessary because it can be replaced by a heterologous promoter.[50] The V region of the sequence can be replaced by a heterologous sequence, a finding suggesting that it is not necessary for targeting hypermutation. Transcription plays a role in hypermutation, possibly by facilitating accessibility of the locus to the mutational machinery. A critical yet unknown aspect of Ig hypermutation is the mechanism that ensures the targeting of lesions to the Ig V region, while sparing the constant domains, which are only a few kilobases downstream from the V region.

Hypermutation of antigen-receptor genes is characterized by mutational hotspots and, in the absence of antigenic-selection, a bias to generate transitions over transversions. The mutational rate and pattern suggest error-prone synthesis by one or more of the polymerases typically involved in the mutagenic bypass of DNA lesions, and evidence strongly implicates their involvement.[51-53] The GC-restricted activation-induced cytidine deaminase (AID) has been demonstrated to be required for both somatic hypermutation and class switch recombination.[54] The molecular mode of action of AID is not fully understood at this time. AID is also required for Ig gene conversion,[55] and it therefore appears to be a critical mediator of all the B-cell–specific mechanisms of Ig gene diversification.

CLASS SWITCH RECOMBINATION: THE ORIGIN OF ISOTYPE DIVERSITY

Class switch recombination occurs exclusively in mature B cells. Mature B cells coexpress surface IgM and IgD antibodies before they encounter antigen, and then they express IgG, IgE, or IgA as memory cells after antigen stimulation. B cells expressing any other isotype originate from precursors that express membrane IgM (mIgM) by a process called *isotype switching*. IgM is expressed first because the Cμ gene is closest to the J genes and the intron between J and Cμ contains important transcriptional enhancers. Two mechanisms are recognized for expression of isotypes whose genes are downstream of Cμ. *Differential splicing* of a transcript including V(D)J-Cμ-Cδ may generate independent messenger RNAs (mRNAs), V(D)J-Cμ, and V(D)J-Cδ, which are translated to μ and δ chains having identical V regions.[56] This mechanism accounts for the large number of B cells that coexpress mIgM and mIgD receptors with identical specificity. The second mechanism, called *switch recombination*, involves translocation of a V(D)J gene from its location upstream of Cμ to a new switch site in the 5′-flanking region of another C$_H$ gene, for example C$_\alpha$1.[57] The receptor/ligand pair, CD40/CD154, plays a major role in the regulation of B- and T-cell interactions.[58] In humans, CD40 triggering is required for the induction of isotype switching. In the hyper-IgM syndrome,[59] a genetic alteration of the CD154 results in a lack of circulating IgG, IgA, and GCs. Soluble factors also influence isotype switching. For example, the cytokines IL-4 and IL-13 induce specific isotype switching toward IgE and IgG4,[60-62] whereas IL-10 induces the switch toward IgG1 and IgG3[63,64] and IgA.[65] Dendritic cells contribute to isotype switching by activating T cells in the extrafollicular areas of secondary lymphoid organs and by directly modulating T-cell–dependent B-cell growth and differentiation by inducing the IgA isotype switch.[66]

IMMATURITY

The molecular basis for the lower titer and poor functional activity of neonatal and infant antibody responses is not well understood. Discovery of the gene defect in X-linked immunodeficiency with hyper-IgM (CD154) showed that this molecule and its associated interaction partners were essential for class switching. Neonatal T cells, like adult T cells, transiently express CD154.[67] Data suggest that either prolonged or repeated signaling through CD40 is required to bring B cells to a state of full differentiation and competence. The lack of such stimulation is a likely partial explanation for the functional immaturity of neonatal B cells. One of the most striking aspects of childhood immunologic immaturity is the inability of young animals and humans to respond to carbohydrate antigens, for example, the polysaccharides of childhood pathogens such as *Haemophilus influenzae* or *Streptococcus pneumoniae*. The molecular basis for this observation has not been determined. The lack of immunogenicity of polysaccharides in this age group can be overcome by conjugation to protein carriers, a strategy that has led to the use of licensed infant vaccines for these pathogens.

TOLERANCE

The immune system has developed many regulatory mechanisms to allow tolerance to self because self-reactive antibodies are inevitably generated in the course of development of the antibody repertoire. B-cell tolerance can be initiated in the bone marrow, a mechanism termed *central tolerance*. Newly emerging immature B cells are highly susceptible to negative selection if they encounter their antigen in the proper context, a phenomenon called *clonal deletion*. Additional mechanisms of tolerance are required, given that not all tissue-specific antigens are present in the bone marrow. These mechanisms, termed *peripheral tolerance*, are principally the result of incomplete activation of B cells that encounter self-antigen outside the bone marrow in sites such as the spleen or lymph node GCs. Incomplete activation of B cells can lead to apoptosis of those B cells or a nonresponsive state in which B cells that recognize the autoantigen are present but unresponsive, termed *anergy*.[68] When the concentration of antigen is low, B-cell development may progress, but immunologic tolerance can be maintained by lack of T-cell reactivity, a state that is called *clonal ignorance*.[69] Finally, secondary rearrangement of the antibody light chain locus, termed *receptor editing*, provides a way for autoreactive B cells destined for deletion or anergy in the periphery to generate a B-cell receptor that is not autoreactive. In summary, the developmental program of B cells provides for multiple mechanisms to promote tolerance of self-antigens.

REFERENCES

1. Kamps WA, Cooper MD: Microenvironmental studies of pre B and B cell development in human and mouse fetuses. J Immunol 129:526, 1982.
2. Bofill M, et al: Human B cell development. II. Subpopulations in the human fetus. J Immunol 134:1531, 1985.
3. Egawa T, et al: The earliest stages of B cell development require a chemokine stromal cell–derived factor/pre-B cell growth-stimulating factor. Immunity 15:323, 2001.
4. Katsura Y: Redefinition of lymphoid progenitors. Nat Rev Immunol 2:127, 2002.
5. Wilson A, et al: Notch 1-deficient common lymphoid precursors adopt a B cell fate in the thymus. J Exp Med 194:1003, 2001.
6. Koch U, et al: Subversion of the T/B lineage decision in the thymus by lunatic fringe-mediated inhibition of Notch-1. Immunity 15:225, 2001.
7. Izon DJ, et al: Eltex1 redirects lymphoid progenitors to the B cell lineage by antagonizing Notch1. Immunity 16:231, 2002.
8. Kitamura D, et al: A critical role of lambda 5 protein in B cell development. Cell 69:823, 1992.
9. Ehlich A, et al: Immunoglobulin heavy and light chain genes rearrange independently at early stages of B cell development. Cell 72:695, 1993.
10. Lassoued K, et al: Expression of surrogate light chain receptors is restricted to a late stage in pre-B cell differentiation. Cell 73:73, 1993.
11. Potter M, Melchers F: Opinions on the nature of B-1 cells and their relationship to B cell neoplasia. Curr Top Microbiol Immunol 252:307, 2000.
12. Schneider, P, et al: BAFF, a novel ligand of the tumor necrosis factor family, stimulates B cell growth. J Exp Med 189:1747, 1999.
13. Moore, PA, et al: BLyS: member of the tumor necrosis factor family and B lymphocyte stimulator. Science 285:260, 1999.
14. Gross, JA, et al: TACI and BCMA are receptors for a TNF homologue implicated in B-cell autoimmune disease. Nature 404:995, 2000.
15. Berek C, et al: Maturation of the immune response in germinal centers. Cell 67:1121, 1991.
16. MacLennan IC: Germinal centers. Annu Rev Immunol 12:117, 1994.
17. Jacob J, et al: Intraclonal generation of antibody mutants in germinal centres. Nature 354:389, 1991.
18. Leanderson T, et al: Expansion, selection and mutation of antigen-specific B cells in germinal centers. Immunol Rev 126:47, 1992.
19. Koopman G, et al: Germinal center B cells rescued from apoptosis by CD40 ligation or attachment to follicular dendritic cells, but not by engagement of surface immunoglobulin or adhesion receptors, become resistant to CD95-induced apoptosis. Eur J Immunol 27:1, 1997.
20. MacLennan IC, et al: The changing preference of T and B cells for partners as T-dependent antibody responses develop. Immunol Rev 156:53, 1997.
21. Lindhout E, et al: Triple check for antigen specificity of B cells during germinal centre reactions. Immunol Today 18:573, 1997.
22. Turner CA Jr, et al: Blimp-1, a novel zinc finger-containing protein that can drive the maturation of B lymphocytes into immunoglobulin-secreting cells. Cell 77:297, 1994.
23. Angelin-Duclos C, et al: Commitment of B lymphocytes to a plasma cell fate is associated with Blimp-1 expression in vivo. J Immunol 165:5462, 2000.
24. Eisenbeis CF, et al: PU.1 is a component of a multiprotein complex which binds an essential site in the murine immunoglobulin lambda 2–4 enhancer. Mol Cell Biol 13:6452, 1993.
25. Reimold AM, et al: Plasma cell differentiation requires the transcription factor XBP-1. Nature 412:300, 2001.
26. Chen-Bettecken U, et al: IgM RNA switch from membrane to secretory form is prevented by adding antireceptor antibody to bacterial lipopolysaccharide-stimulated murine primary B-cell cultures. Proc Natl Acad Sci USA 82:7384, 1985.
27. Matsuda F, et al: The complete nucleotide sequence of the human immunoglobulin heavy chain variable region locus. J Exp Med 188:2151, 1998.
28. Cook GP, Tomlinson IM: The human immunoglobulin VH repertoire. Immunol Today 16:237, 1995.
29. Rao SP, et al: Biased VH gene usage in early lineage human B cells: evidence for preferential Ig gene rearrangement in the absence of selection. J Immunol 163:2732, 1999.
30. Perlmutter RM, et al: Developmentally controlled expression of immunoglobulin VH genes. Science 227:1597, 1985.
31. Schroeder HW Jr, et al: Early restriction of the human antibody repertoire. Science 238:791, 1987.
32. Schroeder HW Jr, Wang JY: Preferential utilization of conserved immunoglobulin heavy chain variable gene segments during human fetal life. Proc Natl Acad Sci USA 87:6146, 1990.
33. Adderson EE, et al: Development of the human antibody repertoire. Pediatr Res 32:257, 1992.
34. Willems van Dijk K, et al: Chromosomal organization of the heavy chain variable region gene segments comprising the human fetal antibody repertoire. Proc Natl Acad Sci USA 89:10403, 1992.
35. Schatz DG, et al: V(D)J recombination: molecular biology and regulation. Annu Rev Immunol 10:359, 1992.
36. Alt FW, et al: VDJ recombination. Immunol Today 13:306, 1992.
37. Cooper MD, Burrows PD: B cell differentiation. In Honjo T, et al (eds): Immunoglobulin Genes. San Diego, Academic Press, 1990, pp 1–21.
38. Tsubata T, Reth M: The products of the pre-B cell specific genes (lambda 5 and VpreB) and the immunoglobulin mu chain form a complex that is transported to the cell surface. J Exp Med 172:973, 1990.
39. Kubagawa H, et al: Light-chain gene expression before heavy-chain rearrangement in pre-B cells transformed by Epstein-Barr virus. Proc Natl Acad Sci USA 86:2356, 1989.
40. Raaphorst FM, et al: Restricted utilization of germ-line VH3 genes and short diverse third complementarity-determining regions (CDR3) in human fetal B lymphocyte immunoglobulin heavy chain rearrangements. Eur J Immunol 22:247, 1992.
41. Mortari F, et al: Human cord blood antibody repertoire: mixed population of VH gene segments and CDR 3 distribution in the expressed Cα and Cγ repertoires. J Immunol 150:1348, 1993.
42. Milili M, et al: The VDJ repertoire expressed in human preB cells reflects the selection of bona fide heavy chains. Eur J Immunol 26:63, 1996.
43. Hillson JL, et al: Emerging human B cell repertoire. Influence of developmental stage and interindividual variation. J Immunol 149:3741, 1992.
44. Cuisinier AM, et al: Mechanisms that generate human immunoglobulin diversity operate from the 8th week of gestation in fetal liver. Eur J Immunol 23:110, 1993.
45. Pascual V, et al: Analysis of Ig H chain gene segment utilization in human fetal liver. J Immunol 151:4164, 1993.
46. Kraj P, et al: The human heavy chain Ig V region gene repertoire is biased at all stages of B cell ontogeny, including early pre-B cells. J Immunol 158:5824, 1997.
47. Brezinschek HP, et al: Analysis of the heavy chain repertoire of human peripheral B cells using single-cell polymerase chain reaction. J Immunol 155:190–202, 1995.
48. Casali P, Notkins AL: Probing the human B cell repertoire with EBV: polyreactive antibodies and CD5+ B lymphocytes. Annu Rev Immunol 7:513, 1989.
49. Hayakawa K, Hardy RR: Development and function of B-1 cells. Curr Opin Immunol 12:346–353, 2000.
50. Storb U, et al: Cis-acting sequences that affect somatic hypermutation of Ig genes. Immunol Rev 162:153, 1998.
51. Zeng X, et al: DNA polymerase eta is an A-T mutator in somatic hypermutation of immunoglobulin variable genes. Nat Immunol 2:537, 2001.
52. Zan H, et al: The translesion DNA polymerase zeta plays a major role in Ig and BCL-6 somatic mutation. Immunity 14:643, 2001.
53. Diaz M, et al: Decreased frequency of somatic hypermutation and impaired affinity maturation but intact germinal center formation in mice expressing antisense RNA to DNA polymerase zeta. J Immunol 167:327, 2001.
54. Muramatsu M, et al: Class switch recombination and hypermutation require activation-induced cytidine deaminase (AID), a potential RNA editing enzyme. Cell 102:553, 2000.
55. Arakawa H, et al: Requirement of the activation-induced deaminase (AID) gene for immunoglobulin gene conversion. Science 295:1301, 2002.
56. Tucker PW: Transcriptional regulation of IgM and IgD. Immunol Today 6:181, 1985.
57. Honjo T: Immunoglobulin genes. Annu Rev Immunol 1:499, 1983.
58. Banchereau J, et al: The CD40 antigen and its ligand. Annu Rev Immunol 12:881, 1994.
59. Callard RE, et al: CD40 ligand and its role in X-linked hyperIgM syndrome. Immunol Today 14:559, 1993.
60. Gascan H, et al: Human B cell clones can be induced to proliferate and to switch to IgE and IgG4 synthesis by interleukin 4 and a signal provided by activated CD4+ T cell clones. J Exp Med 173:747, 1991.
61. Rousset F, et al: Cytokine-induced proliferation and immunoglobulin production in human V-genes triggered through their CD40 antigen. J Exp Med 173:705, 1991.
62. Jabara HH, et al: CD40 and IgE: synergism between anti-CD40 monoclonal antibody and interleukin 4 in the induction of IgE synthesis by highly purified human B cells. J Exp Med 172:1861, 1990.
63. Brière F, et al: Human interleukin 10 induces naive sIgD+ B cells to secrete IgG1 and IgG3. J Exp Med 179:757, 1994.
64. Malisan F, et al: IL-10 induces IgG isotype switch recombination in human CD40-activated naive V-genes. J Exp Med 183:937, 1996.
65. Defrance T, et al: Interleukin 10 and transforming growth factor beta cooperate to induce anti–CD40-activated naive human B cells to secrete immunoglobulin A. J Exp Med 175:671, 1992.
66. Fayette J, et al: Human dendritic cells skew isotype switching of CD40-activated naive B cells towards IgA1 and IgA2. J Exp Med 185:1909, 1997.
67. Splawski JB, et al: CD40 ligand is expressed and functional on activated neonatal T cells. J Immunol 156:119, 1996.
68. Van Parijs L, Abbas AK: Homeostasis and self-tolerance in the immune system: turning lymphocytes off. Science 280:243, 1998.
69. Goodnow CC: Transgenic mice and analysis of B-cell tolerance. Annu Rev Immunol 10:489, 1992.

Mononuclear Phagocyte System

ORIGIN AND DEVELOPMENT OF MONONUCLEAR PHAGOCYTES

Tissue phagocytes have been recognized as fundamental components of host immune defense. The term *mononuclear phagocyte system* (MPS) identifies a specific lineage of phagocytic hematopoietic cells that share certain morphologic, cytochemical, biochemical, genetic, and functional characteristics.[1,2] In this system, mononuclear phagocytes comprise a cell lineage in which tissue macrophages are derived from circulating monocytes and immature bone marrow precursors. Mononuclear phagocytes share common functional characteristics[2,3] including:

1. Phagocytosis and digestion of invading microorganisms and tissue debris
2. Biosynthesis of numerous secretory products
3. Antigen processing and interaction with lymphocytes in development of the primary immune response
4. Generation of a cytotoxic response to tumor cells
5. Performance of specialized tissue functions in concert with functions of other tissue cell types to maintain a homeostatic extracellular environment

Although dendritic cells differ in several morphologic, cytochemical, and functional features from classical cells of the MPS, evidence indicates that at least one population of dendritic cells, the myeloid dendritic cells, derives from the same bone marrow hematopoietic progenitors as circulating monocytes and macrophages.[4] Because dendritic cells and mononuclear phagocytes share a common progenitor pathway, consideration must be given to including dendritic cells as members of the MPS.[5] Dendritic cells exhibit most characteristics just enumerated. First, dendritic cells are phagocytic cells in which captured material enters endosomes for degradation and antigen processing. Second, they synthesize cytokines that direct actions of innate and adaptive immune cells. Third, dendritic cells are highly effective antigen presenting cells. Fourth, dendritic cells provide signals for macrophage and T-cell activation. Finally, dendritic cells exhibit specialized functions to maintain homeostasis of the extracellular environment. In this chapter, myeloid dendritic cells are discussed as components of the MPS.

Overview

The mononuclear phagocyte cell lineage originates from a committed progenitor cell present in the bone marrow (Fig. 156–1). Pluripotent stem cells give rise to progenitor cells committed to a program of proliferation and differentiation. Progenitor cells committed to the myeloid lineage, called colony forming unit granulocyte-macrophages (CFU-GMs), are supported along various myeloid pathways by actions of glycoproteins called colony-stimulating factors (CSFs). CSFs involved in mononuclear phagocyte differentiation include interleukin-3 (IL-3), granulocyte-macrophage colony–stimulating factor (GM-CSF), and monocyte colony–stimulating factor (M-CSF or CSF-1). These factors synergize to support differentiation of CFU-GM into macrophages *in vitro*.[6–8] Addition of M-CSF preferentially induces macrophage differentiation. Inclusion of GM-CSF in combination with IL-4 and tumor necrosis factor-α (TNF-α) generate dendritic cells *in vitro*.[9,10,11,12]

Experiments in which the genes encoding the CSFs have been inactivated *in vivo* through homologous recombination in mice have increased our understanding of the *in vivo* role of the CSFs in regulating MPS cell production. Homologous inactivation of the GM-CSF gene did not appear to have a significant effect on fetal, neonatal, or adult growth and did not alter many aspects of granulocyte and macrophage physiology with one notable exception. Affected mice succumbed to alveolar proteinosis as a result of defective alveolar macrophage function.[13,14] Similar results were observed in affected mice when the common β-subunit for the receptors for GM-CSF, IL-3, and IL-5 was inactivated.[15] Shibata and colleagues[16] identified multiple defects in alveolar macrophage function in GM-CSF–deficient mice, including adhesion, phagocytosis, microbicidal activity, surfactant metabolism, and expression of toll-like receptors (TLRs). Mice suffering from an inherited form of osteopetrosis (op/op) have been shown to have a mutation resulting in M-CSF gene inactivation.[17] Homozygous mutants have a defect in some, but not all macrophage populations. The most profound macrophage derangement is in osteoclast numbers leading to severe bone and tooth abnormalities.[18] As op/op mice age, IL-3 expression increases and any of the deficits in the alveolar macrophage population resolve.[19] These studies confirm the importance of CSF function *in vivo* in MPS development and, in addition, demonstrate the redundancy in these factors.

The identification and characterization of numerous lineage-restricted transcription factors that regulate the pattern of gene expression in hematopoietic cells suggest that transcription factors may play a key role in regulating hematopoietic progenitor cell proliferation and differentiation.[20] One such transcription factor that plays a significant role in MPS development is designated PU.1 (Fig. 156–2). The importance of this factor is underscored by its developmental expression in alveolar macrophages of GM-CSF deletion mice. Defective PU.1 expression in the alveolar macrophages of GM-CSF deficient mice leads to impaired host

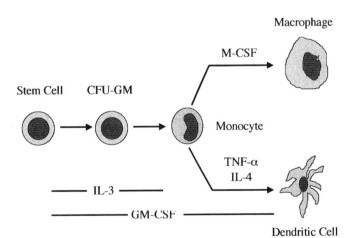

Figure 156–1. Mononuclear phagocyte cell lineage.
CFU-GM = colony-forming units granulocyte macrophage; IL-3 = interleukin-3; GM-CSF = granulocyte-macrophage colony stimulating factor; M-CSF = macrophage-colony stimulating factor; TNF-α = tumor necrosis factor-alpha; IL-4 = interleukin-4.

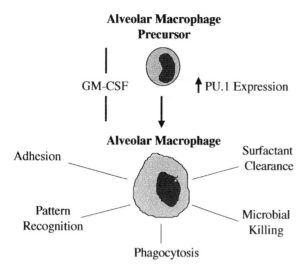

Alveolar Macrophage Precursor

GM-CSF   ↑ PU.1 Expression

Alveolar Macrophage

Adhesion   Surfactant Clearance

Pattern Recognition   Microbial Killing

Phagocytosis

Figure 156–2. Role of granulocyte-macrophage colony stimulating factors (GM-CSF) and PU.1 in regulation of differentiation and function of the alveolar macrophage. GM-CSF induces the transcription factor, PU.1, in macrophage precursors in the lung. PU.1 is required for terminal maturation of alveolar macrophages and it enables these cells to play critical roles in maintenance of lung homeostasis and innate immune responses.

defense functions and surfactant homeostatic mechanisms.[16] These functions are restored using retroviral transduction of the PU.1 gene into alveolar macrophages. Homozygous PU.1 deficient mice also exhibit lack of myeloid dendritic cell development.[21]

Kinetics of Peripheral Blood Monocytes

The normal circulating monocyte count in the healthy human adult is estimated to be between 300 and 450 monocytes/mm³. Peripheral blood monocyte counts have been observed to vary in a cyclic fashion over a 3- to 6-day period.[22,23]

The production and kinetics of circulating human adult mononuclear phagocytes have been studied by *in vivo* pulse labeling of mononuclear phagocytes with tritiated thymidine followed by autotransfusion of radiolabeled leukocytes. The number of promonocytes present in bone marrow has been estimated to be between 3 and 5%, with approximately 40% of the promonocytes actively proliferating.[24] The promonocyte cell cycle rate varies between 30 and 48 hours. These rapidly dividing cells achieve a production rate between 7×10^5 and 7×10^6 monocytes/kg of body weight per hour. After 60 hours of maturation in the bone marrow, mature monocytes move into the intravascular space, where they circulate for approximately 3 days.[24] Van Furth and coworkers[2] calculated that 1.66×10^{10} circulating monocytes leave the intravascular space/hour. Therefore, these investigators estimated the turnover of monocytes to be 0.4×10^9 cells/day. Whitelaw[25] has suggested that the total intravascular monocyte pool is composed of a marginated pool and a circulating pool. He calculated that the marginated pool was 3.3 times greater than the circulating pool. Other investigators have failed to confirm a marginated pool of monocytes in human subjects.[2] Experiments in mice and rats provide evidence for marginated monocyte pools.[26,27]

Kinetics of Macrophages

Analysis of tissue macrophage kinetics is difficult, given that the ultimate fate of tissue macrophages is not precisely known. Alveolar macrophages purportedly move from the respiratory tract to the alimentary tract, where they are eventually cleared.[28] The fate of other tissue macrophages has not been determined.

Tissue macrophages are derived from bone marrow precursors. The first evidence for the bone marrow origin of macrophages was obtained in mouse chimeras[29] and rat parabiosis experiments.[30, 31] Studies in human subjects have confirmed the data observed in animal experiments. In several patients undergoing bone marrow transplantation, isolation and characterization of lung[32] and liver macrophages[33] provided evidence that these cells contained the karyotype of the bone marrow donor. Thus, terminally differentiated macrophages must have been derived from transplanted bone marrow. Furthermore, by following the disappearance of the Y body-containing macrophages from male patients who have received female donor marrow, the half-life of the alveolar macrophage was estimated to be 81 days.

The size of the tissue macrophage compartment is considerable. By some estimates, the number of tissue macrophages is 500 to 1000 times greater than the bone marrow compartment. Some organs, such as the lung and liver, may have particularly large macrophage populations that may account for between 20 and 30% of the total cell number. These cells are long lived and in a number of tissues have been estimated to survive for several months.[28,32,33]

Fetal Period

Embryonic macrophages can be identified early in hematopoietic tissues of the yolk sac. Tissue macrophages present at 3- to 4-weeks' gestation do not appear to be associated with mononuclear phagocyte precursors (promonocytes and monocytes). Determination of the origin of these cells challenges the mononuclear phagocyte concept, in which macrophages are believed to be derived from immature precursors. The true origin of these macrophages remains to be clarified, although some investigators believe that these cells differentiate directly from hemocytoblasts.[34] Cline and Moore[35] have demonstrated that murine macrophages develop *in vitro* from primitive yolk sac precursors. They propose that the macrophage develops from a progenitor in the yolk sac that is proximal to promonocyte and monocyte stages of maturation. Later in gestation when the yolk sac is open to the fetal circulation, promonocytes, monocytes, and macrophages are all readily identifiable.

The liver becomes the predominant hematopoietic organ in the second month of gestation. At 4.5 weeks' gestation, approximately 70% of blood cells present in the liver are morphologically identifiable as macrophages.[36] Over the next 6 weeks, macrophages decrease to approximately 1 to 2% of all differentiated blood cells in the liver, with erythroblasts becoming the most numerous blood cell type in that organ. Primitive hemocytoblasts never account for more than 5% of all hematopoietic cells in the liver.

Although monoblasts and promonocytes may be identified during the period of liver promonopoiesis, true mature monocytes do not appear in the intravascular system of the fetus until the fifth month of gestation.[37] Circulating monocyte numbers remain low until after the sixth month of gestation, at which time bone marrow hematopoiesis predominates. During the first trimester of gestation, monocytes account for 2 to 4% of all hematopoietic cells. At approximately 30 weeks' gestation, monocytes constitute 3 to 7% of all hematopoietic cells.[38]

Analysis of mononuclear phagocyte kinetics has not been possible in the fetal tissue examined. Mitotic figures have been seen in 0.1 to 1.2% of all hematopoietic cells in tissues. However, because of the difficulty in adequate preparation of tissues between delivery and the time of analysis, the number of cells in mitosis might actually be higher.[34] Therefore, the kinetics of mononuclear phagocyte production and distribution to the tissues during the fetal period remain to be determined.

Neonatal Period

Analysis of the origin and development of mononuclear phagocytes in the neonatal period has been limited by the minimal number of approaches available to sample tissue macrophage populations in these patients. The total cellularity of the bone marrow averages 1.36×10^{11} cells/L on the first day of life but declines to 3.5×10^{10} cells/µL by the ninth day of life.[39] Analysis of bone marrow preparations from premature and term infants suggests that there are no significant differences in the differential counts of marrow elements for these populations of newborn infants.

There is a relative monocytosis present throughout the neonatal period. Peripheral blood monocyte counts are highest during the first 24 hours of life and decline over the remainder of the first month of life. Xanthou[40] reported that the peripheral monocyte counts of newborn infants in the first week of life ranges from 300 to 2100 cells/mm³ with a mean of 1000 cells/mm³. Weinberg and colleagues[41] analyzed the peripheral blood monocyte count in newborn infants and found a range between 0 and 1912, with a median of 600 monocytes/mm³ in the first 60 hours of life. They also observed a decline in the upper limit of normal during the first month of life, but the median value of 600 cells/mm³ remained constant. One problem encountered by all of these investigators, which may account for discrepancies in absolute numbers detected, is that mononuclear phagocytes in the newborn period are morphologically heterogeneous. Some monocytes are difficult to differentiate from myelocytes or metamyelocytes belonging to the neutrophil series, whereas other monocytes appear to be morphologically similar to large immature granular lymphocytes.[42]

Analysis of tissue macrophage kinetics in newborn infants has been limited to the examination of pathologic specimens or those gathered at autopsy of cases of stillborn or neonatal death. Alenghat and Esterly[43] performed histologic examination on the lungs of 200 consecutive infants who were stillborn or who died during the neonatal period and reported that the lungs of stillborn infants rarely contained alveolar macrophages. The presence of alveolar macrophages was confirmed in only four of 100 stillborn infants, and evidence of congenital pneumonia was present in several of these cases. In those babies who survived less than 48 hours, alveolar macrophages were observed in 33 of 46 patients. Infants who survived for a period longer than 48 hours uniformly had alveolar macrophages present in their lungs; however, in most of these cases, pneumonic infections were identified. Alveolar macrophages were detected in infants of all gestations (i.e., longer than 30 weeks) who survived longer than 48 hours after birth. These investigators concluded that few alveolar macrophages were present in fetal lungs before birth, but that postnatally, a rapid influx is highly probable.

Experiments in a variety of animal models have confirmed the observation that fetal lung tissue contains few alveolar macrophages.[44-47] Soon after birth in most animal species studied, there are significant increases in the number of alveolar macrophages. Analysis of macrophage kinetics in these studies suggests that macrophage populations in the lungs are replenished both by a continuous monocyte influx and by local proliferation of macrophages.

CHARACTERIZATION OF MONONUCLEAR PHAGOCYTES

Morphology

The morphology of human monocytes and macrophages has been extensively studied at light and electron microscopic levels.[48] The ultrastructure of monocytes is notable for a well-developed Golgi apparatus with a small endoplasmic reticulum containing ribosomes and polysomes. Mitochondria are abundant. Numerous granules containing various lysosomal enzymes are distributed throughout the cytoplasm. The surface membrane of the monocyte includes an extensive system of microvilli. Macrophages are larger than monocytes. The Golgi apparatus, lysosomal granules, and mitochondria are larger than in monocytes. A prominent feature of macrophages is the presence of electron-dense lysosomes along the cell surface. Granules and vacuole are seen along the periphery of the cell, indicating enhanced pinocytosis. Phagosomes are present containing ingested material at various stages of degradation.

Dendritic cells received their name from their distinctive morphology. They are notable for their irregular shape and numerous membrane processes including spiny dendrites, bulbous pseudopods, and lamellipodiae or veils.[49] Distinctive electron microscopic features include prominent mitochondria, endosomes, and lysosomes in the cytoplasm.

Histochemistry

Monocytes and macrophages can be delineated from other leukocytes by cytochemical techniques that detect cellular constituents and biochemical processes. One of the most reliable of these markers is nonspecific esterase, which can be demonstrated using α-naphthyl butyrate as a substrate.[1] Many cell types contain nonspecific esterase, but the isozyme present in monocytes can be identified by inhibition with sodium fluoride.[50] Nonspecific esterase is expressed on the surface of peripheral blood monocytes. As monocytes differentiated into macrophages, additional isozymes of nonspecific esterase are expressed leading to intense cytoplasmic staining.[51] Cord blood monocytes stain positive for nonspecific esterase, however, the proportion of esterase-positive cells is lower than in adult peripheral blood.[52] Peroxidase activity is also prominent in monocytes and diminishes as they mature into macrophages.[53] No differences are observed in peroxidase activity between monocytes from neonates and adults.

Dendritic cells lack many of the enzymes associated with other members of the MPS. Cytochemical reactions show that dendritic cells lack myeloperoxidase and have low levels of 5′ nucleosidase, dipeptidylpeptidase, and cathepsin B activity.[54-57] Other intracellular enzymes, such as nonspecific esterase, acid phosphatase, and lysosomal CD68 may be present in dendritic cells, but their intensity is less than in monocytes or macrophages.[58] Nonspecific esterase decreases with activation of dendritic cells.[59]

Cell Surface Receptors

Numerous cell surface receptors have been identified on human mononuclear phagocytes. Ligands recognized by mononuclear phagocyte receptors include bioactive lipids, carbohydrates, complement components, cytokines, extracellular matrix, growth hormones, pathogen-associated pattern recognition, polypeptide hormones, and lipoproteins.

Fc receptors (FcRs) for immunoglobulin G (IgG) were identified nearly four decades ago with the observation that IgG antibodies could be directly cytophilic for macrophages when opsonized to erythrocytes.[60] Subsequent *in vitro* studies established the role of these receptors in triggering leukocyte effector functions such as macrophage phagocytosis and neutrophil activation by IgG immune complexes.[61, 62] Our current understanding of IgG FcRs has been greatly enhanced by molecular cloning of the murine genes and their human counterparts and by the recently described crystal structures for both receptors.[63-68] Two general classes of FcRs are now recognized: activation receptors characterized by the presence of a cytoplasmic tyrosine activation motif (ITAM) sequence, and an inhibitory receptor, characterized by the presence of a tyrosine inhibition motif (ITIM) sequence.[69,70] Activation and inhibitory receptors bind IgG with comparable affinity and specificity; therefore, co-engagement of both signaling pathways sets the threshold and magnitude for the effector cell response.[71] The balanced function of these receptors has been comprehended through analysis of mice deficient in either the receptor or signaling pathway components.

Activation FcRs include an ITAM motif either intrinsic to the receptor, as in the case of FcγIIA, or as part of an associated subunit, as in FcγI and FcγRIIIA. Cross-linking of the ligand-binding extracellular domain results in tyrosine phosphorylation of the ITAM by members of the src family of molecules. This leads to recruitment of SH2-containing signaling molecules that engage phosphorylated ITAM. Depending on the particular cell type activated by FcR, different kinases are involved in these signaling pathways. Early signaling events include activation of phosphatidyl inositol-3 kinase (PI3 kinase), the enzymatic activity that leads to production of phosphatidyl inositol 3,4,5-tetrakis phosphate (PIP3) and recruitment of binding proteins of the pleckstrin homology (PH) domain class such as phosholipase Cγ (PLCγ).[72-74] Ultimately, activation of PLCγ leads to sustained calcium mobilization. The significance of this activity for FcR function has been determined through analysis of PLCγ2-deficient mice.[75] Cellular processes associated with FcγR activation receptors include degranulation, phagocytosis, antibody-dependent cellular cytotoxicity (ADCC), transcription of cytokine genes, and release of inflammatory mediators.[61,62]

Both activation and inhibitory receptors are present on cells of the MPS, notably monocytes, macrophages, and dendritic cells. In general, activation and inhibitory FcγRs are coexpressed on the same cell, a physiologically important means of establishing a threshold for activating stimuli, because the IgG ligands engage both receptors. The ratio of these two opposing signaling systems determines the cellular response. Importantly, these receptors are modulated in their expression during development and differentiation of effector cells by the cytokine activation of these cells.

Microbes display molecular arrays or patterns that are recognized by pattern recognition molecules. These patterns are shared among groups of pathogens. Representative examples include the lipopolysaccharide (LPS) of gram-negative bacteria, the glycolipids of mycobacteria, peptidoglycans and lipoteichoic acid of gram-positive bacteria, the mannans of yeast, and the double stranded RNA of viruses.[76-78] Important features of these microbial pattern are that 1) they represent invariant structures shared by large groups of microorganisms, 2) they are absolutely essential for the microbe's survival, and 3) they are not produced by the host organism.[79] To limit infection the mammalian host uses an array of pattern recognition molecules. These include complement, the collectins, and a battery of antimicrobial peptides that act with effector cells to combat infectious challenge.

Recognition of LPS is an important function of innate immunity that can have profound consequences for the host. Failure to contain the infection can result in gram-negative sepsis, shock, and death as a result of LPS release. Two LPS-binding proteins have been characterized in mammals; these are the bacterial-permeability increasing protein (BPI) and LPS-binding protein (LBP).[80-82] Binding of LPS by these molecules results in markedly different functional consequences.[83] BPI is a neutrophil granular pattern recognition molecule that exhibits selective toxicity against gram-negative bacteria. BPI has two distinct functional domains, one that binds LPS and is antimicrobial and the other that is opsonic.[84] BPI is most effective at the site of infection and acts in synergy with other antimicrobial peptides such as defensins and the membrane attack complex of complement. In contrast, LBP enhances the sensitivity to LPS by binding to the lipid A moiety of LPS thus allowing triggering of circulating effector at subpicomolar concentrations of LPS. LBP plays a significant role in clearance of bacteria from the circulation. This clearance is mediated by activation of nuclear factor (NF)-kB through the CD14 /TLR 4 signal trans-

duction pathway as illustrated in Figure 156–3. LBP enhances the efficiency of this pathway by binding LPS and shuttling it to the CD14/TLR complex.

Cell Surface Antigens

Morphologic, cytochemical, and enzymatic characteristics have been traditionally used for the identification of mononuclear phagocytes. Monoclonal antibody techniques have provided a more precise description of the mononuclear phagocyte lineage relationships and differentiation sequence.[48] Due to the large number of monoclonal antibodies generated against cell surface antigens of leukocytes, an international workshop was convened to classify and characterize monoclonal antibodies and their leukocyte cell surface antigens. The Human Leukocyte Differentiation Antigen Workshop has evaluated thousands of antibodies to develop common nomenclature.[85] Monoclonal antibodies having similar reactivity patterns to cellular antigens are given a common cluster of differentiation (CD) designation. When only provisional designations are agreed on, these clusters are identified by CDw. Table 156-1 summarizes the CD groupings for the MPS. In some cases, lineage precursor cells and other leukocytes expressing the same cell surface antigens are included. Well-described class I and class II major histocompatibility antigens are not included in the table.

During ontogeny, macrophages in the fetal liver express CD11b as early as 12 weeks' gestation.[86] Another antigenic determinant, CD14, appears to be a more mature antigen. Its expression does not appear until 15- to 21-weeks' gestation. CD14 expression on cord blood and adult blood monocytes is equivalent.[87] In contrast, CD11a, CD11b, and CD11c are expressed at lower density on cord blood monocytes than on cells from adults. Several investigators have reported that human leukocyte antigen (HLA)-DR, HLA-DP, and HLA-DQ are expressed at lower density on neonatal monocytes than on adult monocytes.[52,88-90] Class II histocompatibility antigen density on macrophages has been correlated to antigen presentation capacity *in vitro*.[91] It remains to be determined whether developmental differences in these antigens account for deficient antibody responses to certain foreign antigens in the newborn period.

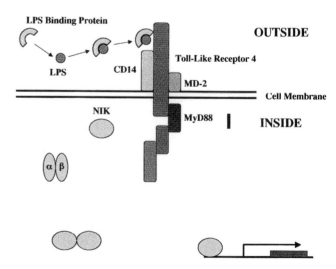

Figure 156–3. The LPS receptor complex consists of CD14, toll-like receptor 4 (TLR4), and MD-2. Lipopolysaccharide (LPS)-binding protein facilitates recognition of LPS by the LPS receptor complex. Signal transduction through TLR4 leads to nuclear translocation of nuclear factor (NF)-kβ and activation of immune response genes.

TABLE 156-1

CD Antigens on Mononuclear Phagocyte Cells

CD	Ligand, Receptor, Associated Molecules	Cell Type	CD	Ligand, Receptor, Associated Molecules	Cell Type
CD1a		Mono, Mac	CD89	IgA1/IgA2	Mono, Mac
CD1b		Mono, Mac	CD91	Alpha2M/LDLs	Mono, Mac
CD1c		Mono, Mac	CD92		Mono, Mac
CD4	MHC Class II, Gp120. IL-16	Mono, DC	CDw93		Mono, Mac
CD9	CD63, CD81, CD82	Mono, Mac	CD95	Fas Ligand	Mono, Mac
CD11a	ICAM 1,2,3	Mono, Mac, Myeloid	CD97	CD55	DC, Mono, Mac
CD11b	iC3b	Mono, Mac, DC, Myeloid	CD98	Actin	Mono, Mac, Leukocytes
CD11c	iC3b	Mono, Mac, DC	CD99		Mono, Mac
CDw12		Mono, Myeloid	CD99R		Mono, Mac
CD13		Mono, Mac	CD100	CD45-serine kinase	Mono, Mac
CD14	LPS	Mono, Mac	CD101		DC, Mono, Mac
CD15	CD62, selectin	Mono	CD102	LFA-1, CD11b/CD18	Mono, Mac
CD15s	E-selectins	Mono	CD104	Laminins (I,II, IV,V), CD49f	Mono, Mac
CD15u	P-selectins	Mono	CD105	TGFβ-1, TGFβ-3	Mono, Mac
CD15su	L-selectins	Mono	CD107a		Mono, Mac
CD16	Fc	Mac	CD111	GD, nectin3, Afadin	Mono, Mac
CD16b	Fc	Mac	CD112	PRR3, Afadin	Mono, Mac
CDw17		Mono, DC	CD114	G-CSF, Jak1, Jak2	Mono, Mac
CD18	CD11a, b, c	Mono, Mac	CD115	CSF-1	Mono, Mac
CD19	CD2, CD81, CD225	DC	CD116	GM-CSF	DC, Mono, Mac
CD29	VCAM-1, MadCAM-1	Mono, Mac	CDw119	IFNγ	DC, Mono, Mac, Leukocytes
CD31	CD38	Mono, Mac	CD120a	TNF, TRADD, TRAF, PiP, LTa	DC, Mono, Mac, Leukocytes
CD32	Phosphatase	Mono, Mac	CD120b	TNF, TRADD, TRAF, PiP, LTa	DC, Mono, Mac, Leukocytes
CD33	Sugar chains	Mono, Mac	Cd121b	IL-1β, IL-1Rα, IL-1α	Mono, Mac
CD35	C3b, C4b, iC3, iC4	Mono, DC	CD122	IL-2, IL-15, CD25, CD132	Mono, Mac
CD36	Thrombospondin	Mono, DC	CD123	IL-3	DC, Mono, Mac
CD37	CD53, CD81, CD82, MHC II	Mono, Mac	CD124	IL-4, IL-13	Mono, Mac
CD38	CD31	Mono, Mac	CD126	IL-6	Mono, Mac
CD39	ATP/ADP	Mac, DC	CD128a	IL-8	Mono, Mac
CD40	CD40L	Mono, Mac, DC	CD128b	IL-8	Mono, Mac
CD43	Hyaluronan	Mono, Mac	CD130	Oncostatin M	Mono, Mac
CD44	Hyaluronan	Mono, Mac	CD131	CD12, CD125, CD116	Mono, Mac
CD45	p56, p59, Src kinases	Mono, Mac, DC, Leukocytes	CD132	IL-12	Mono, Mac
CD45RA	p56, p59, Src kinases	Mono, Mac, DC, Leukocytes	CD135	FL	Mono, Mac
CD45RB	p56, p59, Src kinases	Mono, Mac, DC, Leukocytes	CDw136	MSP, HGFI	Mono, Mac
CD45RC	p56, p59, Src kinases	Mono, Mac, DC, Leukocytes	CDw137	4-1BB ligand	Mono, Mac
CD45RO	p56, p59, Src kinases	Mono, Mac, DC, Leukocytes	CD139		Mono, Mac
CD46	SCR	Mono, Mac	CD140b	PDGF	Mono, Mac
CD47	SIRP	Mono, Mac	CD141	Thrombin, Protein C	Mono, Mac
CD48	CD2, lyn, fyn	Mono, Mac, Leukocytes	CD147		Mono, Mac
CD49b	Collagen, laminin	Mono, Mac	CD148		Mono, Mac
CD49c	Laminin-5, FN, collagen	Mono, Mac	CD150	Tyrosine phosphatase CD45	DC
CD49d	CD106, MadCAM	DC, Mono, Mac	CD155	Polio Virus Receptor	Mono, Mac
CD49e	Fibronectin, Invasin	DC, Mono, Mac	CD156a		Mono, Mac
CD49f	Laminin, Invasin	Mono, Mac	CD156b	Pro-TNF, pro-TGFα, MAD2	DC, Mono, Mac
CD50	LFA-1, Integrin ad/b2	Mono, Mac, Leukocytes	CD157		DC, Mono, Mac
CD51	Arg-Asp-Gly	Mono, Mac	CD162	P-selectin	Mono, Mac
C52		Mono, Mac	CD163		Mono, Mac
CD53	VLA-4, HLA-DR	Mono, Mac, Leukocytes	CD164		Mono, Mac
CD54	LFA-1, Mac1, Rhinovirus	Mono, Mac	CD165		Mono, Mac
CD55	SCR, CD97	Mono, Mac	CD166	Binds CD6	Mono,Mac
CD58	CD2	DC, Mono, Mac, Leukocytes	CD167a	Collagen	DC
CD59	C8a, C9, lck, fyn	Mono, Mac	CD168	CD44	Mono, Mac
CD60a		Mono, Mac	CD169	MUCI, CD206	DC, Mono, Mac
CD60b	9-o-acetyl-GD3	Mono, Mac	CD170	Terminal sialic acid residues	DC, Mono, Mac
CD60c		Mono, Mac	CD171	CD56, CD24	DC, Mono, Mac
CD61		Mono, Mac	CD172	CD47	DC, Mono, Mac
CD62L	CD3, Gly-CAM-1, M	Mono, Mac	CD183	IP-10, IVIG, I-TAC	DC, Mono, Mac
CD63	VLA-3, VLA-6, CD81	Mono, Mac	CD184	HIV-1	DC, Mono, Mac, Leukocytes
CD64	IgG	DC, Mono, Mac	CD195	HIV-1	Mono, Mac
CD65	E-selectin	Mono, Mac	CDw197	SLC, 6 CKine, ELC, MIP3α	DC, Mono, Mac
CD65s	E-selectin or P-selectin	Mono, Mac	CD200	OX2R	DC
CD68	LDL	DC, Mono, Mac, Leukocytes	CD204	LDL	Mono, Mac
CD69		Mono, Mac	CD205	DEC-205	DC, Mono, Mac
CD71	Transferrin	Mono, Mac	CD206	Sialodine sins and CD45	DC, Mono, Mac
CD72	CD5	DC	CD207		DC, Mono, Mac
CD73	AMP	DC	CD208		DC
CD74	HLA-DR, CD44	Mono, Mac	CD209		DC

Table continued on next page

TABLE 156-1

CD Antigens on Mononuclear Phagocyte Cells—Cont'd

CD	Ligand, Receptor, Associated Molecules	Cell Type	CD	Ligand, Receptor, Associated Molecules	Cell Type
CD75		Mono, Mac	CD213a	IL-13	Mono, Mac
CD75s	CD22	Mono, Mac	CDw217	IL-17	Mono, Mac
CD80	CD28/CD152 (CTLA-4)	DC, Mono, Mac	CD220	Insulin	Mono, Mac
CD81	Leu-13, CD19/CD21	DC, Mono, Mac, Leukocytes	CD221	Insulin	Mono, Mac
CD82		Mono, Mac, Leukocytes	CD222	Plasminogen, M6P, IGFII	Mono, Mac
CD83		DC	CD224	GSH	Mono, Mac
CD84		Mono, Mac	CD226	LFA-1	Mono, Mac
CD85a	HLA class I	DC, Mono, Mac	CD227	CD54, CD169	DC, Mono, Mac
CD85d	HLA class I	DC, Mono, Mac	CD230		DC, Mono, Mac
CD85j	HLA class I	DC, Mono, Mac	CD232	CD108	Mono, Mac
CD85k	HLA class I	DC, Mono, Mac	CD234	IL-8, MGSA, RANTES, MCP-1	Mono, Mac
CD86	CD28/CD152 (CTLA-4)	DC, Mono, Mac	CD244	CD48	Mono, Mac
CD87	UPA/Pro-UPA Vitronectin	DC, Mono, Mac	CD245	Lymphocyte receptor	Mono, Mac
CD88	C5a/C5a (desArg)	DC, Mono, Mac			

AMP = Adenosine monophosphate; ATP/ADP = Adenosine triphosphate disodium/adenosine diphosphate sodium; CD = cluster of differentiation; CSF = colony-stimulating factor; CTLA = cytotoxic T lymphocyte-associated antigen; DC = dendritic cell; DEC-205 = dendritic cell and thymic epithelial cell 205 kilodalton protein; DR = deoxyribose; ELC = Epstein-Barr virus-induced gene 1 ligand chemokine; FL = Flt 3 ligand; FN = fibronectin; fyn = protein tyrosine kinase p59-fyn; G-CSF = granulocyte colony-stimulating factor; GD = viral glycoprotein D; GM-CSF = granulocyte-macrophage colony stimulating factor; GSH = growth-stimulating hormone; HGF = human growth factor; HIV = human immunodeficiency virus; HLA = human leukocyte antigen; ICAM = intercellular adhesion molecule; IFN = interferon; IgG = immunoglobulin G; IL = interleukin; IP = interferon-gamma inducible protein; IVIG = intravenous immunoglobulin; lck = lymphocyte-specific protein tyrosine kinase p 56; LDL = low-density lipoprotein; LFA = lymphocyte function-associated antigen; Lta = lymphocyte-transforming activity; Mac = macrophage; MCP = monocyte chemotactic protein; MgP = mucinoglycoprotein; MGSA = melanoma growth-stimulating activity; MHC = major histocompatibility complex; MIP = macrophage inflammatony protein; Mono = monocyte; MSP = murine serum protein; MUC = mucin; OX2R = Orexin receptor 2; PDGF = platelet-derived growth factor; PiP = phosphatidyl inositol phosphate; PRR = poliovirus receptor-related proteins; RANTES = regulation upon activation, normal T-cell expressed and secreted; SCR = Short consensus repeat; SLC = Secondary lymphoid chemokine; I-TAC = interferon-inducible T-cell alpha chemoattractant; TGF = T-cell growth factor; TNF = tumor-necrosis factor; TRADD = tumor necrosis factor receptor-related domain protein; TRAF = tumor necrosis factor receptor-assocciated factor; UPA = urokinase-type plasminogen activator; VCAM = vascular cell adhesion molecule; VLA = virus-like agent.

Dendritic cells lack expression of surface antigens specific for other leukocytes including T cells (CD3), monocytes (CD14), neutrophils (CD16), B cells (CD19), and natural killer (NK) cells (CD56).[92] Myeloid dendritic cells differentiate directly from CD34+ precursors, or indirectly from CD14+ monocytes.[93, 94] They express surface markers associated with myeloid cells, such as CD11b and CD11c.

BIOCHEMISTRY AND METABOLISM OF MONONUCLEAR PHAGOCYTES

Monocyte Metabolism

Metabolic activities of the cells of the MPS vary considerably based on their stage of development, site of origin, and state of activation. Human adult peripheral blood monocytes require an intact glycolytic pathway that is not adversely affected by inhibition of oxidative phosphorylation.[95] Peripheral blood monocytes placed in tissue culture environment demonstrate increased glycolysis with concomitant time-dependent increase in lactate accumulation in the culture media.[96]

Prindull and Prindull[97] compared the glycogen content of mononuclear phagocytes from premature and term newborn infants with that of adult subjects. The glycogen reserves under resting conditions were similar; however, during experimental inflammatory conditions mononuclear phagocytes from adult subjects increased their glycogen content, presumably through pinocytosis of neutrophil glycogen. In contrast, the glycogen content of mononuclear phagocytes from newborn infants decreased. In other studies, investigators compared the glycolytic activity of cord-blood mononuclear cells (preparations included monocytes and lymphocytes) from preterm and term newborn infants with mononuclear cells from adult peripheral blood.[98] Cells from term and premature cord blood mononuclear cells demonstrated decreased glycolysis and little metabolic activity in

response to phytohemagglutinin (PHA) stimulation, whereas cells from adult blood completely converted glucose to lactate and demonstrated a significant increase in glycolysis in response to stimulation with PHA. In addition, cord blood monocyte pyruvate kinase activity and adenosine triphosphate concentrations were significantly diminished compared with measurements obtained from adult peripheral blood monocytes. These investigators proposed that diminished energy metabolism might contribute to the dysfunction in host defense exhibited by newborn infants.

Macrophage Metabolism

Human adult macrophages are capable of using both glycolytic and oxidative phosphorylase pathways to derive their energy requirements. The operative pathway depends on the site of tissue origin. The pulmonary alveolar macrophage exhibits a high degree of oxygen consumption, whereas peritoneal macrophages depend predominantly on anaerobic glycolysis to provide their energy needs.[99] Analysis of the glycolytic enzymes lactate dehydrogenase and pyruvate kinase and the mitochondrial enzyme glutamate dehydrogenase in macrophages suggests that the metabolic activity of tissue macrophages, may be determined by the oxygen tension in the environment. This hypothesis was substantiated by Bar-Eli and colleagues[100] who reported that macrophages derived from a single progenitor cell can develop different metabolic features in response to the oxygen tension in the environment in which they mature. The metabolic state of fetal and neonatal human tissue macrophages has not been determined.

Biosynthesis of Reactive Oxygen Intermediates

Mononuclear phagocytes are capable of either reducing or exciting oxygen molecules to produce highly reactive intermediates, such as superoxide anion, hydrogen peroxide, and the hydroxyl radical. Shortly after the mononuclear phagocyte interacts with stimuli, oxygen consumption increases dramatically. This respiratory burst is associated with enhanced microbicidal activity, particularly in circulating blood monocytes. The respiratory burst and production of reactive oxygen intermediates are discussed in detail in separate studies by Babior[101] and by Nathan and Tsunawaki.[102]

The nitroblue tetrazolium dye (NBT) test is a screening device used to determine deficiencies in oxidative metabolism. The NBT is based on the ability of reactive oxygen intermediates to reduce the soluble yellow NBT dye to a blue-black (formazan) insoluble material that precipitates in the cytoplasm and is readily identified by light microscopy.[103] Cells derived from patients with inherited phagocyte deficiencies of oxidative metabolism fail to reduce NBT.[104] Light emission (chemiluminescence) can also be used to detect the respiratory burst when mononuclear phagocytes generate reactive oxygen intermediates in response to external stimuli. This property provides a semiquantitative assay for the formation of oxygen radicals.

Investigators comparing the respiratory burst generated by cord and adult blood monocytes using the quantitative spectrophotometric NBT assay found no differences in the ability of these cells to reduce NBT *in vitro*.[105] Direct quantitative measurement of oxygen consumption, superoxide anion levels, and hydrogen peroxide production have been performed in parallel studies of cord blood and adult peripheral blood monocytes. These studies suggest that the cord blood monocyte has a respiratory burst that is similar in magnitude to that of adult peripheral blood monocytes.[106]

Macrophages derived from cord blood and adult peripheral blood were found to be equivalent in their capability to generate superoxide in response to soluble stimuli.[107] Treatment of cord blood and adult blood monocyte-derived macrophages with LPS or muramyl dipeptide enhanced production of superoxide anion in response to a soluble stimulus.[108] The superoxide generation by muramyl dipeptide-primed cord blood monocyte-derived macrophages was significantly less than that generated by primed cells from adult blood.[107] These investigators postulated that diminished superoxide generation in response to a priming stimulus indicates that cord blood monocytes may have a diminished capacity to differentiate into activated macrophages.

Biosynthesis of Complement Proteins

The complement (C) system is composed of at least 20 circulating plasma proteins, five membrane-bound proteins that regulate the binding or degradation of complement components, and seven membrane-bound proteins that bind complement components or cleave fragments of components. The complement cascade may be activated through either a classical or an alternative pathway to generate numerous biologically active products. Activation of this cascade through either pathway produces low molecular weight inflammatory peptides (termed anaphylatoxins) and a final large complex of proteins, (termed the membrane attack complex) that inserts into the target cell membrane and results in cell lysis.[109] The anaphylatoxins bind cell surface receptors on many target tissues, which results in release of vasoactive substances, cytokines, arachidonic acid metabolites, and reactive oxygen intermediates. Anaphylatoxins, including opsonic C3b, and chemotactic C5a, stimulate multiple leukocyte functions involved in killing microbial pathogens.[110-112] The significance of the complement system in amplifying the host immune system is demonstrated in animal models and in patients with inherited deficiencies in complement components.[113,114]

The appearance of serum complement components, complement-mediated hemolytic activity, and complement regulatory proteins occurs between 8 and 14 weeks in the human fetus.[115] These components are products of fetal synthesis rather than

maternal components acquired transplacentally.[116,117] In the adult human, complement component synthesis (with the exception of C7) occurs predominantly in the liver.[118] In the embryo and fetus, the major sites of synthesis have not been clearly defined, but extrahepatic sites are thought to predominate. The MPS is likely an important source for complement proteins.[119]

In various animal models, serum complement concentrations and complement-mediated hemolytic activity gradually increase over the course of gestation; however, adult serum concentrations are not achieved until several weeks after delivery.[120,121] In newborn infants, serum complement concentrations are diminished compared with findings in adults. Deficiencies in complement components are more pronounced in infants delivered prematurely.[122,123] Serum complement components generally achieve adult levels by 6 to 18 months of age.

Biosynthesis of Other Secreted Products

Characterization of mononuclear phagocyte secretory products is a major focus of research. Diverse products synthesized by mononuclear phagocytes include polypeptide hormones, complement components, coagulation factors, enzymes, cytokines, extracellular matrix proteins, other binding proteins, bioactive oligopeptides, bioactive lipids, sterol hormones, purine and pyrimidine products, reactive oxygen intermediates, and reactive nitrogen intermediates.

Production of secretory products by mononuclear phagocytes during fetal and neonatal life is limited. Synthesis of the polypeptide hormones interferon (IFN)-α, IL-1, and tumor necrosis factor (TNF) by term cord blood monocytes appears to be quantitatively similar to those of adult peripheral blood monocytes.[124-126] However, TNF production by freshly isolated monocytes derived from the cord blood of premature infants is lower than that of term cord blood and adult peripheral blood monocytes.[126] Other investigators described diminished IL-1 and TNF-α synthesis by preterm and term cord blood monocytes stimulated with LPS.[127] Kaufman and coworkers[128] described a variety of synthetic deficits in LPS-stimulated adherent monocytes from preterm compared with monocytes from full-term infants. These included diminished generation of superoxide, TNF-α, and CD11b/CD18 receptors. They observed no differences in IL-1β or IL-6 production. These investigators postulated that adherence functions such as CD11b/CD18 ligation might be important in modulating subsequent cellular activation and cytokine secretion activities. Synthesis and secretion *in vitro* of several cytokines including G-CSF, GM-CSF, IL-6, IL-8, IL-10, and IL-12 by stimulated monocytes isolated from preterm and term cord blood monocytes are significantly lower at the protein and mRNA level than those measured from stimulated adult blood monocytes.[129-134] Diminished production of GM-CSF by PHA and phorbol myristate acetate (PMA) stimulated newborn mononuclear cells has been determined to be secondary to increased levels of AUF1 isoform (RNA binding proteins) that affect mRNA stability.[129,135] Regulation of IL-10 also appears to be developmentally regulated at the post-transcriptional level.[133]

Goriely and colleagues[136] hypothesize that deficits in neonatal dendritic cell function are responsible in part for impaired T-helper 1 (Th1) function in human newborns. Their investigations of neonatal monocyte-derived dendritic cells revealed diminished expression of HLA-DR and costimulatory molecules CD40 and CD80. In addition they observed a selective defect in IL-12 synthesis at the protein and messenger RNA level in response to LPS, CD40 ligation, or poly-deoxy-inosinic acid:poly-deoxy-cytidylic acid (I:C). Moreover, they found that neonatal dendritic cells were less effective than adult dendritic cells in promoting IFN-γ production by allogeneic adult T cells. This deficit was corrected with addition of recombinant IL-12.

FUNCTIONAL ASPECTS OF MONONUCLEAR PHAGOCYTES

Morphogenesis

Macrophages are critical during morphogenesis of the fetus. In addition to their role in immunity, macrophages participate in modeling organs and engulf debris and apoptotic cells during embryogenesis.[137] For example, they are present in the urogenital ridge, where they clear degenerated cells of the Müllerian duct in the male and the Wolffian duct in the female.[138] They appear to play a similar role in the retina and brain.[139, 140] Macrophages have also been observed in close proximity to areas of apoptosis in the developing fetal mouse footplate.[141]

Movement

Mononuclear phagocytes exhibit both random and directed movement.[142] Random or nondirected movement occurs in the absence of attracting substances. Directed movement along a concentration gradient of chemical attractants is essential for the effective localization of mononuclear phagocytes to sites of infection and inflammation. This directional movement, called *chemotaxis*, is governed by chemoattractant molecules that bind to receptors on the cell surface. Chemotactic substances are produced through activation of the complement, fibrinolytic, and kinin systems or are directly produced by microorganisms. These chemoattractants may also accentuate random migration of mononuclear phagocytes in the absence of a concentration gradient. An entire family of proinflammatory molecules called *chemokines* has been identified and many of its members have been characterized.[143] Several members of this family serve as potent chemoattractants for mononuclear phagocytes. Monocyte chemotactic protein 1, macrophage inflammatory protein 1, and regulation upon activation, normal T-cell expressed and secreted (RANTES) are key regulators of monocyte migration. Dendritic cells migrate to lymphoid organs in response to secondary lymphoid chemokine.[144, 145]

Mononuclear phagocyte migration has been examined in cord blood and neonatal peripheral blood and has been compared with adult peripheral blood monocytes. In most reports, random movement by cord blood monocytes appears to be equivalent to that of adult peripheral blood monocytes.[146-148] To the contrary, several investigators have reported diminished directed movement by cord blood and neonatal peripheral blood compared with that of adult peripheral blood monocytes. Yegin[149] reported that monocyte chemotaxis increased gradually during childhood and was equivalent to adult chemotactic activity after 5 to 6 years of age. These results are consistent with those of other investigators who reported similar chemotactic activity by cord blood and adult peripheral blood monocytes, but dramatically decreased chemotaxis by neonatal peripheral blood monocytes in the first few days of life.[150] Monocyte chemotaxis gradually increased but remained lower than adult peripheral blood monocyte activity over the first 6 months of life. Other groups of investigators report a slightly increased chemotaxis of cord blood monocytes in response to endotoxin-activated adult serum or activated adult lymphocytes.[151, 152] Differences in methods of measurements applied, patient populations examined and monocyte isolation used, likely account for the contradictory results reported by these investigators.

Adherence

Adhesion is a requisite function of mononuclear phagocytes for egress from the circulation, movement through interstitial tissues, and interaction with a wide variety of cell and tissue types. In the systemic circulation, movement of monocytes into tissues occurs in three independent steps. First, monocytes rolling along the vascular endothelium have transient low affinity focal interactions with endothelial cells through adhesion molecules called selectins.[153] L-selectin is constitutively expressed on the cell surface of blood monocytes and interacts with a variety of endothelial cell surface glycoproteins to promote transient monocyte-endothelium contact.[154] E-selectin and P-selectin are adhesion molecules expressed by vascular endothelium after activation.[155, 156] These molecules recognize glycoprotein ligands on the cell surface of monocytes to facilitate monocyte-endothelium adhesion. The second step of monocyte egress from the vascular space involves halting the rolling, shedding of monocyte surface selectins, and firm adhesion of the monocyte to the endothelial cell surface. This firm adhesion is generated by activation of members of the integrin family on the monocyte cell surface. These integrins include CD11a-c and CD18 on monocytes and endothelial cell surface ICAM-1 or ICAM-2.[157] An additional adhesion interaction pathway used by monocytes includes monocyte integrin $\alpha 4 \beta 1$ and endothelial vascular cell adhesion molecule-1 (VCAM-1). Both pathways promote firm adhesion of monocytes to endothelium and enable the final step of extravasation to occur. Monocytes migrate through the endothelium in response to a concentration of chemotactic signals to arrive at a focus of infection or inflammation. People who exhibit moderate to severe deficiency of cell surface integrins or selectins are susceptible to recurrent bacterial infections due to their inability to recruit neutrophils and monocytes to the site of infection. These defects can be visualized using a Rebuck skin window test.[158-160]

Dendritic cells are involved in a number of adhesive interactions that facilitate their migration and interaction with T cells. The initial tethering and rolling may prove to be mediated by selectins. More firm adherence and migration through the endothelium is likely to involve integrins and ICAMs or other immunoglobulin superfamily members. Integrins and CD44 or syndecans may mediate interstitial tissue interactions. Dendritic cell interactions with epithelium probably involve cadherins.

Adhesive properties of fetal and newborn monocytes have been examined to a limited degree. Boner and colleagues reported equivalent adherence cord and adult blood neutrophils and monocytes to glass coverslips.[161] In others studies, Speer and coworkers isolated mononuclear cells from cord and adult subjects and subjected these cells to a nylon-wool packed column.[162] Greater than 85% of esterase positive monocytes from cord and adult blood adhered to the column. Other investigators evaluated the capacity of cord blood monocytes to adhere to denatured collagen and fibronectin coated culture plates.[163] These studies also demonstrated comparable adherence of cord and adult blood monocytes to these substrates. In summary, monocyte adhesiveness appears to be unimpaired in neonatal blood compared to adult blood.

Endocytosis

The ability of mononuclear phagocytes to ingest a variety of materials is crucial to their immunologic function. Endocytosis is important in antimicrobial resistance, removal of old cells, antigen processing, and multiple other functions. Endocytosis is mediated through pinocytosis and phagocytosis. These two processes are believed to use similar mechanisms, however, distinctions have been drawn between them based on size and composition of the particles being ingested. Pinocytosis refers to ingestion of microscopic fluid droplets. Phagocytosis describes ingestion of large particulate matter.[164] Both processes involve internalization of extracellular materials. Phagocytosis is enhanced by opsonization of particulate materials with immunoglobulins or complement components that bind to Fc and C3 receptors on the cell surface of mononuclear phagocytes.

Historically, macrophages and dendritic cells were recognized as separate populations of adherent cells based, in part, on differences in endocytic capabilities. A model of antibody response by mouse spleen cells developed by Mishell and Dutton[165] required cooperation of two populations of cells distinguished by buoyant density and the capacity to adhere to glass or plastic. The high density, non-adherent cells were predominantly lymphocytes, whereas the low density, adherent cells consisted of a macrophage and a non-macrophage (dendritic cell) population.[49, 166] Macrophages had numerous lysosomes and actively internalized any small tracer molecules including microorganisms, antibody-coated particles, soluble horseradish peroxidase, and colloidal carbon. The other adherent cell population called *dendritic cells* based on their morphologic appearance had distinct features, including a paucity of lysosomes, numerous multivesicular vacuoles, and an inability to internalize particulate and fluid phase molecules.[49, 166-168] The multivesicular vacuoles were later recognized to be MHC class II–rich vesicles. A lack of endocytic activity was reported in many of the initial descriptions of dendritic cells.[168-171] After methods were developed to separate dendritic cells from macrophages, several laboratories found that dendritic cells exhibited two features that had not been previously encountered. They expressed high levels of MHC class II products and exhibited remarkable stimulatory capacity for T cell dependent responses (reviewed in Steinman's study[92]). The paucity of lysosomes and weak endocytic activity of dendritic cells, coupled with strong antigen presenting functions were enigmatic to many investigators. The ability to isolate and culture dendritic cells has allowed resolution of certain aspects of this dichotomy.

Macrophages have the ability to internalize a broad spectrum of substrates in digestive lysosomes. Scavenging is a high capacity form of endocytosis that culminates in complete digestion of substrates. In studies applying fluid phase solutes to macrophages, these cells accumulated 10^5 soluble protein molecules per hour (on average) and substrates were digested to the level of amino acids.[172] Adsorptive uptake using Fc receptors enhances clearance properties of macrophages about 1000-fold.[173] In contrast, antigen presentation by dendritic cells requires a relatively small number of MHC-peptide complexes. For example, MHC II-restricted T-T hybrids can respond to presentation of a few hundred specific MHC-peptide complexes.[174, 175] Similarly, naive T-cell stimulation can be achieved by presentation of only a few hundred complexes of MHC and superantigen by dendritic cells.[176]

Dendritic cells, like other antigen presenting cells, have receptors that mediate adsorptive uptake and delivery of peptides to MHC products rather than lysosomes. Dendritic cells can present immune complexes and self-antigens by Fcγ receptors.[177, 178] Furthermore, epidermal Langerhans cells (a specialized tissue macrophage) contain Birbeck granules that can be coated and mediate adsorptive uptake.[179,180] Sallusto and colleagues demonstrated that the mannosyl-fucosyl C-type lectin receptor mediates adsorptive uptake of horseradish peroxidase and FITC-labeled dextran.[181] Other C-type leptin domain containing receptors have been identified and linked to antigen uptake and presentation by dendritic cells.[182,183]

Recycling of internalized membrane is a general feature of endocytosis. Levine and Chain[184] described significant trafficking of endocytic vesicles through endosomes, but not lysosomes, in dendritic cells. They examined endocytic activity using fluorescent solutes and cytofluorography and concluded that a significant portion of the internalized solute was discharged through the recycling process. To the contrary, Sallusto and co-workers[181] showed accumulation and retention of fluorescent solutes for longer periods of time. Their cell population contained more abundant MIIVs (MHC class II compartment vesicles) compared with the cells used by Levine and Chain, thus MIIVs might retain internalized substances longer for the purpose of antigen presentation.

Endocytosis of substrates is limited to discrete stages of the dendritic cell life cycle in response to certain signals. Romani and co-workers[185] and Streilein and Grammer[186] reported that dendritic cells isolated from skin efficiently presented protein antigens, however, after 12 hours in culture this capacity is lost. Splenic dendritic cells also capture antigens on isolation, but lose endocytic activity after overnight culture.[181,187] The proposal that macropinocytosis is increased in dendritic cells by growth factors is consistent with cytokine-induced macropinocytosis in other cell types.[188,189]

During the fetal period, macrophages are capable of immune protection of the fetus. In animal models, primitive macrophages are highly mobile and are capable of ingesting latex particles injected into the yolk sac and carrying them to the mesenchymal stroma and loose connective tissue.[190] Fetal Kupffer cells may detoxify circulating endotoxin. Endotoxin that reaches the amniotic cavity is swallowed by the fetus and gains access to the liver through the portal circulation.[191] Macrophages internalize endotoxin through the LPS receptor. This receptor is present on human fetal Kupffer cells and can be up-regulated as early as 8-weeks' post-conception by IL-3.[192] Later, macrophages contribute to the adaptive immune response as antigen presenting cells and as producers of a variety of cytokines including TNF-α, IL-1, and IL-6.

The kinetics of phagocytosis by monocytes from cord blood and adult peripheral blood have been studied by Schuit and Powell.[193] These investigators found that monocytes isolated from adult peripheral blood ingested all polystyrene particles within 50 minutes. In comparison only 38% of cord blood monocytes had initiated phagocytosis in the same time period. The cord blood monocytes were able to ingest the particles by 100 minutes. These studies were not influenced by the presence of serum or heat-inactivated serum. Other investigators have reported that opsonized (IgG) sheep erythrocytes, *Staphylococcus aureus*, *Escherichia coli*, *Streptococcus pyogenes*, *Toxoplasma gondii*, and type II herpes simplex are ingested by cord blood monocytes as effectively as monocytes derived from adult peripheral blood.[162]

Defective phagocytosis of *Streptococcus agalactiae* by cord blood monocytes has been reported by Marodi and colleagues.[194] Monocytes derived from term cord blood ingested fewer group B Streptococci than monocytes isolated from adult blood. Other studies suggested that the phagocytic defect of group B *Streptococcus* by cord blood monocytes could be overcome by inclusion of adhesive glycoprotein fibronectin in the culture.[195] Although fibronectin alone did not enhance phagocytosis, preopsonizing group B *Streptococcus* with IgG preparation in combination with fibronectin enhanced phagocytosis by cord blood monocytes.

The phagocytic activity of cord blood monocyte–derived macrophages has been compared with that of macrophages derived from adult blood monocytes. After a 10-day culture period, Speer and co-workers[196] determined that cord blood–derived macrophages ingested complement opsonized *S. aureus* to the same extent as macrophages derived from adult blood. Other investigations compared the phagocytic activity of alveolar macrophages from intubated newborns with alveolar macrophages from bronchoalveolar lavage of adult subjects. Phagocytosis of *Candida albicans* by newborn and adult alveolar macrophages was determined to be equivalent with respect to rate and number of organisms ingested.[197]

Dendritic cells derived from cord blood monocytes by culture with IL-4 and GM-CSF exhibited decreased endocytic function compared with adult monocyte-derived dendritic cells.[198] Liu and colleagues[198] suggested that decreased mannose receptor expression might contribute to this developmental deficit. Zheng and coworkers[199] reported that following addition of TNF-α to cultures, monocyte-derived cord blood dendritic cells exhibited equivalent endocytic capacity to adult monocyte-derived dendritic cells. The results of these studies suggest that mononuclear phagocytes in the newborn period have a well-developed endocytic pathway for most microorganisms. Phagocytic activity of mononuclear phagocytes from the fetus and from prematurely born infants has not been reported.

Microbicidal Activity

Several different antimicrobial mechanisms have been identified in mononuclear phagocytes. These are generally divided into oxygen-dependent and oxygen-independent mechanisms. The microbicidal mechanism used by mononuclear phagocytes varies depending on the state of maturation, differentiation, activation, and tissue of origin. The oxygen-dependent mechanism, termed the *respiratory burst*, is initiated with activation of the transmembrane electron transport system involving a reduced nicotinamide adenine dinucleotide, extracellular or phagosomal oxygen, and additional plasma membrane enzymes and cofactors.[101] Superoxide anions are the initial product of the respiratory burst. This molecule is directly toxic to certain proteins and membrane constituents; however, it is often converted to a more powerful antimicrobial agent, hydrogen peroxide, through a reaction catalyzed by superoxide dismutase. Hydrogen peroxide is highly toxic to a number of microorganisms. Hydrogen peroxide toxicity can be further enhanced when it is used as substrate for the oxidation of halides (e.g., iodide, bromide, and chloride) to hypohalous acids and other reactive intermediates.[102] This reaction is catalyzed by the phagocytic enzyme myeloperoxidase. Halide oxidation products are themselves powerful oxidants and probably attack bacterial cell wall components leading to microbial killing. Proposed chemical groups involved in these interactions include amino acids, which are decarboxylated and deaminated; lipid membranes, in which polyunsaturated fatty acids are oxidized; and sulfhydryl groups, which are readily oxidized.[200]

Oxygen-independent antimicrobial mechanisms used by mononuclear phagocytes include acidification of the phagosome and the synthesis and secretion of cationic proteins called *defensins, lipid hydrolases, proteases,* and *nucleases.*[201] The extent to which these mechanisms contribute to antimicrobial activity *in vivo* is uncertain. However, patients with chronic granulomatous disease have provided evidence that, despite a deficient oxygen-dependent antimicrobial system, mononuclear phagocytes from such patients are capable of killing microbial pathogens.[202]

Nitric oxide (NO) is an additional molecule that plays an important role in oxygen-independent macrophage antimicrobial activity.[203] Initially, NO was identified as an antimicrobial and tumoricidal product of activated macrophages, generated from the amino acid L-arginine by the enzymatic activity of *inducible nitric oxide synthase* (iNOS). NO plays many roles in the immune system as well as in other organ systems. In addition to macrophages, several other immune cells produce and respond to NO. Three isoforms of NOs are known: iNOS and two constitutive forms collectively called *constitutive NOS* (cNOS). Although the three isoforms catalyze the same reaction, they differ in their regulation, amplitude and production of NO, and cellular and tissue distribution.[204] NOS activity is determined by several mechanisms, many influenced by immunologic stimuli. The activity of NO is not restricted to the site of its production. It is a highly diffusible gas and can act locally or can be distributed widely in the body through NO vehicles such as S-nitrosothiols, S-nitrosylated proteins, and nitrosyl-metal complexes. Unlike cytokines, the interaction of NO is not restricted to a defined receptor, rather, it can interact with other inorganic molecules (e.g., oxygen or superoxide), structures in DNA (e.g., pyrimidine bases), prosthetic groups (e.g., heme), or proteins leading to S-nitrosylation of thiol groups, nitration of tyrosine residues, or disruption of metal-sulfide clusters (e.g., zinc-finger domains or iron-sulfide complexes). Considering that many targets of NO are regulatory molecules it is evident that NO exerts diverse effects.

NO has a diverse spectrum of activities against infectious pathogens, including antiviral, antimicrobial, immunostimulatory (i.e., proinflammatory), immunosuppressive (i.e., anti-inflammatory), cytotoxic (i.e., cell-damaging), and cytoprotective (i.e., tissue-preserving). The analysis of iNOS-/- mice confirms that most of these effects are mediated by iNOS-derived NO.[205-207] Under different circumstances, depending on the species, strain, infective dose, or route of pathogen entry, iNOS was indispensable or helpful in controlling the infection, had no effect, or worsened the disease.[204] The antimicrobial activity of NO results from a variety of mechanisms including mutation of DNA, inhibition of DNA repair or synthesis, inhibition of protein synthesis, alterations of proteins by S-nitrosylation, adenosine diphosphate (ADP)-ribosylation or tyrosine nitration, or inactivation of enzymes by disruption of Fe-S clusters, zinc-fingers or heme groups, or by peroxidation of lipid membranes.[206, 208] These mechanisms likely account for the most actions against infectious agents. Peroxynitrite (ONOO−), a reaction product of NO and $O_2−$, is a potent antibacterial effector molecule. The nitrating efficiency and production capacity of peroxynitrite by macrophages have been controversial; however, recent investigations have demonstrated that ONOO− might be formed within the microbe by host-derived NO and microbe derived $O_2−$. The significance of ONOO− is underscored by the fact that pathogens such as *Mycobacterium tuberculosis* and *Salmonella typhimurium* have developed mechanisms to detoxify ONOO− to nitrite.[209]

The iNOS-dependent killing of parasites by macrophages can result from depletion of arginine. For certain strains of Leishmania it has been shown that L-hydroxyarginine can inhibit arginase activity in the macrophage or parasite promoting parasite killing. Also, arginine is required for polyamine and DNA synthesis in *Leishmania* and African trypanosomes by the ornithine decarboxylase pathway and by *Trypanosoma cruzi* through the arginine decarboxylase pathway.[210]

Cytotoxic Activity

Under some circumstances mononuclear phagocytes are capable of killing other formed elements of the blood, normal cells, and tumor cells. Mononuclear phagocyte cellular toxicity may occur through means of specific antibodies, called antibody-dependent cellular cytotoxicity (ADCC), or it may occur in the absence of specific antibodies to the target cell.[211] Mononuclear phagocyte-mediated ADCC has been studied extensively. Because antibody specificity is the primary determinant of ADCC reactions, this means of cellular killing is used for disposal of both malignant tissue and normal cells. In ADCC, the immunoglobulin bound target interacts with the Fc receptor on the mononuclear phagocyte. This initial binding is necessary but not sufficient to kill the target. Reactive oxygen intermediates, in particular hydrogen peroxide, are the major secretory products of the mononuclear phagocyte that lyse the target cell.[212] Serine proteases and tumor necrosis factor might also be involved in this lytic mechanism.

Antibody-independent cellular toxicity is highly selective for killing of various types of malignant cells of syngeneic, allogeneic, or xenogeneic origin, without damaging tissue matched nonmalignant cells. This cytotoxicity is mediated through cell-cell contact and is usually highly selective and nonphagocytic in nature. Mononuclear phagocytes may have plasma membrane receptors for certain target cells.[211] TNF, reactive oxygen, NO intermediates, and the putative 40-kDa serine protease have been implicated as major secretory products involved in antibody-independent cellular cytotoxicity.[211]

Cord blood monocytes have been reported to exhibit normal ADCC activity to herpes simplex-infected hepatocytes and to antibody-coated human erythrocytes.[213, 214] Antibody-independent cytotoxicity in term cord blood monocytes has been reported to be diminished by some investigators but to be normal by others.[213, 215] The ontogeny of mononuclear phagocyte cytotoxic functions during fetal development has not been examined.

Antigen Processing and Presentation

The MPS is integral in the establishment of an effective immune system. In addition to the innate immune functions aimed at eradicating invading microorganisms, mononuclear phagocytes are involved in initiating and propagating the adaptive immune response. A complex relationship exists between antigen presenting cells and antigen-specific T cells. The mechanism by which antigen presenting mononuclear phagocytes interact with T cells requires internalization, degradation, and display of antigenic fragments on the cells' surface in association with MHC class II molecules. Macrophages and dendritic cells both participate in this function, although their respective roles likely differ.

Mechanisms of antigen uptake might differ between various cell types in the MPS. Macrophages may be more effective than dendritic cells as scavengers as a result of their extensive repertoire of scavenger receptors.[216] Macrophages also appear to be more effective than dendritic cells at ingestion of large antigenic materials and whole cells.[166] For example, colloidal carbon administered intravenously is predominantly ingested by macrophages. Several investigators have observed limited phagocytosis of large particles such as intact cells, bacteria, and synthetic beads in bone marrow–derived murine dendritic cells.[217-219] Macrophages may contribute to antigen uptake by lysing larger particles such as bacteria, viruses, or tumor cells before transferring the degradation products to dendritic cells.[220, 221]

Dendritic cells are highly active in endocytosis and pinocytosis. This is the process by which small fluid phase particles, usually smaller than 0.5 µm, are internalized.[222] Mouse and human dendritic cells bind antigen at the cell surface and internalize these along with small portions of their plasma membrane.[223] This activated fluid phase endocytosis explains the low density characteristics acquired by dendritic cells *in vitro*. Monocyte-derived dendritic cells generated from peripheral blood mononuclear cells treated with GM-CSF and IL-4 take up extracellular fluid, actively processing approximately 100 times their volume per hour.[181]

Nonspecific inflammatory signals may be required to initiate phagocytosis, endocytosis, and expression of antigen capture receptors. Bacteria express complex carbohydrate molecules on their surface, which may bind to pattern recognition receptors, many of which have lectinlike specificity.[224] Mannose-containing residues bind mannose receptors, thus facilitating phagocytosis by macrophages. Antigen presentation by dendritic cells has been associated with expression of DEC-205 and BDCA-2. DEC-205 is a membrane protein homologous to the macrophage mannose receptor and BDCA-2 is a type II C-type lectin.[182, 183] Down-regulation of these receptors may reduce the risk of extraneous antigen presentation on egress of antigen-presenting cells from the tissue and reprogramming of dendritic cell machinery toward antigen presentation to T cells.

The MHC gene codes for two families of cell surface glycoproteins (classes I and II). Class I MHC molecules include the classical transplantation antigens and are displayed on all cells in the body. Class II MHC molecules are heterodimeric glycoproteins found on the surface of antigen-presenting cells. The MHC gene is polymorphic, therefore a wide variety of class II molecules can be expressed on the surface of antigen-presenting cells.[225]

Endogenous antigen is degraded by intracellular proteases and peptidases to provide peptides in the cytosol. These peptides bind to transporter (TAP) gene products and are delivered to the class I MHC compartment where they are incorporated into the peptide binding groove generated by folding of the class I mole-

cule before moving to the surface. This pathway requires intact proteosome and Golgi transport function. In dendritic cells, additional mechanisms are involved in class I antigen processing. First, dendritic cells internalize antigens through macropinocytosis and then release antigens into the cytosol for classical TAP-dependent MHC class I presentation.[226, 227] Second, peptides produced in high concentrations may be exchanged with peptides on mature MHC class I molecules. Third, carrier molecules or chaperones capture peptides and deliver them through the dendritic cell surface to the endoplasmic reticulum where they are released, processed, and incorporated into MHC class I molecules.

Exogenous antigens including intact organisms, particulates, and soluble antigens are internalized by the phagocytic or endocytic pathway and must undergo degradation and proteolysis before interacting with the MHC class II compartment where peptide loading occurs. Class II α and β chains are synthesized, combined, and transported in association with HLA-DM to the class II compartment. In this compartment HLA-DM dissociates; the class II molecules are membrane bound with their peptide-binding site protected by class II invariant protein (CLIP). Maturation of these vesicles occurs after fusion with the endocytic lysosome pathway.[228] The invariant chains dissociate allowing the appropriate peptides to bind with MHC.[229, 230]

Although expression of class II molecules on antigen-presenting cells is assumed to be a constitutive process in macrophages, studies of antigen processing and presentation in dendritic cells demonstrate the complexity of these mechanisms in this antigen-presenting-cell subtype. During the immature stages of dendritic cell development, cell surface expression of MHC class II and costimulatory molecules is low and endocytic activity is high.[231,232] On encountering inflammatory stimuli or microbial products, these cells undergo a maturational process in which class II and costimulatory molecules are up-regulated and endocytosis is reduced. After this programmatic shift, dendritic cells are capable of effective activation of naive T cells.[233]

Increased expression of MHC class II during dendritic cell maturation is believed to be primarily regulated by the rate of invariant chain proteolysis by cathepsin S and the subsequent binding of antigenic peptides to the newly formed class II $\alpha\beta$ dimer in lysosomes.[234,235] In immature dendritic cells, cathepsin S activity is inhibited by cystatin C, preventing invariant chain (Ii) proteolysis. This leads to sequestration of nonfunctional class II $\alpha\beta$I complexes in the lysosomes. Activation of dendritic cells promotes down-regulation of cystatin C, thus liberating cathepsin S activity. This permits Ii proteolysis and enhanced trafficking of functional class II MHC molecules to the cell surface.

Although Ii proteolysis is assumed to be the primary regulator of class II trafficking during dendritic cell differentiation, additional levels of regulation have recently been identified. Different rates of macropinocytosis and MHC class II recycling have been observed in immature and mature dendritic cells, suggesting that these factors, rather than Ii, proteolysis might control class II MHC surface expression.[236] Macropinocytosis in dendritic cells is controlled by small guanosine triphosphatases such as Rac1 and Cdc42, suggesting molecular mechanisms for regulation of class II transport during dendritic cell maturation.[237] Furthermore, cytokines can modulate class II trafficking in monocytes and can regulate cathepsin activity in dendritic cells.[238,239] It is apparent that antigen-presenting cell function is tightly regulated at the level of MIIC class II transport.

The CD4 subset of T cells recognizes antigen presentation by cells expressing the class II MHC antigens. The density of MHC class II molecules appears to correlate with their ability to present antigens to the CD4-positive T cell. Lymphokines such as IFN-γ increase the expression of MHC class II antigens and enhance antigen presentation. In contrast, prostaglandins of the E class and glucocorticoids inhibit MHC class II antigen expression and antigen presentation.

XX / Developmental Immunobiology

Fetal and Newborn Antigen-Presenting-Cell Capabilities

Investigations of antigen presentation and processing by mononuclear phagocytes from fetal blood have not been reported. Antigen-processing capabilities of monocytes derived from term cord blood have been evaluated by Hoffman and co-workers. [240] In their experiments, maternal and neonatal blood samples were paired so that single-haplotype sharing between mother and child was sufficient to allow for T-cell recognition of cord blood mononuclear phagocytes.[240] When cord blood–adherent mononuclear phagocytes were exposed to tetanus toxoid antigen and cultured with tetanus toxoid–specific T cells, a T-cell proliferative response was observed. This response was equivalent to the response seen when maternal blood adherent mononuclear cells were co-cultured with antigen and T cells. These investigators concluded that newborn mononuclear phagocytes were competent in presenting tetanus toxoid antigen, but they cautioned that additional studies would be required to determine whether antigen processing of other microbial products was as efficient.

Zlabinger and colleagues[241] examined the capacity of cord blood mononuclear phagocytes to present *E. coli* or tetanus toxoid antigen to cord or paternal T cells. In these studies, T cells were co-cultured with either antigen pulsed or control adherent mononuclear phagocytes. When cord blood T cells were co-cultured with pulsed adherent mononuclear phagocytes from cord blood, the proliferative response was significantly less than was seen when paternal T cells were co-cultured with adherent mononuclear phagocytes. However, in experiments in which cord blood adherent mononuclear phagocytes pulsed with *E. coli* were co-cultured with paternal T cells, enhanced T-cell proliferation was of similar magnitude as that seen with adult autologous antigen-presenting mononuclear phagocytes. These investigators also reconfirmed the observations by Hoffman and colleagues that cord blood mononuclear phagocytes were fully capable of processing and presenting tetanus toxoid antigen to antigen-specific T cells.

Few studies of dendritic cells have been done in human neonates, and those that exist were done with dendritic cells differentiated *in vitro* from circulating monocytes with a cocktail of cytokines (i.e., IL-4 in combination with GM-CSF). These cord blood monocyte-derived dendritic cells have limited antigen-presenting cell function[198, 242] and defective IL-12 production.[136] However, it is always difficult to generalize data obtained from these *in vitro* differentiated cells, because they are derived in a static environment containing high concentrations of cytokines and reduced cellular interactions, which might not mimic the physiologic milieu.

Intrinsic functional defects have been identified in immature dendritic cells derived from cord blood monocytes. Hunt and co-workers[243] described low expression of MHC class I and II molecules and adhesion molecules on cord blood–derived dendritic cells. They postulated that this diminished expression contributed to diminished allostimulatory capacity of these dendritic cells compared with adult monocyte-derived dendritic cells. Investigations by Liu and colleagues[198] concurred with findings that cord blood monocyte–derived dendritic cells exhibited reduced CD1a and MHC II expression. They also demonstrated diminished endocytosis related to low mannose receptor expression and reduced allostimulatory activity by cord blood compared with adult dendritic cells.[198]

Mononuclear Phagocyte Activation

The enhanced activity of mononuclear phagocytes against microorganisms and tumor cells requires interaction with sensitized lymphocytes.[244] T lymphocytes stimulated by previous exposure to specific antigens release soluble factors that induce mononuclear phagocytes to enhance microbicidal and tumorici-dal activity.[245] Considerable evidence now exists that IFN-γ is the factor produced by T lymphocytes that induces macrophage activation.[244]

IFN-γ is a highly basic heterogeneous glycoprotein with a molecular weight of 40,000 to 70,000 daltons.[245] The biologically active form of the natural protein consists of dimeric aggregates. Recombinant IFN-γ is not glycosylated and has a molecular weight of 17,000 daltons. The effects of IFN-γ on mononuclear phagocytes are initiated by engagement of IFN-γ with specific receptors on the cell surface.[246] Adams and Hamilton[247] have reviewed the signal transduction mechanism through which IFN-γ binding produces immediate and sustained functional responses. These investigators have proposed that mononuclear phagocyte activation should not refer solely to the effects of a stimulus such as IFN-γ thus leading to a proscribed change in morphology or function, but rather activation may be used to describe a composite of multiple specific capacities that enable the mononuclear phagocyte to perform a complex function.[248]

Mononuclear phagocytes play a key role in the interface between innate and adaptive immunity. Both tissue macrophages and dendritic cells recognize pathogens through a variety of receptors, induce potent stimulatory molecules, and initiate microbicidal pathways. Brightbill and colleagues observed production of IL-12 and NO synthase by macrophages in response to microbial lipoproteins recognized through TLRs.[249] Dendritic cells also produce IL-12, which is capable of inducing T lymphocyte activation and subsequent IFN-γ production.[250, 251]

Marodi and coworkers[252] examined the mechanisms used by cord blood and adult blood monocyte-derived macrophages to ingest and kill *C. albicans*. They determined phagocytosis and killing of *Candida* sp. to be equivalent between cord blood and adult blood monocyte-derived macrophages both in the presence and the absence of serum. Exposure of cord and adult macrophages to IFN-γ resulted in quantitatively different results. Candidacidal activity and superoxide anion generation was maximal for adult macrophages at 100 units/mL interferon-γ, whereas the magnitude of Candidacidal activity and superoxide production by cord blood–derived macrophages remained low at a dose up to 500 units/mL of interferon-γ. The mechanism accounting for this disparity in macrophage activation was not due to differences in interferon-γ receptor density. Recent work by Marodi and co-workers analyzed interferon-γ signaling through STAT-1 in cord blood and adult blood monocytes and monocyte-derived macrophages using flow cytometry. They found comparable expression of STAT-1 between cord and adult cells; however, phosphorylation of STAT-1 in response to interferon-γ was significantly decreased in neonatal monocytes and monocyte-derived macrophages compared with findings in adult cells.[253] These data suggest that defective interferon-γ signaling through STAT-1 in neonatal mononuclear phagocytes might contribute to the unique susceptibility of neonates to intracellular pathogens.

REFERENCES

1. Johnston, R.B., Jr: Current concepts: immunology. Monocytes and macrophages. N Engl J Med, 1988. *318*: pp. 747-52.
2. van Furth, R., et al: Characteristics of human mononuclear phagocytes. Blood, 1979. *54*: pp. 485-500.
3. van Furth, R. and Z.A. Cohn: The origin and kinetics of mononuclear phagocytes. J Exp Med, 1968. *128*: pp. 415-35.
4. Szabolcs, P., et al: Dendritic cells and macrophages can mature independently from a human bone marrow-derived, post-colony-forming unit intermediate. Blood, 1996. *87*: pp. 4520-30.
5. Peters, J.H., et al: Dendritic cells: from ontogenetic orphans to myelomonocytic descendants. Immunol Today, 1996. *17*(6): pp. 273-8.
6. Metcalf, D.: The molecular biology and functions of the granulocyte-macrophage colony-stimulating factors. Blood, 1986. *67*: pp. 257-67.
7. Clark, S.C. and R. Kamen: The human hematopoietic colony-stimulating factors. Science, 1987. *236*: pp. 1229-37.
8. Sieff, C.A.: Hematopoietic growth factors. J Clin Invest, 1987. *79*: pp. 1549-57.

9. Romani, N., et al: Proliferating dendritic cell progenitors in human blood. J Exp Med, 1994. *180*: pp. 83-93.
10. Hagihara, M., et al: Extensive and long-term ex vivo production of dendritic cells from CD34 positive umbilical cord blood or bone marrow cells by novel culture system using mouse stroma. J Immunol Methods, 2001. *253*: pp. 45-55.
11. Szabolcs, P., et al: Growth and differentiation of human dendritic cells from CD34+ progenitors. Adv Exp Med Biol, 1997. *417*: pp. 15-9.
12. Zhang, Y., et al: Induction of dendritic cell differentiation by granulocyte-macrophage colony-stimulating factor, stem cell factor, and tumor necrosis factor alpha in vitro from lineage phenotypes-negative c-kit+ murine hematopoietic progenitor cells. Blood, 1997. *90*: pp. 4842-53.
13. Dranoff, G., et al: Involvement of granulocyte-macrophage colony-stimulating factor in pulmonary homeostasis. Science, 1994. *264*: pp. 713-6.
14. Stanley, E., et al: Granulocyte/macrophage colony-stimulating factor-deficient mice show no major perturbation of hematopoiesis but develop a characteristic pulmonary pathology. Proc Natl Acad Sci U S A, 1994. *91*: pp. 5592-6.
15. Robb, L., et al: Hematopoietic and lung abnormalities in mice with a null mutation of the common beta subunit of the receptors for granulocyte-macrophage colony-stimulating factor and interleukins 3 and 5. Proc Natl Acad Sci U S A, 1995. *92*: pp. 9565-9.
16. Shibata, Y., et al: GM-CSF regulates alveolar macrophage differentiation and innate immunity in the lung through PU.1. Immunity, 2001. *15*: pp. 557-67.
17. Yoshida, H., et al: The murine mutation osteopetrosis is in the coding region of the macrophage colony stimulating factor gene. Nature, 1990. *345*: pp. 442-4.
18. Wiktor-Jedrzejczak, W., et al: CSF-1 deficiency in the op/op mouse has differential effects on macrophage populations and differentiation stages. Exp Hematol, 1992. *20*: pp. 1004-10.
19. Shibata, Y., et al: Alveolar macrophage deficiency in osteopetrotic mice deficient in macrophage colony-stimulating factor is spontaneously corrected with age and associated with matrix metalloproteinase expression and emphysema. Blood, 2001. *98*: pp. 2845-52.
20. Shivdasani, R.A., and S.H. Orkin: The transcriptional control of hematopoiesis. Blood, 1996. *87*: pp. 4025-39.
21. Guerriero, A., et al: PU.1 is required for myeloid-derived but not lymphoid-derived dendritic cells. Blood, 2000. *95*: pp. 879-85.
22. Trubowitz, S. and S. Davies: Pathophysiology of the monocyte-macrophage system. *In* The Human Bone marrow: Anatomy, Physiology, and Pathophysiology. D.S. Trubowitz, Editor. 1982, Boca Raton, CRC Press, pp. 95-126.
23. Douglas, S.D. and M.C. Yoder: The mononuclear phagocyte and dendritic cell systems. *In* Immunologic Disorders in Infants and Children. E.R. Stiehm, Editor. 1996, Philadelphia, WB Saunders Co., pp. 113-132.
24. Meuret, G., et al: Monocytopoiesis in normal man: pool size, proliferation activity and DNA synthesis time of promonocytes. Acta Haematol, 1975. *54*: pp. 261-70.
25. Whitelaw, D.M.: Observations on human monocyte kinetics after pulse labeling. Cell Tissue Kinet, 1972. *5*: pp. 311-7.
26. van Furth, R. and W. Sluiter: Distribution of blood monocytes between a marginating and a circulating pool. J Exp Med, 1986. *163*: pp. 474-9.
27. Meuret, G. and G. Hoffmann: Monocyte kinetic studies in normal and disease states. Br J Haematol, 1973. *24*: pp. 275-85.
28. van Furth, R.: Development and distribution of mononuclear phagocytes. *In* Inflammation: Basic Principles and Clinical Correlates. J.I. Gallin, et al, Editors. 1992, New York, Raven Press: pp. 325-40.
29. Haller, O., et al: Natural, genetically determined resistance toward influenza virus in hemopoietic mouse chimeras. Role of mononuclear phagocytes. J Exp Med, 1979. *150*: pp. 117-26.
30. Parwaresch, M.R., and H.H. Wacker: Origin and kinetics of resident tissue macrophages. Parabiosis studies with radiolabelled leucocytes. Cell Tissue Kinet, 1984. *17*: pp. 25-39.
31. Volkman, A.: The origin and turnover of mononuclear cells in peritoneal exudates in rats. J Exp Med, 1966. *124*: pp. 241-54.
32. Thomas, E.D., et al: Direct evidence for a bone marrow origin of the alveolar macrophage in man. Science, 1976. *192*: pp. 1016-8.
33. Gale, R.P., et al: Bone marrow origin of hepatic macrophages (Kupffer cells) in humans. Science, 1978. *201*: pp. 937-8.
34. Takashina, T.: Haemopoiesis in the human yolk sac. J Anat, 1987. *151*: pp. 125-35.
35. Cline, M.J., and M.A. Moore: Embryonic origin of the mouse macrophage. Blood, 1972. *39*: pp. 842-9.
36. Kelemen, E., and M. Janossa: Macrophages are the first differentiated blood cells formed in human embryonic liver. Exp Hematol, 1980. *8*: pp. 996-1000.
37. Kelemen, E., and W. Calvo: Prenatal hematopoiesis in the human bone marrow and its developmental antecedents. *In* The Human Bone marrow: Anatomy, Physiology, and Pathophysiology. S. Trubowitz and S. Davies, Editors. 1982, Boca Raton, CRC Press: pp. 3-41.
38. Linch, D.C., et al: Studies of circulating hemopoietic progenitor cells in human fetal blood. Blood, 1982. *59*: pp. 976-9.
39. Miller, D.R.: Normal values and examination of the blood: Perinatal period, infancy, childhood, and adolescence. *In* Blood Diseases of Infancy and Childhood. D.R. Miller, Editor. 1984, St. Louis, CV Mosby: pp. 21-45.
40. Xanthou, M.: Leucocyte blood picture in healthy full-term and premature babies during neonatal period. Arch Dis Child, 1970. *45*: pp. 242-9.
41. Weinberg, A.G., et al: Neonatal blood cell count in health and disease. II. Values for lymphocytes, monocytes, and eosinophils. J Pediatr, 1985. *106*: pp. 462-6.
42. Washburn, A.H.: Blood cells in healthy young infants. II. A comparison of routine and special techniques in the differentiation of leukocytes. Am J Dis Child, 1935. *50*: p. 400.
43. Alenghat, E., and J.R. Esterly: Alveolar macrophages in perinatal infants. Pediatrics, 1984. *74*(2): pp. 221-3.
44. Jacobs, R.F., et al: Factors related to the appearance of alveolar macrophages in the developing lung. Am Rev Respir Dis, 1985. *131*: pp. 548-53.
45. Bellanti, J.A., et al: Host defenses in the fetus and neonate: studies of the alveolar macrophage during maturation. Pediatrics, 1979. *64*(5 Pt 2 Suppl): pp. 726-39.
46. Kurland, G., et al: The ontogeny of pulmonary defenses: alveolar macrophage function in neonatal and juvenile rhesus monkeys. Pediatr Res, 1988. *23*: pp. 293-7.
47. Sherman, M., et al: Neonatal lung defense mechanisms: a study of the alveolar macrophage system in neonatal rabbits. Am Rev Respir Dis, 1977. *116*: pp. 433-40.
48. Johnston, R.B.J., and D. Zucker-Franklin: Monocytes and macrophages. *In* Atlas of Blood Cells: Function and Pathology. D. Zucker-Franklin, Editor. 1988, Philadelphia, Lea & Febiger: pp. 323-357.
49. Steinman, R.M., and Z.A. Cohn: Identification of a novel cell type in peripheral lymphoid organs of mice. I. Morphology, quantitation, tissue distribution. J Exp Med, 1973. *137*: pp. 1142-62.
50. Yourno, J., et al: Monocyte nonspecific esterase. Enzymologic characterization of a neutral serine esterase associated with myeloid cells. J Histochem Cytochem, 1986. *34*: pp. 727-33.
51. Kreipe, H., et al: Phenotypic differentiation patterns of the human monocyte/macrophage system. Histochem J, 1986. *18*: pp. 441-50.
52. Stiehm, E.R., et al: Deficient DR antigen expression on human cord blood monocytes: reversal with lymphokines. Clin Immunol Immunopathol, 1984. *30*(3): pp. 430-6.
53. Morris, R.B., et al: Ultrastructure and peroxidase cytochemistry of normal human leukocytes at birth. Dev Biol, 1975. *44*: pp. 223-38.
54. Egner, W., et al: Identification of potent mixed leukocyte reaction-stimulatory cells in human bone marrow. Putative differentiation stage of human blood dendritic cells. J Immunol, 1993. *150*: pp. 3043-53.
55. Buckley, P.J., et al: Human spleen contains phenotypic subsets of macrophages and dendritic cells that occupy discrete microanatomic locations. Am J Pathol, 1987. *128*: pp. 505-20.
56. Knight, S.C., et al: Non-adherent, low-density cells from human peripheral blood contain dendritic cells and monocytes, both with veiled morphology. Immunology, 1986. *57*: pp. 595-603.
57. Thomas, R., L.S. Davis, and P.E. Lipsky: Isolation and characterization of human peripheral blood dendritic cells. J Immunol, 1993. *150*: pp. 821-34.
58. Hart, D.N. and J.L. McKenzie: Isolation and characterization of human tonsil dendritic cells. J Exp Med, 1988. *168*(1): pp. 157-70.
59. MacPherson, G.G., et al: Properties of lymph-borne (veiled) dendritic cells in culture. II. Expression of the IL-2 receptor: role of GM-CSF. Immunology, 1989. *68*: pp. 108-13.
60. Berken, A., and B. Benacerraf: Properties of antibodies cytophilic for macrophages. J Exp Med, 1966. *123*: pp. 119-44.
61. Young, J.D., et al: The increase in intracellular free calcium associated with IgG gamma 2b/gamma 1 Fc receptor-ligand interactions: role in phagocytosis. Proc Natl Acad Sci U S A, 1984. *81*: pp. 5430-4.
62. Anderson, C.L., et al: Phagocytosis mediated by three distinct Fc gamma receptor classes on human leukocytes. J Exp Med, 1990. *171*: pp. 1333-45.
63. Ravetch, J.V., et al: Structural heterogeneity and functional domains of murine immunoglobulin G Fc receptors. Science, 1986. *234*: pp. 718-25.
64. Lewis, V.A., et al: A complementary DNA clone for a macrophage-lymphocyte Fc receptor. Nature, 1986. *324*: pp. 372-5.
65. Hibbs, M.L., et al: Molecular cloning of a human immunoglobulin G Fc receptor. Proc Natl Acad Sci U S A, 1988. *85*: pp. 2240-4.
66. Stengelin, S., et al: Isolation of cDNAs for two distinct human Fc receptors by ligand affinity cloning. Embo J, 1988. 7: pp. 1053-9.
67. Maxwell, K.F., et al: Crystal structure of the human leukocyte Fc receptor, Fc gammaRIIa. Nat Struct Biol, 1999. 6: pp. 437-42.
68. Sondermann, P., et al: The 3.2-A crystal structure of the human IgG1 Fc fragment-Fc gammaRIII complex. Nature, 2000. *406*: pp. 267-73.
69. Daeron, M.: Fc receptor biology. Annu Rev Immunol, 1997. *15*: pp. 203-34.
70. Bolland, S., and J.V. Ravetch: Inhibitory pathways triggered by ITIM-containing receptors. Adv Immunol, 1999. *72*: pp. 149-77.
71. Ravetch, J.V., and S. Bolland: IgG Fc receptors. Annu Rev Immunol, 2001. *19*: pp. 275-90.
72. Salim, K., et al: Distinct specificity in the recognition of phosphoinositides by the pleckstrin homology domains of dynamin and Bruton's tyrosine kinase. Embo J, 1996. *15*: pp. 6241-50.
73. Ferguson, K.M., et al: Structure of the high affinity complex of inositol trisphosphate with a phospholipase C pleckstrin homology domain. Cell, 1995. *83*: pp. 1037-46.
74. Falasca, M., et al: Activation of phospholipase C gamma by PI 3-kinase-induced PH domain-mediated membrane targeting. Embo J, 1998. *17*: pp. 414-22.
75. Wang, D., et al: Phospholipase Cgamma2 is essential in the functions of B cell and several Fc receptors. Immunity, 2000. *13*: pp. 25-35.
76. Ochiai, M., and M. Ashida: A pattern recognition protein for peptidoglycan. Cloning the cDNA and the gene of the silkworm, Bombyx mori. J Biol Chem, 1999. *274*: pp. 11854-8.

77. Levashina, E.A., et al: Constitutive activation of toll-mediated antifungal defense in serpin- deficient Drosophila. Science, 1999. 285: pp. 1917-9.

78. Kim, Y., et al: Gram-negative bacteria binding protein, a pattern recognition receptor for lipopolysaccharide and beta-1,3-glucan, which mediates the signaling for the induction of innate immune genes in Drosophila melanogaster cells. J Biol Chem, 2000. 275: pp. 32721—27.

79. Medzhitov, R., and C.A. Janeway: Innate immunity: the virtues of a nonclonal system of recognition. Cell, 1997. 91: pp. 295-8.

80. Mathison, J.C., et al: Plasma lipopolysaccharide (LPS)-binding protein. A key component in macrophage recognition of gram-negative LPS. J Immunol, 1992. 149: pp. 200-6.

81. Levy, O., et al: Enhancement of neonatal innate defense: effects of adding an N-terminal recombinant fragment of bactericidal/permeability-increasing protein on growth and tumor necrosis factor-inducing activity of gram-negative bacteria tested in neonatal cord blood ex vivo. Infect Immunol, 2000. 68: pp. 5120-5.

82. Horwitz, A.H., et al: Human lipopolysaccharide-binding protein potentiates bactericidal activity of human bactericidal/permeability-increasing protein. Infect Immunol, 1995. 63: pp. 522-7.

83. Wilde, C.G., et al: Bactericidal/permeability-increasing protein and lipopolysaccharide (LPS)-binding protein. LPS binding properties and effects on LPS-mediated cell activation. J Biol Chem, 1994. 269: pp. 17411-6.

84. Gray, P.W., et al: Cloning of the cDNA of a human neutrophil bactericidal protein. Structural and functional correlations. J Biol Chem, 1989. 264: pp. 9505-9.

85. Turni, L., et al: CD guide. In Leucocyte Typing VII. D. Mason and D. Simmons, Editors. 2002, Oxford, Oxford University Press: pp. 747 - 931.

86. Bhoopat, L., et al: The differentiation antigens of macrophages in human fetal liver. Clin Immunol Immunopathol, 1986. 41: pp. 184-92.

87. Marwitz, P.A., et al: Expression and modulation of cell surface determinants on human adult and neonatal monocytes. Clin Exp Immunol, 1988. 72: pp. 260-6.

88. Edwards, J.A., et al: Differential expression of HLA class II antigens on human fetal and adult lymphocytes and macrophages. Immunology, 1985. 55: pp. 489-500.

89. Bulmer, J.N., et al: Expression of class II MHC gene products by macrophages in human uteroplacental tissue. Immunology, 1988. 63: pp. 707-14.

90. Glover, D.M., et al: Expression of HLA class II antigens and secretion of interleukin-1 by monocytes and macrophages from adults and neonates. Immunology, 1987. 61: pp. 195-201.

91. Gonwa, T.A., et al: Antigen-presenting capabilities of human monocytes correlates with their expression of HLA-DS, an Ia determinant distinct from HLA-DR. J Immunol, 1983. 130: pp. 706-11.

92. Steinman, R.M.: The dendritic cell system and its role in immunogenicity. Annu Rev Immunol, 1991. 9: pp. 271-96.

93. Hart, D.N.: Dendritic cells: unique leukocyte populations which control the primary immune response. Blood, 1997. 90: pp. 3245-87.

94. Siena, S., et al: Massive ex vivo generation of functional dendritic cells from mobilized CD34+ blood progenitors for anticancer therapy. Exp Hematol, 1995. 23: pp. 1463-71.

95. Cline, M.J. and R.I. Lehrer: Phagocytosis by human monocytes. Blood, 1968. 32: pp. 423.

96. Cline, M.J.: Metabolism of the circulating leukocyte. Physiol Rev, 1965. 45: pp. 674.

97. Prindull, G., and B. Prindull: Glycogen in inflammatory mononuclear cells of premature and mature newborn infants. J Reticuloendothel Soc, 1970. 7: p. 594.

98. Das, M., et al: Neonatal mononuclear metabolism: Further evidence for diminished monocyte function in the neonate. Pediatr Res, 1979. 13: p. 632.

99. Oren, R.A., et al: Metabolic patterns in three types of phagocytizing cells. J Cell Biol, 1963. 17: p. 487.

100. Bar-Eli, M., et al: The progeny of a single progenitor cell can develop characteristics of either a tissue or an alveolar macrophage. Blood, 1981. 57: pp. 95-8.

101. Babior, B.M.: Oxygen-dependent microbial killing by phagocytes (first of two parts). N Engl J Med, 1978. 298: pp. 659-68.

102. Nathan, C.F., and S. Tsunawaki: Secretion of toxic oxygen products by macrophages: regulatory cytokines and their effects on the oxidase. Ciba Found Symp, 1986. 118: pp. 211-30.

103. Gallin, J.I.: Disorders of phagocytic cells. In Inflammation: Basic Principles and Clinical Correlates. J.I. Gallin, et al, Editors. 1972, New York, Raven Press: pp. 859-74.

104. Hamers, M.N., et al: Complementation in monocyte hybrids revealing genetic heterogeneity in chronic granulomatous disease. Nature, 1984. 307: pp. 553-5.

105. Kretschmer, R.R., et al: Quantitative nitroblue tetrazolium reduction by normal newborn monocytes. J Pediatr, 1977. 91: pp. 306-9.

106. Speer, C.P., et al: Phagocytic activities in neonatal monocytes. Eur J Pediatr, 1986. 145: pp. 418-21.

107. Speer, C.P., et al: Oxidative metabolism in cord blood monocytes and monocyte-derived macrophages. Infect Immunol, 1985. 50: p. 919.

108. Pabst, M.J., and R.B. Johnston, Jr: Increased production of superoxide anion by macrophages exposed in vitro to muramyl dipeptide or lipopolysaccharide. J Exp Med, 1980. 151: pp. 101-14.

109. Muller-Eberhard, H.J.: The membrane attack complex of complement. Annu Rev Immunol, 1986. 4: pp. 503-28.

110. Hugli, T.E., and H.J. Muller-Eberhard: Anaphylatoxins: C3a and C5a. Adv Immunol, 1978. 26: pp. 1-53.

111. Becker, E.L., et al: The ability of chemotactic factors to induce lysosomal enzyme release. I. The characteristics of the release, the importance of surfaces and the relation of enzyme release to chemotactic responsiveness. J Immunol, 1974. 112: pp. 2047-54.

112. Hansch, G.M., et al: Macrophages release arachidonic acid, prostaglandin E2, and thromboxane in response to late complement components. J Immunol, 1984. 133: pp. 2145-50.

113. Linton, S., Animal models of inherited complement deficiency. Mol Biotechnol, 2001. 18: pp. 135-48.

114. Attwood, J.T., et al: Impaired IgG responses in a child with homozygous C2 deficiency and recurrent pneumococcal septicaemia. Acta Paediatr, 2001. 90: pp. 99-101.

115. Lassiter, H.A., et al: Complement system development and disorders during the neonatal period. In Hematopoietic Problems of the Neonate. R.D. Christensen, Editor. 2000, Philadelphia, WB Saunders: pp. 343-64.

116. Gitlin, D., and A. Biasucci: Development of gamma G, gamma A, gamma M, beta IC-beta IA, C 1 esterase inhibitor, ceruloplasmin, transferrin, hemopexin, haptoglobin, fibrinogen, plasminogen, alpha 1-antitrypsin, orosomucoid, beta-lipoprotein, alpha 2-macroglobulin, and prealbumin in the human conceptus. J Clin Invest, 1969. 48: pp. 1433-46.

117. Kohler, P.F., Maturation of the human complement system. I. Onset time and sites of fetal C1q, C4, C3, and C5 synthesis. J Clin Invest, 1973. 52: pp. 671-7.

118. Wurzner, R., et al: Complement component C7. Assessment of in vivo synthesis after liver transplantation reveals that hepatocytes do not synthesize the majority of human C7. J Immunol, 1994. 152: pp. 4624-9.

119. Kai, C., et al: Ontogeny of the third component of complement of Japanese quails. Immunology, 1985. 54: pp. 463-70.

120. Abe, T., et al: Development and genetic differences of complement activity in rabbits. Anim Blood Groups Biochem Genet, 1979. 10: pp. 19-26.

121. Lassiter, H.A., et al: The administration of complement component C9 enhances the survival of neonatal rats with Escherichia coli sepsis. Pediatr Res, 1997. 42: pp. 128-36.

122. Davis, C.A., et al: Serum complement levels in infancy: age related changes. Pediatr Res, 1979. 13: pp. 1043-6.

123. Notarangelo, L.D., et al: Activity of classical and alternative pathways of complement in preterm and small for gestational age infants. Pediatr Res, 1984. 18: pp. 281-5.

124. Bessler, H., et al: Production of interleukin-1 by mononuclear cells of newborns and their mothers. Clin Exp Immunol, 1987. 68: pp. 655-61.

125. Wilson, C.B.: Immunologic basis for increased susceptibility of the neonate to infection. J Pediatr, 1986. 108: pp. 1-12.

126. Weatherstone, K.B., and E.A. Rich: Tumor necrosis factor/cachectin and interleukin-1 secretion by cord blood monocytes from premature and term neonates. Pediatr Res, 1989. 25: pp. 342-6.

127. Peters, A.M., et al: Reduced secretion of interleukin-1 and tumor necrosis factor-alpha by neonatal monocytes. Biol Neonate, 1993. 63: pp. 157-62.

128. Kaufman, D., et al: Decreased superoxide production, degranulation, tumor necrosis factor alpha secretion, and CD11b/CD18 receptor expression by adherent monocytes from preterm infants. Clin Diagn Lab Immunol, 1999. 6: pp. 525-9.

129. Buzby, J.S., et al: Increased granulocyte-macrophage colony-stimulating factor mRNA instability in cord versus adult mononuclear cells is translation-dependent and associated with increased levels of A + U-rich element binding factor. Blood, 1996. 88: pp. 2889-97.

130. Schibler, K.R., et al: Defective production of interleukin-6 by monocytes: a possible mechanism underlying several host defense deficiencies of neonates. Pediatr Res, 1992. 31: pp. 18-21.

131. Schibler, K.R., et al: Diminished transcription of interleukin-8 by monocytes from preterm neonates. J Leukoc Biol, 1993. 53: pp. 399-403.

132. Schibler, K.R., et al: Production of granulocyte colony-stimulating factor in vitro by monocytes from preterm and term neonates. Blood, 1993. 82: pp. 2478-84.

133. Le, T., et al: Regulation of interleukin-10 gene expression: possible mechanisms accounting for its upregulation and for maturational differences in its expression by blood mononuclear cells. Blood, 1997. 89: pp. 4112-9.

134. Lee, S.M., et al: Decreased interleukin-12 (IL-12) from activated cord versus adult peripheral blood mononuclear cells and upregulation of interferon-gamma, natural killer, and lymphokine-activated killer activity by IL-12 in cord blood mononuclear cells. Blood, 1996. 88: pp. 945-54.

135. Buzby, J.S., et al: Developmental regulation of RNA transcript destabilization by A + U- rich elements is AUF1-dependent. J Biol Chem, 1999. 274: pp. 33973-8.

136. Goriely, S., et al: Deficient IL-12(p35) gene expression by dendritic cells derived from neonatal monocytes. J Immunol, 2001. 166: pp. 2141-6.

137. Hinchliffe, J.R., and D.R. Johnson: Development of the Vertebrate Limb. 1980, Oxford, Clarendon Press.

138. De Felici, M., et al: Macrophages in the urogenital ridge of the mid-gestation mouse fetus. Cell Differ, 1986. 18: pp. 119-29.

139. Perry, V.H., et al: Immunohistochemical localization of macrophages and microglia in the adult and developing mouse brain. Neuroscience, 1985. 15: pp. 313-26.

140. Hume, D.A., et al: Immunohistochemical localization of a macrophage-specific antigen in developing mouse retina: phagocytosis of dying neurons

and differentiation of microglial cells to form a regular array in the plexiform layers. J Cell Biol, 1983. 97: pp. 253-7.

141. Hopkinson-Woolley, J., et al: Macrophage recruitment during limb development and wound healing in the embryonic and foetal mouse. J Cell Sci, 1994. 107: pp. 1159-67.

142. Miller, M.E., Phagocytic cells. In Host Defenses in the Human Neonate. M.E. Miller, Editor. 1978, New York, Grune & Stratton: pp. 59-71.

143. Broxmeyer, H.E., and C.H. Kim: Regulation of hematopoiesis in a sea of chemokine family members with a plethora of redundant activities. Exp Hematol, 1999. 27: pp. 1113-23.

144. Sozzani, S., et al: The role of chemokines in the regulation of dendritic cell trafficking. J Leukoc Biol, 1999. 66: pp. 1-9.

145. Chan, V.W., et al: Secondary lymphoid-tissue chemokine (SLC) is chemotactic for mature dendritic cells. Blood, 1999. 93: pp. 3610-6.

146. Marodi, L., et al: Chemotactic and random movement of human newborn monocytes. Eur J Pediatr, 1980. 135: pp. 73-5.

147. Weston, W.L., et al: Monocyte-macrophage function in the newborn. Am J Dis Child, 1977. 131: pp. 1241-2.

148. Klein, R.B., et al: Decreased mononuclear and polymorphonuclear chemotaxis in human newborns, infants, and young children. Pediatrics, 1977. 60: pp. 467-72.

149. Yegin, O.: Chemotaxis in childhood. Pediatr Res, 1983. 17(3): pp. 183-7.

150. Raghunathan, R., et al: Phagocyte chemotaxis in the perinatal period. J Clin Immunol, 1982. 2: pp. 242-5.

151. Pahwa, S.G., et al: Cellular and humoral components of monocyte and neutrophil chemotaxis in cord blood. Pediatr Res, 1977. 11: pp. 677-80.

152. Hawes, C.S., et al: In vitro parameters of cell-mediated immunity in the human neonate. Clin Immunol Immunopathol, 1980. 17: pp. 530-6.

153. Lasky, L.A.: Selectins: interpreters of cell-specific carbohydrate information during inflammation. Science, 1992. 258(5084): pp. 964-9.

154. Hogg, N., and R.C. Landis: Adhesion molecules in cell interactions. Curr Opin Immunol, 1993. 5(3): pp. 383-90.

155. Bevilacqua, M.P., and R.M. Nelson: Selectins. J Clin Invest, 1993. 91: pp. 379-87.

156. Weller, A. S. et al: Cloning of the mouse endothelial selectins. Expression of both E- and P-selectin is inducible by tumor necrosis factor alpha. J Biol Chem, 1992. 267: pp. 15176-83.

157. Carlos, T.M., and J.M. Harlan: Leukocyte-endothelial adhesion molecules. Blood, 1994. 84: pp. 2068-101.

158. Anderson, D.C., and T.A. Springer: Leukocyte adhesion deficiency: an inherited defect in the Mac-1, LFA-1, and p150,95 glycoproteins. Annu Rev Med, 1987. 38: pp. 175-94.

159. Anderson, D.C., et al: The severe and moderate phenotypes of heritable Mac-1, LFA-1 deficiency: their quantitative definition and relation to leukocyte dysfunction and clinical features. J Infect Dis, 1985. 152: pp. 668-89.

160. Freyer, D.R., et al: Modulation of surface CD11/CD18 glycoproteins (Mo1, LFA-1, p150,95) by human mononuclear phagocytes. Clin Immunol Immunopathol, 1988. 46: pp. 272-83.

161. Boner, A. et al: Chemotactic responses of various differential stages of neutrophils from human cord and adult blood. Infect Immunol, 1982. 35: p. 921.

162. Speer, C.P., and R.B.J. Johnston: Phagocyte function. In Neonatal Infections: Nutritional and Immunologic Interactions. P.L. Ogra, Editor. 1984, Orlando, Grune & Stratton: pp. 21-36.

163. Roth, P. P., and R.A. Polin: Adherence of human newborn infants' monocytes to matrix-bound fibronectin. J Pediatr, 1992. 121: pp. 285-8.

164. Gordon, S., and Z.A. Cohn: The macrophage. Int Rev Cytol, 1973. 36: pp. 171-214.

165. Mishell, R.I., and R.W. Dutton: Immunization of dissociated spleen cell cultures from normal mice. J Exp Med, 1967. 126(3): pp. 423-42.

166. Steinman, R.M., et al: Identification of a novel cell type in peripheral lymphoid organs of mice. 3. Functional properties in vivo. J Exp Med, 1974. 139(6): pp. 1431-45.

167. Steinman, R.M., et al: Identification of a novel cell type in peripheral lymphoid organs of mice. V. Purification of spleen dendritic cells, new surface markers, and maintenance in vitro. J Exp Med, 1979. 149(1): pp. 1-16.

168. Schuler, G., and R.M. Steinman: Murine epidermal Langerhans cells mature into potent immunostimulatory dendritic cells in vitro. J Exp Med, 1985. 161: pp. 526-46.

169. Klinkert, W.E., et al: Accessory and stimulating properties of dendritic cells and macrophages isolated from various rat tissues. J Exp Med, 1982. 156: pp. 1-19.

170. Kelly, R.H., et al: Functional anatomy of lymph nodes. II. Peripheral lymph-borne mononuclear cells. Anat Rec, 1978. 190: pp. 5-21.

171. Pugh, C.W., et al: Characterization of nonlymphoid cells derived from rat peripheral lymph. J Exp Med, 1983. 157: pp. 1758-79.

172. Steinman, R.M., and Z.A. Cohn: The interaction of soluble horseradish peroxidase with mouse peritoneal macrophages in vitro. J Cell Biol, 1972. 55(1): pp. 186-204.

173. Steinman, R.M. and Z.A. Cohn: The interaction of particulate horseradish peroxidase (HRP)-anti HRP immune complexes with mouse peritoneal macrophages in vitro. J Cell Biol, 1972. 55: pp. 616-34.

174. Harding, C.V., and E.R. Unanue: Quantitation of antigen-presenting cell MHC class II/peptide complexes necessary for T-cell stimulation. Nature, 1990. 346: pp. 574-6.

175. Demotz, S., et al: The minimal number of class II MHC-antigen complexes needed for T cell activation. Science, 1990. 249: pp. 1028-30.

176. Bhardwaj, N., et al: Small amounts of superantigen, when presented on dendritic cells, are sufficient to initiate T cell responses. J Exp Med, 1993. 178: pp. 633-42.

177. Sallusto, F., and A. Lanzavecchia: Efficient presentation of soluble antigen by cultured human dendritic cells is maintained by granulocyte/macrophage colony-stimulating factor plus interleukin 4 and downregulated by tumor necrosis factor alpha. J Exp Med, 1994. 179: pp. 1109-18.

178. Zaghouani, H., et al: Presentation of a viral T cell epitope expressed in the CDR3 region of a self immunoglobulin molecule. Science, 1993. 259: pp. 224-7.

179. Schuler, G., et al: Coated Langerhans cell granules in histiocytosis X cells. Ultrastruct Pathol, 1983. 5: pp. 77-82.

180. Takigawa, M., et al: The Langerhans cell granule is an adsorptive endocytic organelle. J Invest Dermatol, 1985. 85: pp. 12-5.

181. Sallusto, F., et al: Dendritic cells use macropinocytosis and the mannose receptor to concentrate macromolecules in the major histocompatibility complex class II compartment: downregulation by cytokines and bacterial products. J Exp Med, 1995. 182: pp. 389-400.

182. Jiang, W., et al: The receptor DEC-205 expressed by dendritic cells and thymic epithelial cells is involved in antigen processing. Nature, 1995. 375: pp. 151-5.

183. Dzionek, A., et al: BDCA-2, a novel plasmacytoid dendritic cell-specific type II C-type lectin, mediates antigen capture and is a potent inhibitor of interferon alpha/beta induction. J Exp Med, 2001. 194: pp. 1823-34.

184. Levine, T.P., and B.M. Chain: Endocytosis by antigen presenting cells: dendritic cells are as endocytically active as other antigen presenting cells. Proc Natl Acad Sci U S A, 1992. 89: pp. 8342-6.

185. Romani, N., et al: Presentation of exogenous protein antigens by dendritic cells to T cell clones. Intact protein is presented best by immature, epidermal Langerhans cells. J Exp Med, 1989. 169: pp. 1169-78.

186. Streilein, J.W., and S.F. Grammer: In vitro evidence that Langerhans cells can adopt two functionally distinct forms capable of antigen presentation to T lymphocytes. J Immunol, 1989. 143: pp. 3925-33.

187. Crowley, M., et al: Dendritic cells are the principal cells in mouse spleen bearing immunogenic fragments of foreign proteins. J Exp Med, 1990. 172: pp. 383-6.

188. Brunk, U., et al: Influence of epidermal growth factor (EGF) on ruffling activity, pinocytosis and proliferation of cultivated human glia cells. Exp Cell Res, 1976. 103: pp. 295-302.

189. Racoosin, E.L., and J.A. Swanson: Macrophage colony-stimulating factor (rM-CSF) stimulates pinocytosis in bone marrow-derived macrophages. J Exp Med, 1989. 170: pp. 1635-48.

190. Naito, M., et al: Ontogenic Development of Kupffer Cells. 1982. Amsterdam: Elsevier Biomedical Press.

191. Kutteh, W.H., et al: Regulation of interleukin-6 production in human fetal Kupffer cells. Scand J Immunol, 1991. 33: pp. 607-13.

192. Slayton, W.B., et al: Hematopoiesis in the liver and marrow of human fetuses at 5 to 16 weeks postconception: quantitative assessment of macrophage and neutrophil populations. Pediatr Res, 1998. 43: pp. 774-82.

193. Schuit, K.E., and D.A. Powell: Phagocytic dysfunction in monocytes of normal newborn infants. Pediatrics, 1980. 65: pp. 501-4.

194. Marodi, L., et al: Characteristics and functional capacities of human cord blood granulocytes and monocytes. Pediatr Res, 1984. 18: pp. 1127-31.

195. Jacobs, R.F., et al: Phagocytosis of type III group B streptococci by neonatal monocytes: enhancement by fibronectin and gammaglobulin. J Infect Dis, 1985. 152: pp. 695-700.

196. Speer, C.P., et al: Phagocytosis-associated functions in neonatal monocyte-derived macrophages. Pediatr Res, 1988. 24: pp. 213-6.

197. D'Ambola, J.B., et al: Human and rabbit newborn lung macrophages have reduced anti-Candida activity. Pediatr Res, 1988. 24: pp. 285-90.

198. Liu, E., et al: Decreased yield, phenotypic expression and function of immature monocyte-derived dendritic cells in cord blood. Br J Haematol, 2001. 113: pp. 240-6.

199. Zheng, Z., et al: Generation of dendritic cells from adherent cells of cord blood by culture with granulocyte-macrophage colony-stimulating factor, interleukin-4, and tumor necrosis factor-alpha. J Hematother Stem Cell Res, 2000. 9: pp. 453-64.

200. Klebanoff, S.J.: Oxygen metabolites of phagocytes. In Inflammation: Basic Principles and Clinical Correlates. Gallin, J.I., et al, Editors. 1992, New York, Raven Press: pp. 541-88.

201. Elsbach, P.P., and J. Weiss: Oxygen-independent antimicrobial system of phagocytes. In Inflammation: Basic Principles and Clinical Correlates. Gallin, J.I., et al, Editors. 1992, New York, Raven Press: pp. 603-636.

202. Elsbach, P.P., and J. Weiss: A reevaluation of the roles of the O_2-dependent and O2-independent microbicidal systems of phagocytes. Rev Infect Dis, 1983. 5: pp. 843-53.

203. Hibbs, J.B.J., et al: Synthesis of nitric oxide from L-arginine: a cytokine inducible pathway with antimicrobial activity in mononuclear phagocytes. In Mononuclear Phagocytes. R. van Furth, Editor. 1985, Boston, Kluwer Academic Publishers: pp. 279-92.

204. Bogdan, C.: Nitric oxide and the immune response. Nat Immunol, 2001. 2: pp. 907-16.

205. Nathan, C., and M.U. Shiloh: Reactive oxygen and nitrogen intermediates in the relationship between mammalian hosts and microbial pathogens. Proc Natl Acad Sci U S A, 2000. 97: pp. 8841-8.

206. Bogdan, C., et al: Reactive oxygen and reactive nitrogen intermediates in innate and specific immunity. Curr Opin Immunol, 2000. *12*: pp. 64–76.

207. Hesse, M., et al: NOS-2 mediates the protective anti-inflammatory and antifibrotic effects of the Th1-inducing adjuvant, IL-12, in a Th2 model of granulomatous disease. Am J Pathol, 2000. *157*: pp. 945–55.

208. DeGroote, M.A., and F.V. Fang: Antimicrobial properties of nitric oxide. *In* Nitric Oxide and Infection, F.C. Fang, Editor. 1999, Kluwer Academic / Plenum New York: pp. 231–261.

209. Bryk, R., et al: Peroxynitrite reductase activity of bacterial peroxiredoxins. Nature, 2000. *407*: pp. 211–5.

210. Iniesta, V., et al: The inhibition of arginase by N(omega)-hydroxy-l-arginine controls the growth of Leishmania inside macrophages. J Exp Med, 2001. *193*: pp. 777–84.

211. Adams, D.O., and T.A. Hamilton: The cell biology of macrophage activation. Annu Rev Immunol, 1984. *2*: pp. 283–318.

212. Nathan, C.F: Reactive oxygen intermediates in lysis of antibody-coated tumor cells. *In* Macrophage Mediated Antibody-Dependent Cellular Cytotoxicity. H.S. Koren, Editor. 1983, New York, Marcel Dekker: pp. 79–88.

213. Kohl, S., et al: Human neonatal and maternal monocyte-macrophage and lymphocyte-mediated antibody-dependent cytotoxicity to cells infected with herpes simplex. J Pediatr, 1978. *93*: pp. 206–10.

214. Milgrom, H., and S.L. Shore: Assessment of monocyte function in the normal newborn infant by antibody-dependent cellular cytotoxicity. J Pediatr, 1977. *91*: pp. 612–4.

215. Blaese, R.M., et al: The mononuclear phagocyte system: role in expression of immunocompetence in neonatal and adult life. Pediatrics, 1979. *64*(Suppl): pp. 829–33.

216. Pearson, A.M.: Scavenger receptors in innate immunity. Curr Opin Immunol, 1996. *8*: pp. 20–8.

217. Fanger, N.A., et al: Type I (CD64) and type II (CD32) Fc gamma receptor-mediated phagocytosis by human blood dendritic cells. J Immunol, 1996. *157*: pp. 541–8.

218. Scheicher, C., et al: Uptake of microparticle-adsorbed protein antigen by bone marrow-derived dendritic cells results in up-regulation of interleukin-1 alpha and interleukin-12 p40/p35 and triggers prolonged, efficient antigen presentation. Eur J Immunol, 1995. *25*: pp. 1566–72.

219. Hart, D.N., and J.L. McKenzie: Interstitial dendritic cells. Int Rev Immunol, 1990. *6*: pp. 127–38.

220. Inaba, K., et al: Dendritic cells pulsed with protein antigens in vitro can prime antigen-specific, MHC-restricted T cells in situ. J Exp Med, 1990. *172*: pp. 631–40.

221. McKenzie, J.L., et al: Human dendritic cells stimulate allogeneic T cells in the absence of IL-1. Immunology, 1989. *67*: pp. 290–7.

222. Matsuno, K., et al: A life stage of particle-laden rat dendritic cells in vivo: their terminal division, active phagocytosis, and translocation from the liver to the draining lymph. J Exp Med, 1996. *183*: pp. 1865–78.

223. Takahashi, S., and K. Hashimoto: Derivation of Langerhans cell granules from cytomembrane. J Invest Dermatol, 1985. *84*: pp. 469–71.

224. Ezekowitz, R.A., et al: Molecular characterization of the human macrophage mannose receptor: demonstration of multiple carbohydrate recognition-like domains and phagocytosis of yeasts in Cos-1 cells. J Exp Med, 1990. *172*: pp. 1785–94.

225. Lechler, R.I.: MHC class II molecular structure—permitted pairs? Immunol Today, 1988. *9*: pp. 76–8.

226. Lanzavecchia, A.: Mechanisms of antigen uptake for presentation. Curr Opin Immunol, 1996. *8*: pp. 348–54.

227. Norbury, C.C., et al: Constitutive micropinocytosis allows TAP-dependent major histocompatibility complex class I presentation of exogenous soluble antigen by bone marrow-derived dendritic cells. Eur J Immunol, 1997. *27*: pp. 280–8.

228. Barfoot, R., et al: Some properties of dendritic macrophages from peripheral lymph. Immunology, 1989. *68*: pp. 233–9.

229. Kleijmeer, M.J., et al: MHC class II compartments and the kinetics of antigen presentation in activated mouse spleen dendritic cells. J Immunol, 1995. *154*: pp. 5715–24.

230. Nijman, H.W.: Antigen capture and major histocompatibility class II compartments of freshly isolated and cultured human blood dendritic cells. J Exp Med, 1995. *182*: pp. 163–74.

231. Mellman, I., and R.M. Steinman, Dendritic cells: specialized and regulated antigen processing machines. Cell, 2001. *106*: pp. 255–8.

232. Thery, C., and S. Amigorena: The cell biology of antigen presentation in dendritic cells. Curr Opin Immunol, 2001. *13*: pp. 45–51.

233. Inaba, K., et al: The formation of immunogenic major histocompatibility complex class II-peptide ligands in lysosomal compartments of dendritic cells is regulated by inflammatory stimuli. J Exp Med, 2000. *191*: pp. 927–36.

234. Turley, S.J., et al: Transport of peptide-MHC class II complexes in developing dendritic cells. Science, 2000. *288*: pp. 522–7.

235. Pierre, P.P., and I. Mellman: Developmental regulation of invariant chain proteolysis controls MHC class II trafficking in mouse dendritic cells. Cell, 1998. *93*: pp. 1135–45.

236. Villadangos, J.A., et al: MHC class II expression is regulated in dendritic cells independently of invariant chain degradation. Immunity, 2001. *14*: pp. 739–49.

237. Garrett, W.S., et al: Developmental control of endocytosis in dendritic cells by Cdc42. Cell, 2000. *102*: pp. 325–34.

238. Koppelman, B., et al: Interleukin-10 down-regulates MHC class II alphabeta peptide complexes at the plasma membrane of monocytes by affecting arrival and recycling. Immunity, 1997. 7: pp. 861–71.

239. Fiebiger, E., et al: Cytokines regulate proteolysis in major histocompatibility complex class II-dependent antigen presentation by dendritic cells. J Exp Med, 2001. *193*: pp. 881–92.

240. Hoffman, A.A., et al: Presentation of antigen by human newborn monocytes to maternal tetanus toxoid-specific T-cell blasts. J Clin Immunol, 1981. *1*: pp. 217.

241. Zlabinger, G.J., et al: Cord blood macrophages present bacterial antigen (Escherichia coli) to paternal T cells. Clin Immunol Immunopathol, 1983. *28*: pp. 405–12.

242. Petty, R.E., and D.W. Hunt: Neonatal dendritic cells. Vaccine, 1998. *16*: pp. 1378–82.

243. Hunt, D.W., et al: Studies of human cord blood dendritic cells: evidence for functional immaturity. Blood, 1994. *84*: pp. 4333–43.

244. Murray, H.W.: Interferon-gamma, the activated macrophage, and host defense against microbial challenge. Ann Intern Med, 1988. *108*: pp. 595–608.

245. Gray, P.W.: Molecular analysis of interferon-gamma and lymphotoxin. *In* Mechanisms of Host Resistance to Infectious Agents, Tumors, and Allografts. R.J. North, Editor. 1986, New York, Rockefeller University Press: pp. 441–56.

246. DeMaeyer, E., and J. DeMaeyer-Guignard: Interferons and Other Regulatory Cytokines. 1988, New York, John Wiley & Sons: pp. 67–90.

247. Adams, D.O., and T.A. Hamilton: Molecular transductional mechanisms by which IFN gamma and other signals regulate macrophage development. Immunol Rev, 1987. *97*: pp. 5–27.

248. Adams, D.O., and T.A. Hamilton: Macrophages as destructive cells in host defense. *In* Inflammation: Basic Principles and Clinical Correlates. Gallin, J.I., et al. Editors. 1992, New York, Raven Press: pp. 637–62.

249. Brightbill, H.D., et al: Host defense mechanisms triggered by microbial lipoproteins through toll-like receptors. Science, 1999. *285*: pp. 732–6.

250. Verdijk, R.M., et al: Polyriboinosinic polyribocytidylic acid (poly(I:C)) induces stable maturation of functionally active human dendritic cells. J Immunol, 1999. *163*: pp. 57–61.

251. Schlienger, K., et al: Efficient priming of protein antigen-specific human CD4(+) T cells by monocyte-derived dendritic cells. Blood, 2000. *96*: pp. 3490–8.

252. Marodi, L., et al: Candidacidal mechanisms in the human neonate. Impaired IFN-gamma activation of macrophages in newborn infants. J Immunol, 1994. *153*: pp. 5643–9.

253. Marodi, L., et al: Cytokine receptor signalling in neonatal macrophages: defective STAT-1 phosphorylation in response to stimulation with IFN-gamma. Clin Exp Immunol, 2001. *126*: pp. 456–60.

Elvira Parravicini, Carmella van de Ven, and Mitchell S. Cairo

157 Neonatal Neutrophil Normal and Abnormal Physiology

The neutrophil is a principal component of phagocytic host defense and plays an essential role in the host response to infection and inflammation. Neutrophils are responsible in part for ingesting particles, killing microorganisms, and secreting cytokines and cellular mediators. Neutrophils are derived from bone marrow myeloid-committed progenitor cells, circulate in the peripheral blood, and ultimately migrate to sites of microbial invasion or inflammation. This chapter reviews normal neutrophil physiology, including adherence, activation, chemotaxis, phagocytosis, degranulation, and microbicidal (killing) activity and deficits associated with immature neonatal neutrophils.

ACTIVATION

Circulating neutrophils are continuously and simultaneously exposed to several stimulatory and inhibitory factors that modulate their functions. These agents may be derived directly from bacterial N-formyl peptides, such as N-formyl-methionyl-leucyl-phenylalanine (FMLP), or cell-derived molecules, including activated complement components (C5a), lipids (leukotriene B_4) and platelet-activating factor, eicosanoids, vitamin D–binding protein (γ-globulin), and chemokines that are activated by cytokines. Low doses of one mediator that is not effective for direct activation may enhance the effect of another mediator, so-called *priming*.[1]

To become activated, neutrophils have to be modulated in a strictly coordinated manner by multiple mediators. The balance of concentration of different chemoattractants will determine the sequence of cell function. Cell surface receptors sense for specific chemotactic factors, and intracellular signaling is mediated by an interaction with heterotrimeric G-proteins, which are membrane-bound complexes consisting of a guanosine triphosphate (GTP)–binding α subunit and a βγ unit.[2] On receptor activation, the heterotrimer binds to the receptor mainly by the α subunit, and this induces an exchange of GTP for guanosine diphosphate (GDP) in the α subunit.[3] The subsequent disassociation of the βγ heterodimer[2] activates multiple signaling pathways, resulting in neutrophil adhesion, chemotaxis, and killing activities. Figure 157–1 illustrates some of the better-established pathways.[4] The dissociation of the G-protein subunits mediates activation of phospholipase C and phosphatidylinositol 3-kinase. Phospholipase C catalyzes the hydrolysis of membrane phospholipids giving formation of inositol triphosphate and diacyl-glycerol and release of arachidonic acid. Inositol triphosphate induces calcium release from intracellular stores and diacylglycerol with calcium allows the activation of protein kinase C.[5] On G-protein subunit disassociation, Ras-related proteins of the Rho subfamily are activated as well. Rho family members, which are particularly involved in actin cytoskeleton regulation, are active when bound to GTP and become inactivated with hydrolysis of GTP to GDP. This on-off switch is regulated by several proteins, such as GTPase-activating proteins, guanine nucleotide exchange factor, and guanine nucleotide dissociation inhibitors.[6]

CYTOSKELETON

The cytoskeleton of the neutrophil, the supporting framework of the cell, is a highly complex network composed of microfilaments, microtubules, and regulatory proteins. The microfilaments are perhaps the most dynamic components of the cytoskeleton. They are found close to the plasma membrane, and they comprise actin subunits arranged in highly organized structures. Actin can be present in a monomeric (G-actin) or a filamentous (F-actin) form. In the resting neutrophil, 50% of actin is present in filaments, and the remainder is in the monomeric form. There are cytoplasmic proteins involved in the assembly and disassembly regulation of actin filament. Profilin inhibits or promotes polymerization according to the affinity state, gelsolin decreases the rate of actin-filament elongation and its action is controlled by calcium, and acumentin caps the end of actin filaments. Myosin accounts for 1% of the protein in the neutrophil and possesses binding sites for actin filaments and adenosine triphosphatase (ATPase) activity. F-actin–myosin interaction leads to force generation (at the expense of ATP hydrolysis) and to the contraction of the cytoplasm, which is required for vectorial movements.

Microtubules are long, tubular structures made by helical formation of tubulin molecules. Microtubules may function as a form of skeletal support for microfilaments. Stimulation of neutrophils with chemotactic agents induces a rapid and transient

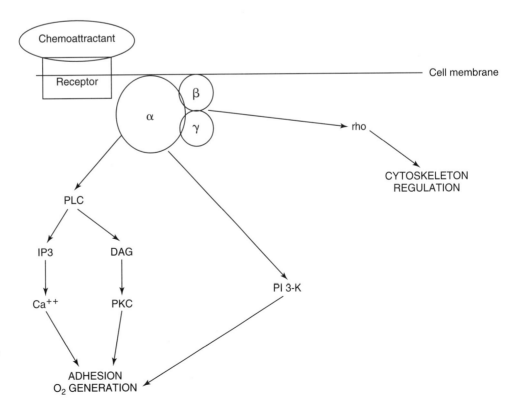

Figure 157–1. Neutrophil activation signaling pathways. Ca++ = calcium ions; DAG = diacylglycerol; IP3 = inositol triphosphate; PI 3-K = phosphatidylinositol 3-kinase; PKC = protein kinase C; PLC = phospholipase C; rho = rho subfamily protein. (Adapted from Burg ND, Pillinger MH: Clin Immunol *99*:7–17, 2001.)

assembly of microtubules, but this does not affect chemotaxis. In locomotion, the microtubule system seems to provide the directional determinant, and microfilaments do the mechanical work.[7]

Directed movement of the neutrophil in a chemotactic gradient depends on cytoskeleton rearrangement and the assumption of polarized morphology by the cell with concentration of F-actin in the anterior lamellipodium and posterior uropod.[8] This is an energy-requiring process, and energy is largely supplied by ATP, generated by anaerobic glycolysis. Oxidative phosphorylation is apparently not required, because the neutrophil has few mitochondria.[9] The rapid polymerization of monomeric G-actin to filamentous F-actin drives modification of cell shape, such as formation of pseudopod and uropod. The cell migrates by repetitive extension of the pseudopod in the direction of the gradient and retraction of the uropod toward the body of the cell.[10]

The relative immaturity of cytoskeleton function in neonatal neutrophils has been evaluated by several investigators. Early studies demonstrated that neonatal polymorphonuclear leukocytes (PMNs) fail to polymerize monomeric G-actin to filamentous F-actin rapidly after stimulation.[11, 12] In addition, reduced microtubule formations have been demonstrated to correlate with the inability of neonatal PMNs to achieve a fully bipolar shape change on stimulation.[13]

Measurement of light-scattering response to FMLP has been used to assess whether defective neonatal neutrophil tubular assembly is a result of impaired signal perception or immature responsiveness of the cytoskeleton. Light-scattering effects are the result of an extremely synchronous and massive rearrangement of organelles in the responding neutrophils. Wolach and colleagues[14] compared the response of neonatal and adult neutrophils with FMLP stimulation. Cell polarization of adult and neonatal neutrophils was similar when they were stimulated with low FMLP concentrations, but with increasing FMLP concentrations, neonatal PMN polarization was reduced compared with adult PMNs. These observations suggest that neonatal neutrophils have a fully functional signal perception, but their cytoskeleton framework fails to comply with the demands of a strong signal.

Taniuchi and associates[15] confirmed these findings by demonstrating differential actin polymerization in adult and neonatal PMN after stimulation with FMLP. No difference was found in binding capacity of FMLP receptors between adult and cord neutrophils, but actin polymerization was significantly decreased in cord blood neutrophils when compared with adults.

Merry and associates[16] investigated the role of actin polymerization and its regulation by protein kinase C and by phosphatases in the defective neutrophil chemotaxis of the human newborn. Neutrophils isolated from adult volunteers and healthy term newborns were studied for assessment of chemotaxis by flow cytometry. Neonatal neutrophils had reduced actin polymerization in response to chemotactic agents that act through cell surface receptors, but not with those that act directly on cytoplasm. This finding suggests that a defect in cell signal transduction may be one of the factors implicated in defective chemotaxis. Phosphatase 1 and 2A inhibitors inhibit chemotaxis, but not actin polymerization. Therefore, phosphatase 1 and 2A can be considered chemotaxis regulators, but not through actin polymerization.

ADHERENCE

The events of phagocytosis begin within minutes of tissue damage or pathogenic invasion with the accumulation and adherence of neutrophils to endothelial surfaces at the site of infection. Recruitment of neutrophils to the site of infection involves a coordinated series of events mediated by three families of adhesion receptors: selectins, integrins, and the immunoglobulin G (IgG) gene superfamily. The initial step in adhesion is rolling of neutrophils along the vessel walls. This process is mediated by three selectins, which have been identified as P- and E-selectins (CD62P, CD62E), induced by inflammatory cytokines on endothelial cells, and L-selectin (CD62L), constitutively expressed on circulating neutrophils.

Selectins are critical in neutrophil transmigration by virtue of their ability to tether leukocytes in a reversible fashion under conditions of shear flow, a process that mediates their rolling on the endothelium of inflamed vessels. Within minutes of activation with certain agonists (phorbol myristate acetate, histamine, thrombin, C5a, or oxidants) or inflammatory mediators (interleukin-8 or platelet-activating factor), selectins are translocated to the plasma membrane, and neutrophil attachment is facilitated by β_2-integrins, leukocyte factor antigen-1 (CD11a/CD18), and Mac-1 (CD11b/CD18). Thus, contact with selectins begins the process of neutrophil adhesion by slowing the velocity of neutrophil flow and increasing the duration of intercellular and membrane contact with the endothelium. Next, firmer attachment is accomplished through the action of the β_2-integrins and intercellular adhesion molecule-1 (ICAM-1) (CD54) and ICAM-2, which mediate neutrophil arrest and transmigration. ICAM-1 (CD54) and ICAM-2 are members of the IgG gene superfamily and are expressed constitutively on endothelial cells, increasing when the endothelium is inflamed. ICAM-1 is the ligand for leukocyte factor antigen-1 and Mac-1 and is required for neutrophil arrest and transmigration.[17] Neutrophil-neutrophil adhesion (aggregation) also involves initial tethering through L-selectin followed by β_2-integrin-dependent firm adhesion.[18]

Neutrophils use various signaling pathways to link receptors for adhesion with effector molecules in the cytoplasm and nucleus. The Rho family of GTPases, members of the Ras superfamily, plays a key role in regulating these responses. The role of the Rho GTPases in phagocyte cell function has been studied. Williams and associates,[19] using a murine model genetically deficient in hematopoietic specific Rho GTPase, Rac-2, demonstrated that Rac-2 plays an essential and unique role in neutrophil rolling by L-selectin, chemotaxis, and phagocytosis.

Several investigators have reported deficient adhesion of neonatal neutrophils to endothelial cells as a result of decreased expression of integrins, diminished expression of L-selectin, and a rigid cytoskeleton that prevents redistribution of adhesion sites. Lorant and associates[20] demonstrated decreased P-selectin expression in endothelial cells lining mesenteric venules and umbilical veins of premature infants compared with term infants. Reports differ regarding the resting and stimulated expression of Mac-1 on neonatal neutrophils. Several groups have demonstrated that the expression of Mac-1 in neonates is equal to that of adults; however, the total cell content of Mac-1 is decreased.[21] Rebuk and associates,[22] however, reported a decrease in baseline expression of neonatal neutrophil Mac-1 and stimulated expression equal to that in adults. Additional studies have shown that neonatal neutrophils fail to up-regulate Mac-1 surface expression to the same extent as adult neutrophils in response to chemotactic stimulation. Mariscalco and associates[21] demonstrated no significant difference in the stimulated expression of Mac-1 in neonatal and adult neutrophils, a significant decrease in the expression of L-selection in neonatal versus adult neutrophils, and a significant decrease in the interaction of neonatal neutrophils with human umbilical vein endothelial cells compared with adult.

Two myeloid-stimulating cytokines, granulocyte colony-stimulating factor (G-CSF) and granulocyte-macrophage colony-stimulating factor (GM-CSF) have been shown to enhance mature neutrophil function. G-CSF improves neutrophil function by increasing adhesion and by stimulating chemotaxis and phagocytosis, and it could improve neutrophil functions that are deficient in the neonate. Ohls and associates[23] reported that in term and preterm neonatal neutrophils, G-CSF significantly increased expression of β_2-integrin to a greater extent than levels observed in adult neutrophils. However, L-selectin expression in term and preterm neonatal neutrophils decreased after G-CSF incubation and decreased further after stimulation.[23] Our laboratory demonstrated that GM-CSF directly up-regulated the expression of the C3bi (complement receptor) in neonatal neutrophils, which resulted in increased aggregation and adherence.[24]

DEFORMABILITY

The movement of adherent neutrophils through vessel walls requires the expansion of pseudopods between endothelial cells, opening a passageway for the remaining portion of the leukocyte. The neutrophil subsequently moves freely in the intercellular spaces under the influence of various chemotactic agents. This movement and diapedesis depends on energy, provided by ATP, and the on neutrophil locomotor apparatus.[9]

Neutrophils from newborn infants, compared with adult PMNs, have been demonstrated to have significantly decreased deformability,[25, 26] especially in immature forms.[27] Immature neutrophils in neonates and adults are both less deformable and larger compared with mature PMNs. During stressful conditions, such as neonatal sepsis, up to 100% of the circulating neutrophils may be immature. In addition, evidence suggests that neutrophils activated *in vivo* or *in vitro* with chemoattractants are much stiffer than unactivated (basal) neutrophils. In particular, pseudopods, which are formed as a result of polymerization and alignment of actin molecules near the surface membrane, are extremely rigid.[28]

Studies of neutrophil transmigration through endothelial monolayers have shown that term neonatal PMNs display about 50% transmigration compared with adult PMNs, and antibody blocking studies have demonstrated that these neonatal PMN abnormalities may be explained, in part, by reduced Mac-1 expression.[29]

Lorant and associates[20] demonstrated that delayed transmigration of neutrophils in the neonatal rat correlates with a defect in the expression of P-selectin on the surface of the endothelial cells. In an animal model of inflammation, radiolabeled neutrophils from adult rats transmigrated into the peritoneum of adult rats five times more efficiently than they did through the peritoneum of neonatal rats. The decreased P-selectin expression was associated with decreased numbers of P-selectin storage granules and decreased P-selectin transcription.

CHEMOTAXIS

Chemotaxis is the directed migration of a cell toward a chemoattractant along a concentration gradient. The ability of neutrophils to undergo chemotaxis implies the possession of a sensory mechanism that must be linked to the locomotor apparatus of the cell. After chemotactic factor-receptor interaction, a complex sequence of events occurs: activation of phospholipases, breakdown of phosphoinositol, activation of protein kinase C, an increase of intracellular calcium, release of eicosanoids and activation of kinases and phosphatases.[5, 30] This sequence of events leads to neutrophil-directed migration.

Since the 1980s, several investigators have studied neonatal neutrophil responses to chemoattractant agents and have determined that neonatal PMNs have normal random migration, but a decreased ability to move toward defined chemoattractant stimuli in comparison with adult PMNs.[31-33]

The neutrophils of clinically stable preterm neonates as immature as 24 weeks' gestation appear functionally very similar to those of term infants.[34] Expression of both L-selectin and Mac-1, after stimulation, is similar to that of term PMNs.[22, 34] However, in a study of preterm neonates, Mac-1 PMN content (both in the cytoplasm and on the cell surface) ranged from 10% of adult levels at 27 weeks' gestation to 48% at 36 weeks' gestation and 57% in term neonates. This study showed a high correlation between Mac-1 PMN content and gestational age.[35]

Sacchi and associates[36] demonstrated that term neonatal PMNs mature to normal adult PMN chemotactic responses by 2 weeks' postnatal age, and preterm neonates (34 and 36 weeks) reach adult values by 40 to 42 weeks' postnatal age. Eisenfeld and associates[37] similarly demonstrated improvement of term neonatal PMN chemotaxis from 40% of adult values at birth to normal adult values between 10 and 32 days' postnatal age. Carr and associates[34] studied preterm infants (24 to 32 weeks' gestational age) over a 2-month period and demonstrated that chemotaxis improved during the second month of life, but it remained abnormal in comparison with adults.

Impaired expression and up-regulation of receptors may additionally contribute to defective chemotaxis. Falconer and associates[38] demonstrated that neutrophils from preterm and stressed neonates have significantly fewer receptors for complement factors C3b and iC3b than term neonates and adults.

Reddy and associates[39] studied CR3 expression in neonatal and adult PMNs. Neonatal neutrophils, on average, expressed less CR3 in comparison with adult PMNs. However, because of the higher concentration of neutrophils in umbilical cord blood versus the adult, the absolute number of neutrophils in cord blood expressing high amounts of CR3 was equivalent to that of adult blood. High proportions of immature PMNs in cord blood may explain the previous findings of deficient CR3 expression. Therefore, the typical neutrophilia of cord blood can be considered a compensatory event in providing the adult concentration of mature neutrophils.

Human complement component C5a is an important mediator of the inflammatory response, neutrophil chemotaxis, and activation. Nybo and associates[40] demonstrated that C5a uptake was significantly lower in neonatal neutrophils compared with adult PMNs. Using FMLP and C5a as stimuli, less migration of neonatal neutrophils was observed in comparison with adult neutrophils.

Various abnormalities of Mac-1 receptors correlate closely with the reduced chemotaxis observed in neonatal neutrophils. In resting neutrophils, Mac-1 receptors are distributed evenly on the cell surface, but during cell locomotion, Mac-1 receptors are translocated to the tail of the cell, whereas new receptors are translocated from stores in cytoplasmic granules to the leading edge of the migrating cell. This process in neonatal neutrophils is not up-regulated to the same extent as in adult PMNs. The defect is thought to be caused by both a reduced total PMN content of preformed Mac-1, which in term neonates is about 60% of adult PMN Mac-1 levels, and a reduced translocation of preformed new receptors from cytoplasmic storage to the PMN surface. The secondary translocation of these receptors to the uropod is also impaired in the neonatal PMN.[41]

Abnormalities in events that follow initial chemotactic factor-receptor interaction have been suggested to contribute to defective PMN chemotaxis. Changes in membrane potential, in the generation of inositol, and in release of calcium ions from intracellular stores have been reported to be impaired in neonatal neutrophils.[42-44] Specific cytoplasmic granules constitute essential supply for the new membrane receptors required for PMN movement. The number of lactoferrin-containing granules appears to be decreased in neonatal neutrophils.[45] Chemoattractant-induced hexose uptake by neonatal neutrophils[46] and release of leukotriene B_4[47] are also decreased when compared with adult PMNs.

Chemotaxis of neonatal and adult neutrophils was compared after stimulation with two chemoattractants: FMLP and DL1.2, a chemotactic monoclonal antibody that binds to a specific neutrophil antigen.[48] Stimulated neonatal neutrophils demonstrated reduced chemotaxis in comparison with adult PMNs, a finding suggesting an aberration in chemoattractant-induced signaling. FMLP induced a rapid increase of intracellular calcium in both adult and neonatal PMNs, but this response was reduced in neonatal PMNs. Moreover, a subpopulation of unresponsive neonatal neutrophils was identified.[48]

Impaired polarization and chemotaxis in neonatal neutrophils may result from insufficient production of hematopoietic growth factors, such as G-CSF and GM-CSF. The in vitro effects of G-CSF and GM-CSF on neutrophil chemotaxis and polarization were studied in isolated PMNs of neonates compared with adults. Both G-CSF and GM-CSF significantly enhanced the chemotaxis of neonatal neutrophils, thus normalizing their chemotactic defect. This effect was more evident when chemotaxis was severely impaired. The reduced polarization, observed in neonatal neutrophils, was corrected after in vitro incubation with both G-CSF and GM-CSF.[49]

PHAGOCYTOSIS

Neutrophils are the predominant mobile phagocytes of the circulating blood. They move from the circulation by adherence to vascular endothelia and migrate through the walls of small blood vessels to the site of infection, where they kill and ingest foreign organisms. Neutrophils possess a selective ability to recognize foreign antigens and have cell surface receptors for the Fc portion of the IgG molecule as well as the C3b complement component. Humoral factors, known as opsonins, coat the foreign antigen and make it more susceptible to phagocytosis after the specific adherence between the opsonized antigen and the neutrophil cell surface receptors. The best-described opsonins are heat-stabile antibodies, immunoglobulins, and complement, particularly the heat-labile component, C3b.[50] Preterm and term neonates have reduced production of immunoglobulins. Because most of the IgG is transferred during the last weeks of gestation, premature infants have decreased levels of circulating IgG. Preterm neonates have significantly lower concentrations of complement components and total hemolytic complement activity compared with term neonates. Thus, decreased IgG and complement components in the neonate may result in deficient opsonization.[51]

Both the Fab and Fc portions of the IgG immunoglobulin molecule enhance phagocytosis. The Fab portion adheres to the bacteria, whereas the Fc portion adheres to receptors on the neutrophil. Neutrophils express three different types of receptors for the Fc component of IgG: FcγRI (CD64), FcγRII (CD32), and FcγRIII (CD16). FcγRII and FcγRIII are low-affinity receptors normally expressed on neutrophils and they bind to polyvalent IgG complexes. However, FcγRI is a high-affinity receptor binding to monomeric IgG and is expressed to a lesser extent on neutrophils. The interaction of these Fc receptors and immunoglobulin initiates the process of phagocytosis, degranulation, and antibody-dependent cellular cytotoxicity (ADCC). Neutrophils from preterm infants express FcγRII and FcγRIII to a significantly lesser extent than neutrophils from term infants and adults.[52,53] Fjaertoft and associates[54] reported that the expression of FcγRI on neutrophils from preterm infants was similar to that in term infants, older infants, children, and adults. However, the expression of FcγRI was significantly increased during bacterial infection. Further, the expression of FcγRI was significantly higher in neutrophils from newborns with bacterial infection than in both noninfected preterm or term newborn infants.[54] Other investigators demonstrated that FcγRI (CD64) expression is a very sensitive marker for diagnosing late-onset nosocomial infection in very low birth weight infants. A significant increase in the expression of CD64 in the very low birth weight neonates was documented at the time of sepsis and remained high 24 hours after the onset of sepsis.[55]

The functional response of the stimulated neutrophil, including the cross-linking of Fcγ receptors, involves a complex cascade of biochemical events. The regulation of phagocytosis

has been associated with the cross-linking of Fcγ receptor by the induction of tyrosine phosphorylation of FcγRII itself. After ligand binding, there is a rapid induction of protein phosphorylation of the several nonreceptor proteins by the activation of multiple kinases, including tyrosine kinase, protein kinase C, and mitogen-activated protein (MAP) kinase. Protein kinase C and Raf-1 have been shown to translocate to the plasma membrane during the first minutes of neutrophil phagocytosis, in which Raf-1 initiates the MAP kinase cascade, activating extracellular signal-regulated protein kinases 1 and 2 (ERK1 and ERK2), which are required for the ingestion of IgG-opsonized particles.[56] Ydrenius and associates[57] reported that cyclic adenosine monophosphate (cAMP) and cAMP-dependent protein kinase (cAPK) regulates F-actin reorganization during IgG-FcR receptor–mediated neutrophil phagocytosis.

The γ subunit of the Fc receptor contains a cell activation motif referred to as immunoreceptor tyrosine-based activation motifs (ITAMs). ITAM tyrosines are phosphorylated after Fcγ clustering, and the phosphorylated ITAMs create sites for the assembly of Src homology 2 (SH2) domains including the Syk tyrosine kinase.[58] The tyrosine kinase, Syk, plays a critical role in the phagocytic pathway mediated by the FcγRs. Matsuda and associates,[59] using antisense oligonucleotides, reported that ablation of Syk expression significantly reduced FcγR-mediated phagocytosis in human monocytes. Further, transfection of Syk into COS1 cells has been shown to enhance FcγR-mediated phagocytosis, and Syk-deficient macrophages do not signal for FcγR-mediated phagocytosis.[60] Hunter and associates[61] determined the regions of Syk that are critical for interaction with the phagocytic pathway and demonstrated that an intact kinase domain is required for facilitating phagocytic signaling by FcγRs.

Activation of the complement system, resulting in the formation of C3b, can be initiated either by the bacteria itself through the alternate complement pathway or by the interaction of specific antibody with microbial antigen and activation of the classical pathway. The complement receptor 3 (CR3, Mac-1, CD11b/CD18) functions as a nonopsonic receptor and is the specific receptor for the complement fragment C3bi. CR3 (a β_2-integrin) is also a receptor for extracellular proteins and, as a lectin, recognizes many different sugars. CR3 is a heterodimer consisting of CD18, the protein common to the β_2-integrins, and CD11b, which contains the C3bi binding site and recognition domain of matrix proteins. An internal peptide sequence in the fibrinogen γ chain has been shown to function as the high-affinity binding site for C3R on neutrophils. Soluble human fibrinogen has been demonstrated to activate neutrophils through a CD11b-dependent mechanism that results in an upregulation of CD11b, enhancement of phagocytosis, and increased degranulation.[62]

C3R is also involved in the selective internalization of pathogenic mycobacteria. The phagocytosis of mycobacteria by neutrophils under nonopsonic conditions elicits the production of superoxide (O_2^-) and the release of specific granule proteins. The mechanism of the nonopsonic phagocytosis is reported to involve CR3, which associates with a glycosylphosphatidylinositol-anchored protein (GPI) and relocates to cholesterol-rich domains in the cell membrane where the mycobacteria are internalized. When CR3 is not associated with a GPI, it remains outside these domains and mediates phagocytosis of opsonized particles.[63]

Once the opsonized microbe and neutrophil establish contact, a cohesive force prevents their separation. The microbe binds to specific receptors on the surface of the neutrophil through microbe-bound opsonins (IgG, C3b). The sequential interaction between opsonins and membrane receptors leads to submembranous activation of neutrophil contractile microfilaments and results in the flow of pseudopods completely surrounding the microbe. The opposed membranes of the pseudopods fuse and then invaginate the captured microbe, enclosing it in an internalized vacuole called a *phagosome.* Ingestion of the foreign particle is an active process requiring ATP glycolysis, glycogenolysis, and oxidative phosphorylation. After the phagosome is formed, degranulation begins, and cytoplasmic azurophilic and specific granules fuse with the phagosome. The granules rupture and discharge toxic chemicals into the phagosome.

Colony-stimulating factors and cytokines have been reported to enhance neutrophil function. Interferon-γ treatment is associated with a significant increase in the expression of the high affinity Fcγ receptor (peaking 48 hours after exposure to the cytokine), as well as a significant increase in neutrophil phagocytosis of opsonized *Staphylococcus aureus.* This increased phagocytosis after interferon-γ treatment correlates with FcγRI expression by the neutrophils.[64] Recombinant GM-CSF and G-CSF have been shown to enhance phagocytic activity of mature neutrophils.[65] *In vitro* studies in our laboratory have demonstrated enhanced neutrophil C3bi expression and bacterial killing in neonatal neutrophils incubated with GM-CSF.[24] Campbell and associates[66] also reported an enhancement of phagocytosis of opsonized type III group B streptococci (III GBS) by neonatal neutrophils after pretreatment with G-CSF and GM-CSF but not tumor necrosis factor-α. They also demonstrated the abrogation of the heightened killing of III GBS by blocking FcγRIII receptors and that phagocytosis was further enhanced by the addition of purified IgG containing III GBS–specific antibody to the GM-CSF–treated neutrophils.[66]

DEGRANULATION

Bacterial killing occurs within a matter of minutes after phagocytosis. The neutrophil makes tight contact with its target, and the plasma membrane flows around the surface until the bacterium is completely enclosed, thus forming a phagosome. The formation of a phagosome limits the amount of extracellular fluid, and the exclusion of external medium allows a new environment to be established that will provide favorable conditions for the biochemistry of oxidant production and bacterial killing. Killing is initiated within seconds of ingestion by two interrelated processes: degranulation, with the release of granule contents into the phagosome; and the respiratory burst, which consists of a series of oxidation-reduction reactions. *Degranulation* begins with the fusion of cytoplasmic azurophilic (or primary) and specific (or secondary and tertiary) granules with the phagosome. The granules then rupture and discharge their contents into the phagosome (Fig. 157-2).[67] Thus, the contents of the cytoplasmic azurophilic and specific granules constitute a significant proportion of the phagosomal volume. These granule contents are generally membrane-active cationic proteins and peptides[67] whose affinity for the negatively charged microbial surface depends not only on electrostatic interactions, but also on their tertiary structure (Table 157-1).[68,69]

Azurophil (primary) granules can be distinguished from specific granules by their affinity for the basic dye, azure A, owing to a high content of acid mucopolysaccharide and myeloperoxidase, which are present only in azurophil granules. Azurophil granules are further characterized by their content of hydrolytic and bactericidal proteins such as elastase, bactericidal permeability-increasing protein (BPI), defensins, and myeloperoxidase. The contents of the azurophil granules are released into the phagosome, thereby exposing ingested microorganisms to high concentrations of hydrolytic enzymes, antimicrobial proteins and peptides, and reactive oxygen intermediates.

Myeloperoxidase, a major constituent of the azurophilic granules, is critical for oxidative killing. It is a classic heme peroxidase that uses hydrogen peroxide (H_2O_2) to oxidize a variety of aromatic compounds and is unique in readily oxidizing chloride ions to the strong nonradical oxidant HOCl. HOCl is the most potent bactericidal oxidant known to be produced by the neutrophil,

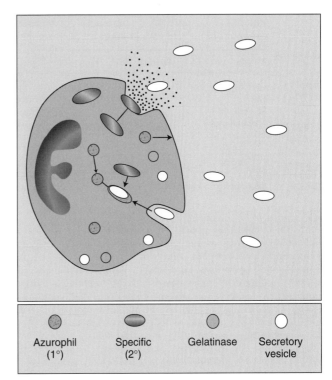

Figure 157–2. Neutrophil degranulation of antibiotic proteins and peptides. An activated neutrophil in the process of phagocytosis of gram-negative bacteria (*open ovals*) is demonstrated. As shown, specific (secondary) granules are more prone to degranulate their contents (including lactoferrin and cathelicidins) into the extracellular space. In contrast, azurophil (primary) granules, containing bactericidal permeability-increasing protein and defensins, are predominantly degranulated into the phagolysosome. To a lesser extent, specific granules also degranulate into the phagolysosome and primary granules to the extracellular space (*arrows*). Neutrophil granule populations, including gelatinase granules and secretory vesicles, are demonstrated at the *bottom* of the figure. (From Levy O: Blood *96*:2664–2672, 2000.)

and many species of bacteria are killed by the myeloperoxidase-H_2O_2-chloride process.[69] Bacterial targets include iron-sulfur proteins, membrane transport proteins, ATP-generating systems, and the origin of replication sites for DNA synthesis. Chloramines are generated indirectly through the reaction of HOCl with amines, and these are also bactericidal. Myeloperoxidase can also generate peroxides and hydroxylated derivatives of phenolics, such as salicylate in the oxidative reactions.[69]

BPI is a 55-kDa cationic protein produced only by precursors of neutrophils and stored in the azurophilic granules. BPI plays a dominant role in the bactericidal activity against gram-negative bacteria and is bactericidal in nanomolar concentrations. The biologic effects of BPI are linked to its high-affinity binding to bacterial lipopolysaccharides, which causes immediate growth arrest; actual killing is accomplished by its interaction with lipid phosphate groups and acyl chains of the membrane lipids perturbing the structures, thereby leading to outer and inner membrane lysis. The antibacterial and antiendotoxin activities of BPI are fully expressed by the amino terminal half of the molecule.[67,70] Further, activated neutrophils release BPI into inflammatory fluids where it is potently bactericidal. Levy and associates[71] reported that neutrophils of newborns are selectively deficient in BPI. These investigators demonstrated that newborn neutrophils from cord blood contain at least three- to fourfold less BPI per cell than adult

TABLE 157-1

Antimicrobial Proteins and Peptides of Neutrophils

Protein	Molecular Weight (kDa)	Neutrophil Granule	Mechanism
Lactoferrin	80	Secondary	Iron-binding/membrane active
BPI	55	Azurophil	Binds lipid A of lipopolysaccharide
Serprocidins	~30	Azurophil	Proteolysis/membrane-active
Cathelicidins	10–20	Secondary	Release of membrane-active peptides
Lysozyme	14.5	Azurophil and secondary	Lysis of peptidoglycan/membrane-active
Defensins	4	Azurophil	Formation of voltage-gated multimeric pores

BPI = bactericidal permeability-increasing protein.

neutrophils, and this deficiency correlated with decreased antibacterial activity of newborn neutrophil extracts against serum-resistant *Escherichia coli*.[71] Further studies reported that supplementing newborn cord blood with recombinant BPI potently inhibited the tumor necrosis factor–inducing activity of gram-negative bacteria and in some cases enhanced bactericidal activity. These results suggest that the administration of recombinant BPI may be of clinical benefit to neonates suffering from gram-negative bacterial infection or endotoxemia.[72]

Serprocidins, 25- to 37-kDa serine proteases localized in the azurophil granules, include elastase, cathepsin G, proteinase 3, and azurocidin/CAP37 (heparin-binding protein) and are related to the granzymes of cytotoxic T cells. The serprocidins exert broad cytotoxic activity against gram-negative and gram-positive bacteria through proteolytic action and direct membrane perturbation.[67] Elastase participates in generating antimicrobial activity during inflammatory responses by cleaving cathelicidin proforms to generate active antimicrobial peptides.[73] Proteinase 3 has the ability to degrade extracellular matrix proteins and also plays an important role in myeloid differentiation. Fractionation of neutrophils has shown that proteinase 3 could be detected not only in azurophil granules, but also in specific granules and in the plasma membrane–enriched fraction containing secretory vesicles.[74]

Defensins, a family of 4-kDa peptides with broad cytotoxic activity against bacteria, fungi, parasites, and viruses, are found in the azurophil granules. The activity of defensins depends on their cationicity and three-dimensional structure. Defensins form multimeric voltage-dependent pores that permeabilize cellular membranes. α-Defensins are expressed in human neutrophils and are characterized by six invariant cysteine residues forming three disulfide bonds. The activity of defensins is limited by monovalent and divalent cations, a finding suggesting that the action of these peptides is limited to prevent indiscriminate cytotoxicity.[67]

Peroxidase-negative specific granules contain distinct antimicrobial proteins and peptides that are deployed toward the leading edge of the chemotaxing neutrophil, thus accomplishing extracellular degranulation.[68] The peroxidase-negative specific granules can be subdivided into secondary granules, defined by the high content of lactoferrin, and tertiary granules, defined by a high concentration of gelatinase. These granules play different functional roles in the process of degranulation. Three novel proteins of specific granules—neutrophil gelatinase-associated lipocalin (NGAL), human cathelicidin (hCAP-18), and SGP28—have been identified to contribute significantly to the function of neutrophils. NGAL is a 25-kDa FMLP-binding protein that may play a role in regulating the inflammatory response by binding small lipophilic mediators such as FMLP, platelet-activating factor, leukotriene B$_4$, and lipopolysaccharide. Synthesis of NGAL has been shown to be induced in peripheral blood neutrophils treated with GM-CSF.[68,75] hCAP-18 is the only human member of the cathelicidin family of bactericidal peptides and is a major protein of specific granules, in which it is co-localized and co-mobilized with lactoferrin.[76,77] The antibacterial and endotoxin-binding domain resides in the C-terminal of hCAP-18 and is believed to be unleashed by the proteases from the azurophil granules. SGP, a glycoprotein with a molecular weight of 28 kDa, is a member of a family of cysteine-rich secretory proteins (CRIPS) and shows high amino acid sequence homology to pathogenesis-related proteins that are believed to be important for resistance to viral, bacterial, and fungal infections.[68]

Lactoferrin, an 80-kDa member of the transferrin family also localized in the secondary granules, exerts a direct microbicidal effect by membrane disruption. It has also been shown to bind to the lipid A moiety of gram-negative bacterial lipopolysaccharide, thus neutralizing its endotoxic activity. Lysozyme is a 14-kDa enzyme that degrades bacterial peptidoglycans by cleaving the glycosidic bond of N-acetyl glucosamine. This enzyme is stored in both the primary and secondary neutrophil granules. The activity of lysozyme is synergistic with other granular proteins including defensins and lactoferrin.[67]

Stimulation of the bacterial tripeptide receptor, FMLP, induces the exocytosis of primary and secondary granules and the process of degranulation. FMLP stimulation has been shown to induce a rapid induction of tyrosine phosphorylation of several intracellular proteins including tyrosine kinases and MAP kinases. Studies of adhesion-dependent degranulation demonstrate that the release of lactoferrin is blocked by a selective inhibitor for the Src family kinases. Additional studies with mice deficient of two Src family kinases, Frg and Hck, have demonstrated the essential role these kinases play in degranulation.[78] Mócsai and associates,[79] using broad-specificity tyrosine kinase inhibitors, reported that FMLP-induced degranulation of primary and secondary granules of neutrophils is mediated by p38 MAP kinase activated by the Src family tyrosine kinases. Degranulation also involves the rapid activation of p38 MAP kinase and phospholipase D after ligand binding to FMLP receptors. Phospholipase D, found primarily in secretory vesicles, is mobilized to the plasma membrane on stimulation and is activated by small GTPases of the ARF and Rho families. Mansfield and associates[80] reported that neutrophil degranulation is regulated by ceramide, an inhibitor of kinase phosphorylation, through the inhibition of phospholipase D. They demonstrated that phospholipase D activity is significantly increased in neutrophils primed with G-CSF and is stimulated with FMLP; however, the activity was completely inhibited by ceramide.[80]

MICROBICIDAL ACTIVITY

Bacterial killing is initiated by two interrelated processes: oxidative and nonoxidative microbicidal activity. The oxygen-dependent mechanism uses a multicomponent enzyme that is dependent on reduced nicotinamide adenine dinucleotide phosphate (NADPH) to convert molecular oxygen into reactive oxygen-derived species, including (O_2^-) and H_2O_2. These molecules, in turn, act in concert with PMN-derived granule components such as myeloperoxidase to exert antimicrobial activity.

Oxidative Microbicidal Activity

The *respiratory burst* is characterized by a severalfold increase in oxygen consumption and a 10-fold increase in glucose utilization by activation of the hexose monophosphate shunt. The respiratory burst results in the production of and release of large quantities of O_2^- and H_2O_2 by the phagocytes into their surroundings. The respiratory burst consists of a series of reactions, all of which depend on the activity of the phagocyte oxidase (PHOX). Current evidence suggests that the PHOX is a complex multicomponent system that catalyzes the one-electron reduction of oxygen to O_2^- at the expense of NADPH. In the resting phagocyte, the PHOX system includes a 91-kDa flavoprotein and a 22-kDa heme protein, usually referred to as flavocytochrome b_{558}. Both are plasma membrane associated, and they act with at least three soluble cytosolic components (p47*phox,* p67*phox,* and rac2). Defective or absent oxidase activity, manifested clinically as chronic granulomatous disease, can be explained on the molecular level as a disorder of flavocytochrome b_{558}, p47*phox,* or p67*phox,* and full activity can be demonstrated using recombinant forms of these factors with added rac2.[81,82] In unstimulated PMNs, each molecule of flavocytochrome b_{558}, with its two heme groups and flavin adenine dinucleotide and NADPH binding sites, is located primarily intracellularly, in the membrane of secretory vesicles and specific granules, with a lesser amount in plasma membrane.[83] The segregation of functionally competent components of the oxidase in intracellular compartments allows resting PMNs, cells with limited synthetic activity, to maintain the response in an inactive but ready-to-be-recruited state.[84] The activation of PMNs triggers degranulation and results in increased surface expression of flavocytochrome b_{558}. Biosynthesis and assembly of mature flavocytochrome require coordinated expression of genes encoding each subunit, because they are located in different chromosomes. For example, clinical evidence indicated that chronic granulomatous disease most commonly has an X-linked pattern of inheritance, and analysis of the X-linked chronic granulomatous disease PMNs demonstrated a membrane defect consistent with the localization of gp91*phox* on the X chromosome, whereas p47*phox* is localized on chromosome 7q11,23 and p67*phox* on 1q25.[85]

The biochemical events of the respiratory burst are the following:

$$2O_2 + \text{NADPH} \xrightarrow{\text{phox}} 2O_2^- + \text{NADP}^+ + \text{H}^+$$

Most of the O_2^- is rapidly converted to H_2O_2 by dismutation either spontaneously or enzymatically by superoxide dismutase (SOD):

$$2O_2^- + 2\text{H}^+ \xrightarrow{\text{SOD}} H_2O_2 + O_2$$

NADPH consumption rises because of the O_2^--forming reaction as well as the detoxification of some of the H_2O_2 by NADPH in a glutathione-dependent process:

$$H_2O_2 + \text{NADPH} + 2\text{GSH} \xrightarrow{\substack{\text{Glutathione} \\ \text{Peroxidase}}} H_2O + \text{GSSG} + \text{NADP}^+ + \text{H}^+$$

The oxidation of glucose by the hexose monophosphate shunt is stimulated by the NADPH consumption and leads to the replenishment of NADPH:

$$\text{Glucose-6-P} + \text{NADP}^+ \xrightarrow{\text{G6PD}} 5\text{-carbon-P} + CO_2 + \text{NADPH}$$

The respiratory burst produces microbicidal agents by the partial reduction of oxygen. However, the most potent of these agents are products from further reactions involving O_2^- and H_2O_2. O_2^- and H_2O_2 react in the presence of iron to form the hydroxyl radical and possibly singlet oxygen.

$$H_2O_2 + O_2^- \xrightarrow{\text{Fe}^{+++}} \text{HO} \bullet + \text{OH}^- + O_2$$

In the best-defined microbicidal system, myeloperoxidase derived from the azurophilic granules catalyzes H_2O_2 in combination with chloride, bromide, or other halide to form HOCl or HOBr:

$$H_2O_2 + 2\text{Cl}^- \xrightarrow{\text{MPO}} 2\text{HOCl}$$

These reactive species halogenate bacterial cell walls, which lose integrity, resulting in cell death. Oxidizing radicals such as O_2^- also contribute significantly to bacterial killing. Microorganisms vary relatively little in their susceptibility to these oxygen-dependent antimicrobial systems.

Several investigators have explored PMN respiratory burst activity in the newborn. The activities of glutathione peroxidase and catalase, the major enzymes responsible for detoxifying H_2O_2 within the cell, were decreased in neonatal neutrophils in comparison with adult PMNs.[86] Neonatal PMN SOD activity, however, was normal[86] or slightly decreased[87] compared with that of adult PMNs.

Adult neutrophils exposed to low concentrations of gram-negative lipopolysaccharides become primed and have increased oxidative response to a second stimulus.[88] Bortolussi and associates[89] demonstrated lipopolysaccharide-deficient priming activity of neonatal PMNs, and Qing and associates[90] identified an association of this reduced priming activity with decreased expression of CD14 on neonatal neutrophils. Subsequently, Bonner and associates[91] investigated the role of ERK1 and ERK2 and found that lipopolysaccharide activated ERK1 and ERK2 in PMNs of adults and newborns, a finding suggesting that the ERK pathway was not responsible for the lack of lipopolysaccharide priming.

In 1986, Allen and associates[92] discovered that activated neutrophils could generate light or chemiluminescence (CL). Sources of this light emission include singlet oxygen, which releases some of its energy as a photon as it decays to the ground state, and carbonyl compounds in excited states. Therefore, CL is a sensitive, noninvasive technique that has been used extensively to measure respiratory burst activity by neutrophils.

Kallman and associates[93] compared the respiratory burst activity of adult and neonatal term and preterm neutrophils after activation and opsonization. Term neonate neutrophils had a CL response identical to that of adults, but preterm (28 to 34 weeks) neutrophils responded with a very much smaller CL peak. The normal CL response of full-term neonates and the reduced respiratory burst activity of preterm infants have been confirmed by others.[94-96]

In contrast to adult PMNs, which tend to increase respiratory burst metabolism in response to sepsis,[97] the respiratory burst of term neonatal neutrophils becomes less active when it is challenged by sepsis or other clinical stress.[98] At the time of diagnosis of sepsis, increased levels of cytokines and intensity of oxidative metabolism were found in serum of newborns by Sikora and associates.[99] Over the course of time, these findings were further accompanied by prolonged neutrophil stimulation and, eventually, by functional exhaustion and diminished oxidative metabolism in PMNs.

Term neonates with GBS sepsis demonstrated neutrophil CL responses of only 50 to 75% compared with uninfected infants, and this was associated with a 10-fold reduction in their ability to kill opsonized GBS *in vitro*.[100] A similar, although less marked, reduction in CL was found in uninfected infants with respiratory distress.[101]

Postnatal maturation of the respiratory burst was studied by Driscoll and associates[102] in 57 premature infants over a 2-month period. During the first week, more immature infants had a lower CL peak. During subsequent maturation, mean PMN CL continued to be lower than in adult controls. The suppression of the respiratory burst seemed to be more closely associated with clinical stress and prolonged intensive care than with low gestational age. Usmani and associates[96] likewise demonstrated suppression of PMN CL at 21 days after preterm birth.

An intriguing aspect of the neonatal respiratory burst is that, although the generation of hydroxyl radicals is reduced, the initial phase of the respiratory burst, O_2^- generation, is increased in neonatal neutrophils compared with adults.[103] Measurement of light scattering in neutrophils from 90 healthy neonates and 96 healthy adults demonstrated that O_2^- generation in response to FMLP of neonates exceeds that of adult PMNs.[14] Ambruso and associates[104] demonstrated that the kinetics of the neonatal NADPH oxidase system, which generates O_2^-, was different from that in adult PMNs, and there was an increase in O_2^- production by cord blood neutrophils collected after labor, in contrast to after cesarean section.[105] The paradoxical findings of reduced bactericidal oxidants and increased generation of O_2^- may be explained by inadequate stores of lactoferrin and myeloperoxidase to catalyze the later stages of the respiratory burst. Lactoferrin, if saturated with iron, enhances the production of hydroxide ions.[106] Neonatal neutrophils contain only half the amount of lactoferrin found in adult cells, and lactoferrin levels in premature neonatal PMNs are even lower.[107] Myeloperoxidase, which is involved in generation of hypochlorous acid from H_2O_2, has been found in normal concentrations in the azurophil granules of term neonatal PMNs,[104] but it is reduced in PMNs from preterm infants.[108]

Reddy and associates[39] studied CR3-dependent respiratory burst activity in neonatal and adult leukocytes. Neonatal neutrophils, on average, expressed less CR3 in comparison with adult PMNs. Because of the higher neutrophil concentration in cord blood versus adult, the calculated number of neutrophils in cord blood expressing high amounts of CR3 was equivalent to that of adult blood. The size of CR3-dependent respiratory burst correlated with CR3 expression; therefore, respiratory burst activities were equivalent in newborn and adult cells. High proportions of immature cells in cord blood may, in part, explain the deficiency in CR3 expression and dependent killing activities.

Nonoxidative Microbicidal Activity

Neutrophil cytoplasmic granules contain antimicrobial agents that are released into phagolysosomes and do not require the production of oxidants for activity. The granules are extremely heterogeneous in terms of shape, size, and content.

The first granule type produced during neutrophil maturation is the azurophilic granule, which contains myeloperoxidase, defensins, cathepsin G, BPI, hydrolases, elastase, and collagenase.[109] Defensins possess antimicrobial activity through their ability to bind to the negatively charged cell surface of the organism and thereby interfere with growth. Cathepsin G microbicidal activity does not depend on proteolysis, but on inhibition of macromolecular synthesis (proteins, RNA, and DNA) of the invading bacteria.[110] BPI contributes to the ability of neutrophils to kill gram-negative bacteria.[111, 112] Elsbach and associates[113] demonstrated no further *E. coli* colony formation within 15 seconds after exposure to BPI. During microbial ingestion, acid hydro-

lases have a digestive role against proteins, complex lipids, polysaccharides, and nucleic acids.

PMN secondary and tertiary granules are produced later in development, and they are twice as abundant as azurophilic granules. They include lysozyme, lactoferrin, gelatinase, and β-glucuronidase. Lysozyme can kill some saprophytic bacteria within the phagocytic vacuole by hydrolyzing the mucopolysaccharides of the bacterial cell walls, as well as by digesting the glycopeptide cell wall debris of dead bacteria. Lactoferrin has bacteriostatic activity by competitively binding the iron required as an essential nutrient for microbial growth.[114] Lactoferrin also makes the bacteria more accessible to lysozyme and thus alters the bacterial cell wall.[115]

To investigate specific deficits in neutrophil microbicidal activity as a risk for neonatal sepsis, Levy and associates[71] compared the relative content of BPI in the neutrophils of neonates and adult. Newborn and adult PMNs contain nearly identical amounts of myeloperoxidase and defensin peptides in their azurophilic granules, but neonatal neutrophils contain three- to fourfold less BPI than adult PMNs. These data suggest a selective deficit of BPI in neonatal neutrophils, which may in part explain the increased incidence of gram-negative sepsis in the neonate.

Studies of bactericidal activity by neonatal neutrophils indicate that phagocytic killing of different microorganisms is normal in most healthy neonates but is reduced in preterm infants.[116, 117] The relevance of reduced microbicidal activity to increased sepsis in preterm infants is supported by *in vitro* studies of bacterial killing. Intracellular killing of *S. aureus* or *E. coli* by neutrophils of term neonates has consistently been demonstrated to be normal,[118-120] whereas killing of staphylococci was impaired in preterm neonates with birth weights less than 2000 g.[121] Various conditions, such as respiratory distress and sepsis, have been associated with decreased bacterial killing.[122] A depression of microbicidal capacity was also demonstrated when neonatal neutrophils were challenged with a large number of *E. coli* organisms.[123] Candidacidal activity has been shown to be normal in neonatal PMNs.[124] However, one study demonstrated that neonatal PMNs were unable to kill *Candida albicans* as efficiently as adult PMNs.[125]

ANTIBODY-DEPENDENT CELLULAR CYTOTOXICITY

Neutrophils are the predominant mobile phagocytes of the circulating blood and provide the first line of defense against infection. However, neutrophils are also active in immunosurveillance against tumor cells.[126-128] The lytic disruption of target cells, cytolysis, is a fundamental immunologic effector function mediated by neutrophils as well as by cytotoxic T cells, natural killer cells, and macrophages. One mechanism of cytolysis is ADCC. Neutrophils exhibit fast recruitment activity *in vivo*, and rapid, potent neutrophil cytotoxicity has been documented toward various tumor targets.[129] Kindzelskii and associates[130] quantitatively and qualitatively studied the kinetics of ADCC on a single-cell level. They demonstrated transient ruptures in tumor cell membranes and multiple small bursts of cytosol observed at specific intervals and at various sites around the perimeter of a target indicating a multihit model of cytolysis.[130]

ADCC requires opsonization of a target cell with immunoglobulin and the engagement of effector cell surface receptors for the Fc domains of immunoglobulin molecules. Neutrophils can trigger ADCC by engagement of FcγRI (CD64), FcγRIα (CD32A), and FcαRI (CD89). FcαRI has been identified as the most effective FcR for neutrophil-mediated tumor cell killing. FcαRI is constitutively expressed on neutrophils and has a medium affinity for both IgA1 and IgA2 that is increased on exposure to G-CSF or GM-CSF.[131, 132] Neutrophil-mediated GM-CSF/Lym-1 cytotoxicity has been reported to require the intervention of FcγRII and CD11b-CD18 integrins.[133] Furthermore, studies with transgenic mice have also demonstrated the requirement of CD11b/CD18 (CR3) for FcαRI-mediated ADCC.[134] The role of CR3 in neutrophil Fc-mediated lysis of tumor cells was further characterized in the CR3-deficient mouse. ADCC was abrogated in CR3-/- neutrophils and in human neutrophils blocked with anti-CR3 monoclonal antibodies.[129] Nagarajan and associates[135] reported that affinity modulation of FcγRIIa is also one of the mechanisms by which neutrophils regulate their FcγR-dependent functions. These studies demonstrate that resting neutrophils express FcγRIIa in a low-affinity state, but on activation, FcγRIIa is converted to a high-affinity state that leads to FcγRIIa-dependent ligand binding and signaling for tumor cell cytotoxicity.[135] Membrane-associated CD45, a protein tyrosine phosphatase essential for antigen receptor kinase–mediated signaling in lymphocytes, has also been shown to regulate and enhance the stimulation and function of neutrophils mediated through Fcγ receptors. Gao and associates[136] demonstrated that neutrophils pretreated with anti-CD45 have a reduced ability to perform ADCC compared with untreated neutrophils.

Antibodies against HLA class II or related epitopes are highly effective in recruiting neutrophils. Whole blood from patients during G-CSF therapy exhibits significantly enhanced lysis of breast cancer target cells in the presence of Her-2/neu antibody, and the extent of tumor killing correlated positively to neutrophil blood counts.[137] Further, separation of whole blood into plasma, mononuclear cells, and neutrophils demonstrated that significant cytotoxicity was found in the neutrophil fraction.[137] Bispecific antibodies contain one specificity against a tumor target and another specificity against selected epitopes of an activating Fc receptor on neutrophils. Preclinical studies of bispecific antibodies and tumor targets have demonstrated that neutrophils are the most active effector cell population in tumor cytolysis. During G-CSF therapy, bispecific antibodies (FcαRI × Her-2/neu) are reported to induce enhanced killing of Her-2/neu+ breast cancer cells.[132] This enhanced cytotoxicity is attributed to the increased neutrophil counts that resulted in higher effector-to-target cell ratios in G-CSF–primed blood.[132] Neutrophils were also found to effectively lyse malignant B cells with an FcαRI × CD20 bispecific antibody.[138] The particular role of extracellular and intracellular domains of CD19 and Her-2/neu for ADCC by neutrophils was examined by creating Her-2/CD19 and CD19/Her-2 chimeric target molecules. Their capacity to trigger ADCC was compared with wild-type Her-2/neu and CD19 targets.[139] Neutrophils predictably killed wild-type Her-2/neu but not CD19 targets; however, neutrophils were also effective against chimeric CD19/Her-2–transfected but not Her-2/CD19–transfected target cells. These results suggest that intracellular domains of target antigens may contribute to effective neutrophil ADCC.[139]

ACKNOWLEDGMENTS

This work is supported in part by a grant from the Pediatric Cancer Research Foundation. We would like to thank Lauren Harrison, R.N., for her assistance in the development of this chapter and Linda Rahl for editorial review of this manuscript.

REFERENCES

1. Hallett MB, Lloyds D: Neutrophil priming: the cellular signals that say "amber" but not "green." Immunol Today 16:264–268, 1995.
2. Hamm HE, Gilchrist A: Heterotrimeric G proteins. Curr Opin Cell Biol 8:189–196, 1996.
3. Bourne HR: How receptors talk to trimeric G proteins. Curr Opin Cell Biol 9:134–142, 1997.
4. Burg ND, Pillinger MH: The neutrophil: function and regulation in innate and humoral immunity. Clin Immunol 99:7–17, 2001.
5. Bokoch GM: Chemoattractant signaling and leukocyte activation. Blood 86:1649–1660, 1995.
6. Baggiolini M: Chemokines and leukocyte traffic. Nature 392:565–568, 1998.
7. Edwards SW: The cytoskeleton: the molecular framework regulating cell shape and the traffic of intracellular component. In Edwards SW (ed): Biochemistry and Physiology of the Neutrophil. Cambridge, Cambridge University Press, 1994, pp 128–148.
8. Stossel TP: The E. Donnall Thomas Lecture, 1993: the machinery of blood cell movements. Blood 84:367–379, 1994.
9. Ward PA: The chemosuppression of chemotaxis. J Exp Med 124:209–226, 1966.
10. Schelonka RL, Infante AJ: Neonatal immunology. Semin Perinatol 22:2–14, 1998.
11. Sacchi F, et al: Abnormality in actin polymerization associated with defective chemotaxis in neutrophils from neonates. Int Arch Allergy Appl Immunol 84:32–39, 1987.
12. Harris MC, et al: Diminished actin polymerization by neutrophils from newborn infants. Pediatr Res 33:27–31, 1993.
13. Anderson DC, et al: Impaired motility of neonatal PMN leukocytes: relationship to abnormalities of cell orientation and assembly of microtubules in chemotactic gradients. J Leukoc Biol 36:1–15, 1984.
14. Wolach B, et al: Neonatal neutrophil inflammatory responses: parallel studies of light scattering, cell polarization, chemotaxis, superoxide release, and bactericidal activity. Am J Hematol 58:8–15, 1998.
15. Taniuchi S, et al: Heterogeneity in F-actin polymerization of cord blood polymorphonuclear leukocytes stimulated by N-formyl-methionyl-leucyl-phenylalanine. Pediatr Int 41:37–41, 1999.
16. Merry C, et al: Phosphorylation and the actin cytoskeleton in defective newborn neutrophil chemotaxis. Pediatr Res 44:259–264, 1998.
17. Ding ZM, et al: Relative contribution of LFA-1 and Mac-1 to neutrophil adhesion and migration. J Immunol 163:5029–5038, 1999.
18. Lynam E, et al: Beta2-integrins mediate stable adhesion in collisional interactions between neutrophils and ICAM-1-expressing cells. J Leukoc Biol 64:622–630, 1998.
19. Williams DA, et al: Dominant negative mutation of the hematopoietic-specific Rho GTPase, Rac2, is associated with a human phagocyte immunodeficiency. Blood 96:1646–1654, 2000.
20. Lorant DE, et al: P-selectin expression by endothelial cells is decreased in neonatal rats and human premature infants. Blood 94:600–609, 1999.
21. Mariscalco MM, et al: P-Selectin support of neonatal neutrophil adherence under flow: contribution of L-selectin, LFA-1, and ligand(s) for P-selectin. Blood 91:4776–4785, 1998.
22. Rebuck N, et al: Neutrophil adhesion molecules in term and premature infants: normal or enhanced leucocyte integrins but defective L-selectin expression and shedding. Clin Exp Immunol 101:183–189, 1995.
23. Ohls RK, et al: Effects of granulocyte colony-stimulating factor on neutrophil adhesive molecules in neonates. J Pediatr Hematol Oncol 23:506–510, 2001.
24. Cairo MS, et al: GM-CSF primes and modulates neonatal PMN motility: up-regulation of C3bi (Mo1) expression with alteration in PMN adherence and aggregation. Am J Pediatr Hematol Oncol 13:249–257, 1991.
25. Miller ME: Phagocyte function in the neonate: selected aspects. Pediatrics 64:709–712, 1979.
26. Dos Santos C, Davidson D: Neutrophil chemotaxis to leukotriene B4 in vitro is decreased for the human neonate. Pediatr Res 33:242–246, 1993.
27. Ruef P, et al: Deformability and volume of neonatal and adult leukocytes. Pediatr Res 29:128–132, 1991.
28. Linderkamp O, et al: Passive deformability of mature, immature, and active neutrophils in healthy and septicemic neonates. Pediatr Res 44:946–950, 1998.
29. Anderson DC, et al: Impaired transendothelial migration by neonatal neutrophils: abnormalities of Mac-1 (CD11b/CD18)-dependent adherence reactions. Blood 76:2613–2621, 1990.
30. Hill HR: Biochemical, structural, and functional abnormalities of polymorphonuclear leukocytes in the neonate. Pediatr Res 22:375–382, 1987.
31. Anderson DC, et al: Abnormal mobility of neonatal polymorphonuclear leukocytes: relationship to impaired redistribution of surface adhesion sites by chemotactic factor or colchicine. J Clin Invest 68:863–874, 1981.
32. Krause PJ, et al: Polymorphonuclear leukocyte adherence and chemotaxis in stressed and healthy neonates. Pediatr Res 20:296–300, 1986.
33. Krause PJ, et al: Polymorphonuclear leukocyte heterogeneity in neonates and adults. Blood 68:200–204, 1986.
34. Carr R, et al: Neutrophil chemotaxis and adhesion in preterm babies. Arch Dis Child 67:813–817, 1992.
35. McEvoy LT, et al: Total cell content of CR3 (CD11b/CD18) and LFA-1 (CD11a/CD18) in neonatal neutrophils: relationship to gestational age. Blood 87:3929–3933, 1996.
36. Sacchi F, et al: Different maturation of neutrophil chemotaxis in term and preterm newborn infants. J Pediatr 101:273–274, 1982.
37. Eisenfeld L, et al: Longitudinal study of neutrophil adherence and motility. J Pediatr 117:926–929, 1990.
38. Falconer AE, et al: Neutrophils from preterm neonates and adults show similar cell surface receptor expression: analysis using a whole blood assay. Biol Neonate 67:26–33, 1995.
39. Reddy RK, et al: A mixed population of immature and mature leucocytes in umbilical cord blood results in a reduced expression and function of CR3 (CD11b/CD18). Clin Exp Immunol 114:462–467, 1998.
40. Nybo M, et al: Reduced expression of C5a receptors on neutrophils from cord blood. Arch Dis Child 78:F129–132, 1998.

41. Carr R: Neutrophil production and function in newborn infants. Br J Haematol *110*:18–28, 2000.
42. Sacchi F, Hill HR: Defective membrane potential changes in neutrophils from human neonates. J Exp Med *160*:1247–1252, 1984.
43. Masuda K, et al: Polymorphonuclear leukocyte heterogeneity of Fc receptor expression and membrane potential in human neonates. Biol Neonate *60*:168–175, 1991.
44. Santoro P, et al: Impaired D-myo-inositol 1,4,5-triphosphate generation from cord blood polymorphonuclear leukocytes. Pediatr Res *38*:564–567, 1995.
45. Gahr M, et al: Diminished release of lactoferrin from polymorphonuclear leukocytes of human neonates. Acta Haematol *77*:90–94, 1987.
46. Abughali N, et al: Impairment of chemoattractant-stimulated hexose uptake in neonatal neutrophils. Blood *82*:2182–2187, 1993.
47. Viggiano D, et al: Impaired leukotriene B₄ release by neonatal polymorphonuclear leukocytes. Pediatr Res *36*:60–63, 1994.
48. Weinberger B, et al: Mechanisms underlying reduced responsiveness of neonatal neutrophils to distinct chemoattractants. J Leukoc Biol *70*:969–976, 2001.
49. Wolach B, et al: Effect of granulocyte and granulocyte macrophage colony stimulating factors (G-CSF and GM-CSF) on neonatal neutrophil functions. Pediatr Res *48*:369–373, 2000.
50. Cairo MS, et al: Phagocytic cells. *In* Rudolph AM, et al (eds): Rudolph's Pediatrics. Norwalk, CT, Appleton & Lange, 1996, pp 1221–1233.
51. Rosenthal J, Cairo MS: Use of hematopoietic cytokines in combination with antibiotics in neonatal sepsis: a review of the role of adjunctive therapy in the management of neonatal sepsis. Int J Pediatr Hematol Oncol *2*:477–487, 1995.
52. Payne NR, et al: Cell-surface expression of immunoglobulin G receptors on the polymorphonuclear leukocytes and monocytes of extremely premature infants. Pediatr Res *33*:452–457, 1993.
53. Smith JB, et al: Expression of the complement receptors CR1 and CR3 and the type III Fc gamma receptor on neutrophils from newborn infants and from fetuses with Rh disease. Pediatr Res *28*:120–126, 1990.
54. Fjaertoft G, et al: Neutrophils from term and preterm newborn infants express the high affinity Fc gamma-receptor I (CD64) during bacterial infections. Pediatr Res *45*:871–876, 1999.
55. Ng PC, et al: Neutrophil CD64 expression: a sensitive diagnostic marker for late-onset nosocomial infection in very low birthweight infants. Pediatr Res *51*:296–303, 2002.
56. Raeder EM, et al: Sphingosine blocks human polymorphonuclear leukocyte phagocytosis through inhibition of mitogen-activated protein kinase activation. Blood *93*:686–693, 1999.
57. Ydrenius L, et al: Activation of cAMP-dependent protein kinase is necessary for actin rearrangements in human neutrophils during phagocytosis. J Leukoc Biol *67*:520–528, 2000.
58. Suzuki T, et al: Differential involvement of Src family kinases in Fc γ receptor–mediated phagocytosis. J Immunol *165*:473–482, 2000.
59. Matsuda M, et al: Abrogation of the Fc gamma receptor IIA-mediated phagocytic signal by stem-loop Syk antisense oligonucleotides. Mol Biol Cell *7*:1095–1106, 1996.
60. Indik ZK, et al: Induction of phagocytosis by a protein tyrosine kinase. Blood *85*:1175–1180, 1995.
61. Hunter S, et al: Structural requirements of Syk kinase for Fc gamma receptor–mediated phagocytosis. Exp Hematol *27*:875–884, 1999.
62. Rubel C, et al: Fibrinogen promotes neutrophil activation and delays apoptosis. J Immunol *166*:2002–2010, 2001.
63. Peyron P, et al: Nonopsonic phagocytosis of *Mycobacterium kansasii* by human neutrophils depends on cholesterol and is mediated by CR3 associated with glycosylphosphatidylinositol-anchored proteins. J Immunol *165*:5186–5191, 2000.
64. Schiff DE, et al: Increased phagocyte Fc γRI expression and improved Fc γ-receptor–mediated phagocytosis after in vivo recombinant human interferon-γ treatment of normal human subjects. Blood *90*:3187–3194, 1997.
65. Cairo MS, et al: Lymphokines: enhancement by granulocyte-macrophage and granulocyte colony-stimulating factors of neonatal myeloid kinetics and functional activation of polymorphonuclear leukocytes. Rev Infect Dis *12*(Suppl 4):S492–497, 1990.
66. Campbell JR, Edwards MS: Cytokines enhance opsonophagocytosis of type III group B *Streptococcus*. J Perinatol *20*:225–230, 2000.
67. Levy O: Antimicrobial proteins and peptides of blood: templates for novel antimicrobial agents. Blood *96*:2664–2672, 2000.
68. Borregaard N, Cowland JB: Granules of the human neutrophilic polymorphonuclear leukocyte. Blood *89*:3503–3521, 1997.
69. Hampton MB, et al: Inside the neutrophil phagosome: oxidants, myeloperoxidase, and bacterial killing. Blood *92*:3007–3017, 1998.
70. Elsbach P: The bactericidal/permeability-increasing protein (BPI) in antibacterial host defense. J Leukoc Biol *64*:14–18, 1998.
71. Levy O: Impaired innate immunity in the newborn: newborn neutrophils are deficient in bactericidal/permeability-increasing protein. Pediatrics *104*:1327–1333, 1999.
72. Levy O, et al: Enhancement of neonatal innate defense: effects of adding an N-terminal recombinant fragment of bactericidal/permeability-increasing protein on growth and tumor necrosis factor-inducing activity of gram-negative bacteria tested in neonatal cord blood ex vivo. Infect Immun *68*:5120–5125, 2000.
73. Shi J, Ganz T: The role of protegrins and other elastase-activated polypeptides in the bactericidal properties of porcine inflammatory fluids. Infect Immun *66*:3611–3617, 1998.
74. Witko-Sarsat V, et al: Presence of proteinase 3 in secretory vesicles: evidence of a novel, highly mobilizable intracellular pool distinct from azurophil granules. Blood *94*:2487–2496, 1999.
75. Axelsson L, et al: Studies of the release and turnover of a human neutrophil lipocalin. Scand J Clin Lab Invest *55*:577–588, 1995.
76. Gudmundsson GH, et al: The human gene FALL39 and processing of the cathelin precursor to the antibacterial peptide LL-37 in granulocytes. Eur J Biochem *238*:325–332, 1996.
77. Sorensen O, et al: The human antibacterial cathelicidin, hCAP-18, is synthesized in myelocytes and metamyelocytes and localized to specific granules in neutrophils. Blood *90*:2796–2803, 1997.
78. Mócsai A, et al: Adhesion-dependent degranulation of neutrophils requires the Src family kinases Fgr and Hck. J Immunol *162*:1120–1126, 1999.
79. Mócsai A, et al: Kinase pathways in chemoattractant-induced degranulation of neutrophils: the role of p38 mitogen-activated protein kinase activated by Src family kinases. J Immunol *164*:4321–4331, 2000.
80. Mansfield PJ, et al: Regulation of polymorphonuclear leukocyte degranulation and oxidant production by ceramide through inhibition of phospholipase D. Blood *99*:1434–1441, 2002.
81. Abo A, et al: Reconstitution of neutrophil NADPH oxidase activity in the cell-free system by four components: p67-phox, p47-phox, p21rac1, and cytochrome b-245. J Biol Chem *267*:16767–16770, 1992.
82. Uhlinger DJ, et al: Reconstitution and characterization of the human neutrophil respiratory burst oxidase using recombinant p47-phox, p67-phox and plasma membrane. Biochem Biophys Res Commun *186*:509–516, 1992.
83. Borregaard N, et al: Subcellular localization of the b-cytochrome component of the human neutrophil microbicidal oxidase: translocation during activation. J Cell Biol *97*:52–61, 1983.
84. DeLeo FR, Quinn MT: Assembly of the phagocyte NADPH oxidase: molecular interaction of oxidase proteins. J Leukoc Biol *60*:677–691, 1996.
85. Yu L, et al: Biosynthesis of the phagocyte NADPH oxidase cytochrome b558: role of heme incorporation and heterodimer formation in maturation and stability of gp91phox and p22phox subunits. J Biol Chem *272*:27288–27294, 1997.
86. Strauss RG, et al: Oxygen-detoxifying enzymes in neutrophils of infants and their mothers. J Lab Clin Med *95*:897–904, 1980.
87. Kugo M, et al: Superoxide dismutase in polymorphonuclear leukocytes of term newborn infants and very low birth weight infants. Pediatr Res *26*:227–231, 1989.
88. Forehand JR, et al: Lipopolysaccharide priming of human neutrophils for an enhanced respiratory burst: role of intracellular free calcium. J Clin Invest *83*:74–83, 1989.
89. Bortolussi R, et al: Deficient priming activity of newborn cord blood-derived polymorphonuclear neutrophilic granulocytes with lipopolysaccharide and tumor necrosis factor-alpha triggered with formyl-methionyl-leucyl-phenylalanine. Pediatr Res *34*:243–248, 1993.
90. Qing G, et al: Diminished priming of neonatal polymorphonuclear leukocytes by lipopolysaccharide is associated with reduced CD14 expression. Infect Immun *63*:248–252, 1995.
91. Bonner S, et al: Activation of extracellular signal-related protein kinases 1 and 2 of the mitogen-activated protein kinase family by lipopolysaccharide requires plasma in neutrophils from adults and newborns. Infect Immun *69*:3143–3149, 2001.
92. Allen RC: Phagocytic leukocyte oxygenation activities and chemiluminescence: a kinetic approach to analysis. Methods Enzymol *133*:449–493, 1986.
93. Kallman J, et al: Impaired phagocytosis and opsonisation toward group B streptococci in preterm neonates. Arch Dis Child *78*:F46–50, 1998.
94. Peden DB, et al: Diminished chemiluminescent responses of polymorphonuclear leukocytes in severely and moderately preterm neonates. J Pediatr *111*:904–906, 1987.
95. Bektas S, et al: Decreased adherence, chemotaxis and phagocytic activities of neutrophils from preterm neonates. Acta Paediatr Scand *79*:1031–1038, 1990.
96. Usmani SS, et al: Polymorphonuclear leukocyte function in the preterm neonate: effect of chronologic age. Pediatrics *87*:675–679, 1991.
97. Babior BM: Oxidants from phagocytes: agents of defense and destruction. Blood *64*:959–966, 1984.
98. Drossou V, et al: Impact of prematurity, stress and sepsis on the neutrophil respiratory burst activity of neonates. Biol Neonate *72*:201–209, 1997.
99. Sikora JP, et al: Proinflammatory cytokine inhibitors, TNF-alpha and oxidative burst of polymorphonuclear leukocytes in the pathogenesis of sepsis in newborns. Arch Immunol Ther Exp (Warsz) *49*:155–161, 2001.
100. Shigeoka AO, et al: Functional analysis of neutrophil granulocytes from healthy, infected, and stressed neonates. J Pediatr *95*:454–460, 1979.
101. Shigeoka AO, et al: Defective oxidative metabolic responses of neutrophils from stressed neonates. J Pediatr *98*:392–398, 1981.
102. Driscoll MS: Longitudinal evaluation of polymorphonuclear leukocyte chemiluminescence in premature infants. J Pediatr *116*:429–434, 1990.
103. Yamazaki M, et al: Increased production of superoxide anion by neonatal polymorphonuclear leukocytes stimulated with a chemotactic peptide. Am J Hematol *27*:169–173, 1988.
104. Ambruso DR, et al: Oxidative metabolism of cord blood neutrophils: relationship to content and degranulation of cytoplasmic granules. Pediatr Res *18*:1148–1153, 1984.

105. Ambruso DR, et al: Increased activity of the respiratory burst in cord blood neutrophils: kinetics of the NADPH oxidase enzyme system in subcellular fractions. Pediatr Res *21*:205–210, 1987.

106. Ambruso DR, Johnston RB, Jr.: Lactoferrin enhances hydroxyl radical production by human neutrophils, neutrophil particulate fractions, and an enzymatic generating system. J Clin Invest *67*:352–360, 1981.

107. Anderson DC, et al: Abnormal stimulated adherence of neonatal granulocytes: impaired induction of surface Mac-1 by chemotactic factors or secretagogues. Blood *70*:740–750, 1987.

108. Rider ED, et al: Myeloperoxidase deficiency in neutrophils of neonates. J Pediatr *112*:648–651, 1988.

109. Edwards SW: The antimicrobial granule enzymes. *In* Edwards SW (ed): Biochemistry and Physiology of the Neutrophil. Cambridge, Cambridge University Press, 1994, pp 54–60.

110. Thomas EL, et al: Human neutrophil antimicrobial activity. Rev Infect Dis *10* (Suppl 2):S450–456, 1988.

111. Cohen MS: Molecular events in the activation of human neutrophils for microbial killing. Clin Infect Dis *18* (Suppl 2):S170–179, 1994.

112. Martin E, et al: Defensins and other endogenous peptide antibiotics of vertebrates. J Leukoc Biol *58*:128–136, 1995.

113. Elsbach P, Weiss J: Oxygen-dependent and oxygen-independent mechanisms of microbicidal activity of neutrophils. Immunol Lett *11*:159–163, 1985.

114. Bullen JJ, et al: The critical role of iron in some clinical infections. Eur J Clin Microbiol Infect Dis *10*:613–617, 1991.

115. Ellison RT, 3rd, Giehl TJ: Killing of gram-negative bacteria by lactoferrin and lysozyme. J Clin Invest *88*:1080–1091, 1991.

116. McCracken GH, Jr., Eichenwald HF: Leukocyte function and the development of opsonic and complement activity in the neonate. Am J Dis Child *121*:120–126, 1971.

117. Marodi L, et al: Characteristics and functional capacities of human cord blood granulocytes and monocytes. Pediatr Res *18*:1127–1131, 1984.

118. Dossett JH, et al: Studies on interaction of bacteria, serum factors and polymorphonuclear leukocytes in mothers and newborns. Pediatrics *44*:49–57, 1969.

119. Forman ML, Stiehm ER: Impaired opsonic activity but normal phagocytosis in low-birth-weight infants. N Engl J Med *281*:926–931, 1969.

120. Mills EL, et al: The chemiluminescence response and bactericidal activity of polymorphonuclear neutrophils from newborns and their mothers. Pediatrics *63*:429–434, 1979.

121. Gahr M, et al: Polymorphonuclear leukocyte function in term and preterm newborn infants. Biol Neonate *48*:15–20, 1985.

122. Wright WC, Jr., et al: Decreased bactericidal activity of leukocytes of stressed newborn infants. Pediatrics *56*:579–584, 1975.

123. Quie PG, Mills EL: Bactericidal and metabolic function of polymorphonuclear leukocytes. Pediatrics *64*:719–721, 1979.

124. Al-Hadithy H, et al: Defective neutrophil function in low-birth-weight, premature infants. J Clin Pathol *34*:366–370, 1981.

125. Xanthou M, et al: Phagocytosis and killing ability of *Candida albicans* by blood leucocytes of healthy term and preterm babies. Arch Dis Child *50*:72–75, 1975.

126. Midorikawa Y, et al: Modulation of the immune response to transplanted tumors in rats by selective depletion of neutrophils in vivo using a monoclonal antibody: abrogation of specific transplantation resistance to chemical carcinogen-induced syngeneic tumors by selective depletion of neutrophils in vivo. Cancer Res *50*:6243–6247, 1990.

127. Matsumoto Y, et al: Recombinant human granulocyte colony-stimulating factor inhibits the metastasis of hematogenous and non-hematogenous tumors in mice. Int J Cancer *49*:444–449, 1991.

128. Colombo MP, et al: Granulocyte colony-stimulating factor gene transfer suppresses tumorigenicity of a murine adenocarcinoma in vivo. J Exp Med *173*:889–897, 1991.

129. van Spriel AB, et al: Mac-1 (CD11b/CD18) is essential for Fc receptor-mediated neutrophil cytotoxicity and immunologic synapse formation. Blood *97*:2478–2486, 2001.

130. Kindzelskii AL, Petty HR: Early membrane rupture events during neutrophil-mediated antibody-dependent tumor cell cytolysis. J Immunol *162*:3188–3192, 1999.

131. Weisbart RH, et al: GM-CSF induces human neutrophil IgA-mediated phagocytosis by an IgA Fc receptor activation mechanism. Nature *332*:647–648, 1988.

132. Valerius T, et al: FcaR$_I$ (CD89) as a novel trigger molecule for bispecific antibody therapy. Blood *90*:4485–4492, 1997.

133. Ottonello L, et al: Monoclonal Lym-1 antibody-dependent cytolysis by neutrophils exposed to granulocyte-macrophage colony-stimulating factor: intervention of FcgR$_{II}$ (CD32), CD11b-CD18 integrins, and CD66b glycoproteins. Blood *93*:3505–3511, 1999.

134. van Egmond M, et al: Human immunoglobulin A receptor (FcaRI, CD89) function in transgenic mice requires both FcRg chain and CR3 (CD11b/CD18). Blood *93*:4387–4394, 1999.

135. Nagarajan S, et al: Cell-specific, activation-dependent regulation of neutrophil CD32A ligand-binding function. Blood *95*:1069–1077, 2000.

136. Gao H, et al: Effects of the protein tyrosine phosphatase CD45 on FcgRIIa signaling and neutrophil function. Exp Hematol *28*:1062–1070, 2000.

137. Stockmeyer B, et al: Preclinical studies with FcgR bispecific antibodies and granulocyte colony-stimulating factor-primed neutrophils as effector cells against HER-2/neu overexpressing breast cancer. Cancer Res *57*:696–701, 1997.

138. Stockmeyer B, et al: Triggering Fc a-receptor I (CD89) recruits neutrophils as effector cells for CD20-directed antibody therapy. J Immunol *165*:5954–5961, 2000.

139. Tiroch K, et al: Intracellular domains of target antigens influence their capacity to trigger antibody-dependent cell-mediated cytotoxicity. J Immunol *168*:3275–3282, 2002.

Jerry A. Winkelstein

158
The Complement System of the Fetus and Neonate

The complement system is composed of a series of soluble proteins and cell membrane receptors that act cooperatively in the host's defense against infection, the production of a normal inflammatory response, the generation of humoral immunity, and the clearance of immune complexes and apoptotic cells. This chapter reviews the biochemistry and biology of the complement system in adult human beings and relates these to the complement system of the fetus and newborn infant.

BIOCHEMISTRY

The majority of the biologically significant effects of the complement system are mediated by the third component (C3) and the terminal components (C5, C6, C7, C8, and C9) (Fig. 158-1; Table 158-1).[1] To effect their biologic functions, however, C3 through C9 must first be activated via either the classic, alternative, or lectin pathways.

Classic Pathway

Activation of the classic pathway is usually initiated by antigen-antibody complexes.[2] Antibodies of the appropriate class or subclass (IgG1, IgG2, IgG3, and IgM) bind to antigen and in doing so create an immune complex, which, in turn, binds and activates the first component of complement (C1). The first component of complement is a macromolecular complex composed of three subcomponents, C1q, C1r, and C1s. The binding of the C1q to the Fc portion of the immunoglobulin leads to the activation of C1r, which, in turn, activates C1s. Activated C1s possesses serine esterase activity and is able to activate the fourth component of complement (C4) by cleaving a small peptide (C4a) from one of its three chains. This exposes an intrachain reactive thiolester in the larger cleavage product (C4b), which allows the nascent C4b to bind covalently to cell surfaces or immunoglobulins through either transacylation of hydroxyl groups or amino groups. The

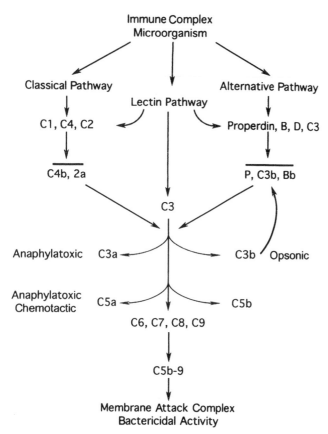

Figure 158–1. The complement system.

Alternative Pathway

Activation of the alternative pathway begins with the C3 molecule.[4] Like C4, native C3 contains an internal thiolester in its alpha-chain. Under normal conditions, the continuous low-grade hydrolysis of this internal thiolester creates a molecule that can bind native factor B and allow its cleavage by a serine protease, factor D. Two cleavage products of factor B are generated: a larger product, Bb, and a smaller product, Ba. The association of the hydrolyzed C3 with Bb then creates a C3-cleaving enzyme, C3,Bb, (termed the *priming* C3-convertase), which is responsible for a continuous, low-grade cleavage of C3 and, hence, the generation of nascent C3b. As with the activation of C4, the cleavage of native C3 exposes a reactive thiolester, which allows the nascent C3b to bind covalently to suitable acceptor molecules on the cell surface. If the nascent C3b binds to a suitable surface, it forms a reversible complex with native factor B, which is then cleaved by factor D to create a highly efficient C3-cleaving enzyme, C3b,Bb (termed the *amplification* C3-convertase).

As with the classic pathway, a number of factors influence the activity of the alternative pathway C3-convertase, C3b,Bb. The enzyme is relatively labile and, under physiologic conditions, rapidly undergoes intrinsic decay through dissociation of the Bb. One of the proteins of the alternative pathway, properdin (P), stabilizes the binding of Bb to C3b and thereby retards its intrinsic decay. Another protein, factor H, competes with factor B for binding to C3b in the assembly of the alternative pathway C3-convertase and can also displace Bb from the C3b,Bb enzyme once it has formed. Factor I inhibits the alternative pathway C3-convertase by inactivating cell-bound C3b through proteolytic cleavage, creating iC3b; its rate of inactivation of C3b is markedly accelerated by factor H.

---

reaction continues with the activation of C2 by C1s. The cleavage of C2 results in the liberation of a small peptide (C2b) and the formation of a bimolecular enzyme, C4b,2a, which is responsible for activating C3 by cleavage and thereby initiating the assembly of the terminal components (C5 through C9) into the membrane attack complex.

If the activation of the classic pathway were to proceed in an uncontrolled fashion, this would result in the generation of excessive amounts of the phlogistic fragments of complement, which, in turn, could cause widespread immunopathologic damage to the host. Fortunately a number of mechanisms act to control the assembly and expression of the classic pathway C3-cleaving enzyme C4b,2a. First, the enzymatic actions of C1r and C1s can be inhibited by a control protein, C1 esterase inhibitor. A second inhibitor, C4-binding protein, inhibits the C4b,2a enzyme by limiting the uptake of C2 by C4b; by accelerating the decay and dissociation of the C2a once it has complexed with C4b; and by enhancing the ability of yet another inhibitor, factor I, to cleave and inactivate C4b. Finally, a fourth inhibitor, decay-accelerating factor, an integral membrane protein found in erythrocytes and a variety of other cells, also accelerates the release of C2a from the C4b,2a enzyme. Thus, in the usual situation, the activation of C3 via the classic pathway proceeds in a controlled fashion.

Activation of the classic pathway is usually initiated by antigen-antibody complexes and therefore is considered to be especially important in acquired immunity. However, some enveloped RNA viruses, some mycoplasma species, and certain species and strains of both gram-negative and gram-positive bacteria can bind C1q directly and activate the classic pathway without a requirement for antibody.[3] Thus, under some circumstances, the classic pathway may also function in natural immunity.

TABLE 158–1

Individual Components of the Human Complement System

Component	Approximate Molecular Weight	Number of Chains
Classic pathway		
C1q	460,000	6A, 6B, 6C
C1r	83,000	Single
C1s	83,000	Single
C4	200,000	1 α, 1 β, 1 γ
C2	102,000	Single
Alternative pathway		
Factor D	25,000	Single
Factor B	93,000	Single
C3 and terminal components		
C3	185,000	1 α, 1 β
C5	190,000	1 α, 1 β
C6	128,000	Single
C7	120,000	Single
C8	163,000	1 α, 1 β, 1 γ
C9	79,000	Single
Control proteins		
C1 inhibitor	105,000	Single
C4-binding protein	550,000	7–8 Identical
Properdin	223,000	4 Identical
Factor H	150,000	Single
Factor I	100,000	1 α, 1 β
Membrane/receptor proteins		
Decay-accelerating factor	70,000	Single
CR1	250,000	Single
CR2	145,000	Single
CR3	250,000	1 α, 1 β

Antibody is not required for the activation of the alternative pathway, and, thus, the alternative pathway is generally viewed as an important mechanism of natural immunity.[3] Antibody can participate functionally, however, in the activation of the alternative pathway by a variety of particles, including virus-infected cells and bacteria. Thus, in some instances, the alternative pathway may participate in acquired immunity.

Two final points regarding the relationship of the classic and alternative pathways to the activation of C3 and C5 through C9 deserve emphasis. First, because C3b is both the product of the alternative pathway C3-convertase and also forms part of the alternative pathway C3-convertase, the activation of C3 via the alternative pathway creates a positive feedback amplification loop (Fig. 158–1). Second, activation of the classic pathway, by creating nascent C3b, can lead to activation of the alternative pathway.

Lectin Pathway

In recent years, evidence has accumulated that a third mechanism exists by which C3 can be activated.[5] Mannose-binding lectin (MBL) is a member of the collectin family of proteins and is composed of identical subunits. MBL is capable of binding to a variety of microorganisms, including bacteria, fungi, and several viruses. MBL interacts with serine proteases, termed MBL-associated serine proteases (MASP1 and MASP2), proteins that share 39% homology with both human C1r and C1s. Like C1s, MASP1 and MASP2 can cleave both C4 and C2, thereby generating C4b,2a, and its C3-cleaving activity. In addition, there is some evidence to support the ability of the MBL-MASP complex to activate C3 via the alternative pathway and directly.

Activation of C3 and the Terminal Components

Whether C3 is activated via the classic, alternative, or lectin pathways, the larger alpha-chain of the C3 is cleaved, generating two fragments of unequal size, C3a and C3b. The activation of C3 by either of the two C3-convertases represents an amplification step because hundreds of C3 molecules can be cleaved by one enzyme. Cleavage of native C3 by either enzyme releases a small peptide (C3a) from the alpha-chain into the fluid phase, where it acts as an anaphylatoxin (see later). Most of the nascent C3b is also released into the fluid phase, where it is rapidly inactivated through hydrolysis of its internal thiolester. Other molecules of C3b, however, bind covalently to cell surfaces or immunoglobulins through the transacylation of hydroxyl groups or amino groups by the reactive thiolester of the nascent C3b.[6] The cell-bound C3b may then be cleaved by factor I and other proteases, yielding a variety of degradation products. Cell-bound C3b is able to act as an opsonin (see later) or combine with either of the two C3-convertases to create two new enzymes, the classic and alternative pathway C5-cleaving enzymes. The classic pathway C5-cleaving enzyme is composed of C4b, 2a, 3b. The alternative pathway C5-cleaving enzyme is composed of (C3b)$_2$, Bb.

Activation of C5 by either the alternative or classic pathway C5-convertases creates a small molecular weight product, C5a, and a larger molecular weight product, C5b. The smaller cleavage product, C5a, is released into the fluid phase, where, as with C3a, it can act as an anaphylatoxin (see later). In addition, C5a possesses potent chemotactic activity (see later). If the C5b combines with native C6 while it is still attached to the C5 convertase, it is stabilized and can initiate formation of the membrane attack complex, a multimolecular assembly of C5b, C6, C7, C8, and C9, which is capable of inserting into cell membranes and thereby expressing cytolytic activity.[7]

Complement Receptors

Receptors for many of the cleavage products of individual components of complement exist on a variety of cells.[8] Receptors for C3a, C4a, and C5a are present on mast cells, and receptors for C5a are also found on neutrophils, monocytes, and macrophages. There are three distinct receptors for C3b and its cleavage products. The CR1 receptor (C3b/C4b receptor) is found on polymorphonuclear leukocytes, eosinophils, monocytes, macrophages, mast cells, glomerular podocytes, B lymphocytes, and some T lymphocytes. In addition, it is found on the erythrocytes of primates, including humans. One of the more important functions of the CR1 receptor is to enhance the phagocytosis of particles opsonized with C3b. In addition, its presence on erythrocytes allows them to bind circulating immune complexes bearing C3b and transport the immune complexes to phagocytic cells of the reticuloendothelial system (see later). The CR2 receptor is found on B lymphocytes and binds C3d,g and C3d as well as iC3b. The functional significance of CR2 on B lymphocytes relates to the role of C3 in humoral immunity (see later). The CR3 receptor is found on the same cells as the CR1 receptor, and its primary ligand appears to be iC3b.

BIOLOGIC CONSEQUENCES OF COMPLEMENT ACTIVATION

Whether C3 and C5 through C9 are activated via the classic or alternative pathways, their activation results in the generation of a variety of biologically significant activities.

Anaphylatoxic Activity

The smaller cleavage products of both C3 and C5 (C3a and C5a) possess anaphylatoxic activity.[9] When compared on a molar basis, C5a is 100 times more potent than C3a. Both of these anaphylatoxins are subject to attack by a serum carboxypeptidase, which rapidly cleaves the C-terminal arginine that is common to both molecules and in each case creates a new molecule (C3a-des Arg and C5a-des Arg) that is significantly less potent than the parent molecule.

Complement-derived anaphylatoxins were originally identified through their ability to cause histamine release from basophils and mast cells, to promote smooth muscle contraction, and to increase vascular permeability. More recently, additional functions of these peptides have been identified.[10] These include the aggregation of platelets and the release of arachidonic acid metabolites. In addition, they can cause leukocytes to aggregate, generate arachidonic acid metabolites, produce toxic oxygen radicals, and discharge their granular enzymes.

Chemotactic Activity

The smaller cleavage product of C5, C5a, is also a potent chemotactic factor, which causes the directed movement of polymorphonuclear leukocytes, monocytes, eosinophils, and basophils.[11] The removal of the terminal arginine by carboxypeptidase not only significantly reduces its anaphylatoxic activity (see previously), but also reduces its chemotactic activity.

Opsonic Activity

The larger cleavage product of C3, C3b, acts as a potent opsonin when fixed to the surface of a particle, such as a red cell or microorganism.[12] As mentioned earlier, nascent C3b fixes covalently to the activating particle, leaving a portion of the bound C3b available to bind to C3b receptors on phagocytic cells. It appears that C3b subserves different opsonic functions depending on the nature of the phagocytic cell and its state of activation. In the case of neutrophils and nonactivated macrophages, C3b promotes attachment of the particle, whereas IgG acts to favor ingestion. In the case of activated macrophages, C3b serves to aid in both attachment and ingestion.

Bactericidal Activity

The generation of complement-mediated serum bactericidal activity requires the participation of the terminal complement components C5b through C9.[13] Only gram-negative bacteria can be killed by complement. Although protoplasts of gram-positive organisms are susceptible to lysis by complement, intact gram-positive organisms are not, suggesting that their thick cell wall interferes with the bactericidal action of the membrane attack complex.

Processing of Immune Complexes

The complement system also appears to play an important role in the processing of immune complexes.[14] The complement system could modify the structure or influence the biologic activities of immune complexes by a number of mechanisms. First, the activation of C3 via the classic pathway can retard the formation of large complexes and prevent their precipitation from serum as well as solubilize them once they are formed. Second, opsonically active C3b can enhance the uptake of immune complexes by phagocytic cells of the reticuloendothelial system and, thus, aid in their clearance. Finally, primates possess receptors for C3b on their erythrocytes, and circulating immune complexes bearing C3b can fix to erythrocytes through these receptors. The erythrocyte-bound complexes are then transported to the liver, where they are stripped from the erythrocytes and cleared from the circulation. In this manner, erythrocytes may serve as a buffer for the disposal of circulating immune complexes in humans.

Role of Complement in Antibody Formation

In vivo studies using animals pharmacologically depleted of C3 or using animals with genetically determined deficiencies of C4 or C3 have clearly shown the complement system to be important in the generation of a normal antibody response.[15] The antibody response to T-dependent antigens is relatively more dependent on an intact complement system than is the response to T-independent antigens. In addition, an intact complement system appears to facilitate the isotype switch from IgM to IgG. The mechanisms by which the complement system participates in antibody formation relate to the fact that B lymphocytes have receptors for C3 cleavage products and that activation of the complement system thereby influences the function of B lymphocytes.

Role of Complement in Clearance of Apoptotic Bodies

Recently, early components of the complement system, especially C1q, have been shown to play an important role in the clearance of apoptotic cells.[16] Apparently, C1q binds directly to blebs on the surface of apoptotic cells. C3 and C4 also bind apoptotic cells, but it is not known whether they are required for clearance.

FETAL SYNTHESIS OF COMPLEMENT COMPONENTS

A number of different approaches have been used to examine the ability of the fetus to synthesize individual components of the complement system.[17] One approach has been to examine the ability of a variety of fetal tissues to synthesize complement components in tissue culture. The synthesis of hemolytically active C1 by segments of fetal small intestine and colon has been demonstrated as early as 19 weeks' gestation[18]; other fetal tissues, such as liver, spleen, lung, and kidney, did not show any significant synthe-

sis of C1.[18] Using radioimmunoassay, the synthesis of the subcomponent C1q has been detected in fetal spleens as early as 14 weeks' gestation.[19] The synthesis of C4, C2, and C3 can be detected as either functional activities or antigenic proteins between 8 and 14 weeks of gestation, and the liver appears to be the major organ responsible for their production.[19-21] Significant synthesis of functionally active C5 can be detected in fetal livers and lungs as early as 8 to 9 weeks' gestation.[19,22] Finally, fetal livers produce functionally active C1 esterase inhibitor in tissue culture as early as 11 weeks after conception.[21]

Some evidence suggests that the synthesis of complement components by cells of the fetus and neonate differs quantitatively and qualitatively from that of adult cells. For example, although the constitutive expression of C3 and factor B by cord blood monocytes is equivalent to that of adult blood monocytes, their ability to increase synthesis of these two complement components in response to stimulation by lipopolysaccharide (LPS) is significantly impaired.[23] It appears that the inability of their monocytes to increase the synthesis of C3 and factor B in response to LPS is limited by pretranslational mechanisms in the fetus and translational mechanisms in the newborn infant.[24]

Other approaches have been used to determine whether the complement components found in fetal and newborn sera are of fetal origin, maternal origin, or both. Many of the individual proteins of the complement system exhibit genetically determined electrophoretic variations (allotypes), some of which occur commonly in the population (>1%).[25] By comparing the allotypes of individual complement components present in cord serum with the allotypes present in maternal serum and paternal serum, one may determine whether a given component in cord serum is of fetal origin or of maternal origin. For example, if a paternal allotype of a given component is present in cord serum but is not present in maternal serum, that is evidence for fetal synthesis. Conversely, if a maternal allotype of a given component is lacking in cord serum of the newborn infant, that is evidence against transplacental passage. Using such allotypic analysis for C4,[26] C3,[27] C6,[28] and factor B,[29] a number of studies have shown that these components in cord blood are of fetal origin and that there has been no transplacental passage of them. Finally, in one instance, a C2-deficient mother gave birth to a child whose cord blood contained C2, which also indicates significant fetal synthesis of this component.[30] Thus, the available data on those components that have been studied suggest that there is significant fetal synthesis of complement components relatively early in gestation and that there is little, if any, transplacental passage of them in humans.

COMPLEMENT LEVELS IN NEONATES

A number of studies have examined levels of individual components of the complement system in normal full-term infants (Tables 158–2 and 158–3). Pregnant women have slightly higher levels of some complement components than do nonpregnant adults.[31-33] Thus, when compared with their mothers, normal full-term infants may appear to have lower levels of individual components than when they are compared with nonpregnant adults.[33-42] For example, the levels of C3 in full-term infants are approximately 40 to 60% of maternal levels but are 60 to 70% of adult levels (Fig. 158–2). Although the levels of most components of either the classic or alternative pathways in full-term infants are at least 50% of adult levels, both C8 and C9 seem to be more severely depressed, with levels in full-term newborn infants as low as 28 and 10% of maternal levels.[37,38]

The serum levels of individual components of complement in premature infants also have been studied. Significant levels of C4, C3, C7, C9, factor B, P, and C1 esterase inhibitor have been detected in fetal serum as early as the end of the first trimester or the beginning of the second trimester.[35,37,43-45] As one might

TABLE 158-2

Classic Pathway of Complement in Full-Term Infants*

	CH_{50}	C1	C1q	C4	C2	C3	C5	C6	C7	C8	C9
Compared with Maternal Sera											
Fireman et al[34]	0.53†			0.56		0.54	0.61				
Adinolfi[35]	0.50†			0.58		0.38					
Sawyer et al[36]	0.60†		0.96	0.74†	0.84†	0.56					
Ballow et al[37]		0.60	0.62	0.50†	0.61†	0.53†	0.50†	0.45†	0.62†	0.28†	0.10†
Compared with Adult Sera											
Adinolfi and Beck[38]									0.67†		0.14
Johnston et al[33]	0.65†					0.74					
Strunk et al[39]	0.81†			0.80		0.60					
Davis et al[40]			0.73	0.60	0.76	0.63	0.75	0.47			

* All values expressed as percentages of either maternal levels or nonpregnant adult levels.
† Functional assays.
Modified from Johnston RB Jr, et al: Pediatrics *64*:S781, 1979.

TABLE 158-3

Alternative Pathway in Full-Term Infants*

	Alternative Pathway Hemolysis	Properdin	Factor B	Factor I	Factor H
Alper et al[29]			0.35		
Feinstein and Kaplan[41]			0.52		
Adinolfi and Beck[38]			0.47		
Minta et al[42]		0.58			
Strunk et al[39]	0.65†	0.71	0.36		
Davis et al[40]		0.53	0.49†	0.55†	0.61†

* All values expressed as percentages of normal, nonpregnant adult levels.
† Functional assays.
Modified from Johnston RB Jr, et al: Pediatrics *64*:S781, 1979.

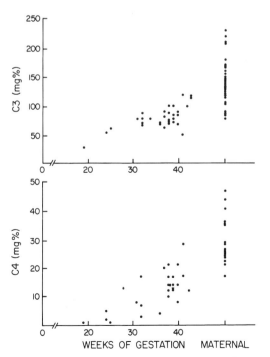

Figure 158–2. The development of serum C3 and C4 in premature and full-term infants. (Modified from Fireman P, et al: J Immunol *103*:25, 1969.)

expect, there is a general tendency for levels of these components to increase with age, but there is also a great deal of scatter at any given age.[34-36, 38, 39, 45] Thus, in some instances, a full-term newborn infant may have a level of C3 or factor B that is lower than that of an infant of 30 weeks' gestation.

The effect of intrauterine growth retardation on serum complement levels also has been examined. It appears that intrauterine growth retardation does not significantly affect the levels of C4, C3, and factor B[46,47], the levels of these three components are more directly related to gestational age than they are to weight.

COMPLEMENT-MEDIATED FUNCTIONS IN NEONATES

In view of the fact that many of the individual components of complement are reduced in concentration in neonatal sera, it is not surprising that those serum activities that depend on the complement system, at least in part, are reduced as well. A number of studies have examined serum opsonic activity in premature and full-term infants.[48-54] Each of these studies has used different species and strains of bacteria as well as different assay systems. Because opsonic requirements differ for different species and even for different strains of bacteria, the results of one study are not always directly comparable with the results of another. For example, some studies have reported reduced serum-opsonizing activity for *Escherichia coli* in full-term infants,[50, 54] whereas others have reported normal opsonizing activity.[51] In one study, serum-opsonizing activity in full-term infants was compared between two different strains of *E. coli* and was normal for a strain of *E. coli* that was opsonized via the classic pathway and reduced for a strain of *E. coli* that was opsonized via the alternative pathway.[52] In the case of *Serratia* and group B streptococci, results also have varied from study to study. In some studies, serum-opsonizing activity for *Serratia*[49] or group B streptococci[50,54] has been normal in full-term infants, whereas in other studies, serum-opsonizing activity for *Serratia*[50] or group B streptococci[53] has been reduced. Most studies have shown that serum-opsonizing activity for staphylococci is normal in full-term infants.[49-51,54]

The results of studies in premature infants appear to be more consistent.[49,51] Serum-opsonizing activity for individual strains of *E. coli*, staphylococci, *Serratia*, and *Pseudomonas* appears to be reduced in premature infants, with a general tendency to increase toward normal with increasing length of gestation.

Serum chemotactic activity also has been studied in neonates. In one study, the ability of serum from normal full-term infants to generate chemotactic activity after activation by bacteria or immune complexes was markedly reduced.[55]

It is not always possible to ascribe the deficient opsonizing or chemotactic activity found in the sera of newborn infants solely to a deficient complement system because deficiencies in other humoral factors important in the generation of these activities may contribute as well. For example, most neonates have low levels of IgM because there is little, if any, transplacental passage of this immunoglobulin class, and fetal synthesis is reduced. Because many antibodies against gram-negative bacteria are of the IgM class, opsonization of some gram-negative bacteria may be reduced in newborns infants because there is insufficient IgM antibody to activate the classic pathway and generate opsonically active C3b. Some studies, however, have directly addressed the functional integrity of the complement system in newborn infants. In one such study, the ability of a variety of bacterial species to activate C3 via the classic or alternative pathways in neonatal sera was examined and found to be diminished.[56] In another study, opsonization of a strain of type 1a group B streptococci that activates the classic pathway without a requirement for antibody was examined and found to be reduced.[53] Thus, it appears that at least part of the decrease in serum-opsonizing and chemotactic activities in neonatal serum is due to a deficient complement system.

ROLE OF COMPLEMENT IN NEONATAL HOST DEFENSE

There is a great deal of evidence, accumulated from studies in experimental animals and from observations in patients, that the complement system plays a critical role in the host's defense against infection. Animals with genetically determined deficiencies of C4,[57] C3,[58] or C5[59] and animals that have been pharmacologically depleted of C3[60] all have an increased susceptibility to infection when challenged with a variety of microorganisms. Similarly, genetically determined deficiencies of nearly all the components of complement have been identified in humans, and many of these individuals have an increased susceptibility to infection.[61]

The complement system has been shown to play an important role in resistance to a variety of bacteria,[60-62] viruses,[63,64] and fungi.[65] It also operates at a number of different anatomic locations, helping defend the host against pneumonia,[66] sepsis,[60,67] and meningitis.[62] It appears to be most critical in the early stages of infection,[60] at least in the case of acute bacterial infections, helping limit bacteria to the initial site of infection[62,66] or participating in the clearance of bacteria from the bloodstream.[57,67] Finally, although the complement system is an important mechanism of resistance to infection in the nonimmune host,[59,60,62] it also plays a significant role in the immune host that possesses antibody.[57,67]

Because so many components of the immune system are reduced in number or in function in the newborn infant, it is

difficult to ascribe the neonates' proclivity for infection solely to a deficient complement system. However, at least one clinical study has shown a strong correlation between low hemolytic complement activity in the serum and an unfavorable prognosis for neonatal sepsis.[68] In addition, when supplemental C9 is added to neonatal serum, the bactericidal capacity of neonatal serum for a number of different strains of *E. coli* is restored to normal.[69] Thus, the deficiencies in the complement system found in some full-term and premature neonates contribute, at least in part, to their increased susceptibility to infection.

REFERENCES

1. Frank MM: The complement system in host defense and inflammation. Rev Infect Dis *1*:483, 1979.
2. Porter RR, Reid KBM: The biochemistry of complement. Nature *275*:699, 1978.
3. Winkelstein JA: Complement and natural immunity. Clin Immunol Allergy *3*:421, 1983.
4. Fearon DT: Activation of the alternative complement pathway. CRC Crit Rev Immunol *1*:1, 1979.
5. Turner MW: Mannose-binding lectin: the pluripotent molecule of the innate immune system. Immunol Today *17*:532, 1996.
6. Hostetter MK, Gordon DL: Biochemistry of C3 and related thioester proteins in infection and inflammation. Rev Infect Dis *9*:97, 1987.
7. Mayer MM, et al: Membrane damage by complement. CRC Crit Rev Immunol *2*:133, 1981.
8. Fearon DT, Wong WW: Complement ligand-receptor interactions that mediate biological responses. Ann Rev Immunol *1*:243, 1983.
9. Hugli TE: The structural basis for anaphylatoxin and chemotactic functions of C3a, C4a, and C5a. CRC Crit Rev Immunol *2*:321, 1981.
10. Vogt W: Anaphylatoxins: possible roles in diseases. Complement *3*:177, 1986.
11. Synderman R, Goetzl EJ: Molecular and cellular mechanisms of leukocyte chemotaxis. Science *213*:830, 1981.
12. Griffin FM: Opsonization. *In* Day NK, Good RA (eds): Biological Amplification Systems in Immunology. New York, Plenum, 1977.
13. Joiner KA: Studies on the mechanism of bacterial resistance to complement-mediated killing and on the mechanisms of action of bactericidal antibody. Curr Top Microb Immunol *121*:99, 1985.
14. Schifferli JA, et al: The role of complement and its receptor in the elimination of immune complexes. N Engl J Med *315*:488, 1986.
15. Ochs HD, et al: Complement, membrane glycoproteins, and complement receptors: their role in regulation of the immune response. Clin Immunol Immunopathol *40*:94, 1986.
16. Navratil JS, Ahearn JM: Apoptosis and autoimmunity. Complement deficiency and systemic lupus erythematosus revisited. Curr Rheumatol Reports *2*:32, 2000.
17. Adinolfi M: Human complement: onset and site of synthesis during fetal life. Am J Dis Child *131*:1015, 1977.
18. Colten HR, et al: Synthesis of the first component of human complement *in vitro*. J Exp Med *128*:595, 1968.
19. Kohler PF: Maturation of the human complement system: I. Onset time and sites of fetal C1q, C4, C3, and C5 synthesis. J Clin Invest *52*:671, 1973.
20. Adinolfi M, et al: Ontogenesis of two components of human complement: B₁E and B₁C globulins. Nature *219*:189, 1968.
21. Colten HR: Ontogeny of the human complement system: *in vitro* biosynthesis of individual complement components by fetal tissues. J Clin Invest *51*:725, 1972.
22. Colten HR: Biosynthesis of the fifth component of complement (C5) by human fetal tissues. Clin Immunol Immunopathol *1*:346, 1973.
23. St. John Sutton MB, et al: Regulation of the synthesis of the third component of complement and factor B in cord blood monocytes by LPS. J Immunol *136*:1366, 1986.
24. Strunk RC, et al: Developmentally regulated effects of LPS on biosynthesis of the third component of complement and factor B in human fibroblasts and monocytes. Immunology *82*:314, 1994.
25. McLean RH, Winkelstein JA: Genetically determined variation in the complement system: relationship to disease. J Pediatr *105*:179, 1984.
26. Bach S, et al: Electrophoretic polymorphism of the fourth component of human complement (C4) in paired maternal and foetal plasmas. Immunology *21*:869, 1971.
27. Propp RP, Alper CA: C3 synthesis in the human fetus and lack of transplacental passage. Science *162*:672, 1968.
28. Alper CA, et al: Polymorphism of the sixth component of complement. *In* Arbuthnott JP, Beely JA (eds): Isoelectric Focusing. London, Butterworth, 1975, p 306.
29. Alper CA, et al: Genetic polymorphism in human glycine-rich beta-glycoprotein. J Exp Med *135*:68, 1972.
30. Ruddy S, et al: Hereditary deficiency of the second component of complement (C2) in man: correlation of C2 hemolytic activity with immunochemical measurements of C2 protein. Immunology *18*:943, 1970.
31. Traub B: The complement activity of the serum of healthy persons, mothers and newborn infants. J Pathol Bacteriol *55*:447, 1943.

32. Ballow M: Phylogenetics and ontogenetics of the complement system. *In* Day NK, Good RA (eds): Biological Amplificiation Systems in Immunology. New York, Plenum, 1977.
33. Johnston RB Jr, et al: Complement in the newborn infant. Pediatrics 64:S781, 1979.
34. Fireman P, et al: Development of the human complement system. J Immunol 103:25, 1969.
35. Adinolfi M: Levels of two components of complement (C4 and C3) in human fetal and newborn sera. Dev Med Child Neurol 12:306, 1970.
36. Sawyer MK, et al: Developmental aspects of the human complement system. Biol Neonate 19:148, 1971.
37. Ballow M, et al: Developmental aspects of complement components in the newborn. Clin Exp Immunol 18:257, 1974.
38. Adinolfi M, Beck SE: Human complement C7 and C9 in fetal and newborn sera. Arch Dis Child 50:562, 1975.
39. Strunk RC, et al: Alternative pathway of complement activation in full-term and premature infants. Pediatr Res 13:641, 1979.
40. Davis CA, et al: Serum complement levels in infancy: age-related changes. Pediatr Res 13:1043, 1979.
41. Feinstein PA, Kaplan SR: The alternative pathway of complement activation in the neonate. Pediatr Res 9:803, 1975.
42. Minta JO, et al: Distribution and levels of properdin in human body fluids. Clin Immunol Immunopathol 5:84, 1976.
43. Adinolfi M, Gardner B: Synthesis of B_1E and B_1C components of complement in human foetuses. Acta Paediatr Scand 56:450, 1967.
44. Giltin D, Biasucci A: Development of gamma G, gamma A, gamma M, beta 1C, beta 1A, C'1 esterase inhibitor, ceruloplasmin, transferrin, hemopexin, haptoglobin, fibrinogen, plasminogen, alpha-1 antitrypsin, orosomucoid, beta-lipoprotein, alpha-2 macroglobulin, and prealbumin in the human conceptus. J Clin Invest 48:1433, 1969.
45. Adamkin D, et al: Activity of the alternative pathway of complement in the newborn infant. J Pediatr 93:604, 1978.
46. Notarangelo LD, et al: Activity of classical and alternative pathways of complement in preterm and small for gestational age infants. Pediatr Res 18:281, 1984.
47. Shapiro R, et al: Serum complement and immunoglobulin values in small for gestational age infants. J Pediatr 99:139, 1981.
48. Miller ME: Phagocytosis in the newborn infant: humoral and cellular factors. J Pediatr 74:255, 1969.
49. Forman ML, Stiehm ER: Impaired opsonic activity but normal phagocytosis in low birth weight infants. N Engl J Med 281:926, 1969.
50. Dossett JH, et al: Studies on interaction of bacteria, serum factors and polymorphonuclear leukocytes in mothers and newborns. Pediatrics 44:49, 1969.
51. McCracken GH Jr, Eichenwald HF: Leukocyte function and the development of opsonic and complement activity in the neonate. Am J Dis Child 121:120, 1971.
52. Mills EL, et al: Deficient alternative complement pathway activity in newborn sera. Pediatr Res 13:1341, 1979.
53. Edwards MS, et al: Deficient classical complement pathway activity in newborn sera. Pediatr Res 17:685, 1983.
54. Marodi L, et al: Opsonic activity of cord blood sera against various species of microorganisms. Pediatr Res 19:433, 1985.
55. Miller ME: Chemotactic function in the human neonate: humoral and cellular aspects. Pediatr Res 5:487, 1971.
56. Winkelstein JA, et al: Defective activation of the third component of complement in the sera of newborn infants. Pediatr Res 13:1093, 1979.
57. Hosea SW, et al: The critical role of complement in experimental pneumococcal sepsis. J Infect Dis 142:903, 1980.
58. Blum JR, et al: The clinical manifestations of a genetically determined deficiency of the third component of complement in the dog. Clin Immunol Immunopathol 34:304, 1985.
59. Shin HS, et al: Heat labile opsonins to pneumococcus: II. Involvement of C3 and C5. J Exp Med 130:1229, 1969.
60. Winkelstein JA, et al: The role of C3 as an opsonin in the early stages of infection. Proc Soc Exp Biol Med 149:397, 1975.
61. Figueroa JE, Densen P: Infectious diseases associated with complement deficiencies. Clin Microbiol Rev 4:359, 1991.
62. Crosson FJ Jr, et al: Participation of complement in the nonimmune host defense against experimental *Haemophilus influenzae* type b septicemia and meningitis. Infect Immunol 14:882, 1976.
63. Hirsch RL, et al: The effect of complement depletion on the course of Sindbis virus infection in mice. J Immunol 121:1276, 1978.
64. Miller A, et al: The role of antibody in recovery from experimental rabies. J Immunol 121:321, 1978.
65. Gelfand JA, et al: Role of complement in host defense against experimental candidiasis. J Infect Dis 138:9, 1978.
66. Bakker-Wondenberg IAJM, et al: Efficacy of antimicrobial therapy in experimental pneumococcal pneumonia: effects of impaired phagocytosis. Infect Immunol 25:366, 1979.
67. Brown EJ, et al: A quantitative analysis of the interaction of antipneumococcal antibody and complement in experimental pneumococcal bacteremia. J Clin Invest 69:85, 1982.
68. Cairo MS, et al: Role of circulating complement and polymorphonuclear leukocyte transfusion in treatment and outcome in critically ill neonates with sepsis. J Pediatr 110:935, 1987.
69. Lassiter HA, et al: Supplemental complement component C9 enhances the capacity of neonatal serum to kill multiple isolates of pathogenic *E. coli* Pediatr Res 35:389, 1994.

Laurie Kilpatrick and Mary Catherine Harris

159

Cytokines and Inflammatory Response in the Fetus and Neonate

CYTOKINE STRUCTURE AND FUNCTION

Inflammation is a protective response to infection or injury and is composed of several different components that mobilize the host defense systems. The inflammatory response is controlled primarily by cytokines, which are endogenous mediators of the immune system. To understand how the inflammatory response is regulated both locally and systemically, it is necessary to examine the production and physiologic function of cytokines.

General Description of Cytokines

Cytokines are multifunctional proteins, often referred to as "hormones of the immune system." Unlike classic hormones, cytokines are produced by various cell types, in response to multiple types of stimuli, and they have overlapping biologic activity.[1-4] Cytokines are potent endogenous mediators whose synthesis and secretion are under tight regulatory control. These endogenous mediators are not stored as preformed molecules in producer cells; rather, new synthesis is required for secretion. Once released, their half-life is relatively short, further limiting biologic activity. Cytokines act in minute quantities (10^{-9} to 10^{-12} mol) by binding to specific cellular receptors that are members of distinct structural families. Most cellular responses to cytokines result in an altered pattern of gene expression that leads to alterations in cellular physiology.

An important function of cytokines is cell-to-cell communication. Cytokines are unusual in that they can communicate in an autocrine, paracrine, or endocrine manner.[3, 4] Most cytokine actions occur on the local level, where cytokines act in a paracrine manner by simple diffusion or by cell-to-cell contact. Some cytokine producer cells also express cytokine receptors, and secreted cytokines can bind to their producer cells and can modulate cell function. Cytokines can also leave the local environment, enter the circulation, interact with different organ systems, and alter host physiology.

A group of cytokines is produced in response to inflammatory stimuli. The function of these *proinflammatory* cytokines is to communicate to surrounding tissue the presence of infection or injury.[2,4] Principal proinflammatory cytokines are tumor necrosis factor-α (TNF-α), interleukin-1 (IL-1), IL-6, IL-8, IL-12, IL-18, and interferon-γ (IFN-γ). TNF and IL-1 are the principal mediators of the inflammatory response and are thought to have a critical role in orchestrating the local response through cell activation and triggering a cytokine cascade.[5] Proinflammatory cytokines can also enter the systemic circulation and can produce immune cell activation and significant alterations in host physiology, such as fever, and the acute phase reaction.[5] Inflammatory stimuli also trigger the synthesis of antiinflammatory cytokines and specific cytokine inhibitors that serve to modify the host inflammatory response.[6-8] Antiinflammatory cytokines limit the inflammatory response by inhibiting proinflammatory cytokine synthesis; key antiinflammatory cytokines include IL-10, IL-13, IL-4, and IL-11. Naturally occurring proinflammatory cytokine inhibitors neutralize proinflammatory cytokine bioactivity by blocking cytokine–cytokine receptor interactions, by binding to either the proinflammatory cytokine itself or to its specific receptor. Naturally occurring inhibitors include soluble proinflammatory cytokine receptors, decoy receptors, receptor antagonists, and cytokine binding proteins. The interplay among these proinflammatory cytokines, antiinflammatory cytokines, and naturally occurring cytokine inhibitors determines the inflammatory response and its effectiveness.

Proinflammatory Cytokines

Tumor Necrosis Factor

TNF-α is one of the principal mediators of the inflammatory response and has a critical role in orchestrating the local inflammatory response through cell activation and initiation of a cytokine cascade. TNF is synthesized as a 26-kDa prohormone, which is processed to a mature form of 17 kDa after cleavage of the residue signal peptide by a matrix metalloproteinase disintegrin.[9-11] The prohormone, with an unusually long leader sequence of amino acids, represents a transmembrane form. TNF can exert activity as a transmembrane cell-associated species as well as in a secreted form.[12]

TNF synthesis is triggered by endotoxin, enterotoxin, toxic shock syndrome toxin-1, viruses, mycobacterial cord factor, C5a, fungal and parasitic antigens, IL-1, and TNF itself.[13] The primary producer cells of TNF are monocytes and tissue macrophages.[14] TNF is also produced by many other cell types, which include lymphocytes, natural killer (NK) cells, neutrophils, mast cells, endothelial cells, keratinocytes, smooth muscle cells, astrocytes, and microglial cells.[13,14]

Tumor Necrosis Factor Receptors. The tight regulation of TNF signaling is important in the control of TNF-induced cellular alterations. Most cell types possess two TNF receptors, a 55- to 60-kDa receptor (TNFR-1 or CD120a) and a 75- to 80-kDa receptor (TNFR-2 or CD120b).[15,16] These two receptors are structurally related and are members of the TNF/NGF receptor superfamily. The extracellular domains of the TNFR-1 and TNFR-2 share 28% homology, but no homology is observed in the cytoplasmic domain.[17,18] The lack of homology of the two receptors suggests that they mediate discrete signaling pathways.[17] The TNFR-1 is largely responsible for proinflammatory cellular responses as well as for regulation of apoptosis.[18-22]

The TNFR-1 (Fig. 159–1) contains a cytoplasmic sequence of approximately 80 amino acids termed the *death domain*. This region regulates apoptosis through its association with effector proteins that activate programmed cell death, but the death domain is also the region in the TNFR-1 that mediates the cell's survival or antiapoptotic pathways.[20] Activation of the TNFR-1 by

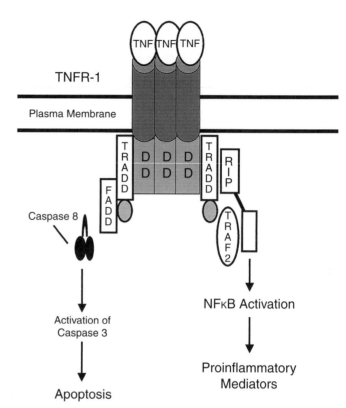

Figure 159–1. The tumor necrosis factor receptor-1 (TNFR-1) signaling complex. Binding of TNF to the TNFR-1 results in the recruitment and formation of a TNFR-1 signaling complex. The TRADD (TNFR-associated death domain) associates with the TNFR-1 through death domain (DD) interactions and serves as a platform for the recruitment of other adaptor proteins including TRAF-2 (TNFR-associated factor-2), RIP (receptor-interacting protein), and FADD (fas-associated death domain). These adaptor proteins recruit additional components necessary for the activation of proinflammatory and apoptotic signaling pathways. Proinflammatory responses are mediated through the activation of transcription factors, such as nuclear factor κ-B (NFκB). Apoptosis is activated through the recruitment of FADD and the subsequent activation of caspases.

TNF results in the formation of a receptor trimer through self-association with the death domains. Receptor trimerization leads to the recruitment of TRADD (TNFR-1 associated death domain protein).[23] TRADD functions as a scaffold protein and subsequently recruits other effector proteins into the receptor complex. TRADD recruits TRAF2 (TNFR-associated factor-2), RIP (receptor-interacting protein), and FADD (Fas-associated death domain) to form the TNFR-1 signaling complex.[24,25] TRAF2 and RIP regulate proinflammatory pathways principally through the activation of the transcription factors NFκB (nuclear factor κ-B) and AP-1 (activator protein-1) that leads to the coordinated expression of proinflammatory cytokines, chemokines, enzymes, and adhesion molecules.[26-28] FADD is essential for TNF-induced apoptosis through its association and activation of caspase 8, thereby initiating apoptosis.[20] Deletion of TNFR-1 results in pronounced immunodeficiency with increased susceptibility to *Listeria monocytogenes* and increased endotoxin and TNF resistance.[21,29] Deletion of TNFR-2 results in modest resistance to TNF and defective scab formation.[30] TNFR-2 may facilitate TNF binding to TNFR-1 by initially binding TNF rapidly and then subsequently passing it to TNFR-1.[19,22]

Interleukin-1

The IL-1 family consists of three structurally related polypeptides: IL-1α, IL-1β, and IL-1 receptor antagonist (IL-ra; see the section on proinflammatory inhibitors).[1,31,32] IL-1α and IL-1β are products of distinct genes located on chromosome 2 and are regulated independently.[33, 34] The two molecules share little sequence homology (22 to 26%) but have similar tertiary structures, bind to the same receptors, and share biologic activities.[31]

Both IL-1α and IL-1β are synthesized as large precursor molecules with molecular weights of 31 kDa. Most of IL-1α remains in the cell cytosol in the proform, where it can function in an autocrine fashion or be transported to the cell surface and participate in cell to cell communication.[1,31] IL-1α is also biologically active when it is cleaved to the 17.5-kDa mature protein by membrane-associated cysteine protease calpains and released from the cell.[1,32] IL-1α is rarely observed in the circulation and appears systemically only during severe disease.[32] In contrast, IL-1β is active only in its cleaved mature form, and after secretion, it is the principle mediator of the systemic effects of IL-1. A cysteine protease, IL-1β–converting enzyme (ICE or Caspase 1), is highly specific for processing IL-1β to the mature, biologically active form.[35,36]

IL-1 synthesis is triggered by many of the same stimuli that activate TNF production (i.e., microbial products or inflammation).[31] IL-1 is synthesized by many different cell types, including monocytes, macrophages, neutrophils, epithelial and endothelial cells, fibroblasts, B and T lymphocytes, smooth muscle cells, microglia, and astrocytes.[32]

Interleukin-1 Receptors. Two different receptors bind IL-1, the Type I IL-1 receptor (IL-1RI) and the Type II IL-1R (IL-1RII). Both receptors are members of the IL-1 receptor/Toll-like receptor (IL-1R/TLR) superfamily (Fig. 159–2).[34,37,38] This receptor family also includes receptors for the proinflammatory cytokine IL-18 and receptors for both gram-negative and gram-positive bacterial products. Most members of this family of receptors contain a conserved cytosolic region termed the Toll–IL-1 receptor (TIR) domain.[38-40] The IL-1RI and IL-1RII have similar extracellular characteristics with three immunoglobulin domains and share 28% sequence homology.[40, 41] The IL-1RII, however, contains a cytoplasmic region of only 29 amino acids that does not contain a TIR domain.[1,37] This receptor may serve as a decoy receptor and may decrease the availability of IL-1b to bind to the functionally active IL-1RI (see the section on cytokine inhibitors).[40] IL-1RI is found on most cell types and is important in transducing the action of IL-1.1, 31 IL-1 binds to IL-1RI with low affinity and requires the recruitment of the IL-1 receptor accessory protein (IL-1RAcP) to the receptor to form a high-affinity receptor complex, a requirement for optimal signal transduction.[34]

IL-1β, similar to TNF, activates the nuclear transcription factors NFκB and AP-1, which trigger the synthesis of numerous proinflammatory mediators. IL-1 binding to IL-1RI elicits the formation of a receptor complex with IL-1RAcP. This trimeric complex then recruits the cytosolic protein MyD88 (myeloid differentiation protein 88).[42] MyD88 acts as an adaptor protein and mediates the association of IRAK (serine/threonine IL-1 receptor–associated kinase) with the receptor complex.[43] IRAK is then phosphorylated, triggering dissociation from MyD88 and subsequent association with TRAF6 (TNF receptor–associated factor 6), which, in turn, initiates signaling, leading to the activation of transcription factors.[44] Although IL-1 and TNF share many of the same postreceptor signaling pathways, they are not totally redundant cytokines. IL-1, unlike TNF, cannot activate cellular programmed cell death pathways.

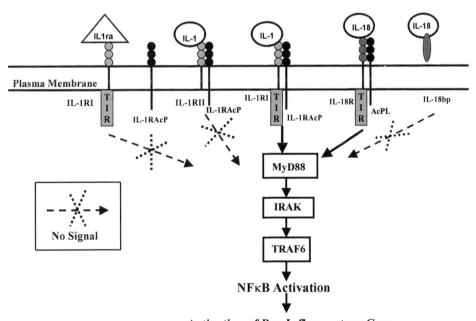

Figure 159–2. Interkeulin-1 (IL-1) and IL-18 receptor family. The IL-1 and IL-18 receptors are members of the interleukin-1/Toll-like receptor family. IL-1 can bind to either the Type I IL-1 receptor (IL-1RI) or the Type II IL-1R (IL 1RII). IL 1 binding to IL-1RI results in the recruitment of the IL-1R accessory protein (IL-1RAcP) to form a complex that activates the MyD88 (myeloid differentiation protein 88) signaling cascade, leading to the activation of the transcription factor nuclear factor κ-B (NFκB) and proinflammatory gene transcription. Members of the IL-1RI signaling complex include MyD88, IRAK (IL-1R associated kinase), and TRAF6 (TNFR-associated factor 6). IL-1ra also binds to the IL-1RI but does not trigger the association of IL-1RAcP and activation of the MyD88 signaling cascade. IL-1RII can bind IL-1, but binding does not result in the formation of a signaling complex. IL-1RII lacks the TIR (Toll/IL-1 receptor) domain and may act as a decoy receptor. IL-18 is also a member of the IL-1/Toll-like receptor family. IL-18 binding to the IL-18R triggers an association with the accessory protein AcPL and activation of the MyD88 signaling cascade. IL-18 can also bind to IL-18bp (IL-18 binding protein) a soluble inhibitor that prevents IL-18 interaction with the IL-18 receptor.

Interleukin-6

IL-6 is a pleiotropic cytokine that can stimulate a multitude of proinflammatory and antiinflammatory cellular alterations. Although IL-6 is a potent inducer of the acute phase response, it also inhibits IL-1 and TNF synthesis and stimulates synthesis of proinflammatory cytokine inhibitors (i.e., sTNFR and IL-1ra).[7,45,46] IL-6 production is stimulated by TNF, IL-1, platelet-derived growth factor, epidermal growth factor, viral and bacterial infections, double-stranded RNA, endotoxin, and cyclic adenosine monophosphate.[47,48] IL-6 is produced by activated monocytes and other cell types, including B and T cells, fibroblasts, endothelial cells, epidermal keratinocytes, and microglia cells.[49]

Interleukin-6 Receptors. The IL-6 receptor system consists of two components. The ligand binding molecule or IL-6R is an 80-kDa glycoprotein (Fig. 159–3).[50] Mutation studies have demonstrated that the cytoplasmic domain of IL-6R is not essential for signal transduction. The second component of the IL-6 receptor system is gp130, a non–ligand binding signal transducer.[51] Both IL-6R and gp130 are members of the cytokine receptor family, which is characterized by four conserved cysteine residues and a tryptophan-serine-X-tryptophan-serine motif above the transmembrane domain.[52, 53] The gp130 is also the common signal transducing subunit for other members of the cytokine receptor family including IL-11, oncostatin-M, ciliary neurotrophic factor, cardiotrophin-1, and leukemia inhibitory factor leading to redundancy in cytokine activity.[54, 55] A soluble form of the IL-6Rα (sIL-6Rα) can also bind IL-6 to form a complex that can then interact with the signal transducing gp130 component in cells that do not express the membrane-bound form of IL-6Rα.[46] Thus, unlike most other soluble cytokine receptors, sIL-6Rα can act as an agonist and can activate cell types that do not respond to IL-6 alone.

Formation of the IL-6 receptor complex leads to activation of gp130 associated tyrosine kinases of the Janus family (JAK) JAK1, JAK2, and Tyk2 resulting in tyrosine phosphorylation of the cytoplasmic domain of gp130.[56-58] These phosphorylated sites serve as docking sites for the transcription factors STAT 1 (signal transducer and activator of transcription-1) and STAT 3. STAT1 and STAT3 are also kinase substrates, and after phosphorylation, they disassociate from the receptor complex and translocate to the cell nucleus, where they initiate expression of target genes. JAK kinases also activate other tyrosine kinases, which, in turn, activate mitogen-activated protein (MAP) kinases and the transcription factors AP-1 and nuclear factor–IL-6 (NF–IL-6).[53, 56, 59]

Interleukin-8 and Chemokines

IL-8 is the prototype of a family of cytokines that are chemotactic for leukocytes. Chemotactic cytokines or chemokines are proinflammatory mediators that orchestrate the recruitment of leukocytes to sites of inflammation. IL-8 is synthesized as a precursor form of 99 amino acids and then, after cleavage of a signal sequence, is secreted in the mature form, with a molecular weight of approximately 8.4 kDa.[60] IL-8 is synthesized by circulating monocytes, macrophages, fibroblasts, endothelial cells, epithelial cells, hepatocytes, keratinocytes, synovial cells, chondrocytes, and some tumor cells.[60, 61] Endotoxin, TNF, and IL-1, but not IL-6, trigger production of IL-8. IL-3, granulocyte-macrophage colony-stimulating factor (GM-CSF), lectins, phorbol esters, immune complexes, and phagocytosis also stimulate IL-8 production.

IL-8 is a member of a supergene family of structurally related 8- to 10-kDa chemotactic cytokines that are characterized by the number and spacing of conserved cysteine residues. The chemokine superfamily contains more than 40 proteins and is divided into 4 subgroups, depending on the position of their conserved cysteine residues, termed CXC, CC, C, and CX₃C.[62-64] The CXC chemokine group contains one amino acid between the first two cysteine residues. CC chemokines contain adjacent cysteine residues. The C chemokine subgroup has a single NH₂-terminal cysteine and contains only one member to date, lymphotactin. The last subgroup CX₃C also contains a single member, fractalkine, which is characterized by separation of the first two cysteine residues by three amino acids.

Members of the family of CXC chemokines arise from different genes clustered around chromosome 4, share sequence homology of between 20 and 50%, and bind to the same receptors.[60,63,64] The CXC chemokine subgroup is further divided into two groups based on the presence or absence of a Glu-Leu-Arg (ELR) motif located before the first cysteine residue and termed ELR⁺CXC and ELR⁻CXC chemokines.[65] ELR⁺CXC chemokines act primarily on neutrophils, whereas ELR⁻CXC chemokines interact with

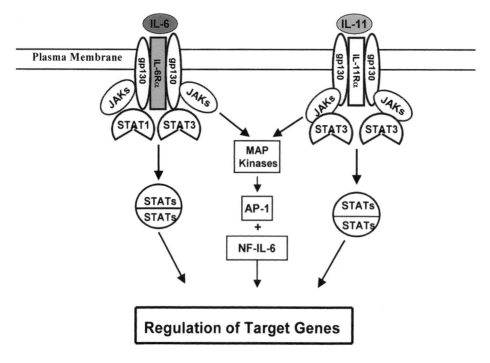

Figure 159–3. Interleukin-6 (IL-6) and IL-11 receptors are members of the IL-6 receptor family and utilize a common signal transducing subunit gp130. IL-6 and IL-11 bind to unique receptor α–chains IL-6Rα and IL-11Rα, respectively. Receptor binding leads to association of gp130 and activation of the JAK/STAT (Janus kinases/signal transducer and activator of transcription) signaling pathway, as well as mitogen-activated protein (MAP) kinases, culminating in activation of gene transcription. AP-1 = activator protein-1; NK = nuclear factor.

mononuclear leukocytes. The ELR+CXC family includes several chemokines with biologic activity similar to that of IL-8, such as GRO-α, GRO-β, GRO-γ, neutrophil activating peptide-2 (NAP-2), epithelial cell–derived neutrophil activating protein-78 (ENA-78), and granulocyte chemotactic protein-2 (GCP-2). CC chemokines act principally on monocytes, basophils, eosinophils, and some lymphocyte subpopulations.[62-64] The best characterized CC chemokine is monocyte chemotactic protein 1 (MCP-1). Other members of the CC chemokine family include MCP-2, MCP-3, RANTES, macrophage inflammatory protein (MIP-1α), and MIP-1β.

Chemokine Receptors. Chemokine receptors are a family of G-protein–coupled receptors composed of at least 10 CC chemokine receptors, 5 CXC chemokine receptors, 1 CX$_3$C chemokine receptor, and 1 C chemokine receptor (Table 159-1).[62,63,66] An unusual feature of this receptor family is their ability to bind more than one chemokine within their particular subclass. An exception is the DARC receptor (Duffy antigen receptor for chemokines) located on erythrocytes and endothelial cells that will bind both CC and CXC chemokines.[62,66] Engagement of this receptor does not appear to activate signal transduction, and DARC may limit leukocyte activation by serving as a chemokine sink.

Two distinct IL-8 receptors (CXCR1 and CXCR2) have been cloned and demonstrate 77% sequence homology.[67,68] CXCR1 binds IL-8 with high affinity and GRO-α and NAP-2 with low

TABLE 159-1
Chemokine Receptors and Their Ligands

Receptors	Ligand
CXC Chemokine Receptors	
CXCR1	IL-8, NAP-2 GROα
CXCR2	ELR+ CXC Chemokines (IL-8, GROα, GROβ, GROγ, NAP-2, ENA-78, GCP-2)
CXCR3	IP-10, MIG, I-TAC
CXCR4	SDF-1
CXCR5	BCA-1
CC Chemokine Receptors	
CCR1	MIP-1α, MCP-3, HCC-2, HCC-4
CCR2	MCP-1, MCP-2, MCP-3, MCP-4
CCR3	Eotaxin, eotaxin-2, eotaxin-3, RANTES, MCP-2, MCP-3, MCP-4
CCR4	TARC, MDC
CCR5	RANTES, MIP-1α, MIP-1β
CCR6	MIP-3α
CCR7	6Ckine, MIP-3β
CCR8	1309, TARC, HCC-4
CCR9	TECK
CCR10	CTACK
CC/CXC Receptor	
DARC Receptor	IL-8, GRO-α, RANTES, MCP-1, MCP-3, MCP-4, eotaxin
C Chemokine Receptor	
CR1	Lymphotactin
CX3C Chemokine Receptor	
CX3CR1	Fractalkine

6Ckine = 6-cysteine chemokine; BCA-1 = B-cell attracting chemokine-1; CTAC = cutaneous T-cell-attracting chemokine; DARC = Duffy antigen receptor for chemokines; ENA-78 = epithelial neutrophil activating protein-78; GCP-2 = Granulocyte chemotactic protein 2; GRO = growth-related oncogene; HCC = hemofiltrate CC chemokine; IP-10 = interferon-γ-inducible protein; I-TAC = interferon inducible T-cell α-chemoattractant; MCP = monocyte chemotactic protein; MDC = macrophage-derived chemoattractant; MIG = monokine induced by interferon-γ; MIP-1 = macrophage inflammatory protein; NAP-2 = neutrophil-activating protein-2; RANTES = regulated on activation normal T cell expressed and secreted; SDF-1 = stromal cell–derived factor-1; TARC = thymus and activation-regulated chemokine; TECK = thymus-expressed chemokine.

affinity, whereas CXCR2 binds most ELR+CXC chemokines.[64] In neutrophils, IL-8 binding to CXCR1 or CXCR2 leads to the activation of G-protein–sensitive phospholipase C, which, in turn, results in the formation of inositol triphosphate and elevation of cytosolic calcium.[60, 61] These receptors also activate other signaling pathways coupled to activation of phosphoinositide 3-kinase, tyrosine kinases, MAP kinase, and low molecular weight proteins Rho and Ras.[69-72] In neutrophils, IL-8 triggers activation and has an important role in the regulation of apoptosis.[61, 73, 74] IL-8 binding also triggers receptor phosphorylation and desensitization, a process thought to be important for continued cellular ability to detect chemotactic gradients.[75]

Interleukin-12

IL-12 is a 74-kDa heterodimer composed of two subunits, an α-chain (p35 subunit) and a β-chain (p40 subunit), which are encoded by separate genes.[76,77] The two subunits are covalently linked by disulfide bonds, a requirement for biologic activity. The p40 subunit of IL-12 contains the receptor binding site, whereas the p30 subunit is required for signal transduction. The two subunits demonstrate little sequence homology, but the p35 subunit shows sequence homology to another proinflammatory cytokine IL-6, whereas the p40 shows homology with the IL-6 receptor.[78, 79] There is speculation that IL-12 may have evolved from a cytokine-cytokine receptor complex that has become covalently linked.[80] IL-12 is produced principally by phagocytic cells, such as monocytes, macrophages, and neutrophils, and by B cells and dendritic cells, in response to bacteria, bacterial products, intracellular pathogens, and viruses.[76,77] The cellular targets of IL-12 are T lymphocytes and NK cells. IL-12 is a potent activator of IFN-γ production, which, in turn, stimulates IL-12 production and creates a positive feedback loop and a strong proinflammatory response but may also lead to uncontrolled cytokine production.[76,77] IL-12 is also essential for Th1 differentiation, which leads to macrophage activation and the production of complement-fixing antibodies.[81]

Interleukin-12 Receptors. IL-12 receptors are expressed primarily on NK and T cells. The receptor is composed of two subunits—IL-12Rβ1 and IL-12Rβ2—and is a member of the gp130 cytokine receptor superfamily.[82] IL-12 signaling is through the JAK/STAT family signal transduction pathway.[83] IL-12 binding to the IL-12 receptor leads to tyrosine phosphorylation of JAK2 and TYK2, subsequent phosphorylation of STAT4, and synthesis of IFN-γ.[76,80,83]

Interferon-γ

IFN-γ is a proinflammatory cytokine produced by activated T cells and NK cells in response to various inflammatory or immune stimuli, including IL-12 and IL-18.[84] T-cell–mediated activation of macrophages is controlled primarily through the production of IFN-γ.[85, 86] In macrophages, IFN-γ triggers cytokine (including TNF) and chemokine synthesis, enhanced superoxide anion generation and nitric oxide (NO) production, and induction of major histocompatibility complex (MHC) class II expression. The biologically active form of IFN-γ is a noncovalent homodimer consisting of two identical polypeptide chains.[86] The cellular targets of IFN-γ are numerous because IFN-γ receptors are present on virtually every cell type, and most of the biologic effects mediated by IFN-γ are through transcriptional regulation of approximately 500 genes.[85,87]

Interferon-γ Receptors. Similar to other cytokine receptor systems, the receptor is composed of two subunits, IFN–γR1, which is necessary for ligand binding, and IFN–γR2, which is involved in signal transduction.[84-86] IFN-γ binding to the IFN–γR1 subunit leads to receptor dimerization and the association of two accessory chains (the IFN–γR2 subunits). Both IFN–γR1 and IFN–γR2 have specific JAK kinases constitutively associated (JAK1 and JAK2, respectively).[88] The formation of the receptor complex results in transphosphorylation of the JAK kinases and subsequent phosphorylation of the IFN–γR1. Tyrosine phosphorylation of the receptor provides a docking site for the cytosolic factor STAT1, which, after receptor phosphorylation, is also phosphorylated. STAT1 phosphorylation results in the formation of STAT complexes, translocation of these complexes to the nucleus, and the regulation of IFN–γ–mediated gene transcription.

Interleukin-18

IL-18 was originally designated the IFN-γ–inducing factor, a factor that stimulated the synthesis of IFN-γ by CD4+ T lymphocytes and had biologic activity similar to that of IL-12.[89] Later studies demonstrated that the IL-18 receptor is a member of the IL-1/Toll-like receptor superfamily,[90, 91] and IL-18 has structural homology with IL-1β. Similar to IL-1β, IL-18 is synthesized in a proform with an unusual signal peptide that lacks the amino acid sequence necessary for secretion.[92,93] Unlike IL-1β, the precursor form of IL-18 has no biologic activity. ProIL-18 is also cleaved by caspase 1 to an 18-kDa nonglycosylated protein. IL-18 is produced by a wide range of cell types including Kupffer cells, macrophages, monocytes, keratinocytes, and osteoblasts in response to inflammatory stimuli, such as lipopolysaccharide (LPS) and exotoxins from gram-positive bacteria.[90,94]

Interleukin-18 Receptors. The IL-18 receptor system is similar to that of the multicomponent IL-1β receptor system (see Fig. 159–2).[34,90,94,95] The IL-18 receptor is composed of two subunits, an IL-18 binding component (IL-18R) and a signal transducing component AcPL that is a homologue of AcP. IL-18 binds to the IL-18R with low affinity that is significantly enhanced with the recruitment of the accessory protein AcPL. Similar to IL-1β receptor system, AcPL does not bind to IL-18; rather, it binds to the IL-18–IL-18R complex. IL-18 binding to the IL-18 receptor complex recruits the same adaptor proteins as IL-1β including MyD88, IRAK, and TRAF-6. These adaptor proteins activate the NFκB, JNK, and MAP kinase signaling pathways. Studies have demonstrated that IL-18 also has an important role in neutrophil migration and activation during inflammation.[96]

Antiinflammatory Cytokines

Interleukin-10

IL-10 was first described as a cytokine synthesis-inhibiting factor and a potent inhibitor of IFN-γ.[97] It is now recognized that IL-10 possesses both potent antiinflammatory and immunosuppressive properties. IL-10 inhibits mononuclear cell synthesis of a wide range of proinflammatory cytokines including TNF, IL-1β, IL-1α, IL-6, IFN-γ, IL-12, IL-18, IL-8, and both CXC and CC chemokines.[7,98-100] In addition to inhibiting the production of proinflammatory cytokines, IL-10 also stimulates the production of natural proinflammatory cytokine inhibitors such as IL-1ra and sTNFRs (see the section on inhibitors of proinflammatory cytokines).[100,101] IL-10 further modulates the proinflammatory response by down-regulating MHC class I expression, oxygen radical production, NO synthesis, and intercellular adhesion molecule-1 (ICAM-1) expression.[7,99-101] These properties make IL-10 a critical factor in the regulation of the magnitude of the inflammatory response and in the prevention of an overwhelming response to inflammation.[99-102] IL-10 is synthesized by numerous cell types including monocytes/macrophages, CD4+ lymphocytes, CD8+ T lymphocytes, B lymphocytes, and epithelial cells in response to bacteria, bacterial products, proinflammatory cytokines, parasites, fungi, and viruses.[100] IL-10 is a homodimer with a molecular weight of 37 kDa whose tertiary structure resembles IFN-γ, a cytokine whose actions are antagonized by IL-10.[100,101]

Interleukin-10 Receptors. IL-10 receptors are members of the class II cytokine receptor family and are expressed predominately on immune cells.[100,103] IL-10R is composed of two subunits, a ligand binding subunit and an accessory subunit. The accessory subunit associates with the receptor after IL-10 binding and is required for signal transduction. Similar to other members of this cytokine receptor family, the receptor complex interacts with members of the JAK family, specifically Jak1 and Tyk2. IL-10 binding triggers tyrosine phosphorylation and activation of the transcription factors Stat3 and Stat1.[104] Critical to its potent antiinflammatory properties, IL-10 inhibits nuclear translocation of the transcriptional factor NFκB and subsequent synthesis of proinflammatory cytokines as well as promoting degradation of mRNA of proinflammatory cytokines.[101,105]

Interleukin-4 and Interleukin-13

IL-4 and IL-13 are products of activated T cells, basophils, and mast cells.[106,107] IL-4 is a 20-kDa glycosylated protein, and IL-13 is a 10-kDa nonglycosylated protein. Although IL-4 and IL-13 have only 20 to 25% amino acid sequence homology, their tertiary structures are highly homologous, and they possess numerous overlapping biologic properties.[7,108-111] Both IL-4 and IL-13 are potent antiinflammatory cytokines that are capable of inhibiting monocyte/macrophage production of proinflammatory cytokines and chemokines. Moreover, IL-4 and IL-13 up-regulate the synthesis of antiinflammatory IL-1ra and promote adherence by increasing expression of adherence molecules. The overlapping biologic properties of these two cytokines are the result of a common component in their respective receptor complexes.[112] However, the two cytokines do not share all biologic properties; most notable is that IL-4, but not IL-13, can promote Th2 lymphocyte differentiation.[109] The functional differences of these cytokines are the result of cell-dependent differential receptor expression.

Interleukin-4 and Interleukin-13 Receptors. The IL-4 receptor consists of two components. The first is a ligand binding chain (IL-4Rα), which it shares with the IL-13 receptor complex and is a member of the hematopoietin receptor superfamily (Fig. 159–4).[109,112-114] The other component is the common γ–signaling chain (γc), which is also an essential component of IL-2, IL-7, IL-9, and IL-15 receptors. IL-4 binds to the IL-4Rα chain with high affinity that triggers heterodimerization of IL-4Rα with the γc chain, a required element for activation of the IL-4 signaling pathway. IL-13 also indirectly interacts with the IL-4Rα. IL-13 binds to a specific binding chain termed IL-13Rα1, which triggers the recruitment of IL-4Rα to the receptor complex and results in enhanced IL-13 binding affinity and the initiation of signaling.[115] A second IL-13 binding component has been identified, IL-13Rα2, which binds IL-13 with higher affinity than IL-13Rα1.[116] The function of IL-13Rα2 has not been fully elucidated, but it may serve as a decoy receptor to down-regulate IL-13 activity. Signaling of both IL-4 and IL-13 is principally mediated through the IL-4Rα chain and involves activation of the transcription factor STAT6.[112-114,117,118] IL-4 binding induces the phosphorylation of the JAK1 associated with the IL-4Rα chain and JAK3 associated with the γc chain. These kinases, in turn, phosphorylate the IL-4Rα chain itself, as well as STAT6, resulting in IL-4–induced gene expression. IL-13 also activates similar signaling pathways. IL-13 binding stimulates phosphorylation of JAK1 associated with the IL-4Rα chain and another member of the JAK family, TYK2, associated with the IL-13Rα1 chain. IL-13 also activates STAT6 presumably via signaling mediated by the IL-4Rα chain. In addition, IL-4 and IL-13 both activate the phosphoinositide 3-kinase pathway, a pathway thought to be critical in IL-4/IL-13 induced cell survival and protection from apoptosis.[113,114,117,119,120]

Interleukin-11

The pleiotropic antiinflammatory IL-11 is a 23-kDa nonglycosylated protein produced by fibroblasts, epithelial cells, and osteoblasts in response to various different stimuli, including

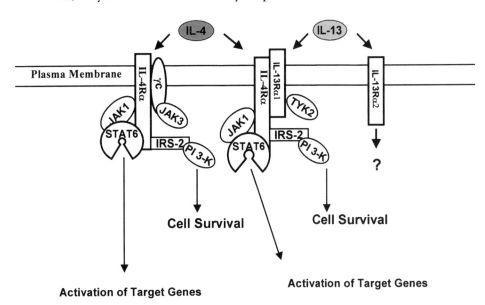

Figure 159–4. Interleukin-4 (IL-4) and IL-13 receptor complexes. The IL-4 receptor (IL-4R) is composed of IL-4Rα and γc subunits, whereas the IL-13 receptor (IL-13R) includes both IL-4Rα and IL-13Rα subunits. IL-4 can bind to both the IL-4 and IL-13 receptor via the common IL-4Rα–chain. In contrast, IL-13 only binds to the IL-13 receptor via the IL-13Rα1 subunit. Both receptors activate STAT6 and IRS-2 (insulin receptor substrate 2) signaling pathways resulting in the induction of gene expression and cell survival pathways. IL-13 also binds to IL-13Rα2 whose function is unclear but may serve as a decoy receptor.

IL-1, TGF-β, TNF, parathyroid hormone, respiratory syncytial virus, rhinovirus, and parainfluenza virus.[121-123] IL-11 is a member of the IL-6 family, proteins that share a four-helix bundle fold motif.[124] Similar to IL-6, IL-11 inhibits production of proinflammatory cytokines and NO, and it is able to induce the acute phase response.[125, 126] IL-11 ablates TNF and IL-1β synthesis through a direct inhibition of gene expression by inhibiting transcription factor NFκB.[127]

Interleukin-11 Receptor. The IL-11 receptor is similar to other members of the IL-6 family of receptors and is composed of an IL-11–specific α chain that binds IL-11 and the gp130 subunit, which is the common receptor β-chain subunit and functions as the signal transduction component of this receptor family (see Fig. 159-3).[128,129] The binding of IL-11 to the IL-11α receptor triggers homodimerization of the gp130 subunit and formation of an IL-11 receptor complex.[130] Signaling through the gp130 receptor is via JAK/STAT pathways.[123, 124] Activation of this signaling pathway by IL-11 is predominantly mediated by JAK1 and STAT3.[131] Other signaling pathways activated by IL-11 include the Ras/MAP kinase pathway, protein kinase C, and Src families.[123]

Inhibitors of Proinflammatory Cytokines

Soluble Tumor Necrosis Factor Receptors

Both the TNFR-1 and TNFR-2 receptors are expressed on the surface of most cell types. In response to various proinflammatory stimuli such as IL-6, IL-1β, IL-2, IFN-γ, and TNF itself, TNFR-1 and TNFR-2 can be proteolytically cleaved and the extracellular cytokine binding domains released from the cell surface.[132, 133] The protease responsible for cleavage of the TNF receptors has yet to be identified, but it is thought to be a membrane-bound nonmatrix metalloproteinase.[134] The shed TNF receptors or soluble TNFRs (sTNFRs) retain their ability to bind TNF and compete with membrane-bound TNF receptors leading to decreased availability of circulating TNF.[135] The shedding of these receptors from the cell surface also serves to decrease a cell's responsiveness to TNF by decreasing the receptor number. sTNFRs are thought to be a part of a negative feedback loop to regulate TNF bioactivity, to control inflammation, and to restore homeostasis. However, sTNFRs can act as agonists as well as antagonists of TNF bioactivity.[132, 136, 137] TNF binding to sTNFRs forms a stable complex and enhances the half-life of circulating TNF.[132] The TNF-sTNFR complex may act as a reservoir and may prolong TNF bioactivity. sTNFRs have been detected in the

plasma and urine of patients with sepsis, and increased TNF/sTNFR ratios are correlated with increased mortality.[138-140]

Interleukin-1ra and Interleukin-1RII

IL-1ra and IL-1RII are two natural regulators of IL-1 biologic activity.[7, 32, 141] Synthesis of IL-1ra is triggered by the same stimuli that trigger IL-1 production, and it is produced by the same cell types. IL-1ra is structurally similar to IL-1α and IL-1β and has a molecular weight similar to that of the mature form of IL-1β. Sequencing studies have shown 26% homology with IL-1β and 19% homology with IL-1α. IL-1ra is a competitive inhibitor and binds to the IL-1RI with similar affinity as IL-1α and IL-1β, but it has no agonist activity (see Fig. 159-2). Structural studies have revealed that IL-1α and IL-1β, in contrast to IL-1ra, bind at multiple sites on the IL-1RI.[142] This type of binding may produce conformational changes in the receptor-ligand complex that permit the association of IL-1RAcP and the activation of signal transduction. IL-1ra binding to the IL-1RI does not trigger the association of IL-1RAcP and the formation of a heterodimer.[143] During the inflammatory response, IL-1ra levels tend to increase later than IL-1, a finding suggesting that IL-1ra functions to block further IL-1 activity and has a role in the termination of the inflammatory response.[144] Administration of IL-1ra to animals reduced inflammation in various different diseases.[7,32,141]

IL-1RII is present as both a membrane-bound receptor and, in a truncated form, as a soluble receptor.[34, 37, 145] The receptor acts as a decoy receptor for IL-1 and is the principal IL-1 receptor on neutrophils, monocytes, macrophages, and B cells.[1,31,40] The extracellular domain of the IL-1RII is similar to that of the IL-1RI and has high affinity for IL-1β but much lower binding affinity for IL-1α and IL-1ra. After IL-1 binding, IL-1RII associates with the IL-1AcP. However, IL-1RII lacks the TIR (Toll/IL-1R) region, and without this domain, the receptor cannot interact with MyD88 and initiate signal transduction (see Fig. 159-2). Thus, the membrane-bound IL-1RII may act as ligand sink by competing for IL-1 binding with the active IL-1RI and by reducing the concentration of available AcP. IL-1RII also exists in a soluble truncated form, and circulating levels are increased during inflammation.[146, 147] The extracellular domain of the IL-1RII is released from the cell surface by proteolytic cleavage by matrix metalloproteases to form a soluble IL-1RII (sIL-1RII).[148] Shedding of the IL-1RII is regulated by two major mechanisms.[145] Antiinflammatory agents, such as IL-4, IL-13, and glucocorticoids, increase gene expression of IL-1RII, enhanced cell surface expression, and subsequent extracellular shedding. Alternatively, rapid shedding of the IL-1RII is triggered by reactive oxygen intermediates, LPS, TNF, and chemoattractants. sIL-1RII binds IL-1β but not IL-1α or IL-1ra and may serve to inhibit the systemic effects of IL-1.

In summary, IL-1 activity is modulated by two different modes of regulation. IL-1ra competitively blocks IL-1 binding to the signaling IL-1RI. A second mechanism of regulation is IL-1RII or decoy receptor, which can bind both IL-1 and IL-1AcP and can prevent their interaction with an active receptor (i.e., IL-1RI). Furthermore, cleavage and release of sIL-1RII into the circulation further serve to modulate systemic IL-1 activity.

Interleukin-18 Binding Protein

Another member of the Toll/IL-1R family is IL-18. IL-18, similar to IL-1 and TNF, has a naturally occurring circulating inhibitor. However, unlike sTNFR or IL-1RII, IL-18 binding protein (IL-18bp) is not a truncated form of the extracellular domain of the IL-18 receptor. Rather, IL-18bp is a naturally occurring antagonist of IL-18 that binds to IL-18 with high affinity and prevents binding to the IL-18 receptor (see Fig. 159–2).[149] The high binding affinity and slow disassociation rate make this a potent inhibitor and not a carrier protein.[150] IL-18bp is composed of a single immunoglobulin domain and lacks a transmembrane and cytoplasmic domain. IL-18bp is not membrane associated and is secreted rather than cleaved from the cell surface.[149, 151] Circulating IL-18bp is present in healthy individuals and is significantly elevated in sepsis.[150] The administration of exogenous IL-18bp protects against lethality in experimental endotoxemia, a finding suggesting an important immunomodulating role for this soluble binding protein.[151, 152]

Inflammation

Inflammation is a protective response after attack by either exogenous agents (microbial, chemical, or physical) or endogenous factors (immunologic or neurologic).[153] The inflammatory response is characterized by the accumulation and subsequent activation of leukocytes in affected tissue. The process is initiated when inflammatory cells at the site of inflammation, such as macrophages, are activated and rapidly produce TNF and IL-1. These cytokines, in turn, activate a cytokine cascade, which generates proinflammatory cytokines IL-6, IL-8, and other chemokines.[1, 2, 5] In addition to proinflammatory cytokines, other mediators such as NO, platelet-activating factor (PAF), prostaglandins, and leukotrienes are also produced. These cascades are responsible for activating complement, coagulation, and kinin cascades as well. As inflammation progresses, antiinflammatory cytokines and cytokine inhibitors are produced, which serve to contain the inflammatory response and to bring about its resolution.

The accumulation of specific subpopulations of leukocytes at the site of inflammation is the result of a series of events: (1) endothelial cell activation and the expression of adhesion molecules; (2) leukocyte expression of adhesion molecules and leukocyte-endothelial cell adhesion; (3) leukocyte transendothelial migration; (4) leukocyte migration along a chemotactic gradient; and (5) the release of reactive oxidants, proteinases, and antimicrobial polypeptides at the site of inflammation.[13] Cytokines are involved at each step of this process and act both locally and systemically to initiate, maintain, and finally resolve the inflammatory response.[1, 5]

Local Effects

At the site of inflammation, the local release of TNF and IL-1 and other proinflammatory cytokines including IL-8, IL-12, IL-18, IL-6, and IFN-γ leads to the activation of endothelial cells and the expression or up-regulation of adhesion molecules such as selectins, ICAMs, platelet-endothelial cell adhesion molecule-1 (PECAM-1), and vascular cell adhesion molecule (VCAM-1).[154–157] This event initiates leukocyte endothelial interaction. Increased endothelial cell surface expression of the adhesion molecules E-selectins and P-selectins (in conjunction with the constitutively expressed L-selectin on leukocytes) mediates the initial adhesive interaction resulting in the leukocyte's rolling along the endothelium.

TNF, IL-1, and IL-18, as well as IFN-γ and IL-4, stimulate the local production of CXC chemokines that promote leukocyte surface expression of the adhesion molecules β₂ integrins and the shedding of L-selectins.[62, 96, 154, 155, 158] The interactions between leukocyte β₂ integrins and endothelial counterligands such as ICAM-1, ICAM-2, and ICAM-3 mediate the firm attachment of the leukocytes to the endothelium and subsequent migration.[66, 155]

Movement of leukocytes to the inflammatory site is directed along a chemotactic gradient, where the strongest concentration of chemoattractants is at the site of inflammation. Local production of chemokines by both immune and nonimmune cells serves as a source for long-lasting chemoattractants. The persistence of chemokines in a stable form ensures prolonged biologic activity for recruitment of neutrophils and monocytes.[60, 156] The movement of specific populations of leukocytes into the inflammatory site depends on the specific stimuli and the resultant type of chemokines synthesized (i.e., CXC chemokines [i.e., IL-8] versus CC chemokines [i.e., MCP-1]).[62, 153] Thus, the movement of leukocytes is a cytokine-mediated process and the result of coordination of endothelial expression of adhesion molecules, leukocyte adherence, and specific chemotactic gradients.[159]

Cytokines are also directly involved in the activation of cells at the inflammatory site. After recruitment of inflammatory cells to the site of inflammation, cytokines can further amplify the inflammatory response through the activation of transcription factors, such as NFκB, which regulate proinflammatory gene expression. Both TNF and IL-1 increase the expression of genes for proinflammatory cytokines, chemokines, adhesion molecules, inducible NO synthase, matrix metalloproteinases, and cyclooxygenase 2.[28] Furthermore, IL-1 and TNF are part of an amplifying loop where these cytokines enhance their own production and prolong local inflammatory responses.

Cytokines and chemokines can also affect the activation of resident and recruited phagocytic cells. Both CXC and CC chemokines are capable of triggering, in their specific target cells, the generation of oxygen radicals. Chemokines also trigger exocytosis of secretory vesicles and specific granules resulting in release of enzymes and other soluble proteins.[60, 61, 66] TNF and IL-1 can prime leukocytes for enhanced phagocytosis, antibody-dependent cytotoxicity, oxygen radical production, and degranulation triggered by a second stimulus such as f-methionine-leucine phenylalanine (fMLP).[32, 160, 161] In adherent neutrophils, TNF triggers the release of oxygen radicals and degradative granule enzymes such as elastase and promotes cytoskeleton reorganization.[162, 163] IFN-γ also acts directly on phagocytic cells and enhances bactericidal activity, phagocytosis, NO synthesis, and oxygen radical production.[80, 87] Studies have demonstrated that IL-18 has a direct role in neutrophil activation and can induce cytokine and chemokine release, increased β₂ integrin expression, and degranulation.[96] Antiinflammatory cytokines can also modulate local activation of phagocytic cells. IL-10, IL-11, IL-4, and IL-13 can inhibit proinflammatory cytokine synthesis, suppress oxygen radical production, and down-regulate NO synthesis, thereby further limiting the local inflammatory response.[101, 105, 108–110, 122, 125]

TNF, IL-1, and IFN-γ also stimulate the release of potent lipid mediators such as PAF, leukotrienes, thromboxane, and prostaglandins.[31, 164–167] These lipid mediators are important in the regulation of vascular tone and permeability. Leukotriene B₄ is a potent chemoattractant, enhances cytokine production, and triggers degranulation and oxygen radical generation. PAF and prostaglandin E₂ (PGE₂) are also potent phagocytic cell activators, but PGE₂ also possesses antiinflammatory properties and down-regulates cytokine production.

Proinflammatory cytokines also play another important role at the site of inflammation. Neutrophils have a relatively short life span in the circulation and undergo spontaneous or constitutive apoptosis within 6 to 10 hours. Neutrophils undergoing apoptosis have decreased oxygen radical production, degranulation, and phagocytosis in response to inflammatory stimuli.[168, 169] TNF and other proinflammatory cytokines delay neutrophil apoptosis, thus prolonging the functional capabilities of neutrophils at the site of inflammation.[170, 171] Thus, cytokines are involved both in trafficking specific populations of leukocytes to the site of inflammation and in the activation process once the leukocytes arrive at their destination.

Coagulation

The coagulation system is activated during the inflammatory response and is an essential component of the host response. Coagulation is initiated by the expression of tissue factor (TF) on the surface of endothelium and monocytes.[172] The proinflammatory cytokines TNF, IL-1, and IL-6 promote the expression of TF and activation of the extrinsic pathway of coagulation resulting in thrombin production and ultimately fibrin deposition.[173-175] Studies have also implicated IL-12, IL-8, and the chemokine MCP-1 as procoagulation mediators.[6, 174, 176, 177] Proinflammatory cytokines further enhance the procoagulation state by also inhibiting key anticoagulation pathways. TNF and IL-1 inhibit the synthesis and release of thrombomodulin, resulting in the impairment of thrombin-mediated protein C activation and the subsequent inhibition of that anticoagulation pathway.[13, 178] Fibrinolysis is suppressed by TNF through the inhibition of tissue-type plasminogen activator release.[179] Tissue-type plasminogen activator is essential for the conversion of plasminogen to the active protease plasmin.[13] Plasmin can dissolve the fibrin network in thrombi. Fibrinolysis is also limited by TNF and IL-1–mediated release of plasminogen-activator inhibitors (e.g., PAI-1), which further inhibit the conversion of plasminogen to plasmin.[13, 179, 180] The stimulation of the extrinsic coagulation pathway, coupled with the inhibition of fibrinolysis, is thought to promote containment and localization of the inflammatory site. However, the activation of the coagulation pathway can further up-regulate the inflammatory response through cross-talk between the two pathways. For example, thrombin binding to its receptor triggers the activation of NFκB, the synthesis of proinflammatory cytokines, and the release of NO.[172, 181] Antiinflammatory cytokines also regulate coagulation. *In vitro*, IL-4, IL-10, and IL-13 modulate TF expression.[182] *In vivo* administration of IL-10 reduced LPS-activation of the coagulation pathway as well as modulated the fibrinolytic system.[183] Although the coagulation system is critical for maintaining homeostasis and the containment of inflammatory stimuli, if it is not adequately regulated, it can lead to the development of disseminated intravascular coagulation and multiple organ failure.

Systemic Effects

Proinflammatory cytokines, either acting alone or synergistically, can produce systemic alterations in host physiology. These systemic alterations include induction of fever, stimulation of hepatic acute phase response, and nonspecific activation of host immune systems.

Fever. IL-1 (previously known as endogenous pyrogen), TNF, and IL-6 are able to raise the temperature set point of an organism and cause fever.[184,185] These cytokines induce the hypothalamic production of prostaglandins, particularly PGE_2, which, through interaction with the EP_3 receptor, stimulates neurotransmitters such as cyclic adenosine monophosphate and increases body temperature.[186] Other proinflammatory cytokines, for example IFN-γ, may indirectly cause fever through induction of IL-1 and TNF synthesis. Cytokines that are members of the same receptor families as pyrogenic proinflammatory

cytokines do not necessarily trigger fever. The IL-18 receptor is a member of the IL-1/Toll-like receptor superfamily, but unlike IL-1 and LPS, it does not trigger PGE_2 synthesis *in vitro* or fever when it is administered *in vivo*.[187] Similarly, IL-11 and IL-6 are both members of the gp130 cytokine family, and both activate the acute phase response.[188] In contrast to IL-6, IL-11 does not produce fever.[189] IL-10 is an endogenous antipyretic cytokine and most likely modulates fever through the inhibition of proinflammatory cytokine synthesis.[190]

Acute Phase Reaction. The synthesis and release of hepatic acute phase proteins are an important mechanism in modulating the inflammatory response and the restoration of homeostasis. Acute phase proteins have diverse biologic activities, and they include antiproteases, antioxidants, activators of the complement system, blood clotting agents, and immune response modulators.[191,192] The hepatic acute phase is regulated principally by IL-6, but other members of the IL-6 family including IL-11, can also induce the acute phase response.[53, 189, 193] TNF, IL-1, IFN-γ, and possibly IL-8 also induce synthesis of various hepatic acute phase proteins.[192, 194, 195] The acute phase reaction is terminated indirectly through the inhibition of proinflammatory cytokine synthesis by IL-4, IL-13, and IL-10.[123, 196] Natural inhibitors of TNF, IL-1, and IL-6, including soluble receptors and receptor antagonists, can also remove excess IL-6, IL-1, and TNF. IL-4, in contrast to other antiinflammatory cytokines, can inhibit synthesis of select hepatic acute phase proteins.[197] Acute phase proteins themselves are also capable of modulating the proinflammatory response through the induction of cytokine antagonists such as IL-1ra.[198] Thus, cross-talk between cytokines and the hepatic acute phase response contributes to the resolution of the inflammatory response.

Inflammatory Diseases

It is now widely believed that proinflammatory cytokines play a central role in inflammatory diseases of infectious or noninfectious origin. TNF triggers a cytokine cascade that initially is composed of the proinflammatory cytokines (IL-1, IL-6, IL-8, IL-12, IFN-γ, IL-18, and TNF itself).[5, 6, 13] These cytokines serve to contain and resolve the inflammatory foci through activation of local and systemic inflammatory responses. TNF also triggers a cytokine cascade of the antiinflammatory cytokines that block proinflammatory cytokine synthesis, as well as cytokine inhibitors that block proinflammatory cytokine actions.[6, 7, 8] In most cases, the inflammatory response is successfully resolved. Overzealous production of cytokines or the inability to shut down proinflammatory cytokine production, however, can lead to increasing concentrations of cytokines in the systemic circulation. This can have a deleterious effect on the host, with the development of hypotension, intravascular thrombosis, pulmonary edema, and hemorrhage, and, if left unchecked, it can lead to multiple organ failure and death. This condition is often referred to as the *systemic inflammatory response syndrome*.[199] This term describes the clinical manifestations of widespread endothelial inflammation that leads to increased vascular permeability.[5, 166] This condition is thought to be the initiating factor in diverse disease disorders, such as bacterial sepsis, ischemia, burn injury, trauma and tissue injury, and hemorrhagic shock.

It has become apparent that interactions between proinflammatory and antiinflammatory mediators regulate the inflammatory response.[4, 6, 7] Antiinflammatory cytokines, in particular IL-10, inhibit proinflammatory cytokine synthesis and adhesion molecule expression while increasing the levels of specific cytokine inhibitors. Excess production of antiinflammatory cytokines, however, can compromise the hosts' ability to clear microorganisms through suppression of immune cell function. If a balance is not maintained, the result is either an excessive proinflammatory response or, alternatively, immunosuppression and increased susceptibility to secondary infection. Thus, although the cytokine cascade triggered by TNF is often beneficial to the host by initiating the inflammatory response, overproduction or underproduction of proinflammatory or antiinflammatory endogenous mediators may actually be deleterious to the host. Studies suggest a genetic predisposition that determines the balance of proinflammatory and antiinflammatory cytokines and, hence, susceptibility to disease.[7, 39, 200] Various polymorphisms have been identified within cytokine and cytokine receptor genes that alter their expression. These cytokine and cytokine receptor polymorphisms may determine the balance of proinflammatory and antiinflammatory cytokines in the inflammatory response.

CLINICAL APPLICATION OF CYTOKINE PHYSIOLOGY IN NEWBORN INFANTS

Cytokine Physiology in Newborn Infants

The newborn period represents a time of increased risk for the development of bacterial infection and increased mortality from sepsis.[201, 202] Among other factors known to increase the risk of bacterial infection is a functional immaturity of newborn immune mechanisms. Both immunoglobulin and complement levels are low, and leukocyte functions, including the secretion of inflammatory mediators, may be deficient.[203-205] Only recently has attention been directed to developmental aspects of the immune response.

The fetus and newborn infant are unique from the standpoint of immunity and infection. The fetus lives in a sterile, immunologically protected environment. However, it is during this time that the development of the immune system is initiated—a highly complex process mediated, at least in part, by the expression of cytokines.[206, 207] Fetal cytokines are known to play a role in the regulation of hematopoiesis and to protect the fetus against rejection. Placental and fetal cytokines also protect the fetus against infection.[206, 207] Evidence suggests that cytokines in the fetus and neonate play a role in the pathophysiology of severe neonatal diseases including sepsis, bronchopulmonary dysplasia (BPD), and necrotizing enterocolitis (NEC).[208-211]

In the past, therapeutic strategies were aimed exclusively at killing the bacteria that caused neonatal infection. It has become evident, however, that many infants die after the sterilization of blood cultures with antimicrobial agents.[212, 213] It is now appreciated that the physiologic derangements that occur during sepsis are secondary to the host response induced by the pathogenic microorganisms. During overwhelming sepsis, the host produces certain proinflammatory cytokines, which initiate a cascade of events resulting in tissue injury at distant sites and generalized multiorgan system failure.[213, 214] This inflammatory response has its origins during the fetal period.[206, 207] Thus, the heightened morbidity and mortality in neonatal sepsis results from physiologic deficiencies in immune function, as well as the pathophysiologic alterations produced by bacterial byproducts.[212, 213] This section discusses the development of the inflammatory response in the fetus and neonate, the production of inflammatory mediators, and their role in the inflammatory response to specific disease processes in newborn infants.

Cytokine Production in Newborn Infants

When compared with the data collected in adults, considerably less is known regarding the production and release of cytokines in the fetus and newborn infant. Data indicate that the proinflammatory cytokines mediate many of the pathophysiologic events during bacterial sepsis. Moreover, there is growing evidence that the fetal inflammatory response plays a major role in the induction of several neonatal diseases. Thus, attention has been focused on determining the capability of monocytes from

newborn infants to produce these cytokines and the balance of proinflammatory and antiinflammatory mediators in the fetus and neonate.

Tumor Necrosis Factor

TNF is an early proximal mediator in the cytokine cascade.[215, 216] This cytokine is produced by human fetal Kupffer cells as well as placental mononuclear cells in response to stimulation by LPS.[217, 218] TNF can be found in amniotic fluid during the second and third trimesters and increases with premature rupture of membranes.[219] Several (but not all) investigators have demonstrated a significant but modest decrease in TNF production by cord blood monocytes.[220-224] In addition, LPS-stimulated cord blood cells from preterm infants secrete significantly less TNF than monocytes obtained from either the term or adult control groups.[222] When analyzed in culture, monocyte/macrophages derived from newborn infants also secreted diminished amounts of TNF when compared with adult cells.[223-225] Kwak and colleagues examined TNF production by cord blood mononuclear cells in response to stimulation by group B streptococci.[226] In contrast to the immediate response to LPS (in which TNF, IL-1β, IL-6, and IL-8 appeared almost simultaneously), stimulation by group B streptococci resulted in increased TNF production but a delayed appearance of the other cytokines.

Abnormalities of TNF production and release, particularly in the preterm infant, may represent a significant factor in the resistance to bacterial infection in this age group. TNF receptor expression may also be diminished. Using flow cytometry and a human recombinant TNF that binds to the 75- and 55-kDa receptors, Chheda and co-workers demonstrated that expression of TNF receptors on cord blood monocytes was also reduced when compared with that of adult cells.[225] Moreover, these findings suggest a dissociation between the production and release of TNF and other cytokines, such as IL-1.

Interleukin-1

IL-1 is also an integral mediator in the cytokine cascade that is produced by fetal Kupffer cells in response to LPS.[217] IL-1 is present in amniotic fluid and increases with premature rupture of membranes.[219] Production of IL-1 by cord blood monocytes is comparable to that in adult controls, even in monocytes obtained from preterm infants.[220-222, 224, 227-230] However, in preterm infants with bacterial sepsis, monocyte IL-1 secretion was lower during the acute infectious phase, but improved significantly during the convalescence period.[231] Bry and co-workers found high levels of the antiinflammatory IL-1ra in the urine of newborn infants, comparable to levels detected in amniotic fluid.[232] Female fetuses have significantly higher urinary IL-1ra levels.[232]

Although monocytes, endothelial cells, and fibroblasts are thought to be the primary sources of cytokine production, neutrophils also possess that capability, albeit in lesser amounts. After stimulation with LPS or TNF, Contrino and associates found significantly increased expression of IL-1 by cord blood neutrophils compared with that in cells from adults.[233] Although neutrophils function primarily as rapid effector cells with little immunoregulatory function, IL-1 secretion by neutrophils may be important in the amplification of the early inflammatory response.

Interleukin-6

IL-6 also plays an important role in mediating the host response to inflammation and infection.[234] The production of IL-6 is induced by other cytokines, notably IL-1 and GM-CSF, and studies have suggested that it may be more of an effector than an initiator of the inflammatory response during sepsis. After stimulation with LPS, IL-6 is produced by human fetal Kupffer cells as early as 13 weeks after conception.[218] This cytokine has also been detected in the amniotic fluid during infection.[235] Several studies have evaluated IL-6 production by monocytes from newborn infants.[220, 227, 235-238] Liechty and colleagues demonstrated equivalent IL-6 production by fetal and maternal mononuclear cells after stimulation with IL-1.[235] However, reduced IL-6 production was demonstrated in cells from preterm neonates, perhaps contributing to their enhanced susceptibility to overwhelming bacterial infection.[235] Despite the fully developed capacity of whole cord blood to synthesize IL-6 after LPS stimulation, Seghaye and associates[220] found that neonatal circulating IL-6 levels were significantly lower than corresponding maternal values. In contrast, Schultz and colleagues,[208] using flow cytometry, found that after LPS stimulation, both term and preterm monocytes displayed a higher percentage of IL-6 positive cells than adults, a finding suggesting an enhanced inflammatory response in these infants.[208, 225]

Zola and associates demonstrated that cord blood lymphocytes express both the gp80 and the gp130 IL-6 receptor, although generally at lower levels than adult cells.[239] The immunofluorescence staining patterns for IL-6 receptors on monocytes were similar for cord and adult cells; however, data are limited.

Interleukin-8

IL-8 is a low molecular weight cytokine that is produced by mononuclear and endothelial cells and attracts and activates neutrophils.[240] Little is known about the expression and function of IL-8 in the fetus. Using cord blood mononuclear cells stimulated with endotoxin, Taniguchi and co-workers found that IL-8 production was significantly greater in neonates born to mothers with chorioamnionitis compared with those born to healthy women.[241] In this study, neonatal mononuclear cells produced IL-8 in a time- and dose-dependent manner; equivalent amounts were produced by mononuclear cells from preterm and term infants. In a similar fashion, Seghaye and associates observed that IL-8 production by cord blood and production by adult blood cultures were similar.[220] Moreover, circulating plasma IL-8 levels were not significantly different in cord and maternal blood. Using flow cytometry to analyze cytokine production at the single cell level, Schultz and colleagues found enhanced IL-8 production by neonatal monocytes after LPS stimulation.[208] In this study, cells from both term and preterm infants displayed a higher percentage of IL-8 positive cells than adults, a finding challenging the existing view of an immature neonatal inflammatory response.[208] Hebra and associates also noted both higher basal and stimulated IL-8 production by fetal (cord blood) monocytes.[227] IL-8 levels in whole cord blood specimens increase in response to the stress of labor and delivery.[242]

Although early studies suggested deficiencies in IL-8 production by neonatal mononuclear cells, more recent literature indicates an intact proinflammatory cytokine pathway.[213, 214, 243, 244] Furthermore, these heightened proinflammatory responses may be detrimental to the host, and elevated levels have been found in several neonatal diseases, including cerebral white matter damage, BPD, and NEC.[208]

Interleukin-10

IL-10 is an antiinflammatory cytokine that decreases the expression and function of proinflammatory cytokines, including TNF, IL-1, and IL-8.[100, 102] In addition, IL-10 limits the participation of helper T cells in delayed hypersensitivity and protects against inflammation. During the fetal period, placental production of IL-10 may prevent immune rejection.[207, 245] Neonates exhibit decreased IL-10 production.[209, 246, 247] Chheda and colleagues demonstrated decreased production of IL-10 by newborn mononuclear cells after LPS stimulation,[225] which may be secondary to abnormal regulatory processes involving TNF and its receptors. Although it is less well explored than other

cytokines, diminished production of IL-10 may contribute to the enhanced proinflammatory state in newborn infants.

Fetal and Neonatal Cytokines in the Inflammatory Response

The fetus and newborn infant are uniquely susceptible to the development of bacterial infection as well as heightened mortality from infectious disease. In adults, cytokines have been implicated as endogenous mediators elaborated during the pathogenesis of sepsis and shock. Work in developmental immunobiology has also suggested that cytokines contribute to the inflammatory response in the fetus and newborn infant with chorioamnionitis, sepsis, NEC, and BPD.

Chorioamnionitis and Brain Injury

Evidence suggests that intrauterine infection is a cause of cerebral palsy in both term and preterm infants. Both clinical and subclinical chorioamnionitis may trigger an inflammatory response in the mother and fetus associated with the elaboration of proinflammatory cytokines. This fetal inflammatory response is thought to contribute to the development of neonatal brain injury and subsequent cerebral palsy.[248-250]

The cytokines TNF, IL-1β, and IL-6 are normally present in amniotic fluid, with levels increasing until term gestation.[248] During the course of intrauterine infection, however, levels of these proinflammatory cytokines are significantly increased and have been correlated with the initiation of preterm labor.[251] Although chorioamnionitis was traditionally considered a maternal infection, more recent evidence suggests that a fetal inflammatory reaction is initiated in response to placental inflammation.[248-250] Observations by Dammann and Leviton support the hypothesis of a fetal vasculitis as part of the response to perinatal infection.[253]

Exposure to LPS during pregnancy is associated with the release of the proinflammatory cytokines TNF, IL-1, and IL-6. Several studies have demonstrated elevations of both amniotic fluid and plasma cytokines as evidence of both maternal and fetal involvement.[254, 255] More recent studies associate these cytokine elevations with the risk of neonatal brain injury and cerebral palsy.[251, 253, 256] In infants who subsequently developed periventricular leukomalacia,[251, 252, 254] Yoon and associates demonstrated higher levels of TNF, IL-1β, IL-6, and IL-8 in amniotic fluid.[251, 257] Chaiwasporangsa and colleagues and Gilstrap and Ramin reported higher umbilical cord plasma IL-6 levels in neonates with white matter damage.[256,258] There were no correlations of plasma TNF, IL-1, and IL-1ra with periventricular leukomalacia.[258, 259] Gomez and colleagues further demonstrated the association between elevated fetal plasma IL-6 levels and several neonatal morbidities, including sepsis, respiratory distress syndrome, BPD, periventricular leukomalacia, and NEC as part of the fetal inflammatory response syndrome.[255]

Shimoya and colleagues measured IL-8 in cord sera from preterm fetuses with and without chorioamnionitis.[260] The IL-8 titers of infected infants were elevated compared with those of infants who were not infected and increased proportionately with the severity of chorioamnionitis graded histologically. The IL-8 elevation, however, was suppressed by the administration of maternal steroid therapy to promote fetal lung maturation. The investigators suggested that the measurement of IL-8 may be more sensitive (97%) and specific (89%) for the diagnosis of chorioamnionitis than conventional markers, such as leukocytes, C-reactive protein, and immunoglobulin M.

Although the mechanism of white matter damage after fetal infection is unclear, several possible hypotheses have been suggested.[249, 261-263] Circulating proinflammatory cytokines may directly induce inflammatory damage to vulnerable areas of the developing brain. Dammann and Leviton proposed that proinflammatory cytokines enter the brain by crossing the blood brain barrier.[261] Cytokines may then cause white matter damage directly, or they may induce further cytokine production by microglia and astrocytes. These brain-derived cytokines, in turn, may injure the developing white matter or germinal matrix.[261] Experimental evidence indicates that inflammatory cytokines are neurotoxic both *in vitro* and *in vivo,* and they inhibit oligodendrocytes in developing white matter.[250] Studies of members of the IL-6 family indicate that the cytokines also shift development of precursor oligodendrocyte cells into astrocytes.[208, 248, 261] Yanowitz and associates further hypothesized that chorioamnionitis and increased levels of proinflammatory cytokines are associated with hemodynamic disturbances in preterm infants.[262] These authors speculated that cytokine-associated systemic hemodynamic disturbances may predispose these infants to perinatal brain injury.

Epidemiologic data suggest that preterm infants exposed to an intrauterine infection are more likely to develop cerebral palsy. There are positive associations between cystic periventricular leukomalacia and intra-amniotic, brain, and umbilical cord cytokine levels.[248, 250, 251, 254, 263] In a meta-analysis of women with histologic and clinical chorioamnionitis, a relative risk of 1.8 (confidence interval, 1.5 to 2.3) was found between chorioamnionitis and cerebral palsy.[250] Although these data do not establish causality between cytokines and perinatal brain injury, they do provide evidence of the association of cerebral palsy with an inflammatory environment at birth.[250]

Genetic polymorphisms in cytokine function and production are likely to be important in the link between chorioamnionitis and the pathogenesis of cerebral palsy.[248, 254] These polymorphisms may, in turn, determine the extent of inflammation after intrauterine infection and may predict which infants will develop brain damage.[248, 250, 253, 264]

Cytokine Levels During Bacterial Sepsis

Sepsis and septic shock are important determinants of morbidity and mortality in the neonatal intensive care unit. Cytokines play a key role in this response in newborn infants. Although the immune system produces cytokines to protect the host when threatened by microbial invasion, overproduction of proinflammatory mediators or an imbalance favoring pro versus antiinflammatory mediators may sometimes occur and may have deleterious effects.[212, 214]

Several investigators examined levels of the proinflammatory cytokines TNF, IL-1, IL-6, and IL-8 during the evolution of bacterial sepsis in newborn infants.[265-269] In an early report, Girardin and associates measured serum TNF levels in 69 neonates at risk of infection.[270] Infants with systemic infection demonstrated significantly higher TNF levels when compared with infants in other patient groups; the highest levels were found in the neonates with circulatory failure, particularly those who died. TNF levels were unrelated to gestational age or to the Gram stain characteristics of the infecting organism. Roman and co-workers demonstrated significantly elevated TNF levels in 23 full-term infants with sepsis at the time of admission to the neonatal intensive care unit.[271] In this study, the degree of elevation seemed related to the severity of sepsis, because the infants who died had the highest levels of TNF. Similarly, Shi and colleagues found that, in neonates with bacterial sepsis, plasma TNF levels directly correlated with severity of illness as judged by pediatric risk of mortality scores.[272]

Miller and colleagues prospectively measured levels of TNF, IL-1, and IL-6 in cord blood samples from neonates born after complicated perinatal courses.[273] In this study, IL-1β levels were significantly elevated in the presence of severe perinatal complications, whereas TNF and IL-6 levels did not reflect the type of delivery or severity of the perinatal course. In infants with strictly defined infectious complications, however, cord blood IL-6 levels were markedly elevated.[273] Similarly, Büscher and associates

measured levels of IL-1β, IL-6, and IL-8 in cord blood from infants with chorioamnionitis, and in this study only IL-6 predicted neonatal infection.[274] In a study of preterm infants of less than 32 weeks' gestation with confirmed or clinical sepsis, Kashlan and colleagues also demonstrated elevations of IL-6 that correlated with histologic chorioamnionitis in these pregnancies.[275]

Numerous studies have demonstrated elevations of IL-6 and IL-8 in infected neonates, although the methodology used to measure cytokine levels has varied, and a group of neonates with "probable" infection is often included.[266, 276-278] Santana and associates found elevated cord blood levels of IL-6 in newborn infants with various infectious and noninfectious conditions, whereas IL-8 was the best predictor of early-onset bacterial infection.[279] Nupponen and co-authors measured neutrophil CD11b expression (in addition to IL-8) as a means to identify infected infants.[276] CD11b expression correlated positively with plasma concentrations of IL-8; both were highly sensitive and specific diagnostic markers. Berner and colleagues measured levels of LPS binding protein and soluble CD 14 in neonates with sepsis.[278] Levels of both LPS binding protein and soluble CD 14 were highly elevated in neonatal sepsis and strongly correlated with IL-1, IL-6, and IL-8 levels. Using chemiluminescence immunoassay that allows results within 1 to 2 hours, Krueger and associates found elevations of IL-6 and IL-8 in preterm infants with culture-proven sepsis.[280] The authors suggested that this method may allow an immediate diagnosis of infection in preterm infants. Using reverse transcriptase polymerase chain reaction, Berner and colleagues also found elevations of IL-8 mRNA to be highly sensitive (86%) and specific (96%) for the detection of neonatal infection.[281]

Lehrnbecher and colleagues extended these findings by measuring both proinflammatory mediators (IL-6, IL-8) as well as sIL-6 receptors in cord blood from infected neonates.[282] Although IL-6 and IL-8 levels were significantly elevated, as predicted from previous studies, sIL-6R levels were significantly reduced in sepsis.[282] This phenomenon has also been described in adults with sepsis, and it is speculated that the reduction of sIL-6R during sepsis may alter the biologic activity of IL-6. Døllner and colleagues found elevated TNF receptors (p 55 and 75) as well as IL-1ra in infected neonates.[283]

Several studies have also followed cytokine levels as a guide to the efficacy of antimicrobial therapy.[284-286] DeBont and associates measured TNF, IL-1, and IL-6 in 18 consecutive newborn infants admitted with a clinical suspicion of sepsis.[284] Plasma TNF and IL-6 levels were significantly increased in the 10 infants with sepsis, although IL-1 levels were only slightly elevated. After the start of antimicrobial therapy and concomitant clinical improvement, TNF, IL-1, and IL-6 levels decreased and normalized within 2 days. Sikora and colleagues found elevations of both proinflammatory (IL-1, IL-6, IL-8) and antiinflammatory (IL-10, IL-13) cytokines early in the course of sepsis that decreased after antimicrobial therapy.[285] Levels of cytokine inhibitors (IL-6sR, sTNFR II) also decreased after treatment.[285] Cytokine elevation has also been demonstrated in newborn infants with nosocomial sepsis. Groll and associates reported elevations of IL-6 in 8 of 10 infants at the onset of proven nosocomial infection; in 7 infants, these values returned to normal on completion of antibiotic therapy.[286]

Given the excessive morbidity and mortality from bacterial sepsis in newborn infants, several investigators have also addressed the predictive value of cytokine measurements in the early diagnosis of bacterial infection.[283, 287-290] In one review, Mehr and Doyle reviewed results of studies published between 1996 and 1999 using TNF, IL-6, and IL-8 as markers of bacterial sepsis in newborn infants.[290] Although the patient populations studied and the cytokines measured varied, several conclusions can be drawn from these data. Of all the cytokines measured, the most consistent results were found using IL-6.[290] Less consistent results were obtained with TNF; however, TNF is an evanescent cytokine, whose levels peak early and decline rapidly during sepsis. IL-1 is an unreliable indicator of bacterial infection. Finally, IL-8 (limited data) may prove most useful for the diagnosis of bacterial infection.

Cytokine Levels During Necrotizing Enterocolitis

NEC is a disease frequently encountered in premature infants in the newborn intensive care unit. Although the manifestations of the illness are quite variable, affected infants not uncommonly develop fulminant sepsis and shock.[291] Similar to the involvement of cytokines in bacterial sepsis, the generation of cytokines in NEC occurs in response to circulating bacteria and their byproducts as well as local mediator release associated with tissue inflammation.[292]

Caplan and associates measured circulating levels of PAF and TNF in 12 newborn infants with NEC and in 8 age-matched control patients.[293] In this pilot study, circulating PAF levels were higher in patients with NEC than in age-matched controls. Feeding alone increased circulating PAF levels, which preceded the development of NEC. Plasma TNF levels were also elevated in affected infants, thereby augmenting the effects of either mediator alone. These studies suggest that both PAF and TNF are important endogenous mediators in the pathogenesis of NEC. Harris and colleagues measured TNF and IL-6 levels in 62 infants with suspected sepsis or necrotizing enterocolitis at presentation of illness and at 12, 24, and 48 hours thereafter.[294] IL-6 levels were highest (10-fold greater) in infants with bacterial sepsis plus NEC, intermediate in infants with bacterial sepsis alone, and lowest in control infants with negative evaluations for infection. Elevated IL-6 levels were also associated with increased mortality. In contrast, plasma TNF levels did not reliably identify infants with sepsis or NEC. These data suggest that increased plasma IL-6 levels in NEC may reflect the combined effects of bacterial invasion of the bloodstream and the systemic response to severe bowel injury. Morecroft and co-workers measured plasma TNF and IL-6 levels in 24 infants with NEC.[295] Although TNF levels were elevated in the majority of samples (71%), there was no correlation between cytokine levels and severity of disease. In contrast, IL-6 levels were significantly increased in infants with definite (Stage II) and advanced (Stage III) NEC. The investigators concluded that although TNF may be an early marker of disease, IL-6 correlates best with disease severity.

Harris and colleagues extended their previous observations and demonstrated elevated plasma IL-8 levels in bacterial sepsis and NEC, which correlated with laboratory markers of inflammation (white blood cell counts, immature to neutrophil ratio).[296] Edelson and colleagues correlated circulatory levels of both pro- and antiinflammatory cytokines with the severity of NEC.[211] At the onset of NEC in infants with severe disease, levels of proinflammatory cytokines (IL-1, IL-8) and counterinflammatory mediators (IL-1ra, IL-10) were increased. Moreover, an IL-1ra concentration higher than 130,000 pg/mL had a high sensitivity (100%) and specificity (92%) for the presence of severe disease.

Viscardi and associates measured inflammatory cytokine (TNF, IL-1, IL-6, IL-8) mRNA in surgical specimens of NEC and normal intestine.[297] Although TNF and IL-1 mRNA levels were higher in intestinal specimens from infants with severe disease, IL-6 and IL-8 mRNA levels did not distinguish between infants with NEC and controls. In contrast, Nadler and colleagues found up-regulation of intestinal IL-8 mRNA in acute NEC; however, elevations of IL-8 did not correlate with mortality.[298] IL-11 mRNA levels were also increased and may represent a protective response to limit the extent of intestinal damage. Levels of IL-8 and IL-11 returned to baseline at the time of stomal closure. Thus, investigations of plasma and intestinal mRNA levels suggest elevations of both proinflammatory and counterinflammatory cytokines in NEC.

Bronchopulmonary Dysplasia

Since the mid-1990s, improvement in neonatal respiratory care has enhanced the survival rate of premature infants who develop chronic lung disease. In these infants the pathogenesis of BPD is complex and likely multifactorial, but evidence suggests the development of an early and persistent inflammatory response in the lung.[209, 299, 300] This inflammatory response may have its origins during the fetal period after intrauterine infection.[209, 301] It has been hypothesized that antenatal inflammation primes the lung so minimal postnatal injury produces an excessive inflammatory response.[210, 302]

Yoon and colleagues reported elevated levels of TNF, IL-1, IL-6, and IL-8 in amniotic fluid from mothers of infants who subsequently developed BPD.[303, 304] Elevated cord blood IL-6 levels suggest that a fetal inflammatory response is an independent risk factor for the development of BPD.[304] Using lung tissue from autopsy specimens from 72 fetuses and neonates (<25 weeks' gestation) who died of amniotic infection or of hyaline membrane disease, Gähler and associates found intense IL-8 staining in neutrophils, in epithelial cells of the terminal airways, and in the connective tissue compartment of the infants who died of hyaline membrane disease.[305] In contrast, in only two of 30 specimens of the amniotic infection group could IL-8 immunoreactivity be demonstrated in the epithelium of alveoli and bronchioli.

In infants who subsequently develop BPD, elevated levels of proinflammatory cytokines have also been detected in bronchoalveolar lavage (BAL) samples within a short time after birth.[301] While IL-1 levels are low on day 1 and then rise through day 14, IL-1 and IL-6 levels are high in BAL samples from ventilated preterm infants during the first week of life. Moreover, IL-6 levels are significantly higher in lung lavage samples from infants who develop chronic lung disease.[306] Kotecha found no differences in IL-6 levels on day 1, but significant elevations at 10 days followed by a decline.[307] In contrast, Kazzi and associates could not identify an increasing trend in IL-1 and IL-6 levels at 5 to 7 days of age in infants at greater risk of developing BPD.[308]

Jones and associates measured IL-8 levels in BAL supernatants from term and preterm infants.[209] Whereas IL-8 levels declined in term infants, elevations persisted in preterm infants over a 96-hour observation period. Kotecha correlated the development of chronic lung disease with increased BAL IL-8 levels in infants with hyaline membrane disease.[307] In another study of preterm infants of 24 to 32 weeks' gestation, a significant increase in IL-8 levels correlated with the duration of intubation.[309] These results are in accord with those reported by Kwong and colleagues, who found the highest IL-8 levels on day 12 of life in preterm infants with diffuse alveolar disease, which then declined to low levels by 28 days of age.[310]

In contrast, Jones and associates found undetectable levels of IL-10 mRNA in BAL samples from preterm infants with respiratory distress syndrome, but measurable levels in term infants with meconium aspiration syndrome.[209] These authors speculated that the susceptibility of the preterm infant to chronic lung disease may in part reflect an inability to generate the antiinflammatory cytokine IL-10.[209, 210] In a more recent study, Blahnik and colleagues found that whereas TNF expression was nearly identical in term and preterm neonates, there was a trend toward diminished levels of IL-10 in the preterm group.[311] In contrast to the foregoing studies, McColm and associates found that IL-10 was readily detectable in BAL samples from ventilated preterm infants with respiratory failure, most of whom developed chronic lung disease.[299] Overall, however, data are consistent with a proinflammatory-antiinflammatory inequality that favors the development of BPD.[301, 311]

Mycoplasmas, particularly *Ureaplasma urealyticum*, have been isolated from the lungs of infants who develop chronic lung disease. These organisms initiate a proinflammatory cytokine response and predispose preterm infants to lung injury.[312-314] Patterson and colleagues found that *U. urealyticum* respiratory tract colonization was associated with elevations of the proinflammatory cytokines TNF and IL-8.[315] Subsequent work by the same group demonstrated that inoculation with *U. urealyticum* partially blocked IL-6 release and reduced IL-10 expression as well.[313] This finding is in contrast to data from Li and associates, who demonstrated increases in both TNF and IL-6 production by macrophages isolated from tracheobronchial fluid after *U. urealyticum* exposure.[316] Baier and associates further demonstrated increased IL-8 and monocyte chemoattractant protein-1 concentrations in BAL from infants who subsequently developed BPD; these authors associated the isolation of *U. urealyticum* with a more robust inflammatory response.[317] In summary, it is hypothesized that *U. urealyticum* alters the host immune balance in favor of the production of proinflammatory mediators and predisposes the preterm infant to prolonged inflammation and lung injury.[313,317]

REFERENCES

1. Pruitt JH, et al: Interleukin-1 and interleukin-1 antagonism in sepsis, systemic inflammatory response syndrome, and septic shock. Shock *3*:235, 1995.
2. Moldawer LL: Biology of pro-inflammatory cytokines and their antagonists. Crit Care Med *22*:S3, 1994.
3. Lowry SF: Cytokine mediators of immunity and inflammation. Arch Surg *128*:1235, 1993.
4. Oberholzer A, et al: Cytokine signaling-regulation of the immune response in normal and critically ill states. Crit Care Med *28*(Suppl 4):N3, 2000.
5. Strieter RM, et al: Role of tumor necrosis factor-α in disease states and inflammation. Crit Care Med *21*:S447, 1993.
6. van der Poll T, van Deventer SJH: Cytokines and anticytokines in the pathogenesis of sepsis. Infect Dis Clin North Am *13*:413, 1999.
7. Opal SM, DePalo VA: Anti-Inflammatory cytokines. Chest *117*:1162, 2000.
8. Blackwell TS, Christman JW: Sepsis and cytokines: current status. Br J Anaesth *77*:110, 1996.
9. Pennica D, et al: Human tumour necrosis factor: precursor structure, expression and homology to lymphotoxin. Nature *312*:724, 1984.
10. Black RA, et al: A metalloproteinase disintegrin that releases tumor necrosis factor-alpha from cells. Nature *385*:729, 1997.
11. Moss ML, et al: Cloning of a disintegrin metalloproteinase that processes precursor tumor necrosis factor-alpha. Nature *385*:733, 1997.
12. Kriegler M, et al: A novel form of TNF/cachectin is a cell surface cytotoxic transmembrane protein: ramifications of complex physiology of TNF. Cell *53*:45, 1988.
13. van der Poll T, Lowry SF: Tumor necrosis factor in sepsis: mediator of multiple organ failure or essential part of host defense? Shock *3*:1, 1995.
14. Vilcek J, Lee TH: Tumor necrosis factor: new insights into the molecular mechanisms of its multiple actions. J Biol Chem *266*:7313, 1991.
15. Loetscher H, et al: Molecular cloning and expression of the human 55 kd tumor necrosis factor receptor. Cell *61*:351, 1990.
16. Schall TJ, et al: Molecular cloning and expression of a receptor for human TNF. Cell *61*:361, 1990.
17. Dembic Z, et al: Two human TNF receptors have similar extracellular, but distinct intracellular domain sequences. Cytokine *2*:231, 1990.
18. Beutler B, van Huffel C: Unraveling function in the TNF ligand and receptor families. Science *264*:667, 1994.
19. Tartaglia LA, Goeddel DV: Two TNF receptors. Immunol Today *13*:151, 1992.
20. Ashkenazi A, Dixit, VM: Death receptors: signaling and modulation. Science *28*:1305, 1998.
21. Pfeffer K, et al: Mice deficient for the 55 kd tumor necrosis factor receptor are resistant to endotoxic shock, yet succumb to *L. monocytogenes* infection. Cell *73*:457, 1993.
22. MacEwan DJ: TNF receptor subtype signaling: differences and cellular consequences. Cell Signal *14*:477, 2002.
23. Hsu H, et al: The TNF receptor-1-associated death domain protein TRADD signals cell death and NFκB activation. Cell *81*:495, 1995.
24. Hsu H, et al: TNF-dependent recruitment of the protein kinase RIP to the TNF receptor-1 signaling complex. Immunity *4*:387, 1996.
25. Hsu H, et al: TRADD-TRAF2 and TRADD-FADD interactions define two distinct TNF receptor 1 signal transduction pathways. Cell *84*:299, 1996.
26. Aggarwal BB: Tumour necrosis factor receptor associated signaling molecules and their role in activation of apoptosis, JNK and NF-κB. Ann Rheum Dis *59*(Suppl I):i6, 2000.
27. Baeuerle PA: Pro-inflammatory signaling: last pieces in the NF-κB puzzle. Curr Biol *8*:R19, 1998.
28. Barnes PJ, Karin M: Mechanisms of disease: nuclear factor- (kappa)B—a pivotal transcription factor in chronic inflammatory diseases. N Engl J Med *336*:1066, 1997.
29. Rothe J, et al: Mice lacking the tumour necrosis factor receptor 1 are resistant to TNF mediated toxicity but highly susceptible to infection by *Listeria monocytogenes*. Nature *364*:794, 1993.
30. Erickson SL, et al: Decreased sensitivity to tumour necrosis factor but normal T-cell development in TNF receptor-2 deficient mice. Nature *372*:560, 1994.
31. Dinarello CA, Wolff SM: The role of interleukin-1 in disease. N Engl J Med *328*:106, 1993.
32. Dinarello CA: Interleukin-1. Cytokine Growth Fact Rev *8*:253, 1997.
33. Webb AC, et al: Interleukin-1 gene (IL1) assigned to the long arm of human chromosome 2. Lymphokine Res *5*:77, 1986.
34. Sims JE: IL-1 and IL-18 receptors, and their extended family. Curr Opin Immunol *14*:117, 2002.
35. Cerretti DP, et al: Molecular cloning of the interleukin-1β converting enzyme. Science *256*:97, 1992.
36. Thornberry NA, et al: A novel heterodimeric cysteine protease is required for interleukin-1β processing in monocytes. Nature *356*:768, 1992.
37. O'Neill LAJ: The interleukin-1 receptor/Toll-like receptor superfamily: signal transduction during inflammation and host defense. Science's Stke (Electronic Resource): Signal Transduction Knowledge Environment 2000(44): REI, 2000.
38. Fitzgerald KA, O'Neill LAJ: The role of the interleukin-1/Toll-like receptor superfamily in host defense and inflammation. Microbes Infect *2*:933, 2000.
39. Dinarello CA: Pro-inflammatory cytokines. Chest *118*:503, 2000.
40. Sims JE, et al: The two interleukin-1 receptors play different roles in IL-1 actions. Clin Immunol Immunopathol *72*:9, 1994.
41. Matsushima K, et al: Properties of a specific interleukin-1 receptor on human Epstein-Barr virus transformed B lymphocytes: identity of the receptors for IL-1α and IL-1β. J Immunol *136*:4496, 1986.
42. Muzio M, et al: IRAK (Pelle) family member IRAK-2 and MyD88 as proximal mediators of IL-1 signaling. Science *278*:1612, 1997.
43. Cao Z, et al: IRAK: a kinase associated with the interleukin-1 receptor. Science *271*:1128, 1996.
44. Cao Z, et al: TRAF6 is a signal transducer for interleukin-1. Nature *383*:443, 1996.
45. Barton BE: IL-6: Insights into novel biological activities. Clin Immunol Immunopathol *85*:16, 1997.
46. Jones SA, et al: The soluble interleukin 6 receptor: mechanisms of production and implications in disease. FASEB J *15*:43, 2001.
47. Sehgal PB: Interleukin 6 in infection and cancer. Soc Exp Biol Med *195*:183, 1990.
48. Mizel SB: The interleukins. FASEB J *3*:2379, 1989.
49. Bluethmann H, et al: Establishment of the role of IL-6 and TNF receptor 1 using gene knockout mice. J Leukoc Biol *56*:565, 1994.
50. Yamasaki K, et al: Cloning and expression of the human interleukin-6 (BSF-2/IFN β) receptor. Science *241*:825, 1988.
51. Taga T, et al: Interleukin-6 triggers the association of its receptor with a possible signal transducer, gp130. Cell *58*:573, 1989.
52. Hirano T: Interleukin-6 and its relation to inflammation and disease. Clin Immunol Immunopathol *62*:S60, 1992.
53. Kishimoto T, et al: Interleukin-6 family of cytokines and gp130. Blood *86*:1243, 1995.
54. Hirano T, et al: Signaling mechanisms through gp130: a model of the cytokine system. Cytokine Growth Fact Rev *8*:241, 1997.
55. Heinrich PC, et al: Interleukin-6-type cytokine signaling through the gp130/JAK/STAT pathway. Biochem J *334*:297, 1998.
56. Taga T, et al: Interleukin-6 triggers the association of its receptor with a possible signal transducer, gp130. Cell *58*:573, 1989.
57. Stahl N, et al: Choice of STATs and other substrates specified by modular tyrosine based motifs in cytokine receptors. Science *267*:1349, 1995.
58. Gerhartz C, et al: Differential activation of acute phase response factor/STAT3 and STAT1 via the cytoplasmic domain of the IL-6 signal transducer gp130. Definition of a novel phosphotyrosine motif mediating STAT1 activation. J Biol Chem *271*:12991, 1996.
59. Nakajima K, et al: Signal transduction through IL-6 receptor: involvement of multiple protein kinases, stat factors, and a novel H7-sensitive pathway. Ann NY Acad Sci *762*:55, 1995.
60. Baggiolini M, Clark-Lewis I: Interleukin-8, a chemotactic and inflammatory cytokine. FEBS Lett *307*:97, 1992.
61. Baggiolini M, et al: Neutrophil activating peptide-1/interleukin 8, a novel cytokine that activates neutrophils. J Clin Invest *84*:1045, 1989.
62. Luster AD: Mechanisms of disease: chemokines—chemotactic cytokines that mediate inflammation. N Engl J Med *338*:436, 1998.
63. Keane MP, Strieter RM: Chemokine signaling in inflammation. Crit Care Med *28*(Suppl 4):N13, 2000.
64. Baggiolini M, et al: Human chemokines: an update. Annu Rev Immunol *15*:675, 1997.
65. Hebert C, et al: Scanning mutagenesis of interleukin-8 identifies a cluster of residues required for receptor binding. J Biol Chem *266*:18989, 1991.
66. Murdoch C, Finn A: Chemokine receptors and their role in inflammation and infectious diseases. Blood *95*:3032, 2000.
67. Holmes WE, et al: Structure and functional expression of a human interleukin-8 receptor. Science *253*:1278, 1991.
68. Murphy PM, Tiffany HL: Cloning of complementary DNA encoding a functional human interleukin-8 receptor. Science *253*:1280, 1991.

69. Curnock AP, et al: Chemokine signaling: pivoting around multiple phospho-inositide 3-kinases. Immunology *105*:125, 2002.

70. Huang R, et al: Neutrophils stimulated with a variety of chemoattractants exhibit rapid activation of p21-activated kinases (Paks): separate signals are required for activation and inactivation of paks. Mol Cell Biol *18*:7130, 1998.

71. Jones SA, et al: A comparison of post-receptor signal transduction events in Jurkat cell transfected with either IL-8R1 or IL-8R2: chemokine mediated activation of p42/p44 MAP-kinase (ERK-2) FEBS Lett *364*:211, 1995.

72. Laudanna C, et al: Role of Rho in chemoattractant-activated leukocyte adhesion through integrins. Science *271*:981, 1996.

73. Norgauer J, et al: Actin polymerization, calcium transient, and phospholipid metabolism in human neutrophils after stimulation with interleukin-8 and N-formyl peptide. J Invest Dermatol *102*:310, 1994.

74. Kettritz R, et al: Interleukin-8 delays spontaneous and tumor necrosis factor-α–mediated apoptosis in human neutrophils. Kidney Internat *53*:84, 1998.

75. Richardson DM, et al: Regulation of human interleukin-8 receptor A: identification of a phosphorylation site involved in modulating receptor functions. Biochemistry *34*:14193, 1995.

76. Colombo MP, Trinchieri G: Interleukin-12 in anti-tumor immunity and immunotherapy. Cytokine Growth Factor Rev *13*:155, 2002.

77. Trinchieri G: Cytokines acting on or secreted by macrophages during intracellular infection (IL-10, IL-12, IFN-γ). Curr Opin Immunol *9*:17, 1997.

78. Merberg DM, et al: Sequence similarity between NKSF and the IL-6/G-CSF family. Immunol Today *13*:77, 1992.

79. Gearling DP, Cosman D: Homology of the p40 subunit of natural killer cell stimulatory factor (NSFK) with the extracellular domain of the interleukin-6 receptor. Cell *66*:9, 1991.

80. Romani L, et al: Interleukin-12 in infectious diseases. Clin Microbiol Rev *10*:611, 1997.

81. Karp CL, Wills-Karp M: Complement and IL-12: yin and yang. Microbes Infect *3*:109, 2001.

82. Presky DH, et al: A functional interleukin 12 receptor complex is composed of two β type cytokine receptor subunits. Proc Natl Acad Sci USA *93*:14002, 1996.

83. Bacon CM, et al: Interleukin 12 (IL-12) induces tyrosine phosphorylation of JAK2 and TYK2: differential use of janus family tyrosine kinases by IL-2 and IL-12. J Exp Med *181*:399, 1995.

84. Dorman SE, Holland SM: Interferon-γ and interleukin-12 pathway defects and human disease. Cytokines Growth Rev *11*:321, 2000.

85. Ramana CV, et al: Stat-1-dependent and -independent pathways in IFN-γ-dependent signaling. Immunol Trends *23*:96, 2002.

86. Bach EA, et al: The IFNγ receptor: a paradigm for cytokine receptor signaling. Annu Rev Immunol *15*:563, 1997.

87. Boehm U, et al: Cellular responses to interferon-γ. Annu Rev Immunol *15*:749, 1997.

88. Darnell JE Jr, et al: JAK-STAT pathways and transcriptional activation in response to IFNs and other extracellular signaling proteins. Science *264*:1415, 1994.

89. Okamura H, et al: Cloning of a new cytokine that induces IFN-γ production by T cells. Nature *378*:88, 1995.

90. Akira S: The role of IL-18 in innate immunity. Curr Opin Immunol *12*:59, 2000.

91. Bazan JF, et al: A newly defined interleukin-1? Nature *379*:591, 1996.

92. Ghayur T, et al: Caspase-1 processes IFN-γ-inducing factor and regulates LPS-induced IFN-γ production. Nature *386*:619, 1997.

93. Gu Y, et al: Activation of interferon-γ–inducing factor mediated by IL-1β converting enzyme. Science *275*:206, 1997.

94. Dinarello CA: Interleukin-18. Methods *19*:121, 1999.

95. Gillespie MT, Horwood NJ: Interleukin-18: perspectives on the newest interleukin. Cytokine Growth Factor Rev *9*:109, 1998.

96. Leung BP, et al: A role for IL-18 in neutrophil activation. J Immunol *167*:2879, 2001.

97. Fiorentino DF, et al: Two types of mouse T-helper cell. IV. Th2 clones secrete a factor that inhibits cytokine production by Th1 clones. J Exp Med *170*: 2081, 1989.

98. Oberholzer A, et al: Interleukin-10: a complex role in the pathogenesis of sepsis syndromes and its potential as an anti-inflammatory drug. Crit Care Med *30*(Suppl 1):S58, 2002.

99. Asadullah K, et al: Interleukin-10 in cutaneous disorders: implications for its pathological importance and therapeutic use. Arch Dermatol Res *291*:628, 1999.

100. Moore KW, et al: Interleukin-10 and the interleukin-10 receptor. Annu Rev Immunol *19*:683, 2001.

101. Opal SM, et al: Interleukin-10: potential benefits and possible risks in clinical infectious diseases. Clin Infect Dis *27*:1497, 1998.

102. Akdis CA, Blaser K: Mechanisms of interleukin-10 mediated immune suppression. Immunology *103*:131, 2001.

103. Ho ASY, et al: A receptor for IL-10 is related to interferon receptors. Proc Natl Acad Sci USA *90*:11267, 1993.

104. Finbloom DS, Winestock KD: IL-10 induces the tyrosine phosphorylation of tyk2 and Jak1 and the differential assembly of STAT1α and STAT3 complexes in human T cells and monocytes. J Immunol *155*:1079, 1995.

105. Wang P, et al: Interleukin (IL)-10 inhibits nuclear factor kappa B (NFkappaB) activation in human monocytes: IL-10 and IL-4 suppress cytokine synthesis by different mechanisms. J Biol Chem *270*:9558, 1995.

106. McKenzie A, et al: Interleukin-13, a T-cell derived cytokine that regulates human monocyte and B-cell function. Proc Natl Acad Sci USA *90*:3735, 1993.

107. Hu-Li J, et al: B cell stimulatory factor-1 (interleukin-4) is a potent costimulant for normal resting T lymphocytes. J Exp Med *165*:157, 1987.

108. Brubaker JO, Montaner LJ: Role of interleukin-13 in innate and adaptive immunity. Cell Mol Biol *47*:637, 2001.

109. Brombacher F: The role of interleukin-13 in infectious diseases and allergy. Bioessays *22*:646, 2000.

110. Koj A: Termination of the acute-phase response: role of some cytokines and anti-inflammatory drugs. Gen Pharmacol *31*:9, 1998.

111. Matsukawa A, et al: Expression and contribution of endogenous IL-13 in an experimental model of sepsis. J Immunol *164*:2738, 2000.

112. Callard RE, et al: IL-4 and IL-13 receptors: are they one and the same? Immunol Today *17*:108, 1996.

113. Nelms K et al: The IL-4 receptor: signaling mechanisms and biologic functions. Annu Rev Immunol *17*:701, 1999.

114. Jiang H, et al: IL-4/IL-13 signaling beyond JAK/STAT. J Allergy Clin Immunol *105*:1063, 2000.

115. McKenzie ANJ: Regulation of T helper type 2 cell immunity by interleukin-4 and interleukin-13. Pharmacol Ther *88*:143, 2000.

116. Caput D, et al: Cloning and characterization of a specific interleukin (IL)-13 binding protein structurally related to the IL-5 receptor alpha chain. J Biol Chem *271*:16921, 1996.

117. Keegan AD, et al: Similarities and differences in signal transduction by interleukin-4 and interleukin-13 analysis of Janus kinase activation. Proc Natl Acad Sci USA *92*:7681, 1995.

118. Lin J-X, et al: The role of shared receptor motifs and common Stat proteins in the generation of cytokine pleiotropy and redundancy by IL-2, IL-4, IL-7, IL-13 and IL-15. Immunity *2*:331, 1995.

119. Zamorano J, et al: IL-4 protects cells from apoptosis via the insulin receptor substrate pathway and a second independent signaling pathway. J Immunol *157*:4926, 1996.

120. Manna SK, Aggarwal BB: Interleukin-4 down regulates both forms of tumor necrosis factor receptor and receptor mediated apoptosis, NF-kappaB, AP-1 and c-Jun N-terminal kinase. Comparison with interleukin-13. J Biol Chem *273*:33333, 1998.

121. Paul SR, et al: Molecular cloning of a cDNA encoding interleukin 11, a stromal cell-derived lymphopoietic and hematopoietic cytokine. Proc Natl Acad Sci USA *87*:7512, 1990.

122. Leng SX, Elias JA: Interleukin-11. Int J Biochem *29*:1059, 1997.

123. Du X, Williams DA: Interleukin-11: review of molecular, cell biology, and clinical use. Blood *89*:3897, 1997

124. Zheng T, et al: IL-11: insights in asthma from overexpression transgenic modeling. J Allergy Clin Immunol *108*:489, 2001.

125. Trepicchio WL, et al: Recombinant human IL-11 attenuates the inflammatory response through down-regulation of pro-inflammatory cytokine release and nitric oxide production. J Immunol *157*:3627, 1996.

126. Baumann H, Schendel P: Interleukin-11 regulates the hepatic expression of the same plasma protein genes as interleukin-6. J Biol Chem *266*:20424, 1991.

127. Trepicchio WL, et al: IL-11 regulates macrophage effector function through the inhibition of nuclear factor-κB. J Immunol *159*:5661, 1997.

128. Zhang XG, et al: Cilary neurotropic factor, interleukin 11, leukemia inhibitory factor, and oncostatin M are growth factors for human myeloma cell lines using interleukin 6 signal transducer gp 130. J Exp Med *179*:1337, 1994.

129. Hilton DJ, et al: Cloning of a murine IL-11 receptor alpha-chain; requirement for gp130 for high affinity binding and signal transduction. EMBO J *13*:4765, 1994.

130. Barton VA, et al: Interleukin-11 signals through the formation of a hexameric receptor complex. J Biol Chem *275*:36197, 2000.

131. Dahmen H, et al: Activation of the signal transducer gp130 by interleukin-11 and interleukin-6 is mediated by similar molecular interactions. Biochem J *331*:695, 1998.

132. Aderka D: The potential biological and clinical significance of the soluble tumor necrosis factor receptors. Cytokine Growth Factor Rev 7:231, 1996.

133. Engelmann H, et al: Two tumor necrosis factor binding proteins purified from human urine: evidence for immunological cross-reactivity with cell surface tumor necrosis factor receptors. J Biol Chem *265*:1531, 1990.

134. Dri P, et al: TNF-induced shedding of TNF receptors in human polymorphonuclear leukocytes: role of the 55-kDa TNF receptor and involvement of a membrane-bound and non-matrix metalloproteinase. J Immunol *165*:2165, 2000.

135. Seckinger P, et al: A human inhibitor of tumor necrosis factor alpha. J Exp Med *167*:1511, 1988.

136. Schluter D, Deckert M: The divergent role of tumor necrosis factor receptors in infectious diseases. Microbes Infect *2*:1285, 2000.

137. Pinckard JK, et al: Constitutive shedding of both p55 and p75 murine TNF receptor in vivo. J Immunol *158*:3869, 1997.

138. VanZee KJ, et al: Tumor necrosis factor soluble receptor circulate during experimental and clinical inflammation and can protect against excessive tumor necrosis factor α in vitro and in vivo. Proc Natl Acad Sci USA *89*:4845, 1992.

139. van der Poll T, et al: Release of soluble receptors for tumor necrosis factor in clinical sepsis and experimental endotoxemia. J Infect Dis *168*:955, 1993.

140. Girardin E, et al: Imbalance between tumor necrosis factor-alpha and soluble TNF receptor concentrations in severe meningococcaemia. Immunology *76*:20, 1992.

141. Arend WP, et al: Interleukin-1 receptor antagonist: role in biology. Annu Rev Immunol 16:27, 1998.
142. Evans RJ, et al: Mapping receptor binding sites in interleukin (IL)-1 receptor antagonist and IL-1β by site directed mutagenesis: identification of a single site in IL-1ra and two sites in IL-1β. J Biol Chem 270:11477, 1995.
143. Greenfeder SA, et al: Molecular cloning and characterization of a second subunit of the interleukin 1 receptor complex. J Biol Chem 270:13757, 1995.
144. Granowitz EV, et al: Production of interleukin-1 receptor antagonist during experimental endotoxemia. Lancet 338:1423, 1991.
145. Mantovani A, et al: Decoy receptors: a strategy to regulate inflammatory cytokines and chemokines. Trends Immunol 22:328, 2001.
146. Giri JG, et al: Elevated levels of shed type II IL-1 receptors in sepsis: potential role for type II receptor in regulation of IL-1 response. J Immunol 153:5802, 1994.
147. Pruitt JH, et al: Increased soluble interleukin-1 type II receptor concentrations in postoperative patients and in patients with sepsis syndrome. Blood 87:3282, 1996.
148. Orlando S, et al: Role of metalloproteases in the release of the IL-1 type II decoy receptor. J Biol Chem 272:31764, 1997.
149. Novick D, et al: Interleukin-18 binding protein: a novel modulator of the Th1 cytokine response. Immunity 10:127, 1999.
150. Novick D, et al: A novel IL-18bp ELISA shows elevated serum IL-18bp in sepsis and extensive decrease of free IL-18. Cytokine 14:334, 2001.
151. Dinarello CA: Targeting interleukin 18 with interleukin 18 binding protein. Ann Rheum Dis 59(Suppl 1):17, 2000.
152. Faggioni R, et al: IL-18 binding protein protects against lipopolysaccharide-induced lethality and prevents development of Fas/Fas ligand–mediated models of liver disease in mice. J Immunol 167:5913, 2001.
153. Baggiolini M, Dahinden CA: CC chemokines in allergic inflammation. Immunol Today 15:127, 1994.
154. Reinhart K, et al: Marker of endothelial damage in organ dysfunction and sepsis. Crit Care Med 30:S302, 2002.
155. Strieter RM, et al: Chemokines in lung injury. Chest 116(Suppl 1):1035, 1999.
156. Dallegri F, Ottonello L: Tissue injury in neutrophilic inflammation. Inflamm Res 46:382, 1997.
157. Bellingan G: Leukocytes: friend or foe. Intensive Care Med 26:S111, 2000.
158. Springer TA: Traffic signals for lymphocyte recirculation and leukocyte emigration: the multistep paradigm. Cell 76:301, 1994.
159. Strieter RM, et al: Cytokines and lung inflammation: mechanisms of neutrophil recruitment to the lung. Thorax 48:765, 1993.
160. Aderem AA: How cytokines signal messages within cells. J Clin Invest 167(Suppl 1):S2, 1993.
161. McLeish KR, et al: Modulation of transmembrane signalling in HL-60 granulocytes by tumour necrosis factor-α. Biochem J 279:455, 1991.
162. Nathan CF: Neutrophil activation on biological surfaces: massive secretion of hydrogen peroxide in response to products of macrophages and lymphocytes. J Clin Invest 80:1550, 1987.
163. Kilpatrick LE, et al: Serine phosphorylation of p60 tumor necrosis factor by PKC-δ in TNF-α-activated neutrophils. Am J Physiol 279:C2011, 2000.
164. Bulger EM, Maier RV: Lipid mediators in the pathophysiology of critical illness. Crit Care Med 28:N27, 2000.
165. Bussolino F, et al: Synthesis and release of platelet-activating factor by human vascular endothelial cells treated with tumor necrosis factor or interleukin 1α. J Biol Chem 263:11856, 1988.
166. Davies MG, Hagen PO: Systemic inflammatory response syndrome. Br J Surg 84:920, 1997.
167. Levy R, et al: Elevated cytosolic phospholipase A2 expression and activity in human neutrophils during sepsis. Blood 95:660, 2000.
168. Kerr JFR, et al: Apoptosis: a basic biological phenomenon with wide-ranging implications in tissue kinetics. Br J Cancer 26:239, 1972.
169. Whyte MKB, et al: Impairment of function in aging neutrophils is associated with apoptosis. J Immunol 150:5124, 1993.
170. Kilpatrick LE, et al: A role for PKC-δ and PI3-kinase in TNF-α–mediated anti-apoptotic signaling in the human neutrophil. Am J Physiol 283:C48, 2002.
171. Akgul C, et al: Molecular control of neutrophil apoptosis. FEBS Lett 487:318, 2001.
172. Marshall JC: Inflammation, coagulopathy, and the pathogenesis of multiple organ dysfunction syndrome. Crit Care Med 29:S99, 2001.
173. Dhainaut J-F, et al: Soluble thrombomodulin, plasma-derived unactivated protein C, and recombinant human activated protein C in sepsis. Crit Care Med 30:S318, 2002.
174. Shebuski RJ, Kilgore KS: Role of inflammatory mediators in thrombogenesis. J Pharmacol Exp Ther 300:729, 2002.
175. Van Gorp ECM, et al: Infectious diseases and coagulation disorders. J Infect Dis 180:176, 1999.
176. Portieje JEA, et al: Interleukin 12 induces activation of fibrinolysis and coagulation in humans. Br J Haematol 112:499, 2001.
177. Neumann F-J, et al: Effect of human recombinant interleukin-6 and interleukin-8 on monocyte procoagulant activity. Arterioscler Thromb Vasc Biol 17:3399, 1997.
178. Cicala C, Cirino G: Linkage between inflammation and coagulation: an update on the molecular basis of the crosstalk. Life Sci 62:1817, 1998.
179. Schleef RR, et al: Cytokine activation of vascular endothelium: effects of tissue-type plasminogen activator and type 1 plasminogen activator inhibitor. J Biol Chem 263:5797, 1988.
180. Levi M, et al: Endothelium: interface between coagulation and inflammation. Crit Care Med 30:S220, 2002.
181. Karima R, et al: The molecular pathogenesis of endotoxic shock and organ failure. Mol Med Today 5:123, 1999.
182. Opal S, et al: Roundtable I: relationships between coagulation and inflammatory processes. Crit Care Med 28:S81, 2000.
183. Pajkrt D, et al: Interleukin-10 inhibits activation of coagulation and fibrinolysis during human endotoxemia. Blood 89:2701, 1997.
184. Dinarello CA, et al: Tumor necrosis factor (cachectin) is an endogenous pyrogen and induces production of interleukin 1. J Exp Med 163:1433, 1986.
185. Netea MG, et al: Circulating cytokines as mediators of fever. Clin Infect Dis 31:S178, 2000.
186. Ushikubi F, et al: Impaired febrile response in mice lacking the prostaglandin E receptor subtype EP3. Nature 395:281, 1998.
187. Gatti S, et al: Effect of interleukin-18 on mouse core body temperature. Am J Physiol 282:R702, 2002.
188. Baumann H, Schendel P: Inerleukin-11 regulates hepatic expression of the same plasma protein genes as interleukin-6. J Biol Chem 266:20424, 1991.
189. Trepicchio WL, Dorner AJ: Interleukin-11-a gp130 cytokine. Ann NY Acad Sci 856:12, 1998.
190. Tatro JB: Endogenous antipyretics. Clin Infect Dis 31:S190, 2000.
191. Bluethmann H, et al: Establishment of the role of IL-6 and TNF receptor 1 using gene knockout mice. J Leukoc Biol 56:565, 1994.
192. Moshage H: Cytokines and the hepatic acute phase response. J Pathol 181:257, 1997.
193. Kopf M, et al: Impaired immune and acute-phase responses in interleukin-6-deficient mice. Nature 368:339, 1994.
194. Gabay C, Kushner I: Mechanisms of disease: acute phase proteins and other systemic responses to inflammation. N Engl J Med 340:448, 1999.
195. Dhainaut J-F, et al: Hepatic response to sepsis: interaction between coagulation and inflammatory processes. Crit Care Med 29:S42, 2001.
196. Jensen LE, Whitehead AS: Regulation of serum amyloid A protein expression during the acute-phase response. Biochem J 334:489, 1998.
197. Loyer P, et al: Interleukin 4 inhibits the production of some acute-phase proteins in human hepatocytes in primary culture. FEBS Lett 336:215, 1993.
198. Tilg H, et al: IL-6 and APPs: anti-inflammatory and immunosuppressive mediators. Immunol Today 18:428, 1997.
199. American College of Chest Physicians/Society of Critical Care Medicine Consensus Conference: Definitions for sepsis and organ failure and guidelines for the use of innovative therapies in sepsis. Crit Care Med 20:864, 1992.
200. van Deventer SJH: Cytokine and cytokine receptor polymorphisms in infectious disease. Intensive Care Med 26:S98, 2000.
201. Klein JO, Marcy SM: Bacterial sepsis and meningitis. In Remington JS, Klein JO (eds): Infectious Diseases of the Fetus and Newborn Infant, 4th ed. Philadelphia, WB Saunders, 1995, pp 835–890.
202. Harris MC, Polin RA: Diagnosis of neonatal sepsis. In Spitzer AR (ed): Intensive Care of the Fetus and Neonate. St. Louis, CV Mosby, 2003.
203. Harris MC, Casey J: Prevention and treatment of neonatal sepsis. In Spitzer AR (ed): Intensive Care of the Fetus and Neonate. St. Louis, CV Mosby, 2003.
204. Philip AGS: Defense mechanisms and deficiencies. In Philip AGS (ed): Neonatal Sepsis and Meningitis. Boston, GK Hall, 1985, pp 29–42.
205. Wilson CB: Immunologic basis for increased susceptibility of the neonate to infection. J Pediatr 108:1, 1986.
206. Nesin M, Cunningham-Rundles S: Cytokines and neonates. Am J Perinatol 17:393, 2000.
207. Slayton W: Development of the immune system in the human fetus. In Christensen RD (ed): Hematologic Problems of the Neonate. Philadelphia, WB Saunders, 2000, pp 21–41.
208. Schultz C, et al: Enhanced interleukin-6 and interleukin-8 synthesis in term and preterm infants. Pediatr Res 51:317, 2002.
209. Jones CA, et al: Undetectable interleukin (IL)-10 and persistent IL-8 expression early in hyaline membrane disease: a possible developmental basis for the predisposition to chronic lung inflammation in preterm newborns. Pediatr Res 39:966, 1996.
210. Speer CP: New insights into the pathogenesis of pulmonary inflammation in preterm infants. Biol Neonate 79:205, 2001.
211. Edelson MB, et al: Circulating pro- and counterinflammatory cytokine levels and severity in necrotizing enterocolitis. Pediatrics 103:766, 1999.
212. Giacoia GP: New approaches for the treatment of neonatal sepsis. J Perinatol 13:223, 1993.
213. Saez-Llorens Z, Lagrutta SF: The acute phase host reaction during bacterial infection and its clinical impact in children. Pediatr Infect Dis J 12:83, 1993.
214. Pennington JE: Therapy with antibody to tumor necrosis factor in sepsis. Clin Infect Dis 17(Suppl 2):S515, 1993.
215. Fong YM, Lowry SF: Tumor necrosis factor in the pathophysiology of infection and sepsis. Clin Immunol Immunopathol 55:157, 1990.
216. Beutler B, Cerami A: Cachectin: more than a tumor necrosis factor. N Engl J Med 316:379, 1987.
217. Kutteh WH, et al: Tumor necrosis factor-α and interleukin-1β production by human fetal Kupffer cells. Am J Obstet Gynecol 165:112, 1991.
218. Kutteh WH, et al: Regulation of interleukin-6 production in human fetal Kupffer cells. Scand J Immunol 33:607, 1991.

219. Romero R, et al: Tumor necrosis factor in preterm and term labor. Am J Obstet Gynecol 166:1576, 1992.
220. Seghaye M-C, et al: The production of pro- and anti-inflammatory cytokines in neonates assessed by stimulated whole cord blood culture and by plasma levels at birth. Biol Neonate 73:220, 1998.
221. Peters AMJ, et al: Reduced secretion of interleukin-1 and tumor necrosis factor-α by neonatal monocytes. Biol Neonate 63:157, 1993.
222. Weatherstone KB, Rich EA: Tumor necrosis factor/cachectin and interleukin-1 secretion by cord blood monocytes from premature and term neonates. Pediatr Res 25:342, 1989.
223. English BK, et al: Production of lymphotoxin and tumor necrosis factor by human neonatal mononuclear cells. Pediatr Res 26:717, 1988.
224. Burchett SK, et al: Regulation of tumor necrosis factor/cachectin and IL-1 secretion in human mononuclear phagocytes. J Immunol 140:3473, 1988.
225. Chheda S, et al: Decreased interleukin-10 production by neonatal monocytes and T cells: relationship to decreased production and expression of tumor necrosis factor-α and its receptors. Pediatr Res 40:475, 1996.
226. Kwak DJ, et al: Intracellular and extracellular cytokine production by human mixed mononuclear cells in response to Group B streptococci. Infect Immun 68:320, 2000.
227. Hebra A, et al: Intracellular cytokine production by fetal and adult monocytes. J Pediatr Surg 36:1321, 2001.
228. Bessler H, et al: IL-1β and IL-3-like activity in preterm infants. Clin Exp Immunol 91:320, 1993.
229. Dinarello CA, et al: Production of leukocytic pyrogen from phagocytes of neonates. J Infect Dis 144:337, 1981.
230. Wilmott RW, et al: Interleukin-1 activity from human cord blood monocytes. Diagn Clin Immunol 5:201, 1987.
231. Srugo I, et al: Interleukin-1 secretion by blood monocytes of septic premature infants. Infection 19:150, 1991.
232. Bry K, et al: Influence of fetal gender on the concentration of interleukin-1 receptor antagonist in amniotic fluid and in newborn urine. Pediatr Res 35:130, 1994.
233. Contrino J, et al: Elevated interleukin-1 expression in human neonatal neutrophils. Pediatr Res 34:249, 1993.
234. Waage A, et al: TNF, IL-1 and IL-6 in human septic shock. Scand J Immunol 28:267, 1988.
235. Liechty KW, et al: Production of interleukin-6 by fetal and maternal cells in vivo during intraamniotic infection and in vitro after stimulation with interleukin-1. Pediatr Res 29:1, 1991.
236. Yachie A, et al: The capability of neonatal leukocytes to produce IL-6 on stimulation assessed by whole blood culture. Pediatr Res 27:227, 1990.
237. Yachie A, et al: Defective production of interleukin-6 in very small premature infants in response to bacterial infection. Infect Immun 60:749, 1992.
238. Saito S, et al: Production of IL-6 (BSF-2/IFN β2) by mononuclear cells in premature and term infants. J Reprod Immunol 17:17, 1990.
239. Zola H, et al: Expression of cytokine receptors by human cord blood lymphocytes: comparison with adult blood lymphocytes. Pediatr Res 38:397, 1995.
240. Van Zee KJ, et al: IL-8 in septic shock, endotoxemia and after IL-1 administration. J Immunol 146:3478, 1991.
241. Taniguchi T, et al: Fetal mononuclear cells show a comparable capacity with maternal mononuclear cells to produce IL-8 in response to lipopolysaccharide in chorioamnionitis. J Reprod Immunol 23:1, 1993.
242. Dembinski J, et al: Cell-associated interleukin-8 in cord blood of term and preterm infants. Clin Diagn Lab Immunol 9:320, 2002.
243. Rowen JL, et al: Group B streptococci elicit leukotriene B₄ and interleukin-8 from human monocytes: neonates exhibit a diminished response. J Infect Dis 172:420, 1995.
244. Schibler KR, et al: Diminished transcription of interleukin-8 by monocytes from preterm neonates. J Leukoc Biol 53:399, 1993.
245. Roth I, et al: Human placental cytotrophoblasts produce the immunosuppressive cytokine interleukin 10. J Exp Med 184:539, 1996.
246. Kotiranta-Ainamo A, et al: Interleukin-10 production by cord blood mononuclear cells. Pediatr Res 41:110, 1997.
247. Vigano A, et al: Differential development of type 1 and type 2 cytokines and β-chemokines in the ontogeny of healthy newborns. Biol Neonate 75:1, 1999.
248. Gaudet LM, Smith GN: Cerebral palsy and chorioamnionitis: the inflammatory cytokine link. Obstet Gynecol Surg 56:433, 2001.
249. Saliba E, Henrot A: Inflammatory mediators and neonatal brain damage. Biol Neonate 79:224, 2001.
250. Wu YW, Colford Jr JM: Chorioamnionitis as a risk factor for cerebral palsy: a meta-analysis. JAMA 284:1417, 2000.
251. Yoon BH, et al: Amniotic fluid inflammatory cytokines (interleukin-6, interleukin-1β, and tumor necrosis factor-α), neonatal brain white matter lesions, and cerebral palsy. Am J Obstet Gynecol 177:19, 1997.
252. Yoon BH, et al: The relationship among inflammatory lesions of the umbilical cord (funisitis), umbilical cord plasma interleukin 6 concentration, amniotic fluid infection, and neonatal sepsis. Am J Obstet Gynecol 183:1124, 2000.
253. Dammann O, Leviton A: Role of the fetus in perinatal infection and neonatal brain damage. Curr Opin Pediatr 12:99, 2000.
254. Yoon BH, et al: Fetal exposure to an intra-amniotic inflammation and the development of cerebral palsy at the age of three years. Am J Obstet Gynecol 182:675, 2000.
255. Gomez R, et al: The fetal inflammatory response syndrome. Am J Obstet Gynecol 179:194, 1998.
256. Chaiworapongsa T, et al: Evidence for fetal involvement in the pathologic process of clinical chorioamnionitis. Am J Obstet Gynecol 186:1178, 2002.
257. Yoon BH, et al: Fetal exposure to an intra-amniotic inflammation and the development of cerebral palsy at the age of three years. Am J Obstet Gynecol 182:675, 2000.
258. Gilstrap LC III, Ramin SM: Infection and cerebral palsy. Semin Perinatol 24:200, 2000.
259. Yoon BH, et al: Interleukin-6 concentrations in umbilical cord plasma are elevated in neonates with white matter lesions associated with periventricular leukomalacia. Am J Obstet Gynecol 174:1433, 1996.
260. Shimoya K, et al: Interleukin-8 in cord sera: a sensitive and specific marker for the detection of preterm chorioamnionitis. J Infect Dis 165:957, 1992.
261. Dammann O, Leviton A: Maternal intrauterine infection, cytokines, and brain damage in the preterm newborn. Pediatr Res 42:1, 1997.
262. Yanowitz TD, et al: Hemodynamic disturbances in premature infants born after chorioamnionitis: association with cord blood cytokine concentrations. Pediatr Res 51:310, 2002.
263. Duggan PJ, et al: Intrauterine T-cell activation and increased pro-inflammatory cytokine concentrations in preterm infants with cerebral lesions. Lancet 358:1699, 2001.
264. Dammann O, et al: Modification of the infection-associated risks of preterm birth and white matter damage in the preterm newborn by polymorphisms in the tumor necrosis factor-locus? Pathogenesis 1:171, 1999.
265. Sullivan JS, et al: Correlation of plasma cytokine elevations with mortality rate in children with sepsis. J Pediatr 120:510, 1992.
266. Kaufman D, et al: Elevations of interleukin-8 in infants with bacterial sepsis. Pediatr Res 39:296A, 1996.
267. Girardin E, et al: Tumor necrosis factor in neonatal listeriosis: a case report. Eur J Pediatr 148:644, 1989.
268. Berner R, et al: Plasma levels and gene expression of granulocyte colony-stimulating factor, tumor necrosis factor-α, interleukin (IL)-1β, IL-6, IL-8, and soluble intercellular adhesion molecule-1 in neonatal early onset sepsis. Pediatr Res 44:469, 1998.
269. Weimann E, et al: G-CSF, GM-CSF and IL-6 levels in cord blood: diminished increase of G-CSF and IL-6 in preterms with perinatal infection compared to term neonates. Perinat Med 26:211, 1998.
270. Girardin EP, et al: Serum tumor necrosis factor in newborns at risk for infections. Eur J Pediatr 149:645, 1990.
271. Roman J, et al: Serum TNF levels in neonatal sepsis and septic shock. Acta Paediatr 82:352, 1993.
272. Shi Y, et al: Plasma nitric oxide levels in newborn infants with sepsis. J Pediatr 123:435, 1993.
273. Miller LC, et al: Neonatal interleukin-1β, interleukin-6 and tumor necrosis factor: cord blood levels and cellular production. J Pediatr 117:961, 1990.
274. Büscher U, et al: IL-1β, IL-6, IL-8 and G-CSF in the diagnosis of early-onset neonatal infections. J Perinat Med 28:383, 2000.
275. Kashlan F, et al: Umbilical vein interleukin 6 and tumor necrosis factor alpha plasma concentrations in the very preterm infant. Pediatr Infect Dis J 19:238, 2000.
276. Nupponen I, et al: Neutrophil CD11b expression and circulating interleukin-8 as diagnostic markers for early-onset neonatal sepsis. Pediatrics 108:12, 2001.
277. Mehr SS, et al: Interleukin-6 and interleukin-8 in newborn bacterial infection. Am J Perinatol 18:313, 2001.
278. Berner R, et al: Elevated levels of lipopolysaccharide-binding protein and soluble CD14 in plasma in neonatal early-onset sepsis. Clin Diagn Lab Immunol 9:440, 2002.
279. Santana C, et al: Cord blood levels of cytokines as predictors of early neonatal sepsis. Acta Paediatr 90:1176, 2001.
280. Krueger M, et al: Cord blood levels of interleukin-6 and interleukin-8 for the immediate diagnosis of early-onset infection in premature infants. Biol Neonate 80:118, 2001.
281. Berner R, et al: Elevated gene expression of interleukin-8 in cord blood is a sensitive marker for neonatal infection. Eur J Pediatr 159:205, 2000.
282. Lehrnbecher T, et al: Immunologic parameters in cord blood indicating early-onset sepsis. Biol Neonate 70:206, 1996.
283. Døllner H, et al: Inflammatory mediators in umbilical plasma from neonates who develop early-onset sepsis. Biol Neonate 80:41, 2001.
284. DeBont ESJM, et al: Tumor necrosis factor-α, interleukin-1β, and interleukin-6 plasma levels in neonatal sepsis. Pediatr Res 33:380, 1993.
285. Sikora JP, et al: Pro-inflammatory cytokines (IL-6, IL-8), cytokine inhibitors (IL-6sR, sTNFRII) and anti inflammatory cytokines (IL 10, IL 13) in the pathogenesis of sepsis in newborns and infants. Arch Immunol Ther Exp (Warsz) 49:399, 2001.
286. Groll AH, et al: Interleukin-6 as early mediator in neonatal sepsis. Pediatr Infect Dis 11:496, 1992.
287. Edgar JDM, et al: Predictive value of soluble immunological mediators in neonatal infection. Clin Sci 87:165, 1994.
288. DeBont ESJM, et al: Diagnostic value of plasma levels of tumor necrosis factor α (TNFα) and interleukin-6 (IL-6) in newborns with sepsis. Acta Paediatr 83:696, 1994.

289. Buck C, et al: Interleukin-6: a sensitive parameter for the early diagnosis of neonatal bacterial infection. Pediatrics 93:54, 1994.

290. Mehr S, Doyle LW: Cytokines as markers of bacterial sepsis in newborn infants: a review. Pediatr Infect Dis J 19:879, 2000.

291. Kliegman RM, Fanaroff AA: Necrotizing enterocolitis. N Engl J Med 310:1093, 1984.

292. Caplan MS, MacKendrick W: Inflammatory mediators and intestinal injury. Clin Perinatol 21:235, 1994.

293. Caplan MS, et al: Role of platelet activating factor and tumor necrosis factor-alpha in neonatal necrotizing enterocolitis. J Pediatr 116:960, 1990.

294. Harris MC, et al: Cytokine elevations in critically ill infants with sepsis and necrotizing enterocolitis. J Pediatr 124:105, 1994.

295. Morecroft JA, et al: Plasma cytokine levels in necrotizing enterocolitis. Acta Paediatr 396(Suppl):18, 1994.

296. Harris MC, et al: Interleukin-8 levels (IL-8) in bacterial sepsis and necrotizing enterocolitis (NEC): correlation with clinical parameters of inflammation. Pediatr Res 51:140A, 2002.

297. Viscardi RM, et al: Inflammatory cytokine mRNAs in surgical specimens of necrotizing enterocolitis and normal newborn intestine. Pediatr Pathol Lab Med 17:547, 1997.

298. Nadler EP, et al: Intestinal cytokine gene expression in infants with acute necrotizing enterocolitis: interleukin-11 mRNA expression inversely correlates with extent of disease. J Pediatr Surg 36:1122, 2001.

299. McColm JR, et al: Measurement of interleukin 10 in bronchoalveolar lavage from preterm ventilated infants. Arch Dis Child 82:F156, 2000.

300. Hallman M: Inflammatory pathways between placenta and foetus. Acta Pædiatr 90:1, 2001.

301. De Dooy JJ, et al: The role of inflammation in the development of chronic lung disease in neonates. Eur J Pediatr 160:457, 2001.

302. Jobe AH: Intrauterine cytokine activation and the role of infection. Biol Neonate 78:244, 2000.

303. Yoon BH, et al: Amniotic fluid cytokines (interleukin-6, tumor necrosis factor-α, interleukin-1, and interleukin-8) and the risk for the development of bronchopulmonary dysplasia. Am J Obstet Gynecol 177:825, 1997.

304. Yoon BH, et al: A systemic fetal inflammatory response and the development of bronchopulmonary dysplasia. Am J Obstet Gynecol 181:773, 1999.

305. Gähler A, et al: Interleukin-8 expression by fetal and neonatal pulmonary cells in hyaline membrane disease and amniotic infection. Pediatr Res 48:299, 2000.

306. Bagchi A, et al: Increased activity of interleukin-6 but not tumor necrosis factor-α in lung lavage of premature infants is associated with the development of bronchopulmonary dysplasia. Pediatr Res 36:244, 1994.

307. Kotecha S: Cytokines in chronic lung disease of prematurity. Eur J Pediatr 155(Suppl 2):S14, 1996.

308. Kazzi SNJ, et al: Serial changes in levels of IL-6 and IL-1β in premature infants at risk for bronchopulmonary dysplasia. Pediatr Pulmonol 31:220, 2001.

309. Huang H-C, et al: Profiles of inflammatory cytokines in bronchoalveolar lavage fluid from premature infants with respiratory distress disease. J Microbiol Immunol Infect 33:19, 2000.

310. Kwong KY, et al: Differential regulation of IL-8 by IL-1β And TNFα in hyaline membrane disease. J Clin Immunol 18:71, 1998.

311. Blahnik MJ, et al: Lipopolysaccharide-induced tumor necrosis factor-α and IL-10 production by lung macrophages from preterm and term neonates. Pediatr Res 50:726, 2001.

312. Papoff P: Infection, neutrophils, and hematopoietic growth factors in the pathogenesis of neonatal chronic lung disease. Clin Perinatol 27:717, 2000.

313. Manimtim WM, et al: *Ureaplasma urealyticum* modulates endotoxin-induced cytokine release by human monocytes derived from preterm and term newborns and adults. Infect Immun 69:3906, 2001.

314. Viscardi RM, et al: Lung pathology in premature infants with *Ureaplasma urealyticum* infection. Pediatr Dev Pathol 5:141, 2002.

315. Patterson AM, et al: *Ureaplasma urealyticum* respiratory tract colonization is associated with an increase in interleukin 1-beta and tumor necrosis factor alpha relative to interleukin 6 in tracheal aspirates of preterm infants. Pediatr Infect Dis J 17:321, 1998.

316. Li Y-H, et al: *Ureaplasma urealyticum*-induced production of pro-inflammatory cytokines by macrophages. Pediatr Res 48:114, 2000.

317. Baier RJ, et al: Monocyte chemoattractant protein-1 and interleukin-8 are increased in bronchopulmonary dysplasia: relation to isolation of Ureaplasma urealyticum. J Invest Med 49:362, 2001.

160

M. Michele Mariscalco

Integrins and Cell Adhesion Molecules

Adhesion is of fundamental importance to cell functioning. Besides providing "anchorage," it also provides cues for migration and signals for growth, differentiation, and cell activation. The two principal types of cell adhesion are cell to extracellular matrix, and cell to cell. Embryonic development, maintenance of tissue architecture, wound healing, hemostasis, inflammation, and the immune response all involve the interaction of cells with extracellular matrices or adjacent cells. The seminal role of adhesion molecules in embryogenesis and tissue morphogenesis cannot be overemphasized. Indeed, much of the understanding of cell adhesion derives from this prolific area of research (reviewed in reference 1). This chapter focuses on the role of cell adhesion in the inflammatory response. In particular, this review outlines the molecular mechanisms necessary for leukocyte localization in inflammation and the immune process, and what is known regarding the changes in these mechanisms in the immature host.

With the use of intravital microscopy, several investigators in the 19th century established white cells adhering to the blood vessel lining as the hallmark of the acute inflammatory response (reviewed in references 2 and 3). In the absence of inflammatory stimuli and under conditions of flow, leukocyte contact with the endothelium is random, and circulating leukocytes do not adhere to the vascular endothelium. With inflammation, leukocytes marginate within the venules, where they are only loosely tethered to the endothelial wall and roll along the surface. After rolling, leukocytes become firmly adherent to the endothelium

and become "activated," i.e., changing shape from a spherical to a flattened configuration. The leukocytes then crawl toward and finally through endothelial cell junctions (also known as transendothelial migration, or diapedesis). Though the initial observations of this phenomenon were made over 150 years ago, only in the past several decades with the identification of specific cell adhesion and chemotactic/activator molecules have the molecular mechanisms of what has been termed the "leukocyte-endothelial cascade" been elucidated. It is important to emphasize that this cascade does not necessarily occur in all areas of the body; other mechanisms appear to be operative in tissues such as the liver, lung, and kidney.

The susceptibility of human neonates to localized soft tissue infections, as well as systemic infections caused by bacterial or fungal agents, has prompted extensive investigations of neonatal host defense mechanisms. Among the most consistently observed functional abnormalities are those related to leukocyte migration. Compared with adult cells, neonatal neutrophils and monocytes have diminished random and directed migration (chemokinesis and chemotaxis, respectively), as well as decreased adhesion to substrates.[4-7] Motile function is affected by gestational age, in that more severe abnormalities have been recognized in premature infants than in term neonates.[8-10]

In vivo studies employing Rebuk "skin windows" in human neonates provide limited data suggesting that inflammatory responses, as reflected by leukocyte exudation, may differ from those in older children and adults.[11] Studies in experimental animals have provided insight into these differences, with diminished localization in response to inflammatory agents in newborn vs. adult animals. The basis for this defect in neonatal leukocyte motility is likely multifactorial and includes diminished decrease in f-actin polymerization,[12] abnormalities of microtubule assembly,[13] and diminished adhesion receptor number and function.[14,15]

CELL ADHESION MOLECULES

Three families of cell adhesion molecules have been found to play a central role in leukocyte-endothelial interactions: the integrins, the immunoglobulin (Ig) gene superfamily, and the selectins.[2,16,17] The ligands for selectins constitute a fourth family of adhesion molecules, though their primary structures have not been well elucidated in all instances (reviewed in reference 18). Newer adhesion molecules identified in the last few years add increasing complexity to this area. These include new members of the Ig superfamily, junctional adhesion molecule-1, 2, 3 (JAM 1, 2, 3)[19] and CD99, whose primary structure has not yet been elucidated.[20] Other molecules found on the cell surface may modulate adhesion and migration, such as platelet endothelial cell adhesion molecule-1 (PECAM-1).[21] PECAM-1, with a structure that originally placed it in the Ig superfamily, appears to have a signaling-inhibitory function, rather than an adhesive function.[21] It is beyond the scope of this chapter to cover each of these molecules in detail; the following will serve as an introduction to the basic elements so that "differences" in neonatal/infant (as compared with mature host) adhesive molecule function can be appreciated.

Integrins

Overview of Structure and Function

As with all cell adhesion molecules, the integrins are transmembrane cell surface proteins. Unlike the other families of cell adhesion molecules, the integrins are heterodimers, consisting of noncovalently associated α and β subunits, generally of 150 and 100 kDa, respectively. Each subunit crosses the membrane once, with most of each polypeptide in the extracellular space (>1600 amino acids) and a short cytoplasmic tail (30 to 50 amino acids). The term *integrin* was originally suggested to describe membrane receptors that "integrate" the extracellular environment (matrix or other cells) with the intracellular cytoskeleton. At present 18 α and 8 β chains have been identified, with the formation of 24 distinct integrins. The adhesion molecules also have a CD, or cluster designation, classification. For example β1, β2 and β3 are also known as CD29, CD18, and CD61, respectively, while β7 has never been given a CD classification (Table 160–1). As seen in Figure 160–1, β subunits define the subfamily of integrin receptors and can associate with more than one α subunit (reviewed in reference 22). Phylogenetically ancient integrins, like the RGD receptors, recognize the tripeptide sequence arginine(R)-glycine (G)-aspartic acid (D) in fibronectin and vitronectin, whereas other integrins mediate the adhesion to the basement membrane laminin (Fig. 160–1). Collagen receptors have inserted I/A domains (α1, α2, α10, α11), which is discussed in more detail in subsequent paragraphs. A pair of related integrins (α4β1, α9β1) recognize both extracellular matrix proteins such as fibronectin as well as an Ig-superfamily cell surface counterreceptor VCAM-1 (vascular cell adhesion molecule). The β2 and β7 integrins (Fig. 160–1) are restricted to leukocytes; their counterreceptors are members of the Ig superfamily. They mediate heterotypic cell-cell interactions, and several mediate adhesion to extracellular matrix proteins. Ligand specificity relies on both subunits of the αβ heterodimer pair. For example, αLβ2 (LFA-1 or CD11a/CD18) binds to intercellular adhesion molecule (ICAM)-1, -2 and -3. αMβ2 (Mac-1 or CD11b/CD18) binds to a different epitope on ICAM-1 and a wide array of other ligands, including iC3b (cell-bound complement fragment), fibrinogen, fibronectin, factor X, β glucan (present on the cell walls of yeast), and even platelet glycoprotein Ibα.[23] Each of the integrins has a specific function, which is mostly nonredundant. The phenotypes of knockout mice, in which the specific integrin is "knocked out" of the genome, details the ligand specificity of these molecules and their various roles.[22, 24] The phenotypes range from a complete block in preimplantation development (β1) to defects in leukocyte (αL, αM, αE, β2, β7) or platelet function (αIIb, β3).

Although integrins appear to have a nonredundant function in regard to their roles in adhesion to extracellular matrix ligands or counterreceptors on adjacent cells, nonetheless they share a number of characteristics. Integrins serve as transmembrane mechanical links from extracellular contacts to the actin microfilament. Integrins affect actin organization and thereby directly influence cell spreading, morphogenesis, and migration. The submembrane cytoskeletal proteins that connect the relatively short cytoplasmic domains of the integrins directly to the cytoskeleton are numerous and complex and include talin, tensin, and α-actinin. However, cytoplasmic tails of integrins also are linked to signal transduction pathways, including tyrosine kinases (e.g., FAK [focal adhesion kinase] and steroid receptor coactivator [SRC]), serine-threonine kinases (e.g., ILK, [integrin-linked kinase], and PKC [protein kinase C]) and other enzymes, e.g., phosphatidyl-inositol 3 kinase. Ligation of integrins triggers a variety of signal transduction events, which affect proliferation, survival/apoptosis, gene expression, and differentiation, in addition to affecting shape, polarity, and motility.[25] What is clear is that integrins are signal transduction receptors, at least as important to cells as more traditional growth factors like epidermal growth factor (EGF), platelet-derived growth factor (PDGF), and transforming growth factor (TGF).

In many instances, integrins are not constitutively "active" and usually exist in an "off" state. When off, integrins do not bind ligand and they do not signal. One of the most important mechanisms of integrin function is the rapid transition from a nonadhesive, low-affinity state to a transient high-affinity state and then return to a low affinity state. This has been termed "inside-out" signaling. For example, the platelet integrin αIIbβ3 is present at high density on circulating platelets, where it is inactive. Activation of the platelet results in activation of αIIbβ3 and binding to its ligands fibrinogen, von Willebrand factor, and fibronectin. This results in aggregation of platelets and adherence to the vessel wall.[26] Members of the β2 integrin subfamily, which are expressed on most leukocytes, are also inactive when the cells are not stimulated. However, β2 integrins become rapidly activated in response to cell activation with low-dose chemokines, cytokines, or shear stress.[27, 28] As with αIIbβ3, the activated β2 integrins may then bind to their ligands on the endothelial surface, other cells, subendothelial matrix, or complement-coated bacteria. Activation of the integrins is transient, with rapid return to an inactive state.[26-29] Clearly, this function of integrins is necessary for maintenance of a "nonthrombotic", "noninflamed" state in the host. In addition, the rapid "turn-on" and "turn-off" of integrin function is of critical importance in the process of the leukocyte-endothelial cascade, discussed in a subsequent section of this chapter.

At least two mechanisms are proposed to explain how integrin activation increases integrin-ligand interactions. One mechanism is conformational changes in integrins (regulating the affinity of the integrin for the ligand) and the other is clustering of integrins and association with the cytoskeleton (regulating the avidity of integrin-ligand binding). That integrin clustering may affect ligand binding is supported by the observations that (1) a proportion of αLβ2 (LFA-1) on cells expressing active αLβ2

TABLE 160-1

Adhesion Molecules in Inflammation and Hemostasis

Name	CD Classification	Primary Cell Expression	Ligand
Integrin Family			
β1 Integrins			
α1β1 (VLA-1)	CD49a/CD29	T- and B-cell subsets, Mono	COL I, COL IV, LN
α2β1 (VLA-2)	CD49b/CD29	T-cell subsets, Mono, PLT, PMN	COL I, COL IV, LN
α3β1 (VLA-3)	CD49c/CD29	T-cell subsets, Mono	FN, COL I, LN
α4β1 (VLA-4)	CD49d/CD29	T-cell, B-cell, Eos, Mono, PMN, Baso	FN, VCAM, Tsp, JAM2
α5β1 (VLA-5)	CD49e/CD29	T-cells, PMN, PLT	FN, Tsp
α6β1 (VLA-6)	CD49f/CD29	T-cells, PMN, PLT, EC	LN
α9β1		PMN, Mono	VCAM-1, OSP, tenascin
β2 Integrins			
αLβ2 (LFA-1)	CD11a/CD18	PMNS, T- and B-cell, Eos, Mono, NK, Macro	ICAM-1, ICAM-2, ICAM-3, JAM-1
αMβ2 (Mac-1)	CD11b/CD18	PMNS, Mono, Eos, NK, Macro, Lymph subset	ICAM-1, iC$_3$b, Fg, FN, factor X, JAM-3?
αXβ2 (p150,95)	CD11c/CD18	PMN, Mono, Eos, Lymph subset	GPIb-IX-V
αDβ2	αD/CD18	LYMPH, Mono, Macro, PMN	iC$_3$b, unknown EC ligand, factor X, ICAM-3, VCAM-1
β3 Integrins			
αIIbβ3 (GPIIbIIIa)	CD41/CD61	PLTS	vWf, FN, Fg, VN, Tsp, COL
αVβ3 (vitronectin receptor)	CD51/CD61	LAK, Macro, Mono, T-cell, PLT, EC, PMN	vWf, VN, FN, Fg, PECAM-1, Tsp, LN, OSP, tenascin, COL
β7 Integrins			
α4β7	CD49d/β7	Gut-associated lymphocytes	VCAM, MAdCAM-1, FN
αEβ7	CD103/β7	Gut-associated lymphocytes	E-CAD
Immunoglobulin Superfamily (IGSF)			
ICAM-1	CD54	T- and B-cell, Mono, EC, pneumocyte, hepatocytes, epithelial cells, fibroblasts	LFA-1, Mac-1
ICAM-2	CD102	EC	LFA-1
ICAM-3	CD50	Lymph, PMN, Mono	LFA-1, αDβ2
VCAM-1	CD106	EC	α4β1, α4β7, α9β
JAM-1		EC, epithelial cells, PMNs, Mono, Lymph, RBC	LFA-1, JAM-1
JAM-2		HEV, EC	JAM-2, JAM-3, α4β1
JAM-3		Lymph	Mac-1?, JAM3
MAdCAM-1		Peyers patch HEV, mesenteric LN	α4β7, L-selectin
PECAM-1*			
Selectins			
L-selectin	CD62-L	Lymph, Mono, Eos, Baso, PMN	CD34, GlyCAM-1, MAdCAM-1, unknown EC ligand, PSGL-1, PNAD, sLe^x-bearing ligands
P-selectin	CD62-P	EC, PLTS	PSGL-1, E-selectin, GPIb-IX-V
E-selectin	CD62-E	EC	PSGL-1, sLe^x-bearing ligand(s), CLA
Selectin Ligands			
PSGL-1	CD162	PMN, Eos, Mono, Lymph	P-selectin, L-selection, E-selectin
GlyCAM-1		Lymph node, lung EC	L-selectin
CD34	CD34	Peripheral LN HEV, leukocyte precursors	L-selectin
"Other"			
CD99	CD99	T-cells, endothelial cells, monocytes	CD99, ?
PECAM-1*	CD31	EC, PMN, PLT, Mono, lymphocyte subsets	PECAM-1, αVβ3

* Though PECAM-1 is now considered a member of the immunoreceptor tyrosine-based inhibitory motif (ITIM) family, by convention it is still listed in the IGSF and "other." Baso = basophil; CLA = cutaneous lymphocyte-associated antigen; COL I = collagen type I; COL IV = collagen type IV; EC = endothelial cell; E-CAD = E-cadherin; Eos = eosinophils; Fg = fibrinogen; FN = fibronectin; GlyCAM-1 = glycosylation-dependent cell adhesion molecule-1; GP1b-IX-V = glycoprotein complex present on the surface of platelets; ICAM = intercellular adhesion molecule; iC3b = inactivated form of complement component C3b; IGSF = immunoglobulin superfamily; JAM = junctional adhesion molecule; LAK = lymphokine-activated killer (cells); LN = laminin; LYMPH = lymphocytes; Macro = macrophages; MAdCAM-1 = mucosal addressin cell adhesion molecule-1; Mono = monocytes; NK = natural killer cells; OSP = osteopontin; PECAM-1 = platelet endothelial adhesion molecule = 1; PLT = platelet; PMN = polymorphonuclear leukocyte; PNAD = peripheral node addressin; PSGL-1 = P-selectin glycoprotein ligand-1; sLe^x = sialylated Lewis X antigen; Tsp = thrombospondin; VCAM = vascular cell adhesion molecule; VLA = very late antigen; Vn = vitronectin; vWf = von Willebrand factor.

is "clustered." (2) αLβ2 became more mobile on the plasma membranes of T cells activated with phorbol esters. (3) αLβ2 activation via intracellular signaling caused αLβ2 clustering, and this clustered form was essential for adhesion of αLβ2 to its primary ligand, ICAM-1.[30] These observations have led to the hypothesis that an inactive integrin (at least αLβ2 and α4β1) is restrained by the cytoskeleton, and an activating agonist causes release of the cytoskeletal tether, which, in turn, leads to integrin mobility on the cell membrane and clustering. It is difficult to know, however, whether clustering triggers ligand binding or is a result of ligand binding after increasing integrin affinity. However, real-time imaging has demonstrated that the formation of visible clusters of integrins in adhering cells occurs after first contacts are made (i.e., within minutes rather than within seconds).[31]

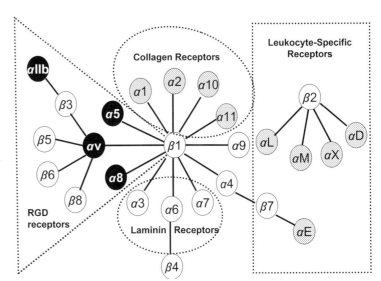

Figure 160–1. The integrin family. Integrins are αβ heterodimers. The figure depicts the mammalian subunits and their αβ associations; β 8 subunits can associate with 18 α subunits to form 24 distinct integrins. α subunits with gray stippling have inserted I/A domains (see text). α subunits with I/A domains are found only in chordates, as are α4 and α9 and subunits β2 to β8. In contrast, α subunits specific for laminin or RGD (black spheres) (see text) are found throughout the metazoa. Note that β2 and β7 integrins are restricted to leukocytes only. (Adapted with permission from Hynes RO: Cell *110*:673, 2002.)

Thus whether clustering and consequently changes in avidity are a major contributor of integrin activation remains controversial.

The second mechanism proposed for increased integrin-ligand binding is activation-dependent changes in integrin conformation. Using crystal structure analysis, electron microscopic images, and electronic magnetic resonance, extensive progress has been made in elucidating conformational regulation of ligand binding by integrins (reviewed in references 22 and 32). The α and β subunit of the integrins are noncovalently associated, and the ligand-binding region is a globular headpiece formed of each subunit. The two long stalk regions containing C-terminal segments from the α and β subunits connect the ligand-binding headpiece to the transmembrane and C-terminal cytoplasmic domains. As seen in Figure 160–2, in the α subunits there are 7 segments of about 60 amino acids each; they have weak homology to each other, but are predicted to fold into a seven-bladed β propeller domain, with Ca^{2+} binding motifs in 4 to 7. As we outlined earlier and show in Figure 160–1, about half of integrin α subunits contain an "inserted" (I) domain, also called a von Willebrand factor A domain (A), since it resembles this structure. The "I/A" domain is the major ligand binding site in those integrins that contain it. An Mg^{2+} binding site is present in the I/A domain. It is inserted between the 2nd and 3rd β sheet. Lee and colleagues[33] identified that glutamine or aspartic acid residue on the ligand, in coordination with divalent cation (Ca^{2+}, Mg^{2+} or Mn^{2+}) participated in increased integrin binding. This region was termed the metal ion–dependent adhesion site (MIDAS). The remainder of the extracellular subunit is predicted to be three β sandwich domains, designated the thigh, calf-1, and calf-2 domains (Fig. 160–2).

The N-terminal cysteine region of the β subunit is termed the *PSI* domain, for plexins, semaphorins, and integrins, since it shares sequence homology with these proteins. The first cysteine of the PSI domain forms a long-range disulfide bond to the C-terminal cysteine-rich region farther down the β-subunit (Fig. 160–2). Although the β subunit lacks a true I domain, it does have a region of about 240 residues, which is highly conserved among species. It has been termed the "I-like" domain since it has a metal-binding motif similar to that of the MIDAS region in the A/I domain, has a weak amino acid sequence homology with the I domain, and a similar secondary structure. The I-like domain appears to directly bind ligands in integrins that lack I/A domains, and indirectly to regulate ligand-binding by integrins that contain I/A domains.[32] Mutations in this region result in lack of association of the integrin β subunit with the α, or loss of

function, resulting in leukocyte adhesion deficiency.[34] As seen in Figure 160–2, the hybrid domain is folded with the I-like domain in the middle, with two covalent connections between the I-like and hybrid domains. There is a cysteine-rich region with four repeats, with structural similarity to epidermal growth factor (integrin-EGF or I-EGF). The cysteine-rich repeats have unique structural properties that make this region rigid and suited for transmission of structural motion in signaling. Many antibodies, which "activate" the integrins or bind only when the integrin is in an activated state, bind to this region.[32]

Several models are proposed for integrin conformational change. One proposal is that there is a global change in conformation. The integrin in the "inactive" conformation is "bent over" (Fig. 160–2C). The ligand-binding headpiece is folded back on the tailpiece and thus is unavailable for binding to ligand. This occurs in the presence of Ca^{2+}. With activation, in the presence of Mn^{2+} or both, the integrin straightens like a switchknife, and the integrin head may then bind to ligand. With the straightening and separation of the "legs" of the integrin, epitopes in the I-EGF and the PSI regions of the β subunit are then "unveiled" and are now available to bind to "activating" antibodies, or alternatively, those antibodies that bind only when the integrin is activated.[35, 36] Separation of the cytoplasmic domains of the legs also permits conformational changes in their structure, allowing them to bind cytoplasmic proteins and signal.

In addition to changes in overall conformation, those integrins with an I/A domain in the α subunit, such as αM and αL, undergo an additional conformational change in the MIDAS binding region, such that in the "open" form, ligands bind.[37, 38] This is hypothesized to occur by a "bell-rope" model.[32] The I-like MIDAS domain of the β subunit becomes "activated" by a conformational change in this subunit, pulls the α helix of the I/A domain of the α subunit "down" (like a bell-rope), converting the I/A domain to a high-affinity conformation. Non-I/A-domain integrins appear to undergo similar conformational changes in which the I-like MIDAS domain of the β subunit is converted from low affinity to high affinity and ready for direct interaction with the acidic residue in the ligand protein.[39, 40]

Several other features are critical for integrin function. Ligand specificity of a particular integrin may be controlled by cell-type specific modulation. The most striking example of this is α2β1, which is a collagen receptor on platelets and a laminin receptor on endothelial cells.[41] α2β1 isolated from either platelets or endothelial cells retains the binding characteristics of its original source. This has not been reported with the β2 integrins. Integrin

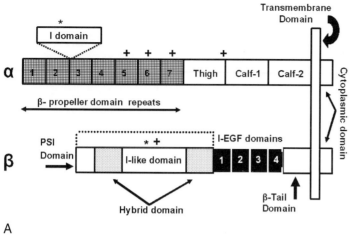

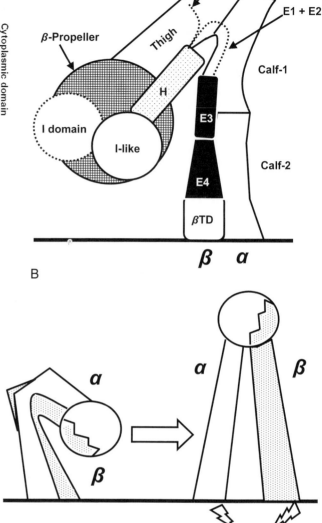

Figure 160–2. Integrin structure. A, General structure of the α and β subunits. Depending on the α subunit, there may also be an inserted "I/A" domain, as outlined in the text. Mg^{2+} and Ca^{2+} binding sites are shown as asterisks (*) and crosses (+) respectively. Only the disulfide bonds within the β chain between the PSI domain and the first I-EGF domain are shown (dotted line). Both chains have numerous disulfide bonds that are not included but account for the complex tertiary structure. I-EGF = integrin-epidermal growth factor-like; PSI = plexin, semiphorins, integrins. **B,** Arrangement of the domains based on the three-dimensional structure of αVβ3 with an added I domain. Domains refer to those listed in **A.** PSI and I-EGF domains 1 and 2 are referenced by a dotted line as they are "out of the plane" of the molecule. The transmembrane and cytoplasmic domains are not included. **C,** Hypothetical model for integrin activation. In the inactive state, the integrin is "bent over" and not available for binding to ligand (*figure on left*). With activation, the integrin "straightens" and the legs separate, permitting binding to ligand. Separation of the legs is also thought to result in "outside-in signaling," demonstrated in this figure by the lightning bolts. (Adapted from Takagi J, Springer TA: Immunol Rev *186:* 141, 2002.)

receptor expression can also be modulated at the transcriptional and translational level. During leukocyte differentiation, the levels of β2 integrins are differentially regulated. αLβ2 appears in early progenitor cells; the expression of αMβ2 (Mac-1) and αXβ2 (p150,95) occurs in later maturational stages.[42] Numerous stimuli up-regulate the level of integrin α4β1 on lymphocytes and macrophages. In contrast, rapid alterations in levels of integrins expressed on the surface of neutrophils and platelets can be achieved by mobilization of intracellular pools of integrins in response to extracellular stimuli and chemotactic factors (Table 160–2). Stimulation of neutrophils or monocytes can increase the αMβ2 and αXβ2 surface expression by ten fold, as they are stored in secretory and tertiary granules.[43] Although not present or present at very low levels under resting conditions, neutrophils that have undergone migration can express large amounts of α2β1, α4β1, α5β1, α6β1 and α9β1, which assist the neutrophil in migrating through extracellular matrix.[44-46] It is unclear whether all these integrins are present in granules or are synthesized de novo. Platelets contain reserves of αIIbβ3 (GPIIB/IIIa, the receptor for fibrinogen, von Willebrand factor, see Table 160–1) in the α granules. With platelet activation, fusion of α granules with the plasma membrane occurs, effectively doubling the number of αIIbβ3 complexes.[47]

β2 Integrins. The β2 subgroup (CD18), found exclusively on leukocytes, are the major contributors to leukocyte motility and function. All members share the common β2 (CD18) subunit (see Figure 160–1 and Table 160–1), but have α unique (CD11) subunits that primarily confer ligand specificity. αLβ2 (LFA-1, CD11a/CD18,) is located on all leukocytes. αMβ2 (Mac-1, CD11b/CD18,) and αXβ2 (p150,95, CD11c/CD18,) are located on neutrophils, monocytes, macrophages, natural killer cells, and some lymphocytes.[16] LFA-1 and Mac-1 appear to interact equally with their endothelial ligand, intercellular adhesion molecule-1 (ICAM-1).[28] However, LFA-1 also binds to both ICAM-2, -3 and JAM-1.[48] Lymphocyte adhesion to the vessel wall involves the interaction of LFA-1 with its endothelial ligands, ICAM-1 and -2. LFA-1 also participates in many other cell-cell interactions, such as T cell activation by antigen-presenting cells, or the killing of virus-infected cells by cytotoxic T lymphocytes.

Mac-1 and p150,95 are capable of binding to a wide range of ligands, including fibrinogen, factor X, denatured albumin, and the complement fragment iC3b. This rather "promiscuous"

TABLE 160-2

Activating Factors for Leukocyte/Platelet Endothelial Adhesion

Activating Agent	Target Cell				
	Endothelial Cell	Neutrophil	Monocyte	Lymphocyte	Platelets
Cytokines					
TNFα	+	+			
IL-1	+	+			
IFN-γ	+	+			
IL-4	+				
Lipids					
Bacterial endotoxin (LPS)	+	+	+	+	
PAF		+	+		
LTB$_4$		+	+		
LTC$_4$	+				
Thromboxane A$_2$					+
Peptide Chemoattractants					
C5a		+	+		
N-formyl peptides (fMLP)		+	+		
C-X-C Chemokines					
CXCL8(IL-8)	+	+		+	
CXCL10 (IP 10)				+	
CXCL5 (ENA 78)	+	+	+	+	
CXCL1 (GRO-α, MGSA-α)	+	+	+	+	
CXCL7 (NAP-2)	+	+	+	+	
CXCL12 (SDF)	+		+	+	+
C-C Chemokines					
CCL3 (MIP-1α)		+	+	+	+
CCL4 (MIP-1β)		+	+	+	
CCL5 (RANTES)			+	+	+
CCL2 (MCP-1)			+	+	
CCL8 (MCP-2),			+	+	+
CCL7 (MCP3)			+	+	+
Others					
Histamine	+	+			
Thrombin	+				+
Hydrogen peroxide	+				
Collagen					+
Adenosine diphosphate					+

C5a = protein produced from cleavage of complement protein C5; ENA 78 = epithelium-derived neutrophil attractant 78; fMLP = N-formyl-methionine-leucine-phenylalanine; GRO-α = growth-regulating protein α; IFN-γ = interferon-γ; IL-1 = interleukin-1; IL-4 = interleukin-4; IL-8 = interleukin-8; IP 10 = γ-interferon-induced peptide; LPS = lipopolysaccharide; LTB$_4$ = leukotriene B$_4$; LTC$_4$ = leukotriene C$_4$; MCP-1, -2, -3 = monocyte chemotactic peptide -1, -2, -3; MGSA = melanocyte growth-stimulating activity; MIP-1α = macrophage inflammatory peptide α; NAP-2 = neutrophil-activating peptide-2; PAF = platelet-activating factor; RANTES = regulated on activation, normal T-cell expressed and secreted; TNFα = tumor necrosis factor α.
Names in parentheses indicate the other names of chemokines.

attachment to a number of native and denatured proteins is important during leukocyte migration over a variety of substrata, and adhesion to and phagocytosis of foreign particles. Neutrophil and monocyte adhesion to endothelium relies mainly on LFA-1 and Mac-1, with only a minor role for p 150,95. A fourth member of the β2 family, αDβ2, has been identified on subsets of human leukocytes, and more strongly on tissue-compartmentalized cells such as the macrophages.[49] It preferentially binds to ICAM-3 and can bind to VCAM-1 if present on lymphocytes.[50]

As with other integrins, both LFA-1 and Mac-1 can participate as classic receptors by generating biochemical signals within the cells. Through such signalling, Mac-1 participates in opsonophagocytosis, release of oxygen species, and antibody-dependent cell cytotoxicity. Similarly, ligation of LFA-1 by monoclonal antibodies has been shown to activate T cells, resulting in homotypic aggregation and stimulation of cytoskeletal rearrangements. Both LFA-1 and Mac-1 can lead to activation of other integrins, particularly the β1 integrins, in a process known as "cross-talk."[30, 51] Thus interaction of LFA-1 or Mac-1 to their

adhesive ligands will activate other integrins on the cell surface for binding to other ligands in the matrix.

β1 and β7 Integrins. The largest number of integrins are members of the β1 (CD29) or VLA subfamily (see Figure 160–1 and Table 160–1). VLA derives from "very late antigen," because the first ones to be identified (VLA-1 and VLA-2) were expressed only at a late stage after T-cell activation. They comprise a series of cellular receptors for extracellular matrix proteins, including fibronectin, collagen, and laminin. α4β1 (VLA-4, CD49d/CD29) is expressed at substantial levels on most mononuclear leukocytes, including lymphocytes, monocytes, eosinophils, basophils, and NK cells, whether the cells are in circulation, within lymphoid organs, or resident in other tissues.[52] α4β1 is also expressed on transmigrated neutrophils.[53] α4β1 binds to vascular cell adhesion molecules -1 (VCAM-1), mucosal addressin cell adhesion molecule-1 (MAdCAM-1), as well as to the alternatively spliced connecting segment (CS-1) of fibronectin. The site of α4β1 binding to VCAM-1 is distinct from that involved in fibronectin binding. α4β1 is important for monocyte and eosinophil trafficking to inflamed tissues, as well as lymphocyte migration and differentiation.[54] Unlike LFA-1 and Mac-1, α4β1 can mediate the initial tether of the leukocyte from the free stream to VCAM-1 and MAdCAM-1.

α1β1, α2β1, α3β1, α5β1, and α6β1 (see Table 160–1) are expressed on T-cell subsets or resting T lymphocytes and generally are of importance to lymphocyte/extracellular matrix interactions. Their ligands include the extracellular matrix proteins collagen, laminin, and fibronectin.[16] Neutrophils also express α2β1, α5β1, α6β1 as they infiltrate lungs, joints, peritoneum, and spleen, and adhere to and migrate through interstitial matrix via pathways that are β2 integrin-independent.[53, 55, 56] α9β1 is expressed extensively on smooth muscle and epithelial cells and mediates adhesion to the extracellular matrix proteins osteopontin and tenascin-C. It is abundantly expressed on neutrophils, modestly expressed on monocytes, but not to lymphocytes. Its ligand is VCAM-1. As with α4β1, α9β1 mediates neutrophil transendothelial migration.[44, 57]

The α4β7 (CD49d/β7) and αEβ7 are expressed primarily on gut-associated T lymphocytes. α4β7 is required for lymphocyte recirculation to specific areas of the gut containing mucosal addressin cell adhesion molecule-1 (MAdCAM-1), which is expressed on Peyer's patch, high endothelial venules, and postcapillary venules in the lamina propria.[54] αEβ7 is expressed on T lymphocytes in the intestinal mucosa, genitourinary tract, lymphocytes derived from the lung and on intraepidermal T cells in some skin disorders. It is also present on 90% of CD8+ T cells. Its primary ligand is E(epithelial)-cadherin.[58]

β3 Integrins. Like Mac-1, αvβ3 (CD51/CD61), also known as the vitronectin receptor, and αIIbβ3 (gp IIb/IIIa) are "promiscuous receptors" and have overlapping ligands, including fibrinogen, von Willebrand factor, fibronectin, collagen, and vitronectin, though each may bind to different regions of the same molecule. αvβ3 is present on a large number of cell types and has been shown to play a role in tumor invasion, proliferation and metastasis, bone resorption, angiogenesis, differentiation, development, and the immune response. It serves as an accessory molecule for T-cell activation and is important for complement deposition on platelets and cells. Additionally, αvβ3 is expressed on macrophages in a maturationally related process, and it mediates recognition of apoptotic cells (both neutrophils and lymphocytes). Thus αvβ3 may represent a mechanism that limits tissue injury through macrophage clearance of leukocytes at an inflamed site.[59]

Many integrins are found on platelets, including α2β1, α5β1, α6β1, and αvβ3 and are important to either stimulatory or adhesive/cohesive phases of platelet function. αIIbβ3 (gp IIb/IIIa) is found exclusively on platelets and is largely responsible for the

final cohesive phase of platelet activation *in vivo*, i.e., platelet aggregation supported by the binding of adhesive proteins, like fibrinogen or von Willebrand factor.[47] Coincident with platelet activation, surface expression of αIIbβ3 increases through release from α granules. Additionally, αIIbβ3 undergoes profound conformational changes, with resultant binding to fibrinogen; resting platelets do not bind fibrinogen. With binding of αIIbβ3, through outside-in signaling, the platelet is stimulated further and can potentiate clot retraction.[47]

Immunoglobulin Gene Superfamily

The immunoglobulin gene (Ig) superfamily encompasses a large group of molecules with multiple immunoglobulin-like domains in the extracellular portion of the molecule, resembling the second domain of the constant region of immunoglobulin (Fig. 160–3). Six members of this family are involved in leukocyte-leukocyte or leukocyte-endothelial interactions. Intercellular adhesion molecule-1 (ICAM-1, CD54), ICAM-2 (CD102), vascular cell adhesion molecule-1 (VCAM-1, CD106), platelet-endothelial cell adhesion molecule-1 (PECAM-1, CD31), and mucosal addressin cell adhesion molecule-1 (MAdCAM-1) all serve as endothelial ligands for leukocytes. Intercellular adhesion molecule-3 (ICAM-3, CD50) is expressed on leukocytes and is important for leukocyte-leukocyte adherence and cell signaling.[16]

ICAM-1, ICAM-2, and ICAM-3 were all initially identified by their ability to interact with LFA-1, and each is the product of distinct though homologous genes. ICAM-1 contains five Ig domains, but ICAM-2 contains two, both domains of which are highly homologous to the two NH2-terminal domains of ICAM-1. ICAM-3 also contains five immunoglobulin domains that are highly homologous to ICAM-1 and -2. The binding site for LFA-1 has been mapped to the first Ig domain for each of the molecules. In contrast, ICAM-1 has been found to bind to Mac-1 through a distinct site in its third immunoglobulin domain.[60] ICAM-1 is constitutively present on endothelial cells as well as on other cell types, including lymphocytes, dendritic cells, fibroblasts, hepatocytes, and epithelial cells such as type I pneumocytes. ICAM-1 is expressed on resting endothelium, but its expression increases dramatically after stimulation with a number of cytokines, including tumor necrosis-α (TNF-α), interleukin-1 (IL-1), and IFN-γ[61] (Fig. 160–4). Similarly, ICAM-1 expression can be induced on lymphocytes. In contrast, ICAM-2 is constitutively present on most cells, is expressed at high levels on resting endothelial cells, and its expression is not augmented by activation. The affinity of ICAM-2 for LFA-1 appears to be weaker than that of ICAM-1, and its role in leukocyte emigration is not well elucidated.[62] ICAM-2 is only modestly present on

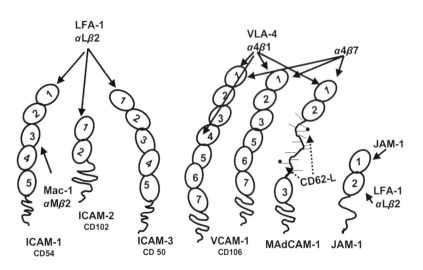

Figure 160–3. Immunoglobulin gene superfamily. The immunoglobulin gene superfamily (IGSF) comprises a large group of molecules, each of which contains multiple extracellular domains resembling the second domain of immunoglobulin (represented here by an oval), a transmembrane domain, and a cytoplasmic tail. Note that there is an alternatively spliced form of VCAM-1 that does not contain domain 4. The sticks and lollipops on MAdCAM-1 refer to the N-linked and O-linked glycosylation sites, respectively. Included also on the structure diagrams are the domains to which specific adhesion molecules bind. ICAM = intercellular adhesion molecule; LFA-1 = lymphocyte function antigen; VCAM = vascular cell adhesion molecule; MAdCAM = mucosal addressin cell adhesion molecule; JAM = junctional adhesion molecule; CD62L = L-selectin; VLA = very late antigen.

leukocytes. ICAM-3 is strongly expressed on resting lympho-cytes, monocytes, and neutrophils.[62] Co-ligand engagement of T cell LFA-1 to ICAM-1, ICAM-2, or ICAM-3 on accessory cells is necessary for full T-cell receptor activation, resulting in cell pro-liferation and IL-2 secretion.[62] All three ICAMs contribute to antigen-specific interactions, so that inhibition with monoclonal antibodies (mAbs) to all three are required to block LFA-1 dependent, antigen-specific T-cell responses completely.

Vascular cell adhesion molecule-1 (VCAM-1) exists predomi-nantly as a 7-domain transmembrane protein in humans, though an alternatively spliced minor form exists (see Figure 160–3). VCAM-1 binds to α4β1 at its first and fourth domains. It also binds to α4β7, α9β1, αDβ2[44, 50, 63] (see Table 160–1). VCAM-1 is ex-pressed constitutively on some nonvascular cells, including den-dritic cells in lymphoid tissues and skin, epithelial cells, some monocyte-derived cells, and bone marrow stromal cells. It was ini-tially identified as an inducible molecule on endothelial cells that mediates adhesion to lymphocytes and monocytes. VCAM-1 is absent on resting endothelial cells but is induced in response to IL-1 and TNF, with maximal expression reached by 6 to 12 hours (see Figure 160–4). VCAM-1 is required for lymphocyte, eosinophil, and monocyte adherence and emigration and appears critical in the initiation of atherosclerosis. Unlike ICAM, it is able to participate in the tethering and rolling of leukocytes.[64]

Platelet endothelial adhesion molecule-1 (PECAM-1, CD31) is a six-Ig domain molecule that mediates both leukocyte- and platelet-endothelial adhesion and leukocyte transendothelial migration. PECAM-1 is present on platelets, bone marrow pre-cursor cells, neutrophils, monocytes, and certain subsets of lym-phocytes. It is highly expressed on endothelial cells, but much less so on neutrophils. With its Ig-like extracellular domains, it was classified initially as a cell adhesion molecule. However, recent work has demonstrated that its cytoplasmic domain may be the "work" end of the molecule.[21] PECAM-1 appears to be a member of the Ig-ITIM (immunoreceptor tyrosine-based inhibitory motif) family. When members of this family are engaged by their extracellular ligand, their cytoplasmic ITIM domain becomes phosphorylated, which serves as a docking site for intracellular lipid and protein phosphatases. Once these cat-alytic enzymes become localized to their cytoplasmic anchors and activated, they affect a wide range of cellular functions, including events that inhibit signaling, proliferation, and cellular activation. In particular, PECAM-1 appears to modulate activation of β1, β2 and β3 integrin function on platelets, lymphocytes, and neutrophils.[21, 50] PECAM-1 participates in *homophilic* (i.e., binds to another PECAM-1 molecule on adjacent cells) and *het-erophilic* interactions (binds to other ligands, such as αvβ3).

An adhesion molecule for lymphocyte recirculation to mucosa is expressed on Peyer's patch high endothelial venules, as well as other venules.[65] Known as mucosal addressin adhesion molecule-1 (MAdCAM-1), it contains three immunoglobulin-like domains and a mucin-like region between domains 2 and 3 (see Figure 160–3). Mucins are serine- and threonine-rich proteins that are heavily glycosylated through an "O" linkage. They are rigid and have an extended structure (see following discussion on selectin-ligands).[17] MAdCAM-1 binds both α4β7 and α4β1.[66] MadCAM-1 is unique in that it is also able to bind L-selectin and mediate lymphocyte rolling with the presence of a mucin-like domain.[67]

Junctional adhesion molecule (JAM)-1, -2, and -3 are the newest additions to the Ig family, and the nomenclature as of 2003 is still nonuniform (see Table 160–1).[68] The JAMs have two extracellular Ig domains and are present on endothelial and epithelial cells at the tight junctions. With stimulation by pro-inflammatory cytokines, JAMs move away from the borders and appear to mediate permeability.[19] JAMs are also present on neutrophils, lymphocytes, and platelets. Recent studies demonstrate that these molecules may play unique roles in leukocyte transendothelial migration as they appear to be ligands for LFA-1 and α4β1.[48, 68]

CD99 does not belong to the Ig superfamily. It is a heavily gly-cosylated transmembrane protein present on many hematopoietic cells and has been shown to increase the presence and activity of LFA-1 and α4β1. Recently it has also been found on endothelial cells, concentrated at the borders between confluent cells. CD99 on monocytes appears to mediate homophilic binding to endothe-lial CD99 and mediate transendothelial migration.[20]

Selectins

There are three members of the selectin (CD62) family of adhe-sion molecules: E- (CD62-E), P- (CD62-P), and L-selectin (CD62-L). This family mediates the earliest events in leukocyte-endothelial adhesion in that they "capture" leukocytes from the free-flowing bloodstream and allow rolling to occur along the blood vessel lining. The name incorporates the term *lectin*, which refers to a wide range of carbohydrate-binding proteins, reflecting the fact that this family of adhesion molecules recognizes carbohydrate ligands. Each is an integral membrane protein with an N-terminal, Ca^{2+}-type lectin domain, followed by an epidermal growth factor (EGF)-like module, multiple copies of the consensus repeat units characteristic of complement-binding proteins, a transmembrane segment, and a short cytoplasmic domain. E-selectin is expressed on activated endothelial cells. With cell activation, P-selectin is rapidly redistributed from secretory granules of endothelial cells and platelets to the plasma membrane. L-selectin is expressed on most leukocytes (see Table 160–1).

L-selectin functions as the peripheral lymph node homing receptor on lymphocytes and binds through its lectin domain to carbohydrate-containing ligands on high endothelial venules in peripheral lymph nodes (see Table 160–1). It also serves as an important adhesion molecule for monocyte, neutrophil, and eosinophil trafficking. The cell surface expression of L-selectin is down-regulated after activation of both lymphocytes and myeloid cells. The process involves the shedding of L-selectin rather than internalization or a conformational change, and it arises through proteolytic cleavage of the molecule at the extra-cellular part, close to the transmembrane region. L-selectin has been demonstrated to be located at the tips of the surface folds of unstimulated neutrophils.[69] In this position, L-selectin would

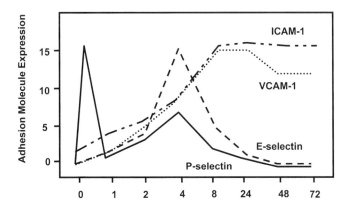

Figure 160–4. Temporal expression of adhesion molecules induced by cytokines. Note that P-selectin has two peaks, at 0.5 hour and 4 to 8 hours. The first peak is due to release of P-selectin from Weibel-Palade bodies; the second is due to protein synthesis. There is constitutive expression of ICAM-1 (intercellular adhesion molecule). VCAM = vascular cell adhesion molecule. (Adapted from Imhof BA, Dunon D: Adv Immunol *58*:345, 1995.)

be in a particularly advantageous position to contact the endothelium in the initial margination of neutrophils. Leukocyte β2 integrin function can be activated via L-selectin ligation in vitro.[2] Inhibition of L-selectin shedding in mice results in decreased leukocyte rolling velocity and an increased number of arrested and transmigrated leukocytes.[70]

P-selectin is constitutively synthesized by megakaryocytes and endothelial cells, but it is sorted into secretory granules (α granules in platelets and Weibel-Palade bodies in endothelial cells). Upon stimulation by thrombin, histamine, hydrogen peroxide, and other secretagogues, P-selectin is rapidly transported to the cell surface by fusion of granule membranes with the plasma membrane (see Table 160–2). Once mobilized, P-selectin usually remains on the cell surface for less than an hour. Lipopolysaccharide and certain other inflammatory cytokines induce P-selectin expression in a manner similar to that of E-selectin. The kinetics for cytokine-induced P-selectin are also similar to those occurring after cytokine-induced E-selectin expression (see Fig. 160–4). P-selectin mediates adhesion between leukocytes and platelets as well as leukocyte-endothelial adhesion (see Table 160–1).

The expression of E-selectin on endothelial cells requires the de novo synthesis of both mRNA and protein. Many stimuli are capable of inducing the expression of E-selectin, including the cytokines IL-1, TNF-α and TNF-β (lymphotoxin), and lipopolysaccharide (LPS) (see Table 160–2). It is also induced on dermal endothelial cells in delayed-type hypersensitivity reactions and in chronically inflamed skin. Maximal expression of E-selectin peaks at 4 to 6 hours and then declines to near basal levels within 24 hours (see Fig. 160–4).

The amino acid sequences of the lectin and EGF domain of all three selectins are highly conserved, suggesting that both domains participate in ligand recognition. The lectin domain of P- and E-selectin have a single Ca^{2+}-binding site, located on the face of the molecule opposite where the EGF domain is attached, and mutagenesis of residues on this surface impairs binding of neutrophils to E- or P-selectin.[71] Although there is strong homology between different selectins in the extracellular domains, there is none in the cytoplasmic tails, suggesting selectin-specific functions for these domains. In particular, the interaction of the cytoplasmic tail of L-selectin with the cytoskeletal actin-binding protein, α-actinin, controls the ability of L-selectin to mediate the binding and rolling of leukocytes to their respective ligands.[72]

Selectin molecules are unique in that interactions with their carbohydrate ligands are dependent on shear stress.[73] They have a very rapid "on" rate, allowing cells to be captured under flowing conditions (as short as 4 milliseconds), but much longer "off" rates, allowing cells to remain attached for longer periods.[74] Recent work has demonstrated that L-selectin–cytoskeletal interactions are required for stabilization of the selectin tether, allowing rolling to occur.[75]

Selectin Ligands

All three selectins bind sialylated and fucosylated oligosaccharides, of which sialyl Lewis^x (sLe^x) is the prototype.[18] Crystal structures of sLe^x bound to lectin domains of P- and E-selectin demonstrate interactions between the fucose and a Ca^{2+} ion. The sialic acid and galactose also interact with the lectin domain.[76] With gene mutation studies in mice, targeted disruption of α1,3 fucosyltransferase eliminates selectin function, suggesting that all relevant interactions require α1,3-linked fucose.[77] P- and L-selectin, but not E-selectin, bind in a Ca^{2+}-independent manner to sulfated glycans. Subsequent studies support that sulfation may occur on either tyrosine residues or on the glycans of a glycoprotein (see Table 160–1). Most, but not all, of the selectin ligand glycoproteins are mucin-like. Mucins are serine- and threonine-rich proteins, heavily O-glycosylated, extended, and rigid.

The mucin P-selectin glycoprotein ligand-1 (PSGL-1) is expressed constitutively by neutrophils, lymphocytes, and eosinophils (see Table 160–1). It is a transmembrane homodimer of disulfide-linked subunits bearing multiple O-glycans on its serine and threonine residues. PSGL-1 mediates rolling of leukocytes to P-selectin, E-selectin, and L-selectin.[78-80] As is the case with L-selectin, PSGL-1 is localized to the tips of the surface folds of unstimulated neutrophils, providing a topographic advantage in the initial interaction of leukocytes with endothelial cells. The N-terminal region of PSGL-1 contains three tyrosine residues, at least two of which are sulfated for high affinity binding for L- and P-selectin.[81] In contrast, the binding of PSGL-1 to E-selectin appears to be mediated primarily by the O-linked glycans.[81, 82] Cutaneous lymphocyte-associated antigen (CLA) is a T-cell glycoprotein containing sLe^x and functions as a ligand for E-selectin. T-cell clones derived from peripheral blood and skin of atopic dermatitis patients differ in their level of CLA from normal hosts. The CLA-epitope is present on PSGL-1 and on skin homing T cells.[83] As is also true for L-selectin, it appears that the cytoplasmic domain of PSGL-1 attaches to cytoskeletal proteins, enabling leukocyte rolling on P-selectin. This occurs through PSGL-1-moesin-F-actin interactions.[84]

Lymphocyte L-selectin recognizes mucins synthesized by the high endothelial veins (HEV) of lymph nodes and Peyer's patches: glycosylation-dependent cell adhesion molecule-1 (GlyCAM-1), CD34 and MAdCAM-1[16] (see Table 160–1). GlyCAM-1 is expressed by the high endothelial venules of peripheral lymph nodes and mesenteric lymph nodes and is secreted.[85] CD34 has a much broader tissue distribution, with constitutive expression on endothelial cells in a diversity of blood vessels. However, its function as an L-selectin ligand is dependent on the glycosylation pattern that is restricted to HEV.[86] The ligand for neutrophil and monocyte L-selectin, which is induced in response to inflammatory mediators such as LPS and TNF, has not yet been elucidated.[87]

LEUKOCYTE, PLATELET, AND ENDOTHELIAL ACTIVATION

Mobilization of leukocytes to sites of acute inflammation is a critical factor in successful host defense. Because activated leukocytes can damage host tissue as well, their localization and activation are tightly controlled. A number of factors have been identified that activate leukocytes or the cells to which they bind, resulting in increased cell adhesion molecule expression and/or chemotactic migratory response (see Table 160–2). Chemoattractants are important in integrin activation and in directing the migration of leukocytes. In chemotaxis, cells move in the direction of an increasing concentration gradient. For example, bacterial peptides (fMLP), anaphylatoxins produced by generation of complement (C5a), lipids such as LTB$_4$, and platelet-activating factor (PAF) all elicit varying leukocyte populations. Leukocytes can sense a chemoattractant concentration difference of 1% across their diameter and therefore migrate in the direction of the attractant. However, the generation of these chemoattractants at sites of inflammation can be diluted rapidly and swept downstream by blood flow unless they are retained at the site of production. PAF is produced by activated endothelial cells when stimulated by histamine, thrombin, and leukotriene C$_4$. Although other cell types release PAF, endothelial cells express and retain PAF on their surfaces under the same conditions that P-selectin occurs.[88]

Chemokines are a group of small (8 to 14 kDa) molecules that regulate cell trafficking of all types of leukocytes. Chemokines interact with a subset of seven-transmembrane spanning, G-protein–coupled receptors (GPCR) on the leukocyte surface. The first chemokines identified were those produced by many cell sources, such as interleukin-8 (IL-8). The latest ones identified are much more tissue- and cell-specific. Table 160-2 includes some of these chemokines.[89,90] Chemokines are subdivided into two major subfamilies based on the arrangement of the two NH_2-terminal cysteine residues, CXC and CC, depending on whether the first two cysteine residues have an amino acid between them (CXC) or are adjacent (CC). Two other groups exist, the CXC3 (or fractalkine) and lymphotactin (XCL) groups. "L" in the name refers to the ligand (i.e., chemokine), and the number is the encoding gene that has previously been established.[89] IL-8, one of the first chemokines identified, is now CXCL-8, as it is in the CXC subfamily and is a ligand (L) encoded on gene 8. The receptors for chemokines are also classified by "R," for receptor. There are two ligands for IL-8 (CXCL8), CXCR1, and CXCR2. Chemokines can share receptors. CXCR1 also binds CXCL1 (Groα/MGSA-α), CXCL6 (GCP-2), and CXCL7 (NAP-2).[89]

Chemokines have a wide array of effects on cell types beyond the immune system—for example, in the central nervous system (CNS) and on the endothelial cells, where they result in either angiogenic or angiostatic effects.[90] Their function in the immune system is important in antigen presentation and development of the immune response. Chemokines are also critical for leukocyte activation and localization. They can induce changes in cell shape, release of intracellular enzymes, formation of bioactive lipids, the respiratory burst, and the activation of integrins and chemotactic migration.[17] Chemokines presented on the surfaces of endothelial cells can participate in the rapid activation of the leukocyte integrin, assisting in the "breaking" mechanism of the rolling leukocyte.[17,91] It appears that chemokines can be "presented" on the surface of endothelial cells by glycosaminoglycans and possibly the Duffy antigen/receptor for chemokines (DARC).[92] In such a manner, chemokine-induced activation of leukocytes can occur.

As previously discussed, cell adhesion molecules may themselves generate biochemical signals within the cells, in a process known as outside-in signaling. The cytoplasmic tails of most of the cell adhesion molecules are relatively short and do not appear to have any intrinsic enzymatic activity generally. Any signals generated, therefore, must occur through coupling of the cytoplasmic tail with cytoplasmic proteins that nucleate the formation of large protein complexes containing both cytoskeletal and catalytic signaling proteins (see Figure 160-2). For neutrophils, ligation of either Mac-1 or LFA-1 results in potentiation of respiratory burst. TNF-induced degranulation and release of proteases is dependent on Mac-1. On lymphocytes, LFA-1 can co-signal along with antigen or anti-CD3 to yield an augmented T-cell response in vitro, with increased calcium flux, cytokine production, and proliferation. One of the most exciting areas of integrin adhesion biology is the observation of adhesion and transmigration of leukocytes in an integrin-dependent manner that results in the expression of a large number of genes associated with the inflammatory response, termed immediate-early (IE) response genes. Many of these genes code for cytokines such as IL-1, TNF, and IL-8.[93] Thus the integrins can modulate not only the response on the adherent cell but also influence the inflammatory milieu by resulting in production of chemokines. Other cell adhesion molecules besides the integrins can also participate in signaling. Endothelial ICAM-1 will signal the cells for oxidative production if ligated through LFA-1.[94] Selectins also can activate leukocyte integrin function and production of oxidative radicals, as well as the production of cytokines and chemokines.[95,96]

"PUTTING IT ALL TOGETHER"—LEUKOCYTE-PLATELET-VESSEL WALL INTERACTIONS

Leukocyte Localization to Inflammatory Sites

Direct observations of microvascular beds have revealed a consistent pattern of leukocyte endothelial interactions.[2] Leukocytes are frequently seen rolling along the walls of small venules but not arteries. Following introduction of inflammatory stimuli, the number of rolling leukocytes increases, and many leukocytes become firmly adherent to the endothelium and change shape from a spherical to a flattened configuration. Leukocyte-leukocyte and leukocyte-platelet aggregates are often seen. Adherent leukocytes then migrate through the endothelial junction and into the region between the endothelium and its basement membrane. After pausing briefly in this location, the leukocytes migrate into the surrounding tissue (Fig. 160-5).

This cascade of events has been divided into a series of steps controlled by specific cell adhesion molecules, cell activators, or chemoattractants. Our understanding of the adhesion cascade has arisen from a variety of experimental techniques protocols: (1) parallel plate flow chambers in which isolated leukocytes are allowed to interact with monolayers of stimulated endothelial cells or transfected cell lines expressing adhesion molecules (or alternatively, purified adhesion molecules adsorbed to glass or plastic) at defined wall shear stresses similar to those found in postcapillary veins; (2) adhesion of leukocytes to substrates in the absence of shear stress; (3) intravital microscopy in which leukocyte behavior can be visualized in vivo; (4) histologic investigation of fixed whole mounts of tissue; (5) animal models of induced inflammation. Genetic defects in cell adhesion molecules in man and the ability to target gene deletion by homologous recombination in mice have contributed greatly to our understanding of this cascade in the past 20 years.[97]

Each of the members of the selectin family can support leukocyte rolling under conditions of flow. Leukocyte L-selectin and PSGL-1 binding to their endothelial ligands, also known as tethering, support the cells as they capture from the free-flowing stream. In inflammatory states, L-selectin ligands and E- and P-selectin are up-regulated (see Table 160-2). Cells then "roll" at a constant shear rate, $α4β1$, constitutively present on all mononuclear leukocytes (as well as all mouse neutrophils and some human neutrophils under specific conditions) can participate in tethering to VCAM, itself up-regulated on the inflamed endothelial cell surface.

Selectins are able to slow, but are insufficient to arrest, rolling leukocytes. Leukocyte arrest requires the activation of the $β2$ integrins and $α4β1$ with adhesion to their respective endothelial ligands (see Table 160-1). Current evidence supports the hypothesis that presentation of chemoattractants such as platelet-activating factor (PAF) and chemokines on the endothelial cell surface, along with tethering, and in the presence of shear stress, permits LFA-1, Mac-1 and $α4β1$ to transition from a low avidity to a high avidity state. The cell may then arrest.[98] It has been estimated that contact duration of more than 25 msec is needed for $β2$ integrin bonds to form.[99] Constitutive endothelial expression of ICAM-1 and ICAM-2 function as ligands for LFA-1 and Mac-1. ICAM-1 expression is augmented by a variety of inflammatory mediators, and even though high levels are found on resting endothelium, inducible expression remains crucial for leukocyte-endothelial interactions. VCAM-1 is present only on inflamed endothelia (see Figure 160-5).

It is generally believed that neutrophils and other leukocytes migrate across the endothelium via penetrating junctions that lie within the intercellular cleft.[3] Within 1 to 2 minutes of contact with a stimulated endothelial monolayer, transendothelial migration is complete.[100] Leukocytes either will stop close to the cell borders or will locomote to the cell border to then complete the transmigration process.[98,101] In vitro, neutrophils preferentially migrate at the tricellular borders of endothelial cells, thus avoiding tight junctions.[102] While patients with genetic defects of $β2$ integrins (leukocyte adhesion deficiency I) have profound defects in leukocyte migration, in vitro experiments and the use of knock-out mice demonstrate that $β2$ integrins only partially mediate transendothelial migration.[97,103] Only recently has progress been made in understanding

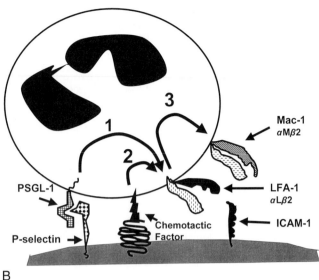

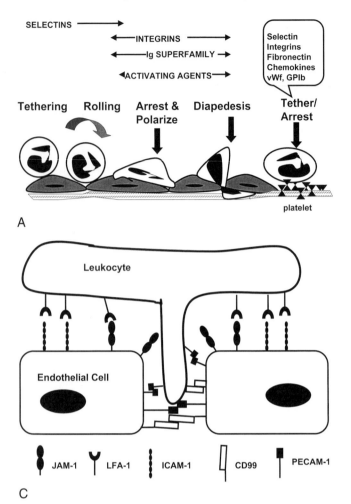

Figure 160–5. Leukocyte localization. A, Leukocytes are captured from the free-flowing stream (tether) and roll on the endothelial lining of the blood vessel. This interaction is mediated by all three members of the selectin family. The leukocyte slows, arrests, and changes shape (polarizes). Integrins and their ligands, the Ig superfamily (IGSF), mediate these steps. The cells then "crawl" or diapedese over the surface of the endothelial surface until they migrate through the endothelium. The integrins, members of the IGSF, and CD99 have a role at this point. A leukocyte also may be tethered by adherent platelets (as shown here) or adherent leukocytes. Platelets through β3 integrins and GPIb-IX-V can bind directly to collagen or fibronectin on exposed basement membrane, or alternatively to von Willebrand factor bound to basement membrane. They can release chemokines that can activate leukocytes directly once tethered. Leukocytes can bind to platelets directly through integrins or to fibrinogen that is bound to platelets. Ig = immunoglobulin; vWf = von Willebrand factor. **B,** Model of leukocyte activation leading to arrest. Leukocytes tether to endothelial cells expressing P-selectin via P-selectin-glycoprotein ligand 1 (PSGL1). In the presence of shear, P-selectin–PSGL-1 interactions can result in leukocyte (and LFA-1) activation (*curved arrow 1*). Chemotactic factors expressed at the endothelial surface also can result in activation of both Mac-1 and LFA-1 (*curved arrow 2*). Finally, LFA-1-ICAM-1 (intercellular adhesion molecule) interactions can augment the adhesivity of Mac-1 (*curved arrow 3*). (Adapted from Smith CW: Microcirculation 7:385, 2000). **C,** Proposed mechanisms for leukocyte transendothelial migration. With stimulation of the endothelial cell, ICAM-1 is up-regulated; JAM-1, which is localized at the interendothelial cleft, appears to be mobilized away from the cleft. With activation of the leukocytes (see **B**), migration across the vascular endothelium can then occur via LFA-1, PECAM-1, JAM-1, and CD99. Leukocyte LFA-1 can bind to JAM-1 and ICAM-1 on the endothelial cell. Leukocytes may then traverse the interendothelial cleft through sequential trans-homophilic interactions of PECAM-1 and CD99. Although CD99 is abundant on lymphocytes and monocytes, it does not appear to be so on neutrophils. JAM = junctional adhesion molecule; PECAM = platelet endothelial adhesion molecule. (Adapted from Aurrand-Lions M, et al: Nature Immunol 3:116, 2002.)

transendothelial migration[104] (see Figure 160–5). JAM-1, which is preferentially located at the interendothelial junction and binds to JAM-1 on neighboring cells, can move away from the junction with endothelial cell activation, though PECAM-1 and CD99 remain.[105] By interaction with LFA-1, JAM-1 may "guide" the leukocyte toward the junction. CD99, which is located toward the basolateral region of the interendothelial cleft, also participates as antibodies against CD99 cause the leukocyte to "hang up" in the interendothelial cleft[20] (Fig. 160–5). The function of PECAM-1 in transendothelial migration remains unclear. Although anti-PECAM-1 monoclonal antibodies inhibit leukocyte emigration *in vivo* and in vitro in some models,[106, 107] its function may be more as a signaling molecule for migration through basement membrane.[21]

Leukocytes also must migrate into the extracellular matrix for localization to inflammatory sites. As outlined in Table 160–1, ECM ligands for integrins include fibrinonectin, laminin, collagen, entactin, tenascin, thrombospondin, and vitronectin. Although Mac-1 and αXβ2 are known to bind fibrinogen after activation, they are not critical for adhesion to and emigration through other ECM proteins. β2 integrin-deficient activated neutrophils adhere to fibronectin, vitronectin, and laminin through α5β1, αvβ3, and α6β1, respectively.[108] β1 integrins, in particular α2β1, but not α4β1 nor α5β1, are critical for leukocyte locomotion in the rat mesentery after chemotactic factor activation.[45, 56] Migratory cells use adhesion receptors and proteolytic enzymes, such as the urokinase/urokinase receptor/plasmin system, to regulate the function of each for the other and migrate through ECM.[109]

Leukocyte Localization in Adaptive Immunity

With inflammation, lymphocytes, like neutrophils and monocytes, extravasate to the affected site.[110] However the mechanism is different in lymphoid organs. Lymphocytes exit from the bloodstream in the postcapillary venules at specialized postcapillary vascular sites called high endothelial venules (HEV). This is the major route for constitutive extravasation, and most recirculating lymphocytes selectively bind to the endothelial cells of the HEV and do not interact with quiescent vascular endothelium. HEV is found in all secondary lymphoid organs (except the spleen). In chronically inflamed nonlymphoid tissue, HEV-like vessels are observed, and they support lymphocyte recruitment. HEVs are found in peripheral lymph nodes (PLNs), mesenteric lymph nodes (MLNs), Peyer's patches, and tonsils.

The controlled expression of adhesion molecules on the lymphocyte and the counter ligands on the specialized endothelial cells of the high endothelial venules (HEVs) of peripheral lymph nodes (draining the skin) and the lymphoid tissues of the mucosa (Peyer's patches, tonsil and appendix) ensures this selectivity of lymphocyte homing. L-selectin is present on virtually all lymphocytes and is required for homing to lymph nodes. Naive lymphocytes have abundant L-selectin, while activated or memory helper T cells lack L-selectin expression but regain it when they transform into fully mature memory cells. L-selectin binds to ligands on PLN, HEV, CD34, and Gly CAM-1. Lymphocytes homing to MLN and Peyer's patch use both L-selectin, and to a lesser extent $\alpha 4\beta 7$ (via binding to MAdCAM-1) to capture from the free-flowing stream.[111] Adhesion and emigration of lymphocytes primarily depend on LFA-1 and endothelial ICAM-1 and -2 on the PLN. For circulation to MLN and Peyer's patch, MAdCAM-1 is responsible for 15% to 90% of firm adhesion through its binding to $\alpha 4\beta 7$. Chemokines specific for lymphoid organs are required to activate the lymphocyte integrins for the transition from a rolling cell to adherent cell capable of transmigration. Although many chemokines specific for lymphocyte integrin activation are produced in inflammatory states, many serve a housekeeping function and are constitutively expressed at high levels in the thymus, lymph nodes, and certain lymphoid tissues.[89, 90]

Cell–Blood Vessel Interactions in the Absence of "the Cascade"

There are many instances in which leukocyte and platelet recruitment to the vascular endothelium does not occur in the sequential manner described earlier. Neutrophils already localized to inflamed endothelium can recruit other neutrophils.[79] In vascular beds where blood flow is diminished either by geometric constraints or by vascular occlusion/vasoconstriction, activation of the $\beta 2$ integrins alone in the presence of a chemotactic gradient may be sufficient for neutrophil transmigration.[3] In the lung, leukocyte sequestration and transmigration appear to occur primarily in the capillaries. Leukocytes appear to "hop" through the capillaries, rather than roll.[112] Neutrophils may spend considerable periods of time in stationary contact with capillary endothelium, and this predisposes to adhesive interactions between the neutrophil and the subjacent endothelium. In inflammatory states such as sepsis, the neutrophils become increasingly less deformable, leading to retention. Though Mac-1 and LFA-1 are not required for the sequestration of neutrophils in the vascular bed of the lungs, they do mediate neutrophil migration. However non-$\beta 2$-integrin–dependent mechanisms are also present.[113] The type of stimulus, the site of administration (lung vs. peritoneum), or the route (intravenous administration vs. intratracheal) will affect the mechanisms required for lung recruitment.[3] Leukocyte localization in the liver and kidney likewise is affected by geometric constraints and specialized endothelia.[114, 115]

In response to vessel injury, platelets translocate on subendothelial von Willebrand factor (vWF) through interactions with platelet GPIb-IX-V, then arrest and recruit additional platelets into the growing thrombi. Stable adhesion requires binding of platelet integrin $\alpha IIb\beta 3$ to immobilized vWF, fibrinogen, and other ligands and by binding of platelet integrin $\alpha 5\beta 1$ to fibrinogen.[116] Neutrophils can tether to and roll on platelet monolayers through neutrophil PSGL-1 and platelet P-selectin.[117] Platelet-derived chemokines and lipid mediators will contribute to leukocyte signaling and integrin activation.[118] Activated leukocytes use Mac-1, and to a lesser extent LFA-1, to adhere firmly to platelets. Although fibrinogen may serve to stabilize leukocyte-platelet adhesion by binding to Mac-1 and $\alpha IIb\beta 3$ simultaneously, leukocyte Mac-1 also may bind directly to GP Ib-IX-V complex on the platelet.[119, 120] Though leukocytes may roll on platelet monolayers in such models, it is likely that little rolling occurs *in vivo*. Instead, neutrophils are directly recruited by immobilized platelets.[121] Leukocytes are critical to the development and maintenance of the hemostatic plug and thrombus, as demonstrated by models in which inhibition of P-selectin function accelerates thrombolysis and prevents reocclusion.[116]

ADHESION MOLECULES AND THE DEVELOPING HOST

As outlined in the beginning of this chapter, several lines of investigation suggest that functional deficits in neonatal leukocyte adhesion increase the infectious susceptibility of the neonate. However, these functional deficits may play a physiologic role in limiting inflammatory responses that are possibly deleterious in immature hosts, such as bronchopulmonary dysplasia (BPD).[122] The remainder of this chapter is devoted to the genetic defects of adhesion molecules, (LAD I, LAD II, and Glanzmann's thrombasthenia) that may present in the neonatal period, and summarizes our understanding of the developmental deficits of adhesion molecule expression and function in the neonate.

Genetic Deficiencies of Adhesion Molecules

Leukocyte Adhesion Deficiency I

Leukocyte adhesion deficiency is an autosomal recessive trait of humans, dogs, and cows, characterized by recurrent, necrotic bacterial infections, impaired pus formation and wound healing, and abnormalities of many adhesion-dependent functions of granulocytes, monocytes, and lymphoid cells[123-125] (Table 160-3). With the targeted mutation of each of the $\beta 2$ integrins in mice, we have found both similarities to and disparities of the syndrome as it occurs in humans and other animals.[24, 97] LAD I is a result of a decrease or absence of the cell surface expression or function of the entire $\beta 2$ integrin family, which is, in turn, a result of heterogeneous mutations of the CD18 gene.[126] The α and β subunits are initially assembled in the cytoplasm of the cell, and only then is the complete 2 integrin heterodimer expressed at the membrane. Both subunits are required for expression. Given the diverse functional characteristics of $\beta 2$ integrins, it is not unexpected that patients with LAD I have profound deficits of acute inflammatory function and specific immunologic defects.[127] Clinical and histopathologic features of LAD I are remarkably similar among human, canine, and bovine subjects. Recurrent necrotic and indolent infections of soft tissues primarily involving the skin, mucous membranes, and intestinal tract are the clinical hallmarks of this disease. Superficial infections on body surfaces may invade locally or systemically. Typical small, erythematous, nonpustular skin lesions often progress to large, well-demarcated ulcerative craters that heal slowly or with a dysplastic scar. Septicemia progressing from omphalitis associated with delayed umbilical cord severance has been observed in several families.[128, 129] Perirectal abscess or cellulitis leading to

TABLE 160-3

Leukocyte Adhesion Deficiencies

	LAD I	LAD II	Rac2 Mutation
Clinical Manifestation			
Recurrent severe infections	+++	+	++
Neutrophilia			
Basal	+	+++	NL
With infection	+++	+++	+++
Gingivitis	++	++	
Skin infections	++	+	+++
Delayed separation of umbilical cord	+++	—	+
Developmental abnormalities	—	+++	—
Laboratory Findings			
β2 integrins	↓, ↓↓, ↓↓↓	NL	NL
sLe^x expression	NL	Absent	NL
Neutrophil rolling	NL	↓↓↓	NL, ↓
Neutrophil adherence	↓↓↓	↓	↓
Neutrophil emigration	↓↓↓	↓↓	NL, ↓↓
Opsonophagocytic activity	↓	NL	↓
Oxidative burst	↓↓	NL	↓↓, ↓↓↓
T- + B-cell function	↓	NL	NL

For LAD 1, minimal (+), moderate (++), and severe (+++) decreases in β2-integrin expression have been described, leading to at least three phenotypes of the disease. Rac2 is a member of the Rho family of GTPases, part of the signaling mechanism for leukocyte function. (See text for details.)
LAD = leukocyte adhesion deficiency; NL = normal.

peritonitis and/or septicemia has been reported, and facial or deep neck cellulitis has been observed to progress from ulcerative mucous membrane lesions of the oral cavity.[130,131] Recurrent invasive candidal esophagitis, erosive gastritis, acute appendicitis, and necrotizing enterocolitis have been reported.[132] Common respiratory infections include severe bacterial laryngotracheitis, recurrent pneumonitis, and sinusitis. Severe gingivitis and/or periodontitis are major features among all patients who survive infancy.

The recurrent infections observed in affected patients appear to reflect the profound impairment of leukocyte mobilization into extravascular inflammatory sites. Skin windows as well as biopsies of infected tissues demonstrate inflammatory infiltrates devoid of neutrophils.[123] This histopathologic feature is particularly striking considering that marked peripheral granulocytosis (5- to 20-fold higher than normal) during episodes of infection is a common finding. Two LAD I phenotypes were originally described. Patients with severe deficiency had essentially undetectable expression of all three complexes on their neutrophils.[123] These patients either died in infancy or demonstrated a susceptibility to severe, life-threatening systemic infections. In contrast, among the six patients with moderate deficiency, life-threatening infections have been observed infrequently. Patients with moderate deficiency expressed 2.5 to 6% of all three β2 complexes.[123] Patients with moderate disease may die in their 2nd to 4th decade of life.[133] In some moderately affected patients, skin lesions may disappear after the first few years of life, recurring only with occasional infections. Severe gingivitis is always observed in these patients and may be the presenting symptom.[134] Several features of the disease have become increasingly clear in the twenty years since the initial description: (1) The variable points of mutation in the β2 subunit affect expression and function of the β2 integrins differently.[126] (2) An increasing number of patients with the phenotype of LAD I have a "normal" expression of β2 integrins on the cell surface, but the integrins do not function "normally," and more than one type of integrin may be affected.[135-137] In these patients, the abnormalities appear to lie in difficulties with integrin signaling and/or activation.

(3) Defects in known cell-signaling systems, such as the Rac2 (a member of the RHO GTPases), have been described in patients with presentations similar to these of LAD I (Table 160-3).[138,139]

Abnormalities of neutrophil or monocyte antibody-dependent cellular cytotoxicity also have been observed in individuals with LAD I.[140] Most patients have normal and self-limiting courses of varicella and other viral infections.[123] The predominance of recurrent bacterial infections in patients with LAD I implies that the functions of neutrophils and monocytes are more profoundly affected than those of lymphocytes. However, T-lymphocyte-mediated killing, proliferative responses, natural killing, and antibody-dependent killing by patient's lymphocytes are deficient compared with adult controls. Nonetheless, delayed cutaneous hypersensitivity reactions are normal in most patients tested, and most individuals demonstrate normal specific antibody synthesis.[123,128]

The diagnosis of severe LAD I is suspected in the neonate (or within the first few months of life) when the infant displays extreme, prolonged neutrophilia associated with recurrent severe infections (see Table 160-3). Delayed separation of the umbilical cord occurs more frequently in patients with the severe phenotype but is not universally found. Delay in cord separation alone does not indicate a child has LAD I. The mean age of umbilical cord separation in normal neonates is reported to be 15.0 ± 7.2 days (SD), with a range of 3 to 67 days.[141] In patients with the severe form of LAD I, prolonged cord retention was associated with omphalitis and extreme neutrophilia. The diagnosis of LAD I is made by immunophenotyping leukocytes with flow cytometry techniques, though other confirmatory testing may be used.[123] With immunophenotyping, in classic LAD I there will be few or no β2 integrins on the neutrophil or lymphocyte surface.[123] Although the patients who were described as having "moderate" LAD I by clinical course had 2.5% to 6% of Mac-1, LFA-1, and p150,95 compared with normal adults,[123] infants with this immunophenotype can still have clinically severe disease and succumb to overwhelming infections within the first year of life.[132] As described earlier, an ever-increasing number of patients with functional defects of β2 integrins have a "normal" expression level. In these patients, clinical course, extreme neutrophilia, and evidence of few if any neutrophils in infected areas should implicate the possibility of neutrophil chemotaxis defect and provoke more sophisticated testing. Treatment for patients with LAD I is limited to surveillance for recurrent infections, prompt institution of antibiotic therapy, and granulocyte transfusions when indicated. Bone marrow transplantation has been advocated for these patients. The European Group for Bone Marrow Transplantation have reported that LAD I patients have good outcomes post-bone marrow transplantation, though graft vs. host disease is a frequent complication.[142] Somatic gene therapy replacement for LAD I may be a possibility but has not yet proved beneficial.

Glanzmann's Thrombasthenia

This relatively rare autosomal recessive disease is characterized clinically by purpura, epistaxis, gingival hemorrhage, and bleeding resulting from qualitative or quantitative defects of platelet αIIbβ3.[143] The diagnosis is virtually assured when there is absence of platelet aggregation in response to all agonists. Platelet αIIbβ3 binds fibrinogen and, under shear, vWF. In Glanzmann's thrombasthenia (GT), platelets attach to exposed subendothelium but do not spread, a process dependent on αIIbβ3. Formation of platelet-fibrinogen and platelet-vWF bridges does not occur, and clot retraction is often defective. In addition, prothrombin, which can bind directly to platelets, is unable to do so in patients with GT, and significantly less thrombin is generated in response to tissue factor. As with LAD I, large series of mutations have been described. However, unlike LAD I in which mutations occur primarily in the β subunit, in GT mutations have been described in genes encoding either the αIIb or β3 gene. Classic GT occurs when there is insufficient or absent expression of αIIbβ3 on the cell surface. Variant GT occurs when there is quantitatively normal expression of αIIbβ3 but it is functionally deficient. Therefore, patient presentation is heterogeneous. Bleeding difficulties range from severe to mild. Patients with either type of GT may be relatively asymptomatic or exhibit profuse bleeding after minor operative or dental procedures. Alternatively, they may present in the newborn period and require frequent blood transfusions.[144,145]

As many of the integrins share common pathways for activation, it is not surprising that individuals are now being described who have defects in β1, β2, and β3. These individuals have normal or near-normal expression of cell surface molecules but have features of both GT and LAD I.[146]

Leukocyte Adhesion Deficiency II LAD II

A new adhesion molecule deficiency was described in 1992. It is characterized by recurrent infections, failure to form pus, gingivitis, and pronounced neutrophilia[147] (see Table 160–3). Although the severity of the infectious complications resembles that of the moderate type of LAD I, the patients express normal levels of the β2 integrins and L-selectin. Additionally, the patients exhibit mental and growth retardation and the rare Bombay blood phenotype. LAD II is due to a congenital defect of endogenous fucose metabolism. This results in an inability to synthesize fucosylated carbohydrate structures, such as sialyl Lewis^x (sLe^x), the carbohydrate ligand recognized both by P- and E-selectin. These patients in fact demonstrate markedly decreased levels of sLe^x on leukocytes and other fucose-containing structures. Neutrophils from these patients bind minimally or not at all to E-selectin and P-selectin, though β2 integrin function is normal.[148] However, *in vivo* they have a marked decrease in migration into skin chambers or skin windows.[149] By means of fluorescein-labeled cells from LAD I and LAD II patients in intravital microscopy (mouse mesenteric preparation after stimulation with TNF), it was observed that (1) LAD I neutrophils demonstrated normal rolling but were unable to stick and emigrate with chemotactic factor stimulation. (2) Neutrophils from LAD II patients rolled very poorly and failed to stick and emigrate under the shear forces provided by flow. However, once flow was reduced, the cells adhered and emigrated in response to LTB$_4$.[150] Like the studies in mice that are deficient in P-selectin and E-selectin,[151] these studies clearly demonstrate the significance in humans of selectin-carbohydrate ligand interactions in initiating low-affinity adhesion manifested by rolling under conditions of flow. When these interactions are not possible, leukocyte emigration cannot occur. Initial studies in infants suggest that high doses of oral fucose supplementation may mitigate some of the clinical effects.[152]

Neonatal Integrin Expression and Function

β2 Integrin Function

It has been known for several decades that neutrophils from cord blood do not adhere to matrix proteins and various substrates and do not migrate to the same extent as adult neutrophils in response to a chemotactic stimulus.[4-6,153] With the identification of the function of the β2 integrins and description of LAD I,[123,128] a molecular basis for diminished neonatal neutrophil adhesion and motility was first detailed.[154]

In resting neutrophils, low levels of Mac-1 are present on the cell surface; during cell locomotion Mac-1 is activated and then may participate in adhesion and translocate to the tail of the cell (uropod).[155] New Mac-1 is released from secretory and secondary granules and locomotion continues.[155,156] Several investigators have demonstrated that neonatal neutrophils do not up-regulate Mac-1 to the same extent as adult cells when stimulated *in vitro*.[9,43,154,157,158] This is likely due to diminished total cell content of preformed Mac-1, which is approximately 60% of adult cells.[14] In addition, it appears that translocation of receptors to the uropod is also diminished.[5] Delays in chemotaxis appear to reverse by 1 month of age.[159] Consistent with this observation, stimulated Mac-1 expression remains depressed until at least 4 weeks of age.[160] The observations that Mac-1 expression on stimulated neonatal neutrophils is diminished compared with adult cells is controversial as others have not found this to be so.[161,162] It is not entirely clear why these discrepancies exist, although possibilities include large variances in expression for the neonatal population, preparation methods, and varying proportions of "immature cells." In premature infants, Mac-1 expression is also diminished compared with adults, which also appears to correlate with a decreased ability to undergo adhesion and chemotaxis.[9] It appears that the more premature the infant, the lower the levels of Mac-1.[163,164] This may be due to greater decreases in the total cell content of Mac-1 in premature neonates than in full-term neonates (30 and 60% of adult values, respectively).[165]

In assays of neutrophil adhesion and transmigration through endothelial monolayers, term neonatal cells display about 50% transmigration compared with adults.[166] The diminished transmigration can be explained almost entirely by reduced Mac-1 expression.[166] LFA-1 expression (and total cell content) is less than adult values before 35 weeks' gestation.[165]

Complementing the *in vitro* studies with neonatal or infant leukocytes, delays in leukocyte localization also have been demonstrated consistently in neonatal animals. The accumulation of leukocytes in the peritoneal cavity is delayed in neonatal animals in response to a variety of chemotactic agents[167,168] and bacteria.[169] Leukocyte extravasation into the lung is also delayed in young animals in response to various bacteria and their products[170,171] and in response to mechanical injury or hyperoxia.[122,172] With a rabbit model, we demonstrated that many of the changes in leukocyte integrins observed in the developing rabbit appear to model what has been described in neonatal human studies.[168] One-day-old rabbit neutrophils have decreased surface expression of the β2 subunit compared with adult and juvenile rabbits (14 days old), and fail to up-regulate Mac-1 (CD11b subunit) with chemotactic factor stimulation to the same extent as adult neutrophils.[168] In addition, neonatal rabbits have diminished neutrophil accumulation in the sterilely inflamed peritoneum compared with adults or juveniles (14 days old) and their extravasated neutrophils exhibit diminished Mac-1 expression.[168] β2 Integrin-dependent neutrophil accumulation in this model was due to LFA-1, as an anti-Mac-1 monoclonal antibody had no effect on blocking leukocyte emigration.[173]

At least in adult humans and in mice, there are distinct roles for Mac-1 and LFA-1 for leukocyte localization in the host response.[2,174] In humans, under conditions in which neutrophils can aggregate with cells expressing ICAM-1 under shear conditions, LFA-1 but not Mac-1 mediated the initial interaction due to shear alone.[28] Chemotactic factor boosted LFA-1–dependent aggregation fourfold. Under the same conditions, Mac-1–dependent aggregation was only one third as efficient.[28] However, Mac-1 was necessary for aggregate stability, particularly at increased shear rates.[28] In assays in which human neutrophils transition from rolling to arrested cells, Mac-1 and LFA each may support the transition independently.[100] Mice deficient in LFA-1 or Mac-1 can use the alternative mechanism to "slow down" the rolling leukocytes, although LFA-1 appears to have a greater role in the transition to firm arrest.[175]

By means of intravital microscopy, we directly examined leukocyte recruitment in rabbit pup mesenteric vessels 6 hours after intraperitoneal injection of IL-1β.[176] Neonatal animals (< 1 week old) have diminished leukocyte arrest and emigration compared with adult animals.[177] Four-week-old pups demonstrated diminished arrest of leukocytes compared with adult animals, though leukocyte emigration was not different. With anti-LFA-1 and anti-Mac-1 antibodies, we demonstrated that in rabbits (1) LFA-1 in animals of all ages was primarily responsible for leukocyte arrest and subsequent emigration. (2) Mac-1–dependent arrest and emigration were not present in neonatal animals, and accounted for about 30% of leukocyte arrest and adhesion in adult animals. (3) Leukocyte arrest in 4-week-old animals was *not* dependent on Mac-1, though Mac-1 accounted for 30% of transmigration.[177] Thus mechanisms for "slowing," "arrest," and subsequent emigration may change with maturation of the host.

The adhesion molecules involved with leukocyte mobility depend on the organ and the inflammatory stimulus used in adult animals; β2-integrins do not appear to be necessary for leukocyte accumulation in the lungs of mice and rabbits infected with *S. pneumoniae*.[113] This appears to be true also for neonatal animals. Term and preterm neonatal rabbits demonstrated increased accumulation of alveolar neutrophils after infection with group B streptococcus.[178] Anti-β2 mAbs failed to inhibit neutrophil influx, though it did inhibit killing of the streptococcus.[178] The age-dependent differences in neutrophil migration appears to be species dependent; neonatal bovine neutrophils have levels of Mac-1, LFA-1, and p150,95 equal to that of adult bovine neutrophils. Furthermore, in this species there were no delays in adhesion to or migration through stimulated bovine endothelial monolayers.[179]

The β2 integrins modulate a number of other events, including phagocytosis of iC3b-coated particles, neutrophil homotypic aggregation, and adhesion-dependent oxidative burst. Phagocytosis of iC3b-coated particles was not different in neutrophils from term or premature infants and adults. Furthermore, the degree of phagocytosis could not be correlated with Mac-1 levels.[180] Phagocytosis of iC3b-opsonized *Candida* or unopsonized candida by monocytes from neonates (in which ingestion occurs via Mac-1) was equal to that of monocytes from adults.[181] Thus it appears that the neonatal neutrophils utilize LFA-1 for adhesion and emigration. Decreased Mac-1 function and/or amount appears to contribute to the deficits in neonatal neutrophil motility. However, other Mac-1 functions may be intact.

β1-Integrin Function

By means of flow cytometry, it has been shown that in healthy 1- to 3-day-old infants there are elevated proportions of total T cells (CD3+), helper T cells (CD3/CD4+) with decreased proportions of CD3/CD8+, and NK cells in the blood compared with adults.[182] The neonates have a higher proportion of immature B cells and CD8+ T cells that express the co-stimulatory molecules CD28 or CD38. Compared with adults, the neonatal blood contains a lower proportion of activated T cells.[182] Such studies and others support the hypothesis that neonatal lymphocytes are naive and prepared to "home" to secondary lymph organs for priming for an immune response, but they do not respond to sites of infection. Those CD4+ cells that are CD45RO+ (memory) have concomitantly increased expression of β1, α5, LFA-1, and CD2, but not necessarily increased α2, α4 and CD44 (another adhesion molecule).[183] Locomotion of T lymphocytes in extracellular matrices appears to be due to both the expression and function of cell adhesion markers, such as α4β1 and α2β1, and loss of L-selectin.[184] Although T cells from children have decreased β1 and α5 compared with adults, they have comparable levels of α4, (probably as α4β7).[185] In addition, child CD45RA+ lymphocytes are β1 integrin "high," while in adults β1^high T cells are CD45R0+.[185] In contrast, lymphocytes from cord blood are uniform for β1 expression; the single peak falls between the two peaks usually seen in adult cells.[185] Thus for cord blood lymphocytes and those from very young infants, α4β1 integrin expression is present at moderate levels and can function as a ligand for VCAM-1.

As with neutrophils, lymphocyte chemotactic responses depend upon chemokine receptor expression. Cord blood lymphocytes in general have diminished chemotactic responses to CCL2 (MCP-1), CCL3 (MIP-1α), CCL5 (RANTES), CXCL9 (MIG), and CXCL10 (IP-10) compared with adult peripheral blood lymphocytes, because they lack the respective chemokine receptor.[186] However, cord blood lymphocytes express both CCR7 and CXCR4, and as such they respond robustly to CCL19 (MIP-3β) and CXCL12 (SDF), respectively, in assays of directed migration. We have shown that cord blood lymphocytes can interact (tether and roll) on cytokine-stimulated endothelial cells to the same extent as do adult peripheral blood cells, and this is dependent on α4β1.[187] In the presence of shear stress, cord blood and adult lymphocytes roll, arrest, and migrate across stimulated endothelial cells when the vascular endothelium bears apical CXCL12 (SDF) (M. Mariscalco, T. Helgason, unpublished results, 2003, and reference 98). Thus neonatal cord blood lymphocytes, though "naive", maintain the capability to localize to an inflammatory response if the signals for localization are present in the microenvironment, i.e., VCAM-1 and chemotactic chemokines for which neonatal cells have receptors.

Neonatal Selectin Function

In assays when L-selectin is known to be operative for the initial tether of flowing neutrophils, neonatal cells are less able to interact with stimulated endothelial cells, compared with adult cells.[188] Neonatal cells have diminished surface expression of L-selectin, and anti-L-selectin monoclonal antibodies have minimal effect on neonatal cell rolling.[188] In contrast, in the presence of anti-L-selectin antibodies, adult cell rolling is decreased to levels comparable to those of neonatal cells.[188] Thus neonatal cells have a relative L-selectin deficiency. Diminished neutrophil L-selectin has been confirmed in other studies of neutrophils and eosinophils from term and preterm infants.[158,161,189] In contrast, neonatal monocytes[158] and fetal neutrophils and eosinophils[157] demonstrate "adult" levels of L-selectin. As L-selectin can be shed from the cell surface, it remains unclear whether the decrease in neutrophil surface L-selectin in the term and preterm neonate is due to activation in utero, or whether it is due to maturational changes in neutrophil content of L-selectin. Though diminished total cellular L-selectin is found in cord neutrophils, soluble L-selectin (that which is cleaved from the cell surface) is also decreased in the serum compared with that of adults.[189] Additionally, cord neutrophils demonstrate diminished down-regulation of L-selectin compared with adult neutrophils with chemotactic peptides and granulocyte-macrophage colony stimulating factor, though the response to IL-8 is equal to that of adult neutrophils.[189]

Do the decreases in neonatal L-selectin result in a decreased ability of neonatal neutrophils to accumulate *in vivo*? Neutrophils from 1-day-old rabbit pups have approximately 60% of adult rabbit levels of L-selectin, and as in human neonatal neutrophils, failed to show a significant decrease after chemotactic factor stimulation.[168] Neutrophil L-selectin expression in the pups remained depressed until about 14 days of age when it was equal to that of adult rabbits. Systemic administration of an anti-L-selectin mAb to rabbits with sterile peritonitis resulted in a significant decrease in peritoneal neutrophil accumulation in both adult and 14-day-old animals. In contrast, there was no effect in the 1-day-old animals.[168] We examined L-selectin–dependent leukocyte localization in the mesenteric vessels of rabbits in response to IL-1β with intravital microscopy.[176] Inhibition of L-selectin had greater effects on arrest and emigration of leukocytes in adult animals than in neonatal animals, especially at those stages in which L-selectin serves as a signaling molecule for integrin activation.[176] Inhibition of L-selectin also had a lesser effect on leukocyte rolling in neonatal than in adult rabbits.

Human neonatal neutrophils appear to have diminished amounts and function of PSGL-1. Neonatal neutrophils demonstrate decreased rolling and arrest compared with adult neutrophils on both E- and P-selectin expressed on either endothelial cells or transfected cell lines.[190-192] Neonatal neutrophils also have decreased interaction to platelet monolayers, and this appears to be due to diminished tether duration of neonatal cell PSGL-1 to platelet P-selectin.[193] As described previously, selectin-ligand interactions have a rapid "on" rate and much longer "off" rate, allowing cells to attach quickly and then remain attached for longer periods, thus facilitating the transition to β2-integrin–mediated arrest.[194] At least for P-selectin, the off rate is much shorter for neonatal cells, thereby requiring these cells to arrest in a shorter period of time than that required by adult cells. As β2 integrin function is depressed in neonatal cells, this puts the neonatal cells at an even greater disadvantage for transition to arrest.

At present there is little understanding of the developmental differences in adhesion molecule expression at the level of the endothelium and other nonleukocytic cells. Human neonatal platelets have decreased up-regulation of P-selectin.[195] However, neonates have increased amounts of more multimerized von Willebrand factor, and as such cord blood platelet deposition on subendothelium may be equal to or exceed that of adult blood.[196]

In the context of the developmental biology of endothelial cell adhesion molecules, it is critical to highlight that much of the *in vitro* work has been performed on human umbilical vein endothelial cells (HUVEC). However, endothelial cells from umbilical veins in culture may not reflect what occurs *in vivo* in either the neonate or mature host. The use of cultured human foreskin has provided some insight as to the relevance of these molecules in the human neonate. Cultured foreskin postcapillary venular endothelium up-regulated ICAM-1 and E-selectin in response to cytokines and growth factors, and the effect was greater than predicted based upon isolated HUVEC assays.[197] Animal models also have been useful, but again there is uncertainty in extrapolating animal (particularly rodent) findings to humans. In neonatal rats subjected to sterile peritonitis, leukocyte accumulation is diminished compared with that of adult animals.[15] However, this did not appear to be due to decreased leukocyte responsiveness, because adult cells injected into neonatal animals also demonstrated decreased localization. Furthermore, there was diminished P-selectin expression on neonatal mesenteric vessels compared with adult animals.[15] That such differences in P-selectin expression are important in human neonates is based upon the following observations: (1) P-selectin expression is diminished on the surfaces of endothelial cells from human newborn mesentery, and expression increases with age. PECAM-1 and ICAM-1 staining was not affected by age. (2) Endothelial cell stores of P-selectin and von Willebrand factor increase with gestational age in humans. (3) There is diminished mRNA in endothelial cells from premature neonates, and decreased P-selectin in endothelial cells from premature neonates is associated with fewer Weibel-Palade bodies.[15]

Adhesion Molecules in Diagnosis and Therapy

Adhesion Molecules as Markers of Inflammation

In 1985, Arnaout and colleagues described eight patients who developed neutropenia while undergoing dialysis. The neutropenia was associated with increased surface expression of MAC-1 on circulating neutrophils.[198] Since this first description, there has been an explosion of studies quantifying the expression of adhesion molecules, either on leukocytes or circulating in the sera, as indications of leukocyte activation/inflammation. An increase in neutrophil Mac-1 expression has been documented in patients undergoing cardiopulmonary bypass,[199] those with sepsis, and at early time points in the adult respiratory distress

syndrome (ARDS).[200] L-selectin is shed from the leukocyte cell surface with cell activation and is thought to occur as the leukocyte transitions from rolling to arrest. Neutrophils deficient in L-selectin cannot localize to an inflammatory site.[201] L-selectin shedding may be a mechanism to release a slowly rolling, activated cell and inhibit it from interacting at a site distant from the original focus. L-selectin expression has been shown to be decreased in neutrophils and monocytes from the cord blood of infants with acute bacterial infection and in adult patients with surgical sepsis.[202, 203] However, L-selectin expression decreases in the neutrophils as they are released from the bone marrow and as they age.[204] In addition, inflammatory mediators, such as glucocorticoids, IL-6, and G-CSF all result in decreased L-selectin on circulating cells, likely as a result of shedding of L-selectin during marrow release.[205] Although soluble L-selectin is found in the plasma, its significance is unclear, though it is present at levels in humans and rodents that potentially can inhibit L-selectin-dependent leukocyte function.[206]

With the observation that there are soluble forms of ICAM-1, L-, E-, and P-selectin in normal human sera or in sera from patients with inflammation, it has been hypothesized that the levels of soluble adhesion molecules could be useful monitors of disease activity (reviewed in references 207 and 208). It is unclear however, whether determining the absolute level of soluble circulating adhesion molecules has the necessary specificity and sensitivity required to predict disease severity or outcome.

Term infants with early-onset sepsis or suspected sepsis have increased Mac-1 expression on circulating neutrophils, compared with those who do not.[164, 209] However, in septic premature infants, increased surface expression of Mac-1 did not occur, though other markers of leukocyte activation (CD33 and CD66b) were present.[210] Furthermore, neutrophil Mac-1 expression was elevated in preterm infants with respiratory distress syndrome, compared with cord blood from full-term infants, and preterm infants not requiring mechanical ventilation.[164, 211] Thus it appears that leukocytes from term infants with sepsis and those with respiratory distress syndrome have evidence of neutrophil activation, at least as demonstrated by Mac-1 expression.

In term infection-free neonates, plasma sL-selectin levels are diminished while sE-selectin level are increased on the second and fifth day of life compared with adult values.[212] From days 2 to 5, there is a decrease in plasma sE-selectin; the baseline level of sL-selectin, which is low compared with that of normal adults, remains unchanged. In a large cohort of infants, with proven on possible infection, plasma levels of C-reactive protein (CRP), IL-6, sICAM-1, and sE-selectin were increased compared with those neonates without infection.[213] However, by means of multiple logistic regression modeling, IL-6 in addition to CRP predicted sepsis, whereas sICAM-1 and sE-selectin did not contribute significantly to the prediction model.

In premature infants, plasma sL-selectin levels were no different between those with respiratory distress and those without respiratory distress.[211] However, bronchoalveolar fluid sL-selectin is increased in premature infants at risk for chronic lung disease compared with more mature infants. Furthermore, those infants who developed chronic lung disease had persistently elevated BAL sL-selectin.[214] Premature infants had increased plasma sP-selectin in cord blood on day 1 of life, regardless of whether or not they developed chronic lung disease.[215] In contrast, plasma sE-selectin was increased in cord blood and in serum samples on days 1 and 3 in those infants who developed chronic lung disease compared with those who did not. Plasma sICAM-1 levels were also increased later in the first week and during the 2nd week of life in those who developed CLD compared with those who did not.[215] Dexamethasone treatment increases the concentration of plasma sL-selectin and decreases sE-selectin.[205, 216] Thus it appears that premature infants who develop CLD have evidence of increased inflammation in their early perinatal and neonatal course, as measured by sE-selectin, sL-selectin, and sICAM-1. It also appears that dexamethasone modulates the inflammatory response as measured by circulating adhesion molecules and those present on circulating cells.

Modulation of Adhesion Molecules as Adjunctive Therapy

A new and exciting era began with the application of antiadhesive strategies to ameliorate tissue injury. Perhaps the most far-reaching has been the use of anti-αIIbβ3 (platelet glycoprotein IIb/IIIa) "chimeric" antibody in patients who have undergone coronary angioplasty for acute ischemic heart disease.[217] Platelets play a large role in ischemic complications of coronary angioplasty, such as abrupt closure of the coronary vessel during or soon after the procedure. At 30 days and 6 months after coronary angioplasty, patients who received the antibody had markedly reduced rates of reinfarction or repeat urgent interventions, compared with patients who did not receive the antibody.[217] The blockade of cell adhesion molecule function with specific murine antibodies is limited in the treatment of human disease because of generation of antimurine antibodies in the recipient. However, the development of chimeras that transform the murine antibodies so they are more human-like may be advantageous in limiting production of antimurine antibodies.

A large number of preclinical studies supported the concept that blocking endothelial-leukocyte interactions would be beneficial in models of ischemia/reperfusion, such as stroke, myocardial infarction, traumatic shock, and cardiopulmonary bypass. However, clinical studies did not support these approaches.[218] In contrast, a humanized antibody against α4 (natalizumab) has been shown to increase rates of clinical remission and quality of life in patients with Crohn disease.[219] Patients with multiple sclerosis treated with this antibody exhibited decreased numbers of new brain lesions, decreased numbers of relapses, and increased quality of life.[220] Humanized anti-LFA-1 antibody has been found to improve patients with severe unremitting psoriasis significantly.[221] Occasionally drugs are developed that appear to have an unexpected antiadhesive effect. This has occurred with HMG-CoA reductase inhibitors like lovastatin. Several of these drugs "lock" LFA-1 into an inactive conformation close to the A/I domain, thereby inhibiting its ability to adhere to ICAM-1.[222] For these patients, inhibition of the inflammatory response in atherosclerosis may have additional beneficial effects in addition to the treatment of hypercholesterolemia.

The experiments in nature, the genetic deficiencies resulting in LAD I, LAD II, and Glanzmann's thrombasthenia, should be a warning to the clinician scientist attempting to manipulate adhesion molecule function without discrimination. For those caring for the premature and full-term neonate, understanding adhesion molecule biology will be crucial in supporting immune function as well as attempting to modulate the effects of inflammatory-mediated injury such as bronchopulmonary dysplasia.

REFERENCES

1. Gumbiner BM: Cell adhesion: the molecular basis of tissue architecture and morphogenesis. Cell 84:345, 1996.
2. Smith CW: Possible steps involved in the transition to stationary adhesion of rolling neutrophils: a brief review. Microcirculation 7:385, 2000.
3. Burns AR, et al: Unique structural features that influence neutrophil emigration in the lung. Physiol Rev 83:1269, 2003.
4. Klein RB, et al: Decreased mononuclear and polymorphonuclear chemotaxis in human newborns, infants, and young children. Pediatrics 60:467, 1977.
5. Anderson DC, et al: Abnormal mobility of neonatal polymorphonuclear leukocytes. Relationship to impaired redistribution of surface adhesion sites by chemotactic factor or colchicine. J Clin Invest 68:863, 1981.
6. Dos Santos C, et al: Neutrophil chemotaxis to leukotriene B₄ in vitro is decreased for the human neonate. Pediatr Res 33:242, 1993.
7. Krause PJ, et al: Polymorphonuclear leukocyte adherence and chemotaxis in stressed and healthy neonates. Pediatr Res 20:296, 1986.
8. Usmani SS, et al: Polymorphonuclear leukocyte function in the preterm neonate: effect of chronologic age. Pediatrics 87:675, 1991.
9. Carr R, et al: Neutrophil chemotaxis and adhesion in preterm babies. Arch Dis Child 67:813, 1992.
10. Carr R: Neutrophil production and function in newborn infants. Br J Haematol 110:18, 2000.
11. Santos JI, et al: Functional leukocyte administration in protection against experimental neonatal infection. Pediatr Res 14:1408, 1980.
12. Harris M, et al: Diminished actin polymerization by neutrophils from newborn infants. Pediatr Res 33:27, 1993.
13. Anderson DC, et al: Impaired motility of neonatal PMN leukocytes: relationship to abnormalities of cell orientation and assembly of microtubules in chemotactic gradients. J Leukoc Biol 36:1, 1984.
14. Abughali N, et al: Deficient total cell content of CR3 (CD11b) in neonatal neutrophils. Blood 83:1086, 1994.
15. Lorant DE, et al: P-selectin expression by endothelial cells is decreased in neonatal rats and human premature infants. Blood 94:600, 1999.
16. Imhof BA, et al: Leukocyte migration and adhesion. Adv Immunol 58:345, 1995.
17. Springer TA: Traffic signals for lymphocyte recirculation and leukocyte emigration: the multistep paradigm. Cell 76:301, 1994.
18. McEver RP: Selectins: lectins that initiate cell adhesion under flow. Curr Opin Cell Biol 14:581, 2002.
19. Aurrand-Lions M, et al: Heterogeneity of endothelial junctions is reflected by differential expression and specific subcellular localization of the three JAM family members. Blood 98:699, 2001.
20. Schenkel AR, et al: CD99 plays a major role in the migration of monocytes through endothelial junctions. Nat Immunol 3:143, 2002.
21. Newman PJ: Switched at birth: a new family for PECAM-1. J Clin Invest 103:5, 1999.
22. Hynes RO: Integrins: bidirectional, allosteric signaling machines. Cell 110:673, 2002.
23. Simon DI, et al: Platelet glycoprotein ibalpha is a counterreceptor for the leukocyte integrin Mac-1 (CD11b/CD18). J Exp Med 192:193, 2000.
24. Hynes RO: Targeted mutations in cell adhesion genes: what have we learned from them? Dev Biol 180:402, 1996.
25. Zamir E, et al: Molecular complexity and dynamics of cell-matrix adhesions. J Cell Sci 114:3583, 2001.
26. Hato T, et al: Complementary roles for receptor clustering and conformational change in the adhesive and signaling functions of integrin αIIbβ3. J Cell Biol 141:1685, 1998.
27. Seo SM, et al: Effects of IL-8, Gro-alpha, and LTB(4) on the adhesive kinetics of LFA-1 and Mac-1 on human neutrophils. Am J Physiol Cell Physiol 281:C1568, 2001.
28. Hentzen ER, et al: Sequential binding of CD11a/CD18 and CD11b/CD18 defines neutrophil capture and stable adhesion to intercellular adhesion molecule-1. Blood 95:911, 2000.
29. Hughes BJ, et al: Recruitment of CD11b/CD18 to the neutrophil surface and adherence-dependent cell locomotion. J Clin Invest 90:1687, 1992.
30. Hogg N, et al: Mechanisms contributing to the activity of integrins on leukocytes. Immunol Rev 186:164, 2002.
31. Plancon S, et al: Green fluorescent protein (GFP) tagged to the cytoplasmic tail of alphaIIb or beta3 allows the expression of a fully functional integrin alphaIIb(beta3): effect of beta3GFP on alphaIIb(beta3) ligand binding. Biochem J 357:529, 2001.
32. Takagi J, et al: Integrin activation and structural rearrangement. Immunol Rev 186:141, 2002.
33. Lee JO, et al: Two conformations of the integrin A-domain (I-domain): a pathway for activation? Structure 3:1333, 1995.
34. Roos D, et al: Hematologically important mutations: leukocyte adhesion deficiency. Blood Cells Mol Dis 27:1000, 2001.
35. Beglova N, et al: Cysteine-rich module structure reveals a fulcrum for integrin rearrangement upon activation. Nat Struct Biol 9:282, 2002.
36. Takagi J, et al: Definition of EGF-like, closely interacting modules that bear activation epitopes in integrin beta subunits. Proc Natl Acad Sci USA 98:11175, 2001.
37. Xiong JP: An isoleucine-based allosteric switch controls affinity and shape shifting in integrin CD11b A-domain. J Biol Chem 275:38762, 2000.
38. Shimaoka M, et al: Reversibly locking a protein fold in an active conformation with a disulfide bond: integrin alphaL I domains with high affinity and antagonist activity in vivo. Proc Natl Acad Sci USA 98:6009, 2001.
39. Emsley J, et al: Structural basis of collagen recognition by integrin alpha2beta1. Cell 101:47, 2000.
40. Xiong JP, et al: Crystal structure of the extracellular segment of integrin alpha Vbeta3 in complex with an Arg-Gly-Asp ligand. Science 296:151, 2002.
41. Kirchofer D, et al: alpha2beta1 Integrins from different cell types show different binding specificities. J Biol Chem 265:615, 1990.
42. Miller IJ, et al: Regulated expression of the Mac-1, LFA-1, p150,95 glycoprotein family during leukocyte differentiation. J Immunol 137:2891, 1986.
43. Kjeldsen L, et al: Granules and secretory vesicles in human neonatal neutrophils. Pediatr Res 40:120, 1996.
44. Taooka Y, et al: The integrin a9b1 mediates adhesion to activated endothelial cells and transendothelial neutrophil migration through interaction with vascular cell adhesion molecule-1. J Cell Biol 145:413, 1999.
45. Werr J, et al: beta1 Integrins are critically involved in neutrophil locomotion in extravascular tissue in vivo. J Exp Med 187:2091, 1998.

46. Dangerfield J, et al: PECAM-1 (CD31) homophilic interaction up-regulates alpha6beta1 on transmigrated neutrophils in vivo and plays a functional role in the ability of alpha6 integrins to mediate leukocyte migration through the perivascular basement membrane. J Exp Med 196:1201, 2002.

47. Calvete JJ: Platelet integrin GPIIb/IIIa: structure-function correlations. An update and lessons from other integrins. Proc Soc Exp Biol Med 222:29, 1999.

48. Ostermann G, et al: JAM-1 is a ligand of the beta(2) integrin LFA-1 involved in transendothelial migration of leukocytes. Nat Immunol 3:151, 2002.

49. Van der Vieren M, et al: A novel leukointegrin, adb2, binds preferentially to ICAM-3. Immunity 3:683, 1995.

50. Van der Vieren M, et al: The leukocyte integrin alpha D beta 2 binds VCAM-1: evidence for a binding interface between I domain and VCAM-1. J Immunol 163:1984, 1999.

51. Werr J, et al: Engagement of beta2 integrins induces surface expression of beta1 integrin receptors in human neutrophils. J Leukoc Biol 68:553, 2000.

52. Hemler ME, et al: Structure of the integrin VLA-4 and its cell- and cell-matrix adhesion functions. Immunol Rev 114:45, 1990.

53. Kubes P, et al: A novel b_1-dependent adhesion pathway on neutrophils: A mechanism invoked by dihydrocytochalasin B or endothelial transmigration. FASEB J 9:1103, 1995.

54. Rose DM, et al: Alpha4 integrins and the immune response. Immunol Rev 186:118, 2002.

55. Loike JD, et al: Differential regulation of b1 integrins by chemoattractants regulates neutrophil migration through fibrin. J Cell Biol 144:1047, 1999.

56. Werr J, et al: Integrin alpha(2)beta(1) (VLA-2) is a principal receptor used by neutrophils for locomotion in extravascular tissue. Blood 95:1804, 2000.

57. Shang T, et al: a9b1 Integrin is expressed on human neutrophils and contributes to neutrophil migration through human lung and synovial fibroblast barriers. J Leukoc Biol 66:809, 1999.

58. Agace WW, et al: T-lymphocyte–epithelial-cell interactions: integrin alpha(E)(CD103)beta(7), LEEP-CAM and chemokines. Curr Opin Cell Biol 12:563, 2000.

59. Byzova TV, et al: Role of integrin alpha(v)beta3 in vascular biology. Thromb Haemost 80:726, 1998.

60. Diamond MS, et al: Binding of the integrin Mac-1 (CD11b/CD18) to the third immunoglobulin-like domain of ICAM-1 (CD54) and its regulation by glycosylation. Cell 65:961, 1991.

61. Pober JS, et al: Overlapping patterns of antigenic modulation by interleukin 1, tumor necrosis factor and immune interferon. J Immunol 137:1893, 1986.

62. de Fougerolles AR, et al: Characterization of the function of intercellular adhesion molecule (ICAM)-3 and comparison with ICAM-1 and ICAM-2 in immune responses. J Exp Med 179:619, 1994.

63. Elices MJ, et al: VCAM-1 on activated endothelium interacts with the leukocyte integrin VLA-4 at a site distinct from the VLA-4/fibronectin binding site. Cell 60:577, 1990.

64. Alon R, et al: The integrin VLA-4 supports tethering and rolling in flow on VCAM-1. J Cell Biol 128:1243, 1995.

65. Streeter PS, et al: Tissue-specific endothelial cell molecule involved in lymphocyte homing. Nature 331:41, 1988.

66. Newham P, et al: Alpha4 integrin binding interfaces on VCAM-1 and MAdCAM-1. Integrin binding footprints identify accessory binding sites that play a role in integrin specificity. J Biol Chem 272:19429, 1997.

67. Berg EL, et al: L-selectin–mediated lymphocyte rolling on MAdCAM-1. Nature 366:695, 1993.

68. Cunningham SA, et al: JAM2 interacts with alpha 4beta 1. Facilitation by JAM3. J Biol Chem 277:27589, 2002.

69. Picker LJ, et al: The neutrophil selectin LECAM-1 presents carbohydrate ligands to the vascular selectins ELAM-1 and GMP-140. Cell 66:921, 1991.

70. Hafezi-Moghadam A, et al: L-selectin shedding regulates leukocyte recruitment. J Exp Med 193:863, 2001.

71. Erbe D, et al: Identification of an E-selectin region critical for carbohydrate recognition and cell adhesion. J Cell Biol 119:215, 1992.

72. Kansas GS, et al: Regulation of leukocyte rolling and adhesion to high endothelial venules through the cytoplasmic domain of L-selectin. J Exp Med 177:833, 1993.

73. Lawrence MB, et al: Threshold levels of fluid shear promote leukocyte adhesion through selectins (CD62L,P,E). J Cell Biol 136:717, 1997.

74. Smith MJ, et al: A direct comparison of selectin-mediated transient, adhesive events using high temporal resolution. Biophys J 77:3371, 1999.

75. Dwir O, et al: Cytoplasmic anchorage of L-selectin controls leukocyte capture and rolling by increasing the mechanical stability of the selectin tether. J Cell Biol 155:145, 2001.

76. Somers WS, et al: Insights into the molecular basis of leukocyte tethering and rolling revealed by structures of P- and E-selectin bound to SLe(X) and PSGL-1. Cell 103:467, 2000.

77. Homeister JW, et al: The alpha(1,3)fucosyltransferases FucT-IV and FucT-VII exert collaborative control over selectin-dependent leukocyte recruitment and lymphocyte homing. Immunity 15:115, 2001.

78. Moore KL, et al: P-selectin glycoprotein ligand-1 mediates rolling of human neutrophils on P-selectin. J Cell Biol 128:661, 1995.

79. Walcheck B, et al: Neutrophil-neutrophil interactions under hydrodynamic shear stress involve L-selectin and PSGL-1. A mechanism that amplifies initial leukocyte accumulation on P-selectin in vitro. J Clin Invest 98:1081, 1996.

80. Xia L, et al: P-selectin glycoprotein ligand-1–deficient mice have impaired leukocyte tethering to E-selectin under flow. J Clin Invest 109:939, 2002.

81. Li F, et al: Post-translational modifications of recombinant P-selectin glycoprotein ligand-1 required for binding to P- and E-selectin. J Biol Chem 271:3255, 1996.

82. Pouyani T, et al: PSGL-1 recognition of P-selectin is controlled by a tyrosine sulfation consensus at the PSGL-1 amino terminus. Cell 83:333, 1995.

83. Fuhlbrigge RC, et al: Cutaneous lymphocyte antigen is a specialized form of PSGL-1 expressed on skin-homing T cells. Nature 389:978, 1997.

84. Snapp KR, et al: Attachment of the PSGL-1 cytoplasmic domain to the actin cytoskeleton is essential for leukocyte rolling on P-selectin. Blood 99:4494, 2002.

85. Lasky LA, et al: An endothelial ligand for L-selectin is a novel mucin-like molecule. Cell 69:927, 1993.

86. Baumhueter S, et al: Binding of L-selectin to the vascular sialomucin CD34. Science 262:436, 1993.

87. Smith CW, et al: Chemotactic factors regulate lectin adhesion molecule 1 (LECAM-1)–dependent neutrophil adhesion to cytokine-stimulated endothelial cells in vitro. J Clin Invest 87:609, 1991.

88. Lorant DE, et al: Coexpression of GMP-140 and PAF by endothelium stimulated by histamine or thrombin: a juxtacrine system for adhesion and activation of neutrophils. J Cell Biol 115:223, 1991.

89. Zlotnik A, et al: Chemokines: a new classification system and their role in immunity. Immunity. 12:121, 2000.

90. Rossi D, et al: The biology of chemokines and their receptors. Annu Rev Immunol 18:217, 2000.

91. Laudanna C, et al: Rapid leukocyte integrin activation by chemokines. Immunol Rev 186:37, 2002.

92. Middleton J, et al: Leukocyte extravasation: chemokine transport and presentation by the endothelium. Blood 100:3853, 2002.

93. Rossetti G, et al: Integrin-dependent regulation of gene expression in leukocytes. Immunol Rev 186:189, 2002.

94. Wang Q, et al: Changes in the biomechanical properties of neutrophils and endothelial cells during adhesion. Blood 97:660, 2001.

95. Simon SI, et al: Neutrophil tethering on E-selectin activates beta 2 integrin binding to ICAM-1 through a mitogen-activated protein kinase signal transduction pathway. J Immunol 164:4348, 2000.

96. Weyrich AS, et al: Monocyte tethering by P-selectin regulates monocyte chemotactic protein-1 and tumor necrosis factor-a secretion. Signal integration and NF-κB translocation. J Clin Invest 95:2297, 1995.

97. Etzioni A, et al: Of man and mouse: leukocyte and endothelial adhesion molecule deficiencies. Blood 94:3281, 1999.

98. Cinamon G, et al: Shear forces promote lymphocyte migration across vascular endothelium bearing apical chemokines. Nat Immunol 2:515, 2001.

99. Taylor AD, et al: Molecular dynamics of the transition from L-selectin- to beta 2-integrin–dependent neutrophil adhesion under defined hydrodynamic shear. Biophys J 71:3488, 1996.

100. Gopalan PK, et al: Preferential sites for stationary adhesion of neutrophils to cytokine-stimulated HUVEC under flow conditions. J Leukoc Biol 68:47, 2000.

101. Burns AR, et al: Neutrophil transendothelial migration is independent of tight junctions and occurs preferentially at tricellular corners. J Immunol 159:2893, 1997.

102. Burns AR, et al: P-Selectin mediates neutrophil adhesion to endothelial cell borders. J Leuk Biol 65:299, 1999.

103. Smith CW, et al: Transendothelial migration of neutrophils (abstract). J Cell Biochem Suppl 17A:327, 1993.

104. Aurrand-Lions M, et al: The last molecular fortress in leukocyte trans-endothelial migration. Nat Immunol 3:116, 2002.

105. Ozaki H, et al: Cutting edge: combined treatment of TNF-alpha and IFN-gamma causes redistribution of junctional adhesion molecule in human endothelial cells. J Immunol 163:553, 1999.

106. Bogen S, et al: Monoclonal antibody to murine PECAM-1 (CD31) blocks acute inflammation in vivo. J Exp Med 179:1059, 1994.

107. Muller WA, et al: PECAM-1 is required for transendothelial migration of leukocytes. J Exp Med 178:449, 1993.

108. Sixt M, et al: Cell adhesion and migration properties of beta 2-integrin-negative polymorphonuclear granulocytes on defined extracellular matrix molecules. Relevance for leukocyte extravasation. J Biol Chem 276:18878, 2001.

109. Chapman HA, et al: Protease crosstalk with integrins: the urokinase receptor paradigm. Thromb Haemost 86:124, 2001.

110. Springer TA: Traffic signals on endothelium for lymphocyte recirculation and leukocyte emigration. Annul Rev Physiol 57:827, 1995.

111. Steeber DA, et al: Molecular basis of lymphocyte migration. The selectins in inflammation. In Gallin JI, Snyderman R (eds): Inflammation: Basic Principles and Clinical Correlates. Philadelphia, Lippincott Williams & Wilkins, 1999, pp 593–605.

112. Lien DC, et al: Neutrophil kinetics in the pulmonary microcirculation during acute inflammation. Lab Invest 65:145, 1991.

113. Doerschuk CM, et al: CD18-dependent and independent mechanisms of neutrophil emigration in the pulmonary and systemic microcirculation of rabbits. J Immunol 144:2327, 1990.

114. Jaeschke H, et al: Cell adhesion and migration III. Leukocyte adhesion and transmigration in the liver vasculature. Am J Physiol 273:G1169, 1997.

115. Rabb H: The T cell as a bridge between innate and adaptive immune systems: implications for the kidney. Kidney Int 61:1935, 2002.

116. McEver RP: Adhesive interactions of leukocytes, platelets, and the vessel wall during hemostasis and inflammation. Thromb Haemost 86:746, 2001.
117. Buttrum SM, et al: Selectin-mediated rolling of neutrophils on immobilized platelets. Blood 82:1165, 1993.
118. Sheikh S, et al: Continuous activation and deactivation of integrin CD11b/CD18 during de novo expression enables rolling neutrophils to immobilize on platelets. Blood 87:5040, 1996.
119. Romo GM, et al: The glycoprotein Ib-IX-V complex is a platelet counter-receptor for P-selectin. J Exp Med 190:803, 1999.
120. Weber C, et al: Neutrophil accumulation on activated, surface-adherent platelets in flow is mediated by interaction of Mac-1 with fibrinogen bound to allbb3 and stimulated by platelet-activating factor. J Clin Invest 100:2085, 1997.
121. Lalor P, et al: Adhesion of flowing leucocytes to immobilized platelets. Br J Haematol 89:725, 1995.
122. Keeney SE, et al: Comparison of pulmonary neutrophils in the adult and neonatal rat after hyperoxia. Pediatr Res 38:857, 1995.
123. Anderson DC, et al: The severe and moderate phenotypes of heritable Mac-1, LFA-1, p150,95 deficiency: their quantitative definition and relation to leukocyte dysfunction and clinical features. J Infect Dis 152:668, 1985.
124. Kehrli ME Jr, et al: Molecular definition of the bovine granulocytopathy syndrome: identification of a deficiency of the Mac-1 (CD11b/CD18) glycoprotein. J Am Vet Med Assoc 51:1826, 1990.
125. Giger U, et al: Deficiency of leukocyte surface glycoproteins Mo1, LFA-1, and Leu M5 in a dog with recurrent bacterial infections: an animal model. Blood 69:1622, 1987.
126. Shaw JM, et al: Characterization of four CD18 mutants in leucocyte adhesion-deficient (LAD) patients with differential capacities to support expression and function of the CD11/CD18 integrins LFA-1, Mac-1 and p150,95. Clin Exp Immunol 126:311, 2001.
127. Anderson DC, et al: Contributions of the Mac-1 glycoprotein family to adherence-dependent granulocyte functions: structure-function assessments employing subunit–specific monoclonal antibodies. J Immunol 137:15, 1986.
128. Anderson DC, et al: Abnormalities of polymorphonuclear leukocyte function associated with a heritable deficiency of high molecular weight surface glycoproteins (GP138): common relationship to diminished cell adherence. J Clin Invest 74:536, 1984.
129. Hayward AR, et al: Delayed separation of the umbilical cord, widespread infections, and defective neutrophil mobility. Lancet 1:1099, 1979.
130. Arnaout MA, et al: Deficiency of a granulocyte-membrane glycoprotein (gp150) in a boy with recurrent bacterial infections. N Engl J Med 306:693, 1982.
131. Bowen TJ, et al: Severe recurrent bacterial infections associated with defective adherence and chemotaxis in two patients with neutrophils deficient in a cell-associated glycoprotein. J Pediatr 101:932, 1982.
132. Rivera-Matos IR, et al: Leukocyte adhesion deficiency mimicking Hirschsprung disease. J Pediatr 127:755, 1995.
133. Weening RS, et al: Defective initiation of the metabolic stimulation of phagocytizing granulocytes: a new congenital defect. J Lab Clin Med 88:757, 1976.
134. Waldrop TC, et al: Periodontal manifestations of the heritable Mac-1, LFA-1 deficiency syndrome—clinical, histopathologic and molecular characteristics. J Periodont 58:400, 1987.
135. Kuijpers TW, et al: Leukocyte adhesion deficiency type 1 (LAD-1)/variant. A novel immunodeficiency syndrome characterized by dysfunctional β2 integrins. J Clin Invest 100:1725, 1997.
136. Hogg N, et al: A novel leukocyte adhesion deficiency caused by expressed but nonfunctional β2 integrins Mac-1 and LFA-1. J Clin Invest 103:97, 1999.
137. Harris ES, et al: A novel syndrome of variant leukocyte adhesion deficiency involving defects in adhesion mediated by beta1 and beta2 integrins. Blood 97:767, 2001.
138. Ambruso DR, et al: Human neutrophil immunodeficiency syndrome is associated with an inhibitory Rac2 mutation. Proc Natl Acad Sci USA 97:4654, 2000.
139. Williams DA, et al: Dominant negative mutation of the hematopoietic-specific Rho GTPase, Rac2, is associated with a human phagocyte immunodeficiency. Blood 96:1646, 2000.
140. Kohl S, et al: The genetic deficiency of leukocyte surface glycoprotein Mac-1, LFA-1, p150,95 in humans is associated with defective antibody-dependent cellular cytotoxicity in vitro and defective protection against herpes simplex virus in vivo. J Immunol 137:1688, 1986.
141. Wilson CB, et al: When is umbilical cord separation delayed? J Pediatr 107:292, 1985.
142. Thomas C, et al: Results of allogeneic bone marrow transplantation in patients with leukocyte adhesion deficiency. Blood 84:1635, 1995.
143. Nurden AT, et al: Inherited defects of platelet function. Rev Clin Exp Hematol 5:314, 2001.
144. Bierling P, et al: Early immunization against platelet glycoprotein IIIa in a newborn Glanzmann type I patient. Vox Sang 55:109, 1988.
145. Boussemart T, et al: Hepatic haematoma related to Glanzmann thrombasthenia in a newborn infant. Br J Obstet Gynecol 103:179, 1996.
146. McDowall A, et al: A novel form of integrin dysfunction involving beta1, beta2, and beta3 integrins. J Clin Invest 111:51, 2003.
147. Etzioni A, et al: Brief report: recurrent severe infections caused by a novel leukocyte adhesion deficiency. N Engl J Med 327:1789, 1992.
148. Phillips ML, et al: Neutrophil adhesion in leukocyte adhesion deficiency syndrome type 2. J Clin Invest 96:2898, 1995.
149. Price TH, et al: In vivo neutrophil and lymphocyte function studies in a patient with leukocyte adhesion deficiency type II. Blood 84:1635, 1995.
150. von Andrian UH, et al: In vivo behavior of neutrophils from two patients with distinct inherited leukocyte adhesion deficiency syndromes. J Clin Invest 91:2893, 1993.
151. Bullard DC, et al: Infectious susceptibility and severe deficiency of leukocyte rolling and recruitment in E-selectin and P-selectin double mutant mice. J Exp Med 183:2329, 1996.
152. Marquardt T, et al: Correction of leukocyte adhesion deficiency type II with oral fucose. Blood 94:3976, 1999.
153. Miller ME: Phagocytic function in the neonate: selected aspects. Pediatrics 64:5709, 1979.
154. Anderson DC, et al: Abnormal stimulated adherence of neonatal granulocytes: impaired induction of surface Mac-1 by chemotactic factors or secretagogues. Blood 70:740, 1987.
155. Mollinedo F, et al: Enhancement of human neutrophil functions by a monoclonal antibody directed against a 19-kDa antigen. J Immunol 149:323, 1992.
156. Bainton DF, et al: Leukocyte adhesion receptors are stored in peroxidase-negative granules of human neutrophils. J Exp Med 166:1641, 1987.
157. Smith JB, et al: Fetal neutrophils and eosinophils express normal levels of L-selectin. Pediatr Res 34:253, 1993.
158. Torok C, et al: Diversity in regulation of adhesion molecules (Mac-1 and L-selectin) in monocytes and neutrophils from neonates and adults. Arch Dis Child 68:561, 1993.
159. Eisenfeld L, et al: Longitudinal study of neutrophil adherence and motility. J Pediatr 117:926, 1990.
160. Kim SK, et al: Comparison of L-selectin and CD11b on neutrophils of adults and neonates during the first month of life. Pediatr Res 53:132, 2003.
161. Rebuck N, et al: Neutrophil adhesion molecules in term and premature infants: normal or enhanced leucocyte integrins but defective L-selectin expression and shedding. Clin Exp Immunol 101:183, 1995.
162. Reddy RK, et al: A mixed population of immature and mature leucocytes in umbilical cord blood results in a reduced expression and function of CR3 (CD11b/CD18). Clin Exp Immunol 114:462, 1998.
163. Smith JB, et al: Expression of the complement receptors CR1 and CR3 and the Type III Fc-gamma receptor on neutrophils from newborn infants and from fetuses with Rh disease. Pediatr Res 28:120, 1990.
164. Nupponen I, et al: Neutrophil activation in preterm infants who have respiratory distress syndrome. Pediatrics 110:36, 2002.
165. McEvoy LT, et al: Total cell content of CR3 (CD11b/CD18) and LFA-1 (CD11a/CD18) in neonatal neutrophils: relationship to gestational age. Blood 87:3929, 1996.
166. Anderson DC, et al: Impaired transendothelial migration by neonatal neutrophils: abnormalities of Mac-1 (CD11b/CD18)-dependent adherence reactions. Blood 78:2613, 1990.
167. Schuit KE, et al: Inefficient in vivo neutrophil migration in neonatal rats. J Leukoc Biol 35:583, 1984.
168. Fortenberry JD, et al: CD18-dependent and L-selectin–dependent neutrophil emigration is diminished in neonatal rabbits. Blood 84:889, 1994.
169. Schuit KE, et al: Kinetics of phagocyte response to group B streptococcal infections in newborn rats. Infect Immun 28:319, 1980.
170. Martin TR, et al: Effects of endotoxin in the lungs of neonatal rats: age-dependent impairment of the inflammatory response. J Infect Dis 171:134, 1995.
171. Martin TR, et al: Lung antibacterial defense mechanisms in infant and adult rats: implications for the pathogenesis of Group B streptococcal infections in the neonatal lung. J Infect Dis 157:91, 1988.
172. Cheung ATW, et al: Host defense deficiency in newborn nonhuman primate lungs. J Med Primatol 15:37, 1986.
173. Graf JM, et al: Contribution of LFA-1 and Mac-1 to CD18-dependent neutrophil emigration in a neonatal rabbit model. J Appl Physiol 80:1984, 1996.
174. Prince JE, et al: The differential roles of LFA-1 and Mac-1 in host defense against systemic infection with Streptococcus pneumoniae. J Immunol 166:7362, 2001.
175. Dunne JL, et al: Control of leukocyte rolling velocity in TNF-alpha-induced inflammation by LFA-1 and Mac-1. Blood 99:336, 2002.
176. Mariscalco MM, et al: Mechanisms of decreased leukocyte localization in the developing host. Am J Physiol Heart Circ Physiol 282:H636, 2002.
177. Mariscalco MM, et al: Ontogeny of Mac-1-dependent localization in a rabbit model (abstract). FASEB J 15:A394, 2001.
178. Sherman MP, et al: The role of pulmonary phagocytes in host defense against group B streptococci in preterm versus term rabbit lung. J Infect Dis 166:818, 1992.
179. Bochsler PN, et al: Transendothelial migration of neonatal and adult bovine neutrophils in vitro. J Leukoc Biol 55:43, 1994.
180. Falconer AE, et al: Impaired neutrophil phagocytosis in preterm neonates: lack of correlation with expression of immunoglobulin or complement receptors. Biol Neonate 68:264, 1995.
181. Marodi L, et al: Candidacidal mechanisms in the human neonate. Impaired IFN-gamma activation of macrophages in newborn infants. J Immunol 153:5643, 1994.

182. O'Gorman MR, et al: Lymphocyte subpopulations in healthy 1–3-day-old infants. Cytometry *34*:235, 1998.
183. Kern F, et al: Discordant expression of LFA-1, VLA-4alpha, VLA-beta 1, CD45RO and CD28 on T-cell subsets: evidence for multiple subsets of "memory" T cells. Int Arch Allergy Immunol *104*:17, 1994.
184. Friedl P, et al: T lymphocyte locomotion in a three-dimensional collagen matrix. J Immunol *154*:4973, 1995.
185. Pilarski LM, et al: Beta 1 integrin (CD29) expression on human postnatal T cell subsets defined by selective CD45 isoform expression. J Immunol *147*:830, 1991.
186. Sato K, et al: Chemokine receptor expressions and responsiveness of cord blood T cells. J Immunol *166*:1659, 2001.
187. Jones DA, et al: A two-step adhesion cascade for T cell/endothelial cell interactions under flow conditions. J Clin Invest *94*:2443, 1994.
188. Anderson DC, et al: Diminished lectin-, epidermal growth factor-, complement binding domain-cell adhesion molecule-1 on neonatal neutrophils underlies their impaired CD18-independent adhesion to endothelial cells in vitro. J Immunol *146*:3372, 1991.
189. Koenig JM, et al: Diminished soluble and total cellular L-selectin in cord blood is associated with its impaired shedding from activated neutrophils. Pediatr Res *39*:616, 1996.
190. Abbassi O, et al: E-Selectin supports neutrophil rolling in vitro under conditions of flow. J Clin Invest *92*:2719, 1993.
191. Mariscalco MM, et al: P-Selectin support of neonatal neutrophil adherence under flow: contribution of L-selectin, LFA-1, and ligand(s) for P-selectin. Blood *91*:4776, 1998.
192. Tcharmtchi MH, et al: Neonatal neutrophil interaction with P-selectin: contribution of P-selectin glycoprotein ligand-1 and sialic acid. J Leukoc Biol *67*:73, 2000.
193. Mariscalco MM, et al: Diminished P-selectin tether duration contributes to depressed neonatal neutrophil-platelet interactions (abstract). FASEB J *16*:A595, 2002.
194. Muller WA: Migration of leukocytes across endothelial junctions: some concepts and controversies. Microcirculation *8*:181, 2001.
195. Rajasekhar D, et al: Neonatal platelets are less reactive than adult platelets to physiological agonists in whole blood. Thromb Haemost *72*:957, 1994.
196. Shenkman B, et al: Increased neonatal platelet deposition on subendothelium under flow conditions: the role of plasma von Willebrand factor. Pediatr Res *45*:270, 1999.
197. Buchsbaum ME, et al: Differential induction of intercellular adhesion molecule-1 in human skin by recombinant cytokines. J Cutane Pathol *20*:21, 1993.
198. Arnaout MA, et al: Increased expression of an adhesion-promoting surface glycoprotein in the granulocytopenia of hemodialysis. N Engl J Med *312*:457, 1985.
199. Finn A, et al: Changes in neutrophil CD11b/CD18 and L-selectin expression and release of interleukin 8 and elastase in pediatric cardiopulmonary bypass. Agents Actions *38*:C44, 1993.
200. Lin RY, et al: Relationships between plasma cytokine concentrations and leukocyte functional antigen expression in patients with sepsis. Crit Care Med *22*:1595, 1994.
201. Kishimoto TK, et al: Neutrophil Mac-1 and MEL-14 adhesion proteins inversely regulated by chemotactic factors. Science *245*:1238, 1989.
202. Hasslen SR, et al: Down-regulation of homing receptors: a mechanism for impaired recruitment of human phagocytes in sepsis. J Trauma *31*:645, 1991.
203. Buhrer C, et al: L-selectin is down-regulated in umbilical cord blood granulocytes and monocytes of newborn infants with acute bacterial infection. Pediatr Res *36*:799, 1994.
204. Van Eeden SF, et al: Polymorphonuclear leukocytes L-selectin expression decreases as they age in circulation. Am J Physiol Heart Circ Physiol *272*:H401, 1997.
205. Nakagawa M, et al: The effect of glucocorticoids on the expression of L-selectin on polymorphonuclear leukocytes. Blood *93*:2730, 1999.
206. Ferri LE, et al: Soluble L-selectin attenuates tumor necrosis factor-alpha-mediated leukocyte adherence and vascular permeability: a protective role for elevated soluble L-selectin in sepsis. Crit Care Med *30*:1842, 2002.
207. Reinhart K, et al: Markers of endothelial damage in organ dysfunction and sepsis. Crit Care Med *30*:S302, 2002.
208. Blake GJ, et al: Novel clinical markers of vascular wall inflammation. Circ Res *89*:763, 2001.
209. Weirich E, et al: Neutrophil CD11b expression as a diagnostic marker for early-onset neonatal infection. J Pediatr *132*:445, 1998.
210. Weinschenk NP, et al: Premature infants respond to early-onset and late-onset sepsis with leukocyte activation. J Pediatr *137*:345, 2000.
211. Sarafidis K, et al: Evidence of early systemic activation and transendothelial migration of neutrophils in neonates with severe respiratory distress syndrome. Pediatr Pulmonol *31*:214, 2001.
212. Giannaki G, et al: Serum soluble E- and L-selectin in the very early neonatal period. Early Hum Dev *60*:149, 2000.
213. Dollner H, et al: Early diagnostic markers for neonatal sepsis: comparing C-reactive protein, interleukin-6, soluble tumour necrosis factor receptors and soluble adhesion molecules. J Clin Epidemiol *54*:1251, 2001.
214. Kotecha S, et al: Soluble L-selectin concentration in bronchoalveolar lavage fluid obtained from infants who develop chronic lung disease of prematurity. Arch Dis Child Fetal Neonatal Ed *78*:F143, 1998.
215. Ramsay PL, et al: Early clinical markers for the development of bronchopulmonary dysplasia: soluble E-selectin and ICAM-1. Pediatrics *102*:927, 1998.
216. Ballabh P, et al: Soluble E-selectin, Soluble L-selectin and soluble ICAM-1 in bronchopulmonary dysplasia, and changes with dexamethasone. Pediatrics *111*:461, 2003.
217. Lefkovits J, et al: Effects of platelet glycoprotein IIb/IIIa receptor blockade by a chimeric monoclonal antibody (abciximab) on acute and six-month outcomes after percutaneous transluminal coronary angioplasty for acute myocardial infarction. EPIC investigators. Am J Cardiol 77:1045, 1996.
218. Harlan JM, et al: Leukocyte-endothelial interactions: clinical trials of anti-adhesion therapy. Crit Care Med *30*:S214, 2002.
219. Ghosh S, et al: Natalizumab for active Crohn's disease. N Engl J Med *348*:24, 2003.
220. Miller DH, et al: A controlled trial of natalizumab for relapsing multiple sclerosis. N Engl J Med *348*:15, 2003.
221. Gottlieb AB, et al: Psoriasis as a model for T-cell–mediated disease: immunobiologic and clinical effects of treatment with multiple doses of efalizumab, an anti-CD11a antibody. Arch Dermatol *138*:591, 2002.
222. Frenette PS: Locking a leukocyte integrin with statins. N Engl J Med *345*:1419, 2001.

161

Helen M. Korchak

Stimulus-Response Coupling in Phagocytic Cells

SIGNAL TRANSDUCTION AND FUNCTIONS IN PHAGOCYTIC CELLS

Interaction of ligands with their specific receptors on phagocytic cells elicits responses such as chemotaxis, cell-cell aggregation, and phagocytosis.[1-7] The generation of active oxygen species such as superoxide (O_2^-) and hydrogen peroxide and the release of granule contents into the phagocytic vacuole contribute to the antimicrobial activities of neutrophils and monocytes.[8-10] In conditions in which these functions are defective, the host may be subject to recurrent infections.[11-14] *Candida* infections are common in neonates, and in the newborn infant, microbicidal activity of monocytes to *Candida* species cannot

be fully activated by interferon-γ (IFN-γ). Growth factors are critical in the production of circulating neutrophils and monocytes; neutropenia in neonates contributes to increased susceptibility to infection. Growth factors trigger signaling pathways for the proliferation and differentiation of stem cells and for the production of circulating phagocytes. An understanding of signaling may allow a targeted control of phagocytic cell numbers and functions.[14, 15] However, the microbicidal mechanism of phagocytes is a double-edged sword; the release of active oxygen species and granule contents and the production of proinflammatory cytokines may contribute to tissue damage during the inflammatory response.[7, 16-21] Phagocytic cells have been implicated in the tissue damage of inflammation in diseases such as asthma, necrotizing enterocolitis, adult respiratory distress syndrome, sepsis, cystic fibrosis, and multiple organ failure.[16,22-25] It is therefore evident that a more precise understanding of the signaling mechanisms for cell activation would be useful in designing strategies to modulate inappropriate neutrophil and monocyte function in neonatal disease.[25-27]

The various receptor types of phagocytic cells can trigger different end responses, which may be signaled by both common and selective signaling pathways. Each signaling pathway possesses the following elements:

ligand/receptor → coupler → transducer → end response

Coupling of the occupied receptor to a signal transduction pathway is triggered by the binding of a specific ligand to its receptor. Two principal coupling mechanisms are used by different receptor types: trimeric G-proteins and protein tyrosine kinase–initiated signaling. Selective activation of a transduction pathway involves activation of specific protein kinases that can be regulated by second messengers or may be part of a protein kinase cascade. In addition, activation of protein kinases results in amplification of the signal, because phosphorylation of multiple proteins results from occupation of a single receptor. Activation of the transduction pathway results in phosphorylation of key protein substrates that elicits activation of end responses, such as chemotaxis, degranulation, cell adherence, and phagocytosis. The turn-off signal for cell responses involves down-regulation of the receptor and activation of phosphatases to dephosphorylate the phosphoproteins.

RECEPTOR TYPES AND COUPLING MECHANISMS

Interaction of the chemoattractant fMet-Leu-Phe (fMLP), the cytokine interleukin-8 (IL-8), the complement component C5a, and leukotriene B_4 with their receptors triggers cell movement, and, at higher concentrations, ligands such as fMLP also trigger cell-cell aggregation, degranulation, and O_2^- generation. The chemotactic receptors are termed *serpentine receptors,* possess seven-transmembrane spanning segments (7TM), and are coupled to the signal transduction pathway by a trimeric G-protein (Fig. 161–1).[2,3,28-30]

Signal transduction can also be initiated by a protein tyrosine kinase–dependent pathway; such receptors are often activated by receptor dimerization or oligomerization.[31] The multimeric Fcγ receptors (FcγRs) interact with immune complexes to trigger phagocytosis, degranulation, and O_2^- generation.[32] Signaling from the FcγRs is not dependent on trimeric G-proteins, but rather it is coupled to the signaling pathway by a tyrosine kinase–dependent mechanism (Fig. 161–2).[33-36] Signaling from the tumor necrosis factor-α (TNF-α), IL-1, IL-6, and granulocyte-macrophage colony-stimulating factor (GM-CSF-1) receptors, and from the integrins CD11a, CD11b, and CD11c, is also initiated by tyrosine kinase.[37-41]

Cross-talk among different signaling pathways has been observed; fMLP acting by a trimeric G-protein–initiated pathway also triggers activation of tyrosine phosphorylation.[13] Receptors for TNF-α, the 55- to 60-kDa TNF receptor type 1 (TNFR1), and the 75- to 80-kDa TNF receptor type 2 (TNFR2), are found in neutrophils, monocytes, and myeloid precursor HL-60 cells.[42]

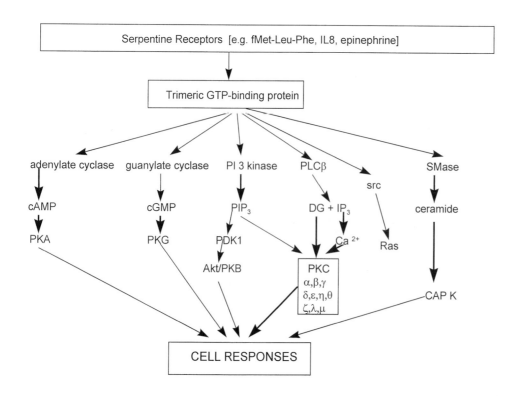

Figure 161–1. Signal transduction pathways triggered by serpentine (7-transmembrane spanning) receptors and trimeric G-proteins. Trimeric G-proteins elicit activation of adenylate cyclase, which generates cyclic adenosine monophosphate (cAMP) and activates protein kinase A (PKA; cAMP-activated kinase). Activation of guanylate cyclase triggers generation of cyclic guanosine monophosphate (cGMP) and activation of protein kinase G (PKG; cGMP-activated kinase). Activation of sphingomyelinase (SMase) triggers generation of ceramide and activation of ceramide-activated protein kinase (CAPK). Trimeric G-proteins also activate phosphatidylinositol-3-kinase (PI-3-kinase), which generates phosphatidylinositol 3,4, 5-tetrakis phosphate (PIP_3), and they activate phospholipase C-β (PLCβ), which generates IP_3, a trigger for Ca^{2+} mobilization, and diglyceride (DG). PIP_3, DG, and Ca^{2+} are cofactors for activation of protein kinase C (PKC) isotypes. Trimeric G-protein signaling can also elicit activation of cytosolic tyrosine kinases (Src) and can trigger signaling via the small G-protein Ras. GTP = guanosine triphosphate; IL8 = interleukin-8.

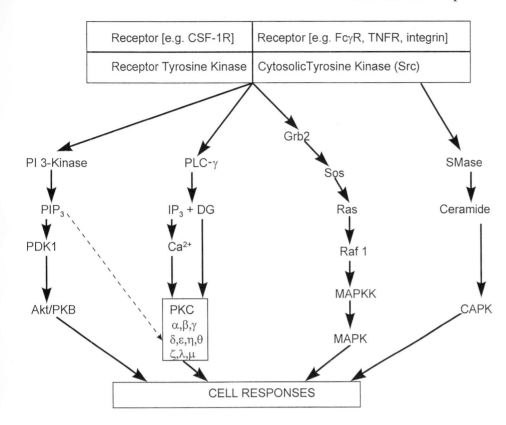

Figure 161–2. Protein tyrosine kinase–initiated signal transduction pathways. Signaling is initiated by receptors that have an intrinsic tyrosine kinase activity or by receptors that lack intrinsic tyrosine kinase activity but associate with Src family cytosolic tyrosine kinases. Activation of tyrosine kinases triggers activation of PI 3-kinase, PLC-γ, and SMase (see Fig. 161–1). Tyrosine kinases trigger activation of the serine/ threonine kinase Raf, via the coupling proteins Grb2 and Shc, the guanine nucleotide exchange factor Sos, and the small G-protein Ras. Raf activates MAP kinase kinase (MAPKK) and MAP kinase (MAPK). CAPK = ceramide-activated protein kinase; CSF = colony-stimulating factor; DG = diglyceride; TNF = tumor necrosis factor.

TNF-α is an incomplete secretagogue. TNF-α can prime neutrophils and HL-60 cells for enhanced O_2^- generation and degranulation triggered by a second stimulus such as fMLP.[43,44] In addition, TNF-α is a secretagogue for adherent, but not for nonadherent, phagocytic cells.[45-47] The dependence of TNF-α–induced responses on adherence involves cross-talk between two signaling pathways, those induced by β_2-integrin and TNF-α.[13,45,47]

Trimeric G-Proteins and Signaling

Ligand occupation of seven-transmembrane spanning receptors activates a group of coupling proteins called *trimeric G-proteins* because they bind guanosine triphosphate (GTP).[28,48-52] These G-proteins regulate certain target enzymes or ion channels called *effectors* because changes in their activity cause alterations in second-messenger levels (e.g., calcium [Ca^{2+}] or cyclic adenosine monophosphate [cAMP]) or ionic composition, which eventually lead to the cell response. Trimeric G-proteins contain three polypeptides—an α-subunit (which binds and hydrolyses GTP), a β-subunit, and a γ-subunit (Fig. 161–3). The β- and γ-subunits dissociate only when denatured and thus form a functional monomer. Functional activity of G-proteins involves a G-protein cycle. When guanosine diphosphate (GDP) is bound, the α-subunit combines with the βγ-subunit to form an inactive trimer that associates with the receptor (see Fig. 161–3). When a ligand occupies the receptor, the receptor is activated and undergoes a conformational change. The GDP-liganded α-subunit responds with a conformational change that decreases the GDP affinity, so the GDP leaves the active site. Because the intracellular concentration of GTP is considerably higher than that of GDP, the departing GDP is replaced by GTP. Binding of GTP induces the active conformation of the α-subunit and causes the activated α-subunit to dissociate from the βγ-subunit and from the receptor. During this activated state, the free α- and βγ-subunits can activate target effectors (Table 161–1; see Fig. 161–1).[48] The activated state continues until the GTP is hydrolyzed to GDP by the intrinsic GTPase activity of the α-subunit. Once the GTP is

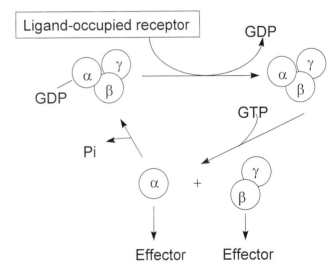

Figure 161–3. The regulatory cycle of heterotrimeric G-proteins. GDP = guanosine diphosphate; GTP = guanosine triphosphate; PI = phosphatidylinositol.

hydrolyzed to GDP, the α-subunits reassociate with the βγ-subunits, become inactive, and reassociate with the receptor. The rate of GTP hydrolysis is a timing mechanism that controls the duration of both α- and βγ-activation. Although the βγ-subunit does not itself bind GTP, its activity is dependent on the hydrolysis of GTP by the α-subunit.

Four subfamilies of α-subunits (see Table 161–1) and multiple β- and γ-subunits have been identified.[49] In neutrophils and monocytes, the principal α-subunits are α_i and α_s.[28,51] Most neutrophil responses induced by chemoattractants such as fMLP are inhibited by pertussis toxin; Gi_2 and Gi_3 are the primary transduction partners associated with these receptors.[28] Both α- and βγ-subunits can positively regulate effectors. The Giα-subunit

TABLE 161-1

Trimeric G-Protein Subunits and Effector Targets

Subunit	Toxin	End Response
α_s	Cholera	Stimulates adenylyl cyclase, regulates Ca^{2+} channels
α_i	Pertussis	Inhibits adenylyl cyclase, regulates K^+ and Ca^{2+} channels
α_q	—	Activates PLCβ
α_{12}	—	Regulates Na^+/K^+ exchange
βγ	—	Activates PLCβ, PLA$_2$, Pl-3-kinase, adenylyl cyclase, K^+ channel

PLA$_2$ = phospholipase A$_2$; PLCβ = phospholipase C$_\beta$.

was originally thought to interact with the effector enzyme, phospholipase C (PLC), in phagocytes; it is now understood that the βγ-subunit regulates PLC-β in phagocytes.[28] Indeed, the βγ-subunit can positively regulate PLC-β, phospholipase A$_2$ (PLA$_2$), phosphatidylinositol-3-kinase (PI-3-kinase), adenylyl cyclase, and the potassium channel.[51] The βγ-subunit may also act through the small molecular weight G-protein ras (see later) (see Fig. 161-2) to activate mitogen-activated protein kinase (MAPK) pathways.[52] The G$_s$ pathway triggers activation of adenylyl cyclase and generation of the second messenger cAMP (see Fig. 161-1). Ligands such as epinephrine, interacting with the β-adrenergic receptor, trigger an α$_s$-transduced increase in cAMP, which is a negative regulator of many phagocytic functions, including O$_2^-$ generation and degranulation, and increases in ligand-induced elevation of cytosolic Ca^{2+}.[53] The pattern of regulation of effectors is very specific.

Tyrosine Kinase–Initiated Signal Transduction

Src Family Protein Tyrosine Kinases

Tyrosine kinase–based signaling can be initiated both by receptors possessing an intrinsic tyrosine kinase and by receptors lacking an intrinsic tyrosine kinase.[54-56] Dimerization of the CSF-1 receptor stimulates an intrinsic tyrosine kinase and leads to downstream signaling (Fig. 161-4).[57] Members of the Src family of cytosolic tyrosine kinases have been found associated with

numerous cell receptors, some with intrinsic tyrosine kinase activity such as the CSF-1 receptor, as well as with receptors possessing no catalytic function (see Fig. 161-4).[56,57] Receptors such as the FcγRs, β$_2$-integrin, TNF-α receptor, and GM-CSF receptor trigger tyrosine kinase–initiated signaling in phagocytic cells. These receptors have no intrinsic tyrosine kinase activity, but they associate with two cytoplasmic tyrosine kinase types, Src and Syk (see Fig. 161-4).[58,59] Src is the prototype for a family of tyrosine kinases that are activated by ligands such as immune complexes and cytokines. However, src is also involved in signaling triggered by trimeric G-protein–initiated signaling.[60-62] There are at least nine members of the Src family: Src, Fyn, Yes, Lyn, Hck, Fgr, Lck, Blk, and Yrk.[56,63] Within the first 15 N-terminal residues, all Src family members bear a signal for myristoylation and, in most cases, a signal for palmitoylation, which direct the association of these tyrosine kinases with cellular membranes (Fig. 161-5). The adjacent domain, the unique domain, is poorly conserved between members of the Src family, and in some cases it is thought to participate in interaction with other proteins. C-terminal to the unique domain is the Src homology 3 (SH3) domain, which promotes protein-protein interactions with proteins that contain left-handed polyproline Type II helices (see Fig. 161-5).[63,64] The domain C-terminal to the SH3 domain is the Src homology 2 (SH2) domain, comprising approximately 100 residues. The SH2 domain is a binding site for phosphotyrosine-containing proteins, and it is frequently found in proteins such as PLC-γ, PI-3-kinase, and Shc, which are involved in tyrosine kinase–based signal transduction.[64-66] The SH2 domains of Src kinases mediate interactions of these proteins with receptor-type protein tyrosine kinases, and they may also mediate the interaction of Src kinases with protein substrates. C-terminal to the SH2 domain is the catalytic domain, which is similar to the catalytic subunit of other protein tyrosine kinases.[56] Phosphorylation of Tyr416 in the catalytic domain is necessary for optimal activity. In the C-terminal tail region of the Src molecule is a conserved tyrosine (Tyr527) that is essential for the phosphorylation-based regulation that is characteristic of Src tyrosine kinases. Phosphorylation of Tyr527 causes interaction of the tail region with the SH2 domain, thus retaining the Src molecule in an inactive conformation. Ligand-initiated signaling triggers dephosphorylation of Tyr(P)527; phosphatases specific for Tyr(P)527 have not been identified. Dephosphorylation of Tyr(P)527 triggers a conformational change in the Src molecule that results in activation of the tyrosine kinase activity.

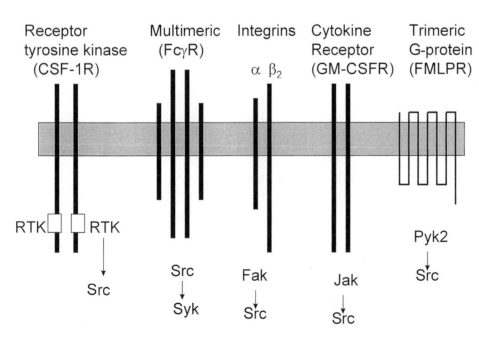

Figure 161–4. Signaling by the cytosolic protein tyrosine kinases Src and Syk. See text for details.

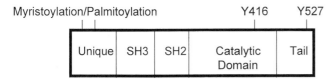

Myristoylation/Palmitoylation   Y416   Y527

| Unique | SH3 | SH2 | Catalytic Domain | Tail |

Figure 161–5. The structure of the Src family of protein tyrosine kinases.

Multiple members of the Src family have been observed in phagocytic cells including Fgr, Fes/Fps, Lyn, Hck, and Fyn.[54,67-71] β_2-Integrin-initiated tyrosine phosphorylation and activation of the Fgr protein tyrosine kinase have been demonstrated in human neutrophils,[67] and they are involved in TNF-α–triggered priming and in TNF-α–triggered adherence-dependent responses.[67,72] Src family members may also be involved in FcγR-initiated signaling.[68-71] A role for Hck and Syk was observed in signaling through FcγRI,[73,74] while physical and functional association of Src-related p59hck, p59fyn, and p56lyn protein tyrosine kinases was noted with FcγRII in a monocytic cell line.[70,71] Considerable redundancy appears to exist in Src-based signaling and the functions of Src family members overlap functionally.[68]

Syk Kinase and Tyrosine Kinase–Mediated Signaling

The SH2 domains of Src family kinases can associate with another tyrosine kinase, termed Syk.[64,68,74,75] Syk is structurally related to the T-cell–specific ZAP70; both Syk and ZAP70 contain two SH2 domains as well as a catalytic domain. Syk is activated after agonist binding to FcγRs (see Fig. 161–4).[59,74-76] Syk binds to short motifs known as tyrosine-activation motifs (TAMs) on the receptor; TAMs contain a conserved $Yx_2Lx_7Yx_2L$ sequence that is phosphorylated on tyrosine and allows ligand-receptor binding. Coordinated tyrosine phosphorylation of the γ-subunit of FcγRs, p72syk, and the cytoskeletal-associated protein paxillin was observed during FcγR-mediated phagocytosis in monocytes and macrophages, and it may be important in integrating signals between the FcγR and the cytoskeleton.[59,74,76]

Cytokine Receptors and the JAK/STAT Signaling Pathway

Cytokine and IFN receptors are constitutively associated with members of the Janus protein kinase (JAK) family of tyrosine kinases: Jak1, Jak2, Jak3, and Tyk2.[77-79] IL-6, IFN-γ, granulocyte CSF (G-CSF), and GM-CSF trigger a JAK/STAT signaling pathway, (Fig. 161–6).[80-83] Ligand binding induces receptor oligomerization and concomitant JAK activation; there are three patterns by which the JAK kinases associate with receptors, depending on the receptor structure (see Fig. 161–6). Cytokines using single-chain receptors such as the G-CSF receptor associate with Jak2; association may be constitutive or enhanced by ligand binding. Receptor aggregation induces aggregation of the Jak2 and allows transphosphorylation of a KEYY site in the kinase activation domain, thus enhancing catalytic activity of the Jak2. The activated Jak2 can then autophosphorylate and phosphorylate cellular substrates recruited to the receptor. A second association pattern is used by receptors that activate two proteins; one protein is used for ligand binding, and the other protein is required for signaling. IL-6 and GM-CSF receptors are typical of this second pattern of signaling. The IL-6 receptor associates with gp130, which associates with and activates Jak1, Jak2, and Tyk2. The GM-CSF receptor associates with a β_c-chain that is common to IL-3 and IL-5 receptors; the membrane proximal domain of the β_c-chain associates with and activates Jak2. The third association pattern in which two receptor chains are required for signaling is used by IFN receptors. In the IFN-γ receptor, the α-chain associates with Jak1, whereas the β-chain associates with Jak2; both Jaks are required for activation of Jak1 and Jak2.

Activation of the JAK pathway results in tyrosine phosphorylation of the receptor signaling subunits that enables binding of SH2-containing proteins such as PLC-γ, PI-3-kinase, and Shc, which are, in turn, phosphorylated by the activated receptor complex. However, the tyrosine kinase substrates most involved in cytokine signaling are the STAT proteins, STATs 1 to 6.[79-81] The STAT proteins are transcription factors that possess SH2 domains through which they bind to the activated receptor and a target tyrosine for JAK kinases just C-terminal to the SH2 domain. Each cytokine receptor selectively binds to and tyrosine-phosphorylates a specific STAT protein, thereby inducing dimerization of the STAT through mutual (P)Tyr-SH2 interactions (see Fig. 161–6). The STAT dimer is translocated to the nucleus, binds to specific promoter elements, and induces gene expression. Receptor selectivity has been demonstrated for the different STATs. STAT1 is specific for IFN and GM-CSF pathways, whereas STAT3 docks to the sequence YXXQ found in the gp130 signaling chain of the IL-6 receptor.[81-84]

DOWNSTREAM SIGNALING MECHANISMS

Low Molecular Weight Guanosine Triphosphate–Binding Proteins as Molecular Switches

Many signal transduction pathways in phagocytes are modulated by low molecular weight (20 to 25 kDa) GTP-binding proteins. These small G-proteins are members of a growing family

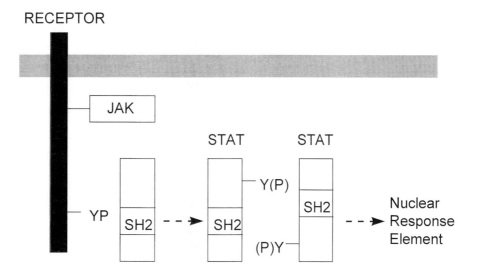

RECEPTOR

Figure 161–6. Interferon/cytokine-initiated signaling by the JAK/STAT pathway.

of GTP-binding proteins known as the Ras superfamily, and they act as molecular switches in regulating a wide range of signaling pathways in virtually all cells.[85-87] The members of the small G-protein superfamily are structurally classified as the Ras, Rho, Rab, Arf, and Ran families and regulate multiple cell functions. Ras G-proteins are regulators of gene expression, Ran proteins regulate nucleocytoplasmic transport, Arf proteins regulate vesicle budding, and Rho proteins (Rho, Rac, and CDC42) regulate the cytoskeleton and assembly of the nicotinamide adenine dinucleotide phosphate (NADPH) oxidase. Like the trimeric G-proteins, small G-proteins are regulated by a mechanism based on the ability to cycle between inactive GDP-bound and active GTP-bound forms. Ligands trigger release of GDP from Ras; the exchange of GDP for GTP is catalyzed by one of the family of regulatory proteins known as guanine nucleotide exchange factors (GEFs).[88, 89] Ras is then inactivated by their intrinsic GTPase activity, which converts the GTP back to GDP; the rate of the GTPase reaction is enhanced by regulator proteins known as GTPase activating proteins (GAPs). Thus, the activity state of a Ras superfamily member is determined by the relative activities of its GEFs and GAPs. Some Ras-related proteins such as Rab and Rho are also regulated by guanine-nucleotide dissociation inhibitors, or GDIs.[87-89] All small G-proteins contain consensus sequences for interaction with GDP and GTP and for GTPase activity. Members of the Ras, Rho, and Rab families have a C-terminal domain that is posttranslationally modified by prenylation and palmitoylation, whereas Arf proteins have an N-terminal myristoylation. The posttranslational modifications allow association of the G-protein with membranes. Localization of small G-proteins is a key element of their function. In addition, the sites of activation of some small G-proteins may be determined by their GEFs. A Ras GEF such as Sos can be recruited to the cytoplasmic tail of a receptor by adaptors such as Grb2/Shc. Rho/Rac/CDC42, which are members of the Rho subfamily, are cytosolic proteins that complex with RhoGDI and are activated by a specific GEF, dbl. Members of the Arf subfamily bind to a GEF termed ARNO, which prefers myristoylated proteins and is activated by membrane-associated phosphatidylinositol-4,5-bisphosphate (PIP$_2$).

Ras proteins are important for downstream signaling from cell surface–associated tyrosine kinases. Receptors with intrinsic tyrosine kinase activity bind the adaptor protein Grb2 by an interaction of the SH2 domain on the Grb2 molecule and an autophosphorylated phosphotyrosine residue on the receptor (Fig. 161-7*A*). Sos, which is named after the *Drosophila* protein Son of Sevenless, is a Ras GEF. Sos is associated with the receptor complex and with Ras, by an interaction between its proline-rich carboxy terminal and the SH3 domain on the Grb2 (see Fig. 161-7*A*). For receptors that lack an intrinsic tyrosine kinase, an additional protein such as Shc is involved; this has been well defined for the T-cell receptor. Shc is a member of a set of tyrosine kinase substrates that substitute for an autophosphorylated receptor as a docking site for Grb2 (see Fig. 161-7*B*). Shc becomes tyrosine-phosphorylated, thus allowing it to bind the SH2 domain of Grb2 and to a tyrosine-phosphorylated residue on the receptor. In this way, a membrane-associated Shc, Grb2, and Sos complex is generated that can lead to Ras activation. Indeed, membrane targeting of Sos alone is sufficient for Ras activation.[52,80,81]

The βγ-subunit of trimeric G-proteins such as Gi has also been connected to tyrosine phosphorylation of Shc and activation of Ras through Grb2/Sos1. This mechanism provides a pathway connecting the serpentine receptors coupled to Gi-proteins such as the fMLP receptor to Ras-mediated signaling (see Fig. 161-7*C*).[2, 90-94] Pyk2, Src kinases, adaptor proteins, and Sos are required for the activation of Ras by serpentine receptors.[90] Ras can then initiate downstream signaling for activation of Raf, MAP kinase, and the trimeric G-protein–activated PI-3-kinase-γ.[92]

MAP Kinases and Ras-Initiated Pathways

The serine/threonine kinase MAPK (for microtubule-associated protein kinase) or ERK (extracellular signaling receptor kinase) is a downstream effector of Ras in multiple signaling systems (see Fig. 161-4). The Ras/Raf/MAPKK/MAPK pathway is one example of a family of MAP kinases that consists of a three-component protein kinase cascade, a serine/threonine protein kinase (MAPKKK), which, in turn, phosphorylates and activates a dual-specificity protein kinase (MAPKK); this, in turn, phosphorylates and activates another serine/threonine protein kinase (MAPK) (see Fig 161-2). MAPK pathways phosphorylate and activate downstream transcription factors and can mediate changes in cell shape, as well as stress responses. More recent work has demonstrated three families of MAPKs—the classic MAPK (or ERKs),

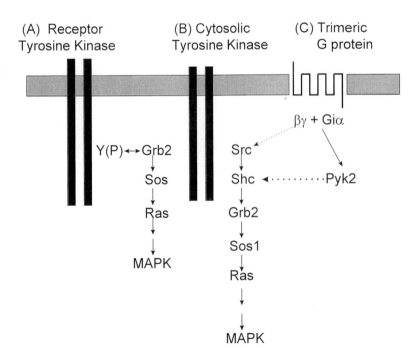

Figure 161–7. Ras signaling from different receptors: receptors with an intrinsic protein tyrosine kinase (**A**); receptors associated with cytosolic protein tyrosine kinases (**B**); and 7-transmembrane spanning receptors coupled to trimeric G-proteins (**C**). MAPK = microtubule-associated protein kinase.

JNK/SAPK, and the HOG cascade; these kinase cascades can be activated by Ras-dependent and Ras-independent pathways.[95,96]

Raf, an MAPKKK, is recruited to the membrane, is phosphorylated, and is activated subsequent to Ras activation[97]; Raf can also be activated by a pathway involving protein kinase C-α (PKC-α). Raf activates an MAPKK (or MEK) by phosphorylation on serine residues. MEK is a dual-specificity kinase capable of phosphorylating MAPK on both tyrosine and threonine residues thus activating MAPK. In phagocytes, activation of MAPK is triggered by the cytokine GM-CSF and by the chemoattractants fMLP and C5a, concomitant with activation of Ras.[98-103] MAPK has been implicated in signaling for bacterial killing, migration, adherence to a substratum, degranulation, and ligand-induced signaling for O_2^- generation in phagocytic cells.[98-103]

LIPID REMODELING AND SIGNALING

Phosphoinositide Remodeling and Signaling

Remodeling of phospholipids is important in the generation of second messengers. Receptors trigger Ca^{2+} mobilization and elicit breakdown of polyphosphoinositides (PPIs) as an initial step in signal transmission.[104-107] Occupation of the receptor activates a phosphoinositide-specific PLC that cleaves plasmalemma-associated PIP_2 to yield diglyceride (DG), an activator of PKC, and inositol-1,4,5-trisphosphate (IP_3), a trigger for the release of intracellular Ca^{2+}.[104-108] The DG can be phosphorylated to generate phosphatidic acid, which, in turn, can be metabolized to phosphatidylinositol (PI), thus completing the PI cycle. Three families of PLC genes have been designated: PLC-β, PLC-γ, and PLC-δ. PLC-β is activated by either α- or βγ-subunits of trimeric G-proteins, whereas PLC-γ is not regulated by trimeric G-protein subunits.[105] The pertussis-sensitive activation of PIP_2 hydrolysis triggered by receptors such as the fMLP receptor is mediated by the βγ-subunit of G_i.[28,106] PLC-γ is activated by tyrosine kinase–mediated signaling pathways.[106]

PIP_2 is a minor constituent of the inner leaflet of the plasmalemma, but it plays a key role in signal transduction, acting as a substrate for both PLC and PI-3-kinase for generation of DG, IP_3, and phosphatidyl inositol-3,4,5-trisphosphate (PIP_3). PIP_2 can also act as a binding site for numerous signaling elements. Synthesis of PIP_2 and regeneration of the PIP_2 depleted by the actions of PLC and PI-3-kinase are required for maintenance of signal transduction and of cell responses such as O_2^- generation. Phosphatidylinositol transfer protein (PITP) plays an important role in phosphoinositide synthesis and in signal transduction via the phosphoinositide-specific PLC (Fig. 161–8).[109,110] PITP is a cytosolic protein that can exchange PI and PC between lipid layers. PITP binds PI in exchange for phosphatidylcholine and presents it to PI-4-kinase to generate PIP; the PIP is then presented to PI-4P,5-kinase to generate PIP_2 (see Fig. 161–8). PITP may also present the substrate PIP_2 to PLC for hydrolysis to the second messengers DG and IP_3. PIP_2 also plays a role in regulating the cytoskeleton and other signaling elements such as phospholipase D (PLD), and the low molecular weight G-protein activating protein, Arf-GAP. Generation of PIP_2 may integrate signals from integrins and other receptors. Integrin-mediated cell adhesion activates PI-5-kinase via the low molecular weight G-protein Rho, and it elevates PIP_2 and thus enhances the ability of PLC to generate DG.

Phosphatidylinositol-3-Kinase and Generation of Phosphatidylinositol 3,4,5-Triphosphate

Activation of PI-3-kinase triggers generation of PIP_3 via phosphorylation of PIP_2 on the 3D position of the inositol ring.[92,106,111,112] PIP_3 plays numerous roles in cell activation;[112-119] PIP_3 has been implicated in regulation of Ca^{2+}-independent PKC isotypes,

protein kinase B (PKB or Akt), low molecular weight G-proteins, O_2^- generation, cytoskeletal rearrangements, and membrane trafficking.[111-115] Activation of PI-3-kinase can be triggered by either trimeric G-protein– or tyrosine kinase–initiated signal transduction.[111] Tyrosine kinase–initiated signaling triggers activation of Class 1A PI-3-kinase, which consists of a p85 regulatory subunit associated with a p110 catalytic subunit.[112] Tyrosine phosphorylation of the p85 translocates the PI-3-kinase to the plasmalemma by binding its regulatory subunit to a receptor associated protein. This increases the activity of the PI-3-kinase and places it in the ideal situation for converting membrane-associated PIP_2 to PIP_3.[112,116-119] Serpentine receptors such as the fMLP receptor activate a novel G-protein–dependent Class 1B PI-3-kinaseγ consisting of a 101-kDa regulatory subunit and a 110-kDa catalytic subunit, that also catalyzes generation of PIP_3.[120] In addition, fMLP receptor ligation also induces activation of the Class Ia PI-3-kinases through Gβγ subunits.[121] Thus, both tyrosine kinase–initiated and G-protein–initiated signaling result in generation of the lipid cofactors DG, IP_3, and PIP_3.

Phospholipase D

Phosphatidylcholine is also a source of lipid second messengers. Activation of PLD triggers hydrolysis of phosphatidylcholine to yield phosphatidic acid, an alternate source of DG.[122-123] A role for the low molecular weight G-protein Arf has been demonstrated in activation of PLD.[124] Phosphatidic acid phosphohydrolase cleaves phosphatidic acid to yield DG. Generation of phosphatidic acid has been implicated in signaling for degranulation and O_2^- generation.

Phospholipase A_2

Cytosolic PLA_2 cleaves the fatty acid arachidonate from the sn2 position on the DG backbone of phospholipids; PLA_2 is a Ca^{2+}-regulated enzyme that contains a CalB domain, which is homologous to the C2 domain found in Ca^{2+}-dependent PKC isotypes.[125,126] Activation of PLA_2 in response to elevated Ca^{2+} is

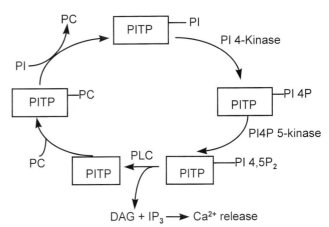

Figure 161–8. A role for phosphatidylinositol transfer protein (PITP) in phosphoinositide synthesis, phosphoinositide remodeling, and generation of second messengers. Phosphatidylinositol (PI) binds to PITP and is phosphorylated on the 4 and 5 positions of the inositol ring by PI-4-kinase and PI-4P 5-kinase to generate $PI-4,5-P_2$ (phosphatidylinositol-4,5-bis phosphate). $PI-4,5-P_2$ is cleaved by phospholipase C (PLC) to yield diacylglyceride (DAG) and inositol-1,4,5-trisphosphate (IP_3), a trigger for Ca^{2+} release from intracellular stores. The PITP then binds phosphatidyl choline (PC), which is exchanged for PI, thus completing the cycle.

accompanied by a CalB-mediated translocation to membranes where the enzyme may interact with its substrates. Arachidonate can also be further metabolized to produce active metabolites 5-hydroxyeicosatetraenoic acid, 5S,12R-leukotriene B$_4$, prostaglandins, and thromboxane.[127] Arachidonic acid may provide a link between surface receptor activity and control of PKC; the PKC isotypes from brain showed differential responsiveness to unsaturated fatty acids, PLC-γ, and Ca^{2+} transients.[125] Free fatty acids are also converted to the fatty acyl coenzyme A ester that can regulate discrete PKC isotypes and can modulate degranulation and O$_2^-$ generation.[128]

Sphingomyelin Metabolism and Signaling

Sphingomyelin is found predominantly in the plasmalemma and is composed of a long chain sphingoid base backbone (predominantly sphingosine), a fatty acid, and a phosphocholine head group.[129] Ligands such as TNF-α, IFNs, and IL-1 trigger activation of a neutral sphingomyelinase that cleaves sphingomyelin to yield ceramide and phosphocholine (see Figs. 161–1 and 161–2).[129-131] Ceramide is structurally analogous to DG and has been shown to activate a proline-directed ceramide-activated protein kinase (CAPK) and a ceramide-activated protein phosphatase related to protein phosphatase 2A (PP2A). TNF-α and fMLP trigger a late generation of ceramide in neutrophils.[132, 133] Ceramide is also generated by agonist-stimulated sphingomyelinase during phagocytosis by neutrophils.[130] The sphingomyelin pathway signals for apoptosis in many cell types including monocytes.[131] The late onset of ceramide generation suggests a role in long-term response such as apoptosis or negative signaling for ligand-initiated cell responses.[130, 131]

SECOND-MESSENGER–REGULATED AND LIPID-REGULATED SERINE/THREONINE KINASES IN SIGNALING

Second-Messenger–Regulated Kinases

Kinases regulated by second messengers and lipids elicit a diverse array of end responses such as gene regulation, ionic movements, cell movements, secretion, O$_2^-$ generation, eicosanoid generation, cell growth, cell differentiation, and apoptosis.[134-137] Serine/threonine kinases such as cAMP-activated kinase (PKA), cGMP-activated kinase (PKG), and Ca^{2+}/calmodulin-activated kinase (CaMK) are activated by the second messengers cAMP, cGMP, and Ca^{2+}, whereas PKC and CAPK are activated by lipids such as DG, phosphatidylserine (PS), PIP$_3$, and ceramide.[2, 3, 28, 136] Second-messenger-regulated and lipid-regulated kinases contain a regulatory domain and a kinase domain. These domains may exist in one protein (e.g., PKC), or they may exist in two separate subunits (e.g., PKA).[135-138]

Catalytic Domains of Kinases

Protein kinases catalyze the reversible phosphorylation of substrate proteins using adenosine triphosphate (ATP) as the donor phosphate source; the ATP binding site is highly conserved in all protein kinases.[139] The catalytic core contains the highly conserved sequence Y-G-X-G-X-[F/Y]-G-X-V, where Y is hydrophobic, and X is less well defined. The glycine-rich sequence is critical for the kinase activity and participates in ATP binding, substrate recognition, enzyme catalysis, and regulation of activity. The sequences determining substrate specificity are less well conserved and exist just outside the ATP-binding domain.

Substrate Specificity of Serine/Threonine Kinases

The kinases PKA, PKC, Akt/PKB, and CaMK phosphorylate serine or threonine residues in the vicinity of the positively charged (basic) residues arginine and lysine.[140-142] For kinases that require basic residues in the substrate sequence, such as PKA, Akt/PKB, PKC, and CaMK II, the substrate binding site of the kinase must contain negatively charged residues. The phosphorylation of serine is generally preferred over threonine. For phosphorylation of a protein by PKA, the presence of basic amino acids N-terminal to the phosphoacceptor serine or threonine is a key factor for substrate recognition by PKA. A substrate recognition sequence for PKA is R-R-X-S(P)-X.

Ca^{2+}/CaMK I, CaMK II, and CaMK III phosphorylate multiple substrates. CaMK catalyzes phosphorylation of synapsin I and regulation of neurotransmitter release; however, a role for CaMK has not been defined in phagocytes. A minimal consensus sequence for phosphorylation by CaMK II is R-X-X-S/T.

Phosphorylation by Akt/PKB requires the presence of basic amino acids N-terminal to the phosphoacceptor serine or threonine. A sequence for potent phosphorylation by Akt/PKB is R-X-R-X-X-T/S.[142]

PKC also requires basic amino acid residues near the phosphoacceptor group of a substrate. The consensus sequence for substrate recognition by PKC is a serine or threonine with positively charged lysine or arginine both upstream and downstream of the target serine/threonine.[140] A sequence for potent phosphorylation by PKC is R-K-X-X-S/T-X-X-R-K.

CAPK is a member of an emerging family of proline-directed serine/threonine kinases that recognize substrates containing the minimal sequence, X-S/T-P-X, in which the phosphoacceptor site is amino-terminal to a proline residue, and X can be any amino acid. The minimal recognition for CAPK is L-T-P, which distinguishes this kinase from other proline-directed kinases including MAPK and cdc-2-kinase.[140]

Targeting of Kinases for Specificity of the Responses

Protein phosphorylation is a primary means of mediating signal transduction events for cell responses; thus, the activities of the kinases must be highly regulated. Regulation may occur by the selective generation of activating cofactors in the correct time frame. A further level of regulation can occur by compartmentalization of the kinase with the appropriate substrate. Targeting of tyrosine kinases of the Src family occurs by SH2 domain binding to phosphotyrosine residues or binding by the SH3 domains.[63-65] Mechanisms for targeting of serine/threonine kinases PKA, PKC, Raf, and protein phosphatases have been demonstrated.[143-147] Stimulus-induced intracellular translocation occurs widely for the protein kinases that constitute cellular signaling networks. Cell stimulation causes translocation of several serine and threonine kinases to new sites, an event that would alter their access to their physiologic substrates. This compartmentalization of kinases is the result of their binding to specific anchoring proteins. Thus, compartmentalization, or targeting, of kinases is critical in relaying signals to the correct downstream molecules.

SECOND MESSENGERS AND KINASE REGULATION

Second-Messenger Generation

Cyclic Adenosine Monophosphate

Ligand-induced activation of adenylate cyclase triggers generation of the second messenger cAMP, a cofactor for the activation of cAMP-activated protein kinase (i.e., PKA). Removal of cAMP is catalyzed by phosphodiesterase and serves to limit the activation of PKA.[148] Ligands such as epinephrine interacting with the β-adrenergic receptor trigger a Gα_s-transduced activation of adenylyl cyclase and an increase in cAMP.[53] The chemotactic peptide fMLP, which triggers signaling via Gα_i, also triggers an increase in cAMP; the mechanism is not fully understood.[149] Elevated cAMP is a negative regulator of many phagocytic functions, including

O_2^- generation, degranulation, phagocytosis, chemotaxis, PLD activation, and Ca^{2+} mobilization.[53,148-152]

Calcium Mobilization

Ligand-induced mobilization of intracellular Ca^{2+} from stores in the endoplasmic reticulum and uptake of extracellular Ca^{2+} play important roles in signal transduction for multiple cell responses.[153] Elevation of cytosolic Ca^{2+} is essential for optimal fMLP-induced O_2^- generation and degranulation.[107,108] Ligands such as fMLP and immune complexes trigger activation of PLC, which cleaves PIP_2 to generate IP_3, a trigger for release of intracellular Ca^{2+} stores, and DG, an activator of DG-dependent PKC.[28,107,108]

Nonexcitable cells such as neutrophils and monocytes lack voltage-gated Ca^{2+} channels.[154] However, ligands such as fMLP trigger Ca^{2+} uptake from the medium into the cytosol through receptor-operated nonselective cation channels that conduct Ca^{2+}, sodium, and potassium.[155,156] Ca^{2+}-activated cation nonselective channels have also been demonstrated in neutrophils and in neutrophilic HL-60 cells.[157,158] In addition, IP_3-initiated depletion of the endoplasmic reticulum Ca^{2+} stores can trigger uptake of extracellular Ca^{2+} via store operated Ca^{2+} channels (SOCC).[159,160] The ligand-induced increase in cytosolic Ca^{2+} is transient, and the Ca^{2+} concentration returns toward resting levels. Ca^{2+} is pumped from the cytosol back into the endoplasmic reticulum by a sarco(endo)plasmic reticulum (SERCA) Ca^{2+}-ATPase and into the extracellular medium by a plasmalemmal Ca^{2+}-ATPase.[161] This Ca^{2+} homeostasis and maintenance of low cytosolic Ca^{2+} are essential for cell survival.

Second-Messenger–Regulated Kinases

Cyclic Adenosine Monophosphate–Activated Protein Kinase A

Elevation of cAMP levels in neutrophils is triggered by ligands such as fMLP, epinephrine, and immune complexes and serves to inhibit signaling and downstream events such as O_2^- generation, and chemotaxis.[53,148-151] cAMP-dependent kinase (PKA) is composed of two distinct subunits—a 49-kDa regulatory (R) subunit and a 38-kDa catalytic (C) subunit.[135] There are at least three forms of C subunits and four forms of R subunits of the cAMP-dependent protein kinase, which together could produce at least 12 forms of protein kinase holoenzyme (R_2C_2). These forms of PKA differ in their sensitivity to cAMP, tissue-specific distribution, autophosphorylation, and targeting to distinct intracellular sites directed by protein-specific binding or possibly by signal sequences. Cα and Cβ have been expressed, and Cγ has only been evaluated at the DNA level. The role of cAMP is to allow dissociation of regulatory and catalytic subunits and to expose the catalytic site.

Pseudosubstrates and Regulation of Protein Kinase A Activity

In the absence of cAMP, PKA exists as a tetramer R_2C_2 and is inactive. In PKA, the regulatory subunit contains a pseudosubstrate sequence R-R-N-A-I, in which the serine (or threonine) of a canonical substrate sequence of PKA is replaced by a nonphosphorylatable alanine.[162] The binding of the pseudosubstrate site in the regulatory subunit to the substrate binding site of the catalytic subunit maintains the holoenzyme in an inactive conformation. The presence of cAMP causes a conformational change in the inhibitory subunit R that allows release of the active catalytic unit.

Targeting of Cyclic Adenosine Monophosphate–Dependent Kinase

Targeting of PKA is critical for an appropriate functional response. Both the catalytic subunit and the type II holoenzyme can be differentially compartmentalized to specific subcellular locations before and after cell stimulation.[143,144,163] Type II PKA is found in the particulate fraction anchored by RII near its protein substrates. This enzyme associates with microtubules, and bind-

ing of cAMP to the holoenzyme releases the catalytic subunit, which can then phosphorylate microtubule-associated proteins. The dissociated catalytic subunits may also translocate to new sites to phosphorylate other substrates. When intracellular cAMP increases, the regulatory subunit is unchanged, whereas the catalytic subunit moves to the cytosol and then to the nucleus.

The proteins that anchor the PKA type II holoenzyme to the cell particulate fraction are termed A kinase anchoring proteins (AKAPs).[144] AKAPs are associated with the cytoskeleton, and many of them are also PKA substrates. These proteins bind the RII subunit as well as calmodulin-dependent protein phosphatase 2B (calcineurin); binding of RII and of the phosphatase occurs at different sites on the AKAP. Binding of PKA and of calcineurin to the same protein may provide coordinate activity of two enzymes that have opposite catalytic activities. It is not known whether these enzymes act on the same substrate. The binding site for RII on AKAP corresponds to an amphipathic helical structure with acidic residues at the hydrophilic face of the helix. Mutations that disrupt this helix reduce RII binding, and a peptide based on this mutated helix prevents PKA regulation of a glutamate receptor-gated channel in other cell types.

Activation of Akt/Protein Kinase B by Phosphatidylinositol-3-Kinase

Akt/PKB, like PKC, is activated by a lipid and comprises a family of isotypes: Akt1 or PKB-α, Akt2 or PKB-β, and Akt3 or PKB-γ.[138] The three genes have 85% sequence identity and share the same structural organization. Binding of 3-phosphorylated phosphoinositides such as PI-3,4,5-P_3 to the pleckstrin homology (PH) domain of Akt induces a conformational change and recruitment to the plasma membrane. This recruitment to the membrane allows phosphorylation of Akt by phosphoinositide-dependent kinase 1 (PDK1) at T308 and subsequent phosphorylation at S473 by PDK2.[164] PDK1 and PKD2 are serine/threonine kinases that are also activated by PI-3-kinase. The first 100 amino acids possess a pleckstrin homology (PH) domain that binds phosphoinositides, and in particular phosphoinositides phosphorylated on the D3 position of the inositol ring. A short glycine-rich region bridges the PH domain and the catalytic domain. The last 70 amino acids of the C-terminus contain a putative regulatory domain. All three isotypes have conserved threonine and serine residues, T308 and S473 in Akt1. These conserved residues together with the PH domain are critical for activation of Akt. Akt/PKB has been implicated in activation of the NADPH oxidase in neutrophils.[165]

Protein Kinase C

PKC, a phospholipid-dependent family of serine/threonine kinases, has been implicated in multiple signal transduction pathways (see Figs. 161–1 and 161–2).[136,137] PKC is a structurally related family of isotypes that possess catalytic and regulatory domains in a single protein which are activated by the lipids PS and DG. The primary sequence can be divided into conserved sequences (C1-C4), which are separated by variable domains (V1-V5). The catalytic domain contains two conserved regions, C3 and C4, which contain the ATP-binding site and the substrate-binding site. Cleavage at the V3 hinge region generates a constitutively active kinase, PKM, which does not require cofactors for activity.

Classic PKC-α, and PKC-β, and PKC-γ are PS, DG, and Ca^{2+} dependent. The regulatory domain in Ca^{2+}-dependent PKC-α, PKC-βI, PKC-βII, and PKC-γ contains two conserved regions, C1 and C2. The βI and βII isoforms are derived by alternate splicing at the C-terminal. The C1 domain is cysteine rich, and it is the binding site for DG and for phorbol esters such as phorbol myristate acetate (PMA); PMA is an activator of PKC. C2 is the Ca^{2+}-binding domain, and it contains a CalB sequence that is also found in PLA_2.

Novel PKC isoforms δ, ε, θ, and η lack the Ca^{2+}-binding domain (C2), and they require PS and DG, but they are not activated by Ca^{2+}. Atypical PKC isotypes, ζ, μ, and λ, also lack the Ca^{2+}-binding domain and have half the zinc finger (C1 domain) responsible for binding DG and PMA; these isotypes require PS for optimal activity, but they are not activated by DG, PMA, or Ca^{2+}.[136, 137] Investigators showed that the novel mediator PIP_3 activates PKC-ζ, PKC-ε, and PKC-δ.[115] Multiple activating cofactors, such as Ca^{2+}, DG, and PIP_3, allow differential control of the PKC isotypes.

Neutrophils contain multiple isotypes of PKC; the major Ca^{2+}-dependent isotype is PLC-β, lesser amounts of PKC-α, plus a novel Ca^{2+}-independent DG-dependent isotype, PKC-n. Neutrophils also possess substantial amounts of the atypical PKC-ζ. A fifth isotype, PKC-δ, is PS and DG dependent and Ca^{2+} independent, and it is found in small amounts in the cytosol of neutrophils. Specific functions for each PKC isotype in phagocytic cells are indicated. PKC-βII and PKC-α have been implicated in O_2^- generation, whereas PKC-ζ plays a role in adherence and PKC-δ phosphorylates and regulates the TNFR1.[166-169]

Pseudosubstrates and Regulation of Protein Kinase C Activity

All PKC isotypes possess a pseudosubstrate region near the N-terminus in the regulatory domain.[162] A pseudosubstrate sequence occurs at residues 19 to 36, RFARKGALRQKN-VHEVKN, in the α, β, and γ isotypes. An alanine residue at position 25, instead of a serine, renders this sequence a potent inhibitor of PKC.[162] Each isotype of PKC contains a related pseudosubstrate sequence. In the absence of cofactors, the PKC is folded so the pseudosubstrate domain binds the substrate binding site in the catalytic domain. Activating cofactors such as PS, DG, and Ca^{2+} cause a conformational change in the molecule so the pseudosubstrate is removed from the catalytic domain and the PKC is able to phosphorylate target peptides.[162]

Receptors for Activated C Kinase and Targeting of Protein Kinase C

A fundamental problem for efficient and selective lipid-based signaling is access of cytosolic enzymes to the membrane-based phospholipids. Enzymes such as PLC-γ are cytosolic, but they must act on the membrane-based lipid substrate PIP_2 to generate the membrane-associated DG. Similarly, cytosolic PKC isotypes must associate with the membrane-bound lipid cofactors PS and DG to be activated. Ca^{2+}-dependent PKC isotypes are translocated from cytosol to membrane in the presence of elevated levels of Ca^{2+}.[146] This Ca^{2+}-driven translocation is reversible and depends on the presence of the C2 or CalB domain. Other enzymes such as PLA_2, which also possess a CalB domain, are similarly translocated to the particulate fraction in the presence of elevated Ca^{2+}.[170] However, all DG-dependent PKC isotypes can be translocated to the particulate fraction by treatment with phorbol esters in a Ca^{2+}-independent manner indicating other mechanisms of translocation.[136,137,146]

Scaffold proteins such as receptor for activated C kinase (RACK) and AKAP are proteins that bind to PKC isotypes and provide localization for greater specificity and efficiency of signaling. RACKs are cytoskeleton and membrane-associated proteins, which have molecular weights of 30 to 36 kDa. RACKs have been shown to associate with the cytoskeleton, to bind selective PH domains, the β–integrin subunit, PLC-γ, and to inhibit Src.[171-174]

Inactive PKC isotypes contain a RACK-binding domain bound to a pseudo-RACK sequence in the regulatory domain; the pseudo-RACK binding site is in the Ca^{2+}-binding domain of PKC-α, β, and γ and in the third variable region of PKC-ζ.[146] A conformational change in PKC induced by cofactors frees the RACK binding site and allows the PKC to bind to RACK. Thus, cofactors simultaneously activate and target PKC isotypes to RACK. RACK also binds PLC-γ, a finding suggesting that RACK serves as an anchor for generation of lipid cofactors and the consequent activation and localization of PKC. It remains to be determined whether RACK also co-localizes the PKC isotype with its substrates as occurs with PKA and AKAP. Peptides based on the pseudo-RACK sequence disrupt the binding of PKC to the RACK and inhibit downstream signaling in heart and brain cells.[146] In neutrophils, RACK1, which is an escort and binding protein for PKC-βII, is involved in negative signaling for O_2^- generation.[175]

Protein Kinase C and Signaling for Superoxide Anion Generation

Activation of different PKC isotypes by lipid mediators has both positive and negative roles in signaling for O_2^- generation. PKC activators such as PMA trigger O_2^- generation by neutrophils and monocytes.[2, 3, 166] Assembly of an active NADPH oxidase and generation of O_2^- requires translocation of cytosolic factors p47phox, p67phox, and rac2 to the plasma membrane, where they interact with the integral membrane protein cytochrome b_{558} (Fig. 161–9).[176] p47phox is a substrate for PKC.[177,178] Akt may also be responsible for phosphorylation of p47phox.[176] It has been proposed that phosphorylation of p47phox may cause a conformational change to reveal the SH3 domain in p47phox and allow it to bind to the membrane-associated cytochrome b_{558} (see Fig. 161–9).[176] A role for PKC-βII has been demonstrated in phosphorylation and translocation of p47phox to the membrane and activation of the NADPH oxidase in neutrophils;[166] in monocytes, a role for PKC-α was indicated.[167]

SUMMARY

Phagocytic cells such as neutrophils, monocytes, and macrophages respond to specific ligands with a variety of responses such as adherence, chemotaxis, microbicidal activity, and generation of inflammatory mediators. Interaction of a ligand with a specific receptor initiates a signal transduction pathway that elicits the end response or responses. Each signaling pathway possesses the following elements: ligand/receptor → coupler → transducer → end response. Each receptor is coupled to specific signaling pathways in a particular cell; however, there may also be cross-talk between different signaling pathways. Receptors can be coupled to the signal transduction pathway by association with a trimeric G-protein or by activation of a tyrosine kinase. Tyrosine kinase–initiated signaling occurs by activation of a tyrosine kinase that is intrinsic to the receptor or by recruitment and activation of cytosolic tyrosine kinases. Different receptors can recruit and activate cytosolic tyrosine kinases of the Src family, Syk kinase, and kinases of the JAK/STAT signaling pathway. Ras proteins are low molecular weight GTP-binding proteins that act as molecular switches in downstream regulation of tyrosine kinase–induced signaling pathways. Trimeric G-proteins and tyrosine kinases also activate lipid remodeling and the generation of second messengers such as Ca^{2+}, DG, PIP_3, ceramide, and cAMP. The second messengers activate specific serine/threonine kinases such as PKC, CAPK, and cAMP kinase, which phosphorylate specific substrates and elicit the cellular responses. Signal transduction is an appropriate target to regulate phagocytic cell function and presents a novel approach to drug development and management of inflammatory diseases such as sepsis, multiple organ failure, adult respiratory distress syndrome, and necrotizing enterocolitis.

Figure 161–9. Signal transduction for assembly of an active nicotinamide adenine dinucleotide phosphate (NADPH) oxidase. The fMet-Leu-Phe (fMLP) receptor coupled to the trimeric G_i-protein, or the p60TNF receptor together with the β_2-integrin (CD11b/CD18) acting via a tyrosine kinase, elicits phospholipid remodeling of phosphatidylinositol-4,5 bisphosphate (PIP$_2$; see Fig. 161–8). Activation of phosphatidylinositol-3-kinase (PI3-K) generates phosphatidylinositol 3,4,5-tetrakis phosphate (PIP$_3$), and activation of phospholipase C (PLC) generates diglyceride (DG) and inositol-1,4,5-trisphosphate (IP$_3$; see Fig. 161–8). DG, Ca^{2+}, and PIP$_3$ are cofactors for activation of protein kinase C (PKC). RACK (*R*eceptor for *A*ctivated *C* *K*inase) co-localizes PLC and PKC. PKC isotypes (αPKC and βPKC) phosphorylate the cytosolic p47phox. The small G-protein rac2, p67phox, and phosphorylated p47phox associate with the membrane-bound cytochrome b$_{558}$ resulting in activation of the NADPH oxidase and reduction of O_2 to O_2^-. PKC can also phosphorylate p60TNFR and can down-regulate tumor necrosis factor-α (TNF-α)–initiated signaling. A phosphorylation site is in the death domain (DD).

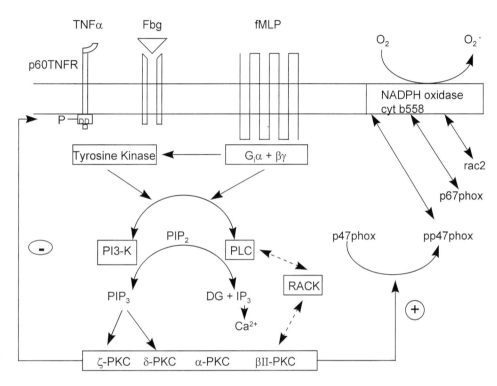

REFERENCES

1. Ben-Baruch A, et al: Signals and receptors involved in recruitment of inflammatory cells. J Biol Chem 270:11703, 1995.
2. Bokoch GM: Chemoattractant signaling and leukocyte activation. Blood 86:1649, 1995.
3. Thelen M, et al: Neutrophil signal transduction and activation of the respiratory burst. Physiol Rev 73:797, 1993.
4. Hunter T: Signaling: 2000 and beyond. Cell 100:113, 2000.
5. Kwiatkowska K, Sobota A: Signaling pathways in phagocytosis. Bioessays 21:422, 1999.
6. Jones G: Cellular signaling in macrophage migration and chemotaxis. J Leukoc Biol 68:593, 2000.
7. Hirsch E, et al: Central role for G protein-coupled phosphoinositide 3-kinase γ in inflammation. Science 287:1049, 2000.
8. Greenberg S, Grinstein S: Phagocytosis and innate immunity. Curr Opin Immunol 14:136, 2002.
9. Yang D, et al: The role of mammalian antimicrobial peptides and proteins in awakening of innate host defenses and adaptive immunity. Cell Mol Life Sci 58:978, 2001.
10. Harrison RE, et al: Microbial killing: oxidants, proteases and ions. Curr Biol 12:R357, 2002.
11. Johnston RB Jr: Clinical aspects of chronic granulomatous disease. Curr Opin Hematol 8:17, 2001.
12. Gao J-L, et al: Impaired antibacterial host defense in mice lacking the N-formylpeptide receptor. J Exp Med 189:657, 1999.
13. Ottonello L, et al: Activation of neutrophil respiratory burst by cytokines and chemoattractants: regulatory role of extracellular matrix glycoproteins. Inflamm Res 47:345, 1998.
14. Goncalves LF, et al: Intrauterine infection and prematurity. MRDD Res Rev 8:3, 2002.
15. Bernstein HM, et al: Use of myeloid colony-stimulating factors in neonates with septicemia. Curr Opin Pediatr 14:91, 2002.
16. Sur S, et al: Sudden-onset fatal asthma: a distinct entity with few eosinophils and relatively more neutrophils in the airway submucosa? Am Rev Respir Dis 148:713, 1993.
17. Spitzer JA, et al: Functional characterization of peripheral, circulating and liver recruited neutrophils in endotoxic rats. J Leukoc Biol 56:166, 1994.
18. Mukaida N, et al: Interleukin-8 (IL-8) and monocyte chemotactic and activating factor (MCAF/MCP-1), chemokines essentially involved in inflammatory and immune reactions. Cytokine Growth Factor Rev 9:9, 1998.
19. Weiss SJ: Tissue destruction by neutrophils. N Engl J Med 320:365, 1989.
20. Schraufstatter IU, et al: Proteases and oxidants in experimental pulmonary inflammatory injury. J Clin Invest 73:1175, 1984.
21. Gao X-P, et al: Role of NADPH oxidase in the mechanism of lung neutrophil sequestration and microvessel injury induced by gram-negative sepsis: studies in p47phox-/- and gp91phox-/- mice. J Immunol 168:3974, 2002.
22. Morel F, et al: The superoxide-generating oxidase of phagocytic cells: physiological, molecular, and pathological aspects. Eur J Biochem 201:523, 1991.
23. DiGiovine B, et al: Bronchoalveolar lavage neutrophilia is associated with obliterative bronchiolitis after lung transplantation: role of IL-8. J Immunol 157:4194, 1996.

24. Tirouvanziam R, et al: Inflammation and infection in naive human cystic fibrosis airway grafts. Am J Respir Cell Mol Biol 23:121, 2000.

25. Sayeed MM: Exuberant Ca²⁺ signaling in neutrophils: a cause for concern. News Physiol Sci 15:130, 2000.

26. Wahl SM, et al: Regulation of leukocyte adhesion and signaling in inflammation and disease. J Leukoc Biol 59:789, 1996.

27. Levitzki A: Signal-transduction therapy: a novel approach to disease management. Eur J Biochem 226:1, 1994.

28. Haribabu B, et al: Function and regulation of chemoattractant receptors. Immunol Res 22:271, 2001.

29. Giannini E, Boulay F: Phosphorylation, dephosphorylation, and recycling of the C5a receptor in differentiated HL60 cells. J Immunol 154:4055, 1995.

30. Klotz KN, Jesaitis AJ: Neutrophil chemoattractant receptors and the membrane skeleton. Bioessays 16:193, 1994.

31. Heldin CH: Dimerization of cell surface receptors. Cell 80:213, 1995.

32. Scott-Zaki P, et al: Neutrophil chemotaxis and superoxide production are induced by cross-linking Fc$_\gamma$RII receptors. Cell Immunol 201:89, 2000.

33. Indik ZK, et al: The molecular dissection of Fcγ receptor mediated phagocytosis. Blood 86:4389, 1995.

34. Coppolino MG, et al: Evidence for a molecular complex consisting of Fyb/SLAP, SLP76, Nck, VASP and WASP that links the actin cytoskeleton to Fc$_\gamma$ receptor signalling during phagocytosis. J Cell Sci 114:4307, 2001.

35. Dusi S, et al: Tyrosine phosphorylation of phospholipase Cγ2 is involved in the activation of phosphoinositide hydrolysis by Fc receptors in human neutrophils. Biochem Biophys Res Commun 201:1100, 1994.

36. Zheng L, et al: Protein tyrosine kinase activity is essential for Fc gamma receptor-mediated intracellular killing of Staphylococcus aureus by human monocytes. Infect Immunol 62:4296, 1994.

37. Chen G, Goeddel DV: TNFR-1 signaling: a beautiful pathway. Science 296:1634, 2002.

38. Miranti CK, Brugge JS: Sensing the environment: a historical perspective on integrin signal transduction. Nat Cell Biol 4:83, 2002.

39. Liu Y, Kao WJ: Human macrophage adhesion on fibronectin: the role of substratum and intracellular signalling kinases. Cell Signal 14:145, 2002.

40. Berton B, Lowell CA: Integrin signalling in neutrophils and macrophages. Cell Signal 11:621, 1999.

41. Schwartz MA, Ginsberg MH: Networks and crosstalk: integrin signalling spreads. Nat Cell Biol 4:E65, 2002.

42. Menegazzi R, et al: Evidence that tumor necrosis factor α (TNF)-induced activation of neutrophil respiratory burst on biologic surfaces is mediated by the p55 TNF receptor. Blood 84:287, 1994.

43. Aderem AA: How cytokines signal messages within cells. J Clin Invest 167(Suppl 1):S2, 1993.

44. McLeish KR, et al: Modulation of transmembrane signalling in HL-60 granulocytes by tumour necrosis factor-α. Biochem J 279:455, 1991.

45. Nathan CF: Neutrophil activation on biological surfaces: massive secretion of hydrogen peroxide in response to products of macrophages and lymphocytes. J Clin Invest 80:1550, 1987.

46. Laudanna C, et al: Effect of inhibitors of distinct signalling pathways on neutrophil O$_2^-$ generation in response to tumor necrosis factor-α, and antibodies against CD18 and CD11a: evidence for a common and unique pattern of sensitivity to Wortmannin and protein tyrosine kinase inhibitors. Biochem Biophys Res Commun 190:935, 1993.

47. Kilpatrick LE, et al: Serine phosphorylation of p60 tumor necrosis factor receptor by protein kinase Cδ in TNF-activated neutrophils. Am J Physiol 279:C2011, 2000.

48. Marinissen MJ, Gutkind JS: G-protein-coupled receptors and signaling networks: emerging paradigms. Trends Pharmacol Sci 22:368, 2001.

49. Neves SR, et al: G protein pathways. Science 296:1636, 2002.

50. Milligan G, White JH: Protein-protein interactions at G-protein-coupled receptors. Trends Pharmacol Sci 22:513, 2001.

51. Sternweis PC: The active role of βγ in signal transduction. Curr Opin Cell Biol 6:198, 1994.

52. Bourne HR: Team blue sees red. Nature 376:727, 1995.

53. Tintinger GR, et al: The antiinflammatory interactions of epinephrine with human neutrophils in vitro are achieved by cyclic AMP-mediated accelerated resequestration of cytosolic calcium. Biochem Pharmacol 61:1319, 2001.

54. Korade-Mirnics Z, Corey SJ: Src kinase-mediated signaling in leukocytes J Leukoc Biol 68:603, 2000.

55. Taniguchi T: Cytokine signaling through nonreceptor protein tyrosine kinases. Science 268:251, 1995.

56. Superti-Furga G: Regulation of the Src protein tyrosine kinase. FEBS Lett 369:62, 1995.

57. Ihle JN: Cytokine receptor signalling. Nature 377:591, 1995.

58. Yan SR, et al: Activation of SRC family kinases in human neutrophils: evidence that p58$^{C\text{-}FGR}$ and p53/56^{LYN} redistributed to a Triton X-100-insoluble cytoskeletal fraction, also enriched in the caveolar protein Caveolin, display an enhanced kinase activity. FEBS Lett 380:198, 1996.

59. Pan X-Q, et al: Activation of three classes of nonreceptor tyrosine kinases following Fcγ crosslinking in human monocytes. Clin Immunol 90:55, 1999.

60. Hall RA, et al: Heptahelical receptor signaling: beyond the G protein paradigm. J Cell Biol 145:927, 1999.

61. Igishi T, Gutkind JS: Tyrosine kinases of the Src family participate in signaling to MAP kinase from both G$_q$ and G$_i$-coupled receptors. Biochem Biophys Res Commun 244:5, 1998.

62. Ma YC, et al: Src tyrosine kinase is a novel direct effector of G proteins. Cell 102:635, 2000.

63. Williams JC, et al: Insights into Src functions: structural comparisons. Trends Biochem Sci 23:179, 1998.

64. Aoki Y, et al: The SH2 domains of Src family kinases associate with Syk. J Biol Chem 270:15658, 1995.

65. Pawson T: Protein modules and signalling networks. Nature 373:573, 1995.

66. Cohen GB, et al: Modular binding domains in signal transduction proteins. Cell 80:237, 1995.

67. Yan SR, Novak MJ: Src-family kinase-p53/p56^{lyn} plays an important role in TNFalpha-stimulated production of O$_2^-$ by human neutrophils adherent to fibrinogen. Inflammation 23:167, 1999.

68. Fitzer-Attas CJ, et al: Fcγ receptor-mediated phagocytosis in macrophages lacking the Src family tyrosine kinases Hck, Fgr, and Lyn. J Exp Med 191:669, 2000.

69. Marcilla A, et al: Identification of the major tyrosine kinase substrate in signaling complexes formed after engagement of Fcγ receptors. J Biol Chem 270:9115, 1995.

70. Ghazizadeh S, et al: Physical and functional association of Src-related protein tyrosine kinases with FcγII in monocytic THP-1 cells. J Biol Chem 269:8878, 1994.

71. Zaffran Y, et al: Zymosan-triggered association of tyrosine phosphoproteins and lyn kinase with cytoskeleton in human monocytes. J Immunol 154:3488, 1995.

72. Forsberg M, et al: Tumor necrosis factor-alpha potentiates CR3-induced respiratory burst by activating p38 MAP kinase in human neutrophils. Immunology 103:465, 2001.

73. Asahi M, et al: Activation of protein-tyrosine kinase p72^{syk} with concanavalin A in polymorphonuclear neutrophils. J Biol Chem 268:23334, 1993.

74. Durden DL, Liu YB: Protein-tyrosine kinase p72^{syk} in FcγRI receptor signaling. Blood 84:2102, 1994.

75. Greenberg S, et al: Tyrosine phosphorylation of the γ subunit of Fc$_\gamma$ receptors, p72^{syk}, and paxillin during Fc receptor-mediated phagocytosis in macrophages. J Biol Chem 269:3897, 1994.

76. Renedo MA, et al: FcγRIIA exogenously expressed in HeLa cells activates the mitogen-activated protein kinase cascade by a mechanism dependent on the endogenous expression of the protein tyrosine kinase Syk. Eur J Immunol 31:1361, 2001.

77. Aronson DS, Horvath CM: A road map for those who don't know JAK-STAT. Science 296:1653, 2002.

78. Ihle JN: The STAT family in cytokine signaling. Curr Opin Cell Biol 13:211, 2001.

79. Al-Shami A, Naccache PH: Granulocyte-macrophage colony-stimulating factor-activated signaling pathways in human neutrophils: involvement of Jak2 in the stimulation of phosphatidylinositol 3-kinase. J Biol Chem 274:5333, 1999.

80. Kishimoto T, et al: Interleukin-6 family of cytokines and gp130. Blood 86:1243, 1995.

81. Brizzi MF, et al: Granulocyte-macrophage colony-stimulating factor stimulates JAK2 signaling pathway and rapidly activates p93, STAT1 p91, and STAT3 p92 in polymorphonuclear leukocytes. J Biol Chem 271:3562, 1996.

82. Durbin JE, et al: Targeted disruption of the mouse Stat1 gene results in compromised innate immunity to viral disease. Cell 84:443, 1996.

83. Kuroki M, O'Flaherty JT: Extracellular signal-regulated protein kinase (ERK)-dependent and ERK-independent pathways target STAT3 on serine-727 in human neutrophils stimulated by chemotactic factors and cytokines. Biochem J 341:691, 1999.

84. Meraz MA, et al: Targeted disruption of Stat1 in mice gene reveals unexpected physiologic specificity in the JAK-STAT signaling pathway. Cell 84:431, 1996.

85. Matozaki T, et al: Small G-protein networks: their crosstalk and signal cascades. Cell Signal 12:515, 2000.

86. Rebollo A, Martinez AC: Ras: recent advances and new functions. Blood 94:2971, 1999.

87. Quinn MT: Low-molecular-weight GTP-binding proteins and leukocyte signal transduction. J Leukoc Biol 58:263, 1995.

88. Sprang S: GEFs: master regulators of G-protein activation. Trends Biochem Sci 26:266, 2001.

89. Feig LA: Guanine-nucleotide exchange factors: a family of positive regulators of Ras and related GTPases. Curr Opin Cell Biol 6:204, 1994.

90. Gawler DJ: Points of convergence between Ca²⁺ and Ras signalling pathways. Biochim Biophys Acta 1448:171, 1998.

91. Ridley AJ: Rho proteins, PI 3-kinases, and monocyte/macrophage motility. FEBS Lett 498:168, 2001.

92. Suire S, et al: Activation of phosphoinositide 3-kinase γ by ras. Curr Biol 12:1068, 2002.

93. Geijsen N, et al: Regulation of p21rac activation in human neutrophils. Blood 94:1121, 1999.

94. Seasholtz TM, et al: Rho as a mediator of G protein–coupled receptor signaling. Mol Pharmacol 55:949, 1999.

95. Worthen GS, et al: FMLP activates Ras and Raf in human neutrophils: potential role in activation of MAP kinase. J Clin Invest 94:815, 1994.

96. Downey GP, et al: Importance of MEK in neutrophil responsiveness. J Immunol 160:434, 1998.

97. Daum G, et al: The ins and outs of Raf kinases. Trends Biochem Sci 19:474, 1994.

98. Yamamori T, et al: Relationship between p38 mitogen-activated protein kinase and small GTPase Rac for the activation of NADPH oxidase in bovine neutrophils. Biochem Biophys Res Commun 293:1571, 2002.

99. Dewas C, et al: The mitogen-activated protein kinase extracellular signal-regulated kinase 1/2 pathway is involved in formyl-methionyl-leucyl-phenylalanine-induced p47phox phosphorylation in human neutrophils. J Immunol 165:5238, 2000.

100. Hii CS, et al: Role of the extracellular signal-regulated protein kinase cascade in human neutrophil killing of Staphylococcus aureus and Candida albicans and in migration. Infect Immunol 67:1297, 1999.

101. Suzuki K, et al: Cytokine-specific activation of distinct mitogen-activated protein kinase subtype cascades in human neutrophils stimulated by granulocyte colony-stimulating factor, granulocyte-macrophage colony-stimulating factor, and tumor necrosis factor-alpha. Blood 93:341, 1999.

102. Karlsson A, et al: Phorbol myristate acetate induces neutrophil NADPH-oxidase activity by two separate signal transduction pathways: dependent or independent of phosphatidylinositol 3-kinase. J Leukoc Biol 67:396, 2000.

103. Winston BW, Riches DWH: Activation of p42mapk/erk2 following engagement of tumor necrosis factor receptor CD120a(p55) in mouse macrophages. J Immunol 155:1525, 1995.

104. Czech MP: PIP₂ and PIP₃: complex roles at the cell surface. Cell 100:603, 2000.

105. Rhee SG, Choi KD: Regulation of inositol phospholipid specific phospholipase C isozymes. J Biol Chem 267:12393, 1992.

106. Zhong L, et al: Roles of PLCβ2 and -β3 and PI3Kγ in chemoattractant-mediated signal transduction. Science 287:1046, 2000.

107. Korchak HM, et al: Activation of the human neutrophil by calcium mobilizing ligands. II. Correlation of calcium, diacyl glycerol and phosphatidic acid generation with superoxide anion generation. J Biol Chem 263:11098, 1988.

108. Jaconi ME, et al: Cytosolic free calcium elevation mediates the phagosome-lysosome fusion during phagocytosis in human neutrophils. J Cell Biol 110:1555, 1990.

109. Cockcroft S: Phosphatidylinositol transfer proteins couple lipid transport to phosphoinositide synthesis. Cell Dev Biol 12:183, 2001.

110. Kular G, et al: Cooperation of phosphatidylinositol transfer protein with phosphoinositide 3-kinase γ in the formylmethionyl-leucylalanine-dependent production of phosphatidylinositol 3,4,5-trisphosphate in human neutrophils. Biochem J 325:299, 1997.

111. Wymann MP, et al: Lipids on the move: phosphoinositide 3-kinases in leukocyte function Immunol Today 21:260, 2000.

112. Fruman DA, et al: Phosphoinositide kinases. Annu Rev Biochem 67:481, 1998.

113. Condliffe AM, et al: Priming of human neutrophil superoxide generation by tumor necrosis factor-alpha is signalled by enhanced phosphatidylinositol 3,4,5-triphosphate but not inositol 1,4,5-triphosphate accumulation. FEBS Lett 439:147, 1998.

114. Liscovitch M, Cantley LC: Signal transduction and membrane traffic: the PITP/phosphoinositide connection. Cell 81:659, 1995.

115. Toker A, et al: Activation of protein kinase C family members by the novel polyphospho-inositides PtdIns-3,4-P₂ and PtdIns-3,4,5-P₃. J Biol Chem 269:32358, 1994.

116. Carpenter CL, et al: Phosphoinositide 3-kinase is activated by phosphopeptides that bind to the SH2 domains of the 85-kDa subunit. J Biol Chem 268:9478, 1993.

117. Corey S, et al: Granulocyte macrophage-colony stimulating factor stimulates both association and activation of phosphoinositide 3OH-kinase and src-related tyrosine kinase(s) in human myeloid derived cells. EMBO J 12:2681, 1993.

118. Vossebeld PJM, et al: Tyrosine phosphorylation-dependent activation of phosphatidylinositide 3-kinase occurs upstream of Ca²⁺-signalling induced by Fcγ receptor cross-linking in human neutrophils. Biochem J 323:87, 1997.

119. Gersuten RE, et al: Role of phosphoinositide 3-kinase in monocyte recruitment under flow conditions. J Biol Chem 276:26, 2001.

120. Stephens LR, et al: Synthesis of phosphatidylinositol (3,4,5)-trisphosphate in permeabilized neutrophils. J Biol Chem 268:17162, 1993.

121. Belisle B, Abo A: N-formyl peptide receptor ligation induces Rac-dependent actin reorganization through Gβγ subunits and class Ia phosphoinositide 3-kinases. J Biol Chem 275:26225, 2000.

122. Reinhold SL, et al: Activation of human neutrophil phospholipase D by three separable mechanisms. FASEB J 4:208, 1990.

123. Frank MO, et al: Inhibition of phospholipase D blocks activation of fibrinogen-adherent neutrophils by tumor necrosis factor. Infect Immunol 62:2622, 1994.

124. Cockcroft S, et al: Phospholipase D: a downstream effector of ARF in granulocytes. Science 263:523, 1994.

125. Leslie CC: Properties and regulation of cytosolic phospholipase A₂. J Biol Chem 272:16709, 1997.

126. Carnevale KA, Cathcart MK: Calcium-independent phospholipase A(2) is required for human monocyte chemotaxis to monocyte chemoattractant protein 1. J Immunol 167:3414, 2001.

127. Degousee N, et al: Groups IV, V and X phospholipases A2s in human neutrophils: role in eicosanoid production and gram-negative bacterial phospholipid hydrolysis. J Biol Chem 277:5061, 2002.

128. Korchak HM, et al: Long chain acyl coenzyme A and signalling in neutrophils: an inhibitor of acyl coenzyme A synthetase, Triacsin C, inhibits superoxide anion generation and degranulation by human neutrophils. J Biol Chem 269:30281, 1994.

129. Liu B, et al: Sphingomyelinases in cell regulation. Cell Dev Biol 8:311, 1997.

130. Hinkovska-Galcheva VT, et al: The formation of ceramide-1-phosphate during neutrophil phagocytosis and its role in liposome fusion. J Biol Chem 273:33203, 1998.

131. Oses-Prieta JA, et al: Molecular mechanisms of apoptosis induced by an immunomodulating peptide on human monocytes. Arch Biochem Biophys 379:353, 2000.

132. Jayadev S, et al: Identification of arachidonic acid as a mediator of sphingomyelin hydrolysis in response to tumor necrosis factor α. J Biol Chem 269:5757, 1994.

133. Nakamura T, et al: Ceramide regulates oxidant release in adherent human neutrophils. J Immunol 269:18384, 1994.

134. Hunter T: Protein kinases and phosphatases: the yin and yang of protein phosphorylation and signaling. Cell 80:225, 1995.

135. Walsh DA, et al: Substrate diversity of the cAMP-dependent protein kinase: regulation based upon multiple binding interactions. Curr Opin Cell Biol 4:241, 1992.

136. Mellor H, Parker PJ: The extended protein kinase C family. Biochem J 332:281, 1998.

137. Gschwendt M: Protein kinase C. Eur J Biochem 259:555, 1999.

138. Chan TO, et al: AKT/PKB and other D3 phosphoinositide-regulated kinases: kinase activation by phosphoinositide-dependent phosphorylation. Annu Rev Biochem 68:965, 1999.

139. Bossemeyer D: The glycine-rich sequence of protein kinases: a multifunctional element. Trends Biochem Sci 19:201, 1994.

140. Kennelly PJ, Krebs EG: Consensus sequences as substrate specificity determinants for protein kinases and protein phosphatases. J Biol Chem 266:15555, 1991.

141. Johnson LN, et al: The structural basis for substrate recognition and control by protein kinases. FEBS Lett 430:1, 1998.

142. Bozinovski S, et al: The synthetic peptide RPRAATF allows specific assay of Akt activity in cell lysates. Analyt Biochem 305:32, 2002.

143. Faux MC, Scott JD: Molecular glue: kinase anchoring and scaffold proteins. Cell 85:9, 1996.

144. Coghlan VM, et al: Association of protein kinase A and protein phosphatase 2B with a common anchoring protein. Science 267:108, 1995.

145. Feliciello A, et al: The biological functions of A-kinase anchor proteins. J Mol Biol 308:99, 2001.

146. Mochly-Rosen D, Kauvar LM: Pharmacological regulation of network kinetics by protein kinase C localization. Semin Immunol 12:55, 2000.

147. Brautigan DL: Protein phosphatases. Recent Prog Horm Res 49:197, 1994.

148. Mikawa K, Akamatsu H: The effect of phosphodiesterase III inhibitors on human neutrophil function. Crit Care Med 28:1001, 2000.

149. Ferretti ME, et al: Modulation of neutrophil phospholipase C activity and cyclic AMP levels by fMLP-OMe analogues. Cell Signal 13:233, 2001.

150. Orlic T, et al: Hypertonicity increases cAMP in PMN and blocks oxidative burst by PKA-dependent and -independent mechanisms. Am J Physiol 282:C1261, 2002.

151. Ydrenius L, et al: Dual action of cAMP-dependent kinase on granulocyte movement. Biochem Biophys Res Commun 235:445, 1997.

152. Kwak J-Y, Uhlinger D: Downregulation of phospholipase D by protein kinase A in a cell-free system of human neutrophils. Biochem Biophys Res Commun 267:305, 2000.

153. Berridge M, et al: Calcium signalling. Curr Biol 9:R157, 1999.

154. Gallin EK: Ion channels in leukocytes. Physiol Rev 71:775, 1991.

155. Schaefer M, et al: Receptor-mediated regulation of the nonselective cation channels TRPC4 and TRPC5. J Biol Chem 275:17517, 2000.

156. Montero M, et al: Activation by chemotactic peptide of a receptor-operated Ca²⁺ entry pathway in differentiated HL60 cells. J Biol Chem 269:29451, 1994.

157. von Tscharner V, et al: Ion channels in human neutrophils are activated by a rise in the free cytosolic calcium concentration. Nature 324:369, 1986.

158. Pittet D, et al: Chemoattractant receptor promotion of Ca²⁺ influx across the plasma membrane of HL-60 cells: a role for cytosolic free calcium elevations and inositol 1,3,4,5-tetrakisphosphate production. J Biol Chem 264:7251, 1989.

159. Putney JW: "Kissin' cousins": intimate plasma membrane-ER interactions underlie capacitative calcium entry. Cell 99:5, 1999.

160. Nusse O, et al: Store-operated Ca²⁺ influx and stimulation of exocytosis in HL-60 granulocytes. J Biol Chem 27:28360, 1997.

161. Korchak HM, et al: Stimulus-response coupling in the human neutrophil. II. Temporal analysis of changes in cytosolic calcium and calcium efflux. J Biol Chem 259:4076, 1984.

162. Kemp BE, et al: Substrate and pseudosubstrate interactions with protein kinases: determinants of specificity. Trends Biochem Sci 19:440, 1994.

163. Klauck TM, et al: Coordination of three signaling enzymes by AKAP79, a mammalian scaffold protein. Science 271:1589, 1996.

164. Belham C, et al: Intracellular signalling: PDK1—a kinase at the hub of things. Curr Biol 9:R93, 1999.

165. Tilton B, et al: G-protein–coupled receptors and Fcγ-receptors mediate activation of Akt/protein kinase B in human phagocytes. J Biol Chem 272:28096, 1997.

166. Korchak HM, et al: Selective role for β-PKC in signaling for O₂⁻ generation but not degranulation or adherence in differentiated HL60 cells. J Biol Chem 273:27292, 1998.

167. Li Q, et al: Protein kinase Cα regulates human monocyte O₂⁻ production and low density lipoprotein lipid oxidation. J Biol Chem 274:3764, 1999.

168. Laudanna C, et al: Evidence of ζ protein kinase C involvement in polymorphonuclear neutrophil integrin-dependent adhesion and chemotaxis. J Biol Chem 273:30306, 1998.
169. Kilpatrick LE, et al: Serine phosphorylation of p60 tumor necrosis factor receptor by protein kinase Cδ in TNF-activated neutrophils. Am J Physiol 279:C2011, 2000.
170. Glaser KB, et al: Phospholipase A₂ enzymes: regulation and inhibition. Trends Pharmacol Sci 14:92, 1987.
171. Rodriguez MM, et al: RACK1, a protein kinase C anchoring protein, coordinates the binding of activated protein kinase C and select pleckstrin homology domains in vitro. Biochem 38:13787, 1999.
172. Liliental J, Chang DD: Rack1, a Receptor for activated protein kinase C, interacts with integrin β subunit. J Biol Chem 273:2379, 1998.
173. Disatnik MH, et al: Phospholipase C-γ1 binding to intracellular receptors for activated protein kinase C. Proc Natl Acad Sci USA 91:559, 1994.

174. Chang BY, et al: RACK1, a receptor for activated C kinase and a homolog of the β subunit of G proteins, inhibits activity of Src tyrosine kinases and growth of NIH 3T3 cells. Mol Cell Biol 18:3245, 1998.
175. Korchak HM, Kilpatrick LE: Roles for βII-PKC and RACK1 in positive and negative signaling for superoxide anion generation in differentiated HL60 cells J Biol Chem 276:8910, 2001.
176. Babior BM, et al: The neutrophil NADPH oxidase. Arch Biochem Biophys 397:342, 2002.
177. El Benna JE, et al: The phosphorylation of the respiratory burst oxidase component p47phox during neutrophil activation. Phosphorylation of sites recognized by protein kinase C and by proline-directed kinases. J Biol Chem 269:23431, 1994.
178. Majumdar S, et al: Protein kinase C isotypes and signal transduction in human neutrophils: selective substrate specificity of calcium dependent β-PKC and novel calcium independent nPKC. Biochim Biophys Acta 1176:276, 1993.

162

N. Scott Adzick

Fetal Wound Healing

Fetal surgical skin wounds heal rapidly, without the scarring and inflammation that accompany adult skin wounds. In all species examined (mice, rats, rabbits, pigs, sheep, and monkeys), the prenatal wound healing process is faster and more efficient than adult repair and produces new tissue rather than scar.[1] Similarly, human fetal surgery has shown that the younger the fetus is at the time of surgery, the less likely he or she will be to be born with surgical scars. A summary of some phenomenologic differences between adult and fetal repair is shown in Table 162-1.

Scarless fetal repair is a consequence of a unique extracellular matrix produced by the fetal fibroblast in the absence of an adult-type inflammatory response to injury. Unraveling the biology of fetal repair has led to novel strategies for the prevention and treatment of scarring and fibrosis. The fetal wound healing process may represent a paradigm for ideal tissue repair. The therapeutic goal is to apply the lessons that the fetus is teaching us to control the quality of healing. This model may provide the necessary tools for the physician to regulate each step of the postnatal wound healing process.

FETAL SKIN

The less-developed state of fetal skin at the time of wounding may be important for scar-free tissue repair. The human fetal epidermis begins with two cell layers, the basal layer and the periderm, at about 4 weeks' gestation. The periderm is the outermost single-cell layer of the fetal skin. Peridermal cells have microvilli and blebs projecting from the surface of the skin into the amniotic fluid. Although the function of the periderm has not been determined, a secretive or absorptive process has been hypothesized. As development continues, an intermediate epidermal cell layer develops. Keratinization begins at 9 to 16 weeks' gestation. During this period, primordial hair follicles and sebaceous glands become evident. By 24 weeks' gestation, the epidermis has completely keratinized and stratifies into adult morphologic layers.

The dermis, which is the location of scar in adult wounds, is similarly undergoing morphologic and biochemical changes. Early in gestation, the fetal dermis is thin and cellular, owing to the paucity of extracellular matrix. As development progresses, dermal collagen is deposited, and sulfated glycosaminoglycans replace nonsulfated glycosaminoglycans, of which hyaluronic acid (HA) is predominant. The rapid growth and the relatively undifferentiated state of fetal skin set the stage for the unique response of fetal skin to injury.

THE FETAL ENVIRONMENT

There are many differences between the fetal and adult environments that may influence wound repair. First, fetal skin wounds are continuously bathed in warm, sterile amniotic fluid that is rich in growth factors. Amniotic fluid is also a fertile source of extracellular matrix molecules (e.g., HA and fibronectin), which are important components in fetal skin wounds.[2] Second, fetal tissue oxygenation is much lower than that of adult tissue. In fetal sheep at midgestation (which is a time when scarless skin healing occurs, tissue PO_2 is only 16 mm Hg, whereas adult tissue PO_2 is 45 to 60 mm Hg.[3] This observation at first seems paradoxical, because wound studies in adults have shown that wound hypoxia may result in delayed healing, impaired leukocyte function, and increased infection.[3] However, the observed differences may relate to differential expression on TGF-β_1 (see subsequent discussion). Finally, the profiles of growth factors in fetal and adult sera are different (e.g., fetal serum contains much higher levels of insulinlike growth factor II and HA-stimulating factor).[4,5]

There are two ways to evaluate the role of the environment in the fetal wound healing process—either put adult skin in the fetal environment, or place fetal skin in the adult environment, then determine the effect of that environment on healing. To investigate the influence of the fetal environment in modulating postnatal wound healing, sheep skin from adult animals was transplanted onto 60-day gestational fetal lambs (term = 145 days).[6] In this experiment, the engrafted adult skin was bathed in amniotic fluid and perfused by fetal blood. The immature fetal immune system does not reject the adult skin graft. The adult grafts were wounded 40 days later (100 days' gestation), at a time that scarless repair occurs in fetal sheep. The wounds were analyzed by collagen immunohistochemistry and were shown to heal with scar formation. Neither an amniotic fluid environment nor perfusion by fetal blood prevented scar formation in the wounded adult skin graft. This study suggests that scarless fetal skin healing properties are intrinsic to fetal skin and are not due to the fetal environment.

Support for this concept comes from the flip-side experiment-fetal tissue healing in the adult environment. Ferguson and Howarth[7] have done these experiments using an opossum called the *Monodelphus domesticus*. At birth, the opossum is physiologically and functionally a fetus and the pouch young remain attached to the mother's nipple for 4 weeks after birth. Therefore, the "fetal" development of this marsupial continues in a nonsterile environment and in the absence of amniotic fluid.

TABLE 162-1

Comparison of Adult and Fetal Skin Wound Healing Characteristics

Wound Healing Characteristics	Adult	Fetus
Scar	Present	Absent
Cell proliferation	Slower	Faster
Speed to closure	Slower	Faster
Scab	Present	Absent
Oxygen tension	Greater	Lesser
Fluid environment	Absent	Present
Sterile environment	Absent	Present
Skin temperature	Cooler	Warmer
Acute inflammation	Greater	Lesser
Matrix deposition	Slower, disorganized	Faster, organized
TGF-β and bFGF	Greater	Lesser
Angiogenesis	Greater	Lesser
Epithelialization	Slower	Faster
Keratinization	Present	Immature

Wounded 2-day-old pouch young heal rapidly and scarlessly outside of the sterile, fluid uterine environment, whereas older animals show extensive scarring.[7] Similarly, using novel *in vitro* systems, both Ihara and Motobayashi[8] and Martin and Lewis[9] in individual studies have shown that isolated fetal rat or mouse tissue grown in organ culture media can heal wounds without scar formation. Thus, amniotic fluid and fetal blood components (e.g., platelets) are not required for scarless repair.

Despite a relatively constant intrauterine environment, fetuses heal without scarring early in gestation and begin to scar late in gestation.[10] There is also a developmentally regulated wound-size threshold beyond which fetal skin heals with scar.[11] We have studied the temporal sequence of repair outcomes in early-, mid-, and late-gestational fetal rhesus monkeys. Early-gestation primate lip wounds heal with regeneration of all skin elements, including collagen, hair follicles, sebaceous glands, and even muscle in the deeper tissue layers. However, as gestation proceeds, the primate fetus first loses its ability to regenerate normal hair follicle and other appendage patterns but remains able to restore a normal, reticular collagen pattern after wounding. This pattern of "transition" wound repair is neither regeneration nor is it classic scarring in that the wound collagen organization is unchanged from that of unwounded skin. By early in the third trimester, a complete switch to adult-type repair occurs, with wounds showing densely packed, disorganized collagen deposition characteristic of scarring.[12]

The experiments described in this section led to the hypothesis that fetal healing must involve different cellular and connective tissue events than adult repair, and that this process is independent of the unique fetal environment. In addition, we have learned that the result of healing in fetal animals also depends on the extent of tissue damage, in that (1) large excisional fetal skin wounds scar earlier in gestation than incisional wounds[13]; (2) the type of tissue that is injured—internal fetal tissues such as diaphragm muscle, stomach, and peritoneum heal with scar formation[14, 15]; and (3) the species of animal—fetal rabbits do not heal excisional skin wounds.[16]

A MODEL OF HUMAN FETAL SKIN REPAIR

An exciting technique to study human fetal skin wound healing in the postnatal environment has been developed. This model has helped delineate the relative importance of fetal tissue properties and the absence of certain inflammatory cytokines in scarless repair. Grafts of human fetal skin placed onto adult athymic mice

retain the morphologic features of normal human fetal skin development. Full-thickness skin grafts from human fetuses at 15- to 22-weeks' gestational age were placed onto athymic mice in two locations: cutaneously onto a fascial bed and thereby exposed to air, and subcutaneously in a pocket under the murine panniculus carnosus (Fig. 162–1).[17] Linear wounds were made in each graft 1 week after transplantation, and grafts were harvested 30 minutes to 30 days after wounding. Wounds made in identical gestational-age human fetal skin grafts healed with scar in cutaneous grafts and without scar in subcutaneous grafts (Fig. 162–2).

Why does the same gestational-age human fetal skin heal with scar in a cutaneous location and without scar in a subcutaneous location? Factors that contribute to this divergent healing response include differences in species-specific extracellular matrix, adult mouse fibroblasts versus fetal human fibroblasts, graft neovascularization, growth factor profile, inflammatory cell recruitment, differentiation, and the presence of an air-tissue interface.[18] *In situ* hybridization with species-specific DNA probes and immunohistochemistry were performed to characterize the healing process of human fetal skin in these two locations. Immunostaining for species-specific fibroblasts, macrophages, and neutrophils was also performed. The cutaneous human fetal grafts healed with scar and demonstrated an influx

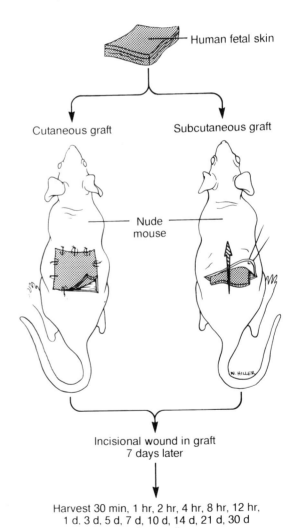

Figure 162–1. Schematic of experimental algorithm of human fetal skin transplantation onto the nude mouse. Each mouse received either two cutaneous or two subcutaneous grafts in dorsolateral flank locations.

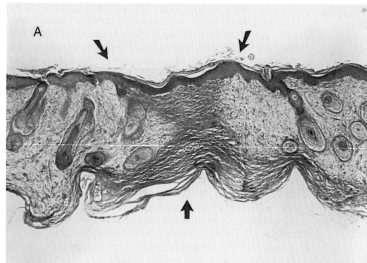
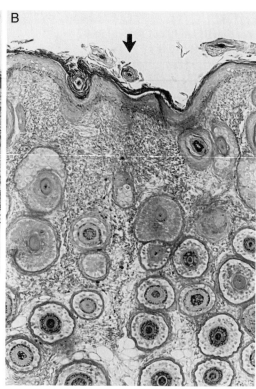

Figure 162–2. Human fetal skin at 19 weeks' gestational age was transplanted onto athymic mice, incisionally wounded and stained with Mallory's trichrome. Cutaneous graft **(A)** healed with scar formation *(arrows)*. Subcutaneous graft **(B)** healed without scar *(arrow)*. The hair follicle and collagen patterns are unchanged from the surrounding unwounded dermis, demonstrating scarless human fetal skin repair. (Original magnification × 50.)

of adult mouse fibroblasts and macrophages. In contrast, the subcutaneous human fetal grafts demonstrated exclusively human fetal fibroblasts in the wound environment, an absence of inflammatory cells, and scar-free repair. We concluded that the highly organized collagen deposition in scarless human fetal wound repair appears to be intrinsic to the human fetal fibroblast and occurs in the absence of an adultlike inflammatory response. The fetal fibroblast appears to be a critical effector cell for scarless repair.

Fetal Fibroblast

In the fetal wound, fibroblasts deposit matrix in an organized fashion similar to that of normal skin, so that the fetal fibroblast may function autonomously. However, this phenomenon changes late in gestation when adultlike healing with scar formation begins. Adult fibroblasts demonstrate a relative excess of cytokines compared with fetal fibroblasts.[19] Important differences in gene regulation have been found between fetal and adult cells, including dermal fibroblasts. For example, prolyl hydroxylase controls an important rate-limiting step in collagen production. Studies comparing early passage human fetal and adult fibroblasts show that prolyl hydroxylase activity in fetal fibroblasts is much greater until approximately 20 weeks' gestation, after which it gradually falls toward adult levels.[20] Regulation of prolyl hydroxylase in fetal cells, unlike adult cells, is controlled by poly-adenosine-5'-diphosphate-ribose synthetase, an enzyme that has been implicated in cell repair and tumorigenesis. Furthermore, early fetal tissues have high endogenous levels of transcription factors called *homeobox genes*.[21] Because a regeneration-specific homeobox gene is expressed during regeneration of newt limbs, it may be that the presence of transcription factors in early fetal cells has a marked effect on the response to wound stimuli.[22]

The identification of cytoskeletal differentiation markers in fibroblasts had led to the recognition of their phenotypic heterogeneity. During wound healing and fibrocontractive diseases in the adult, some fibroblasts acquire morphologic and biochemical features of smooth muscle cells (myofibroblasts), including the expression of α-smooth muscle actin (ASMA).[23] In turn, ASMA expression and myofibroblast function can be modulated by the wound matrix and growth factors,[24] and these interactions change during development. Wound fibroblasts later in gestation acquire more smooth muscle-like elements, suggesting a relationship with the development of scar seen at that time.[25]

We have investigated the role of the myofibroblast in fetal sheep tissue repair, using ASMA immunohistochemistry and transmission electron microscopy for myofibroblast detection. Small excisional wounds in the fetal lamb heal without scar formation or contraction at 75 days' gestation (term = 145 days) when ASMA-positive cells are absent. In contrast, excisional wounds begin to contract and show some scar formation beginning at 100 days' gestation when ASMA-positive myofibroblasts first appear. Transmission electron microscopy studies show that early in development, microfilament bundles in fibroblasts are sparse and disorganized, but as gestation progresses, the bundles become more prevalent and form tightly parallel arrangements characteristic of the contractile machinery of myofibroblasts.[25,26] The acquisition of more smooth muscle–like elements in wound fibroblasts later in gestation implies a relationship to the development of scar seen at that time. Within either the late-gestation fetal wound or the adult wound, the forces of wound contraction generated by myofibroblasts and the "stiffer" matrix that is present may alter the alignment of collagen fibrils and lead to the early establishment of an abnormal, scarlike orientation.

Fetal Wound Matrix

The extracellular matrix is a complex, cross-linked structure of proteins and polysaccharides that surrounds cells and organizes the geometry of normal tissues. Fetal wounds synthesize most matrix molecules present in adult wounds, but there are differences in the timing and pattern of these molecules in fetal wounds.[27] For example, the cell adhesion molecule called *tenascin* is deposited much more rapidly and persists longer in fetal wounds, perhaps accounting for the rapid epithelialization and cellular ingrowth that occur in fetal wound healing.[28]

Collagen is an important component of the extracellular matrix, and a scar is defined as abnormal collagen organization following wound repair in comparison with normal surrounding tissue. Thus, the pattern of collagen deposition in fetal and adult wounds is of particular interest. The orderly deposition of collagen in fetal animal models has been demonstrated using histologic, immunohistochemical, biochemical, and biophysical techniques.[29] The collagen pattern in fetal wounds is reticular and indistinguishable from that of adjacent normal tissue, whereas the adult wound contains large, parallel collagen bundles that are oriented perpendicular to the wound surface.[10] Thus, scarless fetal wound healing reflects the *organization* of collagen, not the absence of collagen in the fetal wound matrix.[30]

Although collagen Types I, III, V, and VI are present in both fetal and adult wounds,[10, 31] there are a few known differences in dermal collagen between the fetus and the adult. The presence of aminopropeptides of Type I collagen in heterogeneous collagen fibrils is more common in the fetus than the adult.[32] The fetal dermis also contains a preponderance of Type III collagen.[33] As the fetus develops, the ratio of Type III/Type I collagen decreases, which may influence collagen fibril size. Small-diameter collagen Type I fibrils with a high turnover and a similar configuration to fetal collagen (in terms of attached Type III collagen and presence of Type I aminopropeptide) occur adjacent to the epidermal-dermal junction in adult skin,[34] which is the region that shows minimal scarring in adult wounds. These minor differences between collagen in the fetal and adult dermis may be important in modulating the nature of the wounding response.

Alterations in the synthesis of proteoglycans and their constituent glycosaminoglycans correlate with the cell proliferation, migration, and collagen synthesis that accompany adult wound healing.[35] Proteoglycans are a heterogeneous group of polyanionic macromolecules consisting of a protein core to which a variable number of linear-sulfated glycosaminoglycan chains are covalently bound. These macromolecules include versican, a large chondroitin sulfate proteoglycan; decorin, a small dermatan-sulfate proteoglycan; and heparan-sulfate proteoglycan. Proteoglycans and glycosaminoglycans have been shown to affect wound collagen organization and fibrillogenesis. By binding to specific binding sites on collagen they control its rate of degradation.[36] The sulfated glycosaminoglycans temporally follow HA in the adult healing process, and the decline of HA levels and the appearance of sulfated glycosaminoglycans have been shown to correlate with the onset of cytodifferentiation in several embryologic systems.[36]

The fetal wound matrix is rich in glycosaminoglycans—in fetal rabbit wounds, the glycosaminoglycan content is approximately three times that of the adult wound during the same time period, and approximately 10 times that found in unwounded fetal skin.[37] HA is the principal glycosaminoglycan present in fetal wounds; it is a large molecule composed of alternating units of glucuronic acid and *N*-acetylglucosamine. An HA-rich matrix permits cell motility and proliferation, and a prolonged presence of HA in fetal wounds may provide the matrix signal that orchestrates healing by regeneration. Mammalian HA also has associated binding proteins, which have been implicated in the biologic activity of HA.[38] HA-receptor expression increases in fetal excisional skin wounds and correlates with fibroplasias.[39] Fibrotic healing of adult and late gestation sheep wounds correlates with increased hyaluronidase activity and removal of HA.[40] Fetal wound fluid, fetal urine, and amniotic fluid have the ability to stimulate and sustain HA synthesis because of a unique "HA-stimulating activity," or HASA. Support for the important role of HA in the fetal wound healing process is provided by the fact that levels of both HA and HASA in fetal lamb wound fluid

decrease significantly during the transition period from fetal- to adultlike healing at 120 days' gestation in fetal sheep.[41] Similarly, there is a gestational age-dependent decrease in both total glycosaminoglycan and HA content in normal fetal sheep skin, and the temporal appearance of extracellular decorin and heparan sulfate proteoglycan coincides with the onset of scarring that begins during late gestation.[42] Chondroitin sulfate proteoglycan is present within fetal mouse wounds at the time of collagen fibril formation, but it is absent at that time in adult mouse wounds.[29] Thus HA and chondroitin sulfate are likely important for scar-free repair, whereas other sulfated glycosaminoglycans may play a role in scar formation. Finally, syndecan-1 and syndecan-4 are induced during wound repair of human neonatal but not fetal skin.[43]

The so-called primary wound scaffolding into which fibroblasts migrate has an important influence on collagen fibrillogenesis. In the fetal wound, fibroblasts can migrate rapidly into a loose honeycomb matrix containing high levels of HA. Conversely, adult wounds exhibit slow fibroblast migration into a denser, more resistant wound matrix. In adult skin, fibroblast migration occurs more easily along the wound margins. These initial differences in the migration and orientation of fibroblasts may establish the pattern of collagen fibrils deposited in the respective wounds, with a loose reticular structure in the fetus and a closely packed, disorganized arrangement in the adult.

Roles of Inflammation and Cytokines in Wound Healing

There are major differences in the degree of inflammation in fetal and adult wounds. Until midgestation, the fetus is significantly neutropenic and has not developed self-nonself immunologic identity.[44] Histologically, there are few, if any, polymorphonuclear leukocytes in fetal wounds,[45] and there may be a defect in immature polymorphonuclear leukocyte chemotactic ability.[46] Some studies have correlated the absence of scarring in fetal wounds with the sparse inflammatory response, as evidenced by markedly reduced macrophage and monocyte infiltrates,[7] the absence of endogenous immunoglobulins at the wound site,[10, 28] reduced angiogenesis, and altered levels of peptide growth factors.[47] The transition of the fetal healing phenotype to a scarring, adult phenotype in the marsupial correlates directly with the amount of inflammatory reaction at the wound site.[48,49] These studies suggest that immature fetal immune cells do not respond to the wounding stimulus in a similar fashion to adult cells.

Peptide growth factors are released by inflammatory cells and help provide a cell-to-cell and cell-to-matrix communication system. These cytokines can affect matrix synthesis, matrix degradation, cell proliferation, and cell recruitment to the wound site. Because of the prominent role that inflammation plays in adult tissue repair, the characteristic inflammatory mediators of adult wound healing may be absent or modified in fetal wounds. For example, fetal platelets release significantly less platelet-derived growth factor (PDGF) and transforming growth factor-β (TGF-β) into serum than adult platelets.[50] In addition, HA inhibits platelet aggregation and cytokine release.[51] A different cytokine profile of fetal wounds, occasioned by the relative lack of inflammatory cells, may cause matrix molecule differences that lead to scar-free healing.

TRANSFORMING GROWTH FACTOR-β AND WOUND HEALING

Of the many cytokines that have been implicated in wound healing, TGF-β affects all phases of the healing process, including the inflammatory response and matrix accumulation.[52] In the adult wound, the macrophage is a crucial inflammatory cell that releases TGF-β, as well as other cytokines. The mammalian TGF-β family consists of three known isoforms, TGF-β_1, -β_2, and -β_3, which are structurally and functionally closely related to one another. Through autocrine and paracrine mechanisms, TGF-β stimulates the deposition of collagen and other matrix components by fibroblasts, inhibits collagenase, blocks plasminogen inhibitor, enhances angiogenesis, and is chemotactic for fibroblasts, monocytes, and macrophages.[53] Thus, TGF-β is capable of stimulating fibrogenesis by the fibroblast.

TGF-β may provide the linkage among states of injury, inflammation, and fibrosis. After tissue injury, activated macrophage-derived TGF-β disturbs the balance of synthesis and degradation of collagens and causes accumulation of extracellular matrix. TGF-β induces α-smooth muscle actin expression in fibroblasts, and this finding correlates with scar formation and pathologic wound contraction.[54] The ability of TGF-β to induce its own production may be crucial for the development of progressive scarring in chronic diseases that lead to eventual obliteration of normal tissue architecture. The correlation between TGF-β levels and scar formation holds true for a variety of fibrotic diseases. Experimental intraperitoneal administration of TGF-β results in adhesion formation.[55] There is enhanced expression of TGF-$β_1$ at the site of scar in the rat brain after localized cerebral injury.[56] In proliferative vitreoretinopathy, total TGF-β levels in intraocular fluid increase as the retinal scarring progresses from mild to moderate to severe.[57] Markedly increased amounts of TGF-β are present in fibrogenic diseases such as cirrhosis,[58] interstitial pulmonary fibrosis,[59] glomerulonephritis,[60,61] and scleroderma.[62]

Exogenously applied TGF-β promotes scar formation in both adult and fetal wounds. Specifically, the addition of TGF-β to polyvinyl alcohol sponges implanted in fetal rabbits produces fibrosis.[63] We have demonstrated that when TGF-β is added to human fetal skin wounds through a slow-release disk, scar formation results.[64] *In vitro* studies have shown that exposure of fetal dermal fibroblasts to TGF-β results in marked up-regulation of collagen gene expression.[65] Thus, the cellular and matrix machinery that is necessary for scar formation exists in fetal wounds.

Not only are fibroblasts capable of responding to the numerous cytokines produced by the immune system, but they can synthesize and secrete growth factors with pleotrophic effects. To test whether fetal and adult fibroblasts have different responses to the low levels of tissue PO_2 in the fetal wound environment, we examined TGF-$β_1$ gene expression in these cells under normoxic and hypoxic conditions. Both fetal and adult fibroblasts showed the potential to produce TGF-$β_1$ at normoxia, but fetal fibroblasts responded to hypoxia with a decrease in TGF-$β_1$ transcription, whereas adult fibroblasts were stimulated by hypoxia to increase TGF-β transcription.[66] Thus, the low fetal wound PO_2 may markedly down-regulate TGF-$β_1$ gene expression.

These studies suggested that scarless fetal wounds may be relatively TGF-β deficient. Indeed, Whitby and Ferguson[47] have performed TGF-β immunostaining studies in fetal mouse wounds and have found that TGF-β was absent, whereas TGF-β staining was abundant in neonatal and adult mouse wounds. We have shown an absence of immunostaining for either TGF-$β_1$ or TFG-$β_2$ from 1 hour to 28 days after wounding human fetal skin.[67] In contrast, wounds in adult human skin grafts demonstrated TGF-$β_1$ at the wound edge at 6 hours through 21 days and TGF-$β_2$ at 12 hours through 7 days. It is possible that TGF-β levels in fetal wounds are below the threshold for detection by immunohistochemical techniques, but compared with adult wounds, fetal wounds are, at least relatively, TGF-β deficient. Although we have detected significant amounts of TGF-β in fetal sheep wound fluid, there may be an alteration or limitation of TGF-β biologic activity by the local fetal wound environment.[68] TGF-β decreases interstitial collagenase in healing human fetal skin.[68] Early gestation fetal mouse fibroblasts contract a collagen gel and secrete and activate TGF-β to a lesser extent than do late gestation fetal and

adult skin fibroblasts.[69] Finally, there is differential expression of fibromodulin and decorin, both TGF-β modulators, in fetal as opposed to adult wounds.[70,71]

Macrophages are the principal source of TGF-β in adult wounds, and the reduced TGF-β levels in fetal wounds may reflect the absent or minimal macrophage infiltrate in these wounds. In adult wounds, TGF-β is also released from the α-granules of activated platelets, so it is possible that fetal platelets may not synthesize or release TGF-β at the fetal wound site. The relative lack of TGF-β, a cytokine known to induce fibrosis, may be an important reason why the fetus heals by regeneration rather than by scarring. TGF-β is likely to be important in adult tissue repair; however, excessive action of this cytokine may be responsible for the tissue damage caused by scarring in many serious diseases. These findings suggest that anti-TGF-β therapeutic strategies may ameliorate scar formation in postnatal fibrotic diseases.

Cytokine Excess in Postnatal Wounds

Ferguson and colleagues mimicked the fetal wound situation within the healing adult rat wound by using an anti-TGF-β polyclonal neutralizing antibody to experimentally reduce TGF-β levels.[72] This manipulation resulted in markedly diminished scarring in adult wounds. The neutralizing antibody-treated wounds had normal tensile strength and a nearly normal dermal architecture compared with untreated wounds, and this salutary effect was accompanied by deposition of less collagen and fibronectin, and infiltration by fewer macrophages and blood vessels. Injection of TGF-β alone had the opposite effects. Application of TGF-β-neutralizing antibody at the time of wounding (and not later) was essential to reduce active TGF-β levels, prevent autoinduction of TFG-β mRNA, and limit macrophage infiltration and further TGF-β release. The effectiveness of this approach has been demonstrated in another fibrotic process, in which administration of either TGF-$β_1$ antiserum or decorin (to neutralize TGF-β biologic activity) suppresses the pathologic increase in matrix synthesis that occurs in an animal model of glomerulonephritis.[72] Thus, the relationship of TGF-β to scar formation fulfills the Koch postulate: TGF-β is absent in scarless fetal wounds, the addition of TGF-β to fetal wounds results in scar formation, the presence of TGF-β after adult injury correlates with the degree of fibrosis observed, and blocking of TGF-β in adult wounds has a potent anti-scarring effect.

Subsequent studies by Shah and Ferguson have shown that neutralization of both TGF-$β_1$ and TGF-$β_2$ isoforms has a much greater, synergistic antiscarring effect than neutralization of either isoform alone.[73] Neutralizing antibodies against PDGF also have some antiscarring effect, but antibodies to epidermal growth factor have no effect on dermal scarring. Although injection of cytokine antibodies into wounds has limited clinical potential because of antigenicity problems, there are other promising ways to reduce wound levels of TGF-$β_1$ and TGF-$β_2$. Addition of the TGF-$β_3$ isoform down-regulates TGF-$β_1$ and -$β_2$ levels and has a pronounced antiscarring effect. The application to rodent wounds of the inexpensive and readily available sugar mannose-6-phosphate also limits scar formation, presumably by blocking the insulin-like growth factor-II/mannose-6-phosphate receptor that is important for TGF-β activation.[74] Various other theoretical anti-TGF-β therapeutic strategies, such as flooding the wound with soluble TGF-β receptors to compete effectively with cellular TGF-β binding sites, or adding antisense oligonucleotides to inhibit TGF-β gene expression, may also make adult wounds heal in a fetal-like manner. Inhibitors of TGF-β may be important future drugs for the control of fibrosis.

Basic fibroblast growth factor (bFGF) is another example of cytokine excess in postnatal wounds. Using immunohistochemical techniques, bFGF can be perceived in neonatal and adult mouse lip wounds, but it is not detected in fetal mouse lip wounds.[46] bFGF is a powerful angiogenesis stimulator, and increased neovascularization is a normal component of adult wound repair.[75] Immunostaining for collagen IV and laminin, normal components of the endothelial basement membrane, shows profuse angiogenesis in adult wounds, whereas fetal wounds have a diminished vascular pattern similar to that of adjacent unwounded fetal tissue.[10,29] An enhanced rate of wound neovascularization in the adult leads to a rapid increase in wound perfusion, thereby delivering more adult serum and inflammatory cells to the site of potential scar formation. Finally, the proinflammatory cytokines interleukin-6 and -8 are diminished in fetal wound healing compared with adult wound repair, which may due to the presence of the anti-inflammatory cytokine interleukin-10 in fetal wounds.[76-78]

In evolutionary terms, it appears that postnatal wounds may be optimized for speed of healing under adverse conditions (e.g., dirt, foreign bodies), and the result is an excessive inflammatory infiltrate and cytokine profile. The potential "fetal" regenerative response in adult wounds may be overwhelmed by an inflammation-induced cytokine surplus, leading to scar formation. This phenomenon is an example of so-called cytokine poisoning, in which the inappropriate reparative response of the patient may prove detrimental to outcome. This paradox is analogous to the pathophysiology of toxic host mediators associated with disease states such as systemic sepsis and multiple organ failure.[79,80]

FUTURE DIRECTIONS

Fetal wound healing studies may help physicians understand what accounts for scarring and, perhaps more importantly, how scar formation can be prevented. There are a number of ways in which the matrix and cellular response of the healing adult wound might be manipulated to reduce scarring: Inhibit the wound inflammatory response by blocking inflammatory cytokines such as TGF-β, bFGF, and PDGF; add exogenous tenascin to facilitate keratinocyte and fibroblast migration into the wound; transplant fibroblasts with fetal characteristics to the adult wound site; provide a more porous wound scaffold by addition of HA or HASA to enhance fibroblast migration and promote regeneration of a normal reticular collagen organization in the wounded dermis. Although all these potential therapeutic strategies require rigorous scientific testing, it may be possible to alter adult wound healing toward a scar-free fetal-like phenotype by modifying one or more of the components that are different between fetal and adult repair.

REFERENCES

1. Adzick NS, Longaker MT (eds): Fetal Wound Healing. New York, Elsevier Scientific Press, 1992.
2. Longaker MT, et al: Studies in fetal wound healing VII. Fetal wound healing may be modulated by elevated hyaluronic acid stimulating activity in amniotic fluid. J Pediatr Surg 25:430, 1991.
3. Jonsson K, et al: Tissue oxygenation, anemia, and perfusion in relation to wound healing in surgical patients. Ann Surg 214:605, 1991.
4. Longaker MT, et al: Studies in fetal wound healing IV. Hyaluronic acid stimulating activity distinguishes fetal from adult wound fluid. Ann Surg 210:667, 1989.
5. Estes JM, et al: Insulin-like growth factor-II in ovine wound fluid: evidence for developmental regulation. Surg Forum 42:659, 1991.
6. Longaker MT, et al: Adult skin wounds in the fetal environment heal with scar formation. Ann Surg 219:65, 1994.
7. Ferguson MWJ, Howarth GF: Marsupial models of scarless fetal wound healing. In Adzick NS, Longaker MT (eds): Fetal Wound Healing. New York, Elsevier Scientific Press, 1992, pp 95-124.
8. Ihara I, Motobayashi Y: Wound closure in foetal rat skin. Development 114:573, 1992.
9. Martin P, Lewis J: Actin cables and epidermal movement in embryonic wound healing. Nature 360:179, 1992.
10. Longaker MT, et al: Studies in fetal wound healing VI. Second and early third trimester fetal wounds demonstrate rapid collagen deposition without scar formation. J Pediatr Surg 25:63, 1990.
11. Cass DL, et al: Wound size and gestational age modulate scar formation in fetal wound repair. J Pediatr Surg 32:41, 1997.
12. Lorenz HP, et al: The ontogeny of scar formation in the non-human primate. Ann Surg 217:391, 1993.
13. Longaker MT, et al: Midgestation fetal lamb excisional wounds contract in utero. J Pediatr Surg 26:942, 1991.
14. Longaker MT, et al: Fetal diaphragmatic wounds heal with scar formation. J Surg Res 50:375, 1991.
15. Meuli M, et al: Scar formation in the fetal alimentary tract. J Pediatr Surg 30:392, 1995.
16. Krummel TM, et al: In vitro and in vivo analysis of the inability of fetal rabbit wounds to contract. Wound Rep Reg 1:15, 1993.
17. Lorenz HP, et al: Scarless wound repair: a human fetal skin model. Development 114:253, 1992.
18. Lin RY, et al: Scarless human fetal skin repair is intrinsic to the fetal fibroblast and occurs in the absence of an inflammatory response. Wound Rep Reg 2:297, 1994.
19. Broker BJ, et al: Comparison of growth factor expression in fetal and adult fibroblasts. Arch Otolaryngol Head Neck Surg 125:676, 1999.
20. Duncan BW, et al: Regulation of prolyl hydroxylase activity in fetal and adult fibroblasts. In Adzick NS, Longaker MT (eds): Fetal Wound Healing. New York, Elsevier Scientific Press, 1992, pp 303-323.
21. Mackenzie A, et al: The homeobox gene Hox 7.1 has specific regional and temporal expression patterns during early murine craniofacial embryogenesis, especially during tooth development in vivo and in vitro. Development 111:269, 1991.
22. Brown R, Brockes JP: Identification and expression of a regeneration-specific homeobox gene in the newt limb blastema. Development 111:489, 1991.
23. Sappino AP, et al: Differentiation repertoire of fibroblastic cells: expression of cytoskeletal proteins as markers of phenotypic modulations. Lab Invest 63:144, 1990.
24. Darby I, et al: Alpha-smooth muscle actin is transiently expressed by myofibroblasts during experimental wound healing. Lab Invest 63:21, 1990.
25. Sappino AP, et al: Colonic pericryptal fibroblasts: differentiation pattern in embryogenesis and phenotypic modulation in epithelial proliferation lesions. Virchows Archiv A Pathol Anat 415:551, 1990.
26. Estes JM, et al: Phenotypic and functional features of myofibroblasts in fetal wounds. Differentiation 56:173, 1994.
27. Cass DL, et al: Epidermal integrin expression is upregulated rapidly in human fetal wound repair. J Pediatr Surg 32:312, 1998.
28. Whitby DJ, et al: Rapid epithelization of fetal wounds is associated with early deposition of tenascin. J Cell Sci 99:583, 1991.
29. Adzick NS, Longaker MT: Scarless wound healing in the fetus: the role of the extracellular matrix. Prog Clin Biol Res 365:177, 1991.
30. Lovvorn HN, et al: Relative distribution and cross-linking of collagen distinguishes fetal from adult sheep wound repair. J Pediatr Surg 34:218, 1999.
31. Whitby DJ, Ferguson MWJ: The extracellular matrix of lip wounds in fetal, neonatal, and adult mice. Development 112:651, 1991.
32. Fleischmajer R, et al: Type I and type III collagen interactions during fibrillogenesis. Ann NY Acad Sci 580:161, 1991.
33. Merkel JR, et al: Type I and type III collagen content of healing wounds in fetal and adult rats. Proc Soc Exp Biol Med 187:493, 1988.
34. Yeo TK, et al: Alterations in proteoglycan synthesis common to healing wounds and tumors. Am J Pathol 138:1437, 1991.
35. Ruoslahti E, Yamaguchi Y: Proteoglycans as modulators of growth factor activities. Cell 64:867, 1991.
36. Bertolami CN, et al: Glycosaminoglycan processing during tissue repair: degradation of hyaluronic acid. In Adzick NS, Longaker MT (eds): Fetal Wound Healing. New York, Elsevier Scientific Press, 1992, pp 215-226.
37. DePalma RL, et al: Characterization and quantification of wound matrix in the fetal rabbit. Matrix 9:224, 1990.
38. Toole BP: Hyaluronan and its binding proteins, the hyaladherins. Curr Opin Cell Biol 2:839, 1991.
39. Lovvorn HN, et al: Hyaluronan receptor expression increases in fetal excisional wounds and correlates with fibroplasias. J Pediatr Surg 33:1062, 1998.
40. West DC, et al: Fibrotic healing of adult and late gestation sheep wounds correlates with increased hyaluronidase activity and removal of hyaluronan. Int J Biochem Cell Biol 29:201, 1997.
41. Estes JM, et al: Hyaluronate metabolism undergoes ontogenetic transition during fetal development: implications for scarless wound healing. J Pediatr Surg 28:1227, 1996.
42. Freund RM, et al: Serial quantification of hyaluronan and sulfated glycosaminoglycans in fetal sheep skin. Biochem Mol Biol Int 29:813, 1993.
43. Gallo R, et al: Syndecans-1 and -4 are induced during wound repair of human neonatal but not fetal skin. J Invest Derm 107:676, 1996.
44. Flake AW, et al: Transplantation of fetal hematopoietic stem cells in utero: the creation of hematopoietic chimeras. Science 223:776, 1986.
45. Adzick NS, et al: Comparison of fetal, newborn, and adult rabbit wound healing by histologic, enzyme-histochemical, and hydroxyproline determinations. J Pediatr Surg 20:315, 1985.
46. Jennings RW, et al: Ontogeny of fetal sheep polymorphonuclear leukocyte phagocytosis. J Pediatr Surg 26:853, 1991.
47. Whitby DJ, Ferguson MWJ: Immunohistochemical localization of growth factors in fetal wound healing. Dev Biol 147:207, 1991.
48. Armstrong J: Healing characteristics of dermal wounds on the pouch young of the short tailed grey opossum. Wound Rep Reg 2:96, 1993.

49. Corvin AJ, et al: Endogenous inflammatory response to dermal wound healing in the fetal and adult mouse. Dev Dyn 212:385–393, 1998.

50. Olutoye OO, et al: Lower cytokine release by fetal porcine platelets: a possible explanation for reduced inflammation after fetal wounding. J Pediatr Surg 31:91–95, 1996.

51. Olutoye OO, et al: Hyaluronic acid inhibits fetal platelet function: implications in scarless healing. J Pediatr Surg 32:1037–1040, 1997.

52. Barnard JA, et al: The cell biology of transforming growth factor β. Biochim Biophys Acta 1032:79, 1990.

53. Sporn MB, Roberts AB: Transforming growth factor-β: recent progress and new challenges. J Cell Biol 119:1017, 1992.

54. Desmouliere A, et al: Transforming growth factor-β1 induces alpha-smooth muscle actin expression in granulation tissue myofibroblasts and in quiescent and growing fibroblasts. J Cell Biol 122:103, 1993.

55. Logan A, et al: Enhanced expression of transforming growth factor β1 in the rat brain after a localized cerebral injury. Brain Res 587:216, 1992.

56. Williams RS, et al: Effect of transforming growth factor β on postoperative adhesion formation and intact peritoneum. J Surg Res 52:65, 1992.

57. Connor TB, et al: Correlation of fibrosis and transforming growth factor-β type 2 levels in the eye. J Clin Invest 83:1661, 1989.

58. Castilla A, et al: Transforming growth factors beta 1 and alpha in chronic liver disease: effects of interferon alfa therapy. N Engl J Med 324:933, 1991.

59. Broekelmann TJ, et al: Transforming growth factor β1 is present at sites of extracellular matrix gene expression in human pulmonary fibrosis. Proc Natl Acad Sci U S A 88:6642, 1991.

60. Border WA, et al: Suppression of experimental glomerulonephritis by anti-serum against transforming growth factor β1. Nature 346:371, 1990.

61. Border WA, Noble NA: Transforming growth factor beta in tissue fibrosis. N Engl J Med 331:1286, 1994.

62. Peltonen J, et al: Evaluation of transforming growth factor β and type I pro-collagen gene expression in fibrotic diseases by in situ hybridization. J Invest Dermatol 94:365, 1990.

63. Krummel TM, et al: TGF-β induces fibrosis in a fetal wound model. J Pediatr Surg 23:647, 1988.

64. Sullivan KM, et al: A model of human fetal skin repair is deficient in transforming growth factor beta. J Pediatr Surg 30:198, 1995.

65. Lorenz HP, et al: Transforming growth factors β1 and β2 synergistically increase collagen gene expression in fetal fibroblasts but not in adult fibroblasts. Surg Forum 44:723, 1993.

66. Chang J, et al: Fetal and adult sheep fibroblast TGFβ1 gene expression in vitro: effects of hypoxia and gestational age. Surg Forum 44:720, 1993.

67. Longaker MT, et al: Regulation of fetal wound healing. Surg Forum 42:654, 1991.

68. Bullard K, et al: Transforming growth factor-beta–1 decreases interstitial colla-genase in healing human fetal skin. J Pediatric Surg 32:1823-1827, 1997.

69. Coleman C, et al: Contractility, transforming growth factor-beta, and plasmin in fetal skin fibroblasts: role in scarless wound healing. Pediatr Res 43:403–409, 1998.

70. Beanes SR, et al: Down-regulation of decorin, a TGF-β modulator, is associated with scarless fetal wound healing. J Pediatr Surg 36:1666–1671, 2001.

71. Soo C, et al: Differential expression of fibromodulin, a TGF-β modulator, in fetal skin development and scarless repair. American J Pathol 157:423–433, 2000.

72. Shah M, et al: Control of scarring in adult wounds by neutralizing antibody to transforming growth factor beta. Lancet 339:213, 1992.

73. Shah M, et al: Neutralizing antibody to TGFβ1,2 reduces cutaneous scarring in adult rodents. J Cell Sci 107:1137, 1994.

74. Shah M, et al: Immunolocalization of TGFβ isoforms in normal and experimen-tally modulated incisional wounds in adult rodents. Wound Rep Reg 2:124, 1993.

75. Folkman J, Shing Y: Angiogenesis. J Biol Chem 267:10931, 1992.

76. Liechty KW, et al: Diminished interleukin-8 production in the fetal wound healing response. J Surg Research 77:80, 1998.

77. Liechty KW, et al: Diminished interleukin-6 production during scarless human fetal wound repair. Cytokine 12:671, 2000.

78. Liechty KW, et al: Fetal wound repair results in scar formation in interleukin-10-deficient mice in a syngeneic murine model of scarless fetal wound repair. J Pediatr Surg 35:866, 2000.

79. Baue AE: The horror autotoxicus and multiple-organ failure. Arch Surg 127:1451, 1992.

80. Deitch EA: Multiple organ failure: pathophysiology and potential future therapy. Ann Surg 216:117, 1992.

Sadhana Chheda, Susan E. Keeney, and Armond S. Goldman

163 Immunology of Human Milk and Host Immunity

Paul Ehrlich reported in 1891 the first evidence that immunity could be transmitted through breast-feeding in experimental animals.[1,2] Few organized studies of that possibility in humans were reported, however, until the 1920s, when Woodbury[3] and Grulee and colleagues[4,5] in separate studies found that the incidence and severity of diarrheal diseases were much lower in breast-fed than cow's milk–fed infants. Those observations were confirmed repeatedly in developing and industrialized countries.[6-14] Furthermore, it was found that the specificity of the protection provided by breast-feeding encompassed bacterial and viral enteric infections due to pathogens such as *Shigella* species,[8-10] *Salmonella* species,[9] *Escherichia coli*,[9] *Vibrio cholerae*,[11] rotavirus,[12-14] and poliovirus.[15]

The following explanations for the protection provided by breast-feeding were advanced:

1. Because human milk was less contaminated with patho-genic microorganisms than formula feedings, fewer infec-tions would be transmitted to the breast-fed infant.

2. Because of the increased spacing of births in lactating women due to contraceptive effects of lactation, the density of children susceptible to common contagious agents would be lower in families where breast-feeding was practiced.[16]

3. In addition, infants who were breast-fed would be less likely to be in group-care facilities and thus would be less exposed to children harboring microbial pathogens.

These propositions were reasonable, but they did not com-pletely explain the protection provided by breast-feeding. In that respect, Wyatt and Mata from Guatemala found that manifesta-tions of infection in breast-fed infants were low even when bac-terial enteropathogens such as *Shigella* were recovered from the nipples and areola of the breast of the mother.[6] Furthermore, some evidence emerged that breast-fed infants may be more resistant to certain common respiratory infections.[17-20]

Despite those earlier studies, the concept, characteristics, and many of the components of the immune system in human milk were not revealed until the last half of the 20th century.[21] By 1973, the following general features of the antimicrobial agents of the immune system in human milk were evident:[22]

1. They are common to mucosal sites.

2. They are adapted to persist in the hostile environment of the gastrointestinal tract.

3. They inhibit or kill certain microbial pathogens synergisti-cally.

4. They are often pluripotent.

5. They protect without triggering inflammatory reactions.

6. The daily production of many factors is inversely related to the ability of the recipient infant to produce those agents at mucosal sites.

The last feature of antimicrobial agents in human milk strongly suggested a relationship between the evolution of the develop-ment of the immune system of the infant and the evolution of the abilities of the mother to produce and secrete immune factors from the lactating mammary gland.[23] Since then, several other somewhat overlapping evolutionary outcomes concerning the relationships between the immune system produced by the mammary gland and the developmental status of the immune system of the infant have been identified.[24] The seven known evolutionary outcomes are as follows:

1. Certain postnatal developmental delays in the immune system are replaced by those same agents in human milk.
2. Other postnatal delays in the immune system are offset by dissimilar agents in human milk.
3. Agents in human milk initiate or augment functions that are otherwise poorly expressed in the infant.
4. Agents in human milk alter the physiologic and biochemical states of the alimentary tract from one suited for fetal life to one that is appropriate for extrauterine life.
5. Defense agents in human milk protect without provoking inflammation, and some agents in human milk inhibit inflammation.
6. Defense agents in human milk have an enhanced survival in the gastrointestinal tract of the recipient infant.
7. Growth factors in human milk augment the proliferation of a commensal enteric bacterial flora.

The realization of many of those evolutionary outcomes came about as a consequence of the discovery of an expanded immune system in human milk that consisted of not only antimicrobial agents but also of anti-inflammatory[25, 26] and immunomodulating agents.[26] The nature and functions of these agents are described in following sections of this chapter.

ANTIMICROBIAL FACTORS

The physical features, functions, and quantities of antimicrobial agents in human milk are summarized in Table 163–1 and are discussed in the following sections.

Proteins

The principal proteins in human milk that are antimicrobial are secretory immunoglobulin A (IgA) antibodies, other immunoglobulins, lactoferrin, lysozyme, mucins, and lactadhedrin. These proteins, except for immunoglobulins other than secretory IgA, are better represented in human milk than other mammalian milks used in human infant nutrition.

Antibodies

The concentrations of IgM are much lower in human milk than in serum.[27] IgM molecules in blood and milk are pentamers. However, unlike serum IgM, some human milk IgM is complexed to secretory component, and the antibody specificities of human milk IgM may be similar to those of secretory IgA in human milk (see later discussion). IgG is also present in human milk, albeit in modest amounts.[27] All IgG subclasses are represented in human milk,[28] but the relative proportion of IgG4 is higher in human milk than serum.[28] Very little IgD is present in human milk.[29] IgE, the immunoglobulin responsible for immediate hypersensitivity reactions, is essentially absent in human milk.[30]

Secretory IgA comprises more than 95% of the immunoglobulins in human milk.[27] This type of IgA consists of two identical IgA monomers united by a 15-kD polypeptide called the joining chain and complexed to a 75-kD glycopeptide, the secretory component.[31, 32] Secretory IgA is assembled when dimeric IgA produced by plasma cells in the stroma of the mammary gland binds to the first domain of polymeric immunoglobulin receptors on the basolateral surface of epithelial cells.[33]

Investigations of the unusual specificities of antibodies in human milk were spurred by epidemiologic evidence that human milk protects against common enteric and respiratory infectious pathogens and the discovery of secretory IgA in human milk by Lars Å Hanson.[34,35] This led to studies of the origins of B cells that are responsible for the production of the immunoglobulin part of those antibodies and mechanism of the assembly of the final molecule, secretory IgA. The specificities of many antibodies were found to be due to immunogen-triggered events in the intestinal tract.[36] It was later ascertained that antigen-stimulated B cells from Peyer patches of the lower small intestinal tract migrated to the mammary gland and that the process was under hormonal control.[37, 38] In addition, a B-cell pathway between lymphoid tissues in the bronchi and the mammary gland was discovered.[39]

This process may be controlled by a mucosal adhesion-cell adhesion system (e.g., mucosal addressin cell adhesion molecule, or MAdCAM[40]), and its counterstructure, $\alpha 4\beta 7$ integrin,[41] and certain cytokines. During mucosal antigenic stimulation, cytokines released from mononuclear cells in Peyer patches induce local B cells to switch from IgM+ to IgA+.[42-45] These isotype-switched B cells then migrate sequentially into local intestinal lymphatic channels and lymph nodes, the thoracic duct, and the vascular circulation. Because of lactogenic hormones and other influences that are poorly understood, the cells move from the vascular compartment to the lactating mammary gland. These IgA+ B cells differentiate to IgA producing-secreting plasma cells that remain in the lamina propria of the mammary gland. In keeping with other mucosal lymphoid tissues, IgA dimers produced by plasma cells in the mammary gland principally contain λ-light chains, whereas κ-light chains predominate in immunoglobulins in human sera.[46]

IgA dimers produced by those plasma cells bind to polymeric immunoglobulin receptors on the basolateral external membranes of mammary gland epithelial cells.[31, 32, 47, 48] The resultant receptor–dimeric IgA complex is transported to the apical side of

---

TABLE 163-1

Primary Functions of Antimicrobial Agents in Human Milk

Agents	Primary Antimicrobial Functions
Proteins	
Lactoferrin	Bacteriostasis produced by Fe^{3+} chelation
	Bacterial killing due to lactoferricin
Lysozyme	Lyses bacterial cell walls by degrading peptidoglycans
Secretory IgA	Binds bacterial adherence sites, toxins, and virulence factors
MUCI	Inhibits the binding of S-fimbriated *Escherichia coli* to epithelial cells
Lactadhedrin	Binds rotavirus and thus prevents its contact with epithelium
Oligosaccharides and glycoconjugates	Receptor analogues inhibit binding of enteric/respiratory pathogens and their toxins to epithelial cells.
Monoglycerides and fatty acids from lipid digestion	Disrupt enveloped viruses, inactivate certain bacteria, defend against infection from *Giardia lamblia* and *Entameoba histolytica*

the cell where the original intracytoplasmic portion of the receptor is cleaved away. The remaining molecule, secretory IgA, is secreted into milk. Thus, enteromammary and bronchomammary pathways protect the immunologically immature infant against the pathogens in the environment of the dyad (Table 163–2). This is important given that secretory IgA antibodies and the antigen-binding repertoire of immunoglobulin molecules are not optimally produced during early infancy.[49] Furthermore, some secretory IgA molecules in human milk are antiidiotypic antibodies and therefore may operate as immunizing agents.[50]

The quantity of secretory IgA declines as lactation proceeds, but a considerable amount of secretory IgA is transmitted to the recipient infant throughout breast-feeding.[51-54] The concentrations of secretory IgA in human milk are highest in colostrum[51] and then gradually decline to a plateau of about 1 mg/mL.[52] The approximate mean intake of secretory IgA per day in healthy full-term breast-fed infants is approximately 125 mg/kg per day at 1 month and approximately 75 mg/kg per day by 4 months.[54]

Secretory IgA is resistant to intestinal proteases such as pancreatic trypsin.[55] Although the first IgA subclass, IgA1, is susceptible to bacterial proteases that attack the hinge region of the molecule,[56] the second subclass, IgA2, is resistant to those proteases and is disproportionally increased in human milk.[27] Furthermore, secretory IgA antibodies against these bacterial IgA proteases are found in human milk.[56] In keeping with those observations, the amount of secretory IgA excreted in the stools of low birth weight infants fed human milk was about 30 times that in infants fed a cow's milk formula.[57] In addition, the urinary excretion of secretory IgA antibodies in the recipients increased as a result of human milk feedings.[58, 59] The origin of secretory IgA antibodies in the urine of infants fed human milk is undetermined. It is improbable that they are from human milk because there is no known mechanism for the transport of the entire molecule from the gastrointestinal tract to the blood or from blood to urine.

Lactoferrin

Lactoferrin is a single-chain glycoprotein with two globular lobes, each of which displays a site that binds ferric iron.[60] In over 90% of lactoferrin in human milk,[61] iron-binding sites are available to compete with siderophilic bacteria and fungal enterochelin for ferric iron.[62-65] The chelation of iron disrupts the proliferation of those microbial pathogens. In addition, the chelation is enhanced by bicarbonate, the principal buffer in human milk.

Lactoferrin also kills some bacteria[66] and fungi,[67] and the responsible part of the molecule (lactoferricin)[67, 68] acts by damaging outer membranes of pathogens.[68] The action is dependent on Ca^{2+}, Mg^{2+}, or Fe^{3+} but not on the ability to chelate Fe^{3+}.[68]

TABLE 163-2

Secretory IgA Antibodies in Human Milk Against Microbial Pathogens

Bacteria-Toxins Virulence Factors	Viruses	Fungi and Parasites
Escherichia coli	Adenovirus	*Giardia lamblia*
Campylobacter sp.	Cytomegalovirus	*Candida* sp.
Clostridium botulinum	Enteroviruses (polio)	
Clostridium difficile	HIV	
Haemophilus influenzae	Influenza virus	
Helicobacter pylori	Respiratory syncytial	
Klebsiella pneumoniae	virus	
Streptococcus pneumoniae	Rotavirus	
Vibrio cholerae		
Salmonella sp.		
Shigella sp.		

There is also evidence that lactoferrin inhibits certain viruses in a manner that is independent of iron chelation.[69-72]

The mean concentration of lactoferrin in human colostrum is between 5 and 6 mg/mL.[51] As the volume of milk production increases, the concentration falls to about 1 mg/ml at 2 to 3 months of lactation.[52] The mean intake of milk lactoferrin in healthy breast-fed full-term infants is about 260 mg/kg per day at 1 month and 125 mg/kg per day by 4 months.[54]

Because of resistance of lactoferrin to proteolysis,[73] the excretion of lactoferrin in the stools is higher in infants fed human milk than in those fed a cow's milk formula.[57,74,75] The quantity of lactoferrin excreted in stools of low birth weight infants fed a human milk preparation is approximately 185 times that excreted by infants fed a cow's milk formula.[57] That estimate, however, may be too high because of the presence of immunoreactive fragments of lactoferrin in the stools of human milk-fed infants.[76] There is also a significant increment in the urinary excretion of intact and fragmented lactoferrin as a result of human milk feedings.[57,76] Stable isotope studies suggest that those increments in urinary lactoferrin and its fragments originate from ingested human milk lactoferrin.[77]

Lysozyme

Lysozyme, a 15-kD single chain protein, lyses susceptible bacteria by hydrolyzing β-1,4 linkages between *N*-acetylmuramic acid and 2-acetylamino-2-deoxy-D-glucose residues in cell walls.[78] High concentrations of lysozyme are present in human milk during all stages of lactation,[51-54] but longitudinal changes in quantities of lysozyme during lactation are unlike most other immune factors in human milk. The mean concentration of lysozyme is about 70 μg/ml in colostrum,[51] 20 μg/ml at 1 month, and 250 μg/ml by 6 months of lactation.[52] The approximate mean daily intake of milk lysozyme in healthy full-term, completely breast-fed infants is 3 to 4 mg/kg per day at 1 month and 6 mg/kg per day by 4 months of age.[54] The high content of lysozyme in human milk and its *in vitro* resistance to proteolysis are in keeping with an eightfold increase in the amount of lysozyme excreted in the stools of low birth weight infants fed human milk compared with findings in infants fed a cow's milk formula.[57] However, in contrast to secretory IgA and lactoferrin, the urinary excretion of this protein is not increased in infants fed human milk.[59]

The lysozyme C gene gave rise some 300 to 400 million years ago to a gene that codes for α-lactalbumin, a protein expressed only in the lactating mammary gland. The protein is a component of lactose synthetase. It is of interest that three domains of this evolutionary descendant of lysozyme are antibacterial.[79] Furthermore, multimeric α-lactalbumin may be antineoplastic.[80]

Fibronectin

Fibronectin, a high molecular weight protein that facilitates the uptake of many types of particulates by mononuclear phagocytes, is present in human milk (mean concentration in colostrum, 13 μg/ml).[81] The *in vivo* effects of this broad-spectrum opsonin in human milk are not known.

Complement Components

All components of the classical and alternative pathways of complement are in human milk, but the concentrations of these components, except for C3, are low.[82,83]

Human Milk Mucin

Milk mucins are high molecular weight proteins that are greatly glycosylated.[84] About two-thirds of the mucin in human milk is membrane bound. The concentration of mucin in human milk is between 50 and 90 mg/ml. A number of milk mucins have been identified. The most prominent one is MUC1. MUC1 has molecular weights between 250 and 450 kDa and is primarily bound to membranes of milk fat globules. In that respect, human milk fat globules and mucin from their membranes inhibit the binding of S-fimbriated *E. coli* to human epithelial cells.[85]

The *in vivo* fate of ingested MUC1 has been investigated. It has been found to be resistant to intragastric digestion in preterm infants.[86] Major fragments of MUC1 are detected in feces of breast-fed infants.[87] Furthermore, mucins from such feces are more able to inhibit bacterial adhesion than feces from formula-fed infants.[88]

Lactadhedrin

It was originally reported that human milk mucin defended against rotavirus, the most common cause of infectious enteritis in human infants, in an experimental murine model.[89] Rotavirus bound not only to the milk-mucin complex, but also to a 49-kDa component of the complex. The active component was later found to be a separate glycoprotein that was designated as lactadherin.[90] Like human MUC1, lactadhedrin is resistant to intragastric digestion.[91]

Oligosaccharides and Glycoconjugates

Oligosaccharides in human milk are produced by glycosyltransferases in the mammary gland. Some of these abundant compounds are receptor analogues that inhibit the binding of certain enteric or respiratory bacterial pathogens and their toxins to epithelial cells.[92-95] Many types of oligosaccharides have been identified in human milk, and new types are still being recognized.[96,97]

Oligosaccharides in human milk are different than those found in commercial milk formulas. Although the quantities of total gangliosides in human and bovine milk are similar, the relative frequencies of each type of ganglioside in milk from these two species are distinct. For example, much more monosialoganglioside 3 and GM_1 are found in human than bovine milk.[97-99]

The chemistry of these compounds dictates the specificity of their binding to the adherence structures of bacterial pathogens. For example, GM_1 gangliosides are receptor analogues for toxins produced by *V. cholerae* and *E. coli*,[93] whereas the globotriaosylceramide Gb3 binds to the β subunits of Shigatoxin.[100] A fucosyloligosaccharide inhibits the stable toxin of *E. coli*,[94] whereas a different one inhibits *Campylobacter jejuni*.[101] Oligosaccharides in human milk also interfere with the attachment of *Haemophilus influenzae* and *Streptococcus pneumoniae*.[95] In that regard, G1cNAc(β1-3) Gal-disaccharide subunits block the attachment of *S. pneumoniae* to respiratory epithelium.

In vivo animal experiments also suggest that oligosaccharides and glycoconjugates in human milk protect against certain enteric bacterial infections.[102] In that regard, certain human milk oligosaccharides survive passage through the alimentary tract[103] and some of the absorbed carbohydrate is then excreted into the urinary tract.[104] Sugars that are present in several glycoconjugates including mucins, lactadherin, and secretory IgA also interfere with the binding of bacterial pathogens to epithelial cells.[105]

In addition to the direct antibacterial effects of the carbohydrates in human milk, nitrogen-containing oligosaccharides, glycoproteins, and glycopeptides in human milk are growth promoters for *Lactobacilli* and *Bifidobacilli*.[106, 107] For example, the growth-promoter activity associated with caseins may reside in the oligosaccharide moiety of those complex molecules.[107]

These factors are responsible to a great extent for the predominance of *Lactobacilli* and *Bifidobacilli* in the bacterial flora of the large intestine of breast-fed infants found in most studies. The bacteria produce large amounts of acetic acid, which aids in suppressing multiplication of enteropathogens. It has also been reported that *Lactobacilli* strain GG aids in the recovery from acute rotavirus infections[108] and may enhance the formation of specific IgG, IgA, and IgM antibodies.[109] In addition, enteric commensal bacteria may stimulate the production of low molecular weight, antibacterial peptides, such as defensins.[101] These types of defense mechanisms may contribute to the comparative paucity in stools of breast-fed infants of bacterial pathogens most often found in urinary tract infections (P-fimbriated *E. coli*).[111]

Lipids

Fatty acids and monoglycerides generated by the enzymatic digestion of lipid substrates in human milk disrupt enveloped viruses.[112-114] These antiviral lipids may aid in prevent coronavirus infections of the intestinal tract[115] and defend against intestinal parasites such as *Giardia lamblia* and *Entameoba histolytica*.[116, 117] Monoglycerides from milk lipid hydrolysis also inactivate certain gram-positive and gram-negative bacteria.[118]

The *in vivo* hydrolysis of ingested milk lipids in early infancy occurs because of two enzymatic mechanisms. The first is due to the action of lingual lipase and the second is due to the activation of human milk bile–salt stimulated lipase in the duodenum. Thus, it is likely that the products of lipid digestion contribute to the defense of the breast-fed infant against enteric infections.

LEUKOCYTES IN HUMAN MILK

Living leukocytes are found in human milk.[119] In contrast to B cells that transform into plasma cells that remain sessile in the mammary gland, other leukocytes attracted to the site traverse the mammary epithelium and become part of the milk secretions. The highest concentrations of leukocytes in human milk occur in the first few days of lactation ($1-3 \times 10^6$/ml).[120] The several types of leukocytes and their major features follow.

Lymphocytes

The relative frequencies of T cells and B cells among lymphocytes in early human milk secretions are 83% and 6%, respectively.[121] The small number of natural killer (NK) cells in human milk[121] is in keeping with the low cytotoxic activity of human milk leukocytes.[122] The small number of B cells is a reflection that most B cells that enter the lamina propria of the mammary gland transform into sessile plasma cells.

Both $CD4^+$ (helper) and $CD8^+$ (cytotoxic/suppressor) T-cell subpopulations are present in human milk,[121, 123] but compared with human blood T cells, the proportion of cytotoxic/suppressor T cells ($CD8^+$) in human milk is increased.[121] Virtually all $CD4^+$ and $CD8^+$ T cells in human milk bear the CD45 isoform, CD45RO, that is indicative of cellular activation.[121,124] In addition, an increased proportion of the T cells displays other phenotypic markers of activation.[121,124]

T cells in human milk produce certain cytokines such as interferon-γ,[124] macrophage migration inhibitory factor,[120] and a monocyte chemotactic factor.[120] The production of interferon-γ is consistent with the CD45RO phenotype of T cells in human milk[121, 123] and the finding that $CD45RO^+$ T cells are the major source of that cytokine.[121] Additional cytokines are produced by human milk leukocytes,[124] but the extents of their production and secretion have not been determined.

Neutrophils and Macrophages

Neutrophils and macrophages in human milk are laden with milk fat globules and perhaps with other membranes that have been phagocytized. Because of these intracytoplasmic bodies, the cells are difficult to identify by common staining methods. They can be identified however by their content of myeloperoxidase (in the case of neutrophils),[120] nonspecific esterase (in the case of macrophages),[120] or by the surface expression of CD14 (in the case of macrophages).[125] Both types of cells in human milk are phagocytic. There is some evidence that the respiratory burst occurs in milk macrophages after stimulation,[126] but their intracellular killing activities appear to be reduced. The macrophages have also been found to process and present antigens to T cells.[127]

After exposure to chemoattractants, human milk neutrophils (compared with blood neutrophils) do not increase their adherence, polarity, directed migration,[128] or deformability.[129] Some of those features appear to be due to agents in human milk. For example, the decreased calcium influx by human milk neutrophils has been duplicated by incubating blood neutrophils in human milk.[130] Unlike human milk neutrophils, the motility of macrophages in human milk is increased compared with their counterparts in blood.[131] These features of neutrophils and macrophages in human milk appear to be due to cellular activation, because these cells display phenotypic markers of activation including an increased expression of CD11b/CD18 and a decreased expression of CD62L (L-selectin).[125]

Potential *in Vivo* Effects

The *in vivo* fate and role of human milk leukocytes in defense of the infant are not well understood. The area about the upper alimentary and respiratory tracts seems to provide potential sites for human milk leukocytes to enter. It is of considerable interest that small numbers of memory T cells are detected in blood in infancy.[132] Thus, it may be possible that maternal memory T cells in milk compensate for the developmental delay in their production in the infant. There is evidence from experimental animal studies that milk lymphocytes enter tissues of the neonate,[120] but that has not been demonstrated in humans. There are also reports of transfer of cellular immunity by breast-feeding.[133] It will be important to ascertain whether those reports will be verified by testing for cellular immunity against many different antigens in young infants who have or have not been breast-fed.

ANTI-INFLAMMATORY AGENTS

Inflammatory agents and systems that give rise to them are poorly represented in human milk.[25] These include (1) the coagulation system, (2) the kallikrein-kininogen system, (3) major components of the complement system, (4) IgE, (5) basophils, mast cells, eosinophils, and (6) cytotoxic lymphocytes. Certain proinflammatory cytokines (see subsequent discussion) are found in human milk, but there is no clinical evidence that they generate inflammatory processes in the recipient.

In contrast to the paucity of inflammatory agents, human milk contains a host of anti-inflammatory agents.[25] They include (1) factors that promote the growth of epithelium and thus strengthen mucosal barriers, (2) antioxidants, (3) agents such as lactoferrin that interfere with certain complement components,[25,134] (4) enzymes that degrade mediators of inflammation, (5) protease inhibitors,[135] (6) agents that bind to substrates such as lysozyme to elastin,[136] (7) cytoprotective agents such as prostaglandins E_1, E_2, and $F_{2\alpha}$,[137,138] and (8) agents that inhibit the functions of inflammatory leukocytes (Table 163–3).[25] Like the antimicrobial factors, many of these factors are adapted to operate in the hostile environment of the alimentary tract.

The main antioxidants in human milk include an ascorbate-like compound,[139] uric acid,[139] α-tocopherol[140,141] and β-carotene.[140,141] In fact, blood levels of α-tocopherol and β-carotene are higher in breast-fed than formula-fed infants not supplemented with those agents.[141]

Mucosal growth factors in human milk include epithelial growth factor,[142] lactoferrin,[143] cortisol,[144] and polyamines.[145,146] Other hormones and growth factors in human milk[147] may also affect the growth, differentiation, and turnover of epithelial cells. These agents may therefore limit the penetration of free antigens and pathogenic microorganisms and affect other barrier functions of the intestinal tract. In keeping with that notion, there are significant differences between the biophysical and biochemical organization and functions of mucosal barriers in adults and

neonates.[148,149] Furthermore, maturation of those functions may be accelerated by human milk.[150,151]

Enzymes in human milk degrade inflammatory mediators that may damage the gastrointestinal tract. In that respect, platelet-activating factor (PAF) plays a role in an intestinal injury in rats induced by endotoxin and hypoxia.[152] Furthermore, an acetylhydrolase that degrades PAF is present in human milk,[153] and the production of human PAF-acetylhydrolase is developmentally delayed.[154] Published results of investigations also indicate that human milk feedings lessen intestinal permeability in young infants.[155-157]

IMMUNOMODULATING AGENTS

Three sets of observations provide the basis of the concept of immunomodulating agents in human milk:

1. Epidemiologic investigations suggest that older children who were breast-fed during infancy may be at less risk for developing certain chronic diseases that are mediated by immunologic, inflammatory, or oncogenic mechanisms. The diseases in question are type 1 diabetes mellitus,[158] lymphomas,[159] acute lymphocytic leukemia,[160] and Crohn's disease.[161] Although preventing or lessening infections by antimicrobial agents or by anti-inflammatory agents in human milk may have long-term consequences, agents that influence the development of systemic or mucosal defenses of the infant may also be responsible for those possible long-term effects.

2. Increased levels of certain immune factors in breast-fed infants cannot be accounted for by passive transfer of those substances from human milk. Breast-feeding primes the recipient to produce higher blood levels of interferon-α in response to respiratory syncytial virus infections.[162] In addition, increments in blood levels of fibronectin achieved by breast-feeding cannot be accounted for by the amounts of that protein in human milk. Moreover, breast-feeding leads to a more rapid development of systemic[163] and secretory[163,164] antibody responses and of secretory IgA in external secretions[57-59] including urine,[58,59] which is far removed from the route of ingestion. Therefore, those increments are not due to absorption of those same factors from human milk.

3. The third line of evidence is the discovery that all leukocytes in human milk are activated (see previous section on leukocytes). Investigations revealed that human milk enhances the movement of blood monocytes *in vitro*. In addition, much of that motility was abrogated by antibodies to tumor necrosis factor-α (TNF-α).[165] Subsequently, TNF-α in human milk was detected immunochemically.[166]

TABLE 163–3

Anti-Inflammatory Factors in Human Milk.

Categories	Examples
Cytoprotectives	Prostaglandins E2, F2α
Epithelial growth factors	Epidermal growth factor, lactoferrin, polyamines
Maturational factors	Cortisol
Enzymes that degrade mediators	PAF-AH
Binders of enzymes	α1-antichymotrypsin
Binders of substrates of enzymes	Lysozyme to elastin
Modulators of leukocytes	Interleukin-10
Antioxidants	Uric acid, α-tocopherol, β-carotene, ascorbate

PAF-AH = Platelet activating factor–acetylhydrolase

Many other cytokines have been found in human milk. They include Th1 cytokines such as interferon-γ,[167] interleukin (IL)-12,[168] and IL-18[169]; proinflammatory cytokines including IL-1β[170] and IL-6[171, 172]; chemotaxins including IL-8,[173] regulated on activation, normal T expressed and secreted (RANTES),[174] and eotaxin[174]; antiinflammatory agents such as transforming growth factor-β (TGF-β)[173, 175] and IL-10[176]; and the cellular growth factors EGF,[142] granulocyte colony-stimulating factor (G-CSF),[177] macrophage-CSF,[178] hepatic growth factor,[179] and erythropoietin[180] (Table 163–4). There are controversies concerning the quantities of some of these agents in human milk. The discrepancies between the results of some of the studies may depend on differences in storage conditions of the specimens and the types of immunoassays. The sites and extents of their effects on the recipient infant are not determined.

Several other immunomodulating agents are in human milk including β-casomorphins,[181] prolactin,[182, 183] antiidiotypic antibodies,[50] α-tocopherol[140, 141] and a host of nucleotides that enhance NK-cell, macrophage, and Th1-cell activities.[184-186]

RELATIONSHIPS BETWEEN THE IMMUNE SYSTEMS IN HUMAN MILK AND THE RECIPIENT

As previously mentioned, seven somewhat overlapping evolutionary outcomes concerning the relationships between the immune status of infants and defense agents in human milk have been recognized.[50, 51] In respect to the first evolutionary outcome, many aspects of the human immune system are incompletely developed at birth, and the immaturity is most marked in very low birth weight infants. These developmental delays include (1) the mobilization and function of neutrophils,[187] (2) the production of lysozyme[188] and secretory IgA[189,190] at mucosal sites, (3) memory T cells that bear CD45RO,[135] (4) the complete expression of the antibody repertoire,[191] and (5) the production of certain cytokines including TNF-α,[192, 193] IL-4,[194] interferon-γ,[194,195] IL-6,[192] IL-10,[193] G-CSF,[196] GM-CSF,[197] and IL-3.[196]

Many of those developmentally delayed defense factors are well represented in human milk (Table 163–5). For example, secretory IgA antibodies in human milk compensate for the low production of secretory IgA at mucosal sites during early infancy. It is also important that the antibody response achieved through this pathway is polyclonal and is directed against not only protein, but also polysaccharide antigens, because infants display a more restricted clonality[198] and do not mount an IgG antibody response to polysaccharide antigens.[199] The problem has been modified by the introduction of conjugate vaccines. Even so, the antibody response to conjugate vaccines is higher in breast-fed than cow's milk-fed infants.[200]

An additional example is the interrelationship between the amount of lysozyme produced by the infant and the quantity secreted into milk. Indeed, the necessity of high lysozyme levels in human milk is coupled to the low production of the protein by mucosal cells during infancy.[188] It is likely that the attainment of normal intraluminal concentrations of lysozyme in infancy is dependent on breast-feeding. This is in keeping with the finding of higher lysozyme activities in stools of breast-fed than in non-breast-fed infants.[57]

The potential *in vivo* effects of immune factors in human milk in the recipient infant depend on the survival of those agents. Although it may be argued that defense agents in human milk would be destroyed by the digestive processes in the gastrointestinal tract, many of these agents may be bioactive in the alimentary and respiratory tracts for the following reasons:

1. Protein components may affect the epithelium, leukocytes, or other cells of proximal parts of the alimentary or respiratory tracts where proteolytic enzymes are not produced.
2. Ingested proteins may escape intragastric-intraduodenal digestion because of developmental delays in the production of gastric HCl and pancreatic proteases.[201] This resistance to digestion may be augmented by the protection provided by the buffering capacity of human milk that shields some acid-labile components of milk, antiproteases in human milk,[135] inherent resistance of many defense agents in human milk to digestive processes, and the protection against digestion of some defense agents in human milk because they are compartmentalized.[166, 172] In that respect, much of the TNF-α in human milk is bound to soluble receptors.[202]

This thesis is borne out as previously discussed by an increased survival of certain human milk defense agents in the alimentary tract of the recipient infant.

PROTECTION OF PREMATURE INFANTS BY HUMAN MILK

Maturational delays of the immune system are generally more profound in premature infants. Furthermore, the potential immunologic problems are compounded by the shortened duration of placental transfer of IgG to the fetus.[203] That predisposes premature infants to certain opportunistic infections. Moreover, major medical problems during the newborn period including pulmonary diseases,[204] nutritional imbalances, and invasive clinical procedures increase the risks of premature infants to infections.

TABLE 163–4

Potential Functions of Certain Cytokines in Human Milk

Cytokines	Possible Functions
Interferon-γ	T-helper 1 cytokine-macrophage activator
Interleukin-1β	Activates T cells and macrophages
Interleukin-6	Enhances IgA production
Interleukin-8	Chemotaxin for neutrophils and CD8+ T cells
Interleukin-10	Th2 cytokine
	Inhibits production of many pro inflammatory cytokines
Interleukin-12	Th1 cytokine
	Enhances production of interferon-γ
TNF-α	Enhances production of polymeric Ig receptors
TGF-β	Enhances isotype switching to IgA+ B cells
G-CSF	Increases granulocyte (neutrophil) production
M-CSF	Increases monocyte production

G-CSF = granulocyte colony stimulating factor; M-CSF = monocyte colony stimulating factor; TGF-β = transforming growth factor-β; TNF-α = tumor necrosis factor-α.

TABLE 163–5

Representative Immune Factors in Human Milk the Production of Which Is Delayed in the Recipient Infant

Agents	Time of Maturation
Secretory IgA	~4–12 mo
Full antibody repertoire	~2 yr
Memory T cells	~2 yr
Lysozyme	~1–2 yr
Lactoferrin	?
Interferon-γ	?
Interleukin-6	?
Interleukin-8	?
Interleukin-10	?
TNF-α	?
PAF-acetylhydrolase	?

PAF-AH = platelet activating factor-acetylhydrolase; TNF-α = tumor necrosis factor-α

Milk from women who have delivered prematurely contains many of the same antimicrobial factors that are found in milk from women who have delivered after a full-term pregnancy.[205] These include secretory IgA, lactoferrin, and lysozyme. The concentrations of those defense agents are higher in preterm than term milk. Those higher concentrations may be in large part due to a lower volume of milk produced by women who have delivered prematurely. That may not be the total explanation for the higher concentrations in that the patterns of the concentrations of some of the antimicrobial factors in preterm and term milk are not exactly the same.[205] Moreover, the concentrations of most anti-inflammatory and immunomodulating factors in preterm milk have not been established.

In addition to the protection against enteric infections and respiratory infections such as otitis media, there are several indications that human milk feedings protect premature infants against systemic infections that are more prone to occur in immature infants. Winberg and his colleagues in Sweden[206] reported that the risk of bacterial sepsis was less in premature newborn infants who were fed human milk. These observations were confirmed by Yu and co-workers in Australia[207] and Nayaryanan and her associates in India,[208] who found that supplemental feedings of expressed human milk were associated with a reduced frequency of infections in low birth weight infants.

Human milk also protects against many cases of necrotizing enterocolitis (NEC).[209] The factors in human milk that are responsible for this protection remain to be elucidated, but evidence from human and experimental animal studies suggests that IgA,[210] erythropoietin,[211,212] PAF-acetylhydrolase,[153] and IL-10[213] are likely possibilities. In each case, there is a developmental delay in the production of the suspected factor, and the agent in question is well-represented in human milk.

Two contrasting experimental animal models of cytokine gene deficiency suggest that anti-inflammatory cytokines in human milk may prevent disorders due to inflammatory processes. Mice homozygous for the TGF-β1 null gene display spontaneous, infiltrations of macrophages and T cells in many organ sites; the lungs, heart, and salivary glands are most prominently involved.[214-216] Furthermore, there is experimental evidence that the effects of the TGF-β1 deficiency are mitigated by the ingestion of that cytokine in murine milk.[216]

In the second animal model, a targeted IL-10 gene deletion was engineered in mice. In those IL-10–deficient animals, a fatal enterocolitis began directly after weaning, and it was dependent on establishment of an enteric bacterial flora.[213] The enterocolitis had some features of Crohn's disease and NEC. Much of the enterocolitis in those animals was prevented by intraperitoneal injections of IL-10 given at the start of weaning.[217]

Although it has not been established whether human milk feedings protect against the pulmonary and vascular effects of hyperoxia, some experimental evidence suggests that one of the anti-inflammatory components of human milk, α_1-antitrypsin, prevents many of those features in hyperoxic neonatal rats including elevations in pulmonary elastolytic activity.[218]

The possible effects of human milk upon the development of atopic diseases have been investigated by many groups, but there is no consensus whether breast-feeding protects against those disorders,[219] except for atopic dermatitis[220] or when food allergens are avoided by complete breast-feeding. Much of the disagreement is probably due to confounding variables including variations in the genetic predisposition to atopic disorders, the sufficiency of breast-feeding, dietary exposures not appreciated by the parents, and exposures to inhalant allergens or irritants that might lead to lung damage. Furthermore, there is evidence that increased exposures to infectious diseases facilitate Th1 responses that lead to the development of cellular immunity, whereas much lower exposures engender Th2 responses that lead to antibody formation and hence to possible IgE-mediated

hypersensitivity. Thus, the effect of breast-feeding on the risk of atopic diseases may well depend on a multiplicity of factors that are not equally represented in all investigated populations.

Moreover, the question is complicated by the transmission of foreign food antigens in human milk[221] and the triggering of allergic reactions by those antigens in some recipient infants.[222] Why only a subpopulation of breast-fed infants develops atopic diseases is unknown. To establish whether a breast-fed infant is reacting to a foreign food antigen in human milk, it is necessary to conduct trials of dietary elimination and oral challenge with the food in question in the mother while she is breast-feeding.[223] If those trials suggest that the infant is reacting to a foreign food antigen in human milk, then the problem may be avoided by eliminating the food allergen from the maternal diet. If the food allergen is a basic food such as cow's milk, the woman must have a diet that supplies the correct types and quantities of nutrients to meet the needs of lactation.[20] If long-term elimination is impractical, then breast-feeding may be stopped and the infant tried on a hypoallergenic formula. In addition, the development of allergic disease in breast-fed infants may be due to alterations in the types of fatty acids found in milks produced by mothers of the allergic infants.[224,225]

The influence of human milk feedings upon the rate of rehospitalizations of premature infants was examined in the 1988 National Maternal and Infant Health Survey conducted by The National Institutes of Child Health and Human Development.[226] Although a cause-effect relationship could not be definitively established, the feeding of human milk was an independent predictor of decreased risk for rehospitalization. Thus, human milk feeding may have beneficial effects on the premature infant that extend beyond the initial hospitalization.

CODA

Human milk contains an array of host resistance factors that are antimicrobial, anti-inflammatory, or immunomodulating. This immune system is adapted to function at mucosal sites and to protect the recipient against a host of infectious and inflammatory processes that are common in the developing infant. In addition, there may be long-term health benefits to the recipient by human milk feedings that apparently are due to alterations in the immune system.

The precise ways in which the immunologic agents in human milk protect the child and how those agents interact with the developing immune system of the recipient are not well understood. These research issues will require the coordinated efforts of neonatologists, immunologists, molecular biologists, and other clinical and basic scientists.

ACKNOWLEDGMENTS

We thank Mrs. Susan C. Kovacevich for her assistance in the preparation of this chapter.

REFERENCES

1. Ehrlich P: Experimentelle Untersuchangen über Immunität. I. ueber ricin. Dtsch Med Wochenschr 1891;32: 1.
2. Ehrlich P: Experimentelle Untersuchangen über Immunität. II. Üeber abrin. Dtsch Med Wochenschr 1891;44: 1.
3. Woodbury RM: The relation between breast and artificial feeding and infant mortality. Am J Hygiene 1922;2: 668.
4. Grulee CG, Sanford HN, Herron PH: Breast and artificially-fed infants. Influence on morbidity and mortality of twenty thousand infants. JAMA 1934;103: 735.
5. Grulee CG, Sandford HN, Schwartz H: Breast and artificially-fed infants. A study of the age incidence in the morbidity and mortality in twenty thousand cases. JAMA 1935;104: 1986.
6. Wyatt RG, Mata LJ: Bacteria in colostrum and milk of Guatemalan Indian women. J Trop Pediatr 1969;15: 159.

7. Mata LJ, Urrutia JJ, Gordon JE: Diarrhoeal disease in a cohort of Guatemalan village children observed from birth to age two years. Trop Geogr Med 1967;19: 247.

8. Mata LJ, Urrutia JJ, García B: Shigella infection in breast-fed Guatemalan Indian neonates. Am J Dis Child 1969;117: 142.

9. Glass RI, Stoll BJ: The protective effect of human milk against diarrhea: a review of studies from Bangladesh. Acta Paediatr Scand (Suppl) 1989;351: 131.

10. Clemens JB, Stanton B, Stoll B, et al: Breast-feeding as a determinant of severity in shigellosis: evidence for protection throughout the first three years of life in Bangladeshi children. Am J Epidemiol 1986;123: 710.

11. Glass RI, Svennerholm AM, Stoll BJ, et al: Protection against Cholera in breast-fed children by antibodies in breast milk. N Engl J Med 1983;308: 1389.

12. Totterdell BM, Chrystie IL, Banatvala JE: Rotavirus infection in a maternity unit. Arch Dis Child 1976;51: 924.

13. McLean BS, Holmes IH: Effects of antibodies, trypsin and trypsin inhibitors on susceptibility of neonates to rotavirus infections. J Clin Microbiol 1981;13: 22.

14. Duffy LC, Riepenhoff-Talty M, Byers TE, et al: Modulation of rotavirus enteritis during breastfeeding. Am J Dis Child 1986;140: 1164.

15. Sabin AB, Fieldsteel AH: Antipoliomyelitic activity of human and bovine colostrum and milk. Pediatrics 1962;29: 105.

16. Thapa S, Short RV, Potts M: Breast feeding, birth spacing and their effects on birth survival. Nature 1988;335: 679.

17. Downham MAPS, Scott, R, Sims DG, et al: Breast-feeding protects against respiratory syncytial virus infections. BMJ 1976;2: 274.

18. Pullan CR, Toms GL, Martin AJ, et al: Breast-feeding and respiratory syncytial virus infection. BMJ 1980;281: 1034.

19. Howie PW, Forsyth JS, Ogston SA, et al: Protective effect of breastfeeding against infection. BMJ 1990;300: 11.

20. Hamosh M, Dewey KG, Garza C, et al: Infant outcomes. Nutrition During Lactation. P 1953-1956. Washington, DC, National Academy Press, 1991.

21. Goldman, AS: The immunological system in human milk: the past—a pathway to the future. In Woodward B, Draper HH (eds): Advances in Nutritional Research. Vol 10. Immunological Properties of Milk. New York, Plenum Publishers, 2001, p 15.

22. Goldman AS, Smith CW: Host resistance factors in human milk. J Pediatr 1973;82: 1082.

23. Goldman AS, Chheda S, Garofalo R: Evolution of immunological functions of the mammary gland and the postnatal development of immunity. Pediatr Res 1998;43: 155.

24. Goldman AS: Modulation of the gastrointestinal tract of infants by human milk. Interfaces and interactions. An evolutionary perspective. J Nutrition 130(2S Suppl) 2000;426S.

25. Goldman AS, Thorpe LW, Goldblum RM, et al: Anti-inflammatory properties of human milk. Acta Paediatr Scand 1986;75: 689.

26. Garofalo RP, Goldman AS: Expression of functional immunomodulatory and antiinflammatory factors in human milk. Clin Perinatol 1999;26: 361.

27. Goldman AS, Goldblum RM: Immunoglobulins in human milk. In Atkinson SA, Lonnerdal B (eds): Protein and Non-Protein Nitrogen in Human Milk. Boca Raton, FL, CRC Press, 1989, p 43.

28. Keller MA, Heiner, DC, Kidd RM, et al: Local production of IgG4 in human colostrum. J Pediatr 1983;130: 1654.

29. Keller MA, Heiner DC, Myers AS, et al: IgD—a mucosal immunoglobulin? Pediatr Res 1984;18: 258A.

30. Underdown BJ, Knight A, Papsin FR: The relative paucity of IgE in human milk. J Immunol 1976;116: 1435.

31. Brandtzaeg P: Polymeric IgA is complexed with secretory component (SC) on the surface of human intestinal epithelial cells. Scand J Immunol 1978;8: 39.

32. Mostov KE, Blobel GA: A transmembrane precursor of secretory component. The receptor for transcellular transport of polymeric immunoglobulins. J Biol Chem 1982: 257: 11816.

33. Bakos M-A, Kurosky A, Goldblum RM, et al: Characterization of a critical binding site for human polymeric Ig on secretory component. J Immunol 1991;147: 3419.

34. Hanson LÅ: Comparative immunological studies of the immune globulins of human milk and blood serum. Int Arch Allergy Immunol 1961;18: 241.

35. Hanson LÅ, Johansson BG: Immunological characterization of chromatographically separated protein fractions from human colostrum. Int Arch Allergy Immunol 1962;20: 65.

36. Goldblum RM, Ahlstedt S, Carlsson B, et al: Antibody forming cells in human colostrum after oral immunisation. Nature (Lond) 1975;257: 797.

37. Roux ME, McWilliams M, Phillips-Quagliata JM, et al: Origin of IgA secretory plasma cells in the mammary gland. J Exp Med 1977;146: 1311.

38. Weisz-Carrington P, Roux ME, McWilliams M, et al: Hormonal induction of the secretory immune system in the mammary gland. Proc Natl Acad Sci USA 1978;75: 2928.

39. Fishaut M, Murphy DS, Neifert M, et al: Broncho-mammary axis in the immune response to respiratory syncytial virus. J Pediatr 1981;99: 186.

40. Streeter PR, Berg EL, Rouse BTN, et al: A tissue-specific endothelial cell molecule involved in lymphocyte homing. Nature 1988;331: 41.

41. Erle DJ, Briskin MJ, Butcher EC, et al: Expression and function of the MAdCAM-1 receptor, integrin α 4β7, on human leukocytes. J Immunol 1994;153: 517.

42. Beagley KW, Fujihasi K, Aicher W, et al: Mucosal homeostasis: role of interleukins, isotype-specific factors and contrasuppression in the IgA response. Immunol Invest 1989;18: 77.

43. Schultz CL, Coffman RL: Control of isotype switching by T cells and cytokines. Curr Opin Immunol 1991;3: 350.

44. Kono YL, Beagley KW, Fujihasi K, et al: Cytokine regulation of localized inflammation. Induction of activated B cells and IL-6 mediated polyclonal IgG and IgA synthesis in inflamed human gingiva. J Immunol 1991;146: 1812.

45. Whitmore AC, Prowse DM, Haughton G, et al: Ig isotype switching in B lymphocytes. The effect of T-cell derived interleukins, cytokines, cholera toxin, and antigen on isotype switch frequency of a cloned B cell lymphoma. Int Immunol 1991;3: 95.

46. Molé CM, Montagne PM, Béné MC, et al: Sequential assay of human milk immunoglobulins show a predominance of lambda chains. Lab Invest 1992;67: 147.

47. Crago SS, Kulhavy R, Prince SJ, et al: Secretory component on epithelial cells is a surface receptor for polymeric immunoglobulins. J Exp Med 1978;147: 1832.

48. Brown WR, Isobe Y, Nakane PK, et al: Studies on translocation of immunoglobulins across intestinal epithelium. II. Immunoelectron microscopic localization of immunoglobulins and secretory component in human intestinal mucosa. Gastroenterology 1976;71: 985.

49. Adderson EE, Johnston JM, Shackerford PG, et al: Development of the human antibody repertoire. Pediatr Res 1992;32: 257.

50. Hahn-Zoric M, Carlsson B, Jeansson S, et al: Anti-idiotypic antibodies to polio virus in commercial immunoglobulin preparations, human serum, and milk. Pediatr Res 1993;33: 475.

51. Goldblum RM, Garza C, Johnson CA, et al: Human milk banking II. Relative stability of immunologic factors in stored colostrum. Acta Paediatr Scand 1982;71: 143.

52. Goldman AS, Garza C, Nichols BL, et al: Immunologic factors in human milk during the first year of lactation. J Pediatr 1982;100: 563.

53. Goldman AS, Garza C, Goldblum RM: Immunologic components in human milk during the second year of lactation. Acta Paediatr Scand 1983;72: 461.

54. Butte NF, Goldblum RM, Fehl LM, et al: Daily ingestion of immunologic components in human milk during the first four months of life. Acta Paediatr Scand 1984;73: 296.

55. Lindh E: Increased resistance of immunoglobulin dimers to proteolytic degradation after binding of secretory component. J Immunol 1985;113: 284.

56. Gilbert JV, Plaut AG, Longmaid B, et al: Inhibition of bacterial IgA proteases by human secretory IgA and serum. Ann NY Acad Sci 1983;409: 625.

57. Schanler RJ, Goldblum RM, Garza C, et al: Enhanced fecal excretion of selected immune factors in very low birth weight infants fed fortified human milk. Pediatr Res 1986;20: 711.

58. Prentice A: Breast feeding increases concentrations of IgA in infants' urine. Arch Dis Child 1987;62: 792.

59. Goldblum RM, Schanler RJ, Garza C, et al: Human milk feeding enhances the urinary excretion of immunologic factors in low birth weight infants. Pediatr Res 1989;25: 184.

60. Anderson BF, Baker HM, Dodson EJ, et al: Structure of human lactoferrin at 3.1-Å resolution. Proc Natl Acad Sci USA 1987;84: 769.

61. Fransson GB, Lonnerdal B: Iron in human milk. J Pediatr 1980;96: 380.

62. Bullen JJ, Rogers HJ, Leigh L: Iron-binding proteins in milk and resistance of Escherichia coli infection in infants. BMJ 1972;1: 69.

63. Spik G, Cheron A, Montreuil J, et al: Bacteriostasis of a milk-sensitive strain of Escherichia coli by immunoglobulins and iron-binding proteins in association. Immunology 1978;35: 663.

64. Stephens S, Dolby JM, Montreuil J, et al: Differences in inhibition of the growth of commensal and enteropathogenic strains of Escherichia coli by lactoferrin and secretory immunoglobulin A isolated from human milk. Immunology 1980;41: 597.

65. Stuart J, Norrel, S., Harrington JP, et al: Kinetic effect of human lactoferrin on the growth of Escherichia coli. J Biochem 1984;16: 1043.

66. Arnold RR, Cole MF, McGhee JR: A bactericidial effect of lactoferrin. Science 1977;197: 263.

67. Bellamy W, Wakabayashi H, Takase M, et al: Killing of Candida albicans by lactoferricin B, a potent antimicrobial peptide derived from the N-terminal region of bovine lactoferrin. Med Microbiol Immunol (Berl) 1993;182: 97.

68. Yamauchi K, Tomita M, Giehl TJ, et al: Antibacterial activity of lactoferrin and a pepsin-derived lactoferrin peptide fragment. Infect Immunol 1993;61: 713.

69. Furmanski P, Li ZP, Fortuna MB, et al: Multiple molecular forms of human lactoferrin. Identification of a class of lactoferrin that possesses ribonuclease activity and lacks iron binding capacity. J Exp Med 1989;170: 415.

70. Andersen JH, Osbakk SA, Vorland LH, et al: Lactoferrin and cyclic lactoferricin inhibit the entry of human cytomegalovirus into human fibroblasts. Antiviral Res 2001;51: 141.

71. Moriuchi M, Moriuchi H: A milk protein lactoferrin enhances human T cell leukemia virus type I and suppresses HIV-1 infection. J Immunol 2001;166: 4231.

72. Arnold D, Di Biase AM, Marchetti M, et al: Antiadenovirus activity of milk proteins: lactoferrin prevents viral infection. Antiviral Res 2002;53: 153.

73. Brines RD, Brock JH: The effect of trypsin and chymotrypsin on the in vitro antimicrobial and iron-binding properties of lactoferrin in human milk and bovine colostrum. Biochim Biophys Acta 1983;759: 229.

74. Spik G, Brunet B, Mazurier-Dehaine C, et al: Characterization and properties of the human and bovine lactotransferrins extracted from the feces of newborn infants. Acta Paediatr Scand 1982;71: 979.

75. Davidson LA, Lonnerdal B: The persistence of human milk proteins in the breast-fed infant. Acta Paediatr Scand 1987;76: 733.

76. Goldman AS, Garza C, Schanler RJ, et al: Molecular forms of lactoferrin in stool and urine from infants fed human milk. Pediatr Res 1990;27: 252.

77. Hutchens TW, Henry JF, Yip TT, et al: Origin of intact lactoferrin and its DNA-binding fragments found in the urine of human milk-fed preterm infants. Evaluation of stable isotopic enrichment. Pediatr Res 1991;29: 243.

78. Chipman DM, Sharon N: Mechanism of lysozyme action. Science 1969; 165: 454.

79. Pelligrini A, Thomas U, Bramaz N, et al: Isolation and identification of three bactericidal domains in the bovine α-lactalbumin molecule. Biochim Biophys Acta 1999;1426: 439.

80. Håkansson A, Andréasson J, Zhivotosky B, et al: Multimeric α-lactalbumin from human milk induces apoptosis through a direct effect on cell nuclei. Exp Cell Res 1999;246: 451.

81. Friss HE, Rubin LG, Carsons S, et al: Plasma fibronectin concentrations in breast fed and formula fed neonates. Arch Dis Child 1988;63: 528.

82. Ballow M, Fang F, Good RA, et al: Developmental aspects of complement components in the newborn. The presence of complement components and C3 proactivator (properdin factor B) in human colostrum. Clin Exp Immunol 1974;18: 257.

83. Nakajima S, Baba AS, Tamura N: Complement system in human colostrum: presence of nine complement components and factors of alternative pathway in human colostrum. Int Arch Allergy Appl Immunol 1977;54: 428.

84. Schroten H: Chemistry of milk mucins and their anti-microbial action. In Woodward B, Draper HH (eds): Advances in Nutritional Research. Vol 10. Immunological Properties of Milk. New York, Plenum Publishers, 2001, pp 231–245.

85. Schroten J, Hanisch FG, Plogmann R, et al: Inhibition of adhesion of S-fimbriated Escherichia coli to buccal epithelial cells by human milk fat globule membrane components: a novel aspect of the protective function of mucins in the nonimmunoglobulin fraction. Pediatr Res 1992;32: 58.

86. Peterson JA, Hamosh M, Scallan CD, et al: Milk fat globule glycoproteins in human milk and in gastric aspirates of mother's milk-fed preterm infants. Pediatr Res 1998;44: 499.

87. Patton S: Detection of large fragments of human milk mucin MUC1 in feces of breast-fed infants. J Pediatr Gastroenterol Nutr 1994;18: 225.

88. Schroten H, Lethen R, Hanish F-G, et al: Inhibition of adhesion of S-fimbriated E coli to epithelial cells by meconium, stool of breast-fed and formula-fed infants—mucins are the major inhibitory component. J Pediatr Gastroenterol Nutr 1992;15: 150.

89. Yolken RH, Peterson JA, Vonderfecht SL, et al: Human milk mucin inhibits rotavirus replication and prevents experimental gastroenteritis. J Clin Invest 1992;90: 1984.

90. Newburg D, Peterson J, Ruiz-Palacios G, et al: Role of human-milk lactadhedrin in protection against symptomatic rotavirus infection. Lancet 1998;351: 1160.

91. Peterson JA, Hamosh M, Scallan CD, et al: Milk fat globule glycoproteins in human milk and in gastric aspirates of mother's milk-fed preterm infants. Pediatr Res 1998;44: 499.

92. Holmgren J, Svennerholm A-M, Ahren C: Inhibition of bacterial adhesion and toxin binding by glycoconjugate and oligosaccharide receptor analogues in human milk. In Goldman AS, Atkinson SA, Hanson LÅ (eds): Human Lactation 3: The Effects of Human Milk on the Recipient Infant. New York and London, Plenum Press, 1987, p 251.

93. Laegreid A, Kolsto Otnaess A-B: Trace amounts of ganglioside GM1 in human milk inhibit enterotoxins from Vibrio cholerae and Escherichia coli. Life Sci 1987;40: 55.

94. Newburg DS, Pickering LK, McCluer RH, et al: Fucosylated oligosaccharides of human milk protect suckling mice from heat-stable enterotoxin of Escherichia coli. J Infect Dis 1990;162: 1075.

95. Andersson B, Porras O, Hanson LA[o], et al: Inhibition of attachment of Streptococcus pneumoniae and Haemophilus influenzae by human milk and receptor oligosaccharides. J Infect Dis 1986;153: 232.

96. Stahl B, Thurl S, Zeng J, et al: Oligosaccharides from human milk as revealed by matrix-associated laser desorption/ionization mass spectrometry. Anal Biochem 1994;223: 218.

97. Newburg DS, Neubauer SH: Carbohydrates in milk: analysis, quantities, and significance. In Jensen RG (ed): Handbook of Milk Composition. San Diego, Academic Press, 1995, p 273.

98. Laegreid A, Kolsto Otnaess A-B, Bryn K, et al: Human and bovine milk: comparison of ganglioside composition and enterotoxin-inhibitory activity. Pediatr Res 1986;20: 416.

99. Newburg DS: Oligosaccharides and glycoconjugates in human milk. J Mammary Gland Biol Neopl 1996;1: 271.

100. Newburg DS, Ashkenazi S, Cleary TG: Human milk contains the Shiga toxin and Shiga-like toxin receptor glycolipid Gb₃. J Infect Dis 1992;166: 832.

101. Newburg DS: Human milk glycoconjugates that inhibit pathogens. Curr Med Chem 1999;6: 117.

102. Newburg DS: Do the binding properties of oligosaccharides in human milk protect human infants from gastrointestinal bacteria? J Nutr 1997;127(5 Suppl): 980S.

103. Chaturvedi P, Warren CD, Buescher CR, et al: Survival of human milk oligosaccharides in the intestine of infants. Adv Exp Med Biol 2001;501: 315.

104. Rudloff S, Dickmann L, Kunz C: Urinary excretion of lactose and complex oligosaccharides in preterm infants. In Allen L, King J, Lonnerdahl B (eds): Nutrient Regulation During Pregnancy, Lactation, and Infant Growth. New York, Plenum Press, 1994.

105. Wold AE, Mestecky J, Tomana M, et al: Secretory IgA carries oligosaccharides for Escherichia coli type 1 fimbrial lectins. Infect Immunol 1990;58: 3073.

106. György P, Jeanloz RW, Von Nicolai H, et al: Undialyzable growth factors for Lactobacillus bifidus var. Pennsylvanicus. Eur J Biochem 1974;43: 29.

107. Bezkorovainy A, Topouzian N: Bifidobacterium bifidus var. Pennsylvanicus growth promoting activity of human milk casein and its derivates. Int J Biochem 1981;13: 585.

108. Isolauri E, Juntunen M, Rautanen T, et al: A human Lactobacillus strain (Lactobacillus GG) promotes recovery from acute diarrhea in children. Pediatrics 1991;88: 90.

109. Kaila M, Isolauri E, Soppi E, et al: Enhancement of the circulating antibody secreting cell response in human diarrhea by a human Lactobacillus strain. Pediatr Res 1992;32: 141.

110. Krisanaprakornkit S, Kimball JR, Weinberg A, et al: Inducible expression of human β defensin 2 by Fusobacterium nucleatum in oral epithelial cells: multiple signaling pathways and role of commensal bacteria in innate immunity and the epithelial barrier. Infect Immunol 2000;68: 2907.

111. Mulvey MA: Adhesion and entry of uropathogenic Escherichia coli. Cell Microbiol 2002;4:257.

112. Welsh JK, Arsenakis M, Coelen RJ, et al: Effect of antiviral lipids, heat, and freezing on the activity of viruses in human milk. J Infect Dis 1979;140: 332.

113. Issacs CE, Thormar H, Pessolano T: Membrane-disruptive effect of human milk: Inactivation of enveloped viruses. J Infect Dis 1986;154: 966.

114. Thromar H, Isaacs CE, Brown HR, et al: Inactivation of enveloped viruses and killing of cells by fatty acids and monoglycerides. Antimicrob Agents Chemother Am Soc Microbiol 1987;32: 27.

115. Resta S, Luby JP, Rosenfeld CR, et al: Isolation and propagation of a human enteric coronavirus. Science 1985;229: 978.

116. Gillin FD, Reiner DS, Wang CS: Human milk kills parasitic protozoa. Science 1983;221: 1290.

117. Gillin FD, Reiner DS, Gault MJ: Cholate-dependent killing of Giardia lamblia by human milk. Infect Immun 1985;47: 619.

118. Issacs CE, Litov RE, Thromar H: Antimicrobial activity of lipids added to human milk, infant formula, and bovine milk. J Nutr Biochem 1995;6: 362.

119. Smith CW, Goldman AS: The cells of human colostrum. I. In vitro studies of morphology and functions. Pediatr Res 1968;2: 103.

120. Goldman AS, Goldblum RM: Transfer of maternal leukocytes to the infant by human milk. In Olding L (ed): Reproductive Immunology/Current Topics in Microbiology and Immunology. Heidelberg, Springer Verlag EMBH, 1997, p 205.

121. Wirt D, Adkins LT, Palkowetz KH, et al: Activated-memory T cells in human milk. Cytometry 1992;13: 282.

122. Kohl S, Pickering LK, Cleary TG, et al: Human colostral cytotoxicity. II. Relative defects in colostral leukocyte cytotoxicity and inhibition of peripheral blood leukocyte cytotoxicity by colostrum. J Infect Dis 1980;142: 884.

123. Bertotto A, Gerli R, Fabietti G, et al: Human breast milk T cells display the phenotype and functional characteristics of memory T cells. Eur J Immunol 1990;20: 1877.

124. Keller MA, Kidd RM, Bryson YJ, et al: Lymphokine production by human milk lymphocytes. Infect Immun 1981;32: 632.

125. Keeney SE, Schmalstieg FC, Palkowetz KH, et al: Activated neutrophils and neutrophil activators in human milk. Increased expression of CD11b and decreased expression of L-selectin. J Leukoc Biol 1993;54: 97.

126. Tsuda H, Takeshige K, Shibata Y, et al: Oxygen metabolism of human colostral macrophages. J Biochem 1984;95: 1237.

127. Osenberg JR, Persitz E, Brautbar C, et al: Cellular immunity in human milk. Am J Reprod Immunol Microbiol 1985;8: 125.

128. Thorpe LW, Rudloff HE, Powell LC, et al: Decreased response of human milk leukocytes to chemoattractant peptides. Pediatr Res 1986;20: 373.

129. Buescher ES: The effects of colostrum on neutrophil function: decreased deformability with increased cytoskeletal-associated actin. In Mestecky J, Blair C, Ogra P (eds): Immunology of Milk and the Neonate. New York, Plenum Press, 1991, p 131.

130. Chacon-Cruz E, Oelberg DG, Buescher ES: Human milk effects on neutrophil calcium metabolism: blockade of calcium influx after agonist stimulation. Pediatr Res 1999;46: 200.

131. Özkaragoz F, Rudloff HE, Rajaraman S, et al: The motility of human milk macrophages in collagen gels. Pediatr Res 1988;23: 449.

132. Chheda S, Palkowetz KH, Rassin DK, et al: Deficient quantitative expression of CD45 isoforms on CD4+ and CD8+ T-cell subpopulations and subsets of CD45RAlowCD45ROlow T cells in newborn blood. Biol Neonate 1996;69: 128.

133. Pabst HF, Spady DW, Pilarsksi AM, et al: Differential modulation of the immune response by breast- or formula-feeding of infants. Acta Paediatr 1997;86: 1291.

134. Kijlstra A, Jeurissen SHM: Modulation of classical C3 convertase of complement by tear lactoferrin. Immunology 1982;47: 263.

135. Lindberg T, Ohlsson K, Westrin B: Protease inhibitors and their relation to protease activity in human milk. Pediatr Res 1982;16: 479.

136. Park PW, Biedermann K, Mecham L, et al: Lysozyme binds to elastin and protects elastin from elastase-mediated degradation. J Invest Dermatol 1996;106: 1075.

137. Shimizu T, Yamashiro Y, Yabuta K: Prostaglandin E₁, E₂, and F₂α in human milk and plasma. Biol Neonate 1992;61: 222.

138. Nen J, Wu-Wang CY, Measel CP, et al: Prostaglandin concentrations in human milk. Am J Clin Nutr 1988;47: 649.
139. Buescher SE, McIlheran SM: Colostral antioxidants: separation and characterization of two activities in human colostrum. J Pediatr Gastroenterol Nutr 1992;14: 47.
140. Chapell JE, Francis T, Clandinin MT: Vitamin A and E content of human milk at early stages of lactation. Early Hum Dev 1985;11: 157.
141. Ostrea Jr EA, Balun JE, Winkler R, et al: Influence of breast-feeding on the restoration of the low serum concentration of vitamin E and β-carotene in the newborn infant. Am J Obstet Gynecol 1986;154: 1014.
142. Carpenter G: Epidermal growth factor is a major growth-promoting agent in human milk. Science 1980;210: 198.
143. Nichols BL, McKee KS, Henry JF, et al: Human lactoferrin stimulates thymidine incorporation into DNA of rat crypt cells. Pediatr Res 1987;21: 563.
144. Kulski JK, Hartmann PE: Changes in the concentration of cortisol in milk during different stages of human lactation. Aust J Exp Biol Med Sci 1981;59: 769.
145. Sanguansermsri J, György P, Zilliken F: Polyamines in human and cow's milk. Am J Clin Nutr 1974;27: 859.
146. Romain N, et al: Polyamine concentration in rat milk and food, human milk, and infant formula. Pediatr Res 32: 58, 1992.
147. Grosvenor CE, Picciano MF, Baumrucker CR: Hormones and growth factors in human milk. Endocrine Rev 1993;14: 710.
148. Pang K, Bresson JL, Walker WA: Development of the gastrointestinal mucosal barrier. III. Evidence for structural differences in microvillus membranes from newborn and adult rabbits. Biochem Biophys Acta 1983;727: 201.
149. Chu SW, Walker WA: Developmental changes in the activities of sialyl- and fucosyltransferases in the rat intestine. Biochem Biophys Acta 1986;740: 170.
150. Teichberg S, Wapnir RA, Moyse J, et al: Development of the neonatal rat small intestinal barrier to nonspecific macromolecular absorption. II. Role of dietary corticosterone. Pediatr Res 1992;32: 50.
151. Heird WC, Schwarz SM, Hansen IH: Colostrum-induced enteric mucosal growth in beagle puppies. Pediatr Res 1984;18: 512.
152. Caplan MS, Kelly A, Hsueh W: Endotoxin and hypoxia-induced intestinal necrosis in rats: the role of platelet activating factor. Pediatr Res 1992;31: 428.
153. Furukawa M, Narahara H, Yasuda K, et al: Presence of platelet-activating factor-acetylhydrolase in milk. J Lipid Res 1993;34: 1603.
154. Caplan MS, Hsueh W, Kelly A, et al: Serum PAF acetylhydrolase increases during neonatal maturation. Prostaglandins 1990;39: 705.
155. Shulman RJ, Schanler RJ, Lau C, et al: Early feeding, antenatal glucocorticoids, and human milk decrease intestinal permeability in preterm infants. Pediatr Res 1998;44: 519.
156. Udall JN, Colony P, Fritze L, et al: Development of gastrointestinal mucosal barrier. II. The effect of natural versus artificial feeding on intestinal permeability to macro-molecules. Pediatr Res 1981;15: 245.
157. Catassi C, Bonucci A, Coppa GV, et al: Intestinal permeability changes during the first month: effect of natural versus artificial feeding. J Pediatr Gastroenterol Nutr 1995;21: 383.
158. Norris JM, Scott FW: A meta-analysis of infant diet and insulin-dependent diabetes mellitus: do biases play a role? Epidemiology 1996;7: 87.
159. Davis MK, Savitz DA, Grauford B: Infant feeding in childhood cancer. Lancet 1988;2: 365.
160. Shu XO, Linet MS, Steinbuch M, et al: Breast-feeding and risk of childhood acute leukemia. J Natl Cancer Inst 1999;91: 1765.
161. Koletzko S, Sherman P, Corey M, et al: Role of infant feeding practices in development of Crohn's disease in childhood. BMJ 1989;298: 1617.
162. Chiba Y, Minagawa T, Mito K, et al: Effect of breast feeding on responses of systemic interferon and virus-specific lymphocyte transformation in infants with respiratory syncytial virus infection. J Med Virol 1987;21: 7.
163. Stephens S, Kennedy CR, Lakhani PK, et al: In-vivo immune responses of breast- and bottle-fed infants to tetanus toxoid antigen and to normal gut flora. Acta Paediatr Scand 1984;73: 426.
164. Stephens S: Development of secretory immunity in breast fed and bottle fed infants. Arch Dis Child 1986;61: 263.
165. Mushtaha AA, Schmalstieg FC, Hughes Jr TK, et al: Chemokinetic agents for monocytes in human milk: possible role of tumor necrosis factor-alpha. Pediatr Res 1989;25: 629.
166. Rudloff HE, Schmalstieg FC, Mushtaha AA, et al: Tumor necrosis factor-α in human milk. Pediatr Res 1992;31: 29.
167. Bocci V, von Bremen K, Corradeschi F, et al: Presence of interferon-gamma and interleukin-6 in colostrum of normal women. Lymphokine Cytokine Res 1993;12: 21.
168. Bryan DL, Hawkes JS, Gibson RA: Interleukin-12 in human milk. Pediatr Res 1999 45(6): 858.
169. Takahata Y, Takada H, Nomura A, et al: Interleukin-18 in human milk. Pediatr Res 2001;50(2): 268.
170. Munoz C, Endres S, van der Meer J, et al: Interleukin-1β in human colostrum. Res Immunol 1990;141: 501.
171. Saito S, Maruyama M, Kato Y, et al: Detection of Il-6 in human milk and its involvement in IgA production. J Reprod Immunol 1991;20: 267.
172. Rudloff HE, Schmalstieg FC, Palkowetz KH, et al: Interleukin-6 in human milk. J Reprod Immunol 1993;23: 13.
173. Palkowetz KH, Royer CL, Garofalo R, et al: Production of interleukin-6 and interleukin-8 by human mammary gland epithelial cells. J Reprod Immunol 1994;26: 57.
174. Bottcher MF, Jenmalm MC, Bjorksten B, et al: Chemoattractant factors in breast milk from allergic and nonallergic mothers. Pediatr Res 2000;47(5): 592.
175. Saito S, Yoshida M, Ichijo M, et al: Transforming growth factor-beta (TGF-β) in human milk. Clin Exp Immunol 1993;94: 220.
176. Garofalo R, Chheda S, Mei F, et al: Interleukin-10 (IL-10) in human milk. Pediatr Res 1994;35: 52.
177. Gilmore HS, McKelvey-Martin VJ, Rutherford S, et al: Human milk contains granulocyte-colony stimulating factor (G-CSF). Europ J Clin Nutr 1994;48: 222.
178. Hara T, Irie K, Saito S, et al: Identification of macrophage colony-stimulating factor in human milk and mammary epithelial cells. Pediatr Res 1995;37: 437.
179. Srivastava MD, Lippes J, Srivastava BI: Hepatocyte growth factor in human milk and reproductive tract fluids. Am J Reprod Immunol 1999;42: 347.
180. Juul SE, Zhao Y, Dame JB, et al: Origin and fate of erythropoietin in human milk. Pediatr Res 2000;48: 660.
181. Brantl V: Novel opioid peptides derived from human β-casein: human β-casomorphins. Eur J Pharmacol 1985;106: 213.
182. Ellis LA, Picciano MF: Bioactive and immunoreactive prolactin variants in human milk. Endocrinology 1995;136: 2711.
183. Ellis LA, Mastro AM, Picciano MF: Milk-borne prolactin and neonatal development. J Mammary Gland Biol Neopl 1996;1:259.
184. Janas IM, Picciano MF: The nucleotide profile of human milk. Pediatr Res 1992;16: 659.
185. Carver JD, Cox WI, Barness LA: Dietary nucleotide effects upon murine natural killer cell activity and macrophage activation. J Parenteral Enteral Nutr 1990;14: 18.
186. Jyonouchi H, Zhang-Shanbhag L, Georgieff M, et al: Immunomodulating actions of nucleotides: enhancement of immunoglobulin production by human cord blood lymphocytes. Pediatr Res 1993;34: 565.
187. Anderson DC, Abbassi O, Kishimoto TK, et al: Diminished lectin-, epidermal growth factor-, complement binding domain-cell adhesion molecule-1 on neonatal neutrophils underlies their impaired CD18-independent adhesion to endothelial cells in vitro. J Immunol 1991;146: 3372.
188. Boat TF: Human tracheobronchial secretions: development of mucous glycoprotein and lysozyme-secreting systems. Pediatr Res 1977;11: 977.
189. Burgio GR, Hanson LÅ, Ugazio AG (eds): Immunology of the neonate. Vienna, Springer, 1987, p 188.
190. Rognum TO, Thrane S, Stoltenberg L, et al: Development of intestinal mucosal immunity in fetal life and the first postnatal months. Pediatr Res 1992;32: 145.
191. Adderson EE, Johnston JM, Shackerford PG, et al: Development of the human antibody repertoire. Pediatr Res 1992;32: 257.
192. Miller LC, Isa S, Lopreste G, et al: Neonatal interleukin-1β, interleukin-6, and tumor necrosis factor: cord blood levels and cellular production. J Pediatr 1990;117: 961.
193. Chheda S, Palkowetz KH, Garofalo R: Decreased interleukin-10 production by neonatal monocytes and T cells: relationship to decreased production and expression of tumour necrosis factor-α and its receptors. Pediatr Res 1996;40: 475.
194. Lewis DB, Yu CC, Meyer J, et al: Cellular and molecular mechanisms for reduced interleukin 4 and interferon-gamma production by neonatal T cells. J Clin Invest 1991;87: 194.
195. Wilson CB, Westfall J, Johnson L, et al: Decreased production of interferon-gamma by human neonatal cells. Intrinsic and regulatory deficiencies. J Clin Invest 1986;77: 860.
196. Cairo MS, Suen Y, Knoppel E, et al: Decreased G-CSF and IL-3 production and gene expression from mononuclear cells of newborn infants. Pediatr Res 1992;31: 574.
197. Cairo MS, Suen Y, Knoppel E, et al: Decreased stimulated GM-CSF expression and GM-CSF gene expression but normal numbers of GM-CSF receptors in human term newborns as compared with adults. Pediatr Res 1991;30: 362.
198. Mortari F, Wang J-Y, Schroeder HW Jr: Human cord blood antibody repertoire. Mixed population of VH gene segments and CDR3 distribution in the expression of Cα and Cγ repertoires. J Immunol 1993;150: 1.
199. Peltola H, Kaayhty H, Virtanen M, et al: Prevention of Haemophilus influenzae type b bacterial infections with the capsular polysaccharide vaccine. N Engl J Med 1994;310: 1561.
200. Pabst HF, Spady DW: Effect of breast-feeding on antibody response to conjugate vaccine. Lancet 1990;336: 269.
201. Koldovsky O: Digestive-absorptive functions in fetuses, infants, and children. In Walker WA, Watkins JB (eds): Nutrition in Pediatrics, Basic Science and Clinical Application. 2nd ed. Hamilton and London, BC Decker, 1996, p 233.
202. Buescher ES, McWilliams-Koeppen P: Soluble tumor necrosis factor-alpha (TNF-alpha) receptors in human colostrum and milk bind to TNF-alpha and neutralize TNF-alpha bioactivity. Pediatr Res 1998;44: 31.
203. Toivanen P, Rossi T, Hirvo T: Immunoglobulins in human fetal sera at different stages of gestation. Experimentia 169;25: 527.
204. Aerde JEE: Acute respiratory failure and bronchopulmonary dysplasia. In Hay WW (ed): Neonatal Nutrition and Metabolism. Chicago, Mosby Year Book Inc, 1991, p 467.
205. Goldman AS, Garza C, Nichols B, et al: The effects of prematurity upon the immunologic system in human milk. J Pediatr 1982;101: 901.
206. Winberg J, Wessner G: Does breast milk protect against septicaemia in the newborn? Lancet 1971;2: 1091.
207. Yu VYH, Jamieson J, Bajuk B: Breast milk feeding in very low birthweight infants. Aust Paediatr J 1981;17: 186.

208. Narayanan I, Prakash K, Bala S, et al: Partial supplementation with expressed breast-milk for prevention of infection in low-birth-weight infants. Lancet 1980;2: 561.

209. Lucas A, Cole TJ: Breast milk and neonatal necrotising enterocolitis. Lancet 1990;336: 1519.

210. Eibl MM, Wolf HM, Furnkranz H, et al: Prevention of necrotizing enterocolitis in low-birth-weight-infants by IgG-IgA feeding. N Engl J Med 1988;319: 1.

211. Kling PJ, Sullivan TM, Roberts RA, et al: Human milk as a potential enteral source of erythropoietin. Pediatr Res 1998;43: 216.

212. Ledbetter DJ, Juul SE: Erythropoietin and the incidence of necrotizing enterocolitis in infants with very low birth weight. J Pediatr Surg 2000;35: 178.

213. Kühn R, Löher J, Rennick D, et al: Interleukin-10-deficient mice develop chronic enterocolitis. Cell 1993;75: 263.

214. Shull MM, Ormsby I, Kier AB, et al: Targeted disruption of the mouse transforming growth factor-β1 gene results in multifocal inflammatory disease. Nature 1992;359: 693.

215. Kulkarni AB, Huh CG, Becker D, et al: Transforming growth factor beta 1 null mutation in mice causes excessive inflammatory response and early death. Proc Natl Acad Sci USA 1993;90: 770.

216. Letterio JJ, Geiser AG, Kulkarni AB, et al: Maternal rescue of transforming growth factor-β1 null mice. Sci 1994;264: 1936.

217. Berg DJ, Davidson N, Kuhn R, et al: Enterocolitis and colon cancer in interleukin-10-deficient mice are associated with aberrant cytokine production and CD4(+) TH1-like responses. J Clin Invest. 1996;98: 1010.

218. Koppel R, Han RN, Cox D, et al: Alpha 1-antitrypsin protects neonatal rats from pulmonary vascular and parenchymal effects of oxygen toxicity. Pediatr Res 1994;36: 763.

219. Dahlgren UI, Hanson LA, Telemo E: Maturation of Immunocompetence in breast-fed vs. formula-fed infants. *In* Woodward B, Draper HH (eds): Advances in Nutritional Research. Vol 10. Immunological Properties of Milk. New York, Plenum Publishers, 2001, p 311.

220. Kramer MS, Chalmers B, Hodnett ED, et al: Promotion of Breastfeeding Intervention Trial (PROBIT): a randomized trial in the Republic of Belarus. JAMA. 2001;285: 413.

221. Kilshaw PJ, Cant AJ: The passage of maternal dietary proteins in human breast milk. Int Arch Allergy Appl Immunol 1984;75: 8.

222. Isolauri K, Tahvanainen A, Peltola T, et al: Breast-feeding of allergic infants. J Pediatr 1999;134: 27.

223. Goldman AS: Association of atopic diseases with breast-feeding: Food allergens, fatty acids, and evolution [editorial]. J Pediatr 1999;134: 5.

224. Wright S, Bolton C: Breast milk fatty acids in mothers of children with atopic eczema. Br J Nutr 1989;62: 693.

225. Duchén K, Yu G, Björksten B: Atopic sensitization during the first year of life in relation to long chain polyunsaturated acids in human milk. Pediatr Res 1998;44: 478

226. Malloy MH, Graubard B: Predictors of rehospitalization among very low birth weight infants (VLBW). Clin Res 1994;41: 791A.

164

Andrew Metinko

Neonatal Pulmonary Host Defense Mechanisms

The lungs are unique internal organs, situated within the body yet interposed between the host and its environment. The development of pulmonary host defense mechanisms capable of restricting the growth of environmental pathogens was therefore an essential step in the evolution of air-breathing animals. To effect gas exchange with the environment, the lungs must be able to buffer the potentially injurious effects to airways and alveoli of multiple substances, including pathogenic organisms, which may be present in the air stream. In a 3.5-kg neonate, with a typical minute ventilation ranging from 100 to 150 ml/(kg • min), this requires the lungs to filter approximately 30 L of inhaled air hourly; a problematic task in that the alveolar surface area requiring protection is 20 times the average neonatal body surface area.[1] Mechanisms must also exist to prevent, or contain, effects of potential pathogens delivered by aspiration of oropharyngeal secretions. Concomitantly, the lungs as reticuloendothelial structures are also responsible for filtering all blood returning to the left atrium via the pulmonary circulation. Thus, the extensive alveolar-capillary membrane, composed of both immune and nonimmune cells, may encounter pathogens by hematogenous routes, as well as by inhalation. Beyond this significant environmental exposure, host defense of the lung presents other unique challenges.[2] Individual alveoli are exposed to the environment in parallel, and thus must be somewhat self-sufficient in initial antigen response. Furthermore, the alveolar-capillary interface, teleologically evolved for gas exchange, offers little barrier to pathogen movement in either direction. Finally, even mild inflammation in this critical location can significantly impair gas exchange, and threaten host survival. Because airways in the lower respiratory tract normally contain few colonies of essentially commensal organisms, evolved pulmonary mechanisms of pathogen containment and clearance, both immunologic and nonimmunologic, are clearly effective.

Available pulmonary host defenses can be broadly categorized as either mechanical or immunologic. Examples of mechanical defenses include the larynx and epiglottis (which are anatomically situated to minimize aspiration of oropharyngeal material) airway angulation, mucus secretion, and mucociliary clearance mechanisms, including the cough reflex. These mechanisms result in progressive filtering of about 99% of inhaled particles as they pass through the conducting airways, so that overall level of antigen exposure at a given site is inversely related to its depth within the respiratory tree. Mechanical barrier components of host defense thus minimize "bulk" exposure to pathogens, and antigens, minimizing the frequency of host immune response activation.

Available immunologic mechanisms are by recent convention broadly categorized as either innate, or adaptive. Innate immune responses are nonspecific, relying on host recognition of "pathogen-associated molecular patterns," such as peptidoglycans, endotoxin, or fungal mannans. Such foreign patterns are recognized, and ligated, either by soluble bioactive substances within the airway (defensins, collectins) or by pattern recognition receptors on macrophages. Subsequent generation of "early response cytokines" (tumor necrosis factor, interleukin [IL]-1) and chemotaxins (leukotrienes, chemokines, split components of complement) leads to recruitment of additional cellular elements of innate immunity, granulocytes and natural killer cells. By means of concurrent cytokine networking with other cells in the alveolar milieu (including epithelia and fibroblasts), alveolar macrophages activate antigen-presenting cells, and lymphocytes move into the alveolar compartment; recruitment of the specialized lymphocytes, T cells and B cells, heralds the onset of the adaptive immune response. These cells manifest specific receptors somatically generated in response to specific antigens, facilitating immunologic "memory" and long-term cell-mediated and humoral immunity. Adaptive immunity thus initiates a targeted response aimed at containment and clearance of a specific antigen, allowing titration of nonspecific, and potentially host injurious, alveolar inflammation. Because of the anatomic location of elements of pulmonary innate immunity, these responses typically precede those of adaptive immunity. However, complex pulmonary immune responses, as seen in pneumonia, require interplay between innate and adaptive elements, rendering such distinctions somewhat arbitrary. A model for how barrier, innate, and adaptive defenses of the lung may interact is depicted in Figure 164–1.

ANATOMIC BARRIER MECHANISMS OF HOST DEFENSE

The neonate is born with an anatomy designed to prevent pulmonary infection; from the nose to the alveoli, multiple nonspecific structural defenses function to prevent penetration of the airway and alveoli by pathogens. Nasal hairs at the nares serve as crude particle filters, and "baffle plates," or turbinates, of the nasal passage catch particles as small as 10 μm. Epiglottic and laryngeal cough reflexes prevent aspiration of oropharyngeal contents. Turbulent flow in upper airways causes mucosal deposition of large particles before they can reach the lower airways, whereas turbulent flow in lower airways induces particle deposition into the mucus blanket overlying the airway epithelium. At sites of airway bifurcation, gas flow is especially turbulent and the rate of particle deposition may be enhanced 100-fold.[3] This tendency for particles to deposit at sites within the upper and lower airways requires specialized anatomic barriers, as well as a mechanism to clear deposited material, if airway colonization and respiratory tract infection is to be prevented. These barrier and clearance functions are provided by specialized epithelial cells of the airway and their mucociliary transport system.

Epithelial Cells

Airway epithelial cells with their apical-tight junctions restrict passive diffusion or pathogen movement across the lateral intracellular space, augmenting local mechanical barriers.[4] A more critical function, however, is for ciliated epithelium to actively expel deposited material derived from the air stream. Excluding regions of the larynx and pharynx where squamous epithelium predominates, ciliated epithelium is present from the upper respiratory tract to the level of the respiratory bronchioles. This ciliated epithelium consists of a number of different cell types, including columnar ciliated cells, mucus-producing goblet cells, serous cells, Clara cells, brush cells, neuroendocrine cells, and basal cells.[5, 6] Ciliated cells are in physical contact at tight junction desmosomes, and in physiologic communication via gap junctions.[7] Columnar ciliated cells may carry up to 200 cilia,

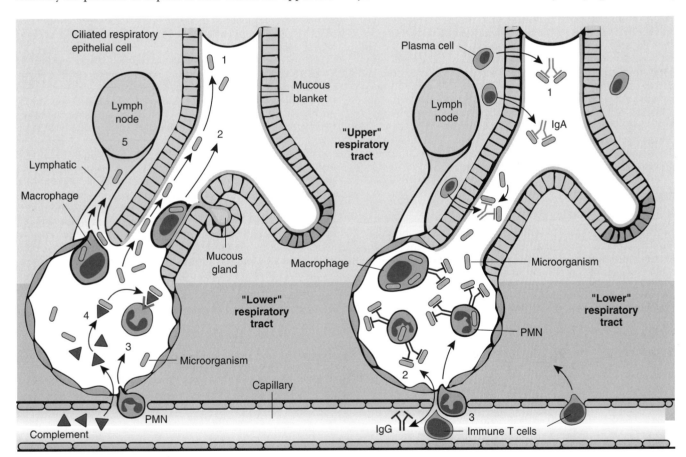

Figure 164–1. Lung defense mechanisms. A, In the nonimmune lung, removal of microbial organisms depends on (1) entrapment in the mucus blanket and removal via the mucociliary elevator, (2) phagocytosis by alveolar macrophages that can kill and degrade organisms and remove them from the air spaces by migrating onto the mucociliary elevator, or (3) phagocytosis and killing by neutrophils recruited by macrophage factors. (4) Serum complement may enter the alveoli and be activated by the alternate pathway to provide the opsonin C3b that enhances phagocytosis. (5) Organisms, including those ingested by phagocytes, may reach the draining lymph nodes to initiate immune responses. **B,** Additional mechanisms operate in the immune lung. (1) Secreted IgA can block attachment of the microorganism to epithelium in the upper respiratory tract. (2) In the lower respiratory tract, serum antibodies (IgM, IgG) are present in the alveolar lining fluid. They activate complement more efficiently by the classic pathway, yielding C3b *(not shown)*. In addition, IgG is opsonic. (3) The accumulation of immune T cells is important for controlling infections by viruses and other intracellular microorganisms. (Adapted from Kobzik L: The lung. *In* Cotran RS, et al [eds]: Robbins Pathologic Basis of Disease, 6th ed. Philadelphia, WB Saunders Co, 1999, p 719.)

ranging from 4 μm in the distal airways to 6 μm centrally. Ciliogenesis commences in the upper trachea early in gestation (week 7) and proceeds distally; by week 24 of gestation, the fetal airway epithelium resembles that of the mature trachea.[8] Although fetal cilia are motile, the function of ciliary activity *in utero* is unknown.

Epithelial cell types responsible for mucus production include the goblet cells, serous cells, and Clara cells. Goblet cells are found predominantly in large airways and are the principal source of mucus. Clara cells are found only in small airways and produce watery secretions; serous cells have similar location and function but have been identified only in fetal tissues. Clara cells also serve as a likely stem cell for regeneration of ciliated epithelium.[9] Submucosal glands located in the cartilaginous portion of the airways also contribute to overall mucus secretion.

Morphologic differences in respiratory epithelium exist between larger and smaller airways. In the trachea and large airways, ciliated columnar epithelium forms an essentially continuous carpet, with a ratio of ciliated cells to goblet cells of 5:1.[10] Ciliated and goblet cell numbers diminish in the peripheral airways until reaching the terminal bronchioles where a ciliated cuboidal epithelium predominates, and Clara cells become the only secretory cells present.[11]

The epithelial surface is protected from direct pathogen contact by a "glycocalyx" layer of mucins tethered to the epithelial cell surface.[12] The products of mucin genes *MUC1* and *MUC4,* these mucins are highly glycosylated and extend up to 1500 nm into the airway lumen. Bacteria introduced into the airway normally become trapped at the tips of cilia and rarely penetrate into the interciliary space or attach alongside cilia. Adhesion of bacteria to the airway epithelium proper is therefore impeded as long as functioning cilia are present and the surrounding epithelium is uninjured and intact.[13] This underscores the crucial role of epithelial integrity and ciliary function in the prevention of bacterial colonization and invasion.

Ciliary Function

Human cilia are composed of nine doublet microtubules (subfibers) surrounding two microtubules. The major microtubular axoneme proteins are dynein, an adenosine triphosphatase (ATPase), and tubulin.[14] At the tip of the cilium, the nine subfibers simplify into nine single fibers that insert into a

common cytoplasmic extension, through which they mechanically engage the overlying mucus sheet during the effective ciliary stroke.[15-17] At the base of the cilium, the nine subfibers end in the basal body, which is anchored to the cytoskeleton (Fig. 164-2).[5] Because all basal bodies of a cell are oriented in approximately the same direction, the effective strokes of all cilia of a given cell have a similar orientation; however, neither the orientation of these structures nor the orientation of the ciliary beats is necessarily identical in adjacent cells.[18,19] During ciliary motion, dynein projections from one subfiber transiently interact with the non–dynein-containing subfiber of an adjacent microtubule doublet and, using energy from dynein-mediated ATP hydrolysis, induce a conformational change resulting in subfiber movement; repetition of this process in adjacent doublets, in a unidirectional front circumferentially, cause the sequential movement of fibers that effect cilia motion.[20,21] From a resting state, a cilium in its recovery stroke swings close to the cell 180° backward, then fully extends and moves through its effective stroke, an arc of approximately 110° in a plane perpendicular to the cell surface.[22] During the effective stroke, the ciliary tip engages the overlying mucus, advancing it in the same direction. Following this, the cilium rests, then repeats this sequence. As a cilium swings backward into its recovery stroke, it engages other resting cilia, stimulating them to begin a recovery stroke; this mechanical recruitment is pivotal for the coordinated beating of airway cilia.[23]

Cilia of human nasal, tracheal, and bronchial mucosa beat at 11 to 15 Hz at body temperature, with progressively slower frequencies noted in proximal bronchi and bronchioles.[24-26] Because the combined surface areas of the distal airways are exponentially greater than those of the central airways, this differential ciliary beat frequency allows efficient handling of the relatively large mucus loads eventually delivered to the trachea. Endogenous mechanisms that allow such local ciliary beat modulation have been described. Local physiologic loads to airway epithelium, such as increased quantities of mucus, can mechanically stimulate increased ciliary beating *in vivo;* this effect appears to be mediated by increased cytosolic calcium[27] and can be reproduced pharmacologically by agents that modulate intracellular calcium levels.[28,29] Ciliary beat frequency is also exquisitely sensitive to alterations in temperature; cilia of the small airways beat optimally near body temperature, decreasing and increasing their beat frequencies in response to decreased and increased body tem-

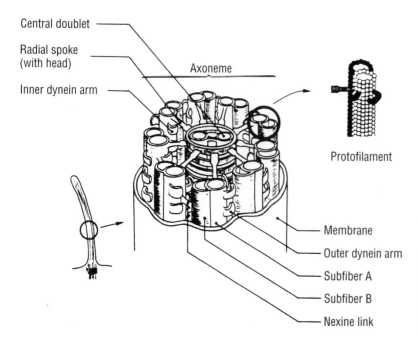

Central doublet
Radial spoke (with head)
Inner dynein arm
Axoneme
Protofilament
Membrane
Outer dynein arm
Subfiber A
Subfiber B
Nexine link

Figure 164–2. Schematic diagram of a cilium. Note the relationship of dynein projections from one subfiber with the adjacent subfiber *(inset).* ATP hydrolysis results in conformational changes of the dynein arm, inducing subfiber movement, and ultimately ciliary movement. (From Guffanti EE, et al: *In* Allegra L, Braga PC [eds]: Bronchial Mucology and Related Diseases. New York, Raven Press, 1990, pp 27-45.)

peratures, respectively.[30] Increased ciliary beat frequency in response to increased ambient air concentrations of nitric oxide (NO) has been described, suggesting that local cellular production of this bioactive substance may modulate ciliary function.[31, 32] These observations are consistent with *in vitro* data demonstrating that ciliated epithelium produces NO, which regulates ciliary beat frequency in an autocrine manner, via a cyclic guanosine monophosphate (GMP) signaling pathway.[33] In addition to the dynein ATPase, a cyclic adenosine monophosphate (AMP)-dependent kinase also facilitates control of ciliary beating.[34, 35] Whether intrinsic neural control of ciliary beat frequency exists is unclear; although acetylcholine increases ciliary beat frequency *in vitro* suggesting a potential role for cholinergic regulation of ciliary "tone,"[36] there is no cholinergic efferent innervation of the superficial airway epithelium, making it unlikely that neural mechanisms regulate lung mucus transport.[37] Finally, recent interest has focused on autocrine and paracrine airway epithelial signals generated by local purinergic pathways.[38] In this emerging model, luminal ATP and uridine triphosphate (UTP) induce increased ciliary beat frequency by binding to G protein–coupled purinoreceptors on the epithelial apical membrane. Nucleotide-hydrolyzing enzymes of the airway surface liberate adenosine, which acts through a separate receptor to sustain the ciliostimulatory effects of ATP, while cilia-derived phosphatases hydrolyze ATP and UTP, down-regulating ciliary beat frequency. Nucleotide release by airway epithelia is induced by shear stress, and possibly other stimuli, so that local mechanical or metabolic perturbations may modulate ciliary activity.[39-41]

Ciliary function may also be affected by a variety of exogenous substances introduced into the airway. Inhaled β-adrenergic agonists may increase ciliary beat frequency by increasing cellular cyclic AMP.[42] Inhaled NO, via metabolism to S-nitrosothiols, may increase ciliary motility.[43] Conversely, ciliary activity may be diminished by a number of anesthetic gases or by exposure to high concentrations of inspired oxygen.[44] Finally, ciliary function may be impaired by substances in the local milieu associated with infection. Specific pathogens, including *Pseudomonas aeruginosa, Streptococcus pneumoniae, Haemophilus influenzae, Mycoplasma pneumoniae,* and *Chlamydia pneumoniae,* produce soluble products inhibiting ciliary function.[45-50] These products may induce ciliary beat slowing, ciliary beat disorientation, ciliostasis, or frank ciliary lysis. Some of these substances are directly ciliotoxic, whereas others act by inducing local macrophages to generate hydrogen peroxide,[51, 52] which has a local cilioinhibitory effect. Lipid-derived inflammatory mediators, such as platelet-activating factor (PAF) induce dose-dependent slowing of ciliary beat, whereas proteins released into the airway lumen during inflammation, such as leukocyte elastase and neutral protease, are also ciliotoxic.[53, 54] Although other inflammatory mediators stimulate ciliary beating *in vitro,* overall mucociliary function is typically diminished during inflammation *in vivo.*[55-57]

Periciliary Fluid

Periciliary fluid is a thin, nonviscous secretion lying just between the epithelial cell and overlying mucus, bathing the basal portion of the cilia and providing an environment of low resistance for the cilia to move during the backstroke portion of their movement cycle. The level of this periciliary fluid layer is critical for effective mucociliary function (Fig. 164-3). If the fluid level is too high, the ciliary tips will not be able to engage the overlying mucus and effect its movement. If the fluid level is too low, the cilia will not be able to disengage from the mucus layer during the recovery stroke and ciliary beating will be impeded;[58] in the extreme, narrowed distance between the epithelial and mucus layers may allow mucins of the epithelial glycocalyx to anneal with those of the mucus layer, effectively paralyzing mucociliary transport and diminishing efficiency of cough propulsion of mucus.[12] Phospholipids from alveoli or secreted from epithelial cells provide an interface between the periciliary fluid and overlying mucus layer, possibly providing an additional "lubricant" function facilitating mucus movement. Periciliary fluid is propulsed up the airway along with the overlying mucus; this effects mucus hydration, lessening its viscosity, and provides a mechanism for clearance of hydrophilic irritants.[59,60]

Periciliary fluid secretion is regulated by active ion transport across the epithelial cells, with concomitant fluid movement that is either passive or aquaporin regulated.[61] Recent *in vitro* work suggests that mature airway epithelium also regulates periciliary fluid secretion in response to external osmolality changes. In this model, evaporative water loss contracts the periciliary layer, increasing tonicity. Passive efflux of water across the apical epithelial membrane results in cell shrinkage, triggering release of epithelial-derived mediators, including NO; these mediators increase blood flow and water content of the submucosa. Movement of water from the submucosa across the basolateral epithelial membrane, possibly regulated by aquaporin 4, restores epithelial cell volume.[62] In contrast, fetal lung fluid results from active secretion of Cl$^-$ by all respiratory tract epithelium, with passive cation and fluid transit into the airway lumen.[63] In the distal airways, these mechanisms persist, providing a source of periciliary fluid and mucus hydration for the rest of lung.[64] Conversely, tracheobronchial epithelium gradually transitions postnatally from Cl$^-$ secretion to Na$^+$ absorption, and Na$^+$ absorption eventually predominates in the larger airways under basal conditions;[65] at the same time, production of mucus components transiently increases. Until this transition is complete, continued Cl$^-$ and fluid secretion by the neonatal respiratory epithelium has significant short-term impacts on ciliary function; in newborns, mucociliary clearance is slow, presumably resulting from increased periciliary fluid secretion and impaired ciliary tip engagement of sparse mucus. As secretory function matures, rates of mucus transport increase, reaching adult values at the same

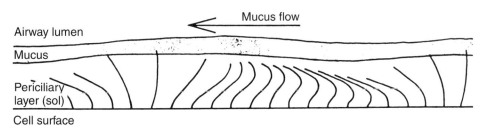

Figure 164–3. The phases of ciliary motion. Note relationship of the periciliary fluid layer and mucus layer as the cilia move through their effective and recovery strokes. Recovery strokes of the cilia occur in the periciliary fluid layer; if this layer is too sparse, the cilia tips will not be able to disengage from the overlying mucus layer, and effective propulsion of mucus will be impeded. (From Mautone AJ, Cataletto MB: *In* Scarpelli EM [ed]: Pulmonary Physiology of the Fetus, Newborn, Child, and Adolescent. Philadelphia, Lea & Febiger, 1990, pp 192-214. Originally adapted from Sanderson SJ, Sleigh MA: J Cell Sci 47:331, 1981.)

time (4 to 8 weeks) as the secretory changes. Of note is that neonatal animal models of diffuse lung injury (e.g., hyperoxic exposure) suggest that during this period of development the airway mucociliary system is particularly vulnerable to damage, and subsequent prolonged malfunction, after pulmonary insult.[66]

Mucins and Mucus

The last components required for mucociliary transport are mucus and the constituent mucins.[67] Mucins are high molecular weight, heavily glycosylated proteins that contribute to the gel-like qualities of mucus. Multiple mucin genes are expressed in the airways, but the primary gene products in mucus are those of MUC5AC and MUC5B.[68] Mucins are formed in the Golgi apparatus, concentrated in vesicles, and released by exocytosis from goblet cells and mucus cells of submucosal glands. On release, the condensed mucin polymers are rapidly hydrated, increasing their volume exponentially; periciliary fluid acts as an electrolyte and water donor in this event.[69] Mucin proteins typically exhibit several hundred sugar side chains that contribute to their structural and barrier functions. Electrostatic repulsion of adjacent sugar chains is thought to result in a rigid "bottle-brush" conformation of mucin molecules, which then cross-link via terminal cysteine residues, imparting gel-like qualities to their mucus milieu.[70] Additionally, owing to the extraordinary density, and diversity of their carbohydrate side chains, mucins are capable of binding virtually any inhaled particle they encounter, facilitating particle entrapment within the mucus layer. Mucin production can be stimulated above basal levels by several mediators of pulmonary inflammation, including histamine, prostaglandins, leukotrienes, platelet-activating factor (PAF), and the cytokines tumor necrosis factor-α (TNF-α) and IL-9, suggesting that mucin barrier function may be up-regulated by local immune response.[71,72]

Apart from mucins, mucus also contains proteoglycans,[73] other proteins, lipids, water, and DNA.[74] DNA is found in significant concentrations only during infection or inflammation of the airways, originating from dead leukocytes or denuded epithelium; large amounts of DNA markedly increase mucus viscosity.[75] Mucus proteins include secretory immunoglobulins and bactericidal proteins such as lysozyme. The dry weight of mucus is 20 to 40 mg/ml and increases dramatically during infection, as mucins and other protein constituents are induced. Mucus is 95% water, and in settings of luminal dehydration the mucus layer can act as a liquid reservoir, preserving volume, and height, of the periciliary layer.[12] Mucus rheology is determined by mucus hydration and by polyionic interactions between mucin molecules. These factors, in turn, depend on the pH and salt content of the periciliary fluid; this may explain the thick, relatively immobile mucus seen with the impaired transepithelial Cl$^-$ secretion and accelerated Na$^+$ absorption characteristic of cystic fibrosis (CF).[76]

Mucus appears in the distal airways as droplets or "patches" secreted at these sites in response to particle deposition. Secreted mucus droplets coalesce as they migrate upward to the bronchi and trachea, where they eventually form a nearly continuous layer; this mucus "blanket" also increases in thickness as it ascends up the large airways. Because of the fast rate at which the cilia tips engage the mucus layer, they encounter the mucus as a solid and are able to effect its transport. A low water content,[77] high glycoprotein content,[78] and purulence resulting in a high DNA content[75] are all associated with increased mucus viscosity and diminished mucus transport rates.

Mucociliary Function

Optimal mucociliary function depends on complex interactions among cilia, the mucus layer, and the intervening periciliary fluid. Both the mucus layer and the periciliary fluid are moved unidirectionally along airway surfaces by ciliary action; cilia effect movement of the mucus layer through direct contact, while frictional interaction with the mucus layer "drags" periciliary fluid. Beyond their propulsive function, cilia also impart vertical movements within the mucus layer; inhaled particles deposited within the airways are effectively "churned" into the mucus layer, facilitating binding by mucins and retention within the mucus layer until forced removal by mucociliary transport.[79] Radioaerosol inhalation techniques to measure mucociliary transport demonstrate rates of 4 to 5 mm/min in the trachea, decreasing in the smaller airways to less than 0.4 mm/min in the bronchioles. Overall mucociliary clearance of the lung is achieved in two phases: (1) an initial rapid phase (half-life of about 4 hours) representing mucociliary clearance of the tracheobronchial tree and (2) a simultaneous slow phase lasting weeks to months, which represents alveolar clearance by non-mucociliary transport mechanisms.[80] Humans exhibit a wide range of mucociliary clearance rates, implying some endogenous control of this process; as noted earlier, purinergic regulatory mechanisms have been postulated, given the demonstrated effect of secreted nucleotides on ciliary beat frequency, goblet cell degranulation, and periciliary fluid secretion.[81,82] Although all aspects of the mucociliary system are established prenatally,[83-85] optimal mucociliary function is not present at birth but continues to develop postnatally, gradually becoming adult-like over several weeks.

Mucociliary function can be disturbed by a change in any of its components, including ciliary activity, periciliary fluid characteristics, mucus secretion, or mucociliary interactions. Relevant environmental influences include temperature and humidity. Nasal mucus transport appears relatively resistant to changes in humidity or temperature, owing to its capacity for warming and humidifying inspired air.[86] However, air of less than 30% relative humidity will produce ciliostasis in the trachea, blunting tracheal mucus transport.[87] Similarly, ciliary beat frequency, and hence mucus transport rates, are diminished at conditions below body temperature. Other potential environmental factors include cigarette smoke,[88] or high inspiratory oxygen concentration,[89] each of which can decrease mucociliary clearance rates. Specific products of pathogenic bacteria may decrease mucociliary clearance rates by decreasing ciliary beat frequency, increasing periciliary fluid levels, and increasing mucus secretion.[90] Numerous pharmacologic agents may also have an impact on mucociliary function. Cholinergic agonists increase mucus clearance by increasing rates of mucus secretion and ciliary beat frequency, whereas atropine decreases mucociliary clearance and transport rates.[91] β-Adrenergic agonists increase intracellular cyclic AMP levels, which increase ciliary beating,[92,34] ion and fluid secretion,[93] and mucus elaboration, resulting in the expected increase in mucociliary transport rates. Methylated xanthines also enhance mucociliary clearance, presumably through similar actions on epithelial cell cyclic AMP levels.[94]

Impaired mucociliary clearance can result from specific types of inherited or acquired ciliary dysfunction. Primary ciliary dyskinesia is a congenital ciliary dysmotility state resulting from the absence of an intermediate chain dynein important in assembly and coordination of heavy chain dyneins of the ciliary shaft;[95] in the 50% of patients with associated situs inversus, these findings define Kartagener's syndrome. Other structural defects, such as abnormal cilia length and orientation, have been described in association with bronchiectasis and recurrent pulmonary infection. Acquired ciliary disorders are most often secondary to inflammatory processes.[96,97] Although a variety of microtubular alterations are reported in the cilia of children with acute viral respiratory infections, diffuse epithelial layer damage by products of bacteria or inflammatory cells remains the sentinel lesion in these states. More than 50% of the ciliated cells of a given area must be injured to affect the mucociliary transport rate, and this degree of involvement is reported in infections with viruses, *Mycoplasma pneumoniae*, and following aspiration of gastric contents.[98-100] In some viral illnesses, diminished mucociliary clearance persists for months, suggesting impaired capacity of epithelium to reestablish normal ciliary structure in the convalescent period.[101, 102]

Abnormalities in airway secretions also result in impaired mucociliary function, and both quantitative and qualitative changes of periciliary fluid and mucus can result from inflammation within the airway. Sustained inflammation at the epithelial cell layer results in decreased ciliation, denudation, goblet cell hyperplasia, and submucosal gland hyperplasia and hypertrophy in the central airways; the net effects are increased mucus production, decreased capacity for mucus propulsion, and ultimately increased mucus accumulation within the airways. Local generation of inflammatory mediators, release of leukocyte enzymes, and secretion of neuropeptides such as substance P have all been implicated as causative factors for these changes.[57, 103-105]

Special situations of mucociliary dysfunction relevant to the neonate are seen in ventilator-associated lung injury and bronchopulmonary dysplasia (BPD). Airway epithelium is exquisitely sensitive to mechanical injury, and manipulations such as endotracheal intubation and/or the use of suction catheters have been shown to cause flattening or denuding of the epithelium, in concert with a local inflammatory response.[106] Both conventional positive-pressure ventilation and high-frequency oscillatory ventilation may engender similar airway epithelial injury, characterized by loss of goblet cells, loss of cilia, and epithelial denudation with squamous metaplasia;[107] if epithelium denudation occurs to the level of the basement membrane, restoration of normal epithelial architecture may take weeks.[108] Similar epithelial changes may be seen when sustained or intense positive-pressure ventilatory support results in BPD. In these neonates, loss of cilia to the levels of the terminal and respiratory bronchioles is described, along with necrosis of the bronchial and bronchiolar mucosa, extensive epithelial denudation, and metaplasia.[109] Goblet cell hyperplasia with mucus hypersecretion may occur; in the setting of concomitant ciliary loss, inability to clear airway secretions ensues.[110] As in other mechanisms of airway injury, restoration of normal epithelial layers and function is gradual and delayed until putative causative agents (positive airway pressure, supplemental oxygen, endotracheal manipulation, inflammatory stimuli) are withdrawn. In the extreme, permanent airway remodeling may occur, characterized by any combination of goblet cell metaplasia, goblet cell hyperplasia, or submucosal gland hypertrophy, resulting in sustained imbalance between mucus production and mucociliary clearance.

AIRWAY REFLEXES

Integration of Breathing and Swallowing

Shared upper pathways for breathing and swallowing require that these functions be closely coordinated to prevent pulmonary contamination with oropharyngeal contents. In the neonate, multiple protective processes functionally separate the respiratory and alimentary tracts during swallowing.[111] The more cranial position of the larynx provides closer approximation of the epiglottis and soft palate, better isolating the oral cavity from the rest of the upper airway. Because newborns have lower resistance across the nasal than the oral passage owing to deficient control of oropharyngeal musculature, nasal breathing is therefore favored, especially by preterm newborns; this may also facilitate functional separation between the upper tracts. Finally, it is well documented that neonatal breathing is interrupted by airway closure during nutritive sucking.[112, 113]

Swallowing has been well described from early in fetal life, and three distinct stages are identified: oral, pharyngeal, and esophageal. In neonates, the oral stage is coincident with nutritive sucking. During the pharyngeal stage, the bolus moves through the pharynx into the esophagus; the larynx is elevated and pulled forward, the epiglottis covers the laryngeal opening, which is further sealed by contraction of the laryngeal adductors, and inhibition of breathing occurs. At the end of the swallow, the airway reopens, and the esophageal phase follows.[114] This transient apneic response is also seen in nonfeeding swallows, which allow the infant to clear the airway of oral secretions or regurgitated materials before resuming breathing.[115, 116] Premature infants typically exhibit incomplete integration of swallowing and breathing functions, such that oral feeding may result in pronounced apneic pauses. Maturation of these functions, whereby swallowing is coordinated to occur at end inspiration, is observed in this population by 35 weeks after conception.[117]

When studied, intact cough reflexes were found in only 50% of term infants, and only 25% of preterm infants; therefore, when challenged by a swallowing misadventure, neonates are more likely to defend the airway by sustained laryngeal closure than by coughing.[118] Reflex laryngeal closure is mediated by stimulation of receptors in the laryngeal mucosa innervated by branches of the superior laryngeal nerves.[119] In newborns, this response can be induced by instillation of liquids into the larynx; sustained apnea occurs until this inciting material is removed.[120] Although potentially pathologic, this response is also adaptive, because attempts to breathe against an obstructed airway are reduced. Conversely, failure of laryngeal closure and premature termination of the apnea before airway clearance has occurred results in aspiration. As maturation occurs, coughing replaces apnea as the primary response to stimulation of these receptors.[121]

Cough and Forced Exhalation

When basal mucociliary transport is inadequate, mucus is cleared from the airways by forced exhalation, or coughing. In each of these mechanisms, energy derived from airflow effects movement of mucus. Interacting with the mucus layer, airflow of sufficient kinetic energy can induce a shear force on the surface of the mucus; the magnitude of this force is proportional to air density and the square of the mean airflow velocity.[122] To move the mucus in the direction of the large airways, the shear force generated by the airflow must overcome mucus viscosity and gravitational forces. At very high airflow velocities (>2500 cm/second), mucus is rended off the surface as droplets, producing the mist flow characteristic of sputum expectoration from the trachea; such airflow velocities can be reached in the small airways during cough or forced exhalation.[123] For a given airflow velocity, a critical mucus depth is required for mucus movement to occur. This critical depth increases with increasing mucus viscosity and decreases with increasing airflow velocity.[124] Because the critical depth for viscous mucus is high, mucus accumulates as a thick layer in the airway before subject to movement by airflow effects.

For a cough maneuver, there is rapid inhalation of a supranormal tidal volume, followed by glottis closure, an intrathoracic pressure increase (50 to 100 mm Hg), and glottis opening with rapid exhalation. With the supramaximal flow and tracheal narrowing described in adults, airflow velocity may reach up to 280 m/s, resulting in efficient upward movement of mucus.[122] The increased compliance of the chest wall and trachea of the normal neonate tend to limit the intrathoracic pressure and airflow velocity attainable, blunting the effectiveness of cough in this population.[125] Coughing is also less effective in settings of respiratory muscle weakness or inability to close the glottis as when endotracheally intubated. However, a cough that is inadequate to generate the required shear forces above may still facilitate mucus clearance by changing secretion of periciliary fluid or by increasing ciliary beating.[126]

A coordinated cough maneuver relies on local chemoreceptors and mechanoreceptors, vagal afferents, signal integration in the doral medulla, and efferent innervation to relevant muscles of inspiration and expiration. The receptors inducing cough are poorly characterized but may be activated by local mediators, including histamine, tachykinins, and substance P.[127, 128] Cough can also be induced by stimulation of other vagally innervated sites, such as the external auditory canal or esophagus. The afferent limb involves the vagus nerve and vagally innervated structures such as the larynx and conducting airways. Of these, the larynx and upper airways seem more sensitive to mechanical stimulation whereas the lower airways are more chemosensitive.[129] Vagal afferents from these sites synapse in the nucleus tractus solitarius of the doral medulla, the putative "cough center." Efferent pathways include the recurrent laryngeal nerve, which stimulates glottic closure, and spinal nerves from C3 to S2, which innervate intercostal, abdominal, and pelvic muscles required to achieve sufficient tidal volume and expiratory pressure. As noted earlier, the cough reflex of premature neonates tends to be "immature," or absent, which is attributed to incomplete myelination of vagal afferents.[130]

In the absence of effective cough, additional airway protective reflexes exist.[131] Mechanical irritation of the epipharynx, via the glossopharyngeal nerve, elicits the sniff-like aspiration reflex, by which foreign particles can be removed from the back of the nose to be either swallowed or expelled by mucociliary clearance. Mechanical stimulation of the vocal folds, by means of the superior laryngeal nerve, elicits a brief expiratory effort without preceding inspiration (the expiration reflex). Lastly, sneezing is an effective clearance mechanism for the nose and nasopharynx. Like coughing, sneezing can be described as having three distinct phases: inspiratory, compressive, and expiratory. In the inspiratory phase, a supranormal tidal volume is rapidly inhaled, followed immediately by closure of both the larynx and pharynx. A powerful expiratory effort follows, with a marked increase of intrathoracic pressure. In the expiratory phase, the pharynx and glottis are opened and high velocity airflow is directed primarily through the nose. Sneezing cannot occur voluntarily and tends to be weak or absent in the early neonatal period.

INNATE IMMUNE MECHANISMS OF HOST DEFENSE

Despite barriers to microbial colonization and invasion discussed earlier, particles of 2 to 10 μm in diameter may still infiltrate to the lower airways and alveoli. Furthermore, anatomic barriers may be inadequate in situations of overwhelming pathogen inoculum via the air stream or ineffective in the situation of lung microbial invasion through hematogenous routes. Immune protective mechanisms are, therefore, frequently employed to contain penetrant microorganisms; such mechanisms may be broadly characterized as either innate or adaptive. Adaptive immunity relies on specialized antigen-presenting cells to activate T cells and B cells, resulting in clonal expansion of lymphocyte pools unique for a specific antigen. Although advantageous for their exquisite specificity and capacity for long-term "memory," such responses are also delayed, owing to the multiple cellular interactions required; this is especially true in the setting of an "immunologically naive" host, such as the newborn. Because delay in this setting may be deleterious to survival, capacity for more immediate immune response must also exist. The soluble and cellular components of this immediate host response constitute innate immunity.

Innate immunity is phylogenetically primitive, nonspecific, immediate, and the primary antimicrobial defense of the naive host. Innate immune responses recognize and target structurally conserved molecular sequences shared among groups of pathogens; these include lipopolysaccharides (LPS) of gram-negative bacteria, lipotechoic acids of gram-positive bacteria,

bacterial lipoproteins or peptidoglycans, mycobacterial glycolipids, fungal mannans, unmethylated bacterial DNA sequences, and double-stranded viral RNAs. These are referred to collectively as "pathogen-associated molecular patterns" (PAMPs) and are recognized and ligated by pattern recognition receptors (PRRs) of the innate immune system. PRRs are nonclonal and do not depend on immunologic memory because they are germline encoded. These receptors are expressed on barrier and effector cells of innate immunity, such as epithelial cells, endothelium, and phagocytes, where binding and activation induces either direct phagocytosis or cellular signals culminating in leukocyte recruitment and nonspecific inflammation.[132] Alternatively, PRRs are also components of soluble or secreted humoral proteins; when present in the airway lining fluid, they constitute an additional "chemical barrier" and essential complement to mucociliary clearance.[12]

Soluble Elements of Innate Immunity

As noted earlier, bacterial clearance from peripheral airways by mucus transport may require up to 6 hours; because bacteria can exhibit doubling times of less than 20 minutes, forced mucociliary clearance alone is potentially inadequate to maintain alveolar and airway sterility. Therefore, concurrent mechanisms to contain bacterial growth must be present. Products of the neonatal lung that may confer innate, or nonspecific, antimicrobial protection include complement, other opsonins such as fibronectin, antimicrobial peptides (defensins, cathelicidins), lysozyme, collectins, and nitric oxide.

Complement

The complement system is a sentinel limb of innate immunity, because it can be directly activated by component recognition of PAMPs. As such, it is a potentially important neonatal host defense, providing a mechanism for direct bacterial lysis in the absence of optimal cellular immune responses. Specific complement components also function as microbial opsonins to facilitate phagocytosis and as chemotaxins to facilitate granulocyte recruitment.[133, 134] The complement system consists of more than 20 proteins synthesized by cells of the liver or reticuloendothelial system. Once activated, most components exhibit a proteolytic function responsible for activation of subsequent components in orderly series. While normally quiescent, circulating and local complement components may be activated by any one of three major pathways.

The classical complement pathway is initiated by the binding of C1q to the Fc portion of either IgG or IgM complexed to antigen. This results in an amplified cascade leading sequentially to activation of C4b2a ("C3 convertase"), generation of C3a and C3b, and formation of the C4b2a3b complex that cleaves C5 into its split components C5a and C5b. The MB lectin pathway is mediated by mannan-binding lectin (MBL), an acute phase protein of the collectin family structurally similar to C1q.[135, 136] MBL possesses domains that recognize and bind membrane glycoproteins of bacteria, yeast, mycobacteria, and certain viruses.[137] Pathogen binding induces an MBL conformational change, exposing two MBL serine proteases that activate C4, ultimately generating classical C3 convertase.[138, 139] The alternative pathway is initiated by a number of substances, including endotoxin, complex polysaccharides, immune complexes, and surface components of intact cells such as certain bacteria and fungi.[140-142] Binding of nascent C3b fragments to these substances protects C3b from inactivation by serum factors H and I. Subsequent cleavage and binding of factor B and the stabilizing protein properdin yield C3bBb, alternative pathway "C3/C5" convertase, which enzymatically cleaves C5 into the active components C5a and C5b. Each pathway ultimately activates terminal components of the complement system to form C5b-9, which inserts into lipid bilayers to form a transmembrane pore, permitting bidirectional solute flow and ultimately cell wall lysis.

Although there is considerable variability in data regarding neonatal complement levels and function, some generalizations can be made. Although many neonates have complement levels within the adult range, the level of components and activity of the alternative pathway are consistently diminished relative to those in the classical pathway. Marked deficiencies of C8 and C9 are seen and appear associated with poor killing of gram-negative bacteria *in vitro*.[143] Poor cross-linking of C3 may contribute to decreased lytic and opsonic activity.[144] Preterm neonates have more consistent impairment of both pathways.[145] Complement levels increase steadily postnatally and reach adult levels by 12 to 18 months of age.[146] Finally, whereas MBL serum levels of term neonates approach those of adults, values in preterm neonates are roughly 60% of levels at term; the absence of increased morbidity or infection suggests only an adjunctive role for the MBL pathway in this population.[147]

Complement components are found throughout the lower respiratory tract and are produced locally by alveolar macrophages, pulmonary fibroblasts, and type II epithelial cells.[148-150] In this milieu, complement activation can be initiated by PAMPs, or in the immune host by IgM or IgG microbial binding. Each pathway results in binding of component C3b, which is recognized by specific receptors on neutrophils and macrophages, facilitating phagocytosis. Generated C3a and C5a are potent neutrophil chemoattractants, whereas C5b initiates the membrane attack complex effecting direct, non–leukocyte-mediated, bacterial killing. Evidence that complement is critical in defending against some pulmonary infections is provided by murine models of acquired and inherited hypocomplementemia, in which pulmonary clearance of *Streptococcus pneumoniae* and *Pseudomonas aeruginosa* is impaired.[151-153]

Fibronectin

Fibronectins are extracellular matrix glycoproteins capable of interacting with a number of macromolecules, as well as cells bearing specific fibronectin receptors.[154] The ability of specific mesenchymal cells such as fibroblasts to elaborate fibronectin during embryogenesis is critical in thoracic development. After birth, basal expression of fibronectin is limited primarily to hepatocytes, which produce circulatory fibronectin, and the respiratory tract, where it is present in saliva, produced by bronchoepithelial cells, and constitutively secreted by alveolar macrophages.[155] Serum concentrations of fibronectin are diminished in neonates (particularly in preterm infants), whereas bronchoalveolar lavage (BAL) levels appear inducible in settings of lung injury.[156-158] Enhanced fibronectin production by pulmonary fibroblasts, alveolar macrophages, and epithelial cells is induced by local production of macrophage-derived cytokines associated with acute inflammation (TNF-α), IL-1β, transforming growth factor-β (TGF-β), and platelet-derived growth factor (PDGF).[159] In acute lung injury, fibronectin stimulates fibroblast and epithelial cell recruitment and endothelial cell proliferation, to facilitate tissue reparative processes. However, the ability of fibronectin to bind certain bacteria, as well as to augment leukocyte adherence and migration, suggest an additional role for this molecule in lung antimicrobial defense.

Fibronectin is bound by a number of pathogenic bacteria (*Staphylococcus aureus*, *Streptococcus pyogenes*, *Escherichia coli*, and *Pseudomonas aeruginosa*), as well as *Mycobacterium* species, *Pneumocystis*, and fungi.[160-165] Because fibronectin binds multiple microorganisms, it may act as a nonimmune opsonin, promoting the binding and internalization of pathogens by phagocytic cells with appropriate receptors; studies demonstrating increased neutrophil and macrophage binding of *S. aureus* tend to support this role.[166, 167] Conversely, this capacity for fibronectin to bind multiple pathogens may provide potential airway adhesion sites if mucociliary clearance is impaired or epithelial cell damage exists, yielding a partial explanation of pulmonary microbial tropism in these settings. In the normal lung, the most important host defense role of fibronectin may be to facilitate binding of, and local colonization by, nonpathogenic organisms.

Iron-Binding Proteins

Iron is an essential element for bacterial growth and survival. Host defenses that have evolved to restrict bacterial colonization or invasion include mechanisms to sequester elemental iron either in cells or complexed to transport proteins.[168] The primary iron-binding protein in serum is transferrin, whereas lactoferrin predominates in mucosal secretions. Because each of these proteins is present in airway mucosal secretions and airway lining fluid, they may be important local protective factors in containing microbial growth. Transferrin is found in BAL fluid in amounts between one and two times greater than matched serum;[169] secretion of this protein in the alveoli by lymphocytes and macrophages is postulated. In contrast, lactoferrin is the predominant iron-binding protein of airway secretions and is rarely present in deep alveolar lavage unless inflammation is actively occurring; it is stored in neutrophil granules, in addition to its secretion on mucosal surfaces.

Iron-binding proteins effectively complex free iron available in mucosal secretions and alveolar lining fluid, thereby limiting the growth of most iron-dependent pathogens; notable exceptions include *Moraxella* and *Neisseria* species, which are able to obtain iron from these proteins.[170] In addition to iron binding, human lactoferrin has other antimicrobial activity against specific bacteria, including *Escherichia coli*, *Streptococcus pneumoniae*, and *Legionella pneumophilia*.[171, 172] Lactoferrin binds to lipopolysaccharide, disrupting gram-negative bacterial membranes, and this effect may be synergistic with the effects of other soluble components of the mucociliary layer such as lysozyme.[173] Lactoferrin also demonstrates antiviral activity, binding to HIV and cytomegalovirus, preventing their uptake by host cells.[174] Cleavage of lactoferrin by either proteases or pepsin yields a small cationic peptide, lactoferricin, with structure and antimicrobial activity similar to those of the defensins.[175] Finally, recent work suggests a unique role for lactoferrin in prevention of bacterial biofilms. Biofilm formation is a growth mode specialized for long-term bacterial colonization of surfaces, as is seen in chronic *Pseudomonas* infection; once established, organisms within biofilms are notoriously resistant to host eradication.[176] By chelating iron, lactoferrin stimulates "twitching," a pili-mediated bacterial motility that deters biofilm formation. Once a biofilm has been established, however, sensitivity to this lactoferrin effect is lost.[177]

Beyond these antimicrobial effects, lactoferrin may also play an important role in modulation of local immune response. As a component of neutrophil secondary granules, lactoferrin is delivered to sites of inflammation. Here, lactoferrin binds LPS, effectively competing with LPS-binding protein and minimizing endotoxin presentation to immune cells.[178] Similarly, lactoferrin also recognizes and binds recurrent "motifs" of bacterial DNA, potentially dampening the broad proinflammatory immune responses that would ordinarily be triggered.[179] Teleologically, this may allow lactoferrin to limit excess immunostimulatory activity at mucosal surfaces with significant microbial exposure.

In summary, transferrin and lactoferrin sequester iron, denying microbial access to this essential element. In addition, lactoferrin has discrete functions as a microbicidal agent, in prevention of bacterial biofilm formation, and in modifying local immune responses. The availability of these iron-binding proteins along epithelial surfaces of the lung constitutes an important component of innate host defense.

Antimicrobial Peptides (Defensins, Cathelicidins, Lysozyme)

Activity of the larger opsonizing or nutrient-binding proteins in maintaining airway sterility is complemented by smaller, endogenous antimicrobial peptides. These peptides act to disrupt cell membranes of a wide range of pathogens, including bacteria, viruses, and fungi; each peptide manifests a broad, but fixed, spectrum of activity, underscoring the need for multiple peptide classes within the airway lining fluid.[180-183] Within the respiratory tree they are produced by epithelial cells, where their expression is both constitutive and inducible, or delivered to vulnerable loci by circulating leukocytes. Apart from their direct antimicrobial activity, which is nearly immediate in onset, these peptides can also activate cellular immunity, amplifying host response as necessary. The major human antimicrobial peptides are lysozyme, cathelicidins, and the defensins.

Defensins are small (3 to 6 kDa, 29–40 amino acids) cationic peptides containing six conserved cysteine residues. They are divided into α and β subclasses on the basis of their secondary structure, but their gene locations imply a common evolutionary origin.[184] Structurally they share a β-sheet conformation that spatially segregates their cationic and hydrophobic amino acid clusters into an amphipathic motif.[185] When secreted, defensins are driven into anionic phospholipid bilayer membranes by electromotive forces where they multimerize into channels, disrupt normal membrane function, and induce cell lysis.[185,186] Although host cells are potential "bystander" targets, their lower anionic lipid content and the presence of cholesterol as a membrane stabilizer imbue significant protection.[187,188] Apart from their structural differences, the α and β defensins differ in their sites of expression and roles in airway defense.

The human α-defensins constitute a subclass of six members: four "human neutrophil peptides" (HNP-1 through HNP-4) and two "human defensins" (HD-5 and HD-6). HD-5 and HD-6 are secreted by Paneth cells of the small intestine and epithelia of the female urogenital tract and are presumed to attenuate local commensal burden; respiratory epithelia is not a source of α-defensins.[189,190] HNPs 1 through 4 are abundant (up to 50% of total protein) in primary granules of neutrophils, where they assist in nonoxidative killing, and are also found in natural killer (NK) cells, monocytes, and lymphocytes.[191,192] Individual α-defensins have unique spectra of antibacterial activity against gram-positive and gram-negative species, as well as activity against enveloped viruses (including *Herpes* species) and activity against *Candida*.[193,182,194] The α-defensins also exhibit both proinflammatory and antiinflammatory activities. As discussed later, they are chemotactic and induce chemotaxins for a variety of immune cells. They also bind to serine protease inhibitors, amplifying PMN-derived elastase activity.[195] Conversely, they can inhibit complement activation by binding to C1q and participate in local wound repair by stimulating epithelial cell proliferation.[196,197] Extracellular α-defensins are scavenged by α2-macroglobulin, which minimizes cytotoxicity to host cells and down-regulates defensin concentration at inflammatory sites.[198] Immunohistochemical analysis has demonstrated HNPs on bronchial epithelial surfaces and in mucinous exudate in the air spaces, presumably derived from PMN granule release within the airway.[199] In adults, α-defensins have been found in BAL fluid of patients with pneumonitis, correlating with chemotaxin concentration and PMN counts.[200]

Unlike the α-defensins, the β-defensins are produced by airway epithelium. This subclass contains four identified human β-defensins (HBD-1 through HBD-4), although more than 20 genes are postulated to exist.[201] As a group, these peptides demonstrate antimicrobial activity against several gram-positive and gram-negative organisms, as well as *Candida* and *Aspergillus* species; however, differences in antimicrobial spectra exist between individual peptides.[189,202] Histologically, β-defensins are expressed in the epithelia of airways and lung, as well as in the serous cells of submucosal glands.[202,203] HBD-1 is found in the BAL specimens of healthy adults; its expression in the airways appears to be constitutive and noninducible.[204] In contrast, the remaining β-defensins are all inducible, with HBD-2 the best characterized. Endotoxin, *Pseudomonas,* and the cytokines TNF-α and IL-1β each induce HBD-2 expression, and this induction may be amplified further by concurrent alveolar macrophage stimulation.[205,206,183] Apart from this interaction with alveolar macrophages, HBDs further interface with cellular immunity by functioning as chemoattractants, or "microchemokines." HBD-1 and HBD-2 are each chemotactic for immature dendritic cells (DCs), as well as memory T cells, by means of ligation of the chemokine receptor CCR6; sustained β-defensin induction by noncontained microbial stimuli may thus invoke cellular and adaptive immune responses.[207] *In vivo,* tracheal aspirates of term and preterm newborns demonstrate similar levels of HBD-2, with increased levels seen in local and systemic infections. These data imply that β-defensin responses are intact even in preterm infants and that neonates may up-regulate some facets of pulmonary innate immunity in the context of a systemic inflammatory response.[208]

Cathelicidins are a diverse family of vertebrate antimicrobial proteins found in leukocytes and on epithelial surfaces where they function like defensins. They are produced as preproproteins, stored as inactive proforms, and require enzymatic cleavage for bioactivity.[209,210] The sole known human cathelicidin is hCAP-18, which requires proteolytic activation by proteinase 3 to liberate the antibacterial peptide LL-37—a 37 amino acid molecule whose amphiphilic α-helical structure facilitates affinity to, and disruption of, bacterial membranes.[211] LL-37 manifests protean effects relevant to host defense. It is a broad-spectrum antimicrobial, with effects against *Actinobacillus, E. coli, P. aeruginosa, E. faecalis,* and *S. aureus* and demonstrates synergy with the defensins.[212,213] LL-37 also directly binds endotoxin and is chemotactic for neutrophils, monocytes, and T lymphocytes.[214,215] LL-37 is found in primary granules of neutrophils and has also been shown in NK cells as well as lymphocytes and monocytes.[192] Expression of LL-37 in the lung is seen in cells of the submucosal glands and surface epithelia of the proximal airway, where its elaboration can be induced by up to 50-fold in states of inflammation.[185,213] Interferon-γ (IFN-γ) has been shown to induce LL-37 release but concurrently down-regulates gene transcription, perhaps balancing antimicrobial effects against host cytotoxicity.[192] At high concentrations, LL-37 can manifest cytotoxicity toward eukaryotic cells, and hosts have scavenging mechanisms as exist for the defensins.[216] *In vivo,* as with the β-defensin data presented earlier, comparable levels of LL-37 are found in the tracheal aspirates of term and preterm newborns, with increased levels seen in local and systemic infections.[208]

Lysozyme is a 14-kDa, very cationic enzyme that hydrolyzes glycosidic bonds of bacterial cell wall peptidoglycan. This peptide is found in the granules of neutrophils and mononuclear phagocytes and is also secreted by airway epithelial cells of the pulmonary tract,[217] where it confers nonspecific antimicrobial protection. Lysozyme is highly active against many streptococci species, but resistance to its enzymatic activity is common among other gram-positive organisms and nearly universal among gram-negative organisms.[218] This is likely caused by variable accessibility of vulnerable glycosidic bonds within the cell wall matrix, with the outer membrane of gram-negative bacteria providing an additional barrier to the penetration of lysozyme. However, in the presence of other membrane-targeting substances such as complement or hydrogen peroxide, lysozyme enhances the destruction of *E. coli* and other gram-negative bacteria.[219,220] Lysozyme is also capable of direct antimicrobial activity toward *S. sanguis* and *S. faecalis* species by virtue of its cationic properties and possesses fungicidal activity against *Candida albicans* by targeting the glycosidic bonds of fungal chitin.[221-223] Although lysozyme may appear redundant in the presence of other antimicrobial peptides, emerging data suggest otherwise. *In vivo,* a transgenic murine model of lysozyme over-expression imbued increased resistance to pulmonary infection from either *P. aeruginosa* or group B *Streptococcus*.[224] Furthermore, lysozyme exhibits important antimicrobial synergy with HBD-2, with LL-37, and with lactoferrin.[213, 225, 226] Together, these findings suggest a critical contribution by lysozyme to airway defense.

Lipopolysaccharide (LPS)-Binding Protein

LPS-binding protein (LBP) is a soluble 60-kDa glycoprotein that recognizes and binds the lipid A moiety of LPS, enhancing host immune response to endotoxin.[227] LBP is homologous to other phospholipid transport proteins and functions as a transport protein that disaggregates soluble LPS and presents it to targets on cellular membranes. LBP:LPS complexes are recognized by inflammatory cells (monocytes/macrophages) expressing the LPS receptor CD14 on their membrane surface; ligation of this receptor facilitates membrane protein interactions that eventually induce the "early response" cytokines TNF-α and IL-1β.[228] Alternatively, LBP can also act as an opsonin for CD14-dependent phagocytosis. LBP is produced primarily in the liver as an acute phase protein, and its plasma concentration increases exponentially during acute inflammatory responses.[229] LBP is also a normal constituent of lung fluid, with alveolar concentrations estimated at 1 μg/ml; these concentrations also increase exponentially with pulmonary inflammation, likely owing to capillary leak of plasma LBP and enhanced local generation.[230] The relevance of LBP to pulmonary host defense is suggested by murine transgenic models of LBP deficiency; such mice exhibit blunted alveolar bacterial clearance, with increased bacteremia and lethality in response to pneumonia.[231] Despite these findings, pulmonary sources of LBP remain a focus of inquiry. Human alveolar type II epithelial cells demonstrate capability *ex vivo* to up-regulate LPB production in response to mediators (TNF-α, IL-1β, IL-6) that similarly induce hepatic acute phase production of LBP.[232] Additionally, animal models suggest that in the neonate, alveolar macrophages may be a concurrent source of LBP in the lung.[233] Although elevated serum levels of LBP have been reported in neonatal sepsis, pulmonary LBP expression in response to respiratory infection remains unquantified in this population.[234]

Pulmonary Collectins

The collectins, or collagenous C-type lectins, are a family of carbohydrate-binding proteins that comprise an innate, constitutive nonclonal defense system. The human collectins include mannan-binding lectin and the pulmonary collectins, surfactant proteins A (SP-A) and D (SP-D). These proteins are characterized by a discrete, four domain primary structure consisting of a cysteine-containing N-terminus, a subsequent collagen-like region, a coiled neck region, and a C-terminal carbohydrate recognition domain (CRD).[235] The basic structural unit of the collectins is a trimer of this polypeptide chain, with triple helical formation at the neck and collagen-like regions; although binding by individual CRDs is relatively weak, trimeric clustering enhances binding affinity by several hundredfold.[236] The capacity for these proteins to interact with spatially separated ligands depends on appropriate oligomerization, and collectins may exhibit different degrees of oligomerization, stabilized by interchain disulfide bonds between the N-terminal cysteine residues.[237] Thus, SP-A preferentially exists as a hexamer of trimeric units, presenting 18 CRDs, whereas SP-D is found in tetrameric form, with 12 CRDs. Collectins function as soluble scavenger receptors, interacting through their lectin CRDs with microbial carbohydrate and glycolipid PAMPs to enhance phagocytosis and pathogen clearance; through this mechanism, collectins exhibit activity against a broad range of bacterial, viral, and fungal pathogens. Beyond these opsonizing qualities, SP-A and SP-D may each exert specific immunomodulatory effects that titrate the magnitude of inflammation and influence pulmonary immune responses.[2, 238]

SP-A and SP-B share many characteristics related to their synthesis and bioactivity. Both collectins are produced by type II alveolar epithelium and Clara cells and secreted into the alveoli and distal airway, probably by a pathway distinct from other surfactant components.[239] Production and secretion of both proteins increases dramatically during the third trimester of fetal lung development and appears to be further inducible *in utero* in response to dexamethasone; both proteins are also up-regulated in response to acute lung injury or epithelial activation by microbial products such as LPS.[240-243] Pathogen encounter with lung collectins results in agglutination and/or opsonization. Agglutination impedes microbial invasion and colonization and facilitates clearance by the mucociliary escalator, whereas agglutination of viruses enhances their internalization by neutrophils.[235, 244] Alternatively, SP-A or SP-D may act as opsonins, by bridging between PAMPs on the microbial surface and collectin receptors on phagocytes.[245] The pulmonary collectins also enhance specific leukocyte functions. Both SP-A and SP-D are chemotactic for neutrophils and macrophages, although SP-D is more potent in this regard.[246] SP-A and SP-D enhance both the phagocytic function of alveolar macrophages, as well as oxyradical production by these cells.[247] Induction of this latter effect requires the collectin CRD(s) to concurrently engage ligand; this presumably minimizes spurious up-regulation of potentially injurious mediators. Finally, SP-A and SP-D have each been shown to inhibit T-cell proliferation.[248] As before, this limits the risk of alveolar inflammatory injury, by titrating the level of T-cell activity in this compartment. Despite these many shared functions, SP-A and SP-D exhibit several biochemical differences that result in distinctive, unshared activities *in vivo*. Relevant differences include solubility, CRD specificity, length of collagen domain, and affinity for available collectin receptors.[235]

SP-D comprises about 30% of the pulmonary collectin pool and is the product of a single gene.[249,250] SP-D exists primarily in a cruciform structure: four homotrimeric subunits radiating from a disulfide-linked hub.[2] SP-D is basic, soluble at physiologic pH, and preferentially distributed within the aqueous phase of surfactant.[235] Unlike SP-A, it is relatively impervious to proteolytic or elastase degradation.[251] Consistent with its presumed role in innate defense, SP-D is up-regulated by LPS-induced cytokines.[235] SP-D binds specifically to carbohydrates containing glucopyranosides, resulting in affinity for the core oligosaccharides of LPS, the mannose-rich oligosaccharides of influenza A hemagglutinin, and fungal cell wall glycoconjugates of *Candida* and *Pneumocystis carinii*.[235, 252-254] SP-D binds to the putative collectin opsonin receptor, gp-340, a macrophage scavenger receptor, and probably other, nonspecific leukocyte receptors; interaction with CD14 has also been postulated.[255, 256] Attempts to further clarify the role of SP-D in host defense have led to the development of transgenic murine models of SP-D deficiency. Such mice exhibit a phenotype of pulmonary alveolar proteinosis, with foamy activated macrophages, hypertrophy of alveolar type II cells, and increased inducible inflammatory response.[257, 258] Diminished uptake and clearance of influenza A virus is noted in this model, but overall microbial clearance is largely unaffected.[259]

In contrast to SP-D, SP-A comprises about 70% of the pulmonary collectin pool.[249] It is the product of two genes, SP-A1 and SP-A2, each producing different chain types; the SP-A subunit can therefore exist as a homotrimer or heterotrimer, introducing heterogeneity to this protein.[260-262] Differential tissue expression has been reported, with SP-A1 expressed in the lower respiratory tract, and SP-A2 expressed in the tracheal and bronchial epithelium and submucosal glands.[239] Its production is up-regulated by interferon-γ (IFN-γ) and also by LPS-induced cytokines.[263,235] SP-A is relatively acidic, insoluble at physiologic pH, and associated with surfactant lipids *in vivo,* where it contributes to the stability of tubular myelin.[2,235] Its short collagen domain and preferred hexameric structure result in a "flower bouquet" pattern, and this clustering of CRDs influences ligand selectivity. SP-A binds specifically to carbohydrates, including fungal wall glycoconjugates and some capsular polysaccharides.[235] It also binds a variety of lipids, including the lipid A moiety of LPS.[264] Relevant pathogens that are ligands for SP-A include *E. coli, Klebsiella pneumoniae, Staphylococcus aureus, Streptococcus pneumoniae, Mycoplasma,* and mycobacteria.[245,264-268] Leukocyte receptors for SP-A include the C1q receptor, SPR210, the 210-kDa receptor specific for SP-A, the gp-340 receptor, and CD14.[2,256,269,270] Engagement of the CD14 receptor allows SP-A to mediate macrophage uptake of LPS in a manner similar to LBP, whereas ligation of the other receptors facilitates internalization of the presented microbe or antigen. Expression of these receptors is regulated by a variety of signals, including LPS, IFN-γ (up-regulation), and granulocyte-macrophage colony-stimulating factor (GM-CSF) (down-regulation), suggesting a more complex immunomodulatory role for SP-A than previously presumed.[271]

SP-A exhibits a variety of immunoregulatory activities within the alveolus. It suppresses IFN-γ, an activator of leukocyte and macrophage inflammatory activity, and an essential mediator for transition to a lymphocyte-mediated adaptive immune response.[272] SP-A may also dampen LPS-dependent cellular activation by competing with LBP.[273] Taken together with the reported SP-A inhibition of T-cell proliferation, these functions suggest that SP-A acts, at least in part, by tempering inflammation that might induce alveolar injury. Such a host-protective role would be consistent with transgenic models of SP-A deficiency, where microbial challenge results in delayed pathogen clearance, increased pathogen dissemination, and enhanced inflammation with increased production of TNF-α, IL-1β, and IL-6.[2,274] This paradigm, however, is complicated by contradictory data regarding SP-A induction of proinflammatory cytokines and up-regulation of inducible NO synthase (iNOS). These disparate findings are reconciled by recent observations that the response to SP-A is determined by the state of cell activation and concurrent stimuli.[275] Thus, SP-A up-regulates iNOS in alveolar macrophages primed by IFN-α, and stimulated by LPS, but conversely inhibits LPS-induced iNOS if IFN-γ priming has not occurred. SP-A, therefore, augments an inflammatory response already underway but dampens similar responses evolving *de novo*.[276] In this context, SP-A induction of iNOS also exerts host protective effects. In a murine model of tuberculosis, exogenous SP-A enhances pathogen entry into alveolar macrophages by almost fivefold. This enhanced entry resulted from SP-A ligation of the SPR210 receptor, with increased endocytosis of the SP-A:BCG complex; SP-A–mediated up-regulation of NO and TNF-α production ensues, achieving increased mycobacterial killing.[277] SP-A similarly enhances *Mycoplasma* killing through analogous NO-dependent mechanisms.[268]

SP-A and SP-D exhibit only partial redundancy of their bacterial specificities, owing to their distinct structures and their differing affinities for specific carbohydrates and lipids. These differences may result in complementary functions that enhance the antimicrobial activity of surfactant *in toto*. One example of such synergy is illustrated by collectin interactions with *Klebsiella,* a pulmonary pathogen that can reversibly switch between encapsulated and unencapsulated phenotypes.[235] Unencapsulated forms of this organism allow optimal adhesion to the epithelial surface, facilitating colonization; these forms predominate early in infection. As noted earlier, SP-A binds to lipid A of LPS whereas SP-D preferentially binds to the LPS core sugars.[253] Because lipid A is embedded within the bacterial cell wall and inaccessible to SP-A, SP-D is the primary collectin ligand for LPS expressed on the surface of unencapsulated forms. Encapsulation limits interaction of SP-D with the underlying LPS but invokes significant binding by SP-A, which recognizes the capsular polysaccharides expressed by this pathogen.[245] In this scenario, SP-A and SP-D thus fulfill distinct, but complementary, opsonizing roles in the innate host response, as depicted in Figure 164-4. Similar complemen-

tary function is illustrated by collectin interaction with influenza A virus (IAV). SP-D binds viral envelope glycoproteins (hemagglutinin and neuraminidase) through its CRD and induces massive agglutination of IAV particles; this agglutination is facilitated by higher-order oligomerization, most achievable by SP-D by virtue of its longer collagen domain.[278,279] Such agglutination generates particle size sufficient for mucociliary clearance and also directly enhances neutrophil uptake and respiratory burst. Alternatively, SP-A activity results from IAV recognition and binding of sialic acid residues on this collectin. SP-A has much less agglutinating capacity but interacts with a broader range of IAV strains, including those that are highly resistant to inhibition by SP-D or serum collectins.[244] SP-A forms much smaller aggregates, resulting in less augmented neutrophil uptake, but enhanced uptake by alveolar macrophages.[280] As before, the differing collectin structures and binding affinities result in a broader range of antimicrobial activity and immune cell activation, which ultimately prove to be beneficial to the host.

In summary, accruing data suggest that the pulmonary collectins participate in every phase of innate pulmonary host defense; they exert direct effects on the invasiveness and viability of pathogens, they facilitate phagocytic uptake of captured organisms, and they modulate leukocyte chemotaxis, respiratory

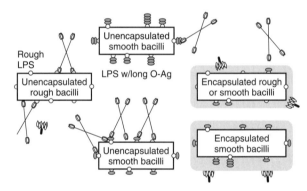

LUNG COLLECTIN INTERACTIONS WITH
LPS AND CAPSULAR POLYSACCHARIDES

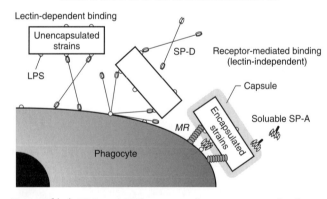

INTERACTIONS WITH GRAM-NEGATIVE BACTERIA

Figure 164–4. SP-A and SP-D are complementary opsonins for gram-negative bacteria. SP-D binds to LPS core sugars exposed by non-encapsulated variants, the phenotype required for colonization and invasion. Encapsulation increases pathogenicity and limits SP-D binding, but allows SP-A recognition and binding of capsular polysaccharides. Subsequent phagocytosis may occur through SP binding to phagocyte surface carbohydrates (lectin-dependent), or may be receptor mediated (lectin-independent), as depicted by SP-A engagement of mannose receptors. (Adapted from Crouch EC: Am J Respir Cell Mol Biol *19*:177-201, 1997.)

burst, and cytokine expression. Although the association of SP-A with tubular myelin places it "on the front line" of antigen encounter, SP-D exhibits nonredundant functions that further augment microbial clearance and complement SP-A activity. As locally synthesized opsonins, the pulmonary collectins are therefore essential for optimal alveolar innate immune response.

Immunomodulating Role of Surfactant

Apart from the specific actions of its collectins, surfactant also exerts a host of immunomodulatory effects within the alveolus. Surfactant enhances phagocytosis, by means of a mechanism separate from the actions of SP-A.[266, 281] Interestingly, this prophagocytic effect is more pronounced for resident alveolar macrophages than for recruited peripheral blood monocytes. Whole surfactant reportedly suppresses mononuclear cell oxyradical production by inhibiting the intracellular assembly of NADPH oxidase, impairing hydrogen peroxide generation.[282] However, specific lipid components of surfactant may exert different modulatory effects. Therefore, although macrophage oxidative burst is blunted by phosphatidylglycerol moieties, it is enhanced by phosphatidylcholine components.[283, 284] Enhanced microbicidal function of phagocytes and downregulation of Fc receptors have each been reported and attributed to the lysophospholipid and free fatty acid components of surfactant.[281, 285, 286] Whole surfactant also modulates phagocyte chemotaxis. Macrophage movement into the alveolus postnatally coincides with increased surfactant synthesis, suggesting a chemotactic effect, possibly SP-A mediated.[247] Conversely, dipalmitoyl phosphatidylcholine (DPCC) treatment of alveolar macrophages *in vitro* decreases their migration in response to serum chemotaxins; this is consistent with a teleologically preferred "default" attenuation of inflammatory response, designed to preserve alveolar function.[287] Lastly, surfactant reportedly

modulates lymphocyte function as well. Lymphocytes exposed *in vitro* to surfactant are less responsive to mitogens and exhibit depressed function; under similar conditions, cytotoxic T cells, B cells, and NK cells are all inhibited to various degrees.[288, 289] As discussed earlier, however, some lipid components (DPCC, phosphatidylglycerol) are more suppressive, whereas less abundant components (cholesterol, sphingomyelin) stimulate lymphocyte proliferation; this suggests that conditions that alter these phospholipids ratios may alter adaptive immune responses.[290] Additionally, the differing effects of SP-A and surfactant lipids on lymphocyte proliferation are consistent with the hypothesis that, in some scenarios, surfactant lipids and proteins may be counterregulatory (summarized in Fig. 164–5).[291]

In contrast to whole surfactant, conventional surfactant analogues (Exosurf, Survanta) contain neither SP-A nor SP-D. Consequently, collectin-mediated immune effects are not provided by exogenous replacement therapies. Moreover, the surfactant replacements are generally immunosuppressive, presumably owing to their nonphysiologic lipid/protein ratios.[247] Both Exosurf and Survanta have been shown to inhibit production of the early response cytokines TNF-α, IL-1β, and IL-6 by stimulated alveolar macrophages, putatively by depressing activation of the nuclear transcription factor NF-κB.[292, 293] Similar suppression of fibroblast-derived IL-6 and prostaglandin E_2 (PGE_2) has also been described, suggesting impairment of those inflammatory responses up-regulated by alveolar cytokine networks. Additionally, Survanta has been shown to blunt lymphocyte proliferation, killer cell cytotoxicity, and adhesion molecule expression, possibly through down-regulation of lymphocyte receptors for IL-2.[294] Much of this is *in vitro* data and must therefore be interpreted cautiously; however, it suggests that available surfactant replacement therapies, although efficacious in normalizing

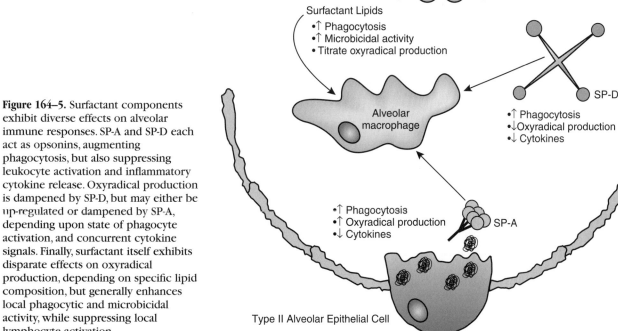

Figure 164–5. Surfactant components exhibit diverse effects on alveolar immune responses. SP-A and SP-D each act as opsonins, augmenting phagocytosis, but also suppressing leukocyte activation and inflammatory cytokine release. Oxyradical production is dampened by SP-D, but may either be up-regulated or dampened by SP-A, depending upon state of phagocyte activation, and concurrent cytokine signals. Finally, surfactant itself exhibits disparate effects on oxyradical production, depending on specific lipid composition, but generally enhances local phagocytic and microbicidal activity, while suppressing local lymphocyte activation.

Surfactant Lipids
- ↑ Phagocytosis
- ↑ Microbicidal activity
- Titrate oxyradical production

Alveolar macrophage

SP-D
- ↑ Phagocytosis
- ↓ Oxyradical production
- ↓ Cytokines

- ↑ Phagocytosis
- ↑ Oxyradical production
- ↓ Cytokines

SP-A

Type II Alveolar Epithelial Cell

pulmonary compliance, may concomitantly attenuate normal alveolar immune cell responses.

Nitric Oxide

Nitric oxide (NO) is a short-lived, oxyradical-related bioactive mediator with potent vasodilatory actions.[295] Basal synthesis of NO seems to occur *in vivo*, implying an important homeostatic role for this molecule. NO is synthesized from L-arginine by the enzyme NO synthase (NOS), which exists in either constitutive or inducible forms. Cells with constitutive NOS include neurons, vascular endothelium, neutrophils, and platelets. Cells with iNOS, and hence recruitable to generate NO, include mononuclear phagocytes, vascular smooth muscle cells, epithelial cells, and hepatocytes.[296-299] Although recognized important actions of NO include vasodilation, smooth muscle relaxation, and inhibition of platelet function, its potent cytotoxic and inflammatory effects also suggest an antimicrobial role for this molecule.

Available data, both circumstantial and specific, implicate NO as playing an important role in nonspecific host response to infection. NO production, from cells containing iNOS, is induced by microbial products such as lipoteichoic acid, endotoxin, and bacterial DNA.[300, 301] NO production is similarly up-regulated by immune activating cytokines such as IFN-γ, TNF-α, IL-1, and IL-2.[302, 303] Specific NO products, such as nitrosylated thiols, may be either bacteriostatic or bacteriocidal, depending on the specific pathogen.[304, 305] Relevant cellular targets of NO products have been identified and include microbial DNA, as well as microbial cysteine proteases, which are critical for virulence or replication of many bacteria, viruses, and parasites.[306, 307] NO products also inhibit viral RNA synthesis, inactivate a broad range of microbial proteins by S-nitrosylation, and induce membrane damage through lipid peroxidation.[300] NO also up-regulates inflammatory cell function; it has been shown to augment macrophage motility, up-regulate surface expression of complement and immunoglobulin Fc receptors, and stimulate leukocyte respiratory burst.[308, 309] Concurrent synthesis of NO increases microbicidal activity of the leukocyte respiratory burst by generating additional cytotoxic radicals such as peroxynitrite, which possesses potent activity against bacteria and *Candida*.[310-312] *In vitro*, phagocytes demonstrate diminished microbicidal activity after NOS inhibition, and this correlates with *in vivo* models in which diminished NOS activity impairs microbial clearance.[309, 313]

Consistent with the previous discussion, there is accruing evidence supporting a role for NO in pulmonary innate immunity. NO is produced along the entire length of the human airway and is present in airway lining fluid at concentrations of about 15 μm.[306, 314] Locally produced NO inhibits sodium uptake from the apical surface of airway epithelial cells, increasing airway hydration and enhancing mucociliary clearance.[315] *In vitro*, iNOS is shown to be expressed by alveolar macrophages and is also inducible in human airway epithelium by proinflammatory cytokines.[316, 317] Therefore, cells of the alveolar capillary membrane (macrophages, endothelium, epithelium) are capable of NO up-regulation in the context of infection, and this is consistent with human findings, where exhaled NO levels are increased in patients with bacterial or viral respiratory infection.[318-320] Multiple *in vitro* studies have demonstrated that iNOS up-regulation is essential for intracellular killing of pulmonary pathogens such as *Mycoplasma*, mycobacteria, or *Legionella pneumophila*.[321-323] Animal studies yield similar results *in vivo*, with NO up-regulation seemingly essential for effective lung microbial clearance.[309] This implied essential role of NO in pulmonary microbial clearance is consistent with recent neonatal data.[324] BAL specimens from preterm (<32 weeks' EGA) infants exposed to intrauterine infection demonstrated a strong association between inability to express iNOS or up-regulate NO, and subsequent development of fulminant pneumonia. Conversely, newborns of similar age

and risk that did not develop pneumonia exhibited iNOS up-regulation and increased NO products on BAL analysis, relative to either their pneumonic cohorts or noninfected controls. A separate retrospective analysis of lung tissue from neonatal autopsies yielded similar findings; alveolar macrophage-derived iNOS could not be detected in specimens from fulminant pneumonia patients but was demonstrable in controls. Taken together, these data suggest that delayed or diminished macrophage-derived NO in the setting of neonatal pulmonary infection correlates with increased morbidity. Etiology of this impaired response is speculative but may result from a paucity of mediators (TNF, IFN-γ) known to up-regulate iNOS expression.

Beyond the functions just detailed, NO exhibits additional immunomodulatory activities relevant to pulmonary host defense. NK cells are specialized cytotoxic lymphocytes and a primary source of IFN-γ within the alveolus; they are normally activated by IL-12. Transgenic iNOS deficiency reportedly induces a phenotype of IL-12 deficiency, despite normal IL-12 levels. This phenotype is characterized by diminished IFN-γ and increased transforming growth factor-β (TGF-β), a cytokine milieu suppressing local macrophage function. Analysis of these data subsequently identified iNOS-derived NO as an essential "cosignal" for IL-12 signal transduction and activation of NK cells.[325] In this model, the signaling role of NO was therefore critical in maintaining a cytokine microenvironment that allowed normal immune cell function. This signaling role is consistent with earlier studies describing NO regulation of gene expression. G proteins and NF-κB may each be activated by NO; NF-κB can, in turn, up-regulate iNOS expression, amplifying local production of NO.[326, 327] Such data have been contradictory, however, with NO variously reported as both inhibiting and enhancing the expression of a variety of immune mediators.[328,329] These data are reconcilable by the finding that NO exerts a biphasic effect on NF-κB activity; via this mechanism, which depends on local NO concentration, NO is able to both up-regulate and down-regulate the expression of a number of inflammatory mediators.[330] In this paradigm, immune activation up-regulates iNOS, generating increased NO. Initial NO activation of NF-κB promotes expression of adhesion molecules and proinflammatory cytokines, facilitating immune cell recruitment. NF-κB up-regulation of iNOS amplifies NO production, eventually generating local NO concentrations sufficient to inhibit NF-κB activity. At this point, both inflammatory cytokine and adhesion molecule expression down-regulate, effectively dampening the component of inflammation sensitive to modulation by NO. In summary, the putative actions of NO in immune cell signal transduction suggest a sentinel role for this molecule in both the initiation and suppression, of cellular immunity.

Carbon Monoxide

As with NO, evolving data suggest a potential role for carbon monoxide (CO) in pulmonary host defense. Endogenous CO derives from degradation of hemoglobin, myoglobin, NOS, and cytochromes, by the enzyme heme oxygenase (HO). HO immunoreactivity is found throughout the airway in respiratory epithelium, alveolar macrophages, seromucous glands, and nose and paranasal sinuses.[331, 332] Like NOS, HO exists in constitutive (HO-2) and inducible (HO-1) isoforms.[333] Whereas HO-2 is basally expressed in most tissues, HO-1 is identified as a heat shock protein inducible by a variety of stimuli, including microbial toxins, proinflammatory cytokines, and reactive oxygen or nitrogen species; both isoforms are substantially expressed in human lungs.[334] Like NO, HO is induced by many infectious agents, and levels of carboxyhemoglobin and/or exhaled CO are reportedly elevated in patients with viral or bacterial respiratory tract infections.[335,336] Unlike NO, however, the direct effects of CO appear less microbicidal, and more antiinflammatory, or host cytoprotective. *In vitro* and *in vivo*, CO has been shown to inhibit endotoxin-induced proinflammatory cytokines, including tumor necrosis factor (TNF), IL-1β, and macrophage inflammatory protein-1β (MIP-1β), while concurrently up-regulating the anti-inflammatory IL-10.[337] Furthermore, in a murine model of influenza A pneumonitis, overexpression of HO-1 resulted in diminished respiratory epithelial cell apoptosis as well as decreased lung inflammation.[338] Outside the context of infection, there is also ample evidence that CO is protective against hyperoxic injury. Transgenic mice deficient in HO-2 are sensitive to hyperoxia, whereas either HO-1 induction or exogenous CO is protective against hyperoxic injury in other rodent models.[333,339] The mechanism(s) of this protection remains incompletely characterized but may involve generation of the antioxidant metabolite bilirubin.[340] Interestingly, NO, like other oxyradical species, is capable of inducing HO-1 activity. The CO subsequently generated then directly inhibits iNOS activity by binding to the heme moiety of this enzyme, suggesting that HO pathways may exert important counter-regulatory effects on NO generation.[306] In summary, both microbial stimuli and the resultant host cytokine response induce HO-1 and endogenous CO production. Despite this association, the protective effects of CO against oxyradical species suggest that its sentinel role may be to minimize host inflammatory injury. Beyond this, it may also serve an important role in innate immune response by titrating the activity and immunomodulatory impact, of iNOS.

To summarize, soluble components of airway lining fluid are essential elements of pulmonary host defense. Fibronectin, complement, and surfactant proteins enhance phagocytosis of bacteria, NO has bacteriostatic and immunomodulatory properties, lactoferrin impairs biofilm formation, and multiple components exhibit direct microbicidal effects. Many of these components can also act to "dampen" or titrate local immune responses, preventing inappropriate inflammation deleterious to pulmonary function and host survival. Finally, each of these components has the capacity to recruit granulocytes, mononuclear cells, or lymphocytes, allowing innate immune mechanisms to initiate cellular responses that may culminate in adaptive immunity.

Cellular Elements of Innate Immunity

As discussed earlier, effective host response to incipient respiratory infection relies primarily on rapid clearance of the offending pathogen(s). When soluble components of innate immunity are insufficient to achieve organism clearance, cellular immune effectors are invoked. Cellular elements of pulmonary innate immunity include resident alveolar macrophages and DCs, as well as neutrophils and monocytes recruited to the air space. The initial interaction of these cells with microorganisms is mediated by soluble and membrane-bound PRRs that recognize and engage the common microbial motifs characteristic of PAMPs. Soluble factors such as the collectins, and LBP, utilize specific cell receptors to "present" organisms for phagocytosis and induce cell activation. Once activated, these cells generate signals that either further amplify innate immune responses or, alternatively, initiate transition to adaptive immunity. Of the cellular PRRs, CD14 appears to be the sentinel receptor for activating alveolar macrophages and inducing cytokines that extend pulmonary immune responses.[229]

CD14 recognizes and binds LPS presented as a complex with LBP; however, for this interaction to induce cell activation, CD14 must interact with a second membrane protein, a member of the Toll family of receptors. Toll-like receptors (TLRs) are highly conserved transmembrane proteins, initially recognized in *Drosophila*, that mediate recognition of microbial products. The cytoplasmic domains of the TLRs are homologous to the IL-1 receptor, suggesting common signal transduction pathways.[341,342] Several TLRs have been identified in humans; TLR4 confers responsiveness to endotoxin; TLR2 confers responsiveness to gram-positive bacteria, mycobacteria, and yeast; TLR3 confers responsiveness to viral double-stranded mRNA; and TLR9 confers responsiveness to bacterial DNA.[343-348] TLRs thus provide specificity to the initial recognition of pathogens, even in the setting of "nonspecific" inflammatory cell response. Engagement of these receptors activates signal transduction pathways that overlap with IL-1β–dependent signaling pathways, generating the "early response" cytokines TNF-α and IL-1β. These cytokines enhance the microbicidal activity of alveolar macrophages and also activate other cells within the alveolus. Whereas this results in immediate amplification of inflammation, it also induces elaboration of pleiotropic cytokines that recruit lymphocytes, activates DCs, and eventually orchestrates the transition to an adaptive immune response.

Macrophages

Macrophages are primary effector cells of innate immunity,[349] serving important functions of phagocytosis, microbial killing, accessory immune function, and regulation of local inflammatory processes through cytokine secretion. Within the lung, pulmonary macrophages constitute a cell population of diverse function and origin. Previously believed to be monocyte derived, fetal pulmonary macrophages have been shown to precede formation of myeloid elements in the liver and bone marrow.[350] Initially present as so-called angular cells within the extravascular stroma, these cells lack the morphologic appearance of differentiated phagocytes but proliferate and differentiate *ex vivo* in response to colony-stimulating factors such as GM-CSF elaborated by lung stromal elements.[351,352] Postnatally, descendants of fetal macrophages likely constitute a self-renewing portion of the alveolar macrophage population, which may be supplemented by cells of myeloid origin.[353] Under conditions of inflammation, peripheral blood monocytes may be recruited to the lungs, where they undergo local differentiation depending on their site of influx.[354] Recruited monocytes, like the angular cells, mature into alveolar macrophages, interstitial macrophages, airway macrophages, or DCs depending on local growth factors and other stimuli; though sharing some functions, each type has slightly different characteristics, perhaps owing to their particular microenvironment.[355,356] The relative number of functional pulmonary macrophages in the neonate is uncertain. Normal resident cell populations are absent from both the airway of stillborn infants and BAL of preterm infants at cesarean section.[357,358] Because true alveolar macrophages are found in infants by 48 hours postnatally, rapid expansion of this cell population clearly occurs. This is consistent with simian models, where alveolar macrophage numbers increase to near adult levels by 48 hours postnatally, temporally associated with increased alveolar surfactant levels.[359] Once macrophage population of the lungs has occurred, the relatively long life span (months) and dual sources of repletion maintain stable lung macrophage numbers, even under conditions of myelosuppression.[360-362]

Phagocytic activity of alveolar macrophages (AM) is essential for clearing air stream particulate matter, macromolecular debris (immune complexes, protease-antiprotease complexes, nonfunctioning surfactant, apoptotic cells), and microbes.[349,363] Redundancy and ruffling of the AM cell membrane provide an expanded surface contact area and facilitate the pseudopodal extensions characteristic of phagocytic "engulfing." AM phagocytosis may be nonspecific or triggered by "pattern-recognition" cell surface receptors that recognize a number of foreign ligands. These include TLRs (TLR2 and TLR4), which bind LPS, and CD14, which recognizes LBP-LPS complexes.[229,364,365] Other pattern-recognition receptors bind mannose, fibronectin, or surfactant proteins, whereas more specific receptors recognize complement components (C1q and C3b) and the Fc portion of most immunoglobulins.[255,270,366-368] If the ingested material is degradable, normal AM surveillance function continues; otherwise, the AM may be removed by upward clearance mechanisms along the respiratory epithelium and mucociliary ladder or through the interstitium by means of regional lymphatic drainage.[369]

After phagocytosis, the plasma membrane–contained particle is internalized by the AM, forming an intracytoplasmic vacuole. This vacuole then fuses with any number of secondary lysosomes to form a phagosome. TLRs may be recruited to phagosomes to sample their contents and initiate an inflammatory response appropriate for the specific organism.[346] Within phagosomes, lysozyme, proteases, and acid hydrolases released from secondary lysosomes will digest most particles; however, because many cell wall–containing bacteria are resistant to enzymatic killing, other mechanisms for their biodegradation must be invoked. In these instances, microbicidal effect is achieved by "oxidative burst" generation of highly cytotoxic reactive species of oxygen[370] and nitrogen,[371] in which electron transfer to the terminal NADPH oxidase in the membrane of the phagolysosome can result in local production of superoxide anion, hydrogen peroxide, hydroxyl radical, singlet oxygen, and NO. AM can also generate NO by expression of iNOS.[372] In the context of these important phagocytic and microbicidal roles, animal and human studies consistently describe depressed levels of neonatal AM function. When neonates of various species are challenged with airway bacterial inoculums, *in vivo,* AM rates of phagocytosis are prolonged, especially in premature subjects; impairment of phagocytosis is also seen *in vitro.*[373-375] Similarly, neonatal AM antimicrobial activity is also diminished; this may correlate with diminished oxidative burst capacity, deficiency of stored lysosomal materials, or other as yet uncharacterized factors.[376-379]

In contrast to commonly encountered bacteria, viruses and other nonviral intracellular pathogens such as mycobacteria have evolved mechanisms to elude macrophage killing and survive within these cells. Relevant intracellular pathogens of the neonate include *Toxoplasma gondii, Listeria monocytogenes,* and herpes simplex virus (HSV); control of infection caused by these organisms therefore relies on mechanisms of enhancing microbicidal activity of the host macrophage. Under most situations of intracellular parasitism, specific cytokines such as IFN-γ, TNF-α, and GM-CSF are generated to stimulate macrophage killing of these organisms.[380, 381] Altered signal transduction in response to IFN-γ has been reported for neonatal AM; however, available data suggest that these cells can be sufficiently activated by IFN-γ to achieve intracellular killing comparable with that achieved by adult macrophages, and similar data exist from animal models of *Listeria* and HSV infection.[382-385] These observations have led to work demonstrating markedly decreased basal and inducible levels of T-cell–derived IFN-γ in neonates,

attributed to lack of priming of the naive T cell by foreign antigen.[386] Decreased IFN-γ secretion by neonatal monocytes has also been reported.[387] This delay in development of antigen-specific memory T cells, coupled with suboptimal capacity for IFN-γ expression by other cells, may account for greater neonatal susceptibility to these pathogens.

In addition to microbial killing by phagocytosis, AM have accessory roles in multiple other immune responses. AM may contribute to infection control by direct or antibody-mediated cytotoxicity for cells expressing microbial antigens.[388] AM can also metabolize complex antigens and "present" small antigen fragments to T cells but lack co-stimulatory signals for T-cell activation, reducing their effectiveness in this role.[389] Finally, their capacity to generate various chemotaxins and cytokines allows the AM to recruit multiple types of inflammatory cells to the alveolus and regulate the ensuing local inflammatory response. Although macrophage-derived IL-1 production for term and preterm neonates corresponds to that of adults, both TNF-α and IL-12 production are less than seen in adults and are markedly depressed (<25%) in premature neonates.[390,391] Moreover, neonatal macrophage-derived TNF-α production is less inducible by IFN-γ than in adults. Deficient production of IFN-γ by neonatal T cells, as previously discussed, may further depress neonatal AM TNF-α production, diminishing AM capacity to fully respond to alveolar pathogens.

In summary, macrophage precursors appear early in lung development. They predate other myeloid elements and may provide an intrinsic, self-renewing local macrophage population, later supplemented as needed by monocyte-derived cells recruited to the lung. Once established, alveolar macrophages function locally to contain and kill microorganisms and to initiate and titrate local inflammatory processes through elaboration of specific cytokines (Fig. 164–6). Available data regarding neonatal AM function correlate with data from other species and suggest that phagocytic function, microbial killing, and antigen presentation may all be compromised relative to AM function in older subjects. The capacity of neonatal AM to elaborate certain cytokines is reduced, correlating with degree of prematurity. Inability of neonatal T cells to express normal levels of IFN-γ may further impact on AM cytokine production, leaving the neonatal alveolus more vulnerable to infection.

PMNs

The pulmonary circulation is a major reservoir for marginated neutrophils, which can be rapidly mobilized for an acute inflammatory response. Emigration of PMNs from the local circulation into the respiratory tract is a dynamic process requiring the generation of signals that sustain PMN contact with the

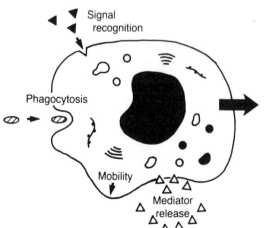

- Scavenge particulates
- Remove macromolecular debris
- Kill microorganisms
- Accessory cell for immune responses
- Recruit and activate other inflammatory cells
- Maintain and repair lung parenchyma
- Surveillance against neoplasms
- Modulate normal lung physiology

Figure 164–6. Summary of alveolar macrophage activity. As depicted, essential functions include mobility, phagocytosis, microbial killing, presentation of antigen to lymphocytes, and ability to respond to specific stimuli (endotoxin, cytokines) by generating mediators to modulate inflammatory processes. The aggregate of these functions allows the macrophage to initiate and direct the evolution of local immune responses, facilitating its central role in pulmonary host defense. (From Crystal RG: *In* Crystal RG, West JB [eds]: The Lung: Scientific Foundations. New York, Raven Press, 1991, pp 527–538.)

vascular endothelium and induce transendothelial diapedesis and chemotactically directed migration to the inflammatory locus. This adherence process is dependent on the expression of specific, corresponding adhesion molecules on both the endothelial cell and PMN surfaces, whereas diapedesis and migration are induced by the local elaboration of specific chemoattractant factors. Once recruited and activated, PMNs, like alveolar macrophages, attempt to contain invading pathogens by means of receptor-mediated phagocytosis. This results in exposure of engulfed pathogens to antimicrobial substances found in primary granules of the PMN (defensins, bactericidal/permeability-increasing protein, serprocidins, lysozyme), as well as reactive oxygen species produced by the PMN "oxidative burst."[370, 392-394] PMNs may also function locally to generate further chemotactic, proinflammatory mediators, such as arachidonate metabolites and IL-8,[395] further amplifying the local inflammatory process.

Several facets of PMN physiology unique to neonates may result in blunted granulocyte recruitment relative to that seen in older children or adults. Systemically, there is diminished capacity to accelerate PMN production in response to infection, owing to both a limited PMN storage pool and already near-maximal baseline levels of PMN production.[396,397] Shorter survival times of neonatal PMNs, suggested by *in vitro* data, may contribute to more rapid depletion, and hence a smaller storage pool. Specific PMN functions are also compromised in the neonate, possibly secondary to diminished LPS binding capacity and hence less endotoxin responsiveness.[398] *In vitro* studies suggest dual defects in neonatal PMN adhesion, resulting in only 40 to 45% binding activity to activated endothelium relative to adult PMNs. Mechanisms identified are a relative deficiency of L-selectin on the neonatal PMN surface[399] and inability of activated PMNs to up-regulate expression of the β2-integrins;[400] the net effect is that neonatal PMNs show impaired binding to activated endothelium and bind less avidly than adult PMNs in the presence of local chemotactic factors. Deficient chemotaxis is also consistently reported in neonatal PMNs, especially in premature infants.[401,402] Because surface receptor density for specific chemotactic factors appears normal, postreceptor binding factors have been implicated. These include a constitutively smaller pool of β2-integrins, whose surface expression is required for PMN binding and diapedesis, and impaired ability of the neonatal PMN to reorganize its cytoskeleton in response to chemotactic stimulation.[402-404] Impaired PMN chemotaxis has also been induced *in vitro* by exposure to indomethacin, suggesting further potential immunologic impairment in premature neonates requiring pharmacologic closure of a patent ductus arteriosus.[405] Finally, important differences in phagocytic activity exist between neonatal and adult PMNs. Although *in vitro* phagocytic activity is comparable, under conditions of decreased opsonization, neonatal PMN phagocytosis is less efficacious;[406] this may be clinically significant in the relatively opsonin-deficient neonatal alveolar milieu. There may also be a diminished capacity to store and release antimicrobial peptides,[392] although other mechanisms (superoxide anion generation, lysozyme release) for intracellular killing of phagocytized organisms appear intact. In summary, identified differences in PMN production, survival time, adhesivity, chemotaxis, and phagocytosis may result in increased vulnerability of the neonate in situations in which pulmonary PMN recruitment is required to contain microbial invasion.

Dendritic Cells

Dendritic cells are a minor (fewer than 1%) pulmonary cell subpopulation but serve a critical role as accessory cells in initiation of primary immune responses. Within the lung, DCs exist as a network of interdigitating cells lying within the alveolar septa and perivascular adventitia and within the airway epithelial cell layer where their contact with air stream particles is enhanced

(Fig. 164-7).[407] DCs express certain membrane antigens characteristic of mononuclear phagocytes yet exhibit poor phagocytic and microbicidal activity. Conversely, DCs are exponentially more potent at T-cell activation than are macrophages.[408] This results from their capacity to present antigen in the context of major histocompatibility complex (MHC) molecules and their surface expression of the B7 ligands CD80 and CD86, which are obligatory second signals for T-cell activation.[409] By virtue of these specialized attributes, DCs are the only antigen-presenting cell capable of activating naive lymphocytes.

As presently characterized, "immature" DCs migrate into the lung, where they sample the environment for particles expressing PAMPs.[410, 411] If encountered, they "acquire" the antigen by receptor-mediated endocytosis.[412] Antigens are degraded in specialized endosomes, where peptide fragments are loaded onto MHC class II molecules for transfer to the cell surface. Concomitantly, the DC chemokine receptor profile is altered, either by microbial products or locally generated cytokines, inducing DC chemotaxis to lung-associated lymph nodes.[413] During this migration, DCs mature from "antigen processors" to antigen presenters, under the influence of locally elaborated GM-CSF.[414] Once in lymphoid tissue, DCs present antigen, stimulate the clonal development of antigen-specific T cells, and activate both cytotoxic and helper T cells; they may also directly interact with B cells to regulate antibody production.[415] Engagement of the DC CD40 surface molecule by the T-cell CD40 ligand induces DC-derived IL-12, which is required for T-cell differentiation and IFN-γ production. DCs can migrate in response to bacterial peptides or LPS, complement cleavage products, early response cytokines such as TNF-α or IL-1, or chemokines; thus, inflammation or infection recruit additional DCs from the peripheral blood.[416] In the basal state, pulmonary DC populations undergo complete turnover every few days, consistent with the robust antigen exposure of the pulmonary tree.[409]

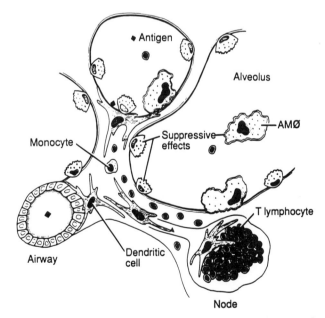

Figure 164–7. Role of pulmonary dendritic cells in the initiation of a local immune response. As depicted, dendritic cells are present in the alveolar septa, underlying airway epithelium, where they encounter antigen present in the air stream. Subsequent processing of antigen and presentation to T cells may initiate an alveolar cellular immune response. As shown, local modulation of the immune response may be exerted by other cellular components of the alveolus. (From Toews GB: *In* Shelhamer JH [moderator]: Ann Intern Med *117*:415, 1992.)

Regulation of DC function is multifactorial, consistent with their central role in titrating pulmonary adaptive immune response. One mechanism of DC regulation is anatomic; although immature DCs can acquire antigen, they cannot present it until they have emigrated to regional lymph nodes. Such strict compartmentalization minimizes (possibly spurious) T-cell activation directly within the alveolus and requires the stimulated T-cell clones to recirculate to the lung in response to additional, "fail-safe" homing signals.[417] DC function is also regulated by secreted products of alveolar macrophages. AM-derived NO inhibits GM-CSF–mediated up-regulation of antigen-presenting activity and directly blunts T-cell activation by interfering with signal transduction.[418,419] AM-derived PGE₂, TGF-β, and IL-10 also suppress antigen processing and MHC class II expression by pulmonary DCs.[420,421] *In vivo*, the role of AM-mediated regulation is shown in murine models of AM depletion, where hyperresponsiveness to aerosolized antigen results.[417] Finally, cytokines produced during early inflammation, including IFN-γ, TNF-α, and GM-CSF, increase MHC class II expression and allow normalization of DC function (depicted in Fig. 164-8).[422]

The prenatal ontogeny of DCs is uncertain; as for alveolar macrophages, animal data suggest early derivation from angular cells of the fetal lung.[423] Postnatally, DCs may be either lymphoid derived or myeloid derived, with each lineage displaying unique characteristics, such as expression of different TLR repertoires for antigen recognition and different profiles of cytokine expression. As DCs mature, TLRs are progressively down-regulated, reflecting transition from antigen recognition to antigen presentation and resulting in greater uniformity of function. However, diminished capacity to generate IL-12 may persist among some DC subsets, limiting the range of T-cell responses that may be invoked.[424] Although mature DCs are a regular part of the human tracheobronchial mucosa after the first year of life, both animal and human data indicate that, at birth, DCs are present in only very small numbers in the respiratory tract.[409,425] Apart from their lower numbers, neonatal DCs also exhibit important functional limitations, including diminished expression of MHC class II antigens and blunted capacity to respond to maturation signals of GM-CSF.[426] Additional *in vitro* data suggest that neonatal DCs have less ability

to modify their chemokine receptor profiles, impairing normal trafficking.[427] Lastly, neonatal DCs exhibit an altered cytokine expression profile relative to adults; specifically, IL-12 production is markedly impaired whereas TNF-α and IL-10 are preserved, resulting in a "skew" toward the effects of the latter two cytokines.[427,428] The net result of these differences is a DC population that is less efficient in both antigen presentation and induction of IFN-γ production, delaying expansion of the memory T-cell pool and contributing to neonatal susceptibility to respiratory infection.

Immunologically Recruitable Pulmonary Structural Cells

Endothelium. Because of its anatomic location at the interface between the vascular and alveolar compartments, the endothelium is uniquely situated to regulate pulmonary immune responses requiring recruitment, and facilitated passage, of intravascular inflammatory cells (Fig. 164-9). Vascular endothelial cells express MHC class II molecules and may act as antigen presenters to T cells.[429] Endothelial cells also participate in immune processes by either elaborating, or responding to, cytokines in the local microenvironment. For example, TNF-α is an endogenous mediator of inflammatory immune responses secreted by alveolar macrophages in response to bacterial endotoxin. Endothelial cells manifest a pleiotropic response to TNF, including increased expression of adhesion molecules, increased prostaglandin production, increased MHC antigen expression, and increased cytokine release, including IL-1, IL-6, IL-8, GM-CSF, and MCP-1.[430-437] The net effect of these signals is an increased chemotactic recruitment and activation of inflammatory cells at the "gate" from the vascular space to the interstitium; the TNF-induced increase in endothelial cell–leukocyte adhesivity further enhances this response. Endothelial cells also express the TLRs TLR4 (constitutive)[438] and TLR2 (inducible by IFN-γ or TNF-α);[439] this allows their direct response to endotoxin, manifested by up-regulation of adhesion molecule expression and induction of IL-1, IL-8, MCP-1, and GM-CSF expression.[429,435,440-443] By responding either to endotoxin directly or to endotoxin-induced macrophage-derived TNF-α, the endothelial cell may either generate an initial immune response or participate in amplifying a local inflammatory cascade.

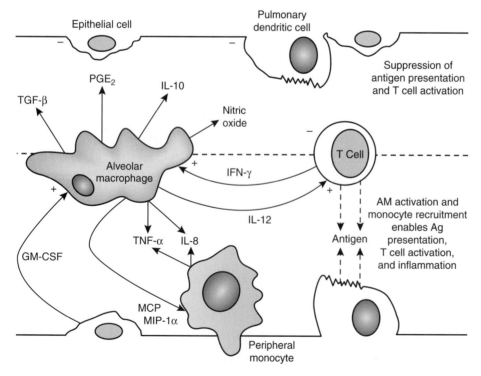

Figure 164–8. Interactions between alveolar macrophages and dendritic cells determine alveolar immune response. Alveolar macrophage-derived mediators (NO, TGF-β, IL-10, PGE₂) suppress antigen processing and presentation by dendritic cells, preventing T cell activation and maintaining a non-inflammatory milieu. This basal state is altered by pro-inflammatory cytokines (TNF, GM-CSF) that activate alveolar macrophages; signals suppressing dendritic cells are dampened, antigen presentation is optimized, and T-cells are activated. Activated T cells and recruited blood monocytes each release mediators that also activate alveolar macrophages, further amplifying alveolar immune response. (Adapted from Riches DWH: *In* Murray JF, Nadel JA [eds]: Textbook of Respiratory Medicine. Philadelphia, WB Saunders, 2000, pp. 385–412.)

Fibroblasts. Whereas most studies of fibroblasts have focused on their production of structural and matrix proteins, it is now evident that fibroblasts may also function as important immune-effector cells at sites of inflammation. When appropriately stimulated, fibroblasts may generate bioactive amounts of multiple cytokines, including IL-6, IL-8, IL-1α, IL-11, colony-stimulating factors, and growth factors such as TGF-β.[444] TNF or IL-1 can each induce fibroblast-derived IL-6, IL-1a, IL-8, and IL-11, and their combined action synergistically further up-regulates fibroblast elaboration of these cytokines.[445, 446] Although fibroblasts and alveolar macrophages are often capable of elaborating the same inflammatory cytokine(s), maximal production of these cytokines typically occurs in response to different signals. This is illustrated by the distinct response of these cells to endotoxin. Endotoxin is a potent stimulator of macrophage-derived TNF and IL-1, while exerting little direct stimulation of fibroblasts. Conversely, pulmonary fibroblasts elaborate inflammatory cytokines in response to IL-1 and TNF,[447] whereas macrophage response to these cytokines is more diverse.[448-451] This suggests that although classical immune cells such as alveolar macrophages produce inflammatory cytokines in a stimulus-specific fashion, fibroblasts produce inflammatory cytokines in response to macrophage-derived TNF or IL-1, independent of the precipitating stimulus. This response serves to amplify local pulmonary inflammation and illustrates the potential immunologic role of the fibroblast, transcending its putative structural function.

Epithelium. Pulmonary epithelial cells serve multiple functions, including maintenance of solute fluxes, production of surfactant, and providing a surface for gas transfer. Beyond these metabolic and barrier functions, pulmonary epithelial cells are capable of augmenting and regulating local innate immunity in response to environmental signals. Alveolar type II cells have collectin receptors, allowing them to internalize microbes presented by these proteins.[2] Epithelial cells also express CD14 and TLR2, allowing them to recognize and respond to endotoxin.[452,453] Endotoxin, or the early response cytokines TNF-α or IL-1β, may each up-regulate epithelial-derived defensins such as HBD-2.[453,454] Airway epithelial cells also exhibit tonic, high-level expression of iNOS with cyto-toxic NO production, directly effecting pulmonary host defense.[455] The cyclooxygenase and lipoxygenase pathways are expressed at high levels in epithelial cells resulting in production of lipid mediators,[456, 457] including the anti-inflammatory prostaglandin E_2 (PGE$_2$)[458] and the neutrophil chemoactivator leukotriene B_4 (LTB$_4$).[459] Infection with respiratory syncytial virus can directly induce epithelial-derived IFN-β, IL-1α, and the chemokines IL-8 and RANTES.[460, 461] Alternatively, pulmonary epithelial cells can also express several cytokines in stimulus-specific fashion, including TGF-β, GM-CSF, IL-5, IL-6, IL-8, and monocyte chemotactic polypeptide-1 (MCP-1);[462-467] expression of these cytokines facilitates chemotaxis and activation of multiple immune cells, including PMNs, mononuclear phagocytes, and T lymphocytes. Airway epithelial cells can titrate local cytokine signal by shedding soluble TNF receptor; this adsorbs available TNF and diminishes its bioactivity.[468] Airway and alveolar epithelial cells *in vivo* also express intercellular adhesion molecule-1 (ICAM-1), a natural ligand for complementary adhesins of PMNs and monocytes, induced in response to IFN-γ, TNF, or IL-1. Increased epithelial expression of ICAM facilitates inflammatory cell migration along epithelial barriers; moreover, antimicrobial activity of phagocytes *in vitro* is enhanced by ICAM-mediated interactions with the alveolar epithelium.[469-471] Finally, airway epithelial cells, in response to specific cytokine stimulation, can express MHC antigens, allowing them to interact directly with T lymphocytes, possibly as antigen-presenting cells.[472] Together, these data suggest that in response to appropriate local stimuli, pulmonary epithelial cells may effect complex immune modulation within the milieu of the alveolus and airway.

CELLULAR MECHANISMS OF ADAPTIVE IMMUNE RESPONSE

In contrast to the broad pattern-recognition triggers of innate immunity, focused cellular or antibody-mediated immune response based on recognition of unique foreign antigen constitutes adaptive immunity. Adaptive immunity requires sensitization to individually encountered antigens; once sensitization

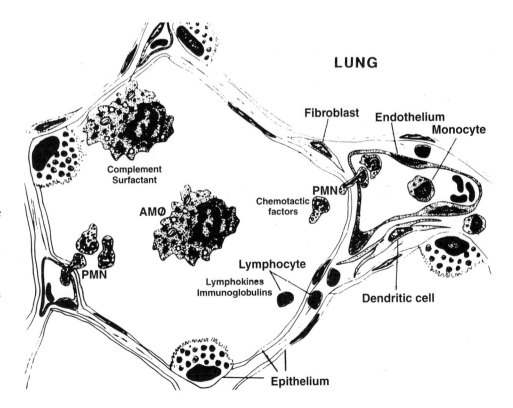

Figure 164–9. Normal alveolar architecture. Note specifically the relative location of structural cells (fibroblasts, epithelial cells, endothelial cells), which may be stimulated to participate in modulating local immune/inflammatory events. As noted in the text, vascular endothelial cells are strategically located to directly facilitate immune cell recruitment to the alveolar space. (From Toews GB: *In* Shelhamer JH [moderator]: Ann Intern Med *117*:415, 1992.)

LUNG

Fibroblast   Endothelium
Monocyte

Complement
Surfactant

PMN

Chemotactic
factors

AMØ

PMN

Lymphocyte

Lymphokines
Immunoglobulins

Dendritic cell

Epithelium

occurs, these immune responses are characterized by their exquisite specificity and long-lasting memory. Although many soluble and cellular components of host defense may link aspects of innate and adaptive immunity, adaptive immune responses are executed by lymphocytes.

Lymphocytes (T cells, B cells, and NK cells) are normally present at multiple sites in the lungs and may participate in complex immune responses to encountered antigens or act directly as effector cells against local microorganisms. Components of the lung lymphocytic system include the intravascular space, the interstitium, and the bronchoalveolar space.[473] The lung intravascular pool of lymphocytes is large (nearly 10 times greater than for the liver on a per gram basis), and increased sequestration of lymphocytes in the pulmonary intravascular space occurs in response to either local inflammatory stimuli or systemic nonspecific inflammatory mediators such as TNF.[474] Lung interstitial lymphocytes are plentiful, with numbers comparable to those of the circulating blood pool, and possess a characteristic size, distribution, subset composition, and cytokine production profile.[475] Large numbers of NK cells are also found in the interstitial space.[476] In the alveolar space, lymphocytes, mostly T cells, comprise approximately 10% of cells recovered from BAL. Alveolar lymphocyte numbers can be augmented in response to intraalveolar stimuli such as endotoxin or other antigenic challenge, suggesting a recruitable pool from either the interstitial or intravascular space.[477, 478] Lymphocytes can depart the bronchoalveolar space by migrating into the interstitium and reach draining lymph nodes through afferent lymphatics.[479]

T Cells

The pulmonary lymphocyte population is made up primarily of T cells.[480,481] Fetal and neonatal T cells express markers found on thymocytes,[482] suggesting that these T cells represent an immature transitional population; alternatively, this may reflect stress-induced release of cortical thymocytes into the circulation. The neonatal T-cell phenotype corresponds closely to that of antigenically naive T cells in the adult.[483, 484] These findings likely reflect a combination of the limited exposure of the neonate to foreign antigen and the limitations of neonatal DC function rather than intrinsic neonatal T-cell dysfunction. T cells recognize foreign peptides that have been modified by antigen-presenting cells and expressed in the context of MHC proteins; several pathways for antigen processing and presentation exist and result in activation of discrete T-cell subsets.[485, 486] Important immunoregulatory functions provided by pulmonary T cells subsets include cytokine production, enhancement of immunoglobulin production, and direct T-cell cytotoxicity.

Cytotoxic T cells mainly express the CD8 coreceptor and act to lyse host cells infected with intracellular pathogens.[487, 488] These T cells recognize small peptide antigens that are presented by MHC class I molecules but also require co-stimulatory interaction between the T-cell CD28 molecule and B7 ligands (CD80 and CD86) expressed by the antigen-presenting cell. In the absence of co-stimulation, the CD8 T cell is rendered either anergic or apoptotic.[485] Activated cytotoxic T cells effect antigen-targeted cell lysis through either release of cytolytic mediators or fas-ligand activation. CD8-mediated cytolysis involves the exocytosis of granules containing perforin, granzyme, and granulysin. Perforin is a glycoprotein that induces pore formation in the target cell membrane, facilitating both osmotic lysis and entry of granzymes and granulysin. Granzymes are serine esterases that activate the caspase cascade, inducing target cell apoptosis. Granulysin is an antimicrobial peptide with broad-spectrum activity against bacteria, mycobacteria, and fungi.[489] Alternatively, T cells can invoke cytolysis by up-regulating their expression of fas ligand, which engages fas molecules on the target cell surface,

initiating the caspase cascade and eventual apoptosis. Cytotoxic lymphocytes are particularly important in host defense against nonlytic viruses, such as cytomegalovirus (CMV), and also appear to be critical in host response to mycobacteria.[490, 491] *Mycobacterium tuberculosis*–specific CD8 cells recovered by BAL demonstrate significant cytolysis of infected macrophages *in vitro*, as well as enhanced secretion of IFN-γ.[492,493] T lymphocytes from newborns are capable of developing into cytotoxic T cells during natural infections postnatally, and *in utero* infection may induce profound CD8 cytotoxic response.[494] In general, however, the incidence of neonatal cytotoxic lymphocyte development and the overall magnitude of the response tend to be diminished, relative to that in older children.[495,496]

Helper T cells, or Th cells, express the CD4 coreceptor, and function to orchestrate B- and T-cell responses. These CD4 cells recognize antigen presented by the MHC class II–dependent pathway and, on activation, may be induced to differentiate into a specific Th phenotype, depending on the concurrent cytokine stimulation they receive. Thus, undifferentiated "Th0" cells, activated in the presence of macrophage-derived IL-12, adopt the Th1 phenotype. Th1 lymphocytes are characterized by their expression of IL-2, IL-12, TNF, and IFN-γ and function to activate macrophages and neutrophils and augment cell-mediated immune responses. Alternatively, in the absence of IL-12, activated Th0 cells are induced by IL-4 to adopt the Th2 phenotype, characterized by secretion of IL-4, IL-5, IL-6, IL-9, IL-10, and IL-13. Th2 lymphocytes function primarily to generate humoral immune responses and antibody production, support B-cell growth and differentiation, and titrate levels of macrophage and neutrophil activity.[497] The Th1 cytokine IFN-γ acts on Th0 cells to induce Th1 differentiation and inhibit Th2 differentiation. Conversely, the Th2 cytokines IL-4 and IL-10 inhibit Th1 differentiation, whereas IL-4 drives further Th2 differentiation. The net result of this cytokine-mediated self-amplification and cross-inhibition is that once a T-cell response begins to develop along one pathway, it becomes progressively "polarized" in that direction; this paradigm, as presently characterized, is summarized in Figure 164–10. In the lung, infectious diseases associated with the need for cell-mediated immunity typically induce Th1 responses, where up-regulation of IFN-γ is critical for macrophage activation and killing of intracellular pathogens. In this context, Th1 response has been shown to be critical for host resistance against a variety of pulmonary pathogens, including *Mycobacterium tuberculosis*, *Legionella pneumophila*, *Chlamydia pneumoniae*, and *Pneumocystis carinii*.[498-501] Under basal conditions, unprimed DCs preferentially secrete IL-10, resulting in an alveolar milieu favoring a default Th2 response that minimizes spurious inflammatory events within this compartment.[417] Such a "Th2 bias" of the lung may be teleologically essential, given its burden of antigen exposure and its vulnerability to immune-mediated injury.

Mature T cells are capable of enhancing antibody secretion by regulating the proliferation and immunoglobulin isotype expression of B cells; this regulation is provided both through contact-dependent mechanisms and through secretion of specific cytokines (Fig. 164–11). Contact-dependent interactions include cognate recognition through MHC antigens or receptor-ligand interactions primarily between the B-cell CD40 molecule and the T-cell CD40 ligand.[502] Activated Th cells markedly up-regulate their surface expression of CD40 ligand, a membrane-bound cytokine with homology to TNF.[503] Subsequent engagement with the B-cell surface CD40 molecule triggers B-cell expression of cytokine receptors. At this point, activated Th cells can begin to secrete cytokines in a directional fashion within the "immunologic synapse." Signals delivered to the B cell via CD40 binding markedly enhance immunoglobulin production and promote immunoglobulin class switching in the presence of coactivation signals provided by specific cytokines; relevant examples include

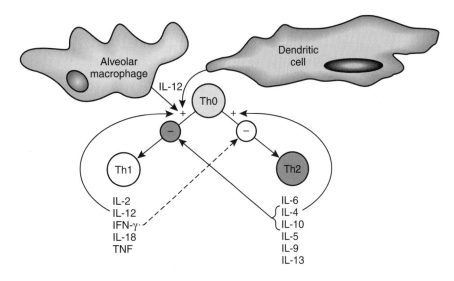

Figure 164–10. The Th1/Th2 paradigm. IL-12, secreted by alveolar macrophages or dendritic cells, induces naïve T helper cells (Th0 phenotype) to differentiate into the Th1 phenotype; Th1 cells are characterized by their secretion of IL-2, IFN-γ, and IL-12. Th1-derived IL-12 induces additional Th1 differentiation, while Th1-derived IFN-γ impairs Th2 differentiation. In the absence of IL-12, IL-4 induces Th0 cells to adopt the Th2 phenotype, characterized by secretion of Th2 cytokines including IL-4, IL-13, and IL-10; these cytokines induce further Th2 differentiation, while suppressing Th1 differentiation. Th1 cells are essential for macrophage activation and maturation of CD8 cells, while Th2 cells promote antibody production.

IL-2, which promotes IgM secretion; IL-4 or IL-13, which facilitates IgE synthesis; IL-10, which induces IgG1 and IgG3 production; and IFN-γ, which promotes IgG2 production.[504-508] The specific cytokine signals may be influenced by the nature of the antigen encountered, as well as the Th phenotype of the activating T cell; however, many cytokines relevant to Ig isotype switching (IL-2, IL-6, IL-10, IL-13) can be expressed by both Th1 and Th2 cells.[509]

With regard to both cytokine elaboration, as well as B-cell stimulation, neonates exhibit important deficiencies related to

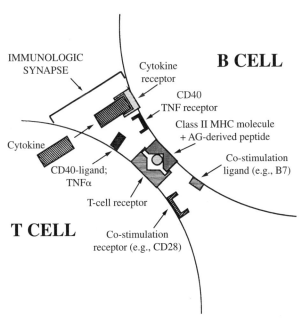

Figure 164–11. B-cell–T-cell interactions that facilitate activation of immune cells: the so-called immunologic synapse. These may be contact-dependent receptor-ligand interactions, as occur between the B cell CD40 receptor and the gp39 (TNF homologue) ligand expressed on activated T cells. Other sites of contact-dependent interaction include MHC presentation of antigen and co-stimulatory receptors, which further upregulate cellular response. Non–contact-dependent mechanisms include local secretion of specific T-cell–derived cytokines, which, in concert with contact activation, direct specific immunoglobulin class switching and elaboration by the B cell. (From Paul WE, Seder RA: Cell 76:241, 1994. Copyright 1994, Cell Press.)

T-cell function. The majority of neonatal T cells present a "naive" phenotype, characterized by decreased expression of the T-cell receptor (TCR), decreased adhesion molecule expression, and diminished expression of the CD40 ligand.[496, 510-511] Neonatal T cells also exhibit diminished cytokine production (notably IL-4, IFN-γ, IL-12, IL-15, GM-CSF), putatively owing to labile posttranscriptional regulation and markedly shortened mRNA half-life.[386, 512-516] Although normal levels of cytokine elaboration are inducible by sustained TCR triggering, the decreased adhesion molecule expression by neonatal T cells impairs interaction with antigen-presenting cells, resulting in co-stimulatory signals insufficient to achieve levels of adult functioning. Similarly, diminished expression of the T-cell CD40 ligand precludes optimal contact-dependent activation of B cells.[511] Finally, neonatal T-cell differentiation appears biased toward a Th2 or Th0 profile under neutral conditions. Factors favoring such a "Th2 bias" include the low MHC-peptide density of neonates (favors priming of Th2 cells), relative dearth of the Th1-inducing cytokines IFN-γ and IL-12, and the greater co-stimulation required to elicit Th1 differentiation.[517, 518] Factors favoring a Th0 state include paucity of the Th2-inducing cytokines IL-4 and IL-10. Interestingly, pregnancy is also associated with a "Th2 bias," with several factors (IL-4, IL-10, TGF-β) present at the maternal-fetal interface that can induce a shift from a Th1 to a Th2 profile.[519] Teleologically, this limits cellular immune responses that might be mounted against the fetus, compromising gestation. In this context, dampened expression of fetal IFN-γ is also teleologically adaptive, and reported mechanisms underlying this persist postnatally, possibly contributing to a blunted neonatal Th1 response.[520] In summary, qualitative differences in both T cells and antigen-presenting cells contribute to the deficient T-cell responses seen in neonates. To overcome a "default Th2 bias" and generate functional Th1 responses, neonatal T cells require greater co-stimulation, in excess of the limited capacities exhibited by antigen-presenting cells of this population. As a result, the ability to mount a cellular immune response to infection acquired perinatally is delayed relative to older hosts; this delayed acquisition of T-cell–dependent, antigen-specific response may account for the more severe clinical course experienced by neonates in response to specific pathogens.[521]

γδ T Cells

T cells expressing the γδ receptor are present on air space epithelial surfaces.[522] These cells do not recirculate and appear to be resident pulmonary lymphocytes. γδ T cells can develop by thymic-independent pathways and can recognize small molecules and intact proteins without the requirement for antigen processing that other T cells exhibit.[523] Small molecule recognition by γδ cells requires cell-cell contact, suggesting that non-MHC molecules may present small antigens to these cells or that co-stimulation from neighboring cells is required.[524] A germline-encoded phosphoantigen binding site enables these cells to respond to mycobacterial pyrophosphate, but they are also activated by antigen from disparate pathogens such as *Listeria monocytogenes*.[525-528] *In vitro*, γδ T cells can be induced to generate IFN-γ, TNF, and IL-4 in stimulus-specific fashion similar to Th0 cells.[529] Although the percentage of γδ T cells is lower in neonates and neonatal γδ T cells lack expression of the serine esterase marker associated with cytotoxicity, decreased γδ T-cell–mediated responses in neonates have not been identified.[530] The precise function of these cells in host defense remains unclear, but their anatomic locale and potential for cytotoxicity suggest a role in rapid initiation of immune reactions at mucosal surfaces of the airway.

B Cells

B cells comprise only a small percentage (<2%) of the lung lymphocyte population, and this proportion of B cells, or their precursors, is attained in the fetal lung by 18 to 22 weeks' gestation.[531] In more mature subjects, B cells of the lung interstitium participate in local humoral responses through elaboration of immunoglobulins in response to specific antigenic stimuli. In the neonate, however, this capacity is limited, attributed in part to the inability of neonatal T cells to provide either the contact-dependent help or cytokine factors required to induce B-cell differentiation into memory B cells.[532, 533] Apart from these differences in T-cell stimulation, neonatal B cells also exhibit phenotypic and functional differences from their adult homologues. A higher percentage of neonatal B cells are so-called B-1 cells, characterized by production mainly of polyreactive, low-affinity IgM, rather than the specific, high-affinity antibodies generated by B-2 cells.[534] Receptor ligation of neonatal B cells induces minimal up-regulation of MHC class II molecules and fails to induce CD86, impairing antigen presentation by these cells.[535] Neonatal B cells also exhibit diminished expression of the complement receptor CD21, limiting their capacity to be stimulated by complement.[536] Although capable of local immunoglobulin production (primarily IgM and IgA), neonatal B cells remain unable to generate antibodies to bacterial capsular polysaccharides; this results in particular vulnerability to organisms such as *Haemophilus influenzae* and group B *Streptococcus*.[537, 538] Neonatal B-cell function and lung humoral defense mechanisms are discussed in further detail later.

NK Cells

NK cells are large granular lymphocytes with cytotoxic function, comprising up to 15% of circulating lymphocytes, but less than 2% of the lung lymphocyte pool. They share a common progenitor with T cells but lack the TCR required for specific antigen recognition.[539] Within the lung, they are found on epithelial surfaces and in the interstitium, and they are also recruitable from the circulation in response to locally generated chemokines.[540] Dormant at baseline, activated NK cells contribute to early innate defense by lysing infected cells and generating cytokines that stimulate T cells and AM.[541] AM-derived IL-12 up-regulates NK cell perforin and granzyme, enhancing activated NK cell lysis of cells infected with bacteria, viruses, or protozoa.[542, 543] Unlike T cells, NK cells cannot recognize specific microbial antigens, responding instead to inappropriately low levels of MHC class I antigen expressed on infected cells.[544] NK cells also possess Fc receptors, allowing them to bind and kill targets coated with IgG (antibody-dependent cellular cytotoxicity [ADCC]); this occurs through combined fas-ligand and perforin/granzyme mechanisms.[545]

Beyond their cytotoxic functions, lung NK cells participate in complex cytokine networks that enhance alveolar immune response (Fig. 164–12). IL-12 is produced locally by AM and other cells in response to microbial stimuli. IL-12 acts in concert with TNF-α or IL-1, IL-2 or IL-15, and NO to induce NK cells to secrete IFN-γ and TNF-α; early in infection, activated NK cells may be the primary source of IFN-γ within the alveolus.[546,547] NK-cell–derived IFN-γ and TNF-α from multiple sources synergistically enhance AM killing of intracellular pathogens.[548] In addition, NK-cell–derived IFN-γ may initiate alveolar T-cell–mediated immunity by inducing differentiation of Th0 cells into a Th1 phenotype.[549] Lastly, NK cells with decreased responsiveness to IL-12 and exhibiting a Th2 cytokine profile have been identified.[550] The role of such cells *in vivo*, if any, is speculative; they may help maintain a less inflammatory "Th2 bias" within the noninfected lung.

The capacity to produce IFN-γ, augment immunity against intracellular pathogens, and effect cytotoxic responses without prior sensitization all imply a sentinel role for NK cells in neonatal host defense. Indeed, NK cell precursors appear early in gestation by thymic-independent mechanisms and reach adult levels by term.[551] NK cytolytic function, however, remains diminished (<50% of adult NK cells) for much of the first year of age, with more pronounced depression in premature neonates.[552, 553] This diminished function corresponds to an immature NK cell subset with impaired perforin/granzyme delivery;[554] this may predispose the neonatal lung to infections with agents such as HSV and cytomegalovirus (CMV).[555,556]

Bronchus-Associated Lymphoid Tissue

Aspects of pulmonary immune function have in the past been attributed to bronchus-associated lymphoid tissue (BALT), which is considered analogous to gut-associated lymphoid tissue as an established site of local antigen uptake and initiation of IgA responses.[557, 558] When present, BALT is localized, abutting the pulmonary arteries near bronchial branch points, and has a microvascular histology, including high endothelial venules, characteristic of lymph node structure.[559] Animal studies reveal that BALT is not constitutively present in all species and that the number and size of BALT appear dependent on antigenic stimulation.[473] Although infections such as chorioamnionitis can induce precocious development of BALT in mid-term human fetuses, BALT is not found in healthy neonates, and most postmortem adult studies demonstrate only isolated instances of BALT.[560-562] This indicates that while the human lung has the capacity to form BALT under certain conditions of antigenic stimulation, persistence of BALT is rare except under conditions of chronic local inflammation.[563] As discussed previously, this

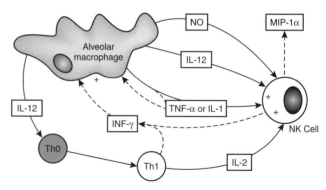

Figure 164–12. NK cells enhance alveolar immune response. Activated alveolar macrophages generate cytokines that induce NK cell activation. Once activated, NK cells may amplify macrophage activity either through elaboration of IFN-γ, or by secretion of MIP-1α, with resultant peripheral mononuclear cell recruitment.

variable presence of BALT in humans does not contradict the presence of large numbers of lymphocytes divided among the lung airway, interstitium, and vascular pool.[475]

Humoral Immune Responses

B lymphocytes bearing surface immunoglobulin of the IgA, IgG, and IgD isotypes appear early in gestation. Although the B-cell immunoglobulin repertoire expands during gestation, at birth it remains limited relative to older hosts.[564, 565] Immunoglobulin-secreting plasma cells appear later in gestation than B cells, between weeks 15 and 30.[566] Typically, neonatal B cells can differentiate into IgM-secreting plasma cells as efficiently as in the adult but do not differentiate into IgG- or IgA-secreting cells until these functions fully mature;[567] as previously discussed, the relative inability to achieve isotype switching in the neonate results at least in part from inadequacy of mutual signaling between neonatal T and B cells.[532,533,535] The antibody response of neonatal B cells to specific antigens develops sequentially, with responsiveness to antigens requiring contact-dependent T-cell help (e.g., protein antigens) preceding the development of responses not requiring such cognate help (e.g., capsular polysaccharides). Although infection of neonates elicits a protective response to most protein antigens, the response to polysaccharide antigens is absent or severely blunted. This has been recently postulated to result from decreased surface expression of CD21 and decreased complement levels, resulting in suboptimal signal transduction via CD21 and inability to achieve the CD21/B cell receptor synergy required for B-cell activation.[536, 568] Alternatively, humoral responses to bacterial capsular polysaccharides are enhanced by specific T-cell–derived cytokines such as IFN-γ, IL-12, and GM-CSF, all of which are relatively deficient in the neonate;[387,569] the limited capacity of naive neonatal T cells to provide these cytokines may thus contribute to the poor antibody responses of neonates to encapsulated bacteria such as group B streptococci. This T-cell immaturity thus combines with differences in antibody repertoire and functional immaturity of B cells to limit the capacity of the fetus or neonate to produce antibodies to certain antigens.

Secretory Immunoglobulins (IgA, IgM)

Secretory component is an epithelial-derived glycoprotein that facilitates transfer of immunoglobulins from subepithelial sites into epithelial-lined lumina by transepithelial transport and secretion.[570,571] By virtue of their ability to form polymeric complexes facilitating transport into epithelial cells and binding by secretory component (Fig. 164–13), IgA and IgM constitute the primary secreted immunoglobulin subclasses of the lung.[572-574] IgM is more abundant in secretions of neonates than in adults. IgM is the first immunoglobulin class to be produced in a primary response to an antigen and is the only immunoglobulin other than IgG that fixes and activates complement. It is secreted as a pentamer, and the resultant 10 antigen-binding sites render it a superb agglutinin. Whereas serum concentrations are low at birth, postnatal IgM concentrations rise rapidly in the first month, reflecting increased antigen exposure; IgM concentrations in premature infants remain lower for the first 6 months of life.[575,576] Secretory IgA is undetectable at birth but found by 1 to 2 weeks in saliva and nasopharyngeal secretions. The earlier expression of secretory IgA relative to serum IgA presumably reflects increased local production in response to encountered antigen.[577] Until capacity for IgA production matures, compensatory protection of the air space mucosa may be provided by increased relative amounts of secretory IgM.[578]

Other Immunoglobulins

IgG is the predominant immunoglobulin isotype at all ages,[575] and passively derived cross-placental transfer of maternal IgG is the primary source of all IgG subclasses detected in the normal

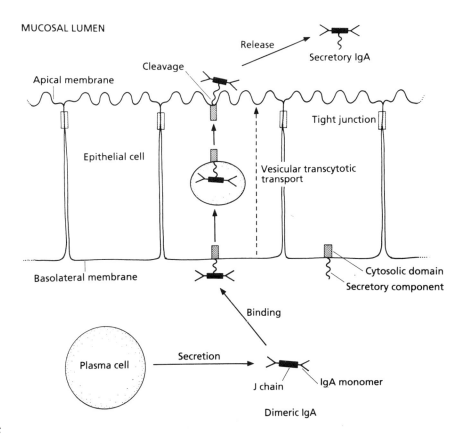

MUCOSAL LUMEN

Figure 164–13. Transfer of multimeric immunoglobulin (here IgA) from the submucosal space across the epithelial cell membrane. This transfer is enabled by binding of the polymeric Ig receptor, whose extracellular portion is secretory component. This polymeric Ig–Ig receptor complex is internalized and passes through the cell; on reaching the luminal membrane, the receptor is cleaved, releasing secretory component bound Ig. (From Sztul E: *In* Barnes PJ, Stockley RA [eds]: Molecular Biology of Lung Disease. London, Blackwell Scientific Publications, 1994, pp 261–278.)

fetus and neonate. Consequently, these levels fall postnatally, reaching a nadir between 3 and 4 months of age when nascent IgG production by the infant is unable to keep pace with utilization of maternally derived IgG. In comparison to term infants, preterm infants have proportionally lower IgG concentrations at birth, demonstrate lower serum IgG nadirs, and manifest lower serum IgG levels throughout the first year of life.[576] While respiratory epithelia possess limited capacity for IgG transfer and secretion, significant quantities of IgG may be found in fluids obtained from bronchoalveolar and airway lavage, likely reflecting passive extravasation across epithelial barriers.[579] In adult models of pneumonitis, both total and relative amounts of IgG are recoverable by BAL, suggesting enhanced intravascular "leakage," as well as local production by IgG-producing B cells recruited to alveolar sites of inflammation.[580] In contrast to IgG, only trace levels of IgD and IgE are present at birth, and passive transfer into neonatal respiratory secretions is negligible.

Recruitment of Lung Immune Cells

Inflammatory Mediators

When constitutive lung defenses are breeched, the capacity to rapidly mobilize immune cells to loci of potential infection must exist. In response to infection of the airway or alveolus, phagocytes may be recruited from the interstitium and intravascular space. PMN and monocyte movement into the lung early in infection is mediated by the local production of a number of chemotactic and proinflammatory signals. Many of these substances are macrophage derived, secreted in response to direct interaction with microbes or microbial products. Release of reactive membrane-derived phospholipids, generation of reactive oxyradical species, and production of proinflammatory peptides constitute available mechanisms for lung cells to amplify local inflammatory responses.

Lipid Mediators

Lipid mediators of inflammation constitute a diverse group of biologically active products liberated from cellular membranes in response to local immune and nonimmune stimuli.[581] In contrast to cytokine synthesis, which requires transcription, translation, and posttranslational processing steps, lipid mediators can be generated within minutes. Endotoxin directly stimulates leukocyte membrane-associated phospholipase A_2 (PLA_2), which metabolizes adjacent membrane phospholipids to release free fatty acid products such as lysophosphatidylcholine and arachidonic acid.[582] Arachidonic acid can be oxidatively metabolized by cyclooxygenase or lipoxygenase pathways to generate a number of bioactive lipid products including thromboxane A_2 (TXA_2), prostacyclin, prostaglandins, and leukotrienes, while lysophosphatidylcholine may be acylated to produce the potent mediator platelet-activating factor (PAF).[582,583]

PAF is synthesized by a number of cells, including mononuclear phagocytes, neutrophils, endothelial cells, platelets, eosinophils, and mast cells, and has demonstrable biologic effects at nanomolar concentrations.[584,585] Known for its induction of platelet aggregation and degranulation, it also stimulates chemotaxis and activation of PMNs and macrophages and augments PMN adhesion to endothelial cells.[585-587] PAF can also stimulate further production of prostaglandins, TXA_2, and leukotrienes, suggesting a capacity to synergistically potentiate the local inflammatory response.[588] Animal models of gram-negative infection suggest a role for PAF in mediating endotoxin-induced inflammation as well as a role in the impaired hypoxic pulmonary vasoconstriction and alveolar capillary leak associated with severe pneumonitis.[589,590] Other studies have linked PAF to transfusion-associated lung injury and reperfusion lung injury.[591,592] In neonates, PAF is implicated in the pathogenesis of septic complications such as disseminated intravascular coagulation and necrotizing enterocolitis.[593] Elevated PAF levels are

documented in the tracheal aspirates of infants in association with meconium aspiration, pneumonia, and intrauterine infection, suggesting a role in neonatal pulmonary inflammation.[594,595]

Arachidonic acids are released from cell membrane phospholipids in response to a variety of inflammatory stimuli.[584] Once liberated, they are primarily metabolized by either the lipoxygenase or the cyclooxygenase pathway. The lipoxygenase pathway produces leukotrienes (LTs), including the potent PMN chemotactic activator LTB_4, and LTC_4 and its cysteinyl degradation products LTD_4 and LTE_4.[596] Of these, LTB_4 appears most critical for generating an inflammatory response. By binding to specific PMN receptors, LTB_4 induces chemotaxis, increases surface expression of the complement receptor CR3, increases secretion of superoxide and lysosomal hydrolases, up-regulates PLA_2 activity, increases synthesis of IL-8 and NO, and diminishes apoptosis.[597-600] In addition, the cysteinyl LTs up-regulate macrophage Fc receptor expression and phagocytic activity. Alveolar macrophages are the primary source of LTs in the lung, but PMNs recruited to the alveolar space can synergize with macrophages to augment LT generation.[601] LT generation is also augmented by cytokines such as IFN-γ and granulocyte colony-stimulating factor (G-CSF), which up-regulate lipoxygenase enzymes above basal levels. The important role of LTs in host response is suggested by a transgenic animal model of LT deficiency; in this model, AM phagocytic function was impaired, intratracheal inoculation of bacteria resulted in increased bacteremia and lethality, and AM function was restorable in vitro by exogenous LTB_4.[602] Leukotriene activity in the human neonatal lung has not been characterized, but animal models suggest that neonatal alveolar macrophages may have diminished capacity to synthesize LTB_4, compared with adults; presumably this results in part from lower inducible levels of IFN-γ and less capacity to up-regulate lipoxygenase pathway enzymes.[603]

Products of the cyclooxygenase pathway include prostacyclin (PGI_2), TXA_2, and prostaglandins. Although TXA_2 increases microvascular tone and activates inflammatory cells, prostaglandin species, particularly the PGE series, are known to block transcription of TNF, suppress leukocyte adhesion, and blunt the generation of other proinflammatory arachidonic acid metabolites.[604,605] Cellular constituents of the lung appear specialized in their generation of arachidonic acid products, with LTB_4, PGE_2, and TXA_2 the primary ones generated by alveolar macrophages. Because inflammatory actions of these mediators may be conflicting, and because alveolar macrophages may produce varying amounts of these mediators at different stages of the inflammatory process, this suggests another mechanism by which the alveolar macrophage may regulate local inflammatory events.

Proteins

Complement. Activation of the complement cascade, by either classical or innate means, results in the eventual generation of multiple components with potent inflammatory activity. C3a, C4a, and C5a all have function as "anaphylatoxins," capable of inducing histamine release and increased vascular permeability; there is evidence that C3a and C5a mediate some of these effects by inducing local production of arachidonic acid metabolites.[606-608] C3a and C5a stimulate PMN lysosomal enzyme release, while C5a is also a potent neutrophil chemotaxin.[609] Subsequent enzymatic hydrolysis of C5a generates the peptide C5a des Arg, which retains potent PMN chemotactic activity.[610,611] When compartmentalized, as within the alveolus, these component effects are dose dependent, resulting in an orderly sequence of PMN recruitment and then activation (Fig. 164-14). Alveolar epithelial surfaces express complement regulatory proteins (decay accelerating factor, membrane cofactor protein)[612] to protect against complement-mediated damage but remain vulnerable to injury from PMNs recruited to, and activated within, the alveolus.

Beyond these well-recognized proinflammatory effects, a more complex role is emerging for complement in immunomodulation

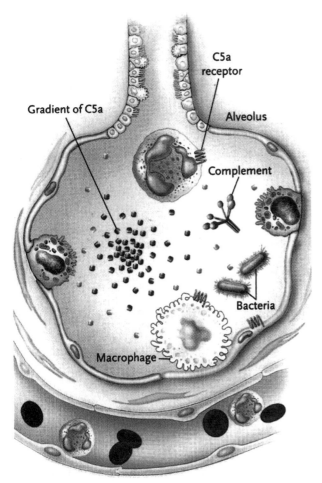

Figure 164–14. Complement components are produced within the alveolus by alveolar macrophages, pulmonary fibroblasts, and type II epithelial cells. Complement activation within this compartment generates a C5a gradient favoring PMN chemotaxis. Increasing local concentrations of C5a arrest chemotaxis and induce PMN respiratory burst and degranulation. Additional local immunomodulation (cytokine induction, IgG receptor upregulation) may occur through C5a interaction with cognate receptors on alveolar epithelium and alveolar macrophages. (Adapted from Gerard C: N Engl J Med *348*:167–169, 2003.)

of the alveolar microenvironment. C3a and C5a may regulate a broad range of inflammatory functions by binding their cognate receptors C3aR and C5aR. Previously recognized only on myeloid cells, both receptors have been demonstrated on human alveolar epithelium and alveolar macrophages, although their function on the former remains unclear.[613] Engagement of the alveolar macrophage C5aR results in increased IgG Fc receptor expression on the AM surface, enhancing AM-derived cytokine production in response to immune complex binding and driving further PMN recruitment.[614] In a murine model of sepsis, putative activation of toll pathways by endotoxin increased C3aR and C5aR expression on alveolar epithelium.[615] In this model, C5a activation of C5aR was implicated in increased expression of TNF-α and IL-6. Conversely, C3a has been shown to depress TNF-α and IL-6 secretion and hence blunt evolution of polyclonal immunity.[616,617] Taken together, these data suggest that C3a and C5a have complex, possibly counterbalancing effects on the inflammatory response.[618] Moreover, by linking complement activation and Fc receptor pathways, C5a may play a broader role in facilitating transition from a purely innate, to a coordinated innate and adaptive, immune response.

Neurokinins. The autonomic nervous system may participate in some aspects of airway inflammation, because stimulated or injured sensory nerves can initiate or amplify leukocyte response. Local axonal reflexes play a role through stimulation of afferent nerve fibers, leading to the release of neurokinins. Neurokinins, such as substance P, are stored in unmyelinated nerve fibers (C fibers) as well as intrinsic airway neurons and released as part of a nociceptive response.[619] Airway surface epithelium and submucosal glands are in proximity to sites of neurokinin release. Once secreted, neurokinins activate the neurokinin-1 receptor (NK-1R), mediating local increases in vascular permeability and leukocyte adherence to airway epithelial surfaces; the ensuing plasma extravasation and leukocyte infiltration constitutes "neurogenic inflammation."[620] The duration and intensity of this response is determined by the rate of neurokinin breakdown by neutral endopeptidase (NEP), an enzyme produced by epithelial cells.[621] Epithelial damage, as caused by inflammation, mechanical injury, or viral infection reduces NEP availability, leading to sustained inflammatory effects of the neurokinins.

Beyond the classic model of neurogenic inflammation, recent work has identified other neurokinin sources within the lung. Resident lung macrophages, as well as circulating leukocytes, have been found to express neurokinin receptors, as well as the preprotachykinin A (PPT-A) gene encoding neurokinins such as substance P.[622,623] This suggests that lung immune cells may use neurokinins for paracrine or autocrine signaling, propagating inflammation beyond the distribution of C fibers and intrinsic neurons.[624] Such a role is supported by animal models of either NK-1R or PPT-A deletion. The injury normally induced by antigen-antibody complexes within the airway is attenuated in a transgenic murine model of NK-1R deletion, suggesting an essential, rather than complementary, function of neurokinins in this type of inflammation.[625] Similarly, PPT-A deficiency blunts immune-complex–mediated inflammation, yielding additional important insights. First, neurokinins intervene very proximally in the inflammatory cascade, because airway TNF-α levels are essentially undetectable in PPT-A–deficient mice. Second, reconstitution of leukocyte PPT-A expression does not alter the blunted inflammatory response in PPT-A–deficient mice; however, transplantation of PPT-A–deficient bone marrow into "wild-type" mice is also protective, underscoring the essential role of leukocyte-derived PPT-A in neurogenic inflammation.[624] These data, taken together, suggest a paradigm in which subepithelial sensory neurons interact synergistically with resident immune cells of the lung to initiate neurogenic inflammation. Secreted neuropeptides are potent chemotaxins and can recruit leukocytes directly or by the induction of cytokines by local interstitial and immune cells.[626] Recruited inflammatory cells then use substance P (or other neurokinins) as an autocrine or paracrine signal, amplifying the inflammatory response. Because of their proximity to surface epithelia and sensory nerve fibers containing substance P, pulmonary macrophages are uniquely suited to regulate neurokinin-mediated events and are postulated to be the critical immune cell in this model.

Apart from their inflammatory actions, other relevant effects of airway neuropeptides relate to alterations in mucus secretion. Substance P stimulates mucin elaboration and increases mucus secretion by stimulating serous cells and goblet cells.[627,628] Both substance P and vasoactive intestinal peptide (VIP) stimulate epithelial cell chloride secretion, increasing periciliary fluid level.[105,629] The net effect is increased local production of mucus, with increased periciliary fluid secretion to maintain mucus hydration and normal viscosity. In the extreme of intense or sustained neurogenic inflammation, however, mucociliary dysfunction may ensue.

Defensins. Apart from their primary antimicrobial activity, defensins also exhibit properties facilitating pulmonary inflammation. *In vitro*, α-defensins have been shown to induce the neutrophil chemoattractant IL-8 from airway epithelial cells, and stimulate alveolar macrophage production of LTB₄ and IL-8.[630,631]

Additionally, HNP-1 and HNP-2 are each directly chemotactic for monocytes and can induce monocyte-derived TNF and IL-1.[632,633] Similar *in vivo* effects are suggested by a murine model in which intravenously administered HNP-1 localized to sites of infection, with increased granulocyte recruitment and bacterial clearance relative to controls.[634] Finally, α-defensins have been shown to induce T-cell–derived IFN-γ, IL-6, and IL-10, whereas β-defensins have chemoattractant effects on immature DCs and naive T cells; this suggests that beyond their antimicrobial and proinflammatory effects, defensins may also facilitate the local transition from innate to adaptive immune response.[635,636]

Proteases. Phagocytic cells (PMNs, mononuclear leukocytes) contain a number of proteolytic enzymes capable of both microbial killing and proteolytic degradation of lung structural elements.[370,637] PMN primary (azurophilic) granules contain serine protease homologues with cytocidal activity (serprocidins); these include neutrophil elastase, cathepsin G, proteinase-3, and azurocidin. The serprocidins are structurally related to the granzymes of cytotoxic lymphocytes and exhibit broad-spectrum microbicidal activity against bacteria, fungi, and protozoa. Proteases contained in primary granules have the capacity to degrade a number of extracellular proteins, including collagen (types I-IV), elastin, fibronectin, laminin, proteoglycans, and complement, contributing to microbicidal action;[638-642] alternatively, many proteases possess antimicrobial activity unrelated to their proteolytic effects.[643] PMN secondary (specific) granules contain collagenase and possibly gelatinase, which facilitate PMN migration.[637,644,645] Stored proteases are released extracellularly in response to various stimuli. Migration of PMN through tissues results in release of specific granule contents; this may be due to the interaction of complement receptors on the specific granule membrane with local complement components directing PMN chemotaxis. In this fashion, specific release of collagenase is induced locally, facilitating PMN navigation through tissues via proteolytic "cleavage planes." Conversely, PMN proteases may seep accidentally into the local milieu during phagocytosis, when primary granules fuse prematurely with incompletely formed phagocytic vacuoles.[646,647] Additionally, certain stimuli, such as endotoxin, induce direct exocytosis of primary granule contents. The local proteolytic actions of secreted proteases is generally controlled by extracellular antiproteases such as α_1-antitrypsin (α_1-AT), α_1-antichymotrypsin, and α_1-protease inhibitor.[648] Under conditions of homeostasis, a balance between proteolytic activity and antiprotease activity exists. However, when antiproteases are deficient, or overwhelmed by the degree of the inflammatory response, diminished regulation of protease activity may ensue. Subsequent proteolytic generation of chemotactic extracellular matrix fragments and complement components can lead to further recruitment of phagocytic cells and intensified local inflammation.

Toxic Oxygen Species

Whereas ambient air provides a metabolic advantage for cellular function, excess molecular oxygen and its metabolic intermediate products can be highly toxic to cells and tissues. This toxicity is exploited by phagocytic cells such as PMNs and macrophages, which have evolved mechanisms to locally generate highly reactive, free radical oxygen species.[649,650] This process is characterized by a rapid uptake of molecular oxygen by the phagocyte (the "oxidative burst") that is triggered by cell membrane signaling before particle ingestion. Activation of cell membrane–associated nicotinamide adenine dinucleotide phosphate (NADPH) oxidase results in shuttling of electrons from cytosolic NADPH to molecular oxygen, initiating a series of reactions responsible for producing multiple oxyradical species (Fig. 164-15). In the presence of activated-membrane NADPH oxidase, molecular oxygen accepts a single donated electron, becoming superoxide ion (O_2^-). Because this radical can either accept or donate an electron, it may be sub-

sequently oxidized or reduced; when two such radicals interact, in the presence of superoxide dismutase, one is oxidized and one is reduced, such that $O_2^- + O_2^- + 2H^+ \rightarrow O_2 + H_2O_2$, generate hydrogen peroxide. Transfer of a second electron to the superoxide ion, via NADPH oxidase, also generates H_2O_2. The majority of the oxygen utilized by phagocytes is metabolized through the superoxide anion, which is not a particularly toxic intermediate and eventually dismutes to hydrogen peroxide either spontaneously or through the actions of superoxide dismutase. Sequential transfer of a third electron reduces hydrogen peroxide to the highly reactive and least stable oxygen intermediate, hydroxyl radical; this electron can be donated by NADPH oxidase or by superoxide anion. Transfer of a fourth electron results in generation of water, the ultimate reduction of molecular oxygen.

Neutrophil granules contain myeloperoxidase, an enzyme capable of generating further antimicrobial oxyradicals. Hydrogen peroxide reacts with myeloperoxidase and available halide species (primarily chloride *in vivo*) to generate hypochlorous acid (HOCl);[651] HOCl is an extremely powerful oxidant, analogous to bleach. Because it is highly reactive, it does not accumulate and is rapidly consumed in further reactions producing new oxidants. An important interaction may be with primary or secondary amines, to produce chloramines; although chloramines are weaker oxidants than HOCl, they tend to be longer lived and remain able to oxidize multiple potential targets.[370]

Activation of phagocytes in the alveolus or the airway can therefore initiate a sequence of reactions locally generating a number of potent, but potentially host injurious, antimicrobials. In particular, the ability of superoxide anion to function as either electron donor or acceptor enables oxyradical species to propagate oxidizing reactions within the cellular milieu, resulting in multiple sites of oxidant injury;[652] this is exemplified by actions of the hydroxyl radical. In a series of steps referred to as the Fenton reaction, superoxide anion reduces cellular iron from the ferric to the ferrous state; ferrous iron subsequently returns to the ferric state by reducing hydrogen peroxide to generate the hydroxyl radical. Once formed, this highly reactive oxyradical interacts with numerous biologic molecules in the immediate environment, resulting in peroxidation of organelle and cell membranes, inactivation of cellular enzymes possessing oxidant vulnerable sulfhydryl groups, depolymerization of carbohydrates, and hydroxylation of nucleic acid bases or so-called nicking of DNA.[653-658] Of note is that any transition metal possessing multivalent capacity catalyzes the Fenton reaction, underscoring the potential host protective role of such acute phase proteins as ceruloplasmin and transferrin in sequestering copper and iron during an inflammatory response. Hydroxyl radical may

$$O_2 \xrightarrow{\text{e-}} O_2^- \qquad \text{(Superoxide anion)}$$

$$O_2 \xrightarrow{\text{e-}} O_2^- \xrightarrow{\text{e- + 2H}^+} H_2O_2 \qquad \text{(Hydrogen peroxide)}$$

$$O_2^- + O_2^- + H_2^+ \longrightarrow O_2 + H_2O_2 \qquad \text{(Hydrogen peroxide)}$$

$$O_2^- + H_2O_2 \xrightarrow{\text{Fe}} O_2 + 2 \cdot OH \qquad \text{(Hydroxyl radical)}$$

Figure 164–15. Available intracellular reactions that reduce molecular oxygen, resulting in sequential generation of specific oxyradical species. Acceptance by molecular oxygen of a single donated electron generates superoxide anion. Hydrogen peroxide is subsequently produced either by further reduction of superoxide species or by superoxide dismutase–driven catalysis of two superoxide anions. Lastly, in a series of electron transfers described as the Fenton reaction, superoxide anion ultimately reduces hydrogen peroxide, in the presence of ferric iron or other multivalent transition metals, to generate the highly reactive hydroxyl radical.

also be generated by reactions between superoxide anion and locally generated nitric oxide.[659]

Beyond their roles as local antimicrobials and mediators of inflammation, oxyradical species may also act locally to augment function of leukocyte proteases in the inflammatory milieu. α_1-antitrypsin, the major protease inhibitor, is vulnerable to oxidation of the methionyl residue at its active site; oxidation of this residue to a sulfoxide group decreases α1-AT activity several thousandfold.[660, 661] Oxidants generated by PMN may therefore provide an oxidant "screen" for preservation of proteolytic enzyme function, allowing generation of both a powerful antimicrobial system and a zone of controlled proteolysis at the inflammatory site. However, when locally generated oxidants become poorly contained or the intensity of oxyradical production overwhelms local antioxidant mechanisms, host injury may occur; this results both from direct cytotoxic effects of oxyradical species as well as continued leukocyte expression of unregulated proteases.[370]

Cytokines

Cytokines play a sentinel role in the recruitment, proliferation, and survival of inflammatory cells within the lung. Cytokines are soluble proteins transiently synthesized by an appropriately stimulated immune or nonimmune effector cell and whose effects are mediated by binding to specific receptors on target cells. A cytokine may have autocrine effect when it modulates the properties of the cell producing it, paracrine effects when modulating the properties of cells proximally, and endocrine effects when it mediates its effects distally. Some cytokines may remain cell associated or membrane bound and exert their effects through cell-to-cell contact; this may facilitate more specific regulation of local inflammatory events. A single cytokine may be produced by many cell types, and a single cell type may produce many cytokines. In general, cytokines are multifunctional molecules, participating in a wide spectrum of immune and nonimmune processes, including inflammation, metabolism, morphogenesis, fibrosis, and hemostasis. The action of a given cytokine may vary depending on its dose, receptor availability, the state of activation of the target cell, and the presence of other cytokines in the local milieu. Additionally, cytokines frequently stimulate target tissues to produce other bioactive cytokines. Accordingly, the biologic effects of cytokines result from their direct effects on target tissues and their ability to interact with one another in regulating target cell function; the eventual response of a cell to these mediators will depend on the sum of the signals received and the cell's state of responsiveness to each of these signals.

Tumor Necrosis Factor

Tumor necrosis factor (TNF) is a phylogenetically primitive mediator, based on its high degree of homology across species. It is produced primarily by monocytes and macrophages in response to LPS, as well as in response to enterotoxin, mycobacterial cell wall products, and components of complement.[662, 663] TNF is also produced by T cells and NK cells.[664, 665] Its local half-life is approximately 6 minutes, with peak levels at 1 to 2 hours after LPS exposure, defining its role as an "early response" mediator in endotoxin-induced inflammatory cascades.[666] It is now clear that TNF is a key mediator of host defense against a wide range of pulmonary pathogens, including *Pseudomonas, Legionella, Klebsiella, Staphylococcus aureus, Streptococcus pneumoniae,* and *Mycobacterium* species.[667-670] Alveolar macrophage–derived TNF remains compartmentalized within the alveolus, where it exerts protean inflammatory effects. TNF acts on PMNs to increase phagocytosis, adhesion molecule expression, and respiratory burst capacity.[671-673] TNF acts on epithelial and vascular endothelial cells to similarly up-regulate

adhesion molecule expression, thereby facilitating inflammatory cell migration.[674, 675] TNF induces IL-1 generation by both endothelial cells and local mononuclear phagocytes, which augments the initial inflammatory signal[676, 677] and can directly induce production of the potent neutrophil activating factor IL-8 from multiple cell types, further amplifying inflammation.[435, 447, 464] TNF also induces IL-6 production by fibroblasts, epithelial cells, and endothelial cells, initiating an acute phase response (detailed later).[434, 446, 678] Neonatal monocytes and T cells have diminished (50 to 60%) capacities to generate TNF relative to adult cells, and these limitations are further pronounced in preterm neonates (25% adult capacity).[391, 512, 679] Despite this, TNF is noted to be significantly induced in neonatal airway fluid, in response to infection or other insult.[680, 681]

Interleukins

Interleukin-1. The IL-1 family consists of two proinflammatory agonists, IL-1α and IL-1β, and the antiinflammatory IL-1 receptor antagonist protein (IL-1ra). IL-1α is primarily membrane bound, whereas IL-1β is secreted. The IL-1 agonists are encoded by separate genes but share the same receptor by virtue of their 23% homology and thus elicit similar effects; because most cells in the body express IL-1 receptors, the effects of this cytokine are pleiotropic.[682, 683] IL-1 binding to its target cell receptor (IL-1R1) activates IL-1 receptor-activating kinase (IRAK), which culminates in liberation, and nuclear translocation, of NF-κB.[684] Of note is that the signal coupling of IL-1 with its receptor is identical to that of LPS on TLR4; this allows IL-1 amplification of host response to endotoxin even by cells that do not express the CD14/TLR4 receptor complex and underscores the critical role of NF-κB activation in the innate immune response.[685] In light of this signal "redundancy" it is perhaps not surprising that IL-1 shares many properties with TNF, including enhancement of adhesion molecule expression by PMNs and endothelial cells, up-regulation of NOS, and neutrophil "priming." Thus, like TNF, IL-1 is an "early response" cytokine, whose generation in response to TNF serves to amplify inflammatory events.[686-688] IL-1 acts on fibroblasts, epithelial cells, and endothelial cells to induce IL-6 and IL-8 production, thereby modulating both enhanced PMN chemoactivation and initiation of the acute phase response.[434, 435, 446, 447, 464, 678] Other actions of IL-1 (reviewed in reference 689) include stimulation of T-cell proliferation, increased IL-2 receptor expression on T and B cells, and increased release of T-cell–derived IL-2.[690, 691] IL-1 actions within the central nervous system are implicated in producing fever.[692] Regulation of IL-1 occurs by either direct IL-1ra antagonism (discussed later) or sequestration of IL-1 by its "decoy" receptor, the IL-1R2. Engagement of this receptor by IL-1 does not induce signal transduction; metalloprotease cleavage of this receptor from cell surfaces releases a soluble IL-1β ligand that blocks IL-1–mediated effects. The IL-1R2 is up-regulated by steroids, IL-4, and other inflammatory cytokines, including IFN-γ and IL-1 itself, the latter, as a presumed compensatory signal to limit scale and duration of an acute inflammatory response.[693]

Cellular sources of IL-1 include mononuclear phagocytes predominantly, endothelial cells, and, to a lesser extent, fibroblasts; consequently, significant amounts of this cytokine are generated within the lung.[433, 694-696] Mononuclear phagocytes do not produce IL-1 constitutively, but its production is induced by multiple stimuli, including viruses, microbial products (endotoxin, peptidoglycans, techoic acid, yeast cell walls), C5a, TNF, and IL-1 itself.[697, 698] Endothelial cells produce IL-1 in response to stimulation by TNF or IL-1.[433, 699] Despite the pleiotropic activities of this cytokine, and its presence in the alveolar compartment, transgenic models of IL-1β deficiency have not supported an essential role for IL-1β in innate pulmonary defenses.[700] In the neonate, however, IL-1β likely serves a critical role as the primary "early response cytokine," owing to the attenuated TNF production of this cohort. Available data suggest that neonates, both term and preterm, possess adult capacity to produce monocyte-derived IL-1 and exceed adult capacity to produce PMN-derived IL-1.[679,701,702]

Interleukin-1 Receptor Antagonist Protein. IL-1ra is an endogenous IL-1 inhibitor that competitively binds to the IL-1R1 without inducing signal.[703] It exists in two intracellular isoforms found in epithelial cells and as a third isoform secreted by monocytes.[704] IL-1ra is synthesized by alveolar macrophages (and other mononuclear cells) in response to LPS or adherent IgG.[705, 706] Intracellular isoforms of IL-1ra are also released by injured or apoptotic cells, possibly limiting further alveolar inflammation after epithelial injury. Emphasizing the potential role of IL-1 in pulmonary inflammation, animal models of endotoxin-induced pneumonitis demonstrate profound anti-inflammatory response to intratracheally instilled IL-1ra, whereas murine models of IL-1ra deficiency show exaggerated and persisting inflammatory response.[707, 708] These data, along with known *in vitro* actions, suggest that IL-1ra may function as an endogenous "down-regulator" of inflammatory cytokine cascading within the alveolar space. Characterization of IL-1ra generation by neonates remains incomplete. IL-1ra is found in tracheal aspirates of preterm infants at risk for bronchopulmonary dysplasia, but this may represent release from injured epithelium rather than *de novo* immune cell production.[709] Serum IL-1ra levels are elevated in healthy newborns, decline within days of birth, and increase in response to infection, indicating capacity for stimulus-specific IL-1ra production.[710,711] However, *in vitro* data show diminished IL-1ra production by stimulated cord blood monocytes from premature infants, suggesting an impaired ability of this cohort to titrate IL-1–driven inflammation.[712]

Interleukin-2. IL-2 is a pleiotropic cytokine produced primarily by T-helper cells and, to a lesser extent NK cells, following antigen-induced activation.[713] This cytokine functions in an autocrine fashion to clonally expand antigen-specific T cells, enhance their production of IFN-γ, and generate memory phenotypes.[714,715] Both Th1 and Th2 subsets may expand in response to IL-2; thus, although IL-2 enhances cellular immune function, it does not specifically favor a Th1 response. IL-2 also acts as a paracrine factor, influencing NK cell, B cell, and phagocyte function. IL-2 enhances NK cell cytotoxicity and stimulates B-cell immunoglobulin production.[716,717] IL-2 also augments macrophage microbicidal activity, cytokine production, and cell surface expression of cytokine receptors.[718] IL-2 appears to be essential for optimal host defense against some intracellular infections, possibly owing to its induction of IFN-γ from T cells and NK cells.[719] Although neonatal leukocytes *in vitro* possess adult capacity to produce IL-2 in response to conventional stimuli, neonatal NK cells are reportedly less responsive to IL-2 stimulation, possibly contributing to impaired cytolytic function within this cohort.[386,720]

IL-2 signaling occurs through the IL-2 receptor (IL-2R), which is composed of three subunits: a unique IL-2Ra component, a β subunit shared with IL-15, and a γ subunit shared with IL-4, IL-7, IL-9, and IL-15. Although heritable IL-2 deficiency is associated with normal T-cell development, IL-2Rγ deficiency results in X-linked severe combined immunodeficiency. This suggests that signals mediated through the IL-2 receptor are essential for T-cell function but may be induced by IL-2–independent means, possibly by some combination of mediators sharing the IL-2Rγ subunit. The IL-2 receptor is up-regulated by IL-2 itself, as well as by IL-1, IL-6, and IL-16.[713,721,722] Soluble forms of this receptor are released by activated T and B cells; these bind free IL-2 and may represent a mechanism of IL-2 regulation.[723]

Interleukin-3 and Interleukin-5. IL-3 is a multipotent hematopoietic growth factor produced by activated T cells, mast cells, monocytes/macrophages, eosinophils, and stromal cells.[724] It is a member of a cytokine superfamily (including IL-5 and GM-CSF) whose overlapping hematopoietic activity results from a shared receptor component. Of note is that at least one variant of pulmonary alveolar proteinosis is attributed to a defect in this common receptor component.[725,726] IL-3 indirectly contributes to pulmonary immune function by stimulating the proliferation of monocyte/macrophage progenitors, acting as a "survival factor" for lymphoid-derived DCs, and enhancing the presentation of exogenous particulate antigen in the context of class I MHC by antigen-presenting cells.[727, 728] IL-3 is considered to be a Th2 cytokine, and it facilitates Th2 response by inhibiting eosinophil apoptosis.[729] While of primary interest in the lung for its potential role in asthma, and the role of its receptor in pulmonary alveolar proteinosis, IL-3 may also facilitate migration and activation of PMNs.[730] In the neonate, leukocyte production of IL-3 is markedly depressed (30%) relative to adult cells, and further *in vitro* suppression is reported in response to corticosteroids.[731,732]

IL-5 is derived from T cells, mast cells, basophils, and eosinophils.[733] In humans, IL-5 is thought to be specific for promoting eosinophil and basophilic maturation and eosinophil survival and chemotaxis.[734] IL-5 appears to be critical for producing tissue eosinophilia and is thus of primary interest for its role in asthma; however, BAL fluid levels of IL-5, and BAL eosinophilia have also been correlated in a wide variety of other conditions.[735] Interestingly, transgenic murine models of modified IL-5 expression suggest that lung-derived IL-5 remains compartmentalized, inducing only air space and not systemic, eosinophilia.[736] The role, if any, of IL-5 in neonatal host response remains uncharacterized. Eosinophilia is reportedly common among premature neonates and considered a marker of occult infection.[737] However, recent evaluation of a small cohort of eosinophilic preterm infants failed to demonstrate any correlation between serum IL-5 levels and presence or degree of eosinophilia. Such data are consistent with earlier studies, in which mRNA analysis reveals markedly diminished expression of this cytokine by neonatal cells.[514]

Interleukin-4 and Interleukin-13. IL-4 is an 18-kDa cytokine produced by activated T cells of the Th2 subset, γδ T cells, mast cells, and basophils. IL-4 has two receptors: a high-affinity receptor that shares signaling components with IL-2 and IL-7 and an alternate receptor that shares components of the IL-13 receptor; cells expressing either receptor can transduce the IL-4 signal. IL-4 stimulation of naive T cells induces their differentiation into Th2 cells, initiating the Th2 response. Concurrently, IL-4 exhibits a number of important functions related to humoral immunity, including B-cell activation and induction of B-cell isotype switching necessary for production of IgE and some IgG subclasses.[738] IL-4 also exerts protean antiinflammatory effects, suppressing cytokine expression by Th1 cells, inhibiting macrophage-derived TNF, IL-1, and IL-8 and inducing macrophage-derived IL-1ra.[509, 739-741] IL-4 directly antagonizes IFN-γ function by inhibiting the expression of many IFN-γ-inducible genes and blunts IFN-γ-augmented microbicidal activity, such as superoxide production.[509,742] Consistent with the Th2 cellular response, IL-4 facilitates the migration of eosinophils, basophils, and monocytes by up-regulating endothelial expression of vascular cell adhesion molecule (VCAM).[743] Neonatal leukocyte production of IL-4 is estimated to be less than 10% of adult capacity, and this correlates with *in vivo* data, in which IL-4 is undetectable in tracheobronchial aspirates of preterm and term newborns.[532,744]

IL-13 shares sequence homology (~30%) and biologic activities with IL-4.[745,746] Primarily expressed by Th2 cells, IL-13 is also inducible from Th1 and Th0 subsets. The activities shared by IL-4 and IL-13 likely result from a shared receptor subunit; however, IL-13-mediated effects are more restricted and IL-13 is generally less potent than IL-4, owing to competitive inhibition resulting from the higher affinity of IL-4 to its receptor.[747] Although IL-13 does not stimulate T cells as IL-4 does, IL-13 can stimulate B-cell proliferation and immunoglobulin isotype switching, synergistically with IL-4.[748] IL-13 exhibits dual effects on monocytes, both stimulatory and inhibitory. IL-13 up-regulates MHC class II molecule expression and monocyte adhesion.[749, 750] Conversely, IL-13 inhibits production of monocyte-derived IL-1, IL-6, TNF, chemokines (IL-8 and MIP-1a), and hematopoietic factors (G-CSF, GM-CSF), while significantly enhancing alveolar macrophage-derived IL-1ra.[750-752] Normal pregnancy is associated with the production of appreciable quantities of IL-13, initially by the placenta and subsequently by the fetus; IL-13 is inducible from cord blood cells by 27 weeks' gestation.[753] Postnatally, higher levels of inducible IL-13 from cord lymphocytes may identify neonates at risk for later development of atopic, or Th2 response-associated, disease processes.[754]

Interleukin-6. IL-6 is the prototype of a multifunctional cytokine. It is primarily produced by mononuclear phagocytes but it is also produced by T and B cells and may be produced by endothelial cells, epithelial cells, and fibroblasts in response to TNF and IL-1.[434,446,678,755] IL-6 production by stimulated neonatal mononuclear cells matches or exceeds that of adults, although diminished production is noted with marked prematurity.[756,757] Its production by mononuclear cells can be induced by LPS and augmented by TNF and IL-1;[448] IL-6 suppresses macrophage-derived TNF and IL-1 production, however, and blunts further activity of these cytokines by inducing soluble TNF receptor and IL-1ra production.[758,759] IL-6 is able to exert effects on a wide range of cells, owing to the unique properties of its receptor. When activated by IL-6, the IL-6 receptor complexes with the gp130 membrane protein, which is required for intracellular signal transduction. IL-6R also circulates in a soluble (sIL-6R) form, which binds secreted IL-6.[760] The IL-6:IL-6R complex may then activate any cell bearing the gp130 membrane protein, allowing IL-6 to activate a wide range of cell types. Functions of IL-6 include providing co-stimulatory signals to enhance T-cell response to IL-2[761] and stimulation of B-cell differentiation and antibody production.[762] IL-6 induces the acute phase response, characterized by hepatocyte production of such proteins as fibrinogen, α_2-macroglobulin, and α_1-antitrypsin and also up-regulates local acute phase protein production by mononuclear phagocytes.[763,764] IL-6 can thus influence the local balance between proteases and antiproteases, dampening protease-induced inflammation. IL-6 is found in BAL specimens of adults with pulmonary inflammation, as well as in BAL specimens of mechanically ventilated, premature neonates; whether IL-6 is a marker, or mediator, of inflammation in either of these scenarios remains unclear.[765-767] In summary, the net effects of IL-6 seem to optimize, or "focus," immune function, given its stimulatory actions on T and B cells, with concomitant down-regulation of TNF- and IL-1-driven inflammation and induced production of host-protective acute phase proteins; in this regard, it may be best thought of as an antiinflammatory cytokine.[768]

Interleukin-9. IL-9 is a pleiotropic cytokine produced primarily by Th2 helper T cells. It supports the growth of activated T-cell subsets and synergizes with IL-3 to induce mast cell proliferation.[769,770] It has also been shown to enhance IL-4-induced IgE and IgG production by human B cells, consistent with the Th2 immune response.[771] Beyond its hematopoietic effects, IL-9 may play a central role in airway defense. IL-9 acts on bronchial epithelial cells *in vitro* to induce eotaxin and the T-cell chemoattractants IL-16 and RANTES.[772,773] IL-9 also acts on airway epithelium *in vitro* to stimulate *MUC5AC* gene transcription and increases mucin secretion *in vivo*.[774] These reactions are exaggerated in asthma, suggesting a sentinel role for IL-9, and this histopathology is found in transgenic murine models of IL-9 overexpression.[775,776] Finally, IL-9 may modulate repair of injured airway epithelium. *In vitro*, IL-9 stimulates goblet cell proliferation and hyperplasia in actively differentiating human airway epithelium, at the expense of ciliated cell repletion; this results in epithelia with diminished ciliation and increased mucus and lysozyme production.[777] These effects may be relevant in repair of ventilator-induced denudation of the airway epithelia, particularly when there is predisposition to a Th2 immune response as

occurs in the neonatal period. Neonatal serum levels of IL-9 have been quantified in one clinical study, where newborns of at least 1500 g birth weight (controls) had mean serum levels of 4.1 pg/ml and stimulated serum levels 4 to 7 times greater.[778] Despite these findings, the presence of IL-9 in the neonatal lung has not been quantified, and its role in either host defense, or pathology, in this age group thus remains speculative.

Interleukin-10. IL-10 is a critical Th2 cytokine produced by T cells, B cells, and mononuclear phagocytes in response to stimuli, including LPS and TNF-α.[449,779-781] Consistent with its role as a Th2 cytokine, IL-10 augments proliferation and differentiation of activated B cells while up-regulating their MHC class II expression.[781] More prominently, however, IL-10 potently suppresses multiple facets of cellular innate immunity. IL-10 inhibits the generation of oxyradicals and NO by macrophages and PMNs, impairing their microbicidal functions.[782,783] IL-10 also suppresses macrophage expression of MHC class II and co-stimulatory molecules CD80 and CD86, diminishing the capacity to present antigen.[784,785] Finally, IL-10 inhibits macrophage-dependent T-cell proliferation and Th1 cytokine production by macrophages, PMNs, Th1 cells, and NK cells.[786,787] Cytokines that are suppressed by IL-10 include TNF, IL-1, IL-2, IL-3, IL-6, IL-12, IFN-γ, and the chemokines IL-8 and MIP-1α.[786-789] Multiple mechanisms underlie these protean suppressive activities, including IL-10 inhibition of NF-κB signal transduction, IL-10–enhanced degradation of TNF and IL-1 mRNA, IL-10–mediated down-regulation of TNF receptor expression, and up-regulation of soluble TNF receptor shedding and IL-1ra expression.[790-793] Conversely, IL-10 also stimulates some aspects of cellular immune function; it up-regulates expression of Fc and PAF receptors, as well as the chemokine receptor CCR5 expressed on monocytes, DCs, Th1 cells, and NK cells.[685] Taken together, these data suggest that IL-10 impairs direct microbial killing but augments macrophage recruitment to sites of inflammation; this may facilitate phagocytic removal of apoptotic granulocytes, preventing inflammation from this source within the alveolus.[794]

There is evidence that IL-10 production in the lungs may be protective in some types of inflammatory injuries, and animal models of pneumonia have helped to clarify this role of IL-10 *in vivo*.[795] Exogenous IL-10, preceding intratracheal bacterial challenge, reduced lung TNF and IFN-γ responses, but increased lung bacterial count, systemic bacteremia, and morbidity in a murine model of *Streptococcus pneumoniae* infection.[796] IL-10 neutralization in this same model resulted in increased lung TNF, diminished lung bacterial counts, and increased survival rates. Similar outcomes have been shown in a murine model of *Klebsiella* pneumonia, treated with systemic anti-IL-10 antibody.[797] The antiinflammatory actions of IL-10 are further demonstrated by transgenic models of IL-10 deficiency.[798] Such animals manifest increased lethality to *Toxoplasma*, coincident with unabated IL-12 production, strong Th1 polarization of lymphocytes, and unbridled systemic inflammatory responses.[799] Given these data, it is thus presumed that in the context of pneumonia, IL-10 acts to modulate the local inflammatory response initiated by the offending pathogen; this preserves alveolar structure, pulmonary gas-exchange function, and host survival.

The data regarding neonatal IL-10 generation is somewhat contradictory but does allow some broad generalizations. First, stimulated neonatal monocytes exhibit only 20 to 40% of the IL-10 production inducible from stimulated adult monocytes.[800,801] Second, available BAL data from mechanically ventilated infants indicates that IL-10 expression in the lung is diminished in preterm infants but increases with advancing gestational age.[802-805] These age-related findings parallel data suggesting differential IL-10 production by lung macrophages *ex vivo* from term and preterm infants.[806] Such differences, if true *in vivo*, suggest that premature infants may be less able to attenuate alveolar inflammation in the setting of a pneumonitis or other inflammatory insult.

Interleukin-11. IL-11 is a 20-kDa, extremely cationic, stromal cell–derived cytokine, considered to be a member of the IL-6 type cytokine family or the neurokines; other members of this family include leukemia inhibitory factor (LIF), ciliary neurotrophic factor, and oncostatin M.[807,808] This family of cytokines is so named due to their ability to regulate neural phenotype.[809] LIF, the prototype of the group, promotes neuronal survival, induces noradrenergic neurons to assume a cholinergic phenotype, and induces the production of tachykinins such as substance P.[810] These cytokines all exhibit some overlapping activities, owing to the shared use of the gp130 subunit in their receptor complexes.[808] Thus, IL-11 regulates the same set of genes in sympathetic neurons as LIF and stimulates immunoglobulin production and the acute phase response much like IL-6.[810,811] Beyond this, IL-11 is a pleiotropic cytokine with many other distinct activities. It augments platelet production, it synergizes with IL-4 in supporting hematopoiesis, and it exhibits antiinflammatory suppression of macrophage-derived TNF, IL-1, and IL-12.[812-815] *In vivo*, it has been shown to attenuate radiation-induced injury to the gastrointestinal mucosa and other structures.[816, 817] A transgenic murine model of IL-11 overexpression results in animals able to tolerate LD_{100} levels of hyperoxia.[818] Interestingly, these effects are not related to up-regulation of antioxidant enzymes but instead result from diminished hyperoxia-induced DNA fragmentation and apoptosis.

Within the lung, IL-11 is also produced by pulmonary fibroblasts and alveolar and airway epithelial cells in response to various stimuli, including IL-1, TGF-β, and histamine.[819, 820] IL-11 has also been identified in neonatal vascular endothelial cells, where its expression is greater than in endothelium from older hosts.[821] Respiratory viruses, including rhinovirus, parainfluenza, and respiratory syncytial viruses have been shown *in vitro* to induce IL-11 from lung fibroblast and epithelial cultures. Furthermore, IL-11 concentrations are elevated in the airway fluid of patients with these viral upper respiratory infections.[822] Given the association of these viruses with reactive airway symptomatology, these data are noteworthy because of unique characteristics of IL-11 that are relevant in the setting of asthma. IL-11 is cationic enough to induce bronchospasm, it can synergize with the Th2 cytokine IL-4 in biologic systems, and, through its neurokine activities, IL-11 can induce tachykinin release and local development of a cholinergic phenotype characteristic of bronchial hyperreactivity. A transgenic murine model of IL-11 overexpression was developed to test the relationship between IL-11 and the asthmatic phenotype. These mice demonstrated peribronchial inflammation, airway remodeling with subepithelial fibrosis, myocyte hyperplasia, and bronchoconstriction on methacholine challenge.[823] Notably, aeroallergen challenge in this model resulted in adhesion molecule down-regulation, decreased inflammation and eosinophilia, and diminished Th2 cytokine gene expression, relative to controls. There was no enhanced Th1 polarization evidenced, and IFN-γ levels were not enhanced.[824] These data suggest that the major role for IL-11 is that of a "repair cytokine," one that mediates cytoprotection, minimizes tissue injury, inhibits tissue inflammation, but induces tissue fibrosis. Like its IL-6 cohort, IL-11 may be best thought of as an antiinflammatory cytokine. IL-11 has not been specifically quantified in neonatal airway surface liquid, but it does not appear to be constitutively expressed. It has been found in the airway secretions of infants with respiratory syncytial virus, rhinovirus, or parainfluenza, however, suggesting that it is inducible in this patient population.[822]

Interleukin-12. IL-12 is a pleiotropic cytokine that influences adaptive immunity by promoting Th1 response.[825] This cytokine is a heterodimeric glycoprotein of two unrelated subunits (p35 and p40); whereas the p35 subunit is constitutively expressed by many cell types, co-expression of the p40 subunit is required for IL-12 bioactivity. The p40 subunit and active IL-12 are produced by macrophages, DCs, neutrophils, and some B cells.[826] IL-12 exhibits multiple proinflammatory functions: it induces Th0 lymphocytes to commit to Th1 differentiation, it increases cytolytic activity of NK cells and cytotoxic T lymphocytes, and it is a potent inducer of the cytokines IFN-γ, TNF-α, GM-CSF, and IL-10 from T cells and NK cells.[827-830] Macrophage-derived IL-12 is induced by microbial (bacteria, fungi) ingestion, intracellular pathogens (bacteria, viruses), or bacterial products such as bacterial DNA or endotoxin; similarly, DCs also generate IL-12 in response to phagocytosis and microbial stimuli.[831-833] Macrophage-derived IL-12 drives NK cells to generate IFN-γ, which in turn enhances phagocyte-derived IL-12, in a powerful proinflammatory loop; this may have evolved in response to those intracellular pathogens, such as mycobacteria, which are relatively poor inducers of IL-12.[834] Regulation of IL-12 activity may occur either at the receptor level or by down-regulation induced by IL-4 or IL-10.[835] Both cytokines inhibit IL-12 production by macrophages and may also inhibit the ability of IL-12 to enhance Th1 differentiation; conversely, IL-12 inhibits both IL-4 and IL-10 expression by their cells of origin. In animal models, p40 subunits form homodimers that compete with IL-12 for binding to its receptor, providing another means of IL-12 regulation.[509] Lastly, IL-12 activity is regulated by its receptor location, which is expressed preferentially on Th1, but not Th2, cells, and induced during T-cell differentiation.[836] Multiple animal models suggest a critical role for IL-12 in host response to pneumonia caused by fungi, intracellular pathogens, and gram-negative bacteria.[837-839] Available *in vitro* data suggest an impaired neonatal capacity to generate IL-12 in response to appropriate stimuli.[390,428,840] Specifically, stimulated cord blood monocytes and monocyte-derived DCs each express markedly diminished IL-12 relative to adult controls; proposed mechanisms include differential posttranscriptional regulation of p40 (monocytes) and suppressed p35 gene expression (DCs). If these data prove true *in vivo*, they suggest that adaptive immune responses in the neonate skew toward a Th2 phenotype and provide an explanation for the diminished IFN-γ production seen in this population.

Interleukin-15. IL-15 is a 15-kDa peptide that shares β-and γ-receptor components with IL-2, resulting in overlapping immune functions including induction of T-cell proliferation and increased T-cell cytotoxic activity.[841] Like IL-2, IL-15 binding requires a distinct α-chain receptor component (IL-15Ra); this component is expressed in a variety of tissues, conferring pleiotropic immune activities distinct from those of IL-2. IL-15 induces NK-cell–derived TNF-α, GM-CSF, and IFN-γ and augments IL-12 up-regulation of T-cell–derived IFN-γ.[842,843] IL-15 also induces NK-cell differentiation, activation, and supports prolonged NK-cell survival.[844] Beyond these effects, IL-15 has also been shown to induce IL-8 expression by T cells and monocytes, as well as up-regulating monocyte-derived MCP-1 and MIP-1β, facilitating phagocyte recruitment and a proinflammatory milieu.[845,846] Finally, IL-15 also directly activates PMNs, inducing membrane "stiffening," enhancing phagocytosis, and delaying apoptosis.[847] Although macrophages are the primary cellular source of IL-15, gene expression of this cytokine has also been identified in lung fibroblast and epithelial cells, DCs, and endothelial cells in response to a variety of bacterial and viral stimuli, indicating a role for IL-15 in pulmonary immune regulation.[848] Such a role is supported by the findings of increased alveolar macrophage–derived IL-15 in patients with active pneumonia and other pulmonary inflammatory processes.[849,850] IL-15 production has not been characterized in the neonatal air space, but stimulated neonatal monocytes *in vitro* exhibit diminished IL-15 mRNA stability and protein expression of only about 30% relative to adult controls.[851] Given this finding, it is reasonable to speculate that attenuated IL-15 production by the neonate may contribute to impaired pulmonary cellular immunity.

Interleukin-16. Originally identified as lymphocyte chemoattractant factor, IL-16 is a potent chemotactic cytokine for CD4 T lymphocytes, monocytes, and eosinophils.[852] Despite its chemoattractant properties, it is not considered a member of the chemokine family. Structurally, it is synthesized in precursor form and cleaved to an active 56-kDa molecule composed of four identical 14-kDa polypeptide subunits; regulation of its function can thus occur at both transcriptional and posttranscriptional levels.[853] Cellular sources of IL-16 include CD8 T lymphocytes, eosinophils, fibroblasts, bronchial epithelial cells, and alveolar type II cells, suggesting a potential role for this cytokine in pulmonary immune function.[852,854-857] Elaboration of IL-16 in response to various signals is cell specific but is typically induced by stimuli including TNF, IL-1β, IL-4, IL-9, serotonin, and histamine.[855-857] Beyond its chemotactic activity, IL-16 also induces expression of the IL-2 receptor on CD4 T cells, enhancing IL-2–dependent T-cell activities, and this may be its most relevant role in the newborn population.[858] The inducibility of IL-16 by allergens, histamine, and Th2 cytokines suggests a primary role in reactive airways disease. However, the low level of IL-16 release seen *in vitro,* absent cytokine stimulation, suggests that this chemoattractant plays only a minor role in immune cell trafficking under basal, noninflammatory conditions. This premise is supported by data from human newborns, in which detectable IL-16 levels in BAL are associated with leukocytic infiltration and eventual progression to chronic lung disease.[859]

Interleukin-17. IL-17 is a proinflammatory cytokine, produced by activated memory CD4 T cells, that facilitates granulopoiesis and pulmonary PMN recruitment in response to local bacterial infection.[860] It is the prototypical member of a cytokine cohort collectively designated IL-17A-F, which also includes IL-25 (IL-17E);[861] this cohort exerts pleiotropic effects on leukocytes and stromal cells through a family of ubiquitously distributed, unique cognate receptors. IL-17 mediates inflammation by up-regulating monocyte-derived TNF, IL-1β, and PGE2, as well as stimulating IL-8 production from fibroblasts, vascular endothelium, and airway epithelial cells.[862-864] IL-17 further supports PMN chemotaxis by up-regulating IFN-γ–induced adhesion molecule expression and putatively enhances PMN activation within airways through its up-regulation of the aforementioned mediators.[865,866] IL-17 is synergistic with TNF in promoting GM-CSF elaboration by fibroblasts and, in a murine model, induced the release of G-CSF and stem cell factor from stromal cells, providing a mechanism for its observed granulopoietic effects.[863,867] Beyond its proinflammatory effects, IL-17 also induces secretion of macrophage-derived IL-1ra, IL-6, and IL-10, each of which potentially quenches TNF and IL-1–driven inflammatory cascades.[862] In the context of these data, it is possible that IL-17 functions as a cross-talk cytokine at the interface between the innate and cellular immune system. At an inflammatory focus, IL-17 secretion by activated T cells could initially accelerate PMN differentiation, recruitment, and activation, while later elaboration of IRAP, IL-10, and IL-6 titrates the inflammatory signal and facilitates transition to a more focused (cellular) immune response. Pulmonary IL-17 has not as yet been quantified in neonatal cohorts but may be negligible given the relative paucity of memory T cells in this population.

Interleukin-18. Initially identified as IFN-γ–inducing factor (IGIF), IL-18 is an approximately 18-kDa protein that enhances IFN-γ production and exhibits other, proinflammatory, functions.[868] IL-18 is similar to IL-1β both in secondary structure and in its secretion as an inactive precursor requiring cleavage by IL-1β–converting enzyme (caspase-1) to become bioactive.[869] IL-18 also shares receptor components and signal transduction mechanisms with IL-1.[870] Binding of IL-18 to its receptor, the IL-1 receptor–related protein (IL-1Rrp), triggers a signaling pathway that requires IL-1 receptor–activating kinase (IRAK) and eventually culminates in the nuclear translocation of NF-κB, and gene transcription. IL-18 may also bind to its alternative ligand, IL-18

binding protein (IL-18bp), an endogenous, soluble, "decoy" receptor that inhibits IL-18 activity; IL-18 bioactivity may thus be titrated either by regulation of cleavage activation or by modulation of IL-18bp levels.[871] IL-18 is present constitutively within the lung, primarily derived from AMs, although also inducible *in vitro* from pulmonary fibroblasts.[872] Like other macrophage-derived cytokines, IL-18 is up-regulated in response to microbial products (LPS, gram-positive bacterial exotoxins) and is also induced by exposure to TNF-α, chemokines (IL-8, MCP-1, MIP-1α), and mycobacteria.[873] As suggested earlier, IL-18 has important IFN-γ–inducing activity. By direct activation of the IFN-γ promoter, IL-18 achieves potent synergy with IL-12 for IFN-γ production by T cells, B cells, and NK cells but only modest induction of IFN-γ in the absence of IL-12; this augmented IFN-γ production may favor a Th1 response within the alveolus.[874] Beyond its IFN-γ–inducing activity, IL-18 exhibits other proinflammatory properties. It enhances proliferation and fas ligand–mediated cytotoxicity of T cells and NK cells, up-regulates TNF-α from T cells and NK cells, and induces T-cell synthesis of IL-2 and GM-CSF.[873-875] IL-18 also induces mononuclear cell expression of IL-1 and IL-6 and indirectly induces chemokine expression (IL-8, MCP-1) by means of its induction of lymphocyte-derived TNF-α.[876] Increased leukocyte and endothelial adhesion molecule expression has also been attributed to this cytokine.[877,878] Consistent with these pleiotropic activities, IL-18 is produced in clinical and various animal models of infection, where it appears protective against fungal, bacterial, and viral pathogens.[879-881] Such a role has been demonstrated *in vivo* in a transgenic model of IL-18 deficiency, where impaired lung bacterial clearance and fulminant progression to systemic infection resulted from intratracheal inoculation with *Streptococcus pneumoniae*.[882] In humans, elevated IL-18 levels are documented in BAL specimens from patients with sarcoidosis or sepsis. IL-18 is also detected in pleural effusions of infants with *Mycoplasma pneumoniae* infection.[883] In neonates, however, the pulmonary expression of IL-18 remains incompletely characterized.

Other Interleukins (IL-7, IL-14). Except where discussed earlier, little is known regarding the actions, if any, of the remaining interleukins on specific pulmonary immune responses; however, to the extent that they are involved in development and interactions of lymphocytes, they may indirectly affect cellular or humoral responses within the lung. IL-7 is produced by stromal cells in the bone marrow, spleen, and thymus primarily but is also found in end organs such as the neonatal gut.[884] IL-7 functions to support growth of B and T cells, possibly by inducing the surface expression of other cytokine receptors involved in early hematopoietic development;[885] IL-7 also augments cytotoxic T-cell generation and NK-cell activity.[886,887] Generation of transgenic IL-7–deficient animals has shed further light on the role of this cytokine. Specifically, IL-7 is required for the maturation, and normal life span, of fetal γδ T cells.[888] Also, IL-7 stimulation allows naive, neonatal T cells to proliferate, without acquiring a more mature phenotype; this enables expansion of the immune system in newborns, while maintaining a naive T-cell pool for subsequent neoantigen exposures throughout life.[884,889] Finally, beyond these findings, IL-7 has also been shown to be essential for the functional development of neonatal T cells and induces the initial expression of IL-4 by activated neonatal T cells.[890] IL-7 gene expression has been identified in adult lung tissue,[891] where its expression may support the maturation and survival of extrathymically derived γδ T cells.[892] The presence, or role, of IL-7 in neonatal pulmonary immune function remains uncharacterized, but similar effects on local γδ T cell and naive T-cell populations are postulated. IL-14 is produced by T cells after stimulation. IL-14 induces proliferation of B cells, and it may have a role in the development and maintenance of B-cell memory; its receptor has been found only on B cells.[893] No studies of IL-14 in specific pulmonary processes, or in the neonatal population, have been reported.

Chemokines

IL-8 and several other structurally homologous proteins comprise the family of cytokines known as chemokines. The chemokine family consists of more than 40 small (70–130 amino acid) cytokines divided into four subfamilies based on the position of one or two conserved cysteine residues located near the N-terminus defining four structural motifs: CXC, CC, C, and CX3C.[894,895] Different leukocyte subsets express a unique "chemokine receptor profile" that defines the response potential of each type of cell. In turn, chemokines can be modified by proteases in the extracellular milieu to become more active (better receptor "fit") or inert.[896] Although most chemokine receptors bind more than one chemokine, CC receptors bind only CC chemokines and CXC receptors bind only CXC chemokines. Chemokines play a critical role in recruitment and activation of inflammatory cells at sites of infection. Both CC and CXC chemokines have positively charged C-terminus residues that bind to negatively charged glycosaminoglycans on matrix proteins in the interstitium and on cell surfaces; this provides a mechanism to stabilize chemokines near sites of generation, achieving relatively fixed local chemotactic gradients. These chemotactic properties are titrated by the variable expression of specific chemokine receptors that are expressed constitutively, or induced by cytokines such as IL-2 or other stimuli.[897] The spectrum of action of a given chemokine is thus a function of its local concentration, its posttranslational processing, and the temporal expression of chemokine receptor(s) on putative target cells. Important representative chemokines implicated in the regulation of pulmonary immune responses include members of the CXC and CC subfamilies.

CXC Chemokine Subfamily. CXC chemokines can be further subdivided into two groups based on the presence or absence of three amino acids (Glu-Leu-Arg: the "ELR" motif) preceding the first cysteine residue. The ELR-CXC chemokines are potent neutrophil chemoattractants and angiogenic agents, whereas non-ELR CXC chemokines are chemoattractant for mononuclear leukocytes and angiostatic. IL-8, the prototypical ELR-CXC chemokine, is produced by a number of pulmonary cells, including mononuclear phagocytes, endothelial cells, fibroblasts, epithelial cells, mesothelial cells, and T cells.[435,447,464,898-900] Chemokine production by these cells can be induced by multiple stimuli, including viruses, bacterial products, TNF, IL-1, C5a, LTB$_4$, and IFN.[901,902] IL-8 accounts for most of the alveolar macrophage-derived chemotactic activity for neutrophils.[903] Actions of IL-8 on PMNs include potent chemoattraction, upregulation of adhesion molecule expression, and enhancement of PMN respiratory burst and degranulation.[904,905] IL-8 also stimulates PMN production of the inflammatory lipid mediators LTB$_4$ and PAF.[906,907] Because LTB$_4$ can directly induce PMN-derived IL-8 generation, the effects of this are twofold; there is both increased LTB$_4$-driven PMN chemotaxis and activation as well as amplified local production of IL-8 leading to further PMN recruitment.[908] Although not chemotactic for monocytes, IL-8 will enhance the respiratory burst of mononuclear phagocytes, suggesting that these cytokines may generate oxyradical species through activation of both PMN and macrophages at inflammatory sites.[909] Recent evidence suggests that IL-8 may also modulate B-cell growth through interactions with IL-2 and IL-4.[910] Novel physical and chemical characteristics of IL-8 include resistance to temperature or pH extremes, slow (hours) inactivation by neutrophil proteinases, and sustained (or enhanced) bioactivity within an inflammatory milieu.[911,912] These features, coupled with its production by multiple immune and nonimmune cells within the lung and its ability to induce its own production through LTB$_4$-neutrophil interactions make IL-8 well suited for its presumed cardinal role in amplifying and sustaining cytokine-driven pulmonary inflammatory responses.

IL-8 is locally expressed in patients with pneumonia, and its critical role in host response is further supported by animal models of bacterial pneumonitis; in these models, depletion of CXC chemokines, or blockade of CXC receptors, attenuates PMN recruitment and blunts pulmonary bacterial clearance.[913-917] A similar role likely exists for IL-8 in neonates, however, data regarding IL-8 production in this population is somewhat contradictory. *In vitro* stimulation of neonatal immune cells has typically demonstrated IL-8 production well below adult levels.[918,919] However, neonatal IL-8 production exceeding adult response has been shown using flow cytometric analysis in an *ex vivo* model of neonatal sepsis.[920] Although challenging to previous conventional wisdom, these findings are consistent with other emerging data showing the presence of significant, inducible IL-8 in the BAL specimens of term and preterm newborns with lung insults such as meconium aspiration syndrome or hyaline membrane disease.[921,922] IL-8 should therefore be considered as a likely relevant mediator both in neonatal pulmonary host defense as well as in inflammatory lung pathology.

CC Chemokine Subfamily. MIP-1α, MCP-1 and other members of the CC chemokine subfamily are derived from multiple pulmonary cells, including PMNs, mononuclear phagocytes, lymphocytes, NK cells, endothelium, fibroblasts, epithelial cells, and mesothelium.[923-929] Stimuli that induce production of the CC chemokines include viruses, bacterial products, TNF, IL-1, C5a, LTB4, and IFN, whereas IL-10 is a potent CC chemokine suppressor. The CC chemokines have specific chemotactic activity for monocytes, lymphocytes, eosinophils, and basophils and tend to have proinflammatory properties.[930-932] Binding of CC chemokines to their corresponding receptors on monocytes produces an increased respiratory burst and induces rapid release of arachidonic acid metabolites.[933,934] Both MIP-1α and MCP-1 regulate monocyte expression of adhesion molecules, preferentially increasing monocyte expression of the β2 integrin CD11/CD18 normally associated with PMNs, rather than the usual monocyte adhesin VLA-4;[935] this enhanced expression of β2 integrins results in augmented monocyte adhesion to endothelium, putatively enhancing monocyte migration to inflammatory loci. The CC chemokines have also been identified in the recruitment of T cells, B cells, and NK cells; however, they appear to lack significant effects on PMNs.[936-939] Elaboration of these chemokines by both immune and nonimmune cells of the lung suggests that they may regulate pulmonary inflammation by recruiting cells (monocytes, T cells) capable of modifying a nonspecific inflammatory response into a focused, adaptive immune response.

While early *in vitro* work demonstrated neonatal monocytes to have decreased inducible MIP-1a relative to adults, recent data have challenged these findings.[940] Basal serum levels of MIP-1α are found to be similar in neonatal and adult cohorts, and monocyte-derived MIP-1a is comparably inducible in these two age groups.[941,942] Levels of MIP-1α are increased in airway fluids of infants with inflammatory pulmonic processes including severe respiratory syncytial virus infection, *Ureaplasma* infection, and respiratory distress syndrome, suggesting local inducibility of this chemokine in response to infection or insult.[943-946] Neonatal levels of MCP-1, in both serum and airway fluid, are found to be similarly inducible in response to appropriate stress.[778,947] Taken together, these data suggest that the CC chemokines, like IL-8, should be considered relevant mediators of both pulmonary host defense and inflammatory lung injury in the neonate.

Interferon-γ

The interferons are a family of glycoprotein mediators synthesized by various cell types in response to viral infection or immune stimulation. Of these, IFN-γ is the most prominent as a mediator of immune cell interactions. Produced by T cells (CD4, CD8, γδ) and NK cells,[948,949] IFN-γ activates mononuclear phagocytes, augmenting phagocytosis and inducing their production of oxyradical species,[950] NO,[951] and cytokines such as TNF, IL-1, and IL-6;[952,953] it also acts synergistically with IL-1 to induce IL-8 expression by pulmonary vascular endothelial cells.[923] IFN-γ up-regulates pulmonary epithelial cell and endothelial cell expression of adhesion molecules, with resultant enhanced PMN adherence.[954,955] This cytokine also increases expression of MHC molecules on epithelial cells and monocytes, enhancing their ability to function as antigen-presenting cells.[956] Finally, proliferation of antigen-stimulated T cells, generation of cytotoxic T cells, and enhanced cytotoxic activity of NK cells is reported in response to IFN-γ.[957] The net outcome of these effects is enhanced leukocyte recruitment and macrophage antimicrobial activity and amplified inflammatory "tone." The enhanced antigen presentation induced by IFN-γ may facilitate later transition from macrophage-driven inflammation to lymphocyte-executed adaptive immune response.

IFN-γ function is regulated both by receptor expression as well as by other cytokines in the alveolar milieu. At the cellular level, TNF-α is synergistic with IFN-γ for macrophage activation. T-cell and NK-cell expressions of IFN-γ are facilitated by monocyte-derived IL-12; IL-12, in turn, acts synergistically with TNF-α, IL-1β, IL-15, and IL-18 to achieve optimal IFN-γ production. Finally, as a sentinel mediator of the Th1 response, IFN-γ is antagonized by the Th2 cytokines IL-4, IL-13, and IL-10. IL-4 suppresses the expression of IFN-γ and other Th1 cytokines. IL-4 and IL-13 each also inhibit the expression of many IFN-γ inducible genes, as well as the ability of IFN-γ to augment microbicidal activities such as superoxide production. IL-10 is similar to IL-4 in its inhibition of IFN-γ synthesis by Th1 cells, NK cells, and macrophages. At the receptor level, Th1 and Th2 cells exhibit differential responses to IFN-γ through their differential expressions of a specific IFN-γ receptor subunit (IFN-γRβ) that transduces suppressive signals.[958] In vivo, mutations of the IFN-γ receptor may increase host susceptibility to mycobacterial infection.[959]

IFN-γ–activated macrophages are capable of restricting the growth of a number of microbes that parasitize macrophages, such as Legionella, mycobacteria, Pneumocystis carinii, pathogenic fungi, and Chlamydia.[960-963] In vivo, IFN-γ replacement has been shown to enhance bacterial clearance in a murine model of Legionella pneumophila, as well as in transgenic IFN-γ–deficient animals challenged with S. pneumoniae or K. pneumoniae.[964-966] Interestingly, in these studies, treatment with IFN-γ did not significantly alter the alveolar inflammatory cell influx, suggesting that benefit derived primarily from direct leukocyte activation. IFN-γ has been demonstrated in the BAL specimens of neonates with respiratory syncytial virus, but the pulmonary expression of this cytokine is generally uncharacterized in this age group.[967] Most likely, the diminished ability of neonatal lymphocytes to generate this cytokine (capacity less than 10% of adult) limits optimal alveolar macrophage activation, compromising neonatal pulmonary immune response.[386,387]

Transforming Growth Factor-β

TGF-β is a cytokine primarily associated with tissue repair and fibrosis, but one that also exerts important immunomodulatory effects. This cytokine is secreted as an inactive disulfide bond–linked dimer, and liberation of the 25-kDa active form occurs in response either to proteolytic activation or acidic conditions.[968] TGF-β is produced by multiple cell lines, including platelets, PMNs, mononuclear cells, fibroblasts, epithelial cells, and endothelial cells, and exerts pleiotropic effects relevant to host immune response.[969] It can directly, or indirectly through IL-6, induce production of acute phase proteins. It can also act as a potent chemoattractant for monocytes and macrophages and can induce these cells to produce TGF-β, thereby amplifying its local effects.[970] Although TGF-β can induce monocyte-derived IL-1 and TNF-α, it inhibits LPS induction of macrophage-derived IL-1, TNF-α, and IFN-γ, thus exhibiting antiinflammatory activity

in settings of immune activation.[971] TGF-β can also down-regulate macrophage NO production and MHC II expression and suppresses macrophage respiratory burst.[972,973] Beyond macrophage deactivation, TGF-β also down-regulates IL-2 receptors, inhibiting IL-2–dependent T-cell proliferation and IL-1–dependent lymphocyte proliferation. Lastly, TGF-β inhibits B-cell differentiation and immunoglobulin isotype switching.[974] The net result of TGF-β activity is impairment of IL-2 effect and inhibition of Th1 response. Within the alveolus, this manifests as impaired antigen presentation and a general suppression of inflammation. In this context, TGF-β may thus contribute to AM titration of alveolar "inflammatory tone." Data defining the role of TGF-β in neonatal pulmonary defense remain incomplete. In vitro, TGF-β production from stimulated neonatal monocytes is only 35 to 40% of that from adult monocytes; this may suggest compromised ability of the neonate to titrate inflammation through TGF production.[975] This is supported by in vivo data showing lower TGF-β levels in the BAL specimens of infants progressing to states of chronic lung disease.[976] Finally, additional studies have shown elevated neonatal BAL levels of TGF-β, suggesting that expression of this cytokine may be more inducible than indicated by in vitro data.[977]

Clara Cell Secretory Protein (CCSP, CC10, CC16)

Clara cell secretory protein (CCSP) is one of the most abundant proteins of the airway lining fluid. It is secreted by Clara cells, as well as by serous and goblet cells of the proximal airways.[978] Structurally, CCSP is a small homodimeric protein consisting of two 8-kDa subunits aligned by disulfide links to form a hydrophobic pocket.[979] This pocket can bind phosphatidylcholine and phosphatidylinositol, and CCSP was thus originally postulated to participate in surfactant metabolism. More recently, CCSP has been noted to modulate inflammatory responses, suggesting a potential immunoregulatory role within the airways and alveoli. In vitro, CCSP has been shown to inhibit PMN chemotaxis, as well as macrophage phagocytosis.[980] Its hydrophobic pocket allows CCSP to "scavenge" phospholipase A_2 within the milieu, further limiting PMN activation.[981] CCSP has also been shown to inhibit the production and bioactivity of IFN-γ.[982] Taken together, these in vitro data suggest that CCSP may function to attenuate "inflammatory tone" within the lung. Murine models of CCSP deficiency have attempted to further clarify the in vivo role of this protein. In a hyperoxic model of lung injury, CCSP-deficient animals exhibited higher lung levels of IL-1β, IL-6, and IL-3, increased lung inflammation, and decreased survival rates.[983] In a model of adenoviral lung infection, CCSP deficiency resulted in earlier, and increased, inflammatory response; this was accompanied by increased expression of TNF, IL-1β, IL-6, and chemokines (MIP-1α and MCP-1).[984] CCSP-deficient animals receiving an antigenic challenge showed increased levels of Th2 cytokines with exacerbated eosinophilic inflammation.[985] Finally, CCSP-deficient mice demonstrate increased expression of IgA.[986] The exaggerated cellular response seen in each of these models is consistent with the putative role of CCSP as an antiinflammatory molecule. Although CCSP secretion is mainly constitutive, it is steroid inducible and is also up-regulated by IFN-γ.[987] Because CCSP itself down-regulates IFN-γ, this constitutes a negative feedback loop that may attenuate IFN-mediated inflammation within the lung. Conversely, LPS depresses CCSP gene expression in a dose-dependent fashion, suggesting that potent signals of infection may dampen CCSP secretion as required to allow an appropriate inflammatory response.[988] Human data tend to support such immunoregulatory roles for CCSP. In newborns, CCSP levels are detected in tracheal/alveolar aspirates obtained at birth and correlate with gestational age. Neonates with clinical signs of infection have increased CCSP levels, correlating inversely with tracheoalveolar fluid leukocyte counts.[989] Similarly, infants who subsequently develop BPD demonstrate diminished inducibility of CCSP and generally lower CCSP levels in their airway fluid, possibly contributing to the increased lung inflammation seen in this process.[990] In summary, CCSP appears to serve a homeostatic role in titrating inflammatory activity within the air spaces of the lung. Although not classically viewed as a cytokine, CCSP meets these criteria because it exhibits receptor-mediated signaling,[978] regulates other cytokines and immune cell function, and is regulated in dose-dependent fashion by relevant biologic stimuli such as IFN and LPS.

Colony-Stimulating Factors

Colony-stimulating factors such as GM-CSF are also identified as participants in pulmonary host defense. These factors, including G-CSF and macrophage-colony stimulating factor (M-CSF), are generated by a number of relevant pulmonary cells, including endothelial cells, epithelial cells, fibroblasts, mononuclear phagocytes, and T lymphocytes; production of these factors may be induced by an array of microbial products and pathogens.[991] Once elaborated at a site of potential infection, these factors exert pleiotropic effects on local immune cells, including increased membrane expression of receptors and adhesion molecules, enhanced motility, increased microbicidal function of phagocytic cells, enhanced phagocyte survival, and stimulation of cytokine secretion by mononuclear phagocytes.[992-996] GM-CSF also acts on macrophages to stimulate their antigen presentation capabilities and directs DC differentiation and distribution in the lung.[997,998] Within the lung, GM-CSF derives from alveolar macrophages, bronchial epithelial cells, and vascular endothelium. It is a potent stimulus for PMN degranulation, and its production by endothelial cells has been implicated in PMN-mediated alveolar injury.[999] Although neonatal T-cell capacity to generate GM-CSF is only 50% of adult T cells, neonatal mononuclear cells possess adult capacity for production of this cytokine and may thus be able to induce local responses dependent on GM-CSF elaboration.[244,245] This premise is supported by data from newborns demonstrating alveolar macrophage generation of GM-CSF.[1000]

Of the colony-stimulating factors, G-CSF appears to be most critical in pulmonary host defense against bacteria. Alveolar macrophages are potent secretors of G-CSF in response to LPS, or when stimulated by TNF or IL-1. AM-derived G-CSF acts locally to recruit, activate, and delay apoptosis of PMNs while acting systemically to induce granulopoiesis and increase the circulating neutrophil count. The importance of G-CSF in this context is underscored by animal studies, where antibody neutralization of G-CSF results in profoundly suppressed PMN recruitment and diminished bactericidal activity against aerosolized *Pseudomonas aeruginosa*.[1001] Of note, G-CSF also induces antiinflammatory mediators such as IL-1ra and soluble TNF receptors, locally titrating the inflammatory response.[1002] Neonatal monocytes can be stimulated to generate near-adult amounts of G-CSF. Preterm infants, however, appear much more compromised in their ability to up-regulate G-CSF production (10 to 30% of adult response), and this may constitute yet another deficiency of pulmonary host defense in this cohort.[1003] Neonatal capacity for production of various cytokines, as presently characterized, is summarized in Figure 164-16.

Adhesion Molecules

Leukocyte migration from the intravascular space to an eventual inflammatory locus within the lung is a multistep process, dependent on mechanisms directing cell movement to the appropriate site; leukocytes must marginate and adhere to the vascular endothelium, followed by diapedesis between endothelial cells and movement from the vascular space. Directed movement along concentration gradients of chemotaxins is one mechanism, while another is haptotaxis, or directed migration along gradients of endothelial adhesiveness. This latter process requires the presence of both leukocyte- and endothelial-derived adhesion molecules and is mediated by three families of molecules: the integrins, the immunoglobulin gene superfamily, and the selectins (Fig. 164-17).

The integrins are a family of proteins involved in cell adhesion and motility. Present on leukocyte membranes, these molecules adhere to specific endothelial ligands and various components of connective tissue matrix. The integrins are expressed as heterodimers, each containing one α and one β chain; subclassification of these adhesins is based on specific α/β chain content. The α4 integrins are expressed at high levels on monocytes, lymphocytes, and eosinophils. Although typically absent from neutrophils, α4 integrin is present on immature PMNs, or on mature forms under conditions of transendothelial migration or chemokine stimulation.[1004] The β1 integrins include VLA-4, found on lymphocytes and monocytes.[1005] The β2 integrins include CD11a/CD18, constitutively expressed on all leukocyte subsets, and CD11b/CD18 and CD11c/CD18, which are prominent adhesins of PMNs.[1006] Because the PMN must deform to navigate the narrow alveolar capillary space, the PMN surface membranes are brought into close contact with those of the

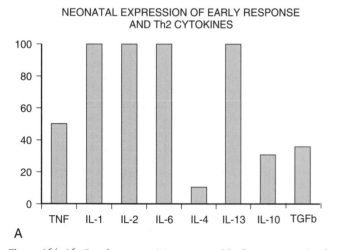

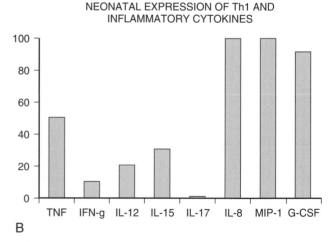

Figure 164–16. Graph summarizing neonatal leukocyte capacity for generation of cytokines relevant in pulmonary host defense. Cytokine levels shown represent percentage of adult response attainable under maximal stimulation. These data are consistent with putative neonatal T cell bias toward a Th2 or Th0 profile, and also suggest impaired neonatal capacity to finely titrate or down-regulate inflammatory responses.

vascular endothelium, inviting adherence interactions.[1007] CD11/CD18 is therefore maintained in an inactive state, until chemotactic activation occurs.[1008] PMN activation results in a CD11/CD18 conformational change to an activated form that recognizes its corresponding endothelial ligand.[1009,1010] PMN activation also results in mobilization of a significant intracellular stored pool of CD11/CD18, facilitating rapid additional surface expression of this molecule,[1006] although the constitutively smaller pool in neonatal PMNs may tend to blunt this response.[402]

The immunoglobulin gene superfamily includes intercellular adhesion molecules 1 and 2 (ICAM-1 and ICAM-2), vascular cell adhesion molecule 1 (VCAM-1) and platelet-endothelial cell adhesion molecule (PECAM). ICAM-1, the endothelial ligand for CD11/CD18, is expressed on endothelial cells constitutively and up-regulated in response to endotoxin, TNF-α, or IL-1β; ICAM-1 is also expressed on the surface of fibroblasts and epithelial cells.[1011] VCAM is similarly up-regulated by TNF-α and IL-1β, recognizes VLA-4 (and other β1 integrins), and binds monocytes and lymphocytes.[1012] PECAM is present constitutively and in the pulmonary vasculature may up-regulate in response to hyperoxia.[1013,1014] Its primary counterreceptor is the P-selectin glycoprotein ligand-1 (PSGL-1), found on a variety of leukocytes, including PMNs.[1015] PECAM-mediated adhesion may be important in transendothelial cell diapedesis of PMNs from the intravascular space.[1016]

The selectin family includes L-selectin, P-selectin, and E-selectin. L-selectin is expressed on the surface of PMNs and is shed shortly after activation *in vitro*.[1017] P-selectin is stored in endothelial cells and rapidly mobilized to the surface after initial endothelial activation.[1018] E-selectin (endothelial-leukocyte adhesion molecule [ELAM]) is expressed on the surface of endothelial cells only after activation by bacterial products, or mediators including C1q, TNF-α, IL-1β, and IL-10.[1019-1022] PMN receptors for the endothelial selectins include PSGL-1 and sialyl Lewis X antigen (sLe^x), an oligosaccharide present on many proteins including the PMN adhesins L-selectin and CD11/CD18.[1023,1024]

The initial step in leukocyte migration to extravascular sites is a slowing of leukocyte movement through the area of inflammation by a series of loose, transient leukocyte-endothelial cell adhesions, characterized as "rolling." This step is mediated through interaction of endothelial selectins with PSGL-1 and L-selectin on the PMN surface;[1025] low L-selectin and sLe^x concentrations on neonatal PMN surfaces have been implicated in impaired chemotaxis but are likely not relevant in the pulmonary circulation where the constrained vascular space obviates the need for this receptor-ligand interaction.[1026,1027] The next step entails binding of local chemotactic activators (C3a, C5a, IL-8, PAF) to the "rolling" PMN, inducing expression and activation of CD11/CD18 and shedding of L-selectin.[1017] Subsequently, the leukocytes firmly attach to the endothelium via CD11/CD18 to ICAM-1 interaction (PMNs) or by means of VLA-4 to VCAM-1 interaction (mononuclear cells, lymphocytes).[1028,1029] The final step is diapedesis of the adherent leukocyte through the vessel wall and migration along a chemotactic gradient to the site of inflammation. Although this process remains incompletely characterized, transendothelial migration appears mediated by the adhesion molecules PECAM and the integrin-associated protein CD47.[1016,1030,1031] Once extravasated, neutrophils appear to follow a fixed chemotactic gradient laid down in the extracellular matrix, migrating along interstitial fibroblasts and eventually squeezing between type I and type II epithelial cells to reach the air spaces of the lung.[1032]

Generation of a Local Immune Response

In animal models of bacterial pneumonia, the influx of inflammatory cells follows a well-orchestrated sequence. First, neutrophils enter the lung within minutes to hours of airway inoculation. PMN accumulation is maximal within 2 days, with cell clearance primarily through apoptosis. By day 2 to 3, monocytes are recruited, with maximal accrual by day 5 to 7 in resolving inflammation. Lymphocyte influx begins by 5 days, often occurring despite clearance of the organism. Although the timing of events is not consistently this rigid, the sequential appearance of each cell type is characteristic, consistent with a transition from acute inflammation to a more specific immune response. Factors unique to the lung that regulate this coordinated host response are now considered.

Intrapulmonary Neutrophil Trafficking

The previously discussed paradigm for neutrophil recruitment is well established for the systemic circulation, where PMN migration typically occurs in postcapillary venules. In contrast, it is

Figure 164–17. The sites of leukocyte-endothelial adhesion molecules. Selectins are expressed on the surface of activated endothelial cells and engage glycoproteins expressed on the neutrophil surface as either selectins (L-selectin) or integrins (CD11/CD18). Chemotactic activation up-regulates surface expression of the neutrophil integrins through a G protein–mediated process and induces conformational changes that facilitate integrin interaction with endothelial adhesion molecules. Adhesion molecules of the immunoglobulin superfamily, constitutively expressed on endothelial surfaces, provide strong complementary ligands for such "activated" neutrophil integrins. (From Collins T: *In* Sirica AE [ed]: Cellular and Molecular Pathogenesis. Philadelphia, Lippincott-Raven, 1996, pp 125–155.)

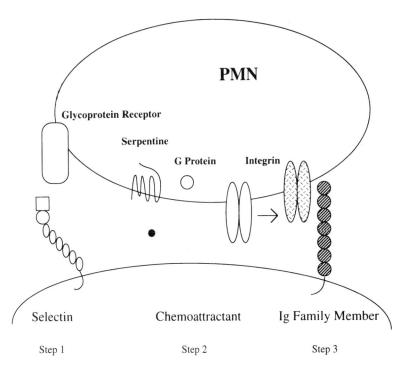

now recognized that alveolar capillaries are the primary sites of PMN extravasation within the lung and that alternative mechanisms of neutrophil recruitment prevail here owing to unique aspects of the pulmonary circulation.[1033] Most marginated neutrophils (up to 50% of intravascular PMN) reside in lung capillaries; thus, compared with other organs, the lungs enjoy a large, readily mobilizable granulocyte pool.[1034] The narrow caliber of these vessels (diameter 5 to 9 μm) does not allow leukocyte rolling but rather requires neutrophils (diameter 6.5 to 8 μm) to deform and slowly "squeeze through" this vascular space; this imposes sustained PMN-endothelial contact, independent of adhesion molecules.[1035] The small distance between pulmonary capillaries and their alveoli facilitates brisk PMN response to alveolar-derived inflammatory signals. In this setting, mediator activation of neutrophils induces cytoskeletal changes that reduce PMN deformability, increasing duration of capillary transit and neutrophil-endothelial contact.[1036] Of note, the impaired deformability of neonatal neutrophils may engender a larger marginated pool of these cells within the newborn lung. Once activated, "stiffened" neutrophils are retained briefly (4 to 7 minutes *in vivo*) near inflammatory sites, until appropriate adhesins can be expressed to facilitate firm attachment and eventual transendothelial diapedesis.[1037]

Beyond the rheologic conditions promoting neutrophil margination, neutrophil trafficking in the pulmonary capillary differs from other vascular sites in the repertoire of adhesive interactions invoked. P-selectin is not expressed on pulmonary capillary endothelium, consistent with spatial constraints that obviate selectin-initiated "rolling" as an initial step in PMN recruitment.[1038] However, once activated, neutrophils are sequestered only transiently and return to the circulation unless firm adhesion to the endothelium occurs. Available data suggest that this adhesion is mediated first by L-selectin, then by CD11/CD18.[1039] Firm adhesion mediated by CD11/CD18 is temporally associated with resolution of neutrophil "stiffening," allowing sufficient PMN surface area to flatten and engage the endothelium.[1036] Once firmly adhered, neutrophil emigration from the vascular space then proceeds in a manner that is either CD11/CD18 dependent or CD11/CD18 independent, depending on the specific stimulus. *Pseudomonas aeruginosa*, *E. coli* (or its endotoxin), IgG immune complexes, and IL-1 each induce PMN emigration mediated by CD11/CD18; because these stimuli also up-regulate endothelial ICAM expression, CD11/CD18 dependent migration may result from critical availability of this counter ligand.[1040,1043] Alternatively, stimuli including hyperoxia, C5a, IL-8, LTB$_4$, and the organisms *Streptococcus pneumoniae*, *Staphylococcus aureus*, and group B *Streptococcus* induce PMN emigration, which is CD11/CD18 independent.[1044-1048] How PMNs emigrate under these conditions remains unclear; binding mediated by various β1-integrins has been postulated, but *in vivo* and *in vitro* data are conflicting.[1046,1049] Integrins of the α4 subclass may be relevant adhesins; they are expressed constitutively on human neutrophils, are up-regulated by transendothelial migration, and support PMN migration in response to chemotaxins such as IL-8.[1050,1051] The α4 integrins also facilitate neutrophil movement through extravascular tissue, providing a mechanism for eventual PMN emigration to the alveolar space.[1052] Like the β1 integrins, however, their actual *in vivo* role in CD11/CD18-independent PMN emigration remains ambiguous.[1053]

In summary, neutrophil trafficking within pulmonary capillaries is regulated by rheologic conditions and adhesive interactions unique to this vascular site. Initial sequestration of PMNs in response to inflammatory stimuli occurs through mediator-induced changes in PMN deformability. Adhesion molecule interaction is then required to maintain the PMN-endothelial contact that precedes active PMN emigration to sites of infection. Subsequent adhesion and emigration can occur through two pathways, one that requires CD11/CD18 and one that does not; the pathway employed appears determined by the specific infec-

tious stimulus and the inflammatory signals generated. This ability of PMNs to adhere and emigrate via integrin-independent means may be critical for allowing the neonate to effectively mount an inflammatory response to inhaled pathogens, despite known limitations of neutrophil adhesion and chemotaxis. Whereas classic multistep PMN migration may still occur in pulmonary postcapillary venules, its relative contribution to overall neutrophil extravasation is uncertain and may vary depending on site and nature of inflammatory stimuli.

Alveolar Macrophage Regulation of Inflammation

The ability of the AM to recruit and regulate other inflammatory cells is the major attribute allowing AMs to locally regulate pulmonary host defenses. In addition to their phagocytic function, the AM can recruit PMNs, eosinophils, interstitial and airway macrophages, and peripheral blood monocytes to the alveolar space; once present in the alveolus, these cells are either activated or suppressed by AM-derived mediators.

Mediators that up-regulate inflammation within the alveolus are not constitutively expressed by alveolar macrophages; their release therefore requires the AM to be in an activated state. Activation typically occurs through engagement of macrophage PRRs and can be titrated by competitive interactions with soluble PRRs within the alveolar milieu. One example of this is the interaction between SP-A, and the CD14 ligand LBP. In the basal, uninflamed state, SP-A is present at much higher concentrations than the acute phase protein LBP and therefore is the primary ligand for any LPS inadvertently deposited from the air stream into the airway surface liquid. This prevents initiation of the LBP/CD14 pathway and dampens inflammatory tone within the alveolus. However, under conditions of inflammation, SP-A concentrations may fall dramatically, owing to degradation by PMN-derived proteases and elastases, whereas LBP is concurrently up-regulated as an acute phase protein. Under these conditions, LBP becomes the dominant LPS-binding protein in the alveolus; this facilitates AM activation via the CD14 receptor, amplifying the bioactivity of LPS and subsequent inflammation severalfold.[229] Alternatively, AM activation can occur in response to GM-CSF elaborated by activated alveolar epithelium or in response to IFN-γ elaborated by local NK or T cells.

The activated AM effects PMN emigration to the alveolus through its production of multiple neutrophil chemotaxins, including the lipid mediators PAF and LTB$_4$, complement components C3a and C5a, and IL-8. Activated AMs also produce TNF-α and IL-1β, which, although not directly chemotactic, can activate PMN and up-regulate local endothelial cell surface adhesins and may thereby facilitate PMN recruitment from the intravascular space. Additionally, AMs have the capacity to recruit and activate other inflammatory cells. AMs can induce chemotaxis and activation of monocytes by secretion of the chemokines MCP-1 and MIP-1α, and in pneumonia this resulting monocyte infiltration typically peaks between days 5 and 7. Mononuclear cell response to either MCP-1 or MIP-1α includes increased respiratory burst, increased chemotaxis, increased monocyte expression of β2 integrins, and increased generation of arachidonic acid products; MCP-1 has also been shown to prime macrophages to respond to LPS, resulting in a proinflammatory amplifying loop. NK cells are also recruited and activated by these chemokines, and AM-derived IL-12 increases NK cell cytoxicity and induces NK-derived IFN-γ, generating another proinflammatory amplifying loop.

Consistent with its role in regulating intraalveolar immune responses, the AM also induces or expresses several mediators capable of honing or down-regulating local inflammatory processes. IL-6 derived directly from AM, or from alveolar cells (fibroblasts, endothelium, epithelium) in response to AM-derived IL-1, induces T- and B-cell proliferation but down-regulates subsequent AM production of TNF or IL-1. More directly,

AM-derived IL-1ra, produced in response to endotoxin or adherent IgG, inhibits local IL-1β effects by competitive binding of the IL-1 receptor. AM release of PGE₂ suppresses chemotaxis and release of inflammatory leukotrienes by PMN and AM, further down-regulating TNF and IL-1 production. AM-secreted TGF-β blunts further AM response to LPS and serves to dampen the proinflammatory amplifying loops noted earlier. Additionally, alveolar macrophages can be induced to generate IL-10, although the most prominent alveolar source of this cytokine may actually be the recruited peripheral monocytes. This cytokine exhibits protean antiinflammatory activity. It suppresses a variety of proinflammatory cytokines and facilitates transition to a T-cell-mediated adaptive immune response. Finally, alveolar macrophages down-regulate inflammation in the air space through clearance of apoptotic neutrophils; this activity is enhanced by the effects of IL-10, which diminishes phagocyte killing capability but up-regulates phagocytic function. This constitutes an antiinflammatory function because failure to clear necrotic PMNs results in protease release, local cell injury, sustained inflammation, and parenchymal destruction, as demonstrated in animal models of pneumonia.[1054]

Intraalveolar Cytokine Networking

Cytokine networking is essential for the normal orchestration of inflammation: the expression of an early response cytokine can activate a variety of immune and structural cells to express more distal cytokines that either sustain the inflammatory response or facilitate its resolution. These processes are particularly evinced by cellular components of the alveolus. Historically, the alveolar-capillary membrane has been viewed only as a barrier for gas exchange, but recent data have altered this concept significantly. This structure is now viewed as a dynamic assembly of immune and nonimmune cells that, via cytokine networking, can simultaneously express a number of immunoregulatory substances, facilitating rapid up-regulation or down-regulation, as needed, of a compartmentalized inflammatory response. These multicellular interactions are complicated and rarely as discrete as the *in vitro* analyses that constitute much of the work in this field. Nevertheless, as presently characterized, cytokine networks can be separated into those involved in initial pathogen response, subsequent amplification of the inflammatory or immune response, or those involved in eventual resolution of inflammation and/or transition to adaptive immunity.

Response Activation. As noted previously, microbial stimulation of alveolar macrophages initiates an innate immune response within the lungs that culminates with recruitment of PMNs and mononuclear phagocytes into alveoli. Engagement of macrophage TLRs, by means of bacterial products presented on CD14, initiates signal transduction that overlaps with IL-1β signaling pathways, resulting in macrophage production of TNF-α and IL-1β. The immediate action of these cytokines is to enhance microbicidal activity of the resident lung macrophages and to prepare the alveolar milieu for recruitment of inflammatory cells. TNF-α and IL-1β induce adhesion molecule expression on vascular endothelial cells and alveolar epithelial cells; this facilitates cell migration into the stimulated alveolus and epithelial activation of inflammatory cells. TNF up-regulates the oxidative burst of adherent PMNs and may therefore activate PMNs during their migration into the lung. PMN activation (and degranulation) during transendothelial migration can increase microvascular permeability, facilitating ease of leukocyte migration, as well as seepage of previously compartmentalized cytokines. Finally, AM-derived TNF-α can stimulate other tissue macrophages and pulmonary capillary endothelium to produce IL-1, thus networking to amplify this "early response." Although these events are best characterized for gram-negative bacteria, they also occur in gram-positive infections, as well as infections by intracellular pathogens such as *Legionella* and *Mycobacterium* species.

Response Amplification. As TNF-α and IL-1 accumulate in the alveolus, they amplify cytokine responses by inducing cytokine production from cells that would not otherwise respond directly to microbial stimuli. A sentinel example of such response amplification is provided by alveolar elaboration of the potent PMN chemoattractant IL-8. The expression of IL-8 by the major cellular constituents of the alveolar-capillary membrane is stimulus specific. Mononuclear phagocytes (alveolar macrophages, blood monocytes) and endothelial cells produce IL-8 in response to endotoxin (LPS), TNF, or IL-1. In contrast, pulmonary fibroblasts and epithelial cells express IL-8 only in response to specific host-derived signals such as locally elaborated TNF or IL-1. These findings are significant in that cells once thought of as purely structural and "targets" of TNF and IL-1 may be enlisted as effector cells in elaborating a potent chemokine and facilitating rapid amplification of local inflammation. In gram-negative pneumonia as an example (Fig. 164–18), the local release of LPS stimulates alveolar or interstitial macrophages to secrete IL-8, TNF, and IL-1. TNF may stimulate proximal endothelial cells to express additional IL-1, amplifying the initial signal. TNF and IL-1 thus present may act in either an autocrine or a paracrine fashion to stimulate contiguous cells to express additional IL-8, resulting in PMN recruitment from the vasculature to the pulmonary interstitium or alveolar space.

Resolution of Inflammation. Because inflammation due to cellular, or Th1, responses may induce local tissue injury, the capacity to appropriately down-regulate inflammation is essential to preserve lung function. Such "counter-balance" is typically provided by networks involving Th2 cytokines, and IL-10 is believed to be a critical mediator in this regard. As noted earlier, IL-10 exhibits protean antiinflammatory effects, including attenuation of phagocytic killing, and inhibition of co-stimulatory molecule expression on antigen-presenting cells. IL-10 is also a potent inhibitor of proinflammatory cytokine production by mononuclear phagocytes, including TNF, IL-1β, chemokines, and the Th1 cytokines IFN-γ and IL-12; significantly, this inhibition is more pronounced for peripheral monocytes than for alveolar macrophages.[1055,1056] *In vitro,* alveolar macrophages stimulated by LPS produce much less IL-10 than TNF or IL-1β, and IL-10 production is delayed by several hours; a similar delay in IL-10 production, relative to IL-12, has been observed *in vivo.*[1057] Temporally, this allows early response cytokines to initiate inflammation, which may be further amplified by local elaboration of chemokines such as IL-8, MCP, and MIP-1α. IL-10 also participates in this amplification step, by up-regulating the chemokine receptor CCR5, facilitating leukocyte recruitment. As peripheral monocytes and DCs are chemotactically recruited into the alveolar space, a "critical mass" of IL-10–responsive cells is eventually achieved within the alveolus. This allows IL-10–mediated suppression of mononuclear cell–derived IL-12, inhibiting "downstream" production of IFN-γ by NK and Th1 cells. This time course of IL-10 generation, and monocyte recruitment, results in delayed suppression of inflammation, putatively allowing sufficient inflammatory response to clear the offending pathogen. This is supported by multiple animal models in which exogenous IL-10 suppresses inflammation too early in host response, resulting in pathogen dissemination and morbid outcome.[796,797] Lastly, IL-10 up-regulates phagocytic function, while suppressing the microbicidal activity of mononuclear cells. This enhances phagocytic clearance of apoptotic PMNs, minimizing inflammation that can result from seepage of granulocyte-derived proteases or chemotaxins.[1058]

Additional cytokine networks may be simultaneously operant in resolution of alveolar inflammation, and, as discussed earlier, these networks may invoke participation of stromal cells. For example, whereas mononuclear phagocytes produce IL-6 in response to LPS, this cytokine is expressed by endothelial cells, epithelial cells, and fibroblasts in preferential response to TNF or

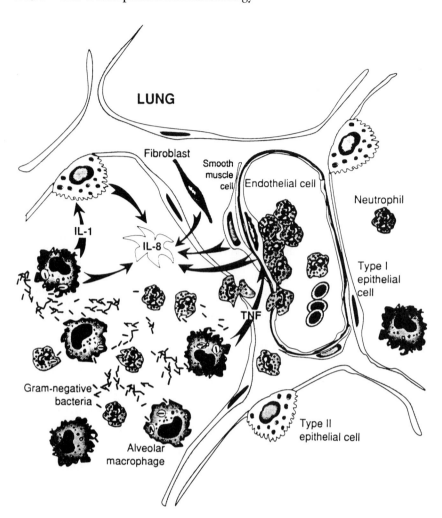

Figure 164–18. Cytokine networking between cells of the alveolar-capillary unit under conditions of gram-negative bacterial invasion. Processing of endotoxin by alveolar macrophages results in release of macrophage-derived IL-8, as well as the early response cytokines tumor necrosis factor (TNF) and IL-1. TNF and IL-1 may act locally to induce further IL-8 secretion from contiguous cells of the alveolar space (fibroblasts, epithelial cells), as well as from the adjacent capillary vascular endothelium. The net effect is rapid amplification of neutrophil chemotactic signals originating from the alveolar-capillary space and brisk up-regulation of an inflammatory response. (Reprinted from Strieter RM, et al: *In* Kelley J [ed]: Cytokines of the Lung. New York, Marcel Dekker, 1993, pp 281–305, by courtesy of Marcel Dekker, Inc.)

IL-1. As previously noted, IL-6 stimulates B-cell antibody production and T-cell proliferation/differentiation while inhibiting LPS-induced mononuclear cell production of TNF and IL-1, removing the stimulus for further stromal-derived IL-8 expression locally. In this fashion, local structural cells (epithelium, fibroblasts, endothelium) of the alveolar capillary membrane may network to down-regulate "cytokine cascading" with local quiescence of a nonspecific, and potentially injurious, inflammatory process. IL-6–mediated B-cell stimulation, in the setting of additional Th2 signals such as IL-10, may herald a transition from nonspecific cellular inflammation to adaptive immunity.

Systemic Cytokine Networking. Pulmonary cytokines generated in response to a local infection ideally, but rarely, remain confined to the alveolar space. Inflammatory disruption of alveolar epithelial integrity allows movement of locally generated cytokines into the intravascular space; this results in systemic cytokine networking, which may be either beneficial or deleterious to the host, depending on the specific cytokine and the context of the infection. For instance, it is likely that lung IL-6 generated during alveolar inflammation reaches the systemic circulation, where it stimulates the hepatic acute phase response. Another example of systemic cytokine networking is provided by alveolar-derived colony-stimulating factors, which are generated as part of the amplification response in pulmonary inflammation. GM-CSF and G-CSF are produced by alveolar macrophages in response to LPS, TNF-α, or IL-1β, whereas GM-CSF is also produced by stimulated epithelial cells and endothelial cells. Alveolar macrophages recovered from patients with pneumonia spontaneously release G-CSF, which acts locally to activate recruited PMNs and delay

their apoptosis.[991] In animal models of pneumonia, levels of G-CSF rise rapidly in the lungs and are measurable in the serum within 24 hours; this response is virtually ablated by antibody neutralization of TNF, underscoring the role of cytokine networking in generating alveolar G-CSF.[1001] Parallel studies have demonstrated that intratracheal deposition of G-CSF induces systemic neutrophilia.[1059] Taken together, these data suggest a model in which the lung, when challenged by bacteria, produces G-CSF in response to locally generated early response cytokines. Alveolar G-CSF easily reaches the circulation, stimulates granulopoiesis, and amplifies the PMN recruitment response initiated by IL-8. This response is associated with higher PMN counts in BAL specimens, more rapid bacterial clearance, and increased host survival.[1001]

Lymphocyte Homing and Response

When nonspecific alveolar inflammatory responses are inadequate to clear local infection, adaptive immune responses are initiated by recruitment and activation of lymphocytes. This process involves chemokine-directed T-cell migration, antigen presentation, and homing of activated lymphocyte to sites of infection within the lung. This intrapulmonary trafficking is complex and reflects the need of T cells to interact with populations of effector cells and antigen-presenting cells in anatomically discrete environments, minimizing spurious inflammation within the alveolus.

This process begins with antigen capture and presentation to T cells, through either MHC class I or MHC class II molecules on the surface of the antigen-presenting cell.[1060] Antigen-presenting cells of the alveolar-capillary interface include alveolar macrophages, DCs, endothelial cells, and recruited peripheral blood monocytes. The antigen-presenting function of recruited peripheral monocytes is intermediate between the marginal effectiveness of alveolar macrophages and the most efficient DCs. Antigen capture by DCs stimulates their maturation and migration to local lymph nodes, where they present antigen to T cells. Migration of both DCs and T cells is guided by locally secreted chemokines that activate the chemokine receptor CCR7; this receptor is expressed on naive T cells and some memory T-cell subsets and is up-regulated during maturation of DCs, facilitating co-localization of these three cell types.[1061]

Antigen processing and display allow DCs, and other lung antigen-presenting cells, to either "prime" antigenically naive T cells or activate memory T cells. Memory T cells have increased expression of adhesion molecules for both the antigen-presenting cells and endothelium, enhancing their rapidity of activation and recruitability to sites of inflammation.[1062] Concomitant with antigen presentation, T cells must also receive a co-stimulatory signal to become activated; such a signal may occur through antigen-presenting cell binding of specific molecules on the T cell (CD28 on naive T cells, CTLA-4 on memory T cells) or may be provided by cytokines such as IL-12 secreted into the local milieu.[1063,1064] Once activated, "effector" T cells reenter the circulation and travel to regions of inflammation in response to local elaboration of specific chemokines. Lung tropism appears to be mediated by a specific chemokine receptor profile, which may be further modified by the state of T-cell activation and its Th phenotype. Thus, for example, Th1 cells preferentially express the chemokine receptor CCR5, rendering them responsive to the CC chemokine MIP-1α.[1065] The differential expression of chemokine receptors, as well as the differential elaboration of chemokines, may orchestrate the trafficking of Th1 and Th2 cells, ultimately determining the phenotype of the local immune response.[1066]

On arrival to the site of infection, activated T cells produce IL-2, which induces clonal expansion of T cells, induces T-cell–derived IFN-γ, and activates macrophages; IFN-γ itself may also activate macrophages, as well as increase the activity of cytotoxic T cells and NK cells. T-cell–derived GM-CSF is also induced, which further activates macrophages, facilitates PMN recruitment, and up-regulates local inflammatory processes such as adhesion molecule expression and cytokine release. Beyond augmentation of local phagocytic responses, T cells also induce and regulate local antibody production. The mucosal IgA response is regulated by T cells, which provide an initial contact-dependent signal to the B cell and subsequently secrete TGF-β, resulting in B-cell switching of IgM expression to IgA expression;[1067] the T-cell cytokines IL-5 and IL-6 are necessary for final differentiation of surface IgA–expressing B cells to IgA-secreting plasma cells. Similarly, elaboration of other cytokines during T-cell–mediated activation induces B-cell switching to other immunoglobulin classes. Ultimately, T-cell–derived cytokines such as IL-4, IL-6, and IL-10 may down-regulate nonspecific local inflammatory responses by depressing both inflammatory cytokine production as well as phagocytic killing activity. Thus, when invoked, the advantages of this lymphocyte-driven immune response are multiple. First, cytokine elaboration by lymphocytes enhances antimicrobial function of macrophages and cytolytic function of NK cells and cytotoxic lymphocytes, thereby optimizing the nonspecific killing response of immune effector cells. Second, the activation of T cells by specific antigenic stimuli "focuses" the immune response by inducing subsequent B-cell production of specific immunoglobulin, resulting in opsonization of the targeted pathogen and enhanced phagocytosis (Fig. 164–19). Finally, when appropriate, expression of specific

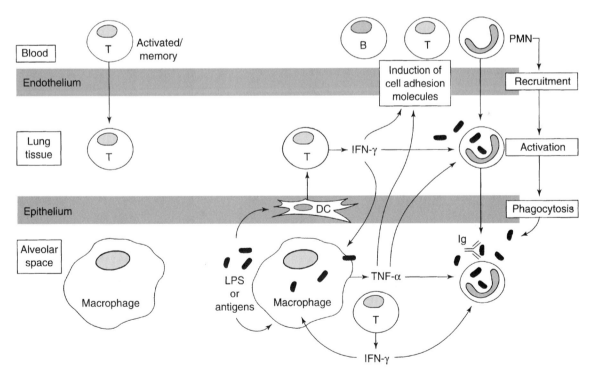

Figure 164–19. The relationship between T lymphocytes and mononuclear phagocytes in generation of a cellular immune response within the lung. Circulating memory T cells home to specific organs, in this case the lung, based on prior antigenic exposure. Subsequent infection in the alveolar space results initially in macrophage activation and production of early response cytokines. Concomitant presentation of antigen by dendritic cells (DC) to T lymphocytes results in elaboration of T-cell–derived interferon-γ (IFN-γ) and other cytokines (TNF-α). Although capable of enhancing phagocytic responses locally, the essential role of activated T cells and their products is to support immunoglobulin isotype switching, thereby focusing the local cellular immune response by inducing B-cell production of specific immunoglobulin directed against the presented antigen. (From Dunkley M, et al: Immunol Today *16*:231, 1995.)

T-cell–derived cytokines may diminish phagocyte activation and cytokine expression, allowing gradual resolution of nonspecific inflammation and restoration of normal alveolar activity.

In the neonate, however, effective pulmonary adaptive immune response is impaired at multiple levels. As noted previously, the phenotype of neonatal T cells is essentially that of antigenically naive adult T cells, presumably caused by limited antigen exposure. These T cells exhibit decreased surface density of TCRs and decreased adhesion molecules. They require sustained receptor stimulation for activation, as well as greater co-stimulation to achieve a Th1 phenotype. Additionally, whereas memory T cells tend to "home" to specific organs based on prior antigenic exposure, neonatal T cells preferentially reside in distal lymphoid tissues, resulting in delayed recruitment. On recruitment, antigen-presenting deficits are exposed. DCs are present in smaller numbers, exhibit less efficient trafficking and antigen presentation, and secrete less IL-12, resulting in an inadequate Th1 response. Neonatal T-cell and B-cell interactions are similarly abnormal, because neonatal T cells demonstrate impaired up-regulation of the CD40 ligand, essential for contact-dependent support of B-cell function, and stimulated neonatal B cells fail to up-regulate CD86, necessary for T-cell co-stimulation. Finally, the presence in the air space of γδ T cells, a potent source of IL-4, may "tip the balance" within the alveolus toward conditions most conducive for Th2 differentiation; under these conditions, diminished T-cell–mediated macrophage activation, decreased inflammatory cytokine expression, and a general decrease in cellular inflammation all ensue. Although such "Th2 bias" is maladaptive in the setting of pulmonary infection, it may be teleologically beneficial in protecting the vulnerable alveolus from indiscriminate inflammatory injury. Finally, it bears noting that Th1 responses can be demonstrated in neonates, although mixed Th1/Th2 responses are more often observed for reasons discussed earlier.[496, 1068] The net effect is a neonatal lymphocyte response that is more delayed, less facile in terms of accessory cell activation, less able to rapidly evolve a Th1 cellular immune response, less focused in regard to specific antibody production, and possibly less efficient in terms of dampening inflammatory responses once initiated.

REFERENCES

1. Longo LD: Fetal gas exchange. *In* Crystal RG, West JB (eds): The Lung: Scientific Foundations. New York, Raven Press, 1991, pp 1699-1710.
2. McCormack FX, Whitsett JA: The pulmonary collectins, SP-A and SP-D, orchestrate innate immunity in the lung. J Clin Invest 109:707-712, 2002.
3. Swift DL: Aerosols and humidity therapy: generation and deposition of therapeutic aerosols. Am Rev Respir Dis 122(Suppl):71-77, 1980.
4. Gumbiner B: Structure, biochemistry and assembly of epithelial tight junctions. Am J Physiol 253:C749-C758, 1987.
5. Plopper CG: Comparative morphologic features of bronchiolar epithelial cells: the Clara cell. Am Rev Respir Dis 128:S37-S41, 1983.
6. Breeze RG, Wheeldon EB: The cells of the pulmonary airways. Am Rev Respir Dis 116:705-777, 1977.
7. Sanderson MJ, et al: Intercellular communication between ciliated cells in culture. Am J Physiol 254:C63-C74, 1988.
8. Morosco GJ, et al: The morphology of ciliogenesis in the developing fetal human respiratory epithelium. Pathol Res Pract 183:403-411, 1988.
9. Johnson NF, Hubbs AF: Epithelial progenitor cells in the rat trachea. Am J Respir Cell Mol Biol 3:579-585, 1990.
10. Rhodin JAG: The ciliated cell: ultrastructure and function of the human tracheal mucosa. Am Rev Respir Dis 93:S1-S15, 1966.
11. Widdicombe JG, Pack RJ: The Clara cell. Eur J Respir Dis 63:202-220, 1982.
12. Knowles MR, Boucher RC: Mucus clearance as a primary innate defense mechanism for mammalian airways. J Clin Invest 109:571-577, 2002.
13. Philippon S, et al: In vitro study of the bronchial mucosa during *Pseudomonas aeruginosa* infection. Virchows Arch 423:39-43, 1993.
14. Hastie AT, et al: Structure and mass of mammalian respiratory ciliary outer arm 19S dynein. Cell Motil Cytoskeleton 11:157-166, 1988.
15. Hastie A, et al: Initial characterization of tektins in cilia of respiratory epithelial cells. Chest 101:47S-48S, 1992.
16. Foliguet B, Puchelle E: Apical structures of human respiratory cilia. Bull Eur Physiopathol Respir 22:43-47, 1986.
17. Rossman CM, et al: Nasal ciliary ultrastructure and function in patients with primary ciliary dyskinesia compared with that in normal subjects and in subjects with various respiratory diseases. Am Rev Respir Dis 129:161-167, 1984.
18. Holley MC, Afzelius BA: Alignment of cilia in immotile-cilia syndrome. Tissue Cell 18:521-529, 1986.
19. Sanderson MJ, Sleigh MA: Ciliary activity of cultured rabbit tracheal epithelium: beat pattern and metachrony. J Cell Sci 47:331-347, 1981.
20. Satir P, et al: The mechanochemical cycle of the dynein arm. Cell Motil 1:303-327, 1981.
21. Gibbons IR: Cilia and flagella of eukaryotes. J Cell Biol 91:107S-124S, 1981.
22. Marino MR, Aiello E: Cinemicrographic analysis of beat dynamics of human respiratory cilia. Cell Motil 80(Suppl):35-39, 1982.
23. Sleigh MA, et al: The propulsion of mucus by cilia. Am Rev Respir Dis 137:726-741, 1988.
24. Yager JA, et al: Human ciliary beat frequency at three levels of the tracheobronchial tree. Am Rev Respir Dis 121:661-665, 1980.
25. Rutland J, et al: Human ciliary beat frequency in epithelium from intrathoracic and extrathoracic airways. Am Rev Respir Dis 125:100-105, 1982.
26. Clary-Meinesz C, et al: Ciliary beat frequency in human bronchi and bronchioles. Chest 111:692-697, 1997.
27. Sanderson MJ, et al: Mechanical stimulation and intercellular communication increase intracellular calcium in epithelial cells. Cell Regul 1:585-596, 1990.
28. Di Benedetto G, et al: Calcium regulation of ciliary beat frequency in human respiratory epithelium in vitro. J Physiol 493:103-113, 1991.
29. Girard PG, Kennedy JR: Calcium regulation of ciliary activity in rabbit tracheal explants and outgrowth. Eur J Cell Biol 40:203-209, 1986.
30. Clary-Meinesz CG, et al: Temperature effect on the ciliary beat frequency of human nasal and tracheal ciliated cells. Biol Cell 76:335-338, 1992.
31. Jain B, et al: Modulation of airway epithelial cell ciliary beat frequency by nitric oxide. Biochem Biophys Res Commun 191:83-88, 1993.
32. Lindberg S, et al: Regulation of mucociliary activity in the upper airways by nitric oxide: clinical implications. *In* Baum GL, et al (eds): Cilia, Mucus, and Mucociliary Interactions. New York, Marcel Dekker, 1998, pp 473-490.
33. Li D, et al: Regulation of ciliary beat frequency by the nitric oxide–cyclic guanosine monophosphate signaling pathway in rat airway epithelial cells. Am J Respir Cell Mol Biol 23:175-181, 2000.
34. Di Benedetto G, et al: Effect of cyclic AMP on ciliary activity of human respiratory epithelium. Eur Respir J 4:789-795, 1991.
35. Wanner A: Effects of methylxanthines on airway mucociliary function. Am J Med 79:16-21, 1985.
36. Ingels KJ, et al: Influence of sympathetic and parasympathetic substances in clinical concentrations on human nasal ciliary beat. Rhinology 30:149-159, 1992.
37. Jeffrey PK: The development of large and small airways. Am J Respir Crit Care Med 157:S174-S180, 1998.
38. Wong LB, Yeates DB: Luminal purinergic regulatory mechanisms of tracheal ciliary beat frequency. Am J Respir Cell Mol Biol 7:447-454, 1992.
39. Morse DM, et al: Differential effects of UTP, ATP, and adenosine on ciliary activity of human nasal epithelial cells. Am J Physiol Cell Physiol 280:C1485-C1497, 2001.
40. Lieb T, et al: Prolonged increase in ciliary beat frequency after short-term purinergic stimulation in human airway epithelial cells. J Physiol 538:633-646, 2002.
41. Knowles MR, Boucher RC: Mucus clearance as a primary innate defense mechanism for mammalian airways. J Clin Invest 109:571-577, 2002.
42. Devalia JL, et al: The effects of salmeterol and salbutamol on ciliary beat frequency of cultured human bronchial epithelial cells, in vitro. Pulmon Pharmacol 5:257-263, 1992.
43. Gaston B: Nitric oxide and thiol groups. Biochim Biophys Acta 1411:323-333, 1999.
44. Wanner A: Clinical aspects of mucociliary transport. Am Rev Respir Dis 116:73-125, 1977.
45. Read RC, et al: Effect of *Pseudomonas aeruginosa* rhamnolipids on mucociliary transport and ciliary beating. J Appl Physiol 72:2271-2277, 1992.
46. Adam EC, et al: *Pseudomonas aeruginosa* II. Lectin stops human ciliary beating: therapeutic implications of fucose. Am J Respir Crit Care Med 155:2102-2104, 1997.
47. Feldman C, et al: The interaction of *Streptococcus pneumoniae* with intact human respiratory mucosa in vitro. Eur Respir J 5:576-583, 1992.
48. Wilson R, et al: Interaction of *Haemophilus influenzae* with mucus, cilia, and respiratory epithelium. J Infect Dis 165:S100-S102, 1992.
49. Shemer-Avni Y, Liebermann D: *Chlamydia pneumoniae*-induced ciliostasis in ciliated bronchial epithelial cells. J Infect Dis 171:1274-1278, 1995.
50. Wilson R, et al: The effects of bacterial products on airway cells and their function. Am J Respir Crit Care Med 154:S197-S201, 1996.
51. Jackowski JT, et al: Effects of *P. aeruginosa*-derived bacterial products on tracheal ciliary function: role of O_2 radicals. Am J Physiol 260:L61-L67, 1991.
52. Kobayashi K, et al: Mechanism of hydrogen peroxide induced inhibition of sheep airway cilia. Am J Respir Cell Mol Biol 6:667-673, 1992.
53. Feldman C, et al: Roxithromycin, clarithromycin, and azithromycin attenuate the injurious effects of bioactive phospholipids on human respiratory epithelium in vitro. Inflammation 21:655-665, 1997.
54. Amitani R, et al: Effects of human neutrophil elastase and *Pseudomonas aeruginosa* pyocyanin on human ciliary beat in vitro. Infect Immun 61:2848-2853, 1993.

55. Jain B, et al: TNFα and IL-1β upregulate nitric oxide–dependent ciliary motility in bovine airway epithelium. Am J Physiol 268:L911-L917, 1995.
56. Wanner A, et al: Effects of chemical mediators of anaphylaxis on ciliary function. J Allerg Clin Immunol 72:663-667, 1983.
57. Hisamatsu K, et al: Platelet activating factor induced respiratory mucosal damage. Lipids 26:1287-1291, 1991.
58. Sleigh MA: Ciliary function in mucus transport. Chest 80:791-795, 1981.
59. Verdugo P: Hydration kinetics of exocytosed mucins in cultured secretory cells of the rabbit trachea: a new model. Ciba Found Symp 109:212-225, 1984.
60. Worlitzsch D, et al: Effects of reduced mucus oxygen concentration in airway Pseudomonas infections of cystic fibrosis patients. J Clin Invest 109:317-325, 2002.
61. Egan M: Ion flux and homeostasis in the lung. In Haddad GG, et al (eds): Basic Mechanisms of Pediatric Respiratory Disease. London, BC Decker, 2002, pp 285-293.
62. Matsui H, et al: Osmotic water permeabilies of cultured, well-differentiated normal and cystic fibrosis airway epithelia. J Clin Invest 105:1419-1427, 2000.
63. Phipps RJ, et al: Developmental changes in the tracheal mucociliary system in neonatal sheep. J Appl Physiol 67:824-832, 1989.
64. Welsh MJ: An apical-membrane chloride channel in human tracheal epithelium. Science 232:1648-1650, 1986.
65. Knowles MR, et al: Bioelectrical properties and ion flow across excised human bronchi. J Appl Physiol 56:868-877, 1984.
66. Harrison G, et al: Bronchiolitis induced by experimental acute and chronic oxygen intoxication in young adult rats. J Pathol 102:115-122, 1970.
67. Lamblin G, et al: Human respiratory mucins. Eur Respir J 5:247-256, 1992.
68. Bernacki SH, et al: Mucin gene expression during differentiation of human airway epithelium in vitro. Am J Respir Cell Mol Biol 20:595-604, 1999.
69. Verdugo P: Mucin exocytosis. Am Rev Respir Dis 144:S33-S37, 1991.
70. Leigh MW: Airway secretions. In Haddad GG, et al (eds): Basic Mechanisms of Pediatric Respiratory Disease. London, BC Decker, 2002, pp 472-488.
71. Lonphre M, et al: Allergen-induced IL-9 directly stimulates mucin transcription in respiratory epithelial cells. J Clin Invest 104:1375-1382, 1999.
72. Louahed J, et al: Interleukin-9 upregulates mucus expression in the airways. Am J Respir Cell Mol Biol 22:649-656, 2000.
73. Strous GJ, Dekker J: Mucin-type glycoproteins. Crit Rev Biochem Mol Biol 27:57-92, 1992.
74. Hubbard RC, et al: A preliminary study of aerosolized recombinant human deoxyribonuclease I in the treatment of cystic fibrosis. N Engl J Med 326:812-815, 1992.
75. Shak S, et al: Recombinant human DNase I reduces the viscosity of cystic fibrosis sputum. Proc Natl Acad Sci U S A 87:9188-9192, 1990.
76. Widdicombe JH, et al: Cystic fibrosis decreases the apical membrane chloride permeability of monolayers cultured from cells of tracheal epithelium. Proc Natl Acad Sci U S A 82:6167-6171, 1985.
77. Tam PY, Verdugo P: Control of mucus hydration as a Donnan equilibrium process. Nature 292:340-341, 1981.
78. Carlstedt I, Sheehan JK: Macromolecular properties and polymeric structure of mucus glycoproteins. Ciba Found Symp 109:157-172, 1984.
79. Worlitzsch D, et al: Effects of reduced mucus oxygen concentration in airway Pseudomonas infections of cystic fibrosis patients. J Clin Invest 109:317-325, 2002.
80. Yeates DB, et al: Mucociliary tracheal transport rates in man. J Appl Physiol 30:487-495, 1975.
81. Knowles MR, et al: Activation by extracellular nucleotides of chloride secretion in the airway epithelia of patients with cystic fibrosis. N Engl J Med 325:533-538, 1991.
82. Davis CW, et al: Goblet cell degranulation in isolated canine tracheal epithelium: response to exogenous ATP, ADP, and adenosine. Am J Physiol 262:C1313-C1323, 1992.
83. Moscoso GJ, et al: The morphology of ciliogenesis in the developing fetal human respiratory epithelium. Pathol Res Pract 183:403-411, 1988.
84. Moscoso GJ, et al: Ciliogenesis and ciliation of the respiratory epithelium in the human fetal cartilaginous trachea. Pathol Res Pract 184:161-167, 1989.
85. Bucher U, Reid L: Development of the mucus-secreting elements in human lung. Thorax 16:219-225, 1961.
86. Andersen, IB, et al: Human mucosal function under four controlled humidities. Am Rev Respir Dis 106:438-439, 1972.
87. Marfatia S, et al: Effect of dry and humidified gases on the respiratory epithelium in rabbits. J Pediatr Surg 10:583-592, 1975.
88. Pettersson B, et al: The inhibitory effect of tobacco smoke compound on ciliary activity. Eur J Respir Dis 66:89-92, 1985.
89. Boat TF: Studies of oxygen toxicity in cultured human neonatal respiratory epithelium. J Pediatr 95:916-919, 1979.
90. Adler KB, et al: Stimulatory effect of Pseudomonas aeruginosa on mucin secretion by the respiratory epithelium. JAMA 249:1615-1617, 1983.
91. Corrsen G, Allen CR: Acetylcholine: its significance in controlling ciliary activity of human respiratory epithelium in vitro. J Appl Physiol 14:901-904, 1959.
92. Tamaoki J, et al: Effect of cyclic AMP on ciliary function in rabbit tracheal epithelial cells. J Appl Physiol 66:1035-1039, 1989.
93. Al-Bazzaz FJ: Role of cyclic AMP in regulation of chloride secretion by canine tracheal mucosa. Am Rev Respir Dis 123:295-298, 1981.

94. Sutton PP, et al: The effect of oral aminophylline on lung mucociliary clearance in man. Chest 80:889-892, 1981.
95. Zariwala M, et al: Germline mutations in an intermediate chain dynein cause primary ciliary dyskinesia. Am J Respir Cell Mol Biol 25:577-583, 2001.
96. Barlocco EG, et al: Ultrastructural ciliary defects in children with recurrent infections of the lower respiratory tract. Pediatr Pulmonol 10:11-17, 1991.
97. Lungarella G, et al: Abnormalities of bronchial cilia in patients with chronic bronchitis: an ultrastructural and quantitative analysis. Lung 161:147-156, 1983.
98. Camner P, et al: Tracheobronchial clearance in patients with influenza. Am Rev Respir Dis 108:131-135, 1973.
99. Biberfeld C, et al: Ultrastructural features of Mycoplasma pneumoniae. J Bacteriol 102:855-861, 1970.
100. Wynne JW, et al: Tracheal mucosa damage after aspiration. Am Rev Respir Dis 124:728-732, 1981.
101. Giorgi PL, et al: Cilia in children with recurrent upper respiratory tract infections: ultrastructural observations. Pediatr Pulmonol 14:201-205, 1992.
102. Konradova V, et al: Ultrastructure of bronchial epithelium in children with chronic or recurrent respiratory diseases. Eur J Respir Dis 63:516-525, 1982.
103. Coles SJ, et al: Potent stimulation of glycoprotein secretion in canine trachea by substance P. J Appl Physiol 57:1323-1327, 1984.
104. Rogers DF, et al: Effects of tachykinins on mucus secretion of human bronchi in vitro. Eur J Pharmacol 174:283-286, 1989.
105. Al-Bazzaz FJ, et al: Substance P stimulation of chloride secretion by canine tracheal mucosa. Am Rev Respir Dis 131:86-89, 1985.
106. Lee RMKW, et al: Trypan blue method for the identification of areas of damage to airway epithelium due to mechanical trauma. SEM 3:1267-1271, 1984.
107. Clark RH, et al: Tracheal and bronchial injury in high-frequency oscillatory ventilation compared with conventional positive pressure ventilation. J Pediatr 111:114-118, 1987.
108. Lundgren R, et al: Respiratory mucosal damage after brush biopsy—an experimental study in rabbits. Eur J Respir Dis 64:9-23, 1983.
109. Bonikos DS, et al: Bronchopulmonary dysplasia: the pulmonary pathologic sequel of necrotizing bronchiolitis and pulmonary fibrosis. Hum Pathol 7:643-666, 1976.
110. Lee RMKW, O'Brodovich H: Airway epithelial damage in premature infants with respiratory failure. Am Rev Respir Dis 136:445-447, 1987.
111. Stevenson RD, Allaire JH: The development of normal feeding and swallowing. Pediatr Clin North Am 38:1439-1453, 1991.
112. Koenig JS: Coordination of breathing, sucking and swallowing during bottle feedings in human infants. J Appl Physiol 69:1623-1629, 1990.
113. Wilson SL, et al: Coordination of breathing and swallowing in human infants. J Appl Physiol 50:851-858, 1981.
114. Miller AJ: Deglutition. Physiol Rev 62:129-184, 1982.
115. Thach BT, Menon A: Pulmonary protective mechanisms in human infants. Am Rev Respir Dis 131:S55-S58, 1985.
116. Menon AP, et al: Airway protective and abdominal expulsive mechanisms in infantile regurgitation. J Appl Physiol 59:716-721, 1985.
117. Mizuno K, Ueda A: The maturation and coordination of sucking, swallowing, and respiration in preterm infants. J Pediatr 142:36-40, 2003.
118. Miller HC, et al: Variations in the gag, cough and swallow reflexes and tone of the vocal cords as determined by direct laryngoscopy in newborn infants. Yale J Biol Med 24:284-291, 1952.
119. Bartlett D: Ventilatory and protective mechanisms of the infant larynx. Am Rev Respir Dis 131:S49-S50, 1985.
120. Perkett EA, Vaughan RL: Evidence for a laryngeal chemoreflex in some human preterm infants. Acta Paediatr Scand 71:969-972, 1982.
121. Leith DE: The development of cough. Am Rev Respir Dis 131:S39-S42, 1985.
122. Wanner A, et al: Mucus clearance: cilia and cough. In Chernick V, Mellins RB (eds): Basic Mechanisms of Pediatric Respiratory Disease: Cellular and Integrative. Philadelphia, BC Decker, 1991, pp 361-382.
123. Leith DE: Cough. In Brain JD, et al (eds): Respiratory defense mechanisms. New York, Marcel Dekker, 1977, pp 545-592.
124. Kim CS, et al: Criteria for mucus transport in the airways by two-phase gas-liquid flow mechanism. J Appl Physiol 60:901-907, 1986.
125. Mautone AJ, Cataletto MB: Mechanical defense mechanisms of the lung. In Scarpelli EM (ed): Pulmonary Physiology of the Fetus, Newborn, Child, and Adolescent. Philadelphia, Lea & Febiger, 1990, pp 192-214.
126. Irwin RS, et al: Managing cough as a defensive mechanism and as a symptom: a consensus panel report of the American College of Chest Physicians. Chest 114:133-181S, 1998.
127. Chang AB, et al: Airway hyperresponsiveness and cough receptor sensitivity in children with recurrent cough. Am J Respir Crit Care Med 155:1935-1939, 1997.
128. Widdicombe JG: Sensory neurophysiology of the cough reflex. J Allergy Clin Immunol 98:84-90, 1996.
129. Bolser DC, et al: Responses of putative nucleus tractus solitarius interneurons in cough reflex pathways during laryngeal and tracheobronchial cough. FASEB J 14:A644, 2000.
130. Fleming PJ, et al: Functional immaturity of pulmonary irritant receptors and apnea in newborn preterm infants. Pediatrics 61:515-518, 1978.
131. Mathew OP, et al: Development of upper airway reflexes. In Chernick V, Mellins RB (eds): Basic Mechanisms of Pediatric Respiratory Disease: Cellular and Integrative. Philadelphia, BC Decker, 1991, pp 55-71.

132. Hoffman JA, et al: Phylogenetic perspectives in innate immunity. Science 284:1313-1318, 1999.

133. Cooper NR: Biology of the complement system. *In* Gallin JI, Snyderman R (eds): Inflammation: Basic Principles and Clinical Correlates. Philadelphia, Lippincott Williams & Wilkins, 1999, pp 281-315.

134. Prodinger WM, et al: Complement. *In* Paul WE (ed): Fundamental Immunology. Philadelphia, Lippincott-Raven, 1999, pp 967-995.

135. Turner MW: Mannose-binding lectin: the pluripotent molecule of the innate. Immunol Today 17:532-540, 1996.

136. Thiel S, et al: The concentration of the C-type lectin, mannan-binding protein, in human plasma increases during an acute phase response. Clin Exp Immunol 90:31-35, 1992.

137. Fraser IP, et al: The serum mannose-binding protein and the macrophage mannose receptor are pattern recognition molecules that link innate and adaptive immunity. Semin Immunol 10:363-372, 1998.

138. Matsushita M, Fujita T: Activation of the classical complement pathway by mannose-binding protein in association with a novel C1s-like serine protease. J Exp Med 176:1497-1502, 1992.

139. Thiel S, Vorup-Jensen T, Stover CM, et al: A second serine protease associated with mannan-binding lectin that activates complement. Nature 386:506-510, 1997.

140. Cooper NR, Morrison DC: Binding and activation of the first component of human complement by lipid A region of lipopolysaccharides. J Immunol 120:1862-1868, 1978.

141. Morrison DC, Kline LF: Activation of the classical and properdin pathways of complement by bacterial lipopolysaccharides (LPS). J Immunol 118:362-368, 1977.

142. Fearon DT, Austen KF: The alternative pathway of complement: a system for host resistance to microbial infection. N Engl J Med 303:259-263, 1980.

143. Lassiter HA, et al: Complement factor 9 deficiency in serum of human neonates. J Infect Dis 166:53-57, 1992.

144. Zach TL, Hostetter MK: Biochemical abnormalities of the third component of complement in neonates. Pediatr Res 26:116-120, 1989.

145. Johnston RB, et al: Complement in the newborn infant. Pediatrics 64:781-786, 1979.

146. Davis CA, et al: Serum complement levels in infancy: age-related changes. Pediatr Res 13:1043-1046, 1979.

147. Lau YL, et al: Mannose-binding protein in preterm infants: developmental profile and clinical significance. Clin Exp Immunol 102:649-654, 1995.

148. Cole FS, et al: Complement biosynthesis by human bronchoalveolar macrophages. Clin Immunol Immunopathol 27:153-159, 1983.

149. Al-Adnani MS, McGee JO: C1q production and secretion by fibroblasts. Nature 263:145-146, 1976.

150. Strunk RC, et al: Pulmonary alveolar type II epithelial cells synthesize and secrete proteins of the classical and alternative complement pathways. J Clin Invest 81:1419-1426, 1988.

151. Gross GN, et al: The effect of complement depletion on lung clearance of bacteria. J Clin Invest 62:373-378, 1978.

152. Toews, GB, Vial WC: The role of C5 in neutrophil recruitment in response to Streptococcus pneumoniae. Am Rev Respir Dis 129:82-86, 1984.

153. Hopken UE, et al: The C5a chemoattractant receptor mediates mucosal defence to infection. Nature 383:86-89, 1996.

154. Limper AH, Roman J: Fibronectin: a versatile matrix protein with roles in thoracic development, repair, and infection. Chest 101:1663-1673, 1992.

155. Villiger B, et al: Human alveolar macrophage fibronectin: synthesis, secretion, and ultrastructural localization during gelatin-coated latex particle binding. J Cell Biol 90:711-720, 1981.

156. Barnard DR, et al: Fibronectin (cold insoluble globulin) in the neonate. J Pediatr 102:453-455, 1983.

157. Dyke MP, Forsyth KD: Plasma fibronectin levels in extremely preterm infants in the first 8 weeks of life. J Paediatr Child Health 30:36-39, 1994.

158. Gerdes JS, et al: Tracheal lavage and plasma fibronectin: relationship to respiratory distress syndrome and development of bronchopulmonary dysplasia. J Pediatr 108:601-606, 1986.

159. Adachi K, et al: Evaluation of fibronectin gene expression by in situ hybridization. Am J Pathol 133:193-203, 1988.

160. Kuusela P: Fibronectin binds to Staphylococcus aureus. Nature 276:718-720, 1978.

161. Speziale P, et al: Fibronectin binding to a Streptococcus pyogenes strain. J Bacteriol 103:34-43, 1984.

162. Abraham SN, et al: Adherence of Streptococcus pyogenes, Escherichia coli, and Pseudomonas aeruginosa to fibronectin coated and uncoated epithelial cells. Infect Immun 41:1261-1268, 1983.

163. Ratliff TL, et al: Attachment of mycobacteria to fibronectin-coated surfaces. J Gen Microbiol 134:1307-1313, 1988.

164. Pottratz ST, Martin WJ: Mechanism of Pneumocystis carinii attachment to cultured rat alveolar macrophages. J Clin Invest 86:1678-1683, 1990.

165. Negre E, et al: The collagen binding domain of fibronectin contains a high affinity binding site for Candida albicans. J Biol Chem 269:22039-22045, 1994.

166. Proctor RA, et al: Fibronectin mediates attachment of Staphylococcus aureus to human neutrophils. Blood 59:681-687, 1982.

167. Eriksen HO, et al: Opsonic activity of fibronectin in the phagocytosis of Staphylococcus aureus by polymorphonuclear leukocytes. Eur J Clin Microbiol 3:108-112, 1989.

168. Finkelstein RA, et al: Role of iron in microbe-host interactions. Rev Infect Dis 5:759-777, 1983.

169. Bell DY, et al: Plasma proteins of the bronchoalveolar surface of the lungs of smokers and non-smokers. Am Rev Respir Dis 124:72-79, 1981.

170. Campagnari AA, et al: Growth of Moraxella catarrhalis with human transferrin and lactoferrin: expression of iron-repressible proteins without siderophore production. Infect Immun 62:4909-4914, 1994.

171. Arnold RR, et al: Bactericidal activity of human lactoferrin: sensitivity of a variety of microorganisms. Infect Immun 28:893-898, 1980.

172. Bortner CA, et al: Bactericidal effect of lactoferrin on Legionella pneumophila. Infect Immun 51:373-377, 1986.

173. Singh PK, et al: Synergistic and additive killing by antimicrobial factors found in human airway surface liquid. Am J Physiol Lung Cell Mol Physiol 279:L799-805, 2000.

174. Swart PJ, et al: Lactoferrin: antiviral activity of lactoferrin. Adv Exp Med Biol 443:205-213, 1998.

175. Ulvatne H, Vorland LH: Bactericidal kinetics of 3 lactoferricins against Staphylococcus aureus and Escherichia coli. Scand J Infect Dis 33:507-511, 2001.

176. Prince AS: Biofilms, antimicrobial resistance, and airway infection. N Engl J Med 347:1110-1111, 2002.

177. Singh PK, et al: A component of innate immunity prevents bacterial biofilm development. Nature 417:552-555, 2002.

178. Elass-Rochard E, et al: Lactoferrin inhibits the endotoxin interaction with CD14 by competition with the lipopolysaccharide binding protein. Infect Immun 66:486-491, 1998.

179. Britigan BE, et al: Lactoferrin binds CpG-containing oligonucleotides and inhibits their immunostimulatory effects on human B cells. J Immunol 167:2921-2928, 2001.

180. Lehrer RI, et al: Interaction of human defensins with Escherichia coli: mechanism of bactericidal activity. J Clin Invest 84:553-561, 1989.

181. Greenwald GI, Ganz T: Defensins mediate the microbicidal activity of human neutrophil granule extract against Acinetobacter calcoacetius. Infect Immun 55:1365-1368, 1987.

182. Daher KA, et al: Direct inactivation of viruses by human granulocyte defensins. J Virol 54:1068-1074, 1985.

183. Travis SM, et al: Antimicrobial peptides and proteins in the innate defense of the airway surface. Curr Opin Immunol 13:89-95, 2001.

184. Ganz T: Defensins and host defense. Science 286:420-421, 1999.

185. Zasloff M: Antimicrobial peptides of multicellular organisms. Nature 415:389-395, 2002.

186. Kagan BL, et al: Antimicrobial defensin peptides form voltage-dependent ion-permeable channels in planar lipid bilayer membranes. Proc Natl Acad Sci U S A 87:210-214, 1990.

187. Lichtenstein AK: Mechanism of mammalian cell lysis mediated by peptide defensins: evidence for an initial alteration of the plasma membrane. J Clin Invest 88:93-100, 1991.

188. Matsuzaki K: Why and how are peptide-lipid interactions utilized for self-defense? Magainins and tachyplesins as archetypes. Biochim Biophys Acta 1462:1-10, 1999.

189. Huttner KM, Bevins CL: Antimicrobial peptides as mediators of epithelial host defense. Pediatr Res 45:785-794, 1999.

190. Ganz T: Antimicrobial peptides in host defense of the respiratory tract. J Clin Invest 109:693-697, 2002.

191. Harwig SS, et al: Neutrophil defensins: purification, characterization, and antimicrobial testing. Methods Enzymol 236:160-172, 1994.

192. Agerberth B, et al: The human antimicrobial and chemotactic peptides LL-37 and α-defensins are expressed by specific lymphocyte and monocyte populations. Blood 96:3086-3093, 2000.

193. Lehrer RI, et al: Defensins: antimicrobial and cytotoxic peptides of mammalian cells. Annu Rev Immunol 11:105-128, 1993.

194. Lehrer RI, et al: Modulation of the in vitro candidacidal activity of human neutrophil defensins by target cell metabolism and divalent cations. J Clin Invest 81:1829-1835, 1988.

195. Panyutich AV, et al: Human neutrophil defensin and serpins form complexes and inactivate each other. Am J Respir Cell Mol Biol 12:351-357, 1995.

196. van den Berg R, et al: Inhibition of the classical pathway of complement by human neutrophil defensins. Blood 92:3898-3903, 1998.

197. Murphy CJ, et al: Defensins are mitogenic for epithelial cells and fibroblasts. J Cell Physiol 155:408-413, 1993.

198. Panyutich A, Ganz T: Activated alpha 2-macroglobulin is a principal defensin-binding protein. Am J Respir Cell Mol Biol 5:101-106, 1991.

199. Zhang P, et al: Innate immunity and pulmonary host defense. Immunol Rev 173:39-51, 2000.

200. Schnapp D, Harris A: Antibacterial peptides in bronchoalveolar lavage fluid. Am J Respir Cell Mol Biol 19:352-356, 1998.

201. Schutte BC, et al: Discovery of five conserved beta-defensin gene clusters using a computational search strategy. Proc Natl Acad Sci U S A 99:2129-2133, 2002.

202. Harder J, et al: Isolation and characterization of human beta-defensin-3, a novel human inducible peptide antibiotic. J Biol Chem 276:5707-5713, 2001.

203. Zhao C, et al: Widespread expression of beta-defensin hBD-1 in human secretory glands and epithelial cells. FEBS Lett 396:319-322, 1996.

204. Singh PK, et al: Production of human beta-defensins by human airway epithelial cells. Proc Natl Acad Sci U S A 95:14961-14966, 1998.

205. Harder J, et al: Mucoid *Pseudomonas aeruginosa,* TNF-α, and IL-1β, but not IL-6, induce human β-defensin-2 in respiratory epithelia. Am J Respir Cell Mol Biol 22:714-721, 2000.

206. Becker MN, et al: CD14 dependent LPS-induced β-defensin-2 expression in human tracheobronchial epithelium. J Biol Chem 275:29731-29736, 2000.

207. Yang D, et al: β-Defensins: linking innate and adaptive immunity through dendritic and T cell CCR6. Science 286:525-528, 1999.

208. Schaller-Bals S, et al: Increased levels of antimicrobial peptides in tracheal aspirates of newborn infants during infection. Am J Respir Crit Care Med 165:992-995, 2002.

209. Zasloff M: Antimicrobial peptides in health and disease. N Engl J Med 347:1199-1200, 2002.

210. Zanetti M, et al: Cathelicidins: a novel protein family with a common proregion and variable C-terminal antimicrobial domain. FEBS Lett 374:1-5, 1995.

211. Sorensen OE, et al: Human cathelicidin, hCAP-18, is processed to the antimicrobial peptide LL-37 by extracellular cleavage with proteinase 3. Blood 97:3951-3959, 2001.

212. Zasloff M: Innate immunity, antimicrobial peptides, and protection of the oral cavity. Lancet 360:1116-1117, 2002.

213. Bals R, et al: The peptide antibiotic LL-37/hCAP-18 is expressed in epithelia of the human lung where it has broad antimicrobial activity at the airway surface. Proc Natl Acad Sci U S A 95:9541-9546, 1998.

214. Larrick JW, et al: Human CAP18: a novel antimicrobial lipopolysaccharide-binding protein. Infect Immun 63:1291-1297, 1995.

215. Yang D, et al: LL-37, the neutrophil granule- and epithelial cell-derived cathelicidin, utilizes formyl peptide receptor-like 1 (FRPL1) as a receptor to chemoattract human peripheral blood neutrophils, monocytes, and T cells. J Exp Med 192:1069-1074, 2000.

216. Johansson J, et al: Conformation-dependent antibacterial activity of the naturally occurring human peptide LL-37. J Biol Chem 273:3718-3724, 1998.

217. Dohrman A, et al: Distribution of lysozyme and mucin (MUC2 and MUC3) mRNA in human bronchus. Exp Lung Res 20:367-380, 1994.

218. Spitznagel JK: Nonoxidative antimicrobial actions of leukocytes. *In* Snyderman R (ed): Contemporary Topics in Immunobiology: Regulation of Leukocyte Function. New York, Plenum Press, 1984, pp 283-343.

219. Wilson L, Spitznagel JK: Molecular and structural damage to *Escherichia coli* produced by antibody, complement, and lysozyme systems. J Bacteriol 96:1339-1348, 1968.

220. Miller TE: Killing and lysis of gram-negative bacteria through the synergistic effect of hydrogen peroxide, ascorbic acid and lysozyme. J Bacteriol 98:949-955, 1969.

221. Laible NG, Germaine GR: Bactericidal activity of human lysozyme, muramidase-inactive lysozyme, and cationic polypeptides against *Streptococcus sanguis* and *Streptococcus faecalis:* inhibition by chitin oligosaccharides. Infect Immun 48:720-728, 1985.

222. Marquis G, et al: Fungitoxicity of muramidase, ultrastructural damage to *Candida albicans.* Lab Invest 46:627-636, 1982.

223. Togbi RS, et al: in vitro susceptibility of *Candida* species to lysozyme. Oral Microbiol Immunol 3:35735-35739, 1988.

224. Akinbi HT, et al: Bacterial killing is enhanced by expression of lysozyme in the lungs of transgenic mice. J Immunol 165:5760-5766, 2000.

225. Bals R, et al: Human β-defensin 2 is a salt-sensitve peptide antibiotic expressed in human lung. J Clin Invest 102:874-880, 1998.

226. Singh PK, et al: Synergistic and additive killing by antimicrobial factors found in human airway surface liquid. Am J Physiol Lung Cell Mol Physiol 279:L799-805, 2000.

227. Schumann RR, et al: Structure and function of lipopolysaccharide binding protein. Science 249:1429-1431, 1990.

228. Ulevitch RJ: Regulation of cellular responses to bacterial endotoxin. *In* Marshall JC, Cohen J (eds): Immune Response in the Critically Ill. New York, Springer, 1999, pp 173-181.

229. Martin TR: Recognition of bacterial endotoxin in the lungs. Am J Respir Cell Mol Biol 23:128-132, 2000.

230. Martin TR, et al: Relationship between soluble CD14, lipopolysaccharide binding protein, and the alveolar inflammatory response in patients with acute respiratory distress syndrome. Am J Respir Crit Care Med 155:937-944, 1997.

231. Fan MH, et al: An essential role for lipopolysaccharide-binding protein in pulmonary innate immune responses. Shock 18:248-254, 2002.

232. Dentener MA, et al: Production of the acute phase protein lipopolysaccharide-binding protein by respiratory type II epithelial cells. Am J Respir Cell Mol Biol 23:146-153, 2000.

233. Lee PT, Holt PG, McWilliam AS: Role of alveolar macrophages in innate immunity in neonates; evidence for selective lipopolysaccharide binding protein production by rat neonatal alveolar macrophages. Am J Respir Cell Mol Biol 23:652-661, 2000.

234. Berner R, et al: Elevated levels of lipopolysaccharide-binding protein and soluble CD14 in plasma in neonatal early-onset sepsis. Clin Diagn Lab Immunol 9:440-445, 2002.

235. Crouch EC: Collectins and pulmonary host defense. Am J Respir Cell Mol Biol 19:177-201, 1998.

236. Brown-Augsburger P, et al: Biosynthesis of surfactant protein D: contributions of conserved NH$_2$-terminal cysteine residues and collagen helix formation to assembly and secretion. J Biol Chem 271:18912-18919, 1996.

237. Kishore U, et al: The alpha-helical neck region of human surfactant protein D is essential for the binding of the carbohydrate recognition domains to lipopolysaccharides and phospholipids. Biochem J 318:505-511, 1996.

238. Bufler P, et al: Surfactant protein A and D differently regulate the immune response to nonmucoid *Pseudomonas aeruginosa* and its lipopolysaccharide. Am J Respir Cell Mol Biol 28:249-256, 2003.

239. Lawson PR, Reid KBM: The roles of surfactant proteins A and D in innate immunity. Immunol Rev 173:66-78, 2000.

240. McCormick SM, Mendelson CR: Human SP-A1 and SP-A2 genes are differentially regulated during development and by cAMP and glucocorticoids. Am J Physiol 266:L367-374, 1994.

241. Dulkerian SJ, et al: Regulation of surfactant protein D in human fetal lung. Am J Respir Cell Mol Biol 15:781-786, 1996.

242. Viviano CJ, et al: Altered regulation of surfactant phospholipids and protein A during acute pulmonary inflammation. Biochim Biophys Acta 1259:235-244, 1995.

243. McIntosh JC, et al: Surfactant proteins A and D increase in response to intratracheal lipopolysaccharide. Am J Respir Cell Mol Biol 15:509-519, 1996.

244. Hartshorn KL, et al: Mechanisms of anti-influenza activity of surfactant proteins A and D: comparison with serum collectins. Am J Physiol 273:L1156-L1166, 1997.

245. Kabha K, et al: SP-A enhances phagocytosis of *Klebsiella* by interaction with capsular polysaccharides and alveolar macrophages. Am J Physiol 272:L344-L352, 1997.

246. Madan T, et al: Binding of pulmonary surfactant proteins A and D to *Aspergillus fumigatus* conidia enhances phagocytosis and killing by human neutrophils and alveolar macrophages. Infect Immun 65:3171-3179, 1997.

247. Wright JR: Immunomodulatory functions of surfactant. Physiol Rev 77:931-962, 1997.

248. Borron PJ, et al: Pulmonary surfactant proteins A and D directly suppress CD3+/CD4+ cell function: evidence for two shared mechanisms. J Immunol 169:5844-5850, 2002.

249. Honda Y, et al: Decreased contents of surfactant proteins A and D in BAL fluids of healthy smokers. Chest 109:1006-1009, 1996.

250. Crouch E, et al: Genomic organization of human surfactant protein D (SP-D). SP-D is encoded on chromosome 10q22.2-23.1. J Biol Chem 268:2976-2983, 1993.

251. Brown-Augsburger P, et al: Site-directed mutagenesis of Cys-15 and Cys-20 of pulmonary surfactant protein D. J Biol Chem 271:13724-13730, 1996.

252. Persson A, et al: Surfactant protein D is a divalent cation-dependent carbohydrate-binding protein. J Biol Chem 265:5755-5760, 1990.

253. Lim BL, et al: Expression of the carbohydrate recognition domain of lung surfactant protein D and demonstration of its binding to lipopolysaccharides of Gram-negative bacteria. Biochem Biophys Res Commun 202:1674-1680, 1994.

254. O'Riordan DM, et al: Surfactant protein D interacts with *Pneumocystis carinii* and mediates organism adherence to alveolar macrophages. J Clin Invest 95:2699-2710, 1995.

255. Holmskov U, et al: Isolation and characterization of a new member of the scavenger receptor superfamily, glycoprotein-340 (gp-340), as a lung surfactant protein-D binding molecule. J Biol Chem 272:13743-13749, 1997.

256. Sano H, et al: Surfactant proteins A and D bind CD14 by different mechanisms. J Biol Chem 275:22442-22451, 2000.

257. Botas C, et al: Altered surfactant homeostasis and alveolar type II cell morphology in mice lacking surfactant protein D. Proc Natl Acad Sci U S A 95:11869-11874, 1998.

258. Wert SE, et al: Increased metalloproteinase activity, oxidant production, and emphysema in surfactant protein D gene-inactivated mice. Proc Natl Acad Sci U S A 97:5972-5977, 2000.

259. LeVine AM, et al: Surfactant protein D enhances clearance of influenza A virus from the lung in vitro. J Immunol 167:5868-5873, 2001.

260. White RT, et al: Isolation and characterization of the human pulmonary surfactant apoprotein gene. Nature 317:361-363, 1985.

261. Floros J, et al: Human SP-A locus: allele frequencies and linkage disequilibrium between the two surfactant protein A genes. Am J Respir Cell Mol Biol 15:489-498, 1996.

262. Voss T, et al: Structural comparison of recombinant pulmonary surfactant protein SP-A derived from two human coding sequences: implications for the chain composition of natural human SP-A. Am J Respir Cell Mol Biol 4:88-94, 1991.

263. Ballard PL, et al: Interferon-gamma and synthesis of surfactant components by cultured human fetal lung. Am J Respir Cell Mol Biol 2:137-143, 1990.

264. Van Iwaarden JF, et al: Binding of surfactant protein A to the lipid A moiety of bacterial lipopolysaccharides. Biochem J 303:407-411, 1994.

265. Geertsma MF, et al: Binding of surfactant protein A to C1q receptors mediates phagocytosis of *Staphylococcus aureus* by monocytes. Am J Physiol 267:L578-584, 1994.

266. Tino MJ, Wright JR: Surfactant protein A stimulates phagocytosis of specific pulmonary pathogens by alveolar macrophages. Am J Physiol 270:L677-688, 1996.

267. Gaynor CD, et al: Pulmonary surfactant protein A mediates enhanced phagocytosis of *Mycobacterium tuberculosis* by a direct interaction with human macrophages. J Immunol 155:5343-5351, 1995.

268. Hickman-Davis J, et al: Surfactant protein A mediates mycoplasmacidal activity of alveolar macrophages by production of peroxynitrite. Proc Natl Acad Sci U S A 96:4953-4958, 1999.

269. Maholtra R, et al: Interaction of C1q receptor with lung surfactant protein A. Eur J Immunol 22:1437-1445, 1992.

270. Chroneos ZC, et al: Purification of a cell-surface receptor for surfactant protein A. J Biol Chem 271:16375-16383, 1996.

271. Chroneos Z, Shepherd VL: Differential regulation of the mannose and SP-A receptors on macrophages. Am J Physiol 269:L721-726, 1995.

272. Wright JR, et al: Surfactant protein A. Regulation of innate and adaptive immune responses in lung inflammation. Am J Respir Cell Mol Biol 24:513-517, 2001.

273. Stamme C, et al: Surfactant protein A inhibits lipopolysaccharide-induced immune cell activation by preventing the interaction of lipopolysaccharide with lipopolysaccharide-binding protein. Am J Respir Cell Mol Biol 27:353-360, 2002.

274. Borron P, et al: Surfactant-associated protein A inhibits LPS-induced cytokine and nitric oxide production in vitro. Am J Physiol Lung Cell Mol Physiol 278:L840-847, 2000.

275. Hickman-Davis JM, et al: Lung surfactant and reactive oxygen-nitrogen species: antimicrobial activity and host-pathogen interactions. Am J Physiol Lung Cell Mol Physiol 281:L517-523, 2001.

276. Stamme C, et al: Surfactant protein A differentially regulates IFN-gamma- and LPS-induced nitrite production by rat alveolar macrophages. Am J Respir Cell Mol Biol 23:772-779, 2000.

277. Weikert LF, et al: Surfactant protein A enhances mycobacterial killing by rat macrophages through a nitric oxide-dependent pathway. Am J Physiol Lung Cell Mol Physiol 279:L216-233, 2000.

278. Hartshorn K, et al: Interactions of recombinant human pulmonary surfactant protein D and SP-D multimers with influenza A. Am J Physiol 271:L753-762, 1996.

279. Crouch E, et al: Collectins and pulmonary innate immunity. Immunol Rev 173:52-65, 2000.

280. Benne CA, et al: Surfactant protein A, but not surfactant protein D, is an opsonin for influenza A virus phagocytosis by rat alveolar macrophages. Eur J Immunol 27:886-890, 1997.

281. O'Neill S, et al: Rat lung lavage surfactant enhances bacterial phagocytosis and intracellular killing by alveolar macrophages. Am Rev Respir Dis 130:225-230, 1984.

282. Geertsma MF, et al: Lung surfactant suppresses oxygen-dependent bactericidal functions of human blood monocytes by inhibiting the assembly of the NADPH oxidase. J Immunol 150:2391-2400, 1993.

283. Juers JA, et al: Enhancement of bactericidal capacity of alveolar macrophages by human alveolar lining material. J Clin Invest 58:271-275, 1976.

284. Hayakawa H, et al: Pulmonary surfactant inhibits priming of rabbit alveolar macrophages. Am Rev Respir Dis 140:1390-1397, 1989.

285. LaForce FM, et al: Inactivation of staphylococci by alveolar macrophages with preliminary observations on the importance of alveolar lining material. Am Rev Respir Dis 108:784-790, 1973.

286. Coonrad JD, et al: Effect of rat surfactant lipids on complement and Fc receptors of macrophages. Infec Immun 54:371-378, 1986.

287. Zeligs BJ, Nerurkar LS, Bellanti JA: Chemotactic and candicidal responses of rabbit alveolar macrophage during postnatal development and the modulating roles of surfactant in these responses. Infect Immun 44:379-385, 1984.

288. Catanzaro A, et al: Immunomodulation by pulmonary surfactant. J Lab Clin Med 112:727-734, 1988.

289. Sitrin RG, Ansfield MJ, Kaltreider HB: The effect of pulmonary surface-active material on the generation and expression of murine B and T lymphocyte effector functions in vitro. Exp Lung Res 85:85-97, 1985.

290. Wilsher ML, et al: Immunoregulatory properties of pulmonary surfactant: influence of variations in the phospholipids profile. Clin Exp Immunol 73:117-122, 1988.

291. Kremlev SG, Umstead TM, Phelps DS: Effects of surfactant protein A and surfactant lipids on lymphocyte proliferation in vitro. Am J Physiol 267:L357-364, 1994.

292. Allen JN, et al: Immunosuppressive properties of surfactant and plasma on alveolar macrophages. J Lab Clin Med 125:356-369, 1995.

293. Antal JM, et al: Surfactant suppresses NF-kappa B activation in human monocytic cells. Am J Respir Cell Mol Biol 14:374-379, 1996.

294. Roth MD, et al: Pulmonary surfactant inhibits interleukin-2-induced proliferation and the generation of lymphokine-activated killer cells. Am J Respir Cell Mol Biol 9:652-658, 1993.

295. Nathan C: Nitric oxide as a secretory product of mammalian cells. FASEB J 6:3051-3064, 1991.

296. Hibbs JB, et al: Nitric oxide: a cytotoxic activated macrophage effector molecule. Biochem Biophys Res Commun 157:87-94, 1988.

297. Shaul PW, et al: Endothelial nitric oxide synthase is expressed in cultured human bronchiolar epithelium. J Clin Invest 94:2231-2236, 1994.

298. Asano K, et al: Constitutive and inducible nitric oxide synthase gene expression, regulation and activity in human lung regulation. Proc Natl Acad Sci U S A 91:10089-10093, 1994.

299. Kobzik L, et al: Nitric oxide synthase in human and rat lung: immunocytochemical and histochemical localization. Am J Respir Cell Mol Biol 9:371-377, 1993.

300. Fang FC: Mechanisms of nitric oxide-related antimicrobial activity. J Clin Invest 99:2818-2825, 1997.

301. Gao JJ, et al: Bacterial DNA and LPS act in synergy in inducing nitric oxide production in RAW 264.7 macrophages. J Immunol 163:4095-4099, 1999.

302. Robbins RA, et al: Inducible nitric oxide synthase is increased in murine lung epithelial cells by cytokine stimulation. Biochem Biophys Res Commun 198:835-843, 1994.

303. Nakayama DK, et al: Cytokines and lipopolysaccharide induce nitric oxide synthase in cultured rat pulmonary artery smooth muscle. Am J Respir Cell Mol Biol 7:471-476, 1992.

304. Morris SL, et al: Identification and characterization of some bacterial membrane sulfhydryl groups which are targets of bacteriostatic and antibiotic action. J Biol Chem 259:13590-13594, 1984.

305. Kaplan SS, et al: Effect of nitric oxide on staphylococcal killing and interactive effect with superoxide. Infect Immun 64:69-76, 1996.

306. Kharitonov SA, Barnes PJ: Exhaled markers of pulmonary disease. Am J Respir Crit Care Med 163:1693-1722, 2001.

307. Saura M, et al: An antiviral mechanism of nitric oxide: inhibition of a viral protease. Immunity 10:21-28, 1999.

308. Fukushima T, et al: Viral respiratory infection increases alveolar macrophage cytoplasmic motility in rats: role of nitric oxide. Am J Physiol 268:L399-L406, 1995.

309. Tsai WC, et al: Nitric oxide is required for effective innate immunity against Klebsiella pneumoniae. Infect Immun 65:1870-1875, 1997.

310. Zhu L, et al: Bactericidal activity of peroxynitrite. Arch Biochem Biophys 298:452-457, 1992.

311. Pacelli R, et al: Nitric oxide potentiates hydrogen peroxide-induced killing of Escherichia coli. J Exp Med 182:1469-1479, 1995.

312. Vazquez-Torres A, et al: Peroxynitrite contributes to the candidacidal activity of nitric oxide-producing macrophages. Infect Immun 64:3127-3133, 1996.

313. MacMicking JD, et al: Identification of NOS2 as a protective locus against tuberculosis. Proc Natl Acad Sci U S A 94:5243-5248, 1997.

314. Gaston B, et al: Endogenous nitrogen oxides and bronchodilator S-nitrosothiols in human airway. Proc Natl Acad Sci U S A 90:10957-10961, 1993.

315. Compeau CG, et al: Endotoxin-stimulated alveolar macrophages impair lung epithelial Na+ transport by an L-Arg-dependent mechanism. Am J Physiol 266:C1330-C1341, 1994.

316. Asano K, et al: Constitutive and inducible nitric oxide synthase gene expression, regulation, and activity in human lung epithelial cells. Proc Natl Acad Sci U S A 91:10089-10093, 1994.

317. Nicholson S, et al: Inducible nitric oxide synthase in pulmonary alveolar macrophages from patients with tuberculosis. J Exp Med 183:2293-2302, 1996.

318. Grasemann H, et al: Metabolites of nitric oxide in the lower respiratory tract of children. Eur J Pediatr 156:575-578, 1997.

319. Murphy AW, et al: Respiratory nitric oxide levels in experimental human influenza. Chest 114:452-456, 1998.

320. Kharitonov SA, et al: Increased nitric oxide in exhaled air of normal human subjects with upper respiratory infections. Eur Respir J 8:295-297, 1995.

321. Hickman-Davis J, et al: Surfactant protein A mediates mycoplasmacidal activity of alveolar macrophages. Am J Physiol Lung Cell Mol Physiol 274:L270-L277, 1998.

322. O'Brien L, et al: Strains of Mycobacterium tuberculosis differ in susceptibility to reactive nitrogen intermediates in vitro. Infect Immunol 62:5187-5190, 1994.

323. Gebran SF, et al: Inhibition of Legionella pneumophila growth by gamma interferon in permissive A/J mouse macrophages: role of reactive oxygen species, nitric oxide, tryptophan, and iron. Infect Immunol 62:3197-3205, 1994.

324. Aikio O, et al: Diminished inducible nitric oxide synthase expression in fulminant early-onset neonatal pneumonia. Pediatrics 105:1013-1019, 2000.

325. Bogdan C, et al: The role of nitric oxide in innate immunity. Immunol Rev 173:17-26, 2000.

326. Lander HM, et al: Nitric oxide signaling: a possible role for G proteins. J Immunol 151:7182-7187, 1993.

327. Adcock IM, et al: Oxidative stress induces NF-κB DNA binding and inducible NOS mRNA in human epithelial cells. Biochem Biophys Res Commun 199:1518-1524, 1994.

328. Lander HM, et al: Activation of human peripheral blood mononuclear cells by nitric oxide-generating compounds. J Immunol 150:1509-1516, 1993.

329. Thomassen MJ, et al: Nitric oxide inhibits inflammatory cytokine production by human alveolar macrophages. Am J Respir Cell Mol Biol 17:279-283, 1997.

330. Connelly L, et al: Biphasic regulation of NF-κB activity underlies the pro- and anti-inflammatory actions of nitric oxide. J Immunol 166:3873-3881, 2001.

331. Andersson JA, et al: Carbon monoxide is endogenously produced in the human nose and paranasal sinuses. J Allergy Clin Immunol 105:269-273, 2000.

332. Lakari E, et al: Expression and regulation of hemeoxygenase 1 in healthy human lung and interstitial lung disorders. Hum Pathol 32:1257-1263, 2001.

333. Otterbein LE, Choi AMK: Heme oxygenase: colors of defense against cellular stress. Am J Physiol Lung Cell Mol Physiol 279:L1029-L1037, 2000.

334. Lim S, et al: Expression of heme oxygenase isoenzymes 1 and 2 in normal and asthmatic airways: effect of inhaled corticosteroids. Am J Respir Crit Care Med 162:1912-1918, 2000.

335. Yasuda H, et al: Increased blood carboxyhemoglobin concentrations in inflammatory pulmonary diseases. Thorax 57:779-783, 2002.

336. Yamaya M, et al: Increased carbon monoxide in exhaled air of subjects with upper respiratory tract infections. Am J Respir Crit Care Med 158:311-314, 1998.

337. Otterbein LE, et al: Carbon monoxide has anti-inflammatory effects involving the mitogen-activated protein kinase pathway. Nat Med 6:422-428, 2000.

338. Hashiba T, et al: Adenovirus-mediated transfer of heme oxygenase-1 cDNA attenuates severe lung injury induced by the influenza virus in mice. Gene Ther 8:1499-1507, 2001.

339. Denery PA, et al: Oxygen toxicity and iron accumulation in the lungs of mice lacking heme oxygenase-2. J Clin Invest 101:1001-1011, 1998.

340. Dailly E, et al: Role of bilirubin in the regulation of the total peroxyl radical trapping antioxidant activity of plasma in sickle cell disease. Biochem Biophys Res Commun 248:303-306, 1998.

341. Ulevitch RJ, Tobias PS: Recognition of gram-negative bacteria and endotoxin by the innate immune system. Curr Opin Immunol 11:19-22, 1999.

342. Medzhitov R, et al: A human homologue of the *Drosophila* Toll protein signals activation of adaptive immunity. Nature 388:394-397, 1997.

343. Lien E, et al: Toll-like receptor 4 imparts ligand-specific recognition of bacterial lipopolysaccharide. J Clin Invest 105:497-504, 2000.

344. Takeuchi O, et al: Differential roles of TLR2 and TLR4 in recognition of gram-negative and gram-positive bacterial cell wall components. Immunity 11:443-451, 1999.

345. Underhill DM, et al: Toll-like receptor-2 mediates mycobacteria-induced proinflammatory signaling in macrophages. Proc Natl Acad Sci U S A 96:14459-14463, 1999.

346. Underhill DM, et al: The Toll-like receptor 2 is recruited to macrophage phagosomes and discriminates between pathogens. Nature 401:811-815, 1999.

347. Alexopoulou L, et al: Recognition of double-stranded RNA and activation of NF-κB by Toll-like receptor 3. Nature 413:732-738, 2001.

348. Bauer S, et al: Human TLR9 confers responsiveness to bacterial DNA via species-specific CpG motif recognition. Proc Natl Acad Sci U S A 98:9237-9242, 2001.

349. Dubois RM: The alveolar macrophage. Thorax 40:321-327, 1986.

350. Sorokin SP, et al: Development of cellular host defense mechanisms. *In* Gaultier C, et al (eds): Lung Development. New York, Oxford University Press, 1999, pp 221-254.

351. Sorokin SP, et al: Macrophage development: III. Transformation of pulmonary macrophages from precursors in fetal lungs and their later maturation in organ culture. Anat Rec 232:415-428, 1992.

352. Sorokin SP, et al: Factors influencing fetal macrophage development: III. Immmunocytochemical localization of cytokines and time-resolved expression of differentiation markers in organ-cultured rat lungs. Anat Rec 248:93-103, 1997.

353. Bitterman PB, et al: Alveolar macrophage replication: one mechanism for the expansion of the mononuclear phagocyte population in the chronically inflamed lung. J Clin Invest 74:460-469, 1984.

354. Blusse van Oud Ablas A, van Furth R: Origin, kinetics and characteristics of pulmonary macrophages in the normal steady state. J Exp Med 149:1504-1518, 1979.

355. Warren JS, et al: Comparative superoxide responses of lung macrophages and blood phagocytic cells in the rat: possible relevance to IgA immune complex induced lung injury. Lab Invest 57:311-320, 1987.

356. Nicod LP, et al: Mononuclear cells in human lung parenchyma: characterization of a potent accessory cell not obtained by bronchoalveolar lavage. Am Rev Respir Dis 136:818-823, 1987.

357. Alenghat E, Esterly JR: Alveolar macrophages in perinatal infants. Pediatrics 74:221-223, 1984.

358. Grigg J, Riedler J: Developmental airway cell biology: the "normal" young child. Am J Respir Crit Care Med 162:S52-S55, 2000.

359. Jackson JC, et al: Postnatal changes in lung phospholipids and alveolar macrophages in term newborn monkeys. Respir Physiol 73:289-300, 1998.

360. Springmeyer SC, et al: Alveolar macrophage kinetics and function after interruption of canine marrow function. Am Rev Respir Dis 125:347-351, 1982.

361. Lin H, et al: Effects of hydrocortisone acetate on pulmonary alveolar macrophage colony-forming cells. Am Rev Respir Dis 125:712-715, 1982.

362. Nakata K, et al: Augmented proliferation of human alveolar macrophages after allogeneic bone marrow transplantation. Blood 93:667-673, 1999.

363. Cox G, et al: Macrophage engulfment of apoptotic neutrophils contributes to the resolution of acute pulmonary inflammation in vitro. Am J Respir Cell Mol Biol 12:232-237, 1995.

364. Arbour NC, et al: TLR4 mutations are associated with endotoxin hypo-responsiveness in humans. Nat Genet 25:187-191, 2000.

365. Haehnel V, et al: Transcriptional regulation of the human Toll-like receptor 2 gene in monocytes and macrophages. J Immunol 168:5629-5637, 2002.

366. Linehan SA, et al: Mannose receptor and scavenger receptor: two macrophage pattern recognition receptors with diverse functions in tissue homeostasis and host defense. Adv Exp Med Biol 479:1-14, 2000.

367. Unkeless JC: Function and heterogeneity of human Fc receptors for immunoglobulin G. J Clin Invest 83:355-361, 1989.

368. Lohmann-Matthes ML, et al: Pulmonary macrophages. Eur Respir J 7:1678-1689, 1994.

369. Thepen T, et al: Migration of alveolar macrophages from alveolar space to paracortical T cell area of the draining lymph node. *In* Kamperdijk A (ed): Dendritic Cells in Fundamental and Clinical Immunology. New York, Plenum Press, 1993, pp 305-310.

370. Weiss SJ: Tissue destruction by neutrophils. N Engl J Med 320:365-376, 1989.

371. Murray HW, Teitelbaum RF: L-Arginine-dependent reactive nitrogen intermediates and the antimicrobial effect of activated human mononuclear phagocytes. J Infect Dis 165:513-517, 1992.

372. Warner RL, et al: Lung sources and cytokine requirements for in vivo expression of inducible nitric oxide synthase. Am J Respir Cell Mol Biol 12:649-661, 1995.

373. Coonrad JD, et al: Impaired pulmonary clearance of pneumococci in neonatal rats. Pediatr Res 22:736-742, 1987.

374. Martin TR, et al: The effect of type-specific polysaccharide capsule on the clearance of group B streptococci from the lungs of infant and adult rats. J Infect Dis 165:306-314, 1992.

375. Sherman MP, et al: Role of pulmonary phagocytes in host defense against group B streptococci in preterm versus term rabbit lung. J Infect Dis 166:818-826, 1992.

376. D'Ambola JB, et al: Human and rabbit newborn lung macrophages have reduced anti-*Candida* activity. Pediatr Res 24:285-290, 1988.

377. Kurland G, et al: The ontogeny of pulmonary defenses: alveolar macrophage function in neonatal and juvenile rhesus monkeys. Pediatr Res 23:292-297, 1988.

378. Sherman MP, Lehrer RI: Oxidative metabolism of neonatal and adult rabbit lung macrophages stimulated with opsonized group B streptococci. Infect Immun 47:26-30, 1985.

379. Ganz T, et al: Newborn rabbit alveolar macrophages are deficient in two microbicidal cationic peptides. Am Rev Respir Dis 132:901-904, 1985.

380. Wang M, et al: Enhancement of human monocyte function against *Candida albicans* by the colony-stimulating factors (CSF) IL-3, granulocyte-macrophage-CSF, and macrophage-CSF. J Immunol 143:671-677, 1989.

381. Smith PD, et al: Granulocyte-macrophage colony-stimulating factor augments human monocyte fungicidal activity for *Candida albicans*. J Infect Dis 161:999-1005, 1990.

382. Marodi L: Deficient interferon-gamma receptor-mediated signalling in neonatal macrophages. Acta Paediatr Suppl 438:117-119, 2002.

383. Bortolussi R, et al: Role of tumor necrosis factor-alpha and interferon-gamma in newborn host defense against *Listeria monocytogenes* infection. Pediatr Res 32:460-464, 1992.

384. Chen Y, Nakane A, Minagawa T: Recombinant murine gamma interferon induces enhanced resistance to *Listeria monocytogenes* infection in neonatal mice. Infect Immun 57:2345-2349, 1989.

385. Kohl S: Protection against murine neonatal herpes simplex virus infection by lymphokine-treated human leukocytes. J Immunol 144:307-312, 1990.

386. Lewis DB, et al: Cellular and molecular mechanisms for reduced interleukin-4 and interferon-gamma production by neonatal T cells. J Clin Invest 87:194-202, 1991.

387. Wilson CB, et al: Decreased production of interferon-gamma by human neonatal cells: Intrinsic and regulatory deficiencies. J Clin Invest 77:860-867, 1986.

388. Stott EJ, et al: Cytotoxicity of alveolar macrophages for virus-infected cells. Nature 255:710-712, 1975.

389. Chelen CJ, et al: Human alveolar macrophages present antigen ineffectively due to defective expression of B7 costimulatory cell surface molecules. J Clin Invest 95:1415-1421, 1995.

390. Joyner JL, et al: Effects of group B streptococci on cord and adult mononuclear cell interleukin-12 and interferon-gamma mRNA accumulation and protein secretion. J Infect Dis 182:974-977, 2000.

391. Burchett SK, et al: Regulation of tumor necrosis factor/cachectin and IL-1 secretion in human mononuclear phagocytes. J Immunol 140:3473-3481, 1988.

392. Ganz T, et al: Defensins. Eur J Haematol 44:1-9, 1990.

393. Levy O: Antibiotic proteins of polymorphonuclear leukocytes. Eur J Hematol 56:263-277, 1996.

394. Iovine NM, et al: An opsonic function of the neutrophil bactericidal/permeability-increasing protein depends on both its N-and C- terminal domains. Proc Natl Acad Sci U S A 94:10973-10978, 1997.

395. Strieter RM, et al: Cytokine-induced neutrophil-derived interleukin-8. Am J Pathol 141:397-407, 1992.

396. Christenson RD: Hematopoiesis in the fetus and neonate. Pediatr Res 26:531-535, 1989.

397. Laver J, et al: High levels of granulocyte and granulocyte-macrophage colony stimulating factors in cord blood of normal full-term neonates. J Pediatr 116:627-632, 1990.

398. Qing G, et al: Lipopolysaccharide binding proteins on polymorphonuclear leukocytes: comparison of adult and neonatal cells. Infect Immun 64:4638-4642, 1996.

399. Smith JB, et al: Expression and regulation of L-selectin on eosinophils from human adults and neonates. Pediatr Res 32:465-471, 1992.

400. Anderson DC, et al: Impaired transendothelial migration by neonatal neutrophils: abnormalities of Mac-1 (CD11b/CD18)-dependent adherence reactions. Blood 76:2613-2621, 1990.

401. Usmani SS, et al: Polymorphonuclear leukocyte function in the preterm neonate. Pediatrics 87:675-679, 1991.

402. Hill HR: Biochemical, structural, and functional abnormalities of polymorphonuclear leukocytes in the neonate. Pediatr Res 22:375-382, 1987.

403. Jones DH, et al: Subcellular distribution and mobilization of MAC-1 (CD11b/CD18) in neonatal neutrophils. Blood 75:488-498, 1990.

404. Anderson DC, et al: Impaired motility on neonatal PMN leukocytes: relationship to abnormalities of cell orientation and assembly of microtubules in chemotactic gradients. J Leukoc Biol 36:1–15, 1984.

405. Kamran S, et al: in vitro effect of indomethacin on polymorphonuclear leukocyte function in preterm infants. Pediatr Res 33:32–35, 1993.

406. Miller ME: Phagocytic function in the neonate: selected aspects. Pediatrics 64:709–712, 1979.

407. Towes GB: Pulmonary dendritic cells: sentinels of lung-associated lymphoid tissues. Am J Resp Cell Mol Biol 4:204–205, 1991.

408. Van Voorhis WC, et al: Relative efficacy of human monocytes and dendritic cells as accessory cells for T cell replication. J Exp Med 158:174–191, 1983.

409. Holt PG: Dendritic cell ontogeny as an aetiological factor in respiratory tract disease in early life. Thorax 56:419–420, 2001.

410. Bauer M, et al: Bacterial CpG-DNA triggers activation and maturation of human CD11c⁻, CD123⁺ dendritic cells. J Immunol 166:5000–5007, 2001.

411. Kadowaki N, et al: Subsets of human dendritic cell precursors express different Toll-like receptors and respond to different microbial antigens. J Exp Med 194:863–869, 2001.

412. Stumbles PA, et al: Resting respiratory tract dendritic cells preferentially stimulate Th2 responses and require obligatory cytokine signals for induction of Th1 immunity. J Exp Med 188:2019–2031, 1998.

413. Sozzani S, et al: Differential regulation of chemokine receptors during dendritic cell maturation: a model for their trafficking properties. J Immunol 161:1083–1086, 1998.

414. Steinman RM: The dendritic cell system and its role in immunogenicity. Annu Rev Immunol 9:271–296, 1991.

415. Wykes M, et al: Dendritic cells interact directly with naïve B lymphocytes to transfer antigen and initiate class switching in a primary T-dependent response. J Immunol 161:1313–1319, 1998.

416. McWilliams AS, et al: Dendritic cells are recruited into the airway epithelium during the inflammatory response to a broad spectrum of stimuli. J Exp Med 184:2429–2432, 1996.

417. Holt PG: Antigen presentation in the lung. Am J Respir Crit Care 162:S151–156, 2000.

418. Holt PG, et al: Downregulation of the antigen-presenting cell functions of pulmonary dendritic cells in vivo by resident alveolar macrophages. J Exp Med 177:397–407, 1993.

419. Bingisser RM, et al: Macrophage-derived nitric oxide regulates T-cell activation via reversible disruption of the Jak3/Stat5 signaling pathway. J Immunol 160:5729–5734, 1998.

420. Roth MD, Golub SH: Human pulmonary macrophages utilize prostaglandins and transforming growth factor β1 to suppress lymphocyte activation. J Leukoc Biol 53:366–371, 1993.

421. Allavena P, et al: IL-10 prevents the differentiation of monocytes to dendritic cells but promotes their maturation to macrophages. Eur J Immunol 28:359–369, 1998.

422. Bilyk N, Holt PG: Inhibition of the immunosuppressive activity of resident pulmonary alveolar macrophages by granulocyte/macrophage colony-stimulating factor. J Exp Med 177:1773–1777, 1993.

423. McCarthy KM, et al: Ontogeny of Ia+ accessory cells in fetal and newborn rat lung. Am J Respir Cell Mol Biol 6:349–356, 1992.

424. Kadowaki N, et al: Subsets of human dendritic cell precursors express different Toll-like receptors and respond to different microbial antigens. J Exp Med 194:863–869, 2001.

425. Tschernig T, et al: Dendritic cells in the mucosa of the human trachea are not regularly found in the first year of life. Thorax 56:427–431, 2001.

426. Nelson DJ, Holt PG: Defective regional immunity in the respiratory tract of neonates is attributable to hyporesponsiveness of local dendritic cells to activation signals. J Immunol 155:3517–3524, 1995.

427. Langrish CL, et al: Neonatal dendritic cells are intrinsically biased against Th-1 immune response. Clin Exp Immunol 128:118–123, 2002.

428. Goriely S, et al: Deficient IL-12(p35) gene expression by dendritic cells derived from neonatal monocytes. J Immunol 166:2141–2146, 2001.

429. Pober JS, et al: Ia expression by vascular endothelium is inducible by activated T cells and by human γ interferon. J Exp Med 157:1339–1353, 1983.

430. Lo SK, et al: Tumor necrosis factor mediates experimental pulmonary edema by ICAM-1 and CD18-dependent mechanisms. J Clin Invest 89:981–988, 1992.

431. Endo H, et al: Additive effects of TNF and IL-1 on induction of prostacyclin synthesis in human vascular endothelial cells. Biochem Biophys Res Commun 156:1007–1014, 1988.

432. Collins T, et al: Recombinant human tumor necrosis factor increases mRNA levels and surface expression of HLA-A,B antigens in vascular endothelial cells and dermal fibroblasts in vitro. Proc Natl Acad Sci U S A 83:446–450, 1986.

433. Libby PJ, et al: Endotoxin and tumor necrosis factor induced interleukin-1 gene expression in adult human vascular endothelial cells. Am J Pathol 124:179–185, 1986.

434. Jirik FR, et al: Bacterial lipopolysaccharide and inflammatory mediators augment IL-6 secretion by human endothelial cells. J Immunol 142:144–147, 1989.

435. Strieter RM, et al: Endothelial cell gene expression of a neutrophil chemotactic factor by TNF, LPS, and IL-1. Science 243:1467–1469, 1989.

436. Broudy VC, et al: Tumor necrosis factor type-α stimulates human endothelial cells to produce granulocyte/macrophage colony-stimulating factor. Proc Natl Acad Sci U S A 83:7467–7471, 1986.

437. Strieter RM, et al: Monocyte chemotactic protein gene expression by cytokine-treated human fibroblasts and endothelial cells. Biochem Biophys Res Commun 162:694–700, 1989.

438. Faure E, et al: Bacterial lipopolysaccharide activates NF-κB through toll-like receptor 4 (TLR-4) in cultured human dermal endothelial cells: differential expression of TLR-4 and TLR-2 in endothelial cells. J Biol Chem 275:11058–11063, 2000.

439. Faure E, et al: Bacterial lipopolysaccharide and IFN-γ induce toll-like receptor 2 and toll-like receptor 4 expression in human endothelial cells: role of NF-κB activation. J Immunol 166:2018–2024, 2001.

440. Meyrick B, et al: Response of cultured human pulmonary artery endothelial cells to endotoxin. Am J Physiol 268:L239–L244, 1995.

441. Bevilacqua MP, et al: Identification of an inducible endothelial leukocyte adhesion molecule, ELAM-1. Proc Natl Acad Sci U S A 84:9238–9242, 1987.

442. Kunkel SL, et al: Endothelial cell-derived novel chemotactic cytokines. In Johnson A, Ferro TJ (eds): Lung Vascular Injury. New York, Marcel Dekker, 1992, pp 213–226.

443. Quesenberry PJ, Gimbrone MA: Vascular endothelium as a regulator of granulopoiesis: production of colony-stimulating activity by cultured human endothelial cells. Blood 56:1060–1067, 1980.

444. Elias JA, et al: Fibroblast immune-effector function. In Phipps R (ed): Pulmonary Fibroblast Heterogeneity. Boca Raton, FL, CRC Press, 1992, pp 295–322.

445. Elias JA, Reynolds MM: Interleukin-1 and tumor necrosis factor synergistically stimulate fibroblast interleukin-1a production. Am J Respir Cell Mol Biol 3:13–20, 1990.

446. Elias JA, Lentz V: IL-1 and tumor necrosis factor synergistically stimulate fibroblast IL-6 production and stabilize IL-6 messenger RNA. J Immunol 145:161–166, 1990.

447. Rolfe MW, et al: Pulmonary fibroblast expression of interleukin-8: a model for alveolar macrophage-derived cytokine networking. Am J Respir Cell Mol Biol 5:493–501, 1991.

448. Kotloff RM, et al: Human alveolar macrophage and blood monocyte interleukin-6 production. Am J Respir Cell Mol Biol 3:497–505, 1990.

449. Wanidworanun C, Strober W: Predominant role of tumor necrosis factor-alpha in human monocyte IL-10 synthesis. J Immunol 151:6853–6861, 1993.

450. Trinchieri G: IL-12 and its role in the generation of Th1 cells. Immunol Today 14:335–338, 1993.

451. Assoian AK, et al: Expression and secretion of type-β transforming growth factor by activated human macrophages. Proc Natl Acad Sci U S A 84:6020–6024, 1987.

452. Fearns C, et al: Murine CD14 gene expression in vivo: extramyeloid synthesis and regulation by lipopolysaccharide. J Exp Med 181:857–866, 1995.

453. Diamond G, et al: The innate immune response of the respiratory epithelium. Immunol Rev 173:27–38, 2000.

454. Singh PK, et al: Production of β-defensins by human airway epithelia. Proc Natl Acad Sci U S A 95:14961–14966, 1998.

455. Guo FH, et al: Continuous nitric oxide synthesis by inducible nitric oxide synthase in normal human airway epithelium in vivo. Proc Natl Acad Sci U S A 92:7809–7813, 1995.

456. Widdicombe JH, et al: Release of cyclyooxygenase products from primary cultures of tracheal epithelia of dog and human. Am J Physiol 256:L361–L365, 1989.

457. Churchill L, et al: Cyclooxygenase metabolism of endogenous arachidonic acid by cultured human tracheal epithelial cells. Am Rev Respir Dis 140:449–459, 1989.

458. Salari H, Chan-Yeung M: Release of 15-hydroxyeicosatetraenoic acid (15-HETE) and prostaglandin E2 (PGE2) by cultured human bronchial epithelial cells. Am J Respir Cell Mol Biol 1:245–250, 1989.

459. Koyama S, et al: Endotoxin stimulates bronchial epithelial cells to release chemotactic factors for neutrophils. J Immunol 147:4293–4301, 1991.

460. Garofalo R, et al: Respiratory syncytial virus infection of human respiratory epithelial cells up-regulates class I MHC expression through the induction of IFN-β and IL-1α. J Immunol 157:2506–2513, 1996.

461. Becker S, et al: RSV infection of human airway epithelial cells causes production of the β-chemokine RANTES. Am J Physiol 272:L512–520, 1997.

462. Marini M, et al: Interleukin-1 binds to specific receptors on human bronchial epithelial cells and upregulates granulocyte/macrophage colony-stimulating factor synthesis and release. Am J Respir Cell Mol Biol 4:519–524, 1991.

463. Levine SJ, et al: Corticosteroids differentially regulate secretion of IL-6, IL-8 and G-CSF by human bronchial epithelial cell line. Am J Physiol 266:L278–L286, 1994.

464. Standiford TJ, et al: Interleukin-8 gene expression by a pulmonary epithelial cell line: a model for cytokine networks in the lung. J Clin Invest 86:1945–1953, 1990.

465. Nakamura H, et al: Interleukin-8 gene expression in human bronchial epithelial cells. J Biol Chem 266:19611–19617, 1991.

466. Paine R, et al: MCP-1 expression by rat type II alveolar epithelial cells in primary culture. J Immunol 150:4561–4570, 1993.

467. Salvi S, et al: Interleukin-5 production by human airway epithelial cells. Am J Respir Cell Mol Biol 20:984–991, 1999.

468. Bader T, Nettesheim P: Tumor necrosis factor-α modulates the expression of its p60 receptor and several cytokines in rat tracheal epithelial cells. J Immunol 157:3089–3096, 1996.

469. Paine R, et al: Regulation of alveolar epithelial cell ICAM-1 expression by cell shape and cell-cell interactions. Am J Physiol 266:L476-L484, 1994.

470. Rothlein R, et al: Induction of intercellular adhesion molecule 1 on primary and continuous cell lines by pro-inflammatory cytokines. J Immunol 141:1665-1669, 1988.

471. O'Brien AD, et al: Role of alveolar epithelial cell intercellular adhesion molecule-1 in host defense against Klebsiella pneumonia. Am J Physiol 276:L961-L970, 1999.

472. Taylor PM, et al: Expression of MHC antigens in normal human lungs and transplanted lungs with obliterative bronchiolitis. Transplantation 48:506-510, 1989.

473. Pabst R: Is BALT a major component of the human lung immune system? Immunol Today 13:119-122, 1992.

474. Johnson J, et al. Morphologic changes in lungs of anesthetized sheep following intravenous infusion of recombinant tumor necrosis factor-alpha. Am Rev Respir Dis 144:179-186, 1991.

475. Pabst R: Compartmentalization and kinetics of lymphoid cells in the lung. Reg Immunol 3:62-71, 1990.

476. Weissler JC, et al: Mononuclear cells in human lung parenchyma. Am Rev Respir Dis 135:941-949, 1987.

477. Sandstrom T, et al: Lipopolysaccharide (LPS) inhalation in healthy subjects increases neutrophils, lymphocytes and fibronectin levels in bronchoalveolar lavage fluid. Eur Respir J 5:992-996, 1992.

478. Gerblich AA, et al: Dynamic T cell changes in peripheral blood and bronchoalveolar lavage after antigen bronchoprovocation in asthmatics. Am Rev Respir Dis 143:533-537, 1991.

479. Pabst R, et al: The physiological role of the lung in lymphocyte migration. Adv Exp Med Biol 237:553-558, 1988.

480. Reynolds HY: Bronchoalveolar lavage. Am Rev Respir Dis 135:250-263, 1987.

481. Erle DJ, et al: Lung epithelial lining fluid T cell subsets defined by distinct patterns of β7 and β-1 integrin expression. Am J Respir Cell Mol Biol 10:237-244, 1994.

482. Wilson M, et al: Ontogeny of human T and B lymphocytes during stressed and normal gestation: phenotypic analysis of umbilical cord lymphocytes from term and preterm infants. Clin Immunol Immunopathol 37:1-12, 1985.

483. Peakman M, et al: Analysis of lymphocyte phenotypes in cord blood from early gestation fetuses. Clin Exp Immunol 90:345-350, 1992.

484. Sanders ME, et al: Human memory T lymphocytes express increased levels of three cell adhesion molecules (LFA-3, CD2, and LFA-1) and three other molecules (UCHL1, CD29, and Pgp-1) and have enhanced IFN-g production. J Immunol 141:1401-1407, 1988.

485. Reiser H, Stadecker MJ: Costimulatory B7 molecules in the pathogenesis of infectious and autoimmune diseases. N Engl J Med 335:1369-1377, 1996.

486. Kersiek KM, Pamer EF: T cell responses to bacterial infection. Curr Opin Immunol 10:471-477, 1998.

487. Stenger S, Modlin RL: Cytotoxic T cell responses to intracellular pathogens. Curr Opin Immunol 10:471-477, 1998.

488. Liu CC, et al: Lymphocyte-mediated cytolysis and disease. N Engl J Med 335:1651-1659, 1996.

489. Stenger S, et al: An antimicrobial activity of cytolytic T cells mediated by granulysin. Science 282:121-125, 1998.

490. Zinkernagel RM: Immunology taught by viruses. Science 271:173-178, 1996.

491. Stenger S, et al: Differential effects of cytolytic T cell subsets on intracellular infection. Science 276:1684-1687, 1997.

492. Oddo M, et al: Fas ligand-induced apoptosis of infected human macrophages reduces the viability of intracellular Mycobacterium tuberculosis. J Immunol 160:5448-5454, 1998.

493. Lalvani A, et al: Human cytolytic and interferon gamma-secreting CD8 T lymphocytes specific for Mycobacterium tuberculosis. Proc Natl Acad Sci U S A 95:270-275, 1998.

494. Hermann E, et al: Human fetuses are able to mount an adultlike CD8 T-cell response. Blood 100:2153-2158, 2002.

495. Lubens RG, et al: Lectin-dependent T-lymphocyte and natural killer cytotoxic deficiencies in human newborns. Cell Immunol 74:40-53, 1982.

496. Adkins B: T-cell function in newborn mice and humans. Immunol Today 20:330-335, 1999.

497. Mosmann TR, Sad S: The expanding universe of T-cell subsets: Th1, Th2 and more. Immunol Today 17:138-146, 1996.

498. Schluger NW, Rom WN: The host immune response to tuberculosis. Am J Respir Crit Care Med 157:679-691, 1998.

499. Susa M, et al: Legionella pneumophila infection in intratracheally inoculated T cell–depleted or non-depleted A/J mice. J Immunol 160:316-321, 1998.

500. Rottenberg ME, et al: Role of innate and adaptive immunity in the outcome of primary infection with Chlamydia pneumoniae, as analyzed in genetically modified mice. J Immunol 162:2829-2836, 1999.

501. Kolls JK, et al: IFN-gamma and CD8+ T cells restore host defenses against Pneumocystis carinii in mice depleted of CD4+ T cells. J Immunol 162:2890-2894, 1999.

502. Noelle RJ, et al: CD40 and its ligand, an essential ligand-receptor pair for thymus-dependent B-cell activation. Immunol Today 13:431-433, 1992.

503. Hollenbaugh D, et al: The human T cell antigen gp39, a member of the TNF gene family, is a ligand for the CD40 receptor: expression of a soluble form of gp39 with B cell co-stimulatory activity. EMBO J 11:4313-4321, 1992.

504. Rousset F, et al: Cytokine-induced proliferation and immunoglobulin production of human B lymphocytes triggered through their CD40 antigen. J Exp Med 173:705-710, 1991.

505. Blackman MA, et al: A model system for peptide hormone action in differentiation: interleukin-2 induces a B lymphoma to transcribe the J chain gene. Cell 47:609-617, 1986.

506. Kuhn R, et al: Generation and analysis of interleukin-4 deficient mice. Science 254:707-710, 1991.

507. Huang S, et al: Immune response in mice that lack the interferon-γ receptor. Science 259:1742-1745, 1993.

508. Moore BB, Towes GB: Humoral immunity in the lung. In Niederman MS, et al (eds): Respiratory Infections. Philadelphia, Lippincott Williams & Wilkins, 2001, pp 27-43.

509. O'Regan A, Center DM: Cytokines in cell-mediated immune responses. In Nelson S, Martin TR (eds): Cytokines in Pulmonary Disease. New York, Marcel Dekker, 2000, pp 83-115.

510. Harris DT, et al: Phenotypic and functional immaturity of human umbilical cord blood T lymphocytes. Proc Natl Acad Sci U S A 89:10006-10010, 1992.

511. Nonoyama S, et al: Diminished expression of CD40 ligand (gp39) by activated neonatal T cells. J Clin Invest 95:66-75, 1995.

512. English BK, et al: Production of lymphotoxin and tumor necrosis factor by human neonatal mononuclear cells. Pediatr Res 24:717-722, 1988.

513. English BK, et al: Decreased granulocyte-macrophage colony-stimulating factor production by human neonatal blood mononuclear cells and T cells. Pediatr Res 31:211-216, 1992.

514. Ehlers S, Smith KA: differentiation of T cell lymphokine gene expression: The in vitro acquisition of T cell memory. J Exp Med 173:25-36, 1991.

515. Buzby JS, et al: Increased granulocyte-macrophage colony stimulating factor mRNA instability in cord versus adult mononuclear cells is translation dependent and associated with increased levels of A+U-rich element binding factor. Blood 88:2889-2897, 1996.

516. Kovarik J, Siegrist CA: Immunity in early life. Immunol Today 19:150-152, 1998.

517. Murray J: How the MHC selects Th1/Th2 immunity. Immunol Today 19:157-163, 1998.

518. Lombardi G, et al: Antigen presentation by interferon-γ-treated thyroid follicular cells inhibits IL-2 and supports IL-4 production by B7 dependent human T cells. Eur J Immunol 27:62-71, 1997.

519. Marzi M, et al: Characterization of type 1 and type 2 cytokine production profile in physiologic and pathologic human pregnancy. Clin Exp Immunol 106:127-133, 1996.

520. White GP, et al: Differential patterns of methylation of the IFN-γ promoter at CpG and non-CpG sites underlie differences in IFN-γ gene expression between human neonatal and adult CD45RO– T cells. J Immunol 168:2820-2827, 2002.

521. Burchett SK, et al: Diminished interferon-γ and lymphocyte proliferation in neonatal and postpartum primary herpes simplex virus infection. J Infect Dis 165:813-818, 1992.

522. Janis EM, et al: Activation of gamma delta T cells in the primary immune response to Mycobacterium tuberculosis. Science 244:713-715, 1989.

523. Chien YH, et al: Recognition by γδ T cells. Annu Rev Immunol 14:511-532, 1996.

524. Hayday AC: γδ T cells: a right time and a right place for a conserved third way of protection. Annu Rev Immunol 18:975-1026, 2000.

525. Borst J, et al: Tissue distribution and repertoire selection of human γδ T cells: comparison with the murine system. Curr Top Microbiol Immunol 173:41-46, 1991.

526. De Libero G, et al: Selection by two powerful antigens may account for the presence of the major population of human peripheral γδ+ T-cells. J Exp Med 173:1311-1322, 1991.

527. Tsuyuguchi I, et al: Increase of T-cell receptor γ/δ-bearing T cells in cord blood of newborn babies obtained by in vitro stimulation with mycobacterial cord factor. Infect Immun 59:3053-3059, 1991.

528. Allison T, et al: Structure of a human γδ T cell antigen receptor. Nature 411:820-824, 2001.

529. Kaufmann SH: γ/δ and other unconventional T lymphocytes: what do they see and what do they do? Proc Natl Acad Sci U S A 93:2272-2279, 1996.

530. Smith MD, et al: Tγδ-cell subsets in cord and adult blood. Scand J Immunol 32:491-495, 1990.

531. Nunez C, et al: B cells are generated throughout life in humans. J Immunol 156:866-872, 1996.

532. Splawski JB, Lipsky PE: Cytokine regulation of immunoglobulin secretion by neonatal lymphocytes. J Clin Invest 88:967-977, 1991.

533. Punnonen J, et al: Induction of isotype switching and Ig production by CD5 and CD10 human fetal B cells. J Immunol 148:3398-3404, 1992.

534. Hannet I, et al: Developmental and maturational changes in human blood lymphocyte subpopulations. Immunol Today 13:215-218, 1992.

535. Marshall-Clarke S, et al: Neonatal immunity: how well has it grown up? Immunol Today 21:35-41, 2000.

536. Griffioen AW, et al: Expression and functional characteristics of the complement receptor type 2 on adult and neonatal B lymphocytes. Clin Immunol Immunopathol 69:1-8, 1993.

537. Adderson EE, et al: Restricted Ig H chain V gene usage in the human antibody response to Haemophilus influenzae type b capsular polysaccharide. J Immunol 147:1667-1674, 1991.

538. Baker CJ, et al: Role of antibody to native type III polysaccharide of group B Streptococcus in infant infection. Pediatrics 68:544-549, 1981.

539. Lanier LL: NK cell receptors. Annu Rev Immunol 16:359-393, 1998.

540. Robinson BWS, et al: Natural killer cells are present in the human lung but are functionally impotent. J Clin Invest 74:942–950, 1984.

541. Weissler JC, et al: Natural killer cell function in human lung is compartmentalized. Am Rev Respir Dis 135:941–949, 1987.

542. Chehimi J, et al: Enhancing effect of natural killer cell stimulatory factor (NKSF/IL-12) on cell-mediated cytotoxicity against tumor-derived and virus-infected cells. Eur J Immunol 23:1826–1830, 1993.

543. Bermudez LEM, Young LS: Natural killer cell–dependent mycobacteriostatic and mycobacterial activity in human macrophages. J Immunol 146:265–270, 1991.

544. Burshtyn DN, Long EO: Regulation through inhibitory receptors: lessons from natural killer cells. Trends Cell Biol 7:473–479, 1997.

545. Eischen CM, et al: Fc receptor–induced expression of Fas ligand on activated NK cells facilitates cell-mediated cytotoxicity and subsequent autocrine NK cell apoptosis. J Immunol 156:2693–2699, 1996.

546. Diefenbach A, et al: Requirement for type 2 NO synthase for IL-12 signalling in innate immunity. Science 284:951–955, 1999.

547. Park DR, Skerrett SJ: Cytokines in Legionella pneumophila infections. In Nelson S, Martin TR (eds): Cytokines in Pulmonary Infectious Disease: Pathogenesis and Therapeutic Strategies. New York, Marcel Dekker, 2000, pp 155–188.

548. Flesch IEA, et al: Growth inhibition of Mycobacterium bovis by IFN-γ stimulated macrophages: regulation by endogenous TNF-α and by IL-10. Int Immunol 6:693–700, 1994.

549. Fearon DT, Locksley RM: The instructive role of innate immunity in the acquired immune response. Science 272:50–53, 1996.

550. Peritt D, Robertson S, Gri G, et al: Differentiation of human NK cells into NK1 and NK2 subsets. J Immunol 161:5821–5824, 1998.

551. Yabuhara A, Kawai T, Komiyama A: Development of natural killer cytotoxicity during childhood: marked increases in number of natural killer cells with adequate cytotoxic abilities during infancy to early childhood. Pediatr Res 68:695–700, 1990.

552. McDonald T, et al: Natural killer cell activity in very low birth weight infants. Pediatr Res 31:376–380, 1992.

553. Phillips JH, et al: Ontogeny of human natural killer (NK) cells: fetal NK cells mediate cytolytic function and express cytoplasmic CD3 epsilon, delta proteins. J Exp Med 175:1055–1066, 1992.

554. Gaddy J, Broxmeyer HE: Cord blood CD16+56– cells with low lytic activity are possible precursors of mature natural killer cells. Cell Immunol 180:132–142, 1997.

555. Harrison CJ, Waner JL: Natural killer cell activity in infants and children excreting cytomegalovirus. J Infect Dis 151:301–307, 1985.

556. Kohl S, et al: Interleukin-2 protects neonatal mice from lethal herpes simplex virus infection: a macrophage-mediated γ interferon–induced mechanism. J Infect Dis 159:239–247, 1989.

557. Bienenstock J, et al: Bronchial lymphoid tissue: I. Morphologic characteristics. Lab Invest 28:686–692, 1973.

558. Bienenstock J, et al: Bronchial lymphoid tissue: II. Functional characteristics. Lab Invest 28:693–698, 1973.

559. Butcher EC, Picker LJ: Lymphocyte homing and homeostasis. Science 272:60–66, 1996.

560. Gould SJ, Isaacson PG: Bronchus-associated lymphoid tissue (BALT) in human fetal and infant lung. J Pathol 169:229–234, 1993.

561. Pabst R, Gehrke I: Is the bronchus-associated lymphoid tissue (BALT) an integral structure of the lung in normal mammals, including humans? Am J Respir Cell Mol Biol 3:131–135, 1990.

562. Delventhal S, et al: Low incidence of bronchus associated lymphoid tissue (BALT) in chronically inflamed human lungs. Virchows Arch 62:271–274, 1992.

563. Tschernig T, Pabst R: Bronchus-associated lymphoid tissue (BALT) is not present in the normal adult lung but in different diseases. Pathobiology 68:1–8, 2000.

564. Schroeder HW, et al: Early restriction of the human antibody repertoire. Science 238:791–793, 1987.

565. Mortari F, et al: Human cord blood antibody repertoire: mixed population of VH gene segments and CDR3 distribution in the expressed Cα and Cγ repertoires. J Immunol 150:1348–1357, 1993.

566. Gathings WE, et al: A distinctive pattern of B cell immaturity in perinatal humans. Immunol Rev 57:107–126, 1981.

567. Durandy A, et al: Phenotypic and functional characteristics of human newborns B lymphocytes. J Immunol 144:60–65, 1990.

568. Carroll MC: The role of complement and complement receptors in induction and regulation of immunity. Annu Rev Immunol 16:545–568, 1998.

569. Peeters CCAM, et al: Interferon-γ and interleukin-6 augment the human in vitro response to the Haemophilus influenzae type b polysaccharide. J Infect Dis 165:S161–S162, 1992.

570. Tomasi TB, et al: Characteristics of an immune system common to certain external secretions. J Exp Med 121:101–124, 1985.

571. Goodman MR, et al: Ultrastructure evidence of transport of secretory IgA across bronchial epithelium. Am Rev Respir Dis 123:115–119, 1981.

572. Brandtzaeg P: Human secretory immunoglobulin M: an immunochemical and immunohistochemical study. Immunology 29:559–570, 1975.

573. Bakos M, et al: Characterization of a critical binding site for human polymeric Ig on secretory component. J Immunol 147:3419–3426, 1991.

574. Mostov KE: Transepithelial transport of immunoglobulins. Annu Rev Immunol 12:63–84, 1994.

575. Stiehm ER, Fudenberg HH: Serum levels of immune globulins in health and disease: a survey. Pediatrics 37:715–726, 1966.

576. Ballow M, et al: Development of the immune system in very low birth weight (less than 1500 g) premature infants: concentrations of plasma immunoglobulins and patterns of infection. Pediatr Res 20:899–904, 1986.

577. Mellander L, et al: Appearance of secretory IgM and IgA antibodies to Escherichia coli in saliva during early infancy and childhood. J Pediatr 104:564–568, 1984.

578. Brandtzaeg P, et al: The clinical condition of IgA-deficient patients is related to the proportion of IgD and IgM-producing cells in their nasal mucosa. Clin Exp Immunol 67:626–636, 1987.

579. Merrill W, et al: Immunoglobulin G subclass proteins in serum and lavage fluid of normal subjects. Am Rev Respir Dis 131:583–587, 1985.

580. Hance AJ, et al: Does de novo immunoglobulin synthesis occur on the epithelial surface of the human lower respiratory tract? Am Rev Respir Dis 137:17–24, 1988.

581. Peters-Golden M, Coffey M: Role of leukotrienes in antimicrobial host defense of the lung. Clin Rev Allergy Immunol 17:261–269, 1999.

582. Bonney RJ, Humes JL: Physiological and pharmacological regulation of prostaglandin and leukotriene production by macrophages. J Leukoc Biol 35:1–10, 1984.

583. Martin TR, et al: Relative contribution of leukotriene B4 to the neutrophil chemotactic activity produced by the resident alveolar macrophage. J Clin Invest 80:1114–1124, 1987.

584. Holtzman MJ: Arachidonic acid metabolism: implications of biological chemistry for lung function and disease. Am Rev Respir Dis 143:188–203, 1991.

585. McManus LM: Platelet activating factor in pulmonary pathobiology. Clin Chest Med 10:107–117, 1989.

586. Hanahan DJ: Platelet activating factor: a biologically active phosphoglyceride. Ann Rev Biochem 55:483–509, 1986.

587. Shaw JO, et al: Activation of human neutrophils with 1-O-hexadecyl/octadecyl-2-acetyl-sn-glyceryl-3-phosphorylcholine (platelet activating factor). J Immunol 127:1250–1255, 1981.

588. Lin AH, et al: Acetyl glyceryl ether phosphorylcholine stimulates leukotriene B4 synthesis in human polymorphonuclear leukocytes. J Clin Invest 70:1058–1065, 1982.

589. Chang SW, et al: Platelet-activating factor mediates hemodynamic changes and lung injury in endotoxin-treated rats. J Clin Invest 79:1498–1509, 1987.

590. Chang SW, et al: Beneficial effect of a platelet-activating factor antagonist, WEB 2086, on endotoxin-induced lung injury. Am J Physiol 258:H153–H158, 1990.

591. Silliman CC, et al: Plasma and lipids from stored packed red blood cells cause acute lung injury in an animal model. J Clin Invest 101:1458–1467, 1998.

592. Minamiya Y, et al: Platelet-activating factor mediates intercellular adhesion molecule-1-dependent radical production in the nonhypoxic ischemia rat lung. Am J Respir Cell Mol Biol 19:150–157, 1998.

593. Caplan MS, et al: Role of platelet-activating factor and tumor necrosis factor-α in neonatal necrotizing enterocolitis. J Pediatr 116:960–964, 1990.

594. Koyama N, et al: Postnatal factors which influence the development of chronic lung disease—the role of chemical mediators. J Jpn Soc Premature Newborn Med 6:62–68, 1994.

595. Koyama N, Ogawa Y: Elevated platelet activating factor in the tracheal aspirate at birth and signs of intrauterine inflammation in infants with neonatal pulmonary emphysema. Eur J Pediatr 158:858–862, 1999.

596. Lewis RA, Austen KF, Soberman RJ: Leukotrienes and other products of the 5-lipoxygenase pathway: biochemistry and relation to pathobiology in human diseases. N Engl J Med 323:645–655, 1990.

597. Wijkander J, et al: 5-Lipoxygenase products modulate the activity of the 85-kDa phospholipase A2 in human neutrophils. J Biol Chem 270:26543–26549, 1995.

598. Marder P, et al: Blockade of human neutrophil activation by LY293 11, a novel leukotriene B4 receptor antagonist. Biochem Pharmacol 49:1683–1690, 1995.

599. Hubbard N, Erickson K: Role of 5-lipoxygenase metabolites in the activation of peritoneal macrophages for tumoricidal function. Mol Immunol 160:115–122, 1995.

600. Hebert MJ, et al: Sequential morphologic events during apoptosis of human neutrophils: modulation by lipoxygenase-derived eicosanoids. J Immunol 157:3105–3115, 1996.

601. Grimminger F, et al: Amplification of LTB4 generation in AM-PMN cocultures: transcellular 5-lipoxygenase metabolism. Am J Physiol 261:L195–203, 1991.

602. Bailie MB, et al: Leukotriene-deficient mice manifest enhanced lethality from Klebsiella pneumonia in association with decreased alveolar macrophage phagocytic and bactericidal activities. J Immunol 157:5221–5224, 1996.

603. Lu MC, et al: Age-related enhancement of 5-lipoxygenase metabolic capacity in cattle alveolar macrophages. Am J Physiol 271:L547–554, 1996.

604. Brigham KL, et al: Prostaglandin E2 attenuation of sheep lung responses to endotoxin. J Appl Physiol 64:2568–2574, 1988.

605. Christman BW, et al: Prostaglandin E2 limits arachidonic acid availability and inhibits leukotriene B4 synthesis in rat alveolar macrophages by a nonphospholipase A2 mechanism. J Immunol 151:2096–2104, 1993.

606. Hugli TE: The structural basis for anaphylatoxin and chemotactic function of C3a, C4a, and C5a. CRC Crit Rev Immunol 1:321–326, 1981.

607. Regal JF, Pickering RJ: C5a-induced tracheal contraction: effect of an SRS-A antagonist and inhibitors of arachidonate metabolism. J Immunol 126:313–316, 1981.

608. Stimler NP, et al: C3a-induced contraction of guinea pig lung parenchyma: role of cyclooxygenase metabolites. Immunopharmacology 5:251-257, 1983.
609. Gerard NP, Gerard C: The chemotactic receptor for human C5a anaphylatoxin. Nature 349:614-617, 1991.
610. Bokisch VA, Muller-Eberhard HJ: Anaphylatoxin inactivator of human plasma: its isolation and characterization as a carboxypeptidase. J Clin Invest 49:2427-2436, 1970.
611. Irvin CG, et al: Airways hyperreactivity and inflammation produced by aerosolization of human C5a des Arg. Am Rev Respir Dis 134:777-783, 1986.
612. Varsano S, et al: Expression and distribution of cell-membrane complement regulatory glycoproteins along the human respiratory tract. Am J Respir Crit Care Med 152:1087-1093, 1995.
613. Drouin SM, et al: Expression of the complement anaphylatoxin C3a and C5a receptors on bronchial epithelial and smooth muscle cells in models of sepsis and asthma. J Immunol 166:2025-2032, 2001.
614. Shushakova N, et al: C5a anaphylotoxin is a major regulator of activating vs. inhibitory FcγRs in immune complex-induced lung disease. J Clin Invest 110:1823-1830, 2002.
615. Riedemann NC, et al: Increased C5a receptor expression in sepsis. J Clin Invest 110:101-108, 2002.
616. Fischer WH, Hugli TE: Regulation of B cell functions by C3a and C3a(desArg): suppression of TNF-α, IL-6, and the polyclonal immune response. J Immunol 159:4279-4286, 1997.
617. Fischer WH, Jagels MA, Hugli TE: Regulation of IL-6 synthesis in human peripheral blood mononuclear cells by C3a and C3a(desArg). J Immunol 162:453-459, 1999.
618. Gerard C: Complement C5a in the sepsis syndrome—too much of a good thing? N Engl J Med 348:167-169, 2003.
619. Fontan JJ, et al: Substance P and neurokinin-1 receptor expression by intrinsic airway neurons in the rat. Am J Physiol 278:L344-355, 2000.
620. McDonald DM, et al: Neurogenic inflammation. A model for studying efferent actions of sensory nerves. Adv Exp Med Biol 410:453-462, 1996.
621. Nadel JA: Neutral endopeptidase modulates neurogenic inflammation. Eur Respir J 4:745-754, 1991.
622. Ho WZ, et al: Human monocytes and macrophages express substance P and neurokinin-1 receptor. J Immunol 159:5654-5660, 1997.
623. Lai JP, et al: Human lymphocytes express substance P and its receptor. J Neuroimmunol 86:80-86, 1998.
624. Chavolla-Calderon M, et al: Bone marrow transplantation reveals an essential synergy between neuronal and hemopoietic cell neurokinin production in pulmonary inflammation. J Clin Invest 112:973-980, 2003.
625. Bozic CR, et al: Neurogenic amplification of immune complex inflammation. Science 273:1722-1725, 1996.
626. Pedersen KE, et al: Neuroimmune interactions in airway inflammation. In Holgate ST (ed): Asthma: Inflammatory Mechanisms. New York, Marcel Dekker, 1998, pp 571-597.
627. Gashi AA, et al: Neuropeptides degranulate serous cells of ferret tracheal glands. Am J Physiol 251:C223-C229, 1986.
628. Kuo HP, et al: Capsaicin and sensory neuropeptide stimulation of goblet cell secretion in guinea pig trachea. J Physiol 431:629-641, 1990.
629. Nathanson I, et al: Effect of vasoactive intestinal peptide on ion transport across dog tracheal epithelium. J Appl Physiol 55:1844-1848, 1983.
630. van Wetering S, et al: Effect of defensins on IL-8 synthesis in airway cells. Am J Physiol 272:L888-896, 1997.
631. Paone G, et al: Human neutrophil peptides stimulate alveolar macrophage production of LTB4 and IL-8. Am J Respir Crit Care Med 159:A511, 1999.
632. Territo MC, et al: Monocyte-chemotactic activity of defensins from human neutrophils. J Clin Invest 84:2017-2020, 1989.
633. Chaly YV, et al: Neutrophil alpha-defensin human neutrophil peptide modulates cytokine production in human monocytes and adhesion molecule expression in endothelial cells. Eur Cytokine Netw 11:257-266, 2000.
634. Welling MM, et al: Antibacterial activity of human neutrophil defensins in experimental infections in mice is accompanied by increased leukocyte accumulation. J Clin Invest 102:1583-1590, 1998.
635. Lillard JW, et al: Mechanisms for induction of acquired host immunity by neutrophil peptide defensins. Proc Natl Acad Sci U S A 96:651-656, 1999.
636. Yang D, et al: Human neutrophil defensins selectively chemoattract naïve T and immature dendritic cells. J Leukoc Biol 68:9-14, 2000.
637. Gabay JE, et al: Antibiotic proteins of human polymorphonuclear leukocytes. Proc Natl Acad Sci U S A 86:5610-5614, 1989.
638. Janoff A: Elastase in tissue injury. Annu Rev Med 36:207-216, 1985.
639. Weiss SJ, Regiani S: Neutrophils degrade subendothelial matrices in the presence of alpha-1-proteinase inhibitor. J Clin Invest 73:1297-1303, 1984.
640. Gadek JE, et al: Human neutrophil elastase functions as a type III collagen "collagenase." Biochem Biophys Res Commun 95:1815-1822, 1980.
641. McDonald JA, Kelley DG: Degradation of fibronectin by leukocyte elastase: Release of biologically active fragments. J Biol Chem 255:8848-8858, 1980.
642. Johnson U, et al: Effects of granulocyte neutral proteases on complement components. Scand J Immunol 5:421-426, 1976.
643. Shafer WM, et al: A spontaneous mutant of Neisseria gonorrhoeae with decreased resistance to neutrophil granule proteins. J Infect Dis 153:910-917, 1986.
644. Travis J: Structure, function, and control of neutrophil proteinases. Am J Med 84:37-42, 1988.
645. Campanelli D, et al: Azurocidin and a homologous serine protease from neutrophils: differential antimicrobial and proteolytic properties. J Clin Invest 85:904-915, 1990.
646. Falloon J, et al: Neutrophil granules in health and disease. J Allergy Clin Immunol 77:653-662, 1986.
647. Wright DG: Human neutrophil degranulation. Methods Enzymol 162:538-551, 1988.
648. Salzet M, et al: Serpins: an evolutionarily conserved survival strategy. Immunol Today 20:541-544, 1999.
649. Babior BM: Oxidants from phagocytes: agents of defense and destruction. Blood 64:959-966, 1984.
650. Cross AR, Jones OTG: Enzymatic mechanisms of superoxide production. Biochim Biophys Acta 1057:281-298, 1991.
651. Klebanoff SJ: Myeloperoxidase-halide-hydrogen peroxidase antibacterial system. J Bacteriol 95:2131-2138, 1968.
652. Halliwell B, Gutteridge JMC: Free Radicals in Biology and Medicine. New York, Oxford University Press, 1989, pp 1-21.
653. Freeman BA, et al: Superoxide pertubation of the organization of vascular endothelial cell membranes. J Biol Chem 261:6590-6593, 1986.
654. Yokota J, et al: Oxygen free radicals affect cardiac and skeletal cell membrane potential during hemorrhagic shock in rats. Am J Physiol 262:H84-H90, 1992.
655. Davies KJA, et al: Protein damage and degradation by oxygen radicals: II. Modification of amino acids. J Biol Chem 262:9902-9907, 1987.
656. Kono Y, Fridovich I: Superoxide radical inhibits catalase. J Biol Chem 257:5751-5754, 1982.
657. Schraufstatter IU, et al: Oxidant injury of cells: DNA strand breaks activate polyadenosine diphosphate-ribose polymerase and lead to depletion of nicotinamide adenine dinucleotide. J Clin Invest 77:1312-1320, 1986.
658. Spragg RG: DNA strand break formation following exposure of bovine pulmonary artery and aortic endothelial cells to reactive oxygen products. Am J Resp Cell Mol Biol 4:4-10, 1991.
659. Beckman JS, et al: Apparent hydroxyl radical production by peroxynitrite: implications for endothelial cell injury from nitric oxide and superoxide. Proc Natl Acad Sci U S A 87:1620-1624, 1990.
660. Matheson NR, et al: Enzymatic inactivation of human alpha-1-proteinase inhibitor by neutrophil myeloperoxidase. Biochem Biophys Res Commun 88:402-409, 1979.
661. Johnson D, Travis J: The oxidative inactivation of human α-1-proteinase inhibitor. J Biol Chem 254:4022-4026, 1979.
662. Beutler B, Cerami A: Cachectin: more than a tumor necrosis factor. N Engl J Med 316:379-385, 1987.
663. Tracey KJ, Cerami A: Tumor necrosis factor: an updated review of its biology. Crit Care Med 21:S415-S422, 1993.
664. Cuturi MC, et al: Independent regulation of tumor necrosis factor and lymphotoxin production by human peripheral blood lymphocytes. J Exp Med 165:1581-1594, 1987.
665. Degliantoni G, et al: Natural killer (NK) cell–derived hematopoietic colony-inhibiting activity and NK cytotoxic factor: relationship with tumor necrosis factor and synergism with immune interferon. J Exp Med 162:1512-1530, 1985.
666. Michie HR, et al: Detection of circulating tumor necrosis factor after endotoxin administration. N Engl J Med 318:1481-1486, 1988.
667. Brieland JK, et al: In vivo regulation of replicative Legionella pneumophila lung infection by endogenous tumor necrosis factor alpha and nitric oxide. Infect Immun 63:3253-3258, 1995.
668. Gosselin D, et al: Role of tumor necrosis factor alpha in innate resistance to mouse pulmonary infection with Pseudomonas aeruginosa. Infect Immun 63:3272-3278, 1995.
669. Laichalk LL, et al: Tumor necrosis factor mediates lung antibacterial host defense in murine Klebsiella pneumonia. Infect Immun 64:5211-5218, 1996.
670. van der Poll T, et al: Passive immunization against tumor necrosis factor-α impairs host defense during pneumococcal pneumonia in mice. Am J Respir Crit Care Med 155:603-608, 1997.
671. Klebanoff SJ, et al: Stimulation of neutrophils by tumor necrosis factor. J Immunol 36:4220-4225, 1986.
672. Gamble JR, et al: Stimulation of the adherence of neutrophils to umbilical vein epithelium by human recombinant tumor necrosis factor. Proc Natl Acad Sci U S A 82:8667-8671, 1985.
673. Tsujimoto M, et al: Tumor necrosis factor provokes superoxide anion generation from neutrophils. Biochem Biophys Res Commun 137:1094-1100, 1986.
674. Tosi MF, et al: Induction of ICAM-1 expression on human airway epithelial cells by inflammatory cytokines: effects of neutrophil-epithelial cell adhesion. Am J Respir Cell Mol Biol 7.214-221, 1992.
675. Pohlman TH, et al: An endothelial cell surface factor(s) induced in vitro by lipopolysaccharide, interleukin-1, and tumor necrosis factor-alpha increases neutrophil adherence by a Cdw18-dependent mechanism. J Immunol 136:4548-4553, 1986.
676. Nawroth PP, et al: Tumor necrosis factor/cachectin interacts with endothelial cell receptors to induce release of interleukin 1. J Exp Med 163:1363-1375, 1986.
677. Bachwich PR, et al: Tumor necrosis factor stimulates interleukin-1 and prostaglandin E2 production in resting macrophages. Biochem Biophys Res Commun 136:94-101, 1986.

678. Crestani B, et al: Alveolar type II epithelial cells produce interleukin-6 in vitro. Regulation by alveolar macrophage secretory products. J Clin Invest 94:731–740, 1994.

679. Weatherstone KB, Rich EA: Tumor necrosis factor/cachectin and interleukin-1 secretion by cord blood monocytes from premature and term neonates. Pediatr Res 25:342–346, 1989.

680. Tullus K, et al: Elevated cytokine levels in tracheobronchial aspirate fluids from ventilator treated neonates with bronchopulmonary dysplasia. Eur J Pediatr 155:112–116, 1996.

681. Viscardi RM, et al: Lung pathology in premature infants with *Ureaplasma urealyticum* infection. Pediatr Dev Pathol 5:141–150, 2002.

682. March CJ, et al: Cloning, sequence, and expression of two distinct human interleukin-1 complementary DNAs. Nature 315:641–647, 1985.

683. Dinarello CA: Interleukin-1 and interleukin-1 antagonism. Blood 77:1627–1652, 1991.

684. Dinarello CA: Interleukin-1, interleukin-18, and the interleukin-1 converting enzyme. Ann NY Acad Sci 856:1–11, 1998.

685. Strieter RM, et al: Cytokines in innate host defense in the lung. J Clin Invest 109:699–705, 2002.

686. Figdor CG, van Kooyk Y: Regulation of cell adhesion. In Harlan JM, Liu DY (eds): Adhesion: Its Role in Inflammatory Disease. New York, WH Freeman, 1992, pp 151–182.

687. Pober JS, et al: Two distinct monokines, interleukin-1 and tumor necrosis factor, each independently induce biosynthesis and transient expression of the same antigen on the surface of cultured human vascular endothelial cells. J Immunol 135:1680–1687, 1986.

688. Ozaki Y, et al: Potentiation of neutrophil function by recombinant DNA-produced interleukin-1-alpha. J Leukoc Biol 43:349–356, 1987.

689. Dinarello CA: Biologic basis for interleukin-1 in disease. Blood 87:2095–2147, 1996.

690. Mizel SB: Interleukin 1 and T-cell activation. Immunol Today 8:330–332, 1987.

691. Dinarello CA: Interleukin-1 and its biologically related cytokines. Adv Immunol 44:153–205, 1989.

692. Breder CD, et al: Interleukin-1 immunoreactive innervation of the human hypothalamus. Science 240:321–324, 1988.

693. Murphy JE, et al: Interleukin-1 and cutaneous inflammation: a crucial link between innate and acquired immunity. J Invest Dermatol 114:602–608, 2000.

694. Nathan CF: Secretory products of macrophages. J Clin Invest 79:319–326, 1987.

695. May LT, et al: Synthesis and secretion of multiple forms of beta 2-interferon/B-cell differentiation factor 2/hepatocyte-stimulating factor by human fibroblasts and monoytes. J Biol Chem 263:7760–7766, 1988.

696. Bochner BS, et al: Interleukin 1 production by human lung tissue: I. Identification and characterization. J Immunol 139:2297–2302, 1987.

697. Dudding LR, et al: Cytomegalovirus infection stimulates expression of monocyte-associated mediator genes. J Immunol 143:3343–3352, 1989.

698. Durum SK, Oppenheim JJ: Proinflammatory cytokines and immunity. In Paul WE (ed): Fundamental Immunology. New York, Raven Press, 1993, pp 801–835.

699. Warner SJC, et al: Interleukin 1 induces interleukin 1: II. Recombinant interleukin 1 induces interleukin 1 production by adult human vascular endothelial cells. J Immunol 139:1911–1917, 1987.

700. Fantuzzi G, et al: Effect of endotoxin in IL-1 beta deficient mice. J Immunol 157:291–296, 1996.

701. Glover DM, et al: Expression of HLA class II antigens and secretion of interleukin-1 by monocytes and macrophages from adults and neonates. Immunology 61:195–201, 1987.

702. Contrino J, et al: Elevated interleukin-1 expression in human neonatal neutrophils. Pediatr Res 34:249–252, 1993.

703. Arend WP, et al: Biological properties of recombinant human monocyte-derived interleukin-1 receptor antagonist. J Clin Invest 85:1694–1697, 1990.

704. Hannum CH, et al: Interleukin-1 receptor antagonist activity of a human interleukin-1 inhibitor. Nature 343:336–340, 1990.

705. Galve-de Rochemonteix B, et al: Characterization of a specific 20–25 kD interleukin-1 inhibitor from cultured human lung macrophages. Am J Respir Cell Mol Biol 3:355–361, 1990.

706. Arend WP, et al: IL-1 receptor antagonist and IL-1 beta production in human monocytes are regulated differently. J Immunol 147:1530–1536, 1991.

707. Ulich TR, et al: The intratracheal administration of endotoxin and cytokines: III. The interleukin-1 (IL-1) receptor antagonist inhibits endotoxin- and IL-1-induced acute inflammation. Am J Pathol 138:521–524, 1991.

708. Hirsch E, et al: Functions of interleukin 1 receptor antagonist in gene knock-out and overproducing mice. Proc Natl Acad Sci 93:11008–11013, 1996.

709. Gupta GK, et al: Effects of early inhaled beclomethasone therapy on tracheal aspirate inflammatory mediators IL-8 and IL-1ra in ventilated preterm infants at risk for bronchopulmonary dysplasia. Pediatr Pulmonol 30:275–281, 2000.

710. Geiger R, et al: Circulating interleukin-1 receptor antagonist levels in neonates. Eur J Pediatr 155:811–814, 1996.

711. Kuster H, et al: Interleukin-1 receptor antagonist and interleukin-6 for early diagnosis of neonatal sepsis 2 days before clinical manifestation. Lancet 352:1271–1277, 1999.

712. Bessher H, et al: Indomethacin and ibuprofen effect on IL-1ra production by mononuclear cells of preterm newborns and adults. Biol Neonate 82:73–77, 2002.

713. Smith KA: Interleukin-2: inception, impact, and implications. Science 240:1169–1176, 1988.

714. Stern JB, Smith KA: Interleukin-2 induction of T-cell G1 progression and c-*myb* expression. Science 233:203–206, 1986.

715. Howard MC, et al: T-cell–derived cytokines and their receptors. In Paul WE (ed): Fundamental Immunology. New York, Raven Press, 1993, pp 763–800.

716. Henney CS, et al: Interleukin-2 augments natural killer cell activity. Nature 291:335–338, 1981.

717. Tigges MA, et al: Mechanism of IL-2 signalling: mediation of different outcomes by a single receptor and transduction pathway. Science 243:781–786, 1989.

718. Espinoza-Delgado I, et al: Interleukin-2 and human monocyte activation. J Leukoc Biol 57:13–19, 1995.

719. Murray HW, et al: Role and effect of IL-2 in experimental visceral leishmaniasis. J Immunol 151:929–938, 1993.

720. Hoshina T, et al: Difference in response of NK cell activity in newborns and adult to IL-2, IL-12, and IL-15. Microbiol Immunol 43:161–166, 1999.

721. Waldmann TA: The structure, function, and expression of interleukin-2 receptors on normal and malignant lymphocytes. Science 240:1169–1176, 1986.

722. Taniguchi T, Minami Y: The IL-2/IL-2 receptor system: a current overview. Cell 73:5–8, 1993.

723. Rubin LA, et al: Soluble interleukin 2 receptors are released from activated lymphoid cells in vitro. J Immunol 135:3172–3177, 1985.

724. Mangi MH, Newland AC: Interleukin-3 in hematology and oncology: current state of knowledge and future directions. Cytokines Cell Mol Ther 5:87–95, 1999.

725. Miyajima A, et al: Receptors for granulocyte-macrophage colony stimulating factor, interleukin-3, and interleukin-5. Blood 82:1960–1974, 1993.

726. Dirksen U, et al: Human pulmonary alveolar proteinosis associated with a defect in GM-CSF/IL-3/IL-5 receptor common β chain expression. J Clin Invest 100:2211–2217, 1997.

727. Grouard G, et al: The enigmatic plasmacytoid T cells develop into dendritic cells with interleukin-3 and CD40-ligand. J Exp Med 185:1101–1111, 1997.

728. Yeh KY, et al: IL-3 enhances both presentation of exogenous particulate antigen in association with class I major histocompatibility antigen and generation of primary tumor-specific cytolytic T lymphocytes. J Immunol 160:5773–5780, 1998.

729. Lloyd CM, et al: Resolution of bronchial hyperresponsiveness and pulmonary inflammation is associated with IL-3 and tissue leukocyte apoptosis. J Immunol 166:2033–2040, 2001.

730. Carlson M, et al: The influence of IL-3, IL-5, and GM-CSF on normal human eosinophil and neutrophil C3b-induced degranulation. Allergy 48:437–442, 1993.

731. Cairo MS, et al: Decreased G-CSF and IL-3 production and gene expression from mononuclear cells of newborn infants. Pediatr Res 31:574–578, 1992.

732. Bessler H, et al: Effect of dexamethasone on IL-2 and IL-3 production by mononuclear cells in neonates and adults. Arch Dis Child Fetal Neonatal Ed 75:F197–201, 1996.

733. Sanderson CJ: Interleukin-5, eosinophils and disease. Blood 79:3101–3109, 1992.

734. Karras JG, et al: Inhibition of antigen-induced eosinophilia and late phase airway hyperresponsiveness by an IL-5 antisense oligonucleotide in mouse models of asthma. J Immunol 164:5409–5415, 2000.

735. Walker C, et al: Cytokine control of eosinophils in pulmonary diseases. J Allergy Clin Immunol 94:1262–1271, 1994.

736. Mould AW, et al: The effect of IL-5 and eotaxin expression in the lung on eosinophil trafficking and degranulation and the induction of bronchial hyperreactivity. J Immunol 164:2142–2150, 2000.

737. Calhoun DA, et al: Granulocyte-macrophage colony-stimulating factor and interleukin-5 concentration in premature neonates with eosinophilia. J Perinatol 20:166–171, 2000.

738. Gascan H, et al: Human B cell clones can be induced to proliferate and to switch to IgE and IgG4 synthesis by interleukin-4 and a signal provided by activated CD4+ T cell clones. J Exp Med 173:747–759, 1991.

739. Gautam S, et al: IL-4 suppresses cytokine gene expression induced by IFN-gamma and/or IL-2 in murine peritoneal macrophages. J Immunol 148:1725–1730, 1992.

740. Essner R, et al: IL-4 down-regulates IL-1 and TNF gene expression in human monocytes. J Immunol 142:3857–3861, 1989.

741. Standiford TJ, et al: IL-4 inhibits expression of IL-8 from stimulated human monocytes. J Immunol 145:1435–1439, 1990.

742. Deng W, et al: Mechanisms of IL-4–mediated suppression of IP-10 gene expression in murine macrophages. J Immunol 153:2130–2136, 1994.

743. Schleimer RP, et al: IL-4 induces adherence of human eosinophils and basophils but not neutrophils to endothelium. J Immunol 148:1086–1092, 1992.

744. Jonsson B, et al: Downregulatory cytokines in tracheobronchial aspirate fluid from infants with chronic lung disease of prematurity. Act Paediatr 89:1375–1380, 2000.

745. McKenzie AN, et al: Interleukin 13, a T-cell–derived cytokine that regulates human monocyte and B-cell function. Proc Natl Acad Sci U S A 90:3735–3739, 1993.

746. Minty A, et al: Interleukin-13 is a new human lymphokine regulating inflammatory and immune responses. Nature 362:248–250, 1993.

747. Zurawski SM, et al: Receptors for interleukin-13 and interleukin-4 are complex and share a novel component that functions in signal transduction. EMBO J 12:2663-2670, 1993.

748. Punnonen J, et al: Interleukin 13 induces interleukin 4-dependent IgG4 and IgE synthesis and CD23 expression by human B cells. Proc Natl Acad Sci USA 90:3730-3734, 1993.

749. Bochner BS, et al: IL-13 selectively induces vascular cell adhesion molecule-1 expression in human endothelial cells. J Immunol 154:799-803, 1995.

750. Calandra T, Heumann D: Inhibitory cytokines. In Marshall JC, Cohen J (eds): Immune Response in the Critically Ill. Berlin, Springer-Verlag, 2000, pp 67-83.

751. de Waal Malefyt R, et al: Effects of IL-13 on phenotype, cytokine production, and cytotoxic function of human monocytes. J Immunol 151:6370-6381, 1993.

752. Yanagawa H, et al: Contrasting effects of interleukin-13 on interleukin-1 receptor antagonist and proinflammatory cytokine production by human alveolar macrophages. Am J Respir Cell Mol Biol 12:71-76, 1995.

753. Williams TJ, et al: Fetal and neonatal IL-13 production during pregnancy and at birth and subsequent development of atopic symptoms. J Allergy Clin Immunol 105:951-959, 2000.

754. Ohshima Y, et al: Dysregulation of IL-13 production by cord blood CD4+ T cells is associated with the subsequent development of atopic disease in infants. Pediatr Res 51:195-200, 2002.

755. Kishimoto T: The biology of interleukin-6. Blood 74:1-10, 1989.

756. Schultz C, et al: Enhanced interleukin-6 and interleukin-8 synthesis in term and preterm infants. Pediatr Res 51:317-322, 2002.

757. Yachie A, et al: Defective production of interleukin-6 in very small premature infants in response to bacterial pathogens. Infect Immun 60:749-753, 1992.

758. Schindler RJ, et al: Correlations and interactions in the production of interleukin-6, IL-1β, and tumor necrosis factor in human blood mononuclear cells: IL-6 suppresses IL-1 and TNFα. Blood 75:40-47, 1990.

759. Tilg H, et al: Interleukin-6 (IL-6) as an anti-inflammatory cytokine: induction of circulating IL-1 receptor antagonist and soluble tumor necrosis factor receptor p55. Blood 83:113-118, 1994.

760. Hirano T: Interleukin 6 and its receptor: ten years later. Int Rev Immunol 16:249-284, 1998.

761. Baroja ML, et al: Cooperation between an anti-T cell (anti-CD28) monoclonal antibody and monocyte-produced IL-6 in the induction of T cell responsiveness to IL-2. J Immunol 141:1502-1507, 1988.

762. Muraguchi A, et al: The essential role of B cell stimulatory factor (BSF-2/IL-6) for the terminal differentiation of B cells. J Exp Med 167:332-344, 1988.

763. Barton BE: IL-6: insights into novel biological activities. Clin Immunol Immunopathol 85:16-20, 1997.

764. Perlmutter DH, et al: Interferon beta 2/interleukin-6 modulates synthesis of alpha 1-antitrypsin in human mononuclear phagocytes and in human hepatoma cells. J Clin Invest 84:138-144, 1989.

765. Martin TR: Lung cytokines and ARDS: Roger S. Mitchell lecture. Chest 116:2S-8S, 1999.

766. Bagchi A, et al: Increased activity of interleukin-6 but not tumor necrosis factor alpha in lung lavage of premature infants is associated with the development of bronchopulmonary dysplasia. Pediatr Res 36:244-252, 1994.

767. Kotecha S, et al: Increase in interleukin-1 beta and IL-6 in bronchoalveolar lavage fluid obtained from infants with chronic lung disease of prematurity. Pediatr Res 40:250-256, 1996.

768. Ulich TR, et al: Intratracheal injection of endotoxin and cytokines: II. Interleukin-6 and transforming growth factor-β inhibit acute inflammation. Am J Pathol 138:1097-1101, 1991.

769. Houssiau FA, et al: Human T cell lines and clones respond to IL-9. J Immunol 150:2634-2640, 1993.

770. Hultner L, et al: Thiol-sensitive mast cell lines derived from mouse bone marrow respond to a mast cell growth enhancing activity different from both IL-3 and IL-4. J Immunol 142:3440-3446, 1989.

771. Dugas B, et al: Interleukin-9 potentiates the interleukin-4-induced immunoglobulin (IgG, IgM and IgE) production by normal human B lymphocytes. Eur J Immunol 23:1687-1692, 1993.

772. Dong Q, et al: IL-9 induces chemokine expression in lung epithelial cells and baseline airway eosinophilia in transgenic mice. Eur J Immunol 29:2130-2139, 1999.

773. Little FF, et al: IL-9 stimulates release of chemotactic factors from human bronchial epithelial cells. Am J Respir Cell Mol Biol 25:347-352, 2001.

774. Longphre M, et al: Allergen-induced IL-9 directly stimulates mucin transcription in respiratory epithelial cells. J Clin Invest 104:1375-1382, 1999.

775. Louahed J, et al: Interleukin-9 upregulates mucus expression in the airways. Am J Respir Cell Mol Biol 22:649-656, 2000.

776. Temann UA, et al: Pulmonary overexpression of IL-9 induces Th2 cytokine expression, leading to immune pathology. J Clin Invest 109:29-39, 2002.

777. Vermeer PD, et al: Interleukin-9 induces goblet cell hyperplasia during repair of human airway epithelia. Am J Respir Cell Mol Biol 28:286-295, 2003.

778. Nelson KB, et al: Neonatal cytokines and coagulation factors in children with cerebral palsy. Ann Neurol 44:665-675, 1998.

779. Del Prete G, et al: Human IL-10 is produced by both type I helper and type II helper T cell clones and inhibits their antigen-specific proliferation and cytokine production. J Immunol 150:353-360, 1993.

780. de Waal Malefyt R, et al: Interleukin-10 (IL-10) inhibits cytokine synthesis by human monocytes: an autoregulatory role of IL-10 produced by monocytes. J Exp Med 174:1209-1220, 1991.

781. Moore KW, et al: Interleukin-10. Annu Rev Immunol 11:165-190, 1993.

782. Laichalk LL, et al: Interleukin-10 inhibits neutrophil phagocytic and bactericidal activity. FEMS Immunol Med Microbiol 15:181-187, 1996.

783. Bogdan C, et al: Macrophage deactivation by interleukin 10. J Exp Med 174:1549-1555, 1991.

784. de Waal Malefyt R, et al: Interleukin-10 (IL-10) and viral IL-10 strongly reduce antigen-specific human T cell proliferation by diminishing the antigen-presenting capacity of monocytes via down regulation of class II major histocompatibility complex expression. J Exp Med 174:915-924, 1991.

785. Ding L, et al: IL-10 inhibits macrophage costimulatory activity by selectively inhibiting the up-regulation of B7 expression. J Immunol 151:1224-1234, 1993.

786. D'Andrea A, et al: Interleukin 10 inhibits human lymphocyte interferon γ-production by suppressing natural killer cell stimulatory factor/IL-12 synthesis in accessory cells. J Exp Med 178:1041-1048, 1993.

787. Ralph P, et al: IL-10, T lymphocyte inhibitor of human blood cell production of IL-1 and tumor necrosis factor. J Immunol 148:808-814, 1992.

788. Fiorentino DF, et al: IL-10 inhibits cytokine production by activated macrophages. J Immunol 147:3815-3822, 1991.

789. de Waal Malefyt R, et al: Interleukin 10. Curr Opin Immunol 4:314-320, 1992.

790. Wang P, et al: Interleukin-10 inhibits nuclear factor κB (NFκB) activation in human monocytes: IL-10 and IL-4 suppress cytokine synthesis by different mechanisms. J Biol Chem 270:9558-9563, 1995.

791. Bogdan C, et al: Contrasting mechanisms for suppression of macrophage cytokine release by transforming growth factor-beta and interleukin-10. J Biol Chem 267:23301-23308, 1992.

792. Dickensheets HL, et al: Interleukin-10 upregulates tumor necrosis factor receptor type II (p75) gene expression in endotoxin-stimulated human monocytes. Blood 90:4162-4171, 1997.

793. Joyce DA, et al: Two inhibitors of pro-inflammatory cytokine release, interleukin-10 and interleukin-4, have contrasting effects on release of soluble p75 tumor necrosis factor receptor by cultured monocytes. Eur J Immunol 24:2699-2705, 1994.

794. Cox G: IL-10 enhances resolution of pulmonary inflammation in vivo by promoting apoptosis of neutrophils. Am J Physiol 271:L566-L571, 1996.

795. Mulligan MS, et al: Protective effects of IL-4 and IL-10 against immune complex-induced lung injury. J Immunol 151:5666-5674, 1993.

796. van der Poll T, et al: Interleukin-10 impairs host defense in murine pneumococcal pneumonia. J Infect Dis 174:994-1000, 1996.

797. Greenberger M, et al: Neutralization of IL-10 increases survival in a murine model of Klebsiella pneumonia. J Immunol 155:722-729, 1995.

798. Rennick DN, et al: Studies with IL-10-/- mice: an overview. J Leukoc Biol 61:389-396, 1997.

799. Gazzinelli RT, et al: In the absence of endogenous IL-10, mice acutely infected with Toxoplasma gondii succumb to a lethal immune response dependent on CD4+ T cells and accompanied by overproduction of IL-12, IFN-γ, and TNF-α. J Immunol 157:798-805, 1996.

800. Cheda S, et al: Decreased interleukin-10 production by neonatal monocytes and T cells: relationship to decreased production and expression of tumor necrosis factor-alpha and its receptors. Pediatr Res 40:475-483, 1996.

801. Kotiranta-Ainamo A, et al: Interleukin-10 production by cord blood mononuclear cells. Pediatr Res 41:110-113, 1997.

802. McColm JR, et al: Measurement of interleukin-10 in bronchoalveolar lavage from preterm ventilated infants. Arch Dis Child Fetal Neonatal Ed 82:F156-159, 2000.

803. Oei J, et al: Decreased interleukin-10 in tracheal aspirates from preterm infants developing chronic lung disease. Acta Paediatr 91:1194-1199, 2002.

804. Huang HC, et al: Profiles of inflammatory cytokines in bronchoalveolar lavage fluid from premature infants with respiratory distress disease. J Microbiol Immunol Infect 33:19-24, 2000.

805. Jones CA, et al: Undetectable interleukin (IL)-10 and persistent IL-8 expression early in hyaline membrane disease: a possible developmental basis for the predisposition to chronic lung inflammation in preterm newborns. Pediatr Res 39:966-975, 1996.

806. Blahnik MJ, et al: Lipopolysaccharide-induced tumor necrosis factor-α and IL-10 production by lung macrophages from preterm and term neonates. Pediatr Res 50:726-731, 2001.

807. Du XX, Williams DA: Interleukin-11: a multifunctional growth factor derived from the hematopoietic microenvironment. Blood 83:2023-2030, 1994.

808. Zhang XG, et al: Ciliary neurotrophic factor, interleukin-11, leukemia inhibitory factor, and oncostatin M are growth factors for human myeloma cell lines using the interleukin-6 signal transducer GP130. J Exp Med 177:1337-1342, 1994.

809. Bazan JF: Neuropoietic cytokines in the hematopoietic fold. Neuron 7:197-208, 1991.

810. Patterson PH, Nawa H: Neuronal differentiation factors/cytokines and synaptic plasticity. Cell 72:123-137, 1993.

811. Baumann H, Schendel P: Interleukin-11 regulates the hepatic expression of the same protein genes as interleukin-6. J Biol Chem 266:20424-20427, 1991.

812. Du X, Williams DA: Interleukin-11: review of molecular, cell biology, and clinical use. Blood 89:3897-3908, 1997.

813. Musashi M, et al: Synergistic interactions between interleukin-11 and interleukin-4 in support of proliferation of primitive hematopoietic progenitors of mice. Blood 78:1448–1451, 1991.

814. Trepicchio WL, et al: Recombinant human IL-11 attenuates the inflammatory response through down-regulation of proinflammatory cytokine release and nitric oxide production. J Immunol 157:3627–3634, 1996.

815. Leng SX, Elias JA: Interleukin-11 inhibits macrophage interleukin-12 production. J Immunol 159:2161–2168, 1997.

816. Du XX, et al: A bone marrow stromal-derived growth factor, interleukin-11, stimulates recovery of small intestinal mucosal cells after cytoablative therapy. Blood 83:33–37, 1994.

817. Redlich CA, et al: IL-11 enhances survival and decreases TNF production after radiation induced thoracic injury. J Immunol 157:1705–1710, 1996.

818. Waxman AB, et al: Targeted lung expression of interleukin-11 enhances murine tolerance of 100% oxygen and diminishes hyperoxia-induced DNA fragmentation. J Clin Invest 101:1970–1982, 1998.

819. Elias JA, et al: Interleukin-1 and transforming growth factor β regulation of fibroblast-derived interleukin-11. J Immunol 152:2421–2429, 1994.

820. Zheng T, et al: Histamine augments cytokine-stimulated IL-11 production by human lung fibroblasts. J Immunol 153:4742–4752, 1994.

821. Buzby J, et al: Coordinate regulation of Steel factor, its receptor (Kit) and cytoadhesion molecule (ICAM-1 and ELAM-1) mRNA expression in human vascular endothelial cells of differing origins. Exp Hematol 22:122–129, 1994.

822. Einarsson O, et al: Interleukin-11: stimulation in vivo and in vitro by respiratory viruses and induction of airways hyperresponsiveness. J Clin Invest 97:915–924, 1996.

823. Tang W, et al: Targeted expression of IL-11 in the murine airway causes airways obstruction, bronchial remodeling, and lymphocytic inflammation. J Clin Invest 98:2845–2853, 1996.

824. Wang J, et al: IL-11 selectively inhibits aeroallergen-induced pulmonary eosinophilia and Th2 cytokine production. J Immunol 165:2222–2231, 2000.

825. Manetti R, et al: Natural killer cell stimulatory factor (interleukin-12) induces T helper type 1 (Th1)-specific immune responses and inhibits the development of IL-4-producing Th cells. J Exp Med 177:1199–1204, 1993.

826. D'Andrea A, et al: Production of natural killer cell stimulatory factor (IL-12) by peripheral blood mononuclear cells. J Exp Med 176:1387–1398, 1992.

827. Hsieh CS, et al: Development of Th1 CD4+ T cells through IL-12 produced by Listeria-induced macrophages. Science 260:547–549, 1993.

828. Gately MK: Interleukin-12: a recently discovered cytokine with potential for enhancing cell-mediated immune responses to tumors. Cancer Invest 11:500–506, 1993.

829. Germann T, et al: Interleukin-12/T cell stimulatory factor, a cytokine with multiple effects on Th1 but not Th2 cells. Eur J Immunol 23:1762–1770, 1993.

830. Kubin M, et al: Interleukin 12 synergizes with B7/CD28 interaction in inducing efficient proliferation and cytokine production of human T cells. J Exp Med 180:211–222, 1994.

831. Cleveland MG, et al: Lipotechoic acid preparations of gram-positive bacteria induce interleukin-12 through a CD14-independent pathway. J Infect Immun 64:1906–1912, 1996.

832. Klinman DM, et al: CpG motifs present in bacterial DNA rapidly induce lymphocytes to secrete interleukin-6, interleukin-12, and interferon gamma. Proc Natl Acad Sci U S A 273:352–354, 1996.

833. Heufler C, et al: Interleukin-12 is produced by dendritic cells and mediates Th1 development as well as IFN-γ production by Th1 cells. Eur J Immunol 26:659–668, 1996.

834. Flesch IEA, et al: Early interleukin-12 production by macrophages in response to mycobacterial infection depends on interferon and tumor necrosis factor-α. J Exp Med 181:1615–1621, 1995.

835. Koch F, et al: High level IL-12 production by murine dendritic cells: up-regulation via MHC class II and CD40 molecules, and down-regulation by IL-4 and IL-10. J Exp Med 184:741–746, 1996.

836. Rogge L, et al: Selective expression of an interleukin-12 receptor component by human T helper 1 cells. J Exp Med 185:825–831, 1997.

837. Cooper AM, et al: The role of interleukin-12 in acquired immunity to Mycobacterium tuberculosis infection. Immunology 84:423–432, 1995.

838. Kawakami K, et al: IL-12 protects mice against pulmonary and disseminated infection caused by Cryptococcus neoformans. Clin Exp Immunol 104:208–214, 1996.

839. Greenberger M, et al: IL-12 gene therapy protects mice in lethal Klebsiella pneumonia. J Immunol 157:3006–3012, 1996.

840. Lee SM, et al: Decreased interleukin-12 from activated cord versus adult peripheral blood mononuclear cells and upregulation of interferon-gamma, natural killer, and lymphokine-activated killer activity by IL-12 in cord blood mononuclear cells. Blood 88:945–954, 1996.

841. Grabstein KH, et al: Cloning of a T cell growth factor that interacts with the β chain of the interleukin-2 receptor. Science 264:965–968, 1994.

842. Carson WE, et al: Interleukin-15 is a novel cytokine that activates human natural killer cells via components of the IL-2 receptor. J Exp Med 180:1395–1403, 1994.

843. Seder RA: High dose IL-2 and IL-15 enhance the in vitro priming of naïve CD4+ T cells for IFN-gamma, but have differential effects on priming for IL-4. J Immunol 156:2413–2422, 1996.

844. Cooper MA, et al: In vivo evidence for a dependence on interleukin-15 for survival of natural killer cells. Blood 100:3633–3638, 2002.

845. Perera LP, et al: IL-15 induces the expression of chemokines and their receptors in T lymphocytes. J Immunol 162:2606–2612, 1999.

846. Badolato R, et al: IL-15 induces IL-8 and monocyte chemotactic protein-1 production in human monocytes. Blood 90:2804–2809, 1997.

847. Girard D, et al: Differential effects of interleukin-15 and IL-2 on human neutrophils: modulation of phagocytosis, cytoskeleton rearrangement, gene expression, and apoptosis by IL-15. Blood 88:3176–3184, 1996.

848. Armitage RJ, et al: IL-15 has stimulatory activity for the induction of B cell proliferation and differentiation. J Immunol 154:483–490, 1995.

849. Zissel G, et al: In vitro release of interleukin-15 by bronchoalveolar lavage cells and peripheral blood mononuclear cells from patients with different lung diseases. Eur Cytokine Netw 11:105–112, 2000.

850. Muro S, et al: Expression of IL-15 in inflammatory pulmonary disease. J Allergy Clin Immunol 108:970–975, 2001.

851. Qian JX, et al: Decreased interleukin-15 from activated cord versus adult peripheral blood mononuclear cells and the effect of interleukin-15 in upregulating antitumor immune activity and cytokine production in cord blood. Blood 90:3106–3117, 1997.

852. Sciaky D, et al: Cultured human fibroblasts express constitutive IL-16 mRNA: Cytokine induction of active IL-16 protein synthesis through a caspase-3-dependent mechanism. J Immunol 163:3806–3814, 2000.

853. Zhang Y, et al: Processing and activation of pro-interleukin-16 by caspase-3. J Biol Chem 273:1144–1149, 1998.

854. Lim KG, et al: Human eosinophils elaborate leukocyte chemoattractants. J Immunol 156:2566–2570, 1996.

855. Laberge S, et al: Secretion of IL-16 from serotonin-stimulated CD8 T cells in vitro. J Immunol 155:310–315, 1996.

856. Arima M, et al: Expression of interleukin-16 by human epithelial cells. Am J Respir Cell Mol Biol 21:684–692, 1999.

857. Cheng G, et al: A549 cells can express interleukin-16 and stimulate eosinophil chemotaxis. Am J Respir Cell Mol Biol 25:212–218, 2001.

858. Cruikshank WW, et al: Lymphokine activation of T4+ T lymphocytes and monocytes. J Immunol 138:3817–3825, 1987.

859. Wang H, et al: Interleukin-16 in tracheal aspirate fluids of newborn infants. Early Hum Dev 67:79–86, 2002.

860. Peng Y, et al: Interleukin-17 and lung host defense against Klebsiella pneumoniae infection. Am J Respir Cell Mol Biol 25:335–340, 2001.

861. Aggarwal S, Gurney AL: IL-17: prototype member of an emerging cytokine family. J Leukoc Biol 71:1–8, 2002.

862. Jovanovic DV, et al: IL-17 stimulates the production and expression of proinflammatory cytokines IL-1β and TNF-α by human macrophages. J Immunol 160:3513–3521, 1998.

863. Fossiez F, et al: T cell interleukin-17 induces stromal cells to produce proinflammatory and hematopoietic cytokines. J Exp Med 183:2593–2603, 1996.

864. Laan M, et al: Neutrophil recruitment by human IL-17 via C-X-C chemokine release in the airway. J Immunol 162:2347–2352, 1999.

865. Kolls JK, et al: Interleukin-17: an emerging role in lung inflammation. Am J Respir Cell Mol Biol 28:9–11, 2003.

866. Hoshino H, et al: Increased elastase and myeloperoxidase activity associated with neutrophil recruitment by IL-17 in airways in vivo. J Allergy Clin Immunol 105:143–149, 2000.

867. Schwarzenberger P, et al: Requirement of endogenous stem cell factor and granulocyte colony-stimulating factor for IL-17–mediated granulopoiesis. J Immunol 164:4783–4789, 2000.

868. Dinarello CA: Interleukin-18, a proinflammatory cytokine. Eur Cytokine Netw 11:483, 2000.

869. Gu Y, et al: Activation of interferon-γ inducing factor mediated by interleukin-1β converting enzyme. Science 275:206–209, 1997.

870. Kojima H, et al: Interleukin-18 activates the IRAK-TRAF6 pathway in mouse EL-4 cells. Biochem Biophys Res Commun 244:183–186, 1998.

871. Novick D, et al: Interleukin-18 binding protein: a novel modulator of the Th1 cytokine response. Immunity 10:127–136, 1999.

872. Jordan JA, et al: Role of IL-18 in acute lung inflammation. J Immunol 167:7060–7068, 2001.

873. Dinarello CA: IL-18: a Th1-inducing, pro-inflammatory cytokine and new member of the IL-1 family. J Allergy Clin Immunol 103:11–24, 1999.

874. Micallef MF, et al: Interferon-γ–inducing factor enhances T helper 1 cytokine production by stimulated human T cells: synergism with interleukin-12 for interferon-γ production. Eur J Immunol 26:1647–1651, 1996.

875. Dao T, et al: Interferon-γ–inducing factor, a novel cytokine, enhances Fas ligand-mediated cytotoxicity of murine T helper cells. Cell Immunol 173:230–235, 1997.

876. Puren AJ, et al: Interleukin-18 induces IL-8 and IL-1β via TNFα production from non-CD14+ human blood mononuclear cells. J Clin Invest 101:711–724, 1998.

877. Kohka H, et al: Interleukin-18/interferon-γ–inducing factor, a novel cytokine upregulates ICAM-1 (CD54) expression in KG-1 cells. J Leukoc Biol 64:519–527, 1998.

878. Morel JC, et al: A novel role for interleukin-18 in adhesion molecule induction through NF kappa B and phosphatidylinositol (PI) 3-kinase–dependent signal transduction pathways. J Biol Chem 276:37069–37075, 2001.

879. Kawakami K, et al: IL-18 protects mice against pulmonary and disseminated infection with Cryptococcus neoformans by inducing IFN-γ production. J Immunol 159:5528–5534, 1997.

880. Bohn E, et al: IL-18 regulates early cytokine production in, and promotes resolution of, bacterial infection in mice. J Immunol 160:299–307, 1998.

881. Fujioka N, et al: Interleukin-18 protects mice against acute herpes simplex virus type 1 infection. J Virol 73:2401–2409, 1999.
882. Lauw FN, et al: IL-18 improves the early antimicrobial host response to pneumococcal pneumonia. J Immunol 168:372–378, 2002.
883. Narita M, et al: Close association between pulmonary disease manifestation in *Mycoplasma pneumoniae* infection and enhanced local production of interleukin-18 in the lung, independent of gamma interferon. Clin Diagn Lab Immunol 7:909–914, 2000.
884. Soares MVD, et al: IL-7 dependent extrathymic expansion of CD45RA+ T cells enable preservation of a naïve repertoire. J Immunol 161:5909–5917, 1998.
885. Moore TA, et al: Inhibition of gamma delta T cell development and early thymocyte maturation in IL-7-/- mice. J Immunol 157:2366–2373, 1996.
886. Goodwin RG, et al: Human interleukin-7: molecular cloning and growth factor activity on human and murine B lineage cells. Proc Natl Acad Sci U S A 86:302–306, 1989.
887. Alderson MR, et al: Interleukin-7 enhances cytolytic T lymphocyte generation and induces lymphokine-activated killer cells from human peripheral blood. J Exp Med 172:577–587, 1990.
888. Laky K, et al: Distinct requirements for IL-7 in development of TCRγδ cells during fetal and adult life. J Immunol 170:4087–4094, 2003.
889. Webb LM, et al: Putative role for interleukin-7 in the maintenance of the recirculating naïve CD4+ T-cell pool. Immunology 98:400–405, 1999.
890. Webb LM, et al: Interleukin-7 activates human naïve CD4+ cells and primes for interleukin-4 production. Eur J Immunol 27:633–640, 1997.
891. Whitehead BF, et al: Cytokine gene expression in human lung transplant recipients. Transplant 56:956–961, 1993.
892. Laky K, et al: The role of IL-7 in thymic and extrathymic development of TCRγδ cells. J Immunol 161:707–713, 1998.
893. Ambrus JL, et al: Identification of a receptor for high molecular weight human B cell growth factor. J Immunol 141:861–869, 1988.
894. Zlotnick A, Yoshie O: Chemokines: a new classification system and their role in immunity. Immunity 12:121–127, 2000.
895. Baggiolini M, Loetscher P: Chemokines in inflammation and immunity. Immunol Today 21:418–420, 2000.
896. Van den Steen PE, et al: Neutrophil gelatinase B potentiates interleukin-8 tenfold by amino-terminal processing, whereas it degrades CTAP-III, PF-4 and GRO-alpha and leaves RANTES and MCP-2 intact. Blood 96:2673–2681, 2000.
897. Loetscher P, et al: Interleukin-2 regulates CC chemokine receptor expression and chemotactic responsiveness in T lymphocytes. J Exp Med 184:569–577, 1996.
898. Strieter RM, et al: Human alveolar macrophage gene expression of interleukin-8 by TNF-α, LPS and IL-1β. Am J Respir Cell Mol Biol 2:321–326, 1990.
899. Goodman RB, et al: Cytokine-stimulated human mesothelial cells produce chemotactic activity for neutrophils including NAP-1/IL-8. J Immunol 148:457–465, 1992.
900. Wechsler AS, et al: Induction of IL-8 expression in T cells uses the CD28 co-stimulatory pathway. J Immunol 153:2515–2523, 1994.
901. Noah TL, Becker S: Respiratory syncytial virus-induced cytokine production by a human bronchial epithelial cell line. Am J Physiol 265:L472–L478, 1993.
902. Lukacs NW, et al: Stimulus and cell-specific expression of CXC and CC chemokines by pulmonary stromal cell populations. Am J Physiol 268:L856–L861, 1995.
903. Goodman RB, et al: Quantitative comparison of C-X-C chemokines produced by endotoxin-stimulated human alveolar macrophages. Am J Physiol 275:L87–95, 1998.
904. Detmers PA, et al: Neutrophil-activating protein 1/interleukin 8 stimulates the binding activity of the leukocyte adhesion receptor CD11b/CD18 on human neutrophils. J Exp Med 171:1155–1162, 1990.
905. Baggiolini M, et al: Activation of neutrophil leukocytes: chemoattractant receptors and respiratory burst. FASEB J 7:1004–1010, 1993.
906. Fogh K, et al: Interleukin-8 stimulates the formation of 15-hydroxy-eicosatetraenoic acid from human neutrophils in vitro. Agents Actions 35:227–231, 1992.
907. Bussolino F, et al: Synthesis of platelet-activating factor by polymorphonuclear neutrophils stimulated with interleukin-8. J Biol Chem 267:14598–14603, 1992.
908. McCain RW, et al: Leukotriene B₄ stimulates human polymorphonuclear leukocytes to synthesize and release interleukin-8 in vitro. Am J Respir Cell Mol Biol 10:651–657, 1994.
909. Walz A, et al: [Ca⁺²]i changes and respiratory burst in human neutrophils and monocytes induced by NAP-1/interleukin-8, NAP-2, and GRO/MGSA. J Leukoc Biol 50:279–286, 1991.
910. Kimata H, Lindley I: Interleukin-8 differentially modulates interleukin-4- and interleukin-2-induced human B cell growth. Eur J Immunol 24:3237–3240, 1994.
911. Peveri P, et al: A novel neutrophil-activating factor produced by human mononuclear phagocytes. J Exp Med 167:1547–1559, 1988.
912. Padrines M, et al: Interleukin-8 processing by neutrophil elastase, cathepsin G, and proteinase-3. FEBS Lett 352:231–235, 1994.
913. Boutten A, et al: Compartmentalized IL-8 and elastase release within the human lung in unilateral pneumonia. Am J Respir Crit Care Med 153:336–342, 1996.
914. Bohnet S, et al: Role of interleukin-8 in community acquired pneumonia: relation to microbial load and pulmonary function. Infection 25:92–100, 1997.
915. Maus U, et al: Expression of pro-inflammatory cytokines by flow-sorted alveolar macrophages in severe pneumonia. Eur Respir J 11:534–541, 1998.
916. Tsai WC, et al: CXC chemokine receptor CXCR2 is essential for protective innate host response in murine *Pseudomonas aeruginosa* pneumonia. Infec Immun 68:4289–4296, 2000.
917. Moore TA, et al: Bacterial clearance and survival are dependent on CXC chemokine receptor-2 ligands in a murine model of pulmonary Nocardia asteroides infection. J Immunol 164:908–915, 2000.
918. Rowen JL, et al: Group B streptococci elicit leukotriene B₄ and interleukin-8 from human monocytes: neonates exhibit a diminished response. J Infect Dis 172:420–426, 1995.
919. Schibler KR, et al: Diminished transcription of interleukin-8 by monocytes from preterm neonates. J Leukoc Biol 53:399–403, 1993.
920. Schultz C, et al: Enhanced interleukin-6 and interleukin-8 synthesis in term and preterm infants. Pediatr Res 51:317–322, 2002.
921. Jones CA, et al: Undetectable IL-10 and persistent IL-8 expression early in hyaline membrane disease: a possible developmental basis for the predisposition to chronic lung inflammation in preterm newborns. Pediatr Res 39:966–975, 1996.
922. Beresford MW, Shaw NJ: Detectable IL-8 and IL-10 in bronchoalveolar lavage fluid from preterm infants ventilated for respiratory distress syndrome. Pediatr Res 52:973–978, 2002.
923. Brown Z, et al: Chemokine gene expression and secretion by cytokine-activated human microvascular endothelial cells: differential regulation of monocyte chemoattractant protein-1 and interleukin-8 in response to interferon-γ. Am J Pathol 145:913–921, 1994.
924. Kasama T, et al: Expression and regulation of human neutrophil-derived macrophage inflammatory protein-1α. J Exp Med 178:63–72, 1993.
925. Standiford TJ, et al: The gene expression of MIP-1α from human blood monocytes and alveolar macrophages is inhibited by IL-4. Am J Respir Cell Mol Biol 9:192–198, 1993.
926. Miller MD, et al: A novel polypeptide secreted by activated human T lymphocytes. J Immunol 143:2907–2916, 1989.
927. Rolfe MW, et al: Expression and regulation of human pulmonary fibroblast-derived monocyte chemotactic peptide (MCP-1). Am J Physiol 263:L536–L545, 1992.
928. Standiford TJ, et al: Alveolar macrophage-derived cytokines induce monocyte chemoattractant protein-1 expression from human pulmonary type II like epithelial cells. J Biol Chem 266:9912–9918, 1991.
929. Antony VB, et al: Pleural mesothelial cell expression of C-C (monocyte chemotactic peptide [MCP-1]) and C-X-C (interleukin-8 [IL-8]) chemokines. Am J Respir Cell Mol Biol 12:581–588, 1995.
930. Leonard EJ, et al: Biological aspects of monocyte chemoattractant protein-1 (MCP-1). Adv Exp Med Biol 305:57–64, 1991.
931. Rot A, et al: RANTES and macrophage inflammatory protein-1 alpha induce the migration and activation of normal human eosinophil granulocytes. J Exp Med 176:1489–1495, 1992.
932. Dahinden CA, et al: Monocyte chemotactic protein 3 is a most effective basophil- and eosinophil-activating chemokine. J Exp Med 179:751–756, 1994.
933. Rollins BJ, et al: Recombinant human MCP-1/JE induces chemotaxis, calcium flux, and the respiratory burst in human monocytes. Blood 8:1112–1116, 1991.
934. Locati M, et al: Rapid induction of arachidonic acid release by monocyte chemotactic protein-1 and related chemokines. J Biol Chem 269:4746–4753, 1994.
935. Vaddi K, Newton RC: Regulation of monocyte integrin expression by β-family chemokines. J Immunol 153:4721–4732, 1994.
936. Carr MW, et al: Monocyte chemoattractant protein-1 acts as a T-lymphocyte chemoattractant. Proc Natl Acad Sci U S A 91:3652–3656, 1994.
937. Taub DD, et al: Monocyte chemotactic protein-1 (MCP-1), -2 and -3 are chemotactic for human T lymphocytes. J Clin Invest 95:1370–1376, 1995.
938. Schall TJ, et al: Human macrophage inflammatory protein alpha (MIP-1α) and MIP-1β chemokines attract distinct populations of lymphocytes. J Exp Med 177:1821–1826, 1993.
939. Maghazachi A, et al: CC chemokines induce the chemotaxis of NK and IL-2–activated NK cells. J Immunol 153:4969–4977, 1994.
940. Chang M, et al: Transforming growth factor β1, macrophage inflammatory protein-1α, and interleukin-8 gene expression is lower in stimulated human neonatal compared with adult mononuclear cells. Blood 84:118–124, 1994.
941. Sullivan SE, et al: Circulating concentrations of chemokines in cord blood, neonates, and adults. Pediatr Res 51:653–657, 2000.
942. Hariharan D, et al: C-C chemokine profile of cord blood mononuclear cells: selective defect in RANTES production. Blood 95:715–718, 2000.
943. Murch SH, et al: Early production of macrophage inflammatory protein-1 alpha occurs in respiratory distress syndrome and is associated with poor outcome. Pediatr Res 40:490–497, 1996.
944. Baier RJ, et al: Monocyte chemoattractant protein-1 and interleukin-8 are increased in bronchopulmonary dysplasia: relation to isolation of *Ureaplasma urealyticum*. J Investig Med 49:362–369, 2001.
945. Baier RJ, et al: Increased interleukin-8 and monocyte chemoattractant protein-1 concentrations in mechanically ventilated preterm infants with pulmonary hemorrhage. Pediatr Pulmonol 34:131–137, 2002.
946. Garofalo RP, et al: Macrophage inflammatory protein-1α (not T helper type 2 cytokines) is associated with severe forms of respiratory syncytial virus bronchiolitis. J Infect Dis 183:393–399, 2001.

947. Inwald DP, et al: High concentrations of GRO-α and MCP-1 in bronchoalveolar fluid of infants with respiratory distress syndrome after surfactant. Arch Dis Child Fetal Neonatal Ed 78:F234-235, 1998.

948. Hardy KJ, Sawada T: Human gamma interferon strongly upregulates its own gene expression in peripheral blood lymphocytes. J Exp Med 170:1021-1026, 1989.

949. Munakata T, et al: Induction of interferon-γ production by human natural killer cells stimulated by hydrogen peroxide. J Immunol 134:2449-2455, 1985.

950. Murray HW: Interferon-gamma, the activated macrophage, and host defense against microbial challenge. Ann Intern Med 108:595-608, 1988.

951. Stuehr DJ, Marletta MA: BCG infection, lymphokine, or IFN-γ induce nitrite/nitrate production by murine macrophages and enhance their synthesis in response to LPS. J Immunol 139:518-525, 1987.

952. Gifford GE, et al: Gamma interferon priming of mouse and human macrophages for induction of tumor necrosis factor production by bacterial lipopolysaccharide. J Natl Cancer Inst 78:121-124, 1987.

953. Jaffe HA, et al: Organ-specific cytokine therapy: local activation of mononuclear phagocytes by delivery of an aerosol of recombinant interferon-γ to the human lung. J Clin Invest 88:297-302, 1991.

954. Look DC, et al: Selective induction of intracellular adhesion molecule-1 by interferon-γ in human airway epithelial cells. Am J Physiol 263:L79-L87, 1992.

955. Dustin ML, et al: Induction by IL-1 and interferon-γ: tissue distribution, biochemistry and function of a natural adherence molecule (ICAM-1). J Immunol 137:245-254, 1986.

956. Koeffler HP, et al: Gamma-interferon induces expression of the HLA-D antigens on normal and leukemic human myeloid cells. Proc Natl Acad Sci U S A 81:4080-4084, 1984.

957. Maraskovsky E, et al: IL-2 and IFN-gamma are two necessary lymphokines in the development of cytolytic T cells. J Immunol 143:1210-1214, 1989.

958. Pernis A, et al: Lack of interferon gamma receptor beta chain and the prevention of interferon gamma signaling in TH1 cells. Science 269:245-247, 1995.

959. Newport MJ, et al: A mutation in the interferon-gamma receptor gene and susceptibility to mycobacterial infection. N Engl J Med 335:1941-1949, 1996.

960. Bhardwaj N, et al: Interferon gamma–activated human monocytes inhibit the intracellular multiplication of Legionella pneumophila. J Immunol 137:2662-2669, 1986.

961. Flynn JL, et al: An essential role for interferon gamma in resistance to Mycobacterium tuberculosis. J Exp Med 178:2249-2254, 1993.

962. Brummer E, et al: Recombinant and natural gamma-interferon activation of macrophages in vitro: different dose requirements for induction of killing activity against phagocytizable and nonphagocytizable fungi. Infect Immun 49:724-730, 1985.

963. Rothermel CD, et al: Oxygen-independent inhibition of intracellular Chlamydia psittaci growth by human monocytes and interferon-γ–activated macrophages. J Immunol 137:689-692, 1986.

964. Skerrett S, Martin T: Intratracheal interferon-γ augments pulmonary defenses in experimental legionellosis. Am J Respir Crit Care Med 149:50-58, 1994.

965. Rubins JB, Pomeroy C: Role of gamma interferon in the pathogenesis of bacteremic pneumococcal pneumonia. Infect Immun 65:2975-2977, 1997.

966. Standiford TJ, et al: Cytokines as mediators of lung innate immunity. In Marshall JC, Cohen J (eds): Immune Response in the Critically Ill. Berlin, Springer-Verlag, 2000, pp 140-154.

967. Mobbs KJ, et al: Cytokines in severe respiratory syncytial virus bronchiolitis. Pediatr Pulmonol 33:449-452, 2002.

968. Laiho M, Keski-Oja J: Transforming growth factors-beta as regulators of cellular growth and phenotype. Crit Rev Oncog 3:1-26, 1992.

969. Munger JS, et al: The integrin alpha v beta 6 binds and activates latent TGF beta 1: a mechanism for regulating pulmonary inflammation and fibrosis. Cell 96:319-328, 1999.

970. McCartney-Francis N, et al: TGF-β regulates production of growth factors and TGF-β by human peripheral blood monocytes. Growth Factors 4:27-35, 1990.

971. Chantry D, et al: Modulation of cytokine production by transforming growth factor-beta. J Immunol 142:4295-4300, 1989.

972. Ding A, et al: Macrophage deactivating factor and transforming growth factors-beta 1, beta 2 and beta 3 inhibit induction of macrophage nitrogen oxide synthesis by IFN-gamma. J Immunol 145:940-944, 1990.

973. Czarniecki CW, et al: Transforming growth factor beta 1 modulates the expression of class II histocompatibility antigens on human cells. J Immunol 140:4217-4223, 1988.

974. Kehrl JH, et al: Transforming growth factor-β suppresses human B lymphocyte Ig production by inhibiting synthesis and switch from the membrane form to the secreted form of Ig mRNA. J Immunol 146:4016-4023, 1991.

975. Chang M, et al: Transforming growth factor-beta 1, macrophage inflammatory protein-1α, and interleukin-8 gene expression is lower in stimulated human neonatal compared with adult mononuclear cells. Blood 84:118-124, 1994.

976. Buron E, et al: Markers of pulmonary inflammation in tracheobronchial fluid of premature infants with respiratory distress syndrome. Allergol Immunopathol 27:11-17, 1999.

977. Kotecha S, et al: Increase in the concentration of transforming growth factor beta-1 in bronchoalveolar lavage fluid before development of chronic lung disease of prematurity. J Pediatr 128:464-469, 1996.

978. Reynolds SD, et al: Secretoglobins SCGB3A1 and SCGB3A2 define secretory cell subsets in mouse and human airways. Am J Respir Crit Care Med 166:1498-1509, 2002.

979. Burmeister R, et al: A two-receptor pathway for catabolism of Clara cell secretory protein in the kidney. J Biol Chem 276:13295-13301, 2001.

980. Mukherjee AB, et al: Uteroglobin: a novel cytokine? Cell Mol Life Sci 55:771-787, 1999.

981. Miele L, et al: Inhibition of phospholipase A_2 by uteroglobin and antiflammin peptides. Adv Exp Med Biol 279:137-160, 1990.

982. Dierynck I, et al: Potent inhibition of both human interferon-γ production and biologic activity by the Clara cell protein CC16. Am J Respir Cell Mol Biol 12:205-210, 1995.

983. Johnston CJ, et al: Altered pulmonary response to hyperoxia in Clara cell secretory protein deficient mice. Am J Respir Cell Mol Biol 17:147-155, 1997.

984. Harrod KS, et al: Clara cell secretory protein decreases lung inflammation after acute virus infection. Am J Physiol 275:L924-930, 1998.

985. Chen LC, et al: Altered pulmonary eosinophilic inflammation in mice deficient for Clara cell secretory 10-kDa protein. J Immunol 167:3025-3028, 2001.

986. Watson TM, et al: Altered lung gene expression in CCSP-null mice suggests immunoregulatory roles for Clara cells. Am J Physiol 281:L1523-1530, 2001.

987. Magdaleno SM, et al: Interferon-gamma regulation of Clara cell gene expression: in vivo and in vitro. Am J Physiol 272:L1142-1151, 1997.

988. Arsalane K, et al: Clara cell specific protein (CC16) expression after acute lung inflammation induced by intratracheal lipopolysaccharide administration. Am J Respir Crit Care Med 161:1624-1630, 2000.

989. Lassus P, et al: Clara-cell secretory protein in preterm infants' tracheal aspirates correlates with maturity and increases in infection. Pediatr Pulmonol 30:466-469, 2000.

990. Ramsay PL, et al: Clara cell secretory protein oxidation and expression in premature infants who develop bronchopulmonary dysplasia. Am J Respir Crit Care Med 164:155-161, 2001.

991. Tazi A, et al: Spontaneous release of granulocyte colony-stimulating factor (G-CSF) by alveolar macrophages in the course of bacterial pneumonia and sarcoidosis: endotoxin-dependent and endotoxin-independent G-CSF release by cells recovered by bronchoalveolar lavage. Am J Respir Cell Mol Biol 4:140-147, 1991.

992. Wang JM, et al: Chemotactic activity of human recombinant granulocyte-macrophage colony-stimulating factor. Immunology 60:439-444, 1987.

993. Weisbart RH, et al: Human granulocyte-macrophage colony-stimulating factor is a neutrophil activator. Nature 314:361-363, 1985.

994. Cox G, et al: Bronchial epithelial cell–derived cytokines (G-CSF and GM-CSF) promote the survival of peripheral blood neutrophils in vitro. Am J Respir Cell Mol Biol 7:507-513, 1992.

995. Zhou X, et al: Human upper airway structural cell–derived cytokines support human peripheral blood monocyte survival: a potential mechanism for monocyte/macrophage accumulation in the tissue. Am J Respir Cell Mol Biol 4:525-531, 1992.

996. Warren MK, Ralph P: Macrophage growth factor CSF-1 stimulates human monocyte production of interferon, tumor necrosis factor, and colony-stimulating activity. J Immunol 137:2281-2285, 1986.

997. Fischer HG, et al: Granulocyte-macrophage colony-stimulating factor-cultured bone marrow-derived macrophages reveal accessory cell function and synthesis of MHC class II determinants in the absence of external stimuli. Eur J Immunol 18:1151-1158, 1988.

998. Tazi A, et al: Evidence that granulocyte-macrophage colony-stimulating factor regulates the distribution and differentiated state of dendritic cells/Langerhans cells in human lung and lung cancers. J Clin Invest 91:566-576, 1993.

999. Gill EA, et al: Bacterial lipopolysaccharide induces endothelial cells to synthesize a degranulating factor for neutrophils. FASEB J 12:673-684, 1998.

1000. Papoff P, et al: Granulocyte colony-stimulating factor, granulocyte-macrophage colony-stimulating factor and neutrophils in the bronchoalveolar lavage fluid of premature infants with respiratory distress syndrome. Biol Neonate 80:133-141, 2001.

1001. Nelson S, Bagby GJ: Granulocyte colony-stimulating factor and modulation of inflammatory cells in sepsis. Clin Chest Med 17:319-332, 1996.

1002. Root RK, Dale DC: Granulocyte colony-stimulating factor and granulocyte-macrophage colony-stimulating factor: comparisons and potential for use in the treatment of infections in nonneutropenic patients. J Infect Dis 179:S342-S352, 1999.

1003. Schibler KR, et al: Production of granulocyte colony-stimulating factor in vitro by monocytes from preterm and term neonates. Blood 82:2478-2484, 1993.

1004. Johnston B, Kubes P: The α4-integrin: an alternative pathway for neutrophil recruitment? Immunol Today 20:545-550, 1999.

1005. Hemler ME, et al: Structure of the integrin VLA-4 and its cell-cell and cell-matrix adhesion functions. Immunol Rev 114:45-65, 1990.

1006. Arnaout MA: Structure and function of the leukocyte adhesion molecules CD11/CD18. Blood 75:1037-1050, 1990.

1007. Worthen GS, et al: Mechanics of stimulated neutrophils: cell stiffening induces retention in capillaries. Science 245:183-186, 1988.

1008. Smith CW, et al: Cooperative interactions of LFA-1 and Mac-1 with intercellular adhesion molecule-1 in facilitating adherence and transendothelial migration of human neutrophils in vitro. J Clin Invest 83:2008-2017, 1989.

1009. Graham IL, Brown EJ: Extracellular calcium results in a conformational change in Mac-1 (CD11b/CD18) on neutrophils: differentiation of adhesion and phagocytosis functions on Mac-1. J Immunol 146:685-691, 1991.

1010. Newton RA, et al: Signalling mechanisms and the activation of leukocyte integrins. J Leukoc Biol 61:422-426, 1997.

1011. Springer TA: Adhesion receptors of the immune system. Nature 346:425-434, 1990.

1012. Elices MJ, et al: VCAM-1 on activated endothelium interacts with the integrin VLA-4 at a site distinct from the VLA-4/fibronectin binding site. Cell 60:577-584, 1990.

1013. Piedboeuf B, et al: Increased endothelial cell expression of platelet endothelial cell adhesion molecule-1 during hyperoxic lung injury. Am J Respir Cell Mol Biol 19:543-553, 1998.

1014. Olsen SL, et al: PECAM expression increases with gestational age. Pediatr Pulmonol 33:255-262, 2002.

1015. Yang J, et al: Targeted gene disruption demonstrates that P-selectin glycoprotein ligand 1 (PSGL-1) is required for P-selectin-mediated but not E-selectin-mediated neutrophil rolling and migration. J Exp Med 190:1769-1782, 1999.

1016. Vaporciyan AA, et al: Involvement of platelet endothelial cell adhesion molecule-1 in neutrophil recruitment in vivo. Science 262:1580-1582, 1993.

1017. Kuhns DB, et al: Loss of L-selectin (CD62L) on human neutrophils following exudation in vivo. Cell Immunol 164:306-310, 1995.

1018. Geng J, et al: Rapid neutrophil adhesion to activated endothelium mediated by GMP-140. Nature 343:757-760, 1990.

1019. Bevilacqua MP, Stengelin S, et al: Endothelial leukocyte adhesion molecule 1: an inducible receptor for neutrophils related to complement regulatory proteins and lectins. Science 243:1160-1165, 1989.

1020. Kawamura N, et al: Lipoteichoic acid-induced neutrophil adhesion via E-selectin to human umbilical vein endothelial cells. Biochem Biophys Res Commun 217:1208-1215, 1995.

1021. Lozada C, et al: Identification of C1q as the heat-labile serum cofactor required for immune complexes to stimulate endothelial expression of the adhesion molecules E-selectin and intercellular and vascular cell adhesion molecules 1. Proc Natl Acad Sci U S A 92:8378-8382, 1995.

1022. Vora M, et al: Interleukin-10 induces E-selectin on small and large blood vessel endothelial cells. J Exp Med 184:821-829, 1996.

1023. Phillips ML, et al: ELAM-1 mediates cell adhesion by recognition of a carbohydrate ligand, sialyl-Le^x. Science 250:1130-1132, 1990.

1024. Vestweber D, Blanks JE: Mechanisms that regulate the function of the selectins and their ligands. Physiol Rev 79:181-213, 1999.

1025. Picker LJ, et al: The neutrophil selectin LECAM-1 presents carbohydrate ligands to the vascular selectins ELAM-1 and GMP-140. Cell 66:921-933, 1991.

1026. Hogg N: Roll, roll, roll your leucocyte gently down the vein. Immunol Today 13:113-115, 1992.

1027. Hogg JC, Doerschuk CM: Leukocyte traffic in the lungs. Annu Rev Physiol 57:97-114, 1995.

1028. Butcher EC: Leukocyte-endothelial cell recognition: three (or more) steps to specificity and diversity. Cell 67:1033-1036, 1991.

1029. Springer TA: Traffic signals for lymphocyte recirculation and leukocyte emigration: the multistep paradigm. Cell 76:301-314, 1994.

1030. Brown E: Neutrophil adhesion and the therapy of inflammation. Semin Hematol 34:319-326, 1997.

1031. Liu Y, et al: The role of CD47 in neutrophil transmigration. J Biol Chem 276:40156-40166, 2001.

1032. Behzad AR, et al: Fibroblasts are in a position to provide directional information to migrating neutrophils during pneumonia in rabbit lungs. Microvasc Res 51:303-316, 1996.

1033. Downey GP, et al: Neutrophil sequestration and migration in localized pulmonary inflammation: capillary localization and migration across the interalveolar septum. Am Rev Respir Dis 147:168-176, 1993.

1034. Carlos TM, Harlan JM: Leukocyte-endothelial adhesion molecules. Blood 84:2068-2101, 1994.

1035. Doerschuk CM, et al: Comparison of neutrophil and capillary diameters and their relation to neutrophil sequestration in the lung. J Appl Physiol 74:3040-3045, 1993.

1036. Motosugi J, et al: Changes in neutrophil actin and shape during sequestration induced by complement fragments in rabbits. Am J Pathol 149:963-973, 1996.

1037. Pecsvarady Z, et al: Kinetics of granulocyte deformability following exposure to chemotactic stimuli. Blood Cells 18:333-352, 1992.

1038. Mulligan MS, et al: Neutrophil-dependent acute lung injury: requirement for P-selectin (GMP-140). J Clin Invest 90:1600-1607, 1993.

1039. Doyle NA, et al: Neutrophil margination, sequestration, and emigration in the lungs of L-selectin deficient mice. J Clin Invest 99:526-533, 1997.

1040. Ramamoorthy C, et al: CD18 adhesion blockade decreases bacterial clearance and neutrophil recruitment after intrapulmonary E coli, but not after S aureus. J Leukoc Biol 61:167-172, 1997.

1041. Qin L, et al: The roles of CD11/CD18 and ICAM-1 in acute Pseudomonas aeruginosa-induced pneumonia in mice. J Immunol 157:5016-5021, 1996.

1042. Mulligan MS, et al: Role of β1, β2 integrins and ICAM-1 in lung injury following deposition of IgG and IgA immune complexes. J Immunol 150:2407-2417, 1993.

1043. Doerschuk CM, et al: Adhesion molecules and cellular biomechanical changes in acute lung injury. Chest 116:37S-43S, 1999.

1044. Keeney SE, et al: Oxygen-induced lung injury in the guinea pig proceeds through CD18-independent mechanisms. Am J Respir Crit Care Med 149:311-319, 1994.

1045. Mulligan MS, et al: Role of leukocyte adhesion molecules in complement-induced lung injury. J Immunol 150:2401-2406, 1993.

1046. Mackarel AJ, et al: Interleukin-8 and leukotriene-B4, but not formylmethionyl leucylphenylalanine, stimulate CD18-independent migration of neutrophils across human pulmonary endothelial cells in vitro. Am J Respir Cell Mol Biol 23:154-161, 2000.

1047. Mizgerd JP, et al: Selectins and neutrophil traffic: margination and Streptococcus pneumoniae-induced emigration in murine lungs. J Exp Med 184:639-645, 1996.

1048. Sherman MP, et al: Role of pulmonary phagocytes in host defense against group B streptococci in preterm versus term rabbit lung. J Infect Dis 166:818-826, 1992.

1049. Burns JA, et al: The α4β1 and α5β1 integrins mediate β2 integrin-independent neutrophil recruitment to endotoxin-induced lung inflammation. J Immunol 166:4644-4649, 2001.

1050. Johnston B, Kubes P: The α4-integrin: an alternative pathway for neutrophil recruitment? Immunol Today 20:545-560, 1999.

1051. Taooka Y, et al: The integrin α9α1 mediates adhesion to activated endothelial cells and transdendothelial neutrophil migration through interaction with vascular cell adhesion molecule-1. J Cell Biol 145:413-420, 1999.

1052. Shang XZ, Isskutz AC: Beta 2 and beta 1 integrin mechanisms in migration of human polymorphonuclear leucocytes and monocytes through lung fibroblast barriers: shared and distinct mechanisms. Immunology 92:527-535, 1997.

1053. Tasaka S, et al: Very late antigen-4 in CD18-independent neutrophil emigration during acute bacterial pneumonia in mice. Am J Resp Crit Care Med 166:53-60, 2002.

1054. Knapp S, et al: Alveolar macrophages have a protective anti-inflammatory role during murine pneumococcal pneumonia. Am J Respir Crit Care Med 167:171-179, 2003.

1055. Armstrong L, et al: Interleukin-10 regulation of tumour necrosis factor alpha from human alveolar macrophages and peripheral blood monocytes. Thorax 51:143-149, 1996.

1056. Park DR, Skerrett SJ: IL-10 enhances the growth of Legionella pneumophila in human mononuclear phagocytes and reverses the protective effects of IFN-γ: differential responses of blood monocytes and alveolar macrophages. J Immunol 157:2528-2538, 1996.

1057. Toews GB: Cytokines and pulmonary host defense against microbes. In Nelson S, Martin TR (eds): Cytokines in Pulmonary Disease. New York, Marcel Dekker, 2000, pp 1-17.

1058. Rubins J: Alveolar macrophages: wielding the double-edged sword of inflammation. Am J Respir Crit Care Med 167:103-104, 2003.

1059. Nelson S, et al: Intratracheal granulocyte colony-stimulating factor enhances systemic and pulmonary host defenses. Am Rev Respir Dis 143S:A398, 1991.

1060. Unanue ER, Allen PM: The basis for the immunoregulatory role of macrophages and other accessory cells. Science 236:551-557, 1987.

1061. Salusto F, et al: The role of chemokine receptors in primary, effector, and memory immune responses. Annu Rev Immunol 18:593-620, 2000.

1062. Pitzalis C, et al: Selective migration of the human helper-inducer memory T cell subset: confirmation by in vivo cellular kinetic studies. Eur J Immunol 21:369-376, 1991.

1063. June CH, et al: Role of the CD28 receptor in T-cell activation. Immunol Today 11:211-216, 1990.

1064. Linsley PS, et al: CTLA-4 is a second receptor for the B cell activation antigen B7. J Exp Med 174:561-569, 1991.

1065. Sallusto F, et al: Flexible programs of chemokine receptor expression on human polarized T helper 1 and 2 lymphocytes. J Exp Med 187:875-883, 1998.

1066. Bonecchi R, et al: Differential expression of chemokine receptors and chemotactic responsiveness of type I T helper cells (Th1s) and Th2s. J Exp Med 187:129-134, 1998.

1067. van Vlasselaer P, et al: Transforming growth factor-β directs IgA switching in human B cells. J Immunol 148:2062-2067, 1992.

1068. Ryan M, et al: Bordetella pertussis respiratory infection in children is associated with preferential activation of type I T helper cells. J Infect Dis 175:1246-1250, 1997.

165

Scott L. Pomeroy and Nicole J. Ullrich

Development of the Nervous System

DEVELOPMENT OF THE CENTRAL NERVOUS SYSTEM

During development, the central nervous system is transformed from a thin layer of undifferentiated tissue into a complex, multilayered system that is capable of processing information and organizing actions. This chapter reviews the major processes of neuronal development as a framework to describe disorders that arise as a result of interruptions in the developmental pathway. The normal developmental sequence and the developmental regulation of gene expression are arranged in approximate chronologic order. An overview of the major events in central nervous system development is provided in Table 165-1.

EARLY CELL DIVISIONS AND CYTOLOGIC SPECIALIZATION

Following division of the fertilized ovum, the two blastomeres retain full developmental potential, as evidenced by the occurrence of identical twins. Within a few cellular divisions, the developmental potential of each cell is determined and becomes restricted. Thus, a degree of specialization is achieved, and the individual cells are no longer capable of giving rise to an intact organism. This progressive specialization of cells, a fundamental aspect of neural development, relates to selective expression of the genome. This selective expression is governed not only by genetic factors, but also by epigenetic influences from the cytoplasm, neighboring cells, or the extracellular environment.[1, 2] Because neural development does not proceed according to an

unalterable plan fixed in the genome, studies of development must take into account both intrinsic and extrinsic influences on the differentiating cells. Similarly, abnormal development can be understood only if the relative contributions of both genetic and epigenetic factors are considered.

FORMATION OF THE BASIC STRUCTURE OF THE NERVOUS SYSTEM (EMBRYOGENESIS)

Early Developmental Events

The rostrocaudal axis of the embryo is initially delineated by the formation of the primitive streak during the two germ cell layer blastula stage. The rostral end of the primitive streak is marked by the Hensen's node. The mesoderm and the notochord arise by an inward migration of cells through the primitive streak, thus creating a third cell layer (Fig. 165-1.) Mesoderm rostral to Hensen's node is referred to as *prechordal mesoderm*, whereas that in close proximity to the notochord is designated *chordal mesoderm*. As the inward migration of presumptive mesoderm progresses to completion, Hensen's node moves caudally, leaving the developing neural plate behind.[1] The transformation of ectoderm into neural epithelium is induced by underlying mesoderm.[3] The inductive process may vary in different regions of the presumptive neural plate, because the brain stem and spinal cord arise under the influence of the chordal mesoderm (dorsal induction), whereas the structurally different forebrain arises under the influence of prechordal mesoderm (ventral induction).[4-6]

Primary and Secondary Neurulation (Dorsal Induction)

Normal Development

During neurulation, the flat sheet of ectoderm is transformed into an elongated tube, the neural tube, by the folding of the neural plate along the rostral-caudal axis. This process is referred to as *primary neurulation*, which refers to events related to formation rostral to the lumbar region, whereas those caudal to the lumbar region are referred to as *secondary neurulation* (Fig. 165-2). During this complex process, many different tissues interact to induce and achieve regional specialization of the neuroectoderm. Induction by chordal mesoderm transforms cuboidal ectoderm into columnar neural epithelium,[7] the first step in the formation of the neural tube. This neural plate is present by 15 days gestation as a midline thickening of the dorsal ectoderm.[8]

Regulatory molecules expressed during neurulation underlie the induction and patterning; despite years of investigation, the

TABLE 165-1

Major Events in Neural Development

Development Event	Peak Time
Primary neurulation	3-4 wk
Prosencephalic cleavage (ventral induction)	5-6 wk
Neuronal proliferation	
Cerebral	2-4 mo
Cerebellar	2-10 mo postnatal
Neuronal migration	
Cerebral	3-5 mo
Cerebellar	4-10 mo postnatal
Neuronal differentiation	
Axon outgrowth	3 mo-birth
Dendritic growth and synapse formation	6 mo-1 yr postnatal
Synaptic rearrangement	Birth-years postnatal
Myelination	Birth-years postnatal

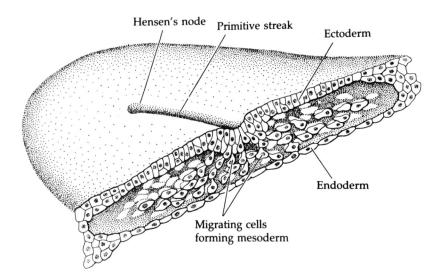

Hensen's node   Primitive streak   Ectoderm

Endoderm

Migrating cells
forming mesoderm

Figure 165–1. Segregation of germ layers, demonstrated in the anterior half of a chick embryo. The invagination of cells through the primitive streak delineates mesoderm from ectoderm and endoderm. Prechordal mesoderm lies anterior to the Hensen's node, whereas chordal mesoderm surrounds the notochord, which will soon form beneath the primitive streak. (From Purves D, Lichtman JW: Principles of Neural Development. Sunderland, MA, Sinauer Associates, 1985, p 12, after Balinsky.[1])

precise molecular basis of this induction remains unknown. Although early investigations focused on neurotransmitters, such as catecholamines or serotonin,[9-12] or other local messengers,[13,14] the molecules follistatin and noggin have emerged as probable neural tube–inducers derived from mesoderm.[15,16]

Neural folds soon appear at the edges of the neural plate as the epithelium continues to thicken and assumes the cytoarchitecture of a pseudostratified epithelium. Although folding of the neural epithelium may occur in part by mechanical forces generated by the expanding neural plate,[17] most experimental evidence indicates that factors intrinsic to the cytoskeleton of the neural epithelial cells are responsible for the process of primary neurulation.[18] By 18 days gestation, a midline groove can be seen in the neural plate.[19] Within the columnar cells, randomly arranged microtubules align themselves with the long axis of the cell, and a ring of actin filaments forms at the cell apex.[20-22] Association of actin with myosin[23] and a protein called spectrin[24] leads to a constriction of the cell apex, which occurs as the cells continue to elongate. Because the apical ends of the neural epithelial cells are joined by tight junctions,[25] the consequence of the cellular forces is a folding of the neural plate such that the edges become approximated at the midline.[17] Primary neurulation occurs with no appreciable cellular proliferation. Not surprisingly, however, the process is arrested by agents that inhibit the formation of microtubules and actin.[20-22,26]

Fusion of the neural folds to form the neural tube begins on day 22 of gestation at the site of the future lower brain stem (see Fig. 165–2). From this point, the fusion progresses rostrally and caudally and results in closure of the anterior neuropore by day 25 of gestation and the caudal neuropore by day 26 of gestation.[6,19] The mechanism of this fusion is incompletely understood, but it may involve nerve cell adhesion molecules (NCAMs)[27] or other components within the extracellular matrix.[28,29] Indirect evidence is from the failure of neurulation following disruption of integrin alpha 6 subunit, which mediates the attachment of neural plate cells to the basal lamina.[30]

As the neural tube closes, cells at the edge of the neural plate separate from the neural epithelium and migrate into the extracellular matrix to become neural crest cells (see Fig. 165–2). This separation is accompanied by a loss of cadherin-mediated cell adhesion from the surrounding neuroepithelium with local decrease in NCAM levels. It is also accompanied by an increase in the cell adhesion to the extracellular matrix with increased expression of fibronectin.[31] Migrating cells extend cellular motile processes to facilitate migration through the embryo in order, ultimately, to reach the final phenotypic sites.[32] Neural

crest cells migrate widely to become neurons and glia in dorsal root and autonomic ganglia. The fate of neural crest derived cells is also to provide innervation for the gastrointestinal tract and become neurons in the sensory ganglia of the cranial nerves (also formed in part by ectodermal placodes)[33] and to become melanocytes, cartilage of the bone and face, and a variety of endocrine and structural tissues.

The ultimate phenotypic and developmental fate of neural crest cells is tied to the timing, mode, and pattern of migration and is in large part controlled by the environment in which they reside. There is complex interplay between the expression of inhibitory extracellular matrix components as well as the dynamic ratio between permissive versus inhibitory components. The most important players in the control of neural crest cell migration are fibronectin, laminin isoforms 1 and 8, aggrecan, and PG-M/versican isoforms V0 and V1.[31] In chick quail chimeras, transplanted crest cells tend to assume the phenotype of the location to which they migrate rather than that of their place of origin.[34-36] Cultured postmitotic crest cells can be induced to change expression of neurotransmitters in myocyte-conditioned medium.[37-39] From these experiments, it can be inferred that the neural crest cells retain a relatively broad developmental potential as they begin migration and that their ultimate fate is strongly influenced by local factors.

Secondary neurulation arises in the conus medullaris, as well as the lower lumbar and sacrococcygeal segments of spinal cord. Given the specific pattern of malformations involving the caudal aspect of the neural tube, it has been postulated that caudal development involves a distinct sequence of cellular and molecular mechanisms.[40] The caudal ends of the neural tube and notochord are contiguous with an undifferentiated group of cells, the caudal cell mass, which extends into the tail fold. By day 30 of gestation, vacuoles coalesce within this mass, become confluent, and contact the central canal of the neural tube. Cellular migration and mesoderm formation in the caudal embryo are influenced by T-box transcription factors and components of the Wnt signaling pathway.[41] As this process of canalization or cavitation progresses during the ensuing weeks, neurons and ependymal cells differentiate to form the caudal end of the spinal cord.[19] Resorption of the tail and other cells of the caudal cell mass leaves the filum terminale, which often contains ependymal cell nests along its length. These nests of ependymal cells that remain can begin to proliferate later in life as a monoclonal population of glial cells. These ependymomas, which are uncommon glial cell tumors, are nonetheless one of the most common tumors of the cauda equina and filum terminale.

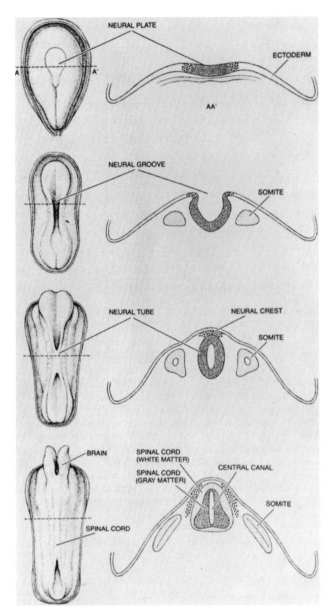

Figure 165–2. Closure of the neural tube in a human embryo during the third and fourth weeks of gestation represented in drawings showing an external view of the embryo (*left*) and a cross-section through the future spinal cord (*right*). As the neural tube forms, cells of the neural crest separate from the neuraxis. (From Cowan WM: The Development of the Brain. Copyright 1979 by Scientific American. All rights reserved.)

Genetic Influences on Neurulation

There have been many recent advances in the study of transcription factors and their role in the control of gene expression during development. Genetic studies defining the molecular signals that govern the development of the fruit fly *Drosophila* have led to the discovery of human homologues and thus have provided new insights into the molecular basis of human central nervous system development. These studies have uncovered a family of genes that direct morphologic development of the fly. At the earliest stages of development, maternal effect genes establish the anteroposterior axis of the embryo and then regulate the expression of genes that establish the boundaries of body segments.[42] These in turn, regulate the expression of *homeotic* genes, which then induce the development of macro-

scopic structures within the boundaries of these segments.[43] Molecular studies have determined that homeotic genes encode a family of transcription factors that are believed to induce the expression of a battery of genes leading to morphologic development of specific body segments and partitioning into morphogenetic units. The homeotic genes were discovered through analysis of mutant forms of *Drosophila*.[43] In some cases, mutations of the homeotic genes were found to promote the anomalous development of macroscopic structures on incorrect segments. One of these genes, *Antennapedia*, normally induces the development of legs on the second thoracic segment. A mutation has been discovered that brings *Antennapedia* under the control of cranial segment promoters, leading to the growth of legs on the fly head.[44]

Mammalian homologues of the *Drosophila* homeotic genes, also called the Hox genes, play key roles in the control of genes that affect embryonic patterning, cell differentiation, and malignant transformation. A vertebrate homologue of the *Drosophila hedgehog* gene, *Sonic Hedgehog (Shh)*, has been found to have a wide variety of activities in vertebrate development. Shh is a soluble factor expressed within the notochord and secreted from the notochord and the floor plate. The receptor Patched (Ptch) is expressed within the presumptive floor plate.[45–47] This regional localization is important for dose-dependent induction during the formation of the floor plate and differentiation of ventral neurons within the spinal cord. Shh is also important for the regulation of some aspects of segmentation and establishing the anteroposterior axis.[48, 49] The cellular response is mediated by receptors as well as transcription factors, which up- and down-regulate activity of Shh in the patterning of diverse cell types.[50–52] Activation of the Shh signal transduction pathway has many other functions; it has been thought to regulate proliferation and inhibit differentiation of spinal cord precursor cells[53] and may thus contribute to tumorigenesis. Mutations of Shh have been associated with holoprosencephaly, with failure of cleavage of midline and frontal structures.[54] These disorders will be discussed in further detail in the section on disorders of prosencephalic development. Members of a family of Hox genes, controlled in part by retinoic acid from the Hensen node, have been found to be critical for specification of hindbrain rhombomeres and segmentally defined development.[55] Exogenous retinoic acid appears to exert teratogenic effects by the anomalous expression of these genes.

Disorders of Structures Derived from Dorsal Induction

Malformations resulting from errors in neural tube formation are among the most severe congenital anomalies. They often are accompanied by alterations in the overlying skeleton, meninges, and skin. Most result in a markedly shortened life span. In general, the more severe anomalies arise earlier in development. The disorders of primary neurulation and failure of neural tube closure are reviewed in order of decreasing severity. This is followed by disorders of secondary neurulation, composed of occult dysraphic states and defects in neural crest migration, both of which are related to neural tube formation.

Neural Tube Defects

Craniorachischisis Totalis. This disorder arises from total failure of neural tube closure and as such is estimated to originate no later than day 22 of gestation.[19, 56] The central nervous system is represented essentially by a neural plate remnant, with no overlying dermal or skeletal covering. Recently, a candidate gene for craniorachischisis was identified in the loop-tail mutant mouse. The human orthologue LPP1 is expressed in the ventral part of the developing neural tube but is excluded from the floor plate where Shh is expressed. Loss of function permits more extensive floor plate induction by Shh and thereby leads to inhibition of midline bending of the neural plate during neurulation.[57] Most embryos with this anomaly are aborted

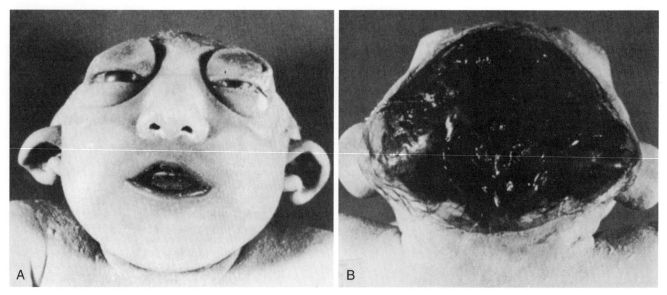

Figure 165–3. A fetus with anencephaly, from frontal **(A)** and dorsal **(B)** views. (Courtesy of Dr. Ronald Lemire.)

spontaneously; only a few survive to term and then typically die within hours.

Anencephaly. This anomaly arises from errors of anterior neural tube closure and is estimated to originate before day 25 of gestation. The defect may extend through the level of the foramen magnum (holoacrania or holoanencephaly) or may be more restricted (meroacrania or meroanencephaly) but characteristically involves the cerebral hemispheres and portions of the brain stem. With no dermal or skeletal covering, the exposed neural tissue appears to degenerate[58] (Fig. 165–3). Genetic and environmental influences both play a role in the development of anencephaly. The incidence of this anomaly is unusually high in some regions of the British Isles.[19, 59] There is an increased incidence with extremes of maternal age, low socioeconomic class, and a positive family history.[59, 60] Most affected fetuses are either spontaneously aborted or stillborn. Of those who survive to term, nearly all die within 1 week without the assistance of mechanical ventilation.

Myeloschisis. This disorder is the result of a failure of posterior neural tube closure and originates no later than 26 days of gestation.[43] The exposed neural plate anomaly extends the length of the spinal cord and has no dermal or skeletal covering. Most affected fetuses are stillborn.

Encephalocele. This disorder probably arises from a restricted disturbance of anterior neural tube closure, although some investigators have failed to find evidence for a dysraphic lesion.[26, 61] The abnormality occurs in the occipital region in 75% of cases in the western hemisphere,[62] though frontal encephaloceles are more common in Southeast Asia.[63] Portions of the brain, the meninges, or both, are herniated through a defect in the skull. The cortical cytoarchitecture of the herniated cerebral tissue is relatively normal, although areas of hemorrhage, necrosis, and focal cortical anomalies are not unusual.[61] The mass is covered with skin and ranges in size from very small to larger than the cranium. Neurologic outcome depends on the size of the defect, the quantity of brain in the protruding lesion, and the presence of other associated anomalies. For example, the Meckel syndrome, inherited in an autosomal recessive pattern, is characterized by an occipital encephalocele, microcephaly, microphthalmia, cleft lip and palate, polydactyly, polycystic kidneys, ambiguous genitalia, and other anomalies.[64] The prognosis with this disorder, understandably, is extremely poor.[65]

Myelomeningocele. This disorder arises from a restricted failure of posterior neural tube closure and therefore is estimated to

arise no later than day 26 of gestation. Approximately 80% of lesions involve the lumbar region. Only a small percentage (fewer than 15%) are restricted to cervical, thoracic, or sacral levels.[66] Within the defect, neural tissue ranges from a neural plate remnant to a variety of abortive neural tube-like structures. The dorsal aspect of the spinal cord tends to be affected to a greater extent than the ventral. Vertebral arches are lacking, although an epithelial covering is sometimes present. Spinal cord lesions above the myelomeningocele, such as syringomyelia, hydromyelia, and diastematomyelia, or split cord, are common.[66,67] Most pathologic evidence indicates that the open lesion arises from a failure of neural tube closure[68, 69] rather than from a reopening of a closed neural tube.[70]

As with anencephaly, the incidence of myelomeningocele is increased in some parts of Great Britain.[71] Neurologic deficits are directly related to the level of the cord lesion and to the presence of associated brain anomalies. Nearly all cases of thoracic myelomeningocele are accompanied by an Arnold-Chiari malformation; as a consequence, hydrocephalus is sometimes present, which usually requires placement of a ventriculoperitoneal shunt. Moreover, as many as one-third of infants experience symptoms consistent with brain stem dysfunction, which is the most common cause of death beyond the neonatal period.[72] There is hypoplasia or aplasia of cranial nerve nuclei in approximately 20% of infants with myelomeningocele who do not survive the neonatal period.[73] Other anomalies of the central nervous system, such as cerebral cortical abnormalities, are associated with myelomeningocele and may account in large part for a higher-than-average incidence of seizures and intellectual impairment.[74] In one careful neuropathologic study of 25 infants, 92% exhibited some degree of cortical dysplasia, 40% of which consisted of polymicrogyria.[73]

Etiology of Neural Tube Defects. Although the cause of most neural tube defects is unknown, a model of multigenetic inheritance with environmental influences is considered best at present.[71,73,75] Evidence for a genetic influence includes ethnic predisposition that persists after relocation to areas of low incidence[71,76] and persistence of a low incidence rate in other ethnic groups despite migration to areas of higher incidence,[71] high prevalence among females,[71] increased incidence with parental consanguinity,[19] increased concordance in monozygotic twins, and increased incidence among close relatives.[77] Environmental influences have been suggested by correlation of incidence with geographic location,[71] association with low socioeconomic status,[71] associations with maternal hyperthermia during the first trimester of pregnancy,[78] maternal diabetes,[79] and the teratogenic effects of drugs,[80] especially maternal valproate ingestion.[81] The teratogenic effects of aminopterin, a folic acid antagonist,[82] have been of particular interest because subsequent studies led to the discovery that folic acid supplementation around the time of conception has a significant preventive effect on the occurrence of neural tube defects.[59,83]

Occult Dysraphic States. Disorders of caudal neural tube formation, that is, secondary neurulation, involve the caudal spinal cord and its coverings. The occult dysraphic states are commonly associated with vertebral anomalies and are usually covered with skin. Elongation of the conus medullaris and shortening and thickening of the filum terminal with "tethering" of these structures may result in traction injuries to the spinal cord. An association of these disorders with primary neural tube malformations is suggested by the occurrence of primary neurulation defects in 4.1% of siblings with occult dysraphic lesions.[84]

The occult dysraphic states are commonly associated with vertebral anomalies and are usually covered with skin. A *myelocystocele* is a localized dilation of the central canal in the caudal spinal cord often associated with severe malformations, including cloacal exstrophy and vertebral anomalies.[18] The caudal cord in *diastematomyelia* is divided by a septum arising from a vertebral body. *Diplomyelia* is a divided, and at times duplicated, spinal cord with no septum. *Meningocele* is an extrusion of subarachnoid space with no gross abnormality of either the brain or spinal cord; when associated with a lipoma, the abnormality is referred to as a *lipomeningocele*. *Lipomata* and other tumors such as *teratomata*, *neuroblastomata*, and *ganglioneuromata* may occur and extend into the dural space. A cutaneous dimple in the lumbosacral region may be contiguous with a *dermal sinus* and a *dermal (dermoid)* or *epidermal (epidermoid) cyst* or may extend into the vertebral canal. Lipoma and dermal sinus are the most common of the occult dysraphic states.[85]

Disorders of Neural Crest–Derived Cells

The group of anomalies consistent with a general defect in neural crest development are known as neurocristopathies. In the piebaldism-Waardenburg syndrome, children have hypoganglionosis, congenital megacolon, abnormalities of the great vessels, sensorineural deafness, and abnormalities of skin, hair, and iris pigmentation.[86] Although this disorder is rare, more restricted abnormalities of neural crest development are considerably more common.

A more common disorder of neural crest cells is colonic aganglionosis (Hirschsprung disease). This disorder is characterized by a congenital lack of neurons in the enteric plexus of the colon as a result of either failure of migration or failure of differentiation of neural crest cells. The rectum is always involved, and more proximal segments are included with decreasing frequency.[87, 88] The anomaly presents in the newborn period as megacolon, the most common cause of neonatal colonic obstruction.[89] A mutation in L1CAM, a gene that encodes a neural cell adhesion molecule, has been described in newborn males with congenital hydrocephalus, aqueductal stenosis, and/or agenesis of the corpus callosum and Hirschsprung disease, suggesting a role for L1CAM-mediated cell adhesion.[90]

Disorders of the spinal and autonomic ganglia are apparently quite rare,[63] but they include congenital insensitivity to pain and familial dysautonomia. Congenital insensitivity to pain with anhidrosis is an autosomal-recessive disorder resulting from defective neural crest differentiation. First-order sensory afferents, which are responsible for pain and temperature sensation, are lacking. In addition, there is neuronal loss in the sympathetic ganglia. Immunohistochemistry with antibodies directed against the S100 protein and neuron-specific enolase, markers of glial and neuronal differentiation, fail to show nerve fibers in the vicinity of the eccrine sweat glands.[91] The presence of multiple coincident neurocristopathies has been reported, specifically with the association between congenital central hypoventilation, long-segment intestinal aganglionosis (Hirschsprung), and autonomic dysfunction and between congenital central hypoventilation, Hirschsprung, and neuroblastoma.[92, 93]

Prosencephalic Cleavage (Ventral Induction)

Normal Development

On day 22 of gestation, as the neural folds begin to close to form the neural tube, the future midbrain and forebrain exist as only a small amount of tissue at the rostral end of the neural plate. The optic vesicles are represented by two thickenings on either side. These thickenings are joined by the optic ridge, the rostral end of the neural plate at this stage, which will later be the site of the optic chiasm.[5] The neural folds close, proceeding both rostrally from the region of the lower brain stem and also caudally from the optic ridge. By day 24 of gestation, closure of the neural folds is nearly complete. Optic vesicles are clearly seen on either side of the rostral neural tube, which is displaced ventrally by the newly formed cranial flexure (Fig. 165–4). The prosencephalon,

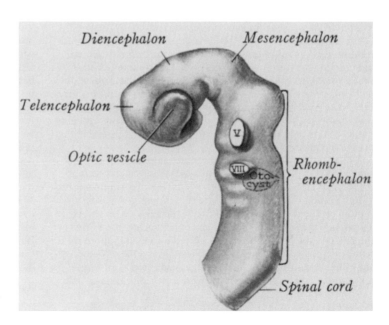

Figure 165–4. A human embryo at approximately 24 days' gestation. The diencephalon and telencephalon (the future cerebral hemispheres) are derived from the prosencephalon. (From Arey LB: Developmental Anatomy. Philadelphia, WB Saunders Co, 1965, p 473.)

which is the rostral portion of the neural tube, soon gives rise to the cerebral hemispheres, olfactory bulbs, and diencephalons under the inductive influence of the ventrally located prechordal mesoderm. These structures are said to arise from ventral induction.[94] This inductive interaction also has an important role in the formation of the face; thus, anomalies of brain development in this region often manifest parallel abnormalities in midline and facial development.

By 35 days' gestation, rudiments of the cerebrum and cerebellum are evident. Both cerebral vesicles begin to evaginate from the neural tube by the end of the fifth week of gestation. As the cerebral vesicles expand, their walls are initially of uniform thickness and are without regional differentiation.[6] By 6 to 8 weeks of gestation, the portion of the neural tube between the cerebral vesicles begins to thicken as it becomes densely populated with cells; this connecting structure constitutes the lamina reuniens. The anterior neural tube, ventral to the lamina reunions, remains thin and sparsely populated with cells and constitutes the lamina terminalis. Over the next 2 weeks, a midline groove forms within the lamina reunions; the groove deepens and then folds so that its walls fuse, forming the commissural plate, through which the cerebral commissures will pass.[95]

Within the neuraxis, clusters of neurons along the midline begin to form nuclei of the brain stem, thalamus, and hypothalamus. Soon afterward, the ganglionic eminence, which is the precursor of the basal ganglia, forms within the wall of the cerebral vesicles. Axons from the olfactory epithelium extend and establish contact with the cerebral wall,[96] which is followed by development of the olfactory bulbs over the sixth and seventh weeks of gestation.[19] Thus, by 6 to 8 weeks of gestation, the basic structure of the central nervous system is formed, concluding embryogenesis. The remarkable expansion of the cerebral hemispheres follows during the remainder of gestation (Fig. 165-5).

Disorders of Structures Derived from Ventral Induction

In the neonate, a wide spectrum of phenotypic expression is seen in association with disorders of structures derived from ventral induction. The range of neurologic abnormalities varies from severe to moderate, and because the malformations usually involve the cerebral hemispheres, mental retardation is very common. The first group of disorders to be discussed, the holoprosencephalies, represents the most common and best-defined group of anomalies related to ventral induction. Other faciotelencephalic malformations, which are either very rare or less clearly related to ventral induction, are considered subsequently.

Holoprosencephaly. Holoprosencephaly is the most common developmental defect of the forebrain and midface in humans; as a group, holoprosencephalies are characterized by fusion (or failure of cleavage) of the cerebral hemispheres into distinct right and left hemispheres. These anomalies occur as a continuum; complete fusion of the cerebral hemispheres is termed *alobar holoprosencephaly*, nearly complete separation of the hemispheres by an interhemispheric fissure is termed *lobar holoprosencephaly*, and intermediate lesions are termed *semilobar holoprosencephalies*. Holoprosencephalic brains with a partial interhemispheric fissure tend to be best developed in the occipital region.[63]

Alobar holoprosencephaly is often accompanied by a significant reduction of brain weight, sometimes to less than one fourth the normal amount.[63] The cerebrum consists of a single sphere with a common ventricle, lacking either a corpus callosum or a septum pellucidum (Fig. 165-6). Deep nuclei, such as the basal ganglia and the structures of the diencephalons, are often fused in the midline. The third ventricle is covered by a membranous roof, which may distend as a large cyst posteriorly, and the optic nerves are either hypoplastic or fused into a single nerve. All forms of holoprosencephaly are associated with a lack of olfactory bulbs

and tracts, which led early investigators to name this group of anomalies *arhinencephaly*. Because this term only partially encompasses the spectrum of malformation, it has been largely discarded. Microscopic examination reveals cortical cytoarchitecture suggestive of the hippocampus or other limbic structures and many areas of cortical disorganization. The most striking aspect of cortical cyctoarchitecture, however, is the marked reduction of neocortex, the hallmark of the human cerebrum.[97]

Clinically, neonates afflicted with alobar holoprosencephaly exhibit apneic episodes, seizures, poikilothermia, and essentially a total lack of higher cortical function. These infants uniformly die within months.[98] Semilobar and lobar holoprosencephalies tend to manifest less reduction of brain weight than does alobar holoprosencephaly.[63] Some cases of lobar holoprosencephaly exhibit only frontal hypoplasia, with hemispheric fusion occurring in the depths of the frontal interhemispheric fissure. These affected children are generally severely mentally retarded and the extent of deficit is directly correlated with the extent of malformation. Those infants with semilobar holoprosencephaly may have slight neurologic development and occasionally survive into childhood. Although most children with lobar holoprosencephaly are severely mentally retarded, they may survive beyond childhood. In less severely afflicted children, the anomaly may escape detection until later in infancy.

Facial anomalies associated with holoprosencephaly vary in severity. The most severe anomaly, cyclopia, is represented by a single midline eye with variable duplication of intrinsic ocular structures. The only nasal structure, a proboscis, may be located above the eye. Marked ocular hypotelorism, with or without a proboscis, is referred to as *ethmocephaly*, and hypotelorism with a flat, single-nostril nose is called *cebocephaly* (after the Cebus monkey). Lesser anomalies include ocular hypotelorism, a flat nose, and midline or bilateral cleft lip and palate. Although the most severe facial anomalies are associated with profound brain anomalies, holoprosencephaly may occur with normal facial development.[19] Conversely, severe facial anomalies of the types observed with holoprosencephaly may occur with normal brain development.[98] Thus, although it is often true that the facial anomaly reflects the brain malformation,[99] this relationship is not entirely consistent. For fetuses with cyclopia, the time of onset of the developmental disturbance is estimated to be no later than 24 days of gestation. Other forms of holoprosencephaly arise by at least day 35 of gestation, when the cerebral hemispheres begin to evaginate from the neural tube.[6, 19] The incidence is about 50-fold greater in aborted embryos than in live births, which indicates that the majority are eliminated prenatally.[100]

Genetically, holoprosencephaly has been associated with a variety of chromosomal abnormalities, most often involving chromosomes 13 to 15 and 18. Autosomal dominant and autosomal recessive as well as X-linked recessive patterns of inheritance have been reported.[101] The genes implicated in holoprosencephaly have recently begun to be identified, and include Shh, ZIC2, SIX3, and TGIF.[102] Holoprosencephaly can be caused by haplo-insufficiency for Shh and by mutations in *ptch*, the gene that encodes the receptor for Shh, which normally acts to repress Shh signaling.[103] Teratogenic causes have also been identified.[104] The incidence is increased in infants of diabetic mothers[105] and has been reported in pregnant ewes that ingest *Veratrum californicum*,[106] which suggests that environmental factors may have a role in the cause of these disorders. The biologically active compound has been identified as cyclopamine, a steroidal alkaloid that may function by antagonism of a post-translationally modified Shh cholesterol moiety.[107] Initially, it was thought that inhibition of cholesterol synthesis could induce holoprosencephaly[108]; however, more recent evidence suggests that compounds that block cholesterol transport by affecting the vesicular trafficking of Niemann-Pick C1 protein

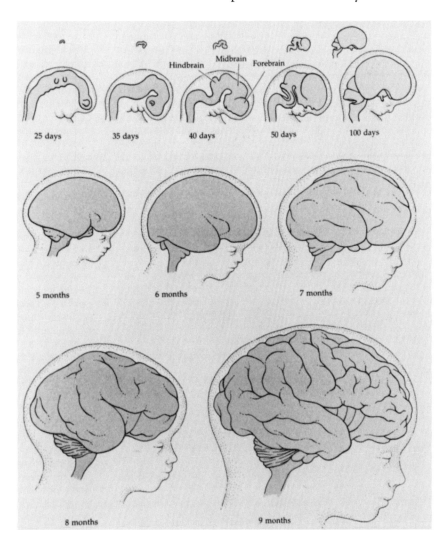

Hindbrain Midbrain Forebrain

25 days   35 days   40 days   50 days   100 days

5 months   6 months   7 months

8 months   9 months

Figure 165–5. Development of the human brain showing the remarkable increase in size of the cerebrum throughout gestation. The five earliest stages are enlarged to show structural detail. (Cowan WM: From Development of the Brain. Copyright 1979 by Scientific American. All rights reserved.)

(NPC1), which is structurally similar to Ptch, are weak Shh antagonists. In fact, NPC1 and Ptch are found to co-localize.[109] Smith-Lemli-Opitz syndrome, an inherited deficiency of the enzyme dehydrocholesterol reductase, has been associated with a less severe form of holoprosencephaly,[108] putatively secondary to the dependence on cholesterol in the biogenesis of Shh and in signal transduction in Shh-responsive cells.[110,111]

Faciotelencephalic Malformations. Other telencephalic malformations with associated facial anomalies result in a spectrum of disturbances of prosencephalic development, which include disorders more severe and less severe than holoprosencephaly. The most severe anomaly, atelencephalic-aprosencephalic microcephaly, is characterized by essentially a total lack of telencephalic and sometimes diencephalic structures. This rare malformation may arise from failure of formation of all or part of the prosencephalon or may be a destructive lesion.[112] Infants thus affected characteristically experience no neurologic development and die in the neonatal period. At the other end of the spectrum, either septo-optic dysplasia or agenesis of the corpus callosum may manifest mild facial involvement with little or no intellectual impairment.

DEVELOPMENT FOLLOWING THE EMBRYONIC PERIOD

After the first 6 weeks of gestation, expansion of the cerebral hemispheres occurs by the proliferation of neurons and glia and then by the growth of neural and glial processes. Over the first 3 months of the postembryogenic period, the full adult complement of neurons proliferates and populates the developing brain. It is a remarkable fact that the neurons formed during this relatively short period may live as long as a century or more. Because differentiated neurons are unable to replicate, they are unable to repopulate the cortex following losses sustained in the perinatal period and beyond.

The differentiation of neurons begins after proliferation of neuronal precursors within specific germinal centers that are always in close proximity to the ventricular or pial surfaces of the developing brain. These young neurons, then, must migrate to the site that they will occupy in the mature brain. As neuronal differentiation proceeds, axons are elaborated and grow to specific sites in the brain to establish synaptic contacts with dendrites and cell bodies of other neurons. Over the course of months to years, a refinement of these synaptic connections occurs, and myelination of axons ensues.

Neuronal and Glial Proliferation

Normal Development

Before the fifth week of gestation, the wall of the early neural tube is a pseudostratified columnar epithelium formed from morphologically identical cells that are actively proliferating. Within the epithelium, the nuclei undergoing deoxyribonucleic acid (DNA) synthesis (the S phase of the cell cycle; Fig. 165-7) are located in the outer half of the ventricular layer. During the postsynthetic gap phase (G2), the cells assume a rounded contour and then undergo mitosis (M phase) at the ventricular luminal surface, followed by a return to the periphery during the G1 phase to again undergo DNA synthesis.[113-115] This interkinetic, "to-and-fro" nuclear migration is repeated with each cell cycle and mitosis. The G1 phase has been defined as the control point for neuronal proliferation.[116] Cell division at this time is symmetric, such that each progenitor cell gives rise to two similar progenitor cells. Cell number, therefore, increases geometrically.[117] The epithelium soon separates into a ventricular zone on the ventricular luminal surface and a cell-sparse marginal zone, representing processes of cells within the

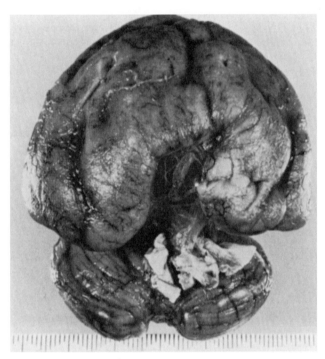

Figure 165-6. Posterior view of a brain exhibiting holoprosencephaly and pachygyria. (From Friede RL: Developmental Neuropathology. New York, Springer-Verlag, 1975, p 284.)

ventricular zone intermingled with the first afferent fibers (Fig. 165-8).[118]

By embryonic day 40, the first neurons form within the ventricular zone. Morphologic analysis and immunohistochemical staining of monkey cerebrum have demonstrated the presence of proliferative units that are composed of both neurons and glial cells within the ventricular zone at this time.[119-121] Progenitor cells become committed to their fundamental phenotype within the germinal epithelium, likely in response to environmental cues.[122] Cell division now becomes asymmetric; each progenitor cell gives rise to two dissimilar daughter cells, one of which becomes a neuron that will migrate to the cortical plate and the other of which remains as a stem cell or dies. With this change in cell division, cell numbers no longer increase geometrically but rather increase arithmetically.[119, 120] Neuronal lineage studies have demonstrated the presence of both multipotential precursor cells as well as committed cells within the cortical germinative zones. A direct transition from a pluripotent cell to a defined phenotype has been postulated for the neural lineage. Clonally related cells may become widely dispersed by tangential or lateral migration and have multiple phenotypes in the mature cortex.[123] The postmitotic neurons become arranged in columns and begin migrating away from the ventricular zone in a radial fashion, initially guided by contacts with surrounding glial cells as well as with neighboring neurons.[119] An intermediate zone containing these migrating neurons forms between the ventricular and marginal zones. By the seventh week of gestation, migrating neurons begin formation of the cortical plate at the junction of the intermediate and marginal zones (see Fig. 165-8).[124-127] Between the ventricular and intermediate zones, the subventricular zone becomes a second site of proliferation, although the cells in this region do not undergo interkinetic movements. This zone is the predominant source of neurons later in the proliferative period.[128]

Neuronogenesis in the cerebral hemispheres ends at midgestation (approximately embryonic day 125).[128] During the period of generation of neurons, most precursor cells are specified to generate a single cell type, and only a few are multipotent; however, there is a growing body of evidence that selective populations of neuronal progenitor cells exist into adulthood. The mechanisms of generation of progenitor cells are largely unclarified; however, their maintenance requires molecules along the Notch pathway.[129, 130] Progenitor cells are also depleted in embryonic brains that are deficient for the presenilin 1 (PS1) gene, which is a key regulator of Notch signaling.[129] Mutations in presenilin 1

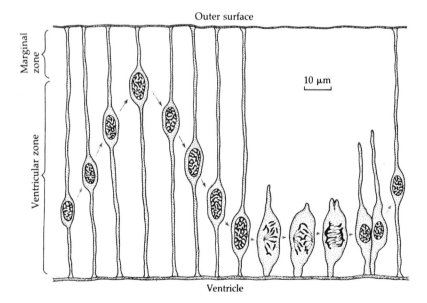

Figure 165-7. Interkinetic nuclear migration during cell proliferation within the ventricular zone. Cell divisions occur at the ventricular surface. Migration outward precedes DNA duplication; the cells then return to the ventricular surface to complete the cell cycle with another division. (From Purves D, Lichtman JW: Principles of Neural Development. Sunderland, MA, Sinauer Associates, 1985, p 19, after Sauer.[98])

are a major cause of familial Alzheimer's disease. Lack of PS1 is thought to be involved in a cell fate decision between postmitotic neurons and neural progenitor cells, as lack of PS1 leads to premature differentiation.[131] Notch signaling is also thought to allow cells that are in direct contact to adopt different fates; thus, local regulation of the notch pathway allows for use of the same signaling mechanism in a variety of different contexts during development.[132] Other genetic and environmental influences are important in the generation and maintenance of progenitor cells. For example, transcription factors such as NeuroD homologues of the helix-loop-helix proteins have been postulated as determination factors, to commit progenitor cells to neuronal fate and alter neuronal differentiation.[133] The role of extracellular signals in regulation of progenitor differentiation is poorly understood, but there is increasing evidence that cell adhesion molecules inhibit cell proliferation and induce differentiation to the neuronal lineage, as indicated by an increase in the number of cells staining positively for microtubule-associated protein 2.[134]

There is growing evidence that neuronogenesis occurs into adulthood, at least in the olfactory cortex and hippocampus.[135-138] Recently, it has also been shown that regions of the adult brain and spinal cord ventricular surface can generate new neurons, as detected by the presence of neural cell adhesion molecules.[139] More recent studies have focused on cortical neurogenesis after injury in adult mammals. After transient middle cerebral artery occlusion, cells with neuron-specific markers are distributed throughout cortex, with the highest density along the border of injury.[140] Ischemic conditions in another experimental paradigm stimulate proliferation of progenitor cells in both young and old rats, but this results in neuronogenesis only in young animals.[141]

Glial proliferation, in contrast to neuronal proliferation, continues regularly throughout life.[127,142,143] Glial cells arise initially early in cortical development. Both glial and neuronal precursors can be found within the ventricular zone,[121] and lineage analysis has demonstrated that neuronal and glial lineages begin to diverge early.[144] The role of extracellular signals in the regulation of differentiation is poorly understood. Clonal analysis indicates that the postnatal cortex produces a diffusible factor that induces progenitor cells to adopt glial fates at the expense of neuronal fates.[145] Laboratory studies have demonstrated that multipotent cerebral progenitor cells grown *in vitro* differentiate into neurons when exposed to platelet-derived growth factor (PDGF) and assume glial phenotype when exposed to ciliary neurotrophic factor (CNTF)[146] or fibroblast growth factor (FGF2).[145] Local factors appear to be important, as cortical progenitors cultured over embryonic cortical slices differentiate into neurons and those cultured over postnatal cortical slices differentiate into glia, suggesting that there are developmentally and environmentally regulated signals.[145]

Following generation within the ventricular zone, glial precursors migrate into the developing cerebral wall, in which they continue to proliferate.[147] Environmental cues also play a role in phenotypic determination during migration to the final destination. Differentiation of glia does not appear to be completely dependent on lineage. Interactions with neurons and other glia, either by direct contact or through soluble factors, are necessary for expression of the adult phenotype.[148-150] Tight clusters of clonally related neurons or glial cells have been found to retain a radially oriented relationship within the mature cortex. Moreover, proliferating progenitor cells in the subventricular zone are in close association with immature astrocytes expressing both vimentin and glial fibrillary acidic protein.[151] The regulation of cycle in glial cells is important both during development and in response to injury, whereas dysregulation of control has been associated with aberrant proliferation and the development of malignant glial tumors.[152] In mammalian cells, the Ras cells, the Ras signaling pathway is an important regulator of cell cycle; uncontrolled Ras signaling has been implicated in human gliomas. In glia, the activation of Ras can either increase or decrease proliferation through its effects on downstream regulators.[153]

Disorders

Because of the rapid pace of neuronal proliferation and its relative restriction in time, it is understandable that an appropriately timed insult could have profound effects on the number of neurons present in the adult brain (Table 165-2). Insults sustained before embryonic day 40, when cells within the neural epithelium are increasing geometrically, would be expected to have a larger impact than those occurring after day 40, when postmitotic neurons already have been formed and neurons are increasing arithmetically. Given the uncertainties in counting large numbers of neurons, it is difficult to define a group of disorders that unequivocally arise from aberrant proliferation. Nonetheless, a number of disorders exist that presumably represent severely deficient production (micrencephaly) or excessive production (macrencephaly) of neurons and glia, because the brain is generally well formed in all respects but size.

Micrencephaly Vera. This heterogeneous group of disorders is defined by the presence of a small brain that does not result from either a destructive event or a derangement of other developmental processes. The timing of onset is, presumably, before the fourth month of gestation; insults incurred earliest in this interval would result in the most severe deficits in brain size. Unlike micrencephaly caused by overt destructive lesions (e.g., cerebral infarctions), neonates with this disorder only rarely exhibit major neurologic signs, such as seizures, although they commonly exhibit mental retardation later.[59]

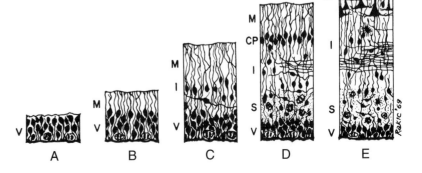

Figure 165–8. Development of the embryonic zones and cortical plate within the cerebral hemispheres. Cortical afferents arrive in the intermediate zone and terminate beneath the cortical plate. CP = cortical plate; I = intermediate zone M = marginal zone; S = subventricular zone; V = ventricular zone. (From Sidman RL, Rakic P: Brain Res *62*:1, 1973.)

TABLE 165-2

Classification of Developmental Disorders by Time of Onset

1. *Induction (3-4 wk)*
   Anencephaly
   Myeloschisis
   Encephalocele
   Myelomeningocele
   Occult dysraphic states
2. *Ventral induction (5-10 wk)*
   Holoprosencephaly
   Septo-optic dysplasia
   Agenesis of corpus callosum
3. *Neuronal proliferation/differentiation (2-5 mo)*
   Micrencephaly vera
   Macrencephaly
   Hemimegalencephaly
   Tuberous sclerosis
4. *Migration (2-5 mo)*
   Schizencephaly
   Lissencephaly
   Pachygyria
   Polymicrogyria
   Heterotopias
5. *Postmigration (>5 mo)*
   Congenital insensitivity to pain
   Mental retardation
   Autism
6. *Myelination (birth-years postnatal)*
   Primary deficiency of myelination
   Hirschsprung disease
   Congenital dysautonomia

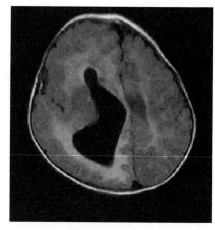

Figure 165–9. Hemimegalencephaly. Axial images reveal marked enlargement of the right cerebral hemisphere as compared to the left. There is straightening of the frontal horn and indistinct gray-white matter distinction in the right frontoparietal region. In addition, the cortices have abnormal gyral patterns. (Courtesy of Drs. Karen Moeller and Richard Robertson.)

It is estimated that as many as 60% of cases of micrencephaly have a genetic cause. The small size is thought to involve either a decrease in the number or in the size of proliferative units.[154] Autosomal recessive, X-linked recessive, and autosomal dominant patterns of inheritance have been described. Several familial patterns, some with associated chorioretinopathy or other ocular disorders, have also been described. Often, no identified cause or pattern of inheritance is found. In the Amish population, a new metabolic disorder characterized by severe, lethal congenital microcephaly and 2-ketoglutaric aciduria has been described, with an unusually high incidence of at least 1 in 500 births.[155] Several environmental factors have been implicated, including irradiation, maternal alcoholism, maternal phenylketonuria, anticonvulsant drugs, organic mercurials, excessive vitamin A, and intrauterine infections (especially rubella and cytomegalovirus).[98]

Macrencephaly. An equally heterogeneous group of disorders is defined by a large but otherwise well-formed brain. The time of onset is less certain than with macrencephaly, but it likely involves or extends beyond the proliferative period. The clinical spectrum ranges from normal function to severe mental retardation with epilepsy. Familial forms include autosomal dominant inheritance, which is thought to be composed of isolated microcephaly and normal intelligence in 50% of cases. In the spectrum of this disorder, macrocephaly is categorized as "idiopathic external hydrocephalus" with prominent extra-axial subarachnoid spaces.[156] The clinical spectrum with autosomal recessive inheritance is associated with a higher incidence of mental retardation.[59, 157]

Other types of macrencephaly are associated with a variety of cutaneous or somatic anomalies. Some neurocutaneous syndromes are notable for excessive proliferation of both neural and glial cells (tuberous sclerosis) or primarily glial cells (neurofibromatosis), whereas others have, in addition, excessive vascular proliferation (Sturge-Weber syndrome, multiple hemangiomatosis). These are often evidenced in the neonatal period

by their cutaneous manifestations, although affected infants also may exhibit seizures.[158, 159] Computed tomography (CT), magnetic resonance imaging (MRI) and ultrasound scanning often are useful to establish the diagnoses. Macrencephaly also can be associated with abnormalities of somatic growth, such as cerebral gigantism and Beckwith syndrome.[160] Lastly, excessive local proliferation of neurons and glia may result in unilateral macrencephaly, with localized enlargement of all or part of one hemisphere. These local anomalies are associated with large and abnormally shaped neurons and glia as well as with heterotopias and abnormally shaped gyri with a thickened cortex. (Fig. 165-9). In some cases, the affected neurons have been found to be heteroploid.[161] Severe seizures may occur in the neonatal period and often continue in association with mental retardation that becomes apparent later in infancy and childhood.[162] This unilateral enlargement of the cerebral hemisphere is present in approximately 50% of children with linear nevus sebaceous, a rare neurocutaneous disorder.[163]

Migration and Determination of Neuronal Fate

Normal Development of Cerebral Cortex

As neurons are generated within the ventricular zone by asymmetric cell divisions, they migrate radially toward the external surface of the neural tube, and thus toward the surface of the developing cortex. The earliest neurons come to reside as horizontally oriented cells within the marginal layer.[115, 164] By the seventh week of gestation, other postmitotic neurons migrate to and aggregate at the junction of the marginal and intermediate zones. At this very early stage, two populations of neurons are apparent in the marginal zone. The more superficial neurons remain within the marginal zone and constitute a transient population called Cajal-Retzius cells. Neurons deep within the marginal zone become displaced beneath the cortical plate to reside as another transient population of neurons within the subcortical plate.[165] Cajal-Retzius and subplate cells, for the most part, exist only during cortical development. The subplate, in particular, has been shown to have a critical role in establishing cortical organization. If subplate neurons of the developing visual cortex are ablated, ocular dominance columns, which are characteristic of mature cortex, fail to develop.[166-168] Defects of subplate neurons also lead to the failure of guidance of thalamocortical inputs and survival of layer IV neurons.[169]

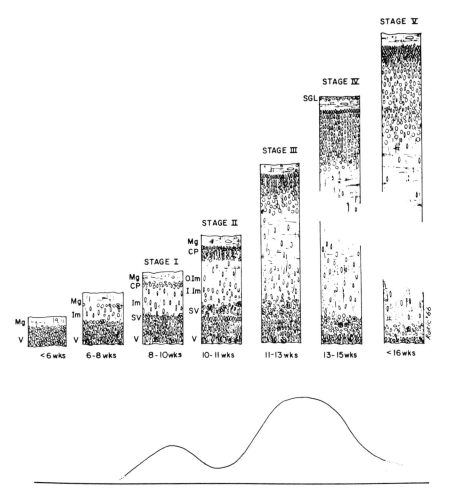

Figure 165–10. Schematic drawing of the human cerebral wall at various gestational stages, indicated below each column. Interruptions of the intermediate zones of the columns on the right indicate a marked thickening of the cortex during this developmental period. The curve below the columns indicates the major waves of neuronal migration. CP = cortical plate; Im = intermediate zone; I.Im and O.Im = inner and outer intermediate zones; Mg = marginal zone; SGL = subpial granular layer; SV = subventricular zone; V = ventricular zone. (From Sidman RL, Rakic P: Brain Res 62:1, 1973.)

The major portion of the cortical plate forms with neuronal migration that occurs in two discrete waves (Fig. 165-10). The first wave consists primarily of ventricular zone cells, which migrate to reside in the deeper layers of the cortical plate. The second wave increasingly involves subventricular zone cells, which migrate to occupy more superficial layers.[170] Thus, with the exception of the earliest neurons (i.e., the precursor of Cajal-Retzius neurons and the neurons of the subcortical plate), the cortex is formed in an inside-out manner.

During the initial phases of cortical plate formation, the path of the neuronal migration is short. Migrating neurons first become arranged in radial columns separated by glial septa. As the intermediate zone thickens, in part because of the arrival of thalamocortical and corticocortical axon terminals (see Fig. 165-8), the distance of migration increases, eventually exceeding the length of migrating neurons by more than tenfold.[171] An orderly pattern over these long distances is retained because migrating neurons follow guides formed by glial cells within the ventricular zone that extend long processes radially to terminate as end-feet on the pial surface (Fig. 165-11).[172, 173] These radial glial cells can be detected by the tenth fetal week.[121] They persist throughout the migratory period and then disappear, probably through a transformation to astrocytes.

During the period of neuronal migration, thalamocortical and corticocortical afferent fibers arrive in the intermediate zone and then extend terminals into the subcortical plate. As migrating neurons pass through the subcortical plate, they intermingle with these nerve terminals. Subcortical plate cells per se transiently express a variety of neuropeptides during this time.[174] The subplate provides guidance for the ingrowth of thalamocortical and corticocortical afferent axons and serves as a waiting site for

these inputs during cortical development.[166] After encountering neurons and afferent axons in the subcortical plate, migrating neurons continue on their path to the cortical plate. The majority of neurons complete migration by midgestation.[175]

The complex organization of cerebral cortex is under tight molecular and environmental control. Mutation of either reelin (*Rln*), an extracellular matrix glycoprotein secreted by Cajal-Retzius cells in the marginal zone as well as by cerebellar granule cells, or disabled-1 (Dab1), the cytoplasmic protein tyrosine kinase adaptor, results in abnormalities in laminar structures and disruption of neuronal layers in the cerebral cortex and hippocampus.[176, 177] Reelin and Dab1, along with a number of other molecules such as VLDL and ApoE2 receptors, provide a regulatory pathway for migration that is required to develop radial cortical organization and to maintain a normal gradient of maturation for the formation of thalamocortical connections.[178-180] Neurotrophin systems, such as brain-derived neurotrophic factor and neurotrophin 4, which are discussed later in more detail, are thought to support regulation of cortical development.

Neuronal lineage analysis has demonstrated the presence of both multipotential precursor cells and neuroepithelial cells with limited developmental potential, which reside within the cortical germinative zones. There is new evidence to suggest that radial glial cells are themselves neuronal progenitor cells.[181-185] This raises the possibility that radial glia and the progenitor cells of the ventricular cells may be one cell class, meaning that the same cell may be responsible for both generation of new neurons and guidance of daughter neurons to their ultimate destinations.[186] Some clonally related cells are found to be widely dispersed and of disparate phenotypes in the mature cortex.[123] These cells from a common lineage are believed to be

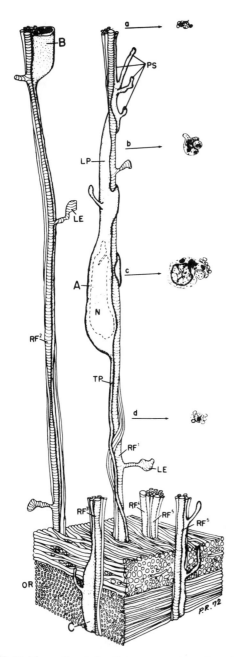

Figure 165–11. Three-dimensional reconstruction of a migrating neuron, based on electron micrographs of semiserial sections. The leading process (LP) of the migrating neuron (A) extends several pseudopodia (PS) as it migrates along the radial glial fiber (RF). Cell bodies of neurons (B) and (C) pass in parallel through the optic radiation (OR). An attenuated trailing process follows. (From Sidman RL, Rakic P: Brain Res *62*:1, 1973.)

derived either from tangential migration of multipotential cells or from lateral movement of multipotential progenitors within the germinal matrix before their radial migration. In other cases, tight clusters of clonally related neurons have been found to retain a radially oriented relationship to one another within the mature cortex.[123, 144] These clusters are believed to be derived from limited potential precursor cells that differentiate in the ventricular or subventricular zone and then migrate outward along radial glial guides.

Transplanation experiments have provided evidence that cell fate may be determined in the germinative zones. Experiments in

which progenitor cells were transplanted from one animal to another at different stages of development have demonstrated that cell fate is specified in a short period of time immediately following the terminal mitosis.[122,187,188] Cells transplanted immediately after mitosis assume a phenotype consistent with the developmental stage of the recipient animal, whereas cells removed from a donor several hours after the terminal mitosis assume the phenotype of the donor rather than the recipient. These results indicate that prospective cortical neurons may become committed to their fundamental phenotype at the time of their final mitosis in the germinative zone, before arrival at the cortical plate. Thus, it appears that the fate of neurons generated within the ventricular zone may, to a degree, already be decided before migration begins.

Normal Development of the Cerebellar Cortex

The cerebellum acts as a center for control of coordination. The cerebellum in the adult contains more than half of all neurons. It receives inputs containing sensory information from the periphery related to position of body parts and control of movements and provides output via the deep cerebellar nuclei to the cerebral cortex. During the second month of gestation, prospective cerebellar neurons are generated within the neuroepithelium lining the rostral half of the fourth ventricle. By 8 weeks of gestation, outward migration of these cells results in the delineation of ventricular, intermediate, and marginal zones.[189] Aggregation of neurons at the boundary between the intermediate and marginal zones is evident by 9 to 10 weeks of gestation. These cells are destined to form both Purkinje cells and neurons of the deep cerebellar nuclei. A third population of neurons is born after the formation of Purkinje cells, which are destined to become the stellate, basket, and Golgi interneurons of the molecular layer. All appear to arise from the subventricular zone, with the full complement of neurons generated by 13 weeks of gestation.[189,190]

Unlike most cell types of the cerebellum, which are generated in the ventricular zone, granule neurons are generated in a second subventricular germinal center called the rhombic lip. This initially small group of cells is evident at 8 weeks of gestation, migrates to a subpial location, and then, by geometric proliferation (i.e., symmetric cell divisions), spreads to cover the entire surface of the developing cerebellum to form the external granular layer. Over the next 3 months, the external granule cell layer increases to a maximum thickness of about nine rows of cells.[191] As postmitotic neurons of the external granule cell layer are generated, they assume a deeper position within the layer. The neurons then extend two processes in opposite directions that are parallel to the outside surface of the cerebellum but perpendicular to the Purkinje dendritic arbor. By 16 weeks of gestation, the cell body begins to migrate inward, leaving behind a vertical process connected to the horizontal processes in a T-shaped configuration. This inward migration is directed by radial glial processes of modified astrocytes called Bergmann glial cells. The migrating neurons pass through Purkinje cell dendrites in the molecular layer and then past the Purkinje cell bodies. After crossing the lamina dissecans—a layer just below the Purkinje cells that is rich in axon terminals of cerebellar afferents, such as the mossy fibers—the migrating neurons form the internal granular layer (Fig. 165-12). Horizontal processes establish synapses with Purkinje cells and become parallel fibers, which are ordered within the molecular layer so that more recently generated fibers lie more superficially.

An unusual feature of the external granule cell layer is that it continues to generate neurons for the remainder of gestation and for as long as 7 to 9 months postnatally.[189] This proliferation is remarkable both in terms of pure numbers as well as the protracted period of development; ultimately, cerebellar granule cells outnumber cerebral cortical neurons by more than 4:1.[190-192] The demonstration that medulloblastoma may arise

Figure 165–12. Schematic drawing of the main events during development of the human cerebellum from the ninth fetal week to 7 postnatal months. The upper row represents outlines of the cerebellum in the midsagittal plane at the same magnification (5-mm scale bar to left). The columns illustrate histogenesis of the cerebellar cortex in the depths of the primary fissure (*asterisk*; 100-μ scale bar at bottom indicates magnification). The major direction of cell migration is indicated by arrows. E = ependyma; EG = external granular layer; G = granular layer; I = intermediate layer; LD = lamina dissecans; M = molecular layer; P = Purkinje layer; V = ventricular zone; W = white matter. (From Sidman RL, Rakic P: Brain Res 62:1, 1973.)

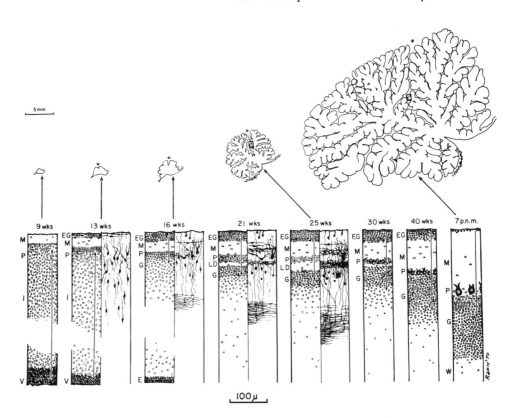

from this layer is, perhaps, understandable given the long period of differentiation, which leaves neurons vulnerable to disruptions in such closely regulated pathways.[193] Multiple genes are thought to be linked to medulloblastoma formation, including Ptch. The Ptch protein is a receptor for Shh, as discussed previously. Ptch normally inhibits signaling, and this inhibition is relieved by binding Shh. This in turn stimulates mitosis of the granule cell precursors. Inactivation of Ptch may therefore lead to the persistent proliferation of granule cell precursors.[194]

There are multiple influences on the complex migrations that take place in the developing cerebellum. Both genetic and environmental cues are important in the establishment of cerebellar cortical migration and organization.[195] Chemoattractive and chemorepulsive signals influence migrations. For example, netrin receptors are differentially expressed on neurons as they reach successive phases of migration.[196] The Notch signaling pathway is also important for neurogenesis in the cerebellum. Notch1 depletion results in premature onset of neurogenesis in the midbrain-hindbrain and Notch1-deficient cells are eliminated by apoptosis and therefore result in a decreased number of neurons in the adult cerebellum.[197] Sonic hedgehog is expressed in the cerebellum throughout life, though it promotes proliferation of developing cerebellar granule cells only in the early postnatal period, suggesting that downstream regulators may be important gatekeepers to the proliferative environment of the external granule cell layer.[198] There is new evidence that zinc finger proteins are involved in the control of cerebellar development. The mouse Zic genes are expressed in developing and mature central nervous system. Mutations in the Zic proteins lead to absent vermis and reduction of proliferation.[199] Lastly, neurotransmitters may be important in the regulation of proliferation and migration of precursor cells via developmentally regulated ligand-gated ion channel receptors.[200]

As these complex migrations occur in the developing cerebellum, critical cellular interactions occur. These interactions are illustrated graphically in three mutant mice (i.e., weaver, reeler, and staggerer),[171, 201] which exhibit alterations in cellular interactions

in the developing cerebellum. For example, an autosomal recessive mutation in the *staggerer* mouse leads to a block in Purkinje cell development, resulting in a reduced number and altered phenotype and ectopic position of surviving cells.[202] In the absence of parallel fiber inputs, Purkinje cells form characteristic dendritic arbors but have a significantly reduced cell volume and truncated dendritic length. This interdependence of neurons for survival and for the expression of their mature form appears to be a fundamental feature of the developing nervous system.[203, 204]

Disorders of Neuronal Migration

Malformations of the cerebral cortex and disorders of neuronal migration are an important cause of developmental disability and seizure formation and may result in profound disturbances of cerebral function. Such disturbances may occur as part of a genetic syndrome, or they may occur in isolation. In the most severe cases, seizures occur in the neonatal period and major motor and other neurologic deficits, including mental retardation, are often evident later in infancy. At the other end of the clinical spectrum, mild aberrations of migration, manifested by isolated neuronal heterotopias, often have no associated neurologic abnormality. Migrational disorders may arise from errors in neurogenesis or from errors in the migrational process itself. Recently, there have been great advances in the molecular genetics and identification of genes and gene products implicated in the development of disorders of cortical migration and in syndromes associated with cortical malformations.

Severe disorders of migration are often accompanied by abnormal development of the cerebral gyri. Although the most rapid development of gyri occurs between 26 and 28 weeks of gestation,[205] which is well beyond the migrational period, normal convolutional development appears to depend on the presence of a normal distribution of cortical neurons with their associated efferent and afferent connections.[206] Convolutions appear as the cortex surface area is expanding rapidly. The folding to produce gyri and sulci appears to relate to the relative surface areas of the outer versus the inner laminae of the cortex.[207] In normal brain, the outer three cortical laminae have a slightly larger surface area than do the inner three cortical laminae, thus resulting in cortical buckling to form gyri and sulci. Abnormal gyral patterns arise with gross disturbances of this relationship. Thus, lissencephalic brains are lacking a full complement of neurons in both inner and outer laminae and form no gyri. Polymicrogyric brains have a reduction of neurons in deeper laminae; the marked reduction of surface area of inner laminae with respect to the outer laminae results in an increased number of convolutions.[207] These disorders of migration result in dramatic abnormalities of the cerebral hemispheres, which often can be detected by CT scanning or MRI.[208] The disorders are discussed in order of decreasing severity.

Schizencephaly. Schizencephaly, or cleft brain, is thought to arise from a restricted but complete failure of cortical genesis.[209, 210] Deep and symmetric clefts classically occur bilaterally in the cerebral hemispheres. Microgyric cortex and neuronal heterotopias are present within these clefts, and ventricular dilation (with or without opening of the clefts) may occur. The demonstration by MRI of unilateral or asymmetric clefts with disordered gyral formation indicates that schizencephalic malformations are not always bilateral or symmetric. Infants with the bilateral classic lesions tend to have severe seizures and mental retardation, but less severe deficits have been described, particularly with unilateral or asymmetric lesions. Schizencephalic lesions probably arise by the second month of gestation, near the onset of migration. Most cases occur sporadically, but a familial occurrence has been documented recently,[211, 212] and heterozygous mutations in the EMX2 homeobox gene have been reported in some patients.[213,214] In the same family, different siblings with the same mutation may experience different clinical severity, suggesting that the pathogenesis is multifactorial. There are several reports of open-lip schizencephaly secondary to cytomegalovirus infection, without the presence of the mutated EMX2 gene.[215]

Lissencephaly (Smooth Brain). This anomaly is defined by the complete lack of gyri and sulci.[63] The cerebral wall consists of an outer hypocellular marginal layer, a middle cellular layer composed of heterotopic neurons, and a thin inner layer of white matter. The disorder arises near the onset of formation of the cortical plate, probably within the first 2 to 3 months of gestation. Different forms of lissencephaly can be distinguished both by radiographic features and by underlying genetic abnormalities, though sporadic inheritance is most common. Posteriorly, predominant gyral abnormalities result from mutations of the LIS1 gene, located on the distal short arm of chromosome 17.[216-218] This gene encodes the beta subunit of platelet-activating factor acetylhydrolase, brain isoform (PAFAH1B1). Mutations of PAFAH1B1 inhibit neuronal migration on an in vitro neuronal migration assay.[219] Deletions of LIS1 greater than 200 kb are associated with the predominantly autosomal dominant Miller-Dieker syndrome (MDS), whereas smaller deletions or point mutations are associated with isolated lissencephaly sequence (ILS).[216,217,220,221] Missense mutations of the LIS1 gene may result in a wider spectrum of clinical sequelae.[222] MDS is characterized by craniofacial abnormalities, malformations of the heart and kidneys, and other somatic anomalies. Anteriorly predominant lissencephaly in hemizygous males and the X-linked subcortical band heterotopia syndrome have been linked to the XLIS or doublecortin (DCX) gene on chromosome 22q,[223-225] which encodes a novel protein of unknown function.

Cobblestone lissencephaly (type II) is most commonly associated with Walker-Warburg syndrome, which is also characterized by communicating hydrocephalus, ocular abnormalities involving both the anterior and posterior chambers of the eye (especially retinal dysplasia), hypotonia, occipital encephalocele (in approximately one third of cases), and muscle histopathologic features compatible with congenital muscular dystrophy.

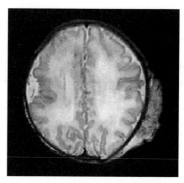

Figure 165–13. Congenital bilateral perisylvian polymicrogyria in a newborn infant who presented with seizures in the first week of life. Axial images show abnormality of the insula and of the parietal cortex, with increased gyrations and a smooth-appearing cortical white matter junction. (Courtesy of Drs. Karen Moeller and Richard Robertson.)

Lissencephaly also occurs in a group of disorders associated with congenital muscular dystrophy, including Fukuyama congenital muscular dystrophy, which is thought to be secondary to mutations of fukutin.[212] Autosomal recessive lissencephaly with cerebellar hypoplasia has been associated with mutations of the reelin gene, which is likely a different phenotype from type 1 lissencephaly.[226] All of these microcephalic infants are markedly hypotonic with severe seizures. Neurologic development is minimal, and most affected babies die in infancy.

Pachygyria. Brains with this anomaly have a few broad gyri. The cerebral wall is composed of an outer marginal layer, a thin superficial layer of unusually shaped neurons, a thick layer of heterotopic neurons apparently arrested in migration, and a thin inner layer of white matter.[63] The cortical plate is represented more fully than in lissencephaly, and thus the malformation is thought to arise somewhat later. Pachygyria has been documented after maternal ingestion of methyl-mercury beginning at 6 to 10 weeks' gestation, suggesting that environmental disturbances can alter migration.[227] Infants with pachygyria usually exhibit severe neurologic disturbance, with seizures, mental retardation, and hypotonicity progressing to spasticity.

Polymicrogyria. The cerebral surface in this anomaly is notable for large numbers of unusually small convolutions (Fig. 165-13). The cerebral wall has five layers. Beneath the marginal layer is an upper dense cell layer. The third layer has a low cell density and a horizontal plexus of myelinated fibers. The fourth layer varies in thickness but tends to remain relatively hypocellular, containing heterotopic neurons arranged in columns and nests. The white matter is relatively well represented compared with the other migrational defects.[63, 228] The disorder generally occurs sporadically, but it has also been described in the Zellweger syndrome, an autosomal recessive disorder associated with lack of peroxisomes, mental retardation, severe hypotonia, hepatomegaly, renal cysts, and facial anomalies.[228, 229] Genetic heterogeneity has been observed in the familial cases of bilateral perisylvian polymicrogyria, a disorder of neuronal migration; onset no later than the fourth to fifth month of gestation is likely.[212] In other cases, it appears that a postmigrational disturbance occurs that is secondary to destruction of deep laminae in otherwise normal cortex. Polymicrogyria has been associated with cortical laminar necrosis resulting from carbon monoxide exposure at approximately 20 to 24 weeks' gestation.[230] In some cases, polymicrogyria is relatively restricted, and neurologic symptoms are related only to the region of cortex involved. For example, focal seizures or dyslexia has been observed with focal polymicrogyria. Widespread polymicrogyria, however, is associated with severe derangement of neurologic development and seizures.

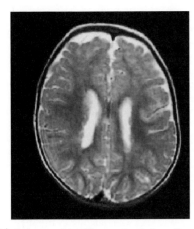

Figure 165–14. Subependymal heterotopia in a 2-year-old girl who presented with new-onset seizures. Axial images reveal multiple nodular masses lining the lateral ventricles. These are isointense, with cortical gray matter on all imaging sequences. (Courtesy of Drs. Karen Moeller and Richard Robertson.)

Heterotopias. These anomalies are small collections of neurons in the white matter that often accompany more severe disorders of migration, but they may also occur without other developmental anomalies. Whether neurologic disturbances accompany isolated neuronal heterotopias has been a controversial issue. Abnormalities of neuronal migration may result in dysmature cells in aberrant locations. Such cells, some with immature features of stem cell precursors, may potentially be a focus of abnormal glial-neuronal proliferation and, ultimately, the site of abnormal, clonal proliferation. Recent studies with MRI have demonstrated heterotopias in patients with seizure disorders, some of adult onset, with or without other neurologic deficits (Fig. 165-14). The thickness of the heterotopic band and the degree of pachygyria may correlate with the severity of seizures. As with other disorders of cortical migration, MRI may broaden the clinical spectrum of neuronal heterotopias. Time of onset is no later than the terminal stages of migration—that is approximately the fifth postnatal month. Recently, truncation of the filamin A, an actin-associated protein, has been reported in several families and in sporadic patients with X-linked bilateral periventricular nodular heterotopias.[231]

Axon Outgrowth

Normal Development

As they migrate along radial glia, many neurons within the cerebral wall extend processes that are soon recognizable as axons. The formation and maintenance of axonal and dendritic arbors is largely under control of environmental cues. The tip of each process is composed of a specialized motile structure, a growth cone, which resembles the head of a club, with microspikes (filopodia) extending in all directions. Living growth cones, when viewed in a microscope, are constantly moving by local extension and retraction. When in contact with an appropriate substrate, they crawl forward and leave behind the elongating axon.[232]

In the developing nervous system, a variety of molecules within the extracellular matrix have been shown to provide this substrate for axon outgrowth. Neurons in culture elongate their axons in a substrate-dependent manner.[233] Two of the most active promoters of growth cone migration, laminin and fibronectin, have been shown to be expressed transiently as components of the extracellular matrix in cortical regions that have particularly active axon growth.[234-236] In addition, responsiveness to laminin

may be developmentally regulated and enhanced by treatments that activate integrin function.[237] Administration of exogenous laminin favors neuronal migration and neurite growth, whereas inhibition or neutralization of laminin results in inhibition of neurite outgrowth. Proteoglycans such as chondroitin sulfate, which are macromolecules composed of core polypeptide and glycosaminoglycan chains, can modulate neurite outgrowth along with laminin.[238, 239] Matrix metalloproteinases, proteases that degrade extracellular matrix molecules, are thought to be involved in stabilization of laminin and cell-matrix interactions.[240] Extracellular matrix proteins, such as collagen, also have been shown in cell culture to suppress apoptosis, or programmed cell death, and thus to provide a more nurturing substrate for neuronal survival and differentiation.[241]

Although extracellular matrix substrates promote axon outgrowth, they alone may not provide all the directional signals required during axon outgrowth. Thus, as growth cones advance, their filopodia extend and appear to explore the local environment, as if to find the path that is most favorable for continued axon growth. Growth-associated protein-43 (GAP-43) is a major growth cone protein whose phosphorylation in response to extracellular guidance cues can secondarily regulate microtube behavior, so that mice lacking GAP-43 fail to form the anterior commissure, hippocampal commissure, and corpus callosum.[242] The axon tends to follow gradients of adhesiveness, as provided by substances within the extracellular matrix[243] and by specific "guide-post" cells along the path of outgrowth.[244] Growth of axons along voltage gradients or diffusible chemical gradients also has been shown to occur.[204]

Specific axon guidance molecules have been identified in the developing nervous system. Some of these molecules, the netrins, for example, have been found to serve as chemoattractants,[245] whereas others, such as the members of the semaphorin/collapsin family,[246] have a chemorepulsive effect on axon guidance. A growing body of evidence indicates, then, that axon guidance is directed by the integrated and summed influence of both attractant and repulsive cues.[247] These cues may be expressed in gradients, and they ultimately lead to the establishment of axon projection maps as found in the projection from the retina to the midbrain tectum. In fact, a family of axon-repulsive molecules, ligands of the *EPH* family of receptor tyrosine kinases, has been identified as the probable positional labels for the retinotectal projection.[248-250]

Within the cerebral hemispheres, some of the earliest elongating axons can be found to cross the commissural plate. By 10 weeks of gestation, the fibers of the anterior commissure are demonstrable in the ventral portion of the lamina reuniens. The dorsal lamina reuniens soon become the site of crossing of axons that form the hippocampal commissure (onset at 11 weeks of gestation) and the corpus callosum (onset at 12 weeks of gestation).[95] These axons extend rapidly and may reach the opposite hemisphere before the migrating neurons from which the axons originate reach the cortical plate.[251] By 20 weeks of fetal life, the shape of the corpus callosum has roughly assumed that of the adult. Careful axon counts in the rhesus monkey indicate, however, that the number of these fibers continues to increase until birth,[252] when the number of callosal axons actually exceeds the adult number by about fourfold. A period of axon elimination then occurs during the first few postnatal months.[252] Excessive numbers of callosal axons have been described in several animals.[253-255] It has been suggested that this early excess represents an initially diffuse projection of cortical neurons that subsequently is refined by axon elimination.

Disorders

Agenesis and hypoplasia of the corpus callosum are the best described lesions of axon outgrowth within the cerebral

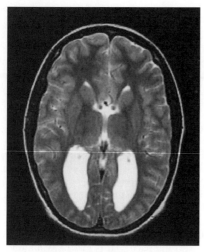

Figure 165–15. Agenesis of the corpus callosum in an 18-year-old girl with a history of psychiatric problems and depression who presented with a new-onset seizure. Axial MRI images show continuity of the third ventricle with the interhemispheric fissure and the lateral convexity of the frontal horns. The bodies of the lateral ventricles are parallel with dilated occipital horns. (Courtesy of Drs. Karen Moeller and Richard Robertson.)

hemispheres. These disorders of callosal formation may arise from a dysgenesis of midline prosencephalic development, involving the commissural and chiasmatic plates, or a dysgenesis of cerebral cortex, as with severe migrational defects. In the latter cases, cortical neurons lack orderly axon outgrowth. With restricted disturbance of the commissural plate, callosal defects may arise as relatively isolated defects in brains with otherwise normal cortical development. In most of these cases, the anterior commissure is intact. As a restricted lesion, lack of the corpus callosum is accompanied by an abnormal gyral pattern on the medial cerebral wall and by a longitudinal bundle of fibers (the Probst bundle) that projects posteriorly and terminates in the ipsilateral hemisphere. Partial agenesis of the corpus callosum usually involves the posterior aspect; the Probst bundle is present only in the region in which the defect occurs.[256,257] The lack of the Probst bundle in normal brain, and its occurrence only in regions in which the corpus callosum is lacking, suggest that the structure represented misdirected fibers of the callosum. The mechanism of this form of agenesis may relate to some abnormality of the dorsal aspect of the lamina reuniens, such as the presence of a mechanical or biochemical impediment or the lack of a molecular signal that normally directs the crossing of the commissural fibers.

Agenesis of the corpus callosum results in a lateral displacement of the lateral ventricles and dilation of the occipital horns, producing a characteristic pattern that can be readily recognized on ultrasound, CT, or MRI scans (Fig. 165–15). Many children with callosal agenesis have a variety of other central nervous system defects, including restricted migrational disturbance and hydrocephalus, reflecting the other important developmental events occurring as the commissures are forming.[256–258] Complete agenesis must originate before 12 weeks' gestation and partial agenesis before 20 weeks' gestation, although more subtle lesions may involve the axons added in the second half of gestation. Most cases occur sporadically, although familial patterns, including autosomal dominant, autosomal recessive, X-linked recessive, and X-linked dominant (the Aicardi syndrome) types have been described.[98] Patients with an isolated callosal defect have no overt neurologic signs, but with careful

testing they can be shown to have defective interhemispheric processing.[259] Children with callosal agenesis may have mental retardation and seizures, but these more pronounced abnormalities probably arise from the other central nervous system defects commonly associated with this disorder.[259,260]

A restricted lesion of axon outgrowth is demonstrable in the optic nerves of children with albinism. This is thought to involve an apparent rerouting of axons from the temporal retina to the contralateral hemisphere instead of to the ipsilateral hemisphere, as occurs normally.[261,262] The cause of this anomaly is not known, but it probably relates to a failure of pigment formation in the optic cup.[263] The axonal disturbance can be detected by testing visual evoked responses.[264, 265] Although the disorder causes abnormal binocular vision, other serious visual defects in albinism decrease the significance of this problem.[262]

Neuronal Death and Trophic Interactions During Development

Normal Development

In the first half of the twentieth century, experimental studies of chick and amphibian embryos demonstrated that removal of a developing limb results in a depletion of limb motor neurons and associated sensory ganglia to a degree that is proportional to the amount of the target tissue removed.[266-268] Although the neuronal depletion initially was considered to be caused by reduced neuronal proliferation, further studies of sensory ganglion neurons after limb bud ablation demonstrated conclusively that a fraction of the neurons that are initially present subsequently die.[269] A similar process of neuronal death also occurs in ganglia during normal development. Subsequent studies have demonstrated neuronal death to be a common, normal event in many regions of the developing neural system, including the neocortex.[270,271] Elimination of cells enable elimination of excessive cells produced during the proliferative and migratory phases of development. The loss can be dramatic and, depending on the region, ranges from 30% to 75%.[267,272]

The causes of neuronal death during development are being investigated actively. One possible explanation is that cell death occurs as a result of a competition among innervating cells for a substance (e.g., trophic factor) available in limited supply from the target; the successful cells thus survive while the others die.[204] The best characterized trophic substance at present is the protein nerve growth factor (NGF), which has been found to be essential for the survival of neurons in the developing autonomic and dorsal root ganglia.[273] NGF is the prototype member of the neurotrophin family of homologous peptide growth factors, which includes brain-derived neurotrophic factor (BDNF), neurotrophin-3 (NT-3), and neurotrophin-4/5 (NT-4/5). Each of these factors has been found to promote the survival and differentiation of diverse neurons of the central and peripheral nervous systems by binding to and activating their specific receptors: NGF interacts with the receptor *TrkA*, BDNF or NT-4/5 with *TrkB*, and NT-3 with *TrkC*. In addition to supporting the survival of neurons, neurotrophins can profoundly affect cell commitment and outgrowth of axons and dendrites.[274] Neuronal outgrowth and survival appear to be at least partially dependent on the presence of BDNF.[275,276] This effect may be mediated, in part, by alterations in intracellular calcium. Other molecules, such as the fibroblast growth factors, have been found to be responsible for promoting the proliferation of uncommitted precursor cells that become neurotrophin-responsive when they commit to a neuronal phenotype.[277,278]

The trophic influences of neurotrophins extend beyond cell survival. Among the surviving neurons, neurotrophins can profoundly affect the extent and direction of axon and dendrite outgrowth independent of the afferent input to the cell.[279-281] In

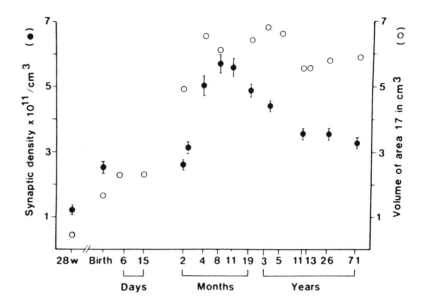

Figure 165–16. Mean synaptic density for all layers of area 17 in the visual cortex is indicated by closed circles (*left hand scale*; vertical bars are standard error of the mean for six synapse counts). Open circles represent the volume of the right area 17 (*right hand scale*). Age is indicated on a logarithmic scale. (From Huttenlocher PR, et al: Neurosci Lett *33:* 247, 1982.)

other cases, trophic effects appear to be mediated in an anterograde manner by afferents. Several investigators have demonstrated that superinnervation enhances and denervation inhibits dendritic growth.[65, 282, 283] The precise mechanism of these influences is not known; in some cases, functional activity appears to be critical. From the studies of trophic interactions, it is becoming increasingly clear in many neural systems that neuronal geometry is influenced by interactions with other neurons. This effect on neuronal geometry, in turn, is likely to have a significant influence on neural connections, producing neural patterns characteristic of the mature nervous system.[203]

In addition to trophic effectors, cell death by "programmed" pathways, or apoptosis, is one mechanism of elimination of cells during embryonic development. Apoptosis is a form of cell death characterized by distinct changes in morphology, including cell shrinkage, bleb formation, pyknosis, and chromatin margination, as well as biochemical changes with DNA fragmentation and degradation of marker proteins. Apoptosis is involved in normal homeostatic processes as well as in many pathologic diseases that are associated with neural cell death. Control of programmed cell death is under the influence of a complex group of molecules, including growth factors, cell cycle regulators, reactive oxygen species, and cytoplasmic proteases.[284]

Disorders

Although no developmental disorders of trophic function have been proven to date, such disorders are probable, in view of the importance of this process. The most likely candidate so far for a human disorder of trophic influence is familial dysautonomia, an autosomal recessive disorder involving primarily peripheral sensory and autonomic neurons.[285] The most consistent neuropathologic finding in this disorder is hypoplasia of autonomic and dorsal root ganglia, which normally contain the cells sensitive to NGF.[286] Deficits of NGF have not yet been demonstrated in these patients.

Disorders that relate to disturbances in normal neuronal death are harder to delineate. Unilateral macrencephaly (see preceding discussion), in which an excess number of neurons is present, is one such developmental disorder. Attempts to clarify the role of apoptosis in normal development may elucidate the mechanism of cell death in pathologic conditions. There is recent evidence that neuronal cell death in diseases such as Alzheimer disease, Parkinson disease, and the inherited ataxias may involve apoptosis.[287-289] Neurotrophins and their receptors, through regulation of differentiation and death of progenitor cells, may be

implicated in the progression of aberrant precursor cells into medulloblastoma. Children with tumors that express low levels of TrkC mRNA have a greater risk of death than children with tumors with high TrkC mRNA expression.[290, 291] Further research clearly is needed in this context.

Dendritic Growth and Synapse Formation

Normal Development

Migrating neurons begin to sprout dendrites as soon as they arrive at the cortical plate. The extension of apical and basilar dendrites occurs first and is followed by the extension of oblique branches off the apical dendrite.[292] As proliferation and migration of neurons generally ceases after the first 5 months of gestation, the increasing size of the cerebral cortex during the latter half of gestation and beyond is brought about by glial proliferation and by the elaboration of neural processes. Golgi-Cox studies of cortical neurons demonstrate that the complexity of dendrites continues to increase for at least 24 months postnatally.[293] Regional differences in rate of development occur, with the rate in association areas being generally slower than that in primary sensory and motor areas.[294, 295] In frontal cortex, the dendritic arbors are rudimentary at birth compared with those in striate cortex.[296] Dendritic length of prefrontal neurons increases as much as five-fold to ten-fold in the first 6 months of life and then continues to increase at a slower rate for months.[297] Some aspects of dendritic form appear to be determined by the neuron itself, as neurons grown in culture often attain a normal, although simplified, dendritic configuration.[298-300]

Synapses appear in the human cerebral cortex as early as the third month of gestation.[301] Their numbers increase coincident with the elaboration of dendritic spines, which are the primary sites onto which synaptic contacts are made.[302, 303] Quantitative determinations by electron microscopy have demonstrated that synapse number increases until 8 months postnatally in the striate cortex and until 24 months after birth in the frontal cortex.[304-306] After reaching these peak values, a slight reduction in numbers occurs over the course of many months (Fig. 165-16).[305] Although patterns of neural connections are initiated by directed axon outgrowth, ultimate cortical organization is effected by specific neuronal interactions. To a considerable degree, these interactions appear to be mediated by molecules on the surface of neurons and neural processes that result in the selective linking of axons to certain neurons by specific chemical affinity (chemoaffinity).[307] N-CAMs have been shown to promote cell-to-cell interactions among neurons.[308] As discussed earlier, the final pattern of synaptic connectivity appears to be shaped by events such as competition for trophic factors and the modulatory effects of neural activity on target cells.[203, 204] Synapse formation and maturation depend on actin filaments and is sensitive to processes that destabilize actin. Increased neuronal activity stabilizes F-actin and associated synaptic proteins, suggesting a correlation between active synapses, actin stability, and the establishment of stable synapses.[309]

Following the establishment of synapses, a period of synaptic rearrangement occurs, which is of fundamental importance for normal neural function. Refinement of redundant connections and elimination of synapses occurs during this process, which is one of the last steps in formation of the neural circuit. In the peripheral nervous system, this phenomenon has been observed in striated muscle and in autonomic ganglia. In both cases, the number of inputs per cell in the neonatal period exceeds that in the adult. Over the course of weeks, synaptic rearrangement decreases the number of inputs per cell, probably by elimination of "weaker" connections and by the strengthening of the remaining connections through successful competition for trophic substances.[310-312] The best-studied example of synaptic rearrangement in the central nervous system involves cerebellar Purkinje cells, which initially have multiple climbing fiber inputs; the inputs subsequently rearrange to the adult pattern of one input per cell.[313-315]

The rearrangement of synapses appears to rely on patterns of neural activity. This has been illustrated most convincingly in the developing striate cortex. In the adult cat, cells in layer IV of the visual cortex are segregated into ocular dominance columns that are alternately driven by one and then the other eye. In the neonatal period, considerable overlap of ocular dominance occurs (Fig. 165-17); the adult arrangement is established gradually over the first few months of life. If the normal pattern of neural activity is interrupted during this period by suturing one eye closed, inputs to the mature cortex are permanently altered, thereby resulting in functionally abnormal binocular vision and decreased visual acuity.[316-319] If, however, the eye is sutured after this critical period, no permanent deficit occurs, even if the suture is left in place for periods as long as months. Similar studies in primates have produced the same result, except that the critical period has been shown to be longer than it is in cats.[320]

Disorders

During the neonatal period, unilateral visual deprivation or persistent strabismus may result in loss of visual acuity in the affected eye. The critical period for these effects in humans appears to be quite long when compared with the critical period in experimental animals. The greatest alteration of acuity occurs with visual deprivation during the first 3 years of life, although subtle abnormalities from deprivation have been detected with onset as late as 10 years of life.[321, 322] Measurable effects have been detected with deprivation as brief as a few weeks, so prompt correction is essential for a good outcome.

Failure of synapse maturation has been postulated as the cause of fragile-X syndrome, the most common single-gene inherited form of mental retardation.[323, 324] Studies of autopsy samples in patients with fragile-X syndrome suggest that dendritic spines fail to assume a normal mature size and shape and that there are more numerous spines per unit length.[324] In the knockout mouse model of fragile-X, cortical spine morphology is more immature, with long, thin spines, in contrast to the more typical stubby, mushroom-shaped spines.[323] This suggests that fragile X mental retardation protein (FMRP), the protein that is absent or reduced in the syndrome, may be important for the process of synapse elimination.

Specific abnormalities of dendritic morphologic characteristics, without other evidence of cortical malformation, have been

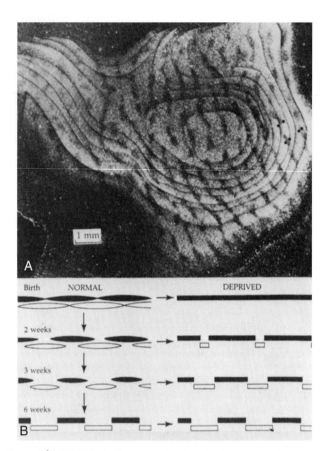

Figure 165-17. Effect of monocular deprivation on ocular dominance columns. **A,** Normally, afferent inputs to layer IV of the visual cortex segregate into ocular dominance columns represented by alternating stripes of approximately equal width. This dark-field autoradiograph is a reconstruction of parallel sections through layer IV of the primary visual cortex of a monkey whose right eye was deprived by lid suture from 2 weeks of age until 18 months, when the animal was sacrificed. Two weeks before death, the normal (*left*) eye was injected with radiolabeled amino acids, which were subsequently transported trans-synaptically to the nerve terminals of the geniculate inputs to the visual cortex. The columns from the nondeprived eye (*white stripes*) are wider than normal. **B,** Probable explanation for the duration of the critical period. Early deprivation alters competition between the projections from the two eyes because they still overlap widely; deprivation at progressively later times produces less obvious effects because the columns have already segregated. The end of the critical period coincides with the completion of the normal process of segregation. (From Purves D, Lichtman JW: Principles of Neural Development. Sunderland, MA, Sinauer Associates, 1985, p 352, after Hubel et al.[222])

found in some children with severe mental retardation, both with and without other evidence for cortical malformation or seizures.[325, 326] The defects often involve a truncation of dendritic length or simplification of dendritic arborization; frequently, dendritic spines are misshapen.[295, 326] In some cases, electron microscopy has demonstrated a disordering of microtubules, which suggests that cytoskeletal disturbances may underlie the morphologic anomalies.[327] The degree to which neurologic disorders with less severe mental retardation involve abnormalities of cortical organization remains to be determined. Such abnormalities have been described in some children with Down syndrome, as well as in children with neurologic disorders

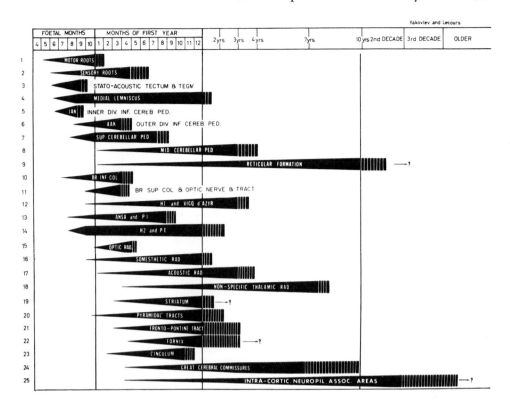

Figure 165–18. Myelogenetic cycles in the human brain. The width and length of the graphs indicate progression in the intensity of staining and the density of myelinated fibers. The vertical stripes at the end of the graphs indicate the approximate age range of termination of myelination. (From Yakovlev PI, Lecours A-R: The myelogenetic cycles of regional maturation of the brain. *In* Minkowski A: Regional Development of the Brain in Early Life. Oxford, Blackwell Scientific, 1967.)

having no definable cause. Because the latter group is such a large one, the data suggest that such abnormalities may underlie an appreciable number of cases.[59] Moreover, the rapid pace of cortical dendritic and synaptic development and the malleability of the neonatal cortex in response to external influences during the neonatal period suggest that the normal neonatal brain may be unusually susceptible to the variety of insults that frequently occur at this critical time. By the same token, because of these developmental capabilities, the infants' brains might be expected to be capable of complexities of recovery from injury—that is, plasticity—not attainable by mature brain.

Myelination

Normal Development

Undifferentiated oligodendrocyte precursor cells arise within the ventricular zone during late embryonic and early postnatal development and soon migrate into the developing cerebral wall. As these precursors migrate, they respond to internal cues as well as to the local influences of the other neurons and glia. These cues determine when progenitor cells exit from the cell cycle, begin to proliferate, and differentiate into mature oligodendrocytes.[328] Oligodendrocyte differentiation is inhibited by the activity of Notch1. In addition, Jagged1, one of the Notch activators, is expressed in unmyelinated axons of the cerebellar molecular layer during normal development.[329] This suggests that the Notch signaling pathway plays a role in axon myelination. The oligodendrocytes align along axons and elaborate cell processes that ultimately form the myelin sheath. Oligodendroglia synthesize myelin-specific proteins and lipids for the assembly of the myelin membrane. In the central nervous system, individual oligodendrocytes may produce myelin for up to 40 parallel axonal segments.[330]

Similar to cortical organization, myelination exhibits pronounced regional variation. These regional features have been defined well in the human cerebrum and are illustrated in Figure 165–18.[97, 331] The earliest myelin is detected within the

roots of motor and then sensory nerves. Myelination soon occurs within the neuraxis, in which sensory systems generally myelinate before motor systems. In cerebrum, primary projection systems begin to myelinate before associative systems. Finally, the cerebral commmissures and other corticocortical projections begin to myelinate and continue to do so for years postnatally.

Disorders

Animal models of myelination have focused on mice deficient of membrane components. The jumpy mutation of the X-linked proteolipid protein (Plp) gene causes dysmyelination and premature death of mice with resultant hypomyelination and increased numbers of dead oligodendrocytes and astrocytes.[332] The primary abnormality in these mice is the inability of oligodendrocytes to associate with and ensheath axons. Animals deficient for Fyn, a tyrosine kinase, show regional differences in myelin deficiency that is equivalent with single amino acid substitutions and with complete absence of Fyn protein.[333]

Children with a primary deficiency of myelination and no other apparent neuropathologic condition have been described by Chattha and Richardson.[334] Affected children demonstrate primary cerebral white matter hypoplasia, which is accompanied clinically by severe but nonprogressive intellectual impairment and spastic quadriparesis evident in infancy. The cause of this disorder is unknown, although a genetic abnormality is suggested by several examples of familial occurrence and by the similarity of neuropathologic features in certain mutant mice. The occurrence of myelin deficiencies in human disorders of amino acid metabolism[335-337] and in malnutrition[338] suggests that decreased synthesis of myelin lipids and proteins may play a major role in disorders of myelination. Inborn metabolic errors that cause neuronal storage, such as beta-galactosidase deficiency in GM1 gangliosidosis, have been associated with dysmature myelination on imaging studies. Evaluation of pathologic specimens from patients with infantile GM1 reveal delayed myelination of later-myelinating structures, suggesting that the metabolic defect has a direct effect on myelin development.[339] Mutations of the SOX100 transcription factor, which is involved in development of neural crest derivatives and glial cell fate determination, have been found in patients with Hirschsprung disease and is associated with several patients with central and peripheral myelin disorders. However, in a cohort of patients with disorders of myelination, no SOX100 mutations were revealed, suggesting an alternative mechanism in those patients with concurrent neurocristopathies.[340]

OVERVIEW

The timing of central nervous system development is a tightly controlled process, regulated by both genetic and epigenetic factors. Defects in brain development may arise at any phase of gestation, affecting cell proliferation, differentiation, migration, formation and pruning of synapses. In addition to genetic events, the timing of the teratogenic events is critical. Insults incurred early in gestation, when the basic structure of the nervous system is being established, tend to have devastating effects on central nervous system structure and function. Later in gestation, the most important developmental events include organization events in the cortex and myelination of axons. Aberrant development during this period results in disorders of cerebral cortical function, which in the least-affected cases may account for learning disorders or other subtle neurologic dysfunction. In this respect, the events of neural development extend over a protracted period, during which the nervous system may be susceptible to a variety of insults.

When does neural development end? In mouse olfactory development, dendritic growth and synapse formation have been shown to continue beyond the age when the animals reach sexual maturity.[341] Other experimental evidence in autonomic ganglia of adult mice suggests an ongoing rearrangement of synapses and of glial cells associated with synapses.[342, 343] This, and other evidence, indicates that neural development continues for months and even years during postnatal life. This may explain the unusual sensitivity of babies and young children to global insults to the nervous system, such as occurs with brain irradiation for tumor therapy,[344] and the unusual ability for children to recover from focal injury to the central nervous system.

REFERENCES

1. Balinsky BI: An Introduction to Embryology, 4th ed. Philadelphia, WB Saunders, 1975.
2. Purves D, Lichtman JW: Principles of Neural Development. Sunderland, MA, Sinauer Associates, 1985.
3. Spemann H: Embryonic Development and Induction. New Haven, CT, Yale University Press, 1938.
4. Eyal-Giladi H: Dynamic aspects of neural induction. Arch Biol 65:180, 1954.
5. Nieuwkoop PD, et al: Activation and organization of the central nervous system in amphibians. I, II, and III. J Exp Zool 120:1, 1952.
6. Sidman RL, Rakic P: Development of the human central nervous system. In Haymaker W, Adams RD (eds): Histology and Histopathology of the Nervous System. Springfield, IL, Charles C Thomas, 1982, pp 3–145.
7. Schoenwolf GC: On the morphogenesis of the early rudiments of the developing central nervous system. Scanning Electron Microsc 1:289, 1982.
8. O'Rahilly R, Gardner E: The initial development of the human brain. Acta Anat 104:123, 1979.
9. Lawrence IE Jr, Burden HW: Catecholamines and morphogenesis of the chick neural tube and notochord. Am J Anat 137:199, 1973.
10. Ignarro LJ, Shideman FE: Appearance and concentrations of catecholamines and their biosynthesis in the embryonic and developing chick. J Pharmacol Exp Ther 159:38, 1968.
11. Schlumpf M, Lichtensteiger W: Catecholamines in the yolk sac epithelium of the rat. Anat Embryol 156:177, 1979.
12. Wallace JA: Monoamines in the early chick embryo: Demonstration of serotonin synthesis and regional distribution of morphogenesis. Am J Anat 165:261, 1982.
13. Davidson EH: Gene Activity in Early Development, 3rd ed. Orlando, FL, Academic Press, 1986, pp 248–249.
14. McMahon D: Chemical messengers in development: a hypothesis. Science 185:1012, 1974.
15. Hemmati-Brivanlou A, et al: Follistatin, an antagonist of activin, is expressed in the Spemann organizer and displays direct neuralizing activity. Cell 77:283, 1994.
16. Lamb TM, et al: Neural induction by the secreted polypeptide noggin. Science 262:713, 1993.
17. Jacobson AG: Morphogenesis of the neural plate and tube. In Connelly TG, et al (eds): Morphogenesis and Pattern Formation. New York, Raven Press, 1981.
18. Gordon R: A review of the theories of vertebrate neurulation and their relationship to the mechanics of neural tube birt defects. J Embryol Exp Morphol 89(Suppl):229, 1985.
19. Lemire RJ, et al: Normal and Abnormal Development of the Human Nervous System. Hagerstown, MD, Harper & Row, 1975.
20. Burnside B: Microtubules and microfilaments in newt neurulation. Dev Biol 26:416, 1971.
21. Karfunkel P: The activity of microtubules and microfilaments in neurulation in the chick. J Exp Zool 181:289, 1972.
22. Karfunkel P: The mechanisms of neural tube formation. Int Rev Cytol 38:245, 1974.
23. Nagele RG, Lee HY: Studies on the mechanism of neurulation in the chick: microfilament-mediated changes in cell shape during uplifting of neural folds. J Exp Biol 213:391, 1980.
24. Sadler TW, et al: A potential for spectrin during neurulation. J Embryol Exp Morphol 94:73, 1986.
25. Revel JP, Brown SS: Cell junctions in development, with particular reference to the neural tube. Cold Spring Harbor Symp Quant Biol 40:443, 1976.
26. Campbell LR, et al: Neural tube defects: a review of human and animal studies on the etiology of neural tube defects. Teratology 34:171, 1986.
27. Thiery JP, et al: Cell adhesion molecules in early chick embryogenesis. Proc Natl Acad Sci USA 79:6737, 1982.
28. Bancroft M, Bellairs R: Differentaition of the neural plate and neural tube in the young chick embryo: a study by scanning and transmission electron microscopy. Anat Embryol 147:309, 1975.
29. O'Shea KS, Kaufman MH: Phospholipase C–induced neural tube defects in the mouse embryo. Experientia 36:1217, 1980.
30. Lallier TE, et al. Integrin alpha 6 expression is required for early nervous system development in Xenopus laevis. Development 122:2539, 1996.
31. Perris R, Perissinotto D: Role of the extracellular matrix during neural crest cell migration. Mech Dev 95:3, 2000.
32. Newgreen D, Gibbins I: Factors controlling the time of onset of the migration of neural crest cells in the fowl embryo. Cell Tissue Res 224:145, 1982.
33. Hamburger V: Experimental analysis of the dual origin of the trigeminal ganglion in the chick embryo. J Exp Zool 148:91, 1961.
34. LeDouarin NM: The ontogeny of the neural crest in avian embryo chimeras. Nature 286:663, 1980.
35. LeDouarin NM: Cell line segregation during peripheral nervous system ontogeny. Science 231:1515, 1986.
36. Noden DM: An analysis of the migratory behavior of avian cephalic neural crest cells. Dev Biol 42:106, 1975.
37. Doupe AJ, et al: Environmental influences in the development of neural crest derivatives: glucocorticoids, growth factors, and chromaffin cell plasticity. J Neurosci 5:2119, 1985.
38. Furshpan EJ, et al: Synaptic functions in rat sympathetic neurons in microcultures. I. Secretion of norepinephrine and acetylcholine. J Neurosci 6:1061, 1986.
39. Furshpan EJ, et al: Chemical transmission between rat sympathetic neurons and cardiac myocytes developing in microcultures: evidence for cholinergic, adrenergic, and dual-function neurons. Proc Natl Acad Sci USA 73:4225, 1976.
40. Catala M: Genetic control of caudal development. Clin Genet 61:89, 2002.
41. Patapoutian A, Reichardt LF: Roles of wnt proteins in neural development and maintenance. Curr Opin Neurobiol 61:392, 2001.
42. Gilbert SF: Developmental Biology. Sunderland, MA, Sinauer, 1994, pp 533–574.
43. Lewis EB: A gene complex controlling segmentation in Drosophila. Nature 276:565, 1978.
44. Struhl G: A homeotic mutation transforming leg to antenna in Drosophila. Nature 292:635, 1981.
45. Echelard Y, et al: Sonic hedgehog, a member of a family of putative secreted signaling molecules, is implicated in the regulation of CNS polarity. Cell 75:1417, 1993.
46. Goodrich LV, et al: Conservation of the hedgehog/patched signaling pathway from flies to mice: induction of a mouse patched gene by hedgehog. Genes Dev 10:301, 1996.
47. Stone DM, et al: The tumour-suppressor gene patched encodes a candidate receptor for Sonic hedgehog. Nature 384:129, 1996.
48. Johnson RL, Tabin C: The long and the short of hedgehog signaling. Cell 81:313, 1995.
49. Smith JC: Hedgehog, the floor plate, and the zone of polarizing activity. Cell 76:193, 1994.
50. Scotting PG, Rex M: Transcription factors in early development of the central nervous system. Neuropathol Appl Neurobiol 22:469, 1996.
51. Litingtung Y, Chiang C: Control of Shh activity and signaling in the neural tube. Dev Dyn 219:143.
52. Patten I, Placzek M: The role of Sonic hedgehog in neural tube patterning. Cell Mol Life Sci 57:1695, 2000.
53. Rowitch DH, et al: Sonic hedgehog regulates proliferation and inhibits differentiation of CNS precursor cells. J Neurosci 19:8954, 1999.

54. Roessler E, et al: Mutations in the human Sonic hedgehog gene cause holoprosencephaly. Nat Genet *14*:357, 1996.

55. Marshall H, et al: Retinoic acid alters hindbrain *Hox* code and induces transformation of rhombomeres 2/3 into a 4/5 identity. Nature *360*:737, 1992.

56. Dekaben AS, Bartelmez GW: Complete dysraphism in 14-somite human embryo. Am J Anat *115*:27, 1964.

57. Murdoch JN, et al: Severe neural tube defects in the loop-tail mouse result from mutation of Lpp1, a novel gene involved in floor plate specification. Hum Mol Genet *10*:2593, 2001.

58. Warkany J: Congenital Malformations. Chicago, Year Book Medical Publishers, 1971.

59. Volpe JJ: Neurology of the Newborn, 4th ed. Philadelphia, WB Saunders, 2001.

60. Fedrick J: Anencephalus: variation with maternal age, parity, social class and region in England, Scotland, and Wales. Ann Hum Genet *34*:31, 1970.

61. Emery JL, Kalhan SC: The pathology of exencephalus. Dev Med Child Neurol *12* (suppl 22):51, 1970.

62. Ingraham FD, Swan H: Spina bifida and cranium bifidum: a survey of 546 cases. N Engl J Med *228*:559, 1943.

63. Friede RL: Developmental Neuropathology. New York, Springer-Verlag, 1975, pp 280–313.

64. Opitz JM: Meckel syndrome. *In* Bergsma D (ed): Birth Defects Compendium. New York, Alan R. Liss, 1979, p 686.

65. Goodman LA, Model PG: Superinnervation enhances the dendritic branching pattern of the Mauthner cell in the developing *Axolotl.* J Neurosci *8*:776, 1988.

66. Emery JL, Lendon RG: The local cord lesion in neurospinal dysraphism (meningomyelocele). J Pathol *110*:83, 1973.

67. Larroch J-C: Malformations of the nervous system. *In* Adams JH, et al (eds): Greenfield's Neuropathology, 4th ed. New York, John Wiley & Sons, 1984, p 392.

68. Dekaben AS: Anencephaly in early human embryos. J Neuropathol Exp Neurol *22*:533, 1963.

69. Osaka K, et al: Myelomeningocele before birth. J Neurosurg *49*:711, 1978.

70. Gardner WJ: Rupture of the neural tube: cause of myelomeningocele. Arch Neurol *4*:1, 1961.

71. Carter CO: Clues to the aetiology of neural tube malformations. Dev Med Child Neurol *32*(Suppl):3, 1974.

72. McLone DG, et al: Concepts in the management of spina bifida. Concepts Pediatr Neurosurg *5*:97, 1985.

73. Gilbert JN, et al: Central nervous system anomalies associated with myelomeningocele, hydrocephalus, and the Arnold-Chiari malformation: reappraisal of theories regarding the pathogenesis of posterior neural tube defects. Neurosurgery *18*:559, 1986.

74. Kawamura T, et al: Cerebral abnormalities in lumbrosacral neural tube closure defect; MR imaging evaluation. Childs Nerv Syst *17*:405, 2001.

75. Kalter H, Warkany J: Congenital malformations. N Engl J Med *308*:424, 491, 1983.

76. Baird PA: Neural tube defects in the Sikhs. Am J Med Genet *16*:49, 1983.

77. Toriello HV, Higgins JV: Occurrence of neural tube defects among first-, second-, and third-degree relatives of probands: results of a United States study. Am J Med Genet *15*:601, 1983.

78. Layde PM, et al: Maternal fever and neural tube defects. Teratology *21*:105, 1980.

79. Zacharias JF, et al: The incidence of neural tube defects in the fetus and neonate of the insulin-dependent diabetic woman. Am J Obstet Gynecol *150*:797, 1984.

80. Taussig HB: A study of the German outbreak of phocomelia: the thalidomide syndrome. JAMA *180*:1106, 1962.

81. Stanley OH, Chambers TL: Sodium valproate and neural tube defects. Lancet *2*:1282, 1982.

82. Thiersch JP: Therapeutic abortions with a folic acid antagonist, 4-aminopteroylglutamic acid (4-amino P.G.A.) administered by the oral route. Am J Obstet Gynecol *63*:1298, 1952.

83. Smithells RW, et al: Apparent prevention of neural tube defects by periconceptual vitamin supplementation. Arch Dis Child *56*:911, 1981.

84. Carter CO, et al: Spinal dysraphism: genetic relation to neural tube malformations. J Med Genet *13*:343, 1976.

85. Anderson FM: Occult spinal dysraphism: a series of 73 cases. Pediatrics *55*:826, 1975.

86. Kaplan P, de Chaderéavian J-P: Piebaldism—Waardenburg syndrome: histopathologic evidence for a neural crest syndrome. Am J Med Genet *31*:679, 1988.

87. Touloukian RJ: Colon aganglionosis. *In* Bergsma D (ed): Birth Defects Compendium. New York, Alan R. Liss, 1979, p 240.

88. Whitehouse FR, Kernohan JW: Myenteric plexus in congenital megacolon: Study of 11 cases. Arch Intern Med *82*:75, 1948.

89. Shandling B: Congenital megacolon. *In* Behrman RE, Vaughan VC (eds): Nelson Textbook of Pediatrics, 13th ed. Philadelphia, WB Saunders, 1987, p 783.

90. Parisi MA, et al: Hydrocephalus and intestinal aganglionosis: is L1CAM a modifier gene in Hirschsprung disease? Am J Med Genet *15*:51, 2002.

91. Sztriha L, et al: Congenital insensitivity to pain with anhidrosis. Pediatr Neurol *25*:63, 2001.

92. Sagel SD, et al: Neonatal Hirschsprung disease, dysautonomia, and central hypoventilation. Obstet Gynecol *93*:834, 1999.

93. Rohrer T, et al: Congenital central hypoventilation syndrome associated with Hirschsprung's disease and neuroblastoma: case of multiple neurocristopathies. Pediatr Pulmonol *33*:71, 2002.

94. Yakovlev PI: Pathoarchitectonic studies of cerebral malformations. III. Arrhinencephalies (holotelencephalies). J Neuropathol Exp Neurol *18*:22, 1959.

95. Rakic P, Yakovlev PI: Development of the corpus callosum and cavum septi in man. J Comp Neurol *132*:45, 1968.

96. Pearson AA: The development of the olfactory nerve in man. J Comp Neurol *75*:199, 1941.

97. Yakovlev PI, Lecours A-R: The myelogenetic cycles of regional maturation of the brain. *In* Minkowski A (ed): Regional Development of the Brain in Early Life. Philadelphia, FA Davis, 1967, pp 3–70.

98. Warkany J, et al: Mental Retardation and Congenital Malformations of the Central Nervous System. Chicago, Year Book Medical Publishers, 1981.

99. DeMyer WE, et al: The face predicts the brain: diagnostic significance of median facial anomalies for holoprosencephaly (arhinencephaly). Pediatrics *34*:256, 1964.

100. Matsunaga E, Shiota K: Holoprosencephaly in human embryos: epidemiologic studies of 150 cases. Teratology *16*:261, 1977.

101. Berry SA, et al: Single incisor in familial holoprosencephaly. J Pediatr *104*:877, 1984.

102. Wallis D, Muenke M. Mutations in holoprosencephaly. Hum Mutat *16*:99, 2000.

103. Ming JE, et al: Mutations in PATCHED-1, the receptor for SONIC HEDGEHOG, are associated with holoprosencephaly. Hum Genet *110*:297, 2002.

104. Cohen MM Jr, Shiota K: Teratogenesis of holoprosencephaly. Am J Med Genet *109*:1, 2002.

105. Barr M Jr, et al: Holoprosencephaly in infants of diabetic mothers. J Pediatr *102*:565, 1983.

106. Binns W, et al: A congenital cyclopian-type malformation in lambs induced by maternal ingestion of a range plant, *Veratrum californicum.* Am J Vet Res *24*:1164, 1963.

107. Incardona JP, et al: The teratogenic *Veratrum* alkaloid cyclopamine inhibits Sonic hedgehog signal transduction. Development *125*:3553, 1998.

108. Kelley RL, et al: Holoprosencephaly in RSH/Smith-Lemli-Opitz syndrome: does abnormal cholesterol metabolism affect the function of Sonic Hedgehog? Am J Med Genet *66*:478, 1996.

109. Incardona JP, et al: Cyclopamine inhibition of Sonic hedgehog signal transduction is not mediated through effects on cholesterol transport. Dev Biol *224*:440, 2000.

110. Incardona JP, Roelink H. The role of cholesterol in Shh signaling and teratogen-induced holoprosencephaly. Cell Mol Life Sci *57*:1709, 2000.

111. Ho KS, Scott MP: Sonic hedgehog in the nervous system: functions, modifications and mechanisms. Curr Opin Neurobiol *12*:57, 2002.

112. Garcia CA, Duncan MC: Atelencephalic microcephaly. Dev Med Child Neurol *19*:227, 1977.

113. Sauer ME, Chittenden AE: Deoxyribonucleic acid content of cell nuclei in the neural tube of the chick embryo: evidence for intermitotic migration of nuclei. Exp Cell Res *16*:1, 1959.

114. Sauer ME, Walker BE: Radioautographic study of interkinetic nuclear migration in the neural tube. Proc Soc Exp Biol NY *101*:557, 1959.

115. Sidman RL, et al: Cell proliferation in the primitive ependymal zone: an autoradiographic study of histogenesis in the nervous system. Exp Neurol *1*:322, 1959.

116. Caviness V, et al: Neocortical malformation as a consequence of nonadaptive regulation of neurogenetic sequence. MRDD Res Rev *6*:22, 2000.

117. Fujita S: Kinetics of cellular proliferation. Exp Cell Res *28*:52, 1962.

118. Marin-Padilla M: Early prenatal ontogenesis of the cerebral cortex (neocortex) of the cat (*Felis domestica*): a Golgi study. I. The primordial neocortical organization. Z Anat Entwick-Gesch *134*:117, 1971.

119. Rakic P: Specification of cerebral cortical areas. Science *241*:170, 1988.

120. Takahashi T, et al: Mode of cell proliferation in the developing mouse neocortex. Proc Natl Acad Sci USA *91*:374, 1994.

121. Levitt P, Rakic P: Immunoperoxidase localization of glial fibrillary acidic protein in radial glial cells and astrocytes of the developing rhesus monkey brain. J Comp Neurol *193*:815, 1980.

122. McConnell SK: Development and decision-making in the mammalian cerebral cortex. Brain Res Rev *13*:1, 1988.

123. Walsh C, Cepko CL: Clonally related cortical cells show several migration patterns. Science *241*:1342, 1988.

124. Angevine JB, Sidman RL: Autoradiographic study of cell migration during histogenesis of cerebral cortex in the mouse. Nature *192*:766, 1961.

125. Berry M, Rogers AW: The migration of neuroblasts in the developing cerebral cortcx. J Anat *99*:691, 1965.

126. Sauer FC: Mitosis in the neural tube. J Comp Neurol *62*:377, 1935.

127. Shimada M, Langman J: Cell proliferation, migration and differentiation in the cerebral cortex of the golden hamster. J Comp Neurol *139*:227, 1970.

128. Lawrence IE Jr, Burden HW: Catecholamines and morphogenesis of the chick neural tube and notochord. Am J Anat *137*:199, 1973.

129. Hitoshi S, et al: Notch pathway molecules are essential for the maintenance, but not the generation, of mammalian neural stem cells. Genes Dev *16*:846, 2002.

130. Schuurmans C, Guillemot F: Molecular mechanisms underlying cell fate specification in the developing telencephalon. Curr Opin Neurobiol *12*:26, 2002.

131. Handler M, et al: Presenilin-1 regualates neuronal differentiation during neurogenesis. Development 127:2593, 2000

132. Justice NJ, Jan YN: Variations on the Notch pathway in neural development. Curr Opin Neurobiol 12:64,2002.

133. Franklin A, et al: NeuroD homologue expression during cortical development in the human brain. J Child Neurol 16:849, 2001.

134. Amoureux MC, et al: N-CAM binding inhibits the proliferation of hippocampal progenitor cells and promotes their differentiation to a neuronal phenotype. J Neurosci 20:3631, 2000.

135. Eriksson PS, et al: Neurogenesis in the adult human hippocampus. Nat Med 11:1313, 1998.

136. Johansson CB, et al: Identification of a neural stem cell in the adult mammalian central nervous system. Cell 96:25, 1999.

137. Roy NS, et al: In vitro neurogenesis by progenitor cells isolated from the adult human hippocampus. Nat Med 6:271, 2000.

138. Kornack DR, Rakic P: Cell proliferation without neurogenesis in adult primate neocortex. Science 294:2127, 2001

139. Alonso G: Neuronal progenitor-like cells expressing polysialylated neural cell adhesion molecule are present on the ventricular surface of the adult rat brain and spinal cord. J Comp Neurol 414:149, 1999.

140. Jiang W, et al: Cortical neurogenesis in adult rats after transient middle cerebral artery occlusion. Stroke 32:1890, 2001.

142. Ichikawa M, Hirata Y: Morphology and distribution of postnatally generated glial cells in the somatosensory cortex of the rat: an autoradiographic and electron microscopic study. Dev Brain Res 4:369, 1982.

143. Mares V, Bruckner G: Postnatal formation of non-neuronal cells in the rat occipital cerebrum: an autoradiographic study of the time and space pattern of cell division. J Comp Neurol 177:519, 1978.

144. Luskin MB, et al: Cell lineage in the cerebral cortex of the mouse studied in vivo and in vitro with a recombinant retrovirus. Neuron 1:635, 1988.

145. Morrow T, et al: Sequential specification of neurons and glia by developmentally regulated extracellular factors. Development 128:3585, 2001.

146. Williams BP, et al: A PDGF-regulated immediate early gene response initiates neuronal differentiation in ventricular zone progenitor cells. Neuron 18:553, 1997.

147. Privat A: Postnatal gliogenesis in the mammalian brain. Int Rev Cytol 40:281, 1975.

148. Skoff RB: Neuroglia: a re-evaluation of their origin and development. Pathol Res Pract 168:279, 1980.

149. Hatten ME, Mason CA: Neuron-astroglia interactions in vitro and in vivo. Trends Neurosci 9:168, 1986.

150. Temple S, Raff RC: Differentiation of a bipotential glial progenitor cell in single cell microculture. Nature 313:223, 1985.

151. Alonso G: Proliferation of progenitor cells in the adult rat brain correlates with the presence of vimentin-expressing astrocytes. Glia 34:253, 2001.

152. Stevens B, Fields RD: Regulation of the cell cycle in normal and pathologic glia. Neuroscientist 8:93, 2002.

153. Scholz H: Control of midline glia development in the embryonic Drosophila CNS. Mech Dev 62:79, 1997.

154. Kornack DR, Rakic P: Changes in cell-cycle kinetics during the development and evolution of primate neocortex. Proc Natl Acad Sci USA 95:1242, 1998.

155. Kelley RI, et al: Amish lethal microcephaly: a new metabolic disorder with severe congenital microcephaly and 2-ketoglutaric aciduria. Am J Hum Genet, 112:318, 2002.

156. Alvarez LA, et al: Idiopathic external hydrocephalus: natural history and relationship to benign familial microcephaly. Pediatrics 77:901, 1986.

157. Gooskins RHJM, et al: Megalencephaly: definition and classification. Brain Dev 10:1, 1988.

158. Kitahara T, Maki U: A case of Sturge-Weber disease with epilepsy and intracranial calcification at the neonatal period. Eur Neurol 17:8, 1978.

159. Nelhaus G, et al: Sturge-Weber disease with bilateral intracranial calcifications at birth and unusual pathologic findings. Acta Neurol Scand 43:314, 1967.

160. DeMeyer W: Megalencephaly in children: clinical syndromes, genetic patterns, and differential diagnosis from other causes of megalocephaly. Neurology 22:634, 1972.

161. Manz HJ, et al: Unilateral megalencephaly, cerebral cortical dysplasia, neuronal hypertrophy and heterotopia: cytomorphometric, fluorometric, cytochemical and biochemical analyses.Acta Neuropathol 45:97, 1979.

162. Taylor DC, et al: Focal dysplasia of the cerebral cortex in epilepsy. J Neurol Neurosurg Psychiatry 34:369, 1971.

163. Gurecki PJ, et al: Developmental neural abnormalities and seizures in epidermal nevus syndrome. Dev Med Child Neurol 38:716, 1996.

164. Marin-Padilla M: Dual origin of the mammalian neocortex and evolution of the cortical plate. Anat Embryol 152:109, 1978.

165. Luskin MB, Shatz CJ: Studies of the earliest generated cells of the cat's visual cortex: cogeneration of subplate and marginal zones. J Neurosci 5:1062, 1985.

166. Ghosh A, et al: Requirement for subplate neurons in the formation of thalamocortical connections. Nature 347:179, 1990.

167. Ghosh A, Shatz CJ: Involvement of subplate neurons in the formation of ocular dominance columns. Science 255:1441, 1992.

168. Ghosh A, Shatz CJ: A role for subplate neurons in the patterning of connections from thalamus to neocortex. Development 117:1031, 1993.

169. Zhou C, et al: The nuclear orphan receptor COUP-TFI is required for differentiation of subplate neurons and guidance of thalamocortical axons. Neuron 24:847, 1999.

170. Rakic P: Neurons in the rhesus monkey visual cortex: systematic relation between time of origin and eventual disposition. Science 183:425, 1974.

171. Sidman RL, Rakic P: Neuronal migration, with special reference to developing human brain: a review. Brain Res 62:1, 1973.

172. Rakic P: Guidance of neurons migrating to the fetal monkey neocortex. Brain Res 33:471, 1971.

173. Rakic P: Mode of cell migration to the superficial layers of fetal monkey neocortex. J Comp Neurol 145: 61, 1972.

174. Chun JJM, et al: Transient cells of the developing mammalian telencephalon are peptide-immunoreactive neurons. Nature 325:617, 1987.

175. Dobbing J, Sands J: Timing of neuroblast multiplication in developing human brain. Nature 226:639, 1970.

176. Rice DS, et al: Disabled-1 acts downstream of Reelin in a signaling pathway that controls laminar organization in the mammalian brain. Development 125:3719, 1998.

177. Quattrocchi CC, et al: Reelin is a serine protease of the extracellular matrix. J Biol Chem 277:303, 2002.

178. Lambert de Rouvroit C, Goffinet AM: A new view of early cortical development. Biochem Pharmacol 56:1403, 1998.

179. Trommsdorff M, et al: Reeler/Disabled-like disruption of neuronal migration in knockout mice lacking the VLDL receptor and ApoE receptor 2. Cell 97:689, 1999.

180. Walsh CA: Genetics of neuronal migration in the cerebral cortex. Ment Retard Dev Disabil Res Rev 6:34, 2000.

181. Malatesta P, et al: Isolation of radial glial cells by fluorescent-activated cell sorting reveals a neuronal lineage. Development 127:5253, 2000.

182. Hartfuss E, et al: Characterization of CNS precursor subtypes and radial glia. Dev Biol 229:15, 2001.

183. Miyata T, et al: Asymmetric inheritance of radial glial fibers by cortical neurons. Neuron 31:727, 2001.

184. Noctor SC, et al: Neurons derived from radial glial cells establish radial units in neocortex. Nature 409:714, 2001.

185. Tamamaki N, et al: Radial glia is a progenitor of neocortical neurons in the developing cerebral cortex. Neurosci Res 41:51, 2001.

186. Noctor SC, et al: Dividing precurosor cells of the embryonic cortical ventricular zone have morphological and molecular characteristics of radial glia. J Neurosci 22:3161, 2002.

187. McConnell SK: Migration and differentiation of cerebral cortical neurons after transplantation into the brains of ferrets. Science 229:1268, 1985.

188. McConnell SK: Fates of visual cortical neurons in the ferret after isochronic and heterochronic transplantation. J Neurosci 8:945, 1988.

189. Rakic P, Sidman RL: Histogenesis of cortical layers in human cerebellum, particularly the lamina dissecans. J Comp Neurol 139:473, 1970.

190. Miale IL, Sidman RL: An autoradiographic analysis of histogenesis in the mouse cerebellum. Exp Neurol 4:277, 1961.

191. Rakic P, Sidman RL: Supravital DNA synthesis in the developing human and mouse brain. J Neuropathol Exp Neurol 27:246, 1968.

192. Williams RW, Herrup K: The control of neuron number. Ann Rev Neurosci 11:423, 1988.

193. Kadin ME, et al: Neonatal cerebellar medulloblastoma originating from the fetal external granular layer. J Neuropathol Exp Neurol 29:583, 1970.

194. Corcoran RB, Scott MP: A mouse model for medulloblastoma and basal cell nevus syndrome. J Neurooncol 53:307, 2001.

195. Wang VY, HY Zoghbi: Genetic regulation of cerebellar development. Nat Rev 2:484, 2001.

196. deDiego I, et al: Multiple influences on the migration of precerebellar neurons in the caudal hindbrain. Development 129:297, 2002.

197. Lutolf S, et al: Notch1 is required for neuronal and glial differentiation in the cerebellum. Development 129:373, 2002.

198. Rubin JB, et al: Cerebellar proteoglycans regulate sonic hedgehog responses during development. Development 129:2223, 2002.

199. Aruga J, et al: Zic2 controls cerebellar development in cooperation with Zic1. J Neurosci 22:218, 2002.

200. Nguyen L, et al: Neurotransmitters as early signals for central nervous system development. Cell Tissue Res 305:187, 2001.

201. Rice DS, Curran T: Mutant mice with scrambled brains: understanding the signaling pathways that control cell positioning in the CNS. Genes Dev 13:2758, 1999.

202. Vogel MW, et al: Purkinje cell fate in staggerer mutants: agenesis versus cell death. J Neurobiol 42:323, 2000.

203. Purves D: Body and Brain: A Trophic Theory of Neural Connections. Cambridge, MA, Harvard University Press, 1988.

204. Purves D, Lichtman JW: Principles of Neural Development. Sinauer, MA, Sunderland, 1985.

205. Chi JG, et al: Gyral development of the human brain. Ann Neurol 1:86, 1977.

206. Goldman-Rakic PS, Rakic P: Experimental modification of gyral patterns. In Geschwind N, Galaburda AM (eds): Cerebral Dominance. Cambridge, MA, Harvard University Press, 1984, pp 179-192.

207. Richman DP, et al: Mechanical model of brain convolutional development. Science 189:18, 1975.

208. Barkovich AJ, et al: MR of neuronal migration anomalies. Am J Neuroradiol 8:1009, 1987.

209. Yakovlev PI, Wadsworth RC: Schizencephalies: a study of the congenital clefts in the cerebral mantle. I. Clefts with fused lips. J Neuropathol Exp Neurol 5:116, 1946.

210. Yakovlev PI, Wadsworth RC: Schizencephalies: a study of the congenital clefts in the cerebral mantle. II. Clefts with hydrocephalus and lips separated. J Neuropathol Exp Neurol 5:169, 1946.

211. Berg RA, et al: Familial porencephaly. Arch Neurol 40:567, 1983.

212. Guerrini R, Carrozzo R: Epilepsy and genetic malformations of the cerebral cortex. Am J Med Genet 106:160, 2001.

213. Faiella A, et al: A number of schizencephaly patients including two brothers are heterozygous for germline mutations in the homeobox gene, EMX2. Eur J Hum Genet 5:186, 1997.

214. Granata T, et al: Familial schizencephaly associated with EMX2 mutation. Neurology 48:1403, 1997.

215. Tannetti P, et al: Cytomegalovirus infection and schizencephaly: case reports. Ann Neurol 43:123, 1998.

216. Dobyns WB et al: Clinical and molecular diagnosis of Miller-Dieker syndrome. Am J Hum Genet 48:584, 1991.

217. Dobyns WB, et al: Differences in the gyral pattern distinguish chromosome 17-linked and X0-linked lissencephaly. Neurology 53:270, 1999.

218. McKusick VA: Mendelian Inheritance in Man. Baltimore, Johns Hopkins University Press, 1986, p 1087.

219. Bix GJ, Clark GD: Platelet-activating factor receptor stimulation disrupts neuronal migration in vitro. J Neurosci 18:307, 1998.

220. Pilz DT, et al: LIS1 and XLIS (DCX) mutations cause most classical lissencephaly, but different patterns of malformation. Hum Mol Genet 7:2029, 1998.

221. Cardoso C, et al: Clinical and molecular basis of classical lissencephaly: mutations in the LIS1 gene (PAFAH1B1). Hum Mutat 19:4, 2002.

222. Leventer RJ, et al: LIS1 missense mutations cause milder lissencephaly phenotypes including a child with normal IQ. Neurology 57:416, 2001.

223. Gleeson JG, et al: Doublecortin, a brain-specific gene mutated in human X-linked lissencephaly and double cortex syndrome, encodes a putative signaling protein. Cell 92:63, 1998.

224. Sossey-Alaoui K, et al: Human doublecortin (DCX) and the homologous gene in mouse encode a putative Ca^{2+} dependent signaling protein which is mutated in human X-linked neuronal migration defects. Hum Mol Genet 7:1327, 1998.

225. Matsumoto N, et al: Mutation analysis of the DCX gene and genotype/phenotype correlation in subcortical band heterotopia. Eur J Hum Genet 9:5, 2001.

226. Hong SE, et al: AR lissencephaly with cerebellar hypoplasia is associated with human RELN mutations. Nat Genet 26:93, 2000.

227. Choi BH, et al: Abnormal neuronal migration, deranged cerebral cortical organization, and diffuse white matter astrocytosis of human fetal brain: a major effect of methylmercury poisoning in utero. J Neuropathol Exp Neurol 37:719, 1978.

228. Volpe JJ, Adams RD: Cerebro-hepato-renal syndrome of Zellweger: an inherited disorder of neuronal migration. Acta Neuropathol 20:175, 1972.

229. Moser HW: Peroxisomal disorders. J Pediatr 108:89, 1986.

230. Bankl H, Jellinger K: Zentralnervose Schaden nach fetaler Kohlenoxyvergiftung. Beitr Path Anat 135:350, 1967.

231. Van der Flier A: Structural and functional aspects of filamins. Biochim Biophys Acta 99:1538, 2001.

232. Bray D: Growth cones: do they pull or are they pushed? Trends Neurosci 10:431, 1987.

233. De-Miguel FF, Vargas J: Steps in the formation of a bipolar outgrowth pattern by cultured neurons, and their substrate dependence. J Neurobiol 50:106, 2002.

234. Chun JM, Shatz CJ: A fibronectin-like molecule is present in the developing cat cerebral cortex and is correlated with subplate neurons. J Cell Biol 106:857, 1988.

235. Hatten ME, et al: Binding of developing mouse cerebellar cells to fibronectin: a possible mechanism for the formation of the external granule layer. J Neurosci 2:1195, 1982.

236. Stewart GR, Pearlman AL: Fibronectin-like immunoreactivity in the developing cerebral cortex. J Neurosci 7:3325, 1987.

237. Ivans JK, et al: Regulation of neurite outgrowth by integrin activation. J Neurosci 20:6551, 2000.

238. Tisay KT, Key B: The extracellular matrix modulates olfactory neurite outgrowth on ensheathing cells. J Neurosci 19:9890, 1999.

239. Bovolenta P, Fernaud-Espinosa I: Nervous system proteoglycans as modulators of neurite outgrowth. Prog Neurobiol 61:113, 2000.

240. Costa S, et al: Astroglial permissivity for neuritic outgrowth in neuron-astrocyte cocultures depends on regulation of laminin bioavailability. Glia 37:105, 2002.

241. O'Connor SM, et al: Survival and neurite outgrowth of rat cortical neurons in three-dimensional agarose and collagen gel matrices. Neurosci Lett 304:189, 2001.

242. Shen Y, et al: Growth-associated protein-43 is required for commissural axon guidance in the developing vertebrate nervous system. J Neurosci 22:239, 2002.

243. Nardi JB: Neuronal pathfinding in developing wings of the moth Manduca sexta. Dev Biol 95:163, 1983.

244. Bentley D, Caudy M: Pioneer axons lose directed growth after selective killing of guidepost cells. Nature 304:62, 1983.

245. Serafini T, et al: The netrins define a family of axon outgrowth-promoting proteins homologous to C. elegans UNC-6. Cell 78:409, 1994.

246. Messersmith EK, et al: Semaphorin III can function as a selective chemorepellent to pattern sensory projections in the spinal cord. Neuron 14:949, 1995.

247. Keynes R, Cook GMW: Axon guidance molecules. Cell 83:161, 1995.

248. Cheng H-J, et al: Complementary gradients in expression and binding of ELF-1 and Mek4 in development of the topographic retinotectal projection map. Cell 82:371, 1995.

249. Drescher U, et al: In vitro guidance of retinal ganglion cell axons by RAGS, a 25 kDa tectal protein related to ligands for Eph-receptor tyrosine kinases. Cell 82:359, 1995.

250. Tessier-Lavigne M: Eph receptor tyrosine kinases, axon repulsion, and the development of topographic maps. Cell 82:345, 1995.

251. Schwartz ML, Goldman-Rakic PS: Some callosal neurons of the fetal monkey frontal cortex have axons in the contralateral hemisphere prior to completion of migration (abstract). Soc Neurosci 12:1211, 1986.

252. LaMantia A-S: The organization and development of the cerebral commissures in the rhesus monkey. Doctoral dissertation, Yale University, 1988.

253. Innocenti GM, et al: Exuberant projection into the corpus callosum from the visual cortex of newborn cats. Neurosci Lett 4:237, 1977.

254. Ivy GO, et al: Differential distribution of callosal projection neurons in the neonatal and adult rat. Brain Res 173:532, 1979.

255. O'Leary DDM, et al: Evidence that the early postnatal restriction of the cells of origin of the callosal projection is due to the elimination of axon collaterals rather than to the death of neurons. Dev Brain Res 1:607, 1981.

256. Loeser JD, Alvord EC Jr: Agenesis of the corpus callosum. Brain 91:553, 1968.

257. Loeser JD, Alvord EC Jr: Clinicopathological correlations in agenesis of the corpus callosum. Neurology 18:745, 1968.

258. Jellinger K, et al: Holoprosencephaly and agenesis of the corpus callosum: frequency of associated malformation. Acta Neuropathol 55:1, 1981.

259. Field M, et al: Agenesis of the corpus callosum: report of two preschool children and review of the literature. Dev Med Child Neurol 20:47, 1978.

260. Grogono JL: Children with agenesis of the corpus callosum. Dev Med Child Neurol 10:613, 1968.

261. Guillery RW, et al: Abnormal visual pathways in the brain of a human albino. Brain Res 96:373, 1975.

262. Witkop CJ Jr, et al: Albinism and other disorders of pigment metabolism. In Stanbury JB, et al (eds): Metabolic Basis of Inherited Disease. New York, McGraw-Hill, 1983, pp 301–346.

263. Guillery RW: Visual pathways in albinos. Sci Am 230:44, 1974.

264. Creel DJ, et al: Abnormalities of the central visual pathways in Prader-Willi syndrome associated with hypopigmentation. N Engl J Med 314:1606, 1986.

265. Creel DJ, et al: Visual system anomalies in human ocular albinos. Science 201:931, 1978.

266. Hamburger V: The effects of wing bud extirpation on the development of the central nervous system in chick embryos. J Exp Zool 68:449, 1934.

267. Oppenheim RW: Neuronal cell death and some related regressive phenomena during neurogenesis: a selective historical review and a progress report. In Cowan WM (ed): Studies in Developmental Neurobiology: Essays in Honor of Viktor Hamburger. New York, Oxford University Press, 1981, pp 74–133.

268. Shorey ML: The effect of destruction of peripheral areas on the differentiation of the neuroblasts. J Exp Zool 7:25, 1909.

269. Hamburger V, Levi-Montalcini R: Proliferation, differentiation and degeneration in the spinal ganglia of the chick embryo under normal and experimental conditions. J Exp Zool 111:457, 1949.

270. Finlay BL, Slattery M: Local differences in the amount of early cell death in neocortex predict local specialization. Science 219:1349, 1983.

271. Pearlman AL: The visual cortex of the normal mouse and the reeler mutant. In Peters A, Jones EG (eds): Visual Cortex, Vol 3. New York, Plenum Press, 1985, pp 1–17.

272. Hamburger V, Oppenheim RW: Naturally occurring neuronal death in vertebrates. Neurosci Comment 1:39, 1982.

273. Levi-Montalcini R: The nerve growth factor: its role in growth, differentiation and function of the sympathetic adrenergic neuron. Prog Brain Res 45:235, 1976.

274. Snider WD: Functions of the neurotrophins during nervous system development: what the knockouts are teaching us. Cell 77:627, 1994.

275. Ghosh A, et al: Requirement of BDNF in activity-dependent survival of cortical neurons. Science 263:1618, 1994.

276. Wiklund P, Ekstrom PA: Axonal outgrowth from adult mouse nodose ganglia in vitro is stimulated by neurotrophin-4 in a Trk receptor and mitogen-activated protein kinase-dependent way. J Neurobiol 45:142, 2000.

277. Ghosh A, Greenberg ME: Distinct roles for bFGF and NT-3 in the regulation of cortical neurogenesis. Neuron 15:89, 1995.

278. Vicario-Abejóan C, et al: Functions of basic fibroblast growth factor and neurotrophins in the differentiation of hippocampal neurons. Neuron 15:105, 1995.

279. Campenot RB: Local control of neurite development by nerve growth factor. Proc Natl Acad Sci U S A 74:4516, 1977.

280. Snider WD: Nerve growth factor enhances dendritic arborization of sympathetic ganglion cells in developing mammals. J Neurosci 8:2628, 1988.

281. Voyvodic JT: Peripheral target regulation of dendritic geometry in the rat superior cervical ganglion. J Neurosci 9:1997, 1989.

282. Benes FM, et al: Rapid dendritic atrophy following deafferentation: an EM morphometric analysis. Brain Res 122:1, 1977.

283. Dietch JS, Rubel EW: Afferent influences on brain stem auditory nuclei of the chicken: the course and specificity of dendritic atrophy following deafferentation. J Comp Neurol 229:66, 1984.

284. Tang DG, Porter AT: Apoptosis: a current molecular analysis. Pathol Oncol Res 2:117, 1996.

285. Menkes JH: Textbook of Child Neurology. Philadelphia, Lea & Febiger, 1985, pp 145–147.

286. Pearson J: Familial dysautonomia (a brief review). J Auton Nerv Syst 1:119, 1979.

287. Gelbard HA, et al: Apoptosis in development and disease of the nervous system: II. Apoptosis in childhood neurologic disease. Pediatr Neurol 16:93, 1997.

288. Burke RE, Kholodilov NG: Programmed cell death: does it play a role in Parkinson's disease? Ann Neurol 44:S126, 1998.

289. Honig LS, Rosenberg RN: Apoptosis and neurologic disease. Am J Med 108:317, 2000.

290. Segal RA, et al: Expression of the neurotrophin receptor TrkC is linked to a favorable outcome in medulloblastoma. Proc Natl Acad Sci USA 91:12867, 1994.

291. Kim JY, et al: Activation of neurotrophin-3 receptor Trk 3 induces apoptosis in medulloblastomas. Cancer Res 59:711, 1999.

292. Juraska JM, Fifkova E: A Golgi study of the early postnatal development of the visual cortex of hooded rats. J Comp Neurol 183:247, 1979.

293. Conel J: The Postnatal Development of the Human Cerebral Cortex. Cambridge, MA, Harvard University Press, 1939.

294. Goldman-Rakic PS, et al: The neurobiology of cognitive development. In Mussen P (ed): Handbook of Child Psychology: Biology and Infancy Development. New York, John Wiley & Sons, 1983, pp 281–344.

295. Purpura DP: Dendritic differentiation in human cerebral cortex: normal and aberrant developmental patterns. In Kreutzberg GW (ed): Advances in Neurology. New York, Raven Press, 1975.

296. Takashima S, et al: Morphology of the developing visual cortex in the human infant. J Neuropathol Exp Neurol 39:487, 1980.

297. Schade JP, van Groenigen DB: Structural organization of the human cerebral cortex. I. Maturation of the middle frontal gyrus. Acta Anat 47:47, 1961.

298. Banker GA, Cowan WM: Further observations on hippocampal neurons in dispersed cell culture. J Comp Neurol 187:469, 1979.

299. Dichter MA: Rat cortical neurons in cell culture: culture methods, cell morphology, electrophysiology, and synapse formation. Brain Res 149:279, 1978.

300. Kriegstein AR, Dichter MA: Morphological classification of rat cortical neurons in cell culture. J Neurosci 3:1634, 1983.

301. Molliver ME, et al: The development of synapses in cerebral cortex of the human fetus. Brain Res 50:403, 1973.

302. Paldino AM, Purpura DP: Quantitative analysis of the spatial distribution of axonal and dendritic terminals of hippocampal pyramidal neurons in immature human brain. Exp Neurol 64:604, 1979.

303. Paldino AM, Purpura DP: Branching patterns of hippocampal neurons of human fetus during dendritic differentiation. Exp Neurol 64:620, 1979.

304. Huttenlocher PR: Synaptic density in human frontal cortex: developmental changes and effects of aging. Brain Res 163:195, 1979.

305. Huttenlocher PR, de Courten C: The development of synapses in striate cortex of man. Hum Neurobiol 6:1, 1987.

306. Huttenlocher PR, et al: Synaptogenesis in human visual cortex—evidence for synapse elimination during normal development. Neurosci Lett 33:247, 1982.

307. Sperry RW: Chemoaffinity in the orderly growth of nerve fiber patterns and connections. Proc Natl Acad Sci U S A 50:703, 1963.

308. Edelman GM: Cell adhesion molecules. Science 219:450, 1983.

309. Zhang W, Benson DL: Stages of synapse development defined by dependence on F-actin. J Neurosci 21:5169, 2001.

310. Lichtman JW: The reorganization of synaptic connections in the rat submandibular ganglion during post-natal development. J Physiol 273:155, 1977.

311. Lichtman JW, Purves D: The elimination of redundant preganglionic innervation to hamster sympathetic ganglion cells in early post-natal life. J Physiol 301:213, 1980.

312. Purves D, Lichtman JW: Elimination of synapses in the developing nervous system. Science 210:153, 1980.

313. Crepel F, et al: Evidence for a multiple innervation of Purkinje cells by climbing fibers in the immature rat cerebellum. J Neurobiol 7:567, 1976.

314. Mariani J, Changeaux J-P: Multiple innervation of Purkinje cells by climbing fibers in the cerebellum of the adult staggerer mutant mouse. J Neurobiol 11:41, 1980.

315. Mariani J, Changeaux J-P: Ontogenesis of olivocerebellar relationships: I. Studies by intracellular recordings of the multiple innervation of Purkinje cells by climbing fibers in the developing rat cerebellum. J Neurosci 1:696, 1981.

316. Hubel DH, Wiesel TN: Receptive fields of cells in striate cortex of very young, visually inexperienced kittens. J Neurophysiol 26:994, 1963.

317. Hubel DH, Wiesel TN: The period of susceptibility to the physiological effects of unilateral eye closure in kittens. J Physiol 206:419, 1970.

318. Wiesel TN, Hubel DH: Single cell responses in striate cortex of kittens deprived of vision in one eye. J Neurophysiol 26:1003, 1963.

319. Wiesel TN, Hubel DH: Comparison of the effects of unilateral and bilateral eye closure on cortical unit responses in kittens. J Neurophysiol 28:1029, 1965.

320. Hubel DH, et al: Plasticity of ocular dominance columns in the monkey striate cortex. Philos Trans R Soc Lond Biol 278:377, 1977.

321. Vaegan TD: Critical period for deprivation amblyopia in children. Trans Ophthalmol Soc UK 99:432, 1979.

322. von Noorden GK: New clinical aspects of stimulus deprivation amblyopia. Am J Ophthalmol 92:416, 1981.

323. Irwin SA, et al: Dendritic spine structural anomalies in fragile-X mental retardation syndrome. Cereb Cortex 10:1038, 2000.

324. Greenough WT, et al: Synaptic regulation of protein synthesis and the fragile X protein. Proc Natl Acad Sci USA 98:7101, 2001.

325. Huttenlocher PR: Dendritic development in neocortex of children with mental defect and infantile spasms. Neurology 24:203, 1974.

326. Purpura DP: Dendritic spine dysgenesis and mental retardation. Science 186:1126, 1974.

327. Purpura DP, et al: Microtubule disarray in cortical dendrites and neurobehavioral failure: I. Golgi and electron microscopic studies. Dev Brain Res 5:287, 1982.

328. Noble M: Glial development and glial-neuronal interaction. In Asbury AK, et al (eds): Diseases of the Nervous System. London, Heinemann, 1986, pp 109–124.

329. Givogri MI, et al: Central nervous system myelination in mice with deficient expression of Notch1 receptor. J Neurosci Res 67:309, 2002.

330. Peters A: Observations on the connections between myelin sheath and glial cells in the optic nerves of young rats. J Anat 98:125, 1964.

331. Gilles FH, et al: Myelinated tracts: growth patterns. In Gilles FH, et al (eds): The Developing Human Brain: Growth and Epidemiologic Neuropathology. Boston, John Wright, 1983, pp 117–183.

332. Thompson CE, et al: The early phenotype associated with the jimpy mutation of the proteolipid protein gene. J Neurocytol 29:207, 1999.

333. Sperber BR, et al: A unique role for Fyn in CNS myelination. J Neurosci 21:2039, 2001.

334. Chattha AS, Richardson EP Jr: Cerebral white-matter hypoplasia. Arch Neurol 34:137, 1977.

335. Malamud N: Neuropathology of phenylketonuria. J Neuropathol Exp Neurol 25:254, 1966.

336. Shuman RM, et al: The neuropathology of the nonketotic and ketotic hyperglycinemias: three cases. Neurology 28:139, 1978.

337. Silberman J, et al: Neuropathological observations in maple syrup urine disease. Arch Neurol 5:351, 1961.

338. Fishman MA, et al: Low content of cerebral lipids in infants suffering from malnutrition. Nature 221:552, 1969.

339. Folkerth RD, et al: Infantile G(M1) gangliosidosis: complete morphology and histochemistry of two autopsy cases, with particular reference to delayed central nervous system myelination. Pediatr Devel Pathol 3:73, 2000.

340. Pingault V, et al: The SOX10 transcription factor: evaluation as a candidate gene for central and peripheral hereditary myelin disorders. J Neurol 248:496, 2001.

341. Pomeroy SL, et al: Postnatal construction of neural circuitry in the mouse olfactory bulb. J Neurosci 10:1952, 1990.

342. Pomeroy SL, Purves D: Neuron/glia relationships observed over intervals of several months in living mice. J Cell Biol 103:1167, 1988.

343. Purves D, et al: Nerve terminal remodeling visualized in living mice by repeated examination of the same neuron. Science 238:1122, 1987.

344. Radcliffe J, et al: Three- and four-year cognitive outcome in children with non-cortical brain tumors treated with whole-brain radiotherapy. Ann Neurol 32:551, 1992.

John Laterra and Gary W. Goldstein

166

Development of the Blood-Brain Barrier

THE MATURE BLOOD-BRAIN BARRIER

The *brain capillary* is a complex of endothelial cells, pericytes, and an associated basement membrane surrounded by foot processes of adjacent astrocytes.[1] All brain capillaries, with the exception of certain distinct regions such as the area postrema of the medulla and the anterior pituitary, express a functional blood-brain barrier. Most, if not all, barrier properties reside in the endothelial cell. The different properties of the barrier, divided into the three categories of anatomic, metabolic, and carrier-mediated transport, are listed in Table 166–1.

The specialized anatomic characteristics of barrier-containing capillaries became defined with the development of electron microscopy. In peripheral capillaries and the nonbarrier capillaries of the central nervous system, bloodborne polar molecules diffuse across the vessel wall through spaces between adjacent endothelial cells and through transcellular routes, namely, endothelial fenestrations and vesicular or tubulovesicular structures (Fig. 166–1). The paracellular pathway and fenestrations are well established, but the contribution from vesicular pathways remains controversial.[2] In contrast, blood-brain barrier capillaries have a low nonspecific permeability to polar substances because these diffusional pathways are sparse or totally lacking.[3-8] The endothelia of barrier-containing brain capillaries are nonfenestrated and are interconnected by a continuous network of complex tight junctions that functionally fuse the plasma membranes of adjacent endothelial cells. These intercellular junctions were definitively demonstrated to be the site of the barrier to passive diffusion of polar plasma solutes by the classic studies of Reese and Karnovsky[8] and of Brightman and Reese,[3] and the distinct structural characteristics of these junctions were confirmed by both transmission electron microscopy and freeze fracture studies. Although tight junctions are found in capillaries of all tissues, they are less extensive and less complex in nonbarrier-forming endothelia and contain intercellular clefts through which passive diffusion occurs. Such clefts are markedly diminished in brain capillaries.

Knowledge of tight junction biochemistry has increased substantially since the identification of the first cytoplasmic (ZO-1) and transmembranous (occludin) tight junction–associated proteins in 1986 and 1993, respectively.[9, 10] Three integral transmembranous proteins and numerous cytoplastic accessory proteins that regulate the junctional complex and link the transmembranous junction proteins to the actin cytoskeleton are now known to comprise tight junctions at the blood-brain barrier (Fig. 166–2). Occludin, a 65-kDa phosphoprotein, has an extracellular domain and four transmembranous domains that mediate calcium-dependent intercellular adhesion activity. The claudins are a multigene (>20 members) family of approximately 22-kDa proteins that also contain four transmembranous domains and reside at the tight junction either adjacent to or complexed with the occludins.[9] Restricted expression of specific claudin family members may confer tissue-specific properties to tight junctions and tissue barriers. Specifically, claudins 1 and 5 have been identified at the blood-brain barrier.[11] Occludin can recruit claudins to tight junctional complexes, and both proteins serve as the principal mediators of interendothelial interaction at the tight junctions and increase junctional complexity and electrical resistance. A third family of transmembranous junctional proteins, the transmembranous junction adhesion molecules, consists of at least three members (JAM-1, JAM-2, JAM-3) of the immunoglobulin superfamily. These molecules also contribute to the high electrical resistance of tight junctions, and they appear to play a special role in inflammatory cell transmigration through junctional complexes.[12]

Several cytoplasmic accessory proteins serve to bridge the transmembranous junctional proteins to the cytoskeleton and contribute to tight junction functions through their regulatory and structural properties.[9] These include the zona occludins proteins ZO-1, ZO-2, and ZO-3, approximately 225-kD proteins that belong to the family of membrane-associated guanylate kinases (MAGUKs). Zona occludins proteins form a scaffold for recruiting regulatory enzymes and couple the occludins and claudins to the actin cytoskeleton. AF6, a target of the guanosine triphosphate (GTP)/GTP exchanger Ras, binds to ZO proteins and may thereby couple cell surface receptor–initiated signaling events to the tight junction. Cingulin is a double-stranded myosinlike protein with binding sites for ZO proteins, junctional adhesion molecule, AF6, and myosin and appears to link the junctional accessory proteins to the cytoskeleton. Junctional protein phosphorylation, proteolytic degradation, and cytoskeletal rearrangement are mechanisms by which tight junction permeability can be altered.

Endothelial pinocytotic vesicles contribute to the movement of substances across peripheral capillaries lacking a blood-brain barrier, and it is generally accepted that endothelia of barrier capillaries contain fewer such vesicles than peripheral capillaries such as those in skeletal muscle.[4, 13] Other vascular beds, such as those in the dura,[13] testis[14] and ciliary processes of the eye,[15] however, also express low densities of cytoplasmic vesicles. An increase in capillary vesicles is seen in some pathologic conditions associated with a loss of blood-brain barrier function.[16-18] Two mechanisms for transendothelial movement of substances through vesicles have been proposed. Palade[19] developed a model in which vesicle formation occurs by endocytosis at the

---

TABLE 166–1

Maturation of the Blood-Brain Barrier

Barrier Property	Developmental Change
Anatomic	
Endothelial-astrocytic association	↑
Complexity of interendothelial tight junctions	↑
Interendothelial clefts	↓↓
Endothelial fenestrations	↓↓
Vesicular transport	↓↓ (?)
Basement membrane	↑
Transport Systems	
Large neutral amino acid transporter (LAT1)	↓
Small neutral amino acid transporter (ATA2)	↑↑
Hexose transporter (GLUT1)	↑ →
Amine	↓
Monocarboxylic acid transporter (MCT1)	↓
Insulin	↓
Metabolism	
Aromatic amino acid decarboxylase	↑
Monoamine oxidase	↑ →
γ-Glutamyl transpeptidase	↑
Alkaline-phosphatase	↓

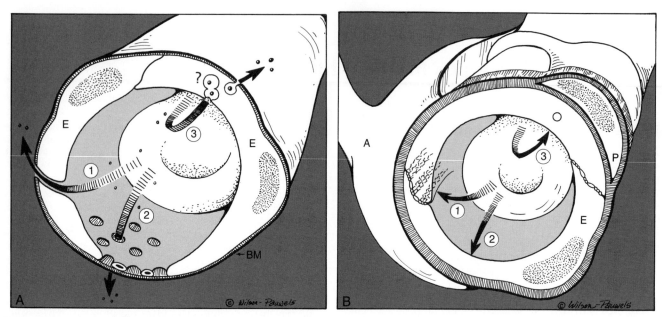

Figure 166–1. Comparative anatomic features of nonbarrier and blood-brain barrier capillaries. **A,** Peripheral capillaries and nonbarrier capillaries of the central nervous system lack an effective barrier to bloodborne polar molecules because of diffusion between endothelial cells *(1),* diffusion through endothelial fenestrations *(2),* and vesicular-tubulovesicular transport *(3).* **B,** Barrier capillaries are ensheathed by astrocytic foot processes, develop complex interendothelial tight junctions that block paracellular diffusion of polar substances, lack fenestrations, and contain a sparse vesicular transport system. A relatively thick basement membrane is interposed among the endothelial cells (E), astrocytic foot processes (A), and pericytes (P).

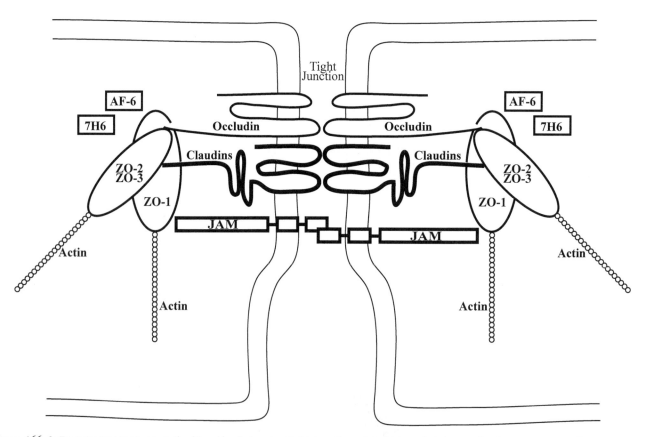

Figure 166–2. Protein interactions at the blood-brain barrier tight junction. A tight junctional complex between two adjacent endothelial cells is shown. Occludin and claudin isoforms are the principal transmembranous tight junction proteins. Occludin accumulation at the tight junction correlates with decreased paracellular permeability to proteins and ions. The cytoplasmic accessory proteins (ZO-1, ZO-2, ZO-3, AF-6, 7H6) spatially organize junctional complexes, serve as enzymatic junctional regulators, and mediate interactions between the cytoplasmic domains of the transmembranous junctional proteins and the cytoskeleton. Junction adhesion molecules (JAM) are tight junction–associated members of the immunoglobulin superfamily that mediate leukocyte transmigration across the blood-brain barrier. (Modified from Huber JD, et al: Trends Neurosci *24:*719, 2001.)

endothelial luminal surface, followed by vesicular transcytoplasmic migration and subsequent release of vesicular contents at the abluminal cell surface. An alternative scheme involves passive transendothelial diffusion of substances within channels formed by the transient fusion of multiple vesicles or by the fusion of vesicles with the endoplasmic reticulum. Transferrin and probably insulin are taken up and are transported across barrier endothelial cells by receptor-mediated vesicular transport systems.[20] A tubulovesicular system connecting the luminal abluminal plasmalemmal surfaces of brain capillary endothelial cells has been described in the developing rat and sheep, but the extent to which such structures exist in humans or provide a route for transcellular diffusion or transport is unresolved.[6,7]

Brain capillary endothelial cells maintain a unique relationship with two other cell types, the pericyte and the astrocyte. The abluminal surfaces of the endothelia of mature brain capillaries are ensheathed by astrocytic foot processes.[1] Historically, the astrocytic end feet were thought to be the site of the blood-brain barrier, but it is now known that the structural and functional barrier properties listed in Table 166-1 are localized in the endothelial cell. However, astrocytes are believed to play a prominent role in the induction of barrier properties in the endothelial cells, as discussed later. Pericytes—cells that are enclosed within the capillary basement membrane—are present in brain capillaries, as they are in nonbarrier capillaries. There is reason to believe that the pericyte is derived from or is developmentally related to the smooth muscle cell, and one proposed role for the pericyte is to regulate capillary diameter and microregional blood flow.[21] Observations from *in vivo* studies suggest that pericytes regulate endothelial growth, and *in vitro* models show that pericytes are able to inhibit endothelial cell division by a transforming growth factor-β–dependent mechanism.[22] Pericytes are closely apposed to the capillary basement membrane and likely synthesize components of the basement membrane. Therefore, the potential exists for the pericyte to influence properties of endothelial differentiation and barrier function by means of direct cell-to-cell signals or by its influence on the composition of the capillary extracellular matrix. Pericytes may express phagocytic functions in response to pathophysiologic states associated with blood-brain barrier breakdown.[23-25] They may also play a normal physiologic role as a second line of defense in the blood-brain barrier. Pericytes are four times as numerous at the blood-retinal barrier, where the capillaries are normally somewhat more permeable to circulating solutes than they are in brain.[15] Loss of retinal pericytes occurs in retinal diseases associated with increased blood-retinal barrier permeability and pathologic retinal endothelial proliferation.

The brain capillary contains a basement membrane that is thicker and more developed than that of nonbarrier capillaries.[26,27] It surrounds the abluminal endothelial surface and physically separates each of the three capillary cell types. Similar to basement membranes in other tissues, it is an extracellular matrix composed of Type IV collagen, proteoglycans, the adhesion proteins laminin and fibronectin, and an uncertain number of other glycoproteins, some of which are likely to be unique to the brain capillary.[28] Aside from the basement membrane's role in the maintenance and compartmentalization of tissue architecture, it provides signals for cell adhesion, polarization, and differentiation. The basement membrane of kidney renal tubules functions as a semipermeable filter to charged macromolecules. There is no evidence for this function in the intact brain capillary; however, some degree of filtering at the level of the basement membrane could take place during conditions that disrupt the interendothelial tight junctions.

Despite the tight barrier to passive diffusion of substances provided by the interendothelial tight junctions, the lack of fenestrations, and low transcellular vesicular transport, certain compounds essential to brain development and function cross the capillary by means of specific carrier-mediated transport systems (Fig. 166-3).[29] The capacity of these transport systems appears to vary with changes in the metabolic requirements of brain and different systemic nutritional states.[30-34] The hexose transporter, GLUT1, is particularly well characterized.[35,36] GLUT1 is a member of a multigene family of seven glucose transporters, GLUT1 to GLUT7. Two forms of GLUT1 exist in brain and are distinguishable by differences in posttranslational glycosylation.[37] The 55-kDa form of GLUT1 is expressed by blood-brain barrier endothelial cells, and the 45-kDa form appears to be primarily expressed by glial cells. GLUT1 is a facilitative, saturable, and stereospecific transporter that functions at both the luminal and abluminal endothelial surfaces. The net flux of glucose into brain is driven by the relatively higher glucose concentration in plasma under normal conditions. Studies show that microvascular endothelial GLUT1 expression increases substantially during early postnatal rat brain development.[38] Inherited defects in the *glut1* gene can impair glucose transport across the blood-brain barrier and can cause abnormally low cerebrospinal fluid glucose (hypoglycorrhachia), neonatal epilepsy, microcephaly, and mental retardation. Sporadic heterozygous mutations in the *glut1* gene (1p35-31.3) are consistent with GLUT1 haploinsufficiency causing this autosomal dominant disorder. A missense mutation (Gly91Asp) in a functionally important cytoplasmic anchor point that is highly conserved among facilitative transport proteins has been identified.[39]

Blood-brain barrier amino acid transport systems have been well characterized by physiologic parameters, and several genes coding for specific blood-brain barrier transporters are now identified. A sodium (Na^+)-independent large neutral amino acid facilitative transport system (L system) is symmetrically located at the luminal and abluminal endothelial surfaces; it selectively transports glutamine, isoleucine, leucine, methionine, phenylalanine, tryptophan, tyrosine, and valine and thus favors essential over nonessential amino acids. This transporter is now identified as a dimeric transmembranous protein member of the heteromeric amino acid transport family consisting of a light chain (LAT1) and a heavy chain (4F2hc).[40,41] Small neutral amino acids, such as alanine, glycine, and serine, are transported asymmetrically from brain to blood by an Na^+-dependent transport system (A system) that is predominantly or exclusively located on the abluminal endothelial cell surface.[42] Because glycine is an inhibitory neurotransmitter that markedly alters brain neuronal activity, the asymmetric function of this transporter is of special significance. The Na^+ dependence of this carrier allows small neutral amino acids such as glycine to be transported up a gradient from brain, in which they are in relatively low concentration, to blood. A small neutral amino acid transporter (ATA2) with functional characteristics similar to the blood-brain barrier A-system transporter and expressed by brain endothelial cells was cloned.[43,44] It is thought that γ-glutamyl transpeptidase, an intracellular compound found in various cell types involved in amino acid transport,[45] may function intracellularly as part of the cystine transport mechanism in brain capillaries.[46-48]

The potassium transporter is ion specific, saturable, and dependent on Na^+,K^+-ATPase.[49] The cytochemical localization of this enzymatic transporter at the abluminal endothelial cell surface is consistent with the active efflux of potassium from brain to blood.[50] The large amount of energy used by this transporter is justified by the need for extremely tight regulation of brain potassium concentrations required for normal neuronal activity. A saturable and stereospecific carrier-mediated transport system for short acids such as lactate, acetate, and propionate was demonstrated by Oldendorf.[51] The ketone bodies β-hydroxybutyrate and acetoacetate also cross the blood-brain barrier by a carrier-mediated transport system.[34,52] A specific monocarboxylic transporter (MCT1) has been cloned, is expressed symmetrically on barrier endothelial luminal and abluminal membranes, and mediates the enhanced uptake and utilization of monocarboxylic acids, the principal neuronal energy source during early brain development and

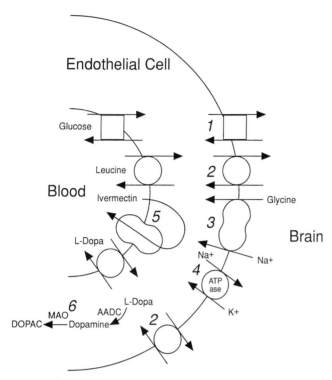

Figure 166–3. Transport and enzymatic properties of blood-brain barrier endothelial cells. Glucose, the primary metabolic substrate for neurons, is transported from blood to brain by a specific facilitative transporter designated GLUT1 (*1*). Large neutral amino acids such as represented by leucine cross endothelial cells through the facilitative L-system transporter LAT1 (*2*). Small neutral amino acids cross antiluminal endothelial membranes through the asymmetrically located energy-dependent A-system transporter ATA2 (*3*) in conjunction with Na+,K+-ATPase (*4*) that also localizes to the endothelial antiluminal membrane. The multiple drug resistance gene product, p-glycoprotein (*5*), serves to pump lipid-soluble compounds such as ivermectin out of barrier endothelial cells. Enzyme systems (*6*) such as aromatic amino acid decarboxylase (AADC) and monoamine oxidase (MAO) serve to inactivate neuroactive compounds such as L-dopa that enter endothelial cells through the L-system transporter LAT1 (*2*).

starvation.[53, 54] Circulating peptides such as insulin, insulin-like growth factors, and transferrin bind specifically and saturably to brain capillaries and are transported across the blood-brain barrier by receptor-mediated transcytosis.[55-57] OATP-A and Oatp2, members of the family of organic anion transporters in human and rat, respectively, are highly expressed by brain endothelial cells and mediate the transport of opioid polypeptides across the blood-brain barrier.[58]

Enzymes present within brain capillary endothelial cells function as a metabolic barrier to certain compounds. The barrier to L-dopa provides the classic example (see Fig. 166–3). L-dopa is transported into capillary endothelial cells by the large neutral amino acid transporter LAT1. Once in the endothelium, it is rapidly metabolized by L-dopa decarboxylase to dopamine, which is unable to cross the abluminal endothelial cell surface and is thus excluded from brain.[59] Brain capillaries are also enriched in monoamine oxidase that likely inactivates toxic amines and catecholamine neurotransmitters.[60] Likewise, endothelial enrichment in γ-glutamyl transpeptidase suggests that glutathione-dependent drug detoxification is especially active in barrier vessels.[61]

The multidrug resistance gene *MDR1* codes for the multidrug resistance gene product, P-glycoprotein, which is up-regulated in brain endothelium.[62, 63] P-glycoprotein was first described in cancer cells, in which it was shown to pump lipophilic substances, including several antineoplastic drugs, actively out of cells.[64, 65] P-glycoprotein is also expressed by normal secretory epithelium and regulates the physiologic secretion of metabolites into bile and urine and directly into the lumen of the gastrointestinal tract.[66] P-glycoprotein forms a protective mechanism that excludes ingested toxins from the brain. This is evidenced by the finding that mice deficient in the homologous *mdr1a* gene display increased sensitivity to the neurotoxic pesticide ivermectin and to the carcinostatic drug vinblastine.[67]

DEVELOPMENTAL ASPECTS

What is known of blood-brain barrier development in vertebrates is derived from a large body of data on a spectrum of organisms ranging from hagfish to sheep. Data derived from human fetal tissue are rare. Comparisons among vertebrate classes indicate that the structural and functional aspects of the blood-brain barrier are remarkably conserved.[68] Because there are significant species differences in the timing of brain growth and differentiation relative to the timing of birth,[69] caution must be exercised when comparing temporal aspects of prenatal or postnatal barrier development among species.

The process of capillary formation in the rat was detailed by Bär and Wolff,[1] and morphometric analyses at various stages of blood-brain barrier development were correlated with capillary permeability to intravascular dyes or horseradish peroxidase (a protein that is easily visualized with the electron microscope by virtue of its ability to form an electron-dense reaction product).[70-72] The earliest vasculature of the rat brain forms a plexus on the surface that is primarily sinusoidal. The endothelial lining of these primitive vessels is fenestrated, as in nonbarrier vessels, and is incompletely surrounded by an undifferentiated mesenchymal layer. At most, an insignificant amount of extracellular matrix material is discernible in a spotty distribution associated with cell surfaces, and the perivascular extracellular space is broad and of variable width. As pericytes begin to differentiate, the endothelial cells become surrounded by pericytes and their processes. The endothelial cells later become invested with astrocytic end-feet, at which point a true capillary-astrocytic complex resembling the mature vessel is formed. The basement membrane becomes recognizable concurrent with these events and appears most developed at regions of closest endothelial-astrocytic contact. There is some suggestion that the basement membrane forms adjacent to the membranes of each cell type and that these membranes become consolidated or fused. Concurrent with astrocytic investment and basement membrane formation are a marked decrease in the width of the perivascular space and a decrease in the fraction of endothelial cell that is surrounded by pericytes or their processes. These events of perivascular consolidation and basement membrane formation in the mouse and rat are most prominent from birth through the first 3 to 4 postnatal weeks. During this period in the mouse, vessel wall thickness decreases by 60%, and the basement membrane thickens from undetectable levels to 71 nm by electron microscopic criteria.[71] Paracellular diffusion diminishes by a factor of 30 during these latter stages of capillary-astrocytic complex formation, basement membrane formation, and perivascular consolidation. Nonbarrier vessels in the area postrema and skeletal muscle do not develop these differentiated features.

As described earlier, the barrier to the diffusion of polar substances across the mature brain capillary is attributed to the presence of very complex interendothelial tight junctions, the lack of fenestrae, and relatively little transendothelial vesicular transport. The establishment of a barrier to diffusion occurs relatively late in

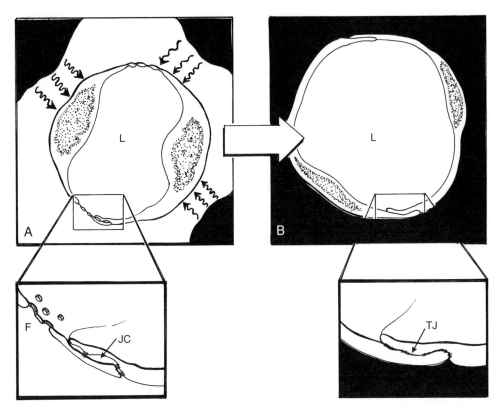

Figure 166–4. Structural changes in blood-brain barrier capillaries during development. Fetal capillaries (**A**) are sinusoid-like, fenestrated vessels with distinct expansions in the junctional clefts suggesting paracellular channels. They are surrounded by loosely arranged neuroepithelial cells (screening). Putative inductive factors (*curved arrows*) from the neuroepithelial cells elicit the formation of mature blood-brain barrier capillary morphology (**B**) and the expression of numerous transport and metabolic endothelial mechanisms detailed in the text. Structurally, the fenestrations disappear and the junctional clefts flatten, suggesting a closure of the paracellular pathways. The capillaries are now completely surrounded by compact neuropil (screening). F = fenestrations; JC = junctional cleft; L = lumen of the vessel; TJ = tight junctional profile.

the developing rodent brain and is most commonly attributed to the maturing of primitive tight junction.[71,73-75] Quantitative morphometric analyses using transmission electron microscopy in the developing mouse[71] and rat[76-78] strongly support this view. Vessels that penetrate the brain from the surface lose their fenestrations within a few days of penetration.[76,77,79] Prebarrier brain capillaries contain tight junctions that are interrupted by clefts that appear to form paracellular channels through which diffusion of polar substances may occur (Fig. 166–4). These clefts decrease in number and width with age, consistent with a maturational process that leads to the closure of the paracellular channel to diffusion.[71] Endothelial junctions in the fetus resemble adult junctions in their size and density,[76,77] but approximately 20% of the junctional clefts are enlarged in the fetus, consistent with a paracellular channel.[76,80] Weinbaum and associates[81] theorized that infrequent large breaks in the junctional strands are the best model to account for small solute permeability in capillaries. The large clefts described in the fetal brain capillaries are infrequent and have approximately the right dimensions to represent the pores modeled by Weinbaum and colleagues. The frequency of expanded junctional clefts decreases late in fetal development and after birth in parallel with declining vascular permeability.[71,78,82] To support the importance of tight junction maturation further are the observations in the mouse that fenestrae disappear much earlier and the density of endothelial vesicles remains very low and unchanged throughout the stage of barrier development.[71] Similar observations have been made in the developing chicken.[83] In certain species, namely, mouse and sheep, a fetal tubulovesicular transendothelial transport system was identified, and the development of the barrier was attributed to its disappearance.[6,84]

Another factor that may contribute to fetal vascular leakiness is the rapid growth of the vascular tree. One of the mechanisms involved in vascular proliferation is the formation of capillary sprouts. Sprouts that form in response to certain pathologic states have structural characteristics of leaky vessels with frank gaps between endothelial cells and a poorly organized basement membrane.[85,86] Interendothelial gaps are probably much less

common, if not lacking, in sprouts of normally developing brain.[87] In any event, blood flow does not begin in capillary sprouts until they make contact with other vessels to form a closed circuit. By this time, the morphologic features associated with leakiness are no longer discernible.

Developmental changes during the first few neonatal weeks also occur in the receptor-mediated carrier systems that control the selective transport of nutrients across the blood-brain barrier and in the enzyme systems that represent the intracapillary metabolic barrier.[30,31,33,34,59,60] The GLUT-1 isozyme of the glucose transporter is expressed by all the cells of the neural tube and the surrounding perineurial vascular plexus before vascular invasion.[88,89] As vessels invade the neural tube, expression of GLUT-1 is maintained in the endothelial cells but is down-regulated in the surrounding neuroepithelium. Oldendorf and colleagues characterized transport changes in developing neonatal rabbit and rat. Brain uptake in newborn rabbits[90] and in rats[32,34] of β-hydroxybutyrate, tryptophan, adenine, and choline is elevated over that of the adult by approximate factors of 3, 1.4, 7, and 3, respectively. The higher Michaelis constant (K_m) and maximum velocity (V_{max}) values in newborns for these protein and neurotransmitter precursors and metabolites are consistent with the requirements of developing brain as well as the relatively high levels of these nutrients presented to suckling neonates in breast milk. Expression of the monocarboxylic acid transporter MCT1 by brain endothelial cells is increased many times in neonatal suckling rats compared with adults, a finding consistent with the greater utilization of monocarboxylates by neurons as a primary energy source in suckling animals.[53,91] In contrast, the K_m and V_{max} for glucose transport are greater in the adult than the newborn rabbit, a finding consistent with differences in glucose and ketone utilization at these ages.[32] In addition, increases in the rate of glucose transport into brain of developing rats correlate with increased brain microvessel GLUT1 expression.[38] The metabolism of toxic amines by monoamine oxidase and L-dopa decarboxylase increases by a factor of 3 during the second postnatal week in the rat. Furthermore, Harik and Kalaria[92] found that the postnatal increase of capillary monoamine oxidase predominantly results from an increase in the monoamine oxidase B isoenzyme, in contrast to a preponderance of the A isoenzyme form in peripheral tissues.

CELLULAR BIOLOGY

Identifying the cellular and biochemical mechanisms that lead to the expression of the blood-brain barrier phenotype in neural capillaries is of considerable interest. A steadily accumulating body of experimental evidence indicates that signals derived from brain parenchyma induce and modulate endothelial blood-brain barrier expression. Transplantation studies in rodent and avian systems show that the commitment to barrier formation is not intrinsic to the endothelial cell, because nonneural endothelium can be induced to form barrier features when it is exposed to the central nervous system tissue environment.[93-95] Furthermore, neural endothelial cells rapidly lose their barrier properties when they are isolated and cultured,[96] but they re-express certain barrier features when they are implanted back into brain.[97] Astrocytes have received the most attention as the source of this inductive influence because they are absent from peripheral tissues, and astrocytic end-feet form an almost continuous ensheathment of neural capillaries to produce a capillary-astrocytic complex (see Fig. 166-1).

A requirement for endothelial-astroglial interactions in endothelial barrier expression *in vivo* is supported by patterns of barrier expression in human and experimental brain tumors. Guerin and colleagues[98,99] showed that barrier-specific proteins are expressed by endothelial cells deep within intracranial astroglial tumors but not by endothelial cells within brain metastases. Thus, certain barrier functions persist in proliferating vessels that retain astroglial associations in the absence of either neurons or oligodendroglia. Destruction of astrocytes using a specific gliotoxin was found to increase blood-brain barrier permeability without causing any changes in the expression of GLUT-1, endothelial barrier antigen (EBA), or γ-glutamyl transpeptidase.[100] Together, these results suggest that multiple environmental cues may selectively influence endothelial barrier expression, and these signals may be different for developing, proliferating, and quiescent brain endothelium.

In vitro studies also support the idea that astroglia-derived environmental signals regulate neural endothelial differentiation. Studies in which endothelial cells are cultured in the presence of astroglial cells or their conditioned medium demonstrate that astrocytes can regulate endothelial organization into microvascular forms and can induce their re-expression of blood-brain barrier phenotypic properties that are typically lost under routine culture conditions. Such barrier properties include the expression of complex interendothelial tight junctions,[101,102] asymmetric amino acid transport,[103] and γ-glutamyl transpeptidase.[104] The induction of interendothelial tight junctions by astrocytes or their conditioned medium is enhanced by cyclic adenosine monophosphate agonists,[102,105] and it specifically increases the P-face association of tight junction particles as defined by freeze fracture analysis.[105] This pattern of tight junction formation *in vitro* mimics tight junction formation *in vivo* as determined by freeze fracture analysis of isolated intact brain microvessels.[105]

It is well established that parenchymal signals regulate microvessel formation, and perivascular astroglia are well positioned to regulate brain endothelial shape and microvessel morphogenesis. This function is supported by *in vitro* studies showing that primary rat brain astrocytes and astroglial tumor cells induce microvascular endothelial cells to differentiate into capillary-like tubular structures.[106] This morphogenic astroglial-endothelial interaction appears to require poorly diffusable cell signals such as extracellular matrix molecules and is tightly regulated by the balance of periendothelial plasminogen activa-

tors and their inhibitors.[107, 108] The regulation of endothelial morphogenic and functional differentiation by perivascular glial cells is consistent with a model in which the perivascular astroglial sheath enhances neuroprotective microvascular mechanisms.

In view of the currently available evidence, it is likely that factors in the neural tissue environment, including those from astrocytes, are responsible for the induction and maintenance of neural endothelial differentiation. Many questions concerning this interaction remain unanswered. The specific determinants of barrier induction have yet to be identified. It is likely that astrocyte-derived nondiffusible extracellular matrix components concurrent with other diffusible signals derived from astrocytes, pericytes, or other more distant glial and neuronal cell types provide a sufficiently inductive influence. At present, available molecular and cellular biologic techniques applied to the characterization and manipulation of *in vivo* models and complex culture systems can be used to test these hypotheses.

REFERENCES

1. Bär T, Wolff JR: The formation of capillary basement membranes during internal vascularization of the rat's cerebral cortex. Z Zellforsch Mikrosk Anat *133*:231, 1972.
2. Bundgaard M: Vesicular transport in capillary endothelium: does it occur? Fed Proc *42*:425, 1983.
3. Brightman M, Reese T: Junctions between intimately apposed cell membranes in the vertebrate brain. J Cell Biol *40*:648, 1969.
4. Coomber BL, Stewart PA: Three-dimensional reconstruction of vesicles in endothelium of blood-brain barrier versus highly permeable microvessels. Anat Rec *215*:256, 1986.
5. Coomber BL, Stewart PA: Morphometric analysis of CNS microvascular endothelium. Microvasc Res *30*:99, 1985.
6. Dziegielewska KM, et al: Studies of the development of brain barrier systems to lipid insoluble molecules in fetal sheep. J Physiol *292*:207, 1979.
7. Lossinsky AS, et al: Characterization of endothelial cell transport in the developing mouse blood-brain barrier. Dev Neurosci *8*:61, 1986.
8. Reese TS, Karnovsky MJ: Fine structural localization of a blood-brain barrier to exogenous peroxidase. J Cell Biol *34*:207, 1967.
9. Huber JD, et al: Molecular physiology and pathophysiology of tight junctions in the blood-brain barrier. Trends Neurosci *24*:719, 2001.
10. Kniesel U, Wolburg H: Tight junctions of the blood-brain barrier. Cell Mol Neurobiol *20*:57, 2000.
11. Lippoldt A, et al: Structural alterations of tight junctions are associated with loss of polarity in stroke-prone spontaneously hypertensive rat blood-brain barrier endothelial cells. Brain Res *885*:251, 2000.
12. Martin-Padura I, et al: Junctional adhesion molecule, a novel member of the immunoglobulin superfamily that distributes at intercellular junctions and modulates monocyte transmigration. J Cell Biol *142*:117, 1998.
13. Stewart PA, et al: Quantitation of blood-brain barrier ultrastructure. J Electron Microsc Tech *27*:516, 1994.
14. Holash JA, et al: Barrier properties of testis microvessels. Proc Natl Acad Sci USA *90*:11069, 1993.
15. Stewart PA, Tuor UI: Blood-eye barriers in the rat: correlation of ultrastructure with function. J Comp Neurol *340*:566, 1994.
16. Nag S, et al: Quantitative estimate of pinocytosis in experimental acute hypertension. Acta Neuropathol (Berl) *46*:107, 1979.
17. Petito CK, et al: Edema and vascular permeability in cerebral ischemia: comparison between ischemic neuronal damage and infarction. J Neuropathol Exp Neurol *41*:423, 1982.
18. Westergaard E, et al: Increased vesicular transfer of horseradish peroxidase across cerebral endothelium, evoked by acute hypertension. Acta Neuropathol (Berl) *37*:141, 1977.
19. Palade GE: Blood capillaries of the heart and other organs. Circulation *24*:368, 1961.
20. Broadwell RD, Banks WA: Cell Biological Perspective for the Transcytosis Of Peptides and Proteins through the Mammalian Blood-Brain Fluid Barriers. Raven Press, New York, 1993.
21. Herman IM, et al: Characterization of microvascular cell cultures from normotensive and hypertensive rat brains: pericyte-endothelial cell interactions in vitro. Tissue Cell *19*:197, 1987.
22. Orlidge A, D'Amore PA: Inhibition of capillary endothelial cell growth by pericytes and smooth muscle cells. J Cell Biol *105*:1455, 1987.
23. Cancilla PA, et al: The reaction of pericytes of the central nervous system to exogenous protein. Lab Invest *26*:376, 1972.
24. Sumner BE: A quantitative study of vascular permeability to horseradish peroxidase, and the subsequent fate of the tracer, in rat brains after portocaval anastomosis. Neuropathol Appl Neurobiol *8*:117, 1982.
25. van Deurs B: Observation on the blood-brain barrier in hypertensive rats, with particular reference to phagocytic pericytes. J Ultrastr Res *56*:65, 1976.

26. Maynard EA: Electron microscopy of the vascular bed of rat cerebral cortex. Am J Anat 100:409, 1957.
27. Wolff J: Beitrage Zur Ultrastruktur der kapillaren in der normalen Grobhirnrinde. Z Zellorsch 60:409, 1963.
28. Timpl R, Dziadek M: Structure, development, and molecular pathology of basement membranes. Int Rev Exp Pathol 29:1, 1986.
29. Pardridge WM, et al: Blood-brain barrier: interface between internal medicine and the brain. Ann Intern Med 105:82, 1986.
30. Cornford EM, et al: Developmental modulations of blood-brain barrier permeability as an indicator of changing nutritional requirements in the brain. Pediatr Res 16:324, 1982.
31. Cornford EM, Cornford ME: Nutrient transport and the blood-brain barrier in developing animals. Fed Proc 45:2065, 1986.
32. Cremer JE, et al: Kinetics of blood-brain barrier transport of pyruvate, lactate and glucose in suckling, weanling and adult rats. J Neurochem 33:439, 1979.
33. Crone C: Facilitated transfer of glucose from blood into brain tissue. J Physiol 181:103, 1965.
34. Moore TJ, et al: Beta-hydroxybutyrate transport in rat brain: developmental and dietary modulations. Am J Physiol 230:619, 1976.
35. Cremer JE, et al: Changes during development in transport processes of the blood-brain barrier. Biochim Biophys Acta 448:633, 1976.
36. Oldendorf WH: Carrier-mediated blood-brain barrier transport of short-chain monocarboxylic organic acids. Am J Physiol 224:1450, 1973.
37. Maher F, et al: Glucose transporter proteins in brain. FASEB J 8:1003, 1994.
38. Vannucci SJ, et al: Glucose transport in developing rat brain: glucose transporter proteins, rate constants and cerebral glucose utilization. Mol Cell Biochem 140:177, 1994.
39. Klepper J: Autosomal dominant transmission of GLUT1 deficiency. Hum Mol Genet 10:63, 2001.
40. Kido Y, et al: Molecular and functional identification of large neutral amino acid transporters LAT1 and LAT2 and their pharmacological relevance at the blood-brain barrier. J Pharm Pharmacol 53:497, 2001.
41. Boado RJ, et al: Selective expression of the large neutral amino acid transporter at the blood-brain barrier. Proc Natl Acad Sci USA 96:12079, 1999.
42. Betz AL, Goldstein GW: Polarity of the blood brain barrier: neutral amino acid transport into isolated brain capillaries. Science 202:225, 1978.
43. Sugawara M, et al: Cloning of an amino acid transporter with functional characteristics and tissue expression pattern identical to that of system A. J Biol Chem 275:16473, 2000.
44. Takanaga H, et al: ATA2 is predominantly expressed as system A at the blood-brain barrier and acts as brain-to-blood efflux transport for L-proline. Mol Pharmacol 61:1289, 2002.
45. Orlowski M, Meister A: The γ-glutamyl cycle: a possible transport system for amino acids. Proc Natl Acad Sci USA 67:1248, 1970.
46. Orlowski M, et al: γ-Glutamyl transpeptidase in brain capillaries: possible site of a blood-brain barrier for amino acids. Science 184:66, 1974.
47. Albert Z, et al: Studies on gamma-glutamyl transpeptidase activity and its histochemical localization in the central nervous system of man and different animal species. Acta Histochem 25:312, 1966.
48. Samuels S, et al: Effect of gamma-glutamyl cycle inhibitors on brain amino acid transport and utilization. Neurochem Res 3:619, 1978.
49. Goldstein GW: Relation of potassium transport to oxidative metabolism in isolated brain capillaries. J Physiol (Lond) 286:185, 1979.
50. Betz A, et al: Polarity of the blood brain barrier: distribution of enzymes between the luminal and antiluminal membranes of brain capillary endothelial cells. Brain Res 182:17, 1980.
51. Oldendorf WH: Brain uptake of radiolabeled amino acids, amines, and hexoses after arterial injection. Am J Physiol 221:1629, 1971.
52. Daniel PM, et al: The transport of ketone bodies into the brain of the rat (in vivo). J Neurol Sci 34:1, 1977.
53. Pellerin L, et al: Expression of monocarboxylate transporter mRNAs in mouse brain: support for a distinct role of lactate as an energy substrate for the neonatal vs. adult brain. Proc Natl Acad Sci USA 95:3990, 1998.
54. Gerhart DZ, et al: Expression of monocarboxylate transporter MCT1 by brain endothelium and glia in adult and suckling rats. Am J Physiol 273:E207, 1997.
55. Pardridge WM, et al: Human blood-brain barrier insulin receptor. J Neurochem 44:1771, 1985.
56. Pardridge WM, et al: Human blood-brain barrier transferrin receptor. Metab Clin Exp 36:892, 1987.
57. Pardridge WM, Oldendorf WH: Transport of metabolic substrates through the blood-brain barrier. J Neurochem 28:5, 1977.
58. Gao B, et al: Organic anion-transporting polypeptides mediate transport of opioid peptides across blood-brain barrier. J Pharmacol Exp Ther 294:73, 2000.
59. Sachs C: Development of the blood-brain barrier for 6-hydroxydopamine. J Neurochem 20:1753, 1973.
60. Hardebo JE, Owman C: Barrier mechanisms for neurotransmitter monoamines and their precursors at the blood-brain barrier. Ann Neurol 8:1, 1979.
61. Sessa G, Perez MM: Biochemical changes in rat brain associated with the development of the blood-brain barrier. J Neurochem 25:779, 1975.
62. Cordon-Cardo C, et al: Multidrug-resistance gene (P-glycoprotein) is expressed by endothelial cells at blood-brain barrier sites. Proc Natl Acad Sci USA 86:695, 1989.
63. Thiebaut F, et al: Immunohistochemical localization in normal tissues of different epitopes in the multidrug transport protein p 170: evidence for localization in brain capillaries and crossreactivity of one antibody with muscle protein. J Histochem Cytochem 37:159, 1989.
64. Riordan JR, et al: Amplification of P-glycoprotein genes in multidrug-resistant mammalian cell lines. Nature 316:817, 1985.
65. Kartner N, et al: Detection of P-glycoprotein in multidrug-resistant cell lines by monoclonal antibodies. Nature 316:820, 1985.
66. Thiebaut F, et al: Cellular localization of the multidrug-resistance gene product P-glycoprotein in normal human tissues. Proc Natl Acad Sci USA 84:7735, 1987.
67. Schinkel AH, et al: Disruption of the mouse mdr1a P-glycoprotein gene leads to a deficiency in the blood-brain barrier and to increased sensitivity to drugs. Cell 77:491, 1994.
68. Cserr HF, Bundgaard M: Blood-brain interfaces in vertebrates: a comparative approach. Am J Physiol 246:R277, 1984.
69. Dobbing J: The development of the blood-brain barrier. Prog Brain Res 29:417, 1968.
70. Delorme P, et al: Ultrastructural study on transcapillary exchanges in the developing telencephalon of the chicken. Brain Res 22:269, 1970.
71. Stewart P, Hayakawa E: Interendothelial junctional changes underlie the developmental "tightening" of the blood brain barrier. Brain Res 429:271, 1987.
72. Wakai S, Hirokawa E: Development of the blood-brain barrier to horseradish peroxidase in the chick embryo. Cell Tissue Res 195:195, 1978.
73. Mollgard K: Lack of correlation between tight junction morphology and permeability properties in developing choroid plexus. Nature 264:293, 1976.
74. Mollgard K, Saunders NR: Complex tight junctions of epithelial and of endothelial cells in early foetal brain. J Neurocytol 4:453, 1975.
75. Mollgard K, Saunders NR: A possible transepithelial pathway via endoplasmic reticulum in foetal sheep choroid plexus. Proc R Soc Lond B Biol Sci 199:321, 1977.
76. Stewart PA, Hayakawa K: Early ultrastructural changes in blood-brain barrier vessels of the rat embryo. Dev Brain Res 78:25, 1994.
77. Bauer HC, et al: Neovascularization and the appearance of morphological characteristics of the blood-brain barrier in the embryonic mouse central nervous system. Brain Res Dev Brain Res 75:269, 1993.
78. Weinstein RS, et al: P-glycoprotein in pathology: the multidrug resistance gene family in humans. Hum Pathol 21:34, 1990.
79. Yoshida Y, et al: Endothelial fenestrae in the rat fetal cerebrum. Brain Res Dev Brain Res 44:211, 1988.
80. Schulze C, Firth JA: Immunohistochemical localization of adherens junction components in blood-brain barrier microvessels of the rat. J Cell Sci 104:773, 1993.
81. Weinbaum S, et al: A three-dimensional junction-pore-matrix model for capillary permeability. Microvasc Res 44:85, 1992.
82. Butt AM, et al: Electrical resistance across the blood-brain barrier in anaesthetized rats: a developmental study. J Physiol 429:47, 1990.
83. Roncali L, et al: Microscopical and ultrastructural investigations on the development of the blood-brain barrier in the chick embryo optic tectum. Acta Neuropathol 70:193, 1986.
84. Lossinsky AS: Ultracytochemical studies of transendothelial transport in cerebral micro-blood vessels during development. J Cell Biol 99:283A, 1984.
85. Ausprunk DH, Folkman J: Vascular injury in transplanted tissues: fine structural changes in tumor, adult and embryonic blood vessels. Virchows Arch B Cell Pathol 21:31, 1976.
86. Schoefl GI: Studies on inflamation. III. Growing capillaries: Their structure and permeability. Virchows Arch A Pathol Anat 337:97, 1963.
87. Nousek-Goebl NA, Press MF: Golgi-electron microscopic study of sprouting endothelial cells in the neonatal rat cerebellar cortex. Brain Res 395:67, 1986.
88. Harik SI, et al: Ontogeny of the erythroid/HepG2-type glucose transporter (GLUT-1) in the rat nervous system. Dev Brain Res 72:41, 1993.
89. Dermietzel R, et al: Pattern of glucose transporter (Glut 1) expression in embryonic brains is related to maturation of blood-brain barrier tightness. Dev Dyn 193:152, 1992.
90. Braun LD, et al: Newborn rabbit blood-brain barrier is selectively permeable and differs substantially from the adult. J Neurochem 34:147, 1980.
91. Leino RL, et al: Monocarboxylate transporter (MCT1) abundance in brains of suckling and adult rats: a quantitative electron microscopic immunogold study. Brain Res Dev Brain Res 113:47, 1999.
92. Kalaria RN, Harik SI: Differential postnatal development of monoamine oxidases A and B in the blood-brain barrier of the rat. J Neurochem 49:1589, 1987.
93. Svendgaard NA, et al: Axonal degeneration associated with a defective blood-brain barrier in cerebral implants. Nature 255:334, 1975.
94. Stewart P, Wiley M: Developing nervous tissue induces formation of blood brain barrier characteristics in invading endothelial cells: a study using quail chick transplantation chimeras. Dev Biol 84:183, 1981.
95. Risau W, et al: Brain induces the expression of an early cell surface marker for blood-brain barrier–specific endothelium. EMBO J 5:3179, 1986.
96. Laterra J, Goldstein GW: Brain Microvessels and Microvascular Cells in Vitro. New York, Raven Press, 1993.
97. Lal B, et al: Endothelial cell implantation and survival within experimental gliomas. Proc Natl Acad Sci USA 91:9695, 1994.
98. Guerin C, et al: The glucose transporter and blood brain barrier of human brain tumors. Ann Neurol 28:758, 1990.
99. Guerin C, et al: Vascular expression of glucose transporter in experimental brain neoplasms. Am J Pathol 140:417, 1992.

100. Krum JM: Experimental gliopathy in the adult rat CNS: effect on the blood-spinal cord barrier. Glia *11*:354, 1994.
101. Tao-Cheng JH, et al: Tight junctions of brain endothelium in vitro are enhanced by astroglia. J Neurosci 7:3293, 1987.
102. Rubin LL, et al: A cell culture model of the blood-brain barrier. J Cell Biol *115*:1725, 1991.
103. Beck DW, et al: Glial cells influence polarity of the blood-brain barrier. J Neuropathol Exp Neurol *43*:219, 1984.
104. DeBault LE, Cancilla PA: γ-Glutamyl transpeptidase in isolated brain endothelial cells: induction by glial cells in vitro. Science *207*:653, 1980.
105. Wolburg H, et al: Modulation of tight junction structure in blood-brain barrier endothelial cells: effects of tissue culture, second messengers and cocultured astrocytes. J Cell Sci *107*:1347, 1994.
106. Laterra J, et al: Astrocytes induce neural microvascular endothelial cells to form capillary like structures in vitro. J Cell Physiol *144*:204, 1990.
107. Wolff JEA, et al: Steroid inhibition of neural microvessel morphogenesis in vitro: Receptor mediation and astroglial dependence. J Neurochem *58*:1023, 1992.
108. Laterra J, et al: Regulation of in vitro glia-induced microvessel morphogenesis by urokinase. J Cell Physiol *158*:317, 1994.

167

Michael V. Johnston and Faye S. Silverstein

Development of Neurotransmitters

The function of the immature brain is determined to a considerable extent by the operational state of the specialized chemical synaptic connections between neurons.[1] The capacity of immature synapses to transfer information determines functions as diverse as hormone release, breathing, and vision. Advances in analyzing and understanding the machinery of chemical neurotransmission are providing a more complete picture of the dynamic events that take place in the fetus and neonate.[2, 3] Conventional biochemical assays for synaptic activities as well as methods with greater spatial resolution (e.g., receptor autoradiography) have been used to assess development of neurotransmitter pathways. These studies indicate that biochemical features of neurotransmission are often markedly different in the immature brain compared with those in the adult brain. Distinct neurotransmitter-specific neuronal groups mature at different rates, so multineuronal networks may have a different functional "balance" at different ages.[1] Moreover, although some components of the synapse, such as neurotransmitter synthetic enzymes, are relatively undeveloped or inactive in the fetus and neonate, others, including certain neurotransmitter receptors and second-messenger systems, are expressed at much higher levels than in adults.[4, 5] These developmental patterns are relevant to understanding normal physiology as well as the effects of disease in the immature brain.

Chemical transfer of messages across synapses depends on coordinated function of several biochemical processes (Fig. 167–1). A neurotransmitter is synthesized by specific enzymes within nerve terminals and may be stored (e.g., catecholamines) in synaptic vesicles awaiting impulse-stimulated release. Specific biochemical uptake processes or "pumps" within axonal nerve terminals may remove transmitter released from the synaptic cleft and may prevent it from having prolonged contact with postsynaptic receptors. Similar uptake processes remove portions of degraded neurotransmitter. For example, acetylcholine is hydrolyzed to yield choline, which is transported into the cholinergic nerve terminal by a high-affinity sodium-dependent uptake process. Stimulation of neurotransmitter release from axons and reuptake is coordinated with electrical impulse flow. In certain groups of synapses, catalytic enzymes are located within the nerve terminal and on the surface of synaptic endings to degrade released neurotransmitter. For example, catecholamines are degraded by the cytoplasmic enzyme monoamine oxidase and by the enzyme catechol-*O*-methyl transferase.

Actions of neurotransmitters are expressed in postsynaptic neurons through specific neurotransmitter receptors. These receptors are generally linked to ionophores (ion channels) or second-messenger systems, or both. Stimulation of receptors linked to ion channels generally produces a change in the membrane potential, such as depolarization in the case of excitatory neurotransmitters (e.g., glutamate) or hyperpolarization produced by inhibitory neurotransmitters such as γ-aminobutyric acid (GABA). Second-messenger systems may stimulate a cascade of intracellular events such as protein phosphorylation or modulation of gene expression. The relative influence of a neurotransmitter pathway during development is determined by the sum of these processes, and differential rates of development in each of them modify the relative influence of pathways markedly at different developmental stages. The separate biochemical processes involved in neurotransmission in a single neuronal group may develop at different rates, and these altered relationships (e.g., among transmitter synthesis, release, and reuptake) determine the pathway's influence.[1]

EARLY BIRTH AND DEVELOPMENT OF THE BRAIN STEM NORADRENERGIC PROJECTION TO CEREBRAL CORTEX

Norepinephrine-containing axons project into the cerebral cortex and other parts of the forebrain from the locus ceruleus in the pons.[6] The noradrenergic axonal network within cerebral cortex is thought to be involved in cortical activation and attention, and axons projected into the diencephalon influence neuroendocrine function. The cell bodies in this pathway are among the earliest to undergo neurogenesis in the developing brain.[7] This finding is consistent with the general pattern that neurons originating in the brain stem are "born" or originate before those in more rostral locations. The cell bodies of this projection originate on gestational days 12 to 14 (total gestational period of 21 days) in rats and on gestational days 27 to 36 in monkeys (total 165 days' gestation).[7] The noradrenergic projection appears to be influential in the immature cortex. In the neonatal rat, approximately one-third of all cortical synapses possess an axonal uptake mechanism for monoamines, a proportion that far exceeds the density in the adult.[8] Some experimental work supports the proposal that noradrenergic axons exert a trophic effect on the developing cortex in fetal and early postnatal life. Development of the visual cortex may be regulated by norepinephrine in the "critical period" of visual plasticity.[9]

Development of the noradrenergic system in cortex has been examined by measuring endogenous levels of the neurotransmitter norepinephrine, the energy-dependent, high-affinity uptake of [³H]norepinephrine into pinched-off nerve endings (synaptosomes), and the activity of the neurotransmitter synthetic enzymes tyrosine hydroxylase and dopamine β-hydroxylase during development.[6, 10–13] Results of these studies have

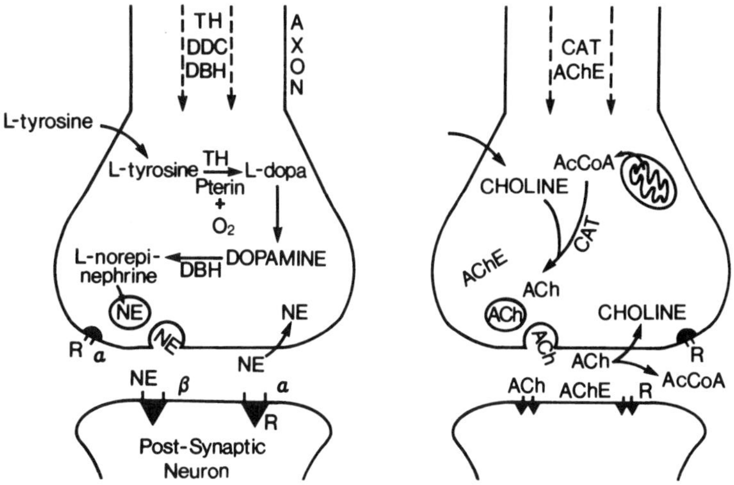

Figure 167–1. Schematic diagrams connected to an axon *(top)* projected from a noradrenergic cell body in the brain stem. The key biochemical markers, which are relatively specific for noradrenergic nerve terminals, are tyrosine hydroxylase (TH) and dopamine β-hydroxylase (DBH), the biosynthetic enzymes, endogenous nor-epinephrine (NE) content, and [³H]NE uptake *in vitro* into sealed-off nerve endings (synaptosomes). The high-affinity uptake pump is shown by the *arrow* directed from the synaptic cleft into the presynaptic terminal. DBH is found only in noradrenergic axons, whereas TH is also found in dopamine nerve terminals. The cortical distributions of noradrenergic and dopamine axons are relatively distinct. β-Adrenergic receptors are found pre-dominantly postsynaptically, whereas α-adrenergic receptors (R) are localized presynaptically and post-synaptically. On the *right,* an acetylcholine synapse is diagrammed, indicating one of the primary markers, choline acetyltransferase (CAT), the enzyme that synthesizes acetylcholine from acetyl coenzyme A (AcCoA) and choline. Endogenous acetylcholine and [³H]choline uptake into synaptosomes are also specific markers. Acetylcholinesterase (AChE) is relatively specifically localized in cholinergic cell bodies in regions such as the basal forebrain but may be non-specific in other regions, including the substantia nigra, and in intrinsic cortical neurons. Muscarinic and nico-tinic acetylcholine receptors (R) are located presynapti-cally and postsynaptically. DDC = L-dopa decarboxylase.

been compared in rodents and subhuman primates. When bio-chemical markers for this neurotransmitter system are studied during development (Fig. 167–2), investigators have noted that the ability of presynaptic nerve terminals to take up [³H]norepi-nephrine develops slightly before endogenous levels of neuro-transmitters and synthetic enzyme activities rise.

Synaptic effects of norepinephrine are expressed at postsynap-tic β-adrenergic and α-adrenergic receptors and at presynaptic α-receptors.[3,14,15] Development of these receptors and of associ-ated second-messenger effects, such as norepinephrine-stimulated cyclic adenosine monophosphate (cAMP) production and phos-phoinositide (PI) hydrolysis, increases rapidly in the postnatal period, as shown in Figure 167–2.[4,16] *In vitro* receptor autoradi-ography has been used to visualize the location and density of these receptors, and these studies have identified specific laminar and regional differences in their development.[3,14,17]

DOPAMINE INNERVATION

Dopamine, the other major catecholamine in the brain, is con-tained within neuronal projections extending from the substantia nigra in the midbrain into the basal ganglia, the hypothalamus, and restricted portions of the cerebral cortex such as the cingu-lum. The neurons from which these projections originate also arise relatively early, at gestational days 13 to 15 in rats and at fetal days 36 to 43 in monkeys.[7] Histofluorescence for dopamine and serotonin has been found in human fetuses as early as 3 months' gestation.[18] The biochemical markers for these axons—the dopamine reuptake system in synaptosomes, the synthetic activ-ity of tyrosine hydroxylase, and endogenous neurotransmitter stores—undergo almost all their maturation in the postnatal period.[1,19] Use of the histofluorescence technique to examine dopamine in the basal ganglia of postnatal animals indicates an early pattern of dopamine islands.[20,21] These islands persist as specialized groupings of axons in the adult brain, although the overall pattern of dopamine is more confluent at that stage. In the adult brain, the specialized compartments extend throughout the

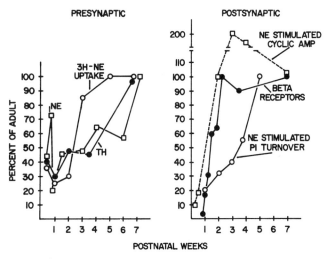

Figure 167–2. Ontogeny of biochemical markers for noradrener-gic axons in rodent cerebral cortex during postnatal develop-ment. Data for the *left panel* are on presynaptic markers in sensorimotor cortex. The *right panel* shows selected receptor and receptor-stimulated second-messenger activities.
AMP = adenosine monophosphate; NE = norepinephrine.
(From Johnston MV: Biochemistry of neurotransmitters in corti-cal development. *In* Peters A, Jones EG [eds]: Cerebral Cortex. New York, Plenum Press, 1988, pp 211–236.)

anteroposterior extent to form a lamellar or "striasomal" pattern. In rodent studies, the turnover of dopamine in the developing brain appears to be relatively high in the postnatal period and exceeds that in the adult. The ratios of homovanillic acid (HVA) and dihydroxyphenylacetic acid, which are products of dopamine oxidation, to endogenous dopamine levels are higher in the brain of immature rodents than in adults. This estimate of turnover suggests that dopamine neurons are active in the early postnatal period.

SEROTONIN PATHWAYS

Serotonin axons emerge from the raphe nuclei in the pons and resemble the widespread projections made by noradrenergic neurons into the forebrain and spinal cord. Serotonin pathways are important for control of hypothalamic and pituitary functions, pain, sleep, appetite, and other behavioral functions. The raphe serotonin neurons also undergo early cell division, with the timing similar to that of catecholamine neurons. Biochemical studies of serotonin turnover indicate that it is relatively high in the neonatal period in rodents, a finding suggesting early establishment of active neuronal impulse flow.[22] In rodents, maturation of serotonergic biochemical markers follows a caudal to rostral gradient with brain stem levels at two-thirds of adult levels at birth and hemisphere activity at 20% of adult levels. In the neonatal rodent, a transient, dense serotonin innervation has been found using an immunohistochemical technique to localize serotonin and autoradiography to image serotonin uptake sites on nerve terminals.[23] In somatosensory cortex, dense patches of serotonin innervation are aligned with specialized cellular aggregates, called *barrels,* before 3 weeks of age. Afterward, the patchy areas of hyperinnervation become more uniform and confluent. The ontogeny of serotonin receptors has been studied in the developing brain, and distinct laminar patterns have been identified.[15] These observations suggest that the pattern of serotonin innervation shares features in common with catecholamine projections from the brain stem. Both systems undergo early neurogenesis and appear to be relatively more densely represented in the neonatal period than later. The axonal arbors of both systems reorganize during postnatal development, and both may influence cortical plasticity.

DEVELOPMENT OF CEREBROSPINAL FLUID LEVELS OF DOPAMINE AND SEROTONIN METABOLITES IN HUMAN INFANTS

Measurement of levels of cerebrospinal fluid (CSF) metabolites of dopamine and serotonin provides an estimate of functional activity of central dopaminergic and serotonergic neurons in humans. The brain is the major site of HVA synthesis, and although up to 30% of the serotonin metabolite, 5-hydroxyindoleacetic acid (5-HIAA), is produced in the spinal cord, the neurons of origin are in the brain stem. A few studies have examined the maturation of catecholamine and serotonin pathways in the perinatal period.[24,25] In one study of neonates, 35 male and 22 female infants (gestational ages ranging from 28 to 42 weeks) were evaluated.[24] They included 38 premature infants (36 weeks or less) and 19 term infants. Common medical problems in these patients included prematurity, asphyxia, respiratory distress, and infection. Examination of the data, however, did not reveal any relationship of these conditions with the monoamine concentrations.

The infants were initially grouped into four age categories for analysis: (1) young premature infants less than 32 weeks' gestational age, (2) premature infants 33 to 36 weeks' gestational age, (3) infants 37 to 42 weeks' gestational age (full term), and (4) older infants up to 6 months of age (Table 167-1). HVA levels increased progressively with maturity ($p < .05$; analysis of variance). Although mean HVA values in girls were slightly higher than those in boys in each age group, these differences were not statistically significant. In contrast to HVA, 5-HIAA levels were similar in these age groups, and there were no significant sex differences. Mean 5-HIAA values in all groups of infants were considerably higher than the values in older children.[25]

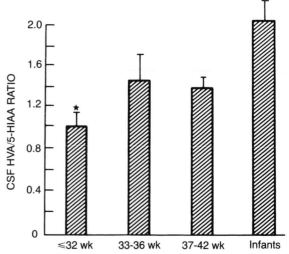

Figure 167–3. Cerebrospinal fluid (CSF) neurotransmitter metabolites in human newborns: (32 weeks or less [$n = 12$], 33 to 36 weeks [$n = 26$], 37 weeks or more [$n = 19$]), and infants 1 to 6 months old ($n = 13$); the *asterisk* indicates $p < .01$, comparing the most immature neonates with the infants using Student *t*-test. 5-HIAA = 5-hydroxyindoleactic acid; HVA = homovanillic acid. (From Silverstein FS, et al: J Neurochem *43*:1769, 1984.)

In Figure 167–3, mean HVA/5-HIAA ratios are plotted for the three groups of neonates and the older infants. The mean HVA/5-HIAA ratio in the most immature infants (28 to 32 weeks' gestation) was 1.0 ± 0.12 (mean ± SEM), whereas in the most mature group (1 week to 6 months old), it was 1.98 ± 0.17 ($p < .01$, comparing these two groups by the Student *t*-test). HVA concentrations increased over the period from the last trimester of pregnancy into early infancy, whereas 5-HIAA levels were relatively stable. Thus, the HVA/5-HIAA ratio changes markedly over this period. The data suggest that the maturation of human dopaminergic neuronal activity lags behind that of serotonin neurons in the perinatal period.

Concentrations of monoamine neurotransmitter metabolites in CSF are determined by the rates of synthesis, release, and degradation of the parent compounds as well as the rate and efficiency of elimination of metabolites from the brain and CSF. Elevated levels in infants may reflect a relatively high monoamine turnover at this age or changes in metabolite clearance from the brain, or both.

TABLE 167-1

Homovanillic Acid and 5-Hydroxyindoleacetic Acid Levels in Cerebrospinal Fluid*

Compares premature and term neonates and older infants			
	n	*5-HIAA* *(ng/mL)*	*HVA* *(ng/mL)*
Group 1 Premature neonates	38	96±10	106±10
Group 2 Term neonates	19	104±7	129±11
Group 3 Infants	13	85±7	159±9†

* Premature neonates range in gestational age from 28 to 36 weeks, term neonates from 37 to 42 weeks. Infants were 1 to 6 months of age. Values are mean ± SEM.
† $p < .05$ using analysis of variance to compare all HVA values in the three groups.
5-HIAA = 5-hydroxyindoleacetic acid; HVA = homovanillic acid.
From Silverstein FS, et al: Concentrations of homovanillic acid and 5-hydroxyindoleacetic acid in cerebrospinal fluid from human infants in the perinatal period. J Neurochem *43*:1769, 1984.

ACETYLCHOLINE PATHWAYS

Acetylcholine serves a variety of important functions in the brain. A major projection from the basal forebrain lateral to the hypothalamus into the cerebral cortex is believed to have a role in cortical activation, learning, memory, and cortical plasticity.[26] Cholinergic circuits in the brain stem and the diencephalon influence autonomic functions and also form part of the control mechanisms for temperature regulation and hormonal release. In the basal ganglia, cholinergic circuits counterbalance the effects of dopamine pathways and serve an important role in controlling motor tone and movement.[19, 21]

The developmental profile of cholinergic neurons has been studied by assaying postnatal endogenous brain concentrations of acetylcholine, [³H]choline uptake into synaptosomes, and the synthetic activity of choline acetyltransferase (ChAT).[11, 16, 27, 28] In the cerebral cortex of rodents, cholinergic markers are present at fairly low levels over the first few postnatal days, and they rise with a sigmoidal pattern during the first postnatal weeks to maturity (Fig. 167–4). Labeling studies with [³H]thymidine autoradiography in rodents indicate that the cell bodies from which this pathway originates in the basal forebrain develop on gestational days 12 to 15.[2, 29] Therefore, the neurons that form the neocortical cholinergic system originate relatively early but differentiate over a more prolonged period than do catecholamine systems.

In the human brain, the nucleus basalis of Meynert in the basal forebrain develops intense acetylcholinesterase (AChE) activity between 12 and 22 weeks' gestation.[29] ChAT activity in human cerebral cortex rises after a gradual developmental pattern during the postnatal period that reaches nearly adult levels in adolescence.[30-32] Histochemical localization of the catabolic enzyme AChE is a marker for cholinergic nerve terminals in cerebral cortex, and this method has been used to examine human postmortem tissue. Kostovic and co-workers[32] found that laminar preferences in AChE staining changed dramatically in the human frontal cortex during the first postnatal year. AChE reactivity of layer 3 pyramidal cell bodies and the surrounding fibrillar network begins to develop after the first postnatal year and increases gradually to its peak intensity in young adults. Studies of ChAT activity and AChE histochemical features point to the coordinated development of cholinergic pathways in the brain with the relatively prolonged development of cognitive skills in humans.

Muscarinic cholinergic receptors that transmit most of the postsynaptic effects of acetylcholine increase in number during postnatal development in rodents, in concert with the development of nerve terminals.[27] In the adult cerebral cortex, a distinct laminar gradient is formed, with more superficial regions relatively enriched.[17] Shaw and associates[17] found that in cats, the laminar gradient is reversed in the postnatal period, with deep layers heavily labeled. During maturation, the receptors progressively reorganize into the adult pattern. Human infant neocortex also demonstrates the inversion of the adult pattern of receptor development noted in kitten cortex. In contrast to the rodent, however, muscarinic receptors in human postmortem neonatal cortex are present at a higher density than in the adult.[3]

One population of muscarinic receptors is coupled to stimulation of the PI turnover second-messenger system.[16] Despite the relatively low levels of muscarinic acetylcholine receptors present in the early postnatal period, these receptors are able to stimulate a vigorous PI turnover response. The magnitude of the PI response stimulated by the muscarinic agonist carbachol increases to a level twice that in the adult at postnatal day 7 in rodents, a finding suggesting that the muscarinic receptors are more tightly coupled to phospholipase C at this age than in the adult. Although presynaptic markers for cholinergic axons and muscarinic receptors are less abundant in the immature brain, enhancement of muscarinic-stimulated second-messenger responses may serve to compensate for this. The studies of muscarinic-stimulated PI turnover and autoradiography of muscarinic receptors suggest that, within certain regions, activities of cholinergic synapses are enhanced in the developing brain.

INHIBITORY GABA-CONTAINING NEURONS

GABA is the predominant inhibitory neurotransmitter in the brain. Important populations of GABA-containing neurons are found in cerebral cortex, in which they are predominantly intrinsic aspinous stellate interneurons, and in the striatonigral projection in the brain stem. GABA-containing neurons are born in the ganglionic eminence of the ventral forebrain, with neurons destined for the cerebral cortex born in the medial ganglionic eminence and those destined for the basal ganglia originating in the lateral ganglionic eminence.[33] Unlike the pyramidal neurons of cerebral cortex that are born in the dorsal forebrain and migrate to their permanent locations

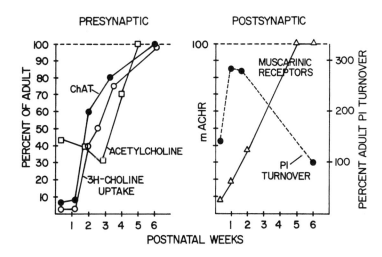

DEVELOPMENT OF CHOLINERGIC INNERVATION

Figure 167–4. Postnatal development of presynaptic and postsynaptic markers for cholinergic synapses in rat neocortex. *Left*, Data for choline acetyltransferase (ChAT), sodium-dependent [³H]choline uptake into synaptosomes, and endogenous acetylcholine are from refs. 11 and 26. The cortical region assayed was the dorsolateral sensorimotor cortex. *Right*, Data on muscarinic receptors are from refs. 16 and 26. The ordinate at *left* is for muscarinic receptors; at the *right*, it is phosphatidylinositol (PI) turnover. mACHR = muscarinic acetylcholine receptors.

radially from the ventricular zone, GABA-containing neurons migrate through the cortex following tangential pathways.[33]

Judged by biochemical assays, GABA-containing synapses reach maturity in rodents at a time midway between the early-developing catecholamine neurons and the later-developing cholinergic systems.[1] The activity of the synthetic enzyme for GABA, L-glutamate decarboxylase, is low in newborn rodent cortex but rises rapidly to achieve adult levels by 3 weeks of age.[34] Maturation of sodium-dependent, high-affinity uptake of [3H]GABA into synaptosomes exhibits a peak at greater than adult levels in cortex at about 3 weeks of age and remains elevated until about 8 weeks of age. The concentration of the neurotransmitter amino acid GABA has already reached approximately 50% of adult levels in neonatal cortex and is at adult levels by 2 weeks of age.

Neurotransmitter receptors for GABA are linked to receptors for benzodiazepine-type drugs, and together they regulate the opening of chloride channels. Stimulation of this ionophore has the effect of hyperpolarizing postsynaptic neurons. Neurotransmitter-binding studies have been used to characterize the ontogeny of both GABA and benzodiazepine receptors.[2] Benzodiazepine receptors are found at relatively high levels in the neonate, and in rodents, levels are almost half the adult level. Significant levels of benzodiazepine receptors have been observed in the human newborn and infant hypothalamus.[35,36] Binding sites for GABA are present at relatively low concentrations at birth and increase slowly in the postnatal period. Studies of postnatal maturation of GABA$_A$ receptors in children using positron emission tomography and [11C]flumazenil indicate that the density is 50% higher in cerebral cortex at 2 years of age than in adults, a finding suggesting age-related pruning in synaptic density with age.[37]

NEUROPEPTIDE-CONTAINING NEURONS

Neuropeptide-containing neurons compose an important, relatively precocious segment of brain circuitry, which is important for a variety of functions in the fetus and newborn. Various neuropeptide-containing neurons found in the brain have been studied from a developmental perspective, mostly in rodents. Neurons containing enkephalin, other opiate peptides, substance P, and thyroid-releasing hormone have been observed in neurons using immunohistochemical techniques in early fetal life in both rodents and humans. Neurons containing cholecystokinin and vasoactive intestinal polypeptide compose important intrinsic groups of neurons.[38-40] In cerebral cortex, these peptides most often coexist with GABA. In rodents, endogenous levels of cholecystokinin, somatostatin, and vasoactive intestinal polypeptide increase relatively slowly to adult levels over the first 7 postnatal weeks.[39-41] In contrast, endogenous levels of substance P reach the adult concentration in the neonatal period and by 3 weeks of age rise to more than three times that level.[2] Opiate systems appear relatively mature in the neonatal period. Metenkephalin-containing neurons and μ-opiate receptors are found in rat entorhinal cortex and hippocampus in neonates. [3H]naloxone-receptor binding in newborn rhesus monkeys demonstrates an adultlike pattern in subcortical structures. Much more remains to be learned about the development of these pathways, especially as they relate to important neuroendocrine function and control of breathing.

EXCITATORY AMINO ACID PATHWAYS

Pathways that use excitatory amino acids are prevalent in the brain and appear to convey information in many intracortical, primary sensory, and cortical projection pathways. For example, the pathways from the cortex into the basal ganglia (corticostriatal pathways), the corticospinal pathways, and the pathways from the eyes to the visual cortex appear to use the excitatory amino acid glutamate or a closely analogous compound as their primary neurotransmitter.[2, 42-44] Electrophysiologic effects of visual stimuli in cerebral cortex are blocked by specific antagonists for glutamate receptors.[45]

In cerebral cortex, high-affinity, sodium-dependent [3H]glutamate synaptosomal uptake into nerve terminals has been used to study development of the visual pathways.[42] [3H]Glutamate uptake, which reflects development of presynaptic nerve terminals in visual cortex of developing rats, increases continuously from birth and reaches adult levels by postnatal day 15 (Fig. 167-5).

Glutamate receptors have been classified into three broad groups determined by their responses to one of three synthetic agonist compounds: N-methyl-D-aspartate (NMDA), α-amino3-hydroxy-5-methyl-4-isoxazolepropionic acid (AMPA), and metabotropic receptors (Fig. 167-6). NMDA and AMPA receptors are linked to ion channels that can admit calcium or sodium, or both, to the neuronal cytoplasm. Ionic receptors that respond to kainic acid are special types of AMPA receptors. Metabotropic receptors stimulated by glutamate regulate levels of the second-messenger molecules cAMP, the polyphosphoinositide IP$_3$, and diacylglycerol. AMPA receptors mostly mediate the "fast" excitatory activity in the nervous system, whereas the other receptors are reserved for more specialized functions. The NMDA receptor channel (Fig. 167-7) opens only when glutamate and glycine stimulate the receptor at the same time that the surrounding membrane potential drops in response to opening of AMPA channels. Under normal circumstances, NMDA receptor-mediated channel opening is reserved for exceptional levels of stimulation mediated by converging stimuli, such as are believed to occur during learning, memory, and other forms of plasticity.

In contrast to the slow rise in biochemical markers for presynaptic glutamate-containing axon terminals, expression of glutamate receptors and of second-messenger systems stimulated by glutamate is enhanced in the perinatal brain.[4,5,43,44-48] The ontogenetic profile of glutamate binding in rodent visual cortex has been shown to rise approximately 10-fold higher than the adult level.[42] After day 15, there is a marked decline in total [3H]glutamate binding that corresponds temporally to the pruning of functional synaptic contacts and the time of eye opening and

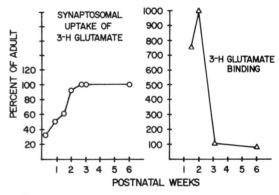

DEVELOPMENT OF GLUTAMATE INNERVATION IN VISUAL CORTEX

Figure 167-5. *Left,* Ontogeny of sodium-dependent synaptosomal uptake activity for [3H]glutamate in synaptosomes prepared from visual cortex of the rat.[42] *Right,* Ontogeny of sodium-independent binding of [3H]glutamate to visual cortex membranes.[45] Although [3H]glutamate uptake approaches adult levels in the third week, total glutamate binding is 10-fold higher than adult levels. This period includes the critical period for cortical visual plasticity.

commencement of activity in visual pathways. A similar over-shoot in glutamate binding has been observed in developmental studies of the rat hippocampus.[5,49] Receptors that make up the NMDA receptor channel complex are overexpressed in the post-natal period.[49] In addition, molecular genetic studies of NMDA receptor subunits indicate that the types of receptor proteins suppressed in the immature brain create receptors and channels that open more easily than adult channels.[50] This finding corresponds to electrophysiologic studies in the kitten visual system and indicates that stimulation mediated by NMDA receptors is enhanced compared with adult cats.[47]

Binding to non–NMDA-preferring [³H]glutamate sites is also markedly increased in several areas of the immature rodent and

human brain in the postnatal period. In the globus pallidus and basal forebrain of the rodent brain, there is marked increase in quisqualate-displaceable [³H]glutamate binding in the perinatal period that declines to relatively low levels in maturity.[51] Similar areas of transiently increased binding are also seen in areas of human fetal brain. Stimulation of PI turnover, the second-messenger system stimulated by a population of quisqualate-preferring glutamate receptors, is also markedly enhanced in hippocampus and striatum in the neonatal period.[4] This response is even larger than the enhanced coupling of PI turnover to muscarinic receptors already described.

The functional enhancement of the effects of the excitatory neurotransmitter systems in developing brain may be related to

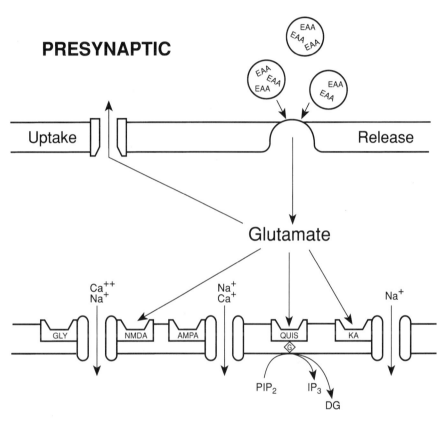

Figure 167–6. Schematic diagram of gluta-mate synapses. Glutamate released from presynaptic nerve terminals can interact with several postsynaptic receptors for glycine (GLY) and glutamate in the N-methyl-D-aspartate (NMDA) conforma-tion linked to a calcium channel. The α-amino3-hydroxy-5-methyl-4-isoxazolepro-pionic acid (AMPA) receptor is linked to a channel that fluxes sodium and some calcium. Glutamate in the conformation of quisqualate (QUIS) can stimulate hydroly-sis of polyphosphoinositides to produce the second messengers inositol-1,4,5 triphosphate (IP₃) and diacylglycerol (DG). The kainate receptor (KA) is a special form of the AMPA receptor. EAA = excita-tory amino acid; PIP₂ = phosphatidylinosi-tol 4,5-bisphosphate.

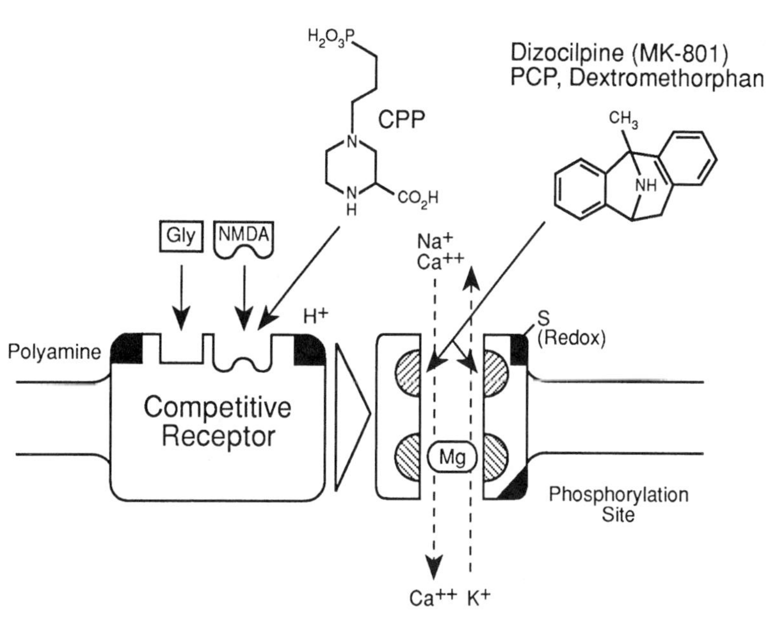

Figure 167–7. The N-methyl-D-aspartate (NMDA) receptor channel complex. Competitive binding sites are present for binding glutamate in the NMDA conformation and glycine (Gly). Antagonists are available to block the competitive sites and the channel. The structure of the channel-blocking drug dizocilpine is shown. Modulatory sites are shown for polyamines, hydrogen ions, redox compounds, and phosphorylation. CPP = NMDA antagonist; PCP = phencyclidine.

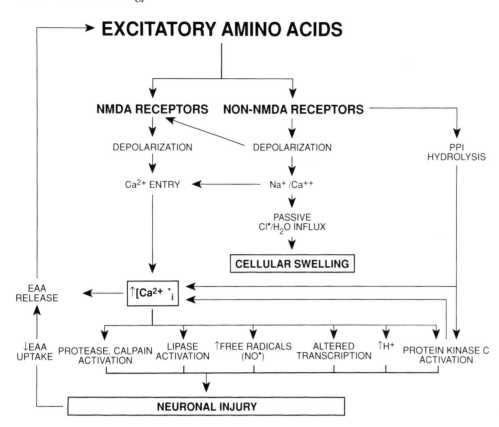

EXCITATORY AMINO ACIDS

Figure 167–8. Schematic of events thought to be triggered by overstimulation of excitatory amino acid receptors in the brain during hypoxia-ischemia and other disorders. EAA = excitatory amino acid; NMDA = N-methyl-D-aspartate; PPI = polyphosphoinositides.

their role in controlling cortical plasticity.[26] *Plasticity* in this context means the remodeling of neuronal connections, which is directly influenced by excitatory input. For example, in the developing visual system, *cortical columns,* defined physiologically, correspond to alternating inputs of each eye to the visual cortex. Closure of one eye during the critical period leads to reduction of function in a series of columns corresponding to that eye in visual cortex, and this change can be observed using physiologic methods as well as autoradiography. The remodeling of *ocular dominance columns* corresponding to one eye can be related to competition among physiologically active axons. Treatment with an NMDA glutamate receptor antagonist can prevent this remodeling in response to amblyopia, a finding suggesting that glutamate receptors mediate activity-dependent plastic changes in developing brain.[52] In this sense, glutamate receptors may mediate a portion of the physiologic activity of sensory stimulation on brain development.

GLUTAMATE-MEDIATED NEUROTOXICITY

Several types of injury in the fetal and neonatal brain appear to be mediated by excessive stimulation of glutamate receptors.[53-55] Hypoxia combined with ischemia leads to release of glutamate from nerve terminals and causes concentrations in the synaptic cleft to reach high levels in the micromolar range. Resulting overstimulation of glutamate receptors, especially the NMDA receptor, causes influx of calcium and sodium into neurons and other cells in the brain (Fig. 167–8). High levels of calcium trigger several intracellular events that can lead to neuronal death. These include activation of proteases, lipases, and protein kinases as well as activation of nitric oxide synthetase, which catalyzes production of nitric oxide. Nitric oxide, a diffusible free radical compound, can cause death of surrounding neurons. Nitric oxide production stimulated by calcium entering through NMDA channels also appears to be a primary signal for increasing cerebral blood flow associated with increased neuronal activity. Nitric oxide and other free

radical compounds can damage mitochondria through *oxidative stress.* Overstimulation of these intracellular events causes cell death by causing necrosis or *apoptosis* (programmed cell death).[55] Glutamate-mediated neurotoxicity seems to be a final common pathway for several forms of injury to the immature brain. Excessive and prolonged blockade of NMDA receptors can also lead to neuronal death, and this my be responsible for the teratogenicity of certain toxins such as ethanol.[56] The developmentally enhanced expression of NMDA receptors and other glutamate receptors in the immature brain plays a role in defining the patterns of selective vulnerability observed in the fetal and neonatal periods.

REFERENCES

1. Coyle J: Biochemical aspects of neurotransmission in the developing brain. Int Rev Neurobiol *20*:65, 1977.
2. Johnston MV: Biochemistry of neurotransmitters in cortical development. *In* Peters A, Jones EG (eds): Cerebral Cortex. New York, Plenum Press, 1988, pp 211–236.
3. Johnston MV, et al: Muscarinic cholinergic receptors in human infant forebrain: ³H-QNB benzilate binding in monogenates and quantitative autoradiography in sections. Dev Brain Res *19*:195, 1985.
4. Nicoletti F, et al: Excitatory amino acid recognition sites coupled with inositol phospholipid metabolism: developmental changes and interactions with alpha 1 adrenoreceptors. Proc Natl Acad Sci USA *83*:1931, 1986.
5. Represa A, et al: Development of high affinity kainate binding sites in human and rat hippocampi. Brain Res *384*:170, 1986.
6. Lidov HGW, et al: Characterization of the monoaminergic innervation of immature neocortex: a histofluorescence study. J Comp Neurol *81*:663, 1978.
7. Levitt P, Rakic P: The time of genesis, embryonic origin and differentiation of the brainstem monoamine neurons in the rhesus monkey. Brain Res *4*:35, 1982.
8. Coyle J, Molliver M: Major innervation of newborn rat cortex by monoaminergic neurons. Science *196*:444, 1977.
9. Bear MF, Singer W: Modulation of visual cortical plasticity by acetylcholine and noradrenaline. Nature *320*:172, 1986.
10. Goldman-Rakic P, Brown R: Postnatal development of monoamine content and synthesis in the cerebral cortex of rhesus monkeys. Brain Res *4*:339, 1982.
11. Johnston M, Coyle J: Ontogeny of neurochemical markers for noradrenergic, GABAergic and cholinergic neurons in neocortex lesioned with methylazoxymethanol acetate. J Neurochem *34*:1429, 1980.

12. Levitt P, Moore RY: Development of the noradrenergic innervation of neocortex. Brain Res *162*:243, 1979.

13. MacBrown R, Goldman PS: Catecholamines in neocortex of rhesus monkeys: Regional distribution and ontogenetic development. Brain Res *124*:576, 1977.

14. Goffinet AM, et al: Autoradiographic study of β₁-adrenergic receptor development in mouse forebrain. Dev Brain Res *24*:187, 1986.

15. Murrin LE, et al: Ontogeny of dopamine, serotonin and spirodecanone receptors in rat forebrain: an autoradiographic study. Dev Brain Res *23*:91, 1985.

16. Heacock AM, et al: Enhanced coupling of neonatal muscarinic receptors in rat brain to phosphoinositide turnover. J Neurochem *48*:1904, 1987.

17. Shaw C, et al: Ontogenesis of muscarinic acetylcholine binding sites in cat visual cortex: reversal of specific laminar distributions during critical period. Dev Brain Res *14*:295, 1984.

18. Nobin A, Bjorklund A: Topography of monoamine neurons systems in the human brain as revealed in fetuses. Acta Physiol Scand Suppl *388*:1, 1973.

19. Johnston MV: Neurotransmitters. *In* Wiggins RC, et al (eds): Developmental Neurochemistry. Austin, TX, University of Texas Press, 1985, pp 193–224.

20. Goldman-Rakic P: Prenatal formation of the cortical input and development of cytoarchitectonic compartments in the neostriatum of the rhesus monkey. J Neurosci *1*:721, 1981.

21. Graybiel A, Ragsdale C: Clumping of acetylcholinesterase activity in the developing striatum of the human fetus and young infant. Proc Natl Acad Sci USA *77*:1214, 1980.

22. Tissari AH: Serotonergic mechanisms in ontogenesis. *In* Boreus L (ed): Fetal Pharmacology. New York, Raven Press, 1973, pp 237–257.

23. D'Amato RJ, et al: Ontogeny of the serotonergic projection to rat neocortex: transient expression of a dense innervation of primary sensory areas. Proc Natl Acad Sci USA *84*:4322, 1987.

24. Silverstein FS, et al: Concentrations of homovanillic acid and 5-hydroxyindoleacetic acid in cerebrospinal fluid from human infants in the perinatal period. J Neurochem *43*:1769, 1984.

25. Seifert WE: Age effect on dopamine and serotonin metabolite levels in cerebrospinal fluid. Ann Neurol *8*:38, 1980.

26. Johnston MV, et al: Sculpting the developing brain. Adv Pediatr *48*:1, 2001.

27. Coyle J, Yamamura H: Neurochemical aspects of the ontogenesis of cholinergic neurons in the rat brain. Brain Res *118*:429, 1976.

28. Hohman CF, Ebner FF: Development of cholinergic markers in mouse forebrain. I. Choline acetyltransferase enzyme activity and acetylcholinesterase histochemistry. Dev Brain Res *23*:225, 1985.

29. Candy JM, et al: Evidence for the early prenatal development of cortical cholinergic afferents from the nucleus of Meynert in the human fetus. Neurosci Lett *61*:91, 1985.

30. Brooksbank BWL, et al: Biochemical development of the human brain. II. Some parameters of the GABAergic system. Dev Neurosci *4*:188, 1981.

31. Brooksbank BWL, et al: Biochemical development of the human brain. I. Some parameters of the cholinergic system. Dev Neurosci *1*:267, 1978.

32. Diebler ML, et al: Developmental changes of enzymes associated with energy metabolism and the synthesis of some neurotransmitters in discrete areas of human neocortex. J Neurochem *32*:429, 1979.

33. Kostovic I, et al: Acetylcholinesterase in the human frontal associative cortex during the period of cognitive development: early laminar shifts and later innervation of pyramidal neurons. Neurosci Lett *90*:107, 1988.

34. Nadarajah, B, Parnavelas, JG: Modes of neuronal migration in the developing cerebral cortex. Nat Rev *3*:423, 2002.

35. Coyle J, Enna S: Neurochemical aspects of the ontogenesis of GABAergic neurons in the rat brain. Brain Res *111*:119, 1976.

36. Najimi M, et al: Regional distribution of benzodiazepine binding sites in the human newborn and infant hypothalamus: a quantitative autoradiographic study. Brain Res *895*:129, 2001.

37. Chugani, DC, et al: Postnatal maturation of human GABAA receptors measured with positron emission tomography. Ann Neurol *49*:618, 2001.

38. Emson PC, et al: Development of vasoactive intestinal polypeptide (VIP) containing neurons in the rat brain. Brain Res *177*:437, 1979.

39. McDonald JK, et al: The morphology and distribution of peptide containing neurons in the adult and developing visual cortex of the rat. II. Vasoactive intestinal peptide. J Neurocytol *11*:825, 1982.

40. McDonald JK, et al: The morphology and distribution of peptide containing neurons in the adult and developing visual cortex of the rat. III. Cholecystokinin. J Neurocytol *11*:881, 1982.

41. McDonald JK, et al: The morphology and distribution of peptide containing neurons in the adult and developing visual cortex of the rat. I. Somatostatin. J Neurocytol *11*:809, 1982.

42. Kvale I, et al: Development of neurotransmitter parameters in lateral geniculate body superior colliculus, and visual cortex of the albino rat. Dev Brain Res *7*:137, 1983.

43. Ritter, LM, et al: Ontogeny of ionotropic glutamate receptor expression in human fetal brain. Brain Res Dev Brain Res *127*:123, 2001.

44. Panigrahy, A, et al: Differential expression of glutamate receptor subtypes in human brainstem sites involved in perinatal hypoxia-ischemia. J Comp Neurol *427*:196, 2000.

45. Schliebs R, et al: Development of glutamate binding sites in the visual structures of the rat brain: effect of visual pattern deprivation. Biomed Biochem Acta *45*:495, 1986.

46. Tsumoto T, et al: NMDA receptors in the visual cortex of young kittens are more effective than those in adult cats. Nature *327*:513, 1987.

47. Tsumoto T, et al: Excitatory amino acid transmitters in neuronal circuits of the cat visual cortex. J Neurophysiol *55*:469, 1986.

48. Sanderson C, Murphy S: Glutamate binding in the rat cerebral cortex during ontogeny. Dev Brain Res *2*:329, 1982.

49. McDonald JW, et al: Differential ontogenic development of three receptors comprising the NMDA receptor/channel complex in the rat hippocampus. Exp Neurol *110*:237, 1990.

50. Sheng M, et al: Changing subunit composition of heteromeric NMDA receptors during development of rat neocortex. Nature *368*:144, 1994.

51. Greenamyre JT, et al: Evidence for a transient perinatal glutamatergic innervation of the globus pallidus. J Neurosci *7*:1022, 1987.

52. Kleinschmidt A, et al: Blockade of "NMDA" receptors disrupts experience-dependent plasticity of striate cortex. Science *238*:355, 1987.

53. Johnston MV, et al: Hypoxic and ischemic central nervous system disorders in infants and children. Adv Pediatr *42*:1, 1995.

54. Johnston, MV, et al: Neurobiology of hypoxic-ischemic injury in the developing brain. Pediatr Res *49*:735, 2001.

55. Johnston, MV, et al: Mechanisms of hypoxic neurodegeneration in the developing brain. Neuroscientist *8*:212, 2002.

56. Ikonomidou, C, et al: Ethanol-induced apoptotic neurodegeneration and fetal alcohol syndrome. Science *287*:1056, 2000.

168

Robert C. Vannucci and Susan J. Vannucci

Perinatal Brain Metabolism

CEREBRAL OXIDATIVE METABOLISM

The oxidative events that operate in the immature brain appear identical to those of adult animals and humans, although quantitative differences certainly exist. *Cellular respiration* is that process whereby an organic substrate is consumed to produce chemical energy (high-energy phosphate bond; ~P), with carbon dioxide and water as the metabolic byproducts. Respiration is a highly efficient process with minimal energy waste. Under physiologic conditions, 1 mol of glucose, the primary cerebral energy fuel, is catabolized in the presence of oxygen to yield 36 mol of adenosine triphosphate (ATP). Other substrates yield proportionately greater or lesser energy, depending on their molecular carbon structure and their entry point into the oxidative pathway.

The biochemical machinery that composes the oxidative pathway is divided into the following three components: glycolysis, a cytoplasmic process; and the tricarboxylic (Krebs) cycle and the cytochrome system, both of which operate within mitochondria (Fig. 168-1).[1-3] Glycolysis proceeds under both aerobic and anaerobic conditions. In the presence of oxygen, glucose is converted to pyruvic acid, which, in turn, enters the Krebs cycle with little or no conversion to lactic acid. When oxygen is not available, metabolites of the Krebs cycle are depleted, and glycolysis is accelerated with the formation of lactic acid in an

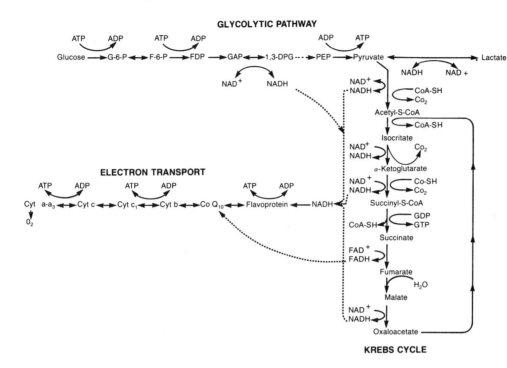

Figure 168–1. Schematic diagram of the oxidative pathway. ADP = adenosine disphosphate; ATP = adenosine triphosphate; CoA = coenzyme A; 1,3-DPG = diphospho-glycerate; FDP = fructose diphosphate; F-6-P = fructose-6-phosphate; GAP = glyceral-dehyde phosphate; GDP = guanosine diphosphate; G-6-P = glucose-6-phosphate; GTP = guanosine triphosphate; NAD^+ = nicotinamide-adenine dinucleotide (oxidized form); NADH = nicotinamide-adenine dinucleotide (reduced form); PEP = phosphoenolpyruvate.

attempt to maintain cerebral energy stores. However, anaerobic glycolysis is an inefficient method to generate energy (2 mol of ATP/mol of glucose); thus, brain function cannot be maintained on this process alone.

Glycolytic control points, that is, those reactions in which the activities of specific enzymes govern the rate of metabolism, include hexokinase, phosphofructokinase (PFK), and possibly pyruvate kinase. Of these enzymes, PFK is predominantly rate limiting for glycolysis in both adult and immature brain.[4-6] Metabolites known to inhibit PFK activity and hence glycolysis include ATP, citrate, and hydrogen ions (H^+), whereas adenosine diphosphate (ADP), adenosine monophosphate (AMP), and inorganic phosphate (P_i) stimulate PFK activity.[2] These glycolytic regulatory mechanisms are important in the cell's response to hypoxia, acid-base imbalance, and other metabolic disturbances.

CEREBRAL HIGH-ENERGY METABOLITES

Metabolites known to exist in brain that can store and transfer energy in the form of anhydride phosphate bonds (~P) include ATP, ADP, and phosphocreatine (PCr).[1,2] Of the three, ATP plays the critical role in the coupling of energy supply to energy demand by substrate and oxidative phosphorylation. PCr acts as a storage metabolite, whereas guanosine triphosphate (GTP) is important in biosynthetic reactions.

Cerebral high-energy metabolites have been measured in perinatal and adult animals by enzymatic, chromatographic, and magnetic resonance (MR) spectroscopic techniques.[4,7-11] Of the nucleotides, ATP predominates and remains stable from term fetal life through adulthood (Table 168-1).[12,13] Lower concentrations have been found in embryonic brain tissue.[11] PCr is lower in the brains of newborn animals than in adults, as is total creatine (PCr + creatine), but the PCr/creatine ratio changes little with postnatal development.[12,13] The lower PCr/creatine ratio in the fetus presumably is the result of a lower brain pH, owing to increased tissue lactate concentrations and hypercapnia (the creatine phosphokinase equilibrium reaction is pH dependent).[12]

MR spectroscopy is a technique whereby the concentration of an organic compound in tissue can be determined by the realignment of selected molecules using a supraconducting magnet.[14] Almost any substance can be analyzed according to the strength,

TABLE 168-1

Cerebral High-Energy Metabolites in Developing Rats*

Metabolite	Fetus	Newborn	1 Wk	Adult
ATP	2.66	2.63	2.64	2.76
ADP	0.43	0.25†	0.53	0.38
AMP	0.03	0.01	0.04	0.03
ATP + ADP + AMP	3.11	2.89	3.21	3.17
PCr	1.74	3.16†	3.33	4.90†
Creatine	5.35	3.83†	4.65†	5.63†
PCr + creatine	7.10	6.99	7.97†	10.53†
PCr/creatine	0.33	0.83†	0.72	0.87

* Values, expressed in mmol/kg wet weight, represent means of four to seven animals in each age group. Fetal, newborn, and 1-week values are from forebrain,[12] whereas adult values are from cerebral cortex.[13]
† $p < .05$ compared with previous age group.
ADP = adenosine diphosphate; AMP = adenodine monophophate; ATP = adenosine triphosphate; PCr = phosphocreatine.

duration, and other characteristics of the magnetic field. The most commonly examined metabolites in brain are the phosphorus-containing compounds, including PCr, ATP, monophosphate and diphosphate esters (includes AMP and ADP, respectively), and P_i.[15-18] Proton MR spectroscopy provides a measurement of numerous hydrogen-containing metabolites, including lactate and creatine.[19-21] Thus, MR spectroscopy is capable of ascertaining the energy status of brain tissue *in vivo* under both physiologic and pathophysiologic conditions, although usually the measurements are semiquantitative (Fig. 168-2).

An investigation using MR spectroscopy in premature and full-term newborn infants confirmed earlier studies in animals that ATP levels remain relatively stable throughout maturation.[17] However, a more recent study suggested that ATP concentrations in the human brain almost double between the newborn period and adulthood.[18] As in animals, levels of PCr, P_i, and the phosphodiesters are low at birth and increase with advancing age. Calculated intracellular pH, as measured from the chemical shift of the P_i peak relative to the PCr peak, is 7.1 in healthy newborn infants. As anticipated, the PCr/P_i and PCr/ATP ratios are lower

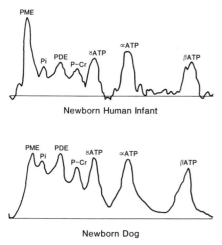

Figure 168–2. Representative phosphorus nuclear magnetic spectra of the brains of a newborn human infant and a newborn dog. δATP, αATP, and βATP = δ, α, and β adenosine triphosphate, respectively; P-Cr = phosphocreatine; PDE = phosphorus diesters; P_i = inorganic phosphate; PME = phosphorus monoesters. (Data for the infant from ref. 17, and data for the dog from ref. 10.)

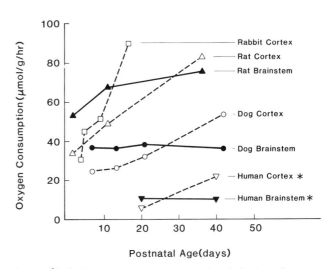

Figure 168–3. *In vitro* oxygen consumption in brains of developing animals and human fetus. Observations on rabbit brain stem are not available. (Data on dog from ref. 23; data on rat from ref. 24; data on rabbit from ref. 25.)

in newborn infants when compared with adult animals. Although the described findings in newborn infants are preliminary, it is anticipated that the continued use and sophistication of MR spectroscopy will contribute substantially to our understanding of the bioenergetics of the perinatal human brain (see later).

QUANTITATIVE ASPECTS OF OXIDATIVE METABOLISM

Measurements of cerebral oxygen consumption give a quantitative estimation of energy production by the brain, because oxygen is required for the oxidative phosphorylation of ADP to ATP in electron transport by the cytochrome system (see previous discussion). Oxygen consumption measurements often are referred to as the *cerebral metabolic rate for oxygen* (CMRO₂), expressed as milliliters per 100 g per minute. Estimates of the CMR in developing animals initially were obtained *in vitro* by the use of the Warburg respirometer to measure the oxygen consumption of brain slices or homogenates in nutrient media. Himwich and associates[22] found that the oxygen consumption (expressed as wet weight of tissue) of minced cerebral tissue with glucose as substrate is 38% lower in 7-day postnatal rats than in adults. Subsequent *in vitro* studies of oxygen consumption in either the whole brain or cerebral cortex of other species, including humans, indicated that the CMR is low at birth and increases with maturation (Fig. 168-3).[22-25] Changes in the rates of glucose utilization during development tend to parallel the increases in oxygen consumption.[24]

Both immature and adult animals exhibit regional differences in brain oxygen consumption *in vitro*.[24, 26, 27] Himwich and Fazekas[27] found that although total oxygen consumption in the brains of 1-week postnatal dogs is 83% of the adult level, there are significant regional differences that change with increasing age. The medulla oblongata exhibits the highest rate of consumption in the immediate newborn period but has the lowest rate of all regions studied in the adult brain (see Fig. 168-3). By contrast, the oxygen consumption of the cerebral cortex is the lowest of all regions analyzed in the newborn period but doubles within 5 weeks of development. These *in vitro* findings of regional differences in brain metabolism between young and adult animals, including humans, have been substantiated by more recent *in vivo* techniques to measure metabolism (see later).

Oxygen consumption can be calculated *in vivo* from the Fick principle by measuring cerebral blood flow (CBF) and the arteriovenous difference for oxygen (A - VO₂) across the brain:

$$CMRO_2 = CBF (A - VO_2)$$

By the use of this technique, oxygen consumption has been determined in immature animals of several species, including humans.[28-38] As shown in Table 168-2, notable species differences exist for the rates of oxygen consumption by brain, differences that reflect the age and functional immaturity of the animal at the time of the measurement as well as species variations in the brain's intrinsic metabolic requirements. Specifically, CMRO₂ is lower in perinatal animals when compared with adults of the same species, and the more immature the animal is at birth, the lower is the rate of oxygen consumption. This assumption is supported by measurements in newborn dogs, a functionally immature animal at birth, in which both CBF and CMRO₂ are 40% of respective values in adult dogs (Table 168-3).[32,33] In contrast, the newborn lamb is relatively mature at birth and already exhibits a CMRO₂ that is equal to or even greater than that of adult sheep.

Oxygen consumption of the brain also has been determined in humans, including newborn infants. The CMRO₂ in young, healthy adults is 3.3 mL/100 g/minute.[37] Oxygen consumption in unanesthetized healthy children aged 3 to 10 years actually is higher by 23% than it is in adults; Kennedy and Sokoloff[39] obtained a value of 5.2 mL/100 g/minute. Settergren and colleagues[38] measured CMRO₂ in children aged 11 days to 15 years who were anesthetized with nitrous oxide. The mean value for CMRO₂ was 3.2 for the entire group, and no age-related differences could be ascertained. Garfunkel and colleagues[36] found CMRO₂ values of 1.1 to 2.1 mL/100 g/minute in three newborn infants anesthetized with barbiturate. However, these low values may not apply to healthy, awake infants, because barbiturates are known to depress the CMRO₂,[40] and the infants had severe central nervous system anomalies.

With the use of positron emission tomography (PET), the CMRO₂ as well as cerebral glucose utilization (CGU; see later) can be ascertained in humans. PET is based on computed tomography, except the source of radiation for external detection is transmitted from within the brain outward rather than passed through the brain as x-rays. In PET, a positron-emitting, rapid-decay isotope,

TABLE 168-2

Cerebral Metabolic Rates for Oxygen in Developing Animals and Humans*

Species	Fetal	Newborn	Adult
Sheep	2.0–3.7	3.9–4.8	4.2
Dog	—	1.1	2.8
Monkey	—	1.1	3.2
Humans	—	1.5	3.2–3.3

* Values are expressed in mL/100 g/minute.
Data for sheep from refs. 28–31; data for dog from refs. 32 and 33; data for monkeys from refs. 34 and 35; and data for humans from refs. 36–38.

TABLE 168-3

Cerebral Blood Flow and Cerebral Metabolic Rates for Oxygen in Newborn and Adult Dogs*

Age	CBF (mL/100 g/min)	A-VO$_2$ (Vol %)	CMRO$_2$ (mL/100 g/min)
Newborn	24 ± 14	5.6 ± 2.5	1.1 ± 0.3
Adult	56 ± 14	$5.0 \pm ?$	2.8 ± 0.8

* Values represent means $\pm$ SD for seven newborn and adult dogs.
A – VO$_2$ = arteriovenous difference for oxygen; CBF = cerebral blood flow; CMRO$_2$ = cerebral metabolic rate for oxygen.
Data for newborn dogs from ref. 33; data for adult dogs from ref. 32.

prepared by a cyclotron, is administered to the subject. The substance circulates to the brain, in which it is metabolized, during which its positrons combine with electrons to form γ-rays. The γ-rays penetrate the brain, skull, and scalp and are recorded externally on a circular array of scintillation detectors. A computer mathematically reconstructs the spatial distribution of the radioactivity within the brain, which either is quantified or is displayed on a cathode-ray screen. Thus, PET offers a noninvasive regional assessment not only of CMRO$_2$ but also of many other biologic processes.

Using PET with ^{15}O-labeled water as the positron-emitting isotope, Altman and associates[41] measured CMRO$_2$ in 11 newborn infants of gestational ages ranging from 26 to 40 weeks. CMRO$_2$ was low in all the infants, and it was beyond the lower range of detection in two. In those infants in whom radioactivity was detectable, CMRO$_2$ ranged from 0.2 to 1.3 mL/100 g/minute, much less than the measured value for human adults of 3.3 mL/100 g/minute. The findings indicate that, as in perinatal animals (see earlier), cerebral oxidative metabolism, especially in small premature infants, is low, a finding reflecting the functional immaturity of the brain.[42] A less likely proposal, offered by Altman and colleagues,[41] is that the energy requirements of the fetal and prematurely newborn brain are met by nonoxidative metabolism, that is, anaerobic glycolysis (see later).

GLYCOLYSIS

As mentioned previously, the rate of glycolysis or the glycolytic flux is controlled by specific, rate-limiting enzymes that are either inhibited or activated by changes in the biochemical milieu of the cytoplasm. Thus, *aerobic glycolysis* is stimulated by those stresses that increase the energy demands of the tissue, specifically, stimulant drugs and hormones, hyperthermia, and seizures. *Anaerobic glycolysis* is stimulated by hypoxia or cerebral ischemia, or both, in an attempt to maintain optimal cellular energy balance despite the oxygen debt. Glycolysis is inhibited by sedative and anesthetic agents, hypothermia, and acidosis, which are conditions that reduce the energy needs of the tissue. Glycolysis cannot cease completely, because at least some energy is always required to maintain ionic gradients across cellular and subcellular membranes, without which cellular integrity is compromised.

The extent to which glycolysis and thus oxidative metabolism can be turned on or off is not entirely known. In adult animals, deep barbiturate anesthesia sufficient to produce an isoelectric electroencephalogram reduces metabolism by no more than 50%,[43] a finding suggesting that up to 50% of cellular energy production is required for maintenance of biochemical and morphologic integrity, whereas the remainder is devoted to the generation of action potentials and to biosynthetic processes. The extent to which glycolysis can be stimulated (*glycolytic capacity*) also is conjectural, although studies in experimental animals suggest that glycolytic flux can be accelerated up to eight- to

ten-fold during extreme metabolic stress, that is, seizures or hypoxia-ischemia.[2] In this regard, both basal glycolytic flux and glycolytic capacity are lower in immature animals than in their adult counterparts, a finding that is in keeping with intrinsically lower rates of oxygen consumption and hence metabolic demands. For example, the calculated rate of cerebral glycolysis of the perinatal rat is approximately 10 μmol glucose/100 g/minute,[44] one-tenth of the calculated rate for adult rat cerebral cortex.[45] During total cerebral ischemia, produced by decapitation, glycolytic flux in newborn rat brain increases fivefold compared with an eightfold increase in adult rat brain.[44, 45] Thus, the ability of perinatal animals to survive a prolonged period of hypoxia or anoxia compared with adults[46] cannot be explained by a heightened capacity of the immature brain to generate energy equivalents through anaerobic glycolysis. Rather, lower cerebral energy demands and hence metabolic requirements underscore the perinatal animal's resistance to hypoxia-ischemia.[9, 44]

MITOCHONDRIAL DEVELOPMENT

Because the mitochondria produce most of the energy used for cellular needs, these "powerhouses" have been investigated during maturation of the brain. Investigators have demonstrated a relative deficiency in the oxidative phosphorylating capacity of mitochondria that characterize the immature brain.[47] Simply put, the immature brain appears less able to synthesize ATP per molecule of oxygen consumed. This coupling of ATP to oxygen, expressed in terms of the ATP/O or P/O ratio, is 3 for the oxidized form of nicotinamide adenine dinucleotide (NAD$^+$)-linked cytochrome components in adult rat brain.[48] Holtzman and Moore[49] measured P/O ratios in several regions of rat brain during maturation. Ratios of 1.5 for NAD$^+$-linked substrates were found in animals 1 to 11 days of postnatal age. Thereafter, ratios increased to 2.4 in pons-medulla and 2.8 in cerebral cortex. The data indicate that the brain cell's increasing efficiency for oxidative phosphorylation (improved coupling) reflects both an increase in the number of mitochondria and an inherent change in their function.

The functional advantage of these mitochondrial changes appears to lie in the pattern of growth of the central nervous system. A striking increase in mitochondrial cell number accompanies neuronal and glial hypertrophy secondary to axonal and dendritic expansion.[50] Furthermore, as individual cells enlarge, the cell surface/volume ratio increases, a circumstance that raises the energy required to maintain ionic gradients across the membrane and to propagate action potentials.[51]

CEREBRAL ENERGY UTILIZATION

Energy utilization by the brain can be inferred from measurements of oxygen or substrate consumption because, under

TABLE 168-4

Cerebral Energy Use Rates and Maximal Glycolytic Capacities of Chick Embryos and Newly Hatched Peeps*

Age (d)	Δ~P	ΔLactate	ΔLactate Δ~P
9	2.84	0.79	0.29
14	3.25	1.51[†]	0.54[†]
16	2.76	2.04[†]	0.78[†]
19	5.76[†]	3.22[†]	0.56[†]
Peeps	8.98[†]	5.09[†]	0.56

* Values, expressed in mmol/kg wet weight, represent means of four to six animals in each age group. The ratio Δlactate/Δanhydride phosphate bond (~P) is an indication of the maximal contribution of anaerobic metabolism to the cerebral metabolic rate.
[†] $p < .05$ compared with the previous age group.
Data from ref. 11.

TABLE 168-5

Substrate Equivalents as Percentage of Total Cerebral Substrate Utilization and Extent of Anaerobic Metabolism in Newborn Animals and Humans

Substrate	Sheep (%)	Dog (%)	Monkey (%)	Human (%)
Glucose	99.5	93.5	70.4	91.1
β-Hydroxybutyrate	0.5	0.5	14.6	5.5
Acetoacetate	0.0	2.0	4.9	3.4
Lactate	0.0	4.0	10.1	0.0
	100	100	100	100
% Glucose → lactate	2.6%	0.0%	0.0%	5.2%

Data for sheep from ref. 56; data for dog from ref. 55, data for monkey from ref. 35; and data for human infant from ref. 38.

steady-state conditions, energy demand and supply are equivalent. Cerebral energy utilization can also be measured directly in the experimental animal by the Lowry decapitation technique.[4] Lowry and associates[4] devised a novel technique to determine the rate of energy use in brain during the total cerebral ischemia that follows decapitation. The investigators assumed that because the isolated head is a closed metabolic compartment (no inflow or outflow), rates of depletion of potential (glucose + glycogen) and endogenous (ATP + ADP + PCr) high-energy stores would be a direct measure of cerebral energy utilization occurring before decapitation. Using this method, investigators showed that the calculated rate of cerebral energy use in perinatal animals, like the CMRO₂, is substantially less than in adults.[4, 9, 44] For example, the energy use rate of the 1-day postnatal rat is 1.3 mmol ~P/kg/minute,[44] 20 times less than the calculated rate of 27 mmol ~P/kg/minute for the adult rat brain.[45]

One can calculate the CMRO₂ from the rate of cerebral energy use if the ADP/O or P/O ratio is known. As already mentioned, P/O ratios for immature rat brain are 1.5 for NAD⁺, and they are 1.2 for the oxidized form of flavin adenine dinucleotide-linked substrates.[49] A source of ATP other than that derived from oxidative phosphorylation of ADP is substrate phosphorylation, which occurs twice in glycolysis and once in the Krebs cycle. Substrate phosphorylation yields 6 mol of ATP for every mole of glucose consumed; 2 mol are required for the initial phosphorylation of glucose and fructose-6-phosphate in glycolysis. Thus, for every mole of glucose consumed, 4 mol of ATP are ultimately generated by a source other than oxidative phosphorylation; this amounts to 20% of the total energy production. Assuming a yield of 3 mol of ~P/mol of oxygen reduced (P/O ratios = 1.5), and taking into account the ATP formed by both oxidative and substrate phosphorylation, the rate of cerebral energy utilization for newborn rats translates to a CMRO₂ of $[1.3 - (1.3 \times 0.2)]/3 = 0.35$ mmol/kg/minute or 0.78 mL/100 g/minute. This value can be compared with a measured CMRO₂ value of 5.4 mL/100 g/minute in adult rat brain,[52] nearly six times greater than that in the perinatal rat. The fetal rat at term exhibits a rate of cerebral energy utilization comparable to that of newborn animals.[44]

The low cerebral energy requirements of most mammals at birth reflect an immaturity of the central nervous system at this stage of development. It has been suggested that cerebral energy demands in the fetal brain are even less well developed than in the newborn brain,[53] and such demands in embryonic life are met predominantly or entirely by anaerobic glycolysis, with only a small contribution from oxidative metabolism.[23, 50] Using the Lowry technique to measure cerebral energy utilization (see earlier), Gonya-Magee and Vannucci[11] measured rates of cerebral metabolism in chick embryos at 9, 14, 16, and 19 days of incuba-

tion and in newly hatched peeps (Table 168-4). Calculated CMRs were not different in the 9-, 14-, and 16-day-old embryos but doubled between 16 and 19 days and doubled again between 19 days and hatching. The extent to which total cerebral energy utilization could be derived from anaerobic glycolysis (Δlactate/Δ~P) increased from a low at day 9 (0.29) to a maximum at day 16 (0.78). The findings of the investigation suggest that cerebral oxidative metabolism becomes progressively lower with decreasing embryonic age, but a nadir is reached below which metabolism can no longer support cerebral function and growth. Furthermore, the data indicate that despite the low metabolic activity of the embryonic brain, at no time during development is anaerobic glycolysis capable of entirely supporting the energy needs of the tissue.

CEREBRAL GLUCOSE UTILIZATION

In all animal species studied, including humans, glucose is the predominant or exclusive organic fuel for cerebral metabolism under physiologic conditions. This dictum also appears to hold true for the fetus and developing postnatal animal. Like CMRO₂, glucose consumption in brain can be measured from a knowledge of CBF and the arteriovenous difference for glucose:

$$CMR_{glucose} = CBF (A - V_{glucose})$$

When $CMR_{glucose}$ (or other organic substrate) and CMRO₂ are measured simultaneously, the substrate-oxygen quotient can be ascertained, which expresses the relative contribution of the substrate to overall oxidative metabolism:

$$Substrate/O_2 = \frac{CMR_{substrate} (No. C \text{ atoms}) \times 100}{CMRO_2}$$

Using these measurements, CGU has been determined in several perinatal animal species as well as in postnatal human infants (Table 168-5).[35, 38, 54-56] As in adult humans,[57, 58] glucose serves as the major organic substrate to support cerebral metabolism in all species studied. Furthermore, most of the glucose consumed is aerobically degraded to carbon dioxide and water or is used in biosynthesis with little or no production of lactic acid (anaerobic glycolysis). Thus, at least under physiologic conditions, glucose is efficiently used to produce the maximal amount of chemical energy possible.

In the past, only global estimates of glucose consumption in brain could be ascertained using the method described earlier. Thanks to the pioneering work of Sokoloff and colleagues,[59, 60] regional CGU (rCGU) now can be determined in both experimental animals and humans. Sokoloff and associates[60] used radioactive 2-[14C]deoxyglucose (2-DG) to measure CGU in 30 or more component structures of adult rat brain. The rationale for the use of 2-DG rather than [14C]glucose relates to the finding that the radioactive analogue of native glucose is lost from the brain as carbon dioxide and water during the course of an experiment; therefore, calculated CGU would underestimate the true CGU value. 2-DG, like glucose, is taken up by brain and is phosphorylated by hexokinase but, unlike glucose, it is unable to be metabolized further along the glycolytic pathway. The theory and application of the 2-DG technique to the experimental animal form the basis for measuring rCGU in humans using PET. Furthermore, because glucose is the predominant cerebral energy fuel, and glucose utilization is stoichiometrically related to oxygen consumption (see previous discussion), the measurement of rCGU is considered to reflect local rates of cerebral energy utilization and intrinsic functional activity.[59]

Using the 2-DG technique, rCGU was investigated in fetal sheep and in newborn rats, lambs, dogs, and monkeys.[61-65] The studies confirmed early *in vitro* experiments (see preceding discussion) that CGU in the perinatal animal is high in brain stem gray matter structures and declines in a caudal to rostral progression through the neuraxis to the cerebral cortex (Table 168–6; Fig. 168–4).[62,63] As in adults, CGU is lowest in subcortical and other white matter structures. Duffy and colleagues[62] equated the hierarchy of rates of glucose consumption to the functional immaturity of the animal with its limited, albeit present, sensory and motor capabilities but with little or no memory or learning abilities at this early stage of development.

Using PET with 18fluoro-2-DG as the positron-emitting isotope, Chugani and Phelps[66,67] measured rCGU in humans from full-term birth through adulthood (Fig. 168–5). In infants 5 weeks of age and younger, glucose utilization was highest in the sensorimotor cerebral cortex, the thalamus, the midbrain–brain stem, and the cerebellar vermis—a distribution of glucose consumption similar to that described in term fetal sheep and in newborn dogs and monkeys (see Fig. 168–4).[61-63] By 3 months of age,

glucose metabolic activity in the infants had increased in the parietal, temporal, and occipital cortices and in the basal ganglia, with subsequent increases in frontal and various association regions of cerebral cortex occurring by 8 months. Little further change in rCGU was observed between 8 and 18 months of postnatal age. The investigators emphasized that the maturational increases in rCGU, measured with PET, are in agreement with the behavioral, neurophysiologic, and anatomic changes known to occur during infant development.

Other investigators measured global and regional rCGU in premature newborn infants using PET.[68,69] Gestational ages ranged from 25 to 37 weeks. Whole brain CGU was less than that seen in full-term infants, when the two age groups were compared.[68] As in full-term infants, glucose utilization was highest in brain stem and cerebellar structures compared with cerebral cortex.

TABLE 168–6

Regional Cerebral Glucose Utilization in Developing Monkeys*

Structure	Newborn	Pubescent	Difference (%)
Frontal cortex	28	50	+44†
Parietal cortex	29	47	+38†
Occipital cortex	32	59	+46†
Hippocampus	25	39	+36†
Corpus callosum	15	11	–36
Caudate nucleus	23	52	+56
Thalamus	35	54	+35†
Substantia nigra	28	29	+3
Inferior colliculus	180	103	–75
Cerebellar hemisphere	22	31	+29

* Values expressed in μmol/100 gm/minute represent means of six to seven animals in each group.
† *p* < .01.
Data from ref. 63.

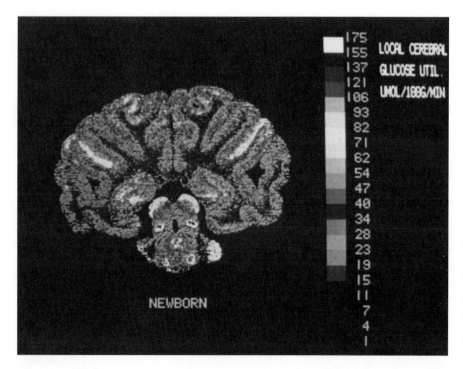

Figure 168–4. Representative [14C]deoxyglucose autoradiogram of brain from a newborn monkey. The *lighter areas* denote regions with higher utilization rates (see scale). Note the high rates of glucose consumption in selected brain stem structures relative to the cerebral hemispheres. (Courtesy of Charles Kennedy, M.D.)

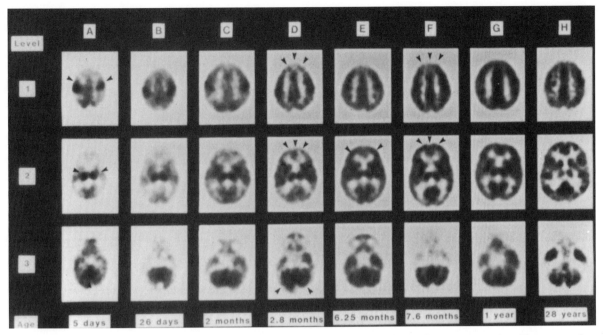

Figure 168–5. Representative ¹⁸fluoro-2-deoxyglucose positron emission tomograms during human maturation. Shown are three horizontal levels of brains at ages ranging from postnatal day 5 through 1 year and adulthood. (From Chugani HT, et al: Ann Neurol *22*:487, 1987.)

The lower rCGU in premature infants correlates with the low $CMRO_2$ observed at similar gestational ages.[41]

RELATIONSHIP BETWEEN CEREBRAL BLOOD FLOW AND GLUCOSE UTILIZATION (FLOW-METABOLISM COUPLE)

With the availability of methods to measure CBF and metabolism in animals and humans, investigators were quick to recognize a quantitative relationship between these two important biologic processes in brain. Further investigation revealed that, under physiologic conditions, CBF was essentially controlled by intrinsic mechanisms that reflect local rates of metabolism, that is, the extent of tissue carbon dioxide and H^+ accumulation. Thus, it is not surprising that CBF and metabolism are tightly linked or coupled. Specifically, when the rate of oxidative metabolism in brain is high, so is CBF, and vice versa. Metabolic diseases are capable of altering this critical relationship, during which neurologic dysfunction occurs, and, if it is severe enough, brain damage supervenes.

The brain *flow-metabolism couple* appears to be a universal phenomenon that encompasses all animal species of all ages and under all physiologic conditions (Fig. 168–6).[28,30-36,38,39,52,58,70-72] In those animals in which CBF and $CMRO_2$ have been measured simultaneously, the relationship has been apparent regardless of age, although differences in the intrinsic rates of metabolism do exist among species. A regional coupling of CBF to metabolism also exists in both adult and immature animals[60,62-64] when rCBF, determined with an inert, radioactive tracer, is compared with rCGU (Fig. 168–7).[64] A visual comparison of the published figures depicting rCBF and rCGU, using PET, also suggests the existence of a regional CBF-metabolism couple in the newborn human infant.[66,67,73] Occasional exceptions to the rule do occur among individual structures (e.g., cerebellum), and this situation may reflect local differences in the contribution of glucose versus alternate substrates to overall

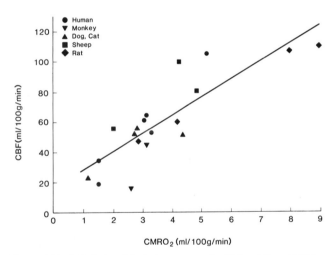

Figure 168–6. Relationship between cerebral blood flow (CBF) and the cerebral metabolic rate for oxygen ($CMRO_2$) in several species of animals. The symbols represent values from animals of varying ages. The *line* denotes the slope of a linear regression analysis with $Y = 12.1X + 16.7$; $r = .85$; $p < .001$. (Data from refs. 28, 30–36, 38, 39, 52, 58, and 70–72.)

metabolism or to the use of glucose in biosynthetic processes (see later).

ALTERNATE SUBSTRATES FOR OXIDATIVE METABOLISM

As mentioned previously, glucose is the predominant or exclusive cerebral energy fuel at all ages under physiologic conditions. However, situations occur in which glucose availability to the brain is limited by hypoglycemia. Under this and other circumstances, the perinatal brain is capable of incorporating and metabolizing substitute organic substrates, the most notable of which are lactic acid and the ketone bodies, β-hydroxybutyrate and acetoacetate. Indeed, the immature brain appears capable of consuming a large number of organic metabolites, also including free fatty acids and amino acids, as long as they are available in reasonable concentrations in blood and the appropriate enzymes for their degradation are present in brain.

The most widely studied substitute fuels for metabolism in perinatal brain have been ketone bodies and lactic acid. Because all developing mammals are nourished with milk with a high-fat content, these animals readily generate ketone bodies through the liver that, in turn, appear in substantial concentrations in blood. Thus, during suckling, ketone bodies partially substitute for glucose to sustain cerebral metabolism and can account for up to 20% of total energy production.[74-76] Likewise, in adults, nutrient fasting induces endogenous ketone body formation, which contributes significantly to overall cerebral metabolism during starvation-induced hypoglyclemia.[77]

Hypoglycemia also is encountered in the immediate newborn period before the initiation of sustained oral or parenteral feeding. During this time, as well as during fetal life, ketone bodies are essentially nonexistent in blood and therefore contribute little to cerebral metabolism.[78,79] In contrast, lactic acid is elevated in late fetal and early postnatal life to the extent that its concentration often exceeds that of glucose.[80-82] Studies in newborn dogs showed that during hypoglycemia, lactic acid not only is incorporated into the perinatal brain but also is consumed to the extent that the metabolite can support up to 58% of total cerebral oxidative metabolism (Fig. 168-8).[55, 83] The versatility of the immature brain to use substitute fuels, thus sparing glucose, undoubtedly contributes to the tolerance of the newborn nervous system to the known deleterious effects of hypoglycemia.

The ability of the immature brain to incorporate and metabolize alternate energy fuels resides, at least in part, in the unique characteristics of its blood-brain barrier. All organic metabolites enter the brain from blood predominantly through a carrier-mediated transport system. Cremer and coworkers[74,84,85] demonstrated the existence of a transport carrier for monocarboxylic acids, including ketone bodies and lactate, in the brains of immature rats, the Michaelis constant (K_m) of which is 10-fold greater than that demonstrated for adult rat brain. The blood-brain uptake capabilities for β-hydroxybutyrate, acetoacetate, and lactate actually exceed those of glucose at an early postnatal age. Thus, alternate substrates can be readily transported into the perinatal brain to support oxidative metabolism during periods of systemic glucose deficiency.

GLUCOSE AND MONOCARBOXYLIC ACID TRANSPORTERS

Relevant to the blood-brain barrier passage of nutrient substrates is the discovery of specific proteins that are required for the transport of such substrates from blood into brain and across cellular membranes (neurons, glia). These integral membrane proteins comprise two distinct families: the facilitative glucose transporter proteins, GLUTs; and the monocarboxylic acid proteins, MCTs, which mediate proton-coupled co-transport. GLUT1 was cloned in 1985, and there are now five proteins, GLUT 1 to GLUT5, with distinct tissue distribution and kinetic characteristics.[86] Although all these proteins have been detected in mammalian brain, GLUT1 and GLUT3 are the isoforms primarily involved in cerebral glucose uptake and CGU.[87] The initial transport of glucose across the endothelial cells of the blood-brain barrier is mediated by a heavily glycosylated form of GLUT1, 55-kDa GLUT1; a less glycosylated product of the same gene, 45-kDa GLUT1, is highly concentrated in choroid plexus, in the ependymal lining of the ventricles, and also in glia. GLUT3 is

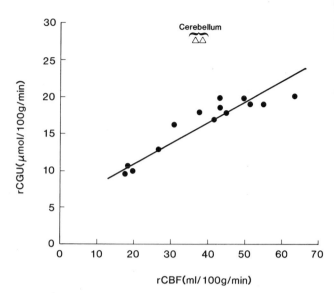

Figure 168–7. Relationship between regional cerebral glucose utilization (rCGU) and regional cerebral blood flow (rCBF) in newborn dogs. The symbols represent values from specific regions of brain. The *line* denotes the slope of a linear regression analysis (excluding cerebellum) with Y = .24X + 7.0; *r* = .93; *p* < .001. (Data from ref. 64.)

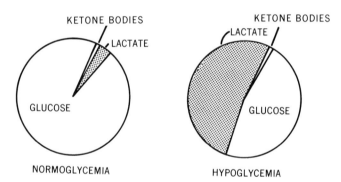

Figure 168–8. Substrate-oxygen quotients as percentage of total cerebral oxidative metabolism in normoglycemic and hypoglycemic newborn dogs. Substrate-oxygen quotients were calculated according to a formula described in the text. (Data from ref. 55.)

the neuronal glucose transporter.[87,88] The MCT family has been cloned only within the past few years and now contains eight members.[89] MCT1 is the most widely distributed; it is detected in several microvessels and appears to be expressed by all neural cells, whereas MCT2 expression is more restricted and is primarily neuronal. Both the GLUTs and the MCTs are developmentally regulated in brain.[90] The concentrations of the glucose transporter proteins are quite low in immature rat brain,[91] in keeping with the well-described low rates of cerebral glucose transport into immature rat brain,[85] and they increase sharply after the second postnatal week (Fig. 168-9). The observation of greatly reduced brain glucose concentrations during hypoxia-ischemia (see later) provides evidence that the concentration of glucose transporter protein is limiting to CGU in animals at this age. Because the delivery of glucose from the blood into the brain is a function of both the substrate concentration in the blood and the transporter concentration, an increase in substrate concentration produced by glucose supplementation maintains a near-normal or even elevated brain glucose level. In addition,

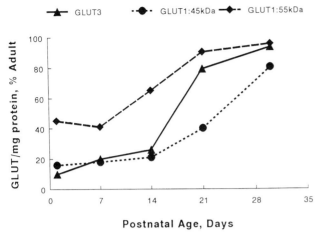

Figure 168–9. Brain glucose transporter proteins during development in the immature rat. Isolated microvessels and cortical membranes were prepared from postnatal rats between birth and 30 days of age and adults. The contents of the facilitative glucose transporter proteins GLUT1 and GLUT3 per milligram membrane protein were determined by Western blot analysis with specific antipeptide antisera to GLUT1 and GLUT3 and [^{125}I]protein A. The figure represents the quantification of four to six animals per age, expressed as a percentage of the adult value.

although calculated intracellular glucose concentrations in immature rats become very low during hypoxia-ischemia, the level of glucose in the cerebrospinal fluid—as a reflection of the concentration in the brain extracellular compartments—does not decrease.[92] Accordingly, it appears that there is a greater limitation imposed at the level of the neurons and glia than at the blood-brain barrier.

The developmental expression of the MCTs shows the reverse pattern. Rodent milk is very high in fat, and suckling pups are naturally ketotic, with circulating levels of β-hydroxybutyrate approaching the millimolar range by the second postnatal week.[90, 93] At this time, cerebral ketone body utilization is also maximal,[93] and this is further reflected in the level and extent of expression of MCT1.[90, 94] Thus, the high levels of ketone body transporter in the blood-brain barrier, as well as in neurons and glia, not only facilitate ketone body transport into the brain but can also aid in the uptake and clearance of lactic acid.

CEREBRAL ENERGY METABOLISM IN HYPOXIA-ISCHEMIA

Hypoxia-acidosis or asphyxia is a frequent cause of acute brain damage in human fetuses and newborn infants and contributes substantially to the chronic neurologic sequelae of cerebral palsy with or without associated mental retardation, epilepsy, or learning disability. Experimental and clinical evidence indicates that hypoxia alone does not produce brain damage, but superimposed cerebral ischemia is a necessary prerequisite for tissue injury to occur. Cerebral ischemia in the setting of asphyxia occurs as a consequence of hypoxic-acidotic cardiovascular depression with secondary systemic hypotension. Cerebral ischemia also occurs as a consequence of occlusive vascular disease of the brain.[95]

Brain hypoxia denotes a cellular oxygen debt, owing to inadequate oxygen delivery (CBF × arterial oxygen saturation through

nutrient arteries). When the tissue (mitochondria) partial pressure of oxygen falls to less than a critical value (<0.1 mm Hg), the cytochrome system of mitochondria becomes unsaturated, and reducing equivalents (reduced forms of NAD [NADH] and flavin adenine dinucleotide) begin to accumulate.[96, 97] ATP production by oxidative phosphorylation is curtailed, with concurrent increases in cellular ADP and AMP, as cytosolic ATP hydrolysis continues to drive endergonic reactions.[2] The elevations in ADP and AMP serve to stimulate glycolysis, through activation of its key regulatory enzyme, PFK (see earlier). Unlike oxidative phosphorylation, which produces 36 mol of ATP for every mole of glucose consumed, glycolysis is an inefficient method to generate ATP by substrate phosphorylation, with net production of only 2 mol of ATP per mole of glucose consumed. To produce the amount of ATP equivalent to that of oxidative phosphorylation, glycolysis would need to increase to a rate of 18 times its basal flux. In reality, glycolysis, even when maximally stimulated, is capable of increasing only four- to fivefold, owing in part to the concurrent accumulation of H$^+$ ions derived from the accumulated NADH, ions that serve to inhibit PFK activity.[4, 44] Thus, glycolysis cannot completely substitute for mitochondrial oxidation, although its stimulation can supplement oxidative phosphorylation under conditions of partial oxygen debt.

Cerebral hypoxia-ischemia severe enough to produce irreversible tissue injury is always associated with major perturbations in the energy status of the brain.[2, 98, 99] Alterations occur not only in the adenine nucleotides but also in PCr, the changes in which actually precede those in ATP, ADP, and AMP. These perturbations were well characterized in an experimental model of perinatal hypoxic-ischemic brain damage.[100] During hypoxia-ischemia, changes in the tissue concentrations of the high-energy phosphate reserves occur early during the course of the metabolic insult and persist well into the recovery period (Fig. 168–10).[101-103] As expected, greater depletions in PCr occur relative to ATP, as the cell attempts to maintain optimal levels of ATP through the CPK equilibrium reaction driven also by the accumulation of ADP and H$^+$ ions. With the eventual decline in tissue ATP, ADP and AMP accumulate in proportion to the loss of ATP. Ultimately, the total adenine nucleotide pool (ATP + ADP + AMP) also decreases, as AMP is catabolized slowly to adenosine and further breakdown products. The concentrations of ATP and the total adenylate compounds do not completely recover after resuscitation, and their persisting partial depletions reflect the presence and severity of tissue destruction (see Fig. 168–10).[101-103]

Of necessity, the loss of cellular ATP during hypoxia-ischemia severely compromises those metabolic processes that require energy for their completion. Thus, ATP-dependent sodium extrusion (efflux) through the plasma membrane in exchange for potassium is curtailed, with a resultant intracellular accumulation of sodium and chloride as well as water (cytotoxic edema). Equally vital to cellular function is the prompt restoration of high-energy phosphate reserves during and after resuscitation. Without regeneration of ATP, endergonic reactions cannot resume, especially those involving the critical event of ion pumping at plasma and subcellular membranes. Intracellular sodium and chloride ions and water continue to accumulate, and electrochemical gradients cannot be re-established. Just how long the cell can survive under this situation is not known, but other factors are called into play that prominently influence ultimate cellular integrity, including the secretion of potentially toxic excitatory amino acids into the synaptic cleft, the intracellular accumulation of free calcium, the intracellular production of nitric oxide, and the production of oxygen free radicals, the last especially during the recovery period.

The mechanism by which ATP disruption persists into the recovery period relates to lingering alterations in the function of mitochondria. In this regard, the classic pathologic studies of

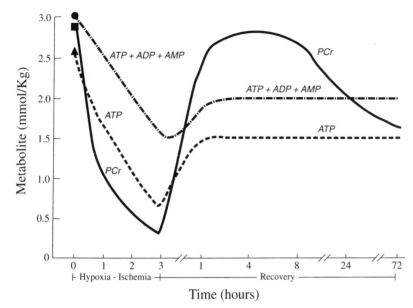

Figure 168–10. Changes in cerebral high-energy phosphate reserves during and after hypoxia-ischemia in the immature rat. Seven-day postnatal rats were subjected to unilateral common carotid artery ligation followed by exposure to systemic hypoxia with 8% oxygen at 37°C. Symbols represent means for adenosine triphosphate (ATP), phosphocreatine (PCr), and total adenine nucleotides (ATP + adenosine diphosphate [ADP] + adenosine monophosphate [AMP]). (Data from refs. 101–103.)

Brown and Brierley[104, 105] indicate that the earliest morphologic alteration of the neuron arising from hypoxia-ischemia is a dilation of mitochondria with an accompanying separation of their cristae. Biochemical studies support the morphologic alterations to the extent that after hypoxia-ischemia, *in vitro* analysis of mitochondria reveals a disturbance in substrate oxidation, a finding suggesting an "uncoupling" of oxidative phosphorylation.[106-108] An *in vivo* investigation in immature rats recovering from cerebral hypoxia-ischemia also suggests the occurrence of an uncoupling of oxidative phosphorylation before or concurrent with the development of morphologically apparent tissue injury.[109] It is assumed that reducing equivalents are oxidized in the presence of oxygen, but ATP is not formed from the energy generated. Such energy is consumed internally (not transferred to the cytosol) or is lost as heat. That oxidative phosphorylation is compromised after hypoxia-ischemia is also confirmed by studies that show that the brain can be well oxygenated concurrent with a persistent depletion in ATP.[102,110,111]

The experimental data regarding the persistent depletion of cerebral high-energy phosphate reserves during recovery from hypoxia-ischemia have relevance to the clinical situation in the asphyxiated newborn human infant. Using MR spectroscopy (see earlier), investigators showed a correlation between lingering alterations in the ratio of PCr to P_i or ATP to P_i and ultimate brain damage as measured by neurodevelopmental status or neurologic assessment.[16, 112, 113] In this regard, PCr/P_i ratios can be normal in the human infant even when brain damage is present,[16, 113] as has also been shown in experimental animals.[101, 103]

A secondary depletion in brain PCr occurs at 18 to 24 hours of recovery from hypoxia-ischemia and beyond in immature experimental animals (see Fig. 168–10),[101-103, 114, 115] and this mimics the late changes in PCr/P_i observed in newborn human infants suffering asphyxial encephalopathy.[16, 112, 113] In newborn pig experiments, PCr/Pi ratios are depressed initially by hypoxia-ischemia only to normalize in the early recovery interval.[114, 115] Thereafter, a secondary decrease in the ratio occurs at 24 and 48 hours of recovery. From human and animal studies, it has been proposed that the secondary failure in cerebral energy status after hypoxia-ischemia is a significant contributor to the ultimate brain damage and neurologic compromise.

However, the secondary decline in PCr does not necessarily denote a delayed energy failure of the brain but rather may reflect a loss of total creatine from the tissue or its conversion to creatinine. The late reduction in PCr, be it in an experimental animal or a human infant, appears to occur as a mass action effect of the CPK equilibrium reaction.[103] Furthermore, the loss of creatine from the brain or its conversion to creatinine, which also would be lost, should result in detectable or increased concentrations of one or both metabolites in cerebrospinal fluid. Possibly, the presence of these compounds in cerebrospinal fluid would serve as a biochemical marker of prior cerebral hypoxia-ischemia in a manner similar to and perhaps more sensitive than the adenine nucleotide derivatives, xanthine and hypoxanthine.[116]

CEREBRAL ACIDOSIS IN HYPOXIA-ISCHEMIA

Hypoxia-ischemia of a severity sufficient to produce brain damage is also associated with tissue acidosis, owing to the accumulation of lactic acid.[2,98,99] The intracellular lactic acidosis results from a shift in glucose utilization from oxidative metabolism to either partial or total anaerobic glycolysis, which occurs during the tissue oxygen debt. Indeed, some investigators have suggested that lactic acidosis is a major contributor to hypoxic-ischemic injury in vulnerable regions of the brain, and a minimum concentration of 15 to 20 mmol lactate/kg brain tissue is required for irreversible damage to occur.[117-119] Furthermore, investigators have shown that the injection of lactic acid into the cerebral cortex of adult rats leads to histologic alterations resembling ischemic infarction, an injury that does not occur after the injection of other organic acids of comparable pH.[120-122] In general, the more severe the tissue lactic acidosis is, the more profound the CBF and metabolic alterations that occur after cessation of the insult,[119,123,124] a finding portending greater ultimate brain damage.

Hypoxia-ischemia leads to cellular acidosis through sources of H^+ ions in addition to lactic acid. Major sources of reducing equivalents include products of the acid hydrolysis of ATP and the formation of NADH + H^+, which accumulates during the cellular energy debt.[125] In this regard, Welsh and co-workers[102] examined the oxidation-reduction (redox) state of immature

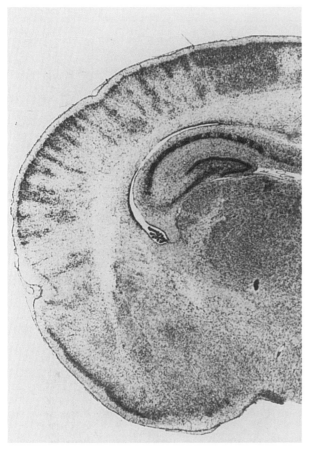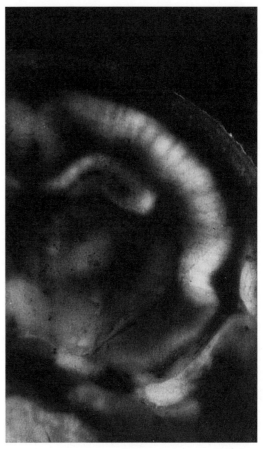

Figure 168–11. Coronal section of immature rat brain showing alterations in reduced nicotinamide adenine dinucleotide (NADH) fluorescence (*right*) during hypoxia-ischemia and histologic alterations (*left*) at 24 hours of recovery. Seven-day postnatal rats were subjected to unilateral common carotid artery ligation followed by systemic hypoxia with 8% oxygen at 37°C.[100] During hypoxia-ischemia, the rat brain was frozen *in situ* and the coronal section was illuminated with ultraviolet light; the fluorescent image then was recorded photographically.[102] Note the columnar pattern of NADH fluorescence (*lighter areas*) in cerebral cortex and the enhanced fluorescence in the CA1 and CA3 sectors of the hippocampus, which correspond closely to the distribution of selective neuronal necrosis seen histologically.

rat brain undergoing hypoxia-ischemia by the technique of reflectance fluorometry (Fig. 168–11). Alterations in regional fluorescence, representing the intracellular accumulation of NADH (+H$^+$), were prominent in the cerebral cortex and in the CA1 sector of the hippocampus during the first hour of hypoxia-ischemia. The pattern of NADH fluorescence closely mimicked the distribution of selective neuronal necrosis observed in this model of perinatal injury. The close correspondence between altered NADH fluorescence and neuropathologic outcome suggests an important role for intracellular acidosis in the pathogenesis of hypoxic-ischemic brain damage. That cellular acidosis occurs during the course of cerebral hypoxia-ischemia in the immature rat is also indicated by a progressive reduction in intracellular pH, calculated from the tissue concentrations of high-energy phosphate reserves.[126]

Using proton MR spectroscopy, several investigators demonstrated a persistent elevation in brain lactate after cerebral hypoxia-ischemia in human newborn infants.[20, 21, 127-129] The persisting lactate concentrations were associated with brain alkalosis. The previously asphyxiated infants uniformly demonstrated severe neurodevelopmental impairment at 1 year of age. Robertson and associates[129] suggested that the persisting cerebral lactic alkalosis is the consequence of a prolonged change in the redox state within neuronal tissue, the presence of phago-

cytic cells, the proliferation of glial cells, or altered buffering mechanisms. We hope that further research will clarify these biochemical abnormalities that linger after cerebral hypoxia-ischemia in newborn human infants.

ACKNOWLEDGMENT

This work is supported by the National Institute of Child Health and Human Development, the National Institute of Neurologic Disease and Stroke, the American Heart Association, and the American Diabetes Association.

REFERENCES

1. McIlwain H, Bachelard HS: Biochemistry and the Central Nervous System. Baltimore, Williams & Wilkins, 1971.
2. Siesjö BK: Brain Energy Metabolism. New York, John Wiley & Sons, 1978.
3. Hawkins R: Cerebral energy metabolism. *In* McCandless DW (ed): Cerebral Energy Metabolism and Metabolic Encephalopathy. New York, Plenum Press, 1985, pp 3–23.
4. Lowry OH, et al: Effect of ischemia on known substrates and cofactors of the glycolytic pathway in brain. J Biol Chem *239*:18, 1964.
5. Lehrer GM, et al: Enzymatic maturation of mouse cerebral neocortex in vitro and in situ. Exp Neurol *26*:595, 1970.
6. Wilson JE: The relationship between glycolytic and mitochondrial enzymes in the developing rat brain. J Biol Chem *239*:223, 1972.
7. Cohen MM, Lim S: Acid soluble phosphate in the developing rabbit brain. J Neurochem *9*:345, 1962.

8. Mandel P, Edel-Harth S: Free nucleotides in the rat brain during postnatal development. J Neurochem *13*:591, 1966.

9. Thurston JH, McDougal DB: Effect of ischemia on metabolism of the brain of the newborn mouse. Am J Physiol *216*:348, 1969.

10. Young RSK, et al: ³¹P NMR study of cerebral metabolism during prolonged seizures in the neonatal dog. Ann Neurol *18*:14, 1985.

11. Gonya-Magee T, Vannucci RC: Ontogeny of cerebral oxidative metabolism in the chick embryo. J Neurochem *38*:1387, 1982.

12. Vannucci RC, Duffy TE: The influence of birth on carbohydrate and energy metabolism in rat brain. Am J Physiol *226*:933, 1974.

13. Duffy TE, Vannucci RC: Perinatal brain metabolism: effects of anoxia and ischemia. *In* Whisnant JP, Sandok BA (eds): Cerebral Vascular Disease. New York, Grune & Stratton, 1975, pp 231–235.

14. Leonard JC, et al: Nuclear magnetic resonance: an overview of its spectroscopic and imaging applications in pediatric patients. J Pediatr *106*:757, 1985.

15. Cady EB, et al: Non-invasive investigation of cerebral metabolism in newborn infants by phosphorus nuclear magnetic resonance spectroscopy. Lancet *1*:1059, 1983.

16. Hamilton PA, et al: Impaired energy metabolism in brains of newborn infants with increased cerebral echodensities. Lancet *1*:1242, 1986.

17. Younkin DP, et al: Unique aspects of human newborn cerebral metabolism evaluated with phosphorus nuclear magnetic resonance spectroscopy. Ann Neurol *16*:581, 1984.

18. Buchli R, et al: Developmental changes of phosphorus metabolite concentrations in the human brain: a ³¹P magnetic resonance spectroscopy study in vivo. Pediatr Res *35*:431, 1994.

19. Ashwal S, et al: ¹H-magnetic resonance spectroscopy–determined cerebral lactate and poor neurologic outcomes in children with central nervous system disease. Ann Neurol *41*:470, 1997.

20. Hanrahan JD, et al: Persistent increases in cerebral lactate concentration after birth asphyxia. Pediatr Res *44*:304, 1998.

21. Barkovich AJ, et al: Proton MR spectroscopy for the evaluation of brain injury in asphyxiated, term neonates. AJNR Am J Neuroradiol *20*:1399, 1999.

22. Himwich HE, et al: The respiratory metabolism of infant brain. Am J Physiol *125*:601, 1939.

23. Himwich HE, et al: Mechanisms for the maintenance of life in the newborn during anoxia. Am J Physiol *135*:387, 1942.

24. Tyler DB, van Harreveld A: The respiration of the developing brain. Am J Physiol *136*:600, 1942.

25. Swaiman KF, et al: Interrelationships of glucose and glutamic acid metabolism in developing rat brain. J Neurochem *10*:635, 1963.

26. Himwich WA, et al: Metabolic studies on perinatal human brain. J Appl Physiol *14*:873, 1959.

27. Himwich HE, Fazekas JF: Comparative studies of the metabolism of brain of infant and adult dog. Am J Physiol *132*:454, 1941.

28. Kjellmer I, et al: Cerebral reactions during intrauterine asphyxia in the sheep. I. Circulation and oxygen consumption in the fetal brain. Pediatr Res *8*:50, 1974.

29. Rosenberg A: Cerebral blood flow and O₂ metabolism after asphyxia in neonatal lambs. Pediatr Res *20*:778, 1986.

30. Rosenberg AA, et al: Role of O₂-hemoglobin affinity in the regulation of cerebral blood flow in fetal sheep. Am J Physiol *251*:H56, 1986.

31. Rosenberg AA, et al: Response of cerebral blood flow to changes in pCO₂ in fetal, newborn, and adult sheep. Am J Physiol *242*:H862, 1982.

32. Brennan RW, et al: Cerebral blood flow and metabolism during cardiopulmonary bypass: evidence of microembolic encephalopathy. Neurology *21*:665, 1971.

33. Hernandez MJ, et al: Cerebral blood flow and oxygen consumption in the newborn dog. Am J Physiol *234*:R209, 1978.

34. Grubb RL, et al: Effects of increased intracranial pressure on cerebral blood volume, blood flow and oxygen utilization in monkeys. J Neurosurg *43*:385, 1975.

35. Levitsky LL, et al: Fasting plasma levels of glucose, acetoacetate, D-β-hydroxybutyrate, glycerol and lactate in the baboon infant: correlation with cerebral uptake of substrates and oxygen. Pediatr Res *11*:298, 1977.

36. Garfunkel JM, et al: The relationship of oxygen consumption to cerebral functional activity. J Pediatr *44*:64, 1954.

37. Kety SS, Schmidt CF: The nitrous oxide method for the quantitative determination of cerebral blood flow in man: theory, procedure, and normal values. J Clin Invest *27*:476, 1948.

38. Settergren G, et al: Cerebral blood flow and exchange of oxygen, glucose, ketone bodies, lactate, pyruvate, and amino acids in anesthetized children. Acta Paediatr Scand *69*:457, 1980.

39. Kennedy C, Sokoloff L: An adaption of the nitrous oxide method to study the cerebral circulation in children, normal values for cerebral blood flow and cerebral metabolic rate. J Clin Invest *36*:1130, 1957.

40. Wechsler RL, et al: Blood flow and oxygen consumption of the human brain during anesthesia produced by thiopental. Anesthesiology *12*:308, 1951.

41. Altman DI, et al: Cerebral oxygen metabolism in newborns. Pediatrics *92*:99, 1993.

42. Yoxall CW, Weindling AM: Measurement of cerebral oxygen consumption in the human neonate using near infrared spectroscopy: cerebral oxygen consumption increases with advancing age. Pediatr Res *44*:283, 1998.

43. Astrup J, et al: Inhibition of cerebral oxygen and glucose consumption in the dog by hypothermia, pentobarbital, and lidocaine. Anesthesiology *55*:263, 1981.

44. Duffy TE, et al: Carbohydrate and energy metabolism in perinatal rat brain: relation to survival in anoxia. J Neurochem *24*:271, 1975.

45. Swabb DF, Boer K: The presence of biologically labile compounds during ischemia and their relationship to the EEG in rat cerebral cortex and hypothalamus. J Neurochem *19*:2843, 1972.

46. Vannucci RC, Plum F: Pathophysiology of perinatal hypoxic-ischemic brain damage. *In* Gaull GE (ed): Biology of Brain Dysfunction, Vol 3. New York, Plenum Publishing, 1975, pp 1–45.

47. Murthy MRV, Rappoport DA: Biochemistry of the developing rat brain. II. Neonatal mitochondrial oxidations. Biochim Biophys Acta *74*:51, 1963.

48. Moore CL, Strasberg PM: Mitochondrial oxidative metabolism. *In* Lajtha A, (ed): Handbook of Neurochemistry, Vol 3. New York, Plenum Press, 1970, pp 53–85.

49. Holtzman D, Moore CL: Oxidative phosphorylation in immature rat mitochondria. Biol Neonate *22*:230, 1973.

50. Davison A, Dobbing J: The developing brain. *In* Davison A, Dobbing J (eds): Applied Neurochemistry. Oxford, Blackwell Scientific, 1968, pp 253–286.

51. Samson FE, et al: Mitochondrial changes in developing rat brain. Am J Physiol *199*:693, 1960.

52. Gjedde A, et al: Cerebral blood flow and oxygen consumption in rat, measured with microspheres or xenon. Acta Physiol Scand *100*:273, 1977.

53. Mayman CI, Tijerina ML: The effect of hypoglycemia on energy reserves of adult and newborn brain. *In* Brierley JB, Meldrum BS (eds): Brain Hypoxia. Philadelphia, JB Lippincott, 1971, pp 242–249.

54. Gregorie NM, et al: Cerebral blood flow and cerebral metabolic rates for oxygen, glucose, and ketone bodies in newborn dogs. J Neurochem *30*:63, 1978.

55. Hernandez MJ, et al: Cerebral blood flow and metabolism during hypoglycemia in newborn dogs. J Neurochem *35*:622, 1980.

56. Jones ME, et al: Cerebral metabolism in sheep: a comparative study of the adult, the lamb, and the fetus. Am J Physiol *229*:235, 1975.

57. Alexander SC, et al: Cerebral carbohydrate metabolism of man during respiratory and metabolic alkalosis. J Appl Physiol *24*:66, 1968.

58. Kety SS: Circulation and metabolism of the human brain in health and disease. Am J Med *8*:205, 1950.

59. Sokoloff L: Localization of functional activity in the central nervous system by measurement of glucose utilization with radioactive deoxyglucose. J Cereb Blood Flow Metab *1*:7, 1981.

60. Sokoloff L, et al: The [¹⁴C]deoxyglucose method for the measurement of local cerebral glucose utilization: theory, procedure and normal values in the conscious and anesthetized albino rat. J Neurochem *28*:897, 1977.

61. Abrams RM, et al: Local cerebral glucose utilization in fetal and neonatal sheep. Am J Physiol *246*:R608, 1984.

62. Duffy TE, et al: Local cerebral glucose metabolism in newborn dogs: effects of hypoxia and halothane anesthesia. Ann Neurol *11*:233, 1982.

63. Kennedy C: Energy metabolism of the brain. *In* Sinclair JC, et al (eds): Perinatal Brain Insult: Mead Johnson Symposium on Perinatal and Developmental Medicine #17. Evansville, IL, Mead Johnson and Company, 1981, pp 30–42.

64. Mujsce DJ, et al: Regional cerebral blood flow and glucose utilization during hypoglycemia in newborn dogs. Am J Physiol *256*:H1659, 1989.

65. Vannucci RC, et al: Regional cerebral glucose utilization in the immature rat: effect of hypoxia-ischemia. Pediatr Res *26*:208, 1989.

66. Chugani HT, Phelps ME: Maturational changes in cerebral function in infants determined by ¹⁸FDG positron emission tomography. Science *231*:840, 1986.

67. Chugani HT, et al: Positron emission tomography study of human brain functional development. Ann Neurol *22*:487, 1987.

68. Kinnala A, et al: Cerebral metabolic rate for glucose during the first six months of life: an FDG positron emission tomography study. Arch Dis Child *74*:F153, 1996.

69. Powers WJ, et al: Cerebral glucose transport and metabolism in preterm human infants. J Cereb Blood Flow Metab *18*:632, 1998.

70. Berntman L, et al: Cerebral oxygen consumption and blood flow in hypoxia: influence of sympathoadrenal activation. Stroke *10*:20, 1979.

71. Dahlquist G, Persson B: The rate of cerebral utilization of glucose, ketone bodies, and oxygen: a comparative *in vivo* study of infant and adult rats. Pediatr Res *10*:910, 1976.

72. Forrester T, et al: Effect of adenosine trisphosphate and some derivatives on cerebral blood flow and metabolism. J Physiol *296*:343, 1979.

73. Volpe JJ, et al: Positron emission tomography in the asphyxiated term newborn: parasagittal impairment of cerebral blood flow. Ann Neurol *17*:287, 1985.

74. Cremer JE, Heath DF: The estimation of rates of utilization of glucose and ketone bodies in the brain of the suckling rat using compartmental analysis of isotopic data. Biochem J *142*:527, 1974.

75. Hawkins RA, et al: Ketone body utilization by adult and suckling rat brain in vivo. Biochem J *122*:13, 1971.

76. Spitzer JJ, Weng JT: Removal and utilization of ketone bodies by the brain of newborn puppies. J Neurochem *19*:2169, 1972.

77. Owen OE, et al: Brain metabolism during fasting. J Clin Invest *46*:1589, 1967.

78. Persson B, et al: Diabetes in pregnancy. *In* Scarpelli EM, Cosmi EV (eds). Reviews in Perinatal Medicine. New York, Raven Press, 1978, pp 1–55.
79. Sann L, et al: Effect of intravenous L-alanine administration on plasma glucose, insulin, and glucagon, blood pyruvate, lactate, and beta-hydroxybutyrate concentrations in newborn infants. Acta Paediatr Scand 67:297, 1978.
80. Goodwin LS, et al: Relationship between cerebrospinal fluid and blood lactate in low birth weight infants. Pediatr Res 14:632, 1980.
81. Stanley CA, et al: Metabolic fuel and hormone responses to fasting in newborn infants. Pediatrics 64:613, 1979.
82. Stemberg ZK, Hodr J: The relationship between the blood levels of glucose, lactic acid, and pyruvic acid in the mother and in both umbilical vessels of the healthy fetus. Biol Neonate 10:227, 1966.
83. Hellman J, et al: Blood-brain barrier permeability to lactic acid in the newborn dog: lactate as a cerebral metabolic fuel. Pediatr Res 16:40, 1982.
84. Cremer JE: Substrate utilization and brain development. J Cereb Blood Flow Metab 2:394, 1982.
85. Cremer JE, et al: Kinetics of blood-brain barrier transport of pyruvate, lactate, and glucose in suckling, weanling, and adult rats. J Neurochem 33:439, 1979.
86. Pessin JE: Mammalian facilitative glucose transporter family: structure and molecular regulation. Am Rev Physiol 54:911, 1992.
87. Vannucci SJ, et al: Glucose transporter proteins in brain: delivery of glucose to neurons and glia. Glia 21:2, 1997.
88. Maher F, et al: Glucose transporter proteins in brain. FASEB J 8:1003, 1994.
89. Price NT, et al: Cloning and sequencing of four new mammalian monocarboxylate transporter (MCT) homologues confirms the existence of a transporter family with an ancient past. Biochem J 329:321, 1998.
90. Vannucci SJ, et al: Developmental expression of the monocarboxylate transporter proteins in rat brain. J Neurochem (in press).
91. Vannucci SJ: Developmental expression of GLUT1 and GLUT3 glucose transporters in brain. J Neurochem 62:240, 1994.
92. Vannucci SJ, et al: Effects of hypoxia-ischemia on GLUT1 and GLUT3 glucose transporters in immature brain. J Cereb Blood Flow Metab 16:77, 1996.
93. Nehlig A, et al: Autoradiographic measurement of local cerebral β-hydroxybutyrate uptake in the rat during postnatal development. Neuroscience 40:871, 1991.
94. Vannucci RC: Hypoxic-ischemic encephalopathy. *In* Fanaroff AA, Martin RJ (eds): Neonatal-Perinatal Medicine. Philadelphia, Mosby-Year Book, 1997, pp 877–891.
95. Vannucci RC: Heterogeneity of hypoxic-ischemic thresholds in experimental animals. *In* Lou HC, et al (eds): Brain Lesions in the Newborn. Copenhagen, Munksgaard, 1994, pp 192–204.
96. LaManna JC, et al: Oxygen insufficiency during hypoxic hypoxia in rat brain cortex. Brain Res 293:312, 1984.
97. Sugano T, et al: Mitochondrial functions under hypoxic conditions: the steady state of cytochrome c reduction and energy metabolism. Biochim Biophys Acta 347:340, 1974.
98. Hossmann K-A: Treatment of experimental cerebral ischemia. J Cereb Blood Flow Metab 2:275, 1982.
99. Raichle ME: The pathophysiology of brain ischemia. Ann Neurol 13:2, 1983.
100. Rice JE, et al: The influence of immaturity on hypoxic-ischemic brain damage in the rat. Ann Neurol 9:131, 1981.
101. Palmer C, et al: Carbohydrate and energy metabolism during the evolution of hypoxic-ischemic brain damage in the immature rat. J Cereb Blood Flow Metab 10:227, 1990.
102. Welsh FA, et al: Columnar alterations of NADH fluorescence during hypoxia-ischemia in immature rat brain. J Cereb Blood Flow Metab 2:221, 1982.
103. Yager JY, et al: Cerebral energy metabolism during hypoxia-ischemia and early recovery in the immature rat. Am J Physiol 262:H672, 1992.
104. Brown AW: Structural abnormalities in neurons. J Clin Pathol 30 (Suppl 11):155, 1977.
105. Brown AW, Brierley JB: The earliest alterations in rat neurones and astrocytes after anoxia-ischaemia. Acta Neuropathol 23:9, 1973.
106. Linn F, et al: Mitochondrial respiration during recirculation after prolonged ischemia in cat brain. Exp Neurol 96:321, 1987.
107. Rehncroná S, et al: Recovery of brain mitochondrial function in the rat after complete and incomplete cerebral ischemia. Stroke 10:437, 1979.
108. Sims NR, Pulsinelli WA: Altered mitochondrial respiration in selectively vulnerable brain subregions following transient forebrain ischemia in the rat. J Neurochem 49:1367, 1987.
109. Vannucci RC: Cerebral glucose and energy utilization during the evolution of hypoxic-ischemic brain damage in the immature rat. J Cereb Blood Flow Metab 14:279, 1994.
110. Dora et, et al: Kinetics of microcirculatory NAD/NADH, and electrocorticographic changes in cat brain cortex during ischemia and recirculation. Ann Neurol 19:536, 1986.
111. Kogure K, et al: The dissociation of cerebral blood flow, metabolism, and function in the early stages of developing cerebral infarction. Ann Neurol 8:278, 1980.
112. Hope PL, et al: Cerebral energy metabolism studied with phosphorus NMR spectroscopy in normal and birth-asphyxiated infants. Lancet 2:366, 1984.
113. Azzopardi D, et al: Prognosis of newborn infants with hypoxic-ischemic brain injury assessed by phosphorus magnetic resonance spectroscopy. Pediatr Res 25:451, 1989.
114. Lorek A., et al: Delayed ("secondary") cerebral energy failure after acute hypoxia-ischemia in the newborn piglet: continuous 48-hour studies by phosphorus magnetic resonance spectroscopy. Pediatr Res 36:699, 1994.
115. Penrice J, et al: Proton magnetic resonance spectroscopy of the brain during acute hypoxia-ischemia and delayed cerebral energy failure in the newborn piglet. Pediatr Res 41:795, 1997.
116. Saugstad OD: Hypoxanthine as an indicator of hypoxia: its role in health and disease through free radical production. Pediatr Res 23:143, 1988.
117. Myers RE: A unitary theory of causation of anoxic and hypoxic brain pathology. *In* Fahn S, et al (eds): Cerebral Hypoxia and Its Consequence. New York, Raven Press, 1979, pp 195–213.
118. Rehncroná S, et al: Excessive cellular acidosis: an important mechanism of neuronal damage in the brain? Acta Physiol Scand 110:435, 1980.
119. Rehncroná S, et al: Brain lactic acidosis and ischemic cell damage. I. Biochemistry and neurophysiology. J Cereb Blood Flow Metab 1:297, 1981.
120. Goldman SA, et al: The effects of extracellular acidosis on neurons and glia *in vitro*. J Cereb Blood Flow Metab 9:471, 1989.
121. Kraig RP, et al: Hydrogen ions kill brain at concentrations reached in ischemia. J Cereb Blood Flow Metab 7:379, 1987.
122. Petito CK, et al: Light and electron microscopic evaluation of hydrogen ion–induced brain necrosis. J Cereb Blood Flow Metab 7:625, 1987.
123. Gardiner M, et al: Influence of blood glucose concentration on brain lactate accumulation during severe hypoxia and subsequent recovery of brain energy metabolism. J Cereb Blood Flow Metab 2:429, 1982.
124. Ginsberg MD, et al: Deleterious effect of glucose pretreatment on recovery form diffuse cerebral ischemia in the cat. I. Local cerebral blood flow and glucose utilization. Stroke 11:347, 1980.
125. Paschen W, et al: Lactate and pH in the brain: association and dissociation in different pathophysiological states. J Neurochem 48:154, 1987.
126. Yager JY, et al: Cerebral oxidative metabolism and redox state during hypoxia-ischemia and early recovery in the immature rat. Am J Physiol 261:H1102, 1991.
127. Penrice J, et al: Proton magnetic resonance spectroscopy of the brain in normal preterm and term infants, and early changes after perinatal hypoxia-ischemia. Pediatr Res 40:6, 1996.
128. Amess PN, et al: Early brain proton magnetic resonance spectroscopy and neonatal neurology related to neurodevelopmental outcome at 1 year in term infants after presumed hypoxic-ischaemic brain injury. Dev Med Child Neurol 41:436, 1999.
129. Robertson NJ, et al: Cerebral intracellular lactic alkalosis persisting months after neonatal encephalopathy measured by magnetic resonance spectroscopy. Pediatr Res 46:287, 1999.

169

Electroencephalography in the Premature and Full-Term Infant

THE CONCEPTS OF STATE AND CONCEPTIONAL AGE

Before addressing the many interesting and complex aspects of the ontogeny of the neonatal electroencephalogram (EEG), an appreciation of the concepts of behavioral state and conceptional age must first be developed. The rhythms of our daily lives are not uniform but are woven into a rich texture of varied activities and behavior. Consider the following illustration. In the early morning we awaken in a relaxed, refreshed, and replenished *state*. Soon we generate activities in preparation to begin the day's work—we are then in a different behavioral *state* of increased activity and heightened physiologic alertness and anticipation. At the peak of the day's work, a *state* of intense concentration, activity, and arousal may exist. By evening, our activity level retraces its steps back through similar behavioral states as we wind down the day. At night a drowsy state heralding the onset of light sleep approaches. Light sleep surrenders to a deeper sleep state until the crisp onset of our first dream *state*. These *sleep states* are organized into patterns that repeat through the night until we awaken the next day and a new cycle begins.

Despite the superficial appearance of disorganization and anarchy that marks a brief and casual inspection of human newborn infants, they display remarkably predictable and recognizable states: constellations or functional clusters of physiologic, behavioral, and neurologic parameters that describe the net condition of the infant.[1,2] It is obvious that an infant's state is the outward and inward expression of neural activity, which can be modified by the environment. The state of a peacefully sleeping infant can be transformed into an aroused or awake state by a sufficiently potent environmental stimulus (light, noise, or touch). State can also fluctuate in response to an internal trigger—a once happy and content infant can quickly dissolve into a frenzy of crying once the pangs of hunger surface. The ability of an infant to display organized and cyclic behavioral states is a useful yardstick to measure the maturity and health of the neonatal brain.[3] Extremely premature infants lack the physical neurologic sophistication required to harmonize and orchestrate the ingredients of recognizable states. Full-term infants do possess the neural equipment for explicit state organization, but this can be altered by the presence of disease. Drugs, medical disorders, unnatural environmental stresses, or neurologic disease consequently may disrupt and distort the normal predictable flow of infantile behavioral states.[4]

Since the presence and organization of electroclinical states are a reflection of neurologic health and maturity, the *conceptional age* (CA) of the infant should be known.[5] Conceptional age is calculated by adding the estimated gestational age (EGA) to the legal age or chronologic age since birth. Thus, a healthy 29-week EGA premature baby with a legal age of 11 weeks has the same CA (29 weeks + 11 weeks = 40 weeks) as a 1-day-old full-term 40-week baby. Although there are some small neurologic-behavioral differences between these 40-week CA babies, they are essentially equivalent in terms of their state of organization and EEG activity.[6]

Early infancy witnesses a period of explosive growth and development unparalleled by any other epoch in the human life span.[7] The clinical changes observable are the outwardly visible signs of underlying anatomic, physiologic, and metabolic central nervous system (CNS) maturation.[8] We now turn our attention to a general description of the ontogeny of infantile states and associated EEG maturation.

OVERVIEW OF THE GENERAL ASPECTS OF THE ONTOGENY OF NEONATAL STATES AND THE ELECTROENCEPHALOGRAM

The cortex of the human fetus has established its foundation by the 8 week of gestation (Table 169-1). Brain function, as measured by the first appearance of an EEG signal, commences shortly thereafter.[9] During the subsequent weeks and months of fetal existence, the anatomic, biochemical, physiologic, and bioelectrical expressions of CNS development mature in concert.[10] Quickening, the first appreciation of fetal motor activity by the mother, is known to be preceded by sustained motor activity (after 8 weeks' gestation) demonstrable by real-time ultrasound. However, at that age, motor activity is almost entirely issued by the brain stem and subcortical structures.[11]

The operational definition of the awake state requires that the eyes be open (Table 169-2). This is not possible before the 24th week of gestation when the eyelids are fused together. Thereafter, it is possible to distinguish an *awake* infant (with eyes open) from an *asleep* infant (with eyes closed). However, except for this eyes open–eyes closed awake-asleep dichotomy, the behavioral state of the infant remains amorphous and primordial. No distinctive EEG changes uniquely discriminate between the aroused and the sleeping infant.[12] By 30 weeks of gestation, the first differences between the EEG in awake and sleeping infants emerges, and the notion of "concordance" arises. Concordance describes the agreement between the electrographic and clinical expression of the infant's state: an awake (eyes open) infant displays a more continuous and low-voltage "aroused" EEG background, whereas a sleeping (eyes closed) infant has a different-appearing EEG that is appropriately matched to the clinical sleep state.

Concordance is only marginally and inconsistently established in the 30-week premature infant. At that age, some segments of the tracing demonstrate fair agreement between the clinical and electrographic expressions of state. Thus, an awake infant who displays eye opening, irregular respirations, and motor activity has a coincident EEG showing a continuous pattern that is in agreement (concordant) with wakefulness. In contrast, in quiet sleep, the eyes are closed, the baby is relatively still, respirations are more regular, and the EEG assumes greater discontinuity than during wakefulness or dream sleep.[13] Within a few more weeks (approximately 32 to 34 weeks' gestation), the healthy premature baby demonstrates much better concordance for longer portions of each tracing. Indeed, at that age, a 1-hour EEG recording might capture several electroclinical behavioral states (see Table 169-1).

At term gestation, a typical sequence of electroclinical states can be demonstrated (see Table 169-2). During wakefulness, the eyes remain open, and the appearance of alert vigilance presides.

TABLE 169-1

Electroclinical Timetable

Age Since Conception	Behavior	EEG
<8 wk	Incomplete cortex; intermittent muscle activity generated by the brain stem	No EEG activity
8+ wk	Periods of more sustained motor activity	First appearance of EEG activity
12-14 wk	Onset of intermittent bursts of regular respiratory muscle activity (breathing movements)	
16-20 wk	Quickening	
24 wk	Eyelids unfuse; operationally, wakefulness (eyes open) alternates with sleep (eyes closed)	Invariant, discontinuous EEG
30 wk	First organization of state: consolidation of physiologic and behavioral parameters that distinguish wakefulness and sleep states	EEG relatively continuous during wakefulness or active sleep; more discontinuous EEG during quiet sleep
32-34 wk	Further consolidation of behavioral state: the child spends most of the time in an indeterminant sleep state; sleep cycle times are brief; better concordance between simultaneous behavior state and the EEG	Clear differences are seen in the awake, transitional sleep; active sleep, and quiet sleep EEGs; the tracing is discontinuous tracé discontinu) mostly during quiet sleep; the EEG can be modified by external stimulation (reactivity)
36-38 wk	At least six distinct behavior states are defined; most of the infant's time is spent asleep; sleep onset begins with active asleep	As concordance improves there is less indeterminant sleep and more quiet sleep; mature continuous slow-wave sleep makes its appearance during quiet sleep; continuous low- to moderate-voltage mixed-frequency activity (activité moyenne) presides during wakefulness and active sleep
40-44 wk	Well-defined behavioral states continue; the infant spends most of the time asleep	Dissolution of many immature EEG patterns (e.g., waning of the Δ brush); emergence of mature quiet sleep states and sleep spindles
4 mo postdelivery	The infant has "settled" through the night and established daytime patterns for eating, naps and play; onset of deliberate volitional motor patterns such as reaching for items of interest; sleep onset is quiet sleep	The percentage of active sleep approaches adult value; longer sleep cycle time and asynchronous sleep spindles in quiet sleep; during wakefulness precursors of α and μ rhythms appear

TABLE 169-2

Electroclinical States at Term

Electroclinical Parameters	Awake	Asleep Active (REM or Dream Sleep)	Asleep Quiet (NREM)
Behavior			
Eyelids	Open	Closed	Closed
Eye movements	Present	REMs	None
Tonic EMG	Variable	Off	On
Phasic EMG	Variable	On	Off
Respirations	Irregular	Irregular, brief apneas	Regular
EEG	Continuous (activité moyenne)	Continuous (activité moyenne)	Discontinuous (tracé alternant) and continuous slow-wave sleep

REM = rapid eye movement; NREM = non-rapid eye movement (sleep).

The level of muscular activity varies from calm quiet to vigorous limb thrashing with crying. The respiratory pattern is irregular. The simultaneous EEG is essentially continuous—there are few interruptions in the nonstop production of low-to moderate-voltage, mixed-frequency cerebral rhythms.[14] The infant may next enter a drowsy state as the harbinger of sleep. The voltage of the continuous EEG pattern increases as more slow activity (Δ) appears. As drowsiness deepens, slow, rolling eye movements begin and the eyelids close. The infant may briefly occupy a transitional or indeterminant sleep state. There are then insufficient criteria to unequivocably classify the electroclinical state as fully developed active or quiet sleep. However, the infant's state soon crystallizes into definite active sleep. Sleep onset that begins with active sleep contrasts sharply with the onset of sleep in healthy older children and adults who usually enter quiet sleep first. Individuals with the sleep disorder narcolepsy also begin their sleep cycle with active or rapid eye movement (REM) sleep. During active sleep, the eyes remain closed. There are bursts of conjugate, jerky, rapid, predominantly horizontal eye movements. REMs are not homogeneously distributed during active sleep but appear in grouped clusters. The coincident EEG mostly resembles that of wakefulness, that is, a continuous low-to-medium-voltage mixture of EEG frequencies. Indeed the cerebral cortex is in a similar "aroused" mode whether the subject is awake or engaged in the mental activities of active sleep. The voltage of the EEG signal attenuates in the setting of

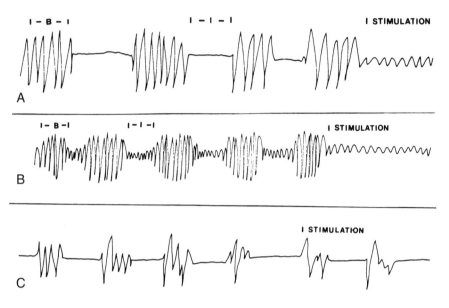

Figure 169–1. Discontinuous EEG activity.
A, Normal quiet sleep in a 33-week preterm baby: During tracé discontinu, the bursts *(B)* are composed of normal EEG patterns; the interbursts (I) represent low-voltage periods of quiescence. Following stimulation, there is behavioral and EEG reactivity and a transition to a more aroused state. **B**, Normal quiet sleep in a full-term baby: During tracé alternant, the bursts *(B)* are composed of normal EEG signals; the interburst voltage is higher (> 25 μV) than tracé discontinu and spectrally resembles the EEG signal during active sleep. Following stimulation, the EEG changes to a continuous, lower-voltage, mixed-frequency signal. **C**, The critically ill premature or full-term infant displays hyporesponsive eye closure signifying lethargy or coma; the bursts of activity are composed of abnormal EEG patterns; the interburst periods are low voltage and tend to be longer than the duration of the interburst during tracé discontinu and tracé alternant. Despite stimulation, there is no EEG reactivity and the fixed, invariant EEG pattern remains.

wakefulness, dreaming, or arousal from quiet sleep because of the removal of the synchronization that exemplifies quiet sleep. The low-voltage EEG is a result of desynchronization of cortical activity.[15]

Once the first active sleep period concludes (the first active sleep state may last only 15 to 25 minutes at that age), the infant again enters transitional or indeterminate sleep that culminates in quiet or non-REM sleep. The baby's body is then "quiet" or motionless except for deep, regular, slow excursions of respiration. The face is expressionless, save for occasional bursts of sucking automatisms. The EEG substantially changes its character as the pattern becomes discontinuous. The voltage of the cortical signal then regularly fluctuates between higher voltage segments of activity and lower voltage periods of quiescence. French electroencephalographers have coined the terms *tracé discontinu* and *tracé alternant* to describe these normal discontinuous quiet sleep patterns (Fig. 169-1). Quiet sleep is a delicate electroclinical state. During mild encephalopathies, more of the EEG may appear as indeterminate sleep at the expense of quiet sleep,[16] that is, the percentage of total sleep time classified as indeterminate sleep increases directly as the percentage of quiet sleep diminishes. Although the EEG may appear normal during wakefulness or active sleep in mild encephalopathies, abnormalities may be confined to quiet sleep.

As term gestation approaches (36 to 38 weeks CA), additional signs of electrographic maturity emerge. Although the circadian rhythms at birth are already set at the adult value (24.8 hours), sleep cycle time at term is 50 minutes and gradually lengthens to mature values of 90 minutes.[17] The EEG pattern of quiet sleep is subtly different from the previous tracé discontinu of the more immature infant. Although the pattern remains discontinuous, the quiescent period is not as low in voltage. The record demonstrates repetitive *alternations* between bursts of higher voltage activity and lower voltage quiescent periods. French investigators designate this alternating tracing as tracé alternant.

At term, quiet sleep is divisible into two distinct patterns. The immature quiet sleep pattern of tracé alternant is the remnant of earlier quiet sleep patterns that evolved from tracé discontinu.

More mature quiet sleep then emerges as continuous slow-wave sleep in which *continuous* high-amplitude θ and Δ activity dominates the record.[18] This resembles in principle the quiet sleep of older infants and children. By 4 to 6 weeks after term, continuous slow-wave sleep also displays, for the first time, the unmistakable sentinel of mature non-REM sleep—the sleep spindle or σ rhythm. Thus, by 6 weeks after term, most healthy infants have cemented the groundwork for the electrocerebral cycles of their future life. By 4 months post-term, the basic architecture of sleep-awake cycles has been transformed from the primitive undifferentiated electroclinical state of the very premature baby to one that basically satisfies the criteria of electroclinical maturity.

By this age, most babies exit wakefulness into non-REM sleep. Furthermore, the proportion of total sleep time occupied by active sleep has fallen from a high value of 50% at term to a mature value of about 20%[18] (Fig. 169-2). During quiet sleep,

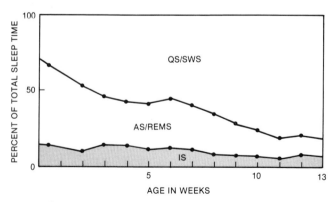

Figure 169–2. Quiet or slow-wave sleep (QS/SWS), active or REM sleep (AS/REMS), and indeterminant sleep (IS) as percentages of total sleep time in normal full-term infants, 1 to 13 weeks old. (From Ellingson RJ, Peters JF: Electroencephalogr Clin Neurophysiol *49*:112, 1980.)

well-formed sleep spindles flourish but do not appear simultaneously in the two hemispheres (i.e., they are asynchronous) until 2 years of age. Poorly developed sleep sharp waves are also visible from the central vertex (C_z) by 4 months of age and are explicit by 6 months of age.[19] During wakefulness, substantial spatial organization of EEG frequencies and rhythms has appeared. The precursors of the well-known μ rhythm (the "idle" rhythm of the motor cortex) and α rhythm (the "idle" rhythm of the visual cortex) dominate the rolandic and occipital areas, respectively.[20] Although at this age the frequency of these waveforms (around 3 to 4 Hz) is too slow for these patterns to be rightfully labeled as a true μ or α rhythm, their morphologic characteristics, rhythmicity, and reactivity to movement or vision impart them with their fundamental characteristics.

The value of an understanding of the concept of state and EEG ontogeny becomes more tangible when discriminating between abnormal and normal EEGs. The EEG is expected to be temporarily low voltage during wakefulness and dream sleep, or after behavioral arousal. However, this normal low-voltage signal is interspersed with higher-voltage EEG segments in quiet sleep. In contrast, the pathologic low-voltage EEG represents a fixed, monotonous, invariant pattern that does not cycle with spontaneous higher voltage activity of quiet sleep. In a similar context, the highly abnormal pattern of "burst suppression" must be distinguished from the normal discontinuity (tracé discontinu and tracé alternant) of immature quiet sleep. The former represents an immutable pattern from which the patient cannot be rescued by the strongest external stimulation (see Fig. 169–1). The cerebral activity during the bursts of burst suppression displays an abnormal morphologic condition, with admixed spikes, sharp waves, or unusual fast (β) activity.

In just a few months, the anatomic, physiologic, synaptogenic, and electrophysiologic properties of the cortex undergo an unparalleled metamorphosis.[8] This introductory overview paints a broad picture of the electroclinical events that encompass early life outside the womb. The next task is to consider the specific details of recording and interpreting the EEG itself.

TECHNICAL ASPECTS OF NEONATAL EEG RECORDINGS

EEGs are recorded in the clinical neurophysiology laboratory or at the infant's cribside in the intensive care nursery.[21] (Fetal EEG refers strictly to EEG sampling during labor and delivery and is comparable to the well-known technique of fetal heart rate monitoring.)[22,23] The recording technologist must exercise great care in order to obtain the most technically acceptable tracing. The EEG is recorded for 40 to 60 minutes to sample EEG activity during several spontaneous state changes. At the conclusion of the EEG, the technologist stimulates the patient with light, sound, and touch to witness arousal patterns that demonstrate reactivity of the EEG signal.

The recording session begins by noting the clinical condition of the baby. The medical and neurologic diagnoses are recorded.[24] The infant's level of consciousness, drugs consumed, respiratory status, arterial blood gas values, and other pertinent laboratory data are noted.

The infant's head is carefully measured from standard bony landmarks (e.g., the inion and nasion) (Fig. 169–3), and the scalp is marked with a crayon at several key locations.[25] When measured properly, these prescribed locations can be reproducibly located by the same or a different technologist on subsequent EEG recordings. Because the scalp surface area of the neonatal skull is small, a limited number of sites is used rather than the full electrode array employed in older individuals. The EEG recording sites are chosen to provide a fair sampling of cortical electrical activity from several representative brain regions. In the International 10/20 system modified for neonates, surface disk electrodes are applied with electrode paste in the following loca-

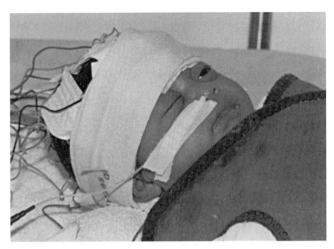

Figure 169–3. Infant undergoing an EEG examination.

tions (Fig. 169-4): FP_3-FP_4 (halfway between the conventional frontal polar [FP_1-FP_2] and frontal [F_3-F_4] regions); C_3-C_4 (central, rolandic, or parasagittal areas); T_3-T_4 (midtemporal or paratemporal); O_1-O_2 (occipital); and F_z (frontal vertex), C_z (central vertex), and P_z (parietal vertex). Additional polygraphic monitors are placed to detect eye movements, nasal airflow, chest wall excursions, and the electrocardiogram (ECG). Altogether, at least 20 recording channels on the electroencephalograph are needed for a complete study. Usually a single montage is used for the whole session.

The neonatal EEG is largely composed of Δ and θ activity, with a relative paucity of faster rhythms (Fig. 169-5). The technique of EEG recording is conducted to exploit the rich presence of this slower activity; the usual EEG recording speed is 30 mm/sec, but neonatal tracings are recorded at a slower paper speed (15 mm/sec). This compresses the signal in the time domain and facilitates visual analysis by enhancing the visibility of the

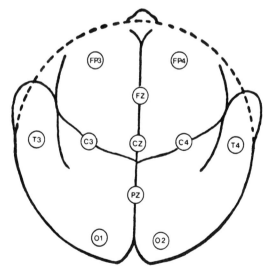

Figure 169–4. Technical specifications. 1. Long interelectrode distances. 2. Multiple polygraphic variables including ECG, eye movements, nasal air flow, chest wall excursion, movement monitor. 3. Recording speed: 15 mm/sec. 4. Recording sensitivity 7 μv/mm. 5. Filters: HLF: 70 Hz, LLF: 0.3 to 1.0 Hz. 6. Montage: Channel: (1) $FP_3 \rightarrow T_3$; (2) $T_3 \rightarrow O_1$; (3) $FP_4 \rightarrow T_4$; (4) $T_4 \rightarrow O_2$; (5) $FP_3 \rightarrow C_3$; (6) $C_3 \rightarrow O_1$; (7) $FP_4 \rightarrow C_4$; (8) $C_4 \rightarrow O_2$; (9) $T_3 \rightarrow C_3$; (10) $C_3 \rightarrow C_z$; (11) $C_z \rightarrow C_4$; (12) $O_4 \rightarrow T_4$; (13) $F_z \rightarrow O_z$; (14) $C_z \rightarrow P_z$ (15) $T_3 \rightarrow C_z$; (16) $T_4 \rightarrow C_z$.

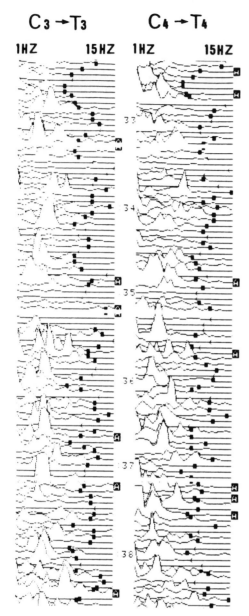

Figure 169–5. Compressed spectral array depicts the distribution of EEG power across frequencies 1 to 15 Hz in the left central-temporal ($C_3 \rightarrow T_3$) and right central-temporal ($C_4 \rightarrow T_4$) regions. Note that most of the power is expressed in the θ- and δ-bandwidth.

Δ activity. The filter settings are also chosen to permit faithful reproduction of the dominantly slow frequency signal. The lower linear frequency is 0.3 to 1 Hz, and the high linear frequency is 70 Hz.

While the tracing is actually being conducted, it is mandatory for the recording technologist to make accurate and copious notations on the unfolding EEG record that describe the patient's behaviour and activity. The presence of eye opening or closure, movements, sucking, hiccups, startles, squirming, and so on all help the encephalographer to understand the behavioral state and identify possible sources of recording artifact.

GENERAL PROPERTIES OF THE NEONATAL EEG

The neonatal EEG is exceptional in many ways. Not only are the specific bioelectric rhythms that compose the signal unique and age-specific but the fundamental *organization* of the signal is confined to infancy. We now consider the infrastructure of neonatal EEG: continuity, synchrony, symmetry, and reactivity.

Continuity and Discontinuity

The property of continuity confers an uninterrupted voltage level to the tracing (Fig. 169–6). There are no substantial voltage breaks or interruptions in a continuous EEG tracing. Continuous EEGs unravel nonstop. Segments of the EEG that show clear-cut interruptions or reductions of voltage are "discontinuous"[26] (Fig. 169–7). The "burst" segments of cerebral electrical activity refer to the active periods in which the EEG voltage is "on." The specific rhythms and patterns that compose the burst activity are then visible. (These specific individual patterns are described later.) Between the bursts of activity are lower voltage interburst periods of relative quiescence. The EEG is "off" in the interburst period. The signal amplitude at a standard recording sensitivity may then fall to zero or a value that is clearly less than the preceding burst activity.

In the extremely young infant (24 to 28 weeks CA), the entire EEG is essentially discontinuous.[27] Whether the child is clinically awake or asleep, active or quiet, the EEG itself is composed almost entirely of a discontinuous background. Stimulation of the patient or spontaneous state changes provoke little qualitative change in the discontinuity.

By 30 weeks of age, more extended periods of relative continuity may appear.[19] The continuous EEG may occasionally persist without interruptions for many minutes as active sleep first materializes and consolidates. By 32 weeks of age, most healthy infants are capable of prolonged, continuous segments of EEG activity during definite active sleep periods. Indeed this is a landmark CA, since for the first time the continuous EEG dominates over the discontinuous portions of the record. Perhaps it is no coincidence that key CNS anatomic and physiologic landmarks mature at the same age.[28]

After 32 weeks of age, EEG discontinuity is mostly confined to quiet sleep. The voltage of the interburst activity, as recorded from the scalp surface with standard recording sensitivity, remains less than 25 µV. This discontinuous quiet sleep tracing (tracé discontinu) resembles the more primitive discontinuity that pervades all states in the very young preterm baby. With advancing maturity, the voltage of the interburst period exceeds 25 µV. The label assigned to this more mature discontinuous quiet sleep activity is tracé alternant, signifying the alternations between the higher voltage bursts and lower voltage interbursts[29] (Fig. 169–8). The distinction between tracé discontinu and tracé alternant is thus somewhat arbitrary. Except for the higher interburst voltage, little else is fundamentally different. A curious feature of the interburst activity of tracé alternant is that it comprises voltages and frequencies that typify the continuous EEG during wakefulness and active sleep.[30] It is as though tracé alternant quiet sleep were composed of brief portions of active sleep (i.e., the interburst segments) separated by bursts of higher voltage slowing.

By 1 month after term, the discontinuous quiet sleep pattern has all but disappeared. Tracé discontinu and tracé alternant gradually yield to the more mature, continuous slow-wave sleep, during which nonstop high-voltage θ and Δ activity dominate the tracing. Eventually the more sophisticated trappings of non-REM sleep (spindles and vertex waves) punctuate the tracing (Fig. 169–9).

Duration of Interbursts

The duration of the burst and interburst periods is maturation (CA)-dependent[12] (Table 169–3). The length of the interburst is relatively longer in the younger preterm infant and decreases near term (Fig. 169–10). Most investigators have reported a range of values for the duration of interburst as a function of CA.[28,31]

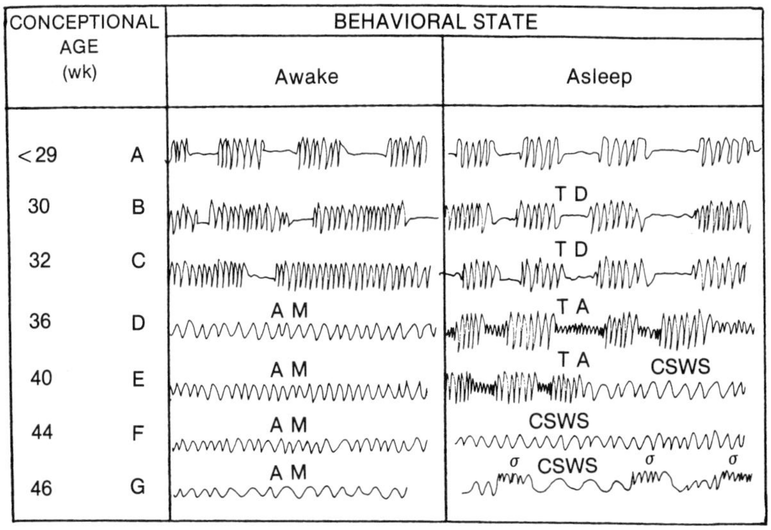

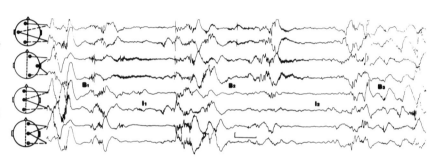

CONCEPTIONAL AGE (wk)		BEHAVIORAL STATE	
		Awake	Asleep
< 29	A		
30	B		T D
32	C		T D
36	D	A M	T A
40	E	A M	T A CSWS
44	F	A M	CSWS
46	G	A M	σ CSWS σ σ

Figure 169–6. Evolution of continuity. *A*, Primordial discontinuity. *B*, Relatively more continuous while awake or during active sleep. Tracé discontinu (TD) during quiet sleep. *C*, Mostly continuous during wakefulness. TD during quiet sleep. *D*, Activité moyenne (AM) continuous low to medium voltage mixed-frequency signal while awake. Tracé alternant (TA) while asleep. *E*, AM during wakefulness. Mixture of immature (TA) and mature continuous slow wave sleep (CSWS) during quiet sleep. *F*, AM during wakefulness. Mostly CSWS during quiet sleep. *G*, AM during wakefulness. Quiet sleep entirely CSWS and sleep spindles (σ) first appear.

Figure 169–7. Tracé discontinu. EEG segment recorded from a 1-week-old (29 weeks EGA) premature infant. The infant is in indeterminant sleep. The background activity is discontinuous and characterized by a series of bursts (B1, B2, B3) separated by lower-voltage periods of quiescence or interbursts (I1, I2). The cerebral electrical activity that makes up the bursts is of normal character, and the duration of the interburst periods is not excessively long for this conceptional age.

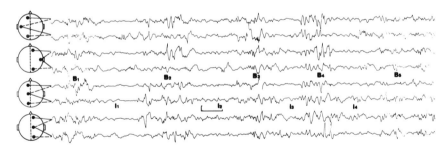

Figure 169–8. Tracé alternant. One-week-old full-term infant in quiet sleep. The cerebral electrical activity is discontinuous and composed of a series of bursts (B1, B2, B3, B4, B5) separated by interburst periods (I1, I2, I3, I4) of lower voltage and brief duration. Compared with tracé discontinu recorded from younger infants, the interburst periods are briefer and higher in amplitude.

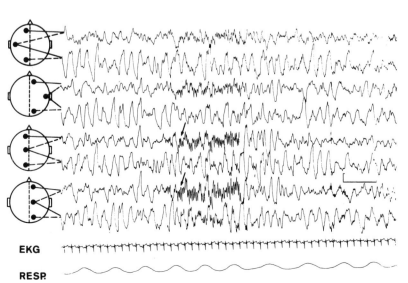

Figure 169–9. Continuous slow wave sleep (CSWS) and spindle. This segment was recorded from a healthy 8-week-old full-term infant during quiet sleep. CSWS is noted with semirhythmic high-amplitude Δ-activity maximally expressed in the bioccipital scalp regions. Twelve-hertz sleep spindles *(arrows)* arise synchronously from the frontocentral regions bilaterally. Although in this segment the spindles arise synchronously, they often do not at this age. Notice that the respiratory pattern is exquisitely regular and that there is a paucity of limb movements during quiet sleep.

EKG

RESP.

TABLE 169-3

The Influence of Conceptional Age on the Duration of the Interburst Period (Quiescence) in Seconds

Sources/Reference	26	27	28	29	30	31	32	33	34	35	Term
Tharp[31]				6-7					4-5		4
Anderson, et al[12]			M = 12 R = 8-16		M = 9 R = 5-14		M = 7 R = 4-11				
Scher[5]			<40		<30						
Parmelee, et al[26]					9.3			6.9			4.7
Eyre, et al[10]	25		25	22		12			10	8	4.0
Mizrahi[24]		8-20									
Lombroso[32]		"Seconds to 2 minutes"									3.6

Conceptional Age (wk)

M̄ = mean; R = range.

The discrepancies in reported values reflect differences in technical recording aspects, EEG criteria that define the boundaries between the burst and interburst intervals, and the clinical condition of the babies.[10] Tharp has shown that concurrent medical conditions of the baby may influence the interburst duration. With relative hypoxia, the interburst period lengthens in parallel[31] (Fig. 169–11). It is probably true that other physically stressful medical conditions (hypoxia, ischemia, hypercapnia, hyponatremia, sepsis, and so on) similarly increase the degree of discontinuity.

Another source of disparity in reported measurements of interburst duration is the selection criteria for individual premature babies. Most "healthy" premature babies have relatively brief interburst periods and eventually mature into developmentally and neurologically normal children. Some sick premature infants have much longer interburst periods and yet fortunately also recover and develop normally. For example, Lombroso[32] has cited "allowable" interburst periods up to 2 minutes, since some of the neonates from whom the measurements were recorded were later developmentally normal. Another perspective is that such excessively long interburst periods are indeed abnormal but do not oblige a permanent adverse outcome in all. The situation is not different from the healthy youngster whose EEG is excessively slow and disorganized following a head injury. The pattern itself is abnormal even though the individual can still enjoy a healthy outcome later.

Excessive Discontinuity

Excessive discontinuity is an electrographic abnormality in which bursts of normally composed EEG signal are separated by longer than normal interburst periods. Mildly excessive discontinuity may reflect a temporary metabolic imbalance or mild encephalopathy. Markedly excessive discontinuity usually connotes more serious metabolic or neurologic abnormalities.[33,34] As the acute encephalopathy passes, the excessive discontinuity gradually subsides.

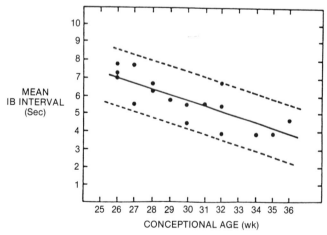

Figure 169–10. Mean interburst intervals (*solid line*) in routine EEGs (30- to 60-minute duration) recorded on 12 newborn infants without evidence of encephalopathy and normal at follow-up. Several infants had more than one tracing. (From Tharp BR: Adv Neurol 46:107, 1986.)

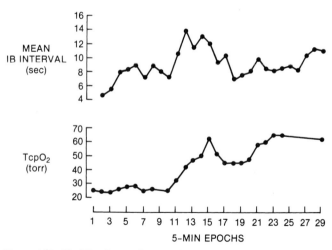

Figure 169–11. The figure depicts the relationship between oxygenation (TcpO$_2$) and mean interburst (IB) intervals/ 5 minutes in a premature infant with a hypoxic-ischemic encephalopathy and pulmonary hypertension. (From Tharp BR: Adv Neurol 46:107, 1986.)

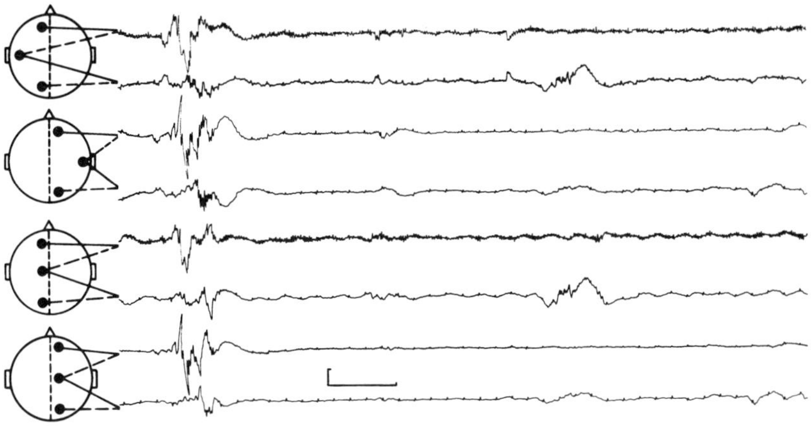

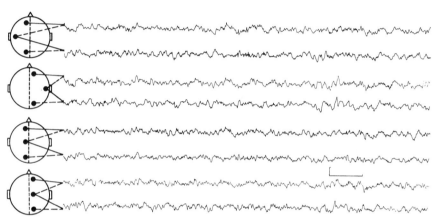

Figure 169–12. Burst suppression. EEG segment recorded from a severely asphyxiated 35-week EGA infant. During the tracing, the child is comatose. The background shows burst suppression. There is a brief burst of erratic cerebral electrical activity that features an atypical bifrontal sharp wave. The burst of activity is followed by a long period of low-voltage suppressed background. There was no reactivity of the EEG to external stimulation.

Figure 169–13. Activité moyenne. Segment of EEG tracing recorded from a 5-day-old full-term infant during wakefulness. During this segment of the record, the child is alert but calm. There is a paucity of movement and muscle artifact. The EEG itself is low-to-medium voltage, is continuous, and represents an average mixture of EEG frequencies (activité moyenne). During active sleep, the EEG has a similar "aroused" appearance.

In the setting of an acute encephalopathy, the term *burst suppression* denotes a markedly abnormal EEG background in which nonreactive, abnormally composed EEG signals are separated by abnormal low-voltage quiescent periods (Fig. 169-12; see also Fig. 169-1).

NORMAL CONTINUITY

By 30 weeks CA, many healthy babies display relatively protracted periods of continuous EEG activity, during which the patient's clinical behavior suggests active sleep. By 32 weeks CA, most records demonstrate definite continuous segments. However, the specific patterns that make up the burst in the discontinuous records appear quite similar to the continuous segments. As term approaches, the actual composition of the continuous segments differs from the discontinuous quiet sleep record. During wakefulness and the active sleep that immediately follows quiet sleep, the continuous EEG is relatively low voltage and represents a rich mixture of frequencies (β, α, θ, and Δ). This continuous "average" background is called *activité moyenne* by French authors (Fig. 169-13). At term, most quiet sleep still displays the immature tracé alternant pattern, which later yields to the more sophisticated *continuous* slow-wave sleep pattern that is the foundation of adult quiet sleep activity.

Although it is apparent that there is a desirable progressive substitution of continuous EEG activity to replace discontinuity, all forms of continuity are not desirable. Some infants electrographically respond to CNS insult with a continuous, but invariant, monotonous EEG that does not display spontaneous-state lability and is unreactive to external stimulation.

Synchrony and Asynchrony

The isolated cerebral cortex generates a discontinuous EEG pattern.[35] Cortex disconnected from deeper pacemakers and remote from intracortical modulation produces a pattern that inherently fluctuates its voltage (high voltage alternating with low voltage). In the discontinuous portion of an EEG, the two cerebral hemispheres can discharge at the same time (i.e., synchronously) or they can fire independently at different times (i.e., asynchronously). Although the temporal relationship of the signal *between* hemispheres is the usual focus of synchrony, the activity *within* each hemisphere can also be examined. Near term, individual regions within each hemisphere discharge simultaneously. For example, at 38 weeks, signals generated in the left frontal, central, temporal, and occipital areas arise together. In the very young premature baby, separate regions within one hemisphere may discharge independently or out of sync. Thus, the temporal regions may be silent while the occipital areas robustly discharge.

Lombroso has proposed an operational definition of interhemispheric synchrony that has been widely adopted.[36] In a synchronous burst, the signal begins in both hemispheres within 1.5 seconds. In an asynchronous burst, one hemisphere leads the other by 1.5 or more seconds. Defined in this fashion, synchrony is a measurable property of the background that evolves with maturity (Table 169-4).

Curiously, in the very young premature infant with primordial discontinuity, interhemispheric synchrony approaches 100%. By 30 to 31 weeks, when the EEG first demonstrates distinguishable state-dependent patterns, synchrony is only about 50% during the discontinuous portions of the recording. It is suspected that

TABLE 169–4

Interhemispheric Synchrony and Conceptional Age

Reference																
	REM						70%–90%									
Lombroso[32]	IS	90%–100%			80%–100%											
	NREM						50%–70%		60%–80%		70%–85%		80%–100%		100%	
Anderson, et al[12]		M̄ = 92% R = 80%–100%			M̄ = 94% R = 79%–100%		M̄ = 94% R = 86%–100%									
		26	27	28	29	30	31	32	33	34	35	36	37	38	39	40
							Conceptional Age (wk)									

M̄ = mean; R = range of values; REM = rapid eye movement sleep; IS = indeterminant sleep; NREM = non–rapid eye movement sleep.

the neurologic substrate that underlies synchrony differs in these two circumstances.[32] With advancing maturity, a greater percentage of the bursts are synchronous until term, when nearly 100% of the bursts of tracé alternant begins simultaneously in the two hemispheres.

Excessive interhemispheric asynchrony for CA is an electrographic abnormality (Fig. 169-14). It is most commonly seen following diffuse encephalopathies (e.g., intraventricular hemorrhage, meningitis, or asphyxia). No unique type of pathologic condition underlies the EEG expression of excessive asynchrony.[37] Excessive interhemispheric asynchrony can also be seen in cerebral dysgenesis, including agenesis of the corpus callosum or Aicardi syndrome. Although it would be tempting to speculate that the corpus callosum is the anatomic prerequisite for synchrony, the situation is probably more complex, since the paired thalami and several commissures also serve as conduits that synchronize activity between the two hemispheres.

Although synchrony is usually intended to describe the temporal unity of the entire hemisphere, some individual EEG signals are also notably synchronous. In the very young premature infant, the occipital regions display remarkably synchronous high-voltage monorhythmic Δ activity. Frontal sharp waves (encoches frontales) and frontal slow transients (anterior dysrhythmia) are also usually synchronous. In contrast, the normal sleep spindles of mature quiet sleep do not achieve full bihemispheric synchrony until 2 years of age.

Symmetry

The average voltage or amplitude of electrical activity in both cerebral hemispheres is generally symmetric.[38] The EEG amplitude and composition are equivalent when a suitably long sample is inspected. Although brief transient asymmetries are common, the overall impression from reading an extended EEG sample should convey the sense that both hemispheres (for that matter, homologous regions of both hemispheres) have equivalent representation of (1) voltage, (2) frequency, and (3) specific background patterns.

The voltage of the background is roughly equal between homologous brain regions and between the two hemispheres. Near term it may be easier to detect voltage asymmetry during quiet sleep, since the naturally higher voltage of tracé alternant exceeds that of wakefulness or active sleep. Care must be exercised in labeling a tracing abnormal because of voltage asymmetry alone (i.e., unaccompanied by a change in the frequency composition of the signal). The voltage at a given scalp location can be reduced by improper electrode placement or electrode gel bridging. Two electrodes accidentally placed too close together "see" the same EEG scalp signal. The differential amplifiers of the electroencephalograph may therefore detect only a modest voltage differential between the two sites, and a low-amplitude output signal results. An artificially low voltage signal also can result from scalp edema, which removes the recording electrode farther from the cortical surface, the generator source of the signal. This can result from edema caused by a dependent head position or the infiltration of a scalp intravenous infusion. However, similar voltage depression can occur with subdural fluid (blood or cerebrospinal fluid) collections.

A transient voltage-frequency asymmetry may be observed occasionally during the transition between tracé alternant and active sleep in some healthy term babies. As the child enters or exits quiet sleep, one hemisphere desynchronizes into a low-

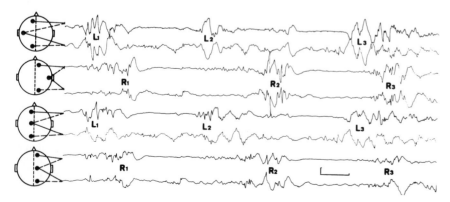

Figure 169–14. Interhemispheric asynchrony. EEG segment recorded during indeterminate sleep in a 3-day-old (37 weeks EGA) infant with congenital heart disease. This EEG segment is discontinuous and shows excessive interhemispheric asynchrony. Notice that discharges from the left central and temporal regions (L1, L2, and L3) are displaced in time from bursts originating from the right central and temporal regions (R1, R2, and R3).

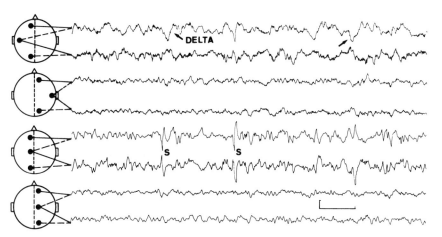

Figure 169–15. Interhemispheric asymmetry. EEG segment recorded from a 4-day-old full-term infant with an unexplained stroke in the distribution of the left middle cerebral artery. In this rhythm strip, there is a clear asymmetry between the two hemispheres. The left temporal and central regions have abundant high-amplitude Δ-activity (*arrows*), which is not present in similar regions in the opposite healthy hemisphere. Furthermore, excessive sharp EEG transients (S) are seen in the left central region.

voltage, continuous, mixed-frequency background, while the other displays the high-voltage tracé alternant quiet sleep pattern. This obvious asymmetry may persist for several minutes until voltage-frequency equality is restored to the two hemispheres. This phenomenon implies that the cycling of sleep and arousal is modulated independently for both hemispheres.

Although symmetry of voltage is the easiest EEG parameter to detect, symmetry of composition is equally important. Localized or lateralized pathologic features may give rise to an asymmetry in the type of EEG signal. There may be a circumscribed paucity of faster or rhythmic waveforms or excessive focal slowing that earmarks a localized cortical functional disturbance (Fig. 169–15). Transient patterns such as Δ brushes or frontal sharp waves are also generally symmetric. For example, an equal number of brushes/minute can be counted from corresponding regions of both hemispheres.

Reactivity

EEG reactivity describes a change in the appearance of the cerebral background activity following a specific provocative stimulus (see Fig. 169–1). Reactivity is both state- and CA-dependent. EEG reactivity should be distinguished from the clinical neurologic reaction to stimulation. The latter may include eye opening, crying, grimacing, limb movement, or a change in the respiratory pattern. These are not always time-locked to a coincident departure from the baseline EEG.

In the very young premature baby, the primordially discontinuous EEG shows no consistent response to external stimulation. However, by 32 to 34 weeks CA, some change can be induced in the EEG background by an arousing stimulus. As such, the quietly sleeping infant whose EEG shows a tracé discontinu pattern can be redirected into an alert state (wakefulness or active sleep) by external stimulation with a corresponding switch to a continuous EEG background.

By term, healthy, quietly sleeping babies show two basic arousal patterns following external stimulation: (1) a temporary increase in discontinuity (longer duration of the interburst period), and (2) attenuation of voltage or desynchronization of the background signals. During quiet sleep, the discontinuous tracé alternant pattern usually displays interburst periods of about 4 to 6 seconds. Following a suitably intense stimulus, the discontinuity of the tracing can temporarily increase, with longer interburst intervals and lower amplitude of interburst activity, thus resembling a brief reversion into tracé discontinu. However, unless the arousal persists and a complete state change ensues, the record soon reverts back to the prior tracé alternant pattern. During either tracé alternant or continuous slow-wave quiet sleep, the second major arousal pattern is an abrupt, widespread voltage reduction and the disappearance of the slowest Δ activity.

Reactivity is best visualized in the EEG of a quietly sleeping infant when increased discontinuity or desynchronization is unmistakable. Stimulation of an awake and alert infant or provocation during active sleep may not produce a dramatic change in the EEG despite a brisk behavioral response.

Nonreactivity

A lack of reactivity is an ominous sign in a suitably mature infant (see Figs. 169–1 and 169–12). Indeed, in the healthy infant, spontaneous-state lability and reactivity to external stimulation are expected markers of health. Infants whose tracings are invariant—lacking spontaneous lability or stimulus-provoked state changes—usually harbor an encephalopathy.

SPECIFIC COMPOSITION OF THE ELECTROENCEPHALOGRAM

The EEG background refers to the collective presence of all ongoing moment-to-moment cerebral electrical patterns. The background can be high or low voltage, continuous or discontinuous, normal or abnormal. The prevailing *ingredients* that collectively constitute the background emerge and fade at different CAs. The background may be considered a foundation or infrastructure. It serves as a stage that is punctuated by short-lived transients, such as sharp waves, or fleeting events, such as electroencephalographic seizures.

During the perinatal period, the infrastructure of the signal is normally dominated by slow activity (θ and Δ) (see Fig. 169–5). With maturity, the frequency of the dominant rhythms increases, with a gradual evolution to higher frequencies.

Many of the specific patterns that make up the EEG background exhibit spatial or state-dependent properties, or both (Table 169–5). For example, bursts of monorhythmic θ activity are spatially maximal in the temporal-occipital regions but are independent of state. Sleep spindles exhibit both spatial and state specificity. They originate from the midline vertex-rolandic regions and are confined to quiet sleep.

Monorhythmic Occipital Δ Activity

The posterior regions of the healthy premature baby are dominated by runs of high-voltage, positive-polarity, slow, biooccipital monorhythmic Δ activity (Fig. 169–16). The runs of Δ activity can last from 2 to 60 seconds and are often synchronously displayed bilaterally, although minor voltage asymmetries are common. This stereotyped Δ activity serves as the most visible dominant posterior rhythm in this age group. It is present in the youngest viable premature infant, peaks between 30 and 33 weeks of age, and clearly begins to recede by 34 weeks of age. It serves as the Δ constituent of occipital brush activity (see the

TABLE 169-5

Summary of General Organization of Electroclinical States

Parameter	27–28 Wk CA	29–30 Wk CA	31–33 Wk CA	34–35 Wk CA	36–37 Wk CA	38–40 Wk CA	41–49 Wk CA
Behavioral states	Primordial; no difference in behavioral states	Some early behavior organized to suggest early states	Behavioral states easier to define; definite periods of AS/QS	Well-defined states	Well-defined states	Well-defined states	Well-defined states
Continuity/discontinuity	Entirely discontinuous	Relatively more continuous during AS	Sustained continuity while awake/ASTD; mostly QS, a little in AS 60%	Continuous in awake/AS; TD in QS only	Well-defined TA; traces of CSWS	TA/CSWS	By 1 mo, AS and QS continuous
Synchrony	80%–90%	50%	60%	70%	80%	100%	
Specific EEG patterns							
Rhythmic occipital Δ	+	++	+++	±	-	-	-
Rhythmic temporal θ	+	++	+++	±	-	-	-
Rhythmic occipital θ	++	++	+	±	-	-	-
Δ brushes	+	++ AS > QS	++ AS > QS	+ QS > AS	+ QS > AS	± QS > AS	± QS only
Irregular central temporal Δ	+	++	+	-	-	-	-
Anterior dysrhythmia (encoches frontales)	-	-	±	+	++	++	+/-
Sleep spindles	-	-	-	-	-	-	- (+ after 44 weeks)
Reactivity	Inconsistent	Inconsistent	Variable	Usually present	Reliably present	Present	Present
Concordance	Poor; awake and asleep EEG are similar	Poor; awake and asleep EEG are similar	Fair; EEG relatively continuous during behavioral AS	Good	Good	Good	Good

AS = active sleep; QS = quiet sleep; TD = tracé discontinu; CSWS = continuous slow wave sleep; TA = tracé alternant; + = present; ++ = abundant; – = absent; ± = variably present.

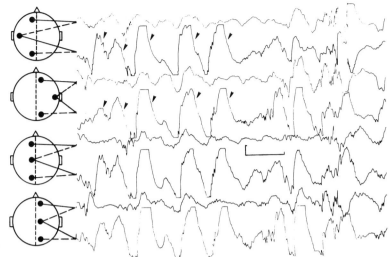

Figure 169–16. Monorhythmic occipital Δ-activity. This EEG segment was recorded from an awake 32-week-old EGA infant. During this relatively continuous segment, the EEG background is dominated by high-amplitude rhythmic occipital Δ-activity (*arrowheads*). Note that the occipital δ-activity on the left arises at the same time (synchronously) with the occipital Δ-activity on the right.

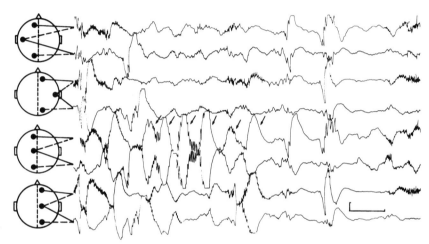

Figure 169–17. Central-temporal Δ-activity. EEG segment recorded from a sleeping 1-week-old (26-week EGA) infant. Note the series of semirhythmic Δ-transients that are best expressed in the left central region (*arrows*). This segment also illustrates intrahemispheric asynchrony. Although there is robust discharging of cerebral electrical activity in the central regions, the temporal and occipital areas are quiet.

discussion on Δ brushes). It is a hardy rhythm; sometimes it is among the last of the "named" EEG background patterns to disappear after a significant encephalopathy.

Central-Temporal Δ Activity

The central and central-temporal regions in the young premature infant show sustained trains of semirhythmic Δ activity that is not nearly as bilaterally synchronous as the monorhythmic occipital Δ activity (Fig. 169–17). It also serves frequently as the Δ foundation for rolandic brush formation. It also fades from the background by 34 weeks of age.

Rhythmic θ Activity (Sawtooth θ)

Short bursts of very rhythmic θ activity arise in the occipital regions of the premature baby less than 30 weeks of age (Fig. 169–18, *A*) and in the temporal-occipital regions in premature infants 30 to 34 weeks of age (Fig. 169–18, *B*). It occurs in all behavioral states. Although rhythmic, the waveform may be sharply contoured. The duration of the burst is variable and may last several seconds. If the burst is very brief, a "larval" discharge can occur, resembling a fragment of sharply contoured activity, and mimic "potentially epileptiform activity" in the temporal areas.

Brushes (Δ Brushes, Spindle-Like Fast Rhythms, Ripples of Prematurity)

The quintessential waveform of prematurity is the Δ brush,[39] a pattern that represents the simultaneous fusion of two subunits: (1) an underlying Δ transient, and (2) superimposed rhythmic fast activity (Fig. 169–19). Brushes occur during wakefulness, active sleep, and quiet sleep. They are not analogous to or the precursor of the conventional sleep spindle (σ rhythm). There are usually no major asymmetries in brush abundance (the number of brushes/hour) compared between homologous regions of the two hemispheres. Brushes are not by nature synchronous.

In the very premature infant, brushes are more common in the rolandic regions[12] (Fig. 169–20). When they achieve their highest expression (32 to 34 weeks CA) brushes are seen in the occipital, rolandic, and temporal regions. Frontal brushes are relatively rare at any age.

Even though brushes occur in all states, their abundance is state-dependent. Up to 34 weeks CA, brushes appear more frequently in active sleep than in quiet sleep.[36] By 34 to 36 weeks CA, the number of brushes in quiet sleep exceeds those in active sleep. By term, brushes are infrequent during wakefulness and may only be seen in quiet sleep, especially tracé alternant. By 1 month after term, brushes have largely vanished as greater maturity emerges.

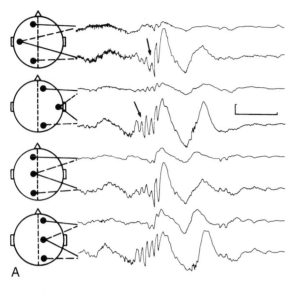

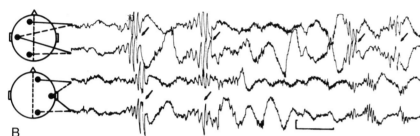

Figure 169–18. Rhythmic θ activity. A, This segment was recorded from a 3-day-old (27-week EGA) premature infant in indeterminate sleep. Notice the appearance of rhythmic bioccipital θ activity (*arrows*) superimposed on high-amplitude monorhythmic bioccipital Δ: activity. **B,** Same patient 2 weeks later. The rhythmic θ activity has largely migrated anteriorly and now principally engages the temporal regions (*arrows*). Rhythmic temporal θ activity is frequently asynchronous between the two temporal regions.

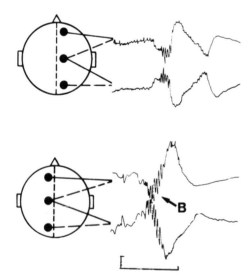

Figure 169–19. Δ-Brush. This segment was recorded from a 4-day-old (33-weeks EGA) infant during probable active sleep. Notice the Δ-brushes in the central regions, composed of an admixture of a Δ-transient with a superimposed "buzz" of β activity (*B*).

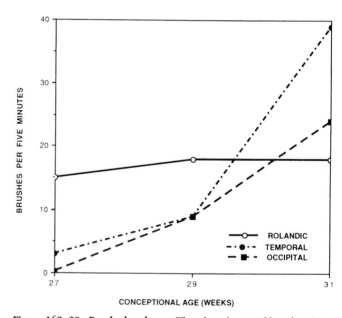

Figure 169–20. Brush abundance. The abundance of brushes is a function of both maturity and location. The graph depicts the abundance (number of brushes/5 minutes of EEG background) seen in the occipital, temporal, and rolandic regions at 27, 29, and 31 weeks of conceptional age.[12]

Anterior Dysrhythmia (Anterior Slowing)

Brief bursts of high-amplitude, relatively symmetric, and synchronous bifrontal rhythmic Δ activity begin between 33 and 34 weeks CA (Fig. 169–21, *A*). Despite the usual pathologic connotation of the prefix *dys-*, this pattern is entirely normal. Anterior dysrhythmia appears in all states but is most abundant

in transitional sleep preceding quiet sleep. In this context it behaves as a "drowsy pattern." It is also very common during quiet sleep but comparatively infrequent in alert wakefulness or dream sleep. Anterior dysrhythmia usually begins to disappear

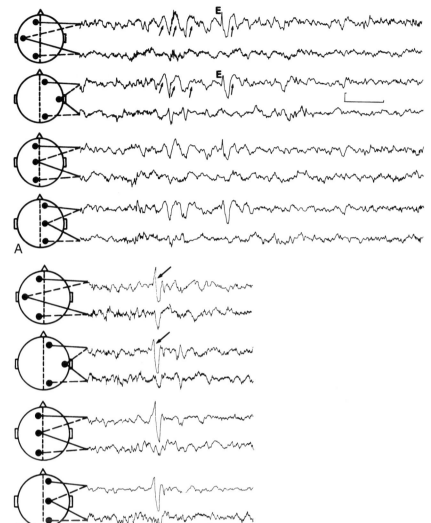

Figure 169–21. **A**, Anterior dysrhythmia. This segment was recorded from a drowsy 1-week-old (39-week EGA) infant. During drowsiness, a run of rhythmic anterior slowing (anterior dysrhythmia [*arrows*]) interrupts the background in the frontal regions. Admixed with the rhythmic anterior slowing is a frontal sharp wave or encoches frontales (E). Note the relative synchrony and symmetry of the anterior dysrhythmia and encoches frontales. **B**, Encoches frontales. EEG segment recorded from a 5-day-old full-term infant during drowsiness. Encoches frontales are recognized as synchronous and symmetric biphasic (negative-positive) bifrontal sharp waves (*arrows*). This pattern often appears simultaneously (i.e., synchronously) between the frontal regions. Frontal sharp waves are most abundant during drowsiness and in quiet sleep and are least evident during alert wakefulness. Sometimes these normal sharp EEG transients are mistaken as "epileptiform" by inexperienced electroencephalographers.

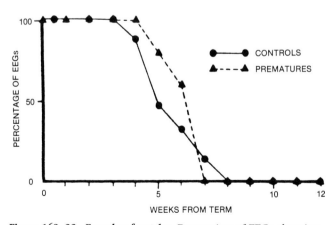

Figure 169–22. Encoches frontales. Proportion of EEGs showing frontal sharp transients in premature and full-term infants. (From Ellingson RJ, Peters JF: Electroencephalogr Clin Neurophysiol *50*:165, 1980.)

by 1 month after term. Although it is a normal pattern, excessive anterior dysrhythmia is abnormal and may be seen in the setting of a mild diffuse encephalopathy.

Encoches Frontales (Frontal Sharp Waves)

The pattern of encoches frontales consists of a biphasic (negative-positive polarity), notched frontal sharp wave that is inextricably entwined with anterior dysrhythmia[40] (Fig. 169-21, *B*). Indeed the two patterns often co-mingle and seem harmonically related, implying they share a common neural generator. They are frontally dominant and usually synchronous and symmetric between the left and right frontal regions. Like anterior dysrhythmia, they first appear in immature form at 33 to 34 weeks CA and in complete form by 35 weeks CA. They start to wane by 1 month after term and decay in parallel with anterior dysrhythmia (Fig. 169-22).

During mild encephalopathies, encoches frontales mildly increase in frequency, and their morphologic characteristics become more variable. Sometimes the pattern shows a sharper (i.e., briefer duration) morphologic appearance. Encoches frontales convey no implication for epileptogenesis. They are an expected normal EEG signal and do not connote a "lowered seizure threshold."

Other Sharp Waves

Healthy babies have occasional sharp EEG transients in the temporal,[41] central, and occipital regions (Fig. 169-23). These transients are most abundant between 37 and 42 weeks CA,

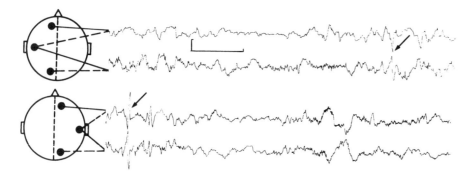

Figure 169–23. Normal sharp EEG transients. This segment was recorded from a healthy 3-day-old full-term infant during active sleep. Occasional sharp EEG transients (SETs) are recorded independently from the temporal regions (*arrows*).

gradually decline in abundance by 4 to 6 weeks after term, and entirely vanish from the background by 10 weeks after term[42] (Fig. 169-24). They are most common in the temporal areas. They are usually sharp waves rather than spikes, arise solitarily rather than in bursts or consecutive runs, and recur with a frequency of about one sharp EEG transient/minute of active sleep (Table 169-6).

Sleep Spindles

By 44 to 46 weeks CA, quiet sleep sheds its immature tracé alternant pattern and establishes its mature foundation as continuous slow-wave sleep. Sleep spindles (about 12 to 14 Hz) then appear from the midline vertex (C_z) or the central regions (C_3 and C_4)[19] (see Fig. 169-9). Sleep spindles are often asynchronous between the two hemispheres and remain so until 2 years of age.

Dominant Rhythmic Patterns of Early Infancy

Soon after the healthy infant leaves the neonatal period, the organization of the EEG begins to resemble, at least in principle, that of the young child. In early infancy, poorly sustained rhyth-

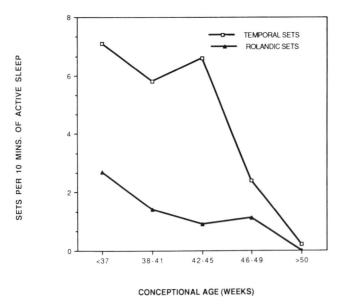

Figure 169–24. SET abundance. The graph depicts the abundance of sharp EEG transients (SETs) in the temporal and central regions during 10 minutes of active sleep. Notice that there are more SETs in the temporal than in the central regions at all ages studied. There is a gradual decline in the frequency of SETs until these patterns disappear from the record near 50 weeks of conceptional age.

mic activity first emerges in the occipital and rolandic regions (Fig. 169-25). The rhythmic occipital patterns are the precursor of the α rhythm. The slow frequency (< 8 Hz) of this dominant occipital rhythm precludes labeling it as "true" α, but its location and reactivity to visual stimuli earmark it as an immature version of the genuine article. The frequency of this pattern gradually increases until it is 8 Hz or faster (usually by age 2 years), at which time the label "α rhythm" can be employed with full justification.

Similarly, runs of central rhythmic patterns appear that resemble an immature μ rhythm, the idle rhythm of the motor cortex. This μ rhythm precursor tends to be about 0.5 Hz faster than its corresponding α precursor in each individual and reaches 8 Hz or faster by age 2 years.

Abnormal EEG Patterns

Newborn infants are exposed to a wide variety of potentially CNS-damaging events. The EEG, a sensitive reflection of cerebral cortical activity, commonly displays an assortment of abnormalities, depending on the injury's severity and topography, and the patient's CA. Most EEG abnormalities are not specific for etiology. Consequently, the tracing does not reveal the cause of the abnormality but rather describes its presence, acuteness, location, and severity. Even though the EEG has little value in revealing the underlying basis of an infant's encephalopathy, it is considered an ideal prognostic indicator.[43-45] Neonates with normal or only mildly abnormal EEGs generally survive and escape permanent brain damage. On the other hand, those with severe abnormalities such as isoelectric or burst-suppression recordings face high mortality and significant morbidity. Those with moderately abnormal EEGs have a mixed outcome: some do well but others later exhibit a chronic static encephalopathy. The prognostic value of the EEG may be particularly important when the design of a neonatal neuroprotection intervention is contemplated. Infants with well-preserved EEGs (good prognosis) may not be suitable candidates for a protection trial since their outcomes are already favorable, even before the intervention or placebo. Those with marked EEG abnormalities (dismal prognosis) may be so profoundly injured that they are beyond the reach of benefit from trial enrollment. Those with moderate EEG abnormalities could "go either way", and the balance might be favorably tipped by help from a neuroprotection intervention. Criteria to assign patients into these mild, moderate, and severe EEG background abnormalities have been proposed by Menache and colleagues.[46]

Clinical seizures are among the most common reasons for neonates to undergo an EEG examination. It is a challenge for all involved in the care of neonates to distinguish epileptic-based neonatal seizures from the wide array of nonepileptic "paroxysmal" behaviors, which may occur in healthy or sick infants. At this point, a brief discussion of pathologic EEG "sharp waves" and electrographic neonatal seizures is in order.

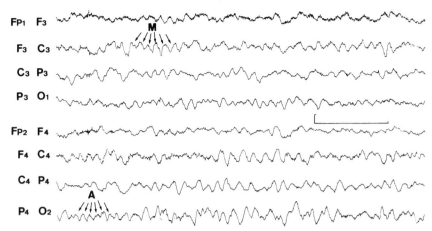

Figure 169–25. Precursors of μ and α rhythms.
This EEG segment was recorded from an awake, alert, and quiet 5-month-old infant. Notice the appearance of rhythmic Δ activity in the central regions that are the precursor of μ activity (M). In the occipital regions, rhythmic θ activity is also noted (A) and is the precursor of α activity.

Pathologic Sharp Waves

Many forms of sharp waves are an expected, normal feature of the EEG background. However, certain characteristics may render them pathologic[47] (Fig. 169-26). For example, contrast the usual behavior of normal temporal sharp waves with pathologic sharp waves recorded *between* seizures in a sick neonate (Table 169-6). The latter transients are often faster (duration ≤ 100 msec), more abundant, and repetitive and may be unusually distributed spatially in a highly localized fashion. Many times, EEGs recorded to "rule out" seizures in a newborn are not fortuitous to actually capture a seizure in progress. Such interictal tracings may still provide evidence that the patient has a "lowered seizure threshold" by revealing an excessive number of negative-polarity spikes and sharp waves. The EEG spikes or sharp waves are not direct proof of seizures but certainly are consistent with their presence.

Positive-polarity sharp waves are different pathologic EEG transients that do not imply a lowered seizure threshold[48] (Fig. 169-27), but rather are a marker for injury to the deep cerebral white matter, such as periventricular leukomalacia. They are usually seen in the midline vertex or rolandic region but can also arise in the temporal areas.[49]

Seizures

In contrast to an isolated sharp wave, which is a fleeting transient EEG pattern, an electrographic neonatal seizure (ENS) unfolds as an *event* with a distinctive beginning and end (Fig. 169-28). A typical ENS lasts about 2 minutes and arises focally from a restricted cortical region.[50] Our knowledge of the relationship between clinical and electrographic seizures has changed over the years, aided by the emergence of video-EEG monitoring. Whereas a routine bedside EEG examination does not capture video and may miss ENSs in a 40-minutes epoch, longer-term video-EEG monitoring may be more revealing in evaluating many neonates with seizures.

The valuable role of video-EEG monitoring for characterizing neonatal seizures was established by Mizrahi and Kellaway,[51] who analyzed video-EEGs from 349 neonates between ages 28 and 44 weeks CA with a clinical suspicion of seizures. Four hundred fifty-one paroxysmal clinical events were recorded in 71 patients, but only 29% of the clinical events in 23 patients had a close temporal association with electrographic seizure activity. In other words, some of the abnormal clinical "seizures" were not *epileptic*, bur rather a type of abnormal brain stem release or postural reflex. Conversely, many electrographic seizures occurred that were not accompanied by any clinical signs of seizure. Such ENSs, termed subclinical or occult, have been identified in other populations. A recent large series from the Neonatal Seizures Clinical Research Centers[52] described 207 infants with video-EEG confirmed seizures. One third of the infants demonstrated only subclinical ENS: despite the definite electrographic seizures, no obvious clinical seizure occurred at the same time. In 10%, all the patients' abnormal-appearing "seizures" were not accompanied by ENS, even though the EEG background was often seriously abnormal, reflecting their acute encephalopathies. Finally, half the patients had one or more electroclinical seizures that feature simultaneous clinical and electrographic seizures. The clinical events in these instances of electroclinical seizures were frequently recurrent, focal, *clonic* twitching of the face, trunk or extremities.

The hallmark of ENSs is the sudden appearance of a repetitive discharge event containing a definite beginning, middle, and end. ENSs evolve in frequency, morphology, and amplitude. Although no two ENSs appear identical, a few simple criteria aid in their recognition: (1) an individual ENS arises from a specific focus. ENSs are rarely, if ever, "generalized" (affecting all brain regions in an organized, synchronized, and symmetric fashion). However, once an ENS originates at its focus, it is free to spread or migrate to other locations. (2) The minimum duration of an ENS is conventionally defined as 10 seconds. Most ENSs are shorter than 2 minutes, but it is common to observe multiple, serial, brief ENSs. (3) The specific shape or morphology of the waveforms that make up the ENS varies widely within and between neonates (Figure 169-29). Any EEG frequency (e.g., theta activity) may compose the seizure. However, the morphology and amplitude of the ENS evolve—the end of the seizure looks different in amplitude and shape from the beginning.

Laroia and colleagues[53] suggested a strategy to target high-risk neonates for video-EEG monitoring. Fifty-one neonates with specific ICU admission diagnoses (e.g., asphyxia, meningitis) underwent a 30 to 60 minute screening EEG, followed by continuous EEG monitoring for 18 to 24 hours. The initial EEG background at admission was classified as normal, immature for age, or mildly, moderately or severely abnormal. Only 1 (4.2%) of 24 infants with normal or immature EEG backgrounds had subsequent ENS. However, 22 of 27 (81%) infants with abnormal EEG backgrounds had ENS. Thus, the initial EEG background significantly predicted the presence or absence of seizures in the subsequent 18 to 24 hours.

Cerebral Function Monitoring

The traditional role of neonatal EEG has been to perform the complete array of electrophysiologic testing under the guidance of a skilled EEG technologist for a brief period of time (i.e., 40 minutes) and *visual* review of the record by a knowledgeable electroencephalographer. Indeed, this remains the mainstay of

TABLE 169-6

Comparison of Sharp EEG Transients (SETs) Recorded in Healthy Infants and Those with Confirmed EEG Seizures

EEG Parameter	Healthy Infants	Infants with Seizures
Background	Normal	Frequently abnormal
SET abundance	Total SETs from left and right central and temporal regions are maximum near term and recur about 1 SET/1.0 min to 1 SET/1.5 min	
Morphologic characteristics	Usually sharp waves (rarely spikes)	Spikes or sharp waves
Repetitive behavior	Isolated, solitary transients	Solitary; runs or bursts of SETs
Pattern of spatial distribution	Temporal > central > occipital during active sleep; no striking asymmetry between left and right hemispheres	Asymmetries may be present between left and right temporal, left and right central, or left and right hemispheres

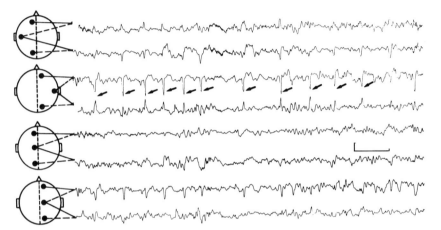

Figure 169–26. Abnormal sharp EEG transients. EEG segment recorded from a 1-week-old (37 weeks EGA) infant with meningitis and seizures. This segment was recorded between electrographic seizures. Note the excessive abundance of sharp EEG transients (*arrows*), which are virtually entirely confined to the right temporal region except for mild spread into the adjacent rolandic area. This type of electrographic abnormality suggests a lowered seizure threshold and is not usually seen in healthy infants.

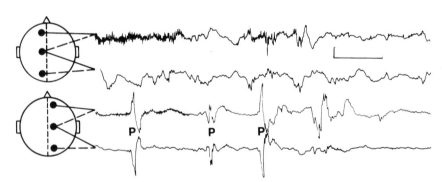

Figure 169–27. Positive rolandic sharp waves. This EEG segment was recorded from a 2-week-old (28 weeks EGA) infant with a right-sided grade IV intraventricular hemorrhage. On subsequent cranial ultrasound examinations, periventricular leukomalacia was noted on the right. Positive rolandic sharp waves (P) are seen as definite sharp EEG transients of positive polarity, which are clearly distinguished from the background activity.

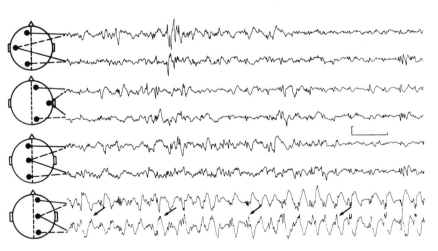

Figure 169–28. Electrographic seizure. This segment was recorded from an asphyxiated 1-day-old full-term infant. An electrographic seizure is in progress (*arrows*). The electrographic seizure is an event with a characteristic evolution of repetitive, stereotyped, rhythmic waveforms or spikes/sharp waves that replace the underlying background rhythms locally. During this particular electrographic seizure, no clinical signs were exhibited by the asphyxiated infant.

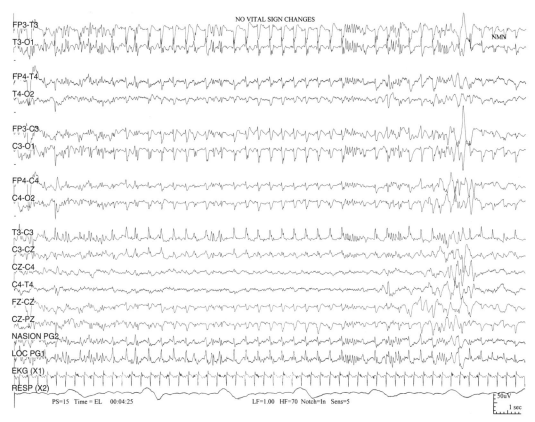

Figure 169–29. An electrographic seizure is recorded from a 42-week CA infant with surgically repaired congenital heart disease. The appearance of the seizure changes during the course of its evolution. No two electrographic seizures appear identical. Rather, it is their electrographic *behavior* that stamps them with the mark of the epileptic process.

contemporary neonatal EEG. There are, nonetheless, circumstances in which immediate bedside testing may be required for which there is insufficient time to summon the technologist or obtain an instantaneous interpretation from the electroencephalographer. The concept of the cerebral function monitor (CFM) is that of a biomedical device that can be applied to one or two scalp locations by the nurse and the "raw" EEG signal processed by computer in a variety of fashions. The CFM, which can be continued for many hours or days, generates a simple output signal that provides useful information of CNS status that can be interpreted by non-neurologists. The CFM can be used to estimate brain functional integrity quickly in the immediate wake of an acute encephalopathy such as hypoxia-ischemia (e.g., deciding which patient is appropriate to enroll in a neuroprotection trial, which typically must be started within a few hours of the insult), screen for electrographic seizures automatically, and show trends of brain status during serious illness or response to treatment.

Although the EEG "signal" is extremely complex, it is still describable in mathematical terms and subject to signal processing, quantitative analyses, and statistical manipulations. Just as an optical prism can separate white light into its component colors, the neonatal EEG can be decomposed into the sum of its component frequencies in the traditional bandwidths of delta (≤ 3 Hz), theta (4–7 Hz), alpha (8–12 Hz) and beta (≥ 13 Hz) frequencies. A CFM based on this principle of analysis[54] simple describes the amount of electrical power (measured in picowatts) that is confined to each of these frequency "bins." In healthy neonates, the robust power of the neonatal EEG is largely relegated to the slow (theta and delta) frequency bins (see Fig. 169-5). Using this relatively simple approach, the EEG of the healthy neonate can be used to develop normative profiles of electrical power distribution across frequency bandwidths in the awake and asleep states, which serve as a benchmark to compare with those demonstrating acute encephalopathy.[55]

Mathematicians may choose from an array of analytical approaches to analyze or quantify the neonatal EEG. The short-time Fourier transform (STFT), higher-order spectral analysis (the so-called bispectrum) and autoregressive segmentation are the names of some of the more popular mathematical tools used to analyze and model complex biologic signals. A unique approach is the application of nonlinear dynamics or chaos theory to neonatal EEG analysis. The principle is quite simple. The normal neonatal EEG is extremely rich in its complexity and inherent "unpredictability". The status or appearance of the background at one moment in time does not predict the next with any probability. The normal neonatal EEG has many "dimensions" of chaos or complexity (unpredictability). In contrast, the EEG of a sick neonate with an extremely low voltage, featureless background or burst suppression (with its regular cycles of "off-signal" and "on-signal") becomes predictable with reduced dimensions of chaos. Finally, CFM may analyze the raw EEG signal by neural networks, constructed to achieve an artificial intelligence approach to "decide" whether a novel *test* EEG segment is normal or not.

The network is first instructed to "learn" the boundaries of the normal EEG, based on input from a wide assortment of normal EEG samples representing many healthy neonates in a variety of biobehavioral states. After the network has "learned" how normal EEG segments appear, a test EEG sample can be submitted for analysis. If the neural network algorithm recognizes the test segment as comparable to prior normal segments in its memory, the analysis designates the test segment as "normal." Thus, this approach does not generate a graphic depiction of EEG function but rather categorical variables, such as a "normal," "moderately abnormal," or "markedly abnormal" EEG.

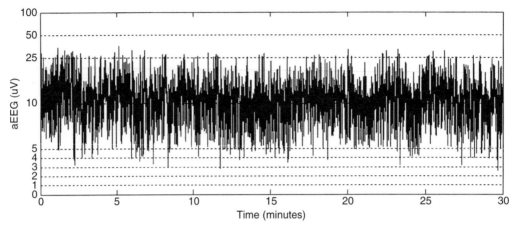

Figure 169–30. This example of a portion of a normal amplitude integrated EEG (aEEG) analyzed "raw" EEG data from a single pair of scalp electrodes (C_3 to C_4). Notice that the graph displays an amplitude *envelope* that modulates between maximum and minimum values.

At present, a very simple method of cerebral function monitoring has reached some clinical application. The approach was developed under the rubric of "amplitude-integrated" EEG or aEEG[56] (Fig. 169-30). One or two scalp locations can be monitored over extended time periods. The recording is obtained with slowly moving chart paper, so that the EEG signal compresses tightly together, providing only an amplitude *envelope* that varies between the largest upper margin and smallest lower margin. In healthy infants, the upper amplitude margin ranges from 30 to 50 μV, and the lower margins range from about 6 to 11 μV. In contrast, an abnormally suppressed aEEG has only ≤ 10 μV for the upper margins and ≤ 5 μV for the lower amplitude margins.[57,58]

CFMs also can be programmed to recognize ENS automatically. Computer-based EEG seizure detection algorithms are highly sensitive in older children and adults, but they are more challenging to design for use in neonates because of their different ictal waveform frequencies and characteristics.[59] Brief, low-amplitude ENSs are especially difficult to detect.

One of the goals of contemporary neonatology is the successful completion of neuroprotection trials. Some trials involve obvious selection criteria of suitable candidates. Premature infants are at high risk for the development of periventricular leukomalacia[60] and have been the subjects of pharmacologic trials with allopurinol, magnesium, steroids, and other agents to reduce its occurrence. Likewise, infants with complex congenital heart disease, requiring surgery that uses deep hypothermic circulatory arrest, commonly experience postoperative seizures and long-term neurocognitive disorders and are easily recognized for enrollment in neuroprotection trials.[61] On the other hand, neuroprotection trials in hypoxic-ischemic encephalopathy (HIE) in the term neonate face difficult challenges. There is currently no simple or universal research definition of hypoxic-ischemic encephalopathy to select candidates for enrollment. For example, two neonates who both have Apgar scores of 3 at 5 minutes may appear entirely different a few hours after birth: one may be alert and orally feeding while the other is stuporous and posturing. In this setting, the time for identification of truly encephalopathic infants is quite short. The window of enrollment into a protection trial, such as deliberate hypothermia, must be determined immediately after birth. Both conventional and aEEG have been proposed to assist in the identification of suitable candidates for neuroprotection trials, since the quality of the EEG signal shortly after birth is one of the best early predictors of mortality and morbidity.[62,63]

REFERENCES

1. Brazelton TB: Neonatal behavioral assessment scale. Clinics in Developmental Medicine, No. 50. London, Heinemann, 1973.
2. Prechtl H: The Neurological Examination of the Full-Term Newborn Infant, 2nd ed. Clinics in Developmental Medicine, No. 63. London, Heinemann, 1977.
3. Scher MS: A developmental marker of central nervous system maturation: Part I. Pediatr Neurol 4:265, 1988.
4. Lombroso CT: Neurophysiological observations in diseased newborns. Biol Psychiatry 10:527, 1975.
5. Scher MS, Barmada MA: Estimation of gestational age by electrographic, clinical, and anatomic criteria. Pediatr Neurol 3:256, 1987.
6. Ellingson RJ, Peters JF: Development of EEG and daytime sleep patterns of low risk premature infants during the first year of life: longitudinal observations. Electroencephalogr Clin Neurophysiol 50:165, 1980.
7. Holmes GL: Morphological and physiological maturation of the brain in the neonate and young child. J Clin Neurophysiol 3:209, 1986.
8. Dorovini-Zis K, Dolman CL: Gestational development of brain. Arch Pathol Lab Med 101:192, 1977.
9. Ellingson RJ, Guenter HR: Ontogenesis of the electroencephalogram. In Himwich WA (ed): Developmental Neurology. Springfield, IL, Charles C Thomas, 1970, pp 441-474.
10. Eyre JA, et al: Quantification of changes in normal neonatal EEGs with gestation from continuous five-day recordings. Dev Med Child Neurol 30:599, 1988.
11. Knuppel RA: Neurological assessment of fetal brain function. Int Pediatr 2:83, 1987.
12. Anderson CM, et al: The EEG of the early premature. Electroencephalogr Clin Neurophysiol 60:95, 1985.
13. Guilleminault C, Souquet M: Sleep states and related pathology. In Korobkin R, Guilleminault C (eds): Advances in Perinatal Neurology. New York, SP Medical and Scientific Books, 1979, pp 225-247.
14. Lombroso CT: Neonatal electroencephalography. In Niedermeyer E, Lopes da Silva F (eds): Electroencephalography. Baltimore, Urban & Schwarzenberg, 1987, pp 725-762.
15. Foote SL, et al: Nucleus locus ceruleus: new evidence of anatomical and physiological specificity. Phys Rev 63:844, 1983.
16. Karch D, et al: Behavioural changes and bioelectric brain maturation of preterm and fulterm newborn infants: a polygraphic study. Dev Med Child Neurol 24:30, 1982.
17. Scher MS, et al: Cerebral neurophysiologic assessment of the high-risk neonate. In Guthrie RD (ed): Neonatal Intensive Care. London, Churchill-Livingstone, 1987, pp 181-220.
18. Ellingson RJ, Peters JF: Development of EEG and daytime sleep patterns in normal full-term infants during the first 3 months of life: longitudinal observations. Electroencephalogr Clin Neurophysiol 49:112, 1980.
19. Tharp BR: Neonatal and pediatric electroencephalography. In Aminoff MJ (ed): Electrodiagnosis in Clinical Neurology. New York, Churchill-Livingstone, 1980, pp 67-117.
20. Pampiglione G: Development of rhythmic EEG activities in infancy (waking state). Rev EEG Neurophysiol 7:327, 1977.
21. Hanley JW: A step-by-step approach to neonatal EEG. Am J EEG Technol 21:1, 1981.
22. Rosen MG, et al: FEEG and organization of fetal brain. In Gluck L (ed): Intrauterine Asphyxia and the Developing Fetal Brain. Chicago, Year Book Medical Publishers, 1977, pp 191-204.
23. Sokol RJ, et al: Fetal electroencephalographic monitoring related to infant outcome. Am J Obstet Gynecol 127:329, 1977.

24. Mizrahi EM: Neonatal electroencephalography: clinical features of the newborn, techniques of recording, and characteristics of the normal EEG. Am J EEG Technol 236:81, 1986.
25. Hellstrom B, et al: Electrode placement in EEG of infants and its anatomical relationship studied radiographically. Am J EEG Technol 4:71, 1964.
26. Parmelee AH, et al: A periodic cerebral rhythm in newborn infants. Exp Neurol 25:575, 1969.
27. Torres F, Anderson C: The normal EEG of the human newborn. J Clin Neurophysiol 2:89, 1985.
28. Hughes JR, et al: Periods of activity and quiescence in the premature EEG. Neuropediatrics 14:66, 1983.
29. Barlow JS: Computer characterization of tracé alternant and REM sleep patterns in the neonatal EEG by adaptive segmentation—an exploratory study. Electroencephalogr Clin Neurophysiol 60:163, 1985.
30. Tharp BR: Neonatal electroencephalography. In Korobkin R, Guilleminault C (eds): Progress in Perinatal Neurology. Baltimore, Williams & Wilkins, 1981, pp 31–64.
31. Tharp BR: Intensive video/EEG monitoring of neonates. Adv Neurol 46:107, 1986.
32. Lombroso CT: Neonatal polygraphy in full-term and premature infants: a review of normal and abnormal findings. J Clin Neurophysiol 2:105, 1985.
33. Clancy R, et al: EEG in premature infants with intraventricular hemorrhage. Neurology 34:583, 1984.
34. Tharp BR, et al: Serial EEGs in normal and abnormal infants with birth weights less than 1200 grams—a prospective study with long-term follow-up. Neuropediatrics 20:64, 1989.
35. Sperling MR, et al: Focal burst-suppression induced by thiopental. Electroencephalogr Clin Neurophysiol 63:203, 1986.
36. Lombroso CT: Quantified electrographic scales on 10 preterm healthy newborns followed up to 40–43 weeks of conceptional age by serial polygraphic recordings. Electroencephalogr Clin Neurophysiol 46:460, 1979.
37. Aso K, et al: Neonatal EEG and neuropathology. J Clin Neurophysiol 6:103, 1989.
38. Aziz SS, et al: Cotside EEG monitoring using computerized spectral analysis. Arch Dis Child 61:242, 1986.
39. Watanabe K, Iwase K: Spindle-like fast rhythms in the EEGs of low birthweight infants. Dev Med Child Neurol 14:373, 1972.
40. Arfel G, et al: Densiteá et dynamique des encoches pointues frontales dans le sommeil du nouveau-neá et du nourrisson. Rev EEG Neurophysiol 7:351, 1977.
41. Karbowski K, Nencka A: Right mid-temporal sharp EEG transients in healthy newborns. Electroencephalogr Clin Neurophysiol 48:461, 1980.
42. Clancy R, Spitzer A: Cerebral cortical function in infants at risk for sudden infant death syndrome. Ann Neurol 18:41, 1985.
43. Cheung PY, Robertson CM: Predicting the outcome of term neonates with intrapartum asphyxia. Acta Paediatrica 89:262, 2000.
44. Hellstrom-Westas L, et al: Early prediction of outcome with aEEG in preterm infants with large intraventricular hemorrhages. Neuropediatrics 32:319, 2001.
45. Holmes GL, Lombroso CT. Prognostic value of background patterns in the neonatal EEG. J Clin Neurophysiol 10:323, 1993.
46. Menache C, et al: Prognostic Value of Neonatal Discontinuous EEG. Pediatr Neurol 27:93, 2002.
47. Clancy RR: Interictal sharp EEG transients in neonatal seizures. J Child Neurol 4:30, 1989.
48. Clancy R, Tharp B: Positive rolandic sharp waves in the electroencephalograms of premature neonates with intraventricular hemorrhage. Electroencephalogr Clin Neurophys 57:395, 1984.
49. Nowack WJ, et al: Positive temporal sharp waves in the neonate. J Clin Neurophysiol 4:315, 1987.
50. Clancy RR, Legido A: The exact ictal and interictal duration of electroencephalographic neonatal seizures. Epilepsia 28:537, 1987.
51. Mizrahi EM, et al: Characterization and classification of neonatal seizures. Neurology. 37:1837, 1987.
52. Mizrahi E, et al: Neurologic impairment, developmental delay and post-natal seizures two-years after video-EEG documented seizures in near-term and full-term neonates: report of the clinical research centers for neonatal seizures. Epilepsia 42(Suppl 7):102, 2001.
53. Laroia N, et al: EEG background as predictor of electrographic seizures in high-risk neonates. Epilepsia 39:545, 1998.
54. Bell AH, et al: Power spectral analysis of the EEG of term infants following birth asphyxia. Dev Med Child Neurol 32:990-8, 1990.
55. Klebermass K, et al: Evaluation of the Cerebral Function Monitor as a tool for neurophysiological surveillance in neonatal intensive care patients. Childs Nerv Syst 17:544, 2001.
56. Toet MC, et al: Amplitude-integrated EEG 3 and 6 hours after birth in full term neonates with hypoxic-ischaemic encephalopathy. Arch Dis Child 81:F19, 1999.
57. al Naqeeb N, et al: Assessment of neonatal encephalopathy by amplitude-integrated electroencephalography. Pediatrics 103:1263, 1999.
58. Hellstrom-Westas L, et al: Predictive value of early continuous amplitude integrated EEG recordings on outcome after severe birth asphyxia in full term infants. Arch Dis Child 72:F34, 1995.
59. Liu A, et al: Detection of neonatal seizures through computerized EEG analysis. Electroencephalog Clin Neurophysiol 82:30, 1992.
60. Fanaroff AA, Hack M: Periventricular leukomalacia—prospects for prevention. N Engl J Med 341:1229, 1999.
61. Clancy RR, et al: Allopurinol neuro-cardiac protection trial in infants undergoing heart surgery utilizing deep hypothermic circulatory arrest. Pediatrics 107:61, 2001.
62. Groenendaal F, de Vries LS: Selection of babies for intervention after birth asphyxia. Semin Neonatol 5:17, 2000.
63. Azzopardi D, et al: Pilot study of treatment with whole body hypothermia for neonatal encephalopathy. Pediatrics 106:684, 2000.

170

Jeffrey M. Perlman

Cerebral Blood Flow in Premature Infants: Regulation, Measurement, and Pathophysiology of Intraventricular Hemorrhage

CEREBRAL BLOOD FLOW AND THE PATHOGENESIS OF INTRAVENTRICULAR HEMORRHAGE

Abnormalities of cerebral blood flow (CBF) may produce germinal matrix hemorrhage and the two major forms of parenchymal hemorrhagic infarction—hemorrhagic venous infarction and hemorrhagic periventricular leukomalacia. These conclusions are based in part on experimental studies in animals. In the newborn beagle puppy, *germinal matrix hemorrhage* can be produced by systemic hypertension (with or without hypotension), and this observation has been applied to the newborn infant with germinal matrix hemorrhage.[1,2] Increased CBF secondary to increases in systemic arterial pressure may occur in

sick asphyxiated infants if the autoregulatory response is perturbed or lost. Impaired autoregulation may occur in association with asphyxia, cranial trauma, and hypercapnia.[3-7] Abrupt increases in systemic arterial blood pressure occur frequently during intensive care nursing of sick preterm infants who require tracheal suctioning or abdominal examination and have been noted after noxious stimulation (placement of intravenous catheters, lumbar puncture).[8] Abrupt increases in systemic arterial blood pressure are also seen after seizures, pneumothorax, and infusions of colloid. Decreased CBF secondary to systemic hypotension is likely to occur if autoregulation is impaired or if the normal preterm arterial blood pressure is close to the downslope of the autoregulatory curve (see later). Systemic hypotension may occur as a consequence of asphyxia and as a complication of a variety of postnatal events, such as sepsis, severe respiratory distress, and myocardial dysfunction.[8]

The primary infarct in *hemorrhagic periventricular leukomalacia* is considered to occur as a consequence of reduced blood flow secondary to systemic hypotension. Support for this hypothesis is obtained from the observation that periventricular white matter has a limited vasodilatory capacity compared with gray matter structures during hypotension in newborn animals.[9] Secondary hemorrhage into infarcted tissue likely occurs with establishment of reperfusion.

In *venous hemorrhagic infarction,* tissue ischemia occurs secondary to elevated venous pressure. The elevation in venous pressure may occur secondary to obstruction of the terminal and medullary veins by either a large germinal matrix hemorrhage or by an acutely distended lateral ventricle (by intraventricular hemorrhage [IVH]).[10, 11] Furthermore, because there are no valves between the right atrium and the major intracranial venous sinuses and veins, abrupt increases in right atrial pressure and intrathoracic pressure are transmitted directly to the intracranial venous system. Therefore, elevated intracranial venous pressure may occur in the following circumstances: during labor and delivery; secondary to postnatal cardiac failure; secondary to tracheal suctioning, pneumothorax, or abnormalities of respiratory mechanics; and secondary to assisted ventilation with high peak inflation pressures and high end-expiratory pressures.[8, 12, 13]

In this chapter, I review the regulation of CBF, the noninvasive and invasive measurements of CBF, the value of these measurements in the assessment of the cerebral circulation, and the relationship of cerebral circulatory changes with the genesis of IVH.

REGULATION OF CEREBRAL BLOOD FLOW

Control of CBF involves the complex interaction of metabolic, chemical, and neural factors that produce their effect by direct action on the cerebral vessels. These vessels also respond to changes in systemic arterial pressure and to normal constituents of the blood such as arterial oxygen content (CaO_2) and carbon dioxide tension ($PaCO_2$). In this section, the control of CBF is reviewed with respect to fluctuations in systemic blood pressure and to changes in systemic factors such as CaO_2, $PaCO_2$, and blood glucose concentration. The complex neural and chemical control of CBF has been reviewed and is beyond the scope of this chapter.[14]

Autoregulation

Autoregulation may be defined as the phenomenon whereby CBF remains constant if cerebral perfusion pressure is varied over a certain range.[4, 15-18] The pressure at which CBF decreases during hypotension is called the *lower limit* of autoregulation, and the pressure at which CBF increases is called the *upper limit* of autoregulation. In adults, CBF is constant over a range of mean arterial blood pressure from 50 to 175 mm Hg.[17, 18] A comparable range of mean arterial blood pressures at which CBF does not vary has not been determined in newborn infants. Because systemic blood pressure is lower in newborn infants than in older children or adults, the range of pressures at which CBF is constant is expected to be lower than in adults. In newborn animals, the range of blood pressures at which CBF is constant is lower than in adult animals.[19, 20] More importantly, in fetal lambs, resting blood pressure is only slightly higher than the lower limit of the autoregulatory curve.[20] If a similar situation existed in newborn infants, moderate hypotension would result in reduced CBF and possible ischemic brain injury.

There is increasing evidence that the autoregulatory response is intact in human neonates who are mildly asphyxiated or who have respiratory distress. Thus, several studies using the xenon washout technique in preterm infants with normal brains have revealed that CBF is unaffected by fluctuations of mean arterial blood pressure within the physiologic range of 25 to 60 mm Hg.[21, 22] These observations were consistent for infants of varying gestational and postnatal ages. In contrast, Lou and colleagues[23] concluded that CBF was impaired in distressed asphyxiated newborns; that is, CBF was significantly related to systolic blood pressure. The conclusions of that study, however, have been questioned because the study group was heterogeneous with regard to gestational age and birth weight, and some infants had an elevated $PaCO_2$ at the time of study.[24] Doppler measurements of flow velocity suggest poorly developed pressure autoregulation in the very premature infant.[25] The limitations of the Doppler technique in this regard are discussed later.

Systemic Factors and Cerebral Blood Flow

Effect of Carbon Dioxide Tension

The cerebral vessels react to both $PaCO_2$ and blood pH. Carbon dioxide has a marked relaxant effect on cerebral vascular muscle, and changes in $PaCO_2$ produce a significant change in CBF. Moderate hypocarbia leads to a reduction in CBF, and moderate hypercarbia leads to an increase in CBF without changes in cerebral oxidative metabolism.[26-28] If the $PaCO_2$ falls to less than 15 to 20 mm Hg, the reduction in CBF is associated with mild reduction in cerebral oxidative metabolism.[29] Although chronic severe hypercarbia elevates CBF, cerebral oxidative metabolism is not altered. Acute elevations in $PaCO_2$, however, may depress cerebral metabolism.[30] Most importantly, hypercarbia abolishes the autoregulatory response because of marked vasodilation, and this disturbance may add to the risk of ischemic brain injury.

The cerebral vessels of fetal and newborn animals are responsive to acute changes in $PaCO_2$, although the reactivity varies as a function of postnatal age and sickness. Thus, spontaneously breathing preterm infants demonstrated appropriate CBF-$PaCO_2$ reactivity shortly after birth,[21, 31] whereas the reactivity was significantly less in mechanically ventilated preterm infants also studied in the first hours of life.[31] The latter infants attained CBF-$PaCO_2$ reactivity similar to that of adults on the second postnatal day.[31] Attenuated CBF-$PaCO_2$ reactivity has similarly been noted in ventilated newborn animals in the immediate postnatal period.[29, 32] The mechanism accounting for this attenuated CBF-$PaCO_2$ reactivity is unclear, and it is considered perhaps to be a consequence of the hypercapnia state *in utero.*[22]

Effect of Arterial Oxygen Content

Arterial hypoxia produces cerebral vasodilation and increases CBF.[33, 34] The effect of hypoxia is related directly to CaO_2 and not to arterial oxygen tension (PaO_2) directly. CaO_2 is determined by the hemoglobin (Hb) concentration in the blood, that is, the oxygen affinity of the Hb and PaO_2. Thus, mild to moderate reductions in PaO_2 that are associated with little change in CaO_2 increase CBF only slightly. A reduction in CaO_2 produces a proportional increase in CBF such that cerebral oxygen delivery (CBF × CaO_2) does not change and cerebral oxygen metabolism is constant. Although the effects of CaO_2 have been studied in detail in experimental animals and in human adults, there are limited data in newborn infants. Both Pryds and Younkin and their colleagues[35, 36] found an inverse relationship between CBF and hematocrit or Hb. The increase in CBF with a lower hematocrit or Hb is presumably the result of a reduced CaO_2, although CaO_2 was not measured in either study.

Effect of Blood Glucose

In adult humans, mild and moderately severe hypoglycemia is not associated with a change in CBF.[37, 38] During hypoglycemic coma, however, CBF increases.[39] In experimental animals, CBF increases during hypoglycemic coma and correlates with a loss of electrical activity on the electroencephalogram.[40-43] The increase in CBF appears to result from increased systemic blood pressure and loss of autoregulation.[44] Thus, if the blood pressure is reduced during hypoglycemic coma, CBF returns to baseline. Pryds and colleagues[45] reported increased CBF in preterm infants with hypoglycemia. Infants with blood glucose levels lower than 30 mg/dL had significantly higher CBF (26 mL/100 g/minute) than did infants with blood glucose levels greater than 30 mg/dL (CBF = 11.8 mL/100 g/minute). None of the infants with low blood glucose levels had signs of hypoglycemia, nor were they in coma. Moreover, no abnormalities of the electroencephalogram were apparent. These data suggest that the response to hypoglycemia in preterm infants is different from that in adults. Furthermore, the data suggest that cerebral glucose metabolism may be critically important to provide the energy requirements of the preterm brain. These data are in agreement with a study in which Altman and colleagues[46] reported that cerebral oxygen metabolism in some preterm infants may be minimal, and cerebral glucose metabolism may provide the necessary energy for preterm cerebral growth and function.

In summary, the newborn circulation shows many of the same characteristics as the adult circulation. The magnitude of the CBF responses and the quantitative relationships of CBF with changes in blood pressure and with a variety of systemic factors have not been fully elucidated. The relationship of these circulatory regulatory responses with the development of IVH and their role in its pathogenesis in sick preterm infants remain to be determined.

MEASUREMENT OF CEREBRAL BLOOD FLOW

Cerebral Arterial Blood Flow Velocity

Cerebral arterial blood flow velocity (CBFV) has been measured in the major intracranial arteries by the Doppler technique. Although this technique does not measure CBF, it has certain advantages; that is, it is noninvasive and is readily available at the bedside.

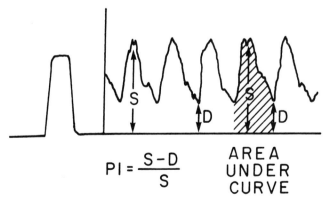

Figure 170–1. Arterial blood flow velocity tracing obtained at the anterior fontanel from the anterior cerebral artery. The deflection of the electronic interval standard is indicated to the *left* of the start of the tracing. S refers to peak systolic velocity, D to end-diastolic velocity, and the *shaded area* to the area under one velocity waveform. The formula for the pulsatility index (PI) is given. (From Volpe JJ: Neurology of the Newborn, 2nd ed. Philadelphia, WB Saunders Co, 1987.)

Principle

The ultrasound technique for the measurement of blood flow velocity makes use of the *Doppler effect;* that is, the frequency of sound waves reflected from a moving object is shifted by an amount proportional to the velocity of the object. When ultrasound is used for measurement of blood flow velocity, the sound waves emitted by the transducer are reflected, and their frequency is shifted by moving red blood cells.[47] The Doppler signals are directly related to the frequency of the transmitted ultrasound and to the cosine of the angle of incidence of the sound beam to the axis of blood flow, and they are inversely related to the velocity of the ultrasound in the tissue. For practical purposes, the frequency of the transmitted ultrasound and the velocity of ultrasound in the tissue are constant from one determination to another; thus, if the angle of incidence is held constant, blood flow velocity will be the main determinant of the Doppler frequency shift.

Attempts to *quantitate* arterial blood flow velocity have used determinations of the pulsatility index (PI) or the area under the velocity curve (Fig. 170–1). The PI is calculated from the formula PI = S – D/S, where S equals the peak systolic velocity and D equals the end-diastolic velocity.[48, 49] Changes in probe angle affect the values for S and D similarly, and thus the PI can be used to minimize the effect of changes in probe angle and to allow meaningful comparisons of serial determinations of CBFV. Measurement of the PI was described initially as a measure of peripheral vascular resistance in large systemic arteries and thus in the current context is assumed to reflect changes in cerebrovascular resistance. Serial measurements of PI may also reflect changes in cerebral perfusion as well as cerebrovascular resistance, especially if either the systolic or diastolic velocity changes individually. However, if both systolic velocity and diastolic velocity change proportionately, serial determinations of the PI will not reveal a change in absolute flow velocity or tissue perfusion. To avoid this problem, determination of the area under the velocity waveforms (determined automatically by most ultrasound machines) has been used. Two types of Doppler systems have been used in the study of the cerebral circulation: continuous-wave and range-gated Doppler systems.

Continuous-Wave Doppler Ultrasound

The continuous-wave system employs a bidirectional, pencil-shaped probe that is placed over the anterior fontanelle and is oriented toward the pericallosal artery (terminal branch of the anterior cerebral artery) as it courses over the genu of the corpus callosum. Alternatively, the right or left middle cerebral artery can be insonated transcranially through the coronal suture. Maximum arterial pulsations of advancing flow are used for measurements.

Range-Gated Doppler Ultrasound

The pulse range-gated Doppler technique selectively detects blood flow in a certain area at a specific distance from the probe. A piezoelectric crystal acts as both a transmitter and a receiver. With this technique, the velocity can be determined from a small area within a specific vessel by adjusting the time between the pulses and the activation of the "gate" for receiving the signal; thus, the depth at which flow signals will be detected can be selected. The range-gated Doppler instrument is usually incorporated into a conventional ultrasound imaging instrument, and the vessel to be insonated can be visualized directly. This visualization provides the capability to determine the angle of insonation and to identify specific arteries (e.g., at the circle of Willis) to be insonated. Present technology, however, does not allow for the measurement of the cross-sectional area of the insonated artery, but if the resolution of the ultrasound instruments can be improved to provide this measurement, a major step toward measurement of total volume of arterial blood flow, rather than only velocity of arterial blood flow, will have been accomplished. Other advantages of this technique are the ability to record the velocity profile of all moving red blood cells in the insonated artery and the ability to compute the instantaneous average blood flow velocity. Because blood flow through a vessel is related to the average velocity and not to the peak velocity, this advantage should help in estimating CBF in situations in which CBF and blood pressure change rapidly.

Relation of Cerebral Arterial Blood Flow Velocity to Cerebral Blood Flow

The degree to which CBFV reflects CBF is of considerable importance because accurate measurement of CBF involves techniques that are complex, expensive, and invasive, whereas measurement of CBFV is a readily available, noninvasive bedside technique. Conventionally, CBF is measured as the volume of blood perfusing a mass of brain tissue per unit of time. The volume of blood flowing in a specified artery is related to the instantaneous average velocity of flow (not peak flow velocity) times the cross-sectional area of the vessel. Thus, measurements of velocity and arterial caliber are essential to provide an estimate of CBF. If the mass of tissue perfused by a given artery and the cross-sectional area of the artery were to remain constant, CBFV would be the major determinant of CBF. However, both the vessel diameter and the mass of tissue supplied by a given artery may change under normal physiologic circumstances and in pathologic conditions. For example, during autoregulation, CBF is maintained constant over a broad range of perfusion pressures by mechanisms that include change of arterial diameter and resistance. Therefore, flow velocity may change inversely relative to vessel diameter even though CBF is unchanged.

In summary, accurate calculation of CBF should be based on average (not peak) CBFV as well as arterial cross-sectional area. Measurements based only on peak CBFV may be misleading. In situations in which it is known that arterial caliber does not change and that a steady state exists, such measurements may provide useful information. However, under conditions of changing arterial blood pressure and CBF, estimation of CBF from peak arterial blood flow velocity is of uncertain value and may not reflect changes in CBF.[14]

Experimental Studies

Several studies have examined the relationship of CBFV with CBF in newborn animals and in the human newborn infant. In experimental animals, CBF was raised or lowered by altering $Paco_2$ or Cao_2.[50-52] CBFV was measured in the anterior cerebral artery, and CBF was determined by either the microsphere technique or autoradiography. All studies were performed under steady-state conditions, and the results were based on measurement of peak, not average, CBFV. Arterial cross-sectional diameter was not measured but can be assumed to change little in the steady state. Changes in CBFV (i.e., systolic velocity, diastolic velocity, area under the velocity curve, and PI) were significantly related to a change in CBF. This result may have been anticipated, because blood flow velocity is one of the major determinants of CBF. However, the degree of correlation in the preceding studies, as determined by the correlation coefficient (r), varied from 0.3 (PI) to 0.9 (area under the velocity curve). In the preceding examples, variation of the PI ($r^2 = 0.09$) accounted for only about 10% of the variation in CBF, whereas variation in the area under the velocity curve ($r^2 = 0.81$) accounted for approximately 80% of the variability of CBF.

Therefore, changes in CBF produced experimentally are associated with a significant change in CBFV. Furthermore, changes in CBFV may account for up to 80% of the variability in CBF *under steady-state conditions*. Because the PI accounts for only

about 10% of the variability of CBF (at least under the conditions studied), it is not prudent to use this index as a general indicator of CBF.

Studies in the Human Newborn

Attempts have been made to correlate CBFV with CBF in human newborn infants. Greisen and coworkers[53] compared CBF, measured by the xenon technique, with anterior cerebral artery and common carotid artery flow velocities. All arterial blood flow velocity variables measured were significantly related to CBF. However, the correlation coefficients varied from 0.4 to 0.8, and diastolic flow velocity exhibited the highest correlation. A similar relationship was found in newborn infants by comparing anterior cerebral artery blood flow velocity with CBF in the frontal region (anterior cerebral artery distribution) measured with positron emission tomography (PET).[54] In 25 premature infants with various neurologic disorders (IVH, asphyxia, hydrocephalus), CBF measured with PET was significantly related to arterial blood flow velocity with a correlation coefficient of 0.7.

Clinical Studies of Cerebral Arterial Blood Flow Velocity and Intraventricular Hemorrhage

Fluctuating Cerebral Arterial Blood Flow Velocity in Infants with Respiratory Distress Syndrome

The measurement of CBFV in ventilated preterm infants with respiratory distress syndrome, infants at high risk of IVH, has led to identification of a specific abnormality of arterial blood flow velocity that is a powerful predictor of the subsequent development of IVH.[55] Serial measurements of CBFV and concomitant measurement of arterial blood pressure in 50 ventilated premature infants weighing less than 1500 g revealed two distinct patterns that developed between 12 and 24 hours of life. The first pattern was designated the *stable pattern* because it was characterized by equal peaks of systolic flow velocity and troughs of diastolic flow velocity (Fig. 170-2). In contrast, the second pattern was designated the *fluctuating pattern* because it was characterized by marked fluctuations in systolic and diastolic blood flow velocity[55] (Fig. 170-3). Simultaneous measurement of arterial blood pressure revealed changes in systolic and diastolic pressure that were identical to those observed in the cerebral circulation. Of the 23 infants with the fluctuating pattern, IVH subsequently developed in 21, whereas the lesion developed in only 7 of 27 infants with a stable pattern. The cause of the fluctuating pattern in these ventilated infants was thought to relate to changes in intrathoracic pressure caused by the infant breathing out of synchrony with the ventilator.[13] These critical observations led to a study designed to prevent IVH by abolishing the fluctuating CBFV (Fig. 170-4).[56] The infant's respiratory effort was abolished by muscle paralysis with pancuronium. In this study, all nonparalyzed infants with fluctuating CBFV (10 of 10) experienced IVH (including 7 infants with severe IVH), whereas only 5 of 14 infants who were paralyzed experienced IVH. Most importantly, none of the paralyzed infants experienced severe IVH.

Changes in Cerebral Blood Flow Velocity with Pneumothorax

Striking changes in CBFV were observed in nine infants in whom IVH developed after pneumothorax.[57] Thus, at the time of the pneumothorax, there was a significant decrease in the PI, which gradually returned to normal after 36 hours. The decrease in PI was in large part accounted for by an increase in the diastolic flow velocity at the time of the pneumothorax. The changes in CBFV were associated with significant changes in systemic blood pressure; that is, mean blood pressure and diastolic blood pressure increased significantly at the time of pneumothorax. As

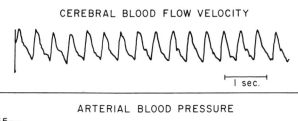

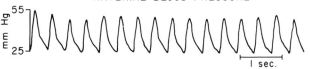

Figure 170–2. Stable arterial blood flow velocity pattern and simultaneously recorded arterial blood pressure in a ventilated premature infant with respiratory distress syndrome. Note the equal peaks and troughs in systolic and diastolic flow velocity and blood pressure. (From Perlman JM, et al: N Engl J Med *312*:1353, 1985; reprinted by permission of the New England Journal of Medicine.)

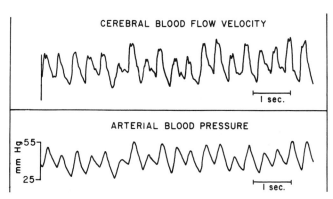

Figure 170–3. Fluctuating arterial blood flow velocity pattern and simultaneously recorded arterial blood pressure in a ventilated premature infant with respiratory distress syndrome. Note the marked fluctuations in systolic and diastolic flow velocity and blood pressure. (From Perlman JM, et al: N Engl J Med *312*:1353, 1985; reprinted by permission of the New England Journal of Medicine.)

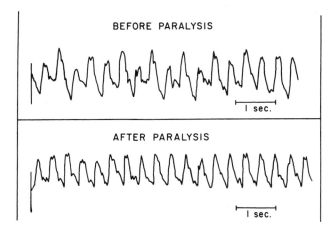

Figure 170–4. Effect of muscle paralysis on fluctuating cerebral blood flow velocity. After paralysis was induced by pancuronium, the fluctuating pattern was eliminated. (From Perlman JM, et al: N Engl J Med *312*:1353, 1985; reprinted by permission of the New England Journal of Medicine.)

discussed previously, changes in PI correlate poorly with changes in CBF. The increase in diastolic flow velocity alone may reflect an increase in cerebrovascular resistance without necessarily any change in CBF. The data suggest that the increase in diastolic flow velocity that occurs with pneumothorax may be important in the genesis of IVH. The precise mechanism is speculative. Does blood flow to the germinal matrix increase and cause capillary rupture? Alternatively, it has been shown that increases in systemic venous pressure occur simultaneously in such infants, and these increases may result in elevated intracranial venous pressure and subsequent ischemic infarction (see earlier discussion).[58]

Cerebral Blood Flow Velocity Changes Under Other Circumstances

After Surfactant Replacement Therapy

As noted earlier, there is a strong association among respiratory distress syndrome, fluctuations in CBFV, and IVH.[55] However, the introduction of surfactant replacement therapy with improvement in respiratory function has not been associated with a reduction in IVH.[59] The mechanisms accounting for this unanticipated finding remain unclear. Cowan and co-workers[60] demonstrated acute changes characterized by a marked decrease in CBFV of 36% within 2 minutes after surfactant administration, with almost complete loss of the diastolic velocity. The decrease in diastolic flow velocity is considered to be secondary to shunting across the patent ductus arteriosus (PDA; see later). In a second study, Jorch and associates[61] demonstrated continuous CBFV variability in treated infants that was comparable to the CBFV variability in untreated infants at 12-hour intervals after surfactant therapy.[61] The significance of these changes to the subsequent development of IVH in infants receiving surfactant therapy has not been determined.

Patent Ductus Arteriosus

CBFV has been measured in infants who develop symptomatic PDA.[62] At the time of the PDA there is a decrease in the PI chiefly as a result of a decrease in the diastolic flow velocity (akin to that observed acutely after surfactant administration). The changes in CBFV reflect similar changes in systemic diastolic blood pressure after development of the PDA. What role these changes may play in the genesis of ischemic infarction in the germinal matrix or periventricular white matter, or both, remains unclear.

Routine Procedures

Marked changes in CBFV have been noted with routine procedures such as endotracheal suctioning.[63] In particular, a prominent increase in diastolic flow velocity has been noted. Concomitant increases in systolic, diastolic, and mean blood pressures also occur. These systemic and cerebral circulatory changes theoretically may predispose the infant to IVH if the systemic arterial pressure increases are transmitted to the germinal matrix (pressure passive circulation) and if the increase in CBFV reflects increased CBF to the area.

Intraventricular Hemorrhage

An initial report of measurements of CBFV in premature infants in whom IVH developed suggested that the PI was low during the first 2 days of life and increased on the third day of life when IVH was thought to develop.[64] However, subsequent studies have failed to show any correlation between CBFV and, specifically, PI and the development of IVH.[65]

In summary, changes in CBFV and blood pressure have been described in premature infants with respiratory distress syndrome, pneumothorax, after surfactant administration, with

PDA, and with routine neonatal procedures. In some of these situations, the CBFV changes have had a temporal relationship with the subsequent development of IVH. The precise mechanism by which these changes lead to IVH is not clear. Moreover, the changes enumerated earlier have been observed in infants with these conditions in whom IVH did not develop. This finding suggests that additional factors are important in the genesis of IVH.

Near-Infrared Spectroscopy

Near-infrared spectroscopy (NIRS) refers to an optical technique that can provide information concerning changes in cerebral oxygen saturation, CBF and volume, cerebral venous oxygen saturation, and cerebral oxygen utilization in the brain.[66] The method is based on two principles: (1) light in the near-infrared range of wavelengths between 700 and 1000 nm can pass through skin, bone, and other tissues relatively easily and illuminates approximately 6 to 8 cm of newborn brain; and (2) there are characteristic absorption bands of oxygenated and deoxygenated Hb and of the mitochondrial enzyme cytochrome oxidase in the near-infrared range. Changes in absorption bands can be used to monitor quantitative changes in the amounts of oxyhemoglobin (HbO_2) and deoxygenated Hb; total Hb (HbO_2 + deoxygenated Hb) is used as an indicator of blood volume. These changes can also be used to monitor the oxidation reduction state of cytochrome oxidase, a critical terminal enzyme of the respiratory mitochondrial electron transport chain, which facilitates electron passage to molecular oxygen for oxidative phosphorylation and adenosine triphosphate synthesis.

When the near-infrared beam is passed through the tissue, a decrease in signal intensity results from the absorbance of a particular chromophore in the medium. Thus, there is a band of maximum absorption at about 810 nm for Hb, above which HbO_2 has greater light absorption, and below which deoxygenated Hb has greater absorption. There is a much smaller peak at about 830 to 840 nm for cytochrome oxidase.

Instrumentation

In general, the spectroscope contains diodes that serve as a source of near-infrared light.[67] The lasers are pulsed sequentially in a rapid on-off fashion. The light from the lasers is captured in glass fiberoptic strands that form a bundle. The end of the bundle is applied to the side of the infant's forehead, commonly against the parietal bone at a point equidistant from the anterior fontanelle and the external auditory meatus (Fig. 170-5). The light traverses the head where a second fiberoptic bundle attached to the opposite side of the head collects the transmitted light photons and conveys them to a photomultiplier tube. The signals are then amplified, expressed as a ratio of a reference signal, and changed into logarithmic form. To prevent interference from background illumination, the infant's head is wrapped in a light-tight bandage.

The attenuation of light by absorption is a measure of the concentration of the chromophore present. The relationship between the absorption and the concentration of the chromophore is best described by a modified Lambert-Beer Law,[68] which, when describing optional absorption in a highly scattered medium, can be expressed as follows:

$$\text{Absorption (OD)} = (acLP) + G$$

where OD = optical density, a = extinction coefficient of the chromophobe (mM × cm), c = concentration of the chromophobe (mM), L = distance between the point of entry and exit (in centimeters), P = "path length factor" to account for scattering of light in the tissue, and G = a factor related to tissue and optode geometry. If one assumes that L, P, and G remain constant during

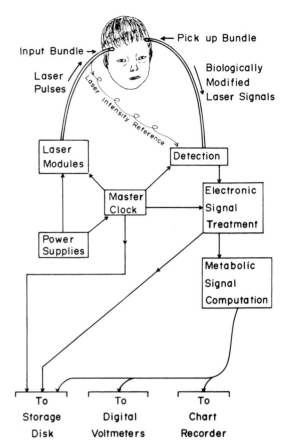

Figure 170-5. Schematic of the NIROSCOPE. (From Brazy JE: *In* Nelson NM [ed]: Current Therapy in Neonatal-Perinatal Medicine, 2nd ed. Toronto, BC Decker, 1990, pp 439-444.)

a study, then changes in chromophore concentration can be expressed as follows:

$$\Delta C = \Delta \frac{OD}{aLP}$$

The chromophore concentration can be calculated because the extinction coefficients (a) of HbO_2, deoxygenated Hb, and cytochrome oxidase have been determined,[68,69] and the value of P in the brains of premature infants measured after death has been determined by the time-of-flight method and found to be 4.39 ± 0.28 (SD). However, the latter determination is not straightforward because of scattering of light within the head.[70] This scattering effect may be modulated by several factors including myelination, bone mineralization, and cell concentration. Moreover, the path length factor (P) is different for the various wavelengths used (775 to 903 nm), with a longer path length at shorter wavelengths.[71]

Clinical Application

Attempts have been made with NIRS to quantitate cerebral blood volume (CBV) and to measure CBF. Wyatt and colleagues obtained a mean CBV value of 2.22 ± 0.40 (SD) mL/100 g in 12 newborn infants born at 25 to 40 weeks of gestation and studied at postnatal ages of 10 to 240 hours with "normal" brains, which is similar to values obtained by PET[72,73] (see later). Mean CBV values were significantly higher, that is, 3.00 ± 1.04 mL/100 g in 10 brain-injured infants ($p < .05$).[72] Similar CBV values were obtained in a subsequent study from the same investigators.[74] In clinical studies, increases in CBV have been observed in association with sharp increases in blood pressure and changes

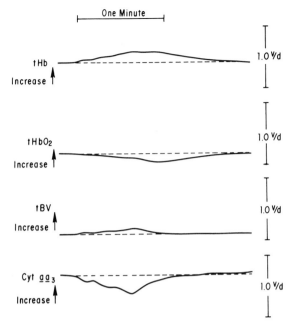

One Minute

tHb
Increase ↑   1.0 V/d

tHbO₂
Increase ↑   1.0 V/d

tBV
Increase ↑   1.0 V/d

Cyt aa₃
Increase ↑   1.0 V/d

Figure 170–6. Typical response to decreased oxygenation: oxyhemoglobin ($tHbO_2$) decreases, whereas deoxyhemoglobin (tHb) rises. There is an overall increase in blood volume (tBV), probably secondary to increased cerebral blood flow in response to hypoxia. Cytochrome a,a₃ (cyt a,a₃) becomes more reduced concurrent with the decrease in oxyhemoglobin. (From Brazy JE: *In* Nelson NM [ed]: Current Therapy in Neonatal-Perinatal Medicine, 2nd ed. Toronto, BC Decker, 1990, pp 439-444.)

in $Paco_2$ (Fig. 170–6).[75-78] By contrast, an increase in CBV accompanied by a decrease in HbO_2 has been noted after endotracheal suctioning; under these conditions, the increase in CBV is consistent with elevated central venous pressure.[79] The response of CBV to $Paco_2$ has been shown to increase with advancing gestational age.[77] Noninvasive measurement of CBF by NIRS employs the Fick principle by determining the rate of increases in cerebral HbO_2 after an increase in arterial oxygen saturation induced by a brief inhalation of oxygen.[80] The mean value of CBF obtained in the 13 premature infants, that is, 18 mL/ 100 g/minute, is comparable to values obtained by the xenon technique and by PET (see later). When estimations of CBF were performed by NIRS and were compared with ^{133}Xe clearance, there was a significant correlation between the two measurements: $r = 0.80, p < .001$ in one study,[81] and $r^2 = 0.84, p < .001$ in a second study.[72] Certain methodologic problems need to be considered: the test-retest variability in the same subject is reported at 15 to 20%; and in one study, up to two-thirds of the NIRS recording was unsuccessful because of inferior quality.[81] NIRS estimation of CBF may be significantly underestimated in the high flow range because of methodologic constraints.

Clinical Studies of Near-Infrared Spectroscopy and Intraventricular Hemorrhage

The relationship between CBF measured in the first 24 hours of life and IVH was determined in 24 premature infants.[82] Infants were classified based on the cranial ultrasound appearance into a normal group, a group with minor IVH, and a third group with moderate to severe IVH. Infants with any form of IVH had lower median CBF (7.0 mL/100 g/minute) than those without IVH (12.2 mL/100 g/minute). On subgroup analysis, those infants

with severe IVH had the lowest CBF values (median 5.8 mL/ 100 g/minute). In a second study, quantitative changes in cerebral concentrations of HbO_2 and deoxygenated Hb coupled with simultaneous measures of arterial oxygen saturation by pulse oximetry and mean arterial pressure were obtained from the first hours of life in 32 premature infants less than 2000 g birth weight.[83] In addition, a measure of cerebral intravascular oxygenation (HbD), that is, HbD = HbO_2 – Hb, which has been shown to be correlated with CBF, was made.[84] Concordant changes in HbD and mean arterial pressure consistent with autoregulation were made in 17 of the 32 infants. Eight of the 17 infants developed either severe IVH or periventricular leukomalacia. Only 2 of the 15 infants with nonconcordant changes developed IVH. These observations are akin to the Doppler findings described earlier.[55]

Near-Infrared Spectroscopy Changes Under Other Circumstances

Surfactant. The acute effects of surfactant replacement therapy on cerebrohemodynamics has also been studied with NIRS.[85] Observations were made before and after surfactant administration in 20 sick premature infants. Surfactant administration caused acute, small transient perturbations in cerebral HbO_2 concentration and CBV.

Treatment of Patent Ductus Arteriosus with Indomethacin. The acute cerebral hemodynamics and oxygen delivery were studied in 13 preterm infants with a PDA who were treated rapidly (over 30 seconds) or by slow infusion (20 to 30 minutes) with indomethacin.[86] Irrespective of rate of administration, indomethacin resulted in a consistent rapid decrease in CBF, oxygen delivery, and reactivity of blood volume to carbon dioxide.

Quantitative Cerebral Blood Flow Measurements

Positron Emission Tomography

Method. The use of PET to measure CBF requires a cyclotron to generate the positron-emitting radionuclides, a PET scan to measure accurately the regional radioactivity *in vivo*, and mathematical models of radiotracer kinetics that relate tissue radioactivity measured by PET to a quantitative value, for example, CBF.[87, 88] These requirements are discussed with special reference to newborn infants.

Emission tomography is a technique that produces an image of the distribution of a previously administered radionuclide in any desired part of the body (e.g., the head). Accurate, quantitative regional measurement of the radionuclide with an external detector is a difficult task for two reasons. First, only a few of the photons emitted from a radioactive source in the sampled region reach the external detectors, because some are absorbed by the tissue. Second, because of Compton scattering, other photons emitted from radioactive sources in regions distant from the sampled region may interact with tissue, change direction, and interact with the external detector. PET largely overcomes these problems by taking advantage of the annihilation radiation generated when positrons are absorbed in matter. Certain radionuclides (e.g., ^{15}O) decay by the emission of a positron, which is a small, positively charged particle. After traveling a few millimeters in tissue, the positron interacts with an electron, with destruction of both. The resultant annihilation event produces two high-energy γ-photons that travel in opposite directions (Fig. 170–7). These photons can then be detected almost simultaneously by a pair of external detectors placed on opposite sides of the positron-emitting source (i.e., 180° apart). If the detector pair is connected by an electronic coincidence circuit so a signal is recorded only when two photons arrive virtually simultaneously, only photons originating from annihilation events between the detector pair will be recorded.[89] Thus, most

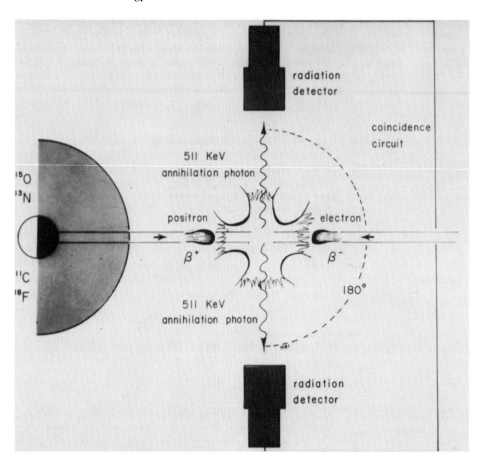

Figure 170–7. Basic principle of positron emission tomography. Isotopes use decay by emission of a positron (β⁺), which travels a few millimeters before colliding with an electron (β⁻), producing an annihilation event. The latter event results in emission of two high-energy photons, which travel at approximately 180° from each other and are detected by radiation detectors, which are linked in coincidence circuits. (From Raichle ME: Annu Rev Neurosci 6:249, 1983; reproduced with permission from the Annual Review of Neuroscience, © 1983 by Annual Reviews, Inc.)

scattered photons are not recorded. To correct for the other problem (i.e., absorption of photons), a correction factor is derived as follows: before performing an individual scan, an external positron-emitting source is placed within the detector field, and the number of coincidences for each detector is recorded. The infant's head is then placed in the detector field (with the external source still in position), and the number of coincidences that each detector now registers is recorded. The difference in recorded coincidences results from absorption (attenuation) of the photons by the infant's head. An attenuation fraction can then be calculated and used to correct data from the subsequent blood flow scans. Failure to correct for attenuation will underestimate the radioactivity present in the sampled tissue and will result in an erroneously low value.

Positron Emission Tomograph. The PET scan is composed of rings of external detectors, connected by coincidence circuits, which surround the head. The multiple rings allow simultaneous reconstruction of multiple transverse slices. The information recorded by the detectors in the multiple rings is used by a computerized system to reconstruct an image that is an accurate quantitative representation of regional tissue radioactivity. The performance characteristics and other technical details of PET design are described in articles and reviews and are not discussed here. However, the one aspect of PET that is especially important to studies of newborn infants and requires special mention is *spatial resolution*. In the PET image, radioactivity from a given region is redistributed or "smeared" over a larger area. As a result of this redistribution, a given region in the reconstructed PET image contains only a portion of the radioactivity actually emitted from that region in the original structure. The remainder of the radioactivity is redistributed into surrounding areas of the image. Similarly, radioactivity from the surrounding regions is redistributed into the region of interest. Thus, the regional radioactivity

measurement made with PET represents the contribution of the radioactivity actually within that region and a contribution from radioactivity in surrounding regions.[87,90-93] This effect is known as *partial volume averaging*. Thus, it is impossible to sample pure cortical gray matter and subcortical white matter because of the small size. In addition, any region that is close to the surface of the brain or to the ventricles will include recording of activity from the cerebrospinal fluid. Inclusion of this physiologically "inactive" fluid will lead to underestimation of the regional measurement for contiguous brain regions.

Measurement of Cerebral Blood Flow with ¹⁵O-labeled Water. The radiotracer employed to measure CBF in infants by PET is ¹⁵O-labeled water. Accuracy of the method has been described in detail and is reviewed briefly.[92-94] ¹⁵O has a half-life of 123 seconds, and this rapid decay of radioactivity allows the absorbed radiation dose to be maintained at a safe, low level. For example, the dose of ¹⁵O-labeled water used to measure CBF in a newborn is 0.7 mCi/kg, which provides a calculated whole body absorbed dose of 57 mrad and an absorbed dose to the brain of 140 mrad. With this method (which is based on a modification of the classic tissue autoradiographic technique), a 40-second PET scan is obtained after the intravenous injection of ¹⁵O-labeled water. There is an essentially linear relationship between regional cerebral radioactivity and regional CBF and, therefore, measured radioactivity in a given region closely approximates mean CBF in that region. Quantitation of absolute values of CBF requires a simultaneous arterial time-activity curve, which is obtained by rapid arterial blood sampling obtained either from a peripheral artery (radial, tibial) or from the descending aorta (through an umbilical arterial catheter).

Although water is a highly desirable tracer for the measurement of CBF (because of its nearly free diffusibility), even the use of water is subject to some error. First, the blood-brain barrier is not completely permeable to water.[94] At high flow, water is incompletely extracted, and consequently blood flow is under-estimated. Fortunately, in the premature infant, quantitative CBF is relatively low, and the permeability of water does not result in a significant error in the calculation of CBF. Another potential source of error with the use of water as a tracer relates to the estimation of the partition coefficient of water in brain. This coefficient is affected by changes in the water content of brain and blood. The newborn brain contains relatively greater amounts of water than does the adult brain, and hence the value of the partition coefficient is different from the adult value. Therefore, an age-appropriate value must be used in the calculation of CBF in the newborn.[95]

PET Measurements of Cerebral Blood Flow in Newborn Infants with Intraventricular Hemorrhage. A single study used PET methodology to measure CBF in premature infants with IVH.[96] Regional CBF was measured in six infants 1 to 15 days after cranial ultrasonography documented IVH associated with a unilateral parenchymal echodensity indicative of hemorrhagic parenchymal infarction. Analysis of the regional CBF images revealed the expected reduction in blood flow in the region of the parenchymal echodensity (Fig. 170–8). However, blood flow was apparently reduced more globally in the affected hemisphere in areas distant to and not involved by the hemorrhage. Neuropathologic studies in these infants revealed hemorrhagic infarction in the region of the parenchymal echodensity and nonhemorrhagic infarction in the periventricular regions distant to the hemorrhagic infarction and apparently corresponding to the areas of reduced blood flow. These findings suggest that the hemorrhagic parenchymal infarct is part of a larger lesion that presumably is ischemic. However, because injured tissue from any cause results in reduced local blood flow, the data do not prove that the cause of the injured periventricular white matter was prior reduction in CBF caused by arterial hypotension or increased intracranial venous pressure. Moreover, other explanations for the apparent

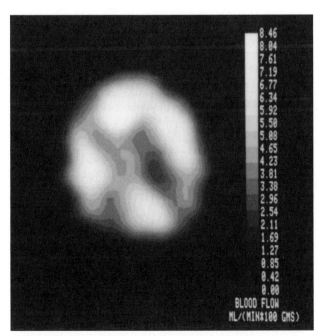

Figure 170–8. Positron emission tomography scan in a premature infant with intraventricular hemorrhage and hemorrhagic parenchymal infarct in the right cerebral hemisphere. Scans represent horizontal section, with the right side of brain at the *right*. The scale is a linear representation of cerebral blood flow (CBF). Extensive impairment of CBF in the hemisphere containing the intracerebral blood is apparent.

wide area of decreased blood flow need to be considered. For example, it is necessary to consider the effect of partial volume averaging (discussed previously), which can be appreciable in the premature infant. This problem may be aggravated if there is ventriculomegaly, a frequent feature in infants with IVH, and parenchymal infarction.[11]

Measurement of Cerebral Blood Flow by Xenon Clearance Techniques

Methodology. The measurement of CBF by xenon techniques is based on the recording of the clearance of ^{133}Xe from the brain by an external detector. The intra-arterial xenon method requires introduction of the tracer directly into the carotid artery. Blood flow is calculated from the clearance curve and the partition coefficient of xenon.[97, 98] This technique is restricted to patients undergoing internal carotid artery catheterization for clinical indications and has not been performed in newborns. Lou and colleagues[99, 100] adapted this technique to the newborn by injecting the radiotracer in the aortic arch, common carotid, or innominate artery through an umbilical artery catheter advanced to the appropriate position for the study.

Because of the invasiveness of administering the radiotracer through an arterial line, some investigators introduced the radiotracer by inhalation or by intravenous administration.[101, 102] In the inhalation method, a tight-fitting mask is placed over the infant's mouth and nose to administer the tracer. If the infant is intubated, the tracer is introduced through the endotracheal tube. Unfortunately, the mask used in the inhalation method is tolerated poorly by some infants, and by provoking considerable movement and a change in the level of consciousness, this technique renders the study difficult to interpret and reproduce. Therefore, the intravenous technique has become the method of choice in the infant who is not intubated.

Detection of Xenon. The clearance of the tracer from the brain is recorded by external detectors placed over the infant's head, and the windows are set to record the rather low-energy γ-waves emitted by the decay of the ^{133}Xe. Certain characteristics of these detector systems may influence the accuracy of measurements of regional CBF in the newborn infant and particularly in the premature newborn.[103, 104] First, the detectors record emissions primarily from a volume of brain that is shaped like a truncated cone. Second, because of Compton scattering of the low-energy γ-waves, radioactive disintegrations from outside the detector field are recorded and may contribute up to 35% of the recorded counts. Third, up to 40% of observed counts in a detector placed over the parietal region will arise from the contralateral hemisphere. This problem makes it difficult to measure regional CBF accurately and to compare hemispheric differences in blood flow. A final factor to be considered is the close proximity of the detectors to the airways of the infant; this feature could result in a significant artifact caused by emissions in these structures after the intravenous or inhalational administration of the radiotracer.

Quantitation of Cerebral Blood Flow. The clearance curves are recorded either linearly or semilogarithmically. Several methods are available to calculate CBF from these curves.[105-108] A two-compartmental analysis has been used to describe the clearances from a fast-flow compartment (considered to represent gray matter) and from a slow compartment (considered to represent white matter). However, under pathologic conditions, especially with infarcts and intracranial hemorrhage, the fidelity of this relationship can change fundamentally (see later). A solution to this problem is provided by a noncompartmental index that represents global CBF and is based on analysis of the washout curve for relatively long periods (e.g., 15 minutes). Another alternative is to analyze only the first part of the clearance curve, that is, the initial slope index. Data from the first 2 minutes of the curve are analyzed, and the value obtained is considered to represent mainly cortical flow, with a small contribution from white matter. Further refinements of this index method are based on performing curve analysis at 1-minute intervals during the early part of the washout curve. There are, however, theoretical limitations for each method when used to detect changes in CBF in infants with cerebrovascular disease. For example, the two-compartmental analyses are not sensitive enough to detect small cortical and subcortical infarcts because of the *look-through phenomenon*; that is, blood flow to normal underlying and surrounding brain is recorded and the flow that is lacking in the infarct is not detected.[109,110] In addition, under such conditions, CBF distribution may not be bimodal, in which case the two-compartmental analysis may give unreliable flow values because of *slippage*, that is, cortical blood flow values in the range of those in the low-flow compartment.[107] The single-compartment, monoexponential analysis of clearance curves will detect a flow change in an infarct, but the reduction of flow may be underestimated markedly.

Finally, the value for the partition coefficient of xenon in the newborn and the changes in the value that may occur with infarcted tissue should be considered. The calculation of quantitative CBF requires the value of the partition coefficient of xenon in gray and white matter. The calculated blood flow is directly proportional to this value. The newborn brain contains less myelin, and hence the value for the partition coefficient is different from that in adults, because xenon is lipid soluble. Griesen[111] measured the partition coefficient for xenon in newborn infants and demonstrated a lower value than that in adults. Accurate measurements of CBF and comparison of values obtained in different studies clearly require this issue to be addressed. In addition, the partition coefficient of xenon may vary in infarcted or hemorrhagic tissue. This variance renders interpretation of changes in CBF especially difficult and indicates that caution should be exercised in interpreting values when marked tissue injury has occurred.

Clinical Studies of Xenon in Cerebral Blood Flow and Intraventricular Hemorrhage. Measurements of CBF with the xenon clearance technique have been performed in term and preterm infants with perinatal asphyxia and respiratory distress.[99,100,112,113] Ment and co-workers[101] reported CBF measurements in 16 infants weighing less than 1250 g at 24 hours, 5 days, and 37 weeks of postconceptual age. IVH was identified by computed tomography (CT) scan performed at 5 days or at autopsy. Nine infants had evidence of IVH, and no infant had a parenchymal infarction. At the time of the first CBF measurement (at 24 hours), five infants exhibited asymmetric hemispheric blood flow: in three cases, the higher flow occurred on the side of the greater IVH; in one case, the higher flow occurred on the side of unilateral subependymal hemorrhage; and in one infant, lower blood flow occurred on the side of maximal IVH. In addition, hemisphere asymmetries in flow were noted in four infants with symmetric IVH. These asymmetries in blood flow were not apparent on the subsequent measurements. The finding of the asymmetry in flow in the infants with symmetric IVH makes it difficult to assign a pathogenetic role to this phenomenon in infants with IVH. The apparent contradictory observations of higher and lower blood flows in the hemispheres with the IVH may be explained in part by the phenomenon of *luxury perfusion*. For example, in adults, blood flow in infarcted brain, although usually reduced, may be higher than resting control values in the acute phase of an infarct. Because the CT scans in the study by Ment and colleagues were performed 4 to 5 days after the initial CBF measurements, it is not clear whether the infants had IVH at the time of the initial measurements. It is possible that, in some infants, the blood flow abnormalities may have preceded the IVH. Perhaps most importantly, limitations of the xenon clearance technique in the newborn should be noted and the regional data interpreted cautiously. As described earlier, hemispheric comparisons in blood flow are

likely to be inaccurate, and alterations of the partition coefficient of xenon in infarcted tissue further complicate interhemispheric comparisons.

In a follow-up study, 31 infants of birth weight less than 1250 g had CBF measurements taken at 6 hours (range, 4 to 11 hours) and on the fifth postnatal day.[114] Cranial ultrasonography, used to document IVH, was performed within 6 hours of birth and then every 12 hours. Infants were divided into three groups: no IVH, early IVH (i.e., present at 6 hours), and interval IVH (appearing after 6 hours but before 5 days). The early IVH group exhibited hemispheric asymmetries in CBF, and five of the infants had reduced CBF to one or both hemispheres. Three of these infants (who had IVH and no initial parenchymal hemorrhagic involvement) progressed to so-called Grade IV hemorrhage (i.e., IVH and a hemorrhagic parenchymal infarct). Thus, one could postulate the following pathogenetic mechanisms to account for development of the hemorrhagic parenchymal infarct in these infants. First, infarction of the hemisphere could have occurred perinatally, as evidenced by the reduced CBF at 6 hours, with secondary hemorrhage into this area between 6 hours and 5 days. Thus, these data could be used to support the theory that the hemorrhagic parenchymal lesion represents hemorrhagic periventricular leukomalacia. Second, the IVH (and germinal matrix hemorrhage) could have caused the reduced CBF. Reduction in CBF has been observed experimentally after introduction of blood and potassium into the lateral ventricles of animals. Third, the IVH and germinal matrix hemorrhage could have obstructed venous return from the periventricular white matter (see earlier), which caused the reduced CBF and subsequent infarction. These hypotheses must be considered with caution; evidence indicates that functional integrity of the newborn brain can be preserved with very low CBF (as low as 5 mL/100 g/minute).[74] Because CBF values in the preceding study were in this range, one cannot assume that infarction had occurred.

In another study by Ment and associates,[115] two premature infants had xenon study results that indicated unilateral reduction in hemispheric CBF at 6 hours of age. These infants also had no evidence of IVH. The first infant, on day 5, was shown to have IVH and hemorrhagic infarcts of the basal ganglia (with later cortical atrophy on CT scan). The second infant, on day 4, experienced bilateral subependymal hemorrhages and an occipital porencephalic cyst. These two cases support further the hypothesis of perinatal cerebral infarction and subsequent IVH.

REFERENCES

1. Goddard J, et al: Moderate rapidly induced hypertension as a cause of intraventricular hemorrhage in the newborn beagle model. J Pediatr 96:1057, 1980.
2. Goddard-Finegold J, et al: Intraventricular hemorrhage following volume expansion after hypovolemic hypotension in the newborn beagle. J Pediatr 100:796, 1982.
3. Freeman J, Ingvar DH: Elimination by hypoxia of cerebral blood flow autoregulation and EEG relationships. Exp Brain Res 5:61, 1968.
4. Harper AM: Autoregulation of cerebral blood flow influence of the arterial blood pressure on the blood flow through the cerebral cortex. J Neurol Neurosurg Psychiatry 29:398, 1966.
5. Reivich M, et al: Effects of trauma on cerebral vascular autoregulation. *In* Toole JF, et al (eds): Seventh Princeton Conference on Cerebral Vascular Disease. New York, Grune & Stratton, 1971, pp 66–89.
6. Paulson OB: Cerebral apoplexy (stroke): pathogenesis, pathophysiology, and therapy as illustrated by regional blood flow measurements in the brain. Stroke 2:327, 1971.
7. Tweed WA, et al: Arterial oxygenation determines autoregulation of cerebral blood flow in fetal lamb. Pediatr Res 17:246, 1983.
8. Volpe JJ: Intraventricular hemorrhage in the premature infant-current concepts. Part I. Ann Neurol 25:3, 1989.
9. Young RSK, et al: Selective reduction of blood flow to white matter during hypotension in newborn dogs: a possible mechanism of periventricular leukomalacia. Ann Neurol 12:445, 1982.
10. Gould SJ, et al: Periventricular intraparenchymal cerebral haemorrhage in preterm infants: the role of venous infarction. J Pathol 151:197, 1987.

11. Guzzetta FF, et al: Periventricular intraparenchymal echodensities in the premature newborn: critical determinant of neurologic outcome. Pediatrics 78:995, 1986.
12. Perlman JM, Volpe JJ: Are venous circulatory abnormalities important in the pathogenesis of hemorrhagic and/or ischemic cerebral injury? Pediatrics 80:705, 1987.
13. Perlman JM, Thach BT: Respiratory origin of fluctuations in arterial blood pressure in premature infants with respiratory distress syndrome. Pediatrics 8:399, 1988.
14. Kontos HA: Validity of cerebral arterial blood flow calculations from velocity measurements. Stroke 20:1, 1989.
15. Heisted DD, Kontos HA: Cerebral circulation. In Sheppard JT, Abboud FM (eds): Handbook of Physiology, Vol 3: The Cardiovascular System. Baltimore, Williams & Wilkins, 1983, pp 137–182.
16. Johnson PC: Review of previous studies and current theories of autoregulation. Circ Res 14-15(Suppl I):2, 1964.
17. Lassen NA: Cerebral blood flow and oxygen consumption in man. Physiol Rev 39:183, 1959.
18. Lassen NA: Autoregulation of cerebral blood flow. Circ Res 14(Suppl I):201, 1964.
19. Hernandez MJ, et al: Autoregulation of cerebral blood flow in the newborn dog. Brain Res 184:199, 1980.
20. Papile LA, et al: Autoregulation of cerebral blood flow in the preterm fetal lamb. Pediatr Res 19:159, 1985.
21. Pryds O, et al: Heterogeneity of cerebral vasoreactivity in preterm infants supported by mechanical ventilation. J Pediatr 115:638, 1989.
22. Pryds O, et al: Cerebral blood flow reactivity in spontaneously breathing preterm infants shortly after birth. Acta Paediatr Scand 79:391, 1990.
23. Lou HC, et al: Impaired autoregulation of cerebral blood flow in the distressed newborn infant. J Pediatr 94:118, 1979.
24. Vannucci RC, Hernandez MJ: Perinatal cerebral blood flow: Mead Johnson Symposium on Perinatal and Developmental Medicine (Baltimore) 17:17, 1980.
25. Jorch G, et al: Failure of autoregulation of cerebral blood flow in neonatal studies by pulsed Doppler ultrasound of the internal carotid artery. Eur J Pediatr 146:468, 1987.
26. Grubb RL, et al: The effects of changes in $PaCO_2$ on cerebral blood volume, blood flow and vascular mean transit time. Stroke 5:630, 1974.
27. Kety SS, Schmidt CF: The effects of active and passive hyperventilation on cerebral blood flow, cerebral oxygen consumption, cardiac output and blood pressure of normal young men. J Clin Invest 25:107, 1946.
28. Reivich M, et al: Reactivity of cerebral vessels to CO_2 in the newborn rhesus monkey. Eur Neurol 6:132, 1971.
29. Wollman H, et al: The effects of extremes of respiratory and metabolic alkalosis on cerebral blood flow in man. J Appl Physiol 24:60, 1968.
30. Kliefoth AB, et al: Depression of cerebral oxygen utilization by hypercapnia in the rhesus monkey. J Neurochem 32:661, 1979.
31. Greisen G, Trojaborg W: Cerebral blood flow, $PaCO_2$ changes, and visual evoked potentials in mechanically ventilated preterm infants. Acta Paediatr Scand 76:394, 1987.
32. Rosenberg AA, et al: Response of cerebral blood flow to changes in $PaCO_2$ in fetal, newborn and adult sheep. Am J Physiol 242:H862, 1982.
33. Jones MD, et al: Effects of changes in arterial O_2 content on cerebral blood flow in the lamb. Am J Physiol 240:H209, 1981.
34. Hudak MC, et al: Effect of hematocrit on cerebral blood flow. Am J Physiol 251:1463, 1986.
35. Pryds O, et al: The effect of $PaCO_2$ and hemoglobin concentration on the day to day variation of CBF in preterm neonates. Acta Pediatr Scand Suppl 360:33, 1989.
36. Younkin DP, et al: The effect of hematocrit and systolic blood pressure on cerebral blood flow in newborn infants. J Cereb Blood Flow Metab 7:295, 1987.
37. Eisenberg S, Seltzer HS: The cerebral metabolic effects of acutely induced hypoglycemia in human subjects. Metabolism 11:1162, 1962.
38. Kety SS, et al: Cerebral blood flow and metabolism in schizophrenia. Am J Psychiatry 104:705, 1948.
39. Della Porta P, et al: Cerebral blood flow and metabolism in therapeutic insulin coma. Metabolism 13:131, 1964.
40. Abdul-Rahman A, et al: Local cerebral blood flow in the rat during severe hypoglycemia, and in the recovery period following glucose injection. Acta Physiol Scand 109:307, 1980.
41. Agardh CD, et al: Endogenous substrates utilized by rat brain in severe insulin-induced hypoglycemia. J Neurochem 36:490, 1981.
42. Anwar M, Vannucci RC: Autoradiographic determination of regional cerebral blood flow during hypoglycemia in newborn dogs. Pediatr Res 24:41, 1988.
43. Hernandez MJ, et al: Cerebral blood and metabolism during hypoglycemia in newborn dogs. J Neurochem 35:622, 1980.
44. Siesjo BK, et al: Regional differences in vascular autoregulation in rat brain in severe insulin-induced hypoglycemia. J Cereb Blood Flow Metab 3:478, 1983.
45. Pryds O, et al: Compensatory increase of CBF in preterm infants during hypoglycemia. Acta Paediatr Scand 77:632, 1988.
46. Altman DI, et al: Cerebral oxygen metabolism in newborn infants measured with positron emission tomography. J Cereb Blood Flow Metab 9:S25, 1989.
47. Strandness DE, Summer DS: Ultrasound Techniques in Angiology. Bern, Hans Huber, 1975.
48. Bada HS, et al: Intracranial pressure and cerebral arterial pulsatile flow measurements in neonatal intraventricular hemorrhage. J Pediatr 100:291, 1982.
49. Pourcelot L: Diagnostic ultrasound for cerebrovascular disease. In Donald J, Levi S (eds): Present and Future Diagnostic Ultrasound. Rotterdam, Kooker Scientific Publications, 1976.
50. Batton DG, Mardis EE: The effect of intraventricular blood on cerebral blood flow in newborn dogs. Pediatr Res 21:511, 1987.
51. Hansen NB, et al: Validity of Doppler measurements of anterior cerebral artery blood flow velocity: correlation with brain blood flow in piglets. Pediatrics 72:526, 1983.
52. Rosenberg AA, et al: Comparison of anterior cerebral artery blood flow velocity and cerebral blood flow during hypoxia. Pediatr Res 19:67, 1985.
53. Greisen G, et al: Cerebral blood flow in the newborn infant. Comparison of Doppler ultrasound and ^{133}xenon clearance. J Pediatr 104:411, 1984.
54. Perlman JM, et al: Cerebral blood flow velocity as determined by Doppler is related to regional cerebral blood flow as determined by positron emission tomography. Ann Neurol 18:407, 1985.
55. Perlman JM, et al: Fluctuating cerebral blood flow velocity in respiratory distress syndrome. N Engl J Med 309:204, 1983.
56. Perlman JM, et al: Reduction of intraventricular hemorrhage by elimination of fluctuating cerebral blood flow velocity in preterm infants with respiratory distress syndrome. N Engl J Med 312:1353, 1985.
57. Hill A, et al: Relationship of pneumothorax to occurrence of intraventricular hemorrhage in the premature newborn. Pediatrics 69:144, 1982.
58. de Lemos RA, Tomosovic JJ: Effects of positive pressure ventilation on cerebral blood flow in the newborn infant. Clin Perinatol 5:395, 1978.
59. Jobe AH: Pulmonary surfactant therapy. N Engl J Med 328:861, 1993.
60. Cowan F, et al: Cerebral blood flow velocity changes after rapid administration of surfactant. Arch Dis Child 66:1105, 1991.
61. Jorch G, et al: Acute and protracted effects of intratracheal surfactant application on internal carotid blood flow velocity, blood pressure and carbon dioxide tension in very low birth weight infants. Eur J Pediatr 148:770, 1989.
62. Perlman JM, et al: The effect of patent ductus arteriosus on flow velocity in the anterior cerebral arteries: ductal steal in the premature newborn infant. J Pediatr 99:767, 1981.
63. Perlman JM, et al: Suctioning in the preterm infant: effects on cerebral blood flow velocity, intracranial pressure and arterial blood pressure. Pediatrics 72:739, 1983.
64. Bada HS, et al: Non-invasive diagnoses of neonatal asphyxia and intraventricular hemorrhage by Doppler ultrasound. J Pediatr 95:775, 1979.
65. Perlman JM, Volpe JJ: Cerebral blood flow velocity in relation to intraventricular hemorrhage in the premature newborn infant. J Pediatr 100:956, 1982.
66. Jobsis FF: Noninvasive infrared monitoring of cerebral and myocardial sufficiency and circulatory parameters. Science 198:1264, 1977.
67. Wyatt JS, et al: Near infrared spectroscopy. In Haddad J, et al (eds): Imaging Techniques of the CNS System of the Neonate. New York, Springer-Verlag, 1991.
68. Cope M: System for longterm measurement of cerebral blood and tissue oxygenation in newborn infants by near infrared transillumination. Med Biol Eng Comput 26:289, 1988.
69. Wray SC, et al: Characterization of the near infrared absorption spectra of cytochrome aa₃ and hemoglobin for the noninvasive monitoring of cerebral oxygenation. Biochim Biophys Acta 933:184, 1988.
70. Cope M, et al: Measurement in optical path length for cerebral near-infrared spectroscopy in newborn infants. Dev Neurosci 12:140, 1990.
71. Delpy DT, et al: Estimation of optimal path length through tissue from direct time of flight measurement. Phys Med Biol 33:1433, 1988.
72. Wyatt JS, et al: Quantitation of cerebral blood flow volume in human infants by near infrared spectroscopy. J Appl Physiol 68:1086, 1990.
73. Altman DI, et al: Cerebral blood flow requirement for brain viability in newborn infants is lower than in adults. Ann Neurol 24:218, 1988.
74. Meek JH, et al: Cerebral blood flow increases over the first three days of life in extremely preterm neonates. Arch Dis Child 78:F33,1998.
75. Brazy JE, et al: Changes in cerebral blood volume and cytochrome aa during hypertensive peaks in preterm infants. J Pediatr 108:983, 1986.
76. Pryds O, et al: Carbon dioxide-related changes in cerebral blood volume and cerebral blood flow in mechanically ventilated preterm neonates: comparison of near infrared spectrophotometry and ^{133}xenon clearance. Pediatr Res 27:445, 1990.
77. Wyatt JS, et al: Response of cerebral blood volume to changes in arterial carbon dioxide tension in preterm and term infants. Pediatr Res 29:553, 1991.
78. Skov LO, et al: Estimating cerebral blood flow in newborn infants: comparison of near infrared spectroscopy and ^{133}Xe clearance. Pediatr Res 27:445, 1991.
79. Shah AR, et al: Fluctuations in cerebral oxygenation and blood volume during endotracheal suctioning in premature infants. J Pediatr 120:769, 1992.
80. Edwards, A. D. et al: Cotside measurement of cerebral blood flow in ill newborn infants by near infrared spectroscopy. Lancet 2:770,1988.
81. Bucher HU, et al: Comparison between near infrared spectroscopy and ^{133}xenon clearance for estimation of cerebral blood flow in critically ill preterm infants. Pediatr Res 33:56, 1993.
82. Meeks JH, et al: Low cerebral blood flow is a risk factor for severe intraventricular haemorrhage. Arch Dis Child 1:F15,1999.
83. Tsuji M, et al: Cerebral intravascular oxygenation correlates with mean arterial pressure in critically ill premature infants. Pediatrics 106:625;2000.
84. Tsuji M, et al: Near infrared spectroscopy detects cerebral ischemia during hypotension in piglets. Pediatr Res 44:591;1998.

85. Edwards AD, et al: Cerebral hemodynamic effects of treatment with modified natural surfactant investigated by near infrared spectroscopy. Pediatr Res 32:532, 1992.

86. Edwards AD, et al: Effects of indomethacin on cerebral haemodynamics in very preterm infants. Lancet 335:1491, 1990.

87. Powers WJ, Raichle ME: Positron emission tomography and its application to the study of cerebrovascular disease in man. Stroke 16:361, 1985.

88. Raichle ME: Positron emission tomography. Annu Rev Neurosci 6:249, 1983.

89. Phelps ME, et al: Application of annihilation coincidence detection to transaxial reconstructive tomography. J Nucl Med 16:210, 1975.

90. Hoffman EJ, et al: Quantitation in positron emission tomography. I. Effect of object size. J Comput Assist Tomogr 3:299, 1979.

91. Mazziotta JC, et al: Quantitation in positron emission computed tomography. V. Physical-anatomical effects. J Comput Assist Tomogr 5:734, 1981.

92. Herscovitch P, et al: Brain blood flow measured with intravenous H2150. I. Theory and error analysis. J Nucl Med 24:782, 1983.

93. Raichle ME, et al: Brain blood flow measured with intravenous H2150. II. Implementation and validation. J Nucl Med 24:790, 1983.

94. Eichling JO, et al: Evidence of the limitations of water as a freely diffusible tracer in brain of the rhesus monkey. Circ Res 35:358, 1974.

95. Herscovitch P, Raichle ME: What is the correct value for the brain-blood partition coefficient of water? J Cereb Blood Flow Metab 5:65, 1985.

96. Volpe JJ, et al: Positron emission tomography in the newborn: extensive impairment of regional cerebral blood flow with intraventricular hemorrhage and hemorrhagic intracerebral involvement. Pediatrics 72:589, 1983.

97. Hoedt-Rasmussen K, et al: Regional cerebral blood flow in man determined by intra-arterial injection of radioactive inert gas. Circ Res 43:237, 1966.

98. Ingvar DH, Lassen NA: Regional blood flow of the cerebral cortex determined by krypton-85. Acta Physiol Scand 54:325, 1962.

99. Lou HC, et al: Low cerebral blood flow in hypotensive perinatal distress. Acta Neurol Scand 56:343, 1977.

100. Lou HC, et al: Low cerebral blood flow: a risk factor in the neonate. J Pediatr 95:606, 1979.

101. Ment LR, et al: Alterations in cerebral blood flow in preterm infants with intraventricular hemorrhage. Pediatrics 68:763, 1981.

102. Younkin DP, et al: Non-invasive method of estimating human newborn regional cerebral blood flow. J Cereb Blood Flow Metab 2:415, 1982.

103. Greisen G: CBF in the newborn infant: issues and methods with special reference to the intravenous 133-xenon clearance technique. rCBF Bull 7:134, 1984.

104. Greisen G, et al: Analysis of cranial 133-xenon clearance in the newborn infant by the two compartment model. Scand J Clin Lab Invest 44:239, 1984.

105. Obrist WD, et al: Regional cerebral blood flow estimated by 133-xenon inhalation. Stroke 6:245, 1975.

106. Olesen J, et al: Regional cerebral blood flow in man determined by the initial slope of the clearance of intra-arterially injected 133-Xe. Stroke 2:519, 1971.

107. Risberg J, et al: Regional cerebral blood flow by 133-xenon inhalation. Stroke 6:142, 1975.

108. Sveinsdottir E, et al: Calculation of regional cerebral blood flow (rCBF) initial-slope index compared to height over area values. In Russell RWR (ed): Brain and Blood Flow. London, Pitman Company, 1971.

109. Bolmsjo M: Hemisphere cross-talk and signal overlapping in bilateral rCBF measurements using Xe-133. Eur J Nucl Med 9:1, 1984.

110. Donley FR, et al: Blood flow measurements and the "look through artefact" in focal cerebral ischemia. Stroke 6:121, 1975.

111. Greisen G: Cerebral blood flow in preterm infants during the first week of life. Acta Paediatr Scand 75:43, 1986.

112. Lou HC, et al: Decreased cerebral blood flow after administration of sodium bicarbonate in the distressed newborn infant. Acta Neurol Scand 57:239, 1978.

113. Ment LR, et al: Postpartum perfusion of the preterm brain: relationship to neurodevelopmental outcome. Child Brain 10:266, 1983.

114. Ment LR, et al: Intraventricular hemorrhage in the preterm neonate: timing and cerebral blood flow changes. J Pediatr 104:419, 1984.

115. Ment LR, et al: Delayed hemorrhagic infarction: a cause of late neonatal germinal matrix and intraventricular hemorrhage. Arch Neurol 41:1036, 1984.

171

Pathophysiology of Intraventricular Hemorrhage in the Neonate

Germinal matrix–intraventricular hemorrhage (IVH) is the most common variety of neonatal intracranial hemorrhage and is characteristic of the premature infant.[1] The *incidence* of IVH in premature infants has declined since the 1970s to a variable degree in most neonatal centers (Fig. 171-1). In well-studied series of premature infants subjected to routine computed tomography (CT) or ultrasound scans and studied in the late 1970s and early 1980s, the incidence of IVH ranged from 34 to 49%.[2-4] During the late 1980s, the incidence had fallen to approximately 20%.[5, 6] During the 1990s, the incidence remained unchanged; one of the largest series, of 19,581 very low birth weight infants in 250 centers collected in the Vermont-Oxford Neonatal Database for 1997, experienced an overall incidence for all IVH of 25%. The incidence of the most severe form of IVH, periventricular hemorrhagic infarction (intraparenchymal echodensity), was 4% and was notably highest at 11% in infants born with a birth weight of less than 750 g.[7] Thus, although there has been a decline in the incidence of all IVH since the early 1980s, it appears that IVH remains a significant problem in the extremely low birth weight infant with a high risk of associated periventricular hemorrhagic infarction.

The *magnitude of the problem* of IVH in the premature infant relates to the relatively high and unchanging incidence of IVH combined with an increase in the absolute number of surviving premature infants. With significant advances in neonatal care since the 1980s,[1] the absolute number of surviving premature infants has increased, most notably the smallest, sickest infants at greatest risk of IVH and its complications. Thus, since the 1980s, in the United States, the proportion of live births weighing less than 1500 g increased from 1.17 to 1.45%.[8] Of the approximately 4 million live births each year in the United States, 55,000 very low birth weight infants will be born, and approximately 85% of these infants will

survive.[9, 10] Thus, in any year in the United States alone, approximately 15,000 premature infants will suffer from IVH, and more than 2000 infants will have periventricular hemorrhagic infarction.

In this chapter, we briefly discuss the background of clinical features and diagnosis of IVH before a more detailed discussion of the neuropathology and pathogenesis of the lesion.

CLINICAL FEATURES

Three basic clinical syndromes are found with IVH: (1) a dramatic *catastrophic* deterioration, which is uncommon and evolves over hours with deep stupor or coma, respiratory abnormalities (arrhythmias, hypoventilation, and apnea), generalized tonic seizures, decerebrate posturing, pupils fixed to light, eyes fixed to vestibular stimulation, and flaccid quadriparesis[11]; (2) a *saltatory* deterioration, the presenting signs of which include an alteration in the level of consciousness, a change (usually a decrease) in spontaneous and elicited motility, hypotonia, and subtle aberrations of eye position and movement[12]; and (3) by far the most common, a *clinically silent* syndrome occurring in 25 to 50% of infants with IVH in whom even careful and serial clinical assessments may fail to reveal any abnormal signs indicative of the lesion.[11, 13]

DIAGNOSIS

The screening procedure of choice in IVH is portable cranial ultrasonography; however, *lumbar puncture* can provide a characteristic cerebrospinal fluid (CSF) profile of intracranial hemorrhage consisting initially of increased red blood cell count and elevated protein content, followed shortly by xanthochromia and depressed glucose content. The degree of elevation of

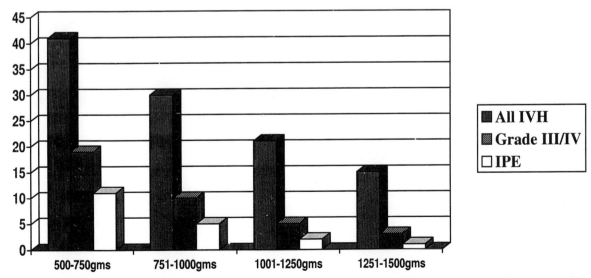

Figure 171–1. The incidence of (percentage of all infants with) all intraventricular hemorrhage (IVH), Grade III/IV IVH, and intraparenchymal echodensity (IPE) in the Vermont-Oxford Network 1997 (*n* = 19,581). (From Horbar JD: Vermont-Oxford Network 1997 Database Summary. Burlington, VT, Vermont-Oxford Network, 1997.)

CSF protein correlates approximately with the severity of the hemorrhage.[14]

Ultrasound

Ultrasound scanning is the procedure of choice in the diagnosis of germinal matrix-IVH in the premature infant. There is vast experience demonstrating the reliability and versatility of cranial ultrasound in this clinical setting for the diagnosis of IVH in the premature infant.[2, 15-21] The grading system using cranial ultrasound for IVH in the infant is based on the presence and amount of blood in the germinal matrix and the lateral ventricles (Table 171-1 and Fig. 171-2). The determination of the presence of blood in the matrix is made best on the coronal cranial ultrasound scan, whereas the determination of the amount of blood in the lateral ventricles is most accurate on the parasagittal cranial ultrasound scan.

Timing of Onset of the Intraventricular Hemorrhage

The *time of onset of IVH* is the first day of life in at least 50% of affected infants, and approximately 90% of the lesions occur by 72 hours.[5, 22] However, *progression* of the lesions occurs in approximately 20 to 40% of the affected infants, with maximal extent of the lesion seen by 3 to 5 days after the initial diagnosis.[23, 24]

Severity of the Intraventricular Hemorrhage

Approximately 25% of the hemorrhages are large, that is, Grade III, with blood usually filling and dilating the lateral ventricles on the parasagittal scan (see Table 171-1). Approximately 15% of all the infants with hemorrhage also have large periventricular echodensity consistent with periventricular hemorrhagic infarction. Of these infants, the severity of the IVH is Grade III in 80% (see Fig. 171-2).

Computed Tomography

CT has the major disadvantage of requiring the sick premature infant to be transported as well as exposing the brain and eyes to ionizing radiation. With these limitations in mind, CT scanning can, however, demonstrate the site and extent of IVH effectively in the premature infant.[3, 4, 25, 26]

Magnetic Resonance Imaging

Magnetic resonance imaging (MRI) has been shown to provide excellent images of IVH, but the advantage of MRI lies in its superior ability to demonstrate the nature and severity of any parenchymal injury.[27-30] However, MRI currently cannot supplant ultrasonography in the evaluation of IVH, because MRI requires transport to the scanner, has a relatively long data acquisition time, precludes the use of metallic materials found on standard neonatal monitoring and support equipment, and is expensive. MRI is particularly useful in the demonstration of the

TABLE 171-1

Grading of Severity of Germinal Matrix–Intraventricular Hemorrhage by Ultrasound Scanning

Severity	Description
Grade I	Germinal matrix hemorrhage with no or minimal intraventricular hemorrhage (10% of ventricular area on parasagittal view)
Grade II	Intraventricular hemorrhage (10–50% of ventricular area on parasagittal view)
Grade III	Intraventricular hemorrhage (>50% of ventricular area on parasagittal view; usually distends lateral ventricle)

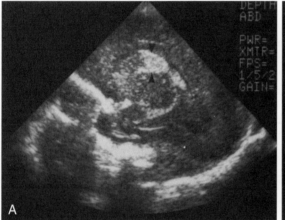
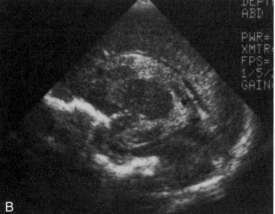
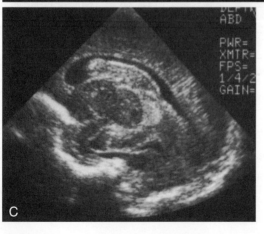

Figure 171–2. Grading of the severity of germinal matrix-intraventricular hemorrhage; parasagittal ultrasound scans. **A,** Grade I. **B,** Grade II. Note the echogenic material filling less than 50% of the ventricular area. **C,** Grade III. Note the large blood clot nearly completely filling and distending the entire lateral ventricle.

parenchymal details of periventricular hemorrhagic infarction (Fig. 171-3).

NEUROPATHOLOGY

The neuropathology of IVH is considered best in terms of the site of origin, that is, primarily the germinal matrix, the spread of the hemorrhage throughout the ventricular system, the neuropathologic consequences of the hemorrhage, and the neuropathologic accompaniments not necessarily related directly to the IVH.

The basic lesion in germinal matrix–IVH is bleeding into the subependymal germinal matrix. Over the final 12 to 16 weeks of gestation, this matrix becomes less and less prominent and is essentially exhausted by term. This region is highly cellular, gelatinous in texture, and richly vascularized (as would be expected for a structure with active cellular proliferation).

Site of Origin

The site of origin of IVH characteristically is the *subependymal germinal matrix* (Fig. 171-4). This cellular region immediately ventrolateral to the lateral ventricle serves initially as the source of cerebral neuronal precursors between approximately 10 to 20 weeks of gestation. Later in the third trimester, the matrix provides glial precursors that will become cerebral oligodendroglia and astrocytes. The matrix undergoes progressive decrease in size, from a width of 2.5 mm at 23 to 24 weeks, to 1.4 mm at 32 weeks, to nearly complete involution by approximately 36 weeks.[31] The many thin-walled vessels in the matrix are a prime source of bleeding. Hemorrhage from the choroid plexus occurs in nearly 50% of infants with germinal matrix hemorrhage and IVH,[32] and, in more mature infants especially, it may be the exclusive site of origin of IVH.

The vascular *site of origin* of germinal matrix hemorrhage within the microcirculation of this region appears to be the prominent endothelial-lined vessels of the matrix and not the arterioles or arteries.[33-36] The vessels in free communication with the venous circulation appear to be of particular importance, such as the capillary-venule junction or small venules. This

has been shown by careful histochemical studies of germinal matrix vessels at the site of hemorrhage[36] and by the emergence of solution into the germinal matrix hemorrhage from postmortem injection into the jugular veins but not from injection into the carotid artery.[35]

Spread of Intraventricular Hemorrhage

In approximately 80% of patients with germinal matrix hemorrhage, blood enters the lateral ventricles and spreads throughout the ventricular system.[34,37] Blood proceeds through the foramina of Magenda and Luschka and tends to collect in the basilar cisterns in the posterior fossa. With substantial collections, the blood may incite obliterative arachnoiditis over days to weeks with impairment in CSF flow. Other sites at which particulate blood clot may lead to impaired CSF dynamics are the aqueduct of Sylvius and the arachnoid villi.

Neuropathologic Consequences of Intraventricular Hemorrhage

Several neuropathologic states occur as apparent consequences of IVH, including, in temporal order of occurrence, germinal matrix destruction, periventricular hemorrhagic infarction, and posthemorrhagic hydrocephalus.

Germinal Matrix Destruction

Destruction of germinal matrix and, perhaps importantly, of its glial precursor cells is a consistent and expected feature of germinal matrix hemorrhage.[33, 34] The hematoma is replaced frequently by a cyst, the walls of which include hemosiderin-laden macrophages and reactive astrocytes. This destruction of glial precursor cells in the germinal matrix may have a deleterious influence on subsequent brain development.

Periventricular Hemorrhagic Infarction

Approximately 15% of infants with IVH also exhibit a characteristic parenchymal lesion, *periventricular hemorrhagic infarction*. The incidence of this lesion increases with decreasing gestational age, such that in infants of 500 to 750 g, periventricular hemorrhagic infarction accounts for approximately one-third

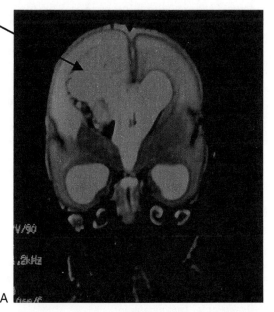
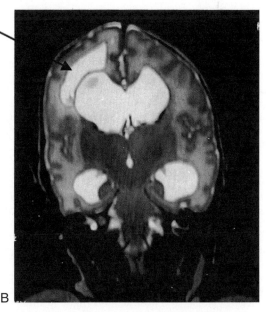

A

B

Figure 171–3. Magnetic resonance imaging (coronal T2-weighted scan) of acute periventricular hemorrhagic infarction. **A,** Note the fan-shaped distribution of increased signal in the parenchyma (*arrow*) and the generalized increased signal in the white matter in the area surrounding the infarct. **B,** Later image of the same infant with cystic transformation of the infarct (*arrow*). Note the ventriculomegaly present in both the acute and the more chronic images.

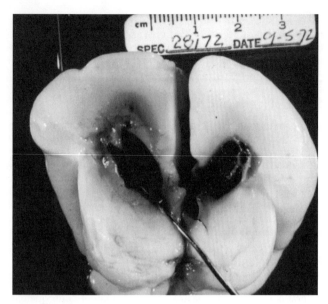

Figure 171–4. Germinal matrix–intraventricular hemorrhage; coronal sections of the cerebrum. The germinal matrix hemorrhage is observable on the right. The probe is in the foramen of Monro.

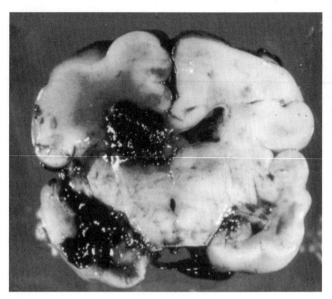

Figure 171–5. Periventricular hemorrhagic infarction with intra-ventricular hemorrhage; coronal section of the cerebrum. Note the evolving hemorrhagic infarction on the same side as the larger germinal matrix–intraventricular hemorrhage.

of all cases of IVH (see Fig. 171-1).[38, 39] The neuropathology of periventricular hemorrhagic infarction consists of a relatively large region of hemorrhagic necrosis in the periventricular white matter, just dorsal and lateral to the external angle of the lateral ventricle (Fig. 171-5). The necrosis is strikingly *asymmetric*—in the largest series reported, 67% of such lesions were exclusively *unilateral,* and in virtually all of the remaining cases, they were grossly asymmetric, even though bilateral.[40] Approximately one-half of the lesions are extensive and involve the periventricular white matter from the frontal to the parieto-occipital regions. Approximately 80% of cases are associated with large IVH, and commonly (and mistakenly), the parenchymal hemorrhagic lesion is described as an "extension" of the hemorrhage. That simple extension of blood into cerebral white matter from germinal matrix or lateral ventricle does *not* account for the periventricular hemorrhagic necrosis has been shown clearly by several neuropathologic studies.[32, 38–42] Microscopic study of this periventricular hemorrhagic necrosis indicates that the lesion is a *hemorrhagic infarction.*[40–43] The careful studies of Gould and associates[41] and Takashima and colleagues[43] emphasize that the hemorrhagic component of the infarction tends to be most concentrated near the ventricular angle where the medullary veins draining the cerebral white matter become confluent and ultimately join the terminal vein in the subependymal region. Thus, it appears likely that periventricular hemorrhagic necrosis occurring in association with large IVH is, in fact, a *venous infarction.*

The pathogenesis of periventricular hemorrhagic infarction appears in most cases to be related directly to the associated germinal matrix-IVH; the association of large asymmetric germinal matrix-IVH and progression to *ipsilateral* periventricular hemorrhagic infarction has been clearly documented.[40, 44, 45] These data raise the possibility that the IVH or its associated germinal matrix hemorrhage may lead to obstruction of the terminal veins with secondary hemorrhagic venous infarction.[40] A similar conclusion was suggested by a neuropathologic study.[41] This pathogenetic formulation received further support from two imaging studies. Doppler determinations of blood flow velocity demonstrated obstruction of flow in the terminal vein by the ipsilateral germinal matrix hemorrhage during the evolution of the infarction in the living premature infant.[46] In addition, an MRI study of acute periventricular hemorrhagic infarction

showed an appearance consistent with a combination of intravascular thrombi and perivascular hemorrhage along the course of the medullary veins within the area of infarction.[47] The pathogenetic scheme that we consider to account for most examples of periventricular hemorrhagic infarction is shown in Figure 171-6.

Hydrocephalus

A third neuropathologic consequence of IVH is progressive posthemorrhagic ventricular dilation, that is, *hydrocephalus.* The likelihood of and the rapidity of evolution of hydrocephalus after IVH is related directly to the quantity of intraventricular blood. Thus, with large IVH, hydrocephalus may evolve over days *(acute* hydrocephalus), and with smaller IVH, the process evolves usually over weeks *(subacute-chronic* hydrocephalus).

Acute hydrocephalus is accompanied by particulate blood clot, which may impair CSF absorption by obstruction of the arachnoid villi. This mechanism may be particularly likely in the newborn with only microscopic arachnoid villi and not larger, later-appearing arachnoid granulations.[48] Other contributing factors to the development of acute hydrocephalus may include an impaired ability to mediate clot lysis with extremely low plasminogen levels and elevations in plasminogen activator inhibitor in the CSF of infants with recent IVH.[49]

Subacute-chronic hydrocephalus relates most commonly either to obliterative arachnoiditis in the posterior fossa resulting in obstruction of fourth ventricular outflow or flow through the tentorial notch or to aqueductal obstruction by blood clot, disrupted ependyma, and reactive gliosis.[33, 50, 51]

Neuropathologic Accompaniments of Intraventricular Hemorrhage

Several neuropathologic states are commonly associated with IVH but are not directly caused by it. The two most common accompaniments are periventricular leukomalacia and pontine neuronal necrosis.

Periventricular Leukomalacia

Periventricular leukomalacia was observed to some degree in 75% of one series of infants who died with IVH.[32] In contrast to

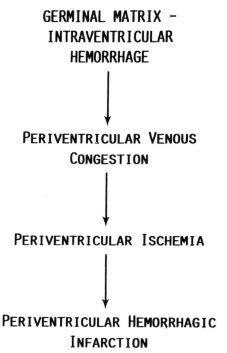

GERMINAL MATRIX -
INTRAVENTRICULAR
HEMORRHAGE

↓

PERIVENTRICULAR VENOUS
CONGESTION

↓

PERIVENTRICULAR ISCHEMIA

↓

PERIVENTRICULAR HEMORRHAGIC
INFARCTION

Figure 171–6. Pathogenesis of periventricular hemorrhagic infarction. The formulation indicates a central role for germinal matrix–intraventricular hemorrhage in causation of the periventricular venous infarction.

parenchymal hemorrhagic infarction, periventricular leukomalacia is a generally symmetric, nonhemorrhagic, and apparently ischemic white matter injury in the arterial end zones (Table 171–2). The frequent association of periventricular leukomalacia with IVH was also emphasized in three other neuropathologic reports.[43, 52] Although it has been reported that approximately 25% of examples of periventricular leukomalacia become hemorrhagic,[32, 53] especially when associated coagulopathy is present, this percentage includes examples accompanied by large IVH and that probably represent the venous infarction discussed earlier as periventricular hemorrhagic infarction. Takashima and colleagues[43] suggested that the two lesions, that is, periventricular hemorrhagic infarction and hemorrhagic periventricular leukomalacia, may be distinguishable in part on the basis of topography. Thus, hemorrhagic periventricular leukomalacia has a predilection for periventricular arterial border zones, particularly in the region near the trigone of the lateral ventricles. Venous infarction, especially its most hemorrhagic component, is particularly prominent more anteriorly; that is, the lesion radiates from the periventricular region at the site of confluence of the medullary and terminal veins and assumes a roughly triangular, fan-shaped appearance in periventricular white matter.

Pontine Neuronal Necrosis

Hypoxic-ischemic neuronal injury may accompany IVH in premature infants, and one subtype of such injury, *pontine neu-*

ronal necrosis, is particularly common. In two carefully studied neuropathologic series,[32, 52] 46 and 71% of infants with IVH exhibited pontine neuronal necrosis. Accompanying neuronal necrosis in the subiculum of the hippocampus was also common.[52, 54, 55] All the infants with IVH accompanied by pontine neuronal necrosis in the series of Armstrong and associates[32] died of respiratory failure. Previous investigations had suggested that pontine neuronal necrosis is related to hypoxic-ischemic insult, hyperoxia, and hypocarbia.[56, 57]

PATHOGENESIS

The pathogenesis of IVH is considered best in terms of intravascular, vascular, and extravascular factors.[1] Clearly, the pathogenesis of IVH is multifactorial, and thus different combinations of these factors are operative in different patients.

Intravascular Factors

Intravascular factors are those that relate primarily to the regulation of blood flow, pressure, and volume in the microvascular bed of the germinal matrix (Table 171–3; Fig. 171–7).

Fluctuating Cerebral Blood Flow

Significant fluctuations in *cerebral blood flow* appear important in the pathogenesis of IVH. It has been shown that a *fluctuating pattern* of arterial blood pressure, characterized by marked, *continuous alterations* in both systolic and diastolic flow velocities, was associated with similar trends in the cerebral blood flow velocity tracings and a high risk of subsequent occurrence of IVH. Smaller fluctuations in arterial pressure of less than 10% (coefficient of variation) did not appear to produce this adverse outcome.[58-60] The cause of the fluctuations in both the systemic and cerebral circulations were related to the mechanics of ventilation,[61,62] as well as to the severity of the infant's illness, with contributing factors of hypercarbia, hypovolemia, hypotension, "restlessness," patent ductus arteriosus, and relatively high inspired oxygen concentrations.[59,62-64]

Increases in Cerebral Blood Flow

The close temporal correlation between the occurrence of IVH and abrupt increases in arterial blood pressure, increases in cerebral blood flow, and cerebral blood flow velocity[65-68] supports the earlier hypothesis[69] that increases in cerebral blood flow play an important pathogenetic role in IVH. One major contributing factor to the premature infant's apparent propensity for dangerous elevations of cerebral blood flow is a pressure-passive state of the cerebral circulation.[70-76]

Elevations of Arterial Blood Pressure and Pressure-Passive Cerebral Circulation. Investigators have shown that intact cerebrovascular autoregulation is found in clinically stable preterm infants and a pressure-passive cerebral circulation is present in sick preterm infants who subsequently develop IVH.[72,77,78] The relationship between a pressure-passive cerebral circulation and the occurrence of IVH was clearly demonstrated in a study of 57 preterm infants[71] in whom ultrasonographic signs of severe IVH developed only in infants with earlier evidence of a pressure-passive cerebral circulation. Those infants with intact cerebrovascular autoregulation developed either no hemorrhage

TABLE 171-2			
Periventricular White Matter Lesions of the Premature Infant			
Term Disturbance	**Symmetry**	**Gross Hemorrhage**	**Probable Site of Circulatory**
Periventricular leukomalacia	Predominantly symmetric	Uncommon	Arterial
Periventricular hemorrhagic infarction	Predominantly asymmetric	Invariable	venous

TABLE 171-3

Pathogenesis of Germinal Matrix Hemorrhage

Intravascular Factors

Fluctuating blood pressure
Increase in cerebral blood flow—systemic hypertension in the setting of a pressure-passive circulation, rapid volume expansion, hypercarbia, decreased hematocrit, decreased blood glucose
Increase in cerebral venous pressure—venous anatomic arrangement, labor and vaginal delivery, respiratory disturbance
Decrease in cerebral blood flow (followed by reperfusion)—systemic hypotension
Platelet and coagulation disturbance

Vascular Factors

Tenous capillary integrity—the germinal matrix is an involuting remodeling capillary bed with deficient vascular lining and a large vascular and luminal area
Vulnerability of matrix capillaries to hypoxic-ischemic injury—the area has a high requirement for oxidative metabolism and lies at a vascular border zone

Extravascular Factors

Deficient vascular support
Excessive fibrinolytic activity

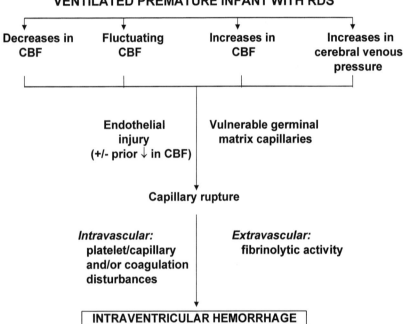

Figure 171–7. Interaction of the major pathogenetic factors for the occurrence of germinal matrix–intraventricular hemorrhage in the premature infant. CBF = cerebral blood flow.

or only mild hemorrhage.[71,74] Consistent with a potential role for arterial hypertension in this setting is the demonstration of a relation between maximum systolic blood pressure above a threshold value and the subsequent occurrence of IVH.[79] The limit for the highest tolerable peak systolic blood pressure was markedly lower for the smaller infants.[79]

Causes of Increased Arterial Blood Pressure in the Human Newborn. Abrupt elevations in arterial blood pressure, which may be accompanied by increased cerebral blood flow velocity, are clearly important to detect and prevent, whenever possible. These causes of elevated arterial blood pressure include the following: such "caretaking" concomitants as inadvertent noxious stimulation, abdominal examination, handling, instillation of mydriatics, and tracheal suctioning; such systemic complications as pneumothorax, exchange transfusion, and rapid infusion of colloid; and such neurologic complications as seizures.[65,66,68,80-86] Pneumothorax has been consistently associated with an elevated risk of IVH.[87, 88] In one study of nine infants, pneumothorax was accompanied consistently by abrupt

elevations of systemic blood pressure and cerebral blood flow velocity, and these circulatory changes were followed within hours by IVH.[89] Studies in newborn dogs documented abrupt increases in arterial blood pressure on rapid evacuation of pneumothorax.[87]

Relevant Experimental Studies: Role of Hypertension. The importance of abrupt increases in systemic blood pressure and cerebral blood flow in the pathogenesis of IVH was demonstrated in *experimental* studies in the newborn beagle puppy[89-93] and in the preterm sheep fetus.[94] A highly predictable and pattern of germinal matrix-IVH hemorrhage clinically similar to that of the human premature infant is produced in the beagle puppy by a sequence of hypotension and hypertension produced by blood removal and volume reinfusion.[95]

Hypercarbia. Careful studies of mechanically ventilated preterm infants show a pronounced reactivity of cerebral blood flow to changes in arterial carbon dioxide tension ($Paco_2$) with an approximately 30% increase in cerebral blood flow per kilopascal increase in $Paco_2$ after the first 24 hours of life.[72, 96, 97]

However, in the first 24 hours of life, the period of greatest risk for IVH, this reactivity is more attenuated, with an approximately 10% increase in cerebral blood flow per kilopascal increase in $Paco_2$ in well premature infants, and most strikingly, this reactivity is *absent* in infants with subsequent severe IVH.[71] This observation suggests that, in the first day of life at least, hypercarbia of at least a moderate degree may not be a major pathogenetic factor for severe IVH in mechanically ventilated infants. A similar lack of correlation between hypercarbia and IVH was apparent in several other studies.[98,99] An increased risk of IVH after hypercarbia, however, is suggested in some reports,[45, 60] including two that employed multivariate analysis.[88,100] In one large study ($n = 463$), hypercarbia (defined as $Paco_2 > 60$ mm Hg) showed a positive relation with IVH.[88] These data suggest that a role for hypercarbia in pathogenesis of IVH may exist with particularly marked elevations of $Paco_2$.

Decreased Hemoglobin. The role of *decreased hematocrit* as a pathogenetic factor for IVH may be greater than previously suspected. There is an inverse correlation in the human infant between hemoglobin concentration and cerebral blood flow.[72,101,102] In one study of premature infants in the first days of life, cerebral blood flow increased by 12% per 1 mmol/L decrease in hemoglobin.[72] Cerebral blood flow presumably increases to maintain cerebral oxygen delivery constant, but with increasing cerebral blood flow, there will be enhanced risk for IVH in those premature infants born anemic.

Decreased Blood Glucose. *Decreased blood glucose* should be considered in the evaluation of pathogenetic factors for IVH in view of the observation that cerebral blood flow increases two- to threefold when blood glucose declines to levels lower than 1.7 mmol/L in the premature infant.[72, 96] Blood glucose levels lower than 1.7 mmol/L in premature infants are not rare in the first days of life in many neonatal intensive care units. More data are needed on a potential contributory role for low blood glucose concentrations in the pathogenesis of IVH.

Increases in Cerebral Venous Pressure

Elevations of cerebral venous pressure may contribute to the occurrence of IVH. Indeed, potential importance of venous factors is suggested by the demonstration that, with postmortem injection of the carotid artery or jugular vein in infants with germinal matrix hemorrhage, the injected material entered the hemorrhage only by venous injections. The *most important causes* of such increases are labor and delivery, asphyxia, and respiratory complications.

Importance of Venous Anatomy. The importance of increased venous pressure in the pathogenesis of IVH relates in part to the *venous anatomy* in the region of the germinal matrix. The direction of deep venous flow takes a peculiar U-turn in the subependymal region at the level of the foramen of Monro, which is the most common site of germinal matrix hemorrhage.

Labor and Delivery. During labor and delivery, marked increases in cerebral venous pressure may occur. Measurement of "fetal head compression pressure" was determined by a compression transducer positioned between the fetal head and the wall of the uterus during labor, with the overall mean pressure found to be 158 mm Hg.[103] Consistent with this hypothesis of increased venous pressure during labor, there appears to be an increased risk of the occurrence of IVH in the premature infant with vaginal delivery and particularly with prolonged labor (>10 to 12 hours).[45, 104-107] Head position, both before delivery and in the neonatal nursery, may also alter cerebral venous drainage. One study documented, using near-infrared spectroscopy, that cerebral venous drainage may be impaired in prone or side positions.[108]

Asphyxia. The importance of increased venous pressure in association with asphyxia in the causation of IVH has been shown in experimental studies of preterm fetal sheep.[94]

Respiratory Disturbances. Data suggest that such factors as positive pressure ventilation with relatively high peak inflation pressure, tracheal suctioning, abnormalities of the mechanics of respiration, and pneumothorax may be major causes of increased cerebral venous pressure in the premature infant.[109-112] Doppler measurements of blood flow velocity in the superior sagittal sinus demonstrated a striking sensitivity of the venous circulation to the level of peak inflation pressure; the smallest infants exhibited the most marked effects.[112]

Tracheal suctioning and pneumothorax have also been shown to produce pronounced changes in venous pressure.[58, 113, 114] Studies of mode of ventilation in premature infants have raised concerns over associations between high-frequency oscillatory ventilation (HFOV) and increased rates of IVH, particularly high-grade IVH.[115] A meta-analysis of the eight randomized controlled studies comparing HFOV and conventional ventilation demonstrated a significant increase in the risk of Grade III or IV IVH (summary relative risk, 1.19 [1.03, 1.38]) with adverse neurodevelopmental outcome in the two trials with follow-up (relative risk, 1.26 [1.01,1.58]).[116] An increased risk of high-grade IVH was documented in a randomized controlled trial of HFOV that documented an increased rate of IVH in those infants who were switched from conventional ventilation to HFOV.[117] The potential mechanism of increased IVH in premature infants receiving HFOV may relate to increased lung volumes with decreased cerebral venous return.[118] However, these findings have led many authors to recommend that conventional ventilation should remain the ventilatory mode of choice in premature infants with respiratory distress syndrome.[116, 117]

Decreases in Cerebral Blood Flow

Importance of Pressure-Passive Cerebral Circulation. Decreases in cerebral blood flow may play an important role in the pathogenesis of IVH. The principal consequence of the decreased cerebral blood flow is injury of germinal matrix vessels, which rupture subsequently on reperfusion. As indicated earlier, hemorrhagic hypotension preceding volume reexpansion is the optimal means to produce IVH experimentally in the newborn beagle puppy. In the premature infant, decreases in cerebral blood flow are most likely with perinatal asphyxia and systemic hypotension. Because of the pressure-passive cerebral circulation in sick premature infants, this hypotension can lead to a parallel decrease in cerebral blood flow.

Perinatal Hypoxic-Ischemic Events. Perinatal hypoxic-ischemic events presumably explain, at least in part, the relationship among low Apgar scores, early acidosis, the early use of bicarbonate, and the subsequent occurrence of IVH, particularly cases that develop in the first 12 hours.[119, 120] The mechanism for provocation of IVH with perinatal asphyxia is complex and includes increases in cerebral venous pressure, changes in cerebral blood flow associated with impaired vascular autoregulation, such as decreases in cerebral blood flow associated with hypotension, and resulting injury to matrix capillaries. Studies of the concentrations of brain-specific creatine kinase isoenzymes in umbilical cord blood or blood samples obtained early in the postnatal period or of the hypoxanthine metabolite, uric acid, in blood samples obtained on the first postnatal day in preterm infants who later developed IVH support the notion that late intrauterine injury (perhaps asphyxia) may be involved in at least some cases of IVH.[121-123] Moreover, the possibility of a perinatal hypoxic-ischemic insult to brain as a predecessor to IVH is suggested also by the finding of electroencephalographic abnormalities before the occurrence of IVH.[124,125]

Postnatal Ischemic Events. The importance of postnatal decreases in arterial blood pressure in the pathogenesis of IVH is indicated by several studies in which arterial blood pressure was monitored continuously from birth or shortly after birth. In a study of approximately 25,000 very low birth weight infants, severe IVH was three times more common in those infants requiring cardiopulmonary resuscitation at delivery (15.3%) than in those not requiring resuscitation (4.9%).[126] A relationship between postnatal arterial hypotension and increased risk of IVH has been frequently documented.[127, 128] Near-infrared spectroscopy in the first 24 hours of life in preterm infants has shown that cerebral blood flow is significantly lower in infants who subsequently develop IVH (median 7.0 mL/100 g/minute) than in those without IVH (median 12.2 mL/100 g/minute).[129] Additionally supportive of a relation between postnatal ischemic events and the occurrence of IVH is the demonstration of decreased cardiac output in the first 36 hours of life in infants who developed the lesion, especially severe IVH.[130] Finally, the potential importance of ischemic injury in pathogenesis is supported further by the demonstration of a marked beneficial effect of administration of superoxide dismutase in prevention of IVH in the beagle puppy model.[131] This enzyme is critical in the defense against free radicals, the formation of which is provoked by hypoxic-ischemic insult.

Platelet and Coagulation Disturbances

Disturbances of platelet-capillary function and coagulation may contribute to the pathogenesis of IVH, although there is a lack of uniformity in results of studies designed to investigate the pathogenetic role of such disturbances.

Platelet-Capillary Function. Forty percent of infants of less than 1500 g birth weight in one study exhibited platelet counts less than 100,000/mm³,[121] and most of these thrombocytopenic infants had abnormal bleeding times. The incidences of IVH in thrombocytopenic versus nonthrombocytopenic infants were 78%, versus 48% for those weighing less than 1000 g. The presence of thrombocytopenia appeared to be an independent pathogenetic factor for causation of IVH. Subsequent work has both confirmed and refuted a role for thrombocytopenia in pathogenesis of IVH.[132, 133] There is also some evidence to suggest that premature infants demonstrate elevated levels of prostacyclin before the occurrence of IVH.[134] Because prostaglandins have an impact not only on platelet function but also on such factors such as cerebral blood flow and free radical production that also may be important in pathogenesis of IVH, it is not clear to what extent effects on platelet-capillary function were independently related to causation of IVH.

Coagulation. Disagreement exists concerning the role of coagulopathy in the causation of IVH.[132,135-137] Because disturbances of coagulation are not uncommon in preterm infants with other provocative factors for IVH (e.g., serious respiratory distress syndrome, asphyxia) or they may occur *secondary* to major hemorrhage, an independent pathogenetic role for such disturbances has been difficult to establish. Although administration of fresh frozen plasma was shown in one study to decrease the incidence of IVH,[138] no effect on coagulation measures accompanied the apparent beneficial effect. Moreover, a later investigation failed to show a beneficial effect of prophylactic early fresh frozen plasma in premature infants.[139,140]

Vascular Factors

Vascular factors that may predispose the blood vessels of the germinal matrix to hemorrhage include the tenuous integrity of matrix capillaries and the vulnerability of these vessels to hypoxic-ischemic injury.

Tenuous Capillary Integrity

Three lines of anatomic evidence suggest that the capillary integrity is tenuous in the germinal matrix. First, these vessels, like the germinal matrix itself, are in a process of involution. Pape

and Wigglesworth[55] characterized the elaborate capillary bed of the germinal matrix as "a persisting immature vascular rete," an immature microvascular network that is remodeled into a mature capillary bed when the matrix disappears. This involuting remodeling capillary bed may be expected to be more susceptible to rupture than would more mature vessels. Second, many studies have emphasized that the matrix microcirculation is composed of simple endothelial-lined vessels, often of a larger size than capillaries but not categorizable as arterioles or venules because of absence of muscle and collagen.[33, 36, 37, 55] Careful studies have documented the absence of muscle[141] and of Type VI collagen.[142] It has been postulated that such vessels are likely to be more susceptible to rupture. Third, an electron microscopic study of cortical and germinal matrix vessels shows a two- to fourfold greater diameter of both the vessels and the lumina of the vessels of the germinal matrix than those of the cortical plate in infants of 25 to 33 weeks of gestation.[143] Thus, in the age range of greatest propensity for occurrence of IVH, the diameters are unusually large, a finding of potential pathogenetic importance because of Laplace's law, which states that the larger the vessel diameter is, the greater the total force on the wall will be at any given pressure.

The possibility should be considered that effects of these maturational deficiencies of germinal matrix vessels underlie the interesting observation that women with a diagnosis of preeclampsia exhibit a much lower risk for an infant with IVH (2.5%) than do women without this diagnosis (17%).[144] This lower risk for IVH has been confirmed.[145, 146] Infants born to preeclamptic mothers exhibit a variety of features suggestive of accelerated maturation of brain and other organs.[135, 147]

Vulnerability to Hypoxic-Ischemic Injury

The matrix capillaries have an increased vulnerability to hypoxic-ischemic injury. Takashima and Tanaka[148] showed that a vascular border zone exists between the end-fields of the striate and thalamic arteries at the usual site for matrix hemorrhage. Thus, it can be postulated that the matrix vessels could be readily injured by ischemia, and, on reperfusion of these injured vessels, hemorrhage could occur. In addition, matrix capillaries, like other brain capillaries, appear to have a high requirement for oxidative metabolism. These brain endothelial cells have been shown to contain three to five times more mitochondria than do systemic capillary endothelial cells.[149] This intense oxidative activity would further enhance the vulnerability of matrix vessels to ischemic insults.

Extravascular Factors

Extravascular factors are those referable to the space surrounding the germinal matrix capillaries. These factors are grouped best into three categories, as discussed in the following subsections.

Deficient Vascular Support

The germinal matrix can be seen by gross examination to be a gelatinous, friable structure and by microscopic examination to be deficient in supporting mesenchymal elements.[33, 69, 150] It appears that the extravascular space provides poor support for the large, endothelial-lined capillaries that course through it and that are the site of the hemorrhage. Gould and Howard[150] assessed astrocytic fibrillary development by immunocytochemical staining for glial fibrillary acidic protein showing minimal astrocytic development as late as 27 weeks of gestation and prominent glial fibrillary acidic protein staining not until 31 weeks in the matrix region. Because of the role of glial fibers in capillary stabilization, these data suggest that deficient astrocytic development may play a role in the pathogenesis of IVH in the premature infant.

Fibrinolytic Activity

An excessive amount of fibrinolytic activity has been defined in the periventricular, germinal matrix region of the human premature infant.[151, 152] Although the source of this activity is not established conclusively, it is likely that the fibrinolytic activity reflects the proteolytic action of a plasmin-generating system involved in developmental remodeling. It is reasonable to suspect that this fibrinolytic activity, an epiphenomenon of the proteolytic system required for remodeling of the germinal matrix, allows the small capillary hemorrhages of the matrix to become the large lesions characteristic of IVH.

MECHANISMS OF BRAIN INJURY

Major Factors

The principal mechanisms of brain injury in the premature infant with IVH relate to one or more of at least the following six major factors (Table 171-4): (1) hypoxic-ischemic injury that may precede the IVH; (2) destruction of germinal matrix with its glial precursors; (3) destruction of periventricular white matter, that is, periventricular hemorrhagic infarction; (4) periventricular white matter injury secondary to intraventricular blood products; (5) a marked increase in intracranial pressure and concomitant defects in cerebral perfusion at the time of severe IVH; and (6) posthemorrhagic hydrocephalus.

Preceding Hypoxic-Ischemic Injury

Neuropathologic studies indicate that infants who die with IVH exhibit two principal lesions related to hypoxic-ischemic insults: periventricular leukomalacia and a subtype of selective neuronal necrosis, pontine and subicular neuronal necrosis. Periventricular leukomalacia has been reported in neuropathologic series in as many as 75% of cases of IVH, and pontine neuronal necrosis is noted in nearly 50%. Moreover, the finding that ventricular dilation correlates strongly with subsequent neurologic and cognitive deficits after IVH, in the absence of progressive hydrocephalus or periventricular hemorrhagic infarction,[153-156] further suggests that concomitant periventricular leukomalacia and cerebral white matter atrophy are common and important in the outcome of infants with IVH.

Destruction of Germinal Matrix and Glial Precursors

One of the consistent neuropathologic consequences of IVH is destruction of germinal matrix with its glial precursor cells. These glial precursor cells are destined to give rise to both oligodendroglia and astrocytes. The loss of the glial precursor cells may affect subsequent cerebral development through the oligodendroglia or astrocytic cell loss. Loss of oligodendroglia cells may lead to a subsequent impairment of myelination after germinal matrix destruction, although evidence to establish such an influence is lacking. The loss of glial precursor cells may also impair subsequent astrocytic development. Gressens and Evrard and their co-workers[157, 158] showed that astrocytes destined for supragranular (upper) cortical layers originate and migrate after the occurrence of neuronal migration and are crucial for normal organizational development of the supragranular cerebral cortex. These astrocytic precursors are likely to be destroyed by germinal matrix hemorrhage, a finding raising the possibility of a subsequent disturbance in cortical development.[158] Such a disturbance would not be detectable by conventional neuropathologic techniques.

TABLE 171-4

Mechanisms of Brain Injury with Germinal Matrix–Intraventricular Hemorrhage

Preceding hypoxic-ischemic injury, especially periventricular leukomalacia
Destruction of glial precursors in germinal matrix—effect on myelination
Destruction of periventricular white matter—periventricular hemorrhagic infarction and subsequent impairment of cortical organization
Periventricular white matter injury secondary to intraventricular, parenchymal, or subarachnoid blood products with vasoconstriction and generation of free radical products
Intracranial hypertension and impaired cerebral perfusion
Posthemorrhagic hydrocephalus

Destruction of Periventricular White Matter: Periventricular Hemorrhagic Infarction

Numerous follow-up studies have correlated cranial ultrasonographic findings in the neonatal period in patients with IVH with the occurrence of subsequent neurologic deficits. These studies confirm that the presence of periventricular hemorrhagic infarction is the single most important determinant of neurologic outcome. Of all survivors of IVH, this lesion accounts for the largest proportion of the subsequent severe neurologic deficits. The deleterious neurologic effects of periventricular hemorrhagic infarction may relate not only to destruction of cerebral white matter per se but also to the effects of the white matter injury on cerebral cortical development. Thus, careful neuropathologic study of cerebral cortical organization in infants who died with major hemorrhagic white matter lesions has shown striking alterations in neuronal axonal and dendritic ramifications in areas overlying the white matter destruction.[159] These abnormalities are postulated to be secondary to disturbances of afferent input to and efferent input from the areas of cortex by disruption of the respective white matter axon. Another potential cause for the cortical abnormalities could be destruction of subplate neurons by the white matter infarction.[160] These neurons are critical for cerebral cortical organization and are abundant in subcortical white matter in the human premature infant. Whatever the mechanism, these *cerebral cortical* abnormalities with periventricular hemorrhagic infarction could be important in determination of subsequent cognitive deficits and seizure disorders.

Periventricular White Matter Injury Secondary to Blood Products

The presence of blood products may have a direct pathogenetic role in the evolution of periventricular white matter injury, as demonstrated by the observation that the presence of IVH is associated with a five- to ninefold increased risk of ultrasonographic correlates (e.g., echolucencies) of white matter injury.[15] Experimental studies suggest that two interacting mechanisms could be operative to produce white matter injury in the presence of IVH: impairment of cerebral blood flow and increased generation of free radicals. *Disturbances of cerebral blood flow* with parenchymal or subarachnoid blood have been demonstrated secondary to local release of vasoconstricting potassium from hemolyzed red blood cells[161] or prostanoids[162] or 5-hydroxytryptamine.[162] Because the walls of cerebral parenchymal vessels do not contain a muscularis necessary for vasospasm in the human premature infant,[141] it seems unlikely that local cerebral blood flow could be affected by this mechanism. However, subarachnoid blood potentially could cause vasoconstriction of major leptomeningeal cerebral vessels, which do contain a muscularis in the human premature.

The more likely mechanism of white matter injury with intraventricular or parenchymal blood involves *increased free radical formation*, provoked by local release of iron from the blood.[163] The presence of blood products is particularly dangerous in the premature infant because the expression of heme oxygenase is especially high in the *immature cerebral white matter*,[164] thus enhancing formation of Fe^{2+} when hemorrhage is present. The Fe^{2+} could then catalyze the generation of the highly reactive and dangerous hydroxyl radical through the Fenton reaction. The early differentiating oligodendroglia has been shown to be exquisitely vulnerable to free radical attack,[165] and thus the enhanced hydroxyl radical generation could accelerate cerebral white matter injury. Although free radical–mediated cellular injury has been proposed as a key pathogenetic factor in cerebral white matter injury in the premature infant, direct evidence heretofore has been lacking. Studies in the premature infant are the first to document an elevation in the early postnatal period in measures of free radical products in the CSF of premature infants with cerebral white matter injury later apparent on MRI at term.[166,167]

Intracranial Hypertension and Impaired Cerebral Perfusion

With massive IVH, intracranial pressure may increase acutely, and, if it is severe enough, the intracranial hypertension may threaten cerebral perfusion. Cerebral perfusion pressure is related to mean arterial blood pressure minus intracranial pressure. In the presence of severe IVH, intracranial pressure as high as 250 to 300 mm of CSF with concomitant systemic hypotension has been observed. This combination is a *rare* occurrence, however, even with large IVH. Experimental studies of the newborn dog demonstrate that instillation of blood into the lateral ventricles can lead to intracranial hypertension, diminished cerebral perfusion pressure, and impaired cerebral blood flow.[87] However, the levels of intracranial pressure in these animal studies, that is, 65 mm Hg, were much higher than expected in the clinical situation. Thus, we consider this mechanism of brain injury with IVH to be rare.

COMPLICATIONS OF INTRAVENTRICULAR HEMORRHAGE

Hydrocephalus

Incidence and Definition

Hydrocephalus, which is a progressive ventricular dilation (PVD) secondary to a disturbance in CSF dynamics, is a not uncommon sequel to IVH (Table 171-5).[2,3,100,168-171] As could be expected, the incidence of posthemorrhagic PVD is related closely to the severity of the initial hemorrhage. A clear clinical distinction between ventriculomegaly secondary to periventricular cerebral atrophy and ventriculomegaly secondary to hydrocephalus with attendant impairment of CSF dynamics can be difficult but is critical for the formulation of appropriate management decisions. In general, the development of ventriculomegaly, secondary to atrophy, occurs slowly, over several weeks, is not associated with the development of increased intracranial pressure or rapid head growth, and evolves to a state of stable ventricular size; that is, ventricular size neither decreases, as in transient hydrocephalus, nor continues to increase, as in persistently progressive hydrocephalus.

Pathogenesis

The pathogenesis of posthemorrhagic hydrocephalus can be considered in terms of either the acute process, apparent within

days, or the subacute-chronic process, apparent within weeks. Acute hydrocephalus appears to be secondary to an impairment of CSF absorption caused by particulate blood clot and demonstrable by ultrasound scan (Fig. 171-8).[172] Subacute-chronic hydrocephalus presumably is related to obliterative arachnoiditis in the posterior fossa where the blood tends to collect.[33] The ventricular dilation may begin essentially with the hemorrhage, especially with marked IVH. More often, definite ventricular dilation and, particularly, the progression thereof begins within 1 to 3 weeks of the hemorrhage.

Relation of Ventricular Dilation to Brain Injury

The precise relation of progressive posthemorrhagic ventricular dilation to brain injury is unclear. This issue is discussed in experimental and clinical studies.

Experimental Studies. The deleterious effects of hydrocephalus on the brain may include disturbances of cerebral white matter, cerebral blood vessels, and cerebral cortex. For *cerebral white matter*, the earliest changes are seen within 1 week after induction of experimental hydrocephalus and involve oligodendrocytes and myelin, with a decrease in myelin-associated enzymes (e.g., ceramide galactosyltransferase) and structural proteins (e.g., myelin basic protein). Later, after several weeks, axonal loss and impaired myelination are apparent. Shunting at 1 week but not at 4 weeks, when axonal loss had occurred, has been shown to allow recovery of myelination.[173] The late occurrence of axonal loss with hydrocephalus was noted in earlier studies.[174-176] Thus, intervention must occur before this stage if prevention of such permanent structural deficits is to be achieved.

A potential role for *cerebral vascular changes and ischemia* in the genesis of the white matter injury in experimental hydrocephalus is demonstrated by morphologic studies that show an alteration in the caliber of major cerebral vessels with a decrease in the secondary and tertiary vessels in the cerebral white matter.[177,178] These changes may explain, at least in part, the decrease in cerebral blood flow and energy metabolism in hydrocephalic animal models.[179-181] Further supportive of cerebral ischemia are the findings in cerebral white matter of increased cerebral rates of glucose metabolism (presumably anaerobic glycolysis), elevated lactate, decreased high-energy phosphates, and elevated free radicals.[182-184] Enhanced free radical production is particularly relevant, in view of the particular vulnerability of differentiating oligodendroglia to free radical attack.[185] These biochemical changes and neurochemical signs of axonal loss have been shown to be prevented by early shunting in the various experimental models.[181,183]

Of additional interest are the documented alterations in *cerebral cortical neurons* in hydrocephalic animal models. Disturbances in catecholaminergic and serotonergic neurotransmitter development and in synaptogenesis with evidence of neuronal degeneration have been delineated.[186-196] These effects may reflect disturbance to ascending and descending axon in cerebral white matter with secondary anterograde and retrograde effects on organizational development of cerebral cortex. Again, these deleterious effects have been shown to be reversible when the hydrocephalic state is corrected early.

Human Studies. Data from studies of infants concerning the deleterious effect of progressive posthemorrhagic ventricular dilation relate to cerebral hemodynamics, neurophysiologic function, morphologic disturbances, biochemical indicators of hypoxia, and clinical outcome. The data are difficult to interpret conclusively because such details as rate of progression, degree and duration of ventriculomegaly, intracranial pressure, preceding parenchymal injury, and neurologic outcome are often not provided.

Concerning *cerebral hemodynamics*, posthemorrhagic hydrocephalus initially has been demonstrated to be associated with *impaired blood flow velocity*,[66,197-200] which can be reversed

TABLE 171–5

Short-Term Outcome of Germinal Matrix-Intraventricular Hemorrhage as a Function of Severity of Hemorrhage

| Grade | Deaths in First 14 Days | | PVD in Survivors > 14 Days Old | | Surgery + Late Death | | Mortality | Surgery in Survivors |
	<750 g (n = 173)	751–1500 g (n = 75)	<750 g (n = 165)	751–1500 g (n = 56)	<750 g (n = 165)	751–1500 g (n = 56)		
I (n = 104)	3/24 (12%)	0/80 (0%)	1/21 (5%)	3/80 (4%)	0 + 4/21 (19%)	0 + 3/80 (0%)	10/104 (10%)	0/94 (0%)
II (n = 65)	5/21 (24%)	1/44 (2%)	1/16 (6%)	6/43 (14%)	0 + 5/16 (31%)	1 + 2/43 (7%)	13/65 (20%)	1/52 (2%)
III (n = 45)	6/19 (32%)	2/26 (8%)	10/13 (77%)	18/24 (75%)	3 + 2/13 (38%)	7 + 4/24 (42%)	14/45 (31%)	10/31 (32%)
IV (n = 34)	5/11 (45%)	5/23 (22%)	5/6 (83%)	12/18 (66%)	1 + 3/6 (66%)	7 + 4/18 (61%)	17/34 (50%)	8/17 (47%)

PVD = progressive ventricular dilation.

with therapy to correct the hydrocephalic state.[66] This disturbance of cerebral blood flow velocity appears to correlate more closely with ventriculomegaly than with increased intracranial pressure.

Concerning *neurophysiologic function,* visual evoked potentials, brain stem auditory evoked potentials, and somatosensory evoked responses have all been shown to be altered by posthemorrhagic ventricular dilation. The studies have demonstrated prolonged latencies of these evoked potentials with posthemorrhagic hydrocephalus in the premature infant.[201-203] Improvement in latencies was demonstrated after CSF removal by placement of a ventriculoperitoneal shunt or direct removal of ventricular fluid.[201-203] These data suggest that an axonal disturbance is caused by ventricular distention, and this disturbance can be reversed by effective therapy.

Concerning *morphologic evidence of brain injury* with posthemorrhagic ventricular dilation, there is a paucity of data from studies of autopsied human infants who do not have markedly advanced disease. Studies of biopsies taken at the time of ventriculoperitoneal shunt placement have shown four major findings: (1) disruption of ependyma, (2) direct evidence of axonal injury ("axonal ballooning"), (3) lipid-laden microglia, and (4) diminished numbers of myelinated axons.[175, 204-207] These findings are consistent with the experimental models of hydrocephalus.

Biochemical evidence of hypoxia has been observed and suggests injury to brain that is reversible by therapy.[208] E*levated CSF levels of hypoxanthine,* a marker for hypoxic tissue, have been found in infants with posthemorrhagic hydrocephalus that

reduced significantly after successful treatment.[208] Although the morphologic effects of hydrocephalus on cerebral vessels and the resulting deleterious cerebral hemodynamic effects are a probable explanation for tissue hypoxia, elevated levels of vasoconstricting eicosanoids (e.g., thromboxanes) or edema-producing eicosanoids (e.g., leukotrienes) appear important. These eicosanoids have been shown to be elevated in CSF of infants with posthemorrhagic hydrocephalus.[209] The source of these compounds remains unclear, and their specific relation to the posthemorrhagic ventricular dilation remains to be established. Biochemical evidence of oxygen deficiency at the mitochondrial level is found with the demonstration by near-infrared spectroscopy of an increase in *brain levels* of *oxidized cytochrome aa_3,* after lumbar puncture in infants with posthemorrhagic hydrocephalus accompanied by increased intracranial pressure.[210,211] This observation is consistent with the demonstration by positron emission tomography of increases in cerebral metabolic rate for oxygen in several infants (one newborn) after treatment of hydrocephalus.[212] More data are needed on these issues.

Natural History

Management of progressive posthemorrhagic ventricular dilation must begin with recognition of the natural history of the disorder.[2, 3, 19, 89, 100, 169-171, 213-229] We undertook a large study of premature infants to reflect the natural history of PVD. In this cohort of 248 very low birth weight infants with IVH (mean gestational age, 27 weeks), 25% of the infants exhibited PVD (Fig. 171–9). Arrest of PVD occurred without treatment in one-

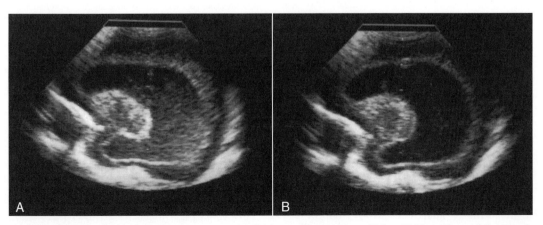

Figure 171–8. **A** and **B,** Acute hydrocephalus with intraventricular hemorrhage. (From Volpe JJ: Neurology of the Newborn, 4th ed. Philadelphia, WB Saunders Co, 2001, p 458.)

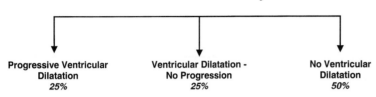

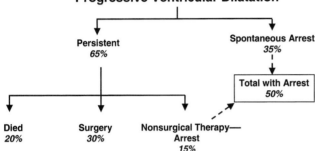

Figure 171–9. Natural history of very low birth weight infants with posthemorrhagic ventricular dilatation.

third of infants with PVD. Of the remaining two-thirds of infants who did not have arrested PVD and thus had persistent PVD, most received nonsurgical therapy consisting of pharmacologic therapy or drainage of CSF by serial lumbar punctures only. Half of the patients with persistent PVD received surgical therapy with insertion of a ventriculoperitoneal reservoir or shunt, and one-third of the infants with persistent PVD died (see Fig. 171-9). The development of PVD after IVH and the occurrence of adverse short-term outcome, such as the requirement for surgical therapy, were predicted most strongly by the severity of IVH (see Table 171-5). These data demonstrate that despite a slight reduction in the overall incidence of PVD, there appears to be a more aggressive course with appreciable mortality and morbidity in the extremely premature infant characteristic of current neonatal intensive care facilities. The major predictor of adverse short-term outcome, defined as death or the need for surgical intervention for PVD, was the severity of IVH (see Fig. 171-9 and Table 171-5).

PROGNOSIS

The prognosis of IVH is considered best in terms of the short-term outcome (mortality rate and development of PVD) and the long-term outcome (neurologic sequelae). The *short-term outcome* relates clearly to the severity of the hemorrhage. The mortality rates and incidences of progressive posthemorrhagic ventricular dilation (i.e., hydrocephalus) are shown in Table 171-5 as a function of the severity of the hemorrhage, documented primarily by ultrasound scan.[3, 15, 230-233] With small lesions, confined to the germinal matrix or accompanied by small amounts of intraventricular blood, mortality rates are low, and the likelihood of PVD in survivors is rare, such that outcome is comparable to that seen in small premature infants without IVH. In contrast, infants with severe lesions, that is, blood filling the ventricles, have high mortality rates (approximately 20%), and more than half of the survivors exhibit PVD. The *long-term outcome* of the infant with IVH depends on the degree of parenchymal injury. Only an approximate relationship exists between the quantity of intraventricular blood and the neurologic outcome (Table 171-6).[19, 40, 44, 171, 215, 216, 226, 228, 230, 233-243] A particular variety of spastic hemiparesis is characteristic of periventricular hemorrhagic infarction. Involvement of the lower extremities is as prominent as involvement of the upper

TABLE 171-6

Long-Term Outcome: Neurologic Sequelae with Germinal Matrix-Intraventricular Hemorrhage as a Function of Severity of Hemorrhage

Severity of Hemorrhage	Incidence of Neurologic Sequelae (%)
Mild	5
Moderate	15
Severe	35
Severe + apparent periventricular hemorrhagic infarction	50-100

extremities. The particular propensity for lesions affecting posterior cerebral white matter to result in cognitive deficits may relate to the presence of fibers crucial for associative functions and integration of visual, auditory, and somesthetic input.

REFERENCES

1. Volpe JJ: Neurology of the Newborn, 4th ed. Philadelphia, WB Saunders Co, 2001.
2. Levene MI, et al: Cerebral structure and intraventricular haemorrhage in the neonate: a real-time ultrasound study. Arch Dis Child 56:416, 1981.
3. Ahmann PA, et al: Intraventricular hemorrhage in the high-risk preterm infant: incidence and outcome. Ann Neurol 7:118, 1980.
4. Papile LA, et al: Incidence and evolution of subependymal and intraventricular hemorrhage: a study of infants with birth weights less than 1,500 gm. J Pediatr 92:529, 1978.
5. Paneth N, et al: Incidence and timing of germinal matrix/intraventricular hemorrhage in low birth weight infants. Am J Epidemiol 137:1167, 1993.
6. Sheth RD: Trends in incidence and severity of intraventricular hemorrhage. J Child Neurol 13:261, 1998.
7. Horbar JD: Vermont-Oxford Network 1997 Database Summary. Burlington, VT, Vermont-Oxford Network, 1997.
8. Guyer B, et al: Annual summary of vital statistics: 1998. Pediatrics 104:1229, 1999.
9. Wilcox AJ, Skjoerven R: Birth weight and perinatal mortality: the effect of gestational age. Am J Public Health 82:378, 1992.
10. McIntire DD, et al: Birth weight in relation to morbidity and mortality among newborn infants. N Engl J Med 340:1234, 1999.
11. Dubowitz LM, et al: Neurologic signs in neonatal intraventricular hemorrhage: a correlation with real-time ultrasound. J Pediatr 99:127, 1981.
12. Volpe JJ: Intracranial hemorrhage in the newborn: current understanding and dilemmas. Neurology 29:632, 1979.

13. Lazzara A, et al: Clinical predictability of intraventricular hemorrhage in preterm infants. Pediatrics 65:30, 1980.
14. Mantovani JF, et al: Failure of daily lumbar punctures to prevent the development of hydrocephalus following intraventricular hemorrhage. J Pediatr 97:278, 1980.
15. Kuban K, et al: White matter disorders of prematurity: association with intraventricular hemorrhage and ventriculomegaly. J Pediatr 134:539, 1999.
16. Babcock DS, Han BK: The accuracy of high resolution, real-time ultrasonography of the head in infancy. Radiology 139:665, 1981.
17. Fleischer AC, et al: The role of sonography and the radiologist-ultrasonologist in the detection and follow-up of intracranial hemorrhage in the preterm neonate. Radiology 139:733, 1981.
18. Grant EG, et al: Real-time ultrasonography of neonatal intraventricular hemorrhage and comparison with computed tomography. Radiology 139:687, 1981.
19. Shankaran S, et al: Sonographic classification of intracranial hemorrhage: a prognostic indicator of mortality, morbidity, and short-term neurologic outcome. J Pediatr 100:469, 1982.
20. Allan WC, Philip AG: Neonatal cerebral pathology diagnosed by ultrasound. Clin Perinatol 12:195, 1985.
21. Levene MI, et al: Ultrasound of the Infant Brain. London, Blackwell Scientific, 1985.
22. Perlman JM, Volpe JJ: Intraventricular hemorrhage in extremely small premature infants. Am J Dis Child 140:1122, 1986.
23. Perlman JM, Volpe JJ: Cerebral blood flow velocity in relation to intraventricular hemorrhage in the premature newborn infant. J Pediatr 100:956, 1982.
24. Levene MI, de VL: Extension of neonatal intraventricular haemorrhage. Arch Dis Child 59:631, 1984.
25. Krishnamoorthy KS, et al: Evaluation of neonatal intracranial hemorrhage by computerized tomography. Pediatrics 59:165, 1977.
26. Rumack CM, et al: CT detection and course of intracranial hemorrhage in premature infants. AJR Am J Roentgenol 131:493, 1978.
27. McArdle CB, et al: Abnormalities of the neonatal brain: MR imaging. I. Intracranial hemorrhage. Radiology 163:387, 1987.
28. Haddad J, et al: Single photon emission computed tomography of the brain perfusion in neonates. In Haddad J, et al (eds): Imaging Techniques Of the CNS Of the Neonates. New York, Springer-Verlag, 1991, pp 161–170.
29. Zuerrer M, et al: MR imaging of intracranial hemorrhage in neonates and infants at 2.35 tesla. Neuroradiology 33:223, 1991.
30. Barkovich AJ: Pediatric neuroimaging, 2nd ed. New York, Raven Press, 1995.
31. Szymonowicz W, et al: Ultrasound and necropsy study of periventricular haemorrhage in preterm infants. Arch Dis Child 59:637, 1984.
32. Armstrong DL, et al: Neuropathologic findings in short-term survivors of intraventricular hemorrhage. Am J Dis Child 141:617, 1987.
33. Larroche JC: Intraventricular hemorrhage in the premature neonate. In Korobkin R, Guilleminault C (eds): Advances In Perinatal Neurology, Vol 1. New York, SP Medical and Scientific Books, 1979, p 115.
34. Rorke LB: Pathology of Perinatal Brain Injury. New York, Raven Press, 1982.
35. Nakamura Y, et al: Germinal matrix hemorrhage of venous origin in preterm neonates. Hum Pathol 21:1059, 1990.
36. Ghazi-Birry HS, et al: Human germinal matrix: venous origin of hemorrhage and vascular characteristics. AJNR Am J Neuroradiol 18:219, 1997.
37. Leech RW, Kohnen P: Subependymal and intraventricular hemorrhages in the newborn. Am J Pathol 77:465, 1974.
38. Golden JA, et al: Frequency of neuropathological abnormalities in very low birth weight infants. J Neuropathol Exp Neurol 56:472, 1997.
39. Fanaroff AA, et al: Very-low-birth-weight outcomes of the National Institute of Child Health and Human Development Neonatal Research Network, May 1991 through December 1992. Am J Obstet Gynecol 173:1423, 1995.
40. Guzzetta F, et al: Periventricular intraparenchymal echodensities in the premature newborn: critical determinant of neurologic outcome. Pediatrics 78:995, 1986.
41. Gould SJ, et al: Periventricular intraparenchymal cerebral haemorrhage in preterm infants: the role of venous infarction. J Pathol 151:197, 1987.
42. Rademaker KJ, et al: Unilateral haemorrhagic parenchymal lesions in the preterm infant: shape, site and prognosis. Acta Paediatr 83:602, 1994.
43. Takashima S, et al: Pathogenesis of periventricular white matter hemorrhages in preterm infants. Brain Dev 8:25, 1986.
44. Perlman JM, et al: Relationship between periventricular intraparenchymal echodensities and germinal matrix-intraventricular hemorrhage in the very low birth weight neonate. Pediatrics 91:474, 1993.
45. Ment LR, et al: Risk factors for early intraventricular hemorrhage in low birth weight infants. J Pediatr 121:776–83, 1992.
46. Taylor GA: Effect of germinal matrix hemorrhage on terminal vein position and patency. Pediatr Radiol 25:S37, 1995.
47. Counsell SJ, et al: Periventricular haemorrhagic infarct in a preterm neonate. Eur J Paediatr Neurol 3:25, 1999.
48. Fawer CL, Levene MI: Elusive blood clots and fluctuating ventricular dilatation after neonatal intraventricular haemorrhage. Arch Dis Child 57:158, 1982.
49. Whitelaw A, et al: Low levels of plasminogen in cerebrospinal fluid after intraventricular haemorrhage: a limiting factor for clot lysis? Acta Paediatr 84:933, 1995.
50. Larroche JC: Post-haemorrhagic hydrocephalus in infancy: anatomical study. Biol Neonate 20:287, 1972.
51. Fukumizu M, et al: Glial reaction in periventricular areas of the brainstem in fetal and neonatal posthemorragic hydrocephalus and congenital hydrocephalus. Brain Dev 18:40, 1996.
52. Skullerud K, Westre B: Frequency and prognostic significance of germinal matrix hemorrhage, periventricular leukomalacia, and pontosubicular necrosis in preterm neonates. Acta Neuropathol (Berl) 70:257, 1986.
53. Armstrong D, Norman MG: Periventricular leucomalacia in neonates: complications and sequelae. Arch Dis Child 49:367, 1974.
54. Torvik A, et al: Affection of the hippocampal granule cells in pontosubicular neuron necrosis. Acta Neuropathol 83:535, 1992.
55. Pape KE, Wigglesworth JS: Haemorrhage, Ischaemia and the Perinatal Brain. Philadelphia, JB Lippincott, 1979.
56. Friede RL. Developmental Neuropathology, 2nd ed. New York, Springer-Verlag, 1989.
57. Ahdab-Barmada M, et al: Pontosubicular necrosis and hyperoxemia. Pediatrics 66:840, 1980.
58. Perlman JM, et al: Fluctuating cerebral blood-flow velocity in respiratory-distress syndrome: relation to the development of intraventricular hemorrhage. N Engl J Med 309:204, 1983.
59. van Bel F, et al: Aetiological role of cerebral blood-flow alterations in development and extension of peri-intraventricular haemorrhage. Dev Med Child Neurol 29:601, 1987.
60. Miall-Allen VM, et al: Blood pressure fluctuation and intraventricular hemorrhage in the preterm infant of less than 31 weeks' gestation. Pediatrics 83:657, 1989.
61. Perlman J, Thach B: Respiratory origin of fluctuations in arterial blood pressure in premature infants with respiratory distress syndrome. Pediatrics 81:399, 1988.
62. Coughtrey H, et al: Variability in cerebral blood flow velocity: observations over one minute in preterm babies. Early Hum Dev 47:63, 1997.
63. Rennie JM: Cerebral blood flow velocity variability after cardiovascular support in premature babies. Arch Dis Child 64:897, 1989.
64. Coughtrey H, et al: Factors associated with respiration induced variability in cerebral blood flow velocity. Arch Dis Child 68:312, 1993.
65. Goldberg RN, et al: The association of rapid volume expansion and intraventricular hemorrhage in the preterm infant. J Pediatr 96:1060, 1980.
66. Hill A, et al: Relationship of pneumothorax to occurrence of intraventricular hemorrhage in the premature newborn. Pediatrics 69:144, 1982.
67. Marshall TA, et al: Physiologic changes associated with ligation of the ductus arteriosus in preterm infants. J Pediatr 101:749, 1982.
68. Funato M, et al: Clinical events in association with timing of intraventricular hemorrhage in preterm infants. J Pediatr 121:614, 1992.
69. Hambleton G, Wigglesworth JS: Origin of intraventricular haemorrhage in the preterm infant. Arch Dis Child 51:651, 1976.
70. Lou HC, et al: Impaired autoregulation of cerebral blood flow in the distressed newborn infant. J Pediatr 94:118, 1979.
71. Pryds O, et al: Heterogeneity of cerebral vasoreactivity in preterm infants supported by mechanical ventilation. J Pediatr 115:638, 1989.
72. Pryds O: Control of cerebral circulation in the high-risk neonate. Ann Neurol 30:321, 1991.
73. Pryds O, Edwards AD: Cerebral blood flow in the newborn infant. Arch Dis Child 74:F63, 1996.
74. Tsuji M, et al: Cerebral intravascular oxygenation correlates with mean arterial pressure in critically ill premature infants. Pediatrics 106:625, 2000.
75. Menke J, et al: Cross-spectral analysis of cerebral autoregulation dynamics in high risk preterm infants during the perinatal period. Pediatr Res 42:690, 1997.
76. Muller AM, et al: Loss of CO_2 reactivity of cerebral blood flow is associated with severe brain damage in mechanically ventilated very low birth weight infants. Eur J Paediatr Neurol 5:157, 1997.
77. Greisen G: Cerebral blood flow in preterm infants during the first week of life. Acta Paediatr Scand 75:43, 1986.
78. Blankenberg FG, et al: Impaired cerebrovascular autoregulation after hypoxic-ischemic injury in extremely low-birth-weight neonates: detection with power and pulsed wave Doppler US. Radiology 205:563, 1997.
79. Perry EH, et al: Blood pressure increases, birth weight–dependent stability boundary, and intraventricular hemorrhage. Pediatrics 85:727, 1990.
80. Goldberg RN: Sustained arterial blood pressure elevation associated with pneumothoraces: early detection via continuous monitoring. Pediatrics 68:775, 1981.
81. Omar SY, et al: Blood pressure responses to care procedures in ventilated preterm infants. Acta Paediatr Scand 74:920, 1985.
82. Perlman JM, Volpe JJ: Suctioning in the preterm infant: effects on cerebral blood flow velocity, intracranial pressure, and arterial blood pressure. Pediatrics 72:329, 1983.
83. Rahilly PM: Effects of sleep state and feeding on cranial blood flow of the human neonate. Arch Dis Child 55:265, 1980.
84. Sonesson SE, et al: Changes in intracranial arterial blood flow velocities during surgical ligation of the patent ductus arteriosus. Acta Paediatr Scand 75:36, 1986.
85. Shah AR, et al: Fluctuations in cerebral oxygenation and blood volume during endotracheal suctioning in premature infants. J Pediatr 120:769, 1992.
86. Anand KJS, et al: Analgesia and sedation in preterm neonates who require ventilatory support: results from the NOPAIN trial. Arch Pediatr Adolesc Med 153:331, 1999.

87. Batton DG, et al: Effect of pneumothorax-induced systemic blood pressure alterations on the cerebral circulation in newborn dogs. Pediatrics 74:350, 1984.

88. Wallin LA, et al: Neonatal intracranial hemorrhage. II. Risk factor analysis in an inborn population. Early Hum Dev 23:129, 1990.

89. Hill A, Volpe JJ: Normal pressure hydrocephalus in the newborn. Pediatrics 68:623, 1981.

90. Goddard-Finegold J, et al: Intraventricular hemorrhage following volume expansion after hypovolemic hypotension in the newborn beagle. J Pediatr 100:796, 1982.

91. Ment LR, et al: Beagle puppy model of intraventricular hemorrhage. J Neurosurg 57:219, 1982.

92. Pasternak JF, Groothuis DR: Regional variability of blood flow and glucose utilization within the subependymal germinal matrix. Brain Res 299:281, 1984.

93. Ment LR, et al: Thromboxane synthesis inhibitor in a beagle pup model of perinatal asphyxia. Stroke 20:809, 1989.

94. Reynolds ML, et al: Intracranial haemorrhage in the preterm sheep fetus. Early Hum Dev 3:163, 1979.

95. Goddard J, et al: Intraventricular hemorrhage: an animal model. Biol Neonate 37:39, 1980.

96. Pryds O, et al: Compensatory increase of CBF in preterm infants during hypoglycaemia. Acta Paediatr Scand 77:632, 1988.

97. Wyatt JS, et al: Response of cerebral blood volume to changes in arterial carbon dioxide tension in preterm and term infants. Pediatr Res 29:553, 1991.

98. Kuban KC, et al: Neonatal intracranial hemorrhage and phenobarbital. Pediatrics 77:4430, 1986.

99. Levene MI, et al: Risk factors in the development of intraventricular haemorrhage in the preterm neonate. Arch Dis Child 57:410, 1982.

100. Szymonowicz W, et al: Antecedents of periventricular haemorrhage in infants weighing 1250 g or less at birth. Arch Dis Child 59:13, 1984.

101. Lipp-Zwahlen AE, et al: Oxygen affinity of haemoglobin modulates cerebral blood flow in premature infants: a study with the non-invasive xenon-133 method. Acta Paediatr Scand Suppl 360:26, 1989.

102. Ramaekers VT, et al: The effect of blood transfusion on cerebral blood-flow in preterm infants: a Doppler study. Dev Med Child Neurol 30:334, 1988.

103. Svenningsen L, et al: Measurements of fetal head compression pressure during bearing down and their relationship to the condition of the newborn. Acta Obstet Gynecol Scand 67:129, 1988.

104. Leviton A, et al: Labor and delivery characteristics and the risk of germinal matrix haemorrhage in low birth weight infants. J Child Neurol 6:35, 1991.

105. Shankaran S, et al: Prenatal and perinatal risk and protective factors for neonatal intracranial hemorrhage. Arch Pediatr Adolesc Med 150:491, 1996.

106. O'Shea M, et al: Prenatal events and the risk of subependymal/intraventricular haemorrhage in very low birthweight neonates. Paediatr Perinat Epidemiol 6:352, 1992.

107. Shaver DC, et al: Early and late intraventricular hemorrhage: the role of obstetric factors. Obstet Gynecol 80:831, 1992.

108. Pellicer A, et al: Noninvasive continuous monitoring of the effects of head position on brain hemodynamics in ventilated infants. Pediatrics 109:434, 2002.

109. Leahy FA, et al: Cranial blood volume changes during mechanical ventilation and spontaneous breathing in newborn infants. J Pediatr 101:984, 1982.

110. Vert P, et al: Intracranial venous pressure in newborns: variation in physiologic state and in neurologic and respiratory disorders. In Stern L, et al (eds): Intensive Care in the Newborn. New York, Masson, 1976, p 185.

111. Vert P, et al: Continuous positive airway pressure and hydrocephalus. Lancet 2:319, 1973.

112. Cowan F, Thoresen M: The effects of intermittent positive pressure ventilation on cerebral arterial and venous blood velocities in the newborn infant. Acta Paediatr Scand 76:239, 1987.

113. Skinner JR, et al: Central venous pressure in the ventilated neonate. Arch Dis Child 67(Suppl 1):374, 1991.

114. Simmons DH, et al: Acute circulatory effects of pneumothorax in dogs. J Appl Physiol 12:255, 1958.

115. HIFI Study Group: High frequency oscillatory ventilation compared with conventional mechanical ventilation in the treatment of respiratory failure in preterm infants. N Engl J Med 320:88, 1989.

116. Henderson-Smart DJ, et al: Elective high frequency oscillatory ventilation versus conventional ventilation for acute pulmonary dysfunction in preterm infants. Cochrane Database Syst Rev CD000104, 2001.

117. Moriette G, et al: Prospective randomized multicentre comparison of high-frequency oscillatory ventilation and conventional ventilation in preterm infants of less than 30 weeks with respiratory distress syndrome. Pediatrics 107:363, 2001.

118. Laubscher B, et al: Haemodynamic changes during high frequency oscillation for respiratory distress syndrome. Arch Dis Child 74:F172, 1996.

119. Leviton A, et al: The epidemiology of germinal matrix hemorrhage during the first half-day of life. Dev Med Child Neurol 33:138, 1991.

120. Tejani N, Verma UL: Correlation of Apgar scores and umbilical artery acid-base status to mortality and morbidity in the low birth weight neonate. Obstet Gynecol 73:597, 1989.

121. Amato M, et al: Correlation of raised cord-blood CK-BB and the development of peri-intraventricular hemorrhage in preterm infants. Neuropediatrics 17:173, 1986.

122. van de Bor M, et al: Serum creatine kinase BB as predictor of periventricular haemorrhage in preterm infants. Early Hum Dev 17:165, 1988.

123. Perlman JM, Risser R: Relationship of uric acid concentrations and severe intraventricular hemorrhage/leukomalacia in the premature infant. J Pediatr 132:436, 1998.

124. Greisen G, et al: EEG depression and germinal layer haemorrhage in the newborn. Acta Paediatr Scand 76:519, 1987.

125. Connell J, et al: Predictive value of early continuous electroencephalogram monitoring in ventilated preterm infants with intraventricular hemorrhage. Pediatrics 82:337, 1988.

126. Finer NN, et al: Cardiopulmonary resuscitation in the very low birth weight infant: The Vermont-Oxford Network Experience. Pediatrics 104:428, 1999.

127. Watkins AM, et al: Blood pressure and cerebral haemorrhage and ischaemia in very low birthweight infants. Early Hum Dev 19:103, 1989.

128. Bada HS, et al: Frequent handling in the neonatal intensive care unit and intraventricular hemorrhage. J Pediatr 117:126, 1990.

129. Meek JH, et al: Low cerebral blood flow is a risk factor for severe intraventricular haemorrhage. Arch Dis Child 81:F15, 1999.

130. Evans N, Kluckow M: Early ductal shunting and intraventricular haemorrhage in ventilated preterm infants. Arch Dis Child 75:F183, 1996.

131. Ment LR: Beagle puppy model of intraventricular hemorrhage: effect of superoxide dismutase on cerebral blood flow and prostaglandins. J Neurosurg 62:563, 1985.

132. Amato M, et al: Coagulation abnormalities in low birth weight infants with peri-intraventricular hemorrhage. Neuropediatrics 19:154, 1988.

133. Lupton BA, et al: Reduced platelet count as a risk factor for intraventricular hemorrhage. Am J Dis Child 142:1222, 1988.

134. Rennie JM, et al: Elevated levels of immunoreactive prostacyclin metabolite in babies who develop intraventricular haemorrhage. Acta Paediatr Scand 76:19, 1987.

135. Kuban K, Volpe JJ: Intraventricular hemorrhage: an update. J Intensive Care Med 8:157, 1993.

136. van de Bor M, et al: Hemostasis and periventricular-intraventricular hemorrhage of the newborn. Am J Dis Child 140:1131 1986.

137. Setzer ES, et al: Platelet dysfunction and coagulopathy in intraventricular hemorrhage in the premature infant. J Pediatr 100:599, 1982.

138. Beverley DW, et al: Prevention of intraventricular haemorrhage by fresh frozen plasma. Arch Dis Child 60:710, 1985.

139. Northern Neonatal Nursing Initiative Trial Group: Randomised trial of prophylactic early fresh-frozen plasma or gelatin or glucose in preterm babies: outcome at 2 years. Lancet 348:229, 1996.

140. Northern Neonatal Nursing Initiative Trial Group: A randomized trial comparing the effect of prophylactic intravenous fresh frozen plasma, gelatin or glucose on early mortality and morbidity in preterm babies. Eur J Pediatr 154:580, 1995.

141. Kuban KC, Gilles FH: Human telencephalic angiogenesis. Ann Neurol 17:539, 1985.

142. Kamei A, et al: Developmental change in type VI collagen in human cerebral vessels. Pediatr Neurol 8:183, 1992.

143. Grunnet ML: Morphometry of blood vessels in the cortex and germinal plate of premature neonates. Pediatr Neurol 5:12, 1989.

144. Kuban KC, et al: Maternal toxemia is associated with reduced incidence of germinal matrix hemorrhage in premature babies. J Child Neurol 7:70, 1992.

145. Perlman JM, et al: Pregnancy-induced hypertension and reduced intraventricular hemorrhage in preterm infants. Pediatr Neurol 17:29, 1997.

146. Leviton A, et al: Maternal receipt of magnesium sulfate does not seem to reduce the risk of neonatal white matter damage. Pediatrics 99:1, 1997.

147. Amiel-Tison C, Pettigrew AG: Adaptive changes in the developing brain during intrauterine stress. Brain Dev 13:67, 1991.

148. Takashima S, Tanaka K: Microangiography and vascular permeability of the subependymal matrix in the premature infant. Can J Neurol Sci 5:45, 1978.

149. Oldendorf WH, et al: The large apparent work capability of the blood-brain barrier: a study of the mitochondrial content of capillary endothelial cells in brain and other tissues of the rat. Ann Neurol 1:409, 1977.

150. Gould SJ, Howard S: An immunohistochemical study of the germinal layer in the late gestation human fetal brain. Neuropathol Appl Neurobiol 13:421, 1987.

151. Gilles FH, et al: Fibrinolytic activity in the ganglionic eminence of the premature human brain. Biol Neonate 18:426, 1971.

152. Takashima S, Tanaka K: Microangiography and fibrinolytic activity in subependymal matrix of the premature brain. Brain Dev 4:222, 1972.

153. Krishnamoorthy KS, et al: Periventricular-intraventricular hemorrhage, sonographic localization, phenobarbital, and motor abnormalities in low birth weight infants. Pediatrics 85:1027, 1990.

154. Whitaker AH, et al: Neonatal cranial ultrasound abnormalities in low birth weight infants: relation to cognitive outcomes at six years of age. Pediatrics 98:719, 1996.

155. Pinto-Martin JA, et al: Cranial ultrasound prediction of disabling and nondisabling cerebral palsy at age two in a low birth weight population. 1995 95:249, 1995.

156. Leviton A, Gilles F: Ventriculomegaly, delayed myelination, white matter hypoplasia, and "periventricular" leukomalacia. How are they related? Pediatr Neurol 15:127, 1996.

157. Gressens P, et al: The germinative zone produces the most cortical astrocytes after neuronal migration in the developing mammalian brain. Biol Neonate 61:4, 1992.

158. Evrard P, et al: New concepts to understand the neurological consequences of subcortical lesions in the premature brain (editorial). Biol Neonate 61:1, 1992.

159. Marin-Padilla M: Developmental neuropathology and impact of perinatal brain damage. II. White matter lesions of the neocortex. J Neuropathol Exp Neurol 56:2195, 1997.

160. Volpe JJ: Subplate neurons: missing link in brain injury of the premature infant? Pediatrics 97:112, 1996.

161. Stutchfield PR, Cooke RW: Electrolytes and glucose in cerebrospinal fluid of premature infants with intraventricular haemorrhage: role of potassium in cerebral infarction. Arch Dis Child 64:470, 1989.

162. Yakubu MA, et al: Hematoma-induced enhanced cerebral vasoconstrictions to leukotriene C₄ and endothelin-1 in piglets: role of prostanoids. Pediatr Res 38:119, 1995.

163. Rehncrona S, et al: Enhancement of iron-catalyzed free radical formation by acidosis in brain homogenates: difference in effect by lactic acid and CO₂. J Cereb Blood Flow Metab 9:65, 1989.

164. Bergeron M, et al: Developmental expression of heme oxygenase-1 (HSP32) in rat brain: an immunocytochemical study. Dev Brain Res 105:181, 1998.

165. Back SA, et al: Maturation-dependent vulnerability of oligodendrocytes to oxidative stress-induced death caused by glutathione depletion. J Neurosci 18:6241, 1998.

166. Inder TE, et al: Elevation of oxidative injury markers in the CNS with periventricular leukomalacia in a premature infant with meningitis. J Pediatr 8:102, 2002.

167. Inder TE, et al: Elevated free radical products in the cerebrospinal fluid of VLBW infants with cerebral white matter injury. Pediatr Res 16:68, 2002.

168. Murphy BP, et al: Posthemorrhagic ventricular dilatation in the premature infant: natural history and predictors ofd outcome. Arch Dis Child 32:110, 2002.

169. Partridge JC, et al: Optimal timing for diagnostic cranial ultrasound in low-birth-weight infants: detection of intracranial hemorrhage and ventricular dilation. J Pediatr 102:281, 1983.

170. Perlman JM, et al: Late hydrocephalus after arrest and resolution of neonatal post-hemorrhagic hydrocephalus. Dev Med Child Neurol 32:725, 1990.

171. Ventriculomegaly Trial Group: Randomised trial of early tapping in neonatal posthaemorrhagic ventricular dilatation. Arch Dis Child 65:3, 1990.

172. Hill AH, et al: A potential mechanism for pathogenesis for early posthemorrhagic hydrocephalus in the premature newborn. Pediatrics 73:19, 1985.

173. DelBigio MR, et al: Myelination delay in the cerebral white matter of immature rats with kaolin-induced hydrocephalus is reversible. J Neuropathol Exp Neurol 56:1053, 1997.

174. Milhorat TH, et al: Structural, ultrastructural, and permeability changes in the ependyma and surrounding brain favoring equilibration in progressive hydrocephalus. Arch Neurol 22:397, 1970.

175. Weller RO, Shulman K: Infantile hydrocephalus: clinical, histological, and ultrastructural study of brain damage. J Neurosurg 36:255, 1972.

176. Rubin RC, et al: Hydrocephalus. I. Histological and ultrastructural changes in the pre-shunted cortical mantle. Surg Neurol 5:109, 1976.

177. Del Bigio MR, Bruni JE: Periventricular pathology in hydrocephalic rabbits before and after shunting. Acta Neuropathol (Berl) 77:186, 1988.

178. Wozniak M, et al: Micro- and macrovascular changes as the direct cause of parenchymal destruction in congenital murine hydrocephalus. J Neurosurg 43:535, 1975.

179. Jones HC, et al: Local cerebral blood flow in rats with congenital hydrocephalus. J Cereb Blood Flow Metab 13:531, 1993.

180. Matsumae M, et al: Energy metabolism in kaolin-induced hydrocephalic rat brain. Childs Nerv Syst 6:392, 1990.

181. Da Silva MC, et al: Reduced local cerebral blood flow in periventricular white matter in experimental neonatal hydrocephalus: restoration with CSF shunting. J Cereb Blood Flow Metab 15:1057, 1995.

182. Chumas PD, et al: Anaerobic glycolysis preceding white matter destruction in experimental neonatal hydrocephalus. J Neurosurg 80:491, 1994.

183. Da Silva MC, et al: High-energy phosphate metabolism in a neonatal model of hydrocephalus before and after shunting. J Neurosurg 81:544, 1994.

184. Braun KPJ, et al: Cerebral ischemia and white matter edema in experimental hydrocephalus: a combined in vivo MRI and MRS study. Brain Res 757:295, 1997.

185. Socci DJ, et al: Evidence that oxidative stress is associated with the pathophysiology of inherited hydrocephalus in the H-Tx rat model. Exp Neurol 155:109, 1999.

186. Lovely TJ, et al: Effects of hydrocephalus and surgical decompression on cortical norepinephrine levels in neonatal cats. Neurosurgery 24:43, 1989.

187. Wright LC, et al: Cytological and cytoarchitectural changes in the feline cerebral cortex during experimental infantile hydrocephalus. Pediatr Neurosurg 16:139, 1990.

188. Miyazawa T, Sato K: Learning disability and impairment of synaptogenesis in HTX-rats with arrested shunt-dependent hydrocephalus. Childs Nerv Syst 7:121, 1991.

189. Miyazawa T, et al: Cortical synaptogenesis in congenitally hydrocephalic HTX-rats using monoclonal anti-synaptic vesicle protein antibody. Brain Dev 14:75, 1992.

190. Suzuki F, et al: Effects of congenital hydrocephalus on serotonergic input and barrel cytoarchitecture in the developing somatosensory cortex of rats. Childs Nerv Syst 8:18, 1992.

191. Suda K, et al: Changes of synapse-related proteins (SVP-38 and Drebrins) during development of brain in congenitally hydrocephalic HTX rats with and without early placement of ventriculoperitoneal shunt. Pediatr Neurosurg 20:50, 1994.

192. Suda K, et al: Early ventriculoperitoneal shunt: effects on learning ability and synaptogenesis of the brain in congenitally hydrocephalic HTX rats. Childs Nerv Syst 10:19, 1994.

193. Miyazawa T, Sato K: Hippocampal synaptogenesis in hydrocephalic HTX-rats using a monoclonal anti-synaptic vesicle protein antibody. Brain Dev 16:432, 1995.

194. Harris NG, et al: Ventricle shunting in young H-Tx rats with inherited congenital hydrocephalus: a quantitative histological study of cortical grey matter. Childs Nerv Syst 10:293, 1994.

195. Zhang YW, DelBigio MR: Growth-associated protein-43 is increased in cerebrum of immature rats following induction of hydrocephalus. Neuroscience 86:847, 1998.

196. Boillat CA, et al: Ultrastructural changes in the deep cortical pyramidal cells of infant rats with inherited hydrocephalus and the effect of shunt treatment. Exp Neurol 147:377, 1997.

197. Alvisi C, et al: Evaluation of cerebral blood flow changes by transfontanelle Doppler ultrasound in infantile hydrocephalus. Childs Nerv Syst 1:244, 1985.

198. van den Wijngaard JA, et al: The blood flow velocity waveform in the fetal internal carotid artery in the presence of hydrocephaly. Early Hum Dev 18:95, 1988.

199. Norelle A, et al: Transcranial Doppler: a noninvasive method to monitor hydrocephalus. J Child Neurol 4(Suppl 1):S87, 1989.

200. Fischer AQ, et al: Pediatric Neurosonography: Clinical, Tomographic, and Neuropathologic Correlates. New York, John Wiley & Sons, 1985.

201. Ehle A, Sklar F: Visual evoked potentials in infants with hydrocephalus. Neurology 29:1541, 1979.

202. McSherry JW, et al: Acute visual evoked potential changes in hydrocephalus. Electroencephalogr Clin Neurophysiol 53:331, 1982.

203. Walker ML, et al: Auditory brain stem responses in neonatal hydrocephalus. Concepts Pediatr Neurosurg 7:142, 1987.

204. Del Bigio MR, Bruni JE: Changes in periventricular vasculature of rabbit brain following induction of hydrocephalus and after shunting. J Neurosurg 69:115, 1988.

205. Weller RO, Mitchel J: Cerebrospinal fluid edema and its sequelae in hydrocephalus. Adv Neurol 28:111, 1980.

206. Weller RO, et al: Brain tissue damage in hydrocephalus. Dev Med Child Neurol Suppl 20:1, 1969.

207. Rowlatt U: The microscopic effects of ventricular dilatation without increase in head size. J Neurosurg 48:957, 1978.

208. Bejar R, et al: Increased hypoxanthine concentrations in cerebrospinal fluid of infants with hydrocephalus. J Pediatr 103:44, 1983.

209. White RP, et al: Eicosanoid levels in CSF of premature infants with posthemorrhagic hydrocephalus. Am J Med Sci 299:230, 1990.

210. du Plessis AJ: Posthemorrhagic hydrocephalus and brain injury in the preterm infant: dilemmas in diagnosis and management. Semin Pediatr Neurol 5:1619, 1998.

211. Casaer P, et al: Cytochrome aa3 and intracranial pressure in newborn infants: a near infrared spectroscopy study (letter). Neuropediatrics 23:111, 1992.

212. Shirane R, et al: Cerebral blood flow and oxygen metabolism in infants with hydrocephalus. Childs Nerv Syst 8:118, 1992.

213. Rumack CM, et al: Timing and course of neonatal intracranial hemorrhage using real-time ultrasound. Radiology 154:101, 1985.

214. Allan WC, et al: Ventricular dilation after neonatal periventricular-intraventricular hemorrhage: natural history and therapeutic implications. Am J Dis Child 136:589, 1982.

215. Papile LA, et al: Relationship of cerebral intraventricular hemorrhage and early childhood neurologic handicaps. J Pediatr 103:273, 1983.

216. Stewart AL, et al: Ultrasound appearance of the brain in very preterm infants and neurodevelopmental outcome at 18 months of age. Arch Dis Child 58:598, 1983.

217. Fleischer AC, et al: Serial sonography of posthemorrhagic ventricular dilatation and porencephaly after intracranial hemorrhage in the preterm neonate. AJR Am J Roentgenol 141:451, 1983.

218. Fishman MA, et al: Progressive ventriculomegaly following minor intracranial hemorrhage in premature infants. Dev Med Child Neurol 26:725, 1984.

219. Papile LA, et al: Posthemorrhagic hydrocephalus in low-birth-weight infants: treatment by serial lumbar punctures. J Pediatr 97:273, 1980.

220. Camfield PR, et al: Progressive hydrocephalus in infants with birth weights less than 1,500 g. Arch Neurol 38:653, 1981.

221. Levene MI, Starte DR: A longitudinal study of post-haemorrhagic ventricular dilatation in the newborn. Arch Dis Child 56:905, 1981.

222. Shankaran S, et al: Outcome after posthemorrhagic ventriculomegaly in comparison with mild hemorrhage without ventriculomegaly. J Pediatr 114:109, 1989.

223. Marro PJ, et al: Posthemorrhagic hydrocephalus: use of an intravenous-type catheter for cerebrospinal fluid drainage. Am J Dis Child 145:1141, 1991.

224. Dykes FD, et al: Posthemorrhagic hydrocephalus in high-risk preterm infants: natural history, management, and long-term outcome. J Pediatr 114:611, 1989.

225. Hanigan WC, et al: Incidence and neurodevelopmental outcome of periventricular hemorrhage and hydrocephalus in a regional population of very low birth weight infants. Neurosurgery 29:701, 1991.

226. Resch B, et al: Neurodevelopmental outcome of hydrocephalus following intra-periventricular hemorrhage in preterm infants: short- and long term results. Childs Nerv Syst 12:27, 1996.

227. Hansen AR, et al: Predictors of ventriculoperitoneal shunt among babies with intraventricular hemorrhage. J Child Neurol 12:381, 1997.
228. Levy ML, et al: Outcome for preterm infants with germinal matrix hemorrhage and progressive hydrocephalus. Neurosurgery 41:1111, 1997.
229. Libenson MH, et al: Acetazolamide and furosemide for posthemorrhagic hydrocephalus of the newborn. Pediatr Neurol 20:185, 1999.
230. McMenamin JB, et al: Outcome of neonatal intraventricular hemorrhage with periventricular echodense lesions. Ann Neurol 15:285, 1984.
231. Kosmetatos N, et al: Intracranial hemorrhage in the premature: its predictive features and outcome. Am J Dis Child 134:855, 1980.
232. Robinson RO, Desai NS: Factors influencing mortality and morbidity after clinically apparent intraventricular haemorrhage. Arch Dis Child 56:478, 1981.
233. Thorburn RJ, et al: Prediction of death and major handicap in very preterm infants by brain ultrasound. Lancet 1:1119, 1981.
234. Ment LR, et al: Neurodevelopmental outcome at 36 months' corrected age of preterm infants in the multicenter indomethacin intraventricular hemorrhage prevention trail. Pediatrics 98:714, 1996.
235. Rushton DI, et al: Structure and evolution of echodense lesions in the neonatal brain: a combined ultrasound and necropsy study. Arch Dis Child 60:798, 1985.

236. Volpe JJ, et al: Positron emission tomography in the newborn: extensive impairment of regional cerebral blood flow with intraventricular hemorrhage and hemorrhagic intracerebral involvement. Pediatrics 72:589, 1983.
237. Catto-Smith AG, et al: Effect of neonatal periventricular haemorrhage on neurodevelopmental outcome. Arch Dis Child 60:8, 1985.
238. van de Bor M, et al: Outcome of periventricular-intraventricular hemorrhage at 2 years of age in 484 very preterm infants admitted to 6 neonatal intensive care units in The Netherlands. Neuropediatrics 19:183, 1988.
239. Roth SC, et al: Relation between ultrasound appearance of the brain of very preterm infants and neurodevelopmental impairment at eight years. Dev Med Child Neurol 35:755, 1993.
240. Ment LR, et al: The eitology and outcome of cerebral ventriculomegaly at term in very low birth weight preterm infants. Pediatrics 104:243, 1999.
241. Krishnamoorthy KS, et al: Neurologic sequelae in the survivors of neonatal intraventricular hemorrhage. Pediatrics 64:233, 1979.
242. Krishnamoorthy KS, et al: Neurodevelopmental outcome of survivors with posthemorrhagic hydrocephalus following Grade II neonatal intraventricular hemorrhage. Ann Neurol 15:201, 1984.
243. Williamson WD, et al: Early neurodevelopmental outcome of low birth weight infants surviving neonatal intraventricular hemorrhage. J Perinat Med 10:34, 1982.

172

Enrico Danzer, Natalie E. Rintoul, Timothy M. Crombleholme, and N. Scott Adzick

Pathophysiology of Neural Tube Defects

Neural tube defects are the most common and most severely disabling malformations of the central nervous system (CNS). They include a wide spectrum of malformations comprising open defects such as myelomeningocele and anencephaly and skin-covered lesions such as encephalocele. The clinical heterogeneity of neural tube defects results from a diversity of underlying mechanisms.[1] In the United States, neural tube defects are one of the most prevalent neonatal anomalies, second only to cardiac malformations. Worldwide, 300,000 or more infants are born each year with neural tube defects.[2] The incidence varies according to geography, ethnicity, and seasonal variation, ranging from 1 to 4 per 1000 live births. The fetal prevalence may well be even higher, because neural tube defects detected by screening amniocentesis and ultrasound often result in elective termination of the pregnancy. The highest incidence of neural tube defects is found in Great Britain, Ireland, Pakistan, northern India, and Egypt. The lowest incidence is observed in Finland, Japan, and Israel. Even within in the United States, a geographic and ethnic distribution of these defects occurs, with the highest incidence in the East and the South, and the lowest in West.[3] There is an increased prevalence of neural tube defects among Hispanics, especially if the mother was born in Mexico.[4] There is also a high incidence of neural tube defects among Sikhs. However, these lesions are frequently restricted to the thoracic level with minimal associated neurologic deficit, suggesting a separate origin.[5] Women in the United States who have had an infant or fetus with a neural tube defect have a 2 to 3% risk of a subsequent affected pregnancy.[6]

In humans, anencephaly and myelomeningocele (spina bifida aperta) are the most common types. Anencephaly is almost always lethal, whereas myelomeningocele, although not usually lethal, has enormous attendant personal, familial, and social costs. The life of most affected children is characterized by recurrent hospitalizations, multiple operations, and physical and cognitive impairments. The associated handicaps are dependent on the level of the spinal lesion, the degree of damage to the exposed neural tissue, and the presence of the Chiari Type II malformation.[7] Less than 20% of neural tube defects are associated with malformation of non-neural tissues, chromosomal defects, or specific genetic syndromes,[8] such as amniotic bands,[9] trisomies 13 and 18, and the autosomal recessive Meckel-Gruber syndrome.

Despite intensive investigation, the etiology of neural tube defects remains unclear, and the controversy over its pathogenesis continues. This chapter focuses on our current understanding of the epidemiologic and environmental factors and reviews recent contributions of experimental and clinical research to the pathophysiology and treatment of neural tube defects.

EMBRYONIC DEVELOPMENT

Normal human brain development can be summarized in six basic stages: (1) primary and secondary neurulation, (2) proencephalic development, (3) neuronal proliferation, (4) neuronal migration, (5) organizational events, and (6) myelination.[10] Understanding the process of CNS development is important to understand the features of the CNS abnormalities in children affected by neural tube defects. Development of the CNS begins prenatally and continues postnatally with overlapping developmental periods (Table 172–1). The embryonic development of the fetal brain and the spinal cord is described in detail in Chapter 165. The embryology, specifically of neural tube formation, is briefly presented here to understand neural tube defects in the context of normal CNS development.

Primary Neurulation

The formation of the neural tube begins on the dorsal aspect of the gastrula stage embryo as a plate of tissue differentiating in the middle of the ectoderm. Neurulation occurs between the third and fourth week of gestation. According to Smith and Schoenwolf,[11] neurulation can be subdivided into four broad morphologic steps: (1) induction of the neural plate, (2) molding of the neural plate, (3) longitudinal bending of the neural plate, and (4) fusion of the neural folds. The stages of primary neurulation are coordinated with progressive and regressive movements of the primitive streak.[12] The critical event in this process is neural induction, which involves interaction between the ectoderm and the underlying mesoderm (notochord). The notochord and chordal mesoderm induce formation of the neural plate, which forms between 16 to 18 days of gestation. The inductive signals are generated by the Hensen node, the avian equivalent of the Spemann organizer.[13,14] Cell proliferation and shape change then result in extension and folding of the primordial neural plate, the precursor of both the brain and the spinal cord. As the notochord forms and elongates, the neural plate enlarges and extends beyond the edges of the notochord. The midline, however, remains tethered to the underlying notochord. The neural plate begins to invaginate along the central axis, to form a longitudinal median groove with neural folds on its sides. In the region of the future spinal cord, this process remains, obliterating the groove and bringing the edges of the plate in apposition. At approximately 22 days of gestation, the neural tube forms by fusion of the opposed neural folds in the region of the future lower brain stem. Fusion progresses rostrally and caudally. The neural tube remains open at both ends (the anterior and the posterior neuropores), and this allows the fluid of the amniotic cavity to communicate with the neural tube lumen. The anterior end of the neural tube closes at approximately 24 days, and the posterior end closes at around 28 days of gestation.[15]

The mechanisms responsible for neural tube formation are not completely understood, but two theories have been advanced, the first being the *zipper closure model,* in which the neural tube closure begins in the cervical region and fusion then proceeds bidirectionally until the neural tube is closed.[16] More recently the *multisite closure model* has been suggested.[17] This model of multisite neural tube closure may provide the best explanation of neural tube formation (Table 172-2).[18,19] In addition, the complex morphologic events of neural tube formation result from the unity of intrinsic and extrinsic features and may also involve nerve cell adhesion molecules[20] or other components within the extracellular matrix.[21] Intrinsic processes include microfilament contraction, actively changing cell shape,[22] and passive folding caused by rapid cell proliferation and underlying membrane tethering.[23] The relationships between the neural plate and the adjacent embryonic tissue constitute the extrinsic forces in neural tube development.

Primary neurulation results in a closed neural tube with its caudal limits in the upper lumbar spinal cord. Secondary neurulation, the process in which the remaining caudal elements of the spinal cord (i.e., conus medullaris, lower lumbar, and sacrococcygeal segments) are fashioned is related to the future vertebral level S2. An open neural tube defect results if closure is not completed during this developmental window.

TABLE 172-1
Normal Human Brain Development and Time of Occurrence

Normal Human Brain Development	Time of Occurrence
Formation of the brain structure	0–20 weeks of gestation
Primary and secondary neurulation	3–4 weeks of gestation
Proencephalic development	4–12 weeks of gestation
Neuronal migration	5–20 weeks of gestation
Neuronal proliferation and brain growth	0 weeks of gestation–12 years of life
Organizational events	12 weeks of gestation–12 years of life
Differentiation, maturation, synaptogenesis	16 weeks of gestation–12 years of life
Apoptosis	24 weeks of gestation–1 month of life
Myelination	13 weeks–30 years of life

Adapted from Volpe JJ: Mental Retard Dev Disabil Res Rev 6:1-5, 2000.

EMBRYONIC AND MOLECULAR MECHANISMS OF NEURAL TUBE DEFECTS
Insights from Mouse Genetic Models

Because neurulation in mouse and human embryos appears to be quite similar anatomically, the mouse has been used as a model for investigating the embryonic mechanisms of neural tube defects. Direct genetic analysis of human neural tube defects has been difficult because of the rarity of familial cases and the lack of specific candidate genes. To date, more than 10 mouse mutant models have been described (i.e., curly tail, loop tail, splotch, vacuolated lens, and *Mlp*-knock-out mice)[24,25] that exhibit a genetic co-segregation of anencephaly, exencephaly, and myelomeningocele analogous to the human condition. However, all these mutants present additional defects that are never, or only infrequently, seen in humans with neural tube defects. For example, the malformations in the mouse mutant splotch are similar to those found in human Waardenburg syndrome Type I[26,27] and Greig cephalopolysyndactyly.[28] Absence of the corpus callosum or thinning of the cerebral cortex and retina is rarely found in humans with neural tube defects, but it is frequently present in the *Mlp*-knock-out mouse.[24] Finally, some knock-outs, such as *Csk*, *Brca1*, and *P53*, show neural tube defects, but they also exhibit growth retardation and other malformations and are associated with a high embryonic lethality.[29-31]

Despite these limitations, investigations in two mouse mutants led to two hypotheses to account for the failure of the posterior neuropore to close, resulting in open defects of the spine. The curly tail (*ct/ct*) mouse mutant, first described by Gruneberg in 1954,[32] exhibits failure of both the anterior and posterior neuropore closure, resembling common forms of human neural tube defects. The basic defect in the curly tail mouse is not within the neuroepithelium; it is in the non-neural tissues.[33] In curly tail (*ct/ct*) mouse mutants, the notochord and the hindgut endoderm demonstrate decreased cell proliferation causing enhanced curvature of the caudal region. This curvature mechanically opposes the closure of the neuropore and leads to the development of open neural tube defects.[34,35] In addition to the altered cell proliferation rates, curly tail mouse embryos exhibit a reduced accumulation of newly synthesized hyaluronate within the extracellular matrix in the notochord and hindgut endoderm.[36] Because hyaluronate significantly contributes to cell proliferation in various cell types, Copp and Bernfield[37] suggested that alteration in hyaluronate synthesis, resulting in suboptimal proliferation of the notochord and hindgut endoderm, may result in neural tube defects.

Curly tail (*ct/ct*) mouse mutants demonstrate an increased level of α-fetoprotein in the amniotic fluid of fetuses with neural tube defects,[38] as well as an incomplete penetrance (60%), which varies with genetic background, a finding supporting the hypothesis of the presence of modifier genes.[39] As in humans,

TABLE 172-2
Multisite Closure Model for Neural Tube Formation

Closure	Region of Fusion at the Neural Tube
1	At the midcervical region and proceeds cranially and caudally
2	At the prosencephalon/mesencephalon boundary and proceeds bidirectionally
3	Proceeds rostally from the stomadeum and convenes cranially with closure 2
4	At the rhombencephalon and proceeds rostrally
5	Unidirectional closure of the caudal end of the neural tube

environmental factors (e.g., retinoic acid, mitomycin C, hydroxyurea, and 5-fluoruracil) are important, with alteration in penetrance and expressivity of the curly tail phenotypes.[40] Although treatment with folate and methionine is effective in reducing the incidence of neural tube defects in humans, these agents have no effect on the incidence or type of neural tube defects in curly tail mice.[41-43] Inositol treatment reduces curly tail neural tube defects by stimulating protein kinase C activity by 70%, a finding suggesting that the curly tail model is a folate-resistant model of neural tube defect phenotypes.[40]

By contrast, homozygous splotch (Sp/Sp) mice were found to have a mutation in the paired domain of the Pax3 gene responsible for the phenotype of these mutants.[44] The failure to express a normal Pax3 protein (a critical embryonic gene in neural tube development in mice and humans) in the neuroepithelial cells appears to impair the ability of the neural plate to undergo folding and fusion during the neurulation process.[44, 45] Although the cellular mechanisms are unknown, Yang and Tarsler[46] and Moase and Tarsler[47] suggested that the failure of Pax3 protein expression affects the cell-cell interaction within the neural plate. Linkage studies of Pax3 and neural tube defects in United States and Dutch families, however, failed to identify the relationship between Pax3 expression and neural tube defects.[48] In addition, mouse models of HOX-deficient mice showed delayed closure and aberrant formation of the neural tube.[49] However, analysis of the four known clusters of HOX genes (A, B, C, D), which play an important role in neural tube development in humans, found no evidence of their involvement in human neural tube defects.[50] A report of linkage between human neural tube defect and the region of the T locus homologue[51] has not been supported by other studies.[52, 53]

In double-mutant mice for splotch and curly tail, the incidence and the severity of spina bifida significantly increase, a finding indicating an additive effect in the disruption of the neurulation process.[54] The neural tube defect phenotypes seen in curly tail mutants resemble those of F52-deficient (also called MacMARCKS) mice, and the F52 gene and ct have both been mapped to distal chromosome 4.[55] The penetrance and severity of ct-gene expression, however, are affected by the modifier genes mapped to murine chromosome 3 and 5.[55] In F52-deficient mice, about 60% are exencephalic, and approximately 10% have spinal neural tube defects.[24] The question that has been raised is whether the curly tail mouse is a mutation of the F52-deficient mouse.[24] However, it is thought that the curly tail mutation addresses cellular defects in the extrinsic forces of neurulation, whereas the MacMARCKS-like protein regulates morphogenesis in various tissues by mediation of cell-cell signaling, changes of actin-cytoskeleton dynamics, and regulation of cytosolic protein expression.[56] Thus, modulations regulated by protein kinase C substrates[56] within the neuroepithelial cells play an integral role as intrinsic forces during neurulation.

To summarize, for most mouse models of neural tube defects, there is still a gap between identifying the gene involved in the development of neural tube defects and the morphogenetic mechanism it contributes to the formation of the neural tube. However, it is possible, and perhaps likely, that neural tube defects in humans result from a combination of common disease-associated alleles in the population or even from a subtle change of function in specialized neurulation genes.

Insights from Teratogenic Models

Various teratogenic neural tube defect models have been examined to understand the mechanisms of abnormal neurulation and to test etiologic and environmental hypotheses suggested by human epidemiologic data. Certain teratogens, such as ethanol, insulin, trypan blue, vitamin A, retinoids, folic acid antagonists,

γ-aminobutyric acid–receptor agonists, and hyperthermia have all been used to induce neural tube defects in vitro and in vivo.[57,58] More than 30 classes of chemicals and drugs are listed in the literature that result in neural tube defects.[59] However, the phenotype of neural tube defects, as well as the development of hindbrain herniation, depends on the timing of administration.[60,61]

Administration of valproic acid on day 8 of gestation in the mouse results in high rates of malformations of the anterior neural tube (i.e., exencephaly),[62] whereas an appropriate dosing regimen of valproic acid on day 9 of gestation results in spina bifida occulta.[63] Studies conducted by Alles and Sulik[64] and by Ehlers and coworkers[65] used retinoic acid to illustrate that teratogenic-induced neural tube defects are dependent on the doses of the teratogenic agent. A dose of 12.5 mg retinoic acid/kg body weight administrated to the dam causes myelomeningocele-like lesions in 58% of fetuses.[65] In contrast, 28.0 mg/kg body weight given to the dam results in myelomeningocele-like lesions in 79% of the fetuses.[64] Histologic examinations of the fetuses revealed a broad spectrum of pathologic alterations of the spine, similar to those seen in humans. Having demonstrated the feasibility of creating a spinal defect resembling a human myelomeningocele with valproic acid, Ehlers and colleagues[66] reported that the administration of methionine (70 mg/kg body weight) to valproic acid–exposed mice fetuses significantly reduced the valproic acid–induced spina bifida rate. The interactions of methionine in neural tube formation are not completely understood. However, methionine may play an important role in normal neural tube formation, because the absence of methionine causes neural tube defects in cultured rat embryos.[67] The most important finding from the teratogenic models, however, is the strain-specific diversity, highlighting the importance of genetic predisposition.[43]

Insights from Mechanical Models

In addition to the genetic and teratogenic models of neural tube defects, newer models of mechanical disruption of normal neural tube development have been described. These models provide further evidence for the two-hit hypothesis. The first "hit" is the failure of neurulation early in gestation. The second "hit" is the spinal cord injury resulting from prolonged exposure of the neural tissue to the intrauterine environment. The first was a primate model[68] in which a fetal lumbar laminectomy (L3-L5) was performed late in gestation. One group of animals was repaired immediately with allogeneic bone paste, whereas a control group had no repair. The unrepaired fetuses showed cystic myelomeningocele-like lesions at birth and showed severe neurologic impairment including paraplegia, incontinence, and somatosensory loss. The repaired group was neurologically normal at birth. Unfortunately, the experiment did not include an initial procedure for creation of the defect with a period of exposure to the intrauterine environment before closure.[68] These results nevertheless support the hypothesis that prolonged exposure of the spinal cord to amniotic fluid causes considerable damage to the neural tissue in a myelomeningocele-like lesion. Heffez and associates[69, 70] reported similar findings in fetal pigs and fetal rats. In both studies, late-gestation fetuses underwent surgical creation of a myelomeningocele-like defect with immediate or delayed (24 hours later) surgical closure resulting in preservation of neurologic function compared with the untreated group. Notably, in some of the animals, dehiscence of their skin closure occurred, resulting in neurologic deficit.[70] Histologic examination of the exposed neural tissue revealed erosion and necrosis, findings similar to those described in children with myelomeningocele. More recently, Correia-Pinto and associates[71] demonstrated, in a surgically created rat model, that late-gestation exposure to meconium increases damage to neural tissue.

These studies show that exposure of the fetal spinal cord to the intrauterine environment results in significant acquired neural tissue damage with corresponding neurologic deficit at birth. In addition, these studies demonstrate that closure of a surgically created myelomeningocele-like lesion is feasible and improves neurologic function at birth. The model that is most similar to human disease is the fetal lamb model of myelomeningocele introduced by Meuli and colleagues in 1994.[72] The myelomeningocele-like defect was surgically created in fetal lambs at 75 days of gestation (term, 145 to 150 days) by excision of skin, paraspinal musculature, and vertebral arches of lumbar vertebrae 1 through 4, exposing the dorsal dura mater. At 100 days of gestation, a reversed latissimus dorsi flap was used to cover the exposed spinal cord, and the animals were delivered by cesarean section just before term.[73,74] As in the primate, rat, and porcine models, the untreated fetuses showed myelomeningo-cele-like lesions at birth with similar neurologic deficits: complete sensorimotor paraplegia, incontinence of stool and urine, and lack of sensory function of the hind limbs.[73,74] Animals that underwent closure of the defect had healed skin wounds and near-normal neurologic function. Despite mild paraparesis, they were able to stand, walk, and perform demanding motor tests, and no signs of incontinence were detected. Furthermore, sensory function of the hind limbs was present clinically and was confirmed electrophysiologically.[73,74]

Hindbrain herniation in children with myelomeningocele is hypothesized to result from leakage of cerebrospinal fluid through the open neural tube at a critical time in posterior fossa formation.[75] Based on this hypothesis, Paek and associates[76] added a myelotomy to the surgically created myelomeningocele in fetal sheep. These investigators demonstrated severe hind-brain herniation in lambs with a myelotomy and an unrepaired myelomeningocele. The brains of lambs that underwent *in utero* repair of the lesion were normal. Bouchard and collagues[77] similarly observed hindbrain disease in 85% of fetuses that underwent myelomeningocele creation with myelotomy (75 days of gestation). The hindbrain anatomy was restored in 88% of the fetuses that underwent fetal myelomeningocele repair (102 days of gestation). In other words, creation of a myelotomy allowed the egress of cerebrospinal fluid from the central hindbrain her-niation. Closure of the myelomeningocele defect, by blocking the leakage of cerebrospinal fluid, is thought to restore the hindbrain anatomy.

To summarize, the fetal sheep model of myelomeningocele demonstrated that a spinal cord lesion could be created *in utero* and repaired at a later time, with improved neurologic function after birth. Unlike the previous animal models,[68,69,70,78] this sheep model more closely resembled that of human myelomeningocele in duration and exposure of the spinal neural tissue to the intrauterine environment as well as in clinical and histologic outcome. Furthermore, brain anomalies (e.g., the hind-brain herniation characteristic of the Chiari II malformation) could be replicated with the addition of a myelotomy to the creation of myelomeningocele.

The results of these studies suggest that the intrauterine envi-ronment plays a considerable role in secondary neural tissue injury, perhaps as much as the primary defect during neural tube formation. In addition, these models establish the feasibility of *in utero* repair and its potential for preserving neurologic function.

NEURAL TUBE DEFECTS AS MULTIFACTORIAL DISORDERS

Genetic Features

Genetic or inherited features are important to understand the origin of neural tube defects. However, as with most congenital defects, the role of genetic and environmental factors in the development of neural tube defects in humans is not completely understood. Several lines of evidence support the existence of a genetic predisposition, including (1) variable incidence among ethnic groups and geographical locations, (2) familial recurrence risks, (3) genetic syndromes associated with neural tube defect, (4) alterations in genes involved in folate metabolism associated with an increased risk for neural tube defects, (5) altered sex ratio, and (6) mouse models with at least 10 mutant gene loci that are associated with neural tube defects. This genetic distri-bution has been interpreted as indicating 60% heritability for human neural tube defects.[79] Neural tube defects, however, have a familial allocation that cannot be accounted for by simple mendelian traits. In addition, the large numbers of mouse models of neural tube defects suggest not only the relative ease with which the neurulation process can be disturbed, but also the genetic heterogeneity of these abnormalities.

Supplementation with folate during early pregnancy signifi-cantly decreases the risk of neural tube defects (see later).[80] The reason for this effect is unknown.[78] Colas and Schoenwolf[12] sug-gested that supplementation of folate only neutralizes a genetic defect in folate homeostasis, such as a metabolic deficiency in its maternal supply[43] or mutations in the methylenetetrahydrofolate reductase gene in the embryo.[82] These genes, however, account only for a small amount of the total genetic environment of neural tube defects.[83] Additionally, folate supplementation reduces the incidence of several congenital malformations,[84] a finding questioning the specificity of its effect in neural tube formation. It appears that the degree and duration of folate deficiency necessary to inhibit DNA synthesis may be greater than the underlying gene defect that is necessary to produce the neural tube defect. In addition, folate deficiency is not itself ade-quate to induce neural tube defects in mice.[85] Because there are folate-resistant neural tube defects, it is necessary to search for new genetic risk factors for neural tube defects.[12]

Environmental Features

Over the years, environmental studies have been instrumental in elucidating the nongenetic causes of neural tube defects in humans. These data suggested that maternal nutrition is impor-tant, and vitamin deficiencies, especially of folic acid, play an essential role in the pathogenesis of neural tube defects.[86-88] A lack of folic acid is a common condition usually caused by a low dietary intake and may be correlated to socioeconomic factors. This may be important during pregnancy, when the folate requirement is increased, but the availability of folate may be reduced by changes in intestinal absorption and renal clear-ance.[89] The risks of neural tube defects and rates of anencephaly are usually higher in groups with lower socioeconomic status.[90]

Identifying specific causal environmental features has proven difficult. In the Collaborative Perinatal Project sponsored by the National Institutes of Health that reviewed the pregnancies of 53,000 women, Myrianthopoulos and Melnick[91] demonstrated that maternal diabetes mellitus, heart disease, and lung disease and the use of diuretics, antihistamines, or sulfonamides were all asso-ciated with an increased risk of neural tube defects. In most cases, the neural tube defect was not associated with other malforma-tions or syndromes. In addition, women who had a short interval between the end of a previous pregnancy and the current preg-nancy had an increased risk of neural tube defect.[91] Maternal dia-betes and other modifications of glucose metabolism such as obesity are well-known risk factors for neural tube defects.[92] The risk ranges from as low as 2% in the United States to as high as 8% in England.[93] Other factors include fever and hyperthermia in early pregnancy,[94] viral infection,[95] parental occupation,[93] and maternal use of some antiepileptic drugs.[96] The role of maternal and paternal age in the origin of neural tube defects is still under debate. For example, McIntosh and associates[97] and Strassburg and colleagues[98] suggested that both maternal age and paternal age are risk factors for neural tube defects. However, other studies have not confirmed this association.[99,100]

NUTRITIONAL STATUS AND PRIMARY PREVENTION

The relation between nutritional status, especially folate intake, and the occurrence of neural tube defects provides a powerful tool for primary prevention of these congenital lesions. However, based on the wide phenotypic spectrum and the multifactorial origin of neural tube defects, it is surprising that only a single agent, folic acid, has been demonstrated to reduce the incidence of neural tube defects significantly. Smithells and colleagues[101] demonstrated that administration of a multivitamin preparation to women who had already one or more affected pregnancies resulted in a marked reduction of recurrence risk for neural tube defects. A subsequent nonrandomized case study and retrospective observational studies supported these initial findings.[102-104] However, the strongest evidence comes from two randomized, double-blind clinical studies. The British clinical trial conducted by the Medical Research Council demonstrated a significant protective effect with periconceptional supplementation of 4 mg folate per day in preventing of neural tube defects.[87] A Hungarian trial[80] revealed that periconceptional multivitamins (containing 12 vitamins, 0.8 mg of folate, 4 minerals, and 3 trace elements) prevented not only recurrences but also the first occurrence of neural tube defects. In addition, a national study of birth certificate data in the United States indicate a 19% decline in the birth prevalence of neural tube defects and a 23% decline in spina bifida incidence among births conceived after folic acid supplementation (October 1998 through December 1999) compared with the neural tube defects reported before folate administration (October 1995 through December 1996).[105]

However, the underlying mechanisms of prevention of neural tube defects are not completely understood. Folic acid is essential as a cofactor for enzymes involved in DNA and RNA synthesis and vitamin B_{12} and vitamin B_6 in the metabolism of methionine.[106] After it was reported that pregnant women with neural tube defects had an elevated blood level of homocysteine,[107] research focused on the homocysteine-methylation cycle. As seen in Figure 172–1, reactions regulating this cycle are dependent on one or more of these vitamins. Inadequate levels of methionine may result from inadequate tissue levels of either the coenzyme, vitamin B_{12}, as methylcobalamin, or folate as 5-methyltetrahydrofolate, of the methionine metabolism. Vitamin B_6 is involved in the first irreversible step in the transsulfuration pathway from methionine to cysteine. Disturbance in the activity of cystathionine β-synthase results in homocysteinemia. Therefore, alterations of the vitamin B_{12}–dependent methionine synthase, folate-dependent methylenetetrahydrofolate-reductase, and vitamin B_6-dependent cystathionine β-synthase may play a causative role in the development of neural tube defects. Treatment with Vitamin B_6 normalizes the hyperhomocysteinemia and hypermethioninemia in approximately 50% of patients,[108] and it may result in a decreased risk of neural tube defects. These hypotheses are supported by experimental studies. For example, neural tube defects are prevented by methionine and folate supplementation in some rodent models.[43,109] The effect of homocysteinemia in the pathogenesis of neural tube defects in chick embryo can be ameliorated by simultaneous folate supplementation.[81] However, the link between common mutations of the genes for methionine synthase, methylenetetrahydrofolate-reductase, and cystathionine β-synthase in humans could not be documented.

To summarize, despite the progress in the research on pathogenesis and approaches to primary prevention, the interpretation of these findings remains difficult. Prevention is not possible in all cases of neural tube defects, but supplementation of folate in a periconceptional dose of 0.36 to 4.0 mg/day can prevent the first occurrence and up to 85% of recurrent neural tube defects.[80,87,110,111]

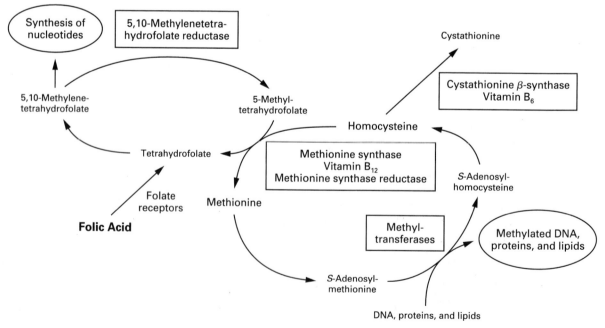

Figure 172–1. The metabolic roles of folic acid. After entering the cell, folic acid, possibly with the aid of folate receptors, is involved in the transfer of carbon atoms that are used to synthesize nucleotides or, through the conversion of homocysteine to methionine, for the methylation of various substrates. These processes are regulated by numerous molecules, including enzymes and vitamins other than folic acid (e.g., vitamins B_6 and B_{12}). The activity of some enzymes, such as methionine synthase, may be influenced by other enzymes, such as methionine synthase reductase. Enzymes and factors that may be important in neural tube development are indicated by *boxes*.

SPECTRUM AND CLINICAL PRESENTATION

Although most studies of neural tube defects deal only with anencephaly and myelomeningocele, the clinical spectrum also includes craniorachischisis totalis, encephalocele, exencephaly, myeloschisis and iniencephaly (Fig. 172–2). Malformations of the normal midline fusion are often referred to as being dysraphic and vary in clinical significance and outcome. Several different schemes are used to categorize neural tube defects; however, the nomenclature is confusing and even contradictory. Most of the lesions involve a failure of neural tube closure. The term *neural tube defect* is used to characterize this entire group of anomalies. Because the varying forms of neural tube defects probably arise by different mechanisms, it is important to describe and classify each defect appropriately. Based on the clinical significance and embryology, neural tube defects should be subdivided into cranial neural tube defects, open spinal neural tube defects, and closed spinal neural tube defects. Disorders of neural tube formation are reviewed next in order of decreasing severity.

Cranial Neural Tube Defects

Craniorachischisis Totalis

Craniorachischisis totalis is characterized by a total failure of neurulation. This is the most severe form of neural tube defects. It occurs before 20 to 22 days of gestation.[112] A neural plate remnant is present throughout, and there is no overlying axial

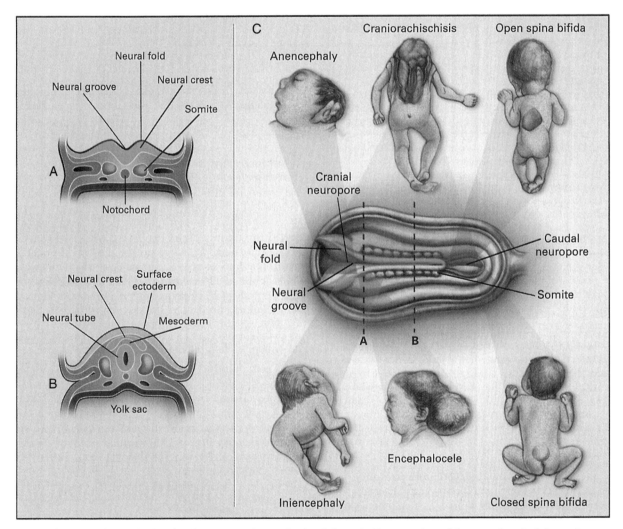

Figure 172–2. Features of neural tube development and neural tube defects. **A,** Cross-section of the rostral end of the embryo at approximately 3 weeks after conception, showing the neural groove in the process of closing, overlying the notochord. The neural folds are the rising margins of the neural tube, topped by the neural crest, and demarcate the neural groove centrally. **B,** Cross-section of the middle portion of the embryo after the neural tube has closed. The neural tube, which will ultimately develop into the spinal cord, is now covered by surface ectoderm (later, the skin). The intervening mesoderm will form the bony spine. The notochord is regressing. **C,** Developmental and clinical features of the main types of neural tube defects. The diagram in the *center* is a dorsal view of a developing embryo, showing a neural tube that is closed in the center but still open at the cranial and caudal ends. The *dotted lines* marked A and B refer to the cross-sections shown in **A** and **B**. *Shaded bars* point to the region of the neural tube relevant to each defect. In anencephaly, the absence of the brain and calvaria can be total or partial. Craniorachischisis is characterized by anencephaly accompanied by a contiguous bony defect of the spine and exposure of neural tissue. In open spina bifida, a bony defect of the posterior vertebral arches (in this case, the lower thoracic vertebrae) is accompanied by herniation of neural tissue and meninges and is not covered by skin. In iniencephaly, dysraphia in the occipital region is accompanied by severe retroflexion of the neck and trunk. In encephalocele, the brain and meninges herniate through a defect in the calvaria. In closed spina bifida, unlike open spina bifida, the bony defect of the posterior vertebral arches (in this case, the lumbar vertebrae), the herniated meninges, and neural tissue are covered by skin. (From Botto LD, et al: N Engl J Med 341:1509, 1999.)

skeleton or dermal covering. Most cases with craniorachischisis totalis are aborted spontaneously, and only a few fetuses have survived to term. The incidence remains unknown.

Anencephaly

Anencephaly (congenital absence of major portion of the brain, skull, and scalp)[113] is the single most common prenatally detected neural tube defect, with an incidence ranging from 1 in 1000 live and stillbirths in the United States to 1 in 100 live and stillbirths in some of the British Isles.[114] In one study, the prevalence of this neural tube defect was noted to change over time because of the impact of prenatal sonographic examination and maternal serum screening. Limb and Holmes[115] reported an incidence of anencephaly that varied between 1.0 and 0.4 per 1000 live and stillbirths during two different study periods (1972 to 1974 and 1979 to 1990). Female fetuses are more commonly affected than males, with a frequency of 3:1 to 4:1.[116] Furthermore, there is an increased incidence of anencephaly in Hispanics, who are 45% more likely than whites to have an affected pregnancy.[117] Anencephaly is associated with maternal hyperthermia as well as with maternal folate, copper, and zinc deficiencies.

In affected fetuses, there is a failure in the development of structures associated with the anterior neural tube closure. The defect is estimated to occur between 24 and 26 days of gestation.[118] The anomaly involves variable amounts of the forebrain and upper brain stem. In some cases, the defect extends through the level of the foramen magnum (holocrania or holoanencephaly, the more severe form), or it may be limited (merocrania or meroanencephaly, the milder form). In addition to the absent cerebral hemispheres, fetuses with anencephaly demonstrate abnormal patterns in the hypothalamus and cerebellum. The frontal, parietal, and squamous parts of the occipital bones fail to develop; instead, the defect may be covered by a variable amount of angiomatous stroma.[9] The exposed neural tissue appears as a hemorrhagic, fibrotic, and degenerated mass of neurons and glia, with no functional cortex.

Anencephaly is uniformly fatal. Most affected fetuses are spontaneously aborted or stillborn. Through reliable prenatal diagnosis, anencephaly is one of the few universally accepted indications for third trimester termination.[119] Survivors are delivered at a mean gestational age of 26.7 ± 5 weeks.[120] The diagnosis of anencephaly can be confirmed on physical examination when the following criteria are met: (1) a large portion of the skull is absent, (2) the scalp is absent over the skull defect, (3) a hemorrhagic fibrotic mass of degenerated brain tissue is exposed to the environment, and (4) no recognizable cerebral hemispheres are present. Because orbits and eyes in anencephalic fetuses are well developed, this malformation imparts a remarkable froglike appearance to the patients. There is no functioning cerebral cortex, but brain stem function is present in varying degrees. Almost all fetuses born with anencephaly die within the first week, but rarely, survival for several months has been reported.[113]

Exencephaly

Exencephaly is a rare fetal anomaly that is incompatible with extrauterine life. This malformation is characterized by partial or complete absence of the calvarium with abnormal development of brain tissue.[121] According to Papp and associates,[122] who screened 36,075 pregnancies for neural tube defects, the incidence of exencephaly is 3 per 10,000 pregnancies. Cox and associates[123] concluded that exencephaly probably represents an embryonic precursor to anencephaly. However, reopening or degeneration of a previously closed neural tube is also possible. Stagiannis and colleagues[124] considered the development of exencephaly related to a failure in mesenchymal migration. The exact pathogenesis remains uncertain.

The absence of the calvarium causes brain destruction by exposing the developing brain to amniotic fluid and repeated trauma. The exposed brain may be destroyed as early as 8 to 10 weeks of gestation.[123] In pathologic studies, the exencephalic brain is covered by a highly vascular epithelial layer. In exencephaly, two relatively equivalent cerebral hemispheric remnants are present within a reddish mass of disorganized tissue, remnants of deep cerebral neural elements, blood vessels, fibrotic tissues, and fluid-filled spaces.[125] In addition, in exencephalic brain tissue, the gyri and sulci are shallowed, flattened, and disorganized.

Experimental studies have demonstrated that hyperglycemia can induce exencephaly in mice,[126] and administration of clomiphene citrate before ovulation in female mice increases the incidence of exencephaly.[127] These effects in mice are similar to the inhibition of neural tube closure seen in newborns of diabetic mothers.

Encephalocele

Encephalocele arises as a failure of fusion of restricted parts of the anterior neural tube closure between 26 and 28 days of gestation, and it demonstrates a variable degree of cerebral herniation through a midline defect of the cranium. However, it is difficult to explain the development of encephalocele merely on embryologic grounds, and its precise pathogenesis remains unknown. Additionally, it has been suggested that the anomaly may occur secondary to herniation of brain through the cranium in the second trimester because of hydrocephalus and is not a primary defect of neural tube closure. In a study in the United States comprising a 17-year survey of births occurring in armed forces hospitals, Wiswell and colleagues,[128] recognized 112 cases of encephalocele in 763,364 live births. This yields an incidence 0.15 per 1000 live births. However, the incidence varies within ethnic groups and geographic regions.[129] In the Western world, 75% of these abnormalities occur in the occipital region, and frontoethmoidal encephaloceles are more common in Malaysia, Thailand, Indonesia, Burma, and parts of Russia.[130-132] The neural tissue within the defect may be relatively normal, although hemorrhage, necrosis, and cortical dysplasia are present in some cases.[133]

Encephaloceles are frequently associated with microcephaly, maternal rubella, maternal diabetes, and genetic syndromes. In addition, encephaloceles are often found with other malformations,[131] including agenesis of the corpus callosum, lissencephaly (in Walker-Walburg syndrome) and craniosynostosis (Apert syndrome), or even renal cystic dysplasia and polydactyly (Meckel-Gruber syndrome). Encephalocele can be produced experimentally by irradiation, trypan blue, or hypervitaminosis.

The prognosis and long-term outcome depend on the associated brain malformations and syndromes. Large size is not important prognostically, because large encephaloceles may not contain neural elements. Microcephaly and the presence of neural tissue in the encephalocele are associated with a poor prognosis.[134] The surgical challenges in affected newborns include closing the anatomic defect in the cranial vault and achieving as near normal a functional outcome as possible with minimal psychomotor defects.[135]

Myeloschisis

The essential defect in *myeloschisis* is failure of posterior tube closure. This anomaly arises not later than 26 days of gestation. The exposed neural plate–like formation involves large portions of the spinal cord and appears as a flat, raw, velvety structure with no vertebrae or dermal covering. Most of these fetuses are stillborn and merge with the category of more restricted anomalies of neural tube development, such as myelomeningocele.

Iniencephaly

Iniencephaly is an abnormality in cervical vertebrae associated with cervicothoracic spinal retroflexion and neural tube defect. Lewis[136] classified iniencephalus into two subtypes: iniencephalus apertus, in which there is involvement of the brain with an encephalocele present; and iniencephalus clauses, in which no malformation of the occipital bone or brain is present. In iniencephaly, developmental disturbances of the neural tube and spine arise very early in embryogenesis, generally between day 26 and day 30 after conception.

Iniencephaly is a rare condition with an estimated incidence between 1 in 1000 and less than 1 in 100,000.[137] Because most iniencephalic fetuses die *in utero,* it is difficult to estimate the true incidence accurately. Experimentally, iniencephaly can be produced with administration of vinblastine, streptonigrin, or triparanol.[138] The pathogenesis of iniencephaly in humans, however, remains unknown. In geographic areas where there is an increased prevalence of anencephaly, there is also an increased prevalence of iniencephaly.[139] Different hypotheses for the pathogenesis of iniencephaly have been developed. It is possible that a primary defect in fetal cervical development resulting in extreme dorsal flexion of the head (lordosis) causes a failure of neural tube closure or even dilation and rupture of a previously closed neural tube.[138] Additionally, iniencephaly may be a primary defect in neural tube formation. Gardner[140] suggested that iniencephaly may be a severe form of the Klippel-Feil syndrome or may belong to the spectrum of malformations of the Dandy-Walker syndrome and the Arnold-Chiari malformation.

In the series of David and Nixon,[141] of 50 fetuses with iniencephaly, 84% had multiple associated malformations. The most frequent malformations were hydronephrosis, cardiovascular malformations, single umbilical artery, diaphragmatic hernia, facial clefts, omphalocele, and clubfoot.[141] Associated abnormalities of the CNS include anencephaly, encephalocele, hydrocephalus, hydromyelia, microcephaly agenesis of the cerebellar vermis, and presence of cerebellar cyst.[138,142] The abnormal fetal growth occurring at such an early stage in gestation may be the reason for the multiple associated malformations, owing to subsequent hindering and cramping of structures related to the retroflexed fetal neck.[141] Despite two case reports that discussed the same surviving iniencephalic patient,[137,139] iniencephaly is almost always lethal.

Open Spinal Neural Tube Defects

Myelomeningocele

Myelomeningocele, or open spina bifida, is a nonlethal neural tube defect with sequelae that affect both the CNS and the peripheral nervous system. The lesion is characterized by the protrusion of the spinal cord and meninges from the spinal canal with an abnormality in the overlying vertebral arches, muscle, and skin. Myelomeningoceles are generally cystic and contain cerebrospinal fluid that drains when the thin sac is disrupted. It is a severe form of spina bifida affecting about 1 of every 2000 children born worldwide.[143,144] Not included in this figure are the 23% of pregnancies ending in elective termination of affected fetuses.[145,146]

More than 80% of children with a neural tube defect can be detected by maternal serum α-fetoprotein screening before birth.[147] Although the determination of amniotic fluid acetylcholinesterase can be helpful, ultrasound is the method of choice in the diagnosis of neural tube defects. Direct visualization of the fetal spine can usually be accomplished by 16 weeks' gestation. Since the 1980s, the sonographic diagnosis of myelomeningocele has been enhanced by the introduction of high-resolution imaging tools and by recognition of specific brain abnormalities.[148] The CNS abnormalities associated with neural tube defects include cerebral ventriculomegaly, microcephaly, abnormalities of the frontal bone, and obliteration of the cisterna magna with anterior curving of the cerebellar hemisphere (banana sign) or an abnormal concavity of the cranium (lemon sign).[149] The abnormal findings of the CNS are thought to be a consequence of the hindbrain herniation (Arnold-Chiari II malformation). First described by Arnold and Chiari at the end of the 19th century,[150,151] the *Arnold-Chiari II malformation* is defined as the maldevelopment of a small posterior fossa and the herniation of the cerebellar vermis and brain stem (including the fourth ventricle) through an enlarged foramen magnum. Additionally, agenesis of the corpus callosum, enlargement of the massa intermedia, cortical heterotopia, and polymicrogyria can be seen. The origin of the Arnold-Chiari II malformation remains in dispute. The predominant hypothesis maintains that an imbalance of hydrodynamic forces occurs secondary to loss of cerebrospinal fluid from the lesion.[76,77,152,153] An alternative theory interprets the hindbrain herniation as the consequence of a traction injury caused by cranial growth imbalance.[152,154-156] Overgrowth of the cerebellum and the brain stem, along with a posterior fossa that is smaller than normal, leads to downward dislodgment of these structures, resulting in Arnold-Chiari II malformation.[157] Despite the controversies about the origin of myelomeningocele-associated hindbrain herniation, these lesions are identifiable in the embryo from as early as 8 weeks of gestation and are established in the fetus by the 12th week.

Pathologic studies of human embryos and fetuses with myelomeningocele in earlier stages of gestation reveal an open neural tube but undamaged neural tissue with almost normal cytoarchitecture.[158] This suggests that neural degeneration occurs at some point later in gestation (the two-hit hypothesis).[65,159] The first hit is the failure of neurulation early in gestation. The second hit is the spinal cord injury resulting from prolonged exposure of the neural tissue to the intrauterine environment. In theory, this secondary event can be prevented if an adequate prenatal covering of the exposed neural tissue can be provided. To have the best outcome, this repair must be fashioned before the onset of irreversible neural damage. There are several observations in human embryos, fetuses, and infants to support this premise.[55,160]

Osaka and associates[161] studied 18 embryos with classic caudal myelodysplasia and found an everted neural plate but preservation of the membranes. Chiari II malformation was not found in any of these embryos, whereas hindbrain herniation was present in two fetuses with caudal myelodysplasia in the same series. Additionally, pathologic signs of ventriculomegaly were not noted in the embryos, but they were found in one fetus with Chiari II malformation.[161]

In a pathologic examination of spinal cords of stillborn human fetuses with myelomeningocele (19 to 25 weeks of gestation), varying degrees of neural tissue loss at the site of the lesion were observed, but the dorsal and ventral horns were normal proximal to the defect.[159] This group was among the first to suggest the two-hit hypothesis because they attributed these alterations to injuries occurring subsequent to the failure of primary neural tube formation. A study of 10 additional fetuses had similar findings.[160]

Marin-Padilla[162] examined numerous human dysraphic malformations and concluded that the primary anomaly was a disturbance of the axial chordomesodermal tissue to support adequate lodging and protection of the developing nervous system and that degeneration and destruction of the neural tissue occur secondarily. Additional support exists for the two-hit hypothesis from *in vitro* studies. Drewek and colleagues[163] reported that damage to open neural tissue appears to be progressive and results from exposure to toxic substances in the amniotic fluid during the third trimester.

Korenromp and colleagues[164] observed that fetuses with myelomeningocele exhibited leg movement at 16 to 17 weeks of gestation. These investigators suggested that the affected fetuses did have good function at that point in gestation. No follow-up could be reported in this series because pregnancies were interrupted. Furthermore, Sival and associates[165] compared the leg movements of 13 fetuses with myelomeningocele prenatally and postnatally. Only one of the 13 had abnormal leg movements before birth, but 11 demonstrated abnormal leg movements postnatally. Two possible explanations for this phenomenon exist. The prenatal leg movements could be secondary to spinal cord reflex rather than of cerebral origin, thus permitting motion without electrical impulses conducted through the damaged spinal cord tissue. In addition, leg movements early in pregnancy could result from cerebral function conducted through an exposed spinal cord that is not yet damaged. However, even extremely experienced sonographers find it difficult to distinguish between spontaneous and reflex-based fetal leg movements.[166]

Most newborns with myelomeningocele show severe neurologic impairment of the lower extremities at birth, a finding suggesting that the neurologic injury may occur later in gestation or even at the time of delivery. It is remarkable that patients with lipomeningomyelocele (in which the neural tissue is covered and protected by skin) often have almost normal lower leg and continence function, despite a neurulation abnormality that is nearly identical to that present in newborns with open neural tube defect. These studies support direct injury as the primary cause of damage and loss of function, because neural tissue is injured exclusively from the protruding spinal cord.[159,160] As the pregnancy progresses, the volume of the amniotic fluid decreases, and this may result in more frequent contact of the exposed neural tissue with the uterine wall. Chick models of oligohydramnios, in which pressure necrosis of prominent areas of the body developed, support this hypothesis.[167]

Closed Spinal Neural Tube Defects

Clinically, closed neural tube defects should be subclassified from open neural tube defects because the embryogenesis appears to differ in most cases. In open defects, there is an essential failure during the primary neurulation, whereas closed neural tube defects appear to result from another form of disturbance during neural tube formation.[168] With few exceptions, the structural malformations of closed neural tube defects are limited to the spinal cord and are not associated with the Arnold-Chiari II malformation or hydrocephalus. In contrast to open defects, newborns with a closed neural tube defect have no exposed neural tissue and do not leak cerebrospinal fluid. Additionally, the prognosis of an infant affected by a closed defect is significantly better than one with an open neural tube defect. Generally, children born with closed defects have an intellectual function that is of the same distribution as the normal population, do not require cerebrospinal fluid–diverting shunts, and have considerably fewer problems with lower extremity sensorimotor function and with bladder and bowel function.[168] Because the clinical manifestations of closed defects can be undetected for days or even years, the origin of this group of neural tube defects is unidentified; no link to genetic, environmental, or dietary factors have been found. The major forms of closed neural tube defect are briefly described in the following sections.

Meningocele

Meningoceles are commonly located in the lumbosacral region in the vertebral arches. These lesions are often covered with skin, and the bony abnormality rarely involves more than two to three vertebrae. The sac of the meningocele consists of both arachnoid and dural meninges and contains cerebrospinal fluid. Most meningoceles also contain neural elements. Meningoceles are an infrequent and heterogeneous group of cystic lesions. The accurate prevalence of meningocele is subject to debate, because meningoceles are often grouped with myelomeningoceles. Furthermore, the pathogenesis remains unknown. The neurologic outcome of affected newborns is normal, but surgical correction and resection of the herniated meninges are indicated.[169]

Lipomatous Malformations

This abnormality includes all the closed neural tube defects with excessive lipomatous tissue present within or attached to the spinal cord or filum terminale. These lesions are called lipomyelomeningocele, lipomyelocele, leptomyelolipoma, lumbosacral lipoma, or lipoma of the filum terminale. The origin of *lipomatous closed neural tube defects* is controversial. Two different theories have been advanced: (1) lipomas arise from cells originating from the somatic mesoderm, and (2) lipomatous closed neural tube defects are a true malformation resulting from defective neurulation.[170] Most affected infants have a good prognosis with nearly normal leg and urologic function.

Dermal Sinus

A *dermal sinus* is a deep squamous epithelium–lined tract found on or near the midline. These lesions are most common in the lumbosacral region (63%),[171] and they sometimes contain hair or occasionally communicate with the dura. Abnormal adhesions between the ectoderm which forms the neural tube and that which is destined to form the skin are discussed as the primary cause of dermal sinuses.[169] Surgical removal of the lesions is indicated, because of the risk of infection and compression of underlying neural elements by the progressive enlargement of the dermal sinus.

Diastematomyelia

The caudal cord in *diastematomyelia* (split cord malformation) is divided by a median septum arising from a vertebral body. Each of the hemicords has a single set of dorsal and ventral nerve roots contained within its own dural sheath. It has been suggested that the defect results from a failure during neurulation and that a second neuroenteric canal becomes advanced with mesenchyme to form an endomesenchymal tract that splits the notochord and neural plate.[172] A few studies have reported that up to 39% of split cord malformations are associated with myelomeningocele.[173,174] Because of a considerable rate of coexistence of these two neural tube defects, Pang and coworkers[172] proposed a common embryogenesis for split cord malformations and myelomeningocele.

BURDEN OF NEURAL TUBE DEFECTS

Anencephaly and myelomeningocele are important contributors to fetal and infant mortality. All newborns affected by anencephaly are stillborn or die shortly after birth, whereas children born with myelomeningocele usually survive. However, the risk of death with neural tube defects varies significantly worldwide, depending not only on the severity of the defect but also on such aspects as availability, use, and acceptance of medical and surgical intervention. For example, in some regions of northern China, nearly 100%,[175] in the Netherlands, 35%,[176] and in the United States, 10%[177] of children affected by neural tube defects die.

For those infants affected by myelomeningocele, the significant lifelong disabilities accompanying this malformation include paraplegia, hydrocephalus,[178] pulmonary dysfunction,[179] sexual dysfunction, skeletal deformations and spinal deformities,[180] incontinence, and cognitive impairment,[181] with approximately 15% of them requiring some form of custodial care.[182,183]

Infants with myelomeningocele almost always have evidence of Chiari II malformation on magnetic resonance imaging (MRI).[184] This represents a caudal displacement of the inferior portion of cerebellar vermis, medulla, and lower pons, and an elongated fourth ventricle through the foramen magnum. Despite aggressive postnatal intervention, nearly 14% of neonates with spina bifida do not survive past 5 years of age, with the mortality rising to 35% in those with symptoms of brain stem dysfunction secondary to the Chiari II malformation.[185]

Clinical symptoms include swallowing difficulty, apnea, and stridor. Strabismus, a nonlethal Chiari II complication, is found in as many as 61% of patients with myelomeningocele.[186] Furthermore, the hindbrain deformity leads to ventriculomegaly in most cases because of impaired circulation of cerebrospinal fluid. Complications of ventriculomegaly probably lead to the impaired cognitive development seen in children with myelomeningocele.[187]

Rintoul and associates[178] performed a retrospective review of 297 patients born with myelomeningocele and described the natural history of ventricular shunting in myelomeningocele patients in relation to radiologic and functional criteria. Most closures (92%) and shunt placements (62%) were performed in the first week of life. The timing of shunt placement and the number of shunt revisions were independent of the level of lesion. The incidence of shunting by functional level was 81%, which is consistent within the generally accepted range of 80 to 85% for an unselected spina bifida population.[188, 189] The rate of ventricular shunting is significantly correlated to the anatomic level of the lesion.[178] One hundred per cent of the patients with thoracic-level lesions required postnatal shunting, compared with 88% of those with lumbar-level lesions and 68% of those with sacral-level lesions.

The availability of newer medical and surgical treatment modalities has significantly decreased the risk of some long-term medical complications, such as renal failure and severe dermatologic problems, affecting the risk of death among adults with myelomeningocele.[190] For example, Shurtleff and associates[191] and Hunt[192] documented that the survival rate to nearly the third decade of life was more than 50% in affected persons in whom the defect was surgically repaired shortly after birth.

The maldevelopment of the spinal cord is generally associated with some degree of weakness and lack of sensation in the lower limbs. Children less than 8 years of age can often walk, sometimes without any assistance. However, as the children get older and heavier, their weight/power ratio increases, and walking becomes more difficult; later, many of the affected children become permanent wheelchair users.

Another, potentially preventable complication of spina bifida is disease-associated latex sensitization.[193, 194] Up to 43% of children with spina bifida are affected.[193] However, it remains unclear whether this association is only a consequence of repeated exposure to latex-containing products (e.g., gloves or catheter material)[195] or is the result of a potential genetic contribution and alteration of the human leukocyte antigen phenotype.[196]

In addition to the emotional impact on the family, the financial burden for family and community are enormous. In the United States, the cost of care for infants born with spina bifida in 1988 was almost 500 million dollars per year (in 1992 dollars) or $294,000 for each infant.[197]

TREATMENT OPTIONS

Standard Treatment

The current standard of care for children born with myelomeningocele is primarily supportive. In an attempt to limit injury of the neural tissue through contact with the uterine wall and birth canal associated with labor and vaginal delivery, fetuses are delivered by elective cesarean section before the onset of labor. This has been shown to result in improved neurologic outcome.[198]

An initial neurologic evaluation of the newborn by the neonatologist and by the pediatric neurologist and neurosurgeon is essential to assess the functional level, the neurologic deficit, and the potential complications (e.g., hydrocephalus, deformities of the lower legs, lower leg movement problems, and future continence problems), and it should include a sensory examination to determine the level of the lesion and prognosis for motor ability.

Surgical repair of the defect is usually performed within the first 24 to 48 hours of life to minimize the risk of infection.[199] The goal of postnatal myelomeningocele repair is to untether the placode and to cover the lesion while preserving function. Because neurologic function typically exists only above the exposed spinal cord, sacrifice of some spinal cord tissue and nerve roots has been considered acceptable.[200]

Fetal Neurosurgical Intervention

Before 1997, fetal surgery was considered only for fetuses with life-threatening anomalies.[201] However, the severe morbidity and significant mortality associated with myelomeningocele combined with the promising results of animal research led to consideration of prenatal intervention for this disorder. In 1997, Bruner and associates[202] reported their preliminary observation from two fetuses with open lumbar myelomeningocele. They described fetoscopic placement of a maternal spit-thickness skin graft over the fetal neural placode. Of the two fetuses reported, one died shortly after surgery, and the other showed no improvement in neurologic function. A full report in 1999[203] revealed that a total of four fetuses were operated on between 22 and 24 weeks of gestation using a maternal skin graft and fibrin glue. Unfortunately, fetal morbidity and mortality by endoscopic coverage were disappointingly high. Two fetal losses occurred; the third infant was delivered by planned cesarean section at 35 weeks' gestation after demonstration of fetal lung maturity. The other infant was delivered by cesarean section at 28 weeks' gestation after preterm labor. The two survivors were 3 years and 6 months old, respectively, at the time of the report. Both required secondary neonatal closure of their myelomeningocele and required ventriculoperitoneal shunting. Both survivors were reported as having only mild motor and somatosensory deficit, but the fate of the maternal skin grafts as patch closure was unclear. The use of maternal skin grafts as patch closure was unsuccessful because glue fixation was inadequate and because the fetus was sufficiently immunocompetent to reject the skin graft at the time of the procedure. After abandoning the endoscopic approach, the same group reported four fetuses that underwent late-gestation (28 to 30 weeks) open repair.[204] None of the reported cases had demonstrable hindbrain herniation at birth, but two required shunts, and their neurologic outcome was not described.

Adzick and colleagues reported an earlier-gestation fetal repair of an open neural tube defect.[205] In this case, a 27-year-old pregnant woman was referred at 23 weeks of gestation for elevated maternal serum α-fetoprotein level. The karyotype was normal. Ultrasound examination showed a thoracolumbar myelomeningocele and good fetal leg movements. With the patient under general anesthesia, a low transverse maternal laparotomy and vertical hysterotomy were performed. The cystic membrane of the lesion was excised, and skin flaps were developed to close the defect. The infant was delivered at 30 weeks of gestation by cesarean section because of preterm labor in which tocolysis failed. The baby briefly required mechanical ventilation (5 days) and showed excellent leg function, except for absent plantar flexion and a right clubfoot.[205] Postnatal MRI revealed that the hindbrain herniation was no longer present.

Sutton and associates[206] reported 10 cases of open fetal surgery for myelomeningocele as a follow-up of the initial report by Adzick and colleagues.[205] Postnatal assessment indicated improved neurologic function and resolution of the hindbrain herniation demonstrated preoperatively by MRI in all patients. One fetus died because of premature delivery at 25 weeks' gestation. The hindbrain herniation (as assessed by serial MRI) improved within 3 weeks after intrauterine closure between 22 and 25 weeks' gestation. No obstetric complications were reported in this small case series. Only one patient required a shunt in the neonatal period, but three other infants required shunts subsequently. It was speculated that fetal repair of myelomeningocele may lead to more normal cerebrospinal fluid pressure gradients with consequent ascent of the hindbrain, reexpansion of the cisterna magna, and improved cerebrospinal fluid circulation. Five patients had leg function at birth that was at least two segments better than expected based on anatomic level, but in two cases, this level of function was lost because of tethering.

Bruner and associates[207] concurrently reported a decreased incidence of hindbrain herniation in 29 patients after open repair between 24 and 30 weeks' gestation. Only 11 (38%) demonstrated any degree of postoperative cerebellar herniation, with moderate herniation present in two infants. In a comparison group of patients repaired postnatally, herniation was present in 95%.[207] Likewise, 17 of the 29 patients (59%) required ventriculoperitoneal shunt placement compared with the control group, which had a 91% shunt placement rate with follow-up of least 6 months. Shunts were placed at a later postnatal age than control patients. Although improved leg function was not found in this group, this group did not exclude fetuses with preoperative evidence of decreased lower extremity function, and repairs were performed later in gestation. The longer *in utero* biochemical and traumatic exposure may have contributed to the lack of improved leg function. There were substantial obstetric complications. In women whose fetuses underwent open *in utero* repair of the myelomeningocele, oligohydramnios was present in 48% versus only 4% of controls, preterm premature rupture of the membranes occurred in 28% versus 4%, preterm uterine contractions occurred in 50% versus 9%, and the gestational age at delivery was significantly lower. Approximately 5 weeks after open fetal surgery, one study patient developed signs and symptoms of a small bowel obstruction. Surgical exploration at 31 weeks' gestation demonstrated hysterotomy dehiscence with adhesions to the small bowel.[207]

More recently, Johnson and associates[208] reported the outcome of 43 fetuses that underwent prenatal repair of myelomeningocele at the Children's Hospital of Philadelphia. The fetuses had thoracic, lumbar, and sacral lesions in 3, 34, and 6 patients, respectively, and all showed the presence of hindbrain herniation. The mean age of surgery was 23 weeks of gestation. Preterm labor resulted in premature delivery and neonatal death of 3 fetuses (7%). The mean gestational age at delivery in survivors was 34 weeks and 3 days. All 40 (100%) surviving fetuses showed reversal of the hindbrain herniation postoperatively by fetal MRI, and only 35% of the infants required postnatal ventriculoperitoneal shunting (1 of 2, 50% thoracic; 12 of 33, 36% lumbar; and 1 of 5, 20% sacral).[208] The ventriculoperitoneal shunt rate compared with the vertebral level in a historical control group of 297 infants collected from the Children's Hospital of Philadelphia Spina Bifida Clinic[178] who underwent neonatal neurosurgical closure was 100% for thoracic, 88% for lumbar, and 68% for sacral lesions.

The initial clinical experience with fetal repair of myelomeningocele, most performed around 24 weeks' gestation, suggests that the need for postnatal ventricular decompression by shunting may be reduced. Earlier repair may improve altered fluid dynamics and subsequently hindbrain herniation, as well as improving lower extremity, bladder, and bowel function. Nevertheless, fetal surgical intervention raises complex ethical and legal issues regarding the risks and benefits for both the fetus and the mother.[209, 210] Furthermore, the current data from *in utero* surgery for myelomeningocele are insufficient to assess the long-term neurologic benefit and risk of this type of intervention.[208,211] Further studies such as the planned prospective randomized clinical trial are essential to determine the risk/benefit ratio of this promising but still experimental approach.

ACKNOWLEDGMENT

This work was supported by a research grant (DA 544/1-1) from the German Research Society (Deutsche Forschungsgemeinschaft), Bonn, Germany.

REFERENCES

1. Dolk H, et al: Heterogeneity of neural tube defects in Europe: the significance of site of defect and presence of other major anomalies in relation to geographic differences in prevalence. Teratology 1991;44:547.
2. Shibuya K, Murray CJL: Congenital anomalies. *In* Marray CJL, Lopez AD (eds): Health Dimensions of Sex and Reproduction: The Global Burden of Sexually Transmitted Diseases, HIV, Maternal Conditions, Perinatal Disorders, and Congenital Anomalies, Vol 3. Boston, Harvard University Press, 1998, p 455.
3. Harmon JP, et al: Prenatal ultrasound detection of isolated neural tube defects: is cytogenetic evaluation warranted? Obstet Gynecol 1995;86:595.
4. Shaw GM, et al: Epidemiologic characteristics of phenotypically distinct neural tube defects among 0.7 million California births 1983–1987. Teratology 1994;49:143.
5. Baird PA: Neural tube defects in the Sikhs. Am J Med Genet 1983;13:511.
6. Little J, Elwood JM: Epidemiology of neural tube defects. *In* Kiley M (ed): Reproductive and Perinatal Epidemiology. Boca Raton, FL, CRC Press, 1991, p 251.
7. Botto LD, et al: Neural tube defects. N Engl J Med 1999;341;1509.
8. Khoury MJ, et al: Etiologic heterogeneity of neural tube defects: clues from epidemiology. Am J Epidemiol 1982;115:538.
9. Goldstein RB, Filly RA: Prenatal diagnosis of anencephaly: spectrum of sonographic appearance and distinction from the amniotic band syndrome. AJR Am J Roentgenol 1988;151:547.
10. Volpe JJ: Overview: normal and abnormal human brain development. Ment Retard Develop Disabil Res Rev 2000;6:1.
11. Smith JL, Schoenwolf GC: Neurulation: coming to closure. Trends Neurosci 1997;20:510.
12. Colas F, Schoenwolf GC: Towards a cellular and molecular understanding of neurulation. Dev Dyn 2001;221:117.
13. Harland R: Neural induction. Curr Opin Genet Dev 2000;10:357.
14. Jessell AG, Sanes JR: Development: the decade of the developing brain. Curr Opin Neurobiol 2000;10:599.
15. DeSesso JM, et al: Apparent lability of neural tube closure in laboratory animals and humans. Am J Med Genet 1999;87:143.
16. Seller MJ: Neural tube defects: are neurulation and canalization forms causally distinct? Am J Med Genet 1990;35:394.
17. Van Allem MI, et al: Evidence of multi-site closure of the neural tube in humans. Am J Med Genet 1993;47:723.
18. Martinez-Frias ML, et al: Epidemiological analysis of multi-site closure failure of the neural tube in humans. Am J Med Genet 1996;66:64.
19. Urioste M, Rosa A: Anencephaly and faciocranioschisis: evidence of complete failure of closure 3 of the neural tube in humans. Am J Med Genet 1998;75:4.
20. Thiery JP, et al: Cell adhesion molecules in early chick embryogenesis. Proc Natl Acad Sci USA 1982;79:6737.
21. O´Shea KS, Kaufman MH: Phospholipase C-induced neural tube defects in the mouse embryo. Experientia 1980;36:1217.
22. Karfunkel P: The mechanisms of neural tube formation. Int Rev Cytol 1974;38:245.
23. Jelinek R, Friebova Z: Influence of mitotic activity on neurulation movements. Nature 1966;209:822.
24. Wu M, et al: Neural tube defects and abnormal brain development in F52-deficient mice. Proc Natl Acad Sci USA 1996;93:2110.
25. Volcik KA, et al: Testing for genetic associations in a spina bifida population: analysis of the HOX gene family and human candidate gene regions implicated by mouse models of neural tube defects. Am J Med Genet 2002;110:203.
26. Tassabehji M, et al: Waardenburg's syndrome patients have mutations in the human homologue of the Pax-3 paired box gene. Nature 1992;355:635.
27. Baldwin CT, et al: An exonic mutation in the HuP2 paired domain gene causes Waardenburg's syndrome. Nature 1992;352:539.
28. Vortkamp A, et al: GLI3 zinc-finger gene interrupted by translocations in Greig syndrome families. Nature 1991;352:539.
29. Gowen LC, et al: Brca1 deficiency results in early embryonic lethality characterized by neuroepithelial abnormalities. Nat Genet 1996;12:191.
30. Imamoto A, Soriano P: Disruption of the csk gene, encoding a negative regulator of Src family tyrosine kinase, leads to neural tube defects and embryonic lethality in mice. Cell 1993;73:1117.
31. Sah VP, et al: A subset of p53-deficient embryos exhibit exencephaly. Nat Genet 1995;10:175.
32. Gruneberg H: Genetical studies on the skeleton of the mouse. VIII Curly tail. J Genet 1954;52:52.
33. Van Straaten HWM, et al: Intrinsic and extrinsic factors in the mechanism of neurulation: effect of curvature of the body axis on closure of posterior neuropore. Development 1993;117:1163.

34. Copp AJ, et al: A cell-type-specific abnormality of cell proliferation in mutant (curly tail) mouse embryos developing spinal neural tube defects. Development 1988;104:285.
35. Brook FA, et al: Curvature of the caudal region is responsible for failure of neural tube closure in the curly tail (ct) mouse embryo. Development 1991;113:671.
36. Copp AJ, Bernfield M: Accumulation of basement membrane-associated hyaluronate is reduced in the posterior neuropore region of mutant (curly tail) mouse embryos developing spinal neural tube defects. Dev Biol 1988;130:583.
37. Copp AJ, Bernfield M: Etiology and pathogenesis of human neural tube defects: insights from mouse models. Curr Opin Pediatr 1994;6:624.
38. Adinolfi M, et al: Levels of alpha-fetoprotein in amniotic fluids of mice (curly-tail) with neural tube defects. J Med Genet 1976;13:511.
39. Letts VA, et al: A curly-tail modifier locus, mct1, on mouse chromosome 7. Genomics 1995;29:719.
40. Greene ND, Copp AJ: Inositol prevents folate-resistant neural tube defects in the mouse. Nat Genet 1997;3:60.
41. Seller MJ: Vitamins, folic acid and the cause and prevention of neural tube defects. Ciba Found Symp 1994;181:161.
42. Van Straaten HW, et al: Dietary methionine does not reduce penetrance in curly mice but causes a phenotype-specific decrease in embryonic growth. J Nutr 1995;125:2733.
43. Fleming A, Copp AJ: Embryonic folate metabolism and mouse neural tube defects. Science 1998;280:2107.
44. Goulding MD, et al: Pax-3, a novel murine DNA binding protein expressed during early neurogenesis. EMBO J 1991;10:1135.
45. Epstein DJ, et al: Splotch (SP2H), a mutation affecting development of the mouse neural tube, shows a deletion within the paired homeodomain of Pas3. Cell 1991;61:767.
46. Yang XM, Tarsler DG: Abnormalities of neural tube formation in pre-spina bifida Splotch-delayed mouse embryos. Teratology 1991;43:643.
47. Moase CE, Trasler DG: Alteration in Splotch neural tube defect mouse embryos. Development 1991;113:1049.
48. Chatkupt S, et al: Absence of linkage between familial neural tube defects and PAX3 gene. J Med Genet 1995;32:200.
49. Lufkin T, et al: Disruption of the Hox-1.6 homeobox gene results in defects in a region corresponding to its rostral domain of expression. Cell 1991;66:1105.
50. Volcik KA, et al: Testing for genetic association in a spina bifida population: analysis of the HOX gene family and human candidate gene region implicated by mouse models of neural tube defects. Am J Med Genet 2002;110:203.
51. Morrison K, et al: Susceptibility to spina bifida: an association study of four candidate genes. Ann Hum Genet 1998;62:379.
52. Trembath D, et al: Analysis of select folate pathway genes, PAX3 and human T in a midwestern neural tube defect population. Teratology 1999;59:331.
53. Speer MC, et al: T locus shows no evidence for linkage disequilibrium or mutation in American Caucasian neural tube defect families. Am J Med Genet 2002;110:215.
54. Estibeiro JP, et al: Interaction between splotch (Sp) and curly tail (Ct) mouse mutants in the embryonic development of neural tube defects. Development 1993;119:113.
55. Neumann PE, et al: Multifactorial inheritance of neural tube defects: localization of major gene and recognition of modifiers in the ct mutant mice. Nat Genet 1994;6:357.
56. Aderem A: The MARCKS brothers: a family of protein kinase C substrates. Cell 1992;71:713.
57. Sulik KK, Sadler TW: Postulated mechanisms underlying the development of neural tube defects: insights from in vitro and in vivo studies. Ann NY Acad Sci 1993;678:8.
58. Briner W: The effect of GABA receptor ligands in experimental spina bifida occulta. BMC Pharmacol 2001;1:2.
59. Copp AJ, et al: The embryonic development of mammalian neural tube defects. Prog Neurobiol 1990;35:363.
60. Duru S, et al: Comparative effects of valproic acid sodium for Chiari-like malformation at 9 and 10 days of gestation in the rat. Childs Nerv Syst 2001;17:399.
61. Alles AJ, Sulik KK: Pathogenesis of retinoid-induced hindbrain malformations in an experimental model. Clin Dysmorphol 1992;1:187.
62. Turner S, et al: Teratogenic effects on the neuroepithelium of the CD-1 mouse embryo exposed in utero to sodium valproate. Teratology 1990;41:421.
63. Nau H, et al: Valproic acid-induced neural tube defects in mouse and human: aspects of chirality, alternative drug development, pharmacokinetics and possible mechanisms. Pharmacol Toxicol 1991;69:310.
64. Alles AJ, Sulik KK: Retinoic acid-induced spina bifida: evidence for a pathogenic mechanism. Development 1990;108:73.
65. Ehlers K, et al: Spina bifida aperta induced by valproic acid and by all-trans-retinoic acid in the mouse: distinct differences in morphology and periods of sensitivity. Teratology 1992;46:117.
66. Ehlers K, et al: Methionine reduces the valproic acid–induced spina bifida rate in mice without altering valproic acid kinetics. J Nutr 1996;126:67.
67. Coelho CND, et al: Whole rat embryos require methionine for neural tube closure. J Nutr 1989;119:1716.
68. Michejda M: Intrauterine treatment of spina bifida: primate model. Z Kinderchir 1984;39:259.
69. Heffez DS, et al: The paralysis associated with myelomeningocele: clinical and experimental data implicating a preventable spinal cord injury. Neurosurgery 1990;26:987.
70. Heffez DS, et al: Intrauterine repair of experimental surgically created dysraphism. Neurosurgery 1993;32:1005.
71. Correia-Pinto J, et al: In utero meconium exposure increases spinal cord necrosis in a rat model of myelomeningocele. J Pediatr Surg 2002;37:488.
72. Meuli M, et al: A new model of myelomeningocele: studies in the fetal lamb. Surg Forum 1994;45:587.
73. Meuli M, et al: In utero surgery rescues neurological function at birth in sheep with spina bifida. Nat Med 1995;1:342.
74. Meuli M, et al: In utero repair of experimental myelomeningocele saves neurologic function at birth. J Pediatr Surg 1996;31:397.
75. McLone DG, Knepper PA: The cause of Chiari II malformation: a unified theory. Pediatr Neurosurg 1989;15:1.
76. Paek BW, et al: Hindbrain herniation develops in surgically created myelomeningocele but is absent after repair in fetal lambs. Am J Obstet Gynecol 2000;183:1119.
77. Bouchard S, et al: Correction of hindbrain herniation and anatomy of the vermis following in utero repair of myelomeningocele in sheep. J Pediatr Surg 2003;38:451.
78. Housley HT, et al: Creation of myelomeningocele in the fetal rabbit. Fetal Diagn Ther 2000;15:275.
79. Emery AEH: Methology in Medical Genetics, 2nd ed. Edinburgh, Churchill Livingstone, 1986.
80. Czeizel AE, Dudas I: Prevention of the first occurrence of neural-tube defects by periconceptional vitamin supplementation. N Engl J Med 1992;327:1832.
81. Lulock M, Daskalakis I: New perspectives on folate status: a differential role for the vitamin in cardiovascular disease, birth defects and other conditions. Br J Biomed Sci 2000;57:254.
82. Shields DC, et al: The "thermolabile" variant of methylenetetrahydrofolate reductase and neural tube defects: an evaluation of genetic risk and the relative importance of genotypes of the embryo and the mother. Am J Hum Genet 1999;64:1045.
83. Gibson KM, Bottiglieri T: Genetic predisposition to neural tube defects? Pediatr Res 2000;48:135.
84. Rosenquist TH, et al: Homocysteine induces congenital defects of the heart and neural tube: effect of folic acid. Proc Natl Scad Sci USA 1996;93:15227.
85. Heid MK, et al: Folate deficiency alone does not produce neural tube defect in mice. J Nutr 1992;122:888.
86. Daly LE, et al: Folate levels and neural tube defects: implication for prevention. JAMA 1995;274:1698.
87. MRC Vitamin Study Research Group: Prevention of neural tube defects: results of the medical research council vitamin study. Lancet 1991;338:131.
88. Abramsky L, et al: Has advice on periconceptional folate supplementation reduced neural-tube defects? Lancet 1999;354;998.
89. Shojania AM: Folic acid and vitamin B12 deficiency in pregnancy and in the neonatal period. Clin Perinatol 1984;11:433.
90. Little J, Elwood JH: Socio-economic status and occupation. In Elwood JM, Little Elwood JH (eds): Epidemiology and Control of Neural Tube Defects, Vol 20 of Monographs in Epidemiology and Biostatistics. Oxford, Oxford University Press, 1992, p 456.
91. Myrianthopoulos MC, Melnick M: Studies in neural tube defects. I. Epidemiologic and etiologic aspects. Am J Med Genet 1987;26:783.
92. Werler MM, et al: Pregnant weight in relation to risk of neural tube defects. JAMA 1996;275:1089.
93. Northrup H, Volcik KA: Spina bifida and other neural tube defects. Curr Probl Pediatr 2000;30;313.
94. Edward MJ, et al: Hyperthermia and birth defects. Reprod Toxicol 1995;9:411.
95. Sharma JB, Gulati N: Potential relationship between dengue fever and neural tube defects in a northern district of India. Int J Gynecol Obstet 1992;39:291.
96. Lammer EJ, et al: Teratogen update: valproic acid. Teratology 1987;35:465.
97. McIntosh GC, et al: Paternal age and the risk of birth defects in offspring. Epidemiology 1995;6 282.
98. Strassburg MA, et al: A population-based case-control study of anencephalus and spina bifida in a low-risk area. Dev Med Child Neurol 1983;25:632.
99. Canfield MA, et al: Hispanic origin and neural tube defects in Houston/Harris County, Texas. I and II. Am J Epidemiol 1996;143:1.
100. Chatkupt S, et al: Study of genetics, epidemiology, and vitamin usage in familial spina bifida in the United States in the 1990s. Neurology 1994;44:65.
101. Smithells RW, et al: Apparent prevention of neural tube defects by periconceptional vitamin supplementation. Arch Dis Child 1981;56:911.
102. Scott JM, et al: The role of nutrition in neural tube defects. Annu Rev Nutr 1990;10:277.
103. Smithells RW, et al: Further experience of vitamin supplementation for prevention of neural tube defect recurrences. Lancet 1983;1:1927.

104. Vergel RG, et al: Primary prevention of neural tube defects with folic acid supplementation: Cuban experience. Prenat Diagn 1990;10:149.
105. Honein MA, et al: Impact of folic acid fortification of the US food supply on the occurrence of neural tube defects. JAMA 2001;285:2981.
106. Finkelstein JD: Methionine metabolism in mammals. J Nutr Biochem 1990;1:228.
107. Mills JL, et al: Homocysteine metabolism in pregnancies complicated by neural-tube defects. Lancet 1995;345:149.
108. Steegers-Theunissen RPM, et al: Maternal hyperhomocysteinemia: a risk factor for neural-tube defects? Metabolism 1994;43:1475.
109. Essien FB, Wannberg SL: Methionine but not folinic acid of vitamin B-12 alters the frequency of neural tube defects in Axd mutant mice. J Nutr 1993;123:27.
110. Berry RJ, et al: Prevention of neural-tube defects with folic acid in China. N Engl J Med 1999;341;1485.
111. Kadir R, Economides DL: Neural tube defects and periconceptional folic acid. CMAJ 2002;167:255.
112. Dekaban AS, Bartelmez GW: Complete dysraphism in 14 somite human embryo. Am J Anat 1964;115:27.
113. Medical Task Force on Anencephaly: The infant with anencephaly. N Engl J Med 1990;332:669.
114. Sanders RC, et al (eds): Structural Fetal Abnormalities, 2nd ed. St. Louis, CV Mosby, 2002, p 20.
115. Limb CJ, Holmes LB: Anencephaly: changes in prenatal detection and birth status, 1972 through 1990. Am J Obstet Gynecol 1994;170:1333.
116. Naidich TP, et al: Cephaloceles and related malformations. AJNR Am J Neuroradiol 1992;13:655.
117. Feuchtbaum LB, et al: Neural tube defects prevalence in California (1990-1994): eliciting patterns by type of defect and maternal race/ethnicity. Genet Test 1999;3:265.
118. Squier MV: Malformation of the nervous system and hydrocephalus. In Jean Keeling (ed): Fetal and Neonatal Pathology, 3rd ed. London, Springer-Verlag, 2001, p 605.
119. Chervenak FA, et al: When is termination of pregnancy during the third trimester morally justifiable? N Engl J Med 1983;309:822.
120. Melnick M, Myrianthopoulos NC: Studies in neural tube defects. II. Pathologic findings in a prospectively collected series of anencephalics. Am J Med Genet 1987;26:797.
121. Casellas M, et al: Prenatal diagnosis of exencephaly. Prenat Diagn 1993;13:417.
122. Papp Z, et al: Exencephaly in human fetuses. Clin Genet 1986;30:440.
123. Cox GG, et al: Exencephaly: sonographic findings and radiologic-pathologic correlation. Radiology 1985;155:755.
124. Stagiannis KF, et al: Exencephaly in autosomal dominant brachydactyly syndrome. Prenat Diagn 1995;15:70.
125. Hendricks SK, et al: Exencephaly: clinical and ultrasonic correlation to anencephaly. Obstet Gynecol 1988;72:898.
126. Sadler TW: Effects of maternal diabetes on early embryogenesis. II. Hyperglycemia-induced exencephaly. Teratology 1980;21:349.
127. Dziadek M: Preovulatory administration of clomiphene causes fetal growth restriction and neural tube defects (exencephaly by an indirect maternal effect. Teratology 1993;47:263.
128. Wiswell TE, et al: Major congenital neurologic malformations. Am J Dis Child 1990;144:61.
129. Lemire RJ: Neural tube defects: clinical correlations. Clin Neurosurg 1983;30:65.
130. Ingraham FD, Swan H: Spina bifida and cranium bifidum: a survey of 546 cases. N Engl J Med 1943;228:559.
131. Chervenak FA, et al: Diagnosis and management of fetal cephalocele. Obstet Gynecol 1984;64:86.
132. David DJ, Proudman TW: Cephaloceles: classification, pathology, and management. World J Surg 1989;13:349.
133. Emery JL, Kalhan SC: The pathology of exencephalus. Dev Med Child Neurol 1970;12(Suppl 22):51.
134. Date I, et al: Long-term outcome in surgically treated encephalocele. Surg Neurol 1993;40:125.
135. Habal MB: Craniofacial correction of the occipital encephalocele. J Craniofac Surg 1993;4:215.
136. Lewis HF: Iniencephalus. Am J Obstet Gynecol 1897;35:11.
137. Gartman JJ, et al: Deformity correction and long-term survival in an infant with iniencephaly. J Neurosurg 1991;75:126.
138. Scherrer CC, et al: Brain stem and cervical cord dysraphic lesions found in iniencephaly. Pediatr Pathol 1992;12:469.
139. Katz VL, et al: Iniencephaly is not uniformly fatal. Prenat Diagn 1989;9:595.
140. Gardner WJ: Klippel-Feil syndrome, iniencephalus anencephalus, hindbrain hernia and mirror movements: overdistension of the neural tube. Childs Brain 1979;5:361.
141. David TJ, Nixon A: Congenital malformations associated with anencephaly and iniencephaly. J Med Genet 1976;13:263.
142. Aleksic S, et al: Iniencephaly: neuropathologic study. Clin Neuropathol 1983;2:55.
143. Edmonds LD, James LM: Temporal trends in the prevalence of congenital malformations at birth based on the birth defects monitoring program, United States, 1979-1987. MMWR Morb Mortal Wkly Rep 1990;39:19.
144. Lary JM, Edmonds LD: Prevalence of spina bifida at birth—United States, 1983-1990: a comparison to two surveillance systems. MMWR Morb Mortal Wkly Rep 1996;45:15.
145. Roberts HE, et al: Impact of prenatal diagnosis on the birth prevalence of neural tube defects, Atlanta 1990-1991. Pediatrics 1995;96:880.
146. Velie EM, Shaw GM: Impact of prenatal diagnosis and elective termination on prevalence and risk estimates of neural tube defects in California, 1989-1991. Am J Epidemiol 1996;144:473.
147. Brock DJH, Sutcliffe RG: Alpha-fetoprotein in antenatal diagnosis of anencephaly and spina bifida. Lancet 1972;2:197.
148. Blumenfeld Z, et al: The early diagnosis of neural tube defects. Prenat Diagn 1993;13:863.
149. Nicolaides KH, et al: Ultrasound screening for spina bifida: cranial and cerebellar signs. Lancet 1986;2:72.
150. Chiari H: Ueber Veraenderungen des Kleinhirns der Pons und der Medulla oblongata in folge von congenitaler Hydrocephalie des Grosshirns. Dtsch Akad Wissenschr Math Natur Klin 1895;63:71.
151. Arnold J: Transposition von Gewebskeimen und Sympodie. Beitr Pathol Anat Allgm Pathol 1894;16:1.
152. McLone DG, Knepper PA: The cause of Chiari II malformation: a unified theory. Pediatr Neurosci 1989;15:1.
153. Padget DH: Spina bifida embryonic neuroschisis—a causal relationship: definition of the postnatal confirmations involving a bifid spine. Johns Hopkins Med J 1968;128:233.
154. Lichtenstein BW: Distant neuroanatomic complications of spina bifida (spinal dysraphism), hydrocephalus, Arnold-Chiari deformity, stenosis of the aqueduct of Sylvius, etc, pathogenesis and pathology. Arch Neurol Psychiatry 1942;47:195.
155. Penfield W, Coburn DF: Arnold-Chiari malformation and its operative treatment. Arch Neurol Psychiatry 1938;40:328.
156. Hoffman HJ, et al: Manifestations and management of Arnold Chiari malformation in patients with myelomeningocele. Childs Brain 1975;1:255.
157. Barry A, et al: Possible factors in the development of the Arnold-Chiari malformation. J Neurosurg 1957;17:238.
158. Patten B: Embryological stages in the establishing of myeloschisis with spina bifida. Am J Anat 1953;93:365.
159. Hutchins GM, et al: Acquired spinal cord injury in human fetuses with myelomeningocele. Pediatr Pathol Lab Med 1996;16:701.
160. Meuli M, et al: The spinal cord lesion in human fetuses with myelomeningocele: implications for fetal surgery. J Pediatr Surg 1997;31:448.
161. Osaka K, et al: Meyelomeningocele before birth. J Neurosurg 1978;49:711.
162. Marin-Padilla M: Spina bifida. In Vinkin EL, Bruyn GW (eds): Handbook of Clinical Neurology. New York, Elsevier, 1978, p 159.
163. Drewek MJ, et al: Quantitative analysis of the toxicity of human amniotic fluid to cultured rat spinal cord. Pediatr Neurosurg 1997;27:190.
164. Korenromp MJ, et al: Early fetal movements in myelomeningocele. Lancet 1986;1:917.
165. Sival DA, et al: Perinatal motor behavior and neurological outcome in spina bifida aperta. Early Hum Dev 1997;50:27.
166. Filly RA: Ultrasound evaluation of the fetal neural axis. In Callen PW (ed): Ultrasonography in Obstetrics and Gynecology. Philadelphia, WB Saunders Co, 1994, p 189.
167. Thévenet A, Sengel P: Naturally occurring wounds and wound healing in chick embryo wings. Roux Arch Dev Biol 1986;195:345.
168. McComb JG: Spinal and cranial neural tube defects. Semin Pediatr Neurol 1997;4:156.
169. McComb JG, Chen TC: Closed spinal neural tube defects. In Tindall GT, et al (eds): The Practice of Neurosurgery. Baltimore, Williams & Wilkins, 1996, p 2753.
170. Catala M: Embryogenesis: why do we need a new explanation for the emergence of spina bifida with lipoma? Childs Nerv Syst 1997;13:336.
171. Powell KR, et al: A prospective search for congenital dermal abnormalities of the craniospinal axis. J Pediatr 1975;87:744.
172. Pang D, et al: Split cord malformation. I. A unified theory of embryogenesis for double spinal cord malformations. Neurosurgery 1992;31:451.
173. Ersahin Y, et al: Split spinal cord malformations in children. J Neurosurg 1998;88:57.
174. Kumar R, et al: Occurrence of split cord malformations in myelomeningocele: complex spina bifida. Pediatr Neurosurg 2002;36:119.
175. Moore CA, et al: Elevated rates of severe neural tube defects in a high-prevalence area in northern China. Am J Med Genet 1997;73:113.
176. den Ouden AL, et al: Prevalenties, klinish beeld en prognose van neural-buidefecten in Netherland. Ned Tijdschr Geneeskd 1996;140:2092.
177. Shurtleff DB, et al: Meningomyelocele: management in utero and post partum. Ciba Found Symp 1994;181:270.
178. Rintoul NE, et al: A new look at myelomeningoceles: functional level, vertebral level, shunting, and the implications for fetal intervention. Pediatrics 2002;109:409.
179. Sherman MS, et al: Pulmonary dysfunction and reduced exercise capacity in patients with myelomeningocele. J Pediatr 1997;131:413.
180. Iborra J, et al: Neurological abnormality, major orthopedic deformities and ambulation analysis in a myelomeningocele population in Catalonia (Spain). Spinal Cord 1999;37:351.
181. Tsai PY, et al: Functional investigation in children with spina bifida: measured by the pediatric evaluation of disability inventory. Childs Nerv Syst 2002;18:48.
182. McLone DG, et al: Concepts in the management of spina bifida. In Humphreys RE (ed): Concepts in Pediatric Neurosurgery. Basel, Karger, 1985, p 97.
183. McLone DG: Care of the neonate with myelomeningocele (abstract). Neurosurg Clin North Am 1998;9:111.

184. Ruge JR, et al: Anatomical progression of the Chiari II malformation. Childs Nerv Syst 1992;8:86.
185. Worley G, et al: Survival at 5 years of a cohort of newborn infants with myelomeningocele. Dev Med Child Neurol 1996;38:816.
186. Biglan AW: Strabismus associated with myelomeningocele. J Pediatr Ophthalmol Strabismus 1995;32:309.
187. McLone DG, Naidich TP: Myelomeningocele: outcome and late complications. *In* McLaurin DL, et al (eds): Pediatric Neurosurgery. Philadelphia, WB Saunders Co, 1989.
188. McLone DG: Results of treatment of children born with a myelomeningocele. Clin Neurosurg 1983;30:407.
189. Caldarelli M, et al: Shunt complications in the first postoperative year in children with myelomeningocele. Childs Nerv Syst 1996;12:748.
190. Kinsman SL, Doehring MC: The cost of preventable conditions in adults with spina bifida. Eur J Pediatr Surg 1996;6(Suppl 1):17.
191. Shurtleff DB, et al: Meningomyelocele: management in utero and postpartum. Ciba Found Symp 1994;181:270.
192. Hunt GM: The medican survival time in open spina bifida. Dev Med Clin Neurol 1997;39:568.
193. Zsolt S, et al: Latex sensitization in spina bifida appears disease-associated. J Pediatr 1999;134:344.
194. Cremer R, A, et al: Latex allergy in spina bifida patients: prevention by primary prophylaxis. Allergy 1998;53:709.
195. Chen Z, et al: Latex allergy correlates with operations. Allergy 1997;52:873.
196. Rihs HP, et al: Molecular analysis of DRB and DQB1 alleles in German spina bifida patients with and with out IgE responsiveness to the latex major aller-gen Hev b1. Clin Exp Allergy 1998;28:175.
197. Waitzman NJ, et al: An assessment of total costs and policy implications. *In* Waitzman NJ, et al (eds): The Cost of Birth Defects: Estimates of the Value of Prevention. Lanham, MD, University Press of America, 1996, p 145.
198. Luthy DA, et al: Cesarean section before the onset of labor and subsequent motor function in infants with myelomeningocele diagnosed antenatally. N Engl J Med 1991;324:662.
199. Guthkelch AN: Aspects of the surgical management of myelomeningocele: a review. Dev Med Child Neurol 1986;28:525.
200. Scott RM, Moore MR: Myelomeningocele repair. *In* Park TS (ed): Contemporary Issues in Neurologic Surgery: Spinal Dysraphism. Boston, Blackwell Scientific, 1992, p 48.
201. Adzick NS, Harrison MR: Fetal surgical therapy. Lancet 1994;343:897.
202. Bruner J, et al: Endoscopic coverage of fetal open myelomeningocele in utero. Am J Obstet Gynecol 1997;176:256.
203. Tulipan N, et al: Reduced hindbrain herniation after intrauterine myelomeningo-cele repair: a report of four cases. Pediatr Neurosurg 1998;29:274.
204. Bruner JP, et al: Endoscopic coverage of fetal myelomeningocele in utero. Am J Obstet Gynecol 1999;180:153.
205. Adzick NS, et al: Successful fetal surgery for spina bifida. Lancet 1998;352:1675.
206. Sutton LN, et al: Improvement in hindbrain herniation demonstrated by serial fetal magnetic resonance imaging following fetal surgery for myelomeningo-cele. JAMA 1999;282:1826.
207. Bruner JP, et al: Fetal surgery for myelomeningocele and the incidence of shunt-dependent hydrocephalus. JAMA 1999;282:1819.
208. Johnson MP, et al: Fetal myelomeningocele repair: short-term clinical out-comes. Am J Obstet Gynecol in press, 2003.
209. Flake AW: Prenatal intervention: ethical consideration for life-threatening and non–life-threatening anomalies. Semin Pediatr Surg 2001;10:212.
210. Chervanak FA, McCullough LB: A comprehensive ethical framework for fetal research and its application to fetal surgery for spina bifida. Am J Obstet Gynecol 2002;10.
211. Mazzola C, et al: Dermoid inclusion cysts and early spinal cord tethering after fetal surgery for myelomeningocele. N Engl J Med 2002;347:256.

173

Jeanette Pleasure and David Pleasure

Trophic Factor and Nutritional and Hormonal Regulation of Brain Development

This chapter reviews advances in understanding the roles of neurotrophic proteins, retinoids, folate, essential fatty acids, and thyroid and steroid hormones in neural development. These molecules play central roles in the epigenetic regulation of neuronal and neuroglial lineages, and when they are not maintained at optimal levels in the developing nervous system, neural structural abnormalities and permanent neurologic dysfunction may result. For example, maternal folate prophylaxis sharply reduces the frequency of neural tube defects (NTDs). We can expect additional therapeutic advances as we learn more about brain metabolism and nutrition.

The development of the nervous system entails the most complex array of cellular migrations and interactions of any organ system. The actions of neural morphogens such as the neurotrophic proteins, retinoids, folate, and thyroid and steroid hormones must be understood within this dynamic context. Actions of these molecules on the nervous system not only depend on their concentrations, but also are stage and location specific. The term *neuropoiesis,* coined by Anderson,[1] is helpful in reminding us of this point, by equating neuronogenesis and gliogenesis with the generation of bone marrow–derived cells, which pass through stages that differ not only in phenotype, responsiveness to exogenous influences, and motility, but also in requirements for growth factors and cofactors.[2,3] Furthermore, just as concentrations of iron and vitamin B_{12} in the bone marrow interact to dictate the size of red blood cells, the epigenetic regulation of neural development must be understood in terms of interacting nutrients, growth factors, and hormones.

NEURAL DEVELOPMENT

This chapter focuses on aspects of neural development directly relevant to the discussion of trophic factor and nutritional and hormonal regulation of brain development. Induction of neuroectoderm, which occurs in the region of ectodermal contact with dorsal mesoderm, is the third major event of embryogenesis, after establishment of embryonic dorsoventral and antero-posterior axes and the formation of mesoderm during gastrulation. The subsequent formation of the forebrain is then induced by mesoderm anterior to the notochord, whereas sonic hedgehog secreted by notochord induces the hindbrain and spinal cord.[4-6]

The neural plate, composed of multipotential neuroectodermal cells destined to form both the central nervous system (CNS) and peripheral nervous system, first appears in the human embryo at 18 days after fertilization. Thereafter, genes begin to be transcribed in this structure that encode adhesion molecules, including neural cell adhesion molecule (N-CAM), L-1, and N-cadherin. Mutations affecting one of these genes, *L1,* which lies on chromosome Xq28, cause X-linked aqueductal stenosis and agenesis of the corpus callosum, which occur with a frequency of 1 in 20,000 births.[7,8] The flat dorsal aspect of the embryo develops lateral furls, and then invagination of the neural plate forms a fold. A tube appears along the length of the fetus by fusion of this fold, proceeding both forward and backward. The anterior neuropore closes at day 24, and the posterior neuropore closes at day 26 to 28.[9,10]

The neural tube initially consists of only a single layer of neuroectodermal cells. These cells proliferate and generate neuroepithelial progenitors for neurons and glia. Radial glia, which appear early during neural tube formation, are stretched as the neural tube enlarges. Neurons originate at the inner lumen border of the neural tube and then migrate outward along the radial glia. Thus, the deepest cortical region contains the ontogenically oldest neurons.[11,12]

Neural crest cells, which form the peripheral and enteric nervous systems, are derived from neuroectoderm of the dorsolateral neural tube. The neural crest cells migrate from the neural tube into the surrounding mesenchyme at about the time of neural tube closure. The cephalic neural crest gives rise to cells that contribute to the formation of the facial skeleton, branchial arches, and, in conjunction with placode-derived cells, the lower cranial nerves. Neural crest cells also migrate from the dorsolateral aspects of the spinal neural tube, there serving as progenitors for the peripheral and enteric nervous systems, the adrenal medulla, and melanocytes.[13-15]

Although the "proper study of mankind is man," (D.H. Lawrence) it is difficult to obtain human neural tissue adequate for study. Therefore, experimental studies of neural development most often use rodent and other experimental animal models.[16] Mouse CNS at birth is at a developmental stage similar to human CNS at 5 to 6 months' gestation. By 10 days post partum, mouse CNS has matured to a stage equivalent to human brain at term. Cerebral cortical neurogenesis is largely completed by birth in both animals, although some new neurons are generated in both mouse and human CNS throughout life, particularly in hippocampus.[17-19] Differentiated oligodendroglia are already present in the human CNS at the time of birth, and CNS myelination in humans commences during the third trimester, whereas in rats and mice, differentiated oligodendroglia first appear at about the time of birth, and myelination is an entirely postnatal process.[20]

NEUROTROPHIC PROTEINS

Various terms are applied to proteins present in extracellular fluids that modulate the behavior of cells, including *hormone, trophic protein, growth factor,* and *cytokine.* In general, hormones are secreted proteins and other molecules that circulate in the bloodstream and act on distant tissues, whereas trophic proteins act on neighboring cells (paracrine factors) or the synthetic cells themselves (autocrine factors).[21,22] The term *trophic,* derived from *trophe,* or sustenance, should properly be assigned to proteins with a nutritive role, but it is usually used to refer to proteins that influence cell survival and differentiation (e.g., neurotrophin-3), rather than to proteins that truly provide nutrients (e.g., plasma lipoproteins). Proteins that enhance proliferation of target cells are referred to as *growth factors,* but many also exert trophic as well as mitogenic effects. The term *cytokine* was initially applied to bioactive proteins released by lymph node– and bone marrow–derived cells, but it is now clear that other cell types, including those derived from neuroectoderm, can also synthesize these proteins. To minimize this semantic confusion, we use the term *neurotrophic protein* to refer to any protein present in extracellular fluid that exerts a paracrine or autocrine effect on the proliferation, differentiation, or survival of neurons or neuroglia.

Rather than attempting a global description of the many neurotrophic protein classes, we briefly mention activin, noggin, and sonic hedgehog, growth factors involved in very early stages of neurogenesis, and then focus on three well-characterized neurotrophic protein families—fibroblast growth factors (FGFs), platelet-derived growth factors (PDGFs), and neurotrophins, which play major roles in neural development. We also touch briefly on yet another neurotrophic protein family, that which includes leukemia inhibitory factor and ciliary neurotrophic growth factor.

Activin, a member of the transforming growth factor protein family, is a negative regulator of the induction of neuroectoderm at the zone of contact of ectoderm with dorsal mesoderm; that is, its concentration or biologic activity must fall in the region of mesoderm-ectoderm contact to permit neuroectoderm to form.[23] *Noggin,* in contrast, exerts a positive effect on this neuroectodermal induction.[24] At a slightly later stage of neurogenesis, *sonic hedgehog,* a protein secreted by notochord, induces the differentiation of motor neurons from the ventral neural tube.[25]

The best-characterized neurotrophic members of the large family of FGFs are basic FGF (FGF-2) and acidic FGF (FGF-1). These proteins are synthesized by both neurons and astroglia.[26,27] It is not clear how, after translation, they are exported to the extracellular space, because they lack amino acid sequences usually required for passage across the plasma membrane. Levels of expression of basic and acidic FGFs are high during CNS development, as well as in the mesenchyme surrounding newly emerged neural crest cells.[28] Later in life, FGF levels in CNS are augmented by trauma.[26,29] The trophic effects of basic and acidic FGF on target cells, including induction of neurogenesis, enhancement of neuronal survival, and inhibition of differentiation of oligodendroglial progenitor cells,[30,31] are mediated by members of the receptor tyrosine kinase family. Binding of basic or acidic FGF to these receptors induces receptor dimerization, activates an intrinsic protein tyrosine kinase resident in an intracellular domain of the receptors, and initiates tyrosine and serine/threonine phosphorylation of other proteins that contribute to transmission of the trophic signal to the cell nucleus.[32,33]

The PDGFs, homodimers or heterodimers of two gene products, PDGF A and PDGF B, are synthesized in neural tissues, as well as in megakaryocytes and other peripheral cell types.[34,35] The PDGFs have mitogenic effects on neuroglia and are survival factors for neurons and the oligodendroglial lineage.[36,37] PDGF signals are transduced by target cell receptor tyrosine kinases.[38]

Much of what is known about the regulation of the early stages of neuronogenesis by protein growth factors pertains to neural crest. Acidic and basic FGFs augment survival of neural crest cells,[28] and brain-derived neurotrophic factor (BDNF) favors neural crest neuronal specification,[39] whereas neuregulin-1 favors their glial specification.[40]

The neurotrophins play leading roles in regulation of the later stages of neuronogenesis.[41] Through activation of their Trk receptors, they stimulate the transition from mitogenically cycling neuroblasts to postmitotic neurons or neuroendocrine cells and enhance neuronal survival.[42,43] Trks A to C, comprising a subgroup of the receptor tyrosine kinase family,[52] are high-affinity neurotrophin receptors. Nerve growth factor (NGF) binds preferentially to TrkA, BDNF and neurotrophin (NT)-4/5 to TrkB, and NT-3 to TrkC.[44,45] Binding of a neurotrophin to the appropriate Trk causes Trk dimerization and stimulates phosphorylation of cytoplasmic Trk tyrosine residues. This initiates a wave of tyrosine and serine/threonine phosphorylations in proteins that associate with phosphotyrosine-containing domains of the Trks through SH2 and other motifs or indirectly through Grb2 and other adaptor proteins. These phosphorylations, in turn, activate ras-dependent and ras-independent signaling pathways to the nucleus.[46-49] Dorsal root ganglion neurons demonstrate a mosaic pattern of expression of trkA, trkB, and trkC mRNAs, with individual neurons typically expressing only one of these mRNAs.[50]

In vivo experiments demonstrate that excess NGF during development causes sympathetic neuronal hyperplasia, whereas NGF depletion results in partial sympathectomy.[51] BDNF supplementation reduces the motor neuron apoptosis that follows nerve transection.[52] Targeted disruption of the trkA, trkB, and trkC genes has helped to reveal the biologic roles of these receptors and their neurotrophin ligands. Numbers of sympathetic and small sensory neurons are reduced in mice lacking TrkA.[53] TrkB knock-out mice have decreased numbers of cranial and dorsal root ganglion neurons and fewer than normal brain stem and spinal cord motor neurons.[54] Mice without TrkC are deficient in large dorsal root ganglion neurons.[55]

Immature or axotomized Schwann cells, and neurons, also express a plasma membrane pan-neurotrophin receptor (p75 neurotrophin receptor [p75NTR])[56] that binds NGF, BDNF, NT-3, and NT-4/5 with lower affinity than do the Trks, but it demonstrates high-affinity binding for the proneurotrophins from which the neurotrophins are generated by proteolytic clipping. Activation of p75NTR can initiate cellular apoptosis.[57]

Another group of proteins, which includes ciliary neurotrophic factor, interleukin-6, oncostatin M, and leukemia inhibitory factor, act on neural stem cells and also influence survival and neurotransmitter phenotype at later stages of neuronal lineages. The effects of this group of proteins are transduced by heteromeric complexes of the common receptor subunit gp130 with other receptor protein subunits.[58-61]

VITAMINS

This section covers vitamin A and folate, two essential cofactors for brain development. There have been advances in understanding their mechanisms of action and in defining the roles of perturbations in their metabolism in the genesis of neural malformations.

Vitamin A and Other Retinoids

Three forms of vitamin A are biologically active: retinol (vitamin A_1 alcohol), which maintains mucous membrane structure and function and is the circulating form of the vitamin; retinal (vitamin A_1 aldehyde), which plays a role in retinal development through conversion to a derivative that incorporates into rhodopsin; and retinoic acid (RA), which contributes to the regulation of pattern formation in the early embryo.[62-64] At least five natural biologically active forms of RA are known: all *trans*-RA; 9-*cis*-RA; 3,4-didehydro-RA; 14-hydroxy-4,14-retroretinol; and 4-oxo-RA. All can act as dysmorphogens.[65] This section focuses on the relevance of vitamin A and the retinoids to the nervous system.

Observations in experimental animals and humans that correlated retinoid exposure with CNS malformations led to recognition of the retinoid receptors and homeodomain-encoded transcription factors as effectors for retinoid actions. Megadoses of retinol and therapeutic oral doses of its analogue, isotretinoin (13-*cis*-RA), elicit teratogenic effects in the human fetus and cause both microcephaly and hydrocephalus.[62, 66, 67] Either vitamin A deficiency or excess can increase intracranial pressure in human infants.[68, 69] The teratogenic potential of retinoids is powerful because malformations resembling RA embryopathy have occurred up to a year after discontinuance of the oral use of the RA analogue etretinate, a form stored in fat and slowly released into the circulation.[70]

The retinoids play important roles during normal neural development at the earliest stages of neurogenesis, at the time of neural plate formation, and, later, when the form of the mature nervous system is established. The neural plate originates from cells in and around Hensen node and the notochord in vertebrate embryos. These three tissues are *zones of polarizing activity,* or restricted regions that contain signals that determine the anteroposterior axis of parts of the embryo.[71] The neural plate binds retinol and is the site for its most efficient conversion to RA.[71] The region most sensitive to RA is the posterior midbrain–anterior hindbrain area of the neural plate.[63] Later in development, retinoids are found in the developing inner ear[72] and the developing neural retina.[73] In retinal tissue, retinoids play a role in cell fate determination by promoting rod photoreceptor development from progenitor cells.[74] Experiments dramatically demonstrating the

effects of retinoids on CNS development were performed in the *Xenopus* embryo, which develops microcephaly and absence of eyes, forebrain, and midbrain after RA or 4-oxo-RA treatment at the late blastula to early neurula stage.[65,75,76] Loss of anterior hindbrain structures also occurs in mammalian embryos with RA exposure.[77] Such exposure, moreover, inhibits migration of cranial neural crest cells in the cultured mouse embryo.[78]

Much of the impetus to pursue RA as an important signaling molecule in the CNS came from the startling and diverse patterns of segmentation defect occurring in both deficiency and excess of retinoids.[79] RA regulates CNS segmentation by inducing the expression of members of a superfamily of genes that contain a conserved homeodomain, the *HOX* and *HOX*-related genes. These genes encode transcription factors that regulate CNS segmentation.[80] Their orderly patterns of spatial interaction are regulated by local concentrations of the retinoids.[64, 82-84] For example, Hox-B2, one of the members of this superfamily, codes for a transcription factor that is expressed in the mouse CNS up to the rhombomere 2/rhombomere 3 border. Studies show that *HOX* genes and RA regulate neural cell adhesion molecule, a key adhesion molecule that modulates cell movement.[85]

Folic Acid

Neural tube closure defects have been firmly linked to folic acid deficiency. The many studies of folate and the brain in animals were prompted by a sentinel study in 1965 by Hibbard and Smithells[86] that showed folate deficiency in 69% of mothers of children with CNS abnormalities compared with 17% of control women. Other observations suggesting an important role for folic acid in the prevention of NTDs included the increased occurrence of anencephaly and meningomyelocele in lower socioeconomic groups with less than adequate nutrition and the increased incidence of defects associated with the use of folic acid inhibitors in pregnant women.

Folate plays an essential role in methyl group transfer reactions. Methylation is cyclic, involving the interchange of methyl groups between homocysteine and methionine, mediated by the enzyme methionine synthase (5-methyltetrahydrofolate-homocysteine *S*-methyltransferase [EC 2.1.1.13]).[87] Methionine, when activated by adenosine triphosphate, becomes *S*-adenosylmethionine. *S*-Adenosylmethionine is a central source for methyl group transfer to proteins, lipids, and nucleic acids. One of the products of methyl transfer is *S*-adenosylhomocysteine, which is then hydrolyzed to homocysteine. In most cells, homocysteine is converted by vitamin B_{12}–dependent methionine synthase back to methionine by remethylation.[87] The latter is the only reaction in the human that requires both folic acid and vitamin B_{12} as cofactors and is responsible for the dependency of cellular folate levels on adequate availability of vitamin B_{12}.[87]

Virtually all cells in all organisms contain folate coenzymes, mediating methyl transfers. A small amount of folate is in nuclei, but there are cellular folate-binding proteins associated both with surface membranes or, intracellularly, within the cytosol and mitochondria. Most of these intracellular folate-binding proteins are enzymes that use folate as a coenzyme in methyl transfer. The placenta and choroid plexus are sites that exhibit folate receptors.[88,89]

Holmes[90] found the prevalence of NTDs in a New England cohort to be 1.2 per 1000; among the 146 cases in his 15-year survey, there were 54 infants with spina bifida, 74 with anencephaly, and 19 with encephalocele. Anencephaly occurs before 24 days' gestation in the human, and approximately 75% of these fetuses die *in utero*. Anencephaly is more common in girls than in boys. There are also ethnic differences in the frequency of NTDs. For instance, in British Columbia, the incidence of NTDs in the Sikh population is about double that in non-Sikhs.[91] Moreover, a recurrence risk of 2.3% between 1958 and 1984 contrasted with 0.24% recurrence risk between 1985 and 1993. This was likely the result of the recommendation of folic acid and multivitamins before conception for at-risk families in British Columbia.[91]

Both RA and folic acid have been studied in several mouse mutants manifesting NTDs. The effect of RA is not uniform; although it increases the incidence of exencephaly (precursor of anencephaly) in four different mutant mouse strains, it also decreases the incidence of caudal spina bifida and tail defects in several of the same strains. Other studies have shown that simple maternal folate deficiency in nongenetically predisposed rodents does not produce NTDs,[92,93] nor does folate treatment prevent NTDs in the genetically predisposed *Axd* mouse, whereas methionine does.[94]

Administration of folate, however, does reduce the incidence of valproate-induced NTDs in the mouse,[95] whereas arachidonic acid and inositol, which contribute to anchoring of folate-binding protein to the plasma membrane, reduce mouse NTDs associated with exposure to phenytoin or hyperglycemia.[96,97] Nau[98] reviewed the effects of phenytoin and valproate on fetal folate metabolism. Epileptic mothers with fetal malformations exhibit low folate levels.[99]

In 1991, the effect of early folic acid supplementation to prevent recurrent NTDs was demonstrated in a multicenter, randomized, double-blind trial.[100] Administration of 4 mg of folic acid daily before conception and during early gestation resulted in a sixfold diminution in risk (0.6% versus 3.6%) of recurrent NTDs.[100] Folic acid supplements were also found key in preventing first occurrences of NTDs.[101]

About that time, the incidence of NTDs was estimated to be 2.5% in 26-day human embryos just completing neurulation, and it decreased to 0.06% at term, owing to fetal loss.[102] It was estimated that 400,000 infants with spina bifida or anencephaly were born yearly throughout the world, and more than half the lesions could be prevented with prenatal folic acid supplements.[103] Since the early 1990s, recommended folic acid doses have been 0.4 mg daily from before conception until 3 months' gestation for the general population and 4 mg daily for women who have already had children with NTDs.[104] The optimal amount of folate appropriate for prophylaxis, however, is still not completely established. One study calculated the effect of supplementation on NTD reduction and, based on 13 published studies, calculated that doubling the serum folate level would halve the risk of NTD. Based on this calculation, a recommendation was made that women planning a pregnancy take 5 mg daily before conception and in early gestation, to lower the risk for NTD by a calculated 85%.[105] Yet another means of prophylaxis was begun in 1996 with the fortification of flour and grains with folic acid. This became mandatory in the United States in January, 1998, with the minimum addition to be 0.14 mg folic acid per 100 g of cereal grain, calculated to increase intake by an average of 0.1 mg/day. This approach was shown to be effective in a Southern California study, which demonstrated that levels of serum and red cell folate greatly exceeded minimal acceptable levels in both socioeconomically disadvantaged and advantaged women.[106] In a survey of multiple states, the NTD prevalence before and after fortification was shown to decrease by 19%, to 30.5 per 100,000 live births[107]; however, no drop occurred in patients with either no or only late prenatal care, a finding confirming the major role of early specific folate prophylaxis.

Most, but not all, cases of spina bifida and anencephaly are preventable with folate supplementation. To investigate this "resistance" to folate, the response to folate loading in women who had had two pregnancies with NTDs was undertaken.[108] Study subjects and controls attained similar serum and red cell folate levels, but no correlation between levels and intake existed in study subjects, a finding implying altered folate metabolism in the women whose folate levels were unpredictable. Homocysteine levels were known to be elevated in women who

had had children with NTDs, although classic homocystinuria is not associated with NTDs.[108,109] Mothers of children with NTDs were also shown to have impaired metabolism of homocysteine when their plasma vitamin B_{12} levels were in the low-normal range.[110,111] Thus, a defect was postulated in the enzyme requiring both vitamin B_{12} and folic acid as cofactors, methionine synthase. Further implication of this enzyme comes from the delay in incorporation of 5-methyltetrahydrofolate into DNA (another methionine synthase catalyzed reaction) in trophoblast cells of women carrying NTD-affected infants.[112]

Abnormality of another enzyme, 5,10-methylenetetrahydrofolate reductase (MTHFR), estimated to be present in 5 to 15% of the general population, is associated with defective transfer of a methyl group to homocysteine to form methionine.[112] Finally, two mutations in the *MTHFR* gene, C677T and A1298C, which lead to increased homocysteine levels, also significantly increase risks for NTDs in children. Homocysteine levels in women with these MTHFR variants can be normalized with large doses of folate.[113,114]

ESSENTIAL FATTY ACIDS

The brain is rich in lipid. Research in animal models shows that brain lipid can be changed, in particular, by alterations in intake of essential fatty acids.[115] The essential fatty acids of the diet are linoleic ($C_{18:2\ \omega-6}$) and linolenic ($C_{18:3\ \omega-3}$) acids. Premature and growth-retarded infants are born with essential fatty acid deficiency, and studies in experimental animals indicate that such deficiency can cause cognitive and visual impairments.[116] Studies of essential fatty acid supplementation in humans have included analyses of the effects of ω-3 fatty acid supplementation or breast milk feedings on premature infants' retinal function,[117] intelligence quotient,[118,119] and visual evoked potentials.[120] Whether supplementation with long chain polyunsaturated fatty acids has a beneficial effect on the rate of neural development in healthy term infants remains controversial.[121,122]

HORMONES

Although the effects of hormonal deficiency or excess on neural function in the adult may be profound, they are in general reversible. In contrast, perturbations in availability of hormones during the critical periods of neuronal and glial development often result in permanent and profound abnormalities in synaptogenesis and myelination. This discussion focuses on thyroid and steroid hormones and emphasizes this special vulnerability of the immature nervous system to deficiencies of these hormones.

Thyroid Hormones

Deficiency of thyroid hormones has major, often devastating, effects on neural development in the fetus and neonate. We discuss the effects of such deficiency on cerebral histogenesis and then explore data on the mechanisms by which thyroid hormones exert their effects on target cells.

Thyroid disorders are the most prevalent endocrinologic derangements in the world, even more common than diabetes mellitus. Endemic hypothyroidism from low dietary iodine consumption still affects almost 400 million people in the world. A study in Guinea, one major center of West Africa's goiter belt, revealed that 70% of the adults in an inland prefecture had goiters.[123] Environmental variables responsible for this high incidence include the low iodine content of the water and soil, excessive intake of goitrogens such as thiocyanate in cassava and flavonoids in millet, and protein malnutrition. Many infants had goiters at birth, and 55% of preschoolers were affected. In a survey of children at puberty, 58% of boys and 80% of girls had goiters.[123] Although the incidence of myxedematous cretinism, manifested by retardation and deafness, was only 2% in this population, this figure is likely to have been markedly lowered because of early death of severely neurologically impaired children in this environment.

The neurologic consequences of early hypothyroidism vary with the degrees of maternal, fetal, and neonatal hypothyroidism.[124] Maternal thyroxine (T_4) is not available to the fetus for brain protection when the mother is iodine deficient, and this accounts for the severe CNS damage of the neurologic endemic cretin, compared with the hypothyroid fetus born to an endocrinologically normal mother.[125]

Sporadic hypothyroidism affects approximately 1 in 4000 live births. Screening programs for this abnormality are widespread among developed countries. Knowledge gained from these programs has made it clear that the fetus is usually unaffected by intrinsic *in utero* hypothyroidism, even when athyrotic. Preservation of brain thyroid status in the hypothyroid human[126] and the rat[127] fetus results from maternal T_4 that crosses the placenta.

Experimentally elicited neonatal hypothyroidism in rodents causes deficiencies in CNS neuronogenesis, synaptogenesis, and myelination.[128-130] Thyroid deficiency can also interfere with the responsiveness of neural tissues to neurotransmitter-mediated and neurotrophic signals.[131,132] For example, adequate supplies of triiodothyronine or T_4 are necessary for normal expression of NT-3 and its receptor, TrkC, by immature rat cerebellar granule cells.[133] Thyroid hormone deficiency also alters the metabolism of the thyroid hormones themselves. The conversion of T_4 to triiodothyronine in the brains of hypothyroid rat fetuses is accelerated, owing to the induction of astroglial type II deiodinase, probably secondary to an elevation in thyrotrophin levels in the fetuses.[134] This homeostatic mechanism helps to preserve brain function in the presence of hypothyroidism in the fetus.

There are important interactions between thyroid hormones and retinoids. Thyroid hormone receptor-α_1 inhibits RA-responsive gene expression,[135] but it cooperates with retinoids in supporting the formation of embryonic mouse cerebral neurons.[136] Moreover, retinoids cause a 200-fold, specific induction in type III deiodinase (the enzyme responsible for degradation of brain T_4) in astroglial cells in culture.[137]

The effects of thyroid hormones on neural and other tissues are transduced by nuclear thyroid receptors-α and β, encoded by genes on chromosomes 17 and 3, respectively.[138,139] These thyroid receptors bind both to thyroid hormone and to thyroid response elements, specific DNA sequences in noncoding regions of thyroid hormone–responsive genes. targeting genes encoding neurotransmitters and cytoskeletal proteins.[140] Thyroid-responsive genes are numerous and are identified frequently.

Thyroid receptors-α and β are homologous to nuclear receptors for steroids, RA, and vitamin D_3 and are detected as early as 10 weeks in the human fetal brain.[141] They are expressed in a spatially and temporally regulated pattern in the CNS. This pattern is of some clinical significance. For example, the anlage of the cochlea is particularly rich in these nuclear receptors. The role of these receptors at a critical period for auditory end-organ development is demonstrated by frequent abnormalities in auditory brain stem responses in hypothyroid children (which tend to persist despite early replacement therapy),[142,143] and it is also shown by the syndrome of isolated deafness in humans with a chromosomal deletion syndrome involving most of the thyroid receptor-β gene.[144] The nuclear thyroid receptors are also subject to mutations that result in inherited thyroid hormone resistance.[141,145]

Environmental exposure of pregnant animals to dioxins and polychlorinated biphenyls leads to behavioral changes similar to those seen after fetal hypothyroidism.[146] These substances are industrial pollutants that have persisted despite their ban in the 1970s. This is especially concerning because of their concentration in fatty tissues and human milk.[147] Several mechanisms for the hypothyroid effects have been postulated: reduction of thyroid hormone at low levels of polychlorinated biphenyls and thyroid receptor-mediated thyromimetic effects at high levels of these toxins.[148] Structural similarity between these two classes of toxins and thyroid hormones permits them to bind to the same transporters and nuclear receptors, thus interfering with the effects of thyroid hormone on the fetal brain.

Steroid Hormones

Glucocorticoids, estrogens, progesterone, androgens, and vitamin D metabolites influence CNS development. A common feature of all these steroids is that their actions are transduced by cytosolic receptors that, on binding of their ligand steroid, are released from complexes with other cytosolic proteins, move to the nucleus, and there modulate transcription of target genes.[149,150] The biologic effects of the steroid hormones on neural tissues are dictated by the distributions of expression and patterns of gene activation of their receptors. These biologic effects include regulation of the secretion of neurotrophins by neuroglia and of the incidence of apoptosis of nascent neurons.[151-154]

Type I adrenal corticosteroid receptors bind both mineralocorticoids and glucocorticoids with high affinity, and they are concentrated largely in the hippocampal system. Type II corticosteroid receptors, which bind glucocorticoids with high affinity, are generalized throughout the brain, but they are most abundant in the anterior pituitary and preoptic region of the hypothalamus.[151-155] In the developing nervous system, glucocorticoids regulate the frequency with which nascent neurons undergo apoptosis.[156] Glucocorticoid excess has complex effects on the immature brain, by stimulating cholinergic neurotransmission through a neurotrophin-dependent mechanism,[157] but also by eliciting neuronal loss in the hippocampus that is associated with life-long impairment of memory.[158]

Receptors for estradiol, progesterone, and androgens are widespread in the developing CNS. Their activation, by maternal steroid hormones and by progesterone, estrogens, and androgens synthesized endogenously in the CNS,[153,159,160] influences the motility of neuroblasts and the development of neurons in sexually dimorphic motor nuclei of the hypothalamus, brain stem, and spinal cord and also exerts effects on synthesis of neurotransmitters.[161-163] Endogenous synthesis of progesterone in the neonatal rat CNS promotes the maturation of cerebellar Purkinje cells.

Activation of CNS neuroglial receptors for the vitamin D metabolite, 1,25-dihydroxyvitamin D_3, stimulates neuroglial neurotrophin synthesis.[164] 1,25-Dihydroxyvitamin D_3 also acts on hippocampal neurons, by down-regulating their expression of L-type calcium channels and thereby protecting these neurons against excitotoxic injury.[165]

REFERENCES

1. Anderson DJ: The neural crest cell lineage problem: neuropoiesis? Neuron *3*:1, 1989.
2. Scheffler B, et al: Marrow-mindedness: a perspective on neuropoiesis. Trends Neurosci *22*:348, 1999.
3. Terskikh AV, et al: From hematopoiesis to neuropoiesis: evidence of overlapping genetic programs. Proc Natl Acad Sci USA *98*:7934, 2001.
4. Yamada T: Caudalization by the amphibian organizer: brachyury, convergent extension and retinoic acid. Development *120*:3051, 1994.
5. Shawlot W, Behringer RR: Requirement for *Lim1* in head-organizer function. Nature *374*:425, 1995.
6. Litingtung Y, Chiang C: Control of Shh activity and signaling in the neural tube. Dev Dyn *219*:143, 2000.
7. Jouet M, Kenwick S: Gene analysis of L1 neural cell adhesion molecule in prenatal diagnosis of hydrocephalus. Lancet *345*:161, 1995.
8. Weller S, Gartner J: Genetic and clinical aspects of X-linked hydrocephalus (L1 disease): mutations in the L1CAM gene. Hum Mutat *18*:1, 2001.
9. Golden JA, Chernoff GF: Multiple sites of anterior neural tube closure in humans: evidence from anterior neural tube defects (anencephaly). Pediatrics *95*:506, 1995.

10. Nakatsu T, et al: Neural tube closure in humans initiates at multiple sites: evidence from human embryos and implications for the pathogenesis of neural tube defects. Anat Embryol (Berl) 201:455, 2000.

11. Rakic P: Mode of cell migration to the superficial layers of the fetal monkey neocortex. J Comp Neurol 145:61, 1972.

12. Noctor SC, et al: Neurons derived from radial glial cells establish radial units in neocortex. Nature 409:714, 2001.

13. Le Douarin NM, et al: Genetic and epigenetic control in neural crest development. Curr Opin Genet Dev 4:685, 1994.

14. Baker CV, Bronner-Fraser M: Vertebrate cranial placodes. I. Embryonic induction. Dev Biol 232:1, 2001.

15. Knecht AK, Bronner-Fraser M: Induction of the neural crest: a multigene process. Nat Rev Genet 3:453, 2002.

16. Juriloff DM, Harris MJ: Mouse models for neural tube closure defects. Hum Mol Genet 9:993, 2000.

17. Cai L, Hayes NL, Nowakowski RS: Synchrony of clonal cell proliferation and contiguity of clonally related cells: production of mosaicism in the ventricular zone of developing mouse neocortex. J Neurosci 17:2088, 1997.

18. Song H, et al: Astroglia induce neurogenesis from adult neural stem cells. Nature 417:39, 2002.

19. Steindler DA, Pincus DW: Stem cells and neuropoiesis in adult human brain. Lancet 359:1047, 2002.

20. Muse ED, et al: Parameters related to lipid metabolism as markers of myelination in mouse brain. J Neurochem 76:77, 2001.

21. Heymach JV Jr, Barres BA: Neuronal self-reliance. Nature 374:405, 1995.

22. Funakoshi H, et al: Muscle-derived neurotrophin-4 as an activity-dependent trophic signal for adult motor neurons. Science 268:1495, 1995.

23. Hemmati-Brivanlou A, Melton DA: Inhibition of activin receptor signaling promotes neuralization in Xenopus. Cell 77:273, 1994.

24. Green JB: Roads to neuralness: embryonic neural induction as derepression of a default state. Cell 77:317, 1994.

25. Johnson RL, Tabin C: The long and short of hedgehog signaling. Cell 81:313, 1995.

26. Huber K, et al: Expression of fibroblast growth factor-2 in hypoglossal motoneurons is stimulated by peripheral nerve injury. J Comp Neurol 382:189, 1997.

27. Chadi G, et al: Temporal and spatial increase of astroglial basic fibroblast growth factor synthesis after 6-hydroxydopamine-induced degeneration of the nigrostriatal dopamine neurons. Neuroscience 61:891, 1994.

28. Bannerman PG, Pleasure D: Protein growth factor requirements of rat neural crest cells. J Neurosci Res 36:46, 1993.

29. Buytaert KA, et al: The temporal patterns of c-Fox and basic fibroblast growth factor expression following a unilateral anteromedial cortex lesion. Brain Res 894:121, 2001.

30. Xu RH, et al: Studies on the role of fibroblast growth factor signaling in neurogenesis using conjugated/aged animal caps and dorsal ectoderm-grafted embryos. J Neurosci 17:6892, 1997.

31. Yasuda T, et al: Apoptosis occurs in the oligodendroglial lineage, and is prevented by basic fibroblast growth factor. J Neurosci Res 40:306, 1994.

32. Stauber DJ, et al: Structural interactions of fibroblast growth factor receptor with its ligands. Proc Natl Acad Sci USA 97:49, 2000.

33. Sung JY, et al: Basic fibroblast growth factor-induced acctivation of novel CREB kinase during the differentiation of immortalized hippocampal cells. J Biol Chem 276:13858, 2001.

34. Yeh HJ, et al: PDGF A-chain gene is expressed by mammalian neurons during development and in maturity. Cell 64:209, 1991.

35. Hardy M, et al: Platelet-derived growth factor (PDGF) and the regulation of Schwann cell proliferation in vivo. J Neurosci Res 31:254, 1992.

36. Cheng B, Mattson MP: PDGFs protect hippocampal neurons against energy deprivation and oxidative injury: evidence for induction of antioxidant pathways. J Neurosci 15:7095, 1995.

37. Grinspan J, et al: Oligodendrocyte maturation and myelin gene expression in PDGF-treated cultures from rat cerebral white matter. J Neurocytol 22:322, 1993.

38. Emaduddin M, et al: Functional co-operation between the subunits in heterodimeric platelet-derived growth factor receptor complexes. Biochem J 341:523, 1999.

39. Sieber-Blum M: Role of neurotrophic factors BDNF and NGF in the commitment of pluripotent neural crest cells. Neuron 6:949, 1991.

40. Paratore C, et al: Survival and glial fate acquisition of neural crest cells are regulated by an interplay between the transcription factor Sox10 and extrinsic combinatorial signaling. Development 128:3949, 2001.

41. Lewin GR: Neurotrophins and the specification of neuronal phenotype. Philos Trans R Soc Lond B Biol Sci 351:405, 1996.

42. Hory-Lee F, et al: Neurotrophin 3 supports the survival of developing muscle sensory neurons in culture. Proc Natl Acad Sci USA 90:2613, 1993.

43. Acheson A, et al: A BDNF autocrine loop in adult sensory neurons prevents cell death. Nature 374:450, 1995.

44. Barbacid M: The Trk family of neurotrophin receptors. J Neurobiol 25:1386, 1994.

45. Jing SQ, et al: Nerve growth-factor mediates signal transduction through homodimer receptors. Neuron 9:1069, 1992.

46. Kaplan DR, Stephens RM: Neurotrophin signal transduction by the Trk receptor. J Neurobiol 25:1404, 1994.

47. Ng NF, Shooter EM: Activation of p21ras by nerve growth factor in embryonic sensory neurons and PC12 cells. J Biol Chem 268:25329, 1993.

48. Suen KL, et al: Molecular cloning of the mouse grb2 gene: differential interaction of the Grb2 adaptor protein with epidermal growth factor and nerve growth factor receptors. Mol Cell Biol 13:5500, 1993.

49. Stephens RM, et al: Trk receptors use redundant signal-transduction pathways involving SHC and PLC-gamma-1 to mediate NGF responses. Neuron 12:691, 1994.

50. Wright DE, Snider WD: Neurotrophin receptor mRNA expression defines distinct populations of neurons in dorsal root ganglia. J Comp Neurol 351:329, 1995.

51. Rice FL, et al: Differential dependency of unmyelinated and A delta epidermal and upper dermal innervation on neurotrophins, trk receptors, and p75LNGFR. Dev Biol 198:57, 1998.

52. Jones KR, et al: Targeted disruption of the BDNF gene perturbs brain and sensory neuron development but not motor neuron development. Cell 76:989, 1994.

53. Smeyne RJ, et al: Severe sensory and sympathetic neuropathies in mice carrying a disrupted Trk/NGF receptor gene. Nature 368:246, 1994.

54. Klein R, et al: Targeted disuption of the trkB neurotrophin receptor gene results in nervous system lesions and neonatal death. Cell 75:113, 1993.

55. Klein R, et al: Disruption of the neurotrophin-3 receptor gene trkC eliminates Ia muscle afferents and results in abnormal movements. Nature 368:249, 1994.

56. Yasuda T, et al: Cultured rat Schwann cells express low affinity receptors for nerve growth factor. Brain Res 436:113, 1987.

57. Lee R, et al: Regulation of cell survival by secreted proneurotrophins. Science 294:1945, 2001.

58. Fan G, Katz DM: Non-neuronal cells inhibit catecholaminergic differentiation of primary sensory neurons: role of leukemia inhibitory factor. Development 118:83, 1993.

59. Masu Y, et al: Disruption of the CNTF gene results in motor neuron degeneration. Nature 365:27, 1993.

60. Ip NY, et al: CNTF and LIF act on neuronal cells via shared signaling pathways that involve the IL-6 signal transducing receptor component gp130. Cell 69:1121, 1992.

61. Shimazaki T, et al: The ciliary neurotrophic factor/leukemia inhibitory factor/gp130 receptor complex operates in the maintenance of mammalian forebrain neural stem cells. J Neurosci 21:7642, 2001.

62. Goodman DS: Vitamin A and retinoids in health and disease. N Engl J Med 310:1023, 1984.

63. Maden M, Holder N: The involvement of retinoic acid in the development of the vertebrate central nervous system. Dev Suppl 2:87, 1991.

64. Langston AW, Gudas LJ: Retinoic acid and homeobox gene regulation. Curr Opin Genet Dev 4:550, 1994.

65. Pijnappel WWN, et al: The retinoid ligand 4-oxo-retinoic acid is a highly active modulator of positional specification. Nature 366:340, 1993.

66. Hall JG, et al: Vitamin A: a newly recognized human teratogen. Harbinger of things to come? J Pediatr 105:583, 1984.

67. Lammer EJ, et al: Retinoic acid embryopathy. N Engl J Med 313:837, 1985.

68. Kasarskis EJ, Bass NH: Benign intracranial hypertension induced by deficiency of vitamin A in infancy. Neurology 32:1292, 1982.

69. Roos RAC, Van Der Blij JF: Pseudotumor cerebri associated with hypovitaminosis A and hyperthyroidism. Dev Med Child Neurol 27:246, 1985.

70. Lammer EJ: Embryopathy in infant conceived one year after termination of maternal etretinate. Lancet 2:1080, 1988.

71. Wagner M, et al: Polarizing activity and retinoid synthesis in floor plate of the neural tube. Nature 345:819, 1990.

72. Represa J, et al: Retinoic acid modulation of the early development of the inner ear is associated with the control of c-fos expression. Development 110:1081, 1990.

73. McCaffrey P, et al: Asymmetric retinoic acid synthesis in the dorsoventral axis of the retina. Development 115:371, 1992.

74. Kelley MW, et al: Retinoic acid promotes differentiation of photoreceptors in vitro. Development 120:2091, 1994.

75. Durston AJ, et al: Retinoic acid causes an anteroposterior transformation in the developing central nervous system. Nature 340:140, 1989.

76. Ruiz I, et al: Retinoic acid modifies the pattern of cell differentiation in the central nervous system of neurula stage Xenopus embryos. Development 112:945, 1991.

77. Morriss-Kay G: Retinoic acid, neural crest, and craniofacial development. Semin Dev Biol 2:211, 1991.

78. Pratt RM, et al: Retinoic acid inhibits migration of cranial neural crest cells in cultured mouse embryo. J Craniofac Gen Dev Biol 7:205, 1987.

79. Gavalas A: Arranging the hindbrain. Trends Neurosci 25:61, 2002.

80. McGinnis W, Krumlauf R: Homeobox genes and axial patterning. Cell 68:283, 1992.

81. Jones FS, et al: Cell adhesion molecules as targets for Hox genes: neural cell adhesion molecule promoter activity is modulated by co-transfection with hox-2.5 and -2.4. Proc Natl Acad Sci USA 89:2086, 1992.

82. Jonk L, et al: Isolation and developmental expression of retinoic-acid-induced genes. Dev Biol 161:604, 1994.

83. Lyn S, Giguere V: Localization of CRABP-I and CRABP-II mRNA in the early mouse embryo by whole-mount in situ hybridization: implications for teratogenesis and neural development. Dev Dyn 199:280, 1994.

84. Balkan W, et al: Transgenic indicator mice for studying activated retinoic acid receptors during development. Proc Natl Acad Sci USA 89:3347, 1992.

85. Colbert MC, et al: Local sources of retinoic acid coincide with retinoid-mediated transgene activity during embryonic development. Proc Natl Acad Sci USA 90:6572, 1993.

86. Hibbard ED, Smithells RW: Folic acid metabolism and human embryopathy. Lancet 1:254, 1965.

87. Scott JM, et al: Folic acid metabolism and mechanisms of neural tube defects. Ciba Found Symp 181:180, 1994.

88. Holm J, et al: High-affinity folate binding in human choroid plexus: characterization of radioligand binding, immunoreactivity, molecular heterogeneity and hydrophobic domain of the binding protein. Biochem J 280:267, 1991.

89. Verma RS, et al: Evidence that the hydrophobicity of isolated, in situ, and de novo-synthesized native human placental folate receptors is a function of glycosyl-phosphatidylinositol anchoring to membranes. J Biol Chem 267:4119, 1992.

90. Holmes LB: Spina bifida: anticonvulsants and other maternal influences. Ciba Found Symp 181:232, 1994.

91. Chambers K, et al: Neural tube defects in British Columbia. Lancet 343:489, 1994.

92. Cockroft DL: Vitamin deficiencies and neural tube defects: human and animal studies. Hum Reprod 6:148, 1991.

93. Heid MK, et al: Folate deficiency alone does not produce neural tube defects in mice. J Nutr 122:888, 1992.

94. Essien FB, Wannberg DL: Methionine but not folinic acid or vitamin B$_{12}$ alters the frequency of neural tube defects in Axd mutant mice. J Nutr 123:27, 1993.

95. Trotz M, et al: Valproic acid-induced neural tube defects: reduction by folinic acid in the mouse. Life Sci 41:103, 1987.

96. Kay ED, et al: Arachidonic acid reversal of phenytoin induced neural tube and craniofacial defects in vivo in mice. J Craniofac Genet Dev Biol 8:179, 1988.

97. Baker L, et al: Myo-inositol and prostaglandins reverse the glucose inhibition of neural tube fusion in cultured mouse embryos. Diabetologia 33:595, 1990.

98. Nau H: Valproic acid-induced neural tube defects. Ciba Found Symp 181:144, 1994.

99. Ogawa Y, et al: Serum folic acid levels in epileptic mothers and their relationship to congenital malformations. Epilepsy Res 8:75, 1991.

100. MRC Vitamin Study Research Group: Prevention of neural tube defects: results of the Medical Research Council vitamin study. Lancet 338:131, 1991.

101. Czeizel AE, Dudas I: Prevention of the first occurrence of neural-tube defects by periconceptional vitamin supplementation. N Engl J Med 327:1832, 1992.

102. Shiota K: Development and intrauterine fate of normal and abnormal human conceptuses. Congenital Anom 31:67, 1991.

103. Oakley GP, et al: Prevention of folic acid-preventable spina bifida and anencephaly. Ciba Found Symp 181:212, 1994.

104. Rush D, Rosenberg IH: Folate supplements and neural tube defects. Nutr Rev 50:25, 1992.

105. Wald NJ, et al: Quantifying the effect of folic acid. Lancet 358:2069, 2001.

106. Caudill MA, et al: Folate status in women of childbearing age residing in Southern California after folic acid fortification. J Am Coll Nutr 20:129, 2001)

107. Honein MA, et al: Impact of folic acid fortification of the US food supply on the occurrence of neural tube defects. JAMA 285:2981, 2001.

108. Wild NJ, et al: Investigation of folate intake and metabolism in women who have had two pregnancies complicated by neural tube defects. Br J Obstet Gynaecol 101:197, 1994.

109. Steegers-Theunissen RPM, et al: Neural tube defects and derangement of homocysteine metabolism. N Engl J Med 324:199, 1991.

110. Kirke PN, et al: Maternal plasma folate and vitamin B$_{12}$ are independent risk factors for neural tube defects. Q J Med 86:703, 1993.

111. Mills JL, et al: Homocysteine metabolism in pregnancies complicated by neural-tube defects. Lancet 345:149, 1995.

112. Habibzadeh N, et al: One-carbon metabolism in pregnancies complicated by neural tube defects. Lancet 345:791, 1995.

113. Van der Put NM, et al: Folate, homocysteine and neural tube defects: an overview. Exp Biol Med 226:243, 2001.

114. Richter B, et al: Interaction of folate and homocysteine pathway genotypes evaluated in susceptibility to neural tube defects (NTD) in a German population. J Hum Genet 46:105, 2001.

115. Innis SM: Insights into possible mechanisms of essential fatty acid uptake into developing brain from studies of diet, circulating lipid, liver, and brain n-6 and n-3 fatty acids. In Dobbing J (ed): Lipids, Learning, and the Brain: Fats in Infant Formulas. Report of the 103rd Ross Conference on Pediatric Research. Columbus, OH, Ross Laboratories, 1993, pp 4–26.

116. Crawford MA, et al: Nutrition and neurodevelopmental disorders. Nutr Health 9:81, 1993.

117. Jeffrey BG, et al: The role of docosahexaenoic acid in retinal function. Lipids 36:859, 2001.

118. Lucas A, et al: Breast milk and subsequent intelligence quotient in children born preterm. Lancet 339:261, 1992.

119. Rao MR, et al: Effect of breastfeeding on cognitive development of infants born small for gestational age. Acta Paediatr 91:267, 2002.

120. Birch DG, et al: Dietary essential fatty acid supply and visual acuity development. Invest Ophthalmol Vis Sci 32:3242, 1992.

121. Gibson RA, Makrides M: n-3 Polyunsaturated fatty acid requirements of term infants. Am J Clin Nutr 71(Suppl 1):251S, 2000.

122. Voigt RG, et al: Relationship between omega 3 long-chain poly-unsaturated fatty acid status during early infancy and neurodevelopmental status at 1 year of age. J Hum Nutr Diet 15:111, 2002.

123. Konde M, et al: Goitrous endemic in Guinea. Lancet 344:1675, 1994.

124. Burrow GN, et al: Maternal and fetal thyroid function. N Engl J Med 331:1072, 1994.

125. Morreale de Escobar G, et al: Effects of iodine deficiency on thyroid hormone metabolism and the brain in fetal rats: the role of the maternal transfer of thyroxin. Am J Clin Nutr 57:280S, 1993.

126. Vulsma T, et al: Maternal-fetal transfer of thyroxine in congenital hypothyroidism due to a total organification defect or thyroid agenesis. N Engl J Med 321:13, 1989.

127. Calvo R, et al: Congenital hypothyroidism, as studied in rats: crucial role of maternal thyroxine but not of 3,5,3'-triiodothyronine in the protection of the fetal brain. J Clin Invest 86:889, 1990.

128. Aniello F, et al: Regulation of five tubulin isotypes by thyroid hormone during brain development. J Neurochem 57:1781, 1991.

129. Nunez J, et al: Regulation by thyroid hormone of microtubule assembly and neuronal differentiation. Neurochem Res 16:975, 1991.

130. Chakraborty M, et al: Thyroidal influence on the cell surface GMi of granule cells: its significance in cell migration during rat brain development. Cell Mol Neurobiol 12:589, 1992.

131. Orford M, et al: Abundance of the alpha-subunits of Gi1, Gi2 and Go in synaptosomal membranes from several regions of the rat brain is increased in hypothyroidism. Biochem J 275:183, 1991.

132. Wong CC, et al: Differential ontogenetic appearance and regulation of stimulatory G protein isoforms in rat cerebral cortex by thyroid hormone deficiency. Dev Brain Res 79:136, 1994.

133. Lindholm D, et al: Neurotrophin-3 induced by tri-iodothyronine in cerebellar granule cells promotes Purkinje cell differentiation. J Cell Biol 122:443, 1993.

134. Saunier B, et al: Evidence for cAMP-independent thyrotropin effects on astroglial cells. Eur J Biochem 218:1091, 1993.

135. Lee LR, et al: Thyroid hormone receptor-alpha inhibits retinoic acid-responsive gene expression and modulates retinoic acid-stimulated neural differentiation in mouse embryonic stem cells. Mol Endocrinol 8:746, 1994.

136. Ved HS, Pieringer RA: Regulation of neuronal differentiation by retinoic acid alone and in cooperation with thyroid hormone or hydrocortisone. Dev Neurosci 15:49, 1993.

137. Esfandiari A, et al: Induction of type III-deiodinase activity in astroglial cells by retinoids. Glia 11:255, 1994.

138. De Nayer P: The thyroid hormone receptors: molecular basis of thyroid hormone resistance. Horm Res 38:57, 1992.

139. Zhang J, et al: The mechanism of action of thyroid hormones. Annu Rev Physiol 62:439, 2000.

140. Oppenheimer JH, et al: Molecular basis of thyroid hormone-dependent brain development. Endocr Rev 18:462, 1997.

141. Ferreiro B, et al: Estimation of nuclear thyroid hormone receptor saturation in human fetal brain and lung during early gestation. J Clin Endocrinol Metab 67:853, 1988.

142. Hebert R, et al: Auditory brainstem response audiometry in congenitally hypothyroid children under early replacement therapy. Pediatr Res 20:570, 1986.

143. Lareau E, et al: Somatosensory evoked potentials and auditory brain-stem responses in congenital hypothyroidism. II. A cross-sectional study in childhood: correlations with hormonal levels and developmental quotients. Electroencephalogr Clin Neurophysiol 67:521, 1987.

144. Bradley DJ, et al: Alpha and beta thyroid hormone receptor (TR) gene expression during auditory neurogenesis: evidence for TR isoform-specific transcriptional regulation in vivo. Proc Natl Acad Sci USA 91:439, 1994.

145. Jaffiol C, et al: Thyroid hormone generalized resistance. Horm Res 38:62, 1992.

146. Jacobstein JL, et al: Intellectual impairment in children exposed to polychlorinated biphenyls in utero. N Engl J Med 335:783, 1996.

147. Greizerstein HB, et al: Comparison of PCB congeners and pesticide levels between serum and milk from lactating women. Environ Res 80:280, 1999.

148. Zoeller RT, et al. Developmental exposure to polychlorinated biphenyls exerts thyroid hormone-like effects on the expression of RC3/neurogranin and myelin basic protein messenger ribonucleic acids in the developing rat brain. Endocrinology 141:181, 2000.

149. Orchinik M, et al: A corticosteroid receptor in neural membranes. Science 252:1848, 1991.

150. Beato M, Klug J: Steroid hormone receptors: an update. Hum Reprod Update 6:225, 2000.

151. Cintra A, et al: Mapping and computer assisted morphometry and microdensitometry of glucocorticoid receptor immunoreactive neurons and glial cells in the rat central nervous system. Neuroscience 62:843, 1994.

152. Diaz R, et al: Distinct ontogeny of glucocorticoid and mineralocorticoid receptor and 11beta-hydroxysteroid dehydrogenase types I and II mRNAs in the fetal rat brain suggest a complex control of glucocorticoid actions. J Neurosci 18:2570, 1998.

153. Bakker J, et al: Quantitative estimation of estrogen and androgen receptor-immunoreactive cells in the forebrain of neonatally estrogen-deprived male rats. Neuroscience 77:911, 1997.

154. Baas D, et al: Rat oligodendrocytes express the vitamin D(3) receptor and respond to 1,25-dihydroxyvitamin D(3). Glia *31*:59, 2000.
155. Welberg LA, Seckl JR, Holmes MC: Prenatal glucocorticoid programming of brain corticosteroid receptors and corticotrophin-releasing hormone: possible implications for behaviour. Neuroscience *104*:71, 2001.
156. Gould E, et al: Adrenal steroids regulate postnatal development of the rat dentate gyrus, II: Effects of glucocorticoids and mineralocorticoids on cell birth. J Comp Neurol *313*:486, 1991.
157. Shi B, et al: Dexamethasone induces hypertrophy of developing medial septum cholinergic neurons: potential role of nerve growth factor. J Neurosci *18*:9326, 1998
158. Brunson KL, et al: Long-term, progressive hippocampal cell loss and dysfunction induced by early-life administration of corticotropin-releasing hormone reproduce the effects of early-life stress. Proc Natl Acad Sci USA *98*:8856, 2001.
159. Schlinger BA, Arnold AP: Circulating estrogen in a male birdsong originates in the brain. Proc Natl Acad Sci USA *89*:7650, 1992.
160. Dakamoto H, et al: Dendritic spine formation in response to progesterone synthesized de novo in the developing Purkinje cell in rats. Neurosci Lett *322*:111, 2002.
161. Kurz EM, et al: Androgens regulate dendritic length of sexually dimorphic mammalian motor neurons in adulthood. Science *232*:395, 1986.
162. Weiland N: Glutamic acid decarboxylase messenger ribonucleic acid is regulated by estradiol and progesterone in the hippocampus. Endocrinology *131*:2697, 1992.
163. Shugrue PJ, Dorsa DM: Estrogen and androgen differentially modulate the growth-associated protein GAP-43 (neuromodulin) messenger ribonucleic acid in postnatal rat brain. Endocrinology *134*:1321, 1994.
164. Neven I, et al: 1,25-Dihydroxyvitamin D$_3$ regulates the synthesis of nerve growth factor in primary cultures of glial cells. Brain Res Mol Brain Res *24*:70, 1994.
165. Brewer LD, et al: Vitamin D hormone confers neuroprotection in parallel with downregulation of L-type calcium channel expression in hippocampal neurons. J Neurosci *21*:98, 2001.

174

Margaret A. Myers

Development of Pain Sensation

Within the past several decades, the field of neonatology has established itself and made vast strides in the reduction of infant morbidity and mortality. Increasingly, this has required that intense and frequently invasive treatments be performed on term and preterm neonates.[1,2] The assessment and treatment of pain has been included only relatively recently in the management of these critically ill neonates. Until the 1980s, newborns infants frequently underwent invasive procedures, including surgery, with no analgesic or anesthetic agent administration. The reasons for this were multifaceted. It was widely believed that the immature neonatal brain could not respond in a manner that perceived or localized painful stimuli.[3,4] Theories about the potential protective aspects of this high-pain threshold during labor and delivery abounded. Clinicians frequently assumed that neonates did not experience pain as severely as adults, nor could they remember painful experiences.[5]

Some of this apparent misconception stems from the fact that neonates and infants lack the ability to communicate verbally.[3] Also, concerns about the potential adverse side effects of analgesic and anesthetic agents in the neonate overwhelmed the perceived benefits.[6] It was not until the radical literature revealed the relative safety of anesthetic agents,[7] and the improved outcomes of patients undergoing surgery with anesthesia,[8-11] that the field of neonatal pain research, both clinical and basic science, blossomed. However, as recently as 1997, a survey of physicians and nurses revealed that though clinicians now believe that infants experience significant procedure-associated pain, they also believe inadequate pain management is provided to these infants.[12] This chapter reviews the development of pain sensation in the fetus and neonate, as well as the clinical markers of pain and the impact of pain treatment on this vulnerable patient population.

THE DEFINITION OF PAIN

The International Association for the Study of Pain defined pain in 1979 as "an unpleasant sensory and emotional response associated with actual or potential tissue damage, or described in terms of such damage."[13] The association also noted that "pain is always subjective," a clearly problematic issue when considering the preverbal nature of the fetus, neonate, and infant. Schechter[3] proposed that pain perception is dependent on two compo-

nents: a sensory component that is neurophysiologically determined, and an emotional component based, among many factors, on affective state, past experience, and development. The following discussion of the development of pain perception in the fetus and neonate concentrates mainly on advances in the understanding of the former component, or nociception, as the complexity of the subjective and emotional aspects of pain perception are poorly understood owing to lack of communication ability in this patient population.

THE DEVELOPMENT OF NOCICEPTION

Pain may be described as a process in which the stimulation of peripheral sensory nociceptors produces responses conducted via the spinal cord neurons to sensory areas of the cerebral cortex. These neural pain pathways, classically thought of as straightforward neuronal "wiring," have been shown to be more complex than originally believed. Wall argued in 1988 that pain pathways contain constantly shifting patterns of interneuronal communication, and that pain pathways are context dependent.[14,15] The basic mechanisms of pain perception in the fetus and neonate are similar to those of adults, though differences obviously exist due to neuroanatomic, neurophysiologic, and neurochemical developmental immaturity. No discussion of pain perception in the human fetus and neonate would be possible without recognizing the groundbreaking works of KJS Anand and colleagues that provide the foundation for much of the research in this field. This massive body of literature has heightened the neonatal practitioner's awareness of pain in this patient population, and has demonstrated improved outcomes in patients receiving adequate treatment for pain.

Neuroanatomy, Neurophysiology, and Neurochemistry

Cutaneous sensory receptors first appear in the perioral area of the human fetus in the 7th week of gestation and spread throughout the fetus by the 20th week of gestation, as outlined in Table 174-1.[16] Evidence suggests that the density of cutaneous nociceptor receptors in the late fetus and neonate is comparable, or may even exceed, that of adult receptor density.[17] Nociceptors may be divided into two broad types: high-threshold mechanoreceptors that respond to pressure, and polymodal

TABLE 174-1

Development of Cutaneous Sensory Receptors in the Human Fetus

Week of Gestation	Location of Receptors
7th	Perioral area
11th	Face, palms, and soles
15th	Trunk, arms, and legs
20th	All cutaneous and mucous surfaces

nociceptors that respond to heat or chemical irritation as well as to pressure.[18] The mechanoreceptor axons are large and myelinated and conduct rapidly (A-delta fibers), providing the rapid onset of sharp localized pain following injury. The polymodal receptor axons are small and unmyelinated, conducting relatively slowly (C-fibers), yielding slow, prolonged, poorly localized pain. These primary afferent fiber signals transmitting the presence of painful stimuli may be amplified or attenuated by activation of local neurons in the affected tissue and spinal cord. Inflammatory mediators such as cytokines, bradykinins, catecholamines, and substance P released from damaged tissues may sensitize both the A and C fibers and other local neurons, causing hyperalgesia.[19]

Cutaneous nociceptor afferents have cell bodies in the dorsal root ganglia of the spinal cord, and there is evidence that sensory fiber-to-dorsal horn interneuron synapse development occurs as early as the 6th week of gestation.[20] The dorsal horn cells are organized in layers that may have significant amplification or attenuation effects upon the afferent nociceptive signals. Development and differentiation of dorsal horn cells begin around 13 weeks' gestation, and the laminar arrangement, as well as synaptic interconnections and neurotransmitter vesicles, matures in some regions of the spinal cord by 30 weeks' gestation.[21] Myelination of the pain pathways of the spinal cord and brain stem is completed during the second and third trimesters of gestation.[22]

Most nociceptive signals to the cerebral cortex travel via second-order neurons in the spinothalamic, spinoreticular, and spinomesoencephalic tracts to synapse in the thalamus. The cerebral cortex neurons develop by 20 weeks' gestation but undergo a process of dendritic branching, or arborization, developing synaptic targets for thalamocortical fibers. Synaptogenesis of thalamocortical connections is established between 20 and 24 weeks' gestation. The cerebral cortex contains no obvious focal pain center; nociception seems to be distributed widely throughout the brain.[23] This overall development and myelination of pain pathways occurs simultaneously with fetal cortical maturation, dendritic arborization, and thalamocortical fiber synaptogenesis, as shown in Figure 174-1.[24] Note that the fetal electroencephalographic patterns suggest some degree of functional maturity of the cerebral cortex prior to 30 weeks' gestation, with continued maturation over the ensuing postconceptual weeks. This idea of functional maturity in the cerebral cortex is supported by studies of neonatal glucose utilization in the sensory regions of the brain, and observations of specific behavioral responses to stimuli in both the fetus and newborn.[24]

The development and function of the various fetal and neonatal neurotransmitters are summarized elsewhere in this text and will not be reviewed here. The complex nature of the pain response is modified by dozens of neurotransmitters within the nervous system.[18] Pain-related neurotransmitters (including the neuropeptide substance P, thought of as the primary afferent nociceptive neurotransmitter) appear in the spinal cord dorsal horn early in gestation. Neurotransmitters such as substance P, calcitonin, and neurokinin have been proposed to amplify pain signals from peripheral sensory neurons. Attenuation of the pain response by endogenous opioid peptides (endorphins), serotonin, monoamines (e.g., glycine), norepinephrine, the neuropeptide enkephalins, and γ-aminobutyric acid (GABA) also occurs. Inhibitory neurotransmitter release from areas of the brain (raphe nucleus, locus coeruleus, periaqueductal gray matter of the midbrain) modulates efferent descending inhibition of the pain response via dorsolateral tracts to inhibit the dorsal horn of the spinal cord. Brief mention must be made of the dorsal horn opioid receptors and their impact on the inhibition of the pain response. Opioids reduce neurotransmitter release into the primary afferent synapses, inhibiting dorsal horn afferent postsynaptic neuronal excitation. This inhibitory activity is evolving to be complex in nature, and research is ongoing to describe further the multiple opioid receptors and their functions.

The foregoing neuroanatomic and neurochemical information leads one to conclude that both the fetus and infant have highly

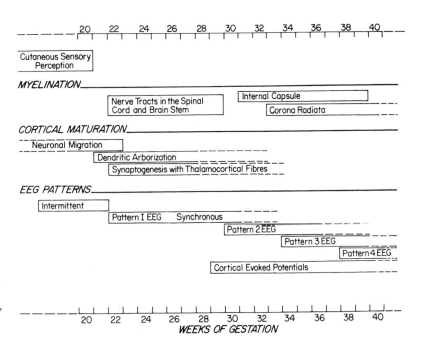

Figure 174–1. Depiction of the maturation of nociceptive pathways and functions during the third trimester of fetal gestation. (From Anand KJS, Hickey PR: N Engl J Med 317:1321, 1987, with permission.)

developed nociceptive systems capable of communicating painful stimuli from the periphery to the cerebral cortex, and regulating the response via efferent inhibitory pathways. The maturation of these systems continues to varying degrees throughout infancy and childhood.

CLINICAL AND PHYSIOLOGIC MARKERS ASSOCIATED WITH PAIN

The physiologic changes associated with pain encompass responses that include those of the cardiovascular, respiratory, endocrine, metabolic, and immune systems.[18]

The hemodynamic and respiratory changes associated with pain frequently have been used as indices of reactivity to assess painful events in preterm and term infants. An increase in an infant's heart rate and blood pressure during and following a painful procedure, such as circumcision or heel lance, has been well documented.[25-28] This presumably reflects increased sympathetic modulation as well as parasympathetic withdrawal.[29] In many cases, this increase can be prevented or attenuated by the use of local or topical anesthetics.[30-33] Whereas infants of all gestational ages demonstrate heart rate reactivity in response to painful stimuli, both gestational age and postconceptual age appear to be factors in determining the magnitude of this physiologic response.[34,35] Infants born at less than 28 weeks' gestational age may be more responsive to painful stimuli as they progress toward term, and they also demonstrate increased heart rate responses to heel lance with increased gestational age at birth. This effect of both gestational age and postconceptual age on the heart rate response to pain is not well understood and may reflect differences in neurologic or cardiovascular development or both.

Neonates undergoing surgery have been observed to experience large fluctuations in measured transcutaneous oxygen tensions.[36,37] Decreases in transcutaneous oxygen tension also were observed during circumcision and could be attenuated or prevented by the use of local anesthetic agents.[33,38] Tracheal intubation, another example of a noxious procedure, caused decreased transcutaneous oxygen tension measurements, as well as increased arterial blood pressure and intracranial pressure in both term and preterm infants.[39,40] These cardiovascular responses could be diminished by the administration of anesthetic agents.[41,42]

The *stress response* is a term used to describe the wide range of hormonal and metabolic changes associated with trauma, both physical and emotional.[43-45] This encompasses the outpouring of pituitary, pancreatic, and adrenal hormones that affect metabolic balance and once may have played a part in allowing injured mammals to catabolize their own body stores, thereby improving survival.[44] The hormonal responses to surgically induced stress in infants have been shown to include increases in catecholamines (both epinephrine and norepinephrine), cortisol, β-endorphins, insulin, glucagon, renin-aldosterone, growth hormone, and prolactin.[46-48] Giannakoulopoulos and colleagues demonstrated that fetuses of 24 to 34 weeks' gestation have shown increases in cortisol and β-endorphin levels in response to intrauterine abdominal needling.[49]

As mentioned earlier, the stress response in neonates has been most closely investigated in response to surgery and relatively minor procedures such as circumcision and venipuncture. Anesthesia generally has been shown to attenuate this stress response, both intra- and postoperatively.[8,10,11] It is interesting that in one study, the neonatal cortisol response to circumcision was not significantly reduced by the administration of a local anesthetic nerve block.[50] Further investigation is needed to confirm this phenomenon. The investigators theorize about the potential problem of awake procedures, (with only regional afferent neuronal blockade) causing a stress response via cortical

and adrenal pathways in infants because of their fear, anxiety, and inability to respond to verbal reassurance.

BEHAVIORAL MARKERS ASSOCIATED WITH PAIN

Anand and Hickey[24] described the behavioral changes associated with pain and divided them into four general categories: simple motor responses, facial expressions, crying, and complex behavioral responses. The simple motor response includes the flexion and adduction of extremities in response to a painful stimulus (e.g., pinprick), found even in preterm infants. Distinct facial expressions have been associated with pain and are the basis for portions of many pain assessment techniques.[51,52] The cry response to painful stimulus has been shown to have specific characteristics and acoustic features that can be differentiated from other crying behavior (e.g., hunger) by adult listeners.[53] The complex responses include such behaviors as altered sleep-wake cycles and irritability following painful stimulus. Changes in complex behavior were noted following circumcision in boy infants; these effects were absent in infants given local anesthesia prior to the painful procedure.[54]

PAIN ASSESSMENT IN THE NEONATE

Assessment of pain in infants is a difficult task given that their preverbal developmental state does not allow communication of their pain in words. Research in the late 1980s and early 1990s established that pain could be assessed in infants by means of cardiorespiratory, neuroendocrine, and behavioral responses to painful stimuli.[55,56] Refinement of infant pain assessment scales continued throughout the 1990s and into the new millennium. Though over three dozen scales have been developed,[57] no single tool has emerged as the "gold standard" for the assessment of neonatal pain.[52,58] The ability to assess pain appropriately has obvious implications on the management of acute procedural and postoperative pain in preterm and term neonates.

PROLONGED EFFECTS OF PAIN

There is a growing body of evidence that pain is associated with more than the relatively short-term effects, such as elevated heart rate, blood pressure, intracranial pressure, and the endocrine/metabolic stress response. Long-lasting effects associated with exposure to pain exist for the neonate and, perhaps, the fetus.

The pain associated with neonatal circumcision and its effect on future behavioral changes has been the focus of several studies.[59,60] Neonatal circumcision was shown to increase the pain response to vaccination at 4 to 6 months of age, implying the presence of memory.[59] Further studies confirmed that there was a stronger pain response to subsequent routine vaccination in circumcised versus uncircumcised infants.[60] Treatment with a topical anesthetic prior to circumcision attenuated this enhanced pain response to 4- to 6-month routine immunizations.

Major surgery performed with preemptive analgesia within the first 3 months of life was not associated with an increased response to pain at later (14-month or 45-month) immunization.[61] This implies that the enhanced pain responses noted earlier diminish over a relatively prolonged period following exposure to the noxious stimulus, or that preemptive analgesia prevented the memory-associated response.

A review of the literature by Mitchell and Boss[62] concluded that infants, especially preterm infants, experience both immediate and long-lasting harmful consequences associated with exposure to severe or repetitive pain, and that structural and physiologic changes occur within the nervous system in response to pain. Bhutta and Anand[63] described an enhanced vulnerability of immature neurons to degenerative changes and noted that repetitive pain during the neonatal period might have a significant impact on neuronal survival. They proposed two mechanisms that lead to neuronal cell death in the immature brain. The first was an *N*-methyl-D-aspartate (NMDA) receptor-mediated neuronal cell calcium influx initiating excitotoxic cell death. The second was enhanced neuronal apoptosis potentially due to maternal separation or metabolic stressors. This conclusion, that there is significant neuronal cell death in response to pain, would seem to be supported by the areas of cortical and subcortical volume loss noted in 8-year-old former preterm children without severe intraventricular hemorrhage.[64] Further research is needed to describe accurately any enhanced neuronal cell death in response to pain in vulnerable fetal and neonatal populations. Prevention or treatment of pain may reduce the potential sequelae of intense, repetitive, and/or prolonged pain and improve outcomes in the vulnerable fetal and neonatal populations.[65]

SUMMARY

Infants have the capacity to perceive pain. The neuroanatomic, neurophysiologic, and neurochemical substrates for pain perception are developed by midgestation and continue to mature throughout late gestation and infancy. Term and preterm infant responses to pain, both physiologic and behavioral, have been well described and are used to perform multidimensional pain assessments. Research supports the concept that behavioral, and perhaps emotional, responses to pain are integrated into the memory and have an impact on subsequent behavior patterns. Also, the effects of severe repetitive or prolonged pain may enhance neuronal cell death with an impact on long-term neurodevelopmental outcome. Adequate pain treatment may alleviate some of these effects.

Recently, attention has focused on the need for all patient populations to be assessed for pain, appropriately treated for pain, and educated about pain. This was emphasized by a Joint Commission on Accreditation of Healthcare Organizations (JCAHO) statement made in 1999: "Recognizing pain as a major, yet largely avoidable, public health problem, JCAHO has developed standards that create new expectations for the assessment and management of pain in accredited hospitals." Infant pain in the neonatal intensive care unit setting has not been well studied from an epidemiologic point of view, but the available information indicates that infants are still exposed to too much potentially preventable or treatable pain. This frequent exposure to pain poses considerable threat to both the immediate and long-term outcomes in this particularly vulnerable population.

REFERENCES

1. Porter FL, Anand KJS: Epidemiology of pain in neonates. Res Clin Forums 20:9, 1998.
2. Barker DP, Rutter N: Exposure to invasive procedures in neonatal intensive care unit admissions. Arch Dis Child 72:F47, 1995.
3. Schechter N: The undertreatment of pain in children: an overview. Pediatr Clin North Am 36:781, 1989.
4. Wallerstein E: Circumcision: the uniquely American medical enigma. Urol Clin North Am 12:123, 1985.
5. Merskey H: On the development of pain. Headache 10:116, 1970.
6. Rees GJ: Anesthesia in the newborn. Br Med J 2:1419, 1950.
7. Robinson S, Gregory GA: Fentanyl-air-oxygen anesthesia for ligation of patent ductus arteriosus in preterm infants. Anesth Analg 60:331, 1981.
8. Anand KJS, et al: Does halothane anaesthesia decrease the metabolic and endocrine stress responses of newborn infants undergoing operation? Br Med J 296:668, 1988.
9. Anand KJS, Aynsley-Green A: Metabolic and endocrine effects of surgical ligation of patent ductus arteriosus in the human preterm neonate: are there implications for further improvement of postoperative outcome? Mod Probl Paediatr 12:123, 1985.
10. Anand KJS, et al: Randomised trial of fentanyl anaesthesia in preterm babies undergoing surgery: effects on the stress response. Lancet 1:62, 1987.
11. Anand KJS, Hickey PR: Halothane-morphine compared with high-dose sufentanil for anesthesia and postoperative analgesia in neonatal cardiac surgery. N Engl J Med 326:1, 1992.
12. Porter FL, et al: Pain and pain management in newborn infants: a survey of physicians and nurses. Pediatrics 100:626, 1997.
13. Merskey H, et al: International Subcommittee for the Study of Pain, Subcommittee on taxonomy: Pain terms: a list with definitions and notes on usage. Pain 6:249, 1979.
14. Wall PD: Stability and instability of central pain mechanisms: Proceedings of the Vth World Congress on Pain, 1988, p 13.
15. Wall PD: The prevention of postoperative pain. Pain 33:289, 1988.
16. Humphrey T: Some correlations between the appearance of human fetal reflexes and the development of the nervous system. Prog Brain Res 4:93, 1964.
17. Gliess J, Stuttgen G: Morphologic and functional development of the skin. In Stave U (ed): Physiology of the Perinatal Period, Vol II, New York, Appleton-Century-Crofts, 1970, p 889.
18. Anand KJS, Carr DB: The neuroanatomy, neurophysiology, and neurochemistry of pain, stress, and analgesia in newborns and children. Pediatr Clin North Am 36: 795, 1989.
19. Dickenson A: Spinal cord pharmacology of pain. Br J Anaesth 75:193, 1995.
20. Okado N: Onset of synapse formation in the human spinal cord. J Comp Neurol 201:211, 1981.
21. Rizvi T, et al: Development of spinal substrate for nociception. Pain 4:195, 1987.
22. Gilles FJ, et al: Myelinated tracts: growth patterns. In Gilles FH, et al (eds): The Developing Human Brain. Boston, Wright & Co, 1983, p 117.
23. Melzack R: Gate control theory on the evolution of pain concepts. Pain Forum 5:128, 1996.
24. Anand KJS, Hickey PR: Pain and its effects in the human neonate and fetus. N Engl J Med 317:1321, 1987.
25. Williamson PS, Williamson ML: Physiologic stress reduction by a local anesthetic during newborn circumcision. Pediatrics 71:36, 1983.
26. Owens ME, Todt EH: Pain in infancy: neonatal reaction to a heel lance. Pain 20:77, 1984.
27. Johnson CC, Strada ME: Acute pain response in infants: a multidimensional description. Pain 24:373, 1986.
28. Olson TL, Downey VW: Infant physiological responses to noxious stimuli of circumcision with anesthesia and analgesia. Pediatr Nurs 24:385, 1998.
29. Oberlander T, Saul JP: Methodological considerations for the use of heart rate variability as a measure of pain reactivity in vulnerable infants. Clin Perinatol 29:427, 2002.
30. Holve RL, et al: Regional anesthesia during newborn circumcision: effect on infant pain response. Clin Pediatr 22:813, 1983.
31. Arnett RM, et al: Effectiveness of 1% lidocaine dorsal penile nerve block in infant circumcision. Am J Obstet Gynecol 163:1074, 1990.
32. Mudge D, Younger JB: The effects of topical lidocaine on infant response to circumcision. J Nurs Midwifery 34:335, 1989.
33. Maxwell LG, et al: Penile block reduces the physiological stress of newborn circumcision. Anesthesiology 65:A432, 1986.
34. Porter FL, et al: Procedural pain in newborn infants: the influence of intensity and development. Pediatrics 104:13, 1999.
35. Craig KD, et al: Pain in the preterm neonate: behavioural and physiological indices. Pain 52:287, 1993.
36. Welle P, et al: Continuous measurement of transcutaneous oxygen tension of neonates under general anesthesia. J Pediatr Surg 15:257, 1980.
37. Venus B, et al: Transcutaneous PO₂ monitoring during pediatric surgery. Crit Care Med 9:714, 1981.
38. Rawlings DJ, et al: The effect of circumcision on transcutaneous pO₂ in term infants. Am J Dis Child 134:676, 1980.
39. Kelly MA, Finer NN: Nasotracheal intubation in the neonate: physiologic responses and effects of atropine and pancuronium. J Pediatr 105:303, 1984.
40. Marshall TA, et al: Physiologic changes associated with endotracheal intubation in preterm infants. Crit Care Med 12:501, 1984.
41. Raju TNK, et al: Intracranial pressure during intubation and anesthesia in infants. Anesth Analg 66:860, 1980.
42. Friesen RH, et al: Changes in anterior fontanel pressure in preterm neonates during tracheal intubation. Anesth Analg 66:874, 1987.
43. Owens ME: Pain in infancy: conceptual and methodological issues. Pain 20:213, 1984.
44. Desborough JP: The stress response to trauma and surgery. Br J Anaesth 85:109, 2000.
45. Goldman RD, Koren G: Biologic markers of pain in the vulnerable infant. Clin Perinatol 29:415, 2002.
46. Anand KJS, et al: Hormonal-metabolic stress responses in neonates undergoing cardiac surgery. Anesthesiology 73:661, 1990.
47. Milne EMG, et al: The effect of intermediary metabolism of open-heart surgery with deep hypothermia and circulatory arrest in infants of less than 10 kilograms' body weight: a preliminary study. Perfusion 1:29, 1986.
48. Chana RS, et al: Serum cortisol and prolactin response to surgical stress in infants and children. J Indian Med Assoc 99:303, 2001.
49. Giannakoulopoulos X, et al: Fetal plasma cortisol and β-endorphin response to intrauterine needling. Lancet 344:77, 1994.
50. Williamson PS, Evans ND: Neonatal cortisol response to circumcision with anesthesia. Clin Pediatrics 25:412, 1986.
51. Grunau RVE, Craig KD: Pain expression in neonates: facial action and cry. Pain 28:395, 1987.
52. Franck LS, et al: Pain assessment in infants and children. Pediatr Clin North Am 47:487, 2000.

53. Porter FL, et al: Neonatal pain cries: effect of circumcision on acoustic features and perceived urgency. Child Dev *57*:790, 1986.

54. Dixon S, et al: Behavioural effects of circumcision with and without anesthesia. J Dev Behav Pediatr *5*:246, 1984.

55. Franck LS: A new method to quantitatively describe pain behavior in infants. Nurs Res *35*:28, 1986.

56. Mathews JR, et al: Assessment and measurement of pain in children. *In* Schechter NL, et al (eds): Pain in Infants, Children and Adolescents. Baltimore, Williams & Wilkins, 1993, p 97.

57. Stevens B, Gibbins S: Clinical utility and clinical significance in the assessment and management of pain in vulnerable infants. Clin Perinatol *29*:459, 2002.

58. Franck LS: Some pain, some gain: reflections on the past two decades of neonatal pain research and treatment. Neonatal Netw *21*:37, 2002.

59. Taddio A, et al: Effect of neonatal circumcision on pain responses during vaccination in boys. Lancet *344*:291, 1994.

60. Taddio A, et al: Effect of neonatal circumcision on pain response during subsequent routine vaccination. Lancet *349*:599, 1997.

61. Peters JW, et al: Major surgery within the first 3 months of life and subsequent biobehavioral pain response to immunization at later age: a case comparison study. Pediatrics *111*:129, 2003.

62. Mitchell A, Boss BJ: Adverse effects of pain on the nervous systems of newborns and young children: a review of the literature. J Neurosci Nurs *34*:228, 2002.

63. Bhutta AY, Anand KJS: Vulnerability of the developing brain neuronal mechanisms. Clin Perinatol *29*:357, 2002.

64. Peterson B, et al: Regional brain volume abnormalities and long-term cognitive outcome in preterm infants. JAMA *284*:1939, 2000.

65. Anand KJS: Consensus statement for the prevention and management of pain in the newborn. Arch Pediatr Adolesc Med *155*:173, 2001.

Special Sensory Systems in the Fetus and Neonate

175

Graham E. Quinn

Retinal Development and the Pathophysiology of Retinopathy of Prematurity

The development of the retina and its functioning components is a complex and highly evolved task. It is also a long-term project composed of many disparate elements that takes months during the gestational period to become functional, but years until differentiation is complete. For example, the optic vesicle is identifiable by the fourth week of gestation, and the vascular supply of the retina is nearly complete by term due date, whereas the development of the macular region continues for the first decade after birth. When an infant is born prematurely, retinal development must proceed in an environment that is, in many ways, alien and results in various insults and perturbations of the orderly, long-term process. The purpose of this chapter is to review retinal development during gestation and the way in which preterm birth may cause changes in the process.

DEVELOPMENT OF THE CELLULAR COMPONENTS OF THE RETINA

Ganglion cells are the first identifiable cells in the developing retina and establish the innermost layer of the retina by the fifth month of gestation or the 130-mm stage. Shortly thereafter, cellular migration into the inner plexiform and inner nuclear layers leads to differentiation of these layers at the 180-mm stage. The development of photoreceptor layer is evident as the outer plexiform layer at the 48-mm stage, and it develops radially from the optic disk and reaches the ora serrata at about 29 weeks' gestation.[1] Kretzer and Hittner[2] defined a four-stage gradient of photoreceptor maturation in which the most mature photoreceptors are present near the optic disk initially and the photoreceptors are increasingly immature as distance from the disk increases. In Stage I of photoreceptor development, the photoreceptor has no outer segment. In Stage II, a small, balloon-like outer segment develops, and disks can be seen in Stage III. By Stage IV, the outer segments are better developed, with stacks of disks evident. Figure 175-1 shows the centrifugal maturation of photoreceptors during the critical 26th to 29th weeks of gestation. The gradient of photoreceptor differentiation is orderly; the first Stage I photoreceptor reaches the ora in the 27th week of gestation, with rapid subsequent maturation.

As the photoreceptor matures, there is an increasing amount of interstitial retinol binding protein present in the region of the receptors. This protein binds both vitamins A and E. By 28 weeks of gestation, the protein is secreted by photoreceptor for more than two-thirds of the way from the disk to the ora serrata, thus

allowing transport of these vitamins to the inner layers of the retina. As shown in Figure 175-1, Stage II or higher photoreceptors are present along approximately 80% of the disk, or the distance at 28 weeks of gestation. As gestation continues, the surface of the retina is increasingly occupied by more mature photoreceptors.[2]

The development of the foveal region takes much longer and is not complete until several years after birth.[3, 4] The mature fovea is avascular and contains the highest density of cones. The fovea can first be identified about the 14th week of gestation, and, later in gestation, there is a central migration of photoreceptor with remodeling of cones to pack into the foveal region. The maturation proceeds very slowly, with ganglion cells still one to two cells thick at term, and there are years of maturation to go before the foveal region reaches adult cone density.[3] There are only scattered ganglion and glial cells in the mature foveolar pit; normal high cone density develops in this area after the age of 10 years. By a complex interaction with bipolar and ganglion cells, the cones create the region of the retina with highest visual acuity and color perception.[4]

DEVELOPMENT OF THE VASCULAR SUPPLY OF THE RETINA

The vascular supply for the retina is composed of two parts: (1) choroidal vessels that underlie the retina and pigment epithelium and (2) retinal vessels that serve the inner retina. The choroidal vasculature in the human appears virtually mature by week 21 of gestation, with mature capillaries and larger vessels by that time.[5] There is little change in this blood supply despite the high rate of growth and development in the retina during mid- to late gestation.

The development of the inner retinal vessels during gestation parallels the complex organization of the maturing retina and is probably driven by the increasing metabolic demands of the fetal retina. If normal maturation is interrupted and retinopathy of prematurity (ROP) occurs, the location where retinopathy develops is determined by the extent of retinal vessel development.[5] For the clinical purpose of assessing retinal vessel development in ROP screenings, the extent of retinal vascularization in the preterm infant is divided into three zones.[6] As shown in Figure 175-2, Zone I is the most posterior and is defined as a circle with the optic nerve as the center and with the radius defined as twice the disk-to-macula distance. Zone II is that area outside Zone I, but within a circle that has a radius of the distance from the disk to the nasal ora serrata. Zone III, the most peripheral zone, is all retinal surface outside Zones I and II. The usefulness of localizing ROP in term of anterior-posterior retinal location has been a major contributing factor in the acceptance of the international classification of ROP.

The early inner retinal vasculature develops from spindle-shaped precursors, beginning at the optic disk and migrating peripherally to the ora serrata. The primordial central retinal artery is derived from a cluster of cells at the base of the hyaloid artery that extends from the optic disk posteriorly to the posterior surface of the lens anteriorly. By week 21 of gestation, vessels are seen 2 to 3 mm around the optic nerve. Development of the retinal vessels proceeds at least twice as fast from week 21 of gestation to week 28 compared with week 28 to term due date.[5] Some investigators have described mesenchymal cells that are vascular precursor cells migrating in advance of the endothelial cells.[5, 7-10] The retinal vessels of the superficial retinal layers reach only about 70% of the distance from the disk to ora serrata at week 27 of gestation, and they gradually advance to near 100% by about term due date. However, among human infants, there are considerable variations in the time course of retinal vascularization. As shown in Figure 175-3, which is based on eye data from 1400 infants who did not develop ROP during the Cryotherapy for Retinopathy of Prematurity Trial,[11] the likelihood that the retinal vessels in a prematurely born infant will have grown into Zone III increases with advancing postconceptional age. For example, among those infants examined at 29 weeks' postconceptional age, there were no eyes with vessels extending into Zone III, whereas by 36 weeks' postconception age, more than half the eyes that did not develop ROP had vascularized into Zone III. However, among the infants who were not observed to develop ROP during the Cryotherapy for Retinopathy of Prematurity Trial, a few eyes had not vascularized into Zone III by 45 to 49 weeks' postconceptional age.[11]

DEVELOPMENT OF ANTIOXIDANT DEFENSE SYSTEMS OF THE RETINA

The retina, in particular photoreceptor membranes, has a high content of polyunsaturated fatty acids,[12] and thus it has a high rate of production of oxygen-derived free radicals. Several systems serve as antioxidant defense systems against oxidative

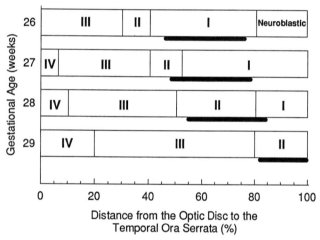

Figure 175–1. Graph shows the gradient of photoreceptor development from 26 to 29 weeks' gestation. *Roman numerals* indicate the stage of photoreceptor development (see text), and the *solid black line* marks the location of the spindle cell apron. (Adapted from Kretzer, FW, Hittner HM: *In* Miguel J, Quintanhilha AT (eds): CRC Handbook of Free Radicals and Antioxidants in Biomedicine. Boca Raton, FL, CRC Press, 1989, pp 315–332.)

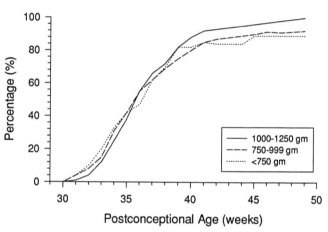

Figure 175–3. Cumulative proportion of infants who did not develop retinopathy of prematurity who retinal vessels terminate in zone III by the postconceptional age of the infant. (Adapted from Palmer EA, et al: Ophthalmology *98*:1628, 1991.)

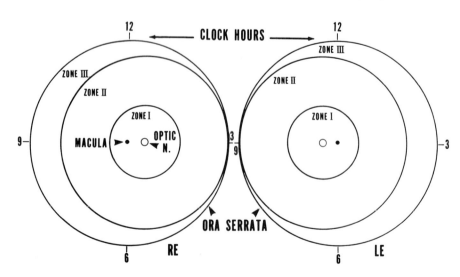

Figure 175–2. Scheme of right and left eyes showing the zone of vascularization to indicate the location and extent of retinopathy of prematurity. (Adapted from ICROP Committee: Arch Ophthalmol *102*:1130, 1984. Copyright © 1984, American Medical Association.)

damage in the cells of the human retina. These antioxidant systems, including vitamins E and C, as well as several enzymatic and nonenzymatic systems, maintain an effective environment for scavenging of oxygen-derived free radicals. For example, reduced glutathione (GSH) and glutathione peroxidase (GSH-P) play important roles in eliminating hydrogen peroxide and lipid hydroperoxides. In addition, GSH, catalyzed by glutathione-S-transferase (GSH-S-ase), covalently binds or initiates peroxidation of electrophilic sites of compounds that could damage cellular membranes.[13]

The most extensively studied antioxidant in the developing human retina is vitamin E, largely because of its investigational use in the treatment of ROP.[14,15] Bhat[16] examined the distribution of vitamin E in the retinas of term and preterm infants with gestational ages ranging from 24 to 40 weeks and with birth weights ranging from 540 to 2900 g. These investigators identified two groups of infants: (1) "unsupplemented" infants, and (2) infants who had received vitamin E supplementation, consisting of 50 mg/kg/day of DL-α tocopherol acetate given within 24 hours after birth and continued until the infant's death. At birth, all infants had low serum α-tocopherol levels, ranging from 0.1 to 0.5 mg/dL, clearly in a deficient range for normal adult levels.[14] As shown in Table 175–1, the retinal levels of vitamin E tended to increase with gestational age, and they were higher in the retina than in the vitreous or the choroid. In addition, supplemented patients had higher levels of vitamin E in the retina, choroid, and vitreous. The retinal levels of vitamin E were also significantly higher in the supplemented group (713 ± 581 µg/g protein, mean ± SD) than in the unsupplemented group (51 ± 57 µg/g protein) ($p < .05$). Thus, it is clear that the retina of the very premature infant has very little reserve antioxidant protection from vitamin E, and vitamin E stores increase with increasing gestational age and with exogenous supplementation of the vitamin.

The regional distribution of antioxidants within the retina may be of importance because the development of the retinal vasculature and photoreceptor, which proceeds from the central to the peripheral retina, leads to increasing demands on the need for antioxidant protection as cells become more metabolically demanding and active. Nielsen and associates[13] measured vitamin E and C levels in vascularized and avascular areas of the retina in eyes of premature infants and in vascularized segments of eyes with mature retinal vascularization. Two groups of eyes were examined: (1) eyes from infants who survived less than 12 hours and who received no vitamin E supplementation and (2) eyes from infants who survived at least 4 days and who received vitamin E supplementation according to the protocol then in place at Baylor College of Medicine (intramuscular injections of 15, 10, and 10 mg/kg on days 1, 2 along with oral tocopheryl acetate at 100 mg/kg/day). These investigators found that the α-tocopherol measured in the avascular region of premature infant retina was only 52% of that measured in the vascularized region of the premature infant retina ($p < .001$). In addition, in both the vascular and avascular retinas of premature infants, the vitamin E content was around 5 to 10% of that measured in the mature retina. It also appeared that infants born after 27 weeks of gestation achieved higher retinal levels of vitamin E than did less mature infants. This finding is in agreement with clinical and pathologic observations of Kretzer and Hittner[1] and of Hittner and associates.[17]

With regard to vitamin C levels, Nielsen and colleagues[13] found that the avascular and vascularized regions of the retina of the premature infant had similar vitamin C levels. They further noted that the vascular region of premature retinas had significantly greater vitamin C content than did the central region of mature retinas ($p < .02$). Therefore, unlike vitamin E, vitamin C content in the avascular and vascularized portions of the premature retina is similar.

Naash and colleagues[18] also examined the regional distribution of GSH-P, GSH-S-ase, and GSH. These investigators found that the activity of GSH-P in the retina of premature infants was about twice that of the retina in mature eyes; both GSH-P and GSH-S-ase showed greater activity in the periphery of premature retinas compared with mature retinas. It appears that, because premature retinas are deficient in vitamin E, antioxidant protection in the preterm infant's eye is largely reliant on GSH-P and GSH-S-ase, along with water-soluble vitamin C.

PATHOPHYSIOLOGY OF RETINOPATHY OF PREMATURITY

ROP is manifest clinically by the abnormal growth of developing retinal vessels and requires two circumstances for its development. The first criterion is incomplete retinal vascularization, and it appears that the more immature the retinal vessels are at a given gestational age, the more likely the eye is to develop

---

TABLE 175-1

Serum, Retinal, Choroidal, and Vitreous Total α-Tocopherol in Unsupplemented and Supplemented Groups

Group and Pt #	Birth Weight (g)	Gestational Age (wk)	Age at Death	α-Tocopherol Levels at Death			
				Serum (mg/dL)	Retina (µg/g protein)	Choroid (µg/g protein)	Vitreous (µg/g protein)
U-1	610	25	48 d	0.2	18.5	14.0	10.0
U-2	624	25	<6 h	0.1	16.0	9.0	1.5
U-3	640	26	6 h	—	17.5	—	—
U-4	640	26	24 h	—	43.0	—	2.5
U-5	700	26	22 d	0.3	40.0	30.0	—
U-6	740	26	24 h	—	47.0	—	—
U-7	2500	36	6 h	0.1	177.0	166.0	268.0
U-8	2500	40	48 h	0.5	969.0	10.0	3.1
S-1	540	24	20 d	1.0	311.0	271.0	144.0
S-2	640	26	45 d	2.1	1130.5	2910.0	22.0
S-3	760	27	34 d	0.7	388.0	291.0	41.0
S-4	930	32	105 d	2.3	1523.0	516.0	351.0
S-5	1250	30	30 d	0.8	211.0	—	—

S = vitamin E supplemented; U = unsupplemented; — indicates missing data.
Adapted by permission from Bhat R: Pediatrics 78:866, 1986. Copyright 1986.

serious forms of ROP.[19] The second criterion is exposure of the developing retina to an abnormal environment. The most likely inciting event is exposure to excess of oxygen-induced free radicals resulting from intrauterine hypoxia, postpartum hypoxia, hyperoxia, or ischemia/reperfusion after premature birth. Postnatally, the insult is probably the result of instability of the infant that leads to a rapidly changing environment for the developing retina, which is already stressed in the relative hyperoxia of the extrauterine world.

Onset

There appears to be a complex interaction between the gestational age of an infant and the onset of ROP. Children who are born very prematurely are at higher risk of developing ROP, including the more severe stages and disease.[20] However, it is also clear that, in terms of postconceptional age, ROP first develops at a predictable time and progresses to more serious stages. As shown in Table 175–2, among children with birth weights of less than 1251 g who were born in 1986 and 1987,[11] the severity of ROP progresses in an orderly fashion from one level to another, with a median value for the earliest stage of ROP, Stage 1, of 34.3 weeks' postconceptional age. With increasing severity of disease, the median postconceptional age at observation is later.

The data shown in Table 175–2 suggest a reasonably tight correlation between gestational age and onset of ROP, and there may be little influence of perinatal events on the onset of ROP. One may also infer from these data that the retinal development must reach a certain threshold level before the clinical manifestations of ROP are apparent.

Further insight into the issue of age at onset of ROP and its relation to gestational age was provided by Quinn and colleagues,[21] using data from a randomized, controlled clinical trial of vitamin E prophylaxis of ROP that was conducted from 1979 to 1981.[22] They tested the hypothesis that perinatal events and stage of retinal development (as a reflection of gestational age) are both important factors in determining the age at onset of ROP by comparing the infant's gestational age at birth with postnatal and postconceptional ages when ROP was first observed. The study population was composed of 111 infants who developed ROP and included infants with birth weights of up to 2000 g and infants with birth weights greater than 2000 g if less than 37 weeks' gestation and receiving more than 23 hours of oxygen supplementation. The inclusion of larger birth weight infants than those shown in Figure 175–3 and Table 175–2 provided a broader range of gestational ages from which to study the impact of gestational age at premature birth on development of ROP. This is important from a theoretical point of view, even

though, at the turn of the 21st century, intensive care nursery, the incidence of ROP in infants with birth weights of more than 1250 g fell dramatically. Figure 175–4 compares the effect of postnatal age when ROP was first noted with gestational age at birth (r = 0.47 with a slope of −0.45, p < .001). As indicated by the negative slope of the regression line, infants born earlier in gestation develop ROP later postnatally than infants born later in gestation. The finding of a slope to the regression line (regardless of whether it is positive or negative) suggests that both gestational age and perinatal events determine the onset of ROP. Quinn and associates[21] suggested that, if only perinatal events were sufficient to determine the onset of ROP, then the age at onset of ROP would be at a constant time after birth, and the regression line would be parallel to the x-axis. If only the stage of retinal development were sufficient to determine when ROP became manifest, then the first examination at which ROP is noted would be at a constant postconceptional age, and the regression line through the data would have a slope of −1 instead of the observed −0.45.

Initiation

The traditional theory about vascular insults that lead to ROP is based on the work of Ashton and associates[23] and Patz and colleagues.[24, 25] In the 1950s and 1960s, these investigators documented vasoconstriction and eventual obliteration of retinal vessels after exposing newborn animals to high concentrations of continuous oxygen. Ashton and colleagues[23, 26, 27] documented endothelial cell death in the kitten model and suggested that the findings in the model could be used to illustrate the course of ROP development in the human infant. They suggested two phases of development of ROP. The first phase is exposure to high oxygen levels, resulting in vasoconstriction of major vessels that produces vasoobliteration of the capillary bed. The second phase is the exuberant growth of new vessels in response to a vasoproliferative substance produced by ischemic peripheral retina on return to a less than high-oxygen environment.

TABLE 175–2

Onset of Various Stages of Retinopathy of Prematurity in Terms of Postconceptional Age in Weeks for Infants with Birth Weights of <1251 g*

	Median	5th percentile	95th percentile
Stage 1 ROP	34.3	*	39.1
Stage 2 ROP	35.4	32.0	40.7
Stage 3 ROP	36.6	32.6	42.9
ROP plus disease	36.3	32.6	42.9
Threshold ROP	36.9	33.6	42.0

* Cannot be determined because 17% of infants had stage 1 ROP at the first eye examination.
ROP = retinopathy of prematurity.
Adapted from Palmer EA, et al: Ophthalmology *98*:1628, 1991.

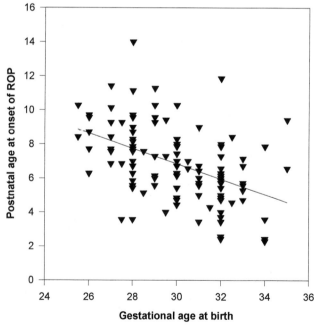

Figure 175–4. The postnatal age (in weeks) at onset of retinopathy of prematurity (ROP) compared with the gestational age for 111 infants who developed ROP. (Adapted from Quinn GE, et al: Br J Ophthalmol *76*:284, 1992.)

Extreme vasoconstriction of the retinal vessels has been observed clinically in human infants exposed to very high oxygen levels that may have existed before modern respirators and oxygen monitoring equipment, but such vasoconstriction is not observed in the neonatal nursery of the late 20th and early 21st centuries. Because most of the support for the theory of vasoconstriction and obliteration is based on animal model work, it may be difficult to make conclusions about human disease. First, as Gole and associates pointed out,[28] in "oxygen-induced retinopathy," ocular neovascularization in the kitten is predominately preretinal, more common in the posterior retina than the peripheral retina, and does not lead to the cicatricial retinal abnormalities that are so prominent in the human. Kremer and colleagues[29] suggested that the extreme vasoobliteration caused by such high oxygen exposures in an effort to induce new vessel formation in the kitten lead to an "acute ischemic vasoproliferative retinopathy caused by total retinal ischemia." This finding is in contrast to the 1977 clinical findings on fluorescein angiography of premature infants with ROP by Flynn and associates,[8] who demonstrated only relatively small areas of vasoobliteration in the region between the vascularized and avascular retina.

D'Amore[30] suggested that growth of microvasculature in the eye is regulated locally by stimulators and inhibitors and that abnormal growth of vessels may be initiated by an imbalance of these factors. Stimulators include a variety of growth factors, including vascular endothelial growth factor (VEGF), vascular permeability factor, basic fibroblast growth factors, and interleukin-8, among others. It appears that relative hypoxia is an essential precursor to the development of retinal neovascularization, leading to the induction or release of an angiogenic factor. Based on the precarious status of the premature infant during the days around birth, it is reasonable to speculate that there are periods of both hypoxia and hyperoxia, both of which would lead to production of oxygen-induced free radicals with subsequent induction of angiogenic factors.

The most likely factor to be implicated in ROP thus far is VEGF. VEGF is a necessary component for the normal development of retinal vasculature.[31-33] The synthesis of VEGF is controlled by oxygen concentration within the cell itself, and its induction is increased by hypoxia in retinal pericytes[34, 35] and by ischemia-induced iris neovascularization.[36] Aiello and colleagues[37] determined the concentration of VEGF obtained from eyes undergoing intraocular surgery for ocular problems including neovascular and nonneovascular disorders. VEGF was detected in 101 of the 178 ocular fluid samples from eyes with diabetic retinopathy, iris neovascularization, or central retinal vein occlusion, compared with only 2 of 31 samples from eyes with no neovascular abnormalities ($\chi^2 = 24.7, p < .0001$). Among eyes with ROP, three samples of aqueous were obtained and showed a elevated mean level of VEGF that was significantly different ($p < .001$) from eyes with no neovascular disorders. Eyes undergoing intraocular surgery for severe ROP are usually in patients who are more than 6 to 9 months old and who have retinal detachments in one or both eyes. Therefore, the evidence that VEGF is a factor that may induce neovascularization seen in the early phases of ROP in humans is provocative, but not certain.

A novel theory of the initiation and progression of ROP was proposed by Hellstrom and colleagues.[38] They presented evidence based on the results of studies in a knock-out mouse model and in a small clinical cohort study of preterm children. They documented the importance of insulin-like growth factor I (IGF-I) in the normal vascularization of the retina. Using the knock-out mouse model, these investigators showed significantly retarded vascular growth in the eyes of IGF-I$^{-/-}$ mice compared with IGF-I$^{+/+}$ mice. Using a measurement of the percentage of distance of vessels from the optic nerve to the retinal periphery, they found that eyes of knock-out animals had a measurement of 58% (4.8SD) compared with a measurement of 70.3% (5.8, $p < .001$. This

finding indicated that IGF-I is essential for vascular development to proceed normally. These investigators also documented that low IGF-I did not suppress VEGF, but rather appeared to permit VEGF to induce vascular development.

Hellstrom and associates[38] also hypothesized that prolonged low IGF-I levels in the newborn preterm infants would be associated with ROP. They obtained weekly IGF-I plasma levels and performed ROP screening examinations in 31 infants with gestational ages of 26 to 30 weeks. ROP Stages 2 to 5[6] were defined as "eyes with ROP" and no ROP observed and Stage 1 ROP as "eyes with no-ROP." Of these 31 infants, 10 developed ROP and 19 did not. When the time from birth to when IGF-I levels reached 30 ng/mL were compared between the ROP and no-ROP groups, the investigators found a mean of 19 days (range, 1 to 79) for those children who developed ROP compared with 58 days (range, 29 to 120) for those children in the no-ROP group ($p < .0001$). In addition, the proliferative phase of the retinopathy was not observed until the IGF-I levels had risen to more than 30 ng/mL. Thus, it appeared that "the development of ROP was strongly associated with a prolonged period of low IGF-I (<30 ng/mL) followed by" the proliferative retinopathy when the IGF-I exceeded this "threshold" level.

It is known that IGF-I is present in sufficient quantities in the placenta and amniotic fluid to promote normal vasculogenesis and that it drops precipitously after preterm birth.[39] Hellstrom and colleagues[38] suggested that the rapid return of IGF-I to near-normal levels quickly will allow normal vascular development and will prevent the development of ROP.

OXYGEN-INDUCED RETINOPATHIES

Other work suggests that further examination of animal models of oxygen-induced retinopathies may be important in understanding the disease in human infants. One of the major problems in dealing with an animal model is that the neonatal animal is essentially healthy and does not have the metabolic instability or respiratory problems that affect the prematurely born infant. This problem may actually be an advantage, because investigators can vary conditions with tight control. The choice of animal model is clearly important. The newborn rat, cat, dog, rabbit, and mouse have all been studied for the possibility of consistent demonstration of oxygen-induced retinopathy.[40]

Using a rat model of ROP, Penn and colleagues[40-42] attempted to duplicate the clinical conditions that produce ROP in the human infant. To produce preretinal neovascularization consistently, they found that a "regimen of systematically varied oxygen" was an essential element and suggested that previous studies using a rat model had produced conflicting results depending on the tightness of control of oxygen administration—meticulous control of constant oxygen levels led to no neovascularization and less consistent control of constant oxygen levels led to new vessel formation. Penn and colleagues[41] demonstrated that preretinal neovascularization was more likely in rats exposed to a 40/80% oxygen cycle than in those rats kept at 80% oxygen alone. In animals that were exposed to cycled 40/80% oxygen with a subsequent period in room air, preretinal neovascularization occurred in 66% (63 of 96), compared with no animals (0 of 50) exposed to constant oxygen followed by room air. This was true even though the 80% exposed rats received a considerably higher oxygen dose over the study period.

In a subsequent report, Penn and colleagues[42] compared 50/10% cycles with 80/40% cycles starting at birth and continuing for 14 days followed by room air for 4 days. In the 50/10% exposed rats, the incidence of preretinal neovascularization was 97% compared with 72% for the 80/40% exposed animals. These studies suggest that range of variation of oxygen administration is not the key to induction of abnormal vascularization. Penn and associates[42] went a step further and attempted to recreate the arterial oxygen tension levels seen in infants who developed serious ROP in a series of studies of newborn rats. These investigators found that prolonged exposures to relative hyperoxia or hypoxia were more likely to result in abnormal vascularization in the rat model than more frequent, less prolonged exposures.

CLINICAL RELEVANCE

The purpose of this chapter is to outline the complex interplay among vascular and retinal elements during gestation and to highlight those factors of fetal development that are most likely to be involved in the pathogenesis of ROP. At our present state of knowledge, it appears that a perinatal insult in the premature infant causes perturbation of normal vasculogenesis. We have just begun to recognize that the stem cells that are the retinal vascular precursors have different behavior when developing in the plane of the retina and when developing into exuberant extraretinal new vessels after penetrating the internal limiting membrane. It may well also be that the rate of return of IGF-I to normal levels is a key indicator of whether a preterm infant is likely to develop ROP. It appears that an increased production of VEGF in the avascular retina leads to the florid new vessel formation that characterizes the early phases of ROP, when a sufficient amount of IGF-I has been produced to allow its expression.

The hypothesis of an oxidant-induced free radical induction of ROP is being or could be tested in various clinical studies that could lead to a reduction of the oxidant-induced free radical insult to the fragile premature newborn infant. The influence of antenatal steroids and surfactant on the development of retinal vascularization remains to be clarified. One may also speculate that supplementation with IGF-I or chemical blockers of VEGF may become available in the future.

ACKNOWLEDGMENT

I gratefully acknowledge the helpful comments of John T. Flynn, MD, in the development of this manuscript, as well as his patient mentoring in understanding ROP since we met more than two decades ago.

REFERENCES

1. Kretzer FL, Hittner HM: Initiating events in the development of retinopathy of prematurity. *In* Silverman WA, Flynn JT (eds): Retinopathy of Prematurity. Boston, Blackwell Scientific Publications, 1985, pp 121–152.
2. Kretzer FW, Hittner HM: Pathogenesis and antioxidant suppression of retinopathy of prematurity. *In* Miquel J, Quintanilha AT (eds): CRC Handbook of Free Radicals and Antioxidants in Biomedicine. Boca Raton, CRC Press, 1989, pp 315–332.
3. Youdelis C, Hendrickson A: A qualitative analysis of the human fovea during development. Vision Res 26:847, 1986.
4. Hendrickson A: A morphological comparison of foveal development in man and monkey. Eye 6:136, 1992.
5. Gariano RF, et al: Vascular development in primate retina: comparison of laminar plexus formation in monkey and human. Invest Ophthalmol Vis Sci 35:3442, 1994.
6. ICROP Committee: International classification of retinopathy of prematurity. Arch Ophthalmol 102:1130, 1984.
7. Ashton M: Oxygen and the growth and development of retinal vessels. Am J Ophthalmol 62:412, 1966.
8. Flynn JT, et al: Retrolental fibroplasia. I. Clinical observations. Arch Ophthalmol 95:217, 1977.
9. Gole GA, et al: Vitamin E and retinopathy of prematurity revisited. Pediatrics 75:1166, 1985.
10. Kretzer FL, Hittner HM: Retinopathy of prematurity: clinical implications of retinal development. Arch Dis Child 63:1151, 1988.
11. Palmer EA, et al: Incidence and early course of retinopathy of prematurity. Ophthalmology 98:1628, 1991.
12. Anderson RE, Risk M: Lipids of ocular tissue. IX. The phospholipids of frog photoreceptor membranes. Vision Res 14:129, 1974.
13. Neilson JC, et al: The regional distribution of vitamins E and C in mature and premature human retinas. Invest Ophthalmol Vis Sci 29:22, 1988.
14. Johnson LH, et al: Vitamin E and ROP: the continuous challenge. *In* Klaus MH, Fanaroff AA (eds): The Yearbook of Neonatal and Perinatal Medicine. St. Louis, CV Mosby, 1993, pp xv–xxiv.
15. Johnson L, et al: Vitamin E and retinopathy of prematurity [letter]. Pediatrics 81:329, 1987.
16. Bhat R: Serum, retinal, choroidal vitreal vitamin E concentrations in human infants. Pediatrics 78:866, 1986.
17. Hittner HM, et al: Suppression of severe retinopathy of prematurity with vitamin E supplementation: ultrastructural mechanism of clinical efficacy. Ophthalmology 91:1512, 1984.
18. Naash MI, et al: The regional distribution of glutathione peroxidase and glutathione-S-transferase in adult and premature human retinas. Invest Ophthalmol Vis Sci 29:149, 1988.
19. Schaffer DB, et al: Prognostic factors in the natural course of retinopathy of prematurity. Ophthalmology 100:230, 1993.
20. Cryotherapy for Retinopathy of Prematurity Cooperative Group: Natural history of retinopathy of prematurity (ROP): the natural ocular outcome of premature birth and retinopathy: status at one year. Arch Ophthalmol 112:903, 1994.
21. Quinn GE: Onset of retinopathy of prematurity as related to postnatal and postconceptional age. Br J Ophthalmol 76:284, 1992.
22. Johnson L, et al: Effect of sustained pharmacologic vitamin E levels on incidence and severity of retinopathy of prematurity: a controlled clinical trial. J Pediatr 114:827, 1989.
23. Ashton N, et al: Role of oxygen in the genesis of retrolental fibroplasia: a preliminary report. Br J Ophthalmol 37:513, 1953.
24. Patz A, et al: Studies on the effect of high oxygen administration I retrolental fibroplasia: a nursery observation. Am J Ophthalmol 35:1248, 1952.
25. Patz A, et al: Oxygen studies in retrolental fibroplasia. II. The production of the microscopic changes of retrolental fibroplasia in experimental animals. Am J Ophthalmol 36:1511, 1953.
26. Ashton N, et al: Effect of oxygen on developing retinal vessels with particular reference to the problem of retrolental fibroplasia. Br J Ophthalmol 38:397, 1954.
27. Ashton N: Some aspects of the comparative pathology of oxygen toxicity in the retina. Br J Ophthalmol 52:507, 1968.
28. Gole GA, et al: Oxygen induced retinopathy: the kitten model reexamined. Aust J Ophthalmol 10:223, 1982.
29. Kremer I, et al: Oxygen-induced retinopathy in newborn kittens: a model for ischemic vasoproliferative retinopathy. Invest Ophthalmol Vis Sci 28:126, 1987.
30. D'Amore PA: Mechanisms of retinal and choroidal neovascularization. Invest Ophthalmol Vis Sci 35:3974, 1994.
31. Pierce EA, et al: Regulation of vascular endothelial growth factor by oxygen in a model of retinopathy of prematurity. Arch Ophthalmol 114:1219, 1996.
32. Stone J, et al: Development of retinal vasculature is mediated by hypoxia-induced vascular endothelial growth factor (VEGF) expression by neuroglia. J Neurosci 15:4738, 1995.
33. Ozaki H, et al: Blockade of vascular endothelial cell growth factor receptor signaling is sufficient to completely prevent retinal neovascularization. Am J Pathol 156:697, 2000.
34. Plouet J, et al: Secretion of VAS/VEGF by retinal pericytes: a paracrine stimulation of endothelial cell proliferation. Invest Ophthalmol Vis Sci 34:900, 1993.
35. Aiello LP, et al: Hypoxic regulation and bioactivity of vascular endothelial growth factor: characterization in retinal microvascular pericytes and pigment epithelial cells. Invest Ophthalmol 35:1868, 1994.
36. Adamis AP, et al: Vascular permeability factor (vascular endothelial growth factor) is produced in the retina and elevated levels are present in the aqueous humor of eye with iris neovascularization. Invest Ophthalmol Vis Sci 34:1440, 1993.
37. Aiello LP, et al: Vascular endothelial growth factor in ocular fluid of patients with diabetic retinopathy and other retinal disorders. N Engl J Med 331:1480, 1994.
38. Hellstrom A, et al: Low IGF-I suppresses VEGF-survival signaling in retinal endothelial cells: direct correlation with clinical retinopathy of prematurity. Proc Nat Acad Sci USA 98:5804, 2001.
39. Lineham JD, et al: Circulating insulin-like growth factor I levels in newborn premature and full-term infants followed longitudinally. Early Hum Dev 13:37, 1986.
40. Penn JS, et al: The range of PaO₂ variation determines the severity of oxygen-induced retinopathy in newborn rats. Invest Ophthalmol Vis Sci 36:2063, 1995.
41. Penn JS, et al: Variable oxygen exposure causes preretinal neovascularization in the newborn rat. Invest Ophthalmol Vis Sci 34:576, 1993.
42. Penn JS, et al: Exposure to alternating hypoxia and hyperoxia causes severe proliferative retinopathy in newborn rats. Invest Ophthalmol Vis Sci 36:724, 1994.

In all vertebrates, the auditory system begins to function before the visual system (Fig. 176–1). In many mammalian species, hearing begins only after birth. In humans, the first responses to sound probably occur by the 24th week of gestation, and by birth, hearing is quite functional, if not adultlike. The finding that human hearing begins prenatally suggests that hearing is very important to human function and survival. The early onset of human hearing also implies that experiences with sound has the potential to influence auditory function and behavior, even in the prenatal period. Because development may capitalize on universally occurring experience with sound to guide its course,[1] it is especially important to recognize the possible effects of early abnormal auditory experiences, as in the case of premature birth.

The prenatal onset of hearing in humans also means that many aspects of early auditory physiology have not been well described in humans. It is difficult to elicit and interpret responses *in utero*. Because of the medical complications associated with premature birth, basic research on premature infants' auditory function is not often a high priority, and of course, there is no guarantee that the development of the auditory system in this special population follows the same course as it would *in utero*. The major landmarks in auditory morphologic development are quite similar in all vertebrates, however. Where structure-function correlations have been established in other species, it is possible to make reasonable predictions about the functional status of the human auditory system even in the prenatal period. At the same time, there are bound to be differences among species, and each auditory capacity depends on many structures, any of which may develop differently in different species. Thus, any conclusions about human auditory physiology based on development in nonhuman species must be recognized as tentative.

This chapter begins with an overview of the morphologic and physiologic development of the human auditory system. Where physiologic data are not available for humans, data from nonhumans are described. The current standard of hearing, however, is auditory behavior; the limited information about the fetal and neonatal development of auditory behavior is reviewed in the second section, and the likely anatomic and physiologic substrates of early auditory behavior are discussed.

EARLY MORPHOLOGY AND PHYSIOLOGY

This section presents in broad outline the course of morphologic development of the auditory system and the physiologic correlates of these events as measured in both humans and nonhumans. In studies of nonhumans, the function of the auditory system is primarily measured as potentials recorded at the site of generation, such as single-unit responses. Gross, scalp-recorded evoked potentials are less frequently used.[2-6] Many of the same auditory capacities—sensitivity, frequency resolution, and temporal resolution—have been measured in human fetuses and neonates. In the case of humans, however, these measurements are largely based on gross, scalp-recorded evoked potentials. Although the same capacities can be measured in this way, it is more difficult to understand the source of immaturity when instruments such as evoked potentials are used. Of course, a satisfactory approach to assessing auditory function in fetuses *in utero* has yet to be developed. Despite these difficulties, many of the developmental trends that have been observed in nonhumans have also been described in human fetuses and neonates.

Peripheral Auditory System: The Ear

The ear is generally divided into three sections: the external ear, including the pinna and ear canal; the middle ear, including the tympanic membrane and ossicles suspended in the tympanic cavity; and the inner ear, including the semicircular canals, vestibule, and cochlea (Fig. 176–2). Functionally, the external and middle ears comprise the conductive component of the ear. They shape the amplitude spectrum of sound arriving at the inner ear. (Every sound can be described as the sum of a series of sinusoids, each with its own frequency, amplitude, and phase; the *amplitude spectrum* of a sound is the function describing amplitude as a function of frequency.) The cochlea is the site of

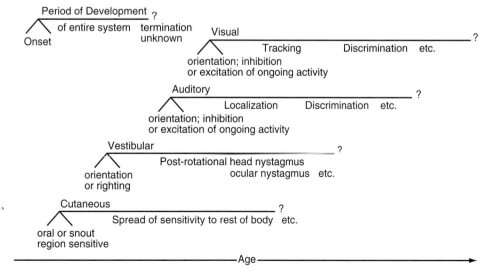

Figure 176–1. The ontogenetic sequence of development of four sensory systems. (From Gottlieb, G., *In* The Biopsychology of Development, E. Tobach, et al, eds. 1971, Academic Press: New York. p. 69.)

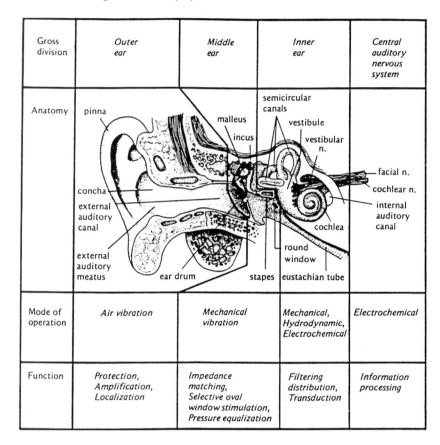

Gross division	Outer ear	Middle ear	Inner ear	Central auditory nervous system
Anatomy				
Mode of operation	Air vibration	Mechanical vibration	Mechanical, Hydrodynamic, Electrochemical	Electrochemical
Function	Protection, Amplification, Localization	Impedance matching, Selective oval window stimulation, Pressure equalization	Filtering distribution, Transduction	Information processing

Figure 176–2. Cross-section of the human ear, showing the external, middle, and inner ear and the major functions of each subdivision. (From Yost, W, *In* Fundamentals of Hearing. 1994, Academic Press: New York. p. 62.)

auditory transduction. Bending of the stereocilia of auditory hair cells resulting from the mechanical displacement of the basilar membrane begins a chain of electrochemical and biochemical events that ends with the generation of an action potential in the neurons of the spiral ganglion (Fig. 176–3). A detailed account of current understanding of sound conduction and transduction in the auditory system can be found in a work by Pickles.[7] Several classic texts describe the embryology and later morphologic development of the peripheral auditory system.[8, 9] More recent texts on this topic are widely accessible.[10, 11]

Conductive Apparatus

The ear canal forms at the dorsal end of the first branchial groove. The cells known as the meatal plug can be identified by 6 gestational weeks; these cells subsequently degenerate to form the ear canal. The distal end of the ear canal closes as it elongates and does not reopen until about the time at which responses to sound can first be recorded. Also at around 6 gestational weeks, six mesenchymal protuberances, the auricular hillocks, appear at the edges of the first branchial groove. The auricular hillocks fuse to form the pinna. Both the ear canal and the pinna continue to grow well into childhood, although in form they are well developed by the time responses to sound can first be recorded.

The mesenchyme that will form the middle ear ossicles is first identifiable at around 5 weeks of gestation. As the ossicles grow and begin ossification, the tympanic cavity expands around them. Eventually, the ossicles will be suspended in the cavity. The tympanic cavity continues to increase in size well into childhood. The linear dimensions and mass of the ossicles are still increasing between 21 and 40 weeks of gestation, and, in fact, they continue to increase somewhat in the postnatal period.[12] The tympanic membrane is derived from the membrane of the first branchial groove. Mesenchyme that grows between the endoderm lining the presumptive tympanic cavity and the surface ectoderm eventually differentiates into the collagenic

fibers that give the membrane its elasticity. As development proceeds, the tympanic membrane thins in cross-section and expands in surface area. The tympanic membrane area is more or less adultlike by about 28 weeks of gestation.[13] It is the ratio of the area of the tympanic membrane to the area of the stapes footplate that allows the middle ear to overcome the impedance mismatch between air and the fluids of the inner ear. Although this ratio has not been followed during development in humans, in cats the ratio changes little over the period when hearing function begins.[14]

Around the time that responses to sound can first be recorded, the conductive mechanism has several characteristics that appear to be common to all mammals.[15] The ear canal and pinna are small. At term birth, the human ear canal is still only 14 to 15 mm long, compared with the adult length of 23 mm.[16-18] The ear canal may not be completely open. The ear canal walls are more compliant in young animals than in adults. The middle ear cavity is also small. The ossicles are not completely ossified, and they are somewhat smaller and lighter than in the adult. The tympanic membrane appears less stiff than in the adult. Many of these characteristics persist in the full-term neonate.

The functional implications of conductive development are quite different for animals who begin to hear *in utero* than they are for animals who begin to hear postnatally. If the neonate first begins to hear airborne sounds, then the external and middle ear will determine the amplitude spectrum of the sound reaching the inner ear. Obviously, the situation *in utero* is quite different. The normal conductive route to the inner ear becomes irrelevant in a fluid environment, and it is likely that little of the sound that reaches the fetus is transmitted through the external and middle ear. (How much sound reaches the fetus is a separate issue reviewed in a subsequent section.) If sound reaches the inner ear, it is most probably conducted through the skull, that is, by bone conduction. The response of the cochlea is the same whether a sound reaches it by conduction through the middle

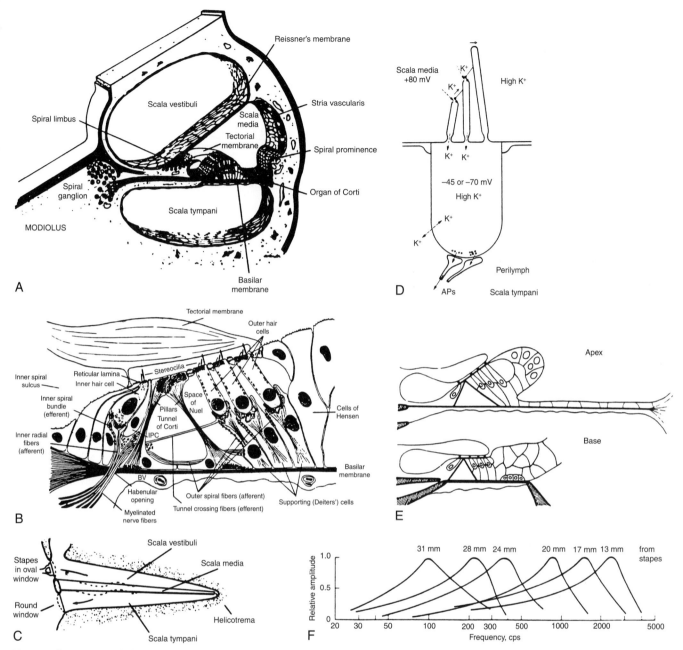

Figure 176–3. Series of drawings illustrating the process by which sound energy is transduced into a neural response by the inner ear. **A**, Cross-section of the cochlear duct. **B**, Schematic cross-section through the organ of Corti. The hair cells are the auditory receptors. **C**, Longitudinal cross-section through the cochlear duct, here represented as if uncoiled. Sound coming through the external and middle ear causes movement of the stapes in the oval window, which results in a traveling wave along the cochlear partition. **D**, Movement of the basilar membrane causes a shearing action across the hair cell stereocilia, opening ion channels in the stereocilia tips, depolarizing the hair cell, and leading to a response in the auditory nerve fiber. **E**, Schematic cross-sections through the organ of Corti near the apex and the base of the cochlea. The basilar membrane is wider and floppier near the apex and narrower and stiffer near the base. **F**, The amplitude of basilar mebrane displacement as a function of frequency at various locations along the basilar membrane, specified in distance from the stapes (cochlear base). The structural differences along the length of the basilar membrane have the results that higher frequencies produce maximum displacements near the base of the cochlea, whereas lower frequencies cause maximum displacements near the apex of the cochlea. Thus, the position of maximum activity along the length of the cochlea provides information about a sound's frequency. (From Pickles, JO. An Introduction to the Physiology of Hearing. 1988: Academic Press: New York. pp. 28, 29, 30, 39, 60.)

ear or through the skull. However, the way the skull shapes the amplitude spectrum of sound reaching the inner ear will be different from the way the external and middle ears do. When sounds are transmitted to the adult inner ear by bone conduc-

tion, using a vibrator placed on the mastoid, much greater sound energy is required to elicit a response. The difference is on the order of 40 dB at 1000 Hz. Furthermore, the response of the skull has a high-frequency emphasis. Compared with air conduction, high frequencies are transmitted relatively more efficiently than low frequencies. For example, for adults, the detection threshold at 1000 Hz is about 15 dB lower than that at 250 Hz for air-conducted tones, but about 22 dB lower for bone-conducted tones. Of course, the fetal skull is not as well ossified as the adult skull, and *in utero* sound is transmitted to the skull from the fluid surrounding the fetus, not from a mechanical vibrator. Thus, although it is clear that the route of sound transmission to the fetal inner ear will have substantial effects on what the fetus hears, the nature of these effects is not entirely predictable from the data on hearing by bone conduction in adults. One clear implication of the differences between air-conducted and bone-conducted sounds is that infants who are born prematurely are exposed to a qualitatively different set of sounds than they would have been *in utero*.

The acoustic consequences of the structural characteristics of the immature conductive apparatus are predictable. The resonance characteristics of a small ear canal and pinna will mean that, for sounds of equal amplitude approaching the listener, high frequencies will reach the middle ear at relatively higher amplitudes than low frequencies. If the ear canal is not fully open, of course, significantly less sound energy will reach the middle ear. Immaturity of the tympanic membrane and ossicles may decrease the efficiency of the middle ear in transmitting sound to the inner ear, and the response of the middle ear may be biased toward lower frequencies. Studies of the acoustic response of the conductive apparatus in nonhuman species confirm these predictions.[19-21]

The acoustics of the external and middle ear have not been described in premature human infants. There are data for 1-month post-term infants. The external ear data are in the form of sound field–to–ear canal transfer functions, which show the level of sound in the ear canal as a function of frequency, when the level of sound in the surrounding field is equal at all frequencies. In adults, this function shows a broad peak of about 10 dB between about 2000 and 5000 Hz as a result of the resonance of the ear canal and pinna (Fig. 176–4A). The peak resonance frequency of the adult external ear is typically given as 2700 Hz. Keefe and his colleagues[18] characterized the acoustic response of the infant external ear. The youngest infants included were 1 month old. The average resonance frequency in this age group was 4000 to 5000 Hz (see Fig. 176–4B), consistent with physical measurements of ear canal length. Thus, relative to adults, the level of sound reaching the neonatal middle ear at frequencies in the 1000- to 3000-Hz range will be lower. Keefe and colleagues also found that the sound field–to–ear canal transfer function is not mature by 24 months' postnatal age, but the age at which the transfer function becomes adultlike is not known.

Keefe and his colleagues[22,23] also published the only comprehensive studies of the acoustic properties of the infant middle ear. Acoustic impedance has three components: resistance, which results from loss of kinetic energy to thermal energy (friction); mass reactance, which results from inertia and is determined by the mass of the medium; and compliant reactance, which results from elasticity and is determined by the stiffness of the medium. In the human middle ear, compliant reactance is the dominant factor. The impedance is said to be compliance dominated, and the sign of the total reactance is negative. Impedance is often discussed in terms of its inverse, that is, in terms of the energy flow rather than the opposition to energy flow. Admittance is inversely related to impedance, conductance is inversely related to reactance, and susceptance is inversely related to resistance.

Keefe and colleagues[22,23] estimated the acoustic conductance, or flow of acoustic energy, by looking into the middle ear in the ear canals of newborns and of 1- to 24-month-old infants. The results for newborns, 1-month-old infants, and adults are shown in Figure 176-5.

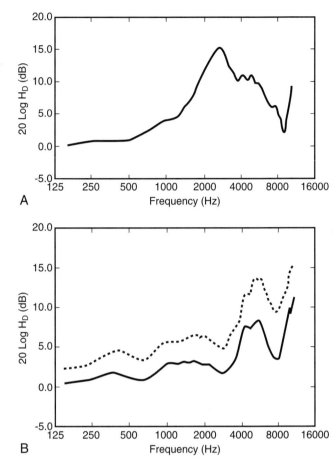

Figure 176–4. Diffuse field transfer functions measured (**A**) in a KEMAR human adult manikin (**B**) for the average 1-month-old infant. The *solid line* is the average; the *dashed line* is the average plus 1 SD. H_D = diffuse field transfer function magnitude. (From Keefe, D, et al: J Acoust Soc Am, 1994. *95*: p. 355.)

The conductance of the infants' middle ear is smaller than that of adults for frequencies higher than 500 Hz, and the greatest difference is at the higher frequencies. For frequencies higher than 1000 Hz, there appears to be some improvement in conductance in the first postnatal month, but at around 4000 Hz, infants would be expected to lose 10 to 15 dB relative to adults. The combined effects of external and middle ear immaturity could lead to a relative loss of 15 to 20 dB in the higher frequencies. At frequencies lower than 500 Hz, both neonates and 1-month-old infants actually appear to generate higher levels of sound in the middle ear than adults. In fact, conductance appears to decline between birth and 1 month and again between 1 month and adulthood in the low frequencies. This result is consistent with the presence of a low-frequency resonance in the neonatal ear canal, perhaps resulting from the greater compliance of the ear canal walls. This could further explain why tympanometry may not be a useful diagnostic tool in young infants.[24]

It is not often appreciated that growth of the pinna, ear canal, and head also has important implications for sound localization. The primary cues to the location of a sound source in the horizontal plane are differences in the phase and intensity of the sound arriving at the two ears.[25] Small heads produce smaller interaural differences. Clifton and associates[26] measured head diameter longitudinally in a group of infants from birth to 22 weeks of age. From these measurements, they estimated that the largest interaural time difference that an infant's head could

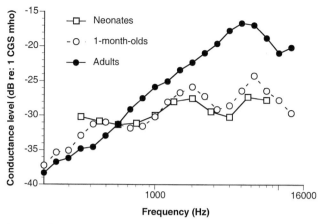

Figure 176–5. Ear canal conductance level, indicating energy flow into the middle ear, as a function of frequency for adults, neonates, and 1-month-old infants. CGS = centimeter-gram-second. (From Keefe, D, et al: J Acoust Soc Am, 1993. *94*: p. 2617; and Keefe, D, et al: Ear Hear, 2000. *21*: p. 443.)

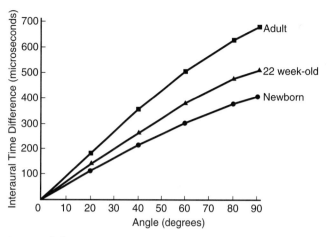

Figure 176–6. Interaural time differences produced by sounds as a function of their position in azimuth, for adults, 22-week-old infants, and newborns. (From Clifton, R.K, et al: Dev Psychol, 1988. *24*: pp. 477–483.)

produce increased from 420 μs at birth to 520 μs at 22 weeks of age. The average adult head, conversely, could produce an interaural time difference on the order of 700 μs. Thus, for any sound source location, the infant must work with a smaller cue (Fig. 176-6). Similar effects would be expected for interaural intensity differences. Interaural differences would also vary with sound frequency differently when the head is small. Interaural phase differences would be useful to fairly high frequencies, but interaural intensity differences in the mid-frequency range would be relatively poor.[27] Finally, the sound field–to–ear canal transfer function changes with the position of the sound source relative to the ear. These spectral cues are used to localize sounds in elevation and to distinguish sound source locations behind the head from those in front of the head. One would expect that smaller pinnas and ear canals would produce poor spectral cues for the localization of sound sources in the mid-frequency range. However, the relative contributions of conductive, cochlear, and neural maturation to the development of sound localization remain to be established.

Cochlea

The earliest structures that can be identified as external, middle, and inner ear arise in close temporal proximity. The otic placode, a thickening of the surface ectoderm at the level of the caudal hindbrain, can be seen early in the fourth week of gestation. The placode invaginates, closes off, and detaches from the epidermal surface to form the otocyst, or otic vesicle, a few days later. Shortly thereafter, the precursors of the spiral ganglion migrate out of the otocyst and come to lie ventromedial to the developing inner ear. As the precursors of the specialized support cells and hair cells are born, the otic cyst elongates, and the older cells are "pushed" toward the distal end of the presumptive cochlea.[28] These undifferentiated cells form a mass along the dorsal wall of the tube. The otocyst coils as it elongates, eventually forming 2.5 turns by the 25th week of gestation. These events are illustrated schematically in Figure 176-7.

The bony labyrinth that contains the cochlea begins to ossify around 16 weeks of gestation. This process must be closely coordinated with cochlear growth and innervation. In fact, Van De Water and his colleagues[29-32] demonstrated that a complex series of interactions between epithelial and mesenchymal tissues regulates the growth, ossification, and differentiation of the inner ear structures. The otic capsule appears to be largely ossified by about 20 weeks' gestational age.[33]

In a series of articles, Lavigne-Rebillard and colleagues[34-42] described, using electron microscopy, the early development of the human cochlea. Their results are quite similar to those reported for nonhuman mammals.[42] As described in other vertebrates, the afferent processes of the spiral ganglion grow into the presumptive cochlea and make contact with undifferentiated cells by 9 weeks of gestation. These cells then separate from their basement membrane and migrate toward the luminal surface of the epithelium. Once the cells have reached the luminal surface, stereocilia form, and other features of hair cells become evident. Efferent processes are not identified in the cochlea until some time later, at about 12 weeks of gestation in humans.[37,43-45] The stria vascularis, which is responsible for maintaining the high resting potential of the cochlea, appears at 9 weeks of gestation, matures slowly between 14 and 20 weeks, and by 34 weeks appears adultlike.[36] The tectorial membrane also appears at about 9 weeks of gestation. Inner hair cells tend to differentiate and mature ahead of outer hair cells. Innervation and differentiation of support cells and hair cells tend to occur earlier at or near the base of the developing cochlea (the base of the cochlea is the end closest to the middle ear; the apex is the end at the top of the cochlear coil).[37,46] These developmental gradients have later functional implications, because inner and outer hair cells play quite different roles in the transduction process and because the frequency eliciting the greatest response decreases progressively along the length of the cochlea from base to apex.

When responses to sound can first be observed, the inner ear is immature in several respects. The fluid spaces within the cochlea are not well developed, the basilar membrane is thick, and the physical arrangement of the support cells and hair cells is immature (Fig. 176-8). Such factors are likely to limit the mechanical response of the cochlea. In addition, the innervation of the hair cells is immature.[35,37,41,47] In mature mammals, afferent endings predominate on inner hair cells, and efferent fibers synapse on afferent fibers, not on the inner hair cell membrane. Around the time that cochlear responses can first be recorded, both afferent and efferent synapses can be found on the inner hair cell membrane. Mature outer hair cells feature massive efferent endings encapsulating their basal membrane and a few small afferent endings. At the onset of hearing, the number of afferent endings contacting outer hair cells is more equal, and both types of endings are rather small and bouton-shaped (Fig. 176-9). The stria vascularis still differs from the adult in several respects, a finding suggesting that the endocochlear potential, the "battery" that

CROSS SECTIONS THROUGH COCHLEAR DUCT

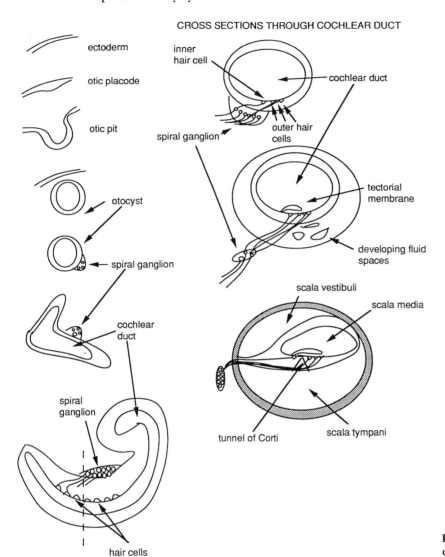

Figure 176–7. Illustration showing major events in the development of the inner ear.

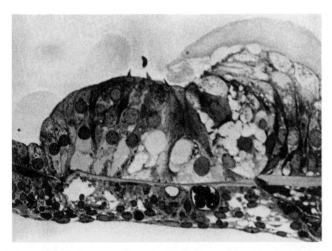

Figure 176–8. Cross-sections through the cochlea of a 20-week-old human fetus, near the upper basal coil. The fluid spaces and mechanical arrangement of cells are underdeveloped. (From Igarashi, Y, Ishii, T: Int J Pediatr Otorhinolaryngol, 1980. *2*: p. 51.)

drives the transduction process, is immature. In electron microscopic studies, Lavigne-Rebillard and her colleagues[34-36] showed that these features are characteristic of the human cochlea approaching 20 to 22 weeks' gestational age.

An obvious implication of the structural immaturity of the cochlea at this stage of development is that sensitivity to sound will be quite poor. More acoustic energy is required to set the basilar membrane in motion, and energy is transferred to the stereocilia less efficiently. Inner hair cells undoubtedly transmit their messages to the central nervous system. The outer hair cells, however, are known to act as effectors, mechanically amplifying the basilar membrane response and increasing the frequency specificity of the response. To the extent that the outer hair cells are immature, sensitivity may be poorer by 30 to 40 dB.

It is well documented in nonhumans that the combination of conductive and cochlear immaturity is reflected in cochlear responses,[48] in single-unit responses in the auditory nerve, brain stem, and cortex,[49-52] and in gross evoked potentials.[3,6,53] When responses to sound are first observed, thresholds are quite high, on the order of 100 dB sound pressure level (SPL). Although the precise time course varies across species, sensitivity improves quite dramatically in the subsequent days or weeks. In humans, this rapid maturation of auditory sensitivity probably occurs

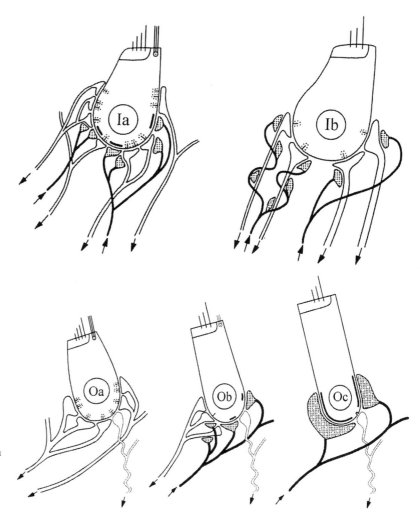

Figure 176–9. Changes in the innervation patterns of inner and outer hair cells around the time that the cochlea begins to function. Efferents are filled fibers with vesiculated profiles and *inward arrows*. Afferents are open fibers with *outward arrows*. (From Pujol, R, et al: *In* Development of the Auditory System, EW Rubel, et al, eds. 1998, Springer-Verlag: New York. pp. 146–192.)

between 24 and 35 weeks' gestational age. Unfortunately, there are no data to document the course of auditory physiologic development before about 28 weeks' gestational age.

Otoacoustic emissions (OAEs) are sounds generated by the action of the outer hair cells that can be recorded in the ear canal to provide a direct measure of cochlear function.[54] OAEs can generally be recorded in normally functioning cochleas, as long as their transmission through the middle ear is not blocked. OAEs have been recorded in infants as young as 30 weeks' conceptional age. Click-evoked OAEs have been recorded in nearly all infants by 33 weeks' conceptional age, at a threshold 10 to 15 dB higher that that of adults.[55] The amplitude of OAE to a fixed-level click also increases between 30 and 40 weeks' conceptional age.[56-58] A frequency-specific OAE can also be recorded when two tones close in frequency, f_1 and f_2, are presented to the ear. In this case, the emission is a pure tone with a frequency equal to $2 f_1-f_2$ and is known as a distortion product OAE (DPOAE). Lasky[59, 60] recorded DPOAE in preterm infants, term infants, and adults. The minimum stimulus level required to elicit a DPOAE was similar across age groups, at least for stimulating tones around 4000 Hz. Lasky concluded that nearly all the observed age-related differences in DPOAE could be accounted for by conductive factors.

The *auditory brain stem response* (ABR) is a scalp-recorded potential reflecting the aggregate response of neurons in the auditory nerve and brain stem. Wave I of the ABR is known to arise from the auditory nerve; the inferior colliculus makes a major contribution to wave V, although it is not clear that it is the sole generator.[61] Adult ABR thresholds for a click are typically about 10 dB normalized hearing level (nHL).[61] The ABR can first be reliably elicited from preterm infants at around 28 weeks' postconceptional age, although there are a few reports of responses at 26 or 27 weeks.[62, 63] Lary and co-workers[63] reported that the average click intensity required to elicit an ABR decreased from about 55 dB nHL at 27 weeks' conceptional age to 21 dB nHL at 38 weeks' conceptional age. Subsequent studies confirmed this result.[64, 65] This pattern is consistent with an improvement in auditory sensitivity on the order of 25 to 30 dB between the onset of the response and term birth, but the relative contributions of conductive, cochlear, and neural sensitivity to the ABR threshold are not known. The latency of wave I decreases between 33 and 44 weeks' conceptional age,[62] but latencies may be prolonged without concomitant sensitivity loss.[66]

One result that seems to be consistent across studies is that, by the time of term birth, thresholds for cochlear responses elicited by broadband sounds are within 10 or 15 dB of adult values. This is the case for wave I of the ABR,[61] OAEs,[55] and electrocochleograms (scalp-recorded cochlear potentials).[67] Because a threshold shift of that magnitude can easily be accounted for by conductive factors,[22] these reports suggest that the cochlea is probably mature by 40 weeks' postconceptional age.

Coincident with the improvement in sensitivity, a dramatic improvement in the frequency selectivity of the cochlear response occurs in nonhumans just after hearing begins. In the mature mammal, each inner hair cell and the afferent fibers connected to it respond over a range of about one-third of an octave (defined as a doubling of frequency). When the cochlea begins to respond to sound, many auditory nerve fibers are essentially "untuned," and the best fibers respond over a range as broad as three octaves (Fig. 176–10).[68] Frequency specificity is closely correlated with sensitivity during development, and its maturation is likely the result of both mechanical maturation of the basilar membrane and the outer hair cells. Many functional consequences of reduced frequency selectivity would be expected, although few of these expectations have been put to the test. Sensitivity to noise is known to be especially poor.[69] The internal representation of the amplitude spectrum of a complex sound is also "fuzzy" to the novice listener, and similar frequencies would be difficult to distinguish.

Frequency selectivity at the cochlear level has been studied with DPOAE. The amplitude of DPOAE can be reduced by presenting external sounds that are close to the emission in frequency; the emission is said to be suppressed. In fact, the better the cochlear frequency selectivity, the narrower the range of frequencies that will suppress the emission. The curve that shows the level of an external tone required to reduce the emission by a criterion amount, as a function of the frequency of the tone, is termed a *suppression tuning curve*. Abdala[70-72] found that preterm and term infants demonstrate sharper suppression tuning curves or better frequency selectivity than adults (Fig. 176–11). Abdala argued that, early in development, the human cochlea "overshoots" the amplification required, as observed in young gerbils by Mills and associates.[73] However, it is also true that suppression tuning curves measured at lower intensity are generally sharper than those measured at higher intensity. Thus, attenuation of the sound reaching the infant cochlea by an immature middle ear could be responsible for the age difference in tuning. The issue remains to be resolved. Of course, neural limitations may effectively limit the frequency selectivity of the system, as discussed later.

As noted earlier, many events in cochlear development tend to occur in structures located at or near the base of the cochlea before they occur in structures located at the apex. Because the mass and stiffness of the basilar membrane vary along its length, in mature vertebrates high-frequency sounds produce greater responses than low-frequency sounds at the base of the cochlea, whereas low-frequency sounds produce greater responses at the apex. Thus, one could predict that responses to high-frequency sounds would appear and mature earlier than those to low-frequency sounds. In fact, just the opposite is typically observed: The initial responses to sound are limited to the low or low-to-middle part of the mature animal's range of hearing. The range of frequencies that elicit responses gradually increases as sensitivity improves during development. The most likely explanation for this apparent paradox is that the basal cochlea is most responsive to relatively low frequencies at the time that it begins to respond.[74-77] Studies suggest that the immature frequency response of the basal cochlea is the result of mechanical properties of the basilar membrane.[73] Although such effects have yet to be demonstrated in humans, they would be predicted to occur between 24 and 37 weeks of gestation.

Central Auditory Nervous System

The limited data concerning the development of the human auditory nervous system are often found in articles dealing with the development of the whole brain.[78] Although this situation has begun to be remedied,[79-86] the available information with respect to human auditory neural development remains sparse. What data are available suggest, however, that there are no substantial differences between humans and nonhumans in the development of the primary auditory pathways. In all vertebrates, the neurons of the auditory pathways undergo final mitosis, migrate to their mature locations, and form appropriate connections in parallel with developmental events at the periphery; by the time the cochlea begins to respond to sound, gross evoked responses can be recorded in the primary auditory cortex.[87,88]

Early sensitivity to sound, however, may be limited by brain stem immaturity. Sininger and Abdala[89] stimulated newborns' frequency-specific ABR thresholds and calibrated their stimuli in the ear canal to control for age differences in ear canal sizes. Their data show that newborns are close to adultlike in sensitivity at 500 Hz, but they are 20 to 25 dB less sensitive than adults at frequencies higher than 4000 Hz. The high-frequency age difference is greater than can be accounted for by middle ear immaturity alone.

Neural immaturities appear to limit the frequency selectivity of the auditory system early in human development. Two studies showed that the ABR to a high-frequency sound is affected by a broader range of interfering frequencies, or "maskers," in 3-month-old infants than in adults.[90,91] This finding suggests that the frequency selectivity of the infant brain stem response is poorer at high frequencies. Because the cochlear response appears to be mature by this age,[92] the source of the immaturity in frequency selectivity is likely to be neural. Presumably, these immaturities will be more pronounced for still younger infants, and the immaturities may extend to lower frequencies as well. Of course, at younger ages, cochlear immaturities may also be present, and it is not known how cochlear and neural immaturities may interact.

The work of Sanes and his colleagues[93-96] has been important to understanding how neural maturation and experience with sound contribute to the development of frequency resolution.

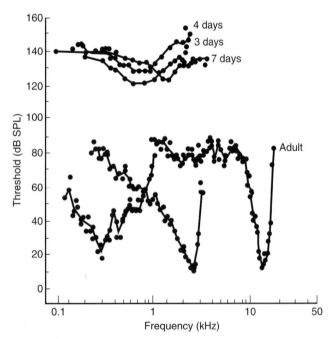

Figure 176–10. Level required to produce a threshold response in fibers of the cat auditory nerve as a function of frequency. Each curve represents the response of a single nerve fiber. Adult responses tend to be "tuned". The fiber tends to respond to very low sound levels within a restricted frequency range. Responses of 3- to 7-day-old kittens require very high sound levels and are not well tuned. SPL = sound pressure level. (From Walsh, EJ and McGee J: Hear Res, 1987. *28*: pp. 97–16.)

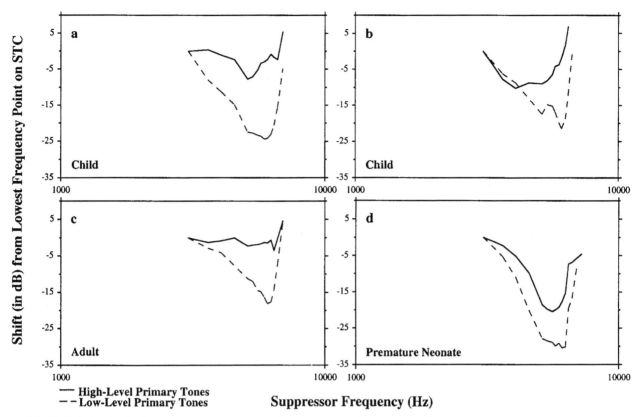

Figure 176–11. Relative level of a suppressor tone required to suppress a distortion product otoacoustic emission, as a function of the frequency of the tone, so-called suppression tuning curves (STC), for high- and low-level stimulating ("primary") tones. Each emission tends to be suppressed with low level tones close to its own frequency. Responses from children 8 to 12 years of age (*a* and *b*). Response from an adult (*c*). Response from a premature infant (*d*). The premature infants' response is sharper than those of other subjects, and the sharpness is maintained at high levels of stimulation. (From Abdala, C: J Acoust Soc Am, 2001. *110*(6): pp. 3155–3162.)

Sanes and Constantine-Paton[93] reported that exposing young mice to repetitive clicks resulted in a reduction in neural frequency selectivity that could not be explained by peripheral effects. The selectivity of neural connections, then, can affect frequency selectivity, and normal experience with sound appears to be necessary to induce or maintain the nervous system's ability to accurately transmit the selective response established at the cochlear level. Sanes and Rubel,[94] moreover, noted that fine frequency selectivity was not characteristic of all neurons in the auditory brain stem. Within a single frequency region, neurons with mature selectivity and neurons with very immature selectivity could be found. Because all these neurons receive their afferent input from the same cochlear location, it is difficult to see how cochlear factors could produce such variability in response. In other studies, Sanes and associates[95] directly measured the increased specificity of neural connections in one auditory brain stem nucleus, and Sanes[96] showed that maturation of structural specificity was reflected in maturation of neural response specificity. Finally, although some neural response patterns appear mature when described on a relative scale, they appear quite immature on an absolute scale. Thus, it is becoming increasingly evident that neural immaturities impose a fundamental limitation on early auditory function, although a detailed description of these immaturities is not yet possible. Certainly in humans, structural maturation of the auditory cortex continues until 11 or 12 years of age.[84, 85]

A commonly reported characteristic of immature auditory neurons is that they cannot sustain a continuous response.[97] In addition, their maximum response rate is quite low.[98] Such response characteristics would have profound influences on all

aspects of acoustic coding. A reduction in the range of intensities that could be processed would be expected, the ability to distinguish a change in intensity would differ, and, of course, sensitivity would be reduced as well. The "fatigability" of young neurons is almost certainly not a result of cochlear limitations, although the reduction in dynamic range may well reflect similar limitations in the cochlear response. Although no data are available in this regard for preterm infants, Durieux-Smith and colleagues[99] reported a similar limitation in the neonatal ABR: Increasing the intensity of a click results in a smaller increase in response amplitude for term neonates than it does for adults (Fig. 176–12). Cornacchia and associates[100] reported that this characteristic of the ABR is adultlike by 6 months after term.

Neural maturation is also clearly reflected in the development of temporal aspects of the neural response. Progressive myelination of neural pathways is noted during development in all vertebrates. It is often stated that myelination of the brain in general, and of the auditory pathway in particular, proceeds in a peripheral-to-central gradient.[78] More recent studies suggested that this gradient holds only on a coarse scale. Moore and colleagues[101, 102] found that, in the human auditory system, the brain stem pathway is myelinated at about the same time along its length, but the brain stem pathway is well myelinated before myelin is observed in the brain stem–to-midbrain pathway. Increased myelination would certainly increase the speed with which information is transmitted through the auditory system. In fact, the latency of both single-unit responses and of gross evoked potentials progressively decreases during development, and the age-related change in response latency is greater in more central nuclei.[5, 52] Increased myelination may also be expected to

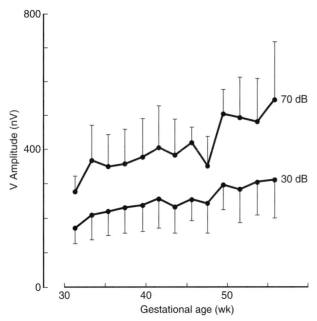

Figure 176–12. Amplitude of wave V of the auditory brain stem response as a function of gestational age for two sound intensities. The effects of increasing intensity are greater at later gestational ages. (From Durieux-Smith, A, et al: J Otolaryngol, 1985. *14*: pp. 12–18.)

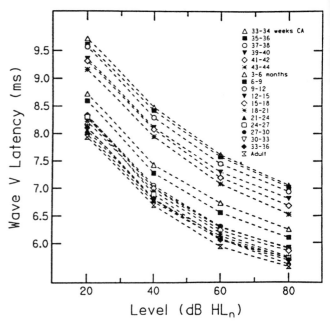

Figure 176–13. Latency of wave V of the auditory brain stem response as a function of sound intensities at various ages. The curves are more or less parallel. HL_n = normalized hearing level. (From Gorga, MP, et al: *J Speech Hear Res*, 1989. *32*: pp. 281–288.)

produce improvements in auditory functions that depend on a precise temporal representation of the stimulus, such as sound localization. Variability in the latencies of action potentials, both within and between neurons, would be reduced in well-myelinated nerve fibers.

Response latency is the most frequently studied characteristic of evoked potentials in humans, and it is one of the few measures that has been made extensively for both preterm and term neonates. Gorga and associates,[62] for example, reported that between 33 and 44 weeks' conceptional age, wave I latency in response to 80-dB nHL clicks decreased from about 1.8 to about 1.6 ms. Wave V latency decreased from 7.0 to 6.5 ms over the same period. The implication of the finding that wave V latency decreases more than wave I latency is that most of the decrease in wave V latency stems from neural maturation. One interesting aspect of these results is that the effects of increasing intensities were no different for the youngest (33 to 34 weeks' conceptional age) and oldest (43 to 44 weeks' conceptional age) infants.[103] In fact, the effects of level on wave V latency were adultlike in the youngest preterms examined (Fig. 176–13). By 40 weeks' conceptional age, wave I latency is close to adult values, but wave V latency continues to decrease into the second postnatal year.[61,104]

Two issues concerning the infant ABR have both developmental and clinical implications. First, there are some reports of rapid improvements in ABR detectability, amplitude, and latency in the first 48 hours after birth.[105-108] Explanations for these rapid postnatal changes vary. The typical explanation is that early postnatal changes result from clearing of fluid or other materials from the middle ear,[108-110] although some argue that cochlear adaptation to extrauterine life is responsible.[110-114] Yamasaki and colleagues[105] found that the wave I-wave V interwave interval, the so-called *central conduction time*, also decreased in the immediate postnatal period. How differences in central conduction time could result from either conductive or cochlear factors is not clear. Thus, although the reason for rapid changes in the ABR after birth are not settled, there seems to be a consensus that stable ABRs are most readily obtained after 48 postnatal hours.

The second issue concerns the use of the ABR in the preterm population. Essentially, the question is whether extrauterine experience affects ABR parameters independently of conceptional age. In other words, is the ABR of a 40-week conceptional age infant whose gestational age is 32 weeks different from the ABR of a 40-week conceptional age infant who was born yesterday? Some studies report no differences between preterm and term infants of equal conceptional age.[115, 116] Eggermont and Salamy[104] found that preterm infants tended to have longer wave latencies, but equivalent interwave latencies. Eggermont and Salamy proposed that this difference arises from the higher incidence of otitis media in the preterm population. Collet and associates,[117] in contrast, reported shorter interwave intervals among preterm infants and concluded that the smaller head size of preterm infants is responsible. In any case, the differences between term and preterm infants of the same conceptional age are small, and there is little evidence of a direct effect of extrauterine experience on the development of the ABR.

At least three factors influence the latency of evoked potentials and are thus potential explanations for developmental changes. First, sensitivity at sites peripheral to the generator of a given wave contributes to its latency. For example, latencies of all ABR waves are longer for lower intensities of sound and in cases of conductive or sensorineural hearing loss.[61] The changes in wave I latency with conceptional age are consistent with about a 20-dB conductive immaturity at 33 to 34 weeks' conceptional age and a 10- to 15-dB conductive immaturity at term birth, as suggested by the middle ear data.[22] To achieve a wave V latency of 7.5 ms, however, the data of Gorga and colleagues[118] indicate that a term infant requires a level about 25 dB higher than an adult (Fig. 176–14). It is clear that neither conductive nor cochlear factors can account for such a large difference. Second, myelinization of the auditory pathway would increase conduction velocity; it is well established that myelinization of the auditory pathways progresses through the postnatal period and into childhood.[78, 102] This is the most clearly established contribution to ABR latency development; by some accounts, conduction time

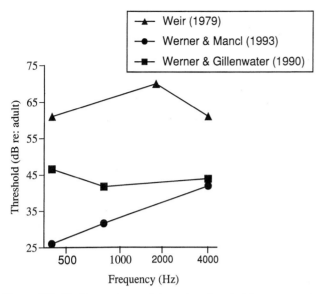

Figure 176–14. Comparison of detection thresholds, expressed relative to adult threshold, at three frequencies from 0- to 1-month-old infants in three studies. (From Werner, LA, and GC Marian: Human Auditory Development. 1995, Westview Press: Boulder, CO.)

improvements can completely account for changes in the latency of the ABR during development.[119] Third, synaptic efficiency may play a role. The number of synapses in the auditory brain stem continues to increase throughout childhood and into adulthood,[120] although the efficiency with which each synapse operates, an unknown quantity, may be more relevant. One finding that suggests that synaptic efficiency may be important is that the wave I–wave V interwave interval is positively correlated with behavioral thresholds in early infancy.[121] There is no evidence that neural latency directly affects sensitivity; in fact, latencies can be very abnormal while sensitivity remains normal.[66] A loss of information resulting from inefficient synaptic transmission could well affect both sensitivity and evoked response latency. Rotteveel and associates[64] also noted an association between ABR threshold and interwave intervals among preterm infants.

Other evoked responses, such as the middle and long latency responses that originate from the midbrain and cortex, have not been studied extensively in neonates.[61] It appears that the difference between infants and adults in threshold for the middle latency response, for example, is greater than the difference in ABR threshold,[122] and middle latency response latencies take longer to reach adult values.[123-126] Cortical responses have been recorded, even in preterm infants,[88] but again, the developmental course of such responses is prolonged. Although the factors that contribute to the delayed maturation of middle latency and late responses have not been delineated, their later development is consistent with the later myelinization of the midbrain and cortical pathway. Other factors may also be involved.

Of course, latency is not the only temporal characteristic of neural responses. Because of the characteristics of the transduction process, auditory neurons tend to fire at the same phase of the stimulus on each cycle of a periodic sound; the neural response is said to be *phase locked*. Phase locking is strong enough and the neural transfer of the phase-locked response is precise enough, that the period, and thus the frequency, of a sound could be estimated on the basis of the interval between action potentials. The precision of neural phase locking is likely to depend on both the efficiency of synaptic transmission and the extent of myelination of nerve fibers. Phase locking is believed to contribute to pitch perception, among other things, and it is the basis of interaural

phase difference processing in sound localization. Of the basic auditory neural response properties, phase locking is the one that takes longest to develop. Brugge and colleagues[50] reported that phase locking in the cat's auditory nerve matured over a 2-week period, with fibers responding to low frequencies achieving mature phase locking earlier. The development of phase locking at the level of the cochlear nucleus followed the same frequency gradient, but it took as long as 2 months to complete.[127] The course of its development in nuclei central to the cochlear nucleus has not been described. The relative contributions of synaptic maturation and increased myelination (see later) to the development of phase locking have not been assessed. The *frequency-following response* is a scalp-recorded response that has the same frequency as the tone used to elicit it. The frequency-following response is believed to reflect the aggregate phase-locked responses in the auditory nerve and brain stem.[61, 128] Two studies examined the frequency-following response in term neonates;[129, 130] in general, the response appeared to be adultlike. Similar measures of phase-locking at more central locations in the nervous system have not been developed. Again, no data on the development of temporal processing are available for preterm infants.

Another property of neurons that has implications for temporal coding is adaptation. Auditory nerve fibers show a characteristic high response rate at stimulus onset, followed by a rapid decrease in response rate to a lower, steady rate. This decrease in response over time is known as *adaptation*. After the offset of the stimulus, there is a recovery period during which it is difficult to elicit responses from the neuron; even spontaneous activity is absent during recovery. There is evidence that the immature auditory system is more susceptible to adaptation than the mature system, and it takes longer to recover from the effects of adaptation. In human infants, increasing the rate of presentation of clicks used to elicit the response has a greater effect on response latency for newborns.[109, 131-133] The size of the latency shift with increasing stimulus rate decreases progressively between 28 and 50 weeks' conceptional age,[134] and the effect is more pronounced for wave V than it is for wave I, a finding suggesting a neural contribution to the effect on wave V. By 3 months of age, the ABR shows rate effects similar to those seen for adults. Responses originating at more central locations, such as the middle latency response, continue to be more susceptible to increased click rate well into childhood.[124]

In a series of studies summarized by Altman and Bayer,[135] the first neurons to undergo their final mitosis, in nearly all auditory nuclei, were the neurons that in adulthood would respond to high-frequency sounds. The same gradient has been reported for at least some aspects of neural differentiation.[136] Although the first cochlear hair cells to undergo final mitosis are apparently the ones that respond to low-frequency sounds,[28] the gradient in neural development mirrors the near-basal to apical gradient of cochlear differentiation and innervation. Thus, the most mature cochlear hair cells would appear to be connected to the most mature neurons in each auditory nucleus. Two studies of the frequency-specific ABR of human infants revealed a similar frequency gradient. The ABR wave I–wave V interwave interval appears to mature first at frequencies of 2 to 4 kHz, and later at both lower and higher frequencies.[137,138] In other words, maturation begins in the middle- to high-frequency range and proceeds to the highest and lowest frequencies simultaneously with development. The first response to mature does so between 1 and 2 years of age, whereas the last is not mature at 2 years.

BEHAVIORAL DEVELOPMENT

An obvious and important question is how the morphologic and physiologic properties of the fetal and neonatal auditory systems are reflected in auditory behavior. It is also one of the more difficult questions to answer.

Sensitivity

Since the 1960s, many studies of fetal motor or cardiac responses to external "sounds" have been published.[139-154] There are numerous methodologic difficulties with these studies. Not the least of these is that a frequently used stimulator is an artificial larynx applied to the maternal abdomen. Much of the energy delivered by such a device is in the frequency range to which tactile receptors are sensitive.[155] Frequently the mother is aware of when stimulus presentations are occurring, so fetal responses to sound may actually represent a response to maternal physiologic state. In any case, the actual sound intensity delivered to the fetus can only be estimated in a very broad fashion, and it is also difficult to estimate the intrauterine level of noise.[149]

Nonetheless, there is a general consensus that the first fetal motor responses to sound occur at about 26 weeks of gestation. This is the case even in studies that used tighter controls on the stimulus and stimulus delivery system.[144] The proportion of fetuses demonstrating responses increases progressively with gestational age,[139, 144] and there is some indication that older fetuses (34 to 39 weeks of gestation) respond to lower sound intensities than do younger fetuses (26 to 28 weeks of gestation).[139, 143] In general, the external SPL required to elicit a fetal response is on the order of 90 to 110 dB. Lecanuet and colleagues,[147] however, reported late-gestation heart rate responses to a syllable played at an external level of only 80 to 90 dB SPL to late-gestation fetuses. Lecanuet and associates[146] showed that late-gestation fetuses responded most often to high-intensity, high-frequency (5000-Hz) sounds. Although responses were recorded to 500- and 2000-Hz stimuli, these were less frequent and tended to occur only at the highest intensities presented. This finding is puzzling in that mammals who begin to hear postnatally respond first to low- to middle-frequency sounds.[156] Differences in the transfer of sound through the maternal abdomen cannot account for the difference: The maternal abdomen appears to attenuate frequencies higher than 1000 Hz rather dramatically.[149] The spectrum of intrauterine noise, however, is weighted toward low frequencies,[149] and so it may mask other low-frequency sounds. Probably the most important factor is that the spectrum of sound delivered to the fetal inner ear is shaped by the skull, rather than by the external and middle ears (see earlier discussion), so the effective level of the high-frequency sound entering the system is higher than that of low frequencies. The apparent sensitivity differences across frequency could be easily accounted for by the acoustic properties of the skull.[157]

If the frequency dependence of the fetal response to sound is determined by how sound is transmitted to the inner ear, then one could predict that preterm infants' responses would be different. However, Gerber and his colleagues[158, 159] reported that both term and 29- to 37-week conceptional age neonates respond motorically to about only 25% of the presentations of a wide-band noise of 90 dB SPL centered at about 3000 Hz. Although Schulman[160] showed that preterm infants' heart rates changed in response to a door bell with a level estimated at about 80 dB SPL, no information about the frequency dependence of the response is available.

Our knowledge of the fetal behavioral response to sound, then, is easily summarized. Fetuses begin to respond to intense external sounds at around 26 weeks of gestation. Late-gestation fetuses appear to respond to somewhat lower intensities, particularly for an appropriate stimulus, and to be more sensitive to high-frequency external sounds. High sound intensities are also required to elicit a motor response from preterm infants at the same conceptional age, but the frequency dependence of the preterm response is unknown .

A few studies estimated thresholds for frequency-specific sounds among term neonates. These data are summarized in Figure 176-14. Weir[161] used a combination of respiratory and motor responses to judge 1- to 8-day postterm infants' sensitivity to pure tones. She found that few infants responded consistently to the stimuli, but those who did respond consistently had thresholds on the order of 30 to 70 dB higher than those of adults. Thresholds were more adultlike at lower frequencies. Subsequent studies using more sensitive measures of behavior in 2- to 4-week-old infants reported more realistic thresholds, 25 to 35 dB higher than those of adults between 0.5 and 4 kHz.[162, 163]

Early threshold immaturity is at least partly accounted for by conductive immaturity. Immature brain stem pathways are also involved, as suggested by the similarity of the behavioral thresholds to those reported for the ABR by Sininger and Abdala.[89] Furthermore, Werner and associates[121] demonstrated a moderately high correlation (about 0.7) between behavioral threshold and ABR wave I–wave V interwave latency among 3-month-old infants, a finding suggesting that some factor such as synaptic efficiency is at least partially responsible for threshold immaturity in early infancy.

Regardless of the mode of sound transmission *in utero*, it is clear that fetuses hear and are affected by the sounds they hear. For example, newborn infants recognize their mother's voice very soon after birth,[164, 165] and they even recognize sounds and speech patterns to which they were exposed only *in utero*.[166-168]

Sound Localization

Among the most widely studied of infant auditory capacities is the ability to localize a sound source. Interest in this topic stems from the observation that sound localization must change postnatally as the head and external ears grow, as well as the recognition that neural development could well involve maturation of the ability to make comparisons between ears and across frequencies. In fact, the precision with which changes in sound source location can be detected improves progressively between term birth and about 5 years of age.[169, 170]

Despite some early controversy on this topic,[171-173] it is now well established that term neonates turn their head and eyes to the left or right toward a sound source.[174-178] Neonates orient toward a sound source slowly, and their heads must be supported to allow the response to occur.[175, 176] The frequency, duration, and repetition rate of the stimulus are important in determining whether a response will occur.[179-183] Muir[184] reported that the orienting response was present in infants as young as 32 weeks' conceptional age.

Sound location is typically specified in terms of angle in azimuth, the horizontal plane intersecting the ears, and angle in elevation above or below that plane. Although nearly all studies of newborns' orientation to sound sources asked infants to make only a left-right discrimination, Muir[184] reported that the extent of the neonate's head turn toward a sound source was related to the position of the sound source in azimuth. The precision with which a newborn can assign a location to a sound source along either dimension has not been established; however, by 1 month of age, infants respond to a change in azimuth on the order of 27°.[185] This figure decreases progressively through infancy and early childhood to a value of 1° to 2°.[169, 170] Similarly, Muir[184] reported that neonates would turn their heads up or down appropriately toward sound sources above or below the azimuthal plane. Morrongiello and her colleagues[186, 187] reported that infants can detect a change in elevation on the order of 15° at 6 months of age; this value decreases to a value of 4° among adults, along a developmental time course similar to that seen for localization in azimuth. Finally, although neonates are able to discriminate left and right sound source locations, they are unable to suppress echoes as adults do,[25] and thus, they would have difficulty in identifying sound source locations in a reverberant environment.[179, 188]

The sources of early immaturity of sound localization are only beginning to be understood. Although physical limitations on head and ear sizes modify and limit the cues available for localization, it is clear that other factors are involved. According to the head size measurements reported by Clifton and colleagues,[26] a newborn would need a change in sound source azimuth of 20° to produce an interaural time difference on the order produced by a 10° change for adults, 10 times the smallest change detected by adults. Actually, newborns cannot detect a change in azimuth as small as 20°. Ashmead and colleagues[189] found that infants could detect interaural time difference changes smaller than those produced by a change in sound source spatial location that they could just barely detect. Both these findings could be taken to mean that the limitation is neither in the physical cue available nor in the coding of the physical cue, but in the assignment of a spatial location to the physical cue. Until additional information on infants' utilization of interaural intensity differences is available, however, it cannot be determined whether interaural intensity cues or their coding also play a role.

To summarize, neonates are capable of distinguishing the location of a sound source on the basis of auditory cues alone to an accuracy of about 25° in both azimuth and elevation. The age at which sound source localization can first be observed is not known. Although the physical size of the neonates' head and ears limit the acoustic information available about sound source location, both the accuracy with which acoustic cues are coded in early infancy and the precision with which values of acoustic cues are mapped onto locations in space are probably greater limitations.

Speech Perception

Some of the most interesting studies of infant auditory perception are those describing the infant's ability to discriminate among speech sounds. Eimas and associates[190] demonstrated that 1-month-old infants discriminated between /b/ and /p/, speech sounds differing in only one phonetic feature. Since that demonstration, the development of speech perception has been one of the most active areas of infant research. The results of these studies are easily summarized, although their interpretation may be more complicated than originally believed. A major finding is that even newborn infants appear to be capable of discriminating between all of the pairs of speech sounds that have been examined to date.[191, 192] Furthermore, this ability appears to extend to the sounds of all spoken languages.[193] Second, although it is clear that the newborn can represent speech sounds sufficiently well to discriminate among sounds under many conditions, the newborn's representation of speech sounds may be less detailed than that of adults or older infants.[194-197] The ability to make fine distinctions among speech sounds probably continues to develop into childhood.[198-206] Abnormal experience with sound may retard this process of refinement.[207] Third, infants appear to be sensitive to many aspects of speech besides phonetic distinctions. For example, they are sensitive to changes in intonation that signal clause boundaries,[208, 209] and they are capable of distinguishing among different languages.[210]

The major events in the development of speech perception during the first year of life involve a progressive specification of native language sounds, sometimes at the cost of losing the ability to discriminate nonnative speech sounds. By 2 months of age, infants appear to recognize the predominant stress pattern that occurs in their native speech.[211] By 6 months of age, they tend to categorize the vowels of their native language in a broader way than they categorize the vowels of other languages.[212, 213] The extent to which these tendencies depend on prenatal experience with speech sounds is not clear; the age when infants first demonstrate these aspects of language-specific perception has not been determined.

By 12 months of age, infants have lost the ability to discriminate among many nonnative consonants.[214-217] Some nonnative consonants appear to be discriminable by infants and remain discriminable into adulthood, such as Zulu "clicks" by American speakers of English.[218] This appears to occur when the nonnative sound is so different acoustically from native sounds that the specification of native speech sounds has no effect on the nonnative speech category. Other speech sounds are discriminable by 6-month-old infants, are not discriminable by 12-month-old children, and remain very difficult for adults to discriminate, such as Nthlakampx (a native American language) glottal stops by Canadian speakers of English.[217] In this case, it appears that as native speech sounds are specified, native speech categories "absorb" acoustically similar nonnative speech categories. Finally, some nonnative vowel sounds are discriminable by 6-month-old infants and not discriminable by 12-month-old children, but they can be discriminated by adults, such as German back-rounded vowels by Canadian speakers of English.[219] Apparently, the refinement of speech perception that occurs during childhood can have the effect of redefining a native speech category in such a way that it no longer includes nonnative speech sounds that may have been "absorbed" early in development.

An important issue for future research in this area is the importance of specific language experience on both the initial specification of native language sounds and the subsequent refinement of speech sound categories. What experience is necessary, how much experience is necessary, and when experience is necessary are not known. Although these are difficult issues to address, they are very important ones for certain populations—preterm infants, infants with congenital hearing loss, and infants with chronic otitis media—whose early experiences with sound are abnormal to varying degrees. Of high interest in this regard are studies that demonstrate that adults exaggerate phonetic differences in the speech they direct to infants.[220-222]

A final note with respect to the development of speech perception is that despite the young infant's sometimes amazing ability to process speech, immature primary auditory processing remains an important constraint on speech processing. Speech is not privileged over other sounds. Six-month-old children require just as much of a boost in SPL to detect and discriminate speech sounds as they do to detect and discriminate pure tones.[223-225] Newborn infants are less sensitive to sound. They may be particularly vulnerable to interference from noise, and their representations of the spectral shape of speech sounds may be "fuzzier" than those of older infants and adults. They may be less capable of following rapid changes in a sound.[226] Thus, it is not surprising that their representations of speech are not detailed[195] or that adults exaggerate many acoustic properties of speech when they speak to infants.[227] Another important issue for future research will be to determine precisely how immature sensory processing limits early speech perception.

SUMMARY AND CONCLUSIONS

Between the time the cochlea begins to function during gestation and the neonatal period, the auditory system undergoes dramatic development. Although there are few data from humans, all indications from the available data from humans and from the non-human literature are that the auditory system of a 28-week fetus is immature indeed: Sensitivity is known to be poor, and both spectral and temporal representations of suprathreshold sounds are likely to be fuzzy. By term birth, hearing has improved dramatically; neonates are capable of discriminating among many complex sounds. Nonetheless, the term neonate is still less sensitive and still less able to process the details of a stimulus than an adult. During very early development, the major contributor to improvements in hearing is probably the maturation of the cochlea. The middle ear and the auditory nervous system, however, continue to develop over a longer period. These are probably the major limitations on hearing in the neonatal period.

Beyond the neonatal period, as the middle ear and auditory nervous system mature, higher-level processes such as attention and memory still limit auditory perception. At some point during infancy, it is likely that these higher-level processes become more important than sensory limitations in determining what infants hear. At present, we do not know when that transition occurs.

ACKNOWLEDGMENTS

Preparation of this chapter was supported by grants from the National Institutes on Deafness and Other Communication Disorders (grant numbers DC00396 and DC04661).

REFERENCES

1. Gottlieb G: Experiential canalization of behavioral development: results. Dev Psychol, 1991. 27: p. 35-39.
2. Blatchley, B.J., W.A. Cooper, and J.R. Coleman, Development of auditory brainstem response to tone pip stimuli in the rat. Brain Res Dev Brain Res, 1987. 32(1): p. 75-84.
3. Smith, D.I. and N. Kraus, Postnatal development of the auditory brainstem response (ABR) in the unanesthetized gerbil. Hear Res, 1987. 27: p. 157-164.
4. Walsh, E.J., J. McGee, and E. Javel, Development of auditory-evoked potentials in the cat. III. Wave amplitudes. J Acoust Soc Am, 1986. 79: p. 745-256.
5. Walsh, E.J., J. McGee, and E. Javel, Development of auditory-evoked potentials in the cat. II. Wave latencies. J. Acoust Soc Am, 1986. 79: p. 725-744.
6. Walsh, E.J., J. McGee, and E. Javel, Development of auditory-evoked potentials in the cat. I. Onset of response and development of sensitivity. J Acoust Soc Am, 1986. 79: p. 712-724.
7. Pickles, J.O., An introduction to the physiology of hearing. Second ed. 1988, San Diego: Academic Press.
8. Bast, T.H. and B.J. Anson, The temporal bone and the ear. 1949, Charles C Thomas: Springfield, IL. 478.
9. Streeter, G.L., On the development of the membranous labyrinth and the acoustic and facial nerves in the human embryo. Am J Anat, 1906. 6: p. 139-165.
10. Moore, K.L. and T.V.N. Persaud, The developing human: clinically oriented embryology. 5th ed. 1993, WB Saunders Co: Philadelphia.
11. Carlson, B.M., Human embryology and developmental biology. 1994, St. Louis: Mosby.
12. Olzsewski, V.J., Morphometry of the auditive ossicles in humans at the conception development. Anat Anz, 1990. 171: p. 187-191.
13. Schonfelder, J.V., P. Rother, and M. Zschackel, Morphological investigation on postnatal changes of the middle ear sound transport apparatus in humans and rabbits. Anat Anz, 1990. 170: p. 213-219.
14. Thomas, J.P. and E.J. Walsh, Postnatal development of the middle ear: Areal ratios in kittens. Otolaryngol Head Neck Surg, 1990. 103(3): p. 427-435.
15. Pujol, R. and D. Hilding, Anatomy and physiology of the onset of auditory function. Acta Otolaryngol (Stockh), 1973. 76: p. 1-10.
16. Feigen, J.A., J.G. Kopun, P.G. Stelmachowicz, and M.P. Gorga, Probe-tube microphone measurements of ear-canal sound pressure levels in infants and children. Ear Hear, 1989. 10(4): p. 254-258.
17. McLellan, J.A. and C.H. Webb, Ear studies in the newborn infant. J Pediatr, 1957. 51: p. 672-677.
18. Keefe, D.H., E.M. Burns, J.C. Bulen, and S.L. Campbell, Pressure transfer function from the diffuse field to the human infant ear canal. J Acoust Soc Am, 1994. 95: p. 355-371.
19. Carlile, S., The auditory periphery of the ferret: Postnatal development of acoustic properties. Hear Res, 1991. 51: p. 265-278.
20. Cohen, Y.E., D.M. Rubin, and J.C. Saunders, Middle ear development. I. Extrastapedius response in the neonatal chick. Hear Res, 1992. 58: p. 1-8.
21. Cohen, Y.E., D.E. Doan, D.M. Rubin, and J.C. Saunders, Middle-ear development. V. Development of umbo sensitivity in the gerbil. Am J Otolaryngol, 1993. 14(3): p. 191-198.
22. Keefe, D.H., J.C. Bulen, K.H. Arehart, and E.M. Burns, Ear-canal impedance and reflection coefficient in human infants and adults. J Acoust Soc Am, 1993. 94: p. 2617-2638.
23. Keefe, D.H., R.C. Folsom, M.P. Gorga, B.R. Vohr, J.C. Bulen, and S.J. Norton, Identification of neonatal hearing impairment: ear-canal measurements of acoustic admittance and reflectance in neonates. Ear Hear, 2000. 21(5): p. 443-61.
24. Bluestone, C.D., T.J. Fria, S.K. Arjona, M.L. Casselbrant, D.M. Schwartz, R.J. Ruben, G.A. Gates, M.P. Downs, J.L. Northern, J.F. Jerger, J.L. Paradise, F.H. Bess, O.T. Kenworthy, and K.D. Rogers, Controversies in screening for middle ear disease and hearing loss in children. Pediatrics, 1986. 77(1): p. 57-70.
25. Blauert, J., Spatial hearing: The psychophysics of human sound localization. Revised ed. 1983, MIT Press: Cambridge, MA. 427.
26. Clifton, R.K., J. Gwiazda, J. Bauer, M. Clarkson, and R. Held, Growth in head size during infancy: Implications for sound localization. Dev Psychol, 1988. 24: p. 477-483.
27. Moore, D.R. and D.R.F. Irvine, A developmental study of the sound pressure transformation by the head of the cat. Acta Otolaryngol (Stockh), 1979. 87: p. 434-440.
28. Ruben, R.J., Development of the inner ear of the mouse: A radioautographic study of terminal mitosis. Acta Otolaryngol (Stockh), 1967. 220: p. 1-44.
29. Van De Water, T.R., P.F.A. Maderson, and T.F. Jaskoll, The morphogenesis of the middle and external ear. Birth defects: Original article series, 1980. 16(4): p. 147-180.
30. Van De Water, T.R., Epithelio-mesenchymal interactions in development of the mammalian inner ear. Anat Rec, 1981. 199: p. 262.
31. Frenz, D.A. and T.R. Van De Water, Epithelial control of periotic mesenchyme chondrogenesis. Dev Biol, 1991. 144: p. 38-46.
32. Noden, D.M. and T.R. Van De Water, The developing ear: Tissue origins and interactions. In The Biology of Change in Otolaryngology, R.J. Ruben, T.R.V.D. Water, and E.W. Rubel, editors. 1986, Elsevier: New York. 15-46.
33. Isaacson, G., M.C. Mintz, and C.T. Sasaki, Magnetic resonance imaging of the fetal temporal bone. Laryngoscope, 1986. 96(December): p. 1343-1346.
34. Lavigne-Rebillard, M. and R. Pujol, Surface aspects of the developing human organ of corti. Acta Otolaryngol (Stockh), 1987. 436: p. 43-50.
35. Lavigne-Rebillard, M. and R. Pujol, Hair cell innervation in the fetal human cochlea. Acta Otolaryngol (Stockh), 1988. 105: p. 398-402.
36. Lavigne-Rebillard, M. and D. Bagger-Sjoback, Development of the human stria vascularis. Hear Res, 1992. 64: p. 39-51.
37. Pujol, R. and M. Lavigne-Rebillard, Early stages of innervation and sensory cell differentiation in the human fetal organ of Corti. Acta Otolaryngol Suppl (Stockh), 1985. 423: p. 43-50.
38. Pujol, R., M. Lavigne-Rebillard, and A. Uziel, Physiological correlates of development of the human cochlea. Semin Perinatol, 1990. 14(4): p. 275-80.
39. Pujol, R. and M. Lavigne-Rebillard, Development of neurosensory structures in the human cochlea. Acta Otolaryngol (Stockh), 1992. 112: p. 259-264.
40. Pujol, R., M. Lavigne-Rebillard, and A. Uziel, Development of the human cochlea. Acta Otolaryngol (Stockh), 1991. 482(Suppl): p. 7-12.
41. Lavigne-Rebillard, M. and R. Pujol, Auditory hair cells in human fetuses: Synaptogenesis and ciliogenesis. J Electron Microsc, 1990. 15: p. 115-122.
42. Pujol, R., M. Lavigne-Rebillard, and M. Lenoir, Development of sensory and neural structures in the mammalian cochlea. In Development of the Auditory System, E.W. Rubel, R.R. Fay, and A.N. Popper, editors. 1998, Springer-Verlag: New York. p. 146-192.
43. Fermin, C.D. and G.M. Cohns, Developmental gradients in the embryonic chick's basilar papilla. Acta Otolaryngol (Stockh), 1984. 97: p. 39-51.
44. Lenoir, M., A. Shnerson, and R. Pujol, Cochlear receptor development in the rat with emphasis on synaptogenesis. Anat Embryol, 1980. 160: p. 253-262.
45. Emmerling, M.R., H.M. Sobkowicz, C.V. Levenick, G.L. Scott, S.M. Slapnick, and J.E. Rose, Biochemical and morphological differentiation of acetylcholinesterase-positive efferent fibers in the mouse cochlea. J Electron Microsc, 1990. 15: p. 123-143.
46. Pujol, R. and A. Sans, Synaptogenesis in the mammalian inner ear. In Advances in Neural and Behavioral Development, R.N. Aslin, editor. 1986, Academic Press: New York. p. 1-18.
47. Pujol, R. and M. Lavigne-Rebillard, Sensory and neural structures in the developing human cochlea. Int J Pediatr Otorhinolaryngol, 1995. 32(Suppl): p. S177-82.
48. Woolf, N.K. and A.F. Ryans, The development of auditory function in the cochlea of the mongolian gerbil. Hear Res, 1984. 13: p. 277-283.
49. Woolf, N.K. and A.F. Ryan, Ontogeny of neural discharge patterns in the ventral cochlear nucleus of the Mongolian gerbil. Dev Brain Res, 1985. 17: p. 131-147.
50. Brugge, J.F., E. Javel, and L.M. Kitzes, Signs of functional maturation of peripheral auditory system in discharge patterns in anteroventral cochlear nucleus of kittens. J Neurophysiol, 1978. 41(6): p. 1557-1579.
51. Brugge, J.F., L.M. Kitzes, and E. Javel, Postnatal development of frequency and intensity sensitivity of neurons in the anteroventral cochlear nucleus of kittens. Hear Res, 1981. 5: p. 217-229.
52. Brugge, J.F., Stimulus coding in the developing auditory system. In Auditory Function: Neurobiological Bases of Hearing, G.M. Edelman, W.E. Gall, and W.M. Cowan, editors. 1988, John Wiley and Sons: New York. p. 113-136.
53. Rebillard, G. and E.W. Rubel, Electrophysiological study of the maturation of auditory responses from the inner ear of the chick. Brain Res, 1981. 229: p. 15-23.
54. Probst, R. and F.P. Harris, Otoacoustic emissions. In Electophysiologic Evaluation in Otolaryngology, B.R. Alford, J. Jerger, and H.A. Jenkins, editors. 1997, Basel: S. Karger AG. p. 182-204.
55. Stevens, J.C., H.D. Webb, M.F. Smith, and J.T. Buffin, The effect of stimulus level on click evoked oto-acoustic emissions and brainstem responses in neonates under intensive care. Br J Audiol, 1990. 24: p. 293-300.
56. Smurzynski, J., Longitudinal measurements of distortion-product and click-evoked otoacoustic emission of preterm infants: Preliminary results. Ear Hear, 1994. 15: p. 210-223.
57. Chuang, S.W., S.E. Gerber, and A.R. Thornton, Evoked otoacoustic emissions in preterm infants. Int J Pediatr Otorhinolaryngol, 1993. 26(1): p. 39-45.
58. Vanzanten, B.G.A., M.R. Kok, M.P. Brocaar, and P.J.J. Sauer, The click-evoked otoacoustic emission, C-Eoae, in preterm-born infants in the post conceptional age range between 30 and 68 weeks. Int J Pediatr Otorhinolaryngol, 1995. 32: p. S187-S197.
59. Lasky, R.E., Distortion product otoacoustic emissions in human newborns and adults. I. Frequency effects. J Acoust Soc Am, 1998. 103(2): p. 981-91.
60. Lasky, R.E., Distortion product otoacoustic emissions in human newborns and adults. II. Level effects. J Acoust Soc Am, 1998. 103(2): p. 992-1000.
61. Hall, J.W.I., Handbook of auditory evoked responses. 1992, Allyn and Bacon: Boston.

62. Gorga, M.P., J.K. Reiland, K.A. Beauchaine, D.W. Worthington, and W. Jesteadt, Auditory brainstem responses from graduates of an intensive care nursery: Normal patterns of response. J Speech Hear Res, 1987. **30**: p. 311-318.

63. Lary, S., G. Briassoulis, L. de Vries, L.M.S. Dubowitz, and V. Dubowitz, Hearing threshold in preterm and term infants by auditory brainstem response. J Pediatr, 1985. **107**: p. 593-599.

64. Rotteveel, J.J., R. de Graaf, E.J. Colon, D.F. Stegeman, and Y.M. Visco, The maturation of the central auditory conduction in preterm infants until three months post term. II. The auditory brainstem responses (ABRs). Hear Res, 1987. **26**: p. 21-35.

65. Guerit, J.M., Applications of surface-recorded auditory evoked potentials for the early diagnosis of hearing loss in neonates and premature infants. Acta Otolaryngol (Stockh), 1985. **421(Suppl)**: p. 68-76.

66. Hendler, T., N.K. Squires, and D.S. Emmerich, Psychophysical measures of central auditory dysfunction in multiple sclerosis: neurophysiological and neuroanatomical correlates. Ear Hear, 1990. **11**(6): p. 403-416.

67. Lieberman, A., H. Sohmer, and G. Szabo, Cochlear audiometry (electrocochleography) during the neonatal period. Develop Med Child Neurol, 1973. **15**: p. 8-13.

68. Walsh, E.J. and J. McGee, Postnatal development of auditory nerve and cochlear nucleus neuronal responses in kittens. Hear Res, 1987. **28**: p. 97-116.

69. Ehret, G., Postnatal development in the acoustic system of the house mouse in the light of developing masked thresholds. J Acoust Soc Am, 1977. **62**: p. 143-148.

70. Abdala, C., A developmental study of distortion product otoacoustic emission (2f1-f2) suppression in humans. Hear Res, 1998. **121**(1-2): p. 125-38.

71. Abdala, C., Maturation of the human cochlear amplifier: Distortion product otoacoustic emission suppression tuning curves recorded at low and high primary tone levels. J Acoust Soc Am, 2001. **110**(3): p. 1465-1476.

72. Abdala, C., DPOAE suppression tuning: Cochlear immaturity in premature neonates or auditory aging in normal-hearing adults? J Acoust Soc Am, 2001. **110**(6): p. 3155-3162.

73. Mills, D., S. Norton, and E. Rubel, Development of active and passive mechanics in the mammalian cochlea. Aud Neurosci, 1994. **1**: p. 77-99.

74. Arjmand, E., D. Harris, and P. Dallos, Developmental changes in frequency mapping of the gerbil cochlea: Comparison of two cochlear locations. Hear Res, 1988. **32**(1): p. 93-96.

75. Harris, D. and P. Dallos, Ontogenetic changes in frequency mapping in a mammalian ear. Science, 1984. **225**: p. 741-743.

76. Lippe, W.R., Shift of tonotopic organization in brain stem auditory nuclei of the chicken during late embryonic development. Hear Res, 1987. **1987**: p. 205-208.

77. Ryals, B.M. and E.W. Rubel, Ontogenetic changes in the position of hair cell loss after acoustic overstimulation in avian basilar papilla. Hear Res, 1985. **19**: p. 135-142.

78. Yakovlev, P.I. and A.-R. Lecours, The myelogenetic cycles of regional maturation of the brain. In Regional Development of the Brain in Early Life, A. Minkowski, editor. 1967, Blackwell: Oxford. p. 3-70.

79. Krmpotic-Nemanic, J., I. Kostovic, Z. Kelovic, D. Nemanic, and L. Mrzljak, Development of the human auditory cortex: Growth of afferent fibers. Acta Anat (Basel), 1983. **116**: p. 69-73.

80. Krmpotic-Nemanic, J., I. Kostovic, Z. Vidic, D. Nemanic, and L. Kostovic-Knezevic, Development of Cajal-Retzius cells in the human auditory cortex. Acta Otolaryngol (Stockh), 1987. **103**: p. 477-480.

81. Krmpotic-Nemanic, J., I. Kostovic, N. Bogdanovic, A. Fucic, and M. Judas, Cytoarchitectonic parameters of developmental capacity of the human associative auditory cortex during postnatal life. Acta Otolaryngol (Stockh), 1988. **105**: p. 463-466.

82. Moore, J.K., C.W. Ponton, J.J. Eggermont, B.J. Wu, and J.Q. Huang, Perinatal maturation of the auditory brain stem response: changes in path length and conduction velocity. Ear Hear, 1996. **17**(5): p. 411-8.

83. Moore, J.K., Y.L. Guan, and S.R. Shi, Axogenesis in the human fetal auditory system, demonstrated by neurofilament immunohistochemistry. Anat Embryol (Berl), 1997. **195**(1): p. 15-30.

84. Moore, J.K. and Y.L. Guan, Cytoarchitectural and axonal maturation in human auditory cortex. Jaro, 2001. **2**(4): p. 297-311.

85. Moore, J.K., Maturation of human auditory cortex: Implications for speech perception. Ann Otol Rhinol Laryngol, 2002. **111**(5): p. 7-10.

86. Arnold, W.J., The spiral ganglion of the newborn baby. Am J Otol, 1982. **3**(3): p. 266-9.

87. Marty, R. and J. Thomas, Réponse l'electro-corticale a la stimulation du nerf cochlaire chez le chat nouveau-né. J Physiol (Paris), 1963. **55**: p. 165-166.

88. Rotteveel, J.J., R. de Graaf, D.F. Stegeman, E.J. Colon, and Y.M. Visco, The maturation of the central auditory conduction in preterm infants until three months post term. V. The auditory cortical response (ACR). Hear Res, 1987. **27**: p. 95-110.

89. Sininger, Y. and C. Abdala, Auditory brainstem response thresholds of newborns based on ear canal levels. Ear Hear, 1996.

90. Abdala, C. and R.C. Folsom, The development of frequency resolution in humans as revealed by the auditory brain-stem response recorded with notched-noise masking. J Acoust Soc Am, 1995. **98**(2 Part 1): p. 921-30.

91. Folsom, R.C. and M.K. Wynne, Auditory brain stem responses from human adults and infants: Wave V tuning curves. J Acoust Soc Am, 1987. **81**: p. 412-417.

92. Bargones, J.Y. and E.M. Burns, Suppression tuning curves for spontaneous otoacoustic emissions in infants and adults. J Acoust Soc Am, 1988. **83**(5): p. 1809-16.

93. Sanes, D.H. and M. Constantine-Paton, The sharpening of frequency tuning curves requires patterned activity during development in the mouse, Mus musculus. J Neurosci, 1985. **5**(5): p. 1152-1166.

94. Sanes, D.H. and E.W. Rubel, The functional ontogeny of inhibition and excitation in the gerbil auditory brain stem. J Neurosci, 1988. **8**: p. 682-700.

95. Sanes, D.H., J. Song, and J. Tyson, Refinement of dendritic arbors along the tonotopic axis of the gerbil lateral superior olive. Dev Brain Res, 1992. **67**: p. 47-55.

96. Sanes, D.H., The development of synaptic function and integration in the central auditory system. J Neurosci, 1993. **13**(6): p. 2627-37.

97. Walsh, E.J. and J. McGee, Rhythmic discharge properties of caudal cochlear nucleus neurons during postnatal development in cats. Hear Res, 1988. **36**: p. 233-248.

98. Sanes, D.H. and E.W. Rubel, The development of stimulus coding in the auditory system. In Physiology of the Ear, A.F. Jahn and J.R. Santos-Sacchi, editors. 1988, Raven Press: New York. p. 431-455.

99. Durieux-Smith, A., C.G. Edwards, T.W. Picton, and B. McMurray, Auditory brainstem responses to clicks in neonates. J Otolaryngol, 1985. **14**: p. 12-18.

100. Cornacchia, L., A. Martini, and B. Morra, Air and bone conduction brain stem responses in adults and infants. Audiology, 1983. **22**: p. 430-437.

101. Moore, J.K., Y.L. Guan, and S.R. Shi, Axogenesis in the human fetal auditory system, demonstrated by neurofilament immunohistochemistry. Anat Embryol, 1997. **195**(1): p. 15-30.

102. Moore, J.K., L.M. Perazzo, and A. Braun, Time course of axonal myelination in human brainstem auditory pathway. Hear Res, 1995. **87**: p. 21-31.

103. Zimmerman, M.C., D.E. Morgan, and J.C. Dubno, Auditory brain stem evoked response characteristics in developing infants. Ann Otol Rhinol Laryngol, 1987. **96**: p. 291-299.

104. Eggermont, J.J. and A. Salamy, Maturational time course for the ABR in preterm and full term infants. Hear Res, 1988. **33**: p. 35-48.

105. Yamasaki, M., H. Shono, M. Oga, K. Shimomura, and H. Sugimori, Changes in auditory brainstem responses of normal neonates immediately after birth. Biol Neonate, 1991. **60**: p. 92-101.

106. Mjoen, S. and E. Qvigstad, Auditory brainstem response in neonates during the first 48 hours after birth. Scand Audiol, 1983. **12**: p. 43-45.

107. Maurizi, M., G. Almadori, L. Cagini, E. Mokini, G. Ottaviani, G. Paludetti, and F. Pierri, Auditory brainstem responses in the full-term newborn: Changes in the first 58 hours of life. Audiology, 1986. **25**: p. 239-247.

108. Adelman, C., H. Levi, N. Linder, and H. Sohmer, Neonatal auditory brain-stem response threshold and latency: 1 hour to 5 months. Electroencephalogr Clin Neurophysiol, 1990. **77**(1): p. 77-80.

109. Morgan, D., M.C. Zimmerman, and J.C. Dubno, Auditory brain stem evoked response characteristics in the full-term newborn infants. Ann Otol Rhinol Laryngol, 1987. **96**: p. 142-151.

110. Thornton, A.R.D., L. Kimm, C.R. Kennedy, and D.C. Cafarelli-Dees, External- and middle-ear factors affecting evoked otoacoustic emissions in neonates. Br J Audiol, 1993. **27**: p. 319-327.

111. Sohmer, H., M. Geal-Dor, and D. Weinstein, Human fetal auditory threshold improvement during maternal oxygen respiration. Hear Res, 1994. **75**: p. 145-150.

112. Sohmer, H., K. Goitein, and S. Freeman, Improvement in sensorineural auditory threshold of the guinea-pig fetus following delivery. Hear Res, 1994. **73**: p. 116-120.

113. Nousak, J.K. and D.R. Stapells, Frequency specificity of the auditory brainstem response to bone-conducted tones in infants and adults. Ear Hear, 1992. **13**: p. 87-95.

114. Sohmer, H. and S. Freeman, Hypoxia induced hearing loss in animal models of the fetus in-utero. Hear Res, 1991. **55**: p. 92-97.

115. Starr, A., R.N. Amlie, W.H. Martin, and S. Sanders, Development of auditory function in newborn infants revealed by auditory brainstem potentials. Pediatrics, 1977. **60**(6): p. 831-838.

116. Despland, P.A. and R. Galambos, Use of the auditory brainstem responses by prematures and newborns infants. Neuropaediatrie, 1980. **11**: p. 99-107.

117. Collet, L., I. Soares, A. Morgon, and B. Salle, Is there a difference between extrauterine and intrauterine maturation on BAEP? Brain Dev, 1989. **11**(5): p. 293-296.

118. Gorga, M.P., J.R. Kaminski, K.L. Beauchaine, W. Jesteadt, and S.T. Neely, Auditory brainstem responses from children three months to three years of age: Normal patterns of response II. J Speech Hear Res, 1989. **32**: p. 281-288.

119. Ponton, C.W., J.K. Moore, E.E. Eggermont, B.J.-C. Wu, and J. Huang. The relation between auditory brainstem size and auditory brainstem response (ABR) interpeak latency during human development. Paper presented at the 17th Midwinter Meeting of the Association for Research in Otolaryngology. 1994. St. Petersburg Beach, FL.

120. Moore, J.K., The human auditory brain stem as a generator of auditory evoked potentials. Hear Res, 1987. **29**: p. 33-43.

121. Werner, L.A., R.C. Folsom, and L.R. Mancl, The relationship between auditory brainstem response latencies and behavioral thresholds in normal hearing infants and adults. Hear Res, 1994. **77**: p. 88-98.

122. Maurizi, M., G. Alamdori, G. Paludetti, F. Ottaviani, M. Rosignoli, and R. Luciano, 40-Hz steady-state responses in newborns and children. Audiology, 1990. **29**: p. 322-328.

123. Moon, C. and W.P. Fifer. Newborn response to a male voice. Paper presented at the International Conference for Infant Studies. 1988. Washington, DC.

124. Jerger, J., R. Chmiel, D. Glaze, and J.D.J. Frost, Rate and filter dependence of the middle-latency response in infants. Audiology, 1987. **26**: p. 269-283.

125. Kraus, N., D. Smith, N.L. Reed, L.K. Stein, and C. Cartee, Auditory middle latency responses in children: effects of age and diagnostic category. Electroencephalogr Clin Neurophysiol, 1985. **62**: p. 343-351.

126. Stapells, D.R., R. Galambos, J.A. Costello, and S. Makeig, Inconsistency of auditory middle latency and steady-state responses in infants. Electroencephalogr Clin Neurophysiol, 1988. **71**: p. 289-295.

127. Kettner, R.E., J.-Z. Feng, and J.F. Brugge, Postnatal development of the phase-locked response to low frequency tones of the auditory nerve fibers in the cat. J Neurosci, 1985. **5**(2): p. 275-283.

128. Kraus, N. and T. McGee, Electrophysiology of the human auditory system. In The Mammalian Auditory Pathway: Neurophysiology, A.N. Popper and R.R. Fay, editors. 1992, Springer-Verlag: New York. p. 335-404.

129. Gardi, J., A. Salamy, and T. Mendelson, Scalp-recorded frequency following responses in neonates. Audiology, 1979. **18**: p. 494-506.

130. Levi, E.C., R.C. Folson, and R.A. Dobie, Coherence analysis of envelope-following responses (EFRs) and frequency-following responses (FFRs) in infants and adults. Hear Res, 1995. **89**: p. 21-27.

131. Dey-Sigman, S.E., R.A. Ruth, and E.W. Rubel. ABR rate/intensity interaction: Developmental effects. Paper presented at meeting of the American Speech-Hearing-Language Association. 1984. Washington, DC.

132. Lasky, R.E., A developmental study on the effect of stimulus rate on the auditory evoked brain-stem response. Electroencephalogr Clin Neurophysiol, 1984. **59**: p. 411-419.

133. Fujikawa, S.M. and B.A. Weber, Effects of increased stimulus rate on brainstem electric response (BER) audiometry as a function of age. J Am Audiol Soc, 1977. **3**(3): p. 147-150.

134. Klein, A.J., E.D. Alvarez, and C.A. Cowburn, The effects of stimulus rate on detectability of the auditory brain stem response in infants. Ear Hear, 1992. **13**(6): p. 401-405.

135. Altman, J. and S.A. Bayer, Time of origin of neurons of the rat inferior colliculus and the relations between cytogenesis and tonotopic order in the auditory pathway. Exp Brain Res, 1981. **42**(3-4): p. 411-23.

136. Smith, Z.D.J., Organization and development of brain stem auditory nuclei in the chicken: Dendritic development in n. laminaris. J Comp Neurol, 1981. **203**: p. 309-333.

137. Teas, D.C., A.J. Klein, and S.J. Kramer, An analysis of auditory brainstem responses in infants. Hear Res, 1982. **7**: p. 19-54.

138. Ponton, C.W., J.J. Eggermont, S.G. Coupland, and R. Winkelaar, Frequency-specific maturation of the eighth-nerve and brain-stem auditory pathway: Evidence from derived auditory brain-stem responses (ABRs). J Acoust Soc Am, 1992. **91**: p. 1576-1587.

139. Birnholz, J.C. and B.R. Benacerraf, The development of human fetal hearing. Science, 1983. **222**(4623): p. 516-8.

140. Gelman, S.R., S. Wood, W.N. Spellacy, and R.N. Abrams, Fetal movements in response to sound stimulation. Am J Obstet Gynecol, 1982. **143**: p. 484-485.

141. Grimwade, J.C., D.W. Walker, M. Bartlett, S. Gordon, and C. Wood, Human fetal heart rate change and movement in response to sound and vibration. Am J Obstet Gynecol, 1971. **109**(1): p. 86-90.

142. Ianniruberto, A. and E. Tajani, Ultrasonographic study of fetal movements. Semin Perinatol, 1981. **5**(2): p. 175-181.

143. Kisilevsky, B.S., D.W. Muir, and J.A. Low, Human fetal responses to sound as a function of stimulus intensity. Obstet Gynecol, 1989. **73**(6): p. 971-976.

144. Kisilevsky, B.S., D.W. Muir, and J.A. Low, Maturation of human fetal responses to vibroacoustic stimulation. Child Dev, 1992. **63**: p. 1497-1508.

145. Lecanuet, J.-P., C. Granier-Deferre, and M.-C. Busnel, Fetal cardiac and motor responses to octave-band noises as a function of central frequency, intensity and heart rate variability. Early Hum Dev, 1988. **18**: p. 81-93.

146. Lecanuet, J.P., C. Granier-Deferre, and M.C. Busnel, Differential fetal auditory reactiveness as a function of stimulus characteristics and state. Semin Perinatol, 1989. **13**(5): p. 421-429.

147. Lecanuet, J.-P., C. Granier-Deferre, A.-Y. Jacquet, and M.-C. Busnel, Decelerative cardiac responsiveness to acoustical stimulation in the near term fetus. Q J Exp Psychol, 1992. **44B**: p. 279-303.

148. Luz, N.P., C.P. Lima, S.H. Luz, and V.L. Feldens, Auditory evoked responses of the human fetus I. Behavior during progress of labor. Acta Obstet Gynecol Scand, 1980. **59**: p. 395-404.

149. Querleu, D., X. Renard, F. Versyp, L. Paris-Delrue, and G. Crepin, Fetal hearing. Eur J Obstet Gynecol Reprod Biol, 1988. **29**: p. 191-212.

150. Schmidt, W., R. Boos, J. Gnirs, L. Auer, and S. Schulze, Fetal behavioral states and controlled sound stimulation. Early Hum Dev, 1985. **12**: p. 145-153.

151. Tanaka, Y. and T. Arayama, Fetal responses to acoustic stimuli. Pract Oto-Rhino-Laryngol, 1969. **31**: p. 269-273.

152. Walker, D., J. Grimwade, and C. Wood, Intrauterine Noise: A Component of the Fetal Environment. Am J Obstet Gynecol, 1971. **109**: p. 91-95.

153. Lecanuet, J.-P., C. Granier-Deferre, H. Cohen, R. Le Houezec, and M.-C. Busnel, Fetal responses to acoustic stimulation depend on heart rate variability pattern, stimulus intensity and repetition. Early Hum Dev, 1986. **13**: p. 269-283.

154. Wedenberg, E., Prenatal tests of hearing. Acta Otolaryngol (Stockh), 1965. **206**: p. 27-31.

155. Iggo, A., Cutaneous sensory mechanisms. In The Senses, H.B. Barlow and J.D. Mollon, editors. 1982, Cambridge University Press: New York. p. 369-408.

156. Rubel, E.W., Ontogeny of structure and function in the vertebrate auditory system. In Handbook of Sensory Physiology: Development of Sensory Systems. Vol. 9. M. Jacobson, editor. 1978, Springer-Verlag: New York.

157. Dirks, D.D., Bone-conduction testing. In Handbook of Clinical Audiology, J. Katz, editor. 1985, Williams & Wilkins: Baltimore. p. 202-223.

158. Gerber, S.E. and G.T. Mencher. Arousal responses of neonates to wide band and narrow band noise. Paper presented at meeting of the American Speech-Language-Hearing Association. 1979. Atlanta, GA.

159. Gerber, S.E., C.G. Lima, and K.L. Copriviza, Auditory arousal in preterm infants. Scand Audiol Suppl, 1983. **19**: p. 88-93.

160. Schulman, C.A., Effects of auditory stimulation on heart rate in premature infants as a function of level of arousal, probability of CNS damage, and conceptional age. Dev Psychobiol, 1969. **2**(3): p. 172-183.

161. Weir, C., Auditory frequency sensitivity of human newborns: Some data with improved acoustic and behavioral controls. Percept Psychophisiol, 1979. **26**: p. 287-294.

162. Werner, L.A. and J.M. Gillenwater, Pure-tone sensitivity of 2- to 5-week-old infants. Infant Behav Dev, 1990. **13**: p. 355-375.

163. Werner, L.A. and L.R. Mancl, Pure-tone thresholds of 1-month-old human infants. J Acoust Soc Am, 1993. **93**: p. 2367.

164. Mehler, J., J. Bertoncini, M. Barriere, and D. Jassik-Gerschenfeld, Infant recognition of mother's voice. Perception, 1978. **7**: p. 491-497.

165. DeCasper, A.J. and W.P. Fifer, Of human bonding: Newborns prefer their mothers' voices. Science, 1980. **208**(June): p. 1174-1176.

166. DeCasper, A.J. and M.J. Spence, Prenatal maternal speech influences newborns' perception of speech sounds. Infant Behav Dev, 1986. **9**: p. 133-150.

167. DeCasper, A.J. and A.D. Sigafoos, The intrauterine heartbeat: A potent reinforcer for newborns. Infant Behav Dev, 1983. **6**: p. 19-25.

168. Panneton, R.K. and A.J. DeCasper. Newborns prefer an intrauterine heartbeat sound to a male voice. In International Conference on Infant Studies. 1984. New York.

169. Litovsky, R.Y. Developmental changes in sound localization precision (MAA) under conditions of the precedence effect. Paper presented at International Conference on Infant Studies. 1992. Miami, FL.

170. Litovsky, R., The influence of the precedence effect on developmental changes in sound localization precision. J Acoust Soc Am, 1993: p. 1-31.

171. Turkewitz, G., H.G. Birch, T. Moreau, L. Levy, and A.C. Cornwall, Effect of intensity of auditory stimulation on directional eye movements in the human neonate. Anim Behav, 1966. **14**: p. 93-101.

172. Wertheimer, M., Psychomotor coordination of auditory and visual space at birth. Science, 1961. **134**: p. 1692.

173. McGurk, H., C. Turnure, and S. Creighton, Auditory-visual coordination in neonates. Child Dev, 1977. **48**: p. 138-143.

174. Muir, D. and T. Field, Newborn infants orient to sounds. Child Dev, 1979. **50**: p. 431-436.

175. Field, T.J., D. Muir, R. Pilon, M. Sinclair, and P. Dodwell, Infants' orientation to lateral sounds from birth to three months. Child Dev, 1980. **51**: p. 295-298.

176. Clifton, R., B.A. Morrongiello, J.W. Kulig, and J.M. Dowd, Developmental changes in auditory localization in infancy. In Development of Perception, R. Aslin, J. Alberts, and M.R. Petersen, editors. 1981, Academic Press: New York. p. 141-160.

177. Clifton, R.K., B. Morrongiello, J. Kulig, and J. Dowd, Auditory localization of the newborn infant: Its relevance for cortical development. Child Dev, 1981. **52**: p. 833-838.

178. Muir, D., R.K. Clifton, and M.G. Clarkson, The development of human auditory localization response: A U-shaped function. Can J Psychol, 1989. **43**: p. 199-216.

179. Clifton, R.K., The development of spatial hearing in human infants. In Developmental Psychoacoustics, L.A. Werner and E.W. Rubel, editors. 1992, American Psychological Association: Washington, DC. p. 135-157.

180. Zelazo, P.R., L.R. Brody, and H. Chaika, Neonatal habituation and dishabituation of head turning to rattle sounds. Infant Behav Dev, 1984. **7**: p. 311-321.

181. Tarquinio, N., P.R. Zelazo, and M.J. Weiss, Recovery of neonatal head turning to decreased sound pressure level. Dev Psychol, 1990. **26**: p. 752-758.

182. Morrongiello, B.A. and R.K. Clifton, Effects of sound frequency on behavioral and cardiac orienting in newborn and five-month old infants. J Exp Child Psychol, 1984. **38**: p. 429-446.

183. Clarkson, M.G. and R.K. Clifton, Acoustic determinants of newborn orienting. In Newborn Attention: Biological Constraints and the Influence of Experience, M.J.S. Weiss and P.R. Zelazo, editors. 1991, Ablex Publishing: Norwood, NJ. p. 99-119.

184. Muir, D., The development of infants' auditory spatial sensitivity. In Auditory Development in Infancy, S.E. Trehub and B.A. Schneider, editors. 1985, Plenum Press: New York. p. 51-84.

185. Morrongiello, B.A., K. Fenwick, and G. Chance, Sound localization acuity in very young infants: An observer-based testing procedure. Dev Psychol, 1990. **26**: p. 75-84.

186. Morrongiello, B.A., Infants' localization of sounds along two spatial dimensions: Horizontal and vertical axes. Infant Behav Dev, 1988. **11**: p. 127-143.

187. Morrongiello, B.A. and P.T. Rocca, Infants' localization of sounds in the median vertical plane: Estimates of minimal audible angle. J Exp Child Psychol, 1987. **43**: p. 181-193.

188. Ashmead, D.H., R.K. Clifton, and E.P. Reese, Development of auditory localization in dogs: Single source and precedence effect sounds. Dev Psychobiol, 1986. **19**(2): p. 91-103.

189. Ashmead, D., D. Davis, T. Whalen, and R. Odom, Sound localization and sensitivity to interaural time differences in human infants. Child Dev, 1991. **62**(6): p. 1211-1226.

190. Eimas, P.D., E.R. Siqueland, P. Jusczyk, and J. Vigorito, Speech perception in infants. Science, 1971. **171**: p. 303–306.

191. Bertoncini, J. and J. Mehler, La perception du langage chez le nourisson: Quelques observations. [Language perception in the newborn infant: Some observations]. Reprod Nutr Dev, 1980. **20**(3B): p. 859–69.

192. Bertoncini, J., R. Bijeljac-Babic, S.E. Blumstein, and J. Mehler, Discrimination in neonates of very short CVs. J Acoust Soc Am, 1987. **82**(1): p. 31–7.

193. Best, C.T., Emergence of language-specific constraints in perception of non-native speech: A window on early phonological development. *In* Developmental Neurocognition: Speech and Face Processing in the First Year of Life, B. de Boysson-Bardies, et al., editors. 1993, Kluwer Academic Publishers: Dordrecht. p. 289–304.

194. Bertoncini, J. and J. Mehler, Syllables as units of infnat speech perception. Infant Behav Dev, 1981. **4**(3): p. 247–260.

195. Bertoncini, J., R. Bijeljac-Babic, P.W. Jusczyk, L.J. Kennedy, and J. Mehler, An investigation of young infants' perceptual representations of speech sounds. J Exp Psychol [Gen], 1988. **117**(1): p. 21–33.

196. Jusczyk, P.W. and C. Derrah, Representation of speech sounds by young infants. Dev Psychol, 1987. **23**: p. 648–654.

197. Jusczyk, P.W., J. Bertoncini, R. Bijeljac-Babic, L.J. Kennedy, and J. Mehler, The role of attention in speech perception by young infants. Cogn Dev, 1990. **5**: p. 265–286.

198. Aslin, R.N., D.B. Pisoni, B.L. Hennessy, and A.J. Perey, Discrimination of voice onset time by human infants: New findings and implications for the effects of early experience. Child Dev, 1981. **52**(4): p. 1135–45.

199. Walley, A.C., More developmental research is needed. J Phonetics, 1993. **21**: p. 171–176.

200. Walley, A.C. and T.D. Carrell, Onset spectra and formant transitions in the adult's and child's perception of place of articulation in stop consonants. J Acoust Soc Am, 1983. **73**: p. 1011–1022.

201. Elliott, L.L., C. Longinotti, D. Meyer, I. Raz, and K. Zucker, Developmental differences in identifying and discriminating CV syllables. J Acoust Soc Am, 1981. **70**: p. 669–677.

202. Elliott, L.L., C. Longinotti, L. Clifton, and D. Meyer, Detection and identification thresholds for consonant-vowel syllables. Percept Psychophysics, 1981. **30**(5): p. 411–416.

203. Elliott, L.L. and L.A. Busse, Syllable identification by children and adults for two task conditions. J Acoust Soc Am, 1985. **77**: p. 1258–1260.

204. Elliott, L.L., L.A. Busse, R. Partridge, J. Rupert, and R. DeGraaff, Adult and child discrimination of CV syllables differing in voicing onset time. Child Dev, 1986. **57**: p. 628–635.

205. Elliott, L.L., M.A. Hammer, M.E. Scholl, and J.M. Wasowicz, Age differences in discrimination of simulated single-formant frequency transitions. Percept Psychophys, 1989. **46**: p. 181–186.

206. Nittrouer, S. and M. Studdert-Kennedy, The role of coarticulatory effects in the perception of fricatives by children and adults. J Speech Hear Res 1987. **30**: p. 319–329.

207. Clarkson, R.L., P.D. Eimas, and G.C. Marean, Speech perception in children with histories of recurrent otitis media. J Acoust Soc Am, 1989. **85**: p. 926–933.

208. Hirsh-Pasek, K., D.G. Kemler Nelson, P.W. Jusczyk, K. Wright Cassidy, B. Druss, and L. Kennedy, Clauses are perceptual units for young infants. Cognition, 1987. **26**: p. 269–286.

209. Jusczyk, P.W., K. Hirsh-Pasek, D.G. Nelson, L.J. Kennedy, A. Woodward, and J. Piwoz, Perception of acoustic correlates of major phrasal units by young infants. Cogn Psychol, 1992. **24**: p. 252–293.

210. Mehler, J., P.W. Jusczyk, G. Lambertz, N. Halsted, J. Bertoncini, and C. Amiel-Tison, A precursor of language acquisition in young infants. Cognition, 1988. **29**: p. 143–178.

211. Jusczyk, P.W., A. Cutler, and N.J. Redanz, Infants' preference for the predominant stress patterns of English words. Child Dev, 1993. **64**: p. 675–687.

212. Grieser, D. and P.K. Kuhl, Categorization of speech by infants: Support for speech-sound prototypes. Dev Psychol, 1989. **25**: p. 577–588.

213. Kuhl, P.K., K.A. Williams, F. Lacerda, K.N. Stevens, and B. Lindblom, Linguistic experience alters phonetic perception in infants by 6 months of age. Science, 1992. **255**: p. 606–608.

214. Werker, J.F., J.H. Gilbert, K. Humphrey, and R.C. Tees, Developmental aspects of cross-language speech perception. Child Dev, 1981. **52**: p. 349–355.

215. Werker, J.F. and R.C. Tees, Developmental changes across childhood in the perception of non-native speech sounds. Can J Psychol, 1983. **37**(2): p. 278–286.

216. Werker, J.F. and R.C. Tees, Cross-language speech perception: Evidence for perceptual reorganization during the first year of life. Infant Behav Dev, 1984. **7**: p. 49–63.

217. Werker, J.F. and C.E. Lalonde, Cross-language speech perception: Initial capabilities and developmental change. Dev Psychol, 1988. **24**: p. 672–683.

218. Best, C.T., G.W. McRoberts, and N.M. Sithole, Examination of perceptual reorganization for nonnative speech contrasts: Zulu click discrimination by English-speaking adults and infants. J Exp Psychol [Hum Percept Perform], 1988. **14**(3): p. 345–60.

219. Werker, J.K. and L. Polka, Developmental changes in speech perception: New challenges and new directions. J Phonetics, 1993. **21**: p. 83–101.

220. Kuhl, P.K., J.E. Andruski, I.A. Chistovich, L.A. Chistovich, E.V. Kozhevnikova, V.L. Ryskina, E.I. Stolyarova, U. Sundberg, and F. Lacerda, Cross-language analysis of phonetic units in language addressed to infants. Science, 1997. **277**: p. 684–686.

221. Burnham, D., C. Kitamura, and U. Vollmer-Conna, What's new, pussycat? On talking to babies and animals. Science, 2002. **296**: p. 1435–1435.

222. Kitamura, C., C. Thanavishuth, D. Burnham, and S. Luksaneeyanawin, Universality and specificity in infant-directed speech: Pitch modifications as a function of infant age and sex in a tonal and non-tonal language. Infant Behav Dev, 2002. **24**(4): p. 372–392.

223. Nozza, R.J., S.L. MIller, R.N.F. Rossman, and L.C. Bond, Reliability and validity of infant speech-sound discrimination-in-noise thresholds. J Speech Hear Res, 1991. **34**: p. 643–650.

224. Nozza, R.J., Infant speech-sound discrimination testing: Effects of stimulus intensity and procedural model on measures of performance. J Acoust Soc Am, 1987. **81**(6): p. 1928–1939.

225. Nozza, R.J., S.L. Miller, R.N.F. Rossman, and L.C. Bond, Reliability and validity of infant speech-sound discrimination in noise thresholds. J Speech Hear Res, 1991. **34**: p. 643–650.

226. Jusczyk, P.W., D.B. Pisoni, M.A. Reed, A. Fernald, and M. Myers, Infants' discrimination of the duration of a rapid spectrum change in nonspeech signals. Science, 1983. **222**: p. 175–177.

227. Fernald, A. and T. Simon, Expanded intonation contours in mothers' speech to newborns. Dev Psychol, 1984. **20**: p. 104–113.

177

Beverly J. Cowart, Gary K. Beauchamp, and Julie A. Mennella

Development of Taste and Smell in the Neonate

This chapter provides a critical overview of the literature on human taste and smell function in the prenatal and neonatal periods, with some consideration of later infancy and early childhood, by integrating and updating our previous reviews and those of our colleagues.[1-7]

Taste and smell share a common stimulus class—chemicals. Functionally, taste is intimately connected to the ingestion or rejection of potential foods and perhaps plays a role in the utilization of ingested foods.[8] Smell also contributes to the identification and acceptance of foods and may be involved in regulating human social interactions (e.g., individual and sexual identification and attraction), as it is in many other animals.[9] Flavor, as an attribute of foods and beverages, is defined as the integration of multiple sensory inputs from the gustatory (taste), olfactory (via retronasal olfaction), and trigeminal (touch, temperature, irritation) systems that a substance elicits in the oral and nasal cavities. In particular, retronasal olfaction, the aromas of substances we put in our mouths, contribute significantly to the complexity of flavor, and a discussion of the ontogeny of flavor perception and preferences is highlighted in the section on smell.

Taste and smell have much in common, but there are major differences as well. Most striking are the apparent differences in the ranges of qualitative experiences aroused by these two senses. Although it is still somewhat controversial, most investigators believe that taste is composed of a restricted set of qualities or categories, namely, sweet, salty, sour, and bitter, with umami, the taste associated with monosodium glutamate (MSG), having more recently gained widespread acceptance as a fifth basic taste after the discovery of taste receptors for L-glutamate.[10,11] It has been hypothesized that this small number of qualities evolved because of the functional importance of the primary stimuli (e.g., sugars, sodium chloride, organic acids, bitter toxins, amino acids) in nutrient selection. A practical consequence of this classification scheme in developmental (as well as other) taste research has been to limit the range of stimuli examined.

In contrast, there is no widely accepted classification scheme for smell stimuli, and this situation has resulted in the absence of an agreed-on set of stimuli to use in sensory tests. Thus, olfactory stimulus selection tends to be based on the availability and presumed safety of single compounds or on ecologically significant odor sources that are not chemically specified (e.g., amniotic fluid, mothers' breast odors).

Human studies can provide data relevant to two aspects of chemical sensation: the sensitivity of the system to chemical stimuli and the hedonic valence of the sensation. In studies in adults, the distinction between these two is usually unambiguous. Measures of sensitivity include thresholds, just-noticeable differences, intensity judgments, sensory adaptation, and so forth, whereas measurements involving a hedonic dimension usually consist of ratings of pleasantness or preference. In studies in infants and young children, these two classes of response to chemical stimuli can be more difficult to distinguish. For taste, very few studies have attempted to evaluate sensitivity specifically; almost all response measures are associated with acceptance or rejection and thus presumably involve a hedonic component. Although published developmental studies on olfaction historically focused more on sensitivity and discrimination, more recent studies have also investigated the hedonic aspects of odors.

TASTE

Prenatal Development

Taste receptors or buds are composed of modified epithelial cells and are found throughout the oral cavity, on the hard and soft palates, the tonsils, the pharynx, the larynx, the epiglottis, and the esophagus;[12] however, they are most numerous on the papillae of the tongue. Peripheral innervation of these cells is via branches of three different cranial nerves: the facial (VII), glossopharyngeal (IX), and vagus (X). Four morphologically distinct types of lingual papillae can be identified in humans, but only three bear taste buds. These are the fungiform, the foliate, and the circumvallate papillae. Fungiform papillae are mushroom-shaped buttons found mainly at the tip and along the front edges of the tongue; many of these may contain no taste buds at any given time, but of those with buds, most have one to three.[13] Most taste buds are found in the foliate and circumvallate papillae. The former consist of parallel folds along the rear edges of the tongue; the latter are flat mounds surrounded by a trench on the posterior dorsal border between the oral and pharyngeal tongue (typically 8 to 12 arranged in an inverted V in humans).

Specialized taste cells first appear in the human fetus at 7 to 8 weeks of gestation, and morphologically mature cells are recognizable at 13 to 15 weeks.[14,15] The taste buds of fetal sheep, whose development parallels that observed in the human fetus, have been shown to respond to chemical stimulation as early as the 80th day of gestation.[16,17] Fetal taste receptors may be stimulated by chemicals present in the amniotic fluid. The fetus begins to swallow episodically at about the 12th week of gestation[18] and may swallow 200 to 760 mL/day by term.[19] Amniotic fluid contains glucose, fructose, lactic acid, pyruvic acid, citric acid, fatty acids, phospholipids, creatinine, urea, uric acid, amino acids, polypeptides, proteins, and salts.[20] Moreover, the chemical composition of the amniotic fluid varies over the course of gestation and may be abruptly altered by fetal urination.[16,21] Reported differential fetal swallowing after injections of sweet or bitter substances into the amniotic fluid of pregnant women suggests that fetuses may show a preference for sweet and a rejection of bitter,[20,22] but a strong demonstration of preferential responding by human fetuses to taste stimuli is lacking.

What may the organism gain from *in utero* taste experience? Swallowing amniotic fluid appears to be necessary for the proper development of the gut, but gustatory stimulation is probably not essential.[23] Neural development of the central and peripheral taste systems could be influenced by the intrauterine chemical milieu, such that acceptance and rejection of substances postnatally may coincide with prior amniotic contents and concentrations.[16,24] Animal model studies support this hypothesis.[25]

Direct studies of taste in the preterm infant are rare, partly because of methodologic limitations. As discussed later, in full-term infants, investigators have monitored facial expressions, autonomic responses, consummatory intake, and sucking behavior when the infants are offered flavored solutions. This is problematic for preterm infants who risk fluid aspiration as a result of immature suck-swallow coordination.

To avoid this problem, nonnutritive sucking was studied in preterm infants (33 to 40 weeks after conception) exposed either to brief, intraoral presentations of very small amounts of glucose solution[26] or to sucrose embedded in a nipple-shaped gelatin medium that released small amounts when mouthed or sucked.[28] Both approaches demonstrated that these infants, who had little or no extrauterine taste experience, possessed the ability to detect sweet and showed an avidity for it by producing stronger and more frequent sucking responses than they did when presented with no-taste controls.

This ability on the part of the preterm infant to respond to sweet gustatory stimulation behaviorally, and presumably physiologically, suggests a possible intervention aimed at stimulating these responses to augment development of the infant. In other words, it may be possible that taste stimulation presented during tube feedings would enhance growth efficiency beyond that achieved by allowing infants to suck on a pacifier during this time.[28-32]

Palatable, sweet-tasting stimuli also promote "calming," analgesic-like reactions in preterm, as well as more mature, infants during heelstick and other invasive procedures. When sweet-tasting sugars are present in the oral cavity, crying is reduced, heart rate increases are attenuated, and facial expressions of pain are blunted in preterm infants as young as 25 weeks after conception.[33] Moreover, this analgesic effect appears to be the result of taste *per se*, because the same sweet solution is ineffective in producing analgesia when administered intragastrically in preterm (32- to 36-week) infants.[34]

These studies indicate that not only are taste buds capable of conveying gustatory information to the central nervous system by the last trimester of pregnancy, but also this information is available to systems organizing changes in sucking, facial expressions, and other affective behaviors.

Sensitivity and Discrimination: Newborns

The principal response measures that have been used to assess neonatal taste perception are tongue movements, autonomic reactivity, facial expressions, and differential ingestion and sucking patterns. With one exception, all these responses are believed to reflect preference or acceptance or pleasure. When infants exhibit affective responses to taste stimuli, it can be inferred that they are sensitive to them; however, failure to observe such responses does not indicate whether the infant failed to detect the stimulus or was simply hedonically indifferent to it.

The single, clear exception to hedonically motivated taste responses is the *lateral tongue reflex*.[35,36] This reflex is elicited by the application of microdrops of fluid to the newborn's tongue, and neither its form nor frequency is affected by qualitative changes in the fluid. Thus, the occurrence of the response appears to be solely dependent on sensory mechanisms. Studies using this measure suggest that newborns possess distinct functional taste receptors for sweet and salty; however, differential responding has only been reliably observed with concentrated taste solutions, for example, 2 mol/L salty, which is undoubtedly a trigeminal as well as a gustatory stimulus, producing irritant sensations.[37-39] Consequently, the utility of this response as a measure of absolute gustatory sensitivity is questionable.

Autonomic reactivity may also provide information on gustatory sensitivity. Crook and Lipsitt[40] and Lipsitt[41] published the only modern studies of infant taste perception using such measures, and their research was limited to sweet taste responsivity. In both studies, heart rate was found to be positively correlated with the concentration of sucrose presented to infants. Lipsitt[41] proposed that the heart rate response is a signal of "the joy that the infant derives from [the] 'pleasure of sensation;'" however, the possibility cannot be discounted that the heart rate response reflects arousal rather than pleasure and could provide a measure of gustatory sensitivity, as opposed to preference, in infancy.

Hedonics: Newborns

Facial expressions, suggestive of contentment and liking or discomfort and rejection, were used to assess the newborn's responsiveness to taste stimuli in some of the earliest investigations of human taste development.[42-44] Steiner and colleagues[45-49] reported that consistent, quality-specific facial expressions can be elicited in the first few hours of life by sweet (sucrose, 0.73 mol/L), sour (citric acid, 0.12 mol/L), and bitter (quinine sulfate, 0.003 mol/L) stimuli. Because the stimuli used to elicit these responses were concentrated, differences among the responses to each taste could be at least partially reflective of differences in the extent of trigeminal involvement. In one study, these investigators examined responses to less concentrated taste stimuli and provided data on the frequency of occurrence of specific facial features.[48] High concentrations of tastes (0.0001 mol/L quinine, 1.0 mol/L sucrose, and 0.25 mol/L urea) elicited more responses than the other stimuli (distilled water, 0.1 mol/L sucrose and 0.15 mol/L urea), and the patterns of response to the quinine and more concentrated urea differed from that elicited by 1.0 mol/L sucrose. However, there was considerable overlap in the frequency distributions of facial features elicited by all the stimuli, and responses elicited by the weaker concentrations of sucrose and urea were similar to those observed after water presentations. Finally, infants displayed distinctive positive facial expressions to soup to which MSG was added when compared with unadulterated soup.[49] MSG alone (i.e., in water) did not appear to elicit these facial responses, however, a finding that raised the question of exactly what it is about the soup-MSG mixture that is of apparent positive hedonic valence.

The most detailed study of newborns' facial responses to taste stimuli was conducted by Rosenstein and Oster.[50] Consistent with the findings of Steiner and colleagues,[45-49] analyses of the patterns of full-face expressions indicated that the newborns discriminated sweet from nonsweet solutions and, among nonsweet solutions, between the sour and bitter taste stimuli. However, such analyses also indicated that taste-elicited facial expressions are not highly stereotyped. There appears to be considerable overlap in the distribution of not only discrete facial actions but also full-face configurations elicited by the different taste stimuli, as well as considerable individual variation in facial responses. Moreover, although hedonically negative facial components were more common in responses to all three nonsweet tastes than in

responses to sweet, untrained observers found only the responses to the bitter tastant to be highly negative. Even with their fine-grained analysis and a concentrated salt stimulus (0.73 mol/L), a distinctive facial response to salt was not identified.

Differential ingestion has been used more frequently than any other response to study taste preference during infancy. There are, however, several limitations associated with this measure. First, because multiple stimuli cannot be presented simultaneously to human infants, thereby providing a true choice situation, the measure should probably be viewed as one of relative acceptance rather than of preference. More critically, the number and range of stimulus concentrations that are either feasible or ethical to present to infants in an unrestricted feeding situation are limited. Finally, the strength of the sucking reflex in young infants is quite strong, and this may mitigate against clear rejection of a taste stimulus.

Intake studies have repeatedly demonstrated strong acceptance of sweet tastes by infants at birth and have shown that newborns respond to even dilute sweet tastes and can differentiate between varying degrees of sweetness.[51-53] However, they have generally failed to demonstrate differential responding to sour or bitter tastes, as well as to salt. In the single exception to this generalization, Desor and colleagues[54] used responses to a mild sweet solution rather than plain water as the baseline measurement (ensuring the infants were capable of responding at levels both higher and lower than baseline) and presented salty (NaCl), sour (citric acid), and bitter (urea) tastes in this sweet base. Under these circumstances, relative suppression of intake was observed with the addition of citric acid concentrations at and above 0.003 mol/L, but no significant changes in intake occurred in response to the addition of either NaCl (0.05 to 0.20 mol/L) or urea (0.18 to 0.48 mol/L). The failure to observe rejection of urea (0.12 to 0.24 mol/L) by newborns, even when presented in a sweet base, has been replicated.[55] In the same study, however, significant rejection of all concentrations of urea was observed in slightly older infants (14 to 180 days, with no difference between responses of infants less than or more than 3 months of age), a finding suggesting an early developmental increase in sensitivity to bitterness.

Absence of differential responding to salt in newborns is consistent with results from the studies of facial expression described earlier, but the apparent indifference to bitter is not. Three points should be noted, however. First, for adults, urea is a much less intensive bitter stimulus than quinine and seems to fall into a separate class of bitter stimuli that may be coded by a different receptor mechanism.[56] Second, although 0.25 mol/L urea elicited facial actions that included apparently negative components similar to those elicited by a quinine stimulus, the urea also elicited more apparently positive facial actions, such as sucking and licking, than did the quinine.[48] Third, when taste stimuli are mixed, the intensity of each of the component tastes tends to be suppressed; sour taste intensity may be less susceptible to suppression than the other primary tastes.[57] Thus, the discrepancy among findings concerning bitter responsivity in newborns could partially reflect differences in the type or intensity of bitter stimuli presented.

Finally, the study of sucking patterns has been used as an alternative to the measurement of intake in full-term newborns, as well as premature infants. Techniques for recording multiple parameters of sucking in response to small stimulus volumes can potentially allow for the study of responses to sapid substances one would be reluctant to have infants consume in any quantity. Conversely, the relative significance of individual parameters of the sucking response and the relationships among different parameters are not well understood. Presentation of minute amounts of sweet solution leads to concentration-dependent increases in the number and length of bursts of sucking activity and to decreases in the time between bursts, all of which are intuitively consistent with a positive hedonic reaction and thus with the results of studies using measures of intake and facial expressions,[58, 59] although seemingly paradoxically, the rate of sucking within bursts after sweet stimulation has been found to decrease.[40, 58] Similarly, the number and strength of sucks in response to urea are relatively depressed in infants older than 2 weeks of age, but not newborns, a result paralleling that seen with intake measures (see earlier).[55]

Responses to sour stimuli have not been formally evaluated using this kind of procedure. In the case of salt, however, sucking parameters seem to reveal a subtle response by newborns not evident in measures of intake or facial expression. Crook[59] reported that even a weak salt solution (0.1 mol/L) significantly decreased the length of sucking bursts. Similarly, Beauchamp and associates[60] found that, relative to water, both 0.2 and 0.4 mol/L NaCl significantly depressed the number of sucks and of sucking bursts produced by newborns, although relative intake of the moderately salty solution (0.2 mol/L) was not significantly depressed.[54]

Each of the measures used in studies of taste responses in very young infants has its limitations, but the convergence of results from different measures of sweet taste perception in newborns gives confidence in the conclusion that infants are quite sensitive to this taste and display an innate preference for it. Similarly, even though sour taste perception has been studied less extensively, measures of intake and facial expression suggest that sour taste perception may be reasonably well developed at birth and that newborns reject substances having this taste. The highly concentrated sour stimuli that have been used to elicit facial expressions do, however, pose some interpretive problems, and additional studies of sour taste responsivity are necessary before strong conclusions can be drawn with regard to sour perception in early development.

Neonatal responses to bitter are more problematic. Newborns respond with highly negative facial expressions to concentrated quinine, but not necessarily to urea. They also do not reject moderately strong urea solutions relative to water as assessed by either intake or sucking measures, although significant rejection seems to appear within a few weeks of birth. As noted, there is evidence of multiple bitter taste transduction sequences.[56, 61] In addition, sensitivity to different bitter compounds may be differentially affected by aging.[62] Thus, the early developmental course of bitter taste perception may also be compound specific.

The newborn's response, or lack thereof, to salt is perhaps most puzzling. Given the subtlety of the responses that have been observed, and the evidence for postnatal development of salt taste reception in other mammalian species,[63-66] it seems likely that humans are relatively insensitive to salt at birth. However, to the extent that this stimulus is perceived, the newborn's hedonic response to it appears to be negative.

Hedonics: Older Infants and Young Children

There are relatively few studies of taste perception in older infants and children as compared with neonates, and many of those that have been reported were based on small samples and not described in detail. For all practical purposes, the measures obtained have been limited to intake (i.e., differential ingestion) and paired comparison or rank ordering of taste stimuli to determine preference, and, with few exceptions, only responses to sweet and salty tastes have been assessed.

Babies beyond the neonatal period (1 to 24 months) have been most neglected in studies of taste development. In part, this is probably because of the lack of clearly appropriate measures of either preference or sensitivity for subjects in this age range. Differential ingestion has been the default option in almost all studies. There are, however, certain problems encountered with older infants that do not arise with neonates. For example, older

infants may be less willing to accept unfamiliar bottles or foods from an unfamiliar person, and, as Filer[67] noted, the amount of any particular food eaten in a natural feeding situation may depend as much on the mother's "mechanical skill... and determination to feed her infant" as on the infant's preference. Finally, because intake has been the only measure obtained from older infants, there is no cross-validation of the meaningfulness of this measure. Nonetheless, a few notable findings, suggestive of developmental or experiential changes in taste preferences during infancy, have been reported.

In the context of studies on effects of protein-calorie malnutrition on taste, sucrose, citric acid, urea, and salt acceptability was evaluated in well-nourished and malnourished Mexican infants from 2 months to 2 years of age.[68] Relative to water, infants less than 1 year of age preferentially ingested 0.1 and 0.2 mol/L NaCl. A preference for sucrose was observed for infants at all ages. The bitter (urea, 0.12 and 0.24 mol/L) and sour (citric acid, 0.006 and 0.012 mol/L) stimuli were tested with the same mild sucrose solution as diluent as used by Desor and colleagues[54] (see earlier). Consistent with findings in newborn infants, citric acid was rejected relative to the diluent. Both concentrations of the bitter urea were also rejected by these infants, as was also found by Kajiura and associates[55] in their group of older infants.

In addition to the classic taste stimuli, a sample of Mexican infants was also tested with a mixture of amino acids and peptides (casein hydrolysate) and with MSG.[69] For these two taste substances, a low-glutamate soup was used as the diluent. Consistent with Steiner's report on newborns,[49] both malnourished and well-nourished infants preferred the soup with MSG (0.4%) to the soup alone. This preference was observed even in the youngest infants tested (2- to 4-month-old infants). In contrast, nutritional state influenced responses to the casein hydrolysate. Infants who were malnourished preferred soup with added casein hydrolysate when compared with soup alone; the opposite response was observed in well-nourished infants[68] and in recovered malnourished infants.[69]

Newborn infants have been found to be indifferent to or to reject salt relative to water, whereas Vazquez and colleagues[68] reported that older infants found salt solutions more acceptable than water. This suggestion of a developmental shift in salt acceptability was supported in studies on a sample of children from the United States. Preferential ingestion of salt water relative to plain water emerged at approximately 4 months of age. Beauchamp and associates[70] and Cowart and Beauchamp[71] argued that experience with salty tastes probably does not play a major role in the shift from apparent indifference to (or rejection of) salt at birth to acceptance in later infancy; rather, this change in response may reflect postnatal maturation of central or peripheral mechanisms underlying salt taste perception, allowing for the expression of a largely unlearned preference for saltiness.

Conversely, there is some evidence that, at least by 6 months of age, frequency of dietary exposure to high-sodium foods (although not total dietary sodium) may affect the degree of preference for salted versus unsalted cereal. In a study of 10 6-month-old infants, Harris and Booth[72] determined the difference between the amount of salted cereal eaten during feedings on 2 days and the amount of unsalted cereal eaten on 2 different days and used that as a measure of salt preference. These investigators found relative preference to be significantly correlated with the number of times the infants were exposed to foods containing at least the amount of sodium in the salted cereal during the week preceding testing; none of the infants actually rejected the salted cereal relative to the unsalted one, however, and all but one exhibited some preference for it by consuming more salted than unsalted cereal.

Effects of early experience on the preference for salt taste are also suggested by the finding that 16-week-old infants of mothers who had experienced extreme morning sickness during pregnancy consumed larger volumes of 0.2 mol/L NaCl than did infants whose mothers had not exhibited this symptom.[73] Moreover, adult children (college students) of mothers who experienced considerable morning sickness during their pregnancies had greater salt preferences than did students whose mothers suffered little or no morning sickness.[73, 74] The proposed mechanism is that morning sickness leads to transient fluid and sodium depletion in a manner analogous to that reported in animal model studies. Consistent with these findings, 12- to 14-year-old children who had been exposed to a chloride-deficient formula during early development showed heightened preferences for salty (but not sweet) foods relative to their unexposed sibling controls;[75] chloride deficiency leads to hormonal alterations that mimic those occurring during sodium deficiency.[76]

Similarly, there is evidence of an effect of experience on the expression of sweet preferences in 6-month-old infants.[77] Intake of sweetened versus unsweetened water was assessed in the same infants at birth and at 6 months. Although the infants preferred sweetened water at both ages, only the 6-month-old infants who had received sugared water as part of their diet continued to exhibit the same degree of preference for sweet in water that they had at birth.

Dietary experience—in particular, familiarity with specific foods and with tastes in specific food contexts—has also been shown to play an important role in the preferences of preschool children.[78-81] The other major finding concerning taste preferences in early childhood has been that children prefer more concentrated sugar and salt than do adults, although the bases for these extreme preferences have yet to be elucidated.[71, 82, 83]

SMELL

Prenatal Development

The human olfactory epithelium lines the roof of the nasal cavity, part of the nasal septum and the superior turbinates, and may extend to the middle turbinates. The olfactory receptor cells are bipolar neurons, with dendrites that bear motile cilia lying in a layer of mucus covering the epithelium. The axons of these cells comprise the olfactory nerve (cranial nerve I) and travel in unmyelinated fascicles through the bony roof of the nasal cavity into the olfactory bulb, where they terminate and synapse with second order cells. The nasal cavity is also innervated by the nasopalantine branch of the trigeminal nerve (cranial nerve V), which mediates pain, touch, temperature, and proprioception and whose receptors also respond to many odorous volatiles.

The ethmoid and nasopalantine branches of the trigeminal nerve have differentiated and respond to tactile stimulation by about the 10th gestational week.[84, 85] The olfactory bulbs and receptor cells have attained adult-like morphology by the 11th week of gestation.[86, 87] Olfactory marker protein, which appears to be a biochemical correlate of olfactory receptor functioning in fetal rats,[88] has been identified in the olfactory epithelium of human fetuses at 28 weeks of gestation.[89] Because the epithelial plugs that obstruct the external nares resolve between gestational weeks 16 and 24,[90] there is a continual turnover of amniotic fluid through the nasal passages. Even in air-breathing organisms, volatile molecules must penetrate the aqueous mucus layer covering the olfactory epithelium to reach receptor sites on the cilia. Thus, there is no fundamental distinction between olfactory detection of airborne and water-borne stimuli.

In fact, amniotic fluid provides a natural, ever-changing olfactory, as well as taste, environment for the fetus.[91-95] In particular, the fetus may learn about the dietary choices of the mother through odorants found in the amniotic fluid that derive from foods eaten by the pregnant mother and reflect their flavors. This was demonstrated experimentally in a study in which amniotic fluid samples were obtained from 10 pregnant women who were undergoing routine amniocentesis and who ingested either garlic or placebo capsules approximately 45 minutes before the procedure.[92] The odor of the amniotic fluid obtained from the women who ingested the garlic, as judged by adult human evaluators, was stronger or more like garlic than amniotic fluid from the women who did not consume garlic.

Several lines of evidence suggest that, at around 28 weeks, the olfactory system is capable of detecting chemical stimuli. Studies in premature newborns demonstrated reactions to odorants (odorous chemicals) in infants as young as 28 weeks of gestation.[42, 96, 97] For example, 8 of 11 sleeping preterm infants (29 to 32 weeks) initiated sucking or displayed arousal-withdrawal within 30 seconds of the presentation of a peppermint extract odorant.[98] Although similar responses were observed in one infant who was 28 weeks' gestation, this was not characteristic of other infants (n = 5) that age. All infants younger than 28 weeks of gestational age failed to respond differentially to the peppermint and control trials, whereas all infants between 32 and 36 gestational weeks did.

Although these data appear to support the hypothesis that functional olfaction has its inception around 28 gestational weeks, three caveats must be put forth. First, the failure of infants who were less than 28 weeks' gestation to respond to an odor stimulus in a reliable manner may reflect a response limitation as opposed to an inability to detect the stimulus. In studies of full-term neonates, change in respiratory rate provides a more reliable measure of the ability to detect odorants than motoric responses,[98, 99] and therefore, it may provide a more sensitive test of the preterm infant's ability to detect odorants. Second, it is not clear whether responses in the aforementioned studies were mediated by the olfactory or trigeminal system. Finally, these studies tested only a small subset of odorants, and it is possible that different odorants could elicit responses in younger preterm infants.

Sensitivity and Discrimination: Newborns

Numerous studies have shown that newborn infants can detect and discriminate various qualitatively distinct odorants.[98, 100-109] In one of the earliest controlled studies, Engen and colleagues[98] compared newborns' responses to odor pairs, the members of which varied in intensity and hedonic valence: 100% acetic acid and phenylethyl alcohol (Experiment 1) and anise oil and tincture of asafoetida (Experiment 2). Odors on cotton swabs were presented to infants during sleep, and general activity, leg withdrawal, respiration (Experiments 1 and 2), and heart rate (Experiment 2) were monitored. The investigators concluded that newborns were sensitive to the odors and that they discriminated among them. The most reliable elicitor of a response was acetic acid, followed in descending order by asafoetida, anise, and phenylethyl alcohol. Because the odors were not equated for perceived intensity, it is unclear whether these differences are best accounted for by differences in quality, intensity, hedonicity, or trigeminal component. For example, 100% acetic acid surely stimulates not only the olfactory receptors but also receptors sensitive to irritation in the nose and in the eyes.

Some evidence suggests that the neonate may be remarkably sensitive to other nonbiologic odors, such as the homologous alcohols.[110-112] The observation that preschoolers[113] and prepubescent school-age children[114] are more likely to be sensitive to a biologic odor, androstenone, than are older children and adults, lends further credence to the possibility that newborns' olfactory acuity may equal or exceed that of adults. Finally, comparisons of olfactory neuroepithelium in fetuses and physiologically normal adults reveals degeneration in adults and a higher ratio of olfactory to respiratory epithelium in fetuses.[115]

Nonetheless, Lipsitt and his colleagues[116] suggested that olfactory sensitivity may increase over the first few days of life. They tested 10 infants' responsiveness to increasing concentrations of asafoetida over the first 4 days of life. Because the concentration step required to produce a response, relative to no-odor control trials, decreased for each of the 10 infants over test days, it was concluded that olfactory threshold decreases during the first 4 days of life.

It is not clear whether this change in response is best explained in terms of (1) a stimulus independent postnatal maturation of peripheral or central neural processes including those that may underlie a shift to more nasal—relative to mouth—breathing, (2) the induction of sensitivity contingent on odor exposure, or merely (3) the development of a more coordinated response system. Although the first and third alternatives are probably the most likely, three findings are consistent with the second alternative. First, newborns tested in a longitudinal design over the first 3 days of life showed more reliable respiratory responses to several odors on the third day of testing than did 3-day-old infants who had not received any prior exposure to the odorants.[100] Second, repeated exposure to one odorant (i.e., androstenone) can induce the ability to detect that odorant in adults.[117] Finally, there are changes in the olfactory system of rodents exposed to odors as either neonates[118-121] or adults.[122] These findings are merely suggestive, and human neonatal studies that directly manipulate odor exposure conditions in relation to age and developing olfactory sensitivity are necessary to discriminate among these alternatives.

Certain other aspects of olfactory function have been examined in infants. Engen and associates[98] reported that exposure to an odorant may result in decreased responsiveness to the odor when assessed as a change in respiratory rate. A subsequent study by the same group provided evidence that this phenomenon is best explained in terms of response habituation, as opposed to sensory fatigue.[99] In infants who showed a decrement in response to a mixture of two odorants (anise oil and asafoetida or amyl acetate and heptanol), the response recovered when they were tested with a component of the mixture at the same concentration as in the mixture. Moreover, the magnitude of the recovery was a function of how perceptually similar (as rated by adults) the component was to the mixture, even when the components were equated for perceived intensity. This finding suggests that perceived similarity among odors is much the same in the newborn as in the adult, although it would be premature to endorse this view without demonstrating similar effects with other odorants. The possibility that odor categories are not dependent on either a language system or much experience with odors is intriguing and is worthy of further study. As yet, there is no agreed-on method for categorizing odors, and the extent to which different schemes of categorization are dependent on experience and language is unclear. Studies of odor similarity in infants could aid in determining "basic" categories for odorous chemicals.

The relationship between perceived intensity and molecular structure of homologous alcohols appears to be much the same in adults and newborns. The likelihood of newborns' responding (using change in respiratory rate as a dependent measure) to each in a series of full-strength homologous alcohols (ethanol to decanol) decreases as the chain length increases, in much the same way as the perceived intensity of these alcohols decreases with increased chain length for adults.[112] Although the short chain alcohols elicit the greatest response when tested at full concentration, the long chain alcohols elicit responses more systematically when threshold concentrations are evaluated. Adult psychophysical data suggest an explanation, showing that the effect of dilution on perceived intensity of these alcohols varies as a function of the chain length: for example, a 50% dilution of a long chain alcohol results in a smaller change in perceived intensity than the same dilution of a short chain alcohol.[112] A subsequent study in which newborns' responses were scaled, using degree of general movement as a measure, revealed a similar relationship between intensity functions and alcohol chain length,[111] a finding confirming an essential similarity between olfactory processing in adults and that in newborns.

The ability to localize an odor source appears to be another perceptual capacity of the newborn. Newborns (1 to 5.5 days old) systematically turn their heads away from a source of ammonium hydroxide located to either the right or left of midline, just below the nostrils.[101] As with many of the foregoing phenomena, it is unclear whether this ability is mediated by the olfactory nerve, the trigeminal system, or both, because ammonium hydroxide is a potent stimulant of the trigeminal nerve. Evaluation of neonates' responses to odorants that appear selectively to stimulate the olfactory nerve, such as phenyl ethyl alcohol or vanillin,[123] could help to distinguish among these possibilities.

Finally, several adult studies have demonstrated that exposure to certain olfactory stimuli can inhibit perception of structurally related chemicals. It is presumed that the interaction of the first odor with many of the same receptors responsive to the second results in a decrement in responsiveness to the second odor. Cross-adaptation studies, like similarity judgments, have been taken as a way to explore basic odor categories. The opposite effect, facilitation of one odor by prior exposure to another, is less common but has been reported.[124] Both cross-adaptation and facilitation have also been observed in human neonates,[111, 125] a further indication of the similarity between infant and adult olfactory function.

In addition to studies of newborns' responses to the odors of arbitrarily chosen, single chemical compounds, there is now a growing body of literature characterizing the neonate's response to odors associated with the mother and her amniotic fluid and breast milk. Most of these studies have used preferential orientation as a response measure and are discussed in the following section on odor hedonics. In this context, however, it is worth noting that within hours after birth, infants can recognize their mothers through the sense of smell alone.[102-104,106-109] Like much of the work discussed earlier, this finding suggests exceptional olfactory acuity in the newborn.

Hedonics: Newborns, Older Infants, and Young Children

Given the striking resemblance between the neonate and the adult in sensitivity and discrimination, as outlined earlier, it is somewhat surprising that the origin of hedonic responses to odors has not been unequivocally traced to the neonatal period; in fact, there is substantial controversy on this issue. This is particularly puzzling because hedonic valence is the most salient psychological attribute of an odor for adults,[126] and anatomically, olfactory structures have relatively direct access to brain structures that govern emotion.[127] Moreover, innately determined hedonic reactions to odors could be hypothesized to play a role in mediating components of food selection and social interaction.

The strongest evidence of affective odor reactions in very early infancy comes from neonatal studies of preferential responses to maternal and milk odors, alluded to earlier.[102-104, 106-109] That these maternal odors have both a calming and feeding preparatory effect on the infant is demonstrated by the findings that newborns spend more time orienting toward a breast pad previously worn by their lactating mothers than one worn by an unfamiliar lactating woman,[106] and infants move the head and arms less, mouth more, and cry less during exposure to their mothers' body odors.[106, 128] Moreover, shortly after birth, infants prefer their mothers' breast unwashed as compared with when it is thoroughly washed and is less odorous.[102] Thus, like other mammalian young, the recognition of and preference for maternal odors may play a role in guiding the infant to the nipple area and facilitating early nipple attachment and breast-feeding. Both early experience and genetic determinants may underlie these preferences.

Several findings suggest that newborns' affective reactions to orthonasally presented odors are influenced by experience. First, unlike breast-feeding infants, bottle-fed infants do not preferentially orient toward their mothers' axillary odors when paired with those of either a nonparturient female or an unfamiliar lactating female.[104] Similarly, breast-feeding infants evidence no recognition of or preference for the axillary odors of their own father relative to another father's.[104] Third, 7-day-old, breast-fed newborns turn toward a perfume that has been worn on the mother's breast during feedings in preference to perfumes worn by other mothers.[129, 130] Fourth, after a 20- to 24-hour period of exposure to an artificial odor (wild cherry or ginger) in the ambient air, female newborns less than 2.5 days old turn their heads in the direction of that odorant (presented on a gauze pad) as opposed to an equally pleasant (to adults) but unfamiliar odorant.[105] A similar preferential response to the familiar odor has been observed in both sexes when testing was delayed for 2 weeks after the initial exposure, thus indicating that neonates retained a memory trace of the exposed scent throughout this period.[131]

Studies also indicate that infants' preferences for retronasally presented odors are mediated by experience. Various volatile flavors (e.g., garlic, alcohol, vanilla, carrot, mint) enter human milk via the mother's diet, altering its smell and, presumably, flavor.[132-136] Both garlic[132] and vanilla[135] in the mother's milk stimulate increased sucking and ingestion by the nursing infant. Enhanced sucking is also observed when the flavor of vanilla is added to bottle-fed infants' formula.[135] Repeated consumption of garlic by nursing mothers modifies their infants' response to garlic-flavored milk, eliminating the enhancement in intake (relative to a day on which a bland diet is consumed) that is seen when mothers have maintained a bland diet for a period of time.[111] Thus, in the case of foods, infants' odor or flavor preferences may largely reflect a positive response to novelty or variety in milk flavor.

Experience with flavor cues in amniotic fluid, mother's milk, or both can lead to enhancement of preferences for the flavors of foods eaten by the mother during pregnancy and lactation. First, day-old infants born to mothers who regularly consumed anise-flavored beverages during pregnancy preferred the odor of anise relative to a control odor, whereas those infants whose mothers did not consume anise displayed aversive or neutral facial reactions to this odor.[94] Second, weaning-aged infants, who had had several weeks of exposure to the flavor of carrots in either amniotic fluid or mothers' milk, consumed significantly more of a carrot-flavored cereal and were perceived by their mothers as enjoying the carrot-flavored cereal more than plain cereal.[95] In contrast, control infants, whose mothers avoided carrots during pregnancy and lactation, exhibited no such preference. Thus, these very early flavor experiences may provide the foundation for cultural and ethnic differences in cuisine.

Early experiences may also result in the generation of olfactory memories through associative learning processes, as suggested by a study on children who were between the ages of 3 and 6 years.[137] Children's hedonic responses to the odor of alcohol were related to the emotional context in which parents experience alcohol and the parents' frequency of drinking. In other words, children of a parent or parents who drank alcohol to change their state of mind or to reduce dysphoric feelings ("escape drinking") were significantly more likely to judge the odor of beer as unpleasant than were similarly aged children whose parents did not drink to escape. This difference between the groups was odor specific: children in the two groups were similar in their preference for the bubble gum and rejection of the pyridine odors. These data support the hypothesis that associative learning in the context of emotionally salient conditions is a powerful mechanism by which odors acquire personal significance and that the emotional context in which children experience an odor can influence subsequent behaviors.

Clearly, experience is important in mediating affective and behavioral responses to odors in infancy and childhood. It has even been argued that all odor preferences and aversions are learned through associational learning processes; even the smell of a skunk would be perceived as pleasant if experienced under appropriate conditions.[130, 138] This view is primarily based on several studies that failed to find adult-like odor preference patterns in children less than 5 years of age.[139, 140] For example, 3- to 4-year-old children have been reported to be as likely to say they like the odors of synthetic sweat and feces as they are to say that they like the smell of amyl acetate (resembling banana or pear).[139] Even 6- to 7-year-old children may differ from adults in their hedonic experience of odors. Although adults and 6- to 7-year-old children have been shown to exhibit similar rank-order preferences for odors,[141-143] children this age were less consistent than the adults in (1) selecting preferred odors in a pair-wise comparison paradigm[141] and (2) classifying odors as "liked" or "disliked."[142]

Methodologic difficulties could contribute to these apparent age-related differences. For example, children as old as 4 years tended to answer questions about odors in the affirmative, saying "yes" whether they were asked whether an odor was pleasant or unpleasant.[131] Perhaps some of the foregoing developmental findings, based on opinion polling, reflect this response bias in young children, rather than developmental changes in olfactory preferences. Furthermore, any method relying on sustained attention or placing demands on memory could yield spurious age differences.

Studies employing more age-appropriate methods provide partial support for this hypothesis. Essentially adult-like odor preference patterns were obtained for a set of nine odorants (carvone, phenylethylmethyl carbinol, methyl salicylate, C-16 aldehyde, eugenol, amyl acetate, androstenone, butyric acid, and pyridine) when 3-year-old children were asked to give "good smells" to a likeable television character (Big Bird) and "bad smells" to a grouchy character (Oscar the Grouch).[113] Although children and adults in this study did differ in their distributions of hedonic ratings for some odorants, the similarities outweighed the differences. Using a similar dichotomous forced-choice task in which children pointed to a smiling face or a frowning face to indicate their odor preferences, Strickland and associates[144] also demonstrated adult-like hedonic classifications of two other odorants (benzaldehyde and dimethyl disulfide) in children as young as 3 years. Together, these studies do not support the conclusion that all odor preferences are learned relatively late in the preschool period and suggest experimental reconsideration of the view that some odors may be inherently pleasant or unpleasant.

REFERENCES

1. Beauchamp GK, et al: The role of flavor in infant nutrition. *In* Heird W (ed): Nutrition During the Second Six Months of Life. New York, Raven Press, 1991, pp 35–47.
2. Beauchamp GK, et al: Development of chemosensory sensitivity and preference. *In* Getchell TV, et al (eds): Smell and Taste in Health and Disease. New York, Raven Press, 1991, pp 405–416.
3. Cowart BJ: Development of taste perception in humans: sensitivity and preference throughout the life span. Psychol Bull 90:43, 1981.
4. Cowart BJ, Beauchamp GK: Early development of taste perception. *In* McBride R, MacFie H (eds): Psychological Basis of Sensory Evaluation. London, Elsevier, 1990, pp 1–17.
5. Mennella JA, Beauchamp GK: Olfactory preferences in children and adults. *In* Laing DG, et al (eds): The Human Sense of Smell. New York, Springer-Verlag, 1992, pp 167–180.
6. Schmidt HJ, Beauchamp GK: Human olfaction in infancy and early childhood. *In* Serby M, Chobor K (eds): Science of Olfaction. New York, Springer-Verlag, 1992, pp 378–395.
7. Mennella JA: Taste and smell. *In* Swaiman KF, Ashwall S (eds): Pediatric Neurology: Principles and Practice, 3rd ed. Philadelphia, CV Mosby, 1999, pp 104–113.
8. Brand JG, et al: Taste and nutrition. *In* Rechcigl M Jr (ed): Handbook of Nutritional Requirements in a Functional Context, Vol 2. Boca Raton, FL, CRC Press, 1981, pp 255–282.

9. Holley A: Neural coding of olfactory information. *In* Getchell TV, et al (eds): Smell and Taste in Health and Disease. New York, Raven Press, 1991, pp 329–343.
10. Chaudhari N, et al: A novel metabotropic glutamate receptor functions as a taste receptor. Nat Neurosci *3*:113, 2000.
11. Nelson G, et al: An amino-acid taste receptor. Nature *416*:199, 2002.
12. Parker GH: Smell, Taste and Allied Senses in the Vertebrates. Philadelphia, JB Lippincott, 1922.
13. Arvidson K: Location and variation in number of taste buds in human fungiform papillae. Scand J Dent Res *87*:435, 1979.
14. Bradley RM: Development of the taste bud and gustatory papillae in human fetuses. *In* Bosma JF (ed): The Third Symposium on Oral Sensation and Perception: The Mouth of the Infant. Springfield, IL, Charles C Thomas, 1972, pp 137–162.
15. Bradley RM, Stern IB: The development of the human taste bud during the foetal period. J Anat *101*:743, 1967.
16. Mistretta CM, Bradley RM: Taste *in utero*: Theoretical considerations. *In* Weiffenbach JM (ed): Taste and Development: The Genesis of Sweet Preference. Washington, DC, US Government Printing Office, 1977, pp 51–64.
17. Mistretta CM, Bradley RM: Taste responses in sheep medulla: changes during development. Science *202*:535, 1978.
18. Conel JL: The Postnatal Development of the Human Cerebral Cortex. I. Cortex of the Newborn. Cambridge, MA, Harvard University Press, 1939.
19. Pritchard JA: Deglutition by normal anencephalic fetuses. Obstet Gynecol *25*:289, 1965.
20. Liley AW: Disorders of amniotic fluid. *In* Assali NS (ed): Pathophysiology of Gestation: Fetal Placental Disorders, vol. 2. New York, Academic Press, 1972, pp 157–206.
21. Mistretta CM, Bradley RM: Taste and swallowing *in utero*: a discussion of fetal sensory function. Br Med Bull *31*:80, 1975.
22. DeSnoo K: Das trinkende Kind im Uterus. Monatsschr Geburtshilfe Gynaekol *105*:88, 1937.
23. Mulvihill SJ, et al: The role of amniotic fluid in fetal nutrition. J Pediatr Surg *20*:668, 1985.
24. Hill DL, Mistretta CM: Developmental neurobiology of salt taste sensation. Trends Neurosci *13*:188, 1990.
25. Hill DL, Prezekop PR Jr: Influences of dietary sodium on functional taste receptor development: a sensitive period. Science *241*:1826, 1988.
26. Tatzer E, et al: Discrimination of taste and preference for sweet in premature babies. Early Human Dev *12*:23, 1985.
27. Maone TR, et al: A new method for delivering a taste without fluids to preterm and term infants. Dev Psychobiol *23*:179, 1990.
28. Bernbaum JC, et al: Non-nutritive sucking during gavage feeding enhances growth and maturation in premature infants. Pediatrics *71*:41, 1983.
29. Ernst JA, et al: Lack of improved growth outcome related to non-nutritive sucking in very low birth weight premature infants fed a controlled nutrient intake: a randomized prospective study. Pediatrics *83*:616, 1989.
30. Field T, et al: Non-nutritive sucking during tube feedings: effects on preterm neonates in an intensive care unit. Pediatrics *70*:381, 1982.
31. Measel CP, Anderson GC: Nonnutritive sucking during tube feedings: effect on clinical course in premature infants. J Obstet Gynecol Neonatal Nursing *8*:265, 1979.
32. Mattes RD, et al: Effects of sweet taste stimulation on growth and sucking in preterm infants. J Obstet Gynecol Neonatal Nursing *25*:407, 1996.
33. Johnston CC, et al: Effectiveness of oral sucrose and simulated rocking on pain response in preterm neonates. Pain *72*:193, 1997.
34. Ramenghi LA, et al: Effect of non-sucrose sweet tasting solution on neonatal heel prick responses. Arch Dis Child *74*:129, 1996.
35. Weiffenbach JM, Thach BT: Elicited tongue movements: touch and taste in the newborn human. *In* Bosma JF (ed): Fourth Symposium on Oral Sensation and Perception: Development in the Fetus and Infant. Washington, DC, US Government Printing Office, 1973, pp 232–244. 33
36. Weiffenbach JM: Sensory mechanisms of the newborn's tongue. *In* Weiffenbach JM (ed): Taste and Development: The Genesis of Sweet Preference. Washington, DC, US Government Printing Office, 1977, pp 205–216.
37. Abrahams H, et al: Gustatory adaptation to salt. Am J Psychol *49*:462, 1937.
38. Kawamura Y, et al: A role of oral afferents in aversion to taste solutions. Physiol Behav *3*:537, 1968.
39. Green BG, Gelhard B: Salt as an oral irritant. Chem Senses *14*:173, 1989.
40. Crook CK, Lipsitt LP: Neonatal nutritive sucking: effects of taste stimulation upon sucking and heart rate. Child Devel *47*:518, 1976.
41. Lipsitt LP: Taste in human neonates: its effect on sucking and heart rate. *In* Weiffenbach JM (ed): Taste and Development: The Genesis of Sweet Preference. Washington, DC, US Government Printing Office, 1977, pp 125–142.
42. Peterson F, Rainey LH: The beginnings of mind in the newborn. Bull Lying-In Hosp *7*:99, 1910–1911.
43. Preyer W: The mind of the child. Brown HW (trans). New York, Appleton, 1901 (originally published, 1882).
44. Shinn MW: The Biography of a Baby. New York, Houghton Mifflin, 1900.
45. Steiner JE: The gustofacial response: observation on normal and anencephalic newborn infants. *In* Bosma JF (ed): Fourth Symposium on Oral Sensation and Perception: Development in the Fetus and Infant. Washington, DC, US Government Printing Office, 1973, pp 254–278.
46. Steiner JE: Facial expressions of the neonate infant indicating the hedonics of food-related chemical stimuli. *In* Weiffenbach JM (ed): Taste and Development: The Genesis of Sweet Preference. Washington, DC, US Government Printing Office, 1977, pp 173–189.
47. Steiner JE: Human facial expression in response to taste and smell stimulation. *In* Reese H, Lipsitt, LP (eds): Advances in Child Development and Behavior, Vol 13. New York, Academic Press, 1979, pp 257–295.
48. Ganchrow JR, et al: Neonatal facial expressions in response to different qualities and intensities of gustatory stimuli. Infant Behav Dev *6*:473, 1983.
49. Steiner JE: What the neonate can tell us about umami. *In* Kawamura Y, Kare MR (eds): Umami: A Basic Taste. New York, Marcel Dekker, 1987, p 97.
50. Rosenstein D, Oster H: Differential facial responses to four basic tastes in newborns. Child Dev *59*:1555, 1988.
51. Desor JA, et al: Taste in acceptance of sugars by human infants. J Comp Physiol Psychol *84*:496, 1973.
52. Desor JA, et al: Preference for sweet in humans: infants, children and adults. *In* Weiffenbach JM (ed): Taste and Development: The Genesis of Sweet Preference. Washington, DC, US Government Printing Office, 1977, pp 161–172.
53. Maller O, Desor JA: Effects of taste on ingestion by human newborns. *In* Bosma JF (ed): Fourth Symposium on Oral Sensation and Perception: Development in the Fetus and Infant. Washington, DC, US Government Printing Office, 1973, pp 279–291.
54. Desor JA, et al: Ingestive responses of human newborns to salty, sour and bitter stimuli. J Comp Physiol Psychol *89*:966, 1975.
55. Kajiura H, et al: Dearly developmental change in bitter taste responses in human infants. Dev Psychobiol *25*:375, 1992.
56. McBurney DH, et al: Gustatory cross-adaptation: sourness and bitterness. Percept Psychophys *11*:228, 1972.
57. Bartoshuk LM: Taste mixtures: is suppression related to compression? Physiol Behav *14*:643, 1975.
58. Crook CK: Modification of the temporal organization of neonatal sucking by taste stimulation. *In* Weiffenbach JM (ed): Taste and Development: The Genesis of Sweet Preference. Washington, DC, US Government Printing Office, 1977, pp 146–160.
59. Crook CK: Taste perception in the newborn infant. Infant Behav Dev *1*:52, 1978.
60. Beauchamp GK, et al: Infant salt taste: developmental, methodological, and contextual factors. Dev Psychobiol *27*:353, 1994.
61. Chandrashekar J, et al: T2Rs function as bitter taste receptors. Cell *100*:703, 2000.
62. Cowart BJ, et al: Bitter taste in aging: compound-specific decline in sensitivity. Physiol Behav *56*:1237, 1994.
63. Ferrel MF, et al: Development of chorda tympani taste responses in the rat. J Comp Neurol *198*:37, 1981.
64. Hill DL, Almli CR: Ontogeny of chorda tympani responses to gustatory stimuli in the rat. Brain Res *197*:27, 1980.
65. Hill DL, et al: Developmental changes in taste response characteristics of rat single chorda tympani fibers. J Neurosci *2*:782, 1982.
66. Mistretta CM, Bradley RM: Neural basis of developing salt taste sensation: response changes in fetal, postnatal and adult sheep. J Comp Neurol *215*:199, 1983.
67. Filer LJ: Studies of taste preference in infancy and childhood. Pediatr Basics *12*:5, 1978.
68. Vazquez M, et al: Flavor preferences in malnourished Mexican infants. Physiol Behav *28*:513, 1982.
69. Beauchamp GK, et al: Dietary status of human infants and their sensory responses to amino acid flavor. *In* Kawamura Y, Kare MR (eds): Umami: A Basic Taste. New York, Marcel Dekker, 1987, pp 125–138.
70. Beauchamp GK, et al: Development changes in salt acceptability in human infants. Dev Psychol *19*:17, 1986.
71. Cowart BJ, Beauchamp GK: Factors affecting acceptance of salt by human infants and children. *In* Kare MR, Brand JG (eds): Interaction of the Chemical Senses with Nutrition. New York, Academic Press, 1986, pp 25–44.
72. Harris G, Booth DA: Infants' preference for salt in food: its dependence upon recent dietary experience. Reprod Infant Psychol *5*:97, 1987.
73. Crystal SR, Bernstein IL: Infant salt preference and mother's morning sickness. Appetite *30*:297, 1998.
74. Crystal SR, Bernstein IL: Morning sickness: impact on offspring salt preference. Appetite *25*:231, 1995.
75. Stein LJ, et al: Increased liking for salty foods in adolescents exposed during infancy to chloride-deficient feeding formula. Appetite *27*:65, 1996.
76. Simopoulos AP, Bartter FC: The metabolic consequences of chloride deficiency. Nutr Rev *38*:201, 1980.
77. Beauchamp GK, Moran M: Dietary experience and sweet taste preference in human infants. Appetite *3*:139, 1982.
78. Birch LL: Dimensions of preschool children's food preferences. J Nutr Ed *11*:77, 1979.
79. Birch LL, Marlin DW: I don't like it; I never tried it: effects of exposure on two-year-old children's food preferences. Appetite *3*:353, 1982.
80. Beauchamp GK, Moran M: Acceptance of sweet and salty tastes in 2-year-old children. Appetite *5*:291, 1985.
81. Cowart BJ, Beauchamp GK: The importance of sensory context in young children's acceptance of salty tastes. Child Dev *57*:1034, 1986.
82. Beauchamp GK, Cowart BJ: Development of sweet taste. *In* Dobbing J (ed): Sweetness. London, Springer-Verlag, 1987, pp 127–140.

83. Beauchamp GK, Cowart BJ: Preference for high salt concentrations among children. Dev Psychol 26:539, 1990.

84. Hogg ID: Sensory nerves and associated structures in the skin of human fetuses of 8 to 14 weeks of menstrual age correlated with functional capability. J Comp Neurol 75:371, 1941.

85. Hooker D: The Prenatal Origin of Behavior. Lawrence, KS, University of Kansas Press, 1952.

86. Humphrey, T: The development of the olfactory and the accessory olfactory formations in human embryos and fetuses. J Comp Neurol 73:431, 1940.

87. Pyatkina GA: Development of the olfactory epithelium in man. Z Mikrosk Anat Forsch (Leipzig) 96:361, 1982.

88. Gesteland RC, et al: Development of olfactory receptor neuron selectivity in the rat fetus. Neuroscience 7:3127, 1982.

89. Chuah MI, Zheng DR: Olfactory marker protein is present in olfactory receptor cells of human fetuses. Neuroscience 23:363, 1987.

90. Schaffer JP: The lateral wall of the cavum nasi in man with special reference to the various developmental stages. J Morphol 21:613, 1910.

91. Hauser GJ, et al: Peculiar odors in newborns and maternal pre-natal ingestion of spicy foods. Eur J Pediatr 44:403, 1985.

92. Mennella JA, et al: Garlic ingestion by pregnant women alters the odor of amniotic fluid. Chem Senses 20:207, 1995.

93. Hepper P: Human fetal olfactory learning. Int J Prenatal Perinatal Psychol 2:147, 1995.

94. Schaal B, et al: Human foetuses learn odours from their pregnant mother's diet. Chem Senses 25:729, 2000.

95. Mennella JA, et al: Pre- and post-natal flavor learning by human infants. Pediatrics 107:88, 2001.

96. Sarnat HB: Olfactory reflexes in the newborn infant. J Pediatr 92:624, 1978.

97. Kussmaul A: Untersuchungen über das Seelenleben des Neugenborenen Menschen. Tubigen, Moser, 1859.

98. Engen T, et al: Olfactory responses and adaptation in the human neonate. J Comp Physiol Psychol 56:73, 1963.

99. Engen T, Lipsitt LP: Decrement and recovery of responses to olfactory stimuli in the human neonate. J Comp Physiol Psychol 59:312, 1965.

100. Self PAF, et al: Olfaction in newborn infants. Dev Psychol 7:349, 1972.

101. Reiser J, et al: Radial localization of odors by human newborns. Child Dev 47:856, 1976.

102. MacFarlane A: Olfaction in the development of social preferences in the human neonate. Ciba Found Symp 33:103, 1975.

103. Russell MJ: Human olfactory communication. Nature 260:520, 1976.

104. Cernoch JM, Porter RH: Recognition of maternal axillary odors by infants. Child Dev 56:1593, 1985.

105. Balogh RD, Porter RH: Olfactory preferences resulting from mere exposure in human neonates. Infant Behav Dev 9:395, 1986.

106. Schaal B: Presumed olfactory exchanges between mother and neonate in humans. In Le Camus J, Conier J (eds): Ethol Psychol. Privat-IEC, Toulouse, 1986, pp 101–110.

107. Porter RH, et al: Breast-fed infants respond to olfactory cues from their own mother and unfamiliar lactating females. Infant Behav Dev 15:85, 1992.

108. Schaal B. et al: Olfactory function in the human fetus: evidence from selective neonatal responsiveness to the odor of amniotic fluid. Behav Neurosci 112:1438, 1998.

109. Varendi H, et al: Does the newborn baby find the nipple by smell? Nature 344:989, 1994.

110. Rovee CK: Olfactory cross-adaptation and facilitation in human neonates. J Exp Child Psychol 13:368, 1972.

111. Rovee CK: Psychophysical scaling of olfactory response to the aliphatic alcohols in human neonates. J Exp Child Psychol 7:245, 1969.

112. Engen T: Psychophysical analysis of the odor intensity of homologous alcohols. J Exp Psychol 70:611, 1965.

113. Schmidt HJ, Beauchamp GK: Adult-like odor preferences and aversions in 3-year-old children. Child Dev 59:1136, 1988.

114. Dorries KM, et al: Changes in sensitivity to the odor of androsterone during adolescence. Dev Psychobiol 22:423, 1989.

115. Nakashima T, et al: Structure of human fetal and adult olfactory neuroepithelium. Arch Otolaryngol 110:641, 1984.

116. Lipsitt LP, et al: Developmental changes in the olfactory threshold of the neonate. Child Devel 34:371, 1963.

117. Wysocki CJ, et al: Ability to smell androstenone can be acquired by ostensibly asnomic people. Proc Natl Acad Sci USA 86:7976, 1989.

118. Wilson DA, et al: Odor familiarity alters mitral cell response in the olfactory bulb of neonatal rats. Dev Brain Res 22:314, 1985.

119. Woo CC, Leon M: Sensitive period for neural and behavioral response development to learned odors. Dev Brain Res 36:309, 1987.

120. Sullivan RM, et al: Good memories of bad events in infancy. Nature 7:38, 2000.

121. Woo CC, et al: Localized changes in olfactory bulb morphology associated with early olfactory learning. J Comp Neurol 263:113, 1987.

122. Wang H-W, et al: Induction of olfactory receptor sensitivity in mice. Science 260:998, 1993.

123. Doty RL, et al: Intranasal trigeminal stimulation from odorous volatiles: psychometric responses from anosmic and normal humans. Physiol Behav 20:175, 1978.

124. Corbit T, Engen T: Facilitation of olfactory detection. Percept Psychophys 10:433, 1971.

125. Engen T, Bosack TN: Facilitation in olfactory perception. J Comp Physiol Psychol 68:320, 1969.

126. Schiffman S: Physicochemical correlates of olfactory quality. Science 185:112, 1974.

127. Kandel ER, Schwartz JH: Principles of Neural Science. New York, Elsevier, 1985.

128. Sullivan RM, Toubas P: Clinical usefulness of maternal odor in newborns: soothing and feeding preparatory responses. Biol Neonate 74:402, 1998.

129. Schleidt M, Genzel C: The significance of mother's perfume for infants in the first weeks of their life. Ethiol Sociobiol 11:145, 1990.

130. Engen T: The acquisition of odour hedonics. In Van Toller S, Dodd GH (eds): Perfumery: The Psychology and Biology of Fragrance. London, New York, Chapman & Hall, 1988.

131. Davis LB, Porter RH: Persistent effects of early odor exposure on human neonates. Chem Senses 16:169, 1991.

132. Mennella JA, Beauchamp GK: Maternal diet alters the sensory qualities of human milk and the nursling's behavior. Pediatrics 88:737, 1991.

133. Mennella JA, Beauchamp GK: The effects of repeated exposure to garlic-flavored milk on the nursling's behavior. Pediatr Res 34:805, 1993.

134. Mennella JA, Beauchamp GK: The transfer of alcohol to human milk: effects on flavor and the infant's behavior. N Engl J Med 325:981, 1991.

135. Mennella JA, Beauchamp GK: The human infant's response to vanilla flavors in mother's milk and formula. Infant Behav Dev 19:13,1996.

136. Mennella JA, Beauchamp GK: Smoking and the flavor of breast milk. N Engl J Med 339:1559, 1998.

137. Mennella JA, Garcia PL: The child's hedonic response to the smell of alcohol: effects of parental drinking habits. Alcohol Clin Exp Res 24:1167, 2000.

138. Engen T: The Perception of Odors. New York, Academic Press, 1982.

139. Stein M, et al: A study of the development of olfactory preferences. AMA Arch Neurol Psychiatry 80:264, 1958.

140. Peto E: Contribution to the development of smell feeling. Br J Med Psychol 15:314, 1986.

141. Engen T: Method and theory in the study of odor preferences. In Johnston J, et al (eds): Human Response to Environmental Odors. New York, Academic Press, 1974, pp 121–141.

142. Kniep EH, et al: Studies in affective psychology. Am J Psychol 43:406, 1931.

143. Moncreiff RW: Odour Preferences. London, Leonard Hill, 1966.

144. Strickland M, et al: A procedure for obtaining young children's reports of olfactory stimuli. Percept Psychophys 44:379, 1988.

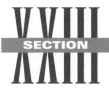

178

Bulent Erol, Kathrin V. Halpern, and John P. Dormans

The Growth Plate: Embryologic Origin, Structure, and Function

Bone formation and skeletal growth constitute a fascinating process of unique morphologic and biochemical changes that occur during fetal development and are capitulated on a daily basis throughout adolescent development. During development, bone tissue may grow or form directly from mesenchymal tissue (intramembraneous ossification), or it may form from replacement of a cartilaginous model (endochondral ossification). Intramembraneous bone formation occurs at the periosteal surfaces of all bones and in parts of the pelvis, scapula, clavicles, and skull. Alternately, endochondral ossification occurs at the base of the skull, the vertebrae, and the appendicular skeleton. It is not clear why certain bones preform in cartilage and others in membrane.

Cartilage, in contrast to bone tissue, may continue to grow interstitially. Such proliferating cartilage constitutes the basis for much of the size increase of bones as organs. In the long bones of the limbs, the proliferating cartilage is located at the ends and may be referred to as a *growth plate* or *physis*. Growth plate cartilage is unlike hyaline or articular cartilage because of its unique blood supply, zonal structure, biochemistry, and process of matrix mineralization. Proliferating cartilage of different configurations is located in the skull (sutures and the base), the spine (end plates and synchondroses), the pelvis (triradiate cartilages), and the carpus and tarsus. A discussion of the growth plate, however, usually focuses on the structure of a typical long bone growth plate such as the distal femur or proximal tibia because of its highly organized histology and great activity.

DEVELOPMENT OF THE GROWTH PLATE

Limb development has been studied in various organisms. Chick studies provided a wealth of information in the past because of the accessibility of the limb bud *in ovo*. However, molecular studies have focused largely on the mouse embryo. Cross-species transplants have indicated that many of the same signals control limb formation in both organisms. Additional information about limb patterning has been derived from the study of regenerating amphibian limbs.

In all vertebrates, the formation of the developing limb bud is initiated by the mesenchyme. Two sources of mesenchyme contribute to the formation of the limb: somites give rise to all the limb muscle cells, whereas cells from the lateral plate mesoderm give rise to connective tissue and cartilage.[1,2] Of these two cell populations, it is the connective tissue-cartilage precursors that

determine the primary limb pattern. In the absence of somites, the lateral plate mesoderm forms a limb with normal skeletal structure and tendons, but devoid of any musculature.

During the fourth week of gestation, the embryonic limb bud formation is initiated by the lateral plate mesoderm as a small projection on the ventrolateral body wall (Fig. 178-1).[3] There is a craniocaudal time gradient, with the upper limb bud appearing and progressing slightly ahead (1 to 2 days) of the lower limb bud. However, the events in upper and lower limb buds are similar in character and sequence. This mesenchymal projection is covered by ectoderm, the tip of which thickens and becomes the *apical ectodermal ridge* (AER) (see Fig. 178-1). Underlying the AER are rapidly proliferating, undifferentiated mesenchymal cells that are called the *progress zone* (PZ). Proliferation of these cells causes limb outgrowth. The interaction between the AER and the undifferentiated mesenchymal cells underlying it is crucial for limb development. When all limb elements have differentiated, the AER disappears.

As the limb bud grows, it develops asymmetries along the proximodistal (flank to digit tip), anteroposterior (thumb to small finger), and dorsoventral (back of hand to palm) axes (Fig. 178-2). These three major limb axes appear to be set up at different times and by different mechanisms. Some of the important signals for initiating and maintaining these axes have been worked out in detail. The genes that initiate and potentiate signals in different axes often interact and feed back, resulting in effects that are not confined to one direction of growth.

Limb Bud Outgrowth and Proximodistal Patterning

Limb bud development is dependent on signals emanating from the AER; removal of the AER stops limb bud growth and leads to limb truncation, or a graft of an AER to an ectopic site on the bud leads to extra limb growth in the ectopic location. Limb bud outgrowth can be sustained after excision of the AER, by insertion of beads carrying fibroblast growth factors (FGFs) FGFs comprise a group of similar proteins that affect cell proliferation, differentiation, and motility. FGF-2, FGF-4, and FGF-8 are expressed in the AER, and each is able to sustain limb bud outgrowth.[4,5] FGF-10 and FGF-8 are the critical FGFs expressed during the initiation of limb bud outgrowth, and the expression of each supports and promotes the expression of the other.[6] It was shown that WNT-2b (*Wnt*; mammalian homolog of drosophila segment

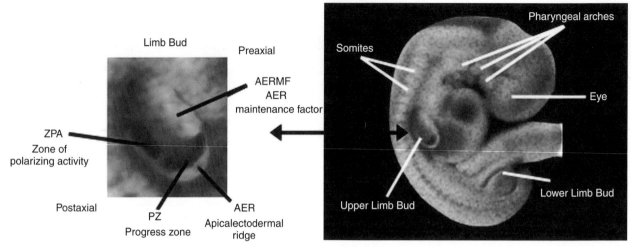

Figure 178–1. A 5-week-old human embryo and enlargement of the upper and lower limb buds. The limb bud at this time is a jacket of ectoderm (AER; apical ectodermal ridge) covering undifferentiated mesenchymal cells (PZ; progress zone). The zone of polarizing activity (ZPA), which is involved in anteroposterior patterning of the limb, is localized in a small area of mesoderm along the posterior border of the limb bud.

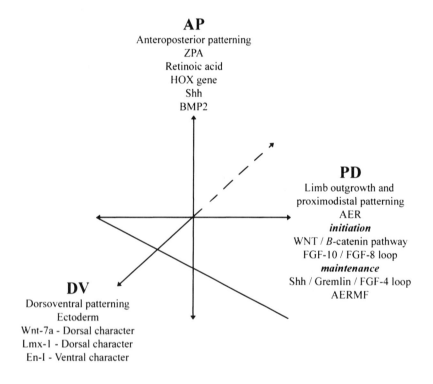

AP
Anteroposterior patterning
ZPA
Retinoic acid
HOX gene
Shh
BMP2

PD
Limb outgrowth and
proximodistal patterning
AER
initiation
WNT / *B*-catenin pathway
FGF-10 / FGF-8 loop
maintenance
Shh / Gremlin / FGF-4 loop
AERMF

DV
Dorsoventral patterning
Ectoderm
Wnt-7a - Dorsal character
Lmx-1 - Dorsal character
En-1 - Ventral character

AER (apical ectodermal ridge); Wnt (wingless); FGF (fibroblast growth factor); Shh (sonic hedgehog); AERMF (AER maintenance factor), ZPA (zone of polarizing activity); HOX (homeobox-containing gene); BMP (bone morphogenic protein); En (engrailed)

Figure 178–2. Three major limb axes. As the limb bud grows, it develops asymmetries along the proximodistal (PD), anteroposterior (AP), and dorsoventral (DV) axes. The genes encoding the important signals that initiate and maintain these axes often interact and feed back, resulting in effects that are not confined to one direction of growth. AER = apical ectodermal ridge; AERMF = AER maintenance factor; BMP = bone morphogenic protein; En = engrailed; *Fgf* = fibroblast growth factor; *Hox* = homeobox-containing gene; *Shh* = sonic hedgehog; *Wnt* = wingless; ZPA = zone of polarizing activity.

polarity gene-wingless) and WNT-8c proteins, through β-catenin (WNT/β-catenin pathway), mediate the FGF-8/FGF-10 loop that controls limb initiation.[7]

A protein called sonic hedgehog (*shh*) seems to act in a regulatory loop with FGFs expressed in the AER to maintain cell growth and proliferation in the mesenchyme and to maintain the integrity of the AER. The formin gene, which encodes several proteins thought to function as cytokines, is required to establish this Shh/FGF-4 feedback loop. Studies have implicated bone

morphogenic proteins (BMPs), members of the transforming growth factor-β (TGF-β) superfamily, in the negative regulation of the AER. The formin gene appears to interact with a BMP antagonist, gremlin, in the regulation of the Shh/FGF-4 feedback loop.[8] The existence of an AER maintenance factor was proposed based on classic embryologic studies in the chick embryo. It has been proposed that FGF-10 may be the AER maintenance factor, because it can induce both FGF-8 expression and thickening of nonridge ectoderm.[8]

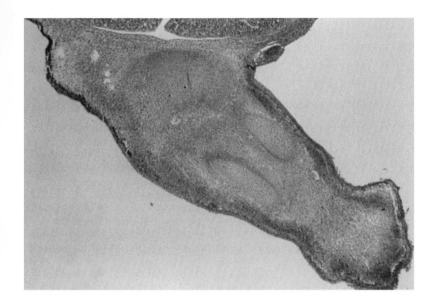

Figure 178-3. Longitudinal section of the developing hindlimb from a 13-day mouse embryo (H&E, ×40). Mesenchymal condensations of the skeletal anlagen have begun to form. (From Zaleske DJ: The growth plate: embryologic origin, structure, and function. *In* Polin RA, et al [eds]: Fetal and Neonatal Physiology, 2nd ed. Philadelphia, WB Saunders Co, 1998, pp 2351-2359.)

Anteroposterior Axis Determination

Anteroposterior axis determination is under the control of an area of tissue in the posterior aspect of the limb bud called the *zone of polarizing activity* (ZPA) (see Fig. 178-1). The experiments initially suggested that a morphogenic gradient of a diffusible signal originating from the ZPA determines the anteroposterior axis. Although early studies showed that exogenous application of retinoic acid to the anterior border of a normal limb could mimic results from ZPA transplant studies,[9] retinoic acid is not a simple morphogen acting through a gradient. It appears that retinoic acid acts by regulating the cells that can express SHH protein.[10] It is likely that a homeobox-containing (*HOX*) gene is an intermediate that is stimulated by retinoic acid, and its expression specifies the Shh-expressing cells. SHH stimulates the gene for BMP2.

Dorsoventral Axis Determination

The dorsoventral axis is under the control of both the mesoderm and ectoderm of the limb bud at different stages of development. The mesoderm specifies the axis initially, but very early after limb bud formation, the ectodermal orientation becomes prominent. Evidence suggests that WNT-7a, a secreted signaling protein, confers the dorsal character to the ectoderm and stimulates Lmx-1.[11] Lmx-1 is a *HOX* gene that encodes a transcription factor (LMX-1) that dorsalizes mesoderm. The ventral limb expresses a transcription factor called *engrailed* (EN-1), which appears to suppress Wnt-7a expression, thereby limiting the activity of LMX-1 to the dorsal mesenchyme.[12]

Both the AER and the ZPA activate *HOXA* and *HOXD* genes. *HOX* genes have specifically been shown to affect the growth of cartilage and precartilaginous condensations. They may be important in determining the length, segmentation, and branching of limb elements. *HOX* genes are not expressed strictly along anteroposterior or dorsoventral axes, and their position of expression differs in various areas of the limb.

Bone and Growth Plate Development

The first sign of future potential bone formation occurs in the early embryonic period as a localized condensation of the mesenchyme. Cellular condensations may arise as a result of either increased mitotic activity or an aggregation of cells drawn toward a specific site.[13] As the mesenchyme begins to condense, the cells become more rounded, concomitant with a reduction in the amount of intercellular substance. This stage is referred to as the *precartilage blastema*. As the tissue continues to mature, the mesenchymal condensations differentiate into chondrocytes that form a template, or anlagen (skeletal anlagen), of the future bone (Fig. 178-3). This transformation occurs during the sixth week of gestation. The expression of some specific molecular markers, such as aggrecan and Type II collagen, distinguishes differentiating chondrocytes from the undifferentiated mesenchymal cells remaining at the periphery of the skeletal element that form a structure called the *perichondrium*.[14] During the seventh week of gestation, the innermost chondrocytes of the anlagen further differentiate into hypertrophic chondrocytes. At the same time as the chondrocyte hypertrophy, perichondrial cells start to differentiate into osteoblasts to form, around the cartilaginous core, a mineralized structure, termed the *bone collar*.[15] Once fully differentiated, hypertrophic chondrocytes become surrounded by a calcified extracellular matrix that favors, through a vascular endothelial growth factor–dependent pathway, vascular invasions from the bone collar. This process brings in chondroblasts that will degrade the extracellular matrix surrounding the hypertrophic chondrocytes and provides progenitors of osteoblasts derived from the bone collar.[16] The osteoblasts produce an osteoid matrix on the surfaces of the calcified cartilaginous bars and form the primary trabeculae; and this process is called *endochondral ossification*. This initial site of ossification is known as the *primary ossification center*, and most of these appear in the late fetal period (Fig. 178-4).

This sequential process of chondrocyte proliferation, hypertrophy, and replacement by osteoblasts becomes organized into the growth plate at each end of the expanding bone. The growth plates are apposed to the metaphyses at either end of the long bone. The histologic elements of the growth plate are well defined. Chondrocyte division is well organized into zones that can be demonstrated autoradiographically using tritiated thymidine.[17-19] Once the growth plate has been formed, longitudinal growth of the bone occurs by appositional growth of cells from within the growth plate, and new bone is formed in the metaphyseal side of each growth plate through a process that recapitulates the stages that occurred in the central portion of the original cartilaginous anlage. The rate at which this growth occurs is different at different anatomic positions; proliferating cartilage is arranged differently at different anatomic locations.[20]

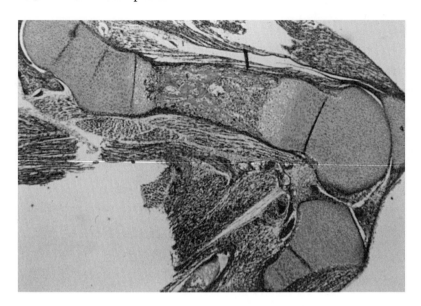

Figure 178–4. Longitudinal section of the femur and proximal tibia from an 18-day mouse fetus (H&E, ×40). The primary center of ossification has formed at the midshaft of the femur. The proximal (*left,* hip) and distal (*right,* knee) chondroepiphyses are visible, as are part of the cartilaginous patella and the proximal tibial chondroepiphysis. (From Zaleske DJ: The growth plate: embryologic origin, structure, and function. *In* Polin RA, et al [eds]: Fetal and Neonatal Physiology, 2nd ed. Philadelphia, WB Saunders Co, 1998, pp 2351–2359.)

This process continues until closure of the growth plates at skeletal maturity.

At specific times in the postnatal development of each long bone, a secondary center of ossification (epiphysis) forms at the end of each bone. The secondary center of ossification is another zone of proliferating cartilage beneath the articular cartilage and is responsible for growth of the chondroepiphysis cartilage surrounding the epiphysis (Fig. 178–5).[21] The processes of chondrocyte proliferation and hypertrophy, matrix calcification, vascular invasion, and osteoblastic new bone formation occur in the same sequence as in the growth plate associated with the primary ossification center. However, the epiphyseal end of the long bone enlarges as a result of radial apposition of cells around the secondary ossification center.

Molecular Biology of Chondrocyte Differentiation

To divide chondrocytes into two subgroups, nonhypertrophic (resting and proliferating) and hypertrophic, is helpful to understand their differentiation processes. Several growth factors have been demonstrated to control nonhypertrophic chondrocyte differentiation *in vivo.* FGF receptor-3 (FGFR3) is expressed in proliferating chondrocytes of the growth plate, and it functions to restrain chondrocyte division (negative regulatory effect).[22] Indian hedgehog (Ihh), a mammalian homologue of the *Drosophila* hedgehog, is another factor regulating nonhypertrophic chondrocyte proliferation. The studies have shown the marked decrease in nonhypertrophic chondrocyte proliferation in Ihh-deficient mice.[15] An interesting link between the Ihh pathway and the FGF pathway is indicated by data showing that FGFR3 signaling can inhibit Ihh expression.[22]

The hypertrophic chondrocytes comprise two subpopulations: the prehypertrophic chondrocytes and the fully differentiated hypertrophic chondrocytes. Parathyroid hormone (PTH)–related peptide (PTHrP) binds to the PTH/PTHrP receptor present in prehypertrophic chondrocytes, and it plays a critical role in regulating hypertrophic chondrocyte differentiation. PTHrP expression is under the control of Ihh; Ihh upregulates the synthesis of PTHrP by prehypertrophic chondrocytes, thereby indirectly slowing down the process of chondrocyte hypertrophy.[15] Wnt signaling also plays an important role in the regulation of hypertrophic chondrocyte biology. Studies have shown that misexpression of Wnt-4 accelerates the nonhypertrophic to hypertrophic transition and results in slightly advanced ossification, whereas misexpression of Wnt-5a causes a delay in the transition from prehypertrophic to hypertrophic

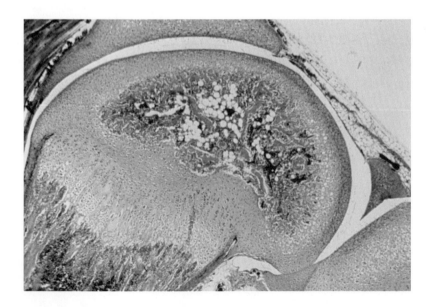

Figure 178–5. Longitudinal section of the distal femur from a 10-day postnatal mouse (H&E, ×40). The secondary center of ossification has now formed within the distal femoral chondroepiphysis. The growth plate or physis is clearly defined between the secondary center of ossification and the metaphysis. (From Zaleske DJ: The growth plate: embryologic origin, structure, and function. *In* Polin RA, et al [eds]: Fetal and Neonatal Physiology, 2nd ed. Philadelphia, WB Saunders Co, 1998, pp 2351–2359.)

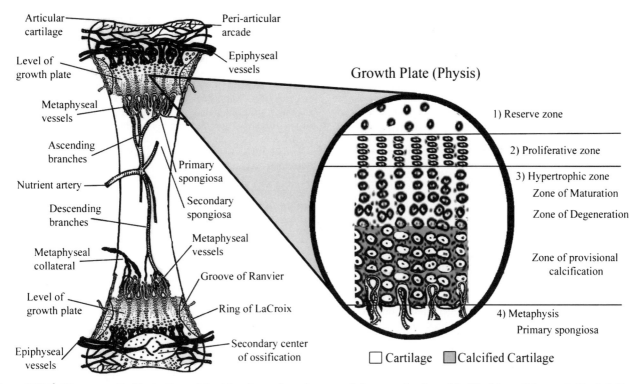

Figure 178–6. Diagrammatic illustration of the blood supply and zones of the growth plate. (Modified from Scheuer L, Black S: Bone development. *In* Scheuer L, Black S, [eds]: Developmental Juvenile Osteology. London, Academic Press, 2000, pp 18-31.)

chondrocyte and results in a mild delay in ossification.[22] Core-binding factor-α subunit 1 (CBFA1), a member of the runt family of transcription factors, is expressed in prehypertrophic chondrocytes, and its constitutive expression in nonhypertrophic chondrocytes induces hypertrophic chondrocyte differentiation, Ihh expression, and, eventually, endochondral bone formation.[23] These functions, along with its role during osteoblast differentiation and vascular invasion, identify CBFA1 as the most pleiotropic regulator of skeletogenesis.

GROWTH PLATE

The growth plate of a long bone provides an exceptional correlation among histology, ordered cytodifferentiation, molecular biology, and physical function. The growth plate is composed of a cartilaginous component that is surrounded by a fibrous component and bounded by a bony metaphyseal component. Each component has a unique structure, biochemistry, and function; together, these result in longitudinal and latitudinal growth and remodeling of the developing skeleton. The vascular supply of the growth plate results in unique biochemical properties and is integral to normal function.

Vascular Supply

The normal growth and development of a bone are inextricably linked to its vascular, and in particular its arterial, supply. In fact, the onset and maintenance of ossification depend on a constant supply of nutrients. There are three major vascular suppliers to the growth plate: the epiphyseal arteries, the nutrient arteries, and the perichondrial arteries (Fig. 178-6). The epiphyseal arteries are derived from periarticular vascular arcades that form on the nonarticular bone surfaces. These arteries send branches through the cartilaginous epiphysis within cartilage canals to supply the reserve and proliferative zones of the growth plate.[24] Thus, the overall viability of the growth plate to maintain normal

bone growth and development depends on the integrity of these vessels. Any damage to these arteries will result in growth arrest.

The metaphyseal supply is primarily derived from the nutrient arteries, also known as diaphyseal arteries. The nutrient arteries are generally derived from an adjacent major systemic artery. A nutrient artery enters a bone through its nutrient foramen, which leads into a nutrient canal, and once the vessel reaches the medullary cavity, it divides into ascending and descending medullary branches.[24, 25] The ascending and descending medullary branches anastomose with the metaphyseal collaterals at the metaphyseal zone. The metaphyseal supply induces blood-borne precursors that promote ossification and remodeling at the hypertrophic zone (HZ) of the growth plate.[24,26] The physeal cartilage itself maintains a separation between these two circulations throughout normal human growth. The perichondrial arteries supply the ring of LaCroix and the groove of Ranvier. Capillaries from this system communicate with the epiphyseal and metaphyseal capillaries in addition to the vessels of the joint capsule.

Cartilaginous Component

Within the growth plate, the various subpopulations of chondrocytes (zones)—reserve (resting), proliferative (proliferating), hypertrophic—are arranged in columns (see Fig. 178-6). These chondrocytes regulate longitudinal growth of the skeleton until their disappearance at the end of puberty in humans. Each zone has characteristic histologic and biochemical features that define its formation. The zone farthest away from the diaphysis and closest to the epiphysis is the *reserve zone* (RZ). In this zone, the chondrocytes are small, round, and randomly distributed. The chondrocytes in the RZ replicate rarely; the ratio of matrix volume to cell volume is the highest of any layer of the growth plate.[27] The matrix contains randomly oriented fibrils of Type II collagen, which inhibits calcification and acts as a barrier to the advancing front of the secondary center of ossification.[14] The chondrocytes in this zone receive a vascular supply from the epiphyseal vessels; however, the epiphyseal vessels do not actually arborize in the RZ, and hence the oxygen tension in this zone is relatively low. The precise function of the RZ remains ill defined. Two likely functions are (1) physical separation between the osseous tissue of the secondary center and the remainder of the growth plate and (2) synthesis and storage of nutrients and raw materials (i.e., glycogen, lipid, and protein) that will be used by other chondrocytes in the lower zones of the growth plate.

In the adjacent *proliferative zone*, the chondrocytes are tightly bound in columns parallel to the axis of the length of the bone. The cytoplasm contains glycogen stores and is rich in endoplasmic reticulum, features suggesting a rich source of nutrients for aerobic glycolysis and a high capacity for protein synthesis. Of the three zones, this zone has the highest rate of proteoglycan synthesis and turnover. The proteoglycans (aggrecans) in this zone are large aggregates consisting of glycosaminoglycans attached to core proteins.[28] Such aggregates inhibit calcification. The chondrocytes replicate rapidly in the proliferative zone, and they become flattened and slightly irregular in shape. The rate of duplication of cells is closely regulated and usually constant.[29] The binding matrix is contiguous with the matrix of the RZ and has the same biochemical composition. The Type II collagen fibrils are oriented longitudinally, surrounding the columns of chondrocytes. The epiphyseal vessels that crossed the RZ terminate in the proliferative zone, thereby resulting in the highest oxygen concentration in the growth plate. The presence of rich glycogen stores and a high oxygen tension supports aerobic metabolism in the proliferative zone chondrocyte. The functions of the proliferative zone — matrix production and cellular division — together contribute to longitudinal growth.

The HZ has traditionally been divided into two parts: the upper, or zone of maturation; and the lower, or zone of degeneration. The lowest portion of the HZ is also called the zone of provisional calcification. In the zone of maturation, the chondrocytes start to hypertrophy. There is a change in the proteoglycans of the matrix in this zone, with the size of the aggrecan decreasing. This decrease results from an active degradation mediated by physeal enzymes, including metalloproteases (i.e., collagenase, stromelysin, and neutral growth plate proteases).[30, 31] There is also a marked decrease in Type II collagen synthesis. In moving down the cellular column and away from the epiphyseal vessels, the chondrocytes are exposed to an environment of increasingly lower oxygen tension.

The major energy source for production of adenosine triphosphate (ATP) in the HZ chondrocytes is anaerobic glycolysis of glucose from endogenous glycogen stores. Glycogen is stored in the RZ and proliferative zone and is then consumed in the HZ. Metabolic activity in the HZ cells differs from that in most animal cells. In most cell types, glucose is oxidized to pyruvate in the cytoplasm, and the pyruvate then enters the mitochondria (by glycerol phosphate shuttle) to be further oxidized by the Krebs cycle. The Krebs cycle is an important additional energy source for most cells. In the growth plate, pyruvate continues to enter the mitochondria but at a much reduced rate, and glycerol phosphate does not enter the mitochondria because the growth plate zones lack the glycerol phosphate shuttle. Thus, even in the presence of oxygen, the growth plate cartilage metabolizes glucose relatively anaerobically. The mitochondria of the chondrocytes in the proliferative zone are capable of conducting the Krebs cycle and generating ATP. However, in the HZ, owing to lower oxygen tension, there is a switch in the function of the mitochondria from ATP production to calcium accumulation. These mitochondrial stores allow buffering of the ionized intracellular calcium in the already high concentrations of the HZ.[32]

In the zone of degeneration, there is a further diminution in proteoglycan size. The proteoglycan, which in aggrecan form is an inhibitor of calcification, no longer serves such a role because

it is increasingly degraded.[30, 31] Biochemical analysis shows that the chondrocytes in this zone are very active metabolically. They synthesize alkaline phosphatase, neutral proteases, and Type X collagen, thereby participating in matrix mineralization. The mitochondria of the chondrocytes here begin to disgorge the calcium previously accumulated. This calcium apparently is packaged in vesicles of cellular membrane and is deposited into the surrounding matrix.[33] The hypertrophic chondrocytes do not synthesize Type II collagen in the lower HZ, but instead they synthesize Type X collagen, a unique protein associated with endochondral ossification.[34, 35] Active changes in chondrocytic activity occur at this site and lead to degeneration and cell death at the last intact transverse septum forming the interface with the metaphysis.[36] The longitudinal septa begin to calcify in this region of the growth plate; hence this zone is also termed the *zone of provisional calcification.* This is where the last transverse septa are ultimately degraded.

Metaphysis

The metaphysis begins distal to the last intact transverse septum of each cartilaginous cell column of the HZ (see Fig. 178-6). It functions in the removal of the mineralized cartilaginous matrix of the HZ and in the formation of the primary spongiosa. Bone formation begins with the invasion of the hypertrophic lacunae by vascular loops, bringing with them osteoblasts that begin the synthesis of bone. The osteoblasts progressively lay down bone on the cartilage template. Subsequently, the initial woven bone and cartilage bars of the primary spongiosa are resorbed by osteoblasts and are replaced by lamellar bone to produce the secondary spongiosa.[37]

Perichondral Ring of LaCroix and Groove of Ranvier

Surrounding the periphery of the physis are a wedge-shaped structure, the *groove of Ranvier,* and a ring of fibrous tissue, the *ring of LaCroix* (see Fig. 178-6). The cells in the groove of Ranvier are active in cell division and contribute to an increase in the diameter, or latitudinal growth, of the growth plate. The basic structure of the perichondral ring of LaCroix is a fibrous collagenous network that is continuous with the fibrous portion of the groove of Ranvier and the periosteum of the metaphysis. The perichondral ring functions as a strong mechanical support at the bone-cartilage junction of the growth plate.

GROWTH AND ITS CONTROL

The endocrine control of the growth plate is a complex and important aspect of growth. Numerous factors have been identified as important regulators of bone and cartilage (Table 178-1). Some of these factors (systemic hormones, vitamins, and growth factors) are produced at a site distant from the growth plate and therefore act on the chondrocytes through a classic endocrine mechanism. Other factors both are produced and act within the growth plate and therefore function as paracrine or autocrine factors. Each zone of the growth plate may be specifically targeted by one or more agents to affect a particular stage in the cell maturation phenomenon.

Growth hormone (GH) is a peptide hormone secreted by the pituitary gland, and its absence leads to pituitary dwarfism. GH acts throughout the growth plate and primarily affects cellular proliferation. GH does not directly stimulate the growth plate; rather, it stimulates production of a group of peptide growth factors termed *somatomedin* or *insulin-like growth factor* (IGF). The effects of GH mainly result from the production of serum-derived IGF by the liver, but there is also a direct GH effect to induce chondrocytes to produce IGF locally (paracrine or autocrine effect). IGF-I (somatomedin C) is the potent stimulator

TABLE 178-1

Growth Plate Control

Agent	Effect
Specific endocrine hormones	
Thyroid hormones	↑ Chondrocyte proliferation, ↑ chondrocyte maturation
Growth hormones	Secreted by pituitary, converted to somatomedin (IGF-I); IGF-I interacts with local factors
IGF-I	↑ Chondrocyte proliferation
Insulin	Interacts with IGF-I receptor, ↑ chondrocyte proliferation
PTH-related peptide	Binds to PTH receptor → ↑ cAMP → ↑ chondrocyte proliferation and matrix synthesis, also works through inositol triphosphate and protein kinase C
Androgens	Anabolic but pharmacologic doses may promote growth plate closure
Estrogens	Inhibit bone resorption but may be important agent in plate closure
Local agents	
Growth factors	
Cytokines	
Other small, molecules autocrine, paracrine	
Fibroblast growth factor	↑ Chondrocyte proliferation, interacts with IGF-I
Transforming growth factor-β	Relatively weak and variable effects depending on other agents present, ↑ chondrocyte proliferation and maturation
Interleukin-1	↑ Matrix degradation through metalloproteinases
Prostaglandin	↑ Proteoglycan, ↓ collagen, alkaline phosphatase
Vitamins	
Vitamin A	Required for chondrocyte maturation
Vitamin C	Necessary cofactor for collagen synthesis
Vitamin D and metabolites	Required for calcification of matrix, deficiency leads to failure of calcification and marked elongation of the hypertrophic zone (rickets)

↑ = up-regulates; ↓ = down-regulates; cAMP = cyclic adenosine monophosphate; IGF-I = insulin-like growth factor-I; PTH = parathyroid hormone.

of postnatal growth mediating chondrocyte proliferation and matrix synthesis, whereas IGF-II is the fetal somatomedin.[38] Immunohistochemical studies have localized the highest concentration of IGF-I receptors to the PZ of the growth plate.[39] IGF-I increases cellular proliferation, probably by two mechanisms: by direct IGF-I effects; and, perhaps more important, through the modulation of other growth factor effects. The synergistic interactions of IGF-I with FGF and TGF-β are specific for DNA synthesis, a finding that confirms the central role of IGF-I on mitogenesis in the growth plate.[38] Insulin can cross-react with the IGF-I receptors and therefore may have some minor anabolic effect at physiologic insulin levels.[32]

The thyroid hormones, thyroxine and triiodothyronine, are peptide hormones produced by the thyroid gland. The thyroid hormones act on the PZ and upper HZ chondrocytes through a systemic endocrine mechanism. Thyroxine enhances cartilage growth by two functions: (1) it increases DNA synthesis in cells from the proliferative zone and (2) it increases glycosaminoglycan and collagen synthesis and alkaline phosphatase activity. Its effect on cartilage growth is mediated by synergy between thyroxine and IGF-I. These two agents together restore both growth and maturation. Triiodothyronine also increases cartilage growth by interacting with IGF-I. It promotes the cytodifferentiation from proliferative to hypertrophic chondrocyte, independently from IGF-I, however.

PTH is produced by the parathyroid glands. It acts primarily on the proliferative zone and upper HZ chondrocytes, and it has a direct agonist role in the cellular metabolism of the growth plate. There is a complex relationship among PTH, the intracellular calcium concentration, and regulation of growth plate.[40] In the growth plate chondrocyte, PTH stimulates the production of inositol triphosphate from phosphoinositol 4,5-biphosphate. Inositol triphosphate induces the release of calcium from an intracellular store, which causes a transient increase in the cytosolic ionized calcium concentration. PTH also mediates an increase in proteoglycan synthesis through the breakdown of membrane phosphoinositides and subsequent activation of protein kinase C. The regeneration of membrane phosphoino-

sitides can result in the stimulation of prostaglandin synthesis, which also appears to have a small stimulatory effect on proteoglycan synthesis.

The effects of sex steroids (androgens and estrogens) on proliferating cartilage are complex. Although androgens and estrogens may increase chondrocyte division, they may also interact with adrenal steroids and many other factors. Androgens function primarily in the lower portion of the growth plate to stimulate mineralization. Their anabolic effect is manifested as an increased deposition of glycogen and lipids in cells and an increase in proteoglycans in cartilage matrix.[32] Androgens can also stimulate DNA synthesis in chondrocytes. Supraphysiologic doses of androgens depress growth and accelerate growth plate closure.

Besides FGFs (see the earlier discussion of the development of the growth plate), several other growth factors have been demonstrated to contribute to the regulation of growth plate development. Platelet-derived growth factor stimulates DNA synthesis and cell replication of chondrocytes as well as protein synthesis. TGF-β is a multifunctional peptide that controls cell replication and differentiation. It is involved in cartilage formation during the first step of endochondral bone formation. Release of TGF-β is stimulated by PTH, but the overall effect of TGF-β appears to depend on constituent growth factors in the cell. Therefore, its effects may be stimulatory or inhibitory, depending on the hormonal environment when TGF-β is introduced to the chondrocytes.[32] For example, TGF-β can inhibit progression of growth plate chondrocytes to the full hypertrophic phenotype, but this can be overcome by the thyroid hormones.[20] TGF-β is a potent inhibitor of a lymphocyte-activating factor called *interleukin-1,* which induces degradation in growth plate chondrocytes.[41]

Several vitamins are required for normal growth plate function.[42] The active metabolites of vitamin D (1,25 and 24,25-dihydroxyvitamin D) are produced in the liver and kidney. Vitamin D deficiency results in an elongation of the cell columns of the growth plate. This effect is considered to be secondary to a vitamin D–induced decrease in systemic calcium and

TABLE 178-2

Molecular Basis of Some Abnormalities of the Growth Plate

Condition	Molecule	Human Chromosome Location

Achondroplasia
  Hypochondroplasia
  Thanatophoric dysplasia
	Fibroblast growth factor receptor-3 (FGFR3)	4

Diastrophic dysplasia	Diastrophic dysplasia sulfate transporter	5

Stickler syndrome
  Spondyloepiphyseal dysplasia congenita
  Kniest dysplasia
	Type II collagen	12

Pseudoachondroplasia Multiple epiphyseal dysplasia	Cartilage oligomeric matrix protein (COMP)	19
Jansen metaphyseal chondrodysplasia	PTH-PTHrP receptor	3

PTH = parathyroid hormone; PTHrP = parathyroid hormone-related peptide.

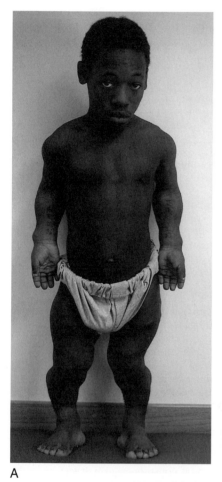
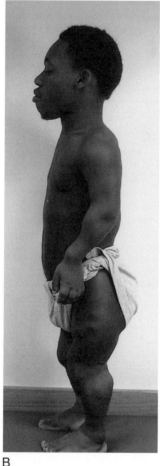
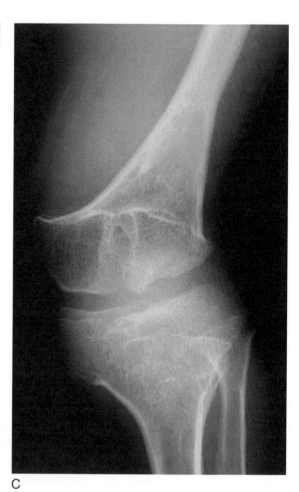

A   B   C

Figure 178–7. A 19-year-old patient with spondyloepiphyseal dysplasia congenita. **A** and **B**, Note the markedly short stature with short trunk and limbs. There are angular deformities of the lower limbs. **C**, An anteroposterior radiograph of the knee shows abnormally flattened and broad femoral and tibial epiphyses, causing angular deformities.

phosphorus and the subsequent inhibition of mineralization. The vitamin D metabolites are bound to cells in all growth plate zones except the HZ. The highest levels are found in the PZ. A deficiency state leads to rickets, which at the histologic level of the growth plate manifests itself as a failure of calcification of the matrix and marked elongation of the HZ. Histologically, the RZ and PZ are normal, but the HZ is greatly expanded, and this results in widening of the growth plate.

Vitamin C is a necessary cofactor for the synthesis of collagen. Deficiency of vitamin C leads to scurvy. The greatest deficiency in collagen synthesis is seen in the metaphysis. The microscopic appearance of the cartilaginous portion of the growth plate is normal, but that of the metaphysis is quite abnormal. The physeal-metaphyseal junction is particularly disrupted, with persistence of calcified cartilage and sparse bony trabeculae. Vitamin A is essential for epiphyseal cartilage cell metabolism.

A deficiency state results in impairment of the chondrocyte maturation.

CORRELATED CLINICAL CONDITIONS

It is important to review some skeletal dysplasias (osteochondrodysplasias), a group of genetic disorders characterized by generalized disorders of growth and development of bone and cartilage. The generalized disturbance in the development of the skeleton affects the skull, spine, and extremities in varying degrees resulting in disproportionate short stature (short-trunk or short-limb dwarfism). The pathogenesis of many of these conditions is slowly being discovered, teaching us little by little about the growth of the skeleton (Table 178–2).

Achondroplasia, the most frequent form of short-limb dwarfism, is an autosomal dominant condition, although two-thirds of cases arise by spontaneous new mutations that have been mapped to chromosome 4, in a region encoding *Fgfr-3.*[43,44] The activating mutations in the *Fgfr-3* gene lead to a retardation in chondrocyte proliferation resulting in abnormal endochondral ossification. *Hypochondroplasia* is an autosomal dominant allelic variant of achondroplasia with similar phenotypic and genotypic features, and the mutation in the *Fgfr-3* gene occurs in a different region (in the tyrosine kinase domain, in contrast to the transmembrane domain in achondroplasia).[44] A mutation in *Fgfr-2* underlies the *Crouzon syndrome,* in which the cranial sutures are disrupted.[45] In the *Pfeiffer* and *Jackson-Weiss syndromes* (both of which are characterized by craniosynostoses and limb defects), there are mutations in both *Fgfr-1* and *Fgfr-2.*[46] The coordination of the various *Fgfrs* and receptors appears to be responsible for proportional growth.

Diastrophic dysplasia is a rare autosomal recessive condition characterized by short-limb dwarfism with spinal deformities and specific hand, foot, and ear abnormalities. The responsible gene has been mapped to chromosome 5 and encodes a sulfate transporter protein (diastrophic dysplasia sulfate transporter).[47] Impaired function of this protein is thought to lead to undersulfation of proteoglycans in the cartilage matrix, thus affecting hydration of cartilage.

Mutations in the gene encoding Type II collagen, the predominant protein of cartilage, underlie several skeletal dysplasias: Stickler syndrome, spondyloepiphyseal dysplasia congenita, Kniest dysplasia, and Langer-Saldino achondrogenesis.[48,49] These conditions are characterized by short-trunk dwarfism and severe involvement of the vertebrae and epiphyseal centers (Fig. 178–7). The gene defect has been linked to a deletion in the *COL2A1* gene on chromosome 12.

Pseudoachondroplasia and *multiple epiphyseal dysplasia* are frequent, autosomal dominant disorders characterized by short-limb dwarfism and epiphyseal and metaphyseal changes. The gene responsible for these disorders has been localized to chromosome 19 and appears to encode the cartilage oligomeric matrix protein, a glycoprotein found in matrix surrounding chondrocytes.[50]

Jansen metaphyseal chondrodysplasia is a rare autosomal dominant disorder characterized by abnormal growth plate maturation and laboratory findings that are indistinguishable from hyperparathyroidism. This disorder is caused by activating mutations in PTH/PTHrP receptors.[51] This receptor is important both in calcium metabolism and in regulation of chondrocyte maturation.[52] By somatic cell hybrid analysis, the mutations in the PTH receptor gene have been mapped to chromosome 3 in humans.

REFERENCES

1. Chevallier A, et al: Developmental fate of the somitic mesoderm in the chick embryo. *In* Ede DA (eds): Vertebrate Limb and Somite Morphogenesis. Cambridge, Cambridge University Press, 1977, pp 421–432.

2. Christ B, et al: Experimental analysis of the origin of the wing musculature in avian embryos. Anat Embryol *150*:171, 1977.
3. Sledge CB, Zaleske DJ: Developmental anatomy of joint. *In* Resnick D, Niwayama G (eds): Diagnosis of Bone and Joint Disorders, 2nd ed. Philadelphia, WB Saunders Co, 1988, pp 604–624.
4. Ohuchi HTN, et al: An additional limb can be induced from the flank of the chick embryo by FGF-4. Biochem Biophys Res Commun *209*:809, 1995.
5. Cohn MJ, et al: Fibroblast growth factors induce additional limb development from the flank of chick embryos. Cell *80*:739, 1995.
6. Ohuchi H, et al: The mesenchymal factor, FGF10, initiates and maintains the outgrowth of the chick limb bud through interaction with FGF8, an apical ectodermal factor. Development *124*:2235, 1997.
7. Kawakami Y, et al: WNT signals control FGF-dependent limb initiation and AER induction in the chick embryo. Cell *104*:891, 2001.
8. Capdevila J, Izpisua Belmonte JC: Patterning mechanisms controlling vertebrate limb development. Annu Rev Cell Biol *17*:87, 2001.
9. Summerbell D: The effect of local application of retinoic acid to the anterior margin of the developing chick limb. J Embryol Exp Morphol 78:269, 1983.
10. Thaller C, Eichele G: Retinoid signaling in vertebrate limb development. *In* Crombrugghe B, et al (eds): Molecular and Developmental Biology, Vol 1. New York, New York Academy of Sciences, 1996, p 785.
11. Dealy CN, et al: Wnt-5a and Wnt-7a are expressed in the developing chick limb bud in a manner suggesting roles in pattern formation along the proximodistal and dorsoventral axes. Mech Dev *43*:175, 1993.
12. Loomis CA, et al: Analysis of the genetic pathway leading to formation of ectopic apical ectodermal ridges in mouse engrailed-1 mutant limbs. Development *125*:1137, 1998.
13. Hall BK, Miyake T: The membranous skeleton: the role of cell condensations in vertebrate skeletogenesis. Anat Embryol *186*:107, 1992.
14. Horton WA, Machado MM: Extracellular matrix alterations during endochondral ossification in humans. J Orthop Res 6:793, 1988.
15. St-Jacques B, et al: Indian hedgehog signaling regulates proliferation and differentiation of chondrocytes and is essential for bone formation. Genes Dev *13*:2072, 1999.
16. Vu TH, et al: MMP-9/gelatinase B is a key regulator of growth plate angiogenesis and apoptosis of hypertrophic chondrocytes. Cell *93*:411, 1998.
17. Kember NF: Cell population kinetics of bone growth: the first ten years of autoradiographic studies with tritiated thymidine. Clin Orthop 76:213, 1971.
18. Kember NF: Cell kinetics and the control of growth in long bones. Cell Tissue Kinet *11*:477, 1978.
19. Diao E, et al: Kinetic and biochemical heterogeneity in vertebrate chondroepiphyseal regions during development. J Orthop Res 7:502, 1989.
20. Zaleske DJ: The growth plate: embryologic origin, structure, and function. *In* Polin RA, et al (eds): Fetal and Neonatal Physiology, 2nd ed. Philadelphia, WB Saunders Co, 1998, pp 2351–2359.
21. Scheuer L, Black S: Bone development. *In* Scheuer L, Black S, (eds). Developmental Juvenile Osteology. London, Academic Press, 2000, pp 18–274.
22. Karsenty G, Wagner EF: Reaching a genetic and molecular understanding of skeletal development. Dev Cell *2*:389, 2002.
23. Takeda S, et al: Continuous expression of Cbfa1 in non-hypertrophic chondrocytes uncovers its ability to induce hypertrophic chondrocyte differentiation and partially rescues Cbfa1-deficient mice. Genes Dev *15*:467, 2001.
24. Brooks M, Rewell WJ: Blood Supply of Bone: Scientific Aspects, 2nd ed. London, Springer-Verlag, 1998.
25. Crock HV: An Atlas of Vascular Anatomy of the Skeleton and Spinal Cord. London, Dunitz, 1996.
26. DeSimone DP, Reddi AH: Vascularization and endochondral bone development: changes in plasminogen activator activity. J Orthop Res *10*:320, 1992.
27. Robertson WW: Newest knowledge of the growth plate. Clin Orthop *253*:270, 1990.
28. Buckwalter JA: Proteoglycan structure in calcifying cartilage. Clin Orthop *172*:207, 1983.
29. Kember NF: Aspects of the maturation process in growth cartilage in the rat tibia. Clin Orthop 95:288, 1973.
30. Ehrlich MG, et al: Patterns of proteoglycan degradation by a neutral protease from human growth-plate epiphyseal cartilage. J Bone Joint Surg Am *64*:1350, 1982.
31. Ehrlich MG, et al: Partial purification and characterization of a proteoglycan-degrading neutral protease from bovine epiphyseal cartilage. J Orthop Res *2*:126, 1984.
32. Iannotti JP, et al: Growth plate and bone development. *In* Simon SR (ed): Orthopaedic Basic Science. Washington, DC, American Academy of Orthopaedic Surgeons, 1994, pp 185–217.
33. Iannotti JP, et al: Growth plate matrix vesicle biogenesis. Clin Orthop *306*:222, 1994.
34. Burgeson RE, Nimni ME: Collagen types: molecular structure and tissue distribution. Clin Orthop *282*:250, 1992.
35. Sandell LJ, et al: Expression of collagens I, II, X, and XI and aggrecan mRNAs by bovine growth plate chondrocytes in situ. J Orthop Res *12*:1, 1994.
36. Breur GJ, et al: Linear relationship between the volume of hypertrophic chondrocytes and the rate of longitudinal bone growth in growth plates. J Orthop Res *9*:348, 1991.
37. Dietz FR, Morcuende JA: Embryology and development of the musculoskeletal system. *In* Morrisy RT, Weinstein SL (eds): Lowell and Winter's Pediatric Orthopaedics, 5th ed. Philadelphia, Lippincott Williams & Wilkins, 2001, pp 1–31.

38. O'Keefe RJ, et al: Effects of transforming growth factor-B1 and fibroblast growth factor on DNA synthesis in growth plate chondrocytes are enhanced by insulin-like growth factor-I. J Orthop Res 12:299, 1994.
39. Makover A-M, et al: Binding of insulin-like growth factor-I (IGF-I) to primary cultures of chondrocytes from rat rib growth cartilage. Cell Biol Int Rep 13:655, 1989.
40. Iannotti JP, et al: Mechanism of action of parathyroid hormone-induced proteoglycan synthesis in the growth plate chondrocyte. J Orthop Res 8:136, 1990.
41. Chandrasekhar S, Harvey AK: Transforming growth factor-beta is a potent inhibitor of IL-1 induced protease activity and cartilage proteoglycan degradation. Biochem Biophys Res Commun 157:1352, 1988.
42. Mankin HJ: Metabolic bone disease. J Bone Joint Surg Am 76:760, 1994.
43. Shiang R, et al: Mutations in the transmembrane domain of FGFR3 cause the most common genetic form of dwarfism, achondroplasia. Cell 78:335, 1994.
44. Le Merrer M, et al: A gene for achondroplasia-hypochondroplasia maps to chromosome 4p. Nat Genet 6:318, 1994.
45. Reardon W, et al: Mutations in the fibroblast growth factor receptor 2 gene cause Crouzon syndrome. Nat Genet 8:98, 1994.
46. Jabs EW, et al: Jackson-Weiss and Crouzon syndromes are allelic with mutations in fibroblast growth factor receptor 2. Nat Genet 8:275, 1994.
47. Hastbacka J, et al: The diastrophic dysplasia gene encodes a novel sulfate transporter: positional cloning by fine-structure linkage disequilibrium mapping. Cell 78:1073, 1994.
48. Prockop DJ: Mutations in collagen genes as a cause of connective-tissue diseases. N Engl J Med 326:540, 1995.
49. Kuivaniemi H, et al: Mutations in collagen genes: causes of rare and some common diseases in humans. FASEB J 5:2052, 1991.
50. McKusick VA: Online Mendelian Inheritance in Man, OMIM™. McKusick-Nathans Institute for Genetic Medicine, John Hopkins University (Baltimore, MD) and National Center for Biotechnology Information, National Library of Medicine (Bethesda, MD), 2000. World Wide URL://www.ncbi.nlm.nih.gov/omim/
51. Schipani E, et al: A constitutively active mutant PTH-PTHrP receptor in Jansen-type metaphyseal chondrodysplasia. Science 268:98, 1995.
52. Erlebacher A, et al: Toward a molecular understanding of skeletal development. Cell 80:371, 1995.

179

Kathrin V. Halpern, Bulent Erol, and John P. Dormans

Common Musculoskeletal Conditions Related to Intrauterine Compression: Effects of Mechanics on Endochondral Ossification

Intrauterine compression syndromes are a group of conditions caused by abnormal pressures placed on the growing fetus in the uterus (Table 179-1). Although some of the physical manifestations of these conditions are obvious to the naked eye at birth, others are subtle and are detected only on thorough physical examination. Most compression syndromes are mild, with a favorable natural history, and are easily treated (e.g., metatarsus adductus, medial tibial torsion). However, a few conditions affect the fetus severely and often require invasive treatment (e.g., congenital constriction band syndrome). Compression syndromes cannot be attributed to intrinsic germ plasm defects, metabolic or enzyme disorders, mechanical disruptions of normal tissue, or exogenous mutagens. Although their origin is not fully understood, it is clear that both genetic and environmental factors are involved in most of these conditions.

ETIOLOGY OF INTRAUTERINE COMPRESSION SYNDROMES

It is important to review the etiologic factors causing intrauterine compression syndromes, because such a review provides an understanding of the pathogenesis and natural history of these conditions. An extreme condition that is thought to be related to intrauterine compression is *congenital constriction band syndrome* (amniotic band syndrome).[1] The clinical presentation of this condition is quite variable; the three main manifestations are syndactyly, superficial or deep constriction bands involving a digit or extremity, and intrauterine amputation (Fig. 179-1). Although two main conflicting theories focus on whether the band formation is the result of factors intrinsic or extrinsic to the embryo or fetus, the disorder may be more heterogeneous than considered in the past. The extrinsic theories have the widest acceptance. It has been proposed that entanglement of the limbs in defects or in free strands of amnion results in constriction band syndrome.[2, 3] The lack of hereditary factors, the ultrasonographic demonstration of prenatal amniotic bands, the involvement of the longer digits, and the histologic demonstration of amnion in constriction bands also support the extrinsic theory. Conversely, the intrinsic theory proposes that a defect of the subcutaneous germ plasm causes soft tissue necrosis and subsequent healing, with the formation of constriction bands.[4]

Rotational deformities, also known as torsional deformities, of the lower limbs (i.e., femoral anteversion, medial tibial torsion, metatarsus adductus) are also related to intrauterine environmental conditions and can be considered in a discussion of compression syndromes. Rotation of limbs is part of the normal developmental process; the upper limb bud rotates externally, and the lower limb bud rotates internally, resulting in externally rotated upper extremities and internally rotated lower limbs. Based on the previous studies focused on various etiologic factors causing rotational abnormalities, one can make the assumption that rotational deformities arise in the prenatal period and are a natural outcome of embryologic process.[5-9] They are a multifactorial result of fetal development, with evolution, heredity, mechanical forces, and intrauterine position all playing various roles in affected infants.

TABLE 179-1

Common Musculoskeletal Conditions Related to Intrauterine Compression

Congenital constriction band syndrome
Rotational deformities: femoral anteversion, medial tibial torsion
Congenital dislocation of the knee
Torticollis
Metatarsus adductus
Calcaneovalgus foot
Congenital idiopathic clubfoot
Developmental dysplasia or dislocation of the hip
Teratologic hip dysplasia, clubfoot (syndromic clubfoot)

Most compression syndromes present with varying degrees of severity. *Congenital dislocation of the knee* (CDK) is a relatively rare deformity that varies from simple hyperextension to anterior dislocation of the tibia on the femur. Although most cases are sporadic, some reports of occurrence within families suggest a possible genetic basis.[10, 11] Additionally, the association of CDK with some congenital foot deformities (clubfoot and vertical talus) that have polygenic modes of inheritance is another factor suggesting a genetic origin.[12, 13] Milder forms of CDK are believed to be positional deformities, occurring in association with breech position *in utero*.[13] However, severe CDK is a pathologic deformity, and it often occurs in the presence of muscle imbalance or ligamentous laxity.[12-14]

Compression syndromes may involve multiple body parts, such as in torticollis, hip dysplasia, and metatarsus adductus. However, some studies have shown that the association among these conditions is not as strong as once thought.[15-17] *Congenital muscular torticollis,* the most common cause of torticollis in infancy and childhood, is an asymmetric deformity of the neck and head resulting from contracture of the sternocleidomastoid muscle, with the head tilted toward the involved site and the chin rotated toward the opposite shoulder (Fig. 179-2). The exact cause is not known, and there are several theories. Because of the birth history, one theory is that of compartment syndrome resulting from soft tissue compression of the neck at the time of delivery.[18] Currently, a more widely accepted theory is *in utero* crowding, because three of four children with congenital muscular torticollis have the lesion on the right side,[19] and up to 20% have developmental hip dysplasia.[20] The finding that this condition can occur in children with normal birth histories or in children born by cesarian section also supports the *in utero* crowding theory over the perinatal compartment syndrome theory. A genetic predisposition has also been described;[21] however, familial occurrence is rare, given that the development of the condition is influenced by other factors.[22]

Metatarsus adductus, medial deviation of the forefoot on the hindfoot, with neutral (normal) alignment of the hindfoot, is the most common congenital foot deformity (Fig. 179-3). Although earlier studies[23,24] indicated an association of metatarsus adductus with hip dysplasia, more recent studies[15, 16] have shown no significant association between these two conditions. The theory that metatarsus adductus is the result of *in utero* positioning is supported by the high rate of spontaneous resolution[25] and the strong association with twin pregnancies.[26, 27] Conversely, some anatomic studies propose the cause to be muscle imbalance[28, 29] or abnormality in shape of tarsal bones.[30, 31] It may be that the position theory applies to those feet that correct spontaneously, and the anatomic theories apply to those that do not.

Congenital idiopathic clubfoot (congenital talipes equinovarus) is a complex, three-dimensional foot deformity that consists of plantar flexion, inversion, and adduction of the foot. (Fig. 179-4A). This condition is probably etiologically heterogeneous (i.e., multifactorial). The incidence of clubfoot varies widely with respect to race and gender and increases with the number of affected relatives, a finding suggesting that the origin is at least partly influenced by genetic factors.[32] Environmental factors may modulate the genetic expression of the disorder. Intrauterine positioning is one of the many possible factors (i.e., histologic, vascular, neurologic, and muscular anomalies) proposed as a causative mechanism for this disorder.

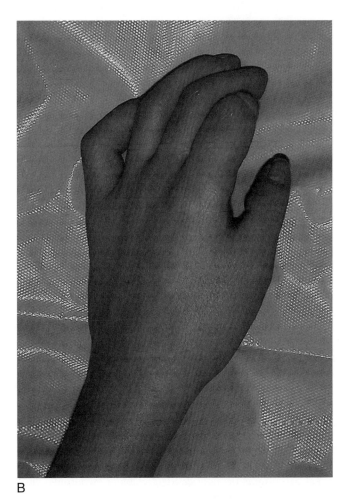

A   B

Figure 179–1. A and B, A 6-year-old girl with congenital constriction band syndrome. Clinical photographs demonstrate autoamputation of the long and index digits through the distal and middle phalanges, respectively. Also note a superficial constriction band in the distal segment of the ring finger.

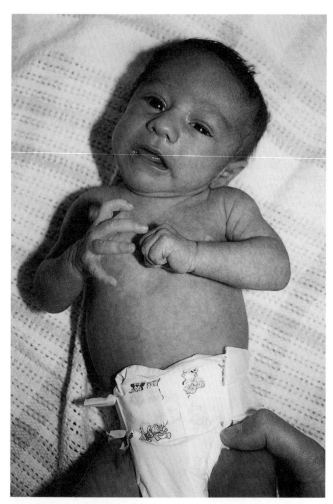

Figure 179–2. A 1-month-old infant with congenital muscular torticollis. The clinical photograph shows asymmetric deformity of the neck and head resulting from contracture of the sternocleidomastoid muscle, with the head tilted toward the involved side and the chin rotated toward the opposite shoulder.

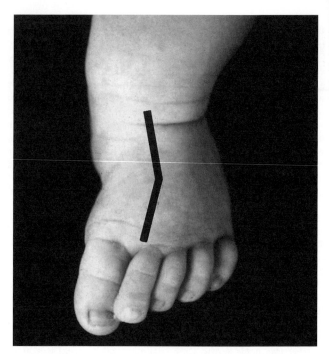

Figure 179–3. A 6-month-old child with metatarsus adductus. The clinical photograph shows medial deviation of the forefoot on the hindfoot, with neutral alignment of the hindfoot.

Developmental dysplasia or *dislocation of the hip* (DDH), terminology that replaces the older term congenital dysplasia or dislocation of the hip, includes all cases that are clearly congenital and those that are developmental, and it incorporates dysplasia, subluxation, and dislocation of the hip (Fig. 179-5). The genetic effects on the hip joint in patients with DDH are revealed in primary acetabular dysplasia, various degrees of joint laxity, or a combination of both. Intrauterine molding, breech position, oligohydramnios, and neuromuscular mechanisms, such as meningomyelocele, can profoundly influence genetically determined intrauterine growth.[33-35] The association of DDH with other intrauterine compression syndromes (torticollis and metatarsus adductus), although the results of current studies make it questionable, still lends some support to the *in utero* crowding theory in the pathogenesis of this condition.[8, 20, 24]

It is important to make a distinction between deformities that occur relatively late in fetal development and those that occur earlier (i.e., in the first trimester). The descriptor for long-standing deformities is *teratologic,* deriving its meaning from the Greek word *teras* or monster. Rigid clubfoot (syndromic clubfoot) and hip dislocation, associated with arthrogryposis or spina bifida, are often described as teratologic. These severe conditions are the result of an imbalance in the musculature surrounding the joint that causes displacement of bony structures

early in fetal development. There is no spontaneous correction of teratologic deformities, as there may be with some deformities occurring in the latter stages of fetal development. The treatment principles of positional deformity and teratologic deformity mostly vary from one another.

Theoretical Basis

The formation of the musculoskeletal system depends on several important guiding factors.[36] It is imperative that the proper genetic information be present in the cells, to form the necessary bone, cartilage, muscle, and fibrous tissues from the primitive mesenchymal cell layer.[37, 38] Furthermore, motion is needed for the proper formation and orientation of joints. It has also been shown that mechanically or chemically induced electrical currents are important in the development of a structurally intact musculoskeletal system.[8, 39] It is therefore possible that some deformities in a genetically normal fetus can be caused by abnormalities of other formative mechanisms. Assuming that all these elements have properly coordinated in the development of a fetus, one must look to external forces applied to the fetus to explain the occurrence of deformities. The abnormal external forces exerted by amniotic bands, a nulliparous uterus, uterine wall malformations, high fetal weight, or oligohydramnios may cause the fetus to assume abnormal positions in which tissues are compressed, movement is restricted, and thus normal development and remodeling are slowed or even halted.

Once a fetal bone anlage is formed in cartilage under the influence of genetic and hormonal factors (endochondral ossification [see Chap. 178]), its growth and shape are determined largely by the physical forces acting thereon.[40] One need only look to Wolff's law, first described in 1892, to understand the importance of external forces on bone growth. This theory simply states that bone elements place or displace themselves in the direction of functional forces and increase or decrease their masses to reflect the strength of these forces. The distribution of bone matrix and calcification, both in the cortices and in the medullary trabeculae, are probably guided by microelectrical

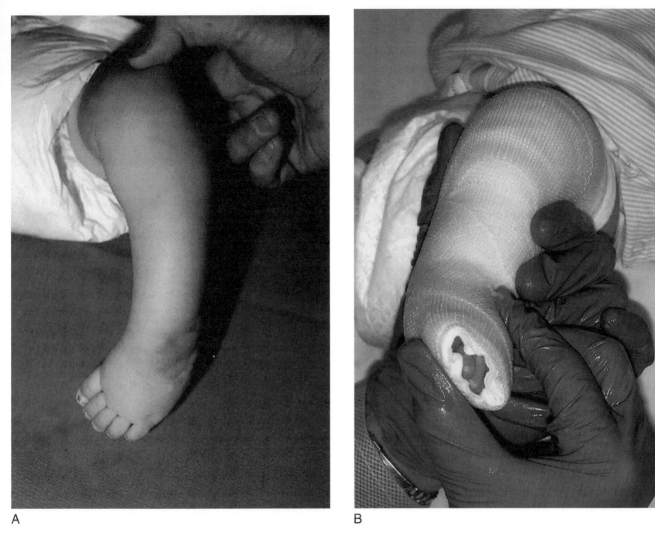

A
B

Figure 179–4. A 3-week-old infant with congenital idiopathic clubfoot. **A,** Clinical photograph demonstrates three-dimensional foot deformity consisting of plantar flexion, inversion, and adduction of the foot. **B,** This patient was successfully treated with manipulation and casting.

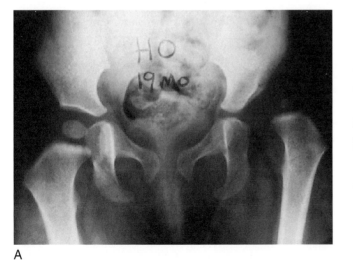
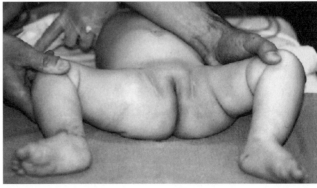

A
B

Figure 179–5. A 19-month-old girl with developmental dysplasia of the left hip. **A,** An anteroposterior plain radiograph of the pelvis shows a dislocated left hip with a poorly developed acetabulum. **B,** Physical examination of the hips shows limited abduction on the left side, which is a common clinical finding associated with hip dislocation in this age group. This patient was successfully treated with adductor tenotomy, closed reduction, and spica casting.

currents generated by stresses and movement within the bone. Bone is seen to add itself to areas of electronegativity and to remove itself from areas of electropositivity.[41]

Longitudinal bone growth is governed by pressure phenomena. When the physis of a tubular bone is under greater than normal force, it does not grow as rapidly as in areas of normal force distribution. Depending on the amount of force applied, the bone may either slow or completely stop its growth. Asymmetric forces produce asymmetric growth, which consequently leads to bony deformity.[42]

Normal remodeling occurs in the region of a joint by the shear and compression forces that are exerted through the joint. These forces determine the shape of the joint and are modulated by the initial shape of the joint (hinge, ball and socket, or gliding), the strength of muscular contraction about the joint, and the constraining ligamentous structures about the joint. Carter and Wong[43] demonstrated the importance of proper forces to the development of normal joint structure. These investigators showed that the placement and time of appearance of the ossific nucleus in the epiphyses of long bones are determined by the mechanical stresses placed on the epiphysis. Intermittently applied shear stresses promote endochondral ossification and thereby the formation of the ossific nucleus in the epiphysis. Intermittently applied hydrostatic compression retards or prevents cartilage degeneration and ossification and therefore maintains the thickness of articular cartilage on the surface of the joint. Abnormal shear forces and hydrostatic pressures can lead to irregularities in hyaline cartilage thickness and misshapen epiphyses with delayed or aberrant epiphyseal nuclear ossification.[43]

This etiologic model can be applied to some positional abnormalities, such as DDH. Assuming that at an early phase of gestation, a normal acetabulum, femoral head, and capsule are externally compressed by abnormal pressures in a position of adduction and flexion, the capsule will become elongated, and the femoral head will be posteriorly and inferiorly displaced in the acetabulum. The acetabulum, which is still cartilaginous, will not ossify normally because of the hydrostatic pressure. As a result, the acetabulum will not contour normally to the femoral head. Additionally, because of external constriction of limb motion, the necessary normal movement is unable to occur. The muscles, specifically the hip flexors, become contracted, and this further perpetuates the abnormal positioning. The elongated capsule and the pliant posterior acetabulum will allow the femoral head to slide out of joint (subluxation or dislocation). As a result of prolonged dislocation, secondary acetabular and soft tissue changes occur.

NATURAL HISTORY AND TREATMENT OF INTRAUTERINE COMPRESSION SYNDROMES

A relationship clearly exists between the duration of compression causing a deformity and the ease with which the deformity may be treated. Based on this relationship, it is a matter of ease to create a three-tiered classification of intrauterine compression syndromes as they relate to prognosis and treatment (Table 179-2). The first tier of this classification relates to all those deformities thought to be caused by short-term exposure to abnormal external forces during development or those that are a result of low abnormal external pressure. These deformities usually correct spontaneously; examples include medial tibial torsion, calcaneovalgus foot positioning, and mild metatarsus adductus. The deformities are corrected by the existence of forces in the extrauterine environment that counteract those that caused the deformity *in utero*. Stretching exercises may help to speed resolution, but bracing and surgery are not indicated.

More severe deformities that resolve to some degree, but often leave behind residual abnormalities, should be considered as the second tier of the classification. In some cases, the residual abnormality can be treated in a preemptive manner. In severe metatarsus adductus deformities, proposed nonoperative management includes manipulation and serial casting. The efficacy of splints and braces or corrective shoes in treating foot deformities has never been shown. Surgery is very rarely indicated.[44] Congenital muscular torticollis can also be a subject of the second tier. Treatment of congenital muscular torticollis initially consists of conservative measures.[45, 46] Good results can be expected with stretching exercises alone. These results also may reflect, in part, the favorable natural history of many of these children. The exact role of the efficacy of these stretching measures, versus a natural history of spontaneous resolution, is not known; there are many anecdotal cases of spontaneous resolution. Stretching measures are usually unsuccessful after 1 year of age, and surgery is recommended.[46] Milder forms of CDK, such as hyperextension or recurvatum, usually can be managed with conservative treatment. Treatment begins with gentle stretching and then continues with serial casts and removable splints. These knees often show rapid improvement with this treatment protocol.

The third tier of the classification is composed of compression deformities that usually do not correct spontaneously to any degree. The deformities in this group may progress after birth because of physical changes in the anatomy and function of the area involved, and they usually require intervention by means of

---

TABLE 179-2

Classification of Intrauterine Compression Syndromes Based on Natural History and Treatment

Classification	Example	Natural History	Treatment
Tier 1	Medial tibial torsion Calcaneovalgus foot Mild metatarsus adductus	Spontaneously correcting	Observation
Tier 2	Severe metatarsus adductus Congenital muscular torticollis Mild congenital dislocation of the knee	Spontaneously correcting with residual deformity	Treatment indicated; mostly conservative, rarely surgical
Tier 3	Congenital constriction band syndrome Severe congenital dislocation of the knee Idiopathic congenital clubfoot Developmental dysplasia of the hip Teratologic hip dysplasia, clubfoot (syndromic clubfoot)	No spontaneous correction; progression without intervention	Intervention required; conservative or surgical

conservative or surgical treatment. An extreme example of this sort of deformity is congenital constriction band syndrome. Although superficial, asymptomatic constriction bands do not require treatment, the bands extending to the deep subcutaneous tissue or fascia may require surgical intervention, particularly in the presence of vascular insufficiency or neurologic deficit.[44] Moderate or severe forms of CDK (subluxation or dislocation), particularly those occurring in association with neuromuscular or genetic syndromes, usually do not respond to conservative treatment, and these patients should be considered for surgical treatment.[12,47]

In most infants with idiopathic congenital clubfoot, the condition does not resolve fully without intervention and persists as a rigid, unsightly deformity. The goal of treatment is to achieve a plantigrade, painless foot that looks normal, although it is not normal, and provides adequate function. The initial treatment of clubfoot, regardless of its severity or rigidity, is nonoperative. Modalities include serial manipulation and casting,[48,49] taping, physical therapy and splinting,[50] and continuous passive motion with a machine.[51] The combination of manipulation and casting is the technique used most frequently in the United States, based on experience, practicality, and cost. The technique of manipulation and casting, described by Ponseti,[49] is now becoming the standard of treatment (see Fig. 179-4B). Surgery is indicated if there is failure to achieve satisfactory clinical and radiographic evidence of deformity correction by nonoperative methods.

The natural history of untreated DDH may demonstrate a wide spectrum, but it has been proved that most patients with untreated DDH will have symptomatic hip joint problems (i.e., degenerative joint disease), requiring complex surgical procedures, in their adult life. The fundamental treatment goals in DDH are the same, regardless of age: to obtain reduction and maintain that reduction, to provide an optimal environment for femoral head and acetabular development. Children diagnosed in the newborn period and until 6 months of age can be successfully treated with conservative treatment by using a Pavlik harness (Fig. 179-6). Children 6 months to 2 years of age are usually treated with closed reduction (reduction with closed methods). In children older than 2 years of age at the time of diagnosis of DDH, open reduction (reduction with open-surgical methods) is usually necessary. Open reduction may be accompanied by other surgical procedures (i.e., femoral shortening or pelvic osteotomy), showing that with increasing age, the treatment becomes more complex.[44]

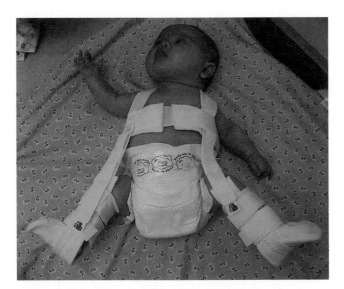

Figure 179-6. Newborn with developmental dysplasia of the hip. This patient was successfully treated with a Pavlik harness.

Most intrauterine compression syndromes are multifactorial in origin. It is believed that genetic factors play important roles in the development of most of these conditions, and environmental factors may modulate the genetic expression of these disorders. Intrauterine compression is one of the most commonly proposed environmental factors, and it is believed that the degree of deformity is directly related to the extent and duration of intrauterine compression. Improvements in genetics will provide a better understanding of the pathogenesis of these conditions and will result in more effective treatment options.

REFERENCES

1. Walter JH Jr, et al: Amniotic band syndrome. J Foot Ankle Surg 37:325, 1998.
2. Torpin R: Amniochorionic mesoblastic fibrous strings and amniotic bands: associated constricting fetal malformations or fetal death. Am J Obstet Gynecol 91:65, 1965.
3. Torpin R: Fetal Malformations Caused by Amnion Rupture During Gestation. Springfield, IL, Charles C Thomas, 1968.
4. Streeter GL: Focal deficiencies in fetal tissues and their relationship to intrauterine amputation. Contrib Embryol 22:1, 1930.
5. Staheli LT, et al: Lower-extremity rotational problems in children: normal values to guide management. J Bone Joint Surg Am 67:39, 1985.
6. Katz K, et al: Rotational deformities of the tibia and foot in preterm infants. J Pediatr Orthop 10:483, 1990.
7. Wilkinson JA: Breech malposition and intra-uterine dislocations. Proc R Soc Med 59:1106, 1966.
8. Dunn PM: Congenital postural deformities. Br Med Bull 32:71, 1976.
9. Carter DR: Mechanical loading history and skeletal biology. J Biomech 20:1095, 1987.
10. Curtis BH, Fisher RL: Congenital hyperextension with anterior subluxation of the knee: surgical treatment and long-term observations. J Bone Joint Surg Am 51:255, 1969.
11. McFarland BL: Congenital dislocation of the knee. J Bone Joint Surg 11:281, 1929.
12. Curtis BH, Fisher RL: Heritable congenital tibiofemoral subluxation: clinical features and surgical treatment. J Bone Joint Surg Am 52:1104, 1970.
13. Johnson E, et al: Congenital dislocation of the knee. J Pediatr Orthop 7:194, 1987.
14. Vedantam R, Douglas DL: Congenital dislocation of the knee as a consequence of persistent amniotic fluid leakage. Br J Clin Pract 48:342, 1994.
15. Gruber MA, Lozano JA: Metatarsus varus and developmental dysplasia of the hip: is there a relationship? Orthop Trans. 15:336, 1991,.
16. Kollmer CE, et al: Relationship of congenital hip and foot deformities: a national Shriner's Hospital survey. Orthop Trans 15:96, 1991.
17. Walsh JJ, Morrissy RT: Torticollis and hip dislocation. J Pediatr Orthop 18:219, 1998.
18. Davids JR, et al: Congenital muscular torticollis: sequela of intrauterine or perinatal compartment syndrome. J Pediatr Orthop 13:141, 1993.
19. Ling CM, Low YS: Sternomastoid tumor and muscular torticollis. Clin Orthop 86:144, 1972.
20. Weiner DS: Congenital dislocation of the hip associated with congenital muscular torticollis. Clin Orthop 121:163, 1976.
21. Engin C, et al: Congenital muscular torticollis: is heredity a possible factor in a family with five torticollis patients in three generations? Plast Reconstr Surg 99:1147, 1997.
22. McKusick VA: Online Mendelian Inheritance in Man. McKusick-Nathans Institute for Genetic Medicine, Johns Hopkins University (Baltimore, MD) and National Center for Biotechnology Information, National Library of Medicine (Bethesda, MD), 2000. World Wide Web URL: http://www.ncbi.nlm.nih.gov/omim/
23. Jacobs JE: Metatarsus varus and hip dysplasia. Clin Orthop 16:203, 1960.
24. Kumar SJ, MacEwen GD: The incidence of hip dysplasia with metatarsus adductus. Clin Orthop 164:234, 1982.
25. Rushforth GF: The natural history of hooked forefoot. J Bone Joint Surg Br 60:530, 1978.
26. Hunziker UA, et al: Neonatal metatarsus adductus, joint mobility, axis and rotation of the lower extremity in preterm and term children 0-5 years of age. Eur J Pediatr 148:19, 1988.
27. Wynne-Davies R, et al: Aetiology and interrelationship of some common skeletal deformities. (Talipes equinovarus and calcaneovalgus, metatarsus varus, congenital dislocation of the hip, and infantile idiopathic scoliosis). J Med Genet 19:321, 1982.
28. Kite JH: Congenital metatarsus varus. J Bone Joint Surg Am 49:388, 1967.
29. Ghali NN, et al: The management of metatarsus adductus et supinatus. J Bone Joint Surg Am 66:376, 1984.
30. Reimann I, Werner HH: The pathology of congenital metatarsus varus. A postmortem study of a newborn infant. Acta Orthop Scand 54:847, 1983.
31. Morcuende JA, Ponseti IV: Congenital metatarsus adductus in early human fetal development: a histologic study. Clin Orthop 333:261, 1996.
32. Wynne-Davies R: Family studies and the cause of congenital clubfoot. J Bone Joint Surg Br 46:445, 1964.

33. Strayer LM Jr: Embryology of he human hip joint. Clin Orthop 74:221, 1971.
34. Walker JM: Morphological variants in the human fetal hip joint. J Bone Joint Surg Am 62:1073, 1980.
35. Walker JM, Goldsmith CH: Morphometric study of the fetal development of the human hip joint: significance for congenital hip disease. Yale J Biol Med 54:411, 1981.
36. Murray PDF: Bones: A Study of the Development and Structure of the Vertebrate Skeleton, 2nd ed. New York, Cambridge University Press, 1985, p 70.
37. Hall BK: The role of tissue interactions in the growth of bone. In Dixon AD, Sarnat BG (eds): Factors and Mechanisms Influencing Bone Growth. New York, Alan R Liss, 1982, p 205.
38. Singh IJ, et al: Modulation of osteoblastic activity by sensory and autonomic innervation of bone. In Dixon AD, Sarnat BG (eds): Factors and Mechanisms Influencing Bone Growth. New York, Alan R Liss, 1982, p 535.
39. Becker RO: The bioelectric factors in amphibian-limb regeneration. J Bone Joint Surg Am 43:643, 1961.
40. Guidera KJ, et al: The embryology of lower-extremity torsion. Clin Orthop 302:17, 1994.
41. Friedenberg ZB, Brighton CB: Bioelectric potentials in bone. J Bone Joint Surg Am 48:915, 1966.
42. Arkin AM, Katz JF: The effects of pressure of epiphyseal growth. J Bone Joint Surg Am 38:1056, 1956.
43. Carter DR, Wong M: Mechanical stresses and endochondral ossification in the chondroepiphysis. J Orthop Res 6:148, 1988.
44. Morrissy RT, Weinstein SL (eds): Lovell and Winter's Pediatric Orthopaedics, 5th ed. Philadelphia, Lippincott Williams & Wilkins, 2001.
45. Binder H, et al: Congenital muscular torticollis: results of conservative management with long-term follow-up in 85 cases. Arch Phys Med Rehabil 68:222, 1987.
46. Canale ST, et al: Congenital muscular torticollis: a long-term follow-up. J Bone Joint Surg Am 64:810, 1982.
47. Ferris B, Aichroth P: The treatment of congenital knee dislocation: a review of nineteen knees. Clin Orthop 216:135, 1987.
48. Morquende J, et al: Plaster cast treatment of clubfoot: the Ponseti method of manipulation and casting. J Pediatr Orthop B 3:161, 1994.
49. Ponseti IV: Congenital clubfoot: Fundamentals of Treatment. New York, Oxford University Press, 1996.
50. Bensahel H, et al: Results of physical therapy for idiopathic clubfoot: a long-term follow-up study. J Pediatr Orthop 10:189, 1990.
51. Dimeglio A, et al: Orthopaedic treatment and passive motion machine: consequences for the surgical treatment of clubfoot. J Pediatr Orthop B 5:173, 1996.

180

Walid K. Yassir, Benjamin A. Alman, and Michael J. Goldberg

Defective Limb Embryology

LIMB EMBRYOLOGY

The formation of the embryonic limb involves a complex sequence of histologic and biochemical changes.[1-4] Cells change position and shape (thereby bringing a basic form), and, in turn, they undergo cytodifferentiation and acquire specialized structures and functions. In the 1940s, Streeter devised a staging system for the events that take place beginning with the one-cell fertilized egg and ending with the *embryonic period,* the time when all body parts and organ systems are formed. This embryonic period is divided into 23 stages, lasts 56 days, and, by convention, ends when there is penetration of the nutrient artery into the humerus. The staging or timing of events is important in establishing relationships among organ systems. However, important biochemical alterations occur in cells before alterations in their structure become visible. Progress has been made in clarifying the biochemical signals that determine limb patterning. Broadly stated, limb patterning occurs in four phases: (1) the cells that constitute the limb field are established; (2) signals produced from specialized centers within the field allow for positional determination; (3) positional information is recorded by specific gene expression; and (4) cells differentiate into limb components based on encoded positional data.[5] Alterations in these various stages are recognized as causes of human limb malformation.

PATHOGENESIS OF LIMB ABNORMALITIES

A distinction needs to be made between cause and mechanism.[6, 7] The causes of many syndromes or specific defects are well known. For example, the cause of Down syndrome is the genetic information contained on the extra chromosome 21. This extra genetic information is responsible for the disturbances in morphogenesis and is also responsible for the endocrine, malignant, and infectious diseases and for the premature aging seen in this syndrome. Nothing is yet known, however, about the underlying biochemical mechanisms. Similarly, the cause of certain specific limb abnormalities such as the thrombocytopenia-absent radius syndrome is precisely known. It is an abnormal, mutant, autosomal recessive gene. Yet the mechanism by which

this genetic aberration produces total absence of the radius bilaterally, with preservation of the thumb, is not known. Pathogenesis is a broader term that covers both cause and mechanism. Unfortunately, at this stage, little can be said with certainty about the pathogenesis of limb abnormalities. The causes of birth defects that involve the limb can be broadly grouped as follows: (1) environmental, agents that affect the fetus; (2) genetic, chromosomal and classic mendelian disorders; and (3) collaborating, a combination of environmental and genetic factors.[6,8] At least half of the recognizable limb abnormalities are of unknown cause.

1. Environmental. In a few conditions, a single exogenous insult, a specific environmental factor, can be identified. Thalidomide is such an example. Thalidomide stands almost alone, however, among the proved teratologic agents in humans. Although other drugs and even occupational hazards have been suggested, careful epidemiologic studies are needed to confirm an increased risk of limb abnormalities in children born to women exposed to such substances. The experience in animals is, for the most part, irrelevant to humans, and as a generalization, humans seem to be more resistant to the teratogenic effects of drugs than are other animals.

2. Genetic. Certain syndromes caused by chromosomal defects have limb abnormalities. The polydactyly observed in trisomy 13 and the absent thumb in ring chromosome 4 are examples. Similarly, isolated limb abnormalities such as syndactyly and malformation syndromes with limb defects such as thrombocytopenia-absent radii are transmitted as single genetic traits; the former is autosomal dominant, and the latter is autosomal recessive.

3. Collaborating. In these instances, causation is the complex combination of genetic and environmental factors. This cause, common to so many limb abnormalities, is often arrived at by default. One must also recognize that embryogenesis is so complicated that there is room for an accident.

Many data are available regarding the mechanisms responsible for limb defects; however, much of that information is derived from animal studies and cannot always be generalized to humans. Vascular compromise as a mechanism for the production of congenital limb deficiencies has gained considerable support.[6, 7, 9-14] Vascular compromise may produce tissue ischemia, alterations in cell metabolism, or cell death. Vasoconstrictive drugs administered to the pregnant animal can produce vasospasm in the placenta or the embryo. Inadequate blood supply may be caused by placental insufficiency or maternal vascular disease, such as hypertension, toxemia, or diabetes. Vascular mechanisms may be relevant to certain clinical situations in humans. There is an increasing body of evidence that thalidomide mediates its teratogenicity by inhibiting the ingrowth of new blood vessels in selective thalidomide-sensitive pathways. This feature has led to its experimental uses, notably in the treatment of multiple myeloma and plexiform neurofibromas.[15-20] Thrombi originating in the placenta can pass into the fetus and have been postulated as a cause of congenital amputations.[13] In addition, it is believed that amniotic bands produce limb deficiency by disruption of the vascular supply. It has been argued that limb-reduction anomalies may be related to mechanical compression of the early embryo that, in turn, causes ischemia and arrest of limb development.[7, 13] Mechanical compression may occur with abnormalities in the shape of the uterus, such as a bicornuate or fibromatous uterus.

Congenital limb anomalies are often part of a syndrome. Identification of syndromes is important not only for the purpose of genetic counseling, but also because associated malformations may directly affect management of the limb deformity. Limb deformities, furthermore, may be the clue to more serious, initially occult malformations elsewhere. Indeed, it is appropriate to think of limb anomalies as a symptom and not as a diagnosis. No meaningful discussion of limb anomalies can take place without first discussing normal limb embryology.

Normal Limb Embryology

When observed under the low-power microscope, implantation of the zygote occurs on day 6, and 20 days later (late in the fourth week of embryonic life), the limb buds appear as lateral swellings. Because of the early dominance of the head, the arm buds seem to be located further down the body. The leg buds appear 2 days after the arms, which is characteristic of embryonic development; cranial structures develop before caudal ones, and proximal structures differentiate sooner than those distal. The entire process of limb development takes only 4 weeks: marginal blood vessels are evident by day 31, the nerves enter on day 36, and the finger rays develop by day 41; individual muscle groups can be observed by day 44 and joints by day 47; with the start of skeletal ossification on day 56, the process is complete. The limbs initially project outward, almost at right angles to the body wall. Subsequently, they bend at the elbow and knee so the palm and the sole face the trunk, with the thumb and the great toe pointing cephalad. Then, in a rapid and remarkable fashion, both sets of limbs undergo a torsion of 90° about their long axes, but in opposite directions. This change causes the elbows to point caudad (the arms in a "surrender" posture) and the knees cephalad (the legs in a "frog" position). At that time, just 8 weeks after fertilization, the embryonic period is complete, all parts have formed, and the crown-rump length is 3 cm.

Under high-power magnification, one sees intense cellular activity and cytodifferentiation. As the limb buds enlarge, the similar-appearing mesenchymal cells condense, forming identifiable primitive anlagen of skeletal elements. These primitive elements then, in an orderly fashion, become cartilage. At 8 weeks, ossification begins with the appearance of a bone collar around the central portion of the primitive bone.

Where the primitive cartilage and skeletal anlagen meet, a condensation of the intervening tissue called the *interzone* occurs. The interzones are the future joints, and from the interzones, articular cartilage, synovium, ligaments, and menisci develop.

Although joint interzones are apparent during the embryonic period, cavitation of the joint requires motion, which does not occur until after the eighth week. If the embryo, or fetus, becomes paralyzed, the articular surface flattens, the joint capsule thickens, and the joint cavity fills with fibrous tissue, bringing some understanding to the creaseless, fusiform, rigid limbs of newborns with arthrogryposis multiplex congenita.

The process by which the vascular system is formed in the embryo and fetus is poorly understood, but it appears to play an important role in the development of many congenital malformations. Coincident with the appearance of the limb bud is the appearance of scattered thin-walled vessels. These vessels ultimately develop into arteries and veins, some permanent and some transient. It is entirely unknown, however, what directs these combinations and replacements. A border vein develops first and is located along the periphery of the limb on its postaxial (ulnar, fibular) side. It is functional for only 10 days, and then the adult venous pattern appears. During the fifth week of embryonic life, a major artery (axillary, femoral) enters the limb bud and extends as a large median artery on the volar surface of the limb bud. Then, in swift order, preaxial and postaxial arteries appear, but rather than maintaining a three-branched vascular tree, the large mainstem, median interosseous artery undergoes a decrease in size and for the most part disappears, its function assumed by the two peripheral arteries. The persistence of primitive vascular patterns that include the median artery raises questions about the cause of congenital anomalies such as agenesis of the tibia and fibula and clubfoot.[10, 11, 14, 21]

On the 36th day of embryonic life, the nerve trunks enter the limb, with the anterior division of the nerve to supply the flexor muscles and the posterior division to supply the extensors. It is unknown, however, what guides the nerves to their target. Some investigations have postulated that it is the neural crest, or the muscles themselves, whereas others have pointed to a curious condensation of nerve cells at the leading edge of ingrowth called the pioneer growth cone.

Myoblasts develop in limb bud mesenchyme and form a dorsal and volar mass that is destined to be the extensor and flexor muscles. By day 44, individual muscle groups begin to surround the cartilaginous skeleton. The tendons develop independently, seemingly quite autonomous from the muscles they soon join. The tendons insert into the bone, but if the normal site of skeletal attachment is not formed, they attach to the next available bone, to the fascia, or to another tendon. In the event no muscle is formed, the tendon degenerates.

Microsurgical manipulation of the limb bud and molecular studies of its development are beginning to shed light on the control mechanisms of limb development.[4, 5, 21-23] A limb's three axes develop simultaneously. Each axis appears to be more or less under the control of a dominant set of genes that necessarily interact with genes in the other two axes.[24] Understanding of these pathways is increasing at a rapid pace, and a familiarity with their novel nomenclature becomes necessary as the identification of pathway alterations leading to human limb anomaly increases.

At day 24, the Wolff crest, a mesodermal ridge rich in RNA, develops along the lateral wall of the embryo. The ectoderm overlying the ridge becomes thickened in four specific areas, one for each limb. A limb bud develops at each of these sites. Three regions, each with its own specific function, develop at the distal end of the bud.[3] The thickened ectoderm becomes the apical ectodermal ridge (AER). Proliferating mesodermal cells just deep to the AER become the progress zone (PZ), and mesodermal cells located just posterior to the PZ become the zone of polarizing activity (ZPA). Interaction between the AER and PZ is necessary for maintenance of these regions. The AER is responsible for controlling the general development of the PZ. Removing the AER results in only the most proximal limb development (e.g., only the proximal humerus). Grafting a leg AER to an arm PZ results in the arm bud's developing into a leg. AER transplanted between species causes the recipient animal to develop the limb of the donor. The ZPA is located posteriorly and orients the developing limb. In the human hand, the little finger is on the posterior side. If the ZPA is grafted to the anterior side of the limb, a duplicate limb, with opposite orientation, develops. Control of limb development can be thought of as proceeding simultaneously along three axes: proximodistal, anteroposterior, and dorsoventral.

Proximodistal Axis

This axis is under the control of the fibroblast growth factor (FGF) pathway. A complex relationship between FGF-8 and FGF-10 appears to be necessary for limb bud inititation.[5] FGF-10 is expressed in cells fated to become leg or wing in the developing chick.[25] FGF-8, however, appears to act at some distance from the limb bud and may be an early initiator, related to FGF-10 in an as yet unelucidated feedback pathway.[5] FGF-2, FGF-4, and FGF-8 are expressed in the AER. When FGF-4 is applied to a limb bud stripped of its AER, it causes formation of a normal-length, although malformed, limb.[23] Although no human limb anomalies are known to be secondary to defects in FGF synthesis, several have been well described in relation to defective FGF receptors. Mutations in FGFR3 cause achondroplasia, hypochondroplasia, or thanatophoric dwarfism, depending on which portion of the receptor is involved.[26,27]

Anteroposterior Axis

Sonic hedgehog gene (*SHH*) is important for establishing the anteroposterior polarity of limbs. This gene gives the ZPA its morphogenetic properties. The expression of this gene is inducible by retinoic acid. When applied to the opposite side of the limb bud, it produces a duplicate limb identical to that produced by grafting the ZPA.[22] Furthermore, *SHH* deletion experiments suggest not only that the SHH gene product is crucial to anteroposterior polarizing activity, but also that this polarizing activity is essential to proper anteroposterior and proximodistal development.[5] A complex series of controls restricts SHH to the ZPA. *SHH* mutation has yet to be demonstrated in human limb anomaly; however, it is implicated in the polydactyly that often accompanies the Smith-Lemli-Opitz syndrome. SHH protein becomes covalently linked to cholesterol during its maturation. Smith-Lemli-Opitz syndrome, characterized by hypocholesterolemia secondary to a defect in the 7-cholesterol reductase, may lead to SHH dysfunction and the clinically apparent limb anomalies of this syndrome.[24] SHH action is believed to be mediated by other gene families, PTC, GLI, BMP, and HOX proteins, among others. *GLI3* mutations have been encountered in Greig cephalopolysyndactyly, Pallister-Hall syndrome, and postaxial polydactyly type A.[27] SHH pathway malfunction mediated through GLI may be related to the VACTERL (vertebral, anal, cardiac, tracheal, esophageal, renal, and limb) association.[28]

Dorsoventral Axis

The AER forms at the boundary between the dorsal and ventral portions of the limb. *Wnt-7a* and radical fringe (*r-Fng*) are two genes expressed in the dorsal ectoderm. *Wnt-7a* apparently induces expression of *LMX-1* in dorsal mesoderm. Engrailed-1 (*EN-1*), expressed in the ventral ectoderm, appears necessary for the restriction of *Wnt-7a* and *r-Fng* expression to the dorsal ectoderm and to the establishment of the dorsoventral boundary.[27] *LMX1b* mutations have been identified in the nail-patella syndrome, in which abnormalities are noted in nails, patellae, elbows, and renal parenchyma (Fig. 180-1).

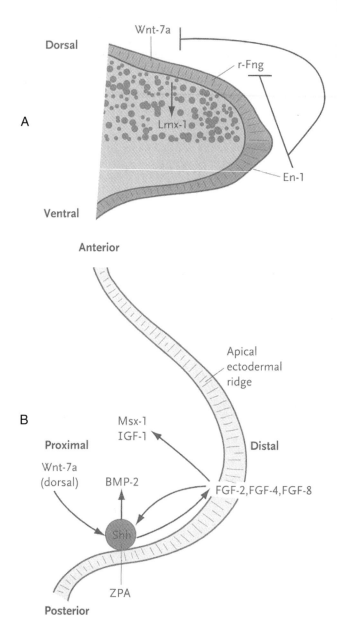

Figure 180–1. Schematic representations of molecular control of limb development. **A,** Molecular control of the dorsoventral axis. Engrailed-1 (*EN-1*) inhibits both *Wnt-7a* and radical fringe (*r-Fng*). **B,** Molecular control along the anteroposterior and proximodistal axes. BMP-2, bone morphogenic protein 2; FGF = fibroblast growth factor; IGF-1 = insulin-like growth factor-I; ZPA = zone of polarizing activity. (From Carlson BM: Human Embryology and Developmental Biology, 2nd ed. St. Louis, CV Mosby, 1999.)

Other Patterning

Several other genes involved in limb bud patterning have been implicated in human limb malformation.[24] The *TBX* genes are so named because they share a region of homology to the DNA binding domain (T-box) of the murine Brachury or T gene. At least five *TBX* genes (*TBX2, TBX3, TBX4, TBX5,* and *TBX15*) are expressed in the vertebrate developing limb.[29,30] Loss of function mutations have been identified in *TBX3* and *TBX5*, both located at 12q24. *TBX5* mutations are the cause of the *Holt-Oram syndrome,* an autosomal dominant disorder with variable expression. The syndrome is characterized by radial ray malformations and cardiac anomalies.[24] Studies have suggested that the specific residue involved in the loss of function mutation leads to a preponderance of cardiac malformations, limb anomalies, or both.[31] *TBX3* mutations cause the *ulnar-mammary syndrome,* characterized by ulnar ray alterations in upper and lower limbs along with hypoplasia of the mammary and sweat glands, transmitted in an autosomal dominant fashion.

Within the PZ, the homeobox, or *HOX,* gene family seems to play an important role. *HOX* genes are a highly conserved set of transcription factor genes found in all animal species. Certain *HOXa* and *HOXd* genes are expressed in the developing limb in three phases, corresponding roughly to the appearance of the stylopod (femur or humerus), zeugopod (radius/ulna and tibia/fibula), and autopod. Two human syndromes are known to be caused by *HOX* mutations. *Synpolydactyly,* in which third and fourth digit syndactyly is seen in upper or lower extremities along with digital duplication, is caused by a gain of function mutation in *HOXD13.* Inactivation of the last *HOX* gene to be expressed (*HOXD-13*) leads to a small but normally formed limb, illustrating that each of the *HOX* genes is responsible for a certain sequence of limb development, rather than for a particular anatomic portion of the limb.[21] The *hand-foot-genital syndrome,* affecting both digital and genitourinary development, is caused by a premature stop codon in the homeodomain of *HOXA13.* The rate of proliferation of mesodermal cells may control the sequence of *HOX* gene expression because the cells

with the highest proliferative rate (the posterior cells) express this series of genes first.

Morphogenesis of the limb seems to be a combination of genetic programming from some cells (e.g., the AER) and the end result of stimulation in other cells (e.g., the sequence of *HOX* gene expression determined by proliferative rate). The control of differentiation of the mesodermal cells into muscle, bone, and cartilage is still unclear, although several specific growth factors are expressed in the cells during differentiation into osteoblasts, myocytes, and chondrocytes. Despite the data from these studies, much remains to be learned about the molecular mechanisms underlying normal limb development. Other genes that control cell proliferation, differentiation, and even death may be identified.

Regardless of whether the limb abnormality has an environmental, genetic, or collaborating cause, molecular mechanisms clearly play a key role in abnormal development. This is currently an area of intense study. One can imagine how a defect in the genes involved in limb development could lead to an abnormal limb. As we have described, several human syndromes are now known or are strongly believed to result from genetic defects (Table 180-1).

Congenital anomalies of the limbs are not uncommon. Precise estimates of the birth prevalence rate or such abnormalities, however, are difficult to determine. Different nomenclature and classifications are employed, further obscuring precise data.[8]

TABLE 180-1

Genetics of Limb Anomalies

Syndrome	Limb Anomaly	Gene Implicated
Proximodistal Axis		
Apert syndrome	Limbs	*FGFR1*
	Synostosis of radius and humerus	
	Fusion of carpal bones, especially capitate and hamate	
	Hands	
	Symmetric osseous and/or cutaneous syndactyly of hands and feet	
	Broad distal phalanx of thumb	
	Feet	
	Broad distal hallux	
Pfeiffer syndrome	Limbs	*FGFR1* and *FGFR2*
	Radiohumeral synostosis of elbow	
	Hands	
	Broad thumb	
	Partial syndactyly of fingers and toes	
	Brachymesophalangy of hands and feet	
	Feet	
	Broad great toe	
Achondroplasia	Limbs	*FGFR3*
	Rhizomelic shortening	
	Trident hand	
	Brachydactyly	
	Short femoral neck	
	Metaphyseal flaring	
	Limited elbow and hip extension	
	Generalized joint hypermobility	
Hypochondroplasia	Limbs	*FGFR3*
	Shortened limbs	
	Short tubular bones with mild metaphyseal flare	
	Limited extension at elbows	
	Genu varum	
	Bowleg	
	Hands	
	Lack of trident hand helps distinguish it from achondroplasia	
	Brachydactyly	
Thanatophoric dysplasia	Limbs	*FGFR3*
	Marked shortness and bowing of long bones	
	"French telephone receiver" femurs	
	Flared and irregular metaphyses	

Table continued on next page

TABLE 180-1

Genetics of Limb Anomalies—Cont'd

Syndrome	Limb Anomaly	Gene Implicated
Anteroposterior Axis		

Smith-Lemli-Opitz syndrome	Limbs
	  Limb shortening
	Hands
	  Short thumbs
	  Postaxial polydactyly
	  Proximally placed thumbs
	Feet
	  Syndactyly of second and third toes
	  Postaxial polydactyly
	  Talipes calcaneovalgus
	  Short, broad toes
	  Overriding toes
	  Metatarsus adductus
		?*SHH* via 7-cholesterol reductase

Greig syndrome and
  cephalopolysyndactyly
	Limbs
	  Syndactyly
	  Polysyndactyly
	  Bifid thumb and great toe terminal phalanges
		GLI3

Pallister-Hall syndrome	Limbs
	  Distal shortening of limbs
	  Radial subluxation
	Hands
	  Postaxial polydactyly
	  Oligodactyly
	  Short fourth metacarpals
	  Syndactyly
	Feet
	  Syndactyly
	  Postaxial polydactyly
		GLI3

Postaxial polydactyly type A	Limbs
	  Postaxial polydactyly
	  Well-formed articulating extra digit in Type A
	  Pedunculated postminimi in Type B
		GLI3

Dorsoventral Axis		

Nail-patella syndrome	Limbs
	  Elongated radius with hypoplasia of radial head
	  Elbow deformities (60–90%) with limited range of motion
	  Hypoplastic or absent patella (60–90%)
	  Patellar dislocation
	  Disproportionate prominence of the femoral medial condyle
	Hands
	  Fifth finger clinodactyly
	Feet
	  Talipes equinovarus
		LMX1b

Other Patterning		

Holt-Oram syndrome	Limbs
	  Absent thumb
	  Bifid thumb
	  Triphalangeal thumb
	  Carpal bone anomalies
	  Upper extremity phocomelia
	  Radial-ulnar anomalies
	  Asymmetric involvement
		TBX5

Ulnar mammary syndrome	Limbs
	  Hypoplastic/absent/deformed ulna
	  Hypoplastic/absent/deformed radius
	  Hypoplastic humerus
	Hands
	  Absent third, fourth, and fifth ulnar rays
	  Postaxial polydactyly
	Feet
	  Short fourth and fifth toes
		TBX3

REFERENCES

1. Beatty E: Upper limb tissue differentiation in the human embryo. Hand Clin *1*:391, 1985.
2. Hinchliffe JR, Johnson DR: The Development of the Vertebrate Limb. Oxford, Clarendon Press, 1980.
3. Wolpert L: Pattern formation in biological development. Sci Am *239*:154, 1978.
4. Zaleske DJ: Development of the upper limb. Hand Clin *1*:383, 1985.
5. Johnson RL, Tabin CJ: Molecular models for vertebrate limb development. Cell *90*:979, 1997.
6. Goldberg MJ, Bartoshesky LE: Congenital hand anomaly: etiology and associated malformations. Hand Clin *1*:405, 1985.
7. Graham JM, et al: Limb reduction anomalies and early in utero limb compression. J Pediatr *96*:1052, 1980.
8. Temtamy SA, McKusick VA: The genetics of hand malformations. Birth Defects Orig Artic Ser *14*:1, 1978.
9. Hootnick DR, et al: Congenital arterial malformations associated with clubfoot: a report of two cases. Clin Orthop 1982:160, 1982.
10. Hootnick DR, et al: Vascular dysgenesis associated with skeletal dysplasia of the lower limb. J Bone Joint Surg Am *62*:1123, 1980.
11. Hoyme HE, et al: Vascular pathogenesis of transverse limb reduction defects. J Pediatr *101*:839, 1982.
12. Hoyme HE, et al: The vascular pathogenesis of some sporadically occurring limb defects. Semin Perinatol 7:299, 1983.
13. Miller, ME: Structural defects as a consequence of early intrauterine constraint: limb deficiency, polydactyly, and body wall defects. Semin Perinatol 7:274, 1983.
14. Van Allen MI, et al: Vascular pathogenesis of limb defects. I. Radial artery anatomy in radial aplasia. J Pediatr *101*:32, 1982.
15. Sauer H, et al: Thalidomide inhibits angiogenesis in embryoid bodies by the generation of hydroxyl radicals. Am J Pathol *156*:151, 2000.
16. Stephens TD: Proposed mechanisms of action in thalidomide embryopathy. Teratology *38*:229, 1988.
17. Stephens TD, et al: Mechanism of action in thalidomide teratogenesis. Biochem Pharmacol *59*:1489, 2000.
18. Stephens TD, Fillmore BJ: Hypothesis: thalidomide embryopathy-proposed mechanism of action. Teratology *61*:189, 2000.
19. Waage A, Seidel C: Thalidomide: a dreaded drug with new indications. Tidsskr Nor Laegeforen *121*:2954, 2001.
20. Wolpert L: Vertebrate limb development and malformations. Pediatr Res *46*:247, 1999.
21. Duboule D: How to make a limb? Science *266*:575, 1994.
22. Johnson RL, et al: Sonic hedgehog: a key mediator of anterior-posterior patterning of the limb and dorso-ventral patterning of axial embryonic structures. Biochem Soc Trans *22*:569, 1994.
23. Tickle C: Molecular basis of limb development. Biochem Soc Trans *22*:565, 1994.
24. Manouvrier-Hanu S, et al: Genetics of limb anomalies in humans. Trends Genet *15*:409, 1999.
25. Ohuchi H, et al: The mesenchymal factor, FGF10, initiates and maintains the outgrowth of the chick limb bud through interaction with FGF8, an apical ectodermal factor. Development *124*:2235, 1997.
26. Bonaventure J, et al: Common mutations in the gene encoding fibroblast growth factor receptor 3 account for achondroplasia, hypochondroplasia and thanatophoric dysplasia. Acta Paediatr Suppl *417*:33, 1996.
27. Innis JW, Mortlock DP: Limb development: molecular dysmorphology is at hand! Clin Genet *53*:337, 1998.
28. Kim J, et al: The VACTERL association: lessons from the Sonic hedgehog pathway. Clin Genet *59*:306, 2001.
29. Bamshad M, et al: Mutations in human TBX3 alter limb, apocrine and genital development in ulnar-mammary syndrome. Nat Genet *16*:311, 1997.
30. Bamshad M, et al: Reconstructing the history of human limb development: lessons from birth defects. Pediatr Res *45*:291, 1999
31. Schneider MD, Schwartz RJ: Heart or hand? Unmasking the basis for specific Holt-Oram phenotypes. Proc Natl Acad Sci USA *96*:2577, 1999.

SUGGESTED READING

Carlson BM: Human Embryology and Developmental Biology, 2nd ed. St. Louis, CV Mosby, 1999.
McKusick-Nathans Institute for Genetic Medicine and National Center for Biotechnology Information, National Library of Medicine (Bethesda, MD), Online Mendelian Inheritance in Man, 2000.

181

Harvey B. Sarnat

Ontogenesis of Striated Muscle

HISTORICAL BACKGROUND

The timing and sequence of striated muscle maturation are as precise and predictable as in the nervous system. Interest in neuromuscular ontogeny began with the studies of MacCallum in the late nineteenth century.[1] The account of histologic changes in developing human muscle published in 1917 by Tello in Spain[2] remains as accurate and valid today as any subsequent studies by light microscopy. Ultrastructural studies of developing muscle by transmission electron microscopy began in the 1950s and was later supplemented by the use of the scanning electron microscope two decades later. Histochemical techniques to demonstrate biochemical constituents and enzymatic activities in developing muscle were introduced in the 1960s and 1970s; the 1980s was a decade for the introduction of immunocytochemistry to identify other molecules of subcellular components. The late 1980s and early 1990s saw a major breakthrough in the understanding of muscle differentiation by the discovery of myogenic regulatory genes and their transcription products. Studies of the complex interactions of these genes, their translated proteins, and the role of various trophic factors continue to be the focus of current investigations in muscle ontogenesis. Modern embryology, an integration of classic descriptive morphogenesis and the molecular genetic regulation of myogenesis, is the foundation for understanding the pathogenesis of congenital myopathies.[3]

EMBRYONIC ORIGIN OF MUSCLE

Muscle originates even before the three definitive germ layers are differentiated from the gastrula. The epiblast, the uppermost layer of the bilayered blastula, contains primordial mesodermal cells. Epiblastic cells migrate toward a line formed between parallel ridges that converge at one end; this line is known as the *primitive streak*, and the convergence of the parallel ridges is designated "anterior" and termed the *primitive node*. The axis thus formed establishes bilateral symmetry and a cephalocaudal gradient as the fundamental body plan.

From the primitive node and streak, epiblastic cells stream into the space between the two layers to form paired columns of prospective mesoderm. The primitive node is the future notochord. It is positioned beneath the future neural plate, which is of ectodermal origin. The mesodermal columns are composed of undifferentiated mesenchymal cells extending the entire length of the primitive streak. These cells migrate laterally and rostrally to fill the space between the overlying surface ectoderm, which includes the neural plate, and the deeper endodermal layer, except for an area on either side of the notochord beneath the neural plate.

Further development subdivides the layer of primitive mesenchyme. A thickened band of mesoderm condenses on either side of the primitive streak, from which primordial somites will differentiate. The myotomal plates within these still-unsegmented somite columns are anatomically distinct from the broad lateral expanse and a smaller intermediate strip of mesoderm. Elongation of the embryo is accompanied by regression of the primitive node (notochordal process) and streak caudally. As the node moves posteriorly, paired blocks of somites become segmentally condensed from the originally continuous somitic plate on either side of the developing neural tube. In addition, the lateral mesoderm splits into two layers: the upper or *somatopleure* forms the body wall, whereas the lower or *splanchnopleure* forms the mesenteries of the internal organs. A lateral palisading of paraxial mesenchyme against the lateral aspects of the notochord precedes overt segmentation, but once formed, the boundaries between somites are stable and provide no opportunity for cellular mixing.[4]

Segmentation of the myotomal plate occurs along a rostrocaudal gradient. As the more caudal segments are still in the process of separating, segregated anterior somites are already changing in size and arrangement. In transverse section, the somites are composed of high columnar cells arranged radially around a small central cavity. The dorsal part of the somite, the *dermatome*, retains this columnar structure and forms a flat plate beneath the surface ectoderm. Cells of the ventral portion of each somite disperse to form a loose network known as the *sclerotome*. The small myocele cavity of the somite is transitory and becomes obliterated by cellular proliferation.

The myotome that differentiates at the medial end of the dermatome as a ventral extension near the neural tube differentiates into the axial (i.e., paraspinal) muscles and also into the muscles of the extremities as the limb buds form. The contractile elements of the developing muscle are of somitic origin, whereas the tendons, interstitial connective tissue, blood vessels, and epimysial sheaths are somatopleural derivatives.

The notochord and floor plate ependyma of the neural plate synthesize retinoic acid[5] and express a gene known in vertebrates as *Sonic hedgehog (SHH)*.[6] These factors are important in the dorsoventral patterning not only of the developing neural tube but also of the somites. Overexpression of these factors has a powerful ventralizing influence so that an ectopic length of notochord or a section of neural tube floor plate transplanted ventral to the newly formed segmental somite causes the excessive differentiation of sclerotome (the ventral part of the somite) and deficient formation of the myotome and dermatome, the dorsal part of the somite.[6-9] As the fetus matures, the loss of balanced antagonism between ventralizing genes, such as *SHH*, and dorsalizing genes, such as those of the *bone morphogenic protein (BMP)* and *paired homeobox (PAX)* families, may result in segmental amyoplasia at the level of the notochordal or floor plate implant, a disturbance of *somitic induction*. Notochordal signals also regulate the transcriptional cascade of myogenic bHLH genes in the somite for myoblastic differentiation.[10] In a genetic mutant mouse in which somites form after notochordal degeneration, there is accelerated apoptosis of epaxial myotomes.[11]

MYOGENIC REGULATORY GENES

A family of four proto-oncogenes directs the differentiation of striated muscle from any undifferentiated or incompletely differentiated mesodermal cell by blocking the methylation of DNA.[12] The molecular mechanism of myoblast differentiation requires the activation and suppression of specific genes in a temporal and spatial sequence controlled by a complex array of regulatory transcription factors. Each of these genes can activate the expression of another and, under certain circumstances, can autoactivate as well.[13-16] The four myogenic regulatory genes are a "family" not only because of their closely related functions in myogenesis but also because they all share encoding transcription factors of the *basic helix-loop-helix* (bHLH) protein, a

molecular structure so fundamental in evolution that it is even found in some bacteria. These four genes or *myogenic regulatory factors (MRFs)* that control the specification and differentiation of striated muscle lineage are *Myf5, myogenin, MRF4* (also known as *herculin* and *Myf6*), and *myoblast-differentiating factor*, also known as *MyoD* or *MyoD1*.[13,17-25] Several other genes influence these MRFs or interact with them in ways that augment or impair their expression. *Myogenin* mainly mediates myoblast fusion, and, without this factor, an abundance of myoblasts may form but they do not fuse to form myotubes. The expression of *Myf5* and *MRF4* is transient in early ontogenesis and returns much later in fetal life to persist into adult life.[23]

One of the most remarkable and complex features of all myogenic genes is their intimate interactions with one another. After the discovery of this family of genes, initially it was thought that they all were redundant and any could substitute for another if one were deleted. Some indeed do have overlapping functions, such as *Myf5* and *MyoD*, that allow normal muscle development if one, but not both, of these two is defective.[26,27] A similar overlap or redundancy exists between *MRF4* and *MyoD*.[28] In general, despite these partial redundancies, each gene regulates a different aspect of myogenesis, however, and they do not easily compensate for each other either in the embryo and fetus or in myoblast precursor cells in adults for the regeneration of muscle.[29] *MyoD* cannot compensate for an absence of myogenin expression.[30] *MRF4* has functions similar to those of myogenin but not of *MyoD*[31] and can substitute for myogenin early in development.[32] *Myf5* similarly may be redundant with myogenin but less efficiently.[33,34] In *MRF4-* or in myogenin-deficient mice, there are particularly severe impairments in the development of the thoracic myotomes for intercostal muscle development, and rib fusions and sternal defects result, but these are probably secondary because neither of these two genes is expressed in rib cartilage or sternum.[35]

Myogenic factor 5 (Myf5) is the earliest muscle-specific bHLH gene activated in the developing embryo.[14,19] Its expression is restricted to the medial aspect of the myotome, adjacent to the least mature myocytes.[9] *Myf5* alone cannot support myogenesis without the other three bHLH genes, however.[36] *Myf5* also seems to be mitogenic in inducing the proliferation of myoblast precursors. *Myf5* requires some activation by *MRF4*, and murine *MRF4-*null mutants show extremely reduced expression of *Myf5*, similar to *Myf5* knockout mice.[27] *Myogenin* can substitute for *Myf5* but is less efficient in this function.[33]

Myogenin does not serve a proliferative function in the genesis of myoblasts but is essential to myoblast fusion in the formation of myotubes, and it is expressed before fusion begins.[37] *Myogenin* inactivation in mice results in a normal number of myoblasts, but they become arrested in terminal differentiation.[27] Wild-type myoblasts can rescue *myogenin*-null myoblasts and cause them to fuse *in vivo*.[38] *Myogenin* is a specific transcriptional target of mitochondrial activity, unlike *Myf5* and *MyoD*.[39]

MyoD1 is the last of the genes to become activated.[23,24] *Myf5* expression is normally suppressed by *MyoD*.[26] Despite its late expression, fetal mouse myoblasts express both *myogenin* and *MyoD* on day 1 in culture, but adult myoblats (satellite cells) have a delay in expression of these genes and of myoblast fusion,[40] though satellite cells co-express proliferating cell nuclear antigen and *MyoD* upon entering the mitotic cycle, and *MyoD* is critical for the programming of satellite cells into *myogenin*-differentiating cells.[41] The transition from proliferation to differentiation is delayed in mice lacking *MyoD*. Though co-expressed, *MyoD* and *Myf5* act at different times in the cell cycle: *Myf5* is maximally expressed in the G2 phase and is minimal in G1; *MyoD* is maximal in G1 and minimal in S-phase; it is re-expressed in G2, but not as strongly as in G1.[42] Another bHLH muscle–restricted transcription factor, *MyoR*, which antagonizes *MyoD*, has been identified recently.[43] *MyoD* and *myogenin* are expressed not only during fetal ontogenesis but also in adult life and are essential to the function of myogenic stem cells (i.e., satellite cells) in normal adults and also in the regenerating muscle in muscular dystrophies.[44,45] The myogenic regulatory genes, particularly *MyoD*, are so dominant that they are able to convert fibroblasts, chondroblasts, and other partially differentiated mesodermal lineages into myoblasts.[46]

The human locus of the *MyoD1* gene is on chromosome 11, very near the domain associated with embryonal rhabdomyosarcoma.[25] The genes encoding *Myf5* and *MRF4* are on chromosome 12 and that for *myogenin* is on chromosome 1. *MyoD* and *myogenin* are strongly expressed in human rhabdomyosarcoma cell lines.[47-49]

In addition to the family of four bHLH genes, *Pax3* has important interactions. It is redundant with *Myf5*: an absence of both *Pax3* and *Myf5* in embryonic mice results in generalized total amyoplasia and death; an isolated *Myf5* mutation causes milder, partial amyoplasia. Upregulation of *Pax3* in chick embryos, by contrast, leads to precocious muscle development and arrested migration of myoblast precursor cells. *Pax3* and *Lbx1* both induce myoblast proliferation.[50] Other genes that *Pax3* induces include *Dach2*, *Eya2*, and *Six1*.[51,52] *Myogenin* is another key regulator of *Six1*.[53] *Pax3* is essential for the migration but not differentiation of limb muscle precursors.[54] Additional important functions of *Pax3* are the development of the eyes and the differentiation and maintenance of Bergmann glial cells of the cerebellum.

Other important genes or gene families that influence the bHLH myogenic genes are BMP2, which inhibits terminal differentiation of myogenic cells by suppressing *MyoD* and *myogenin*[55] and LIM protein, which promotes myogenesis by enhancing the activity of *MyoD*.[56] Wnt signaling also plays a role in regulating the functions of *MyoD* and *myogenin*.[57]

Myostatin is a negative regulator gene of muscle maturation.[58,59] It is a member of the TGFβ family, similar to BMP. It has the latest expression in somites, after all other myogenic genes and desmin are already expressed. It also is co-expressed with *MyoD* but has a wider extent, also involving nonmuscular tissues such as the dermis. *Myostatin* inhibits transition from proliferation to differentiation but does not destroy myoblasts or alter mitotic cycling. *Myostatin* has recently received attention in the lay press because of its potential use to enhance athletic performance.[60,61] There is also a business interest in it to augment the muscular bulk of cattle and swine.

In later stages of muscle ontogenesis, the selective accumulation of *MyoD1* and *myogenin* mRNA transcripts is not purely under genetic control but is modulated and modified by innervation of the muscle and by hormonal influences.[62-64] These effects begin earlier than the stage of histochemical differentiation of muscle fiber types at midgestation. Insulin-like growth factor (IGF) regulates normal *myogenin* expression[65] and influences muscle differentiation both upstream and downstream of *myogenin*.[66] IGF also augments proliferation that precedes differentiation.[67] Basic fibroblast growth factor (bFGF) similarly has a regulating influence on myoblast proliferation and differentiation.[68] Tumor necrosis factor-a, a cytokine, and bFGF differentially inhibit IGF-I-induced expression of *myogenin* in myoblasts.[69,70] IGF-I has early inhibitory and late stimulatory effects on *myogenin* transcription.[71] Other families of genes whose transcription factors influence myodifferentiation include the POU homeodomain,[72] RHO proteins,[73] and SOX proteins.[74] A small number of neuroepithelial cells of the mouse neural tube co-express neuronal markers and also *Myf5* and myosin *in vitro*, suggesting a potential for myogenesis from the neural tube itself.[75]

CYTODIFFERENTIATION OF MUSCLE CELLS

The presumptive myoblast is a morphologically undifferentiated mesenchymal cell that divides mitotically, lacks the distinctive myofilaments of muscle cells, and does not fuse with neighboring cells of the same type.[76] The myoblast differs from its precursor, the presumptive myoblast, by synthesizing myosin and actin and assembling these proteins into thick and thin myofilaments, indicating a commitment to further differentiation as a muscle cell.[77] Although sarcomeres do not form in myoblasts, irregularly scattered clusters of myofilaments are loosely organized into interdigitating arrays. The cytoplasm of myoblasts is sparse. Adjacent myoblasts fuse by extending their contractile myofilaments across the plasma membranes of both cells and aligning the myofilaments produced by a row of several fused myoblasts (Fig. 181–1). Myoblast fusion is enhanced by

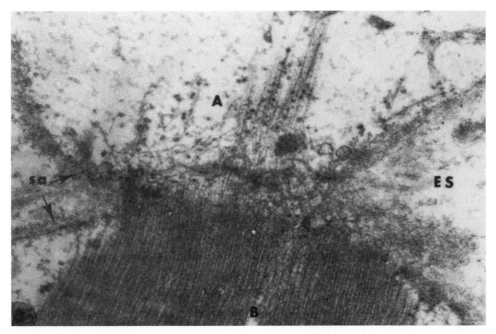

Figure 181–1. Myoblast (**A**) fusing with early myotube (**B**) in the vastus lateralis muscle of a 12-week fetus. Filaments from the myotube are seen extending into the neighboring cell. ES = extracellular space; sa = sarcolemma. (×50,000.) (From Tomanek RJ, Colling-Saltin A-S: Am J Anat *149*:227, 1977.)

isoforms of the neural cell adhesion molecule that mediates interactions of apposed plasma membranes.[78]

The multinucleated syncytium of the row of fused myoblasts forms the myotube. Early myotubes continue to fuse with myoblasts and also with other early myotubules[79] (Fig. 181-2). Circumferentially distributed myofilaments align themselves parallel to the longitudinal axis of the row of fused myoblasts as the filaments grow in length to extend through several fused myoblasts. Myotubular nuclei are enclosed within the center of the newly formed myotube as a single row within a central core of cytoplasm containing the membranous organelles and cytoplasmic particles. Cytoplasm is abundant, and contractile myofilaments are sparse in myotubes in comparison with more mature myocytes, but myofilaments and myofibrils are much more numerous in late myotubes than in early myotubes. Early myotubes predominate until the time of innervation at about 11 weeks' gestation, and late myotubes are dominant during the second half of the myotubular stage from 11 to 16 weeks' gestation.

Intermediate filaments, thinner but longer than the contractile myofilaments, appear in fusing myoblasts and myotubes.[80] These intermediate filaments, such as vimentin and desmin, are cytoskeletal proteins that help organize the cytologic structure of the muscle cell and spatial relationships of organelles, including the orientation and alignment of myofilaments (see later).

A basal lamina (i.e., basement membrane) appears as an indistinct, electron-dense thickening around the developing myotube. It usually encloses several myotubes and a number of less-differentiated myoblasts and presumptive myoblasts in the vicinity.[76, 80, 81] Mast cells, fibroblast-like cells, and other "unclassified" cells also may be included within the basal lamina.[82] Isolated myoblasts lack a basal lamina.[81]

Further maturation of the myotube to become a myocyte involves the synthesis of more contractile myofilaments and more numerous myofibrils, displacing the central nuclei to the peripheral subsarcolemmal region and dispersing the sarcoplasm (i.e., cytoplasm) and its organelles between myofibrils. The Z-bands of several myofibrils within each maturing myotube are not "in register" with each other and do not become aligned consistently until approximately 30 weeks' gestation.[76] The sar-

cotubular system begins forming in the late myotube but is not mature until after 30 weeks' gestation.

After the myofiber achieves morphologic maturity in the relative positions and orientations of the various subcellular components, the next phase consists of the myofiber achieving greater length, an increase in the number of myofibrils in a cross-sectional field of the myofiber, and the development of histochemical fiber types. Although the number of myofibers and their morphologic maturation are mainly genetically determined, metabolic differentiation into fiber types is principally under neural control. Metabolic fiber types also exhibit subtle morphologic differences in the relative number of mitochondria and glycogen granules and in variation in the width of the Z-band.

Spindle-shaped mononucleated cells with abundant polyribosomes and endoplasmic reticulum persist in close apposition to the myotube and myocyte (i.e., multinucleated myofiber) enclosed within the same basal lamina. Such cells are presumptive myoblasts (Fig. 181-3). In mature muscle, they are redesignated *satellite cells* (Fig. 181-4). Although they are dormant and inactive, they are capable of mitotic proliferation and myogenesis even in the adult and are the basis of regeneration of injured muscle.[83-87]

No stage of fetal muscle development is "pure" in the sense of muscle cells exhibiting the same degree of maturation uniformly. Transitions among periods of development are gradual. At 5 to 8 weeks' gestation, presumptive and true myoblasts predominate, but scattered myotubes are already evident at 6 weeks' gestation. The period of 8 to 16 weeks' gestation is regarded as the myotubular stage of development, and myotubes are indeed the most numerous types of muscle cells. However, many myoblasts are still identified, presumptive myoblasts frequently undergoing mitosis are encountered, and a few maturing myocytes beyond the myotubular stage are scattered during the latter weeks of this period. From 16 to 20 weeks' gestation, there is a progressive maturation of myotubes to the cytologic structure of the mature myocyte, but a few myotubes persist. Histochemical differentiation of muscle occurs mainly between 20 and 30 weeks' gestation. From 30 weeks' gestation to term, myofibers undergo several more subtle morphologic adjustments to maturity, such as alignment of Z-bands of adjacent myofibrils to attain "register" and further development of the sarcotubular system.

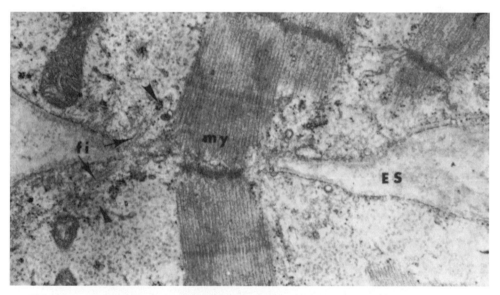

Figure 181–2. Fusion of two myotubes, more advanced in development than the myocytes shown in Figure 181-1, from the soleus muscle of a 16- to 17-week fetus. A well-formed myofibril (*my*) extends between two cells, which are joined by a narrow channel of sarcoplasm. Polyribosomes (*arrowheads*) and unassembled filaments (*fi*) are present in both cells. ES = extracellular space. (×19,500.) (From Tomanek RJ, Colling-Saltin A-S: Am J Anat *149*:227, 1977.)

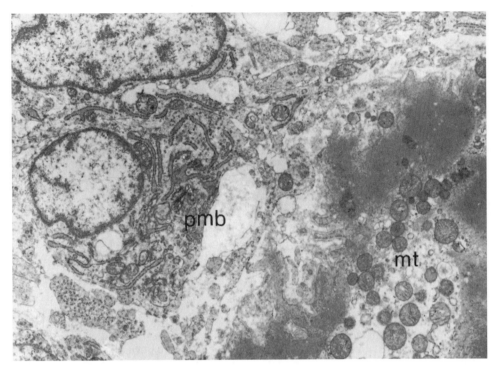

Figure 181–3. Presumptive myoblast (pmb) associated with a myotube (mt) in the quadriceps femoris muscle of a 14-week human fetus. An extensive rough endoplasmic reticulum and many free ribosomes are present, but no contractile filaments or T tubules are developed. Mitochondria also are seen, both in the presumptive myoblast and in the central core of sarcoplasm of the adjacent myotube. (Electron micrograph, ×12,000.)

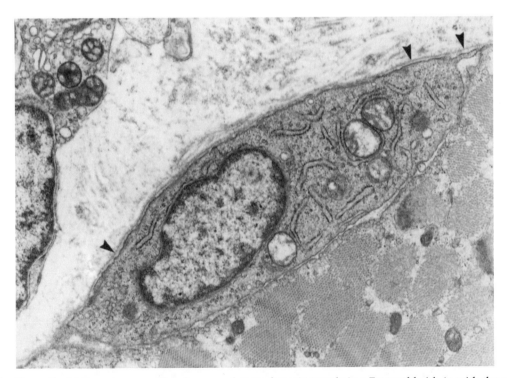

Figure 181–4. Satellite cell of fully mature myofiber from quadriceps femoris muscle in a 7-year-old girl. As with the presumptive myoblast of fetal muscle (see Fig. 181–3), the satellite cell contains mitochondria, rough endoplasmic reticulum, and free ribosomes but no contractile proteins or T tubules and is enclosed within the same basal lamina *(arrowheads)* as the adjacent myofiber. The satellite cell is capable of mitosis and differentiation to become a true myoblast and then mature further and is the cell responsible for regeneration of injured muscle at any age. (Electron micrograph, uranyl acetate and lead citrate, ×20,000.)

A 427-kD cytoskeletal protein known as *dystrophin* is encoded by a large gene at the Xp21.2 locus. This subsarcolemmal protein attaches to the sarcolemmal membrane overlying the A-band and M-band of the myofibrils and consists of four distinct regions or domains: the amino-terminus (N-terminus) contains 250 amino acids and is related to the binding site of α-actinin; the second domain is the largest with 2800 amino acids and contains many repeats, giving it a characteristic rod shape; a third domain is rich in cysteine and is related to the carboxyl-terminus (C-terminus) domain of 400 amino acids, unique to dystrophin and to a dystrophin-related protein encoded by chromosome 6.[88] Dystrophin may be demonstrated in striated muscle by its immunoreactivity, either by immunoperoxidase reaction (Fig. 181–5) or by fluorescence microscopy, and is detected in developing human fetal muscle at 11 weeks' gestation.[89,90] Dystrophin mRNA normally is detected in cardiac and smooth muscle in striated muscle and in the brain. The dystrophin gene encodes a 14-kb messenger ribonucleic acid (mRNA) of about 80 exons. Defective dystrophin is the biologic basis of Duchenne and Becker muscular dystrophies.

Several dystrophin-related glycoproteins also form in this same general period. *Adhalen* (alpha-sarcoglycan) becomes expressed before 14 weeks' gestation. The other sarcoglycans (β, γ, δ) are expressed shortly thereafter. Dysferlin and caveolin-3 are other sarcolemmal membrane proteins at different sites from dystrophin and the sarcoglycans. Caveolin-3 is first detected on day 10 in developing human somites.[91]

Cadherins are another group of transmembrane proteins that mediate calcium-dependent cell-cell adhesion by means of homophilic binding; M(muscle)-cadherin is a recently detected cell type–specific member of this family. In regenerating muscle and in developing fetal muscle, reactivity for M-cadherin is restricted to the plasma membrane of myoblasts and satellite cells and is most intense at the membrane areas facing adjacent myotubes or myofibers.[92-94] M-cadherin is genetically expressed but appears to be neurally regulated;[95] it is not expressed in denervated muscle.[93] The mechanism by which increased cadherin promotes early steps in muscle differentiation is by upregulation of *myogenin*.[96,97]

Merosin is an extracellular matrix protein forming the heavy chain of the skeletal muscle basement membrane protein *laminin* and is important for maintaining the integrity of the sarcolemma. Defective merosin is implicated in the pathogenesis of one form of congenital muscular dystrophy,[98-100] and the chromosomal site of the disease gene is at the 6q2 locus.[100] The merosin (laminin-M) gene maps to chromosome 6q22-23.[101] Merosin may be detected prenatally in the human placenta.[102] Type XIX collagen is a transient extracellular matrix protein that contributes to the the formation of fetal basal lamina and closely follows the expression of *Myf5*.[103] Extracellular matrix is required for muscle differentiation and for the fusion of myoblasts to form myotubes, independent of *myogenin*.[104] Inhibition of fibrillar collagen production in avian and mammalian embryos results in abnormal somite formation and perturbed myogenesis.[105-107]

The innervation of muscle fibers occurs at about 11 weeks' gestation, in the middle of the myotubular stage. Muscle spindles and Golgi tendon organs form after the myotubular stage as the general fascicular organization of the muscle evolves.

The development of joints in the extremities begins at about 5 weeks' gestation within the early mesenchymal condensations of precartilaginous bone. Joint spaces are already apparent by 7 weeks. Motion is probably essential for the development of joints, and some auricular motion is evident as early as 8 weeks, before myotubes are innervated. These small-amplitude movements probably result from spontaneous contractions of newly formed sarcomeres. Active fetal movements are well established after 11 weeks, with the innervation of skeletal muscle, and increase progressively in both force and range of motion around articulations until birth.

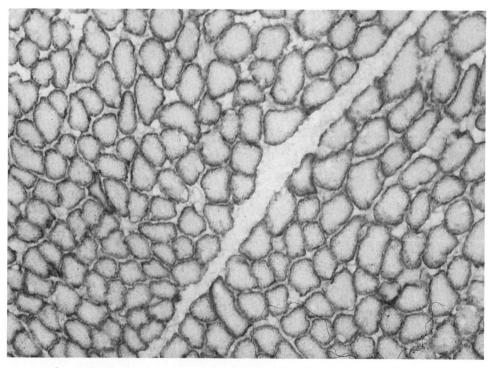

Figure 181–5. Immunocytochemical stain demonstrating dystrophin outlining the sarcolemma of normal quadriceps femoris muscle fibers in a biopsy of a full-term male neonate. The monoclonal antibodies shown are specific for the rod domain of the dystrophin molecule; other antibodies demonstrate only the C-terminus or N-terminus. Dystrophin immunoreactivity is first detected in developing human muscle at 11 weeks' gestation. (×250.)

MORPHOLOGIC STRUCTURE OF MYOTUBES AND MYOCYTES

Sarcolemmal Nuclei

Myoblasts and myotubes have large, vesicular, ovoid nuclei. The chromatin is finely dispersed throughout the nucleoplasm, with a thin condensation against the nuclear membrane. One or often two prominent nucleoli are present (Fig. 181-6). Ultrastructurally, the ribonucleoprotein of these nucleoli forms coarse, electron-dense strands (nucleolonemata) rather than the more massive nucleolar sphere of the mature sarcolemmal nucleus (Fig. 181-7). These features of the nucleoli and of the finely dispersed deoxyribonucleic acid (DNA) are characteristic of active transcription of RNA needed for the synthesis of contractile proteins. The nuclei of regenerating myofibers of children and adults have a similar appearance. The nuclear membrane of fetal myotubes contains pores, similar to the mature state. In the term neonate, some sarcolemmal nuclei are still vesicular and ovoid as are seen in less-mature stages, but most nuclei have acquired the elongated shape with dense chromatin that characterizes the mature state (Fig. 181-8). The nuclei of myotubes are arranged in a single-file row within the central core of sarcoplasm. Nuclei may be tightly packed and in contact with neighboring nuclei, or they may be separated by intermediate segments of sarcoplasm of variable lengths (Fig. 181-9). Both arrangements occur simultaneously within the same muscle, and contiguous as well as widely spaced nuclei occur within different segments along the same myofiber. Closely spaced nuclei are generally more characteristic of early myotubes than of late myotubes. Intranuclear lamin A/C is expressed in differentiating myoblasts.[108] Lamin A/C, lamin B1, and emerin are defective in certain hereditary myopathies, highlighting the importance of myonuclear membrane proteins, as well as sarcolemmal plasma membranes, in the integrity of normal muscle development and maintenance.

Sarcoplasmic Organelles

The abundant sarcoplasm (i.e., cytoplasm) within the core of the myotube between and around nuclei contains membranous organelles. These are mitochondria with well-formed cristae, Golgi apparatus generally at the end of a nucleus, and single-membrane vesicles. Most vesicles have dense cores and probably are lysosomes. Notably lacking from the core of sarcoplasm in myotubes are transverse tubules and sarcoplasmic reticulum (SR) (i.e., endoplasmic reticulum), including their diads and triads that are so common in the intermyofibrillar sarcoplasm of more mature myocytes. Mitochondria are almost the only organelles found in the subsarcolemmal sarcoplasma of myotubes. The septae of sarcoplasm that separate the myofibrils of myotubes contain few organelles, unlike the intermyofibrillar sarcoplasm of mature myofibers, although mitochondria may already begin to redistribute themselves between myofibrils of late myotubes.[81]

Glycogen

Free glycogen particles are numerous in the central core of sarcoplasm and in the subsarcolemmal region of myotubes but are less concentrated between myofibrils. In older fetuses (after 30 weeks' gestation) and in the first postnatal month, double-membrane vesicles or membranous fragments containing glycogen are commonly seen in the intermyofibrillar sarcoplasm. These vesicles are probably derived from lysosomes. Free glycogen particles are notably lacking from the regions of vesicle-enclosed glycogen.[76]

Contractile Myofilaments

In the myoblast, randomly oriented thin and thick myofilaments occur sparsely in the cytoplasm without parallel alignment or evidence of even rudimentary sarcomere formation. Z-band material is not condensed. The early myotube shows poorly aligned thin

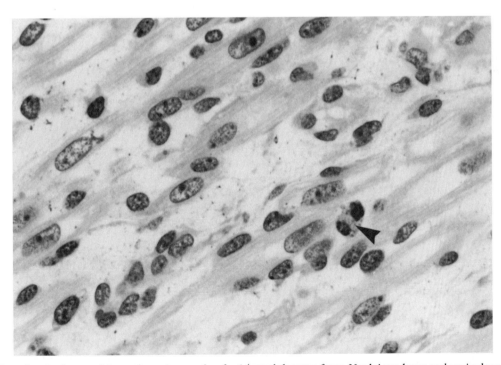

Figure 181-6. Myotubes in the quadriceps femoris muscle of a 14-week human fetus. Nuclei are large and vesicular with finely dispersed chromatin and one or two prominent nucleoli. Mitotic figures of presumptive myoblasts *(arrowhead)* are common. (Hematoxylin-eosin, ×1000.)

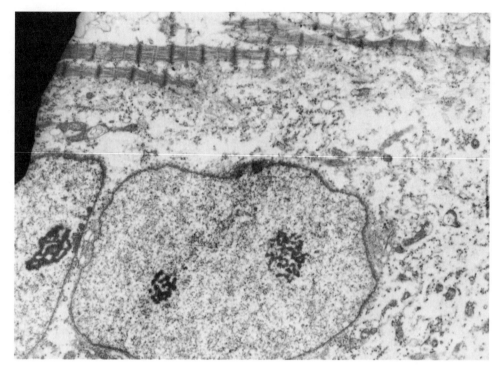

Figure 181–7. Myotube in the quadriceps femoris muscle of a 14-week human fetus. Nuclei exhibit finely dispersed chromatin and strands of ribonucleoprotein-forming nucleoli. Newly formed sarcomeres of contractile proteins are seen at the top of the figure. The sarcoplasmic core contains many mitochondria. (Electron micrograph, uranyl acetate and lead citrate, ×10,000.)

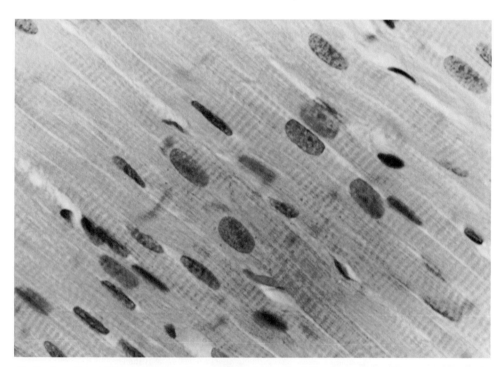

Figure 181–8. Longitudinal section of the quadriceps femoris muscle from a full-term neonate. Many sarcolemmal nuclei retain the ovoid, vesicular appearance of the immature myofiber, but others are elongated and hyperchromatic, characteristic of mature myocytes. (Hematoxylin-eosin, ×1000.)

myofilaments in the periphery of the cytoplasm, near the inner cell membrane; clusters of thick myofilaments with their associated ribosomes are in close proximity.[76] Lattice formation involving alternating thick and thin filaments in a hexagonal array and Z-bands become evident with the synthesis of even a small number of myofilaments. Haphazardly oriented thin filaments are peripheral to the lattice structure, suggesting their assembly even as new myosin filaments are synthesized. However, filament assembly and lattice formation may not depend on the presence of Z-band material because clusters of thin and thick filaments without

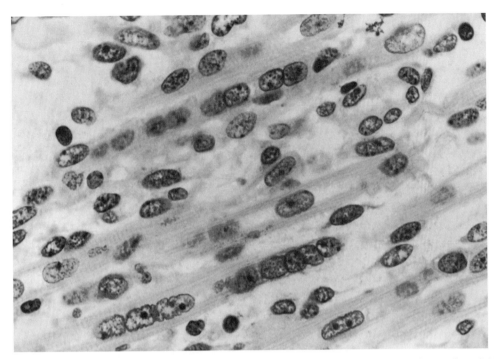

Figure 181–9. Myotubes in the quadriceps femoris muscle of a 12-week human fetus. The spacing of central nuclei is variable. Rows of closely spaced, contiguous nuclei without intervening sarcoplasm are seen, or segments of internuclear sarcoplasm, often several nuclear diameters in length, are found. (Hematoxylin-eosin, ×1000.)

associated Z-material are commonly encountered. The Z-bands that are seen always show fine filaments extending in either direction, and the earliest appearance of Z-bands is consistently observed in foci of thin filament formation.[76] Z-material may form when thick myofilaments are either present or lacking, and it appears to be unrelated to myosin.

Thick filaments are synthesized in different sites of the early myotube cytoplasm than are thin filaments. Although thin filaments first appear in the periphery of the cytoplasm, thick filaments appear nearer the central core of sarcoplasm. Thin filaments also appear earlier than thick filaments.[109] Ribosomes are attached along the thick filaments but decrease in number as these myosin filaments are incorporated into the lattice structure of the sarcomere.

As more thin and thick myofilaments are assembled into a lattice structure, and repeating sarcomeres form as the myotube lengthens, the contractile filaments form a denser tubular structure enclosing the core of sarcoplasm and central nuclei (Fig. 181–10). The wall of this tube of contractile filaments thickens, and the diameter of the myotube increases. Progressive conversion of the myotube to a mature myofiber involves continued synthesis and arrangement of myofilaments, encroachment on the central sarcoplasmic core, and squeezing of the sarcoplasm between groups of myofilaments as the septa that isolate groups of myofilament lattices from adjacent groups. In addition, the central nuclei "migrate" between the forming myofibrils to the subsarcolemmal position that they occupy in the mature myofiber.

Growth of the myofiber near term and postnatally involves mostly a continued synthesis of contractile proteins and an increased number of myofibrils, associated with a corresponding increase in the amount of sarcoplasm and organelles, as well as the addition of more sarcomeres as the muscle grows in length.

Intermediate Filaments

Intermediate filaments are fibrous cytoskeletal polymers intermediate in size between 6-nm actin filaments and 23-nm microtubules that form the structural framework of nearly all eukaryotic cells. These scaffold proteins anchor cells against mechanical stress and function as bridges between linkage proteins and other cytoskeletal components.[109, 110] Perinuclear regions of myotubes characteristically include nonoriented filaments, intermediate in diameter to thick 15-nm and thin 8-nm contractile filaments and measure 10 to 12 nm.[76, 80] Muscle intermediate filaments also are found distal to regions of sarcomere formation. These intermediate filaments are cytoskeletal proteins that help maintain the positions of nuclei and organelles in all cells and help organize the alignment of contractile elements but are not contractile themselves. They may be important in determining the polarity of the early myotube.

Intermediate filament proteins have specific immunoreactivity in differentiating cells and mature cells of various types. The development of intermediate filaments has been less studied in muscle than in the nervous system, and most studies have focused on maturing muscle in tissue culture rather than on animal or human fetuses *in vivo*. Vimentin is largely a transitory fetal intermediate protein that disappears from most cells with maturation. In the fetal central nervous system, vimentin is demonstrated in primitive neuroectodermal cells but is replaced by either neurofilament protein or glial fibrillary acidic protein in cells differentiating along neuronal or glial lines, respectively. Vimentin is prominent in myoblasts,[111-114] and some investigators find that it disappears after myoblast fusion.[113] It continues to be expressed in fetal myotubes and has stronger immunoreactivity in late myotubes than in early myotubes, (Fig. 181–11) but it is not demonstrated in mature striated muscle (see Fig. 181–11). However, even in adult life it persists in smooth muscle cells, including the muscular walls of blood vessels.

Another important muscular intermediate filament, desmin, is responsible for maintaining the register of Z-bands between adjacent myofibrils by forming links between Z-bands.[115] Desmin is thus the third protein, in addition to actinin and actin, to be localized at the Z-band using immunocytochemical techniques.

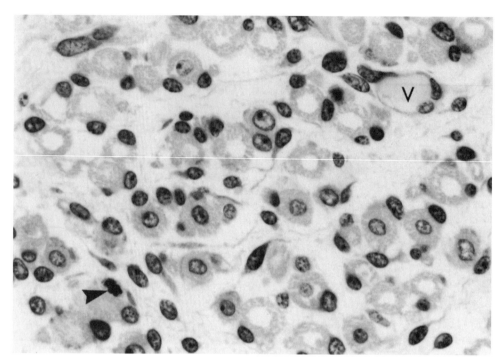

Figure 181–10. Transverse section of the quadriceps femoris muscle in a 12-week human fetus. Late myotubes are a thick cylinder of myofibrils, surrounding central nuclei and the central core of sarcoplasm, seen as a clear space at levels between nuclei. Early myotubes have much thinner cylinders of myofibrils. The peripheral nuclei associated with some myotubes are myoblasts or presumptive myoblasts; one of the latter is undergoing mitosis *(arrowhead)*. Blood vessels (*V*) are a thin endothelium without smooth muscular walls. (Hematoxylin-eosin, ×1000.)

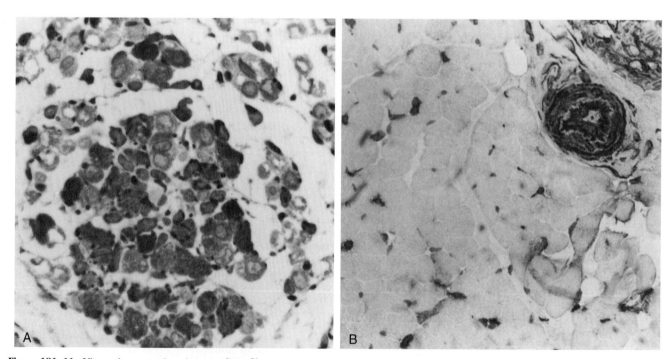

Figure 181–11. Vimentin, a transient intermediate filament protein, is strong in fetal myotubes (dark-staining immunoreactive product), particularly late myotubes, but is no longer seen in striated myofibers of the term neonate, although it is still strongly reactive in smooth muscle of vascular walls and also in endothelial cells. **A**, 14-week fetus. **B**, Full-term neonate. (1:200 dilution; ×1000.)

Desmin synthesis is initiated at the time of myoblast fusion and is prominent in fetal myotubes, especially late myotubes (Fig. 181-12*A*), having the same distribution as vimentin.[111, 112] Early myotubes contain three times as much desmin as vimentin,[114]

but this is difficult to demonstrate in mature muscle by immunocytologic reaction (see Fig. 181-12*B*). Desmin filaments begin to redistribute transversely at the time of sarcomere formation.[113] Nevertheless, desmin is still demonstrated in adult muscle by

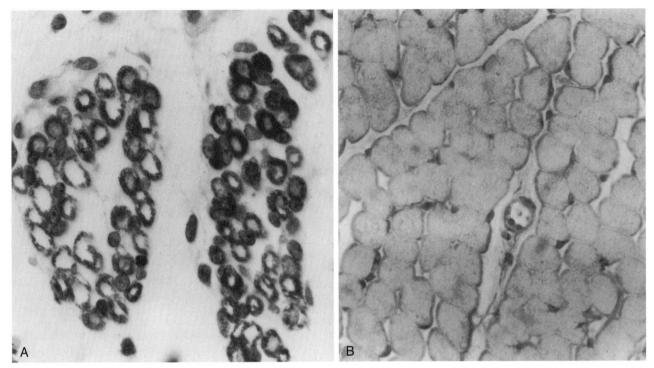

Figure 181–12. Desmin (dark-staining product) is abundant in myotubes and has the same distribution as vimentin. It is no longer demonstrated by immunoreactivity in term neonatal muscle, although it persists in small amounts to maintain the registry of adjacent Z-bands. **A**, 14-week fetus. **B**, Full-term neonate. (1:800 dilution; ×1000)

electrophoretic and special immunologic methods.[112-118] The sparse strands of desmin in adult muscle connect myofibrils at the level of the Z-bands to adjacent sarcolemma, mitochondria, and nuclei to maintain the relative positions of these structures, but they do not attach to the T-tubule systems.[118] Desmin also is associated with the neuromuscular junction site.[119] Immunocytochemistry demonstrates both vimentin and desmin in human striated muscle fibers until about 36 weeks' gestation, although neither is as strongly expressed as in myotubes.[120] In the term neonate, vimentin is not normally demonstrable in myofibers but is prominent in the endothelial cells of blood vessels. Desmin shows only trace or no immunoreactivity in myofibers unless incubated with highly concentrated antibodies (1:50 dilution used for tumors is not appropriate; 1:1200 dilution should be employed.[121] As with vimentin, desmin continues to be strongly expressed by immunocytochemical methods in mature smooth muscle cells, in which these intermediate filaments appear to be associated with the plasma membrane but are not connected to either the actin or myosin filaments.[122] Desmin is closely associated with αB-crystallin, and is augmented in certain human myopathies in a general category as "myofibrillar myopathies."[123]

Microtubules

Microtubules that are approximately 25-nm in diameter are characteristic in regions of myofilament synthesis and early assembly, but they are lacking in regions of more advanced myofibril formation.[76] Their orientation is usually oblique, and they are situated near the ends of developing sarcomeres. A microtubular network is present in both mononucleated myoblasts, in which they radiate from a juxtanuclear center toward the cell periphery, and multinucleated myotubes, in which microtubules are numerous and are arranged in parallel longitudinal orientation.[115,116]

Ribosomes

Ribosomes are abundant in regions of myofilament assembly and sarcomere formation.[80] They may be single and free in the cytoplasm, may occur in clusters as polyribosomes, or may be membrane associated. Ribosomes are structurally related to the formation of thick myosin filaments but not to the formation of thin filaments. Polyribosomes of about 15 individual ribosomes are consistently clustered near both ends of the thick filaments, nearest to the I-band, and single ribosomes also occur along the length of the myosin filament.[124] Ribosomes decrease in number and virtually disappear as the sarcomeres form, and they are rare in mature muscle. They reappear in regenerating myofibers at any age. The high RNA content in fetal myotubes and regenerating myofibers of injured mature muscle, and the lack of demonstrable RNA in mature normal myocytes, are well demonstrated by acridine orange fluorochrome studies.[125]

Sarcotubular System

In myotubes and mature myofibers, the endoplasmic reticulum of less-differentiated myoblasts and presumptive myoblasts is called the SR. Early myotubes exhibit multiple vesicular structures that probably are a primordial stage in the formation of SR. Irregular tubules show branching as the myotube matures, and these tubules are found in regions of cytoplasm containing myofilaments and forming sarcomeres. Numerous Z-bands are in continuity with the SR, but this is not a constant feature. Some studies suggest that the SR tubules completely encircle the Z-band,[81] but my observations agree with those of Tomanek and Colling-Saltin[76] that this is an inconsistent feature. The SR does not appear essential in the assembly of myofilaments. The alignment of Z-bands in register with those of adjacent myofibrils, a late development after 30 weeks' gestation, may be a function of SR tubules associated with Z-bands, however.[76] The SR of both developing and mature myocytes is mostly smooth, without attached ribosomes. Short segments of rough endoplasmic reticulum are also encountered in myotubes but not in mature myofibers.

The T-system develops by invaginations of the sarcolemma (i.e., cell membrane) of the myotube in cultured chick embryonic muscle.[126] Observations of human fetal muscle suggest a similar process of T-tubule formation.[76] Diads, a close association of an SR tubule and a T-tubule, and triads, a T-tubule between a pair of dilated terminal cisternae of SR, are seen only in the periphery of myotubes, often associated with the sarcolemmal membrane[76, 126-128] (Fig. 181-13). Diads and triads occur in deeper regions of the myofiber only after sarcoplasmic septa separate the myofibrils as the central core of cytoplasm becomes dispersed with advanced maturation of the myotube. Membranes of SR and T-tubules first become apposed with no visible structure between them; tenuous connections next traverse the space between apposed membranes, and well-developed bridges finally form.[128] Cisternae of the SR expand to form their characteristic structure after contacting T-tubules.[126] SR cisternae contain electron-dense material that consists of mucopolysaccharides or glycoproteins to provide sites for calcium binding.

The observation that during early fetal development SR cisternae seldom show connections to other SR components suggests either that they develop independently or that they form on short fragments of SR that eventually unite with other SR tubules.[76] Triads have a predominantly longitudinal orientation relative to the long axis of the myofiber until about 28 weeks' gestation, after which time they rotate to the mature transverse orientation (see Figure 181-13).[126-129]

Spherical vesicles with bristles on their outer surface in the periphery of the myotube are probably components of SR terminal cisternae rather than T-tubules because they also are found in satellite cells. Presumptive myoblasts of fetal muscle and satellite cells of mature muscle possess an extensive endoplasmic reticulum, but T-tubules are not evident and do not appear until the myotubular stage of development.[76]

PHYSIOLOGIC CELL DEATH OF MYOTUBES

Degenerating myotubes occur singly or in small groups among normal myotubes in fetuses of 10 to 14 weeks' gestation.[130-132] Mononuclear phagocytic cells may be numerous around degen-

erating myocytes. Electron microscopy reveals nonartifactual extensive necrotic and degenerative changes in both nuclei and sarcoplasm, loss of cell membranes, amorphous condensation of myofibrils, and extrusion of cellular contents into the endomysial extracellular space. This process of physiologic cell death is similar to that observed in the central nervous system and other body systems. An even earlier phase of apoptosis occurs among myoblasts still in the somitic myotome, before migrating into the sites of axial and appendicular muscles.[11]

GROWTH OF MYOFIBERS

The size of an individual muscle is determined by the number and size of its constituent myofibers and also by the amount of connective tissue that forms septa separating fascicles (i.e., perimysium). The diameter of individual muscle fibers is affected by many factors, including age, nutrition, exercise, and the effects of hormones, drugs, and disease. However, the number of muscle fibers in a particular muscle is relatively constant after birth and is genetically programmed.[133,134] A few studies have suggested a postnatal increase in total myofibers of particular muscles such as those of mastication.[133] Protein-calorie malnutrition during fetal development may alter the final number of muscle fibers in animals,[135] but this phenomenon has not been adequately studied in human infants who have suffered intrauterine growth retardation or who are born to undernourished mothers. Ratios of histochemical fiber types within the muscle are under neural control, by contrast, and are mutable in either fetal or adult life, being altered by abnormal innervation patterns (see further on). The average cross-sectional diameter of muscle fibers in the term neonate is 15 μm; the adult mean diameter of 65 μm is achieved at about 13 years of age. A standard curve plotted in 1969 for quantitative measurement in muscle biopsies of children remains valid and widely used by pathologists.[136]

Between 9 and 16 weeks' gestation in the human embryo, myotubes contain about 35 myofibrils in a transverse section of the tube of contractile filaments. Mature muscle fibers each contain about 80 to 110 myofibrils in transverse section. Initially, myotubes are larger in cross-sectional diameter than other myofibers, but the situation is later reversed; as myotubes lengthen, their diameter actually decreases. Although the ratio of myotubes to maturing myofibers reverses, hypertrophy of individual myofibers replaces hyperplasia (i.e., increased number of

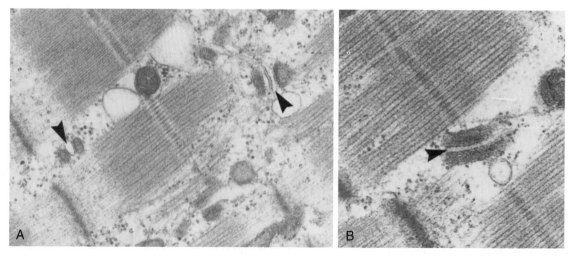

Figure 181–13. Triad formation in full-term neonatal muscle. The triads *(arrowheads)* are formed by a T-tubule with a pair of dilated terminal cisternae of sarcoplasmic reticulum. They generally occur at or near the Z-band and are perpendicular to the long axis of the myofiber in the mature state (**A**), although they initially have a more parallel orientation in relation to the myofiber axis (**B**) until about 28 weeks' gestation. (Electron micrographs, uranyl acetate and lead citrate. **A**, ×25,000; **B**, ×35,000.)

myofibers) as the principal factor contributing to the total increase in the transverse area of the whole muscle.

Myofibril number is not related to myotube size, although it does increase at a declining rate. The total proliferation in number of sarcolemmal nuclei with longitudinal growth of the myofiber is accomplished by mitosis of presumptive myoblasts and their conversion to true myoblasts, rather than by proliferation of existing sarcolemmal nuclei, because the latter are incapable of mitosis. This process slows in late gestation.[132]

Between 20 and 24 weeks' gestation, about 10% of total myofibers in a cross-sectional field are noted to be about twice as large as the remaining 90%. These hypertrophic fibers are scattered uniformly throughout the fascicles and are never grouped. They were first identified by Wohlfart in 1937 and were designated by him as b-fibers; the majority population of smaller fibers were termed a-fibers,[137] a terminology still used. The Wohlfart b-fibers were also later shown to be distinguishable from the a-fibers (see further on) by histochemical reactivity. Between 24 and 30 weeks' gestation, as histochemical differentiation proceeds, the Wohlfart a-fibers increase in diameter to achieve the same size as the b-fibers that do not grow as fast, until the two populations of myofibers can no longer be distinguished by size after 30 weeks.

Growth of myofibers during late gestation is mainly in length rather than diameter, but the latter accelerates in the postnatal period. Some increase in the number of myofibers in late gestation and postnatally may occur because of longitudinal splitting; an explanation of this splitting down the middle of the growing myofiber is that when a fiber achieves a critical size, the oblique pull of peripheral actin filaments is strong enough to cause the Z-band to rupture.[138] Postnatally, linear growth of skeletal myofibers is greatest in the first 2 years and is accomplished mainly by adding sarcomeres rather than by extending the distance between Z-bands.

METABOLIC DIFFERENTIATION OF MYOFIBERS

After nearly all fetal myotubes have become myocytes with peripheral sarcolemmal nuclei and an intermyofibrillar distribution of sarcoplasm and organelles, the next major maturational development is the differentiation of the uniform population of myofibers into a heterogeneous population of two distinct metabolic types and subtypes of at least one of these. Neural influence is first expressed in muscle maturation in the further growth and morphologic reorganization of myotubes and plays no role in the fusion of myoblasts to become myotubes. However, the expression of metabolic differences between muscle fibers is strongly controlled by innervation, and myofibers retain the capacity to change metabolic type with changes in innervation, as with denervation-reinnervation of muscle. This mutability is retained in human striated muscle not only during fetal life and infancy but also in the adult.

Metabolic differences between myofibers are expressed as relative differences in various enzymatic activities of the oxidative and glycolytic pathways, differences in calcium-mediated myofibrillar adenosine triphosphatase (ATPase) isozymes that are expressed maximally at various pH ranges, in heavy-chain myosin, and in relative numbers or concentrations of mitochondria, lipid droplets, and glycogen particles within the sarcoplasm. These features are well demonstrated in frozen tissue section by histochemical methods and, more recently, by immunocytochemical reactivity for heavy-chain myosin that distinguishes fiber types in formalin-fixed, paraffin-embedded sections.[139] The histochemical differentiation of developing muscle in humans was studied by numerous investigators in the 1960s and 1970s, and their similar conclusions are confirmatory.

The period of histochemical differentiation is between 20 and 30 weeks' gestation in humans, but some differences among myofibers in their metabolic profiles may be seen as early as 18 weeks. Before that time, all myofibers appear histochemically uniform with all enzymatic stains; using myofibrillar ATPase stains, they correspond to IIc fibers, which are considered the least differentiated subtype in mature muscle.

The early phase of histochemical differentiation, generally 20 to 24 weeks, coincides with the appearance of Wohlfart b-fibers, the 10% of total myofibers that are larger than the rest and are scattered evenly throughout the fascicles without being grouped.[137,140] These Wohlfart b-fibers are uniformly type I (i.e., strong ATPase activity at acid pH of preincubation, strong oxidative enzymatic activity and weaker glycolytic activity, less glycogen than type II); the 90% remaining Wohlfart a-fibers react histochemically as type II (i.e., strongest ATPase activity at alkaline pH of preincubation, weaker oxidative and stronger glycolytic enzymatic activity, and more glycogen than type I) and correspond almost exclusively to subtype IIc of mature muscle (Fig. 181–14).

As maturation proceeds, and especially during the later phase of histochemical differentiation from 24 to 30 weeks' gestation, there is progressive conversion of many type II fibers (Wohlfart a-fibers) to type I fibers; however, growth of the population of smaller fibers at a greater rate than growth of the Wohlfart b-fibers obliterates the distinction of these populations by either size or their reactivity as type I. By 30 weeks' gestation, most muscles of the human body have relatively equal numbers of types I and II myofibers, and they are distributed in a mosaic or checkerboard pattern without large groups of either type, although small groups of three to five fibers of the same type may occur. Type II fibers may predominate in the single line of myofibers along the edges of fascicles.

During the later period of histochemical differentiation (after 30 weeks' gestation), type II fibers become distinguished by myofibrillar ATPase stains as subtypes defined by their degree of inhibition of reaction at varying pH of preincubation.[140] Thus, at high pH, such as 9.8 or 10.4, all type II fibers are uniformly stained darker than type I fibers. At pH 4.6 or 4.7, type I fibers are dark, whereas some type II fibers are intermediate in intensity and others are totally inhibited and unstained. The inhibited fibers are designated IIa, and the intermediate fibers are designated IIb and IIc. At a still lower pH of preincubation (4.3), IIa fibers remain completely inhibited, IIb fibers are either totally inhibited or very light, and IIc fibers are intermediate—darker than IIb fibers but not as dark as type I fibers. At maturity, about 65% of total type II fibers are designated IIa, 30% are designated IIb, and only 5% are designated IIc. In the term neonate, however, 15 to 20% of type II fibers are IIc or "undifferentiated" fibers (see Figure 181–14).[140–142] Differentiation of the soleus muscle, with a higher percentage of type I fibers, is not complete until 9 to 12 months of age in the human infant and is accompanied by slowing of contractile properties that correspond to the functional use of this muscle as the infant stands more and prepares to walk.[142]

The oxidative enzymatic activity of the mitochondria and SR has a characteristic histochemical distribution using stains of the electron transport chain (e.g., nicotine adenine dinucleotide [reduced form]–tetrazolium reductase) and of the tricarboxylic acid (Krebs) cycle (e.g., succinate dehydrogenase; malate dehydrogenase, isocitrate dehydrogenase). In myotubes, the activity follows the distribution of mitochondria and is seen only in the central core of sarcoplasm and in the subsarcolemmal region (Fig. 181–15A). As the myofiber matures, the mitochondria become redistributed in the intermyofibrillar sarcoplasm. Therefore, type I fibers, which have more mitochondria than type II fibers, appear darker (see Fig. 181–15B). Oxidative enzymatic stains used to be regarded only in relative ratio of activity to glycolytic enzyme stains, but it is now recognized that each is a marker for the specific mitochondrial respiratory chain

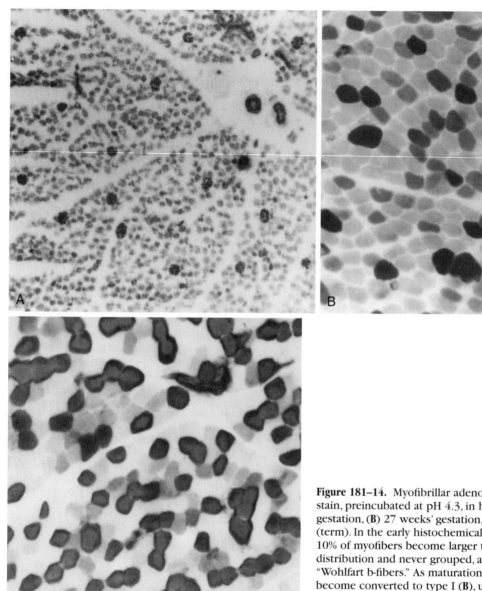

Figure 181–14. Myofibrillar adenosine triphosphatase (ATPase) stain, preincubated at pH 4.3, in human fetuses at *(A)* 24 weeks' gestation, **(B)** 27 weeks' gestation, and **(C)** 40 weeks' gestation (term). In the early histochemical stage of development **(A)**, about 10% of myofibers become larger than the others, are scattered in distribution and never grouped, and react as type I fibers, the "Wohlfart b-fibers." As maturation proceeds, more type II fibers become converted to type I **(B)**, until there is a relatively equal number of the two types at term **(C)**. There is still a greater proportion of subtype IIc fibers (intermediate intensity of staining) at birth than in the adult. (×250.)

complexes, and they have assumed an even greater value in interpreting some muscle biopsies, as well as in developmental studies of muscle.

Myophosphorylase activity also may be histochemically demonstrated in unfixed frozen sections of striated muscle. A fetal form of myophosphorylase is replaced by the mature form of the enzyme after birth. In addition to myophosphorylase, phosphofructokinase and other enzymes of the glycolytic Embden-Meyerhof pathway may also be demonstrated in fetal muscle as early as the late myotubular stage. Distinction between histochemical fiber types is not evident until after 24 weeks' gestation, however. The myogenic genes may also play a role in muscle fiber–type differentiation, even though this phase of ontogenesis is considerably later than the primary period of expression of these genes. In transgenic mice, myogenin induces, or at least accompanies, a shift from glycolytic (type II fibers) to oxidative (type I fibers) metabolism.[143, 144] With aging in adult life, there are also changes in levels of expression of *myogenin* and *MyoD* proteins in muscle.[145]

FASCICULAR ORGANIZATION OF DEVELOPING MUSCLE

As the paired longitudinal somitic plates on either side of the neural plate begin to segment into somites, the space between somites contains looser, less densely cellular mesenchyme than the more compact somites. The mesenchymal cells in this looser tissue differentiate into fibroblasts and soon secrete collagen into the intercellular space as the more compact mesenchymal cells of the somites predominantly become myoblasts and primordial dermal cells. During growth of the limb buds, the individual muscles of the extremities are derived from the somites, whereas the collagenous muscle capsules (i.e., epimysium), blood vessels, and tendons are somatopleural derivatives.

Individual muscles consist of loose arrays of presumptive and true myoblasts and differentiating myotubes without the connective tissue septa that subdivide more mature muscle into fascicles. During the myotubular stage of myogenesis, myotubes and myoblasts cluster in small groups of three to as many as eight

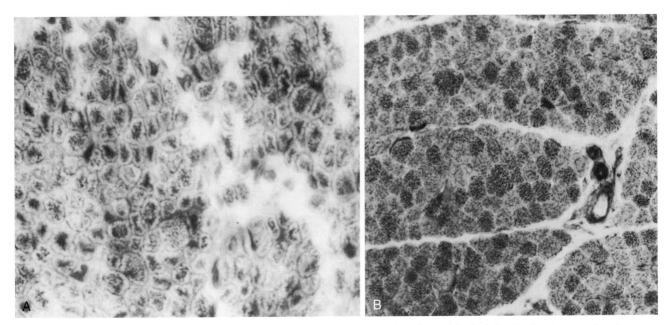

Figure 181–15. **A,** Oxidative enzymatic (mitochondrial) activity has a characteristic histochemical distribution in myotubes: intense staining confined to the central core of sarcoplasm and a thin rim in the subsarcolemmal region, the cylinder of myofibrils remaining unstained. Fiber types cannot be distinguished. **B,** In term neonatal muscle, the oxidative enzymatic activity is now redistributed uniformly in the intermyofibrillar sarcoplasm. Dark points of activity are mitochondria. The darker-staining fibers are type I, and the lighter-stained fibers are type II, as in the adult. (Nicotinamide adenine dinucleotide, tetrazolium reductase [NADH-TR]: **A,** ×1000; **B,** ×250.)

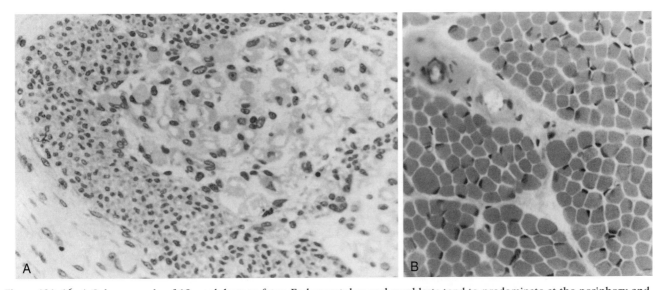

Figure 181–16. **A,** Soleus muscle of 12-week human fetus. Early myotubes and myoblasts tend to predominate at the periphery, and late myotubes are more frequent in the interior of the muscle. Perimysial connective tissue septa have not yet developed. **B,** Term neonate, quadriceps femoris muscle. The fascicular organization of the muscle is well developed, with a well-defined perimysium that includes arterioles, venules, and intramuscular nerves. (Hematoxylin-eosin; **A,** ×400; **B,** ×250.)

cells, but mostly three to five myotubes, surrounded by a single common basal lamina.[141, 146] Single myotubes enclosed within their own individual basal lamina and isolated myoblasts without a basal lamina also appear.[76] Independent myotubes become more numerous in later stages of development, and by the end of the myotubular stage, clusters of myotubes within a common basal lamina are no longer seen, although single myotubes continue to be closely associated with myoblasts and presumptive myoblasts.[146] Myoblasts and early myotubes tend to predominate

at the periphery of the developing muscle, and maturation of the myotubes in the center of the muscle is more advanced (Fig. 181-16A).

Fibroblasts also are included within developing muscle and produce delicate reticular and collagen fibers. Thin collagenous septa (i.e., perimysium) divide the muscle into fascicles, particularly in association with the growth of blood vessels. This process begins in the late myotubular stage, occurring mainly as myotubes are converted to myocytes with peripheral nuclei and continuing during the early phase of histochemical differentiation. By 30 weeks' gestation, the fascicular organization of muscle is well established. Perimysial connective tissue then thickens, and by term the perimysium is well developed and includes all arterioles, venules, and nerves that penetrate the muscle (see Fig. 181-16B). Endomysial collagen fibers between individual myofibers within a fascicle are thinner, sparser, and much more delicate in the term neonate than in the older child; the endomysium mainly develops postnatally.

Blood vessels within developing muscle are seen as early as 6 weeks' gestation in humans. During the myotubular stage of development, vessels consist of delicate channels or sinuses with thin endothelial cells and wide lumina (Figs. 181-17 and 181-18). With growth of the perimysium, the feeding vessels develop smooth muscular walls and a thicker endothelium. The capillary network becomes denser as myofibers mature and contraction becomes more forceful. By term, both capillaries and larger arterioles and venules are well developed (see Figure 181-16B).

MUSCLE SPINDLES AND TENDON ORGANS

Intrafusal fibers are already forming during the myotubular stage of development, but they are difficult to recognize histologically because they closely resemble extrafusal fibers at this time. The distinctive connective tissue capsule of the spindle does not form until later.[147-149] Spindles may be readily identified after 20 weeks' gestation in humans, and they appear fully mature at 30 weeks, including well-developed nuclear bag and nuclear chain forms of intrafusal fibers (Fig. 181-19) with their mature histochemical characteristics.

Intrafusal fibers enclosed by a delicate collagenous capsule may be recognized as early as 14 weeks' gestation in human fetuses, so spindles actually begin forming late in the myotubular stages.

In the rat, the earliest detectable spindles in hindlimb muscles are seen less than 2 days before birth and consist of a single myotube bearing simple nerve terminals of the large primary afferent axon from nearby unmyelinated intramuscular nerve

trunks. The capsule forms by an extension of the perineurium of the supplying nerve fasciculus and is confined initially to the innervated zone.[147-150] Myoblasts are present within the capsule of the spindle throughout its development and fuse to form a smaller and less-differentiated myotube. This myotube matures in close association with the initial fiber, and by birth it has formed the smaller, intermediate nuclear bag fiber identified in the adult. Nuclear chain fibers develop in the same way, but myoblast fusion forms satellite myotubes in apposition to more mature fibers within the same basal lamina. By 4 days postnatally, the adult complement of four intramuscular muscle fibers is present. Fusiform innervation begins at birth and is not complete until the twelfth postnatal day (rat) when the myofibrillar ultrastructure is fully mature.[149] The periaxial space appears at the same time. The afferent innervation thus precedes the efferent nerve supply to the intrafusal spindle fibers. Morphogenesis of the rat muscle spindle is complete at 25 days after birth.[150]

As with the differing morphologic features between extrafusal and intrafusal muscle fibers, mature intrafusal fibers exhibit histochemical characteristics that are unique and do not correspond to the histochemical types of extrafusal fibers.[151-154] These histochemical subpopulations appear somewhat later than the differentiation of fiber types of extrafusal myofibers, with some overlap.

Golgi tendon organs are stretch receptors found between muscle and tendon and less frequently within the tendon itself. They also are distributed in the intermuscular connective tissue and in the capsules of joints. Tendon organs are almost as numerous as muscle spindles, although infrequently seen in muscle biopsies.[155] Tendon organs lie in series with the main mass of muscle, so they are sensitive to any sudden change in muscle length, active or passive, or to a summation of active and passive stretch. Their afferent nerve fibers all belong to group Ib, with widespread central connections that allow for patterned and sequential engagement of synergistic and antagonistic muscles as integrated movements. Golgi tendon organs develop after the myotubular stage and are well formed by 28 weeks' gestation.

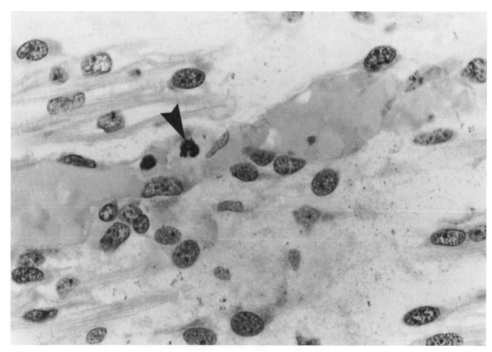

Figure 181–17. Intramuscular blood vessel in quadriceps femoris muscle of a 14-week fetus. The vessel is thin walled, and the lumen is wide and dilated. The mitotic figure *(arrowhead)* may be an endothelial cell or a presumptive myoblast. (Hematoxylin-eosin, ×1000.)

Numerous pacinian corpuscles similar to those of the dermis also occur near the myotendinous junction, mainly within the tendon (Fig. 181–20), but they also occur in the perimysium between muscle fascicles at distal ends of muscles.

Unlike extrafusal myofibers that characteristically undergo atrophy and disappear after loss of their motor nerve supply, intrafusal spindle fibers continue to develop normally during the first 3 weeks after de-efferentation of immature neonatal rat

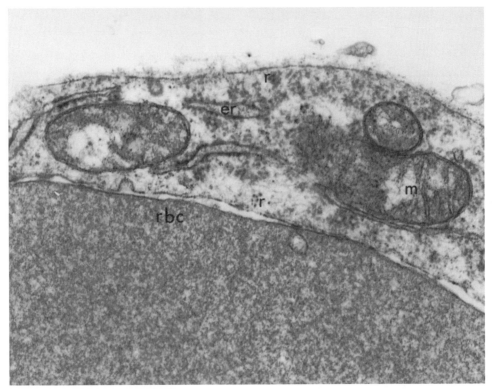

Figure 181–18. Endothelial cell of intramuscular blood vessel of a 14-week fetus. Mitochondria (*m*), rough endoplasmic reticulum (*er*), and free ribosomes (*r*) are seen in the cytoplasm. A red blood cell (*rbc*) is seen in the lumen of the vessel. (Electron micrograph, uranyl acetate and lead citrate, ×25,000)

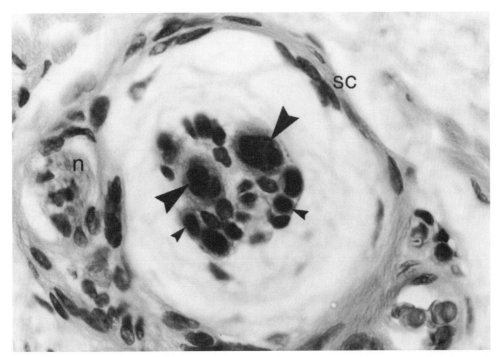

Figure 181–19. Muscle spindle within the quadriceps femoris muscle of a term neonate. Both nuclear bag fibers *(large arrowheads)* and nuclear chain fibers *(small arrowheads)*, as well as the spindle capsule (*sc*) and associated nerve (*n*), are well developed at birth. (Hematoxylin-eosin, ×1000)

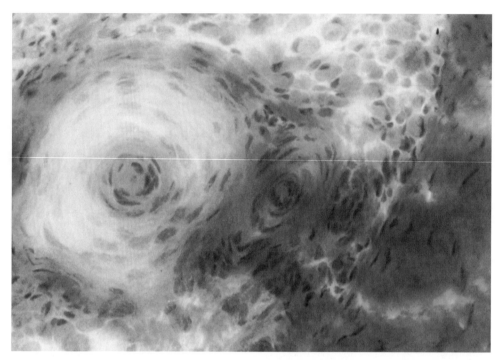

Figure 181–20. Pacinian corpuscle near myotendinous insertion of the quadriceps femoris muscle in a 36-week premature infant. The fibrous epimysial muscle capsule is seen on the right. (Gomori trichrome, ×1000.)

muscle, but only if their afferent sensory nerve supply and dorsal root ganglia are preserved, even if the spinal cord segment is extirpated. Intrafusal fibers then actually proliferate at 3 to 5 weeks after denervation with the supernumerary fibers forming from the fusion of myoblasts derived from activated intrafusal satellite cells, and also from longitudinal splitting of pre-existing intrafusal myofibers.[155-159] New intrafusal fibers originate from both nuclear bag and nuclear chain fibers but mainly from the latter.[156] The ratio of myosin heavy chain isoforms is altered under these circumstances.[152, 159] The total efferent and afferent denervation of muscle spindles, by contrast, results in atrophy and numeric reduction of intrafusal myofibers.[159, 160] In sum, intrafusal muscle fibers are much more dependent on sensory than on motor nerve supply to preserve their integrity and they proliferate as a delayed response to de-efferentation, rather than undergo atrophy.[161]

TENDON DEVELOPMENT

Tendons are dense fibrous bands that attach striated muscles to bones, as either the proximal origin or the distal insertion of the muscle. In *traction tendons*, in which the line of action corresponds to that of the muscle, few blood vessels are uniformly distributed within the tendon tissue. In *gliding tendons*, which change their direction of pull, an avascular zone normally forms in the region where the tendon wraps around the pulley.[162] The angiogenic peptide vascular endothelial growth factor (VEGF) is present in both endothelial cells and tenocytes (a fibroblast derivative) of human fetal tendons exposed to traction, but not in the avascular zone of gliding tendons that are predominantly exposed to compressive and shearing forces. The avascular zone of tendons might be caused by a mechanically induced downregulation of VEGF expression.[163] Tendons begin forming at the time of the differentiation of the fascicular organization of muscle. The transitional zone is a mixture of perimysial fibrous bands and myofibers that may show cytoarchitectural differences from the same fibers in the main belly of the muscle, and hence can

easily be misinterpreted as myopathic findings in muscle biopsies taken too near the insertion, as during "heel cord" (Achilles tendon) lengthening procedures.

MEMBRANE EXCITABILITY AND INNERVATION OF FETAL MUSCLE

The resting membrane potential of mature muscle, about 90 mV, is actively maintained by continuous energy production derived from Na$^+$,K$^+$-ATPase (calcium-mediated ATPase and creatine kinase are the energy sources for the contractile mechanism of myofibrils). This energy-generating system for maintaining membrane excitability develops early in myogenesis; even early myotubes already have a continuously polarized membrane. Spontaneous subthreshold potentials may be recorded anywhere along the sarcolemmal membrane, but their site of origin is in the middle of the fiber at the point at which end plates are eventually formed.[163] They resemble the miniature end-plate potentials of adult fibers but occur at a lower frequency and with a slower time course. The plasma membrane of myoblasts also is excitable, although it may easily fatigue. The compound that most strongly and consistently provokes membrane depolarization is acetylcholine (ACh), the transmitter secreted at the neuromuscular junction of mature striated muscle in humans, all vertebrates, and some invertebrates.

ACh receptors are among the first membrane proteins to appear during the development of striated muscle. In the larval amphibian *Xenopus*, functional ACh receptors begin to form within 2 hours after the myotomes begin to appear, which is much earlier than nerve contacts muscle.[164,165] In the rat, peripheral nerves and functional ACh receptors both appear when developing muscle cells are first identified,[166] but functional innervation is not required for the development of ACh receptors, and myoblasts isolated in tissue culture continue to develop them.[167] The expression of ACh receptors in living rat embryos is unaltered after destruction of their motor neurons.[168]

Although innervation is not essential for the initial formation of functional ACh receptors, innervation of muscle leads to a major redistribution of receptors, eventually resulting in their aggregation at the points of nerve contact.[165,168,169] After the concentration of receptors at the synapse point, there is a decrease in the density of receptors in portions of the sarcolemmal membrane not directly contacted by nerve endings.[165,170,171] The decreased density of ACh receptors is accompanied by a low sensitivity of nonsynaptic membrane to ACh, a characteristic of adult muscle fibers. Aggregates of synaptic junction receptors remain following denervation; removal of the nerve results in a return of high levels of extrajunctional receptors.[172,173]

Innervation of human striated muscle occurs in the middle of the myotubular stage of development, maximally at about 11 weeks' gestation, but motor end plates begin to form as early as 9 weeks' gestation and continue to develop and mature until 20 weeks' gestation.[174] The primitive motor end plate contains a few axons always covered by one Schwann cell. It does not change either in number or in structure between 10 and 20 weeks' gestation, although continuous modification of the postsynaptic membrane is observed throughout this period.[175] The axon contains a few synaptic vesicles and is in close contact with the unfolded plasma membrane of the primary myotube. The first morphologic change indicative of end-plate formation is seen at the junction of the sarcolemma with the axolemma, the former having a distinct thickening in the small junctional zone. This thickening of the postsynaptic membrane may already be evident when the axon is 20 to 30 nm away from the muscle cell.[175] At the mature myotubular stage, at about the 14th week of gestation, synaptic gutters and primary synaptic clefts form. Secondary synaptic clefts are first seen in the 16th week of gestation. The characteristic convolutions of the mature postsynaptic membrane are thus well established by midgestation and are fully mature at birth.

Myotubes initially are innervated from several nerves. The mature single-nerve supply to each myofiber results from retraction of all but one nerve as development proceeds. Fidziańska found several synaptic axonal terminals grouped together and filled with synaptic vesicles at the motor end plate of human fetuses of 10 to 20 weeks' gestation; these axonal terminals did not seem to change in either ultrastructural appearance or number during this period and were always covered by a single Schwann cell.[175] Silver impregnations of nerve fibers also show a single motor end plate on each fetal myofiber supplied by more than one axon.[176] It may be concluded from these data that each developing myofiber has just one end plate but that this end plate is supplied by two or more axons, a conclusion consistent with other electrophysiologic and morphologic data that suggest polyneural innervation of fetal muscle fibers. Scanning electron microscopy of nerve-muscle cultures also confirms that a single embryonic muscle fiber may be contacted by as many as five different nerves arising from different motor neurons.[177] Physiologic cell death of a spinal neuroblast is unrelated to the change from polyneuronal to mononeuronal innervation of muscle,[178] but functional neuromuscular innervation is probably one factor that regulates the natural process of cell death among embryonic motor neurons of the spinal cord, because the number of motor neurons undergoing natural cell death is closely related to muscular activity.[179]

"Myotube satellite cells" with long cytoplasmic processes extending beyond the basal lamina into the endomysial space are seen in developing extraocular muscles. They contact free cells of similar appearance, as well as axon-surrounding Schwann cells, often forming an extensive network. These myotube satellite cells resemble Schwann cells in all respects except for the lack of an associated axon, and they may be Schwann cells disposed to promote axonal growth toward differentiating myofibers not yet innervated.[180]

Spinal motor nerve roots begin their myelination cycle at about 16 weeks' gestation, and roots and peripheral nerves are well myelinated by late gestation.[181] In the phrenic nerve, one and a half turns of myelin are seen around nerve fibers at 15 weeks' gestation;[182] the vagal nerve begins its myelination cycle at about 24 weeks' gestation in humans[183] and at a corresponding age in fetal lambs.[184] Myelination of axons innervating extraocular muscles is reported by some investigators as early as 18 weeks' gestation.[185]

SUPRASEGMENTAL NEURAL INFLUENCES ON MUSCLE MATURATION

The importance of innervation to muscle fiber maturation beyond the myotubular stage is well demonstrated both *in vivo* and *in vitro*. Neonatal neurectomy in rats prevents further development of the myocyte.[186] In humans, the effects of perinatal denervation on the morphologic features of muscle are well demonstrated in progressive spinal muscular atrophy, a degenerative motor neuron disease beginning in fetal life and continuing after birth.[187]

Suprasegmental centers in the cerebrum, cerebellum, and brain stem may alter the discharge pattern of motor neurons and change the course of muscle maturation. Classic studies document that excessive nerve stimulation experimentally causes a conversion of type II fibers to type I in the rat,[188,189] and abnormal suprasegmental stimulation of lower motor neurons in the human fetus may have a similar influence on histochemical differentiation.

Histochemical abnormalities in the muscle biopsy specimens from infants with cerebral malformations have been noted by several researchers.[190-193] Similar aberrations in the sizes and ratios of histochemical fiber types occur in the muscles of neonates with congenital contractures after fetal immobilization (i.e., arthrogryposis multiplex congenita).[193] Prospective study of the muscles of infants with various types of cerebral dysgenesis documented by imaging procedures or by postmortem examination demonstrates that three categories of disorders in muscle maturation may be identified: (1) delayed maturation in term infants, the muscle being morphologically normal but incompletely differentiated histochemically; (2) fiber–type predominance of more than 80% of either type I or type II fibers; and (3) the classic "congenital muscle fiber–type disproportion," defined as a predominance and uniform hypoplasia of type I fibers, often with secondary hypertrophy of type II fibers.[194,195]

An equally dramatic finding is the presence of normal and histochemically mature neonatal muscle in infants with normal spinal cords but severely hypoplastic brains, or with such severe dysplasias that few if any descending pathways exist to relay suprasegmental impulses.[194] This finding in the human is supported by observations in the stage 13 or 14 (day 2) chick embryo that extirpation of several cervical segments of spinal cord does not alter the development of motor end-plate distribution or histochemical differentiation by ATPase of muscles innervated by more caudal segments.[196] The relatively isolated human spinal cord with normal muscle maturation demonstrates that the motor unit is capable of maturing normally without cerebral influence, and the aberrant patterns found in infants with cerebral dysgenesis suggest that abnormal descending upper motor neuron influences may alter the course of muscle ontogenesis, probably by interfering with the discharge pattern of the lower motor neuron.

The most common malformation of the brain associated with abnormal muscle development is cerebellar hypoplasia as an isolated anomaly or in conjunction with cerebral dysplasias.[194,195] Abnormal development of brainstem structures is also associated with aberrant muscle maturation, but congenital lesions confined to suprasegmental structures, even when severe, do not seem to affect muscle development. Descending brainstem pathways become myelinated during the period of histochemical differentiation of muscle, between 20 and 30 weeks' gestation,[181] and are functional during this period. The corticospinal tract, by contrast, is unmyelinated until much later, after muscle maturation is complete, and probably subserves several functions in the term neonate.[197, 198] It is therefore likely that suprasegmental influences on muscle maturation are mediated by the numerous small bulbospinal (i.e., "subcorticospinal") pathways, such as the tectospinal, rubrospinal, olivospinal, vestibulospinal, and reticulospinal tracts, than by the much larger but late-myelinating corticospinal tract.

REFERENCES

1. MacCallum JB: On the histogenesis of the striated muscle fibre and the growth of the human sartorius muscle. Johns Hopkins Hosp Bull *9*:208, 1898.
2. Tello JF: Génesis de las terminaciones nerviosas motrices y sensitivas. I. En el sistema locomotor de los vertebrados superiores. Histogénesis muscular. Trab Lab Invest Biol Univ Madrid *15*:101, 1917.
3. Sarnat HB: New insights into the pathogenesis of congenital myopathies. J Child Neurol *9*:193, 1994.
4. Wood A, Thorogood P: Patterns of cell behavior underlying somitogenesis and notochord formation in intact vertebrate embryos. Dev Dynam *201*:151, 1994.
5. Wagner M, et al: Polarizing activity and retinoid synthesis in the floor plate of the neural tube. Nature *345*:819, 1990.
6. Fan C-M, Tessier-Lavigne M: Patterning of mammalian somites by surface ectoderm and notochord: evidence for sclerotome induction by a hedgehog homolog. Cell *79*:1175, 1994.
7. Pourquié O, et al: Control of dorsoventral patterning of somitic derivative by notochord and floor plate. Proc Natl Acad Sci U S A *90*:5242, 1993.
8. Brand-Saberi B, et al: The ventralizing effect of the notochord on somite differentiation in chick embryos. Anat Embryol *188*:239, 1993.
9. Venters SJ, et al: Early development of the myotome in the mouse. Dev Dynam *216*:219, 1999.
10. Pownall ME, et al: Notochord signals control the transcriptional cascade of myogenic bHLH genes in somites of quail embryos. Development *122*(suppl):1475, 1996.
11. Asakura A, Tapscott SJ: Apoptosis of epaxial myotome in Danforth's short-tail (Sd) mice in somites that form following notochord degeneration. Dev Biol *203*:276, 1998.
12. Lucarelli M, et al: The dynamics of myogenin site-specific demethylation is strongly correlated with its expression and with muscle differentiation. J Biol Chem *276*:7500, 2001.
13. Braun TE, et al: Differential expression of myogenic determination genes in muscle cells: possible autoactivation by the *Myf* gene products. EMBO J *8*:3617, 1989.
14. Braun T, et al: A novel human muscle factor related to but distinct from *MyoD1* induces myogenic conversion in 10T1/2 fibroblasts. EMBO J *8*:701, 1989.
15. Thayer MJ, et al: Positive autoregulation of the myogenic determination gene *MyoD1*. Cell *58*:241, 1989.
16. Yee S-P, Rigby PWJ: The regulation of myogenin gene expression during the embryonic development of the mouse. Genes Dev *7*:1277, 1993.
17. Rhodes SJ, Konieczny SF: Identification of *MRF4*: a new member of the muscle regulatory factor gene family. Genes Dev *3*:2050, 1989.
18. Miner JH, Wold B: Herculin, a fourth member of the *MyoD* family of myogenic regulatory genes. Proc Natl Acad Med U S A *87*:1089, 1990.
19. Ott M-O, et al: Early expression of the myogenic regulatory gene *Myf-5*, in precursor cells of skeletal muscle in the mouse embryo. Development *111*:1097, 1991.
20. Wright WE, et al: Myogenin, a factor regulating myogenesis, has a domain homologous to *MyoD*. Cell *56*:607, 1989.
21. Braun TE, et al: *Myf-6*, a new member of the human gene family of myogenic determination factors: evidence for a gene cluster on chromosome 12. EMBO J *9*:821, 1990.
22. Bober E, et al: The muscle regulatory gene *Myf-6*, has a biphasic pattern of expression during early mouse development. J Cell Biol *113*:1255, 1991.
23. Hinterberger TJ, et al: Expression of the muscle regulatory factor *MRF-4* during somite and skeletal myofiber development. Dev Biol *147*:144, 1991.
24. Hannon K, et al: Temporal and quantitative analysis of myogenic regulatory and growth factor gene expression in the developing mouse embryo. Dev Biol *151*:137, 1992.
25. Weintraub H, et al: The *myoD* gene family: nodal point during specification of the muscle cell lineage. Science *251*:761, 1991.
26. Rudnicki MA, et al: Inactivation of *MyoD* in mice leads to up-regulation of the myogenic HLH gene *Myf-5* and results in apparently normal muscle development. Cell *71*:383, 1992.
27. Arnold HH, Braun T: Targeted inactivation of myogenic factor genes reveals their role during mouse myogenesis: a review. Int J Dev Biol *40*:345, 1996.

28. Rawls A, et al: Overlapping functions of the myogenic bHLH genes *MRF4* and *MyoD* revealed in double mutant mice. Development *125*(suppl):2349, 1998.
29. Sabourin LA, Rudnicki MA: The molecular regulation of myogenesis. Clin Genet *57*:16, 2000.
30. Myer A, et al: *MyoD* cannot compensate for the absence of myogenin during skeletal muscle differentiation in murine embryonic stem cells. Dev Biol *229*:340, 2001.
31. Sumariwalla VM, Klein WH: Similar myogenic functions for myogenin and *MRF4* but not MyoD in differentiated murine embryonic stem cells. J Genet Devel *30*:239, 2001.
32. Zhu Z, Miller JB: *MRF4* can substitute for myogenin during early stages of myogenesis. Dev Dynam *209*:233, 1997.
33. Wang Y, Jaenisch R: Myogenin can substitute for *Myf5* in promoting myogenesis but less efficiently. Development *124*(suppl):2507, 1997.
34. Wang Y, et al: Functional redundancy of the muscle-specific transcription factors *Myf5* and myogenin. Nature *379*:823, 1996.
35. Vivian JL, et al: Thoracic skeletal defects in myogenin- and *MRF4*-deficient mice correlate with early defects in myotome and intercostal musculature. Dev Biol *224*:29, 2000.
36. Valdez MR, et al: Failure of *Myf5* to support myogenic differentiation without myogenin, *MyoD* and *MRF4*. Dev Biol *219*:287, 2000.
37. Andres V, Walsh K: Myogenin expression, cell cycle withdrawal and phenotypic differentiation are temporally separable events that precede cell fusion upon myogenesis. J Cell Biol *132*:657, 1996.
38. Myer A, et al: Wild-type myoblasts rescue the ability of myogenin-null myoblasts to fuse *in vivo*. Dev Biol *185*:127, 1997.
39. Rochard P, et al: Mitochondrial activity is involved in the regulation of myoblast differentiation through myogenin expression and activity of myogenic factors. J Biol Chem *275*:2733, 2000.
40. Yablonka-Reuveni Z, Paterson BM: *MyoD* and myogenin expression patterns in cultures of fetal and adult chicken myoblasts. J Histochem Cytochem *49*:455, 2001.
41. Yablonka-Reuveni Z, et al: The transition from proliferation to differentiation is delayed in satellite cells from mice lacking *MyoD*. Dev Biol *210*:440, 1999.
42. Kitzmann M, et al: The muscle regulatory factors *MyoD* and *Myf5* undergo distinct cell cycle-specific expression in muscle cells. J Cell Biol *142*:1456, 1998.
43. Lu J, et al: *MyoR*: a muscle-restricted basis helix-loop-helix transcription factor that antagonizes the actions of *MyoD*. Proc Natl Acad Sci U S A *96*:552, 1999.
44. Megeney LA et al: *MyoD* is required for myogenic stem cell function in adult skeletal muscle. Genes Devel *10*:1173, 1996.
45. Jin Y, et al: Expression of *MyoD* and myogenin in dystrophic mice, *mdx* and *dy*, during regeneration. Acta Neuropathol *99*:619, 2000.
46. Davis RL, et al: Expression of a single cDNA converts fibroblasts to myoblasts. Cell *37*:879, 1987.
47. Sonobe H et al: A new human pleomorphic rhabdomyosarcoma cell-line, HS-RMS-1, exhibiting *MyoD1* and myogenin. Int J Oncol *17*:119, 2000.
48. Cessna MH, et al: Are myogenin and *myoD1* expression specific for rhabdomyosarcoma? A study of 150 cases, with emphasis on spindle cell mimics. Am J Surg Pathol *25*:1150, 2001.
49. Astolfi A, et al: Identification of new genes related to the myogenic differentiation arrest of human rhabdomyosarcoma cells. Gene *274*:139, 2001.
50. Mennerich D, Braun T: Activation of myogenesis by the homeobox gene *Lbx1* requires cell proliferation. EMBO J *20*:7174, 2001.
51. Ohto H, et al: Cooperation of *Six* and *Eya* in activation of their target genes through nuclear translocation of *Eya*. Mol Cell Biol *19*:6815, 1999.
52. Ridgeway AG, Skerjanc IS: *Pax3* is essential for skeletal myogenesis and the expression of *Six1* and *Eya2*. J Biol Chem *276*:19033, 2001.
53. Spitz F, et al: Expression of myogenin during embryogenesis is controlled by *Six*/sine oculis homeoproteins through a conserved *MEF3* binding site. Proc Natl Acad Sci U S A *95*:14220, 1998.
54. Daston G, et al: *Pax-3* is necessary for migration but not differentiation of limb muscle precursors in the mouse. Development *122*(suppl):1017, 1996.
55. Katagiri T, et al: Bone morphogenic protein-2 inhibits terminal differentiation of myogenic cells by suppressing the transcriptional activity of *MyoD* and myogenin. Exp Cell Res *230*:342, 1997.
56. Kong Y, et al: Muscle LIM protein promotes myogenesis by enhancing the activity of *MyoD*. Mol Cell Biol *17*:4750, 1997.
57. Ridgeway AG, et al: *Wnt* signaling regulates the function of *MyoD* and myogenin. J Biol Chem *275*:32398, 2000.
58. Ríos R, et al: Myogenin is an inhibitor of myogenic differentiation. Am J Physiol – Cell Physiol *282*:C993, 2002.
59. Lin J, et al: Myostatin knockout in mice increases myogenesis and decreases adipogenesis. Biochem Biophys Res Commun *291*:701, 2002.
60. Jesper I, et al: Muscle, genes and athletic performance. Sci Am *283*:48, 2000.
61. Sharma M, et al: Myostatin in muscle growth and repair. Exer Sport Sci Rev *29*:155, 2001.
62. Hughes SM, et al: Selective accumulation of *MyoD* and myogenin mRNAs in fast and slow adult skeletal muscle is controlled by innervation and hormones. Development *118*:1137, 1993.
63. Esser K, et al: Nerve-dependent and -independent patterns of mRNA expression in regenerating skeletal muscle. Dev Biol *159*:173, 1993.
64. Larson PF, et al: Morphologic relationship of polyribosomes and myosin filaments in developing and regenerating skeletal muscle. Nature *222*:1168, 1969.

65. Xu Q, Wu Z: The insulin-like growth factor phosphatidylinositol 3-kinase-Akt signaling pathway regulates myogenin expression in normal myogenic cells but not in rhabdomyosacroma-derived RD cells. J Biol Chem 275:36750, 2000.

66. Tureckova J, et al: Insulin-like growth factor-mediated muscle differentiation: collaboration between phosphatidylinositol 3-kinase-Akt signaling pathways and myogenin. J Biol Chem 276:39264, 2001.

67. Engert JC, et al: Proliferation precedes differentiation in IGF-I-stimulated myogenesis. J Cell Biol 135:431, 1996.

68. Funakoshi Y, et al: An immunohistochemical study of basic fibroblast growth factor in the developing chick. Anat Embryol 187:415, 1993.

69. Szalay K, et al: TNF inhibits myogenesis and downregulates the expression of myogenic regulatory factors MyoD and myogenin. Eur J Cell Biol 74:391, 1997.

70. Layne MD, Farmer SR: Tumor necrosis factor-alpha and basic fibroblast growth factor differentially inhibit the insulin-like growth factor-I induced expression of myogenin in C2C12 myoblasts. Exp Cell Res 249:177, 1999.

71. Adi S, et al: Opposing early inhibitory and late stimulatory effects of insulin-like growth factor-I on myogenin gene transcription. J Cell Biochem 78:617, 2000.

72. Dominov JA, Miller JB: POU homeodomain genes and myogenesis. Dev Genet 19:108, 1996.

73. Takano H, et al: The Rho family G proteins play a critical role in muscle differentiation. Mol Cell Biol 18:1580, 1998.

74. Beranger F, et al: Muscle differentiation is antagonized by SOX15, a new member of the SOX protein family. J Biol Chem 275:16103, 2000.

75. Tajbakhsh S, et al: A population of myogenic cells derived from the mouse neural tube. Neuron 13:813, 1994.

76. Tomanek RJ, Colling-Saltin A-S: Cytological differentiation of human fetal skeletal muscle. Am J Anat 149:227, 1977.

77. Holtzer HK, et al: Thick and thin filaments in postmitotic, mononucleated myoblasts. Science 188:943, 1975.

78. Peck D, Walsh FS: Differential effects of over-expressed neural cell adhesion molecule isoforms on myoblast fusion. J Cell Biol 123:1587, 1993.

79. Fidziańska A: Human ontogenesis. I. Ultrastructural characteristics of developing human muscle. J Neuropathol Exp Neurol 39:476, 1980.

80. Kelly DE: Myofibrillogenesis and Z-band differentiation. Anat Rec 163:403, 1969.

81. Minguetti G, Mair WGP: Ultrastructure of developing human muscle. Biol Neonate 40:276, 1981.

82. Ontell M: Neonatal muscle: an electron microscopic study. Anat Rec 189:669, 1977.

83. Mauro A: Satellite cell of skeletal muscle fibres. J Biophys Biochem Cytol 9:493, 1961.

84. Muir AR, et al: The ultrastructure of the satellite cells in skeletal muscle. J Anat 99:435, 1965.

85. Ishikawa H: Electron microscopic observations of satellite cells with special reference to the development of mammalian skeletal muscles. Z Anat Entw Gesch 125:43, 1966.

86. Church JCT: Satellite cells and myogenesis: a study in the fruit-bat web. J Anat 105:419, 1969.

87. Allam Ali M: Myotube formation in skeletal muscle regeneration. J Anat 128:553, 1979.

88. Pons F, et al: Dystrophin and dystrophin-related protein (utrophin) distribution in normal and dystrophin-deficient skeletal muscle. Neuromusc Disord 3:507, 1993.

89. Prelle A, et al: Appearance and localization of dystrophin in normal human fetal muscle. Int J Dev Neurosci 9:607, 1991.

90. Martin J-J, et al: Duchenne muscular dystrophy. Immunohistochemistry of foetal muscles. Acta Neurol Belg 93:130, 1993.

91. Biederer CH, et al: The basic helix-loop-helix transcription factors myogenin and Id2 mediate specific induction of caveolin-3 gene expression during embryonic development. J Biol Chem 275:26245, 2000.

92. Donalies M, et al: Expression of M-cadherin, a member of the cadherin multigene family, correlates with differentiation of skeletal muscle cells. Proc Natl Acad Sci U S A 88:8024, 1991.

93. Moore R, Walsh FS: The cell adhesion molecule M-cadherin is specifically expressed in developing and regenerating but not denervated skeletal muscle. Development 117:1409, 1993.

94. Bornemann A, Schmalbruch H: Immunocytochemistry of M-cadherin in mature and regenerating rat muscle. Anat Rec 239:119, 1994.

95. Hahn CG, Covault J: Neural regulation of N-cadherin gene expression in developing and adult skeletal muscle. J Neurosci 12:4677, 1992.

96. Seghatoleslami MR, et al: Upregulation of myogenin by N-cadherin adhesion in three-dimensional cultures of skeletal myogenic BHK cells. J Cell Biochem 77:252, 2000.

97. Goichberg P, et al: Recruitment of beta-catenin to cadherin-mediated intercellular adhesion is involved in myogenic induction. J Cell Sci 114:1309, 2001.

98. Friday BB, et al: Calcineurin activity is required for the inititiation of skeletal muscle differentiation. J Cell Biol 149:657, 2000.

99. Tomé FMS, et al: Congenital muscular dystrophy with merosin deficiency. C R Acad Sci III 317:351, 1994.

100. Sunada Y, et al: Deficiency of merosin in dystrophic dy mice and genetic linkage of laminin M-chain. J Cell Biol 269:13729, 1994.

101. Hillaire D, et al: Localization of merosin-negative congenital muscular dystrophy to chromosome 6q2 by homozygosity mapping. Hum Mol Genet 3:1657, 1994.

102. Vuolteenaho R, et al: Human laminin-M chain (merosin): complete primary structure, chromosomal assignment and expression of the M and A chain in human fetal tissues. J Cell Biol 124:381, 1994.

103. Voit T, et al: Prenatal detection of merosin expression in human placenta. Neuropediatrics 25:332, 1994.

104. Sumiyoshi H, et al: Embryonic expression of type XIX collagen is transient and confined to muscle cells. Dev Dynam 220:155, 2001.

105. Osses N, Brandan E: ECM is required for skeletal muscle differentiation independently of muscle regulatory factor expression. Am J Physiol – Cell Physiol 282:C383, 2002.

106. Melo F, et al: Extracellular matrix is required for skeletal muscle differentiation but not myogenin expression. J Cell Biochem 62:227, 1996.

107. Chernoff EA, et al: The effects of collagen synthesis inhibitory drugs on somitogenesis and myogenin expression in cultured chick and mouse embryos. Tissue Cell 33:97, 2001.

108. Muralikrishna B, et al: Distinct changes in intranuclear lamin A/C organization during myoblast differentiation. J Cell Sci 114:4001, 2001.

109. Allen ER, Pepe F: Ultrastructure of developing muscle cells in the chick embryo. Am J Anat 116:115, 1965.

110. Graf WD, Sarnat HB: Intermediate filament proteinopathies. From cytoskeletons to genes to functional nosology. Neurology 58:1451, 2002.

111. Gard DL, Lazarides E: The synthesis and distribution of desmin and vimentin during myogenesis in vitro. Cell 19:263, 1980.

112. Tokuyasu KT, et al: Distribution of vimentin and desmin in developing chick myotubes in vivo. I. Immunofluorescence study. J Cell Biol 98:1961, 1984.

113. Tassin A-M, et al: Unusual organization of desmin intermediate filaments in muscular dysgenesis and TTX-treated myotubes. Dev Biol 129:37, 1988.

114. Sarnat HB: Myotubular myopathy: arrest of morphogenesis of myofibres associated with persistence of fetal vimentin and desmin. Four cases compared with fetal and neonatal muscle. Can J Neurol Sci 17:109, 1990.

115. Lazarides E: Intermediate filaments as mechanical integrators of cellular space. Nature 283:249, 1980.

116. Tassin A-M, et al: Fate of microtubule organizing centers during myogenesis in vitro. J Cell Biol 100:35, 1985.

117. Tokuyasu KT, et al: Distributions of vimentin and desmin in developing chick myotubes in vivo. II. Immunoelectron microscopic study. J Cell Biol 100:1157, 1985.

118. Tokuyasu KT, et al: Immunoelectron microscopic studies of desmin (skeletin) localization and intermediate filament organization in chicken skeletal muscle. J Cell Biol 96:1727, 1983.

119. Askanas V, et al: Immunocytochemical localization of desmin at human neuromuscular junctions. Neurology 40:949, 1990.

120. Sarnat HB: Vimentin and desmin in maturing skeletal muscle and developmental myopathies. Neurology 42:1616, 1992.

121. Sarnat HB: Technical note: Dilatuions of anti-desmin and anti-vimentin antibodies in the immunocytochemical examination of human muscle biopsies. Ped Dev Pathol, 2003, in press.

122. Cooke P: A filamentous cytoskeleton in vertebrate smooth muscle fibres. J Cell Biol 68:539, 1976.

123. Goebel HH, Warlo HT: Progress in desmin-related myopathies. J Child Neurol 15:565, 2000.

124. Larson PF, et al: Morphological relationship of polyribosomes and myosin filaments in developing and regenerating skeletal muscle. Nature 222:1168, 1969.

125. Sarnat HB: L'acridine-orange: un fluorochrome des acides nucléiques pour l'étude des cellules musculaires et nerveuses. Rev Neurol (Paris) 141:120, 1985.

126. Ezerman EB, Ishikawa H: Differentiation of the sarcoplasmic reticulum and T-system in developing chick skeletal muscle in vitro. J Cell Biol 35:405, 1967.

127. Ishikawa H: Satellite cells in developing muscle and tissue culture. In Mauro A, et al (eds): Regeneration of Striated Muscle and Myogenesis. Amsterdam, Excerpta Medica, 1970, pp 167–179.

128. Edge MB: Development of apposed sarcoplasmic reticulum at the T-system and sarcolemma and the change in orientation of triads in rat skeletal muscle. Dev Biol 23:634, 1970.

129. Walker SM, et al: Relationship of the sarcoplasmic reticulum to fibril and triadic junction development in skeletal muscle fibers of fetal monkeys and humans. J Morphol 146:97, 1975.

130. Hayes VE, Hikida RS: Naturally occurring degeneration in chick muscle development: ultrastructure of the M. complexus. J Anat 122:67, 1976.

131. Webb JN: The development of human skeletal muscle with particular reference to muscle cell death. J Pathol 106:221, 1972.

132. Lindon C, et al: Cell density-dependent induction of endogenous myogenin (MRF4) gene expression by Myf5. Dev Biol 240:574, 2001.

133. Rayne J, Crawford GNC: Increase in fibre numbers of the rat pterygoid muscles during postnatal growth. J Anat 119:347, 1975.

134. Stickland NC, Goldspink G: A possible indicator muscle for the fibre content and growth characteristics of porcine muscle. Anim Prod 16:135, 1973.

135. Stickland NC, et al: Effects of severe energy and protein deficiencies on the fibres and nuclei in skeletal muscle of pigs. Br J Nutr 34:421, 1975.

136. Brooke MH, Engel WK: The histographic analysis of human muscle biopsies with regard to fiber types. 4. Children's biopsies. Neurology 19:591, 1969.

137. Wohlfart G: Über das Vorkommen verschiedener Arten von Muskelfasern in der Skelettmuskulatur des Menschen und einiger Saugetiere. Acta Psychiatr Neurol Scand (Suppl 12), 1937.

138. Goldspink G: The proliferation of myofibrils during muscle fibre growth. J Cell Sci 6:593, 1970.

139. Behan WMH, et al: Validation of a simple, rapid, and economical technique for distinguishing type 1 and 2 fibres in fixed and frozen skeletal muscle. J Clin Pathol 55:375, 2002.

140. Fenichel GM: The B fiber of human fetal skeletal muscle. Neurology 13:219, 1963.

141. Colling-Saltin A-S: Enzyme histochemistry on skeletal muscle of the human foetus. J Neurol Sci 39:169, 1978.

142. Kumagai T, et al: Development of human fetal muscles: a comparative histochemical analysis of the psoas and the quadriceps muscles. Neuropediatrics 15:198, 1984.

143. Elder GCB, Kakulas BA: Histochemical and contractile property changes during human muscle development. Muscle Nerve 16:1246, 1993.

144. Hughes SM, et al: Myogenin induces a shift of enzyme activity from glycolytic to oxidative metabolism in muscles of transgenic mice. J Cell Biol 145:633, 1999.

145. Hu P, et al: Correlations between MyoD, myogenin, SERCA1, SERCA2 and phospholamban transcripts during transformation of type-II to type-I skeletal muscle fibers. Pflugers Arch–Eur J Physiol 434:209, 1997.

146. Alway SE, et al: The effects of age and hindlimb suspension on the levels of expression of the myogenic regulatory factors MyoD and myogenin in rat fast and slow skeletal muscles. Exp Physiol 86:509, 2001.

147. Russell RG, Oteruelo FT: An ultrastructural study of the differentiation of skeletal muscle in the bovine fetus. Anat Embryol 162:403, 1981.

148. Cuajunco F: Development of the neuromuscular spindle in human fetuses. Carnegie Inst Contrib Embryol 28:95, 1940.

149. Milburn A: The early development of muscle spindles in the rat. J Cell Sci 12:175, 1973.

150. Kucera J, et al: Motor and sensory innervation of muscle spindles in the neonatal rat. Anat Embryol 177:427, 1988.

151. Zelená J: The morphological influence of innervation of the ontogenetic development of muscle-spindles. J Embryol Exp Morphol 5:283, 1957.

152. Khan MA, Soukup T: A histoenzymatic study of rat intrafusal muscle fibres. Histochemistry 62:179, 1979.

153. Spiro AJ, Beilin RL: Human muscle spindle histochemistry. Arch Neurol 20:271, 1969.

154. Kucera J, Dorovini-Zis K: Types of human intrafusal muscle fibres. Muscle Nerve 2:437, 1979.

155. Stuart DG, et al: Properties and central connections of Golgi tendon organs with special reference to locomotion. In Banker BQ, et al (eds): Research in Muscle Development and the Muscle Spindle. Amsterdam, Excerpta Medica, 1972, pp 437–464.

156. Zelená J, Soukup T: The differentiation of intrafusal fiber types in rat muscle spindles after motor denervation. Cell Tissue Res 153:115, 1974.

157. Zelená J, Soukup T: Increase in the number of intrafusal muscle fibres in rat muscles after neonatal motor denervation. Neuroscience 52:207, 1993.

158. Kucera J, Walro JM: The effect of neonatal deafferentation or deefferentation on myosin heavy chain expression in intrafusal muscle fibers of the rat. Histochemistry 90:151, 1988.

159. Soukup T, et al: Influence of neonatal motor denervation on expression of myosin heavy chain isoforms in rat muscle spindles. Histochemistry 94:245, 1990.

160. Novotová M, Soukup T: Neomyogenesis in neonatally de-efferented and postnatally denervated rat muscle spindles. Acta Neuropathol 89:85, 1995.

161. Zelená J: Morphogenetic influence of innervation on the ontogenetic development of muscle spindles. J Embryol Exp Morphol 5:283, 1957.

162. Soukup T, et al: Differentiation of supernumerary fibres in neonatally de-efferented rat muscle spindles. Differentiation 53:35, 1993.

163. Petersen W, et al: Angiogenesis in fetal tendon development: spatial and temporal expression of the angiogenic peptide vascular endothelial cell growth factor. Anat Embryol 205:263, 2002.

164. Siegelbaum SA, et al: Single acetylcholine-activated channel currents in developing muscle cells. Dev Biol 104:366, 1984.

165. Kullberg RW, et al: Development of the myotomal neuromuscular junction in Xenopus laevis: an electrophysiological and fine-structural study. Dev Biol 60:101, 1977.

166. Chow I, Cohen MW: Developmental changes in the distribution of acetylcholine receptors in the myotomes of Xenopus laevis. J Physiol 339:553, 1983.

167. Dennis MJ, et al: Development of neuromuscular junctions in rat embryos. Dev Biol 81:266, 1981.

168. Braithwaite AW, Harris AJ: Neural influence on acetylcholine receptor clusters in embryonic development of skeletal muscles. Nature 279:549, 1979.

169. Role LW, et al: On the mechanism of acetylcholine receptor accumulation at newly formed synapses on chick myotubes. J Neurosci 5:2197, 1985.

170. Steinbach JH: Developmental changes in acetylcholine receptor aggregates at rat skeletal neuromuscular junctions. Dev Biol 84:267, 1981.

171. Smith MA, Slater CR: Spatial distribution of acetylcholine receptors at developing chick neuromuscular junctions. J Neurocytol 12:993, 1983.

172. Dwyer DS, et al: Immunological properties of junctional and extrajunctional acetylcholine receptor. Brain Res 217:23, 1981.

173. Brehm P, Henderson L: Regulation of acetylcholine receptor channel function during development of skeletal muscle. Dev Biol 129:1, 1988.

174. Kelly AM, Zacks SJ: The fine structure of motor end-plate morphogenesis. J Cell Biol 42:154, 1969.

175. Fidziańska A: Human ontogenesis. II. Development of the human neuromuscular junction. J Neuropathol Exp Neurol 39:606, 1980.

176. Riley DA: Multiple axon branches innervating single end-plates of kitten soleus myofibres. Brain Res 110:158, 1976.

177. Shimada V, Fischbach DA: Scanning electron microscopy of nerve-muscle contacts in embryonic cell culture: temporal and spatial relations of synaptic members. In Milhorat AT (ed): Exploratory Concepts in Muscular Dystrophy. Amsterdam, Excerpta Medica, 1974, pp 619–636.

178. Oppenheim RW, Majors-Willard C: Neuronal cell death in the brachial spinal cord of the chick is unrelated to the loss of polyneuronal innervation in wing muscle. Brain Res 154:148, 1978.

179. Pittman R, Oppenheim RW: Cell death of motoneurons in the chick embryo spinal cord. IV. Evidence that a functional neuromuscular interaction is involved in the regulation of naturally occurring cell death and the stabilization of synapses. J Comp Neurol 187:425, 1979.

180. Gamble HJ, et al: Electron microscope observations on human fetal striated muscle. J Anat 126:567, 1978.

181. Richardson EP Jr: Myelination in the human central nervous system. In Haymaker W, Adams RD (eds): Histology and Histopathology of the Nervous System, Vol 1. Springfield, IL, Charles C Thomas, 1982, pp 146–173.

182. Wozniak W, et al: Myelination of the human phrenic nerve. Acta Anat 112:281, 1982.

183. Sachis PN, et al: Myelination of the human vagus nerve from 24 weeks postconceptional age to adolescence. J Neuropathol Exp Neurol 41:466, 1982.

184. Hasan SU, et al: Vagal nerve maturation in the fetal lamb: an ultrastructural and morphometric study. Anat Rec 237:527, 1993.

185. Martínez AJ, et al: Extraocular muscles: morphogenic study in humans. Light microscopy and ultrastructural features. Acta Neuropathol 38:87, 1977.

186. Engel WK, Karpati G: Impaired skeletal muscle maturation following neonatal neurectomy. Dev Biol 17:713, 1968.

187. Fidziańska-Dolot A, Hausmanowa-Petrusewicz I: Morphology of the lower motor neuron and muscle. In Gamstorp I, Sarnat HB (eds): Progressive Spinal Muscular Atrophies. New York, Raven Press, 1984, pp 55–89.

188. Kugelberg E: Adaptive transformation of rat soleus motor units during growth: histochemistry and contraction speed. J Neurol Sci 27:269, 1976.

189. Salmons S, Sréter FA: Significance of impulse activity in the transformation of skeletal muscle type. Nature 263:30, 1976.

190. Fenichel GM: Abnormalities of skeletal muscle maturation in brain damaged children: a histochemical study. Dev Med Child Neurol 9:419, 1967.

191. Curless RG, et al: Histological patterns of muscle in infants with developmental brain abnormalities. Dev Med Child Neurol 20:159, 1978.

192. Farkas-Bargeton E, et al: Delay in the maturation of muscle fibres in infants with congenital hypotonia. J Neurol Sci 39:17, 1978.

193. Fenichel GM: Cerebral influence on muscle fibre typing. The effect of fetal immobilization. Arch Neurol 20:644, 1969.

194. Sarnat HB: Le cerveau influence-t-il le développement musculaire du foetus humain? Can J Neurol Sci 12:111, 1985.

195. Sarnat HB: Cerebral dysgeneses and their influence on fetal muscle development. Brain Dev 8:495, 1986.

196. Laing NG, Lamb AH: Muscle fibre types and innervation of the chick embryo limb following cervical spinal cord removal. J Embryol Exp Morphol 89:209, 1985.

197. Sarnat HB: Do the corticospinal and corticobulbar tracts mediate functions in the human newborn? Can J Neurol Sci 16:157, 1989.

198. Sarnat HB: Functions of the corticospinal and corticobulbar tracts in the human newborn. J Pediatr Neurol 1:3, 2003.

PITUITARY

Adda Grimberg and Jessica Katz Kutikov

182

Hypothalamus: Neuroendometabolic Center

Enabled by its strategic anatomy, the hypothalamus uniquely serves the interface between the neural and endocrine systems. It is at the same time a part of the brain, an intrinsic component of neural pathways, and an endocrine gland, specially connected to the pituitary gland to form the "master gland" unit of the body. The multiple functions of the hypothalamus ultimately involve regulation of the body's energy status and the maintenance of *homeostasis,* or bodily equilibrium. It has been long understood that to refine this regulation, the hypothalamus responds to information from the brain and to the levels of the peripheral hormones and body fluids it is controlling. There is a growing appreciation that the hypothalamus also receives input from the gut and fat stores, in essence closing the loop of metabolic regulation. All these incoming factors are compared to intrinsic set points, and outgoing messages are then released to enact modifications that will match the body to the appropriate set point. We have reviewed pediatric disorders of the neuroendocrine system, both congenital and acquired, elsewhere;[1] this chapter focuses on normal anatomy, embryology, and physiology of the hypothalamus.

ANATOMY

Despite the importance of the hypothalamus for multiple homeostatic functions, the structure is less than 1% of human brain volume; its various parts total approximately 4 g of the 1200 to 1400 g of an adult human brain.[2] Many of the borders of the hypothalamus are difficult to distinguish and are semi-arbitrary. The hypothamalus lies at the base of the third ventricle, immediately posterior to the optic chiasm.[2-4]

Because of its many eminences, the hypothalamus is an irregular structure that roughly forms a diamond. It is composed of four main structures:[2] the tuber cinereum, the median eminence, the infundibulum, and the mamillary bodies. The tuber cinereum lies centrally on the inferior aspect of the hypothalamus. The median eminence, a central swelling located on the tuber cinereum, forms the floor of the third ventricle. The infundibulum is a stalk that connects the median eminence to the posterior lobe of the pituitary, and the mamillary bodies are two round protuberances at the posterior end of the inferior surface of the hypothalamus.[4]

The hypothalamus can be difficult to describe because of its lack of landmarks. Of the many systems devised to divide the hypothalamus into discrete areas, two are particularly helpful. One describes nine zones, determined by their mediolateral and anteroposterior locations;[2, 3] it is shown in Figure 182-1. The second system defines discrete clusters of cell bodies (nuclei)

that have characteristic anatomic positions and functions (Table 182-1). Hypothalamic nuclei are not well circumscribed in adult brains. Examination of developing brains, in which cell groups are more discrete, has led to a greater understanding of hypothalamic architecture. Nonetheless, this schema is also semi-arbitrary and is divided in many ways, depending on the source.

An area of particular controversy involves reports of sexual structural differences in several hypothalamic nuclei.[5] In both rats and human adults, the sexually dimorphic nucleus of the preoptic area is larger in males than in females.[6,7] Another preoptic cell group was found to be larger in men.[8-10] The bed nucleus of the stria terminalis is male predominant,[5, 11] whereas the massa intermedia (interthalamic adhesion) is female predominant.[12] Age-related changes in neuronal health and sex hormone activity can affect these differences. For example, because the cell loss of human senescence in the sexually dimorphic nucleus of the preoptic area follows different time courses in men and women, the magnitude of the structural difference is age dependent.[5, 13] Sexual functional differences have also been shown in the hypothalamus by immunocytochemistry staining for various neuronal products (e.g., somatostatin and vasopressin) and hormone receptors (e.g., androgen and estrogen receptors).[5] Speculation and controversy surround the implications for sexually dimorphic behaviors and psychological phenomena. Most relevant to neonatologists is the debate about imprinting of the brain by androgens *in utero* and its consequences for therapeutic outcomes in patients with various intersex conditions including ambiguous genitalia.

A final anatomic feature that is integral to hypothalamic functioning is its blood supply. The hypothalamus communicates with the anterior pituitary gland through a special portal circulation that not only is fenestrated (the exception to the blood-brain barrier), but also transmits information bidirectionally. This feature enhances the ability of the hypothalamus to receive both signals from the general circulation and feedback from the pituitary. Furthermore, the hypothalamohypophyseal portal system ensures that high concentrations of hypothalamic factors reach the pituitary, often at concentrations that far surpass those in the general circulation.[14]

EMBRYOLOGY

Early in nervous system development, three primary brain vesicles form from the neural tube: the prosencephalon or forebrain, the mesencephalon or midbrain, and the rhombencephalon or hindbrain.[15] Secondary vesicles then form from the prosencephalon during the fourth to fifth weeks of gestation. The

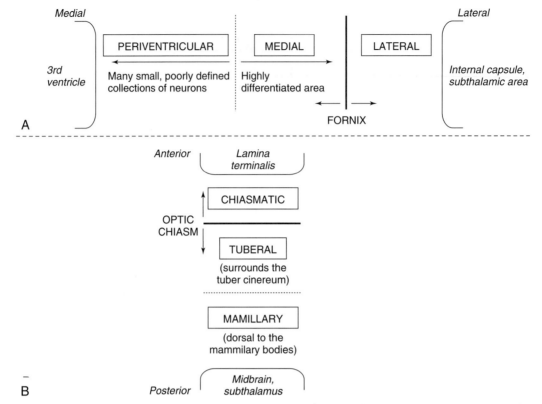

Figure 182–1. Nine anatomic areas of the hypothalamus. Three mediolateral (**A**) and three anteroposterior zones (**B**) form a grid that divides the hypothalamus into 9 anatomic areas. Defining features and boundaries of each zone are shown. The chiasmatic region can be further subdivided into preoptic (anterior to optic chiasm) and supraoptic (superior to optic chiasm) areas.

TABLE 182–1

Hypothalamic Nuclei

Anteroposterior Region	Nuclei	Anatomy	Function
Chiasmatic	Preoptic area	Small nuclear groups, anterior to optic chiasm	Controls blood pressure, body temperature, hormonal release, reproductive activity
	Suprachiasmatic nucleus	Midline nucleus above optic chiasm	Sets circadian rhythm and sleep wake cycles, regulates body temperature, hormonal control
	Paraventricular nucleus	Medial half = parvocellular neurons; lateral half = magnocellular neurons	Produces oxytocin and antidiuretic hormone (magnocellular neurons); regulates anterior pituitary function (parvocellular neurons); regulates autonomic responses
	Supraoptic nucleus	Superior to optic chiasm; also contains magnocellular neurons	Produces oxytocin and antidiuretic hormone
	Anterior nucleus	Between the paraventricular and supraoptic nuclei	Less differentiated; role ill-defined
Tuberal	Dorsomedial nucleus	Dorsal part of medial zone; projects locally and to periaqueductal gray matter	Feeding, growth, maturation, reproduction; parvocellular neurons regulate anterior pituitary function
	Ventromedial nucleus	Ventral part of medial zone; projects locally and to periaqueductal gray matter	Feeding, growth, maturation, reproduction; parvocellular neurons regulate anterior pituitary function
	Arcuate nucleus	Basal portion of tuber cinereum	Parvocellular neurons regulate anterior pituitary function; dopaminergic neurons
	Lateral hypothalamic nucleus	Large neurons lateral to ventromedial nucleus	Signals hunger
Mamillary	Posterior nucleus	Prominent nucleus, medial	Controls autonomic function
	Mamillary nuclei	Complex of three or four nuclei	Hippocampus→mamillary nuclei→thalamus; Papez circuit possibly involved in emotion and memory

secondary vesicles are termed the telencephalon, or endbrain, and the diencephalon. The telencephalon grows to cover all other brain structures and eventually becomes the cerebral hemispheres. The diencephalon also grows, forming a roof plate and two alar plates. During the sixth embryonic week, neuroblasts in the inferior portion of the alar plates of the diencephalon proliferate, forming the human hypothalamus.[15, 16] Hypothalamic development occurs in two main stages: forebrain induction by early signals before or during gastrulation and then cell type differentiation by ventralizing and rostralizing signals from the axial mesendoderm. Axial mesendoderm induction of hypothalamic development is necessary for eye separation, and its failure causes holoprosencephaly.[17]

Distinct cell groups are easier to distinguish in the fetal hypothalamus than in the adult hypothalamus. The fetal hypothalamic nuclei become recognizable between 6 and 12 weeks of gestation. At this same time, the hypothalamic fiber tracts develop, and many hypothalamic factors become detectable. For example, somatostatin, dopamine, and thyrotropin-releasing hormone are detectable as early as the 10th week of gestation.[16] At 9 to 10 weeks of gestation, little differentiation of the hypothalamic nuclei has taken place. By 24 to 33 weeks, the hypothalamus contains an increased number of better-defined structures and more closely resembles an adult hypothalamus. By the immediate postnatal period, the neonatal hypothalamic cell groups are remarkably similar to those structures in a mature adult.[18]

Information about the embryology of the hypothalamohypophyseal portal system is limited. There is evidence that the primary plexus begins to develop as early as 11.5 weeks' gestation.[16] Capillary penetrance of the median eminence is not evident until more than 16 weeks' gestation.[19] Further development throughout gestation is indicated by the greater number of capillary loops and the more mature vasculature present at birth.[16]

Our understanding of hypothalamic embryology has progressed from the morphologic to the genetic level. Development of the hypothalamus and pituitary gland is coordinated through parallel actions of genes expressed in both organs; extrinsic signals activate repertoires of transcription factors in a well-defined spatiotemporal pattern that lead to cellular differentiation into the various cell types that assume the distinct functions of the mature organs.[17,20,21] Some of these genes are summarized in Table 182-2.

NEUROLOGIC FUNCTIONS

Like other brain centers, the hypothalamus participates in neural pathways by synthesizing and secreting neurotransmitters, chemical messengers used for synaptic transmission, signaling, and neuromodulation. Different pathways control various functions of the hypothalamus, although for some functions, discrete areas or nuclei are not identifiable as the control centers. Some of the neurotransmitters are summarized in Table 182-3. Other neurotransmitters are also involved in hypothalamic functioning, such as the excitatory amino acids in a pathway connecting to the hippocampus and limbic system, but their actions are less well understood.

Circadian Rhythms

The suprachiasmatic nucleus sets the clock for the body's circadian rhythms, adaptations to the reproducible 24-hour day/night cycle of life on earth.[22] Neurons of the suprachiasmatic nucleus oscillate in a synchronized fashion *in vitro* with a period close to 24 hours.[23] *In vivo*, these oscillations become entrained to the solar day/night cycle by light; signals from the retina are transmitted by the retinohypothalamic tract to the suprachiasmatic nucleus. In the suprachiasmatic nucleus, these signals affect gene

expression for at least four transcription factors that act in a transcription/transduction feedback loop to determine the oscillations.[22, 23] Suprachiasmatic neurons contain somatostatin, vasoactive intestinal polypeptide, vasopressin or antidiuretic hormone (ADH), and neurotensin. Efferent pathways, including one that controls pineal function, then regulate various endocrine, cardiovascular, temperature, and behavioral circadian rhythms.[2, 22, 24]

In humans, the suprachiasmatic nucleus is recognized by mid-gestation and the retinohypothalamic tract by 80% gestation.[22, 25] Fetuses show 24-hour rhythms in hormones, cardiovascular function, and behavior. Rather than being synchronized with the time of day, their rhythms are set by maternal signals, including the maternal cortisol rhythm.[22]

Autonomic Nervous System Function

A topographic arrangement of autonomic function exists in the hypothalamus; parasympathetic control stems mainly from anterior and medial regions, whereas the lateral and posterior areas control sympathetic responses. Parasympathetic activity results in slowing of the heart rate, peripheral vasodilation, and increased gastrointestinal motility. Alternatively, sympathetic stimulation results in pupillary dilation, increased heart rate and blood pressure, and other responses associated with increased emotional stress.[2]

Heart rate, heart rate variability, and other cardiac measures are often used as markers when assessing fetal and neonatal autonomic function.[26,27] Fetuses at 20 weeks' gestational age demonstrate heart rate stability and differences among individuals. Fetal heart rate, beginning at 24 weeks' gestation, may be predictive of postnatal heart rate, but fetal heart rate variability does not become predictive of postnatal heart rate variability until 6 weeks later. This finding likely reflects a later maturation of the neuroregulatory system that controls heart rate variability.[26] The reduction in heart rate variability in fetuses with increasing gestational age also suggests that the autonomic nervous system continues to develop throughout gestation.[27]

Autonomic activity in fetuses varies over the course of a day. For instance, in normal fetuses, the fetal autonomic activity that controls heart rate follows a 12-hour cycle, as opposed to the maternal 24-hour rhythm. This 12-hour rhythm disappears immediately after birth, although the 24-hour circadian rhythm does not become established until 2 to 4 weeks later.[28]

Temperature Regulation

Like autonomic control, temperature regulation occurs regionally, rather than in discrete nuclei. The preoptic anterior hypothalamus contains thermosensitive neurons that detect increases in blood temperature and cool the body by heat dissipation, whereas the posterior hypothalamus conserves heat when decreased body temperature is detected.[2, 29] The temperature control centers of the hypothalamus coordinate behavioral, autonomic, and endocrine responses of the body to regulate body temperature, including panting and peripheral vasodilation in response to increased body temperature, shivering and peripheral vasoconstriction in response to decreased body temperature,[30] and modulation of thyroid hormone–stimulated thermogenesis.[31] Hypothalamic injury can produce prolonged hypothermia resulting from alterations in the temperature set point or defects in heat production mechanisms. Fever results from an elevation of the temperature set point by inflammatory cytokines, such as interleukin-1, that raise prostaglandin E levels in the hypothalamus; normal physiologic mechanisms then maintain body temperature at this elevated set point.[29]

The fetal environment is stable at about 37°C; the temperature gradient, wherein fetal temperature is about 0.5 to 1.0°C higher

TABLE 182-2

Genes in Hypothalamic Development

Gene	Normal Function	Consequences of Mutation or Deletion
Rpx/Hesx1	Expressed during gastrulation in the midline endoderm-mesoderm (prechordal plate precursor), to induce anterior head structures Afterward, expression is restricted to Rathke pouch Ventral→dorsal down-regulation of expression coincides with pituitary cell differentiation	Deletions: absence of infundibulum and Rathke pouch (most severe); hypothalamic floor expansion and abnormal bifurcation of Rathke pouch Homozygous missence mutations (*R53C*) cause septo-optic dysplasia, which is frequently associated with hypothalamic/pituitary dysfunction
Shh (sonic hedgehog)	Expressed by oral ectoderm Induces its own expression and that of other genes (e.g., *Nkx2.1*) in ventral midline neural cells Suppresses *Pax6* expression in the midline Required for resolution of the single retinal field into two separate primordia	Holoprosencephaly Hypothalamic/pituitary absence or dysfunction
Six3	Transcription factor Expressed in Rathke pouch and hypothalamus Involved in early induction of the pituitary gland	Holoprosencephaly Hypothalamic/pituitary absence or dysfunction
Gli3	Represses *Shh* signaling	Pallister-Hall syndrome (hypothalamic hamartomas)
Nkx2.1/Tebp/TTF-1	Dorsoventral gradient of expression (higher in ventral region and posterior pituitary; none in Rathke pouch) Required for development of Rathke's pouch	Absence of entire pituitary gland Absence of selective hypothalamic nuclei (premamillary nucleus, arcuate nucleus, mamillary body, supramamillary nucleus)
Brn-2	Coexpressed with *Brn-4* in presumptive paraventricular and supraoptic nuclei Required for terminal differentiation and survival of magnocellular and parvocellular neurons in these nuclei	Magnocellular and parvocellular neurons fail to project axons into the posterior pituitary Complete loss of posterior pituitary
Sim1	Expressed in paraventricular and supraoptic nuclei	Paraventricular and supraoptic nuclei fail to express *Brn-2*, oxytocin, antidiuretic hormone, thyrotropin-releasing hormone, corticotropin-releasing hormone, somatostatin Homozygous deletion: perinatal lethal from complete development defect of paraventricular nucleus Haploinsufficiency: isolated hyperphagia, early-onset obesity, increased linear growth, no decrease in energy expenditure
Nhlh2	Expressed in developing hypothalamus Expressed in both embryonic and adult pituitary	Hypogonadism and progressive adult obesity Reduction of pro-opiomelanocortin–producing cells in the arcuate nucleus (increased leptin resistance)
SF-1/Ftz-F1	Expressed in developing adrenal glands, gonads, and diencephalon Regulates both androgens and müllerian inhibiting factor (i.e., male differentiation)	Absence of adrenal glands Absence of gonads Absence of pituitary gonadotropes (no luteinizing hormone, follicle-stimulating hormone, and gonadotropin-releasing hormone)
Gsh-1	Binds to growth hormone–releasing hormone promoter	Hypoplastic pituitary gland Dwarfism; growth hormone deficiency (from absence of growth hormone–releasing hormone in arcuate nucleus) Sexual infantilism and infertility
Necdin	Paternal monoallelic expression in developing hypothalamus	Decreased number of oxytocin-producing cells in paraventricular nucleus Decreased number of gonadotropin-releasing hormone–producing cells in preoptic region Mutant mice show neonatal lethality with reduced penetrance Maps to the critical region of Prader-Willi syndrome
Peg3	Paternal monoallelic expression in developing hypothalamus	Decreased number of oxytocin-producing cells in paraventricular nucleus Abnormal maternal behavior leading to perinatal lethality of offspring mice

Data from Kioussi C, et al: Mech Dev *81*:23, 1999; and Michaud JL: Clin Genet *60*:255, 2001.

TABLE 182-3

Hypothalamic Neurotransmitters

Category	Neurotransmitter	Pathway	Function
Monoamines			
Catecholamines	Dopamine	Incertohypothalamic tract Mesencephalic tract Tuberoinfundibular tract Median eminence	Influences secretion of pituitary hormones Primary inhibitor of prolactin L-DOPA stimulates GH release
	Norepinephrine	Lateral tegmental system Dorsal tegmental system Can be localized to all hypothalamic nuclei; highest concentrations in the arcute nucleus and median eminence	Regulates emotional and motivated behavior Stimulates GH and gonadotropin release Inhibits secretion of oxytocin, vasopressin, and ACTH
	Epinephrine	Cell bodies near the locus ceruleus	Inhibits secretion of vasopressin and oxytocin
Indoleamines	Serotonin	Most of the hypothalamic nuclei Highest concentrations in the arcuate and suprachiasmatic nucleus	Involved in cyclic release of some hypothalamic hormones Stimulates GH and PRL release
	Histamine	Tuberomamillary nucleus in the posterior lateral hypothalamus	May help maintain arousal Stimulates oxytocin, vasopressin, and GH release
Cholinergic	Acetylcholine	Large amount present in median eminence	Stimulates secretion of vasopressin, oxytocin, ACTH and gonadotropin release Inhibits somatostatin; stimulates GH release Inhibits TSH release
Amino acid (inhibitory)	γ-Aminobutyric acid (GABA)	Synthesized from glutamate Basal gangliar system	In anterior hypothalamus, helps induce sleep Inhibits oxytocin, vasopressin, ACTH, PRL, and TSH release Stimulates GH and gonadotropin release
Peptides	Angiotensin II	Renin (from kidneys) cleaves angiotensinogen (made by liver) to angiotensin I; angiotensin I cleaved by angiotensin converting enzyme in lungs in angiotensin II	Stimulates secretion of vasopressin Stimulates ACTH and luteinizing hormone and inhibits PRL and GH release Induces thirst, drinking behavior Involved in regulation of water balance
	Atrial natriuretic peptide	Left atrium Anterior tip of third ventricle Many neuronal endings in the median eminence	Opposes vasopressin secretion Involved in regulation of water balance
	β-Endorphins	Arcuate nucleus and basal tuberal area in the rat Project through the anterior hypothalamic area and innervate the median eminence	Released during stress Stimulate ACTH, PRL, and GH release

ACTH = corticotropin; GH = growth hormone; PRL = prolactin; TSH = thyroid-stimulating hormone.

than maternal temperature, results in fetal heat dissipation. Heat loss occurs through the placenta, fetal skin, amniotic fluid, and uterine wall. The hypothalamus most likely controls this higher fetal temperature *in utero.* After birth, the neonate has tremendous heat losses through the skin that require functioning thermoregulatory mechanisms to prevent hypothermia. Premature infants are often unable to maintain appropriate body temperature and behave like poikilotherms rather than homeotherms. How the hypothalamus matures to the environmental conditions after birth is still unknown.[32]

Emotional Expression and Behavior

Selective stimulation or lesions of various areas in the hypothalamus elicit different behavioral and emotional responses such as aggression, anger, fear, pleasure, and sexual gratification. Although the hypothalamus is important for integrating and expressing emotion, other areas of the brain, including the cortex, limbic system, and thalamus, interact with the hypothalamus to bring about the varied types of responses.[2,33,34]

The hypothalamus participates in the two physiologic stress response systems, the sympathetic-adrenal-medullary system and the hypothalamic-pituitary-adrenal system. The sympathetic-adrenal-medullary system causes the well-known stress-induced release of epinephrine. Sympathetic-adrenal-medullary activation, which is dependent on characteristics of both the situation and the individual, occurs in response to challenges with a faster onset than activation of the hypothalamic-pituitary-adrenal axis.[35] Hypothalamic-pituitary-adrenal axis function culminates in cortisol release, which is described in detail in Chapters 186 and 187. Stress induction of the hypothalamic-pituitary-adrenal axis is active in newborns. When neonates are exposed to noxious stimuli (e.g., circumcision, heel stick blood sampling), cortisol levels rise and can be associated with how much the baby cries. Once the noxious stimulus is removed, healthy neonates quickly return to basal cortisol concentrations. Soothing procedures such as the use of a pacifier can reduce crying in response to noxious stimuli, but they do not affect the hypothalamic-pituitary-adrenal response to the stimuli.[36]

ENDOCRINE FUNCTIONS

The hypothalamus also serves as an endocrine organ, synthesizing and releasing hormones into the circulation to effect changes in target tissues. Hypothalamic endocrine activity can be divided into two distinct categories as established by the anatomy of the hypothalamopituitary unit. Because the posterior pituitary gland, or neurohypophysis, is composed of axonal projections from the hypothalamus, the hormones released into the circulation by the posterior pituitary are actually made in cell bodies of the hypothalamus. In contrast, the anterior pituitary gland, or adenohypophysis, is a distinct gland. The hypothalamus secretes various releasing and inhibiting factors that regulate anterior pituitary hormone synthesis and release. These factors are made in hypothalamic neurons and are carried down axons to the median eminence. They then reach the anterior pituitary by the special hypothalamohypophyseal portal circulation, whereas the anterior pituitary hormones reach their target organs by the peripheral circulation.[24]

Hypothalamic hormone production and release are primarily regulated by humoral feedback. There are three levels of feedback regulation to the hypothalamus. *First-order feedback* involves one hormone, as exemplified by oxytocin and ADH. These hormones act on target cells (breast, uterus, kidney) but do not stimulate the release of secondary hormones. Oxytocin and ADH levels, together with nonhormonal signals (e.g., plasma osmolality and hypovolemia or hypotension for ADH), directly regulate their own production and release. Close proximity of oxytocin and ADH neurons and co-localization of receptors for the hormones on the neurons that produce those hormones allow local concentrations of oxytocin and ADH within the supraoptic and paraventricular nuclei to refine further activity of the neurons that produce them.[37-39] *Second-order feedback* involves a second hormone produced by the pituitary, such as prolactin (PRL). Hypothalamic hormones stimulate or inhibit anterior pituitary release of a hormone, and the circulating levels of the pituitary hormone feed back to regulate hypothalamic hormone release. For example, increases in circulating PRL concentrations stimulate hypothalamic secretion of dopamine (PRL-inhibiting factor) into the hypothalamohypophyseal portal circulation to prevent excessive PRL release by the pituitary; high PRL levels also inhibit hypothalamic release of vasoactive intestinal polypeptide, a hormone that stimulates PRL release.[40] In a *third-order feedback* loop, a third endocrine gland (e.g., adrenals, gonads, thyroid) is involved in addition to the hypothalamus and pituitary. Within a third-order feedback pathway, multiple types of feedback loops exist: long, short, and ultrashort feedback. Long-loop feedback occurs when hormones from peripheral endocrine target cells or substances from tissue metabolism influence the production of hypothalamic hormones. This type of feedback is most often negative, although it can be positive. Short-loop feedback is second-order feedback within a third-order feedback system. For instance, certain pituitary hormones (e.g., corticotropin, luteinizing hormone, thyroid-stimulating hormone) not only stimulate target gland hormone production, but also feed back to limit or terminate hypothalamic releasing hormone production (corticotropin-releasing hormone, gonadotropin-releasing hormone, and thyrotropin-releasing hormone, respectively). When hypothalamic hormone release affects its own synthesis, ultrashort feedback has occurred. This is similar to first-order feedback within a third-order system. The mechanism of this ultrashort feedback is either through neurotransmission between two cells in the

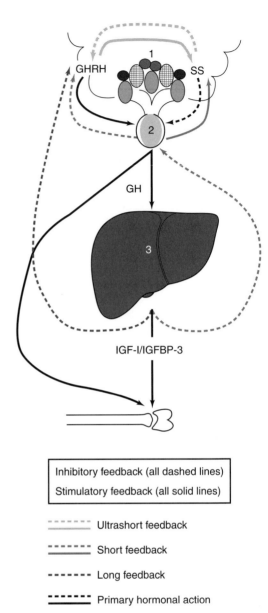

| Inhibitory feedback (all dashed lines) | |
| Stimulatory feedback (all solid lines) | |

-------	Ultrashort feedback
-------	Short feedback
------	Long feedback
▬▬▬	Primary hormonal action

Figure 182–2. The growth hormone (GH) axis exemplifies a third-order feedback loop. A third-order feedback loop involves hormonal production by three endocrine glands: (*1*) the hypothalamus produces growth hormone releasing hormone (GHRH) and somatostatin (ss); (*2*) the pituitary gland produces GH; and (*3*) the liver acts as an endocrine gland, producing insulin-like growth factor-I (IGF-I) and its binding protein (IGFBP-3). Stimulatory feedback is depicted as a solid arrow, inhibitory feedback as a dashed arrow. Ultrashort feedback is colored in *red,* short feedback in *blue,* and long feedback in *black.* Primary hormonal action is shown in *green.* Among the final end-organs of this system is the growth plate of growing bones. (See also color plates).

hypothalamus or through pituitary tanycyte release of the hormone into cerebrospinal fluid, which can regulate hypothalamic activity because the hypothalamus is located at the base of the third ventricle.[24] The growth hormone pathway (reviewed in detail elsewhere[41,42]) is an excellent example of a third-order system and is shown in Figure 182–2.

Two neurosecretory systems produce hypothalamic hormones (summarized in Table 182–4): magnocellular and parvo-

TABLE 182-4

Hypothalamic Hormone Axes

Neurosecretory System	Hormone	Hormone Gene Locus	Hypothalamic Nucleus of Origin	Secondary Pituitary Hormone	Pituitary Action	Final Axis Gland	Axis Function
Magnocellular	ADH	20p13	Supraoptic and paraventricular	NA	V1b receptors: stimulate ACTH release	NA	Enhances renal free water retention; vasoconstriction
	Oxytocin	20p13	Supraoptic and paraventricular	NA	NA	NA	Stimulates uterine contractions at parturition; milk let-down reflex for lactation
Parvocellular	GHRH	20q11.2	Arcuate	GH	Stimulatory	Liver	Somatic growth
	ss	3q28	Paraventricular; also in neocortex, basal ganglia, limbic system; endocrine pancreas and gut (D cells)	GH, PRL, TSH, ACTH	Inhibitory	Liver	Regulation of pituitary function, especially somatic growth; neurotransmitter; gut function and pancreatic endocrine regulation (locally produced ss)
	CRH	8q13	Paraventricular	ACTH	Stimulatory	Adrenals	Maintenance of normal blood pressure and glucose; stress response
	TRH	3q13.3-q21	Paraventricular	TSH	Stimulatory	Thyroid	Regulates overall metabolic rate; effects on heart, bone, gut and other organ functions
	GnRH	GnRH1 = 8p21-p11.2; GnRH2 = 20p13	Arcuate	LH, FSH	Stimulatory	Gonads	Reproduction
	Dopamine	—	Arcuate	PRL	Inhibitory	NA	Lactation

ACTH = corticotropin; ADH = antidiuretic hormone or vasopressin; CRH = corticotropin-releasing hormone; FSH = follicle-stimulating hormone; GH = growth hormone; GHRH = growth hormone-releasing hormone; GnRH = gonadotropin-releasing hormone; LH = luteinizing hormone; PRL = prolactin; ss = somatostatin; TRH = thyrotropin-releasing hormone; TSH = thyroid-stimulating hormone (thyrotropin).

cellular. The *magnocellular system* consists of specialized, large-celled (magnocellular) neurons, the hypothalamoneurohypophysial tract, and the neurohypophysis (posterior pituitary). Its principal products are ADH and oxytocin. Most of the magnocellular neurons are located in the supraoptic and paraventricular nuclei, but additional small nuclei also contain these neurons.[3] Apart from projections to neurohypophysis, some magnocellular neurons project to the median eminence and some ADH-containing fibers project to the choroid plexus in the lateral ventricles and brain stem regions.[14]

In contrast, the *parvocellular secretory cells* are small neurons, mostly in the region of the tuber cinereum below the third ventricle, that produce the hypophysiotropic hormones.[3] The parvocellular neurons are found in various hypothalamic nuclei, including the arcuate and paraventricular nuclei, and project to the median eminence.[24] Their hormonal products (all peptide hormones except dopamine) are carried by the hypothalamohypophyseal portal system to the anterior pituitary, where they regulate adenohypophyseal function. Because the hormonal systems of the anterior pituitary are reviewed in detail in other chapters of this book, we focus on the magnocellular system.

Adult numbers of oxytocin- and ADH-producing cells in the supraoptic and paraventricular nuclei exist as early as the second half of gestation, which is earlier than development of some other nuclei.[43] Oxytocin and ADH can be detected as early as the 10th gestational week. Vasopressinergic neurons appear 1 week earlier in the supraoptic than in the paraventricular nucleus. Although an adult organization of vasopressinergic neurons can be identified early in the second trimester, the number of those neurons seems to increase until the 26th week of gestation. The vasopressinergic system of neurons is also highly active in the perinatal period.[44]

The synthetic pathways of oxytocin and ADH are very similar.[45] Both are synthesized from protein precursors (prohormones) that are encoded by single-copy genes located near each other on chromosome 20. Both genes are composed of three exons; the entire mature hormone is encoded within the first exon. The remainder of the oxytocin gene encodes neurophysin I, whereas the longer ADH gene also encodes neurophysin II and the glycoprotein, copeptin.[46] The prohormones are transported down the axons and are stored in colloid-filled vesicles. Proteolytic enzymes in these neurosecretory granules cleave oxytocin and ADH from the neurophysins, which are presumed to primarily serve as their carriers during axonal transport. When the magnocellular cell bodies are properly stimulated, oxytocin, ADH, and the neurophysins are released from the axonal terminals by calcium-dependent exocytosis.[3] In addition to oxytocin and ADH, magnocellular secretory granules contain many other peptides but in much smaller amounts. These include dynorphin, enkephalins, galanin, and cholecystokinin, and although they are secreted along with oxytocin and ADH, the role of many of these peptides is unknown.[47]

Oxytocin

Oxytocin secretion is prompted by mechanical vaginal distention and, in lactating women, by suckling and nipple stimulation; there is no recognized stimulus for its secretion in men. Cholinergic and α-adrenergic fibers carry the stimulatory inputs, whereas β-adrenergic fibers provide inhibition of oxytocin release. Oxytocin serves two physiologic functions: it aids in parturition by stimulating uterine contractions, and it facilitates nursing by stimulating contraction of myoepithelial cells in the lactating mammary gland (milk "let-down" reflex). In fact, nursing cannot occur without oxytocin, and maternal and fetal stress during labor and delivery can reduce oxytocin release, thereby impairing lactation.[48] Oxytocin action at parturition is primed by two major changes. Oxytocin release, which occurs in brief secretory bursts, increases in both the fetus and the mother during labor.[49, 50] Meanwhile, the increase in uterine oxytocin receptors at term makes the uterus particularly sensitive to the hormone.[49] Oxytocin secretion is suppressed by relaxin, an ovarian peptide that suppresses uterine contractions and relaxes pelvic connective tissue during parturition.[51] Therapeutically, oxytocin and its analogues are used to induce labor (or to augment labor in uterine dysfunction), to prevent postpartum uterine atony or hemorrhage, and to promote milk let-down in lactation.

Antidiuretic Hormone

The two names of this hormone, vasopressin and ADH, reflect its two main actions, which are mediated by two different classes of receptors. V1 receptors stimulate vasoconstriction, glycogenolysis, platelet aggregation, and vascular smooth muscle hypertrophy. A subclass of V1 receptors (V1b) is located in the anterior pituitary and stimulates corticotropin release. V2 receptors increase water permeability of the renal collecting ducts by inducing aquaphorins; this results in greater water retention and decreased urine volume. Neural input for ADH secretion can elicit newly synthesized hormone within 30 minutes, but it also exhibits fatigue with high frequencies or prolonged duration.[52] The main stimulus for the antidiuretic effects of ADH is an elevation in plasma osmolality, primarily the extracellular fluid concentration of sodium chloride, as detected by osmoreceptor cells within the hypothalamus. Baroreceptor (carotid sinuses, aortic arch, cardiac atria, and great veins) sensing of hypovolemia or hypotension leads to ADH levels superseding those required for maximal urine concentration and causes vasoconstriction.[14] In most cases, the two mechanisms act in concert; dehydration leads to both hypernatremia and hypovolemia. However, the two ADH responses may become dissociated in disease states involving intravascular volume depletion despite total body fluid overload and hyponatremia (e.g., congestive heart failure, cirrhosis, and nephrotic syndrome).[53] Deficiency of ADH hormone production and resistance to ADH action cause central and nephrogenic diabetes insipidus, respectively;[54] both disorders are characterized by polyuria, polydipsia, and a tendency to dehydration. In contrast, the syndrome of inappropriate ADH secretion (SIADH) is characterized by diminished urine output and free water intoxication.

During development, ADH aids in regulating the proliferation and morphogenesis of target cells in the brain, pituitary, kidney, and liver. Because the fetus contributes significantly to modulation of fluid fluxes among the maternal, fetal, and amniotic fluid compartments, fetal ADH action is an important component of adaptive responses to changes in the environment *in utero*.[55] The ADH system also plays an essential role in fetal adaptation to the stresses of labor.[44, 55] In the perinatal period, ADH is integral in establishing body fluid homeostasis, by providing the brain, pituitary, heart, and adrenals with increased blood flow and aiding in regulation of the cardiovascular system, water reabsorption, gluconeogenesis, and glycogenolysis after delivery.[44]

METABOLIC REGULATION

The hypothalamus plays a crucial role in regulating the body's metabolic state by controlling both feeding behavior and energy expenditure rates. The regulation is so precise that, under reasonably steady-state conditions, deflections in the body weight and fat mass of mammals remain within 0.5 to 1%.[56] The importance of the hypothalamus to this system has long been appreciated because of the hyperphagia and obesity syndromes that result from hypothalamic lesions. The ventromedial nucleus of the hypothalamus has been identified as a satiety center, whereas the lateral hypothalamic area stimulates feeding.[2] More recent investigations have focused on the peripheral hormones that feed metabolic information back to the hypothalamus.

Leptin

The *OB* gene, located on chromosome 7q31.1 and encoding the hormone leptin, was cloned and sequenced in 1994.[57] Leptin is produced by white adipose tissue[58, 59] and is secreted into the circulation in proportion to the body's fat mass. Circulating both freely and protein bound, leptin crosses the blood-brain barrier and binds to leptin receptors in the central nervous system. Many of these receptors are located in the hypothalamus and control pathways involved in the regulation of appetite and thermogenesis.[58] Thus, leptin serves as the hypothalamic index of body fat mass.[59] Leptin has other neuroendocrine functions, including regulation of fertility and the secretion of growth hormone, corticotropin-releasing hormone, thyrotropin-releasing hormone, and PRL.[58]

The exact mechanism of leptin uptake into the central nervous system has yet to be elucidated. One possibility involves the neurons of the median eminence, which not only project outside the blood-brain barrier but also express leptin receptors. Once inside the central nervous system, leptin can bind to receptors present in many hypothalamic nuclei, especially the arcuate, dorsomedial, ventromedial, and ventral premammillary nuclei.[60] Leptin binding to its receptor signals the body's energy status to two opposing classes of neurons. Pro-opiomelanocortin (POMC) neurons (catabolic pathways) are stimulated by leptin, whereas neuropeptide Y (NPY) neurons (anabolic pathways) are inhibited.[59]

Leptin directly stimulates POMC neurons, which are located in the arcuate nucleus as well as outside the hypothalamus in the nucleus of the tractus solitarius. POMC is a precursor to many polypeptides termed melanocortins, including α-melanocyte-stimulating hormone. When the hypothalamic melanocortin receptors MC3-R and MC4-R are stimulated by α-melanocyte-stimulating hormone, food intake is decreased and energy expenditure is increased.[56, 59] Agouti gene-related peptide

(AGRP) is an endogenous melanocortin system antagonist that is also expressed in the arcuate nucleus.[61]

AGRP mRNA is highly co-localized with mRNA of NPY,[62] the system opposing POMC. A member of the pancreatic polypeptide family, the anabolic, orexigenic hormone NPY is widely distributed in the human brain. NPY potently stimulates feeding, is capable of overriding the body's satiety and weight control mechanisms,[56] and reduces energy expenditure by decreasing nonshivering thermogenesis in brown adipose tissue.[56,58] Leptin inhibits NPY activity. NPY can inhibit POMC neurons directly at the cell body or postsynaptically through the release of AGRP.[56] Thus, leptin stimulates POMC neurons both directly and indirectly, by eliminating the POMC inhibition by NPY,[59] and the two opposing systems are coordinated toward an overall negative effect on energy balance. Many other substances have been implicated in energy homeostasis, but not all are understood as well as the POMC/NPY systems. Those also under leptin regulation include orexins,[56] cocaine- and amphetamine-regulated transcript, glucagon-like peptide-1, melanin-concentrating hormone, and cholecystokinin.[58,60]

Leptin is secreted in a rhythmic pattern that correlates to meals (leptin levels are reduced by fasting). Leptin's actions on the hypothalamus probably serve a long-term regulatory system that sets a point of satiety; short-term regulatory systems that control single meal intake are more likely determined by leptin actions on the brain stem. Obesity more frequently results from leptin resistance than from leptin deficiency. Leptin levels in females are almost double those in males with the same body mass index or fat reserve. This finding not only has implications for leptin physiology, but also supports the role of leptin in reproductive and gonadal function.[58] The gender difference in leptin levels is found at birth, which suggests that the process begins *in utero*.[58,63]

The role of leptin in the fetus is unknown. Leptin has been identified in fetal cord blood in the 18th week of gestation. Adipose tissue development occurs during the second trimester, and consistent with this finding, leptin levels dramatically increase at 34 weeks' gestation.[61] Leptin is also produced by the placenta, but in very small amounts that are unlikely to contribute significantly to cord blood levels.[63] The level of leptin for body weight is disproportionately high in neonates.[58,63] The reason for this is unknown, but it normalizes toward adult levels around 2 weeks of life.[58] Neonatal leptin levels have been shown to predict weight gains in infancy.[58,64]

Ghrelin

Ghrelin is an orexigenic peptide that was first identified in 1999 as the endogenous ligand for the growth hormone secretagogue receptor.[65] Its central role in the stimulation of feeding was not appreciated until 2001.[66] Ghrelin is produced primarily in the stomach (X/A-like cells of the oxyntic glands), but also in the duodenum, jejunum, pituitary, kidney, placenta, and hypothalamus.[67] Although it is accepted that ghrelin-producing neurons exist in the hypothalamus, it is still controversial whether ghrelin is produced there in physiologically relevant amounts.[66,67] Regardless of the source, ghrelin can reach the mediobasal and mediolateral hypothalamus through the general circulation. It is unknown whether peripherally produced ghrelin can reach areas of the hypothalamus protected by the blood-brain barrier. Once ghrelin reaches the hypothalamus, the peptide targets ghrelin receptors present in various hypothalamic nuclei. Ghrelin then exerts its energy homeostatic effects through a central mechanism involving NPY[67,68] and AGRP.[67]

The effects of ghrelin on body metabolism are opposite to those of leptin. However, ghrelin appears to be regulated more acutely, unlike the more chronic regulation of leptin. During food deprivation, leptin levels fall, POMC production decreases, NPY and AGRP levels rise, and ghrelin levels increase.[69] In this situation, ghrelin serves as a hunger signal, trying to restore the body to a state of positive energy balance. Ghrelin levels drop after feeding, are decreased in obesity, and are increased in anorexia nervosa.[67,70]

Apparently independent of its orexigenic effects, ghrelin stimulates growth hormone release. Because they work through different receptors (growth hormone secretagogue receptor and growth hormone-releasing hormone receptor, respectively), ghrelin and growth hormone-releasing hormone stimulation of growth hormone secretion are synergistic.[71] Much remains to be learned about ghrelin physiology and involvement in pathologic conditions, but this relatively new hormone exemplifies how neurologic pathways, hormonal activities, and metabolic control can be integrated through the hypothalamus.

REFERENCES

1. Moshang Jr T, Grimberg A: Neuroendocrine Disorders in Children. *In* McMillan JA, et al (eds): Oski's Pediatrics: Principles and Practice, 3rd ed. Philadelphia, Lippincott Williams & Wilkins, 1999, pp 1787–1793.
2. Parent A: Carpenter's Human Neuroanatomy, 9th ed. Baltimore, William & Wilkins, 1996.
3. Burt AM: Textbook of Neuroanatomy. Philadelphia, WB Saunders Co, 1993.
4. Nolte J: The Human Brain, 4th ed. Philadelphia, CV Mosby, 1999.
5. Swaab DF, et al: Structural and functional sex differences in the human hypothalamus. Horm Behav 40:93, 2001.
6. Gorski RA, et al: Evidence for a morphological sex difference within the medial preoptic area of the rat brain. Brain Res 148:333, 1978.
7. Swaab DF, Fliers E: A sexually dimorphic nucleus in the human brain. Science 228:1112, 1985.
8. Allen LS, et al: Two sexually dimorphic cell groups in the human brain. J Neurosci 9:497, 1989.
9. LeVay S: A difference in hypothalamic structure between heterosexual and homosexual men. Science 253:1034, 1991.
10. Byne W, et al: The interstitial nuclei of the human anterior hypothalamus: an investigation of sexual variation in volume and cell size, number and density. Brain Res 856:254, 2000.
11. Allen LS, Gorski RA: Sex difference in the bed nucleus of the stria terminalis of the human brain. J Comp Neurol 302:697, 1990.
12. Allen LS, Gorski RA: Sexual dimorphism of the anterior commissure and massa intermedia of the human brain. J Comp Neurol 312:97, 1991.
13. Hofman MA, Swaab DF: The sexually dimorphic nucleus of the preoptic area in the human brain: a comparative morphometric study. J Anat 164:55, 1989.
14. Reichlin S: Neuroendocrinology. *In* Wilson JD, et al (eds): Williams Textbook of Endocrinology, 9th ed. Philadelphia, WB Saunders Co, 1998, pp 165–388.
15. Moore KL, Persaud TVN (eds): The Developing Human, 6th ed. Philadelphia, WB Saunders Co, 1998.
16. Fuse Y: Development of the hypothalamic-pituitary-thyroid axis in humans. Reprod Fertil Dev 8:1, 1996.
17. Michaud JL: The developmental program of the hypothalamus and its disorders. Clin Genet 60:255, 2001.
18. Koutcherov Y, et al: Organization of human hypothalamus in fetal development. J Comp Neurol 446:301, 2002.
19. Hyyppa M: Hypothalamic monoamines in human fetuses. Neuroendocrinology 9:257, 1972.
20. Scully KM, Rosenfeld MG: Pituitary development: regulatory codes in mammalian organogenesis. Science 295:2231, 2002.
21. Kioussi C, et al: A model for the development of the hypothalamic-pituitary axis: transcribing the hypophysis. Mech Develop 81:23, 1999.
22. Seron-Ferre M, et al: The development of circadian rhythms in the fetus and neonate. Semin Perinatol 25:363, 2001.
23. van Esseveldt KE, et al: The suprachiasmatic nucleus and the circadian time-keeping system revisited. Brain Res Rev 33:34, 2000.
24. Genuth SM: The endocrine system. *In* Berne RM, Levy MN (eds): Physiology, 4th ed. Philadelphia, CV Mosby, 1998, pp 779–1013.
25. Hao H, Rivkees SA: The biological clock of very premature primate infants is responsive to light. Proc Natl Acad Sci USA 96:2426, 1999.
26. DiPietro JA, et al: Antenatal origins of individual differences in heart rate. Dev Psychobiol 37:221, 2000.
27. Ursem NTC, et al: An estimate of fetal autonomic state by spectral analysis of human umbilical artery flow velocity waveforms. Cardiovasc Res 37:601, 1998.
28. Suzuki T, et al: Detection of a biorhythm of human fetal autonomic nervous activity by a power spectral analysis. Am J Obstet Gynecol 185:1247, 2001.

29. Boulant JA: Role of the preoptic-anterior hypothalamus in thermoregulation and fever. Clin Infect Dis *31*(Suppl 5):S157, 2000.

30. Kupfermann I, et al: Motivational and addictive states. *In* Kandell ER, et al (eds): Principles of Neural Science, 4th ed. New York, McGraw-Hill, 2000, pp 998–1013.

31. Freake HC, Oppenheimer JH: Thermogenesis and thyroid function. Annu Rev Nutr *15*:263, 1995.

32. Okken A: Postnatal adaptation in thermoregulation. J Perinatol Med *19* (Suppl 1):67, 1991.

33. Canteras NS: The medial hypothalamic defensive system: hodological organization and functional implications. Pharmacol Biochem Behav *71*:481, 2002.

34. DiMicco JA, et al: The dorsomedial hypothalamus and the response to stress: part renaissance, part revolution. Pharmacol Biochem Behav *71*:469, 2002.

35. Bauer AS, et al: Associations between physiological reactivity and children's behavior: advantages of a multisystem approach. J Dev Behav Pediatr *23*:102, 2002.

36. Gunnar MR: Reactivity of the hypothalamic-pituitary-adrenocortical system to stressors in normal infants and children. Pediatrics *90*:491, 1992.

37. Hurbin A, et al: The vasopressin receptors colocalize with vasopressin in the magnocellular neurons of the rat supraoptic nucleus and are modulated by water balance. Endocrinology *143*:456, 2002.

38. Moos F, et al: New aspects of firing pattern autocontrol in oxytocin and vasopressin neurones. Adv Exp Med Biol *449*:153, 1998.

39. Richard P, et al: Rhythmic activities of hypothalamic magnocellular neurons: autocontrol mechanisms. Biol Cell *89*:555, 1997.

40. Sarkar DK: Evidence for prolactin feedback actions on hypothalamic oxytocin, vasoactive intestinal peptide and dopamine secretion. Neuroendocrinology *49*:520, 1989.

41. Cuttler L: The regulation of growth hormone secretion. Endocrinol Metab Clin North Am *25*:541, 1996.

42. Grimberg A, De Leon D: Growth. *In* Moshang Jr T (ed): Requisites in Pediatrics: Endocrinology. St. Louis, CV Mosby, 2003.

43. Swaab DF: Neurohypophyseal peptides in the human hypothalamus in relation to development, sexual differentiation, aging, and disease. Regul Pept *45*:143, 1993.

44. Ugrumov MV: Magnocellular vasopressin system in ontogenesis: development and regulation. Microsc Res Tech *56*:164, 2002.

45. Brownstein M J, et al: Synthesis, transport, and release of posterior pituitary hormones. Science *207*:373, 1980.

46. Sausville E, Carney D, Battey J: The human vasopressin gene is linked to the oxytocin gene and is selectively expressed in a cultured lung cancer cell line. J Biol Chem *260*:10236, 1985.

47. Morris JF, Pow DV: New anatomical insights into the inputs and outputs from hypothalamic magnocellular neurons. Ann NY Acad Sci *689*:16, 1993.

48. Dewey KG: Maternal and fetal stress are associated with impaired lactogenesis in humans. J Nutr *131*:3012S, 2001.

49. Chard T: Fetal and maternal oxytocin in human parturition. Am J Perinatol *6*:145, 1989.

50. Theodosis DT: Oxytocin-secreting neurons: a physiological model of morphological neuronal and glial plasticity in the adult hypothalamus. Front Neuroendocrinol *23*:101, 2002.

51. Schwabe C, Bullesbach EE: Relaxin: structures, functions, promises, and nonevolution. FASEB J *8*:1152, 1994.

52. Leng G, et al: Mechanisms of vasopressin secretion. Horm Res *37*:33, 1992.

53. Haycock GB: The syndrome of inappropriate secretion of antidiuretic hormone. Pediatr Nephrol *9*:375, 1995.

54. Knoers NV, Deen PM: Molecular and cellular defects in nephrogenic diabetes insipidus. Pediatr Nephrol *16*:1146, 2001.

55. Ervin MG: Perinatal fluid and electrolyte regulation: role of arginine vasopressin. Semin Perinatol *12*:134, 1988.

56. Williams G, et al: The hypothalamus and the control of energy homeostasis. Physiol Behav *74*:683, 2001.

57. Zhang Y, et al: Positional cloning of the mouse obese gene and its human homologue. Nature *372*:425, 1994.

58. Casanueva FF, Dieguez C: Neuroendocrine regulation and actions of leptin. Front Neuroendocrinol *20*:317, 1999.

59. Rahmouni K, Haynes WG: Leptin signaling pathways in the central nervous system: interactions between neuropeptide Y and melanocortins. Bioessays *23*:1095, 2001.

60. Elmquist JK: Hypothalamic pathways underlying the endocrine, autonomic, and behavioral effects of leptin. Physiol Behav *74*:703, 2001.

61. Ollmann MM, et al: Antagonism of central melanocortin receptors in vitro and in vivo by agouti-related protein. Science *278*:135, 1997.

62. Broberger C, et al: The neuropeptide Y/agouti gene–related protein (AGRP) brain circuitry in normal, anorectic, and monosodium glutamate-treated mice. Proc Natl Acad Sci USA *95*:15043, 1998.

63. Tome MA, et al: Sex-based differences in serum leptin concentrations from umbilical cord blood at delivery. Eur J Endocrinol *137*:655, 1997.

64. Ong KKL, et al: Cord blood leptin is associated with size at birth and predicts infancy weight gain in humans. J Clin Endocrinol Metab *84*:1145, 1999.

65. Kojima M, et al: Ghrelin is a growth-hormone–releasing acylated peptide from stomach. Nature *402*:656, 1999.

66. Nakazato M, et al: A role for ghrelin in the central regulation of feeding. Nature *409*:194, 2001.

67. Horvath TL, et al: Minireview: ghrelin and the regulation of energy balance—a hypothalamic perspective. Endocrinology *142*:4163, 2001.

68. Shintani M, et al: Ghrelin, an endogenous growth hormone secretagogue, is a novel orexigenic peptide that antagonizes leptin action through the activation of hypothalamic neuropeptide Y/Y1 receptor pathway. Diabetes *50*:227, 2001.

69. Toshinai K, et al: Upregulation of ghrelin expression in the stomach upon fasting, insulin-induced hypoglycemia, and leptin administration. Biochem Biophys Res Commun *281*:1220, 2001.

70. Ariyasu H, et al: Stomach is a major source of circulating ghrelin, and feeding state determines plasma ghrelin-like immunoreactivity levels in humans. J Clin Endocrinol Metab *86*:4753, 2001.

71. Hataya Y, et al: A low dose of ghrelin stimulates growth hormone (GH) release synergistically with GH-releasing hormone in humans. J Clin Endocrinol Metab *86*:4552, 2001.

183

Diva D. De León, Pinchas Cohen, and Lorraine E. Levitt Katz

Growth Factor Regulation of Fetal Growth

Growth during fetal life is characterized by an early period of cell division and formation of the major organ systems, followed by a more prolonged period of growth and refinement of organ development. Growth factors are peptides or proteins that serve as key regulators of cell proliferation and differentiation. They exert their effects by binding to specific receptors, which mediate signal transduction across cell membranes. The binding triggers a cascade of responses, including those involving second messengers, which ultimately result in cell mitogenesis or differentiation. Over the last decade the scientific literature has witnessed an explosion of information regarding the physiology of these agents. It is evident that a variety of growth factors are expressed in diverse tissues during embryonic life, and they may have endocrine as well as autocrine-paracrine effects.

INSULIN-LIKE GROWTH FACTOR AXIS

The primary regulator of postnatal somatic growth is growth hormone (GH). In the liver and other target cells, GH induces the production of somatomedins, also called insulin-like growth factors (IGF-I and IGF-II).[1] The somatomedins, particularly IGF-I, have direct (endocrine) effects on somatic growth and on the proliferation of many tissues and cell types. This cascade of growth control is known as the *somatomedin hypothesis*. Both IGF-I and IGF-II are expressed during fetal development in a GH-independent fashion. In addition to their anabolic effects, IGFs are also thought to be significant autocrine-paracrine factors involved in cellular and tissue function.[2] Locally produced IGFs have been demonstrated in nearly all tissue types, where they are considered to be responsible for cell growth and differentiation. GH is thought to play only a minor role in fetal growth that is limited to the third trimester. This chapter presents evidence that the IGFs and their regulatory proteins play a central role in the regulation of fetal growth.

Insulin-like Growth Factors

IGF-I and IGF-II are two closely related peptide hormones of approximately 7 kD molecular weight that share a high degree of structural similarity with proinsulin.[2] Like proinsulin, they are composed of A, B, and C domains; however, they also include a D domain. Together, these components form the mature IGF peptide. The IGFs are synthesized with an additional extension peptide known as the *E peptide*, which is removed during post-translational processing. Both IGF-I and IGF-II are encoded by a single gene each, which results in several mRNA species, owing to alternative splicing. The IGF-I gene spans 95 kb (containing 6 exons) on the long arm of chromosome 12, and the IGF-II gene has a total genomic size of 35 kb and is made up of 9 exons. The IGF-II gene is located on the short arm of chromosome 11 (near the insulin gene), in an area that is paternally imprinted in all mammalian species. This phenomenon may be related to the fact that IGF-II is a major fetal growth factor.

Insulin-like Growth Factor Receptors

The IGFs interact with specific receptors, designated as type I and type II IGF receptors, as well as with the insulin receptor, which can bind IGF-I and IGF-II, but with much lower affinity than insulin.[3,4] The type I IGF receptor binds IGF-I with high affinity, IGF-II with slightly lower affinity, and insulin with low affinity. This receptor mediates the known mitogenic effects of the IGFs. The type I IGF receptor and the closely related insulin receptor are heterotetramers composed of two pairs of α and β subunits, the result of post-translational processing of a single gene product that encodes for the entire receptor. The two α subunits, which are involved in ligand binding, are linked by disulfide bonds and are primarily extracellular. The β subunits are connected to the α subunit by disulfide bonds and function as intracellular tyrosine kinases. Upon ligand binding, they undergo a conformational change, which enables them to bind ATP and become autophosphorylated. Subsequently, these kinases appear to phosphorylate cytoplasmic molecules known as the insulin-responsive substrates (IRS-1 and -2), which are involved in mediating many of the effects of insulin and IGFs.[5] IRS proteins couple insulin/IGF receptors to the PI 3-kinase and extracellular signal-regulated kinase (ERK) cascades. Products of PI 3-kinase, including phosphatidylinositol-3,4-biphosphate and phosphatidylinositol-3,4,5-triphosphate, attract serine kinases to the plasma membrane, including the phosphoinositide-dependent kinase (PDK1 and PDK2) and at least three protein kinase B (PKB or AKT) isoforms. During co-localization at the plasma membrane, PDK1 or PDK2 phosphorylates and activates PKB1,-2, or -3. The activated PKB or AKT phosphorylates many substrates to control various biologic signaling cascades, including glucose transport, protein synthesis, glycogen synthesis, cell proliferation, and cell survival, in various cells and tissues.[6]

The type II IGF receptor is structurally distinct from the type I receptor and the insulin receptor; it primarily binds IGF-II.[5] Unlike the insulin receptor and the type I IGF receptor, the type II IGF receptor is not a tyrosine kinase. Instead, it is a monomeric receptor with a large extracellular domain made up of 15 repeat sequences and a small region homologous to the collagen-binding domain of fibronectin. The type II IGF receptor is 270 kD in size and functions also as the cation-independent mannose-6-phosphate receptor.[7] The receptor does not have a signaling domain and is thought to be recycled between the plasma membrane and intracellular compartments. It has also been suggested that the type II IGF receptor targets excess IGF-II for lysosomal destruction during fetal life.[4] The type II receptor is maternally imprinted in mice but not in humans.[8]

Additional members of the class of receptors for the IGF/insulin family are less well characterized. One receptor has biologic properties intermediate between the insulin and the type I IGF receptor; it binds both insulin and IGFs with high affinity. Analysis of tissues where this receptor appears to be common (such as placenta), as well as transfection experiments, has demonstrated that it is composed of one insulin receptor α-β dimer and one type I IGF receptor α-β dimer: it has thus been labeled the hybrid receptor. Its physiologic role in the placenta remains elusive, but it may explain the potent insulin-like effects seen with intravenous administration of IGF-I to humans.[9] The cDNA for an additional receptor has been cloned, and because of its high homology with the insulin receptor, it has been designated as the insulin receptor–related receptor or IRR.[10] IRR is an orphan receptor of the insulin receptor family that does not bind insulin or insulin-like peptide and can be expressed as variably spliced isoforms. IRR may have a role in fetal development, because its expression occurs specifically in developing renal and neural tissues. IRR is also expressed in pancreatic islets, but the lack of this receptor in mice does not affect β-cell development and function.[11] An additional atypical IGF receptor with altered ligand binding also has been described. This may represent a post-translationally modified type I IGF receptor of unclear function.

Insulin-like Growth Factor Binding Proteins

The IGF binding proteins (IGFBPs), a family of proteins with high affinity for the IGFs, have been shown to be involved in the modulation of the mitogenic effects of IGFs on cells. *In vivo*, the IGFs are bound to this family of six structurally and evolutionarily related IGFBPs (IGFBP-1 through IGFBP-6). In serum, the majority (70% to 80%) of the IGFs exist in a 150-kDa complex composed of one IGF molecule, IGFBP-3, and the acid-labile subunit (ALS). A smaller proportion (~20%) of the IGFs are associated with other serum IGFBPs within a 50-kDa complex, and less than 5% of the IGFs are found in the free form of 7.5 kDa. ALS is a protein that binds to the IGF/IGFBP-3 binary complex, primarily in serum, prolonging the $t_{1/2}$ of serum IGFs and facilitating their endocrine actions. These IGFBPs appear to regulate the availability of free IGFs for interaction with the IGF receptors, as well as to interact directly with cell function.[12] They are part of a superfamily that comprises six high-affinity IGFBPs and at least four other low-affinity IGF binders, termed insulin-like growth factor binding protein-related proteins (IGFBP-rP).[13] In addition, there is limited evidence that the cell surface proteoglycan glypican-3, mutations of which cause the overgrowth syndrome known as Simpson-Golabi-Behmel type I, also binds IGF-II and may modulate its function.[14]

IGFBP-1 is a 25-kD protein that is found in high concentrations in amniotic fluid; it is also secreted by hepatocytes under negative regulation by insulin. IGFBP-2 is a 31-kD molecular weight protein found in serum, cerebrospinal fluid, and seminal plasma. It is expressed in many fetal and adult tissues. IGFBP-3 is the major binding protein in postnatal serum and is synthesized by hepatocytes and other cells. In plasma, IGFBP-3 is found as part of a 150 kD complex, which also includes an acid-labile subunit and an IGF molecule, all of which are GH dependent. IGFBP-4 is a 24-kD protein that has been identified in serum, seminal plasma, and numerous cell types. IGFBP-5 appears to be an IGF-enhancing protein that is found in cerebrospinal fluid and serum. It is also observed in rapidly growing fetal tissues. IGFBP-6 has relative specificity for IGF-II over IGF-I. It is found in cerebrospinal fluid and serum and is produced by many cells. The six cloned cDNAs for the IGFBPs show a high degree of structural similarity and sequence conservation across species. IGFBPs are tightly regulated by various endocrine factors and are uniquely expressed during ontogeny.[15]

Three possible models for the interaction of the IGFBPs with the IGFs and their receptors have been proposed.[16] The first is that these molecules limit the availability of free IGFs for interaction with the IGF receptors. For example, the addition of IGFBPs to many cell cultures *in vitro* results in the inhibition of IGF actions within these experimental systems.[17] In other systems, however, IGFBPs have been demonstrated to enhance IGF action, under circumstances that may involve cellular processing of the IGFBPs.[18] Finally, as has been shown in several *in vitro* systems, IGFBPs may inhibit cell growth in an IGF-independent fashion, acting via their own receptors.[16,17]

IGFBP-3 is a mediator of apoptosis under the control of a number of cell cycle regulators.[19] Using specific antisense oligonucleotides and neutralizing anti-IGFBP-3 antibodies to block IGFBP-3 expression and action, IGFBP-3 was identified as the mediator of apoptosis induced by retinoic acid and TGF-β in multiple cell types.[20-23]

Insulin-like Growth Factor Binding Protein Proteases

A group of enzymes that are capable of cleaving IGFBPs have been recognized as potential modulators of IGF action.[24] First identified in pregnancy serum, IGFBP-3 proteolytic activity is responsible for the disappearance of intact IGFBP-3 from the serum of pregnant individuals, with no change in IGFBP-3 immunoreactivity and an increase in lower molecular weight fragments.[25,26] IGFBP proteases also have been reported in the serum of severely ill patients in states of cachexia, in critically ill neonates; in patients with GH receptor deficiency, in prostate cancer patients, and in patients with other malignancies.[27-29] Prostate-specific antigen was the first kallikrein protein demonstrated to be an IGFBP protease.[30] Subsequently, it has been determined that other members of the kallikrein family, such as nerve growth factor (NGF), also serve as specific IGFBP proteases.[31] Cathepsins are another class of IGFBP proteases, which have been shown to be active in acid pH.[32] Finally, matrix metalloproteinases, which are known to cleave collagen and other extracellular matrix components, are emerging as a new group of IGFBP proteases.[33] It has been speculated that the IGFBP proteases are important modulators of IGF bioavailability and bioactivity through their modification of the IGF carrier proteins.

The proteolytic activity may play a role in regulating IGF availability at the tissue level by decreasing the affinity of the binding proteins for the growth factors, releasing free IGFs and allowing increased receptor binding.[30,34] Together, all these interrelated molecules act in a coordinated fashion to control growth and differentiation. This system of molecules has been termed the *IGF axis*, and it is summarized in Figure 183–1.

ADDITIONAL GROWTH-REGULATING PEPTIDES

Fibroblast Growth Factor Family of Peptides and Receptors

Fibroblast growth factors (FGFs) are a family of peptide cytokines that are important in the regulation of many tissues. At least 7 different FGFs (FGF-1 through -7) have been identified, including the best-characterized acidic FGF (aFGF or FGF-1), basic FGF (bFGF or FGF-2), and keratinocyte growth factor (KGF or FGF-7). The FGFs exert their actions by binding to at least three receptors, FGFR1, FGFR2, and FGFR3, which have distinct tissue distributions. FGFs appear primarily to have autocrine-paracrine functions in organ growth and differentiation, as well as in carcinogenesis. It has also been shown that the genetic form of dwarfism known as achondroplasia is caused by a mutation in the FGFR3 gene.[35] Additionally, a human mutation in the FGFR2 gene caused craniosynostosis, a disease characterized by abnormal closure of the bones in the skull but normal long bone growth. These data suggest that normal FGFR signaling is essential for normal osteogenic growth. Thus far, targeted disruptions of murine FGF-2 and FGF-5 genes have been reported, and the phenotypes associated with them do not include growth abnormalities, but the animals do exhibit limb maldevelopment. Future studies will further define the role that different components of the FGF systems play in somatic and tissue growth.

Nerve Growth Factors

The complex array of cells that comprise the nervous system is under the regulatory influence of specific growth factors, such as nerve growth factor (NGF), neurotensin, and the neural derived growth factors (NDGFs). NGF is synthesized in peripheral cells and transported retrograde up the neuronal axis to the cell body—this process suggests that NGF is a neurotropic agent

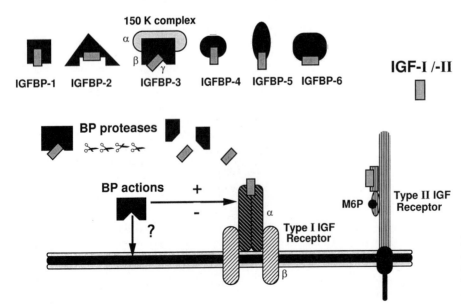

Figure 183–1. The insulin-like growth factor axis, including the IGFs, IGFBPs, and IGFBP proteases. The relationship of the components of the IGF axis is depicted in this figure.

directing neurons to sites of innervation.[36] NGF exerts its effects on cells derived from the neural crest, including central nervous system and peripheral nervous system neurons, and some non-neurons, such as immune cells and endocrine cells. NGF stimulates mitosis in some cell types and is capable of inducing differentiation events in neural tissue. NGF synthesis is controlled in part by hormones, such as testosterone and thyroxine. It also has been demonstrated that the γ subunit of NGF serves as an IGFBP protease.[31] Further research will better elucidate the interactions between NGF and the IGF axis components in the regulation of cellular growth.

Epidermal Growth Factor System

Epidermal growth factors (EGFs) and their receptors are widespread in many tissues and participate in developmental processes such as neonatal eyelid opening and tooth eruption. EGFs have potent mitogenic actions that have been extensively explored in cell culture systems. The receptor for EGFs was characterized as a prototype model for signal transduction involving tyrosine kinases. EGFs have been identified in most body fluids of mammals, and the now extensive *in vitro* data indicate multiple cellular functions of EGFs. The EGF family of growth factors appears to be important in mammalian development and function, although the precise roles and significance are not yet clear. Members of the EGF family may have a role in embryogenesis and fetal growth because receptors have been identified in fetal tissues. The mouse fetus expresses EGF receptors from 12 days onward.[37] EGFs can induce tracheal branching morphogenesis in chick lung rudiments and stimulate epithelial maturation in the lung and other tissues in rabbits.[38] Neither EGF antibody administration to newborn animals nor gene targeting of EGF, however, has caused major deleterious effects, as might be expected from the *in vitro* studies. Furthermore, EGF transcripts have not been detected in the fetus. It is unclear whether similar molecules may be involved in somatic growth. Transforming growth factor alpha (TGF-α) is a peptide that displays 30% homology with EGF and exerts effects through the EGF receptor.[39, 40] It has been shown to be expressed in pre-implantation mouse embryos and decidua of rat and thus may be important in fetal development.[41, 42] A targeted mutation of the EGF receptor demonstrated its significance in fetal development and growth.[39]

Other Growth-Promoting Peptides

A growing number of new growth factors are being recognized as having growth-promoting activities in certain cell types. In general, these molecules appear to play important autocrine-paracrine as well as endocrine roles. Notable among these are groups of growth factors that have tissue-specific effects. Endothelin, platelet-derived growth factor (PDGF), and vascular-epithelial growth factor (VEGF) regulate angiogenesis and other vascular processes in addition to modulating the function of numerous cultured cells. PDGF acts in sequence with other growth factors to regulate entry into the cell cycle.[43] A variety of hematopoietic growth factors such as granulocyte colony-stimulating factor (G-CSF), macrophage colony–stimulating factor (M-CSF), erythropoietin, and thrombopoietin promote the growth of the different lineages of the precursor cells in the bone marrow. Growth of immune system cells is stimulated by an array of cytokines, including interleukins and interferons. Other growth factors that have been attributed to specific tissues (such as hepatocyte growth factor [HGF]) are being recognized as having general growth-promoting effect in numerous tissues. Additional organ-specific growth regulatory molecules are being described in the gastrointestinal tract and kidneys.

Although these growth factors have potent effects on cellular growth, they appear to have little effect on somatic growth.

Growth Inhibitory Peptides

A particularly interesting class of cytokines that can negatively modulate cellular growth are members of the TGF-β family, which are structurally distinct from TGF-α. TGF-β can either act to mediate cellular growth and malignant transformation, or act as a growth inhibitory substance with the potential of arresting the growth of normal and neoplastic cells. TGF-β transcripts have been detected in preimplantation embryos.[41] This peptide is involved in mesodermal differentiation and organogenesis. It may stimulate some mesenchymal mitosis, while inhibiting the proliferation of epithelial cells. Transforming growth factor-βs have both autocrine and paracrine effects. The response depends on the origin of the cell. In some cell types (i.e., hepatocytes, hematopoitic cells) cell growth is stimulated, whereas in other cell types (i.e., osteoblasts, granulocytes) growth is inhibited. During pregnancy, transforming growth factors are important in the regulation of trophoblast invasion, decidualization, and placentation.[44] Mutations in the TGF-β family ligands are responsible for a number of human diseases, including hereditary chondrodysplasia.[45] Retinoic acid and other steroid hormones also have been shown to have inhibitory effects on cell growth. Tumor necrosis factors (TNF) and other compounds have been described to have similar effects. These molecules may regulate the entry to cells into programmed cell death (apoptosis).

GROWTH FACTORS IN FETAL GROWTH: ANIMAL MODELS

Insulin-like Growth Factor Axis Expression

The embryo establishes its own IGF axis very early in gestation, providing evidence that this axis plays a functional role in fetal growth. mRNA for IGF-II, the type II IGF receptor, and IGFBP-2, -3, and -4 are among the earliest of fetal mouse transcripts and are detectable in two cell murine embryos by reverse transcriptase polymerase chain reaction.[46-48] These transcripts become more abundant as gestation progresses. The distribution of the type II IGF receptor in tissues corresponds to that of IGF-II mRNA. IGF-I expression occurs somewhat later, by 7 to 8 days' gestation in mouse embryos.[49, 50] The type I IGF receptor is expressed in 8-cell rat embryo, and its mRNA is widely distributed in various tissues by midgestation.[51] Regulation of IGF expression in fetal life is not fully defined. Postnatal IGF synthesis is controlled by GH and by nutritional status, but IGF regulation in intrauterine life is less well understood and does not appear to be GH dependent. Furthermore, there is evidence that IGFs not only stimulate proliferation, but also can induce differentiation events in some cells during organogenesis in an autocrine or paracrine manner. These actions, with regard to organ differentiation, are probably tightly regulated within specific tissues and developmental stages during intrauterine life.

Overexpression of the Growth Hormone Insulin-like Growth Factor Axis in Transgenic Animals

Overexpression of GH, IGF-I, and IGF-II

The creation of transgenic mice overexpressing GH-IGF axis molecules has furthered the understanding of the control of IGF-I secretion and actions in fetal and postnatal growth (Table 183-1). Mice with GH overexpression display increased postnatal linear growth and dramatic weight gain to as much as twice normal body weight with selective organ hypertrophy.[52, 53] Acceleration of growth correlates with the onset of GH-dependent IGF-I

TABLE 183-1

Physical and Biochemical Features of Various GH/IGF-I Transgenic Mouse Models

Transgene	Postnatal Growth (% Normal Weight)	GH	IGF-I	IGFBP-3	Brain Size	Liver Size
GH	200	↑↑	↑↑	----------	Normal	↑↑
IGF-I	130	↓	↑	↑	↑↑	↑
GH⁻	60	↓↓	↓↓	↓↓	↓	↓↓
GH⁻/IGF-I⁺	Normal	↓	Normal	Normal or ↓	↑	↓

GH = growth hormone; IGF-I = insulin-like growth factor-I; IGFBP-3 = IGF-binding protein-3; GH⁻ = growth hormone deficient.

expression during the second to third postnatal week, suggesting that the growth-promoting properties of the transgene are mediated via the induction of IGF-I expression postnatally. IGF-I transgenic mice are also larger than normal, but their weight increase (30% over control mice), which occurs after 4 to 6 weeks of postnatal life, is more modest compared with that of the GH transgenic mice, which is likely related to the lower IGF levels seen with the former.[54] The brains and other organs of these animals demonstrate a large increase in weight relative to overall growth. IGF-I levels in these mice are elevated but are lower than those seen in the GH transgenic mice; endogenous GH and hepatic IGF-I expression are suppressed by 60% to 75% (Table 183-2).[55] IGF-II transgenic mice are not bigger than normal, but in the existing models, the majority of IGF-II expression occurs postnatally.[56]

To separate out more completely the effects of endogenous GH and IGF-I expression, IGF-I transgenic mice were mated with a GH-deficient mouse strain.[57,58] The offspring displayed normal body weight and linear growth. Some non-GH dependent effects of IGF-I were present, including a disproportionate increase in brain weight, implying that these are local effects of IGF-I. The

livers of these mice were hypoplastic (an effect seen in GH-deficient mice), an abnormality that was only partially corrected with IGF-I. Overall, the transgenic animal data confirm the role of GH and/or IGF-I in postnatal growth and suggest that IGF-I mediates the majority of GH effects, but that variations in local expression IGF-I can result in altered growth of specific tissues.

Overexpression of IGFBPs

Mice overexpressing IGFBP-1 are similar (or slightly smaller) in size to the wild type at birth.[59,60] Brain weights are decreased in these transgenic mice compared with the wild type.[61] It is generally believed that IGFBP-1 functions to inhibit IGF-I action and thus may contribute to the impaired fetal brain development seen in these transgenic animals. Overexpression of IGFBP-2 in mice did not result in a different birth weight and only a reduction of body weight gain at an age later than 3 weeks postnatally.[62]

In two different IGFBP-3 transgenic mouse models, transgene expression resulted in organomegaly that develops in places different from the major expression sites.[63,64] Total body weight in transgenic mice overexpressing IGFBP-4 is indistinguishable

TABLE 183-2

Physical and Biochemical Features of the Various GH/IGF-I Knockout Mouse Models

Knockout	Birth Weight (% of birth weight)	Other Features	Postnatal Course
IGF-I	60	Normal placenta; decreased brain size	Slow growth; die before adulthood
IGF-II	60	Small placenta	Normal growth rate
IGF-I + IGF-II	30	Small placenta; no respirations	Immediate postnatal death
LID	Normal	75% reduction in serum IGF-I	Normal growth
ALS	Normal	65% reduction in serum IGF-I	10% reduction in body weight
LID + ALSKO	Normal	85%–90% reduction in serum IGF-I; increased GH levels	30% reduction in body weight and length
IGF-I receptor	45	No respirations	Immediate postnatal death
IGF-II receptor	130	Edema, large placenta	Death *in utero*
IGF-I receptor + IGF-II receptor	100	Large placenta	Normal growth rate
IGF-I receptor + IGF-II	30	Small placenta	
IGF-II receptor + IGF-II	80	Small placenta	
IGF-I receptor + IGF-II receptor + IGF-II	30	Small placenta	
IGF-I + GH receptor	17		Postnatal growth retardation
IRS-1	50–70	Insulin resistance	Survive with normal growth rate but remain small with no catch-up growth
IRS-2	90	Insulin resistance, β-cell failure	Develop diabetes
AKT-1	80	Normal glucose tolerance	Partial neonatal mortality Persistent small size in surviving pups
Insulin genes (Ins1 + Ins2)	80–85	Diabetes	Normal growth rate; early death from diabetes
Insulin receptor	90	Diabetes; hypotrophy of subcutaneous fat	Normal growth rate; early death from diabetes

GH = growth hormone; IGF-I = insulin-like growth factor-I; IRS-1 = insulin-responsive substrate-1; LID = liver IGF-I deficient mice; ALSKO = ALS knockout mice; LID + ALSKO = double-knockout for LID and ALS.

from that of control animals.[65] No transgenic models overexpressing IGFBP-5 or IGFBP-6 have been reported so far.

Insulin and Insulin-like Growth Factor Axis Null Mutations

Studies of null mutations (knockouts) created by homologous recombination in the genes encoding insulin, IGF-I, IGF-II, and the IGF receptors have enabled scientists to explore the role of the IGF axis in fetal growth. In all the null mutations, body proportions are qualitatively normal.

IGFs and IGF Receptor Mutations

Mice in which the IGF-II gene has been eliminated by targeted disruption are severely growth retarded *in utero* (60% normal size at birth), with small placentas.[66, 67] After birth, however, IGF-II-lacking mice have normal survival and grow at a near-normal rate, although their size remains small relative to normal littermates. In the heterozygous state, the IGF-II knockout can manifest itself only if the paternal allele is targeted, elegantly demonstrating the paternal imprinting of the IGF-II gene.[68] IGF-I gene-targeted mice are also small (60% of normal) at birth, whereas the placentas are of normal size.[66,69,70] Furthermore, they display dramatic growth arrest postnatally (30% of normal). These mice have an increase in death rate during the neonatal period, which may be related to poorly developed diaphragms and lungs.

Postnatal development of surviving IGF-I knockout mice has been analyzed in detail. At 2 months of age, IGF-I deficient mice show extensive reductions of brain size, consistent with a role of IGF-I in axon growth.[71] Morphologic and morphometric analysis of long bones in mice lacking IGF-I indicate that IGF-I promotes bone development by increasing cellular proliferation, without affecting differentiation. The growth plates are uniformly affected, with reductions in the resting, proliferative, and hypertrophic chondrocytes. As a result, the formation of secondary ossification centers is delayed.[72] At present, only one human homozygous partial deletion of the IGF-I gene has been described, in a 15-year-old boy. This patient had severe prenatal and postnatal growth failure, sensorineural deafness, and mental retardation.[73] Mice with null mutations of both IGF-I and IGF-II displayed further intrauterine growth retardation (to 30% normal size), and all these mice died after birth from respiratory failure. Thus, IGF-I and -II appear to have independent growth-promoting activities that are additive when both are absent. The results of the studies confirm that both IGF-I and IGF-II appear to be critical for fetal growth, whereas IGF-I promotes postnatal growth, as well. IGF-II may dictate the size of the placenta and consequently affect fetal size.

Liver IGF-I deficient (LID) mice grow normally, despite a 75% reduction in serum IGF-I levels. In these mice, expression of IGF-I in nonhepatic tissues is normal, suggesting that the normal growth exhibited by these animals was mediated by autocrine/paracrine actions of IGF-I, as well as by some nonhepatic sources of circulating IGF-I.[74] Similarly, ALS knockout (ALSKO) mice demonstrate only a 10% reduction in body weight despite a 65% reduction in circulating IGF-I levels.[75] These findings are consistent with the idea that locally synthesized IGF-I plays a prominent role in somatic growth. A more recent mouse model, double knockout for LID+ALS, showed serum levels of IGF-I reduced to about 10% to 15% of normal levels. In these animals, GH levels were markedly increased and linear growth was severely attenuated (30% reduction in body length and weight starting at 2 to 3 weeks of age). Thus, the double gene disruption LID + ALSKO mouse model demonstrates that a threshold concentration of circulating IGF-I is necessary for normal growth.[76]

Gene targeting of the type I IGF receptor[70] results in severe intrauterine growth retardation, with a phenotype similar to that seen in double IGF-I + IGF-II gene-targeting. These mice also die

after birth, apparently from inadequate respiration. The results indicate that the mitogenic effects of IGF-I and IGF-II are mediated primarily through the type I IGF-receptor. The fact that only the mice missing IGF-II displayed decreased placental growth (independent of the type I and type II receptor), however, suggests that an additional receptor mediates IGF-II actions in fetal life. Gene targeting of the type II receptor[77] results in mice that are 30% larger than littermates, compatible with its negative growth-modulating effect. This gene is maternally imprinted in mice, but not in humans. Thus, those inheriting the maternal IIR allele lack functional IIR receptors and die shortly after birth. The levels of lysosomal enzymes in amniotic fluid are increased, and there is selective organ enlargement. It has been hypothesized that mice lacking the type IIR accumulate toxic levels of IGF-II.

These studies provide supportive evidence that IGF-II/Man-6-P receptor may function primarily as a degradative pathway to remove IGF-II from the extracellular environment. The opposite imprinting of IGF-II and the type II IGF receptor may modulate fetal demand and maternal supply of nutrients.[78] The phenotype of mice lacking both type I IGF receptor and type II IGF receptor provides evidence for the ability of IGF-I to signal through the insulin receptor, since these mice have normal embryonic and postnatal growth. It has been shown that mice lacking the type II IGF receptor are rescued from perinatal lethality and undergo near-normal postnatal development when they carry null mutations of the type I IGF receptor. Triple mutants lacking IGF-II and both IGF receptors exhibit only about 30% normal weight, phenotypically indistinguishable from double mutants lacking IGF type I receptor and IGF-II (see Table 183–2).[79] Genetic evidence indicates that the receptor supporting growth of the type I/type II IGF receptor double mutants is the insulin receptor, since mice lacking all three genes (insulin receptor, type I IGF receptor, type II IGF receptor) are nonviable 30% dwarfs.[80] Thus, embryonic growth of type I/type II IGF receptor knockout mice must be sustained through IGFs binding to the insulin receptor, since this is an existing embryonic growth pathway.

To address the issue of the role of GH and IGF-I in growth, Lupu and colleagues[72] have generated mice lacking both IGF-I and growth hormone receptor. Double knockout mice are more growth retarded (17% of normal) than mice lacking either gene alone, indicating that the two genes act both independently and synergistically to promote growth. Whereas IGF-I promotes both prenatal and postnatal growth, GH appears to be required exclusively for postnatal growth, since the growth defect in GH receptor-deficient mice becomes apparent only after postnatal day 20.

Insulin and Insulin Receptor Mutations

The generation of mice bearing insulin receptor mutations has been instrumental in dissecting the pathogenesis of insulin resistance, diabetes, and obesity. In terms of somatic growth, mice lacking the insulin receptor are born at term with slight growth retardation (approximately 10%);[80] inactivation of the two insulin genes also results in a slight impairment of embryonic growth, with a 15% to 20% decrease of birth weight.[81] The growth impairment observed in mice lacking the insulin genes indicates that the effect of insulin to promote mouse embryo growth is paltry compared with that of IGF-I and IGF-II. Mutations of the insulin receptor in humans are phenotypically heterogeneous in terms of the metabolic consequences. As in mice, lack of the insulin receptor in humans is compatible with embryonic development and term birth. Most strikingly, humans lacking the insulin receptor are severely growth retarded at birth and gain little if any weight thereafter.[82] The likeliest explanation of the difference between insulin receptor–deficient mice and children is that embryonic growth of humans and rodents follows different patterns. During the last trimester of human gestation, corresponding to the first weeks of postnatal life in mice, there is a significant increase in adipose mass. The adipose organ is exquisitely sensitive to insulin, as demonstrated by the excessive adiposity of fetuses exposed to high insulin concentrations *in utero* who are born large for gestational age as a result of maternal diabetes,[83,84] or hyperinsulinism.[85] Thus, in contrast to mice, insulin is a fetal growth factor in humans. There have been no reports of null mutations of the human insulin gene.

Insulin-like Growth Factor Binding Protein Mutations

When the knockout approach has been applied to the IGFBP, the results are rather disappointing: in IGFBP-2 knockout mice, a reduction in spleen weight of adult males was the only morphologic alteration.[86] IGFBP-4 mutants appear to be slightly smaller than normal counterparts, and the genetic ablation of IGFBP-6 has not resulted in any apparent phenotypical manifestation.[87] It has been speculated that functional compensation by other members of the IGFBP family (including the recently described IGFBP-rPs) may prevent the appearance of dramatic phenotypes.[88]

Insulin-Responsive Substrate and AKT Mutations

Two IRS proteins, called IRS-1 and IRS-2, mediate many insulin and IGFs responses, especially those that are associated with somatic growth and carbohydrate metabolism. The IRS-1 branch of the pathway plays a significant role to mediate the effects of IGF-I on growth. Deletion of the IRS-1 gene in mice reduces embryonic and neonatal growth, whereas deletion of IRS-2 barely reduces prenatal and early postnatal growth by 10%. The IRS-1 knockout mouse has been described with the phenotype of fetal growth retardation as 50% to 70% normal size in the homozygous state. Postnatally, these mice continue to be small (50% to 70% of normal weight), and catch-up growth does not occur. The offspring display no obvious developmental abnormalities and have normal bone development. Gene targeting of IRS-1 results in impairment of both growth and carbohydrate metabolism, compatible with its role in mediating both insulin and IGF-I effects.[89,90] Growth is reduced 40% in IRS-2$^{-/-}$ mice that are also haploinsufficient for IRS-1, whereas growth is reduced 70% in IRS-1$^{-/-}$ mice also haploinsufficient for IRS-2. Thus IRS-2 cannot fully replace IRS-1 in this process. IRS-2$^{-/-}$ mice exhibit a diabetic phenotype with peripheral insulin resistance and β-cell failure.[6]

Downstream from IRS, AKT-1 and AKT-2 gene deletion also results in different phenotypes. Although AKT-2 knockout mice exhibit insulin resistance, at birth AKT-1 knockout mice have a 20% reduction in body weight compared with wild-type mice. The decrease in body weight persists throughout postnatal development regardless of sex. These mice have normal glucose tolerance. These data demonstrate that AKT-1 is most important to the growth of the organism, both *in utero* and after birth, whereas AKT-2 is critical to insulin-dependent control of carbohydrate metabolism.[91,92]

IGF axis gene knockouts are summarized in Table 183–2.

GROWTH FACTORS IN HUMAN FETAL GROWTH

Pregnancy

During pregnancy, circulating levels of IGFs rise in maternal serum and significantly in fetal serum.[93,94] Placental GH, human placental lactogen (HPL), and nutritional factors may regulate maternal IGF-I levels during pregnancy.[95,96] Placental GH is not detected in the fetus, but HPL stimulates IGF-I and IGF-II production in fetal tissue.[97] Maternal IGFBP-1 levels rise fivefold to tenfold during gestation,[26,93] probably as a manifestation of the insulin resistance of pregnancy. IGFBP-1 levels are substantial in amniotic fluid, where they may have a fetal renal or hepatic source. A negative correlation exists between term IGFBP-1 levels in maternal serum or IGFBP-1 levels in amniotic fluid at 16 weeks' gestation and fetal weight.[98] Thus, the elevated IGFBP-1 concen-

trations (10 to 100 ng/L) in amniotic fluid may modulate fetal IGF action. It has also been suggested that elevated maternal IGFBP-1 levels may limit trophoblast invasion and negatively affect placental growth.

Pregnancy-associated IGFBP-3 protease activity, which has been shown to appear after 6 weeks' gestation, is responsible for the decrease and progressive disappearance of intact IGFBP-3 by Western ligand blot (without a change in IGFBP-3 immunoreactivity) and the appearance of lower molecular weight fragments of IGFBP-3 with a lower affinity to IGFs.[26,99,100] It has been demonstrated that IGFBP-2, IGFBP-4, and IGFBP-5 also undergo proteolysis during pregnancy.[26,101] The significance of the pregnancy-associated protease remains unclear. Some have postulated that IGFBP proteolysis may play a role in facilitating trophoblastic invasion.[102] It has been demonstrated that the pregnancy serum protease may play a role in regulating IGF bioactivity by making IGFs more available to the cells.[103] Thus, it is possible that this proteolytic activity could affect placental and consequently fetal growth, by releasing free IGFs and allowing increased receptor binding.

Insulin-like Growth Factor Axis Expression by the Fetus

Few data are available regarding the earliest expression of the IGF axis in the human embryo. In the trophoblast, however, IGF-II mRNA is detected by days 12 to 18,[104,105] and soon after type I and II receptor mRNA can also be found.[106] The animal data demonstrating IGF-II expression before that of IGF-I indicate the importance of IGF-II in early embryogenesis. There is widespread expression of IGFs in all human tissues during the second trimester.[107] Western immunoblotting techniques have demonstrated that type II IGF receptors are present in most human fetal tissues at 23 weeks.[108] The widespread expression and action of IGFs in embryogenesis are mostly autocrine/paracrine and GH independent. Although the control of IGF levels in the fetus is not well understood, it is thought that IGF actions occur in concert with other hormones and growth factors and are greatly influenced by the presence and distribution of IGFBPs. Techniques of immunocytochemistry, *in situ* hybridization, and Northern analysis have identified IGFBP-1 through IGFBP-6 in most fetal tissues.[109,110] Synthesis and secretion of IGFBPs are tissue-specific.[108]

In the third trimester, fetal serum IGF-I concentrations steadily increase, correlating with the time of peak fetal weight gain. Although fetal serum IGF-I levels are low compared with those in adults, several investigators have reported that maternal and fetal cord serum IGF-I levels correlated with birth weight,[111-114] suggesting co-regulation by nutritional factors. This correlation, however, has not been a consistent finding in every study.[93] Insulin levels appear to affect IGF levels as well, although this may be a secondary effect. Fetal IGF-II levels have shown a correlation with birth weight in some studies but not in others.[113,114] The animal studies presented in the previous section indicate that IGFs are not under endocrine control prenatally and that GH deficiency, although affecting postnatal growth, does not result in significant prenatal growth retardation. Nevertheless, data from humans with idiopathic hypopituitarism do support a role of GH in third trimester fetal growth because these infants, although still within the normal growth curves, often have mean birth lengths 0.8 to 1.7 standard deviation scores below the mean.[115,116] Furthermore, neonates with GH insensitivity (Laron syndrome) are also small at birth (−1.59 mean height standard deviation score), and their serum levels of IGF-I and IGF-II are also low at birth.[117] A case of severe intrauterine growth retardation in a patient with a homozygous partial deletion of the IGF-I gene proves that

IGF-I plays a critical part in human fetal growth, independently of GH.[73]

The IGFBP profile in cord serum reveals a pattern that is different from adult serum. IGFBP-3 is low, with relative prominence of IGFBP-2.[111] Furthermore, IGFBP-1 levels in cord serum are up to tenfold higher than levels seen in adults and decline markedly during the first week of life. IGFBP-1 levels show a negative correlation with birth weight. Several authors have reported a lack of correlation of cord IGFBP-1 levels with cord insulin and C-peptide levels, but a recent paper demonstrated significantly elevated insulin levels associated with decreased IGFBP-1 levels in large for gestational age infants (born to nondiabetic mothers).[118] A reverse trend was seen in intrauterine growth retardation (IUGR) levels in this same study.

Intrauterine Growth Retardation

IUGR refers to infants with birth weights and/or length equal to or lower than 2 standard deviations below the mean (≤ -2 SD) in relation to gestational age for the same sex, a cut-off point that corresponds approximately to the 3rd percentile for gestational age. There were 4,058,814 infants born in the United States in 2000; applying a 2.3% defination of IUGR, one can calculate an incidence of approximately 93,400 infants born with IUGR in the United States.[119]

IUGR may result from diverse genetic and environmental influences on the developing fetus: chromosomal defects, maternal nutrition, genetics, or decreased uteroplacental blood flow. Disproportional IUGR can result from circulatory changes in the fetus that favor redistribution of blood flow to the heart and brain. In severe IUGR, the head size is compromised as well. Endocrine factors appear to play a role in the process of IUGR. Decreased levels of placental GH and maternal IGF-I have been demonstrated in IUGR.[120] In both preterm and term infants, low birth weight is associated with low cord serum IGF-I and IGFBP-3 and high IGFBP-1.[118,121,122] In infants with IUGR, IGF expression has been shown to be decreased.[111,114,118,123] Some investigators, however, have demonstrated more variable IGF levels in infants with IUGR,[93] so this one marker may underestimate the complexity of IUGR, including the multitude of etiologic factors. It also has been demonstrated that IUGR infants have elevated IGFBP-1 levels, decreased IGF-II levels, and decreased IGFBP-3 levels compared with appropriate for gestational age infants.[114,118,123] IGFBP-2 levels may be higher as well, similar to what is seen in postnatal hypopituitary patients.[118] The increase in IGFBP-1 (mostly of hepatic origin) appears to be the result of inadequate nutrient supply, with resultant hypoinsulinemia.

It has been speculated that the elevated IGFBP-1 levels in these infants may sequester IGFs, thus restricting fetal growth. Not only are there alterations in IGF levels in children with IUGR but also the IGF type I receptor affinity was reduced in a subgroup of patients with IUGR.[124] The finding of a homozygous partial deletion of the IGF-I gene in a patient with severe IUGR[73] implicates IGF-I in the etiology of this disorder, but larger studies looking for mutations in the IGF-I gene in several groups of children with IUGR have failed to identify them, suggesting that mutations of these genes are not a common cause of IUGR.[125,126] Conversely, an association between a polymorphism of the IGF-I gene and low serum IGF-I levels was found in a recent study involving children with short stature born small for gestational age (SGA), suggesting that genetically determined low serum IGF-I levels may lead not only to reduction in birth length, weight, and head circumference but also to persistent short stature.[127] Transforming growth factor-β has also been implicated in the pathogenesis of IUGR. Transforming growth factor-β cord blood levels were found to be significantly lower in pregnancies complicated by IUGR when compared with the levels appropriate for gestational age (AGA) controls.[44]

The majority of children born with IUGR will experience adequate catch-up growth in length during the first 2 years of life. Postnatal catch-up usually begins immediately after birth, and in fact, most of the increases in height standard deviation score (SDS) occur by 6 months of age.[128,129] McCowan and coworkers showed that 40 of 203 (20%) infants born small for gestational age remained short and 31 (16%) remained light at 6 months.[130] After about 2 years of age, most children born small for gestational age tend not to exhibit further catch-up growth, and about 10% will remain ≤ -2 SD for height throughout childhood and adolescence and into adulthood, indicating a persistent failure to achieve normal linear growth. In one study, a large population of neonates was followed until adulthood and measured at the age of 20 to 21 years. Compared with the appropriate for gestational age control population, the small for gestational age subjects were 4 to 6 cm shorter as adults.[131]

Growth retardation during the fetal period has been associated with a higher prevalence of such conditions as hypertension, cardiovascular disease, and type 2 diabetes in adult life. These findings have led to the "fetal origins" of adult disease hypothesis advocated by Barker.[132] This theory proposes that *in utero* insults lead to "reprogramming" of the endocrine system that eventually predisposes those born small for gestational age to the above-mentioned conditions and other adverse health outcomes. It is important to note that life-long programming of the IGF system by the intrauterine hormonal and nutritional environment has also been suggested to be a key mediator of the link between small size at birth and cardiovascular disease in adulthood.[133]

Insulin resistance and type 2 diabetes are more prevalent among persons who were born with low birth weight, and insulin resistance has been linked to thinness at birth followed by obesity in adulthood.[134,135] An increased prevalence of syndrome X (or metabolic syndrome: obesity, cardiovascular disease, hypertension, and type 2 diabetes) has been reported among adults who were born small for gestational age.[136]

Growth hormone therapy recently has been approved for the long-term treatment of growth failure in children born small for gestational age who fail to manifest catch-up growth by age 2 years. Different studies have proved the efficacy of growth hormone therapy in promoting catch-up growth in IUGR children. Some of these studies have also demonstrated positive effects of growth hormone therapy on body composition, blood pressure, and lipid metabolism.[137-139] The evidence that growth hormone therapy has an impact on final height in IUGR children is limited.[140-142] Further studies are required.

Table 183-3 summarizes these findings.

Macrosomia

Alterations in the IGF axis also have been demonstrated in infants who are large for gestational age, including those born to diabetic mothers (see Figure 183-2 and Table 183-3). IGF-I, insulin, and IGFBP-3 levels are increased in large for gestational age infants, whereas IGFBP-1 levels are significantly decreased.[118] Fetal hyperinsulinemia secondary to maternal diabetes mellitus

TABLE 183-3

Insulin-like Growth Factor Axis Findings Seen in Extremes of Human Fetal Growth

	IGF-I	IGF-II	IGFBP-1	IGFBP-3	IGFBP-2
Intrauterine growth retardation	↓	↓	↑	↓	↑
Large for gestational age	↑	Normal or ↑	↓	↑	Normal

IGF-I = insulin-like growth factor-I; IGFBP-1 = IGF binding protein-1.

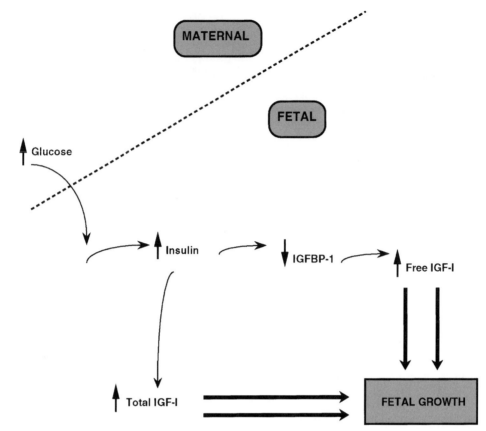

Figure 183–2. A schematic model of illustrating the interrelationships between maternal and fetal glucose, insulin, IGF-I, and IGFBP-1 levels in the regulation of fetal growth and the evolution of macrosomia.

results in increased body fat with a more modest increase in body length. Insulin promotes fetal growth by permitting nutrient uptake, and increased IGF-I production may be a result of the nutritional state of these infants.[143] The alterations in IGFBP-1 also appear to be secondary to the higher insulin levels, but IGF-I levels and nutritional status also may play a role. It has been speculated that the lower IGFBP-1 levels result in less inhibition of IGF-I effects, resulting in greater growth.

Infants with the Beckwith-Wiedemann syndrome have a doubling in IGF-II gene dosage as a result of alterations in chromosome 11p15.5. These infants are macrosomic and often demonstrate evidence of congenital hyperinsulinism. Placental hypertrophy is seen as well.[144] In the limited studies that have been performed, levels of IGF-II are not increased in cord serum in these infants, but it is possible that IGF-II gene dosage may increase fetal growth through the stimulation of placental growth.[102, 145] These infants are also predisposed to develop IGF-II–dependent neoplasms, such as Wilms' tumor. In fact, when birth weights of over 1800 patients with Wilms' tumor were analyzed, the mean was significantly greater than the national average, especially for those with Beckwith-Wiedemann syndrome or hemihypertrophy, suggesting the presence of systemic growth effects of IGF-II on both fetal size and the development of Wilms' tumor.[146]

SUMMARY

In recent years, the medical and scientific literature has witnessed an explosion of information regarding the physiology of growth and growth factors in prenatal life, and the various components of the IGF axis in particular. Local IGFs and IGFBPs are of prime importance with regard to fetal and placental growth.

Genetic manipulations of IGF axis components in fetal mice have further clarified the roles of these agents. Undoubtedly, the coming years will bring even more new information on the physiology and pathology of these key cellular regulators. Furthermore, these discoveries are likely to lead to the increasing use of diagnostic tests, and the recognition of genetic mutations of GH-IGF axis in cases of IUGR, as well as to therapeutic applications of these agents.

REFERENCES

1. Rotwein P: Structure, evolution, expression and regulation of insulin-like growth factors I and II. Growth Fact 5:3, 1991.
2. LeRoith D, et al: Insulin-like growth factors. Biol Signals 1:173, 1992.
3. Nielsen FC: The molecular and cellular biology of insulin-like growth factor II. Prog Growth Fact Res 4:257, 1992.
4. Oh Y, et al: New concepts in insulin-like growth factor receptor physiology. Growth Regul 3:113, 1993.
5. Nissley P, Lopaczynski W: Insulin-like growth factor receptors. Growth Fact 5:29, 1991.
6. White MF: IRS proteins and the common path to diabetes. Am J Physiol Endocrinol Metab 283:E413, 2002.
7. Nakae J, et al: Distinct and overlapping functions of insulin and IGF-I receptors. Endocr Rev 22:818, 2001.
8. Kalscheuer VM, et al: The insulin-like growth factor type-2 receptor gene is imprinted in the mouse but not in humans. Nat Genet 5:74, 1993.
9. Moxham CP, et al: Insulin-like growth factor-I receptor β-subunit heterogeneity: evidence for hybrid tetramers composed of insulin-like growth factor I and insulin receptor heterodimers. J Biol Chem 264:13238, 1989.
10. Zhang B, Roth RA: The insulin receptor–related receptor. Tissue expression, ligand binding specificity, and signaling capabilities. J Biol Chem 267:18320, 1992.
11. Kitamura T, et al: Preserved pancreatic β-cell development and function in mice lacking the insulin receptor-related receptor. Mol Cell Biol 21:5624, 2001.
12. Lamson G, et al: Insulin-like growth factor binding proteins: structural and molecular relationships. Growth Fact 5:19, 1991.

13. Baxter RC, et al: Recommendations for nomenclature of the insulin-like growth factor binding proteins superfamily. Endocrinology 139:4036, 1998.
14. Pilia G, et al: Mutations in GPC3, a glypican gene, cause the Simpson-Golabi-Behmel overgrowth syndrome. Nat Genet 12:241, 1996.
15. Donovan SM, et al: Ontogeny of serum insulin–like growth factor binding proteins in the rat. Endocrinology 125:2621, 1989.
16. Cohen P, et al: Transfection of the human insulin-like growth factor binding protein-3 gene into Balb/c fibroblasts inhibits cellular growth. Mol Endocrinol 7:380, 1993.
17. Valentinis B, et al: The human insulin-like growth factor binding protein-3 inhibits the growth of fibroblasts with a targeted disruption of the IGF-I receptor gene. Mol Endocrinol 9:361, 1995.
18. Clemmons DR: Insulin-like growth factor binding proteins: roles in regulating IGF physiology. J Dev Physiol 15:105, 1991.
19. Grimberg A, Cohen P: Role of insulin-like growth factors and their binding proteins in growth control and carcinogenesis. J Cell Physiol 183:1, 2000.
20. Erondu NE, et al: Regulation of endothelial IGFBP-3 synthesis and secretion by IGF-I and TGF-beta. Growth Regul 6:1, 1996.
21. Gucev ZS, et al: Insulin-like growth factor binding protein 3 mediates retinoic acid and transforming growth factor β2-induced growth inhibition in human breast cancer cells. Cancer Res 56:1545, 1996.
22. Han GR, et al: All-trans-retinoic acid increases transforming growth factor-β2 and insulin-like growth factor binding protein-3 expression through a retinoic acid receptor-alpha-dependent signaling pathway. J Biol Chem 272:13711, 1997.
23. Rajah R, et al: Insulin-like growth factor (IGF)–binding protein-3 induces apoptosis and mediates the effects of transforming growth factor-β1 on programmed cell death via a p53- and IGF-independent mechanism. J Biol Chem 272:12181, 1997.
24. Lamson G, et al: Proteolysis of IGFBP-3 may be a common regulatory mechanism of IGF action in vivo. Growth Reg 3:91, 1993.
25. Davenport ML, et al: Regulation of serum insulin-like growth factor-I (IGF-I) and IGF binding proteins during rat pregnancy. Endocrinology 127:1278, 1990.
26. Giudice LC, et al: Insulin-like growth factor binding proteins in maternal serum throughout gestation and in the puerperium: effects of a pregnancy-associated serum protease activity. J Clin Endocrinol Metab 71:806, 1990.
27. Cotterill AM, et al: The insulin-like growth factor (IGF)-binding proteins and IGF bioactivity in Laron-type dwarfism. J Clin Endocrinol Metab 74:56, 1992.
28. Cohen P, et al: Clinical aspects of insulin-like growth factor binding proteins. Acta Endocrinol [Copenh] 124:74, 1991.
29. Bhala A, et al: Insulin-like growth factor axis parameters in sick hospitalized neonates. J Pediatr Endocrinol Metab 11:451, 1998.
30. Cohen P, et al: Prostate-specific antigen (PSA) is an IGF binding protein-3 (IGFBP-3) protease found in seminal plasma. J Clin Endocrinol Metab 75:1046, 1992.
31. Rajah R, et al: 7S nerve growth factor is an insulin-like growth factor-binding protein protease. Endocrinology 137:2676, 1996.
32. Conover CA, De Leon DD: Acid-activated insulin-like growth factor-b. J Biol Chem 269:7076, 1994.
33. Fowlkes JL, et al: Matrix metalloproteinases degrade insulin-like growth factor–binding protein-3 in dermal fibroblast cultures. J Biol Chem 269:25742, 1994.
34. Cohen P, et al: Biological effects of prostate-specific antigen as an insulin-like growth factor binding protein-3 protease. J Endocrinol 142:407, 1994.
35. Velinov M, et al: The gene for achondroplasia maps to the telomeric region of chromosome 4p. Nature Genet 6:314, 1994.
36. D'Ercole AJ: Growth factors and development. In Polin R, Fox W (eds): Fetal and Neonatal Physiology. Philadelphia, WB Saunders, 1991, pp 1820–1828.
37. Adamson ED, Meek J: The ontogeny of epidermal growth factor receptors during mouse development. Dev Biol 103:62, 1984.
38. Goldin GV, Opperman LA: Induction of supernumerary tracheal buds and the stimulation of DNA synthesis in the embryonic chick lung and trachea by epidermal growth factor. J Embryol Exp Morphol 60:235, 1980.
39. Miettinen PJ, et al: Epithelial immaturity and multi-organ failure in mice lacking EGF receptor. Nature 376:337, 1985.
40. Lee DC, et al: Cloning and sequence analysis of a cDNA for rat transforming growth factor-alpha. Nature 313:489, 1985.
41. Rappolee DA, et al: Developmental expression of PDGF, TGF-alpha, and TGF-beta genes in preimplantation mouse embryos. Science 241:1823, 1988.
42. Han VK, et al: Expression of rat transforming growth factor alpha mRNA during development occurs predominantly in the maternal decidua. Mol Cell Biol 7:2335, 1987.
43. Ross R, et al: The biology of platelet-derived growth factor. Cell 46:155, 1986.
44. Östlund E, et al: Transforming growth factor-β1 in fetal serum correlates with insulin-like growth factor-I and fetal growth. Obstet Gynecol 100:567, 2002.
45. Attisano L, Wrana JL: Signal transduction by TGF-β superfamily. Science 296:1646, 2002.
46. Hahnel A, Schultz GA: Insulin-like growth factor binding proteins are transcribed by preimplantation mouse embryos. Endocrinology 134:1956, 1994.
47. Adamson ED: Activities of growth factors in preimplantation embryos. J Cell Biochem 53:280, 1993.
48. Kaye PI, et al: Insulin and the insulin-like growth factors in preimplantation development. Reprod Fertil Dev 4:373, 1992.
49. D'Ercole AJ: The insulin-like growth factors and in utero growth. Growth Genet Horm 8:1, 1992.
50. Rappolee DA, et al: IGF-II acts through an endogenous pathway regulated by imprinting in early mouse embryos. Genes Dev 6:939, 1992.
51. Smith RM, et al: Mouse preimplantation embryos exhibit receptor-mediated binding and transcytosis of maternal IGF-I. Biol Reprod 49:1, 1993.
52. Palmiter RD, et al: Dramatic growth of mice that develop from eggs microinjected with metallothionein–growth hormone fusion genes. Nature 300:611, 1982.
53. Palmiter RD, et al: Metallothionein–human GH fusion genes stimulate growth of mice. Science 222:809, 1983.
54. Matthews LS, et al: Expression of IGF-I in transgenic mice with elevated levels of growth hormone is correlated with growth. Endocrinology 123:433, 1988.
55. Camacho-Hubner C, et al: Regulation of insulin-like growth factor binding proteins in transgenic mice with altered expression of growth hormone and IGF-I. Endocrinology 129:1201, 1991.
56. Wolf E, et al: Consequences of postnatally elevated insulin-like growth factor-II in transgenic mice: endocrine changes and effects on body and organ growth. Endocrinology 135:1877, 1994.
57. Behringer RR, et al: Dwarf mice produced by genetic ablation of growth hormone expressing cells. Genes Dev 2:453, 1988.
58. Behringer R, et al: Expression of IGF-I stimulates normal somatic growth in growth hormone transgenic mice. Endocrinology 127:1033, 1990.
59. Murphy LJ, et al: Hormonal regulation of insulin-like growth factor binding protein-1 expression and the development of transgenic mouse models to study IGFBP-1 function. Adv Exp Med Biol 343:279, 1993.
60. Dai Z, et al: Human insulin-like growth factor-binding protein-1 (hIGFBP-1) in transgenic mice: characterization and insights into the regulation of IGFBP-1 expression. Endocrinology 135:1316, 1994.
61. D'Ercole AJ, et al: Brain growth retardation due to expression of human insulin-like growth factor binding protein-1 in transgenic mice: an in vivo model for the analysis of IGF function in the brain. Brain Res Dev Brain Res 82:213, 1994.
62. Hoeflich A, et al: Overexpression of insulin-like growth factor-binding protein-2 in transgenic mice reduces postnatal body weight gain. Endocrinology 140:5488, 1999.
63. Murphy LJ, et al: Expression of human insulin-like growth factor–binding protein-3 in transgenic mice. J Mol Endocrinol 15:293, 1995.
64. Neuenschwander S, et al: Involution of the lactating mammary gland is inhibited by the IGF system in a transgenic mouse model. J Clin Invest 97:2225, 1996.
65. Wang J, et al: Overexpression of insulin-like growth factor-binding protein-4 (IGFBP-4) in smooth muscle cells of transgenic mice through a smooth muscle α-actin-IGFBP-4 fusion gene induces smooth muscle hypoplasia. Endocrinology 139:2605, 1998.
66. Baker J, et al: Role of insulin-like growth factors in embryonic and postnatal growth. Cell 75:73, 1993.
67. DiChiara T, et al: A growth deficiency phenotype in heterozygous mice carrying an insulin-like growth factor II gene disrupted by targeting. Nature 345:78, 1990.
68. DiChiara T, et al: Parental imprinting of the mouse insulin-like growth factor-II gene. Cell 64:849, 1991.
69. Powell-Braxton L, et al: IGF-I is required for normal embryonic development in mice. Genes Dev 7:2609, 1993.
70. Liu JP, et al: Mice carrying null mutations of the genes encoding insulin-like growth factor I (IGF-I) and type I IGF receptor. Cell 75:59, 1993.
71. Beck KD, et al: IGF-I gene disruption results in reduced brain size, CNS hypomyelination, and loss of hippocampal granule and striatal parvalbumin-containing neurons. Neuron 14:717, 1995.
72. Lupu F, et al: Roles of growth hormone and insulin-like growth factor I in mouse postnatal growth. Dev Biol 229:141, 2001.
73. Woods KA, et al: Intrauterine growth retardation and postnatal growth failure associated with deletion of the insulin-like growth factor I gene. N Engl J Med 335:1363, 1996.
74. Yakar S, et al: Normal growth and development in the absence of hepatic insulin-like growth factor I. Proc Natl Acad Sci U S A 96:7324, 1999.
75. Ueki I, et al: Inactivation of the acid-labile subunit gene in mice results in mild retardation of postnatal growth despite profound disruptions in the circulating insulin-like growth factor system. Proc Natl Acad Sci U S A 97:6868, 2000.
76. Yakar S, et al: Circulating levels of IGF-I directly regulate bone growth and density. J Clin Invest 110:771, 2002.
77. Wang ZQ, et al: Regulation of embyonic growth and lysosomal targeting by the imprinted IGF-2/MPR gene. Nature 372:464, 1994.
78. Haig D, Graham C: Genomic imprinting and the strange case of the insulin-like growth factor-II receptor. Cell 64:1045, 1991.
79. Ludwig T, et al: Mouse mutants lacking the type 2 IGF receptor (IGF2R) are rescued from perinatal lethality in IGF2 and IGF1r null backgrounds. Dev Biol 177:517, 1996.
80. Louvi A, et al: Growth-promoting interaction of IGF-II with the insulin receptor during mouse embryonic development. Dev Biol 189:33, 1997.
81. Duvillie B, et al: Phenotype alterations in insulin-deficient mutant mice. Proc Natl Acad Sci U S A 94:5137, 1997.
82. Hone J, et al: Homozygosity for a null allele of the insulin receptor gene in a patient with lepreuchanism. Hum Mutat 6:17, 1995.

83. Tyrala EE: The infant of the diabetic mother. Obstet Gynecol Clin North Am 23:221, 1996.

84. DeBaun MR, et al: Hypoglycemia in Beckwith-Wiedemann syndrome. Semin Perinatol 24:164, 2000.

85. Reinecke-Luthge A, et al: The molecular basis of persistent hyperinsulinemic hypoglycemia of infancy and its pathologic substrates. Virchows Arch 436:1, 2000.

86. Pintar JE, et al: Genetic approaches to the function of insulin-like growth factor-binding proteins during rodent development. Horm Res 45:172, 1996.

87. Pintar J, et al: Genetic disruption of IGF binding proteins. In Takano K, et al (eds): Molecular Mechanism to Regulate the Activities of Insulin-like Growth Factors. Amsterdam, Elsevier Science, 1998, pp 65–70.

88. Schneider MR, et al: Transgenic mouse models for studying the functions of insulin-like growth factor-binding proteins. FASEB J 14:629, 2000.

89. Tamemoto H, et al: Insulin resistance and growth retardation in mice lacking insulin receptor substrate-1. Nature 372:182, 1994.

90. Araki E, et al: Alternative pathway of insulin signalling in mice with targeted disruption of the IRS-1 gene. Nature 372:186, 1994.

91. Cho H, et al: AKT1/PKBα is required for normal growth but dispensable for maintenance of glucose homeostasis in mice. J Biol Chem 276:38349, 2001.

92. Cho H, et al: Insulin resistance and diabetes mellitus–like syndrome in mice lacking the protein kinase AKT2 (PKB beta). Science 292:1728, 2001.

93. Gargosky S, et al: Circulating levels of IGFs increase and molecular forms of their serum binding protein change with human pregnancy. Biochem Biophys Res Commun 170:1157, 1990.

94. Hall K, et al: Serum levels of somatomedins and somatomedin-binding proteins in pregnant women with type I or gestational diabetes and their infants. J Clin Endocrinol Metab 63:1300, 1986.

95. Scippo ML, et al: Syncytiotrophoblast localization of the human growth hormone variant mRNA in the placenta. Mol Cell Endocrinol 92:R7, 1993.

96. Caufriez A, et al: Regulation of maternal IGF-I by placental GH in normal and abnormal human pregnancies. Am J Physiol 265:E572, 1993.

97. Handwerger S: The physiology of placental lactogen in human pregnancy. Endocrinol Rev 12:329, 1991.

98. Drop SLS: Correlation between fetal IGFBP-1 levels and birthweight. Int Growth Monitor 4:26, 1994.

99. Holly J, et al: Proteases acting on IGFBPs; their occurrence and physiologic significance. Growth Regul 3:88, 1993.

100. Hossenlopp P, et al: Evidence of enzymatic degradation of IGFBPs in the 150kD complex during pregnancy. J Clin Endocrinol Metab 71:797, 1990.

101. Claussen M, et al: Proteolysis of insulin-like growth factor binding protein-5 by pregnancy serum and amniotic fluid. Endocrinology 4:1964, 1994.

102. Deal C, Guyda HJ: Regulation of fetal growth and the GH-IGF axis: lessons from mouse to man. Int Growth Monitor 4:1, 1995.

103. Blat C, et al: In vivo proteolysis of serum IGFBP-3 results in increased availability of IGF to target cells. J Clin Invest 93:2286, 1994.

104. Brice AL, et al: Temporal changes in the expression of the insulin-like growth factor II gene associated with tissue maturation in the human fetus. Development 106:532, 1989.

105. Ohlsson R, et al: IGF-II and short range stimulatory loops in control of human placental growth. EMBO J 9:1993, 1989.

106. Ohlsson R, et al: Blastocyst implantation precedes induction of insulin-like growth factor-II gene expression in human trophoblasts. Development 106:555, 1989.

107. Han VKM, et al: Cellular localization of IGF messenger RNA in the human fetus. Science 236:193, 1987.

108. Funk B, et al: Expression of the IGF-II, M6P receptor in multiple human tissues during fetal life and early infancy. J Clin Endocrinol Metab 75:424, 1992.

109. Hill DH, Clemmons J: Similar distribution of IGFBPs 1,2,3 in human fetal tissues. Growth Factors 6:315, 1992.

110. Delhanty PJD, et al: IGFBP 4,5,6 mRNA in the human fetus; localization to sites of growth and differentiation. Growth Regul 3:8, 1993.

111. Lassarre C, et al: IGFs and their binding proteins in human fetal serum; relationships with growth in normal subjects and in subjects with IUGR. Pediatr Res 29:219, 1991.

112. Gluckman PD, et al: Studies of insulin-like growth factor I and II by specific radio ligand assays in umbilical cord blood. Clin Endocrinol (Oxf) 19:405, 1983.

113. Bennett A, et al: Levels of insulin-like growth factors I and II in human cord blood. J Clin Endocrinol Metab 57:609, 1983.

114. Verhaege J, et al: C-peptide, the insulin-like growth factors I and II and IGF binding protein 1 in umbilical cord serum: correlations with birthweight. Am J Obstet Gynecol 169:89, 1993.

115. Wit JM, van Unen H: Growth of infants with neonatal growth hormone deficiency. Arch Dis Child 67:920, 1992.

116. Gluckman PD, et al: Congenital idiopathic GH deficiency associated with prenatal and postnatal growth failure. J Pediatr 121:920, 1992.

117. Savage MO, et al: Clinical features and endocrine status in patients with GH insensitivity (Laron syndrome). J Clin Endocrinol Metab 77:1465, 1993.

118. Guidice LC, et al: Insulin-like growth factors and their binding proteins in the term and preterm human fetus and neonate with normal and extremes of intrauterine growth. J Clin Endocrinol Metab 80:1548, 1995.

119. Martin JA, et al: Births: final data for 2000. Natl Vital Stat Rep 50:1, 2002.

120. Mirlesse V, et al: Placental GH levels in normal pregnancy and in pregnancies with intrauterine growth retardation. Pediatr Res 34:439, 1993.

121. Kajantie E, et al: Markers of type I and type III collagen turnover, insulin-like growth factors and their binding proteins in cord plasma of small premature infants: relationships with fetal growth, gestational age, preeclampsia, and antenatal glucocorticoid treatment. Pediatr Res 49:481, 2001.

122. Verhaeghe J, et al: C-peptide, insulin-like growth factors I and II, and insulin-like growth factor binding protein-1 in umbilical cord serum: correlations with birth weight. Am J Obstet Gynecol 169:89, 1993.

123. Wang HS, et al: The concentration of insulin-like growth factor I in human umbilical cord serum at delivery: relation to fetal weight. J Endocrinol 129:459, 1991.

124. Ducos B, et al: IGF type I receptor ligand binding characteristics are altered in a subgroup of children with intrauterine growth retardation. J Clin Endocrinol Metab 86:5516, 2001.

125. Lajara R, et al: Low prevalence of insulin-like growth factor-I gene mutations in human growth disorders. J Clin Endocrinol Metab 70:687, 1990.

126. Mullis PE, et al: Constitutionally short stature: analysis of the insulin-like growth factor-I gene and the human growth hormone gene cluster. Pediatr Res 29:412, 1991.

127. Arends N, et al: Polymorphism in the IGF-I gene: clinical relevance for short children born small for gestational age (SGA). J Clin Endocrinol Metab 87:2720, 2002.

128. Ong KL, et al: Association between postnatal catch-up growth and obesity in childhood: prospective cohort study. BMJ 320:967, 2000.

129. Albertsson-Wikland K, Karlberg J: Postnatal growth of children born small for gestational age. Acta Paediatr (Suppl) 423:193, 1997.

130. McCowan L, et al: Perinatal predictors of growth at six months in small for gestational age babies. Early Hum Dev 56:205, 1999.

131. Leger J, et al: Prediction factors in the determination of final height in subjects born small for gestational age. Pediatr Res 43:808, 1998.

132. Barker DJ: Fetal origins of cardiovascular disease. Ann Med 31 (Suppl)1:3, 1999.

133. Kajantie E, et al: IGF-I, IGF binding protein (IGFBP)-3, phosphoisoforms of IGFBP-1, and postnatal growth in very low birth weight infants. J Clin Endocrinol Metab 87:2171, 2002.

134. Lithell HO, et al: Relation of size at birth to non-insulin dependent diabetes and insulin concentrations in men aged 50–60 years. BMJ 312:406, 1996.

135. Hattersley AT, Tooke JE: The fetal insulin hypothesis: an alternative explanation of the association of low birthweight with diabetes and vascular disease. Lancet 353:1789, 1999.

136. Barker DJP, et al: Type 2 (non-insulin-dependent) diabetes mellitus, hypertension, and hyperlipidemia (syndrome X): relation to reduced fetal growth. Diabetology 36:62, 1993.

137. de Zegher F, et al: High-dose growth hormone treatment of short children born small for gestational age. J Clin Endocrinol Metab 81:1887, 1996.

138. Sas T, et al: Body composition, blood pressure, and lipid metabolism before and during long-term growth hormone (GH) treatment in children with short stature born small for gestational age either with or without GH deficiency. J Clin Endocrinol Metab 85:3786, 2000.

139. Leger J, et al: Human growth hormone treatment of short-stature children born small for gestational age: effect on muscle and adipose tissue mass during a 3-year treatment period and after 1 year's withdrawal. J Clin Endocrinol Metab 83:3512, 1998.

140. Coutant R, et al: Short stature associated with intrauterine growth retardation: final height of untreated and growth-hormone treated children. J Clin Endocrinol Metab 83:1070, 1998.

141. Zucchini S, et al: Final height of short subjects of low birth weight with and without growth hormone treatment. Arch Dis Child 84:340, 2001.

142. Ranke MB, Lindberg A: Growth hormone treatment of short children born small for gestational age or with Silver-Russell syndrome: results from KIGS (Kabi International Growth Study), including the first report on final height. Acta Paediatr (Suppl) 417:18, 1996.

143. Gluckman PD: The endocrine regulation of fetal growth in late gestation: the role of insulin-like growth factors. J Clin Endocrinol Metab 80:1047, 1995.

144. Takayama M, et al: Abnormally large placenta associated with Beckwith-Wiedemann syndrome. Gynecol Obstet Invest 22:165, 1986.

145. Weksberg R, et al: IGF-II serum levels are normal in patients with Beckwith-Wiedemann syndrome. Am J Hum Genet (Suppl), Abstract 323, 1990.

146. Leisenring WM, et al: Increased birthweight of national Wilms' tumor study patients suggests growth factor excess. Cancer Res 5423:4680, 1994.

Growth Hormone and Prolactin

This chapter examines the roles of the diverse and varied functions of growth hormone (GH) and prolactin (PRL) in fetal development and the perinatal period. These are evolutionarily related hormones of the lactogenic superfamily, and, while their concentrations are high in fetal life, the functional significance of these high concentrations is unclear. The placenta is also a rich source of lactogenic hormones secreted into the maternal circulation, where they play an important role in maternal metabolic adaptations and in preparation of the mammary gland. A thorough discussion of GH or PRL could easily extend beyond the scope of this chapter. We will instead focus on recent advances in the GH-PRL field, with emphasis on their roles during fetal development and the perinatal period.

THE DEVELOPMENT OF HYPOTHALAMOPITUITARY CONTROL

The differentiation of adenohypophyseal cell lineages within Rathke's pouch is dependent on a series of transcriptional factors that generate spatial and temporal patterns of gene expression (for review, see reference 1). Gene deletions or mutations of some of these signaling molecules (i.e., Pit-1, Six6, and Pax6) have been shown to result in pituitary abnormalities or altered numbers of pituitary cell types. Pit-1, in particular, is required for the development of somatotrophs, lactotrophs, and thyrotrophs.[1] Dominant and recessive mutations in Pit-1 lead to absent or diminished GH, PRL, and thyroid-stimulating hormone (TSH) secretion. Pit-1 regulates the respective transcription of GH, PRL, and TSH, acting as a gene activator or repressor, depending on which cell type these genes are expressed in. Pit-1 interacts with cell type–specific transcriptional co-regulators, and this interaction may be determined by slight structural changes in their otherwise highly homologous 5′ flanking regions. A 2-bp sequence variation in the Pit-1 binding site of the GH promoter can induce a conformational change in the DNA structure that may be critical to the transcriptional machinery distinguishing between the GH and PRL regulatory regions. Thus, several mechanisms are in place to ensure specificity of pituitary cell-type transcriptional control.

In mice, differentiation of the thyrotrope occurs around embryonic day 12.5 (E12.5),[1] making TSH one of the first pituitary gene products observed. Somatotrophs and lactotrophs develop last (in mice, approximately E16), and can comprise up to half of the pituitary cell-type population.[1,2] In sheep, in which brain development is largely completed before birth, both somatotrophs and lactotrophs can be identified by 60 days' post-conception (PC; term is 146 days).[3] In humans, GH is first detectable in the fetal pituitary by immunocytochemistry at 8 weeks PC. PRL-secreting cells can be detected by 12 weeks PC, but their number is low until after 26 weeks PC, when there is a considerable hyperplasia of lactotrophs.[4]

Some pituitary tumors secrete both GH and PRL from a single cell, and it has been suggested that there may be a common bihormonal-secreting precursor. In studies of primary pituitary cultures derived from neonatal rats[5] and cultured human fetal pituitary cells,[6] one third of the GH- or PRL-synthesizing cells secrete both GH and PRL simultaneously. As PRL secretion inevitably commences at a later stage of development than GH secretion, it has been suggested that lactotrophs may be derived from this putative somatomammotroph.[6] More recently, it has been shown that an immortalized cell line—GHFT[7]—has properties of somatomammotrophs and is able to differentiate to PRL-secreting lactotrophs after treatment with FGF-2.[8]

The development of the hypothalamic–pituitary adenohypophyseal circulation has been reviewed elsewhere.[9] The portal circulation matures early in development and is not a rate-limiting step in the development of functional control of adenohypophyseal secretion in fetal life. Instead, the development of neuroregulatory control over hypothalamic release and inhibitory factors, as well as the development of hormone receptors, makes way for negative feedback loops to appear. Additionally, the unique milieu of the fetus exposes it to placental neuromodulators, such as prostanoids and estrogen, which play a part in the changing pattern of circulating fetal and perinatal hormone concentrations.

The mechanisms for GH release and inhibition develop progressively from early gestation. Somatostatin (SS), which is inhibitory to GH release, is detectable in the human fetal hypothalamus by 11 weeks PC,[10,11] and SS-staining neurons terminate in the median eminence by 16 weeks.[12] Growth hormone-releasing hormone (GHRH)-staining neurons are detected in the median eminence by 18 weeks.[13] Less is known of the development of the other hypothalamic GH-releasing factor, ghrelin, which will be discussed later. The dominant stimulator of PRL release is the tripeptide, thyrotropin-releasing factor (TRF). However, in contrast to GH release, which is low in the absence of hypothalamic influences, PRL release is under tonic inhibition by dopamine (DA) of hypothalamic origin.[14] DA is present in the human fetal hypothalamus by 10 weeks' gestation, at concentrations higher than those observed in the adult hypothalamus.[15,16] Dopaminergic regulation of PRL release can be demonstrated in the fetal sheep by the beginning of the third trimester. Additionally, DA inhibition may derive from non-neuronal sources.[14,17,18]

GROWTH HORMONE

Growth hormone (GH) promotes postnatal somatic growth by stimulating paracrine and endocrine production of IGF-1 and also has IGF-1 independent effects on metabolism. The pulsatile release of pituitary GH is primarily due to the opposing influences of hypothalamic GHRH and SS. Circulating GH and IGF-1, in turn, can influence their own expression by negative feedback mechanisms to the hypothalamus and pituitary.

Growth hormone is detectable in human fetal plasma by at least 10 weeks PC.[19] In species with long gestations, such as the human and sheep, high levels of GH relative to postnatal concentrations are established by midgestation. The pattern of secretion can be shown to be pulsatile *in utero* with both elevated peaks and nadirs, and sexually dimorphic.[20] Concentrations fall gradually in late gestation and precipitously within hours of birth.[20] This pattern appears to be due to early maturation of responsivity of the fetal somatotroph to GHRH, plus later development of inhibitory control accelerated by endocrine and metabolic events surrounding birth. The release of SS and GHRH is under control of a variety of neuromodulators and neurotransmitters. These include dopamine, which is inhibitory[21]; opiates[22]; serotonin[23]; γ-aminobutyric acid (GABA)[24]; and β-adrenergic stimuli.[25] The development of these neuro-transmitter controls appears progressively during the late phase of pregnancy.[20] Immaturity of inhibitory control by SS and IGF-1[9,26] contribute to the high concentration of GH observed in the fetus. Both SS and GHRH influence the sheep fetal pituitary from at least 75 days PC,[27,28] though the data suggest that *in vitro* and *in vivo*, SS is less effective in inhibiting GH secretion prenatally than it is postnatally.[29,30] IGF-I levels are low in the fetal circulation because of the relative immaturity of GH receptors (GHR), thus failing to induce the negative feedback loop that would prevent GH hypersecretion.[31] Hence, the fetal pituitary is "gated" to remain in a hypersecretory state.

Ghrelin, an endogenous ligand for the GH secretagogue receptor, has potent GH-secreting properties.[32] Ghrelin is primarily produced in the stomach but is also detected in the pituitary, hypothalamus, and placenta.[32] Several reports have indicated a role for ghrelin in pregnancy and fetal development. Ghrelin levels are higher in women with pregnancy-induced hypertension than in normotensive pregnant women,[33] which is supported by observations of ghrelin-binding studies in heart and blood vessels.[34] Ghrelin levels are high in the neonate, in whom it may have a role in the initiation of feeding and protect against neonatal hypoglycemia.[35] Ghrelin also has been detected in fetal and infant lung, where its expression peaks in the first 18 weeks of gestation and decreases thereafter.[36] The role of ghrelin in controlling fetal GH secretion, however, is unknown.

In the sheep, the mechanism of the rapid decline in GH secretion at birth has been studied in detail. Free fatty acid infusions inhibit GH secretion almost totally by a direct action on the somatotroph.[26] Free fatty acid concentrations are low until birth, when they rise rapidly within a few minutes owing to the onset of nonshivering thermogenesis (NST). In a series of experiments in which the individual events of birth have been mimicked without delivering the fetus, it has been possible to show that the initiation of NST is dependent on oxygenation of the fetus and removal of a presumed placental inhibitor.[37,38] Data in other species are limited, but in the human term infant, thermogenesis is initiated soon after birth[39] and increases more slowly in the premature infant, offering one explanation for the slower GH decline in preterm infants.[40]

The functional significance of elevated GH concentrations in the fetus remains uncertain—the phenotype of the child with isolated GH deficiency is rather unremarkable: generally restricted to hypoglycemia, micropenis, and perhaps a small reduction in birth length. Indeed, it had generally been considered that GH had no significant role in promoting fetal skeletal growth. However, recent clinical studies show a small effect of GH in late gestation on linear growth.[41] In turn, these small effects on linear growth have been attributed to the late appearance of the GH receptor (GHR) in musculoskeletal tissues.

The physiology of the GHR has been reviewed elsewhere.[42-44] Data suggest that the concentration of GHR in hepatic tissue is low until after birth, as determined in sheep,[45,46] bovine,[47,48] pig,[49] and rat,[50] and GHR appears to be induced by the peripartum glucocorticoid surge.[51] If extrapolated to the human, it would suggest that GH-dependent growth first appears after the 34th week of pregnancy.

In sheep, GHR mRNA can be detected as early as embryonic day 51, albeit at levels 30% of what can be detected postnatally.[52] Pantaleon and colleagues[53] have reported that transcripts encoding GH, GHR, and GH-binding protein (GHBP) have been detected in mouse preimplantation embryos from E1 to 4, fol-

lowed by detection of GH protein at the 2-cell stage. GHR is presumed to be functional at this stage in that exogenous GH administration to blastocysts promotes glucose transport and glycogen breakdown and increases protein synthesis.[53] Waters and Kaye[54] suggest that the increased glucose transport and glycogen breakdown promote the formation of ATP that fuels the Na+ pumps and ionic gradients required for blastocoele formation and resulting cell proliferation. There are also reports of immunoreactive GHR in the human fetus from the second trimester.[55,56] Whether GHR is fully functional at these early developmental stages remains to be determined. GHR can be alternatively spliced to give rise to transcript variants, though not much is known about their function.[52] One variant, in particular, has been observed only in the human placenta and is an individual-specific polymorphism that leads to deletion of exon 3.[57,58]

GH may play a role in fetal metabolism. The hypophysectomized fetal lamb retains excess adiposity, and this is reversed by the administration of GH.[59] Similarly, GH has been shown in the fetal lamb to affect glucose/insulin metabolism[60] in a manner analogous to its postnatal diabetogenic action. In the rabbit, GH has been suggested as a stimulator of fetal hepatic glycogen synthesis.[61,62] This may be the basis of the hypoglycemia seen in human neonates with isolated GH deficiency.[63,64]

PROLACTIN

PRL is synthesized by lactotrophs in the pituitary, but it may also be produced in other tissues (i.e., mammary gland, ovary, decidua, pancreas, kidney, osteoblasts, lymphocytes, and so on) where it is synthesized locally (for review, see references 18, 65, and 66). In the mother, PRL is best understood for its role in milk secretion, but more recently it has been associated with the development of maternal behavior.[18] In the fetus, PRL has been associated with lung maturation and may have osmoregulatory properties.[18] The PRL gene is present as a single copy on human chromosome 6.[18] Several transcriptional and translational modifications of PRL have been described that may contribute to its ability to mediate diverse functions.

PRL is detected in both the maternal and fetal circulation. In the first trimester of human pregnancy, maternal PRL levels begin to rise in response to increasing estrogen and by term reach a level ten times that of a nonpregnant woman.[67] As PRL does not cross the placenta, the fetus produces its own PRL from early on in gestation.[68,69] PRL is first detected by 12 weeks PC[70-72] when levels are low; after 26 weeks PC, they rise sharply. PRL in cord blood is markedly elevated at 170 ng/mL compared with less than 20 ng/mL in adults. There is a positive correlation between cord blood PRL levels and gestational age.[73,74] PRL levels decline by more than 60% in the first week following birth,[75] and this decline is delayed in premature infants.[76]

A similar pattern is observed in experimental animals. In sheep, PRL levels rise by 135 days' gestation (term = 146 d) and decline after birth.[77,78] Data are similar for the rhesus.[79] However, in most altricial species such as the rat, plasma PRL is low at birth and levels do not rise until 15 days after birth and peak prior to puberty.[80,81]

Estrogen is the primary contributor to the prenatal rise in PRL levels. Estrogen acts directly on the pituitary to promote the synthesis and release of PRL.[18] It increases the number of TRH-binding sites on the lactotroph and reduces DA secretion and antagonism of DA action.[82-85] A temporal correlation between the rise in PRL and estrogen levels late in gestation shows a lag in the rise in PRL compared with estrogen in both humans[6] and sheep. Further, at least in sheep, the interanimal variation in PRL concentrations and the seasonal and diurnal variations are difficult to reconcile, with a dominant role for estrogen in short-term regulation of fetal PRL secretion. It seems likely that estrogen exerts a long-term tonic influence on the maturation of the lactotroph and synthesis of PRL, rather than having short- or inter-mediate-term regulatory effects. It may be that chronic exposure to estrogen is the mechanism by which the pituitary in the second half of gestation switches from secreting virtually no PRL to maintaining a significant and progressive hyperprolactinemia.

PRL levels are also influenced by seasonal patterns.[18] They fluctuate in fetal sheep according to the length of the photope-riod, with higher concentrations secreted in longer, rather than shorter, photoperiods. It has been determined that maternal melatonin during the dark phase plays a key role in relaying this information to the sheep fetus.

PRL exerts its biologic activity by binding to the PRL receptor (PRLR), which like GHR, is a member of the cytokine receptor superfamily.[65] PRLR protein can be detected in the human fetus as early as 7.5 weeks' gestation, and like PRL, it is distributed in nearly all tissues.[86] Structurally, the receptor transverses the cell membrane, once with a single, short transmembrane domain, and extracellular and intracellular domains that are conserved across the cytokine receptor superfamily.[65] A single gene encodes hPRLR, which is localized to chromosome 5 in close proximity to the GHR gene.[65] Human GH and PL (to be described) also bind to the hPRLR with high affinity,[87] in contrast to many other species. The PRLR is alternatively spliced to generate several short (s) and one long (l) variant, differing by length and sequence in their cytoplasmic tail.[65] In general, binding to PRLR causes activation of the JAK/STAT cell-signaling pathways and STAT-1 and -5 are directly activated by PRL.[65] The l-PRL receptor transmits a com-plete intracellular signal, whereas the s-PRL receptor may be a clearance form.[65] It is interesting that s-PRLR may act in a domi-nant negative fashion over PRLR dimerization by forming inactive s- and l-PRL heterodimers.[88] The administration of cortisol to the fetal sheep stimulates the expression of l- and s-PRLR.[89] The mechanism of cortisol action on the PRLR is unclear at this time, as glucocorticoid response elements have not been identified in the PRLR gene promoter.[90]

It has been suggested that PRL plays a role in the development of brown fat. In placentally restricted sheep, the l-PRL receptor is reduced in fetal adipose tissue,[91] which may have an impact on NST after birth, whereas enhanced maternal nutrition results in increased levels of l-PRL receptor in adipose tissue, as well as an increase in uncoupling protein-1 (UCP-1), a protein involved in thermoregulation.[92]

Lower levels of fetal/neonatal PRL correlate with increased risk of respiratory distress syndrome, and PRL may play a role in enhancing fetal lung maturation.[73,74,93] Lactogenic receptors are present in the fetal lung,[94] though a group has reported an inabil-ity of labeled hPRL to bind human lung preparations.[95] Infusion of PRL alone to the fetal rabbit or lamb did not appear to alter surfactant production.[96] However, PRL is synergistic with corti-sol and thyroid hormones in promoting lung maturation in the sheep *in vivo*,[97] and this is supported by *in vitro* data.[98]

PRL has long been recognized as an osmoregulatory hormone in teleost fish and amphibia.[18] Fetal PRL secretion is dramatically affected by changes in the osmolality of fetal cerebrospinal fluid,[99] and it has been suggested that the perinatal changes in PRL secretion relate to changes in sodium homeostasis.[100] Manipulation of PRL levels in the newborn rabbit suggests that PRL enhances water retention, and that the loss of total body water in the first few days after birth could be due to the decline in plasma PRL concentrations.[101] Decidual PRL has been sug-gested to play a role in the regulation of amniotic fluid volume and osmolarity,[102] and it can be demonstrated to alter the per-meability of the human fetal membranes to water.[103,104]

It has also been suggested that in the rodent, PRL may regulate somatic growth in the early neonate,[105,106] but no comparable data exist in larger mammals. The earlier speculation that PRL may be adrenocorticotropic *in utero*[74] has not been confirmed in more direct observations.[107,108]

PLACENTAL LACTOGENIC HORMONES

The placentas of all species secrete multiple members of the lac-togenic family, suggesting an important role in maintaining preg-nancy. However, this role is poorly understood. In humans, members of this family include a variant form of GH and an evo-lutionarily and structurally related class of hormones, the pla-cental lactogens (PLs). In humans, the genes encoding pituitary GH (GH-N), placental GH (GH-V), PL-A, PL-B, and PL-*like* (PL-L) are clustered on the same chromosome, 17q22–24. PL-A and PL-B have slightly divergent cDNA sequences, but after process-ing of their respective prehormones, they give rise to an iden-tical PL hormone product. PL-L has been suggested as a pseudogene, but transcripts from all three PL genes can be detected at varying abundance in the placenta.[109] There are, however, many species differences on the evolution of placental growth hormone and PLs. For instance, PRL mRNA is reported to be present in the baboon placenta, but in women, the decidua appears to be the major source of extrapituitary PRL production, followed by its release into amniotic fluid.[110]

PL is detected in both the maternal and fetal circulation, but its role within the fetus is largely unknown.[109] In humans, PL is first detected in the maternal circulation beginning at 6 weeks' ges-tation where its levels progressively rise to a concentration range of 200 to 300 nM at term. In a species-specific fashion, PL is func-tionally similar to PRL or GH: in sheep, PL is primarily soma-totropic; in humans, it is primarily lactogenic. PL stimulates mammogenesis and promotes maternal insulin resistance and, thus, maternal lipolysis, to ensure adequate reserves of glucose and free fatty acids for the fetus.[109] PL may also enhance mater-nal appetite.[111] In sheep, PL levels rise in response to maternal starvation, leading some to suggest that it stimulates repartition-ing of maternal nutrients to the fetus, as well as stimulates the fetus to use its own substrates.[112-114] In the fetus, PL may indi-rectly promote growth by stimulating amino acid uptake, DNA synthesis, and IGF-1 production.[109]

While hPL is functionally more like hPRL, its sequence is similar to that of hGH. In humans and primates, the PL and GH gene families are clustered on the same respective chromosome. Human PL has more sequence identity to hGH-N (85%) than to hPRL (17%).[109] In contrast, PL in rodents and ruminants is most similar to PRL. Analogous to humans, the mouse and ovine (o) PL genes are contiguous with their PRL counterpart and share more sequence similarity with the PRL coding region than with GH (oPL vs. oPRL: 48% homology; oPL vs. oGH: 27% homology).[115,116] Mice also have two variants of PL: mPL-1 and mPL-2, that can sub-stitute for pituitary PRL secretion during pregnancy. mPL-1 is first detected after implantation, when pituitary PRL expression ceases, where it assumes maintenance of the corpus luteum. By midgestation, mPL-1 expression declines and is replaced by mPL-2 for the remainder of pregnancy.[117,118] This redundancy of func-tion bares some resemblance to the onset of hGH-V, another unique placental hormone that will be discussed later.

The search for a specific PL receptor has uncovered another example of redundancy of function within the GH-PL-PRL family. There is no definitive evidence for a distinct PL receptor. Instead, PL is capable of binding to either homo- or heterodimers of GH and PRL receptors. In sheep, oPL binds the GH receptor with higher affinity than oGH.[45,119,120] It has been shown in mice that mPL-1 and -2 exert their biologic activity by binding to PRL receptors (PRLR),[121-123] whereas in sheep, oGH and oPL may bind a common receptor that is either composed of a monomeric GH receptor (GHR) or a heterodimer of GHR and PRLR.[119,124] It is unknown whether an analogous heterodimer of GHR and PRLR occurs in humans.

A second gene for GH encodes a variant form found only in the placenta. Placental GH (GH-V) is synthesized by syncytiotro-phoblasts beginning at around 24 weeks PC, and gradually replaces GH expression from the pituitary (for review, see references 125 and 126). GH-V is synthesized by the placenta until term and is secreted in a continuous fashion, unlike pulsatile pituitary GH secretion. However, it would appear that unlike PL, secretion of GH-V is solely into the maternal circulation.[125,126] GH-V is not subject to regulation by GHRH but is suppressed by elevated maternal glucose.[125,126] GH-V exerts its biologic activity by binding primarily to the GH receptor, as it does not have the Zn^+ binding site required for interaction with the PRL receptor.[127] A clear definitive role for GH-V has not been determined, but in pregnancies complicated by intrauterine growth retardation, GH-V levels are decreased.[125,126] GH-V may have a part in inducing insulin resistance in the mother to ensure adequate glucose reserves for the fetus, thereby contributing indirectly to fetal growth.[125,126]

REFERENCES

1. Scully KM, Rosenfeld MG: Pituitary development: regulatory codes in mammalian organogenesis. Science 295:2231, 2002.
2. Hadley ME: Pituitary hormones. In Hadley ME (ed): Endocrinology. Englewood Cliffs, NJ, Prentice-Hall, 1994, pp 85–111.
3. Webb PD: The pars distalis (anterior pituitary) in the fetal sheep: an ultrastructural study. J Dev Physiol 3:319, 1981.
4. Asa SL, et al: Human fetal adenohypophysis: histologic and immunocytochemical analysis. Neuroendocrinology 43:308, 1986.
5. Hoeffler JP, et al: Ontogeny of prolactin cells in neonatal rats: initial prolactin secretors also release growth hormone. Endocrinology 117:187, 1985.
6. Mulchahey JJ, et al: Hormone production and peptide regulation of the human fetal pituitary gland. Endocrine Rev 8:406, 1987.
7. Lew D, et al: GHF-1-promoter-targeted immortalization of a somatotropic progenitor cell results in dwarfism in transgenic mice. Genes Dev 7:683, 1993.
8. Lopez-Fernandez J, et al: Differentiation of lactotrope precursor GHFT cells in response to fibroblast growth factor-2. J Biol Chem 275:21653, 2000.
9. Gluckman PD, et al: The neuroendocrine regulation and function of growth hormone and prolactin in the mammalian fetus. Endocrinol Rev 2:363, 1981.
10. Aubert ML, et al: The ontogenesis of human fetal hormones. IV. Somatostatin, luteinizing hormone releasing factor, and thyrotropin releasing factor in hypothalamus and cerebral cortex of human fetuses 10–22 weeks of age. J Clin Endocrinol Metab 44:1130, 1977.
11. Bugnon C, et al: Immunocytochemical study of the ontogenesis of the hypothalamic-somatostatin-containing neurons in the human fetus. Metabolism 27:1161, 1978.
12. Bugnon C, et al: Immunocytologic study of hypothalamic LH-RH neurons of the human fetus. Brain Res 128:249, 1977.
13. Bresson JL, et al: Ontogeny of the neuroglandular system revealed with HPGRF 44 antibodies in human hypothalamus. Neuroendocrinology 39:68, 1984.
14. Ben-Jonathan N, Hnasko R: Dopamine as a prolactin (PRL) inhibitor. Endocr Rev 22:724, 2001.
15. Bertler A: Occurrence and localization of catecholamines in the human brain. Acta Physiol Scand 51:97, 1961.
16. Hyyppa M: Hypothalamic monoamine in human fetuses. Neuroendocrinology 9:257, 1972.
17. Gluckman PD, et al: Hormone ontogeny in the ovine fetus. VI. Dopaminergic regulation of prolactin secretion. Endocrinology 105:1173, 1979.
18. Freeman ME, et al: Prolactin: structure, function, and regulation of secretion. Physiol Rev 80:1523, 2000.
19. Kaplan SL, Grumbach MM: Nonspecific inhibitors in serum and the immunoassay of human growth. J Clin Endocrinol Metab 22:1153, 1962.
20. Gluckman PD, et al: The functional maturation of the somatotropic axis in the perinatal period. In Kunzel W, Jensen A (eds): The Endocrine Control of the Fetus. Berlin, Springer-Verlag, 1988, pp. 201–209.
21. Marti-Henneberg C, et al: Hormone ontogeny in the ovine fetus. XII. The dopaminergic regulation of growth hormone (oGH) and chorionic somatomammotropin (oCS) release. Endocrinology 109:1355, 1981.
22. Gluckman PD, et al: Hormone ontogeny in the ovine fetus. X. The effects of beta endorphin and naloxone on circulating growth hormone, prolactin, and chorionic somatomammotropin. Endocrinology 107:76, 1980.
23. Marti-Henneberg C, et al: Hormone ontogeny in the ovine fetus. XI. The serotoninergic regulation of growth hormone (GH) and prolactin (PRL) secretion. Endocrinology 107:1273, 1980.
24. Gluckman PD: The ontogenesis of GABA-mediated inhibition of growth hormone release in sheep. J Dev Physiol 4:227, 1982.
25. Gluckman PD: The development of β-adrenergic mediated inhibition of growth hormone secretion in the ovine fetus. J Dev Physiol 4:207, 1982.
26. Bassett NS, Gluckman PD: The effect of fatty acid infusion on growth hormone secretion in the ovine fetus: evidence for immaturity of pituitary responsiveness in utero. J Dev Physiol 9:301, 1987.
27. Gluckman PD: Changing responsiveness to growth hormone releasing factor in the perinatal sheep. J Dev Physiol 6:509, 1984.
28. Gluckman PD, et al: Hormone ontogeny in the ovine fetus. III. The effect of exogenous somatostatin. Endocrinology 104:974, 1979.
29. de Zegher F, et al: Hormone ontogeny in the ovine fetus and neonate. XXII. The effect of somatostatin on the growth hormone (GH) response to GH-releasing factor. Endocrinology 124:1114, 1989.
30. Silverman BL, et al: Regulation of growth hormone (GH) secretion by GH-releasing factor, somatostatin, and insulin-like growth factor I in ovine fetal and neonatal pituitary cells in vitro. Endocrinology 124:84, 1989.
31. Gluckman PD, Butler JH: Parturition-related changes in insulin-like growth factors-I and -II in the perinatal lamb. J Endocrinol 99:223, 1983.
32. Horvath TL, et al: Minireview: ghrelin and the regulation of energy balance—a hypothalamic perspective. Endocrinology 142:4163, 2001.
33. Makino Y, et al: Alteration of plasma ghrelin levels associated with the blood pressure in pregnancy. Hypertension 39:781, 2002.
34. Nagaya N, et al: Hemodynamic and hormonal effects of human ghrelin in healthy volunteers. Am J Physiol 280:R1483, 2001.
35. Chanoine J-P, et al: Immunoreactive ghrelin in human cord blood: relation to anthropometry, leptin, and growth hormone. J Pediatr Gastroenterol Nutr 35:282, 2002.
36. Volante M, et al: Ghrelin expression in fetal, infant, and adult human lung. J Histochem Cytochem 50:1013, 2002.
37. Gluckman PD, et al: Maturation of thermoregulatory and thermogenic mechanisms in fetal sheep. In Kunzel W, Jensen A (eds): The Endocrine Control of the Fetus. Physiologic and Pathophysiologic Aspects. Heidelberg, Springer Verlag, 1988, pp 300–305.
38. Power GG, et al: Oxygen supply and the placenta limit thermogenic responses in fetal sheep. J Appl Physiol 63:1896, 1987.
39. Schubring C: Temperature regulation in healthy and resuscitated newborns immediately after birth. J Perinat Med 14:27, 1986.
40. Hull D: Thermal control in very immature infants. Br Med Bull 44:971, 1988.
41. Gluckman PD, et al: Congenital idiopathic growth hormone deficiency associated with prenatal and early postnatal growth failure. The International Board of the Kabi Pharmacia International Growth Study. J Pediatr 121:920, 1992.
42. Kopchick JJ, Andry JM: Growth hormone (GH), GH receptor, and signal transduction. Mol Genet Metab 71:293, 2000.
43. Roupas P, Herington AC: Cellular mechanisms in the processing of growth hormone and its receptor. Mol Cell Endocrinol 61:1, 1989.
44. Gluckman PD, Breier BH: The regulation of the growth hormone receptor. In Heap RB, et al (eds): Biotechnology in Growth Regulation. London, Butterworths, 1988, pp 27–33.
45. Freemark M, et al: Placental lactogen and GH receptors in sheep liver: striking differences in ontogeny and function. Am J Physiol 251:E328, 1986.
46. Gluckman PD, et al: The ontogeny of somatotropic binding sites in ovine hepatic membranes. Endocrinology 112:1607, 1983.
47. Breier BH, et al: Plasma concentrations of insulin-like growth factor-1 and insulin in the infant calf: ontogeny and influence of altered nutrition. J Endocrinol 119:43, 1988.
48. Badinga L, et al: Covalent coupling of bovine growth hormone to its receptor in bovine liver membranes. Mol Cell Endocrinol 52:85, 1987.
49. Breier BH, et al: Somatotrophic receptors in hepatic tissue of the developing pig. J Endocrinol 123:25, 1989.
50. Maes M, et al: Ontogeny of liver somatotropic and lactogenic binding sites in male and female rats. Endocrinology 113:1325, 1983.
51. Breier BH, et al: The induction of hepatic somatotrophic receptors after birth in sheep is dependent on parturition-associated mechanisms. J Endocrinol 141:101, 1994.
52. Klempt M, et al: Tissue distribution and ontogeny of growth hormone receptor messenger ribonucleic acid and ligand binding to hepatic tissue in the midgestation sheep fetus. Endocrinology 132:1071, 1993.
53. Pantaleon M, et al: Functional growth hormone (GH) receptors and GH are expressed by preimplantation mouse embryos: a role for GH in early embryogenesis? Proc Natl Acad Sci U S A 94:5125, 1997.
54. Waters MJ, Kaye PL: The role of growth hormone in fetal development. Growth Horm IGF Res 12:137, 2002.
55. Hill DJ, et al: Localization of the growth hormone receptor, identified by immunocytochemistry, in second trimester human fetal tissues and placenta throughout gestation. J Clin Endocrinol Metab 75:646, 1992.
56. Werther GA, et al: Growth hormone (GH) receptors are expressed on human fetal mesenchymal tissues—identification of messenger ribonucleic acid and GH-binding protein. J Clin Endocrinol Metab 76:1638, 1993.
57. Urbanek M, et al: Expression of a human growth hormone (hGH) receptor isoform is predicted by tissue-specific alternative splicing of exon 3 of the hGH receptor gene transcript. Mol Endocrinol 6:279, 1992.
58. Stallings-Mann ML, et al: Alternative splicing of exon 3 of the human growth hormone receptor is the result of an unusual genetic polymorphism. Proc Natl Acad Sci U S A 93:12394, 1996.
59. Stevens D, Alexander G: Lipid deposition after hypophysectomy and growth hormone treatment in the sheep fetus. J Dev Physiol 8:139, 1986.
60. Parkes MJ, Bassett JM: Antagonism by growth hormone of insulin action in fetal sheep. J Endocrinol 105:379, 1985.
61. Jost A, Picon L: Hormonal control of fetal development and metabolism. Adv Metab Disord 4:123, 1970.
62. Jost A, et al: Plasma growth hormone in the rabbit fetus. Relation to maturation of the liver and lung. C R Seances Acad Sci Serie D Sci Naturel 288:347, 1979.

63. Goodman HG, et al: Growth and growth hormone. II. A comparison of isolated growth-hormone deficiency and multiple pituitary-hormone deficiencies in 35 patients with idiopathic hypopituitary dwarfism. N Engl J Med 278:57, 1968.

64. Lovinger RD, et al: Congenital hypopituitarism associated with neonatal hypoglycemia and microphallus: four cases secondary to hypothalamic hormone deficiencies. J Pediatr 87:1171, 1975.

65. Bole-Feysot C, et al: Prolactin (PRL) and its receptor: actions, signal transduction pathways and phenotypes observed in PRL receptor knockout mice. Endocrinol Rev 19:225, 1998.

66. Ben-Jonathan N, et al: Extrapituitary prolactin: distribution, regulation, functions, and clinical aspects. Endocr Rev 17:639, 1996.

67. Jaffe RB: Integrative maternal-fetal endocrine control systems. *In* Yen SSC, Jaffe RB (eds): Reproductive Endocrinology, 2nd ed. Philadelphia, WB Saunders, 1986, pp 770–788.

68. Gluckman PD, et al: Hormone ontogeny in the ovine fetus. XIV. The effect of estradiol-17B infusion on fetal plasma gonadotropins and prolactin. Endocrinology 112:1618, 1983.

69. McMillen IC, et al: Concentrations of prolactin in the plasma of fetal sheep and in amniotic fluid in late gestation and during dexamethasone-induced parturition. J Endocrinol 99:107, 1983.

70. Suganuma N, et al: Ontogenesis of pituitary prolactin in the human fetus. J Clin Endocrinol Metab 63:156, 1986.

71. Aubert ML, et al: The ontogenesis of human fetal hormones. III. Prolactin. J Clin Invest 56:155, 1975.

72. Winters AJ, et al: Fetal plasma prolactin levels. J Clin Endocrinol Metab 41:626, 1974.

73. Gluckman PD, et al: Prolactin in umbilical cord blood and the respiratory distress syndrome. J Pediatr 93:1011, 1978.

74. Hauth JC, et al: A role of fetal prolactin in lung maturation. Obstet Gynecol 51:81, 1978.

75. Sultan C, et al: Evolution de la prolactine plasmatique chez l'enfant normal, de la naissance à l'adolescence. C R Soc Biol Fil 171:131, 1976.

76. Perlman M, et al: Prolonged hyperprolactinemia in preterm infants. J Clin Endocrinol Metab 47:894, 1978.

77. Phillips ID, et al: The relative roles of the hypothalamus and cortisol in the control of prolactin gene expression in the anterior pituitary of the sheep fetus. J Neuroendocrinol 8:929, 1996.

78. Mueller PL, et al: Hormone ontogeny in the ovine fetus. V. Circulating prolactin in mid and late gestation. Endocrinology 105:129, 1979.

79. Shambaugh GE III, et al: Characterization of rat placental TRH-like material and the ontogeny of placental and fetal brain TRH. Placenta 4:329, 1983.

80. Dussault JH, et al: The development of the hypothalamo-pituitary axis in the neonatal rat: sexual maturation in male and female rats as assessed by hypothalamic LHRH and pituitary and serum LH and FSH concentrations. Can J Physiol Pharmacol 55:1091, 1977.

81. Oliver C, et al: Developmental changes in brain TRH and in plasma and pituitary TSH and prolactin levels in the rat. Biol Neonate 37:145, 1980.

82. Ajika K, et al: Effect of estrogen on plasma and pituitary gonadotropins and prolactin, and on hypothalamic releasing and inhibiting factors. Neuroendocrinology 9:304, 1972.

83. Cramer OM, et al: Estrogen inhibition of dopamine release into hypophysial portal blood. Endocrinology 104:419, 1979.

84. Lieberman ME, et al: Estrogen control of prolactin synthesis in vitro. Proc Natl Acad Sci U S A 75:5946, 1978.

85. Raymond V, et al: Potent antidopaminergic activity of estradiol at the pituitary level on prolactin release. Science 200:1173, 1978.

86. Freemark M, et al: Ontogenesis of prolactin receptors in the human fetus in early gestation. J Clin Invest 99:1107, 1997.

87. Lowman HB, et al: Mutational analysis and protein engineering of receptor-binding determinants in human placental lactogen. J Biol Chem 266:10982, 1991.

88. Berlanga JJ, et al: The short form of the prolactin (PRL) receptor silences PRL induction of the beta-casein gene promoter. Mol Endocrinol 11:1449, 1997.

89. Phillips ID, et al: Hepatic prolactin receptor gene expression increases in the sheep fetus before birth and after cortisol infusion. Endocrinology 138:1351, 1997.

90. Hu Z, et al: Multiple and tissue-specific promoter control of gonadal and nongonadal prolactin receptor gene expression. J Biol Chem 271:10242, 1996.

91. Symonds ME, et al: Prolactin receptor gene expression and foetal adipose tissue. J Neuroendocrinol 10:885, 1998.

92. Budge H, et al: Effect of maternal nutrition on brown adipose tissue and its prolactin receptor status in the fetal lamb. Pediatr Res 47:781, 2000.

93. Smith YF, et al: Serum prolactin and respiratory distress syndrome in the newborn. Pediatr Res 14:93, 1980.

94. Mendelson CR, Boggaram V: Hormonal control of the surfactant system in fetal lung. Annu Rev Physiol 53:415, 1991.

95. Labbe A, et al: Comparative study of the binding of prolactin and growth hormone by rabbit and human lung cell membrane fractions. Biol Neonate 61:179, 1992.

96. Ballard PL, et al: Failure to detect an effect of prolactin on pulmonary surfactant and adrenal steroids in fetal sheep and rabbits. J Clin Invest 62:879, 1978.

97. Schellenberg JC, et al: Synergistic hormonal effects on lung maturation in fetal sheep. J Appl Physiol 65:94, 1988.

98. Quirk JGJ, et al: Role of fetal pituitary prolactin in fetal lung maturation. Semin Perinatol 6:238, 1982.

99. Figueroa JP, et al: Osmotic regulation of prolactin secretion in the fetal sheep. J Dev Physiol 13:339, 1990.

100. Ertl T, et al: Postnatal development of plasma prolactin level in premature infants with and without NaCl suppression. Biol Neonate 44:219, 1983.

101. Coulter DM: Prolactin: a hormonal regulator of the neonatal tissue water reservoir. Pediatr Res 17:665, 1983.

102. Josimovich JB, et al: Amniotic prolactin control over amniotic and fetal extracellular fluid water and electrolytes in the rhesus monkey. Endocrinology 100:564, 1977.

103. Holt WF, Perks AM: The effect of prolactin on water movement through the isolated amniotic membrane of the guinea pig. Gen Comp Endocrinol 26:153, 1975.

104. Tyson JE, et al: Studies of prolactin secretion in human pregnancy. Am J Obstet Gynecol 113:14, 1972.

105. Nicoll CS: Comparative aspects of prolactin physiology: is prolactin the initial growth hormone in mammalian species also? *In* Harter RC (ed): Progress in Prolactin Physiology and Pathology. Proceedings of the International Symposium on Prolactin. Nice, France, 1977. North Holland, The Netherlands, Elsevier Biomedical Press, 1978, pp 175–187.

106. Sinha YN, Vanderlaan WP: Effect on growth of prolactin deficiency induced in infant mice. Endocrinology 110:1871, 1982.

107. Laatikainen T, et al: Fetal and maternal serum levels of steroid sulfates, unconjugated steroids, and prolactin at term pregnancy and in early spontaneous labor. J Clin Endocrinol Metab 50:489, 1980.

108. Takahashi K, et al: Lack of relationship between prolactin and adrenal steroidogenesis in the ovine fetus. Am J Obstet Gynecol 139:427, 1981.

109. Handwerger S, Freemark M: The roles of placental growth hormone and placental lactogen in the regulation of human fetal growth and development. J Pediatr Endocrinol Metab 13:343, 2000.

110. Reis FM, Petraglia F: The placenta as a neuroendocrine organ. Front Horm Res 27:216, 2001.

111. Min SH, et al: Growth-promoting effects of ovine placental lactogen (oPL) in young lambs: comparison with bovine growth hormone provides evidence for a distinct effect of oPL and food intake. Growth Reg 6:144, 1996.

112. Gluckman PD: The role of pituitary hormones, growth factors and insulin in the regulation of fetal growth. *In* Clarke JR (ed): Oxford Reviews of Reproductive Biology, 8th ed. Oxford, Clarendon Press, 1986, pp 1–60.

113. Gluckman PD, Barry TN: Relationships between plasma concentrations of placental lactogen, insulin-like growth factors, metabolites, and lamb size in late gestation ewes subject to nutritional supplementation and in their lambs at birth. Domest Anim Endocrinol 5:209, 1988.

114. Anthony RV, et al: The growth hormone prolactin gene family in ruminant placenta. J Reprod Fertil 49:83, 1995.

115. Soares MJ, et al: The uteroplacental prolactin family and pregnancy. Biol Reprod 58:273, 1998.

116. Colosi P, et al: Cloning and expression of ovine placental lactogen. Mol Endocrinol 3:1462, 1989.

117. Faria TN, et al: Localization of placental lactogen-I in trophoblast giant cells of the mouse placenta. Biol Reprod 44:327, 1991.

118. Faria TN, et al: Ontogeny of placental lactogen-I and placental lactogen-II expression in the developing rat placenta. Dev Biol 141:279, 1990.

119. Breier BH, et al: Characterization of ovine growth hormone (oGH) and ovine placental lactogen (oPL) binding to fetal and adult hepatic tissue in sheep: evidence that oGH and oPL interact with a common receptor. Endocrinology 135:919, 1994.

120. Breier BH, et al: Physiological responses to somatotropin in the ruminant. J Dairy Sci 74:20, 1991.

121. Colosi P, et al: Purification and partial characterization of two prolactin-like glycoprotein hormone complexes from the midpregnant mouse conceptus. Endocrinology 120:2500, 1987.

122. Harigaya T, et al: Hepatic placental lactogen receptors during pregnancy in the mouse. Endocrinology 122:1366, 1988.

123. Haro LS, Talamantes FJ: Interaction of mouse prolactin with mouse hepatic receptors. Mol Cell Endocrinol 41:93, 1985.

124. Anthony RV, et al: Placental-fetal hormonal interactions: impact on fetal growth. J Anim Sci 73:1861, 1995.

125. Lacroix MC, et al: Human placental growth hormone—a review. Placenta 23:587, 2002.

126. Zumkeller W: The role of growth hormone and insulin-like growth factors for placental growth and development. Placenta 21:451, 2000.

127. Ray J, et al: Human growth hormone-variant demonstrates a receptor binding profile distinct from that of normal pituitary growth hormone. J Biol Chem 265:7939, 1990.

Leona Cuttler and Mark R. Palmert

185

Luteinizing Hormone and Follicle-Stimulating Hormone Secretion in the Fetus and Newborn Infant

The pituitary gonadotropins, luteinizing hormone (LH) and follicle-stimulating hormone (FSH), influence the function of the differentiated gonad *in utero* and regulate gonadal function in later life. LH and FSH are secreted by the same pituitary cell, the gonadotroph, under the influence of hypothalamic and other hormones. LH and FSH are glycoproteins, as are thyroid-stimulating hormone (TSH) and human chorionic gonadotropin (hCG). Each of these four glycoproteins consists of an α and β subunit. Although the α subunits are identical, the β subunits differ and thereby confer biologic specificity. The biologic activity of hCG, a placental glycoprotein, is similar to that of LH. This chapter reviews the anatomic development of key components of the gonadotropin regulatory axis (including the hypothalamus, pituitary, and portal circulation), the role of gonadotropins in the fetus and neonate, the factors that control gonadotropin secretion, and disorders in the development of the gonadotropin regulatory system.

DEVELOPMENT OF THE HYPOTHALAMUS AND PITUITARY

Hypothalamus

The hypothalamus (Table 185–1) develops from the primitive forebrain (prosencephalon), the most cephalad part of the neural tube. By approximately the fifth week after conception, the forebrain differentiates into the cerebral hemispheres and the diencephalon; the ventral aspect of the diencephalon then develops into the hypothalamus. By 14 to 16 weeks of gestation, hypothalamic nuclei and fiber tracts have differentiated.[1-5]

Gonadotropin-releasing hormone (GnRH; also termed luteinizing hormone–releasing hormone [LRF, LHRH]), a hypothalamic peptide, is the major physiologic secretagogue of gonadotropins in mature animals. It is released by specific hypothalamic neurons and is carried by the portal circulation to the pituitary. Several aspects of GnRH ontogeny are noteworthy. First, during early embryologic development, GnRH neurons originate in the nasal region near the developing olfactory bulbs, and later extend caudad and migrate to the hypothalamus,[6,7] achieving an adult distribution by midgestation.[8] The product of the Kallmann syndrome gene (KAL1) plays a critical role during this stage of development, explaining some instances of the association between impaired olfactory function and GnRH deficiency seen in this syndrome[9] (see later section on conditions associated with abnormalities of gonadotropins).

Second, complex molecular mechanisms are responsible for tissue-specific transcriptional activity of the GnRH gene. Available evidence indicates that the GnRH gene is targeted to hypothalamic neurons by enhancer and promoter elements acting in concert with transcription factors such as Otx2, Brn-2, and Oct-1.[10,11] There is also evidence that the orphan nuclear receptors DAX-1 and SF-1 are important for the proper development and function of the entire hypothalamic-pituitary-gonadal axis.[9]

Third, the GnRH gene is expressed and the protein found in the hypothalamus during early stages of development. GnRH protein has been detected by radioimmunoassay of whole brain extract as early as 4.5 weeks' gestation.[12] GnRH has been identified within the hypothalamus by 8 to 13 weeks' gestation.[12-17] By 16 weeks'

gestation, GnRH-containing neurons are known to terminate on portal vessels.[18] In lower animals, GnRH has been localized primarily to the nervus terminalis during early embryogenesis and only later appears within the hypothalamus.[19,20]

Most studies of fetal hypothalamic GnRH content have involved fetuses from a relatively brief developmental window during early gestation to midgestation, and thus comprehensive developmental trends have been difficult to establish. The hypothalamic content of GnRH has been reported by some investigators[15,21] to rise during the first half of gestation, although others report little relationship to gestational age during this period.[12,17,22] Hypothalamic GnRH content generally has been reported to be similar in male and female fetuses,[13,15,17,21] with some exceptions.[22] Little is known about the early postnatal development of hypothalamic GnRH in humans, although Bugnon and associates[14] noted an increase in immunoreactive GnRH neurons in hypothalami of human neonates compared with those of late gestational fetuses.

Pituitary

The pituitary gland arises from ectoderm, with the adenohypophysis (anterior pituitary) originating from oral ectoderm and the neurohypophysis (posterior pituitary) deriving from the neuroectoderm.[23] In humans, Rathke pouch, the precursor of the anterior pituitary, develops as an evagination of the primitive stomodeum at approximately the fourth week of gestation[24-26] and separates from the stomodeum by the fifth week of gestation. The floor of the sella turcica forms by the seventh week of gestation, and, by the eighth week, the connection of the pouch with the oral cavity fully disappears.[23]

The anterior pituitary is eventually populated by at least five highly differentiated cell types that emerge in a temporally and spatially specific fashion and include the corticotrophs (which secrete adrenocorticotropic hormone [ACTH]), the somatotrophs (which secrete growth hormone), the lactotrophs (which secrete prolactin), the thyrotrophs (which secrete thyroid-stimulating hormone) and the gonadotrophs (which secrete LH and FSH).[27,28] Investigation has focused on the molecular mechanisms responsible for the differentiation of the specific cell types, and two important principles have emerged from these ongoing studies—namely, that the differentiation of specific cell types in the pituitary follows a highly ordered sequence, and that the coordinated expression and down-regulation of homeodomain transcription factors plays a critical role in controlling the differentiation.[23,27,28] For example, rodent studies indicate that differentiation of all cell types requires transient expression of Rpx (also called Hesx1), but then, on approximately embryonic day 10, the cells divide into Lhx3 dependent and independent lineages (Fig. 185–1). The main population of corticotrophs is Lhx3 independent and appears by embryonic day 12 or 13; the other cell lineages appear to be Lhx3 dependent. Under the influence of Prop-1, the Lhx3 dependent lineage further bifurcates into Pit-1 dependent and independent pathways. The Pit-1 dependent pathway leads to the differentiation of somatotrophs, lactotrophs, and thyrotrophs by embryonic day 16. The Pit-1 independent pathway, under the influence of other factors, including SF-1, leads to differentiation of the gonadotrophs by embryonic day 17. In addition to intrinsic pitu-

TABLE 185-1

LH and FSH in the Human Fetus and Neonate: Early Milestones in the Anatomic Development of the Hypothalamus and Pituitary Unit

	Week of Gestation	Comment	References
Hypothalamus			
Forebrain differentiates into cerebral hemispheres and diencephalon; the latter then develops into hypothalamus	3-5		2-5
GnRH identified in whole brain extract	4.5		12
GnRH neurons found in olfactory placode	5.5		66
GnRH identified in hypothalamus	8-13		12,13,15-17
Pituitary			
LH and FSH identified within the pituitary	9.5-11	Pituitary secretes LH and FSH *in vitro* 5-7 wk	29-37,66
Pituitary releases gonadotropins into circulation	11-12		66
Portal Circulation			
Intact	11.5-12		52

GnRH = gonadotropin-releasing hormone; LH = luteinizing hormone; FSH = follicle-stimulating hormone.

itary factors, there is evidence that, at distinct developmental stages, inductive processes from adjacent tissue are also important for proper cell differentiation and expansion of the pituitary cell lineages.[23] (The reader is referred to references 23, 27, and 28 for detailed discussion of this complex developmental sequence.)

The importance of these basic components of pituitary development to human physiology is emphasized by identification of human mutations that cause predictable phenotypes.[23, 27, 28] For example, mutations in Rpx lead to inherited forms of septo-optic dysplasia and congenital hypopituitarism. A homozygous Lhx3 defect has been identified in individuals with combined pituitary hormone deficiency of all anterior pituitary hormones except ACTH. Similarly, mutations in Prop-1 have been associated with abnormalities of somatotroph, lactotroph, thyrotroph, and gonadotroph function. Conversely, Pit-1 gene mutations are associated with deficient somatotroph, lactotroph, and thyrotroph function, with relative preservation of gonadotropin secretion.

Once formed, the gonadotroph secretes LH and FSH early in embryogenesis. The fetal pituitary secretes LH and FSH in culture at 5 to 7 weeks' gestation according to some investigators,[29, 30] although some investigators disagree.[18] The amount of hormone secreted increases with advancing age of the fetus.[18]

LH and FSH have been detected in the pituitary by immunoassay and immunocytochemistry as early as 9.5 to 11 weeks' gestation.[31-38] The pituitary content of LH and FSH then rises sharply,[32, 38] with pituitary LH and FSH content peaking at 25 to 29 weeks' gestation in female fetuses and at 35 to 40 weeks' gestation in males.[38] The pituitary content of LH and FSH is higher in female fetuses than in males between approximately 10 and 25 weeks' gestation, as assessed by radioimmunoassay[32, 37-39] and immunocytochemistry.[33] This sexual dimorphism may reflect testosterone production by the male fetus, with resulting inhibition of pituitary gonadotropin production.[40]

Early in gestation, the predominant pituitary glycoprotein fraction is the α subunit.[14, 34, 36, 41] As gestation progresses, the relative amount of β subunit and intact gonadotropin appears to rise.[14, 33, 41, 42] Relatively little is known about postnatal pituitary gonadotropin development. Kaplan and colleagues[17] found that the content and concentration of pituitary LH and FSH in 2- to 6-month-old infants were higher than in late gestational female fetuses. In five male infants, pituitary LH and FSH content (but not concentration) was higher than that of midgestational male fetuses.[17]

It is not clear to what extent GnRH normally contributes to the functional development of the gonadotroph. Because pituitaries of anencephalic fetuses have reduced gonadotropin content[17] as well as persistent predominant secretion of the α subunit of glycoproteins,[34, 41] one may infer that GnRH normally contributes to gonadotroph development and function. This concept is supported by the observation that GnRH can stimulate differentia-

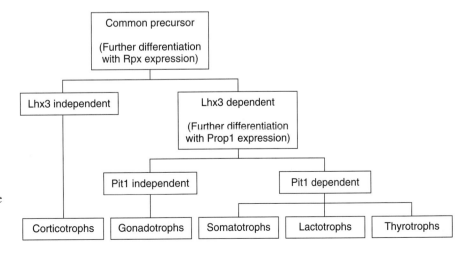

Figure 185–1. Schematic summary of the development of anterior pituitary cell types (for full details, see references 23, 27, and 28).

tion of fetal rat gonadotrophs *in vitro*[43,44] and LH synthesis in cultured fetal human pituitary cells.[45] The observations, however, that (1) anencephalic human fetuses have differentiated gonadotrophs,[46-48] that (2) the primitive rat pituitary can synthesize LH when transplanted to the kidney of an adult host,[49] and that (3) the primitive rat pituitary can synthesize LH *in vitro*[49,50] suggest that the fetal pituitary has potential for some differentiation in the absence of direct hypothalamic influences.[51]

Portal Circulation

Work using vascular casts suggests that the hypothalamic pituitary portal system is intact by 11.5 to 12 weeks of gestation,[52] earlier than originally estimated.[53-55] It has been suggested that local diffusion may allow communication between the hypothalamus and pituitary before that time.[17]

ROLE OF PITUITARY GONADOTROPINS IN THE FETUS AND NEONATE

Fetal pituitary LH and FSH are not required for sexual and gonadal differentiation. Pituitary gonadotropins, however, are required for normal function of the differentiated gonad. Because human chorionic gonadotropin (hCG) can activate LH receptors, placental hCG leads to production of testosterone early in gestation,[40,56] and this testosterone production leads to normal formation of male external genitalia by 12 to 14 weeks' gestation. However, later in gestation, testosterone production by the fetal testes depends on fetal LH, and this LH-induced testosterone production is responsible for growth of the formed phallus during the later stages of pregnancy. The increased incidence of normally formed but small phallus (microphallus) and cryptorchidism in male infants with anencephaly or gonadotropin deficiency[57-60] supports the concept that pituitary gonadotropins influence testicular growth and function later in gestation, as does the finding that the testes of anencephalic fetuses are hypoplastic, with decreased numbers of testicular Leydig cells.[59-63] In females, anencephalic fetuses have been reported to show small ovaries with hypoplasia of the primary follicles.[62] Some reports suggest that the ovaries are relatively normal until 34 to 36 weeks' gestation and only later show evidence of maldevelopment.[63]

REGULATION OF PITUITARY LUTEINIZING HORMONE AND FOLLICLE-STIMULATING HORMONE SECRETION IN THE FETUS AND NEONATE

Factors That Regulate Pituitary Luteinizing Hormone and Follicle-Stimulating Hormone Secretion in Adults

In adults, the secretion of pituitary LH and FSH involves the finely balanced interplay of several regulatory agents (Fig. 185–2). The major elements involved in this interplay are the hypothalamus, pituitary, and gonad (a unit referred to as the hypothalamic-pituitary-gonadal [HPG] axis). The main stimulus for pituitary gonadotropin secretion is the hypothalamic decapeptide GnRH. Until recently, only one GnRH gene and one GnRH receptor had been identified. Now more than 10 GnRH molecules and several GnRH receptors have been identified in mammals and nonmammalian vertebrates.[64] At least two forms of GnRH and two GnRH receptors are expressed in humans. The function and tissue specificity of these various molecules is still being elucidated, but the regulation of LH and FSH secretion seems to reside primarily with the originally identified molecular species.[64] The factors that regulate synthesis and release of GnRH from the hypothalamus are subjects of intense investigation but remain largely enigmatic. There is evidence for involvement of a wide range of

factors, including stress, health, and nutritional status; gonadal steroids; endogenous opioids; prostaglandins; growth factors; leptin; neuropeptides (such as neuropeptide Y); and central neurotransmitters (such as norepinephrine, serotonin, dopamine, acetylcholine, glutamate, and γ-aminobutyric acid).[65-68]

The normal pulsatile secretion of LH is believed to be mediated directly by episodic release of GnRH. The pulsatile release of GnRH is critical for the maintenance of gonadotropin secretion in adults; continuous administration of exogenous GnRH to adults leads to an initial increase in gonadotropin secretion, followed by prolonged suppression of gonadotropin secretion owing to downregulation of the pituitary gonadotroph.[43,69-71] GnRH acts on the gonadotroph to stimulate gonadotropin release by binding to specific cell surface receptors.[72-75] Through secondary messenger systems, GnRH receptor binding leads to the mobilization of intracellular calcium (which affects the initial burst of LH secretion) and an influx of extracellular calcium that is necessary to maintain sustained gonadotropin secretion.[67] There is evidence *in vitro* for involvement of a guanosine triphosphate (GTP)–binding protein, phosphoinositide metabolism, and protein kinase C in the intracellular signaling processes.[75,76]

Gonadal secretions are also major physiologic regulators of LH and FSH secretion in adults. Gonadal steroids exert negative feedback (inhibitory) effects on gonadotropin release, and in mature premenopausal women, estrogens exert positive feedback,

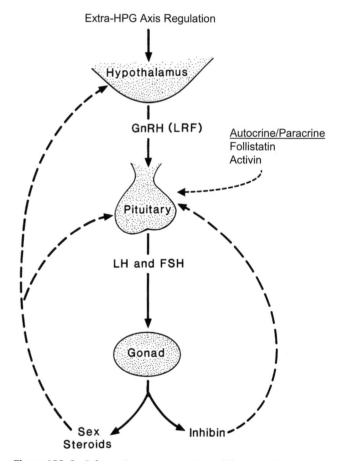

Figure 185–2. Schematic representation of the gonadotropin control system in adults. Dashed lines indicate feedback loops. HPG = hypothalamic-pituitary-gonadal; GnRH = gonadotropin-releasing hormone; LRF = luteinizing releasing factor. The principal sex steroids in females are estradiol and progesterone; in males, the principal sex steroid is testosterone. For detailed discussion of regulatory mechanisms, see references 66 to 68.

mediating the ovulatory surge of gonadotropins. In addition to steroids, the gonads produce peptides, such as inhibins A and B, that selectively modulate FSH-secreting cells. Although other regulators, such as activins and follistatin, are present in the peripheral circulation, these factors probably act in an autocrine/paracrine fashion, with activin stimulating FSH release and follistatin inhibiting FSH release by binding to activin. (For complete reviews of the regulation of gonadotropin secretion in adults, the reader is referred to references 67, 68, and 76 through 83.)

In developing animals, the roles of the various components of this complex system are not fully understood. In the next section, current knowledge regarding each of these regulatory influences in the fetus and newborn infant is reviewed.

Factors That Regulate Pituitary Luteinizing Hormone and Follicle-Stimulating Hormone Release in the Fetus and Newborn Infant

Gonadotropin-Releasing Hormone (GnRH)

GnRH is present in the human fetal hypothalamus by 8 to 11 weeks' gestation.[12-18, 21] Although the secretory pattern of GnRH during human fetal and early neonatal development is not known, embryonic GnRH neurons from nonhuman primates secrete their peptide in a pulsatile manner *in vitro*—suggesting an intrinsic pulsatile secretion of GnRH that may be independent of non-GnRH neuronal synaptic input.[66, 84]

GnRH appears to influence gonadotropin release early in gestation. The human fetal pituitary *in vitro* releases LH or FSH, or both, in response to GnRH by approximately 13 to 19 weeks' gestation (Figs. 185–3 through 185–6).[85-88] By the second trimester, pretreatment with estradiol enhances the sensitivity of human fetal pituitaries to GnRH.[89] GnRH appears capable of influencing LH synthesis as well as secretion at this period of development.[45]

The findings of Takagi and associates[90] suggest that the human fetal pituitary releases gonadotropins in response to exogenous GnRH *in vivo* by the second trimester, and that the increment in

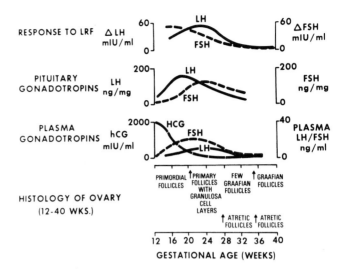

Figure 185–4. Graphic comparison of gonadotropin response to LRF (GnRH), pituitary and plasma gonadotropins, and plasma hCG, with histologic changes in the ovary of the human female fetus during gestation. (From Gluckman PD, et al: *In* Tulchinsky LD, Ryan KJ [eds]: Maternal-Fetal Endocrinology. Philadelphia, WB Saunders, 1980, p 2423.)

LH and FSH levels following GnRH administration is greater in the second than in the third trimester. These findings are supported by studies in monkeys[39, 91, 92] and sheep[93] that show the fetal gonadotroph to be responsive to GnRH or its analogues *in vivo* and that demonstrate a decline in gonadotroph response to GnRH with advancing gestational age.[93, 94, 95]

In human neonates[89, 90, 96] and infants,[97-101] exogenous GnRH also stimulates gonadotropin release. Limited data suggest that the responsiveness of the gonadotroph to GnRH varies with age during infancy. Tapanainen and colleagues[101] administered GnRH (50 µg/m² intravenously) to infant boys who had undescended but palpable testes and who ranged in age from 3 to 390 days. GnRH stimulated LH and FSH release in all age groups, but peak gonadotropin release occurred at 1 to 3 months of age, with a subsequent decline from 3 to 12 months of age. A similar age-dependent change in LH response to GnRH was found in infant monkeys.[91]

Gonadotropin secretion is episodic in rhesus monkey[102] and ovine[62, 103] fetuses, as well as in human, ovine,[104] and rhesus[105] infants. In the ovine fetus, administration of a GnRH antagonist decreases LH pulse frequency.[103] Because pulsatile secretion of LH is believed to depend on pulsatile release of GnRH, these findings also suggest a role for endogenous GnRH in the regulation of LH release in the perinatal period.

The ontogeny of gonadotroph GnRH receptors in humans is not known. However, the observation that the fetal pituitary releases gonadotropins in response to GnRH by the second trimester[18, 85, 87, 88, 90] suggests the presence of hypophyseal GnRH receptors by that time. In rats, pituitary binding sites for GnRH have been detected by 13 days gestation (term = 22 days),[106] with the pituitary GnRH receptor number increasing in the late prenatal and early postnatal period.[107] Postnatally, the concentration of GnRH receptors in rodents is highest between 15 and 20 to 30 days of age and decreases thereafter to reach adult levels by approximately 60 days of age.[72]

Although GnRH has been detected in the placenta[64, 108] as well as the hypothalamus, the role of the placental material in the physiologic regulation of pituitary gonadotropin release is uncertain. Anencephalic and gonadotropin-deficient fetuses are deficient in hypothalamic—but presumably not in placental—GnRH. That these infants generally have subnormal quantities of

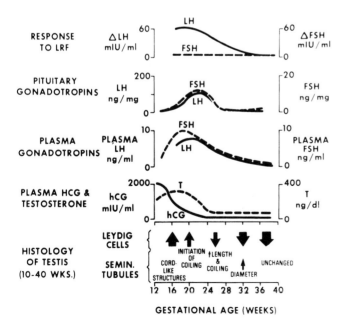

Figure 185–3. Graphic comparison of gonadotropin response to LRF (GnRH), pituitary and plasma gonadotropins, and plasma hCG and testosterone, with histologic changes in the testis of the human male fetus during gestation. (From Gluckman PD, et al: *In* Tulchinsky LD, Ryan KJ [eds]: Maternal-Fetal Endocrinology. Philadelphia, WB Saunders, 1980, p 2423.)

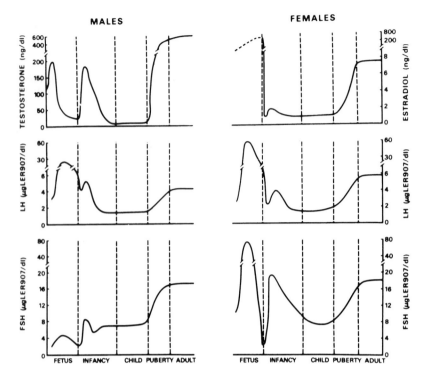

Figure 185–5. Mean concentrations of serum LH, FSH, and estradiol during human pregnancy and postnatal development. (From Winter JS, et al: J Clin Endocrinol Metab *42*:679, 1976.)

pituitary gonadotropins[17, 42] suggests that placental GnRH may not be an important factor for the normal regulation of gonadotropin release *in utero*.

The overall influence of neurotransmitters on gonadotropin release in the human fetus and neonate is not known, although some animal studies suggest that specific neurotransmitters such as glutamate and endogenous opioids may be involved in the fetal regulation of gonadotropin release.[109,110]

Taken together, the available data indicate that the pituitary gonadotroph is responsive to hypothalamic GnRH during fetal life, and that endogenous GnRH stimulates gonadotropin release in the fetus and neonate.

Gonadal Steroids

There is indirect evidence that the capacity of gonadal steroids, especially testosterone, to inhibit gonadotropin release develops

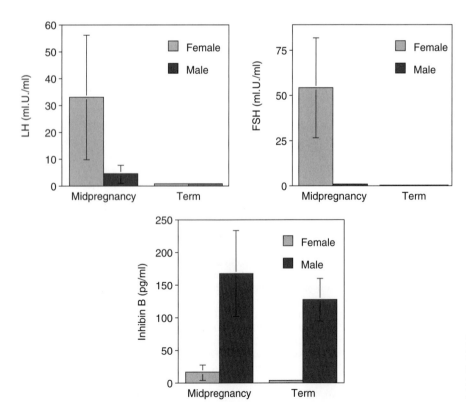

Figure 185–6. LH, FSH, and inhibin B levels in human fetal female and male serum at midpregnancy and term (mean ± SD. (From Debieve et al: J Clin Endocrinol Metab *85*:270, 2000.)

during fetal development. This concept is derived largely from animal experiments. For example, castration of male rhesus fetuses at approximately midgestation results in elevation of gonadotropin levels,[66, 111-113] and early testosterone or dihydrotestosterone replacement prevents the rise of gonadotropins following castration.[112] These results suggest that functional negative feedback between the testes and the hypothalamic-pituitary axis is present by midgestation in rhesus fetuses. The role of fetal ovarian estrogen in regulating gonadotropin secretion is less clear, in part because both male and female fetuses develop in an environment that is rich in estrogens of feto-placental origin. In female rhesus fetuses, gonadectomy has had variable results on gonadotropin secretion.[111-113] Estradiol infusions blunt LH release in the late gestational ovine fetus.[114] Gonadotropin levels, which rise in the early postnatal period, may reflect, in part, a release from negative feedback as sex steroids are removed from the fetal circulation.

By the newborn period, gonadal steroids appear to suppress gonadotropin secretion in both sexes. Castration of newborn female rhesus monkeys results in elevation of FSH and, to a lesser extent, LH levels.[115] Orchiectomy of male monkey neonates also results in elevation of LH and FSH, suggesting that testosterone may influence early postnatal gonadotropin secretion in males.[113, 115-117] The specific gonadotropin secretion pattern differs between neonatal castrated male and female monkeys, and it has been suggested that this reflects intrinsic sexual dimorphism of hypothalamic GnRH secretion.[115] Similarly, gonadal failure in human neonates leads to elevated gonadotropin levels,[118] indicating that gonadal products normally suppress gonadotropin secretion even in the neonatal period. Further evidence for negative feedback by gonadal steroids derives from the observation that administration of estrogen and progesterone to extremely premature female infants suppresses LH and FSH secretion.[119]

Castration-induced elevation of circulating gonadotropins, however, is not fully sustained into late childhood, and gonadotropin levels in both experimental orchiectomy and in naturally occurring gonadal failure decline during infancy or early childhood (only to rise again in the peripubertal period).[56,113,116,118] However, the gonadotropin levels do not reach levels as low as those in children with normal gonads.[120] Taken together, these findings suggest that although gonadal steroids influence gonadotropin secretion in neonates, they are not the sole mediators of changing gonadotropin levels in infancy. The eventual decline in gonadotropin levels in late infancy and early childhood is due primarily to extragonadal and presumably central hypothalamic-pituitary factors in combination with some gonadal derived inhibition.[113,116,117]

Inhibin

Inhibins are polypeptides secreted by the Sertoli cells in the testis and by the granulosa cell in the ovary, which inhibit the release of FSH but not LH from the pituitary. Inhibin is also synthesized by the placenta.[121] Biologically active inhibin is present in the fetus, and administration of inhibin suppresses serum FSH.[122] In newborn male rats, inhibin production is high, and administration of inhibin antiserum to male newborn rats causes a rise in serum FSH.

A recent study reported no measurable inhibin A in human fetuses but found inhibin B in male and female fetuses at midgestation, with higher levels in males than females (Figs. 185–6 through 185–8). Circulating inhibin levels are higher in premature than in term infants.[123] Inhibin B levels are higher in boys than in girls after birth.[124] In boys, levels peak at approximately 3 to 12 months of age and remain elevated until approximately 15 months of age.[124, 125] One report notes a more complex pattern with considerable interindividual variation in female infants.[124]

Although the precise role of inhibins in the fetus and neonate is not clear, these findings suggest that endogenous inhibin may play a physiologic role in suppressing FSH in fetal and neonatal animals.[122,126]

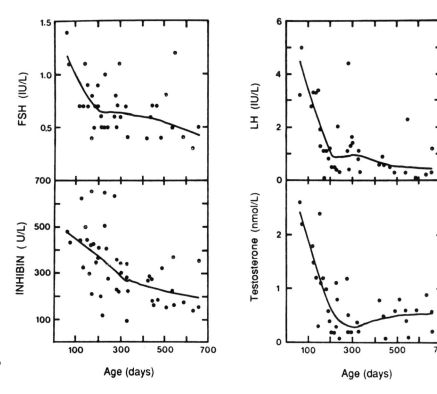

Figure 185–7. Scatterplot matrix of hormone changes with age in boys. The *continuous line* represents the robust, locally weighted regression. (From Burger HG, et al: J Clin Endocrinol Metab *72*:682, 1991.)

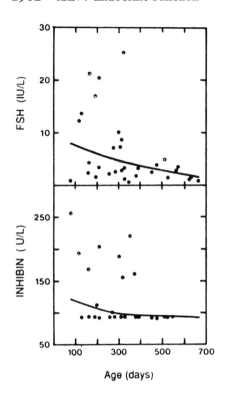

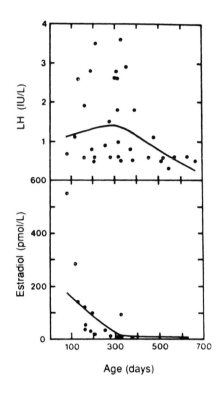

Figure 185–8. Scatterplot matrix of hormone changes with age in girls. The *continuous line* represents the robust, locally weighted regression. (From Burger HG, et al: J Clin Endocrinol Metab 72:682, 1991.)

PLASMA GONADOTROPINS IN THE FETUS AND NEONATE

General Pattern (Figs. 185–3 through 185–8)

Little is known about plasma gonadotropin levels in human fetuses before 10 to 14 weeks' gestation. Circulating immunoreactive FSH is detectable by the 10th to 13th week of gestation in human fetuses and rises to peak levels at approximately midgestation (see Figures 185–3 through 185–6).[38, 40] At that time, FSH concentrations are comparable to those of castrated animals. FSH levels then decline; by birth, FSH levels are low, similar to those of prepubertal children.[17,38,95,127,128] Circulating LH concentrations in the fetus follow a similar pattern.[32,38,40,128] Studies in premature infants are consistent with studies in fetuses and show a decline in serum LH and FSH levels with advancing gestational age.[123]

Soon after birth, LH and FSH levels rise (see Figure 185–5). Although reported patterns vary somewhat, this increase is sustained for weeks to months and is followed by a decline to prepubertal levels (see Figures 185–5, 185–7, and 185–8).[111, 129, 130] The specific patterns also differ between boys and girls, as discussed in detail later.[130–132]

Pulsatile secretion of gonadotropins is a hallmark feature of the mature hypothalamic-pituitary axis. Studies in the primate[102] and ovine[103, 133] fetuses suggest that pulsatile secretion of gonadotropins may develop *in utero*. There is evidence that gonadotropin secretion in the 1- to 3-month-old human infant is also episodic.[134,135] In the lamb[104] and castrated newborn male rhesus monkey,[105] gonadotropin secretion also appears to be episodic.

Circulating hCG, the placental glycoprotein, declines from high levels at 13 to 17 weeks' gestation to low levels at term (see Figures 185–3 and 185–4)[32,38,90] and falls to undetectable levels by the fifth postnatal day.[90,132] The α glycoprotein subunit is the predominant glycoprotein component in fetal plasma and cord blood and in the pituitary gland. Plasma levels of free α subunit are high at midgestation and decline near term.[34, 41, 127] The α glycoprotein hormone subunit may originate from cells that secrete LH, FSH, hCG, or TSH. The finding that α subunit declines postnatally[36, 136] whereas plasma LH and FSH rise, suggests that most of the α subunit that circulates in the fetus is derived from hCG.

Sexual Dimorphism

Sexual dimorphism characterizes both the prenatal and postnatal patterns of gonadotropin secretion. In the fetus, FSH levels peak at midgestation in both sexes, but FSH levels at this time are higher in female fetuses than in male fetuses (see Figures 185–3 through 185–6).[17,32,40,56,90,127,128,137] LH levels have also been reported to be higher at midgestation in females than in males[32,127,128] but not in all studies.[38, 90] The subsequent decline in LH and FSH levels with advancing gestational age occurs in both sexes, and by term, the low FSH levels are similar in males and females (see Figures 185–3 through 185–6). Cord blood concentrations of both LH and FSH are low.[40,90,132,138,139]

Reports of gonadotropin levels in the postnatal period and early infancy have varied somewhat, but some generalization seems valid. After birth, FSH levels rise markedly in girls to peak at approximately 3 months of age and usually decline to prepubertal levels by 6 to 9 months,[66] although elevated levels can persist up to 2 years.[124] In contrast, FSH levels of male infants have been reported to rise less briskly, peak at 1 week to 3 months of age at levels lower than those of females,[35, 66, 84, 124, 132, 140] and more uniformly decline to prepubertal levels by about 4 to 9 months after birth.[124,132] LH peaks in boys at approximately 1 to 3 months of age and declines to prepubertal levels by about 4 to 9 months.[66,124,132,137] Girls exhibit a similar pattern, but, in contrast to FSH, peak LH levels are generally lower than those of boys.[35, 132, 140] Similar patterns of gonadotropin secretion have been found in the ovine fetus[141] and in neonatal subhuman primates.[132,142,143]

Mechanisms Postulated to Be Responsible for Characteristic Patterns of Gonadotropin Levels in the Fetus and Neonate

The mechanisms underlying the characteristic changes in gonadotropin levels in the fetus and neonate are not fully elucidated. In the fetus, it has been suggested that rising levels of LH and FSH at midgestation reflect autonomous or unrestrained release of gonadotropins.[38, 40] The later decline in gonadotropin levels with advancing gestational age may reflect increased sensitivity to the inhibitory effects of gonadal steroids (especially in boys)[38, 40]; rising levels of circulating fetal estrogen in both sexes[40]; and reduced GnRH secretion owing to central neuro-inhibitory influences or maturation of sensitivity to sex steroids, or both.[40] Recent data from the study of 46,XY infants with androgen insensitivity syndrome (AIS) suggest that the withdrawal from the negative feedback of androgens during the neonatal transition may play a critical role in the postnatal LH and testosterone surge.[144] In a longitudinal study, infants with partial AIS mounted the expected postnatal surges, but LH and testosterone levels failed to increase in infants with complete AIS.[144] The early postnatal rise in gonadotropin levels had been postulated to reflect the loss of the negative feedback effect previously exerted by maternal estrogens. This mechanism now seems less likely in 46,XY infants, but the roles that estradiol and androgens play in regulation of the postnatal surge in 46,XX infants remains unclear.[145] After the postnatal surge, the reproductive endocrine axis enters a long period of relative, but not absolute, quiescence (often referred to as the "juvenile pause") until GnRH secretion re-emerges, leading to pubertal maturation. The factors causing the postnatal decline in gonadotropin levels are not clear. Several regulatory processes likely are involved, including central neuroinhibitory processes[116,117] and the potentially increased sensitivity of the hypothalamus and pituitary to the negative feedback effect of gonadal steroids.[40] Factors that may mediate the central inhibition include the relative predominance of γ-aminobutyric acid versus glutamate neurotransmitter activity and the inhibitory action of neuropeptide Y (NPY).[66,146] Although not fully understood, it is becoming increasingly likely that the factors responsible for the juvenile pause are not simply the mirror image of the factors that lead to reactivation of GnRH secretion with puberty.[147]

CONDITIONS ASSOCIATED WITH ABNORMALITIES OF GONADOTROPIN SECRETION IN THE FETUS AND NEONATE

Anencephaly

Anencephaly is a severe defect of neural tube development that is incompatible with long-term survival. Major portions of the nervous system are absent, usually including the hypothalamus. The pituitary gland is present but small. Although the number and size of pituitary cells appear normal at week 17 or 18 of gestation, by term gonadotrophs are almost absent.[148] The pituitary content of LH and FSH appears reduced,[17,42] and is comparable to that of 10- to 20-week fetuses.[17] The α subunit appears to be the dominant glycoprotein factor.[41,42]

Anencephalic male infants often have normally formed but small external genitalia and undescended testes. This likely reflects reduced testosterone synthesis in the latter part of gestation owing to gonadotropin deficiency. The testes have reduced numbers of Leydig cells, and the epididymis is underdeveloped.[59-61, 63] Anencephalic female fetuses have normal external genitalia, consistent with the concept that gonadotropins and ovarian secretion products are not essential for female sexual differentiation. The ovaries are small, with reduced numbers of primary follicles.[62]

In anencephalic newborn infants, basal plasma LH and FSH levels are generally low compared with normal neonates,[17, 138] and, in a limited number of studies, LH and FSH levels failed to rise after administration of exogenous GnRH.[17,98,149]

Together, these characteristics of infants with anencephaly suggest that pituitary differentiation may occur even in the absence of normal GnRH production, but that full activity and maintenance of the immature gonadotroph normally requires endogenous GnRH.

Congenital Hypothalamic and Pituitary Abnormalities

GnRH deficiency can stem from lack of GnRH secretion or from lack of pituitary responsiveness secondary to, for example, mutations in the GnRH receptor.[9] The hypogonadotropic hypogonadism can be an isolated hormonal abnormality (e.g., Kallmann syndrome and idiopathic hypogonadotropic hypogonadism) or occur in association with deficiency of other pituitary-hypothalamic hormones. As discussed previously, Kallmann syndrome is characterized by the combination of hypogonadotropic hypogonadism and anosmia (or hyposmia). Absence or abnormalities of the olfactory bulbs have been described in this condition[150] and failure of GnRH neurons to migrate from the olfactory placode to the hypothalamus during embryonic development appears to account for hypogonadotropic hypogonadism in these patients.[20] Kallmann syndrome can occur sporadically or be transmitted through X-linked, autosomal dominant, or autosomal recessive inheritance, with some cases of X-linked transmission stemming from mutations in the KAL1 gene.[151, 152] Aside from anosmia, patients with Kallmann syndrome also can exhibit mirror movements and unilateral renal agenesis in addition to physical (genital) manifestations of hypogonadotropic hypogonadism (described later in this section).[152] Rare cases of other genetic abnormalities (such as mutations in DAX-1, PC-1, leptin, and the leptin receptor) also have been associated with GnRH deficiency.[9]

Gonadotropin deficiency (LH and FSH deficiency) also can arise from abnormalities of the pituitary gland. Congenital hypopituitarism, often involving multiple pituitary hormones, may be idiopathic or associated with underlying defects, such as midline defects and/or optic nerve hypoplasia. As discussed previously, rare mutations in critical developmental factors underlie some cases of hypopituitarism.[23, 27, 28] In addition, FSH and LH deficiency can derive from mutations in either the β subunit of these hormones or in the LH and FSH receptors.[9]

Many features of gonadotropin deficiency will not be apparent in the neonatal period. At birth, girls with congenital GnRH or gonadotropin deficiency have normal external genitalia because, as noted, female sexual differentiation does not appear to require GnRH, LH-FSH, or ovarian hormones. Males with congenital GnRH or gonadotropin deficiency (whether isolated or associated with other pituitary hormone deficiencies), tend to have microphallus and undescended testes.[57,58] Infants with Kallmann syndrome and other forms of gonadotropin deficiency have been reported to show low basal gonadotropin levels and subnormal gonadotropin responses to GnRH,[17,57,58] although some variability has been noted.[57,58] Male infants with LH receptor abnormalities are unable fully to stimulate testosterone production in response to LH or hCG signaling and can present with phenotypes ranging from complete failure of virilization to hypospadias and/or microphallus.[9] Of note, because neonates with congenital growth hormone and adrenocorticotropic hormone (ACTH) deficiency are prone to develop hypoglycemia, the association of hypoglycemia and microphallus—particularly in a full-term infant—should alert the physician to the possibility of congenital panhypopituitarism.

Gonadal Failure

Gonadal differentiation and its abnormalities are described in another chapter. In this section, we refer to gonadal failure as absence of normal gonadal development or inability of the gonad to produce sex steroid, and we discuss the effects of such failure on gonadotropin secretion.

Elevated circulating levels of gonadotropins have been found in neonates and infants with gonadal failure.[118, 120] In these conditions, the elevation of gonadotropins represents an appropriate response to the primary deficiency of gonadal products. For example, in the syndrome of gonadal dysgenesis (Turner syndrome), levels of FSH and, to a lesser extent, LH are elevated above the normal range during infancy.[118] This finding is consistent with the concept that the negative feedback loop between the gonad and the hypothalamic-pituitary unit is intact in the newborn infant. In Turner syndrome, gonadotropin levels decline somewhat after age 4 years, even despite continuing gonadal failure,[118] suggesting that both central processes and gonadal factors contribute to the inhibition of gonadotropin secretion in the prepubertal child.

Similarly, elevation of basal and stimulated gonadotropin levels has been described in male infants with anorchia, rudimentary testes,[153] and other forms of primary testicular failure.[154] Interpretation of the normality of basal gonadotropin levels must be related to the age of the child. Boys with anorchia have elevated concentrations of basal gonadotropins, particularly FSH, from infancy to 4 years. The levels of gonadotropins then decrease somewhat until 9 years of age, at which time they rise and remain elevated during adulthood. The levels of FSH are lower than those seen in girls with gonadal dysgenesis. This may be attributable to the effect of fetal testosterone on the fetal hypothalamus.[73] Male infants with certain forms of androgen resistance may have elevation of LH.[155] Although many congenital disorders are associated with ambiguous genitalia or hypogonadism, information regarding associated perinatal gonadotropin secretion is often lacking.

Prematurity and Small-for-Gestational Age Status

The effects of prematurity on gonadotropin secretion are not fully understood. In preterm females, cord blood levels of LH and FSH were found to be elevated and declined with advancing gestational age to term.[156, 157] A similar but less striking pattern was observed by some[156] but not all[157, 158] studies of male newborn infants. For the first 10 postnatal weeks, serum levels of LH and FSH are higher in premature infant girls than in full-term girls; no difference in gonadotropin levels between premature and term male infants has been noted.[156, 159] Hypersecretion of FSH has been reported in infants born small for gestational age.[160]

REFERENCES

1. Hyyppa M: Hypothalamic monoamines in human fetuses. Neuroendocrinology 9:257, 1972.
2. Kuhlenbeck H: The Human Diencephalon—A Summary of Development, Structure, Function, and Pathology. New York, Karger, 1954.
3. Lemire RJ: Embryology of the central nervous system. In Davis JA, Dobbins J (eds): Scientific Foundations of Paediatrics. Philadelphia, WB Saunders, 1974, p 547.
4. O'Rahilly R, Gardener E: The timing and sequence of events in the development of the human nervous system during the embryonic period proper. Z Anat Entwicklungsgesch 134:1, 1971.
5. Papez JW: The embryologic development of the hypothalamic area in mammals. Res Publ Assoc Nerv Ment Dis 20:31, 1940.
6. Ronnekleiv OK, Resko JA: Ontogeny of gonadotropin-releasing hormone-containing neurons in early development of rhesus Macaques. Endocrinology 126:598, 1990.
7. Schwanzel-Fakuda M, Pfaff DW: Origin of luteinizing hormone–releasing hormone neurons. Nature 338:161, 1989.
8. Kim KH, et al: Gonadotropin-releasing hormone immunoreactivity in the adult and fetal human olfactory system. Brain Res 826:220, 1999.
9. Achermann JC, et al: Genetic causes of human reproductive disease. J Clin Endocrinol Metab 87:2447, 2002.
10. Kelley CG, et al: The Otx2 homeoprotein regulates expression from the gonadotropin-releasing hormone proximal promoter. Mol Endocrinol 14:1246, 2000.
11. Wolfe A, et al: Identification of a discrete promoter region of the human GnRH gene that is sufficient for directing neuron-specific expression: a role for POU homeodomain transcription factors. Mol Endocrinol 16:435, 2002.
12. Winters AJ, et al: Concentration and distribution of TRH and LRH in the human fetal brain. J Clin Endocrinol Metab 39:960, 1974.
13. Aubert ML, et al: The ontogenesis of human fetal hormones: IV. somatostatin, luteinizing hormone releasing factor, and thyrotropin releasing factor in hypothalamus and cerebral cortex of human fetuses 10-22 weeks of age. J Clin Endocrinol Metab 44:1130, 1977.
14. Bugnon C, et al: Cyto-immunological study of the ontogenesis of the gonadotropic hypothalamo-pituitary axis in the human fetus. J Steroid Biochem 8:565, 1977.
15. Clements JA, et al: Ontogenesis of gonadotropin-releasing hormone in the human fetal hypothalamus. Proc Soc Exp Biol Med 163:437, 1980.
16. Gilmore DP, et al: Presence and activity of LHRH in the mid-term human fetus. J Reprod Fertil 52:355, 1978.
17. Kaplan SL, et al: The ontogenesis of pituitary hormones and hypothalamic factors in the human fetus: maturation of central nervous system regulation of anterior pituitary function. Recent Prog Horm Res 32:161, 1976.
18. Asa SL, et al: Human fetal adenohypophysis: morphologic and functional analysis in vitro. Neuroendocrinology 53:562, 1991.
19. Schwanzel-Fukuda M, et al: Ontogenesis of neurons producing luteinizing hormone–releasing hormone (LHRH) in the nervus terminalis of the rat. J Comp Neurol 238:348, 1985.
20. Schwanzel-Fukuda M, et al: Luteinizing hormone–releasing hormone (LHRH) expressing cells do not migrate normally in an inherited hypogonadal (Kallmann) syndrome. Mol Brain Res 6:311, 1989.
21. Aksel S, Tyrey L: Luteinizing hormone–releasing hormone in the human fetal brain. Fertil Steril 28:1067, 1977.
22. Siler-Khodr TM: Studies in human fetal endocrinology: I. luteinizing hormone–releasing factor content of the hypothalamus. Am J Obstet Gynecol 130:795, 1978.
23. Mullis PE: Transcription factors in pituitary development. Mol Cell Endocrinol 185:1, 2001.
24. Atwell WJ: The development of the hypophysis cerebri in man, with special reference to the pars tuberalis. Am J Anat 37:159, 1926.
25. Conklin JL: The development of the human fetal adenohypophysis. Anat Rec 160:79, 1968.
26. Daikoku S: Studies on the human foetal pituitary: 2. on the form and histological development, especially that of the anterior pituitary. Tokushima J Exp Med 5:214, 1958.
27. Cohen LE, et al: Transcription factors and hypopituitarism. Trends Endocrinol Metab 10:326, 1999.
28. Scully KM, et al: Pituitary development: regulatory codes in mammalian organogenesis. Science 295:2231, 2002.
29. Piereson M, et al: Etude de la secretion hypophysaire du foetus humain: corrélations entre morphologie et activité secretoire. Ann Endocrinol 34:418, 1973.
30. Siler-Khodr TM, Khodr GS: Hormone synthesis and release from human fetal adenohypophyses in vitro. J Clin Endocrinol Metab 39:891, 1974.
31. Baker BL, Jaffe RB: The genesis of cell types in the adenohypophysis of the human fetus as observed with immunocytochemistry. Am J Anat 143:137, 1975.
32. Clements JA, et al: Studies on human sexual development: III. fetal pituitary and serum, and amniotic fluid concentrations of LH, CG, and FSH. J Clin Endocrinol Metab 42:9, 1976.
33. Currie RW, et al: An immunocytochemical and routine electron microscopic study of LH and FSH cells in the human fetal pituitary. Am J Anat 161:281, 1981.
34. Hagen C, McNeilley AS: Identification of human luteinizing hormone, follicle-stimulating hormone, luteinizing hormone beta-subunit and gonadotrophin alpha-subunit in foetal and adult pituitary glands. J Endocrinol 67:49, 1975.
35. Hammond GL, et al: Serum steroids and pituitary hormones in infants with particular reference to testicular activity. J Clin Endocrinol Metab 49:40, 1979.
36. Kaplan SL, et al: Alpha and beta glycoprotein hormone subunits (hLH, hFSH, hCG) in the serum and pituitary of the human fetus. J Clin Endocrinol Metab 42:995, 1976.
37. Skebelskaya YB, Kuznetsova LV: Comparative data of radioimmunological and biological activity of luteinizing hormone in the hypophysis and blood serum of human fetuses. Probl Endocrinol 24:47, 1978.
38. Kaplan SL, Grumbach MM: The ontogenesis of human foetal hormones: II. luteinizing hormone (LH) and follicle stimulating hormone (FSH). Acta Endocrinol 81:808, 1976.
39. Siler-Khodr TM, Khodr GS: Studies in human fetal endocrinology: II. LH and FSH content and concentration in the pituitary. Obstet Gynecol 56:176, 1980.
40. Gluckman PD, et al: The human fetal hypothalamus and pituitary gland. In Tulchinsky D, Ryan KJ (eds): Maternal-Fetal Endocrinology. Philadelphia, WB Saunders, 1980, pp 196-232.

41. Hagen C, McNeilly AS: The gonadotropins and their subunits in foetal pituitary glands and circulation. J Steroid Biochem 8:537, 1977.
42. Dubois PM, et al: Immunocytological localization of LH, FSH, TSH and their subunits in the pituitary of normal and anencephalic human fetuses. Cell Tissue Res 191:249, 1978.
43. Begeot M, et al: Influence of gonadoliberin on the differentiation of rat gonadotrophs: an in vivo and in vitro study. Neuroendocrinology 38:217, 1984.
44. Kudo A, et al: Effects of gonadotropin-releasing hormone (GnRH) on the cytodifferentiation of gonadotropes in rat adenohypophyseal primordia in organ culture. Cell Tissue Res 276:35, 1994.
45. Castillo RH, et al: Luteinizing hormone synthesis in cultured fetal human pituitary cells exposed to gonadotropin-releasing hormone. J Clin Endocrinol Metab 75:318, 1992.
46. Matwijiw I, Faiman C: Control of gonadotropin secretion in the ovine fetus: the effects of a specific gonadotropin-releasing hormone antagonist on pulsatile luteinizing hormone secretion. Endocrinology 121:347, 1987.
47. Salazer H, et al: The human hypophysis in anencephaly: I. ultrastructure of the pars distalis. Arch Pathol 87:201, 1969.
48. Satow Y, et al: Electron microscopic studies of the anterior pituitaries and adrenal cortices of normal and anencephalic human fetuses. J Electron Microsc 21:29, 1972.
49. Gash D, et al: Comparison of gonadotroph, thyrotroph and mammotroph development in situ, in transplants and in organ culture. Neuroendocrinology 34:222, 1982.
50. Watanabe YG, Daikoku S: Immunohistochemical study on adenohypophyseal primordia in organ culture. Cell Tissue Res 166:407, 1976.
51. Mulchahey JJ, et al: Hormone production and peptide regulation of the human fetal pituitary gland. Endocrine Rev 8:406, 1987.
52. Thliveris JA, Currie RW: Observations on the hypothalamo-hypophyseal portal vasculature in the developing human fetus. Am J Anat 157:441, 1980.
53. Niemineva K: Observations on the development of the hypophyseal portal system. Acta Paediatr Scand 39:366, 1950.
54. Raiha N, Hjelt L: The correlation between the development of the hypophyseal portal system and the onset of neurosecretory activity in the human fetus and infant. Acta Paediatr Scand 72:610, 1957.
55. Rinne UK: Neurosecretory material passing into the hypophyseal portal system in the human infundibulum, and its foetal development. Acta Neurovegetativa 25:310, 1963.
56. Reyes FI, et al: Studies on human sexual development: II. fetal and maternal serum gonadotropin and sex steroid concentrations. J Clin Endocrinol Metab 38:612, 1974.
57. Evain-Brion D, et al: Diagnosis of Kallmann's syndrome in early infancy. Acta Paediatr Scand 71:937, 1982.
58. Lovinger RD, et al: Congenital hypopituitarism associated with neonatal hypoglycemia and microphallus: four cases secondary to hypothalamic hormone deficiencies. J Pediatr 87:1171, 1975.
59. Zondek LH, Zondek T: The influence of complications of pregnancy and of some congenital malformations on the reproductive organs of the male foetus and neonate. In Forest MG, Bertrand J (eds): Endocrinologie sexuelle de la periode perinatal Paris. INSERM 32:79, 1974.
60. Zondek LH, Zondek T: Observations on the testis in anencephaly with special reference to the Leydig cells. Biol Neonate 8:329, 1965.
61. Bearn JG: Anencephaly and the development of the male genital tract. Acta Paediatr Acad Sci Hung 9:159, 1968.
62. Ch'in KY: The endocrine glands of ancephalic foetuses. Chin Med J 2(Suppl):63, 1938.
63. Zondek LH, Zondek T: Ovarian hilar cells and testicular Leydig cells in anencephaly. Biol Neonate 43:211, 1983.
64. Neill JD: Minireview: GnRH and GnRH receptor genes in the human genome. Endocrinology 143:737, 2002.
65. McCann SM, Krulich L: Role of transmitters in control of anterior pituitary hormone release. In deGroot LJ (ed): Endocrinology. Philadelphia, WB Saunders, 1989, pp 117–130.
66. Terasawa EI, et al: Neurobiological mechanisms of the onset of puberty in primates. Endocr Rev 22:111, 2001.
67. Marshall JC: Regulation and gonadotropin synthesis and secretion. In Degroot J, et al (eds): Endocrinology. Philadelphia, WB Saunders, 2001, pp 1916–1925.
68. Rosenfield RL: Puberty in the female and its disorders. In Sperling MA (ed): Pediatric Endocrinology. Philadelphia, WB Saunders, 2002, pp 455–518.
69. Belchetz PE, et al: Hypophysial responses to continuous and intermittent delivery of hypothalamic gonadotropin releasing hormone. Science 202:631, 1978.
70. deKoning JA, et al: Refractoriness of the pituitary gland after continuous exposure of luteinizing hormone releasing hormone. J Endocrinol 79:311, 1978.
71. Smith MA, Vale W: Desensitization to gonadotropin-releasing hormone observed in superfused pituitary cells on cytodex beads. Endocrinology 108:752, 1981.
72. Clayton RN, Catt KG: Gonadotropin-releasing hormone receptors: characterization, physiological regulation, and relationship to reproductive function. Endocr Rev 2:186, 1981.
73. Lustig RH, et al: Ontogeny of gonadotropin secretion in congenital anorchism: sexual dimorphism versus syndrome of gonadal dysgenesis and diagnostic considerations. J Urol 138:587, 1987.
74. Marian J, et al: Regulation of the rat pituitary gonadotropin-releasing hormone receptor. Mol Pharmacol 19:399, 1981.
75. Stojilkovic SS, Catt KJ: Expression and signal transduction pathways of gonadotropin-releasing hormone receptors. Rec Prog Horm Res 50:161, 1995.
76. Conn PM: GnRH regulation of gonadotropin release and target cell responsiveness. In de Groot LJ (ed): Endocrinology. Philadelphia, WB Saunders, 1989, pp 284–295.
77. Bourguinon JP, Frandrimont P: The gonadotropins. In De Groot LJ (ed): Endocrinology. Philadelphia, WB Saunders, 1989, pp 296–317.
78. Karsch FJ: Central actions of ovarian steroids in the feedback regulation of pulsatile secretion of luteinizing hormone. Annu Rev Physiol 49:365, 1987.
79. Reichlin S: Neuroendocrinology. In Wilson JD, Foster DW (eds): Williams Textbook of Endocrinology. Philadelphia, WB Saunders, 1985, pp 492–567.
80. Hall JE, Crowley WF: Gonadotropins and the gonad: normal physiology and their disturbances in clinical endocrine diseases. In de Groot L (ed): Endocrinology, 3rd ed. Philadelphia, WB Saunders, 1995, pp 242–258.
81. Lincoln DW: Luteinizing hormone–releasing hormone. In de Groot LJ (ed): Endocrinology, 3rd ed. Philadelphia, WB Saunders, 1995, pp 218–229.
82. Hayes FJ, et al: Aromatase inhibition in the human male reveals a hypothalamic site of estrogen feedback. J Clin Endocrinol Metab 85:3027, 2000.
83. Hayes FJ, et al: Differential regulation of gonadotropin secretion by testosterone in the human male: absence of a negative feedback effect of testosterone on follicle-stimulating hormone secretion. J Clin Endocrinol Metab 86:53, 2001.
84. Grumbach MM: The neuroendocrinology of human puberty revisited. Horm Res 57(suppl 2):2, 2002.
85. Dumesic DA, et al: Estradiol sensitization of cultured human fetal pituitary cells to gonadotropin-releasing hormone. J Clin Endocrinol Metab 65:1147, 1987.
86. Goodyer CG, et al: Human fetal pituitary in culture: hormone secretion and response to somatostatin, luteinizing hormone releasing factor, thyrotrophin releasing factor and dibutyryl cyclic AMP. J Clin Endocrinol Metab 45:73, 1977.
87. Groom GV, Boyns AR: Effect of hypothalamic releasing factors and steroids on release of gonadotropins by organ cultures of human fetal pituitaries. J Endocrinol 59:511, 1973.
88. Pasteels JL, et al: Synthesis and release of gonadotropins and their subunits by long-term organ cultures of human fetal hypophyses. Mol Cell Endocrinol 9:1, 1977.
89. Delitala G, et al: Effect of LRH on gonadotropin secretion in newborn male infants. J Clin Endocrinol Metab 46:689, 1978.
90. Takagi S, et al: Sex differences in fetal gonadotropins and androgens. J Steroid Biochem 8:609, 1977.
91. Huhtaniemi IT, et al: Stimulation of pituitary-testicular function with gonadotropin-releasing hormone in fetal and infant monkeys. Endocrinology 105:109, 1979.
92. Sopelak VM, Hodgen GD: Infusion of gonadotropin-releasing hormone agonist during pregnancy: maternal and fetal responses in primates. Am J Obstet Gynecol 156:755, 1987.
93. Mueller PL, et al: Hormone ontogeny in the ovine fetus: IX. luteinizing hormone (LH) and follicle-stimulating hormone responses to LH-releasing factor in mid- and late gestation and in the neonate. Endocrinology 108:881, 1981.
94. Yonekura ML, et al: Changing pituitary response to gonadotropin releasing hormone in fetal and infant primates (Abstract 208). In Scientific Abstracts of the Twenty-Seventh Annual Meeting of the Society for Gynecology Investigation, Denver, 1980.
95. Gennser G, et al: Pituitary hormone levels in plasma of the human fetus after administration of LRH. J Clin Endocrinol Metab 43:470, 1976.
96. Dunkel L, et al: Responsiveness of the pituitary-testicular axis to gonadotropin-releasing hormone and chorionic gonadotropin during the first week of life. Pediatr Res 18:1085, 1984.
97. Betend B, et al: Étude de la fonction gonadotrope hypophysaire par le test à la LH-RH pendant la première année de la vie. Ann Endocrinol (Paris) 36:325, 1975.
98. Furuhashi N, et al: Effects of synthetic LH-RH and TRH on pituitary function in anencephalic infants. Gynecol Obstet Invest 11:231, 1980.
99. Garnier PE, et al: Effect of synthetic luteinizing hormone–releasing hormone (LH-RH) on the release of gonadotrophins in children and adolescents: VI. relations to age, sex and puberty. Acta Endocrinol 77:422, 1974.
100. Suwa S, et al: Serum LH and FSH responses to synthetic LH-RH in normal infants, children and patients with Turner's syndrome. Pediatrics 54:470, 1974.
101. Tapanainen J, et al: Effect of gonadotropin-releasing hormone on pituitary-gonadal function of male infants during the first year of life. J Clin Endocrinol Metab 55:689, 1982.
102. Jaffe RB, et al: Peptide regulation of pituitary and target tissue function and growth in the primate fetus. Rec Prog Horm Res 44:431, 1988.
103. Marian J, Conn PM: Subcellular localization of the receptor for gonadotropin-releasing hormone in pituitary and ovarian tissue. Endocrinology 112:104, 1983.
104. Savoie S, et al: Perinatal activity of the hypothalamic-pituitary-gonadal axis in the lamb: III. LH, testosterone and prolactin secretory pattern in newborn lambs. Horm Res 15:167, 1981.

105. Plant TM: Pulsatile luteinizing hormone secretion in the neonatal male rhesus monkey. J Endocrinol *93*:71, 1982.
106. Jennes L: Prenatal development of gonadotropin-releasing hormone receptors in the rat anterior pituitary. Endocrinology *126*:942, 1990.
107. Aubert ML, et al: Ontogeny of hypothalamic luteinizing hormone–releasing hormone (GnRH) and pituitary GnRH receptors in fetal and neonatal rats. Endocrinology *116*:1565, 1985.
108. Siler-Khodr TM, Khodr GS: Content of luteinizing hormone–releasing factor in the human placenta. Am J Obstet Gynecol *130*:216, 1978.
109. Bettendorf M, et al: A neuroexcitatory amino acid analogue, *N*-methyl-D, L-aspartate (NMDA), elicits LH and FSH release in the ovine fetus by a central mechanism (Abstract 1071). 70th Annual Meeting of the Endocrine Society, 1988.
110. Cuttler L, et al: Hormone ontogeny in the ovine fetus: XVIII. the effect of an opioid antagonist on luteinizing hormone secretion. Endocrinology *116*:1997, 1985.
111. Ellinwood WE, et al: The effects of gonadectomy and testosterone treatment on luteinizing hormone secretion in fetal rhesus monkeys. Endocrinology *110*:183, 1982.
112. Resko JA, Ellinwood WE: Negative feedback regulation of gonadotropin secretion by androgens in fetal rhesus macaques. Biol Reprod *33*:346, 1985.
113. Winter JS, et al: The role of gonadal steroids in feedback regulation of gonadotropin secretion at different stages of primate development. Acta Endocrinol *114*:257, 1987.
114. Gluckman PD, et al: Hormone ontogeny in the ovine fetus: XIV. the effect of 17 beta-estradiol infusion on fetal plasma gonadotropins and prolactin and the maturation of sex steroid–dependent negative feedback. Endocrinology *112*:1618, 1983.
115. Plant TM: A striking sex difference in the gonadotropin response to gonadectomy during infantile development in the rhesus monkey (*Macaca mulatta*). Endocrinology *119*:539, 1986.
116. Plant TM: The effects of neonatal orchidectomy on the developmental pattern of gonadotropin secretion in the male rhesus monkey (*Macaca mulatta*). Endocrinology *106*:1451, 1980.
117. Plant TM: A study of the role of the postnatal testes in determining the ontogeny of gonadotropin secretion in the male rhesus monkey (*Macaca mulatta*). Endocrinology *116*:1341, 1985.
118. Conte FA, et al: A diphasic pattern of gonadotropin secretion in patients with the syndrome of gonadal dysgenesis. J Clin Endocrinol Metab *40*:670, 1975.
119. Trotter A, et al: Effects of postnatal estradiol and progesterone replacement in extremely preterm infants. J Clin Endocrinol Metab *84*:4531, 1999.
120. Ropelato MG, et al: Gonadotropin secretion in prepubertal normal and agonadal children evaluated by ultrasensitive time-resolved immunofluorometric assays. Horm Res *48*:164, 1997.
121. Petraglia F, et al: Localization, secretion, and action of inhibin in human placenta. Science *237*:187, 1987.
122. Albers N, et al: Hormone ontogeny in the ovine fetus: XXIV. porcine follicular fluid "inhibins" selectively suppress plasma follicle-stimulating hormone in the ovine fetus. Endocrinology *125*:675, 1989.
123. Massa G, et al: Serum levels of immunoreactive inhibin, FSH, and LH in human infants at preterm and term birth. Biol Neonate *61*:150, 1992.
124. Andersson AM, et al: Longitudinal reproductive hormone profiles in infants: peak of inhibin A levels in infant boys exceeds levels in adult men. J Clin Endocrinol Metab *83*:675, 1998.
125. Byrd W, et al: Regulation of biologically active dimeric inhibin A and B from infancy to adulthood in the male. J Clin Endocrinol Metab *83*:2849, 1998.
126. Rivier C, et al: Age-dependent changes in physiological action, content, and immunostaining of inhibin in male rats. Endocrinology *123*:120, 1988.
127. Beck-Peccoz P, et al: Maturation of hypothalamic-pituitary-gonadal function in normal human fetuses: circulating levels of gonadotropins, their common α-subunit and free testosterone, and discrepancy between immunological and biological activities of circulating follicle-stimulating hormone. J Clin Endocrinol Metab *73*:525, 1991.
128. Debieve F, et al: Gonadotropins, prolactin, inhibin A, inhibin B, and activin A in human fetal serum from midpregnancy and term pregnancy. J Clin Endocrinol Metab *85*:270, 2000.
129. Tseng MT, et al: Effects of fetal decapitation on the structure and function of Leydig cells in rhesus monkeys (*Macaca mulatta*). Am J Anat *143*:349, 1975.
130. Burger HG, et al: Serum gonadotropin, sex steroid, and immunoreactive inhibin levels in the first two years of life. J Clin Endocrinol Metab *72*:682, 1991.
131. Winter JSD, et al: Pituitary-gonadal relations in infancy: 2. patterns of serum gonadal steroid concentrations in man from birth to two years of age. J Clin Endocrinol Metab *42*:679, 1976.
132. Winter JSD, et al: Pituitary-gonadal relations in infancy: 1. patterns of serum gonadotropin concentrations from birth to four years of age in man and chimpanzee. J Clin Endocrinol Metab *42*:545, 1975.
133. Clark SJ, et al: Hormone ontogeny in the ovine fetus: XVII. demonstration of pulsatile luteinizing hormone secretion by the fetal pituitary gland. Endocrinology *115*:1774, 1984.
134. Waldhauser F, et al: Pulsatile secretion of gonadotropins in early infancy. Eur J Pediatr *137*:71, 1981.
135. de Zegher F, et al: Pulsatile and sexually dimorphic secretion of luteinizing hormone in the human infant on the day of birth. Pediatr Res *32*:605, 1993.
136. Styne DM, et al: Plasma glycoprotein hormone alpha-subunit in the neonate and in prepubertal and pubertal children: effects of luteinizing hormone-releasing hormone. J Clin Endocrinol Metab *50*:450, 1980.
137. Gendrel D, et al: Simultaneous postnatal rise of plasma LH and testosterone in male infants. J Pediatr *80*:600, 1980.
138. Furuhashi N, et al: Concentrations of luteinizing hormone–human chorionic gonadotropin, beta subunit of human chorionic gonadotropin, follicle-stimulating hormone, estradiol, cortisol, and testosterone in cord sera and their correlations. Am J Obstet Gynecol *143*:918, 1982.
139. Penny R, et al: Follicle stimulating hormone (FSH) and luteinizing hormone–human chorionic gonadotropin (LH-HCG) concentrations in paired maternal and cord sera. Pediatrics *53*:41, 1974.
140. Forest MG, et al: Hypophyso-gonadal function in humans during the first year of life. J Clin Invest *53*:819, 1974.
141. Sklar CA, et al: Hormone ontogeny in the ovine fetus: VII. circulating luteinizing-hormone and follicle-stimulating hormone in mid- and late gestation. Endocrinology *108*:874, 1981.
142. Frawley LS, Neill JD: Age-related changes in serum levels of gonadotropins and testosterone in infantile male rhesus monkeys. Biol Reprod *20*:1147, 1979.
143. Fuller GB, et al: Sex-dependent gonadotropin concentrations in infant chimpanzees and rhesus monkeys. Proc Soc Exp Biol Med *169*:494, 1982.
144. Bouvattier C, et al: Postnatal changes of T, LH, and FSH in 46,XY infants with mutations in the AR gene. J Clin Endocrinol Metab *87*:29, 2002.
145. Quigley CA: Editorial: The postnatal gonadotropin and sex steroid surge—insights from the androgen insensitivity syndrome. J Clin Endocrinol Metab *87*:24, 2002.
146. Majdoubi ME, et al: Neuropeptide Y: a hypothalamic brake restraining the onset of puberty in primates. Proc Natl Acad Sci U S A *97*:6179, 2000.
147. Majdoubi ME, et al: Changes in hypothalamic gene expression associated with the arrest of pulsatile gonadotropin-releasing hormone release during infancy in the agonadal male rhesus monkey (*Macaca mulatta*). Endocrinology *141*:3273, 2000.
148. Pilavdzic D, et al: Pituitary morphology in anencephalic human fetuses. Neuroendocrinology *65*:164, 1997.
149. Cavallo L, et al: Endocrine function in four anencephalic infants. Horm Res *15*:159, 1981.
150. De Morsier G: Etudes sur les dysraphes cranio-encephaliques. Schweiz Arch Neurol Psychiatr *74*:309, 1954.
151. Oliveira LM, et al: The importance of autosomal genes in Kallmann syndrome: genotype-phenotype correlations and neuroendocrine characteristics. J Clin Endocrinol Metab *86*:1532, 2001.
152. Quinton R, et al: Idiopathic gonadotrophin deficiency: genetic questions addressed through phenotypic characterization. Clin Endocrinol (Oxf) *55*:163, 2001.
153. Acquafredda A, et al: Rudimentary testes syndrome revisited. Pediatrics *80*:209, 1987.
154. Dunkel L, et al: Hypergonadotropic hypogonadism in newborn males with primary testicular failure. Acta Paediatr Scand *73*:740, 1984.
155. Lee PA, et al: Diagnosis of the partial androgen insensitivity syndrome during infancy. JAMA *255*:2207, 1986.
156. Shinkawa O, et al: Changes of serum gonadotropin levels and sex differences in premature and mature infants during neonatal life. J Clin Endocrinol Metab *56*:1327, 1987.
157. Tapainen J, et al: Hormonal changes during the perinatal period: FSH, prolactin and some steroid hormones in the cord blood and peripheral serum of preterm and fullterm female infants. J Steroid Biochem *20*:1153, 1984.
158. Tapainen J: Hormonal changes during the perinatal period: serum testosterone, some of its precursors, and FSH and prolactin in preterm and full-term male infant cord blood and during the first week of life. J Steroid Biochem *18*:13, 1983.
159. Tapanainen J, et al: Enhanced activity of the pituitary-gonadal axis in premature human infants. J Clin Endocrinol Metab *52*:235, 1981.
160. Ibanez L, et al: Hypersecretion of FSH in infant boys and girls born small for gestational age. J Clin Endocrinol Metab *87*:1986, 2002.

James C. Rose, Jeffrey Schwartz, and Sharla Young

Development of the Corticotropin-Releasing Hormone–Corticotropin/β-Endorphin System in the Mammalian Fetus

Corticotropin-releasing hormone (CRH) and AVP (AVP) are two hypothalamic factors that stimulate the corticotrophs of the anterior pituitary to secrete corticotropin (ACTH) and other peptides derived from the protein pro-opiomelanocortin (POMC) (Figs. 186-1 and 186-2). Together, these components are part of a system, the importance of whose development extends beyond its nominal role in postnatal physiology. During gestation, timely activation of this system is required for the maturation of other organs. In contrast, inappropriate activity of this system during development is associated with fetal programming, that is, subtly adverse changes that increase the emergence of disease later in life. In this chapter, we add more recent observations on the development of the CRH-ACTH system to the information presented in the previous edition of this book.[1]

POMC, the ultimate biosynthetic precursor of ACTH, is initially cleaved to pro-ACTH and β-lipotropin (β-LPH). Pro-ACTH is subsequently cleaved to yield other biologically active peptides, including ACTH and N-POMC(1-77); both these peptides are thought to play key roles in the development and function of the fetal adrenal cortex. In corticotrophs of the anterior pituitary, the enzyme prohormone convertase 1 (PC1, also sometimes called PC3) is responsible for the generation of β-LPH, pro-ACTH, N-POMC(1-77), and ACTH from POMC. In intermediate lobe melanotrophs of some species, a second enzyme, PC2, is found, and it is responsible for further cleavage of ACTH into α-melanotropin and corticotropin-like intermediate lobe peptide (CLIP). Although β-LPH is also precursor to other peptides, the biologic relevance of these during development is largely unknown, and little emphasis is placed on them here.

Two incidental points on POMC-derived peptides are worth noting for the interpretation of results presented in this chapter and elsewhere. Immunoreactive β-endorphin (β-End) is often secreted 1:1 with ACTH and is under similar regulatory control. As such, at times β-End has been measured as an index of corticotroph activity. Immunoassays for ACTH use antibodies raised against ACTH(1-39) or portions thereof. Because these amino acid sequences are present in other peptides (e.g., POMC), which react to a greater or lesser extent with the antibodies, *immunoreactive* ACTH may not always refer to ACTH(1-39) only.

DEVELOPMENTAL ANATOMY, BIOCHEMISTRY, AND REGULATION

Corticotropin-Releasing Hormone

The neurovascular link between the hypothalamus and pituitary is present by 12 weeks of gestation (0.30 G term = 40 weeks) in the human fetus, and by 16 weeks (0.40 G), nerve fibers weakly stained by antiserum to CRH are present in the rostral part of the median eminence. The CRH fibers increase in number between 18 and 30 weeks of gestation, and terminal dilatations in perivascular areas can be observed by mid-gestation. Cell bodies containing CRH are difficult to identify and are not observed before 19 weeks (0.48 G).[1]

In some areas of the fetal hypothalamus, there is a very similar distribution of fibers containing CRH and projections containing AVP, and certain fibers stain with antisera to both peptides. Thus, it is possible that CRH and AVP are co-localized in fetal hypothalamic neurons in a fashion similar to that observed in adults.[1]

The placenta is another source of CRH for the human fetus. Immunoreactive and bioactive CRH-like activity has been identified in the placenta,[1,2] and immunoreactive CRH has been localized to the syncytiotrophoblast and intermediate trophoblast layers.[1,2] Moreover, CRH mRNA is also present in the human placenta, and levels increase over the last 5 weeks of gestation.[2,3] Several factors may play a role in regulating the expression of CRH in the placenta, including glucocorticoids, progesterone, and possibly estrogen. In humans, the CRH gene is found on chromosome 8, and there is substantial conservation in the promoter region among different species.[2,4] Regulatory sequences identified on the promoter include cyclic adenosine monophosphate (cAMP), half estrogen, and ecdysone regulatory elements. The cAMP element appears functional because both forskolin (which increases cAMP) and the cAMP analogue 8-Br-cAMP increase the expression of CRH in syncytiotrophoblast cells; deletion or mutation of the consensus cAMP regulatory element in placental cells transfected with the CRH promoter attenuates the response to cAMP.[2] Whereas glucocorticoids decrease expression of CRH in the hypothalamus, they increase expression in the placenta. This positive effect on expression appears mediated by the cAMP regulatory element because mutation of this regulatory element abolishes the stimulatory effect of dexamethasone on promoter activity in transfected placental cells.[2]

The physiologic role of placental CRH is a topic of active investigation and debate. CRH is a more potent vasodilator than prostacyclin in the human fetal placental circulation, and the peptide may act through a nitric oxide–mediated path.[5] The high levels of CRH in maternal blood in conditions associated with poor umbilical or placental perfusion suggest a role for CRH in mediating the vascular tone of the placenta during hypoxia or ischemia.[5] CRH has several important interactions with other peptides and prostanoids found in the placenta. For example, prostaglandins F_{2a} and E_2, which play an important role in labor, are both stimulated by and potentiate CRH release. The effects of oxytocin on myometrial contractility are potentiated by CRH, and the peptide causes the release of oxytocin from placental cells.

CRH exerts its effect by binding to two different types of receptors: CRH-R1 and CRH-R2. Both these receptors have isoforms, and evidence suggests both types are found in placental tissue.[5] The CRH-R2 type has also been identified in myometrium from pregnant but not from nonpregnant women.[5] Agents including certain cytokines, glucocorticoids, neurotransmitters, and peptides stimulate CRH release, whereas nitric oxide and progesterone inhibit release from placental tissues.[6]

In humans, immunoreactive CRH is in fetal cord blood. The levels of CRH are higher in the umbilical vein than in the umbilical artery, and the CRH concentration in fetal plasma is significantly lower than, but correlated with, maternal plasma

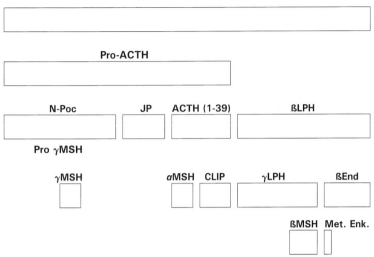

Figure 186–1. Schematic representation of the pro-opiomelanocortin (POMC). N-Poc (also called pro γMSH) is the aminoterminal end of POMC. CLIP = corticotropin-like intermediate lobe peptide; JP = joining peptide; LPH = lipotropic hormone; Met. Enk. = methionine enkephalin; MSH = melanocyte-stimulating hormone.

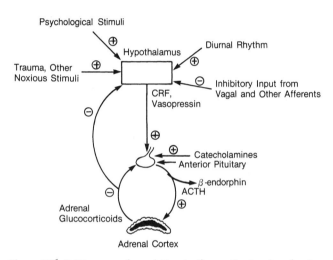

Figure 186–2. Diagram of regulation in the corticotropin-releasing factor (CRF)/corticotropin (ACTH)/β-endorphin (β-End) axis. (Redrawn from Gannog W: Review of Medical Physiology, 13th ed. Norwalk, CT, Appleton & Lange, 1987, p 314.)

concentrations.[1] Plasma levels of CRH are low in pregnant women (<50 pg/mL) and increase 15- to 18-fold in late pregnancy. After delivery, maternal plasma levels of the peptide decline rapidly.[5] Maternal and umbilical cord plasma CRH levels are greater in preterm deliveries, intrauterine growth retardation, and preeclampsia.[5] Taken together, these observations imply that the placenta secretes CRH into the fetal and maternal circulation and that plasma levels of CRH may be an index of the well-being of the fetus.

The observation that women in the last trimester of pregnancy have very high levels of plasma CRH, whereas ACTH and cortisol levels remain in the normal range, was a paradox until the existence of a binding protein for CRH was reported. This binding protein inhibits the ACTH-releasing activity of CRH. In humans, CRH binding protein (CRH-BP) is synthesized in the liver, placenta, and brain. After association with CRH, the binding protein dimerizes. In the presence of low concentrations of CRH, only a single protein molecule is bound to the binding protein; however, in the presence of a large excess of CRH, the dimer is able to bind two CRH molecules. During the last few weeks of pregnancy, the concentration of this binding protein

decreases, resulting in an increase in the levels of free CRH. The proposed function of the CRH-BP is to modulate the action of placental, hypothalamic, and other CRH secretory sites in the brain.[1]

In the placenta, CRH-BP is produced by the external layer of the placental villi, the target cells of locally produced CRH. CRH-BP mRNA and protein expression are also localized in the amnion, chorion, and maternal decidua; all these tissues also produce CRH. This local production of CRH-BP in the placenta suggests an important role in the autocrine and paracrine regulation of CRH. Although CRH-BP has been found to be important in the regulation of free CRH during pregnancy, the binding protein is also found in men and in nonpregnant women.[1] This observation has led to the suggestion that CRH-BP may bind a new family of CRH-like proteins that may be important in peripheral or immunologic functions.

In the ovine fetal hypothalamus, CRH-containing neurons have also been identified. Although it was initially thought that they appear much later in development than they do in humans, it now seems the CRH-containing neurons appear at a similar stage in gestation in both species (0.38 G versus 0.34 G, respectively). Neurons containing AVP are identified by 0.29 G in the external layer of the ovine median eminence. Thus, there does not appear to be a significant difference in the time of appearance of these two peptides in the developing ovine hypothalamus.

Both CRH peptide and mRNA levels are increased close to term (Fig. 186–3) in the fetal sheep hypothalamus. Within the paraventricular nucleus, a region-specific change in CRH mRNA expression has been noted. In other regions of the fetal brain (hippocampal-amygdala complex and frontal cortex), CRH mRNA levels remain relatively constant, but the peptide increases in late gestation. In the brain stem, where CRH is important for autonomic functions, CRH mRNA expression does not change during gestation, but the polyadenylation pattern of CRH mRNA in the hypothalamus does change.[1] The physiologic significance of this increase in poly A tail length is not known for certain, but it may be related to an increase in the stability or translatability of the message.

Manipulations such as adrenalectomy and glucocorticoid implants have led to further understanding of the physiologic mechanisms underlying the regulation of CRH peptide and gene expression in the fetal hypothalamus. These experiments led to the conclusion that, in the fetus, CRH expression is regulated by glucocorticoid negative feedback, similar to the regulation found in adults. However, the efficacy of glucocorticoid negative feedback may decrease with increasing gestational age. This decrease

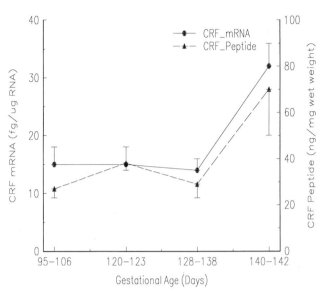

Figure 186–3. Changes in hypothalamic corticotropin-releasing factor (CRF) mRNA and peptide during development in the fetal sheep. Both message and peptide increase at term. (Redrawn from Keiger CJ, et al: Mol Brain Res 27:103, 1994.)

in negative feedback efficacy could explain why, in spite of high plasma cortisol levels, the hypothalamic drive stimulating ACTH secretion does not decrease in the late-gestation fetus. Any link between CRH message levels and peptide secretion remains unclear.

Corticotropin/β-Endorphin

Bearing in mind the potential problems with immunohistochemical localization of components of the protein POMC, cells containing ACTH, α-melanocyte–stimulating hormone (α-MSH), β-LPH, and β-End have been identified in the human fetal pituitary. The cells containing ACTH, β-End, and β-LPH appear by 8 weeks of gestation, whereas cells staining for α-MSH have been reported at 13 weeks (0.32 G). As one would expect, because of the common parent molecule, it has been possible to co-localize ACTH, β-End, and β-LPH. Cells containing these peptides are also found in the pituitaries of anencephalic fetuses, a finding suggesting that the hypothalamus is not essential for the expression of these hormones in early development. Indeed, the observation that mice lacking either CRH or the CRH-R1 receptor have a normal complement of corticotrophs further emphasizes that corticotroph development can occur without CRH action on the pituitary.[7]

Similar localization studies have been conducted with the fetal sheep pituitary, and corresponding results have been obtained. Anterior lobe cells staining positive for ACTH and β-End/β-LPH have been identified by 0.26 G, and the same cells react with antisera to the three peptides; that is, the peptides are co-localized. There are developmental changes in the morphology of ovine fetal pituitary corticotrophs possibly analogous to the changes described in corticotrophs in the human fetal pituitary.

As noted earlier, PC1 and PC2 are the enzymes in the pituitary responsible for the posttranslational cleavage of POMC.[8] These enzymes are serine proteases of the subtilisin/kexin type that cleave at basic amino acids. PC1 is present in anterior lobe corticotrophs, and its actions ultimately produce N-POMC(1–77),

ACTH(1–39), and a sequence found between these peptides called joining peptide (JP) (see Fig. 186–1). Removal of further amino acids from N-POMC(1–77) means that it is sometimes found as N-POMC(1–76) and N-POMC(1–74). PC2 and its associated binding protein 7B2 are present in intermediate lobe melanotrophs. The ontogeny of PC1 and PC2 is of critical importance because the activity of these enzymes in the endocrine cells determines the biologic activity of the secretory product.

There is some controversy in the literature regarding developmental changes in the posttranslational processing of the POMC molecule in the human fetal pituitary. Initially, it was thought that small amounts of ACTH and large amounts of α-MSH and CLIP were present between 12 and 38 weeks of gestation (0.30 to 0.95 G). However, these results have not been confirmed. Other investigators have reported that when pituitary extracts from fetuses of between 12 and 22 (0.30 to 0.55 G) weeks were subjected to gel filtration chromatography and the fractions obtained were analyzed by radioimmunoassay, the levels of ACTH were always higher than the α-MSH concentrations. The concentrations of β-End and β-LPH were also substantial in the fetal pituitary. Using high-performance liquid chromatography for the separation of the various components of the POMC molecule in combination with radioimmunoassay for the measurement of ACTH, α-MSH, and β-End, Brubaker and colleagues[9] demonstrated no correlation between gestational age and fetal pituitary content of ACTH and α-MSH. In contrast, the content of β-End increased as gestational age increased. These studies were done with pituitaries from fetuses between 11 and 19 weeks (0.28 to 0.48 G) of gestation. A similar age-related increase in β-End was also noted by Fachinetti and colleagues.[10] It has been reported that, in human anterior pituitaries, the proportion of immunoreactive ACTH of molecular weight 4500, likely ACTH(1–39), is higher in adults than fetuses, and the proportion of high molecular weight ACTH, likely POMC, falls progressively from fetuses to infants to adults.[11] Therefore, the majority of evidence indicates that some changes in POMC processing occur during development, and ACTH and β-End are found in the human fetal pituitary from early in gestation. Thus, ACTH could provide tropic and trophic stimulation to the fetal adrenal, at least from the beginning of the second trimester.

The pituitary is not the only potential source of ACTH and β-End available for the human fetus. There is compelling evidence that the placenta contains these peptides and other components of the POMC molecule. Although several investigators have demonstrated, using both radioimmunoassay and bioassay, the presence of ACTH and β-End in extracts of human placenta and fetal membranes, the relative amounts of peptides present are 100- to 1000-fold less than the quantities found in the fetal pituitary. The biosynthesis of immunologically identified ACTH and β-End has been demonstrated, and immunohistochemical staining has revealed the presence of these peptides in the syncytiotrophoblast. Additional evidence that the placenta actually synthesizes POMC-derived peptides is furnished by the report that POMC-like mRNA is present in the human placenta.

The role, if any, of these placentally derived fragments of the POMC molecule in the human fetus is unknown. The finding that the placenta can synthesize and secrete CRH, ACTH, β-End, and large quantities of steroids suggests that paracrine interactions may exist among these hormones, and some findings indicate that such is the case.

In the ovine fetus, as in the human fetus, there is evidence suggesting maturational changes in the posttranslational processing of the POMC molecule. Immunoreactive ACTH, β-End, and β-LPH have been identified in extracts of ovine fetal pituitaries after chromatographic separation of peptides of various sizes. In addition to those peptides identified according to elution profile and immunoreactivity, three major peaks of large molecular weight material with ACTH immunoreactivity are present. The relative amounts of these peaks are greater in pituitaries obtained at 0.83 G than in pituitaries obtained at 0.98 G. The changing pattern of POMC processing is not likely the result solely of the appearance of PC1.[12] Studies indicate that PC1 appears at a stage of development when processing occurs at a relatively low rate, and the levels of PC1 change little across a period of markedly increasing processing activity. In addition, glucocorticoids, which alter the *type of ACTH* that is secreted by pituitary cells,[13] have no effect on fetal pituitary levels of PC1 or PC2.[14] Together, these data suggest that the posttranslational processing of POMC depends on numerous factors in addition to the prohormone convertases.

The physiologic implications of this change in the pattern of ACTH-like peptides are potentially quite significant. These large molecular weight peptides, which cross-react with ACTH in radioimmunoassays, could have little or no biologic activity in terms of steroidogenic capacity. Thus, as the proportion of this material changes relative to the proportion of native ACTH(1–39), the ratio of bioactive to immunoreactive ACTH should change in the fetal pituitary, and this has been reported.[1] If this change in processing in the pituitary is also reflected by a change in the secretion of bioactive ACTH by the fetal corticotroph, it could explain how increased drive to fetal adrenal steroid secretion occurs before the detection of any marked change in plasma immunoreactive ACTH concentration.

Another potential effect of high molecular weight forms of ACTH is their action to inhibit ACTH induced-steroidogenesis. Some evidence suggests that this can occur. Earlier studies on possible steroidogenic actions or high molecular weight ACTH were followed by more recent assessments of biologic activity *in vivo* and *in vitro*. POMC inhibits the cortisol response to ACTH in calves *in vivo*. Moreover, POMC and pro-ACTH are both potent inhibitors of the cortisol response to ACTH in adrenal cells prepared from fetal, but not adult, sheep (Fig. 186–4).[1]

REGULATION OF CORTICOTROPIN AND β-ENDORPHIN IN THE FETUS

β-Endorphin: Studies in Humans

There have been numerous reports of the plasma concentrations of β-End in umbilical cord obtained from human fetuses at the time of delivery. Although some discrepancies regarding absolute quantities exist, there have been three consistent findings. First, when chromatography of plasma samples has been employed to separate members of the POMC family, β-End and β-LPH (see Fig. 186–1) are found in fetal plasma in higher concentrations than those observed in physiologically normal adults. Second, the fetal plasma β-End concentration when measured after chro-

matography, or β-End–like activity when measured without chromatography, is always elevated in cases of fetal distress. The third consistent finding is a reasonable correlation between ACTH and β-End concentrations when both hormones are measured simultaneously in fetal plasma. This finding suggests that the secretion of these two hormones, at least from the anterior pituitary, is under similar regulatory mechanisms in the fetus and the adult.[1] Additional support for the coordinate release of both β-End and ACTH is the observation that CRH stimulates the secretion of both peptides from human fetal pituitaries *in vitro*.

The source of the β-End circulating in fetal plasma is not known. Although there is one report that umbilical arterial levels are greater than umbilical venous levels, a finding suggesting a fetal site of origin, others have been unable to establish that such a gradient exists. Thus, a placental source for the peptide cannot be excluded. The finding that β-End does not disappear from the circulation in the newborn after delivery suggests that the fetal pituitary must make some contribution to the plasma concentrations observed in the fetus. Any β-End from the placenta should disappear from the neonatal circulation fairly rapidly, owing to the relatively short half-life of the peptide. It seems unlikely that β-End from the mother crosses the placenta to enter the fetal circulation because there is no correlation between maternal and fetal plasma concentrations of the hormone.[1]

β-Endorphin: Studies in Fetal Sheep

The regulation of β-End secretion in the fetal lamb closely resembles that of ACTH. For example, hypoxemia with or without simultaneous changes in pH increases both β-End and β-LPH concentrations. These findings are also quite consistent with those in humans concerning the effects of hypoxemia on β-End and β-LPH concentrations. When animals are studied at different stages of gestation, the β-End responses to the same hypoxemic stimulus increase as gestation progresses. A negative feedback relationship also appears to exist between cortisol and β-End because bilateral adrenalectomy, which reduces fetal plasma cortisol after 0.84 G, also increases plasma β-End at this time.[1]

Corticotropin: Studies in Humans

ACTH is found in fetal plasma by 16 weeks of gestation (0.40 G). The plasma concentration of the peptide does not change significantly between 0.40 and 0.60 G when it is measured in samples obtained at fetoscopy from fetuses later proved to be normal. However, after 0.85 G, fetal plasma ACTH levels tend to decline. This is of interest because the plasma concentrations of cortisol in the fetus tend to increase over this same period.

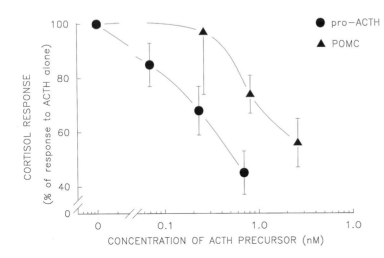

Figure 186–4. Effects of pro-corticotropin (pro-ACTH) (*circles*) and pro-opiomelanocortin (POMC) (*squares*) on the cortisol responses to ACTH(1–39) (*solid symbols* = 10^{-10}; *open symbols* = 10^{-11} M) in cultured fetal sheep adrenal cells. (Data from Schwartz J, et al: Am J Physiol *268*:E623, 1995.)

Generally, fetal plasma ACTH levels tend to be equivalent to or higher than maternal plasma concentrations.[1]

The available evidence indicates all the ACTH circulating in fetal blood originates from the pituitary. Allen and associates[15] reported undetectable levels of ACTH (<15 pg/mL) in two anencephalic infants. Similarly, Miyakawa and colleagues[16] were unable to detect ACTH in cord plasma from two anencephalic fetuses. Little ACTH appears to cross the placenta from mother to fetus because below-normal plasma ACTH concentrations have been found in fetuses whose mothers received intravenous infusion of the peptide to elevate maternal plasma concentrations two- to tenfold.[16]

In vitro studies have been conducted to determine the ontogeny of the fetal pituitary ACTH/β-End responses to various secretagogues. Using a superfusion system, Gibbs and associates[17] showed that CRH stimulated the release of ACTH and β-End from pituitaries obtained from fetuses older than 20 weeks of gestation (0.50 G). No responses to CRH were observed when pituitaries from fetuses younger than 0.50 G were examined. In contrast, in both superfusion and static incubation systems, CRH increased ACTH output from pituitary cells obtained from fetuses at 14 weeks of gestation (0.35 G). The explanation for the discrepancy between these two studies is unknown.[1]

AVP also stimulates ACTH release from the fetal pituitary, and AVP and CRH exert a synergistic effect. Incubation of pituitary cells in the presence of dexamethasone for 24 hours suppresses the basal release of ACTH from the cells, and the synthetic glucocorticoid also inhibits CRH-induced ACTH secretion. These observations suggest that ACTH secretion in the human fetus in early gestation is regulated by AVP and CRH, and negative feedback of adrenal glucocorticoids on ACTH secretion exists.

Corticotropin: Studies in Fetal Sheep

By far, most of what we know concerning regulation of the CRH-ACTH/β-End system has been derived from studies in fetal sheep. The plasma immunoreactive ACTH levels in the fetal lamb remain relatively low over the last third of gestation; however, in the 24 to 48 hours preceding parturition, a marked increase in ACTH occurs. This increase in ACTH is unique because it occurs in spite of the high levels of fetal plasma cortisol that exist at this time. The explanation for this increment in ACTH is unknown.

Studies have also examined the changing ratios of other POMC-derived peptides, such as N-POMC(1–77) and pro-ACTH (as well as POMC itself), to ACTH(1–39) as a function of gestational age and stimulation by CRH or AVP. The picture emerging is that the increase in total immunoreactive ACTH that may occur toward term is paralleled by, if not the direct result of, a small but definite increase in the concentration of ACTH(1–39) relative to either N-POMC(1–77) (Fig. 186–5) or the biosynthetic precursors POMC and pro-ACTH. A complementary finding has been observed *in vitro* with slices of anterior pituitary of fetal sheep secreting increasing amounts of ACTH(1–39) relative to precursors as a function of gestational age; these findings suggest an increasing capacity of pituitary corticotrophs to synthesize, process, and secrete ACTH(1–39) as development progresses. Indeed, when a sensitive bioassay is used to measure ACTH activity in fetal plasma, levels increase between 100 and 140 days of gestation.[18]

Although there is little compelling evidence indicating that a diurnal rhythm exists in resting fetal plasma ACTH concentrations, significant variations in plasma ACTH levels are observed when multiple blood samples are obtained from the same animal through long-term indwelling catheters. This could indicate episodic secretion or that the repetitive removal of small samples of blood is a stimulus to ACTH release in the fetus.

By mid-gestation, the fetus responds to various stimuli by increasing plasma ACTH concentrations, and there are matura-

tional changes in the ACTH responses to stress. For example, hemorrhage of 15% of estimated fetal blood volume increases plasma ACTH concentration after 0.69 G; at earlier times, this magnitude of blood loss does not activate ACTH secretion.

Drug-induced arterial hypotension has also been used to examine developmental changes in fetal ACTH responses to stress. When stimulus intensity is kept constant, there is a larger increase in fetal plasma ACTH concentration between 0.83 and 0.88 G than at earlier or later periods of development. These observations are consistent with the developmental change in β-End release after hypoxemia described earlier and suggest that mechanisms governing the responses of these two hormones to stress mature at similar rates.

Some evidence suggests that the fetal ACTH response to certain stimuli is proportional to the magnitude of the stimulus, as is the response in adults. Hemorrhage of 5% of estimated fetal blood volume causes no change in mean arterial pressure and no change in plasma ACTH concentration, whereas hemorrhage of 15% of blood volume elicits a fall in mean arterial pressure and an increase in plasma ACTH in fetuses older than 0.68 G. When mean arterial pressure is reduced in fetuses between 0.81 and 0.92 G by vena cava obstruction, plasma ACTH increases as mean arterial pressure declines. However, partial caval obstruction, which does not lower mean arterial pressure, also does not increase fetal plasma ACTH. No changes in fetal blood gases or pH were observed in these experiments. Therefore, the data indicate that fetal ACTH responses are related to the magnitude of the reduction in mean arterial pressure produced by the two manipulations.[1]

Highlighting the complexity of the regulation of ACTH secretion are studies that examined qualitative as well as quantitative changes in plasma ACTH concentration or secretion. Castro and colleagues[19] measured changes in late-gestation fetal sheep plasma ACTH in terms of biologic and immunologic activities. These investigators found that, with stressors of increasing severity, the bioactive/immunoactive (B/I) ratio increases, a finding suggesting the mobilization of relatively more bioactive ACTH with increasing stress input.[19]

Arterial hypoxemia has also been used to test responsiveness of the fetal CRH-ACTH/β-End system. Reductions in fetal arterial oxygen tension are associated with significant increases in plasma ACTH concentrations, a finding suggesting that hypoxemia is a potent stimulus to fetal ACTH secretion. However, fetal hypoxemia is frequently accompanied by a fall in fetal arterial pH and,

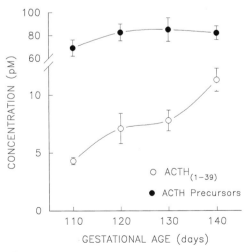

Figure 186–5. Plasma concentrations of corticotropin (ACTH) precursors and ACTH(1–39) during development in the fetal sheep. (Redrawn from Carr GA, et al: Endocrinology *136*:520, 1995.)

when this occurs, ACTH release may be a consequence of the reduction in oxygen tension, pH, or a combination of the two.

Presumably, ACTH responses to various stresses are mediated by secretagogues that act at the level of the pituitary. The impact of CRH on ovine fetal ACTH secretion has been studied by several investigators. With one exception, all agree that CRH stimulates ACTH secretion in chronically cannulated fetal lambs from approximately 0.65 G. The fetal ACTH responses to CRH vary with age, and most data indicate that responses are attenuated close to term.[1]

Age-related changes in responsiveness have also been found *in vitro*, with the largest increments in ACTH release occurring from pituitary cells obtained early in gestation. ACTH responses to CRH can be found in pituitaries obtained from ovine fetuses at 0.43 G. This approximates the period of development when CRH can first be shown to have an effect on ACTH release from human fetal pituitary cells.

Another potential regulator of ACTH release in the fetal lamb is AVP. AVP stimulates ACTH secretion from the ovine fetal pituitary both *in vitro* and *in vivo*. In addition, there is a synergistic effect of CRH and AVP on fetal ACTH release. Such a synergism has also been observed in studies in adults and may reflect the ability of these peptides to activate different intracellular pathways leading to ACTH release from corticotrophs.

The bioactive to immunoreactive B/I ratio of ACTH is also influenced by both CRH and AVP. Administration of either increases the B/I ratio, a finding that implies that both secretagogues promote the release of ACTH(1–39) over other POMC-derived peptides.[20]

Evidence implicating CRH and AVP as mediators of stress-induced increments in ACTH is found in the report of McDonald and associates.[1] These workers placed bilateral electrolytic lesions in the fetal paraventricular nucleus. After a 4-day period for recovery, the chronically instrumented fetal lambs were subjected to a brief period of arterial hypotension or hypoxemia to stimulate ACTH secretion. In sham-lesioned animals, there was the expected increase in ACTH after either stress; however, in the lesioned animals, the ACTH response was absent (Fig. 186–6). Thus, destruction of the cell bodies whose axons release CRH and AVP into the hypophysial portal vessels blocks the ACTH response to stress in the fetus.

In contrast to the possible importance for AVP in stress-induced stimulation of ACTH, its role in maintaining basal levels of ACTH in the fetus seems less pronounced. It has been hypothesized that endogenous AVP could play an obligatory role in maintaining basal ACTH release in fetal sheep of 0.9 to 1.0 G. Injection of an AVP antagonist in sufficient quantity to block the effects of exogenous AVP had no effect on basal ACTH levels, a finding leading these investigators to conclude that AVP is not obligatory.[1]

Other studies have extended our knowledge into the supplementary role on ACTH secretion played by metabolites of arachidonic acid. In one, a thromboxane mimetic was shown to increase fetal plasma ACTH when it was administered into a carotid, but not a systemic, artery. In another, intracerebroventricular prostaglandin E_2 also increased plasma ACTH.

It is not clear whether catecholamines have a role in regulating ACTH release in the ovine fetus. Infusions of epinephrine caused ACTH to increase fivefold in fetal lambs at 0.77 gestation, but fetal arterial pH also fell. Therefore, it is not clear whether the ACTH response was directly related to the catecholamine infusion or to the ensuing acidosis. When epinephrine was used to stimulate ACTH release from short-term cultures of sheep fetal pituitary cells, no consistent responses were observed.[1]

Do glucocorticoids exert negative feedback effects on the CRH-ACTH/β-End system in the fetus? This question is really composed of two separate issues: one related to regulation of basal levels and one concerning modulation of stress responses.

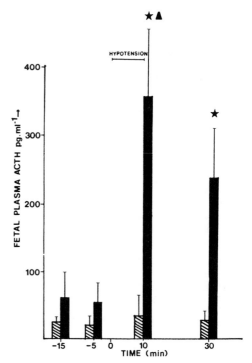

Figure 186–6. Plasma corticotropin (ACTH) responses (mean ± SD) of paraventricular nucleus lesioned fetuses (*n* = 4) and sham-lesioned controls (*n* = 3) to nitroprusside-induced hypotension from 0 to 10 minutes at 112 to 117 days' gestation. *Asterisk* = $p < .01$ when lesioned and sham groups are compared at a given time point; Δ = significantly greater than resting concentration ($p < .05$). (From McDonald TJ, et al: J Dev Physiol *10*:191, 1988.)

For glucocorticoids to affect either basal or stress-related increases in activity in the CRH-ACTH/β-End axis, glucocorticoid receptors should be present in the fetal pituitary or in brain regions thought to be important for regulation of the system. The presence of specific glucocorticoid binding sites has been reported in cytosol preparations of fetal pituitary, hypothalamus, and hippocampus. Receptors are present as early as midgestation in all three tissues, and the concentration of binding sites does not vary uniformly with gestational age. However, receptor levels are higher in the fetus than in the adult. The association constants calculated by Scatchard analysis of the data indicate that a high-affinity binding site and sucrose density gradient profiles of the ligand-binding site complex are characteristic of a glucocorticoid receptor. Thus, at least a portion of the biochemical machinery essential for glucocorticoid modulation of the CRH-ACTH/β-End system is present by 0.5 G.[1]

In most instances in which it has been studied, administration of cortisol or synthetic glucocorticoids inhibits the basal plasma concentration of ACTH. The ability to observe suppression of resting levels of ACTH may be related to the sensitivity of the assays used to measure the hormone. If plasma ACTH concentrations are close to the sensitivity of the assay used for measurement, suppression would be difficult to demonstrate. Another approach to establish whether cortisol regulates basal ACTH secretion is to reduce fetal plasma cortisol concentrations and to determine whether plasma ACTH increases coincidentally with the fall in cortisol. Blockade of steroid biosynthesis in fetal sheep causes a fall in fetal plasma cortisol and an increase in fetal plasma ACTH close to term (Fig. 186–7). Surgical adrenalectomy during this period produces comparable results. At earlier periods of development, inhibition of cortisol synthesis in

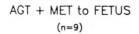

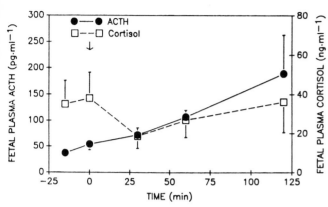

Figure 186–7. Plasma corticotropin (ACTH) and cortisol levels before and after aminoglutethimide (AGT) and metyrapone (MET) given to nine fetal lambs at 0.90 ± 01 gestation. The means are denoted by *circles* or *squares* and the SEM by *vertical bars.* The *arrow* indicates when the drugs were given. When no *vertical bar* is shown, the SEM is enclosed in the symbol. There was a fall in fetal plasma cortisol ($p < .01$) and an increase in ACTH ($p < .02$). (From Rose JC, et al: Endocrinology *123*:1307, 1988.)

pregnant ewes reduces fetal plasma cortisol concentration and increases ACTH levels. Cortisol infusions into fetuses prevent the decline in steroid concentrations and the increases in plasma ACTH. In addition, the mRNA for POMC is elevated in fetal sheep in response to adrenalectomy. These observations are consistent, and they indicate that cortisol circulating in fetal plasma tonically inhibits resting fetal plasma ACTH secretion by 0.70 G.[1]

Glucocorticoids block stress-induced increments in fetal plasma ACTH levels. This effect is present as early as 0.65 G. At term, increased drive to the CRH-ACTH/β-End system associated with the onset of labor may reduce the efficacy of glucocorticoids in inhibiting stress-induced ACTH secretion.

Consistent with the ability of glucocorticoids to inhibit basal and stress-related ACTH secretion is their ability to block ACTH release in response to CRH. Infusions of cortisol block ACTH responses to injections of CRH in the fetus. The ACTH responses to injections of AVP are also blocked by synthetic glucocorticoids in the ovine fetus, and dexamethasone inhibits ACTH release after the simultaneous injection of CRH and AVP. The ability of glucocorticoids to inhibit CRH- and AVP-stimulated release of ACTH *in vivo* has been confirmed *in vitro,* and suppression of responses is observed in pituitaries obtained from animals from 0.43 G until term.[1]

Responses to CRH are also attenuated because endogenous levels of plasma cortisol increase in late gestation, and a highly significant inverse correlation has been observed between fetal plasma cortisol levels and ACTH responses to CRH.

Cortisol infusion also changes the B/I ratio. Infusion of physiologically relevant doses of cortisol reduces the ratio in fetal plasma, thereby indicating a selective inhibitory action on the secretion of ACTH(1–39).[13] The effect of cortisol may be primarily on CRH-responsive corticotrophs.[21]

As mentioned earlier, there is a change in ACTH responsiveness to secretagogues during development. Cultures of pituitary cells from immature fetuses (100 to 115 days of gestation) respond robustly to CRH and very modestly to AVP. In contrast, cultured cells from mature fetal pituitaries have minor responses to CRH but pronounced response to AVP. This developmental change in the ability of these secretagogues to increase ACTH release is not found in cells from mature fetuses adrenalectomized at about 120 days of gestation. These cells show a pattern of secretion resembling that of cells from immature fetuses. A probable explanation for these observations is that the increase in cortisol normally seen at the end of gestation promotes the change in ACTH secretory responses to CRH and AVP; when the cortisol increase does not occur late in gestation, then the corticotrophs maintain an immature profile of responsiveness.[22]

The developmental changes in the overall secretory pattern are found at the level of single cells; that is, whereas CRH causes more corticotrophs to secrete ACTH in pituitaries from immature fetuses, AVP recruits more cells to secrete ACTH in mature pituitaries.[23] There is also evidence of further maturation of the response of corticotrophs. In the immature fetal pituitary, ACTH-secretory responses to CRH or AVP can be totally accounted for by the recruitment of erstwhile nonsecreting cells to secrete. In term pituitaries, as in those of adults, the response to AVP involves both recruitment and an increase in the average amount of ACTH secreted per cell.[23] As noted, the decrease in CRH responsiveness late in gestation is associated with no further recruitment of corticotrophs to secrete ACTH.[23] It is likely that this change in CRH responsiveness is the result of a decease in CRH receptor levels present in the pituitary. CRH-R1 receptor mRNA and protein decrease throughout late gestation and in response to cortisol treatment.[24]

In summary, the major regulators of ACTH release in the ovine fetus, at least after mid-gestation, appear to be CRH and AVP. By 0.65 G, small physiologic increases in plasma cortisol levels block stress-induced activation of the CRH-ACTH/β-End system, and the majority of evidence indicates that glucocorticoids modulate activity in this system over the last third of gestation.

SIGNIFICANCE

In contrast to the paucity of information concerning the role of β-End in the fetus, there is convincing evidence that the primary role of ACTH in fetal life is the regulation of adrenal steroid secretion. All the available data indicate that, in the absence of ACTH, normal adrenal maturation does not occur, and the spontaneous development of adrenal steroidogenic function can be induced precociously by administering ACTH to the fetus. In fact, hypophysectomized fetal sheep or fetuses with the hypothalamus disconnected from the pituitary, receiving constant rate infusions of ACTH, demonstrate a typical term surge in cortisol concentration and are delivered on time. Consequently, the major significance of ACTH in the fetus is derived from its biologic effects on the fetal adrenal.

During intrauterine development, the normal maturation of many organ systems including the pulmonary, gastrointestinal, and central nervous systems depends on adrenocortical steroids, and the marked increase in cortisol that occurs in fetuses of several species appears essential for survival of the neonate.[1] This is clearly demonstrated by the results of the studies in mice with targeted disruption of the CRH or CRH receptor gene (*knock-out mice*). Knock-outs not only of CRH but also of CRH receptor type 1 (CRH-R1, the predominant CRH receptor in the pituitary) display problems with development. The fetuses are delivered normally but die within 24 hours of birth because of insufficient lung maturation. This developmental problem occurs only if both the mother and the fetus are homozygous knock-outs,[25, 26] a finding suggesting that these fetuses have insufficient corticosteroid levels late in development. Because CRH knock-out fetuses develop normally as long as the mother is heterozygous, the dam can compensate for this deficit in glucocorticoids, presumably by placental transfer. However, when the dam is also CRH deficient, she cannot compensate for the fetal deficit unless glucocorticoids are supplemented in the drinking water during pregnancy.[25, 26] This effect appears to be specific to CRH action at CRH-R1 receptors because CRH-R2 knock-out mice develop normally.[27] Thus, timely development of the fetal CRH-ACTH/β-End system is a prerequisite for the successful transition from intrauterine to extrauterine life.

N-POMC(1–77) and possibly other peptides derived from the amino terminal of POMC may be important regulators of adrenal development.[28, 29] This peptide, also known as 16K fragment and pro-γ-MSH, has been implicated in compensatory adrenal growth.[30, 31] Immunoneutralization of this peptide is associated with impaired compensatory growth.[30] Studies with infusions in fetal sheep have demonstrated a role for the peptide in adrenal growth and steroidogenic capacity.[28, 29] Circulating N-POMC (1–77) is believed to be cleaved at the adrenal to N-POMC (1–52), which is the active mitogen, and an adrenal receptor for the mitogenic peptide has been described.[30, 31]

As outlined in this chapter, numerous factors influence the activity of the fetal corticotrophs, thereby regulating adrenal steroidogenic activity. The importance of these factors extends well beyond fetal physiology and even fetal development. The concept of *fetal programming* has been elaborated, and evidence is rapidly accumulating that fetal adjustments to adverse environmental factors may result in permanent changes, albeit subtle ones, that render the fetus more susceptible to some diseases in adult life. The programming concept has its origin in human epidemiologic studies that link small birth weight and the later emergence of disease.[32] Virtually all animal models of fetal programming indicate that elevated or precocious activity of the pituitary-adrenal axis in fetal life is associated with programming. Thus, observations such as altered ACTH or cortisol responses in fetal sheep that were subject to an adverse environment at some stage of gestation may represent important physiologic adaptations with permanent implications.

Finally, abundant evidence indicates that the timing of the initiation of labor in several species depends on orderly maturation of the fetal adrenal. If this maturation is directed by the CRH-ACTH/β-End system, then the brain-pituitary-adrenal axis must be considered a pivotal endocrine system for the fetus in coordinating preparation for birth with the onset of parturition.

REFERENCES

1. Rose JC, et al: Development of the corticotropin-releasing factor adrenocorticotropic hormone/beta-endorphin system in the mammalian fetus. *In* Polin RA, Fox WF (eds): Fetal and Neonatal Physiology, Vol 2. Philadelphia, WB Saunders Co, 1998, p 2431.
2. King BR, et al: The regulation of human corticotrophin-releasing hormone gene expression in the placenta. Peptides *22*:795, 2001.
3. Majzoub JA, Karalis KP: Placental corticotropin-releasing hormone: function and regulation. Am J Obstet Gynecol *180*:S242, 1999.
4. Nicholson RC, King BR: Regulation of CRH gene expression in the placenta. Front Horm Res *27*:246, 2001.
5. Karteris E, et al: The role of corticotropin-releasing hormone receptors in placenta and fetal membranes during human pregnancy. Mol Genet Metab *72*:287, 2001.
6. Fadalti M, et al: Placental corticotropin-releasing factor. An update. Ann NY Acad Sci *900*:89, 2000.
7. Smith GW, et al: Corticotropin releasing factor receptor 1–deficient mice display decreased anxiety, impaired stress response, and aberrant neuroendocrine development. Neuron *20*:1093, 1998.
8. Seidah NG, et al: The subtilisin/kexin family of precursor convertases: emphasis on PC1, PC2/7B2, POMC and the novel enzyme SKI-1. Ann NY Acad Sci *885*:57, 1999.
9. Brubaker PL, et al: Corticotropic peptides in the human fetal pituitary. Endocrinology *111*:1150, 1982.
10. Sacedon R, et al: Partial blockade of T-cell differentiation during ontogeny and marked alterations of the thymic microenvironment in transgenic mice with impaired glucocorticoid receptor function. J Neuroimmunol *98*:157, 1999.
11. Parker CR, Porter JC: Developmental changes in molecular forms of immunoreactive adrenocorticotropin in the anterior pituitary gland of humans. Endocr Res *25*:397, 1999.
12. Bell ME, et al: Expression of proopiomelanocortin and prohormone convertase-1 and -2 in the late gestation fetal sheep pituitary. Endocrinology *139*:5135, 1998.
13. Zehnder TJ, et al: Cortisol infusion depresses the ratio of bioactive to immunoreactive ACTH in adrenalectomized sheep fetuses. Am J Physiol *274*:E391, 1998.
14. Holloway AC, et al: Effects of cortisol and estradiol on pituitary expression of proopiomelanocortin, prohormone convertase-1, prohormone convertase-2, and glucocorticoid receptor mRNA in fetal sheep. Endocr J *14*:343, 2001.
15. Allen JP, et al: Maternal-fetal ACTH relationship in man. J Clin Endocrinol Metab *37*:230, 1973.
16. Miyakawa I, et al: Transport of ACTH across human placenta. J Clin Endocrinol Metab *39*:440, 1974.
17. Gibbs DM, et al: Synthetic corticotropin-releasing factor stimulates secretion of immunoreactive beta-endorphin/beta-lipotropin and ACTH by human fetal pituitaries in vitro. Life Sci *32*:547, 1983.
18. Castro MI, et al: The ratio of plasma bioactive to immunoreactive ACTH-like activity increases with gestational age in the fetal lamb. J Dev Physiol *18*:193, 1992.
19. Castro MI, et al: Bioactive-to-immunoreactive ACTH activity changes with severity of stress in late-gestation ovine fetus. Am J Physiol *265*:E68, 1993.
20. Zehnder TJ, et al: Regulation of bioactive and immunoreactive ACTH secretion by CRF and AVP in sheep fetuses. Am J Physiol *269*:E1076, 1995.
21. Butler TG, et al: Functional heterogeneity of corticotrophs in the anterior pituitary of the sheep fetus. J Physiol *516*:907, 1999.
22. Fora MA, et al: Adrenocorticotropin secretion by fetal sheep anterior and intermediate lobe pituitary cells in vitro: effects of gestation and adrenalectomy. Endocrinology *137*:3394, 1996.
23. Perez FM, et al: Developmental changes in ovine corticotrophs in vitro. Endocrinology *138*:916, 1997.
24. Green JL, et al: Corticotropin-releasing hormone type I receptor messenger ribonucleic acid and protein levels in the ovine fetal pituitary: ontogeny and effect of chronic cortisol administration. Endocrinology *141*:2870, 2000.
25. Muglia LJ, et al. The physiology of corticotropin-releasing hormone deficiency in mice. Peptides *22*:725, 2001.
26. Venihaki M, Majzoub JA: Animal models of CRH deficiency. Front Neuroendocrinol *20*:122, 1999.
27. Preil J, et al: Regulation of the hypothalamic-pituitary-adrenocortical system in mice deficient for CRH receptors 1 and 2. Endocrinology *142*:4946, 2001.
28. Coulter CL, et al: *N*-Proopiomelanocortin (1–77) suppresses expression of steroidogenic acute regulatory protein (StAR) mRNA in the adrenal gland of the fetal sheep. Endocr Res *26*:523, 2000.
29. Coulter CL, et al: Role of pituitary POMC-peptides and insulin-like growth factor II in the developmental biology of the adrenal gland. Arch Physiol Biochem *110*:99, 2002.
30. Bicknell AB, et al: Characterization of a serine protease that cleaves pro-gamma-melanotropin at the adrenal to stimulate growth. Cell *105*:903, 2001.
31. Bicknell AB, et al: Identification of a putative adrenal receptor for the N-POMC mitogenic peptide. Presented at the 84th Annual Meeting of the Endocrine Society, San Francisco, CA, June 19–22, 2002.
32. Barker DJP (ed): Fetal origins of cardiovascular and lung disease. *In* Lung Biology in Health and Disease, Vol 151. New York, Marcel Dekker, 2000.

187

Jeremy S. D. Winter

Fetal and Neonatal Adrenocortical Physiology

The adrenal cortex during prenatal and neonatal life demonstrates remarkable changes in size, structure, and steroidogenic function, phenomena that have excited the curiosity and imagination of investigators since the early years of the 20th century. As can be seen in Figure 187–1, the fetal adrenal by term reaches adult size and is, in relation to body weight, about 20 times larger than the adult gland. By the end of pregnancy, it is producing 100 to 200 mg of steroids daily, a rate several times higher than that of a resting adult.[1]

The bulk of this material consists of Δ^5-3β-hydroxysteroids, such as dehydroepiandrosterone (DHA), which, although biologically inactive, can undergo further hepatic and placental metabolism to produce estrogens. After parturition, the neonatal adrenal cortex rapidly involutes, and these Δ^5-3β-hydroxysteroids almost disappear from the circulation, not to reappear until late childhood and puberty.[2,3] It is obvious that the remarkable growth and activity of the fetal adrenal cortex must be a response to some factors unique to the intrauterine environment; what is less clear is to what degree these phenomena are essential for the maintenance of pregnancy and eventual parturition.

EMBRYOGENESIS AND HISTOLOGIC DEVELOPMENT OF THE ADRENAL CORTEX

The primordium of the adrenal cortex appears at about 25 days' gestation in an area of dorsal celomic epithelium at the cranial edge of the developing mesonephros. Initially, this adrenocortical blastema is composed of rapidly dividing undifferentiated cells containing small mitochondria with scanty laminar cristae and minimal endoplasmic reticulum. The gland rapidly enlarges; by 6 to 8 weeks' gestation, cells of the inner cortex differentiate to form a distinct fetal zone, and an outer subcapsular rim of immature cells remains as the so-called definitive zone.

Thereafter, although the gland continues to grow almost exponentially,[4,5] mitotic activity is limited to the outer subcapsular layer, just as in postnatal life.[6,7] The immature basophilic cells of this definitive zone are characterized by scanty cytoplasm containing elongated mitochondria with shelflike cristae and scarce tubules of smooth endoplasmic reticulum. They divide rapidly and contribute centripetally by an indistinct transitional zone to an enlarging fetal zone that eventually occupies more than 80% of the gland.[8] As the adrenal enlarges, it assumes an extended, flattened shape, which permits growth but limits cortical thickness to less than 1.5 mm. During the 9th to 12th weeks of fetal life, sinusoids carrying blood from subcapsular arterioles to the central adrenal vein develop, and this provides the framework for postnatal organization of the zona fasciculata.

The large eosinophilic cells of the fetal zone, in contrast to those of the definitive zone, are well differentiated for active steroidogenesis.[9] Their abundant cytoplasm is packed with a convoluted network of smooth and rough endoplasmic reticulum containing granular areas of nucleoprotein that may, in part, represent signal recognition particles[10] responsible for the insertion and orientation of microsomal steroidogenic enzymes. The mitochondria are large with tubular or vesicular cristae; lipid droplets may occur, and some cells show a prominent Golgi apparatus. The plasma membrane bears numerous microvilli, and cell-to-cell attachments are present.

By term gestation, each adrenal weighs about 4 g, but after parturition, rapid involution occurs. In the first 4 days of life, each gland loses 25% of its mass and by 1 month is reduced to half its fetal size. The adrenal gland of a 1-year-old infant weighs less than 1 g, and its cortical thickness has shrunk to about 0.6 mm. Early studies of neonatal autopsy material described extensive degeneration and necrosis within the fetal zone, with hemorrhage, interstitial edema, and heterophagocytosis, but it seems likely that these were artifacts caused by disease and agonal events.[11] Because involution causes the cells of the postnatal adrenal to become smaller and to resemble fetal definitive zone cells, an erroneous conclusion was reached from cross-sectional histologic studies that suggested that the fetal zone disappears and is replaced by inward extension of the definitive zone to form the adult zona fasciculata. Such disappearance of the fetal zone, however, does not occur under normal circumstances, and one cannot observe within the definitive zone the increased mitotic activity necessary to permit this apparent enlargement. Instead, what happens during the first weeks and months after birth is a gradual reduction in size and remodeling of fetal zone cells, which assume the appearance and organization typical of zona fasciculata. McNulty[12] studied this process in healthy neonatal monkeys and observed a centripetal wave of transformation of fetal zone cells to zona fasciculata, with only rare mitotic figures and no evidence of necrosis or collapse. There is every reason to assume that a similar process of postnatal adrenocortical involution occurs in humans.

FUNCTIONAL MATURATION OF THE FETAL ADRENAL

Molecular Biology of the Adrenocortical Cell

The human adrenal cortex can produce at least 50 steroids, but only 2, cortisol and aldosterone, are essential for independent life and health, and only these have defined feedback systems with tropic hormones to regulate their secretion. The adrenal cortex of the fetus and the adult also produces large amounts of 19-carbon steroids, such as DHA, which can be metabolized elsewhere to biologically active androgen or estrogen. Because the human placenta does not express cytochrome $P450_{C17}$ (17-hydroxylase and 17,20-desmolase) activity, it depends on preformed C_{19} steroids of either maternal or fetal adrenal origin as substrate for estrogen biosynthesis.

Figure 187–2 summarizes the pathways of steroidogenesis in a typical adrenocortical cell. Most of the enzymes involved in cortisol and aldosterone synthesis are members of the ubiquitous cytochrome P450 family of heme-containing mixed-function oxidases.[13] The rate-limiting step in steroidogenesis is delivery of substrate cholesterol from cellular stores to the cholesterol side chain cleavage complex ($P450_{scc}$), which is located on the mitochondrial inner membrane; this process is mediated by a steroidogenesis acute regulatory protein (StAR), expression of which is regulated by cyclic adenosine monophosphate (cAMP).[14] Other proteins, such as sterol carrier protein 2 and steroidogenesis

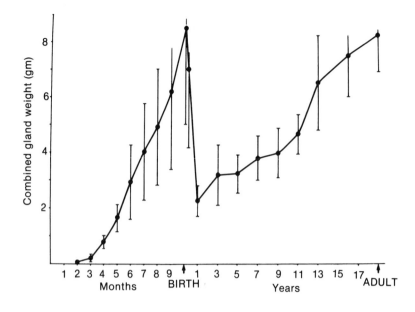

Figure 187–1. Adrenal gland weights during human development. (From Neville AM, O'Hare MJ: The Human Adrenal Cortex. Berlin, Springer-Verlag, 1982, p 12.)

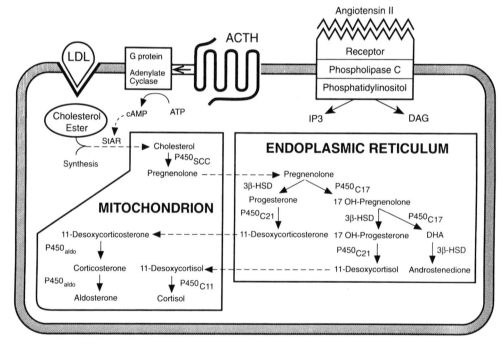

Figure 187–2. Pathways of steroid biosynthesis in an adrenocortical cell, showing the intracellular locations of the steroidogenic enzymes: $P450_{SCC}$ (cholesterol side chain cleavage); $P450_{C17}$ (17-hydroxylase and 17,20-desmolase); $P450_{C21}$ (21-hydroxylase); $P450_{C11}$ (11β-hydroxylase); $P450_{aldo}$ (18-hydroxylase and aldosterone synthetase); and 3β-HSD (3β-hydroxysteroid dehydrogenase and Δ5-3-ketosteroid isomerase). The rate-limiting step appears to be delivery of substrate cholesterol derived from low-density lipoprotein (LDL) to $P450_{scc}$ on the mitochondrial inner membrane, a process that is mediated by a novel steroidogenesis acute regulatory protein (StAR). Expression of this protein is regulated by corticotropin (ACTH) and cyclic adenosine monophosphate (cAMP). Actions of angiotensin II are mediated by inositol triphosphate (IP_3) and 1,2-diacylglycerol (DAG). ATP = adenosine triphosphate.

activator peptide, may also play a role in this rate-limiting process. The mitochondrial enzymes $P450_{scc}$, $P450_{C11}$, and $P450_{aldo}$ are the terminal components of an electron transport chain involving reduced nicotinamide-adenine dinucleotide phosphate (NADPH), a flavoprotein (adrenodoxin reductase), and an iron-sulfur protein (adrenodoxin). The genes for $P450_{c11}$ and $P450_{aldo}$ both lie on chromosome 8, and their sequences are 93% identical.[15] $P450_{c11}$ is normally expressed in the cortisol-producing zona fasciculata and is positively regulated by corticotropin (ACTH), whereas $P450_{aldo}$ is expressed in the zona glomerulosa and mediates aldosterone synthesis under the influence of angiotensin II.

The two microsomal P450 enzymes $P450_{c17}$ (with 17-hydroxylase and 17,20-desmolase activities) and $P450_{c21}$ (with 21-hydroxylase activity) use NADPH and an intermediary flavoprotein NADPH-cytochrome P450 reductase as coenzymes. The final enzyme, 3β-HSD (with both 3β-hydroxysteroid dehydrogenase and Δ5-3-ketosteroid isomerase activities), uses NAD as a cofactor.

It can be seen from Figure 187–2 that two branch points for steroidogenesis exist that determine the relative amounts of aldosterone, cortisol, and DHA secreted by any adrenal cell. Each of these involves the interaction of 3β-HSD and $P450_{c17}$ with a

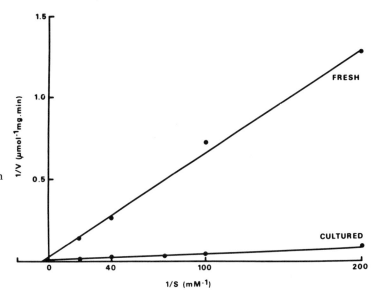

Figure 187–3. Double reciprocal plot of 3β-hydroxy-steroid dehydrogenase (3β-HSD) activity (V) as a function of dehydroepiandrosterone substrate concentration (S) in human fetal adrenal cells before and after 6 days of tissue culture. The decrease in the slope of the regression reflects a marked increase in 3β-HSD activity after culture. (From Winter JSD: *In* D'Agata R, Chrousos GP [eds]: Recent Advances in Adrenal Regulation and Function. New York, Raven Press, 1987, pp 51–66.)

common substrate, either pregnenolone or 17OH-pregnenolone. In the fasciculata, both enzymes are expressed; pregnenolone is converted to 17-hydroxysteroids such as 17OH-pregnenolone, which can then be transformed to cortisol or DHA. In the zona glomerulosa, $P450_{c17}$ is not expressed; therefore, only 17-desoxysteroids such as progesterone and aldosterone are produced.

The second branch point, which determines relative production of cortisol and DHA within the fasciculata or reticularis, also depends on the relative activities of 3β-HSD and $P450_{c17}$ and their ability to transform 17OH-pregnenolone. One level of control for this interaction is gene expression: If 3β-HSD is not expressed, the secretion products of that cell are Δ^5-3β-hydroxysteroids such as DHA. Additional controls may exist, however, including the availability of critical cofactors. There is some evidence that the P450 reductase/$P450_{c17}$ ratio may influence electron availability and thus determine whether this enzyme can accomplish the second step of 17,20-bond scission to produce DHA.[13] In similar fashion, changes in the redox state of $NADH/NAD^+$ may influence the activity of 3β-HSD and may promote adrenal secretion of DHA. Studies have demonstrated that 3β-HSD exists not only in the endoplasmic reticulum, but also in the mitochondrial inner membrane.[16] Differential activities in these two sites, together with mechanisms to regulate interorganelle steroid transfer, could profoundly influence relative cortisol and DHA secretion rates.

Regulated steroidogenic gene transcription seems to be the mechanism that underlies zone-specific enzyme expression and probably some chronic developmental shifts in steroid secretion.[17, 18] This process involves both discrete 5′-flanking DNA promoter elements and DNA-binding nuclear proteins whose actions are regulated by hormonal factors, in particular, ACTH and angiotensin II. The adrenal response to ACTH is initiated by binding to a specific high-affinity membrane receptor,[19] followed by activation of adenylate cyclase and release of cAMP. cAMP, primarily through its impact on protein kinase A,[20] serves both to stimulate delivery of cholesterol substrate to $P450_{scc}$ (by peptides such as StAR) and to promote expression of all steroidogenic enzymes. It is possible that other cellular second messengers such as calcium or diacylglycerol mediate some actions of ACTH.[21,22]

Angiotensin II acts through its own unique membrane receptors, found primarily on zona glomerulosa cells, to regulate intracellular calcium concentrations and protein kinase C. This process is complex,[23] but one major effect of angiotensin II is to inhibit $P450_{c17}$ expression. In addition, together with local factors such as insulin-like growth factor-II (IGF-II), epidermal growth

factor, and basic fibroblast growth factor, angiotensin II promotes division of undifferentiated subcapsular cells and thus adrenocortical growth. It can be seen, therefore, that ACTH and angiotensin II act in concert, through cAMP and protein kinase C, to regulate adrenal growth, differentiation, and zone-specific function.

Unique Aspects of Fetal Adrenal Steroidogenesis

There are important differences in the relative activities of steroidogenic enzymes in the human fetal adrenal that cause marked differences in the pattern of steroids produced. The steroidogenically active fetal zone expresses abundant amounts of $P450_{scc}$ and $P450_{c17}$ but no 3β-HSD mRNA or protein[24-27]; thus, its major secretion product is DHA. In early gestation, the outer definitive zone expresses only small amounts of $P450_{scc}$ and probably produces little steroid; later in pregnancy, this zone does express some $P450_{scc}$ and 3β-HSD (but not $P450_{c17}$) and comes to resemble adult zona glomerulosa. Mesiano and colleagues[26] identified a transitional zone of cells between the definitive and fetal zones that expresses all the enzymes necessary for cortisol biosynthesis, including 3β-HSD, and that may be the precursor of the postnatal zona fasciculata. *In vitro* exposure of fetal zone cells to ACTH quickly induces 3β-HSD activity and stimulates cortisol secretion (Fig. 187–3). Clearly, therefore, there must be other factors unique to the fetal environment that block ACTH-induced expression of 3β-HSD in the fetal zone of the adrenal.

The major substrate for fetal adrenal steroidogenesis is cholesterol, derived from circulating low-density lipoprotein (LDL) by a process that involves binding to specific membrane LDL receptors, followed by absorptive endocytosis and hydrolysis to release free cholesterol.[28, 29] Cholesterol sulfate may also be derived from this process, some of which can be metabolized directly to sulfated pregnenolone and DHA.[30] Fetal serum LDL concentrations are considerably lower than those of adults,[31] presumably because of utilization for steroidogenesis because levels are much higher in anencephaly.[32] In addition to this circulating LDL cholesterol, additional cholesterol substrate can be provided by *de novo* adrenal synthesis.[33] As befits its active steroidogenic role, the fetal zone contains more LDL-binding sites per cell and shows a higher rate of *de novo* cholesterol synthesis than the definitive zone.[34]

The fetal zone also possesses a potent steroid sulfotransferase.[35,36] Thus, its major products are DHA sulfate, pregnenolone sulfate, and several free Δ^5-3β-hydroxysteroids, with lesser amounts of active Δ^4-3-ketosteroids, such as cortisol.[37] Fetal adrenal cells *in vitro* can use preformed progesterone to synthesize cortisol and corticosterone, in addition to small amounts of aldosterone.[38-40] Although there is a negative arteriovenous gradient in umbilical cord progesterone, suggesting some fetal metabolism,[41,42] this pathway is not enhanced by ACTH.[43] Studies in nonhuman primates demonstrate conclusively that cholesterol, rather than progesterone, is the primary precursor for fetal cortisol synthesis.[44,45]

Fetoplacental Steroid Metabolism

Δ4-3-Ketosteroids

The effect of gestational age on cord serum total cortisol concentrations is shown in Figure 187–4. Levels rise from about 20 nmol/L (0.7 μg/dL) at 13 weeks' gestation to 150 nmol/L (4.5 μg/dL) at term, with even higher values after spontaneous delivery. These values represent the net result of input from both fetal and maternal sources and clearance through fetal and placental metabolism. Fetal serum levels of corticosteroid-binding globulin (transcortin) are low in relation to maternal values.[46] Furthermore, progesterone, the concentrations of which are high, competes for corticosteroid-binding globulin–binding sites and tends to increase levels of free steroid. Mean serum free or unbound cortisol concentrations increase severalfold during the latter half of pregnancy but remain lower than those in the maternal circulation.[47]

The metabolic clearance of cortisol from the fetal compartment is extremely rapid, with about 80% oxidized in fetal tissues and placenta to cortisone and its further metabolites.[48] About 60% of the total cortisol in the fetal compartment is ultimately transferred to the mother, either as cortisol or as cortisone, and under normal circumstances the human fetus appears to be a net exporter of cortisol.[49] When fetal cortisol secretion fails, however, as in the hypopituitary or hypoadrenal fetus, contributions from the maternal compartment appear to be sufficient to maintain fetal health and development.

The fetal adrenal is the major source of cortisol production, as evidenced by the positive arteriovenous gradient in cord serum cortisol levels, which persists throughout pregnancy.[50,51] In an effort to maintain cortisol levels in the presence of rapid metabolic clearance, the fetal adrenal must secrete cortisol at rates that, per unit weight, equal or exceed those of the adult.[52,53] Beitins and coworkers[54] calculated that 60 to 75% of the cortisol in the fetal compartment represents direct fetal adrenal secretion, whereas the remainder derives from placental transfer or metabolic conversion of cortisone.

Maternal cortisol readily crosses the placenta, but during transit most of it is oxidized by placental 11β-hydroxysteroid dehydrogenase to cortisone. Some tissues, such as chorion, liver, and lung, express 11-ketosteroid reductase activity,[55-57] and thus the opportunity exists for local conversion of cortisone back to cortisol within target cells. It is possible that the balance of cortisol-cortisone interconversion is regulated during fetal life by factors such as thyroid hormones.[58]

In vitro human adrenal cells can secrete aldosterone and mineralocorticoid intermediates such as corticosterone and 11-desoxycorticosterone (DOC).[59] In addition, some fetal tissues, including kidney, can convert placental progesterone into DOC by an independent process, but most of this material is quickly conjugated to DOC sulfate. Fetal plasma aldosterone levels are high in relation to maternal and nonpregnant values,[60-63] a finding indicating that the fetal adrenal does secrete aldosterone *in vivo*. Beitins and colleagues[61] found that the offspring of sodium-depleted mothers had higher than normal plasma aldosterone levels; however, it is not clear at what stage of development fetal aldosterone secretion comes under the influence of the renin-angiotensin system, because the fetal lamb shows little aldosterone response to angiotensin. Aldosterone can affect renal tubular function in fetal lamb,[64,65] but similar studies have not been carried out in humans. The newborn human kidney is relatively unresponsive to exogenous aldosterone,[66,67] possibly because basal aldosterone levels are already high.

Δ5-3β-Hydroxysteroids

The paradox of human fetal adrenal steroidogenesis is that although the gland is obviously under maximal stimulatory drive in an effort to maintain fetal cortisol levels, the actual major products of this process are biologically inactive Δ5-3β-hydroxysteroids such as pregnenolone, 17OH-pregnenolone, and DHA and their sulfate conjugates. The fetal pituitary-adrenal axis responds to stress, such as hypoxemia, by dramatically increasing adrenal steroid production. Because of the rate-limiting deficiency of 3β-HSD activity, there is little or no capacity to increase cortisol levels; rather, fetal stress leads to increased production of DHA, DHA sulfate, and their metabolites.[68] This confronts the fetus with the additional problem of how to deal metabolically with these steroids, at least some of which otherwise could be converted to testosterone and cause inappropriate virilization. Both the fetal adrenal and the liver have high levels of 16α-hydroxylase and sulfotransferase activity, but little sulfatase activity. Thus, the bulk of the DHA produced is converted to 16α-hydroxy-DHA sulfate,

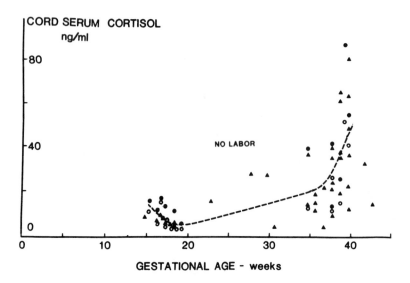

Figure 187–4. Cortisol concentrations in human umbilical arterial (*closed circles*), venous (*open circles*), and mixed (*solid triangles*) cord serum obtained at cesarean section without labor. Results of ng/mL can be converted to nmol/L by multiplying by 2.8. (From Murphy BEP: Am J Obstet Gynecol *144*:276, 1982.)

which then undergoes placental metabolism to inert estriol conjugates. Some fetal DHA sulfate is aromatized by the placenta to active estradiol and estrone; indeed, because the placenta lacks $P450_{c17}$, it must receive preformed 19-carbon steroids from maternal or fetal sources to synthesize estrogens (Fig. 187-5). In clinical situations, however, such as congenital adrenal hypoplasia or placental sulfatase deficiency, in which fetal DHA is for some reason not available, the placenta seems to be able to make sufficient estrogen from maternal DHA and androstenedione. In the situation of genetic StAR protein deficiency (so-called lipoid congenital adrenal hyperplasia), in which the fetoplacental unit is incapable of any estrogen formation, pregnancy proceeds normally to term.[69] This observation casts doubt on the traditional notion that the fetoplacental collaborative arrangement for estrogen biosynthesis plays an essential role in the maintenance of pregnancy.

REGULATION OF ADRENAL FUNCTION IN THE FETUS AND NEONATE

Corticotropin

Because ACTH does not cross the placenta, fetal plasma ACTH concentrations depend entirely on the integrity of the fetal hypothalamic-pituitary unit. Immunoreactive ACTH and related peptides derived from pro-opiomelanocortin (POMC) can be detected in the pituitary by 5 to 8 weeks' gestation.[70] Even the earliest pituitary specimens show capillary connections to the developing hypothalamus;[71] fetal pituitary ACTH secretion may respond to neurohumoral factors such as corticotropin-releasing factor and arginine vasopressin as early as 14 weeks' gestation,[72-74] and it is certainly responsive by mid-gestation.[75,76] There is evidence that the placenta can also synthesize ACTH and other POMC-derived peptides;[77,78] this material may contribute to maternal ACTH levels, but there is as yet no evidence of an effect on fetal adrenal function.

The acute effect of ACTH on the adrenal is to stimulate total steroidogenesis by promoting delivery of cholesterol substrate to mitochondrial cytochrome $P450_{scc}$.[79] In addition, ACTH has long-term stimulatory effects on the expression of steroidogenic enzymes, the number of LDL receptors, and the rate of *de novo* cholesterol synthesis. ACTH also stimulates adrenal growth by promoting both cellular hypertrophy and proliferation; the latter is a biphasic effect, with initial short-term protein kinase C–mediated inhibition of mitosis and then subsequent cAMP-mediated stimulation of cell division.[80,81] It seems likely that ACTH stimulates local production of some growth factors, such as IGF-II, which, in turn, induces adrenal cell division by a paracrine effect.[82,83] Other mitogenic factors, possibly of placental origin, have also been suggested as regulators of fetal adrenal growth.[84]

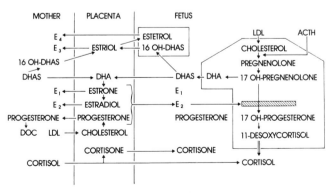

Figure 187–5. Fetoplacental and maternoplacental steroidogenic interactions during pregnancy. ACTH = corticotropin; DHA = dehydroepiandrosterone; DOC = 11-desoxycorticosterone; LDL = low-density lipoprotein.

In the absence of ACTH, as in anencephaly, the fetal adrenal is reduced in size even in the youngest specimens (15 weeks' gestation) studied.[85] The steroidogenic fetal zone is characteristically absent in anencephaly, but its development can be induced by administration of ACTH.[8] Because of a marked reduction in fetal DHA sulfate production,[86] placental estrogen production becomes dependent solely on maternal C19 steroid substrate and is reduced to about 10% of normal. The anencephalic adrenal *in vitro* shows low levels of adenylate cyclase activity,[87] but these and other steroidogenic functions return after exposure to ACTH.[88]

The involution of the adrenal cortex after parturition reflects the normal reduction in plasma ACTH levels that occurs once the influence of the placenta on cortisol metabolic clearance is removed and circulating free cortisol levels rise. Anything that reduces ACTH secretion before parturition, such as fetal hypophysectomy or dexamethasone administration, causes precocious involution and transformation of the fetal adrenal, whereas postnatal infusion of ACTH permits preservation and even expansion of the fetal zone.[12] A histologic appearance similar to that of the fetal zone has been described in older children with untreated congenital adrenal hyperplasia[89] and in adults administered large amounts of ACTH.[90]

Fetal adrenal cells are exquisitely sensitive to ACTH stimulation, responding to concentrations as low as 1 pg/mL.[59] For comparison, mid-gestation fetal plasma ACTH concentrations are around 250 pg/mL,[91] a level at which adrenal stimulation is maximal. Although the fetal pituitary produces a whole family of POMC-derived peptides, including β-endorphin, β-lipotropin, α-melanocyte–stimulating hormone, and corticotropin-like intermediate lobe peptide, none of these has any adrenocorticotropic effect at physiologic concentrations.[92] Because co-culture of adrenal and pituitary cells elicits responses identical to those of ACTH alone,[59] it seems unlikely that the pituitary secretes any other adrenocorticotropic factor in significant amounts. Although fetal plasma ACTH levels decline somewhat toward term, they remain much higher than those of postnatal life;[91,93,94] in the fetal sheep, ACTH secretion reaches the remarkable rate of about 5 ng/kg/minute.[95] Fetal pituitary ACTH secretion appears to be pulsatile,[96] but little is known about circadian variations in response to maternal cortisol rhythms.

It is not entirely clear at what stage of fetal development feedback regulation of ACTH secretion by cortisol becomes fully operative.[97] The common clinical observation, however, that large doses of dexamethasone[98] (which crosses the placenta without oxidation) can act by 4 to 6 weeks' gestation to block adrenal androgen production by the 21-hydroxylase–deficient fetus[99] suggests that normal pituitary-adrenal feedback relationships are operative in the first trimester, as soon as the adrenal cortex becomes functional. In the ovine fetus, one can readily demonstrate the presence of pituitary and hypothalamic glucocorticoid receptors and feedback inhibition of ACTH release by day 60 of pregnancy.[100,101] The human fetal pituitary-adrenal axis at term can be suppressed by exogenous glucocorticoid,[102,103] but the effect is readily overcome by the stress of labor and delivery.[104,105]

Other Tropic Factors

Numerous peptides of either pituitary or placental origin have been suggested as regulators of fetal adrenal steroidogenesis, but only for ACTH is the evidence compelling or reproducible. The fetal pituitary produces several other POMC-derived peptides; however, none of these or other pituitary hormones such as growth hormone, prolactin, or thyrotropin has a stimulatory effect on adrenal steroidogenesis at physiologic concentrations.[92] There is, however, some evidence that *N*-terminal POMC fragments may stimulate adrenal growth and may potentiate the actions of ACTH.[106,107] It has been tempting to suggest that placental hormones, such as chorionic gonadotropin or somatomammotropin, may stimulate fetal adrenal DHA production because this would provide a ready explanation for the transition to Δ^4-3-ketosteroid secretion after parturition. Careful studies using pure preparations of these factors, however, indicate no such effect on adrenal function.[53,92]

After birth, angiotensin II is an important regulator of adrenal growth and enzyme expression,[23] but in fetal life, it appears to have little effect.[108] Both definitive zone and fetal zone cells are deficient in angiotensin II receptors, and neither responds effectively in terms of aldosterone, cortisol, or DHA production. Perhaps this reflects a relative lack of insulin or IGF-I effect because these hormones influence angiotensin II receptor expression.[109] Another hormonal factor that may contribute to deficient 3β-HSD expression is the relative absence of triiodothyronine during fetal life.[110]

Considerable attention has been directed to the role of local growth factors, in particular IGF-II, in regulating fetal adrenal growth and development. IGF-II is highly expressed in human fetal adrenal cells, is mitogenic for adrenal cells, and is up-regulated by ACTH and other activators of the protein kinase A signal transduction pathway.[83,111] In the fetal sheep adrenal, IGF-II is co-localized to cells that express 3β-HSD activity,[112] but it is not yet clear how this relates to the relative 3β-HSD deficiency characteristic of the human fetal adrenal. *In vitro*, IGF-II appears to augment ACTH-stimulated fetal adrenal production of both cortisol and DHA. Other paracrine factors have been implicated in the regulation of adrenal growth and differentiation, including tumor necrosis factor-α, interferon-γ, transforming growth factor-β, epidermal growth factor, and basic fibroblast growth factor. Similarly, prostaglandin[2] has been shown to induce development of ACTH receptors and expression of 3β-HSD and P450$_{c17}$ activities.[113] The genes for inhibin synthesis are also expressed in human fetal adrenal cells,[114] but it is not clear whether bioactive dimeric inhibins and activins are produced and have a paracrine role.

Various neuropeptides, including vasopressin and vasoactive intestinal polypeptide, have been implicated as minor regulators

of adrenal growth and function.[115] Finally, there is evidence that catecholaminergic and peptidergic autonomic neural input can stimulate adrenocortical growth and steroidogenesis, but the implications for the fetal adrenal are unclear.[116]

Steroid Effects

When definitive zone or fetal zone cells are removed from the fetal environment and are exposed to ACTH, they rapidly express 3β-HSD[117] and secrete steroids, including cortisol, in a pattern identical to that of the adult adrenal (Fig. 187–6). It is well established that various steroids can inhibit 3β-HSD activity[118,119] and thus influence relative activities of 3β-HSD and P450$_{c17}$ (Fig. 187–7). *In vitro* exposure of fetal adrenal cells to a combination of ACTH and estradiol (Fig. 187–8) can induce the typical steroidogenic secretion pattern seen *in utero*. Although these steroid-induced effects are seen at physiologic concentrations of ambient steroids,[120,121] and they can be reproduced *in vitro* even with adult adrenal cells,[88] it is not at all clear that this accounts for the 3β-HSD deficiency of the human fetal adrenal. Placental steroids such as estradiol appear to inhibit preformed 3β-HSD enzyme, but there is no evidence that they block 3β-HSD gene expression, although they may enhance expression of P450$_{c17}$.[122] Furthermore, fetal zone cells express only small amounts of estrogen or progesterone receptor,[123] so a receptor-mediated effect on gene transcription seems unlikely. The fetal adrenal does have glucocorticoid receptors, and there is some evidence that cortisol itself may exert an autocrine effect on adrenal cell proliferation, enzyme induction, and ACTH responsiveness.[124,125]

ADAPTATION TO EXTRAUTERINE LIFE

By term, the adrenal cortex is secreting steroids, including not only DHA, but also cortisol and aldosterone, at high rates, primarily under the influence of ACTH, although the renin-angiotensin system may also be operative. Comparison of cord plasma ACTH

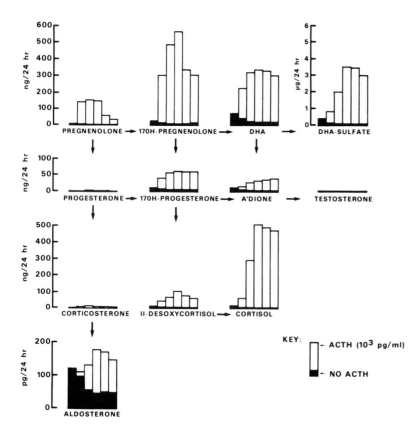

KEY:
☐ ← ACTH (10^3 pg/ml)
■ ← NO ACTH

Figure 187–6. The pattern of daily steroid production by human fetal adrenal cells during 6 days of culture in the presence or absence of corticotropin (ACTH). DHA = dehydroepiandrosterone. (From Fujieda K, et al: J Clin Endocrinol Metab 53:34, 1981.)

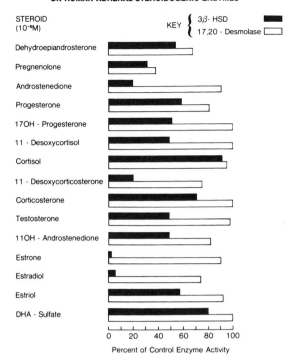

EFFECT OF AMBIENT STEROIDS ON HUMAN ADRENAL STEROIDOGENIC ENZYMES

STEROID (10⁻⁶M)   KEY { 3β- HSD ▮ / 17,20 - Desmolase ▯ }

Percent of Control Enzyme Activity

Figure 187–7. Effect of ambient steroids (10⁻⁶ M) on the activities of 3β-hydroxysteroid dehydrogenase (3β-HSD) and 17,20-desmolase in human adrenal microsomes. DHA = dehydroepiandrosterone. (From Winter JSD: *In* D'Agata R, Chrousos GP [eds]: Recent Advances in Adrenal Regulation and Function. New York, Raven Press, 1987, pp 51–66.)

concentrations after vaginal delivery (~1500 pg/mL) with those during cesarean section (~30 pg/mL) demonstrates that the hypothalamus and pituitary can respond to the stress of labor.[126] Plasma levels of corticotropin-releasing factor are also markedly increased at this time,[127, 128] as are levels of vasopressin. This perinatal surge of ACTH secretion is accompanied by parallel increases in other POMC-derived peptides, such as β-endorphin and β-lipotropin,[129,130] and it elicits an immediate response in fetal adrenal secretion of cortisol, DHA, and pregnenolone.[131, 132] Although prenatal administration of glucocorticoid can suppress the pituitary-adrenal axis throughout the first week of life,[133] this does not block the cortisol response either to labor[104, 105] or to exogenous ACTH.[134]

The changes in mean circulating levels of various steroids of adrenal or placental origin during the neonatal period are summarized in Table 187–1. Unconjugated placental steroids such as progesterone or estradiol are cleared rapidly after parturition, but the clearance of sulfate conjugates is noticeably prolonged. At birth, because of the stress of labor, serum concentrations of cortisol are quite high; in full-term infants, these fall by about half over the first 1 to 3 days of life, although values may be higher in premature infants.[135] Levels of free or unbound cortisol show a similar pattern but in the absence of illness remain relatively stable after 3 days of age.[136] Very small (<27 weeks' gestation) newborns may show lower levels of serum cortisol throughout the neonatal period.[137] Although this probably reflects general immaturity of the hypothalamic-pituitary-adrenal axis, there appears to be a component of adrenocortical enzymatic immaturity because serum levels of cortisol precursors, such as 17-hydroxypregnenolone, 17-hydroxyprogesterone, and 11-desoxycortisol, are elevated in such infants.[138]

From birth, ACTH and cortisol are secreted in pulsatile fashion, with secretory bursts at intervals of 1 to 2 hours.[139] The basal cortisol production rate of term and premature neonates is about 20 μmol/M² per day, similar to that of adults. Separation from the placenta reduces the metabolic clearance rate of cortisol,

Figure 187–8. The influence of added estradiol on the pattern of steroids produced by human fetal adrenal cells in the presence of corticotropin (ACTH). Each *bar* represents the mean total steroid production during 5 days of tissue culture. The symbols are as follows: control (*white*); ACTH 100 pg/mL alone (*dotted*); and ACTH plus estradiol 1 μg/mL (*cross-hatched*). DHA = dehydroepiandrosterone. (From Fujieda K, et al: J Clin Endocrinol Metab *54*:89, 1982.)

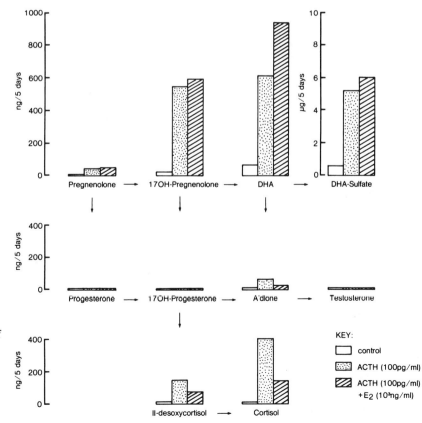

TABLE 187-1

Mean Plasma Concentrations of Pituitary, Adrenal, and Placental Hormones During Fetal and Neonatal Life*

	Midpregnancy	Birth	1 Day	1 Week	3 Months	6 Months	Adult Male
ACTH (pmol/l)	55	32	14	8	9	4	<16
Renin activity (pmol/l S)	NA	2.4	5.1	3.2	2.6	2.1	.1-.6
Δ^4-3-Ketosteroids (nmol/l)							
Progesterone	240	1920	40	1.6	1	0.8	<2
16αOH-progesterone	50	100	3	2	NA	NA	NA
17OH-progesterone	50	100	3	3	2	1	<6
11-desoxycorticosterone	NA	19	3.4	0.3	0.1	0.1	<.4
Corticosterone	NA	29	2.2	1.4	0.8	1.1	1-50
Aldosterone	2	1	1	0.4	0.4	0.8	.1-.8
Androstenedione	3	15	6	1	1	0.4	1.7-6.9
Cortisol	20	530	100	96	91	174	50-700
Cortisone	90	380	113	60	55	NA	NA
Estradiol	11	32	NA	0.04	0.04	0.04	<.18
Estrone	23	38	NA	NA	0.1	0.1	<.2
Estriol	145	350	NA	NA	NA	NA	NA
Δ^5-3β-Hydroxysteroids (nmol/l)							
Pregnenolone	NA	4290	NA	NA	5	1.7	1.3-7.3
DHA	NA	32	12	12	5	1	6.2-24.2
16αOH-DHA	18	15	4	3	NA	NA	NA
Steroid sulfates (nmol/l)							
Pregnenolone sulfate	NA	2750	2150	1350	650	92	133
DHA sulfate	3200	5200	3600	640	145	83	2600-10400
16αOH-DHA sulfate	3600	8300	NA	NA	NA	NA	NA
Estrone sulfate	22	28	NA	NA	NA	NA	NA
Estradiol sulfate	6	13	NA	NA	NA	NA	NA
Estriol sulfate	420	4100	2570	1475	NA	NA	NA

* NA indicates suitable data are not available or levels are negligible. Steroid concentrations can be converted approximately to ng/ml by multiplying by 0.3; plasma ACTH can be converted to pg/ml by multiplying by 44; plasma renin activity can be converted to ng/ml/h by multiplying by 4.7.
ACTH = adrenocorticotropic hormone.
From Winter JSD: *In* Anderson DC, Winter JSD (eds): Adrenal Cortex. London, Butterworths, 1985.

however, leaving the neonate with a considerable excess of adrenal secretory capacity. In the absence of ACTH stimulation, the fetal zone, which constitutes 80% of the adrenal cortex, involutes rapidly. This process involves primarily a reduction in cell size and architectural remodeling to form zone fasciculata,[140] but in some circumstances focal necrosis may occur.[141]

As adrenal involution occurs, with a gradual reduction in cortical thickness and intra-adrenal steroid concentrations, there is a striking improvement in adrenal 3β-HSD activity and a corresponding increase in the capacity to secrete cortisol. This process is reflected in a gradual reduction in plasma and urinary levels of DHA and other Δ^5-3β-hydroxysteroids.[142] Immediately after birth, administration of exogenous ACTH elicits a three- to fourfold rise in plasma cortisol levels, with a similar increase in DHA sulfate.[134, 143, 144] In sharp contrast, ACTH stimulation between 1 and 4 months of age produces a 30-fold increase in plasma cortisol[145] but only small increments in DHA sulfate.[146] As the adrenal cortex continues to involute, however, there is a corresponding reduction in cortisol secretory capacity. By 1 year of age, cortisol responses are similar to those of adults, but ACTH still elicits only minimal increases in DHA sulfate.[95] Secretion of ACTH and cortisol is normally pulsatile in infancy; it would appear that the usual circadian rhythm is established by at least 6 months of age.[147] Plasma renin activity and aldosterone levels are quite high during the first few days of life and remain higher than those of adults through infancy.

FUNCTIONS OF THE ADRENAL CORTEX DURING FETAL AND NEONATAL LIFE

One has only to observe the rapid deterioration of an infant with adrenal insufficiency to understand how vital normal glucocorticoid and mineralocorticoid function is to the neonate. It is less clear, however, to what extent the fetal adrenal cortex plays a necessary role in prenatal development and parturition. As has already been discussed, the major fetal adrenal secretion products are inactive Δ^5-3β-hydroxysteroid conjugates such as DHA sulfate. This material can undergo placental conversion to estrogen, but when this mechanism is not available, as in placental sulfatase deficiency or fetal adrenal hypoplasia, there is little deleterious effect on the course of pregnancy. Similarly, it seems unlikely that mineralocorticoids of fetal origin plan an important role in fetal or amniotic fluid electrolyte dynamics, given the high circulating concentrations of placental progesterone and its metabolites such as DOC that would compete for the aldosterone receptor.

There is considerable evidence that glucocorticoids can induce specific proteins and influence maturation of various systems (hepatic, intestinal, pulmonary) in the developing fetus.[148] In concert with other adrenal factors,[149] glucocorticoids affect adrenomedullary catecholamine synthesis. Studies in several species show that glucocorticoids accelerate alveolar differentiation and enhance surfactant synthesis, with important effects on lung pressure-volume relationships and permeability.[150]

There is also evidence of a role for endogenous adrenal steroids in normal fetal lung development. The developing lung contains glucocorticoid receptors, and there is a close temporal correlation between fetal cortisol levels and various indices of lung maturation.[151] In fetal sheep, pituitary ablation retards lung development, but this can be restored with ACTH. In the human fetus, anencephaly is associated with histologic evidence of delayed lung maturation;[152] however, live-born infants with deficient pituitary or adrenal function do not commonly develop hyaline membrane disease, perhaps because they are born at or after term and have time for adequate lung development despite low cortisol levels. The human fetus, because of the maternal contribution, can never be totally deficient in cortisol.

The use of exogenous corticosteroids for either maternal or fetal indications during pregnancy has raised concerns about possible adverse effects on fetal growth, immunologic function, or eventual neurologic development. Studies in various species, including nonhuman primates, have confirmed that high doses of glucocorticoid can retard both fetal and placental growth.[153] These observations may not be relevant to the short courses of dexamethasone used in respiratory distress syndrome prevention or to the situations in which pregnant women receive corticosteroids for conditions such as asthma.[154] They do raise important questions, however, about the use of high-dose dexamethasone therapy throughout pregnancy, as for the prevention of fetal virilization in congenital adrenal hyperplasia.

The observation that, in some species, prenatal administration of glucocorticoid causes premature delivery has focused attention on the role of the fetal adrenal cortex in the initiation of parturition.[155] In sheep during the last 72 hours of pregnancy, there is a brisk rise in fetal cortisol secretion, followed by marked changes in placental production of estrogen and progesterone and subsequent effects on uterine prostaglandin synthesis and contractility. There is evidence that this glucocorticoid effect involves induction of aromatase and 17-hydroxylase activities in the term placenta.[156]

The evidence of a role of the fetal adrenal in the onset of parturition is less convincing in primates than it is in sheep.[157] Although dexamethasone administration causes increased placental estrogen synthesis in sheep, the opposite occurs in humans because of suppression of the fetal DHA contribution. There is disagreement in the literature about whether anencephaly or fetal adrenal hypoplasia regularly prolongs gestation.[158, 159] Fetal hypophysectomy prolongs gestation,[160] but attempts to accomplish the same end by fetal adrenalectomy were inconclusive.[161] As noted earlier, in the complete absence of any fetal adrenal function, pregnancy and parturition are quite normal. Pepe and colleagues[162] showed that placental estrogens can enhance fetal pituitary ACTH expression (and presumably fetal adrenal steroidogenesis), but it remains to be seen whether this has any impact on the timing of parturition. Therefore, although it seems probable that some fetoplacental communication system involving not only steroids, but also cytokines and prostaglandins, exists to coordinate the events of human parturition, the details of such an interrelationship remain unclear.[163]

Once parturition has occurred, the neonate is immediately dependent on normal adrenal cortisol and aldosterone secretion for survival. Although cortisol has a bewildering multitude of biologic effects, they can be classified under three main headings:

1. Maintenance of blood glucose levels through stimulation of hepatic gluconeogenesis, reduction of extrahepatic protein synthesis, and inhibition of insulin secretion.
2. Inhibition of inflammatory and allergic reactions through effects on lymphokines and other cellular mediators.
3. Facilitation of renal free water excretion.

Obviously, the first action is most important for the neonate; in the absence of normal pituitary-adrenal function, hypoglycemia can occur within a few hours of birth.

Aldosterone and, to a lesser extent, other mineralocorticoids such as DOC stimulate active sodium reabsorption and promote excretion of potassium and hydrogen in the distal tubule of the kidney and in sweat glands, intestinal mucosa, and salivary glands. This process requires initial binding to a mineralocorticoid receptor, followed by mRNA-dependent protein synthesis and functional changes in the epithelial cells that enhance sodium transport across the mucosal surface membrane. In the neonate, one can see signs of mineralocorticoid insufficiency either because of insufficient aldosterone secretion or because of blockade of renal tubular mineralocorticoid receptors by com-

peting steroids such as 17OH-progesterone. In infants with adrenal insufficiency, the earliest evidence of electrolyte disturbance is rising levels of serum potassium and plasma renin activity at 4 or 5 days of age. By the second week of life, urinary sodium loss is sufficient to trigger compensatory vasopressin-mediated water retention, and one can see the typical picture of hyponatremia, hyperkalemia, and acidosis.

REFERENCES

1. Siiteri PK, MacDonald PC: Placental estrogen biosynthesis during human pregnancy. J Clin Endocrinol Metab 26:751, 1966.
2. Winter JSD: Functional changes in the adrenal gland during life. In D'Agata R, Chrousos GP (eds): Recent Advances in Adrenal Regulation and Function. New York, Raven Press, 1987, pp 51–66.
3. Winter JSD: Development of the pituitary-adrenal axis in childhood and adolescence. In Savage MO, et al (eds): Frontiers in Paediatric Neuroendocrinology. London, Blackwell, 1994, pp 51–60.
4. Carr BR, Casey ML: Growth of the adrenal gland of the normal human fetus during early gestation. Early Hum Dev 6:121, 1982.
5. Rocian-Sobkowska J, et al: Cytological aspects of the human adrenal cortex development in the course of intra-uterine life. Histol Histopathol 8:725, 1993.
6. Crowder RE: The development of the adrenal gland in man, with special reference to origin and ultimate location of cell types and evidence in favor of the cell migration theory. Carnegie Contrib Embryol 36:193, 1957.
7. Zajicek G, et al: The streaming adrenal cortex: direct evidence of centripetal migration of adrenocytes by estimation of cell turnover rate. J Endocrinol 111:477, 1986.
8. Johannison E: The foetal adrenal cortex in the human: its ultrastructure at different stages of development and in different functional states. Acta Endocrinol 58:130, 1968.
9. Nussdorfer GG: Cytophysiology of the adrenal cortex. Int Rev Cytol 98:211, 1986.
10. Sakaguchi M, et al: Signal recognition particle is required for co-translational insertion of cytochrome P-450 into microsomal membranes. Proc Natl Acad Sci USA 81:3361, 1984.
11. DeSa DJ: Stress responses and its relationship to cystic pseudofollicular change in the definitive cortex of the adrenal gland in stillborn children. Arch Dis Child 53:769, 1978.
12. McNulty WP: Postnatum evolution of the adrenal glands of rhesus macaques. In Novy MJ, Resko JA (eds): Fetal Endocrinology. New York, Academic Press, 1981, pp 53–64.
13. Miller WL: Molecular biology of steroid hormone synthesis. Endocr Rev 9:295, 1988.
14. Clark BJ, et al: The purification, cloning, and expression of a novel luteinizing hormone-induced mitochondrial protein in MA-10 mouse Leydig tumor cells. J Biol Chem 269:28314, 1994.
15. Kawamoto T, et al: Cloning and expression of a cDNA for human cytochrome P450 aldo as related to primary aldosteronism. Biochem Biophys Res Commun 173:309, 1990.
16. Sauer LA, et al: Topology of 3β-hydroxy-5-ene-steroid dehydrogenase/Δ5-Δ4-isomerase in adrenal cortex mitochondria and microsomes. Endocrinology 134:751, 1994.
17. Moore CCD, Miller WL: The role of transcriptional regulation in steroid hormone biosynthesis. J Steroid Biochem Mol Biol 40:517, 1991.
18. Parker KL, Schimmer BP: Transcriptional regulation of the adrenal steroidogenic enzymes. Trends Endocrinol Metab 4:46, 1993.
19. Cone RD, Mountjoy KG: Molecular genetics of the ACTH and melanocyte-stimulating hormone receptors. Trends Endocrinol Metab 4:242, 1993.
20. Durand PL, et al: Changes in protein kinase activities in lamb adrenals at late gestation and early postnatal stages. Mol Cell Endocrinol 53:195, 1987.
21. Carr BR, et al: The role of calcium in steroidogenesis in fetal zone cells of the human fetal adrenal gland. J Clin Endocrinol Metab 63:913, 1986.
22. Farese RV: Phosphoinositide metabolism and hormone action. Endocr Rev 4:78, 1983.
23. McAllister JM, Hornsby PJ: Dual regulation of 3β-hydroxysteroid dehydrogenase, 17α-hydroxylase, and dehydroepiandrosterone sulfotransferase by adenosine 3′,5′-monophosphate and activators of protein kinase C in cultured human adrenocortical cells. Endocrinology 122:2012, 1988.
24. Doody KM, et al: 3β-Hydroxysteroid dehydrogenase/isomerase in the fetal zone and neocortex of the human fetal adrenal gland. Endocrinology 126:2487, 1990.
25. Dupont E, et al: Ontogeny of 3β-hydroxysteroid dehydrogenase/Δ5-Δ4 isomerase (3β-HSD) in human adrenal gland performed by immunocytochemistry. Mol Cell Endocrinol 74:R7, 1990.
26. Mesiano S, et al: Localization of cytochrome P450 cholesterol side-chain cleavage, cytochrome P450 17-hydroxylase/17,20-lyase, and 3β-hydroxysteroid dehydrogenase isomerase steroidogenic enzymes in human and rhesus monkey fetal adrenal glands: reappraisal of functional zonation. J Clin Endocrinol Metab 77:1184, 1993.
27. Milewich L, et al: 3β-Hydroxysteroid dehydrogenase activity in glandular and extraglandular human fetal tissues. J Clin Endocrinol Metab 73:1134, 1991.

28. Carr BR, et al: Metabolism of low density lipoprotein by human fetal adrenal tissue. Endocrinology *107*:1034, 1980.

29. Higashijima M, et al: Studies on lipoprotein and adrenal steroidogenesis. I. roles of low density lipoprotein and high density lipoprotein cholesterol in steroid production in cultured human adrenocortical cells. Endocrinol Jpn *34*:635, 1987.

30. Mason JI, Hemsell PG: Cholesterol sulfate metabolism in human fetal adrenal mitochondria. Endocrinology *111*:208, 1982.

31. McConathy WJ, Lane DM: Studies on the apolipoproteins and lipoproteins of cord serum. Pediatr Res *14*:757, 1980.

32. Parker CR Jr, et al: Inverse relationship between LDL-cholesterol and dehydroisoandrosterone sulfate in human fetal plasma. Science *208*:512, 1980.

33. Carr BR, Simpson ER: De novo synthesis of cholesterol by the human fetal adrenal gland. Endocrinology *108*:2154, 1981.

34. Carr BR, et al: Low density lipoprotein binding and de novo synthesis of cholesterol in the neocortex and fetal zones of the human fetal adrenal gland. Endocrinology *110*:1994, 1982.

35. Hobkirk R: Steroid sulfotransferases and steroid sulfate sulfatases: characteristics and biological roles. Can J Biochem Cell Biol *63*:1127, 1985.

36. Korte K, et al: Sterol sulfate metabolism in the adrenals of the human fetus, anencephalic newborn and adult. J Clin Endocrinol Metab *55*:671, 1982.

37. Mason JI, et al: Steroidogenesis in dispersed cells of the human fetal adrenal. J Clin Endocrinol Metab *56*:1057, 1983.

38. Branchaud CL, et al: Contribution of exogenous progesterone to human adrenal cortisol synthesis in vitro: a comparison of early gestational fetal and adult tissues. Steroids *47*:269, 1986.

39. Dufau ML, Villee DB: Aldosterone biosynthesis by human fetal adrenal in vivo. Biochem Biophys Acta *176*:637, 1969.

40. Yoshida N, et al: Biosynthetic pathways for corticoids and androgen formation in human fetal adrenal tissue in vivo. Endocrinol Jpn *25*:191, 1978.

41. Hagemanas FC, Kittinger GW: The influence of fetal sex on the levels of plasma progesterone in the human fetus. J Clin Endocrinol Metab *36*:389, 1973.

42. Harbert GM Jr, et al: Concentration of progesterone in newborn and maternal circulation at delivery. Obstet Gynecol *23*:413, 1964.

43. Macnaughton MC, et al: The effect of synthetic ACTH on the metabolism of [4-^{14}C] progesterone by the previable human fetus. J Steroid Biochem *8*:499, 1977.

44. Ducsay CA, et al: Maternal and fetal production rates of progesterone in rhesus macaques: placental transfer and conversion to cortisol. Endocrinology *117*:1253, 1985.

45. Pepe GJ, Albrecht ED: The utilization of placental substrates for cortisol synthesis by the baboon fetus near term. Steroids *35*:591, 1980.

46. Hadjian AJ, et al: Cortisol binding to proteins in plasma in the human neonate and infant. Pediatr Res *9*:40, 1975.

47. Campbell AL, Murphy BEP: The maternal-fetal cortisol gradient during pregnancy and at delivery. J Clin Endocrinol Metab *45*:435, 1977.

48. Pasqualini JR, et al: Cortisol and cortisone metabolism in the human foeto-placental unit at midgestation. J Steroid Biochem *1*:209, 1970.

49. Mitchell BF, et al: Cortisol production and metabolism in the late gestation rhesus monkey fetus. Endocrinology *108*:916, 1981.

50. Leong MKH, Murphy BEP: Cortisol levels in maternal venous and umbilical cord arterial and venous serum at vaginal delivery. Am J Obstet Gynecol *126*:471, 1976.

51. Murphy BEP: Steroid arteriovenous differences in umbilical cord plasma: evidence of cortisol production by the human fetus in mid-gestation. J Clin Endocrinol Metab *35*:678, 1973.

52. Jaffe RB, et al: Regulation and function of the primate fetal adrenal gland and gonad. Proc Prog Horm Res *37*:41, 1981.

53. Walsh SW, et al: In utero regulation of rhesus monkey fetal adrenals: effects of dexamethasone, adrenocorticotropin, thyrotropin-releasing hormone, prolactin, human chorionic gonadotropin and α-melanocyte stimulating hormone on fetal and maternal plasma steroids. Endocrinology *104*:1805, 1979.

54. Beitins IZ, et al: The metabolic clearance rate, blood production, interconversion and transplacental passage of cortisol and cortisone in pregnancy near term. Pediatr Res 7:509, 1973.

55. Lugg MA, Nicholas TE: The effect of dexamethasone on the activity of 11β-hydroxysteroid dehydrogenase in foetal rabbit lung during the final stage of gestation. J Pharm Pharmacol *30*:587, 1978.

56. Michaud NJ, Burton AF: Maternal-fetal relationships in corticosteroid metabolism. Biol Neonate *32*:132, 1977.

57. Smith BT: The role of pulmonary corticosteroid 11-reductase activity in lung maturation in the fetal rat. Pediatr Res *12*:12, 1978.

58. Monder C, Shackleton CHL: 11β-Hydroxysteroid dehydrogenase: fact or fancy? Steroids *44*:383, 1984.

59. Fujieda K, et al: The control of steroidogenesis by human fetal adrenal cells in tissue culture. I. responses to adrenocorticotropin. J Clin Endocrinol Metab *53*:34, 1981.

60. Bayard F, et al: Transplacental passage and fetal secretion of aldosterone. J Clin Invest *49*:1389, 1970.

61. Beitins IZ, et al: Plasma aldosterone concentration at delivery and during the newborn period. J Clin Invest *51*:386, 1972.

62. Brown EH, et al: Aldosterone, corticosterone, cortisol, 11-deoxycortisol and 11-deoxycorticosterone in the blood of chronically cannulated ovine foetuses: effect of ACTH. Acta Endocrinol *88*:364, 1978.

63. Wintour EM, et al: Potassium: aldosterone relationships in pregnant ewes and chronically cannulated ovine fetuses. Pediatr Res *13*:265, 1979.

64. Lingwood B, et al: Effect of aldosterone on urine composition in the chronically cannulated ovine foetus. J Endocrinol *76*:553, 1978.

65. Siegel SR, et al: Transplacental transfer of aldosterone and its effects on renal function in the fetal lamb. Pediatr Res *15*:163, 1981.

66. Greenberg AJ, et al: Renal tubular unresponsiveness to mineralocorticoids in normal infants and children with adrenal disorders. J Clin Endocrinol Metab *27*:1197, 1967.

67. Stark P, et al: Control of plasma aldosterone in infancy and childhood. Helv Paediatr Acta *30*:349, 1973.

68. Shepherd RW, et al: Fetal and maternal endocrine responses to reduced uteroplacental blood flow. J Clin Endocrinol Metab *75*:301, 1992.

69. Saenger P, et al: Prenatal diagnosis of congenital lipoid adrenal hyperplasia. J Clin Endocrinol Metab *80*:200, 1995.

70. Asa SL, et al: Human fetal adenohypophysis: histological and immunocytochemical analysis. Neuroendocrinology *43*:308, 1986.

71. Thliveris JA, Currie RW: Observations on the hypothalamo-hypophyseal portal vasculature in the developing human fetus. Am J Anat *157*:441, 1980.

72. Blumenfeld Z, Jaffe RB: Hypophysiotropic and neuromodulatory regulation of ACTH in the human fetal pituitary gland. J Clin Invest *78*:288, 1986.

73. Faucher DJ, et al: Increased fetal secretion of ACTH and cortisol by arginine vasopressin. Am J Physiol *254*:R410, 1988.

74. Hargrave BY, Rose JC: By 95 days of gestation CRF increases plasma ACTH and cortisol in ovine fetuses. Am J Physiol *13*:E422, 1986.

75. Gibbs DM: Effects of synthetic corticotropin-releasing factor and dopamine on the release of immunoreactive β-endorphin/β-lipotropin and α-melanocyte-stimulating hormone from human fetal pituitaries in vitro. J Clin Endocrinol Metab *55*:1149, 1982.

76. Goodyer CG, et al: Ontogeny of the human fetal pituitary-adrenal axis. *In* Saez JM, et al (eds): Ontogenesis of the Endocrine System. Paris, Editions INSERM, 1983, pp 163–187.

77. Demura R, et al: Placental secretion of prolactin, ACTH and immunoreactive β-endorphin during pregnancy. Acta Endocrinol *100*:114, 1982.

78. Laatikainen T, et al: Localization and concentrations of β-endorphin and β-lipotrophin in human placenta. Placenta *8*:381, 1987.

79. Waterman MR, Simpson ER: Cellular mechanisms involved in the acute and chronic actions of ACTH. *In* Anderson DC, Winter JSD (eds): Adrenal Cortex. London, Butterworth, 1985, pp 57–85.

80. Arola J, et al: Role of adenylate cyclase-cyclic AMP–dependent signal transduction in the ACTH-induced biphasic growth effect of rat adrenocortical cells in primary culture. J Endocrinol *139*:451, 1993.

81. Arola J, et al: Protein kinase C signal transduction pathway in ACTH-induced growth effect of rat adrenocortical cells in primary culture. J Endocrinol *141*:285, 1994.

82. Feige JJ, Baird A: Growth factor regulation of adrenal cortex growth and function. Prog Growth Factor Res *3*:103, 1991.

83. Voutilainen R, Miller WL: Developmental and hormonal regulation of mRNAs for insulin-like growth factor II and steroidogenic enzymes in human fetal adrenals and gonads. DNA *7*:9, 1988.

84. Simonian M, et al: Placental-derived mitogenic factor for human fetal adrenocortical cell cultures. In Vitro Cell Dev Biol *23*:57, 1987.

85. Gray ES, Abramovitch DR: Morphologic features of the anencephalic adrenal gland in early pregnancy. Am J Obstet Gynecol *137*:491, 1980.

86. Easterling WE, et al: Neutral C_{19}-steroids and steroid sulfates in human pregnancy: II. dehydroepiandrosterone sulfate, 16α-hydroxydehydroepiandrosterone sulfate in maternal and fetal blood of pregnancies with anencephalic and normal fetuses. Steroids *8*:157, 1966.

87. Carr BR: Adenylate cyclase activity in membrane fractions of adrenal tissue of human anencephalic fetuses. J Clin Endocrinol Metab *63*:51, 1986.

88. Winter JSD, Smail PJ: Effects of ACTH and estradiol on steroid production by cultured adrenal cells from an anencephalic fetus and from normal adults. Steroids *42*:677, 1984.

89. Padalko NL: Morphology of the adrenal cortex in the adrenogenital syndrome with salt loss. Arch Pathol *48*:51, 1986.

90. Symington T, et al: Effect of exogenous corticotropin on the histochemical pattern of the human adrenal cortex and a comparison with the changes during stress. J Clin Endocrinol Metab *16*:580, 1956.

91. Winters AJ, et al: Plasma ACTH levels in the human fetus and neonate as related to age and parturition. J Clin Endocrinol Metab *39*:269, 1974.

92. Fujieda K, et al: The control of steroidogenesis by human fetal adrenal cells in tissue culture. III. the effects of various hormonal peptides. J Clin Endocrinol Metab *53*:690, 1981.

93. Csontos K, et al: Elevated plasma β-endorphin levels in pregnant women and their neonates. Life Sci *25*:835, 1979.

94. Wardlaw AL, et al: Plasma β-endorphin and β-lipotropin in the human fetus at delivery: correlation with arterial pH and PO_2. J Clin Endocrinol Metab *49*:888, 1979.

95. Forest MG, et al: Developmental patterns of the plasma levels of testosterone, Δ^4-androstenedione, 17α-hydroxyprogesterone dehydroepiandrosterone and its sulfate in normal infants and prepubertal children. *In* James VHT, et al (eds): The Endocrine Function of the Human Adrenal Cortex. London, Academic Press, 1978, pp 561–582.

96. Jones CT: Normal fluctuations in the concentration of corticosteroids and ACTH in the plasma of foetal and pregnant sheep. Horm Metab Res *11*:237, 1979.

97. Charnvises S, et al: Adrenal steroids in maternal and cord blood after dexamethasone administration at midterm. J Clin Endocrinol Metab 61:1220, 1985.

98. Althaus ZR, et al: Transplacental metabolism of dexamethasone and cortisol in the late gestational age rhesus monkey (Macaca mulatta). Dev Pharmacol Ther 9:332, 1986.

99. David M, Forest MG: Prenatal treatment of congenital adrenal hyperplasia resulting from 21-hydroxylase deficiency. J Pediatr 105:799, 1984.

100. Rose JC: Regulation of pituitary adrenal function in the fetus. In Albrecht ED, Pepe GJ (eds): Perinatal Endocrinology. Ithaca, NY, Perinatology Press, 1985, pp 21–53.

101. Yan K, et al: Changes in glucocorticoid receptor number in the hypothalamus and pituitary of the sheep fetus with gestational age and after adrenocorticotropin treatment. Endocrinology 126:11, 1990.

102. Ohrlander SAV, et al: Impact of betamethasone load given to pregnant women on endocrine balance of feto-placental unit. Am J Obstet Gynecol 123:228, 1975.

103. Strecker JR, et al: Suppression of the maternal and fetal pituitary-adrenocortical axis by administration of betamethasone during pregnancy (abstract). Acta Endocrinol 215(Suppl):33, 1978.

104. Dorr HG, et al: Antenatal betamethasone therapy: effects on maternal, fetal and neonatal mineralocorticoids, glucocorticoids, and progestins. J Pediatr 108:990, 1986.

105. Kauppila A, et al: ACTH levels in maternal, fetal and neonatal plasma after short-term prenatal dexamethasone therapy. Br J Obstet Gynaecol 84:124, 1976.

106. Durand P, et al: Effects of proopiomelanocortin-derived peptides, methionine-enkephalin and forskolin on the maturation of ovine fetal adrenal cells in culture. Biol Reprod 31:694, 1984.

107. Saphier PW, et al: Elevated levels of N-terminal pro-opiomelanocortin peptides in fetal sheep plasma may contribute to fetal adrenal gland development and the preparturient cortisol surge. Endocrinology 133:1459, 1993.

108. Siegel SR, Fisher DB: Ontogeny of the renin-angiotensin-aldosterone system in the fetal and newborn lamb. Pediatr Res 14:99, 1980.

109. Penhoat A, et al: Characterization of insulin-like growth factor I and insulin receptors on cultured bovine adrenal fasciculata cells: role of these peptides on adrenal cell function. Endocrinology 122:2518, 1988.

110. Simonian MH: ACTH and thyroid hormone regulation of 3β-hydroxysteroid dehydrogenase activity in human fetal adrenocortical cells. J Steroid Biochem 25:1001, 1986.

111. Voutilainen R, et al: Parallel regulation of parentally imprinted H19 and insulin-like growth factor-II genes in cultured human fetal adrenal cells. Endocrinology 134:2051, 1994.

112. Han VKM, et al: Insulin-like growth factor-II (IGF-II) messenger ribonucleic acid is expressed in steroidogenic cells of the developing ovine adrenal gland: evidence of an autocrine/paracrine role for IGF-II. Endocrinology 131:3100, 1992.

113. Rainey WE, et al: Prostaglandin E₂ is a positive regulator of adrenocorticotropin receptors, 3β-hydroxysteroid dehydrogenase, and 17α-hydroxylase expression in bovine adrenocortical cells. Endocrinology 129:1333, 1991.

114. Voutilainen R, et al: Hormonally regulated inhibin gene expression in human fetal and adult adrenals. J Clin Endocrinol Metab 73:1026, 1991.

115. Malendowicz IK: Involvement of neuropeptides in the regulation of growth, structure and function of the adrenal cortex. Hist Histopathol 8:173, 1993.

116. Holzwarth MA, et al: The role of adrenal nerves in the regulation of adrenocortical functions. Ann NY Acad Sci 512:449, 1987.

117. Fujieda K, et al: The control of steroidogenesis by human fetal adrenal cells in tissue culture. II. Comparison of morphology and steroid production in cells of the fetal and definitive zones. J Clin Endocrinol Metab 53:401, 1981.

118. Byrne GC, et al: Kinetic analysis of adrenal 3β-hydroxysteroid dehydrogenase activity during human development. J Clin Endocrinol Metab 60:934, 1985.

119. Byrne GC, et al: Steroid inhibitory effects upon human adrenal 3β-hydroxysteroid dehydrogenase activity. J Clin Endocrinol Metab 62:413, 1986.

120. Couch RM, et al: Regulation of the activities of 17-hydroxylase and 17,20-desmolase in the human adrenal cortex: kinetic analysis and inhibition by endogenous steroids. J Clin Endocrinol Metab 63:613, 1986.

121. Dickerman Z, et al: Intra-adrenal steroid concentrations in man: zonal differences and developmental changes. J Clin Endocrinol Metab 59:1031, 1984.

122. Mesiano S, Jaffe RB: Interaction of insulin-like growth factor-II and estradiol directs steroidogenesis in the human fetal adrenal toward dehydroepiandrosterone sulfate production. J Clin Endocrinol Metab 77:754, 1993.

123. Hirst JJ, et al: Steroid hormone receptors in the adrenal glands of fetal and adult rhesus monkeys. J Clin Endocrinol Metab 75:308, 1992.

124. Arola J, et al: Corticosterone regulates cell proliferation and cytochrome P450 cholesterol side-chain cleavage enzyme messenger ribonucleic acid expression in primary cultures of fetal rat adrenals. Endocrinology 135:2064, 1994.

125. Darbeida H, et al: Glucocorticoid induction of the maturation of ovine fetal adrenocortical cells. Biochem Biophys Res Commun 145:999, 1987.

126. Pohjavuori M, Fyhrquist F: Vasopressin, ACTH and neonatal haemodynamics. Acta Paediatr Scand Suppl 305:79, 1983.

127. Nagashima K, et al: Cord blood levels of corticotropin-releasing factor. Biol Neonate 51:1, 1987.

128. Sasaki A, et al: Immunoreactive corticotropin-releasing factor is present in human maternal plasma during the third trimester of pregnancy. J Clin Endocrinol Metab 59:812, 1984.

129. Facchinetti F, et al: Plasma opioids in the first hours of life. Pediatr Res 16:95, 1982.

130. Goland RS, et al: Human plasma β-endorphin during pregnancy labor and delivery. J Clin Endocrinol Metab 52:74, 1981.

131. Arai K, Yanaihara T: Steroid hormone changes in fetal blood during labor. Am J Obstet Gynecol 127:879, 1977.

132. Predine J, et al: Unbound cortisol in umbilical cord plasma and maternal plasma: a reinvestigation. Am J Obstet Gynecol 135:1104, 1979.

133. Sippell WG, et al: Development of endogenous glucocorticoids, mineralocorticoids and progestins in the human fetal and perinatal period. Eur J Clin Pharmacol 18:90, 1980.

134. Ohrlander S, et al: ACTH test to neonates after administration of corticosteroids during gestation. Obstet Gynecol 49:691, 1977.

135. Kraiem Z, et al: Serum cortisol levels: the first 10 days in full-term and preterm infants. Isr J Med Sci 21:170, 1985.

136. Rokicki W, et al: Free cortisol of human plasma in the first three months of life. Biol Neonate 57:21, 1990.

137. Scott SM, Watterberg KL: Effect of gestational age, postnatal age, and illness on plasma cortisol concentrations in premature infants. Pediatr Res 37:112, 1995.

138. Hingre RV, et al: Adrenal steroidogenesis in very low birth weight preterm infants. J Clin Endocrinol Metab 78:266, 1994.

139. DeZegher F, et al: Properties of thyroid-stimulating hormone and cortisol secretion by the human newborn on the day of birth. J Clin Endocrinol Metab 79:576, 1994.

140. Sucheston ME, Cannon MS: Development of zonular patterns in the human adrenal gland. J Morphol 126:477, 1968.

141. Ducsay CA, et al: Endocrine and morphological maturation of the fetal and neonatal adrenal cortex in baboons. J Clin Endocrinol Metab 73:385, 1991.

142. Shackleton CHL, et al: Steroids in newborns and infants: the changing pattern of urinary steroid excretion during infancy. Acta Endocrinol 74:157, 1973.

143. Barnhart BJ, et al: Adrenal cortical function in the postmature fetus and newborn infant. Pediatr Res 14:1367, 1980.

144. Pintor C, et al: The first 48 hours of life: cortisol and dehydroepiandrosterone sulphate under basal conditions and after ACTH stimulation. In LaCauza C, Root AW (eds): Problems in Pediatric Endocrinology. London, Academic Press, 1980, pp 305–310.

145. Forest MG: Age-related response in plasma testosterone, Δ⁴-androstenedione and cortisol to adrenocorticotropin in infants, children and adults. J Clin Endocrinol Metab 47:931, 1978.

146. Noguchi A, Reynolds JW: Serum cortisol and dehydroepiandrosterone sulfate responses to adrenocorticotropin stimulation in premature infants. Pediatr Res 12:1057, 1978.

147. Onishi S, et al: Postnatal development of circadian rhythm in serum cortisol levels in children. Pediatrics 72:399, 1983.

148. Ballard PL: Hormones and Lung Maturation. Berlin, Springer-Verlag, 1986.

149. Cheung CY: Enhancement of adrenomedullary catecholamine release by adrenal cortex in fetus. Am J Physiol 247:E693, 1984.

150. Ikegami M, et al: Corticosteroids and surfactant change lung function and protein leaks in the lung of ventilated premature rabbits. J Clin Invest 79:1371, 1987.

151. Murphy BEP: Conjugated glucocorticoids in amniotic fluid and fetal lung maturation. J Clin Endocrinol Metab 47:212, 1978.

152. Naeye RL, et al: Adrenal gland structure and the development of hyaline membrane disease. Pediatrics 47:650, 1971.

153. Johnson JW, et al: Long-term effects of betamethasone on fetal development. Am J Obstet Gynecol 141:1053, 1981.

154. Fitzsimons R, et al: Outcome of pregnancy in women requiring corticosteroids for severe asthma. J Allergy Clin Immunol 78:349, 1986.

155. Thorburn GD, Challis JRG: Endocrine control of parturition. Physiol Rev 59:863, 1979.

156. France JT, et al: The regulation of ovine placental steroid 17α-hydroxylase and aromatase by glucocorticoid. Mol Endocrinol 2:193, 1988.

157. Challis JRG, Hooper S: Birth: outcome of a positive cascade. Clin Endocrinol Metab 3:781, 1989.

158. Davies IJ, Ryan KJ: The comparative endocrinology of gestation. Vitam Horm 30:223, 1972.

159. Swaab DFK, et al: Influence of the fetal hypothalamus and pituitary on the onset and course of parturition. In Knight J, O'Connor M (eds): Ciba Foundation Symposium: The Fetus and Birth. Amsterdam, Elsevier, 1977, p 379.

160. Chez RA, et al: Some effects of fetal and maternal hypophysectomy in pregnancy. Am J Obstet Gynecol 108:643, 1970.

161. Mueller-Heubach E, et al: Effect of adrenalectomy on pregnancy in the rhesus monkey. Am J Obstet Gynecol 112:221, 1972.

162. Pepe GJ, et al: Activation of the baboon fetal pituitary-adrenocortical axis at midgestation by estrogen: enhancement of fetal pituitary proopiomelanocortin messenger ribonucleic acid expression. Endocrinology 135:2581, 1994.

163. Olson DM, et al: Control of human parturition. Semin Perinatol 19:52, 1995.

THYROID

Daniel H. Polk and Delbert A. Fisher

188

Fetal and Neonatal Thyroid Physiology

EMBRYOGENESIS AND HISTOLOGIC DEVELOPMENT OF THE THYROID GLAND

The human *thyroid gland* is a derivative of the primitive buccopharyngeal cavity.[1-3] It develops from contributions of two types of anlagen: a midline thickening of the pharyngeal floor (median anlage) and paired caudal extensions of the fourth pharyngobranchial pouch (lateral anlagen). All these structures are discernible by day 16 to 17 of gestation; by 24 days' gestation, the median anlage has developed a thin, flasklike diverticulum, extending from the floor of the buccal cavity down to the fourth branchial arch. At 40 days' gestation, the median and lateral anlagen have fused, and by 50 days' gestation, the buccal stalk has ruptured. During this period, the thyroid gland migrates caudally to its definitive location in the anterior neck, helped in part by its relationship with developing cardiac structures.

The early histologic development of the thyroid gland has been divided into three phases: (1) precolloid (7 to 13 weeks' gestation), (2) early colloid (13 to 14 weeks' gestation), and (3) follicular (>14 weeks' gestation) phases.[4] In the precolloid phase, the thyroid cells contain an intracellular canaliculus derived from the smooth endoplasmic reticulum. As these canaliculi mature, they migrate toward the cell apex and begin to discharge their contents extracellularly. In the early follicular stage, these canaliculi fuse, and desmosomes define the borders of these spaces, thus allowing for the central accumulation of colloid. At this time (~70 days' gestation), iodide concentration and thyroglobulin synthesis can be demonstrated within the gland. During the final follicular phase, there is a further increase in the size of the colloid spaces, as well as progressive cell growth and accumulation of thyroid hormones.

The *parathyroid glands* develop between 5 and 12 weeks' gestation from the third and fourth pharyngeal pouches. The third pouches encounter the migrating thyroid anlage, and the parathyroid anlagen are carried caudally with the thyroid gland. They finally come to lie at the lower poles of the thyroid lobes as the inferior parathyroid glands. The fourth pouches encounter the thyroid anlage later and come to rest at the upper poles of the thyroid lobes as the superior parathyroid glands. The individual parathyroid glands increase in size from less than 0.1 mm diameter at 14 weeks to 1 to 2 mm at birth. The fifth pouches contribute paired ultimobranchial bodies that become incorporated into the developing thyroid gland as the parafollicular C cells, the calcitonin-secreting cells.[5,6]

Hypothalamic maturation proceeds from the fifth week through 30 to 35 weeks' gestation.[2] Most of the hypothalamic nuclei and fibers of the supraoptic tract are visible histologically by 12 to 14 weeks. Thyrotropin-releasing hormone (TRH), gonadotropin-releasing hormone, and somatostatin are detectable in hypothalamic tissue by 10 to 12 weeks. Between 10 and 35 weeks, continuing histologic maturation of the hypothalamus takes place.

The anterior *pituitary gland* is a derivative of the primitive buccal cavity (Rathke pouch), and its embryologic development parallels that of the thyroid anlagen.[2] By the fifth week in the human embryo, the Rathke pouch makes contact with a funnel-shaped ventral diverticulum of the third cerebral ventricle, the infundibular process. By 12 weeks, the buccal connection is obliterated by the developing sphenoid bone, and the pituitary gland becomes partially encapsulated within a bony cavity, the sella turcica. Between 9 and 12 weeks, many pituitary cell types appear, each more or less specialized for secretion of one of the anterior pituitary hormones. Secretory granules can be identified within these cells at 10 to 12 weeks, and thyrotropin (TSH) is identifiable by bioassay and immunoassay at this time.

Abnormalities of hypothalamic or pituitary gland embryogenesis can be associated with TSH deficiency and secondary hypothyroidism. Developmental abnormalities of the thyroid gland usually represent defects in early morphogenesis resulting from aberrant thyroid tissue migration. The most common anomaly is the persistence of the thyroglossal duct. This is not usually associated with altered thyroid status in the newborn, but it may present in later life as an infected fistulous tract. Abnormalities of thyroid embryogenesis (thyroid dysgenesis) include agenesis or ectopic tissue in sublingual, cervical, mediastinal, or even intracardiac locations. Failure of fusion of median and lateral anlagen may produce cystic masses of cells in various locations in the neck. Although ectopic thyroid tissue may manifest some function, infants with these anomalies usually exhibit some degree of hypothyroidism. Calcitonin deficiency also is present in children with congenital hypothyroidism.[7] Hypoparathyroidism, however, is not associated with thyroid dysgenesis, although the parathyroid glands may be ectopic.

THYROID HORMONE SYNTHESIS

Circulating plasma iodide enters the thyroid follicular cells and is combined with tyrosine through a series of enzymatically mediated reactions to form the active thyroid hormones 3,5,3'−triiodothyronine (T_3) and thyroxine (T_4). The steps in synthesis and release of thyroid hormones include the following:

1. Active transport of inorganic iodide from plasma to thyroid cell.
2. Synthesis of tyrosine-rich thyroglobulin, which acts as the intermediate iodine acceptor.
3. Organification of trapped iodide as iodotyrosines.
4. Coupling of monoiodotyrosines (MIT) and diiodotyrosines (DIT) to form the iodothyronines, T_3 and T_4, with storage of iodotyrosines and iodothyronines in follicular colloid.
5. Endocytosis and proteolysis of colloid thyroglobulin to release MIT, DIT, T_3, and T_4.
6. Deiodination of released iodotyrosines within the thyroid cell with reuse of the iodine. These steps and their inhibitors are outlined in Table 188–1 and are pictorially represented in Figure 188–1.

Iodide Concentration

The first and rate-limiting step in the synthesis of thyroid hormones involves the concentration of iodide by the thyroid follicular cell. The thyroid iodide transporter is located in the follicular cell plasma membrane.[8,9] Extrathyroidal tissues (gastric mucosa,

TABLE 188-1	
Biochemical Steps to Thyroid Hormone Synthesis	
Step	**Inhibitor**
1. Iodide transport	DNP, ouabain
2. Thyroglobulin synthesis	Protein synthesis inhibitors
3. Organization of iodide	PTU, MMI
4. MIT, DIT coupling	PTU, MMI
5. Thyroglobulin endocytosis and proteolysis	Lithium, colchicine, cytochalasin B
6. Deiodination	Dinitrotyrosine

DIT = diiodotyrosines; DNP = dinitrophenol; MIT = monoiodotyrosines; MMI = methimazole; PTU = propylthiouracil.

salivary gland, mammary gland, choroid plexus, placenta, and skin) also concentrate iodide, but these tissues are not able to organify iodide. Iodide transport requires energy and is inhibited by dinitrophenol or ouabain, implying requirements for oxidative metabolism and phosphorylation. Iodide transport is linked to sodium (Na$^+$) transport and to Na$^+$, potassium–adenosine triphosphatase (Na$^+$,K$^+$-ATPase) activity, but the actual mechanism of transport remains uncertain. In basal conditions, the thyroid/serum ratio of iodide is 30 to 40:1. This ratio reaches several hundredfold in circumstances of iodine deficiency and TSH stimulation.

Thyroglobulin Synthesis and Iodide Organification

Thyroglobulin contains the tyrosyl residues that provide the substrate for organification of iodide.[10, 11] It is a large glycoprotein (molecular weight 660,000 daltons, sedimentation coefficient of 19S) with two subunits, each of which is composed of several peptide chains. Thyroglobulin is the predominant protein in thyroid colloid, and about 3% of the thyroglobulin protein is composed of tyrosine residues. Iodination of these tyrosyl residues requires an activated, reactive iodine molecule. This is provided via a thyroid peroxidase enzyme complex that produces hydrogen peroxide as the oxidizing agent. The iodination occurs at the cell-colloid interface and is linked to the process of exocytosis of thyroglobulin. These processes of oxidation, iodination, and exocytosis are rapid; half the intracellular iodide is incorporated into thyroglobulin colloid within 2 minutes after the iodide is trapped by the follicular cell.[10, 11] Thyroid peroxidase also is involved in the coupling of MIT and DIT to form T$_3$ and T$_4$. The peroxidase enzyme complex is inhibited by the antithyroid drugs propylthiouracil and methimazole. A defect in the iodide trapping process, a defect in thyroglobulin synthesis, or a defect in the peroxidase enzyme complex can produce hypothyroidism.

Coupling of Iodotyrosines

Although it is not known whether T$_4$ formation *in vivo* involves predominantly intramolecular or intermolecular coupling of MIT and DIT residues, the coupling process itself has been well characterized. As indicated earlier, thyroid peroxidase also catalyzes the coupling of MIT and DIT residues, although nonenzymatic coupling is theoretically possible. The relative proportions of T$_3$ and T$_4$ formed depend on the influence of several factors, including TSH and iodine availability, which modulate the relative proportions of MIT and DIT. Under basal conditions, in the absence of iodine deficiency or excessive TSH stimulation, 70% of the total thyroglobulin iodoprotein is in the form of iodotyrosines, with the remainder as iodothyronines in a T$_4$/T$_3$ ratio of 10 to 20:1.[10, 11] Hypophysectomy and iodine deficiency are known to impair the efficiency of coupling, probably by decreasing the efficiency of

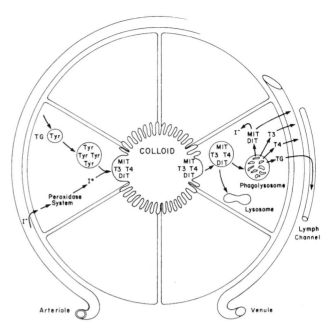

Figure 188–1. Biochemical steps in the production of thyroid hormone. DIT = diiodotyrosine; MIT = monoiodotyrosine; T$_3$ = triiodothyronine; T$_4$ = thyroxine; TG = thyroglobulin.

thyroglobulin iodination. The thioureylene drugs (propylthiouracil, methimazole, carbimazole), through their action as thyroid peroxidase inhibitors, act to decrease both iodination and iodotyrosine coupling in the thyroid. Propylthiouracil also inhibits the peripheral metabolism of thyroid hormones. It is not clear whether specific defects in the coupling process lead to clinical disease. Most of the patients for whom coupling defects have been proposed are either iodine deficient or have organification defects that lead to inefficient coupling.

Thyroglobulin Proteolysis and Thyroid Hormone Secretion

Thyroglobulin, stored in colloid after iodination at the apical thyrocyte cell membrane, must reenter the cell and undergo proteolysis to release the bound and stored thyroid hormones.[10, 11] This process, which is modulated to a great degree by TSH, involves endocytosis of colloid as phagosomes, fusion of phagosomes with lysosomes to form phagolysosomes, and subsequent proteolysis. Hydrolyzed free MIT, DIT, T$_3$, and T$_4$ are then released from the lysosomes into the follicular cell cytoplasm from which T$_3$ and T$_4$ can diffuse into thyroidal capillary blood. The follicular cell also contains an outer (phenolic) ring iodothyronine deiodinase that converts T$_4$ to T$_3$. Activity of this deiodinase is under TSH control such that the amounts of secreted T$_3$ and T$_4$ in relation to the ratio of T$_3$/T$_4$ stored in thyroglobulin increase during TSH stimulation. Thyroid-stimulating antibodies may mimic these effects of TSH and contribute to the increased levels of T$_3$ secretion seen in patients with Graves disease.

Microtubular function is necessary for proper transport of vesicles within the follicular cell.[11] Thus, colchicine and cytochalasin B have inhibitory effects on the secretion of thyroid hormones. High doses of iodide also inhibit the release of thyroid hormones, at least in part via endocytosis and colloid resorption; in addition, there may be an inhibiting effect on lysosomal protease activity. There is ample evidence to indicate that exposure of neonates to relatively high concentrations of iodide or organic iodine-containing compounds can produce transient hypothyroidism.

Iodotyrosine Deiodination and Recycling of Intrathyroidal Iodide

Although proteolytic cleavage of thyroglobulin results in the liberation of free iodotyrosines as well as iodothyronines, only small amounts of MIT and DIT leave the follicular cell.[11] Thyroid follicular cells contain an iodotyrosine deiodinase, which catalyzes the rapid deiodination of MIT or DIT. This enzyme is inhibited by dinitrotyrosine. The iodide generated from deiodination of iodotyrosines is principally reused for iodination of thyroglobulin, although some diffuses from the thyrocyte (the so-called *iodide leak*).

FETOPLACENTOMATERNAL THYROID INTERACTION

The relative independence of the maternal and fetal hypothalamic-pituitary thyroid hormone systems is suggested by several clinical observations. The placenta is impermeable to TSH and is largely impermeable to the thyroid hormones. These data are summarized in Table 188–2.[12] Direct evidence of placental transfer of thyroid hormones is provided by studies using various thyroid hormone analogues and tracers. Human studies have shown limited transfer from mother to fetus. Large doses of T_4 given to women produced only minor changes in cord serum concentrations of hormonal iodine.[13] Supraphysiologic doses of T_3 administered on a long-term basis to pregnant women several weeks before delivery significantly increased maternal serum T_3 levels but only minimally lowered fetal T_4 values.[14, 15] Studies in rats have shown low but significant levels of thyroid hormones in fetal tissues before the time of fetal thyroid hormone production.[16, 17]

The thioureylene antithyroid drugs cross the placenta and may compromise fetal and neonatal thyroid function.[18, 19] The placenta also is permeable to selected synthetic thyroid hormone analogues such as 3′,5′-dimethyl,5-isopropyl thyronine (DIMIT). There is no current rationale for use of these analogues, however, owing to their low biologic activity. Finally, the placenta is permeable to the hypothalamic peptide TRH. Both primate and human fetuses early in the third trimester respond to pharmacologic doses of exogenous TRH with an increase in serum TSH.[20, 21] Little endogenous TRH is normally detected in adult humans, owing to the presence of TRH-degrading enzyme systems in the blood. Although the sera of pregnant women contain somewhat lower levels of these enzymes than do nonpregnant sera, the nearly immeasurable levels of TRH in the maternal circulation have little effect on fetal thyroid function.[18]

The unique fetal environment, by contrast, includes many extrahypothalamic sources of TRH. Fetal gut tissues, particularly pancreas, produce TRH, and this pancreatic TRH has been isolated and found to be identical to hypothalamic TRH. In newborn rat pups, pancreatectomy, but not encephalectomy, is associated with reduced circulating TRH levels.[22] The placenta also produces an immunoreactive TRH, which appears to be identical to hypothalamic pyroGlu-His-ProNH$_2$.[23] Other forms of TRH that have TSH-releasing activity have been reported in the placenta.[24] These substances presumably derive from alternative cleavage of the prepro-TRH molecule. The high circulating level of TRH in the fetus results from increased production in extrahypothalamic tissues and from low or absent levels of TRH-degrading activity in fetal blood.[25, 26] Human cord values of TRH are also elevated.[27] Administration of anti-TRH antibodies to neonatal rats does not alter serum TSH levels, a finding suggesting that TRH is not required for TSH secretion at this early stage of thyroid development.[28] The significance of TRH in human cord blood is not clear.

In addition to TRH, the placenta produces TSH-like activity. The α-subunit of TSH is identical to that of human chorionic gonadotropin (hCG), and the β-subunit of hCG has structural homology with the β-subunit of TSH; thus, hCG has some TSH-like bioactivity.[29, 30] The biologic potency of hCG, however, is only about 0.01% that of TSH, and hCG normally has little influence on fetal thyroid system development or function. The large increase in maternal serum hCG activity that occurs early in pregnancy may account for the slight, transient suppression of maternal TSH levels seen early in the first trimester.[29, 30]

Placental permeability to maternal molecules may be a factor affecting fetal thyroid function as a result of maternal pathophysiologic states (acute iodide administration, autoimmune thyroid disease, pharmacotherapy of thyrotoxicosis). The fetal pituitary-thyroid axis, however, normally develops independently of maternal thyroid axis influence. The placenta and selected fetal tissues may serve as a source of TRH, but the extent of this influence on fetal thyroid function is uncertain. The limited maternofetal transfer of thyroid hormones may be important for fetal development, particularly brain growth and differentiation, in circumstances of fetal hypothyroidism.

CONTROL OF THYROID HORMONE PRODUCTION

The pattern of human perinatal thyroid hormone secretion is shown in Figure 188–2. Maturation of thyroid system control can be considered in three phases: hypothalamic, pituitary, and thyroidal. Changes in these systems are complex and are superimposed on the increasing production and increasing serum

TABLE 188–2

Placental Permeability for Substances Affecting Thyroid Function

Substance	Placental Permeability
I⁻	+ + + +
TRH	+ + +
Thioureylenes	+ + +
IgG antibodies	+ + +
T_3	0
T_4	+
TSH	0

I⁻ = iodide; T_3 = triiodothyronine; T_4 = thyroxine; TRH = thyrotropin-releasing hormone; TSH = thyroid-stimulating hormone.

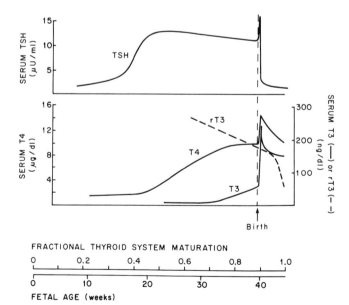

Figure 188–2. Patterns of circulating levels of thyroid-stimulating hormone (TSH), reverse triiodothyronine (rT$_3$), thyroxine (T$_4$), and triiodothyronine (T$_3$) in the human fetus.

concentration of serum thyroid hormone–binding globulin (TBG), as well as the changing pattern of fetal tissue iodothyronine deiodination during gestation. Maturation of these latter systems is described in the next section.

Although the fetal thyroid gland is able to concentrate iodide and to synthesize thyroglobulin at 70 to 80 days' gestation, little thyroid hormone synthesis occurs until about 18 weeks' gestation. At this time, thyroid follicular cell iodine uptake increases, and T_4 becomes measurable in the serum. Both total and free T_4 concentrations then increase steadily until the final weeks of pregnancy.[31,32] This pattern differs from the pattern of development of serum T_3 levels in the fetus. The fetal serum T_3 concentration is low (<15 ng/dL) until 30 weeks and then increases slowly in two distinct phases: a prenatal and a postnatal phase. Prenatally, serum T_3 increases slowly after 30 weeks' gestation to reach a level of approximately 50 ng/dL in term cord serum.[31-34] Postnatally, both T_3 and T_4 serum concentrations increase fourfold to sixfold within the first few hours of life, and they peak 24 to 36 hours after birth. These levels then gradually decline to adult values over the first 4 to 5 weeks of life. The prenatal increase in serum T_3 seems to be largely the result of progressive maturation of hepatic Type I (phenolic) outer ring iodothyronine deiodinase activity and increasing hepatic conversion of T_4 to T_3, although other tissue sources of deiodinase such as brown fat and kidney may be involved.[34]

Fetal serum TSH increases rapidly from a low level at 18 weeks to a peak value at 24 to 28 weeks' gestation, and then it gradually declines until term.[31,32] At the time of parturition, partly in response to cold stress, there is an acute release of TSH (the TSH surge), resulting in an elevated level by 30 minutes of life.[35] The level of circulating TSH remains modestly elevated for 2 to 3 days after birth. The increases in thyroid hormone that occur immediately after birth are not totally dependent on TSH and may represent other influences on the thyroid gland at the time of parturition. The high postnatal T_3 level in the days after birth results from TSH stimulation of thyroidal T_3 secretion as well as further rapid maturation of tissue outer ring monodeiodinase activity in the neonatal period.[36,37]

There are progressive increases in fetal serum T_4, free T_4, and TSH during the latter half of gestation, with an increasing free T_4/TSH ratio.[32,33,38] The pituitary gland contains a Type II outer ring iodothyronine deiodinase that converts T_4 to T_3, which, in turn, binds to the nuclear T_3 receptor to modulate TSH production. In most circumstances, it is circulating T_4 that is most important in TSH control. Thus, even when the circulating T_3 level is low (as in mid-gestation), there may be significant negative feedback control (by T_4) of pituitary TSH secretion. The progressive increase in the free T_4/TSH ratio in the late-gestation fetus, however, results more from the increase in free T_4 than from a decrease in TSH; a progressive maturation of thyroidal response to TSH has been shown in fetal sheep and seems likely in the human fetus.[33,38] An additional cause of the progressive increase in the free T_4/TSH ratio with a minimal change in TSH is a progressive increase in feedback sensitivity of the pituitary to thyroid hormone inhibition of TSH production. The mechanism for this is not yet clear. Changes in pituitary thyrotroph T_3 or TRH receptors, a decrease in thyrotroph outer ring iodothyronine deiodinase activity, or decreasing T_3 receptor action on TSH biosynthesis may be involved.

The ontogeny of TRH secretion and function in the fetus remains somewhat obscure. TRH immunoactivity is detectable in the hypothalamus by mid-gestation, and it increases markedly in the third trimester after the peak in serum TSH activity is noted. The premature infant (<30 to 32 weeks' gestation) is characterized by low levels of T_4 and free T_4, a normal or low level of TSH, and a normal or prolonged TSH response to TRH, indicating a state of physiologic TRH deficiency.[39,40] The full-term human fetus responds to pharmacologic maternal doses of TRH with a somewhat prolonged increase in TSH, a finding suggesting a degree of relative hypothalamic (tertiary) hypothyroidism.[21] Peripheral sources of TRH (placenta and pancreas) probably contribute to the elevated circulating levels of fetal and cord blood TRH and presumably account for the high circulating TSH level characteristic of the mid-gestation fetus. This TRH may be responsible for the high fetal serum TSH level before the increase in hypothalamic TRH concentration. The significance of ectopic TRH to the development of thyroid system control, however, remains to be investigated.

The control of fetal thyroid hormone secretion can be characterized as a balance among increasing hypothalamic TRH secretion, increasing thyroid follicular cell sensitivity to TSH, and increasing pituitary sensitivity to thyroid hormone inhibition of TSH release.[32,37,40] The fetus progresses from a state of both primary (thyroidal) and tertiary (hypothalamic) hypothyroidism in mid-gestation through a state of mild tertiary hypothyroidism during the final weeks of pregnancy and to fully mature thyroid function in the perinatal period.

FETAL THYROID HORMONE METABOLISM

The thyroid gland is the sole source of T_4, whereas most of the T_3 that circulates in the adult is derived from conversion of T_4 to T_3 via monodeiodination in peripheral tissues.[12,41,42] Deiodination of the iodothyronines is the major route of metabolism, and monodeiodination may occur either at the outer (phenolic) ring or the inner (tyrosyl) ring of the iodothyronine molecule. Outer ring monodeiodination of T_4 produces T_3, the active form of thyroid hormone with greatest affinity for the nuclear receptor. Inner ring monodeiodination of T_4 produces rT_3, an inactive metabolite. In mature humans, 70 to 90% of circulating T_3 is derived from peripheral conversion of T_4, and 10 to 30% results from direct glandular secretion. Nearly all the circulating rT_3 derives from peripheral conversion, with only 2 to 3% coming directly from the thyroid gland. T_3 and rT_3 are progressively metabolized to diiodo, monoiodo, and noniodinated forms of thyronine, none of which possesses biologic activity.

Two types of outer ring iodothyronine monodeiodinase (5'-MDI) have been described. Type I 5'-MDI, predominantly expressed in liver and kidney, is a high–dissociation constant (K_m) enzyme, inhibited by propylthiouracil, and its activity is stimulated by thyroid hormone. Type II 5'-MDI, predominantly located in brain, pituitary, and brown adipose tissues, is a low-K_m enzyme insensitive to propylthiouracil, and its activity is inhibited by thyroid hormone.[41] Type I 5'-MDI activity in liver and perhaps kidney and muscle probably accounts for most of the circulating T_3. Type II 5'-MDI acts primarily to increase local intracellular levels of T_3 in the brain and pituitary and is important to brown adipose tissue function during the immediate postnatal period. The outer ring iodothyronine deiodinase also deiodinates reverse T_3 to diiodothyronine.

Both Type I and Type II 5'-MDI are present in third trimester fetuses.[42-45] In sheep, a species in which thyroid hormone system maturation closely resembles that in humans, hepatic Type I 5'-MDI activity increases threefold to fourfold, and brain Type II 5'-MDI activity increases about 50% over the last third of gestation.[42] Both deiodinase species are thyroid hormone responsive. Hepatic Type I 5'-MDI activity, however, becomes thyroid hormone responsive (e.g., activity decreases with hypothyroidism) only during the final weeks of gestation. Brain Type II activity, in contrast, is responsive (increases with hypothyroidism) throughout the final third of gestation.[45,46] Thus, Type II deiodinase probably plays an important role to provide a source of intracellular T_3 to those tissues (e.g., pituitary and, in some species, brown fat and brain) dependent on T_3 during fetal life, whereas the ontogeny of the Type I enzyme (to provide increased serum T_3 levels) increases only during the final weeks of gestation and during postnatal life.[42]

An inner (tyrosyl) ring iodothyronine monodeiodinase (Type III 5'-MDI) has been characterized in most fetal tissues, including the placenta.[21,42] This enzyme system catalyzes the conversion of T_4 to rT_3 and T_3 to diiodothyronine. The maturation of these enzyme systems has been studied primarily in the rodent and sheep. Fetal thyroid hormone metabolism is characterized by a predominance of Type III enzyme activity, particularly in liver, kidney, and placenta, and this accounts in part for the increased circulating levels of rT_3 observed in the fetus.[41-43] Placental Type III deiodinase contributes to amniotic fluid rT_3 levels and presumably also contributes to circulating fetal rT_3.[12] The persistence of high circulating rT_3 levels for several weeks in the newborn, however, indicates that Type III 5'-MDI activities expressed in nonplacental tissues are also important to the maintenance of high circulating rT_3 levels.[12]

Studies have shown high concentrations of sulfated iodothyronine analogues in human and ovine fetal serum.[47-51] These include T_4 sulfate (T_4S), reverse T_3 sulfate (rT_3S), T_3 sulfate (T_3S), and T_2 sulfate (T_2S). To understand fetal iodothyronine metabolism better and to assess the significance of the several iodothyronine analogues in the fetus, plasma clearance and production rates were measured in the fetal sheep model using steady-state, constant infusion kinetic analysis of radioiodine-labeled hormones.[50] Average production rates, calculated as the product of basal hormone concentrations and clearances, are shown in Table 188-3. Several studies demonstrated T_4 production rates of 20 to 50 µg/kg/day at 120 to 130 days' gestation. Production rates for rT_3 and T_3 were approximately 5 and 2 µg/kg/day. Average production rates for T_4S, rT_3S, and T_3S were estimated to be 10, 12, and 2 µg/kg/day, respectively.[50]

Current information suggests that rT_3 and the sulfate conjugates have low affinity for the nuclear T_3 receptors and minimal biologic activity.[52] Thus, the production of inactive thyroid hormone analogues in the fetus (rT_3, T_4S, rT_3S = 29 µg/kg/day) greatly exceeds the production of active T_3 (2 µg/kg/day). Clearly, most of the T_4 in the fetus is metabolized to inactive metabolites via the Type I and Type III iodothyronine monodeiodinase and sulfotransferase enzyme systems in fetal tissues. There is suggestive evidence that T_3S can be metabolized *in vivo* to T_3.[53] T_3S production is quite limited, however, and the combined average production rate for T_3 and T_3S (4 µg/kg/day) in the fetal sheep is low. It appears from these data that peripheral thyroid hormone metabolism in the sheep fetus, in contrast to the adult, is shunted to inactivation, rather than to production of active hormone.

The alanine side chain of the inner ring of the iodothyronines also may undergo decarboxylation or transamination.[54] Although the acetic acid derivatives of T_4 have some biologic activity *in vitro*, their rapid degradation *in vivo* precludes much physiologic significance. Pyruvate and lactate derivatives also have been isolated, both with minimal biologic activity. Thyroid hormones also are excreted as both free and glucuronide or sulfuronide conjugates in urine and stool; some of these forms can undergo hydrolysis and enterohepatic recirculation. In general, gut excretion accounts for less than 15% of the total amount of metabolized T_3 or T_4 after birth.

Both T_3 and T_4 in blood are associated with various plasma proteins, including TBG, T_4-binding prealbumin (TBPA), and albumin.[54] TBG serves as the primary transport protein for both T_3 and T_4; about 70% of the total T_4 and 40 to 60% of total T_3 are bound to TBG. The remaining thyroid hormones are distributed about equally between TBPA and albumin. The binding affinities of these proteins are such that adult free T_4 and T_3 concentrations are about 0.03 and 0.3% of the total hormone concentrations. TBG, TBPA, and albumin are produced by the liver, and production of these proteins increases progressively during the final half of gestation. Hepatic TBG production is stimulated by estrogen, and the increasing levels of estrogens during pregnancy

TABLE 188-3

Average Iodothyronine Production Rates in Fetal Sheep

	Production Rate (µg/kg/d)	
Iodothyronine	**Fetus***	**Newborn†**
T_4	20–50	35
rT_3	5	2
T_3	2	16
T_4S	10	0.6
rT_3S	12	8
T_3S	2	0.4

* 120–135 days' gestation; pregnancy 150 days' duration in sheep.
† 7–14 postnatal days.
rT_3 = reverse triiodothyronine; rT_3S = reverse T_3 sulfate; T_3 = triiodothyronine; T_4 = thyroxine; T_3S = T_3 sulfate; T_4S = T_4 sulfate.
Data from reference 42.

account, at least in part, for the T_4 concentration, which increases progressively from mid-gestation until 34 to 35 weeks' gestation.[12,33] The free T_4 level, however, also increases, owing to progressively increasing T_4 production.[33,37] The T_3 concentration also increases, from a barely detectable level before 30 weeks' gestation to 50 ng/dL in the term fetus, and the free T_3 concentration probably increases in parallel.

Fetal thyroid hormone metabolism is largely oriented to production of inactive metabolites via production of sulfate conjugates and predominant T_4 inner ring monodeiodination to rT_3. The type 2 deiodinase activity in fetal brain and brown adipose tissues serves to protect these tissues in the event of fetal T_4 deficiency.

Thyroid System Effects and Adaptation to Extrauterine Life

In general, much of the fetal thyroid development is preparatory, providing for the relatively large amounts of thyroid hormones required for normal postnatal development. The production of active thyroid hormones is markedly increased in association with the events of parturition (see Fig. 188-2). During the first hours after birth, there is an abrupt threefold to sixfold increase in circulating T_4 and T_3 levels, coincident with an increase in serum TSH concentration.[32] The initial increases in circulating thyroid hormone levels largely result from increased hormone secretion from the thyroid gland.[35,36] The TSH surge (which is likely a response to the thermal stimuli coincident with birth), however, can be obtunded in the neonatal sheep by warm bath immersion without complete inhibition of the increments in T_3 or T_4.[3] Other substances that may modulate the acute increases in circulating thyroid hormones include catecholamines. A postnatal increase in serum catecholamine concentrations also occurs at the time of parturition,[55] and the thyroid gland is adrenergically innervated. Stimulation of thyroidal adrenergic receptors may augment TSH-induced changes in the T_4/T_3 ratio of secreted thyroid hormones. Because TBG concentrations remain relatively constant throughout the newborn period, free T_4 and T_3 levels rise abruptly after birth in association with increases in hormone production rates. The cold-stimulated TSH surge is short-lived, and the decrease in TSH that follows during the 72 to 96 hours after birth results from feedback inhibition by T_4 at either the hypothalamic or the pituitary level (or both).[32,37] The serum TRH concentration is elevated in cord blood and falls in the days after birth. A clear increase in the serum TRH value coincident with the increase in TSH after parturition has not been reported, but the parallel increases in both TSH and prolactin levels in the early hours after birth support the view that the TSH surge is mediated by TRH.[32,37] Thyroid hormone levels in the newborn gradually return to adult levels by about 1 month of age. The high level of circulating rT_3 characteristic of the fetus persists after birth and gradually declines to the adult range by 4 to 6 weeks of age.[44]

The metabolic significance of the neonatal thyroid hormone surge is not entirely clear. Physiologic processes known to be modulated by thyroid hormone in adults, such as thermogenesis and cardiovascular responses, clearly are important in the transition from intrauterine to extrauterine life, and it is tempting to link these with the changes in thyroid hormone metabolism that occur during transition. Several studies have attempted to establish such a link. Brown adipose tissue is the major site for newborn thermogenesis.[56] Hypothyroidism induced during the final weeks of gestation is associated with impaired brown adipose tissue thermogenesis, largely owing to the effects of T_4 on brown adipose tissue iodothyronine monodeiodinase activity and mitochondrial uncoupling protein (thermogenin).[57] Obtundation of the postnatal T_3 surge (by acute thyroidectomy in newborn sheep), however, does not accentuate transient neonatal hypothermia, a finding indicating that the prenatal T_4 level is more important in neonatal thermogenesis than is the early postnatal T_3 surge.[36]

A similar relationship between thyroid system function and neonatal cardiovascular adaptation has been described in neonatal sheep; normal fetal thyroid function in the final weeks of gestation is required for the increases in myocardial performance associated with the transition to extrauterine life. Obtundation of the acute increase in serum T_3 at birth, however, does not alter neonatal cardiovascular adaptation.[58] These observations support the view that in the sheep, the level of thyroid function during the final weeks of gestation is more important than the neonatal increases in T_3 and T_4 for successful neonatal transition. The situation in the human neonate may be somewhat different. Neonates with congenital thyroid agenesis have few, if any, signs or symptoms of thyroid hormone deficiency, and their postnatal environmental adaptation usually is not impaired.[32, 59] The fetal sheep is relatively more mature at birth, presumably accounting for this difference. The precise timing of maturation of thyroid hormone effects on thermogenesis and cardiovascular function in the human neonate has not been defined. It is clear that most (95%) infants with congenital hypothyroidism at birth have few manifestations of thyroid hormone deficiency and develop normally when replacement therapy is begun in the neonatal period. Serum TSH levels are elevated, and there may be a 3- to 6-week retardation in bone maturation.[32] The posterior fontanelle may be relatively large, and the physiologic hyperbilirubinemia of the newborn may be more marked and prolonged. Growth is not impaired, however, and other metabolic alterations usually are not evident.

The ontogenesis of various thyroid actions has been characterized in rodents. These include tissue thermogenesis, carcass and muscle growth, skeletal maturation, skin and brain maturation, and hormone and growth factor production and action. Some of these effects represent thyroid hormone actions on specific gene products, probably mediated via thyroid hormone receptor control of gene transcription.[42, 60] Other thyroid hormone actions represent complex events, the mechanisms of which are not yet understood, such as the effects on growth, skeletal maturation, and brain development.

The thyroid hormone dependency of these growth and metabolic events in rodents is manifest in the postnatal period, in general during the second and third postnatal weeks. Nuclear thyroid hormone receptors appear in most rodent tissues during the last week *in utero* and the first postnatal week.[61] Thus, there is a discrepancy between the timing of appearance of selected thyroid hormone actions and the appearance of thyroid nuclear receptors, and it is possible that at least some of the variation in timing of appearance of thyroid hormone actions in the rodent relates to maturation of events beyond the step of T_3 binding to the nuclear receptors. Other thyroid hormone receptors have

been identified, including mitochondrial and plasma membrane receptors, but the significance of these is not yet clear.[60] Most of the effects described previously are believed to be mediated via the nuclear receptors.

A similar delay in appearance of selected thyroid hormone actions has been observed in developing sheep.[42,60] The sheep, like the human and in contrast to the rodent, is a precocious species and is relatively mature at birth. In fetal sheep, effects of thyroid hormones on various parameters of brain development appear as early as 0.5 to 0.6 of thyroid system development. Thyroid effects on skin maturation and growth also appear relatively early in gestation, whereas effects on heart, lung, kidney, and liver are delayed until the final few weeks before birth. In the sheep, as in the rodent, the appearance of selected thyroid hormone actions late in gestation, such as the effects on hepatic malic enzyme activity and hepatic epidermal growth factor receptor concentrations, is not accountable on the basis of appearance of thyroid hormone nuclear receptors; hepatic receptors are present by 0.5 of gestation.[42] The effect of thyroid hormone on lung β-adrenergic receptor binding also occurs well after the appearance of thyroid hormone nuclear receptors in the lung.[62] Thus, the timing of maturation of thyroid hormone actions is variable in both rodent and sheep species and relates to the ontogenesis of nuclear thyroid hormone receptors as well as to maturation of postnuclear mechanisms.

In humans, thyroid nuclear receptors have been reported in fetal lung, brain, heart, and liver at 13 to 19 weeks' gestation.[63,64] The only thyroid hormone actions that have been characterized in the fetus are the effects of hypothyroidism on serum TSH and bone maturation. Most effects of thyroid hormone on perinatal developmental processes occur postnatally (Fig. 188–3).

Thyroid hormones affect important developmental processes, including growth, thermogenesis, and development. The largely successful transition of athyrotic infants to extrauterine life reflects the limited importance of fetal thyroid hormones in all but the final weeks of gestation. An exception to this may be the fetal brain, a major site of Type II iodothyronine monodeiodinase activity in the fetus. The presence of this enzyme system in the brain early in development and its demonstrated response to fetal hypothyroidism in the rat and sheep suggest that intracellular conversion of T_4 to T_3 in brain is important in these species for normal development and differentiation of the central nervous system. The critical period for this effect in the sheep is the last trimester of gestation; in the rat, the critical period is the

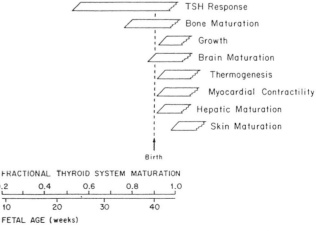

Figure 188–3. Onset of actions of thyroid hormone in the developing human. The *left edge of the bar* indicates the initiation of thyroid hormone responsiveness of the indicated parameter. TSH = thyroid-stimulating hormone.

first 3 postnatal weeks. Precise data are not available for the human fetus, but early treatment of congenital hypothyroidism in the neonate prevents mental retardation, a finding suggesting that the period of thyroid dependency of the human brain begins in the postnatal period. Early and adequate postnatal thyroid hormone replacement in athyrotic infants also normalizes growth and development.

Low-T$_3$ Syndrome in Premature Infants

In the preterm infant, changes in thyroid function parameters during neonatal adaptation are qualitatively similar to those in term infants but are quantitatively obtunded.[32, 33] The neonatal TSH surge and the neonatal T$_4$ and T$_3$ peak responses decrease with decreasing gestational age, and the transient low-T$_3$ state that follows probably is related to the state of relative undernutrition in the neonatal period.[32] Premature infants have an increased susceptibility to neonatal morbidity, including birth trauma, acidosis, hypoxia, hypoglycemia, hypocalcemia, and infection, all superimposed on feeding disorders and relative malnutrition. All these factors tend to inhibit conversion of T$_4$ to T$_3$ in the neonatal period and aggravate the extent of the low-T$_3$ state characteristic of prematurity.[32, 65-67] Serum T$_3$ values may remain low in these infants for 1 to 2 months.

Features of the *low-T$_3$ syndrome* in premature infants include a low serum T$_3$ concentration secondary to a decreased rate of conversion of T$_4$ to T$_3$, variable but usually elevated serum rT$_3$ levels, and normal or low total serum T$_4$ concentrations.[32, 33] Free T$_4$ levels usually are in the range of values for healthy premature infants of matched gestational age and weight. TSH values are low in these infants. Preterm infants presenting with low or borderline-low thyroid hormone levels and elevated TSH values should be carefully evaluated for hypothyroidism, including assays of thyroid-blocking immunoglobulins. A course of T$_4$ replacement therapy may be warranted in these infants.

There are remaining concerns regarding ultimate cognitive function in preterm infants with low thyroid hormone values. Early (first week of life) low T$_4$ levels have been associated with neuralgic dysfunction at 5 years of life and poor school performance at 9 years of age.[68] This finding prompted several studies examining the effect of T$_4$ supplementation in very preterm infants. Randomized, placebo-controlled T$_4$ replacement in preterm infants less than 30 weeks' gestation resulted in improved neurologic function in very preterm infants (25 to 26 weeks' gestation) but worsened cognition and behavioral development in infants born after 29 weeks' gestation.[69] Moreover, results from various antenatal TRH exposure trials (preterm fetuses exposed to maternal TRH treatment in an attempt to improve subsequent postnatal lung function) also suggest that early alterations in thyroid system function may be associated with deleterious intellectual outcomes.[70, 71] Thus, the use of thyroid hormones in nonhypothyroid preterm infants should be restricted to those infants enrolled in approved studies.

REFERENCES

1. Pintar JE, Toran Allerand CD: Normal development of the hypothalamic-pituitary-thyroid axis. In Braverman LE, Utiger RD (eds): The Thyroid, 6th ed. Philadelphia, JB Lippincott, 1991, pp 7-21.
2. Grumbach MM, Gluckman PD: Fetal hypothalamus and pituitary gland: the maturation of neuroendocrine mechanisms controlling the secretion of fetal growth hormone, prolactin, gonadotropins, adrenocorticotropin-related peptides, and thyrotropin. In Tulchinsky D, Little AB (eds): Maternal-Fetal Endocrinology, 2nd ed. Philadelphia, WB Saunders Co, 1994, pp 194-261.
3. Fisher DA, et al: Ontogenesis of hypothalamic-pituitary-thyroid function and metabolism in man, sheep and rat. Recent Prog Horm Res 33:59, 1977.
4. Shepard TH: Onset of function in the human fetal thyroid: biochemical and radioautographic studies from organ culture. J Clin Endocrinol Metab 27:945, 1987.
5. Pearse AGE, Carvalheira AF: Cytochemical evidence for an ultimobranchial origin of rodent thyroid C cells. Nature 214:929, 1967.
6. Moseley JM, et al: The ultimobranchial origin of calcitonin. Lancet 1:108, 1968.
7. Kruse K, et al: Monomeric serum calcitonin and bone turnover during anticonvulsant treatment in congenital hypothyroidism. J Pediatr 111:57, 1987.
8. Nillson M, et al: Iodide transport in primary cultured thyroid follicle cells: evidence of a TSH regulated channel mediating iodide selectively across the apical domain of the plasma membrane. Eur J Cell Biol 52:270, 1990.
9. Wolff J: Congenital goiter with defective iodide transport. Endocr Rev 4:240, 1983.
10. Lissitzky S: Iodine metabolism in the thyroid, thyroid hormone formation, and biosynthesis and structure-function relationship of thyroglobulin. In DeGroot LJ, et al (eds): Endocrinology. Philadelphia, WB Saunders Co, 1989, pp 512-522.
11. Gentile F, et al: Biosynthesis and secretion of thyroid hormones. In DeGroot LJ, et al (eds): Endocrinology, 3rd ed. Philadelphia, WB Saunders Co, 1995, pp 517-542.
12. Burrow GN, et al: Maternal and fetal thyroid function. N Engl J Med 331:1072, 1994.
13. Fisher DA, et al: Placental transport of thyroxine. J Clin Endocrinol 24:393, 1964.
14. Dussault J, et al: Studies of serum triiodothyronine across the human placenta. J Clin Endocrinol 29:595, 1969.
15. Raiti S, et al: Evidence for the placental transfer of triiodothyronine in human beings. N Engl J Med 277:456, 1967.
16. Morreale de Escobar G, et al: Effects of iodine deficiency on thyroid hormone metabolism and the brain in fetal rats: the role of the maternal transfer of thyroxine. Am J Clin Nutr 52(Suppl):2805, 1993.
17. Escobar del Rey F, et al: Effects of maternal iodine deficiency on the L-thyroxine and 3,5,3'-triiodo-L-thyronine contents of rat embryonic tissues before and after onset of fetal thyroid function. Endocrinology 118:1259, 1986.
18. Roti E, et al: The placental transport synthesis and metabolism of drugs which affect thyroid function. Endocr Rev 4:131, 1983.
19. Marchant B, et al: The placental transfer of propylthiouracil, methimazole, and carbimazole. J Clin Endocrinol Metab 45:1187, 1977.
20. Jacobsen BB, et al: Pituitary-thyroid responsiveness to thyrotropin-releasing hormone in preterm and small-for-gestational-age newborns. Acta Paediatr Scand 66:541, 1977.
21. Roti E, et al: Human cord blood concentrations of thyrotropin, thyroglobulin and iodothyronines after maternal administration of thyrotropin-releasing hormone. J Clin Endocrinol Metab 53:813, 1981.
22. Engler P, et al: Thyrotropin releasing hormone in the circulation of the neonatal rat is derived from the pancreas and other extraneural tissues. J Clin Invest 67:800, 1981.
23. Shambaugh G, et al: Thyrotropin-releasing hormone activity in human placenta. J Clin Endocrinol Metab 48:483, 1979.
24. Youngblood WW, et al: Thyrotropin-releasing hormone like bioactivity in placenta: evidence for the existence of substances other than pyroglu-hisproNH (TRH) capable of stimulating pituitary thyrotropin release. Endocrinology 106:541, 1980.
25. Neary JT, et al: Lower levels of thyrotropin-releasing hormone degrading activity in human cord and maternal sera than in the serum of euthyroid nonpregnant adults. J Clin Invest 62:1, 1978.
26. Araten-Spire S, Czernichow P: Thyrotropin releasing hormone degrading activity of neonatal human plasma. J Clin Endocrinol Metab 50:88, 1980.
27. Perelman AH, et al: Cord blood thyrotropin releasing hormone. Clin Res 29:111A, 1981.
28. Theodoropoulas T, Braverman LE: Thyrotropin releasing hormone is not required for thyrotropin secretion in the perinatal rat. J Clin Invest 63:588, 1979.
29. Kimura M, et al: Physiologic thyroid activation in normal early pregnancy is induced by circulating hCG. Obstet Gynecol 75:775, 1990.
30. Ballabio M, et al: Pregnancy induced changes in thyroid function: role of human chorionic gonadotropin as putative regulator of maternal thyroid. J Clin Endocrinol Metab 73:824, 1991.
31. Fisher DA: Thyroid hormone and thyroglobulin synthesis and secretion. In Delange F, et al (eds): Pediatric Thyroidology. Basel, Karger, 1985, pp 44-56.
32. Fisher DA, Klein AH: Thyroid development and disorders of thyroid function in the newborn. N Engl J Med 304:702, 1981.
33. Klein AH, et al: Developmental changes in pituitary-thyroid function in the human fetus and newborn. Early Hum Dev 6:321, 1982.
34. Wu SY, et al: Maturation of thyroid hormone metabolism. In Wu SY (ed): Thyroid Hormone Metabolism. Boston, Blackwell Scientific, 1991, pp 293-320.
35. Fisher DA, Odell WD: Acute release of thyrotropin in the newborn. J Clin Invest 48:1670, 1969.
36. Polk DH, et al: Serum thyroid hormone and tissue 5'-monodeiodinase activity in acutely thyroidectomized newborn lambs. Am J Physiol 14:E151, 1986.
37. Roti E: Regulation of thyroid-stimulating hormone (TSH) secretion in the fetus and neonate. J Endocrinol Invest 11:145, 1988.
38. Fisher DA, et al: Maturation of human hypothalamic-pituitary-thyroid function and control. Thyroid 10:229, 2000.
39. Fisher DA: Euthyroid low T$_4$ and T$_3$ status in prematures and sick infants. Pediatr Clin North Am 37:1297, 1990.
40. Delange F, et al: Transient disorders of thyroid function and regulation in preterm infants. In Delange F, et al (eds): Pediatric Thyroidology. Basel, Karger, 1985, pp 369-393.
41. Leonard JL: Biochemical basis of thyroid hormone deiodination. In Wu SY (ed): Thyroid Hormone Metabolism. Boston, Blackwell Scientific, 1991, pp 1-28.

42. Fisher DA, et al: Fetal thyroid metabolism, a pluralistic system. Thyroid 4:367, 1994.
43. Chopra IJ, et al: 3,3′5′–Triiodothyronine (reverse T$_3$) in fetal and adult sheep: studies of metabolic clearance rate, production rate, serum binding, and thyroidal content relative to thyroxine. Endocrinology 967:1080, 1975.
44. Oddie TH, et al: Comparison of T$_4$, T$_3$, rT$_3$ and TSH concentrations in cord blood and serum of infants up to 3 months of age. Early Hum Dev 3:239, 1979.
45. Polk DH, et al: Ontogeny of thyroid hormone effect on tissue 5′–monodeiodinase activity in fetal sheep. Am J Physiol 254:E337, 1988.
46. Kaplan MM, Yaskoski KA: Effects of congenital hypothyroidism and partial and complete food deprivation on phenolic and tyrosyl ring iodothyronine deiodination in rat brain. Endocrinology 110:761, 1982.
47. Chopra IJ, et al: A radioimmunoassay for measurement of 3,5,3′ triiodothyronine sulfate (T3S): studies in thyroidal and non thyroidal diseases, pregnancy and neonatal life. J Clin Endocrinol Metab 75:189, 1992.
48. Chopra IJ, et al: A radioimmunoassay for measurement of thyroxine sulfate. J Clin Endocrinol Metab 76:145, 1993.
49. Wu SY, et al: Thyroxine sulfate is a major thyroid hormone metabolite and potential intermediate in the monodeiodination pathways in fetal sheep. Endocrinology 131:1751, 1992.
50. Polk DH, et al: Metabolism of sulfoconjugated thyroid hormone derivatives in developing sheep. Am J Physiol 266:E892, 1994.
51. Wu SY, et al: Identification of 3,3′-T2S as a fetal thyroid hormone derivative in maternal urine in sheep. Am J Physiol 268:E33, 1995.
52. Spaulding SW, et al: Studies on the biological activity of triiodothyronine sulfate. J Clin Endocrinol Metab 74:1062, 1992.
53. Santini F, et al: Thyromimetic effects of 3,5,3′-triiodothyronine sulfate in hypothyroid rats. Endocrinology 133:105, 1993.
54. Refetoff S, Nicoloff JT: Thyroid hormone transport and metabolism. In DeGroot LJ, et al (eds): Endocrinology, 3rd ed. Philadelphia, WB Saunders Co, 1995, pp 560–582.
55. Padbury JF, et al: Neonatal adaptation: greater sympathoadrenal response in preterm than full-term fetal sheep at birth. Am J Physiol 11:E443, 1985.
56. Polk DH: Thyroid hormone effects on neonatal thermogenesis. Semin Perinatol 12:151, 1988.
57. Polk DH, et al: Effect of fetal thyroidectomy on newborn thermogenesis in lambs. Pediatr Res 21:453, 1987.
58. Breall JA, et al: Role of thyroid hormone in postnatal circulatory and metabolic adjustments. J Clin Invest 73:1418, 1985.
59. Fouron JC, et al: Cardiac dimensions and myocardial function of infants with congenital hypothyroidism. Br Heart J 47:584, 1982.
60. Fisher DA, Polk DH: Maturation of thyroid hormone actions. In Delange F, et al (eds): Research in Congenital Hypothyroidism. New York, Plenum Publishing, 1989, pp 61–77.
61. Perez-Castillo A, et al: The early ontogenesis of thyroid hormone receptors in the rat fetus. Endocrinology 117:2457, 1985.
62. Ballard PL: Thyroid hormones: effects and binding. In Ballard PL (ed): Hormones and Lung Maturation. Monographs on Endocrinology, Vol 20. Berlin, Springer-Verlag, 1986, pp 197–235.
63. Bernal J, Pekonen F: Ontogenesis of nuclear 3,5,3′–triiodothyronine receptors in human fetal brain. Endocrinology 114:677, 1984.
64. Gonzales LA, Ballard PL: Identification and characterization of nuclear 3,5,3′-triiodothyronine binding sites in fetal human lung. J Clin Endocrinol Metab 53:21, 1981.
65. Eggermont E, et al: The thyroid system function in preterm infants of postmenstrual ages of 31 weeks or less: evidence for a "transient lazy thyroid system." J Helv Paediatr Acta 39:220, 1984.
66. Franklin R, O'Grady C: Neonatal thyroid function: effects of nonthyroidal illness. J Pediatr 107:599, 1985.
67. Chopra IJ: Euthyroid sick syndrome: is it a misnomer? J Clin Endocrinol Metab 82:329, 1997.
68. Den Ouden AL, et al: The relation between neonatal thyroxine levels and neurodevelopmental outcome at age 5 and 9 years in a national cohort of very preterm and/or low birthweight infants. Pediatr Res 39:142, 1996.
69. Briet JM, et al: Neonatal thyroxine supplementation in very preterm children: developmental outcome evaluated at early school age. Pediatrics 107:712, 2001.
70. Crowther C, et al: Australian collaborative trial of antenatal thyrotropin-releasing hormone: adverse effects at 12 month follow-up. Pediatrics 93:311, 1997.
71. Briet JM, et al: Outcome after antenatal thyrotropin-releasing hormone treatment. Pediatrics 110:249, 2000.

Ovary and Testis

189

Robert P. Erickson and Stan R. Blecher

Genetics of Sex Determination and Differentiation

The classic paradigm of mammalian, including human, sexual development postulates an initially "indifferent" (sexually undifferentiated) state. The primordial, indifferent gonad is situated in the gonadal ridge region of the intermediate mesoderm of the fetus. In genetic males, the indifferent gonad is induced to become a testis; in the uninduced (female) state, an ovary develops; all other sexual dimorphism results from the action of hormones produced in males by the testis or from the lack of these hormones in females.[1] Mesenchymal cells of the gonadal (genital) ridge and the neighboring metanephros are destined, in males, to give rise to androgen-producing Leydig cells of the testis or, in females, to the theca cells of the ovary and to connective tissue. The adjacent celomic epithelium grows into the mesodermal mass to produce the Sertoli cells of the testicular seminiferous tubules or the follicle cells of the ovary. In addition, primordial germ cells migrate to the developing gonad to give rise to sperm or egg cells.

Current knowledge builds on this framework. It is now known that *genetic maleness* in mammals normally depends on the presence of a sex-determining region of the Y chromosome, and femaleness depends on its absence. This commitment of the organism to the pathway of either male or female development is called *sex determination;* subsequent development of sex-specific organs, with establishment of sexual phenotype,[2] is called *sexual differentiation.*

The effect of the sex-determining region of the Y chromosome in formation of the testis is not direct, but rather is mediated by other, so-called *downstream,* genes. Moreover, the action of the Y-chromosomal region is preceded by *upstream* gene action that is evidently a prerequisite for the Y-chromosomal function. Finally, some Y-chromosomal (male-specific) gene action may itself influence sexual phenotype before gonadal development, that is, at a *pregonadal* juncture. Many genetic pathways interact in a complex and, in part, overlapping and redundant manner, to execute the genetic control of sexual development. The following section describes this dynamic, sequential program as occurring in four stages: Y-chromosomal sex determination, established at conception; pregonadal sexual development and sexual dimorphism; gonadal stage of sexual development; and secondary sexual differentiation.

Y-CHROMOSOMAL SEX DETERMINATION

Sex-Determining Role of the Mammalian Y Chromosome

In 1923, it was demonstrated cytologically that humans have X and Y chromosomes.[3] By analogy with *Drosophila,* it was assumed that sex determination in mammals would be mediated by the ratio of the number of X chromosomes to the number of sets of autosomes (i.e., chromosomes other than the sex chromosomes). However, in 1959, it was discovered that an X0 sex chromosome karyotype (i.e., absence of the Y chromosome) produced a predominantly female phenotype both in mice[4] and in humans (Turner syndrome),[5] and XXY produced predominant maleness in humans (Klinefelter syndrome).[6, 7] These observations demonstrated that the presence of a Y chromosome, independent of the number of X chromosomes, resulted in the development of a mammalian embryo as a male, whereas in the absence of the Y chromosome it developed as a female. Thus, the Y chromosome appeared to possess a gene or genes the presence or absence of which determined the destiny of the bipotential gonad as a testis or an ovary, respectively and, through this, the development of the dimorphic secondary sex characteristics.[1] In the human, the hypothetical Y-chromosomal gene was named *TDF* (testis-determining factor), and in mice, it was called *Tdy* (testis-determining gene on the Y). The minor deviations of Klinefelter and Turner syndromes from the normal male and female phenotype, respectively, probably result from the influence of other (non-*TDF*) sex-chromosomal factors (see later) on the sex differentiation pathway.

Early Y-Chromosomal Candidate Sequences: H-Y Antigen, *Bkm* Sequences, and *Zfy*

Many candidate genes for *TDF* have been studied, taking into account biochemical differences between males and females and the evolutionary conservation expected in genes involved in sex determination. Investigators proposed that the highly conserved, male-specific molecule, H-Y antigen (originally identified in skin transplantation experiments), was the product of *TDF*.[8] For more than 10 years, this proposal was considered valid. However, the findings of phenotypically male XX*Sxr* male mice that did not express H-Y,[9] and of XY humans of female phenotype who were H-Y positive,[10] excluded this hypothesis. Another candidate for *TDF* was the repetitive sequence *Bkm* (banded krait minor) that was originally isolated from the snake *Bungarus fasciatus*[11] and that, in some vertebrates, was found only in the sex chromosomes. This hypothesis was rejected because, in humans, these sequences are dispersed in the genome and are not concentrated in the sex-specific region of the Y chromosomes.[12]

The discovery that 46,XX males usually have *translocations* (transfers of chromosomal material) of Yp (where p indicates the short arm of a chromosome) to one of their Xps was a major breakthrough in mapping *TDF* on the Y chromosome.[13, 14] The X and Y chromosomes have *homologous* (genetically equivalent) segments at the ends of their respective p (and of) arms, and these segments pair at meiosis. Because of genetic exchange between these segments, genes located in this region appear to be neither X nor Y linked; that is, they appear to be inherited as if on autosomes. Accordingly, these regions are called *pseudoautosomal*. The occurrence of abnormal cross-overs adjacent to the pseudoautosomal region can result in the illegitimate transfer of *TDF* to the X chromosome.[15, 16] Molecular analyses in such patients permitted the construction of a deletion map of the Y chromosome,[17, 18] and these studies showed that a small region of Yp adjacent to the pseudoautosomal region is essential for testicular differentiation. Finer mapping continued, and one candidate gene was mistakenly identified: Page and associates[19] found a highly conserved sequence that seemed to map with a male-determining Y fragment and named it *ZFY*. However, one of their XX males did not have *ZFY*, and the finding of more such patients[20, 21] suggested that *ZFY* could not be *TDF*.

SRY Gene

The resumed search for *TDF* was targeted on 35 kB of DNA between the proximal (i.e., toward the centromere of the chromosome) limit of the pseudoautosomal region of the Y chromosome and the breakpoint in XX males lacking *ZFY*. A subclone selected for its male specificity in mammals was found to encode an 80–amino acid segment that was homologous to the mating-type protein in *Schizosaccharomyces pombe* and also to a conserved 80–amino acid, DNA-binding motif present in the HMG1 (*high mobility group*) transcription-regulating proteins.[22] Further analyses of various tissues disclosed a transcript of this gene, only in the testes. It was proposed that this gene, designated *SRY* (sex-determining region, Y chromosome) was *TDF*.[22] Soon thereafter, mutations in the *SRY* were found in some cases of XY, pure gonadal dysgenesis.[23, 24, 25, 26] The mouse *Sry* gene was cloned at the same time as *SRY*.[27] (In accordance with standard convention, gene symbols are italicized; gene product symbols are not. Human genes are indicated by upper-case letters, whereas their mouse homologues are in lower-case except for the first letter, which for dominant genes is capitalized). Much information on human *SRY* has been obtained indirectly from studies on mouse *Sry*. In the following, these symbols are used specifically for their respective species, or *SRY/Sry* is used for situations applying to both.

Mice transgenic for a fragment containing *Sry* showed 40,XX sex reversal; that is, mice otherwise destined to be female had a male appearance (although they were sterile).[28] Testes of these mice were histologically similar to those of human XX males. However, sex reversal did not always occur. This incomplete penetrance may be related to the influence of genetic background on *Sry* transgene expression.[29] Genetic modifiers may also be the explanation for the multiple phenotypes seen with particular mutations in *SRY*. The human gene *SRY* does not cause sex reversal in transgenic mice; that is, it is not nearly as conserved in function as some human genes, a few of which can work even in *Drosophila*. The HMG boxes of *SRY* and its mouse homologue, *Sry*, are examples of so-called *generalized HMG boxes*.[30] It has been demonstrated that the *SRY* HMG box binds to synthetic DNA fragments of the sequence AACAAAG.[31]

The principal evidence to support that *SRY* is *TDF* is the following:

1. It is localized in the smallest region of chromosome Y capable of inducing testicular differentiation in humans[22] and in mice.[27]
2. Some cases of XY, pure gonadal dysgenesis present *de novo* mutations in the *SRY* gene.[23-26]
3. In the mouse, expression correlates with the initiation of testicular determination in the gonadal ridge,[32] and, in both

mice and humans, its expression in the blastocyst corresponds to the faster growth of the Y-bearing blastocyst (see later).[33-36]
4. A fragment of DNA that includes the mouse gene is able to induce male-type development in transgenic XX mice.[28]
5. It is an evolutionarily conserved gene on the Y chromosome of metatherian and eutherian mammals.[22, 37]

PREGONADAL SEXUAL DEVELOPMENT AND SEXUAL DIMORPHISM

In humans, although the sex chromosome complement and therewith the sex-determining genes are established at fertilization, it is not until about 42 days that differentiation of the indifferent gonads into testes in the male or, slightly later, their development into ovaries in the female can be detected. However, very early male and female embryos, and possibly even zygotes, do differ phenotypically, and in the previous edition of this book we argued that differential gene expression at pregonadal stages influences or sets the scene for subsequent gonadal sex determination and differentiation. Sex differences that are evident in early developmental stages, but for which the detailed genetic basis is not yet determined, include the time of occurrence of the first cleavage division, the rate of early embryonic cell division, the rate of accumulation of proteins, and differences in external genitalia. There is now evidence that pregonadal expression of genes upstream to *Sry* influences the sex-determining pathway. Some of these upstream genes are autosomal, although, as discussed later, pregonadal Y-chromosomal gene expression, including expression of *Sry* itself, also occurs.

Phenotypic Pregonadal Sexual Dimorphism for which Specific Genes Have Not Yet Been Identified

First Cleavage Division of the Zygote

Yadav and colleagues,[38] studying *in vitro* fertilized and cultured bovine embryos, found that early cleaving embryos were significantly more likely to be male than female. This sexual dimorphism suggests the possibility that differential expression of Y- or X-linked genes is present in the zygote, shortly after fertilization.

Rates of Cell Division in Early Embryos

Scott and Holson[39] reported that male rat fetuses are larger than female, and they have a higher protein content, at 12.5 days after coitus. Preimplantation XY mouse embryos have been reported to be more advanced than XX,[40] as have cattle embryos.[41, 42] Thornhill and Burgoyne[43] argued that the paternal X has a retarding effect on postimplantation mouse embryos. However, Burgoyne[44] found an accelerating effect of the Y chromosome on preimplantation mouse embryos, although the trait appeared to be polymorphic. Peippo and Bredbacka[45] found that in day 3 *in vivo* mouse embryos, females were found to be more advanced; during a subsequent 24-hour *in vitro* culture period, the increase in cell number was greater in male embryos. These authors proposed that previous results suggesting increased rates of cell division in male embryos may be an artifact of *in vitro* culture. Mittwoch has long maintained[46] that fast growth rate actually leads to testis formation and slow rate to ovary formation.

Pregonadal, Genetically Determined Development of Male External Genitalia

An important brick in the structure of current understanding of pregonadal expression of sex-determining genes emerged from studies on some marsupials, such as the tammar wallaby. In these animals, some features of sexual dimorphism, including the scrotum in the male and the mammary glands in the female, appear before development of the gonads and independently of hormones.[47] Although these organs develop mainly under hormonal influence in true (eutherian) mammals, evolutionary conservation of some pregonadal sex-determining gene expression has been shown to occur in mice. The XX*Sxr* pseudomale mouse is a chromosomal female (XX) that is masculinized by transposition of *Sry* and neighboring genes to an X but lacks the rest of the Y chromosome. The anogenital space, the size of which is a measure of masculinization (and which is also the region in which the scrotum develops) is smaller in prepubertal and adult pseudomales than in their normal, XY brothers.[48]

Genes Known to Be Transcribed Pregonadally

Early Transcription of Zfy and SRY

Transcripts of *Sry* and *Zfy* are present in the mouse embryo at the blastocyst stage,[33] and in the human embryo *SRY* and *ZFY* have been found to be transcribed at the one cell stage—the earliest genes yet found to be transcribed in the human embryo.[34, 35] These data suggest that *SRY/Sry* could be involved in the initiation of the genetic cascade that leads to sex determination.[49]

Expression of H-Y Antigen by Early Embryos

As mentioned earlier, evidence of the existence of a male-specific molecule, subsequently named H-Y, originally emerged from skin transplantation experiments in inbred mice. One epitope of human H-Y, called *SMCY*, has been cloned.[50] A serologically detectable counterpart of H-Y, now called SMA (serologically detected male antigen) has been extensively used as a method of exploring genetic sex. Studies on early embryos have shown that H-Y antigen is detectable as early as at the eight-cell stage.[51] Although the genetics of sex-specific antigens is far from clear, this finding does further underscore that sex-specific gene expression commences at an early stage in embryogenesis.

Genes Functioning Upstream of SRY/(Sry)

For the orderly function of the sex-determining gene *SRY/Sry*, normal operation of two other sets of genes must first occur. These two sets are those genes controlling the establishment of the cells and tissues (mentioned earlier) that are precursors of the gonads and those genes that directly influence *SRY/Sry*.

Genes that Act On Precursor Cells and Tissues. Several genes of this type are known. Some of these are expressed at early developmental stages, and others are expressed in the gonadal ridge shortly before the activation of *SRY/Sry* that immediately precedes gonadal differentiation.

Of *genes that function at early stages of development*, members of the *Lhx* family may be near the "top" of the cascade. *Lhx* refers to the LIM homeobox gene family, which contains transcription factors.[52] Genetic knock-out (KO) (experimental inactivation) of the mouse gene *Lhx1*, which has a role in gastrulation, causes absence of kidneys and gonads.[53] KOs of *Lhx-9* also fail to form gonads because somatic cells of the genital ridge fail to proliferate. Mice with KO of *Emx2* do not have kidneys, ureters, gonads, and genital tracts.[54]

Gene action in the gonadal ridge before sex-specific gonadal differentiation includes the following. Steroidogenic factor-1 (SF-1/*Sf-1*; homologous to the *Drosophila* gene *Fushi tarazu* 1 factor, sometimes referred to as *Ftz* F1), a key regulator of steroidogenic enzymes in adrenocortical cells,[55] is expressed in the urogenital ridge at embryonic day 9 to 9.5 in the mouse. This occurs before the expression of *Sry*[56]; this result has been confirmed in humans.[57] KO of *Sf-1* resulted in mice that died 8 days after birth.[58, 59] The KO mice lacked adrenal glands and gonads and had a resulting deficiency in corticosterone that was the likely cause of death.

Erickson and colleagues[60] predicted that human mutations in *SF-1* would lead to "a phenotype associated with predominantly

female appearance and severe neonatal problems due to lack of steroid hormones." Such a patient has now been described. A 46,XY female with adrenal failure at 2 weeks of life was found to have a heterozygous, adjacent two–base pair mutation.[61] The region of 9q33 to which *SF-1* maps[62] has not yet been associated with cytogenetic abnormalities and problems of sexual differentiation.

Other genes that are expressed in mouse gonadal ridge at day 9.5, before *Sry* and before sexual determination become evident, may have a role in preparing the gonad for sexual differentiation. These include *Dmrt-1* and *Dmrt-2* and *Wt-1*. DMRT-1, a mammalian homologue of a gene shared between *C. elegans* and *Drosophila*, maps to distal (i.e., toward the tip of the chromosome arm) 9p.[63] It has long been known that deletions at distal 9p are frequently associated with 46,XY sex reversal. *DMRT-1* is expressed in the genital ridge at day 9.5.[64] Initially, expression is equal in genital ridges of both sexes but gradually it becomes limited to expression in the 40,XY mouse gonad. The avian homologue of *DMRT-1* is also expressed in the genital ridge and wolffian duct (a precursor of internal sex organs) before sexual differentiation in the avian embryo; the same is not true of the *SRY* homologue.[64] Thus, as may be expected for a gene with homology to *Caenorhabditis elegans* and the *Drosophila* gene involved in sex determination, *DMRT-1* may have a more conserved role in sexual determination in vertebrates than does *SRY*.

The association between the Wilms' tumor 1 (*WT-1*) gene and testis development was recognized from investigations into the Denys-Drash and the WAGR syndromes. In Denys-Drash syndrome, caused by point mutations of the *WT-1* gene, patients have complex nephropathy and sexual ambiguity. Male patients with Denys-Drash syndrome may have female or ambiguous external genitalia with dysgenic gonads. WAGR syndrome, caused by deletions of 11p13, consists of *W*ilms' tumor, *a*niridia, *g*enitourinary anomalies, and mental *r*etardation. Patients with the WAGR syndrome may have undescended testes and hypospadias. The deletions suggest a tumor suppressor in this region related to Wilms' tumor.[65] It has been proposed that the *WT-1* gene is involved in mesenchymal-epithelial interactions,[66] for example between Sertoli cells and Leydig cells. Such interactions are crucial in both the developing kidney and the gonad. *WT-1* has at least 24 different isoforms, that is, different forms of the gene, simultaneously present and that arise through alternative splicing of the messenger RNA of the gene. Of these many isoforms, particular interest has focused around two that are highly conserved in evolution[67] and are caused by alternative splice donor sites at the end of exon 9 of the gene. The two isoforms, respectively, either possess or lack the three amino acids K (lysine), T (threonine) and S (serine). Children with Frasier syndrome, a variant of Denys-Drash syndrome, are mostly mutant for the splice site that creates the KTS insertion and therefore have a deficiency of the +KTS isoform.[68] Homozygous mice lacking the Wt-1 +KTS isoforms also show a complete XY sex reversal resulting from a dramatic reduction of *Sry* expression.[69] However, some conflicting data exist; thus, whereas interactions between *Sry* and *Wt-1* in the developing mouse gonad are clearly important, their relative roles in control of sexual determination are not yet clear.

Genes that Directly Influence SRY/Sry. Two known mutants in mice suggest the possibility that chromatin changes could be the initial stage in sex determination. One possible mechanism for this could be "release" of *SRY* from an autoinhibition that this gene may normally undergo, through a receptor on the gene to which the gene's own product can bind. The gene *M33* is the mouse homologue of the *Drosophila* gene *Polycomb*, which regulates chromatin structure. KO of *M33* caused failure of growth of the primordial gonad at the normal time of *Sry* expression, a finding suggesting that *M33* may be upstream of *Sry*. The mutants show hermaphroditism with intersex genitalia or complete male-to-female sex reversal.[70] Moreover, the gene for the syndrome ATR-X (α-*t*halassemia (sometimes), mental *r*etardation, mapping to the *X*), which also shows sexual ambiguity,[71] interacts with heterochromatin proteins and modifies DNA. Fibroblast growth factor 9 (FGF-9) may be an important mediator of *SRY* action.[72] The *Fgf9* KO shows deficient mesonephric cell migration into the gonad, deficient mesenchymal proliferation, decreased Sertoli cell function, and frequent sex reversal.

GONADAL STAGE

The data on transcription of *SRY* in human and mouse blastocysts, discussed previously, suggest the possibility that earlier events set in motion biochemical pathways related to the visible event of gonadal ridge differentiation. Furthermore, for normal female sex determination to occur and for the primitive gonad to differentiate to an ovary, homozygosity of at least one X-chromosomal locus appears to be essential. Relatively little is known about genetic control of ovarian development. A possible candidate gene for a role is *DSS*,[73] discussed later.

The components of the human bipotential gonadal primordium are described earlier in this chapter. Migration of the primordial germ cells is completed in the sixth week of gestation, when the embryonic female or male gonads are indistinguishable. The absence of primordial germ cells is not compatible with ovarian differentiation but does not prevent testicular seminiferous tubule morphogenesis.[74] Evidence suggests that the initial stages of gonadal differentiation are realized in the supporting cells (pre-Sertoli or prefollicular),[75] but cell-to-cell interactions are critical for the function of *SRY* and, in general, for gonadal differentiation.[76]

Genes Acting Downstream of *SRY/Sry*

Although *SRY/Sry* appears to be the Y-chromosomal sex-determining switch, it is not the ultimate, masculinizing gene of the sex determination pathway. First, it is not essential in all mammals. The males of several species of voles[77] and spinous country rats[78] develop appropriately without it. Second, investigations into the XX true hermaphrodites frequently seen among South African Bantus have also not detected Y-chromosomal sequences.[79] Thus, mammalian male sex determination can certainly occur in the absence of *SRY*, and in normal human development several genes downstream of *SRY* are involved.

It has been proposed that the HMG domain of the gene product *SRY* binds to regulatory DNA sequences of a hypothetical negative regulator of male sex determination, gene "Z."[80] Interaction of *SRY* with the Z gene is postulated to inhibit the regulatory effect of Z, resulting in a male phenotype. One possible inhibitory target for *SRY* is *SOX3*,[81] a member of the *SOX* gene family, described later. *SOX3* is more abundantly expressed in female than in male genital ridges.[82] Gene Z was thought to be located on Xp21.[80] Some 46,XY individuals with sex reversal have partial duplications of Xp and an intact *SRY* gene. They usually have female external and internal genitalia with partial gonadal dysgenesis.[73] Bernstein and colleagues[83] presented two cases and concluded that "testis-determining genes of the Y chromosome may be suppressed by regulatory elements of the X." The X homologue of *ZFY*, *ZFX*, which escapes inactivation, may be one candidate.[84] XXY (Klinefelter syndrome) patients do develop testes but they are not normal, and these patients do have partially feminized phenotypes. Furthermore, some XXY triploids have shown sexual ambiguity;[85] lack of X-inactivation in the triploids may be the cause.[86] Bardoni and colleagues[73] hypothesized a single gene in the Xp region of interest and named it *DSS* (*d*osage *s*ensitive *s*ex reversal). This region includes *DAX1* (*d*osage-sensitive sex reversal, *a*drenal hypoplasia congenita gene on the *X* chromosome gene *1*), gene defects of

which cause adrenal hypoplasia congenita.[87, 88] *DAX1* is a candidate for *DSS*. Capel[89] argued that an increased dosage of *DAX1* would override the *SRY* signal for testis development. Indeed, *DAX1* is normally down-regulated in the developing testis, whereas its expression persists in the developing ovary.[90] Overexpression in *Dax1* transgenics delays testicular development and can result in sex reversal in the presence of a weakly functioning (hypomorphic) *Sry*.[91]

Another gene involved in dosage-dependent 46,XY sex reversal is *WNT-4*, which maps to distal 1p, duplications of which sometimes cause male pseudohermaphroditism.[92] The *Wnt-4* KO does not affect male sexual development, but the females are masculinized.[93] The overexpression of *WNT-4* (in transfection experiments with cultured Sertoli and Leydig cells) appears to result in up-regulation of *DAX-1*, linking these two dosage-dependent pathways that enhance the female sexual development program.[94]

A family of genes with homology greater than 60% to the HMG box of *SRY* was discovered and was designated *SOX* (*SRY* box-related) genes).[95, 96] These genes are evolutionarily conserved. The relationship between *SRY* and the *SOX* genes has aroused great interest from the point of view of the origin and evolution of *SRY* in mammals.[97] *SOX3* is mentioned earlier. In camptomelic dysplasia, resulting from haploinsufficiency of *SOX9*, partial sex reversal of XY individuals may occur.[98] Increased dosage of *SOX9*, resulting from a chromosomal duplication, strongly masculinized a fetus.[99] In mice, *Sox9* transgenics develop a normal male appearance in the absence of *Sry*[100] and 40,XX, *Sry* minus mice (i.e., genetic females) carrying the deletion *Odsex*, which maps about 1 million base pairs upstream of *Sox9*, up-regulate *Sox9* expression in fetal gonads and develop as phenotypic males.[101] Investigators have shown that the HMG box of *SRY* recognizes the promoter elements of the gene for müllerian-inhibitory substance (MIS; discussed later), but this binding is insufficient to regulate transcription in *in vitro* systems. It also binds to the promoter of aromatase P450.[102] Thus, *SRY* could contribute, along with *SOX9*, to transcription of these target genes. Because no evidence of a role of *SRY* in *SOX9* expression has come to light, *SRY* is postulated to be the deinhibitor of a yet to be identified inhibitor of *SOX9* in mammals, in which species MIS is a presumptive target of *SOX9* regulation.[103] The relationships of *SOX9/Sox 9* and MIS may be different in *SRY*-negative male mammals and in nonmammalian species. Co-stimulators, with *SOX9*, of MIS may include SF-1 and other gene products. MIS and testosterone appear at this time to be the major, downstream masculinizers in the sex determination pathway.

SECONDARY SEXUAL DEVELOPMENT

The classic paradigm of sexual development, mentioned earlier, was formulated in principle by Alfred Jost[1] at the end of the 1940s, to explain the results of his observation that extirpation of the gonads (ovaries or testes) of rabbits before sexual differentiation had occurred invariably resulted in the development of a female-type pattern in the fetuses.[104] This established that, although sex-determining genes are evidently responsible for directing the development of the gonad, secondary sexual differentiation of *internal duct systems* and *external genitalia* is under hormonal control in humans and other eutherian mammals.

Indifferent (bipotential) external structures are initially present in males and females. The testis produces androgens, which masculinize the labioscrotal folds to form a scrotum and the genital tubercle to form the penis. In the absence of the testis, and therewith of high levels of androgen molecules, the labioscrotal folds fail to fuse and form labia, and the genital tubercle becomes the clitoris. Internally, the mesonephric (wolffian) and paramesonephric (müllerian) ducts develop into male or female structures, respectively. Testicular androgen promotes development of the wolffian ducts into epididymides, vasa deferentia, and seminal vesicles, and the absence of androgens leads to degeneration of the wolffian ducts. Also produced in the testis is MIS, which causes disintegration of the müllerian duct. In the female, in the absence of MIS, the müllerian duct becomes the uterine tubes, uterus, and the upper part of the vagina.

The possible place of the gene for MIS in the sequence of events downstream of *SRY*[105] is discussed earlier. Information on genes controlling female secondary sexual development are beginning to emerge from studies on patients with female pseudohermaphroditism with caudal dysplasia. Patients with female pseudohermaphroditism have ambiguous or male-type external genitalia with female karyotype. Perloff and colleagues[106] and others[107-110] described a distinct form of female pseudohermaphroditism associated with malformations of the internal genital, urinary, and gastrointestinal tracts. These defects include atresia or duplication of the uterus and vagina, fistulas between the urinary and gastrointestinal and genital tracts, urethral stenosis or atresia, and skeletal anomalies including vertebral and radial defects. They may occur in the apparent absence of testosterone or *SRY*.[111] Possible causes include a disturbance of a specific caudal developmental field,[108] a primary defect in the cloacal membrane,[110] or failed fusion of the urorectal septum with the cloacal membrane.[112]

Some cases of penoscrotal transposition,[113, 114] and some cases of prune belly sequence and of bilateral renal agenesis,[107, 115] have similar patterns of caudal malformations. Furthermore, this pattern of dysmorphism, but without female pseudohermaphroditism, is found in the VACTERL (*v*ertebral-*a*nal-*c*ardiac-*t*racheal-*e*sophageal fistula–*r*adial [or *r*enal]-other *l*imb), and MURCS (*m*üllerian duct aplasia-*r*enal aplasia, *c*ervicothoracic *s*omite dysplasia) associations, and Rokitansky syndrome, caudal dysplasia, and exstrophy of the bladder and cloaca sequences. These three conditions usually occur sporadically in families. In most cases, the cause is unknown. Autosomal dominant inheritance of multiple caudal anomalies has also been described.[116] Searches for the genes are more easily performed in mice.

The role of growth factors in the differentiation of the genital tubercle has been explored in mice. The possible role of *Fgf9* in gonadal differentiation was mentioned previously. *Fgf8* and *Fgf10* are implicated in external sexual differentiation; KO of *Fgf10* has quite marked sexual ambiguity.[117] A pathway initiated by sonic hedgehog (Shh), and its interactions with some of these factors, has been studied in organ cultures of murine genital tubercles.[118] *Shh* KO embryos showed no external genitalia at 12.5 days' gestation and showed down-regulation of *Fgf8*. Cultured genital tubercle explants treated with antibody to Shh also showed marked down-regulation of *Fgf10*. These findings are also relevant to the hypospadias seen in Smith-Lemli-Opitz syndrome; part of the developmental defects seen in this cholesterol synthesis deficiency may result from altered Shh signaling. Holoprosencephaly, sometimes seen in Smith-Lemli-Opitz syndrome), occurs with *Shh* haploinsufficiency, whereas hypospadias does not. Shh is also required for prostate development.[119] In contrast, desert hedgehog is required to maintain germ cells in the testis.[120]

Although *Wnt4* is implicated in gonadal differentiation (see earlier), *Wnt5a* has also been implicated in genital tubercle development.[121] Moreover, the role of MIS in development seems quite dependent on the signaling molecule *Wnt-7a*. In *Wnt-7a* KO, males fail to undergo regression of the müllerian duct, whereas females show abnormal oviduct or uterine development.[122, 123] The MIS receptor is not expressed in the males;[122] thus, *Wnt-7a* is essential for MIS function.

Multiple *Hox* genes, including the *Hoxa* and *Hoxd* groups, are involved in sexual differentiation. For example, compound double homozygous deficiency of *Hoxa-13* and *Hoxd-13*

showed a complete absence of external genitalia.[124] Haploinsufficiency of the *HOXD* complex caused genital anomalies of a small phallus and no palpable testes in one case and penoscrotal transposition with micropenis in another, with multiple limb and other abnormalities.[125] Hand-foot-genital syndrome with male cryptorchidism and hypospadias results from mutations in *HOXA13*.[126]

CONCLUSION

The sex-determination pathway, like most developmental pathways, has a strong tendency to maintain its function; that is, it is homeostatic. Redundancy in pathways may be part of the mechanism by which the homeostatic continuation of sexual development occurs. One can surmise that certain genes in the pathway may be up-regulated or down-regulated to compensate for deficiencies in other members of the pathway. Further understanding of the sex-determination pathway will come from studies of altered gene expression in deficient states and the location and identification of modifier genes that alter the pathway.

REFERENCES

1. Jost A, et al: Studies on sex differentiation in mammals. Recent Prog Horm Res *29*:1, 1973.
2. George FW: Sexual differentiation. *In* Griffin MD, Ojeda SR (eds): Textbook of Endocrine Physiology, 2nd ed. New York, Oxford University Press, 1992, pp 117.
3. Painter TS: Mammalian spermatogenesis. J Exp Zool *137*:291, 1923.
4. Welshons WJ, Russell LB: The Y-chromosome as the bearer of male determining factors in the mouse. Proc Natl Acad Sci USA *45*:560, 1959.
5. Ford CE, et al: A sex chromosome anomaly in a case of gonadal dysgenesis (Turner's Syndrome). Lancet *1*:711, 1959.
6. Jacobs PA, Strong JA: A case of human intersexuality having a possible XXY sex-determining mechanism. Nature *183*:302, 1959.
7. Ford CE, et al: The chromosomes in a patient showing both mongolism and the Klinefelter syndrome. Lancet *1*:709, 1959.
8. Wachtel SS, et al: Possible role for H-Y antigen in the primary determination of sex. Nature *257*:235, 1975.
9. McLaren A, et al: Male sexual differentiation in mice lacking H-Y antigen. Nature *312*:552, 1984.
10. Simpson E, et al: Separation of the genetic loci for the H-Y antigen and for testis determination on human Y chromosome. Nature *326*:876, 1987.
11. Jones KW, Singh L: Conserved repeated DNA sequences in vertebrate sex chromosomes. Hum Genet *58*:46, 1981.
12. Kiel-Metzger K, et al: Evidence that the human Y chromosome does not contain clustered DNA sequences (Bkm) associated with heterogametic sex determination in other vertebrates. N Engl J Med *313*:242, 1985.
13. Evans HS, et al: Heteromorphic X chromosomes in 46,XX males: evidence for the involvement of X-Y interchange. Hum Genet *49*:11, 1979.
14. Magenis RE, et al: Translocation (X:Y) (p22.33; p11.2) in XX males: etiology of male phenotype. Hum Genet *62*:271, 1989.
15. Gueallaen G, et al: Human XX males with Y single copy DNA fragments. Nature *307*:172, 1984.
16. Stalvey JRD, et al: Sex vesicle "entrapment": translocation or nonhomologous recombination of misaligned Yp and Xp as alternative mechanisms for abnormal inheritance of the sex-determining region. Am J Med Genet *32*:546, 1989.
17. Vergnaud G, et al: A deletion map of the human Y chromosome based on DNA hybridization. Am J Hum Genet *38*:109, 1986.
18. Nakahori Y, et al: Molecular cloning and mapping of 10 new probes on the human Y chromosome. Genomics *9*:765, 1991.
19. Page DC, et al: The sex-determining region of the human Y chromosome encodes a finger protein. Cell *51*:1091, 1987.
20. Palmer CG, et al: Genetic evidence that ZFY is not the testis-determining factor. Nature *342*:937, 1989.
21. Verga V, Erickson RP: An extended long-range restriction map of the human sex-determining region on Yp, including ZFY, finds marked homology on Xp and no detectable Y sequences in an XX male. Am J Hum Genet *44*:756, 1989.
22. Sinclair AH, et al: A gene from the human sex-determining region encodes a protein with homology to a conserved DNA-binding motif. Nature *346*:240, 1990.
23. Berta P, et al: Genetic evidence equating SRY and the testis-determining factor. Nature *348*:448, 1990.
24. Jager RJ, et al: A human XY female with a frame shift mutation in the candidate testis-determining gene SRY. Nature *348*:452, 1990.
25. Hawkins JR, et al: Evidence for increased prevalence of SRY mutations in XY females with complete rather than partial gonadal dysgenesis. Am J Hum Genet *51*:979, 1992.

26. Affara NA, et al: Analysis of SRY in 22 sex-reversed XY females identifies four new point mutations in the conserved DNA binding domain. Hum Mol Genet 2:785, 1993.

27. Gubbay J, et al: A gene mapping to the sex-determining region of the mouse Y chromosome is a member of a novel family of embryonically expressed genes. Nature 346:245, 1990.

28. Koopman P, et al: Male development of chromosomally female mice transgenic for Sry. Nature 351:117, 1991.

29. Hacker A, et al: Expression of Sry, the mouse sex-determining region gene. Development 121:1603, 1995.

30. Bianchi ME, et al: The DNA binding site of HMG1 protein is composed of two similar segments (HMG boxes), both of which have counterparts in other eukaryotic regulatory proteins. EMBO J 11:1055, 1992.

31. Harley VR, et al: DNA binding activity of recombinant SRY from normal males and XY females. Science 225:453, 1992.

32. Koopman P, et al: Expression of a candidate sex-determining gene during mouse testis differentiation. Nature 348:450, 1990.

33. Zwingman T, et al: Transcription of the sex-determining region genes Sry and Zfy in the mouse preimplantation embryo. Proc Natl Acad Sci USA 90:814, 1993.

34. Ao A, et al: Transcription of paternal Y-linked genes in the human zygote as early as the pronucleate stage. Zygote 2:281, 1994.

35. Fiddler M, et al: Expression of SRY transcripts in preimplantation human embryos. Am J Med Genet 55:80, 1995.

36. Pergament E, et al: Sexual differentiation and preimplantation cell growth. Hum Reprod 9:1730, 1994.

37. Foster JW, et al: Evolution of sex determination and the Y chromosome: SRY-related sequences in marsupials. Nature 359:531, 1992.

38. Yadav BR, et al: Relationships between the completion of first cleavage and the chromosomal complement, sex, and developmental rates of bovine embryos generated in vitro. Mol Reprod Dev 36:434, 1993.

39. Scott WJ, Holson JF: Weight differences in rat embryos prior to sexual differentiation. J Embryol Exp Morphol 40:259, 1977.

40. Tsunoda, et al: Altered sex ratio of live young after transfer of fast- and slow-developing mouse embryos. Gamete Res 12:301, 1985.

41. Avery, et al: Sex and development in bovine in-vitro fertilised embryos. Theriogenology 35:953, 1991.

42. Xu KP, et al: Sex-related differences in developmental rates of bovine embryos produced and cultured in vitro. Mol Reprod Dev 31:249, 1992.

43. Thornhill AR, Burgoyne PS: A paternally imprinted X chromosome retards the development of the early mouse embryo Development 118:171, 1993.

44. Burgoyne PS: A Y-chromosomal effect on blastocyst cell number in mice. Development 117:341, 1993.

45. Peippo J, Bredbacka P: Sex-related growth rate differences in mouse preimplantation embryos in vivo and in vitro. Mol Reprod Dev 40:56, 1995.

46. Mittwoch U: Blastocysts prepare for the race to be male. Hum Reprod 8:1550, 1993.

47. Renfree MB, Short RV: Sex-determination in marsupials: evidence for a marsupial-eutherian dichotomy. Phil Trans R Soc Lond 322:41, 1988.

48. Atkinson TG, Blecher SR: Aberrant anogenital distance in XXSrx ("sex-reversed") pseudomale mice. J. Zool Lond 233:581, 1994.

49. Boyer TR, Erickson RP: Detection of circular and linear transcripts of Sry in pre-implantation mouse embryos: differences in requirements for reverse transcriptase. Biochem Biophys Res Commun 198:492, 1994.

50. Kent-First MG, et al: Gene sequence and evolutionary conservation of human SMCY. Nat Genet 14:128, 1996.

51. Epstein CJ, et al: Expression of H-Y antigen on preimplantation mouse embryos. Tissue Antigens 15:63, 1980.

52. Hobert O, Westphal H: Functions of LIM-homeobox genes. Trends Genet 16:75, 2000.

53. Shawlot W, Behringer RR: Requirement for Lim1 in head-organizer function. Nature 374:425, 1995.

54. Miyamoto N, et al: Defects of urogenital development in mice lacking Emx2. Development 124:1653, 1997.

55. Lala DS, et al: Steroidogenic factor 1, a key regulator of steroidogenic enzyme expression, is the mouse homolog of fushi tarazu factor 1. Mol Endocrinol 6:1249, 1992.

56. Ikeda Y, et al: Developmental expression mouse steroidogenic factor 1, an essential regulator of the steroid hydrolaxes. Mol Endocrinol 8:654, 1994.

57. de Santa Barbara P, et al: Direct interaction of SRY-related protein SOX9 and steroidogenic factor 1 regulates transcription of the human anti-müllerian hormone gene. Mol Cell Biol 18:6653, 1998.

58. Luo X, et al: A cell-specific nuclear receptor is essential for adrenal and gonadal development and sexual differentiation. Cell 77:481, 1994.

59. Sadovsky Y, et al: Mice deficient in the orphan receptor steroidogenic factor 1 lack adrenal glands and gonads but express P450 side-chain-cleavage enzyme in the placenta and have normal embryonic serum levels of corticosteroids. Proc Natl Acad Sci USA 92:10939, 1995.

60. Erickson RP, et al: Genetic Disorders of Human Sexual Development. New York, Oxford University Press, 1999, pp 11–38.

61. Achermann JC, et al: A mutation in the gene encoding steroidogenic factor-1 causes XY sex reversal and adrenal failure in humans. Nat Genet 22:125, 1999.

62. Taketo M, et al: Homologs of Drosophila fushi-tarazu factor 1 map to mouse chromosome 2 and human chromosome 9q33. Genomics 25:565, 1995.

63. Raymond CS, et al: Evidence for evolutionary conservation of sex-determining genes. Nature 391:691, 1998.

64. Raymond CS, et al: Expression of Dmrt1 in the genital ridge of mouse and chicken embryos suggests a role in vertebrate sexual development. Dev Biol 215:208, 1999.

65. Hastie ND: Life, sex, and WT1 isoforms: three amino acids can make all the difference. Cell 106:391, 2001.

66. van Heyningen V, Hastie ND: Wilms' tumor: reconciling genetics and biology. Trends Genet 8:16, 1992.

67. Kent J, et al: The evolution of WT1 sequence and expression pattern in the vertebrates. Oncogene 11:1781, 1995.

68. Little M, et al: WT1: what has the last decade told us? Bioessays 21:191, 1999.

69. Hammes A, et al: Two splice variants of the Wilms' tumor 1 gene have distinct functions during sex determination and nephron formation. Cell 106:319, 2001.

70. Katoh-Fukui Y, et al: Male-to-female sex reversal in M33 mutant mice. Nature 393:688, 1998.

71. Gibbons RJ, et al: Mutations in a putative global transcriptional regulator cause X-linked mental retardation with α-thalassemia (ATR-X syndrome). Cell 80:837, 1995.

72. Colvin JS, et al: Male-to-female sex reversal in mice lacking fibroblast growth factor 9. Cell 104:875, 2001.

73. Bardoni B, et al: A dosage sensitive locus at chromosome Xp21 is involved in male to female sex reversal. Nat Genet 7:497, 1994.

74. Merchant-Larios H: Germ and somatic cell interactions during gonadal morphogenesis. In: "Ultrastructure of reproduction." Van Blerkom J and Motta PM (eds). Amsterdam Martinus Nijhoff, 1984, p 19.

75. Bogan JS, Page DC: Ovary? Testis? A mammalian dilemma. Cell 76:603, 1994.

76. Goodfellow PN, Lovell-Badge R: SRY and sex determination in mammals. Annu Rev Genet 27:71, 1993.

77. Just W, et al: Absence of Sry in species of the vole Ellobius. Nat Genet 11:117, 1995.

78. Sotou S, et al: Sex determination without the Y chromosome in two Japanese rodents Tokudaia osimensis osimensis and Tokudaia osimensis spp. Mamm Genome 12:17, 2001.

79. Ramsay M, et al: XX true hermaphroditism in southern African blacks: an enigma of primary sexual differentiation. Am J Hum Genet 43:4, 1988.

80. McElreavy K, et al: A regulatory cascade hypothesis for mammalian sex determination: SRY represses a negative regulator of male development. Proc Natl Acad Sci USA 90:3368, 1993.

81. Marshall Graves JA: Interactions between SRY and SOX genes in mammalian sex determination. Bioessays 20:264, 1998.

82. Collignon J, et al: A comparison of the properties of Sox-3 with Sry and two related genes, Sox-1 and Sox-2. Development 122:590, 1996.

83. Bernstein R, et al: Female phenotype and multiple abnormalities in sibs with a Y chromosome and partial X chromosome duplication: H-Y antigen and Xg blood group findings. J Med Genet 17:291, 1980.

84. Scherer G, et al: Duplication of an Xp segment that includes the ZFX locus causes sex inversion in man. Hum Genet 81:291, 1989.

85. Graham JM Jr, et al: Triploidy: pregnancy complications and clinical findings in seven cases. Prenat Diagn 9:409, 1989.

86. Petit P, et al: Full 69,XXY triploidy and sex-reversal: a further example of true hermaphrodism associated with multiple malformations. Clin Genet 41:175, 1992.

87. Muscatelli F, et al: Mutations in the DAX-1 gene give rise to both X-linked adrenal hypoplasia congenita and hypogonadotropic hypogonadism. Nature 372:672, 1994.

88. Zanaria E, et al: An unusual member of the nuclear hormone receptor superfamily responsible for X-linked adrenal hypoplasia congenita. Nature 372:635, 1994.

89. Capel B, et al: Circular transcripts of the testis-determining gene Sry in adult mouse testis. Cell 73:1019, 1993.

90. Swain A, et al: Mouse Dax1 expression is consistent with a role in sex determination as well as in adrenal and hypothalamus function. Nat Genet 12:404, 1996.

91. Swain A, et al: Dax1 antagonizes Sry action in mammalian sex determination. Nature 391:761, 1998.

92. Garcia-Heras J, et al: De novo partial duplications 1p: report of two new cases and review. Am J Med Genet 82:261, 1999.

93. Vainio S, et al: Female development in mammals is regulated by Wnt-4. Nature 397:405, 1999.

94. Jordan BK, et al: Up-regulation of WNT-4 signaling and dosage-sensitive sex reversal in humans. Am J Hum Genet 68:1102, 2001.

95. Denny P, et al: A conserved family of genes related to the testis determining gene, SRY. Nucleic Acids Res 20:2887, 1992.

96. Stevanovic M, et al: SOX3 is an X-linked gene related to SRY. Hum Mol Genet 2:2013, 1993.

97. Foster JW, Marshall GJA. An SRY-related sequence on the marsupial X chromosome: implications for the evolution of the mammalian testis-determining gene. Proc Natl Acad Sci USA 91:1927, 1994.

98. Tommerup N, et al: Assignment of an autosomal sex reversal locus (SRA1) and campomelic dysplasia (CMPD1) to 17q24.3-q25.1. Nat Genet 4:170 1993.

99. Huang B, et al: Autosomal XX sex reversal caused by duplication of SOX9. Am J Med Genet 87:349, 1999.

100. Vidal VPI, et al: Sox9 induces testis development in XX transgenic mice. Nat Genet 28:216, 2001.

101. Bishop CE, et al: A transgenic insertion upstream of *Sox9* is associated with dominant XX sex reversal in the mouse. Nat Genet *26*:490, 2000.
102. Haqq CM, et al: *SRY* recognizes conserved DNA sites in sex-specific promoters. Proc Natl Acad Sci USA *90*:1097, 1993.
103. Oreal E, et al: Early expression of AMH in chicken embryonic gonads precedes testicular SOX9 expression. Dev Dyn *212*:522, 1998.
104. Jost A: Problems of fetal endocrinology: the gonadal and hypophyseal hormones. Recent Prog Horm Res *8*:379, 1953.
105. Haqq CM, et al: Molecular basis of mammalian sexual determination: activation of müllerian inhibiting substance gene expression by SRY. Science *266*:1494, 1994.
106. Perloff WH, et al: Female pseudohermaphroditism: a description of two unusual cases. J Clin Endocrinol *13*:783, 1953.
107. Carpentier PJ, Potter EL: Nuclear sex and genital malformation in 48 cases of renal agenesis, with special reference to non-specific female pseudohermaphroditism. Am J Obstet Gynecol *78*:235, 1959.
108. Lubinsky MS: Female pseudohermaphroditism and associated anomalies. Am J Med Genet *6*:123, 1980.
109. Hokamp HG, Muller KM: Prune belly syndrome and female pseudohermaphroditism. Pathol Res Pract *117*:76, 1983.
110. Robinson Jr HB, Tross K: Agenesis of the cloacal membrane: a possible teratogenic anomaly. Perspect Pediatr Pathol *8*:79, 1984.
111. Erickson RP, et al: Molecular and clinical studies of three cases of female pseudohermaphroditism with caudal dysplasia suggest multiple etiologies. Clin Genet *51*:331, 1997.
112. Escobar LF, et al: Urorectal septum malformation sequence. Am J Dis Child *141*:1021, 1987.
113. MacKenzie J, et al: Penoscrotal transposition: a case report and review. Am J Med Genet *49*:103, 1994.
114. Parida SK, et al: Penoscrotal transposition and associated anomalies: report of five new cases and review of the literature. Am J Med Genet *59*:69, 1995.
115. Reinberg Y, et al: Prune belly syndrome in females: a triad of abdominal muscular deficiency and anomalies of the urinary and genital systems. J Pediatr *118*:395, 1991.
116. Erickson RP, et al: Use of a probe for the putative sex determining gene, zinc finger Y, in the study of patients with ambiguous genitalia and XY gonadal dysgenesis. Am J Med Genet *36*:232, 1990.
117. Haraguchi R, et al: Molecular analysis of external genitalia formation: the role of fibroblast growth factor (FGF) genes during genital tubercle formation. Development *127*:2471, 2000.
118. Haraguchi R, et al: Unique functions of sonic hedgehog signaling during external genitalia development. Development *128*:4241, 2001.
119. Podlasek CA, et al: Prostate development requires sonic hedgehog expressed by the urogenital sinus epithelium. Dev Biol *209*:28, 1999.
120. Bitgood MJ, et al: Sertoli cell signaling by desert hedgehog regulates the male germline. Curr Biol *6*:298, 1996.
121. Yamaguchi TP, et al: A Wnt5a pathway underlies outgrowth of multiple structures in the vertebrate embryo. Development *126*:1211, 1999.
122. Parr BA, McMahon AP: Sexually dimorphic development of the mammalian reproductive tract requires *Wnt-7a*. Nature *395*:707, 1998.
123. Miller C, Sassoon DA: Wnt-7a maintains appropriate uterine patterning during the development of the mouse female reproductive tract. Development *125*:3201, 1998.
124. Kondo T, et al: Of fingers, toes and penises. Nature *390*:29, 1997.
125. Del Campo M, et al: Monodactylous limbs and abnormal genitalia are associated with hemizygosity for the human 2q31 region that includes the *HOXD* cluster. Am J Hum Genet *65*:104, 1999.
126. Mortlock DP, Innis JW: Mutation of *HOXA-13* in hand-foot-genital syndrome. Nat Genet *15*:179, 1997.

Anne Grete Byskov and Lars Grabow Westergaard

190 Differentiation of the Ovary

DEVELOPMENT OF A FUNCTIONAL OVARY

Three major events, namely, initiation of meiosis, formation of follicles, and differentiation of steroid-producing cells, are prerequisites for development of a functional ovary. In the human, as in many other mammalian species, these events begin during fetal life, at a time when germ cells and somatic cells have populated the ovarian anlage.

In both sexes, the human gonads are closely connected to the mesonephros throughout early differentiation. Mesonephric cells as well as cells from the ovarian surface epithelium migrate simultaneously with the primordial germ cells to form the future gonadal tissue at the ventrocranial aspect of the mesonephros.[1, 2] In the fetal mouse, cells from mesonephros form an *adrenogenital primordium* characterized by activity for steroidogenic factor 1 (SF-1).[3] This primordium may be the progenitor of the hormone-producing somatic cells of the differentiated gonad of both sexes and of the adrenal gland.[3]

Meiosis and follicle formation are interrelated processes, the first being the prerequisite for the second, which, conversely, secures survival of the oocyte. The steroid-producing theca cells form later, around the growing follicles. Whether differentiation of steroid-producing cells in the stroma is connected to the foregoing two events is less clear.

The follicles constitute the functional part of the ovary. Within the follicle, a unique micromilieu forms that secures oocyte growth and maturation. However, intraovarian and interovarian regulatory mechanisms as well as systemic interrelationships participate in controlling the fate of female germ cells.

Gonadal Sex Determination

In contrast to some other vertebrate classes (e.g., amphibians and fish), spontaneous sex reversal has never been reported in mammals.[4] In most vertebrate classes, gonadal differentiation is the result of the genetic sex. In mammals, the testis is formed when a Y chromosome is present, and an ovary develops if this chromosome is absent, irrespective of additional sex chromosomes.[5] During the 1970s and 1980s, a testis-determining region of the Y chromosome was located in smaller and smaller parts of the chromosome. In 1990, the sex-determining region Y—a single gene—was found.[6-8] It is believed that if the *Sry* gene is not activated, ovarian development will take place. Sex determination is a complex process, and a screen for genes that may be involved in gonadal and sex duct formation revealed that at least 72 genes seem to be involved.[9]

EARLY OVARIAN DIFFERENTIATION

In the human, the invasion of primordial germ cells into the gonadal ridge is completed around the ninth week of fetal life.[10] The invading mesonephric cells accumulate in the central part of the ovary and form the intraovarian rete in the medulla (Fig. 190-1). The growing medulla gradually pushes the germ cells toward the periphery, to form the cortex with a high density of germ cells (Fig. 190-2).

The ovary is usually recognizable by morphologic criteria at a later stage of gonadal differentiation than the testis. The first signs signifying that the indifferent gonad is becoming a testis

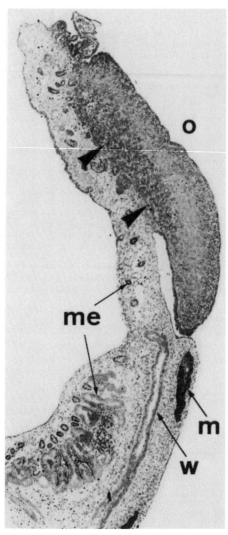

Figure 190–1. Ovarian-mesonephric complex of an 11-week-old human fetal ovary. The mesonephric cells that invade the ovary are recognized as the dark cell mass *(arrowheads)* in the basal part of the ovary (O). The Wolffian duct (w), the müllerian duct (m), and mesonephric tubules (me) are seen. (×200.) (From Byskov AG, Høyer PE: *In* Knobil E, Neil J [eds]: The Physiology of Reproduction. New York, Raven Press, 1988.)

are the formation of the testicular cords enclosing the germ cells[11] and the rounding up of the organ.[12] In the human testis, these events take place at the sixth week of fetal life.

Cords enclosing the germ cells are, however, also seen at early stages of ovarian differentiation in some mammalian species (e.g., the pig and the sheep). In other species (e.g., the mouse and the hamster), the germ cells are more evenly distributed throughout the ovary. These different patterns of germ cell location within the ovary are closely related to the onset of meiosis. Meiosis begins only after a "delay period" in species in which germ cell cords are formed (delayed meiosis), and earlier in species without ovarian cord formation (immediate meiosis).[13] During the delay period, transitory ovarian steroidogenesis takes place (see later). This is analogous to early testicular differentiation, in which steroidogenesis begins immediately after testicular cords are formed.[14, 15] It has been proposed that enclosure of germ cells into specific germ cell compartments, either as temporarily formed cords or as follicles, is a prerequisite for the start of steroid production in the developing gonads.[13]

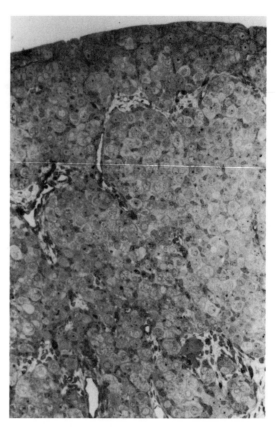

Figure 190–2. Human fetal ovary, 21st week, showing the cortex packed with oocytes. (×300.)

Morphologically and functionally, the human fetal ovary represents an intermediate type between cord formation and noncord formation. Although germ cells are clustered during fetal life, well-defined cords are not formed (Fig. 190–3; see Fig. 190–2).[16] Nonetheless, the delay period lasts for a relatively long period, from the onset of sex differentiation around the sixth week of gestation until the 11th week, when meiosis starts.[17] Few or no steroids are produced by human ovaries during the delay period, although the aromatizing enzyme system is present by the sixth week of fetal life.[18] Interstitial cells with ultrastructural resemblance to steroid-producing cells have been recognized from the 13th week of fetal life (Fig. 190–4).[19]

The origin of the somatic cell population of the cortex is uncertain, and different theories have been proposed. Generally, the following sources for their origin have been suggested: the surface epithelium,[20] the mesonephros, or a combination of the two.[16, 21]

In vitro experiments attempted to trace the origin of gonadal somatic cells by culturing fetal mesonephric tissue from one mouse strain carrying a cellular marker together with fetal gonads from another strain without a marker[22, 23] and vice versa.[24] However, results of the first studies indicated that mesonephric cells almost entirely migrated to the testis, not to the ovary, whereas the later study showed that cells moved in both directions in both sexes. Thus, the origin of the somatic cells of the gonads is still uncertain.

MEIOTIC PROPHASE OF OOCYTES

By the end of the 10th week of gestation, the human ovarian cortex contains numerous mitotically dividing germ cells called *oogonia*. When the oogonia stop dividing and enter meiosis, they are termed *oocytes*. The first oocytes in the human ovary are seen during the 11th week of fetal life. Transformation of an

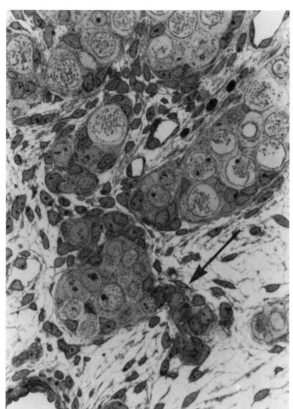

Figure 190–3. Human fetal ovary, 21st week, with clusters of oocytes in different stages of meiosis in the inner part of the cortex, in connection with an intraovarian rete cord *(arrow)*. (×600.)

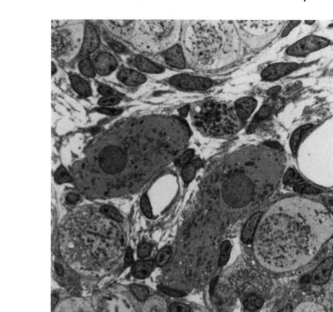

Figure 190–4. Two interstitial cells in the inner part of the ovarian cortex from a fetal human ovary, 21 weeks old. (×900.)

oogonium into an oocyte and then into an ovum with a haploid number of chromosomes denotes *oogenesis*.

The number of oogonia increases exponentially by mitotic division from around 20,000 in the 6-week-old human fetus to around 250,000 in the 10th week,[25] and it reaches a maximum of 7 million in the 20th week (Fig. 190–5).[26] Certain genes and transcription factors are involved in multiplication of the oogonia, such as DAX-1[27] and expression of Kit protein.[28, 29] Extensive degeneration, however, reduces the number of germ cells drastically during the rest of fetal life, and around birth only 1 to 2 million oocytes are left.[26, 30]

Process of Meiosis

Meiosis begins with premeiotic DNA synthesis, followed by the transitory stages of the first meiotic prophase: preleptotene-leptotene-zygotene-pachytene and diplotene stages. When the diplotene stage is reached, the process is arrested (Fig. 190–6). During this first meiotic prophase, the maternal and paternal genes are exchanged between the homologous chromosomes. The diplotene stage, sometimes named the dictyate stage, is maintained until the oocyte resumes meiosis (just before ovulation) or degenerates and may thus last for the whole fertile life span. Oocyte degeneration may occur at any time during development. At resumption of meiosis, the first meiotic prophase is completed, and the oocyte proceeds through the first meiotic division, the reduction division, in which the homologous chromosomes are separated into the daughter cells, now each containing 1n chromosomes and 2c (i.e., copy) DNA. The second meiotic division, which takes place by fertilization, is not preceded by the usual DNA synthesis, and the

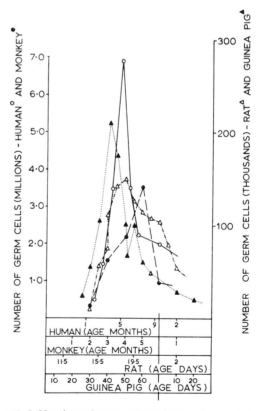

Figure 190–5. Number of germ cells in fetal and neonatal ovaries of human, monkey, rat, and guinea pig. (From Baker TG: *In* Balin H, Glasser SR [eds]: Reproductive Biology. Amsterdam, Excerpta Medica, 1973.)

DNA content is therefore halved to 1c. In the human, the meiotic divisions result in gametes with 23 chromosomes (1n) and 1c DNA.

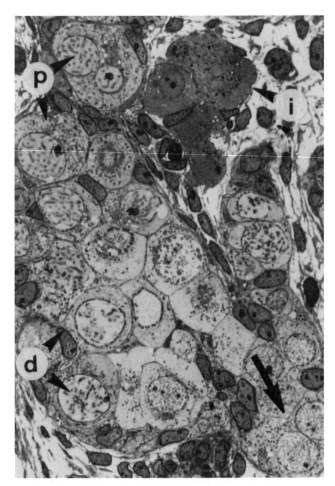

Figure 190–6. Inner part of the ovarian cortex of a human ovary, 21-week-old fetus, showing different stages of meiosis and interstitial cells *(arrow)*. d = early diplotene; i = interstitial cells; p = pachytene. (×900.)

Meiotic Prophase: Morphologic Features and Genetic Control

The different transitory stages of meiosis are recognized by the configuration of the chromosomes. In the preleptotene and leptotene stages, the chromosomes become condensed and are seen as thin coiled threads, each thread consisting of identical sister chromosomes. The chromosomes coil increasingly during progression through the zygotene to pachytene stages. The synaptonemal complexes begin to form in the zygotene and are completed in the pachytene stage. These structures represent the pairing of homologous chromatids. It seems that proper formation of the synaptonemal complexes ensures normal chromosome segregation in the reduction division of meiosis.[31] Passing into the diplotene stage, the chromosomes decoil, and chiasmata or crossing-over may be recognized. At this stage, the paternal and maternal chromatids exchange gene material. The amount of exchanged gene material can be evaluated in the metaphase of the second meiotic division after labeling of premeiotic oogonia in S phase with bromine deoxyuridine.[32] During the diplotene stage, the oocyte and its nucleus enlarge. The chromosomes decondense, thus making the nucleus faintly stainable.

Only few genes with functions specific for the early meiotic processes are known. One of these is *Dazla,* which encodes for a protein with RNA-binding element and is found in human oogonia.[33] *Dazla*-deficient mice are infertile because the oocytes

are lost when passing through meiosis.[34] Other genes are needed for the structural organization of chromosomes during assembly of the synaptonemal complexes and recombination, Scp1-3.[35-37]

As discussed earlier, meiosis begins with premeiotic DNA synthesis and ultimately leads to the 4c DNA content of the leptotene stage.[38,39] This DNA must last until ovulation ceases, which in the human can occur up to 50 years later. In other mammalian species, it has been shown by DNA labeling that no neoformation of oocytes takes place later in life; that is, the entire pool of oogonia is transformed into oocytes early in life.[40-43] However, there seems to be at least one exception to this rule, because DNA synthesis appears to occur in oogonia-like germ cells in the ovaries of adult prosimians (lower primates).[44,45]

In contrast to somatic cells, the DNA synthesis of germ cells is not strictly confined to the S phase. By flow cytometric sorting of rabbit oogonia and oocytes, it was found that DNA synthesis extends into the leptotene stage.[46] Therefore, it seems that the premeiotic DNA synthesis is a part of the early meiotic process itself.

In the early stages of fetal ovarian development, oogonia and oocytes are often interconnected by cytoplasmic bridges[47] forming so-called *germ cell cysts.*[48] These bridges may be important for exchange of intercellular signals and may explain why groups of germ cells divide synchronously and enter meiosis in clusters (see Fig. 190–6).[49]

Initiation and Regulation of Meiosis

In the human ovary, meiosis is initiated in the 11th week of fetal life.[17] The first leptotene stages appear in the central part of the ovary, as in ovaries of all other mammalian species. Gradually, meiosis proceeds toward the periphery of the cortex. Around the 32nd week of fetal life, all oogonia have been transformed into oocytes,[50] and by the time of birth, almost all oocytes are in the diplotene stage.[51]

The time of onset of meiosis in the female varies among different mammalian species but occurs always at an early stage of development, often in fetal life. In the testis, by contrast, initiation of meiosis is postponed until puberty in all species. These discrepancies have led to the hypothesis that an internal clock of the germ cells determines the onset of meiosis, independent of external factors.[52] However, the male germ cells can be induced to enter meiosis prematurely, for example, if the cells are located in the adrenal gland of the human fetus[53] or if they are exposed to a meiosis-inducing substance before the testis is sex differentiated.[13] Thus, it seems uncertain whether a germ cell clock governs the switch from mitosis to meiosis or it is triggered by paracrine or other external stimuli (see later). Genes that are specifically involved in transformation of the mitotically dividing oogonia into the meiotic direction are not yet identified.

Meiosis-Regulatory Substances

A characteristic feature of the developing mammalian ovary is that the germ cells first entering meiosis are those situated in the central part of the ovary,[54] in close connection with the mesonephric-derived rete ovarii.[21] It has therefore been proposed that the mesonephric-derived cells in the ovary trigger the onset of meiosis.[21] *In vitro* experiments with gonads of fetal mouse[55] and hamster[56] suggest that the mesonephros produces a substance that promotes and induces meiosis in male as well as in female germ cells. This substance was termed *meiosis-inducing substance.*[57] Meiosis-inducing substance is produced by gonadal tissues—ovaries and testes—in which meiosis is ongoing, including preovulatory human follicles.[58] In contrast to the developing ovary, meiosis of prespermatogonia in the differentiating testis is prevented when they become enclosed in testicular cords. It was proposed that meiosis-preventing substance within the testicular cords is responsible for meiotic prevention: meiosis-inducing substance and meiosis-preventing substance interact in the control of the meiotic process. The critical factor for determining whether meiosis is induced, resumed, or prevented may be the ratio between meiosis-inducing substance and meiosis-preventing substance.[13]

Meiosis-inducing substance or meiosis-preventing substance activity has been detected in fetal and adult gonadal tissues collected from numerous mammalian species (Table 190-1). Meiosis-inducing substance and meiosis-preventing substance are not species specific, because meiosis is induced or prevented in fetal mouse germ cells by spent culture media prepared from gonadal tissues of other species.[13]

The presence of Meiosis-inducing substance in gonads in which meiosis is initiated and its role in this process have been questioned. One study showed that fetal male mouse germ cells are "passively" entering meiosis when they are mixed and cultured with lung cells.[59] Thus, as mentioned, the control of onset of meiosis may be built into the germ cell lines, in females as well as in males, but meiosis is prevented in the male germline (meiosis-preventing substance?) by enclosure in testicular cords.

The chemical structures of meiosis-activating sterols, which are able to induce resumption of meiosis in mammalian oocytes, have been identified.[60] Meiosis-activating sterols were extracted from gonads of different species in which meiosis is ongoing, such as human preovulatory follicular fluids and bull testicular tissue.[61] It is uncertain at present whether meiosis-activating sterols are identical to the previously described meiosis-inducing substance.

FOLLICULOGENESIS

Folliculogenesis is the process during which the diplotene oocyte becomes surrounded by a single layer of granulosa cells and enclosed by an intact basal lamina, thus forming a specific germ cell compartment (Fig. 190-7). Whether a follicular arrangement of granulosa cells and basal membrane can occur without the presence of an oocyte has been disputed, because it has not yet been possible to create gonads completely devoid of germ cells, such as by selective destruction by drugs.[62]

The separation of the diplotene oocyte from the surrounding tissue secures its survival and creates a unique micromilieu, which sustains further growth and differentiation. If the oocyte in the diplotene stage fails to be enclosed in a follicle, it invariably degenerates. Some follicles die as a result of specific programmed cell death, or *apoptosis*.[63-65] In the fetal human ovary, *naked oocytes* (diplotene oocytes without a granulosa layer) are often seen, but they always appear to be degenerating. Such oocytes are never seen later in life.[66]

The first follicles are encountered in the human ovary around the 16th week of fetal life, and folliculogenesis is completed immediately after birth.[67] The appearance and growth of the first

follicles coincide with the increase of fetal gonadotropins. Whether these two events are causally related is uncertain. The mechanisms that control folliculogenesis are not clarified. Investigators found that the factor in germline α (Figα), which is a transcription factor, is mandatory for follicle formation in the mouse,[68] but a similar factor in the human has not yet been described.

Formation of the Granulosa Layer

The first follicles are formed in the inner part of the cortex, where oocytes first reach the diplotene stage.[69] In the newborn mouse ovary, programmed breakdown of the germ cell cysts may serve as a prerequisite for follicle formation.[70] It has been observed that the granulosa cells of the first and always centrally placed follicles are initially connected with the intraovarian rete cords.[71] This finding supports the assumption that granulosa cell precursors are of mesonephric origin. In fact, transplant experiments of fetal mouse ovaries showed that when invasion of mesonephric cells into the ovary is prevented, follicles are not formed.[72] It has also been proposed that the surface epithelium may give rise to granulosa cells, because proliferation of this epithelium into the cortex takes place during early stages of ovarian differentiation, before folliculogenesis.[21] One morphologic study of the formation of ovarian follicles during fetal sheep development suggested that almost all granulosa cells originate from the ovarian surface epithelium.[73] It is thus possible that mesonephric-derived cells as well as cells of the surface epithelium contribute to the granulosa cell population.

Across mammalian species, the first generation of follicles appears to differ from later ones, exhibiting a different pattern of growth and differentiation (Fig. 190-8).[74] The granulosa cells of these follicles seem to arise as a result of migratory processes of the extraovarian rete cells into the intraovarian rete that are in contact with the oocytes.[72, 75] Growth of later generations of follicles, which are no longer connected to the intraovarian rete, depends on proliferation of the fixed population of granulosa cells already enclosed in the follicle.[76, 77]

The granulosa layer of the first generation of follicles that starts to grow often differs compared with later generations. The basal membrane does not always enclose the granulosa layer. It forms a tail-like extension (see Fig. 190-8), which is sometimes connected to the intraovarian rete tubules. The first generation of follicles in the human fetal ovary may contain several oocytes of varying size and even oogonia. Sometimes one oocyte is larger than the others (see Fig. 190-8*B*). Small oocytes—not enclosed in follicles—may also be seen in

TABLE 190-1

Female Tissues from Which Meiosis-Inducing Substance or Meiosis-Preventing Substance Has Been Harvested

		MIS	MPS
Human	Fetal ovaries, 8-12 wk	+	–
	Preovulatory follicles	++	–
Mouse	Fetal ovaries, 13-14 d postconception	+	–
Rat	Newborn	–	++
Cow	Preovulatory follicles	++	–

MIS = meiosis-inducing substance; MPS = meiosis-preventing substance.

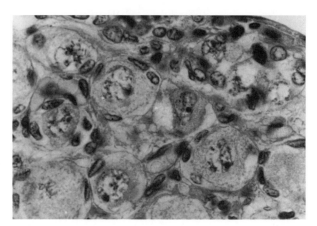

Figure 190–7. Primordial follicles in the ovarian cortex of a 30-week-old human fetus. (×560.)

clusters densely packed with somatic cells (see Fig. 190–8). It seems that, early in development, the interaction between the oocyte and the granulosa cells is not yet fully established for the control of follicular formation.

INITIATION OF FOLLICULAR GROWTH

As soon as follicles are formed, some of them begin to grow. Thereafter, initiation of follicular growth from the pool of small resting follicles continues until the pool is exhausted at menopause. It is not certain whether follicular growth is initiated in the oocyte, in the granulosa cells, or simultaneously in both. In the immature mouse ovary, the number of granulosa cells of small follicles increases before the oocyte begins to grow.[78] At the same time, the oocyte nucleolar RNA polymerase activity increases,[78] and the nucleus enlarges.[79] Therefore, it seems that initiation of growth in the oocyte and the granulosa cells is closely related.[80]

Once initiated, follicular growth continues until the follicle either ovulates or degenerates.[81] It is unknown what events trigger the initiation of growth. Exogenous gonadotropins have been reported to initiate follicular growth in the infant mouse ovary.[82] Follicular growth is also sustained by gonadotropins *in vitro* as well as *in vivo*.[83–85] Moreover, retardation of follicular growth is seen in hypophysectomized fetal monkeys,[86] in anencephalic human fetuses,[67] and in infant mice treated with antigonadotropins.[87] Conversely, follicles begin to grow in cultures of fetal mouse[83,88] and hamster[84] ovaries, even in the absence of gonadotropins and steroid hormones.

It is therefore likely that factors other than gonadotropins control initiation of follicular growth. In the 1990s, numerous growth factors and other local acting factors or hormones as well as their receptors were identified in the mammalian ovary during early stages of folliculogenesis. However, folliculogenesis and early follicle growth seem to be controlled differently in different species. In primates, androgens stimulate insulin-like growth factor I of the small oocyte and initiate follicular development, but this process does not occur in rodents.[89] Growth differentiation factor-9 (GDF-9), a distant member of the transforming growth factor-β superfamily, is specifically expressed in the oocyte of all sizes in different species,[90,91,92] and mice with inactivated GDF-9 are infertile and lack growing follicles.[93]

Whether GDF-9 is also needed for early follicular growth in other species is not yet clarified. In the human fetal and adult ovary, transforming growth factor-β and its receptor are expressed in granulosa cells of nongrowing follicles and may be involved in growth initiation.[94]

OVARIAN STEROIDOGENESIS

Early Steroid Production by the Ovary

In species with delayed meiosis, such as the sheep,[95] rabbit,[96] and cow,[97] considerable amounts of estradiol are secreted during a limited premeiotic period (the delay period) of fetal life. In the rabbit, it has been shown by quantitative cytochemistry that the intraovarian rete cells of the medulla exhibit activity of 3β-hydroxysteroid dehydrogenase during the delay period.[98] It is likely that these cells are responsible for the synthesis of the steroids.[99] However, in other species (i.e., those with immediate meiosis), steroid production is low or undetectable during early stages of development. In the human, no ovarian estradiol synthesis can be detected until late in fetal life.[100, 101] This is striking when one considers the following: (1) the human fetal ovary possesses aromatizing enzyme systems for conversion of androgens to estrogens beginning with the eighth week of gestation;[18] (2) cells with ultrastructural characteristics of steroid production potentials are noted from the 12th week of gestation[1]; and (3) the activity of 3β-hydroxysteroid dehydrogenase is present in such cells from the 20th week of fetal life.[99] In the human, the early interstitial cells are located in the inner part of the ovarian cortex close to the developing follicles, but they never make contact with the oocytes (see Fig. 190–4).

The mechanisms that trigger differentiation of the steroid-producing cells and initiation of steroid production are unknown. In the human fetus, the production of luteinizing hormone (LH) and follicle-stimulating hormone reaches a peak between the 16th and 20th weeks of gestation and then levels off and remains low until puberty.[102,103] Thus, the peak production of gonadotropins occurs several weeks before the start of ovarian steroidogenesis. Moreover, once started, a slight increase of ovarian steroidogenesis (i.e., estrogen production) is seen throughout late fetal life when fetal gonadotropin secretion decreases. It therefore seems unlikely that pituitary gonadotropins regulate fetal ovarian steroidogenesis.

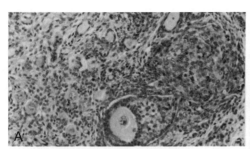
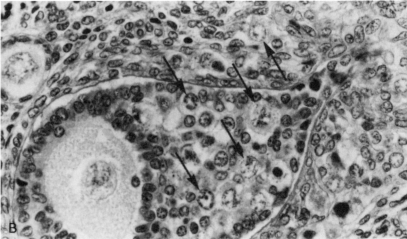

Figure 190–8. A, Abnormal follicle of a human fetal ovary, 33 weeks old. Besides a large oocyte, the granulosa layer contains numerous small oocytes, some of which are degenerating. The granulosa layer opens up into a "nest" of small oocytes tightly packed with somatic cells. (×400.) **B,** Higher magnification of **A.** The *arrows* point at some of the small oocytes.

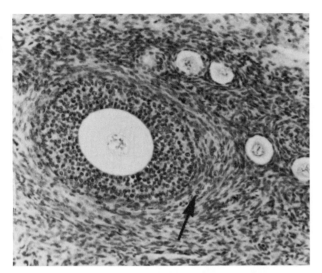

Figure 190–9. Inner part of the ovarian cortex of a 32-week-old human fetus showing a growing preantral follicle with a differentiating theca layer *(arrow)* and some primordial follicles. (×450.)

Formation of the Theca Layer and Early Follicular Steroidogenesis

In the human ovary from late fetal life and until follicles are exhausted from the senile ovary, theca cells differentiate around the late preantral or early antral follicles (Fig. 190–9).[76] Spindle-shaped hypotrophic cells encircle the basement membrane delineating the follicle together with blood vessels and nerves. Soon the theca cells acquire the ultrastructural and biochemical characteristics of steroid-producing cells. The origin of the theca cells is not established, but a pool of cells with potential for differentiating into theca cells must be present at all times, because every growing follicle sooner or later during its development requires a theca layer.

In the adult ovary, estrogen production by the follicle is the result of a synergism between the theca cells and the granulosa cells.[104] As soon as the theca cells differentiate around the follicle, the granulosa cells acquire 3β-hydroxysteroid dehydrogenase activity,[99] and by that time the follicular unit should be able to produce steroids. The late fetal ovary and the ovary during childhood contain numerous small antral follicles with well-differentiated theca cells. However, throughout childhood, serum levels of estrogens and other steroids remain low, probably because of lack of sufficient gonadotropic stimulation during this period.

FORMATION OF THE OVARIAN STROMA

During early fetal life, the main cell types that contribute to the ovarian stroma are mesenchyme and fibroblasts. Later in development, remnants of degenerating small follicles add to the stroma mass. Although some cells are equipped with enzymes necessary for steroidogenesis, it is uncertain to what extent these cells participate in ovarian hormone production. Typically luteinized interstitial tissue is not seen until after the first ovulation has occurred. Apart from a supportive role, the function of the stromal tissue in the fetal and immature ovary is obscure.

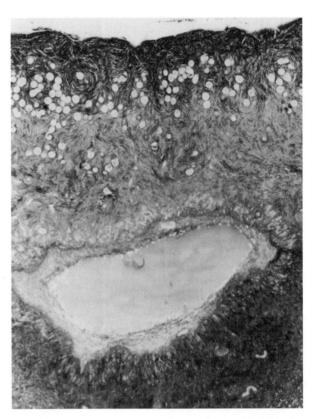

Figure 190–10. Cortex of an ovary from a 4-year-old child. Many small oocytes populate the area below the dense tunica albuginea. Remnants of a collapsing antral follicle occupy the *lower part of the figure.* (×280.)

FOLLICULAR GROWTH DURING CHILDHOOD

Birth itself is not a landmark in ovarian development and differentiation. Follicular growth starts around the 18th week of fetal life, and antral follicles are often seen 1 month before birth. Therefore, the ovaries of the female newborn infant contain preantral and antral follicles, at different stages of growth and atresia, in addition to a large pool of primordial follicles.[30] Follicular growth is the normal finding in the ovary of the newborn infant (see Fig. 190–8B).[66, 105] Absent or retarded growth of follicles at the time of birth is seen only in ovaries of diseased children.[106] The perinatal and postnatal increases in human chorion gonadotropin, which only decline after the third months of age, sometimes cause development of ovarian cysts a few months later. If the cysts are larger than 5 cm in diameter, intervention may be needed to prevent adnexal torsion.[107]

All follicles that start to grow during childhood are destined to undergo atresia at some stage of development, because there are no ovulations before menarche (Fig. 190–10). Although follicles may reach 6 mm in diameter during childhood, the size of the largest healthy, growing follicle does not generally exceed 1 mm.[108] The number of antral follicles also increases with age. In the newborn infant, three to five follicles larger than 1 mm in diameter may be present, whereas in 8-year-old girls, the number is often 10 or more (Fig. 190–11). This increase in the number of antral follicles is probably caused by the simultaneous increase in the basal levels of follicle-stimulating hormone and luteinizing hormone.[109]

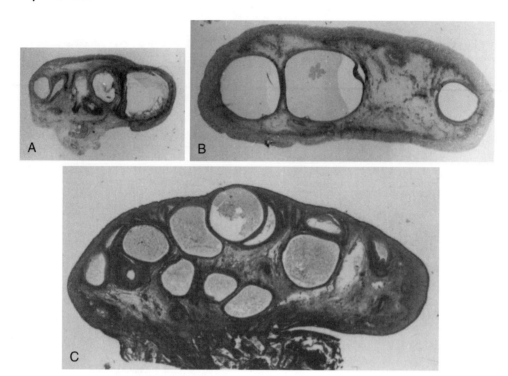

Figure 190–11. Human ovaries of young children, all with several antral follicles, none of which exceed 6 mm in diameter. (×5.) **A,** 2 months old. **B,** 4 years old. **C,** 7 years old.

REFERENCES

1. Byskov AG, Høyer PE: Embryology of mammalian gonads and ducts. *In* Knobil E, Neill JD (eds): The Physiology of Reproduction. New York, Raven Press, 1994, pp 487–540.
2. van Wagenen G, Simpson ME: Embryology of the ovary and testis: *Homo sapiens* and *Macaca mulatta*. New Haven, CT, Yale University Press, 1965, pp 1–256.
3. Hatano O, et al: Identical origin of adrenal cortex and gonad revealed by expression profiles of Ad4BP/SF-1. Genes Cells *1*:663, 1996.
4. Chan ST: Natural sex reversal in vertebrates. Philos Trans R Soc Lond B Biol Sci *259*:59, 1970.
5. Polani PE: Sex chromosome anomalies in man. *In* Hamerton JL (ed): Chromosomes in Medicine. London, Heinemann, 1962, pp 73–139.
6. Sinclair AH, et al: A gene from the human sex-determining region encodes a protein with homology to a conserved DNA-binding motif. Nature *346*:240, 1990.
7. Gubbay J, et al: A gene mapping to the sex-determining region of the mouse Y chromosome is a member of a novel family of embryonically expressed genes. Nature *346*:245, 1990.
8. Koopman P, et al: Male development of chromosomally female mice transgenic for Sry. Nature *351*:117, 1991.
9. Wertz K, Herrmann BG: Large-scale screen for genes involved in gonad development. Mech Dev *98*:51, 2000.
10. Witschi E: Migration of the germ cells of human embryos from the yolk sac to the primitive gonadal folds. Contrib Embryol *209*:67, 1948.
11. Clermont Y, Huckins C: Microscopic anatomy of the sex cords and seminiferous tubules in growing and adult albino rats. Am J Anat *180*:79, 1961.
12. Byskov AG, et al: Dependence of the onset of meiosis on the internal organization of the gonad. *In* McLaren A, Wylie CC (eds): Current Problems in Germ Cell Differentiation. Cambridge, Cambridge University Press, 1983, pp 215–224.
13. Byskov AG: Regulation of meiosis in mammals. Ann Biol Anim Bioch Biophys *19*:1251, 1979.
14. Catt KJ, et al: LH-hCG receptors and testosterone content during differentiation of the testis in the rabbit embryo. Endocrinology *97*:1157, 1975.
15. Wartenberg H: Differentiation and development of the testis. *In* Burger H, Kretser DD (eds): The Testis, Comprehensive Endocrinology. New York, Raven Press, 1981, pp 39–80.
16. Wartenberg H: Development of the early human ovary and role of the mesonephros in the differentiation of the cortex. Anat Embryol (Berl) *165*:253, 1982.
17. Gondos B, et al: Initiation of oogenesis in the human fetal ovary: ultrastructural and squash preparation study. Am J Obstet Gynecol *155*:189, 1986.
18. George FW, Wilson JD: Conversion of androgen to estrogen by the human fetal ovary. J Clin Endocrinol Metab *47*:550, 1978.
19. Gondos B, Hobel CJ: Interstitial cells in the human fetal ovary. Endocrinology *93*:736, 1973.
20. Witschi E: Embryogenesis of the adrenal and the reproductive glands. Horm Res *6*:1, 1951.
21. Byskov AG: The role of the rete ovarii in meiosis and follicle formation in the cat, mink and ferret. J Reprod Fertil *45*:201, 1975.
22. Martineau J, et al: Male-specific cell migration into the developing gonad. Curr Biol *7*:958, 1997.
23. Tilmann C, Capel B: Mesonephric cell migration induces testis cord formation and Sertoli cell differentiation in the mammalian gonad. Development *126*:2883, 1999.
24. Nielsen M, Byskov AG: Somatic cell exchange occurs between mouse fetal gonads and mesonephri during in vitro culture. Cells Tissues Organs *169*:325, 2001.
25. Bendsen E, et al: Number of germ cells in human fetal gonads from the 4th to the 10th week in vivo, and after culture of gonads with octylphenol (abstract). Hum Reprod *15*:162, 2000. 2001.
26. Baker T: Oogenesis and ovarian development. *In* Balin H, Glasser S (eds): Reproductive Biology. Amsterdam, Excerpta Medica, 1973, pp 398–437.
27. Swain A, et al: Dax1 antagonizes Sry action in mammalian sex determination. Nature *391*:761, 1998.
28. Manova K, Bachvarova R: Expression of c-kit encoded at the W locus of mice in developing embryonic germ cells and presumptive melanoblasts. Dev Biol *146*:312, 1991.
29. Tisdall DJ, et al: Stem cell factor and c-kit gene expression and protein localization in the sheep ovary during fetal development. J Reprod Fertil *116*:277, 1999.
30. Block E: Quantitative morphological investigations of the follicular system in women. Acta Anat *14*:108, 1952.
31. Mahadevaiah SK, et al: Tdy-negative XY, XXY and XYY female mice: breeding data and synaptonemal complex analysis. J Reprod Fertil *97*:151, 1993.
32. Polani PE: An experimental approach to female mammalian meiosis: differential chromosome labeling and an analysis of chiasmata in the female mouse. *In* Vogel H, Jagiello G (eds): P & S Biological Sciences Symposia: Bioregulators of Reproduction. New York, Academic Press, 1981, pp 59–87.
33. Brekhman V, et al: The DAZL1 gene is expressed in human male and female embryonic gonads before meiosis. Mol Hum Reprod *6*:465, 2000.
34. Ruggiu M, et al: The mouse Dazla gene encodes a cytoplasmic protein essential for gametogenesis. Nature *389*:73, 1997.
35. Meuwissen RL, et al: A coiled-coil related protein specific for synapsed regions of meiotic prophase chromosomes. EMBO J *11*:5091, 1992.
36. Offenberg HH, et al: SCP2: a major protein component of the axial elements of synaptonemal complexes of the rat. Nucleic Acids Res *26*:2572, 1998.
37. Yuan L, et al: The murine SCP3 gene is required for synaptonemal complex assembly, chromosome synapsis, and male fertility. Mol Cell *5*:73, 2000.

38. Peters H, Crone M: DNA synthesis in oocytes of mammals. Arch Anat Microsc Morphol Exp 56:160, 1967.

39. Peters H, et al: DNA synthesis in oocytes of mouse embryos. Nature 195:915, 1962.

40. Crone M, et al: The duration of the premeiotic DNA synthesis in mouse oocytes. Exp Cell Res 39:678, 1965.

41. Franchi LL, et al: The development of the ovary and the process of oogenesis. In Zuckerman S (ed): The Ovary. London, 1962, pp 1–88.

42. Kennelly JJ, Foote RH: Oocytogenesis in rabbits: the role of neogenesis in the formation of the definitive ova and the stability of oocyte DNA measured with tritiated thymidine. Am J Anat 118:573, 1966.

43. Mintz B: Continuity of the female germ cell line from embryo to adult. Arch Anat Microsc Morphol Exp 48:155, 1959.

44. Ioannou JM: Oogenesis in adult prosimians. J Embryol Exp Morphol 17:139, 1967.

45. Kumar TCA: Oogenesis in lorises: Loris tardigradus lydekkerianus and Nycticebus coucang. Proc R Soc Lond B 169:167, 1968.

46. Larsen JK, et al: Flow cytometry and sorting of meiotic prophase cells of female rabbits. J Reprod Fertil 76:587, 1986.

47. Gondos B, Zamboni L: Ovarian development: the functional importance of germ cell interconnections. Fertil Steril 20:176, 1969.

48. Pepling ME, et al: Germline cysts: a conserved phase of germ cell development? Trends Cell Biol 9:257, 1999.

49. Russe I: Oogenesis in cattle and sheep. Bibl Anat 24:77, 1983.

50. Baker TG: A quantitative and cytological study of germ cells in human ovaries. Philos Trans R Soc Lond B 158:417, 1963.

51. Wagenen G, Simpson ME: Embryology of the Ovary and Testis (Homo sapiens and Macaca mulatta). New Haven, CT, Yale University Press, 1965.

52. McLaren A: The fate of germ cells in the testis of fetal Sex-reversed mice. J Reprod Fertil 61:461, 1981.

53. Zamboni L, Upadhyay S: Germ cell differentiation in mouse adrenal glands. J Exp Zool 228:173, 1983.

54. Winiwarter H: Recherche sur l'ovogenèse de l'ovaire des mammifères (lapin et homme). Arch Biol 17:33, 1901.

55. Grinsted J, et al: Induction of meiosis in fetal mouse testis in vitro by rete testis tissue from pubertal mice and bulls. J Reprod Fertil 56:653, 1979.

56. Fajer AB, et al: The induction of meiosis by ovaries of newborn hamsters and its relation to the action of the extra ovarian structures in the mesovarium (rete ovarii). Ann Biol Anim Biochim Biophys 19:1273, 1979.

57. Byskov AG, Saxén L: Induction of meiosis in fetal mouse testis in vitro. Dev Biol 52:193, 1976.

58. Westergaard L, et al: Is resumption of meiosis in the human preovulatory oocyte triggered by a meiosis-inducing substance (MIS) in the follicular fluid? Fertil Steril 41:377, 1984.

59. McLaren A, Southee D: Entry of mouse embryonic germ cells into meiosis. Dev Biol 187:107, 1997.

60. Byskov AG, et al: Chemical structure of sterols that activate oocyte meiosis. Nature 374:559, 1995.

61. Byskov AG, et al: Role of meiosis activating sterols, MAS, in induced oocyte maturation. Mol Cell Endocrinol 187:189, 2002.

62. Merchant H: Rat gonadal and ovarian organogenesis with and without germ cells: an ultrastructural study. Dev Biol 44:1, 1975.

63. Hughes FM Jr, Gorospe WC: Biochemical identification of apoptosis (programmed cell death) in granulosa cells: evidence for a potential mechanism underlying follicular atresia. Endocrinology 129:2415, 1991.

64. Tilly JL, et al: Involvement of apoptosis in ovarian follicular atresia and postovulatory regression. Endocrinology 129:2799, 1991.

65. Morita Y, Tilly JL: Oocyte apoptosis: like sand through an hourglass. Dev Biol 213:1, 1999.

66. Peters H, et al: Follicular growth in fetal and prepubertal ovaries of humans and other primates. Clin Endocrinol Metab 7:469, 1978.

67. Baker TG, Scrimgeour JB: Development of the gonad in normal and anencephalic human fetuses. J Reprod Fertil 60:193, 1980.

68. Soyal SM, et al: FIGalpha, a germ cell-specific transcription factor required for ovarian follicle formation. Development 127:4645, 2000.

69. Waldeyer W: Eierstock und Ei. Leipzig: Engleman, 1870.

70. Pepling ME, Spradling AC: Mouse ovarian germ cell cysts undergo programmed breakdown to form primordial follicles. Dev Biol 234:339, 2001.

71. Byskov AG, Lintern-Moore S: Follicle formation in the immature mouse ovary: the role of the rete ovarii. J Anat 116:207, 1973.

72. Byskov AG, et al: Influence of ovarian surface epithelium and rete ovarii on follicle formation. J Anat 123:77, 1977.

73. Sawyer HR, et al: Formation of ovarian follicles during fetal development in sheep. Biol Reprod 66:1134, 2002.

74. Mossman HW, Duke KL: Comparative Morphology of the Mammalian Ovary. Madison, WI, University of Wisconsin Press, 1973.

75. Stein LE, Anderson CH: A qualitative and quantitative study of rete ovarii development in the fetal rat: correlation with the onset of meiosis and follicle cell appearance. Anat Rec 193:197, 1979.

76. Peters H: Folliculogenesis in mammals. In Jones RE (ed): The Vertebrate Ovary. New York, Plenum Press, 1978, pp 121–144.

77. Pedersen T: Follicle growth in the immature mouse ovary. Acta Endocrinol (Copenh) 62:117, 1969.

78. Lintern-Moore S, Moore RM: Follicular development in the neonatal mouse ovary. Biol Reprod 96:123, 1979.

79. Byskov AG, et al: Differentiation, growth and maturation of oocytes. In Haseltine FP, Findlay JK (eds): Growth Factors in Fertility Regulation: WHO/NICHD Symposium Proceedings. Cambridge, Cambridge University Press, 1989, pp 3–12.

80. Hirshfield AN: Development of follicles in the mammalian ovary. Int Rev Cytol 124:43, 1991.

81. Peters H, McNatty KP: The Ovary: A Correlation of Structure and Function in Mammals. London, Granada Publishing, 1980.

82. Lintern-Moore S: Initiation of follicular growth in the infant mouse ovary by exogenous gonadotrophin. Biol Reprod 17:635, 1977.

83. Baker TG, Neal P: Initiation and control of meiosis and follicular growth in ovaries of the mouse. Ann Biol Anim Bioch Biophys 13:137, 1973.

84. Challoner S: Studies of oogenesis and follicular development in the golden hamster. III. The initiation of follicular growth in vitro. J Anat 119:157, 1975.

85. Greenwald G, Roy SK: Follicular development and its control. In Knobil E, Neill JD (eds): The Physiology of Reproduction. New York, Raven Press, 1994, pp 629–724.

86. Gulyas BJ, et al: Effects of fetal or maternal hypophysectomy on endocrine organs and body weight in infant rhesus monkeys (Macaca mulatta): with particular emphasis on oogenesis. Biol Reprod 16:216, 1977.

87. Eshkol A: Ovarian development in infant mice: dependence on gonadotrophic hormones. In Butt WR (ed): Gonadotrophins and Ovarian Development. Edinburgh, Livingstone, 1970, pp 249–258.

88. Nikitin AI, Byskov AG: Mesonephric influence on the survival of fetal mouse germ cells: preliminary results. In Byskov AG, Peters H (eds): Development and Function of Reproductive Organs. Amsterdam, Excerpta Medica, 1981, pp 51–57.

89. Monget P, Bondy C: Importance of the IGF system in early folliculogenesis. Mol Cell Endocrinol 163:89, 2000.

90. McGrath SA, et al: Oocyte-specific expression of growth/differentiation factor-9. Mol Endocrinol 9:131, 1995.

91. Elvin JA, et al: Molecular characterization of the follicle defects in the growth differentiation factor 9–deficient ovary. Mol Endocrinol 13:1018, 1999.

92. McNatty KP, et al: Growth and paracrine factors regulating follicular formation and cellular function. Mol Cell Endocrinol 163:11, 2000.

93. Dong J, et al: Growth differentiation factor-9 is required during early ovarian folliculogenesis. Nature 383: 531, 1996.

94. Gougeon A, Busso D: Morphologic and functional determinants of primordial and primary follicles in the monkey ovary. Mol Cell Endocrinol 163:33, 2000.

95. Mauleon P, et al: Very early and transient secretion of oestradiol-17β by foetal sheep ovary in vitro. Ann Biol Anim Bioch Biophys 17:399, 1977.

96. Grinsted J, et al: Influence of mesonephros on foetal and neonatal rabbit gonads. I. Sex-steroid release by the testis in vitro. Acta Endocrinol (Copenh) 99:272, 1982.

97. Shemesh M: Estradiol-17 beta biosynthesis by the early bovine fetal ovary during the active and refractory phases. Biol Reprod 23:577, 1980.

98. Byskov AG, et al: Origin and differentiation of the endocrine cells of the ovary. J Reprod Fertil 75:299, 1985.

99. Høyer PE: Histoenzymology of the human ovary: dehydrogenases directly involved in steroidogenesis. In Motta P, Hafez ESE (eds): Biology of the Ovary. The Hague, Martinus Nijhoff, 1980, pp 52–67.

100. Reyes FI, et al: Studies on human sexual development. I. Fetal gonadal and adrenal sex steroids. J Clin Endocrinol Metab 37:74, 1973.

101. Taylor T, et al: Human foetal synthesis of testosterone from perfused progesterone. J Endocrinol 60:321, 1974.

102. Winter JSD, et al: Sex steroid production by the human fetus: its role in morphogenesis and control by gonadotropins. In Blandau RJ, Bergma D (eds): Morphogenesis and Malformation of the Genital System. New York, Alan R. Liss, 1977, pp 41–58.

103. Bidlingmaier F, Knorr D: Plasma estrogens in childhood and adolescence. Acta Paediatr Scand 62:8, 1973.

104. Falck B: Site of production of oestrogen in rat ovary as studied in microtransplants. Acta Physiol Scand 163:1, 1959.

105. Gougeon A: Regulation of ovarian follicular development in primates: facts and hypotheses. Endocr Rev 17:121, 1996.

106. Peters H, et al: The development of the ovary during childhood in health and disease. In Coutts JRT (ed): Functional Morphology of the Human Ovary. Edinburgh, MTP Press, 1981, pp 26–34.

107. Dolgin SE: Ovarian masses in the newborn. Semin Pediatr Surg 9:121, 2000.

108. Himelstein-Braw R, et al: Follicular atresia in the infant human ovary. J Reprod Fertil 46:55, 1976.

109. Faiman C, Wirth J: Gonadotropins and sex hormone pattern in puberty, clinical data. In Grumbach MM, et al (eds): The Control of the Onset of Puberty. London, John Wiley & Sons, 1974, pp 32–61.

191

Testicular Development

Until the seventh week after conception, primordial cells that ultimately develop into Sertoli cells, germ cells, and Leydig cells form not a testis, but a morphologically undifferentiated gonad.[1] The most important insight into testicular development was proposed by Jost in 1973. Without the benefit of current genetic knowledge, Jost suggested that these undifferentiated cells will develop into testes based on the "genetic sex," and in the absence of a genetic sex-determining factor, ovarian structures will result.[2] Furthermore, his paradigm suggested that the testis itself was the critical determinant of the male phenotype.

EMBRYOLOGY OF TESTICULAR STRUCTURES

The germ cells may be seen on the 24th day after conception in the caudal part of the embryonic yolk sac, and they migrate into the wall of the yolk sac and gut by the fifth week. During this time, mitotic division results in an increase in cell numbers. It is during the sixth week that the germ cells reach the mesentery, the mesonephros, and, finally, the genital ridge.[3] What stimulates the germ cells to migrate is not known. However, because they are responsible for gonadal differentiation, their failure to reach the genital ridge may result in *gonadal agenesis* or *gonadal indifferentiation.*

During the sixth week, the genital ridge thickens, and by the seventh week, it connects with the mesonephros.[4] Also during the sixth week, the seminiferous cords are noted to arise from the epithelium, and the germ cells migrate into the mesenchyme within these cords. There are also somatic cells within the cords that develop into fetal Sertoli cells. The seminiferous cords and the overlying epithelium begin to separate at the end of the sixth week when fibroblastic cells that will give rise to the tunica albuginea appear and an obvious large arteriole develops. The rete testis develops in the region of mesorchium and extends into the mesonephric ridge by the ninth week to join the tubules. The seminiferous tubules will later connect to the mesonephric duct via the ductuli efferentes.

The differentiation of the indifferent gonad to a testis occurs around the seventh to eighth weeks and is mediated by a DNA-binding protein called SRY (sex-determining region Y). Its presence has been demonstrated in humans and other mammals,[5, 6] and it is the product of a gene located on the short arm of the Y chromosome.[7] It is now clear that XY mice with a deletion of SRY develop ovaries and female phenotypes, and XX transgenic mice with an expression of SRY develop testes and male phenotypes.[8] In the mouse, SRY is expressed only in cells that will eventually become Sertoli cells and for only a few hours, but it appears to up-regulate a similar protein, SOX-9 (SRY HMG box gene-9).[9] Knock-out and transgenic studies for SRY have shown that SOX-9 is the critical downstream gene for testis development.[10] SOX-9 induces the undifferentiated cells that can form either ovarian or testicular tissue to form testes. After inducing Sertoli cell differentiation and in concert with certain nuclear hormone receptor genes that are also involved at different stages of testicular development (most prominently *M33, LHX, GATA-4, WT1,* and *SF1*), SOX-9 stimulates Sertoli cells, germ cells, Leydig cells, and myoid cells to form a testis.[11] There has only been one gene currently identified that acts as an "antitesticular gene." *DAX-1,* when overexpressed in XY mice, can result in an ovary and a female phenotype.[12] Today we know with certainty that gonadal sex is determined by genetic sex, and without the influence of SRY and SOX-9, ovarian structures will result.

Histologically, the first evidence of differentiation in the gonad is the differentiation of Sertoli cells. They are located in seminiferous cords with the germ cells and are likely of coelomic origin. Although the cells that ultimately develop into Sertoli, germ, and Leydig cells can also develop into their ovarian counterparts, the peritubular myoid cells are seen only in testes. They separate the tubules from the interstitium and likely play an important role in Sertoli cell differentiation. The interstitium contains Leydig cells, endothelial cells, macrophages, and fibroblasts (Fig. 191–1). Leydig cells, which are derived from fibroblastic elements in the gonadal mesenchyme, are critical to developing a male phenotype. The testis (and not the ovary) develops a large arteriole early in development that, via capillaries, drains into venules in the mesonephros. It has been suggested that the arteriole serves to carry central hormones (e.g., luteinizing hormone [LH] and human chorionic gonadotropin [hCG]) to the testis, and the venules carry testicular hormones (e.g., testosterone and müllerian-inhibiting substance [MIS]) to other parts of the body, thus allowing the testis to be the principal determinant of the male phenotype.

LEYDIG CELL DEVELOPMENT

Differentiation of fibroblasts to Leydig cells occurs around the eighth week of gestation. They are steroidogenic cells, and their function is the production of testosterone. The initial stimulus to form Leydig cells is unclear, but suppression of the gene *WNT-4* seems to be critical.[13] Ultimately, their differentiation is dependent on the stimulation of LH and hCG secretion. From the 14th to the 18th week of fetal life, there is a peak in Leydig cell development.[14, 15] The morphologic changes seen at this time have been well described. The cells have an ovoid contour with prominent nucleolar development, and the formation of smooth endoplasmic reticulum is seen in the expanding cytoplasm. The number of fetal Leydig cells decreases dramatically in late pregnancy (coincident with a decrease in LH and hCG), but another increase occurs 2 to 3 months after birth in response to an increase in LH.[16] A second decrease at around the fourth to sixth postnatal month results in a diversity of cell populations including fibroblast-like cells, fetal Leydig cells, degenerating fetal Leydig cells, and infantile Leydig cells. The term *infantile type* has been used to describe the cells with a multilobated nucleus and moderately developed smooth endoplasmic reticulum. This cell population increases in number during childhood.[16, 17] Some investigators find the terminology inappropriate and suggest the term *immature* rather than *infantile*.[18] According to the generally accepted *biphasic model,* the fetal-type Leydig cells are precursors of the adult-type Leydig cells. The adult cells have the characteristics of other steroid-secreting cells such as a large polygonal configuration, eccentric nuclear position, and a specific "organelle association" of anastomosing tubules of smooth endoplasmic reticulum, pleomorphic mitochondria, and well-developed Golgi apparatus (Fig. 191–2). Morphologically, the adult cells can be differentiated from the fetal cells by the presence of Reinke crystals. Although the function of Reinke crystals is not known, their appearance is specific for mature Leydig cells.[19]

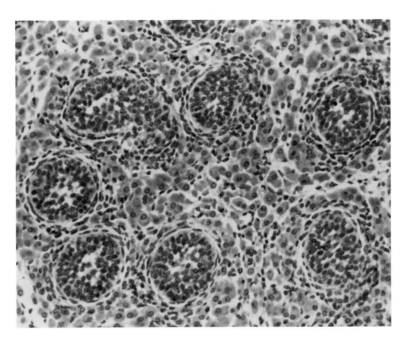

Figure 191–1. Human fetal testis at 12 weeks' gestation with seminiferous cords and interstitial tissue including numerous Leydig cells. (×250.)

One theory about Leydig cell development suggests that, in humans, a third phase of Leydig cell differentiation exists between the fetal and the adult configuration. It has been suggested that this differentiation takes place during the second increase in Leydig cell number in the first few postnatal months.[20] Histologically, there are intermediate types of cells showing decreased numbers of smooth endoplasmic reticulum with prominent cytoplasmic filaments. The regression of the cells and the diversity of cell populations in the infant testis have been considered evidence of the continuity of development by supporters of the triphasic theory.

Endocrinologic Correlates

The first appearance of Leydig cells correlates with the onset of testosterone production.[21] Testosterone is essential for masculinization of the male genitalia,[2] and it reaches its peak level in the early second trimester.[22] Similarly, the decrease in testosterone levels around the 16th to 18th week of gestation correlates with the regression of fetal-type Leydig cells. Testosterone secretion is regulated by hCG and LH via receptors on the cell surface of Leydig cells.[23] Placental hCG stimulates testosterone synthesis in the fetus *in vitro*[24] and reaches its peak concentration shortly before testosterone[25] and LH.[26] Molecular studies have confirmed these findings. The expression of genes responsible for the steroidogenic enzymes is most prominent around 14 to 16 weeks of gestation and diminishes thereafter.[27, 28] The molecular findings also correlate with the serum concentrations of testosterone and hCG.

The secretion of FSH and LH is regulated by gonadotropin-releasing hormone (GnRH) via the hypothalamic-pituitary axis.[29] GnRH is found in large amounts in the fetal hypothalamus between 8 and 18 weeks of gestation.[30] Pituitary gonadotropin (both LH and FSH) and serum testosterone levels rise in response to GnRH.[29] After an increase in these levels shortly after birth, the levels of gonadotropins and testosterone are quite low until they increase at puberty (Fig. 191-3). In addition to the presence of Reinke crystals, an important difference between the fetal-type and adult-type Leydig cells is their response to gonadotropins. Presumably because of the loss of LH and hCG receptors and a decrease in the steroidogenic enzymes, adult Leydig cells exhibit a more limited response to gonadotropins.[31]

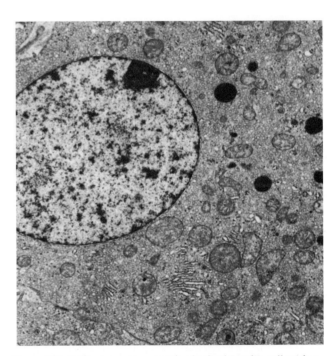

Figure 191–2. Electron micrograph of a fetal Leydig cell with a round, eccentric nucleus, well-developed smooth endoplasmic reticulum, and prominent tubulovesicular mitochondria. (×9000.)

This relative lack of sensitivity has not been observed in either animal[32] or human[33] fetal Leydig cells.

SERTOLI AND GERM CELL DEVELOPMENT

The Sertoli cells and germ cells are the two components of the fetal seminiferous cords (Fig. 191-4). There is a close anatomic and functional relationship between these two cell types. In particular, it appears that many germ cell functions are highly regulated by the Sertoli cells. Although the Sertoli cells are dominant in number in the initial embryonic testis, the ratio of germ cells

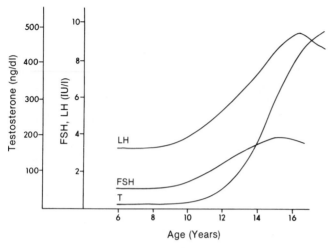

Figure 191–3. Testosterone, follicle-stimulating hormone (FSH), and luteinizing hormone (LH) levels in boys during childhood and pubertal development. (From Gondos B: *In* Gondos B, Riddick DH [eds]: Pathology of Infertility. New York, Thieme, 1987, p 226.)

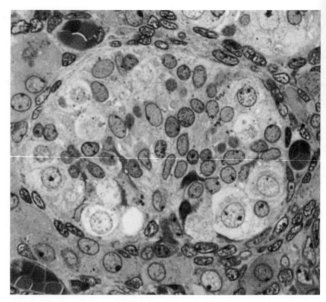

Figure 191–4. Fetal seminiferous cord with columnar-shaped Sertoli cells and large, round germ cells at the periphery. (Toluidine blue, ×500.)

to Sertoli cells varies widely at different stages of development. For example, there are only a few gonocytes in the undifferentiated gonad as a result of limited mitotic activity. Thereafter, germ cell mitotic activity is likely stimulated by testosterone from the Leydig cells. In the human testis, the ratio of germ cells to immature Sertoli cells changes in favor of the germ cells from the 8th to the 22nd week of gestation. This is followed by a continuous decrease in relative germ cell number through the remainder of fetal life, when testosterone levels decrease, but a slight increase through the first 4 months of life, when testosterone levels increase. At 6 months of age, the ratio is reversed because of both the high proliferation rate of Sertoli cells and the pause in the development of germ cells.[34] Although the testis remains relatively quiescent until puberty, an increase in germ cell mitotic activity between the ages of 7 to 9 years equalizes the ratio of the germ cells to Sertoli cells.[35]

Different types of germ cells are present at different phases of development (Table 191-1). The round to oval gonocytes are located centrally in the tubules. Later, the gonocytes are seen in the periphery of the tubules, close to the basal lamina. At this point, they are classified as *prespermatogonia*.[36] In this peripheral location within the cord, cytoplasmic bridges may be seen between prespermatogonia, resulting from incomplete cytokinesis during germ cell mitosis.[37] After the onset of spermatogenesis, the importance of these interconnections between differentiating spermatogonia becomes obvious because they allow the synchronization of germ cell maturation. Two types of spermato-

gonia are identified in humans: A and B. Type A spermatogonia are also divided into Ad (dark type A) and Ap (pale type A) groups. The identification of the different types of spermatogonia is based on morphology and variations in chromatin precipitation within the nucleus.[38] Studies in adults who underwent orchidopexy before the age of 2 years showed that the presence of Ad spermatogonia in infancy is a good predictor of future fertility.[39] The development of germ cells is a continuous process, and many different types of germ cells are located simultaneously among the Sertoli cells. Early spermatogonia are found along the basement membrane, and mature forms are present closer to the tubular lumen. Sertoli cells remain close to the basement membrane of the seminiferous tubule and have cytoplasmic connections with the lumen. During spermatogenesis, numerous forms of germ cells can be identified, including, from the least to the most mature form, Ad spermatogonia, Ap spermatogonia, type B spermatogonia, primary spermatocytes (leptotene, zygotene, and pachytene, in order of development), secondary spermatocytes, Sa, Sb1, Sb2, Sc, Sd1, and Sd2 spermatids, and, finally, spermatozoa.

The mechanisms that result in germ cell differentiation are being elucidated. In rodents, the gonocytes proliferate for a few days after reaching the genital ridge, and shortly after birth, they differentiate to A type spermatogonia.[40] This differentiation can be prevented by many factors, such as cryptorchidism, irradiation, vitamin A deficiency, and mutations in the genes that

TABLE 191-1

Types of Germ Cells Present at Different Stages of Development

Type	Stage	Activity	Shape	Location
Prespermatogenesis	Fetus-child			
Gonocytes		Mitosis*	Round	Central
Prespermatogonia		Mitosis*	Round	Peripheral
Spermatogensis	Puberty-adult			
Spermatogonia		Mitosis	Round	Basal
Spermatocytes		Meiosis	Round	Adluminal
Spermatids		Maturation	Round to elongated	Adluminal
Spermatozoa		Transport	Elongated	Luminal

* Limited mitotic activity.

encode either the c-kit receptor or its ligand SCF (stem cell factor) in the testicular germ cell. The role of c-kit is interesting. *In situ* hybridization studies in mouse embryos showed that c-kit is expressed in the germ cells before and after migration to the genital ridge.[41] Studies with the administration of anti–c-kit monoclonal antibody have demonstrated that the c-kit receptor and its ligand SCF have a role in the proliferation of the differentiated type A spermatogonia. Undifferentiated type A spermatogonia are not affected, showing that spermatogonial stem cell proliferation is not regulated by the c-kit/SCF system in the mouse.[42] Further evidence comes from stem cell transplantation studies. Germ cells obtained from GFP (green fluorescent fusion protein) transgenic mice were used for transplantation, and these studies confirmed that SCF is necessary for proliferation of differentiated germ cells, but not for undifferentiated type A spermatogonia.[43]

With the current renewed interest in stem cell research, an interesting question is whether the fetal gonocytes are the only source of the adult germ cells. Although germ cells are the principal cells involved in the developmental process called *prespermatogenesis* during fetal life and childhood, actual spermatogenesis does not occur until puberty. Primordial germ cells are accepted as stem cells because they are capable of forming typical colonies (that resemble embryonic stem cells) in culture.[44] Varying models exist among different species to explain the proliferation of spermatogonia and the stem cell renewal. A widely accepted model in rats and mice theorizes that the different types of undifferentiated A type spermatogonia are the source of the renewal for spermatogenic stem cells.[45] The undifferentiated spermatogonia are divided into three groups based on their location in relation to the basement membrane: A single, A paired, and A aligned. The A single type cells are thought to be the stem cells for spermatogenesis, because some of them undergo self-renewal whereas others differentiate. However, the ratio of the cell types and the regulatory mechanism of these changes are not well understood.[46,47]

Totipotential primitive germ cells may be related to testicular cancer. Fetal germ cells and the cells of intraepithelial germ cell neoplasia have many histologic and ultrastructural similarities.[48] Because of the evidence that intraepithelial germ cell neoplasia cells may be the origin of germ cell tumors in the adult testis, some authors have suggested that persistent undeveloped germ cells (or regression of differentiated germ cells to primitive totipotential germ cells) may give rise to germ cell tumors of the testis.[49] Hence, a failure of normal germ cell development could be the basis for the increased risk of testicular neoplasia in patients with abnormal testes.

The development of germ cells is interrelated with the development of Sertoli cells. Histologically, fetal Sertoli cells have round to elliptical nuclei, small nucleoli, and a relatively small amount of smooth endoplasmic reticulum.[50] They are rich in ribosomes and rough endoplasmic reticulum that are the likely source of MIS (Fig. 191-5). These cells are present in seminiferous cords until puberty. Their numbers stay steady, but the ratio of Sertoli cells to tubule diminishes in time because of the elongation and enlargement of the tubules. An important feature of the cytoarchitecture of Sertoli cells is the presence of tight junctions between adjacent cell membranes (Fig. 191-6). This unique characteristic is thought to allow the Sertoli cells to create a microenvironment for controlling the biochemical milieu within the cords, as well as to allow them to direct the migration of germ cells within the seminiferous tubules. This anatomic feature results in the blood-testis barrier, discussed in more detail later.

In addition to supporting the germ cells, Sertoli cells also play a role in the production and secretion of various proteins, some of which act outside the testis. Sertoli cells secrete MIS, also often called antimüllerian hormone. This hormone is a member of the transforming growth factor-β (TGF-β) superfamily, is pro-

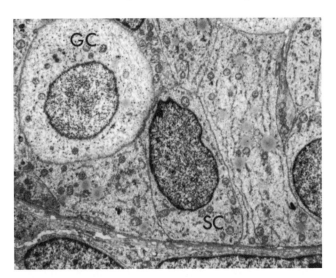

Figure 191–5. Fetal Sertoli cells (SC) with prominent polyribosomes and strands of rough endoplasmic reticulum. GC = gonocyte. (×6000.)

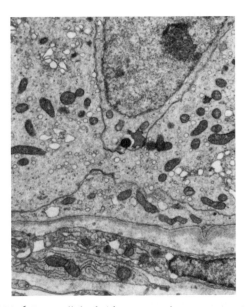

Figure 191–6. Intercellular bridge connecting prespermatogonia in postnatal seminiferous cord. (×6500.)

duced exclusively by Sertoli cells, and is responsible for the regression of müllerian duct structures in males. Indeed, mutations of MIS or its type II receptor have been shown to be responsible for persistent müllerian duct and hernia uteri inguinale syndrome. MIS is detectable in fetal serum by the eighth week of gestation and, as such, is good evidence of the presence of testicular tissue.[51] After an increase toward the end of the second trimester, serum MIS drops to a low, but measurable level in the third trimester.[52] The reason for the presence of MIS at all in the third trimester is uncertain. However, it has been suggested that MIS may play a role in delaying lung maturation. Respiratory distress syndrome is seen more in male than in female newborns. Furthermore, incubating female rat lungs with MIS results in the suppression of phosphatidylcholine accumulation, and this, in turn, causes surfactant deficiency and inhibition of lung maturation.[53] MIS levels remain significant during childhood, and, in general, levels of MIS are inverse to those of testosterone, a finding suggesting a feedback loop in which MIS has an inhibitory effect on the function of Leydig cells.

Another regulatory protein secreted by Sertoli cells is inhibin. Inhibin provides negative feedback to the hypothalamic-pituitary axis and thereby reduces FSH secretion. This glycoprotein is also a member of the TGF-β superfamily and has two subunits: inhibin A and inhibin B.[54] Although both have been shown effective in suppressing FSH secretion,[55] only inhibin B has been found to be physiologically important in humans.[56] It is theorized that inhibin may also play a role locally in regulating germ cell development, but data to support this concept are limited.

Blood-Testis Barrier

A unique feature of the developed testis is a barrier between the bloodstream and the testicular tubules. This likely serves to maintain the microenvironment needed for spermatogenesis and may prevent autoimmune destruction of differentiating germ cells. Anatomically, the blood-testis barrier is a consequence of the tight junctions between Sertoli cells. This allows the Sertoli cells to separate the adluminal components of the seminiferous tubules from the basal components, the basement membrane, and, hence, the interstitium.[57] Functionally, it was shown that these tight junctions prevent the passage of tracers from the interstitium to the adluminal compartment of the seminiferous tubules.[58,59] Some of the mechanisms by which the Sertoli cells maintain the barrier have been elucidated. In the rat testis, inhibitors of protein phosphatase disrupt the barrier, whereas pretreatment of Sertoli cells with a protein tyrosine kinase inhibitor *in vitro* prevents this effect.[60] Similarly, both protein kinase A activator and protein kinase C inhibitors also perturb the Sertoli cell tight junctions, a finding showing that the barrier mechanism is at least partially regulated by protein kinases. More studies of this complex and important feature of the testis are ongoing.

The age at which the blood-testis barrier becomes fully functional in humans is not known. In rats, it is clear that the barrier does not develop completely until puberty.[61] Spermatogonia and preleptotene spermatocytes are located close to the basement membrane, whereas differentiating spermatocytes and spermatids are found in the adluminal compartment.[62] Migration of the spermatocytes occurs during meiosis, which begins around the time of puberty. The findings that the barrier develops around the time of puberty and that diethylstilbestrol can postpone the formation of these tight junctions suggest that the development of the barrier is at least partially under hormonal control.[63]

PERITUBULAR STRUCTURES

In humans, at least three layers separate the seminiferous tubules from the interstitium.[64] The outer layer is made up of fibroblastic cells that form the adventitia and provide most of the structural integrity of the tubules. The middle layer contains myoid cells that have contractile ability and may therefore play a significant role in movement of spermatozoa through the tubules to the rete testis and may also be important for spermatogenesis. In experimentally created cryptorchidism, there is thickening in peritubular structures that most likely interrupts the movement of differentiating germ cells.[65] There is also evidence that the peritubular myoid cells have steroidogenic functions and induce Sertoli cells to secrete substances that form the basement membrane.[66] Hence, the myoid cells are critical for testicular development. The innermost layer is rich in collagen and is positioned immediately adjacent to the basal membrane of the tubules. It has also been demonstrated that these cells secrete substances that likely play a role as paracrine factors. One of these substances is P-Mod-S, a protein that has been found to induce Sertoli cell differentiation *in vitro*.[67]

CELL-CELL INTERACTIONS

Many different types of interactions have been identified among the different cell types in the testis. These interactions were highlighted in a review by Skinner.[68] Sertoli cell–germ cell interaction is the best-recognized interaction, and the regulatory role of Sertoli cells in spermatogenesis has been examined extensively. Sertoli cells also have a close interrelationship with Leydig cells and peritubular cells. Many proteins are exchanged, including growth factors (TNF-α, TGF-β, insulin-like growth factor I, interleukin 1), transport proteins (albumin-binding protein, transferrin, ceruloplasmin), extracellular matrix components (laminin, collagens, proteoglycans), protease inhibitors (α_2-macroglobulin, plasminogen activator) and regulatory proteins (inhibin, MIS). Similar agents are also secreted by Leydig cells and peritubular cells and are essential to maintain control at extracellular, intercellular, and molecular levels.

TESTICULAR APOPTOSIS

Apoptosis is important in many organ systems during development, probably as a means of removing embryologic remnants that are no longer needed to allow space for further development of more mature structures. Most studies of apoptosis in the testis have focused on germ cells in the adult testis. More recently, studies of the developing testis have highlighted an important role for apoptosis in the developing testis. In immature rats, hypophysectomy induced DNA fragmentation (a marker of apoptosis) in both interstitium and seminiferous tubules. Treatment with hCG suppressed hypophysectomy-induced apoptosis by 77% in interstitial cells and by 46% in tubular cells, whereas FSH suppressed apoptosis by 90% in both compartments.[69] In another rat study, apoptotic DNA fragmentation was found in germ cells, but not in Sertoli and Leydig cells, after the administration of a GnRH antagonist.[70] The same study demonstrated that the germ cell apoptosis was detected in rats only between 16 and 32 days of age, a finding showing that gonadotropin dependence is age related. Treatment with a GnRH antagonist caused a decrease in serum FSH, but not in LH. Because FSH receptors are primarily on Sertoli cells, it can be inferred that FSH seems to stimulate germ cells via their relationship with Sertoli cells. One article reported some striking results in quantitative analysis of both germ cells and somatic cells in the human fetal testis.[71] After analyzing 17 male fetuses, the authors concluded that apoptotic cell death occurred in all cell types and at all gestational ages. Leydig cells were found to undergo apoptosis more than the other cell populations in every stage of gestation, but the reason was unclear.

Current studies have focused on the identification of factors that control testicular apoptosis. In particular, the Fas-Fas ligand system has been found to regulate apoptosis in human germ cells.[72] Tumor necrosis factor-α, a cytokine highly expressed in Sertoli cells, was found to inhibit germ cell apoptosis in humans.[73] These studies were done in adult testes, and results in developing testes could be different.

REFERENCES

1. van Wagenen G, et al: Embryology of the ovary and testis in *Homo sapiens* and *Macaca mulatta*. New Haven, CT, Yale University Press, 1965.
2. Jost A, et al: Studies on sex differentiation in mammals. Recent Prog Horm Res 29:1, 1973.
3. Witschi E: Migration of the germ cells of human embryos from the yolk sac to the primitive gonadal folds. Contrib Embryol Carnegie Inst 32:67, 1948.
4. Pinkerton JHM, et al: Development of the human ovary: a study using histochemical techniques. Obstet Gynecol 18:152, 1961.
5. Sinclair AH, et al: A gene from the human sex-determining region encodes a protein with homology to a conserved DNA-binding motif. Nature 346:240, 1990.

6. Daneau I, et al: Bovine SRY gene locus: cloning and testicular expression. Biol Reprod *52*:591, 1995.

7. Page DC, et al: The sex-determining region of the human Y chromosome encodes a finger protein. Cell *51*:1091, 1987.

8. Koopman P, et al: Male development of chromosomally female mice transgenic for Sry. Nature *351*:117, 1991.

9. Hacker A, et al: Expression of Sry, the mouse sex determining gene. Development *121*:1603, 1995.

10. Morais da Silva S, et al: Sox9 expression during gonadal development implies a conserved role for the gene in testis differentiation in mammals and birds. Nat Genet *14*:62, 1996.

11. Kent J, et al: A male-specific role for SOX9 in vertebrate sex determination. Development *122*:2813, 1996.

12. Swain A, et al: Dax1 antagonizes Sry action in mammalian sex determination. Nature *391*:761, 1998.

13. Jordan BK, et al: Up-regulation of WNT-4 signaling and dosage-sensitive sex reversal in humans. Am J Hum Genet *68*:1102, 2001.

14. Kuopio T, et al: Developmental stages of fetal-type Leydig cells in prepubertal rats. Development *107*:213, 1989.

15. Waters BL, et al: Development of the human fetal testis. Pediatr Pathol Lab Med *16*:9, 1996.

16. Codesal J, et al: Involution of human fetal Leydig cells: an immunohistochemical, ultrastructural and quantitative study. J Anat *172*:103, 1990.

17. Nistal M, et al: A quantitative morphological study of human Leydig cells from birth to adulthood. Cell Tissue Res *246*:229, 1986.

18. Prince FP: The triphasic nature of Leydig cell development in humans, and comments on nomenclature. J Endocrinol *168*:213, 2001.

19. Gupta SK, et al: Intranuclear Reinke's crystals in a testicular Leydig cell tumor diagnosed by aspiration cytology: a case report. Acta Cytol *38*:252, 1994.

20. Prince FP: Ultrastructure of immature Leydig cells in the human prepubertal testis. Anat Rec *209*:165, 1984.

21. Siiteri PK, et al: Testosterone formation and metabolism during male sexual differentiation in the human embryo. J Clin Endocrinol Metab *38*:113, 1974.

22. Reyes FI, et al: Studies on human sexual development. II. Fetal and maternal serum gonadotropin and sex steroid concentrations. J Clin Endocrinol Metab *38*:612, 1974.

23. Catt KJ, et al: LH-hCG receptors and testosterone content during differentiation of the testis in the rabbit embryo. Endocrinology *97*:1157, 1975.

24. Huhtaniemi IT, et al: HCG binding and stimulation of testosterone biosynthesis in the human fetal testis. J Clin Endocrinol Metab *44*:963, 1977.

25. Clements JA, et al: Studies on human sexual development. III. Fetal pituitary and serum, and amniotic fluid concentrations of LH, CG, and FSH. J Clin Endocrinol Metab *42*:9, 1976.

26. Hagen C, et al: Identification of human luteinizing hormone, follicle-stimulating hormone, luteinizing hormone beta-subunit and gonadotrophin alpha-subunit in foetal and adult pituitary glands. J Endocrinol *67*:49, 1975.

27. Voutilainen R, et al: Developmental expression of genes for the steroidogenic enzymes P450scc (20,22-desmolase), P450c17 (17 alpha-hydroxylase/17,20-lyase), and P450c21 (21-hydroxylase) in the human fetus. J Clin Endocrinol Metab *63*:1145, 1986.

28. Greco TL, et al: Ontogeny of expression of the genes for steroidogenic enzymes P450 side-chain cleavage, 3 beta-hydroxysteroid dehydrogenase, P450 17 alpha-hydroxylase/C17-20 lyase, and P450 aromatase in fetal mouse gonads. Endocrinology *135*:262, 1994.

29. Goodyer CG, et al: Human fetal pituitary in culture: hormone secretion and response to somatostatin, luteinizing hormone releasing factor, thyrotropin releasing factor and dibutyryl cyclic AMP. J Clin Endocrinol Metab *45*:73, 1977.

30. Clements JA, et al: Ontogenesis of gonadotropin-releasing hormone in the human fetal hypothalamus. Proc Soc Exp Biol Med *163*:437, 1980.

31. Catt KJ, et al: Regulation of peptide hormone receptors and gonadal steroidogenesis. Recent Prog Horm Res *36*:557, 1980.

32. Warren DW, et al: Hormonal regulation of gonadotropin receptors and steroidogenesis in cultured fetal rat tests. Science *218*:375, 1982.

33. Leinonen PJ, et al: Leydig cell desensitization by human chorionic gonadotropin does not occur in the human fetal testis. J Clin Endocrinol Metab *61*:234, 1985.

34. Hilscher B, et al: Histological and morphometric studies on the kinetics of germ cells and immature Sertoli cells during human prespermatogenesis. Andrologia *24*:7, 1992.

35. Muller J, et al: Quantification of germ cells and seminiferous tubules by stereological examination of testicles from 50 boys who suffered from sudden death. Int J Androl *6*:143, 1983.

36. Gondos B, et al: Ultrastructure of germ cell development in the human fetal testis. Z Zellforsch Mikrosk Anat *119*:1, 1971.

37. Dym M, et al: Further observations on the numbers of spermatogonia, spermatocytes, and spermatids connected by intercellular bridges in the mammalian testis. Biol Reprod *4*:195, 1971.

38. Clermont Y: Kinetics of spermatogenesis in mammals: seminiferous epithelium cycle and spermatogonial renewal. Physiol Rev *52*:198, 1972.

39. Hadziselimovic F, et al: Importance of early postnatal germ cell maturation for fertility of cryptorchid males. Horm Res *55*:6, 2001.

40. Huckins C, et al: Evolution of gonocytes in the rat testis during late embryonic and early post-natal life. Arch Anat Histol Embryol *51*:341, 1968.

41. Orr-Urtreger A, et al: Developmental expression of c-kit, a proto-oncogene encoded by the W locus. Development *109*:911, 1990.

42. Yoshinaga K, et al: Role of c-kit in mouse spermatogenesis: identification of spermatogonia as a specific site of c-kit expression and function. Development *113*:689, 1991.

43. Ohta H, et al: Regulation of proliferation and differentiation in spermatogonial stem cells: the role of c-kit and its ligand SCF. Development *127*:2125, 2000.

44. Resnick JL, et al: Long-term proliferation of mouse primordial germ cells in culture. Nature *359*:550, 1992.

45. Oakberg EF: Spermatogonial stem-cell renewal in the mouse. Anat Rec *169*:515, 1971.

46. de Rooij DG, et al: Feedback regulation of the proliferation of the undifferentiated spermatogonia in the Chinese hamster by the differentiating spermatogonia. Cell Tissue Kinet *18*:71, 1985.

47. de Rooij DG, et al: Arrest of spermatogonial differentiation in jsd/jsd, Sl17H/Sl17H, and cryptorchid mice. Biol Reprod *61*:842, 1999.

48. Gondos B: Ultrastructure of developing and malignant germ cells. Eur Urol *23*:68, 1993.

49. Massad CA, et al: Morphology and histochemistry of infant testes in the prune belly syndrome. J Urol *146*:1598, 1991.

50. Nistal M, et al: Morphological and histometric study on the human Sertoli cell from birth to the onset of puberty. J Anat *134*:351, 1982.

51. Josso N, et al: Anti-mullerian hormone in early human development. Early Hum Dev *33*:91, 1993.

52. Schwindt B, et al: Serum levels of mullerian inhibiting substance in preterm and term male neonates. J Urol *158*:610, 1997.

53. Catlin EA, et al: Mullerian inhibiting substance depresses accumulation in vitro of disatured phosphatidylcholine in fetal rat lung. Am J Obstet Gynecol *159*:1299, 1988.

54. Ying SY: Inhibins, activins, and follistatins: gonadal proteins modulating the secretion of follicle-stimulating hormone. Endocr Rev *9*:267, 1988.

55. Good TE, et al: Isolation of nine different biologically and immunologically active molecular variants of bovine follicular inhibin. Biol Reprod *53*:1478, 1995.

56. Anawalt BD, et al: Serum inhibin B levels reflect Sertoli cell function in normal men and men with testicular dysfunction. J Clin Endocrinol Metab *81*:3341, 1996.

57. Chemes HE, et al: Patho-physiological observations of Sertoli cells in patients with germinal aplasia or severe germ cell depletion: ultrastructural findings and hormone levels. Biol Reprod *17*:108, 1977.

58. Flickinger C, et al: The junctional specializations of Sertoli cells in the seminiferous epithelium. Anat Rec *158*:207, 1967.

59. Dym M, et al: The blood-testis barrier in the rat and the physiological compartmentation of the seminiferous epithelium. Biol Reprod *3*:308, 1970.

60. Li JC, et al: The inter-Sertoli tight junction permeability barrier is regulated by the interplay of protein phosphatases and kinases: an in vitro study. J Androl *22*:847, 2001.

61. Setchell BP, et al: Development of the blood-testis barrier and changes in vascular permeability at puberty in rats. Int J Androl *11*:225, 1988.

62. Russell LD: Observations on the inter-relationships of Sertoli cells at the level of the blood-testis barrier: evidence for formation and resorption of Sertoli-Sertoli tubulobulbar complexes during the spermatogenic cycle of the rat. Am J Anat *155*:259, 1979.

63. Toyama Y, et al: Neonatally administered diethylstilbestrol retards the development of the blood-testis barrier in the rat. J Androl *22*:413, 2001.

64. Hermo L, et al: Arrangement of connective tissue components in the walls of seminiferous tubules of man and monkey. Am J Anat *148*:433, 1977.

65. Suvanto O, et al: Effect of experimental cryptorchidism and cadmium injury on the spontaneous contractions of the seminiferous tubules of the rat testis. Virchows Arch B Cell Pathol *4*:217, 1970.

66. Richardson LL, et al: Basement membrane gene expression by Sertoli and peritubular myoid cells in vitro in the rat. Biol Reprod *52*:320, 1995.

67. Skinner MK, et al: Testicular peritubular cells secrete a protein under androgen control that modulates Sertoli cell functions. Proc Natl Acad Sci USA *82*:114, 1985.

68. Skinner MK: Cell-cell interactions in the testis. Endocr Rev *12*:45, 1991.

69. Tapanainen JS, et al: Hormonal control of apoptotic cell death in the testis: gonadotropins and androgens as testicular cell survival factors. Mol Endocrinol *7*:643, 1993.

70. Billig H, et al: Apoptosis in testis germ cells: developmental changes in gonadotropin dependence and localization to selective tubule stages. Endocrinology *136*:5, 1995.

71. Helal MA, et al: Ontogeny of human fetal testicular apoptosis during first, second, and third trimesters of pregnancy. J Clin Endocrinol Metab *87*:1189, 2002.

72. Pentikainen V, et al: Fas regulates germ cell apoptosis in the human testis in vitro. Am J Physiol *276*:E310, 1999.

73. Pentikainen V, et al: TNFalpha down-regulates the Fas ligand and inhibits germ cell apoptosis in the human testis. J Clin Endocrinol Metab *86*:4480, 2001.

Ahmet R. Aslan and Barry A. Kogan

Testicular Descent

Testicular maldescent in the newborn is one of the easiest diagnoses to make, yet understanding the mechanism of testicular descent continues to be one of the most challenging topics in pediatric urology. Because the testis develops in the abdomen and travels along the inguinal canal to reach the scrotum, many anatomic structures are involved, including the epididymis, gubernaculum, vas deferens, and processus vaginalis. Further, when we consider the number of hormonal factors, cytokines, and neurotransmitters that are involved, the complexity of testicular descent is clear.

Research in this area has been done in both humans and animal preparations. Human fetal studies have obvious limitations, so most work has been done in animals. Of course, the major pitfall of animal studies is the anatomic differences among species. For example, rats have a saclike cremaster muscle that is important for development of the processus vaginalis, whereas humans and other large mammals have a striplike cremaster.[1] The rat cremaster results in a pouchlike processus vaginalis; hence, the rat testis can travel between the abdomen and the scrotum easily. Rat testes also differ from larger mammals in timing of descent, because descent is normally completed postnatally, usually around day 21 after birth. Despite these problems, much is known about testicular descent, and the following discussion highlights the most important anatomic and hormonal factors in testicular descent.

PHASES OF HUMAN TESTICULAR DESCENT

The path that the testis follows during its migration is well defined; however, the phases of testicular descent are still debatable. Some investigators have divided the process into three phases: intra-abdominal, transinguinal, and scrotal. Early in gestation, the position of the testis is at the level of the lower pole of the kidney. Whether a transabdominal phase of "descent" exists is controversial. It has been suggested that the testis retains a stable position while the abdomen grows cephalad. Although some investigators do not acknowledge a transabdominal phase, others claim that the gubernaculum, processus vaginalis, and cremasteric muscle are involved in this phase of descent. If transabdominal migration does occur, it takes place somewhere between the 8th and 26th weeks of gestation. Before inguinal descent starts around 26 weeks of gestation,[2] the testis lies at the level of anterior iliac supine. Although the passage through the inguinal canal takes only a few days,[3] the descent from external ring to the bottom of the scrotum requires about 4 weeks more. In most cases, the entire process is completed by the 32nd week, but it can be as late as 9 months postnatally.

FACTORS IN TESTICULAR DESCENT

Gubernaculum

This jellylike structure has,[4] ever since its discovery, been thought to be important in testicular descent. The origin of the term is *gubernare*, which means "to control" in Latin. The term was probably originally used by Hunter,[5] to explain its leading role in testicular descent. However, its exact contribution remains controversial. One of the first theories of testicular descent was that traction of the gubernaculum on the testis

plays a major role in the process. The presence of the cremaster muscle intertwined with the gubernaculum supports this theory. In humans, the gubernaculum increases in size from the 15th to the 24th week of gestation. It has been suggested that this growth is responsible for moving the testis from the abdomen into the inguinal canal. This gubernacular growth is characterized by hyperplasia and hypertrophy of the mesenchymal cells and an increase in extracellular matrix, in particular, hyaluronic acid. The increase in hyaluronic acid seems to cause a secondary inflow of water that results in gubernacular enlargement. What triggers this mechanism is not clear, but androgens seem to be involved.[6, 7] Indeed, when pregnant rats were treated during this phase of development with either flutamide (an antiandrogen) or finasteride (a 5α-reductase inhibitor), testicular descent was prevented.[8] Other investigators have suggested that a substance called *descendin* may also be involved. This low molecular weight substance is secreted by the testis, independent of androgens, at ages corresponding to the first phase of testicular descent.[9] Evidence for this is based on the finding that gubernacular cell proliferation was stimulated by testicular extracts (descendin), whereas ovarian extracts and androgens did not have any effect.[10]

Another substance that plays a role in gubernacular development is an insulin-like peptide isolated from the Leydig cells.[11] In the mouse, the Insl3/relaxin-like factor (RLF) gene is specifically expressed in Leydig cells, and it likely has an important function in the transabdominal phase of the testicular descent. Zimmermann and colleagues[12] showed that male mice with a disruption of the *Insl3* gene had bilateral cryptorchidism, abnormal spermatogenesis, and infertility. Examination of these animals revealed an underdeveloped gubernaculum and nonregressed cranial suspensory ligaments. These data suggest that *Insl3* is involved in the development of these structures in the mouse. However, human studies have shown that the rate of mutations of this gene is the same in cryptorchid children as in control subjects.[13, 14]

The period of growth in the gubernaculum is followed (between the 25th and 32nd weeks of gestation) by a phase of regression.[3] It has been suggested that this regression leaves a space, something like a vacuum, that brings the testis through the inguinal canal into the scrotum. Although this phase is also under hormonal control, the androgens probably act as paracrine factors and activate catabolic enzymes, such as acid phosphatase, that result in gubernacular regression.[15]

These theories are supported by the existence of cremasteric muscle that theoretically could pull the testis into position. Conversely, it is unclear whether the testis is actually attached to the gubernaculum.[16] Indeed, in both humans and animals, there are instances of a maldescended testis associated with a descended epididymis.[17, 18] Moreover, division of the gubernacular attachment to the testis or epididymis in rats fails to prevent development of the processus vaginalis and, in most studies, descent of the testis.[19] Confusing this picture is the finding that, in rats, division of the distal gubernaculum prevents testicular descent. However, studies have shown that division of the distal gubernaculum also prevents development of the scrotum and the processus vaginalis, likely as a result of mechanical disruption of the scrotum and division of the genitofemoral nerve.[20] Hence, division of the distal gubernaculum is suboptimal for studying testicular descent.

Investigators have become interested in the role of *cranial suspensory ligaments* in testicular descent. These structures regress in males, but are present in females, a finding suggesting that their presence may play a role in preventing full intra-abdominal testicular descent. For example, human patients with androgen insensitivity syndrome have abdominal testes and persistent gonadal ligaments.[21] Similar findings are seen in androgen-insensitive testicular feminizing mice (Tfm) (although the testes descend to the lower abdomen in both humans and mice), again suggesting that regression of these ligaments is likely under androgenic control.[22] Further evidence comes from the finding that, when antiandrogen treatment was given to male rats prenatally, these cranial suspensory ligaments failed to regress.[23] Conversely, female newborn rats treated with androgens had regression of the ligaments, and the ovaries were located caudal to the kidney.[24] It is clear that androgens play a role in the regression of these ligaments and the ligaments are important in testicular descent.

In summary, the literature suggests that the gubernaculum does not pull the testis into the scrotum, but it does have an important role in guiding the testis along the correct path into the scrotum. Indeed, an ectopic testis likely results when the gubernaculum itself has a primary attachment separate from the scrotum (usually in the femoral area or perineum) and therefore guides the testis to an abnormal position.

Genitofemoral Nerve and Calcitonin Gene–Related Peptide

The genitofemoral nerve also seems to be important for testicular descent. Indeed, animal experiments demonstrate that when the genitofemoral nerve is divided early in gestation, gubernacular regression and an undescended testis result.[25] The genitofemoral nerve likely acts via calcitonin gene–related peptide (CGRP), a neuropeptide that is located in many sites in the nervous system.[26] It mediates both motor and sensory nerves as well as some autonomic functions.[27, 28] CGRP has been localized within the motor nucleus of genitofemoral nerve, and CGRP receptors have been shown within the cremasteric muscle of the rat gubernaculum. Further, these receptors are up-regulated after denervation of the genitofemoral nerve.[29, 30] Additional evidence comes from data showing that exogenous treatment with CGRP stimulates gubernacular development, whereas CGRP 8-37 (a synthetic CGRP antagonist) delays testicular descent.[31, 32] Finally, *in vivo*, CGRP causes contraction in the rat gubernaculum.[33]

Although it is thought that CGRF acts in an androgen-mediated way, the antiandrogen flutamide alters the sensory, but not the motor, nucleus of the genitofemoral nerve.[34-36] An explanation for this finding is that the androgens act to influence CGRP via the central nervous system, which is clearly sexually dimorphic. In one study, castration increased CGRP in the spinal nucleus of the genitofemoral nerve and led to an increased number of motor neurons containing CGRP.[37] Hence, abnormalities of the autonomic nervous system may result in maldescent of the testis.[38] In summary, it is likely that the genitofemoral nerve is a source of CGRP and that CGRP plays a role in gubernacular development.

Intra-Abdominal Pressure

Because the gubernaculum does not seem to pull the testis into the scrotum, another factor must be involved. It has been suggested that intra-abdominal pressure is that factor. If a regression of the gubernaculum results in a patent processus vaginalis, it is reasonable to accept that intra-abdominal pressure would push the testis into this empty space. Indeed, children with prune belly syndrome and gastroschisis usually have undescended testes. It appears, however, that they also have central nervous system abnormalities that could affect pituitary function, and this situation, in turn, could interfere with testicular descent.[39, 40] In an animal study to test the role of intra-abdominal pressure, testicular descent occurred in rats in spite of a surgically created abdominal wall defect that likely reduced intra-abdominal pressure.[41] In addition, because the intra-abdominal pressure theory fails to explain the occurrence of unilateral maldescended testes, it seems highly unlikely that intra-abdominal pressure has a major role in testicular descent.

Hormones

Since 1932, when Engle first reported treating monkeys with maldescended testes by using an extract from urine of pregnant monkeys (ultimately proven to be hCG), it has been clear that hormones must have a significant role in testicular descent in mammals.[42] Indeed, any factor that interferes with the hypothalamic-pituitary-testicular axis affects testicular descent. A prime example of this is seen in patients with Kallmann syndrome, in whom the rate of maldescended testes is increased greatly. Another example of the importance of androgens is seen in patients with various forms of androgen insensitivity. Patients with complete androgen insensitivity (previously termed *testicular feminization*), for example, uniformly have intra-abdominal testes.

Numerous animal studies have also demonstrated the hormonal dependency of testicular descent.[43, 44] Juenemann and associates demonstrated that estrogen treatment prevented testicular descent in newborn rats.[45, 46] Moreover, there are now good data showing that both inguinal descent and intra-abdominal descent are under androgenic control. For example, in the dog, bilateral orchiectomy performed after the completion of gubernacular outgrowth prevents gubernacular regression, but testosterone treatment can induce the regression despite orchiectomy. Timing is important in this stimulation because testosterone is unable to restore the gubernacular outgrowth prevented by early orchiectomy.[47, 48] The role of dihydrotestosterone is more controversial. 5α-Reductase activity is present in the rat gubernaculum, which is also rich in androgen receptor protein.[49, 50] Furthermore, testosterone is as effective as dihydrotestosterone in reversing the inhibitory effect of estradiol on testicular descent.[51] Similarly, finasteride, a 5α-reductase inhibitor, has little effect on testicular descent, a finding suggesting that dihydrotestosterone is not more important than testosterone in the process of testicular descent.[8]

Endocrine studies in children have been used to elucidate the role of hormones in testicular descent. The newborn period seems to be the best time for hormonal measurements, because normal male infants have relatively high plasma testosterone levels during the first 6 months of life.[52] Lower testosterone levels have been detected in cryptorchid infants,[53] and it has been suggested that this is because LH levels are reduced also.[54, 55] Some cryptorchid children have been shown to have antipituitary antibodies, but unfortunately, on a case-by-case basis, the presence of these antibodies did not correlate with low testosterone levels.[55] Other studies have emphasized the impairment in testosterone synthesis in undescended testes.[56] We have performed similar studies, but in contrast with the findings of Gendrel and colleagues,[54] we have demonstrated hormonal differences only between infants with bilateral cryptorchidism and those with normally descended testes. No differences were seen in neonates with unilateral undescended testis (Figs. 192–1 through 192–3).

Müllerian-Inhibiting Substance

Müllerian-inhibiting substance (MIS) is secreted from the Sertoli cells in boys, and its primary function is to cause regression of the müllerian duct in the fetus. The idea that MIS may be

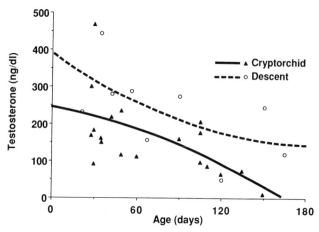

Figure 192–1. Second-order linear regression curves of testosterone values during the first 6 months of life in cryptorchid patients with and without spontaneous postnatal testicular descent. Generally, those with postnatal descent had higher values, but the difference is small. For cryptorchid patients, $y = 239 - .67x - .005x^2$, $r' = .60$; for patients with spontaneous descent, $y = 385 - 2.69x + 008x^2$, $r = .60$.

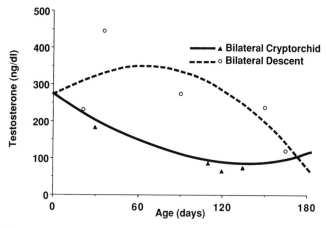

Figure 192–2. Second-order linear regression curves of testosterone values during the first 6 months of life in bilaterally cryptorchid patients with and without spontaneous testicular descent. There is a large difference between groups, with higher values in those patients having spontaneous descent. For cryptorchid patients, $y = 252 - 2.58 + .009x^2$, $r = .99$; for patients with spontaneous descent, $y = 265 + 2.50x - .020x^2$, $r = .75$.

involved in testicular descent is based on studies showing that boys with maldescended testes have lower levels of MIS than do normal boys.[57] In addition, because there were significant differences in MIS levels between patients with bilateral maldescent and those with unilateral maldescent, it has been suggested that MIS may be responsible for the transabdominal phase of descent.[58] Further support for this concept is the finding that the highest levels of MIS are detected *in utero* during the first two trimesters, and this coincides with the time of migration of the testes through the abdomen to the inguinal canal. However, there are also serious conflicts about the role of MIS. One strong piece of evidence against a role for MIS comes from a study of female rats that had been immunized against MIS. Although male offspring of these rats had müllerian duct remnants as expected, they nonetheless had descended testes, a finding suggesting that MIS is not required for testicular descent.[59]

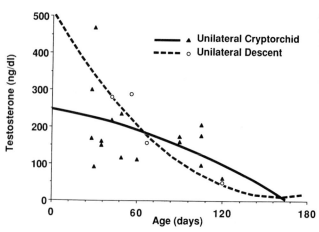

Figure 192–3. Second-order linear regression curves of testosterone values during the first 6 months of life in unilaterally cryptorchid patients with and without spontaneous testicular descent. There is no real difference between the groups. For cryptorchid patients, $y = 241 - .60x - .005x^2$, $r = .54$; for patients with spontaneous descent, $y = 536 - 6.48x + .02x^2$, $r = .94$.

Epidermal Growth Factor

In rats, the salivary glands are the major source of epidermal growth factor (EGF), and removal of these glands results in maldescended testes. Furthermore, extrinsic EGF was able to reverse cryptorchidism induced by flutamide.[60] The mechanism of action of EGF is unclear, but one theory is that EGF acts to stimulate the placental-gonadal axis, and any increase in the placental gonadotropins would enhance androgen production. In addition, EGF can both stimulate the androgen-binding capacity of male reproductive cells and bind to the androgen receptor to virilize the genitalia, even in the absence of androgens.[61] In summary, it seems that EGF has a role in testicular descent, but its exact function remains unclear.

DIAGNOSIS AND INCIDENCE OF CRYPTORCHIDISM

It is difficult to determine the exact incidence of cryptorchidism because of the difficulty in differentiating truly maldescended testes from those that are retractile. All normal males older than 6 months of age have a cremasteric reflex that is thought to be protective for the testes. It is triggered when the scrotum is exposed to cold temperature or in times of stress and fear. Unfortunately, these events are common during a typical medical office visit and often lead to misdiagnosis on routine physical examination. One study demonstrated only 13.5% complete agreement on testicular position between two experienced observers.[62] Normally descended testes can be misdiagnosed as maldescended, or may even be impalpable, depending on the strength of the reflex and the skill of the examiner. It is striking that not only is the true incidence of maldescended testis difficult to determine, but also many children undergo an unnecessary operation as a result of this misdiagnosis.[63] Further, the classification of retractile testes as "undescended" may be a cause of underestimating the complications of true cryptorchidism.

The best time to make the initial diagnosis is the neonatal period, because the cremasteric reflex is not prominent before 6 months of age. Based on Scorer's study performed in 3612 consecutive newborns,[64] the incidence of maldescended testis at birth is 4.2%. Using 2500 g of birth weight as a cut-off value for prematurity, the incidence is 21% in premature infants and 2.7% in full-term infants. By the end of the 9 months, most of these testes descend spontaneously, resulting in an incidence rate of 0.8%. Because the incidence is 0.73% in adults, any further spontaneous testicular descent should not be expected after 9 months of age.[65]

When testes are impalpable, the problem becomes more complex. In the past, radiologic tests were used to localize impalpable testes. Herniography, angiography, and testicular venography were used in distant past but are highly invasive and have a high false-positive rate. Ultrasound is noninvasive, but early hopes for the usefulness of the technique have not been realized. In practice, the test is not helpful unless the testes are located superficially.[66] Computed tomography and magnetic resonance imaging scans are the most accurate localizing techniques, but they generally require sedation or anesthesia and are expensive.[67, 68] Moreover, operative exploration needs to be done whether or not these tests demonstrate the testis. Diagnostic laparoscopy is now the first choice in the diagnosis of impalpable testis.[69-71] Beyond the high success rate of this approach for locating the testis, a major benefit of laparoscopy is the ability to use laparoscopic techniques to bring down the testis during the same procedure.

COMPLICATIONS OF MALDESCENDED TESTES

Maldescended testes are associated with several serious problems. Some may be corrected by treatment, but others may persist. For example, there is a high rate of *inguinal hernia* in patients with maldescended testes. Surgical orchiopexy corrects this. Similarly, there is a higher rate of *testicular torsion* in patients with maldescended testes. Surgery corrects this as well. The two major complications of maldescended testes are *infertility* and *malignancy*. Of interest, the data supporting the concept that bringing the testis down into the scrotum helps to prevent these complications are controversial.

Fertility can be evaluated in many ways. Studying fertility based on semen analysis shows significant abnormalities in these patients, despite successful treatment. For example, a review of 11 studies showed normal semen analysis in only 50% of patients with a history of unilateral cryptorchidism and in 28% of those with a history of bilateral cryptorchidism.[68] Despite this gloomy outlook based on semen analysis, the effect on paternity is considerably less. Some older studies suggested that patients with unilateral maldescended testis had normal fertility,[72] but those with bilateral cryptorchidism had more significant problems.[68, 73] More recent studies showed a paternity rate of 90% (versus 93% of controls) in patients with a history of unilateral cryptorchidism and a rate of 65% in those with bilateral cryptorchidism.[74, 75] A fascinating and as yet unresolved issue is whether early treatment can improve the fertility potential. Several early studies looked at paternity in adults who had undergone unilateral orchiopexy previously. Semen analyses performed after unilateral vasectomy of the unoperated side revealed that the previously maldescended testis contributed virtually no sperm.[76] Of course, these patients were treated in a previous era, and only limited data are available for patients treated at approximately age 1 year, which is the current standard. A few limited studies suggested that treatment with LH-releasing hormone analogues after orchidopexy is beneficial in the improvement of spermatogenesis and therefore of fertility.[77] These authors suggested that the transformation of gonocytes to Ad (adult dark) spermatogonia is crucial for future fertility.[77, 78] Because of these findings, they also recommended testicular biopsy in every maldescended testis and hormonal treatment of such testes that have less than 0.2 Ad spermatogonia per tubule.[78]

There appears to be an increased risk of testicular neoplasia in patients with cryptorchidism. For example, about 10% of testicular neoplasms arise from a maldescended testis, even though the incidence of maldescended testes is only 0.8%.[79, 80] Other studies have also calculated an increased risk that varies from 4.7-fold to 48-fold, and these studies suggest that abdominal testes have a risk of malignancy four times higher than that of inguinal testes.[81] Furthermore, in bilateral cryptorchidism, if one of the testes has malignant disease, there is a 15% chance of developing a contralateral tumor, and this rate is 30% if the testes are intra-abdominal.[80] Even in unilateral cryptorchidism, there seems to be an increased risk of malignant disease in the contralateral testis. Unfortunately, no data support or refute the idea that early treatment lowers the risk.

REFERENCES

1. Wensing CJ: Testicular descent in the rat and a comparison of this process in the rat with that in the pig. Anat Rec *214*:154, 1986.
2. Scorer CG: The natural history of testicular descent. Proc R Soc Med *58*:933, 1965.
3. Heyns CF: The gubernaculum during testicular descent in the human fetus. J Anat *153*:93, 1987.
4. Backhouse KM: The gubernaculum testis hunteri: testicular descent and maldescent. Ann R Coll Surg Engl *35*:15, 1964.
5. Hunter J: Observations on Certain Parts of the Animal Economy. London, Longmans, Green & Co, 1785.
6. Heyns CF, et al: Hyperplasia and hypertrophy of the gubernaculum during testicular descent in the fetus. J Urol *135*:1043, 1986.
7. Heyns CF, et al: The glycosaminoglycans of the gubernaculum during testicular descent in the fetus. J Urol *143*:612, 1990.
8. Spencer JR, et al: Effects of flutamide and finasteride on rat testicular descent. Endocrinology *129*:741, 1991.
9. Fentener van Vlissingen JM, et al: In vitro model of the first phase of testicular descent: identification of a low molecular weight factor from fetal testis involved in proliferation of gubernaculum testis cells and distinct from specified polypeptide growth factors and fetal gonadal hormones. Endocrinology *123*:2868, 1988.
10. Visser JH, et al: Proliferation of gubernaculum cells induced by a substance of low molecular mass obtained from fetal pig testes. J Urol *153*:516, 1995.
11. Adham IM, et al: Cloning of a cDNA for a novel insulin-like peptide of the testicular Leydig cells. J Biol Chem *268*:26668, 1993.
12. Zimmermann S, et al: Targeted disruption of the Insl3 gene causes bilateral cryptorchidism. Mol Endocrinol *13*:681, 1999.
13. Koskimies P, et al: A common polymorphism in the human relaxin-like factor (RLF) gene: no relationship with cryptorchidism. Pediatr Res *47*:538, 2000.
14. Tomboc M, et al: Insulin-like 3/relaxin-like factor gene mutations are associated with cryptorchidism. J Clin Endocrinol Metab *85*:4013, 2000.
15. Levy JB, et al: The hormonal control of testicular descent. J Androl *16*:459, 1995.
16. Gier HT, et al: Development of mammalian testes and genital ducts. Biol Reprod *1*(Suppl 1):1, 1969.
17. Scorer CG: The anatomy of the testicular descent: normal and incomplete. Br J Surg *49*:357, 1962.
18. Bedford JM: Anatomical evidence for the epididymis as the prime mover in the evolution of the scrotum. Am J Anat *152*:483, 1978.
19. Frey HL, et al: Role of the gubernaculum and intraabdominal pressure in the process of testicular descent. J Urol *131*:574, 1984.
20. Clarnette TD, et al: The genitofemoral nerve may link testicular inguinoscrotal descent with congenital inguinal hernia. Aust NZ J Surg *66*:612, 1996.
21. Barthold JS, et al: Testicular position in the androgen insensitivity syndrome: implications for the role of androgens in testicular descent. J Urol *164*:497, 2000.
22. Hutson JM, et al: The hormonal control of testicular descent. Endocr Rev *7*:270, 1986.
23. van der Schoot P, et al: Androgen-induced prevention of the outgrowth of cranial gonadal suspensory ligaments in fetal rats. J Androl *13*:534, 1992.
24. Lee SM, et al: Effect of androgens on the cranial suspensory ligament and ovarian position. Anat Rec *255*:306, 1999.
25. Beasley SW, et al: Effect of division of genitofemoral nerve on testicular descent in the rat. Aust NZ J Surg *57*:49, 1987.
26. Rosenfeld MG, et al: Production of a novel neuropeptide encoded by the calcitonin gene via tissue-specific RNA processing. Nature *304*:129, 1983.
27. New HV, et al: Calcitonin gene–related peptide regulates muscle acetylcholine receptor synthesis. Nature *323*:809, 1986.
28. Sigrist S, et al: Specific receptor and cardiovascular effects of calcitonin gene–related peptide. Endocrinology *119*:381, 1986.
29. Yamanaka J, et al: Demonstration of calcitonin gene–related peptide receptors in the gubernaculum by computerized densitometry. J Pediatr Surg *27*:876, 1992.
30. Yamanaka J, et al: Testicular descent. II. Ontogeny and response to denervation of calcitonin gene–related peptide receptors in neonatal rat gubernaculum. Endocrinology *132*:280, 1993.
31. Samarakkody UK, et al: Intrascrotal CGRP 8-37 causes a delay in testicular descent in mice. J Pediatr Surg *27*:874, 1992.
32. Griffiths AL, et al: Exogenous calcitonin gene–related peptide causes gubernacular development in neonatal (Tfm) mice with complete androgen resistance. J Pediatr Surg *28*:1028, 1993.

33. Park WH, et al: The gubernaculum shows rhythmic contractility and active movement during testicular descent. J Pediatr Surg 26:615, 1991.
34. Barthold JS, et al: Lack of feminization of the cremaster nucleus by prenatal flutamide administration in the rat and pig. J Urol 156:767, 1996.
35. Hrabovszky Z, et al: Undescended testis is accompanied by calcitonin gene related peptide accumulation within the sensory nucleus of the genitofemoral nerve in trans-scrotal rats. J Urol 165:1015, 2001.
36. Hrabovszky Z, et al: Does the sensory nucleus of the genitofemoral nerve have a role in testicular descent? J Pediatr Surg 35:96, 2000.
37. Popper P, et al: The effect of castration on calcitonin gene–related peptide in spinal motor neurons. Neuroendocrinology 50:338, 1989.
38. Bingol-Kologlu M, et al: A comparative histopathologic and immunohistopathologic evaluation of cremaster muscles from boys with various inguinoscrotal pathologies. Eur J Pediatr Surg 11:110, 2001.
39. Hadziselimovic F, et al: Omphalocele, cryptorchidism, and brain malformations. J Pediatr Surg 22:854, 1987.
40. Orvis BR, et al: Testicular histology in fetuses with the prune belly syndrome and posterior urethral valves. J Urol 139:335, 1988.
41. Quinlan DM, et al: Abdominal wall defects and cryptorchidism: an animal model. J Urol 140:1141, 1988.
42. Engle ET: Experimentally induced descent of the testis in the Macacus monkey by hormones from the anterior pituitary and pregnancy urine. Endocrinology 16:513, 1932.
43. Husmann DA, et al: Time-specific androgen blockade with flutamide inhibits testicular descent in the rat. Endocrinology 129:1409, 1991.
44. Husmann DA, et al: Reversal of flutamide-induced cryptorchidism by prenatal time-specific androgens. Endocrinology 131:1711, 1992.
45. Juenemann KP, et al: Fertility in cryptorchidism: an experimental model. J Urol 136:214, 1986.
46. Kogan BA, et al: Fertility in cryptorchidism: further development of an experimental model. J Urol 137:128, 1987.
47. Baumans V, et al: The effect of orchidectomy on gubernacular outgrowth and regression in the dog. Int J Androl 5:387, 1982.
48. Baumans V, et al: The role of a non-androgenic testicular factor in the process of testicular descent in the dog. Int J Androl 6:541, 1983.
49. George FW, et al: Partial characterization of the androgen receptor of the newborn rat gubernaculum. Biol Reprod 39:536, 1988.
50. George FW: Developmental pattern of 5 alpha-reductase activity in the rat gubernaculum. Endocrinology 124:727, 1989.
51. Spencer JR, et al: Studies of the hormonal control of postnatal testicular descent in the rat. J Urol 149:618, 1993.
52. Forest MG, et al: Hypophyso-gonadal function in humans during the first year of life. I. Evidence for testicular activity in early infancy. J Clin Invest 53:819, 1974.
53. Gendrel D, et al: Reduced post-natal rise of testosterone in plasma of cryptorchid infants. Acta Endocrinol (Copenh) 89:372, 1978.
54. Gendrel D, et al: Simultaneous postnatal rise of plasma LH and testosterone in male infants. J Pediatr 97:600, 1980.
55. Pouplard A, et al: Antigonadotropic cell antibodies in the serum of cryptorchid children and infants and of their mothers. J Pediatr 107:26, 1985.
56. Farrer JH, et al: Impaired testosterone biosynthesis in cryptorchidism. Fertil Steril 44:125, 1985.
57. Donahoe PK, et al: Mullerian inhibiting substance in human testes after birth. J Pediatr Surg 12:323, 1977.
58. Yamanaka J, et al: Serum levels of Mullerian inhibiting substance in boys with cryptorchidism. J Pediatr Surg 26:621, 1991.
59. Tran D, et al: Persistence of mullerian ducts in male rabbits passively immunized against bovine anti-mullerian hormone during fetal life. Dev Biol 116:160, 1986.
60. Cain MP, et al: Alterations in maternal epidermal growth factor (EGF) effect testicular descent and epididymal development. Urology 43:375, 1994.
61. Gupta C, et al: Activation of androgen receptor in epidermal growth factor modulation of fetal mouse sexual differentiation. Mol Cell Endocrinol 123:89, 1996.
62. Olsen LH: Inter-observer variation in assessment of undescended testis: analysis of kappa statistics as a coefficient of reliability. Br J Urol 64:644, 1989.
63. Cooper BJ, et al: Orchidopexy: theory and practice. BMJ 291:706, 1985.
64. Scorer C: The descent of the testis. Arch Dis Child 39:605, 1964.
65. Baumrucker G: Incidence of testicular pathology. Bull US Army Med Dept 5:312, 1946.
66. Madrazo BL, et al: Ultrasonographic demonstration of undescended testes. Radiology 133:181, 1979.
67. Lee JK, et al: Utility of computed tomography in the localization of the undescended testis. Radiology 135:121, 1980.
68. Fritzsche PJ, et al: Undescended testis: value of MR imaging. Radiology 164:169, 1987.
69. Silber SJ, et al: Laparoscopy for cryptorchidism. J Urol 124:928, 1980.
70. Sutherland RS, et al: Therapeutic laparoscopy for the nonpalpable testicle. Tech Urol 2:142, 1996.
71. Bogaert GA, et al: Therapeutic laparoscopy for intra-abdominal testes. Urology 42:182, 1993.
72. Gilhooly PE, et al: Fertility prospects for children with cryptorchidism. Am J Dis Child 138:940, 1984.
73. Fallon B, et al: Long-term follow-up of fertility in cryptorchid patients. Urology 25:502, 1985.
74. Miller KD, et al: Fertility after unilateral cryptorchidism: paternity, time to conception, pretreatment testicular location and size, hormone and sperm parameters. Horm Res 55:249, 2001.
75. Lee PA, et al: Fertility after bilateral cryptorchidism: evaluation by paternity, hormone, and semen data. Horm Res 55:28, 2001.
76. Alpert PF, et al: Spermatogenesis in the unilateral cryptorchid testis after orchiopexy. J Urol 129:301, 1983.
77. Hadziselimovic F, et al: Treatment with a luteinizing hormone-releasing hormone analogue after successful orchiopexy markedly improves the chance of fertility later in life. J Urol 158:1193, 1997.
78. Hadziselimovic F, et al: The importance of both an early orchidopexy and germ cell maturation for fertility. Lancet 358:1156, 2001.
79. Campbell H: The incidence of malignant growth of the undescended testicle: a reply and re-evaluation. J Urol 81:563, 1959.
80. Gilbert JBHaJB: Incidence and nature of tumors in ectopic testes. Surg Gynecol Obstet 71:731, 1940.
81. Giwercman A, et al: Testicular cancer risk in boys with maldescended testis: a cohort study. J Urol 138:1214, 1987.

INDEX

Note: Page numbers followed by f refer to figures; those followed by t indicate tables.

A

Abdominal wall, thermoreceptors in, 552
Abortion
  induced, for multifetal reduction, 170f,
    170-171, 171f
  spontaneous
    alcohol consumption and, 235
    early, in multiple pregnancy, 171
Abruptio placentae
  alcohol consumption and, 235
  in multiple pregnancy, 168
Acardia, in multiple pregnancy, 174, 174f
Acclimation, thermal, 560
Acetaminophen
  during lactation, 255
  half-life of, 186t
Acetylcholine
  airway innervation and, 842
  as neurotransmitter, 1709, 1709f, 1875t
  cardiac conduction and, 682, 683f, 684
  umbilicoplacental circulation mediation by,
    752t
Achondroplasia, 1836t, 1837, 1857t
Acid-base balance
  potassium homeostasis and, 1281
  regulation of, 1361-1364
    extracellular buffer system and, 1361,
      1363
    in fetus, 1362
    in neonates, 1363-1364
    intracellular buffer system and, 1361, 1363
    renal compensatory mechanisms and,
      1362
    research compensatory mechanism and,
      1362
  renal tubular function and, prenatal, 1236
  status of, calcium transport and, 1288
Acidemia, cardiac function and, 654
Acidification of urine. See Urinary
  acidification.
Acidosis
  cerebral, in hypoxia-ischemia, 1722-1723,
    1723f
  lactic, 1212t
    in hypoxemia, fetal, 773
  metabolic
    cardiac function and, 654
    fetal, 1362
    neonatal, 1363-1364
    potassium homeostasis and, 1281, 1285
    with hypothermia, 587
  respiratory
    fetal, 1362
    metabolic compensation for, 1329-1330
    neonatal, 1364

Aciduria, arginosuccinic, 595
Acinar buds, 786
Acinar tubules, 786
Acinus(i)
  organization of, 1177
  pancreatic, 1142-1143
ACTH. See Adrenocorticotropic hormone.
Actin filaments, 635
Action potential, cardiac. See Cardiac action
  potential.
Activated partial thromboplastin time
  in adults, 1436t
  in children, 1441t
  in fetuses, 1436t
  in full-term infants, 1436t, 1438t
  in neonates, 1449
  in premature infants, 1437t
  systems for, 1435, 1442t
Activating mutations, 21
Activation potential, 671
Active transport, placental
  of amino acids, 512
  of calcium, 314t, 314-316, 315f
  of drugs, 179, 207
Activin, brain development and, 1786
Activiteá moyenne, 1733
Acute phase reaction, 1563
Acute renal failure, 1335-1339
  causes of, 1338, 1339t
  intrinsic, 1335
  pathophysiologic mechanisms of,
    1335-1338, 1336f
    glomerular transcapillary hydraulic
      pressure difference and, 1337-1338,
      1338f
    golmerular capillary ultrafiltration
      coefficient and, 1338
    plasma colloid osmotic pressure and,
      1338
    plasma flow rate and, 1336-1337
  postrenal, 1335
  prerenal, 1335
  prognosis of, 1339
Acute tubular necrosis, 1335
Acyclovir, during lactation, 256
ADCC. See Antibody-dependent cellular
  cytotoxicity.
Adenosine
  calcium transport and, 1289
  chemoreceptor-mediated cardiovascular
    responses and, 722
  renal blood flow and, 1244
  thermogenesis and, neonatal, 547t
  umbilicoplacental circulation mediation by,
    752t

Adenosine monophosphate, cyclic
  as second messenger, 1598-1599
  pulmonary liquid transport regulation by,
    826-827, 828f
Adenosine triphosphate
  availability of, apoptosis versus necrosis
    and, 75
  calcium transport and, 1289
ADH. See Vasopressin.
Adhalen, 1854
Adhesion molecules. See Cell adhesion
  molecules; Immunoglobulin gene
  superfamily; Integrins; Selectin(s).
Adipose tissue
  brown, 404-412
    5'-deiodinase and thyroid and, 410f,
      410-411, 411f
    depots of, 405
    development of, prolactin and, 1893
    diseases affecting, 412
    in newborns, 404-405
    recruitment of, 411
    thermogenesis and, 405
      clinical implications of, 411-412
      substrates for, 408-410
    thermogenesis in. See Thermogenesis,
      nonshivering.
    UCP1 and, 405f, 405-408, 406f
      acute regulation of, 406-407, 407f
      adaptive regulation of, 407-408, 408f
      semiacute regulation of, 407
      UCP gene and, 406
  lipids in, 601t
  lipolysis in, 419-420, 420f, 421f
    hypoglycemia and, 495
  white, 405
Admixture lesions, in congenital heart
  disease, 711-712
  single-ventricle physiology with, 711-712
  systemic arterial oxygen saturation
    determinants with, 711
  systemic arterial oxygen saturation versus
    systemic oxygen transport in, 711, 712f
Adrenal cortex, 1915-1923, 1916f. See also
  Corticosteroids; Glucocorticoids;
  Mineralocorticoids; specific
  corticosteroids, e.g. Cortisol.
  adaptation of, to extrauterine life,
    1920 1922, 1922t
  embryogenesis of, 1915
  functional maturation of, fetal, 1915-1919
  fetoplacental steroid metabolism and,
    1918f, 1918-1919, 1919f
  molecular biology of adrenocortical cell
    and, 1915-1917, 1916f
  steroidogenesis and, 1917f, 1917-1918

Adrenal cortex *(Continued)*
    functions of, 1922-1923
    histologic development of, 1915
    regulation of, in fetus and neonate,
        1919-1920
        steroids in, 1920, 1920f, 1921f
        tropic factors in, 1919-1920
Adrenal insufficiency, bronchopulmonary
    dysplasia and, 956
Adrenergic agents, 227-232
    pharmacodynamics of, 228, 229-232, 230f,
        231f
    pharmacokinetics of, 228f, 228-229, 229f
    in neonates, 229
β-Adrenergic agents, for preterm labor, 108,
    109t
β-Adrenergic agonists, lung liquid and, 830
β-Adrenergic blockers, during lactation, 256
Adrenergic nervous system, renal blood flow
    and, 1246-1247
Adrenergic receptors, down-regulation of, in
    shock, neonatal, 775-776
α-Adrenergic receptors, in lower airway, 844
β-Adrenergic receptors
    in brown adipose tissue, 408
    in lower airway, 844
    polymorphisms of, 205
Adrenocorticotropic hormone
    adrenal adaptation to extrauterine life and,
        1921-1922, 1922t
    adrenal regulation by, 1919
    fetal regulation of
        human studies of, 1910-1911
        in fetal sheep, 1911-1913, 1911f-1913f
    pattern during pregnancy, 1909-1910
    placental, 124
    plasma concentration of, fetal and neonatal,
        1922t
    significance of, fetal, 1913-1914
    source of, 1909
Adrenomedullin, umbilicoplacental
    circulation mediation by, 752t
Adsorption reservoirs, 1027, 1027f
Aerobic glycolysis, 1716
Afferent(s), of lower airway, 842, 843f
Afferent thermosensitive pathways, 552
Afterload
    decreased, cardiovascular physiology and,
        714
    fetal, 650-651, 652f
    increased
        cardiovascular physiology and, 713-714
        congenital cardiac lesions causing, 714
    myocardial contractility and, 638
Age
    conceptional, 1726
    developmental, apoptosis versus necrosis
        and, 74
    gestational, respiratory water and
        evaporative heat loss related to, 577,
        581t
    of neonate, glucose metabolism in, 458,
        458f
    standard metabolic rate and, 549-550,
        550f
    thermoregulation and, 557, 557f
Agonists, 188-189
Air-blood barrier, 783, 787-788
    nutrition and, 808
Airflow mechanics, measurement of, 923-924,
    924f
Airway(s)
    distending airway pressure applied to, for
        hyaline membrane disease, 932-933,
        933f

Airway(s) *(Continued)*
    fetal
        contractions of, lung liquid flow and, 822
        surgical obstruction of, lung liquid flow
            and, 822
    lower, 842-847, 843f
        in neonatal lung injury, function of,
            846-847, 847f
        innervation of, 842-846
            afferents and, 842, 843f
            cholinergic, 842-843, 844f
            nonadrenergic noncholinergic,
                844-846, 845f
            sympathetic, 843-844
        physiologic responses of, maturational
            changes in, 846
    reactivity of, measurement of, 838-839
    resistance of, 963, 965f
        in bronchopulmonary dysplasia,
            established, 957-958
    upper, 834-840
        embryology of, 834
        function of
            clinical assessment of, 837-840, 839f
            mechanical ventilation and, 836-837,
                837f
        injury of
            endoscopic evaluation of, 839-840
            radiographic evaluation of, 839
        mechanics and regulation of, 834f,
            835-836, 836f
        muscles of, in apnea, 911-912, 911f-913f
        reflexes of, in apnea, 912-914, 914f
        structure of, 834-835
Airway reflexes, in neonatal pulmonary host
    defense, 1625-1626
Alanine
    fetal accretion of, 531t
    fetal uptake of, 520
    in parenteral amino acid mixtures, 533t, 534t
    normal plasma and urine levels of, 1296t
    requirements for, of low birth weight
        infants, 530t-532t
β-Alanine, normal plasma and urine levels of,
    1296t
Albinism, 591-592
    oculocutaneous, 592, 592t
    optic nerve lesion associated with, 1690
Albumin, serum, in neonatal nutritional
    assessment, 297
Albuterol, during lactation, 255
Alcohol (ethanol)
    amino acid transport and, 517
    contraindication to, for nursing mothers, 255
    for preterm labor, 108, 109t
    maternal use/abuse of, 234-237
        alcohol pharmacology and, 235
        clinical management of, during
            pregnancy, 236t, 236-237
        fetal and neonatal effects of, 234-236, 235t
    pharmacology of, 235
Aldosterone
    functions of, 1923
    plasma concentration of, fetal and neonatal,
        1922t
    potassium homeostasis and, 1285
    renal tubular function and, 1237
    sodium transport in distal renal tubule and,
        1273t, 1273-1274
Alkalemia, potassium homeostasis and, 1281
Alkalosis
    metabolic
        fetal, 1362
        neonatal, 1364
        potassium homeostasis and, 1285

Alkalosis *(Continued)*
    respiratory
        fetal, 1362
        metabolic compensation for, neonatal,
            1329-1330
        neonatal, 1364
Allantois, 1108
    definition of, 114t
Alobar holoprosencephaly, 1680, 1682f
Alpha-tocopherol. *See also* Vitamin E.
    protection during antioxidant stress, 355
    γ-tocopherol versus, 356-357
Aluminum, accumulation of, in cholestasis,
    1220
Alveolar capillary dysplasia, 792
Alveolar dead space, in hyaline membrane
    disease, 931
Alveolar epithelium, 1034-1040
    air-liquid interface establishment and,
        1038-1039
    basal lamina and, gestational changes in,
        1037
    historical perspective on, 1034, 1035f
    in utero development of, 1034-1036, 1036f
    postnatal maturation of, 1039f, 1039-1040,
        1040f
    secretory event and, 1038, 1038f
    surfactant desorption and recycling and,
        1039
    surfactant metabolism and, 1036, 1037f,
        1037t
    transition to air breathing and, 1037, 1038f,
        1039, 1039f
    type II, organization during development,
        1036-1037
Alveolar instability, in hyaline membrane
    disease, 930, 931f
Alveolar stability, surfactant and, 1021-1023,
    1022f
Alveolar wall, structure of, 795
Alveolar-capillary respiratory membrane, 783,
    787-788
    diffusion through, pulmonary gas exchange
        and, 879
    nutrition and, 808
Alveolarization, 794-800, 795, 796f, 799t, 818
    alveolar wall structure and, 795
    lung development and, phases of, 795
    regulation of, 796-799
        estrogens and, 798-799
        fibroblast growth factor and, 799
        glucocorticoids and, 797-798
        growth factors and, 799
        inflammation and, 799
        nutrition and, 799
        oxygen and, 799
        platelet-derived growth factor and, 797
        retinoic acid and, 798
        testosterone and, 798, 799
        thyroid hormone and, 799
        vascular endothelial growth factor and,
            796-797
Alveologenesis, 789
Alveolus(i)
    basal lamina of, gestational changes in,
        1037
    formation of, 789
        impairment of, after lung injury in
            premature lung, 946-947
    surfactant and. *See* Surfactant, pulmonary;
        Surfactant proteins; Surfactant therapy.
Amino acid(s). *See also* Protein(s).
    absorption of, 1156-1157
    accretion of, changing rates of, 530
    balance of, 522-523, 523f, 523t

Amino acid(s) (Continued)
  blood-brain barrier transport systems for,
    1701
  branched-chain, fetal uptake of, 519-520
  chemistry of, 527-528
  dietary, classification of, 528, 528t
  essential, 528, 528t
    requirements for, 506-507, 507f
  excitatory, 1710f, 1710-1712, 1711f
  fetal utilization of, 456
  free, tracer studies of, 507
  homeostasis of, imbalances and, 517
  kinetics of, 504-506, 505f, 506f
  metabolism of
    fetal
      in skeletal muscle, 522
      oxidation and, 520-521
    in fetal growth restriction pregnancies,
      262-265, 264f
    in mid-gestation, 521
    whole body, models for, 501-502, 502f
  placental consumption of, 517
  placental transport of. See Placental
    transfer/transport, of amino acids.
  requirements for, 506-507, 507f, 529-532,
    530t-532t
    for parenteral nutrition, 532-534, 533t,
      534t
  transport of, 1294-1298, 1295f
    developmental aspects of, 1295, 1296t,
      1297-1298
    in fetal growth restriction pregnancies,
      262-265, 264f
  uptake of
    in brown adipose tissue, 410
    umbilical, 517-520, 518f
      placentofetal amino acid cycling and,
        518-520, 519f
    uterine, 517
Aminoacidopathies, 1212t
Aminoaciduria, developmental, 1295
Aminogram, plasma, in neonatal nutritional
  assessment, 297
Aminophylline
  for apnea, 914-915
  for preterm labor, 109t
Amniocentesis, microbial recovery during,
  133-134
Amnion, definition of, 114t
Amniotic epithelium, 95
Amniotic fluid, aspiration of, 937
AMP. See Adenosine monophosphate.
Amphetamines, maternal use of, 244, 245
  contraindication to, for nursing mothers, 255
Amphipathic molecules, 1018
Amplitude spectrum, of sound, 1803
Amylase
  pancreatic, in neonates, 1152
  salivary
    in neonates, 1152
    prenatal, 1152
Anaerobic glycolysis, 1716
Anal regions, embryology of, 36-37, 37f
Analgesics. See also specific drugs and drug
    types.
  during lactation, 255
Anaphylatoxins, complement-derived, 1551
Anchoring villi, 85, 92
Androgens. See also Testosterone.
  brain development and, 1789
  growth plate control by, 1835
  plasma concentration of, fetal and neonatal,
    1922t
Androstenedione, plasma concentration of,
  fetal and neonatal, 1922t

Anemia
  hypoproliferative, 1413-1417
  maternal, in multiple pregnancy, 168
  of bronchopulmonary dysplasia, 1417
  of prematurity, 1413-1416
    erythropoietin for
      clinical trials in, 1414, 1415t
      pharmacokinetics and, 1414, 1416
      side effects of, 1416
    nutritional supplementation in, 1416
  of Rh disease, late, 1416-1417
  oxygen delivery to tissues and, 888, 888f
  with congenital anomalies requiring
    surgery, 1417
  with congenital heart disease, 1417
Anencephaly, 1678, 1678f, 1777f, 1778, 1780
  gonadotropic secretion abnormalities
    associated with, 1903
Anergy, 1516
Anesthesia
  in infants, thermogenesis and, 411
  local, uteroplacental blood flow and, 763
Aneuploidy, 9
Ang-1/Ang-2, vascular development and, 624f,
  624-625, 625f
Angelman syndrome, 10
Angioblast(s), 35, 35f
  hepatic, 1176
Angioblastic clusters, 35, 35f
Angiogenesis, 79-83, 80f, 622, 623f, 623-624,
  624f, 625f, 1444-1445
  angiogenic growth factors and receptors
    and, 81-82
  biomechanical force and, 55
  defects in, of skin, 594
  definition of, 622
  embryonic, 80
  extracellular matrix and, 54-56
  extracellular matrix-dependent changes in
    cell shape and, 55-56
  integrins and, 55
  matrix metalloproteinases and, 55
  placental, 80-81
  pulmonary, 818
Angiopoietins, 81-82
Angiotensin II
  adrenal regulation by, 1920
  adrenocortical development and, 1917
  arterial baroreflex and, 720-721
  as growth factor, 1254t, 1254-1255
  blood pressure and, 1252-1253, 1253f
  chorionic, 127
  fluid and electrolyte balance and, 1254
  glomerular filtration rate and, 1257
  hypoxia and, 655
  maturational changes in, 1251
  molecular biology of, 1249
  receptors for
    maturational changes in, 1251-1252,
      1252f
    molecular biology of, 1249-1250
  renal hemodynamics and, 1244-1245,
    1253-1254
  sodium transport in distal renal tubule and,
    1273t, 1273-1274
  umbilicoplacental circulation and, 752t,
    754f
  uteroplacental blood flow and, 99-100,
    100f, 101f
Angiotensin-converting enzyme
  inhibitors of
    during lactation, 256
    glomerular filtration rate and, 1265
  maturational changes in, 1251
  molecular biology of, 1249

Angiotensinogen
  activity of, maturational changes in, 1250
  molecular biology of, 1249
Annular pancreas, 1103
Anorectal motility, 1135
  in neonates, 1135
Anserine, normal plasma and urine levels of,
  1296t
Antagonists, 188-189
Antennapedia gene, in central nervous system
  development, 1677
Anterior dysrhythmia, on
  electroencephalography, 1736t,
  1738-1739, 1739f
Anterior nucleus, hypothalamic, 1872t
Anteroposterior axis
  determination of, 1831
  in limb development, 1846, 1848t
Anthropometry, neonatal, 293-296
Antiasthma agents, during lactation, 255
Antibodies. See Immunoglobulin(s); specific
    immunoglobulins.
Antibody-dependent cellular cytotoxicity,
  1532-1533
  in host defense against viruses, 1500
  neonatal, 1505-1506
  of neutrophils, 1546-1547
Anticipation, 7
Anticoagulants, contraindication to, for
    nursing mothers, 253t, 253-254
Anticodons, 4
Anticonvulsants, during lactation, 256
Antidiuretic hormone. See Vasopressin.
Antigen(s), of fetal erythrocytes, 1409-1410
Antigen-presenting cells, 1533-1534
  fetal and newborn capabilities of, 1534
Antihypertensive agents
  during lactation, 256
  for preeclampsia, 154
Antiinfective agents, during lactation, 255-256
Antiinflammatory components, in human
    milk, 281, 1614, 1614t
Antimetabolites, contraindication to, for
    nursing mothers, 253, 253t
Antimicrobial agents
  during lactation, 255-256
  natural, 1479-1480
Antioxidants
  deficiency of, in prematurity, 939
  in human milk, 1614
  retinal development of, 1798-1799, 1799t
  vitamin E as, 354-355
Antiplasmin
  in children, 1442t
  in full-term infants, 1440t
  in premature infants, 1440t
Antithrombin
  in adults, 1436t
  in children, 1441t
  in fetuses, 1436t
  in full-term infants, 1436t, 1439t
  in premature infants, 1439t
Antitrypsin
  in children, 1441t
  in full-term infants, 1439t
  in premature infants, 1439t
  α_1-Antitrypsin deficiency, 1215
Anus, imperforate, 1109
Aorta, coarctation of, afterload increase with,
  714
Aorta-gonad-mesonephros region,
  hematopoiesis in, 1377, 1388
Aortic blood flow, fetal, during labor, 762
Aortic regurgitation, cardiovascular
    physiology and, 714

Aortic stenosis, afterload increase with, 714
Apert syndrome, 48, 786, 790, 1857t
Apgar scoring, resuscitation and, 766, 766t
Apical ectodermal ridge, 1829-1830, 1830f
  in limb development, 1845-1846
Apical membrane, of mammary alveolar cell,
  transport across, 286
Apnea
  central, 906
  continuum from infant to child and adult
    and, 915-916
  idiopathic, 907, 916
  in neonates, 895-896, 896f, 897f
  mixed, 905-906, 906f
  obstructive, 906
  of prematurity, 905-917
    classification of, 905-906, 906f
    definition of, 905
    epidemiology of, 907, 909f
    initiation of, 916
    neurodevelopmental outcome of,
      915-916
    physiologic effects of, 906-907,
      907f-909f
    physiologic factors in, 907-914
      alteration in central drive as, 907-909,
        910f
      chemoreceptor and mechanoreceptor
        responses as, 910f, 910-911
      gastrointestinal reflux as, 914
      periodic breathing as, 911, 911f
      sleep state as, 909-910
      upper airway and chest wall muscle
        responses as, 911-912, 911f-913f
      upper airway reflexes as, 912-914,
        914f
    sudden infant death syndrome and, 915
    termination of, 916-917
    therapeutic interventions for, 914-916
      body position and, 915
      continuous positive airway pressure
        as, 914, 914f
      pharmacologic, 914-915, 915t
Apneic threshold level, 892
Apolipoprotein E, in high density lipoprotein,
  of fetus and newborn, 360
Apoptosis, 72-74
  activation through death receptors, after
    tissue injury, 74
  choice between necrosis and, factors
    determining, 74-75
  following brain injury, molecular evidence
    of, 73-74
  following hypoxia-ischemia, 73
  in cerebral injury, relation between necrosis
    and, 73
  in folliculogenesis, 1945
  in morphologic development of embryo
    and fetus, 72
  in neuronal damage, 73
  mitochondria in, 75-77
    Bcl-2 family members and, 76-77
    mitochondrial permeability transition
      and, 75-76, 76f, 77
  modes of cell death in tissue injury and, 73
  of malignant cells, α-lactalbumin and, 280
  of stem cells, 1369
  preeclampsia and fetal growth impairment
    and, 153
  prevention or suppression of, by
    hypothermia, 586
  T cell, in host defense against viruses,
    neonatal, 1504-1505
  testicular, 1954
  trophoblastic invasion and, 93-94

Apoptosomes, 72
Apoptotic cells, clearance of, complement
  and, 1552
Apparent life-threatening events, 915
Apparent volume of distribution, 192-193
aPTT. See Activated partial thromboplastin
  time.
Aquaporins
  in fetus, urinary concentration and, 1311
  urinary concentration and, 1307t,
    1307-1309
  in neonates, 1314-1316, 1315f
Aqueous pores hypothesis, 198
Arachidonic acid. See also Fatty acids, long
  chain.
  accumulation of, maternal influences on,
    430
  in neonatal pulmonary host defense, 1642
  renal blood flow and, 1246
Arcuate nucleus, hypothalamic, 1872t
ARF. See Acute renal failure.
Arginine
  fetal accretion of, 531t
  in parenteral amino acid mixtures, 533t,
    534t
  normal plasma and urine levels of, 1296t
  requirements for, of low birth weight
    infants, 530t-532t
Arginine vasporessin. See Vasopressin.
Arginosuccinic aciduria, 595
Arm fat area assessment, in neonatal
  nutritional assessment, 295
Arm muscle measurement, in neonatal
  nutritional assessment, 295
Arousal, essential fatty acid deficiency and,
  433
Arterial baroreflex
  humoral interactions on, 720-721
  neonatal, function of, 721
  resetting of, 719-720
  sensitivity of, mechanisms regulating, 718,
    719f
Arterial blood flow, cerebral. See Cerebral
  arterial blood flow velocity.
Arterial oxygen content, cerebral blood flow
  and, 1746
Arteries, trophoblastic invasion of, 94
Artificial ventilation. See Mechanical
  ventilation.
Arylamine N-acetyltransferase 2
  polymorphism, 214-215
Asparagine, requirements for, of low birth
  weight infants, 530t
Aspartate
  fetal accretion of, 531t
  in parenteral amino acid mixtures, 533t,
    534t
  requirements for, of low birth weight
    infants, 530t-532t
Aspartic acid, normal plasma and urine levels
  of, 1296t
Asphyxia
  birth, hyperinsulinism in, 495-496
  glomerular filtration rate and, 1265
  intraventricular hemorrhage and, 1763
Aspirin
  during lactation, 255
  for preterm labor, 109t
Assist/control ventilation, 974
Assisted ventilation. See High-frequency
  ventilation; Liquid ventilation; Mechanical
  ventilation.
Asymmetric cellular division, 57
Atelectasis, prevention of, patient-triggered
  ventilation for, 936

Atenolol, during lactation, 256
Atopic disease, breast-feeding and, 281
Atosiban
  for preterm labor, 109t
  placental transfer of, 207
ATP. See Adenosine triphosphate.
Atria, septation of, 616
Atrial natriuretic peptide
  as neurotransmitter, 1875t
  chorionic, 127
  glomerular filtration rate and, 1258
  renal blood flow and, 1245
  renal hemodynamics and, 1233
  renal sodium transport regulation by, 1276,
    1276f
  renal tubular function and, 1238
  umbilicoplacental circulation mediation by,
    752t
Atrial septal defects, 715
Atrioventricular canal, septation of, 616
Atrioventricular conduction
  atrioventricular conduction system
    formation and, 678-680, 680f, 680t
  before atrioventricular conduction system
    formation, 678, 679f
  physiology of, 680-682, 681f, 682f
Auditory brain stem response, 1809, 1810,
  1812
Auditory system, 1803f, 1803-1816
  behavioral development and, 1813-1815
    sensitivity and, 1814
    sound localization and, 1814-1815
    speech perception and, 1815
  central auditory nervous system and,
    1810-1813, 1812f, 1813f
  ear and, 1803-1810, 1804f
    cochlea of, 1807-1810, 1808f-1811f
    conductive apparatus of, 1804-1807,
      1806f, 1807f
Augmentation gene therapy, 15
Autonomic nervous system
  cardiac conduction and, 682
  hypothalamic control of, 1873
Autoregulation
  hypoxia and, 654
  of cerebral blood flow, 1746
  of glomerular filtration rate, 1258
  of organ blood flow, 776
  of renal blood flow, 1258
    postnatal, 1242-1243
  pressure-flow, 703
AVP. See Vasopressin.
Axons, outgrowth of, 1689-1690
  disorders of, 1689-1690, 1690f
  normal, 1689
Azurophilic granules, 1543, 1543f
  in neonatal pulmonary host defense, 1644

B

B cells
  development of, 1518-1521
    anatomic sites of, 1518
    class switch recombination and, 1521
    commitment to B-cell lineage and,
      1518-1519
    diversification after V(D)J recombination
      and, 1521
    germinal centers and, 1519-1520
    immaturity and, 1521
    ontogeny of V-gene expression and, 1520
    physiological functions of CD5+ B cells,
      1520-1521
    plasma cell differentiation and, 1520

B cells (*Continued*)
  postcommitment, 1519, 1519f
  receptor diversity and, 1520
  tolerance and, 1521
  in host defense, 1478, 1482-1483
    against viruses, 1500
    neonatal, 1505-1506
  in human milk, 1613
  in neonatal pulmonary host defense, 1640
  proliferation of, T-cell signal for, 1517
Bacteria
  colonization by
    of gut, necrotizing enterocolitis and, 1170
    of skin, skin cleansing and, at birth, 602-603, 603t
  normal flora and, in host defense, 1476
Bacterial infection(s)
  changing nature of, 1475-1476
  host defense against, 1476-1483
    B and T lymphocytes in, 1478
    components of, 1480-1483
      B lymphocytes as, 1482-1483
      colony-stimulating factors as, 1482
      interferons as, 1482
      interleukins as, 1481-1482
      natural killer cells as, 1482
      T lymphocytes as, 1480-1481
      tumor necrosis factor as, 1481
    epithelial cells, mucosal barriers, and normal bacterial flora in, 1476
    mast cells in, 1477-1478
    monocytes, macrophages, and dendritic cells in, 1477
    natural antimicrobial agents in, 1479-1480
    natural opsonins in, 1478-1479
    neonatal, complement in, 1554
    neutrophils in, 1476-1477
    pathogen-associated receptors in, 1479
Bacterial lipopolysaccharide, in host defense, 1479
Bacterial permeability-increasing factor, 1479
Bacterial sepsis, cytokine levels during, 1566-1567
Bactericidal actions
  complement-mediated, 1552
  of mononuclear phagocytes, 1532
  of neutrophils, 1544-1546
    nonoxidative, 1546
    oxidative, 1545-1546
Bag and mask ventilation, for resuscitation, limitations of, 769, 770f
Balanced translocation carriers, 7
BALT. *See* Bronchus-associated lymphoid tissue.
Barbiturates, maternal use of, 245
Bardet-Biedl syndrome, 20
Baroreflex, arterial
  humoral interactions on, 720-721
  neonatal, function of, 721
  resetting of, 719-720
  sensitivity of, mechanisms regulating, 718, 719f
Basal cell layer, of skin, 589
Basal lamina, alveolar, gestational changes in, 1037
Basal metabolic rate, 549
Basal plate, 92
Base deficit, resuscitation and, 768, 769f
Base pairing, 1
Basement membrane, of brain capillaries, 1701
Basic helix-loop-helix protein, 1850
Basolateral membrane, calcium transport across, 1287

Bayley Scales of Infant Development, docosahexaenoic acid and, 436
B-cell activating factor, 1519
Bcl-2 protein, apoptotic inhibition by, 76-77
Beckwith-Wiedemann syndrome, 1888
Beds, heated, heat exchange between infant and environment in, 572
Behavior, essential fatty acid deficiency and, 431-433
Behavioral fever, 567
Behavioral markers, for pain, 1794
Behavioral regulation, of heat loss, 559
Behavioral states
  concept of, 1726
  electroencephalography and, 1726-1729, 1727t, 1728f, 1728t
Benzodiazepines, maternal use of, 244-245
Beta-adrenergic agents, for preterm labor, 108, 109t
Beta-adrenergic agonists, lung liquid and, 830
Beta-adrenergic blockers, during lactation, 256
Beta-adrenergic receptor polymorphisms, 205
Beta-endorphins, 1875t
  fetal regulation of, 1910
  pattern during pregnancy, 1909-1910
  source of, 1909
Beta-lipotropin
  pattern during pregnancy, 1909-1910
  source of, 1909
Betamethasone, protein binding of, 205t
Bicarbonate
  potassium homeostasis and, 1281
  renal bicarbonate threshold and, 1328
  tubular reabsorption of
    developmental aspects of, 1329
    in mature kidney, 1327-1328
Bile
  composition of, 1188-1189, 1189f
  flow of
    cholestasis and. *See* Cholestasis.
    inadequate, consequences of, 1220
    ontogeny of, 1218-1219
    transporters and, 1190-1192
      basolateral, 1190-1191
      canalicular, 1191-1192
      developmental expression of, 1192
      regulation of, 1190-1192, 1191f
    formation of, 1187-1188, 1189
    neonatal, 1192-1193
Bile acids, 1158, 1179-1184
  chemical structure and properties of, 1179-1180
  conjugated, placental transfer of, 208
  enterohepatic circulation of, 1181-1182, 1182f, 1189-1190, 1190f
    alteration in, 1183-1184
    during development, 1183, 1184f
  in bile, 1188
  metabolism of, 1182-1183
    altered, 1183-1184, 1184t
    placental role in, 1183
  physiologic function of, 1179, 1180f, 1180t
  synthesis of, 1180f, 1180-1181, 1181f
    alteration in, 1184
    disorders of, 1193-1194
    during development, 1182t, 1182-1183, 1183f
    regulation of, 1181, 1181f
Bile ducts
  development of, 1176-1177
  intrahepatic, formation of, 1188
Bile salt export pump, 1191-1192
Bile salt-stimulated lipase, 1157
Biliary tree, development of, 1188, 1188t, 1189f

Bilirubin, 1199-1204
  conjugation of, 1199-1200
    genetic variations in, 1200
  elevation of, in neonatal hyperbilirubinemia, 1199, 1200-1201
  excretion of, 1200
  light absorption by, 1206-1207, 1207f
  photochemistry of, 1207-1209
    configurational isomerization and, 1207-1208, 1208f
    photo-oxidation and, 1208-1209
    structural isomerization and, 1208, 1209f
  photoproduct formation by, 1209, 1209f
  phototherapy and. *See* Phototherapy, for jaundice.
  production of, 1199
  structure of, 1205-1206, 1206f
  transport and uptake of, 1199
  unconjugated, toxicity of, 1201-1202
    affinity for nerve cells and, 1202-1203
    bilirubin entry into brain and, 1201-1202, 1202f
    cellular, 1203-1204
    clinical aspects of, 1204
Bilirubin encephalopathy, 1201, 1204
Biliverdin reductase, 1199
Bioavailability, of drugs, 180-181
Biochemical markers
  in neonatal nutritional assessment, 296-298
  of glomerular filtration rate, 1258-1259, 1259f, 1260f, 1260t
  of inflammation, 1587-1588
  of nonshivering thermogenesis, 544-545, 546t
  of preterm labor, 107
Bioelectrical impedance analysis, total body, for body water measurement, 1352-1353
Biomechanical force, angiogenesis and, 55
Biopsychosocial model, anemia of, 1417
Biotransformation, of drugs, 182-184, 183t
  in liver, factors affecting, 184
  phase I reactions in, 182-183, 183t
  phase II reactions in, 183t, 184
Biotrauma, 964
Bipotent stem cells, 1365
Birth. *See also* Delivery; Labor.
  adaptation to extrauterine life and
    adrenal, 1920-1922, 1922t
    thyroid hormones and, 1930-1932, 1931f
  establishment of continuous breathing at, 893-894, 894f, 895f
  glomerular filtration rate at, 1262-1263, 1263f
  lung injury at, mechanical, 935
  lung liquid flow after, 823
  myocardial function and, 652-653, 653f
  preterm. *See* Preterm labor.
  skin transition at, 600t, 600-604, 601t
    acid mantle development and, 601-602, 603f
    bacterial colonization and skin cleansing and, 602-603, 603t
    cutaneous immunosurveillance and, 603-604, 604f, 604t
    water loss, temperature control, and blood flow and, 601, 601f-603f
  surfactant pool size changes after, 1057-1058, 1058f
  sympathetic nervous system activity of, 722-724, 723f, 724f
  thermoregulatory system maturity at, 563-565, 564f
  thyroid system and, 1930-1932, 1931f
  transition to air breathing at, 1037, 1038f

Birth (Continued)
   surfactant changes associated with, 1039,
      1039f
   umbilicoplacental circulation closure at,
      754
   vitamin A at
      plasma status of, 349
      storage of, 349
Birth weight. See also Low birth weight
      infants.
   maternal marijuana use and, 241
Bitter taste, newborn responses to, 1822
Blastema, precartilage, 1831
Blastocyst, 29, 30f, 58
   placental development and. See Placenta,
      development of.
Blastomeres, 29
Bleeding. See Coagulation entries; Factor
      entries; Hemorrhage; Hemostasis.
Bleeding disorders, neonatal, 1447-1457
   in liver disease, 1454
   inherited, 1450-1452
      combined factor deficiencies as, 1452
      factor XIII deficiency as, 1452
      factors I, V, and X deficiencies as,
         1451-1452
      hemophilia as, 1450-1451, 1452t
      von Willebrand's disease as, 1452
   intracerebral hemorrhage and, 1454-1455
   normal hemostasis and, 1447-1448
   patient evaluation in, 1448f, 1448-1450
      clinical laboratory evaluation for,
         1448-1449
      for risk of hemorrhagic complications,
         1450, 1451t
      limitations of clinical laboratory for,
         1449-1450, 1450f
   qualitative platelet disorders and, 1455
   thrombocytopenia as, 1455-1457, 1456t
      alloimmune, 1457
      autoimmune, 1457
      primary, 1455-1456
      secondary, 1456-1457
   vitamin K deficiency and, 1452-1454, 1453f
Bleeding time, in neonates, 1444, 1449
Blood. See also specific components, e.g.
      Erythrocytes.
   coagulation of. See also Coagulation
      factors; Factor entries; Hemostasis.
      animal models of, 1444
      intraventricular hemorrhage and, 1764
      vitamin K and, 369
   deficiency of. See Ischemia.
   differential counts in, 1397, 1399t
   oxygenation of, deficient. See Hypoxemia.
   volume of, 1341, 1342t, 1343t, 1402
      during labor and delivery, 1345
      maternal, in pregnancy, 143, 143t
      measurement of, 1346t, 1346-1347
Blood flow. See also Circulation;
      Hemodynamics.
   cerebral. See Cerebral blood flow.
   cerebral artery. See Cerebral arterial blood
      flow velocity.
   fetal
      circulatory failure and, 657-659, 660f,
         661f
      with congenital malformation of heart,
         657, 658f, 659f
      heat loss and, 559, 560f
      in fetal growth restriction pregnancies,
         260-261
         umbilical blood flow and, 260-261, 261f
         uterine blood flow and, 260
      placental, 223-224

Blood flow (Continued)
   pulmonary
      effective versus ineffective, 707
      ratio to systemic blood flow, 707
   redistribution of, hypoxia and, 655-656
   regional, maternal, in pregnancy, 143t, 144
   renal. See Renal blood flow.
   systemic
      ratio to pulmonary blood flow, 707
      reduction of, reduction of oxygen
         transport due to, 706-707
      resuscitation and, 769-770, 770f
   umbilical. See Umbilical blood flow.
   uterine, during pregnancy
      anatomic changes in, 144-145, 145f
      functional and molecular changes in,
         145-146
   uteroplacenta. See Uteroplacental blood flow.
   uteroplacental. See Uteroplacental blood
      flow.
Blood islands, 35, 35f
Blood pressure
   arterial, fetal, maintenance of,
      umbilicoplacental circulation in,
      753-754
   during apnea, 907, 909f
   elevated. See Hypertension; Hypertension,
      pulmonary.
   low
      glomerular filtration rate and, 1265
      pressor-resistant, in neonates, 777
   maternal, in pregnancy, 143t, 144. See also
      Preeclampsia/eclampsia.
   regulation of, 717-724
      angiotensin II in, 1252-1253, 1253f
      cardiopulmonary reflexes and, 721-722
      chemoreflex responses and, 722
      neural modulation of basal hemodynamic
         state and, 717-721, 719f
         arterial baroreflex and, 719-721
      sympathetic activity at birth and,
         722-724, 723f, 724f
   systemic, neonatal, 776
Blood vessels. See Pulmonary vasculature;
      Vasculature; specific types of vessels, e.g.
      Capillaries.
Blood-brain barrier, 1699-1704
   cellular biology of, 1704
   development of, 1702-1704, 1703f
   fetal, 226
   mature, 1699, 1699t, 1700f, 1701-1702, 1702f
Blood-testis barrier, 1954
Blot hybridization, 11f, 11-12
BMP4, in lung development, 817-818
Body composition, neonatal, assessment of,
      292-293, 293f, 293t, 294t
Body length, in neonatal nutritional
      assessment, 294
Body mass, standard metabolic rate and,
      549-550, 550f
Body position, apnea and, 915
Body temperature. See also Fever; Heat;
      Hyperthermia; Hypothermia;
      Thermogenesis.
   as nonshivering thermogenesis marker, 546t
   classes of organisms and, 548
   deep (core), stability during ontogenesis,
      562, 562f, 563f
   maternal, changes of, 542-543
   normal, 554
   standard metabolic rate and, 550, 550f
Body water, 1351-1355
   compartmentation of, 1351, 1352f
   extracellular, 1351
      measurement of, 1353

Body water (Continued)
   intracellular, 1351
      measurement of, 1353
   loss of
      neonatal, 570-571
         through skin, 601, 601f
      respiratory, 571, 576-577, 580f, 580t
         during mechanical ventilation, 577
         during phototherapy, 577, 581t
         gestational age and, 577, 581t
         intubation and, 577
      through skin
         determination of, 570-571
         during first day and first 4 postnatal
            weeks, 572-573, 574f, 575t
         nonionizing radiation and, 575-576,
            579f
   maturational changes in volume of,
      1353-1355, 1354f
   placental transfer of, 118-119
   postnatal changes in, 1355, 1355f
   reabsorption of, fetal, maturation of, 1309,
      1309f, 1310f
   total body, measurement of, 1351-1353,
      1352f
   transcellular, 1351
Body weight. See also Birth weight; Low birth
      weight infants.
   gain in, maternal, in multiple pregnancy,
      169
   genetic obesity and, 412
   in neonatal nutritional assessment, 294
   loss of, neonatal, 1345
Bohr effect, 883-884
Bombesin, pancreatic secretion and, 1148
Bone(s). See also Musculoskeletal entries.
   formation of, 1831f, 1831-1832, 1832f
   growth plate of. See Growth plate.
Bone collar, 1831
Bone marrow
   differential counts in, 1397, 1399t
   hematopoiesis in, 1377
Bone marrow transplantation, 1369-1370
Bone mineralization measurements, in
      neonates, 299, 299t
Bone morphogenic protein, 1850
BPD. See Bronchopulmonary dysplasia.
BPI, neutrophil, 1543-1544, 1544t
Bradycardia, during apnea, 906-907
Bradykinin
   glomerular filtration rate and, 1258
   renal blood flow and, 1245
   umbilicoplacental circulation mediation by,
      752t
Bradymetabolic organisms, 548
Brain. See also Central nervous system.
   bilirubin entry into, 1201-1202, 1202f
   capillaries of, 1699. See also Blood-brain
      barrier.
   basement membrane of, 1701
   development of, 1785-1789
      embryonic, 32, 33t
      essential fatty acids and, 1788-1789
      fetal, 389-390
         biochemical development and
            myelination and, 389
         fatty acid deficiency and, 389f,
            389-390
         lipid composition changes during, 390
      maternal alcohol consumption and, 236
      neural, 1785-1786
      neurotrophic proteins and, 1786-1787
      vitamins and, 1787-1788
   electroencephalography and. See
      Electroencephalography.

Brain (Continued)
  energy status of, resuscitation and, 771, 771f
  glucose transporters in, 491
  lipid composition of, change in, during fetal
      development, 390
  neonatal, ketone bodies in, 426
  oxidative metabolism in. See Cerebral
      metabolism.
  oxygenation of, resuscitation and, 771
  smooth, 1688
Brain injury
  apoptosis in
      hypothermia and, 586
      molecular evidence for, 73-74
      relation between necrosis and, 73
  cerebral metabolism and, 586
  chorioamnionitis and, 1565-1566
  excitotoxins and, 583, 586
  free radicals and, 586
  inflammatory second messengers in,
      suppression of, 586
  latent phase of, intracellular pathways in, 586
  necrosis in, relation between apoptosis
      and, 73
  neuroprotection for, hypothermia for. See
      Hypothermia, neuroprotection using.
  pathophysiologic phases of, 583, 583f, 584f
Brain natriuretic peptide, umbilicoplacental
      circulation mediation by, 752t
Brain stem, thermoreceptors in, 552
Branchial arch code, hindbrain and, 45
Branching morphogenesis, 783
  in lung development, 812, 815-816
      molecular mechanisms regulating,
          786-787
Breast
  developmental anatomy of, 285, 285f
  zinc metabolism in, 344
Breast-feeding. See also Human milk;
      Lactation.
  cognitive function and, 282
  formula versus, gastrointestinal tract
      growth and, 1096-1097
  infant growth related to, 277
  late effects of, 281
  protective effects of, against necrotizing
      enterocolitis, 1171
Breathing
  artificial. See Mechanical ventilation.
  continuous, establishment at birth,
      893-894, 894f, 895f
  control of, 890-899
      conceptual perspective on, 890
      establishment of continuous breathing at
          birth and, 893-894, 894f, 895f
      fetal, 890-893
          agents modifying, 891-893, 892f, 893f
          breathing pattern at rest and, 890, 891f
          fetal state and, 890-891, 891f, 892f
      historical perspective on, 890
      neonatal, 894-899
          breathing pattern at rest and, 894-895,
              895f
          chemical, 896-898, 898f
          periodic breathing and apnea and,
              895-896, 896f, 897f
          pulmonary reflexes and, 898
          respiratory muscles and, 898-899
  coordination with swallowing, 1126-1127
  host defense and, 1625
  energetics of, 868-869, 869f
  fetal breathing movements and
      diaphragm and, 855, 856f
      lung development and, 805
      lung liquid flow and, 822

Breathing (Continued)
  mechanics of, 864-869, 865t
      active, 866-868
          expiratory time constant and, 867-878
          of chest wall distortion, 866-867, 868f
          energetics of breathing and, 868-869,
              869f
      passive, 864-866
          during artificial ventilation, 864-865
          during spontaneous breathing,
              865-866, 866f, 867f
      terminology related to, 865t
  neurochemical control of, 962, 962t
  of air, transition to, at birth, 1037, 1038f
  periodic, 905. See also Apnea.
      apnea related to, 911, 911f
      in neonates, 895-896, 896f, 897f
  regulation of, 768-769
  resuscitation and
      bag and mask ventilation for, limitations
          of, 769, 770f
      first inflations and, 769, 770f
      in premature infants, 769
      insufflation pressure and, 769
      time to first breath and, 767, 768t
  spontaneous, mechanics of, 864
      passive, 865-866, 866f, 867f
  tidal, airway function measurements during,
      838
Breathing movements, fetal
  diaphragm and, 855, 856f
  lung development and, 805
  lung liquid flow and, 822
Brn-2 gene, in hypothalamic development,
      1874t
Bronchial atresia, 790
Bronchial stenosis, 790
Bronchiolar cysts, 792
Bronchogenic cysts, congenital, 791
Bronchomalacia, 790
Bronchopulmonary dysplasia, 949
  after initial respiratory failure, 934-935
  airway function measurements in, 838, 839f
  airway reactivity measurements in, 838-839
  cardiovascular function in, 959
  cytokine levels during, 1567-1568
  following hyaline membrane disease,
      926-927
  following respiratory distress syndrome,
      945-946
  pathogenesis of, 834
  pathophysiology of, 954-959, 955f, 956f
  pulmonary function in, 956-959
      gas exchange and, 958-959
      in early bronchopulmonary dysplasia,
          956-957
      in established bronchopulmonary
          dysplasia, 957f, 957-958, 958f
      long-term, 959
Bronchopulmonary sequestration, 785-786,
      790-791
Bronchoscopy
  flexible, 840
  rigid, 840
Bronchus-associated lymphoid tissue, in
      neonatal pulmonary host defense,
      1640-1641
Brown adipose tissue. See Adipose tissue,
      brown.
Brown oculocutaneous albinism, 592
BSEP deficiency, 1193
Buffer systems
  extracellular, 1361
      fetal, 1361
      neonatal, 1363

Buffer systems (Continued)
  intracellular, 1361
      fetal, 1361
      neonatal, 1363
Bupivacaine
  placental transfer of, 202t
  protein binding of, 205t
Burst-forming unit-erythroid, 1388, 1397
Burst-forming unit-megakaryocyte, 1421

C

Cadherins, 1854
Caffeine
  for apnea, 914, 915t
  half-life of, 186t
Cajal-Retzius cells, 1684
Calcitonin
  biochemistry of, 310, 311f
  biosynthesis of, 310
  calcium homeostasis and, 309-311, 310f
      neonatal, 326
  calcium transport and, 1288
  metabolism of, 310
  physiologic actions of, 309-310
  placental calcium transport and, 318
Calcitonin gene-related peptide
  calcium homeostasis and, 310-311
  testicular descent and, 1957
  umbilicoplacental circulation mediation by,
      752t
Calcium, 303-311
  calcium handling by, 1286
  calcium-sensing receptor and, 303f,
      303-304
  cellular metabolism of, 304f, 304-305
  cytosolic, contraction and, 637
  distribution in body, neonatal, 323, 324t
  excitation-contraction coupling and,
      638-639
  gastrointestinal transport of, neonatal,
      328-332, 329f, 330f
  homeostasis of, 305-311, 325-327,
      1286-1289
      calcitonin and, 309-310, 310f, 311f, 326
      calcitonin gene-related peptide and,
          310-311
      calcium transport and, 1288
          fetal and neonatal aspects of, 1289
          paracellular, 1286-1287
          regulation of, 1287-1289
          transcellular, 1287, 1287f
      mechanism of, 305
      parathyroid hormone and, 305f, 305-306,
          325-326
      parathyroid hormone-related protein
          and, 306-307
      renal handling and, 1286
      vitamin D and, 307-308, 308f, 326f,
          326-327
  intracellular, ligand-induced mobilization of,
      1599
  maternal plasma concentration of, placental
      calcium transport and, 317
  muscle fiber sensitivity to, in diaphragm,
      861
  myofilament sensitivity to, 637
  placental transport of. See Placental
      transfer/transport, of calcium.
  renal handling of, 1286
  sarcolemmal function and, 646
  transport of
      fetal and neonatal aspects of, 1289
      paracellular, 1286-1287

Calcium (Continued)
   regulation of, 1287-1289
   transcellular, 1287, 1287f
Calcium-channel blockers, for preterm labor, 108, 109t
Calcium-induced calcium release, 638-639
Calcium-sensing receptor, calcium transport and, 1288
Calcium/sodium exchange system, 317
Calorimetry, in neonates, 298
cAMP. See Adenosine monophosphate, cyclic.
Cancer
   apoptosis of malignant cells and, α-lactalbumin and, 280
   childhood, maternal smoking and, 240
   hematopoietic reconstitution in, 1370
   pancreatic, proto-oncogenes and, 1148-1149
   with maldescended testes, 1959
Candidate gene approach, 14
Candidiasis
   invasive, host defense against, 1488-1489
      deficient anticandidal activities of neonatal monocytes and macrophages and, 1488-1489
      phagocytes in, 1488
   mucocutaneous, host defense against, 1487-1488
      deficient T-cell immunity in newborns and, 1488
      virulence factors and surface host defense and, 1487
Cap, in transcription, 3
Capillaries
   integrity of, intraventricular hemorrhage and, 1764
   of brain, 1699. See also Blood-brain barrier.
      basement membrane of, 1701
Capillary membrane, volume loading and, 1348
Capsular chorion frondosum, 95
Capsular decidua, 95
Captive bubble tensiometer, 1023
Captopril, during lactation, 256
Carbamazepine
   during lactation, 256
   half-life of, 186t
Carbohydrates. See also specific carbohydrates, e.g. Glucose.
   digestion of, 1152-1154
      disaccharides and, 1152-1154
         postnatal, 1153-1154
         prenatal, 1152-1153, 1153f
      pancreatic enzymes in, 1146
      polysaccharides and, 1152
         postnatal, 1152, 1152f
         prenatal, 1152
   metabolism of
      cold exposure and, 543
      disorders of, 1212t
      during pregnancy, 464
      fetal
         energy requirements and, 465-466
         energy substrates and, 469-472, 470t-471f
         metabolic rate and, 467-469, 468t, 469t
         oxygen consumption and, 466t, 466-467, 467f, 468f
      in fetal growth restriction pregnancies, 261-262, 263f, 264f
Carbon balance, 523, 523t
Carbon dioxide
   fetal breathing and, 892, 893
   intraventricular hemorrhage and, 1762-1763
   neonatal breathing and, 896-897

Carbon dioxide gradient, gas exchange and, 871-872
Carbon dioxide tension, cerebral blood flow and, 1746
Carbon monoxide
   in neonatal pulmonary host defense, 1632-1633
   umbilicoplacental circulation mediation by, 752t
γ-Carboxylation system, vitamin K-dependent, 370, 370f
   development of, regulation of, 372, 372f
   maturation of, 371f, 371-372, 372f
Cardiac action potential, 669t, 669-676, 670f, 671t, 672f-674f, 673t
   atrial, 677-678, 678f
   developmental changes in, 673-676
      phase 0 and, 675
      phase 1 and, 675f, 675-676
      phases 2 and 3 and, 676, 676t, 677f
      resting membrane potential and, 673-675
   phase 0 of, 671, 672f
      developmental changes in, 675
Cardiac conduction, 676-687
   atrioventricular
      atrioventricular conduction system formation and, 678-680, 680f, 680t
      before atrioventricular conduction system formation and, 678, 679f
      physiology of, 680-682, 681f, 682f
   autonomic innervation-modulation of, 682
   from sinus node to atrioventricular node, 677-678, 678f
   parasympathetic nervous system and, 682, 683f, 684, 684f
   sympathetic nervous system and, 684-687, 686f
Cardiac function, 635-663. See also Myocardial entries.
   hypoxic stress and, 653-657
      acidemia and, 654
      circulation and, 654-656
         flow redistribution and, 655-656
         hematologic adjustments and, 654-655
         humoral responses and, 655
         local response and, 654
         metabolism and, 656
         reflex responses and, 655
      failure of adaptation to, 657
      maladaption to, 656
      myocardial contraction and. See Myocardial contraction.
      ventricular. See Ventricular function.
Cardiac jelly, 615
Cardiac looping, 34
Cardiac malformations, congenital, fetal blood flow patterns with, 657, 658f, 659f
Cardiac muscle. See also Myocardial contraction.
   embryology of, 35
Cardiac neural crest, 614-615
Cardiac output
   maternal, in pregnancy, 143, 143t
   neonatal, 776
   oxygen transport and, 881
   resuscitation and, 770
Cardiac tube, formation and looping of, 615
Cardiomegaly, fetal, 659
Cardiomyocyte, 635, 636f, 637f
Cardiopulmonary reflexes, 721-722
Cardiovascular disease
   drug elimination and, 185
   maternal. See Maternal cardiovascular disease.

Cardiovascular drugs. See also Antihypertensive agents.
   during lactation, 256
Cardiovascular system
   fetal, maternal cocaine use and, 238
   high-frequency ventilation and, 984
   hypothermia and, 586-587
   in bronchopulmonary dysplasia, 959
   in shock. See Shock, cardiovascular compromise and.
   intestinal circulation and, 702-703
   maternal. See Maternal cardiovascular disease; Maternal cardiovascular system.
   respiratory function and, 975-976
   with liquid ventilation, 990
Carnosine, normal plasma and urine levels of, 1296t
Cartilage
   of growth plate, 1833-1834
   of upper airway, 834-835
k-Casein, in human milk, 280
Caspases, 72
Catabolic activator protein, 41
Catecholamines
   in hypoxemia, fetal, 773-774
   neonatal glucose metabolism and, 479
   regulation of renal sodium transport by, 1275f, 1275-1276
   ventilation-perfusion matching and, 878
Cathelicidins
   in neonatal pulmonary host defense, 1628
   neutrophil, 1544, 1544t
Cathepsins, 528
Cation-Cl cotransporters, 1273
Caudal neuropore, 31
C4b-BP
   in adults, 1436t
   in fetuses, 1436t
   in full-term infants, 1436t
CBF. See Cerebral blood flow.
CC chemokines, in neonatal pulmonary host defense, 1650
CCK. See Cholecystokinin.
CCSP, in neonatal pulmonary host defense, 1651-1652
CD antigens, on mononuclear phagocytes, 1526, 1527t-1528t, 1528
CD4 T cells
   antigen processing and presentation and, 1533
   cytolytic, in host defense against viruses, 1496-1497
      neonatal, 1503
   IFN-γ production by, in host defense against viruses, neonatal, 1503
   in host defense against viruses, 1490, 1495
      neonatal, 1502-1503
   in human milk, 1613
CD5 B cells, 1520-1521
CD8 T cells
   in host defense against viruses, 1490, 1497f, 1497-1499, 1498f
      neonatal, 1503-1504
   in human milk, 1613
CD11b protein, 1542
CD18 protein, 1542
CD28, in host defense against viruses, 1499
CD40, in host defense against viruses, 1496, 1496f
   neonatal, 1503
CD40-ligand, in host defense against viruses, 1496, 1496f
   neonatal, 1503
CD80-86, in host defense against viruses, 1499

CD99 protein, 1574t, 1579
cDNA, 12
Cebocephaly, 1680
Cell adhesion, 1572-1573
Cell adhesion molecules, 1573-1588. See also
  Immunoglobulin gene superfamily;
  Integrins; Selectin(s).
  as inflammation markers, 1587-1588
  in neonatal pulmonary host defense,
    1652-1653, 1653f
  modulation of, as adjunctive therapy, 1588
  neonatal expression and function of,
    1585-1586
Cell columns, 85, 86f
Cell cycle, 5
Cell death, programmed. See Apoptosis.
Cell islands, 94
Cell membranes
  apical, of mammary alveolar cell, transport
    across, 286
  cardiac, developmental changes in,
    644-645, 645f
Cell morphology, extracellular matrix-
  dependent changes in, 55-56
Cell replacement therapies, 63-64
Cell signaling, in disseminated intravascular
  coagulation, 1462
Cell surface receptors, on mononuclear
  phagocytes, 1525-1526, 1526f
Cell type, apoptosis versus necrosis and, 74
Cell-cell adhesion junctions, of skin, 590
Cell-cell interactions, testicular, 1954
Cell-matrix adhesion system, of skin, 590
Cellular respiration, 1713
Cellular retinoic acid-binding protein, 348, 348f
Cellular retinol-binding protein type II, 350,
  350f
Central auditory nervous system, 1810-1813,
  1812f, 1813f
Central conduction time, 1812
Central inspiratory drive, alteration in, apnea
  and, 907-909, 910f
Central nervous system. See also Brain; Spinal
  cord.
  development of, 1675t, 1675-1694
    axon outgrowth in, 1689-1690
      disorders of, 1689-1690, 1690f
      normal, 1689
    cytologic specialization in, 1675
    dendritic growth and synapse formation
      in, 1691-1693
      disorders of, 1692-1693
      normal, 1691f, 1691-1692, 1692f
    early cell divisions in, 1675
    embryonic, 1675-1681
      early events in, 1675, 1676f
      primary and secondary neurulation in,
        1675-1679, 1677f, 1678f
      prosencephalic cleavage in, 1679f,
        1679-1681, 1681f, 1682f
    migration and determination of neuronal
      fate in, 1684-1689
      disorders of, 1687-1689, 1688f, 1689f
      normal, 1684-1687, 1685f-1687f
    myelination in, 1693-1694
      disorders of, 1693-1694
      normal, 1693, 1693f
    neuronal and glial proliferation in,
      1681-1684
      disorders of, 1683-1684, 1684f, 1684t
      normal, 1681-1683, 1682f, 1683f
    neuronal death and trophic interactions
      during, 1690-1691
      disorders of, 1691
      normal, 1690-1691

Central nervous system (Continued)
  gastrointestinal contractions and,
    1111-1112, 1112f
  high-frequency ventilation and, 984
Central tolerance, 1521
Centroacinar cells, 1143
Centromeres, 5
Cephalopolysyndactyly, 1848t
Cerebral acidosis, in hypoxia-ischemia,
  1722-1723, 1723f
Cerebral arterial blood flow velocity
  clinical studies of, 1748-1749
    after surfactant replacement therapy,
      1749
    in intraventricular hemorrhage, 1749-1750
    in patent ductus arteriosus, 1749
    in respiratory distress syndrome, 1748,
      1749f
    with pneumothorax, 1748-1749
    with routine procedures, 1749
  hydrocephalus and, 1766-1767
  measurement of, 1747f, 1747-1748
  relation to cerebral blood flow, 1748-1749
    experimental studies of, 1748-1749
    in human newborn, 1748-1749
Cerebral blood flow
  decreases in, intraventricular hemorrhage
    and, 1763-1764
  fetal
    during labor, 762
    maternal cocaine use and, 238
  fluctuating, intraventricular hemorrhage
    and, 1761
  glucose utilization and, 1719, 1719f, 1720f
  in premature infant, 1745-1754
    intraventricular hemorrhage and,
      1745-1746
    measurement of, 1747-1754
      cerebral arterial blood flow velocity
        and. See Cerebral arterial blood
        flow velocity.
      near-infrared spectroscopy for, 1750f,
        1750-1751, 1751f
      quantitative, 1751-1754, 1752f, 1753f
    regulation of, 1746-1747
      arterial oxygen content and, 1746
      autoregulation and, 1746
      blood glucose and, 1747
      carbon dioxide tension and, 1746
  increases in, intraventricular hemorrhage
    and, 1761-1763
  neonatal, 776
  resuscitation and, 771
Cerebral cerebellar development, normal,
  1686-1687, 1687f
Cerebral circulation, pressure-passive,
  intraventricular hemorrhage and,
  1761-1762, 1763
Cerebral cortex
  development of
    disorders of, 1687-1689, 1688f, 1689f
    normal, 1684-1686, 1685f, 1686f
  neurons of, changes in, hydrocephalus and,
    1766
Cerebral functioning,
  electroencephalographic monitoring of,
  1741-1744, 1744f
Cerebral metabolic rate for oxygen, 1715
Cerebral metabolism, 1713-1723, 1714f
  cerebral energy utilization and, 1716-1717,
    1717t
  cerebral glucose utilization and, 1717t,
    1717-1719, 1718f, 1718t, 1719f
    cerebral blood flow related to, 1719,
      1719f, 1720f

Cerebral metabolism (Continued)
  cerebral injury and, 586
  glucose and monocarboxylic acid
    transporters and, 1720-1721, 1721f
  glycolysis and, 1716
  high-energy metabolites and, 1714t,
    1714-1715, 1715f
  in hypoxia-ischemia, 1721-1723, 1722f,
    1723f
  mitochondrial development and, 1716
  quantitative aspects of, 1715f, 1715-1716,
    1716f
Cerebral palsy, preeclampsia and, 154
Cerebral vascular changes, hydrocephalus
  and, 1766
Cerebral venous pressure, increases in,
  intraventricular hemorrhage and, 1763
Cervical effacement, preterm labor and,
  106-107
Cervical incompetence, intra-amniotic
  infection with, 133
Cervicitis, Chlamydia trachomatis, 132
Cesarean section, neonatal thermogenesis
  and, 545-546
CFTR. See Cystic fibrosis transmembrane
  conductance regulator.
CFTR gene, 5
CGRP. See Calcitonin gene-related peptide.
Checkpoints, in cell cycle, 6
Chédiak-Higashi syndrome, 592, 592t
Chemokines
  characteristics of, 1558-1559
  in host defense against viruses, 1492
  in neonatal pulmonary host defense, 1650
  leukocyte mobilization to inflammatory
    sites and, 1580-1581
  receptors for, 1559, 1559t
Chemoreceptors
  in apnea, 910f, 910-911
  in cardiovascular regulation, 722
Chemotactic receptors, viral antigen-specific T
  cell expression of, in host defense against
  viruses, 1499
  neonatal, 1504
Chemotaxis, 1530
  complement-derived, 1551
  of neutrophils, 1541-1542
Chenodeoxycholic acid, 1180. See also Bile
  acids.
Chest wall
  distortion of, mechanics of, 866-867, 868f
  muscles of, in apnea, 911-912, 911f-913f
Chiasmatic nuclei, hypothalamic, 1872t
Chief cells, 1123
Chlamydia trachomatis infection,
  intrauterine infection, 132
Chloramphenicol
  during lactation, 256
  half-life of, 186t
Chloride
  total body, measurement of, 1353
  transepithelial transport of, pulmonary,
    824-825
  transport of, neonatal respiratory disorders
    and, 831
Chloride channels, urinary concentration and,
  1309
Chlorothiazide, during lactation, 256
Chlorpropamide, during lactation, 257
Cholecystokinin
  gastrointestinal tract growth and, 1098
  pancreatic secretion and, 1146, 1147-1148
Cholestasis , 1183-1184
  acquired, 1194
  coagulopathy in, 1454

Cholestasis (Continued)
    congenital, 1193-1194
    hepatic manifestations of, 1216t
    in metabolic disorders, 1214
    neonatal, 1218-1220
        hepatic injury in, mechanisms of,
            1219-1220
        ontogeny of bile flow and, 1218-1219
Cholesterol. See also Lipoprotein(s).
    adrenal steroidogenesis and, 1917
    biosynthesis of, 1180, 1181f
        congenital defects and, 381, 382f, 383f
    fetal development and, 380-384
    fetal sources of, 381, 384
    in bile, 1188, 1189f
    metabolism of, 1180-1181
        fetal development and, 441-442, 442f
        postnatal development and, 443
    serum concentrations of
        in fetal development, 440-441
            in experimental animals, 441
            in humans, 440-441, 441f, 441t
        in postnatal development, 442-443
            in experimental animals, 443
            in humans, 442f, 442-443
        perinatal disease and, 443
Cholic acid, 1180, 1180f. See also Bile acids.
Cholinergic innervation, of lower airway,
    842-843, 844f
Chondrocytes, 1833-1834
    differentiation of, 1831f, 1831-1832, 1832f
    molecular biology of, 1832-1833
Chordal mesoderm, 1675
Chorioamnionitis, 949-951
    animal models of, 950-951, 951f
    brain injury and, 1565-1566
    fetal lung injury due to, 950
    lung maturation and, 950
    preterm birth associated with, 133
    viral, 132
Chorion, definition of, 114t
Chorion frondosum, capsular, 95
Chorionic connective tissue, 95
Chorionic corticotropin-releasing hormone,
    placental, 126f, 126-127
Chorionic gonadotropin-releasing hormone,
    placental, 126
Chorionic plate, 94
Chorionic somatostatin, placental, 126
Chorionic thyrotropin-releasing hormone,
    placental, 126
Chorionicity, 166
    determination of, 166f, 166-167, 167f
Chromatin, 1-2
Chromium-51 ethylenediaminetetra-acetic
    acid, as glomerular filtration rate marker,
    1259
Chromosomal anomalies, in multiple
    pregnancy, 171
Chromosomal deletions, terminal, 7, 7f
Chromosomal disorders, 9-10
Chromosomal mutations, 7, 7f
Chromosomes, 1-2
    nonmendelian disease and, 22, 23f, 24f
Chymotrypsin
    postnatal, 1155
    prenatal, 1155
Chymotrypsinogen, prenatal, 1155
Cigarette smoking, maternal, 239-240
Ciliary function, in neonatal pulmonary host
    defense, 1622f, 1622-1623
Cimetidine, during lactation, 257
Ciprofloxacin, during lactation, 256
Circadian rhythms, hypothalamic control of,
    1873

Circulation. See also Blood flow; Blood
        pressure; Hemodynamics; Hypertension.
    cerebral, pressure-passive, intraventricular
        hemorrhage and, 1761-1762
    fetal
        fetal plasma concentration of drugs and,
            225
        velocimetry in fetal growth restriction
            and, 260
    gastrointestinal. See Intestinal circulation.
    hypoxic effects on, 654-675
        flow redistribution and, 655-656
        hematologic adjustments and, 654-655
        humoral responses and, 655
        local response and, 654
        metabolic, 656
        reflex responses and, 655
    intestinal. See Intestinal circulation.
    maternal, drug transfer into breast milk
        from, 250-251, 251f
    neonatal, physiology of, 776
    placental. See Placental circulation.
    prenatal nutrition and, 727-731
        environmental stimuli and, 728
            transduction of, 730-731
        epidemiologic observations on, 727
        fetal adaptations and, 728-729
        genetics versus environment and, 727-728
        maternal adaptations and, 730
        nutrients and, 728, 728f, 729f
        postnatal adaptations and, 729-730
        timing and, 728
    umbilicoplacental, 749
        anatomy of, 749f, 749-750
        closure of, at birth, 754
    uterine, definition of, 114t
    uteroplacental, maternal adaptations to
        pregnancy and, 143t, 144
Citrulline, normal plasma and urine levels of,
    1296t
Clara cell secretory protein, in neonatal
    pulmonary host defense, 1651-1652
Cleavage, 29
Clinical description of shock, 777
Cloaca, persistent, 1109
Cloacal membrane, 1109
Clonal deletion, 1521
Clonal ignorance, 1521
Cloning, 12, 12f, 16
Clubfoot
    idiopathic, congenital, 1839, 1841f
    rigid, 1840
Coagulation. See also Hemostasis.
    animal models of, 1444
    inhibitors of, consumption of, in
        disseminated intravascular coagulation,
        1462
    intraventricular hemorrhage and, 1764
    vitamin K and, 369
Coagulation factors. See also Factor entries.
    deficiencies of, inherited, 1450-1452
        combined, 1452
        hemophilia as, 1450-1451, 1452t
        of factor XIII, 1452
        of factors II, V, and X, 1451-1452
Coagulation system
    activation of, during inflammatory
        response, 1563
    maternal, in multiple pregnancy, 168
Coagulopathy, consumptive, in disseminated
    intravascular coagulation, 1463
Coarctation of the aorta, afterload increase
    with, 714
Cocaine
    amino acid transport and, 517

Cocaine (Continued)
    detection in fetus, 238-239
    maternal use of, 237-239
        contraindication to, for nursing mothers,
            255
    pharmacology of, 237
Cochlea, 1807-1810, 1808f-1811f
Codons, 3
Cognitive development
    maternal alcohol consumption and, 236
    maternal smoking and, 240
Cognitive function
    breast-feeding and, 282
    essential fatty acid deficiency and, 432
    in offspring, preeclampsia and, 154
Cold exposure
    carbohydrate metabolism and, 543
    thermogenesis and, 543
Colinearity, 45
Collagen(s)
    development of, nutrition and, 808
    hematopoiesis and, 1389-1390
Collagenase, in neonatal pulmonary host
    defense, 1644
Collectins
    in host defense, 1479
    in neonatal pulmonary host defense,
        1629-1631, 1630f
    in pulmonary surfactant, 1008-1012, 1009f,
        1009t, 1011f
Collodion babies, 591
Colloid oncotic pressure, plasma, in acute
    renal failure, 1338
Colonic aganglionosis, 1109, 1114-1115, 1679
Colonic motility, 1134f, 1134-1135, 1141
Colony-forming unit(s), 1388
Colony-forming unit-erythrocyte, 1397
Colony-forming unit-erythroid, 1397, 1400f
Colony-forming unit-granulocyte, 1397
Colony-forming unit-macrophage, 1397
Colony-forming unit-megakaryocyte, 1397,
    1421
Colony-forming units-erythroid, 1388
Colony-stimulating factors
    in host defense, 1482
    in neonatal pulmonary host defense, 1652,
        1652f
Compartments, drug distribution to, 186, 186f
    multicompartment, 187, 187f
    single-compartment, 186
Complement proteins
    biosynthesis of, 1529
    components of, in human milk, 1612
    in host defense, 1478
        against viruses, 1500
        neonatal, 1505-1506
        neonatal, pulmonary, 1626-1627,
            1642-1643, 1643f
Complement receptors, 1542, 1551
Complement system, 1549-1554
    activation of, 1551-1552
        anaphylatoxic activity and, 1551
        antibody formation and, 1552
        apoptotic body clearance and, 1552
        bactericidal activity and, 1552
        chemotactic activity and, 1551
        immune complex processing and, 1552
        opsonic activity and, 1551-1552
    alternative pathway of, 1550-1551
        in neonates, 1552, 1553t
    biochemistry of, 1549-1551, 1550f, 1550t
    C3 and terminal component activation and,
        1551
    classic pathway of, 1549-1550
        in neonates, 1552, 1553t

Complement system (Continued)
complement receptors and, 1551
fetal synthesis of components of, 1552
lectin pathway of, 1551
neonatal
component levels and, 1552-1553, 1553f, 1553t
functions mediated by, 1553-1554
host defense and, 1554
Compression isotherm, 1019
Compression reservoirs, 1027
Computed tomography, in intraventricular hemorrhage, 1758
Concentration, in isotope studies, 450
Conceptional age, 1726
Congenital anomalies
cholesterol biosynthesis and, 381, 382f, 383f
in multiple pregnancy, 171
requiring surgical repair, anemia with, 1417
Congenital constriction band syndrome, 1838, 1839f
Congenital cystic adenomatoid malformations, 792
Congenital heart disease, 705-716
admixture lesions and, 711-712
single-ventricle physiology with, 711-712
systemic arterial oxygen saturation determinants with, 711
systemic arterial oxygen saturation versus systemic oxygen transport in, 711, 712f
anemia with, 1417
bidirectional shunting and, 710-711
left-to-right shunting and
at atrial level, 708
at ventricular or great artery level, 707-708, 709f
effects of, on cardiac physiology, 714-715
lesions with, 715
phenotypic effects of
duration of, 707
no appreciable effect and, 706
reduction of oxygen transport as, 706-707
physiological effects of, 713-714
afterload and, 714
left-to-right shunting and, 714-715
restriction of ventricular filling and, 715-716
right-to-left shunting and, 715
valve regurgitation and, 714
with adequate pumping capacity, 713-714
pulmonary vascular resistance and, 707
right-to-left shunting and, 708, 710-711
isolated, 710
lesions with, 715
systemic arterial oxygen saturation determinants with, 708, 710f-711f
systemic oxygen delivery with, 708, 710
transposition physiology in, 712-713, 713f
Conjoined twins, 172, 172f
Connective tissue disorders, 593, 593t
Connexins, 590
Constitutive nitric oxide synthase, 1532
Constriction band syndrome, congenital, 1838, 1839f
Contiguous gene syndromes, 9-10
Continuous positive airway pressure, 969, 970t
for apnea, 914, 914f
inadvertent PEEP and, 972
to prevent lung injury, 935
Contractile myofilaments, 1855-1857, 1858f
Contractile proteins, 615

Copper, accumulation of, in cholestasis, 1220
Cor pulmonale, in bronchopulmonary dysplasia, 959
Cord blood, platelets in, 1443-1444
Cornified cell envelope, 589
Corona radiata, 27
Coronary heart disease, adult, fetal origins of, 160-164
adult living standards related to, 163-164, 164t
biologic mechanisms of, 162-163
congenital heart disease epidemics and, 164
developmental plasticity and, 161
growth and, 161f, 161t, 161-162, 162f, 162t
hypertension and type 2 diabetes and, 162, 163t
maternal nutrition and, 164
Corpus callosum, agenesis of, 1689-1690, 1690f
Corticosteroids. See also Glucocorticoids; Mineralocorticoids; specific corticosteroids, e.g. Cortisol.
brain development and, 1789
fetal lung development and, 807
prenatal, surfactant therapy with, 1083f, 1083-1084
Corticosterone, plasma concentration of, fetal and neonatal, 1922t
Corticotropin. See Adrenocorticotropic hormone.
Corticotropin-releasing hormone
actions of, 1907
binding protein for, 1908
hypothalamic secretion of, 1877, 1877t
levels during pregnancy, 1908-1909
sources of, 1907
umbilicoplacental circulation mediation by, 752t
Cortisol
adrenal adaptation to extrauterine life and, 1921-1922, 1922t
arterial baroreflex and, 720
fetoplacental steroid metabolism and, 1918, 1918f
functions of, 1923
plasma concentration of, fetal and neonatal, 1922t
renal tubular function and, 1238
umbilicoplacental circulation mediation by, 752t
Cortisone, plasma concentration of, fetal and neonatal, 1922t
Co-stimulation, 1516
in host defense against viruses, 1499
neonatal, 1504
Co-stimulatory molecules, 1516
Cotyledons
definition of, 114t
placental, 90, 92f
Cough, host defense and, 1625-1626
CPAP. See Continuous positive airway pressure.
Cranial neuropore, 31
Craniofacial morphogenesis, 44-48
growth factors and their cognate receptors and, 46-47, 47f
hindbrain and branchial arch code and, 45
retinoids and, 47-48
transcriptional factors and, 45-46, 47f
Craniorachischisis totalis, 1677-1678, 1777f, 1777-1778
Creatinine
as glomerular filtration rate marker, 1258-1259, 1259f, 1260f, 1260t
clearance of, 1260-1261

CRH. See Corticotropin-releasing hormone.
Crigler-Najjar syndrome, types I and II, 1200
Cross-bridges, cycling kinetics of, diaphragmatic contractile properties and, 860-861
Crouzon syndrome, 48, 786, 790, 1837
Cryptorchidism, diagnosis and incidence of, 1958-1959
CT. See Computed tomography.
Cutaneous receptors, 606-607, 607f, 607t
thermal, neonatal, 550-551, 551f
Cutis laxa, 593
CXC chemokines, in neonatal pulmonary host defense, 1650
Cyclic adenosine monophosphate
as second messenger, 1598-1599
pulmonary liquid transport regulation by, 826-827, 828f
Cyclins, 6
Cyclooxygenase
renal blood flow and, 1246
umbilicoplacental circulation and, 754t
Cystathionine, normal plasma and urine levels of, 1296t
Cystatin C, abnormal glomerular filtration rate detection by, 1262, 1262f
Cystic fibrosis, hepatic manifestations of, 1214
Cystic fibrosis transmembrane conductance regulator
bile formation and, 1187-1188
pulmonary ion transport and, 825
Cyst(e)ine
fetal accretion of, 531t
in parenteral amino acid mixtures, 533t, 534t
normal plasma and urine levels of, 1296t
requirements for, of low birth weight infants, 530t-532t
Cytidylyltransferase, surfactant phospholipid and, 1041, 1042, 1044-1047
Cytochrome aa_3, brain levels of, in hypoxia, 1767
Cytochrome P450
adrenocortical development and, 1916f, 1916-1917
CYP2C9 polymorphism and, 214
CYP2C19 polymorphism and, 214
CYP2D6 polymorphism and, 213-214, 214t
drug biotransformation and, 183, 183t
Cytogenetics, 21-22
Cytokine(s), 1555-1568. See also specific cytokines, e.g. Tumor necrosis factor.
acute phase reaction and, 1563
antiinflammatory, 1560-1561
interleukin-4 as, 1560, 1561f
interleukin-10 as, 1560
interleukin-11 as, 1560-1561
interleukin-13 as, 1560, 1561f
chorionic, 127
description of, 1555-1556
excess, in postnatal wounds, 1608-1609
fever and, 1563
in host defense against viruses, 1491-1492
neonatal, 1501
in megakaryocytopoiesis, 1422-1424, 1423f
in neonates, 1564-1568
inflammatory response and, 1565-1568
physiology of, 1564
production of, 1564-1565
in wound healing, 1607
inhibiting hematopoiesis, 1377
intraalveolar networking of
in neonatal pulmonary host defense, 1655-1656
resolution of inflammation and, 1655-1656

Cytokine(s) (Continued)
　　response activation and, 1655
　　　response amplification and, 1655, 1656f
　　systemic, 1656
　　lung development and, 951-952
　　maternal, trophoblastic invasion and, 94
　　placental transfer of, preeclampsia and fetal
　　　growth impairment and, 151
　　proinflammatory, 1556-1560, 1562-1563,
　　　1563-1564
　　chemokines as, 1558-1559, 1559t
　　inhibitors of, 1561-1562
　　interferon-γ as, 1559-1560
　　interleukin-1 as, 1557, 1557f
　　interleukin-6 as, 1558, 1558f
　　interleukin-8 as, 1558
　　interleukin-12 as, 1559
　　interleukin-18 as, 1560
　　tumor necrosis factor as, 1556, 1556f
　　with intrauterine infection, labor onset
　　　and, 136f, 136-137
　　receptors for, 1377-1378, 1378f, 1379f
　　　JAK/STAT signaling pathway and, 1595,
　　　1595f
　　T-cell development and, 1512, 1513t
　　Th1, in host defense against viruses, 1495f,
　　　1495-1496
Cytokinesis, 6
Cytolytic CD4 T cells, in host defense against
　　viruses, 1496-1497
　　neonatal, 1503
Cytoplasmic inheritance, 10
Cytoskeleton
　　cardiac, developmental changes in, 643-644
　　of neutrophils, 1539-1540
Cytosolic pathway, of ketone body utilization,
　　424
Cytotrophoblast, 29, 85, 86f, 87, 95

D

D cells, 1122
Dazla gene, 1944
Death domain, 1556
Death receptors, apoptotic activation
　　through, after tissue injury, 74
Decidua, capsular, 95
Defensins, 1480, 1532
　　in neonatal pulmonary host defense, 1628,
　　　1643-1644
　　neutrophil, 1544, 1544t
Degranulation, neutrophils and, 1543f,
　　1543-1544, 1544t
Dehydroepiandrosterone, plasma
　　concentration of, fetal and neonatal,
　　1922t
Dehydroepiandrosterone sulfate, plasma
　　concentration of, fetal and neonatal,
　　1922t
5'-Deiodinase, in brown adipose tissue,
　　410-411
　　internal action of, 410, 410f
　　perinatal recruitment of, 411, 411f
　　regulation of, 410-411
　　systemic action of, 410
Delayed rectifier, 671-672
Delivery
　　cerebral venous pressure elevation during,
　　　intraventricular hemorrhage and, 1763
　　fluid changes during, 1345
　　lung liquid during, 823
Delta activity, on electroencephalography,
　　monorhythmic, occipital, 1735, 1736t,
　　1737, 1737f

Delta brushes, on electroencephalography,
　　1736t, 1737, 1737f
Delta T cells, in host defense against viruses,
　　1500
　　neonatal, 1505
Dendrites, growth of, 1691-1693
　　disorders of, 1692-1693
　　normal, 1691f, 1691-1692, 1692f
Dendritic cells, 1531-1532
　　antigen processing and presentation and,
　　　1533
　　in host defense, 1477
　　　against viruses, neonatal, 1502-1503
　　in neonatal pulmonary host defense, 1635f,
　　　1635-1636, 1636f
　　myeloid, in host defense against viruses,
　　　1493
Densitometry, for body water measurement,
　　1351
Deoxyribonucleic acid. See DNA entries.
Dermal sinus, 1679, 1780
Dermal-epidermal junction, 594
　　clinical relevance of, 594, 594t
Dermatome, 1850
Dermis, 592-594
　　blood vessels, lymphatics, and nerves of,
　　　593
　　clinical relevance of, 593t, 593-594
Dermoid cysts, spinal, 1679
Dermopathy, restrictive, 593
Descendin, 1956
Desiccation method, for body water
　　measurement, 1351
N-Desmethyl diazepam, protein binding of,
　　205t
Desmin, 1857-1859, 1859f
Desmosomes, 590
Desoxycorticosterone, plasma concentration
　　of, fetal and neonatal, 1922t
Development
　　definition of, 4
　　genes and, 4-5, 5f
Developmental age, apoptosis versus necrosis
　　and, 74
Developmental plasticity, 161
Dexamethasone
　　placental transfer of, 207
　　prenatal, toxicity of, 1072-1073
Diabetes mellitus, type 2, growth and, 162,
　　163t
Diabetic pregnancy, mineral transfer in, 320
Diaphragm, 848-862, 849f
　　contractile properties of, 857-862
　　developmental changes in, 861-862
　　excitation-contraction coupling and, 857,
　　　858f
　　fiber type and MHC isoform composition
　　　and, 857, 858f-861f, 860
　　MCH isoform expression and calcium
　　　sensitivity and, 861
　　MHC isoform expression and cross-
　　　bridge cycle kinetics and, 860-861
　　crural, gastroesophageal reflux and,
　　　1163-1164, 1164f, 1165f
　　embryologic origins of, 851-852
　　innervation of, 852-855, 852f-858f
　　myogenesis of, 849-851, 850f
　　myosin and, heavy chain, 851
Diaphragmatic hernias, congenital, 792
　　lung hypoplasia and, 806-807
　　pulmonary hypoplasia due to, treatment of,
　　　809
Diastematomyelia, 1679, 1780
Diastolic runoff, 708
Diastrophic dysplasia, 1836t, 1837

Diazepam
　　floppy infant syndrome and, 205
　　for benzodiazepine withdrawal, 245
　　protein binding of, 205t
Diazoxide, for preterm labor, 109t
DIC. See Disseminated intravascular
　　coagulation.
Dideoxynucleosides, placental transfer of, 207
Diet. See also Malnutrition; Nutrition.
　　pancreatic secretion and, 1146-1147
Differential splicing, 1521
Differentiation, 4
　　apoptosis versus necrosis and, 74
Diffusion
　　facilitated, of drugs, 179-180
　　transplacental, 207
　　passive, of drugs, 179, 220-221, 221f, 222f,
　　　223
Diffusion coefficient, 880
DiGeorge syndrome, 20, 619
Digestion, 1151-1158. See also specific classes
　　of nutrients.
Digestive system, embryology of, 36-38
Digoxin
　　during lactation, 256
　　half-life of, 186t
Dipalmitoylphosphatidylcholine, 1015, 1016,
　　1018, 1019f, 1019-1020, 1020f, 1021,
　　1022f
　　for surfactant therapy, 1075
　　selective adsorption of, 1026, 1026f, 1026t
2,3-Diphosphoglycerate
　　blood-oxygen hemoglobin affinity and, 884,
　　　885f, 885-886, 886t
　　metabolism of, 1408, 1408f
Diplomyelia, 1679
Direct calorimetry
　　in neonates, 298
　　nonshivering thermogenesis and, 546-547
Disaccharides, digestion of, 1152-1154
　　postnatal, 1153-1154
　　prenatal, 1152-1153, 1153f
Discrimination
　　of smells, in neonates, 1823-1824
　　taste, in neonates, 1820-1821
Disopyramide, during lactation, 256
Disseminated intravascular coagulation, 1452t
　　neonatal, 1460-1466
　　diagnosis of, 1465, 1465t
　　pathophysiology of, 1460f, 1460-1465,
　　　1461f, 1463f, 1464t
　　cell signaling and, 1462
　　cellular activation in, 1462
　　coagulation activation in, 1462
　　coagulation inhibitor consumption
　　　and, 1462
　　consumptive coagulopathy and
　　　multiple organ failure and, 1463
　　fibrinolysis suppression and, 1463
　　vascular permeability and tissue
　　　damage and, 1462-1463
　　treatment of, 1465-1466, 1466t
Distending airway pressure, for hyaline
　　membrane disease, 932-933, 933f
Diuretics
　　calcium transport and, 1289
　　during lactation, 256
DNA
　　recombinant, 11, 12, 16, 17t
　　structure of, 1, 2f, 3f
DNA chips, 17, 18f
DNA libraries, 12, 16
DNA ligase, 11
Dobutamine
　　for shock, in neonates, 778-779

Dobutamine (Continued)
  pharmacodynamics of, 231, 231f
  in neonates, 231-232, 232f
  pharmacokinetics of, 228f, 228-229, 229f
Docosahexaenoic acid. See also Fatty acids, long chain.
  accumulation of
    in lower brain, behavioral changes with, 433
    maternal influences on, 430
  functional effects of, studies of, 434-436
Dominant negative mutations, 21
Dopamine, 1707-1708
  as neurotransmitter, 1875t
  for shock, in neonates, 778-779
  hypothalamic secretion of, 1877, 1877t
  metabolites of, cerebrospinal fluid levels of, 1708, 1708f, 1708t
  pharmacodynamics of, in neonates, 231-232, 232f
  pharmacokinetics of, 228-229, 229f
Doppler ultrasound
  continuous-wave, for cerebral arterial blood flow velocity measurement, 1747
  for uteroplacental blood flow measurement, 759-761, 761f
  physical principle of, 759-760, 760f
  range-gated, for cerebral arterial blood flow velocity measurement, 1747-1748
  velocity waveform analysis and, 760f, 760-761, 761f
  volume flow estimation and, 760
Dorsomedial nucleus, hypothalamic, 1872t
Dorsoventral axis
  determination of, 1831
  in limb development, 1846, 1846f, 1848t
Dosage compensation, 9
Double helix of DNA, 1, 3f
Doubly labeled water method, for energy consumption measurement, 452-453
Down syndrome, 9
Downstream genes, 1935
Doxapram, for apnea, 915
Drug(s). See also Pharmacodynamics; Pharmacogenetics; Pharmacokinetics; specific drugs and drug types.
  action of, localization of, 188
  active, 223, 224f, 225f
  agonist, 188
  antagonist, 188
  capacity-limited, 184
  clearance of, fetal, fetal plasma concentration of drugs and, 225
  delivery using fluid ventilation, 998-999
  distribution of, fetal, 218-226
    clinical applications of, 226
    placental transfer and. See Placental transfer/transport, of drugs.
    plasma concentration and. See Drug(s), fetal plasma concentration of.
    tissue, 226
  dose of
    delivered in breast milk, 252
    dose-response relationship and, 188-189, 189f
    multiple
      accumulation after multiple intravenous boluses and, 195
      accumulation after multiple short-duration infusions and, 195
    single, administration by short-duration infusion, 194, 194f
  elimination of
    fetal, fetal plasma concentration of drugs and, 225-226

Drug(s) (Continued)
  urinary, fetal, fetal plasma concentration of drugs and, 226
  excretion of, in breast milk. See Breast-feeding, drug excretion into breast milk and.
  fetal breathing and, 892-893
  fetal plasma concentration of
    determinants of, 218, 219f
    fetal circulation and, 225
    fetal drug clearance and, 225
    fetal elimination mechanisms and, 225-226
    maternal plasma concentration and, 218
    two-compartment model and, at steady state, 225
  first-order kinetics of, 180
  flow-limited, 184
  half-lives of, 186t
  interaction with receptors, 188-189, 189f
  ionization of, placental transfer and, 201-203, 202t, 203t
  lipid solubility of, placental transfer and, 199-201, 201f
  loading dose of, 186
  maintenance dose of, 186-187
  maximal efficacy of, 188
  molecular weight of, placental transfer and, 205-206, 206f
  optimal dosing schedule for, 187
  over-the-counter, during lactation, 257
  plasma concentration of
    fetal. See Drug(s), fetal plasma concentration of.
    maternal, 218
  potency of, 188
  protein binding of, placental transfer and, 203-205, 204f-206f, 204t, 205t
  psychoactive
    maternal use of, during lactation, 253t, 254, 256
    pharmacology of, 244
  stereoselectivity of, placental transfer and, 206-207
  therapeutic index of, 188-189
  toxicity of, 188
Dubin-Johnson syndrome, 1193
Duct cells, pancreatic, 1143
Ductus arteriosus, patent, 743-747
  anatomic closure of
    histologic changes and, 744-745
    vasoconstriction related to, 746
  bronchopulmonary dysplasia associated with, 954, 955, 955f
  hemodynamic and pulmonary alterations in, 746-747
  in hyaline membrane disease, 928-929, 929f
  incidence of, 743
  indomethacin treatment of, cerebral blood flow measurement with, 1751
  lung injury associated with, 936
  vasoconstriction/vasorelaxation balance and, 743-744
Ductus venosus blood flow, fetal
  during labor, 762
  in fetal growth restriction pregnancies, 261, 262f
Duodenal atresia, 1103, 1103f
Duodenal stenosis, 1103, 1103f
Duodenum
  embryogenesis of, anomalies of, 1103, 1103f
  embryology of, 37
  organogenesis of, 1103
Duplications, chromosomal, 7, 7f

Dwarfism, 1836f, 1836t, 1837
Dynamic mutations, 7
Dystrophin, 1854, 1854f

E

E peptide, 1881
Ear(s), 1803-1810, 1804f
  cochlea of, 1807-1810, 1808f-1811f
  conductive apparatus of, 1804-1807, 1806f, 1807f
  embryology of, 33, 34f
ECG. See Electrocardiogram.
Eclampsia. See Preeclampsia/eclampsia.
ECM. See Extracellular matrix.
Ectodermal dysplasia, hypohidrotic, 596
Edema, 1357-1360
  fetal, 1360
  intravenous protein infusions and, 1359-1360
  lymph flow modulation of, 1359
  protein movement across microvascular border and, 1359
  transvascular fluid filtration and, 1357-1359
  with hydrops, 1360
EEG. See Electroencephalography.
EGF. See Epidermal growth factor.
Ehlers-Danlos syndrome, 593, 593t
Eicosanoids
  placental, 128
  shock and, neonatal, 775
Elastin
  development of, nutrition and, 808
  mutations of, 593
Electrical response activity, gastrointestinal, 1111, 1111f
Electrocardiogram
  fetal, during labor, 763-764
  resuscitation and, 771
Electroencephalography, neonatal, 1726-1744
  composition of, 1735, 1736t, 1737-1744
    abnormal patterns in, 1740, 1741f, 1741-1744
    anterior dysrhythmia in, 1736t, 1738-1739, 1739f
    central-temporal delta activity in, 1736t, 1737, 1737f
    delta brushes in, 1736t, 1737, 1738f
    dominant rhythmic patterns of early infancy in, 1740, 1741f
    encoches frontales in, 1736t, 1737, 1737f
    monorhythmic occipital delta activity in, 62t, 1735, 1737, 1737f
    rhythmic theta activity in, 1736t, 1737, 1738f
    sharp waves in, 1736t, 1739-1740, 1740f, 1741t
    sleep spindles in, 1736t, 1740
  continuity and discontinuity in, 1730, 1731f
    excessive discontinuity in, 1732-1733, 1733f
    interburst duration in, 1730, 1732, 1732f, 1732t
    normal continuity in, 1733f, 1733-1735
      nonreactivity and, 1735
      reactivity and, 1735
      symmetry and, 1734-1735, 1735f
      synchrony and asynchrony and, 1733-1734, 1734f, 1734t
  ontogeny of neonatal states and, 1726-1729, 1727t, 1728f, 1728t
  technical aspects of, 1729f, 1729-1730, 1730f

Electrolyte balance. *See also specific electrolyges, e.g. Sodium.*
  angiotensin II and, 1254
Electrophiles, 182
Embden-Meyerhof pathway, erythrocyte glucose metabolism via, 1406
Embryo, 29, 30f
  angiogenesis in, 80
  glucose transporters in, 490
  ketone bodies and, 426
  morphologic development of, apoptosis in, 72
Embryoblast, 85, 86f
Embryogenesis. *See also specific organs.*
  regulation of, 41–50, 42f
    craniofacial morphogenesis and, 44–48
    craniosynostosis and, 48
    molecular determinants for timing and positional information and, 43–44
    principles of, 41–43, 43f
    signal transduction mechanisms and, 48f, 49f, 49–50
  thyroid, 1926
  zinc in, 344
Embryology, 25–39
  fertilization and, 28–29, 29f
  growth and maturation and, 38–39, 39f
  morphogenesis and, 29–31, 30f
  of digestive system, 36–38
  of ear, 33, 34f
  of eye, 32–33, 33f
  of gametes, 25–28
  of heart, 33–35, 34f
  of musculoskeletal system, 35, 36f
  of nervous system, 31f, 31–32, 32f
  of respiratory system, 36, 37f
  of skeletal system, 35–36
  of urinary system, 38
  of vessels, 35, 35f
Embryonic germ cells, 60–62, 1365
Embryonic stem cells, 1365
  human, 1366–1367
  murine, 1366
Emotional expression/behavior, hypothalamic control of, 1875–1876
Emphysema, lobar, congenital, 791
Encephalocele, 1678, 1777f, 1778
Encephalopathy, bilirubin, 1201, 1204
Encoches frontales, on electroencephalography, 1736t, 1739, 1739f
Endocardial cushions, 616
Endochondral ossification, 36, 1831, 1832f
Endocrine drugs, during lactation, 256–257
Endocrine function. *See also specific hormones.*
  maternal, in multiple pregnancy, 168
Endocytosis
  by mononuclear phagocytes, 1530–1532
  in placental transfer, 118
Endogenous pyogen, 566
Endometrium, definition of, 114t
Endomitosis, 1421
Endonucleases, as restriction enzymes, 11, 11f
Endoreduplication, 1421
ß-Endorphins, 1875t
  fetal regulation of, 1910
  pattern during pregnancy, 1909–1910
  source of, 1909
Endoscopy, of upper airway, 839–840
Endothelial cells
  in neonatal pulmonary host defense, 1636, 1637f
  vascular, origin of, 621–623, 622f
Endothelial-derived relaxing factor, hypoxia and, 655

Endothelin
  glomerular filtration rate and, 1258
  renal blood flow and, 1245
  renal hemodynamics and, 1233–1234
Endothelin-1
  hypoxia and, 655
  intestinal circulation and, 704
  umbilicoplacental circulation mediation by, 752t
  ventilation-perfusion matching and, 878
Energy consumption, measurements of, 452–453
  doubly labeled water method for, 452–453
  open-circuit indirect respiratory calorimetry for, 452, 452f
Energy intake, protein utilization and, 536, 536t
Energy metabolism, cerebral
  energy utilization and, 1716–1717, 1717t
  high-energy metabolites and, 1714t, 1714–1715, 1715f
  in hypoxia-ischemia, 1721–1723, 1722f
Energy requirements, fetal, 465–466
Energy status, of brain, resuscitation and, 771, 771f
Energy substrates, fetal, 469
  uptake of, 469–472
    of carbohydrate, 470f, 470–471, 471f
    of glucose, 471–472
    oxygen quotient and, 469–470, 470t
    respiratory quotient and, 470
    substrate use and, 470
Enrichment, in isotope studies, 451
Enteral alimentation, necrotizing enterocolitis and, 1170–1171
Enteral nutrition, vitamin A and, 349–350
Enteric nervous system
  development of, 1114
  gastrointestinal contractions and, 1112, 1113f
Enterochromaffin-like cells, 1122
Enterocolitis, necrotizing. *See Necrotizing enterocolitis.*
Enterohepatic circulation, of bile acids, 1181–1182, 1182f, 1189–1190, 1190f
  alteration in, 1183–1184
  during development, 1183, 1184f
Environmental temperature, thermoregulation and, 555–556, 557f
Enzymes. *See also specific enzymes, e.g. Lactase.*
  blood-brain barrier and, 1702
  drug metabolizing, 183, 183t
    fetal plasma concentration of drugs and, 225
  in human milk, 281, 282t, 1614
  ketone body utilization and, 425, 425t
  matrix-degrading, with intrauterine infection, labor onset and, 137
  pancreatic, secretion of, 1144–1146, 1145f
  regulating placental endocrine and paracrine activities, 128
Eph-B4, vascular patterning and, 625
Ephrin-B2, vascular patterning and, 625
Epicardium, development of, 615
Epidermal growth factor
  chorionic, 127
  fetal growth and, 1883
  gastrointestinal tract growth and, 1098
  liver growth and development and, 1178
  pancreatic secretion and, 1147, 1148
  testicular descent and, 1958
Epidermal stem cells, 1371
Epidermis. *See Skin, epidermis of.*
Epidermoid cysts, spinal, 1679

Epidermolysis bullosa, 594, 594t
Epinephrine
  as neurotransmitter, 1875t
  endotracheal, pharmacokinetics of, in neonates, 229
  for anemia due to Rh hemolytic disease, 1416–1417
  for shock, in neonates, 779
  glomerular filtration rate and, 1258
  neonatal glucose metabolism and, 479
Epiphyses, 1832, 1832f
Epithelial cells
  in host defense, 1476
  in neonatal pulmonary host defense, 1621–1622
Epithelial sodium channel, 1273
EPO. *See Erythropoietin.*
Ergot alkaloids, contraindication to, for nursing mothers, 253t, 254
Erythroblasts, primitive, 1377
Erythrocytes, 1397–1417
  anemia and. *See Anemia.*
  fetomaternal transfer of, 1402
  hemoglobin and. *See Hemoglobin.*
  metabolism of, 1405–1408, 1406t
    2,2–diphosphoglycerate metabolism and, 1408, 1408f
    Embden-Meyerhof pathway and, 1406
    glycolysis and, 1405, 1407f
    pentose phosphate pathway and, 1406–1407, 1408f
  neonatal, physical properties of, 1408–1410
  oxygen transport by, 1410f, 1410–1411, 1411t, 1412t, 1413f
  production of
    control of, 1400
    extraembryonic, 1397
    intraembryonic, 1397, 1398f
    regulation of, 1398, 1400
    sites and stages of, 1397–1398, 1398f, 1399t, 1400f
  red blood cell indices in fetus and neonate and, 1400–1402, 1401t, 1402t
  volume of, 1341, 1342t, 1343t
Erythroid growth factors, 1398
Erythroid progenitors, 1397
  concentration of, 1397–1398, 1400f, 1400t
  fetal, unique features of, 1398, 1400
  ontogeny of, 1397
Erythropoietin
  as hematopoietic growth factor, 1376t, 1378f
  for anemia of bronchopulmonary dysplasia, 1417
  for anemia of prematurity
    clinical trials of, 1414, 1415t
    pharmacokinetics of, 1414, 1416
    side effects of, 1416
  for anemia with congenital heart disease, 1417
Escherichia coli, 1482–1483
Esophageal atresia, 1101, 1102f
Esophageal duplication, 1101
Esophageal motility, 1127, 1128f, 1129, 1139
  esophageal body and, 1127
  gastrointestinal reflux and, sphincteric mechanisms of, 1129, 1130f
  lower esophageal sphincter and, 1127, 1129
  upper esophageal sphincter and, 1127
Esophageal ring, 1101
Esophageal stenosis, 1101
Esophagus. *See also Gastroesophageal reflux.*
  embryogenesis of, anomalies of, 1101–1102, 1102f
  embryology of, 37
  organogenesis of, 1101

Esophagus (Continued)
  separation from trachea, 824, 825t
  short, congenital, 1102
Esterase inhibitor
  in children, 1441t
  in full-term infants, 1439t
  in premature infants, 1439t
Estradiol, plasma concentration of, fetal and
    neonatal, 1922t
Estradiol sulfate, plasma concentration of, fetal
    and neonatal, 1922t
Estriol, plasma concentration of, fetal and
    neonatal, 1922t
Estriol sulfate, plasma concentration of, fetal
    and neonatal, 1922t
Estrogens
  alveolarization and, 798-799
  brain development and, 1789
  growth plate control by, 1835
  plasma concentration of, fetal and neonatal,
    1922t
  prolactin levels and, 1892-1893
  surfactant phospholipid biosynthesis and,
    1046
Estrone, plasma concentration of, fetal and
    neonatal, 1922t
Estrone sulfate, plasma concentration of, fetal
    and neonatal, 1922t
Ethanol. See Alcohol (ethanol).
Ethanolamine, normal plasma and urine levels
    of, 1296t
Ethmocephaly, 1680
Ethosuximide, during lactation, 256
Etidocaine, placental transfer of, 202t
Ex vivo gene therapy, 15, 15f
Exchange transfusions, oxygen delivery to
    tissues and, 888f, 888-889
Excitation-contraction coupling, 638-639
  diaphragm and, 857, 858f
Excitotoxins, cerebral injury and, 583, 586
Exencephaly, 1778
Exhalation, forced, host defense and, 1625-1626
Exocytosis
  in placental transfer, 118
  lactation and, 286
Exons, 2, 3f
Expiratory reserve volume, 919
Expiratory time constant, 867-868
Expressed sequence(s), 2, 3f
Expressed sequence tags, 16
Extracellular buffer system
  fetal, 1361
  neonatal, 1363
Extracellular matrix, 52-56
  angiogenesis and, 54-56
  cardiac, developmental changes in, 643, 644
  enzymes degrading, with intrauterine
      infection, labor onset and, 137
  functions of, genetic approaches to dissect,
      53
  hematopoiesis and, 1389
  multifunctional nature of, 52
  receptors of, 53-54
  renal, remodeling of, 1227
  structural diversity of, 52-53
Extracellular water, 1351
Extralobar sequestrations, 790, 791
Eye, embryology of, 32-33, 33f

F

Facial responses, of neonates, taste and, 1821
Facilitated diffusion, of drugs, 179-180
  transplacental, 207

Facilitated glucose transporters, 487-489, 488f
  structure and properties of, 489-490
Faciotelencephalic malformations, 1681
F-actin, 635
Factor assays, in neonates, 1449
Factor I, in fetuses, 1436t
Factor II
  deficiency of, 1451-1452
  in fetuses, 1436t
Factor IIc
  in adults, 1436t
  in children, 1441t
  in full-term infants, 1436t, 1438t
  in premature infants, 1437t
Factor V
  deficiency of, 1451-1452
  in adults, 1436t
  in children, 1441t
  in fetuses, 1436t
  in full-term infants, 1436t, 1438t
  in premature infants, 1437t
Factor VII
  in adults, 1436t
  in children, 1441t
  in fetuses, 1436t
  in full-term infants, 1436t, 1438t
  in premature infants, 1437t
Factor VIII
  deficiency of, 1450, 1451, 1452, 1452t
  in adults, 1436t
  in children, 1441t
  in fetuses, 1436t
  in full-term infants, 1436t, 1438t
  in premature infants, 1437t
Factor IX
  deficiency of, 1450, 1452t
  in adults, 1436t
  in children, 1441t
  in fetuses, 1436t
  in full-term infants, 1436t, 1438t
  in premature infants, 1437t
Factor X
  deficiency of, 1451-1452
  in adults, 1436t
  in children, 1441t
  in fetuses, 1436t
  in full-term infants, 1436t, 1438t
  in premature infants, 1437t
Factor XI
  deficiency of, 1450, 1452t
  in adults, 1436t
  in children, 1441t
  in fetuses, 1436t
  in full-term infants, 1436t, 1438t
  in premature infants, 1437t
Factor XII
  in adults, 1436t
  in children, 1441t
  in fetuses, 1436t
  in full-term infants, 1436t, 1438t
  in premature infants, 1437t
Factor XIII
  in children, 1441t
  in full-term infants, 1438t
  in premature infants, 1437t
Factor XIII deficiency screen, in neonates, 1449
Factorial method, for protein metabolism
    assessment, 529
FAS. See Fetal alcohol syndrome.
Fascicles, in developing muscle, 1862-1864,
    1863f-1865f
Fasting
  glucose kinetics during, 458
  maternal, carbohydrate metabolism and, 464
  protein metabolism and, fetal, 522, 522f

Fasting systems
  development of, delayed, in neonates, 495,
    496t
  hormonal regulation of, 495, 495t
Fat. See Lipid(s); Lipoprotein(s); specific lipids,
    e.g. Cholesterol.
Fatty acids
  as nonshivering thermogenesis markers,
    544, 545, 546t
  deficiency of, fetal brain development and,
    389f, 389-390
  essential
    brain development and, 1788
    deficiency of, effects of, 432-433
    maternal, hyperlipoproteinemia and, 375
  free, placental transfer of, 377-379, 379f
  from circulation, as thermogenesis
    substrate, 408-409
  hyperlipidemia as source of, for fetus,
    375-376, 376f
  in plasma, maternal versus fetal, 361
  intracellularly derived, as thermogenesis
    substrate, 408
  intrauterine accretion of, 390, 391f
  long-chain, 429-437, 430f
    accumulation during development,
        430-431
      dietary influences on, 431
      maternal influences on, 430
      synthesis and, 430-431
    cognitive effects of, 435-436
    deficiency of, behavioral effects of,
        431-433
    fetal metabolism of, growth restriction
        and, 154
    functional effects of, experimental
        studies of, 434-436
    gastrointestinal tract growth and, 1098
    global tests of infant development and,
        436
    in developing infant, 433-434
    polyunsaturated, cognitive function and,
        282
    retinal and visual effects of, 434-435
  oxidation of, defects of, 1212t
    neonatal hypoglycemia and, 498
  polyunsaturated, cord, placental transfer
    and, 392
  postnatal utilization of, 392-393
  short-chain, gastrointestinal tract growth
    and, 1097-1098
  surfactant, biosynthesis of, 1041-1042, 1042f
  synthesis of, in brown adipose tissue,
    409-410
  vitamin requirement and, 363t, 363-365,
    363f-365f, 364t
Fatty liver of pregnancy, acute, in multiple
    pregnancy, 168-169
Feedback, hypothalamus and, 1876
Fenoprofen, for preterm labor, 109t
Fertility
  maternal, lactation and, 288
  with maldescended testes, 1959
Fetal alcohol syndrome, 234-235, 235t
  maternal marijuana use and, 241
Fetal antigen 1, 1148
Fetal breathing movements
  diaphragm and, 855, 856f
  lung development and, 805
  lung liquid flow and, 822
Fetal burst pattern, of small bowel
    contraction, 1133
Fetal fibronectin, as preterm labor marker, 107
Fetal growth restriction. See Intrauterine
    growth restriction.

Fetal heart rate
  during labor, 763
  umbilical artery blood flow and, during
    labor, 762
Fetal inflammatory response syndrome,
  137-138, 138f
Fetal loss
  in multiple pregnancy, 171, 174-175
  intrauterine, of one twin, 174-175
Fetal lung maturity, in multiple pregnancy, 171
Fetal membranes
  definition of, 114t
  development of, 95
Fetal tissues, ketone bodies in, 426
Fetoacinar protein, 1148
Fetus papyraceus, 171
Fever
  behavioral, 567
  in neonates, 565f, 565-567
  mechanism of, 566
  pathogenesis of, 566-567
  with inflammatory response, 1563
FGF. See Fibroblast growth factor.
FGR. See Intrauterine growth restriction.
Fibrinogen
  in children, 1441t
  in full-term infants, 1438t
  in premature infants, 1437t
Fibrinolytic activity
  intraventricular hemorrhage and, 1765
  suppression of, in disseminated
    intravascular coagulation, 1463
Fibrinolytic system, 1442-1443, 1443t
Fibroblast(s), fetal, 1606
Fibroblast growth factor
  alveolarization and, 799
  brain development and, 1786
  fetal growth and, 1882
  gastrointestinal tract growth and, 1099
  hepatogenesis and, 1176
  in lung development, 812-813, 816, 818
  in postnatal wounds, 1608-1609
  lung development and, 786-787, 789
  receptors for, mutations in, clinical
    implications of, 48
Fibronectin
  fetal, as preterm labor marker, 107
  hematopoiesis and, 1389, 1390
  in host defense, 1478-1479
  in human milk, 1612
  in neonatal pulmonary host defense, 1627
  lung development and, 787
FIC1 deficiency, 1193
Fick's principle, 1351
First-order feedback, 1876
First-pass effect, 180
Fistulas, tracheoesophageal, 790
Flecainide, during lactation, 256
Floppy infant syndrome, 205
Flow limitation, in placental transfer,
  114-115
Flow probe techniques, for uteroplacental
  blood flow measurement, 759
Flow-metabolism couple, 1719, 1719f, 1720f
Fluid(s). See also specific fluids, e.g. Body
    water.
  blood, plasma, and red blood cell volumes
    and, 1341, 1342t, 1343t
  distribution of, 1341-1344
  during labor and delivery, 1345
  edema and. See Edema.
  interstitial, 1351
    volume of, 1341-1343
  lymph and lymph flow and, 1343-1344,
    1344f

Fluid(s) (Continued)
  lymphatics and capillary membrane and,
    1348-1349
  neonatal weight loss and, 1345
  periciliary, in neonatal pulmonary host
    defense, 1614f, 1623-1624
  perinatal changes in, 1345
  placenta and, 1349
  placental transfusion and, 1345
  plasma and interstitial fluid volumes and,
    1341-1343
  prelabor changes in, 1345
  regulation of, 1345-1348
    hemorrhage and, 1347-1348
    hypoxia and, 1348
    measurement of fluid volumes and,
      1346t, 1346-1347
    volume loading and, 1348
    volumes under steady-state conditions
      and, 1347, 1347f, 1348f
  special fluid compartments and, 1344
  total body, 1341, 1342f
  transvascular filtration of, 1357-1359
    intravenous protein infusions and,
      1359-1360
Fluid and electrolyte balance, angiotensin II
    and, 1254
Fluid resuscitation, for shock, in neonates,
  777-778
Focal adhesion, 54
Folic acid, brain development and,
  1787-1788
Follicle(s), ovarian, growth of, initiation of,
  1946
Follicle stem cells, 1371-1372
Follicle-stimulating hormone
  deficiency of, 1903
  functions of, 1898
  Leydig cells and, 1951, 1951f
  patterns of, in fetus and neonate
    general, 1902
    mechanisms responsible for, 1903
  regulation of, 1898-1901
    in adults, 1898f, 1898-1899
    in fetus and neonate, 1899-1901
  sexual dimorphism and, 1902
Follicular cells, development of, 27, 28t, 29f
Folliculogenesis, 1945f, 1945-1946
Foramen primum, 34
Forced expiratory flow, measurement of, 838,
  839f, 923-924, 924f
Forkhead box transcription factors, lung
    development and, 785
Formulas, for preterm infants, lipids in,
  394-395
foxa1, in lung development, 817
foxb1, in lung development, 817
foxf1, in lung development, 818-819
Fragile-X syndrome, 1692
Frameshift mutations, 6-7, 7f
Frank-Starling relationship, 636-637, 637f
Free radicals, cerebral injury and, 586
Fructose intolerance, hereditary,
  1214-1215
FSH. See Follicle-stimulating hormone.
Functional residual capacity, 919, 962
  in hyaline membrane disease, 930
Fungi, host defense against, 1487-1489
  against invasive candidiasis,
    1488-1489
  against mucocutaneous candidiasis,
    1487-1488
  neonatal, complement in, 1554
Funisitis, 950
Fusogenic properties, 1025

G

G cells, 1120-1122, 1121f, 1122f
Galactosemia, 1214
Gametes, 25-28
  female, development of, 25-27, 27f, 28t
  male, development of, 27-28
  organization of, 25
  origin of, 25, 26f
Gamma T cells, in host defense against
    viruses, 1500
  neonatal, 1505
Gamma-aminobutyric acid, 1709-1710
  as neurotransmitter, 1875t
Gamma-carboxylation system, vitamin K-
    dependent, 370, 370f
  development of, regulation of, 372, 372f
  maturation of, 371f, 371-372, 372f
Gamma-tocopherol
  in human nutrition, 357-358
  α-tocopherol versus, 356-357
Ganglioneuromata, spinal, 1679
Gap junctions, of skin, 590
Gas exchange, 870-879, 871f
  diffusion and, 879
  in bronchopulmonary dysplasia, 958-959
  mechanisms of, with high-frequency
    ventilation, 980-982
    asymmetric velocity profiles as, 981, 981f
    bulk flow as, 980
    entrainment as, 982
    molecular diffusion as, 982
    pendelluft as, 980-981, 981f
    Taylor-type dispersion as, 981f, 981-982
    ventilation-perfusion relationships and. See
      Ventilation-perfusion relationships.
  with liquid ventilation, 989-990
Gastric acid
  protein digestion and
    postnatal, 1154-1155, 1155f
    prenatal, 1154
  secretion of, regulation of, 1122-1123
Gastric atresia, 1102
Gastric duplication, 1102
Gastric lipase, 1123
Gastric motility, 1129, 1131
  control of gastric emptying and, 1129
  in neonates, 1131
  liquid emptying and, 1129, 1131
  solid emptying and, 1131
Gastric motor function, 1139-1140
Gastric secretion, 1117-1123
  chief cell function and, 1123
  D-cell function and, 1122
  enterochromaffin-like cells and, 1122
  G-cell function and, 1120-1122, 1121f, 1122f
  of lipase, 1123
  organogenesis and cell differentiation and,
    1118, 1118f
  parietal cell function and, 1119-1120
  regulation of, in adults, 1118-1119, 1119f
Gastrin, 1121-1122
  gastric acid secretion and, 1121
  G-cell secretion of, 1121, 1121f
  pancreatic secretion and, 1147, 1148
Gastroesophageal reflux, 1163-1166
  antireflux mechanism and, 1163-1164
    high-pressure zone and, 1163-1164,
      1163f-1165f
  free, spontaneous, 1165-1166
  mechanisms of, 1164-1166
    high-pressure zone relaxation as,
      1164-1165, 1166f, 1167f
    intra-abdominal pressure gradients as,
      1165, 1167f

Gastroesophageal reflux (Continued)
  spontaneous free gastroesophageal reflux
    as, 1165-1166
  neonatal, 1166
  sphincteric mechanisms of, 1129, 1130f
Gastrointestinal circulation. See Intestinal
  circulation.
Gastrointestinal contractions, 1111-1116
  intestinal motility and, 1115-1116
  intestinal motor activity and, 1115, 1115f
    development of, 1115-1116
  myogenic control of, 1111, 1111f
  neural control of, 1111-1114
    central nervous system and, 1111-1112,
      1112f
    enteric nervous system and, 1112, 1113f
    neurotransmitters and, 1112-1114
Gastrointestinal drugs, during lactation, 257
Gastrointestinal function, maternal, in
  multiple pregnancy, 168-169
Gastrointestinal hormones, gastrointestinal
  tract growth and, 1098
Gastrointestinal motility, 1125-1135
  anorectal, 1135
    in neonates, 1135
  colonic, 1134f, 1134-1135, 1141
  development of, 1135, 1136f
  esophageal, 1127, 1128f, 1129, 1139
    esophageal body and, 1127
    gastrointestinal reflux and, sphincteric
      mechanisms of, 1129, 1130f
    lower esophageal sphincter and, 1127,
      1129
    upper esophageal sphincter and, 1127
  gastric, 1129, 1131, 1139-1140
    control of gastric emptying and, 1129
    in neonates, 1131
    liquid emptying and, 1129, 1131
    solid emptying and, 1131
  necrotizing enterocolitis and, 1170
  small intestinal, 1131-1134, 1132f,
    1140-1141
    coordination of, 1132, 1132f
      ontogeny of, 1132-1134, 1133f
  suck and swallowing and, 1125-1127, 1126f
    coordination of swallowing with
      breathing and, 1126-1127
    oral phase of swallowing and,
      1125-1126, 1126f, 1127f
    pharyngeal swallowing and, 1126
Gastrointestinal reflux, apnea and, 914
Gastrointestinal tract. See also specific organs.
  calcium transport in, 328-332, 329f, 330f
  development of, 1095-1099
    environmental influences on, 1095-1096,
      1097f
    nature of growth and, 1095, 1096f
    trophic factors in, 1096-1098
      gastrointestinal hormones as, 1098
      glucocorticoids as, 1099
      nutrients and, 1096-1098
      thyroid hormones as, 1099
      tissue growth factors as, 1098-1099
  embryonic development of, homeobox
    genes and, 69-70
  lipolytic activities of
    postnatal, 1157-1158
    prenatal, 1157
  magnesium transport in, 334-338,
    335f-337f
  phosphorus transport in, 332-334, 333f
  potassium homeostasis and, 1285
Gastroschisis, 1106, 1107f
Gastrulation, 30, 30f
  skin development and, 590

GATA-6, lung development and, 789
G-CSF. See Granulocyte colony-stimulating
  factor.
Gelatinase, in neonatal pulmonary host
  defense, 1644
Gene(s). See also specific genes.
  development and, 4-5, 5f
  developmental, disease and, 19-20
  expression of
    apoptosis and, 74
    regulation of, 4
  function of, 2-5
  in hypothalamic development, 1873, 1874t
  regulation and development of
    oxygen-sensing via, 903-904, 904t
    pharmacogenetics and, 215-216
  structure of, 2, 3f
  transcription of, 2-3
  translation of, 3-4
Gene mapping, 13-14, 18-19
Gene mutations, disease-associated, 19-21
  atypical inheritance and, 20
  complex inheritance and, 20-21
  developmental genes and, 19-20
  identification of, 19
Gene therapy, 14-15, 15f, 63-64
Gene transfer, for stem cell therapy, 1370
Genetic code, 3
Genetic disorders, 7-11. See also specific
  disorders.
  chromosomal, 9-10
  heterogeneity in, 10-11
  Mendelian, 7-9
    autosomal dominant, 8, 8f
    autosomal recessive, 7-8, 8f
    X-linked, 8f, 9
  mitochondrial, 10
  multifactorial, 10
  of skin
    of appendages, 595-596
    of dermal-epidermal junction, 594, 594t
    of dermis and subcutis, 593t, 593-594
    of nonkeratinocytes, 591-592, 592t
    prenatal diagnosis of, 596
Genetic engineering, 11
Genetic heterogeneity, 20
Genetics, 1-15. See also Gene(s); specific
  genes.
  cell division and recombination and, 5-6
  genomic organization and, 1-2
  molecular. See Molecular genetics.
  mutation and, 6-7, 7f
  nucleic acid structure and, 1, 2f, 3f
Genitalia. See also specific organs, i.e. Testes.
  male, external, development of, 1936-1937
Genitofemoral nerve, testicular descent and,
  1957
Genome, organization of, 1-2
Genome project, 13
Genomic libraries, 12
GER. See Gastroesophageal reflux.
Germ cell(s)
  development of, 1951-1954, 1952f, 1952t,
    1953f
  embryonic, 1365
Germ cell cysts, 1944
Germinal centers, B-cell development in,
  1519-1520
Germinal matrix
  hemorrhage of, 1745
    intraventricular, 1759, 1765
  subependymal, as site of origin of
    intraventricular hemorrhage, 1759,
    1760f
Germline mosaicism, 8

Gestation. See Pregnancy.
Gestational age, respiratory water and
  evaporative heat loss related to, 577, 581t
Gestational hypertension, 146, 147t
  in multiple pregnancy, 169
Gestational thrombocytopenia, 1429
GFR. See Glomerular filtration rate.
GH. See Growth hormone.
Ghrelin, 1879, 1892
Gilbert syndrome, 1200
Glanzmann's thrombasthenia, 1584-1585
Gli3 gene, in hypothalamic development,
  1874t
Glia, proliferation of, normal, 1683
Glial precursor cells, destruction of,
  intraventricular hemorrhage and, 1765
Gliding tendons, 1866
Globin chain synthesis, 1403-1404, 1404f
Globin genes, 1402-1403, 1403f
Glomerular capillary hydraulic pressure, in
  acute renal failure, 1337-1338, 1338f
Glomerular capillary ultrafiltration coefficient,
  in acute renal failure, 1338
Glomerular filtration, of drugs, 184
Glomerular filtration rate
  abnormal, cystatin C detection of, 1262,
    1262f
  at birth, 1262-1263, 1263f
  autoregulation of, 1258
  clearance and, 1258
  glomerular markers and, 1258-1259, 1259f,
    1260f, 1260t
  in acute renal failure, 1335, 1336, 1336f
  in neonates
    clinical assessment of, 1259-1262
      estimation without urine collection
        for, 1261-1262
      standard clearances for, 1259-1261
    development of, 1256-1265
    factors impairing, 1264-1265, 1265f
    increase in, determinants of, 1263-1264,
      1264t
    maturation during first month of life,
      1263, 1263f, 1264f
    physiology of, 1257f, 1257-1258
    prenatal development of, 1234, 1234f, 1235f
    vasoactive agents and, 1257-1258
Glomerular plasma flow rate, in acute renal
  failure, 1336-1337
Glomerulotubular balance, 1254
Glucagon
  calcium transport and, 1288
  neonatal glucose metabolism and, 479
Glucagon peptide 2, gastrointestinal tract
  growth and, 1098
Glucoamylase, 1152
Glucocorticoids. See also Corticosteroids;
  specific glucocorticoids, e.g. Cortisol.
  alveolarization and, 797-798
  antenatal, lung development and, 952-953
  arterial baroreflex and, 720-721
  brain development and, 1789
  gastrointestinal tract growth and, 1099
  neonatal glucose metabolism and, 479
  neonatal growth and, 272
  pancreatic secretion and, 1147
  preeclampsia and fetal growth impairment
    and, 151-152, 152f
  pulmonary liquid and ion transport
    regulation by, 827-828
  surfactant phospholipid biosynthesis and,
    1044-1045
  therapeutic, during pregnancy, 1923
Gluconeogenesis
  acetone as precursor for, 424, 425f

Gluconeogenesis *(Continued)*
  defects in, neonatal hypoglycemia and, 497-498
  fetal, 474
  hypoglycemia and, 494-495
  in newborn, 459-461, 460f, 460t
  in utero, 455
Glucose
  amino acid metabolism and, in fetal skeletal muscle, 522
  as thermogenesis substrate, 409
  calcium transport and, 1288
  cerebral blood flow and, 1747
  cerebral utilization of, 1707f, 1707t, 1709f, 1717t, 1717-1719
    cerebral blood flow and, 1719, 1719f, 1720f
  decreased, intraventricular hemorrhage and, 1763
  fetal uptake of, 470f, 470-471, 471f
  homeostasis of, fasting, physiology of, 494-495
  placental transfer of, 116
  renal tubular function and, prenatal, 1236
  storage of, fetal, 472-474
    as glycogen, 472, 473f, 474
Glucose metabolism, 449-461. *See also* Hyperglycemia; Hypoglycemia.
  by erythrocytes, 1405-1406, 1407f
  energy consumption measurement and, 452-453
    doubly labeled water method for, 452-453
    open-circuit indirect respiratory calorimetry for, 452, 452f
  fetal, 453-457
    gluconeogenesis and, 455
    glucose sources and, 454f, 454-455, 457, 457f
    glucose utilization and, 455
    glycogen metabolism and, 457, 457f
    maternal-fetal glucose relationship and, 453, 453f
    placental glucose transport and, 453-454
    regulation of, 456-457
    substrate utilization and, 455-456, 456f
  in fetal growth restriction pregnancies, 261-262, 263f, 264f
  isotopic tracer studies of, 449-452
    cost of, 449
    ideal tracer for, 449-452
    isotope abundance and, 449
    quantification of substrate metabolic fate and, 451-452
    quantification of substrate rate of appearance and disappearance and, 450f, 450-451, 451f
  ketone bodies and, 425-426
  neonatal, 457-461
    age and, 458, 458f
    gluconeogenesis and, 459-461, 460f, 460t
    glucose kinetics and, 457-458
    hormones and, 478-486
      glucagon and, 479
      insulin and, 479
      kinetic analyses of, 479-482, 480f-482f
      neonatal insulin resistance and sensitivity and, 482-484, 483f-485f
      neonatal substrate availability and, 484-486
    in very low birth weight infants, 461
    regulation of glucose production and, 458-459, 459f
    substrate availability and, 484-486

Glucose transporters, 487-492, 1720-1721, 1721f
  facilitated, 487-489, 488f
    structure and properties of, 489-490
  localization and regulation of, 490-492
    in brain, 491
    in embryo, 490
    in kidney, 492
    in liver, 491
    in lung, 491
    in muscle, 492
    in placenta, 490-491
  novel, 490
  sodium-dependent, 487
  structure and properties of, 489-490
Glucose-6-phosphatase, deficiency of, neonatal hypoglycemia and, 497-498
Glucose-6-phosphate translocase, deficiency of, neonatal hypoglycemia and, 497-498
Glucuronidation, 184
Glutamate
  as neurotransmitter, 1710f, 1710-1712, 1711f
  fetal accretion of, 531t
  fetal uptake of, 519
  gastrointestinal contractions and, 1113-1114
  in parenteral amino acid mixtures, 533t, 534t
  neurotoxicity mediated by, 1712, 1712f
  placental transfer of, 117
  requirements for, of low birth weight infants, 530t-532t
Glutamate hydrogenase hyperinsulinism, 497
Glutamic acid, normal plasma and urine levels of, 1296t
Glutamine
  fetal uptake of, 518, 519
  gastrointestinal tract growth and, 1097
  normal plasma and urine levels of, 1296t
  requirements for, of low birth weight infants, 530t
Glycerol
  as nonshivering thermogenesis marker, 544-545, 546t
  placental transfer of, 379-380, 380f
Glycine
  fetal accretion of, 531t
  fetal uptake of, 518-519
  in parenteral amino acid mixtures, 533t, 534t
  normal plasma and urine levels of, 1296t
  requirements for, of low birth weight infants, 530t-532t
Glycoconjugates, in human milk, 280, 280t, 1613
Glycogen
  fetal, 472, 473f, 474
  in myotubes, 1855
  metabolism of, fetal, 457, 457f
  sources of, in fetus, 457
Glycogen storage diseases, neonatal hypoglycemia and, 498
Glycogenolysis
  fetal, 472
  hypoglycemia and, 494
Glycolysis
  aerobic, 1716
  anaerobic, 1716
  erythrocyte, 1405. 1407f
  in cerebral metabolism, 1713-1714, 1716
Glycolytic capacity, 1716
Glycolytic control points, 1714
Glycosaminoglycans, hematopoiesis and, 1390
Glycosylation defects, hepatic pathology due to, 1215

GM-CSF. *See* Granulocyte-macrophage colony-stimulating factor.
GnRH. *See* Gonadotropin-releasing hormone.
Gold compounds, contraindication to, for nursing mothers, 253t, 254
Golgi tendon organs, 1864-1866, 1866f
Goltz syndrome, 593
Gonadal agenesis, 1950
Gonadal differentiation, 1898
Gonadal failure, 1904
Gonadal indifferentiation, 1950
Gonadal steroids
  follicle-stimulating hormone regulation by, 1900-1901
  luteinizing hormone regulation by, 1900-1901
Gonadotropin(s). *See also specific gonadotropins, e.g.* Follicle-stimulating hormone.
  abnormal secretion of, conditions associated with, 1903-1904
  plasma levels of
    in fetus and neonate, 1902-1903
    patterns of
      general, 1902
      mechanisms responsible for, 1903
      sexual dimorphism and, 1902
Gonadotropin-releasing hormone
  deficiency of, 1903
  follicle-stimulating hormone regulation by, 1899f, 1899-1900, 1900f
  hypothalamic secretion of, 1877, 1877t
  luteinizing hormone regulation by, 1899f, 1899-1900, 1900f
  placental, 126
G-proteins, trimeric, signaling and, 1593f, 1593-1594, 1594t
Granulocyte antigens, fetal, 1392-1393, 1393t
Granulocyte colony-stimulating factor
  as hematopoietic growth factor, 1377-1378, 1378f, 1379f, 1380-1385
  fetal growth and, 1883
  in host defense, 1482
  in neonatal pulmonary host defense, 1652, 1652f
  neutrophil adherence and, 1540-1541
Granulocyte-macrophage colony-stimulating factor
  as hematopoietic growth factor, 1376t
  in host defense, 1482
  in neonatal pulmonary host defense, 1652
  neutrophil adherence and, 1540-1541
Granulocytopoiesis, 1388-1395
  accelerated neutrophil production in fetus and neonate and, 1393-1395, 1394t
  circulating and marginated blood neutrophil pools and, 1390-1392, 1391t, 1392t
  fetal granulocyte progenitors and, 1388-1389
  fetal hematopoietic environment and, 1389f, 1389-1390
  fetal neutrophil antigens and, 1392-1393, 1393t
  neutrophil proliferative and storage pools and, 1390, 1391f
Granulosa layer, of ovarian follicles, formation of, 1945-1946, 1946f
Great arteries, transposition of, physiology of, 712-713, 713f
Greig syndrome, 1848t
Griscelli syndrome, 592, 592t
Groove of Ranvier, 1834

Growth
    coronary heart disease and, 161f, 161t,
        161-162, 162f, 162t
        biologic mechanisms and, 162-163
    hypertension and, 162, 163t
    neonatal. See Neonatal growth.
    retardation of, maternal opioid use and, 242
    type 2 diabetes mellitus and, 162, 163t
Growth discordancy, in multiple pregnancy,
    170, 170f
Growth factors, 1786, 1880-1888. See also
        specific factors, e.g. Insulin-like growth
        factors.
    adrenal regulation by, 1920
    affecting pluripotent progenitor cells, 1377
    alveolarization and, 799
    angiogenic, 81-82
    angiotensin II as, 1254t, 1254-1255
    chorionic, 127
    cross-talk between integrins and, 54
    embryogenesis and, 46-47, 47f
    erythroid, 1398
    fetal growth and, 1880-1888
        animal models of, 1883-1886
        human, 1886-1888
    gastrointestinal tract growth and,
        1098-1099
    growth plate control by, 1834-1835, 1835t
    hematopoietic. See Hematopoietic growth
        factors.
    in human milk, 1614
    in wound healing, 1607
    lineage-specific, 1377
    liver growth and development and, 1177t,
        1177-1178
    lung development and, 785, 786-787
    placental, preeclampsia and fetal growth
        impairment and, 151
    renal organogenesis and, 1231
Growth hormone, 267-271, 1891-1892
    deficiency of
        genetic forms of, 269
        isolated, 269
    fetal growth and, 1880
    neonatal growth and, insulin-like growth
        factors and, 270-271
    overexpression of, in transgenic animals,
        1883-1884, 1884t
    phosphate transport and, 1292
    protein utilization and, 537
    receptors for, 269
    release of, 267-268
    therapeutic use of, fir intrauterine growth
        restriction, 1887
Growth hormone-releasing hormone,
    267-268
    hypothalamic secretion of, 1877, 1877t
Growth plate, 1829-1837
    cartilaginous component of, 1833-1834
    control of, 1834-1837, 1835t
    development of, 1829-1833
        anteroposterior axis determination in,
            1831
        bone formation in, 1831f, 1831-1832,
            1832f
        chondrocyte differentiation in,
            1832-1833
        dorsoventral axis determination in, 1831
        limb bud outgrowth and proximodistal
            patterning in, 1829-1830, 1830f
    groove of Ranvier of, 1834
    metaphysis of, 1834
    perichondral ring of LaCroix of, 1834
    skeletal dysplasias and, 1836f, 1836t, 1837
    vascular supply of, 1833, 1833f

Growth restriction, fetal. See Intrauterine
    growth restriction.
Gsb-1 gene, in hypothalamic development,
    1874t
GTPase, in signal transduction, 1381
Guanosine triphosphate
    low molecular weight GTP-binding
        proteins and, as molecular switches,
        1595-1596, 1596f
    trimeric G-protein binding of, 1593, 1593f,
        1594t
Gubernaculum, 1956-1957

H

H+, K+-ATPase, parietal cell function and,
    1120
Hair, 594-595
    genetic disorders of, 595
Hair follicles, stem cells for, 1371-1372
Hand-foot-genital syndrome, 19, 20f, 1847
Haploinsufficiency, 21
Haplotypes, 14
Harlequin fetus, 591
hCG. See Human chorionic gonadotropin.
Head circumference, in neonatal nutritional
    assessment, 294-295
Healing. See Wound healing.
Heart. See also Cardiac entries; Cardiovascular
        entries; Myocardial entries.
    development of, 613f, 613-619
        cardiac tube formation and looping and,
            615
        coronary circulation development and,
            615
        electrical activity and contractility and,
            615
        epicardial development and, 615
        failure of, in multiple pregnancy, 174,
            174f
        hemodynamics and, 619
        innervation and, 619, 619f
        precursors of, 613-615
            epicardium as, 615
            neural crest as, 614-615
            primary heart fields as, 613-614
            secondary hear field as, 614, 614f
            vestibular spine as, 614
        septation and, 615-619
            endocardial cushions and, 616
            of atrioventricular canal and atria, 616
            outflow tract and, 616f-618f, 616-619
            ventricular, 619
    embryology of, 33-35, 34f
Heart disease. See Congenital heart disease;
    Coronary heart disease.
Heart rate
    fetal, 648-649, 648f-650f
        during labor, 763
        umbilical artery blood flow and, during
            labor, 762
    maternal, in pregnancy, 143, 143t
    resuscitation and, 766-767, 767f, 767t
Heat. See also Body temperature;
        Temperature; Thermoregulation.
    elimination of, 542-543
        maternal temperature and, 542-543
        placental transfer and, 542, 542f
        through skin and uterine wall, 542, 543f
    exchange between infant and environment,
        571-580
        calculation of, 571-572
        in heated beds, 572
        in incubators, 572

Heat (Continued)
        skin-to-skin care and, 577-578
        through respiratory tract, 571-572,
            576-577, 580f, 580t
            during mechanical ventilation, 577
            during phototherapy, 577, 581t
            gestational age and, 577, 581t
            intubation and, 577
        through skin, 572-576
            during first day after birth, 573-575,
                576f-578f
            during first hours after birth, 572, 573f
            during first weeks after birth, 575,
                579f
            nonionizing radiation and, 575-576,
                579f
            total, 575
            under radiant heaters, 572
    loss of. See Thermoregulation, heat loss and.
    production of. See Thermogenesis.
Heated beds, heat exchange between infant
    and environment in, 572
Helium dilution technique, for functional
    residual capacity measurement, 920, 922f
Hematologic function
    hypoxia and, 654-655
    maternal, in multiple pregnancy, 168
Hematopoiesis, 1374-1385, 1375f
    hepatic, 1177, 1388, 1389
    ontogeny of, 1376-1377
        growth factors and. See Hematopoietic
            growth factors.
    progenitor cells and, 1375-1376, 1376t
    stem cells and, 1374
Hematopoietic growth factors, 1376, 1376t,
    1377-1385
    cytokine, 1377-1378, 1378f, 1379f
    influencing hematopoietic stem cells, 1377
    influencing multipotent progenitor cells,
        1377
    inhibitory, 1377
    interaction with hematopoietic
        progenitors, 1384-1385
        developmental differences, between
            adult and fetal progenitors and, 1384
        prenatal growth factor effects on
            nonhematopoietic tissues and,
            1384-1385
    lineage-specific, 1377
    placental transport of, 1383-1384
    pleiotropy and, 1382, 1382t
    production of
        by mature effector cells, developmental
            differences in, 1385
        placental, 1383
    receptors for, 1377-1380
        cytokine, 1377-1378, 1378f, 1379f
        soluble, 1378, 1379t, 1380
    redundancy and, 1382-1383
    signal transduction and, 1380f, 1380-1382
        downstream signaling mechanisms and,
            1381-1382, 1382f, 1383f
        JAK protein tyrosine kinases as,
            1380-1381
        SRC protein tyrosine kinases as, 1381
    soluble, 1378, 1379t, 1380
Hematopoietic stem cells, 1374, 1375-1376,
    1376t
    fetal versus adult, 1388-1389
    growth factors affecting, 1377. See also
        Hematopoietic growth factors.
    hematopoietic growth factor interaction
        with, developmental differences
        between adult and fetal progenitors
        and, 1384

Heme oxygenase, umbilicoplacental
circulation and, 754t
Hemidesmosomes, 590
Hemodynamics. *See also* Blood flow;
Circulation.
cardiac, development of, 619
of umbilical blood flow, 750
mean blood flow and, 750, 750f
pulsatile blood flow and, 750
pulmonary, 708
renal, control of, 1231-1234
by atrial natriuretic factor, 1233
by endothelin, 1233-1234
by kallikrein-kinin system, 1233
by nitric oxide, 1233
by prostaglandins, 1233
by renal sympathetic nervous system,
1232-1233
vascular development and, 627, 627f
with patent ductus arteriosus, 746-747
Hemoglobin
affinity for oxygen, 881, 882-883, 883f
2,3-diphosphoglycerate and, 884, 885f,
885-886, 886f
factors altering, 883-884, 1410-1411,
1411t
concentration during gestation, 1400-1401,
1401t, 1402t
decreased, intraventricular hemorrhage
and, 1763
structure of, 881f, 881-882, 882f
synthesis of, 1402-1405
globin chain synthesis and, 1403-1404,
1404f
globin genes and, 1402-1403, 1403f
hypoxia and, 655
Hemonectin, hematopoiesis and, 1390
Hemophilia, 1450-1451, 1452t
Hemorrhage
fluid volume and, 1347-1348
germinal matrix, 1745
intracranial, 1454-1455
intraventricular. *See* Intraventricular
hemorrhage.
risk of, assessment of, 1450, 1451t
Hemorrhagic disease of the newborn, 1453
Hemorrhagic infarction, periventricular
intraventricular hemorrhage and, 1765
with intraventricular hemorrhage,
1759-1760, 1760f, 1761f
Hemorrhagic periventricular leukomalacia,
1746
Hemostasis, 1435-1445
angiogenesis and, 1444-1445
animal models of coagulation and, 1444
blood vessel wall and, 1444
coagulation system and, 1435-1436,
1436t-1442t, 1442
coagulant proteins and, 1435-1436
thrombin regulation and, 1436, 1442
fibrinolytic system and, 1442-1443, 1443t
normal, 1447-1448
platelets and, 1443-1444
in cord blood, 1443-1444
megakaryocyte precursors of, 1443
neonatal platelet function and, 1444
primary, 1447
Henderson-Hasselbalch equation, 223, 1361
Heparin, for thrombosis, neonatal, 1470t
Heparin cofactor II
in adults, 1436t
in children, 1441t
in fetuses, 1436t
in full-term infants, 1436t, 1439t
in premature infants, 1439t

Hepatic blood flow, 1186, 1187f
fetal, in fetal growth restriction
pregnancies, 261
Hepatic stem cells, 1371
Hepatocellular inflammation, 1216t
Hepatocellular necrosis, 1214-1215, 1216t
Hepatocyte(s), 1186, 1187f
membrane domains of, 1186-1187
polarity of, 1186, 1187f
Hepatocyte growth factor
fetal growth and, 1883
gastrointestinal tract growth and, 1099
in hepatogenesis, 1176
liver growth and development and,
1177-1178
Hepatogenesis. *See* Liver, development of.
Herbal medicines, during lactation, 257
Herculin, 1850-1851
Hereditary hemorrhagic telangiectasia, 594
Hering-Breuer reflex, 842, 911, 912
fetal breathing and, 892
neonatal breathing and, 898
Hermansky-Pudlak syndrome, 592, 592t
Hernias
diaphragmatic, congenital, 792
lung hypoplasia and, 806-807
pulmonary hypoplasia due to, treatment
of, 809
inguinal, with maldescended testes, 1959
Heroin, 241. *See also* Opioids.
contraindication to, for nursing mothers,
255
Herpes simplex virus, host defense against,
1490
Herpesviruses
biology of, 1490
vaccination for, 1505-1506
Heterodimers, obligate, 590
Heterotopia, 1689, 1689f
Heterotopic mucosal tissue, 1101, 1103
HFV. *See* High-frequency ventilation.
HIF-1
hypoxia and, 655
oxygen-sensing via, 903-904, 904t
vascular development and, 628f, 628-629
High mobility group proteins, 46
High-density lipoprotein, of fetus and
newborn, apolipoprotein E in, 360
High-frequency ventilation, 979-984
advantages of, 982-983
theoretical, 982f, 982-983
animal studies of, 983
cardiovascular effects of, 984
central nervous system effects of, 984
clinical studies of, 983
differences between devices used for, 979
disadvantages of, 983-984
gas exchange mechanisms with, 980-982
asymmetric velocity profiles as, 981,
981f
bulk flow as, 980
entrainment as, 982
molecular diffusion as, 982
pendelluft as, 980-981, 981f
Taylor-type dispersion as, 981f, 981-982
inadvertent hyperventilation with, 983
jet, 979, 981f
lung expansion with, 983-984
monitoring of, 983
oscillatory, 979, 980f
oxygenation with, 979-980
pressure distribution with, 982, 982f
to prevent lung injury, 936
types of, 979, 980f, 981f
ventilation with, 980

High-pressure zone, 1163f, 1163-1164
crural diaphragm and, 1163-1164, 1164f,
1165f
lower esophageal sphincter and, 1163,
1164f
transient relaxation of, 1164-1165, 1166f,
1167f
Hindbrain, branchial arch code and, 45
Hindgut
embryogenesis of, anomalies of, 1109
organogenesis of, 1108-1109, 1109f, 1110f
Hip, developmental dysplasia (dislocation) of,
1840, 1841f
natural history and treatment of, 1843
Hirschsprung disease, 1109, 1114-1115, 1679
Histamine
gastric acid secretion and, 1122
umbilicoplacental circulation mediation by,
752t
Histidine
fetal accretion of, 531t
in parenteral amino acid mixtures, 533t, 534t
normal plasma and urine levels of, 1296t
requirements for, of low birth weight
infants, 530t-532t
Histidine decarboxylase activity, 1122
Histone, 1
Holoprosencephaly, 1680-1681, 1682f
Holt-Oram syndrome, 19, 1846-1847, 1848t
HOM-C complex, 65
Homeobox genes, 65-70
anomalies of, human diseases associated
with, 70, 70t
intestinal development and, 69-70
liver development and, 68
lung development and, 67-68
pancreas and, 1149
pancreas development and, 68-69
Homeostasis, hypothalamic maintenance of,
1871
Homeothermic organisms, 548
Homing receptors, viral antigen-specific T cell
expression of, in host defense against
viruses, 1499
neonatal, 1504
Homocystine, normal plasma and urine levels
of, 1296t
Homovanillic acid, cerebrospinal fluid levels
of, 1708, 1708f, 1708t
Hormones, 1786. *See also* Corticosteroids;
Glucocorticoids; Mineralocorticoids;
specific hormones, e.g. Estrogens.
amino acid transport and, 516-517
counterregulatory, deficiencies of, neonatal
hypoglycemia and, 497
gastrointestinal, gastrointestinal tract
growth and, 1098
in hypoxemia, fetal, 773-774
liver growth and development and, 1177,
1177t
placental. *See* Placental hormones.
potassium homeostasis and, 1281
protein utilization and, 537
pulmonary ion and liquid transport
regulation by, 826-828, 828f
steroid. *See* Steroid hormones.
testicular descent and, 1957
thyroid. *See* Thyroid hormones.
Host defense
against bacteria. *See* Bacteria, host defense
against.
against fungi, 1487-1489
against invasive candidiasis, 1488-1489
against mucocutaneous candidiasis,
1487-1488

Host defense (Continued)
    neonatal, complement in, 1554
  against viruses. See Viruses, host defense
    against.
  human milk and. See Human milk, immune
    protection provided by.
  intestinal, necrotizing enterocolitis and,
    1169–1170
  neonatal, complement in, 1554
  pulmonary, neonatal, 1620–1658, 1621f
    adaptive, 1637–1658
      adhesion molecules in, 1652–1653,
        1653f
      alveolar macrophage regulation of
        inflammation and, 1654–1655
      B cells in, 1640
      bronchus-associated lymphoid tissue
        in, 1640–1641
      chemokines in, 1650
      Clara cell secretory protein in,
        1651–1652
      colony-stimulating factors in, 1652,
        1652f
      complement in, 1642–1643, 1643f
      defensins in, 1643–1644
      humoral immune responses in, 1641f,
        1641–1642
      inflammatory mediators in, 1642
      interferon-γ in, 1650–1651
      interleukins in, 1645–1649
      intraalveolar cytokine networking and,
        1655–1656
      intrapulmonary neutrophil trafficking
        in, 1653–1654
      lymphocyte homing and response in,
        1656–1658, 1657f
      natural killer cells in, 1640, 1640f
      neurokinins in, 1643
      proteases in, 1644f, 1644–1645
      T cells in, 1638–1640, 1639f
      toxic oxygen species in, 1644f,
        1644–1645
      transforming growth factor-β in,
        1651
      tumor necrosis factor in, 1645
    airway reflexes and, 1625–1626
    anatomic barrier mechanisms of,
      1621–1625
      ciliary function as, 1622f, 1622–1623
      epithelial cells as, 1621–1622
      mucins and mucus as, 1624
      mucociliary function as, 1624–1625
      periciliary fluid as, 1614f, 1623–1624
    innate, 1626–1637
      antimicrobial peptides in,
        1628–1629
      carbon monoxide in, 1632–1633
      collectins in, 1629–1631, 1630f
      complement in, 1626–1627
      dendritic cells in, 1635f, 1635–1636,
        1636f
      endothelial cells in, 1636, 1637f
      epithelial cells in, 1637
      fibronectin in, 1627
      iron-binding proteins in, 1627
      lipopolysaccharide-binding protein in,
        1629
      macrophages in, 1633–1634, 1634f
      nitric oxide in, 1632
      polymorphonuclear neutrophils in,
        1634–1635
      surfactant in, 1631f, 1631–1632
    surfactant and, 1066–1067
Hox genes, 19, 41–42
  limb development and, 1846–1847

Human chorionic gonadotropin
  functions of, 1898
  patterns of, in fetus and neonate, general,
    1902
  placental, 123, 123f
Human chorionic gonadotropin-releasing
  hormone, placental, 126
Human chorionic somatotropin, placental, 123
Human Genome Project, 13, 17–19
  genetic and physical map and, 19
  linkage analysis and, 18–19
  polymorphic markers and, 17–18
Human milk, 275–282. See also Breast-feeding.
  bile salt-stimulated lipase in, 1157
  composition of, 250, 275–282, 276t
    antiinfective properties and, 278
    atopic disease and, 281
    bioactive components and, 277–278
    cognitive function and, 282
    immunoglobulins as, 278
    infant growth and, 277
    late effects of breast-feeding and,
      281–282
    lipids in, 393–394
    nonimmune protection and, 278t,
      278–281, 279t
  drug excretion into, 249–257
    clinical implications of, 252–253
    dose estimation and, 252
    drug contraindications due to, 253t,
      253–255
    drug transfer into milk and, 250–251,
      251f
    drug transfer to infant and, 251–252
    drugs commonly used during lactation
      and, 255–257
  immune protection provided by,
    1610–1616
    antiinflammatory agents and, 1614, 1614t
    antimicrobial factors and, 1611t,
      1611–1613
    immune status of infant related to, 1615,
      1615t
    immunomodulating agents and,
      1614–1615, 1615t
    in premature infants, 1615–1616
    leukocytes and, 1613–1614
  lipoprotein lipase in, 1157
  production of, 250
  secretion of. See Lactation.
  synthesis of, cellular mechanisms for,
    285–287, 286f
  volume of, 275
  volume produced, 287
Humoral control, of intestinal circulation,
  703–704, 704t
Humoral immune responses, in neonatal
  pulmonary host defense, 1641f,
  1641–1642
H-Y antigen, 1937
Hyaline membrane disease, 926–933, 927f
  hypoxemia in, 929f, 929–930
    extrapulmonary shunting and, 929–930
    intrapulmonary shunting and, 929
  ischemic damage in, 928
  lung fluid in, 928, 928f
  nitric oxide in, 737
  patent ductus arteriosus in, 928–929, 929f
  pathology of, 927
  pulmonary function in, 930–931, 931f
  surfactant deficiency in, 928
  treatment of, 931–933
    airway distention and, 932–933, 933f
    fraction of inspired oxygen and, 932,
      932f

Hybridization, of DNA, 1
Hydrocephalus, with intraventricular
  hemorrhage, 1760, 1766–1768
  incidence and definition of, 1766, 1767t
  natural history of, 1767–1768, 1768f
  pathogenesis of, 1766, 1767f
  ventricular dilation related to brain injury
    and, 1766–1767
Hydrochlorothiazide, during lactation, 256
Hydrocortisone, pancreatic secretion and,
  1147, 1148
Hydrogen ion excretion
  by mature kidney, 1328
  developmental aspects of, 1328–1329
Hydronephrosis, congenital, 1332–1333
Hydrophilic groups, in surfactant, 1018
Hydrophilic molecules, placental transfer of,
  112, 114, 116t
Hydrophobic groups, in surfactant, 1018
Hydrops fetalis
  edema formation in, mechanisms of,
    1360
  nonimmune, 657–659, 660f, 661f
Hydroxybutyrate, ketone body utilization and,
  424
Hydroxyeicosatetraenoic acids, with
  intrauterine infection, labor onset and,
  136
Hydroxyindoleacetic acid, cerebrospinal fluid
  levels of, 1708, 1708f, 1708t
Hydroxysteroids
  fetoplacental steroid metabolism and,
    1918–1919, 1919f
  plasma concentration of, fetal and neonatal,
    1922t
Hyperbilirubinemia, neonatal, 1199,
  1200–1201
  phototherapy for. See Phototherapy, for
    jaundice.
Hypercalcemia, calcium transport and, 1288
Hypercarbia, intraventricular hemorrhage
  and, 1762–1763
Hyperemia, postprandial, 703
Hyperglycemia, maternal, fetal effects of, 475t,
  475–476
Hyperinsulinism
  congenital, 496–497
    dominant, 497
    focal, 497
    glutamate dehydrogenase, 497
    insulin secretion in, 496, 497f
    potassium channel, 496–497
  in birth asphyxia and small for gestational
    age infants, 495–496
Hyperlipidemia
  in cholestasis, 1220
  maternal, fetal vitamin E nutrition and,
    363–365
  of pregnancy, 360f, 360–361
Hyperlipoproteinemia, in pregnancy, 375–376,
  376f
Hyperoxia, lung injury due to, 846–847, 847f
Hypertension
  arterial
    causes of, in newborn, 1761–1762
    intraventricular hemorrhage and,
      1761–1762
  gestational, in multiple pregnancy, 169
  growth and, 162, 163t
  in bronchopulmonary dysplasia, 959
  in offspring, preeclampsia and, 154–155
  intracranial, 1766
  maternal. See also Preeclampsia/eclampsia.
    gestational, 146, 147t
  pulmonary. See Pulmonary hypertension.

Hyperthermia, in sudden infant death
  syndrome, 565
Hyperthyroidism, neonatal, 272
Hypertrophic zone, of growth plate, 1833,
  1834
Hyperventilation
  inadvertent, with high-frequency
    ventilation, 983
  respiratory alkalosis due to, 1329
Hypervitaminosis A, 351
Hypocalcemia, calcium transport and, 1288
Hypochondroplasia, 1836t, 1837, 1857t
Hypofibrinogenemia, 1452t
Hypoglycemia, 494-498
  characteristics of, 494, 494t
  fasting glucose homeostasis and, physiology
    of, 494-495
  maternal, fetal effects of, 476
  neonatal
    congenital disorders presenting with,
      496-498
    transient, 495-496, 496t
Hypohidrotic ectodermal dysplasia, 596
Hypokalemia, with hypothermia, 587
Hypometabolism, adaptive, 541, 542f
Hypopituitarism, genetic forms of, 269
Hypotension
  glomerular filtration rate and, 1265
  pressor-resistant, in neonates, 777
Hypothalamus, 1871-1879
  anatomy of, 1871, 1872f, 1872t
  congenital abnormalities of, 1903
  control by, development of, 1891
  development of, 1896, 1897t
  embryology of, 1871, 1873, 1874t
  endocrine functions of, 1876f, 1876t,
    1876-1878
    antidiuretic hormone and, 1878
    oxytocin and, 1878
  in metabolic regulation, 1878-1879
    ghrelin and, 1879
    leptin and, 1878-1879
  neurologic functions of, 1873, 1875t,
    1875-1876
    anatomic nervous system and, 1873
    circadian rhythms and, 1873
    emotional expression and behavior as,
      1875-1876
    temperature regulation as, 1873, 1875
  thermoreceptors in, 551-552, 552f
Hypothermia
  neuroprotection using, 582-587
    cooling during resuscitation and
      reperfusion and, 583-584
    duration of, 585
    long-term effectiveness of, 585
    mechanisms of action of, 586
    pathophysiologic phases of cerebral
      injury and, 583, 583f, 584f
    prolonged cooling and, 584
    selective cooling of head and, 585-586
    temperature for, 585
    timing of, 584, 585f
  systemic effects of, 586-587
Hypothyroidism, neonatal, 271-272
Hypovolemia
  glomerular filtration rate and, 1265
  shock and, neonatal, 776-777
Hypoxanthine, cerebrospinal fluid levels of,
  elevated, in hypoxia, 1767
Hypoxemia
  cardiovascular response to, 722
  fetal, 474t, 474-475
    cardiovascular function and, 774
    renal responses to, 774

Hypoxemia (Continued)
  fetal response to, 773-774
  glomerular filtration rate and, 1265
  in hyaline membrane disease, 929f, 929-930
    extrapulmonary shunting and, 929-930
    intrapulmonary shunting and, 929
  myocardial ischemia with tricuspid
    regurgitation and, in neonates, 662f,
    662-663, 663f
  neonatal vulnerability to, 870
  oxygen delivery to tissues and, 887
  reduction of oxygen transport due to, 706
Hypoxia
  acute and chronic, 566f, 567, 567f
  arterial, cerebral blood flow and, 1746
  biochemical evidence of, 1767
  cardiac function and. See Cardiac function,
    hypoxic stress and.
  cerebral, 1722-1723, 1723f
  cerebral energy metabolism in, 1721-1723,
    1722f
  fetal, effects on neonate, 567-568
  neonatal thermogenesis and, 546, 546f
  perinatal, intraventricular hemorrhage and,
    1763
  preceding, intraventricular hemorrhage
    and, 1765
  pulmonary vasoconstriction in, ventilation-
    perfusion matching and, 875f,
    875-876, 876f
  thermoregulation and, 567-568
  vascular development and, 627-629, 628f,
    631-632, 632f
  volume loading and, 1348
  vulnerability to, intraventricular
    hemorrhage and, 1764
Hysteresis, 1016

I

Ichthyoses, 591
IGF. See Insulin-like growth factor.
Iintrons, 2, 3f
Immune complexes, complement processing
  of, 1552
Immunity
  adaptive, leukocyte localization in, 1583
  human milk and. See Human milk, immune
    protection provided by.
  humoral, in neonatal pulmonary host
    defense, 1641f, 1641-1642
  skin defenses and, 603-604, 604f, 604t
  T-cell-mediated, deficient, in newborns,
    1488
Immunoglobulin(s)
  antimicrobial, in human milk, 1611-1613,
    1612t
  formation of, complement and, 1552
  in host defense
    against viruses, 1500
      neonatal, 1505-1506
    natural antibodies and, 1478
  in human milk, 278
  natural, in host defense, 1478
  secretory, in neonatal pulmonary host
    defense, 1641, 1641f
Immunoglobulin A
  in human milk, 1611
  in neonatal pulmonary host defense, 1641,
    1641f
Immunoglobulin G
  in neonatal pulmonary host defense,
    1641-1642
  placental transfer of, 118

Immunoglobulin gene superfamily, 1574t
  in neonatal pulmonary host defense, 1652,
    1653, 1653f
Immunomodulating agents, in human milk,
  1614-1615, 1615t
Immunomodulation, to prevent lung injury,
  938-939
Immunoreceptor tyrosine-based activation
  motifs, 1542
Imprinting, 10
  genetic disease and, 22, 23f
In neonatal pulmonary host, epithelial cells
  in, 1637
In vitro gene therapy, 15
In vivo gene therapy, 15, 15f
Inadvertent PEEP, 972
Inborn errors of metabolism, hepatic
  disorders in, 1211-1213
  categories of, 1211, 1212t-1213t, 1213
  presentation of, timing of, 1211
Incomplete penetrance, 8
Incubators, heat exchange between infant and
  environment in, 572
Indicator amino acid oxidation method,
  506-507, 507f
Indicator dilution method, for body water
  measurement, 1351-1352, 1352f, 1353
Indirect calorimetry
  in neonates, 298
  respiratory, open-circuit, for energy
    consumption measurements, 452, 452f
Indomethacin
  for patent ductus arteriosus, cerebral blood
    flow measurement with, 1751
  for preterm labor, 109t
  half-life of, 186t
  uteroplacental blood flow and, 763
Inducible nitric oxide synthase, 1532
Inert gases, for ventilation-perfusion matching
  assessment, 872-873, 874f
Infant-childhood-pubertal growth charts, 266,
  268f
Infarction, hemorrhagic, venous, 1746
Infection(s)
  antenatal, postnatal lung development and,
    952, 952f, 953f
  bacteria. See Bacterial infection(s).
  glucocorticoid impact on, 1070-1071
  host defense against. See Bacteria, host
    defense against; Host defense; Human
    milk, immune protection provided by;
    Viruses, host defense against.
  intrauterine. See Intrauterine infection.
  lower genital tract, preterm labor and, 107
  Ureaplasma urealyticum
    intrauterine
      amniocentesis detection of, 133-134
      detection with sequence-based
        techniques, 135
    lung injury due to, 937, 937f
Infertility, with maldescended testes, 1959
Inflammation, 1562-1563
  adhesion molecules as markers of,
    1587-1588
  alveolar macrophage regulation of, in
    neonatal pulmonary host defense,
    1654-1655
  alveolarization and, 799
  cytokines in, 1562-1563
    coagulation and, 1563
    local effects of, 1562-1563
    systemic effects of, 1563
  hepatocellular, 1216t
  in wound healing, 1607
  neonatal lung injury and, 937-939, 938f

Inflammation (Continued)
    duration of inflammation and, 938
    interrupting to prevent, 938–939
    interruption of lung development and,
        938–939
Inflammatory cascade, necrotizing
        enterocolitis and, 1171–1172, 1172f,
        1172t
Inflammatory diseases, cytokines in,
        1563–1564
Inflammatory mediators
    in neonatal pulmonary host defense, 1642
    intestinal circulation and, 704
    with intrauterine infection, preterm birth
        associated with, 135–137
Inguinal hernia, with maldescended testes,
        1959
Inhibin
    chorionic, 127
    follicle-stimulating hormone regulation by,
        1901, 1901f, 1902f
    luteinizing hormone regulation by,
        1900–1901
Iniencephaly, 1777f, 1778–1779
Inner cell mass, 29, 30f
Inotropy, fetal heart and, 651–652
Inspiratory/expiratory ratio, mechanical
        ventilation and, 973, 974t
Insufflation pressure, for resuscitation, 769
Insulin
    amino acid metabolism and, in fetal skeletal
        muscle, 522
    amino acid transport and, 516–517
    calcium transport and, 1288
    5′-deiodinase activity and, 410–411
    excess of. See Hyperinsulinism.
    maternal metabolism of, conceptus' effect
        on, 464
    neonatal glucose metabolism and, 479
    neonatal growth and, 271
    placental transfer of, 207
    protein utilization and, 537
    receptors for, mutations of, animal models
        of, 1885–1886
    secretion of, in congenital hyperinsulinism,
        496, 497f
    sensitivity to, in neonates, 482–484,
        483f–485f
Insulin resistance, in neonates, 482–484,
        483f–485f
Insulin-like growth factor, 1880–1882
    adrenal regulation by, 1920
    chorionic, 127
    expression of, animal models of, 1883
    fetal expression of, 1886–1887
    fetal growth and, 1880–1882
    gastrointestinal tract growth and,
        1098–1099
    growth hormone and, 270–271
    growth plate control by, 1834–1835
    IGF binding protein proteases and, 1882,
        1882f
    IGF binding proteins and, 1881–1882
        levels during pregnancy, 1886
        mutations of, animal models of, 1886
        overexpression of, animal models of,
            1884–1885
    in intrauterine growth restriction, 1887,
        1887t
    in macrosomia, 1887–1888, 1888f
    overexpression of, in transgenic animals,
        1883–1884, 1884t
    preeclampsia and fetal growth impairment
        and, 152–153
    protein utilization and, 537

Insulin-like growth factor (Continued)
    receptors for, 1881
        mutations of, animal models of, 1885
    retinopathy of prematurity and, 1801
Insulin-responsive substrate, mutations of,
        animal models of, 1886
Integrins, 53–54, 1573–1578, 1574t, 1575f,
        1576f, 1577t
    β1 and β7 subgroups of, 1574t, 1577–1578
    β1 subgroup of, 1574t, 1577–1578
        neonatal expression and function of,
            1586
    β2 subgroup of, 1574t, 1576–1577
        neonatal expression and function of,
            1585–1586
    β3 subgroup of, 1574t, 1578
    β7 subgroup of, 1574t, 1577–1578
    angiogenesis and, 55
    cross-talk between growth factors and, 54
    ductus arteriosus smooth muscle and, 745
    in acute renal failure, 1337
    in neonatal pulmonary host defense,
        1652–1653, 1653f
    in trophoblastic invasion, 93
    ligand binding by, 1573–1575
    neonatal expression of, 1585–1586
    signaling through, 54
Intercellular adhesion molecules, 1574t,
        1578f, 1578–1579
Intercellular domain, 1187
Interfacial tension, 1019
Interferon(s)
    in host defense, 1482
        against viruses, 1491
    receptors for, JAK/STAT signaling pathway
        and, 1595, 1595f
Interferon-γ
    acute phase reaction and, 1563
    CD4 T cell production of, in host defense
        against viruses, neonatal, 1503
    characteristics of, 1559
    in neonatal pulmonary host defense,
        1650–1651
    inflammation due to, 1562
    mononuclear phagocyte activation by, 1534
    receptors for, 1559–1560
    T-cell development and, 1513t
Interleukin(s)
    as hematopoietic growth factors, 1376t,
        1377, 1378, 1378f, 1379f, 1380–1385
    in host defense, 1481–1482
        against viruses, 1491–1492
    in neonatal pulmonary host defense,
        1645–1649
    T-cell development and, 1512, 1513t
Interleukin-1
    acute phase reaction and, 1563
    characteristics of, 1557
    fever and, 1563
    growth plate control by, 1835
    in neonatal pulmonary host defense,
        1645–1646
    inflammation due to, 1562
    inhibitors of, 1561–1562
    production of, in neonates, 1564
    receptors for, 1557, 1557f
Interleukin-1 receptor antagonist protein, in
        neonatal pulmonary host defense, 1646
Interleukin-2, in neonatal pulmonary host
        defense, 1646
Interleukin-3, in neonatal pulmonary host
        defense, 1646
Interleukin-4
    acute phase reaction and, 1563
    characteristics of, 1560

    in neonatal pulmonary host defense, 1646
    receptors for, 1560, 1561f
Interleukin-5, in neonatal pulmonary host
        defense, 1646
Interleukin-6
    acute phase reaction and, 1563
    characteristics of, 1558
    fever and, 1563
    in neonatal pulmonary host defense, 1647
    inflammation due to, 1562
    production of, in neonates, 1564–1565
    receptors for, 1558, 1558f
Interleukin-7, in neonatal pulmonary host
        defense, 1649
Interleukin-8
    acute phase reaction and, 1563
    characteristics of, 1558
    in neonatal pulmonary host defense, 1650
    inflammation due to, 1562
    production of, in neonates, 1565
Interleukin-9, in neonatal pulmonary host
        defense, 1647
Interleukin-10
    acute phase reaction and, 1563
    characteristics of, 1560
    in neonatal pulmonary host defense, 1647
    production of, in neonates, 1565
    receptors for, 1560
Interleukin-11
    acute phase reaction and, 1563
    characteristics of, 1560–1561
    in neonatal pulmonary host defense, 1648
    receptors for, 1561
Interleukin-12
    characteristics of, 1559
    in neonatal pulmonary host defense, 1648
    inflammation due to, 1562
    receptors for, 1559
Interleukin-13
    acute phase reaction and, 1563
    characteristics of, 1560
    in neonatal pulmonary host defense,
        1646–1647
    receptors for, 1560, 1561f
Interleukin-14, in neonatal pulmonary host
        defense, 1649
Interleukin-15, in neonatal pulmonary host
        defense, 1648
Interleukin-16, in neonatal pulmonary host
        defense, 1649
Interleukin-17, in neonatal pulmonary host
        defense, 1649
Interleukin-18
    characteristics of, 1560
    in neonatal pulmonary host defense, 1649
    inflammation due to, 1562
    receptors for, 1560
Interleukin-18 binding protein, 1562
Intermediate filaments, of myotubes,
        1857–1859, 1858f, 1859f
Intermittent mandatory ventilation, 972,
        973–974
    synchrony on, 973–974
International normalized ratio, 1435
International sensitivity index, 1435
Interphase, mitotic, 5
Interstitial cells of Cajal, 1131
Interstitial fluid, 1351
    measurement of, 1353
    volume of, 1341–1343
        measurement of, 1346–1347
        regulation of, 1345–1348
Intervening sequences, 2, 3f
Intervillous space, 85, 91
Intestinal atresia, congenital, 1106

Intestinal blood flow, regulation of, necrotizing enterocolitis and, 1170
Intestinal circulation, development of, 701-704
blood flow control and, 702-704
cardiovascular function and, 702-703
humoral, 703-704, 704t
local, 704
neural, 703, 703t
clinical considerations in, 704
microcirculation and, 702, 703f
venous drainage and, 702
Intestinal duplications, 1106, 1108, 1108f
Intestinal motility, development of, 1115-1116
Intestinal motor activity, 1115, 1115f
Intestinal rotation, incomplete, 1103
Intestinal stenosis, congenital, 1106
Intestines, absorption in, of vitamin E, 356
Intracellular buffer system
fetal, 1361
neonatal, 1363
Intracellular water, 1351
measurement of, 1353
Intracranial hemorrhage, 1454-1455
Intracranial hypertension, 1766
Intralobar sequestrations, 790-791
Intrauterine compression syndromes, 1838t, 1838-1843
etiology of, 1838-1842, 1839f-1841f
theoretical basis for, 1840, 1842
natural history and treatment of, 1842t, 1842-1843, 1843f
Intrauterine fetal demise, of one twin, 174-175
Intrauterine growth restriction, 259-265, 266-267, 268f
amino acid transport changes in, 516
blood flow measurements and, 260-261
fetal hepatic and ductus venosus, 261, 262f
umbilical, 260-261, 261f
uterine, 260
fetal velocimetry changes and, 260
growth factors in, 1887, 1887t
metabolic changes associated with, 261-265
amino acids and, 262-265, 264f
carbohydrates and, 261-262, 263f, 264f
mineral transfer in, 320
placental development and, 259-260
umbilical blood flow in, 755
Intrauterine infection, 132-138
ascending
pathways of, 132
stages of, 132
chronic, 133-135
amniocentesis detection of, 133-134
preterm labor associated with, 134-135
sequence-based techniques for detecting, 135
etiology of, 138
fetal inflammatory response syndrome with, 137-138, 138f
maternal host response to, 138
microbiology of, 132
preterm labor associated with, 132-133
molecular mechanisms for, 135-137
inflammatory cytokines in, 136f, 136-137
matrix-degrading enzymes in, 137
prostaglandins and, 1
with chronic infection, 134-135
Intrauterine tissues, placental integration with, 128-129

Intravascular volume, maternal, in multiple pregnancy, 167-168
Intraventricular hemorrhage, 1454, 1455, 1757f, 1757-1768
cerebral arterial blood flow and, 1749-1750
cerebral blood flow measurement in
with positron-emission tomography, 1753, 1753f
with xenon clearance tehcniques, 1754-1755
clinical features of, 1757
complications of, 1766-1768
hydrocephalus as, 1766-1768, 1767f, 1767t, 1768f
diagnosis of, 1757-1759
computed tomography in, 1758
magnetic resonance imaging in, 1758-1759, 1759f
ultrasound in, 1758, 1758f, 1758t
mechanisms of brain injury in, 1765-1766
germinal matrix destruction and glial precursors as, 1765
intracranial hypertension and impaired cerebral perfusion as, 1766
major factors in, 1765, 1765t
periventricular white matter injury as, 1765-1766
preceding hypoxic-ischemic injury as, 1765
neuropathology of, 1759-1761
germinal matrix destruction and, 1759
hydrocephalus and, 1760
periventricular hemorrhagic infarction and, 1759-1760, 1760f, 1761f
periventricular leukomalacia and, 1760-1761, 1761t
pontine neuronal necrosis and, 1761
site of origin and, 1759, 1760f
spread of hemorrhage and, 1759
pathogenesis of, 1761-1765
extravascular factors in, 1764-1765
intravascular factors in, 1761-1764, 1762f, 1762t
vascular factors in, 1764
pathophysiology of, cerebral blood flow and, 1745-1746
prognosis of, 1768, 1768t
Intrinsic factor, parietal cell secretion of, 1120
Intubation, respiratory water and evaporative heat exchange and, 577
Inulin
as glomerular filtration rate marker, 1258
clearance of, 1259-1260
method for, without urine collection, 1261-1262
constant infusion of, without urine collection, for glomerular filtration rate estimation, 1261
Inversions, chromosomal, 7, 7f
Inward rectifier, 672
Iodide(s)
concentration of, thyroid hormone synthesis and, 1926-1927
intrathyroidal, recycling of, 1928
organification of, 1927
Iodide leak, 1928
Iodine, in human milk, 276t, 277
Iodine-containing compounds, contraindication to, for nursing mothers, 253t, 254
Iodotyrosines
coupling of, 1927
deiodination of, 1928
Iohexol, as glomerular filtration rate marker, 1259

Ion(s)
alterations in, oxygen-sensing via, 901-903
transport of, in lung liquid. See Lung liquid, ion transport and.
Ion channels, 669
voltage-gated, 671, 673t
Ionization, of drugs, placental transfer and, 201-203, 202t, 203t
Iothalamate sodium, as glomerular filtration rate marker, 1259
Iron
lung injury in, 939
placental transfer of, 207
Iron storage disease, neonatal, 1214-1215
Iron-binding proteins, in neonatal pulmonary host defense, 1627
Ischemia
cerebral acidosis in, 1722-1723, 1723f
cerebral energy metabolism in, 1721-1723, 1722f
hydrocephalus and, 1766
perinatal, intraventricular hemorrhage and, 1763
postnatal, intraventricular hemorrhage and, 1763-1764
preceding, intraventricular hemorrhage and, 1765
vulnerability to, intraventricular hemorrhage and, 1764
Ischemic necrosis, in hyaline membrane disease, 928
Islets, pancreatic, 1143
Isohydric principle, 1361
Isolated growth hormone deficiency, 269
Isoleucine
fetal accretion of, 531t
in parenteral amino acid mixtures, 533t, 534t
normal plasma and urine levels of, 1296t
requirements for, of low birth weight infants, 530t-532t
Isoniazid, during lactation, 256
Isotope studies. See Stable isotope tracer studies.
Isotype switching, 1521
Isoxsuprine hydrochloride, for preterm labor, 109t
Ito cells, development of, 1177
IUGR. See Intrauterine growth restriction.
IVH. See Intraventricular hemorrhage.

J

Jackson-Weiss syndrome, 1837
JAK protein tyrosine kinases, signal transduction by, 1380-1381
Jansen metaphyseal chondrodysplasia, 1836t, 1837
Jaundice
neonatal, 1199, 1200-1201
phototherapy for. See Phototherapy, for jaundice.
Jet, placentomes and, 91
Junctional adhesion molecules, 1574t, 1579
Junctional zone, 92

K

Kallikrein-kinin system
renal hemodynamics and, 1233
renal tubular function and, 1238
Kallmann syndrome, 1957
Keratinization, 591

Keratinocytes, 589–590
Keratodermas, palmoplantar, 591
Keratohyaline granules, 589
Kernicterus, 1201, 1202, 1204
Ketogenesis, hepatic. *See* Liver, ketogenesis in.
Ketone bodies, 419–426
  availability of, 419, 420t
  placental transfer of, 380
  production of
    extrahepatic, 419–420, 420f, 421f
    intrahepatic, 420–423, 421f
      fatty acid catabolism pathway and,
        420–421
      insulin and glucagon in, 422–423, 423t
      malonyl-CoA and, 422, 422f
      neonatal fatty acid catabolism and, 423
      neonatal hepatic changes and, 421–422
    regulation of, 419–423
  utilization of, 423–426, 424f
    acetone as gluconeogenic precursor and,
      424, 425f
    cytosolic pathway of, 424
    enzyme activity and, 425, 425t
    glucose metabolism and, 425–426
    hydroxybutyrate utilization and, 424
    in neonatal tissues, 426
    mitochondrial pathway of, 423–424
Ketonemia
  in neonatal period, 419
  in pregnancy, 419
Ketosteroids
  fetoplacental steroid metabolism and, 1918,
    1918f
  plasma concentration of, fetal and neonatal,
    1922t
Kidney(s). *See also* Renal *entries*.
  amino acid transport by, 1294–1298, 1295f
    developmental aspects of, 1295, 1296t,
      1297–1298
  architectonics of, 1223–1224, 1224f–1226f
  calcium homeostasis and, 1286–1289
    fetal and neonatal aspects of, 1289
    paracellular calcium transport and,
      1286–1287
    regulation of calcium transport and,
      1287–1289
    transcellular calcium transport and, 1287,
      1287f
  compensatory growth of, with nephron
    loss, stimuli for, 1331–1332
  development of, *in utero*, 1229–1238
    concentration capacity and, 1237
    glomerular filtration and, 1234, 1234f,
      1235f
    hemodynamics and, 1231–1234
    molecular and cellular regulation of
      organogenesis and, 1229–1231, 1230f
    nephron formation and, 1229, 1230f
    renal blood flow and, 1231, 1232f
    tubular function and. *See* Renal tubular
      function.
  drug excretion by, 184–185
  embryogenesis of, 1223
  failure of. *See* Acute renal failure.
  glucose transporters in, 492
  hypoxemia and, fetal, 774
  multicystic, unilateral, 1332
  nephrons of. *See* Nephrogenesis;
    Nephron(s).
  organic acid transport by, 1200t,
    1299–1302, 1300f
  organogenesis of, 1225–1226
    molecular and cellular regulation of,
      1229–1231, 1230f
  phosphate transport and, 1290–1292

Kidney(s) *(Continued)*
    factors influencing, 1291–1292
    nephron sites of, 1290, 1290f
    transcellular, 1291, 1291f
  phosphorus handling by, 1290
  potassium homeostasis and, 1282f,
    1282–1285
    acid-base balance and, 1285
    distal sodium delivery and transepithelial
      voltage and, 1284
    hormones and, 1284–1285
    potassium intake and cellular potassium
      content and, 1284
    potassium transport along nephron and,
      1282–1284, 1283f, 1283t
    tubular flow rate and, 1284
  sodium transport in. *See* Sodium, renal
    transport of.
  urinary concentration and. *See* Urinary
    concentration.
Kinetochores, 6
Kininogen, high molecular weight
  in adults, 1436t
  in children, 1441t
  in fetuses, 1436t
  in full-term infants, 1436t, 1438t
  in premature infants, 1437t
Klieber equation, 549
Klinefelter syndrome, 9, 1935
Knee, congenital dislocation of, 1839
Kneeometry, 266
Kneist dysplasia, 1836t, 1837
Krebs cycle, in cerebral metabolism, 1713
Kupffer cells, development of, 1177

L

Labor
  cerebral venous pressure elevation during,
    intraventricular hemorrhage and, 1763
  fluid changes during, 1345
  lung liquid and, 823, 823f, 830
  onset of, 104
    at term, 104, 105t
    prostanoids and, 128
  preterm. *See* Preterm labor.
  uteroplacental blood flow during. *See*
    Uteroplacental blood flow, during
    labor.
Lactadhedrin, in human milk, 1613
α-Lactalbumin, in human milk, 280
Lactase
  postnatal, 1153
  prenatal, 1152, 1153f
Lactase phlorizin hydrolase, 1152–1153
Lactate
  fetal utilization of, 456, 456f
  in neonates, 607
Lactation, 284–290. *See also* Breast-feeding.
  definition of, 285
  developmental anatomy of breast and, 285,
    285f
  maternal effects of, 287–288
  milk ejection and
    oxytocin and, 287
    regulation of, 287
    suckling and, 287
  milk synthesis and secretion and, 285–287
    cellular mechanisms for, 285–287, 286f
    milk volume produced and, 287
    regulation of, 287
  secretory activation of, 288–290
    delays in, 289–290
    hormonal requirements for, 289, 289f

Lactation *(Continued)*
    initial milk volume and, 288f, 288–289,
      289f
Lactic acidosis, 1212t
  in hypoxemia, fetal, 773
Lactoferrin
  in human milk, 278–280, 279t, 1612
  in neonatal pulmonary host defense, 1627
  neutrophil, 1544, 1544t
Lactogen(s), placental, 1893–1894
Lactogenesis, stage II. *See* Secretory activation.
Lactose
  digestion of, 1153
  in human milk, 275, 276t
Lamellar bodies, 598–599
  composition of, 1008
  epidermal versus pulmonary, 599, 600t
  secretion of, 1038, 1038f, 1055
Lamellar granules, 589
Lamina propria, 95, 835
Laminin, 1854
  lung development and, 787
Langerhans cells, 591
Langer-Saldino achondrogenesis, 1837
Langmuir-Blodgett films, 1020
Langmuir-Wilhelmy balance, 1023
Laron syndrome, 1886
Laryngotracheal sulcus, 783
Laryngotracheoesophageal cleft, 1101
Lateral hypothalamic nucleus, 1872t
Lectins, collagenous C-type, in neonatal
    pulmonary host defense, 1629–1631,
    1630f
Left-to-right shunting
  at atrial level, 708
  at ventricular or great artery level, 707–708,
    709f
  effects of, on cardiac physiology, 714–715
  lesions with, 715
Leptins
  chorionic, 127
  metabolic regulation by, 1878–1879
  neonatal growth and, 271
  preeclampsia and fetal growth impairment
    and, 153
  thermogenesis and, 544
    neonatal, 547t
Lesch-Nyhan syndrome, 10
Let-down, 287
Leucine
  catabolism of, 505, 505f
  fetal accretion of, 531t
  in parenteral amino acid mixtures, 533t, 534t
  normal plasma and urine levels of, 1296t
  requirements for, of low birth weight
    infants, 530t–532t
Leukocyte(s)
  activation of, to inflammatory sites,
    1580–1582, 1582f, 1583
  in human milk, 1613
  lung injury mediated by, 937–938, 938f
  migration of, in neonatal pulmonary host
    defense, 1652–1653
Leukocyte adhesion deficiency I, 1583–1584,
    1584t
Leukocyte adhesion deficiency II, 1585
Leukomalacia, periventricular
  hemorrhagic, 1746
  with intraventricular hemorrhage,
    1760–1761, 1761t
Leukotrienes
  umbilicoplacental circulation mediation by,
    752t
  with intrauterine infection, labor onset and,
    136

Levcromakalin, for preterm labor, 109t
Levothyroxine, during lactation, 256-257
Leydig cells, development of, 1950-1951, 1951f
  endocrinologic correlates of, 1951, 1952f
LH. See Luteinizing hormone.
Lidocaine
  placental transfer of, 202t
  protein binding of, 205t
Ligament of Treitz, 1105
Ligandin, 1199
Limb(s), embryology of, 1844-1847,
  1847t-1848t
  anteroposterior axis and, 1846, 1848t
  dorsoventral axis and, 1846, 1846f, 1848t
  normal, 1845-1846
  proximodistal axis and, 1846, 1847t
Limb buds, development of, 1829-1830, 1830f
Linkage analysis, 18-19
Linkage disequilibrium, 14
Linkage mapping, 13-14
Lipases
  bile salt-stimulated, 1157
  gastric, 1123
  hormone-sensitive, as protein kinase
    substrate, 408
  lipoprotein, 1157
  milk, 1158
  pancreatic, 1157-1158
  preduodenal, 1157
  prenatal, 1157
Lipid(s). See also Hyperlipidemia;
  Lipoprotein(s); Phospholipids; specific
  lipids, e.g. Cholesterol.
  absorption of, 1158
  as neonatal energy source, 415-418
    fat oxidation in utero and at birth and,
      415-416
    fat oxidation rate in growing infants and,
      416t, 416-418, 417t
    medium chain triglycerides and,
      416-417, 417t
    total parenteral nutrition and, 417f,
      417-418, 418t
  dietary, for postnatal infants, 399
  digestion of, 1157-1158
    postnatal, 1157-1158
    prenatal, 1157
  in human milk, 276, 276t, 280-281, 281t,
    1613
    synthesis and secretion of, 286
  in skin, 600, 601t
  in surfactant. See Phospholipids, surfactant.
  metabolism of
    brain development and, 389-390
    fetal, 388-390
    maternal, placental lipid transfer and,
      376-380, 377f, 378f
  parenteral, for postnatal infants, 399-400
  plasma, pattern in newborn, 358-361, 359t,
    360f
  postnatal accretion of, 392-398
    absorption and, 395-397
      of medium and long chain
        triglycerides, 396-397
      physiologic phases of, 395-396, 397t
    fatty acid utilization and, 392-393
    intake and, 393-395
      human milk and, 393-394
      preterm infant formula and, 394-395
    metabolism and, 397-398
      accretion and, 397-398
      oxidation and, 397
  preterm infant requirements for, 398-399
  remodeling of, signaling and, 1597f,
    1597-1598

Lipid bilayers, 220
Lipid hydrolases, 1532
Lipid solubility, of drugs, placental transfer
  and, 199-201, 201f
Lipolysis, in adipose tissue, hypoglycemia and,
  495
Lipomata, spinal, 1679
Lipomatous malformations, 1780
Lipomeningocele, 1679
Lipopolysaccharide-binding protein, in
  neonatal pulmonary host defense, 1629
Lipoprotein(s)
  excess, in pregnancy, 375-376, 376f
  metabolism of
    fetal development and, 441-442, 442f
    postnatal development and, 443
  plasma, 358
    pattern in newborn, 358-361, 359t, 360f
    tocopherol distribution in plasma and,
      358, 359f
    tocopherol transfer to tissues and, 358
    vitamin E transport and, 358
  serum concentrations of
    fetal development and, long-term
      consequences of nutrition on,
      443-444
    in fetal development, 440-441
      in experimental animals, 441
      in humans, 440-441, 441f, 441t
    in postnatal development, 442-443
      in experimental animals, 443
      in humans, 442f, 442-443
    perinatal disease and, 443
    postnatal development and, long-term
      consequences of nutrition on,
      443-444
Lipoprotein lipase, 1157
  maternal, hyperlipoproteinemia and, 375
  pathology related to, 409
  perinatal recruitment of, 409, 409f
  regulation of, in brown adipose tissue,
    408-409
β-Lipotropin
  pattern during pregnancy, 1909-1910
  source of, 1909
Lipoxygenase products, with intrauterine
  infection, labor onset and, 136
Liquid ventilation, 985-999
  biomedical applications for, 995-999
    for drug and tracer delivery, 998-999
    for respiratory insufficiency, 995-998
      animal studies of, 995-997, 996f, 997f
      perfluorochemicals and, 997-998, 998f
  fluid-filled lung and, 986-990, 988f
    biochemical findings in, 991-993, 992t,
      992f-994f
    cardiovascular responses and, 990
    cellular findings in, 993, 995
    gas exchange and, 989-990
    histologic and morphologic findings in,
      993, 994f, 995f
    metabolic responses and, 990
    pulmonary mechanics and, 987-989, 989f
    structure and function of, 986-987,
      988f
  perfluorochemical liquids for, 985-986,
    986f, 986t, 987f, 987t
  saline for, 985
  techniques for, 990t, 990-991, 991f
  tidal, 989, 991
Lissencephaly, 1688
Lithium
  contraindication to, for nursing mothers,
    253t, 254
  during lactation, 254

Liver
  acinar organization of, 1177
  bile acids and. See Bile acids.
  bile formation in. See Bile.
  biliary duct development and, 1176-1177
  cellular composition of, 1186
  development of, 1095-1099, 1188, 1188t,
    1189f
    environmental influences on, 1095-1096,
      1097f
    nature of growth and, 1095, 1096f
    regulation of, 1177t, 1177-1178
    specific interactions promoting, 1176,
      1176t
    trophic factors in, 1096-1098
      gastrointestinal hormones as, 1098
      glucocorticoids as, 1099
      nutrients and, 1096-1098
      thyroid hormones as, 1099
      tissue growth factors as, 1098-1099
    vascular, 1176
  differential counts in, 1397, 1399t
  drug biotransformation in, factors affecting,
    184
  embryogenesis of, 1175-1176
  embryology of, 37, 37f
  embryonic development of, homeobox
    genes and, 68
  fetal, hematopoiesis in, 1377
  glucose transporters in, 491
  hematopoiesis and, 1177, 1388, 1389
  hepatic blood flow and, 1186, 1187f
    fetal, in fetal growth restriction
      pregnancies, 261
  hepatic stem cells and, 1371
  hepatocellular inflammation and, 1216t
  hepatocellular necrosis, 1214-1215, 1216t
  hepatocytes and. See Hepatocyte(s);
    Hepatocyte growth factor.
  inborn errors of metabolism and,
    1211-1213
    categories of, 1211, 1212t-1213t, 1213
    presentation of, timing of, 1211
  injury/enlargement of, 1213-1217
    glycosylation defects and, 1215
    hereditary fructose intolerance and, 1214
    in α₁-antitrypsin deficiency, 1215
    in cystic fibrosis, 1214
    in galactosemia, 1214
    in neonatal iron storage disease, 1214
    in peroxisomal disease, 1215
    in tyrosinemia, 1215
    in urea cycle enzyme disorders,
      1214-1215
    mitochondrial depletion and, 1215-1216
    steatosis and, 1215
    storage disorders and, 1216t, 1216-1217
  ketogenesis in
    hypoglycemia and, 495
    regulation of, 420-423, 421f
      fatty acid catabolism pathway and,
        420-421
      insulin and glucagon and, 422-423,
        423t
      malonyl-CoA and, 422, 422f
      neonatal fatty acid catabolism and,
        423
      neonatal hepatic changes and,
        421-422
  membrane domains of, 1186-1187
  sinusoidal cells of, 1177
  vascular anatomy of of, 1176
  vascular development of, intrahepatic,
    1176
  vitamin K metabolism in, 369-371, 370f

Liver disease
 coagulopathy in, 1452t, 1454
 drug elimination and, 185
Lobar emphysema, congenital, 791
Lobar holoprosencephaly, 1680
Local anesthetics, uteroplacental blood flow
  and, 763
Local control, of intestinal circulation, 704
LOD score, 19
Loricin, 589
Low birth weight infants
 amino acid requirements for, 529-532,
   530t-532t
 energy intake of, protein utilization and,
   536, 536t
 protein intake of, quality of protein and,
   535
Low molecular weight heparin, for
  thrombosis, neonatal, 1470t
Lower esophageal sphincter, 1127, 1129
 gastroesophageal reflux and, 1129, 1130f,
   1163, 1164f
Lower genital tract infections, preterm labor
  and, 107
Low-pass filters, 982, 982f
Lumbar puncture, in intraventricular
  hemorrhage, 1757-1758
Lung(s). See also Pulmonary entries;
  Respiratory entries.
 canalicular phase of, 1034
 derecruitment of
  in hyaline membrane disease, 930
  to prevent lung injury, 935, 935f
 development of, 783-792, 784t
  abnormal, 789-792
   distal parenchymal malformations and,
     791-792
   tracheobronchial tree malformations
     and, 790-791
  adrenal steroids in, 1922
  alveolar development in, 818
  alveolar stage of, 784t, 789, 813t
   molecular mechanisms regulating, 789
  antenatal factors influencing
   chorioamnionitis as, 949-951
   cytokines as, 951-952
   infection as, 952, 952f, 953f
  branching morphogenesis in, 812,
    815-816
  canalicular stage of, 784t, 787-788, 795,
    813t
  corticosteroids and, 807
  cytokines and, 951-952
  disorders of, treatments for, 808-809
  early, 812
  embryonic stage of, 783-786, 788t, 813t
   homeobox genes and, 67-68
   malformations and, 786
   molecular mechanisms regulating,
     784-786
  epithelial differentiation in, 816-818,
    817f
  esophageal-tracheal separation in,
    814-815t
  fetal breathing movements and, 805
  fetal lung expansion and, 802-805
   increased, effects of, 804
   mechanotransduction mechanisms
     and, 805-806, 806f
   physiologic control of, 802-803, 803f,
     804f
   reduced, effects of, 803-804
  fetal lung hypoplasia and, physical causes
    of, 806-807
  glandular phase of, 1034

Lung(s) (Continued)
  interruption by inflammatory processes,
    938
  left-right asymmetry and, 814-815, 815f
  lung bud and lobe formation in,
    molecular basis of, 812-814, 813f
  metabolic factors in, 807-808
  nitric oxide in, 733-741
   as selective pulmonary vasodilator,
     735-737, 736f-738f
   in persistent pulmonary hypertension
     of the newborn, 737-740, 739f,
     740f
   in premature neonates, 740-741, 741f
   nitric oxide synthases and, 733-735,
     735f
   vasoregulation by, 733, 734f
  prolactin in, 1893
  pseudoglandular stage of, 784t, 786-787,
    795, 813t
   molecular mechanisms regulating,
     786-787
  saccular stage of, 784t, 788, 795, 813t, 1034
  vascular, 818-819
 expansion of, 802-805
  increased, effects of, 804
  mechanotransduction mechanisms and,
    805-806, 806f
  overexpansion and, 936
  physiologic control of, 802-803, 803f, 804f
  reduced, effects of, 803-804
  with high-frequency ventilation, 983-984
 fluid-filled, liquid ventilation and. See Liquid
   ventilation, fluid-filled lung and.
 gas exchange in. See Gas exchange;
   Ventilation-perfusion relationships.
 glucose transporters in, 491
 growth of, abnormal, 695-696, 697f
 host defense and. See Host defense,
   pulmonary.
 hyaline membrane disease and. See Hyaline
   membrane disease.
 maturity of, in multiple pregnancy, 171
 neonatal, ketone bodies in, 426
 overexpansion of, 936
 premature, 942-947
  adult lung structure and function and,
    942
  injury of, 945-947
   acute, 945-946
   alveolar function impairment after,
     946-947
   chronic, 945-946
   structure of, 942, 943f, 944
   vulnerabilities of, 934-935
  structure of, of distal lung, 942
 surfactant and. See Surfactant, pulmonary;
   Surfactant proteins; Surfactant therapy.
Lung compliance, 963
 during artificial ventilation, 864-865
 during spontaneous breathing, 865-866,
   866f
 in bronchopulmonary dysplasia,
   established, 957, 958f
 in hyaline membrane disease, 930
Lung disease
 antenatal factors influencing, 949-953
 in preterm infants, spectrum of, 949, 950f
Lung hypoplasia, fetal, physical causes of,
   806-807
Lung injury
 fetal, 950
 mechanical ventilation causing, in
   respiratory distress syndrome,
   1060-1061, 1061f-1064f, 1063

Lung injury (Continued)
 neonatal, 934-940, 940f
  aspiration, 937
  humoral, 936-937, 937f
  inflammation and, 937-939, 938f
   duration of inflammation and, 938
   interrupting to prevent, 938-939
   interruption of lung development and,
     938-939
  leukocyte-mediated, 937-938, 938f
  lower airway function in, 846-847
  mechanical mechanisms of, 935-936
  sequelae of, 934-935
  vulnerabilities of premature lung and, 934
 of premature lung
  acute. See Respiratory distress syndrome.
  chronic. See Bronchopulmonary
    dysplasia.
  with mechanical ventilation, etiology of,
    963-965
Lung liquid, 822-831, 823f, 1344
 flow of
  during fetal life, 822
  perinatal changes in, 822-823
 formation of, during fetal life, 822
 in neonatal respiratory disease, 829f,
   829-830
 ion transport and, 831, 831f
  airway ion transport studies and, 830, 830f
  hormonal regulation of, 826-828, 828f
  in neonatal respiratory disease, 830f,
    830-831
  mechanisms of, 823-826, 824f
   chloride and, 824-825
   sodium and, 825-826, 826f, 827f
  oxygen regulation of, 828f, 828-829
 lung injury associated with, 936
 secretion of, during fetal life, 822
 volume of, decrease before labor, 823
Lung resistance, in hyaline membrane disease,
   930
Lung transplantation, for surfactant protein
   deficiency, 1091
Lung volumes
 dynamic, in neonates, 922
 in bronchopulmonary dysplasia,
   established, 957, 957f
 static, in neonates, 919-921, 921f, 922f
Lung water. See Lung liquid.
Luteinizing hormone
 deficiency of, 1903
 functions of, 1898
 Leydig cells and, 1951, 1951f
 patterns of, in fetus and neonate
  general, 1902
  mechanisms responsible for, 1903
 regulation of, 1898-1901
  in adults, 1898f, 1898-1899
  in fetus and neonate, 1899-1901
 sexual dimorphism and, 1902
Lymph
 drainage of, outflow pressure and, 1359
 flow of, 1344, 1344f
  edema modulation by, 1359
 volume of, 1343-1344
Lymphangiectasis, pulmonary, congenital, 792
Lymphangiogenesis, in skin, 594
Lymphatics
 fluid volume and, 1348-1349
 of skin, 593
Lymphocytes. See also B cells; T cells.
 homing and response of, in neonatal
   pulmonary host defense, 1656-1658,
   1657f
 maternal, trophoblastic invasion and, 94

Lysine
   fetal accretion of, 531t
   in parenteral amino acid mixtures, 533t, 534t
   normal plasma and urine levels of, 1296t
   requirements for, of low birth weight
      infants, 530t–532t
Lysozyme, 1480
   in human milk, 280, 1612
   in neonatal pulmonary host defense,
      1628–1629
   neutrophil, 1544, 1544t

M

M₂ receptors, in lower airway, 842–843
M₃ receptors, in lower airway, 843
Macrencephaly, 1684, 1684f
Macroglobulin
   in children, 1441t
   in full-term infants, 1439t
   in premature infants, 1439t
Macronutrients, gastrointestinal tract growth
   and, 1097
Macrophage(s)
   alveolar, regulation of inflammation by, in
      neonatal pulmonary host defense,
      1654–1655
   antigen processing and presentation and,
      1533
   fetal, 1524
   in host defense, 1477
   in human milk, 1613–1614
   in neonatal pulmonary host defense,
      1633–1634, 1634f
   kinetics of, 1524
   metabolism of, 1528
   neonatal, 1525
      deficient anticandidal activities of,
         1488–1489
Macrophage colony-stimulating factor
   as hematopoietic growth factor, 1376t,
      1377, 1381–1384
   fetal growth and, 1883
Macrophage inflammatory protein-1α, as
   hematopoietic growth factor, 1376t
Macrosomia, 1887–1888, 1888f
Magnesium
   calcium transport and, 1288
   distribution in body, neonatal, 324–325
   gastrointestinal transport of, neonatal,
      334–338, 335f–337f
   homeostasis of, regulation of, 327–328
   placental transport of, 319t, 319–320
      control of, 320
      hormonal regulation of, 320
      in diabetic pregnancy, 320
      in intrauterine growth restriction, 320
      mechanisms of, 320
Magnesium sulfate
   for preeclampsia, 154
   for preterm labor, 108, 109t
Magnetic resonance imaging, in intraventricular
   hemorrhage, 1758–1759, 1759f
Magnocellular system, 1877, 1877t
Major histocompatibility complex
   antigen processing and presentation and,
      1533
   T-cell receptor interaction of, 1514
Malignancies
   childhood, maternal smoking and, 240
   hematopoietic reconstitution in, 1370
   pancreatic, proto-oncogenes and,
      1148–1149
   with maldescended testes, 1959

Malignant cells, apoptosis of, α-lactalbumin
   and, 280
Malnutrition
   in cholestasis, 1220
      thermogenesis and, 411–412
Malrotations, midgut, 1106
Mamillary nuclei, hypothalamic, 1872t
Manganese, accumulation of, in cholestasis,
   1220
Mannose-binding protein, in host defense,
   1479
Marfan syndrome, 593
Marijuana
   maternal use of, 240–241
      contraindication to, for nursing mothers,
         255
   pharmacology of, 240
Mast cells, in host defense, 1477–1478
Maternal cardiovascular disease, 146–155
   adaptive changes mimicking, 146
   fetal growth and development and,
      149–154
      growth excess and, 151
      growth restriction and, 150f, 150–151
      mechanisms of impairment of, 151–154
   future risks for offspring, 154–155
   hypertensive, 146, 147t, 147–149, 154–155.
      See also Preeclampsia/eclampsia.
   treatment of, 154
Maternal cardiovascular system, 142–155
   adaptations to pregnancy, 143t, 143–144
      in multiple pregnancy, 167
   blood flow and
      regional, uteroplacental circulation and,
         144, 144f
      uterine
         anatomic changes during pregnancy,
            144–145, 145f
         functional and molecular changes
            during pregnancy, 145–146
   disease of. See Maternal cardiovascular
      disease.
Maternal cotyledons (lobes; lobules), 90, 92f
Maternal disorders
   cardiovascular. See Maternal cardiovascular
      disease.
   fetal effects of, 474–476
      fetal hypoxemia as, 474t, 474–475
      of hyperglycemia, 475t, 475–476
      of hypoglycemia, 476
Maternal drug abuse, 234–245. See also
   specific drugs.
   of alcohol, 234–237, 235t, 236t
   of cocaine, 237–239
   of marijuana, 240–241
   of nicotine, 239–240
   of opioids, 241–244, 242t
   of psychotherapeutic drugs, 244–245
   prevalence of, 234
Maternal hydration, fetal fluid volume and,
   1349
Maternal inheritance, 10
Maternal nutrition, fetal development and,
   164
Maternal temperature, changes of, 542–543
Maternal thrombocytopenia, 1427–1429,
   1429t
Maternofetal barrier
   development of, 86–87, 87f, 88t
   integrity of, 89
Maternofetoplacental unit, steroidogenesis
   and, 124f, 124–125, 125f
Matrix metalloproteinases
   angiogenesis and, 55
   in nephrogenesis, 1227

Maturation, thermoregulation and, 560,
   561–562
Maturation compartments, 1390–1392, 1391t,
   1392f
Maximum expiratory flow-volume curves, 838
M-CSF. See Macrophage colony-stimulating
   factor.
MDR3 deficiency, 1193
MDR3 gene, bile flow and, 1192
Mean airway pressure, 972–973, 973f
Mean cell volume, 1401
Mean platelet volume, in neonates, 1448
Measured peak concentration, 195
Measured trough concentration, 195
Mechanical ventilation, 961–984
   adjuncts to, 975–976
   airway function and, 836–837, 837f
   breathing mechanics during, 864
      passive, 864–865
   control variables in, 967t, 967–973
      continuous positive airway pressure as,
         969, 970t
      inspiratory/expiratory ratio as, 973, 974t
      mean airway pressure as, 972–973, 973f
      oxygen therapy as, 967–969, 968f
      peak inflating pressure as, 969–971, 970f,
         971t
      rate effects as, 971–972, 972f, 972t
   conventional, 966t, 966–967, 967f
      advances in, 973–975
   decision to use, 965–966
   for respiratory distress syndrome, 945
      lung injury due to, 1060–1061,
         1061f–1064f, 1063
   glomerular filtration rate and, 1265
   high-frequency. See High-frequency
      ventilation.
   intraventricular hemorrhage and, 1763
   lung injury with, etiology of, 963–965
   patient-triggered, for atelectasis prevention,
      936
   pulmonary physiology and
      pathophysiology and, 961–962, 962f,
         963t, 964f, 965f, 965t
   respiratory water and evaporative heat loss
      during, 577
   to prevent lung injury, 936
   waveforms in, 970, 971t
   with surfactant therapy, 1082–1083
Mechanoreceptors, in apnea, 911
Mechanotransduction, 964
Meckel diverticulum, 1108f
Meconium
   aspiration of, 937
   bile acids in, 1182, 1182t
   maternal marijuana use and, 241
Medium chain acyl coenzyme A
   dehydrogenase, deficiency of, neonatal
   hypoglycemia and, 498
Medium chain triglycerides, as neonatal
   energy source, 416–417, 417t
Megacolon, aganglionic, congenital, 1109,
   1114–1115, 1679
Megakaryocytes, 1421–1430
   neonatal thrombocytopenia and,
      1427–1430
      alloimmune, 1429
      congenital, 1429–1430
      infection associated with, 1429, 1429t
      maternal causes of, 1427–1429, 1429t
      platelet counts in, 1427, 1427f, 1427t,
         1428f
   platelet production and, 1443
   site of, 1426–1427
   production of, 1421–1424, 1422f

Megakaryocytes (Continued)
    cytokine effects on, 1422-1424, 1423f
    fetal and neonatal, 1424-1425, 1425t, 1426f
    megakaryocytes and, 1421-1422, 1422t
    progenitors for, 1421, 1422f, 1425-1426
    transitional cells in, 1421
Meiosis, 6
    prophase of oocytes and. See Ovary(ies), meiotic prophase of oocytes and.
Meiosis-inducing substances, 1944-1945
Melanocytes, 591
MELAS syndrome, 10
Meloxicam, for preterm labor, 109t
Membrane(s). See also Cell membranes; Premature rupture of membranes.
    semipermeable, 220
Membrane excitability, in striated muscle, 1866
Membrane transporters, 180
Memory T cells, postnatal development of, 1516-1517
Mendelian disorders, 7-9
    autosomal dominant, 8, 8f
    autosomal recessive, 7-8, 8f
    X-linked, 8f, 9
Meningocele, 1679, 1780
Menkes kinky hair syndrome, 595
Mental Developmental Index, docosahexaenoic acid and, 436
Meperidine, half-life of, 186t
Mepivacaine
    placental transfer of, 202t
    protein binding of, 205t
MERFF syndrome, 10
Merkel cells, 591
Merosin, 1854
Mesenchyme, 30
    splanchnic, 783
Mesoderm
    chordal, 1675
    prechordal, 1675
Messenger RNA, 2-3
Metabolic acidosis
    cardiac function and, 654
    fetal, 1362
    neonatal, 1363-1364
    potassium homeostasis and, 1281, 1285
    with hypothermia, 587
Metabolic alkalosis
    fetal, 1362
    neonatal, 1364
    potassium homeostasis and, 1285
Metabolic clearance rate, in isotope studies, 450
Metabolic rate
    fetal, integration of, 467-469, 468t, 469t
    in bronchopulmonary dysplasia, 959
    standard, 549-550
        body mass and age and, 549-550, 550f
        body temperature and, 550, 550f
        thermoregulation and, 554-555
Metabolic reduction, law of, 549
Metabolic responses, with liquid ventilation, 990
Metabolism. See also specific substances and sites, e.g. Bile acids, metabolism of and Cerebral metabolism.
    hypothalamic regulation of, 1878-1879
        ghrelin in, 1879
        leptin in, 1878-1879
    inborn errors of, hepatic disorders in, 1211-1213
        categories of, 1211, 1212t-1213t, 1213
        presentation of, timing of, 1211

Metabolites, of drugs, fetal plasma concentration of drugs and, 226
Metals, metabolism of, disorders of, 1213t
Metanephric mesenchyme, 1223, 1226
    ureteric bud growth and branching regulation by, 1226-1227
Metanephros, formation of, 1223
Metaphase, mitotic, 6
Metatarsus adductus, 1839, 1840f, 1841f
Methadone, 241
    for opioid withdrawal, 244
    pharmacology of, 242
Methionine
    fetal accretion of, 531t
    in parenteral amino acid mixtures, 533t, 534t
    normal plasma and urine levels of, 1296t
    requirements for, of low birth weight infants, 530t-532t
1-Methylhistidine, normal plasma and urine levels of, 1296t
3-Methylhistidine
    in neonatal nutritional assessment, 297-298
    normal plasma and urine levels of, 1296t
Methylxanthines, for apnea, 914-915, 915t
Metronidazole, during lactation, 256
Mevalonate pathway, 381, 382f
Mexiletine, during lactation, 256
MHC. See Major histocompatibility complex.
Micelles, in bile, 1189
Microcephaly vera, 1683-1684
Microcirculation, intestinal, 702, 703f
Microdeletion syndromes, 9-10
Microgastria, 1102
Microsomes, drug biotransformation by, 182-183, 183t
Microtubule-associated protein kinases, Ras-initiated pathways and, 1596-1597
Microtubules, 1859
Microvilli, of upper airway, 834
Midarm circumference, in neonatal nutritional assessment, 295, 295f
Midarm/head circumference ratio, in neonatal nutritional assessment, 295-296, 296f
Midchildhood growth spurt, 267
Midgut
    embryogenesis of, anomalies of, 1106, 1107f, 1108, 1108f
    organogenesis of, 1104-1105, 1105f, 1106f
Migratory motor complexes, 1140
Milk, human. See Breast-feeding; Human milk; Lactation.
Milk lipase, 1158
Mineral(s)
    accumulation of, in cholestasis, 1220
    trace, in human milk, 276t, 277
Mineralocorticoids. See also Corticosteroids; specific mineralocorticoids, e.g. Aldosterone.
    calcium transport and, 1288
    functions of, 1923
    potassium homeostasis and, 1284-1285
Minimal enteral feeding, 1096
Minute ventilation, 922, 971
Missense mutations, 6, 7f
Mitochondria
    depletion of, hepatic pathology due to, 1215-1216
    development of, cerebral metabolism and, 1716
    in apoptosis and necrosis, 75-77
        Bcl-2 family members and, 76-77
        mitochondrial permeability transition and, 75-76, 76f, 77
    ketone body utilization in, 423-424

Mitochondrial disorders, 10
    of energy production, 1212t
Mitosis, 5-6
MMPs. See Matrix metalloproteinases.
Molecular genetics, 11-15, 16-24
    blot hybridization and, 11f, 11-12, 16-17, 17f, 18f
    clinically useful protein production by, 13
    cloning and, 12, 12f, 16
    disease inheritance and molecular pathogenesis and, 21
    disease-association mutations and, 19-21
    gene mapping and, 13-14, 18-19
    gene therapy and, 14-15, 15f
    genomics and, 13
    Human Genome Project and, 13, 17-19
    library construction and, 17
    nucleic acid hybridization and, 16-17, 17f, 18f
    polymerase chain reaction and, 12-13, 13f, 17
    recombinant DNA technology and, 16, 17t
    restriction enzymes and, 11, 11f
    traditional and molecular cytogenetics and, 21-22
Molecular size, drug permeability and, 223
Molecular weight, of drugs, placental transfer and, 205-206, 206f
Monilethrix, 595
Monoamniotic twins, 171, 172f
Monocarboxylic acid transporters, 1720, 1721
Monocytes
    in host defense, 1477, 1482
    metabolism of, 1528
    neonatal, deficient anticandidal activities of, 1488-1489
    peripheral blood, kinetics of, 1524
Mononuclear cells, in host defense, 1482
Mononuclear phagocytes, 1523-1534
    activation of, 1534
    adherence of, 1530
    antigen processing and presentation and, 1533-1534
    cell surface antigens on, 1526, 1527t-1528t, 1528
    cell surface receptors on, 1525-1526, 1526f
    complement protein biosynthesis and, 1529
    cytotoxic activity of, 1532-1533
    development of, 1523f, 1523-1525, 1524f
        during fetal period, 1524
        during neonatal period, 1525
        macrophage kinetics and, 1524
        peripheral blood monocyte kinetics and, 1524
    endocytosis and, 1530-1532
    histochemistry of, 1525
    in host defense against viruses, 1492-1493
    macrophage metabolism and, 1528
    microbicidal activity of, 1532
    monocyte metabolism and, 1528
    morphogenesis of, 1530
    morphology of, 1525
    movement of, 1530
    reactive oxygen intermediate biosynthesis and, 1528-1529
    secretory product biosynthesis and, 1529
Monooxygenase, 183
Monosaccharides, absorption of, 1154
    postnatal, 1154, 1154f
    prenatal, 1154
Monozygotic twins, 165-166
Morphine. See also Opioids.
    fetal breathing and, 893f
    pharmacology of, 241-242
Morphogen(s), lung development and, 785

Morphogenesis, 29–31, 30f
Mosaicism
  germline, 8
  skin in, 593
Motivation, essential fatty acid deficiency and, 433
MR spectroscopy, cerebral high-energy metabolites and, 1714–1715, 1715f
MRI. See Magnetic resonance imaging.
mRNA, 2–3
MRP2 gene, bile flow and, 1192
MRP3 gene, bile flow and, 1190–1191
Mucins
  in human milk, 1612–1613
  in neonatal pulmonary host defense, 1624
Mucociliary function, in neonatal pulmonary host defense, 1624–1625
Mucosa
  barrier function of, in host defense, 1476
  of upper airway, 835
Mucus, in neonatal pulmonary host defense, 1624
Müllerian-inhibiting substance, testicular descent and, 1957–1958
Multicomparment drug distribution, 187, 187f
Multifactorial genetic disorders, 10
Multifetal gestations. See Multiple pregnancy.
Multifetal reduction, 170f, 170–171, 171f
Multiple epiphyseal dysplasia, 1836t, 1837
Multiple inert gas elimination technique, 872
Multiple organ failure, in disseminated intravascular coagulation, 1463
Multiple pregnancy, 165–176
  chorionicity and, 166
    determination of, 166f, 166–167, 167f
  dizygotic, 166
  fetal physiology and, 169f, 169–175
    fetal lung maturity and, 171
    fetal pathophysiology and, 171–175, 172f–174f
    growth and, 169–170, 170f
    multifetal reduction and, 170f, 170–171, 171f
  incidence of, 165
  intra-amniotic infection with, 133
  maternal physiology and, 167–169
    cardiovascular, 167
    endocrine, 168
    gastrointestinal, 168–169
    hematologic, 168
    hypertension and, 169
    intravascular volume and, 167–168
    nutrition and, 169
    pulmonary, 168
    renal, 168
    uterine, 167
  monozygotic, 166
  zygosity and, 165–166
Multiple-frequency bioelectrical impedance analysis, for body water measurement, 1353
Multipotent adult stem cells, 1371–1372
Muscle(s)
  cardiac. See also Myocardial entries.
    embryology of, 35
  chest wall, in apnea, 911–912, 911f–913f
  contraction of. See also Gastrointestinal contractions; Myocardial contraction.
    force development and, 635–636, 637f
  glucose transporters in, 492
  myogenesis of, 849–851, 850f
  respiratory. See Diaphragm; Respiratory muscle(s).

Muscle(s) (Continued)
  striated, 1849–1868
    cellular cytodifferentiation and, 1851–1852, 1851f–1854f, 1854
    contractile myofilaments of, 1855–1857, 1858f
    embryonic origin of, 1849–1850
    fascicular organization of, 1862–1864, 1863f–1865f
    glycogen in, 1855
    historical background of, 1849
    intermediate filaments of, 1857–1859, 1858f, 1859f
    membrane excitability and innervation of, fetal, 1866–1867
    microtubules of, 1859
    muscle spindles and tendon organs and, 1864–1866, 1865f, 1866f
    myofiber differentiation in, metabolic, 1861–1862, 1862f, 1863f
    myofiber growth in, 1860–1861
    myogenic regulatory genes and, 1850–1851
    myotubule degeneration in, 1860
    ribosomes of, 1859
    sarcolemmal nuclei of, 1855, 1855f–1857f
    sarcoplasmic organelles of, 1855
    sarcotubular system of, 1859–1860, 1860f
    suprasegmental neural influences on, 1867–1868
    tendon development and, 1866
  thermoreceptors in, 552
  upper airway, in apnea, 911–912, 911f–913f
Muscle fibers, type of, diaphragmatic contractile properties and, 857, 858f–861f, 860
Muscle spindles, in developing muscle, 1864–1866, 1865f, 1866f
Muscular torticollis, congenital, 1839, 1840f
Musculoskeletal disorders
  intrauterine compression and, 1838t, 1838–1843
  etiology of, 1838–1842, 1839f–1841f
    theoretical basis for, 1840, 1842
  natural history and treatment of, 1842t, 1842–1843, 1843f
  lung hypoplasia and, 807
Musculoskeletal system, embryology of, 35, 36f
Mutations, 6–7
  activating, 21
  chromosomal, 7, 7f
  dominant negative, 21
  dynamic, 7
  frameshift, 6–7, 7f
  missense, 6, 7f
  nonsense, 7, 7f
  point, 6
  single-gene, 6–7, 7f
Myelin, tubular, 1016, 1017f, 1038f, 1038–1039, 1063
Myelination
  in central nervous system, 1693–1694
    disorders of, 1693–1694
    normal, 1693, 1693f
  of brain, fetal, 389
Myelocystocele, 1679
Myeloid dendritic cells, in host defense against viruses, 1493
Myelomeningocele, 1678, 1779–1782
  burden of, 1780–1781
  treatment of, 1781–1782
Myeloperoxidase, 1480
  neutrophil, 1543
Myeloschisis, 1678, 1778

Myoblast(s)
  cytodifferentiation of, 1851–1852, 1851f–1854f, 1854
  in limb development, 1845
  in myogenesis, 849–851, 850f
Myoblast-differentiating factor, 1850
Myocardial contraction, 635–639
  maternal, in pregnancy, 143, 143t
  maturation and, 639–647, 640f
    membrane systems and, 644–645, 645f
    myocardial sympathetic nervous system and, 646–647
    passive mechanical properties and, 644
    sarcolemmal function and, 645–646
    structure and, 639–644
      contractile proteins and, 641–643, 643f
      cytoskeleton and extracellular matrix and, 643–644
      hyperplasia and physiologic hypertrophy and, 639–640, 641f
      myofibrillar, 641
  myofilament and cell structure and, 635, 636f, 637f
    afterload effects and, 638
    excitation-contraction coupling and, 638–639
    force development and, 635–636, 637f
    length and preload effects and, 636–638, 637f
    sarcomere proteins and active force development and, 635
Myocardial function
  birth effects on, 652–653, 653f
  disorders of, shock and, neonatal, 777
  resuscitation and, 769–770
Myocardial ischemia, with tricuspid regurgitation and hypoxemia, in neonates, 662f, 662–663, 663f
Myocytes, 1855–1860
  contractile myofilaments of, 1855–1857, 1858f
  developmental changes in, 639, 640f
  ribosomes of, 1859
  sarcotubular system of, 1859–1860, 1860f
  structure of, developmental changes in, 641
Myofibers
  growth of, 1860–1861
  metabolic differentiation of, 1861–1862, 1862f, 1863f
Myofibrils, structure of, developmental changes in, 641
Myofilaments, 635, 636f
  contractile, 1855–1857, 1858f
  sensitivity of, to calcium, 637
Myogenesis, 849–851, 850f
Myogenic regulatory factors, 1850–1851
Myogenic response, to hypoxic stress, 654
Myogenin, 1850–1851, 1854
Myosin, 635
  developmental changes in, 641–642
  heavy chain, 851
  isoforms of, 851
    diaphragmatic contractile properties and, 857, 858f–861f, 860–861
Myostatin, 1851
Myotubes, 1855–1860
  glycogen in, 1855
  innervation of, 1867
  intermediate filaments of, 1857–1859, 1858f, 1859f
  microtubules of, 1859
  sarcoplasmic organelles of, 1855
  sarcotubular system of, 1859–1860, 1860f

N

Na-Cl cotransporter, 1274
Nail-patella syndrome, 596, 1848t
Nails, development of, 595
Na+,K+-ATPase
   para-aminohippurate transport and, 1300-1301
   potassium homeostasis and, 1279
   pulmonary ion transport and, 825, 827-828
   sarcolemmal function and, 645-646
   sodium transport and, 1271
Na-K-Cl cotransporters, 1274
Naked oocytes, 1945
Nalidixic acid, during lactation, 256
NANC innervation, of lower airway, 844-846, 845f
Naproxen, for preterm labor, 109t
Natural killer cells
   in host defense, 1482
      against viruses, 1500
         neonatal, 1501-1502, 1505
   in host defense against viruses, 1494f, 1494-1495
   in neonatal pulmonary host defense, 1640, 1640f
Near-infrared spectroscopy, for cerebral blood flow measurement, 1749f, 1750-1751, 1751f
   in intraventricular hemorrhage, 1751
   with indomethacin treatment of patent ductus arteriosus, 1751
   with surfactant therapy, 1751
Near-miss SIDS, 915
Necdin gene, in hypothalamic development, 1874t
Necrosis
   choice between apoptosis and, factors determining, 74-75
   following hypoxia-ischemia, 73
   in cerebral injury, relation between apoptosis and, 73
   ischemic, in hyaline membrane disease, 928
   mitochondria in, 75-77
      Bcl-2 family members and, 76-77
      mitochondrial permeability transition and, 75-76, 76f, 77
Necrotizing enterocolitis
   cytokine levels during, 1567
   neonatal, 1169-1172
      inflammatory cascade and, 1171-1172, 1172f, 1172t
      prematurity and, 1169t, 1169-1171
         bacterial colonization and, 1170
         enteral alimentation and, 1170-1171
         gastrointestinal motility and, 1170
         host defense and, 1169-1170
         intestinal blood flow regulation and, 1170
Neonatal growth, 266-272
   breast-feeding and, 277
   glucocorticoids and, 272
   growth hormone and, 267-271
      deficiency of
         genetic forms of, 269
         isolated, 269
      insulin-like growth factors and, 270-271
   hormonal control of, 267, 268f
   insulin and, 271
   leptin and, 271
   maternal alcohol consumption and, 236
   pattern of, 266-267
   sex steroids and, 272
   thyroid hormone and, 271-272

Neoplastic disease
   apoptosis of malignant cells and, α-lactalbumin and, 280
   childhood, maternal smoking and, 240
   hematopoietic reconstitution in, 1370
   pancreatic, proto-oncogenes and, 1148-1149
   with maldescended testes, 1959
Nephrogenesis, 1224-1228, 1230f, 1239
   control and modulation of, 1225-1226
   epithelialization in, 1227
   extracellular matrix remodeling and cell adhesion in, 1227
   mesoderm differentiation in, 1226
   morphogenesis in, 1227
   stages of, 1225, 1226f
   ureteric bud in, 1226
      regulation by metanephric mesenchyme, 1226-1227
   vascularization in, 1227-1228
Nephron(s)
   fluid transport in, urinary concentration and, in neonates, 1312
   long, urinary concentration and, in neonates, 1317, 1317t
   loss of, 1330-1333
      adaptation versus maladaptation to, 1332
      long-term reduction in renal mass and, 1330-1332, 1331t
      postnatal adaptation to, 1333
      prenatal adaptation to, 1332-1333
      renal function with, prediction of, 1333
      renal response to, clinical aspects of, 1332-1333
      short-term reduction in renal mass and, 1330
   number of, renal mass and, 1330-1331, 1331t
   phosphate transport and, 1290, 1290f
   short, urinary concentration and, in neonates, 1317, 1318f, 1319, 1319t
   urinary concentration and, 1304-1306, 1305f
Nerve(s)
   cardiac, 619, 619f
   of skin, 593
   umbilicoplacental circulation and, 754-755
Nerve cells, bilirubin affinity for, 1202-1204
Nerve development, of limbs, 1845
Nerve growth factor
   brain development and, 1786
   fetal growth and, 1882-1883
Nervous system
   adrenergic, renal blood flow and, 1246-1247
   auditory, central, 1810-1813, 1812f, 1813f
   autonomic
      cardiac conduction and, 682
      hypothalamic control of, 1873
   central. *See* Brain; Central nervous system; Spinal cord.
   embryology of, 31f, 31-32, 32f
   enteric
      development of, 1114
      gastrointestinal contractions and, 1112, 1113f
   parasympathetic, cardiac conduction and, 682, 683f, 684, 684f
   sympathetic. *See* Sympathetic nervous system.
Net protein balance, 503
Net protein gain, 503
Neural control
   of basal hemodynamic state, 717-721, 719f
   of intestinal circulation, 703, 703t

Neural crest
   cardiac, 614-615
   cell derived from, disorders of, 1679
Neural crest cells, 1786
Neural plate, 31, 1785
Neural stem cells, 1370-1371
   clinical utility of, 63-64
Neural tube
   development of, 1786
   dorsal induction of, 1675-1679, 1677-1679
      disorders of, 1677-1679, 1678f
      normal, 1675-1676, 1677f
   ventral induction of, 1679-1681
      disorders of, 1679-1681, 1682f
      normal, 1679, 1679f, 1681f
Neural tube defects, 1677-1679, 1772-1782
   as multifactorial disorders, 1775-1776
      environmental features and, 1775-1776
      genetic features and, 1775
   burden of, 1780-1781
   cranial, 1777f, 1777-1779
   embryonic development and, 1772-1773, 1773t
      primary neurulation and, 1772-1773, 1773t
   etiology of, 1678-1679
   folic acid and, 1776, 1776f, 1787-1788
   mechanisms of, 1773-1775
      mechanical models and, 1774-1775
      mouse genetic models and, 1773-1774
      teratogenic models and, 1774
   occult dysraphic states as, 1679
   prevention of, 1776, 1776f
   spectrum of, 1777, 1777f
   spinal
      closed, 1777f, 1780
      open, 1777f, 1779-1780
   treatment of, 1781-1782
      fetal neurosurgical intervention as, 1781-1782
      standard, 1781
Neuroblastomata, spinal, 1679
Neurodevelopmental disorders, in offspring, preeclampsia and, 154
Neurodevelopmental interface, skin as, 606-609
   cutaneous receptors and electrical maturation and, 606-607, 607f, 607t
   skin as information rich surface and, 607-609, 608f
Neurodevelopmental tests, docosahexaenoic acid and, 436
Neuroendocrine bodies, 786
Neurogenesis, 1370
Neurohumoral reflexes, hypoxia and, 655
Neurokinins, in neonatal pulmonary host defense, 1643
Neurologic disorders
   maternal opioid use and, 242-243
   neonatal
      maternal cocaine use and, 237-238
      maternal marijuana use and, 241
Neurons
   damage to, apoptosis in, 73
   death of, during development, 1690-1691
      disorders of, 1691
      normal, 1690-1691
   GABA-containing, 1709-1710
   migration and determination of fate of, 1684-1689
      disorders of, 1687-1689, 1688f, 1689f
      normal

Neurons (Continued)
cerebral cerebellar development and, 1686-1687, 1687f
cerebral cortex development and, 1684-1686, 1685f, 1686f
necrosis of, pontine, periventricular, 1761
neuropeptide-containing, 1710
proliferation of, 1681-1684
disorders of, 1683-1684, 1684f, 1684t
normal, 1681-1683, 1682f, 1683f
Neuropeptide(s)
adrenal regulation by, 1920
chorionic, 127
Neuropeptide Y
cardiac conduction and, 685-686, 686f
umbilicoplacental circulation mediation by, 752t
Neurophysiologic function, with hydrocephalus, 1767
Neuropoiesis, 1370-1371, 1785
Neuropores, 31
Neuroprotection, hypothermia for. See Hypothermia, neuroprotection using.
Neurorestoration, 63
Neurotransmitters, 1706-1712, 1707f. See also specific neurotransmitters, e.g. Dopamine.
gastrointestinal contractions and, 1112-1114
hypothalamic, 1875t
noradrenergic projection to cerebral cortex and, 1706-1707, 1707f
Neurotrophins, brain development and, 1786-1787
Neurulation, 1675-1676, 1677f
genetic influences on, 1677
Neutrophil(s)
accelerating production in fetus and neonate, 1393-1395, 1394t
in host defense, 1476-1477
in human milk, 1613-1614
intrapulmonary trafficking of, in neonatal pulmonary host defense, 1653-1654
neonatal, 1538-1547
activation of, 1539, 1539f
adherence of, 1540-1541
antibody-dependent cellular cytotoxicity of, 1546-1547
chemotaxis of, 1541-1542
cytoskeleton of, 1539-1540
deformability of, 1541
degranulation and, 1543f, 1543-1544, 1544t
microbicidal activity of, 1544-1546
nonoxidative, 1546
oxidative, 1545-1546
phagocytosis by, 1542-1543
Neutrophil antigens, fetal, 1392-1393, 1393t
Neutrophil proliferative pool, 1390
Neutrophil storage pools, 1390-1392, 1391t, 1392f
NFATc1, vascular patterning and, 625-626
Nhlh2 gene, in hypothalamic development, 1874t
Nicardipine, for preterm labor, 109t
Nicotine
amino acid transport and, 517
maternal use of, 239-240
contraindication to, for nursing mothers, 255
pharmacology of, 239
Nifedipine
for preterm labor, 108, 109t
uteroplacental blood flow and, 763

Nitric oxide
calcium transport and, 1289
gastrointestinal contractions and, 1112-1113
glomerular filtration rate and, 1258
hypoxia and, 655
in neonatal pulmonary host defense, 1632
in pulmonary development, 733-741
as selective pulmonary vasodilator, 735-737, 736f-738f
in persistent pulmonary hypertension of the newborn, 737-740, 739f, 740f
in premature neonates, 740-741, 741f
nitric oxide synthases and, 733-735, 735f
vasoregulation by, 733, 734f
intestinal circulation and, 704
renal blood flow and, 1245-1246, 1246f
renal hemodynamics and, 1233
shock and, neonatal, 775
umbilicoplacental blood flow and, 102, 752t
uteroplacental blood flow and, 102
ventilation-perfusion matching and, 878, 878f
Nitric oxide synthases, 1532
constitutive, 1532
in host defense against viruses, 1492-1493
in pulmonary development, 733-735, 735f
inducible, 1532
umbilicoplacental circulation and, 754t
Nitrofurantoin, during lactation, 256
Nitrogen. See also Amino acid(s); Protein(s).
accretion of, intrauterine growth and, 509-512, 510f, 511t, 512t
losses of, stress and, 534-535
metabolism of, turnover of individual components of, 504-506, 505f, 506f
Nitrogen balance, 501, 502f, 503, 523, 523t
operative stress and, 535
Nitrogen gradient, gas exchange and, 871
Nitrogen washout technique, for functional residual capacity measurement, 920-921
Nitroglycerine, for preterm labor, 109t
Nkx2.1/Tebp/TTF-1 gene, in hypothalamic development, 1874t
Nociception, 1792-1794
neuroanatomy, neurophysiology, and neurochemistry of, 1792-1794, 1793f, 1793t
Nonadrenergic noncholinergic innervation, of lower airway, 844-846, 845f
Nonhistone chromosomal protein, 1, 2
Nonionizing radiation, heat exchange and water loss and, under radiant heaters, 575, 579f
Nonsense mutations, 7, 7f
Nonsteroidal anti-inflammatory drugs, during lactation, 255
Norepinephrine
as neurotransmitter, 1875t
for shock, in neonates, 779
glomerular filtration rate and, 1258
neonatal glucose metabolism and, 479
noradrenergic projection to cerebral cortex and, 1706-1707, 1707f
thermogenesis and, neonatal, 547t
umbilicoplacental circulation mediation by, 752t
Norfloxacin, during lactation, 256
Normal bacterial flora, in host defense, 1476
Northern blotting, 12, 16
NTCP gene, bile flow and, 1190-1191
Nucleases, 1532
Nucleic acid, primary structure of, 1, 2f, 3f
Nucleic acid hybridization, 11f, 11-12, 16-17, 17f, 18f

Nucleolus, 3
Nucleosomes, 1
Nucleotides, 1, 2f
gastrointestinal tract growth and, 1097
in human milk, 281
Nucleus tractus solitarii, gastrointestinal contractions and, 1111-1112
Null alleles, 21
Nutrient balance studies, in neonates, 298
Nutrition
alveolarization and, 799
enteral. See Enteral nutrition.
fetal, long-term consequences on lipoprotein concentrations, 443-444
fetal lung development and, 807-808
gastrointestinal tract growth and, 1096
maternal
in multiple pregnancy, 169
lactation and, 287-288
neonatal, long-term consequences on lipoprotein concentrations, 443-444
neonatal growth and, 272
parenteral. See Parenteral nutrition.
prenatal, circulation and. See Circulation, prenatal nutrition and.
vitamin A in, guidelines for, 351
Nutritional assessment, neonatal, 291-299
anthropometric, 293-296, 295f, 296f
biochemical, 296-298
body composition and, 292t, 292-293, 293f, 294t
bone mineralization measurements for, 299, 299t
medical history and, 291, 292t
nutrient balance studies for, 298
nutritional intake and, 291-292, 292t
physical examination and, 291, 292t
stable isotope studies for, 298-299

O

OAEs, 1809, 1810
Obesity, genetic, 412
Obligate heterodimers, 590
Oculocutaneous albinism, 592, 592t
Ofloxacin, during lactation, 256
15O-labeled water, for cerebral blood flow measurement, 1753
Oligohydramnios, 792
lung hypoplasia and, 806
Oligosaccharides
digestion of, postnatal, 1152
in human milk, 280, 280t, 1613
Omphalocele, 1106
Omphaloileal fistula, 1106
Omphalomesenteric duct, 1104-1105, 1106
Oncoproteins, 42
Ontogeny, interaction with pharmacogenetics, 216
Oocytes
meiotic prophase of. See Ovary(ies), meiotic prophase of oocytes and.
naked, 1945
Oogenesis, 1943
Oogonia, development of, 25-27, 27f, 28t
Operative stress, protein utilization and, 534-535
Opioids
contraindication to, for nursing mothers, 255
maternal abuse of, 241-244
pharmacology of, 241-242
withdrawal from, 243-244

Opsonins
  complement component C3b as, 1551–1552
  natural, in host defense, 1478–1479
Optic nerve, hypoplasia of, maternal alcohol
  consumption and, 236
Oral cavity, embryology of, 36–37, 37f
Oral contraceptives, contraindication to, for
  nursing mothers, 253t, 254
Organ blood flow, neonatal, autoregulation of,
  776
Organic acids
  renal tubular function and, prenatal, 1236
  transport of, 1200t, 1299–1302, 1300f
Organic acidurias, 1212t
Organic anion transporting peptide proteins,
  bile flow and, 1190–1191
Organic bases, renal tubular function and,
  prenatal, 1236
Organic ion transporter, 1299
Organoaxial volvulus, 1103
Ornithine, normal plasma and urine levels of,
  1296t
Osler-Weber-Rendu syndrome, 594
Osmoregulation, prolactin in, 1893
Ossification, endochondral, 36
Osteogenesis imperfecta, 593
Osteonectin, hematopoiesis and, 1389
Osteopenia, bone mineralization studies for,
  299, 299t
Osteum primum, 34
Otoacoustic emissions, 1809, 1810
Outflow tract, cardiac, 616f–618f, 616–619
Ovarian-placental shift, 125
Ovary(ies), 1941–1947
  development of, 1941
    gonadal sex determination and, 1941
  early differentiation of, 1941–1942, 1942f,
    1943f
  follicular growth and
    during childhood, 1947, 1947f, 1948f
    initiation of, 1946
  folliculogenesis and, 1945f, 1945–1946
    granulosa layer formation and,
      1945–1946, 1946f
    meiotic prophase of oocytes and,
      1942–1945, 1943f
    genetic control of, 1944
    initiation of, 1944
    morphological features of, 1944
    process of, 1943, 1944f
    regulation of, 1944–1945, 1945t
  steroidogenesis in, 1946–1947
    theca layer formation and, 1947, 1947f
    stroma formation and, 1947
Overfeeding, thermogenesis and, 412
Over-the-counter drugs, during lactation, 257
Oxidant risk, to neonate, 365–366
Oxidative stress
  apoptosis versus necrosis and, 75, 75t
  lung injury due to, 939
Oximetry, pulse Doppler, 872
Oxygen
  alveolarization and, 799
  lung injury due to, 846–847, 847f
  neonatal breathing and, 897–898
  partial pressure of
    alveolar, gas exchange and, 870–871,
      872f, 873f
    arterial, gas exchange and, 870–871, 872f,
      873f
  placental transfer of, 114–115, 116t
  pulmonary ion and liquid transport
    regulation by, 828f, 828–829
  retinopathy induced by, 1801–1802
  toxicity of, 967

Oxygen consumption
  fetal, 466–467
    measurement of, 466t, 466–467, 467f, 468f
    shock and, 773
  fetal heat production and, 541, 542f
  neonatal, thermoregulation and, 601, 602f
  of brain, determination of, 1715, 1716f
Oxygen delivery
  deficient. See Hypoxia.
  fetal, 885, 885f
    shock and, 773
  physiological alterations and, 887–889
  systemic, with right-to-left shunting, 708, 710
Oxygen extraction, fetal, shock and, 773
Oxygen quotient, fetal, 469–470, 470t
Oxygen saturation
  arterial
    determinants of
      with admixture lesions, 711
      with right-to-left shunting, 708,
        710f–711f
    systemic oxygen transport versus, with
      admixture lesions, 711, 712f
  fetal, developmental changes in, 773
  resuscitation and, 767–768, 768f, 768t
Oxygen sensing, 900–904
  via gene regulation, 903–904, 904f
  via membrane proteins, 901–903
Oxygen tension
  alveolar, gas exchange and, 870–871, 872f,
    873f
  arterial, gas exchange and, 870–871, 872f,
    873f
Oxygen therapy, 967–969, 968f
  for hyaline membrane disease, 932, 932f
Oxygen transport, 880–889
  erythrocyte 2,3-diphosphoglycerate and,
    884, 885f, 885–886, 886t
  erythrocytes and, 1410f, 1410–1411, 1411t,
    1412t, 1413f
  fetal, 884f, 884–889
    erythrocyte 2,3-diphosphoglycerate and,
      885f, 885–886, 886t
    oxygen delivery and, 885, 885f
  hemoglobin and. See Hemoglobin.
  oxygen delivery and. See Oxygen delivery.
  postnatal changes in, 886f, 886–887, 887f
  reduction of, in congenital heart disease,
    706
  systemic, systemic arterial oxygen
    saturation versus, with admixture
    lesions, 711, 712f
  transport system and, 880–881
Oxygenation
  of brain, resuscitation and, 771
  surfactant therapy effects on, 1078, 1078f
  with high-frequency ventilation, 979–980
Oxyhemoglobin saturation curve, 882–883,
  883f
Oxytocin
  hypothalamic secretion of, 1877, 1877t,
    1878
  milk ejection and, 287
  placental, 127
  synthesis of, 1877–1878
  umbilicoplacental circulation mediation by,
    752t

P

Pacemaker, cardiac, 676–677
Pachygyria, 1688
Pacinian corpuscles, 1865, 1866f
PAF. See Platelet activating factor.

Pain, 1792–1795
  assessment of, in neonates, 1794
  behavioral markers associated with, 1794
  clinical and physiologic markers associated
    with, 1794
  definition of, 1792
  nociception and, 1792–1794
    neuroanatomy, neurophysiology, and
      neurochemistry of, 1792–1794,
      1793f, 1793t
  prolonged effects of, 1794–1795
Pallister-Hall syndrome, 786, 1848t
Palmitoylphosphatidylcholine, in pulmonary
  surfactant, 1007, 1007t
Palmoplantar keratodermas, 591
Pancreas
  agenesis of, 1104
  annular, 1104, 1104f
  embryogenesis of, anomalies of, 1104, 1104f
  embryonic development of, 37
    homeobox genes and, 68–69
  exocrine, 1142–1149
    diet and weaning and, in rodents,
      1146–1147
    embryology and histogenesis of, 1142f,
      1142–1143
    fetal antigens and, 1148
    homeobox genes and, 1149, 1149f
    nonhuman, ontogeny of, 1143–1144
    proto-oncogenes and, 1148–1149
    regulation of, 1147–1148
    secretion by, 1144
      ontogeny in human, 1144–1146, 1145f
      ontogeny in rodents, 1146
  organogenesis of, 1104, 1104f
Pancreatic amylase, in neonates, 1152
Pancreatic anlagen, 1104, 1104f
Pancreatic ducts, variations of, 1104
Pancreatic enzymes, 1157–1158
  in neonates, 1152
  proteolytic
    postnatal, 1155
    prenatal, 1155
Pancreatic lipases, 1157–1158
Paneth cells, 1371–1372
Para-aminohippurate, transport of,
  1299–1301, 1300f
Paracellular pathway, in lactation, 286–287
Parasympathetic nervous system, cardiac
  conduction and, 682, 683f, 684, 684f
Parathyroid glands, 1926
Parathyroid hormone
  calcium homeostasis and, 305f, 305–306
    neonatal, 325–326
  calcium transport and, 1287
  cellular actions of, 306
  growth plate control by, 1835
  mechanism of action of, 306
  metabolism of, 306
  phosphate transport and, 1291
  placental calcium transport and, 318
  placental magnesium transport and, 320
  placental phosphorus transport and, 319
  secretion of, 305–306
  umbilicoplacental circulation mediation by,
    752t
Parathyroid hormone-related peptide
  calcium homeostasis and, 306–307
  calcium transport and, 318, 1288
  physiologic effects of, 307
  structure of, 307
  umbilicoplacental circulation mediation by,
    752t
Paraventricular nucleus, hypothalamic, 1872t
Paregoric, for opioid withdrawal, 243

Parenteral nutrition
    amino acid requirements for, 532–534,
        533t, 534t
    cholestasis associated with, 1194
    for postnatal infants, lipid emulsions for,
        399–400
    lipid emulsions for, for neonates, 417f,
        417–418, 418t
    vitamin A and, 350
Parietal cells
    diminished function of, in neonates, 1120
    secretion by, 1119–1120
    of intrinsic factor, 1120
Partial expiratory flow-volume curves, 838
Parturition, adrenal role in initiating, 1923
Parvocellular system, 1877, 1877t
Passive diffusion, of drugs, 179, 220–221, 221f,
    222f, 223
Patent ductus arteriosus. See Ductus
    arteriosus, patent.
Pax genes, 19
PC. See Phosphatidylcholine.
PCR. See Polymerase chain reaction.
PDGF. See Platelet-derived growth factor.
Peak concentration, measured, 195
Peak inflating pressure, 969–971, 970f, 971t
PEEP. See Continuous positive airway
    pressure.
Peg3 gene, in hypothalamic development,
    1874t
Pendelluft, with high-frequency ventilation,
    980–981, 981f
Penetrance, incomplete, 8
Pentose phosphate pathway, of erythrocytes,
    1406–1407, 1408f
Peptidase, activity of, in small intestine,
    1155–1156
Peptide(s). See also specific peptides, e.g.
        Atrial natriuretic peptide.
    antimicrobial, in neonatal pulmonary host
        defense, 1628–1629
Peptide YY, gastrointestinal tract growth and,
    1098
Perfluorochemicals, for liquid ventilation,
    985–986, 986f, 986t, 987f, 987t, 988–989
    in respiratory distress syndrome, 997–998,
        998f
    uptake of, 991–993, 992f–994f, 992t
Perfusion. See also Reperfusion; Ventilation-
        perfusion relationships.
    matching of, to optimize maternal/fetal
        exchange, 753
    placental, reduced, preeclampsia and fetal
        growth impairment and, 151
    regional, hypoxia and, 654–655
    systemic, low, in neonates, 661f, 661–662,
        662f
Perichondral ring of LaCroix, 1834
Perichondrium, 1831
Periciliary fluid, in neonatal pulmonary host
    defense, 1614f, 1623–1624
Periodic breathing, 905
    apnea related to, 911, 911f
    in neonates, 895–896, 896f, 897f
Peripheral tolerance, 1521
Peripheral vascular resistance, vasoactive
        mediators influencing, ventilation-
        perfusion matching and, 877f, 877–878,
        878f
Periventricular hemorrhagic infarction, with
        intraventricular hemorrhage, 1759–1760,
        1760f, 1761f
Periventricular leukomalacia, with
        intraventricular hemorrhage, 1760–1761,
        1761t

Permeability, of placental tissue, 220–221
Peroxisomal disease, hepatic pathology due
    to, 1215
Peroxisomes, synthesis of, disorders of, 1213t
Persistent truncus arteriosus, 618
PET. See Positron emission tomography.
Pethidine, uteroplacental blood flow and,
    763
PFA-100, in neonates, 1449
Pfeiffer syndrome, 48, 786, 790, 1837, 1857t
P-glycoprotein, 1702
Phagocyte(s), in host defense, against invasive
    candidiasis, 1488
Phagocyte oxidase, 1545
Phagocytic cells, stimulus-response coupling
        in, 1591–1600
    downstream signaling mechanisms and,
        1595–1597
        low molecular weight guanosine
            triphosphate-binding proteins and,
            1595–1596, 1596f
        MAP kinases and Ras-initiated pathways
            and, 1596–1597
    lipid remodeling and signaling and,
        1597–1598
        phosphatidylinositol-3-kinase and, 1597
        phosphoinositide, 1597, 1597f
        phospholipase A_2 and, 1597–1598
        phospholipase D and, 1597
        sphingomyelin and, 1598
    receptor types and, 1592f, 1592–1595,
        1593f
        trimeric G-proteins and, 1593f,
            1593–1594, 1594f
        tyrosine kinase-initiated signal
            transduction and, 1594f, 1594–1595,
            1595f
    second-messenger-regulated, 1598–1600
        protein kinase C and, 1599–1600, 1601f
        second-messenger generation and,
            1598–1599
        second-messenger-regulated kinases and,
            1598, 1599
    signal transduction and, 1591–1592
Phagocytosis
    by mononuclear phagocytes, 1530, 1531
        in neonatal pulmonary host defense,
            1633–1634, 1634f
    by neutrophils, 1542–1543
    in placental transfer, 118
Pharmacodynamics, 188–189, 189f
    dose-response relationship and, 188–189,
        189f
    of adrenergic agents, 229–232, 230f, 231f
        in neonates, 231–232, 232f
    pharmacogenetics and, 213t, 215
    receptor classification and, 188
    receptor regulation and, 188
Pharmacogenetics, 211–216, 212t, 213t
    gene regulation and development and,
        215–216
    interaction with ontogeny, 216
    pediatric, clinical, 216
    pharmacodynamics related to, 213t, 215
    pharmacokinetics related to, 212t, 212–213
    phase I drug oxidation polymorphisms and,
        213–214
        CYP2C9, 214
        CYP2C19, 214
        CYP2D6, 213–214, 214t
    phase II drug oxidation polymorphisms
        and, 214–215
        NAT2, 214–215
        TMPT, 215
Pharmacogenomics, 211

Pharmacokinetics, 190–197
    apparent volume of distribution and,
        192–193
    bioavailability and, 180–181
    dose adjustments and
        bedside, examples of, 196–197
        mathematical, examples of, 195–196
    drug absorption and, 179–180
        factors affecting, 180
        kinetics of, 180
        membrane transporters and, 180
        transport mechanisms and, 179–180
    drug clearance and, 187, 193, 193f
        first-pass, 193
    drug distribution and, 181–182, 186, 186f
        factors affecting, 181–182, 182t
        multicompartment, 187, 187f
        single-compartment, 186
    drug elimination and, 182–186
        biotransformation and, 182–184, 183t
        disease effects on, 185–186
        first-order, 191f, 191t, 191–192
        multicompartment, 191–192, 192f
        renal, 184–185
        zero-order, 192
    half-lives and, 186, 186t, 187f
    models in, 190–191
    multiple-dose administration and, 194–195
    of adrenergic agents, 228f, 228–229, 229f
        in neonates, 229
    of maternofetal drug exchange, 199, 199f,
        199t, 200t
    pharmacogenetics and, 212t, 212–213
    single-dose administration and, by short-
        duration infusion, 194, 194f
    steady-state conditions and, 193, 194t
    zero-order kinetics of, 187–188
Pharmacologic agents. See Drug(s);
        Radiopharmaceuticals; specific drugs and
        drug types.
Phencyclidine, contraindication to, for nursing
        mothers, 255
Phenobarbital
    contraindication to, for nursing mothers,
        253t, 254
    during lactation, 256
    for opioid withdrawal, 243
    half-life of, 186t
    protein binding of, 205t
Phenylalanine
    fetal accretion of, 531t
    in parenteral amino acid mixtures, 533t,
        534t
    normal plasma and urine levels of, 1296t
    requirements for, of low birth weight
        infants, 530t–532t
Phenylbutazone, half-life of, 186t
Phenytoin
    during lactation, 256
    half-life of, 186t
    protein binding of, 205t
Phosphate
    calcium transport and, 1288
    dietary, phosphate transport and, 1292
    renal tubular function and, prenatal,
        1236–1237
Phosphatidylcholine
    biosynthesis of, rate of, 1055
    in pulmonary surfactant, 1006–1008, 1007f,
        1007t, 1008t
    surfactant, biosynthesis of, 1041, 1042f
        developmental changes in, 1042–1044,
            1043f, 1043t
        hormone-induced changes in, 1044–1046
        regulation of, mechanism of, 1046–1048

Phosphatidylglycerol
in pulmonary surfactant, 1007, 1007f, 1007t
surfactant, biosynthesis of, 1041, 1042f
unsaturated, for surfactant therapy, 1075
Phosphatidylinositol, surfactant, biosynthesis
of, 1041, 1042f
Phosphatidylinositol 3,4,5-triphosphate,
generation of, 1597
Phosphatidylinositol-3-kinase, remodeling of,
signaling and, 1597
Phosphoinositides, remodeling of, signaling
and, 1597, 1597f
Phospholipase A_2 remodeling of, signaling
and, 1597-1598
Phospholipase D, remodeling of, signaling
and, 1597
Phospholipids
adsorption of, surfactant proteins and,
1024-1025
in bile, 1188, 1189f
pulmonary, 1006-1008, 1007f, 1007t, 1008t
surfactant, 1018-1019, 1019f, 1041-1050
biosynthesis of, 1041, 1042f, 1042-1048
developmental changes in, 1042-1044,
1043f, 1043t
hormone-induced changes in,
1044-1046
regulation of, mechanism of,
1046-1048
secretion of, 1048f, 1048-1050, 1049f
ventilation-perfusion matching and,
877-878
Phosphorus
distribution in body, neonatal, 323-324
gastrointestinal transport of, neonatal,
332-334, 333f
homeostasis of, 1289-1292
phosphate transport and, 1290-1292
factors influencing, 1291-1292
nephron sites of, 1290, 1290f
transcellular, 1291, 1291f
regulation of, 327
renal phosphorus handling and, 1290
placental transport of, 318t, 318-319
hormonal regulation of, 319
mechanisms of, 319, 319f
Phototherapy
for jaundice, 1205-1210
bilirubin light absorption and,
1206-1207, 1207f
bilirubin photochemistry and,
1207-1209
configurational isomerization and,
1207-1208, 1208f
photo-oxidation and, 1208-1209
structural isomerization and, 1208,
1209f
bilirubin photoproduct formation and,
1209, 1209f
bilirubin structure and, 1205-1206,
1206f
mechanism of, 1209-1210, 1210f
heat exchange and water loss and, through
skin, 575-576
respiratory water and evaporative heat loss
during, 577, 581t
Phrenic nerve, 852, 852f
Physical therapy, in neonates, 1449
Physiologic dead space, in hyaline membrane
disease, 931
Physis. See Growth plate.
Piebaldism, 592, 592t
Pinocytosis
by mononuclear phagocytes, 1530
in placental transfer, 118, 207

Pituitary gland, 1926
congenital abnormalities of, 1903
control by, development of, 1891
development of, 1896-1898, 1897f,
1897t
hormones secreted by. See specific
hormones, e.g. Follicle-stimulating
hormone.
Placenta
amino acid consumption of, 517
angiogenesis in, 80-81, 82, 83f
bile acid metabolism of, 1183
cell islands of, 94
circulation of. See Placental circulation.
corticotropin-releasing hormone from,
1907
development of, 85-95
cell islands and, 94
chorionic plate and, 94
early, 85-87, 86f
implantation and lacunar period of, 85,
86f
maternofetal barrier and, 86-87, 87f,
88t
villous, 85-86, 86f
fetal growth restriction and, 259-260
fetal membranes and, 95
septa and, 94
structural, drug transport and, 218-219,
219f
trophoblastic invasion in, 91-94
arterial, 94
interstitial, 92-94, 93f
umbilical cord and, 94-95
fluid volume and, 1349
glucose transporters in, 490-491
heat production in, 541-542
hematopoietic growth factor production
by, 1383
lipid metabolism of, 391
lipid transport by, 391-392
metabolism of, 224-225
perfusion of, in vitro, for study of umbilical
circulation, 751
preeclampsia origin in, 147-149
scintigraphy of, for uteroplacental blood
flow measurement, 759
septa of, 94
thyroid-stimulating hormone produced by,
1928
villi of, 87f, 87-91
anchoring, 85, 92
cotyledons and villous trees and, 90-91,
92f
development of, 85-86, 86f
fetal endothelium and, 87
fetoplacental angioarchitecture and, 90
intermediate, immature, 90, 91f
intermediate, mature, 90
intervillous space and, 91
maternofetal barrier integrity and, 89
mesenchymal, 90
stem, 90
terminal, 90, 90f
tertiary, 86
trophoblast and, 87-89, 89f
types of, 89-90, 90f, 91f
villous stroma and, 87
zinc metabolism in, 343
Placental abruption
alcohol consumption and, 235
in multiple pregnancy, 168
Placental barrier, 220
Placental bed, 92
Placental blood flow, 223-224

Placental circulation, 97-102
nitric oxide and, 102
prostaglandins and, 100-101
regulation of, 97
steroid hormones and, 102
vascular bed development and, 97-99, 98f,
99f
vasoconstrictors and, 99-100, 100f, 101f
Placental clock, 127
Placental hormones, 122-129
enzymes regulating, 128
hypophyseal-like, 123f, 123-124
hypothalamic-like releasing and inhibiting
activities of, 125-127, 126f
placental integration with intrauterine
tissues and, 128-129
steroidogenesis and, 124f, 124-125, 125f
Placental lactogens, 1893-1894
Placental perfusion, reduced, preeclampsia
and fetal growth impairment and, 151
Placental transfer/transport, 111-119, 112f,
113t, 114t, 115f, 117f, 119
diffusional, 111-112, 114-115
flow limitation and, 114-115
hydrophilic permeability and, 112, 114,
116t
endocytosis and exocytosis and, 118
fetal growth and, 119, 120t
gestational changes in, 119
of amino acids, 116-117, 512-517
active, 512
development of transport capacity and,
515-516
drugs and toxins and, 517
hormones and, 516-517
in intrauterine growth restriction, 516
transport systems and, 512-514, 513t
transporter proteins and, 514t, 514-515
anionic, 515
cationic, 515
neutral, 514-515
of calcium, 314-318
active, 314t, 314-316, 315f
bidirectional, 316
control of, 317
hormonal regulation of, 317-318
in diabetic pregnancy, 320
in intrauterine growth restriction, 320
maternal calcium concentration and, 317
mechanisms of, 316-317
of drugs, 197-208, 218-225
active, 224
active drug and, 223, 224f, 225f
by facilitated diffusion, 224
by pinocytosis, 224
clinical applications of, 208
ionization and, 201-203, 202t, 203t
lipid solubility and, 199-201, 201f
methodologic approaches to, 198
models of, 220, 220f
molecular weight and, 205-206, 206f
passive, 220-221, 221f, 222f, 223
pharmacokinetic models of, 199, 199f,
199t, 200t
placental blood flow and, 223-224
placental metabolism and, 224-225
protein binding and, 203-205, 204t,
204f-206f, 205t
selective transport mechanisms and,
207-208
stereoselectivity and, 206-207
structural development of placenta and,
218-219, 219f
of erythrocytes, 1402
of free fatty acids, 377-379, 379f

Placental transfer/transport (Continued)
of glycerol, 379–380, 380f
of heat, 542, 542f
of hematopoietic growth factors, 1383–1384
of ketone bodies, 380
of lipids, 391–392
of magnesium, 319t, 319–320
control of, 320
hormonal regulation of, 320
mechanisms of, 320
of phosphorus, 318t, 318–319
hormonal regulation of, 319
mechanisms of, 319, 319f
of substrates, preeclampsia and fetal growth impairment and, 151
of water, 118–119
or magnesium
in diabetic pregnancy, 320
in intrauterine growth restriction, 320
transporter protein-mediated, 115–117
amino acids and, 116–117
glucose transfer and, 116
Placental transfusion, during delivery, neonatal fluid volumes and, 1345
Placentomes, 91
Plasma, volume of, 1341–1343, 1342t, 1343t
during labor and delivery, 1345
measurement of, 1346–1347
regulation of, 1345–1348
Plasma clearance rate, in neonates, 231–232
Plasma colloid oncotic pressure, in acute renal failure, 1338
Plasma transport, of vitamin A, 347–348, 348f
Plasma water volume measurement, 1353
Plasmids, 16
Plasminogen
in children, 1442t
in full-term infants, 1440t
in premature infants, 1440t
Plasminogen activator inhibitor-1
in children, 1442t
in full-term infants, 1440t
in premature infants, 1440t
Plasticity
developmental, 161
of stem cells, 1366, 1372
Platelet(s), 1443–1444
activation of, during birth process, 1444
disorders of. See also Thrombocytopenia.
qualitative, 1455
in cord blood, 1443–1444
leukocyte mobilization to inflammatory sites and, 1580–1582, 1582f
megakaryocyte precursors of, 1443
morphology of, in neonates, 1448
neonatal platelet function and, 1444
production of, by megakaryocytes, site of, 1426–1427
Platelet activating factor
in neonatal pulmonary host defense, 1642
intestinal circulation and, 704
necrotizing enterocolitis and, 1171
shock and, neonatal, 775
Platelet aggregation testing, in neonates, 1449
Platelet count, in neonates, 1448
Platelet endothelial adhesion molecule-1, 1574t, 1579
Platelet flow cytometry, in neonates, 1449
Platelet-capillary function, intraventricular hemorrhage and, 1764
Platelet-derived growth factor
alveolarization and, 797
brain development and, 1786
fetal growth and, 1883

Platelet-derived growth factor (Continued)
growth plate control by, 1835
lung development and, 787, 789
Pleiotropy, 8
of cytokine function, 1382, 1383f
Pluripotent stem cells, 58, 1365
growth factors affecting, 1377
Pneumotachography, for tidal volume measurement, 922
Pneumothorax, intraventricular hemorrhage and, 1763
Poikilothermic organisms, 548
Point mutations, 6
Polydactyly, postaxial, type A, 1848t
Polymerase chain reaction, 12–13, 13f, 16
amniotic fluid microorganism detection by, 135
Polymicrogyria, 1688, 1688f
Polymorphonuclear neutrophils, in neonatal pulmonary host defense, 1634–1635
Polypeptides, placental transfer of, 207
Polyploidization, 1421
Polysaccharides, digestion of, 1152
postnatal, 1152, 1152f
prenatal, 1152
Ponderal index, in neonatal nutritional assessment, 295–296
Pontine neuronal necrosis, periventricular, 1761
Portal circulation, development of, 1898
Portal vein, preduodenal, 1103
Positive end-expiratory pressure. See Continuous positive airway pressure.
Positron emission tomography, 1715–1716
cerebral glucose utilization on, 1718f, 1718t, 1718–1719, 1719f
cerebral blood flow and, 1719
for cerebral blood flow measurement, 1751–1753, 1752f, 1753f
Posterior nucleus, hypothalamic, 1872t
Postmitotic compartments, 1390–1392, 1391t, 1392f
Postprandial hyperemia, 703
Potassium
blood-brain barrier transporter for, 1701–1702
homeostasis of, 1279–1285, 1280f
external, regulation of, 1282–1285
gastrointestinal tract and, 1285
renal contribution to, 1282f, 1282–1285, 1283f
internal, regulation of, 1279, 1281t, 1281–1282
acid-base balance and, 1281
hormones and, 1281
plasma potassium concentration and, 1281
with hypothermia, 587
ionic flux of, oxygen-sensing via, 901, 902f, 903f
renal tubular function and, prenatal, 1236
Potassium channel hyperinsulinism, neonatal, 496–497
Potassium currents, voltage-gated, 676, 676t
Power spectral analysis, of baroreflex function, 721
Prader-Willi syndrome, 10
Prealbumin, serum, in neonatal nutritional assessment, 297
Prebiotics, in human milk, 281
Precartilage blastema, 1831
Prechordal mesoderm, 1675
Preconditioning, 904
Preeclampsia/eclampsia, 147t, 147–149
fetal growth and development and, 149–154

Preeclampsia/eclampsia (Continued)
growth excess and, 151
growth restriction and, 150f, 150–151
mechanisms of impairment of, 151–154
future risks for offspring and, 154–155
in multiple pregnancy, 169
maternal pathophysiology of, 149, 150t
placental origin of, 147–149
risk factors for, 147, 147t
treatment of, 154
Pregnancy. See also Maternal entries.
carbohydrate metabolism during, 464
complicated, glucocorticoids and, 1071
corticotropin-releasing hormone levels during, 1908
insulin-like growth factor levels during, 1886
ketonemia in, 419
length of, maternal marijuana use and, 241
loss of
alcohol consumption and, 235
early, in multiple pregnancy, 171
maternal adaptation to, in multiple pregnancy, 167–169
maternal cardiovascular system during. See Maternal cardiovascular disease; Maternal cardiovascular system.
maternal drug abuse during. See Maternal drug abuse; specific drugs.
multiple. See Multiple pregnancy.
outcome of, maternal marijuana use and, 240–241
twin. See Multiple pregnancy.
vitamin E requirements during, 361, 361f, 362f
Pregnenolone, plasma concentration of, fetal and neonatal, 1922t
Pregnenolone sulfate, plasma concentration of, fetal and neonatal, 1922t
Pre-kallikrein
in adults, 1436t
in children, 1441t
in fetuses, 1436t
in full-term infants, 1436t, 1438t
in premature infants, 1437t
Preload
fetal, 649–650, 650f, 651f
myocardial contractility and, 636–638, 637f
Premature infants. See Preterm infants.
Premature labor. See Preterm labor.
Premature rupture of membranes
intra-amniotic infection with, 133
respiratory distress syndrome with, glucocorticoids and, 1071
Prematurity, ripples of, on electroencephalography, 1736t, 1737, 1737f
Preoptic area, hypothalamic, 1872t
Preprotachynin A gene, in neonatal pulmonary host defense, 1643
Prespermatogenesis, 1953
Prespermatogonia, 1952
Pressure gradients, intra-abdominal, gastroesophageal reflux and, 1165, 1167f
Pressure-flow autoregulation, 703
Pressure-support ventilation, 974
Pressure-volume curve, surfactant therapy effects on, 1075–1076, 1075f–1077f
Preterm infants. See also Low birth weight infants; Preterm labor.
anemia in
erythropoietin for
clinical trials in, 1414, 1415t
pharmacokinetics and, 1414, 1416
side effects of, 1416
nutritional supplementation in, 1416

Preterm infants (Continued)
apnea in. See Apnea, of prematurity.
complications in, glucocorticoid effect on, 1070, 1071f
dietary fat composition for, 399
fat requirements of, 398–399
formula for, lipids in, 394–395
formulas for, composition of, 529, 530t
gonadotropin secretion in, 1904
hyaline membrane disease in. See Hyaline membrane disease.
low-T_3 syndrome in, 1932
lung disease in, spectrum of, 949, 950f
lung of. See Lung(s), premature.
necrotizing enterocolitis in. See Necrotizing enterocolitis.
neonatal growth in, 266–267
nitric oxide in, inhaled, 740–741, 741f
parenteral lipid emulsions for, 399–400
patient ductus arteriosus in. See Ductus arteriosus, patent.
protection by human milk, 1615–1616
respiratory distress syndrome in, lung structure in, 1055, 1056f
resuscitation of, first inflations for, 769
retinopathy of prematurity in, 1799–1801
initiation of, 1800–1801
onset of, 1800, 1800f, 1800t
shock in, abnormal peripheral vasoregulation and, 777
surfactant in, quality of, 1065–1066
zinc requirement of, early postnatal, 345
Preterm labor, 103–108. See also Preterm infants.
definition of, 103
etiology of, 104–105, 106f
intrauterine infection associated with, 108, 132–133
causal relationship and, 134–135
chronic, 134
fetal infection and, 133
histologic chorioamnionitis and, 133
molecular mechanisms of, 135–137, 136f
with acute cervical incompetence, 133
with intact membranes, 132–133
with PROM, 133
with twin gestations, 133
obstetric management of, 107–108, 108t, 109t
prediction of, 105–107, 107t
prevention of, 107, 107t
Prilocaine, placental transfer of, 202t
Primary chorionic plate, 85
Primary energy failure, 771, 771f
Primary neuroendocrine cells, differentiation of, 816–817, 817f
Primary neurulation, 1675
Primary ossification center, 1831, 1832f
Priming, of neutrophils, 1539
Primitive node, 1849
Primitive respiratory diverticulum, 783
Primitive streak, 1849
Probiotics, in human milk, 281
Procainamide, during lactation, 256
Proctodeum, 1109
Profilaggrin, 589
Progastrin, 1121, 1122f
pancreatic secretion and, 1147
Progenitor cells, hematopoietic, 1375–1376, 1376t
Progesterone
lactation and, 289, 289f
plasma concentration of, fetal and neonatal, 1922t
Programmed cell death. See Apoptosis.

Programming, developmental, 161
Progress zone
in limb development, 1845–1846
of growth plate, 1829
Prolactin, 1892–1893
lactation and, 289, 289f
placental, 123
receptor for, 1893
surfactant phospholipid biosynthesis and, 1046
Proliferating cell nuclear antigen, 1143
Proliferative zone, of growth plate, 1834
Proline
fetal accretion of, 531t
in parenteral amino acid mixtures, 533t, 534t
normal plasma and urine levels of, 1296t
requirements for, of low birth weight infants, 530t–532t
PROM. See Premature rupture of membranes.
Pronephros, 1223
Pro-opiomelanocortin, 1907, 1908f, 1909
Prophase, mitotic, 5–6
Proportional-assist ventilation, 975
Prostacyclin
in neonatal pulmonary host defense, 1642
shock and, neonatal, 775
thermogenesis and, neonatal, 547t
Prostaglandin(s)
glomerular filtration rate and, 1257–1258, 1265
in neonatal pulmonary host defense, 1642
labor onset and, with intrauterine infection, 136
regulation of renal sodium transport by, 1275
renal blood flow and, 1246
renal hemodynamics and, 1233
renal tubular function and, 1238
umbilicoplacental blood flow and, 100–101
urinary concentration and, in neonates, 1316
uteroplacental blood flow and, 100–101
Prostaglandin E_2
calcium transport and, 1289
fever and, 566
shock and, neonatal, 775
thermogenesis and, neonatal, 547t
umbilicoplacental circulation mediation by, 752t
Prostaglandin F, umbilicoplacental circulation mediation by, 752t
Prostaglandin I_2, umbilicoplacental circulation mediation by, 752t
Prostanoids, placental, 128
Proteases
in neonatal pulmonary host defense, 1644f, 1644–1645
insulin-like growth factor binding protein, 1882, 1882f
levels during pregnancy, 1886
lung injury mediated by, 939
Protein(s). See also Amino acid(s).
absorption of, 528, 1156–1157
balance studies of, 1156
test meal analysis of, 1156f, 1156–1157
antimicrobial, in human milk, 1611
balance of, 523
chemistry of, 527–528
clinically useful, production using molecular genetics, 13
coagulant, 1435–1436
complement. See Complement proteins.
degradation of, 528
measurement of, 507–508
digestion of, 528, 1154–1156

Protein(s) (Continued)
gastric acidity and, 1154–1155
postnatal, 1154–1155, 1155f
prenatal, 1154
in small intestine, 1155–1156
pancreatic proteolytic enzymes and, 1155
proteolytic activity and, 1155
glucose transporter. See Glucose transporters.
in human milk, 275–276, 276t, 278–280, 279t
in surfactants, 1014–1015
intravenous infusions of, transvascular fluid filtration changes with, 1359–1360
iron-binding, in neonatal pulmonary host defense, 1627
lipopolysaccharide-binding, in neonatal pulmonary host defense, 1629
metabolism of, 501–508
fetal, fasting and, 522, 522f
measurement of, 502–508, 503t
amino acid requirements and, 506–507, 507f
degradation of specific proteins in, 507–508
end-product approach to, 503–504, 504f, 504t, 505f
free labeled amino acids in, 507
kinetics of individual components in, 504–506, 505f, 506f
synthesis of specific proteins in, 507
nitrogen balance and, 501, 502f
whole body, models for, 501–502, 502f
movement across microvascular barrier, 1359
neurotrophic, brain development and, 1786–1787
quality of, protein utilization and, 535–536
requirements for, 529, 530t
study methods for, 529
surfactant. See Surfactant proteins.
synthesis of, 528
fetal, 521f, 521t, 521–522
tracer studies of, 507
transporter. See Transporter proteins.
turnover of, 528–529
fetal, 521
utilization of, 534–537
clinical status and, 534–535
concomitant intake of other nutrients and, 536–537
concomitant protein intake and, 536, 536t
hormones and, 537
quality of protein intake and, 535–536
Protein binding, of drugs, placental transfer and, 203–205, 204t, 204f–206f, 205t
Protein C
in adults, 1436t
in children, 1441t
in fetuses, 1436t
in full-term infants, 1436t, 1439t
in premature infants, 1439t
Protein kinase(s)
JAK/STAT family of, signal transduction and, 1595, 1595f
substrate for, in brown adipose tissue, 408
Protein kinase A
activation of, 1599
CAMP-activated, 1599
regulation of, 1599
Protein kinase C, 1599–1600
receptors for, 1600
regulation of, 1600

Protein kinase C (Continued)
  signaling for superoxide anion generation
      and, 1600, 1601f
  targeting of, 1600
Protein phosphorylation, 188
Protein S
  in adults, 1436t
  in children, 1441t
  in fetuses, 1436t
  in full-term infants, 1436t, 1439t
  in premature infants, 1439t
Proteoglycans
  development of, nutrition and, 808
  hematopoiesis and, 1390
Proteolysis
  in small intestine, 1155-1156
  in stomach, 1154-1155
      postnatal, 1154-1155, 1155f
      prenatal, 1154, 1155
  postnatal, 1155
  prenatal, 1155
Proteomes, 4
Proteomics, 4
Proteus syndrome, 593
Prothrombin time
  in adults, 1436t
  in children, 1441t
  in fetuses, 1436t
  in full-term infants, 1436t, 1438t
  in premature infants, 1437t
Proto-oncogenes, 42
  pancreas and, 1148-1149
Proximodistal axis, in limb development,
      1846, 1847t
Proximodistal patterning, 1829-1830
Pseudoachondroplasia, 1836t, 1837
Pseudoautosomal regions, 6, 1936
Psychoactive drugs
  maternal use of, 244-245
      during lactation, 253t, 254, 256
  pharmacology of, 244
Psychomotor Developmental Index,
      docosahexaenoic acid and, 436
PU.1, in mononuclear phagocyte
      development, 1523-1524, 1524f
Pulmonary acinus, 786, 788
Pulmonary agenesis, 791
Pulmonary aplasia, 791
Pulmonary arterial pressure
  vasoactive mediators increasing, 877f,
      877-878, 878f
  ventilation-perfusion matching and,
      874-875
Pulmonary blood flow, resuscitation and, 770,
      770f
Pulmonary circulation, development of,
      818-819
Pulmonary compliance
  dynamic, 922
  measurement of, 922-923
      during tidal breathing, 838
  static, 922
Pulmonary energetics, measurement of, 923
Pulmonary epithelium
  differentiation of, in lung development,
      816-818, 817f
  ion transport across, 823-826, 824f
Pulmonary function. See also Lung entries;
      Respiratory entries.
  cardiovascular function and, 975-976
  dynamic, surfactant therapy effects on,
      1077-1078, 1078f
  evaluation of
      in neonates, 919-925
      airflow mechanics in, 923-924, 924f

Pulmonary function (Continued)
      clinical applications of, 924-925
      dynamic lung volumes in, 922
      instrumentation for, 919, 920t, 921f
      normal values for, 924, 924t
      physiologic background for, 919,
          920f
      pulmonary compliance in, 922-923,
          923f
      static lung volumes in, 919-921, 921f,
          922f
  pulmonary function profiles and,
      837-840, 839f
  with mechanical ventilation, 975
  in bronchopulmonary dysplasia, 956-959
      early, 956-957
      established, 957f, 957-958, 958f
      gas exchange and, 958-959
      long-term, 959
  maternal, in multiple pregnancy, 168
Pulmonary gas exchange. See Gas exchange;
      Ventilation-perfusion relationships.
Pulmonary hemorrhage, with surfactant
      therapy, 1080
Pulmonary host defense. See Host defense,
      pulmonary.
Pulmonary hypertension
  experimental pathophysiology of, 698-699,
      699f
  hypothermia and, 587
  in bronchopulmonary dysplasia, 959
  of newborn, persistent, nitric oxide in,
      737-740, 739f, 740f
  pathophysiology of, experimental, 698-699,
      699f
  reversal of, 695
      failure of, 696
Pulmonary hypoplasia, 791
  liquid ventilation for, 997
Pulmonary lymphangiectasis, congenital,
      792
Pulmonary mechanics, measurement of, 923,
      923f
Pulmonary overinflation, 791
Pulmonary reflexes
  fetal breathing and, 892
  neonatal breathing and, 898
Pulmonary regurgitation, cardiovascular
      physiology and, 714
Pulmonary resistance, measurement of,
      922-923
  during tidal breathing, 838
Pulmonary stenosis, afterload increase with,
      714
Pulmonary surfactant. See Surfactant,
      pulmonary; Surfactant proteins;
      Surfactant therapy.
Pulmonary vascular resistance
  cardiac function and, 878
  in congenital heart disease, 707
  resuscitation and, 770, 770f
Pulmonary vasculature. See also Pulmonary
      hypertension.
  development of, 629-633, 630f-632f,
      690-699
      abnormal, 695-696, 697f
          induction of, 696, 698
      clinical implications of, 699
      decreased growth of vascular bed and, 699
      elevated resistance and, failure to
          reverse, 696
      fetal morphology and, 690f-692f,
          690-695
          cellular mechanisms and, 692,
              694-695, 694f-696f

Pulmonary vasculature (Continued)
      microscopic features and, 691-692,
          693f, 694f
      venous, 699
  regulation of, nitric oxide in, 733
Pulmonary vasoconstriction, hypoxic,
      ventilation-perfusion matching and, 875f,
      875-876, 876f
Pulmonary venous connection, total
      anomalous, 716
Pulsating bubble surfactometer, 1023
Pulse Doppler oximetry, 872
Purpura fulminans, neonatal, 1466f,
      1466-1467
  coagulation findings in, 1467, 1467t
  therapy for, 1467
Pyloric stenosis, 1102
Pyogen, endogenous, 566

Q

Quinidine, during lactation, 256
Quinine, during lactation, 256
Quinolones, during lactation, 256

R

Radiant heaters
  heat exchange between infant and
      environment under, 572, 575, 579f
  water loss under, 575, 579f
Radiation, nonionizing, heat exchange and
      water loss and, under radiant heaters,
      575, 579f
Radioangiography, for uteroplacental blood
      flow measurement, 759
Radiopharmaceuticals, contraindication to, for
      nursing mothers, 254, 254t
Random concentration, 195
Ranitidine, during lactation, 257
RDS. See Respiratory distress syndrome.
Reactive oxygen species
  biosynthesis of, 1528-1529
  lung injury due to, 939
  shock and, neonatal, 775
Rearrangement, in antigen receptor
      development, 1513
Receptor down-regulation, 188
Receptor editing, 1521
Receptor occupancy theory, 188
Receptor tyrosine kinases, vascular
      development and, 623-625, 624f, 625f
Receptor up-regulation, 188
Recombinant DNA, 11, 12, 16, 17t
Recombination, 6
Recreational chemicals, contraindication to,
      for nursing mothers, 253t, 255
Rectoanal reflex, 1135
Red blood cells. See Anemia; Erythrocytes.
Reduction division, 6
Redundancy, of cytokine function, 1382-1383
Reflexes. See specific types of reflexes, e.g.
      Pulmonary reflexes.
Regulatory metabolic rise, 550
Relaxin, chorionic, 127
Renal agenesis, 1332
Renal blood flow
  angiotensin II in, 1253-1254
  control of, 1231-1234
  nephron loss and, 1331
  postnatal, 1242-1247
      autoregulation of, 1242-1243
      intrarenal, 1242

Renal blood flow (Continued)
    regulation of, 1234f, 1243-1247
        anatomic development and, 1243-1244
        renal nerves and adrenergic system
            and, 1246-1247
        vasoactive factors in, 1244-1246
        total, 1242, 1243f
    prenatal development of, 1231, 1232f
    urinary concentration and, in neonates, 1320
Renal compensatory mechanisms, 1362
    fetal, 1362
Renal disease, drug elimination and, 185
Renal dysplasia, 1332
Renal function. See also Kidney(s).
    maternal, in multiple pregnancy, 168
Renal hypoplasia, 1332
Renal pelvis, urinary concentration and, in
    neonates, 1320, 1321f
Renal sympathetic nerve activity, blood
    pressure regulation and, 718, 719f, 721,
    722, 723-724
Renal tubular function
    aldosterone and, 1237
    atrial natriuretic peptide and, 1238
    cortisol and, 1238
    kallikrein-kinin system and, 1238
    prenatal development of, 1234-1237
        acid-base homeostasis and, 1236
        glucose and, 1236
        organic acids and bases and, 1236
        phosphate and, 1236-1237
        potassium and, 1236
        sodium and, 1234-1236, 1235f
    prostaglandins and, 1238
    renin-angiotensin system and, 1237-1238
Renal tubules
    collecting, fluid transport in, 1312, 1312t
    distal, sodium transport in, 1273f,
        1273-1274
        aldosterone and angiotensin II and,
            1273t, 1273-1274
        epithelial sodium channel and, 1273
    drug reabsorption by, 185
    drug transport by, 184-185
    medullary, inner, urinary concentration and,
        in neonates, 1319-1320, 1319f-1321f
    proximal, sodium transport in, 1271-1273
        sodium bicarbonate co-transporter and,
            1272-1273
        sodium reabsorption and, 1271-1272
        sodium/hydrogen transporter and, 1271
Renin
    activity of, maturational changes in,
        1250-1251, 1251t
    molecular biology of, 1249
    plasma concentration of, fetal and neonatal,
        1922t
Renin-angiotensin system, 1249-1255, 1250f.
    See also Angiotensin II.
    components of
        maturational changes in activity of,
            1250-1252, 1252f
        molecular biology of, 1249-1250
    renal tubular function and, 1237-1238
    urinary concentration and, in neonates,
        1316-1317
Renin-angiotensin-aldosterone system,
    regulation of renal sodium transport by,
    1274-1275, 1275f
Reperfusion
    cooling during, for neuroprotection,
        583-584
    in cerebral injury, cerebral metabolism,
        excitotoxins, and free radicals during,
        586

Replacement gene therapy, 15
Repolarization, cardiac, 676, 676t
Reserve zone, of growth plate, 1833
Residual volume, 919
Respiratory acidosis
    fetal, 1362
    metabolic compensation for, neonatal,
        1329-1330
    neonatal, 1364
Respiratory alkalosis
    fetal, 1362
    metabolic compensation for, neonatal,
        1329-1330
    neonatal, 1364
Respiratory burst, 1532, 1545
Respiratory compensatory mechanisms, 1362
    fetal, 1362
Respiratory disease. See also specific
        disorders, e.g. Hyaline membrane
        disease.
    neonatal, lung liquid in
        airway ion transport studies and, 820, 820f
        ion transport and, 829f, 829-831
        treatment and, 830-831
Respiratory distress syndrome, 944-945,
    1055-1067. See also Hyaline membrane
    disease.
    glucocorticoids for prevention of,
        1069-1073, 1070t
        combined with other hormones, 1073
        dexamethasone-specific toxicity and,
            1072-1073
        effectiveness of, 1070-1072
            complications associated with preterm
                birth and, 1070, 1071f
            in complicated pregnancies, 1071
            neonatal and maternal infection and,
                1070-1071
            NIH recommendations for, 1072, 1072t
            premature rupture of membranes and,
                1071
            respiratory distress syndrome
                incidence and, 1070, 1071f
            repeated courses and, 1072
            synergism with surfactant therapy, 1073,
                1073t
    in preterm infant, lung structure and, 1055,
        1056f
    infants surviving, chronic disease in,
        945-946
    initial events in, model for, 1067, 1067f
    maternal alcohol consumption and, 236
    mechanical ventilation for
        liquid ventilation as, 995-996, 996f, 997f,
            997-998, 998f
        lung injury due to, 1060-1061,
            1061f-1064f, 1063
    nitric oxide in, 736
        in premature infants, 740-741, 741f
    surfactant and. See Surfactant, pulmonary;
        Surfactant proteins; Surfactant therapy.
Respiratory diverticulum, primitive, 783
Respiratory epithelium, of upper airway, 834,
    835-836
Respiratory muscle(s). See also Diaphragm.
    fatigue of, in preterm infants, 962
    neonatal breathing and, 898-899
    unloading of, 975
Respiratory primordium, 783
Respiratory quotient, fetal, 470
Respiratory system, 783. See also Lung(s);
    Pulmonary entries.
    embryology of, 36, 37f
    heat exchange through, 571-572, 576-577,
        580f, 580t

Respiratory system (Continued)
        during mechanical ventilation, 577
        during phototherapy, 577, 581t
        gestational age and, 577, 581t
        intubation and, 577
    hypothermia and, 587
    resistance of
        during artificial ventilation, 865
        during spontaneous breathing, 866
    water loss through, in neonates, 571,
        576-577, 580f, 580t
        during mechanical ventilation, 577
        during phototherapy, 577, 581t
        gestational age and, 577, 581t
        intubation and, 577
Resting energy expenditure, measurement of,
    291
Resting membrane potential
    developmental changes in, 673-675
    of mature muscle, 1866
Restriction enzymes, 11, 11f
Restriction fragment length polymorphisms,
    14
Restrictive dermopathy, 593
Resuscitation, 765-771
    brain oxygenation and, 771
    breathing and
        first inflations and, 769, 770f
        regulation of, 768-769
    cerebral electrophysiological changes
        during, 771
    cooling during, for neuroprotection,
        583-584
    energy status in brain and, 771, 771f
    hemodynamic changes during, 769-771
        cerebral blood flow and, 771
        pulmonary blood flow and, 770, 770f
        systemic blood flow and myocardial
            function and, 769-770, 770f
    metabolic changes during, 768, 769f
    physiologic changes during, 765-766, 766f
    response to, 766-768
        Apgar scoring and, 766, 766t
        heart rate and, 766-767, 767f, 767t
        oxygen saturation and, 767-768, 768f,
            768t
        time to first breath and, 767, 768t
Retina, 1797-1802
    development of, 1797-1799
        clinical relevance of, 1802
        of antioxidant defense systems,
            1798-1799, 1799t
        of cellular components, 1797, 1798f
        vascular, 1797-1798, 1798f
    docosahexaenoic acid and, 434-435
    retinopathy and, 1799-1802
        of prematurity, 1799-1801
            initiation of, 1800-1801
            onset of, 1800, 1800f, 1800t
            oxygen-induced, 1801-1802
Retinaldehyde (retinal), 347
Retinoic acid
    alveolarization and, 798
    in lung development, 814
    lung development and, 785-786, 808
Retinoic acid receptor(s), 348, 348f
Retinoic acid receptor elements, 348, 348f
Retinoid(s). See also Vitamin A.
    brain development and, 1787
    embryogenesis and, 47-48
Retinoid x receptors, 349
Retinol
    lung development and, after lung injury in
        premature lung, 947
    placental transfer of, 207

Retinol-binding protein, 347–348, 348f
  in neonatal nutritional assessment, 297
Retinopathy, 1799–1802
  of prematurity, 1799–1801
    initiation of, 1800–1801
    onset of, 1800, 1800f, 1800t
    oxygen-induced, 1801–1802
Retroviruses, 12
Reverse transcriptase, 12
Rh hemolytic disease, anemia due to, late,
  1416–1417
Ribonucleic acid, structure of, 1, 2f
Ribosomal RNA, 3
Ribosomes, of myocytes, 1859
Rieger syndrome, 46–47
Right-to-left shunting, 708, 710–711
  bidirectional, 710–711
  isolated, 710
  lesions with, 715
  systemic arterial oxygen saturation
    determinants with, 708, 710f–711f
  systemic oxygen delivery with, 708, 710
Ripples of prematurity, on
  electroencephalography, 1736t, 1737,
  1737f
Ritodrine, uteroplacental blood flow and, 763
Ritodrine hydrochloride, for preterm labor,
  109t
RNA
  ribosomal, 3
  structure of, 1, 2f
RNA polymerases, 2–3
Rotational deformities, in intrauterine
  compression syndromes, 1838
Rpx/Hesx1 gene, in hypothalamic
  development, 1874t
rRNA, 3

S

Salbutamol, for preterm labor, 109t
Salicylates
  during lactation, 255
  for preterm labor, 109t
  half-life of, 186t
  protein binding of, 205t
Saline, for liquid ventilation, 985, 988
Salivary amylase
  in neonates, 1152
  prenatal, 1152
Salt taste
  newborn responses to, 1821
  older infants' and children's responses to,
    1822–1823
Sarcolemmal function, developmental changes
  in, 645–646
Sarcomeres, 635
  contractile proteins of
    developmental changes in, 641
    isoforms of, 641–643, 643f
  length of, 637
  proteins of, 635
  structure of, developmental changes in, 641
Sarcoplasmic organelles, of myotubes, 1855
Sarcoplasmic reticulum, cytosolic calcium
  concentration and, 637
Sarcosine, normal plasma and urine levels of,
  1296t
Sarcotubular system
  of myocytes, 1859–1860, 1860f
  of myotubes, 1859–1860, 1860f
Satellite cells, 1852, 1853f
Saturation kinetics, 192
Schizencephaly, 1688

Schwann cells, 852, 853f
Scintigraphy, placental, for uteroplacental
  blood flow measurement, 759
Sclerotome, 1850
Sebaceous glands, 595, 599
  lipids in, 601t
Second messengers
  inflammatory, cerebral injury and, 586
  kinases regulated by, 1598–1600
    protein kinase C as, 1599–1600, 1601f
    second-messenger regulation and,
      1598–1599
Secondary neurulation, 1675, 1676
Secondary ossification, center, 1832, 1832f
Second-order feedback, 1876
Secretin, pancreatic secretion and, 1147
Secretory activation, 288–290
  delays in, 289–290
  hormonal requirements for, 289, 289f
  initial milk volume and composition and,
    288f, 288–289, 289f
Seizures, electroencephalography with,
  1741–1744, 1742f–1744f
Selectin(s), 1574t
  in host defense, 1479
  in neonatal pulmonary host defense, 1652,
    1653, 1653f
  neonatal expression and function of,
    1586–1587
  neutrophil adherence and, 1540
Selectin ligands, 1574t, 1580
Selective serotonin reuptake inhibitors,
  during lactation, 256
Semilobar holoprosencephaly, 1680
Seminiferous tubules, development of, 1954
Semipermeable membranes, 220
Sensitivity
  to smells, in neonates, 1823–1824
  to sound, 1814
  to taste, in neonates, 1820–1821
Sensory function
  essential fatty acid deficiency and, 432
  neonatal, 607–609, 608f
Sepsis
  bacterial, cytokine levels during, 1566–1567
  cholestasis associated with, 1194
  oxygen delivery to tissues and, 888
  shock and, 777
Septation, of heart, 615–619
  endocardial cushions and, 616
  of atrioventricular canal and atria, 616
  outflow tract and, 616f–618f, 616–619
  ventricular, 619
Serine
  fetal accretion of, 531t
  fetal uptake of, 518, 519
  in parenteral amino acid mixtures, 533t,
    534t
  normal plasma and urine levels of, 1296t
  requirements for, of low birth weight
    infants, 530t–532t
Serine protease homologues, in neonatal
  pulmonary host defense, 1644
Serine/threonine kinases
  catalytic domains of, 1598
  second-messenger-regulated, 1598
  substrate specificity of, 1598
  targeting of, for specificity of responses,
    1598
Serotonin, 1708
  as neurotransmitter, 1875t
  metabolites of, 1708, 1708f, 1708t
  umbilicoplacental circulation mediation by,
    752t
Serpentine receptors, 1592, 1592f

Serprocidins
  in neonatal pulmonary host defense, 1644
  neutrophil, 1544, 1544t
Sertoli cells, development of, 1951–1954,
  1952f, 1953f
Set point, 554
  displacement of, fever and, 566
Severity of injury, apoptosis versus necrosis
  and, 74–75, 75t
Sex determination
  gonadal, 1941
  Y-chromosomal, 1935–1936
    early Y-chromosomal candidate
      sequences and, 1935–1936
    SRY gene and, 1936
Sex steroids. See also Androgens; Estrogens;
  Testosterone.
  neonatal growth and, 272
Sexual development
  gonadal stage of, 1938
  pregonadal, 1936–1938
    for which specific genes are known,
      1937–1938
    for which specific genes haven not been
      identified, 1936–1937
  secondary, 1938–1939
Sexual differentiation, 1898
SF-1/Ftz-F1 gene, in hypothalamic
  development, 1874t
Sharp waves, in neonatal
  electroencephalography, 1736t,
  1739–1740, 1740f, 1741t
  pathologic, 1741, 1742f
Shear stress, vascular development and,
  632–633
Shock, 772–779
  cardiovascular compromise and
    in fetus, 773–774
      developmental changes in fetal gas
        parameters and, 773
      hypoxemia and, 773–774
      oxygen delivery, oxygen consumption,
        and oxygen extraction and, 773
    in neonate, 774–779
      cellular and molecular factors in,
        775–776
      definition and phases of shock and,
        774–775
      pathogenesis of, 776–777
      physiology of circulation and, 776
      treatment of, 777–779
  clinical description of, 777
  warm, 777
Short esophagus, congenital, 1102
Shunting
  bidirectional, 710–711
  left-to-right
    at atrial level, 708
    at ventricular or great artery level,
      707–708, 709f
    effects of, on cardiac physiology,
      714–715
    lesions with, 715
  right-to-left, 708, 710–711
    isolated, 710
    lesions with, 715
    systemic arterial oxygen saturation
      determinants with, 708, 710f–711f
    systemic oxygen delivery with, 708, 710
Side-population profiles, 1369
SIDS. See Sudden infant death syndrome.
Signal sequences, 13
Signal transduction
  hematopoietic growth factors and, 1380f,
    1380–1382

Signal transduction (Continued)
    by JAK protein tyrosine kinases,
        1380-1381
    by SRC protein tyrosine kinases, 1381
    downstream signaling mechanisms and,
        1381-1382, 1382f, 1383f
    in phagocytic cells. See Phagocytic cells,
        stimulus-response coupling in.
    mechanisms of, 48f, 49f, 49-50
Signaling, through integrins, 54
Sim 1 gene, in hypothalamic development,
    1874t
Single-compartment drug distribution, 186
Single-injection technique, for glomerular
    filtration rate estimation, 1261
Single-ventricle physiology, 711-712
Sinusoidal cells, development of, 1177
Six3 gene, in hypothalamic development, 1874t
Skeletal muscle. See also Diaphragm.
    amino acid metabolism in, fetal, 522
    embryology of, 35, 36f
Skeletal system. See also Bone(s);
    Musculoskeletal entries.
    embryology of, 35-36
Skin, 589-596, 597t, 597-609
    appendages of, 594-596
        clinical relevance of, 595-596
        hair as, 594-595
        nails as, 595
        sebaceous glands as, 595
        sweat glands as, 595
    as neurodevelopmental interface, 606-609
        cutaneous receptors and electrical
            maturation and, 606-607, 607f, 607t
        skin as information rich surface and,
            607-609, 608f
    as primary care interface, 609, 609t
    dermal-epidermal junction of, 594
        clinical relevance of, 594, 594t
    dermis and subcutis of, 592-594
        blood vessels, lymphatics, and nerves of,
            593
        clinical relevance of, 593t, 593-594
    development of, 589, 590f
    diseases of, 591, 593t, 593-594, 594t
        pigmentary, 591-592, 592t
        prenatal diagnosis of, 596
    epidermis of, 589-592
        clinical relevance of, 591
        cornified envelope and lamellar body of,
            597-599, 598f
        development of, 590-591, 597-600, 598t
        differentiation of, 591
        in very low birth weight infant, strategies
            for maturation/repair of, 604-606,
            605t
        morphogenesis of, 591
        nonkeratinocytes in, 591-592, 592t
        specification of, 590
        vernix and, biology of, 599f, 599-600,
            600f, 600t
    fetal, 1604
    heat conductance through, 542, 543f
    heat exchange between infant and
        environment through, 572-576
        during first day after birth, 573-575,
            576f-578f
        during first hours after birth, 572, 573f
        during first weeks after birth, 575, 579f
        nonionizing radiation and, 575-576, 579f
        total, 575
    of very low birth weight infant, 604-606
        epidermal barrier repair strategies for,
            604-606, 605t
        ineffectiveness as barrier, 604, 605f

Skin (Continued)
    repair of, model of, 1605f, 1605-1607, 1606f
    thermoreceptors in, neonatal, 550-551,
        551f
    transition at birth, 600t, 600-604, 601t
        acid mantle development and, 601-602,
            603f
        bacterial colonization and skin cleansing
            and, 602-603, 603t
        cutaneous immunosurveillance and,
            603-604, 604f, 604t
        water loss, temperature control, and
            blood flow and, 601, 601f-603f
    water loss through
        in neonates, 570-571
            determination of, 570-571
            during first day and first 4 postnatal
                weeks, 572-573, 574f, 575t
            nonionizing radiation and, 575-576,
                579f
        neonatal, 601, 601f
Skin conductance, neonatal, 608, 608f
Skinfold thickness, in neonatal nutritional
    assessment, 295
Skin-to-skin care, heat exchange and, 577-578
Sleep
    in fetus, 890-891, 891f, 892f
    neonatal, maternal cocaine use and, 238
Sleep apnea syndrome, 916
Sleep spindles, on electroencephalography,
    1736t, 1740
Sleep state
    apnea and, 909-910
    in fetus, 890-891, 891f, 892f
Slow response action potentials, 671
Small for gestational age infants, 259, 267
    birth, 495-496
    body fluid compartments in, 1355
    gonadotropin secretion in, 1904
Small intestinal motility, 1131-1134, 1132f,
    1140-1141
    coordination of, 1132, 1132f
    ontogeny of, 1132-1134, 1133f
Small intestine, protein digestion in,
    1155-1156
Smell sense, 1819-1820, 1823-1825
    preferences of older infants and young
        children and, 1824-1825
    sensitivity and discrimination and, in
        neonates, 1823-1824
Smith-Lemli-Opitz syndrome, 1848t
Smoking, maternal, 239-240
Smooth brain, 1688
Smooth muscle
    ductus arteriosus, 745
    embryology of, 35, 36f
    of lower airway, mechanical strain and, 846
    of upper airway, 834, 835
Socioeconomic status, neonatal growth and,
    272
Sodium
    ionic flux of, oxygen-sensing via, 901-903
    perinatal lung liquid clearance and,
        825-826, 826f
    placental transfer of, 112, 114
    reabsorption of, in proximal renal tubule,
        1271-1272
    renal transport of, 1267-1276
        clearance studies and
            in animals, 1267-1268
            in neonates, 1268-1271, 1269f, 1270f,
                1270t
        fractional sodium excretion and, 1267,
            1268f, 1268t, 1269f
        in distal tubule, 1273f, 1273-1274

Sodium (Continued)
    aldosterone and angiotensin II and,
        1273t, 1273-1274
    epithelial sodium channel and, 1273
    in proximal tubule, 1271-1273
        sodium bicarbonate co-transporter
            and, 1272-1273
        sodium reabsorption and, 1271-1272
        sodium/hydrogen transporter and,
            1271
    Na-K-ATPase and, 1271
    regulation of, 1274-1276
        by atrial natriuretic peptides, 1276,
            1276f
        by catecholamines, 1275f, 1275-1276
        by prostaglandins, 1275
        by renin-angiotensin-aldosterone
            system, 1274-1275, 1275f
    renal tubular function and, prenatal,
        1234-1236, 1235f
    transport in lung, 825-826, 826f
        knock-out models of, 826, 827f
    transport of, neonatal respiratory disorders
        and, 830-831
Sodium bicarbonate co-transporter,
    1272-1273
Sodium channels
    cardiac action potential and, 670f, 671, 673f
    epithelial, pulmonary ion transport and,
        825, 827f
Sodium chloride, urinary concentration and,
    1303
Sodium, potassium, chloride co-transporter,
    825
Sodium-dependent glucose transporters, 487
Sodium/hydrogen transporter, 1271
Solubility, drug permeability and, 223
Somatic stem cells, 1365
Somatomedin. See Insulin-like growth factor.
Somatomedin hypothesis, 1880-1881
Somatopleure, 1850
Somatosensory evoked potentials,
    resuscitation and, 771
Somitic induction, 1850
Sonic hedgehog gene
    in central nervous system development, 1677
    in hypothalamic development, 1874t
    in lung development, 813-814, 817
    striated muscle and, 1850
Sound
    amplitude spectrum of, 1803
    localization of, 1814-1815
Sour taste, newborn responses to, 1822
Southern blotting, 11f, 11-12, 16
Spare receptors, 188-189
Specific activity, in isotope studies, 450-451
Specific dynamic action, 549
Spectroscopy, near-infrared, for cerebral blood
    flow measurement, 1749f, 1750-1751,
    1751f
    in intraventricular hemorrhage, 1751
    with indomethacin treatment of patent
        ductus arteriosus, 1751
    with surfactant therapy, 1751
Speech perception, 1815
Sphingomyelin, metabolism of, signaling and,
    1598
Spike potentials
    gastrointestinal, 1111, 1111f
    in small intestinal contraction, 1131-1132,
        1132f
Spina bifida, 1779-1781
Spinal cord. See also Central nervous system.
    embryogenesis of, 32, 32f
    thermoreceptors in, 552

Spindle-like fast rhythms, on electroencephalography, 1736t, 1737, 1737f
Splanchnic mesenchyme, 783
Splanchnopleure, 1850
Spondyloepiphyseal dysplasia congenita, 1836f, 1836t, 1837
Spurt, placentomes and, 91
SRC protein tyrosine kinases, signal transduction by, 1381
SRY protein, 1
SRY/sry gene, 1936
  early transcription of, 1937
  genes acting downstream of, 1938
  genes acting upstream of, 1937-1938
SSRIs. *See* Selective serotonin reuptake inhibitors.
Stable isotope tracer studies
  for protein metabolism assessment, 529
  nutritional, in neonates, 298-299
  of amino acid kinetics, 504-506, 505f, 506f
  of fetal substrate use, 470
  of glucose metabolism, 449-452
    cost of, 449
    ideal tracer for, 449-452
    isotope abundance and, 449
    quantification of substrate metabolic fate and, 451-452
  of labeled amino acids, 507
  of protein synthesis, 507
  terminology used in, 450-451
Standard metabolic rate, 549-550
  body mass and age and, 549-550, 550f
  body temperature and, 550, 550f
Staphylococcus epidermidis, 1482-1483
  skin colonization by, skin cleansing and, 602
Starch, digestion of, postnatal, 1152
Steady-state conditions, 193, 194t
Steady-state system, in isotope studies, 450
Steatorrhea, in cholestasis, 1220
Steatosis, 1215, 1216t
Stem cell(s), 57-64, 58f, 59f, 1365-1372
  adult, 1365-1366, 1367-1372
    clinical uses of, 1369-1370
    epidermal, 1371
    fetal progenitors compared with, 1384
    follicle, 1371-1372
    hematopoietic
      human, 1369-1370
      murine, 1367-1369
    hepatic, 1371
    intestinal epithelial, 1372
    multipotent, 1372
    neural, 1370-1371
  apoptosis of, 1369
  B-cell precursors and, 1518-1519
  bipotent, 1365
  clinical utility of, 63-64
  definition of, 1365
  embryo-derived, 58-62
    embryonic development and, 58-59, 59f
    embryonic germ cells as, 60-62
      of human origin, 60, 61, 62f
      of mouse origin, 59-60
    embryonic, 1365, 1366-1367
      clinical uses of, 1367
      human, 1366-1367
      migration of, 1368-1369
      murine, 1366
  erythropoietic, 1397
  fetal, adult progenitors compared with, 1384
  germ cell development and, 1953
  hematopoietic, 1374

Stem cell(s) *(Continued)*
  mononuclear phagocyte progenitors and, 1523f, 1523-1524, 1524f
  plasticity of, 63, 1366, 1372
  pluripotent, 58, 1365
  somatic, 1365
  T-cell precursors and, 1512, 1513t
  terminology related to, 1365-1366
  tissue-derived or tissue-resident, 62-63
  totipotent, 1365
  unipotent, 1365
Stem cell factor, as hematopoietic growth factor, 1376f, 1377, 1378, 1384
Stem cells, hematopoietic, 1375-1376, 1376t
  fetal versus adult, 1388-1389
  growth factors affecting, 1377. *See also* Hematopoietic growth factors.
  hematopoietic growth factor interaction with, developmental differences between adult and fetal progenitors and, 1384
Stereoselectivity, of drugs, placental transfer and, 206-207
Steroid hormones. *See also* Corticosteroids; Glucocorticoids; Mineralocorticoids; *specific hormones, e.g.* Cortisol.
  brain development and, 1789
  for shock, in neonates, 779
  gonadal
    follicle-stimulating hormone regulation by, 1900-1901
    luteinizing hormone regulation by, 1900-1901
  ovarian production of, 1946-1947, 1947f
  placental synthesis of, 124f, 124-125, 125f
  umbilicoplacental blood flow and, 102
  uteroplacental blood flow and, 102
Stickler dysplasia, 1837
Stomach. *See also* Gastric *entries.*
  antrum of, 1139
  embryogenesis of, anomalies of, 1102-1103
  embryology of, 37
  fluid in, 1344
  fundus of, 1139
  organogenesis and cell differentiation and, 1118, 1118f
  organogenesis of, 1102
  proteolysis in, 1154-1155
    postnatal, 1154-1155, 1155f
    prenatal, 1154, 1155
Storage disorders, 1212t
  hepatic pathology due to, 1216t, 1216-1217
Stratum corneum, 589-590, 591, 599f
  development of, 597-598, 598f
  lipids in, 601t
Stratum granulosum, 589, 591
Stratum spinosum, 589
Streptococci, Group B, 1482-1483
Stress, protein utilization and, 534-535
Stress response, pain and, 1794
Stroke volume, maternal, in pregnancy, 143, 143t
Stroma, ovarian, formation of, 1947
Subcutis, 592-594
  blood vessels, lymphatics, and nerves of, 593
  clinical relevance of, 593t, 593-594
Subependymal germinal matrix, as site of origin of intraventricular hemorrhage, 1759, 1760f
Substance abuse. *See* Maternal drug abuse; *specific drugs.*
Substance P
  cardiac conduction and, 685, 686
  umbilicoplacental circulation mediation by, 752t

Sucking, 1125, 1126f
  nonnutritive, 1140
  of neonates, taste and, 1821-1822
Suckling. *See also* Breast-feeding; Human milk.
  lactation and, 287
Sucrase, prenatal, 1152, 1153f
Sucrase-isomaltase, prenatal, 1152
Sudden infant death syndrome
  apnea related to, 915
  hyperthermia in, 565
  maternal cocaine use and, 238
  maternal opioid use and, 242t, 242-243
  maternal smoking and, 240
Sulcus limitans, 32
Sulfisoxazole, kernicterus and, 1202
Sulfonamides, during lactation, 256
Summit metabolism, 544
Superoxide anion, generation of, protein kinase C and signaling for, 1600, 1601f
Suprachiasmatic nucleus, hypothalamic, 1872t
Supraoptic nucleus, hypothalamic, 1872t
Surface tension, 1016-1019, 1017f-1019f
  at alveolar-capillary interface, 987
  lung mechanics and, 1016-1017, 1017f
  reduction by pulmonary surfactant, 1019-1021, 1020f-1022f
  surfactant proteins and
    during film compression, 1025-1026
    during film expansion, 1026
    evidence to classical model of, 1026-1028
Surfactant, pulmonary, 962, 1003-1091, 1055-1067, 1057f
  alveolar stability and, 1021-1023, 1022f
  composition of, 1006-1012, 1007f, 1014-1016, 1055-1056
    lipid components in. *See* Phospholipids, pulmonary.
    of natural surfactants, 1014, 1015f, 1015t
    of therapeutic surfactants, 1015-1016
    proteins in. *See* Surfactant proteins.
  deficiency of
    in hyaline membrane disease, 928
    in premature infants, 740
  desorption of, 1039
  development of, nutrition and, 808
  forms of, 1005, 1006f, 1063, 1064f
  historical perspective on, 1003-1004
  in liquid ventilation, 987, 988
  in neonatal pulmonary host defense, 1631f, 1631-1632
  inactivation of, 1028-1029, 1063, 1064t, 1065, 1065f, 1066f
  initial events in respiratory distress syndrome and, model for, 1067, 1067f
  initiation of air breathing at birth and, 1039, 1039f
  innate host defenses and, 1066-1067
  isolation of, 1005-1006
  life cycle of, 1005, 1006f
  lung biology of, 1016, 1016f, 1017f
  mechanical ventilation and, lung injury with, 1060-1061, 1061f-1064f, 1063
  metabolism of, 1058-1060, 1059f-1061f
  phospholipids in. *See* Phospholipids, surfactant.
  physicochemical functions of, 1023-1028
    adsorption as, 1024-1025
    surface tension and
      during film compression, 1025-1026
      during film expansion, 1026
      evidence to classical model of, 1026-1028
  quality of, in preterm infant, 1065-1066
  recycling of, 1039

surfactant, pulmonary (Continued)
 surface tension and, 1017–1019,
  1017f–1019f
  lung mechanics and, 1016–1017, 1017f
  reduction by surfactant, 1019–1021,
   1020f–1022f
 surfactant forms and, 1063, 1064f
 surfactant inactivation and, 1063, 1064t,
  1065, 1065f, 1066f
 surfactant pool size and, 1056–1057, 1057f
  after birth, 1057–1058, 1058f
 surfactant treatment and, 1066, 1066f
 technical approaches for studying, 1023
 to prevent lung injury, 935
Surfactant proteins, 1008–1012, 1009f, 1009t,
  1011f, 1014–1015, 1023–1028,
  1085–1091
 adsorption and, 1024–1025
 deficiency of
  of SP-B, 1086–1091
   clinical aspects of, 1086
   evaluation of infants with, 1090
   laboratory findings in, 1087–1088,
    1088f, 1089f
   molecular genetics and epidemiology
    of, 1086, 1087f
   of SP-B variants, 1088–1090
   partial and transient, 1088
   treatment of, 1090–1091
  of SP-C, 1091
 in host defense, 1479
  against viruses, 1492
  in neonatal pulmonary host defense,
   1629–1631, 1630f
  immunomodulating role of, 1631f,
   1631–1632
 secretion of, 1050–1051
 specific proteins and, 1085–1086
 surface tension and
  during film compression, 1025–1026
  during film expansion, 1026
  evidence to classical model of,
   1026–1028
Surfactant therapy, 975, 1074–1084
 administration of, 1081
 cerebral blood flow measurement with,
  1751
 clinical trials of, 1078–1079, 1079f
 complications of, 1080, 1080t
 dynamic lung function and, 1077–1078,
  1078f
 for respiratory distress syndrome, 945
 historical perspective on, 1004
 interaction with maternal corticosteroids,
  1083f, 1083–1084
 limitations of, 736
 oxygenation response to, 1078, 1078f
 prenatal glucocorticoid combined with,
  1073, 1073t
 pressure-volume curves and, 1075–1076,
  1075f–1077f
 repetition of, 1079–1080
 response to, ventilation effects on,
  1082–1083
 routine clinical use of, 1080f, 1080–1081
 surfactant function with, 1066, 1066f
 surfactants for use in, 1074–1075
 timing of, 1079
 variables influencing surfactant distribution
  and, 1081–1082, 1082f
Swallowing, 1125–1127, 1126f
 coordination with breathing, 1126–1127
  host defense and, 1625
 oral phase of, 1125–1126, 1126f, 1127f
 pharyngeal, 1126

Swallowing center, 1126
Sweat glands, development of, 595
Sweat secretion, heat loss and, 559
Sweet taste
 newborn responses to, 1821, 1822
 older infants' and children's responses to,
  1823
Symmetrical cellular division, 57
Sympathetic nervous system
 activity of, at birth, 722–724, 723f, 724f
 cardiac conduction and, 684–687, 686f
 glomerular filtration rate and, 1258
 intestinal circulation and, 703, 703t
 lower airway innervation and, 843–844
 myocardial, 646–647
 renal, hemodynamics and, 1232–1233
Symporters, 1271
Synaptonemal complex, 6
Synaptosomes, bilirubin affinity for,
  1202–1204
Synchronized intermittent mandatory
  ventilation, 974
Syncytial fusion, trophoblastic invasion and,
  93
Syncytiotrophoblast, 29, 85, 86f, 87–89, 89f
Synpolydactyly, 19, 1847
Systemic inflammatory response syndrome,
  1563

T

T cells
 apoptosis of, in host defense against
  viruses, neonatal, 1504–1505
 cytotoxic, in neonatal pulmonary host
  defense, 1638
 development of, 1512–1517
  antigen designations and, 1512, 1513t
  antigen receptor generation and,
   1512–1514
  B cells and, 1517
  commitment to T-cell lineage and, 1512
  cytokines and, 1512, 1513t
  extrathymic, 1514
  functional responses of fetal T cells and,
   1515–1516
  other T-lineage specific molecule
   expression and, 1514–1515
  postnatal, of memory T cells, 1516–1517
  T-cell phenotypes and antigen receptors
   and, 1515, 1515t, 1516t
  T-cell receptor/major histocompatibility
   complex interactions in, 1514
  thymus colonization and, 1512
 expressing γδ receptor, in neonatal
  pulmonary host defense, 1639–1640
 fetal, functional responses of, 1515–1516
 helper, in neonatal pulmonary host defense,
  1638, 1639f
 in host defense, 1478, 1480–1481
 in human milk, 1613
 in neonatal pulmonary host defense,
  1638–1640, 1639f
 mature, in neonatal pulmonary host
  defense, 1638–1639, 1639f
 mediated immunity mediated by, deficient,
  in newborns, 1488
 memory, postnatal development of,
  1516–1517
 receptors for
  generation of, 1512–1514
  major histocompatibility complex
   interaction of, 1514
  T-cell phenotypes and, 1515, 1515t, 1516t

Tachymetabolic organisms, 548
Taste sense, 1819–1823
 facial responses of newborns and,
  1821–1822
 preferences of older infants and young
  children and, 1822–1823
 prenatal development of, 1820
 sensitivity and discrimination in newborns
  and, 1820–1821
Taurine
 normal plasma and urine levels of, 1296t
 placental transfer of, 117
Tay syndrome, 595
T-box genes, 19–20
TDF gene, 1, 1935
Technetium-99m diethylaminetriaminepenta-
  acetic acid, as glomerular filtration rate
  marker, 1259
Telophase, mitotic, 6
Temperature
 body. See Body temperature; Fever; Heat;
  Hyperthermia; Hypothermia;
  Thermogenesis.
 environmental
  thermogenesis and, 411
  thermoregulation and, 555–556, 557f
 threshold, for thermoregulatory effector
  action elicitation
  adjustment of, 563, 564f
  long-term displacement of, 560f,
   560–561, 561f
  short-term displacement of, 561
Tendon(s), development of, 1866
Tendon organs, 1864–1866, 1866f
Teratomata, spinal, 1679
Terbutaline sulfate, for preterm labor, 109t
Term
 definition of, 103
 labor onset at, 104
Terminal chromosomal deletions, 7, 7f
Tertiary active transport, 1299
Tertiary villi, 86
Testes
 descent of, 1956–1959
  calcitonin gene-related peptide and, 1957
  complications of maldescended testes
   and, 1959
  cryptorchidism and, diagnosis and
   incidence of, 1958–1959
  epidermal growth factor and, 1958
  genitofemoral nerve and, 1957
  gubernaculum in, 1956–1957
  hormones influencing, 1957, 1958f
  intra-abdominal pressure and, 1957
  Müllerian-inhibiting substance and,
   1957–1958
  phases of, 1956
 development of, 1950–1954
  apoptosis in, 1954
  cell-cell interactions in, 1954
  embryologic, 1950, 1951f
  Leydig cells in, 1950–1951, 1951f
   endocrinologic correlates of, 1951,
    1952f
  peritubular structures in, 1954
  Sertoli cells and germ cells in,
   1951–1954, 1952f, 1952t, 1953f
   blood-testis barrier and, 1954
Testicular feminization, 1957
Testicular torsion, with maldescended testes,
  1959
Testosterone
 alveolarization and, 798, 799
 follicle-stimulating hormone regulation by,
  1900–1901

Testosterone *(Continued)*
    Leydig cells and, 1951
    luteinizing hormone regulation by,
        1900-1901
Tetracycline, during lactation, 255-256
Tetrahydrocannabinol, maternal use of,
    240-241
    contraindication to, for nursing mothers,
        255
TGFß. *See* Transforming growth factor ß.
Th1 cytokines, in host defense against viruses,
    1495f, 1495-1496
Thanatophoric dysplasia, 1857t
Theca cells, formation of, 1947, 1947f
Theophylline
    during lactation, 255
    for apnea, 914-915, 915t
    half-life of, 186t
Thermistor method, for uteroplacental blood
    flow measurement, 759
Thermogenesis, 405
    clinical implications of, 411-412
    fetal
        alterations in, 541, 542f
        basal, 541
        regulation of, 545, 545f, 546f, 546t, 547t
    mechanisms of, 543-544
    modes of, 556-557
    neonatal
        cesarean section and, 545-546
        hypoxia and, 546, 546f
        metabolic processes and, 548-550
            standard metabolic rate and, 549-550,
                550f
        nonshivering, 543, 556-557, 558f
            activation and regulation of, 543-544,
                544f
            during cooling, 587
            indicators of, 544-546
            lack of, 557
            loss of, 557, 558f
            neural control of, 558-559
            sites of, 557
            threshold for, 556f
        placental, 541-542
        shivering, 543, 556, 557-558, 558f, 559f
            neural control of, 558
            threshold for, 556f
        substrates for, 408-410
        UCP1 and. *See* UCP1.
        uterine wall, 541-542
Thermoneutral zone, 555-556
Thermoreceptors
    hypothalamic, 551-552, 552f, 553f
    in abdominal wall, 552
    in brain stem, 552
    in muscle, 552
    in spinal cord, 552
    neonatal, 550-552
        afferent thermosensitive pathways and,
            552
        cutaneous, location and properties of,
            550-551, 551f
        internal, location and properties of,
            551-552, 552f, 553f
Thermoregulation
    heat exchange and
        in incubators. *See* Incubators.
        routes of, 571-572
        with heated beds, 572
        with radiant heaters, 572
    heat loss and, 559, 560t
        behavioral regulation of, 559
        through, sweat secretion, 559
        vasomotor control of, 559, 560f

Thermoregulation *(Continued)*
    hypothalamic control of, 1873, 1875
    neonatal, 548-568
        adaptive and developmental changes in,
            559-565
            acclimation versus maturation and, 560
            changes in passive system and,
                562-563, 563f, 564f
            effector threshold temperature
                adjustment and, 563, 564f
            long-term threshold temperature
                displacement and, 560f, 560-561,
                561f
            maturation and, 561-562
            maturity of thermoregulatory system
                at birth and, 563-565, 564f
            short-term threshold temperature
                displacement and, 561
            stability of deep body temperature
                during ontogenesis and, 562, 562f,
                563f
        heat loss and, 559, 560f
        heat production and. *See* Thermogenesis,
            neonatal.
        integration of thermal inputs and,
            552-554, 554f, 555f
        metabolic rate and environmental
            temperature and, 554-556, 557f
        metabolism and heat production and,
            548-550
            standard metabolic rate and, 549-550,
                550f
        models for, 548, 549f
        normal body temperature and, 554
        oxygen consumption and, 601, 602f
        pathophysiology related to, 565-568
            fever and, 565f, 565-567
            hypoxia and, 566f, 567-568
            sudden infant death syndrome and, 565
        principles of, 548
        set point and, 554
        thermoreceptors and, 550-552
            afferent thermosensitive pathways
                and, 552
            cutaneous, location and properties of,
                550-551, 551f
            internal, location and properties of,
                551-552, 552f, 553f
        water exchange and, routes of, 570-571
Theta activity
    central-temporal, on electroencephalography,
        1736t, 1737, 1737f
    rhythmic, on electroencephalography,
        1736t, 1737, 1737f
Thigh circumference, in neonatal nutritional
    assessment, 296
Thigh/head circumference ratio, in neonatal
    nutritional assessment, 296
Thiopurine *S*-methyltransferase
    polymorphism, 205
Third-order feedback, 1876
Thoracic gas volume, 919
Threonine
    fetal accretion of, 531t
    in parenteral amino acid mixtures, 533t,
        534t
    normal plasma and urine levels of, 1296t
    requirements for, of low birth weight
        infants, 530t-532t
Threshold potential, in small intestinal
    contraction, 1131, 1132f
Thrombin
    generation of, 1447
    in neonates, 1448
    regulation of, 1436, 1442

Thrombin time, in neonates, 1449
Thrombin-clotting time
    in adults, 1436t
    in fetuses, 1436t
    in full-term infants, 1436t, 1438t
    in premature infants, 1437t
Thrombocytopenia
    gestational, 1429
    maternal, 1427-1429, 1429t
    neonatal, 1427-1430, 1455-1457, 1456t
        alloimmune, 1429, 1457
        autoimmune, 1457
        congenital, 1429-1430
        infection associated with, 1429, 1429t
        maternal causes of, 1427-1429, 1429t
        platelet counts in, 1427, 1427f, 1427t,
            1428f
        primary, 1455-1456
        secondary, 1456-1457
        severe, 1452t
Thrombocytopenia-absent radius syndrome,
    1430
Thromboelastography, in neonates, 1449
Thrombophilia, fetal, growth restriction and,
    153
Thrombopoietin, 1423
    as hematopoietic growth factor, 1376t
Thrombosis
    neonatal, 1467-1470
        coagulation testing in, 1468-1469
        pathophysiology of, 1467t, 1467-1468
        therapy of, 1469t, 1469-1470, 1470t
        thrombus formation and, 1447
Thromboxane, 128
    umbilicoplacental circulation mediation by,
        752t
Thromboxane A_2, in neonatal pulmonary host
    defense, 1642
Thymic stromal lymphoprotein, T-cell
    development and, 1512, 1513t
Thyroglobulin
    proleolysis of, 1927
    synthesis of, 1927
Thyroid gland, 1926-1932. *See also* Thyroid
    hormones.
    embryogenesis of, 1926
    histologic development of, 1926
Thyroid hormones
    adaptation to extrauterine life and,
        1930-1932, 1931f
    alveolarization and, 799
    brain development and, 1788-1789
    calcium transport and, 1289
    fetal metabolism of, 1929-1930, 1930t
    fetoplacentomaternal thyroid interaction
        and, 1928, 1928t
    gastrointestinal tract growth and, 1099
    growth plate control by, 1835
    low-T_3 syndrome and, in premature infants,
        1932
    neonatal glucose metabolism and, 479
    neonatal growth and, 271-272
    phosphate transport and, 1292
    prenatal glucocorticoid combined with, for
        respiratory distress syndrome
        prevention, 1073
    pulmonary liquid and ion transport
        regulation by, 827, 828f
    secretion of, 1927
    surfactant phospholipid biosynthesis and,
        1045
    synthesis of, 1926-1928, 1927f, 1927t
        control of, 1928f, 1928-1929
        intrathyroidal iodide recycling and, 1928
        iodide concentration and, 1926-1927

Thyroid hormones (Continued)
    iodide organification and, 1927
    iodotyrosine coupling and, 1927
    iodotyrosine deiodination and, 1928
    thyroglobulin proteolysis and, 1927
    thyroglobulin synthesis and, 1927
Thyroid transcription factor-1, in lung
    development, 814, 817
Thyroid-stimulating hormone, placental
    production of, 1928
Thyrotropin-releasing hormone
    G-cell secretion of, 1120–1121
    hypothalamic secretion of, 1877, 1877t
    prenatal glucocorticoid combined with, for
        respiratory distress syndrome
        prevention, 1073
    surfactant phospholipid biosynthesis and,
        1045
Thyroxine. See also Thyroid hormones.
    pancreatic secretion and, 1148
Tidal flow:volume relationship, measurement
    of, 923, 924f
Tidal liquid ventilation, 989, 991
Tidal volume, 922
Tidal volume-guided ventilation, 974–975
Tie1 and Tie2, vascular development and,
    624f, 624–625, 625f
Tight junctions, in lactation, 286–287
Tissue factor pathway inhibitor
    in adults, 1436t
    in fetuses, 1436t
    in full-term infants, 1436t
Tissue growth factors, gastrointestinal tract
    growth and, 1098–1099
Tissue injury
    apoptotic activation after, through death
        receptors, 74
    cell death in, modes of, 73
Tissue-type plasminogen activator
    for thrombosis, neonatal, 1470t
    in children, 1442t
    in full-term infants, 1440t
    in premature infants, 1440t
Titin, 635
TNF. See Tumor necrosis factor.
Tobacco use, maternal, 239–240
Tocolytic therapy
    for preterm labor, 108, 109t
    uteroplacental blood flow and, 763
α-Tocopherol. See also Vitamin E.
    protection during antioxidant stress, 355
    γ-tocopherol versus, 356–357
γ-Tocopherol
    in human nutrition, 357–358
    α-tocopherol versus, 356–357
Tolbutamide, during lactation, 257
Tolerance, B cells and, 1521
Torsional deformities, in intrauterine
    compression syndromes, 1838
Torticollis, muscular, congenital, 1839, 1840f
Total anomalous pulmonary venous
    connection, 716
Total body bioelectrical impedance analysis,
    for body water measurement, 1352–1353
Total body chloride content, for body water
    measurement, 1353
Total body electrical conductivity, for body
    water measurement, 1353
Total lung capacity, 919
Total parenteral nutrition. See Parenteral
    nutrition.
Totipotent stem cells, 1365
Toxic oxygen species, in neonatal pulmonary
    host defense, 1644f, 1644–1645
tPA. See Tissue-type plasminogen activator.

TPN. See Parenteral nutrition.
Trabeculae, placental, 85, 86f
Trace minerals, in human milk, 276t, 277
Tracers. See also Stable isotope tracer
    studies.
    nonrecycling, 451
    reversible (recycling), 451
Trachea
    embryology of, 834
    structure of, 834–835
Tracheal diverticulum, 1101
Tracheal genesis, 790
Tracheal stenosis, 790
Tracheal suctioning, intraventricular
    hemorrhage and, 1763
Tracheobronchial tree, 783
    congenital malformations of, 790–791
Tracheoesophageal fistulas, 790, 1101, 1102f
Tracheoesophageal septum, formation of, 824,
    825t
Tracheomalacia, 790
Traction tendons, 1866
Transcription, 2–3
Transcription factors, 45–46, 47f
    lung development and, 784–786
    mutations in, clinical implications of, 48
Transcytosis, lactation and, 286
Transdifferentiation, 63
Transferrin
    in neonatal pulmonary host defense, 1627
    serum, in neonatal nutritional assessment,
        297
Transforming growth factor ß
    embryogenesis and, 42
    fetal growth and, 1883
    gastrointestinal tract growth and, 1099
    growth plate control by, 1835
    in lung development, 816
    in neonatal pulmonary host defense, 1651
    in postnatal wounds, 1608
    in wound healing, 1607–1609
    lung development and, 787
    T-cell development and, 1513t
Translation, genetic, 3–4
Translational developmental biology, 57
Translocations, chromosomal, 7, 7f
Transporter(s)
    blood-brain, 1701–1702
    cation-Cl cotransporters as, 1273
    glucose. See Glucose transporters.
    membrane, 180
    monocarboxylic acid, 1720, 1721
    Na-Cl cotransporter as, 1274
    Na-K-Cl cotransporters as, 1274
    organic ion, 1299
    sodium bicarbonate co-transporter as,
        1272–1273
    sodium, potassium, chloride co-transporter
        as, 825
    sodium/hydrogen transporter, 1271
Transporter genes, bile flow and, 1190–1192,
    1191f
Transporter proteins
    light chain
        anionic, placental transport of amino
            acids and, 515
        cationic, placental transport of amino
            acids and, 515
        neutral, placental transport of amino
            acids and, 514–515
    placental transfer mediated by, 115–117
    placental transport of amino acids and,
        514t, 514–515
Transposition of the great arteries, physiology
    of, 712–713, 713f

Transthyretin, serum, in neonatal nutritional
    assessment, 297
Trefoil factors, gastrointestinal tract growth
    and, 1099
Treitz, ligament of, 1105
TRH. See Thyrotropin-releasing hormone.
Triallelic inheritance, 20
Trichothiodystrophy, 595
Tricuspid regurgitation, myocardial ischemia
    with hypoxemia and, in neonates, 662f,
    662–663, 663f
Triglycerides. See also Lipoprotein(s).
    as thermogenesis substrates, 408–409
    long chain, postnatal absorption of,
        396–397
    medium chain
        in infant formula, for steatorrhea, 1220
        postnatal absorption of, 396–397
    metabolism of
        fetal development and, 441–442, 442f
        postnatal development and, 443
    serum concentrations of
        in fetal development, 440–441
            in experimental animals, 441
            in humans, 440–441, 441f, 441t
        in postnatal development, 442–443
            in experimental animals, 443
            in humans, 442f, 442–443
        perinatal disease and, 443
Triiodothyronine. See also Thyroid hormones.
    deiodinase and, 410
    thermogenesis and, neonatal, 547t
Triiodothyronine (T₃), para-aminohippurate
    transport and, 1300, 1300f
Trimeric G-proteins, signaling and, 1593f,
    1593–1594, 1594t
tRNA, 3
Trophic feeding, 1096
Trophoblast, 85, 86f, 87–89, 89f
    definition of, 114t
Trophoblast invasion, 91–94
    arterial, 94
    failed, preeclampsia due to, 148, 148f
    interstitial, 92–94, 93f
Trophoblastic cell column, 92
Trophoblastic shell, 85
Tropomyosin, developmental changes in, 642
Troponins, 635
    developmental changes in, 642–643, 643f
Trough concentration, measured, 195
Truncus arteriosus, persistent, 618
Trypsin, postnatal, 1155
Trypsinogen, prenatal, 1155
Tryptophan
    fetal accretion of, 531t
    in parenteral amino acid mixtures, 533t,
        534t
    normal plasma and urine levels of, 1296t
    requirements for, of low birth weight
        infants, 530t–532t
TSH. See Thyroid-stimulating hormone.
T-system
    cardiac, 645
    in striated muscle, 1860, 1860f
Tuberal nuclei, hypothalamic, 1872t
Tubular myelin, 1016, 1017f, 1038f,
    1038–1039, 1063
Tubuloglomerular feedback, 1253–1254
Tumor necrosis factor
    acute phase reaction and, 1563
    as hematopoietic growth factor, 1376t
    characteristics of, 1556
    fetal growth and, 1883
    fever and, 1563
    in host defense, 1481

Tumor necrosis factor (Continued)
  in neonatal pulmonary host defense, 1645
  inflammation due to, 1562
  production of, in neonates, 1564
  receptors for, 1556, 1556f
  soluble, 1561
Turner syndrome, 1935
Turnover, in isotope studies, 450
Turnover time, in isotope studies, 450
Twin(s). See also Multiple pregnancy.
  conjoined, 172, 172f
  dizygotic, 166
  monoamniotic, 171, 172f
  monozygotic, 165-166, 166
  vanishing, 171
Twin reversed arterial perfusion syndrome,
    174, 174f
Twin-to-twin transfusion syndrome, 172-174,
    173f, 174f
Two-compartment model, of placental drug
    transport, 200, 220f
  at steady state, fetal plasma concentration
    of drugs and, 225
Tyrosine
  fetal accretion of, 531t
  in parenteral amino acid mixtures, 533t, 534t
  normal plasma and urine levels of, 1296t
  requirements for, of low birth weight
    infants, 530t-532t
Tyrosine kinases
  protein
    JAK, in signal transduction, 1380-1381
    SRC, in signal transduction, 1381
  signal transduction initiated by, 1594-1595
  Src family of, signal transduction initiated
    by, 1594f, 1594-1595, 1595f
  Syk family of, signal transduction initiated
    by, 1595
Tyrosinemia, 1215
  coagulopathy in, 1454

U

UCP1, 405f, 405-408, 406f
  acute regulation of, 406-407, 407f
  adaptive regulation of, 407-408, 408f
  in altricial species, 407, 408f
  in human newborn, 408
  in immature newborn species, 407
  in precocial newborn species, 407-408
  perinatal expression of, 407-408, 543-544,
    544f
  semiacute regulation of, 407
  thermogenesis and, neonatal, 547t
  UCP gene and, 406
Ulnar-mammary syndrome, 1847, 1848t
Ultrafiltration, renal, 1257
Ultrasound
  Doppler. See Doppler ultrasound.
  in intraventricular hemorrhage, 1758,
    1758f, 1758t
  of umbilical blood flow, 750-751, 751f
Umbilical artery blood flow, during labor,
    761-762
Umbilical blood flow, 748-757
  hemodynamics of, 750
    mean blood flow and, 750, 750f
    pulsatile blood flow and, 750
  in intrauterine growth restriction, 755
  regulation of, 753-755
    closure of umbilicoplacental circulation
      at birth and, 754
    fetal arterial blood pressure maintenance
      and, 753-754

Umbilical blood flow (Continued)
  fetal growth and, 753
  innervation in, 754-755
  perfusion/perfusion matching to
    optimize maternal/fetal exchange
    and, 753
  vasoactive mediators in, 754, 754t
  wall shear stress in, 755
  study methods for, 750-751
    implanted instrumentation as, 751
    perfused placenta in vitro as, 751
    ultrasound as, 750-751, 751f
    umbilicoplacental vessels in vitro as,
      751, 752t
  umbilicoplacental anatomy and, 749f,
    749-750
Umbilical circulation
  amino acid uptake by, 517-520, 518f
    placentofetal amino acid cycling and,
      518-520, 519f
  definition of, 114t
Umbilical cord
  development of, 94-95
  glucose uptake by, regulation of, 456-457
  polyunsaturated fatty acids in, placental
    transfer and, 392
Umbilical cord blood, as graft source, 1370
Umbilical polyps, 1106
Umbilical sinus, 1106
Umbilicoplacental blood flow
  nitric oxide and, 102
  prostaglandins and, 100-101
  steroid hormones and, 102
  vasoconstrictors and, 100
Umbilicoplacental circulation, 749
  anatomy of, 749f, 749-750
  closure of, at birth, 754
Umbilicoplacental vascular bed, development
  physiologic functions of, 97-99, 98f, 99f
Umbilicoplacental vessels, in vitro study of,
  751, 752t
Uniparental disomy, 10, 22
Unipotent stem cells, 1365
Upper esophageal sphincter, 1127
Urea, urinary concentration and, 1303,
    1304-1306, 1305f
  in neonates, 1312-1313, 1313f, 1313t
Urea cycle enzyme disorders, 1212t,
    1214-1215
Ureaplasma urealyticum infection
  intrauterine
    amniocentesis detection of, 133-134
    detection with sequence-based
      techniques, 135
    lung injury due to, 937, 937f
Ureteric bud, 1223, 1224, 1229
  outgrowth of
    induction of, 1226
    regulation by metanephric mesenchyme,
      1226-1227
Uric acid, renal transport of, 1301f,
    1301-1302, 1302f
Urinary acidification, 1327-1330
  bicarbonate reabsorption and
    developmental aspects of, 1329
    in mature kidney, 1327-1328
  developmental aspects of, 1328
  hydrogen ion excretion and
    by mature kidney, 1328
    developmental aspects of, 1328-1329
  metabolic compensation for respiratory
    acidosis/alkalosis and, neonatal,
    1329-1330
  net acid excretion and, 1328
  renal bicarbonate threshold and, 1328

Urinary concentration
  concentrating mechanism and, 1303-1309,
    1304f
    aquaporins in, 1307t, 1307-1309
    chloride channels and, 1309
    medullary gradient development and,
      1303-1304, 1304f
    renal pelvis and, 1306-1307
    short-loop nephrons and urea in,
      1304-1306, 1305f
    vasa rectae in, 1306, 1306f
  in fetus, 1309-1311
    aquaporins and, 1311
    maturation of fetal water reabsorption
      and, 1309, 1309f, 1310f
    vasopressin and, 1310-1311
  in neonates, 1311-1320, 1312t
    anatomic factors limiting ability for, 1317,
      1317t, 1318f-1321f, 1319-1320
    physiologic factors limiting ability for,
      1312t-1314t, 1312-1320, 1313f,
      1315f
Urinary diluting mechanism, physiology of,
    1320-1324, 1322f
  in fetus, 1322-1323
  in neonates, 1323f, 1323-1324
Urinary system, embryology of, 38
Urine, formation of, 1257
Urocortin, umbilicoplacental circulation
  mediation by, 752t
Urorectal septum, 1109, 1109f
Urotensin-1, umbilicoplacental circulation
  mediation by, 752t
Uterine blood flow, during pregnancy
  anatomic changes in, 144-145, 145f
  functional and molecular changes in,
    145-146
Uterine circulation, definition of, 114t
Uterine wall
  heat conductance through, 542, 543f
  heat production in, 541-542
Uteroplacental blood flow, 758-764
  during labor, 758, 759f, 761f, 761-764
    fetal aortic blood flow and, 762
    fetal cerebral blood flow and, 762
    fetal electrocardiogram and, 763-764
    fetal heart rate and, 763
    pharmacologic effects on, 763
    umbilical artery flow and, 761-762
  nitric oxide and, 102
  recording methods for, 759-761
  steroid hormones and, 102
  vasoconstrictors and, 99-100, 100f, 101f
Uteroplacental circulation, maternal
  adaptations to pregnancy and, 143t, 144
Uteroplacental vascular bed
  development physiological functions of,
    97-99, 98f, 99f
  maternal adaptations to pregnancy and,
    development physiological functions
    of, 97-99, 98f, 99f
Uterus
  amino acid uptake by, 517
  in multiple pregnancy, 167

V

Vaccines, for herpesvirus infections,
    1505-1506
VACTERL syndrome, 790
Valine
  fetal accretion of, 531t
  in parenteral amino acid mixtures, 533t,
    534t

Valine (Continued)
  normal plasma and urine levels of, 1296t
  requirements for, of low birth weight
    infants, 530t-532t
Valproic acid
  during lactation, 256
  protein binding of, 205t
Valvular regurgitation, cardiovascular
  physiology and, 714
Vanishing twin, 171
Vasa rectae, urinary concentration and, 1306,
  1306f
Vascular beds, umbilicoplacental and
  uterplacental, development physiological
  functions of, 97-99, 98f, 99f
Vascular cell adhesion molecule-1, 1574t,
  1579, 1579f
Vascular development, 621-633
  angiogenesis and. See Angiogenesis.
  during pseudoglandular lung development,
    molecular mechanisms regulating, 787
  endothelial cell origin and, 621-623, 622f
    mechanisms of new blood vessel
      formation and, 622, 623f
    primary vascular plexus formation and,
      622-623
  epigenetic events during, 626-629
    hemodynamic forces and, 627, 627f
    hypoxia and, 627-629, 628f
  future research on, 633
  of limbs, 1845
  of lung, 818-819
  of pulmonary vessels, 629-633, 630f-632f
  receptor tyrosine kinases and ligands in,
    623-625, 624f, 625f
  retinal, 1797-1798, 1798f
  vascular patterning and, 625-626, 626f
Vascular endothelial growth factor
  alveolarization and, 796-797
  angiogenesis and, 81, 82, 83f
  fetal growth and, 1883
  gastrointestinal tract growth and, 1099
  in lung development, 818
  lung development and, 787
    after lung injury in premature lung,
      946-947
  receptors for
    lung development and, 787
    vascular development and, 621-622, 629,
      630-631, 632
  retinopathy of prematurity and, 1801
  vascular development and, 621-622, 622f,
    623-624, 624f, 625f, 629, 632
Vascular support, deficient, intraventricular
  hemorrhage and, 1764-1765
Vascularization, of nephrons, 1227-1228
Vasculature. See also Cardiovascular entries;
  Maternal cardiovascular disease; specific
  vessels, e.g. Capillaries.
  embryology of, 35, 35f
  of growth plate, 1833, 1833f
  of skin, 593
  permeability of, in disseminated
    intravascular coagulation, 1462-1463
  thermoregulation and, neonatal, 601, 603f
  umbilicoplacental, in vitro study of, 751, 752t
  walls of
    hemostasis and, 1444
    leukocyte mobilization to inflammatory
      sites and, 1580-1582, 1582f, 1583
Vasculogenesis, 79
  definition of, 622
  primary vascular plexus formation in,
    622-623, 623f
  pulmonary, 818

Vasoactive agents, glomerular filtration rate
  and, 1257-1258
Vasoactive intestinal peptide
  adrenal regulation by, 1920
  cardiac conduction and, 687
  umbilicoplacental circulation mediation by,
    752t
Vasoactive peptides
  chorionic, 127
  ventilation-perfusion matching and,
    877-878
Vasoconstriction
  patent ductus arteriosus and, 743-744, 746
  thermoregulation and, neonatal, 601, 603f
Vasodilation
  heat loss and, 559, 560f
  pulmonary, nitric oxide and, 735-737,
    736f-738f
Vasopressin
  adrenal regulation by, 1920
  arterial baroreflex and, 720
  calcium transport and, 1289
  hypothalamic secretion of, 1877, 1877t,
    1878
  hypoxia and, 655
  renal blood flow and, 1244
  synthesis of, 1877-1878
  umbilicoplacental blood flow and, 100, 752t
  urinary concentration and
    in fetus, 1310-1311
      endogenous vasopressin and, 1310
      exogenous vasopressin and, 1310,
        1310t
    in neonates, 1313-1314, 1314t
  uteroplacental blood flow and, 100
Vasoregulation
  peripheral, neonatal shock and, 777
  pulmonary, nitric oxide in, 733
Vasorelaxation, patent ductus arteriosus and,
  743-744
VEGF. See Vascular endothelial growth factor.
Velocardiofacial syndrome, 619
Venous hemorrhagic infarction, 1746
Ventilation
  assisted. See Mechanical ventilation.
  distribution of, ventilation-perfusion
    matching and, 878, 879t
  in bronchopulmonary dysplasia,
    established, 957
  in hyaline membrane disease, 930-931
  with high-frequency ventilation, 980
Ventilation-perfusion relationships, 870-878
  alveolar and arterial oxygen tension and,
    870-871, 872f
  carbon dioxide gradient and, 871-872
  distribution of ventilation and, 878, 879t
  hypoxic pulmonary vasoconstriction and,
    875f, 875-876, 876f
  inert gases for assessing, 872-873, 873f
  nitrogen gradient and, 871
  pulmonary arterial pressure and, 874-875
  vasoactive mediators influencing, 877f,
    877-878, 878f
  with liquid ventilation, 990
Ventricles
  of brain, dilation of, in hydrocephalus, brain
    injury and, 1766-1767
  of heart
    filling of, restriction of, congenital cardiac
      lesions with, 715-716
    septation of, 619
Ventricular function, of heart
  impaired, manifestations of, 657-663
    fetal, 657-659, 658f, 660f, 661f
    neonatal, 659-663, 661f-663f

Ventricular function, of heart (Continued)
  of immature heart, 647-653
    afterload and, 650-651, 652f
    birth effects on, 652-653, 653f
    heart rate and, 648-649, 648f-650f
    inotropy and, 651-652
    preload and, 649-650, 650f, 651f
Ventromedial nucleus, hypothalamic, 1872t
Verapamil, for preterm labor, 109t
Vernix, biology of, 599f, 599-600, 600f, 600t
Very low birth weight infants
  glucose metabolism in, 461
  skin of, 604-606
    epidermal barrier repair strategies for,
      604-606, 605t
    ineffectiveness as barrier, 604, 605f
Vesicles, transsyncytial movement of, 118
Vestibular spine, in cardiac development, 614
Villi
  definition of, 114t
  intestinal, 1371-1372
Vimentin, 1857, 1858f, 1859
VIP. See Vasoactive intestinal peptide.
Viral antigen-specific T cells, chemotactic and
  homing receptor expression by, in host
  defense against viruses, 1499
Viruses
  host defense against, 1490-1506
    adaptive, 1490, 1495-1500
      B cells, antibody, ADCC, and
        complement and, 1500
      CD4 T cell-mediated, 1495
      CD8 T cell-mediated antiviral immunity
        and, 1497f, 1497-1499, 1498f
      CD28/CD80-86 co-stimulation and,
        1499
      CD40-ligand/CD40 interactions and,
        1496, 1496f
      chemotactic and homing receptor
        expression by viral antigen-
        specific T cells and, 1499
      cytolytic CD4 T cell-mediated
        mechanisms and, 1496-1497
      gamma/delta T cells and, 1500
      NK T cells and, 1500
      Th1 cytokine production and, 1495f,
        1495-1496
    against herpes simplex virus, 1490
    innate, 1490-1495
      chemokines in, 1492
      cytokines in, 1491-1492
      interferons in, 1491
      mononuclear phagocytes and
        inducible nitric oxide synthase
        and, 1492-1493
      myeloid dendritic cells and, 1493
      natural killer cells and, 1494f,
        1494-1495
      surfactant proteins in, 1492
    neonatal, 1501-1506
      B cells, antibody, ADCC, and
        complement in, 1505-1506
      CD4 T cell IFN-γ production and, 1503
      CD4 T cells and dendritic cells in,
        1502-1503
      CD8 T cells in, 1503-1504
      CD40-ligand/CD40 interactions in,
        1503
      chemotactic and homing receptor
        expression and, 1504
      complement in, 1554
      co-stimulation and, 1504
      cytokines in, 1501
      cytolytic CD4 T cells in, 1503
      gamma/delta T cells in, 1505

Viruses (Continued)
  NK T cells in, 1505
  NL cells in, 1501-1502
  T cell apoptosis and, 1504-1505
  intrauterine infection caused by, 132
Visual attention, docosahexaenoic acid and, 435
Visual function
  docosahexaenoic acid and, 434-435
  neonatal, maternal marijuana use and, 241
Vitamin(s)
  fat-soluble, deficiency of, in cholestasis, 1220
  in human milk, 276t, 276-277
  water-soluble, placental transfer of, 207
Vitamin A, 347f, 347-351. See also Retinoid entries; Retinol entries.
  brain development and, 1787
  bronchopulmonary dysplasia and, 956
  deficiency of, 350-351
  digestion and absorption of, 350, 350f
  enteral nutrition and, 349-350
  excretion of, 349
  fetal acquisition of, 349
  growth plate control by, 1837
  guidelines for, 351
  lung development and, 808
  metabolism of, 347f, 347-351
    in cell, 348, 348f
    nuclear processing and, 348-349
    transport and, in plasma, 347-348, 348f
  parenteral nutrition and, 350
  plasma status at birth, 349
  storage at birth, 349
  toxicity of, 351
Vitamin C, growth plate control by, 1837
Vitamin D
  biologic actions of, 309
  biologic concentration of, 309
  brain development and, 1789
  calcium homeostasis and, 307-309
    neonatal, 326f, 326-327
  calcium transport and, 1288
  growth plate control by, 1835, 1837
  lung development and, 808
  metabolism of, 308, 308f
  molecular mechanism of action of, 308-309
  placental calcium transport and, 318
  placental phosphorus transport and, 319
  regulation of, 308
Vitamin D receptor, 309
Vitamin E, 353-366
  antioxidant functions of, 354-355
  deficiency, 355
  early studies of, 353-354, 354f
  excretion of, 356
  fetal accumulation of, 361, 361f, 362t
  functional requirements for, 355
  in human nutrition, 357-358
  in newborn and young infant, patterns of membrane content and, 361-363, 362f
  intestinal absorption of, 356
  maternal hyperlipidemia and, 363-365
  maternal requirement for
    dietary, 363
    fatty acid composition effects on, 363t, 363-365, 363f-365f, 364t

Vitamin E (Continued)
  membrane content of, protection of, 355-356
  non-antioxidant functions of, 355
  oxidant risk and, 366
  plasma transport of, 358
    apolipoprotein influence on, 358, 359f
  sources and activity of, 356t, 356-357
  transfer to tissues, 358
Vitamin K, 369-372
  blood coagulation and, 369
  γ-carboxylation system dependent on, 370, 370f
    development of, regulation of, 372, 372f
    maturation of, 371f, 371-372, 372f
  deficiency of, 1452t, 1452-1454, 1453f
  hepatic function and metabolism of, 369-371, 370f
Vitelline arteries, 702
Vitelline veins, 702
Voltage-gated ion channels, 671, 673t
Volume loading, responses to, 1348
Volume of distribution, 226
  apparent, 192-193
  in isotope studies, 450
Volume reserve, of neonatal heart, 714-715
Volume status, calcium transport and, 1288
Volume-guarantee ventilation, 974-975
Volvulus, 1102-1103
von Willebrand disease, 1452
von Willebrand factor
  in full-term infants, 1438t
  in neonates, 1449
  in premature infants, 1437t

W

Waardenburg syndrome, 19, 592, 592t
Wakefulness, in fetus, 890, 891
Warm shock, 777
Water. See Body water.
Weaning, pancreatic secretion and, 1146-1147
Wedging, cardiac tube looping and, 615
Weight
  gain in, maternal, in multiple pregnancy, 169
  in neonatal nutritional assessment, 294
  loss of, neonatal, 1345
Western blotting, 12
White matter
  cerebral, hydrocephalus and, 1766
  periventricular
    destruction of, intraventricular hemorrhage and, 1765
    injury to, secondary to blood projects, intraventricular hemorrhage and, 1765-1766
Window current, 671
Wolff crest, development of, 1845
Wound healing, 1604-1609, 1605t
  fetal
    fetal environment and, 1604-1605
    fetal skin and, 1604
    future research directions for, 1609
    model of, 1605f, 1605-1607, 1606f

Wound healing (Continued)
    fetal fibroblast and, 1606
    fetal wound matrix and, 1606-1607
    transforming growth factor-ß and, 1607-1609
  model of, 1605f, 1605-1607, 1606f
    inflammation and cytokines in, 1607
  postnatal, cytokine excess and, 1608-1609
  transforming growth factor-ß and, cytokine excess in postnatal wounds and, 1608-1609
Wound matrix, fetal, 1606-1607
WT1 gene, renal organogenesis and, 1229-1231, 1230f

X

Xanthenes, for apnea, 914-915, 915t
Xenon clearance techniques, cerebral blood flow measurement using, 1753-1754
X-linked disorders, 8f, 9

Y

Y chromosome
  sex-determining role of, 1935
  SRY gene and, 1936
Yolk sac, hematopoiesis in, 1376-1377, 1388
Yolk sac placenta, definition of, 114t

Z

Z-bands, in striated muscle, 1859-1860
Zero-order kinetics, 187-188
Zfy gene, early transcription of, 1937
Zinc, 342-345
  biochemistry of, 342
  biology of, 342-343
  deficiency of, 344-345
    during infancy, 344-345
    embryogenesis and, 344
    fetal development and, 344
  homeostasis of, whole body, 344
  metabolism of
    fetal, 343-344
    in mammary gland, 344
    intracellular, 343
    maternal, 343
    placental, 343
  postnatal requirements for, in preterm infant, 345
Zinc finger transcription factors, lung development and, 785
Zinc supplements, for breast-fed infants, 276t, 277
Zona pellucida, 26-27
Zone of degeneration, of growth plate, 1834
Zone of polarizing activity
  in limb development, 1845, 1846
  of growth plate, 1831
Zone of provisional calcification, of growth plate, 1834
Zygosity, 165-166

P/N 9997628314

9 789997 628312